CANCER EPIDEMIOLOGY AND PREVENTION

Second Edition

Edited by

DAVID SCHOTTENFELD, M.D.

John G. Searle Professor of Epidemiology
University of Michigan School of Public Health
Ann Arbor, Michigan

JOSEPH F. FRAUMENI, JR., M.D.

Director, Division of Cancer Epidemiology and Genetics
National Cancer Institute
Bethesda, Maryland

New York Oxford
OXFORD UNIVERSITY PRESS
1996

Oxford University Press

Oxford New York
Athens Auckland Bangkok Bogota Bombay Buenos Aires
Calcutta Cape Town Dar es Salaam Delhi Florence Hong Kong
Istanbul Karachi Kuala Lumpur Madras Madrid Melbourne
Mexico City Nairobi Paris Singapore Taipei Tokyo Toronto

and associated companies in
Berlin Ibadan

Published by Oxford University Press, Inc.,
198 Madison Avenue, New York, New York 10016

Oxford is a registered trademark of Oxford University Press

Library of Congress Cataloging-in-Publication Data
Cancer epidemiology and prevention /
edited by David Schottenfeld, Joseph F. Fraumeni, Jr.—2nd ed.
p. cm. Includes bibliographical references and index.
ISBN 0-19-505354-0
1. Cancer—Prevention.
2. Cancer—Epidemiology.
I. Schottenfeld, David.
II. Fraumeni, Joseph F.
[DNLM: 1. Neoplasms—epidemiology.
2. Neoplasms—prevention & control.
QZ 200 C215127 1996] RC268.C354 1996 616.99'4—dc20
DNLM/DLC for Library of Congress 95-34524

9 8 7 6 5 4 3 2 1

Printed in the United States of America
on acid-free paper

To Rosalie and Tricia

Preface

Of all deaths caused by either cancer or cardiovascular disease in the United States, more than 70 percent occur in persons aged 65 years or older. However, the past three decades have witnessed dramatic decreases in age-specific mortality rates for heart disease and stroke, surpassing 50 percent, while adult cancer mortality rates, even after excluding deaths due to lung cancer, have declined by only 10 to 15 percent. In recent years the age-adjusted death rate for all malignant neoplasms was more than 90 percent of the rate for diseases of the heart. If these trends continue, cancer will emerge within five to ten years as the leading cause of death in the United States and other industrialized nations.

The discipline of epidemiology, which addresses societal concerns for disease prevention and health promotion, lies at the foundation of preventive medicine and the strategic targeting of public health practices and policies. Over the past fifty years, the application of increasingly sophisticated observational and experimental research methods in cancer epidemiology has led to the characterization of high- and low-risk populations throughout the world and to the identification of a spectrum of chemical, physical, and microbial carcinogens, as well as agents that may inhibit carcinogenesis. More recently, epidemiologic approaches have contributed to the elucidation of genetic and other mechanisms of susceptibility to cancer.

Compelling epidemiologic data indicate that a substantial fraction of cancer mortality and morbidity can be prevented by life-style changes such as avoiding tobacco products, limiting consumption of alcohol and exposure to ultraviolet radiation, consuming optimal amounts of fresh fruits and vegetables, and controlling dietary energy consumption while increasing physical activity. Reductions in mortality may also be achieved by periodic screening examinations, especially those aimed at the early detection of breast, cervical, and colorectal cancers. Globally, infectious agents probably account for 10 to 15 percent of cancer deaths, which eventually may be avoided by immunization or antimicrobial therapy, as well as targeted surveillance and early detection in high-risk populations. While 5 to 10 percent of cancer mortality in industrial nations may result from exposures in the workplace, it is noteworthy that many of the chemical and physical agents currently viewed as environmental carcinogens were originally identified through epidemiologic studies in occupational settings. A relatively smaller proportion of cancers may be attributed to pharmaceutical agents, including hormones, but these established relationships have generated important insights into mechanisms of cancer causation.

This new edition of *Cancer Epidemiology and Prevention* represents a systematic updating and provides a critical review of information that has been gathered since the first edition was published in 1982. The chapters in both editions are grouped into five major sections: Basic Concepts, Magnitude of Cancer, Causes of Cancer, Cancer by Tissue of Origin, and Cancer Prevention and Control. However, new chapters appear in the various sections of this edition. In the section on Basic Concepts these include chapters on the molecular and genetic events in neoplastic transformation, molecular epidemiology, quantitative risk assessment, and mathematical models. In the section on Magnitude of Cancer, a chapter on incidence, mortality, and survival based on the United States SEER data reviews patterns among racial and ethnic minority groups. The section on Cancer by Tissue of Origin has been expanded to include a chapter on cancers of the vulva and vagina, and a segment on cancer of the anus in the chapter on large intestine. In the concluding section on Cancer Prevention and Control, a new introductory chapter on principles and applications of cancer prevention offers a bridge from the scientific discoveries of epidemiologic research to the translational interventions that have an impact on cancer incidence and mortality.

The task of completing this edition was challenging because of the rapid succession of major advances that have taken place in cancer epidemiology and prevention, molecular genetics, and other aspects of cancer biology and carcinogenesis. The goal of preparing a comprehensive and authoritative new edition was achieved through the collective efforts of a distinguished group of contributing authors and consulting editors.

The introductory chapters dealing with Basic Concepts encompass conceptual issues of causal inference in epidemiology, the applicability of animal experimental studies, the morphologic classification of cancer and its natural history from precursor to invasive lesions, the succession of genetic and epigenetic events underlying cellular transformation and progression to metastatic cancer, and the application of biostatistical methods in quantitative risk assessment and mathematical models for predicting risk. The chapter on molecular epidemiology reviews the enhanced potential for discovering causal relationships and elucidating carcinogenic mechanisms when laboratory and epidemiologic methods are conceptually integrated.

The section on Magnitude of Cancer reviews the remarkable variations in cancer incidence around the world and the major shifts in cancer risk among migrant populations that have provided important leads concerning the role of cultural and life-style risk factors, including diet and nutrition. Cancer incidence, mortality, and survival patterns in the United States are reviewed overall and for selected racial and ethnic minority groups. A chapter on the economic impact of cancer estimates the direct medical costs of treating specific types of cancer, costs to the family and community in providing rehabilitative services or palliative care, and costs to society as a result of premature death or lost productivity.

The section on the Causes of Cancer provides the foundation for appreciating the complex and multifactorial origins of human cancer. Whereas the neoplastic process may be viewed as genetic perturbations in the regulation of cellular proliferation and differentiation, these events are triggered or propagated by life-style risk factors and exposures to environmental agents that are critically evaluated in this section. Emphasis is given to the interactive relationship of familial and genetic factors and their potential impact on susceptibility to carcinogenic agents. This section also reviews the salient developments in AIDS-related malignancies that have taken place since the first edition.

The section on Cancer by Tissue of Origin strives to provide a comprehensive epidemiologic profile of each form of cancer. Wherever possible, efforts are made to develop a unifying concept of pathogenesis or rationale for prevention, and to highlight promising areas of future research.

The concluding section on Cancer Prevention and Control addresses the opportunities for translating the results of epidemiologic, clinical, and laboratory research into interventions designed to reduce the cancer burden in populations. Such efforts may focus on altering the behavior of high-risk individuals or reducing the distribution of risk factors in a population. Various behavioral models are guiding community-based programs or clinical practices that are designed to facilitate adherence to cost-effective screening interventions or otherwise enhance health promotion and disease prevention. These models are reviewed, as is the rationale for the use of synthetic or natural chemopreventive agents to suppress or block the carcinogenic process among individuals at increased risk of cancer. Major potential advances in the prevention and control of cancer are discussed—advances that may only be achieved through the shared responsibility of an informed public, a supportive health care system, and a cooperative network of national and international agencies.

Ann Arbor, Michigan D. S.
Bethesda, Maryland J.F.F.

Acknowledgments

Because of delays in the preparation of this volume, we were compelled to ask the contributing authors to update their chapters. It is only through their extraordinary collective efforts that we are able to publish a textbook that is both comprehensive and current. We take this opportunity to thank them publicly for all the work they have put into their chapters. In addition, the editors are grateful to Jeffrey W. House and Susan Hannan at Oxford University Press for their encouragement and skillful guidance throughout the development of this volume. We also thank Mrs. Christine Wenner and Mrs. Angela Reid of the University of Michigan School of Public Health for their organizational skills in communicating with authors and scrutinizing manuscripts.

Contents

Part IV Cancer by Tissue of Origin

Contributors

Christopher I. Amos, PhD
Department of Epidemiology
M.D. Anderson Hospital and Tumor Institute
Houston, Texas

Kristin E. Anderson, PhD
Division of Epidemiology
School of Public Health
University of Minnesota
Minneapolis, Minnesota

Bruce K. Armstrong, MBBS, DPhil
Australian Institute of Health and Welfare
Canberra, Australia

Donald F. Austin, MD
Oregon Health Division
Center for Disease Prevention and Epidemiology
Portland, Oregon

John A. Baron, MD
Departments of Medicine and Community and Family Medicine
Dartmouth Medical School
Hanover, New Hampshire

Helmut Bartsch, PhD
Division of Toxicology
German Cancer Research Center
Heidelberg, Germany

Marshall H. Becker, PhD†
Department of Health Behavior and Health Education
The University of Michigan
School of Public Health
Ann Arbor, Michigan

John W. Berg, MD
Department of Pathology
University of Colorado
School of Medicine, and
Colorado Department of Public Health and Environment
Denver, Colorado

Leslie Bernstein, PhD
Department of Preventive Medicine
Norris Comprehensive Cancer Center
University of Southern California
Los Angeles, California

†Deceased.

William J. Blot, PhD
International Epidemiology Institute, Ltd.
Rockville, Maryland

John D. Boice, Jr., ScD
Radiation Epidemiology Branch
National Cancer Institute
Bethesda, Maryland

Louise A. Brinton, PhD
Environmental Epidemiology Branch
National Cancer Institute
Bethesda, Maryland

Martin L. Brown, PhD
Applied Research Branch
Division of Cancer Prevention and Control
National Cancer Institute
Bethesda, Maryland

Jonathan Buckley, MBBS, PhD
Department of Preventive Medicine
University of Southern California
School of Medicine
Los Angeles, California

Linda Burhansstipanov, DrPH
AMC Cancer Research Center
Denver, Colorado

Julie E. Buring, ScD
Channing Laboratory
Harvard Medical School
and Brigham and Women's Hospital
Boston, Massachusetts

Kenneth P. Cantor, PhD
Environmental Epidemiology Branch
National Cancer Institute
Bethesda, Maryland

Raymond A. Cartwright, MD
Leukemia Research Fund
Centre for Clinical Epidemiology
University of Leeds
Department of Pathology
Leeds, England

Clair Chilvers, MSc
Department of Public Health in Medicine and Epidemiology
University of Nottingham Medical School
Queens Medical Center
Nottingham, England

Wong-Ho Chow, PhD
International Epidemiology Institute, Ltd.
Rockville, Maryland

Noreen M. Clark, PhD
Department of Health Behavior and Health Education
The University of Michigan
School of Public Health
Ann Arbor, Michigan

Linda S. Cook, PhD
Fred Hutchinson Cancer Research Center
Seattle, Washington

Pelayo Correa, MD
Department of Pathology
Louisiana State University Medical Center
New Orleans, Louisiana

Rochelle E. Curtis, MA
Radiation Epidemiology Branch
National Cancer Institute
Division of Cancer Epidemiology and Genetics
Bethesda, Maryland

Janet R. Daling, PhD
Fred Hutchinson Cancer Research Center
Division of Public Health Sciences
Epidemiologic Research Unit
Seattle, Washington

Nicholas E. Day, PhD (Consulting Editor)
MRC Biostatistics Unit
Institute of Public Health
Cambridge University
Cambridge, England

Susan S. Devesa, PhD
Epidemiology and Biostatistics Program
Division of Cancer Epidemiology and Genetics
National Cancer Institute
Bethesda, Maryland

Dallas R. English, PhD
Department of Public Health
The University of Western Australia
Nedlands, Perth, Western Australia

Virginia L. Ernster, PhD
Department of Epidemiology and Biostatistics
University of California School of Medicine
San Francisco, California

Alfred S. Evans, MD†
Department of Epidemiology and Public Health
Yale University School of Medicine
New Haven, Connecticut

†Deceased.

Marianne Ewertz, MD
Finsencentret, Rigshospitalet
Copenhagen, Denmark

Diana C. Farrow, PhD
Department of Epidemiology
University of Washington
Fred Hutchinson Cancer Research Center
Seattle, Washington

Thomas R. Fears, PhD
Biostatistics Branch
National Cancer Institute
Bethesda, Maryland

Joseph F. Fraumeni Jr., MD (Editor)
Division of Cancer Epidemiology and Genetics
National Cancer Institute
Bethesda, Maryland

Gary D. Friedman, MD
Division of Research
Kaiser Permanente
Oakland, California

Deborah Grady, MD
San Francisco Veterans Affairs Medical Center
General Internal Medicine
San Francisco, California

Raymond S. Greenberg, MD, PhD
Medical University of South Carolina
Charleston, South Carolina

Benjamin F. Hankey, ScD
Cancer Statistics Branch
National Cancer Institute
Bethesda, Maryland

Angela Harras, BA
Cancer Statistics Branch
National Cancer Institute
Bethesda, Maryland

Brian E. Henderson, MD (Consulting Editor)
Department of Preventive Medicine
Norris Comprehensive Cancer Center
University of Southern California
Los Angeles, California

Charles H. Hennekens, MD, DrPH
Channing Laboratory
Harvard Medical School
and Brigham and Women's Hospital
Boston, Massachusetts

Lisa J. Herrinton, PhD
Division of Research
Kaiser Permanente
Oakland, California

Thomas A. Hodgson, PhD
National Center for Health Statistics
Centers for Disease Control and Prevention
Hyattsville, Maryland

John W. Horm, MSc
National Center for Health Statistics
Centers for Disease Control and Prevention
Hyattsville, Maryland

Syed S. Islam, MBBS, DrPH
Institute of Occupational and Environmental Medicine
West Virginia University
School of Medicine
Morgantown, West Virginia

Ole Møller Jensen, MD†
Danish Cancer Registry
Institute of Cancer Epidemiology
Copenhagen, Denmark

John M. Kaldor, PhD
The University of New South Wales
St. Vincent's Hospital Medical Center
Sydney, New South Wales, Australia

Margaret R. Karagas, PhD
Program in Epidemiology
Fred Hutchinson Cancer Research Center
Seattle, Washington

Leo J. Kinlen, MD
CRC Cancer Epidemiology Research Group
University of Oxford
The Radcliffe Infirmary
Oxford, England

Kenneth H. Kraemer, MD
Laboratory of Molecular Carcinogenesis
National Cancer Institute
Bethesda, Maryland

Charles E. Land, PhD
Radiation Epidemiology Branch
National Cancer Institute
Bethesda, Maryland

Lester B. Lave, PhD
Graduate School of Industrial Administration
Carnegie-Mellon University
Pittsburgh, Pennsylvania

Frederick P. Li, MD
Dana-Farber Cancer Center
Boston, Massachusetts

†Deceased.

Jonathan M. Liff, PhD
Rollins School of Public Health
Emory University
Atlanta, Georgia

Martha S. Linet, MD
Biostatistics Branch
National Cancer Institute
Bethesda, Maryland

W. Thomas London, MD
Fox Chase Cancer Center
Philadelphia, Pennsylvania

Thomas M. Mack, MD
Department of Preventive Medicine
University of Southern California
Los Angeles, California

Wendy J. Mack, PhD
Department of Preventive Medicine
University of Southern California
Los Angeles, California

Susan Preston-Martin, PhD
Department of Preventive Medicine
University of Southern California
Los Angeles, California

Katherine A. McGlynn, PhD
Fox Chase Cancer Center
Philadelphia, Pennsylvania

Joseph K. McLaughlin, PhD
International Epidemiology Institute, Ltd
Rockville, Maryland

Anthony J. McMichael, MBBS, PhD
London School of Hygiene and Tropical Medicine
Department of Epidemiology and Population Sciences
London, England

Anthony B. Miller, MD, DrPH
NCIC Epidemiology Unit
University of Toronto
Toronto, Ontario, Canada

Robert W. Miller, MD, DrPH
Genetic Epidemiology Branch
National Cancer Institute
Bethesda, Maryland

Richard R. Monson, MD
Department of Epidemiology
Harvard School of Public Health
Boston, Massachusetts

Alan S. Morrison, MD, ScD†
Department of Epidemiology
Brown University Health Sciences Center
Providence, Rhode Island

Nancy E. Mueller, ScD
Department of Epidemiology
Harvard School of Public Health
Boston, Massachusetts

Calum S. Muir, MB, PhD†
Information and Statistics Division
Common Services Agency for the Scottish Health Services
Edinburgh, Scotland

Nubia Muñoz, MD
International Agency for Research on Cancer
Lyon, France

J. Nectoux
Descriptive Epidemiology Program
International Agency for Research on Cancer
Lyon, France

Abraham Nomura, MD
Japan-Hawaii Cancer Study
Honolulu, Hawaii

Andrew F. Olshan, PhD
Department of Epidemiology
University of North Carolina
School of Public Health
Chapel Hill, North Carolina

Sally L. Paine, MPH
London School of Hygiene and Tropical Medicine
Department of Epidemiology and Population Sciences
London, England

Frederica P. Perera, DrPH
Division of Environmental Health Sciences
Columbia University
School of Public Health
New York, New York

Malcom C. Pike, PhD
Department of Preventive Medicine
University of Southern California
Los Angeles, California

Henry C. Pitot, MD, PhD (Consulting Editor)
McArdle Laboratory for Cancer Research
University of Wisconsin
Madison, Wisconsin

†Deceased.

Charles Poole, ScD
Department of Epidemiology and Biostatistics
Boston University School of Public Health
Boston, Massachusetts

John D. Potter, MBBS, PhD
Cancer Prevention Research Program
Fred Hutchinson Cancer Research Center
Seattle, Washington

Dale L. Preston, PhD
Department of Statistics
Radiation Effects Research Foundation
Minami-Ku, Hiroshima, Japan

Peggy Reynolds, PhD
California Department of Health
Environmental Epidemiology Services
Emeryville, California

Dorothy P. Rice, BA
Department of Social and Behavioral Sciences
School of Nursing
University of California
San Francisco, California

Lynn A. Gloeckler Ries, MS
Cancer Statistics Branch
National Cancer Institute
Bethesda, Maryland

Thomas E. Rohan, MD
National Cancer Institute of Canada
Department of Preventive Medicine and Biostatistics
University of Toronto
Toronto, Ontario, Canada

Elaine Ron, PhD
Radiation Epidemiology Branch
National Cancer Institute
Bethesda, Maryland

Karin A. Rosenblatt, PhD
Department of Epidemiology
University of Washington
Fred Hutchinson Cancer Research Center
Seattle, Washington

Ronald K. Ross, MD
Department of Preventive Medicine
Norris Comprehensive Cancer Center
University of Southern California
Los Angeles, California

Kenneth J. Rothman, DrPH
Section of Preventive Medicine and Epidemiology
Department of Medicine
Boston University School of Medicine
Boston, Massachusetts

George C. Roush, MD
Cancer Prevention Research Institute
New York, New York

Raymond W. Ruddon, Jr., MD, PhD
Eppley Institute for Research in Cancer and Allied Diseases
University of Nebraska Medical Center
Omaha, Nebraska

Paul A. Scherr, PhD, ScD
Division of Chronic Disease Control and Community Intervention
Centers for Disease Control and Prevention
Atlanta, Georgia

Mark H. Schiffman, MD
Environmental Epidemiology Branch
National Cancer Institute
Bethesda, Maryland

David Schottenfeld, MD (Editor)
Department of Epidemiology
The University of Michigan
School of Public Health
Ann Arbor, Michigan

Joseph Scotto, MS
Biostatistics Branch
National Cancer Institute
Bethesda, Maryland

Joseph V. Selby, MD
Division of Research
Kaiser Permanente
Oakland, California

Karen J. Sherman, PhD
Division of Public Health Sciences
Fred Hutchinson Cancer Research Center
Epidemiologic Research Unit
Seattle, Washington

Carl M. Shy, MD, DrPH
Department of Epidemiology
School of Public Health
University of North Carolina
Chapel Hill, North Carolina

Debra T. Silverman, ScD
Environmental Epidemiology Branch
National Cancer Institute
Bethesda, Maryland

Janet L. Stanford, PhD
Program in Epidemiology
Fred Hutchinson Cancer Research Center
Seattle, Washington

Louise C. Strong, MD (Consulting Editor)
Dept. of Experimental Pediatrics/Genetics
M.D. Anderson Hospital and Tumor Institute
Houston, Texas

David B. Thomas, MD, DrPH
Program in Epidemiology
Fred Hutchinson Cancer Research Center
Seattle, Washington

Lorenzo Tomatis, MD
International Agency for Research on Cancer
Lyon, France

Margaret A. Tucker, MD
Genetic Epidemiology Branch
National Cancer Institute
Bethesda, Maryland

Noel S. Weiss, MD, DrPH (Consulting Editor)
Department of Epidemiology
University of Washington
School of Public Health
Seattle, Washington

Alice S. Whittemore, PhD
Epidemiology and Biostatistics
Department of Health Research and Policy
Stanford University School of Medicine
Stanford, California

Louise Wideroff, PhD
Environmental Epidemiology Branch
National Cancer Institute
Bethesda, Maryland

Walter C. Willett, MD, DrPH
Department of Nutrition
Harvard School of Public Health
Boston, Massachusetts

Sidney J. Winawer, MD
Department of Medicine
Gastroenterology and Nutrition Service
Memorial Sloan-Kettering Cancer Center
New York, New York

Mimi C. Yu, PhD
Norris Comprehensive Cancer Center
University of Southern California
Los Angeles, California

Shelia Hoar Zahm, ScD
Environmental Epidemiology Branch
National Cancer Institute
Bethesda, Maryland

PART I | Basic Concepts

1 Causation and causal inference

KENNETH J. ROTHMAN
CHARLES POOLE

CAUSATION

The Evolution of the Concept of Causation

The understanding of causation has evolved in tandem with our knowledge about causal relations in nature. Aristotle, whose scientific views lingered dominant over Western thought for centuries, had described four different types of cause for each object: (1) *material cause*, which was the matter of the object; (2) *formal cause*, which was the pattern imposed on the matter; (3) *efficient cause*, which was the force producing the object; and (4) *final cause*, which was the purpose of the object. All these aspects of "causal" inquiry raised searching questions concerning the nature of how things came to be as they were.

The prevailing doctrine of scientific philosophy at the apex of ancient Greek civilization and in most centuries since was *rationalism*, a doctrine that regarded reason as the source of all knowledge of the physical world. For Aristotle, as for many of the other thinkers of his time, the answers to searching questions about nature were available to any serious thinker. Rationalism, combined with the weighty traditionalism that flourished in the long era when religious principles overshadowed science and the central authority of the church went unchallenged, fostered a predominance of authoritarian and to a large extent Aristotelian views about nature. With the rise of Protestantism in Europe, however, it became possible to challenge existing doctrines.

As modern science took root in the seventeenth century, *empiricism* replaced rationalism as the dominant philosophy of science. Empiricism substituted observation for reason, or rather combined observation with reason in a new methodology, which came to be called *induction*. According to the inductive principle of empiricism, causation was an inferred relation between two events that were repeatedly observed to occur in the same time sequence. To infer causation required observation, prediction, and additional observation to verify the prediction. This profound change in scientific thought characterized the rise of modern science.

Empiricism was not without its critics. Foremost among them was David Hume, who argued that the mere temporal conjunction of two events, or the reported conjunction of such events, cannot impart to an observer any knowledge about a causal connection between these events. Hume revealed the process of inductive inference to be a logically faulty process: without direct evidence for a causal connection, which was impossible, induction could lead to incorrect inferences. Inductive logic, therefore, was not really a "logic" at all. For him, induction became a psychological process by which a person's convictions about causal relations between events are modified by observations. With this simple but profound skepticism, Hume shook the new foundation of empiric science.

Ever since Hume, defenders of empiricism have attempted to answer his criticism of inductive "logic" and his relegation of induction to the psychological realm. A notable defender of induction was Immanuel Kant, whose answer to Hume was imbedded in his concept of the *synthetic a priori*. Kant distinguished between two types of judgments: *analytic*, which were logical truisms unrelated to empirical judgments, and *synthetic*, which were judgments that extended knowledge. Kant believed that some synthetic judgments are made without reference to experience. For him, the explanation of the existence of these *synthetic a priori* judgments was the central issue in metaphysics. The concept of causation was one of Kant's *synthetic a priori* judgments: that events had causes was simply assumed to be known, and induction was merely the process of identifying the causes.

Hume died before Kant's arguments were published, but Reichenbach (1951) provided a response that Hume might have given to Kant:

> How does it help us to know that there is a cause if we wish to know what the cause is? It is true, if we knew there were no cause it would be nonsensical to search for one; but that is not our situation. We do not know whether there is a cause; in this situation we make inductive inferences, based on observation, and conclude, say, that the moon is the cause of the tides. This inductive inference is

what I question; and it would remain just as questionable if you could prove the general statement that there is a cause.

Reichenbach proposed a different solution to "Hume's problem" (as Kant described it), a solution that Reichenbach contended could not have been proposed before the development of probability theory and quantum mechanics. He argued that Heisenberg's principle of uncertainty, by which individual atomic phenomena are explainable only in probabilistic terms, shows that a concept of "strict causality" is not tenable. According to Reichenbach's view, natural laws are, in effect, only idealized statistical laws, and causality is not an ultimate principle, but only a substitute for statistical regularity. He proposed that " . . . . the idea of a strict causality is to be abandoned, and that the laws of probability take over the place once occupied by the law of causality."

Reichenbach concluded that scientific philosophy has led us to the truth that empirical knowledge can never be certain. Hume's objection to the use of inductive logic was the inconsistency of a "logic" that is uncertain. For Hume, such a methodology was invalid; for Reichenbach, it is the best we can achieve, and this status of superiority validates it. Carnap (1962) took Reichenbach's argument further by attempting to formalize inductive logic in a set of probability laws intended to quantify the degree of confirmation of a hypothesis. The notion of probabilistic causality has continued to be a major theme in the modern philosophy of science (Good, 1983; Suppes, 1984).

Yet another answer to "Hume's problem" was proposed by Popper (1968), who accepted Hume's repudiation of induction as a logic. Popper argued that the view that the validity of scientific statements can be quantified by probabilities is an evasion of Hume's criticism. Whereas other philosophers believe that induction is necessary and therefore tried to substantiate it, Popper found it quite dispensable. He maintained that, as a matter of logic, scientific statements are in principle conclusively decidable only in the negative. They can logically be falsified but not verified. Falsification, unlike verification, requires no inductive inference, only deductive logic. Observable deductions are drawn from hypotheses. If the observation is made, and it is valid, the hypothesis is corroborated. If the observation conflicts with the deduction, and the observation is valid, the hypothesis is refuted. Popper acknowledged that all empirical observations are fallible, so that empirical refutation is not conclusive, but he emphasized the *logical* distinction between falsification and verification. Popper's view coincides with the historical view of science: widely accepted theories have been subsequently replaced, after falsification, with new theories. No conclusive verification has ever occurred, even though in every era there are theories that are "accepted" as having been "established" by "conclusive" observations.

Popper and his followers have emphasized the importance of attempting to refute theories, and have argued that this attempt is a more productive path than the attempt to confirm or verify theories. Magee (1985) has illustrated this point with the following example: If one has a theory that water boils at 100°C, one can attempt to confirm this theory with repeated experiments. Nevertheless, no number of confirmations can prove the theory to be true, or even increase its probability of being true. If one searches for conditions that may show the theory to be false, one may learn that water in a closed vessel will not boil at 100°C. Such refuting observations, if valid, will ideally lead to reformulation of the theory or to a new theory altogether. The new theory will explain more observations than the former one, and on that basis will be clearly preferable, but no more capable of being proven true than was the initial theory. Thousands of confirmations of the original theory would not have increased its probability of being correct one bit, and would not have led to the insights that enabled a more encompassing theory to be formulated. In this way, science progresses rapidly with attempts at refutation, whereas it might cease entirely if only attempts at confirmation were to be made.

The practical ramifications of the distinction between searching for verification and attempting to refute theories can profoundly affect the way in which scientists approach their work. The popular image of a scientist doggedly pursuing a favorite thesis becomes an objectionable model from the standpoint of refutation because this image encourages scientists to consider their pet theories as their own intellectual property, to be defended, confirmed, proven, and when all the evidence is in, cast in stone as "established knowledge." Such attitudes foster little interest in criticism, especially of one's own research, and can condemn scientists to defensive and unproductive labors. In pursuit of verification scientists may become personally identified with, and attached to, the theories toward which their research is directed. The concern in evaluating competing theories may then devolve into the degree of belief that scientists have, individually and collectively, for competing theories. In this way authoritarianism blossoms, because the weight to be attached to a given scientist's beliefs must be based on his or her reputation and credentials as an authority.

It was to guard against zeal in clinging to theories, and to promote zeal in criticizing them, that Medawar (1979) sagely warned: "I cannot give any scientist of any age better advice than this: the intensity of the conviction that a hypothesis is true has no bearing on whether it is true or not."

Whereas Reichenbach and Carnap attempted to modify and formalize inductive logic, and Popper resolved Hume's problem not by rescuing induction but by arguing that scientific progress does not involve inductive logic at all, all would agree that scientific knowledge is uncertain in two senses, empirical and logical. The empirical uncertainty of scientific observations themselves is almost universally accepted. For Reichenbach and Carnap the nature of the logical uncertainty was that of probability, the probability that a hypothesis is true; for Popper, the logical uncertainty was that of tentativeness, in particular, the tentative survival of a hypothesis after all attempts thus far to refute it. Reichenbach and Carnap believed that if knowledge could not be made certain, at least it could be made more probable. Popper argued that knowledge can be made neither certain nor more probable and that all we ever have is a set of theories that have not yet been refuted and replaced by superior theories. Whereas the inductivist approach is a Lamarckian process of learning from repetitive instruction by empirical observations, the refutationist approach is a Darwinian process in which the fittest hypotheses survive in the place of those that cannot stand up to empirical tests.

The lack of scientific content of unfalsifiable statements does not mean that such statements have no place in science. Indeed, unfalsifiable hypotheses such as Lamarck's and Darwin's theories of evolution may have utility as guiding principles of scientific research programs (Lakatos, 1978). Lack of scientific content simply means that there is no sense in conducting empirical research *about* an unfalsifiable hypothesis. If a hypothesis prohibits nothing, every observation that can be made will be consistent with it. It is thus a waste of time and effort to gather data that can only confirm such "infinitely confirmable" hypotheses.

Popper's emphasis on the falsifiability of a theory has implications for current thought in carcinogenesis, as we shall see: the multi-stage theory, which is much discussed, is so general a statement that it cannot be falsified; it therefore has no scientific content. Specific variants of the theory, however, such as Knudson's (1971) two-mutation model, are more easily falsifiable and therefore of greater scientific interest.

An Epidemiologic Concept of Causation

Philosophers of science have improved our understanding of the logic of causal inference, but there remains a need, at least in epidemiology, to formulate a general and coherent model of causation to facilitate the conceptualization of epidemiologic problems. A first step in the development of one such model is to distinguish conceptually between *sufficient causes* and *components* of sufficient causes (Rothman, 1976). A sufficient cause of an occurrence of disease is the set of conditions and events *without any one of which* the occurrence would not have taken place. Precisely because a sufficient cause implies inevitability of the effect, sufficient causes are impossible to identify in their entirety. A component of a sufficient cause, however, implies by its presence only the possibility of the effect; the actual outcome depends on the occurrence of the complementary component causes that are needed to complete that sufficient cause. The conditions and events that epidemiologists study as "exposures" or "potential risk factors" are hypothetical component causes. Blocking the action of a component cause will render an otherwise sufficient cause insufficient, and thereby prevent the effect, at least through one mechanism. It is still possible that the effect will occur anyway through another mechanism, i.e., a different sufficient cause, that does not include as a component cause the factor that has been blocked.

Consider, as an example, cigarette smoking as a cause of lung cancer. The estimates from hundreds of epidemiologic studies indicate that most cases of lung cancer are attributable to sufficient causes (i.e., causal mechanisms) that involve smoking as a component cause. By avoiding smoking, or by making a noncarcinogenic cigarette, we could prevent most cases of lung cancer. It would not be necessary to block any other component of any sufficient cause that involves smoking in order to prevent these cases of lung cancer from occurring. A few cases of lung cancer would still occur, though, because there are other sufficient causes of lung cancer that do not involve smoking, as evinced by the occurrence of lung cancer among nonsmokers.

When two conditions or events are components of the same sufficient cause, they interact synergistically. Thus the effect of joint exposure to the two complementary component causes will be greater than the sum of their independent effects (Rothman, 1974). Synergism between cigarette smoking and asbestos exposure in the causation of lung cancer, therefore, implies that four kinds of biological mechanisms (sufficient causes) potentially produce lung cancer among smokers who are exposed to asbestos: (*1*) mechanisms that involve neither asbestos nor smoking; (*2*) mechanisms that involve smoking but not asbestos; (*3*) mechanisms that involve asbestos but not smoking; and (*4*) mechanisms that involve both smoking and asbestos. Lung cancer cases of the fourth type can be prevented by avoiding smoking *or* by avoiding asbestos exposure. Epidemiologic measures exist to estimate the number of cases or the incidence rate attributable to each type of sufficient cause, either in absolute terms or as a proportion of the total number of cases or the entire rate in a group of people exposed to two or more complementary causes (Rothman, 1986).

Some component causes of a sufficient cause may be thought of as "passive" components, those that contribute appropriate conditions for the other components causes to act. Genetic characteristics that are risk factors fall into this category of component causes. Nearly every complete cause has components that are genetic, and these can be thought of as "susceptibility factors." Nongenetic component causes also may contribute to the effect in a similar way by providing the right conditions for other component causes to act. Ingested nitrite, for example, may cause cancer if it is chemically converted to nitrosamine in the stomach. The reaction is dependent on pH, with the highest yield occurring at a pH of 3.4, and lesser yields at a lower or higher pH (Mirvish, 1970). Very little conversion occurs below a pH of 1.5 or above a pH of 5.0. The pH of stomach contents depends on the type and quantity of food consumed; it is usually much lower than 3.4 when the stomach is empty, but may be near 3.4 after a large meal. Sufficient alkalinity of the gastric contents may be thought of as a passive component cause of cancer, permitting dietary nitrite to be converted to an active carcinogen, which may then induce cancer.

Generally speaking, only "active" component causes of cancer are considered carcinogens. Active causes produce transitions between stages under conditions created by passive component causes. The passive role of the latter group of component causes corresponds to that of a susceptibility factor, but not to what is usually meant by a carcinogen. This distinction between carcinogenic agents and other component causes of cancer is obviously not conceptually rigorous, but rather only a distinction that derives from common usage. In principle, under the sufficient cause model, there is no important distinction to be drawn between component causes that are "active" and those that are "passive," because a component cause may be *either* a condition (passive) or an event (active).

CARCINOGENESIS

The Multistage Theory of Carcinogenesis

The precise number of stages in a causal path cannot be determined meaningfully, because the causal sequence can always be described in finer detail, and the designation of stages is ultimately an arbitrary classification. Even a single abrupt transition event could be dissected into many gradations. Often, however, the transitions in a causal path appear to be reasonably categorized into one or more distinct events. In the development of general carcinogenic theories, attention has focused almost exclusively on heritable intracellular changes as opposed to extracellular conditions and events or intracellular changes that are not passed on from one cell to its progeny. Carcinogenesis has at least two and possibly many heritable, intracellular transitions, which have come to be called *stages*. Carcinogenic agents are considered *initiators* if they act in early stages, and *promotors* if they act in later stages.

A formalization of the implications of sequentially acting component causes as applied to carcinogenesis has been discussed in terms of the *multistage theory of carcinogenesis*. Under this theory, the development of a cancer is the last stage in a sequence of stochastic heritable cellular events, for which the transition probabilities from one stage to the next are usually assumed to be constant over time. Although theoreticians have not reached any consensus as to which form or forms of such a theory might actually apply in carcinogenesis, the consequences of various forms of the general theory have been examined in detail and compared with epidemiologic evidence. (For reviews, see Peto [1977], and Freedman and Navidi [1989].) Such comparisons of theory and observations are difficult to interpret, because time trends in incidence, inaccuracies in reporting, non-heritable cellular events, and multiple etiologies, among other concerns, all work to distort the observations predicted by the theory. As Freedman and Navidi (1989) have indicated, one variation of the model or another can be made to fit almost any set of pertinent data. The mathematical assumptions and approximations for some forms of the theory have also been widely misunderstood (Moolgavkar, 1978).

Despite these reservations, many scientists have been attracted to the multistage theory because of its generality and the close correspondence between age-incidence curves predicted from the theory and those actually observed (Cook et al. 1969). The precise value of the theory is debatable, however, in view of the difficulty with which the theory might be falsified. Indeed, the multistage theory in a general form could be used, as already indicated, as a general model of causation to apply to all etiologic situations. What gives any theory scientific content are the restrictions that are incorporated into it for any given situation. On these grounds, theories that are less general than the multistage theory ought to attract greater attention from the standpoint of research *about* a theory as opposed to research *under* a theory. For example, Moolgavkar and Venzon (1979) have shown that a two-stage model can generate age-incidence curves similar in shape to those generated from more complicated multistage models, thus extending the applicability of Knudson's (1971) two-stage model for embryonal tumors to include adult tumors. They argue that biologic interpretation (i.e., initiation and promotion) can be given to no more than two distinct stages, making their two-stage model more acceptable than alternatives that posit three or more stages.

Induction Period and Latent Period

Some scientists use the terms *induction period* and *latent period* interchangeably (*incubation period* is also used), but the time interval between exposure to an etiologic agent and appearance of disease symptoms can be meaningfully partitioned in a way that suggests a distinction between these terms. The Oxford English Dictionary (1971) defines *latent* as "hidden," whereas *induction* is defined as the "act of causing or producing." Conceptually, then, the *induction period* is the time interval during which a sufficient cause is completed. In reference to a particular component cause, the induction period would begin at the time of action of the component cause and end when all the other component causes that constitute a sufficient cause have completed their action to cause the disease. At the time of disease causation, when the induction period ends, the *latent period* begins. In principle, the latent period could be reduced to near zero with more accurate means to detect presymptomatic disease; the length of the latent period is simply the time interval from the occurrence of a disease to detection.

The latent period is conceptually part of the causal process only to the extent that during the latent period, disease may "spontaneously" disappear or fail to progress, in which case clinical disease would not occur. Logically, however, such alterations in the progression of disease should be considered part of the causal process of *clinical* disease, thus implying that where the natural history of disease is not that of inevitable progression, the latent period is subsumed within the induction period, which accordingly would end not at the occurrence of preclinical disease, but at the start of symptoms. For diseases that progress inevitably to become clinically apparent, the latent period would follow the induction period. It is impossible, of course, to determine when the induction period ends and the latent period begins for any individual case, though these time periods can be estimated for large groups of people. The conceptual distinction between induction period and latent period is worth maintaining because these two time periods define the intervals during which primary prevention (i.e., blocking a sufficient cause) and secondary prevention (i.e., preclinical detection and treatment) would be applicable.

For exposures that are continuous or intermittent, there remains the difficulty in determining when the exposure acts etiologically. Customarily, epidemiologists measure induction periods from the time of first exposure, because the relevant time of action is unknown, whereas the time of first exposure can usually be determined. A better practice, however, is to choose an arbitrary accumulation of exposure, and determine the time at which that level is reached. It is possible to vary the estimates for the sufficient dose of exposure and learn from the epidemiologic analysis which estimate is most appropriate. This procedure can also incorporate variations in exposure dose with time.

Some carcinogens have lengthy induction periods for certain cancers; an example is the occurrence of adenocarcinoma of the vagina 15 to 30 years after exposure of female fetuses to diethylstilbestrol. It appears, on the basis of the age distribution of cases, that the sufficient cause is usually completed during puberty or adolescence for women who develop this disease; therefore the time before puberty or adolescence would be the induction period, and the interval following that period until symptoms appear would be the latent period.

Frequently some types of cancer are described as diseases of lengthy induction period, the implication being that the action of any carcinogen causing that cancer precedes the development of the tumor by a long interval. The disease itself, however, should not be classified as having a lengthy induction period; the induction period refers to the interval between the action of a specific component cause and the disease initiation. Because a component cause might act at any "stage" during carcinogenesis, the length of the induction period for a specific component or carcinogen would depend on the point during the causal sequence at which the carcinogen acted. Carcinogens acting during a late stage (promotors) would have a short induction period, even if the complete causal chain involves a long sequence of stages requiring many years or decades to complete. From animal experiments it appears that estrogens act as late-stage carcinogens; this finding has been confirmed from epidemiologic research on replacement estrogen therapy and endometrial cancer, which indicates that estrogens have relatively brief (3 to 10 year) induction and latent periods before the occurrence of endometrial cancer (Jick et al. 1979). In addition, it has been found that the risk for endometrial cancer increases with the length of time estrogens have been used, but drops quickly if estrogen therapy is discontinued, a pattern that also agrees with the results from animal studies of promotors.

The Implications of Epidemiologic Observations

One prediction from certain multistage models is that each of two carcinogens acting at different stages in the causal process will have effects that are, under some conditions, proportional to the effect of the other; i.e., the effects are interactive according to a "multiplicative" pattern. Asbestos and smoking seem to interact in exactly this way in causing lung cancer (Saracci, 1977); the implication, given the appropriateness of the multistage model, is that asbestos and smoking act at different stages. No attempt, however, has been made to contrast this hypothesis with competing alternatives, such as reduced mucociliary clearance of asbestos fiber from the smokers' lungs (Cohen et al., 1979) or enhancement by asbestos of the transport of chemical carcinogens in cigarette smoke across cell membranes (Lakowicz et al., 1980). Thus, a need exists to test variants of the multistage theory of carcinogenesis not only against each other, but also against hypothetical mechanisms of synergism that do not involve heritable cellular transitions. Smoking and alcohol also show an interaction that may be multiplicative in causing cancer of the mouth and pharynx (Rothman and Keller, 1972).

Some epidemiologic evidence is consistent with a single cause affecting more than one stage of the carcinogenic process. One example, described by Peto (1977), is smoking and lung cancer. Ex-smokers maintain a constant incidence of lung cancer from the time of cessation, whereas continuing smokers show a steadily increasing incidence. According to Peto, this pattern implies that smoking affects the penultimate stage of carcinogenesis. Other data, however, indicate that new smokers do not exhibit a change in incidence from their smoking for many years, indicating that smoking affects an early stage. Of course, other interpretations might be given to these findings, but the implication that smoking affects both an early and a late part of the carcinogenic process for lung cancer is both interesting and plausible.

The time distribution of disease after occurrence has implications for the stage at which a carcinogen acts. Land and Norman (1978), analyzing the distribution of induction periods for various cancers after exposure to ionizing radiation, concluded that if a two-stage model is assumed, radiation affects only the first stage for lung and breast cancer (resulting in a typically long induction period), but the second stage for chronic granulocytic leukemia (resulting in a short induction period).

CAUSAL INFERENCE

The preceding sections describe the theoretical basis for scientific inference and a conceptual model of causation that can be modified as needed to describe carcinogenesis. Here we consider in more specific terms how causal inference proceeds. Because most scientific knowledge outside of the physical sciences represents a collection of causal statements, we shall consider the problem of scientific inference and causal inference to be equivalent in this discussion.

The process of generalizing beyond a set of observations has often been construed to involve a judgment about what features of the observations may be extrapolated to a target zone (in epidemiologic studies, a target population). Such extrapolation is thought to require an understanding of which conditions are relevant and which are irrelevant to the generalization. For example, a study of smoking and lung cancer in men might be generalized to a target population of women. To do so would require a presumption that being male is irrelevant to the carcinogenic action that smoking has on lung tissue, a presumption based on theories about the mechanism of carcinogenesis and the biologic similarity between male and female lungs. On the other hand, a study of diet and breast cancer in women might not be considered generalizable to men, because physiologic differences between the sexes may play a role in the causal process.

This model of scientific inference as a generalization of observations is a descendant of the inductivist approach that ushered in the era of modern science. The conventional wisdom in this approach is that generalization from a study group to a target population depends upon the degree to which the study group is representative of the target population. "Representativeness," the crucial concept for generalization, has been given various interpretations. The most orthodox interpretation is for "representativeness" to mean statistical representativeness, in the sense of a sample. With this interpretation for representativeness, generalization would be confined literally to those individuals who might have been included as study subjects. This type of generalization corresponds to statistical inference, but it is not scientific inference. If it were scientific inference, there would be no application to humans of any results obtained from research with other species. Every human population would require its own set of epidemiologic studies, and these studies would have to be repeated for every new generation!

Part of the difficulty in understanding scientific inference seems to be the tendency to equate it with the more mechanical process of statistical inference with which many people are familiar. The superficial similarities between epidemiologic work and that of poll-taking (for example, both can involve finding people, interviewing them, and worrying about bias from non-response) may explain in part why statistical inference, which is important in poll-taking, has often been seen as the crucial inferential process in epidemiology and related biological sciences. Epidemiologic study designs are usually stronger if the subject selection is guided by the need for making a valid comparison, which may call for severe restriction of admissible subjects to a narrow range of characteristics, rather than a generally futile attempt to make the subjects statistically representative of the potential target populations.

Despite its obvious flaws, the influence of inductivism remains strong, and it has led some scientists to the adoption of specific guidelines for generalization. These guidelines are usually posited as criteria by which an observation of an association in a study population might be judged to reflect a causal association. It is ironic that the most widely discussed set of causal criteria is that of Hill (1965), because Hill explicitly cautioned against using characteristics of associations (such as their strength, consistency and coherence) as "hard and fast rules of evidence." Nevertheless, committees of the U.S. Surgeon General (U.S. Department of Health, Education, and Welfare, 1964, 1982) and, more recently, Susser (1988) have extended and elaborated these characteristics as criteria for causal judgment.

The problem with causal criteria is the same problem as with any positivist approach to inference in empirical science, namely that there can be no criteria to make an algorithm out of inference (Lanes and Poole, 1984). Empirical science will always be making corrections to previous inferences—some being small refinements, other being major revisions in thinking. This process occurs by trial and error: testable hypotheses are developed and from them, potentially falsifiable observations are deduced and then tested against empirical experience. This focus on the hypothesis and the observations that might refute or corroborate it contrasts starkly with the focus on associations and the characteristics that would make them more or less "likely" to be causal.

Superior alternatives to the statistical interpretation of "representativeness" have fostered the attitude that scientific inference is a more abstract concept than the plain mechanics of statistical sampling. The model for scientific inference is intellectually less confining than the model for statistical inference. Rather than construe scientific inference as a process of moving from a study population to a target population, we can construe it as the process of formulating an abstract scientific explanation (that is, hypothesis, conjecture or theory) for the observations in hand and for future observations that might be made to test an explanation against its competing alternatives. Generalization in this sense is the formulation of a general theory, which depends not on statistical representativeness of the study subjects but rather on the integration of the scientific findings from a particular study into the larger fabric of scientific knowledge (Pearce, 1990; Renton, 1994). Data on study populations provide a way of testing such generalized explanations. Under this model, generalizations need not spring from observations: indeed, since they involve creative thought and data are mute, it is arguable whether one can claim that any hypothesis can be "generated by the data." Scientific generalizations are generated by the minds of the scientists who interpret the data. Statistical generalization from a sample to the population from which the sample was drawn does not merit the dignity of being called a scientific inference.

REFERENCES

CARNAP R. 1962. Logical Foundations of Probability, 2nd ed. Chicago, University of Chicago Press.

COHEN D, ARAI SF, BRAIN JD. 1979. Smoking impairs long-term dust clearance from the lung. Science 204:514–515.

COOK PJ, DOLL R, FELLINGHAM SA. 1969. A mathematical model for the age distribution of cancer in man. Int J Cancer 4:93–112.

FREEDMAN DA, NAVIDI WC. 1989. On the multistage model for carcinogenesis. Environ Health Perspect 81:169–188.

GOOD IJ. 1983. Good Thinking. The Foundation of Probability and its Applications. Minneapolis, University of Minnesota Press, pp. 197–236.

HILL AB. 1965. The environment and disease: association or causation? Proc Soc Med 58:295–300.

JICK H, WATKINS RN, HUNTER JR, et al. 1979. Replacement estrogens and endometrial cancer. N Engl J Med 300:218–222.

KNUDSON AG. 1971. Mutation and cancer: statistical study of retinoblastoma. Proc Natl Acad Sci USA 68:820–823.

LAKATOS I. 1978. The Methodology of Scientific Research Programmes. Philosophical Papers, Vol. I. Cambridge, Cambridge University Press.

LAKOWICZ JR, BEVAN DR, RIEMER SC. 1980. Transport of a carcinogen, benzo[a]pyrene, from particulates to lipid bilayers. Biochim Biophys Acta 629:243–258.

LAND CE, NORMAN JE. 1978. The latent periods of radiogenic cancers occurring among Japanese A-bomb survivors. *In* International Atomic Energy Agency Symposium on the Late Biological Effects of Ionizing Radiation. Hiroshima, Radiation Effects Research Foundation; and Washington, D.C., Medical Follow-up Agency, National Academy of Sciences.

LANES SF, POOLE C. 1984. "Truth in Packaging?" The unwrapping of epidemiologic research. J Occup Med 26:571–574.

MAGEE B. 1985. Philosophy and the Real World. An Introduction to Karl Popper. La Salle, IL, Open Court.

MEDAWAR PB. 1979. Advice to a Young Scientist. New York, Basic Books, p. 39.

MIRVISH SS. 1970. Kinetics of dimethyl nitrosation in relation to nitrosamine carcinogenesis. J Natl Cancer Inst 44:633–639.

MOOLGAVKAR SH. 1978. The multistage theory of carcinogenesis and the age distribution of cancer in man. J Natl Cancer Inst 61:49–52.

MOOLGAVKAR SH, VENZON DJ. 1979. Two-event models for carcinogenesis: incidence curves for childhood and adult tumors. Math Biosci 47:55–77.

OXFORD ENGLISH DICTIONARY, OXFORD UNIVERSITY PRESS, 1971.

PEARCE, N. 1990. White swans, black ravens, and lame ducks: necessary and sufficient causes in epidemiology. Epidemiology 1:47–50.

PETO R. 1977. Epidemiology, multistage models, and short-term mutagenicity tests. *In* Hiatt H, Watson JD, Winsten JA, et al. (eds): Origins of Human Cancer. New York, Cold Spring Harbor Publications.

POPPER KR. 1968. The Logic of Scientific Discovery. New York, Harper & Row.

REICHENBACH H. 1951. The Rise of Scientific Philosophy. Berkeley, University of California Press.

RENTON A. 1994. Epidemiology and causation: a realist view. J Epidemiol Community Health 48:79–85.

ROTHMAN KJ. 1974. Synergism and antagonism in cause-effect relationships. Am J Epidemiol 99:385–388.

ROTHMAN KJ. 1976. Causes. Am J Epidemiol 104:587–592.

ROTHMAN KJ. 1986. Modern Epidemiology, Boston, Little, Brown, and Co.

ROTHMAN KJ, KELLER AZ. 1972. The effect of joint exposure to alcohol and tobacco on risk of cancer of the mouth and pharynx. J Chron Dis 25:711–716.

SARACCI R. 1977. Asbestos and lung cancer: an analysis of the epidemiological evidence on the asbestos-smoking interaction. Int J Cancer 20:323–331.

SUPPES P. 1984. Probabilistic Metaphysics. Oxford: Basil Blackwell.

SUSSER M. 1988. Falsification, verification, and causal inference in epidemiology: reconsiderations in the light of Sir Karl Popper's philosophy. *In* Rothman KJ (ed): Causal Inference, Epidemiology Resources Inc. Newton, MA, pp. 33–57.

U.S. DEPARTMENT OF HEALTH, EDUCATION, AND WELFARE. 1964. Smoking and Health. Report of the Advisory Committee to the Surgeon General. U.S. Government Printing Office, Washington, D.C., Public Health Service Publication No. 1103.

U.S. DEPARTMENT OF HEALTH, EDUCATION, AND WELFARE. 1982. The Health Consequences of Smoking: Cancer. A Report of the Surgeon General. Rockville, Maryland, Public Health Service, Publication No. 82–50179.

2 Experimental studies in the assessment of human risk

LORENZO TOMATIS
JOHN M. KALDOR
H. BARTSCH

An assessment of the number or of the proportion of cancers that could be prevented by measures of primary prevention would obviously be of paramount importance. It would be difficult, however, and probably impossible to make an accurate quantification of what could be achieved today in terms of primary prevention of cancers. Even in the most qualified, and quoted, attempt the authors could not go beyond a range of acceptable estimates that, for a certain class of factors, first of all diet, is quite wide (Doll and Peto, 1981). While it is reasonable to assume that a considerable proportion of cancer cases are allocated to environmental agents, etiological factors have not yet been identified for cancers that occur at some of the most frequent target organs, such as prostate and colon in men, and breast and colon in women. The identification of etiological agents of cancer has depended on the availability of at least two forms of evidence: the high incidence of a relatively rare disease in well defined population groups, and the results of experimental carcinogenicity tests.

The identification of cancer-causing agents has therefore been conditioned by the observational nature of the epidemiological approach and its consequent potential for bias, and by the forcibly simplified cause-effect relationship and schematism underlying long-term carcinogenicity tests, in which tumors are taken to occur as a direct consequence of the exposure to one single agent. This characteristic of long-term tests directly descends from the experiments of Yamagiwa and Ichikawa in 1915 (Yamagiwa and Ichikawa, 1915), which marked the beginning of experimental carcinogenesis. These experiments were followed a few years later by those of M. Tsutsui (1918), who described the induction of benign and malignant skin tumors in mice using a method that was adopted all over the world and remained one of the most popular for many decades. It was almost inevitable that the search for carcinogenic agents would become oriented toward those agents that these two approaches could most easily and reliably identify and that were mostly chemical or chemical mixtures.

At present, there are over 4 million organic and inorganic chemicals in the computerized registry of the Chemical Abstracts Service (CAS) of the American Chemical Society; the structures of 3.4 million of these are fully defined. Although the number of chemicals in the register increases at a rate of 6,000 per week, only a minority are used widely: the CAS has estimated that 63,000 are in common use (Maugh, 1978). This number may not be entirely accurate, but it certainly gives an indication of the magnitude of the problem. The fact that acute and chronic toxicity data are available for only a minority of these chemicals can be explained by the fact that the industry developed rapidly during a period in which health problems related to chemicals were not receiving adequate attention. We are therefore now faced with a backlog accumulated over many decades. Since a greater effort to investigate the possible toxicity of environmental chemicals has been initiated only in recent years, it is not surprising that an increasing number of reports have indicated toxic effects for chemicals (Tomatis, 1979).

It is not unreasonable to assume that other chemicals among the thousands to which we are exposed will eventually be identified as carcinogenic to humans, besides those for which a positive association with the occurrence of cancer in humans has already been proven.

Although it is unlikely that in this way a satisfactory etiological justification to all or perhaps even most human cancers will be provided, we will, however, acquire the possibility of implementing an efficient primary prevention on an increasing fraction of human tumors.

AGENTS RECOGNIZED AS HUMAN CARCINOGENS

One of the first authoritative lists of cancer-causing agents, and probably the best at that time, was prepared by a WHO Expert Committee in 1964 (WHO, 1964). Exposure to sunlight; tobacco smoking; chewing of betel, nass, and tobacco; consumption of alcohol; atmospheric pollution; some medicaments; ionizing radiation; and several specific industrial cancer hazards were listed among the recognized etiological factors susceptible to control.

That report, which is still well worth reading today, gave large credit to experimental carcinogenesis and to the results obtained from long-term carcinogenicity testing. Testing was, in fact, extensively recommended, with the implication that the results obtained could serve as a basis for preventive measures, and would support or confirm, in some instances, epidemiological observations. The further testing of tobacco smoke was, for instance, recommended, in spite of the overwhelming epidemiological evidence for carcinogenicity in humans. Such an attitude was not much different from that prevailing when Passey (1922) painted the skin of mice with coal tar, using the method developed by Tsutsui (1918), and obtained results that were regarded as providing final confirmation of the observations made by Percival Pott on humans a century and a half before.

It was around the time of the publication of the WHO list, under the pressure of the overwhelming epidemiological evidence of the carcinogenicity of tobacco smoke on the one hand, and the difficulty of reproducing the striking human findings in animal studies on the other, that an attitude began to prevail that encouraged epidemiologists to lay down certain criteria for assessing causation for chronic diseases in humans which could essentially stand on the epidemiological evidence alone (Bradford Hill, 1971; Doll, 1967). The attitude prevailing today is that only epidemiological studies may provide unequivocal evidence that an exposure is carcinogenic to humans. This had as a consequence that the experimental evidence, in particular that obtained in long-term animal tests, has been often regarded as a sort of second-rate type of evidence: it is claimed that chemicals proven to be carcinogenic in animals cannot be considered human carcinogens until there is epidemiological proof. The IARC recommends, however, that in the absence of adequate human data, it is biologically plausible and prudent to regard agents for which there is sufficient evidence of carcinogenicity in experimental animals as if they presented a carcinogenic risk to humans (IARC, 1987b). The IARC thus attempts to reconcile a scientifically objective analysis of the data with an interpretation of the evidence of carcinogenicity provided by experimental data that is biologically plausible, is public health oriented, and takes into account the principles of primary prevention. The possibility, as well as the limitations, of using mechanistic information in the evaluation of carcinogenicity have been considered in a critical review of the available knowledge on mechanisms of carcinogenesis (IARC, 1991; Vainio et al,

TABLE 2–1. *Industrial Processes Causally Associated with Human Cancer*

Exposure	*Target Organ*	
	Human	*Animal*
Aluminum production	Lung, bladder (lymphoma, esophagus, stomach)[a]	No relevant data
Auramine, manufacture of	Bladder	Mouse, rat: liver (auramine, technical grade)
Boot and shoe manufacture and repair	Leukemia, nasal sinus (bladder, digestive tract)	No relevant data
Coal gasification	Skin, lung, bladder	No relevant data
Coke production	Skin, lung, kidney	No relevant data
Furniture and cabinet making	Nasal sinus	Inadequate evidence (wood dust)
Hematite mining, underground, with exposure to radon	Lung	Inadequate evidence (hematite) Rat, dog: lung (radon)
Iron and steel founding	Lung (digestive tract, genito-urinary tract, leukemia)	No relevant data
Isopropyl alcohol manufacture, strong-acid process	Nasal sinus (larynx)	Inadequate evidence (isopropyl oils)
Magenta, manufacture of	Bladder	Inadequate evidence (magenta)
Painters, occupational exposure as	Lung (esophagus, stomach, bladder)	No relevant data
Rubber industry	Bladder, leukemia (lymphoma, lung, renal tract, digestive tract, skin, liver, larynx, brain, stomach)	Inadequate evidence
Strong-inorganic acid mists containing sulfuric acid	Lung, nasal sinus, larynx	No relevant data

[a]Suspected target organs in parentheses.

TABLE 2–2. *Chemicals, Groups of Chemicals, or Mixtures Carcinogenic to Humans (Group 1) for which Exposures Are Mostly Occupational*

Exposure	*Target Organ(s) (Suspected Target Organs)*	
	Human	*Animal*[a]
4-Aminobiphenyl	Bladder	M, liver, bladder; R, mammary gland, intestine; D/Rb, bladder
Arsenic and arsenic compounds	Lung, skin (liver, kidney, gastrointestinal tract)	M/H, (lung, larynx)
Asbestos	Lung, pleura, peritoneum	M, peritoneum; R, lung, pleura, peritoneum
Benzene	Leukemia	M, lung, lymphoma, leukemia, zymbal gland; R, oral cavity, zymbal gland, skin, mammary gland, forestomach
Benzidine	Bladder	M, liver; R, mammary gland, zymbal gland; H, liver; D, bladder
Beryllium and beryllium compounds	Lung	R, lung; Rb, bone
Bis (chloromethyl)ether and chloromethyl methyl ether (technical-grade)	Lung	M, lung, skin; R, lung, nasal cavity; H, lung
Cadmium and cadmium compounds	Lung (prostate ?)	R, lung leukemia, testis, prostate, local
Chromium [VI] compounds	Lung (nasal cavity)	M/R, lung, local
Coal-tar pitches	Skin, lung, bladder	M, skin
Coal tars	Skin, lung	M/Rb, skin; R, lung
Ethylene oxide[b]	(Lymphatic and hematopoietic system)	M, lung, Harderian gland, uterus, ma R, forestomach, leukemia, brain, peritoneal mesothelioma
Mineral oils, untreated and mildly treated	Skin (lung, bladder)	M/Rb/Mk, skin
Mustard gas (Sulfur mustard)	Pharynx, lung	M, (lung, local)
2-Naphthylamine	Bladder	M, lung, liver; R/H/D/Mk, bladder
Nickel compounds	Nasal cavity, lung	R, lung, local
Shale oils	Skin	M/Rb, skin
Soots	Skin, lung	M, skin; R, lung
Talc containing asbestiform fibers	Lung (pleura)	—
Vinyl chloride	Liver, lung, blood vessels	M, liver, lung, mammary gland, blood vessels; R, liver, zymbal gland, blood vessels; H, liver, blood vessels, skin

[a]M, mouse; R, rat; D, dog; Rb, rabbit; H, hamster; Mk, monkey; F, fish.
[b]Upgraded on the basis of mechanistic data.

1992). It was concluded that an agent for which there is sufficient evidence of carcinogenicity in experimental systems, but less than sufficient epidemiological evidence, could be evaluated as being carcinogenic to humans (Group 1 of the IARC Monographs) when there is convincing evidence that in exposed humans the agent acts on a relevant mechanism of carcinogenesis. At the opposite end, it is conceivable that an agent for which there is sufficient evidence of carcinogenicity in experimental animals could be evaluated as not classifiable as to its carcinogenicity to humans (Group 3 of the IARC Monographs), when there is strong convincing evidence that the mechanism of carcinogenicity in animals does not operate in humans (IARC, 1991; Vainio et al, 1992).

Some 25 years after the report of the WHO Expert Committee of 1964 (WHO, 1964) the list of etiological factors of human cancer is considerably longer, but it still reflects the absolute preponderance of environmental chemical agents. Twelve of the cancer-causing agents of the WHO 1964 list were environmental chemicals or complex chemical mixtures, and so are 58 of the 66 exposures recognized today as carcinogenic to humans. This large majority of chemical agents may lead one to assume that cancer is a disease predominantly related to environmental chemicals. One may then ask if the chemical agents so far identified are actually the most important ones and, consequently, if the tests used for their identification were suitable to identify the important agents responsible for human cancer. These points will be discussed making use of the data base of the IARC Monograph Program (IARC, 1981–1992; IARC, 1987a; IARC, 1987b), from which the lists of human carcinogens in Tables 2–1 through 2–3 and in part of Table 2–4 have been derived.

For convenience, the recognized agents evaluated as being carcinogenic to humans are presented in separate lists of industrial processes (Table 2–1), chemicals and groups of chemicals for which exposures have been mostly occupational (Table 2–2), drugs causally asso-

TABLE 2–3. *Drugs Carcinogenic to Humans (Group 1)*

Exposure	Target Organ(s) (Suspected Target Organs)	
	Human	Animal[a]
Analgesic mixtures containing phenacetin	Kidney, bladder	R, kidney
Azathioprine	Lymphoma, hepatobiliary system, skin	M (lymphoma); R (zymbal gland)
N,N-Bis (2-chloroethyl)-2-naphthylamine (Chlornaphazine)	Bladder	M (lung); R (local)
1,4-Butanediol dimethanesulfonate (Myleran)	Leukemia	M, lymphoma/leukemia, ovary
Chlorambucil	Leukemia	M (lung); R, lymphoma/leukemia
1-(2-Chloroethyl)-3-(4-methylcyclohexyl)-1-nitrosourea (Methyl-CCNU)	Leukemia	R (lung)
Cyclosporin	Lymphoma, skin	M (leukemia)
Cyclophosphamide	Leukemia, bladder	M, leukemia, lung, mammary gland; R, bladder, leukemia
Diethylstilbestrol	Cervix/vagina, breast (endometrium)	M, mammary gland, cervix, uterus, ovary, lymphoma; R, mammary gland, pituitary; H, kidney, cervix, uterus
Estrogen replacement therapy	Uterus	H, (kidney)
Estrogens, nonsteroidal	Cervix/vagina, breast (endometrium)	—
Estrogens, steroidal	Uterus (breast)	—
Melphalan	Leukemia	M, lymphoma, lung
8-Methoxypsoralen (Methoxsalen) plus ultraviolet radiation	Skin	M, skin
MOPP and other combined chemotherapy including alkylating agents	Leukemia	—
Oral contraceptives, combined[b]	Liver	—
Oral contraceptives, sequential	Uterus	—
Thiotepa	Leukemia	M/R, leukemia
Treosulfan	Leukemia	—

[a]M, mouse; R, rat; D, dog; Rb, rabbit; H, hamster; Mk, monkey; F, fish.
[b]There is also conclusive evidence that these agents have a protective effect against cancers of the ovary and endometrium.

TABLE 2–4. *Environmental and Biological Agents and Cultural Risk Factors Carcinogenic to Humans (Group 1)*

Exposure	Target Organ(s) (Suspected Target Organs)	
	Human	Animal[a]
Aflatoxins	Liver	M, lung; R, liver, kidney, colon; H/F/Mk, liver
Alcohol drinking	Oral cavity, pharynx, larynx, esophagus, liver	—
Betel quid with tobacco	Oral cavity	M (skin); H (forestomach)
Erionite	Pleura	M, local; R, pleura, local
Helicobacter pylori (infection with)	Stomach	—
Hepatitis B virus (chronic infection with)	Liver	—
Hepatitis C virus (chronic infection with)	Liver	—
Opistharcis viverrini (infection with)	Bile duct	H (bile duct)
Radon and its decay products	Lung	R/D, lung
Salted fish (Chinese style)	Nasopharynx	R (nasal cavity)
Schistosoma haematobium (infection with)	Bladder	Mk bladder
Solar radiation	Skin	M, skin
Tobacco products, smokeless	Oral cavity (pharynx, esophagus)	—
Tobacco smoke	Lung, bladder, oral cavity, pharynx, larynx, esophagus, pancreas	R/H, lung; M/Rb, skin

[a]M, mouse; R, rat; D, dog; Rb, rabbit; H, hamster; Mk, monkey.

ciated with cancer in humans (Table 2–3), and environmental and biological agents and culturally determined risk factors (Table 2–4).

These lists reflect the point made above, that most recognized carcinogens (as well as most of the probable human carcinogens) are chemicals to which humans have begun to be exposed only within the last 150 years. The human species has in fact been confronted with the massive presence of man-made chemicals in the general and working environment and with the expansion of the most carcinogenic cultural habit (tobacco smoking) only since the middle of the last century. This holds true also for the chemicals, groups of chemicals, or complex exposures that have been evaluated as probably or possibly carcinogenic to humans (Groups 2A and 2B, respectively, in the categorization used within the IARC Monographs Program) (Tables 2–5 through 2–7), as well as for the chemicals for which there are no epidemiological data and the experimental data available are inadequate for an evaluation of carcinogenicity (Group 3 within the IARC Monograph Program).

A striking feature of the present lists of recognized carcinogenic agents is their imbalance in relation to cancers in men and women; they relate more to cancers occurring frequently in men. This can be partly explained by the facts that males have been much more frequently exposed to carcinogenic hazards through their occupation, took up the habit of smoking earlier than females, and, where the habit of drinking alcoholic beverages is common, they drink more than do females.

TABLE 2–5. *Industrial Processes, Chemicals, Groups of Chemicals, or Mixtures Probably Carcinogenic to Humans (Group 2A) for Which Exposures are Mostly Occupational*

	Target Organ(s) (Suspected Target Organs)	
Exposure	*Human*	*Animal*[a]
INDUSTRIAL PROCESSES		
Art glass (manufacture of)	(Lung)	—
Hairdresser or barber (occupation as)	(Bladder)	—
Nonarsenical insecticides (occupational exposures in spraying and application of)	(Lung, myeloma)	—
Petroleum refining (occupational exposures in)	(Leukemia, skin)	—
CHEMICALS, GROUPS OF CHEMICALS, OR MIXTURES		
Arylamide[b]	—	R, peritoneum, thyroid, mammary gland, brain, oral cavity, uterus
Acrylonitrile	(Lung, prostate, lymphoma)	R, zymbal gland, nervous system, mammary gland
Benzidine-based dyes[b]	—	R, liver, mammary gland, bladder
1,3 Butadiene	(Leukemia, lymphoma)	M, heart, lung, lymphoma, mammary gland, forestomach, ovary; R, mammary gland, thyroid, pancreas
para-Chloro-*ortho*-toluidine and its strong acid salts	(Bladder)	M, blood vessels
Creosotes	(Skin)	M, skin, lung
Diethyl sulfate	—	R, forestomach, local, nervous system
Dimethylcarbamoyl chloride	—	M, skin, local; R/H, nasal cavity
Dimethyl sulfate	—	R, nasal cavity, local, nervous system
Epichlorohydrin	—	R, forestomach, nasal cavity, lung
Formaldehyde	(Nasopharynx)	R, nasal cavity
4,4′-Methylene bis(2-chloroaniline) (MOCA)	(Bladder)	M, liver, blood vessels; R, liver, lung, mammary gland, blood vessels; D, bladder
Polychlorinated biphenyls	(Liver, bile ducts, leukemia, lymphoma)	M/R, liver
Silica, crystalline	(Lung)	R, lung, lymphoma
Styrene-7,8-oxide	—	R, forestomach
Tris(2,3-dibromopropyl)phosphate	—	M, forestomach, lung, liver, kidney
Vinyl bromide	—	R, liver, zymbal gland

[a]M, mouse; R, rat; D, dog; Rb, rabbit; H, hamster; Mk, monkey; F, fish.
[b]Upgraded on the basis of mechanistic data.

TABLE 2–6. *Drugs and Pesticides Probably Carcinogenic to Humans (Group 2A)*

Exposure	Target Organ(s) (Suspected Target Organs)	
	Human	Animal[a]
Drugs		
Adriamycin[b]	—	R, mammary gland
Androgenic (anabolic) steroids	(Liver)	R, prostate
Azacitidine[b]	—	M, lung, lymphoma, leukemia
Bischloroethyl nitrosourea (BCNU)	(Leukemia)	R, lung, nervous system
Chloramphenicol	(Leukemia)	—
1-(2-Chloroethyl)-3-cyclohexyl-1-nitrosourea (CCNU)[b]	—	R, lung
Chlorozotocin[b]	—	R, peritoneum
Cisplatin[b]	—	M, lung; R, leukemia
5-Methoxypsoralen	—	M, skin
Nitrogen mustard	(Skin)	M, lung, skin
Phenacetin	(Kidney, bladder)	M, kidney; R, kidney, bladder, nasal cavity
Procarbazine hydrochloride[b]	—	M, lung, leukemia; R, mammary gland, brain, leukemia; Mk, leukemia
Pesticides		
Captafol[b]	—	M, heart, intestine, liver, kidney; R, liver, kidney
Ethylene dibromide[b]	—	M, forestomach, lung, skin; R, forestomach, liver, blood vessels, nasal cavity, peritoneum, mammary gland, skin

[a]M, mouse; R, rat; D, dog; Rb, rabbit; H, hamster; Mk, monkey; F, fish.
[b]Upgraded on the basis of mechanistic data.

TABLE 2–7. *Environmental and Biological Agents and Cultural Habits Probably Carcinogenic to Humans (Group 2A)*

Exposure	Target Organ(s) (Suspected Target Organs)	
	Human	Animal[a]
Benz[*a*]anthracene[b]	—	M, lung, liver, skin bladder
Benzo[*a*]pyrene[b]	—	M, forestomach, lung, skin; R, forestomach, mammary gland; H, forestomach; Rb, skin
Clonorchis sinensis (infection with)	(Bile duct)	D (bile duct)
Dibenz[*a,h*]anthracene[b]	—	M, forestomach, lung, skin, mammary gland
Diesel engine exhaust	(Lung, bladder)	M, lung, skin; R, lung
Hot maté drinking	(Esophagus)	
IQ (2-amino-3-methylimidazo-[4,5-f]quimoline)[b]	—	M, liver, lung, forestomach; R, liver, intestine, zymbal gland, mammary gland, skin
N-Nitrosodiethylamine	—	M/R/H, liver, lung, esophagus, forestomach, nasal cavity; Rb/M/F, liver
N-Nitrosodimethylamine	—	M, liver, lung, kidney, blood vessels; R, liver/bile duct, blood vessels, kidney, lung, nasal cavity; H, bile duct, blood vessels; G, liver/bile duct; F, liver
Sunlamps and sunbeds (use of)	(Skin)	M, skin
Ultraviolet radiation A	(Skin)	M, skin
Ultraviolet radiation B	(Skin)	M, skin
Ultraviolet radiation C	(Skin)	M, skin

[a]M, mouse; R, rat; D, dog; Rb, rabbit; H, hamster; Mk, monkey; F, fish.
[b]Upgraded on the basis of mechanistic data.

It may also, however, reflect the bias of our society to show concern about matters involving men. The second limitation refers to the fact that the etiological agents of human cancer so far identified are predominantly associated with tumors occurring at certain sites such as lung, bladder, skin, bone marrow, while there is little or no indication that they are of etiological relevance to cancer occurring at the uterine cervix, breast (DES and other estrogens are here the exception), ovary, colon-rectum, stomach, and prostate.

QUALITATIVE CORRELATIONS BETWEEN CARCINOGENICITY IN EXPERIMENTAL ANIMALS AND IN HUMANS

An important support for the value of experimental data in predicting a qualitatively similar effect in humans comes from the fact that experimental evidence of carcinogenicity has on several occasions been obtained before the epidemiological evidence. This happened, for instance, in the cases of 4-aminobiphenyl, aflatoxins, diethylstilbestrol, melphalan, 8-methoxypsoralen + UV radiation, mustard gas, radon gas, and vinyl chloride (IARC, 1987b).

The qualitative concordance between human and experimental carcinogenicity data may be defined in terms of sensitivity and specificity. Sensitivity measures what proportion of human carcinogens may be detected by long-term carcinogenicity testing.

Of the 66 agents recognized as human carcinogens in the first 61 volumes of the IARC Monographs, 13 are industrial complex exposures and 6 therapeutic combinations, which cannot be included in assessing concordance, as they could not be submitted to proper experimental tests. For treosulfan no experimental data on carcinogenicity have been published, and for smokeless tobacco products, all published studies were inadequate for evaluation. Of the remaining 35 chemicals, for 23 (68%) the results provided sufficient evidence of carcinogenicity (i.e., they were usually carcinogenic in at least two animal species). For nine chemicals or groups of chemicals, namely analgesic mixtures containing phenacetin, azathioprine, arsenic and arsenic compounds, chlornaphazine, ciclosporin, mustard gas, myleran, betel quid with tobacco, and methyl-CCNU, the evidence provided by long-term carcinogenicity tests was limited (i.e., evidence of carcinogenicity was less than sufficient but pointing to a carcinogenic activity). The three chemicals with inadequate evidence of carcinogenicity in animals were ethanol, soots, and talc containing asbestiform fibers. For alcoholic beverages, one adequate study was available, and did not provide evidence of carcinogenicity.

For six of the eight chemicals for which there was limited evidence of carcinogenicity (azathioprine, betel quid with tobacco, chlornaphazine, mustard gas, myleran, and methyl-CCNU), the limitations are mainly related to an incomplete or improper testing design and/or reporting of the results, while for one (analgesic mixtures containing phenacetin) the results of the experimental tests provided limited evidence for the mixture although sufficient evidence for phenacetin alone. For arsenic, recent results on its possible mechanism of action (gene amplification) may explain why traditional long-term tests have so far provided only limited evidence for carcinogenicity (Lee et al, 1988).

The fact that concordance is imperfect between data in humans and results in experimental animals (namely, for 11 of the 35 human carcinogens tested in experimental animals the evidence for carcinogenicity is less than sufficient) has often been taken as an argument to downgrade the value of results from experimental animals in predicting similar effects in humans. It could, however, equally well be interpreted to support an opposite view—i.e., that even limited experimental evidence of carcinogenicity provides a serious warning that a chemical could be carcinogenic to humans. If we combine the animal results providing sufficient evidence with those providing limited evidence of carcinogenicity, then the sensitivity of long-term carcinogenicity studies to detect human carcinogens increases to 91%.

The specificity of long-term animal assays, i.e., the proportion of human noncarcinogens that are negative in animal studies, is difficult to assess since noncarcinogenicity is very difficult to prove. Also, much less effort has been put—for understandable reasons—into studies of noncarcinogenicity. In Supplement 7 of the IARC Monographs (1987b), one chemical only, caprolactam, has been classified solely on experimental evidence as "probably not carcinogenic to humans." From the public health point of view, the specificity is in general much less important than the sensitivity.

Ennever et al (1987) examined 29 chemicals for which at least one epidemiological study was available indicating lack of carcinogenicity and found that animal carcinogenesis experiments had found positive results in a high proportion, thereby implying poor specificity of the animal bioassay. However, this conclusion was based in a number of cases on weak epidemiological evidence of lack of carcinogenicity. Indeed, Goodman and Wilson (1991) have shown that quantitative risk prediction from the positive animal experiments would, for most of the agents tested, indicate that the epidemiological studies used to assert lack of carcinogenicity had very little probability of detecting a significant carcinogenic effect, because human exposure levels were too low or sample sizes too small.

Since extrapolation from experimental animal data to humans is just a form of interspecies comparison, it may be relevant to examine the level of consistency between data obtained in different rodent species. Indeed, it has been argued that the concordance between humans and rodents cannot exceed that between mice and rats (Lave et al, 1988). The basis for this argumentation is that rodents are closer to each other, in several physiological and biochemical parameters, than they are to humans. It should be noted, however, that the interindividual variation between humans may be extremely wide, in comparison to standard laboratory rodents; it could even exceed the variation between rodent species (Lave et al, 1988; Sabadie et al, 1980; Sabadie et al, 1981). When a large number of humans are exposed to a chemical agent, it is therefore at least possible that some of them are equally sensitive to the carcinogenic action of that chemical as is the most sensitive rodent species.

In a 1981 review, Purchase (1981) made a comparison between the carcinogenic activity of 250 chemicals in the mouse and the rat, and found an overall concordance between the two species of 85%, for both the positive and the negative results. A similar percentage was found in a previous survey (Tomatis et al, 1973) and a slightly lower percentage of concordance was found within the U.S. National Toxicology Program (NTP) results. A first survey of the latter results, made in 1984 (Haseman et al, 1984) on 86 chemicals tested, showed that 63% of chemicals carcinogenic in the rat were also carcinogenic in the mouse and 74% of those negative in the rat were also negative in the mouse. In a further survey (Huff et al, 1988) on 266 chemicals adequately tested, the percentages were 68% and 78%, respectively.

Of some interest is also that only around 50% of the chemicals tested in the National Toxicology Program were proven to have a carcinogenic activity even though the chemicals were primarily selected because of a suspicion of carcinogenicity. It is not enough, therefore, to submit a suspect chemical to a long-term carcinogenicity test, even at the Maximum Tolerated Dose (MTD) level, which is included routinely by the NTP in its testing procedures, for it to become automatically a carcinogen.

For most of the chemicals showing both animal and human carcinogenicity, an increased incidence of tumors in the organ(s) that are the target organ(s) in humans has been observed in at least one animal species following at least one route of administration (Tables 2–1 through 2–4). This concordance of target organs could be largely a result of the thorough testing to which chemicals have been subjected when there is epidemiological evidence of carcinogenicity. There is in fact a total absence of concordance of target organs only for two agents, chlornaphazine and methyl-CCNU, both of which were submitted to only a limited number of tests with possibly inadequate test designs.

While a concordance in target organs could be seen as further supporting the biological similarity between experimental animals and humans, it should not be seen as a requirement for the application of experimental results to human hazard evaluation. The experimental evidence of carcinogenicity of 2-naphthylamine, BCME, and cyclophosphamide, for example, was first provided by tumors found in target organs other than those observed in humans. In the case of BCME, a demand for the induction of tumors in experimental animals similar to those observed in humans actually led to a delay in implementing measures to reduce human exposure (Tomatis, 1978). In the case of cyclophosphamide, more than ten years elapsed between the first demonstration of its carcinogenic effect in the lung, liver, testis, and mammary gland (Tokuoka, 1965) and the studies demonstrating the induction of tumors of the bladder (Schmähl and Habs, 1979). The bladder was initially thought to be the only target in humans until a leukemogenic effect of the drug was demonstrated in patients treated for cancers of the breast and ovary (IARC, 1987a).

The validity of experimental tests in demonstrating the carcinogenicity of many chemicals is beyond doubt, but they cannot be expected to provide evidence, at least when used in the traditional manner, for the carcinogenicity of every causative factor of human cancer. The development of tests capable of demonstrating the promoting or modulating activity of certain exposures (Ito et al, 1988; Semple et al, 1987; Yamasaki, 1988), as well as the use of short-term tests, may help to complete and refine results obtained in animal tests and contribute to making them more efficient as well as more specific. Similarly, the methodology that is being developed for distinguishing between so-called spontaneous and induced tumors (Wiseman et al, 1986; You et al, 1989) may also help to clarify some of the results of long-term carcinogenicity tests that have been until now difficult to interpret (such as an increased incidence in treated animals of tumors occurring at various sites in treated animals). There is, inevitably, a temporal gap between the expansion of knowledge in the mechanisms of carcinogenesis and its application or applicability to the routine implementation of carcinogenicity test as well as most epidemiological surveys, but it is important that the gap does not widen because of an avoidable inertia.

QUANTITATIVE CORRELATIONS BETWEEN CARCINOGENICITY IN EXPERIMENTAL ANIMALS AND IN HUMANS

The primary goal of an animal cancer bioassay is to determine whether a chemical tested is carcinogenic or not. However, since assay results are quantitative, they can also be used to estimate the increase in cancer risk over background associated with each dose level tested. Based on these estimates, carcinogenic potency can be defined as the increase in cancer risk per unit dose, or inversely, as the dose required to increase cancer risk by a specified amount. Potency estimates of this kind have been suggested by several authors (Meselson and Russel, 1977; Crouch and Wilson, 1979; Peto et al, 1984) as a means of summarizing in a single number the quantitative information from an animal cancer test. Although potency estimates are conceptually appealing, there are considerable practical problems involved in deriving them from experimental data and in applying them to predict human carcinogenic risk.

First of all, the requirement of a single number to summarize the quantitative results of a bioassay imposes some strong assumptions, the most important of which is linearity, on some defined scale, in the relationship between dose and tumor rate. While some chemicals appear to increase tumor rate in a manner that is proportional to dose, others do so at a rate proportional to a higher power of dose. The use of a single potency figure clearly cannot fully represent the potency of both classes of agents across a wide range of doses (Kodell et al, 1991). Estimation of potency also involves assumptions about the time pattern of tumor induction. For example, the TD_{50} (Peto et al, 1984) is estimated assuming that the pattern is proportional among dose groups, and that the only effect of exposure to the test compound is to increase incidence by the same proportion at each age. An agent whose effect was to advance the appearance time of each naturally occurring tumor rather than to increase tumor yield could not conform to the proportionality model, and its potency estimate under the model would not adequately reflect its tumorigenic potential.

Even if these mathematical assumptions could be shown to be satisfied, the application of potency estimates to the prediction of human cancer risk poses even more formidable problems. Human exposure to chemical compounds rarely corresponds to the constant daily dose typically applied over the lifetime of the test animals in laboratory experiments. If potency estimates are to be used to quantify human risk, it is usually necessary to assume that only cumulative or average dose is relevant, ignoring the possible effect of dose fractionation, breaks in exposure, and periods when exposure was more intense. Another difficulty lies in the choice of sites from animal experiments to be used in the prediction of human risk. Some rodent carcinogens produce an increase in tumor incidence at multiple sites, some of which do not even correspond to human organs. For example, cyclophosphamide is carcinogenic to the lung, mammary gland, and bone marrow of mice, and the bladder, mammary gland, and bone marrow in rats (see Table 2–3). Should the potency figure used for humans be the one estimated from all sites, all sites at which a dose-related increase was observed, or only the site(s) for which human risk prediction is required? In addition, should the rat or the mice data be used, an average of the two, or the higher of the two?

Questions of this kind can only be answered empirically, by validating the quantitative predictions from animal experiments against the corresponding estimates obtained from studies in humans. Here we encounter the final stumbling block: there are very few carcinogenic agents for which reliable estimates of human dose-effect relationships can be obtained, either because of the poor quality of exposure measurements, the small number of cancer cases observed, or confounding owing to exposures other than the one under study. The most important and best-quantified human chemical carcinogen, tobacco smoke, does not have a strictly comparable rodent model, and a similar situation applies for alcoholic beverages. There remain for validation of animal potency estimates the few dozen industrial chemicals and pharmaceutical drugs for which human carcinogenesis studies are available. Although these studies are, to varying degrees, all subject to one or more of the limitations of exposure measurement, sample size, or confounding, they provide the only data base for comparing human and animal potency estimates.

The first attempt at such a comparison was the survey carried out by the United States National Academy of Sciences (1975), in which a reasonable correlation was shown between simple measures of carcinogenic potency for experimental animals and humans. Several other undertakings of this kind have been completed since then, the most comprehensive probably being the recent study by Allen et al (1988). Using a database on 23 substances identified as carcinogenic to humans, experimental animals, or both, they estimated several indices of potency. For humans, the basic index used was the dose in mg/kg body weight estimated to cause a 25% increase over the background tumor mortality, if exposure took place daily between the ages of 20 and 65. Estimation was carried out under a number of the assumptions described above, including linearity of the dose-response curve and the equating of risk for individuals with the same cumulative dose, regardless of how it was delivered over time. An attempt was made to quantify uncertainty in exposure estimates and the resulting imprecision in the potency estimates. A comparable index was estimated from the results from animal experiments on the 23 substances. The rank correlation between the human and animal potency estimates was very high and did not materially depend on the rodent species used, whether or not the estimates were the same tumor site in animals and humans, or the way in which dose was calculated. The potency esti-

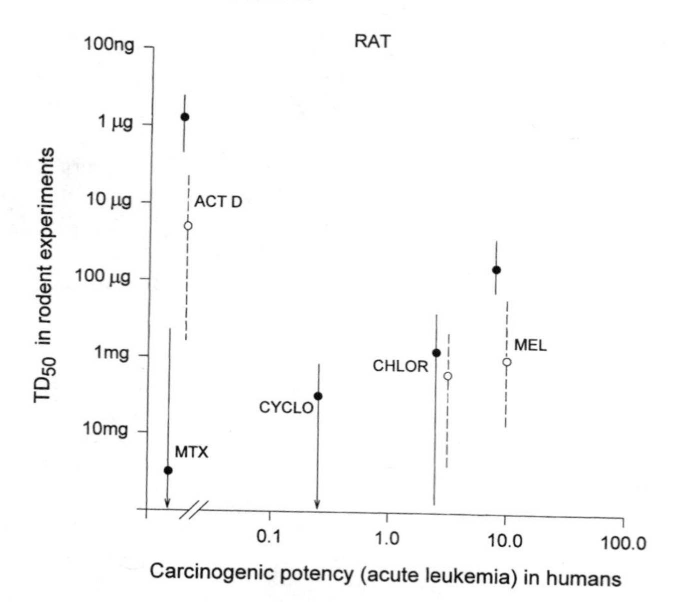

FIG. 2–1. TD_{50}s with 99% confidence intervals for carcinogenic potency in rats (*y*-axis) plotted against leukemogenic potency in humans (*x*-axis). — All tumors; – – – hematopoietic system tumors. Abbreviations: ACT D = actinomycin D; CHLOR = chlorambucil; CYCLO = cyclophosphamide; MEL = melphalan; MTX = methotrexate. (From Kaldor J et al, 1988).

mates and confidence intervals from one of these analyses resulted in the highest correlation between the two sets of estimates (.90; $p = .0001$). The lowest correlation (0.49; $p = .015$) resulted from an analysis restricted to substances for which the experimental results were over at least 80% of the test animals' lifetime (Allen et al, 1988).

It is impressive that quantitative estimation of carcinogenic effect can produce such good concordance between humans and animals, given the fundamental problems in the quality of the basic information and the definition of potency, and the disparate nature of the substances involved. A study of potency correlation for alkylating chemotherapy agents demonstrated a similarly good rank correlation, based on a much smaller group of closely related nitrogen mustard compounds, chlorambucil, melphalan, and cyclophosphamide (Kaldor et al, 1988). The potency estimates are shown in Figure 2–1. These findings suggest that quantitative production of carcinogenic potency is feasible if one is prepared to accept broad bands of uncertainty, often ranging over several orders of magnitude.

The meaning of potency correlations between animal species has been questioned by Bernstein et al. (1985), who showed that correlations in toxicity could lead to apparent correlations in potency, since the highest dose levels tested in an experiment, which depend on the toxicity, constrain to within about one and a half orders of magnitude the possible estimates of potency that can be obtained from the experiment. Phenomena of this kind could be operating in the study of human-animal potency correlations involving pharmaceutical drugs, if dose levels of drugs administered therapeutically depend on their toxicity.

However, Kodell et al. (1991) have pointed out that the constraint on potency estimates may be largely imposed by the linearity assumption implicit in their estimation; if alternative dose-response shapes were permitted in the estimation, it may be possible to examine the human-animal potency correlation more critically.

The chapter in this volume by Whittemore considers in detail the practical issue of quantitative prediction of human carcinogenicity from animal studies, and the implication for the establishment of exposure standards.

USE OF SHORT-TERM TESTS

Short-term tests (STTs) for the detection of chemical carcinogens and mutagens can be divided broadly into the following categories: (a) induction of DNA damage/repair, (b) gene mutations or cytogenetic changes in submammalian/mammalian cells and organisms, and (c) in vitro transformation of cultured mammalian cells. The utility, limitations, and deployment of STT have been reviewed extensively (Montesano et al, 1986; Rosenkranz, 1988). Any test system must incorporate some aspects of mammalian metabolism; this is done in vitro either by adding a rodent or human liver fraction or by using metabolically competent cells, like rodent embryo cells or rodent/human hepatocytes (Bartsch et al, 1982). Microbial mutagenicity tests can also be adapted to test body fluids or excreta from exposed animals or humans. Some methods, such as the host-mediated assay, in vivo cytogenetics and mutation assays (lymphocytes) that monitor genotoxic damage in the intact mammalian organism, or tests in *Drosophila melanogaster*, involve in vivo activation.

STTs alone or in combination have been in use for almost two decades, for the screening of chemicals for potential carcinogenicity and genotoxicity. Often, positive results obtained in such assays have resulted in a reduction in human exposure or the introduction of substitutes, thus contributing to the prevention of chemical carcinogenesis in humans. Successful applications of such rapid screening assays also included the analysis of environmental mixtures or body fluids, which made it possible to isolate and identify individual carcinogenic agents in complex matrices, and to discover new naturally occurring and man-made agents in the environment.

Several STTs for the detection of carcinogens as mutagens have been validated with a variety of chemical of known carcinogens and noncarcinogens for sensitivity (the percentage of substances found to be both carcinogenic and mutagenic), specificity (the percentage of substances found to be both noncarcinogenic and nonmutagenic), accuracy or concordance (the percentage of correct matches), and predictive value (the percentage of carcinogens among the tested substances found to be mutagenic). For one of the most widely used STT, the *Salmonella*/microsome assay, average figures of 90% for its predictive value and 80% for accuracy (concordance) have been reported (Kier et al, 1986). Increasing demand for quantitative carcinogenicity data, for the purposes of risk assessment, has stimulated the examination of whether there is a quantitative relationship between the potency of a carcinogen in animals (humans) and its biologic activity in an STT. At present, such a correlation between quantitative aspects of an activity in any STT—e.g., mutagenicity and carcinogenicity in animals exists for certain groups of structurally related carcinogens—is not sufficiently established for all classes of carcinogens to allow its general use (McCann et al, 1988).

Recently, the results of a validation study of short-term in vitro tests for mutagenicity against rodent carcinogenicity have been published by Tennant et al (1987). The results were surprising in several ways: none of the STT were as predictive of carcinogenicity as had been expected on the basis of many previous studies; all four assays studied were judged to be almost equally effective; no combination of STTs predicted carcinogenicity significantly better than a single STT; and the three most potent carcinogens were uniformly negative in all four STTs. These widely discussed results (Brockman and DeMarini, 1988; Heddle, 1988; Shelby, 1988; Zeiger, 1987) reporting an accuracy of as low as ~60% can be largely explained by the inclusion in the database of an increased number of chemicals that were found to be carcinogenic in rodents and apparently do not act via mutagenic/electrophilic intermediates, and that are today often termed nongenotoxic carcinogens. These results have important implications for the use of STTs, the main aim of which has been to detect carcinogens, but how relevant is this validation study for the detection of human carcinogens? It would therefore be of the greatest importance, for public health aspects and for adopting future testing strategies in genetic toxicology, to determine whether genotoxic and nongenotoxic carcinogens contribute similarly to the cancer burden in humans.

For this purpose we have analyzed a total of 180 human and/or animal carcinogens, evaluated in the IARC Monographs (volumes 1 to 42), for their carcinogenic effects and their activities in STT (excluding in vitro cell transformation assays). Data on these compounds have recently been updated and published in Supplements 6 and 7 to the IARC Monographs on the Evaluation of Carcinogenic Risks to Humans (IARC, 1987a; 1987b). Similar analyses on the performance of STTs were done previously for a smaller number of chemicals evaluated in IARC Monographs volumes 1–20, and on human carcinogens (Tomatis et al, 1982; Kuroki and Matsushima, 1987; Shelby et al, 1988). In the following, we present a brief summary of our analyses; full details are published elsewhere (Bartsch and Malaveille, 1989). Similar conclusions have also been reached by other authors (Shelby and Zeiger, 1990).

PREVALENCE OF GENOTOXIC AGENTS AMONG HUMAN CARCINOGENS

The agents considered in Supplements 6 and 7 of the IARC Monographs comprise chemicals, groups of chemicals, industrial processes, occupational exposures, and cultural habits, and when broken down contained 50 established human carcinogenic agents (Group 1), 37 probable human carcinogens (Group 2A), 159 possible human carcinogens (Group 2B), and 383 agents that cannot be classified (Group 3). Either because of nonavailability of data or because the exposures were complex, the number of agents on which this analysis on the prevalence of genotoxic agents among human carcinogens could be performed had to be reduced. It now comprises 30 agents in Group 1, 37 agents in Groups 2A, and 113 in Groups 2B, which include mostly individual chemicals and a few complex mixtures. The criteria for evaluating the degree and strength of evidence for carcinogenicity in humans and in experimental animals, and for making the overall evaluation of carcinogenicity in humans, are those described in full in the preamble to Supplement 7 (IARC, 1987a). These were based on standard terms that are described briefly below. In parentheses are given the abbreviations used for categorization of the agents in Table 2–1.

Human Carcinogenicity Data

Sufficient Evidence of Carcinogenicity: A causal relationship has been established between exposure to the agent and human cancer. *Limited evidence of carcinogenicity*: A positive association has been observed between exposure to the agent and cancer for which a causal interpretation is considered to be credible, but chance, bias, or confounding could not be ruled out with reasonable confidence. *Inadequate evidence of carcinogenicity*: The available studies are of insufficient quality, consistency, or statistical power to permit a conclusion regarding the presence or absence of a causal association.

Experimental Carcinogenicity Data

Sufficient Evidence of Carcinogenicity ($A^{S}S$): A causal relationship has been established between the agent and an increased incidence of malignant neoplasms or of an appropriate combination of benign and malignant neoplasms in (a) two or more species of animals or (b) in two or more independent studies in one species carried out at different times or in different laboratories or under different protocols. *Limited evidence of carcinogenicity (A^L)*: The data suggest a carcinogenic effect but are limited for making a definite evaluation. *Inadequate evidence of carcinogenicity (A^I)*: The studies cannot be interpreted as showing either the presence or absence of a carcinogenic effect because of major qualitative or quantitative limitations.

Overall Evaluation

The total body of evidence from human and experimental studies was finally taken into account and the agent was classified in Supplement 7 (IARC, 1987a) in one of the following categories, and the designated group was given:

Group 1—The agent is carcinogenic to humans (H^1): This category is used only when there is sufficient evidence of carcinogenicity in humans. *Group 2*—This category includes agents for which the degree of evidence of carcinogenicity in humans is almost sufficient, as well as agents for which there are no human data, but for which there is experimental evidence of carcinogenicity. Agents are assigned to either 2A (probably carcinogenic H^{2A}) or 2B (possibly carcinogenic H^{2B}) on the basis of epidemiological, experimental, and other relevant data.

Group 3—The agent is not classifiable as to its carcinogenicity to humans: Agents are placed in this category when they do not fall into any other group.

Genotoxicity Data from STTs

For the purpose of this analysis, the evidence relating to genotoxic activity in STT, which is described in Supplement 6 and the Monographs (Volumes 1–42), was also classified into one of the following categories. *Sufficient evidence of genotoxicity (ST^+)* is provided when an agent exhibited activity in at least three tests for DNA damage, mutations, and chromosomal effects, one of which must involve mammalian cells in vitro or in vivo and which must include at least two or three endpoints: DNA damage, mutation, and chromosal effects. *Limited evidence of genotoxicity (ST^L)* is provided when an agent was active in at least one validated STT, which is indicative of DNA damage or chromosomal effects. *Inadequate evidence of genotoxicity (ST^I)* is provided when an agent produced controversial and thus uninterpretable results in various STT. Six of these compounds (in Group 3) were excluded from this analysis. *Sufficient evidence for lack of genotoxicity (ST^-)* is provided when an agent was inactive in a spectrum of genotoxicity assays. The abbreviations given in parentheses here, are used to indicate the biological properties of an agent according to the different categories.

The prevalence of agents that show activities in STTs for genotoxicity in Groups 1, 2A, and 2B agents are summarized in Table 2–1. Among Group 1 agents, 80% (24 with $H^1A^SST^+$ and $H^1A^LST^+$ combined) showed sufficient evidence for activity in genotoxicity assays. If one includes those agents with limited evidence of activity in short-term tests ($H^1AS^ST^L$), the figure rises to 93%. Thus, among the 30 identified human carcinogens, only 7% are animal carcinogens, but gave consistently negative results in short-term tests for genotoxicity (H^1, A^S, ST^-). These two compounds belong to the class of hormones that are present in contraceptives and steroidal estrogens (cf. Table IX). When the same analysis was performed for agents in Group 2A, termed probable human carcinogens, the picture that emerged was very similar to that for Group 1: 84% (31 $H^{2A}A^SST^+$) had sufficient evidence for genotoxicity. This figure rises to 95% when $H^{2A}A^SST^+$ and H^{2A} A^S ST^L are combined (35/37). Only two agents (5%) are nongenotoxic animal carcinogens: an adrogenic steroid and polychlorinated biphenyls. Group 2B (possible human carcinogens) comprises a total of 113 agents. Fifty percent (57 agents with H^{2B} A^S ST^+ and H^{2B} A^L ST^+ combined) of these carcinogens can be classified as agents with sufficient evidence for activity in STTs. This prevalence is lower than that in Groups 1 and 2A because fewer data from STTs were available. But when agents with limited evidence for activity in STTs (45 agents with H^{2B} A^S ST^L and HH^{2B} A^L ST^L combined) are included in the calculation, again a 90% prevalence of genotoxic carcinogens was obtained.

In Supplement 7, 17 agents were reclassified from the previous Group 2B into Group 2A, and 2 agents from Group 3 to Group 2B on the basis of other relevant biological data. Because the prevalence of genotoxic substances in Groups 2A and 2B is similar, this reclassification did not affect the present analyses: similar prevalence figures were obtained when they were calculated from groups of agents before reclassification.

The results from the analysis reveal a prevalence for genotoxic carcinogens ranging from 80% to 93% in Group 1, 84% to 90% in Group 2A, and 50% to 90% in Group 2B. The higher estimates include those agents that were tested and found active in only one validated genotoxicity assay—i.e., had, according to our criteria, limited evidence of genotoxicity in STT.

The present database does not permit analysis of the performance of STT either singly or as a battery, because only one compound (caprolactam) was identified in the IARC Monographs Program as having evidence suggesting lack of carcinogenicity in humans and animals. Thus, specificity and accuracy (concordance) cannot be determined. Results from this analysis clearly indicate that there is no obvious relationship between the degree of evidence of human carcinogenicity and the prevalence of genotoxic animal carcinogens in Groups 1A and 1B, most of which are active in several species and/or tissues (Wilbourn et al, 1986).

In order to exclude the possibility that the high preponderance of genotoxic carcinogens in Group 1 is due to a selection bias of agents chosen for epidemiological studies, a similar analysis was performed with Group 3 agents. These agents cannot be classified for their carcinogenicity to humans and may represent a more random sample. Among the 334 substances in this group, only 149 were assayed in STTs. In a subset of 66 agents with limited evidence for carcinogenicity in animals and with sufficient or limited evidence for activity in STTs combined ($A^L ST^+$ and $A^L ST^L$), again a 90% prevalence of genotoxic agents was found. As this prevalence figure is the same as in Group 1, as well as Groups 2A and 2B, this argues against at least one of the possible selection bias acting for agents in Group 1. It thus appears more likely that the unequal distribution of genotoxic and nongenotoxic animal carcinogens (i.e., a 9-fold excess of genotoxic carcinogens) would thus not be a special characteristic of our database; it could therefore possibly indicate that the universe of carcinogenic chemicals to which humans are exposed may likewise contain only a minor proportion of nongenotoxic chemicals. This assumption, although speculative at the time, is derived from the analyses of agents to which humans are or were actually exposed, which is a prerequisite for their inclusion in the IARC Monographs Program, and represent the best data set that can be used for such an analysis.

There may be several reasons why epidemiological studies have been able to reveal human carcinogenicity in Group 1 substances more clearly than in other groups. One reason certainly can be that exposure levels were so extreme as to cause cancer in a high proportion of the exposed individuals, and another that these substances were potent human carcinogens. This latter question cannot be directly addressed, since there are few quantitative data on potency available for humans. Instead it was examined by plotting histograms for the TD^{50} values in rodents (Fig. 2–2) of agents in Groups 1, 2A, and 2B, assuming a similar ranking of carcinogenic potency in humans, this procedure supported by the observed reasonable correlation in potency ranking of several antineoplastic drugs in humans and rodents (Kaldor et al, 1988) (and this chapter).

Although for Group 1 the number of entries is low (see legend for Fig. 2–2) the similarity of the three histograms that was found for each of the Groups 1, 2A,

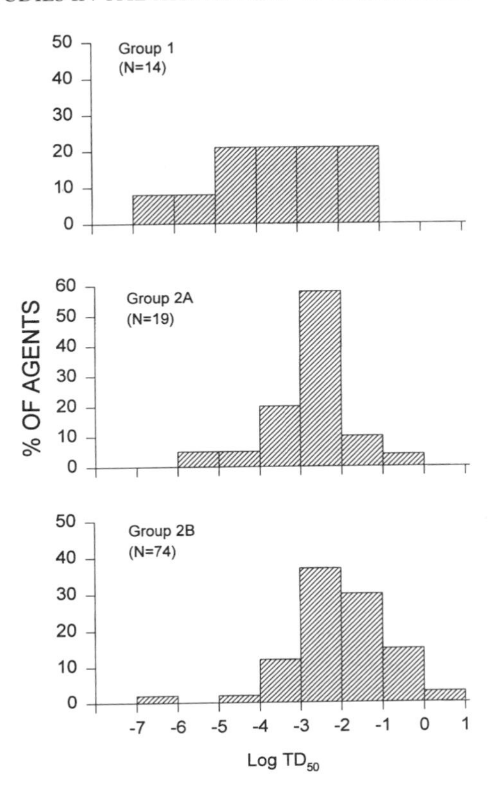

FIG. 2–2. TD_{50} values, defined as the daily dose (in g/kg b.w.) necessary to halve the percentage of tumor-free animals, were taken from an article by Gold et al (1984). When several estimates were reported, the lowest TD_{50} values in rodents were used. For 14/30 agents in Group 1, 19/37 agents in Group 2A, and 74/112 agents in Group 2B, TD_{50} values were available. (Reproduced from Bartsch and Malaveille, 1989).

and 2B for a total of 107 chemicals reveals that the carcinogenic potency (TD_{50}) in rodents does not constitute a criterion to distinguish Group 1 carcinogens from those in Groups 2A and 2B.

These data indicate that neither the prevalence of genotoxic carcinogenic nor the distribution of carcinogenic potency in rodents reveals any specific characteristics of the human carcinogens in Group 1 that differentiates them from agents in Groups 2A and 2B (or from many in Group 3). This suggests that carcinogens in Groups 2A and 2B, and possibly several in 3, are carcinogenic to humans provided that the conditions of exposure exist. Consequently one has to assume that the level of human exposure is an important variable that determines which animal carcinogens, now listed in Groups 2A and 2B, end up in Group 1.

Although in no case is the exact mechanism by which these apparently nongenotoxic agents induce tumors in animals known, it appears that several of them compete with endogenous ligands for binding to cellular receptors that regulate cell growth and differentiation in mammals. It is therefore reasonable to assume that only relatively few chemicals can fortuitously interact with such receptors, because of the specificity of the complex structures that have evolved during evolution so as to minimize interference with regulatory processes in mammalian cells. In contrast, genotoxic intermediates are produced from many xenobiotics as a consequence of biotransformation reactions by phase I and phase II drug-metabolizing enzymes that act with a rather low substrate specificity on virtually any foreign compound. This hypothesis could explain why a large excess of genotoxic carcinogens is found among the established, probable, and possible human carcinogens that were identified in the IARC Monographs Program.

From this analysis on the prevalence of genotoxic carcinogens among three groups of agents to which humans were or are exposed, consisting of established human carcinogens (Group 1, N = 30), probable human carcinogens (Group 2A, N = 37), possible human carcinogens (Group 2B, N = 113), we can conclude that: (1) The high prevalence on the order of 80% to 90% of genotoxic carcinogens that was found in each of the Groups 1, 2A, and 2B implies that genotoxic carcinogens as a group add more to the cancer burden in man than the nongenotoxic counterpart. We must here stress, however, that the preponderance of genotoxic over nongenotoxic carcinogens in Group 3, and possibly in Groups 2B and 2A, may have resulted in part from the type of approaches used for the identification of carcinogenic agents. The type of tests used may indeed have favored the identification of agents operating through a particular mechanism. Even if the tests presently used would miss agents that are carcinogenic by a different mechanism, the identification and subsequent lowering of exposure to genotoxic carcinogens in the external and internal environment of man would still remain an important goal for primary cancer prevention. (2) An agent with unknown carcinogenic potential, but showing sufficient evidence for activity in genotoxicity assays (as defined in this article) may represent a hazard to humans if sufficient exposure exists. In contrast, an agent that shows a lack of activity in a spectrum of genotoxicity assays must still be tested in a rodent bioassay for carcinogenicity, in view of the present nonavailability of validated STT for nongenotoxic carcinogens. (3) The validation of STT for detection of potential carcinogens should be done with agents whose carcinogenicity (and lack of it) has been carefully assessed, preferably using the same criteria as defined in the IARC Monographs, i.e., with agents having sufficient evidence of carcinogenicity in animals. Most of the genotoxic carcinogens in Groups 1, 2A, and 2B are multispecies carcinogens (Wilbourn et al, 1986), which appears to be an intrinsic biological feature of human carcinogens that this IARC Monograph Program has identified so far. In contrast, the database of rodent carcinogens by the NTP and NCI of the U.S. contained a high proportion of agents that were carcinogenic in one species or one tissue only (Ashby and Tennant, 1988). It was the inclusion of such agents in the validation study of Tennant et al (1987) that has lead to a much poorer test performance on STTs than that reported by many other previous studies. Thus, the relevance of STTs should be judged on their ability to predict human hazards and not on their perfect correlation to rodent carcinogenicity.

Although many short-term tests are still being refined and better defined in terms of their usefulness, there is little doubt that they will continue to play a major role in identifying new carcinogens and mutagens in complex internal and external environment of man; this task cannot be tackled only by epidemiological studies and animal tests, in view of the time, expense, and the difficulty of dealing with complex mixtures and the limitations in sensitivity.

CONCLUSIONS

The variations in different countries in the incidence of cancer that occur at the most common target organs fluctuate between 4- and 100-fold (Parkin et al, 1987; IARC, 1990). This observation, together with the results of studies in migrant populations, showing that migrants tend to acquire cancer characteristics of the host countries, are among the strongest arguments to support the important role played by environmental factors in the development of human tumors. A decisive argument is obviously that a certain number of environmental factors have indeed been identified as being causally related to human cancer. Historically, observations in humans have by far preceded evidence provided by experimental results, but both the epidemiological and experimental approaches, at least since the beginning of this century, have contributed to the identification of human carcinogens.

We are at present aware of 66 agents or mixtures or exposure circumstances causally related to human cancer, the majority of which are environmental chemicals. The human exposure to most of these chemicals is rather recent—that is, it goes back to last century when the synthesis of new chemicals, as well as the massive exploitation of naturally occurring chemicals, such as certain metals and asbestos, underwent a considerable expansion and the industrial production of cigarettes began.

It would be illusory to pretend that complete prevention of human cancer could be achieved solely by controlling these relatively new carcinogenic agents, but it would be similarly deceptive to deny the importance of trying to control them and of continuing to do so. The new hazards, which have been added to much older ones, such as ionizing and nonionizing radiations, mycotoxins, certain combustion products, and possibly viruses, contributed to deep social injustices that have only recently been largely overcome in most industrialized countries, but certainly not in all regions and countries of the world. Certain developing countries are, in terms of occupational hazards, in a situation similar to that of industrialized countries 50 to 70 years ago. Similarly, developing countries are today faced with the same threat of a massive penetration, supported by the tobacco corporations, of the habit of smoking that occurred many decades ago in industrialized countries.

The carcinogenicity tests still have an irreplaceable role to play in the prevention of the emission into our environment of new hazardous chemicals, as well as in warning about the presence of carcinogens among the chemicals already in our environment. It is not unreasonable to assume, in fact, that other chemicals among the thousands to which we are exposed will eventually be identified as carcinogenic to humans, or in some way related to an increased frequency of human cancer.

Even if the experimental tests for carcinogenicity, as presently used, may not be apt to identify all important human carcinogens, they still provide useful predictions about the similar effects in humans for a considerable number of environmental exposures. Past experience showed that the experimental evidence of carcinogenicity indeed preceded evidence in humans for certain chemicals, and it could have been used to discontinue exposure before a confirmation from studies in humans would become available. This was the case of 4-aminobiphenyl, aflatoxins, mustard gas, DES, melphalan, 8-methyoxypsoralen + UV radiation, and vinyl chloride (Tomatis et al, 1989).

The high prevalence (80%–90%) of genotoxic agents among the identified human carcinogens justifies the continued use of short-term tests that use DNA, mutational, and chromosomal damage as endpoint. If an agent is clearly active in several of those tests, it should be considered as a potential human carcinogens, if sufficient exposure exists. These tests do and will play a major role in isolating and characterizing carcinogenic components in complex mixtures.

The role of carcinogenicity tests in the quantitative estimation of risks is still questionable, but examples given in this chapter indicate that, in at least certain instances, there is a rather good concordance between human and animal data. Moreover, advances in our understanding of the mechanisms of carcinogenesis may make them more helpful in evaluating risks from low levels of exposure and in allowing direct interspecies extrapolations. Information on relevant mechanisms of carcinogenesis can—indeed, already are at present—be of some use in the evaluation of carcinogenicity and in interpreting the significance of experimental data in predicting human risks (IARC, 1991; Vainio et al, 1992).

REFERENCES

ALLEN BC, CRUMP KS, SHIPP AM. 1988. Correlation between carcinogenic potency of chemicals in animals and humans. Risk Anal 8 (4):531–544.

ASHBY J, TENNANT RW. 1988. Chemical structure, *Salmonella* mutagenicity and extent of carcinogenicity as indicators of genotoxic carcinogenesis among 222 chemicals tested in rodents by the U.S. NCI/NTP. Mutat Res 204:7–115.

BARTSCH H, KUROKI T, ROBERFROID M, MALAVEILLE C. 1982. Metabolic activation systems *in vitro* for carcinogen/mutagen screening tests. In de Serres FJ, Hollaender A (eds): Chemical Mutagens—Principles and Methods for their Detection, Vol. 7. New York and London: Plenum Press, pp. 95–161.

BARTSCH H, MALAVEILLE C. 1989. Prevalence of genotoxic chemicals among animal and human carcinogens evaluated in the IARC Monograph series. Cell Biol Toxicol 5:115–127.

BERNSTEIN L, GOLD LS, AMES BN, PIKE MC, HOEL DG. 1985. Some tautologous aspects of the comparison of carcinogenic potency in rats and mice. Toxicol Appl Pharmacol 5:79–86.

BRADFORD HILL A. 1971. Principles of Medical Statistics. London: The Lancet Limited, pp. 313–323.

BROCKMAN HE, DEMARINI DM. 1988. Utility of short-term tests for genetic toxicity in the aftermath of the NTP's analysis of 73 chemicals. Environ Mol Mutagen 11:421–435.

CROUCH E, WILSON R. 1979. Interspecies comparison of carcinogenic potency. J Toxicol Environ Health 5:1095–1118.

DOLL R. 1967. Prevention of cancer: pointers from epidemiology. London: The Nuffield Provincial Hospital Trust and Rock Carling Fellowship.

DOLL R, PETO R. 1981. The causes of cancer. J Natl Cancer Inst 66:1101–1308.

ENNEVER FK, NOONAN TJ, ROSENKRANZ HS. 1987. The predictivity of animal bioassays and short-term genotoxicity tests for carcinogenicity and noncarcinogenicity to humans. Mutagenesis 2:73–78.

GOLD LS, SAYER CB, MAGAW R, BACKMAN GM, DE VECIANA M, LEVINSON R, HOOPER NK, HAVENDER WR, BERNSTEIN L, PETO R, PIKE MC, AMES BN. 1984. A carcinogenic potency database of the standardized results of animal bioassays. Environ Health Perspect 58:9–319.

GOODMAN G, WILSON R. 1991. Predicting the carcinogenicity of chemicals in humans from rodent bioassay data. Environ Health Perspect 94:195–218.

HASEMAN JK, CRAWFORD DD, HUFF JE, BOORMAN GA, MCCONNELL EE. 1984. Results from 86 two-year carcinogenicity studies conducted by the National Toxicology Program. J Toxicol Environ Health 14:621–639.

HEDDLE JA. 1988. Prediction of chemical carcinogenicity from *in vitro* genetic toxicity. Mutagenesis 3 (4):287–291.

HUFF JE, MCCONNELL EE, HASEMAN JK, BOORMAN GA, EUSTIS SL, SCHWARTZ BA, RAO GN, JAMESON CK, HART LG, RALL DP. 1988. Carcinogenesis studies: results of 398 experiment on 104 chemicals from the US National Toxicology Program. Ann NY Acad Sci 534:1–30.

IARC. 1981–1992. IARC Monographs on the Evaluation of Carcinogenic Risks to Humans, Volumes 1–54. Lyon, France: International Agency for Research on Cancer.

IARC. 1987a. IARC Monographs on the Evaluation of Carcinogenic Risks to Humans. Overall Evaluations of Carcinogenicity: An updating of IARC Monographs. Volumes 1–42, Supplement 7.

IARC. 1987b. IARC Monographs on the Evaluation of Carcinogenic Risks to Humans. Genetic and Related Effects: An Updating of Selected IARC Monographs from Volumes 1–42, Supplement 6, Lyon, France.

IARC. 1990. Cancer: Causes, Occurrence and Control (L. Tomatis, ed). Lyon, France: International Agency for Research on Cancer.

IARC. 1991. Consensus Report on Mechanisms of Carcinogenesis in Risk Identification. IARC Internal Technical Report No 91/002, Lyon, France.

ITO N, IMAIDA K, TSUDA H, SHIBATA M, AOKI T, DE CAMARGO JLV, FUKUSHIMA S. 1988a. Wide-spectrum initiation models: possible applications to medium-term multiple organ bioassays for carcinogenesis modifiers. Gann 79:413–417.

ITO N, TSUDA H, TATEMATSU M, INOVE T, TAGAWA Y, AOKI T, UWAGAWA S, KAGAWA M, OGISO T, MASUI T, IMAIDA K, FUKUSHIMA S, ASAMOTO M. 1988b. Enhancing effects of various hepatocarcinogens on induction of preneoplastic glutathione S-transferase placenta forum positive foci in rats—an approach for a new medium-term bioassay system. Carcinogenesis 9:387–394.

KALDOR JM, DAY NE, HEMMINKI K. 1988. Quantifying the carcinogenicity of antineoplastic drugs. Eur J Cancer Clin Oncol 24 (4):703–711.

KIER LD, BRUSICK DJ, AULETTA AE, VON HALLE ES, BROWN MM, SIMMON VF, DUNKEL V, MCCANN J, MORTELMANS K, PRIVAL M, RAO TK, RAY V. 1986. The *Salmonella typhimurium*/mammalian microsomal assay. A report of the U.S. Environmental Protection Agency Gene-Tox Program. Mutat Res 168:9–240.

KODELL RL, GAYLOR DW, CHEN JJ. 1991. Carcinogenic potency correlations: real or artifactual? J Toxicol Env Health 32:1–9.

KUROKI T, MATSUSHIMA T. 1987. Performance of short-term tests for detection of human carcinogens. Mutagenesis 2 (1):33–37.

LAVE LB, ENNEVER FK, ROSENKRANZ HS, OMENN GS. 1988. Information value of the rodent bioassay. Nature 336:431–433.

LEE T-C, TANAKA N, LAMB PW, GILMER TM, BARRETT JC. 1988. Induction of gene amplification by arsenic. Science 241:79–81.

MAUGH TH. 1978. Chemicals: How many are there? Science 199:162.

MCCANN J, GOLD S, HORN L, MCGILL R, GRAEDEL TE, KALDOR J. 1988. Statistical analysis of Salmonella test data and comparison to results of animal cancer tests. Mutat Res 205:183–196.

MESELSON M, RUSSEL K. 1977. Comparisons of carcinogenic and mutagenic potency. In Hiatt HH, Watson JD, Winsten JA (eds): Origins of Human Cancer. New York: Cold Spring Harbor Laboratory, pp. 1473–1481.

MONTESANO R, BARTSCH H, VAINIO H, WILBOURN J, YAMASKI H (eds). 1986. Long-term and short-term assays for carcinogens: a critical appraisal. IARC Scientific Publications No. 83, International Agency for Research on Cancer.

NATIONAL ACADEMY OF SCIENCES. 1975. Pest Control: An assessment of present and alternative technologies. Volume 1: Contemporary pest control practices and prospects. Washington, D.C.

PARKIN DM, LÄÄRÄ E, MUIR CS. 1987. Estimates of the worldwide frequency of sixteen major cancers in 1980. Int J Cancer 41:184–197.

PASSEY RD. 1922. Experimental soot cancer. Br Med J 2:1112–1113.

PETO R, PIKE MC, BERNSTEIN L, GOLD LS, AMES BN. 1984. The TD^{50}: a proposed general convention for the numerical description of the carcinogenic potency of chemicals in chronic exposure animal experiments. Environ Health Perspect 58:9–319.

PURCHASE IF. 1981. Interspecies comparisons of carcinogenicity. Br J Cancer 41:454–468.

ROSENKRANZ HS (ED). 1988. Genotoxic Toxicology Testing and Biomonitoring of Environmental or Occupational Exposure. Mutat Res 205:1–426.

SABADIE N, MALAVEILLE C, CAMUS AM, BARTSCH H. 1980. Comparison of the hydroxylation of benzo(a)pyrene with the metabolism of vinyl chloride, *N*-nitrosomorphiline and *N*-nitroso-*N*-methylpiperazine to mutagens by humans and rat liver microsomal fractions. Cancer Res 40:119–126.

SABADIE N, RICHTER-REICHHELM HB, SARACCI R, MOHR U, BARTSCH H. 1981. Interindividual differences in oxidative benzo(a)pyrene metabolism by normal and tumorous surgical lung specimens from 105 lung cancer patients. Int J Cancer 27:417–425.

SCHMÄHL D, HABS M. 1979. Carcinogenic action of low-dose cyclophosphamide given orally to Sprague-Dawley rats in a lifetime experiment. Jpn J Cancer Res 23:706–712.

SEMPLE E, HAYS MA, PURCHASE TH, HAINES L, FARBER E. 1987. Mitogenic activity in platelet-poor plasma from rats with persistent liver nodules or liver cancer. Biochem Biophys Res Commun 148:449–455.

SHELBY MD. 1988. The genetic toxicity of human carcinogens and its implications. Mutat Res 204:3–15.

SHELBY MD, ZEIGER E, TENNANT RW. 1988. Commentary on the status of short-term tests for chemical carcinogens. Env Mol Mutagen 11:437–441.

SHELBY MD, ZEIGER E. 1990. Activity of human carcinogens in the Salmonella and rodent bone-marrow cytogenetics tests. Mutat Res 234:257–261.

TENNANT RW, MARGOLIN BH, SHELBY MD, ZEIGER E, HASEMAN JK, SPALDING J, CASPARY W, RESNICK M, STASIEWICZ S, ANDERSON B, MINOR R. 1987. Prediction of chemical carcinogenicity in rodents from in vitro genetic toxicity assays. Science 236:933–941.

TOKUOKA S. 1965. Induction of tumours in mice with N,N-bis(2-chloroethyl)-N′,O-propylenephosphoric acid ester diamide (cyclophosphamide). Gann 56:537–541.

TOMATIS L, PARTENSKY C, MONTESANO R. 1973. The predictive value of mouse liver tumour induction in carcinogenicity testing: a literature survey. Int J Cancer 12:1–20.

TOMATIS L. 1978. The value of long-term testing for the implementation of primary prevention. In Hiatt HH, Watson JD, Winsten FA (eds): Origins of Human Cancer, New York: Cold Spring Harbor Laboratory, pp. 1339–1357.

TOMATIS L. 1979. The predictive value of rodent carcinogenicity tests in the evaluation of human risks. Annu Rev Pharmacol Toxicol 19:511–530.

TOMATIS L, BRESLOW NE, BARTSCH H. 1982. Experimental studies in the assessment of human risk. In Schottenfeld D, Fraumeni, JF Jr (eds): Cancer Epidemiology and Prevention. Philadelphia: W. B. Saunders, pp. 44–73.

TOMATIS L, AITIO A, WILBOURN J, SHUKER L. 1989. Human carcinogens so far identified. Jpn J Cancer Res 80:795–807.

TSUTSUI H. 1918. Über das künstlich erzeugte Cancroid bei der Maus. Gann 12:17–21.

VAINIO H, MAGEE P, MCGREGOR D, MCMICHAEL AJ (EDS). 1992. Mechanisms of Carcinogenesis in Risk Identification. IARC Scientific Publication 116, Lyon, France: International Agency for Research on Cancer.

WILBOURN J, HAROUN L, HESELTINE E, KALDOR J, PARTENSKY C, VAINIO H. 1986. Response of experimental animals to human carcinogens: an analysis based upon the IARC Monographs programme. Carcinogenesis 7 (11):1853–1863.

WISEMAN RW, STOWERS SJ, MILLER EC, ANDERSON MW, MILLER JA. 1986. Activating mutations of the c-Ha-ras protooncogene in chemically induced hepatomas of the male B6C3 F1 mouse. Proc Natl Acad Sci USA 83:5825–5829.

WORLD HEALTH ORGANIZATION. 1964. Prevention of Cancer, Tech. Rep. Series No. 276, Geneva, Switzerland.

YAMAGIWA K, ICHIKAWA K. 1915. Über die künstliche Erzeugung von Papillom. Verh Jpn Path Ges 5:142–148.

YAMASAKI H. 1988. Multistage carcinogenesis: implications for risk estimation. Cancer Metastasis Rev 7:5–18.

YOU M, CANDRIAN U, MAROUPOT RR, STONER GD, ANDERSON MW. 1989. Activation of the k-ras protooncogene in spontaneously occurring and chemically induced lung tumours of the strain A mice. Proc Natl Acad Sci USA, 86:3070–3074.

ZEIGER E. 1987. Carcinogenicity of mutagens: predictive capability of the *Salmonella* mutagenesis assay for rodent carcinogenicity. Cancer Res 47:1287–1296.

3 Morphologic classification of human cancer

JOHN W. BERG

Morphologic classification of cancer refers primarily to the histologic classification made by the pathologist based on microscopic examination. Besides providing the clinician with information necessary to determine treatment and prognosis, the diagnosis should be of importance to the epidemiologist since it is the way to separate cancers of a site into different diseases, including diseases with different etiologies.

Compared with its potential, very little use is made currently by epidemiologists of histologic or other pathologic information. For only a few cancers is the epidemiologic importance of histology generally appreciated. Perhaps the best known, as well as the earliest example, is Kreyberg's separation of the histologic types of lung cancer closely associated with cigarette smoking from the others (Kreyberg, 1962). Other epidemiologic implications of specific histologic types of cancers do not seem to be as widely known. Probably the association between radiation and mixed mesodermal tumors of the uterus will be better known to epidemiologists than to pathologists, while the latter may be more aware than the former of the special etiologic implications of lymphomas of the thyroid or small intestine. Although both groups should know that a cluster of rare cancers can point to a new cause (angiosarcomas of the liver to vinyl chloride, mesotheliomas to asbestos, among others), to date, epidemiologists have failed to exploit this fact by examining incoming cancer registry data; they generally passively await handouts from perceptive pathologists. Better acquaintance with morphology could remedy this. It also could enable epidemiologists to identify many new entities to study by indicating which cancers are most likely to have special etiologies or to have developed from different precursor lesions.

Also, it should be pointed out that epidemiologists need to know something about morphology simply for the purpose of communication. Suppose epidemiologists wish to look at local data after seeing the report that woodworkers are at special risk for adenocarcinoma of the nasal sinuses. When they request the cases of adenocarcinoma of this site from the cancer registry or the local pathologist's files, they are in danger of being taken literally and getting exactly those cases whose diagnosis is adenocarcinoma. The epidemiologist needs to understand that in these files the term *adenocarcinoma* is used in a generic sense and includes, in addition to adenocarcinomas as a specific diagnosis, all types of gland-like or gland-derived carcinomas of the site, including adenoid cystic carcinomas (more than twice as common as adenocarcinoma) and the half dozen or so other kinds of adenocarcinomas originating in the sinuses.

SOURCES OF THE MORPHOLOGIC DIVERSITY OF CANCERS

Of the 71 major categories into which the *International Classification of Diseases*, 1975 revision (ICD–9, World Health Organization, 1977) divided invasive human cancer, 10 were histologically defined (leukemias, lymphomas, and melanomas) and 7 were categories for cancers whose origins were unknown or uncertain. Of the 54 sites listed, 48 were important cancer sites because of their epithelium and only 6 primarily because of cancers arising in other kinds of tissue. This alone suggests the importance of epithelium as a source of cancer. Put another way, 85% of all registered cancers will be carcinomas, i.e., cancers of epithelium; another 2% will be the closely related melanomas, and about 1% will be mixtures of epithelial and nonepithelial elements or unclassifiable, so only 12% of cancers will be proven noncarcinomas. *Epithelium* is the term applied to the cells that cover the external surface of the body or that line the internal cavities, plus those cells derived from the linings that form glands. These cells are the first point of contact of the body with environmental substances. The epithelial cells include the cells that secrete or otherwise process the body's chemicals and so come into

I wish to thank the SEER program staff and especially Mrs. Constance Percy for providing me with many sets of special tabulations.

particular contact with circulating carcinogens or precarcinogens. As they metabolize these chemicals, they produce a wide variety of derivative compounds, including ultimate (immediate) carcinogens. In addition, epithelial cells and blood cells are the major dividing cells in adults. This is important because most cancers become invasive and clinically important only after the cells originally damaged by a carcinogen have undergone several divisions. Muscle or fat, with a low rate of cell division, although exposed to radiation or some other carcinogen, will be less likely than epithelium to undergo sufficient proliferation for latent malignant changes to be manifested clinically. The other subgroups of cancers in an epithelium-containing organ are sarcomas arising from the connective tissue (fat, fibrous tissue, vessels, nerves, and muscles) and lymphomas. In most organs, lymphoid tissue is not a normal component but is present as part of a pathologic reaction.

Besides carcinomas, sarcomas, and lymphomas, occasionally one may encounter (in an organ) cancers of a primitive or mixed-cell type. These may have arisen from multipotential stem cells remaining in the organ or by dedifferentiation; the choice between the two explanations remains a matter of debate. Regardless of their origin, these tumors help explain why almost any type of cancer can be found in almost any site upon occasion, and why a discussion like this must contain so many qualifications.

Carcinomas fall into four major groups: (*1*) *epidermoid (pavement cell) carcinomas*, which in the broadest sense include transitional cell carcinomas as well as squamous cell (keratinizing) carcinomas; (*2*) *adenocarcinomas* (carcinomas secreting mucins or hormones or at least forming gland-like structures); (*3*) *special site-specific types*, such as hepatomas, or travesties of normal liver cells, or seminomas, which are cancers arising from germinal epithelium; and (*4*) *undifferentiated carcinomas* with neither epidermoid nor glandular features. Small cell carcinomas of the lung and medullary carcinomas of the breast could be put in this last group as well as tumors diagnosed only as carcinoma because they are too primitive (undifferentiated) to show what sort of epithelium they had arisen from. In some instances one is forced to put cancers with mixed characteristics in group 3 out of ignorance, but many mixed types can be characterized more explicitly. The sarcomatous component of some larynx cancer has been shown to be metaplastic squamous cell carcinoma; a mixed papillary and follicular carcinoma of the thyroid is clinically and epidemiologically a variety of papillary carcinoma, not follicular carcinoma, while a mixed hepatoma-cholangiocarcinoma epidemiologically is a cholangiocarcinoma, not hepatoma.

Epidemiologically one can make two generalizations about the diversity of carcinomas found at any site. First of all, the further apart in appearance two types of carcinoma are, the more likely it is that they will have different epidemiologic characteristics. For example, the epidemiology of squamous cell carcinoma of a particular site would be expected to differ more from adenocarcinoma at that site than for the adenocarcinomas to differ from one another. In the oral cavity almost all squamous cell carcinomas, whether from surface epithelium or from salivary glands, are linked in the United States with smoking or drinking. By contrast, the several kinds of adenocarcinomas of the mouth all arise from salivary glands, and none have any demonstrated relation to tobacco and alcohol intake.

Secondly, the morphology of the carcinoma may give clues to its origin. Squamous cell carcinoma has been the most common type of lung cancer. This may be surprising at first glance because there is no squamous epithelium in the normal lung. What happens is that smoking, like other forms of lung injury, often changes the normal glandular ciliated epithelium to metaplastic squamous epithelium. This metaplastic epithelium is especially prone to further cancerous change. Also, noxious materials accumulate in regions of metaplasia. Hence most cancers of the lung produced by tobacco arose from metaplastic squamous epithelium and retained features of that epithelium. Now, however, adenocarcinomas are becoming more common while squamous cell carcinomas are less common (Beard et al., 1988), and the most likely explanation, though one not verified to my knowledge, is that perhaps because of better nutrition, or the changing composition of cigarette tobacco smoke (e.g., tobacco-specific nitrosamines) squamous metaplasia has become less frequent (Wynder and Hoffmann, 1994).

In other organs, too, the morphology of a carcinoma should reflect the particular metaplasia from which it arose or show which cells in the epithelium responded to the carcinogen. This in turn is determined, if only in a probabilistic sense, by the nature of the carcinogen and its mode of contact. Deducing etiology from morphology is still a dream for most cancers but recent advances are closing the gap. It is now clear that the morphology of a cancer reflects the pattern of chromosome changes (translocations and deletions) which have activated particular oncogenes or led to inactivation of cancer suppressor genes (Sandberg, 1994; Weinberg, 1994). For the clinician such correlation explains why morphology implies behavior. For the epidemiologist there is the hope that differences in appearance can be traced back to different causes of genetic alteration.

Undifferentiated carcinomas represent a major but generally unrecognized problem for epidemiology. The word *undifferentiated* (or *anaplastic*) is used as a description of the grade of a particular type of carcinoma, such as adenocarcinoma or squamous cell carcinoma. It also is used as the basic name for cancers that lack clues as to the cell of origin, i.e., no mucin secretion or squamous differentiation. As mentioned previously, some of these latter cancers, such as oat cell carcinoma and medullary carcinoma, still have quite specific and recognizable morphologies. Other cancers are given this name because they have no distinguishing features or structural features at all. Still others really may not belong in the undifferentiated category but are put there because the pathologist sees no pattern in the submitted material. It may have been crushed or burned in removal; it might simply be a very small sample, even a cytologic preparation of isolated cells.

As interest in specific morphologic types increases, there is recurrent need to describe these types in terms of age-adjusted incidence rates as one does for cancers of a standard site. Unfortunately, as one can see in Appendix A, cancers of unspecified type may comprise an important fraction of the proven cancers at a site. In a combined tabulation of lung cancers from the *Third National Cancer Survey* (Cutler and Young, 1975) and the first 5 years of the National Cancer Institute's *Surveillance, Epidemiology and End Results* (SEER, Young et al., 1981) over 25% of the proven cancers were not typed, despite the epidemiologic as well as clinical importance of such typing. Hence histologically specific incidence rates that omit these cancers can be ignoring a major component. On the other hand, simple proportional allocation of the unspecified cancers to specific types is incorrect whenever the specific types have different age distributions. They usually do because the unspecified diagnoses are made preferentially in older patients. Having other pathologists relook at the material rarely will justify its cost. However, major reductions in nonspecific diagnoses may be achieved by reabstracting the case records in search of additional, more specific pathologic diagnoses or descriptions. (Only recently has it become the norm for cancer registrars to use descriptive terms as well as diagnoses when assigning the morphologic code number.) The alternative is proportional allocation of nonspecific diagnoses in proportion to specific ones separately for each age–sex–race stratum before morphologically specific incidence rates are calculated. This recommendation is based partly on the fact that allowing for age, sex, and racial distributions, nonspecific cases look more like a representative mix than dedifferentiation of one particular cancer type. For this chapter the percentages of specific types of cancer in Appendix A were calculated after exclusion of the nonspecific diagnoses noted at the end of each site listing.

Morphology as discussed thus far has referred only to histologic typing of cancers. However, morphology also could mean the "gross" appearance to the naked eye and in fact, some macroscopic growth patterns have prognostic implications. Two examples would be the better prognosis of (1) circumscribed as opposed to stellate, scirrhous breast cancers, and (2) papillary as opposed to ulcerated, infiltrating cancers of the digestive and urinary tracts. As yet, such growth differences have not been shown to have etiologic implications; if such differences are demonstrated, the best solution would be to use a separate field to describe gross morphology as we now describe stage and grade in registry data.

Cancer *Grade* refers to the degree to which the cancer cells are or are not uniform and do or do not resemble corresponding normal cells. (The two properties are different but are mixed in various proportions in most grading schemes.) Grade usually has been considered important only with regard to prognosis (see Henson, 1988). It may have epidemiologic implications as well. Bladder and prostatic cancers appear to be different diseases in blacks and whites and the difference is marked not so much by different histologies but by different grade distributions at the time of diagnosis (for transitional cell carcinomas of the bladder, Hankey and Myers, 1987) or even before (adenocarcinoma of the prostate, Guilegardo et al., 1980). Grade is not mentioned as such in their results but as they point out, their classification is close to that used by Gleason for grading. Discovering the causes for higher grade (worse) cancers of these sites in blacks is particularly challenging epidemiologically because similar grade differences definitely are *not* seen at most other sites. Other possible epidemiologic differences associated with grade are mentioned in Appendix A.

Finally, a broad definition of *morphology* includes details of where the cancer arose within the organ or tissue. This separation usually is presented in statistical tabulations only for segments of the large intestine. However, at a number of other sites, the subsites are less alike than histologically different cancers of any one subsite. One vivid example of this is the major epidemiologic differences between cancers of the various components of the "gallbladder and extrahepatic bile ducts" category. Within each of the subsites, even the separation of squamous cell cancers from adenocarcinomas is not epidemiologically justified.

THE CURRENT CLASSIFICATION OF CANCER

This chapter is written under the assumption that optimal use of pathologic information requires some understanding not only of pathological nomenclature but also of the classification system that currently is generally accepted for use in cancer registries and its relation to the classification used in vital statistics. For more than two decades a general stability of nomenclature in the United States has been matched by a similar relative stability of the coding classification. This classification grew out of the conviction of Drs. Cuyler Hammond,

Arthur Wells, and others, that pathologic information was too complex to be handled adequately by a one-dimensional code such as the World Health Organizations *International Classification of Diseases* (ICD) or even the mixed concepts of the then standard, two-dimensional code of the *Standard Nomenclature of Diseases and Operations* (Thompson and Hayden 1961). Instead, a committee built upon the concept of separate fields for different kinds of information. One field was for the site of the pathologic lesion; a second, for the morphologic change; a third, for the etiology of the lesion; and a fourth, for its functional disturbance (e.g., abnormal hormone secretion by a lung cancer). This concept of separate fields for different types of information was developed into the *Systematized Nomenclature of Pathology* (SNOP) (College of American Pathologists, 1965) and has been maintained and expanded into the *Systematized Nomenclature of Medicine* (SNOMED) (College of American Pathologists, 1979)—the two classifications and coding schemes generally accepted and promoted by pathologists and their organizations in the U.S.

The SNOP and SNOMED codes are general purpose and while they do have separate sections in morphology for neoplasms, their site codes are not optimal for cancer. On the other hand, the neoplasm section of the various revisions of ICD was primarily, though far from purely, a site code. Hence the American Cancer Society replaced an outdated and unwieldy *Manual of Tumor Nomenclature and Coding–1951* with a new MOTNAC–1968 (American Cancer Society, 1968) version that wedded a site code derived from the cancer section of ICD–8 to the (morphologic) neoplasm section of SNOP. The identity explains why ICD–Oncology morphology begins with 8000.

This proved a success in that the morphologic rubrics corresponded well with then current pathological nomenclature, and the topographic rubrics permitted a fairly simple conversion to the ICD code. By the time the 9th revision of the ICD appeared, there was enough international consensus among cancer registries on the merit of this approach that together the ICD and SNOP codes from MOTNAC–1968 were expanded and updated by an international committee to produce the first *International Classification of Diseases—Oncology* (ICD–O) (World Health Organization 1976). Reciprocally, the morphology section of the ICD–O served as the neoplasm section of SNOMED.

This history is given in some detail partly to facilitate communication between epidemiologists and pathologists with their apparently quite different coding schemes. The history is also important for working with data collected over time. Each new version of the code introduces changes, especially new categories. Older data may be "converted," but except for an unusual case-by-case review, cases that should have been or even were diagnosed as a type, e.g., as *tubular carcinoma*, before that term was given a separate code number in the ICD–O (1978), will have been coded to some general category of MOTNAC and so be lost. Hence the sudden appearance of tubular carcinomas of the breast in 1978 is artificial, not the manifestation of a new carcinogen.

A new version of the ICD, ICD–10, has been created and presumably will eventually come into use in all countries. Because many specialties felt they needed more categories, the format has been completely changed from numeric to alpha-numeric. Cancers are in section C; other neoplasms are in section D. Some important cancer sites, such as ovary, have their own major category. Some reordering into more logical sequences has been done: retroperitoneal cancers (though not mediastinal ones) are now with other soft tissue cancers. To make death certificate data more useful for epidemiologists, mesotheliomas and Kaposi's sarcomas have their own code numbers. In anticipation of ICD–10, ICD–O was updated and the site codes changed to alpha-numeric (ICD–O–2, World Health Organization, 1990). As before, the histologic categories of ICD were not used, and as a result, the site *concepts* are essentially unchanged. Except for the lymphomas which, as usual, have a new classification, the major (3-digit) morphology categories remain unchanged, although about 70 new 4-digit categories have been added. These new codes have been adopted by many U.S. cancer registries for 1992 data and earlier data converted, meriting the caution mentioned above.

Much of the success of SNOP and MOTNAC–1968 was due to the committees that created them eschewing personal and idiosyncratic terminology, and relying instead on generally accepted authority, especially on the fascicles from the Armed Forces Institute of Pathology (1949–1963). In turn, ICD–O utilized both newer volumes from that series and the volumes comprising the *International Histological Classification of Tumors* (IHCT, World Health Organization,) also sponsored by the World Health Organization (see in particular Sobin et al., 1978). Descriptions of most morphologic entities can be found in these volumes and perhaps should be preferred to those from other sources.

The current classification scheme provides relative ease of coding and a more or less hierarchical organization of terms. It is not as satisfactory with regard to consistency of coding. Too often there is more than one rubric in the histology code for diagnoses that at that site should refer to the same entity. For most sites, more than 30 histologies will appear in a registry file of any size and for some sites, such as lung, there will be over 50 "different" kinds of cancer reported. This contrasts with a median number of only six histologies a site in a current comprehensive but practical analytic scheme. Only nine of the more than 40 sites have more than ten specific types of importance. A part of this excess of histologic diagnoses is due to the occasional use of some outdated or idiosyncratic terms, but mostly the problem reflects the fact that terms can be synonyms at one site but not at another so they need separate code numbers. For example, for cancers of the bowel and ovary *papillary carcinoma* (8050), *papillary adenocarcinoma* (8260) and *adenocarcinoma, not otherwise specified* (8140) appear epidemiologically equivalent. In the breast, of course, papillary (adeno)carcinoma is a special entity, while plain *adenocarcinoma* indicates that no classification of the cancer has been attempted. On the other hand, papillary carcinoma in the mouth, pharynx, or larynx means a clinical and epidemiologically special type of squamous cell cancer, while in the urinary tract it implies a low-grade transitional cell carcinoma particularly unlike squamous cell cancers of the same site. With nothing in the classification to assist one in the understanding of these nuances, proper and complete retrieval or organization of histologic data is difficult even for most pathologists.

There also are problems with site and particularly subsite definitions. When there are six or seven partly overlapping subsites for the tongue, it is likely that many cancers will cross boundary lines. Such cancers are likely to be coded to the *overlapping* .8 rubric or to the *not otherwise specified* (NOS) .9 rubric.

Another problem is that some cancers are particularly susceptible to be coded to an assortment of sites. An example would be the assignment of a primary site for a liposarcoma involving the parotid gland and adjacent structures. Some will call it a sarcoma of the parotid, others, a sarcoma of the cheek. In the latter case, the coder has the choice of coding it to the cheek mucosa, to the skin of the cheek (actually "skin of the outer parts of the face") if skin fixation is mentioned, to connective tissues of the head, face, and neck, or to the wastebasket category, "other and ill-defined sites of the head, face and neck."

Epidemiologists should be aware that, despite the existence of a standard classification, pathological nomenclature and classification properly remains in a state of flux. Molecular biology in particular offers many new criteria for pathologists to apply. Also, there continue to be new insights on the relation of microscopic appearance to clinical prognosis and response to particular treatments. The difficulty is that not all new classifications are improvements and not all prove to be reproducible by other pathologists. In the new revisions of ICD and ICD–O, the aims were to drop outdated terms but not to accept too soon new proposals that may prove ephemeral. Whatever decisions are made, one can be sure that some histologic diagnoses will be missing and some will have meanings not acceptable to a particular pathologist. Experience suggests that temporary, local solutions be found for these problems rather than expecting frequent modification of the standard classification.

ORGANIZATION OF ICD–O CODED DATA FOR EPIDEMIOLOGY

Table 3–1 presents a standard way of organizing cancer cases from any one site. It is safe to say that cancers in groups I–III, even at the same site, will have different epidemiologies. Further, we know that carcinomas of different sites have little in common epidemiologically even when they are histologically similar. The same can be confidently said for lymphomas arising in organs (non-nodal lymphomas). It is less likely to be true for sarcomas and may not be true at all for other cancers such as neuroblastomas. Hence it is suggested that can-

TABLE 3–1. *Principal Separations for Cancers**

Cancer Type by Group Number	*ICD–O Numbers*
I. Carcinomas	
A. Epidermoid carcinomas[a]	8051-813
B. Adenocarcinomas	814, 816, 818–822, 825–850, 852–855, 857, 894[b]
C. Other specific carcinomas	803–804, 815, 817, 823, 824, 851, 856, 858–867
D. Unspecified ("Carcinoma NOS")	801–802
II. Lymphomas	959–971, (975 for ICD–O–1 only)
III. Sarcomas and other soft tissue tumors	868–871, 880–892, 899, 904, 912–934[c], 937, 954–958
IV. Leukemia	980–994
V. Other specified types of cancer	872–879, 893, 895–898, 900–903, 905–911, 918–936[c], 938–953, 972–974, (976 for ICD–O–2 only)
VI. Unspecified types of cancer	800, (999 ICD–O–1 only)

*Definitions in terms of ICD–O rubrics. First 3 digits of ICD–O numbers usually suffice to describe the range of the definitions and, with the exception noted in footnote a, also serve as definitions.

[a]ICD–O number 8050, Papillary carcinoma NOS (805 in SNOP and MOTNAC–68), is a term of variable meaning. When an organ contains an appreciable number of other epidermoid carcinomas, this term also is assumed to mean a papillary epidermoid carcinoma. Where the organ is the site of many adenocarcinomas and few epidermoid carcinomas, the term is assumed to refer to papillary adenocarcinomas.

[b]"Malignant mixed tumor," 894, for practical purposes, is a diagnosis applied only to major and minor salivary gland cancers. As such, it is epidemiologically, clinically, and pathologically an adenocarcinoma that has arisen from a benign "mixed tumor" ("pleomorphic adenoma").

[c]918–934 are in group III if they arise in soft tissue, in group V if they arise in bone.

cers of groups III and V be treated as one does leukemias and studied by histologic category across all sites.

This approach contradicts that of the ICD wherein all lymphomas regardless of origin are grouped, while the cancers of groups III and V are assigned to the organ of origin whenever that is known. The reason for this, of course, is that before chemotherapy, treatment was determined mostly by the site of the cancer as it still is in many cases today (the removal of organ lymphomas to a common collective is illogical by this reasoning, since many can be treated by the same kind of local or regional therapy appropriate for carcinomas of the site).

Table 3–1 has served as the starting point for the definition of multiple primary cancers (International Agency for Research on Cancer, 1994) and for the basic tabulations in the 1995 supplement to the journal *Cancer* (Percy, 1995) describing histologic aspects of the first 15 years of cancer data submitted to the National Cancer Institute's Surveillence, Epidemiology and End Results (SEER) program (Percy et al., in press).

Since carcinomas make up such a large percentage of cancers, it is usually desirable to subdivide them. Ideally this should be done on the basis of epidemiologic differences. The prototype for this as mentioned earlier was Kreyberg's division of lung cancers into type I (squamous cell and small cell carcinomas), or those almost entirely caused by cigarette smoking, and type II (the adenocarcinomas and other specific types), or those less closely related or unrelated to smoking. The division is too simple since adenocarcinomas now comprise an important subset of lung cancers, while small cell carcinomas in women are epidemiologically more like adenocarcinomas than squamous cell cancers, but the clear linkage of morphology and epidemiology is a milestone.

The difficulty in applying this concept to cancers of other organs is that relatively few definite correspondences between morphology and etiology are known. However, it is possible to utilize the lung analogy in another way. When cigarette smoking was primarily a habit of men, the sex ratio for each type of lung cancer was an excellent guide to the significance of the cigarette link. Totally unrelated cancers such as carcinoids had a M/F ratio of less than one, whereas the ratio for type I cancers was about 10:1, and for adenocarcinomas about 3:1.

In other instances, age differences indicate epidemiologic differences. Leukemia is perhaps the best known example, but age differences also separate the major groups of ovarian cancer (Berg and Lampe, 1981). Race, too, can be a good epidemiologic surrogate for the differences in uterine cancer epidemiology. Whites are at increased risk for the hormone-related adenocarcinomas, blacks for the radiation and genetically linked sarcomas.

From these examples it has seemed reasonable to generalize: If the patients who develop two different cancer types differ significantly in their age, sex, or racial distributions, then the two cancer types are more likely to have different etiologies or different pathogenesis than if the demographic characteristics of the two populations are similar.

This concept of demographic difference or similarity can be quantified in two ways (Berg, 1985). An overall statistical test of the null hypothesis of no age, sex, or racial differences can be performed. Because the three variables often are correlated, the subtest on each should be done with the data stratified by the other two variables and usually by time as well, since both incidence and diagnostic fashions can change. Secondly, the differences between two groups can be translated to an overall standardized distance measurement (Gordon, 1981; Sneath and Sokal, 1973). The latter measure is particularly useful when large data sets are involved, since statistical "significance" may be due to only small differences. If the two tests agree that the populations are similar, the groups probably should be merged in the absence of strong reasons to the contrary. If they agree that the differences are important, then the cancer types should be studied separately. If the distance is large but the null hypothesis not rejected, the size of at least one group probably is too small to merit separate treatment. If the distance is small, the groups probably should be merged, except in very large studies, regardless of the statistical significance.

Based on this concept, Appendix A indicates which subsites or histological types within major categories of cancer seemed to be the best candidates for epidemiologic separation because they occurred in different groups of people or at different ages. These recommendations resulted from a comprehensive survey of the 1978–1982 cases (coded using ICD–O 1) reported to the National Cancer Institute's SEER program. All histologic, grade, and subsite categories that had 15 or more cases were compared. It should be emphasized that the *demographic distance* concept is an arbitrary one and is in no way to be considered more authoritative than what appears in the other chapters of this book. Moreover, such a listing never can be complete or up-to-date. Categories that had few cases at the time may well have become more popular and so prove to be epidemiologically different. More importantly, a new carcinogen can appear and preferentially produce cancers of a type not previously recognized epidemiologically. Often the table groupings will serve only to indicate which cancers should be excluded from a study of the dominant type. Percentages of confirmed cases are given so that the size of the data pool needed for a study of less common cancers can be estimated.

AFTERWORD

While this chapter is concerned with pathologist–epidemiologist interactions, present experience suggests that one expensive type of collaboration is invoked unnecessarily often, namely, review of all pathologic material from a study by an individual or panel (Kempson, 1985; Gilchrist et al., 1988). In most cases nothing important will be added, and on occasion the "fine tuning" can worsen correlations if the criteria used are idiosyncratic or not epidemiologically relevant. Review is of value primarily in two situations. It obviously is necessary if the classification is a new one familiar only to a few (see the discussion in Wolf et al., 1988). It also is advisable when time trends in histology are being studied, but then the reviewer should be blinded as to dates—a precaution usually not mentioned in reports. Otherwise, the more specific the original diagnosis, the more likely it is that the pathologist used mainstream criteria and that review will add nothing.

Where then should epidemiologists look for remediable problems among pathologic diagnoses? They should look first in both nonstandard diagnoses (those not found in standard references) and in the overly general diagnoses such as cancer and carcinoma. The former group should be rare enough to simply omit or lump into a miscellaneous category, the latter should benefit most by reabstracting. If no more specific diagnosis is found, it should mean that there was not enough readable material for better classification.

The other major problem for pathologists is making a reproducible diagnosis that relies on quantitation of properties. This includes not only grading but, for example, diagnosing acute leukemia when it is defined as a leukemia with more than 20% blasts in blood or bone marrow. Such definitions produce countless arguments both about the exact percentage point to be used for separation and about the methods of counting and classifying cells. If quantitative definitions must be used, one hopes the dividing line can be placed in regions for which examples are uncommon. In the preceding example, 20% blasts would be a far better definition if patients usually had less than 10% or more than 50% than if 15% to 25% blast counts were common. In the latter case, reproducibility will be low, and perhaps the statistically oriented epidemiologist could nudge pathologists towards better separation criteria.

When there are conflicting classification schemes, how can the epidemiologist choose? First one could look for the scheme best correlated with epidemiologic or at least with demographic variables. Secondly, the scheme must be validated by more than one group. Only thus can any reported correlations be verified and, equally important, the transportability of the diagnostic criteria from one pathologist to another be demonstrated. The Lukes-Butler classification of Hodgkin's disease was an example of a generally reproducible and epidemiologically useful scheme.

As time goes on we can expect more and more examples where epidemiologic and pathologic specificity are inseparable. The rate of discovery should accelerate as epidemiologists and pathologists make greater use of each others' information.

REFERENCES

AMERICAN CANCER SOCIETY. 1968. Manual of Tumor Nomenclature and Coding, 1968 ed. New York, American Cancer Society.

ARMED FORCES INSTITUTE OF PATHOLOGY 1949-1963. Atlas of Tumor Pathology Washington D.C., Armed Forces Institute of Pathology.

BEARD CM, JEDD MB, WOOLNER LB, et al. 1988. Fifty-year trend in incidence rates of bronchogenic carcinoma by cell type in Olmsted County, Minnesota. J Natl Cancer Inst 80:1404–1407.

BERG JW. 1985. The epidemiologic meaning of histology in lung cancer. *In* Mizell M, Correa P (eds): Lung Cancer: Causes and Prevention. Deerfield Beach, Verlag Chemie Intl, pp. 104–117.

BERG JW, LAMPE JG. 1981. High risk factors in gynecological cancer. Cancer 48:429–441.

COLLEGE OF AMERICAN PATHOLOGISTS. 1965. Systematized Nomenclature of Pathology. Chicago, College of American Pathologists.

COLLEGE OF AMERICAN PATHOLOGISTS. 1979. Systematized Nomenclature of Medicine. Skokie, College of American Pathologists.

CUTLER SJ, YOUNG JL JR. 1975. Third National Cancer Survey: Incidence Data. Natl Cancer Inst Monogr 41. Bethesda, MD, U.S. Public Health Service, DHEW Publication No. (NIH) 75-787.

GILCHRIST KW, HARRINGTON DP, WOLF BC, NEIMAN RS. 1988. Statistical and empirical evaluation of histopathologic reviews for quality assurance in the Eastern Cooperative Oncology Group. Cancer 62:861–868.

GORDON AD. 1981. Classification. London, Chapman and Hall.

GUILEGARDO JM, JOHNSON WP, WELSH RA, et al. 1980. Prevalence of latent prostate cancer in two US populations. J Natl Cancer Inst 65:311–316.

HANKEY BF, MYERS MH. 1987. Black/White differences in bladder cancer patient survival. J Chron Dis 40:65–73.

HENSON DE. 1988. The histological grading of neoplasms. Arch Pathol Lab Med 112:1091–1096.

INTERNATIONAL AGENCY FOR RESEARCH ON CANCER. 1994. Multiple Primaries. Lyon, France: International Agency for Research on Cancer, Internal Report No. 94/003.

KEMPSON RL. 1985. Pathology quality control in the cooperative clinical cancer trial programs. Cancer Treat Rep 69:1207–1210.

KREYBERG L. 1962. Histological Lung Cancer Types. Oslo, Norwegian Universities Press.

PERCY C, YOUNG JL, MUIR C et al. 1995. Histology of cancer. incidence and prognosis: SEER population-based data, 1973-1987. Cancer (Suppl), 75:139-422.

SANDBERG AA. 1994. Cancer cytogenetics for clinicians. CA Cancer J Clin 44:136–159.

SNEATH PHA, SOKAL RR. 1973. Numerical Taxonomy. San Francisco, W.H. Freeman.

SOBIN LH, THOMAS LB, PERCY C, et al. 1978. A Coded Compendium of the International Histological Classification of Tumors. Geneva, World Health Organization.

THOMPSON ET, HAYDEN A. 1961. Standard Nomenclature of Diseases and Operations. Fifth Edition, New York, McGraw-Hill.

WEINBERG RA. 1944. Oncogenes and tumor suppressor genes. CA: Cancer J Clin 44:160–170.

WOLF BC, GILCHRIST KW, MANN RB, NEIMAN RS. 1988. Evaluation of pathology review of malignant lymphomas and Hodgkin's disease in cooperative clinical trials. Cancer 62:1301–1305.

WORLD HEALTH ORGANIZATION: INTERNATIONAL CLASSIFICATION OF DISEASES, 1975 Revision. Geneva, World Health Organization, 1977.

WORLD HEALTH ORGANIZATION. 1990. ICD–O. International Classification of Diseases for Oncology. Geneva, World Health Organization, 1976; 2nd ed.

WORLD HEALTH ORGANIZATION: INTERNATIONAL HISTOLOGICAL CLASSIFICATION OF TUMORS. Geneva, World Health Organization, 1976.

WYNDER EL, HOFFMANN D. 1994. Smoking and lung cancer: scientific challenges and opportunities. Cancer Res 54:5284–5295.

YOUNG JL JR, PERCY CL, ASIRE AJ, eds. 1981. Surveillance, Epidemiology, and End Results. Incidence and Mortality Data 1973–77. Natl Cancer Inst Monogr 57. Bethesda, MD, U.S. Dept. Health and Human Services, NIH Publication 81-2330.

APPENDIX A. *Suggested Separations and Groupings of Invasive Cancers for Epidemiologic Purposes*

Subsite Frequencies from SEER 1978–82, Histologic frequencies from SEER 1973–87. (Histologic and anatomic entities that are separated appeared to occur in different subsets of the SEER population. Entities that are grouped did not.)	*Frequency*
LIP, 140/C00 (1st/2nd edition ICD–O site codes)	
Histology as in Table 3–1	
Upper lip, 140.0/C00.0 Patient characteristics and histologies differ from 140.1/C00.1.	7%
Lower lip, 140.1/C00.1 99.8% are squamous cell carcinomas. Keratinizing squamous cell cancers, 8071 and grades 3–4, occur in older patients.	86%
Mucosa of lower lip, 140.4/C00.4	5%
? related to cancers of oral mucosa.	
Other specified sites	2%
Overlapping and unspecified subsites, 140.8, 140.9/C00.8, C00.9,	
SALIVARY GLANDS 142/C07–08 (better 141–149/C01–08)	
Carcinomas of minor salivary glands appear as various kinds of adenocarcinomas of all of the oral and pharyngeal sites. Resemblances for each histologic type across all sites are closer than are resemblances of various types within a site.	
Mucoepidermoid carcinomas, 843, 848 Low-grade carcinomas occurred in younger patients.	30%
Adenoid cystic carcinomas, 820	22%
Epidermoid carcinomas, 807–812 (major glands only)	10%
Acinar cell carcinomas, 855	7%
Malignant mixed tumors, 894	5%
Adenocarcinoma NOS, 814	14%
Lymphomas	6%
Other specified types Duct carcinomas, 850, 852, and malignant monomorphic adenomas, 819, 829, 831, 839, 856, are interesting but rare.	5%
Unspecified types, 800–802, 5% of proven cancers	
OTHER MOUTH, 141, 143–145/C01–06 Adenocarcinomas are minor salivary gland cancers (above).	
Lymphomas of the base of tongue, 141.0, 141.6/C01, C02.4 should be grouped with lymphomas of other parts of Waldeyer's ring, 146.0, 147/C09, C11, C14.2.	
Sarcomas and odontogenic cancers should be merged with corresponding tumors of the soft tissues and bones, respectively, of the head and neck.	
Remaining cancers (squamous cell, melanoma, unspecified) differ at different subsites as indicated. Papillary cancers, 805 and grade 4 cancers can be separated if frequent enough.	
Base of tongue and lingual tonsil, 141.0, 141.6/C01, C02.4	18%
Other specified tongue sites	18%
Tongue NOS[a], 141.8, 141.9/C02.8, C02.9	7%
Upper gum and cheek, 143.0, 145.0, 145.1/C03.0, C06.0, C06.1	6%
Lower gum, 143.1/C03.1	5%
Gum NOS[a], 143.8, 143.9/C03.9	1%
Floor of mouth and retromolar area, 144, 145.6/C04, C06.2	33%
Hard palate, 145.2/C05.0	1%
Soft palate and uvula, 145.3, 145.4/C05.1, C05.2	9%
Palate NOS[a], 145.5/C05.8, C05.9	1%
Mouth, overlapping and unspecified, 145.8, 145.9/C06.8, C06.9, 4% of proven cancers.	

(*continued*)

Subsite Frequencies from SEER 1978–82, Histologic frequencies from SEER 1973–87. (Histologic and anatomic entities that are separated appeared to occur in different subsets of the SEER population. Entities that are grouped did not.)	*Frequency*
NASOPHARYNX, 147/C11	
Subsites were infrequently used.	
Squamous cell and transitional cell carcinomas, 807, 812	69%
Lymphoepitheliomas, 808	16%
Lymphomas (group with others of Waldeyer's ring, see above).	8%
Other specified types	8%
Unspecified histologies, 800–802, 16% of proven cancers	
OTHER PHARYNX, 146, 148, 149.0/C09, C10, C12–C14.0	
Histologic divisions as above for Other Mouth	
Tonsil, 146.0/C09 (lymphomas were 15% of typed cancers)	25%
Other oropharynx, 146.1–146.9/C10	32%
Hypopharynx, 148/C12, C13 (patients much like those in preceding group)	43%
Pharynx etc., unspecified, 149.0/C14.0, 16% of proven cancers	
ESOPHAGUS, 150/C15	
Histology divisions as in Table 3–1 except that adenocarcinomas of the lower esophagus, 150.2, 150.5/C15.2, C15.5, usually are related to Barrett's esophagus and so should be separated from other adenocarcinomas. Merging them with cancers of the gastric cardia may be useful.	
Upper third and cervical esophagus, 150.0, 150.3/C15.0, C15.3 (96% squamous)	16%
Middle third and thoracic esophagus, 150.1, 150.4/C15.1, C15.4 (92% squamous)	45%
Lower third and abdominal esophagus, 150.2,150.5/C15.2, C15.5 (63% squamous)	39%
Overlapping and unspecified esophagus, 150.8, 150.9/C15.8, 15.9, 17% of proven cancers	
STOMACH, 151/C16	
Histologically the epidemiologic terms "intestinal" and "diffuse" were uncommon. A. Hanai, Osaka, has suggested the following equivalents: intestinal: 8050, 8143, 8144, 8210, 8211, 826, 848, 851, and grades 1–2 for 8010 and 8140; diffuse: 8012, 802, 803, 804, 8141, 8142, 8145, 8221, 8231, 849, 855, grades 3–4 for 800, 801, 8140, and grade 4 for 8230. Other carcinomas would be placed in a miscellaneous category. Lymphomas comprised 5% of typed cancers, and leiomyosarcomas, 889, 2%.	
Gastric cardia, 151.0/C16.0	29%
Fundus, body, lesser curvature, 151.3–151.5/C16.1, C16.2, C16.5	35%
Gastric antrum, 151.2/C16.3	30%
Pylorus 151.1/C16.4 (Patients resembled those with cancers of the fundus, etc., though sites are not contiguous.)	6%
Other and unspecified sites, 151.6–151.9/C16.6–16.9, 43% of confirmed cancers	
SMALL INTESTINE, 152/C17	
Histology as in Table 3–1	
Duodenum, 152.0/C17.0 (85% adenocarcinomas)	26%
Jejunum, 152.1/C17.1 (54% adenocarcinomas)	25%
Ileum, 151.2/C17.2 (16% adenocarcinomas, 54% malignant carcinoids, 20% lymphomas)	48%
Overlapping and unspecified, 151.8, 151.9/C17.8, 17.9, 23% of confirmed cancers	
LARGE INTESTINE, 153, 154.0, 154.1/C18–20	
Histologies as in Table 3–1 except that carcinoma in familial polyposis, 8220, and signet ring cell carcinoma, 849, should be separated from other adenocarcinomas. Squamous cell carcinomas and melanomas of the rectum should be merged with those of the anus.	
Appendix, 153.5/C18.1	1%
Cecum and ascending colon, 153.4, 153.6/C18.0, C18.2	25%
Hepatic flexure, 153.0/C18.3 (Patient characteristics appear a mixture of those with cancers of the ascending and transverse colon.)	3%
Transverse colon, 151.1/C18.4	7%
Splenic flexure and descending colon, 153.7, 153.2/C18.5, 18.6	9%
Sigmoid colon and rectosigmoid, 153.3, 154.0/C18.7, C19	36%
Rectum, 154.1/C20	20%
Overlapping and unspecified, 153.8, 153.9/C18.8, C18.9, 2% of confirmed cancers	

(*continued*)

Subsite Frequencies from SEER 1978–82, Histologic frequencies from SEER 1973–87. (Histologic and anatomic entities that are separated appeared to occur in different subsets of the SEER population. Entities that are grouped did not.)	*Frequency*
ANUS, 154.2–154.8/C21	
Histology as in Table 3–1; epidermoid carcinomas 77%, adenocarcinomas 21%, melanoma 1%	
LIVER, 155/C22	
Cholangiocarcinomas: all cancers from site 155.1/C22.1 plus histologies 8050, 814, 816, 818, 826, 844, 848, 850	23%
Hepatomas, 817, 819	72%
Hepatoblastomas, 894, 897, 898	2%
Angiosarcomas, 912, 913	1%
Other specified histologies	2%
Unspecified histologies, 800–802, 6% of confirmed cancers	
GALLBLADDER AND EXTRAHEPATIC BILE DUCTS, 156/C23, C24	
No histologic separation of carcinomas appeared justified.	
Gallbladder, 156.0/C23	58%
Extrahepatic bile ducts, 156.1/C24.0	30%
Ampulla of Vater, 156.2/C24.1 (Patients with carcinomas resembled those with duodenal carcinomas.)	13%
Overlapping and unspecified, 156.8, 156.9/C24.8, C24.9, 4% of confirmed cancers	
PANCREAS, 157/C25	
No subsite separations seemed useful.	
"Usual" duct carcinomas, 814, 804, 805, 807, 821, 826, 843, 848, 849, 850, 856, 857	96%
Islet cell carcinomas, 815	2%
Other specific types	2%
(Acinar carcinomas, 855, and cystadenocarcinomas, 844–847, were interesting but rare.)	
Unspecified types, 800–802, 15% of confirmed cancers	
RETROPERITONEUM AND PERITONEUM 158/C48	
These (properly) are no longer grouped within cancers of the digestive tract.	
Histology separation as in Table 3–1	
Lymphomas merge with those of 196/C77.	
Other specific noncarcinomas: combine across all sites.	
Carcinomas: consider of unknown primary site.	
INTERNAL NOSE, 160.0/C30.0	
Histology as in Table 3–1	
Epidermoid carcinomas, 62%	
Merge esthesioneuroblastomas, 952, across sites.	
MIDDLE EAR, 160.1/C30.1	
Too few cancers to analyze.	
NASAL SINUSES, 160.2–160.9/C31	
Histology as in Table 3–1	
Merge esthesioneuroblastomas across sites.	
Maxillary sinus, 160.2/C31.0	79%
Ethmoid sinus, 160.3/C31.1 (Cancer frequency may be increasing.)	12%
Other specified sinuses	9%
Overlapping and unspecified, 160.8, 160.9/C31.8, C31.9, 8% of confirmed cancers	
LARYNX, 161/C32	
Histology as in Table 3–1	
Grade 1 squamous cell cancers and supraglottic cancers differed from other types because of a special predilection for men.	
Glottis, 161.0/C32.0	61%
Supraglottis, 161.1/C32.1	37%
Other specified sites	2%
Overlapping and unspecified, 161.8, 161.9/C32.8, C32.9, 13% of confirmed cancers	

(continued)

APPENDIX A. *Suggested Separations and Groupings of Invasive Cancers for Epidemiologic Purposes (Continued)*

Subsite Frequencies from SEER 1978–82, Histologic frequencies from SEER 1973–87. (Histologic and anatomic entities that are separated appeared to occur in different subsets of the SEER population. Entities that are grouped did not.)	*Frequency*
TRACHEA, 162.0/C33	
Too few to subdivide. The demographic properties were not like lung cancers of similar histology.	
BRONCHUS AND LUNG, 162.1–162.9/C34	
Each subsite has a (significantly) different mix of histologies and these determined much of the demographic differences between subsites. This is not to say that further study of subsites for specific types may not prove epidemiologically rewarding.	
Squamous cell carcinomas, keratinizing, 8071	2%
Squamous cell carcinoma, large cell nonkeratinizing, 8072	1%
Squamous cell carcinoma, other and NOS, 8070, 8073–8076	37%
Small cell carcinoma[b], 804	21%
Adenocarcinomas[b], 814, 820, 823, 829, 831, 832, 843, 848, 849, 851, 855, 856, 857	33%
Bronchiolar carcinomas, 825, 826	5%
Malignant carcinoids, 824	1%
Giant cell carcinoma, 8031	0.3%
Other specified types	0.7%
Unspecified types, 800–802, 21% of confirmed cancers Large cell carcinoma, 8012, is a useful diagnosis clinically but not epidemiologically.	
PLEURA, 163/C38.4	
Subsites were coded infrequently and were not used in ICD–10.	
Mesotheliomas, 905, 98% of typed cancers, should be looked at across all sites.	
Subtypes of mesothelioma were uncommonly coded.	
THYMUS, 164.0/C37	
Thymomas, 858, 79% of typed cancers	
Carcinoids are of possible interest but rare.	
HEART AND MEDIASTINUM, 164.1–164.9/C38.0–38.3, 38.8	
Subsites were coded infrequently through heart, 164.1/C38.0 is of interest.	
Germ cell tumors, 906–910: merge across soft tissue sites by type and sex.	35%
Soft-part sarcomas: merge with those of thorax.	29%
Neuroblastomas, 949, 950: merge across all sites.	17%
Other specified types (mostly lymphomas)	19%
Unspecified type, 800, 11% of confirmed cancers	
BONE MARROW, 169.1/C42.1	
Used almost entirely for myelomas, 973, and leukemias, 980–994. See the SEER Monograph (Young et al., 1981) and NCI's annual "Cancer Statistics Review" for the characteristics of the more common particular types of leukemia.	
SPLEEN, 169.2/C42.2	
84% are lymphomas, but these probably are not primary unless the stage is localized.	
Angiosarcomas are of epidemiologic interest but rare.	
RETICULOENDOTHELIAL SYSTEM, 169.3/C42.3	
86% were reticuloendothelial cancers, 974 in ICD–0–1, 972 in ICD–O–2.	
BONES, 170/C40, C41	
Histology seems a better basis for separation than subsite.	
Osteogenic sarcomas, 918, 919 Subtypes were too uncommon to analyze.	35%
Chondrosarcomas, 922, 924	25%
Ewing's sarcoma, 9260	16%
Lymphomas, as in Table 3–1	7%

(*continued*)

APPENDIX A. *(Continued)*

Subsite Frequencies from SEER 1978–82, Histologic frequencies from SEER 1973–87. (Histologic and anatomic entities that are separated appeared to occur in different subsets of the SEER population. Entities that are grouped did not.)	*Frequency*
Other specific types of epidemiologic interest but uncommon in most series	19%
Chordoma, 937. Merge across all (bone, soft tissue, etc.) sites. Malignant giant cell tumors, 925 Malignant fibrous histiocytomas, 883 Fibrosarcomas (of bone), 881 Malignant odontogenic tumors, 927–934 Angiosarcomas, 912, 913 Monostotic myelomas, 973	
Unspecified, 800, 880, 3% of confirmed cases	
CONNECTIVE AND OTHER SOFT TISSUE, 171/C47, C49	
(Should also include 158/C48, 164.1–164.9/C38, and soft-part sarcomas coded to 195/C76 and 199/C80.)	
Histology appears a better basis for separation than subsite. Except for leiomyosarcomas, 889, merging across all sites may be desirable.	
Malignant fibrous histiocytomas[c], 883	24%
Liposarcomas[c], 884, 885	22%
Malignant neurilemmomas[c,d], 956	5%
Fibrosarcomas[d], 881	10%
Rhabdomyosarcomas[e], 890	4%
Hemangiosarcomas[e], 912, 913	4%
Leiomyosarcomas, 889	10%
Synoviomas, 904	5%
Neurofibrosarcomas, 954	3%
Unspecified[d,e], 880, 11% of confirmed cancers	
Lymphomas should be grouped with those in 196/C77. Other cancers also excluded from the above counts: neuroblastomas, 949, 950; Kaposi's sarcoma, 914; mesotheliomas, 905; and germ cell tumors, 906–910, should be merged across all sites.	
SKIN, 173/C44	
Basal cell and squamous cell carcinomas, 805–809, usually are not collected by cancer registries.	
Melanomas 872–879	74%
Melanomas of different skin subsites are known to have different epidemiologies determined largely by degree of skin pigmentation and amount of sun exposure. Finer site divisions than those in ICD–O probably could be used. Superficial spreading melanoma, 8743, 38% of melanomas Melanoma in Hutchinson's freckle, 8742, 6% of melanomas	
Amelanotic melanoma, 873, 1%	
Other and unspecified melanomas, 55%	
Skin appendage carcinomas, 810, 814–855	3%
Dermatofibrosarcomas, 8832	3%
Kaposi's sarcoma, 9140 More common in more recent series	7%
Other soft-part sarcomas, as in Table 3–1	1%
Mycosis fungoides, 9700, 9701	3%
Other cutaneous lymphomas (especially 9702–9709 in ICD–O–2)	2%
BREAST, 174, 175/C50	
Subsite differences were not great and seemed due to modest differences in histologic distribution.	
Duct and lobular carcinomas, 8500, 8502, 852[f], 814, 853, 854, 801, 8481, 819, 820, 821, 823, 825, 831, 832, 835, 840, 849, 855	92%
Comedocarcinomas, 8501	1%
Medullary carcinomas with lymphoid stroma, 8512	0.2%
Medullary carcinoma NOS, 8510	3%

(continued)

Subsite Frequencies from SEER 1978–82, Histologic frequencies from SEER 1973–87. (Histologic and anatomic entities that are separated appeared to occur in different subsets of the SEER population. Entities that are grouped did not.)	*Frequency*
Colloid carcinomas, 8480	2%
Papillary carcinomas, 8050, 826, 844, 845, 8503–4	1%
Other specified types Adenosquamous carcinomas, 856, 857; squamous cell carcinomas, 807; small cell carcinomas, 804; malignant cytosarcoma phillodes, 902; angiosarcomas, 912, 913; stromal sarcomas (most other soft part sarcomas); and lymphomas all may have different epidemiologies, but are uncommon.	0.9%
Cancer NOS, 800, 0.2% of confirmed cancers.	
UTERUS NOS, 179/C55	
Practically, squamous cell carcinomas can be assigned to cervix, 180/C53, and all other cancers merged with Other Uterus, below.	
CERVIX UTERI, 180/C53	
Subsites differ only on the basis of histology.	
Microinvasive squamous cell carcinomas, 8076	7%
Other epidermoid carcinomas, 8070–8075, 812, 801, 802, 804, 843, 856, 857	81%
Papillary squamous cell carcinomas, 805	0.4%
Mucinous carcinomas, 848	1%
Clear cell (mesonephroid) carcinomas, 831, 911	0.55%
Other adenocarcinomas, 814, 820, 821, 826, 838	9%
Other specified cancers	1%
Unspecified cancers, 800, 0.4% of confirmed cancers	
OTHER UTERUS, part 179/C55, 181/C58, 182/C54	
(Choriocarcinomas, ideally coded to 181, were found at all 3 sites.)	
Papillary adenocarcinomas, 8050, 826	6%
Clear cell carcinomas, 831, 911	1%
Other adenocarcinomas[g], 814, 821, 832, 838, 844, 846, 848, 856, 857	86%
Choriocarcinomas, 910	0.6%
Mullerian mixed tumors, 895	2%
Carcinosarcomas, 898, (8960 ICD–O–1, 8933 ICD–O–2)	1%
Stromal sarcomas, 880, 8930, 8931	1%
Leiomyosarcomas, 889	2%
Other specific types Epidermoid carcinomas, 8052, 807, 812, 813, and embryonal rhabdomyosarcomas, 890, 891, 8991, are interesting but rare.	0.5%
Unspecified cancers, 800–802, 2% of confirmed cancers	
OVARY, 183.0/C56	
Serous cystadenocarcinomas[h], 8441, 846, 9014, (8442 ICD–O–2)	40%
Endometrioid carcinomas, 838, 857	14%
Mucinous cystadenocarcinomas, 847, 9015	14%
Cystadenocarcinoma NOS[h], 8440, 845	11%
Clear cell carcinomas, 831, 911	5%
Dysgerminomas and embryonal carcinomas, 906, 907, 9100	2%
Malignant teratomas, 908, 909, 824, 9101, 9102	2%
Malignant Brenner tumors, 900, 807, 812, 813, 856	1%
Malignant sex cord tumors, 859–866	3%
Mucinous carcinoma NOS, 8480	4%
Carcinosarcomas, 895, 898, 9010–9013 (8960 ICD–O–1, 8933 ICD–O–2)	2%
Other specified types	1%
Nonspecific cancers, 800–802, 8050, 814, 826, 8481, 849, 37% of confirmed cancers	
FALLOPIAN TUBE, 183.2/C57.0	
96% are carcinomas; no subdivisions appear justified.	

(*continued*)

Subsite Frequencies from SEER 1978–82, Histologic frequencies from SEER 1973–87. (Histologic and anatomic entities that are separated appeared to occur in different subsets of the SEER population. Entities that are grouped did not.)	*Frequency*
OTHER FEMALE GENITAL TRACT, 183.3–183.9, 184.8, 184.9/C57.1–57.9	
Too few cancers to subdivide or analyze.	
VAGINA, 184.0/C52	
Histology as in table 3–1; 76% are epidermoid cancers. Adenocarcinomas in younger women of course are of special interest.	
VULVA, 184.1–184.4/C51	
Among the specific subsites the labia major have most of the basal cell carcinomas and adenocarcinomas, but only 22% of the cancers were assigned a subsite.	
Basal cell carcinomas, 809	6%
Papillary epidermoid carcinomas, 805	3%
Other epidermoid carcinomas[i], 807, 808, 75%	812
Adenocarcinomas, as in Table 3–1	7%
Melanomas, 872–879	7%
Other specified types	2%
Unspecified, 800–802, 4% of confirmed cancers	
PROSTATE, 185/C61	
Histology as in Table 3–1. Although transitional cell carcinomas, 812, 813 occur in larger ducts while the adenocarcinomas basically are acinar cancers, both occurred at the same ages and with about the same racial distribution.	
Grade 1 carcinomas occurred in younger men.	
TESTIS, 186/C62	
Anaplastic seminomas, 9062	5%
Spermatocytic seminomas, 9063	1%
Seminoma NOS, 9061	45%
Malignant teratomas, 908	18%
Embryonal carcinomas and choriocarcinomas 907, 910	28%
Sarcomas, as in Table 3–1	1%
Lymphomas	3%
Other specific cancers	0.4%
PENIS, 187.1–187.4/C60	
94% of typed cancers are epidermoid.	
Grade 1 cancers occur in younger patients.	
SCROTUM, 187.7/C63.2	
Epidermoid carcinomas, 805, 807	41%
Basal cell carcinomas, 809	17%
Adenocarcinomas, as in Table 3–1	18%
Soft-part sarcomas, as in Table 3–1	20%
Other specified types	3%
Unspecified, 800–801, 3% of confirmed cancers	
OTHER MALE GENITAL, 187.5, 187.6, 187.8, 187.9/C63.0, C63.1, C63.7–63.9	
Too uncommon to analyze	
BLADDER, 188/C67	
Subsite differences largely due to differences in histology.	
Papillary transitional cell carcinomas[j], 813, 8050	59%
Transitional cell carcinoma NOS[j], 812	37%
Squamous cell carcinomas, 807, 8052	2%
Adenocarcinomas (non-urachal)[k], 814, 826, 8310, 8323, 857	1%
Other specific cancers	1%
Urachal adenocarcinomas, 8470, 848, 849 are interesting but rare.	
Unspecified, 800–802, 2% of confirmed cancers	

(continued)

APPENDIX A. *Suggested Separations and Groupings of Invasive Cancers for Epidemiologic Purposes (Continued)*

Subsite Frequencies from SEER 1978–82, Histologic frequencies from SEER 1973–87. (Histologic and anatomic entities that are separated appeared to occur in different subsets of the SEER population. Entities that are grouped did not.)	*Frequency*
KIDNEY, 189.0, 189.1/C64, C65	
The separation of the pelvis from the rest of the kidney often was not used: 16% of the transitional cell and squamous cell carcinomas of the pelvis are coded to kidney NOS.	
Papillary adenocarcinomas, 826	1%
Other adenocarcinomas, as in Table 3–1	79%
Transitional cell and squamous cell carcinomas[l], 8052–813	16%
Nephroblastomas, 896	3%
Other specified types	1%
Unspecified types, 800–802, 8050 (of kidney NOS), 3% of confirmed cancers.	
URETER, 189.2/C66	
Transitional cell carcinomas, 812–3	97%
Squamous cell carcinoma, 807	2%
Adenocarcinomas	1%
URETHRA, 189.3, 189.4/C68.0, C68.1	
Papillary transitional cell carcinomas, 813	23%
Transitional cell carcinoma NOS, 812	35%
Squamous cell carcinomas[m], 8051–807	22%
Adenocarcinomas[m], as in Table 3–1	18%
Other specified types	2%
Unspecified types, 800–802, 4% of confirmed cancers	
EYE, 190/C69	
Epidermoid cancers, 8052–813 (mostly conjunctiva and cornea, 190.3–4/ C69.0–.1)	7%
Melanomas, 872–879[n]	66%
Retinoblastomas, 951	12%
Adenocarcinomas (lacrimal gland and duct, (190.2, 190.7/C69.5)	2%
Lymphomas (orbit, 190.1/C69.6)	10%
Soft-part sarcomas, as in Table 3–1 (orbit)	3%
Unspecified types, 800–801, 1% of confirmed cancers	
BRAIN, 191/C71	
Subsite differences largely accounted for by histology.	
Protoplasmic and gemistocytic astrocytomas, 941	2%
Fibrillary astrocytomas, 9420	2%
Pilocytic astrocytomas, 9421	1%
Anaplastic astrocytoma, 9401	4%
Astrocytoma, NOS and astroblastomas[o], 9400, 943	33%
Giant cell glioblastoma, 9441	0.4%
Glioblastoma multiforme, 9440	42%
Ependymomas and related tumors, 939	2%
Oligodendrogliomas, 945	4%
Medulloblastomas and cerebellar sarcomas, 947, 948	4%
Mixed gliomas[o], 9382	2%
Lymphomas	3%
Other specified types	2%
Unspecified types, 800, 9380, 4% of confirmed	
OTHER CENTRAL NERVOUS SYSTEM, 192/C70, C72	
Cranial nerves, 192.0/C72.2–72.5 Most malignant tumors were gliomas and should be merged with those of the brain.	14%
Meninges, 192.1, 192.3/C70	35%
Spinal cord, 192.2/C72.0, 72.1 Different from brain sites. Too few cases to subdivide by histology.	51%
Overlapping and unspecified, 192.8, 192.9/C72.8, 72.9, 10% of 192, 0.2% of 191–192 Most were lymphomas.	

(continued)

Subsite Frequencies from SEER 1978–82, Histologic frequencies from SEER 1973–87. (Histologic and anatomic entities that are separated appeared to occur in different subsets of the SEER population. Entities that are grouped did not.)	*Frequency*
THYROID, 193/C73	
Papillary carcinomas, 8050, 826, 834, 835, 845	74%
Follicular carcinomas, 833	16%
Medullary carcinomas, 851	3%
Giant cell carcinomas, 8030–8033	1%
Hurthle cell carcinomas and adenocarcinomas NOS, 829, 814	3%
Lymphomas	2%
Other specified types	1%
Unspecified types, 800–802, 3% of confirmed cancers	
ADRENAL, 194.0/C74	
(Adrenal cortical) carcinomas, 837, 801, 802, 814	57%
Malignant pheochromocytomas, 870	8%
Neuroblastomas, 949, 950 (merge across all sites)	30%
Other specified types	4%
Unspecified type, 800, 2% of confirmed cancers	
PARATHYROID GLAND, 194.1/C75.0	
Use Table 3–1, grouping all carcinomas.	
PITUITARY GLAND, 194.3/C75.1	
Use Table 3–1, grouping all carcinomas.	
PINEAL GLAND, 194.4/C75.3	
Cancers were too rare to analyze properly.	
Germ cell tumors, 906–910	63%
Pineoblastomas, 9362	30%
Gliomas, 938–948	7%
Unspecified types, 800–802, 6% of confirmed cases	
CAROTID BODY AND OTHER PARAGANGLIA, 194.5, 194.6/C75.4, C75.5	
Malignant tumors too uncommon to analyze.	
ILL-DEFINED SITES, 195/C76	
Recode carcinomas to 199.9/C80, unknown primary	
Recode soft-part sarcomas to appropriate place in 171/C49.	
Recode melanomas to appropriate place in 173/C44.	
Recode bone tumors to appropriate place in 170/C40, C41.	
Other types should be collected in across-site analyses.	
LYMPH NODES, 196/C77	
Essentially used only for lymphomas. Subsites mainly reflect Hodgkin's–non-Hodgkin's differences.	
Hodgkin's disease, 965, 966 Nodular sclerosis, 9656, 9657 (9663–9667 in ICD–O–2), 53% of HD Lymphocytic predominance, 9651 (9657–9659 in ICD–O–2), 4% of HD Other and unspecified HD, 43%	28%
Other lymphomas, 9591–964, 969, 975 (9591–9595, 967–971 in ICD–O–2)	72%
The classification of non-Hodgkin's lymphomas used in 1978–82 is no longer relevant. A special analysis was done on SEER 1986 lymphoma data coded according to the newer terminology, including the Working Formulation (WF), used in ICD–O–2 (see page xxxiii of that book).	
Groups A, D, E, F of the WF and "diffuse cleaved large cell lymphomas," 9670^{P}, 9671–9676, 9681, 9697, 9698 in ICD–O–2	41%
Group B (part) follicular small cleaved cell lymphoma, 9693–9695	4%
Group B (part) poorly differentiated nodular lymphocytic lymphoma, 9696	11%
Group C mixed small cleaved and large cell follicular lymphoma, 9691, 9692	6%
Group G (part) diffuse large cell lymphoma, 9680	27%
Group G (part) diffuse large cell noncleaved lymphoma, 9682	2%
Group H immunoblastic large cell lymphoma, 9684	3%

(continued)

APPENDIX A. *Suggested Separations and Groupings of Invasive Cancers for Epidemiologic Purposes (Continued)*

Subsite Frequencies from SEER 1978–82, Histologic frequencies from SEER 1973–87. (Histologic and anatomic entities that are separated appeared to occur in different subsets of the SEER population. Entities that are grouped did not.)	*Frequency*
Group I lymphoblastic lymphoma, 9685	1%
Group J (part) small cell noncleaved lymphoma, 9686	2%
Group J (part) Burkitt's lymphoma, 9687	1%
T-cell lymphomas, 970	0.5%
Nonspecific non-Hodgkin's lymphomas, 9591–9595, 9690, 6% of non-Hodgkin's lymphomas	
Malignant lymphoma, not otherwise specified, 9590, 7% of all malignant lymphomas	
UNKNOWN PRIMARY SITE, 199.9/C80	
Papillary adenocarcinomas, 826	2%
Other adenocarcinomas, as in Table 3–1	51%
Squamous cell carcinomas, 807	9%
Small cell carcinomas, 804	2%
Other specified carcinomas	3%
Soft-part sarcomas, as in Table 3–1, move to 171.9/C49.9	1%
Other specific types, group across sites	1%
Carcinoma, type unspecified, 801, 802	24%
Cancer, type unspecified, 800	7%

[a]These NOS sites tend to be used for older patients and so are much alike.
[b]These cancers occurred in fairly similar groups of people.
[c,d,e]Sarcomas with the same letter (c,d,e) occurred in similar patients.
[f]Lobular carcinoma is less common in blacks and rarely diagnosed in men, but epidemiologic studies have shown no difference in risk factors between duct and lobular carcinomas in white women.
[g]Grade increased significantly with age.
[h]Grade 1 cancers occur in younger women as will borderline tumors (made malignant in ICD–O–2).
[i]Grade 1 cancers occurred in younger patients.
[j]If grade is available, grade 1 cancers from these two sets are similar and separable, as are grade 2 cancers. Grades 3–4 papillary transitional cell cancers are rare but do differ from other transitional cell grades 3–4 cancers and from the lower grade cancers.
[k]Demographically these are midway between 812 and 807 cases, while pathologically they, like squamous cell cancers, are metaplastic variants of the basic transitional cell cancers.
[l]Grade 1 papillary transitional cell carcinomas, 813, occurred in younger patients.
[m]These cancers occurred in the same types of patients.
[n]Spindle cell melanomas, 8772, occurred in a different patient set than the other 877 melanomas.
[o]These patients resembled those with glioma NOS, 9380.
[p]The cell type of chronic lymphatic leukemia resembles that of small lymphocytic lymphoma, 9670 but the leukemia cases were older and more often men.

4 Morphology and natural history of cancer precursors

PELAYO CORREA

It has been known for more than a century that human cancer often arises in areas of an organ that show previous (precancerous) histologic abnormalities. Recamier in 1829 noted that cancer develops in irritated moles (Ewing, 1928). For many years these abnormalities were considered *heterotopias* and formed the basis for Cohnheim's hypothesis that tumors developed from misplaced embryonal rests. The interpretation of these changes remains controversial even today, but considerable knowledge has accumulated to help us better understand their natural history.

Part of the controversy is semantic and arises because the meaning of the term *precancerous* is understood according to the needs of the users. For the clinicians concerned about each individual patient's diagnostic and therapeutic needs, precancerous means "obligate antecedents of invasive carcinoma" (Koss, 1975). This interpretation of the term often leads to a pragmatic decision: if it "inevitably becomes cancer," all attempts to remove the lesion should be made; if it only "sometimes" becomes cancer, no immediate therapeutic measures are usually warranted (Rosai and Ackerman, 1978). On the other hand, researchers interested in a better understanding of the cellular alterations that precede the invasion of tissues by neoplasia use the term to describe morphologic and chemical cellular alterations that begin at the earlier phases of the process, even if in many cases they do not lead to invasive cancer (Lipkin, 1977). These semantic difficulties were recognized by Stout, who in 1932 wrote as follows in his introduction to *Human Cancer*, referring to the term precancerous:

> In some ways it has been an unfortunate term because it has connoted in many minds an inevitable sequence of events. Such, of course, is very far from the truth . . . . By precancerous, therefore, is meant simply a condition which may be associated with development of cancer.

For the purposes of epidemiology and primary prevention of cancer, Stout's definition is more applicable and is therefore adopted for our purposes.

Several similar terms have been used in the medical literature in an effort to avoid the semantic confusion: *precancerous* and *premalignant* may lead to misinterpretation because they imply a need for intervention; the terms *antecedent* and *precursor* have been used to encompass lesions that might precede cancer chronologically but do not inevitably lead to it (Burdette, 1970; Haenszel et al, 1976). Since in our opinion the term *precursor* better fits the latter concept, we have preferred it in our discussion. For practical purposes lesions are generally divided into two categories: (a) *less advanced lesions* that share morphologic characteristics with other benign processes and do not involve the proliferation of cell clones with neoplastic phenotype, as in the case of the inflammatory, hyperplastic, and metaplastic lesions of the cervix, stomach, and bronchus; and (b) *more advanced lesions* or *dysplasias*, which include abnormal clones and are considered dangerous if untreated.

The theoretical as well as pragmatic implications of the precursor phenomenon have in general been underestimated. Some points that justify their study are briefly summarized below:

1. Precursor cellular changes hold the clue to an understanding of the mechanisms of carcinogenesis. Changes in cell kinetics and DNA synthesis have been detected in the initial carcinogenic process, long before the cells are committed to autonomous behavior (Lipkin, 1977). Recent advances in carcinogenesis and molecular biology have underscored the value of precursors in the identification of abnormal genes (Fearon et al 1990; Harris 1991).
2. Abnormal proteins formed by precursor lesions can help in the exploration of the neoplastic process as well as in the identification of individuals at high risk of developing certain cancers.
3. Precursor lesions may be used to identify individuals in a community who are either susceptible or resistant to carcinogenic influences that may be ubiquitous in their environment. This could be useful for secondary cancer prevention and for the study of genetic markers of susceptibility or resistance to cancer.
4. Studies of the progression of precursors can help

determine if etiologic factors under study influence the initiation or the promotion of the neoplastic process.

5. For epidemiologists, precursor lesions offer a solution to the problem of the prolonged latency period that frequently puts the researcher in the difficult position of trying to obtain information about events that occurred 30 or more years earlier in the life of the individual.

6. The identification of precursor changes offers hope of inducing the regression of lesions which, if untreated, would lead to invasion and death of the host (Wattenberg et al, 1977). This concept is being explored at the present time in chemoprevention trials.

MARKERS OF PRENEOPLASIA AND EARLY NEOPLASIA

The scientific tools available to study cancer precursors have increased considerably in number and improved in recent years. An extensive discussion of them is not intended in this chapter, but a brief enumeration is warranted. They will be further discussed below in relation to specific models.

Classical histologic techniques have provided most of the original descriptions of the carcinogenic process and they continue to be of great value. From observations in humans, precursor lesions have been characterized by several degrees of architectural distortion and nuclear atypia, which could in theory be organized to cover the spectrum from normalcy to invasive cancer. By logical inference, it has been assumed that these stages, or degrees, represent a continuum of progressive changes. The observational setting, requiring microscopic visualization of tissue and its removal from the body, has not allowed a direct confirmation of this theory. It is also customary to separate the different stages of the spectrum into artificial groups, the most frequent of which are the mild, moderate, and marked dysplasia categories. However, such divisions are arbitrary and difficult to reproduce in inter-observer testing. They represent a pathologist's opinion which, it is assumed, might help the clinician in reaching decisions relating to patient care. If the degrees of dysplasia are to be used for the building of epidemiologic models, a special effort should be made to minimize the inter- and intra-observer variation in diagnoses.

Autoradiographic techniques, after incubation of fresh human tissue with tritiated thymidine, have contributed considerably to our understanding of the precancerous process by defining the bounds of the proliferative zone in each organ. Such a zone is expanded in specific ways in each organ studied, which allows the identification of high-risk populations and individuals (Lipkin, 1988). The proliferative zone can be also identified with techniques not requiring radioactive isotopes, such as the bromodeoxiuridine (BRDU) and proliferative nuclear antigens (cyclins) (PCNA) (Sarraf et al, 1991). The highly proliferative state observed in such cases is amenable to intervention and in theory could be a marker of the expected effects of chemoprevention trials.

Studies of flow cytometry are now possible not only in fresh tissue but also in paraffin embedded tissue. They allow the estimation of DNA content of individual cells and identify subpopulations of cells with abnormal DNA content. Of particular interest is the detection of aneuploidy, a clear indication of abnormal cell replication.

Nuclear abnormalities can also be identified through the presence of micronuclei. These are fragments of DNA that become separated from the main nucleus during the replication cycle and are observed as separate, small nuclear fragments in the cytoplasm. They are indicators of relatively recent clastogenic events, have the same organ-specificity of the carcinogen under study, and have been successfully used as markers of carcinogen exposure in human cytology specimens (Wargovich et al, 1983; Fontham et al, 1986).

Recent study of *nucleolar organizer regions (NORs)* has led to their consideration as a marker of abnormal cell replication. NORs are chromosomal fragments in which ribosomal DNA is encoded and they are responsible for the development of the nucleolus into which NORs project as large loops of DNA (De Capoa et al, 1985; Leong and Gilham, 1989; Rosa et al, 1990). During cell division they are located in the short arms of acrocentric chromosomes 13, 14, 15, 21, 22. Theoretically, 20 NORs should be demonstrable in human normal diploid nuclei, but they are tightly aggregated within one or two nucleoli so that the individual units are not discernible. In tissue sections of normal diploid cells, as opposed to chromosome spreads, only one or two NORs are seen. The number of "histologic NORs" can increase considerably if dispersion of the NORs throughout the nucleus takes place (as in hyperproliferative states), if an increase of transcriptional activity makes otherwise inconspicuous NORs prominent, or if cell ploidy increases, in which case a real increase in the number of NORs takes place. NORs are therefore markers of abnormal cell proliferation and may be helpful in characterizing the precursor stages (Fig. 4–1).

Chromosome analysis of cells in the state of division has identified abnormalities not only in tumor cells but also in somatic cells of the host. This allows linking of specific abnormalities to specific tumors and identifies the location of the abnormal genes. A recent example of the usefulness of this technique is the deletion in subband 13q 14.1 of chromosome 13, location of the retinoblastoma (*Rb*) gene (Yunis and Ramsay, 1978). This gene apparently carries a growth-suppressing function

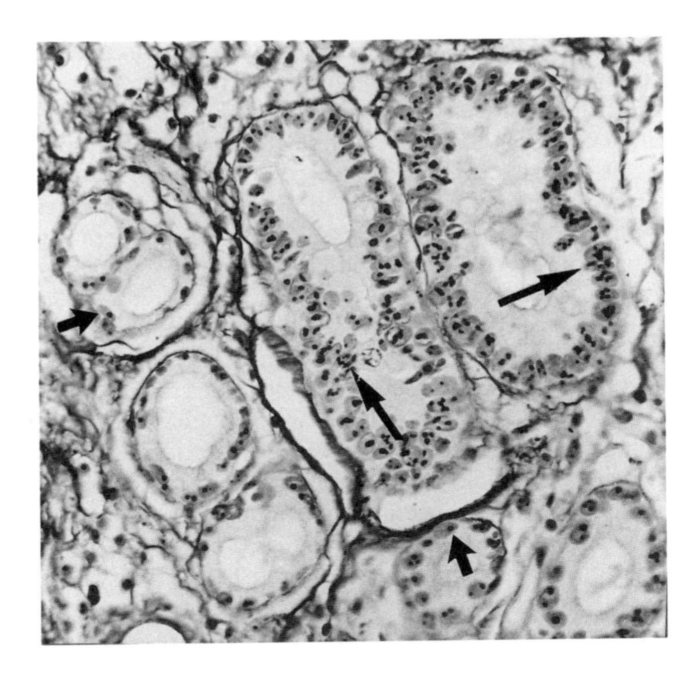

FIG. 4–1. Nucleolar organizer regions (NORs) as indicators of hyperproliferative state in chronic atrophic gastritis. One NOR per nucleus (*short arrows*) is the rule in the glands on the lower and left side of the photograph, contrasting with numerous NORs per nucleus in the two glands in the center of the microphotograph (*long arrows*) which are in a state of hyperproliferation.

(or anti-oncogene), and its absence allows the neoplastic proliferation of epithelial cells in the retina and possibly other tissues (Friend et al, 1986).

The growth suppressor role of the *Rb* gene contrasts with the growth stimulator role of classical oncogenes whose amplification may result from somatic mutations. Recent advances in molecular biology have thrown much light on the study of pre-neoplastic nuclear abnormalities, especially through the use of restriction enzymes (which allow the study of specific segments of the DNA molecule) and of DNA amplification techniques which multiply the number of DNA copies available for study.

Another source of information on the precancerous process comes from the study of secretions or cytoplasmic components of cells. It is well known that neoplastic cells may secrete abnormal products that may reflect fetal or embryonal cell functions. Such markers as the alpha-feto-protein and the carcinoembryonic antigen are good examples. Preneoplastic changes are also frequently detected by the presence of such products. Changes in the chemical composition of mucus secretions in gastrointestinal precancerous states as well as the appearance of abnormal digestive enzymes in such cells are good examples of these phenomena. Many of these abnormal products are antigenic and detected by immunologic techniques which identify "fetal antigens" whose function is not well known. Such antigens tend to be organ specific and have been developed for a variety of tissues.

One interesting group of such antigenic markers is the complex of the so-called blood group antigens, whose presence is not restricted to blood cells. These antigens are carbohydrate moieties, components of glycoproteins and glycolipids present in many tissues, especially of epithelial type. ABH antigens are present in red blood cells of human adults. In the fetus they are present in endothelial cells and in the epithelium of many organs, especially the gastrointestinal tract. They disappear from these tissues during the stage of functional maturation. The Lewis antigenic system has a pattern of distribution in tissues which is specific for organs, segments of organs, and stages of fetal development. It is possible, therefore, to utilize these antigens as markers of loss of differentiation in epithelial preneoplastic conditions. There are indications that changes in blood group antigen distribution take place before other morphologic alterations are observable in cells undergoing neoplastic transformation (Sakamoto et al, 1989; Itzkowitz, 1986; Torrado et al, 1989; Torrado et al, 1992).

Observations of markers of cell replication and differentiation in humans have shown that cancer precursor lesions may regress to normality. Some models suggest that the proportion of regression to normality decreases as the precursor state becomes more advanced. We will summarize work concerning the morphology and natural history of lesions considered to be precursors of carcinomas of the uterine cervix, the female breast, the stomach, and the large bowel.

UTERINE CERVIX AND RELATED EPITHELIA

Morphology

Cancer precursors in the uterine cervix have been recognized for many years, especially since the pioneering work of George Papanicolaou made it possible to identify them in cytologic specimens and apply measures of secondary prevention. Most carcinomas and precursor lesions start at the squamocolumnar junction, the point of contact of two very different microenvironments: the glandular endocervix and the desquamating exocervix. Chronic inflammatory changes at this point are extremely prevalent, especially in sexually active women, most of whom display changes of squamous metaplasia characterized by replacement of the glandular by squamous type of epithelium.

Most of the time, this metaplasia is mature in the sense that it displays the normal orderly differentiation of squamous epithelial surfaces. Up to this point, the described lesions are considered nonspecific reactions to injury without a premalignant significance.

In the squamous epithelium, partial loss of differentiation can be observed, and this change is referred to as *dysplasia*. In some cases it is manifested by the fact that cells with large nuclei and scanty cytoplasm, normally confined to the basal and parabasal layers, appear in more superficial areas of the epithelium but do not interfere with the polarization and maturation of the more superficial epithelial cells. This constitutes *mild dysplasia* and represents a borderline lesion between inflammatory hyperplasia and early preneoplasia. In cases considered to be more advanced, the abnormal cells with large nuclei migrate upward toward the surface and are more abundant in number, but still allow a moderate degree of differentiation and polarization of the epithelium. These are usually called *moderate dysplasias*. Still more advanced cases show most of the thickness of the epithelium occupied by large cells with a minimum degree of polarization and differentiation. These constitute *severe* or *marked dysplasia*. Any of the degrees of dysplasia just described may extend into the lumen of the endocervical glands.

When maturation is completely lost and all cells are immature, the lesion is called *carcinoma in situ*. There are no clear-cut morphologic characteristics to allow a sharp separation between the various degrees of dysplasia and carcinoma in situ. These terms are used because the pathologist needs to give an educated assessment of the degree of the lesion's progression. Some investigators have proposed the term *intraepithelial neoplasia* (CIN) to encompass all degrees of dysplasia and to express the concept of a continuum of change within the same disease category (Richart, 1967). In this nomenclature, *CIN I* and *CIN II* correspond to mild and moderate dysplasia, while *CIN III* corresponds to severe dysplasia, which is practically synonymous with carcinoma in situ (CIS) and should be treated as one entity. A real problem exists for the epidemiologist trying to measure disease frequency, since most cancer registries include carcinoma in situ and exclude dysplasias. The real frequency of intraepithelial neoplasia, therefore, requires special efforts in data gathering.

Papilloma Viruses. Considerable progress has been made recently in this field since it has been recognized that human papilloma viruses (HPV) play a central role in epithelial abnormalities of the cervix. Papilloma viruses have been known to infect humans and many other animal species as superficial infections leading mostly to benign, self-limited, papillomatous lesions of the skin and the external genitalia. In 1980 Jenson and co-workers reported that bovine papilloma viruses (which can be sustained in tissue culture) had common antigenic properties with HPV. Broad spectrum antisera were developed which soon detected the presence of viral capsular proteins in human cervical smears and biopsies (Morin et al, 1981). Viral particles from human condylomas and warts were then used to produce broad spectrum antisera. The peroxidase–antiperoxidase immunochemical techniques were then used to demonstrate the presence of viral products in human cervical tissue, which were reported in 50% of suspect tissues with CIN (Meisels et al, 1984). Such first generation immunologic techniques did not detect HPV in malignant tumors.

It was then recognized that HPV induced characteristic histopathologic changes, the most typical of which had been previously described as "Koilocytotic atypia" by Koss and Durfee in 1956 as a possible "stepping stone in the genesis of cervix cancer."

Molecular biology techniques were then applied in the study of HPV infections that were being discovered with an unexpected frequency in female genital lesions. Hybridization techniques indicated that HPV was a conglomerate of many related viruses: using an arbitrary cut-point of 30% or less cross-hybridization, more than 60 types have been described. The pathologic potential of these types has been studied to some extent, but at this point our knowledge is still nebulous. It is becoming clear that some types are associated with benign lesions which usually do not progress to malignancy but rather regress "spontaneously" as in the case of most cutaneous warts associated with types 1–4, 5, 10, 36, 37, and 39. In the case of the female genital tract, such "benign" HPV's are mainly types 6 and 11 (Fig. 4–2). They are mostly found in condyloma acuminata and flat condylomas; but such lesions occasionally contain HPV 16, which seems to be the most common type with malignant potential (Fig. 4–3). Other types associated with carcinomas of the genital tract are numbers

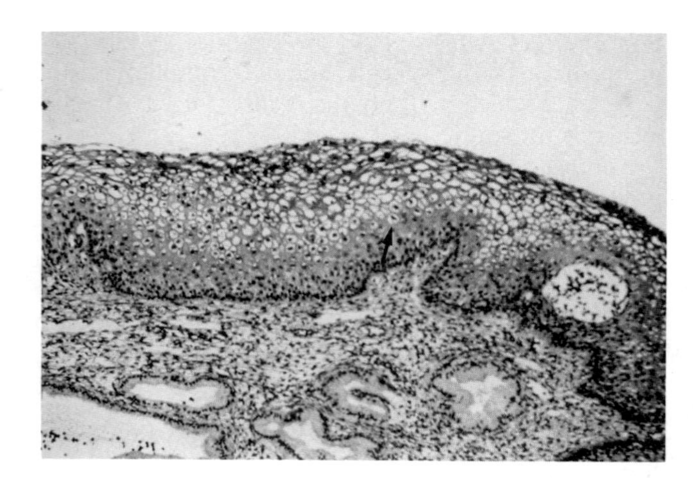

FIG. 4–2. Microphotograph of uterine cervical tissue with extensive koilocytosis. The tissue has been stained for HPV 6-11 with peroxidase–antiperoxidase techniques. The darkly stained virus particles appear in the center of the koilocytotic vesicle in the upper layers of the epithelium. (Photograph courtesy of Dr. Miguel Pedraza.)

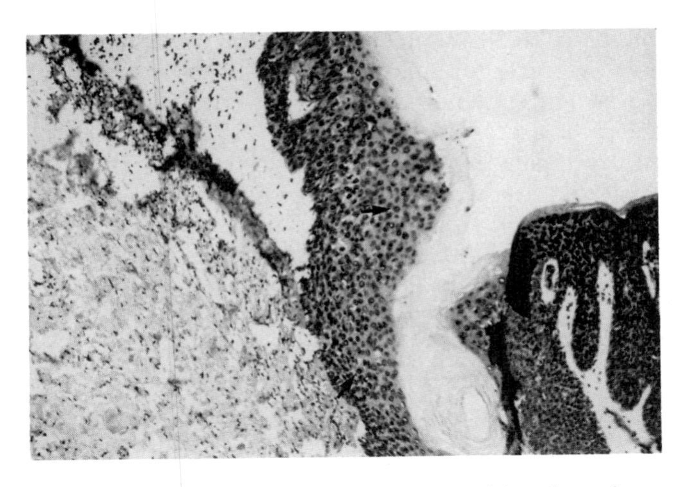

FIG. 4–3. Microphotograph of carcinoma in situ of the vulva and cervix showing positive staining for HPV types 16–18. (Photograph courtesy of Dr. Miguel Pedraza.)

18, 31, 33–35, and 52. HPV 18 has been particularly associated with adenocarcinomas and aggressive cervical carcinomas. HPV 16 has consistently been found in Bowenoid papulosis, a benign genital lesion of young men and women, to which findings convey a likely premalignant role (Wilczynski et al, 1988; Yajima et al, 1988; Ikenberg et al, 1989).

International studies based on PCR technology have reported a relative risk of invasive cancer higher than 20 for HPV types 16, 18, 31, 33, and 35 (Muñoz et al, 1992). It has been proposed that herpesviruses may be the initiators and that HPV play the role of promoters (Zur Hausen, 1987). The germinal layer of the squamous epithelia is believed to be the target of HPV infection, and the integration of viral genes with the host cells results in increased cellular proliferation. In approximately 85% of the cases, cervical cancer is associated with infection of the oncogenic types of HPV (mainly types 16 and 18). In such cases it has been shown that E6 oncogene product of the virus binds to the most ubiquitous suppressor gene, namely, *p53*. Similarly, the E7 product binds to the other major suppressor gene, namely, the retinoblastoma gene. It thus appears that infection of cervical epithelial cells with oncogenic strains of HPV blocks the major proteins in charge of regulating the normal cell cycle. The immortality of HeLa cells, originally obtained from a cervical carcinoma, appears to be linked to its being infected with HPV 18. In the 15% of tumors not infected with HPV, a mutation of the *p53* suppressor gene has been reported (Howley et al, 1989; Munger et al, 1989; Levin et al, 1990).

What makes some HPV types induce only benign lesions (such as 6 and 11) is not clear. In the experimental model of the cotton tail rabbit papilloma as well as in human carcinomas arising in patients with epidermodysplasia verruciformis, large numbers of episomal molecules persist in malignant cells.

Reassessment of the evidence for a morphologic continuum of cervical intraepithelial lesions suggests that mild or low-grade dysplasia may be a different entity from severe or high-grade dysplasia. The former may be self-healing infections associated with the "low-risk" HPV's, while the latter may progress to a more advanced lesion and be linked to the "high-risk" HPVs (Kiviat et al, 1992).

Epidemiologic studies done before the role of HPV was suspected had indicated that cervical cancer was a venereal disease, which has been confirmed by virologists. Other factors, however, had been identified as playing an etiologic role, such as hormonal influences, tobacco products, and other venereal infections such as herpes genitalis. These findings have led to the postulations of etiologic models such as the one proposed by Koss (1987) outlined in Fig. 4–4.

Flow cytometry and related techniques usually show that proliferative lesions have euploid or polyploid DNA patterns. Aneuploidy is suspected as an indicator of neoplastic clones and is a marker of aggressive behavior in tumors. Well-differentiated carcinomas, however, may occasionally display euploid patterns.

The new technology has opened new avenues of research and new clinical horizons. It is now possible to determine if a clinically or colposcopically suspect genital lesion is associated with the "benign" viruses (i.e., 6, 11) or with potentially carcinogenic types (i.e., 16, 18). Preliminary results of cohorts of Finnish women with HPV infection followed over two years have shown that the rate of progression to more advanced CIN lesions, or CIS, is highest for HPV 16 infection

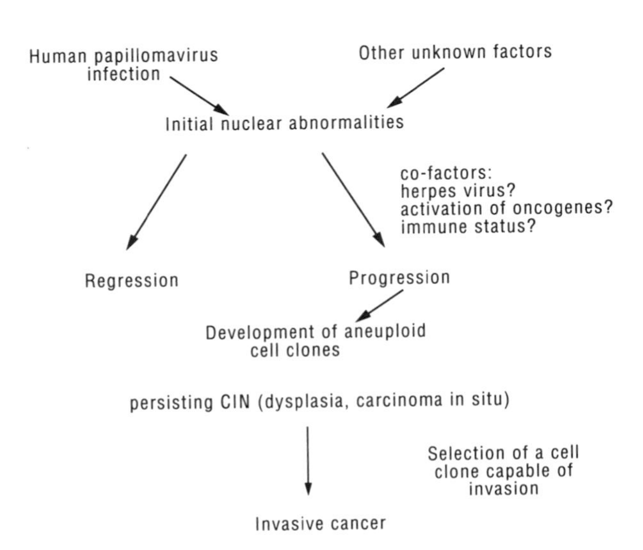

FIG. 4–4. Outline of etiologic model of carcinogenesis of the uterine cervix proposed by Koss (1987). (Reproduced with permission from Springer Verlag.)

(33.3%), which also shows the smallest rate of spontaneous regression (5.6%). The rate of regression for HPV 6/11 is greater: 25.6%. All lesions recurring after conization contained HPV 16 DNA. The rate of progression for HPV 6/11, however, was relatively high: 25.6%. These data suggest that HPV 6/11 types do represent a risk (Syrjänen et al, 1985a, b; Syrjänen, 1991). It is hoped that longer follow-up of this and similar cohorts will clarify the situation. Co-infection with several HPV types is well documented (Vila et al, 1989). Also well documented is the infection without clinically manifested lesions, which probably reflects a latency period, the length of which is so far undetermined. Subclinical infections are more frequent in men than in women.

Cancer Prevention through Screening. Following Papanicolaou's development of cervical cytology as a clinical tool, there was hope that this method could eventually eradicate invasive cervical cancer. In subsequent years, eradication has not been accomplished, and it has been pointed out that the drop in cervical cancer incidence rates had begun in many countries before vaginal cytology was used as a screening method. Questions were then raised as to the value of cervical cytology in secondary prevention of invasive cervical carcinoma. The latter observation called for a closer scrutiny of the hypothetical cause-and-effect relationship between the advent of vaginal cytology and the drop in mortality rates for cervical cancer.

Conceivably the precytology drop in incidence could have been due to improved social and economic conditions. The fact that the reported incidence of carcinoma in situ is not decreasing suggests that the factors responsible for the decreasing rate before cytology screening do not fully account for the totality of the present drop in incidence and mortality rates for carcinoma of the cervix. Cramer (1974) has reported a positive interstate correlation between the drop in cervical cancer incidence and mortality on the one hand and the rate of women screened by cytology on the other. This suggests that screening has contributed to the decline in incidence and mortality of invasive cancer, presumably through the identification and treatment of precursor lesions. Similar analyses in other communities have also provided evidence in the same direction (Miller et al, 1976). Supporting evidence for the role of screening was further provided by Johannesson et al (1978), who were able to link records of cervical cancer patients with previous histories of cytology as provided by accurate independent sets of records. They found that the deaths from cervical cancer were largely confined to women who had never been screened. The average annual death rate for women who had a negative reading on cytology screening during the previous 10 years was 2.6/100,000, compared to 29.5 and 23.5/100,000 in two consecutive time intervals for women who were never screened. Case-control studies to test retrospectively cervical cytology as a protective factor have shown that the risk of developing invasive carcinoma is at least 10 times greater in non-screened as in screened women (Aristizabal et al, 1984; Berrino et al, 1986).

In view of the accumulated international evidence, only partially reviewed here, it seems reasonable to conclude that screening has indeed led to the prevention of deaths from cervical cancer. The argument that this has been accomplished only by removing the risk organ from the population is irrelevant in light of the clear pragmatic gains obtained in terms of prevention.

Based on the results of programs of screening in eight countries over a period of over 20 years, the percentage reduction in the cumulative rate of invasive cervical cancer over the age range of 35–65 with different frequencies of screening has been calculated, assuming a screen at age 35 and a previous negative screen (Hakama et al, 1986) (see table below).

Screening frequency	*% reduction*
1 year interval	93.3
2	92.5
3	91.4
5	83.9
10	64.2

On the basis of this type of data, it is considered safe to screen every 3 years after a negative screen. This point is somewhat controversial because it is argued that a yearly check-up is more convenient. Most of the better data on screening come from Canada and European countries where centralized, usually government sponsored, programs are in place. Such is rarely the case in the United States and it is alleged that the decentralized, mostly private, structure for cervical cancer screening conveys a higher rate of false-negative results (20%–40%) compared to such rates in centrally organized European programs (less than 10%). Small laboratories with less volume may have more relaxed quality control mechanisms. The main reasons for failure of the screening programs have been identified in Europe, in order of importance, as follows: (*1*) failure to reach all women (especially high-risk women); (*2*) inadequate follow-up of abnormal smears; (*3*) long interval (more than 5 years) since last smear; and (*4*) false-negative results (Chamberlain, 1986). Tumors with a rapid evolution (very short "sojourn" time) account for a very small proportion (2%–3%) of failures.

Temporal Relationships. A consistent pattern of greater average age of patients with more advanced lesions has been reported. A compilation of data from 12 large studies (Langley and Compton, 1973) indicates the following mean ages: dysplasia, 36.0; carcinoma in situ, 39.2; and invasive carcinoma, 49.8.

The proportion of epithelial abnormalities (relative to each other) varies with age in such a way as to suggest that they represent a continuum of atypia that increases in severity with age, as can be seen in Table 4–1, taken from Johnson et al (1968). Since the rate of total abnormalities does not increase with age, this may be interpreted as the slow progression of one disease complex in a subsegment of the population that is probably either more susceptible or represents the group most intensely exposed to environmental factors. This disease would be manifested by mild dysplasia shortly after the beginning of active sexual life and would progress to cancer if left untreated for 20 or more years.

Contrary to expectations, the prevalence rate of precursor lesions in autopsy specimens did not increase with age, parity, or lower socioeconomic status in Cali, Colombia (Duque et al, 1979). This suggests that promotional factors result in a faster transformation from mild atypia to cancer in susceptible populations.

Based on cross-sectional data, many estimates have been made of the duration of each stage (Langley and Compton, 1973). Most authors estimate the dysplastic phase to last from 2 to 3 years and the carcinoma in situ phase from 5 to 10 years. It is questionable whether these estimates reflect the true situation, but the consistency of the pattern in different populations strongly supports the concept that these stages are indeed sequential in time. The transit time is believed to vary drastically with age: Coppleson and Brown (1975) have estimated that the average transit time from carcinoma in situ to invasive carcinoma is 17 years at age 25 but only 4 years at age 70. Our findings in Colombia indicate an increase in the surface area covered by dysplastic lesions with age (Duque et al, 1979). A similar finding has been reported for carcinoma in situ (Boyes et al, 1962).

TABLE 4–1. *Distribution of Dysplasia, Carcinoma in Situ, and Invasive Cancer in Relation to Age of Discovery in Los Angeles Populations*

		Percent Distribution		
Age in Years	*Rate/1000 Patients*	*Dysplasia*	*Carcinoma In Situ*	*Invasive Cancer*
20–29	15.3	71.2	19.0	9.8
30–39	14.0	50.7	44.3	5.0
40–49	12.0	35.8	49.2	15.0
50–59	11.0	38.2	40.0	21.8
60–69	15.3	31.4	35.3	33.3
70+	11.9	25.2	8.4	66.4

[a]Calculated from the rates for dysplasia, carcinoma in situ, and invasive cancer reported by Stern and Neely (1964).

Most data also indicate that the time spent in each successive stage becomes shorter as the more advanced stages are reached. In Barron and Richart's (1968) study, the predicted estimated mean time (in months) spent in each stage is approximately as follows: very mild dysplasia, 70; mild dysplasia, 37; moderate dysplasia, 29; severe dysplasia, 11. Marked discrepancies in such estimates have been reported. Regression of preneoplastic cervical lesions has been well documented but the estimates vary considerably (from 5% to 65%) not only with age and stage but also between populations. Several mathematical models of the natural history of cervical carcinogenesis have been proposed, and have been critically reviewed by Prorok (1986). The estimates of the proportion of progression and regression, as well as the calculations on transition times, were made before the HPV era. It is possible that part of the discrepancies in earlier reports will be resolved when the HPV type associated with the lesions is taken into consideration.

BREAST CANCER PRECURSORS

An understanding of the precancerous process of the female breast is needed for the prevention of one of the most common cancers in our community. A large proportion of adult women have in their breasts histologic changes of various degrees which in the past have been known by the all-encompassing term *fibrocystic disease*. Controversial views have been expressed as to the possible role of such benign changes in the carcinogenesis process. Recent progress in this area has come from two disciplines: experimental carcinogenesis and epidemiology.

An experimental animal model with direct implications for the human situation has been developed by Russo and co-workers (Russo and Russo, 1980, 1987, 1988; Russo et al, 1987a, b, 1988). It examines in detail the effects of 7,12 dimethylbenz (a) anthracene (DMBA) on the mammary epithelium of the rat. The carcinogenic effect of DMBA is inhibited by pregnancy-induced differentiation of the gland. The normal glandular epithelium evolves from a primary main lactiferous duct which branches into multiple secondary ducts which sprout further until reaching sixth generation branches. These end in club-shaped terminal end buds (TEB) that are composed of 3 to 6 layers of medium-sized epithelial cells (Fig. 4–5). After the age of 21 days, TEBs begin to cleave into 3 to 5 small alveolar buds (AB) which later differentiate further to form the lobular structures. The progressive differentiation of TEBs into ABs is accentuated by each estrous cycle. DMBA administration at the time when TEBs are being differentiated into ABs

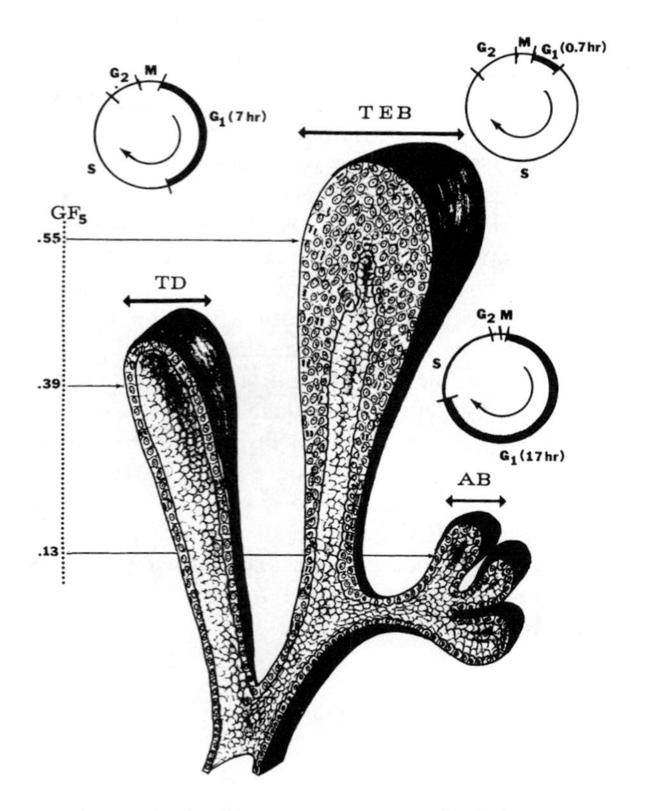

FIG. 4–5. Schematic representation of terminal structures of the mammary gland of virgin rats and diagrams of cell cycle of each structure. *TD* = terminal duct; *TEB* = terminal end buds; *AB* = alveolar buds. (Reproduced with permission, Russo and Russo, 1980.)

prevents such differentiation and induces instead large numbers of transformed structures that grow in the form of intraductal proliferations (IDP). These become larger and coalesce to form intraductal adenocarcinomas (Fig. 4–6). DMBA effects on already differentiated ABs do not result in carcinomatous transformation; they may remain unmodified, become cystic, or form adenomas (Fig. 4–6). The effects of the carcinogen DMBA, therefore, depend on the timing of the insult because it determines the type of the target epithelium. The more differentiated the structure at the time of the insult, the more benign and organized the lesions will be that develop. Several reasons account for the abovementioned results. One is that the length of the cell cycle (Tc) for TEB epithelial cells is 13 hours, compared to 34 hours for the AB and lobular cells, which explains the high rate of binding of DMBA to DNA and lower DNA repair activity. Ductal and alveolar cells also differ in their chemical handling of the carcinogen. Ductal cells produce more polar and less phenolic compounds than lobular cells, which results in greater production of epoxides, resulting in even higher DNA-DMBA binding. Further, ductal cells remove adducts less efficiently than lobular cells. This is attributed to the shorter G1 phase of the cell cycle rather than to a lack of DNA reparative enzymes.

Full-term pregnancy and lactation are needed for the complete differentiation of the mammary epithelium and convey a permanent protective effect against the carcinogenic influence of DMBA. Administration of the carcinogen after pregnancy interruption results in the same high incidence of tumors observed in virgin rats, or much higher than that observed in parous animals (Russo and Russo, 1980).

These experimental results fit very well with epide-

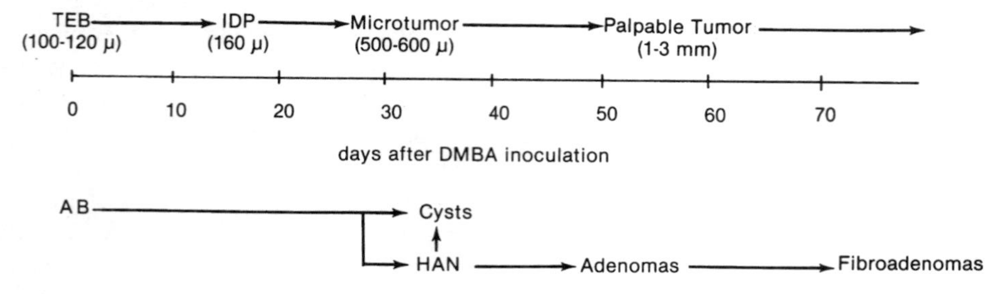

FIG. 4–6. Diagrammatic representation of the two different pathogenic pathways for benign and malignant lesions. Malignant lesions originate from terminal end buds (*TEB*) and appear earlier than benign lesions, which originate from alveolar buds (*AB*). The earliest lesion detected after DMBA administration is the intraductal proliferation (*IDP*). Hyperplastic alveolar nodules (*HAN*) precede benign adenomas. (Reproduced with permission from Russo and Russo, 1987.)

miological findings pointing out that full-term pregnancy during the first part of the reproductive cycle of women lowers considerably the subsequent risk of breast cancer (Mac Mahon et al, 1979). This indicates that the early reproductive age of women is a crucial time when reproductive and environmental events may convey permanent protection (a "protective window") or permanent high risk (a "risk window") (De Ward and Trichopoulos, 1988). The longer the "window" lasts before a full-term pregnancy, the greater the chances of proliferative changes in the ductal epithelium because less differentiation of alveolar and lobular structures takes place.

The ductal epithelium can be induced to differentiate into alveolar and lobular structures by means of pregnancy-related hormones. Chorionic gonadotropin (HcG) induces differentiation of the mammary epithelium and inhibits tumor development. Placental lactogen fails to stimulate gland differentiation and increases the incidence of tumors. Estrogens stimulate growth (but not differentiation) of mammary epithelium while progesterone stimulates differentiation of alveolar structures. Some of these hormones are being consumed by millions of women as contraceptives (Russo and Russo, 1988). Differences in the timing and the chemical composition of contraceptive prescriptions may have very different effects on the mammary epithelium and may account for some of the discrepant results of epidemiologic studies on the effect of contraceptives on breast cancer. Experimental models indicate that the contraceptive norethynol mestranol (Enovid) at low doses reduces cancer risk, probably because it reduces the proportion of ductal cells by inducing differentiation of alveolar structures (Russo and Russo, 1988). It may be then possible to prevent breast cancer in women by hormonal administration early in the reproductive cycle. The effect may not be the same at later ages because greater proportions of (undifferentiated) ductal cells are present.

The human female breast epithelium follows a developmental process which has been studied in mastectomy specimens. It is somewhat similar to that of the rat. Four different types of lobular structures have been identified (Russo and Russo, 1987a). Type 1, or virginal lobules, contain 5–6 alveoli (Fig. 4–7). Type 2 contains about 47 (Fig. 4–8), and type 3 contains about 81 alveoli per lobule (Fig. 4–9). Type 4 are those seen during pregnancy and contain approximately 180 alveoli per lobule. Women with a history of abortion or who had developed ductal carcinoma in the contralateral breast had ductal structures but not type 3 lobules in their breasts (Russo and Russo, 1987b; Russo et al, 1988). Women with a history of full-term pregnancy had glands almost exclusively composed of type 3 alveoli. Intralobular terminal ducts in human breasts have the highest levels of

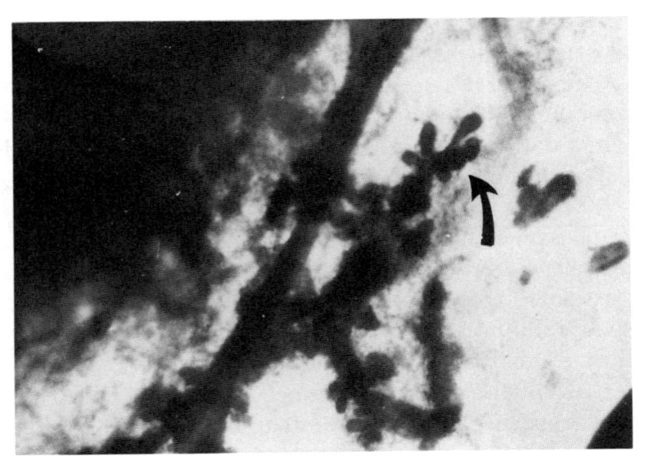

FIG. 4–7. Whole mount preparation of breast tissue of a 30-year-old nulliparous woman containing type I lobules composed of six alveolar buds (*arrow*). (Reproduced with permission from Russo et al, 1988.)

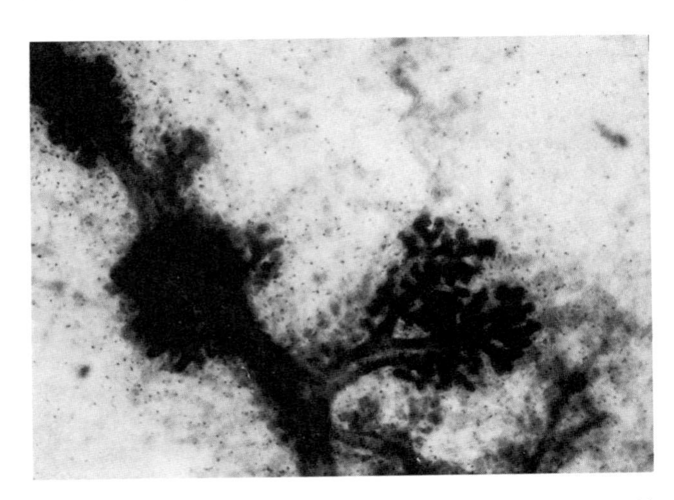

FIG. 4–8. Whole mount preparation of breast tissue of a 44-year-old female containing type II lobules. (Reproduced with permission from Russo and Russo, 1988.)

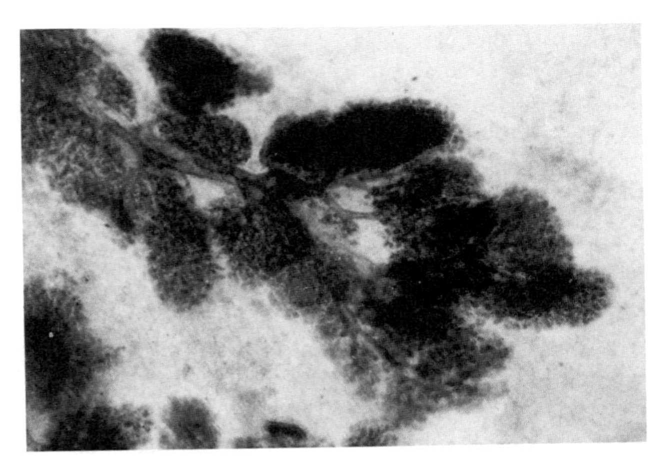

FIG. 4–9. Whole mount preparation of breast tissue of a 30-year-old parous woman containing type III lobules. (Reproduced with permission from Russo and Russo, 1988.)

tritiated thymidine incorporation and are known sites of origin of breast carcinomas.

Human breast epithelial cells can be grown in culture for a limited time and can be transformed when incubated with carcinogens if the donors have poor gland development and no history of pregnancy (Russo et al, 1988). The ultimate manifestation of the transformed state, namely in vitro immortality and tumorigenesis in xenogeneic hosts, has not been achieved. It has been postulated that the permanent growth of transformed cells is inhibited by coexistent nontransformed cells in the culture. They may exert their influence by the transfer of growth inhibitor substances through so-called gap junctions. Such gap junctions can be decreased in their capacity to establish intercellular communications by a low calcium medium. Cancer inhibitors such as retinoic acid tested in other cell culture systems increase communications between transformed and surrounding normal cells, which diminishes the number of transformed foci (Yamasaki and Katoh, 1988; Bertram et al, 1991). Modulation of gap junction communications can, therefore, be an important factor in human breast carcinogenesis as well as in other organs.

The interaction between chemical carcinogens and activation of oncogenes in mammary tissue is the subject of contemporary research. In human breast cancer *ras p21* expression is enhanced in 70% of the cases (Thor et al, 1986). This expression is observed in rats treated with methyl nitroso urea (MNU) but not with DMBA (Russo et al, 1987b). It appears that *ras* oncogenes can transform established rodent cell lines but not primary cultures. The carcinogen(s) of pertinence to the human situation are unknown but it would appear that they are related to *ras* gene activation. Amplification of the *erb2* (*neu*) oncogene product is more prominent in poorly differentiated tumors that carry a worse prognosis (Slamon et al, 1987). A susceptibility gene has been proposed in chromosome 17q 12-21 (Hall et al, 1992; Narod et al, 1991).

The role of benign breast lesions as indicators of cancer risk has been clarified to a great extent by the work of Page, Dupont and co-workers (Page et al, 1978; Dupont and Page, 1985) who combined pathology and epidemiology techniques. Retrospective (historical) cohort studies of women who had a previous biopsy were identified. After exclusions due to previous breast cancer diagnoses, fibroadenomas, inadequate tissue for evaluation, and nonproliferative lesions, a cohort of 3398 women was assembled. Their postbiopsy experience was ascertained for an average period of 17 years with a successful follow-up rate of 84.4%. Histologically the lesions were classified according to the presence and type of ductal hyperplasia. An overall relative risk of 1.5 (95% confidence intervals [C.I.] 1.3–1.8) was found for all proliferative lesions combined, compared with 0.89 (0.62–1.3) for nonproliferative lesions. When the proliferative lesions were associated with atypia (namely atypical hyperplasia), a significantly elevated cancer relative risk of 3.5 was observed. Atypical hyperplasia in patients with a family history of breast cancer carried a relative risk of 8.9. The overall increase in the risk is, therefore, due mainly to atypical hyperplasia and is considerably enhanced by family history of breast cancer. Atypical hyperplasia is a true precursor of breast cancer in women and the one lesion which requires careful follow-up of patients for secondary prevention. Other lesions are so prevalent and carry such a low risk of cancer that large-scale patient follow-up is unwarranted. Atypical hyperplasia is approximately equivalent to the intraductal proliferation of the rat model.

GASTRIC CARCINOMA

Morphology of Precursor Lesions

There are two main epidemiologic types of gastric carcinoma (Lauren, 1965). The *diffuse* or *endemic* type displays little intercountry variation in frequency. Although certain lesions have been described as precursors of such tumors (Borchard et al, 1979; Bordi, 1982; Gandur-Manaymneh et al, 1988), epidemiologic information at the present time is insufficient to make a judgment about their role in cancer prevention. The *intestinal* or *epidemic* type accounts for the excess of gastric cancer in populations at high risk and is usually found against a background of chronic atrophic gastritis (CAG), an inflammatory change associated with chronic and progressive loss of gastric glands, presumably preceded by nonspecific superficial gastritis. CAG is a multifocal phenomenon that starts in the antral-body junction and spreads to extensive areas as the foci become confluent (Correa et al, 1970). The atrophic glands are replaced by tubular structures lined by cells that are foreign to the normal stomach but normally present in the intestine: goblet cells, absorptive cells, and Paneth cells. The gastric mucosa then gradually becomes intestinalized. The lesion is called *intestinal metaplasia* (IM) (Figs. 4–10, 4–11). From the histopathologic point of view, the lesions just described are "mature" and "benign." They may be precursors of cancer in the epidemiologic sense but at present are not a clinical indication for specific surveillance or therapeutic measure for the patient. A small proportion of patients with intestinal metaplasia develop more advanced lesions. Research on the prevention of more advanced lesions is being conducted. Atypical changes in the metaplastic epithelium represent the critical steps requiring identification.

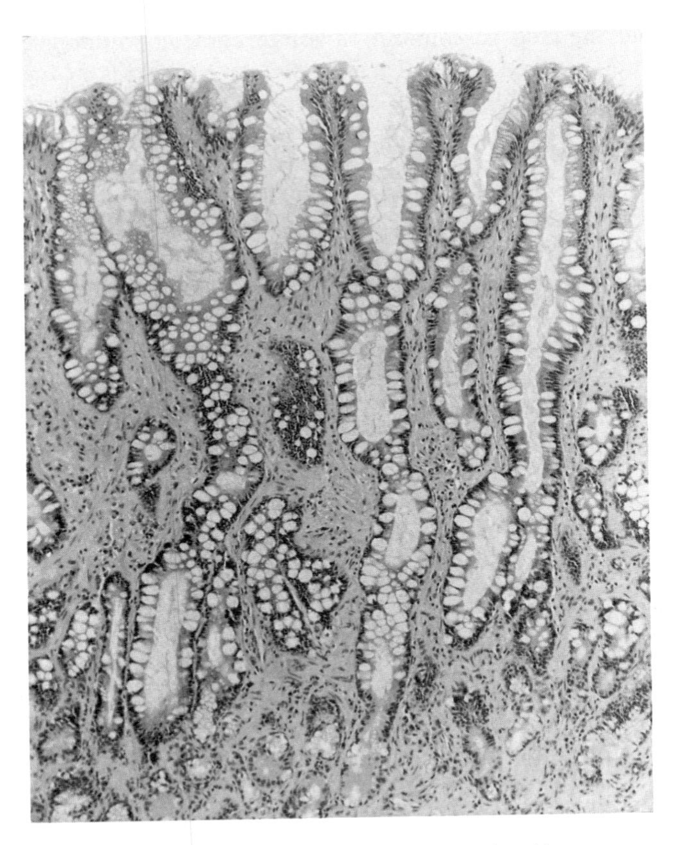

FIG. 4–10. Microphotograph of gastric mucosa replaced by structures resembling small intestinal glands lined by eosinophilic enterocytes with brush borders alternating with goblet cells. Small intestinal metaplasia.

It appears from the available morphologic and experimental evidence that intestinal metaplasia resembles small intestine when it first appears and retains such a phenotype for most of the life of the individual (Fig. 4–10). The phenotype is characterized by pseudovilli lined by columnar absorptive cells with prominent brush border (enterocytes) alternating with goblet cells which secrete acid nonsulfated mucin (sialomucin). The absorptive cells have the complete battery of small intestinal digestive enzymes: sucrase, alkaline phosphatase, leucine amino peptidase, etc. This type of metaplasia has received the names of *Type I, complete*, or *small intestinal type*. In some patients the digestive enzymes are gradually lost, the mucin secretion is changed to include sulfomucin (typical of the normal colon and rectum), and the architecture becomes simplified with loss of absorptive cells. Instead of as well-defined goblets, the mucin secretion is expressed as multiple vacuoles which distend the cytoplasm. The brush border is lost because only a few microvilli persist in the surface of the glandular epithelial cells. This type of metaplasia has been called *Type III*, or *colonic* (Fig. 4–11). It is more frequently found in older patients around the incisura angularis and is the predominant type around areas of dysplasia or small carcinomas.

The dysplastic changes follow one of two routes. One consists of the proliferation and branching of glandular elements, resulting in irregularly distorted lumens reminiscent of hyperplastic epithelial changes, and is called *hyperplastic dysplasia*, or *Type I* (Cuello et al, 1979; Jass, 1983). The dysplastic changes, measured in terms of nuclear atypias and architectural irregularities, vary from mild to severe. The more advanced cases of these lesions are sometimes called *carcinoma in situ* because, although the cells themselves are morphologically neoplastic, they are still bound by the basement membrane of the original metaplastic gland. Carcinomas arising in hyperplastic dysplasias are often poorly differentiated intestinal type adenocarcinomas.

The second route of metaplastic dysplasia is characterized by the proliferation of multiple, small, closely packed tubular glands reminiscent of the adenomatous

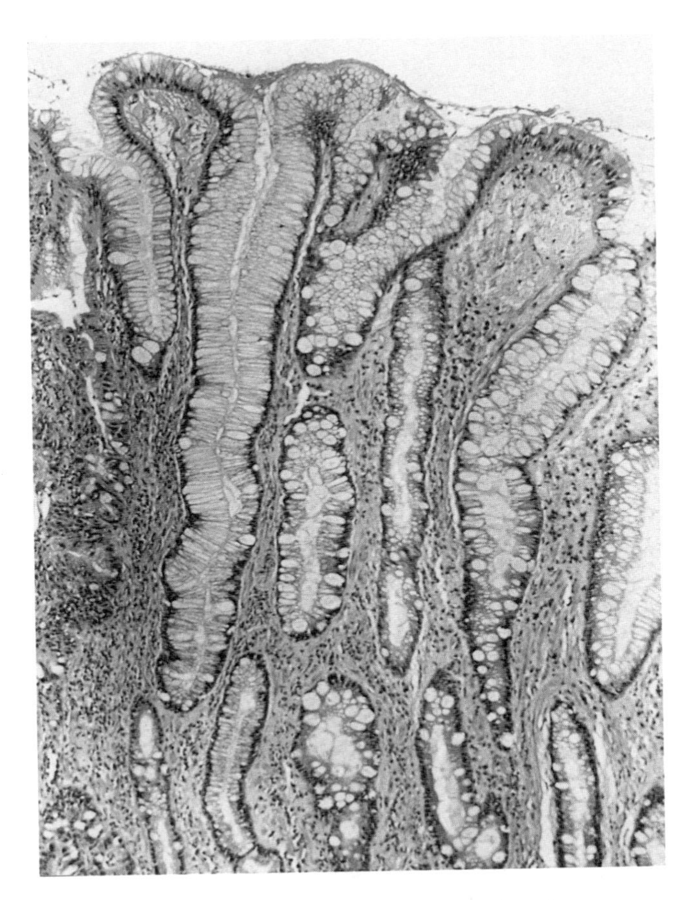

FIG. 4–11. Microphotograph of gastric mucosa replaced by structures resembling colonic gland lined by columnar cells distended by numerous mucus vacuoles of different sizes. Enterocytes and brush border are absent. Colonic metaplasia is present.

polyps of the colon; for that reason, these lesions are called *adenomatous dysplasias* (Fig. 4–12). Several degrees of nuclear and architectural abnormalities are seen in the adenomatous glands, from mild to severe. When the glandular proliferation becomes exuberant, they may give rise to adenomatous polyps, which carry a high premalignant potential.

The steps identified above with morphologic and histochemical techniques suggest a gradual change in the gastric epithelium with increased cell replication and decreased differentiation. Other techniques have identified additional markers of the process.

A gradual appearance of fetal antigens has been documented in human gastric biopsies, representing progressively more advanced lesions. A human second trimester fetal antigen has been found in 10% of superficial gastritis, 38% of chronic atrophic gastritis, 50% of intestinal metaplasia, and 86% of dysplasia (Higgins et al, 1984). Alterations in the expression of the Lewis system of blood group antigens resembling the fetal pattern of their expression have been documented in gastric carcinoma cells and in normal appearing cells surrounding overt carcinomas (Sipponen and Lindgren, 1986; Torrado et al, 1989, 1992a). Mucin-associated antigens have been detected in gastric carcinomas and in metaplastic cells that surround them. The pattern seen in the latter cells resembles fetal duodenum, which contains antigens found in adults in the colon, duodenum, and small intestine (Bara et al, 1981; Nardelli et al, 1983).

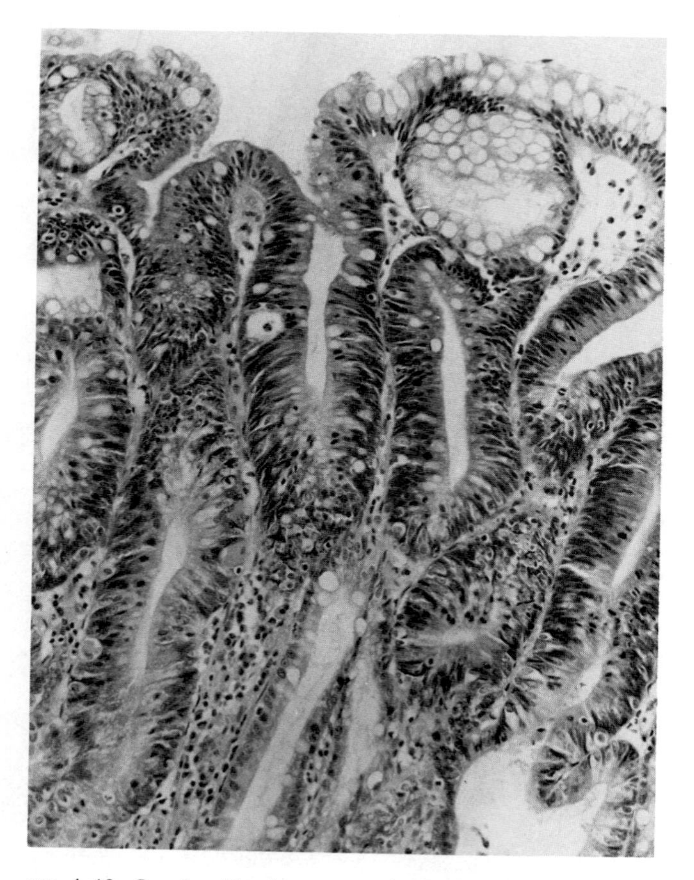

FIG. 4–12. Gastric with adenomatous dysplasia originating in previously metaplastic epithelium. The nuclei are large, elongated, crowded, hyperchomatic, and not circumscribed to the base of the cells.

Autoradiographic studies in precursor lesions have shown expansion of the replication zone incorporating tritiated thymidine. When such studies have been done in conjunction with fetal antigens, their abnormal expression has been found in the expanded replication zone (Lipkin et al, 1985).

Products of abnormal oncogene amplification have been found in intestinal metaplasia but their significance is not yet understood (Noguchi et al, 1980; Ciclitira et al, 1987).

Screening High-Risk Populations. Gastric cancer is the second most frequent neoplasm in the world (Parkin et al, 1993). Screening for gastric cancer has been practiced mostly in Japan and has coincided with a decrease in mortality rates and with an increase in the proportion of "early" cancers. The techniques are costly and their efficiency has not been documented (Oshima et al, 1986). All high-risk populations display a very high prevalence of gastric precursors in the adults—mainly chronic atrophic gastritis and intestinal metaplasia. Gastroscopic techniques are excellent diagnostic tools and have become available to large numbers of individuals. They are, however, cumbersome and costly. They could become even more useful in the diagnosis of premalignant lesions and early cancer if some less invasive method of screening were available. Screening methods are being evaluated at the present time but none is yet widely used for screening large populations. One method being tested is the measure of pepsinogens (PG) in the blood. There are two main classes of pepsinogens: *PG I*, which is primarily produced by the chief cells of the gastric corpus, and *PG II*, which is also produced by the antral glands. Since the gastric precancerous process leads to progressive atrophy of the corporal mucosa, a very low *PG I* and a very low *PG I/II* ratio are associated with a high risk of gastric cancer. *PG I* blood levels below 20 μg/l are good indicators of very high risk (Samloff et al, 1982; Stemmermann et al, 1987; Miki et al, 1987).

Biomarkers of risk based on biopsy material are being developed and may allow categorization of patients at very high risk. Two markers which are widely available are sulfomucins and Lewis antigen alterations. They have been studied in high-risk populations of Colombia both in cross-sectional and cohort follow-up studies. Table 4–2 shows the relative risk of colonic metaplasia

TABLE 4–2. *Estimated Relative Risk (R.R.) of Colonic Metaplasia and Dysplasia Associated with Abnormal Phenotypic Expression of Two Markers*

Markers		*R.R. Cross-Sectional Study*		*R.R. Prospective Study*	
Sulfomucin	*Lewis*	*Colonic Metaplasia*	*Dysplasia*	*Colonic Metaplasia*	*Dysplasia*
–	–	1.0	1.0	1.0	1.0
+	–	4.0	1.0	4.9	11.0
–	+	3.2	1.7	6.9	5.8
+	+	48.0	11.2	32.7	13.0

and dysplasia observed with each marker alone and in combination. The potential of such techniques appears convincing. Other markers are being developed in other laboratories (Correa et al, 1990; Correa, 1992).

Statistical Association between Cancer and Precursors. Intestinal metaplasia of the gastric mucosa was described by Kupffer in 1883 and interpreted as displaced embryonic rests, or heterotopia. The microscopic observation that carcinoma arose in areas of metaplasia was emphasized by Jarvi and Lauren in 1951 and later corroborated by investigators in several countries (Morson, 1955; Ming et al, 1967; Correa et al, 1970; Grundmann, 1975; Oehlert et al, 1975).

The prevalence of metaplasia in the gastric mucosa of the autopsy series was positively correlated with the frequency of gastric carcinoma in the same populations (Bonne et al, 1938; Imai et al, 1971). Studies of internal migrants in Colombia showed that this positive correlation was maintained in migrants after many years of residence outside of the high-risk environment (Correa et al, 1970). The presence of long-standing metaplasia, therefore, offered an explanation for the previous observation by Haenszel and Segi (1967) that the gastric cancer risk in migrants to the United States was determined by their earlier premigration experience in the high-risk environment of their native country.

Temporal Relationships. Precursors of gastric carcinoma can be found in the gastric mucosa beginning in the second decade of life. At this age, however, they are represented only by small foci of mucosal atrophy that do not alter gastric function significantly. Mathematical models of the precancerous process suggest that within each population there is a subgroup that develops gastritis and is selected around the age of 20. After that age, the curve becomes asymptotic; the lesions may increase in extension and severity, but the prevalence of unaffected individuals remains constant (Correa et al, 1976). The proportion of individuals affected is considerably larger in high-risk than in low-risk populations. Since second generation migrants in a low-risk environment acquire the low risk of the host country, an interaction between genetics and environment appears to take place. This was explored in a segregation analysis of 110 Colombian families comprising 557 individuals (Bonney et al, 1986). Transmission of a recessive autosomal gene with penetrance dependent on age and maternal status was found, indicating the interaction of genetic and environmental etiologic factors. Fig. 4–13 summarizes the model and shows that homozygous individuals with affected mothers develop CAG at an earlier age than other groups. Homozygous individuals with unaffected mothers have a slightly lower prevalence in the first decades than the above group but show the same prevalence after age 50. Heterozygous individuals have a much lower prevalence and are practically free of CAG up to age 60. Genetic forces, therefore, determine the age at which environment factors succeed in inducing atrophic gastritis, which then starts the precancerous process.

CAG and intestinal metaplasia are present in the gastric mucosa for many years (most probably more than two decades in most cases). The surface area covered by these lesions increases with age, and foci of dysplasia begin to appear usually when atrophy and metaplasia are very extensive. The next biologic step is what has been called "early" cancer in the Japanese literature. This is characterized by a superficial spread within the mucosa and submucosa and presumably loss of cancer cells via desquamation into the gastric lumen. At this stage, cell kinetics studies have shown that the generation time (T) is 4 to 15 days but that the doubling time of the tumor (D) is 2 to 3 years (Fujita and Hattori,

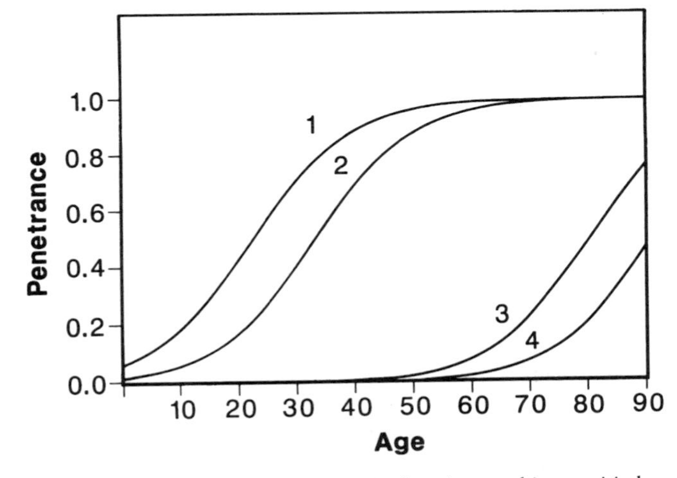

FIG. 4–13. Prevalence of (*penetrance*) chronic atrophic gastritis by age. Homozygous recessive subjects (*1*) with affected mother reach plateau levels at earlier age than homozygous recessive without affected mothers (*2*). Carriers with affected mother (*3*) and carriers without affected mothers (*4*) show atropic gastritis only very late in life and do not reach high prevalence. (From Bonney et al, 1986.)

1977). The tumor may be growing for many years without attaining a large size and without becoming invasive. In the Japanese experience, early or intramucosal carcinoma has a post-gastrectomy 5-year survival rate of more than 90%. This situation changes radically when the tumor penetrates the muscular layer of the stomach (muscularis propria), where loss of tumor cells by desquamation is not a factor. In such cases, T is the same (4 to 15 days), but D is considerably shorter—0.6 to 2 months. These cell kinetics data correlate well with the poor prognosis of more advanced gastric carcinoma.

Sex Ratios. The well-known male predominance in the incidence of gastric cancer is not found in precursor lesions as reported in Finland (Siurala et al, 1968) and Colombia (Haenszel et al, 1976), where prevalence rates of precursors are similar in both sexes. This seems to indicate that initiator factors are equally potent in both sexes but that promoters are more effective in males. This seems supported by the fact that dysplastic changes in intestinal metaplasia are more frequent and more advanced in males (Cuello et al, 1979). Recent findings in nutritional epidemiologic studies provide a hypothetical explanation for the above (see below).

Diet. Populations with a high risk of gastric cancer are very dissimilar in their dietary patterns and do not have too many specific food items in common. Most of them, however, have a high starch, low fat, low protein intake, as well as a low intake of fruits and fresh leafy vegetables. Dietary epidemiologic studies of cancer precursors have been reported for Colombia, Japan, and the United States (Correa et al, 1983; Nomura et al, 1982; Fontham et al, 1986). The common theme of the findings has been an excessive intake of irritants, mostly salt and alcohol, and a low intake of fresh fruits and vegetables, which appear to act as protectors. A cross-sectional study of serum micronutrients in Colombian populations with precursor lesions found that the blood levels of beta-carotene (and to a lesser degree alpha-tocopherol) were significantly lower in patients with dysplasia than in subjects with normal gastric mucosa or with the less advanced precursors CAG and IM (Haenszel et al, 1985). The data then point to a preventive effect in the late stages of the carcinogenic process, mostly promotion and perhaps progression. Surveys of micronutrients have shown that the blood levels of carotene are usually higher in females than in males (U.S. Department of Health, Education, and Welfare, 1982). Carotene levels may therefore offer at least a partial explanation for why the M/F ratio is 1 for the incidence of CAG-IM and >1 for dysplasia and carcinoma.

As discussed above, diet may provide protectors against stomach cancer. Other dietary components enhance the risk of gastric cancer. Excessive salt intake is one of these enhancing factors, as concluded from cross-sectional, case-control, and experimental studies. In addition to being an irritant that leads to cell destruction and excessive replication, salt enhances the effectiveness of well-known gastric carcinogens such as N-methyl-N-nitroso-N′-nitroguanidine (Correa, 1988).

Another potential factor in gastric carcinogenesis in *Helicobacter pylori*, recently recognized as the most frequent cause of chronic gastritis (Blaser, 1987). The role of such bacterial infection in human gastric carcinogenesis is supported by 3 recent, nested case-control studies showing that subjects with antibodies to the bacterin in serum collected years before, had a relative risk of carcinoma from 2.6 to 6 times that of non-infected individuals (Nomura et al, 1991; Parsonnett et al, 1991; Forman et al, 1991). The infection is practically always present in diffuse antral gastritis, apparently the forerunner of duodenal ulcer. There is no indication that the duodenal ulcer syndrome increases gastric cancer risk. *Helicobacter pylori* is also frequently found in multifocal chronic atrophic gastritis intestinal metaplasia and dysplasia (Correa et al, 1989) and it is conceivable that the bacterial infection plays an adjuvant etiologic role under such circumstances. The infection induces a state of hyper-proliferation which favors the carcinogenic process (Brenes et al, 1993).

Patients with precursor lesions have excessive gastric juice nitrite, mostly formed by bacteria in the gastric cavity. Nitrites are well-known precursors of potent carcinogens that may be involved in gastric carcinogenesis. Nitrosation of Japanese fish has been used to induce gastric carcinoma in rats (Weisburger et al, 1980). Nitrosation of food frequently eaten by high-risk populations, especially fava beans and Chinese cabbage, has resulted in the formation of potent mutagens, mostly nitroso-indols (Yang et al, 1984; Wakabayashi et al, 1987).

Conclusions. The gastric precancerous process appears to be represented by sequential changes in the gastric mucosa involving first phenotypic alterations only (atrophy and reparative hyperplasia) and later genotypic alterations (metaplasia and dysplasia). These changes appear modulated by dietary items belonging to three basic groups: irritants, genotoxic agents, and protectors. The most ubiquitous irritant appears to be excessive salt intake. The genotoxic agent(s) is unknown but suspected to be a nitroso compound(s). The protectors so far identified are mostly antioxidants: beta-carotene, ascorbic acid, and alpha-tocopherol. These factors appear to interact with some intricacy as outlined in Fig. 4–14. The entire process is initiated much earlier in susceptible individuals selected by a CAG gene transmitted autosomally with penetrance depending on age and on having an affected mother.

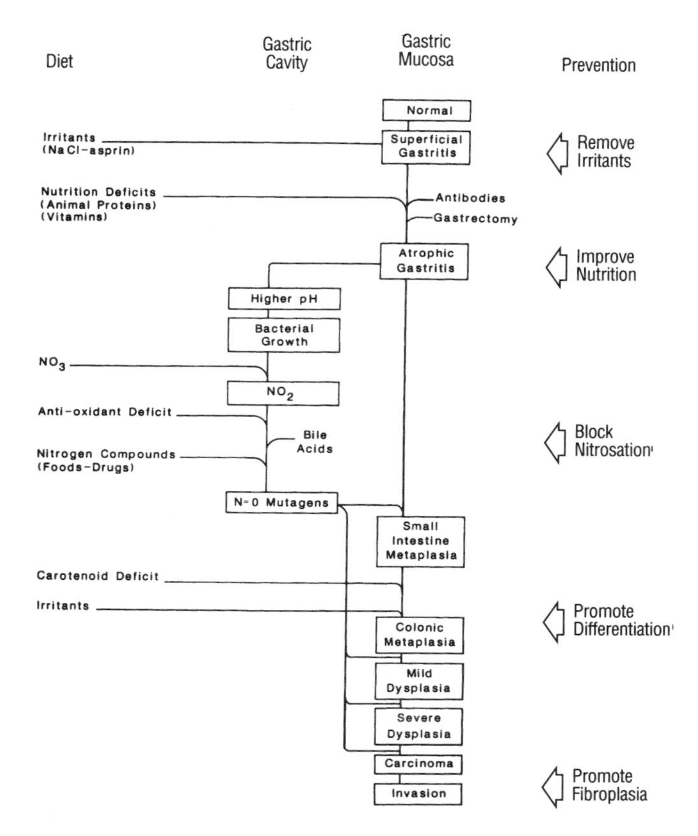

FIG. 4–14. Etiologic model of gastric carcinogenesis showing the presumed timing of etiologic factors and their interaction with the presumed precursor lesions of the gastric mucosa.

LARGE BOWEL CARCINOMA

Morphology of Precursor Lesions

The great majority of colorectal carcinomas are thought to arise in adenomatous polyps (Morson and Bussey, 1970; Lane et al, 1978). Hyperplastic and juvenile polyps have no proven premalignant role (Correa et al, 1972). Premalignant changes have also been identified in the flat (not polypose) mucosa in cases of ulcerative colitis. A small proportion of carcinomas arise in flat colorectal mucosa without apparent premalignant changes (Spratt and Ackerman, 1962).

Although dysplasias in ulcerative colitis (UC) account for less than 1% of colon carcinomas, they constitute an important problem for the patient, the clinician, and the pathologist. Cancer risk in UC patients increases with time and is especially high after 10 years of active disease. Areas of dysplasia are small and multifocal, and carcinomas associated with them are usually poorly differentiated and very aggressive. For such reasons, a definitive diagnosis of dysplasia usually leads to total colectomy. Separating true dysplasias from active regenerative hyperplasia may be a difficult task. To overcome the difficulties in diagnosis a classification has been developed and illustrated by an international group of experts (Riddel et al, 1983). Criteria for dysplastic vs. regenerative changes were extensively defined and a new category to accommodate lesions of uncertain nature was created. Table 4–3 shows the categories and the suggested management policy. It is recommended that the diagnosis of dysplasia be made by two independent pathologists on biopsy material obtained in two endoscopic examinations. The histologic criteria for the diagnosis are based on architectural distortion of crypts, irregular or absent maturation towards the surface, partial or complete loss of mucin secretion, and nuclear abnormalities.

It has been recognized for some time that the colorectal mucosa adjacent to carcinomas often shows histochemical abnormalities (Filipe and Branfoot, 1974). A decrease in secretion of sulfomucins, the most abundant rectal mucin, is replaced by an increase in the secretion of sialomucin, the most abundant mucin of the small intestine. Similar changes have also been found in patches of mucosa distant from the tumor. These changes have been called *transitional mucosa* and are interpreted as a regression to the pattern of mucus secretion observed in the human fetal gut. It is not clear if such patches of transitional mucosa are forerunners of more advanced cancer precursors. A simple and inexpensive test has been proposed to detect abnormal sugar moieties in rectal mucus samples obtained with digital examination. These abnormal moieties are present in patients with colorectal cancer and it has been

TABLE 4–3. *Provisional Schema of Patient Management Related to Classification of Dysplasia*[*]

Biopsy Classification	*Implications for Patient Management*
NEGATIVE	
Normal mucosa	
Inactive (quiescent) colitis	Continue regular follow-up.
Active colitis	
INDEFINITE	
Probably negative	
Unknown	Institute short-interval follow-up.
Probably positive	
POSITIVE	
Low-grade dysplasia	Institute short-interval follow-up or consider colectomy, especially with gross lesion, after dysplasia is confirmed.
HIGH-GRADE DYSPLASIA	Consider colectomy after dysplasia is confirmed.

*From Riddel et al, 1983.

suggested that they may be detected in precancerous states (Shamsuddin and Elsayed, 1988; Kristal et al, 1992).

Adenomatous polyps are proliferations of the large bowel epithelium, which, in their more mature form, are composed of closely packed tubular glands, resulting in a small mass that protrudes into the intestinal lumen (Fig. 4–15). In the great majority of subjects bearing these polyps, tubular adenomas remain mature and small, are not associated with clinical manifestations, and are not transformed into carcinomas (Correa et al, 1972; Morson, 1974). In a small proportion of cases (around 5% according to Morson) these lesions lead to carcinoma and in such cases go through a process of dysplasia manifested by architectural and cellular abnormalities. Architecturally, these dysplastic changes result in primary and secondary branchings of the originally straight glands (Kosuka, 1975) and in the formation of elongated projections which constitute a variable proportion of tubulovillous adenomas (Morson and Sobin, 1976). The greater the proportion of villous elements in a polyp, the greater the chances of malignant transformation. Pure villous adenomas have a very high risk of malignant transformation (around 40% according to Morson, 1974). Cellular abnormalities are measured in terms of increased nuclear size and staining quality, irregular shape, presence of prominent nucleoli, frequency of mitoses, and stratification.

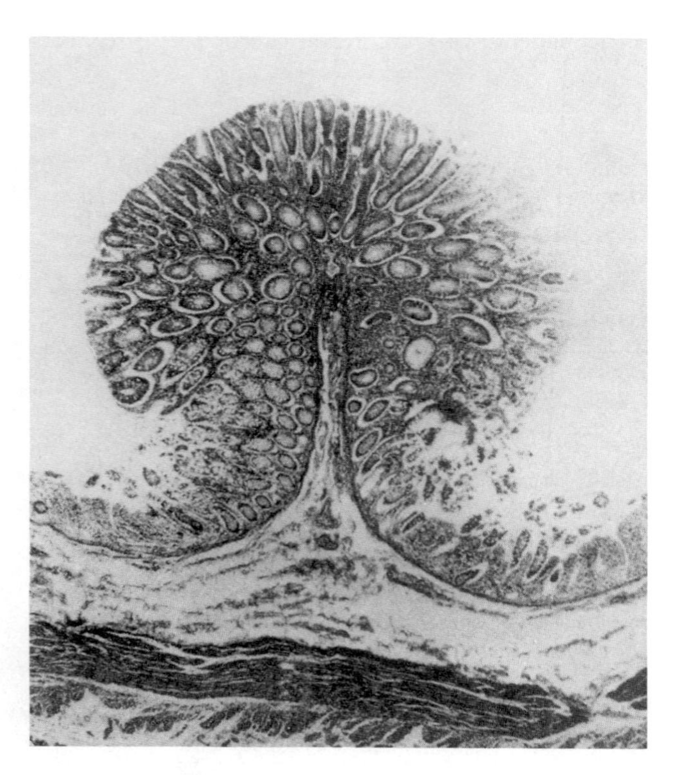

FIG. 4–15. Low-power photograph of adenomatous polyp of the colon.

Phenotypic and genetic alterations as potential markers of cancer risk in adenomatous polyps have been investigated. Blood group antigens have received considerable attention, and various degrees of reversion to fetal patterns, as well as expression of antigens that would be incompatible in normal adult cells, have been reported. Examples of such findings are the abnormal expression of H substance (Compton et al, 1987), Lex antigens, and their sialylated derivatives, disialosyl Lea (Itzkowitz et al, 1988) and Ley (Lundy et al, 1988). Carcinoembryonic antigen has been detected in adenomatous polyps and in the serum of patients of such lesions (Amanti et al, 1985). Abnormalities of cytokeratins, an exceptionally complex group of intermediate filaments, have been detected in colon carcinomas and in villous adenomas but only to a minimal degree in hyperplastic or adenomatous polyps (Chesin et al, 1986). The above phenotypical markers have not yet reached the state of clinical usefulness and have not been tested in prospective studies.

Genotypic alterations have also been detected in adenomatous polyps. Approximately 40% of colon cancers have mutated *ras* genes and similar mutations have been detected in some polyps, especially the c-K-*ras* mutation. Some polyps with atypical changes, however, do not show such mutation (Forrester et al, 1987). Similarly, c-*myc* antigen has been detected in 70% of colon cancers and in villous adenomas. Its expression in adenomatous polyps is intermediate between what is observed in cancers and in normal colonic mucosa. There seems to be some cooperation between these oncogenes: c-*myc* gene transfers rodent cells in culture only when activated *ras* genes are also present (Stewart et al, 1986). Vogelstein and co-workers have studied the molecular alterations in the different stages of the precancerous process. They have proposed a model in which the following key events accumulate in successive generations of cells: (1) a mutation of the familial adenomatous polyposis gene *(FAP)* in chromosome 5q which may be responsible for the hyperproliferative state observed; (2) hypomethylation present in very small adenomas which may lead to aneuploidy and loss of suppressor genes; (3) *ras* gene mutation (usually K-*ras*) which, through clonal expansion, may lead to large adenomas and dysplastic changes; (4) deletion of the *DCC* gene (deleted in colon carcinoma) in chromosome 18q; and (5) allelic deletion in chromosome 17p, usually seen in later stages of the tumor (*p53* suppressor gene deletion or mutation). The progressive accumulation of these molecular lesions, rather than their order with respect to one another, seems to determine the biologic behavior of the tumor and its invasiveness. (Vogelstein et al, 1989; Fearon and Vogelstein, 1990).

Statistical Association between Carcinoma and Adenomatous Polyps. There is a close correlation between the incidence of colon cancer and the prevalence of adenomatous polyps at autopsy in populations for which such data are available. Both entities display a socioeconomic gradient in populations at low or intermediate risk (Haenszel et al, 1975). In developed countries the socioeconomic gradient for colon cancer is not observed consistently. Recent rises in the frequency of both conditions have been reported in blacks in the UnitedStates.

Greater size and multiplicity of polyps correlate positively with colon cancer incidence in interpopulation comparisons. The prevalence and severity of dysplasia in adenomatous polyps are greater in populations at greater risk (Sato et al, 1976). More advanced dysplastic changes have been reported from the sigmoid than from the proximal colon segments, replicating the higher frequency of carcinomas located in the sigmoid as compared to in the more proximal colon segments in most populations (Haenszel and Correa, 1971).

Genetic Susceptibility. There are several indications of the influence of genetic mechanisms in colon cancer causation. Hereditary colonic carcinoma has been classified into three main categories: (1) familial polyposis (including Gardner's syndrome), transmitted as an autosomal dominant condition in which thousands of adenomas cover the large bowel surface; (2) cases with common (but less numerous) adenomas, also transmitted as an autosomal dominant trait, with carcinomas being diagnosed at ages similar of those of the general population; and (3) cases not associated with multiple colonic polyps, the non-polyposis colorectal cancer syndrome. The latter category includes Lynch syndrome I with tumors confined to the large bowel and Lynch syndrome II, which is associated with other cancers, most frequently of the ovary and endometrium (cancer family syndrome) (Lynch et al., 1988). Studies of thymidine incorporation in the colon mucosa of subjects with sporadic adenomas show an expansion of the proliferative zone when compared with normal mucosa of subjects belonging to low-risk families. This method may be a marker of familial susceptibility in the "flat" mucosa, indicating an alteration of cell kinetics previous to the formation of adenomas (Lipkin, 1988).

Follow-Up of Patients with Polyps. A few patients have refused operations to resect adenomatous polyps diagnosed by biopsy. Morson (1974) reports that three such patients later were found to have carcinomas in the same location of the previous polyp. The carcinomas appeared 5, 6, and 13 years after the discovery of the polyps. In another case, the polyp was resected 11 years after diagnosis and was still histologically benign (Prager et al, 1974; Brahme et al, 1974; Olsen et al, 1988). These studies indicate that resection of polyps decreases the risk of subsequent colon cancer in the segment where the polyps were resected but not in more proximal segments not visualized at the time of the original endoscopy. A recently reported study of 500 patients with 1,240 polyps removed by colonoscopy followed by an average of 53 months formed a recurrence rate of 26%, of which approximately 7% demonstrated malignant change. In patients with more than 4 polyps the recurrence rate was 59%. It has been recommended therefore, that after a first polyp resection, colonoscopy be carried out yearly until the colon is cleared of recurrent lesions, followed by colonoscopy at 3-year intervals (Olsen et al, 1988). Removal of adenomatous polyps is one of the strategies for reduction of colorectal cancer incidence through screening (Winawer et al, 1991).

REFERENCES

AMANTI C, MIDIRI G, BENEDETTI M, et al. 1985. Tissue CFA detection by immunoperoxidase (PAD) test in colorectal polyps: correlation with the degree of dysplasia. J Surg Oncol 28:222–290.

ARISTIZABAL N, CUELLO C, CORREA P, et al. 1984. The impact of vaginal cytology on cervical cancer risks in Cali, Colombia. Int J Cancer 34:5–9.

BARA J, HAMELIN L, MARTIN E, et al. 1981. Intestinal M3 antigen, a marker of intestinal-type differentiation of gastric carcinomas. Int J Cancer 28:711–719.

BARRON BA, RICHART RM. 1968. A statistical model of the natural history of cervical carcinomas based on a prospective study of 557 cases. J Natl Cancer Inst 41:1343–1353.

BERRINO F, GATTA G, D'ALTO M, et al. 1986. Efficacy of screening in preventing invasive cervical cancer: a case-control study in Milan, Italy. *In* Hakama H, Miller AB, Day NE (eds): Screening for Cancer of the Uterine Cervix. International Agency for Research on Cancer, Scientific Publication No. 76, Lyon, France, pp. 111–124.

BERTRAM JS, PUNG A, CHURLEY M, KAPPOCK JJ, WILKENS LR, COONEY RV. 1991. Diverse carotenoids protect against chemically induced neoplastic transformation. Carcinogenesis 12:671–678.

BLASER MJ. 1987. Gastric Campylobacter-like organisms, gastritis, and peptic ulcer disease. Gastroenterology 93:371–383.

BONNE C, HARTZ PH, H KLERKS IV, et al. 1938. Morphology of the stomach and gastric secretion in Malays and Chinese and the different incidence of gastric ulcer and cancer in these races. Am J Cancer 33:265–279.

BONNEY GE, ELSTON R, CORREA P, et al. 1986. Genetic etiology of gastric carcinoma. I. Chronic atrophic gastritis. Genet Epidemiol 3:213–224.

BORCHARD F, MITTELSTAEDT A, STUX G. 1979. Dysplasien in resektionmagen und klassifikation problems verschiedener dysplasienformen. Verh Dtsch Ges Pathol 63:250–257.

BORDI C. 1982. I precursori del carcinoma gastrico. Istocitopatologia 3:51–58.

BOYES DA, FIDLER HK, LOCK OR. 1962. Significance of in situ carcinoma of the uterine cervix. Br Med J 1:203–205.

BRAHME F, EKELUND GR, NORDEN JG, et al. 1974. Metachromous colorectal polyps. A comparison between the development of colorectal polyps and carcinoma in persons with and without polyps in their history. Dis Colon Rectum 17:166–171.

BRENES F, RUIZ B, CORREA P, HUNTER FM, et al. 1993. Helicobacter pylori causes hyperproliferation of the gastric epithelium. Pre- and post-eradication indices of proliferating cell nuclear antigen. Am J Gastroenterol 88:1870–75.

BURDETTE W. 1970. Carcinoma of the Colon and Antecedent Epithelium. Springfield, Illinois, Charles C Thomas.

CHAMBERLAIN J. 1986. Reasons that some screening programs fail to control cervical cancer. In Hakama H, Miller AB, Day NE (eds): Screening for Cancer of the Uterine Cervix. International Agency for Research on Cancer, Scientific Publication No. 76, Lyon, France, pp. 161–168.

CHESIN PG, RETTIG WJ, MELAMED MR. 1986. Expression of cytokeratins in normal and neoplastic colonic epithelial cells. Am J Surg Pathol 10:829–835.

CICLITIRA PJ, MACARTNEY JC, EVAN G. 1987. Expression of c-myc in non-malignant and pre-malignant gastrointestinal disorders. J Pathol 151:293–296.

COMPTON C, WYATT R, KONUGRES A. 1987. Immunohistochemical studies of blood group substance H in colorectal tumors using a monoclonal antibody. Cancer 59:118–127.

COPPLESON LW, BROWN B. 1975. Observations on a model of the biology of carcinoma of the cervix: a poor fit between observation and theory. Am J Obstet Gynecol 122:127–136.

CORREA P. 1988. A human model of gastric carcinogenesis. Cancer Res 48:3554–3560.

CORREA P. 1992. Human gastric carcinogenesis. A multi-step and multi-factorial process. Cancer Res 52:6735–6740.

CORREA P, CUELLO C, DUQUE E. 1970. Carcinoma and intestinal metaplasia of the stomach in Colombian migrants. J Natl Cancer Inst 44:297–306.

CORREA P, CUELLO C, DUQUE E, et al. 1976. Gastric cancer in Colombia. III. Natural history of precursor lesions. J Natl Cancer Inst 57:1027–1035.

CORREA P, CUELLO C, FAJARDO LF, et al. 1983. Diet and gastric cancer: nutrition survey in a high risk area. J Natl Cancer Inst 70:673–676.

CORREA P, DUQUE E, CUELLO C, et al. 1972. Polyps of the colon and rectum in Cali, Colombia. Int J Cancer 9:86–96.

CORREA P, HAENSZEL W, CUELLO C, et al. 1990. Gastric precancerous process in a high risk population. I. Cross-sectional studies. II. Cohort follow-up. Cancer Res 50:4731–4740.

CORREA P, MUÑOZ N, CUELLO C, et al. 1989. The role of Campylobacter pylori in gastroduodenal disease. Prog Surg Pathol 10:551–567.

CRAMER DW. 1974. The role of cervical cytology in the declining morbidity and mortality of cervical cancer. Cancer 34:2018–2027.

CUELLO C, CORREA P, ZARAMA G, et al. 1979. Histopathology of gastric dysplasias. Correlations with gastric juice chemistry. Am J Surg Pathol 3:341–500.

DECAPOA A, BALDIN A, MARIEKA P, et al. 1985. Hormone regulated rRNA gene activity is visualized by selective staining of NORs. Cell Biol Int Rep 9:791.

DEWARD F, TRICHOPOULOS D. 1988. A unifying concept of etiology of breast cancer. Int J Cancer 41:666–669.

DUPONT WD, PAGE DL. 1985. Risk factors of breast cancer in women with proliferative breast disease. N Engl J Med 312:146–151.

DUQUE E, CUELLO C, ARISTIZIBAL N, et al. 1979. Premalignant lesions of the cervix in Cali, Colombia. J Natl Cancer Inst 63:953–963.

EWING J. Neoplastic Diseases. Philadelphia, W.B. Saunders, 1928, p. 97.

FEARON E, VOGELSTEIN SA. 1990. A genetic model of colorectal tumorigenesis. Cell 61:709–767.

FILIPE MI, BRANFOOT AC. 1974. Abnormal patterns of mucus secretion in apparently normal mucosa of large intestine with carcinoma. Cancer 34:282–290.

FONTHAM E, CORREA P, RODRIGUEZ E, et al. 1986. Validation of smoking history with the micronuclei test. *In* Hoffman D and Harris C (eds): Mechanisms of Tobacco Carcinogenesis. Cold Spring Harbor Laboratory, pp. 113–119.

FONTHAM E, ZAVALA D, CORREA P, et al. 1986. Diet and chronic atrophic gastritis: a case-control study. J Natl Cancer Inst 76:621–627.

FORMAN D, NEWELL DG, FULLERTON F, et al. 1991. Association between infection with Helicobacter pylori and risk of gastric cancer: evidence from a prospective investigation. Br Med J 302:1302–1305.

FORRESTER K, ALMOGUERA C, HAN K, et al. 1987. Detection of high incidence of k-ras oncogenes during human colon carcinogenesis. Nature 327:298–303.

FRIEND SH, BERNARDS R, ROGELJ S, et al. 1986. A human DNA segment with properties of the gene that predisposes to retinoblastoma and osteosarcoma. Nature 323:643–646.

FUJITA S, HATTORI I. 1977. Cell proliferation, differentiation and migration in the gastric mucosa: a study of the background of carcinogenesis. *In* Farber E, Kawachi T, Nagayo T, et al. (eds): Pathophysiology of Carcinogenesis in Digestive Organs. Baltimore, University Park Press, pp. 21–36.

GANDUR-MANAYMNEH L, PAZ J, ROLDAN E, et al. 1988. Dysplasia of nonmetaplastic gastric mucosa. A proposal for its classification and its possible relationship to diffuse-type gastric carcinoma. Am J Surg Pathol 12:96–114.

GRUNDMANN E. 1975. Histologic types and possible initial stages of early gastric carcinoma. Beitr Pathol Bd 154:256–280.

HAENSZEL W, CORREA P. 1971. Cancer of the colon and rectum and adenomatous polyps. A review of epidemiologic findings. Cancer 28:14–24.

HAENSZEL W, CORREA P, CUELLO C. 1975. Social class differences in large bowel cancer in Cali, Colombia. J Natl Cancer Inst 54:1031–1035.

HAENSZEL W, CORREA P, CUELLO C, et al. 1976. Gastric cancer in Colombia. II. Case-control epidemiologic study of precursor lesions. J Natl Cancer Inst 57:1021–1026.

HAENSZEL W, CORREA P, LOPEZ A, et al. 1985. Serum micronutrient levels in relation to gastric pathology. Int J Cancer 36:43–48.

HAENSZEL W, SEGI M. 1967. Stomach Cancer Among the Japanese. UICC Monograph Series, Vol. 10. Berlin, Springer-Verlag, pp. 55–63.

HAKAMA H, MILLER AB, DAY NE. 1986. Screening for squamous cervical cancer. The duration of low risk following negative results in cervical cytology tests. IARC Working Group Summary. International Agency for Research on Cancer, Scientific Publication No. 76, Lyon, France, pp. 133–142.

HALL JM, FRIEDMAN L, GUENTHER C, et al. 1992. Closing in on breast cancer on chromosome 17q. Am J Hum Genet 50:1235–1242.

HARRIS CC. 1991. Chemical and physical carcinogenesis: Advances and perspectives in the 1990's. Cancer Res (Suppl) 51:5023–5044.

HIGGINS PJ, CORREA P, CUELLO C, et al. 1984. Fetal antigens in the precursor stages of gastric cancer. Oncology (Basel) 41:73–76.

HOWLEY PM, MUNGER K, WERNESS VA, et al. 1989. Molecular mechanisms of transformation by the human papillomaviruses. Int Symp Princess Takamatsu Cancer Res Fund 20:199–206.

IKENBERG H, GISSMAN L, GROSS G, et al. 1989. Human papillomavirus type 16 related DNA in general Bowen's disease and bowenoid papulosis. Int J Cancer 32:563–565.

IMAI T, KUBO T, WATANABE H. 1971. Chronic gastritis in Japanese with reference to high incidence of gastric carcinoma. J Natl Cancer Inst 47:179–195.

ITZKOWITZ SH, YUAN M, FERRELL LU, et al. 1986. Cancer associated alteration of blood group antigen expression in human colorectal polyps. Cancer Res 46:5976–5984.

ITZKOWITZ SH, YUAN M, FOKUSHI Y, et al. 1988. Immunohistochemical comparison of Lea, monosialosyl Lea (CA19-9) and disialosyl Lea antigens in human colorectal and pancreatic tissues. Cancer Res 48:3834–3842.

JARVI O, LAUREN P. 1951. On the role of heterotopias of the intestinal epithelium in the pathogenesis of gastric cancer. APMIS 29:26–44.

JASS J. 1983. A classification of gastric dysplasia. Histopathology 7:181–193.

JENSON AB, ROSENTHAL JR, OLSON C, et al. 1980. Immunological relatedness of papillomaviruses from different species. J Natl Cancer Inst 64:495–500.

Johannesson G, Geirsson G, Day N. 1978. The effect of mass screening in Iceland, 1965–74, on the incidence and mortality of cervical carcinoma. Int J Cancer 21:418–425.

Johnson L, Nickerson RJ, Easterday CC, et al. 1968. Epidemiologic evidence for the spectrum of change from dysplasia through carcinoma in situ to invasive cancer. Cancer 22:901–914.

Kiviat NB, Critchlow CW, Kurman RJ. 1992. Reassessment of the morphological continuum of cervical intraepithelial lesions: Does it reflect different stages in the progression to cervical carcinoma? IARC Sci Publ 119:59–66.

Koss LG. Precancerous lesions. *In* Fraumeni J (ed) 1975. Persons at High Risk of Cancer. New York, Academic Press, pp. 85–102.

Koss LG. 1987. Carcinogenesis in the uterine cervix and human papillomavirus infection. *In* SyrjÑnen K, Gissmann L, Koss LG (eds): Papillomaviruses and Human Disease. Berlin, Springer Verlag, pp. 235–266.

Koss LG, Durfee GR. 1956. Unusual patterns of squamous epithelium of uterine cervix; cytologic and pathologic study of koilocytotic atypia. Ann NY Acad Sci 63:1245–1261.

Kosuka S. 1975. Premalignancy of the mucosal polyp in the large intestine: I. Histologic gradation of the polyp on the basis of epithelial pseudostratification and glandular branching. Dis Colon Rectum 18:483–493.

Kristal AR, Baker MS, Feld AD, et al. 1992. Evaluation of a test for abnormal rectal mucus for earlyl detection of colon cancer. Cancer Epidemiol Biomarkers Prev 1:303–306.

Lane N, Fenoglio CM, Kaye GL, et al. 1978. Defining the precursor tissue of ordinary large bowel carcinoma: implications for cancer prevention. *In* Lipkin M and Good RA (eds): Gastrointestinal Tract Cancer. New York, Plenum Medical Book Co., pp. 295–324.

Langley FA, Compton AC. 1973. Epithelial abnormalities of the cervix uteri. Recent Results Cancer Res 40:86–107.

Lauren P. 1965. The two histological main types of gastric carcinoma: diffuse and so-called intestinal type carcinoma. APMIS 64:31–49.

Leong A, Gilham P. 1989. Silver staining of nucleolar organizer regions in malignant melanoma and melanotic nevi. Hum Pathol 20:257–262.

Levin TJ, Manley MW. 1990. Tumor suppressor genes: the p53 and retinoblastoma sensitivity genes and gene products. Biochim Biophys Acta 1032:119–136.

Lipkin M. 1977. Growth kinetics of normal and premalignant gastrointestinal epithelium. The University of Texas System Cancer Center M.D. Anderson Hospital and Tumor Institute 29th Annual Symposium of Fundamental Cancer Research. Baltimore, Williams and Wilkins, pp. 569–589.

Lipkin M. 1988. Biomarkers of increased susceptibility to gastrointestinal cancer: new application to studies of cancer prevention in human subjects. Cancer Res 48:235–245.

Lipkin M, Correa P, Mikol B, et al. 1985. Proliferative and antigenic modifications in human epithelial cells in chronic atrophic gastritis. J Natl Cancer Inst 75:613–619.

Lipkin M, Newmark H. 1988. Application of intermediate biomarkers and the prevention of cancer of the large intestine. *In* Steele G, Burt RW, Winawer SJ, Kan JP (eds): Basic and Clinical Perspectives of Colorectal Polyps and Cancer. Alan R Liss, New York, pp. 135–150.

Lundy J, Chen J, Wang P, et al. 1988. Phenotypic and genetic alterations in precancerous cells in the colon. Anticancer Res 9:1005–1014.

Lynch HT, Watson P, Lanspa S, et al. 1988. Clinical nuances of Lynch syndromes I and II. *In* Steele G, Burt RW, Winawer SJ, Kan JP (eds): Basic and Clinical Perspectives of Colorectal Polyps and Cancer. Alan R Liss, New York, pp. 177–188.

Mac Mahon B, Cole P, Lin TM, et al. 1979. Age at first birth and breast cancer risk. Bull World Health Organ 43:209–211.

Meisels A, Morin C, Casas-Cordero M. 1984. Lesions of the uterine cervix with papillomaviruses and their clinical consequences. *In* Koss L, Coleman DU (eds): Advances in Clinical Cytology, Vol. 2 New York, Masson, pp. 1–32.

Miki K, Ichinose M, Shimuzu A. 1987. Serum pepsinogens as a screening test of extensive chronic gastritis. Gastroenterol Jpn 22:133–141.

Miller AB, Lindsey J, Hill GB. 1976. Mortality from cancer of the uterus in Canada and its relationship to screening for cancer of the cervix. Int J Cancer 17:602–612.

Ming SC, Goldman H, Freiman DG. 1967. Intestinal metaplasia and histogenesis of carcinoma in human stomach. Cancer 20:1418–1429.

Morin C, Braun I, Casas-Cordero M. et al. 1981. Confirmation of papillomavirus etiology of condylomatons cervix lesions by the peroxidase-antiperoxidase technique. JNCI 66:831–835.

Morson B. 1955. Carcinoma arising from areas of intestinal metaplasia in the gastric mucosa. Br J Cancer 9:377–385.

Morson B. 1974. The polyp-cancer sequence in the large bowel. Proc R Soc Med 67:451–457.

Morson B, Bussey HIR. 1970. Predisposing Causes of Intestinal Cancer. Chicago, Year Book Medical Publishers.

Morson BC, Sobin LH. 1976. Histological typing of intestinal tumors. *In* World Health Organization: International Classification of Tumors. Geneva World Health Organization.

Munger K, Phelps UC, Bubb U, Howley PM. 1989. The E6 and E7 genes of the human papillomavirus type 16 together are necessary for transformation of primary human keratinocyte. J Virol 63:4417–4421.

Muñoz N, Bosch FX, Sanjosé S, et al. 1992. The causal link between HPV and invasive cervical cancer: A population based case-control study in Colombia and Spain. Int J Cancer 52:743–749.

Nardelli J, Bara J, Rosa B, et al. 1983. Intestinal metaplasia and carcinomas of the human stomach: an immunologic study. J Histochem Cytochem 31:366–375.

Narod SA, Feunteun J, Lynch HT, et al. 1991. Familial breast-ovarian cancer locus on chromosome 17q 12–23. Lancet 338:82–83.

Noguchi M, Hirohashi S, Shimosato Y, et al. 1980. Histologic demonstration of antigens reactive with anti p21-ras monoclonal antibody (RAP-5) in human stomach cancers. J Natl Cancer Inst 77:379–385.

Nomura A, Stemmermann GN, Chgou PH, et al. 1991. *Helicobacter pylori* infection and gastric carcinoma in a population of Japanese-Americans in Hawaii. N Engl J Med 325:1132–1136.

Nomura A, Yamakawa H, Ishidate T. 1982. Intestinal metaplasia in Japan: association and diet. J Natl Cancer Inst 68:401–405.

Oehlert W, Keller P, Henke M, et al. 1975. Die dysplasien der magenschleimhaut. Dtsch Med Wochenschr 100:1950–1956.

Olsen WH, Lawrence WA, Snook CW. 1988. Review of recurrent polyps and cancer in 500 patients with initial colonoscopy for polyps. Dis Colon Rectum 31:222–227.

Oshima A, Hirata N, Ubukata T. 1986. Evaluation of a mass screening program of stomach cancer. Int J Cancer 38:829–833.

Page DL, Vander Zwaag R, Rogers LW, et al. 1978. Relation between component parts of fibrocytic disease complex and breast cancer. J Natl Cancer Inst 61:1055–1063.

Parkin M, Pisani P, Ferlay J. 1993. Estimates of world incidence of 12 major cancers in 1985. Int J Cancer 54:594–606.

Parsonnet J, Friedman GD, Vandersteen DT, et al. 1991. Helicobacter pylori infection and risk of gastric cancer. N Eng J Med 325:1127–1131.

Prager ED, Swinton NW, Young J, et al. 1974. Follow-up study of patients with benign mucosal polyps discovered by rectosigmoidoscopy. Dis Colon Rectum 17:322–330.

PROROK PC. 1986. Mathematical models and natural history in cervical cancer screening. *In* Hakana H, Miller AB, Day NE (eds): Screening for Cancer of the Uterine Cervix. International Agency for Research on Cancer, Scientific Publication No. 76, Lyon, France, pp. 185–196.

RICHART RM. 1967. Natural history of cervical intraepithelial neoplasia. Clin Obstet Gynecol 10:748.

RIDDEL R, GOLDMAN H, RANSCHOFF DF, et al. 1983. Dysplasia in inflammatory bowel disease: standardized classification with provisional clinical application. Hum Pathol 14:931–968.

ROSA J, METHA A, FILIPE M. 1990. Nucleolar organizer regions in gastric carcinoma and its precursor stages. Histopathology 16:265–269.

ROSAI J, ACKERMAN LV. 1978. The pathology of tumors: Part precancerous and pseudomalignant lesions. CA Cancer J Clin 28:331–342.

RUSSO J, CALAF G, ROI L, et al. 1987. Influence of age and gland topography on cell kinetics of normal human breast tissue. J Natl Cancer Inst 78:413–418.

RUSSO J, REINA D, FREDERICK J, RUSSO IH. 1988. Expression of phenotypical changes by human breast epithelium cells treated with carcinogens in vitro. Cancer Res 48:2837–2857.

RUSSO IH, RUSSO J. 1988. Hormonal prevention of mammary carcinogenesis: a new approach in anticancer research. Anticancer Res 8:1247–1264.

RUSSO J, RUSSO IH. 1980. Influence of differentiation and cell kinetics on the susceptibility of the rat mammary gland to carcinogenesis. Cancer Res 40:2677–2687.

RUSSO J, RUSSO IH. 1987a. Development of human mammary gland. *In* Neville MC, Daniels CH (eds): The Mammary Gland. New York, Plenum Publishing Corp., pp. 67–93.

RUSSO J, RUSSO IH. 1987b. Biology of disease. Biological and molecular basis of mammary carcinogenesis. Lab Invest 57:112–137.

SAKAMOTO J, WATENABE T, TOKUMARU T, et al. 1989. Expression of Lewisa, Lewisb, Lewisx, Lewisy, Sialyl Lewisa, and sialyl Lewisx blood group antigens in human gastric carcinoma and in normal gastric tissue. Cancer Res 49:745–752.

SAMLOFF M, VARIS K, IHAMAKI T, et al. 1982. Relationship among serum pepsinogen I, serum pepsinogen II and gastric mucosal histology. A study in relatives of patients with pernicious anemia. Gastroenterology 83:204–209.

SARRAF CE, MCCORMICK F, BROWN GR, et al. 1991. Proliferating cell nuclear antigen immunolocalization in gastrointestinal epithelia. Digestion 50:85–91.

SATO E, OUCHI A, SASANO N, et al. 1976. Polyps and diverticulosis of large bowel in autopsy population of Akita prefecture, compared with Miyagi. Cancer 37:1316–1321.

SHAMSUDDIN A, ELSAYED A. 1988. A test for detection of colorectal cancer. Hum Pathol 19:7–10.

SIPPONEN P, LINDGREN J. 1986. Syalitated Lewis determinant CA19-9 in benign and malignant gastric tissue. APMIS 94:305–311.

SIURALA M, ISOKOSKI M, VARIS K, et al. 1968. Prevalence of gastritis in a rural population. Scand J Gastroenterol 3:211–223.

SLAMON DJ, CLARK GM, WONG SG, et al. 1987. Human breast cancer: correlation of relapse and survival with amplification of HER-2/neu oncogene. Science 235:177–182.

SPRATT JS, ACKERMAN LV. 1962. Small primary adenocarcinomas of the colon and rectum. JAMA 279:337–346.

STEMMERMANN GN, SAMLOFF IM, NOMURA AMY, et al. 1987. Serum pepsinogen I and II and stomach cancer. Clin Chim Acta 163:191–198.

STERN E, NEELY PM. 1964. Dysplasia of the uterine cervix. Incidence of regression, recurrence and cancer. Cancer 17:508–512.

STEWART J, EVAN G, WATSON J, et al. 1986. Detection of the c-myc oncogene product in colonic polyps and carcinoma. Br J Cancer 53:1–6.

STOUT AP. (1932). Human Cancer. Philadelphia, Lea and Febiger, p18.

SYRJÄNEN KJ. 1991. Epidemiology of human papillomavirus (HPV) infections and their association with genital squamous cell cancers. Eur J Cancer 27:989–992.

SYRJÄNEN K, PARKINEN S, MANTYJARVI R, et al. 1985a. Human Papillomavirus type as an important determinant of the natural history of HPV infections in uterine cervix. Eur J Epidemiol 227:180–187.

SYRJÄNEN K, VAYRYNEN M, MANTYJARRI R, et al. 1985b. Natural history of cervical human papillomavirus infections based on prospective follow-ups. Br J Obstet Gynaecol 92:1086–1092.

THOR A, OHUCHI N, HORAND H, et al. 1986. Ras gene alterations and enhanced levels of ras p21. Expression in a spectrum of benign and malignant human mammary tissues. Lab Invest 55:603–615.

TORRADO J, BLANCO E, COSME A, et al. 1989. Expression of Type I and Type II blood groups related antigens in normal and neoplastic gastric mucosa. Am J Clin Pathol 91:249–254.

TORRADO J, CORREA P, RUIZ B, et al. 1992a. Lewis antigen alterations in gastric cancer precursors. Gastroenterology 102:424–430.

TORRADO J, CORREA P, RUIZ B, et al. 1992b. Prospective study of Lewis antigen alterations in the gastric precancerous process. Cancer Epidemiol Biomarkers Prev 1:199–205.

VILA LL, FRANCO EL. 1981. Epidemiologic correlates of cervical cancer neoplasia and risk of human papilloma infection in asymptomatic women in Brazil. J Natl Cancer Inst 81:332–340.

US DEPARTMENT OF HEALTH, EDUCATION, AND WELFARE: Ten state nutrition survey. Washington, DC, Publication No. HSM 72-8132, IV 165–IV 174, 1982.

VOGELSTEIN B, FEARON ER, KERN SE, et al. 1989. Allelotype of colorectal carcinomas. Science 244:207–211.

WAKABAYASHI K, NAGAO M, OCHIAI M, et al. 1987. Recently identified nitrite-reactive compounds in food: occurrence and biological properties of the nitrosated products. *In* Bartsch H, O'Neill I, Schutte-Herman R (eds): Relevance of N-Nitroso Compounds to Human Cancer. New York, Oxford University Press, 1987, pp. 287–291.

WARGOVICH MJ, GOLDBERG H, NEWMARK H, et al. 1983. Nuclear aberrations as a short-term test for carcinogenicity to the colon: evaluation of 19 agents in man. J Natl Cancer Inst 71:113–139.

WATTENBERG LW, LAM LKT, SPEIER JL, et al. 1977. Inhibitors of chemical carcinogenesis. Cold Spring Harbor Conferences of Cell Replication. *In* Hiatt HH, Watson JD, Winsten JA (eds.): Origins of Human Cancer. Cold Spring Harbor Laboratory, pp. 785–799.

WEISBURGER JH, MARGUART H, HIROTA N. 1980. Induction of cancer of the glandular stomach in rats by extract of nitrite treated fish. J Natl Cancer Inst 64:163–167.

WILCZYNSKI SP, BERGEN S, WALKER J, et al. 1988. Human papilloma viruses and cervical cancer: analysis of histopathologic features associated with different viral types. Hum Pathol 19:697–704.

WINAWER S, SCHOTTENFELD D, FLEHINGER B. 1991. Colorectal cancer screening. J Natl Cancer Inst 83:243–253.

YAJIMA H, NODA T, DE VILLIERS EM, et al. 1988. Isolation of a new type of human papillomavirus (HPV526) with transforming activity from cervical cancer tissue. Cancer Res 48:7164–7772.

YAMASAKI H, KATOH F. 1988. Further evidence of gap-functional intercellular communication in induction and maintenance of transformed foci in BHLB/c 3t3 cells. Cancer Res 48:3490–3495.

YANG D, TANNENBAUM SR, BUCHI G, et al. 1984. 4-chloro-6-methoxyindole is the precursor of a patent mutagen that forms during nitrosation of the Java bean *(Vicia faba)*. Carcinogenesis (London) 5:1219–1224.

YUNIS JJ, RAMSAY N. 1978. Retinoblastoma and subband deletion of chromosome 13. Am J Dis Child 132(2):161–163.

ZUR HANSEN H. 1987. Papillomaviruses in human cancers. Cancer 59:1692–1696.

5 Stages in neoplastic development

HENRY C. PITOT

Neoplasia, like most disease states, is characterized by a period of latency between the initial etiologic insult and the clinical appearance of the disease itself. In the case of infectious disease, the initial insult is the entrance of the offending organism into the host, and the latent period is the time during which the infectious organism multiplies and alters the host's capacity for response until this combination of factors disrupts the normal homeostasis of the host; this is then manifested as the clinically apparent disease. Other disease states resulting from such problems as autoimmunity, dietary deficiencies, cardiovascular disorders, endocrine abnormalities, and genetic defects exhibit similar latent periods before there is obvious evidence of disease.

The same sequence occurs in neoplastic development, and the evidence for latency here was first noted in the development of specific human neoplasms. Among the first to describe a latency period in human neoplasia was Ramazzini (cf. Wright, 1964), who observed a high incidence of breast cancer in Catholic nuns and reasoned that the causative factor was the lack of parity in this population. This implied a latency period between the lack of pregnancy in the early years of life and the development of mammary carcinoma in later years. An even more direct association was the observation by Percival Pott (1775) of the occurrence of cancer of the scrotum in a number of adult males, all of whom had been chimney sweeps as young boys. From this common factor of their histories, Pott, with remarkable insight, concluded (1) that the occupation of these men as young boys was directly and causally related to their later neoplastic disease and (2) that the soot to which they were exposed in excessive amounts in their work as chimney sweeps was the causative agent of the cancer. Here again, there was a latency period between their work as chimney sweeps and the development of skin cancer many years later.

Many other observations have been made in humans with respect to both chemical carcinogenesis (Miller, 1978) and radiation carcinogenesis (cf. Shimkin, 1977). These, along with the experimental demonstration of chemically induced cancer of the skin in rodents, first observed by Yamagiwa and Ichikawa (1915), all demonstrate the existence of an extensive latent period between the initial exposure to the carcinogenic insult and the appearance of observable neoplasms. However, it was not until the 1940s that a systematic study of the latency period of neoplastic development was undertaken. The pioneering studies of several investigators (Rous and Kidd, 1941; Mottram, 1944; Berenblum and Shubik, 1947) demonstrated that in one model system, epidermal carcinogenesis in the mouse, the latency period of neoplastic development could be divided into at least two separate processes or stages. The first, which occurred at the time of the initial application of the carcinogenic agent, was referred to as *initiation*; the period following that until the appearance of an observable neoplasm, usually stimulated by a second agent, was termed the stage of *promotion*. Little more than a decade later, Foulds (1954) proposed that the stage of initiation, which established "a persistent region of incipient *neoplasia* whence tumors of varied kinds emerge at a later time" (Foulds, 1965), was followed by a process he termed *progression*, which included all of the remainder of neoplastic development. The basis for this latter concept was experimental mammary adenocarcinoma in the mouse. Today these two concepts of the latency period of neoplastic development may be combined into one multistage model, which includes at least three defined stages of development: initiation, promotion, and progression.

IDENTIFICATION AND CHARACTERIZATION OF THE STAGES OF NEOPLASTIC DEVELOPMENT FROM ANIMAL STUDIES

The stages of initiation and promotion, as exemplified by the natural history of epidermal carcinogenesis in the mouse, were studied for many years with relatively little emphasis on the latency period of the development of other histogenetic types of neoplasms. The original two-stage concept was modified by several authors to suggest that the stage of promotion could be divided into at least two phases (Boutwell, 1964; Kinzel et al, 1986; Slaga et al, 1980). The active component of croton oil, which had been used in most experiments on tumor promotion during the first two decades after its discovery, was purified and shown by Hecker (1971) to reside in the chemical, tetradecanoylphorbol acetate (TPA). However, it was not until 1975, with the demonstration of a two-stage development in the natural history of hepatic carcinogenesis in the rat by Peraino and his associates, that a much greater application of the multistage concept of carcinogenesis began to develop.

Today it is apparent that many examples of initiation and promotion occur in the development of a variety of different neoplasms in a number of different species. Some examples are shown in Table 5–1. This list is not meant to be an exhaustive compilation of all examples of the two-stage phenomenon in experimental carcinogenesis, but it does show that this phenomenon is ubiquitous and in all likelihood, under appropriate circumstances, can be demonstrated in the natural history of development of many, if not all, histogenetic types of neoplasm in animals.

Characterization of the Stages of Initiation, Promotion, and Progression from Animal Studies

Of the various examples of two-stage carcinogenesis in animals depicted in Table 5–1, two model systems in

TABLE 5–1. *Animal Systems Exhibiting the Stages of Initiation and Promotion during Carcinogenesis**

Tissue	*Neoplasm*	*Species*	*Initiator*	*Promoter*	*Reference*
Bladder	Papilloma, carcinoma	Dog	2-Naphthylamine	*D*, *L*-tryptophan	Radomski et al, 1978
Bladder	Papilloma, Carcinoma	Rat Rat	MNU, FANFT BBN	Saccharin BHA Urolithiasis	Imaida et al, 1983; Shirai et al, 1987; Cohen, 1983; Hicks, 1980
Colon	Adenoma Adenocarcinoma	Rat Rat	MNNG DMH	Lithocholate Na barbiturate	Reddy and Watanabe, 1979 Pollard and Luckert, 1979
Dermis	Fibrosarcoma	Mouse	3-MC	TPA	Devens et al, 1984
Embryo cells (in vitro)	Foci of altered morphology	Hamster	BP, MNNG	TPA, $1,25\text{-(OH)}_2$	Jones et al, 1984
Epidermis	Papilloma, carcinoma	Mouse, rat, hamster	BP, DMBA, 3-MC, 7-BrMeBA, TEM, Trp-P-2	TPA, skin abrasion, Telcocidin B, Aplysiatoxin, Okadiac acid, Pristane, Chrysartoxin, Dioctanoylglycerol	Slaga et al, 1982; Scribner and Scribner, 1980; Perrella and Boutwell, 1983; Takahashi et al, 1986; Argyris and Slaga, 1981; Sugimura, 1982; Horton et al, 1981; DiGiovanni et al, 1985; Verma, 1988; Suganuma et al, 1988; Schweizer et al, 1982
Epidermis	Melanoma	Hamster, mouse	DMBA	TPA Croton oil	Goerttler et al, 1984 Berkelhammer and Oxenhandler, 1987
Esophagus	Carcinoma Carcinoma	Rat Rat	AMN NNP	TPA NaCl	Matsufuji et al, 1987 Konishi et al, 1986
Forestomach	Papilloma, carcinoma Carcinoma	Rat Rat	MNNG MNNG	BHA Histamine	Shirai et al, 1984 Tatsuta et al, 1983
Liver[a]	Neoplastic nodule, adenoma, hepatocellular carcinoma	Rat	AAF, DMH DEN, DMN DAB, or NNM	PB PB αHCH, CPA, Nafenopin PenCDF Wy-14,643 Choline deficiency Dietary tryptophan TCDD DDT BHT Ethinyl estradiol Mestranol Orotic acid $CHCl_3$ Deoxycholic acid Polyhalogenated biphenyls Dibromoethane	Peraino et al, 1971; Pitot et al, 1978; Schulte-Hermann et al, 1981; Nishizumi and Masuda, 1986; Glauert et al, 1986a; Reddy and Rao, 1978; Shinozuka et al, 1979; Sidransky et al, 1985; Pitot et al, 1980; Peraino et al, 1975; Peraino et al, 1977; Maeura and Williams, 1984; Yager et al, 1984; Rao et al, 1984; Deml and Oesterle, 1985 Cameron et al, 1982; Kimura et al, 1976; Jensen et al, 1982; Milks et al, 1982; Moore et al, 1983

(*continued*)

TABLE 5–1. *(Continued)*

Tissue	Neoplasm	Species	Initiator	Promoter	Reference
Liver	Hepatocellular carcinoma	Hamster	BHP	PB	Makino et al, 1986
					Makino et al, 1986
	Cholangiocarcinoma			DCA	
	Adenomas		DMN	CCl_4	Tanaka et al, 1987
Liver	Hepatocellular adenoma Hepatocellular carcinoma	Mouse (C3H, DBA, CD-1, B6C3F1)	DEN	PB, BHA, DEHP Polychorinated biphenyls TCPOBOP	Hagiwara et al, 1986; Diwan et al, 1986; Anderson et al, 1983; Della Porta et al, 1987
Liver	Hepatoma	Trout	Aflatoxin	Me-sterculate	Lee et al, 1971
Lung	Pulmonary adenomas	Mouse	Urethan 4NQO	BHT Glycerol	Witschi, 1983; Inayama, 1986
Mammary gland	Adenoma/carcinoma	Rat	DMBA	Prolactin, dietary fat, caloric content, and energy utilization	Ip et al, 1980; Ip et al, 1985; Boissonneault et al, 1986;
			NMU	Dietary fat	Cohen et al, 1986
Pancreas	Adenoma, acinar; adenocarcinoma, acinar	Rat	Azaserine	Unsaturated fat	Roebuck et al, 1981;
	Ductular carcinoma	Rat	HAQO	Testosterone	Hayashi and Katayama, 1981
Prostate	Adenocarcinoma	Rat	NMU	Testosterone	Pollard and Luckert, 1987
Stomach, glandular	Adenomas and carcinomas	Rat	MNNG	Nataurocholate	Kobori et al, 1984
	Adenocarcinoma	Rat	MNNG	Formaldehyde	Takahashi et al, 1986
	Adenocarcinoma	Rat	MNNG	p-Methylcatechol	Hirose et al, 1989
	Adenocarcinoma	Rat	MNNG	Somatostatin	Tatsuta et al, 1989
	Adenocarcinoma	Rat	MNNG	Meth and Leu enkephalins	Iishi et al, 1992
Thyroid	Adenomas	Rat	DHPN DEN NMU	PB, AT PB, EPH I_2-deficient diet	Hiasa et al, 1983; Hiasa et al, 1982; Diwan et al, 1988; Ohshima and Ward, 1984
Vagina	Stromal polyp Papilloma, carcinoma	Rat Mouse	NMU DMBA	Estradiol TPA	Sheehan et al, 1982; Goerttler et al, 1980

*Abbreviations used in this table are as follows: MNU, N-methyl-N-nitrosourea; FANFT, N[4-(5-nitro-2-furyl)-2-thiazoyl]formamide; BBN, N-butyl-N-(4-hydroxybutyl)nitrosamine; BHA, butylated hydroxyanisole; MNNG, N-methyl-N[1]-nitro-N-nitrosoguanidine; DMH[1,2], dimethylhydrazine; TPA, tetradecanoyl phorbol acetate; 3-MC, 3-methylcholanthrene; BP, benzo[a]pyrene; 1,25-$(OH)_2$-D_2, 1α,25-dihydroxycholecalciferol; DMBA, 7,12-dimethylbenzanthracene; 7-BrMeBA, 7-bromomethyl benzanthracene; TEM, triethylene melamine; Trp-P-2,3-amino-1-methyl-5H-pyrido[4,3-b]-indole; AMN, N-amyl-N-methylnitrosamine; AAF, 2-acetylaminofluorene; DEN, diethylnitrosamine; DMN, dimethylnitrosamine; DAB, dimethylaminoazobenzene; NNM, N-nitrosomorpholine; αHCH, αhexachlorocyclohexane; PenCDF, 2,3,4,7,8-pentachlorodibenzofuran; CPA, cyproterone acetate; PB, phenobarbital; TCDD, 2,3,7,8-tetrachlorodibenzo-p-dioxin; DDT, dichlorodiphenyltrichloroethane; BHT, butylated hydroxytoluene; DCA, deoxycholic acid; DEHP, di(2-ethylhexyl)-phthalate; TCPOBOP, 1,4-bis[2-(3,5-dichloropyridyloxy)]benzene; 4NQO, 4-nitroquinoline-1-oxide; NMU, N-nitrosomethylurea; HAQO, 4-hydroxyaminoquinoline 1-oxide; DHPN, N-bis(2-hydroxypropyl)nitrosamine; AT, 3-amino-1,2,4-triazole; EPH, 5-ethyl-5-phenylhydantoins; AOM, azoxymethane; PB, phenobarbital.

vivo, epidermal carcinogenesis in the mouse (DiGiovanni, 1992) and hepatocarcinogenesis in the rat (Goldsworthy et al, 1986), have been studied most extensively from the view of their multistage nature. From these two systems it has been possible to characterize the stages of initiation, promotion, and progression, at least to the extent that such characterization may be useful in future experimental studies directed toward understanding the cellular and molecular biologic nature of the latency period in neoplastic development.

Table 5–2 shows the characteristics of the stages of initiation, promotion, and progression that have been found primarily from studies on the mouse skin and rat liver systems. However, it should be noted that these characteristics, with or without some modifications, are potentially applicable to the natural history of the development of any neoplasm in animals and, as we shall see later in this chapter, to a significant extent also in human carcinogenesis.

Initiation. The process of initiation, the first stage in the natural history of neoplastic development, is permanent and irreversible, as demonstrated in several experiments (cf. Boutwell, 1964; Pitot et al, 1978) on the extended time that may occur between initiation and subsequent promotion with virtually no loss in the appearance of lesions. However, the effectiveness of initiation appears to depend on its relationship in time to cellular repli-

TABLE 5–2. *Biological Characteristics of the Stages of Initiation, Promotion, and Progression in Carcinogenesis**

Initiation	*Promotion*	*Progression*
Irreversible, with constant "stem cell" potential.	Reversible increase in replication of progeny of the initiated cell population.	Irreversible. Measurable and/or morphologically discernible alteration in cell genome's structure.
Efficacy sensitive to xenobiotic and other chemical factors.	Reversible alterations in gene expression.	Growth of altered cells sensitive to environmental factors during early phase.
Spontaneous (fortuitous) occurrence of initiated cells can be demonstrated.	Promoted cell population existence dependent on continued administration of the promoting agent.	Benign and/or malignant neoplasms characteristically seen.
Requires cell division for "fixation".	Efficacy sensitive to dietary and hormonal factors.	"Progressor" agents act to advance promoted cells into this stage but may not be initiating agents.
Dose response does not exhibit a readily measurable threshold.	Dose response exhibits measurable threshold and maximal effect dependent on dose of initiating agent.	Spontaneous (fortuitous) progression can be demonstrated.
Relative effect of initiators depends on quantitation of focal lesions following defined period of promotion.	Relative effectiveness of promoters depends on their ability with constant exposure to cause an expansion of the progeny of the initiated cell population.	

*Adapted from Pitot et al (1987a), with permission.

cative DNA synthesis and cell division (Ying et al, 1982; Ishikawa et al, 1980; Hennings et al, 1978). Furthermore, the process of DNA synthesis itself is critical for the "fixation" and thus the irreversibility of initiation (Warwick, 1971; Frei and Ritchie, 1963; McCormick and Bertram, 1982; Borek and Sachs, 1968). Since "spontaneous" neoplasms occur ubiquitously in the human and all experimental animal species, "spontaneous" initiation must have occurred as well. "Spontaneously" or "fortuitously" initiated cells have been identified in the tissues of experimental animals (Emmelot and Scherer, 1980; Popp et al, 1985; Ethier and Ullrich, 1982) and in the human (van Bogaert, 1984). The total number of cells developing from such spontaneous initiation increases with the age of the animal (Schulte-Hermann et al, 1983; Ogawa et al, 1981) as well as after the administration of promoting agents (Pitot et al, 1985). Thus it is not surprising that promoting agents, while exhibiting no demonstrable interaction with macromolecules, can, on extended chronic administration, promote cell growth from spontaneously initiated cells. This process may then ultimately result in malignancy.

The stage of initiation can also be altered as a result of the environmental modification of the metabolism of initiating agents to their ultimate forms (cf. Wattenberg, 1978; Wattenberg et al, 1983; Thompson et al, 1984). The presence or absence of a threshold or no-effect level of the action of initiating agents has been determined only by extrapolation. Such investigations rely on the appearance of neoplasms as a measure of the process of initiation in the majority of instances (Ehling et al, 1983). Furthermore, the direct measurement of initiation in systems such as multistage hepatocarcinogenesis, which allow the quantitative evaluation of the early clones of initiated cells, also demonstrates that initiation is a linear, dose-related phenomenon not exhibiting a readily measurable threshold (Scherer and Emmelot, 1975; Pitot et al, 1987b). In this latter system it is possible to evaluate quantitatively the relative potency of agents as initiators of multistage hepatocarcinogenesis (Pitot et al, 1987b).

Promotion. The characteristic of the stage of promotion that clearly distinguishes it from the stages of initiation and progression is reversibility or instability. In the model systems of multistage carcinogenesis studied most extensively, this characteristic of promotion is evident (Tatematsu et al, 1983; Glauert et al, 1986b; Stenbäck, 1978; DiPaolo et al, 1981). Furthermore, in both multistage hepatocarcinogenesis (Hendrich et al, 1986) and multistage epidermal carcinogenesis (Reddy et al, 1987), focal lesions that disappear when application of the promoting agent is discontinued will reappear on readministration of the promoting agent. The exact mechanism of the loss of cell populations during the period of promotion on removal of the promoting agent is not clear, although in multistage hepatocarcinogenesis it may be due to individual cell death (Bursch et al, 1984). Furthermore, studies by Hanigan and Pitot (1985) demonstrated that hepatic cells in the stage of promotion are actually dependent on the presence of the promoting agent in vivo for their continued existence. This phenomenon is completely analogous to the "dependent" neoplasms of endocrine tissues described by Furth (1968).

Unlike initiation, the stage of promotion can be continually modulated by a variety of environmental alterations, including the frequency with which the promoting agent is administered (Boutwell, 1964), the aging process (Van Duuren et al, 1975), and the composition and amount of the diet (Hendrich et al, 1988; Boutwell, 1964). In concert with the reversible aspect of the stage of promotion, the dose response of promoting agents exhibits a threshold or no-effect level and a maximal response, the latter resulting from the fact that a finite number of cells were initiated and the promoting agent possesses no initiating activity itself (Verma and Boutwell, 1980; Goldsworthy et al, 1984).

Boutwell (1974) has also proposed that the principal molecular action of promoting agents is the alteration of gene expression, an effect also reversed on withdrawal of the promoting agent. Many promoting agents exert their effects on gene expression through the mediation of receptor mechanisms (cf. Pitot, 1986). The regulation of the expression of many genes is altered by the chronic administration of promoting agents such as ornithine decarboxylase (O'Brien et al, 1975), many enzymes of xenobiotic metabolism (cf. Williams, 1984), γ-glutamyl transpeptidase (Kitagawa et al, 1980; Sirica et al, 1984), transglutaminase (Lichti and Yuspa, 1988), and others. Finally, the relative potency of promoting agents may be related to their effectiveness in expanding the population of initiated cell clones, as seen in multistage hepatocarcinogenesis (Pitot et al, 1987b).

Progression. The term *progression* was originally employed by Leslie Foulds (1965) to signify all periods of development of neoplasia beyond the stage of initiation. With the clear demonstration of the stages of initiation and promotion as critical components in the development of a variety of different histogenetic types of neoplasms, such a concept is no longer tenable. However, it is also clear that the appearance of irreversible, aneuploid malignant neoplasms is a component of a stage distinct from that of initiation and promotion (cf. Schulte-Hermann, 1985; Pitot, 1989). As can be seen from the characteristics of this irreversible stage listed in Table 5–2, readily demonstrable changes in the structure of the genome of the neoplastic cell in the stage of progression are evident. Furthermore, such changes are directly related to the increased growth rate, invasiveness, metastatic capability, and biochemical changes in the neoplastic cell during this stage. These latter characteristics of progression had been emphasized by Foulds, but with a greater understanding of the molecular nature of changes in the cell genome and their effects on the structure and function of the cell, a relationship as defined above can now be made. That such changes continue to evolve (progress) during the stage of progression has now been shown in the development of a number of different types of neoplasms, including experimental epidermal carcinogenesis (Aldaz et al, 1987), leukemia and lymphomas (cf. Nowell, 1986), and recently in our own laboratory during multistage hepatocarcinogenesis (Sargent et al, 1989).

Although the usual course of events in the stage of progression is toward greater karyotypic instability (Kraemer et al, 1974), cells in the stage of progression may be induced by treatment with specific chemicals to differentiate terminally, thereby removing them from continued progression to an even more malignant state (Reiss et al, 1986). Other environmental alterations, however, may produce changes in gene expression, growth rate, and functional processes within cells during this stage (Horsfall et al, 1986; Noble, 1977). Chemical agents that act on a cell in the stage of promotion to convert it to the stage of progression exist in the form of complete carcinogens (cf. Pitot, 1986; Pitot, 1991a) and, at least theoretically, as chemical agents exhibiting only such "progressor" activity (Pitot et al, 1987a). Few, if any, agents have been definitively characterized as "progressors" in multistage carcinogenesis, although studies by O'Connell et al (1986) indicate that the free radical generator, benzoylperoxide, may be such an agent. Theoretically, progressor agents must be capable of inducing the genetic changes characteristic of the stage of progression and thus should exhibit some degree of clastogenic activity. That putative progressor agents can act in this manner has now been demonstrated with an "initiation-promotion-initiation" format such as that proposed earlier by Potter (1981) and experimentally demonstrated in the mouse epidermis by Hennings et al (1985). These latter investigators showed that, when the usual initiation-promotion format was followed by the application of a second complete carcinogen, such as an alkylating agent, a rapid and high incidence of carcinomas resulted, unlike that seen in the standard initiation-promotion format in mouse epidermis, which results primarily in benign neoplasms during the timespan of the experiment. With experimental multistage hepatocarcinogenesis in the rat, a similar regimen has been used to induce "foci-within-foci"; these have been proposed as representing the earliest morphologic, discernible beginning of the stage of progression in this tissue (Scherer, 1987; Farber, 1973; Hirota and Yokoyama, 1985). The occurrence of foci-within-foci in many initiation-promotion protocols for rat liver, such as that described by Pitot et al (1978), is relatively infrequent. However, this would be expected if the alteration actually represents the earliest demonstrable lesion at the interface of the stages of promotion and progression, since in this latter model system few malignant neoplasms result, despite the large number of altered hepatic foci seen during the stage of promotion. Thus, the occasional focus-in-focus in this system probably represents spontaneous or fortuitous progression, analogous to spontaneous initiation, in both instances resulting in a genetically new population. Furthermore, specific morphologic markers can be correlated during the natural history of neoplastic development with the stages of promotion and progression in many instances, in both the animal and the human, as we will discuss in the next section.

Conclusions from Animal Experiments. Based on the existence and characteristics of the stages of initiation, promotion, and progression during carcinogenesis in animal systems, the classification of carcinogenic agents may be related to the stage(s) at which they exert their principal effects on the carcinogenic process (cf. Pitot and Dragan, 1991). Such a classification may be seen in Table 5–3, which lists agents that may act primarily at one of the three stages (initiating, promoting, or progressor agents), as well as complete carcinogens with properties to effect any and all of the three stages of carcinogenesis. Not shown in the table are noncarcinogens, which, it is hoped, represent the majority of agents with which humans and animals come in contact during their life spans. Noncarcinogens do not effect any of the stages of carcinogenesis, and thus acute or chronic exposure does not lead to the development of neoplasia. On the other hand, since promoting agents have as their principal mechanistic effect the alteration of genetic expression, a wide variety of substances may exhibit this characteristic and thus could be considered as potential promoting agents.

From the characteristics of the three stages of neoplastic development as seen in animals, it is the stages of initiation and progression that involve changes in the structure of the genome of the cell. Such genetic changes are clearly demonstrable during the stage of progression, and there is overwhelming evidence that initiation results in alterations of the genetic material of the cell as well (Miller, 1978). Thus the natural history of the development of neoplasia in the multistage concept is quite analogous to the two-hit theory of Knudson (1986), developed from studies of neoplasms in the human that exhibit a clear Mendelian pattern of autosomal dominant inheritance. Therefore, with the biology of neoplastic development in the animal becoming somewhat clarified, it is appropriate to apply such knowledge to the natural history of neoplastic development in the human in order (1) to determine whether such conclusions developed from model systems have application to human carcinogenesis and (2) to utilize knowledge gained from both animal and human studies toward the prevention and control of cancer in the human and in animals.

TABLE 5–3. *Classification of Carcinogenic Agents in Relation to Their Action on One or More Stages of Carcinogenesis*

Initiating agent (incomplete carcinogen)—capable only of initiating cells
Promoting agent—capable of causing the expansion of initiated cell clones
Progressor agent—capable of converting an initiated cell or a cell in the stage of promotion to a potentially malignant cell
Complete carcinogen—possessing the capability of inducing cancer in normal cells; usually possessing properties of initiating, promoting, and progressor agents

MULTISTAGE CARCINOGENESIS IN THE HUMAN

Within a decade after the demonstration of the multistage nature of epidermal carcinogenesis in the mouse, epidemiologists and biostatisticians began to consider carcinogenesis in the human as a multistage phenomenon. Nordling (1953) and Armitage and Doll (1954), attempting to explain the increase in cancer in the human with age, proposed models in which the development of neoplasms in the human was a result of a number of separate and stable changes in the preneoplastic and neoplastic cell. The model proposed by the latter authors further suggested that these changes occurred in a definite sequence; this model has been utilized in a consideration of the development of several different types of human neoplasms (cf. Moolgavkar, 1986). Somewhat more recently, Peto (1977) discussed the Armitage and Doll model, considering it in a closer relationship to the biology of the neoplastic process. In addition, Whittemore (1977) expanded on a similar multistage model for human carcinogenesis, also related to the age distribution of human cancer. Perhaps the most significant and biologically applicable multistage model is that of Moolgavkar (1978; 1986), in which two specific events lead to the ultimate development of a malignant cell. This model coincides well with the two-hit model of Knudson (1986) discussed above, as well as with the irreversible nature of the stages of initiation and progression in multistage carcinogenesis, also discussed above.

Evidence for a multistage process in human carcinogenesis comes from a number of sources. One of these is the demonstration in the development of a number of different human histogenetic types of neoplasms of latent preneoplastic and/or premalignant lesions characteristically seen in many patients. Some of the more common of these lesions are listed in Table 5–4. Interestingly, most of these lesions have their counterparts in the development of the same neoplasms in lower forms of life, particularly rodents (Pitot and Dragan, 1993). A text edited by Henson and Albores-Saavedra (1986) details the pathology of such lesions in the human. Several

TABLE 5–4. *Preneoplastic and/or Premalignant Lesions in the Human*

Tissue	Human
Skin	Keratoacanthoma (Haber, 1966)
Tracheobronchial epithelium	Atypical metaplasia (Trump et al, 1978)
Esophagus	Moderate to severe dysplasia (Correa, 1982)
Stomach	Intestinal metaplasia (Saito and Shimoda, 1986)
Colon	Polyp (Day, 1984)
Pancreas	Focal acinar cell dysplasia (Longnecker et al, 1980)
Liver	Liver cell dysplasia (Watanabe et al, 1983) Focal nodular hyperplasia (Knowles and Wolff, 1976)
Bladder	Moderate to severe dysplasia (Murphy and Soloway, 1982)
Adrenal	Adrenocortical nodules (Cohen 1966) In situ neuroblastoma (Beckwith and Perrin, 1963)
Mammary gland	Atypical lobule type A (van Bogaert, 1984) Juvenile papillomatosis (Rosen et al, 1985)
Uterus	Cervical dysplasia (Chi et al, 1977)

characteristics of many of these lesions indicate that they represent cells in the stage of promotion; for example, (1) the numbers of such premalignant lesions far outnumber the number of malignancies that ultimately develop in any single individual, e.g., prostatic carcinoma, neuroblastoma of the adrenal, renal cell carcinoma, and colon carcinoma (cf. Tulinius, 1984); (2) many of these lesions spontaneously disappear with time, e.g., in situ neuroblastoma (Beckwith and Perrin, 1963), and upon withdrawal of the carcinogenic or inciting stimulus, e.g., focal nodular hyperplasia of the liver (Edmondson et al, 1977) and cervical dysplasia (Chi et al, 1977); and (3) the appearance of a malignant lesion arising within a preexisting preneoplastic or benign neoplasm, e.g., carcinoma of the breast (Rosen et al, 1985) and of the gastrointestinal tract (cf. Grundmann, 1983).

Evidence of the Multistage Nature of Human Carcinogenesis—Epidemiologic Studies

The conclusions from epidemiologic investigations with respect to the multistage nature of the development of neoplasia in the human have been closely correlated with several multistage models of carcinogenesis, especially those patterned after the Armitage and Doll model (1954). In this and related models the effect of carcinogenic agents is seen to be primarily in altering the rates at which cells pass from one stage to the next. By such formulations, some agents would affect transitions primarily at an early stage, whereas others would affect the process at a later stage. On the basis of such conclusions, one can then crudely separate carcinogens into "early stage" and "late stage" carcinogens, depending on their primary site of action as evidenced from epidemiologic investigations. Obviously a number of factors are very important in attempting to determine such actions by carcinogens, the most useful relating exposure to time and age. In particular, the time since the initial exposure, the duration of exposure, the time following cessation of exposure, and the age at first exposure to the agent are all important in these considerations, although in many cases it may not be possible to determine each of these parameters with confidence. If the agent is an "early stage" carcinogen, both the increase in incidence beginning with and during exposure and the decrease in incidence following cessation of exposure will be delayed. However, when a late stage is affected, responses both to starting and ceasing exposure will be much more rapid. Such relationships have been discussed by Day and Brown (1980). By this type of reasoning, ionizing radiation may be considered as an early stage carcinogen in the induction of a number of solid neoplasms in the human. In several such instances (Boice et al, 1985), an increased risk of cancer tends to rise only about 10 years after exposure and continues to increase for several decades thereafter. In contrast, the marked excess of reticulum-cell sarcomas after organ transplantation is evident within 6 months after the procedure, indicating that the process may be considered a "late stage" carcinogen by reasoning as above (Kinlen, 1982). On the other hand, the exposure to sunlight and its relation to nonmelanoma skin cancer in the average individual would classify it as an early stage carcinogen, but exposure of patients with the genetic disease xeroderma pigmentosum to the same agent would classify sunlight as a late-stage carcinogen, in view of the extremely rapid appearance of skin neoplasms in such individuals (cf. Berry, 1984). Such a finding points out the critical nature of the genetic background of the individual when such a classification is used. Thus the terms "early" and "late," as used in attempting to correlate multistage models with epidemiologic findings, may not necessarily relate directly to the stages of initiation, promotion, and progression as discussed here.

The incidence of cancer in the human clearly increases with age, but different neoplasms exhibit different peak incidences during the life span of the human (cf. Anisimov, 1983). The incidence of many cancers that exhibit a Mendelian type of inheritance occurs in early childhood, whereas the peak incidence of breast and cervical cancer is usually in the fourth and fifth decades, and that of prostatic cancer after the age of 65. With the possible exception of those neoplasms exhibiting a genetic basis and appearing very early in life, the data argue for extended latent periods in the most common human neoplasms and the likely presence of a multistage nature in the development of these cancers. Even those neoplasms exhibiting an autosomal dominant pattern of inheritance may be considered to have a multistage nature in their development. In this model, all cells of the organism may be considered as initiated, exhibiting a single genetic alteration or "hit," as proposed by Knudson (1986); the second hit, which has now been shown to result from chromosomal or other major genetic changes resulting in homozygosity of the genetic locus associated with tumor development, is comparable to the stage of progression (Murphree and Benedict, 1984).

In considerations of the relationship of age, exposure, and the clinical incidence of malignant neoplasia, the classification of some well-known human chemical agents was proposed by Day (1983), as shown in Table 5–5. In this table, several known human chemical carcinogens are characterized as to whether they are early or late stage carcinogens on the basis of epidemiologic findings. It will be of interest to determine how such a classification relates to the effects, known and proposed, of these agents on the specific stages of carcinogenesis in the development of human neoplasia.

Evidence of the Multistage Nature of Human Carcinogenesis—Action of Carcinogens at Specific Stages of Carcinogenesis

From the viewpoint of pathology and the pathogenesis of human neoplasia as well as epidemiologic studies, the multistage nature of much human cancer is highly probable. On this basis and the findings in numerous animal systems concerning the multistage nature of neoplastic development and the effects of specific carcinogens on specific stages, it is reasonable to propose that known human carcinogenic agents may also exert their effects at specific stages. The epidemiologic classification of human carcinogens briefly noted in Table 5–5 may be considered a forerunner of such an attempt.

TABLE 5–5. *Epidemiologic Classification of Stages in the Development of Several Human Neoplasms**

Carcinogenic Agent	*Site Affected*	*Proposed Stage Affected*
Tobacco smoke	Lung	Early and late
Arsenic	Lung	Late
Nickel	Nasal sinuses	Late
Estrogens	Endometrium	(Very) late
	Breast	Late
Chloromethyl ether	Lung	Early
Ionizing radiation	Breast, thyroid	Early
	Other sites (e.g., leukemia)	Early and other effects
Asbestos	Pleura, peritoneum	Early
	Lung	Early (?) and late
Sunlight	Melanoma	Early (?) and late

*Adapted and modified from Day (1983), with permission.

Table 5–6 lists chemicals and chemical mixtures for which there is sufficient evidence of carcinogenicity to humans on the basis of the findings of the International Agency for Research on Cancer (cf. Vainio et al, 1985). This table does not include a variety of chemical mixtures and processes also known to be carcinogenic, nor does it include infectious agents such as the Epstein-Barr virus, the hepatitis B virus, and the human papillomavirus, all of which have been shown, primarily by epidemiologic investigations, to be carcinogenic in the human (cf. Pitot, 1986).

The table also lists the evidence of carcinogenicity for these agents in animal systems. It should be noted that several chemicals, such as arsenic compounds, benzene, and smokeless tobacco products, are listed as exhibiting either limited or inadequate evidence of carcinogenicity. In smokeless tobacco products, however, *N*-nitrosamines, known to be carcinogenic to animals, have been isolated (Hoffmann and Adams, 1981). The proposed classification of these agents in relation to their effects on the stages of carcinogenesis is related to their known actions on the cellular genome as well as the effects of chronic administration. Thus those agents with known initiating activity are capable of inducing mutations in prokaryotic and related systems, whereas those labeled as progressor agents in this classification exhibit demonstrable clastogenic or chromosome-damaging properties, in line with the characteristics of progression and progressor agents as discussed earlier in this chapter. The presence of question marks indicates a lack of knowledge on the basis of either experimental or human data. This is true because most of these agents have not been tested for their promoting action, and one cannot assume that agents having both initiating and progressor activities would also have promoting action, since at sufficiently high doses initiation and progression may occur simultaneously, leading directly to the development of a malignant neoplasm. For a summary of most of this information, the reader is referred to the discussion by Shelby (1988) on the genetic toxicity of human carcinogens. However, in certain cases, other information is necessary. In analogy to other aromatic amine carcinogens, the designation that 4-aminobiphenyl, benzidine, and 2-naphthylamine have promoting action is reasonable (Schwarz et al, 1984; Saeter et al, 1988). The promoting action of coal tars and tobacco smoke can be demonstrated from data with mouse epidermal carcinogenesis and epidemiologic data in humans (cf. Boutwell, 1964; Loeb et al, 1984). Ultraviolet light of wave lengths 320–360 nm (UVA) has been shown to

TABLE 5–6. *Chemicals and Chemical Mixtures for Which There Is Sufficient (S) Evidence of Carcinogenicity for Humans**

	Evidence of Carcinogenicity[a]		*Proposed Classification in Relation to Effects on the Stages of Carcinogenesis*[b]		
	HUMAN	ANIMAL	INITIATOR	PROMOTER	PROGRESSOR
4-Aminobiphenyl	S	S	+	+	+
Analgesic mixtures containing phenacetin	S	L	±	+	+
Arsenic and certain arsenical compounds	S	I	−	?	+
Asbestos	S	S	−	+	+
Azathioprine	S	L	+	?	+
Benzene	S	L	−	?	+
Benzidine	S	S	+	+	+
N,N′-bis(2-chloroethyl)-2-naphthylamine (chlornaphazine)	S	L	+	?	+(?)
Bis(chloromethyl)ether and technical grade chloromethyl methyl ether	S	S	+	?	+
1,4-Butanediol dimethylsulfonate (Myleran)	S	L	+	?	+
Chlorambucil	S	S	+	?	+
Chromium and certain chromium compounds	S	S	+	?	+
Coal tars	S	S	+	+	+
Conjugated estrogens	S	I	−	+	?
Cyclophosphamide	S	S	+	?	+
Diethylstilbestrol	S	S	−	+	+
Melphalan	S	S	+	?	+
Methoxsalen with UVA therapy (PUVA)	S	S	+	+	+
Mineral oils (certain)	S	S	−	+(?)	−
Mustard gas	S	L	+	?	+
2-Naphthylamine	S	S	+	+	±
Smokeless tobacco products (oral use)	S	I	+	?	?
Tobacco smoke	S	S	+	+	+
Treosulphan	S	ND	+	?	+
Vinyl chloride	S	S	+	+	+

*This table is modified from the article by Vainio et al (1985) and based on the publications of the International Agency for Research on Cancer.

[a]S = sufficient; L = limited; I = inadequate; ND = no data.

[b]+ = evidence for such an action; − = no evidence for such an action; ? = no data available; (?) = data available only problematic.

exhibit promoting action on the development of skin cancer in rodents (Staberg et al, 1983), and thus it is reasonable to suggest that its effect in association with psoralens would combine to result in the complete carcinogenicity of this process. That mineral oils are promoting agents has been shown in rodents by the administration of specific long-chain aliphatic hydrocarbons in the promotion of epidermal carcinogenesis (Baxter and Miller, 1987; Horton et al, 1981) and the development of plasma cell myelomas (Anderson and Potter, 1969). Vinyl chloride is indicated as a complete carcinogen on the basis of its clastogenic and mutagenic effects, although in rodents this agent has the ability both to initiate and to promote focal hepatic lesions (Laib et al, 1985).

Thus, while a number of question marks remain in this proposed classification, future studies in animals and careful epidemiologic investigations may allow us to make a more definitive classification of human carcinogenic agents on the basis of their effects on specific stages in the development of cancer.

IMPLICATIONS OF THE MULTISTAGE DEVELOPMENT OF HUMAN CANCER IN RELATION TO THE NATURE OF CARCINOGENIC AGENTS

Up to the present time, concepts of the action of carcinogenic agents have been generally limited to the general hypothesis that all agents which induce neoplasia act irreversibly on the cellular genome. Although an understanding of the multistage nature of neoplastic development does not radically change this view, it does present new avenues of approach to cancer prevention from a mechanistic, regulatory, and even social viewpoint.

Although the process of initiation is irreversible, it is also, by itself, relatively unimportant, compared with the stages of promotion and progression in relation to the ultimate appearance of cancer as a disease. As pointed out earlier from animal studies and the obvious nature of many human neoplasms, spontaneous or fortuitous initiation is ubiquitous throughout the animal kingdom. Some studies in animals have suggested that this background initiation increases with the age of the animal (Schulte-Hermann et al, 1983), while other investigations have suggested a plateau effect in certain species (Pitot et al, 1985). In the human some epidemiologic evidence argues that initiation must occur early in life in relation to certain childhood neoplasms (cf. Miller, 1978), as well as some seen in the adult (Moolgavkar et al, 1980). In any event, it is later factors in the multistage nature of cancer development that are critical for initiated cells to develop into malignant neoplasms. This is not to diminish the importance of the process of initiation and of attempts to decrease the exposure of humans to initiating agents, but rather to place this stage of neoplastic development in the human in proper perspective in relationship to the stages of promotion and progression.

Based on our knowledge of promoting agents in animals as well as some epidemiologic evidence for their action in the human, the proposal that tumor promotion is quantitatively the most important stage in the genesis of human cancer is not unrealistic. The abuse of tobacco products accounts for more than 30% of human malignant neoplasms in Western society (Doll and Peto, 1981). Although tobacco smoke is a complete carcinogen, epidemiologic evidence argues that it is the stage of tumor promotion, as represented by the continued chronic abuse of tobacco products over many years, that finally results in the development of malignant disease. Cessation of smoking results in a prompt reduction of risk of developing lung cancer, the risk decreasing as the time from cessation increases. This reversibility of the action of this complete carcinogen is that of a promoting agent. Dietary factors have also been implicated in a large percentage of human neoplasms, possibly as high as 25% or 30% (Doll and Peto, 1981). Not only are major dietary constituents such as fat and protein implicated, but abuse of dietary intake has also been related to increased cancer incidence in animals and humans (cf. Willett and MacMahon, 1984). Virtually all of these mechanisms appear to act during the stage of promotion, exhibiting both reversibility and the absence of direct effects on the genome. Finally, endogenous hormones, many of which are promoting agents (Pitot, 1991b), appear to play significant roles in the development of at least two major human cancers—of the breast (Miller, 1981) and of the prostate (Donn and Muir, 1985).

Since the stage of promotion is reversible upon cessation of the chronic exposure to the promoting agent and there is no evidence for a direct effect of promoting agents on genetic structure, preventive effects aimed at this stage are likely to be most efficacious. Furthermore, a number of studies have now demonstrated (cf. Wattenberg, 1985) that chemicals administered to animals during the stage of promotion can actually prevent further action of the promoting agent(s). The active prevention of cancer by the administration of specific chemicals (chemopreventive agents) is a realistic method for the control of a number of human cancers in the future.

It is the stage of progression in which malignant disease appears, which is irreversible, and which is most directly associated with the development of cancer as a disease in the human that directly involves cancer therapy. The activation of a variety of proto-oncogenes, by both mutational and gene amplification mechanisms (Field and Spandidos, 1990; Brison, 1993), has been described in most if not all human neoplasms. On the one hand, while generally multiple genes are involved, in some types of neoplasms a very high percentage of one activated proto-oncogene may occur (Pellegata et al, 1994; Brison, 1993). In a few instances, evidence for the existence of such mutations very early during the development of neoplasia has also been presented (Burmer and Loeb, 1989). On the other hand, mutational alteration of tumor suppressor genes involving both alleles may be even more frequently seen in neoplasia as predicted by Knudsen's hypothesis. Such has been the case with substantial evidence for the involvement of multiple tumor suppressor genes in malignant neoplasms (cf. Yokota and Sugimura, 1993). Thus, as predicted from the characteristics of the stage of tumor progression (Table 5–2), multiple mutations can be expected and are to be found in malignant human neoplasia. Furthermore, with increasing evidence that our environment contains agents—progressor agents—that specifically act to induce this stage, it behooves regulatory agencies to develop assays for such agents and to monitor more closely for their presence in the human environment. This is particularly important in view of the evidence implicating tumor promotion as the stage at which the risk for the development of human cancer increases most. Those progressor agents that are incapable of initiation may act on cells in the stage of promotion and thus become greater potential risks to humans for the development of malignant neoplasms.

Our knowledge and understanding of the multistage development of human neoplasia thus becomes critical in our understanding and rational development of preventive measures for the control of human cancer. A molecular understanding, in all its facets, of the nature of the stage of progression may also lead us to a more rational therapy of this disease in individuals in whom the stages of initiation and promotion have already occurred.

REFERENCES

ALDAZ CM, CONTI CJ, KLEIN-SZANTO AJP, et al. 1987. Progressive dysplasia and aneuploidy are hallmarks of mouse skin papillomas: relevance to malignancy. Proc Natl Acad Sci USA 84:2029–2032.

ANDERSON LM, VAN HAVERE K, and BUDINGER JM. 1983. Effects of polychlorinated biphenyls on lung and liver tumors initiated in suckling mice by *N*-nitrosodimethylamine. J Natl Cancer Inst 71:157–163.

ANDERSON PN, POTTER M. 1969. Induction of plasma cell tumours in BALB/c mice with 2,6,10,14-tetramethylpentadecane (pristane). Nature 222:994–995.

ANISIMOV VN. 1983. Carcinogenesis and aging. Adv Cancer Res 40:365–424.

ARGYRIS TS, SLAGA TJ. 1981. Promotion of carcinomas by repeated abrasion in initiated skin of mice. Cancer Res 41:5193–5195.

ARMITAGE P, DOLL R. 1954. The age distribution of cancer and a multi-stage theory of carcinogenesis. Br J Cancer 8:1–12.

BAXTER CS, MILLER ML. 1987. Mechanism of mouse skin tumor promotion by *n*-dodecane. Carcinogenesis 8:1787–1790.

BECKWITH JB, PERRIN EV. 1963. In situ neuroblastomas: a contribution to the natural history of neural crest tumors. Am J Pathol 43:1089–1104.

BERENBLUM I, SHUBIK P. 1947. A new, quantitative approach to the study of the stages of chemical carcinogenesis in the mouse's skin. Br J Cancer 1:383–386.

BERKELHAMMER J, OXENHANDLER RW. 1987. Evaluation of premalignant and malignant lesions during the induction of mouse melanomas. Cancer Res 47:1251–1254.

BERRY CL. 1984. Temporal variations in carcinogenic effects. Hum Toxicol 3:3–6.

BOICE JD JR, DAY NE, ANDERSEN A, et al. 1985. Second cancers following radiation treatment for cervical cancer. An international collaboration among cancer registries. J Natl Cancer Inst 74:955–975.

BOISSONNEAULT GA, ELSON CE, PARIZA MW. 1986. Net energy effects of dietary fat on chemically induced mammary carcinogenesis in F344 rats. J Natl Cancer Inst 76:335–338.

BOREK C, SACHS L. 1968. The number of cell generations required to fix transformed state in x-ray-induced transformation. Proc Natl Acad Sci USA 59:83–85.

BOUTWELL RK. 1964. Some biological aspects of skin carcinogenesis. Prog Exp Tumor Res 4:207–250.

BOUTWELL RK. 1974. The function and mechanism of promoters of carcinogenesis. CRC Crit Rev Toxicol 2:419–443.

BRISON O. 1993. Gene amplification and tumor progression. Biochim Biophys Acta 1155:25–41.

BURMER GC, LOEB LA. 1989. Mutations in the *KRAS2* oncogene during progressive stages of human colon carcinoma. Proc Natl Acad Sci USA 86:2403–2407.

BURSCH W, LAUER B, TIMMERMANN-TROSIENER I, et al. 1984. Controlled death (apoptosis) of normal and putative preneoplastic cells in rat liver following withdrawal of tumor promoters. Carcinogenesis 5:453–458.

CAMERON RG, IMAIDA K, TSUDA H, et al. 1982. Promotive effects of steroids and bile acids on hepatocarcinogenesis initiated by diethylnitrosamine. Cancer Res 42:2426–2428.

CHI CH, RUBIO CA, LAGERLÖF B. 1977. The frequency and distribution of mitotic figures in dysplasia and carcinoma *in situ*. Cancer 39:1218–1223.

COHEN LA, THOMPSON DO, MAEURA Y, et al. 1986. Dietary fat and mammary cancer. I. Promoting effects of different dietary fats on *N*-nitrosomethylurea-induced rat mammary tumorigenesis. J Natl Cancer Inst 77:33–42.

COHEN RB. 1966. Observations on cortical nodules in human adrenal glands. Their relationship to neoplasia. Cancer 19:552–556.

COHEN SM. 1983. Promotion in urinary bladder carcinogenesis. Environ Health Perspect 50:51–59.

CORREA P. 1982. Precursors of gastric and esophageal cancer. Cancer 50:2554–2565.

DAY DW. 1984. The adenoma-carcinoma sequence. Scand J Gastroenterol 19(Suppl 104):99–107.

DAY NE. 1983. Time as a determinant of risk in cancer epidemiology: the role of multi-stage models. Cancer Surv 2:577–593.

DAY NE, BROWN CC. 1980. Multistage models and primary prevention of cancer. J Natl Cancer Inst 64:977–989.

DELLA PORTA G, DRAGANI TA, MANENTI G. 1987. Two-stage liver carcinogenesis in the mouse. Toxicol Pathol 15:229–233.

DEML E, OESTERLE D. 1985. Dose-dependent promoting activity of chloroform in rat liver foci bioassay. Cancer Lett 29:59–63.

DEVENS BH, LUNDAK RL, BYUS CV. 1984. Induction of murine fibrosarcomas by low dose treatment with 3-methylcholanthrene followed by promotion with 12-O-tetradecanoyl-phorbol-13-acetate. Cancer Lett 21:317–324.

DIGIOVANNI J. 1992. Multistage carcinogenesis in mouse skin. Pharmacol Ther 54:63–128.

DIGIOVANNI J, DECINA PC, PRICHETT WP, et al. 1985. Mechanism of mouse skin tumor promotion by chrysarobin. Cancer Res 45:2584–2589.

DIPAOLO JA, DEMARINIS AJ, EVANS CH, et al. 1981. Expression of initiated and promoted stages of irradiation carcinogenesis *in vitro*. Cancer Lett 14:243–249.

DIWAN BA, RICE JM, OHSHIMA M, et al. 1986. Interstrain differences in susceptibility to liver carcinogenesis initiated by N-nitrosodiethylamine and its promotion by phenobarbital in C57BL/6NCr, C3H/HeNCr^{MTV-} and DBA/2NCr mice. Carcinogenesis 7:215–220.

DIWAN BA, RICE JM, NIMS RW, et al. 1988. P-450 enzyme induction by 5-ethyl-5-phenylhydantoin and 5,5-diethylhydantoin, analogues of barbiturate tumor promoters phenobarbital and barbital, and promotion of liver and thyroid carcinogenesis initiated by *N*-nitrosodiethylamine in rats. Cancer Res 48:2492–2497.

DOLL R, PETO R. 1981. *The Cause of Cancer*. New York, Oxford University Press.

DONN AS, MUIR CS. 1985. Prostatic cancer: some epidemiological features. Bull Cancer (Paris) 72:381–390.

EDMONDSON HA, REYNOLDS TB, HENDERSON B, et al. 1977. Regression of liver cell adenomas associated with oral contraceptives. Ann Intern Med 86:180–182.

EHLING UH, AVERBECK D, CERUTTI PA, et al. 1983. Review of the evidence for the presence or absence of thresholds in the induction of genetic effects by genotoxic chemicals. Mutat Res 123:281–341.

EMMELOT P, SCHERER E. 1980. The first relevant cell stage in rat liver carcinogenesis. A quantitative approach. Biochim Biophys Acta 605:247–304.

ETHIER SP, ULLRICH RL. 1982. Detection of ductal dysplasia in mammary outgrowths derived from carcinogen-treated virgin female BALB/c mice. Cancer Res 42:1753–1760.

FARBER E. 1973. Hyperplastic liver nodules. Methods Cancer Res 7:345–375.

FIELD JK, SPANDIDOS DA. 1990. The role of *ras* and *myc* oncogenes in human solid tumours and their relevance in diagnosis and prognosis (review). Anticancer Res 10:1–22.

FOULDS L. 1954. The experimental study of tumor progression: a review. Cancer Res 14:327–339.

FOULDS L. 1965. Multiple etiologic factors in neoplastic development. Cancer Res 25:1339–1347.

FREI JV, RITCHIE AC. 1963. Diurnal variation in the susceptibility of mouse epidermis to carcinogen and its relationship to DNA synthesis. J Natl Cancer Inst 32:1213–1220.

FURTH J. 1968. Hormones and neoplasia. *In* Engel A, Larson T (eds). Thule International Symposia on Cancer and Aging, pp. 131–151. Stockholm, Nordiska Bokhandelns Förlag.

GLAUERT HP, BEER D, RAO MS, et al. 1986a. Induction of altered hepatic foci in rats by the administration of hypolipidemic peroxisome proliferators alone or following a single dose of diethylnitrosamine. Cancer Res 46:4601–4606.

GLAUERT HP, SCHWARZ M, PITOT HC. 1986b. The phenotypic stability of altered hepatic foci: effect of the short-term withdrawal of phenobarbital and of the long-term feeding of purified diets after the withdrawal of phenobarbital. Carcinogenesis 7:117–121.

GOERTTLER K, LÖHRKE H, HESSE B. 1980. Two-stage carcinogenesis in NMRI mice: intravaginal application of 7,12-dimethylbenz[a]anthracene as initiator followed by the phorbol ester 12-O-tetradecanoylphorbol-13-acetate as promoter. Carcinogenesis 1:707–708.

GOERTTLER K, LOEHRKE H, HESSE B, et al. 1984. Skin tumor formation in the European hamster (*Cricetus cricetus* L.) after topical initiation with 7,12-dimethylbenz[a]anthracene (DMBA) and promotion with 12-O-tetradecanoylphorbol-13-acetate (TPA). Carcinogenesis 5:521–524.

GOLDSWORTHY T, CAMPBELL HA, PITOT HC. 1984. The natural history and dose-response characteristics of enzyme-altered foci in rat liver following phenobarbital and diethylnitrosamine administration. Carcinogenesis 5:67–71.

GOLDSWORTHY T, HANIGAN MH, PITOT HC. 1986. Models of hepatocarcinogenesis in the rat—contrasts and comparisons. CRC Crit Rev Toxicol 17:61–89.

GRUNDMANN E. 1983. Classification and clinical consequences of precancerous lesions in the digestive and respiratory tracts. Acta Pathol Jpn 33(2):195–217.

HABER H. 1966. The skin. *In* Wright GP, Symmers WStC (eds): Systemic Pathology, Vol. II. New York, Elsevier Publishing Co., pp. 1479–1481.

HAGIWARA A, DIWAN BA, WARD JM. 1986. Modifying effects of butylated hydroxyanisole, di(2-ethyl-hexyl)phthalate or indomethacin on mouse hepatocarcinogenesis initiated by *N*-nitrosodiethylamine. Jpn J Cancer Res 77:1215–1221.

HANIGAN M, PITOT HC. 1985. Growth of carcinogen-altered rat hepatocytes in the liver of syngeneic recipients promoted with phenobarbital. Cancer Res 45:6063–6070.

HAYASHI Y, KATAYAMA H. 1981. Promoting effect of testosterone propionate on experimental exocrine pancreatic tumors by 4-hydroxyaminoquinoline 1-oxide in rats. Toxicol Lett 9:349–354.

HECKER E. 1971. Isolation and characterization of the cocarcinogenic principles from croton oil. Methods Cancer Res 6:439–484.

HENDRICH S, GLAUERT HP, PITOT HC. 1986. The phenotypic stability of altered hepatic foci: effects of withdrawal and subsequent readministration of phenobarbital. Carcinogenesis 7:2041–2045.

HENDRICH S, GLAUERT HP, PITOT HC. 1988. Dietary effects on initiation and promotion of hepatocarcinogenesis in the rat. J Cancer Res Clin Oncol 114:149–157.

HENNINGS H, MICHAEL D, PATTERSON E. 1978. Croton oil enhancement of skin tumor initiation by *N*-methyl-*N'*-nitro-*N*- nitrosoguanidine: possible role of DNA replication. Proc Soc Exp Biol Med 158:1–4.

HENNINGS H, SHORES R, MITCHELL P, et al. 1985. Induction of papillomas with a high probability of conversion to malignancy. Carcinogenesis 6:1607–1610.

HENSON DE, ALBORES-SAAVEDRA J. 1986. *The Pathology of Incipient Neoplasia.* Philadelphia, W.B. Saunders Company.

HIASA Y, OHSHIMA M, KITAHORI Y, et al. 1982. Promoting effects of 3-amino-1,2,4-trazole on the development of thyroid tumors in rats treated in *N*-bis(2-hydroxypropyl)nitrosamine. Carcinogenesis 3:381–384.

HIASA Y, KITAHORI Y, KONISHI N, et al. 1983. Effect of varying the duration of exposure to phenobarbital on its enhancement of *N*-bis(2-hydroxypropyl)nitrosamine-induced thyroid tumorigenesis in male Wistar rats. Carcinogenesis 4:935–937.

HICKS RM. 1980. Multistage carcinogenesis in the urinary bladder. Br Med Bull 36:39–46.

HIROSE M, YAMAGUCHI S, FUKUSHIMA S, HASEGAWA R, TAKAHASHI S, ITO N. 1989. Promotion by dihydroxybenzene derivatives of *N*-methyl-*N'*-nitro-*N*-nitrosoguanidine-induced F344 rat forestomach and glandular stomach carcinogenesis. Cancer Res 49:5143–5147.

HIROTA N, YOKOYAMA T. 1985. Comparative study of abnormality in glycogen storing capacity and other histochemical phenotypic changes in carcinogen-induced hepatocellular preneoplastic lesions in rats. Acta Pathol Jpn 35(5):1163–1179.

HOFFMANN D, ADAMS JD. 1981. Carcinogenic tobacco-specific *N*-nitrosamines in snuff and in the saliva of snuff dippers. Cancer Res 41:4305–4308.

HORSFALL DJ, TILLEY WD, ORELL SR, et al. 1986. Relationship between ploidy and steroid hormone receptors in primary invasive breast cancer. Br J Cancer 53:23–28.

HORTON AW, BOLEWICZ LC, BARSTAD AW, et al. 1981. Comparison of the promoting activity of pristane and *n*-alkanes in skin carcinogenesis with their physical effects on micellar models of biological membranes. Biochim Biophys Acta 648:107–112.

IISHI H, TATSUTA M, BABA M, OKUDA S, TANIGUCHI H. 1992. Enhancement by methionine- and leucine-enkephalin of gastric carcinogenesis, induced by *N*-methyl-*N'*-nitro-*N*-nitrosoguanidine in Wistar rats. Oncology 49:407–410.

IMAIDA K, FUKUSHIMA S, SHIRAI T, et al. 1983. Promoting activities of butylated hydroxyanisole and butylated hydroxytoluene on 2-stage urinary bladder carcinogenesis and inhibition of γ-glutamyl transpeptidase-positive foci development in the liver of rats. Carcinogenesis 4:895–899.

INAYAMA Y. 1986. Promoting action of glycerol in pulmonary tumorigenesis model using a single administration of 4-nitroquinoline 1-oxide in mice. Jpn J Cancer Res 77:345–350.

IP C, YIP P, BERNARDIS LL. 1980. Role of prolactin in the promotion of dimethylbenz[*a*]anthracene-induced mammary tumors by dietary fat. Cancer Res 40:364–378.

IP C, CARTER CA, IP MM. 1985. Requirement of essential fatty acid for mammary tumorigenesis in the rat. Cancer Res 45:1997–2001.

ISHIKAWA T, TAKAYAMA S, KITAGAWA T. 1980. Correlation between time of partial hepatectomy after a single treatment with diethylnitrosamine and induction of adenosinetriphosphatase-deficient islands in rat liver. Cancer Res 40:4261–4264.

JENSEN RK, SLEIGHT SD, GOODMAN JI, et al. 1982. Polybrominated biphenyls as promoters in experimental hepatocarcinogenesis in rats. Carcinogenesis 3:1183–1186.

JONES CA, CALLAHAM MF, HUBERMAN E. 1984. Enhancement of chemical-carcinogen-induced cell transformation in hamster embryo cells by 1α,25-dihydroxycholecalciferol, the biologically active metabolite of vitamin D_3. Carcinogenesis 5:1155–1159.

KIMURA NT, KANEMATSU T, BABA T. 1976. Polychlorinated biphenyl(s) as a promoter in experimental hepatocarcinogenesis in rats. Z Krebsforsch 87:257–266.

KINLEN LJ. 1982. Immunosuppressive therapy and cancer. Cancer Surv 1:565–583.

KINZEL V, FÜRSTENBERGER G, LOEHRKE H, et al. 1986. Three-stage tumorigenesis in mouse skin: DNA synthesis as a prerequisite for the conversion stage induced by TPA prior to initiation. Carcinogenesis 7:779–782.

KITAGAWA T, WATANABE R, SUGANO H. 1980. Induction of γ-glutamyl transpeptidase activity by dietary phenobarbital in "spontaneous" hepatic tumors of C3H mice. Gann 71:536–542.

KNOWLES DM, WOLFF M. 1976. Focal nodular hyperplasia of the liver. Hum Pathol 7:533–545.

KNUDSON AG JR. 1986. Genetics of human cancer. Annu Rev Genet 20:231–251.

KOBORI O, SHIMIZU T, MAEDA M, ATOMI Y, WATANABE J, SHOJI M, MORIOKA Y. 1984. Enhancing effect of bile and bile acid on stomach tumorigenesis induced by *N*-methyl-*N*′-nitro-*N*-nitrosoguanidine in Wistar rats. J Natl Cancer Inst 73:853–861.

KONISHI N, KITAHORI Y, SHIMOYAMA T, TAKAHASHI M, HIASA Y. 1986. Effects of sodium chloride and alcohol on experimental esophageal carcinogenesis induced by N- nitrosopiperidine in rats. Jpn J Cancer Res 77:446–451.

KRAEMER PM, DEAVEN LL, CRISSMAN HA, et al. 1974. On the nature of heteroploidy. Cold Spring Harbor Symp Quant Biol 38:133–144.

LAIB RJ, PELLIO T, WÜNSCHEL UM, et al. 1985. The rat liver foci bioassay: II. Investigations on the dose-dependent induction of ATPase-deficient foci by vinyl chloride at very low doses. Carcinogenesis 6:69–72.

LEE DJ, WALES JH, SINNHUBER RO. 1971. Promotion of aflatoxin-induced hepatoma growth in trout by methyl malvalate and sterculate. Cancer Res 31:960–963.

LICHTI U, YUSPA SH. 1988. Modulation of tissue and epidermal transglutaminases in mouse epidermal cells after treatment with 12-O-tetradecanoylphorbol-13-acetate and/or retinoic acid *in vivo* and in culture. Cancer Res 48:74–81.

LOEB LA, ERNSTER VL, WARNER KE, et al. 1984. Smoking and lung cancer: an overview. Cancer Res 44:5940–5958.

LONGNECKER DS, SHINOZUKA H, DEKKER A. 1980. Focal acinar cell dysplasia in human pancreas. Cancer 45:534–540.

MAEURA Y, WILLIAMS GM. 1984. Enhancing effect of butylated hydroxytoluene on the development of liver altered foci and neoplasms induced by *N*-2-fluorenylacetamide in rats. Food Chem Toxicol 22:191–198.

MAKINO T, OBARA T, URA H, et al. 1986. Effects of phenobarbital and secondary bile acids on liver, gallbladder, and pancreas carcinogenesis initiated by *N*-nitrosobis(2-hydroxypropyl)amine in hamsters. J Natl Cancer Inst 76:967–975.

MATSUFUJI H, UEO H, MORI M, et al. 1987. Enhancement of esophageal carcinogenesis induced in rats by *N*-amyl-*N*-methylnitrosamine in the presence of 12-*O*-tetradecanoylphorbol-13-acetate. J Natl Cancer Inst 79:1123–1129.

MCCORMICK PJ, BERTRAM JS. 1982. Differential cell cycle phase specificity for neoplastic transformation and mutation to ouabain resistance induced by *N*-methyl-*N*′-nitro-*n*-nitrosoguanidine in synchronized C3H10T1/2 C18 cells. Proc Natl Acad Sci USA 79:4342–4346.

MILKS MM, WILT SR, ALI I, et al. 1982. Dibromoethane effects on the induction of γ-glutamyl-transpeptidase positive foci in rat liver. Arch Toxicol 51:27–35.

MILLER AB. 1981. Breast cancer. Cancer 47:1109–1113.

MILLER RW. 1978. Environmental causes of cancer in childhood. *In* Barness LA (ed.): Advances in Pediatrics, Vol. 25 Chicago Year Book Medical Publishers, Inc., pp. 97–119.

MOOLGAVKAR S. 1978. The multistage theory of carcinogenesis and the age distribution of cancer in man. J Natl Cancer Inst 61:49–52.

MOOLGAVKAR SH. 1986. Carcinogenesis modeling: from molecular biology to epidemiology. Annu Rev Public Health 7:151–169.

MOOLGAVKAR SH, DAY NE, STEVENS RG. 1980. Two-stage model for carcinogenesis: epidemiology of breast cancer in females. J Natl Cancer Inst 65:559–569.

MOORE MA, HACKER H-J, KUNZ HW, et al. 1983. Enhancement of NNM-induced carcinogenesis in the rat liver by phenobarbital: a combined morphological and enzyme histochemical approach. Carcinogenesis 4:473–479.

MOTTRAM JC. 1944. A developing factor in experimental blastogenesis. J Pathol Bacteriol 56:181–187.

MURPHREE AL, BENEDICT WF. 1984. Retinoblastoma: clues to human oncogenesis. Science 223:1028–1033.

MURPHY WM, SOLOWAY MS. 1982. Urothelial dysplasia. J Urol 127:849–854.

NISHIZUMI M, MASUDA Y. 1986. Enhancing effect of 2,3,4,7,8-pentachlorodibenzofuran and 1,2,3,4,7,8-hexachlorodibenzofuranon diethylnitrosamine hepatocarcinogenesis in rats. Cancer Lett 33:333–339.

NOBLE RL. 1977. Hormonal control of growth and progression in tumors of Nb rats and a theory of action. Cancer Res. 37:82–94.

NORDLING CO. 1953. A new theory on the cancer-inducing mechanism. Br J Cancer 7:68–72.

NOWELL PC. 1986. Mechanisms of tumor progression. Cancer Res 46:2203–2207.

O'BRIEN TG, SIMSIMAN RC, WILLIAMS-ASHMAN HG. 1975. Induction of the polyamino-biosynthetic enzymes in mouse epidermis and their specificity for tumor promotion. Cancer Res 35:2426–2433.

O'CONNELL JF, KLEIN-SZANTO AJP, DIGIOVANNI DM, et al. 1986. Enhanced malignant progression of mouse skin tumors by the free-radical generator benzoyl peroxide. Cancer Res 46:2863–2865.

OGAWA K, ONOE T, TAKEUCHI M. 1981. Spontaneous occurrence of gamma-glutamyl transpeptidase-positive hepatocytic foci in 105-week-old Wistar and 72-week-old Fischer 344 male rats. J Natl Cancer Inst 67:407–412.

OHSHIMA M, WARD JM. 1984. Promotion of *N*-methyl-*N*-nitrosourea-induced thyroid tumors by iodine deficiency in F344/NCr rats. J Natl Cancer Inst 73:289–296.

PELLEGATA NS, SESSA F, RENAULT B, et al. 1994. *K-ras* and *p53* gene mutations in pancreatic cancer: ductal and nonductal tumor progress through different genetic lesions. Cancer Res 54:1556–1560.

PERAINO C, FRY RJM, STAFFELDT EF. 1971. Reduction and enhancement by phenobarbital of hepatocarcinogenesis induced in the rat by 2-acetylaminofluorene. Cancer Res 31:1506–1512.

PERAINO C, FRY RJM, STAFFELDT. E, et al. 1975. Comparative enhancing effects of phenobarbital, amobarbital, diphenylhydantoin, and dichlorodiphenyltrichloroethane on 2-acetylaminofluorene-induced hepatic tumorigenesis in the rat. Cancer Res 35:2884–2890.

PERAINO C, FRY RJM, STAFFELDT E, et al. 1977. Enhancing effects of phenobarbitone and butylated hydroxytoluene on 2-acetylaminofluorene-induced hepatic tumorigenesis in the rat. Food Cosmet Toxicol 15:93–96.

PERRELLA FW, BOUTWELL RK. 1983. Triethylenemelamine: an initiator of two-stage carcinogenesis in mouse skin which lacks the potential of a complete carcinogen. Cancer Lett 21:37–41.

PETO R. 1977. Epidemiology, multistage models and short-term mutagenicity tests. *In* Hiatt HH, Watson JD, Winsten JA (eds): Origins of Human Cancer. Cold Spring Harbor Laboratory, 1403–1428.

PITOT HC. 1986. Fundamentals of Oncology, 3rd ed. New York, Marcel Dekker.

PITOT HC. 1989. Progression: the terminal stage in carcinogenesis. Jpn J Cancer Res 80:599–607.

PITOT HC. 1991a. Characterization of the stage of progression in hepatocarcinogenesis in the rat. *In*: Sudilovsky O, Lotta L, Pitot HC (eds): Boundaries Between Promotion and Progression, New York, Plenum Press, pp. 3–18.

PITOT HC. 1991b. Endogenous carcinogenesis: the role of tumor promotion. Proc Soc Exp Biol Med 198:661–666.

PITOT HC, BARSNESS L, GOLDSWORTHY T, et al. 1978. Biochemical characterization of stages of hepatocarcinogenesis after a single dose of diethylnitrosamine. Nature 271:456–458.

PITOT HC, GOLDSWORTHY T, CAMPBELL HA, et al. 1980. Quantitative evaluation of the promotion by 2,3,7,8-tetrachlorodibenzo-*p*-dioxin of hepatocarcinogenesis from diethylnitrosamine. Cancer Res 40:3616–3620.

PITOT HC, GROSSO LE, GOLDSWORTHY T. 1985. Genetics and epigenetics of neoplasia: facts and theories. Carcinogenesis 10:65–79.

PITOT HC, BEER DG, HENDRICH S. 1987a. Multistage carcinogenesis of the rat hepatocyte. *In* Butterworth BE *Banbury Report 25: Nongenotoxic Mechanisms in Carcinogenesis*. Cold Spring Harbor, New York, Cold Spring Harbor Laboratory, pp. 41–53.

PITOT HC, GOLDSWORTHY TL, MORAN S, et al. 1987b. A method to quantitate the relative initiating and promoting potencies of hepatocarcinogenic agents in their dose-response relationships to altered hepatic foci. Carcinogenesis 8:1491–1499.

PITOT HC, DRAGAN YP. 1991. Facts and theories concerning the mechanisms of carcinogenesis. FASEB J 5:2280–2286.

PITOT HC, DRAGAN YP. 1993. Stage of tumor progression, progressor agents and human risk. Proc Soc Exp Biol Med 202:37–43.

POLLARD M, LUCKERT PH. 1979. Promotional effect of sodium barbiturate on intestinal tumors induced in rats by dimethylhydrazine. J Natl Cancer Inst 63:1089–1092.

POLLARD M, LUCKERT PH. 1987. Autochthonous prostate adenocarcinomas in Lobund-Wistar rats: a model system. Prostate 11:219–227.

POPP JA, SCORTICHINI BH, GARVEY LK. 1985. Quantitative evaluation of hepatic foci of cellular alteration occurring spontaneously in Fischer-344 rats. Fundam Appl Toxicol 5:314–319.

POTT P. 1775. Chirurgical observations relative to the cataract, the polypus of the nose, the cancer of the scrotom, the different kinds of ruptures, and the mortification of the toes and feet. London, Hawes, Clark, and Collins.

POTTER VR. 1981. A new protocol and its rationale for the study of initiation and promotion of carcinogens in rat liver. Carcinogenesis 2:1375–1379.

RADOMSKI JL, KRISCHER C, KRISCHER KN. 1978. Histologic and histochemical preneoplastic changes in the bladder mucosae of dogs given 2-naphthylamine. J Natl Cancer Inst 60:327–333.

RAO PM, NAGAMINE Y, ROOMI MW, et al. 1984. Orotic acid, a new promoter for experimental liver carcinogenesis. Toxicol Pathol 12:173–178.

REDDY AL, CALDWELL M, FIALKOW PJ. 1987. Studies of skin tumorigenesis in PGK mosaic mice: many promoter-independent papillomas and carcinomas do not develop from pre-existing promoter-dependent papillomas. Int J Cancer 39:261–265.

REDDY BS, WATANABE K. 1979. Effect of cholesterol metabolites and promoting effect of lithocholic acid in colon carcinogenesis in germ-free and conventional F344 rats. Cancer Res 39:1521–1524.

REDDY JK, RAO MS. 1978. Enhancement by Wy-14,643, a hepatic peroxisome proliferator, of diethylnitrosamine-initiated hepatic tumorigenesis in the rat. Br J Cancer 38:537–543.

REISS M, GAMBA-VITALO C, SARTORELLI AC. 1986. Induction of tumor cell differentiation as a therapeutic approach: preclinical models for hematopoietic and solid neoplasms. Cancer Treat Rep 70:201–218.

ROEBUCK BD, YATER JD JR, LONGNECKER DS, et al. 1981. Promotion by unsaturated fat of azaserine-induced pancreatic carcinogenesis in the rat. Cancer Res 41:3961–3966.

ROSEN PP, HOLMES G, LESSER ML, et al. 1985. Juvenile papillomatosis and breast carcinoma. Cancer 55:1345–1352

ROUS P, KIDD JG. 1941. Conditional neoplasms and subthreshold neoplastic states. A study of tar tumors in rabbits. J Exp Med 73:365–376.

SAETER G, SCHWARZE PE, NESLAND JM, et al. 1988. 2-Acetylaminofluorene promotion of liver carcinogenesis by a non-cytotoxic mechanism. Carcinogenesis 9:581–587.

SAITO K, SHIMODA T. 1986. The histogenesis and early invasion of gastric cancer. Acta Pathol Jpn 36:1307–1318.

SARGENT L, XU Y-H, SATTLER GL, et al. 1989. Ploidy and karyotype of hepatocytes isolated from enzyme altered foci in two different protocols of multistage hepatocarcinogenesis in the rat. Carcinogenesis, 10:387–391.

SCHERER E. 1987. Relationship among histochemically distinguishable early lesions in multistep-multistage hepatocarcinogenesis. Arch Toxicol (Suppl) 10:81–94.

SCHERER E, EMMELOT P. 1975. Kinetics of induction and growth of precancerous liver-cell foci, and liver tumour formation by diethylnitrosamine in the rat. Eur J Cancer 11:689–696.

SCHULTE-HERMANN R. 1985. Tumor promotion in the liver. Arch Toxicol 57:147–158.

SCHULTE-HERMANN R, OHDE G, SCHUPPLER J, et al. 1981. Enhanced proliferation of putative preneoplastic cells in rat liver following treatment with the tumor promoters phenobarbital, hexachlorocyclohexane, steroid compounds, and nafenopin. Cancer Res 41:2556–2562.

SCHULTE-HERMANN R, TIMMERMANN-TROSIENER I, SCHUPPLER J. 1983. Promotion of spontaneous preneoplstic cells in rat liver as a possible explanation of tumor production by nonmutagenic compounds. Cancer Res 43:839–844.

SCHWARZ M, PEARSON D, PORT R, et al. 1984. Promoting effect of 4-dimethylaminoazobenzene on enzyme altered foci induced in rat liver by *N*-nitrosodiethanolamine. Carcinogenesis 5:725–730.

SCHWEIZER J, LOEHRKE H, HESSE B, et al. 1982. 7,12-demethylbenz[a]anthracene/12-O-tetradecanoyl-phorbol-13-acetate-mediated skin tumor initiation and promotion in male Sprague-Dawley rats. Carcinogenesis 3:785–789.

SCRIBNER NK, SCRIBNER JD. 1980. Separation of initiating and promoting effects of the skin carcinogen 7-bromomethylbenz(a) anthracene. Carcinogenesis 1:97–100.

SHEEHAN DM, FREDERICK CB, BRANHAM WS, et al. 1982. Evidence for estradiol promotion of neoplastic lesions in the rat vagina after initiation with *N*-methyl-*N*-nitrosourea. Carcinogenesis 3:957–959.

SHELBY MD. 1988. The genetic toxicity of human carcinogens and its implications. Mutat Res 204:3–15.

SHIMKIN, MB. 1977. Contrary to Nature. Washington D. C., United States Government Printing Office.

SHINOZUKA H, SELLS MA, KATYAL SL, et al. 1979. Effects of a choline-devoid diet on the emergence of γ-glutamyltranspeptidase-positive foci in the liver of carcinogen-treated rats. Cancer Res 39:2515–2521.

SHIRAI T, FUKUSHIMA S, OHSHIMA M, et al. 1984. Effects of butylated hydroxyanisole, butylated hydroxytoluene, and NaCl on gastric carcinogenesis initiated with *N*-methyl-*N*′-nitro-*N*-nitrosoguanidine in F344 rats. J Natl Cancer Inst 72:1189–1198.

SHIRAI T, TAGAWA Y, FUKUSHIMA S, et al. 1987. Strong promoting activity of reversible uracil-induced urolithiasis on urinary bladder carcinogenesis in rats initiated with *N*-butyl-*N*-(4-hydroxybutyl)nitrosamine. Cancer Res 47:6726–6730.

SIDRANSKY H, GARRETT CT, MURTY CN, et al. 1985. Influence of dietary tryptophan on the induction of γ-glutamyltranspeptidase-positive foci in the livers of rats treated with hepatocarcinogen. Cancer Res 45:4844–4847.

SIRICA AE, JICINSKY JK, HEYER EK. 1984. Effect of chronic phenobarbital administration on the gamma-glutamyl transpeptidase activity of hyperplastic liver lesions induced in rats by the Solt/Farber initiation: selection process of hepatocarcinogenesis. Carcinogenesis 5:1737–1740.

SLAGA TJ, FISCHER SM, NELSON K, et al. 1980. Studies on the mechanism of skin tumor promotion: evidence for several stages in promotion. Proc Natl Acad Sci USA 77:3659–3663.

SLAGA TJ, FISCHER SM, WEEKS CE, et al. 1982. Studies on the

mechanism involved in multistage carcinogenesis in mouse skin. J Cell Biochem 18:99–119.

STABERG B, WULF HC, KLEMP P, et al. 1983. The carcinogenic effect of UVA irradiation. J Invest Dermatol 81:517–519.

STENBÄCK F. 1978. Tumor persistence and regression in skin carcinogenesis. Z Krebsforsch 91:249–259.

SUGANUMA M, FUJIKI H, SUGURI H, et al. 1988. Okadaic acid: an additional non-phorbol-12-tetradecanoate-13-acetate-type tumor promoter. Proc Natl Acad Sci USA 85:1768–1771.

SUGIMURA T. 1982. Potent tumor promoters other than phorbol ester and their significance. Gann 73:499–507.

TAKAHASHI M, HASEGAWA R, FURUKAWA F, et al. 1986. Effects of ethanol, potassium metabisulfite, formaldehyde and hydrogen peroxide on gastric carcinogenesis in rats after initiation with *N*-methyl-*N'*-nitro-*N*-nitrosoguanidine. Jpn J Cancer Res (Gann) 77:118–124.

TAKAHASHI M, FURUKAWA F, MIYAKAWA Y, et al. 1986. 3-Amino-1-methyl-*5H*-pyrido[4,3-^{b}]-indole initiates two-stage carcinogenesis in mouse skin but is not a complete carcinogen. Jpn J Cancer Res 77:509–513.

TANAKA T, MORI H, WILLIAMS GM. 1987. Enhancement of dimethylnitrosamine-initiated hepatocarcinogenesis in hamsters by subsequent administration of carbon tetrachloride but not phenobarbital or *p,p'*-dichlorodiphenyltrichloroethane. Carcinogenesis 8:1171–1178.

TATEMATSU M, NAGAMINE Y, FARBER E. 1983. Redifferentiation as a basis for remodeling of carcinogen-induced hepatocyte nodules to normal appearing liver. Cancer Res 43:5049–5058.

TATSUTA M, IISHI H, BABA M, TANIGUCHI H. 1989. Enhancement by somatostatin of experimental gastric carcinogenesis induced by *N*-methyl-*N'*-nitro-*N*-nitrosoguanidine in Wistar rats. Cancer Res 49:5534–5536.

TATSUTA M, YAMAMURA H, ICHII M, TANIGUCHI H. 1983. Promotion by histamine of carcinogenesis in the forestomach and protection by histamine against carcinogenesis induced by *N*-nitroso-*N*-methylnitroguanidine in the glandular stomach in W rats. J Natl Cancer Inst 71:361–364.

THOMPSON HJ, CHASTEEN ND, MEEKER LD. 1984. Dietary vanadyl(IV) sulfate inhibits chemically-induced mammary carcinogenesis. Carcinogenesis 5:849–851.

TRUMP BF, MCDOWELL EM, GLAVIN F, et al. 1978. The respiratory epithelium. III. Histogenesis of epidermoid metaplasia and carcinoma in situ in the human. J Natl Cancer Inst 61:563–575.

TULINIUS H. 1984. Late determinants of cancer. Pathol Res Pract 179:74–80.

VAINIO H, HEMMINKI K, WILBOURN J. 1985. Data on the carcinogenicity of chemicals in the *IARC Monographs* programme. Carcinogenesis 6:1653–1665.

VAN BOGAERT L-J. 1984. Mammary hyperplastic and preneoplastic changes: taxonomy and grading. Breast Cancer Res Treat 4:315–322.

VAN DUUREN BL, SIVAK A, KATZ C, et al. 1975. The effect of aging between primary and secondary treatment in two-stage carcinogenesis on mouse skin. Cancer Res 35:502–505.

VERMA AK. 1988. The protein kinase C activator *L*-α-dioctanoylglycerol: a potent stage II mouse skin tumor promoter. Cancer Res 48:1736–1739.

VERMA AK, BOUTWELL RK. 1980. Effects of dose and duration of treatment with the tumor-promoting agent, 12-O-tetradecanoylphorbol-13-acetate, on mouse skin carcinogenesis. Carcinogenesis 1:271–276.

WARWICK GP. 1971. Effect of the cell cycle on carcinogenesis. Federation Proc. 30:1760–1765.

WATANABE S, OKITA K, HARADA T, et al. 1983. Morphologic studies of the liver cell dysplasia. Cancer 51:2197–2205.

WATTENBERG LW. 1978. Inhibition of chemical carcinogenesis. J Natl Cancer Inst 60:11–18.

WATTENBERG LW. 1985. Chemoprevention of cancer. Cancer Res 45:1–8.

WATTENBERG LW, BORCHERT P, DESTAFNEY CM, et al. 1983. Effects of *p*-methoxyphenol and diet on carcinogen-induced neoplasia of the mouse forestomach. Cancer Res 43:4747–4751.

WHITTEMORE AS. 1977. The age distribution of human cancer for carcinogenic exposures of varying intensity. Am J Epidemiol 106:418–432.

WILLETT WC, MACMAHON B. 1984. Diet and cancer—an overview. Part I and II. N Engl J Med 310:633–638 and 697–701.

WILLIAMS GM. 1984. Modulation of chemical carcinogenesis by xenobiotics. Fundam Appl Toxicol 4:325–344.

WITSCHI HP. 1983. Promotion of lung tumors in mice. Environ Health Perspect 50:267–273.

WRIGHT WC. 1964. Diseases of Workers. New York, Hafner Publishing Co.

YAGER JD, CAMPBELL HA, LONGNECKER DS, et al. 1984. Enhancement of hepatocarcinogenesis in female rats by ethinyl estradiol and mestranol but not estradiol. Cancer Res 44:3862–3869.

YAMAGIWA K, ICHIKAWA K. 1915. Experimentelle Studie über die Pathogenese der Epithelialgeschwulste. Mitteilungen Med. Facultat Kaiserl Univ. Tokyo 15(2):295–344.

YING TS, ENOMOTO K, SARMA DSR, et al. 1982. Effects of delays in the cell cycle on the induction of preneoplastic and neoplastic lesions in rat liver by 1,2-dimethylhydrazine. Cancer Res 42:876–880.

YOKOTA J, SUGIMURA T. 1993. Multiple steps in carcinogenesis involving alterations of multiple tumor suppressor genes. FASEB J 7:920–925.

6 Molecular and genetic events in neoplastic transformation

RAYMOND W. RUDDON, JR.

Cancer is a complex family of diseases and carcinogenesis is a complex process. From a clinical point of view, cancer is a large group of diseases, perhaps up to a hundred or more, that vary in their age of onset, rate of growth, state of cellular differentiation, diagnostic detectability, invasiveness, metastatic potential, prognosis, and response to various therapeutic modalities. From a molecular and cell-biological point of view, however, cancer may be a relatively small number of diseases in that the molecular lesions which induce cancer seem to result from certain common types of alterations to a cell's genetic apparatus. Ultimately, cancer is a disease of abnormal gene expression. There are several possible mechanisms by which the altered gene expression observed in cancer cells is achieved. This chapter will attempt to define what these mechanisms are.

The field of cancer genetics originated with Boveri's somatic mutation hypothesis for the origin of cancer (Boveri, 1914). He postulated that the abnormality of a cancer cell is caused by "a wrongly combined chromosomal complex" and that this leads to the abnormal proliferation of cancer cells. This trait becomes fixed such that the defect is passed on to all cellular descendents of the original cancer cell. The field of molecular biology has given us new insights into the genetic alterations of cancer cells, and we can now define in elegant detail some of the biochemical aspects of the process that Boveri described. Surprisingly, his ideas turned out to be quite perspicacious.

CANCER AS A CELLULAR DISEASE

Phenotype of the "Typical" Cancer Cell

Cancer cells, in general, have a number of morphological and biochemical features in common. Frequent morphological features are their large nuclei, prominent nucleoli, undifferentiated appearance, and high mitotic index compared to their normal tissue counterparts. The cellular properties that malignant cancer cells have in common include their unregulated cellular proliferation, invasiveness, and metastatic potential. The general characteristics of transformed malignant cells are listed in Table 6–1. A number of these changes may be characteristic of certain rapidly proliferating cell populations and not be specific for the malignant state. No single criterion is adequate, as there are many exceptions both ways: some nontransformed cells have one or more of these characteristics and some transformed cells lack one or more of them. Taken together, however, these criteria appear to define a cell that will produce a tumor when injected into an appropriate host animal. A number of these properties relate only to malignant cells growing in cell culture. However, a number of the properties of transformed cells in culture are characteristic of cancers growing in an animal or a patient.

The evidence that these properties are found in transformed cells and that they are related to malignancy is discussed in the following sections.

Cell Surface Alterations

Malignant transformation of mammalian cells is accompanied by multiple changes in the cell surface or plasma membrane of cells (Hakomori, 1985; Feizi, 1985; Yamashita et al, 1985; Hanski et al, 1991). These alterations are morphological, functional, and immunological in nature. For instance, changes in membrane fluidity, cell surface ionic charge, lectin binding affinity, cell permeability and transport mechanisms, intercellular communication, cell surface associated enzymes and receptors, turnover and shedding of cell surface components, activity of cell surface associated proteases, cellular adhesion to extracellular matrix, and reactivity with antibodies, have all been observed in one or more types of malignantly transformed cells.

While the biochemical basis for all these changes is often not clear, several generalizations can be made. One fact that is clear is that there are compositional

I thank Joan Amato for her careful preparation of the manuscript.

TABLE 6–1. *Properties of Transformed Malignant Cells Growing in Cell Culture and/or In Vivo**

1. Cytologic changes resembling those of cancer cells in vivo, including increased cytoplasmic basophilia, increased number and size of nuclei, increased nuclear: cytoplasmic ratio, and formation of clusters and cords of cells.
2. Alteration in growth characteristics:
   a. "Immortality" of transformed cells in culture. Transformed malignant cells become "immortal" in that they can be passaged in culture indefinitely.
   b. Decreased density-dependent inhibition of growth or loss of "contact inhibition." Transformed cells frequently grow to a higher density than their normal counterparts, and they may pile up in culture rather than stop growing when they make contact.
   c. Decreased serum requirement. Transformed cells usually require lower concentrations of serum or growth factors to replicate in culture than do nontransformed cells.
   d. Loss of anchorage dependence and acquisition of ability to grow in soft agar. Transformed cells may lose their requirement to grow attached to surfaces and can grow as free colonies in a semisolid medium.
   e. Loss of cell cycle control. Transformed cells fail to stop in G_1 or at the G_1/S boundary in the cell cycle when they are subject to metabolic restriction of growth.
   f. Resistance to apoptosis (programmed cell death).
3. Changes in cell membrane structure and function, including increased agglutinability by plant lectins, alteration in composition of cell surface glycoproteins, proteoglycans, glycolipids, and mucins, appearance of tumor-associated antigens, and increased uptake of amino acids, hexoses, and nucleosides.
4. Loss of cell-cell and cell–extracellular matrix interactions that foster cell differentiation.
5. Loss of response to differentiation-inducing agents and altered cellular receptors for these agents.
6. Altered signal transduction mechanisms, including constitutive rather than regulated function of growth factor receptors, phosphorylation cascades, dephosphorylation mechanisms.
7. Increased expression of oncogene proteins due to chromosomal translocation, amplification, or mutation.
8. Loss of tumor suppressor gene protein products due to deletion or mutation.
9. Genetic imprinting errors that lead to overproduction of growth promoting substances, e.g., IGF-2.
10. Increased or unregulated production of growth factors, e.g., TGF-α, tumor angiogenesis factors, PDGF, hematopoietic growth factors (e.g., CSFs, interleukins).
11. Genetic instability leading to progressive loss of regulated cell proliferation, increased invasiveness, and increased metastatic potential. "Mutator" genes may be involved in this effect.
12. Alteration in enzyme patterns. Transformed cells have increased levels of enzymes involved in nucleic acid synthesis and produce higher levels of lytic enzymes, e.g., proteases, collagenases, glycosidases.
13. Production of oncodevelopmental gene products. Many transformed malignant cells growing in culture or in vivo produce increased amounts of oncofetal antigens (e.g., carcinoembryonic antigen), placental hormones (e.g., chorionic gonadotropin), or placental-fetal type isoenzymes (e.g., placental alkaline phosphatase).
14. Ability to produce tumors in experimental animals. This is the sine qua non that defines malignant transformation in vitro. If the cells believed to be transformed do not produce tumors in appropriate animal hosts, they cannot be defined as "malignant." However, failure to grow in an animal model does not rule out the fact that they may be tumorigenic in a different type of animal.
15. Ability to avoid the host's antitumor immune response.

*From Ruddon, 1995a, with permission.

changes in cell surface glycoproteins, glycolipids, and mucins that occur, and many of these may help explain the differences between cancer and normal cells noted above. It is becoming increasingly clear that many changes occurring on the cell surface of cancer cells are related to changes in cell surface carbohydrates. One of the commonly observed alterations in cell surface carbohydrates is a shift to higher molecular weight glycans caused by one or more of the following: increased branching on the trimannosyl core of asparagine-linked oligosaccharides, increased polylactosaminoglycan chain formation, and increased sialylation (Easton et al, 1991). These changes in carbohydrates have also been associated with reduced cellular adhesion to the extracellular matrix and with increased invasiveness and metastatic potential of tumor cells.

Recently, the enzymatic basis for some of these changes has been found. There are several glycosyltransferase activities in mammalian cells that are responsible for the synthesis and processing of oligosaccharides on cell surface glycoproteins and glycolipids. One important family of these are the N-acetyl-glucosaminyl (GlcNAc) transferases (Fig. 6–1) (Yamashita et al, 1985; Mizuochi et al, 1983). Six of these have been identified: GlcNAc transferases I through VI. The activities of certain of these are altered during transformation of cells by oncogenic viruses or in cancer tissues. Examples include an increase in GlcNAc transferase V in baby hamster kidney (BHK) cells transformed with polyoma vi-

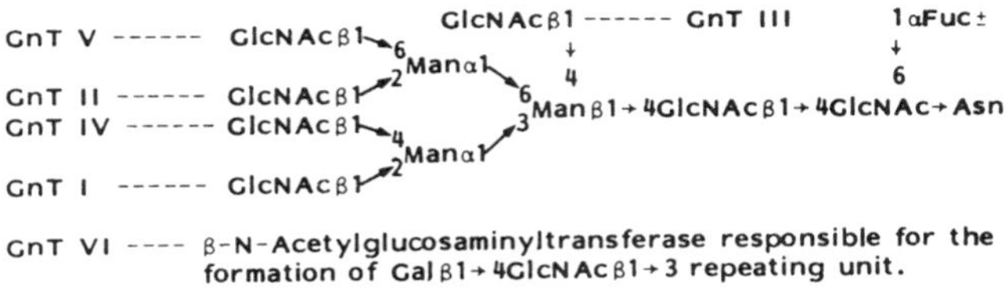

FIG. 6–1. A structure showing the possible β-N-acetylglucosamine residues that can be attached to the trimannosyl cores of the complex-type asparagine-linked sugar chains. The different β-N-acetylglucosaminyltransferases (abbreviated as *GnT*) responsible for the addition of each β-N-acetylglucosamine residue are indicated by the Roman numerals *I* through *VI*. [from Yamashita, 1985, with permission].

ruses or Rous sarcoma virus, increases in GlcNAc transferase III in hepatomas, and increases of both GlcNAc III and V in *ras* transformed NIH 3T3 cells (Easton et al, 1991). In addition, alterations in the levels of oligosaccharide elongating enzymes have been found in virally transformed cells. These changes in enzyme activities appear to explain the increased branching of N-linked oligosaccarides, the elongated polylactosaminoglycan chains, and the increased sialylation of carbohydrates often observed in cancer cells. This in turn explains, at least in part, the altered antigenicity of tumor cells and the fact that many monoclonal antibodies made against animal and human tumor cells recognize a carbohydrate-determined epitope. Many of these tumor antigens have turned out to be modifications of blood group–specific antigens that reflect an earlier stage of cellular differentiation of the tissue from which the cancer was derived (Feizi, 1985; Yamashita et al, 1985). As yet, many of the genes for these carbohydrate synthesis and processing enzymes have not been cloned and their regulatory mechanisms are yet to be clarified.

Extracellular Matrix. The extracellular matrix (ECM) is the complex structure of carbohydrate and protein-containing components that make up the basement membranes underlying epithelial tissues and that support structural tissues such as bone and muscle. The ECM forms sheet-like structures that appear early in the differentiation steps of development and that serve as a support and a barrier for cell layers (Yurchenco and Schittny, 1990). It is now apparent that the basement membranes of epithelial tissues, first seen in the light microscope years ago, serve a complicated role in cell-cell adhesion and in the regulation of cell proliferation and differentiation. The ECM that makes up basement membranes is a target for the lytic enzymes secreted by metastatic cancer cells (see below). The biochemical components of the ECM of epithelial tissues include laminin, type IV collagen, heparin sulfate proteoglycan, entactin, and fibronectin, as well as other components that contribute to the ECM of specific tissues, e.g., osteonectin in bone.

ECM components are produced early in the development of multicellular organisms by cells in tissues undergoing differentiation. It is now known that the ECM is not an inert structural element in tissues but that it provides important signals that regulate gene expression, cell proliferation, and cell differentiation. Cells' interactions with the ECM are mediated by cell surface receptors that link the ECM to the internal cellular skeletal network via a transmembrane component of the receptors. One of the important ECM components in this transmembrane signaling process is laminin, which is a large (450,000 molecular weight) glycoprotein, cruciate in structure, and with multiple binding domains for cell surface receptors and other components of the ECM (Mecham, 1991). Several types of laminin binding proteins have been identified on cell surface membranes. Those include a high affinity 67 kDA "receptor," galactoside binding lectins, galactosyltransferase, sulfatides, and integrins, a family of cell surface receptors that bind various ECM components, including fibronectin, vitronectin, thrombospondin, collagen, and von Willebrand factor as well as laminin.

The interactions of tumor cells with the ECM are important in determining the invasiveness and metastatic potential of cancer cells, and the ability of cancer cells to attach to laminin correlates with their metastatic potential (Cioce et al, 1991). The 67 kDa high affinity laminin receptor has been particularly associated with a cancer cell's metastatic capability, in that highly metastatic cells express higher levels of laminin receptors on their surface than do less metastatic or benign tumor cells of the same tissue type. A number of examples can be cited: the number of laminin receptors on breast carcinoma cells correlates with the extent of lymph node metastases in patients; the number of 67 kDa laminin receptors also correlates with the degree of invasiveness and metastasis of colon carcinoma cells in patients with that disease (Cioce et al, 1991).

Thus for cancer cells to be invasive and metastatic they apparently need to attach to the ECM, locally degrade it to slip into the blood stream or lymphatic channels, and circulate to distant organs, attach to endothelium, invade again, and set up housekeeping in the new target organ. (This process will be described in greater detail in the next section.) Attachment of cells via laminin receptors is thus important for at least two of the steps involved in metastasis: initial attachment to the ECM and attachment to the endothelium in target organs.

Other attachment factors, however, are also important in the metastatic process. One of these attachment factors is a type of cell-cell adhesion molecule (CAM) called E-cadherin. It acts as a calcium-dependent adhesion factor for cell-cell interactions of epithelial cells and plays a key role in the normal development of epithelial tissues (Vleminckx et al, 1991). Loss or aberrant expression of E-cadherin has been implicated in the invasive and metastatic potential of tumor cells. *ras*-transformed, invasive Madin-Darby canine kidney (MDCK) cells lack E-cadherin expression, but if the E-cadherin cDNA is transfected into these cells, they lose their invasiveness (Vleminckx et al, 1991). Similarly, noninvasive clones of *ras*-transformed MDCK cells are rendered invasive by transfection of a plasmid encoding E cadherin–specific antisense RNA. Moreover, human cancer cell lines from bladder, breast, lung, and pancreas carcinomas were found to be noninvasive by an in vitro assay if they expressed E-cadherin and invasive if they did not (Frixen et al, 1991). The former could be rendered invasive if treated with monoclonal antibodies to E-cadherin, and the latter could be made noninvasive by transfection with E-cadherin cDNA.

Taken together, these data indicate the importance of cell adhesion to the ECM and of cell-cell adhesion molecules (CAMs) in the expression of the metastatic phenotype. Strategies, then, to increase the expression of normal CAMs in tumor tissue might be thought of as ways to modulate this phenotype.

Tumor Metastasis

For the most part, the reason that cancer is a fatal disease is because cancer cells can invade through tissues and metastasize to distant organs in the body. Not all the cells in a tumor mass have equal metastatic potential, but those that do represent a significant population of the cells in a malignant tumor that has reached a progressive stage (Liotta et al, 1983; Fidler, 1990). Invasion and metastasis are facilitated by attachment factors that tumor cells use to attach to the ECM and endothelium of blood vessels as noted above, by lytic enzymes such as proteases, collagenases, and glycosidases that allow tumor cells to penetrate through tissue barriers, by an increased motility, and possibly by tissue chemoattractants that may play a role in the selective "homing" of tumor cells to certain organs (Liotta et al, 1983).

Proteases and Collagenases. The invasive and metastatic potential of tumor cells has been correlated in a number of studies with the activity of various protease activities, including serine proteases such as plasmin (activated by plasminogen activator), thiol proteases such as the cathepsins, and metalloproteases such as type IV collagenase (Liotta et al, 1991). These proteolytic activities do not go unabated in tissues, even tumor tissues, because there are a number of tissue protease inhibitors that keep them in check under normal conditions. Proteases, after all, are needed for a number of natural processes such as normal tissue repair, tissue remodeling during development, and implantation of the blastocyst and growth of the placenta during normal pregnancy. In these instances, as opposed to highly malignant tumors, the proteases and anti-proteases are kept in a tightly regulated balance, the mechanisms for which are not entirely clear, but probably involve the local release of growth factors, feedback from the ECM, etc. For example, metalloproteases are induced by interleukin-1, epidermal growth factor (EGF), and platelet-derived growth factor (PDGF) (Matrisian, 1990), whereas transforming growth factor beta (TGF-ß) has been shown to induce the production of plasminogen activator inhibitor type 1 and to decrease the degradation of the ECM by human fibrosarcoma cells in culture (Cajot et al, 1990). Thus normally there is a stringently regulated process that controls the release of proteases and their inactivation once they have done their job. Tumor cells of the metastatic variety have lost or do not respond to this control mechanism.

Another important concept for understanding the biology of tumor metastasis is the interaction of cancer cells with the surrounding stroma in which they grow. Cross-talk among the cancer cells, the ECM, and the supporting stroma occurs. As an epithelial tumor grows and breeches the ECM, the tumor cells come into contact with the fibroblasts and other mesenchymal cells in the supporting stroma. Via production and secretion of various growth factors and cytokines and interaction among tumor cells, stromal cells, and ECM components, the process of invasion and metastasis goes on. This is also, apparently, part of the process by which tumors become vascularized. They secrete factors called *tumor angiogenesis factors* that induce the growth of vascular endothelial channels through the stroma and ECM to reach the tumor, and that appears to be the time in the life cycle of a malignant neoplasm when it undergoes a spurt of growth and becomes more aggressive (Folkman et al, 1989).

Interestingly, Chambon and his colleagues (Basset et al, 1990) have isolated a gene of the ECM-degrading metalloprotease family (which they have called *stromolysin-3*) which is expressed in stromal cells of invasive breast carcinomas but not in less advanced in situ breast carcinomas. Furthermore, the fact that the gene is expressed at high levels in the stromal cells of invasive breast carcinomas, but not in carcinoma cells themselves, suggests that release of a factor from the carcinoma cells induces the expression of the stromolysin-3 gene and that this event is related to tumor progression.

An important family of metalloprotease inhibitors found in tissues are the tissue inhibitors of metalloprotease (TIMPs). Two of these have been identified: TIMP-1 and TIMP-2. In some animal models, administration of TIMP-1 inhibits metastasis, and transfection of antisense TIMP-1 RNA induces oncogenicity in murine 3T3 cells (Liotta et al, 1991). Addition of TIMP-2 to the cell culture medium has been shown to block the invasiveness of human fibrosarcoma cells in an in vitro assay (Albini et al, 1991).

The cathepsins are a family of cysteine proteases that also appear to be involved in the metastatic process. Cathepsin B activity is elevated in a variety of human and animal tumors and is found at higher levels in metastatic as opposed to nonmetastatic B16 melanoma cells (Rozhin et al, 1990). Cathepsin L is expressed at higher levels in a wide variety of human cancers than in their normal counterpart tissues (Chauhan et al, 1991). Other proteases and protease inhibitors have been found in tumor tissue, including tumor-associated trypsinogen-2 (TAT-2) and a corresponding inhibitor (TATI) (Koivunen et al, 1991). Undoubtedly, more tumor-associated proteases and tissue protease inhibitors will be found in the future, and this whole area is a fertile ground for learning more about the biology of tumor metastasis.

Another way that cancer cells may disrupt the normal architecture of the ECM is by producing an incomplete or faulty ECM in the area of a growing tumor. There is evidence, for example, of altered biosynthesis and deposition of ECM components by human (Frenette et al, 1988) as well as animal (Dulbecco et al, 1988) malignant neoplasms. Again, the number of genes involved in ECM production and their control is only poorly understood, but this area is beginning to undergo intense scrutiny.

Cancer Metastasis Genes. Cell fusion experiments, similar to those described for the discovery of tumor suppressor genes (see below), have shown that when metastatic tumor cells are fused with nonmalignant cells, the resulting hybrid cells that are tumorigenic are not metastatic (Sidebottom and Clark, 1983), suggesting the presence of metastasis suppressor genes. Such genes have now been found.

A metastasis suppressor gene, called *nm*23, was identified by mRNA "subtraction" experiments comparing the content of mRNA found in metastatic vs. nonmetastatic murine melanoma cells (Steeg et al, 1988). The levels of *nm*23 mRNA were ten-fold lower in melanoma cell lines of high metastatic potential compared to those with low potential. Subsequently, a similar gene has been found in human cells and low levels of its expression have been correlated with metastasis and poor patient prognoses in breast cancer (Hennessy et al, 1991). However, in human colon tissue, *nm*23 mRNA levels were increased in colon carcinoma cells compared to normal colonic mucosa (Haut et al, 1991), suggesting that *nm*23 gene expression is controlled differently in different tissues.

The function of the *nm*23 gene has recently been identified. There is a gene in the fruitfly *Drosophila* that, when mutated, causes morphologically deformed wing discs in the larval stage. This gene, called *awd,* for abnormal wing discs gene, has been cloned and sequenced. After the *nm*23 gene sequence was determined, a gene database search revealed that it was 78% homologous to the *awd* gene. A further clue came when the cDNA clones for nucleoside diphosphate kinase (NDP kinase) were isolated from the slime mold *Dictyostelium* and from a *Myxococcus* microorganism. These cDNA clones were found to be highly homologous to the *nm23/awd* gene, and the *awd* gene product was subsequently shown to be a NDP kinase (Biggs et al, 1990).

NDP kinases are an ubiquitous family of enzymes that catalyze the transfer of the terminal phosphate group of 5′-triphosphate nucleoside donors to diphosphate nucleoside acceptors, e.g., guanosine disphosphate (GDP) to guanosine triphosphate (GTP) via adenosine triphosphate (ATP). These kinases participate in functions that could affect tumor cell proliferation and metastasis by an action on G protein–coupled signal transduction mechanisms that regulate microtubule assembly, since GTP is required for this function. The NDP kinase coded for by the *awd* gene is associated with microtubules in *Drosophila* larvae (Biggs et al, 1990). What role this might have in tumor metastasis is speculative at this point, but since microtubules are important for cell locomotion and for response to external signals mediated by the ECM, loss of regulatory mechanisms mediated by NDP kinases could result in loss of normal matrix-cell interactions.

Another putative metastasis suppressor gene has been identified in human mammary epithelial cells (Zou et al, 1994). The product of this gene, called *maspin,* is related to the serpin family of protease inhibitors (*ser*ine *p*rotease *in*hibitors) (Potempa et al, 1994). Maspin is expressed in normal mammary epithelial cells but not in most mammary carcinoma cell lines. Transfection of the maspin gene into a human mammary carcinoma cell line did not alter the cells' growth properties in vitro, but reduced the ability of the transfected cells to induce tumors and metastasize in nude mice. These cells also had a reduced ability to invade through a basement membrane matrix in vitro. Maspin expression was also reduced or lost in advanced breast cancer specimens from patients, suggesting that maspin is a tumor metastasis suppressor in vivo.

Types of Genetic Alterations That Occur in Cancer Cells

Most, if not all, of the phenotypic characteristics that typify a malignant cancer cell are the result of some alteration of gene readout. Thus in addition to the crucial cell surface events described above, the enhanced state of proliferation, decreased differentiation, altered enzyme patterns, increased production of growth factors and their receptors, as well as other cancer cell–associated phenotypic characteristics, result from changes in expression of nuclear genes.

Several alterations in the regulation of gene expression have been observed in malignant cells. These include chromosomal alterations manifest by changes in ploidy, translocation events, and deletions; changes in gene copy number (amplification); and alterations in gene transcription, due to mutations in promoter or enhancer regions of genes as well as to rearrangements and insertions of regulatory sequences that alter the transcription of structural genes.

Chromosomal Abnormalities in Cancer. The discovery of the Philadelphia chromosome (Ph^1) by Nowell and

Hungerford (1960) in patients with chronic myelogenous leukemia (CML) was one of the first definitive chromosomal abnormalities described for human cancer. Ph[1] turned out to be a shortened chromosome 22 resulting from a translocation of a piece of chromosome 22 to chromosome 9 (Rowley, 1973). More than 90% of patients with CML have this alteration, and the fact that it occurs only in the leukemia cells argues that it is related to the malignant transformation of these cells.

Numerous other chromosomal breakages and rearrangements have also been observed in human cancer cells (reviewed in Rowley, 1990; Solomon et al, 1991). The observation that many of these alterations involve a relatively limited number of breakpoints suggests that certain regions of human chromosomes are more susceptible to damage by carcinogenic agents than others. Indeed, the location and "fragility" of such sites appears to be heritable, and several of these sites correspond to breakpoints frequently observed in the chromosomal rearrangements seen in cancer cells (Yunis, 1983). A number of fragile sites have been detected in the human genome. In one study, 7 of 17 fragile sites were found to occur at chromosomal sites involved in rearrangements or deletions seen in human cancer cells. In addition, 12 of 13 chromosomes containing fragile sites have been observed to be altered in cancer tissue (Le Beau and Rowley, 1984). That at least some of these fragile sites are targets for chemical carcinogens is suggested by the fact that a deletion of a specific part of chromosome 7 is seen in patients who develop acute nonlymphocytic leukemia after a history of exposure to radiation, alkylating agents, or pesticides (Yunis, 1983).

Of approximately 329 chromosomal sites detected by chromosomal banding techniques in the human genome, 90 breakpoints have been observed in a review of over 3,800 cases of cancer (Mitelman, 1984). These aberrations were distributed over all chromosomes except number 19 and the sex chromosomes. Of these, the most common alterations involved breakpoints on chromosomes 11, 5, 1, 3, 9, 8, 17, 22 and 6, in order of decreasing number detected per chromosome. A number of these frequently affected chromosomes contain genes coding for enzymes involved in nucleic acid synthesis or intermediary metabolism and contain the genetic loci of cellular oncogenes (Rowley, 1990; Solomon et al, 1991).

Translocations and Inversions. Reciprocal translocations are typical of leukemias and lymphomas. More than 100 commonly occurring translocations have been observed (Solomon et al, 1991). The fact that many of these occur consistently in certain specific cancer types argues strongly that they are involved in a key way in generating the malignant phenotype.

As noted above, the first constant translocation observed was the reciprocal translocation between the long arm (called q) of chromosome 9, band 34 and band 11 of the q arm of chromosome 22 (for the location of the band, the short arm p above the centromere and long arm q below the centromere are divided numerically). The shorthand used by cytogeneticists to describe this is t(9;22)(q34;q11).

Later it became apparent that the t(9;22) translocation in CML involved a breakpoint near the Abelson (*abl*) protooncogene. Indeed, as it turned out, this was just one of many such translocations involving protooncogenes in leukemia and lymphoma. In fact, the common involvement of protooncogenes in these breakpoints is strong evidence for the involvement of these genes in the malignant process of leukemia and lymphoma. The first translocation junction involving a protooncogene to be analyzed was actually the t(8;14) translocation seen in Burkitt's lymphoma (Dalla-Favera et al, 1982; Taub et al, 1982) (Fig. 6–2). This translocation results in the translocation of the *myc* cellular protooncogene from chromosome 8 to chromosome 14 near the immunoglobulin heavy chain Cμ *(Ig-Cμ)* gene, resulting in the activation of the *myc* gene.

The genes involved in the breakpoint junction of CML were the next to be identified. In 1982 Hagemei-

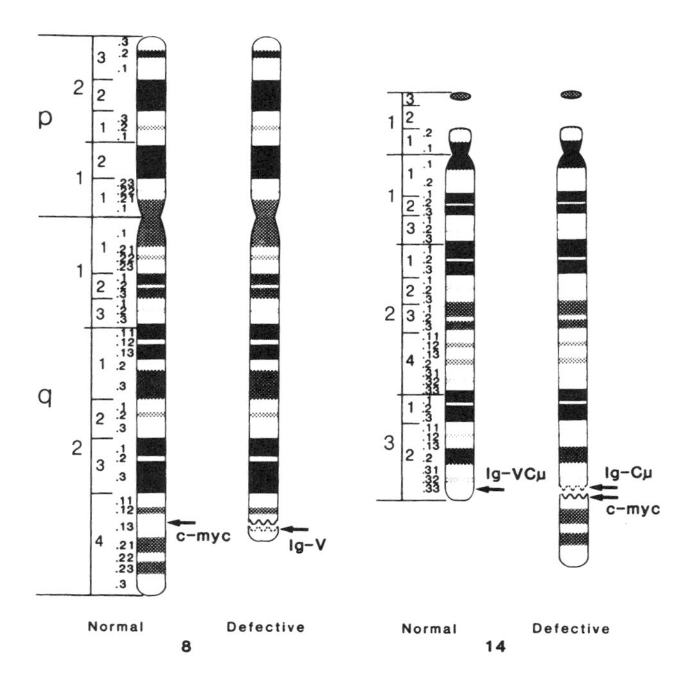

FIG. 6–2. Location of *c-myc* oncogene and heavy-chain immunoglobulin variable (*V*) and constant μ (C_μ) genes on normal and defective chromosomes 8 and 14 in Burkitt's lymphoma, represented at the 1200-Giesma band stage. The defective chromosome 8 loses the *c-myc* and gains *V* genes. The defective chromosome 14 gains *c-myc* from chromosome 8, becoming contiguous or near to C_μ. *Arrows* point to the normal and rearranged location of these genes. *Broken ends* of defective chromosomes indicate breakpoint sites. [From Yunis, 1983, with permission].

jier et al. showed that the c-*abl* gene was translocated from chromosome q to the Ph[1] chromosome (chromosome 22). This was identified because of its homology to the viral oncogene v-*abl* isolated from a mouse pre-B-cell leukemia. Using a probe derived from the v-*abl* gene, Heisterkamp et al. (1985) identified by chromosomal "walking" (see below) across the translocation junction sequences that were derived from chromosome 22, thus proving a reciprocal translocation event. The breakpoints on chromosome 22 in 17 out of 17 CML patients examined occurred within a 5.8 kilobase segment, which they called the breakpoint cluster region, or *bcr*. The breakpoints in *abl* on chromosome 9 occur at variable sites, but always in introns. As a result of the translocation, the *abl* gene piece containing exon II through to its 3′ terminus is moved to the midpoint of the *bcr* gene, which encodes a GTPase activating protein (GAP), forming a fusion gene, which codes for a chimeric Bcr-Abl protein. This protein has high tyrosine kinase activity, a signal transduction mechanism often deregulated in cancer cells.

Another well-defined translocation (t(11;14)) involves the *bcl*1 gene, originally defined by its rearrangement with the immunoglobin heavy chain locus (IgH) in B-cell chronic lymphocytic leukemia (B-CLL), diffuse B cell lymphoma, and multiple myeloma (Tsujimoto et al, 1984). *bcl*2 is another oncogene identified by translocation, in this case by the t(14;18) translocation observed in follicular lymphoma (Haupt et al, 1991). *bcl*2 is involved in regulation of lymphocyte proliferation and differentiation and acts to prolong cell survival.

Genes encoding transcriptional regulatory factors are frequently involved in translocation breakpoints seen in hematologic malignancies. For example, two related helix-loop-helix (HLH) type transcriptional regulators LYL1 and TCL5 are rearranged in T-cell acute lymphoblastic leukemia (T-ALL) (Solomon et al, 1991). Myc is an HLH protein that is translocated and deregulated in both B- and T-cell neoplasms. The TCL3 locus identified in the t(10;14) of some T-ALLs codes for a homeobox protein, HOX11, also a transcriptional regulator.

The multiplicity of translocation events in various cancers strongly suggests that they have a causal relationship in inducing the cancer phenotype. However, some of them may occur as secondary events in the evolution of more aggressive phenotypic changes. The inherent genetic instability of malignant cells leads to further karyotypic abnormalities as the disease progresses, reflecting additional genetic alterations that increase growth potential.

Evidence that malignant transformation of cells doesn't usually result from single translocation events comes from patients with ataxic telangiectasia, who have an increased likelihood of developing leukemia. These patients may have T-lymphocytes with a translocation present for several years before leukemia develops (Russo et al, 1989). Similarly, some patients with benign follicular hyperplasia have *bcl*2 gene rearrangements (Limpens et al, 1991). Thus additional genetic mutation events must occur to trigger the development of the full-blown malignant phenotype.

Chromosomal Deletions. A driving force for the detection of genetic abnormalities in cancer cells is the application of the techniques of molecular biology, e.g., gene cloning, in situ hybridization, restriction endonuclease mapping of gene sequences, and polymerase chain reaction (PCR) analysis of gene transcription. The use of these techniques has led to the conclusion that a given chromosomal abnormality may be associated with a variety of neoplasms, and that a given oncogene can be activated in a variety of human cancers.

Certain general statements can be made about the kinds of chromosomal abnormalities seen. The most common defects observed in solid tumors are deletions in specific gene sequences sometimes observed as loss of a part of a banding region or the loss of heterozygosity of a specific genetic allele (Fearon et al, 1985). Reciprocal translocations between two chromosomes are also observed; however, in the case of solid tumors, as contrasted with leukemia and lymphoma, few of these translocation breakpoints have been cloned. Gene amplifications are sometimes observed as homogeneously staining regions on chromosome banding patterns or as small chromosome-like fragments in cells called *double-minute chromosomes.* Single base substitutions or point mutations also occur in a variety of cancers (see below). As in the case of the translocations discussed above, many of the genetic changes seen in solid tumors result in activation of a cellular oncogene. In tumors with genetic deletions, a tumor suppressor gene may be lost.

Deletion of genetic material in a cancer cell suggests loss of function that regulates cell proliferation or differentiation. More than 20 human solid tumors have been shown to have some type of chromosomal deletion (Table 6–2) and the number is growing as more tumors are analyzed by molecular techniques. Some chromosome deletions appear to be specific for certain tumor types. These include deletion del(13)(q14q14) seen in retinoblastoma that results in loss of the *RB* (retinoblastoma) tumor suppressor gene, the 11p13 deletion in Wilms' tumor, and the deletion of the *DCC* (deleted in colon cancer) gene in colon carcinoma (see below). Deletions in the long arm of chromosome 5 (del 5q) are seen in a number of hematologic diseases, including acute nonlymphocytic leukemia and chronic myeloproliferative disorders. These deletions commonly involve the 5q21-31 region that contains genes encoding growth

TABLE 6–2. *Deletion and Loss of Heterozygosity in Solid Tumors**

Tumor	Chromosomal Deletion in Tumor	Allele Loss
	Cloned	
Retinoblastoma	13q14	13q
Colorectal carcinoma	17p 18q	5q; 17p; 18q
Wilms' tumor	11p13	11p
	Noted	
Bladder adenocarcinoma	1q21-23 Monosomy 9	9q; 11p; 17
Breast adenocarcinoma	1p11-13 3p11-13 3q11-13	1p; 1q; 3p; 11p; 13q; 16q; 17p; 17q; 18q
Glioma	1p32-36 6p15-q27 7q22-q34 8p21-23 9p24-p13	17
Leiomyosarcoma (intestine)	1p12-12	NT[a]
Leiomyoma (uterus)	6p21 7q21-31	NT
Lipoma	13q12-13	NT
Lung adenocarcinoma	3p13-23	3p; 13q; 17p
Lung small cell carcinoma	3p13-23	3p; 13q; 17p
Mesothelioma	3p21-25	NT
Mesothelioma (pleura)	1p11-13	NT
Malignant fibrous histiocytoma	1q11	NT
Melanoma	1p11-22 6q11-27	1p
Meningioma	Monosomy 22 22q12-13	22q12-qter
Neuroblastoma	1p32-36	1p
Ovarian adenocarcinoma	3p13-21 6q15-23	3p; 6q; 11p; 17q
Prostatic adenocarcinoma	7q22 10q24	10; 16
Renal cell carcinoma	3p13-21	3p
Uterine adenocarcinoma	1q21-23	3p

Source: Reprinted with permission from Solomon et al., Chromosome aberrations and cancer. *Science* 254:1153. Copyright 1991 by the American Association for the Advancement of Science.

[a]NT, not tested.

factors and growth factor receptors involved in myeloid cell differentiation (Wasmuth et al, 1989). The *p53* tumor suppressor gene–containing region of chromosome 17p is deleted or mutated in a wide variety of human cancers.

The fact that there is such commonality among cancer cell types in the loss of chromosomal material strongly suggests that these regions contain genes coding for regulatory factors involved in cell proliferation and/or differentiation of a wide variety of cell types. Many of these regions contain genes involved in cell cycle regulation through interaction with factors called *cyclins* or in signal transduction pathways that regulate response elements of particular growth regulatory genes.

Induction of the malignant neoplastic process is thought to involve at least two genetic "hits." In the case of genetically predisposed tumors, the first genetic alteration may be inherited through the germline, with the second alteration occuring after birth. In genetically predisposed cells, the remaining single normal allele may be sufficient to maintain normal growth regulation, and a second deletion or mutation is required to inactivate the remaining normal allele. In the case of a tumor suppressor gene, both alleles are then, in effect, lost or inactivated.

Loss of heterozygosity at a genetic locus has frequently been the mechanism for detecting deletion or mutation of genes involved in cancer causation. This is detectable by a technique called *restriction fragment length polymorphism* (RFLP).

Gene Amplification. Gene amplification can occur at different levels. A gene that is usually present in a single copy in normal cells may be duplicated or undergo a small increase in copy number. This is ordinarily difficult to detect by molecular or cytogenetic techniques. A second level of amplification may involve ten- to 100-fold or so increases in copies of a genetic locus containing certain genes (the amplified region is sometimes called an *amplicon*). This level of amplification may be manifest by homogeneously staining regions (HSRs) or extrachromosomal double-minute chromosomes (DMs) (Alitalo et al, 1983; Alitalo, 1985). A third level of amplification can result from the duplication of whole chromosomes leading to a trisomy of an individual chromosome or in some cases to increases in a number of chromosomes (polyploidy).

Amplifications of genes observed in human cancers include amplification of the N-*myc* gene in stage III and IV neuroblastoma, of the epidermal growth factor receptor–regulated gene *her-2/neu* in advanced breast and ovarian carcinomas, and of the *int*-2, *hst*1, and *prad*1 oncogenes in breast and squamous cell carcinomas and in melanoma.

Trisomy of chromosome 8 has been observed in acute myelocytic leukemia (AML), acute lymphocytic leukemia (ALL), and myeloproliferative disease. Trisomy of chromosome 9 has been seen in myeloproliferative disorders and of chromosome 12 in malignant lymphoma and lymphoproliferative disorders. Some malignant lymphomas have a trisomy of 3, and a trisomy of 7 has been found in some carcinomas and neurogenic tumors (reviewed in Solomon et al, 1991).

Aneuploidy. The genetic instability manifested during tumor progression is characterized by a variety of aberrations in the genome, including point mutations; gene deletions, rearrangements, and amplifications; chromosome translocations; and abnormal chromosome number, known as *aneuploidy*. Although the more subtle changes in the genome—namely, point mutations, gene deletions, and gene rearrangements—may be associated with initiation of the malignant transformation process, gross changes in the number of chromosomes usually occur as tumors progress in malignancy. As noted earlier, certain chromosomal deletions, translocations, and trisomies are characteristically associated with a particular form of cancer; these are called *nonrandom chromosomal alterations*. Changes in cell ploidy, however, are associated with a variety of tumor types in their advanced stages and may be random in the sense that no definitive pattern of chromosome number is associated with a given tumor type. In advanced cancers, both random and nonrandom chromosomal alterations may be found. These continuing genomic changes bring about tumor heterogeneity and the natural selection of more highly invasive and metastatic cancers. Thus tumor progression, in a sense, may be viewed as a highly accelerated evolutionary process (Sager et al, 1985).

Disomy. An unusual type of inheritance pattern has been observed in patients with a genetically determined large fetus syndrome called Beckwith-Wiedemann syndrome (BWS). In these patients there is a propensity to develop malignant neoplasms, particularly Wilms' tumor of the kidney, but hepatoblastomas and rhabdomyosarcomas also occur. These patients have a uniparental paternal disomy for the 11p15.5 region of chromosome 11 and a loss of the maternal allele of this locus in the tumors that they develop (Henry et al, 1991). In an analogous fetal overgrowth syndrome in the mouse, a region of chromosome 7 homologous to human chromosome 11p15.5 also contains a paternal disomy (Ferguson-Smith et al, 1991). Interestingly, this locus contains the gene for insulin-like growth factor 2 (IGF-2), and an increased level of IGF-2 mRNA is seen in the tumors of BWS patients. Since the maternal allele of this locus is lost in these tumors, it suggests that overexpression of growth promoting genes (IGF-2) and loss of a tumor suppressor function on the maternal chromosome locus 11p15 combine to cause the malignant tumors in these individuals.

Genomic Imprinting. Genomic imprinting, which is the selective repression of expression of a genetic allele from either the maternal or paternal gene set, is a known phenomenon in *Drosophila* and mice, but was until recently not observed in humans. It is now known to be the likely cause of loss of regulation of some genes in human cancer. For example, as noted above, in patients with Beckwith-Wiedemann syndrome, who have a high propensity to develop Wilms' tumors of the kidney, there is loss of heterozygosity at the chromosome 11p15 locus that contains two genes, H19 and IGF-2 that are genetically imprinted in the mouse. Paternal uniparental expression of IGF-2 and maternal monoallelic expression of H19 occur in the mouse. Both of these genes have the same type of monoallelic expression in humans (Rainier et al, 1993). In contrast, about 70% of Wilms' tumors, of those without heterozygosity at this locus, have biallelic-expression of H19 and/or IGF-2, suggesting loss of imprinting of these genes in the tumors. It is likely that more examples of loss of genomic imprinting will be found in human cancers. The mechanism for genetic imprinting appears to involve methylation of specific DNA sequences (Feinberg et al, 1995).

Trinucleotide Expansion. In the human genome there are interspersed repeated DNA sequences widely dispersed throughout the genome. These interspersed repeats are frequently close to or even within structural genes. And while structural genes in general have a low mutation rate (e.g., about 1 amino acid out of 400 per 200,000 years) (Alberts et al, 1983), repeated sequences have much higher mutation frequencies (Richards et al, 1992). Since they are usually in noncoding regions of the genome, these mutations are tolerated by the organism and indeed may even be beneficial by allowing genetic recombination and alternate splicing events to produce new gene arrangements that help an organism adopt to new environments.

The interspersed repeated DNA sequences can undergo a unique form of mutation, namely, variation in copy number. This form of mutation, sometimes called *dynamic mutation,* (Richards et al, 1992) results from an increase in copy number of repeated trinucleotide sequences, hence the term *trinucleotide expansion*. This form of mutation has now been linked to a number of genetic diseases, including the fragile X syndrome, in which a CGG trinucleotide is amplified (Kremer et al, 1991; Fu et al, 1991); myotonic dystrophy and spinal bulbar muscularatrophy, in which the amplified repeat is trinucleotide CAG (reviewed in Richards et al, 1992); and Huntington's chorea, in which the amplified repeat is also CAG (The Huntington's Disease Collaborative Research Group, 1993). While normal individuals may have 6–60 copies of these repeats, unaffected transmitting individuals may have 60–200 copies, and severely affected persons may have more than 1,000 copies of a trinucleotide repeat. An unusual feature of this type of mutation is that the copy number increases with succeeding generations, explaining the phenomenon of "genetic anticipation," in which asymptomatic carriers in earlier generations pass on the mutant chromosome to their offspring such that, in successive generations, the repeat length and the severity of the disease increase.

Sequencing studies have revealed that the trinucleotide repeats occur in the 3′ untranslated regions of certain genes. In the case of the CAG repeat in myotonic dystrophy, for example, the repeat occurs near a region coding for a cyclic AMP-dependent protein kinase-like sequence. It isn't apparent why these amplified trinucleotide repeats in uncoded regions near a gene would so dramatically affect function, but the data suggest that these sequences have some regulatory action. In the case of the fragile X syndrome, the amplification blocks transcription of a gene called *FMR-1* (Pieretti et al, 1991). If one scans the human GenBank, more than 30 sequences with 5 or more copies of trinucleotide repeats can be found. For example, at least 10 human genes contain p(CCG)n repeats of five or more copies, including at least one protooncogene (Richards et al, 1992).

While no such mutations have as yet been reported in human cancer, it seems likely that similar genetic changes will be identified in individuals with a susceptibility to develop cancer, especially since some protooncogenes and other regulatory genes contain such trinucleotide repeats.

Point Mutations. Point mutations that lead to single base changes in a DNA sequence are frequently involved in chemical carcinogenesis and in activation of protooncogenes. Reaction of DNA with carcinogenic chemicals can lead to formation of base adducts that can cause base mispairing during DNA replication or loss of an adducted nucleic acid base producing an abasic site in the DNA chain. Such abasic sites may then produce an inappropriate base in the daughter strand during DNA repair or replication, leading to a point mutation. If this mutation is in a regulatory element of a gene, loss or alteration of regulation of gene expression can occur. If the mutation is in a coding region of a gene, an altered protein may be formed.

Microsatellite Instability. DNA sequences termed *microsatellites* are one to six nucleotide motifs randomly repeated numerous times in the human genome. For example, about 100,000 (CA)n dinucleotide repeats are found scattered throughout the human genome and many of these exhibit genetic polymorphisms in the length of the repeats. In colorectal cancer, a number of studies have shown differences in the repeat (CA)n length between tumor and normal DNA from colon specimens from the same patient (reviewed in Yee et al, 1994). This microsatellite instability (MSI) correlated with tumor location in the ascending colon, with increased patient survival, and inversely, with loss of heterozygosity for chromosomes 5q, 17p, and 18q. MSI has been found in both "sporadic" and familial colorectal cancers. Similarly, MSI has now been reported in breast cancer (Yee et al, 1994), small cell lung cancer (Merlo et al, 1994), non–small cell lung cancer (Shridhar et al, 1994), urinary bladder cancer (Gonzalez-Zulueta et al, 1994), and gastric cancer (Mironov et al, 1994). Thus the data suggest that MSI is a common genetic alteration in human cancer.

Mismatch DNA Repair Defects. The frequent occurrence of MSI and other genetic alterations suggests a generalized defect in human cancer. For instance, the genome of patients with hereditary non-polyposis colorectal cancer (HNPCC) syndrome contains frequent alterations within (CA)n and other simple repeated sequences. This syndrome, which affects as many as 1 out of 200 individuals in the Western world, predisposes affected persons to cancers of the colon, endometrium, ovary, and other organs, often before age 50 (Lynch et al, 1993). Such alterations in the stability of (CA) in sequences indicate a DNA replication error called the *RER phenotype*. RER^+ tumor cells display a biochemical defect in mismatch DNA repair analogous to a similar defect in bacteria and yeast. A gene responsible for this DNA repair defect has been found and maps to chromosome 2p. This gene, called *hMSH2* (human *mut*S homologue 2), is homologous to the bacterial gene *mut*S, which is responsible for strand specific mismatch repair (Fishel et al, 1993; Parson et al, 1993).

Oncogenes

Since many of the genetic alterations described above lead to changes in expression of cellular oncogenes or tumor suppressor genes, they will be discussed in some detail.

Oncogenes and their normal cellular counterparts, the protooncogenes, can be classified by their function into several different categories as reviewed by Hunter (Table 6–3) (Hunter, 1991). A number of these genes encode growth factors, e.g., *sis* (PDGF B-chain), *int*-2 and *hst* (fibroblast growth factor [FGF]-like factor). These oncogene growth factors can stimulate tumor cell proliferation by paracrine or autocrine mechanisms, but by themselves may not be sufficient to sustain the transformed phenotype.

A second type of oncogene codes for altered growth factor receptors, many of which have associated tyrosine kinase activity. These include the *src* family of oncogenes, *erb* B (EGF receptor), and *fms* (colony stimulating factor [CSF-1] receptor). For some of these receptor-like, tyrosine kinase–associated membrane proteins, the actual ligand is not known (e.g., *trk*, *met*, and *ros*). A third type is another receptor class, but without associated tyrosine kinase activity. This class is represented by the *mas* gene product (angiotensin receptor) and the $\alpha_{1\beta}$ adrenergic receptor.

TABLE 6–3. *Functions of Cell-Derived Oncogenic Proteins**

Oncogene	*Transforming Protein*	*Location*	*Function*
CLASS 1—GROWTH FACTORS			
sis (V)	p28$^{env\text{-}sis}$	Secreted	PDGF-like growth factor
int-2 (T)	p34$^{int\text{-}2}$	Secreted?	FGF-related growth factor
hst (KS3)(T)	p22^{hst}	Secreted	FGF-related growth factor
FGF-5 (T)	p27	Secreted	FGF-related growth factor
wnt-1 (T)	gp40$^{wnt\text{-}1}$	Membranes/secreted	Growth factor?
IL-3	p15	Secreted	Cytokine
CLASS 2—RECEPTOR AND NONRECEPTOR PROTEIN-TYROSINE KINASES			
src (V)	p60$^{v\text{-}src**}$	Plasma membrane	Activated nonreceptor PTK
yes (V)	P90$^{gag\text{-}yes}$	Plasma membrane?	Activated nonreceptor PTK
fgr (V)	P70$^{gag\text{-}fgr}$	?	Activated nonreceptor PTK
lck (T)	p56^{lck}	Plasma membrane	Nonreceptor PTK
fps/fes (V)	P140$^{gag\text{-}fps}$	Cytoplasm	Activated nonreceptor PTK
abl/bcr-abl (V/T)	P160$^{gag\text{-}abl}$ P210$^{bcr\text{-}abl}$	Membrane and cytoskeleton	Activated nonreceptor PTK
ros (V)	p68$^{gag\text{-}ros}$	Membrane associated	Truncated receptor PTK
erbB (V)	gp68/74$^{erb\text{-}B}$	Plasma and cytoplasmic membranes	EGF receptor PTK domain
neu (T)	p185^{neu}	Plasma membrane	Mutant receptor PTK
tel-PDGRF (T)	?	Cytoplasm?	Tel Ets-family protein—PDGFR PTK domain fusion
fms (V)	gP180$^{gag\text{-}fms}$	Plasma and cytoplasmic membranes	Mutant CSF-1 receptor protein-tyrosine kinase
met	P65$^{tpr\text{-}met}$	Cytosol	HGF receptor protein-tyrosine kinase domain
trk (T)	P70$^{TM\text{-}trk}$	Cytosol	Nonmuscle tropomyosin-NGF receptor PTK domain fusion
kit (V)	P80$^{gag\text{-}kit}$	?	Truncated stem cell factor receptor PTK
sea (V)	gP155$^{env\text{-}sea}$	Plasma membrane	Mutant receptor PTK
ret (T)	p96^{ret}	?	Mutant receptor PTK
CLASS 3—RECEPTORS LACKING PROTEIN-TYROSINE KINASE ACTIVITY			
mas (T)	p65^{mas}	Plasma membrane?	Angiotensin receptor
mpl (V)	p45$^{env\text{-}mpl}$	Plasma membrane?	Activated cytokine family receptor
int-3 (T)	p60$^{int\text{-}3}$	Plasma membrane?	Activated notch receptor?
tan-1 (T)	p60$^{tan\text{-}1}$	Plasma membrane?	Activated notch receptor?
CLASS 4—MEMBRANE-ASSOCIATED G PROTEINS AND REGULATORS			
H-ras (V/T)	p21$^{H\text{-}ras}$	Plasma membrane	Activated small G protein
K-ras (V/T)	p21$^{K\text{-}ras}$	Plasma membrane	Activated small G protein
N-ras (T)	p21$^{N\text{-}ras}$	Plasma membrane	Activated small G protein
gsp (T)		Plasma membrane	Activated mutant $G\alpha_s$
gip (T)		Plasma membrane	Activated mutant $G\alpha_i$
dbl (T)	p66^{dbl}	Cytoplasm	GTP exchange factor for CDC42Hs
vav (T)	p91^{vav}	Cytoplasm?	SH2 signal regulator/GTP exchange factor?
CLASS 5—CYTOPLASMIC PROTEIN-SERINE KINASES			
raf/mil (V)	P90$^{gag\text{-}raf}$	Cytoplasm	Activated protein-serine kinase
pim-1 (T)	p36$^{pim\text{-}1}$	Cytoplasm	Protein-serine kinase
mos (V)	p37$^{v\text{-}mos}$	Cytoplasm	Protein-serine kinase
cot (T)	p52^{cot}	?	Protein-serine kinase
akt (V)	p105$^{gag\text{-}akt}$	Cytoplasm/membranes?	Activated protein-serine kinase
CLASS 6—CYTOPLASMIC REGULATORS			
crk (V)	P47$^{gag\text{-}crk}$	Cytoplasm	SH2/SH3 signal regulator
shc	p52/46^{shc}	Cytoplasm?	SH2 signal regulator
nck	p47^{nck}	Cytoplasm	SH2/Sh3 signal regulator

(*continued*)

TABLE 6–3. *(Continued)*

Oncogene	*Transforming Protein*	*Location*	*Function*
CLASS 7—NUCLEAR TRANSCRIPTION FACTORS			
myc (V/T)	$P110^{gag\text{-}myc}$	Nucleus	bHLH-LZ[a] transcription factor
N-myc (T)	$p66^{N\text{-}myc}$	Nucleus	bHLH-LZ transcription factor
L-myc (T)	$p64^{L\text{-}myc}$	Nucleus	bHLH-LZ transcription factor
lyl-1 (T)	$p29^{lyl\text{-}1}$	Nucleus?	bHLH transcription factor
tal-1/scl (T)	$pp42^{tal\text{-}1}$	Nucleus	bHLH transcription factor
myb (V)	$P48^{gag\text{-}myb\text{-}env}$	Nucleus	Transcription factor
fos (V)	$p55^{v\text{-}fos}$	Nucleus	Mutant bZIP[b] transcription factor: AP-1 subunit
jun (V)	$p65^{gag\text{-}jun}$	Nucleus	Mutant bZIP transcription factor: AP-1 subunit
maf (V)	$p45^{v\text{-}maf}$	Nucleus	Mutant bZIP transcription factor
pml-RAR	$p110^{pml\text{-}RAR}$	Nucleus	Chimeric Pml-RARa protein
erbA	$P75^{gag\text{-}erb\text{-}A}$	Nucleus	Dominant negative mutant thyroxine (T_3) receptor
rel (V)	$p59^{v\text{-}rel}$	Nucleus/cytoplasm	Dominant negative mutant NF-$_k$B-related protein
bcl-3 (T)	$p46^{bcl\text{-}3}$	?	I_kB NF-$_k$B inhibitor and transactivator
ets (V)	$P135^{gag\text{-}myb\text{-}ets}$	Nucleus	Mutant transcription factor
spi-1/PU-1 (T)	$p42^{spi\text{-}1}$	Nucleus	Ets-family transcription factor
ski (V)	$p125^{gag\text{-}ski}$	Nucleus	Sequence-specific DNA-binding protein
evi-1 (T)	$p120^{Evi\text{-}1}$	Nucleus?	Mutant zinc finger transcription factor?
E2A-pbx-1 (T)	$p77P^{E2A\text{-}pbx\text{-}1}$	Nucleus	Chimeric E2A-homeobox transcription factor
trx (T)	?	Nucleus	Mutant Drosophila Trithorax-like homeobox protein
hox11 (T)	$p40^{hox11}$	Nucleus?	Overexpressed homeobox transcription factor
hox2.4 (T)	$p37^{hox2.4}$	Nucleus?	Overexpressed homeobox transcription factor
qin (V)	$P85^{gag\text{-}qin}$	Nucleus	Mutant forkhead family transcription factor
CLASS 8—CELL CYCLE REGULATORS			
bcl-1	cyclin D1	Nucleus	Activating subunit of Cdk4 and Cdk6
ΔN-cyclin A	ΔN-cyclin A	Nucleus	Mutant activating subunit of Cdc2 and Cdk2
CLASS 9—ANTI-APOPTOSIS FACTORS			
bcl-2 (T)	$p25^{bcl\text{-}2}$	Cytoplasm	Blocks apoptosis of B cells

From Hunter (SALK Institute), 1995, with permission.
*This table is not an exhaustive list, but describes the best characterized oncogenes. (V) and (T) indicate viral or tumor cell oncogenes, respectively.
**The approximate sizes of the proteins are given in kDa in the protein name, e.g., $p60^{v\text{-}src}$ is a 60 kDa protein. By convention a capital P is used for viral oncoproteins that are fusion proteins with the viral gag structural protein.
[a]bHLH = basic region/helix-loop-helix DNA-binding domain; LZ = leucine zipper DNA-binding domain.
[b]bZIP = basic region/leucine zipper DNA-binding domain.

A fourth class of oncogene products are membrane-associated, guanine nucleotide binding proteins such as the Ras family of proteins. These proteins bind GTP, have associated GTPases, and act as signal transducers for cell surface growth factor receptors. The transforming *ras* oncogenes have been mutated in such a way as to render them constitutively active by maintaining them in a GTP binding state, most likely because of a defect in the associated GTPase activity.

A fifth category are the cytoplasmic oncoproteins with serine/threonine protein kinase activity. These include the products of the *raf, pim*-1, *mos,* and *cot* genes. A prototype of this class is the c-Raf protein which is activated by a variety of tyrosine kinase-associated receptors (see above). There is some evidence that c-Raf can translocate to the nucleus and may act as a "shuttle" to convey membrane-activated cytoplasmic signals to the nucleus (Hunter, 1991). The oncogenic form of Raf has lost part of its regulatory amino terminal sequence and appears to be constitutively active. c-Crk, a sixth type, is also a cytoplasmic protein, and it appears to act by stabilizing tyrosine kinases associated with the Src family of oncoproteins. A seventh, large class of oncogenes are those that code for nuclear transcription factors such as *myc, myb, fos, jun, erb-A,* and *rel.* For a number of these, the oncogenic alteration that makes them transforming oncoproteins is a mutation that leads to loss of negative regulatory elements (e.g., for *jun, fos,* and *myb*), and in other cases (e.g., *erb-A* and *rel*), the activating mutations cause the loss of their active domains, producing a mutant protein that prevents the activity of the normal gene product—a so-called dominant negative mutation. It is interesting that mutations of the tumor suppressor gene *p53*, in sort of a "reverse twist," produce a dominant negative effect by producing a protein that in this case prevents the action of a tumor suppressor function (see below).

A number of oncogenes have been implicated in human cancer, and their mechanisms of activation are shown in Table 6–4. It has been noted that the detection of activated or mutated oncogenes in human cancers could have diagnostic and therapeutic implications, a sort of "oncogenes at the bedside" approach (Bishop, 1991). For example, the detection of the *bcr/abl* gene in leukemic cells could confirm the diagnosis of chronic myelogenous leukemia. The levels of the *neu* oncogene product has been used to determine the prognosis in breast cancer. Loss or damage to the *RB* or *p53* genes can be used to determine susceptibility to certain cancers, and so on.

Tumor Suppressor Genes

Knowledge about the existence of tumor suppressor genes came about from somatic cell hybridization experiments in which tumor cells were fused with normal cells and their malignant phenotype examined (Harris, 1988; Sager, 1989). The resulting cell hybrids were usually, though not always, nontumorigenic, and this loss of tumorigenicity was found to be associated with the presence of certain chromosomes. If these chromosomes were lost during subsequent passage of the cultured hybrid cells, they reverted to a malignant phenotype. These results suggested the presence of a tumor suppressor function coded for by genes on the lost chromosomes. This evidence was greatly strengthened by experiments utilizing the transfer of the missing putative suppressor chromosome into malignant cells and showing that the phenotype reverted to normal (Stanbridge, 1990).

Evidence supporting the two-hit hypothesis of Knudson (1985) (see below) also strengthened the argument for the loss of some genetic function being important in carcinogenesis. The two-hit theory states that at least two genetic mutations are necessary for a cell to become malignant. In the case of hereditary cancers, such as the hereditary form of retinoblastoma, one mutation would be present in the germ line and a second one would occur sometime after conception. The identification of the retinoblastoma (*Rb*) gene and the demonstration that both alleles are lost or inactivated in retinoblastoma definitively showed that tumor suppressor genes exist.

TABLE 6–4. *Protooncogenes and Human Tumors: Some Consistent Incriminations**

Protooncogene[a]	*Neoplasm(s)*	*Lesion*
ABL	Chronic myelogenous leukemia	Translocation
ERBB-1	Squamous cell carcinoma; astrocytoma	Amplification
ERBB-2 (NEU)	Adenocarcinoma of breast, ovary and stomach	Amplification
GIP	Carcinoma of ovary gland and adrenal gland	Point mutations
GSP	Adenoma of pituitary gland; carcinoma of thyroid	Point mutations
MYC	Burkitt's lymphoma	Translocation
	Carcinoma of lung, breast and cervix	Amplification
L-MYC	Carcinoma of lung	Amplification
N-MYC	Neuroblastoma; small cell carcinoma of lung	Amplification
H-RAS	Carcinoma of colon, lung and pancreas; melanoma	Point mutations
K-RAS	Acute myelogenous and lymphoblastic leukemia; carcinoma of thyroid; melanoma	Point mutations
N-RAS	Carcinoma of genitourinary tract and thyroid; melanoma	Point mutations
RET	Carcinoma of thyroid	Rearrangement
ROS	Astrocytoma	?
K-SAM	Carcinoma of stomach	Amplification
SIS	Astrocytoma	?
SRC	Carcinoma of colon	?
TRK	Carcinoma of thyroid	Rearrangement

*From Bishop, 1991, with permission.

[a]The list is intended to be representative but not exhaustive. It includes loci that suffer demonstrable damage and loci that are abnormally expressed for reasons not yet known.

TABLE 6–5. *Suppressor Genes in Human Tumors**

Chromosomal Location	*Tumor Type*
DETECTED BY CELL HYBRIDIZATION OR CHROMOSOME TRANSFER	
1p	Neuroblastoma
3p	Renal ca.
6	Endometrial ca.
9	Endometrial ca.
11	Neuroblastoma; cervical ca.; Wilms' tumor
DETECTED THROUGH LOSS OF HETEROZYGOSITY OR DIRECT MOLECULAR PROBING	
1p	Melanoma; MEN[a] type 2; neuroblastoma; medullary thyroid ca; pheochromocytoma; ductal cell ca.
1q	Breast ca.
3p	SCLC[a]; adeno ca. of lung; cervical ca; von Hippel-Lindau disease, renal cell ca.
5q	Familial adenomatous polyposis; colorectal ca.
9q	Bladder ca.
10q	Astrocytoma; MEN type 2
11p	Wilms' tumor; rhabdomyosarcoma; breast ca.; hepatoblastoma; transitional cell bladder ca.; lung ca.
11q	MEN type 1
13q	Retinoblastoma; osteosarcoma; SCLC; ductal breast ca.; stomach ca.; bladder ca.; colon ca.
17p	SCLC; colorectal ca; breast ca.; osteosarcoma; astrocytoma; squamous cell lung ca.
17q	NF[a] type 1
18q	Colorectoral ca.
22q	NF type 2; meningioma; acoustic neuroma; pheochromocytoma

*Source: Reprinted with permission from Weinberg, Tumor suppressor genes. *Science* 254:1138. Copyright 1991 by the American Association for the Advancement of Science.

[a]MEN, multiple endocrine neoplasia; SCLC, small cell lung carcinoma; NF, neurofibromatosis.

It is now known that a number of other gene deletions or allelic inactivations occur in a wide variety of human cancers, and a number of additional putative tumor suppressor genes have been localized to specific chromosomes (Table 6–5) (Weinberg, 1991).

The first tumor suppressor gene that was cloned was the *Rb* gene that is the defective gene in retinoblastoma. Cavenee et al used restriction fragment length polymorphisms (RFLPs) to map the defective gene to chromosome 13q14 and showed that a loss of heterozygosity at this locus in the tumor was due to loss of the normal allele from the unaffected parent (Cavenee et al, 1985). This indicated a germline mutation, uncovered by the loss of heterozygosity, and helped substantiate the Knudson hypothesis. The *Rb* gene was subsequently cloned by Friend et al (1986). It is now known that a variety of other human cancers have inactivated *Rb* alleles, including sarcomas, small-cell lung, bladder, and a few breast carcinomas (reviewed in Marshall, 1991), although the role of *Rb* loss of heterozygosity (LOH) in these tumors is not clear.

A number of other tumor suppressor genes or candidate tumor suppressor genes have been cloned and are being characterized (Table 6–6) (Marx, 1993). This almost certainly is only the tip of the iceberg and many more will likely be discovered as more is learned about cancer cell genetics and the map of the human genome. At this point, however, a number of generalizations can be made (Table 6–7), and a comparison with activation of oncogenes is instructive (Levine, 1993). A single mutation can be sufficient to activate an oncogene (e.g., *ras*); a second is not crucial since there would not necessarily be any particular selective pressure to sustain it. Mutations in *onc* genes are gain of function events and lead to increased cell proliferation and decreased cell differentiation. Oncogene mutations do not appear to be inherited through the germline since their dominant effects could disrupt normal development. Oncogenes

TABLE 6–6. *Some Known or Candidate Tumor Suppressor Genes**

Gene	*Cancer Types*	*Product Location*	*Mode of Action*	*Hereditary Syndrome*
APC	Colon carcinoma	Cytoplasm?	?	Familial adenomatous polyposis
DCC	Colon carcinoma	Membrane	Cell adhesion molecule	—
NF1	Neurofibromas	Cytoplasm	GTPase-activator	Neurofibromatosis type 1
NF2	Schwannomas and meningiomas	Inner membrane?	Links membrane to cytoskeleton?	Neurofibromatosis type 2
p53	Colon cancer: many others	Nucleus	Transcription factor	Li-Fraumeni syndrome
Rb	Retinoblastoma	Nucleus	Transcription factor	Retinoblastoma
RET	Thyroid carcinoma: pheochromocytoma	Membrane	Receptor tyrosine kinase	Multiple endocrine neoplasia type 2
VHL	Kidney carcinoma	Membrane?	?	von Hippel-Lindau disease
WT-1	Nephroblastoma	Nucleus	Transcription factor	Wilms' tumor

*Source: Reprinted with permission from Marx. Learning how to suppress cancer. *Science* 261:1385. Copyright 1993 by the American Association for the Advancement of Science.

TABLE 6–7. *Properties of Oncogenes and Tumor Suppressor Genes**

Property	*Oncogenes*	*Tumor Suppressor Genes*
Mutational events involved in cancer	One	Two
Function of mutation	Gain of function ("dominant")	Loss of function ("recessive")
Germline inheritance	No	Yes
Somatic mutations	Yes	Yes
Effect on growth control	Activate cell proliferation	Negatively regulate growth-promoting genes
Effects of gene transfection	Transform partly abnormal fibroblasts (e.g., NIH3T3)	Suppress malignant phenotype in malignant cells
Genetic alterations	Point mutations, gene rearrangements, amplification	Deletions, point mutations

*From Ruddon, 1995b, with permission.

are mutated in a wide variety of human cancers (e.g., *ras, myc*). In contrast, tumor suppressor gene inactivations are loss of function events, usually require a mutational event in one allele followed by loss or inactivation of the other allele, are recessive in nature, and mutations may be inherited through the germline. One point of similarity is that somatic mutational events can occur both in oncogenes and in tumor suppressor genes and may accumulate over a lifetime.

A point should be made about the terms "dominant" and "recessive." In the classical Mendelian sense, the terms refer to an inheritance pattern resulting from the interplay between one paternal and one maternal allele in a diploid offspring. In cancer cells, this principle often does not hold. Chromosomal duplications, loss, and rearrangements often occur such that normal ploidy is disrupted. Thus a cancer cell may often be something other than diploid. It is clear from experimental studies that the balance between oncogene expression and tumor suppressor gene expression is a gene dosage effect (Harris, 1988). For example, hybrid cell formation between a normal fibroblast and a malignant cell will usually produce a nontumorigenic hybrid if one malignant chromosome set is present, but not if there are two malignant sets. Furthermore, hybrids containing two copies of a chromosome bearing a tumor suppressor gene show more stable suppression of the malignant phenotype than cells having only one copy.

The *p53* tumor suppressor gene was discovered by a totally different route (Weinberg, 1991). The p53 protein was initially found in SV40 virus transformed cells in association with the SV40 large T antigen, which is a critical protein for cell transformation by SV40. It was also found that cotransfection of rodent cells with *ras* and *p53* genes produced cell transformation. Thus p53 originally was thought to be an oncoprotein or at least a co-factor to an oncoprotein. It was later found that the p53 protein that had transforming capability was in fact a mutated form of the protein and that the wild type protein had a tumor suppressor function in that it inhibited cell transformation and cell proliferation. It has also been found that there are germline mutations of the *p53* gene in Li-Fraumeni syndrome, a genetically inherited trait that makes individuals susceptible to certain cancers such as rhabdomyosarcomas, leukemias, melanomas, and carcinomas of the brain, breast, lung, larynx, colon, and adrenal cortex at an early age (Malkin, et al, 1990). Somatic mutations in the *p53* gene have now been implicated in a wide variety of human cancers, including leukemias, lymphomas, sarcomas, and carcinomas of the lung, breast, colon, esophagus, liver, bladder, ovary, and brain (Hollstein et al, 1991).

The ubiquitous nature of alterations of p53 in human cancer indicates that p53 has a central role in transformation of cells to a malignant phenotype. The function of p53 isn't exactly clear, but it, like the RB protein, appears to play a central role in cell cycle events: it appears to be a substrate for cyclin/cdc2 kinase; it has a DNA binding domain that implies a transcriptional regulatory function; and it is bound up by certain transforming oncoproteins such as SV40 large T, adenovirus E1B, and papilloma virus E6. Interestingly, the p53 protein is also found intracellularly in complexes with the heat shock cognate protein Hsc 70, a "chaperonin" that may be involved in the assembly of p53 subunits, which is a necessary event for p53 to function normally. Mutant p53 appears to bind normal (wild type) p53 into a tight complex with Hsc 70, preventing the normal assembly and release of functional p53 oligomers. This may explain how one mutated allele of the *p53* gene can function in a "dominant negative" way to inhibit the function of the normal protein.

One might ask how the activation of oncogenes and the inactivation of tumor suppressor genes act in concert to bring about cancer. One interesting model of how this occurs has been proposed by Vogelstein and his colleagues (Fearon and Vogelstein, 1990) (Fig. 6-3).

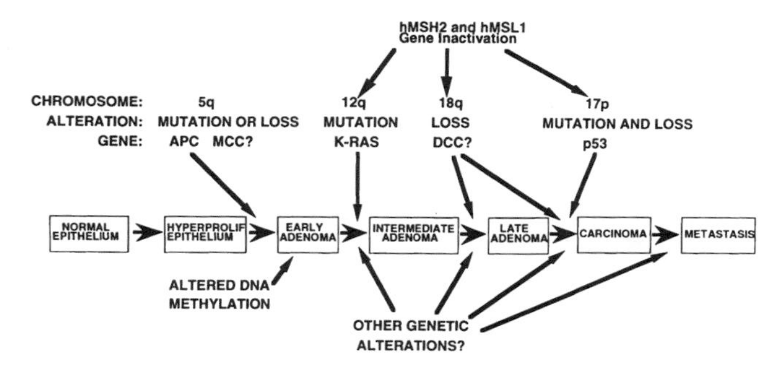

FIG. 6–3. Genetic alterations that occur during the progression of colorectal adenocarcinoma [From Fearon and Vogelstein, 1990, with permission].

In this model, the loss of certain tumor suppressor genes and the activation of oncogenes occur at various steps in the progression from normal colonic epithelium to metastatic carcinoma. For example, the activation of the K-*ras* gene by mutation occurs at the transition from early to intermediate adenoma, and the loss of the *p53* gene occurs during the progression from late adenoma to carcinoma (Baker et al, 1990).

THE PROCESS OF CARCINOGENESIS

Tumor Initiation and Promotion/Progression

The concept that the development of cancer is a multistage process came about from studies done in the early 1940s with viral and chemical carcinogens. Peyton Rous and his colleagues found that certain virus-induced skin papillomas in rabbits would regress and then could be induced to reappear and undergo malignant transformation by the application of irritant substances such as turpentine or chloroform. They coined the terms *initiation* and *promotion* to describe these distinct events (Friedewald and Rous, 1944). Sall and Shear (1940) and Berenblum (1941) used the mouse skin-painting model to show that if mice received a single application of a polycyclic aromatic hydrocarbon (PAH), such as benzo(a)pyrene or methylcholanthrene, and were subsequently painted chronically with creosote or croton oil, a high proportion of the animals developed skin carcinomas, whereas those animals painted with a single application of the PAH alone or the continued application of croton oil alone did not develop carcinomas. Taken together, these early studies suggested a multistage mechanism for carcinogenesis. Multistage carcinogenesis has also been observed for other tissues in experimental animal studies and, indeed, the data appear to fit with what is known about the carcinogenic process in humans (see *Chapter 5*). The molecular genetic and biochemical events that occur during the two stages appear to be overlapping but distinct.

Mechanisms of Tumor Initiation

Initiation of the malignant transformation process in cells by a carcinogenic agent requires a permanent and heritable change in gene expression in the transformed cell. Using the principle of Ockham's razor as well as a lot of experimental evidence, the best bet for the cause of the initiating events is a direct mutational interaction of the carcinogenic agent with the cell's DNA.

Evidence supporting the mutational theory comes from a number of areas. First, agents that damage DNA are frequently carcinogenic. Chemical carcinogens almost invariably have to be activated to electrophilic agents that react with DNA in order to be carcinogenic (Miller and Miller, 1981). The type of adduct formation with DNA bases correlates well with the carcinogenicity of a number of chemical agents. Second, most carcinogenic agents are mutagens. Employing short-term bacterial mutagenesis assays, Ames and his colleagues (McCann et al, 1975) as well as others (Lave and Omenn, 1986; Zeiger, 1987; Tennant et al, 1987) estimate that about 80% of all known chemical carcinogens are mutagenic. Finally, the incidence of cancer in patients with genetically inherited DNA-repair defects is much higher than in non-affected individuals. Examples of this include the high incidence of skin cancers in individuals with xeroderma pigmentosum, a condition characterized by extreme sensitivity to the ultraviolet irradiation of sunlight; patients with ataxia telangiectasia, a cerebellar degenerative disease for which there is an associated high propensity to develop leukemia and other cancers; and patients with Fanconi's anemia, who have developmental abnormalities, hematologic insufficiency, and an increased risk to develop cancer.

Initiating chemical carcinogens have been shown to activate c-*onc* genes. Weinstein and his colleagues have found that murine and rat neoplasms induced by chemical carcinogens have a high level of expression of endogenous retroviral-like *onc* gene sequences (reviewed by Weinstein, 1988). For example, during the course of azomethane-induced and high fat diet–promoted colon carcinogenesis in rats, increased expression of c-*myc*, c-Ha-*ras*, and an endogenous rat retroviral sequence (RALV) was observed (Guillem et al, 1988). Activation of the c-*ras* oncogene has been noted in a number of human and animal tumors, the "classic" human case being that of a point mutation in the 12th codon of c-*ras* in human bladder cancer cells, resulting in the incorporation of a valine instead of a glycine in the encoded *p21* gene product (Tabin et al, 1982; Reddy et al, 1982). This results in a p21 protein that lacks GTPase activity, which may explain its role as a constitutively turned-on activator of G-protein coupled systems in transformed cells.

In support of the idea that chemical carcinogens can activate cellular *onc* genes by mutation, Barbacid and his colleagues have shown that nitrosomethylurea (NMU), a potent mammary gland carcinogen, induces an activated c-Ha-*ras* in carcinogen-induced mammary carcinoma cells by a G → A base transition in the 12th codon (Sukumar et al, 1983; Zarbl et al, 1985). Similarly, dimethylbenzanthracene (DMBA), during induction of mammary tumors in rats, appears to activate c-*ras* by a mutation in codon 61 (Zarbl et al, 1985). Point mutations in activated c-Ki-*ras* have also been found in γ irradiation–induced lymphomas (Guerrero et al, 1984), suggesting that physical carcinogens, like chemical carcinogens, can act by activating c-*onc* genes. These data strengthen the concept of common molecular targets for various kinds of carcinogenic agents.

As discussed above, oncogenic viruses can interact in a number of ways with the host's genome to initiate carcinogenic events. Similarly, X- and γ-irradiation, in doses that initiate carcinogenesis, also damage DNA. Thus the evidence is quite compelling that the molecular events that cause the initiation process of tumorigenesis involve direct interaction with the genome (Harris, 1991). There is also evidence for genetic "drift" that leads to increasing genetic alterations as cancer progresses. This may be caused by a "mutator phenotype" that has been associated with multistage carcinogenesis (Loeb, 1991).

Mechanisms of Tumor Promotion

Tumor promotion, on the other hand, does not appear to involve irreversible and heritable damage to cells and is at least partially reversible. The "gold standard" of tumor promoting agents is the phorbol ester tetradecanoyl phorbol acetate (TPA). This agent and other promoters of different chemical structure share several features in common (reviewed by Ruddon, 1995c). First of all, they act as mitogens for target cells altered by initiating agents. A number of enzyme activities are elevated in promoter-treated cells, including ornithine decarboxylase, ATPase, and plasminogen activator. TPA and other tumor-promoting phorbol esters stimulate Na^+/H^+ exchange across cell membranes, leading to a transient intracellular alkalinization that precedes mitogenesis. Other membrane effects of TPA include inhibition of gap-junction formation, phosphorylation of certain growth factor receptors, and cytoskeletal alterations.

In the case of phorbol esters and certain similar analogs, the mitogenic and other cellular events appear to be triggered by activating a Ca^{2+}-, phospholipid-dependent phosphoprotein kinase called protein kinase C (PKC). PKC, in turn, can phosphorylate a variety of cellular substrates, some of which may activate the transcription of genes involved in cellular proliferation. To relate the total tumor promoting activity of TPA to its action on PKC, however, is most likely an oversimplification. TPA causes cell damage, edema, and acute inflammation in the epidermis when applied in doses at which it acts as a promoting agent. Thus the promoting mitogenic events may be secondary to a hyperplastic response caused by chronic tissue damage. Indeed, there is evidence that TPA can generate oxygen-free radicals in cells and that TPA-induced tumor promotion can be inhibited by free radical scavengers (reviewed by Cerutti, 1985).

The "Two-Hit" Model of Carcinogenesis

Most cancer biologists agree that carcinogenesis is a multistage process involving an initiating mutational event(s), followed by the clonal expansion of a damaged cell lineage via the action of tumor promoters. The clonal expansion/selection phase may take many cell population doublings (and many years in humans) to progress into a detectable malignant neoplasm. During the promotion/progression phase, there is most likely a telescoped evolutionary process involving the generation of new subclones and the loss of old subclones of cells due to genetic instability and selection pressures of the growth environment. This leads to the appearance of cells programmed to survive in an autonomous fashion unregulated by normal growth regulatory mechanisms (Nowell, 1976). The frequent end result is a highly invasive, undifferentiated cell type with an abnormal karyotype. It is important, however, to note the fact that the cause of certain cancers clearly has a strong hereditary input. Retinoblastoma, neuroblastoma, and Wilms' tumor in children, as well as colon carcinoma in adults with familial polyposis, are examples of inherited neoplasms. Even in the hereditary form of these cancers, however, it is clear that inheritance of the "cancer gene(s)" is not sufficient, at the cellular level, to produce a cancer, because, of the several millions of cells at risk, only a very few become malignant. For example, although the presence of the retinoblastoma susceptibility trait bears with it a 95% chance of getting the disease, only 3 or 4 tumors, on the average, occur in the retina, which has several million cells. Thus some second, rare event must occur in the susceptible cell population to induce the ultimate malignant transformation.

Knudson (reviewed in Moolgavkar and Knudson, 1981) has utilized this sort of information to postulate the two-stage or two-hit model of carcinogenesis. Briefly, it states that malignant transformation requires two genetic events: both are irreversible and most likely mutational in origin. A clone of initiated, "one-hit" cells is expanded via mitogenic events (promotion), increasing the population of damaged cells (and in some cases producing a benign tumor). Promotion also increases the population of cells in which a second mutational hit can occur that leads to the final steps of malignant transformation. In the case of the dominantly inherited hereditary cancers, the first hit is passed on in germ line cells and the second hit occurs some time after birth in a somatic cell that already contains the first hit. In nonhereditary forms of cancer, both hits occur in somatic cells after birth.

There is significant, though circumstantial, evidence to support the two-hit hypothesis. Children with the genetically inherited form of retinoblastoma, for example, have a greatly increased risk of developing osteogenic sarcoma after receiving irradiation (Knudson, 1977). These individuals already have an increased risk via a germ line mutation, and exposure to a second mutagenic agent, i.e., irradiation, increases the chance for the second mutational event necessary for malignant transformation.

One conundrum is how can a dominantly inherited trait at the population level appear to be a recessive trait at the cellular level, e.g., as in the case of the chromosomal deletions seen in retinoblastoma and Wilms' tumor cells. The explanation appears to be that the inherited trait is due to a heterozygous deletion of one allele of a gene, the *Rb* gene in the case of retinoblastoma, and that the second mutation occurs at the same site on the homologous chromosome, leading to a complete or homozygous deletion. In such a situation, the heterozygous deletion present in the germ line would have to produce a state of high susceptibility for the second mutational event. Thus segregation analysis would be consistent with an autosomal dominant inheritance with high penetrance.

There are several implications of this model for experimentally induced carcinogenesis (Moolgavkar and Knudson, 1981). In the classical mouse skin-painting experiments, for instance, the initiating agents interact with genomic DNA, producing an initiated, one-hit cell. Continuous application of the promoting agent phorbol ester leads to a proliferation of cells in an initiated intermediate stage and produces the preneoplastic papillomas. If promoter application is stopped, the papillomas regress, unless one of the papilloma cells sustains a second hit and assumes malignant characteristics. If promoter application, however, is continued, proliferation of the one-hit intermediate cells continues, thus creating an expanded cell population with enhanced probability of sustaining a second hit and thus of becoming malignant. As noted above, promoters themselves may damage DNA by oxygen radical formation and increase the likelihood of such genetic events as altered DNA repair or homologous chromosome exchanges. In this scheme, the papillomas would bear a heterozygous mutation and the ultimate squamous cell carcinomas would be homozygous. It should be remembered, of course, that some carcinogens are complete carcinogens and have both initiating and promoting activity if tissues are exposed to them chronically. Complete carcinogens include certain polycyclic aromatic hydrocarbons, and other powerful mutagenic agents for which there is experimental evidence that continued administration of them as single agents can produce tumors in experimental animals. Most likely, cigarette smoke contains complete carcinogens or a mixture of initiators and promoters.

CONCLUSIONS

The hallmarks of cancer at the cellular level are unregulated proliferation, invasiveness, and metastatic potential. Cancer cells within a malignant tumor are a heterogeneous population, yet malignant cells have a number of biochemical and genetic characteristics in common. Several changes at the cell membrane of cancer cells may explain their antisocial behavior: they shed a variety of lytic enzymes such as proteases and collagenases, they bear altered cell surface glycoproteins and glycolipids, they may produce a faulty extracellular matrix. At the genomic level, also, several types of alterations may be seen. These include chromosomal deletions or rearrangements, gene amplification, altered gene packaging and transcription, point mutations, activation of cellular oncogenes, inactivation or loss of tumor suppressor genes, or a combination of these events. The end result, however, is the same: the expression of genes involved in cell proliferation, invasion, and metastasis and the suppression of genes favoring cell differentiation.

REFERENCES

ALBERTS B, BRAY D, LEWIS J, et al. 1983. Molecular Biology of the Cell. New York: Garland Publishing, pp. 214–215.

ALBINI A, MELCHIORI A, SANTI L, et al. 1991. Tumor cell invasion inhibited by TIMP-2. J Natl Cancer Inst 83:775–779.

ALITALO K. 1985. Amplification of cellular oncogenes in cancer cells. Trends Biochem Sci 10:194–197.

ALITALO K, SCHWAB M, LIN CC, et al. 1983. Homogeneously staining chromosomal regions contain amplified copies of an abundantly expressed cellular oncogene (c-*myc*) in malignant neuroendocrine cells from a colon carcinoma. Proc Natl Acad Sci USA 80:1707–1711.

BAKER SJ, PREISINGER AC, JESSUP JM, et al. 1990. p53 gene mutations occur in combination with 17p allelic deletions as late events in colorectal tumorigenesis. Cancer Res 50:7717.

BASSET P, BELLOCQ JP, WOLF C, et al. 1990. A novel metalloproteinase gene specifically expressed in stromal cells of breast carcinomas. Nature 348:699–704.

BERENBLUM I. 1941. The mechanism of carcinogenesis: A study of the significance of carcinogenic action and related phenomena. Cancer Res 1:807–814.

BIGGS J, HERSPERGER E, STEEG PS, et al. 1990. A Drosophila gene that is homologous to a mammalian gene associated with tumor metastasis codes for a nucleoside diphosphate kinase. Cell 63:933–940.

BISHOP JM. 1991. Molecular themes in oncogenesis. Cell 64:235–248.

BOVERI T. 1914. Zur Frage der Erstehung Maligner Tumoren. Jena: Fischer.

CAJOT JF, BAMAT J, BERGONZELLI GE, et al. 1990. Plasminogen-activator inhibitor type 1 is a potent natural inhibitor of extracellular matrix degradation by fibrosarcoma and colon carcinoma cells. Proc Natl Acad Sci USA 87:6939–6943.

CAVENEE WK, HANSEN MF, NORDENSKJOLD M, et al. 1985. Genetic origin of mutations predisposing to retinoblastoma. Science 228:501.

CEDAR H. 1988. DNA methylation and gene activity. Cell 53:45–46.

CERUTTI PA. 1985. Prooxidant states and tumor promotion. Science 227:375–381.

CHAUDHURI JP, VOGEL W, VOICULESCU I, WOLF U. 1971. A simplified method of demonstrating Giemsa band pattern in human chromosomes. Humangenetik 14:83–84.

CHAUHAN SS, GOLDSTEIN LJ, GOTTESMAN MM. 1991. Expression of cathepsin L in human tumors. Cancer Res 51:1478–1481.

CIOCE V, CASTRONOVO V, SHMOOKLER BM, et al. 1991. Increased expression of the laminin receptor in human colon cancer. J Natl Cancer Inst 83:29–36.

DALLA-FAVERA R, BREGNI M, ERIKSON J, et al. 1982. Human c-*myc onc* gene is located on the region of chromosome 8 that is translocated in Burkitt lymphoma cells. Proc Natl Acad Sci USA 79:7824–7827.

DAYTON AI, SELDEN JR, LAWS G, et al. 1984. A human c-*erb* A oncogene homologue is closely proximal to the chromosome 17 breakpoint in acute promyelocytic leukemia. Proc Natl Acad Sci USA 81:4495–4499.

DE TAISNE C, GEGONNE A, STEHELIN D, et al. 1984. Chromosomal localization of the human proto-oncogene c-*ets*. Nature 310:581–583.

DECAPRIO JA, LUDLOW JW, FIGGE J, et al. 1988. SV40 large tumor antigen forms a specific complex with the product of the retinoblastoma susceptibility gene. Cell 54:275–283.

DRABKIN HA, BRADLEY C, HART I, et al. 1985. Translocation of c-*myc* in the hereditary renal cell carcinoma associated with a t(3;8) (p14.2q24.13) chromosomal translocation. Proc Natl Acad Sci USA 82:6980–6984.

DULBECCO R, ARMSTRONG B, ALLEN R. 1988. Reversion toward an earlier stage of differentiation and loss of polarity during progression of N-methyl-N-nitrosourea-induced rat mammary tumors. Proc Natl Acad Sci USA 85:9292–9296.

EASTON EW, BOLSCHER JGM, EIJNDEN DHVD. 1991. Enzymatic amplification involving glycosyltransferases forms the basis for the increased size of asparagine-linked glycans at the surface of NIH 3T3 cells expressing the N-ras proto-oncogene. J Biol Chem 266:21674–21680.

FEARON ER, FEINBERG AP, HAMILTON SH, VOGELSTEIN B. 1985. Loss of genes on the short arm of chromosome 11 in bladder cancer. Nature 318:377–380.

FEARON ER, VOGELSTEIN B. 1990. A genetic model for colorectal tumorigenesis. Cell 60:759–767.

FEINBERG AP, RAINIER S, DEBAUN MR. 1995. Genomic imprinting, DNA methylation, and cancer. Natl Cancer Inst Monogr No. 17:21–26.

FEIZI T. 1985. Demonstration by monoclonal antibodies that carbohydrate structure of glycoproteins and glycolipids are oncodevelopmental antigens. Nature 314:53–57.

FERGUSON-SMITH AC, CATTANACH BM, BARTON SC, et al. 1991. Embryological and molecular investigations of parental imprinting on mouse chromosome 7: Nature 351:667–670.

FIDLER IJ. 1990. Critical factors in the biology of human cancer metastasis: Twenty-eighth G.H.A. Clowes Memorial Award Lecture. Cancer Res 50:6130–6138.

FISHEL R, LESCOE MK, RAO MRS, et al. 1993. The human mutator gene homolog MSH2 and its association with hereditary nonpolyposis colon cancer. Cell 75:1027–1038.

FOLKMAN J, WATSON K, INGBER D, HANAHAN D. 1989. Induction of angiogenesis during the transition from hyperplasia to neoplasia. Nature 339:58–61.

FRENETTE GP, CAREY TE, VARANI J, et al. 1988. Biosynthesis and secretion of laminin and laminin associated glycoproteins by non-malignant and malignant human keratinocytes: A comparison of cell lines from primary and secondary tumors in the same patient. Cancer Res 48:5193–5202.

FRIEDEWALD WF, ROUS P. 1944. The initiating and promoting elements in tumor production: An analysis of the effects of tar, benzpyrene, and methylcholanthrene on rabbit skin. J Exp Med 80:101–126.

FRIEND SH, BERNARDS R, ROGELJ S, et al. 1986. A human DNA segment with properties of the gene that predisposes to retinoblastoma and osteosarcoma. Nature 323:643–646.

FRIXEN UH, BEHRENS J, SACHS M, et al. 1991. E-Cadherin-mediated cell-cell adhesion prevents invasiveness of human carcinoma cells. J Cell Biol 113:173–185.

FU Y-H, KUHL DPA, PIZZUTI A, et al. 1991. Variation of the CGG repeat at the fragile X site results in genetic instability: Resolution of the Sherman Paradox. Cell 67:1047–1058.

GONZALEZ-ZULUETA M, RUPPERT JM, TOKINO K, et al. 1994. Microsatellite instability in bladder cancer. Cancer Res 53:5620–5623.

GROUDINE M, WEINTRAUB H. 1982. Propagation of globin DNase I-hypersensitive sites in absence of factors required for induction: A possible mechanism for determination. Cell 30:131–139.

GUERRERO I, VILLASANTE A, CORCES V, PELLICER A. 1984. Activation of a c-K-*ras* oncogene by somatic mutation in mouse lymphomas induced by gamma radiation. Science 225:1159–1162.

GUILLEM JG, HSIEH LL, O'TOOLE KM, et al. 1988. Changes in expression of oncogenes and endogenous retroviral-like sequences during colon carcinogenesis. Cancer Res 48:3964–3971.

HAGEMEIJER A, BOOTSMA D, SPURR NK, et al. 1982. A cellular oncogene is translocated to the Philadelphia chromosome in chronic myelocytic leukemia. Nature 300:765–767.

HAKOMORI S-I. 1985. Aberrant glycosylation in cancer cell membranes as focused on glycolipids: overview and perspectives. Cancer Res 45:2405–2414.

HANSKI C, SHEEHAN J, KIEHNTOPF M, et al. 1991. Increased number of accessible sugar epitopes defined with monoclonal antibody AM-3 on colonic mucins is associated with malignant transformation of colonic mucosa. Cancer Res 51:5342–5347.

HARRIS CC. 1991. Chemical and physical carcinogenesis: Advances and perspectives for the 1990's. Cancer Res 51:5023s–5044s.

HARRIS H. 1988. The analysis of malignancy by cell fusion: The position in 1988. Cancer Res 48:3302–3306.

HAUPT Y, ALEXANDER WS, BARRI G, et al. 1991. Novel zinc finger gene implicated as *myc* collaborator by retrovirally accelerated lymphomagenesis in Eμ-*myc* transgenic mice. Cell 65:753–763.

HAUT M, STEEG PS, WILLSON JKV, MARKOWITZ SD. 1991. Induction of nm23 gene expression in human colonic neoplasms and equal expression in colon tumors of high and low metastatic potential. J Natl Cancer Inst 83:712–716.

HEISTERKAMP N, STAM K, GROFFEN J. 1985. Structural organization of the *bcr* gene and its role in the Ph^1 translocation. Nature 315:758–761.

HEISTERKAMP N, STEPHENSON JR, GROFFEN J, et al. 1983. Localization of the c-able oncogene adjacent to a translocation breakpoint in chronic myelocytic leukemia. Nature 306:239–242.

HENNESSY C, HENRY JA, MAY FEB, et al. 1991. Expression of the antimetastatic gene nm23 in human breast cancer: An association with good prognosis. J Natl Cancer Inst 83:281–285.

HENRY I, BONAITI-PELLIÉ C, CHEHENSSE V, et al. 1991. Uniparental paternal disomy in a genetic cancer-predisposing syndrome. Nature 351:665–667.

HOLLSTEIN M, SIDRANSKY D, VOGELSTEIN B, HARRIS CC. 1991. p53 mutations in human cancers. Science 253:49–53.

HUNTER T. 1991. Cooperation between oncogenes. Cell 64:249–270.

KNUDSON AG JR. 1977. Genetic predisposition to cancer: *In* Hiatt HH, Watson JD, Winsten JA (eds): Origins of Human Cancer. Cold Spring Harbor, NY: Cold Spring Harbor Laboratory, pp. 45–52.

KNUDSON, AG JR. 1985. Hereditary cancer, oncogenes, and antioncogenes. Cancer Res 45:1437–1443.

KOIVUNEN E, RISTIMAKI A, ITKONEN O, et al. 1991. Tumor-associated trypsin participates in cancer cell-mediated degradation of extracellular matrix. Cancer Res 51:2107–2112.

KONOPKA JB, WATANABE SM, SINGER JW, et al. 1985. Cell lines and clinical isolates derived from Ph^1-positive chronic myelogenous leukemia patients express *c-abl* proteins with a common structural alteration. Proc Natl Acad Sci USA 82:1810–1814.

KREMER EJ, PRITCHARD M, LYNCH M, et al. 1991. Mapping of DNA instability at the fragile X to a trinucleotide repeat sequence p(CCG)n. Science 252:1711–1714.

LAVE LB, OMENN GS. 1986. Cost-effectiveness of short-term tests for carcinogenicity. Nature 324:29–34.

LE BEAU MM, ROWLEY JD. 1984. Heritable fragile sites in cancer. Nature 308:607–608.

LEE EY-HP, TO H, SHEW J-Y, et al. 1988. Inactivation of the retinoblastoma susceptibility gene in human breast cancers. Science 241:218–221.

LEVINE AJ. 1993. The tumor suppressor genes. Annu Rev Biochem 62:623–651.

LIMPENS J, DE JONG D, VAN KRIEKEN JHJM, et al. 1991. *Bcl-2*/J_H rearrangements in benign lymphoid tissues with follicular hyperplasia. Oncogene 6:2271–2276.

LIOTTA LA, RAO CN, BARSKY SH. 1983. Tumor invasion and the extracellular matrix. Lab Invest 49:636–649.

LIOTTA LA, STEEG PS, STETLER-STEVENSON WG. 1991. Cancer metastasis and angiogenesis: An imbalance of positive and negative regulation. Cell 64:327–336.

LOEB LA. 1991. Mutator phenotype may be required for multistage carcinogenesis. Cancer Res 51:3075–3079.

LYNCH HT, SMYRK TC, WATSON P, et al. 1993. Genetics, natural history, tumor spectrum and pathology of hereditary nonpolyposis colorectal cancer: An updated review. Gastroenterology 104:1535–1549.

MAKOS M, NELKIN BD, LERMAN MI, et al. 1992. Distinct hypermethylation patterns occur at altered chromosome loci in human lung and colon cancer. Proc Natl Acad Sci USA 89:1929–1933.

MALKIN D, LI FP, STRONG LC, et al. 1990. Germ line p53 mutations in a familial syndrome of breast cancer, sarcomas, and other neoplasms. Science 250:1233–1238.

MARSHALL CJ. 1991. Tumor suppressor genes. Cell 64:313–326.

MARX J. 1993. Learning how to suppress cancer. Science 261:1385–1387.

MATRISIAN LM. 1990. Metalloproteinases and their inhibitors in matrix remodeling. Trends Genet 6:121–125.

MCCANN J, CHOI E, YAMASAKI E, AMES BN. 1975. Detection of carcinogens as mutagens in the *Salmonella*/microsome test: Assay of 300 chemicals. Proc Natl Acad Sci USA 72:5135–5139.

MECHAM RP. 1991. Receptors for laminin on mammalian cells. FASEB J 5:2538–2546.

MERLO A, MABRY M, GABRIELSON E, et al. 1994. Frequent microsatellite instability in primary small cell lung cancer. Cancer Res 54:2098–2101.

MILLER EC, MILLER JA. 1981. Searches for ultimate chemical carcinogens and their reactions with cellular macromolecules. Cancer 47:2327–2345.

MIRONOV NM, AGUELON MA-M, POTAPOVA GI, et al. 1994. Alterations of $(CA)_n$ DNA repeats and tumor suppressor genes in human gastric cancer. Cancer Res 54:41–44.

MITELMAN F. 1984. Restricted number of chromosomal regions implicated in aetiology of human cancer and leukemia. Nature 310:325–327.

MIZUOCHI T, NISHIMURA R, DERAPPE C, et al. 1983. Structures of the asparagine-linked chains of human chorionic gonadotropin produced in choriocarcinoma: Appearance of trianternary sugar chains and unique bianternary sugar chains. J Biol Chem 258:14126–14129.

MOOLGAVKAR SH, KNUDSON AG JR. 1981. Mutation and cancer: A model for human carcinogenesis. J Natl Cancer Inst 66:1037–1052.

NOWELL PC. 1976. The clonal evolution of tumor cell populations. Science 194:23–28.

NOWELL PC, HUNGERFORD DA. 1960. A minute chromosome in chronic granulocytic leukemia. Science 132:1497.

PARSON R, LI G-M, LONGLEY MJ, et al. 1993. Hypermutability and mismatch repair deficiency in RER^+ tumor cells. Cell 75:1227–1237.

PETERS G, BROOKES S, SMITH R, DICKSON C. 1983. Tumorigenesis by mouse mammary tumor virus: Evidence for a common region for provirus integration in mammary tumors. Cell 33:369–377.

PIERETTI M, ZHAN F, FU Y-H, et al. 1991. Absence of expression of the FMR-1 gene in fragile X syndrome. Cell 66:817–822.

POTEMPA J, KORZUS E, TRAVIS J. 1994. The serpin superfamily of proteinase inhibitors: structure, function, and regulation. J Biol Chem 269:15957–15960.

RAINIER S, JOHNSON LA, DOBRY CJ, et al. 1993. Relaxation of imprinted genes in human cancer. Nature 362:747–749.

REDDY EP, REYNOLDS RK, SANTOS E, BARBACID M. 1982. A point mutation is responsible for the acquisition of transforming properties by the T24 human bladder carcinoma oncogene. Nature 300:149–152.

RICHARDS RI, SUTHERLAND GR. 1992. Dynamic mutations: A new class of mutations causing human disease. Cell 70:709–712.

ROWLEY JD. 1973. A new consistent chromosomal abnormality in chronic myelogenous leukemia identified by quinacrine fluorescence and Giemsa staining. Nature 243:290–293.

ROWLEY JD. 1990. Molecular cytogenetics: Rosetta stone for understanding cancer—Twenty-ninth G.H.A. Clowes Memorial Award Lecture. Cancer Res 50:3816–3825.

ROZHIN J, GOMEZ AP, ZIEGLER GH, et al. 1990. Cathepsin B to cysteine proteinase inhibitor balance in metastatic cell subpopulations isolated from murine tumors. Cancer Res 50:6278–6284.

RUDDON RW. 1995a. Phenotypic characteristics of cancer cells. *In* Cancer Biology, 3rd ed. New York: Oxford University Press, pp. 96–140.

RUDDON RW. 1995b. Tumor suppressor genes. *In* Cancer Biology, 3rd ed. New York: Oxford University Press, pp. 318–340.

RUDDON RW. 1995c. Causes of cancer. *In* Cancer Biology, 3rd ed. New York: Oxford University Press, pp. 231–276.

RUSSO G, ISOBE M, GATTI R, et al. 1989. Molecular analysis of a t(14;14) translocation in leukemic T-cells of an ataxia telangiectasia patient. Proc Natl Acad Sci USA 86:602–606.

SAGER R. 1989. Tumor suppressor genes: The puzzle and the promise. Science 246:1406–1412.

SAGER R, GADI IK, STEPHENS L, GRABOWY CT. 1985. Gene amplification: An example of an accelerated evolution in tumorigenic cells. Proc Natl Acad Sci USA 82:7015–7019.

SALL RD, SHEAR MJ. 1940. Studies in carcinogenesis. XII. Effect of the basic fraction of creosote oil on the production of tumors in mice by chemical carcinogens. J Natl Cancer Inst 1:45–51.

SHRIDHAR V, SIEGFRIED J, HUNT J, et al. 1994. Genetic instability of microsatellite sequences in many non-small cell lung carcinomas. Cancer Res 54:2084–2087.

SHTIVELMAN E, LIFSHITZ B, GALE RP, CANAANI E. 1985. Fused transcript of *abl* and *bcr* genes in chronic myelogenous leukaemia. Nature 315:550–554.

SIDEBOTTOM E, CLARK SR. 1983. Cell fusion segregates progressive growth from metastasis. Br J Cancer 47:399–405.

SLAMON DJ, CLARK GM, WONG SG, et al. 1987. Human breast cancer: Correlation of relapse and survival with amplification of the HER-2/neu oncogene. Science 235:177–182.

SMITH HS, LIOTTA LA, HANCOCK MC, et al. 1985. Invasiveness and ploidy of human mammary carcinomas in short-term culture. Proc Natl Acad Sci USA 82:1805–1809.

SODROSKI JG, ROSEN CA, HASELTINE WA. 1984. Trans-acting transcriptional activation of the long terminal repeat of human T lymphotropic viruses in infected cells. Science 225:381–385.

SOLOMON E, BORROW J, GODDARD AD. 1991. Chromosome aberrations and cancer. Science 254:1153–1160.

STANBRIDGE EJ. 1990. Human tumor suppressor genes. Annu Rev Genet 24:615–657.

STRAUSS BS. 1992. The origin of point mutations in human tumor cells. Cancer Res 52:249–253.

STEEG PS, BEVILACQUA G, KOOPER L, et al. 1988. Evidence for a novel gene associated with low tumor metastatic potential. J Natl Cancer Inst 80:200–204.

SUKUMAR S, NOTARIO V, MARTIN-ZANCA D, BARBACID M. 1983. Induction of mammary carcinomas in rats by nitroso-methylurea involves malignant activation of H-*ras*-1 locus by single point mutations. Nature 306:658–661.

TABIN CJ, BRADLEY SM, BARGMANN CI, et al. 1982. Mechanism of activation of a human oncogene. Nature 300:143–149.

TAUB R, KIRSCH I, MORTON C, et al. 1982. Translocation of the c-*myc* gene into the immunoglobulin heavy chain locus in human Burkitt lymphoma and murine plasmacytoma cells. Proc Natl Acad Aci USA 79:7837–7841.

TENNANT RW, MARGOLIN BH, SHELBY MD, et al. 1987. Prediction of chemical carcinogenicity in rodents from in vitro genetic toxicity assays. Science 236:933–941.

THE HUNTINGTON'S DISEASE COLLABORATIVE RESEARCH GROUP. 1993. A novel gene containing a trinucleotide repeat that is expanded and unstable on Huntington's disease chromosomes: Cell 72:971–983.

TRONICK SR, POPESCU NC, CHEAH MSC, et al. 1985. Isolation and chromosomal localization of the human *fgr* protooncogene, a distinct member of the tyrosine kinase gene family. Proc Natl Acad Sci USA 82:6595–6599.

TSUJIMOTO Y, YUNIS J, ONORATO-SHOWE L, et al. 1984. Molecular cloning of the chromosomal breakpoint of B-cell lymphomas and leukemias with the t(11;14) chromosome translocation. Science 224:1403–1406.

VLEMINCKX K, VAKAET, L JR, MAREEL M, et al. 1991. Genetic manipulation of E-Cadherin expression by epithelial tumor cells reveals an invasion suppressor role. Cell 66:107–119.

WASMUTH JJ, PARK C, FERRELL RE. 1989. Report of the committee on the genetic constitution of chromosome 5. Cytogenet Cell Genet 51:137–148.

WEINBERG RA. 1991. Tumor suppressor genes. Science 254:1138–1146.

WEINSTEIN IB. 1988. The origins of human cancer: Molecular mechanisms of carcinogenesis and their implications for cancer prevention and treatment—Twenty-seventh G.H.A. Clowes Memorial Award Lecture. Cancer Res 48:4135–4143.

WHYTE P, BUCHKOVICH KJ, HOROWITZ JM, et al. 1988. Association between an oncogene and an anti-oncogene: the adenovirus E1A proteins bind to the retinoblastoma gene product. Nature 334:124–129.

YAMASHITA K, TACHIBANA Y, OHKURA T, KOBATA A. 1985. Enzymatic basis for the structural changes of asparagine-linked sugar chains of membrane glycoproteins of baby hamster kidney cells induced by polyoma transformation. J Biol Chem 260:3963–3969.

YEE CJ, ROODI N, VERRIER CS, PARL FF. 1994. Microsatellite instability and loss of heteroxygosity in breast cancer: Cancer Res 54:1641–1644.

YUNIS JJ. 1983. The chromosomal basis of human neoplasia. Science 221:227–235.

YURCHENCO PD, SCHITTNY JC. 1990. Molecular architecture of basement membranes. FASEB J 4:1577–1590.

ZARBL H, SUKUMAR S, ARTHUR AV, et al. 1985. Direct mutagenesis of Ha-*ras*-1 oncogenes by *N*-nitroso-*N*-methylurea during initiation of mammary carcinogenesis in rats. Nature 315:382–385.

ZEIGER E. 1987. Carcinogenicity of mutagens: Predictive capability of the *Salmonella* mutagenesis assay for rodent carcinogenicity. Cancer Res 47:1287–1296.

ZOU Z, ANISOWICZ A, HENDRIX MJC, et al. 1994. Maspin, a serpin with tumor-suppressing activity in human mammary epithelial cells. Science 263:526–529.

7 Molecular epidemiology in cancer prevention

FREDERICA P. PERERA

The impetus behind molecular epidemiology is the awareness that as much as 80% of cancer is theoretically preventable because the controlling causative factors are exogenous rather than inborn or inherent. We can estimate that in the absence of external carcinogenic exposures resulting from lifestyle, occupation, and the ambient environment, 400,000 of the annual 500,000 deaths in the United States could be averted. More effective methods are needed to identify groups and individuals at greatest risk of cancer at a stage where intervention is possible. Molecular epidemiology offers a potentially powerful tool in cancer prevention by combining biomarkers (measurements of carcinogenic dose, biologic response and susceptibility) with epidemiologic methods.

The challenge is formidable. A large variety of carcinogens are present in cigarette smoke, the workplace, indoor and ambient air, drinking water and the food supply. Although there is controversy over the relative contribution of natural vs. synthetic carcinogens to cancer risk, both are important. A number of carcinogens of natural origin are found in the diet and significant contamination by industrial or man-made chemicals, pesticides, metals, and fibers occurs across all media (Perera and Boffetta, 1988; Ames and Gold, 1990; Landrigan, 1992). Therefore, prevention of environmentally related cancer must address both lifestyle and nonlifestyle factors. It is increasingly recognized that "gene-environment" interactions are significant determinants of cancer risk (Harris, 1989). However, because exogenous factors can be manipulated readily—in contrast to genetic factors—elimination or reduction of carcinogenic exposures must be a priority in cancer prevention.

Cigarette smoking accounts for an estimated 30% of all cancer (American Cancer Society, 1993); yet even if smoking and other exposures now known to cause cancer were eliminated, cancer incidence would remain high because risk factors have not been established for most of the prevalent cancers such as cancers of the breast, prostate, and colon (Weinstein et al, 1993). The task of identifying environmental risk factors is enormous, given that few of the 50,000 chemicals already in commerce have been tested sufficiently for carcinogenicity and thousands of new chemicals are introduced into production each year (National Research Council, 1993b). Therefore, increased efforts are needed to screen existing and new chemicals for carcinogenicity and to monitor populations for early indicators of risk.

Traditionally, the two major tools in identifying and assessing carcinogenic risks have been epidemiology and quantitative risk assessment. Both have serious limitations. In determining whether a causal relationship exists between a specific environmental exposure and cancer, epidemiology has been severely handicapped by the long latency of the disease and problems in estimating past exposure. It is also insensitive to modest increases in common cancers and cannot serve as an early warning system. Interactions between exposures and lifestyle factors further complicate the job of the epidemiologist. It has therefore been difficult to attribute increases in cancer incidence or mortality to specific agents, much less to establish dose–response relationships. As a result, conclusive epidemiologic data exist only for certain occupational cancers, drugs, cigarette smoking, and rare cancers in humans. For most environmental sources of carcinogens, epidemiologic data are either limited (e.g., chlorination by-products in drinking water) or lacking altogether (e.g., pesticide residues in the diet).

Quantitative risk assessment for environmental carcinogens has, therefore, largely relied upon extrapolation from results of chronic bioassays in rodents rather than on human data. It is encouraging that in the instances where one can compare human risk estimates for the same carcinogen based on experimental and hu-

Support for this research was provided by Public Health Service Grants R01CA-53772, R01CA-43013 and 5 R01CA-39174 from the National Cancer Institute; by NIEHS grants CA51196 and P01-ES05294; by a grant from the American Cancer Society, PDT373, and by grants from Fogarty International Center, March of Dimes Birth Defects Foundation, the Colette Chuda Environmental Fund, and the Noreen T. Holland Breast Cancer Foundation.

man data (asbestos, benzene, gasoline, and cadmium) the resulting risk estimates are comparable (see Perera et al, 1989 for review). A recent review has reaffirmed the validity of the chronic bioassay (National Research Council, 1993a). Nonetheless, quantitative risk assessment is an uncertain exercise, involving a number of assumptions about interspecies relationships and the nature of the carcinogenic process itself.

The potential contribution of molecular epidemiology to cancer prevention is multifaceted (Hulka et al, 1990; Schulte and Perera, 1993). Relevant to risk assessment is the possibility of using biomarkers to identify potential risks (hazards) to humans and to provide comparative molecular dosimetry and response data in experimental animals and humans, facilitating quantitative extrapolation between species. Another potential contribution is the molecular documentation of human interindividual variation in the biologic response and susceptibility to carcinogens, which then could be factored explicitly into quantitative risk assessment and regulatory policy (Perera et al, 1991a).

With respect to epidemiology, biologic markers can be incorporated into analytic studies (cohort and case-control) in such a way as to increase the power of such studies to identify a causal relationship between exposure to a specific agent and increased risk of cancer. For example, plasma cotinine, urinary mandelic acid, and aflatoxin B_1 (AFB_1) in urine can be considered reliable indicators of exposure to and internal dose of tobacco smoke, styrene, and dietary AFB_1, respectively. Carcinogen–DNA adducts can provide even more mechanistically relevant information on the interacted or biologically effective dose of carcinogens. As such, both types of markers can serve to assign subjects to "exposed" and "unexposed" groups on a more meaningful basis than self-reported exposure, job history, or environmental monitoring, thereby increasing the power of a study by reducing random exposure misclassification. Moreover, certain biologic markers of preclinical response or biologic effect (once established as correlated with cancer and occurring before progression to malignancy were inevitable) might ultimately replace clinical disease as an endpoint. Possible candidates include specific alterations of specific oncogenes or tumor suppressor genes and signal chromosomal aberrations. By providing an earlier and a more commonly occurring outcome, such markers would mitigate the latency problem in cancer epidemiology, increase study power, and allow effective intervention. Finally, a combination of such biologic measures of molecular dose and effect with biomarkers of susceptibility could identify subgroups at highest potential risk for epidemiologic investigation.

Implicit in the above discussion is the anticipation that biomarkers will significantly expand our knowledge of the mechanisms or stage at which individual carcinogens exert their effect. Such information would permit us to design effective intervention and prevention strategies, and to monitor their efficacy. For example, biomarkers might be used to identify persons who would benefit most from chemoprevention and to provide intermediate endpoints in clinical trials of chemopreventive agents (Lippman et al, 1990; Reynolds, 1991).

Despite this potential, most biomarkers are in the validation stage, so that the field is at an intermediate stage of development. As illustrated by studies summarized in Tables 7–1 through 7–3, there exist numerous biomonitoring studies where persons with known (usually high) exposures to genotoxic compounds have been sampled. There are relatively few examples of molecular epidemiologic studies in which a hypothesis regarding cancer causation has been tested. There are still fewer well-developed applications of molecular epidemiology to quantitative risk assessment, such as that for ethylene oxide (Ehrenberg et al, 1986; Hogstedt, 1986). In addition, as can be clearly seen from Tables 7–1 through 7–3, there is a dearth of methods to detect carcinogens that do not interact efficiently with the genetic material. This is a significant problem since many environmental carcinogens, such as dioxin and other chlorinated organics, fall into this category.

On the other hand, the feasibility of biomonitoring and molecular epidemiology has been demonstrated. The diversity of methods now being validated and the increasing interest in seriously addressing problems posed by the fusion of laboratory technology and epidemiology are both highly encouraging. For review see Perera, 1987; International Agency for Research on Cancer, 1988; Vineis et al, 1990b; Harris, 1991; Hulka, 1991; Sugimura et al, 1991; Schulte and Perera, 1993.

The purpose of this chapter is to provide an overview of biologic markers and their current application in human biomonitoring and molecular cancer epidemiology. Methodologic problems will then be discussed, followed by recommendations for future research.

OVERVIEW OF METHODS AND RECENT STUDIES

Carcinogenesis is a complex, multistep process. The term *biomarker* is used to describe the application of chemical, physical, radiologic, and immunobiologic tests to human biologic samples, such as blood, urine, and tissue. These tests indicate the extent of an individual's exposure to an agent of interest, resultant biologic effects, inherent or acquired genetic susceptibility, or disease status of the host. The term *disease status* is used broadly and encompasses the continuum from normal to preclinical to clinical disease.

Tables 7–1 through 7–4 provide examples of each category of biologic marker. Four classes of markers are discussed, differing in terms of the point at which they occur or operate along the continuum between initial exposure to an environmental agent and overt clinical disease. The first category of ***internal dose*** refers to the measurement of the amount of a carcinogen or its metabolites present in cells, tissues, or body fluids. Examples of internal dosimeters include DDT and PCBs in serum and adipose tissue from environmental contamination, plasma or salivary cotinine from cigarette smoke, urinary aflatoxin indicative of dietary exposure, *N*-nitroso compounds in urine from dietary sources and cigarette smoke, and mutagenicity of urine reflective of exposure to various genotoxicants (see Table 7–1). Such internal dosimeters have the advantage of being comparatively easy to monitor, and they demonstrate that exposure has resulted in uptake and bioactivation of carcinogens. They cannot provide quantitative data about interactions with cellular targets; however, as will be discussed, an association has been seen between a marker of internal dose (AFB_1 metabolites in stored urine samples) and risk of liver cancer (Ross et al, 1992). Table 7–1 provides examples of compounds and exposure sources analyzed using each type of internal dosimeter as well as biologic samples and populations studied.

By contrast, markers of ***biologically effective dose*** reflect the amount of carcinogen that has interacted with cellular macromolecules (e.g., DNA, RNA, or protein) at a target site or a surrogate. As such, this class of markers is more mechanistically relevant to carcinogenesis than internal dose is, but it poses more challenging analytical problems. Examples include carcinogen–DNA adducts and their potential surrogate, carcinogen-protein adducts. (See Table 7–2 for examples of exposures and populations studied to date.) The biological basis for measuring DNA adducts derives from extensive experimental data supporting their role in the initiation and possibly in the progression of cancer (Miller and Miller, 1981; Weinstein et al, 1984; Harris et al, 1987; Yuspa and Poirier, 1988). Despite this impressive body of information, however, much remains to be uncovered about the quantitative relationship between adduct formation (as a necessary but not sufficient event) and cancer risk. At present, inferences about risk based on measurement of carcinogen–DNA adducts can be made only on a population basis and are at best semiquantitative. Factors that are likely to play a role in individual cancer risk include the specific type and biological effectiveness of adducts formed (e.g., location in tissue, cell type, site of binding on the genome and persistence), the existence of modulating factors (both ge-

TABLE 7–1. *Examples of Biomarkers of Internal Dose**

Compound Analysed	*Exposure Source*	*Biologic Sample*	*Population*	*References*
Aflatoxin B_1	Diet	Urine	Chinese residing in areas of low and high cancer risk; liver cancer cases and controls	Zhu et al, 1987; Ross et al, 1992
Benzene, Toluene	Cigarette smoke	Blood	Smokers, nonsmokers	Hajimiragha et al, 1989
CFA	Occupational exposure	Urine	Workers	Cadsforth et al, 1988
Cotinine	Cigarette smoke	Plasma	Smokers and nonsmokers, children and adults	Crawford et al, 1994
Glu-P-1, Glu-P-2	Diet	Plasma	Uremic patients and controls	Manabe et al, 1987
1-Hydroxypyrene	Coal tar products coal tar treated	Urine	Workers, smokers, patients	Jongeleen et al, 1989; Tolos et al, 1990; Bos et al, 1988
3-Hydroxy-BP	Coal tar products	Urine	Coal tar treated patients	Jongeleen et al, 1986
MeIQx	Diet	Urine	Consumers of fried beef	Berggren and Sjostedt, 1983
Mutagens	Cigarette smoke, various occupational exposures	Urine	Smokers, workers	reviewed in Everson, 1986; Vainio et al, 1984
Nitrosamino acids	N-nitroso compounds in diet	Urine	Chinese residing in areas of low and high cancer risk	Lu et al, 1986
N-nitrosoproline	Cigarette smoke	Urine	Smokers, nonsmokers; unexposed	Garland et al, 1986; Hoffmann and Hecht, 1985
Trp-P-1, Trp-P-2	Diet	Plasma	Volunteers	Manabe and Wada, 1988
Trp-P-1, Trp-P-2	Diet	Bile	Patients	Manabe and Wada, 1990
Thymine glycol	Agents that cause oxidative damage to DNA	Urine	Volunteers	Cathgart et al, 1984

*CFA, 3-chloro-4-fluoroaniline; Glu-P-1, 2-amino-6-methyldipyrido[1,2-a:3′,2′-d] imidazole; Glu-P-2, 2-aminodipyrido[1,2-a:3′,2′-d] imidazole; 3-Hydroxy-BP, 3 hydroxybenzo(a)pyrene; MeIQx, 2-amino-3,8-dimethylimidazo[4,5-f]quinoxaline; Trp-P-1, 3-amino-1,4-dimethyl-5H-pyrido [4,3-b] indole; Trp-P-2, 3-amino-1-methyl-5H-pyrido[4,3-b] indole.

TABLE 7–2. *Examples of Markers of Biologically Effective Dose**

Endpoint	*Exposure Source*	*Biologic Sample*	*Population*	*References*
4-ABP-Hb	Cigarette smoke	RBC	Smokers, nonsmokers	Bryant et al, 1987, 1988; Maclure et al, 1990; Vineis et al, 1990a
AFB_1-albumin	Diet	Plasma	China	Wild et al, 1990; Gan et al, 1988
Alkylated Hb	Propylene oxide	RBC	Workers	Osterman-Golkar et al, 1984
BP and CHRY-Hb	Cigarette smoke	RBC	Smokers	Day et al, 1990
Cisplatinum-protein	Cisplatin chemotherapy	Plasma, RBC	Chemotherapy patients	Fichtinger-Schepman et al, 1987; Mustonen et al, 1988; Parker et al, 1991; Perera et al, 1992b
Hydroxyethylhistidine Hydroxyethylvaline	Ethylene oxide	RBC	Workers, smokers, volunteers	Calleman et al, 1978; van Sittert et al, 1985; Farmer et al, 1986; Tornqvist et al, 1986; Mayer et al, 1991
NNK, NNN-Hb	Cigarette smoke	RBC	Smokers	Carmella et al, 1990
PAH-albumin	PAH in workplace, in cigarette smoke	Plasma	Workers, smokers	Weston et al, 1988; Sherson et al, 1990; Lee et al, 1991
4-ABP-DNA	Cigarette smoke and occupation	Lung tissue	Volunteers	Wilson et al, 1989
Acrolein-DNA	Cyclophosphamide chemotherapy	WBC	Chemotherapy patients	McDiarmid et al, 1991
AFB_1-guanine	Diet	Urine	Chinese and Kenyans residing in a high exposure and high and low risk area respectively; cases and controls	Autrup et al, 1983; Groopman et al, 1985; Ross et al, 1992
AFB_1-DNA	Diet	Liver tissue	Taiwanese	Hsieh et al, 1988; Zhang et al, 1991
Cisplatinum-DNA	Cisplatin chemotherapy	WBC	Chemotherapy patients	Reed et al, 1986, 1988; Perera et al, 1992
O^4-Ethylthymine	Methylating agents	Liver tissue	Liver cancer patients	Huh et al, 1989
3-Methyladenine	Methylating agents	Urine	Unexposed volunteers	Shuker et al, 1988; Prevost et al, 1990
O^6-Methyldeoxy-guanosine	Nitrosamines in diet, smoking, chemotherapy	Esophageal and stomach mucosa, placenta, WBC	Chinese and European cancer patients, smokers	Umbenhauer et al, 1985; Wild et al, 1986; Foiles et al, 1988; Sonlibtis et al, 1990; Hall et al, 1991
8-MOP-DNA	8-Methoxypsoralen chemotherapy	Skin	Psoriasis patients	Santella et al, 1988
5-OH-methyl uridine	Diet	WBC	Low fat and normal diet	Djuric et al, 1991
PAH-DNA	PAH in cigarette smoke, in workplace, in polluted air, and diet	WBC, lung tissue, placenta	Lung cancer patients smokers, workers, volunteers	Reviewed in Calleman, 1982; Perera et al, 1988; Santella, 1988; Hemminki et al, 1990; Santella et al, 1991; Rothman et al, 1992
Spectrum of DNA adducts	Betel and tobacco chewing, smoking, industrial exposures, wood smoke	Placenta, lung tissue, oral mucosa WBC, bone marrow, colonic mucosa	Smokers, workers, volunteers	Reviewed in Santella et al, 1991

*4-ABP, 4-aminobiphenyl; AFB_1, aflatoxin B_1; CHRY, chrysene; Hb, hemoglobin; NNK, 4-(methylnitrosamino)-1-(3-pyridyl)-1-butanone; NNN, N^1-nitrosonornicotine; PAH, polycyclic aromatic hydrocarbons; RBC, red blood cells; WBC, white blood cells; 5-OH-methy uridine, 5-hydroxymethyluradine.

netic and acquired) and the presence of endogenous or exogenous promoting agents or cocarcinogens. Studies are ongoing to address these questions, as well as to determine whether DNA adducts measured in tissue, such as peripheral blood cells, are a reasonable surrogate for target tissue such as the lung or breast.

As an example of a marker of biologically effective dose, polycyclic aromatic hydrocarbons (PAH)–DNA adducts have been associated with workplace exposure to PAHs, and with exposure to air pollution and cigarette smoke (Perera et al, 1988; Hemminki et al, 1990; Herbert et al, 1990; Perera et al, 1992a; Crawford et al,

TABLE 7–3. *Examples of Markers of Early Biologic Effect or Response**

Endpoint	*Exposure Source*	*Biologic Sample*	*Population*	*References*
Chromosomal aberrations	Occupational exposure, radiation	WBC	Workers	Evans, 1982; Sarto et al, 1984[a]; van Sittert et al, 1985; Galloway et al, 1986
DNA hyperploidy	Aromatic amines	Bladder and lung cells	Workers	Hemstreet et al, 1988
GPA mutation	Chemotherapeutic agents, radiation	RBC	Patients, Japanese atom bomb survivors	Jensen et al, 1986; Langlois et al, 1987; Kyoizumi et al, 1989; Bigbee et al, 1990
HPRT mutation	Chemotherapeutic agents, radiation	WBC	Workers, patients	Messing et al, 1986; O'Neill et al, 1987; McGinniss et al, 1990; Ostrosky-Wegman et al, 1990
Micronuclei	Organic solvents, heavy metals, cigarette smoke, betel quid	WBC, oral mucosa	Workers	Hogstedt et al, 1983; Stich and Dunn, 1988
Mutation in tumor suppressor genes	AFB_1	Tumor tissue	Patients	Bressac et al, 1991; Hsu et al, 1991
Oncogene activation	PAH, cigarette smoke	Serum	Patients, workers	Kirk-Othmer, 1979; Brandt-Rauf and Niman, 1988; Perera et al, 1988
Single strand breaks	Styrene	WBC	Workers	Walles et al, 1988
Sister chromatid exchange	Occupational exposure, radiation	WBC	Workers	Carrano and Moore, 1982; Kelsey, 1989; Wilcosky and Rynard, 1990
Unscheduled DNA synthesis	Propylene oxide	WBC	Workers	Pero et al, 1982

*AFB_1, aflatoxin B_1; GPA, glycophorin A; HPRT, hypoxanthine guanine phosphoribosyl transferase; PAH, polycyclic aromatic hydrocarbons; RBC, red blood cells; WBC, white blood cells.

1994; Mooney et al, in press [b]). They have also been associated with lung cancer in several case–control studies (Sinopoli et al, 1990; Tang et al, 1993). A recent study of their persistence in ex-smokers indicates that in total leukocytes, PAH-DNA adducts have a half-life of approximately 16 weeks (Mooney et al, in press [b]).

Since chemical carcinogens bind to proteins as well as to DNA, determination of protein adducts is being increasingly used as an alternate marker of biologically effective dose (reviewed in Skipper and Tannenbaum, 1990). However, the relationship between protein adducts and DNA adducts may vary for each compound of interest and must be determined. Because of the large amounts in blood, both hemoglobin and albumin have been used for determination of biologically effective dose. Both proteins provide information on relatively recent exposure since the lifespan of the red blood cell is 4 months and the half-life of albumin is 21 days. Ethylene oxide-hemoglobin adducts resulting from occupational exposure were the first protein adducts to be measured by gas chromatography/mass spectrometry (GC/MS) (van Sittert et al, 1985; Tornqvist et al, 1986). Elevated ethylene oxide-hemoglobin adduct levels have been seen in workers as well as smokers by GC/MS and immunoassay (Tornqvist et al, 1986; Wraith et al, 1988; Mayer et al, 1991). 4-Aminobiphenyl-hemoglobin adducts have been measured by GC/MS in heavy smokers before and after smoking cessation (Bryant et al, 1987; Maclure et al, 1990; Mooney et al, in press [b]) and in fetal blood of infants of mothers who smoked (Coghlin et al, 1991). Serial sampling of smokers following cessation indicates that 4-ABP-hemoglobin adducts are highly smoking related, with a half-life of approximately 10 weeks (Mooney et al, in press [b]). Hemoglobin adducts of the tobacco-specific nitrosamines have also been measured by GC/MS in snuff dippers and smokers (Carmella et al, 1990). Table 7–2 provides examples of measurement of carcinogen-protein adducts.

The third category comprises markers that indicate

TABLE 7–4. *Examples of Markers of Genetic Susceptibility*

Gene[a]	Population	Reference
CYP 2D6	Lung cancer cases and controls	Ayesh et al, 1984; Vahakangas and Pelkonen, 1989; Caporaso et al, 1990; Kanajiri et al, 1990 (applies to CYP 2D6, CYP 1A1, CYP 2E1)
CYP 1A1	Lung cancer cases and controls	
CYP 2E1	Lung cancer cases and controls	
GSTM 1 (μ)	Lung, stomach, colon cancer	Seidegard and Pero, 1988; Strange et al, 1991
NAT	Smokers, colon	Ilett et al, 1987; Minchin et al, 1993
DNA repair genes		Reviewed in Friedberg, 1985
Tumor suppressor genes, Rb, p53	Retinoblastoma, Li-Fraumeni syndrome	Reviewed in Marshall, 1991; Li, 1990

[a]CYP, cytochrome P450; GST, glutathione-s-transferase; NAT, N-acetyltransferase; Rb, retinoblastoma.

an irreversible ***biologic effect*** resulting from a toxic interaction, either at the target or an analogous site, which is known or believed to be pathogenically linked to cancer. A wide variety of biomarkers fall into this category, from DNA single strand breaks to gene and chromosomal mutation to alterations in target oncogenes or tumor suppressor genes. Table 7–3 provides examples of exposures and populations biomonitored for these endpoints. It is readily apparent that few of these markers are chemical- or exposure-specific (in contrast to the molecular dosimetry markers). Hence there is the need for extensive information on other factors (lifestyle and environmental) that could affect these endpoints and act as confounding variables in a molecular epidemiologic study.

One extremely promising approach to establishing causality is to combine knowledge of the type or pattern of mutations induced by specific DNA-damaging agents with patterns of mutations that are frequently seen in human tumors (Harris, 1991). For example, there is a correspondence between the point mutation induced in experimental systems by AFB_1 (substitution of T for G) and the predominant point mutation seen in the *p53* tumor suppressor gene in hepatocellular carcinomas from cases living in regions of China where AFB_1 is a known risk factor (Jones et al, 1991). Similarly, in lung cancer cases the most common base substitution in the *p53* gene is the G-to-T transversion. The G-to-T mutation has been found in approximately half of all non–small cell lung cancers and has been associated with lifetime cigarette use (Suzuki et al, 1992). In vitro mammalian cell assays also have shown the ability of benzo(a)pyrene (BP) diol epoxide to predominantly cause this type of substitution (Harris, 1990), a finding that supports a hypothesis of tobacco-induced mutagenesis. The same G-to-T mutations also were found in the *K-ras* protooncogene in about 40% of human lung adenocarcinomas studied, as well as in BP-induced rodent lung tumors. The ability of BP to bind to DNA and preferentially cause this type of mutation in critical genes supports the hypothesis that smoking-related mutations are instrumental in lung carcinogenesis by activating oncogenes and inactivating tumor suppressor genes.

Biomarkers of *susceptibility* constitute the fourth category. Individual susceptibility to cancer may result from genetic and acquired factors, including differences in metabolism, DNA repair, inherited mutations in tumor suppressor genes, and nutritional deficiencies. In addition, stage of development may be a factor, as in the case of the infant and young child who may receive a proportionally greater exposure than the adult and whose physiologic immaturities may confer heightened susceptibility (Whyatt, 1995). For example, many carcinogens are metabolically activated or detoxified by P450 enzymes before binding to DNA. Thus a number of studies indicate that elevated metabolic activity of specific cytochrome P450 (CYP1A1, CYP2D6) enzymes is associated with lung cancer risk (reviewed in Ayesh et al, 1984; Vahakangas and Pelkonen, 1989; Caporaso et al, 1990; Kawajiri et al, 1990). Another metabolic phenotype related to increased cancer risk is the ability to detoxify aromatic amines via N-acetylation. Thus "slow" acetylators have been reported to be at increased risk for bladder cancer (Cartwright et al, 1982; Evans et al, 1983; Karkaya et al, 1986; Mommsen and Aagaard, 1986). "Phase II" enzymes detoxify carcinogens via conjugation of metabolites with glucuronide, glutathione or sulfate to produce hydrophilic products for excretion. Some, but not all studies, have shown that individuals lacking in activity of the phase II detoxifying enzyme glutathione-S-transferase M_1 (GSTM1) had an elevated risk of developing lung adenocarcinoma (Seidegard and Pero, 1988; Strange et al, 1991).

Genetic predisposition to cancer induction may also result from inherited mutations in tumor suppressor genes (e.g., retinoblastoma or *p53*) which regulate cell growth and terminal differentiation (for review see Marshall, 1991). For example, in Li-Fraumeni syndrome, patients with inherited mutations in the *p53* gene are at as much as 1000-fold increased risk for cancers at multiple sites including the breast (Li, 1990). Deficiencies in the ability to repair DNA damage also increase risk. Xeroderma pigmentosa patients lack the ability to repair DNA damage from ultraviolet (UV) radiation; these individuals are at elevated risk for the development of skin cancer from exposure to sunlight (reviewed in Friedberg, 1985).

Another factor that may influence susceptibility to certain cancers is nutritional status, resulting from intake of dietary fat and vitamins (Cohen, 1987; Willett, 1990; Marx, 1991; Block, 1992). An association has been seen between dietary fat and various cancers (Cohen, 1987; Willett, 1990); and some (but not all) studies have shown a protective effect of certain vitamins such as beta-carotene, vitamin C, vitamin E, and retinol (Willett, 1984; National Research Council, 1989).

The use of biomarkers—and particularly those indicative of susceptibility with their potential for stigmatization of the individual—engender significant ethical concerns (Ashford, 1986; Schulte, 1989 for review). These must be addressed before biomarkers are applied to screen populations or test individuals to determine risk of cancer.

As shown in Tables 7–1 through 7–4, biologic markers have been studied in four types of populations: (1) those with defined environmental exposures to carcinogens (cigarette smokers, workers, persons with certain ambient or dietary exposures); (2) clinical populations with exposure to carcinogenic drugs; (3) cancer patients; and (4) controls without exposure or disease. With respect to Tables 7–1 through 7–3, each one of the biomarkers listed has been elevated in at least one of the exposed (at-risk) populations. Two consistent findings in these studies have been (1) significant interindividual variation in levels of markers among persons with comparable exposure and (2) a measurable contribution of background exposures in so-called unexposed controls. These points will be discussed in greater detail below in the context of criteria for validation of biologic markers.

These studies have demonstrated that most of the methods are adequately sensitive for human studies. However, the results have often been limited by technical variability in the assays, small sample size, lack of appropriate controls, failure to account for confounding variables, and a paucity of data on exposure. Nonetheless, significant progress has been made in substantiating laboratory methods and addressing problems posed by the union of laboratory technology and epidemiology (Perera, 1987; International Agency for Research on Cancer, 1988; Schulte, 1989; Vineis et al, 1990; Harris, 1991; Hulka, 1991; Sugimura et al, 1991; Schulte and Perera, 1993).

Most of the research summarized in Tables 7–1 through 7–4 has consisted of *transitional* studies (Hulka, 1991; Schulte et al, 1993) that are largely cross-sectional in design. They have investigated the relationship between particular exposures to carcinogens and levels of biologic markers as well as to what degree these levels effect modification by susceptibility factors. Cross-sectional and longitudinal transitional studies are a first step in applying biomarkers in etiology studies but do not allow causal inferences to be drawn.

Descriptive molecular epidemiologic studies have been useful in generating hypotheses regarding cancer causation. Examples include an early ecological study exploring the correlation between a biological marker (AFB_1-guanine concentration in urine) and liver cancer incidence in Kenya (Autrup et al, 1983). Another is the comparison of O^6-methyldeoxyganosine adducts (presumably from dietary nitrosamines) in esophageal and stomach tumors from Chinese and European patients (Umbenhauer et al, 1985; Wild et al, 1986). Although the results of such ecological studies are limited by the lack of information about individual exposure, they are useful in providing clues for further, more hypothesis-testing, molecular epidemiologic studies (Hogstedt, 1988). An analogy is the well-known, conventional ecologic study relating industry concentration data to county rates of lung cancer mortality (Blot and Fraumeni, 1976). This led to a case–control study which confirmed the hypothesis that lung cancer in certain coastal areas was associated with the ship-building industry, possibly through asbestos exposure (Blot et al, 1978).

Another category of molecular epidemiologic research, *analytic or hypothesis-testing studies*, comprises cross-sectional, retrospective (case-control), and prospective longitudinal studies, or a combination thereof. Their purpose is to produce a valid estimate of a hypothesized cause–effect relationship between a suspected risk factor and cancer. A number of case–control studies have evaluated the association between various biomarkers and cancer. For example, various markers of biologically effective dose (carcinogen–DNA adducts), markers of biologic effect (Sister chromatid exchanges and oncogene activation) and markers of susceptibility (GSTM1) have been compared in cancer cases and controls (Sinopoli et al, 1990; van Schooten et al, 1990; Perera et al, 1991b; Shields et al, 1993; Tang et al, 1993). PAH-DNA adduct levels in peripheral blood cells of lung cancer patients who were current smokers were significantly higher than levels in current smokers without cancer, and a significant association was seen between adduct formation and lung cancer after controlling for smoking (odds ratio, 6.8, confidence intervals, 1.6–29.6) (Tang et al, 1993). These results suggest a constitutional factor operating to modulate risk of lung cancer from environmental exposures such as cigarette smoke.

In retrospective case–control studies, ideally one would want a permanent marker left decades earlier by the initiating carcinogen. Unfortunately, in the case of discontinued past exposures, even the most long-lived markers will be diluted by cell turnover, thereby underestimating the true past or cumulative dose. Only if exposure had been continuous and had not changed significantly during the past decades (and only if the disease had not altered metabolism) would current levels of the marker be directly representative of critical prior exposure. However, even short-lived markers can indicate the individual's responsiveness to carcinogenic exposures, provided that metabolism were unchanged by disease. Therefore, a finding of elevated adducts, oncogene activation, or chromosomal aberrations in cases with comparable current exposure to that of controls provides valuable, albeit circumstantial, evidence that these markers play a role in cancer risk.

An elegant juxtaposition of results from a conventional case–control study of bladder cancer and from biomonitoring of individuals who were representative of the same source population has provided evidence that adduct formation is causally related to cancer risk. The data have also provided insights into the mechanisms of bladder cancer causation. In the case–control study, the risk of bladder cancer in Turin, Italy, was 2.5 times higher among smokers of black tobacco than among smokers of blond tobacco (Vineis et al, 1988). A subsequent study of volunteers from Turin showed correspondingly higher levels of 4-aminobiphenyl hemoglobin (4-ABP-Hb) adducts in the blood of smokers of black tobacco compared to smokers of blond tobacco (Bryant et al, 1988). The differences in adduct levels were approximately proportional to the relative risk of each group. Urinary mutagenicity was also twice as high in smokers of black tobacco as in smokers of blond tobacco (Malaveille et al, 1989). These findings were not surprising since aromatic amines, including 4-ABP, are more concentrated in smoke from black tobacco than from blond tobacco. An extension of this research has linked a marker of genetic susceptibility (acetylation phenotype) and formation of 4-ABP-Hb adducts with bladder cancer. In smokers, the slow acetylator phenotype was linked both to higher risk of arylamine-induced bladder cancer and to formation of 4-ABP-Hb adducts derived from cigarette smoke (Vineis and Terracini, 1990).

The most definitive approaches to establishing the relationship between biomarkers and risk are the prospective cohort, nested case–control or case–cohort study designs (Schulte et al, 1993). Examples include a prospective study investigating the relationship between biomarkers in blood samples drawn just after chemotherapy to subsequent cases of second malignancy (Kaldor and Day, 1988). Another is the Nordic study of the predictive value of cytogenetic markers for cancer risk (Brogger et al, 1990). The nested case-control design combines the advantages of the retrospective and prospective study designs. Biologic samples and data are collected at the initiation of a cohort study and are stored. Incident cases are matched to controls and samples are then retrospectively assayed to determine the relative risk. For example, in a recent study of AFB_1 and hepatitis B in Shanghai, China, analysis of stored urine samples from 22 cases and 140 matched controls has revealed relative risks of 2.4 for any AFB_1 metabolite in urine and 4.9 for AFB_1-guanine adducts (Ross et al, 1992). A multiplicative effect of AFB_1 and hepatitis B was also observed.

METHODOLOGIC ISSUES: CRITERIA AND STRATEGIES FOR VALIDATION

Validation of a biomarker involves the systematic identification of factors that influence the ability of the marker to predict exposure or outcome in a test population (Hulka et al, 1990; Schulte and Perera, 1993; Mooney et al, in press [b], for discussion). During the validation process, evidence is weighed to determine whether or not a biomarker measures what it claims to measure, whether it be exposure, disease, or susceptibility. Validation can be considered a two-stage process involving first laboratory and then epidemiologic studies, although many of the steps require iteration as new information becomes available. The ultimate goal of the validation effort is to allow biomarkers to be used in appropriate epidemiologic and clinical applications, which will require their assessment with respect to the characteristics listed in Table 7–5. The first step, *laboratory validation*, involves ascertainment of such factors as the shape of the dose–response curve, low-dose sensitivity, exposure specificity, and reproducibility of the assay. In the second step, *epidemiologic validation*, the population sensitivity and specificity, intra- and interindividual variation in biomarker response, persistence, background occurrence, positive predictive value, as well as biological relevance and feasibility, are all evaluated.

Human exposures are complex and dynamic in nature, and the human metabolic and pharmokinetic processes in humans may not be known for each xenobiotic. Epidemiologic validation does not require exhaustive knowledge of these factors, but does demand sufficient knowledge of potential confounding factors on which to base a consistently reproducible exposure–biomarker or biomarker–disease relationship. If confounders are not adequately assessed, the biomarker will be incorrectly attributed to the exposure/disease under study.

A major goal of molecular epidemiology is to elucidate the factors and mechanisms that explain why persons vary in their risk of disease. Therefore, central to the validation of biomarkers is the assessment of the factors, including effect modifiers, which contribute to interindividual variation in these measurements. As discussed above, interindividual variation in response is attributable to differences in a variety of factors, including

TABLE 7–5. *Characterization of Biomarkers Required for Molecular Epidemiologic Validation*

Laboratory	*Epidemiologic*
Dose-response curve	Background levels in "unexposed" people
Reproducibility of the assay:	Intraindividual variation over time:
From run to run	Without altering exposure
From day to day	When exposure is removed (persistence/half-life)
From one laboratory to another	Interindividual variation:
Detection limit (low-dose sensitivity)	Response to a given exposure
Exposure specificity	Persistence of biomarker
	Levels in surrogate vs. target tissue
	Biologic relevance to disease
	Positive predictive value (yield of high-risk individuals)
	Feasibility:
	Amount and availability of tissue
	Cost
	Time required for each assay

personal exposure and genetic and acquired susceptibility. Therefore, persons with the same apparent exposure can vary widely in their biomarker response. Not surprisingly, marked interindividual variation has been observed in virtually all molecular epidemiologic and biomonitoring studies of populations having occupational or environmental exposure to mutagens/carcinogens (Harris, 1989). For example, PAH-DNA adducts measured in persons cotinine-verified as having recent exposure to cigarette smoke were found to vary by 40-fold (Mooney et al, in press [a]), while adducts in coke oven workers and Polish residents varied by 50-fold and 90-fold respectively (Hemminki et al, 1990; Perera et al, 1992a). Studies are ongoing to distinguish the relative contributions of laboratory variability, and intraindividual variability from biologic variation in biomarkers.

Prevention: The Use of Biomarkers in Health Interventions

Once biomarkers have been validated they can be used to determine populations at increased risk of cancer in order to target interventions to those who would most benefit. Persons identified as being at high risk of disease could be removed from the exposure; medical surveillance could be increased; and/or chemoprevention could be initiated. Biological markers have the potential to provide feedback during the intervention and to monitor its efficacy. For example, Gritz has proposed using biomarkers in feedback studies to encourage smoking cessation by increasing the smoker's perceived risk of cancer, changing attitudes about smoking, and by increasing adherence to cancer prevention protocols (Gritz, 1992). Biological markers could be used to emphasize the negative effects of exposure (i.e., continued smoking), and to show the biological benefit of quitting smoking.

With respect to chemoprevention, studies of baseline levels of serum vitamins and biomarkers indicate a protective effect of certain antioxidant micronutrients. For example, a cross-sectional study of 63 heavy smokers (one or more packs per day for at least 10 years) has shown that serum concentrations of alpha-tocopherol and vitamin C were inversely related to the levels of PAH-DNA adducts in lymphocytes measured in the same individuals (Grinberg-Funes et al, 1994). These associations were limited to the subjects with the GSTM1 null genotype, which is consistent with prior studies indicating a protective effect of both antioxidant micronutrients and GSTM1 genotype in lung cancer.

Biologic markers already play an important role in the evaluation of chemopreventive agents, specifically in Phase II trials (Benner et al, 1992; Freedman et al, 1992; Kelloff et al, 1992). For example, current trials involving lung and upper aerodigestive tract tumors are evaluating micronuclei, DNA content, genetic alteration in oncogenes, as well as markers of proliferation, growth regulation and differentiation (Benner et al, 1992). Research suggests that additional biomarkers of genetic damage such as carcinogen–DNA adducts can be useful as intermediate endpoints in intervention studies of exposed or at-risk populations.

CONCLUSION AND RECOMMENDATIONS

The field of molecular cancer epidemiology has experienced rapid progress in the past ten years and should be capable of significantly improving strategies for cancer prevention. It is, however, at a critical point in its development and validation where laboratory experts and epidemiologists must work closely together to lay the necessary groundwork for definitive etiologic and intervention studies (Hulka et al, 1990; Schulte and Perera, 1993). Specific recommendations are as follows:

1. Collaborative studies involving exchange of standards and biologic samples and using corroborative methods. One such effort, involving three different laboratories, helped to resolve inconsistencies in results of immunoassays for PAH-DNA adducts (Santella et al, 1988). Others have established the identity of carcinogen–DNA damage in placental tissue and blood using a combination of laboratory techniques (Weston et al, 1988, 1989).
2. Further development and validation of methods capable of distinguishing exposure-specific patterns of molecular damage such as signal lesions in target genes.
3. Development of biologic markers for carcinogens such as dioxin and other organochlorines which are widespread and are of concern with respect to breast and testicular cancer, but which would not be detected by available biomarkers that largely reflect direct damage to DNA.
4. Research to characterize the extent and nature of intra- and interindividual variability and background levels of markers in humans. Variability in human response and preexisting damage are key considerations in risk assessment of environmental carcinogens and can be ascertained by serial sampling of exposed and unexposed populations.
5. Pharmacokinetic modeling and time-course studies in humans to define the persistence of markers in various cell types as a basis for designing the optimal sampling strategy and for interpreting dose–response data.
6. Sample banks to archive human biologic samples from well-selected cohorts or focused surveys. These could provide blood, urine, breast milk, saliva, semen,

placentae, autopsy samples, or biopsy samples for retrospective analysis.

7. The use of batteries of biologic markers reflecting complementary mechanisms and varying time periods of exposure. The battery should include chemical-specific and "generic" markers and those which reflect recent and past exposures, markers of preclinical effect and susceptibility. For example, a battery designed to assess the role of occupational exposure to aromatic amines in bladder cancer might include acetylator status as a marker of susceptibility, immunoassays to aromatic amine–DNA adducts in leukocytes, cytogenetic effects in lymphocytes, and measurement of ras p21 protein products in plasma or urine. Studies of environmental causes of breast cancer might include concentrations of organochlorine residues in serum, carcinogen–DNA adducts formed by aromatic compounds including PAH, alterations in P450 enzymes, and mutations in the *p53* gene.

8. Parallel studies in humans and experimental animals using the same biologic markers to compare mechanisms, response to exposure, and risk in different species. The relationships between dose and effect markers and tumor incidence can most feasibly be evaluated in the experimental model as a first step in understanding their biologic significance in humans. Ultimately, prospective studies in both species are needed to answer important questions facing risk assessors about the validity of interspecies extrapolation to estimate risks of low-level human exposures.

9. Longitudinal studies in model populations, especially those in whom cancer latency is expected to be short. Examples are cancer patients treated with high-dose chemotherapy who experience a high rate of secondary cancer ($\leq$10%) or heavily exposed worker groups being monitored pursuant to workplace regulations.

10. "Case–case" studies using biomarkers to differentiate cancer cases by tumor characteristics and exposure patterns (Taylor, 1990) and retrospective or "nested" case–control studies in humans.

11. A national database to enable researchers to share data on biologic markers from experimental and molecular epidemiologic studies.

12. Standardization of methods in all aspects of molecular epidemiology: laboratory methods, criteria for identifying individual vs. population effects, methods of data analysis, reporting terminology, and questionnaires (Schulte and Perera, 1993).

Validation of molecular epidemiology requires a concerted interdisciplinary research effort. However, the promise of molecular epidemiology in preventing cancer and the rapid progress to date in developing and applying biomarkers provide strong incentives to meet this challenge.

REFERENCES

AMERICAN CANCER SOCIETY. 1993. Cancer Facts and Figures—1993. Atlanta, American Cancer Society.

AMES BN, GOLD LS. 1990. Dietary carcinogens, environmental pollution, and cancer: some misconceptions. Med Oncol Tumor Pharmacother 7:69–85.

ASHFORD NA. 1986. Policy considerations for human monitoring in the workplace. J Occup Med 28:563–568.

AUTRUP H, BRADLEY KA, SHAMSUDDIN AKM, WAKHISI J, WASUNNA A. 1983. Detection of putative adduct with fluorescence characteristics identical to 2,3-dihydro-2-(7-guanyl)-3-hydroxyaflatoxin B1 in human urine collected in Murang'a District, Kenya. Carcinogenesis 4:1193–1195.

AYESH R, IDLE J, RICHIE J, CROTHERS M, HETZEL M. 1984. Metabolic oxidation phenotypes as markers for susceptibility to lung cancer. Nature 312:169–170.

BENNER SE, HONG WK, LIPPMAN SM, LEE JS, HITTELMAN WM. 1992. Intermediate biomarkers in upper aerodigestive tract and lung chemoprevention trials. J Cell Biochem (Suppl.) 16G:33–38.

BERGGREN G, SJOSTEDT S. 1983. Preinvasive carcinoma of the cervix uteri and smoking. Acta Obstet Gynecol Scand 62:593–598.

BIGBEE WL, WYROBECK AW, LANGLOIS RG, JENSEN RH, EVERSON RB. 1990. The effect of chemotherapy on the in vivo frequency of glycophorin A "null" variant erythrocytes. Mutat Res 240:165–175.

BLOCK G. 1992. The data support a role for antioxidants in reducing cancer risk. Nutr Rev 50(7):207–13.

BLOT WJ, FRAUMENI JF. 1976. Geographical patterns of lung cancer: Industrial correlations. Am J Epidemiol 103:539–550.

BLOT WJ, HARRINGTON JM, TOLEDO A, HOOVER R, HEATH CW, FRAUMENI JF. 1978. Lung cancer after employment in shipyards during World War II. New Engl J Med 299:620–624.

BOS RP, JONGENEELEN FJ. 1988. Nonselective and selective methods for biological monitoring of exposure to coal tar products. *In* Bartsch K, Hemminki K, O'Neill IK (eds): Methods for Detecting DNA Damaging Agents in Humans: Applications in Cancer Epidemiology and Prevention. IARC Sci Publ 89. Lyon, France, International Agency for Research on Cancer, 389–395.

BRANDT-RAUF PW, NIMAN HL. 1988. Serum screening for oncogene proteins in workers exposed to PCB's. Br J Ind Med 45:689–693.

BRESSAC B, KEW M, WANDS J, OZTURK M. 1991. Selective G to T mutations of *p53* gene in hepatocellular carcinoma from southern Africa. Nature 350:429–430.

BROGGER A, HAGMAR L, HANSTEEN IL, HEIM S, HOGSTEDT B, KNUDSEN L, LAMBERT B, LINNAINMAA K, MITELMAN F, NORDENSON I, REUTERWALL C, SALOMAA S, SKERFVING S, SORSA M. 1990. An inter-Nordic prospective study on cytogenetic endpoints and cancer risk. Cancer Genet Cytogenet 45:1264–1272.

BRYANT MS, SKIPPER PL, TANNENBAUM SR, NIURE M. 1987. Hemoglobin adducts of 4-aminobiphenyl in smokers and nonsmokers. Cancer Res 47:612–618.

BRYANT MS, VINEIS P, SKIPPER P, TANNENBAUM SR. 1988. Hemoglobin adducts of aromatic amines: Association with smoking status and type of tobacco. Proc Natl Acad Sci USA 85:9788–9791.

CALLEMAN CJ. 1982. In vivo dosimetry by means of alkylated hemoglobin: A tool in the design of tests for genotoxic effects. *In* Bridges BA, Butterworth BE, Weinstein IB (eds): Indicators of Genotoxic Exposure, Banbury Report No. 19, Cold Spring Harbor, New York, Cold Spring Harbor Laboratory, pp. 157–167.

CALLEMAN CJ, EHRENBERG L, JANSSON B, OSTERMAN-GOLKAR S,

SEGERBACK D, SVENSSON K, WACHTMEISTER CA. 1978. Monitoring and risk assessment by means of alkyl groups in hemoglobin in persons occupationally exposed to ethylene oxide. J Environ Pathol Toxicol 2:427–442.

CAPORASO NE, TUCKER MA, HOOVER RN, HAYES RB, PICKLE LW, ISSAQ HJ, MUSCHIK GM. 1990. Lung cancer and the debrisoquine metabolic phenotype. J Natl Cancer Inst 82:1264–1272.

CARMELLA SG, KAGAN SS, KAGAN M, FOILIES PG, PALLADINO G, QUART E, HECHT SS. 1990. Mass spectrometric analysis of tobacco-specific nitrosamine hemoglobin adducts in snuff dippers, smokers, and nonsmokers. Cancer Res 50:5438–5445.

CARRANO AV, MOORE DH. 1982. The rationale and methodology for quantifying sister chromatid exchange frequency in humans. *In* Heddle JA (ed): Mutagenicity: New Horizons in Genetic Toxicology. New York, Academic Press, pp. 267–304.

CARTWRIGHT RA, GLASHAN RW, ROGERS HJ, BARHAM-HALL D, AHMAD RA, HIGGINS E, KAHN MA. 1982. Role of N-acetyltransferase phenotypes in bladder carcinogenesis: A pharmacokinetic epidemiological approach to bladder cancer. Lancet 2:842–846.

CATHGART R, SCHWEIRS E, SAUL RL, AMES BN. 1984. Thymine glycol and thymidine glycol in human and rat urine: A possible assay for oxidative DNA damage. Proc Natl Acad Sci USA 81:5633–5637.

COGHLIN J, GANN PH, HAMMOND SK, SKIPPER PL, TAGHIZADEH K, PAUL M, TANNENBAUM SR. 1991. 4-Aminobiphenyl hemoglobin adducts in fetuses exposed to the tobacco smoke carcinogen in utero. J Natl Cancer Inst 83:274–280.

COHEN L. 1987. Diet and cancer. Sci Am 257:42–48.

CRAWFORD FG, MAYER J, SANTELLA RM, COOPER T, OTTMAN R, TSAI WY, SIMON-CEREIJIDO G, WANG M, TANG D, PERERA FP. 1994. Biomarkers of environmental tobacco smoke in preschool children and their mothers. J Natl Cancer Inst 86:1398–1402.

DAY BW, NAYLOR S, GAN LS, SAHALI Y, NYUGEN TT, SKIPPER PL, WISHNOK JS, TANNENBAUM SR. 1990. Molecular dosimetry of polycyclic aromatic hydrocarbon epoxides and diol epoxides via hemoglobin adducts. Cancer Res 50:4611–4618.

DJURIC Z, HEILBURN LK, READING BA, BOOMER A, VALERIOTE FA, MARTINO S. 1991. Effects of a low-fat diet on levels of oxidative damage to DNA in human peripheral nucleated blood cells. J Natl Cancer Inst 83:766–769.

EADSFORTH CV, COVENEY PC, SJOE WHA. 1988. An improved analytical method, based on HPLC with electrochemical detection, for monitoring exposure to 3-chloro-4-fluoroaniline. J Anal Tox 12:330–333.

EHRENBERG L, OSTERMAN-GOLKAR O, TORNQVIST M. 1986. Macromolecule adducts, target dose, and risk assessment. *In* Ramel C, Lambert B, Magnusson J (eds): Genetic Toxicology of Environmental Chemicals, Part B: Genetic Effects and Applied Mutagenesis. New York, Alan R. Liss, pp. 253–260.

EVANS DAP, EZE LC, WHIBLEY EJ. 1983. The association of the slow acetylator phenotype with bladder cancer. J Med Genet 20:330–333.

EVANS HJ. 1982. Cytogenetic Studies on industrial populations exposed to mutagens. *In* Bridges BA, Butterworth BE, Weinstein IB (eds): Indicators of Genotoxic Exposure, Banbury Report No. 19. Cold Spring Harbor, New York, Cold Spring Harbor Laboratory, pp. 325–340.

EVERSON RB. 1986. Detection of occupational and environmental exposures by bacterial mutagenesis assays of human body fluids. J Occup Med 28:647–655.

FARMER PB, BAILEY E, GORF SM, TORNQVIST M, OSTERMAN-GOLKAR S, KAUTIIAINEN A, LEWIS-ENRIGHT DP. 1986. Monitoring human exposure to ethylene oxide by the determination of haemoglobin adducts using gas chromatography-mass spectrometry. Carcinogenesis 7:637–640.

FICHTINGER-SCHEPMAN AMJ, VAN OOSTEROM AT, LOHMAN PHM, BERENDS F. 1987. Interindividual human variation in cisplatinum sensitivity, predictable in an in vitro assay? Mutat Res 190:59–62.

FOILES PG, MIGLIETTA LM, AKERKAR SA, HECHT SS. 1988. Detection of O-Methyldeoxyguanosine in human placental DNA. Cancer Res 48:4184–4188.

FREEDMAN LS, SCHATZKIN A, SCHIFFMAN MH. 1992. Statistical validation of intermediate markers of precancer for use as endpoints in chemoprevention trials. J Cell Biochem (Suppl.) 16G:27–32.

FRIEDBERG EC. 1985. DNA Repair. New York, W.H. Freeman and Company.

GALLOWAY SM, BERRY PK, NICHOLS WW, WOLMAN SR, SOPER KA, STOLLEY PD, ARCHER P. 1986. Chromosome aberrations in individuals occupationally exposed to ethylene oxide and in a large control population. Mutat Res 170:55–74.

GAN LS, SKIPPER PL, PENG X, GROOPMAN JD, CHEN JS, WOGAN GN, TANNENBAUM SR. 1988. Serum albumin adducts in the molecular epidemiology of aflatoxin carcinogenesis: Correlation with aflatoxin B1 intake and urinary excretion of aflatoxin M1. Carcinogenesis 9:1323–1325.

GARLAND WA, KUENZIG W, RUBIO F, KORNYCHUK H, NORKUS EP, CONNEY AH. 1986. Urinary excretion of nitrosodimethylamine and nitrosoproline in humans: Interindividual differences and the effect of administered ascorbic acid and tocopherol. Cancer Res 46:5392–5400.

GRINBERG-FUNES RA, SINGH VN, PERERA FP, BELL DA, YOUNG TL, DICKEY C, WANG LW, SANTELLA RM. 1994. Polycyclic aromatic hydrocarbon–DNA adducts in smokers and their relationship to micronutrient levels and glutathione-S-transferase M1 genotype. Carcinogenesis 15:2449–2454.

GRITZ ER. 1992. Paving the road from basic research to policy: Cigarette smoking as a prototype issue for cancer control science. Cancer Epidemiol Biomarkers Prev 1:427–434.

GROOPMAN JD, DONAHUE PR, ZHU J, CHEN J, WOGAN GN. 1985. Aflatoxin metabolism and nucleic acid adducts in urine by affinity chromatography. Proc Natl Acad Sci USA 82:6492–6496.

HAJIMIRAGHA H, EWERS U, BROCKHAUS A, BOETTGER A. 1989. Levels of benzene and other volatile aromatic compounds in the blood of non-smokers and smokers. Int Arch Occup Environ Health 61:513–518.

HALL N, BADAWI AF, O'CONNOR PJ, SAFFHILL R. 1991. The detection of alkylation damage in the DNA of human gastrointestinal tissues. Br J Cancer 64:59–63.

HARRIS C. 1991. Chemical and physical carcinogenesis: Advances and perspectives for the 1990s. Cancer Res (Suppl) 51:50235–50445.

HARRIS CC. 1989. Interindividual variation among humans in carcinogen metabolism, DNA adduct formation and DNA repair. Carcinogenesis 10(9):1563–1566.

HARRIS CC, WESTON A, WILLEY J, TRIVERS G, MANN D. 1987. Biochemical and molecular epidemiology of human cancer: Indicators of carcinogen exposure, DNA damage and genetic predisposition. Environ Health Perspect 75:109–119.

HEMMINKI K, GRZYBOWSKA E, CHORAZI M, TWARDOWSKA-SAUCHA K, SROCZYNSKI JW, PUTMAN KL, RANDERATH K, PHILLIPS DH, HEWER A, SANTELLA RM, YOUNG TL, PERERA FP. 1990. DNA adducts in humans environmentally exposed to aromatic compounds in an industrial area of Poland. Carcinogenesis 11:1229–1231.

HEMSTREET GP, SCHULTE PA, RINGEN K, STRINGER W, ALTEKRUSE EB. 1988. DNA hyperploidy as a marker for biological response to bladder carcinogen exposure. Int J Cancer 42:817–820.

HERBERT R, MARCUS M, WOLFF MS, PERERA FP, ANDREWS L, GODBOLD JH, RIVERA M, STEFANIDIS M, QUING LU X, LANDRIGAN PJ, SANTELLA RM. 1990. Detection of adducts of deoxyribonicleic acid in white blood cells of roofers by ^{32}P-postlabeling. Scand J Work Environ Health 16:135–143.

HOFFMANN D, HECHT SS. 1985. Nicotine-derived N-nitrosamines and tobacco-related cancer: Current status and future direction. Cancer Res 45:935–944.

HOGSTEDT B, AKESSON B, AXELL K, GULLBERG B, MITELMAN F, PERO RW, SKERVING S, WELINDER H. 1983. Increased frequency of lymphocyte micronuclei in workers producing reinforced polyester resin with low exposure to styrene. Scand J Work Environ Health 49:271–276.

HOGSTEDT LC. 1986. Future perspectives, needs and expectations of biological monitoring of exposure to genotoxicants in prevention of occupational disease. *In* Sorsa M, Norppa H (eds): Monitoring of Occupational Genotoxicants. Progress in Clinical and Biological Research. New York, Alan R. Liss, pp. 231–243.

HOGSTEDT LC. 1988. Summary: Epidemiological applications. *In* Bartsch H, Hemminki K, O'Neill IK (eds): Methods for Detecting DNA Damaging Agents in Humans: Applications in Cancer Epidemiology and Prevention. IARC Sci Publ 89. Lyon, France, pp. 21–22.

HSIEH L, HSU SW, CHEN DS, SANTELLA RM. 1988. Immunological detection of aflatoxin B1-DNA adducts formed in vivo. Cancer Res 48:6328–31.

HSU IC, METCALF RA, SUN T, WELSH JA, WANG NJ, HARRIS CC. 1991. Mutational hotspot in the p53 gene in human hepatocellular carcinomas. Nature 350:427–428.

HUH NH, SATOH MS, SHIGA J, RAJEWSKY MF, KUROKI T. 1989. Immunoanalytical detection of 04-ethylthymine in liver DNA of individuals with or without malignant tumors. Cancer Res 49:93–97.

HULKA BS. 1991. Epidemiological studies using biological markers: Issues for epidemiologists. Cancer Epidemiol Biomarkers Prev 1:13–19.

HULKA BS, GRIFFITH JD, WILCOSKY TC (EDS). 1990. Biologic Markers in Epidemiology. New York, Oxford University Press.

INTERNATIONAL AGENCY FOR RESEARCH ON CANCER. 1988. IARC Monograph on the Evaluation of Carcinogenic Risk to Humans: Genetic and Related Effects. An Update of Selected IARC Monographs, Vols. 1–42, Suppl. 6. Lyon, France, International Agency for Research on Cancer.

ILETT KF, DAVID BM, DETHON P, CASTELEDEN WM, KWA R. 1987. Acetylator phenotype on colorectal carcinoma. Cancer Res 47:1466–1469.

JENSEN RH, LANGLOIS RG, BIGBEE WL. 1986. Determination of somatic mutations in human erythrocytes by flow cytometry. *In* Ramel C, Lambert B, Magnusson J (eds): Genetic Toxicology of Environmental Chemicals, Part B: Genetic Effects and Applied Mutagenesis. New York, Alan R. Liss, pp. 177–184.

JONES PA, BUCKLEY JD, HENDERSON BE, ROSS RK, PIKE MC. 1991. From gene to carcinogen: A rapidly evolving field in molecular epidemiology. Cancer Res 51:3617–3620.

JONGELEEN FJ, ANZION RBM, THEUWS JLG, BOS RP. 1989. Urinary 1-hydroxypyrene levels in workers handling petroleum coke. J Toxicol Environ Health 26:133–136.

JONGELEEN FJ, BOS RP, ANZION RBM, THEUWS JLG, HENDERSON PT. 1986. Biological monitoring of polycyclic aromatic hydrocarbons metabolites in urine. Scand J Work Environ Health 12:137–143.

KALDOR J, DAY NE. 1988. Epidemiological studies of the relationship between carcinogenicity and DNA damage. *In* Bartsch H, Hemminki K, O'Neill IK (eds): Methods for Detecting DNA Damaging Agents in Humans: Applications in Cancer Epidemiology and Prevention. IARC Sci Publ 89. Lyon, France, International Agency for Research on Cancer, pp. 460–468.

KARKAYA AE, COK L, SARDAS S, GOGUS O, SARDAR OS. 1986. N-acetyltransferase phenotype of patients with bladder cancer. Hum Toxicol 5:333–335.

KAWAJIRI K, NAKACHI K, IMAI K, YOSHII A, SHINODA N, WATANABE J. 1990. Identification of genetically high risk individuals to lung cancer by DNA polymorphisms of the cytochrome P4501A1 gene. FEBS Lett 263:131–133.

KELLOFF GJ, MALONE WF, BOONE CW, STEELE VE, DOODY LA. 1992. Intermediate biomarkers of precancer and their application in chemoprevention. J Cell Biochem (Suppl.) 16G:15–21.

KELSEY KT, WIENCKE JK, LITTLE FF, et al. 1989. Sister chromatid exchange in painters recently exposed to solvents. Environ Res 50:248–255.

KIRK RE, OTHMER DF. 1979. Encyclopedia of Chemical Technology. New York, Willey.

KYOIZUMI S, NAKAMURA N, HAKODA M, AWA AA, BEAN MA, JENSEN RH, AKIYAMA M. 1989. Detection of somatic mutations at the glycophorin A locus in erythrocytes of atomic bomb survivors using a single beam flow sorter. Cancer Res 49:581–588.

LANDRIGAN PJ. 1992. Commentary: Environmental disease—A preventable epidemic. Am J Public Health 82:941–943.

LANGLOIS RG, BIGBEE WL, KGOIZUMI S, NAKAMURA N, BEAN MA, AKIYAMA M, JENSEN RH. 1987. Evidence for increased somatic cell mutations at the glycophorin A locus in atom bomb survivors. Science 236:445–448.

LEE BM, BAOYUN Y, HERBERT R, HEMMINKI K, PERERA FP, SANTELLA RM. 1991. Immunologic measurement of polycyclic aromatic hydrocarbon-albumin adducts in foundry workers and roofers. Scand J Work Environ Health 17:190–194.

LI FP. 1990. Familial cancer syndromes and clusters. Curr Probl Cancer 49:75–113.

LIPPMAN SM, LEE JS, LOTAN R, HITTLEMAN W, WARGOVICH MJ, HONG WK. 1990. Biomarkers as intermediate endpoints in chemoprevention trials. J Natl Cancer Inst 82:555–560.

LU SH, OHSHIMA H, FU HM, TIAN Y, LI FM, BLETTNER M, WAHRENDORF J, BARTSCH H. 1986. Urinary excretion of N-nitrosamino acids and nitrate by inhabitants of high- and low-risk areas for esophageal cancer in northern China: Endogenous formation of nitrosoproline and its inhibition by vitamin C. Cancer Res 46:1485–1491.

MACLURE M, BRYANT MS, SKIPPER PL, TANNENBAUM SR. 1990. Decline of the hemoglobin adduct of 4-aminobiphenyl during withdrawal from smoking. Cancer Res 50:181–184.

MALAVEILLE C, VINEIS P, ESTEVE J, OSHIMA H, BRUN G, HAUTEFEVILLE A, GALLET P, RONCO G, TERRACINI B, BARTSCH H. 1989. Levels of mutagens in the urine of smokers of black and blond tobacco correlate with their risk of bladder cancer. Carcinogenesis 10:577–586.

MANABE S, WADA O. 1988. Analysis of human plasma as an exposure level monitor for carcinogenic tryptophan pyrolysis products. Mutat Res 209:33–38.

MANABE S, WADA O. 1990. Identification of carcinogenic tryptophan pyrolysis products in human bile by high-performance liquid chromatography. Environ Mol Mutagen 15:229–235.

MANABE S, YANAGISAWA H, ISHIKAWA S, KITAGAWA Y, KANAI Y, WADA O. 1987. Accumulation of 2-amino-6-methyldipyridol[1,2-a:3′,2′-d]imidazole and 2-aminodipyrido[1,2-a:3′,2′-d]imidazole, carcinogenic glutamic acid pyrolisis products, in plasma of patients with uremia. Cancer Res 47:6150–6155.

MARSHALL CJ. 1991. Tumor suppressor genes. Cell 64:313–326.

MARX J. 1991. Zeroing in on individual cancer risk. Science 253:612–616.

MAYER J, WARBURTON D, JEFFREY A, PERO R, WALLES S, ANDREWS L, TOOR M, LATRIANO L, WAZNEH L, TANG D, TSAI WY, KURODA M, PERERA FP. 1991. Biologic markers in ethylene oxide-exposed workers and controls. Mutat Res 248:163–176.

MCDIARMID MA, IYPE PT, KOLODNER K, JACOBSON-KRAM D, STRICKLAND PT. 1991. Evidence for acrolein-modified DNA in peripheral blood leukocytes of cancer patients treated with cyclophosphamide. Mutat Res 248:93–99.

MCGINNISS MJ, FALTA MT, SULLIVAN LM, ALBERTINI RJ. 1990.

In vivo hprt mutant frequencies in T-cells of normal human newborns. Mutat Res 240:117–126.

MESSING K, SEIFERT AM, BRADLEY WEC. 1986. In vivo mutant frequency of technicians professionally exposed to ionizing radiation. *In* Sorsa M, Norppa H (eds): Monitoring of Occupational Genotoxicants. New York, Alan R. Liss, pp. 87–97.

MILLER EC, MILLER JA. 1981. Mechanisms of chemical carcinogenesis. Cancer 47:1055–1064.

MINCHIN RF, KADLUBAR FF, ILETT KF. 1993. Role of acetylation in colorectal cancer. Mutat Res 290:35–42.

MOMMSEN S, AAGAARD J. 1986. Susceptibility in urinary bladder cancer: Acetyltransferase phenotypes and related risk factors. Cancer Lett 32:199–205.

MOONEY LA, BELL DA, SANTELLA RM, VAN BENNEKUM A, OTTMAN R, PAIK M, BLANER W, LUCIER GW, COVEY L, YOUNG T-L, COOPER TB, GLASSMAN AH, PERERA FP. 1995a. The contribution of genetic and nutritional factors to DNA damage in heavy smokers. Submitted.

MOONEY LA, SANTELLA RM, COVEY L, JEFFREY A, BIGBEE W, RANDALL MC, COOPER TB, OTTMAN R, TSAI WY, WAZNEH L, GLASSMAN AH, YOUNG T-L, PERERA FP. 1995. Decline of DNA damage and other biomarkers in peripheral blood following smoking cessation. Cancer Epidemiol Biomarkers Prev 4:627–634.

MUSTONEN R, HEMMINKI K, ALHONEN A, HIETANEN P, KIILUNEN M. 1988. Determination of cis-Diamminedichloroplatinum (II) in blood compartments of cancer patients. *In* Bartsch H, Hemminki K, O'Neill IK (eds): Methods for Detecting DNA Damaging Agents in Man: Applications in Cancer Epidemiology and Prevention. IARC Sci Publ 89. Lyon, France, International Agency for Research on Cancer, pp. 329–332.

NRC DIET AND HEALTH. 1989. Implications for Reducing Chronic Disease Risk. Washington, D.C.: National Academy Press.

NATIONAL RESEARCH COUNCIL. 1993a. Issues in Risk Assessment. Washington, D.C., National Academy Press.

NATIONAL RESEARCH COUNCIL. 1993b. Toxicity Testing and Strategies to Determine Needs and Priorities. Washington, D.C., National Academy Press.

O'NEILL JP, MCGINNISS MJ, BERMAN JK, SULLIVAN LM, NICKLAS JA, ALBERTINI RJ. 1987. Refinement of a T-lymphocyte cloning assay to quantify the in vivo thioguanine-resistant mutant frequency in humans. Mutagenesis 2:87–94.

OSTERMAN-GOLKAR S, BAILEY E, FARMER PB, GORF SM, LAMB JH. 1984. Monitoring exposure to propylene oxide through the determination of hemoglobin alkylation. Scand J Work Environ Health 10:99–102.

OSTROSKY-WEGMAN P, MONTERO R, PALAO A, CORTINAS DE NAVA C, HURTADO F, ALBERTINI RJ. 1990. 6-Thioguanine-resistant T-lymphocyte autoradiographic assay: Determination of variation frequencies in individuals suspected of radiation exposure. Mutat Res 12:1253–1258.

PARKER RJ, GILL I, TARONE R, VIONNET JA, GRUNBERG S, MUGGIA FM, REED E. 1991. Platinum-DNA damage in leukocyte DNA of patients receiving carboplatin and cisplatin chemotherapy, measured by atomic absorption spectrometry. Carcinogenesis 12:1253–1258.

PERERA FP. 1987. Molecular cancer epidemiology: A new tool in cancer prevention. J Natl Cancer Inst 78:887–898.

PERERA FP, BOFFETTA P. 1988. Perspectives on comparing risks of environmental carcinogens. J Natl Cancer Inst 80:1282–1293.

PERERA FP, BOFFETTA P, NISBET I. 1989. The role of man-made chemicals in the etiology of human cancer. *In* De Vita VT, Hellman S, Rosenberg SA, (eds): Important Advances in Oncology. Philadelphia, J.B. Lippincott Co., pp. 249–265.

PERERA FP, HEMMINKI K, GRZYBOWSKA E, MOTYKIEWICZ G, MICHALSKA J, SANTELLA RM, YOUNG TL, DICKEY C, BRANDT-RAUF P, DEVIVO I, BLANER W, TSAI WY, CHORAZY M. 1992a. Molecular and genetic damage from environmental pollution in Poland. Nature 360:256–258.

PERERA FP, HEMMINKI K, YOUNG TL, BRENNER D, KELLY G, SANTELLA RM. 1988. Detection of polycyclic aromatic hydrocarbon-DNA adducts in white blood cells of foundry workers. Cancer Res 48:2288–2291.

PERERA FP, MAYER J, SANTELLA RM, BRENNER D, JEFFREY A, LATRIANO L, SMITH S, WARBURTON D, YOUNG TL, TSAI W-Y, HEMMINKI K, BRANDT-RAUF P. 1991a. Biologic markers in risk assessment for environmental carcinogens. Environ Health Perspect 90:247–254.

PERERA FP, MOTZER RJ, TANG D, REED E, PARKER R, WARBURTON D, O'NEILL P, ALBERTINI R, BIGBEE W, JENSEN RH, SANTELLA RM, TSAI WY, SIMON-CEREIJIDO G, RANDALL C, BOSL G. 1992b. Multiple biologic markers in germ cell patients treated with platinum-based chemotherapy. Cancer Res 52:3558–3565.

PERERA FP, SANTELLA RM, BRANDT-RAUF P, KAHN S, JIANG W, MAYER J. 1991b. Molecular epidemiology of lung cancer. *In* Brugge J, Curran T, Harlow E, McCormick F (eds): Origins of Human Cancer: A Comprehensive Review. Cold Spring Harbor, New York, Cold Spring Harbor Laboratory, pp. 219–236.

PERO RW, BRYNGELSSON T, HOGSTEDT B, AKESSON B. 1982. Occupational and in vitro exposure to styrene assessed by unscheduled DNA synthesis in resting human lymphocytes. Carcinogenesis 3:681–685.

PREVOST V, SHUKER DEG, BARTSCH H, PASTORELLI R, STILLWELL WG, TRUDEL LJ, TANNENBAUM SR. 1990. The determination of urinary 3-methyladenine by immunoaffinity chromatography-monoclonal antibody-based ELISA: Use in human biomonitoring studies. Carcinogenesis 11:1747–1751.

REED E, OZOLS RF, TARONE R, YUSPA SH, POIRIER MC. 1988. The measurement of cisplatin-DNA adduct levels in testicular cancer patients. Carcinogenesis 9:1909–11.

REED E, YUSPA SH, ZWELLING LA, OZOLS RF, POIRIER MP. 1986. Quantitation of cis-diamminedichloroplatinum II cis-platin-DNA-intrastrand adducts in testicular and ovarian cancer patients receiving cisplatin chemotherapy. J Clin Invest 77:545–550.

REYNOLDS T. 1991. Biomarkers help advance chemoprevention research. J Natl Cancer Inst 83:1368–1370.

ROSS RK, YUAN JM, YU MC, WOGAN GN, QIAN GS, TU JP, GROOPMAN JD, GAO YT, HENDERSON BE. 1992. Urinary aflatoxin biomarkers and risk of hepatocellular carcinoma. Lancet 339:943–946.

ROTHMAN N, POIRIER MC, CORREA-VILLASENOR A, FORD DP, HANSEN JA, O'TOOLE T, STRICKLAND PT. 1993. Association of PAH-DNA adducts in peripheral white blood cells with dietary exposure to PAHs. Environ Health Perspect 99:265–267.

SANTELLA RM. 1988. Application of new techniques for detection of carcinogen adducts to human population monitoring. Mutat Res 205:271–282.

SANTELLA RM, WESTON A, PERERA FP, TRIVERS GT, HARRIS CC, YOUNG TL, NGUYEN D, LEE BM, POIRIER MC. 1988. Interlaboratory comparison of antisera and immunoassays for benzo(a)pyrene-diol-epoxide-I-modified DNA. Carcinogenesis 9:1265–1269.

SANTELLA RM, YANG XY, DE LEO V, GASPARRO FP. 1988. Detection and quantification of 8-methoxypsoralen-DNA adducts. *In* Bartsch H, Hemminki K, O'Neill IK (eds): IARC Sci Publ No. 89. Methods for Detecting DNA Damaging Agents in Humans: Applications in Cancer Epidemiology and Prevention. Lyon, France, International Agency for Research on Cancer, 333–340.

SANTELLA RM, ZHANG YJ, HSIEH LL, YOUNG TL, LU XQ, LEE BM, YANG GY, PERERA FP. 1991. Immunologic methods for monitoring human exposure to benzo(a)pyrene and aflatoxin B1: Measurement of carcinogen adducts. *In* Vanderlaan M (ed): Immunoassays for Monitoring Human Exposure to Toxic Chemicals. Washington, D.C., American Chemical Society, pp. 229–245.

SARTO F, COMINATO I, PINTON AM, BROVEDANI PG, FACCIOLI CM, BIANCHI V, LEVIS AG. 1984. Cytogenetic damage in workers exposed to ethylene oxide. Mutat Res 138:185–195.

SCHULTE PA. 1989. A conceptual framework for the validation and use of biologic markers. Environ Res 48:129–144.

SCHULTE PA, PERERA FP (eds). 1993. Molecular Epidemiology: Principles and Practices. New York, Academic Press.

SCHULTE PA, ROTHMAN N, SCHOTTENFELD D. 1993. Design considerations in molecular epidemiology. *In* Schulte PA, Perera FP (eds): Molecular Epidemiology: Principles and Practices. San Diego, Academic Press, pp. 159–198.

SEIDEGARD J, PERO RW. 1988. The genetic variation and the expression of human glutathione transferase mu. Klin Wochenschr 66(11):125–126.

SHERSON D, SABRO P, SIGSGAARD T, JOHANSEN F, AUTRUP H. 1990. Biological monitoring of foundry workers exposed to polycyclic aromatic hydrocarbons. Br J Ind Med 47:448–453.

SHIELDS PG, CAPORASO NE, FALK RT, SUGIMURA H, TRIVERS GE, TRUMP BF, HOOVER RN, WESTON A, HARRIS CC. 1993. Lung cancer, race, and a CYP1A1 genetic polymorphism. Cancer Epidemiol Biomarkers Prev 2:481–485.

SHUKER DEG, FARMER PB. 1988. Urinary excretion of 3-methyladenine in humans as a marker of nucleic acid methylation. *In* Bartsch H, Hemminki K, O'Neill IK (eds): Methods for Detecting DNA Damaging Agents in Humans: Applications in Cancer Epidemiology and Prevention. IARC Sci Publ 89. Lyon, France, International Agency for Research on Cancer, pp. 92–96.

SINOPOLI NT, TRIVERS GE, FICORELLA C, TOMAO S, MARTELLI M, CAGNAZZO P, SAMA N, HARRIS CC, FRATI I. 1990. Immunoassay detection of carcinogen–DNA adducts in tumor and noninvolved lung tissue from lung cancer patients. Proc Am Assoc Cancer Res 31:97.

SKIPPER PL, TANNENBAUM SR. 1990. Protein adducts in the molecular dosimetry of chemical carcinogens. Carcinogenesis 11:507–518.

SOULIOTIS VL, KAILA S, BOUSSIOTIS VA, PANGALIS GA, KYRTOPOULOS SA. 1990. Accumulation of 6-methylguanine in human blood leukocyte DNA during exposure to procarbazine and its relationships with dose and repair. Cancer Res 50:2759–2764.

STICH HF, DUNN BP. 1988. DNA adducts, micronuclei and leukoplakias as intermediate endpoints in intervention trials. *In* Bartsch H, Hemminki K, O'Neill IK (eds): Methods for Detecting DNA Damaging Agents in Humans: Applications in Cancer Epidemiology and Prevention. IARC Sci Publ 89. Lyon, France, International Agency for Research on Cancer, pp. 137–145.

STRANGE RC, MATHAROO B, FAULDER GC, JONES P, COTTON W, ELDER JB, DEAKIN M. 1991. The human glutathione S-transferases: A case–control study of the incidence of the GST1 O phenotype in patients with adenocarcinoma. Carcinogenesis 12:25–28.

SUGIMURA H, WESTON A, CAPORASO NE, SHIELDS PG, BOWMAN ED, METCALF RA, HARRIS CC. 1991. Biochemical and molecular epidemiology of cancer. Biomed Environ Sci 4:73–92.

SUZUKI H, TAKAHASHI T, KUROISHI T, SUYAMA M, ARIYOSHI Y, TAKAHASHI T, UEDA R. 1992. *p53* mutations in non–small cell lung cancer in Japan: Association between mutations and smoking. Cancer Res 52:734–736.

TANG DL, SANTELLA RM, BLACKWOOD MA, WARBURTON D, LUO J, YOUNG TL, MAYER J, TSAI W-Y, PERERA FP. 1993. A case–control molecular epidemiology study of lung cancer. Proc Am Assoc Cancer Res 34:5.

TAYLOR TA. 1990. Oncogenes and their applications in epidemiologic studies. Am J Epidemiol 130:6–13.

TOLOS WP, SHAW PB, LOWRY LK, MACKKENZIE BA, DENG JF, MARKEL HL. 1990. [1]-Pyrenol: A biomarker for occupational exposure to policyclic aromatic hydrocarbons. Appl Occup Environ Hyg 5:303–309.

TORNQVIST M, MOWERS J, JENSEN S, EHRENBERG L. 1986. Monitoring of environmental cancer initiators through hemoglobin adducts by a modified Edman degradation method. Anal Biochem 154:255–266.

UMBENHAUER D, WILD CP, MONTESANO R, SAFFHILL R, BOYLE JM, HUH N, KIRSTEIN U, THOMALE J, RAJEWSKY MF, LU SH. 1985. O-methyldeoxyguanosine in oesophageal DNA among individuals at high risk of oesophageal cancer. Int J Cancer 36:661–665.

VAHAKANGAS K, PELKONEN O. 1989. Host variations in carcinogen metabolism and DNA repair. *In* Lynch HT, Hirayama T (eds): Genetic Epidemiology of Cancer. Boca Raton, Florida, CRC Press, pp. 35–54.

VAINIO H, SORSA M, FALCK K. 1984. Bacterial urinary assay in monitoring exposure to mutagens and carcinogens. *In* Berlin A, Draper M, Hemminki K, Vainio H (eds): Methods of Monitoring Human Exposure to Carcinogenic and Mutagenic Agents. IARC Sci Publ 59. Lyon, France, International Agency for Research on Cancer 247–258.

VAN SCHOOTEN FJ, HILLEBRAND MJX, VAN LEEUWEN FE, LUTGERINK JT, VAN ZANDWIJK N, JANSEN HM, KRIEK E. 1990. Polycyclic aromatic hydrocarbon-DNA adducts in lung tissue from lung cancer patients. Carcinogenesis 11:1677–1681.

VAN SITTERT NJ, DE JONG G, GARNER RC, DAVIES R, DEAN BJ, WREN LJ, WRIGHT AS. 1985. Cytogenetic, immunological, and hemotological effects in workers in an ethylene oxide manufacturing plant. Br J Ind Med 42:19–26.

VINEIS P, CAPORASO N, TANNENBAUM SR, SKIPPER PL, GLOGOWSKI J, BARTSCH H, CODA M, TALASKA G, KADLUBAR F. 1990a. Acetylation phenotype, carcinogen-hemoglobin adducts, and cigarette smoking. Cancer Res 50:3002–3004.

VINEIS P, ESTEVE J, HARTGE P, HOOVER R, SILBERGMAN DT, TERRACINI B. 1988. Effects of timing and type of tobacco in cigarette-induced bladder cancer. Cancer Res 48:3849–3852.

VINEIS P, FAGGIANO F, TERRACINI B. 1990b. Biochemical epidemiology: Uses in the study of human carcinogenesis. Teratogenesis Carcinog Mutagen 10:231–237.

VINEIS P, TERRACINI B. 1990. Biochemical epidemiology of bladder cancer. Epidemiology 1:448–452.

WALLES SAS, NORPPA H, OSTERMAN-GOLKAR S, MAKI-PAAKKANEN J. 1988. Single-strand breaks in DNA of peripheral lymphocytes of styrene-exposed workers. *In* Bartsch H, Hemminki K, O'Neill IK (eds): Methods for Detecting DNA Damaging Agents in Humans: Applications in Cancer Epidemiology and Prevention. IARC Sci Publ 89. Lyon, France: International Agency for Research on Cancer pp. 223–226.

WEINSTEIN IB, GATTONI-CELLI S, KIRSCHMEIER P, LAMBERT M, HSIAO W, BACKER J, JEFFREY A. 1984. Multistage carcinogenesis involves multiple genes and multiple mechanisms. *In* Cancer Cells: The Transformed Phenotype. Cold Spring, New York, Cold Spring Harbor Laboratory, pp. 229–237.

WEINSTEIN IB, SANTELLA RM, PERERA FP. 1995. The molecular biology and molecular epidemiology of cancer. *In* Greenwald P, Kramer BS, Weed DL (eds): The Science and Practice of Cancer Prevention and Control. New York, Marcel-Dekker, 83–110.

WESTON A, MANCHESTER DK, POIRIER MC, CHOI JS, TRIVERS GE, MANN DL, HARRIS CC. 1989. Derivative fluorescence spectral analysis of polycyclic aromatic hydrocarbon-DNA adducts in human placenta. Chem Res Toxicol 2:104–108.

WESTON A, WILLEY JC, MANCHESTER DK, WILSON VL, BROOKS BR, CHOI JS, POIRIER MC, TRIVERS GE, NEWMAN MJ, MANN DL, HARRIS CC. 1988. Dosimeters of human exposure to carcinogens: polycyclic aromatic hydrocarbon-macromolecular adducts. *In* Bartsch H, Hemminki K, O'Neill IK (eds): Methods for Detecting DNA Damaging Agents in Humans: Applications in Cancer Epidemiology and Prevention. IARC Sci Publ 89. Lyon, France, International Agency for Research on Cancer, pp. 181–189.

WHYATT RM, PERERA FP. 1995. Application of biologic markers to studies of environmental risks in children and the developing fetus. Environ Health Perspect 103 (Suppl 6):105–110.

WILCOSKY TC, RYNARD MR. 1990. Sister chromatid exchange. *In* Hulka BS, Wilcosky TC, Griffith JD (eds): Biological Markers in Epidemiology, New York, Oxford University Press, pp. 105–124.

WILD CP, JIANG YZ, SABBIONI G, CHAPOT B, MONTESANO R. 1990. Evaluation of methods for quantitation of aflatoxin-albumin and their application to human exposure assessment. Cancer Res 50:245–251.

WILD CP, UMBENHAUER D, CHAPOT B, MONTESANO R. 1986. Monitoring of individual human exposure to aflatoxins (AF) and N-nitrosamines (NNO) by immunoassays. J Cell Biol 30:171–179.

WILLETT WC. 1990. Vitamin A and lung cancer. Nutrition Reviews 48:201–211.

WILLETT WC, MACMAHON B. 1989. Diet and cancer: An overview (Part I). National Research Council. New Engl J Med 310:633–638.

WILSON VL, WESTON A, MANCHESTER DK, TRIVERS GE, ROBERTS DW, KADLUBAR FF, WILD CP, MONTESANO R, WILLEY JC, MANN DL, HARRIS CC. 1989. Alkyl and aryl carcinogen adducts detected in human peripheral lung. Carcinogenesis 10:2149–2153.

WRAITH MJ, WATSON WP, EADSFORTH CV, VAN SITTERT NJ, TORNQVIST M, WRIGHT AS. 1988. An immunoassay for monitoring human exposure to ethylene oxide. *In* Bartsch H, Hemminki K, O'Neill IK (eds): Methods for Detecting DNA Damaging Agents in Humans: Applications in Cancer Epidemiology and Prevention. IARC Sci Publ 89. Lyon, France, International Agency for Research on Cancer, pp. 271–274.

YUSPA SH, POIRIER MC. 1988. Chemical carcinogenesis: From animal models to molecular models in one decade. Adv Cancer Res 50:25–70.

ZHANG YJ, CHEN CJ, LEE CS, HAGHIGHI B, YANG GY, WANG LW, FEITELSON M, SANTELLA RM. 1991. Aflatoxin B1-DNA adducts and hepatitis B virus antigens in hepatocellular carcinoma and non-tumorous liver tissue. Carcinogenesis 12:2247–2252.

ZHU J, ZHANG L, HU X, XIAO Y, CHEN J, XU Y, CHU JF, CHU FS. 1987. Correlation of dietary aflatoxin B1 levels with excretion of aflatoxin M1 in human urine. Cancer Res 47:1848–1852.

8 Quantitative risk assessment

ALICE S. WHITTEMORE

Since publication of the first edition of this volume in 1982, there has been heated debate in the U.S. about the use of quantitative risk assessment in the development of regulatory priorities and policies for environmental carcinogens (Ashford et al, 1983; Wildavsky, 1984; Efron, 1984; Freedman and Zeisel, 1988). Hardly an arcane argument among ivory-tower theoreticians, the debate has involved the Congress, the courts, and to an increasing extent the public. It has centered not on how many angels can dance on the head of a pin, but rather on how many molecules of a chemical can cause human cancer. To some, the two questions bear a disquieting resemblance.

The controversy has raged over the relevance to humans of positive cancer data in laboratory animals, the need for regulation in the absence of positive human data, the value of statistical models fitted to limited animal data obtained at high dose rates to predict human response at low ones, and the appropriateness of a regulatory distinction between "genotoxic" and "nongenotoxic" chemicals. The intractability of these issues has tempted scientists to shun quantitative risk assessment as unscientific, if not impossible. This avoidance behavior is understandable in a profession wherein career and sense of accomplishment are built not on unsuccessful attempts to address difficult questions, but rather on innovative approaches to well-posed, answerable questions. Yet the scientific community has an obligation to consider the problem and to share its insights with regulators because quantitative risk assessment cannot be avoided. The extremes of banning a chemical (regardless of its value) or of permitting unlimited exposures to a chemical (regardless of its danger) both involve implicit risk assessment. Scientific expertise is needed to find a satisfactory middle road between these extremes.

Cancer prevention through regulation of environmental carcinogens involves risk analysis and risk management. Risk analysis has three components: hazard identification, exposure assessment, and quantitative risk assessment. *Hazard identification* is the qualitative decision that a substance may pose a cancer threat to humans. *Exposure assessment* evaluates the distribution and intensity of exposure to the substance in human populations. *Quantitative risk assessment* estimates the magnitude of cancer probability associated with specified patterns of exposure to the substance. In contrast to the scientific considerations of risk analysis, risk management is the social process of specifying maximum exposure limits, including no limits, to the substance, based on its risks and benefits to society.

Hazard identification and exposure assessment are relatively straightforward tasks that will not be discussed here. In contrast, quantitative risk assessment (involving the scientific evaluation of data) and risk management (involving social and political judgment) are difficult and controversial tasks, distinct in theory but overlapping in practice. The overlap is occasioned by lack of conclusive data to reach a clear scientific consensus. Indeed, the term *science policy* has emerged to describe issues that are grounded in scientific analysis but for which data are insufficient to support an unequivocal conclusion, and whose resolution depends on determinations of social policy (Ashford et al, 1983).

Several chapters in this book discuss quantitative risk assessment. In particular, Chapter 2 ("Experimental studies in the assessment of the human risk") reviews the use of animal experiments and short-term laboratory tests in determining human cancer risks, and discusses statistical models for risk extrapolation from high to low doses in animals, and from animals to humans. Chapter 67 ("Environmental regulation and policy making") reviews the history of environmental regulation in the U.S. in the twentieth century, and describes the U.S. legal framework for regulating carcinogens and the mandates of U.S. regulatory agencies.

This chapter does not duplicate that material. Instead, it focuses on subsequent progress and setbacks in evaluating human risk from environmental carcinogens. The section on quantitative risk assessment describes recent perspectives on the use of epidemiological and laboratory data in risk assessment, with emphasis on the potential for more informed, less conflict-ridden assessment provided by new developments in molecular biology. The regulation of formaldehyde, a carcinogen

This research was supported by NIH grant CA47448 and by a grant to SIMS from the Environmental Protection Agency.

that is nevertheless useful to society, provides a paradigm for many of the issues raised. The section on formaldehyde contains a brief review of formaldehyde and its regulatory history. That story dramatizes the susceptibility of risk assessment to the pragmatic exigencies and political pressures of risk management described in the section on policy problems. The last section concludes with future challenges in the assessment and management of cancer risks.

FORMALDEHYDE

Discovered in 1859, formaldehyde has been produced commercially since the early 1900s. It is a versatile chemical used in the manufacture of plastics and resins, particle board, plywood, paper, home insulation, leather and agricultural products, permanent-press fabrics, preservatives, embalming fluids, drugs, and cosmetics. As such, it contributes in many ways to the benefits enjoyed by industrialized society. Formaldehyde also occurs as a pollutant of indoor air because of urea-formaldehyde foam insulation and particle board used in building construction, and of outdoor air because of the natural photooxidation of hydrocarbons emitted from automobile and airplane exhaust, power plants, oil refineries, and incinerators.

The U.S. produced about six billion pounds of formaldehyde in 1979, making the compound the 26th largest volume chemical produced by this country (Environmental Protection Agency, 1981). An estimated 1.4 million U.S. workers are exposed to formaldehyde in the diverse occupations listed in Table 8–1. About 11 million are thought to breathe formaldehyde vapors released in buildings by construction and insulation materials, and virtually everyone has some exposure to the ubiquitous chemical in polluted air or in consumer products. Formaldehyde also occurs endogenously in humans (Hutson, 1970).

TABLE 8–1. *Occupations with Potential Exposure to Formaldehyde**

Anatomists	Fungicide workers
Agricultural workers	Furniture dippers and sprayers
Bakers	Fur processors
Beauticians	Glass etchers
Biologists	Glue and adhesive makers
Bookbinders	Hexamethylenetetramine makers
Botanists	Hide preservers
Crease-resistant textile finishers	Histology technicians (assumed to include necropsy and autopsy technicians)
Deodorant makers	Ink makers
Disinfectant makers	Lacquerers and lacquer makers
Disinfectors	Medical personnel (assumed to include pathologists)
Dress-goods shop personnel	Mirror workers
Dressmakers	Oil-well workers
Drugmakers	Paper makers (Particleboard makers)
Dyemakers	Pentaerythritol makers
Electrical insulation makers	Photographic film makers
Embalmers	Plastic workers
Embalming-fluid makers	Resin makers
Ethylene glycol makers	Rubber makers
Fertilizer makers	Soil sterilizers and greenhouse workers
Fireproofers	Surgeons
Formaldehyde resin makers	Tannery workers
Formaldehyde employees	Taxidermists
Foundry employees	Textile mordanters and printers
Fumigators	Textile waterproofers
	Varnish workers
	Wood preservers

*From International Agency for Research on Cancer (1982), Volume 29.

Formaldehyde has a simple chemical structure and formula (HCHO). Its biological effects, however, are complex. The compound is a rodent carcinogen, producing nasal tumors in rats (Fig. 8–1). Its carcinogenicity is consistent with its toxicity to the genome of mammalian cells. Formaldehyde forms N-hydroxymethyl DNA adducts and cross-links between DNA and proteins in human cells (Craft et al, 1987). It inhibits the resealing of single strand breaks in DNA caused by ionizing radiation, inhibits the unscheduled DNA synthesis occurring after exposure to ultraviolet radiation and certain chemical carcinogens, and inhibits the repair of DNA damage caused by other compounds (Grafstrom et al, 1983, 1985). Formaldehyde is itself a mutagen, causing mutations at the hprt locus in human lymphoblasts exposed in vitro (Crosby et al, 1988; Liber et al, 1989).

At the epigenetic level, formaldehyde causes cell degeneration, necrosis, inflammation, and increased cell proliferation in the nasal epithelium of rodents exposed to its vapors. As discussed in the next section, increased cell proliferation may itself play an important role in formaldehyde's carcinogenicity. In humans, formaldehyde at high exposure levels may on rare occasions induce bronchial asthma (Bardana and Montanaro, 1991).

Epidemiologic data implicating formaldehyde as a human carcinogen are conflicting and inconclusive. Elevated risks for cancers of the brain, lymphatic system, hemopoietic system, and skin have been noted among embalmers, pathologists, and anatomists (Harrington and Shannon, 1975; Walrath and Fraumeni, 1983; Stroup et al, 1986). By contrast, a deficit of cancers of

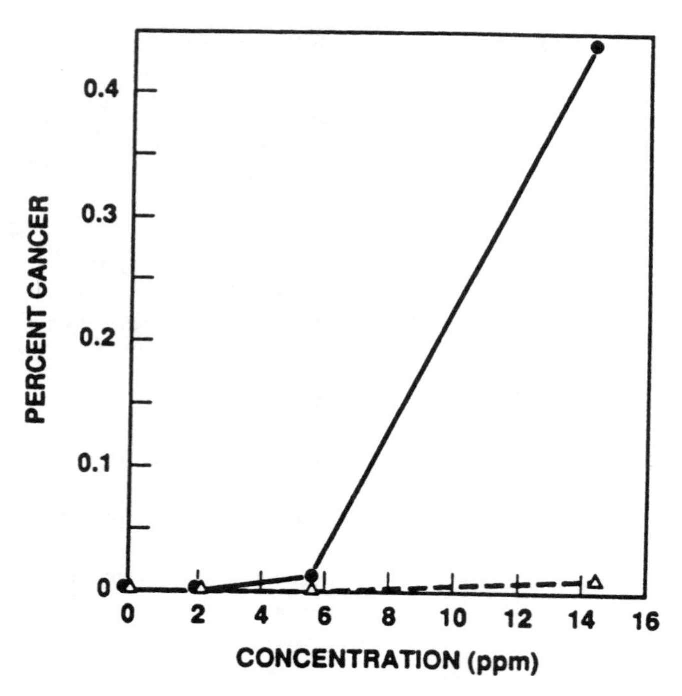

FIG. 8–1. Incidence of squamous-cell carcinoma of the nasal cavity among Fischer-344 rats and C57BL/6XCH3F$_1$ mice vs. airborne formaldehyde concentration. Animals were exposed to 0, 2.0, 5.6, and 14.3 ppm of formaldehyde gas 6 hr/day, 6 days/week, for 24 months. (From Kerns et al, 1983, with permission.)

the lung, esophagus, or mouth was found among British physicians working in scientific research, pathology, or biochemistry (Doll and Peto, 1977). Moreover, a cohort mortality study of 26,000 workers employed in ten industries producing or using formaldehyde found no excesses for leukemia, brain cancer, or nasal cancer (Blair et al, 1986). Although slight excesses were seen for Hodgkin's disease and cancers of the lung and prostate, they were not consistently related to estimated formaldehyde exposure levels. Interestingly, the investigators did find a sharp but not statistically significant exposure–response trend for nasopharyngeal cancer (Blair et al, 1987). These studies had limited (<20%) power to detect increases in mortality specifically from nasal cancer (the neoplasm seen in rats) because of its infrequent occurrence in humans. However, the studies generally had good (>70%) statistical power to detect twofold or greater increases in lung cancer. More complete reviews of the epidemiologic data for formaldehyde are provided elsewhere (e.g., Nelson et al, 1986; Smith, 1992). Overall, the International Agency for Research on Cancer (IARC) has judged that the epidemiologic data provide inadequate evidence to assess the carcinogenicity of formaldehyde in humans (IARC, 1982).

Its genotoxicity, its carcinogenicity in rats, and its adverse noncarcinogenic effects in humans have prompted the recommendation or promulgation of occupational exposure limits for formaldehyde by at least 18 countries. These limits are listed in Table 8–2. Additionally, the U.S. Environmental Protection Agency (EPA) has recommended an exposure limit of .123 mg/m^3 (.1 ppm) in outdoor ambient air. Four European countries have recommended exposure limits for indoor air. The EPA has identified formaldehyde as a toxic waste and requires that persons who generate, transport, treat, store, or dispose of it comply with the regulations of the federal hazardous waste management program. Anyone discharging more than 1000 pounds of formaldehyde into waterways must notify the EPA. Canada has banned the use of urea-formaldehyde foam insulation in home construction.

Yet no country has banned all formaldehyde production. Indeed, the EPA has registered the compound for use as a volatile fumigant in nonfood agricultural applications, and for the control of mold and mildew. Many states in the U.S. require the use of formaldehyde in embalming.

The history of formaldehyde regulation in the U.S. has not been without controversy. In October 1979 the Chemical Industry Institute for Toxicology (CIIT) reported bioassay data showing that formaldehyde is carcinogenic to rats at 5.6 and 14.3 ppm, and carcinogenic to mice at 14.3 ppm (Fig. 8–1). This report prompted the EPA, the Occupational Safety and Health Administration (OSHA), and the Consumer Product Safety Commission to convene a federal panel on formaldehyde. The panel concluded that "formaldehyde should be presumed to pose a carcinogenic risk to humans" (Federal Panel on Formaldehyde, 1984). The responses of the three regulatory groups to this conclusion illustrate how science and policy interact in the regulation of compounds with important benefits and potentially serious risks.

In March 1981 the EPA considered formaldehyde under Section 4(f) of the Toxic Substances Control Act, which requires the agency to act promptly when any data suggest that people are exposed to a carcinogen. Two months later, however, a new administrator took office at the EPA and delayed action on the chemical. In February 1982 the EPA Assistant Administrator for Pesticides and Toxic Substances formally recommended against considering formaldehyde as a priority candidate for regulation on the grounds that ". . . rats seem to be particularly sensitive to formaldehyde; and that long human experience does not seem to indicate any pressing concerns . . ." (Todhunter, 1982). The Natural Resources Defense Council then brought suit against the EPA to reverse its decision not to act. In April 1987, more than seven years after the CIIT report, the EPA reversed itself, concluding on the basis of the CIIT bioassay that formaldehyde is "a probable human carcinogen."

TABLE 8–2. *National Occupational Exposure Limits for Formaldehyde**

Country	Year	Concentration		Interpretation[b]	Status
		mg/m³	PPM		
Australia	1978	3	2	Ceiling	Guideline
Belgium	1978	3	2	Ceiling	Regulation
Bulgaria	1971	1	—	Maximum	Regulation
Czechoslovakia	1976	2	—	TWA	Regulation
		5	—	Ceiling (10 min)	
Finland	1975	3	2	Ceiling	Regulation
German Democratic Republic	1979	2	—	Maximum (30 min)	Regulation
		2	—	TWA	
Federal Republic of Germany	1979	1.2	1	TWA[c]	Guideline
Hungary	1974	1	—	TWA[d]	Regulation
Italy	1978	1.2	1	TWA	Guideline
Japan	1978	2.5	2	Ceiling	Guideline
The Netherlands	1978	3	2	Ceiling	Guideline
Poland	1976	2	—	Ceiling	Regulation
Romania	1975	4	—	Maximum	Regulation
Sweden	1978	3	2	Maximum (15 min)	Guideline
Switzerland	1978	1.2	1	TWA	Regulation
U.S.A.[a]					
OSHA	1987	1.5	1	TWA	Regulation
		3	2	Ceiling (15 min)	Regulation
ACGIH	1981	3	2	Ceiling	Guideline
		1.5	1	TWA	
NIOSH	1976	1.2	1	Ceiling (30 min)	Guideline
U.S.S.R.	1977	0.5	1	Maximum	Regulation
Yugoslavia	1971	1	0.8	Ceiling	Regulation

*From International Agency for Research on Cancer (1982), Volume 29.
[a]OSHA, Occupational Safety and Health Administration; ACGIH, American Conference of Governmental Industrial Hygienists; NIOSH, National Institute for Occupational Safety and Health.
[b]TWA, time-weighted average.
[c]Skin irritant.
[d]May be exceeded 5 times per shift as long as average does not exceed value.

Upon receipt of the federal panel's report, OSHA and the National Institute for Occupational Safety and Health prepared a joint current intelligence bulletin recommending that formaldehyde be handled as a potential carcinogen and that appropriate controls be used to reduce worker exposure. In March 1981, shortly after the arrival of a new Assistant Secretary of Labor for OSHA, the agency withdrew its sponsorship of this bulletin. In June 1981, OSHA attempted to fire Peter F. Infante, Director of its Office of Carcinogen Identification and Classification, in connection with his outspoken opinion that formaldehyde is a human carcinogen (Sun, 1981). Infante's notice came soon after OSHA's receipt of an angry letter assailing his conduct from an attorney for the Formaldehyde Institute, an association of formaldehyde producers and users. At hearings of the House Science and Technology Investigations Subcommittee, Representative Albert Gore (D-Tenn.) remarked, "if OSHA succeeds in firing Dr. Infante, it will be a clear message to all civil servants who are charged with protecting the public health that those who do their job will lose their job" (Sun, 1981).

Although OSHA rescinded its notice to Infante, the heat over formaldehyde did not abate. The agency denied an October 1981 petition by the United Auto Workers and 13 other labor unions for an emergency standard for formaldehyde under Section 6(c) of the Occupational Safety and Health Act (Young, 1981). Section 6(c) specifies that OSHA shall set such a standard if it determines that workers are exposed to grave danger from a hazard.

The Formaldehyde Institute argued against federal regulation of the chemical on the grounds that the animal bioassay data do not provide a sufficient basis to regard formaldehyde as a likely human carcinogen, and that federal regulatory agencies should await the development of conclusive epidemiological data before taking protective action. This position outraged those who felt it contradicts the established regulatory principle that confirmed positive animal data are presumptive evidence of carcinogenicity in humans, and that conclusive human data are not necessary for regulatory action. In 1984 the United Auto Workers brought suit against OSHA to reduce the existing 3 ppm workplace limit. On December 4, 1987 OSHA did so, reducing it to 1 ppm.

In the spring of 1982 the Consumer Product Safety Association responded to the federal panel's report with a ban on urea-formaldehyde foam insulation, effective August 1982. Earlier that spring the Formaldehyde Institute filed suit to challenge the ban, and in April 1983 the Fifth Circuit District Court overturned it on the grounds that reliance on a single study (the CIIT bioassay) did not represent good science.

To some, the responses of EPA and OSHA under leadership appointed by an Administration committed to "deregulation" suggested sympathy for the concerns of the Formaldehyde Institute at the expense of the agencies' mandate to protect the public health (Perera, 1982; Ashford et al, 1983). Clearly, the responses digressed from the Regulatory Council's 1979 policy statement on the regulation of chemical carcinogens, which specified: (1) negative epidemiological studies will not be presumed to indicate that a substance is not carcinogenic; (2) sites exposed by routes other than those tested will be presumed to be at risk; (3) negative bioassay results for some animal species, even in well-conducted tests, will not be said to detract from well-established, positive evidence for other species; and (4) a no-effect threshold level will not be assumed to exist for carcinogenic substances (Regulatory Council, 1979). Two scientific questions formed the heart of the controversy. The first concerns the relevance to low (less than 1 ppm) exposures of carcinogenicity observed at the high experimental dose rates of 5.6 ppm and 14.3 ppm. The second concerns the relevance to humans of nasal cancer in rats, and the need for positive human data to regulate a chemical found carcinogenic in animals. We turn first to these scientific questions, before addressing the science–policy confusion surrounding them.

QUANTITATIVE RISK ASSESSMENT—A NECESSARY RISK

The story of formaldehyde highlights an important feature of quantitative risk assessment—its necessity. Like it or not, we cannot avoid it. A society that takes no action to regulate formaldehyde makes a quantitative risk assessment: existing levels of the chemical carry risks so low (compared to its benefits) that the society is prepared to accept them. At the other extreme, a society choosing to ban formaldehyde production also makes a quantitative risk assessment: any exposure level carries a risk so high that the society is prepared to forego the chemical's benefits. Clearly the assessment of formaldehyde-induced cancer risks lies between these extremes.

The formaldehyde problem underscores several key issues characterizing quantitative risk assessment. Some of these are scientific issues, some are social policy issues, and some are hybrids, involving subtle mixtures of both science and policy. This section reviews the scientific issues, which center on (1) the validity of extrapolation from the high dose rates used in animal experiments to the low limits considered for population exposures, and (2) the validity of animal experiments as markers for human risk.

How Many Molecules: Low Dose Extrapolation

The dose rates in the formaldehyde bioassay shown in Figure 8–1 range from 2 ppm to 14.3 ppm. Formaldehyde concentrations exceeding 14.3 ppm were measured in the U.S. workplace as recently as 1970 (National Institute for Occupational Safety and Health, 1976; National Research Council, 1980), and concentrations of .1 to 3.4 ppm have been measured in houses insulated with urea-formaldehyde foam (National Research Council, 1980). Thus the bioassay dose rates are comparable to human exposures. More commonly, rodent bioassays at dose rates as low as human exposures are not feasible, because too many animals are needed to detect the resulting small risks that nevertheless are of concern to society. Therefore assumptions are required to relate cancer probability at experimental dose rates to cancer probability at proposed human exposure limits. A dose–response model is a set of such assumptions, together with some specification of variability in cancer occurrence among individuals. Even in the case of formaldehyde, a dose–response model is needed to extrapolate the risk to the current U.S. occupational exposure limit of 1 ppm because no carcinomas were observed in the laboratory animals at dose rates below 5.6 ppm.

The Carcinogen Assessment Group of the EPA has used a linear dose–response model to estimate cancer probability at proposed human exposure limits (Carcinogen Assessment Group, 1980). This model assumes that cancer probability at low dose rates is proportional to dose rate. One scientific defense for the model is evidence that mutations are critical events in carcinogenesis, together with evidence that the chance of mutation is proportional to the number of mutagenic molecules reaching the cell. Another defense is the so-called additivity argument (Peto, 1978), which runs as follows.

A carcinogen causing the same type of cell damage as do other carcinogens already present in the environment induces additional cancers in proportion to its amount, regardless of any low-dose nonlinearities it may exhibit in isolation. That is, low-dose nonlinearities are irrelevant if the population is already exposed to moderate dose rates of essentially the same agent.

Perhaps the most politically potent defense raised for the linear model is the belief that it is "conservative" (i.e., health protective), erring on the side of overestimating, rather than underestimating, the cancer probability attached to a given exposure limit. This defense sounds comforting, but its consequence could be the effective ban of many valuable chemical products.

Table 8–3 shows "safe" formaldehyde dose rates estimated by various dose–response models. (Here a safe dose rate is one producing a lifetime risk of one in a million for nasal cancer in rats exposed to formaldehyde.) These dose–response models are described in detail elsewhere (e.g., Zeise et al, 1987). The linear model gives an unacceptable fit to these highly nonlinear data, and those models involving high enough powers of dose to fit adequately, give estimated safe dose rates of about 1000 times higher than that of the linear model. The disparities in these estimates, though large, are dwarfed by those seen when risks are extrapolated to human exposures several orders of magnitude lower than the bioassay dose rates (as is true for example, for saccharin (Occupational Safety and Health Administration, 1980; Whittemore, 1986).

We cannot afford the loss of benefits implied by the linear model when that model is inappropriate. We must sharpen our tools to better weed out the genuine threats while enjoying the benefits of those with little or no threat. To increase the accuracy of low-dose risk estimates, we must first identify critical determinants of the dose–response relationship, and then measure how the determinants change between high and low exposures. Possible determinants include the amount of compound that is absorbed rather than eliminated, the tissues to which the compound is distributed, the amount of compound transformed to active metabolites (if metabolic activation is needed), the amount detoxified to noncarcinogenic metabolites, and the amount of macromolecular damage that is repaired.

TABLE 8–3. *Dose Rates Estimated to Produce a 10^{-6} Lifetime Risk of Nasal Cancer in Rats Exposed to Formaldehyde Vapor*[*]

Dose–Response Model	*Dose Rate (PPM)*
Linear	0.66×10^{-3}
Multistage	0.66
Multihit	1.47
Logit	0.87
Weibull	0.76
Probit	2.08

[*]From Gibson (1983).

To accomplish the task of identifying critical determinants of the dose–response relationship, recent attention has focused on measuring the molecular dose of a carcinogen, defined as the amount reaching a critical target site such as DNA. Since metabolic activation and detoxification are saturable (and therefore nonlinear) processes, cancer probability should be more nearly proportional to molecular dose than to external exposure. Formaldehyde, for example, is detoxified to formate via a saturable glutathione-dependent pathway. Only the remaining free formaldehyde reacts with cellular macromolecules. Saturation of this detoxification pathway by glutathione depletion may explain some of the nonlinearity observed in Figure 8–1. Measurements of formaldehyde in the cells of animals exposed to both the bioassay dose rates and the lower human ones might serve as "dose" in the linear dose–response model to produce risk estimates consistent with the observed data.

The use of molecular dosimetry in quantitative risk assessment is not without difficulties. One difficulty is the appropriate choice of dosimeter. Many carcinogens (like formaldehyde) react at more than one site on DNA, producing several types of DNA adducts. Formaldehyde-induced–N-hydroxymethyl adducts and DNA–protein cross-links may have different efficiencies in causing mutations that lead to carcinogenesis. Another difficulty is the instability of some adducts, due perhaps to reaction reversibility or DNA repair. This instability complicates the task of obtaining reliable measurements. Despite these difficulties, information of critical importance in low-dose extrapolation can derive from molecular dosimetry at the applied dose rates of the bioassay and at the lower levels considered as limits for human exposures.

Another important determinant of the dose–response relationship is the rate of cell proliferation induced by the carcinogenic agent. Cell proliferation is considered a critical component of the carcinogenic process. It is believed necessary for the conversion of promutagenic lesions into heritable mutations, for selective clonal expression of initiated cell populations, and for the irreversible progression from benign clones to malignant tumors.

Cell proliferation is quantified by administering an agent that selectively labels only cells in DNA synthesis. The label may either be a radioactive one, such as [^{3}H]thymidine, or one detected by antibodies, such as bromodeoxyuridine. The principle is the same. Animals previously exposed to, say, formaldehyde, are injected with the labelling agent and then sacrificed. The numbers of labelled cells in the target tissues are counted and used to quantify the proliferation rates induced by the formaldehyde exposure.

Figure 8–2 shows the percent of labelled cells in the nasal epithelium of rats and mice exposed to formaldehyde (Swenberg et al, 1986). Cell proliferation is seen to be a highly nonlinear response, with nonlinearities similar to those of the bioassay shown in Figure 8–1. Because these cell proliferation data were obtained after acute (3 day) rather than chronic formaldehyde exposures, they are not completely comparable to the chronic bioassay data. New antibody-based methods facilitate measurement of cell proliferation rates after months of exposure, providing the bioassay with a marker to link chronically applied dose rate to tumor occurrence.

In summary, recent advances in toxicology now make it possible to measure several potentially critical determinants of carcinogenesis. Measurement of these determinants (which are intermediate between external exposure and cancer occurrence) at high experimental dose rates and at lower human exposures will enhance the utility of existing data for more accurate low-dose extrapolation of risk.

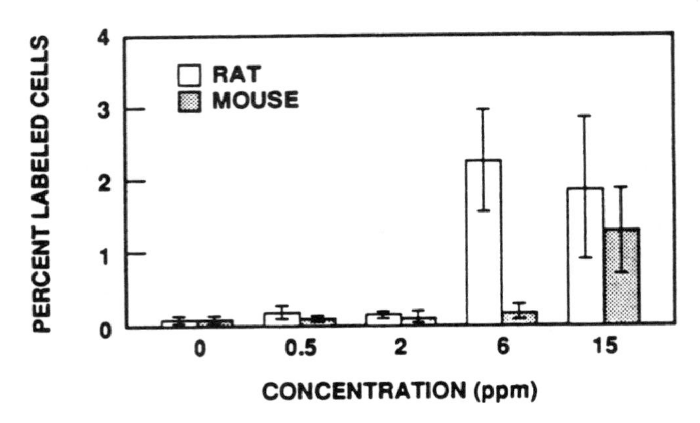

FIG. 8–2. Percent of labelled cells (± standard error) in level 2 of the nasal passages of Fischer-344 rats and C57BL/6XCH3F$_1$ mice exposed to formaldehyde gas 6 h/day for 3 days. [^{3}H]thymidine was administered 2 hours after the third exposure. (From Swenberg et al, 1986, with permission.)

Of Mice and Men: Interspecies Extrapolation

Risk assessment in the 1970s evolved from hopes that human risks from environmental carcinogens could be controlled by eliminating chemicals that test positive in animal experiments. The Ames Salmonella test showed that carcinogens are mutagens, raising the further possibility that short-term tests for mutagenicity and other genotoxic effects could screen for carcinogens. Animal experiments could be supplemented or even replaced by rapid and inexpensive test batteries that would detect human carcinogens with high sensitivity and specificity. Ideally, human data never would be needed.

These hopes have not panned out. Laboratory experiments are still imperfect tools for detecting human cancer. The IARC has determined that there is sufficient evidence from human observations, but limited, inadequate, or nonexistent evidence from animal experiments to classify as carcinogens the substances listed in Table 8–4. The fact that many of these substances have tested positive in one or more of the short-term tests reflects not the sensitivity of the test battery, but rather the intense scrutiny the substances have received, relative to those for which no human data are available.

Thus human data continue to be needed, despite the obvious desirability of discovering hazards before human exposure to them. Consequently, exposed populations should be monitored routinely for cancer occurrence, as described in the concluding section. The most promising developments in the monitoring of exposed populations involve the use of exposure markers in biological samples, as discussed in Chapter 7 of this volume. Such markers have the potential to document exposure levels, identify and quantify unusual susceptibility to environmental toxicants, detect neoplastic precursors, and provide etiologically supportive links between exposure and disease. But first they must be validated as reliable correlates of both disease and exposure, particularly of past exposure. Laboratory experiments are needed to provide this validation under controlled conditions.

As a chemical whose carcinogenicity has inadequate support from human data, yet sufficient support from laboratory animal data, formaldehyde represents the situation converse to that of Table 8–4. The formaldehyde situation is far more common. Studies of cancer risk in exposed humans do not exist for many environ-

TABLE 8–4. *Chemicals or Chemical Mixtures with Sufficient Evidence for Carcinogenicity in Humans But Not in Experimental Animals**

Analgesic mixtures containing phenacetin
Arsenic and certain arsenic compounds
Azathioprine
Betel quid
N,N$^{\text{-bis}}$*(2-chloroethyl)-2-naphthylamine*
1,4-butanediol dimethanesulphonate
Mustard gas
Certain combined chemotherapy regimens for lymphomas
Conjugated estrogens
Smokeless tobacco products
Treosulphan

*As defined by the International Agency for Research on Cancer (1982).

mental chemicals. Epidemiological studies are not feasible, either because it is too difficult to define exposures (which occur in conjunction with other exposures), or because insufficient time has elapsed to detect an increased risk. Human data are lacking for major classes of chemicals such as the N-nitrosamines, which are animal carcinogens, and which are widespread in the human environment. We have no choice but to regulate such chemicals on the basis of the animal data.

Few would argue the critical importance and utility of the formaldehyde bioassay data to risk assessment for this compound. Yet Figure 8–1 illustrates great interspecies variability even within rodents: the mouse is substantially less susceptible to formaldehyde than is the rat. When the linear model described above was fit to the mouse data, the resulting safe dose rate was increased by about two orders of magnitude. This large variability casts doubt on the reliability of risk extrapolation from rodent to humans. It raises several questions about interspecies extrapolation. What are the consequences of the current policy of using the most sensitive species to predict human risk? What should be the relative importance of epidemiological data and animal experiments in the quantitative risk assessment of chemicals like formaldehyde, for which the human data show no clear risk and yet the animal data are demonstrably positive?

These questions defy simple answers. Clearly, an important distinction separates chemicals such as the nitrosamines, which lack reliable epidemiological data, and chemicals such as formaldehyde and saccharin, for which well-designed and well-conducted human studies have not shown a demonstrable risk. Such studies provide upper bounds on risk that can be used in setting priorities for regulation. There is hope that the same technical advances offering help in low-dose extrapolation also will help to reconcile conflicts in response among different species. The cell proliferation data for formaldehyde illustrate this point.

Returning to Figures 8–1 and 8–2, we see parallel responses in the two species: more tumors in the rat than the mouse, and more cell proliferation in the rat than the mouse. Other data on DNA cross-linking and cell proliferation in the rat and monkey (Swenberg et al, 1986; Heck et al, 1989; Monticello et al, 1989; Morgan et al, 1991; Monticello and Morgan, 1994) bring us closer to reliable estimates for response in humans. To use these data for human risk estimation, we must assume that cell proliferation rates in the monkey are reliable surrogates for those in humans. We also must assume that information on cell proliferation and molecular dosimetry can be combined to form a reliable marker for carcinogenesis. With these assumptions, we may ultimately predict the extent and location of the human cancer response on the basis of the extent and location of active metabolite and cell proliferation in the monkey. In so doing, we may find that apparent inconsistencies in cancer occurrence among mouse, rat, and humans are quite consistent with interspecies differences in DNA dose and cell proliferation rates. Furthermore, the tissues exhibiting increased proliferation in the monkey can guide site-specific analyses of epidemiological data. For example, rats and mice breathe only nasally. By contrast, the monkey, like humans, breathes both orally and nasally. Therefore, those respiratory tissues showing increased proliferation in the monkey may be the most likely sites of cancer occurrence in humans. Moreover, the rodent–primate breathing differences render the absence of excess nasal cancers among formaldehyde-exposed humans less inconsistent with the bioassay data than would appear at first glance.

In summary, new techniques for measuring intermediate markers for carcinogenic response offer potential to reconcile conflicts between animal species and between animals and humans (Swenberg, 1987; Hulka et al, 1990; Starr, 1990; Horton et al, 1992; Conolly and Anderson, 1993). The measurement of such markers in rodents, in nonhuman primates, and in humans promises more reliable prediction of human risks. Through the use of such markers, animal experiments and epidemiological studies can work synergistically to put quantitative risk assessment on a firmer scientific base, leaving less room for policy conflicts.

POLICY PROBLEMS

Formaldehyde is a useful compound with no readily available, safe substitute. Banning its production (explicitly, or implicitly by imposing restrictive exposure limits) carries a heavy price. Clearly a tradeoff is required to arrive at exposure limits. Scientific and social issues are inextricably interwoven in this tradeoff. To deal with it, we need to know the human health risks incurred by specific exposures. With this information, we must then decide how much burden should be placed on the occupationally exposed so that society can benefit. We do not yet have the technical means to address the first issue, or the procedural mechanisms to reach a consensus for the second one. Lack of these tools aggravates the confusion of science and policy.

The absence of unequivocal data concerning human risks permits a broad spectrum of interpretation. Value judgements drive the most forceful of these interpretations, as evidenced by the furor over formaldehyde. Nevertheless, the interpretations are presented, criticized, and defended as scientific conclusions. This tendency for political and philosophical differences to masquerade as scientific disputes is also manifested by the overkill in critiques of completed studies whose results have undesirable implications for the interests of one or another faction in a regulatory issue. For example, the lack of strong positive findings among formaldehyde workers in an important study (Blair et al, 1986) triggered criticism of the investigators' scientific competence and integrity sufficient to warrant a congressional hearing (Occupational Safety and Health Administration, 1986). While constructive peer review is a useful process, critiques that exaggerate a study's flaws and overlook its strengths for the purpose of discrediting its findings are counterproductive and a poor use of resources.

The fusion of facts and values in the masquerade of politics as science contradicts the prevailing notion that risk assessment for toxic substances is (or should be) entirely objective and scientific. For example, the National Academy of Sciences Committee on the Institutional Means for Assessment of Risks to Public Health recommended "that regulatory agencies . . . maintain a clear distinction between assessment of risks and consideration of the risk management alternatives; that is, the scientific findings and policy judgements embodied in risk assessments should be explicitly distinguished from the political, economic and technical considerations that influence the design and choice of regulatory strategies" (National Academy of Sciences, 1983).

While it is useful to call attention to the desirability of such a distinction, in practice it is often an unrealistic and unattainable goal. Values enter risk assessment in many covert ways. They determine the quantity and quality of information obtained about a chemical, influence explicit and implicit assumptions used to analyze data, affect the interpretation of data, and influence the weights used to combine disparate sets of data (see Whittemore, 1983 for examples).

Our failure to recognize and confront the inseparable fusion of facts and values in toxicant risk analysis has contributed to the frequent occurrence of regulatory impasses requiring costly and time-consuming litigation. The task of resolving these complex science–policy issues has overwhelmed the courts which lack the mandate and expertise to tackle it. Science advisory panels have been proposed to improve the courts' technical expertise (Whittemore, 1983). However, the creation of such panels would treat symptoms instead of causes and would foster inappropriate use of the judiciary by excluding the public from the decision-making process.

FUTURE CHALLENGES

The major challenge is to develop more efficient regulatory procedures that rely less on the courts. Regulatory litigation consumes valuable human resources and should be the exception rather than the rule. One antidote for the negative side-effects of politicization on scientific research is awareness of the hybrid nature of risk assessment. We need to recognize that separation of regulatory policy into matters of fact and value is illusory, and to sensitize ourselves to value judgments when they occur. They will and must occur because setting standards for hazards at work and in the environment is a social and political process.

Another antidote is to allocate resources sufficient to insure the conduct of sound studies and to incorporate into the studies the advice of experts chosen to represent the concerns of all sides in sensitive issues. Also helpful are consensus conferences to evaluate and synthesize existing data, such as that convened to evaluate the toxicity of formaldehyde (Consensus Workshop on Formaldehyde, 1984).

Ultimately, the usefulness of quantitative risk assessment to regulatory policy will depend on the development of new public participation mechanisms, and development of improved ways for scientists and regulators to communicate with the public. Leone (1986) argues that in our action-oriented society there is a political bias toward regulation, and that what is needed is "the art of doing nothing." Risk managers need to create the credibility and authority to avoid taking action when they feel the costs far outweigh the benefits. The implementation of California's Proposition 65, the Safe Drinking Water and Toxic Enforcement Act of 1986, entailed regular meetings of the public, the California Department of Health Services, regulators, special interest groups, and a panel of scientists. The exchange at such meetings provided a model for public participation in resolving the complex issues surrounding risk assessment (Kizer et al, 1988).

Finally, improved regulatory procedures require more informative data on which to base scientific judgements. Well-designed and well-conducted epidemiological studies continue to be needed. The absence of reliable laboratory screens for human carcinogens mandates aggressive monitoring of occupationally exposed populations. Early detection of occupational carcinogens requires annually updated and linkable medical, job, and smoking histories for all current and former employees. Continued morbidity and mortality monitoring after retirement is particularly important in view of increasing trends in cancer rates among older age groups that cannot be explained by increased diagnostic accuracy (Davis et al, 1986). This monitoring makes sense from the industrial point of view because most such studies would reveal no excess risk, and the accumulated negative human evidence, coupled with estimates of exposure levels for various agents, would be useful in resisting overzealous regulation. The monitoring also makes sense from the workers' point of view because real hazards would be detected earlier than they otherwise might be. Finally, it makes sense for the public who would learn that prolonged exposure to many agents feared harmful have not produced observable human hazards.

In the interim, we must rely on laboratory experiments to assess risk for those compounds distributed widely in the human environment and for which epidemiological studies do not exist. We also need laboratory data for chemicals, such as formaldehyde, that do not show a clear risk in epidemiological studies. The formaldehyde experimental data contribute the following important information: (1) formaldehyde is a carcinogen; (2) susceptibility to formaldehyde's carcinogenicity varies substantially with dose rate and species; and (3) DNA binding and increased cell proliferation correlate well with carcinogenicity across dose rate and species. The epidemiological data contribute the following important information: prolonged exposure to formaldehyde has not produced respiratory cancer risks in humans of the magnitude seen for asbestos, arsenic, radon, or tobacco.

These complementary contributions can be linked on a firmer scientific basis with data on preneoplastic markers. Biologically motivated mathematical theories can be tested against species- and dose-rate–specific data on dose to the target tissue, on biologically active dose to the target cells, on specific types of chromosome aberrations in the target cells, on cell proliferation rates, and on extent of dysplasia, hyperplasia, and metaplasia in the target tissue. Such theories, when consistent with the data, can provide more realistic estimates and help to reconcile interspecies differences. The opportunities to collect and analyze these new data are the most encouraging events in quantitative risk assessment in the past decade. Despite the obstacles ahead, we are now a giant step closer to risk assessments based on a real understanding of carcinogenesis.

REFERENCES

Ashford NA, Ryan CW, Calart CC. 1983. Law and science policy in federal regulation of formaldehyde. Science 222:894–900.

Bardana EJ Jr, Montanaro A. 1991. Formaldehyde: an analysis of its respiratory, cutaneous, and immunologic effects. Ann Allergy 66:441–452.

Blair A, Stewart P, O'Berg M, et al. 1986. Mortality among industrial workers exposed to formaldehyde. JNatl Cancer Inst 76:1071–1084.

Blair A, Stewart PA, Hoover RN, Fraumeni JF. 1987. Cancers of the nasopharynx and oropharynx and formaldehyde exposure (letter). JNatl Cancer Inst 78:191–192.

Carcinogen Assessment Group. 1980. Method for determining the unit risk estimate for air pollutants. Washington, D.C., Office of Health and Environmental Assessment, Environmental Protection Agency.

Conolly RB, Andersen ME. 1993. An approach to mechanism-based cancer risk assessment for formaldehyde. Environ Health Perspect 101 (Suppl) 6:169–76.

Consensus Workshop on Formaldehyde. 1984. Report on the consensus workshop on formaldehyde. Environ Health Perspect 58:323–381.

Craft TR, Bermudez E, Skopek TR. 1987. Formaldehyde mutagenesis and formation of DNA-protein crosslinks in human lymphoblasts in vitro. Mutat Res 176:147–155.

Crosby RM, Richardson KK, Craft TR, et al. 1988. Molecular analysis of formaldehyde-induced mutations in human lymphoblasts and *E. coli*. Environ Mol Mutagen 12:155–166.

Davis DL, Lilienfeld AD, Gittelsohn A, Scheckenbach ME. 1986. Increasing trends in some cancers in older Americans: Fact or artifact? Toxicol Ind Health 2:127–144.

Doll R, Peto R. 1977. Mortality among doctors in different occupations. BMJ 1:1433–1436.

Efron E. 1984. The Apocalyptics. New York, Simon and Schuster.

Environmental Protection Agency, Office of Toxic Substances. 1981. Options Paper on Formaldehyde. Washington, D.C., Office of Toxic Substances, U.S. Environmental Protection Agency.

Federal Panel on Formaldehyde. 1984. Report of the federal panel on formaldehyde. Environ Health Perspect 43:139–168.

Freedman DA, Zeisel H. 1988. From mouse to man: the quantitative assessment of cancer risks. Stat Sci 3:3–56.

Gibson JE. 1983. Risk assessment using a combination of testing and research results. *In* Gibson JE (ed.): Formaldehyde Toxicity, New York, Hemisphere Publishing.

Grafstrom RC, Fornace AJ Jr, Autrup H, et al. 1983. Formaldehyde damage to DNA and inhibition of DNA repair in human bronchial cells. Science 220:216–218.

Grafstrom RC, Curran RD, Yang LL. 1985. Genotoxicity of formaldehyde in cultured human bronchial fibroblasts. Science 22:89–91.

Harrington JM, Shannon HS. 1975. Mortality study of pathologists and medical laboratory technicians. BMJ ii:329–332.

Heck H d'A, Casanova M, Steinhagen WH, et al. 1989. Formaldehyde toxicity—DNA-protein cross-linking studies in rats and nonhuman primates. *In* Feron V-J (ed): Nasal Carcinogens in Rodents: Relevance to Human Risk. The Netherlands, Pudoc Wageningen Publisher.

Horton VL, Higuchi MA, Rickert DE. 1992. Physiologically based pharmacokinetic model for methanol in rats, monkeys and humans. Toxicol Appl Pharmacol 117:26–36.

Hulka BS, Wilcosky TC, Griffith JD (eds). 1990. Biological Markers in Epidemiology. New York, Oxford, Oxford University Press.

Hutson DH. 1970. Mechanisms of biotransformation. *In* Hathway DE (ed): Foreign Compound Metabolism in Mammals, Vol. 1. London, The Chemical Society, pp. 314–395.

International Agency for Research on Cancer. 1982. IARC Monographs on the Evaluation of Carcinogenic Risk of Chemicals, Suppl. 4. Chemicals Industrial Processes and Industries Association with Cancer in Humans. IARC Monographs Vols. 1–29. Lyon, International Agency for Research on Cancer.

Kizer KW, Warriner TE, Book SA. 1988. Sound science in the implementation of public policy: a case report on California's Proposition 65. JAMA 260:951–955.

Leone RA. 1986. Risk management: A strategic perspective on the art of doing nothing. *In* Meyer RW, Lee H (eds): Environmental Risk Management: Research Needs and Opportunities. Cambridge, Massachusetts, Energy and Environmental Policy Center, John F. Kennedy School of Government, Harvard University, pp. 103–119.

Liber HL, Benferado K, Crosby RM, et al. 1989. Formaldehyde-induced and spontaneous alterations in human hrpt DNA sequence and mRNA expression. Mutat Res 226:31–37.

Monticello TM, Morgan KT. 1994. Cell proliferation and formaldehyde-induced respiratory carcinogenesis. Risk Anal 14:313–319.

MONTICELLO TM, MORGAN KT, EVERITT JI, POPP JA. 1989. Effects of formaldehyde gas on the respiratory tract of rhesus monkeys. Am J Pathol 134:515–527.

MORGAN KT, KIMBELL JS, MONTICELLO TM, et al. 1991. Studies of inspiratory airflow patterns in the nasal passages of the F344 rat and rhesus monkey using nasal molds: relevance to formaldehyde toxicity. Toxicol Appl Pharmacol 110:223–240.

NATIONAL ACADEMY OF SCIENCES, Committee on the Institutional Means for Assessment of Risks to Public Health. 1983. Risk Assessment in the Federal Government: Managing the Process. Washington, D.C., National Academy Press.

NATIONAL INSTITUTE FOR OCCUPATIONAL SAFETY AND HEALTH. 1976. Criteria for a Recommended Standard. Occupational Exposure to Formaldehyde. DHEW (NIOSH) Publ. no. 77-126. Washington, D.C., U.S. Government Printing Office.

NATIONAL RESEARCH COUNCIL. 1980. Formaldehyde—An Assessment of Its Health Effects. Prepared for the Consumer Products Safety Commission. Washington, D.C., Academy of Sciences, pp. 1–38.

NELSON N, LEVINE RJ, ALBERT RE, et al. 1986. Contribution of formaldehyde to respiratory cancer. Environ Health Perspect 70:23–35.

OCCUPATIONAL SAFETY AND HEALTH ADMINISTRATION. 1980. Identification, Classification and Regulation of Potential Occupational Carcinogens. Federal Register 45(15):5002.

OCCUPATIONAL SAFETY AND HEALTH ADMINISTRATION. 1986. Occupational Exposure to Formaldehyde. Federal Register 51(239):44796.

PERERA F, PETITO C. 1982. Formaldehyde: A question of cancer policy? Science 216:1285–1291.

PETO R. 1978. Carcinogenic effects of exposure to very low levels of carcinogenic substances. Environ Health Perspect 22:155–159.

REGULATORY COUNCIL. 1979. Statement on Regulation of Chemical Carcinogens; Policy and Request for Public Comment. Federal Register 44(60):600038.

SMITH AE. 1992. Formaldehyde. Occup Med 42:83–88.

STARR TB. 1990. Quantitative cancer risk estimation for formaldehyde. Risk Anal 10:85–91.

STROUP NE, BLAIR A, ERIKSON GE. 1986. Brain cancer and other causes of death in anatomists. J Natl Cancer Inst 77:1217–1224.

SUN M. 1981. A firing over formaldehyde. Science 213:630–631.

SWENBERG JA. 1987. High-to-low dose extrapolation. Environ Health Perspect 76:57–63.

SWENBERG JA, GROSS EA, RANDALL HW. 1986. Localization and quantification of cell proliferation following exposure to nasal irritants. *In* Barrow CS (ed): Toxicology of the Nasal Passages. New York, Hemisphere Publishing Corp., pp. 291–300.

TODHUNTER J. 1982. Review of data available to the Administrator concerning formaldehyde and di(2-ethylhexyl)phthalate (DEHP). Memorandum to AM Gorsuch.

WALRATH J, FRAUMENI JF, JR. 1983. Mortality patterns among embalmers. Int J Cancer 31:407–411.

WHITTEMORE AS. 1983. Facts and values in risk analysis for environmental toxicants. Risk Anal 3:23–33.

WHITTEMORE AS. 1986. Epidemiology in risk assessment for regulatory policy. J Chron Dis 39:1157–1168.

WILDAVSKY A. 1984. Letter to the Editor. Science 224:550–556.

YOUNG H. 1981. United Auto Workers petition for emergency temporary standard on formaldehyde. Sent to T Auchter.

ZEISE L, WILSON, CROUCH EAC. 1987. Dose–response relationships for carcinogenesis: a review. Environ Health Perspect 73:259–308.

9 Mathematical models in cancer epidemiology

JOHN M. KALDOR
NICHOLAS E. DAY

Human cancers are rare diseases with long latent periods and multifactorial etiologies. As such, their study has naturally inspired the development of mathematical models, which involve probabilistic relationships between the risk of disease and various environmental, constitutional, and temporal variables. Such models are behind most of the inferences made in cancer epidemiology, although they are not always stated explicitly. Even the simple assertion "agent X causes cancer in humans" can only be interpreted by restating it in the form "individuals who have been exposed to agent X have a higher risk of cancer than individuals who have not" or "the risk of cancer increases with increasing exposure to agent X." Both of these restatements in turn require mathematical models to define what is meant by the risk of cancer for an individual, and the second requires a definition of exposure that can be used as a scale to rank individuals.

The goal of this chapter is to examine critically the mathematical models that have been used in cancer epidemiology. We first consider the process by which models are obtained, and their role in studying human cancer. We then discuss in detail some of the mathematical models that have been proposed, the ways in which they have been applied in studying specific types of cancer, and their strengths and limitations as tools in scientific inference.

WHERE DO THE MATHEMATICAL MODELS IN CANCER EPIDEMIOLOGY COME FROM?

Formal definition of a mathematical model is beyond the scope of this chapter, and ultimately leads into questions in the philosophy of science. For the present purposes, it is sufficient to define a mathematical model for cancer risk as an equation or equations expressing the dependence of cancer incidence (or some other measure of the disease) on a set of observable variables and a set of quantities known as parameters, whose true values may be unknown. Thus defined, a model has mathematical properties that can be explored in the absence of any epidemiological or other data. Any process by which the values of unknown parameters are estimated from suitable data is known as fitting the model to the data, a terminology that can seem somewhat inappropriate, since the model may in fact fit rather poorly.

Two quite different classes of mathematical models have been used in cancer epidemiology. They may be broadly distinguished as biomathematical models and statistical models. The biomathematical models, of which the best known today are probably those originally proposed by Armitage and Doll (1954) and Moolgavkar and Knudson (1981), are derived by translating series of hypotheses about the biological processes involved in carcinogenesis into mathematical terms. The statistical models, on the other hand, draw on well-established mathematical structures such as linear regression equations, which have been applied in many other areas of scientific inference, as a means of expressing relationships between cancer risk and other variables.

The two model classes differ not only in their origin but also in the role they have played in cancer research. The biomathematical models have been used primarily as the basis for discussion about the mechanisms of carcinogenesis, and have not had a place in the routine statistical analysis of most studies. They have in a few carefully chosen cases been compared with epidemiological data, but usually in a rather informal way, either to lend support to or refute one or more of the biological hypotheses that have gone into the derivation of the model. The statistical models, on the other hand, function more as the basic tools of cancer epidemiology, for summarizing and interpreting the massive amount of numerical information obtained in epidemiological studies.

There are several reasons for these differences in role. In general, the biomathematical models can only express rather specific relationships, albeit often having complicated structures. Although they may be well understood as mathematical entities, procedures for estimating their unknown parameters from epidemiological data are far from standardized, and are certainly not widely available on computer software. In contrast, estimation methods for the statistical models have properties that have been investigated in detail, and they can be implemented using a variety of commercially distributed computer programs.

Despite these differences, the two classes do have features in common. The biomathematical models are refined or modified on the basis of epidemiological data, just as the statistical ones are, even if further biological hypotheses are invoked to justify the changes, and the statistical models are not developed without reference to the biological meaning of the measurements involved. Both types of models have been used as the basis for making predictions about cancer risk in specific populations. Ideally, there would be a convergence in solutions provided by the two approaches for any given problem. In practice, however, a choice is made of a class of models, and a particular model within a class, using criteria that we consider in the next section.

CRITERIA FOR IDENTIFYING A GOOD MODEL

The way in which a model is judged depends entirely on the use to which it is to be put. A scientist may formalize his or her conception of some aspect of carcinogenesis by using a mathematical model, simply as a way to communicate the idea to others. At this stage of the scientific process, the criterion by which the model is judged is simply the degree to which it reproduces its proposer's theory. At the other extreme, a mathematical model used to predict the increase in human cancer risk following exposure to a specific environmental agent for the purpose of government regulation must be subject to the most stringent possible experimental and observational validation, and finally should be judged largely by the degree to which the errors associated with its assumptions can be quantified.

The assumptions behind models are usually dealt with in one of three ways. Some are evaluated rather formally, using the statistical framework of hypothesis testing and confidence-interval estimation. Others are treated more informally, although still with the use of observational or experimental data. The remainder are taken on faith, either because they are accepted as being true through a collective suspension of disbelief, or because it is recognized that their evaluation would require data that are not, and may never be, available. A simple example may serve to illustrate these distinctions. Consider the problem of estimating a confidence interval for the increase in lung cancer risk due to occupational exposure to a carcinogen in a particular industry. The model to be used may involve assumptions about similarity of effect in smokers and nonsmokers, which could be formally tested if information on smoking habits were available for study subjects. The model is also likely to involve the assumption that employment in a certain work area entails exposure to the agent for which the risk is being estimated. This assumption may be checked using environmental measurements in the workplace, but is unlikely to be verifiable for each worker in the area. In the third category might be implicit assumptions concerning the representativeness of the study subjects, with regard to any unmeasured determinants of lung cancer risk acting in addition to age, smoking status, and other factors that have been investigated in the study.

Errors associated with the first two kinds of assumptions can in general be quantified in a reasonable way. Error due to the third kind of assumption is by definition not assessed, and often one cannot even say whether it is a trivial component of the overall model error, or its most important part. Furthermore, this difficulty grows with the model's complexity: For a given amount of data, the extent to which assumptions can be verified decreases as the number of assumptions increase.

From a purely statistical viewpoint, mathematical models are evaluated by two sets of criteria, which may be in direct conflict. One is the closeness of fit of the model to available data, and the other is the simplicity of the model. Increasing the complexity of a model by adding extra parameters of various kinds can certainly improve the degree to which it conforms to observations, but ultimately leads back to a structure that is indistinguishable from the observations themselves in its ability to summarize or describe the phenomena under study. Formal statistical hypotheses tests may be used to evaluate whether increases in a model's complexity are justified by the observations, but after a certain point, which depends on how much and what kind of data are available, it is no longer possible to distinguish whether extra parameters are improving the fit or not. This phenomenon is known in statistical terms as nonidentifiability, and may also find its expression in large confidence intervals on the parameters concerned or an inability to reject simpler models due to low power. Too often in the development of either biomathematical or statistical models, nonidentifiability remains unrecognized, and a model that appeals to the modeler is approved (or accepted, in the classical hypothesis-testing terminology) simply because it cannot be excluded, even when the evidence against a wide range of other models is no stronger.

A controversial issue in the evaluation of models assumptions is the weight that should be placed on what might be called biological good intentions. Some authors have argued that a model which involves mathematical representations of proposed biological phenomena is in some sense a priori better than one which does not, even before the process of model fitting begins. In fact, if one accepts the necessity of taking an equally critical attitude to all model assumptions, biological hypotheses would be examined in exactly the same way as seemingly more arbitrary statistical ones, and the question should not arise. However, biological assumptions are often based on an accumulation of different kinds of information from a variety of sources, and may be difficult to evaluate in the formal way demanded by statistical theory. Furthermore, scientists differ substantially among themselves in the criteria that they apply for criticizing model assumptions, whether biological or otherwise. Thus, even if the goal of modeling is clear, which itself is not always the case, we are still far from being able to propose a unified and generally agreed procedure for arriving at the best model to describe a given body of data.

With this somewhat abstract background, we now turn to consider some of the specific mathematical models that have been used in cancer epidemiology.

THE BIOMATHEMATICAL MODELS

In this section, we outline some of the major developments that have occurred in the evolution of biomathematical models for human cancer. In doing so, we have tried to indicate the degree to which model validation has taken place. For mathematical details, the reader should consult the original papers. Other critical reviews of the biomathematical models are also available (Peto, 1977; Moolgavkar, 1986; Kaldor and Day, 1987).

Early Developments: The Multistage Model

In a series of experiments that began during the 1940s, experimental scientists demonstrated that some chemical agents, referred to as promoters, were apparently incapable of causing cancer on their own, but could substantially increase tumor yield when applied to animals that had been first exposed to certain carcinogens (Berenblum and Shubik, 1947; Mottram, 1944). The proposed explanation for this phenomenon was that the promoters could only act on cells that had already been partially transformed toward malignancy by the previous action of the so-called initiator, suggesting that there was an intermediate state between normalcy and malignancy.

Concurrently, improvements in national vital statistics showed that for most types of cancer, the mortality rate increased sharply with age. This observation stimulated the search for a mathematical form that could reproduce the age-mortality curves and that was based on biological assumptions about tumor development. Fisher and Holloman (1951) proposed that transformation of a minimum number of cells was the essential requirement for cancer development, and Nordling (1953) and Armitage and Doll (1954) countered with the idea of a single cell undergoing a minimum number of changes, each of which was heritable and could be passed on to daughter cells, before becoming malignant. When translated into mathematical expressions, and assuming that individual cells are affected independently and with low probabilities of transition that do not change with time (Moolgavkar, 1978), both these hypotheses predict that cancer occurrence increases as an integer power of age. The power depends on the required minimum number of cells or stages, and the relationship is linear on a doubly logarithmic plot, with a slope equal to the integer power. Armitage and Doll pointed out that the model involving a minimum number of cells also implied an integer power relationship between exposure level and cancer, and they contended that this prediction was inconsistent with animal carcinogenesis experiments. At the time when these papers were published, there may well have been no evidence for upward curvature in dose-response curves for carcinogenesis. However, several experimental and epidemiological studies have since demonstrated relationships of this kind. Among animal carcinogens thiotepa and orthotoluidine are only two examples of agents that induce tumors at a rate that increases more rapidly as the dose increases (Gold et al, 1984), and cigarette smoking increases lung cancer risk according to a relationship that has been interpreted to include a quadratic term to convey upward curvature (Doll and Peto, 1978). No attempt was made formally to evaluate the power model's agreement with the age-incidence curve for cancer until Cook, et al (1969) carried out an extensive analysis using information that was newly available in the first volume of Cancer Incidence in Five Continents (Doll et al, 1966). This publication, like its successors (Cancer Incidence in Five Continents, Volumes II–VI), listed cancer incidence rates over a limited time period from a number of geographical areas broken down by site, sex, and age. For each of 24 types of cancer, Cook and her colleagues examined the extent to which the relationship between age and incidence followed the curve

$$I_t = At^{k-1}$$

where I_t is the cancer incidence at age t, and A and k are unknown constants. If the Armitage-Doll model were valid, k would represent the number of stages that a cell has to pass through as it is transformed to malignancy, and A would be proportional to the product of the transition rates. Their conclusion was that for a number of types of cancer the power relationship seemed to hold. Furthermore, the crucial parameter k for each cancer type did not vary substantially across sex or registries, and it ranged across cancer types from 2 (melanoma) to 12 (prostatic cancer). However, there was sufficient departure from the relationship for the authors to also conclude that "the simple power relationship between cancer incidence and age is inadequate to explain the greater part of the observed data." In fact, as they themselves made clear in an extensive discussion of their results, even if carcinogenesis indeed follows a multistage process of the kind proposed, a number of further conditions must be satisfied for it to be manifested as a simple power relationship between age and cancer incidence in a population at any given time.

In general, these conditions relate to the constancy of A, the product of the transition rates. If these rates are dependent on external factors in the environment, they may be modified as individuals are exposed to changing environments. These changes may occur in a way that is strongly related to year of birth, such as the sharp increase in cigarette smoking that occurred in British men born around the turn of the century. On the other hand, they may equally affect all age groups in a particular time period: consider, for example, the human population's ultraviolet exposure. Another possibility is that host factors whose level changes with age, such as hormones, may modify the transition rates, and consequently their product A. Finally, transition rates may have a genetic component leading to population heterogeneity regardless of environmental and endogenous variations in time. It would indeed be surprising if all of these factors had no effect on A, either by being absent or somehow canceling each other out.

Soon after proposing their model, Armitage and Doll (1957) recognized that by allowing for a growth advantage of intermediate cells, the desired shape of the age-incidence curve could be generated by a model with only two stages, and Pike (1966) showed that the power curve could be derived under rather general assumptions about the mechanism of carcinogenesis. Peto (1977) pointed out that different hypotheses about the duration of time required for a single malignant cell to grow into a clinically detectable tumor could also result in curves with essentially the same shape, provided k was varied appropriately. There is nothing unique about the biological hypotheses that can produce age-incidence curves that are exactly or approximately linear on a double logarithmic scale. Furthermore, the fundamental assumptions about the number of stages and the independence of individual cells in their likelihood of making the transition between stages remain completely unverified by experimental or epidemiological findings.

The Multistage Model and Specific Carcinogens

By the late 1970s information from epidemiological studies had accumulated to the extent that for several carcinogens, quantitative statements could be made about various temporal aspects of their carcinogenic effect and the shape of the carcinogenesis dose-response curve. A number of authors (Whittemore, 1977; Day and Brown, 1980; Peto et al, 1982; Siemiatycki and Thomas, 1981) began to examine the predictions of the multistage model with regard to these factors, and to compare the predictions with the epidemiological findings. These activities were not so much aimed at evaluating the model itself as using the model as a basis for distinguishing or classifying the known human carcinogens. It was proposed that a carcinogen acted by increasing one or more of the transition rates between stages over the spontaneous or background rate, a suggestion that received substantial support from contemporary studies showing an apparently high correlation between the carcinogenic activity of a chemical agent and its ability to cause mutations or other forms of heritable genetic damage in in vitro assays (Ames et al, 1975). The mathematical consequences of an increase in transition rates were used to derive relationships between cancer risk and such variables as age at exposure, duration of exposure, time since cessation of exposure, and the interaction between two carcinogenic agents. Table 9–1summarizes the relationships predicted, considering various stages affected, and assuming that the number of susceptible normal cells is constant with age, and only the exposure under study can modify transition rates. Most of them are intuitively quite logical: for example, if a carcinogen affects only the first transition rate, the excess number of cancers will not depend on age because the pool of normal cells does not increase; in contrast, an agent capable of increasing the rate of later transitions has a larger pool of partially trans-

TABLE 9–1. *Predictions of the Multistage Model for Early and Late Stage Carcinogens*

Variable for Which Effect is Predicted	*Effect on Excess Cancer Risk if Agent acts as*		
	Early Stage Only	*Late Stage Only*	*Early and Late Stages*
Age at exposure	None	Increase	Small increase
Time since first exposure	Slow increase	Rapid increase	Slow increase
Time since last exposure	Little or none	Plateau	Plateau
Dose-response	Linear	Linear	Quadratic or higher power
Interaction between two carcinogens	Additive	Additive	Multiplicative[a]

[a]Assuming one agent acts at an early stage and the other at a late stage.

formed cells to affect in older as compared to younger individuals, simply owing to a greater number of spontaneous transitions between stages having occurred over time.

In order to classify carcinogens according to these different characteristics, various statistical approaches were adopted. Some authors (Day and Brown, 1980; Peto et al, 1982) made informal comparisons of observed relationships between cancer risk and variables of the kind listed in Table 9–1, and the relationships predicted under different multistage assumptions, while Brown and Chu (1983) and Kaldor et al (1986) used the techniques of multiple regression to statistically test predicted relationships. Thomas (1983) fitted the multistage model in its strict mathematical form (to data on lung cancer among asbestos workers), but in doing so, he found it necessary to make a priori assumptions about which stages might be affected by the carcinogens under study. Table 9–2 summarizes some of the conclusions that have been reached about human carcinogens regarding their characteristics under the multistage model. It is worth noting that, regardless of the validity of the model itself, the variables suggested by the model and used in the classification of carcinogens are often of substantial interest in themselves. For example, it is important to know what happens to lung cancer risk when smokers give up their habit, even if the relevance of the information to carcinogenic mechanisms is not proven.

Incorporation of Cellular Kinetics

It has long been recognized that for several types of cancer, the age-incidence curve is inconsistent with the simple multistage prediction of a power law, in ways that are too extreme to be attributed to chance or the effects of temporal changes in environmental or host factors. Striking examples are the cancers of childhood, which by definition exhibit a peak of the early years of life, and breast cancer, with its characteristic change in slope around the menopause years. Pike (1983) suggested that the breast cancer age-incidence curve could be explained by viewing the time scale not as chronological age but as breast tissue aging, which began at menarche, continued through the years of fertility with possible modifications due to pregnancies, and declined at menopause. With tissue age defined in this way, and making certain assumptions about hormonal influences on the rate of aging, the model succeeds well in reproducing the age-incidence curve for breast cancer. A similar approach, but discussing breast cancer epidemiology more broadly, is given by Moolgavkar et al (1980).

A more general approach, which can be used to explain the age-incidence curve of breast, childhood, and other cancers, has been proposed by Moolgavkar and Knudson (1981). Like Armitage and Doll (1957) over

TABLE 9–2. *Human Carcinogens: Classification under the Multistage Model*

Agent	*Type of Cancer*	*Observed Patterns of Risk*
Cigarette smoke	Lung	• No effect of age at exposure on excess risk • Constant or decreased excess risk after cessation of exposure • Superlinear dose-response
Ionizing radiation	Solid tumors	• Increased excess risk with age at exposure • Increased excess risk with time since exposure • Linear dose-response
	Leukemia	• Increased excess risk for exposure in childhood and with age in adults • Excess risk increases rapidly, then drops
Asbestos	Lung	• Increased excess risk with age at exposure • Decreased relative risk after cessation of exposure
	Mesothelioma	• No effect of age at exposure on excess risk • Increased excess risk with time since exposure
Exposures in nickel refining	Nasal sinus	• Increased excess risk with age at exposure • Increased excess risk with time since exposure
	Lung	• No effect of age at exposure on excess risk • Decreased relative risk after cessation of exposure
Arsenic	Lung	• Increased excess risk with age at exposure • Constant excess risk after cessation of exposure
Aromatic amines	Bladder	• No effect of age at exposure on excess risk • Increased excess risk after cessation of exposure
Hormones	Breast	• Flattening of age-incidence curve after cessation of endogenous estrogen exposure at menopause
	Endometrium	• Slow decrease in risk after cessation of estrogen use

two decades earlier, they adopted a model in which there was only a single intermediate stage on the pathway to malignancy, and which took into account cellular growth kinetics. As well as a growth advantage for intermediate over normal cells, the proposed model incorporated information about the division and death rates of the normal cells that are the targets for the first transition. Their model was largely inspired by the work of Knudson (1971) on retinoblastoma, a rare tumor of the retinal cells that occurs almost exclusively in children age 4 years old or less. Susceptibility to the disease appears to be subject to dominant inheritance in about 40% of cases, and for children with a family history of retinoblastoma, it is very likely to appear in both eyes.

Knudson et al (1975) had already postulated that familial cases arise through the inheritance of a single constitutional mutation, followed by a second random mutation in the retinal cells, but that the nonfamilial or sporadic cases required two random mutations. He used information from a case series to compare the observed distribution of onset times with that predicted by the theory. Moolgavkar and Venzon (1979) developed the mathematical basis of the two-stage model with growth kinetics, and Moolgavkar and Knudson (1981) showed that by making suitable assumptions about the net division rates of normal and intermediate cells, age-incidence curves appropriate for childhood cancer and breast cancer (Moolgavkar et al, 1980) could be generated, as could the usual power-type relationship. The shape for childhood cancers including retinoblastoma was produced by assuming that the number of susceptible normal cells increases sharply in the early years of life and then decreases rapidly to zero before adolescence. For tissues such as the retina this pattern fits closely with what is known about organ development. However, there are other childhood tumors, including acute lymphocytic leukemia, for which there is no evidence for growth kinetics of this kind in the ostensible target organ. For breast cancer, the number of susceptible normal cells is supposed to be under hormonal control, in a way that closely parallels the model of Pike (1983), and describes the observed age-incidence curves equally well (Moolgavkar et al, 1980).

Apart from its ability to mimic the empirical age-incidence curves for most types of human cancer, the two-stage model with growth kinetics has attracted attention because of its ability to incorporate the effect of so-called nongenotoxic carcinogens. Under the model, a carcinogen may be assumed to act by increasing the rate of transitions rate between stages, as is supposed in the classical multistage model, but it may also be postulated to increase the net division rate of normal or intermediate cells. Defined in this way, an increase in the division rate of intermediate as compared to normal cells corresponds closely to the experimentalist's notion of a promoting effect: partially transformed cells are given a growth advantage in the presence of the promoter, which increases the number of such cells and hence the probability that one or more will undergo malignant transformation. The model can also be used to represent a carcinogenic effect of mitogens that increase the division rate and hence the number of susceptible cells in normal tissue. Moolgavkar (1983) discusses in detail the model's predictions with regard to the effect of duration of exposure, time since cessation of exposure, and other variables under different assumptions about the mechanism of carcinogenic action. In the first serious attempt to fit the model formally to epidemiological carcinogenesis data, Moolgavkar et al (1989) ran into the identifiability problem: although the model described the observed relationship between smoking and lung cancer mortality in British doctors (Doll and Peto, 1978), the available data were "incapable of distinguishing among various hypotheses regarding the relative roles of the two mutation rates and the kinetics of intermediate cell growth."

As a simple yet unifying theory, the model proposed by Moolgavkar and Knudson has had enormous value in facilitating communication among the experimentalists, epidemiologists, and geneticists working on the problem of human cancer. It is consistent with much available experimental and observational information, but nonetheless remains largely a theory, and is far from being validated as a description of the mechanisms. Advances in cytogenetics (Benedict et al, 1983) and molecular biology (Cavanee et al, 1983; Koufos et al, 1984) have confirmed the presence of two characteristic chromosomal changes (deletions in the same region of both copies of chromosome 13) in retinoblastoma tumor cells, and a single change in all cells of individuals who suffer from the familial form of the disease. However, Matsunaga (1979) has reported a study suggesting that in bilateral (and presumably familial) cases, the time of occurrence of the tumor is more highly correlated between the two eyes than would be predicted by the model. Investigation of Wilms' tumor, a cancer of the kidney whose epidemiological and genetic features closely parallel those of retinoblastoma, has indicated that the tumor preferentially retain the affected chromosome that originated with the father (Schroeder et al, 1987; Williams et al, 1989). This finding suggests that loss of function at the homologous loci, or "antioncogenes" in the terminology proposed by Knudson (1985), is not sufficient for tumor development, and that some other factor related to the father's chromosome is playing a role.

For other kinds of cancer, there is no indication that exactly two genetic changes distinguish malignant from normal cells in the same tissue. Mutations in up to five oncogenes, the DNA sequences that are known to be capable of inducing tumors when transfected into experimental animals, have been found in colon tumor tissue (Vogelstein et al, 1988). Whether all of those mutations are necessary for malignancy, or even independent, remains to be demonstrated, but neither is their presence clearly consistent with a two-mutation model. Premalignant lesions such as colon polyps or dysplastic naevi have also been suggested to represent clones of partially transformed cells (Moolgavkar and Knudson, 1981), but again, it is unknown how many genetic changes separate them from normal or malignant cells.

Since oncogenes can be activated by point mutations (Bos, 1988), and many carcinogens are known to be mutagens (Ames et al, 1975), it is certainly plausible that a carcinogen may act by increasing transition rates between stages, although there is no direct evidence for this phenomenon from human or in vivo animal studies. The direct increase in cellular proliferation rates implied by the two-stage model is one, but not the only, nongenotoxic mechanism that has received support from in vitro studies (Trosko and Changa, 1983).

Epidemiological Evidence: What More Can Be Obtained?

Since mathematical models for carcinogenesis were first proposed, their relationship to the practice of cancer epidemiology has never been firmly established. Certainly, the models have been useful in suggesting variables for epidemiological analyses, which, as noted above, are of importance in their own right, whatever the results may tell us about carcinogenic mechanisms. Close examination of epidemiological data by modelers in search of support for their theories has also led to improvements in the methodology of data collection and statistical analyses.

It is even harder to define the contribution of epidemiology to furthering the understanding of the mechanism of carcinogenesis. Although epidemiological studies have clearly shown that simplistic biological hypotheses are untenable, they have been less successful in demonstrating the existence of more complex mechanisms, and it may well be asking too much of epidemiology to expect illumination of subcellular and even molecular processes. Nevertheless, there have been examples to the contrary: it is unlikely that the significance of the chromosomal deletions in retinoblastoma would have been so rapidly appreciated if the epidemiological characteristics of the disease had not already been well understood through the use of mathematical modeling. At another level, the epidemiological association between cervical cancer and sexual behavior justified the search for a sexually transmitted vector with transforming capacity, which eventually led to the human papillomavirus being identified as the most likely candidate (Zur Hausen, 1976).

Can epidemiologists actively contribute to an understanding of the biological basis of carcinogensis, and in particular to those aspects that would together lead to a mathematical model of the process? The emergence of a subspecialty named molecular epidemiology (Perera and Weinstein, 1982) shows that the intention is there, even if the field is still too new to have had a chance to prove itself. There are several types of study that could eventually lead to a clarification of the assumptions behind the mathematical models for carcinogenesis:

1. Investigation of oncogene mutations in normal, precursor, and malignant cells from the same individual. These studies are being carried out by many research centers, but often involve small numbers of subjects sampled in a way that is not clearly stated, and would benefit from a more epidemiological approach.
2. Sample banking. As techniques become available to identify partially transformed cells or their markers, epidemiological studies in which cancer occurrence is evaluated in the donors of stored tissue will help to identify genetic changes on the pathway to malignancy.
3. Epidemiological studies that focus on the implications of specific mechanistic hypotheses. Questions such as the effect of smoking cessation on cancer risk remain only partly resolved, because the studies on which inference is currently based were implemented with other goals in mind. Specially designed investigations of this kind may be viewed by some as a waste of resources, but will ultimately produce clearer answers, albeit to fewer questions, than many of the all-purpose multivariable studies that continue to dominate cancer epidemiology today.

THE STATISTICAL MODELS

The other major class of models has had much wider application in cancer epidemiology than the biomathematical models, and has received closer scrutiny from statisticians. In describing the role they have played, we again avoid mathematical details and concentrate on the underlying principles involved.

The History of Statistical Models in Cancer Epidemiology

The major methodological problems that have confronted observational cancer epidemiology have been bias in the selection of study subjects, imprecision due to small numbers of subjects, and confounding arising through associations among the risk factors being investigated and other determinants of the disease. Selection bias has largely been eliminated through the use of cancer registries and other sources of population information as sampling frames, and account is taken of the number of study subjects explicitly in the framework of hypothesis testing and confidence-interval estimation. The problem of confounding, however, has been addressed largely through the use of statistical models.

Consider initially the problem of determining whether or not exposure to a particular factor—say, an industrial agent— increases cancer risk, and suppose that a second factor—smoking, for example—is suspected of being associated with both disease risk and the first factor; in other words, of being a confounder. The most direct way in which smoking can be controlled for in the evaluation of the industrial agent's carcinogenicity is to estimate whether the agent produces an increased cancer risk separately for smokers and nonsmokers. If the results are not concordant for the two groups, explanations would be sought in random variation or confounding due to a third factor, and if both of those possibilities could be excluded, the conclusion would be drawn that smokers and nonsmokers differ in their response to the agent under study.

This approach to confounding requires little in the way of mathematical structure, but is ultimately untenable. In most studies there are simply too many potential confounding variables, and too few study subjects in each group created by cross-classification of the variables, to attempt within-group estimation of the carcinogenic effect due to the factor of interest.

The first solution to this problem was to use stratification, adopting a model under which the risk factor was assumed to have the same but unknown carcinogenic effect, no matter what the value of the confounding variables. The imprecise within-group estimates of the effect could then be added up across groups, to give a summary estimate that was reasonably precise, and adjusted for confounding. The classic paper by Mantel and Haenszel (1959) proposed this idea, which was only later provided with a formal theoretical basis. The crucial model assumption of equality of effect can be critically evaluated by comparing the estimate of carcinogenic effect between broad classes of the confounding variables. For example, suppose that in addition to smoking, age and sex are suspected of potentially confounding an estimate of the industrial agent's carcinogenicity. After cross-classifying the study subjects into small categories of smoking status, age, and sex, the summary estimate of effect would be calculated, first overall, and then separately for each sex, broad age groups, and smokers and nonsmokers.

Again, however, this solution came to be viewed as impractical. Stratification according to many variables inevitably produced groups in which all subjects were either exposed or unexposed to the agent of primary interest, and which could of course contribute nothing to the summary effect estimate. Furthermore, the approach did not lend itself to the exploration of functional relationships among variables, and was seen as clumsy for the analysis of so-called exploratory studies, in which the effects on cancer risk of a large number of often speculative factors are examined simultaneously.

The next development required a major leap in terms of model complexity. The advent of high-speed computers made it possible to estimate multiple regression parameters, and theoretical advances had shown how to use regression equations in the study of dichotomous outcome variables (Cox, 1970) and then survival (Cox, 1972). Application to epidemiological case-control (Prentice and Pyke, 1979) and cohort (Breslow et al, 1983) studies soon followed. It was rapidly recognized that if the factor of interest and the confounding variables combined in the specific, simple way specified by a regression equation, the confounding factor could be controlled for by simultaneous estimation of the parameters in the equation. Regression adjustment has since taken over as the preferred method of confounding control in cancer epidemiology.

Multiple Logistic Regression

For a combination of historical reasons, the regression model applied to epidemiological, and in particular case-control, data became known as multiple logistic regression. The originators of the method were no doubt well aware of its underlying assumptions and the possible biases that may result when they do not hold, but in routine use they are more often than not forgotten, or at least ignored.

As it is most frequently applied, the model supposes that the risk of cancer is the multiplicative product of the risks due to certain factors. These factors are identified by testing the null hypothesis that after accounting for other risk factors, they have no effect on risk. The factors that do show evidence for an effect are retained, and their associations with disease risk are declared to be real and not due to chance or confounding by the other factors. If there is only a single potentially confounding variable and it has relatively few categories, the logistic regression estimate of effect for a factor of interest will generally differ little from the summary estimate that would be calculated using the stratification method. If, on the other hand, there are many variables, the results can differ substantially, because of the use of a multiplicative model not only for the interaction between the risk factor and the confounding variables, but also for all interactions among the confounding variables. The stratification method is vulnerable to the same error, but the required estimation of the carcinogenic effect separately for each subgroup along the way

TABLE 9–3. *Estimation of the Relative Risk of Leukemia Due to Chemotherapy for Ovarian Cancer*

		Including All Subjects		Excluding All Subjects Treated with More than One Drug	
Agent	Dose[a]	Treated Cases/Controls	Relative Risk (Standard Error)	Treated Cases/Controls	Relative Risk (Standard Error)
Melphalan	Low	10/24	4.4[b] (1.9)	9/18	5.2[b] (2.0)
	High	22/18	23.0[b] (2.0)	17/18	9.8[b] (1.8)
Chlorambucil	Low	2/4	2.9 (2.7)	2/2	6.8 (3.0)
	High	10/6	9.0[b] (1.9)	6/2	16.0[b] (2.4)
Thiotepa	Low	6/9	2.6 (1.9)	4/6	4.8[b] (2.3)
	High	5/10	2.3 (2.1)	5/6	4.6[b] (2.1)
Cyclophosphamide	Low	10/19	1.8 (1.6)	4/14	1.3 (1.8)
	High	9/19	2.2 (1.7)	8/15	2.5 (1.7)

[a]As defined by the median dose in control subjects.
[b]$p < .05$ (two-sided).

before calculation of the summary measurement would most likely have produced warnings of the inappropriateness of the simple model. In contrast, logistic regression tends to be used as a black box to produce "adjusted" effect estimates, without critical examination of the underlying hypotheses.

At the root of the problem lies a paradox: the more the complexity of a study seems to call for logistic regression to solve the confounding problem, the less the assumptions of multiplicativity that justify its use can be evaluated. An example drawn from a case-control study of leukemia following ovarian cancer (Kaldor et al, 1990) shows a situation where the available data are too sparse to permit the evaluation of any model assumptions (Table 9–3).When the relative risk is estimated separately for women who received only one kind of drug during the course of this treatment for ovarian cancer, the results are coherent. When logistic regression is used to estimate the relative risk for all drugs simultaneously, including in the process women who had been treated with several drugs, the estimates become less clear. Statistical significance at the .05 level is only attained for two rather than all four drugs, and the increase in risk between the low- and high-dose categories of these two drugs is very sharp, in contrast to the simple twofold increase in the preceding analysis. In the analysis of many epidemiological studies, we do not have the luxury of being able to carry out checks of this kind, and may well be in the position represented by the second set of estimates based on logistic regression. Some kind of adjustment has been achieved, but its effect on the results is not clear.

The two sets of estimates in Table 9–3 illustrate another important point about statistical model-building. Some of the estimates calculated by logistic regression have smaller nominal standard errors than those calculated after exclusion of subjects treated by several drugs, because they are based on more observations. On the other hand, we can be more confident in the whole process by which the second set of estimates was obtained, because it is not so dependent on unverifiable assumptions of multiplicativity. This trade-off between validity and precision is one of the major themes of statistical inference, and preferable solutions clearly represent compromises between the two goals.

Alternatives to Regression Models

There are several general strategies to confounding control that may be adopted in preference to uninterpretable regression adjustments. For future studies, a few principal questions of interest should be delineated, and the sample size should be calculated so that these questions can be answered clearly using stratification methods. Where appropriate, matching should be used to maximize the precision of effect estimates within strata. Small, inconclusive epidemiological studies are no more justifiable than small, inconclusive clinical trials (Peto et al, 1976). Logistic and other regression methods clearly retain a role when functional relationships are being explored, but their use should never be automated.

In general, statistical analyses or reanalyses of studies for which data collection is already complete should be carried out with the recognition that a certain degree of adjustment for confounding cannot be made convincingly, and that corresponding questions must, for the moment, remain unanswered.

CONCLUDING REMARKS

The two broad classes examined in this chapter do not by any means include all the mathematical models that have been proposed in the context of cancer epidemiology. Some other important applications have been in the study of cancer screening (Walter and Day, 1983), the evaluation of temporal and spatial clustering of cancer cases (Mantel, 1967; Smith, 1982), and the genetic transmission of cancer susceptibility (Bishop and Gardner, 1980; Williams and Anderson, 1984).

In discussing the ways in which mathematical models are and have been used in cancer epidemiology, we have taken a critical rather than a simply descriptive perspective. Models are a fundamental tool of scientific interest, and will remain so in any field where relationships are being investigated. However, they often take on a life of their own, which can come to guide their use more than the phenomena that they are intended to represent. This fate has to a certain extent befallen the multiple logistic model in cancer epidemiology, and may be appropriate now to reevaluate both the way in which it has been applied and the substantial results it has yielded. The biomathematical cancer models could perhaps also be evaluated in a more rigorous way than they have been in the past.

On the other hand, the adoption of a model can be viewed as a kind of gamble, which if successful will lead to increased understanding of the phenomena under study. An overly critical attitude to model assumptions through an insistence on absolute proof at every step is tantamount to scientific paralysis.

The most recent developments in statistical modeling have been mainly in random effects regression models and the concept of frailty (Gilks et al, 1993; Breslow and Clayton, 1993). With more powerful computing techniques, more complex models are now being elaborated. Further elaboration of biomathematical models has not received much attention, perhaps owing to the increasing insight into the molecular changes involved in the carcinogenic process.

REFERENCES

AMES BN, MCCANN J, YAMASAKI E. 1975. Methods for detecting carcinogens and mutagens with the Salmonella/mammalian microsome mutagenicity test. Mutat Res 32:347.

ARMITAGE P, DOLL R. 1954. The age distribution of cancer and a multistage theory of carcinogenesis. Br J Cancer 8:1.

ARMITAGE P, DOLL R. 1957. A two-stage theory of carcinogenesis in relation to the age distribution of human cancer. Br J Cancer 11:161–169.

BENEDICT WF, MURPHREE AL, BANERJEE A, SPINA CA, SPARKES MC, SPARKES RS. 1983. Patient with 13 chromosome deletion: Evidence that the retinoblastoma gene is a recessive cancer gene. Science 219:973.

BERENBLUM I, SHUBIK P. 1947. A new, quantitative, approach to the study of the stages of chemical carcinogenesis in the mouse's skin. Br J Cancer 1:383.

BISHOP DT, GARDNER EJ. 1980. Analysis of the genetic predisposition to cancer in individual pedigrees. In Banbury Report 4: Cancer Incidence in Defined Populations." New York: Cold Spring Harbor Laboratory.

BOS JL. 1988. The ras gene family and human carcinogenesis. Mutat Res, 195:255.

BRESLOW NE, CLAYTON DG. 1993. Approximate inference in generalized linear mixed models. JASA 88:9–25.

BRESLOW NE, DAY NE. 1987. Statistical Methods in Cancer Research. Vol. II: The Design and Analysis of Cohort Studies. IARC Scientific Publications No. 82. Lyon, France: International Agency for Research on Cancer.

BROWN CC, CHU KC. 1983. Implications of the multistage theory of carcinogenesis applied to occupational arsenic exposure. J Natl Cancer Inst 70:455.

CAVANEE WK, DRYJA TP, PHILLIPS RA, BENEDICT WF, GODBOUT R, GALLIE BL, MURPHREE AL, STRONG LC, WHITE RL. 1983. Expression of recessive alleles by chromosomal mechanisms in retinoblastoma. Nature 305:779.

CLAYTON D, SCHIFFLERS E. 1987a. Models for temporal variation in cancer rates. I. Age-period and age-cohort models. Stat Med 6:449–467.

CLAYTON D, SCHIFFLERS E. 1987b. Models for temporal variation in cancer rates. II. Age-period-cohort models. Stat Med 6:469–481.

COOK PJ, DOLL R, FELLINGHAM SA. 1969. A mathematical model for the age distribution of cancer in man. Int J Cancer 4:93.

COX DR. 1970. The Analysis of Binary Data. London: Methuen.

COX DR. 1972. Regression models and life tables. J R Stat Soc B 34:187–220.

DAY NE, BROWN CC. 1980. Multistage models and the primary prevention of cancer. J Natl Cancer Inst 64:977.

DOLL R, PAYNE P, WATERHOUSE J. (EDS.). 1966. Cancer Incidence in Five Continents. A Technical Report. Geneva: International Union Against Cancer.

DOLL R, PETO R. 1978. Cigarette smoking and bronchial carcinoma: dose and time relationships among regular smokers and lifelong non-smokers. J Epidemiol Community Health 32:303.

FISHER JC, HOLLOMAN JH. 1951. A new hypothesis for the origin of cancer foci. Cancer 4:916–918.

GILKS WR, CLAYTON DG, SPIEGELHALTER DJ, BEST NG, MCNEIL AJ, SHARPLES LD, KIRBY AJ. 1993. Modelling complexity: applications of Gibbs sampling in medicine (with discussion). J R Stat Soc B 55:39–52.

GOLD LS, SAWYER CB, MAGAW R, BACKMAN GM, DE VECIANA M, LEVISON R, HOOPER NK, HAVENDER WR, BERNSTEIN L, PETO R, PIKE MC, AMES BN. 1984. A carcinogenic potency database of the standardized results of animal bioassays. Environ Health Perspect 58:9–319.

KALDOR J, PETO J, EASTON D, DOLL R, HERMON C, MORGAN L. 1986. Models for respiratory cancer in nickel refinery workers. J Natl Cancer Inst 77:841–848.

KALDOR J, DAY NE. 1987. Interpretation of epidemiological studies in the context of the multi-stage model of carcinogenesis. In Barrett JC (ed.): Mechanisms of Environmental Carcinogenesis, Vol. II, Multistep Models of Carcinogenesis. Boca Raton, FL: CRC Press. pp 21–58. N.D.

KALDOR JM, DAY NE, PETTERSSON F, CLARKE EA, PEDERSEN D, MEHNERT W, BELL J, HOST H, PRIOR P, KARJALAINEN S, NEAL F, KOCH M, BAND P, CHOI W, POMPE KIRN V, ARSLAN A, ZARÉN B, BELCH AR, STORM H, KITTELMANN B, FRASER P, STOVALL M. 1990. Leukemia following chemotherapy for ovarian cancer. N Engl J Med 322:1–6.

KNUDSON AG. 1971. Mutation and cancer: Statistical study of retinoblastoma. Proc Natl Acad Sci USA, 68:820–823.

KNUDSON AG. 1985. Hereditary cancer, oncogenes, and antioncogenes. Cancer Res 45:1437–1443.

KNUDSON AG, HETHCOTE HW, BROWN BW. 1975. Mutation and childhood cancer: A probabilistic model for the incidence of retinoblastoma. Proc Natl Acad Sci USA 72:5116–5120.

KOUFOS A, HANSEN MF, LAMPKIN BC, WORKMAN ML, COPELAND

NG, JENKINS NA, CAVENEE WK. 1984. Loss of alleles at loci on human chromosome 11 during genesis of Wilms' tumour. Nature 309:170.

MANTEL N. 1967. The detection of disease clustering and a generalized regression approach. Cancer Res 27:209–220.

MANTEL N, HAENSZEL W. 1959. Statistical aspects of the analysis of data from retrospective studies of disease. J Natl Cancer Inst 22:719–748.

MATSUNAGA E. 1979. Hereditary retinoblastoma: Host resistance and age at onset. J Natl Cancer Inst 63:933–939.

MOOLGAVKAR SH. 1978. The multistage theory of carcinogenesis and the age distribution of cancer in man. J Natl Cancer Inst 61:49–52.

MOOLGAVKAR SH. 1983. Model for human carcinogenesis: Action of environmental agents. Environ Health Perspect 50:285.

MOOLGAVKAR SH. 1986. Carcinogenesis modeling: From molecular biology to epidemiology. Ano Rev Public Health 7:151–169.

MOOLGAVKAR SH, VENZON DJ. 1979. Two-event models for carcinogenesis: Incidence curves for childhood and adult tumors. Math Biosci 47:55.

MOOLGAVKAR SH, DAY NE, STEVENS RG. 1980. Two-stage models for carcinogenesis: Epidemiology of breast cancer in females. J Natl Cancer Inst 65:559.

MOOLGAVKAR SH, KNUDSON AG. 1981. Mutation and cancer: A model for human carcinogenesis. J Natl Cancer Inst 66:1037.

MOOLGAVKAR SH, DEWANJI A, LÜBECK G. 1989. Cigarette smoking and lung cancer: Reanalysis of the British doctors' data. J Natl Cancer Inst 81:415–420.

MOTTRAM JC. 1944. A developing factor in experimental blastogenesis. J Pathol Bacteriol 56:181.

MUIR C, WATERHOUSE J, MACK T, POWELL J, WHELAN S. 1987. Cancer Incidence in Five Continents, Vol. V. Lyon, France: International Agency for Research on Cancer.

NORDLING CO. 1953. A new theory on the cancer inducing mechanism. Br J Cancer 7:68.

PERERA FP, WEINSTEIN IB. 1982. A pilot project in molecular cancer epidemiology: Determination of benzo(a)pyrene-DNA adducts in animal and human tissues by immunoassays. Carcinogenesis 3:1405–1410.

PETO R. 1977. Epidemiology, multistage models and short-term mutagenicity tests. In Hiatt HH, Watson JD, Winsten JA (eds): Origins of Human Cancer, New York: Cold Spring Harbor Laboratory, p. 1403.

PETO R, PIKE MC, ARMITAGE P, BRESLOW NE, COX DR, HOWARD SV, MANTEL N, MCPHERSON K, PETO J, SMITH PG. 1976. Design and analysis of randomized clinical trials requiring prolonged observation of each patient. I. Introduction and design. Br J Cancer 34:585–613.

PETO J, SEIDMAN H, SELLIKOFF IJ. 1982. Mesothelioma mortality in asbestos workers: Implications for models of carcinogenesis and risk assessment. Br J Cancer 45:124.

PIKE MC. 1966. A method of analysis of a certain class of experiments in carcinogenesis. Biometrics 22:142.

PIKE MC. 1983. "Hormonal" risk factors, "breast tissue age" and the age-incidence of breast cancer. Nature 303:767.

PRENTICE RL, PYKE R. 1979. Logistic disease incidence models and case-control studies. Biometrika 66:403–411.

SCHROEDER WT, CHAO LY, DAO DD, et al. 1987. Nonrandom loss of maternal chromosome 11 alleles in Wilms' tumor. Am J Hum Genet 40:413–420.

SIEMIATYCKI J, THOMAS D. 1981. Biological models and statistical interactions: An example from multistage carcinogenesis. Int J Epidemiol 10:383–387.

SMITH PG. 1982. Spatial and temporal clustering. In Schottenfeld D, and Fraumeni JF eds: Cancer Epidemiology and Prevention. W.B. Saunders, pp. 391–407.

THOMAS DC. 1983. Statistical methods for analyzing effects of temporal patterns of exposure on cancer risks. Scand J Work Environ Health 9:353.

TROSKO JE, CHANG CC. 1983. Potential role of intercellular communication in the rate-limiting step in carcinogenesis. In JA Cimo ed: Cancer and the Environment: Possible Mechanisms of Thresholds for Carcinogens and Other Toxic Substances. New York: Mary Ann Liebert, Inc., pp. 5–21.

VOGELSTEIN B, FEARON ER, HAMILTON SR, et al. 1988. Genetic alterations during colorectal-tumor development. N Engl J Med, 319:525–532.

WALTER SD, DAY NE. 1983. Estimation of the duration of a preclinical disease state using screening data. Am J Epidemiol 118:865–886.

WHITTEMORE AS. 1977. The age distribution of human cancer for carcinogenic exposures of varying intensity. Am J Epidemiol 106:418.

WILLIAMS WE, ANDERSON WE. 1984. Genetic epidemiology of breast cancer: Segregation analysis of 200 Danish pedigrees. Genet Epidemiol 1:7–20.

WILLIAMS JC, BROWN KW, MOTT MG, et al. 1989. Maternal allele loss in Wilms' tumor. Lancet i:283–284.

ZUR HAUSEN H. 1976. Condylomata acuminata and human genital cancer. Cancer Res 36:794.

PART II | The Magnitude of Cancer

10 International patterns of cancer

C. S. MUIR
J. NECTOUX

The existence of differing patterns of cancer occurrence throughout the world has been known for many years, as perusal of the first chapter of Clemmesen's book *Statistical Studies in Malignant Neoplasms* (1965) and of the fascinating, if little known monograph, *The Mortality from Cancer throughout the World*, published in 1915 by Hoffman, the actuary to the Prudential Insurance Company, reveals. Yet it was not until 1984 that an estimate was made of the world cancer burden and of the relative importance of the more common cancers (Parkin et al, 1984). This estimate, for the year 1975, not only assessed the burden and relative importance of the various sites of cancer for the world as a whole but also did so for each of the 24 demographic regions recognized by the United Nations. This exercise has been repeated twice and comparable estimates have been produced for 1980 and 1985 (Parkin et al, 1988a, 1993): the top ten cancers around 1985 are given in Figure 10–1.

The global total number of new cancers in 1985 was estimated at 7.62 million, almost exactly divided between the sexes and between developed (48%) and developing countries (52%), although two-thirds of the world's population are represented in the latter (Fig. 10–2). These estimates are regrettably not uniformly based on incidence data collected by cancer registries but depend on a variety of sources of information, including cancer incidence from cancer registries, extrapolation of incidence from mortality data, and initially, in large areas of the world, supplemental figures from relative frequency data largely obtained from the monograph *Cancer Occurrence in Developing Countries* (Parkin, 1986) (Fig. 10–2). The methods used, notably for the developing countries, have been refined over the years and are discussed in the original publications.

Despite the caveats given in these papers, the information presented is likely to reflect the relative burden and site-specific pattern in many parts of the world. For both sexes the regional patterns are very diverse. A few of the 24 demographic regions have been selected for graphic presentation for 1985 (Figs. 10–3 to 10–10) and comment. Globally, for both sexes the first five ranking sites account for close to 60% of the cancers and, females in China excepted, for over half of the cancers in any region.

The rankings of these estimates have changed over the past 10 years. For both sexes the relative importance of stomach cancer has tended to fall and that of lung cancer to rise nearly everywhere. Breast cancer did not fall within the first five ranking sites in China around 1975 but is now considered to be in third place.

In their latest paper, Parkin et al (1993) also provide estimates of age-standardized incidence rates, which provide a measure of the differences in risks between populations.

DATA SOURCES

The sixth volume of the *Cancer Incidence in Five Continents* monograph series (Parkin et al, 1992), which covers the period 1983–1987, contains good quality incidence data for 137 populations from over 100 cancer registries, and *this material forms the basis for the description of international cancer incidence patterns which follows*. On occasion, data from volume V of *Cancer Incidence in Five Continents* (Muir et al, 1987) are cited: such rates are denoted by [V]. There are many sources of bias in incidence data and differences must therefore be assessed with some caution; several indices of the reliability of these data are presented and discussed in Parkin et al (1992). Although the data appearing in this publication are presented in as standard a form as possible, there are differences in registry practices and the reader should always consult the source. Thus some registries include the so-called benign papilloma of bladder with the overtly malignant lesions; others, the benign and unspecified tumors of brain and nervous system with the malignant. Wherever possible, "deviations" from standard practice are signalled in Parkin et al (1992).

This rather selective presentation of data means that large portions of the globe are not covered. For several cancers such as lung and stomach, the more widely

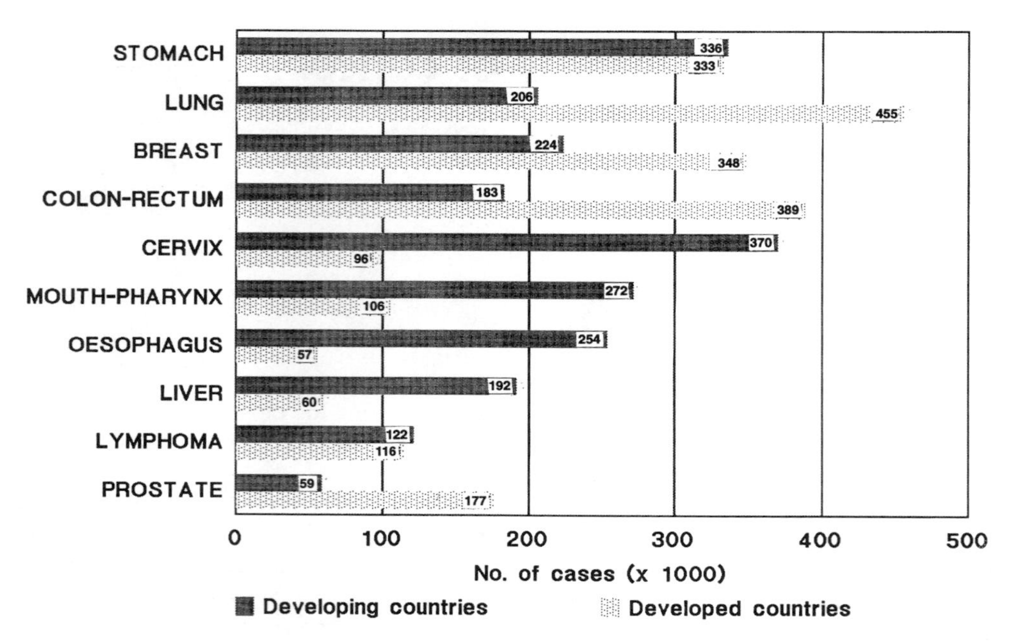

FIG. 10–1. Ten most common cancers (numbers in thousands) in developed and developing countries around 1985.

available cancer mortality figures can be used as a surrogate measure of incidence due to the relatively poor survival, but for others the death rate can be influenced by differences in availability and effectiveness of therapy. There are many problems of accuracy of death certification and although international comparability has improved, national differences in the coding of death certificates still pose problems (Percy and Muir, 1989).

For cancer mortality statistics, the most useful recent compilations are those by Kurihara et al (1984), the World Health Organization ([WHO], 1988), and Aoki et al (1992). WHO has ceased to routinely publish detailed compendia of cancer mortality statistics but is normally willing to make a magnetic tape of the more complete data available. The successive volumes of the *World Health Statistics Annual* contain information for the somewhat restricted list of sites in the Basic Tabulation List (WHO, 1988). Many useful compilations of local, national (Napalkov et al, 1983; Sharp et al, 1993), regional (Estève et al, 1993), and international

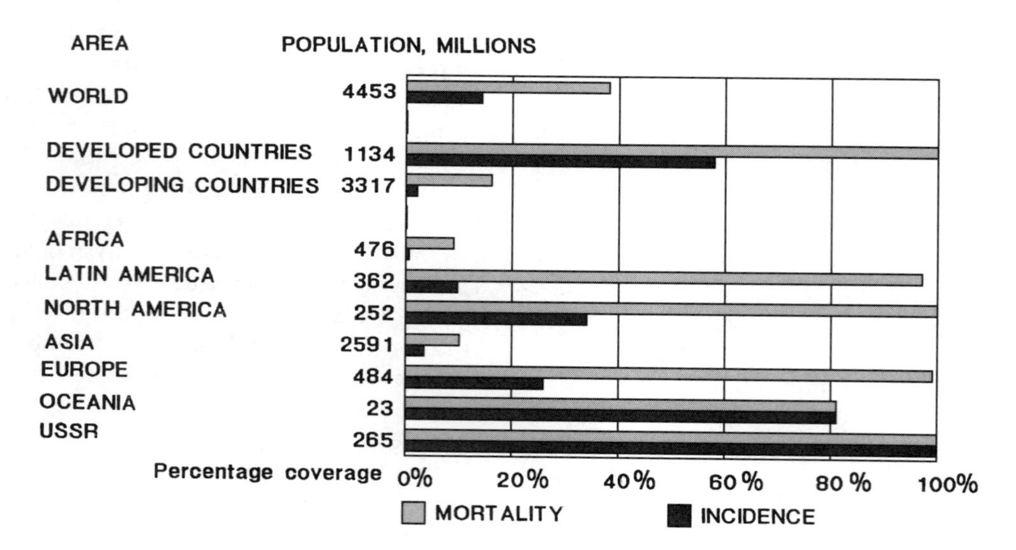

FIG. 10–2. Availability of cancer mortality and incidence data by United Nations geographic area, 1980.

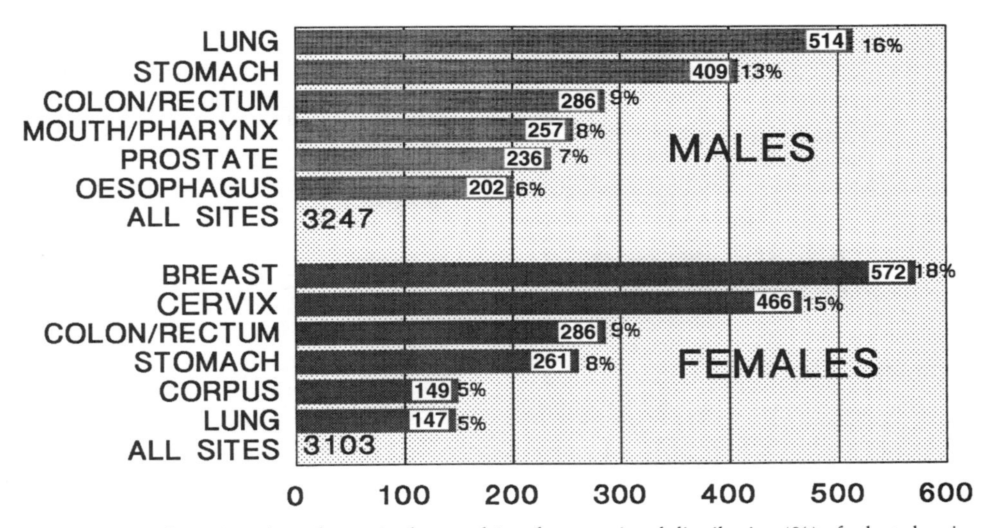

FIG. 10–3. Incidence (number of cases in thousands) and proportional distribution (%) of selected major cancer sites throughout the world, in males and females, 1985.

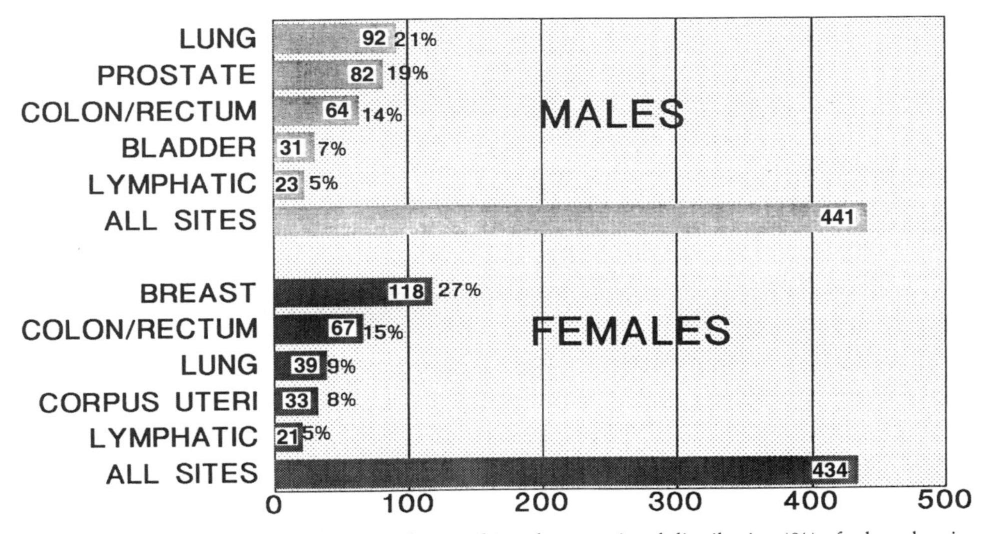

FIG. 10–4. Incidence (number of cases in thousands) and proportional distribution (%) of selected major cancer sites in North America, in males and females, 1985.

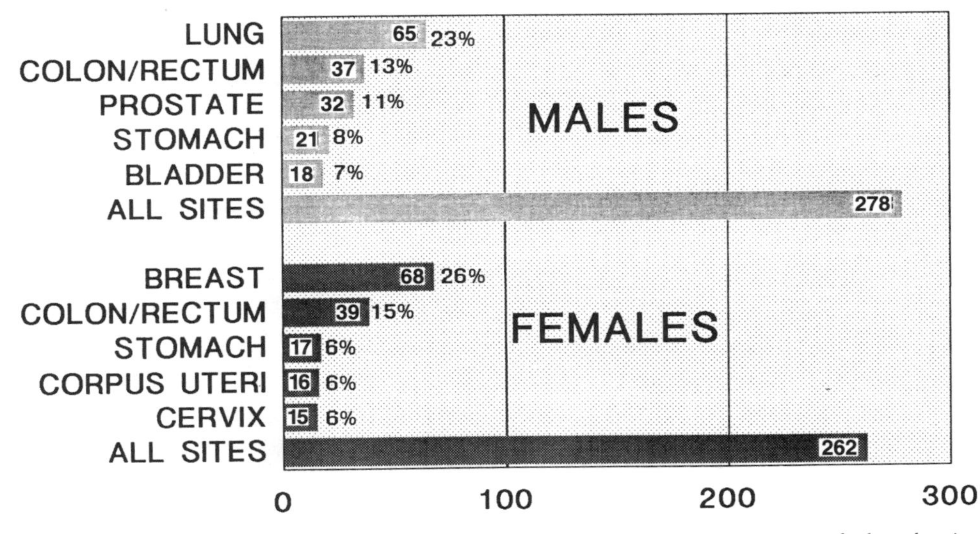

FIG. 10–5. Incidence (number of cases in thousands) and proportional distribution (%) of selected major cancer sites in Western Europe, in males and females, 1985.

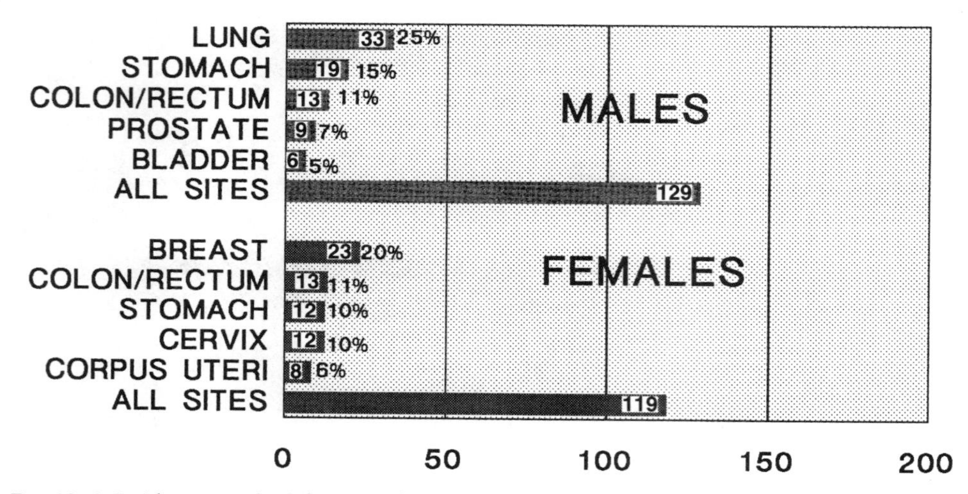

FIG. 10–6. Incidence (number of cases in thousands) and proportional distribution (%) of selected major cancer sites in Eastern Europe, in males and females, 1985.

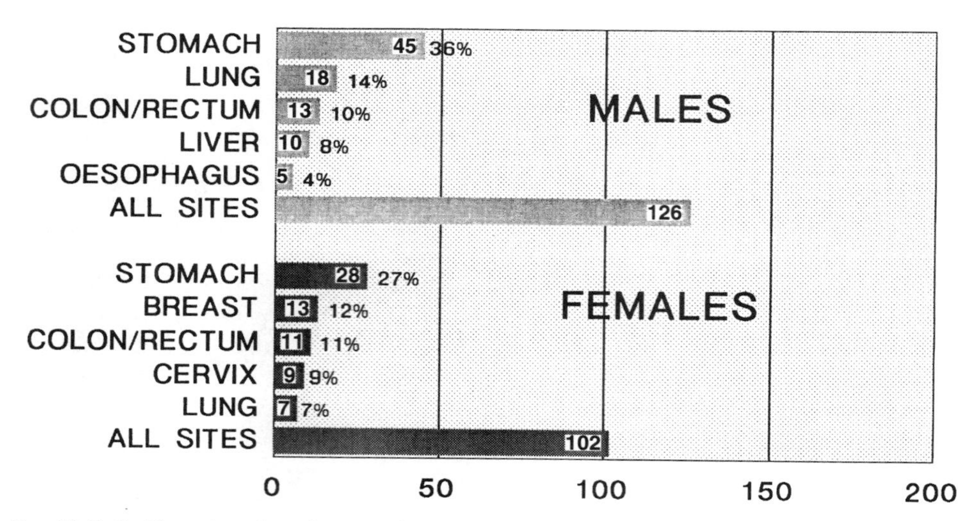

FIG. 10–7. Incidence (number of cases in thousands) and proportional distribution (%) of selected major cancer sites in Japan, in males and females, 1985.

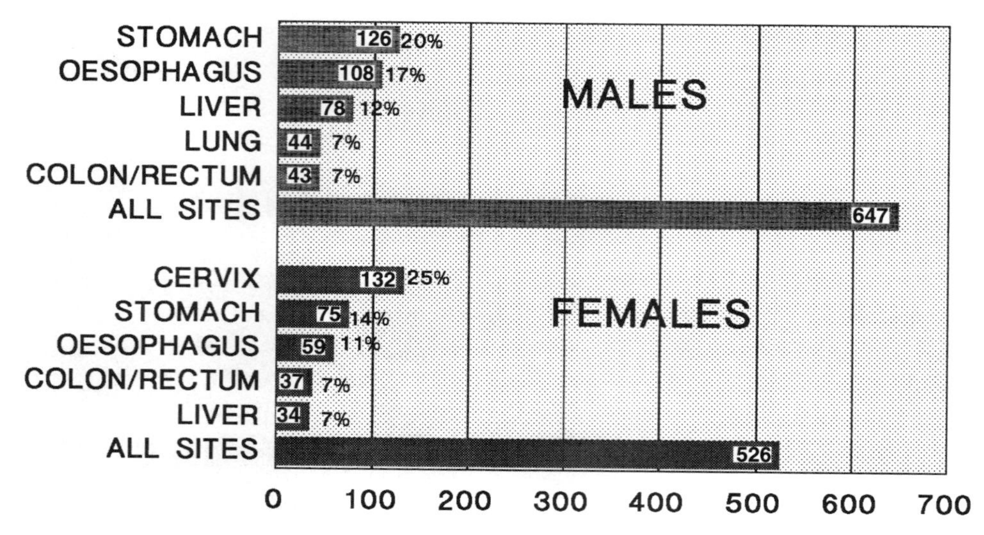

FIG. 10–8. Incidence (number of cases in thousands) and proportional distribution (%) of selected major cancer sites in China, in males and females, 1985.

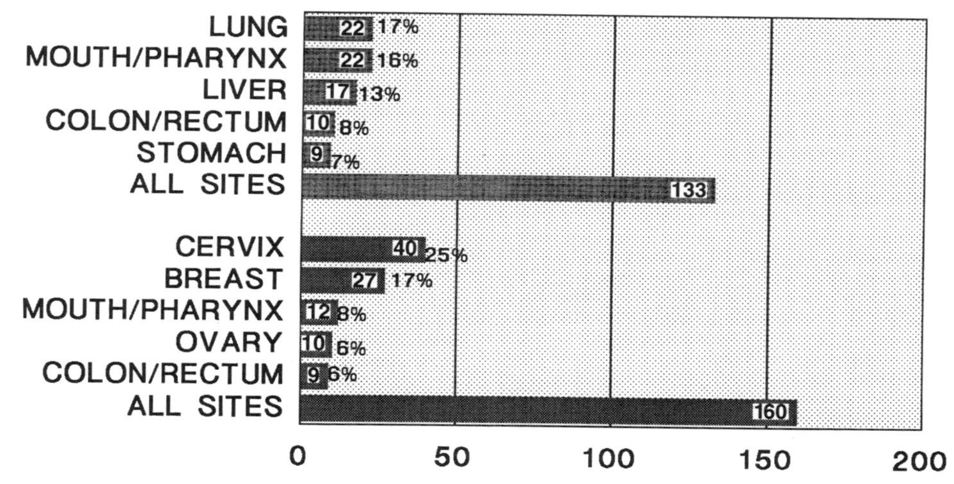

FIG. 10–9. Incidence (number of cases in thousands) and proportional distribution (%) of selected major cancer sites in Southeast Asia, in males and females, 1985.

cancer data (Boring et al, 1994) exist. While the annual *Cancer Statistics Review* provides a wealth of information about the areas within the U.S. covered by the Surveillance, Epidemiology and End Results (SEER) Program of the U.S. National Cancer Institute (NCI) (Sondik et al, 1986; NCI, 1988; Miller et al, 1993), data from other U.S. registries are given in the *Cancer Incidence in Five Continents* monographs. Further, the presentation of data in the *Cancer Statistics Review* does not lend itself to easy international comparison.

Attention is drawn to contrasts in risk between different ethnic groups living within the same country and to the rates for Chinese and Japanese dwelling in their country of origin and in the United States. Unfortunately, unlike the pioneering studies of Haenszel and Kurihara (1968) on mortality, the data in the *Cancer Incidence in Five Continents* monographs do not distinguish between Japanese born in Japan and now resident in the United States, and US-born Japanese. Such information is, however, available in great detail for the Chinese populations of Singapore (Lee et al, 1988) and for various groups migrating to Australia, notably from the United Kingdom, Italy, Greece, and Yugoslavia (for example, Bonett and Roder [1988]). Geddes et al (1993) provide data on migrants from Italy. The most comprehensive study of change in risk on migration is probably that from Israel (Steinitz et al, 1989), which covers the period 1961 to 1981 and which examines the problems inherent in the analysis and interpretation of such data.

For several sites comment is made on changes in incidence over time. If not specifically referenced, these values have been calculated at the International Agency for Research on Cancer (IARC), and if a time period is not specified, the reader should refer to the years cov-

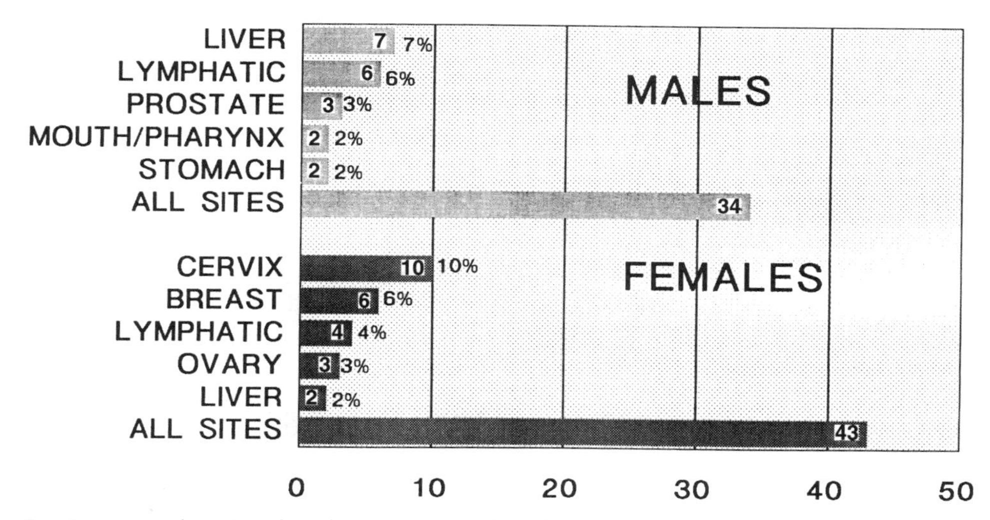

FIG. 10–10. Incidence (number of cases in thousands) and proportional distribution (%) of selected major cancer sites in West Africa, in males and females, 1985.

ered by volumes V and VI of *Cancer Incidence in Five Continents, 1978–1982* (Muir et al, 1987) and *1983–1987* (Parkin et al, 1992). Time trends in both incidence and mortality have recently been extensively reviewed (Coleman et al, 1993; Doll et al, 1994).

Time trends in the United States are largely derived from Miller et al (1993). It should be noted that incidence (1973–1990) is restricted to the 10% of the U.S. population covered by the SEER program, whereas mortality is for the entire U.S. for the same period (see also Devesa et al, 1987).

PRESENTATION OF INCIDENCE AND MORTALITY DATA

Incidence and mortality rates are usually published for each site of cancer as a series of age-specific rates. To facilitate comparisons, synoptic age-standardized rates per 100,000 population per year are normally provided. Although corrected for differences in population age structures, such indices can conceal quite substantial variations between age-groups; thus, primary liver cancer was 50 times more common overall in Mozambique than in the United States, but only twice as common in older age-groups. An unusual age distribution for an uncommon cancer can result in distorted age-standardized rates. Such an occurrence may be suspected when the crude and age-standardized rates diverge substantially.

In the text which follows, most of the incidence rates are age-standardized to the world population distribution as devised by Segi Institute of Cancer Epidemiology (1964), and simplified by Doll et al (1966, 1976), which represents the age distribution of 46 countries around 1950. Rates are average annual per 100,000 population per annum. Standardization to this population results in values which are lower than the crude incidence rate in developed countries and higher than the crude rate in developing countries. Thus the crude rates of lung cancer in males in Scotland and Bombay for the period 1983–1987 were 131.6 and 7.0, whereas the age-standardized rates were 88.1 and 14.0, respectively. The crude rate permits comparison of the burden per 100,000 population; the age-standardized rate reflects the risk.

Actual rates quoted are given to one decimal place. Ranges are given as integers. When a range of incidence is mentioned, on occasion a few values may lie outside that range. If *sex is not specified then rates are for males*. For many sites, male rates are frequently about twice those for females with the exception of colon where incidence rates tend to be about the same, and cancers of gall bladder and thyroid which predominate in females.

Another measure of the impact of cancer is the cumulative risk or the risk an individual would have of developing or dying from a given cancer (or other disease) during a certain age span if no other causes of death were operative. The cumulative rate, which is a good approximation of cumulative risk up to 75 years of age, is very easy to calculate, being the sum over each year of age of the age-specific incidence rates (Day, 1976). Many find this measure, usually given as a percentage, to be more readily understandable than age-standardized rates, as no arbitrary standard population is used. It can also be considered as a directly age-standardized rate with the same size of population in each age group.

Comparison of cumulative rates for the age spans 0–64 and 0–74 shows that many cancers exert much of their effect during the decade between 65 and 74 years of age. The cumulative rate for prostatic cancer in Sweden is 1.25% at 0–64 but 5.77% at 0–74. Comparable figures from the United States for blacks in Atlanta are 3.32% and 12.49%; in Miyagi, Japan, the figures are 0.13% and 0.82%. In many developed countries, where the average age of the population is high, about one-third of incident cancers are diagnosed in persons 75 years of age and over.

Some of the most intriguing international differences known are based on relative frequency data (Dunham and Bailar, 1968; Cook and Burkitt, 1971; Parkin et al, 1988a)—that is, the proportion of a given cancer in relation to all cancers in a clinical or pathology series. Such frequencies are subject to many biases and are rarely referable to a defined population. Historically, many elevated frequencies have been confirmed when cancer registration was introduced; for example, cancer of the nasopharynx in Chinese in Singapore was first suspected to be frequent around 1911 (Muir and Shanmugaratnam, 1967). The significance of a low frequency, particularly of cancer of internal organs, is much more difficult to assess, as it may be due to underdiagnosis.

For the many regions of the world, where neither incidence nor mortality data are available, the reader can nonetheless obtain a feel for cancer patterns and levels in such areas from Parkin et al (1984, 1988a, 1993). In this chapter, most of this information has not been taken into account.

In general, the etiological implications of the many differences in cancer patterns are not mentioned, these being considered in other chapters. Nonetheless, variations in the occurrences of cancer have given rise to causal hypotheses.

International Differences by Site

The content of each of the cancer sites discussed is as defined by the 9th revision of the *Manual of the Inter-*

national Statistical Classification of Diseases (WHO, 1977), hereafter referred to as ICD–9, which was issued in 1979. The anatomical site approach used by the ICD is much less pertinent for the tumors of childhood which tend to be tissue-rather than organ-specific. The monograph *International Incidence of Childhood Cancer*, edited by Parkin et al (1988b), uses a more appropriate histological classification and is cited when appropriate.

As noted previously, owing to the very large gaps in cancer registration coverage, it is quite possible that significant geographic and ethnic variations remain to be discovered. However, even the most superficial examination of the available figures shows that there are substantial geographic differences in the incidence of cancer at nearly all sites. For example, site-specific ratios for males range from 140 for nasopharynx to 130 for prostate, 80 for liver, and 15 for bladder and, for females, 95 for liver, 30 for breast, and 20 for cervix uteri.

It could be argued that the extremes are atypical, but as will be seen there is geographically a wide range of incidence rates for many cancers. When comparing such international data, there is always the possibility that low rates are due to underreporting. Yet it is unlikely that the low rate for cancer of the larynx in Norwegian women or that for cancer of the cervix uteri in that part of the Jewish population of Israel born in Europe or North America is artifactual.

It will be noted that, from time to time, high age-standardized rates may be observed for generally uncommon tumors in small populations. For example, in volume V of *Cancer Incidence in Five Continents* (Muir et al, 1987), eye cancer in male Pacific Polynesian islanders resident in New Zealand had an incidence of 4.4, which is substantially higher than that of the non-Maori (white) population of that country, or 1.2. However, the former rate is based on four cases, the latter on 92. Such rates may indeed reflect a true excess, may be the result of statistical instability, or represent a failure to match the numerator with the correct denominator. (It is possible that the numerator was inflated by persons coming to New Zealand specifically for treatment.) A degree of caution is thus called for when comparing rates, but nonetheless, there are wide differences based on adequate numbers in the occurrence of many cancers—differences which demand an explanation in causal terms.

Lip (ICD–9 140)

The highest rate of lip cancer in males recorded is from South Australia (13.5), and fairly high incidence levels are also seen in several parts of Canada—11.0 in Newfoundland and 10.6 in Saskatchewan. Other relatively high rates occur in Tasmania (8.4) and the Australian Capital Territory (8.0), and in parts of eastern and southern Europe such as Nowy Sacz, Poland (7.2), Belarus (6.7), rural Cluj, Romania (6.2), Granada (11.4), Zaragoza (10.1) and Murcia (10.0) in Spain, and Ragusa in Sicily (6.2).

Most populations have rates of less than 5, with the lowest, in the range nil to 0.9, occurring in Asia. Within Israel the incidence among males born in that country is 5.2 in contrast to 1.4 observed in those born in Africa or Asia. The black populations of the United States exhibit very low or nil rates.

Lip cancer is very unusual in women. In Khon Kaen, Thailand, rates for women (3.8) exceed those for males (0.1). (This is consonant with the higher relative frequency among females observed earlier in Chiang Mai [Menakanit et al, 1971]). The highest rate elsewhere is that observed in South Australia (2.5).

The risk of lip cancer seems to be falling virtually everywhere, Israel excepted, where an annual increase of 8% was observed among males and of 12% among females between 1975 and 1980.

Most lip cancers occur on the lower lip. It may not always be possible to distinguish between cancers arising on the lip proper and those originating in the skin of the lip: by definition, basal cell carcinomas arise from the skin of the lip.

Tongue (ICD–9 141)

The highest recorded rate of cancer of the tongue, based on small numbers, is among blacks in the Bahamas (16.3). Elevated rates for these cancers also occur in India and are associated with the chewing of the betel quid (Ahmedabad males, 14.0). High levels ranging from 7 to 10 are also recorded among males in parts of France, in the departments of the Doubs, Bas-Rhin and Calvados. Rates in the 3 to 5 range are found in Switzerland, parts of Spain, and in Slovenia. Incidence in the black populations of the United States, namely around 4, is usually double that in whites. Elsewhere, incidence is usually below 2. For females rates are much lower, except for in Ahmedabad, Bombay, Manila, and Rizal (Philippines) (2.2, 2.5, 2.3, and 1.7, respectively).

The incidence of lingual cancer is falling nearly everywhere. A modest rise among young U.S. males, perhaps linked to increasing use of snuff and chewing tobacco, has been noted (Davis and Severson, 1987).

Oral Cavity (ICD–9 143–145)

Cancer of the oral cavity shows fairly large geographical differences. The highest male rates occur in France (13.4 in Bas-Rhin and 10.5 in Calvados). Lower levels, in the 5 to 7 range, are recorded in other parts of that country, these being close to incidence in the French-speaking cantons of Switzerland. Within the United States rates among blacks are from 30 to 50% greater than among whites, the latter being around 4.

A sex differential for mouth cancer incidence is conspicuous in most Caucasian populations, as rates among females tend to be very low. In contrast, in India in Bangalore (9.6) and Madras (8.3), higher rates are commonly recorded among women who chew betel quid, which frequently contains tobacco. Corresponding rates for males in these cities are 4.4 and 6.9, respectively. Among Singapore Indians the rate for oral cancer in males is 5.7.

Although anatomically, surgically, and functionally distinct, the cancers of the sites that make up the oral cavity and pharynx share the same etiologic factors, namely, tobacco and alcohol. While they are frequently tabulated by ICD rubric, their importance as a group, which may approach that of lung cancer, may not be evident. Globally, cancers of the mouth and pharynx (ICD–9 140–149) ranked 5th among males and 7th among females around 1985 (Parkin et al, 1993), accounting for 270,000 and 143,000 new cases, respectively.

Nasopharynx (ICD–9 147)

Signal ethnic and geographic differences can be seen in the incidence of nasopharyngeal cancer (Shanmugaratnam, 1982). This disease is rare in most of the world, with rates usually below 1 per 100,000, whereas higher levels are observed in Southeast Asia and southeast China. The rates for females are usually half those for males.

The highest incidence rates are found in Hong Kong—28.5 for males and 11.2 for females. For the Singapore Chinese population rates are 18.1 and 7.4, respectively: those for U.S. Chinese are in the 7 to 9 range in males, or levels comparable to those in the Philippines. Algerians resident in Sétif, Singapore Malays, and residents of north Thailand and of the Northwest Territories and Yukon of Canada exhibit rates in the 4 to 6 range. Lanier et al (1976) reported incidence levels of up to 25 in Inuit populations of northern Canada, Greenland, and Alaska. Rates in the 5 to 10 range have been recorded in Algeria, Morocco, and Tunisia (Sasco et al, 1985).

While the Chinese have the highest rates of this cancer there are significant and persistent risk variations between Chinese communities. The Cantonese in Singapore (M, 29.9; F, 11.4) constantly have a higher risk than in Hokkien (M, 16.6; F, 6.3) and Teochew (M, 17.4; F, 6.4). There has been no significant change in incidence among Singapore Chinese over the period 1968–1982 (Lee et al, 1988), in contrast to cancers at other sites. Downward changes in risk over the past decade for U.S. Chinese are difficult to interpret, as data are not published by dialect group.

Esophagus (ICD–9 150)

In global terms, esophageal cancer was ranked 7th among males and 10th among females around 1985 (Parkin et al, 1993), accounting for 196,000 and 108,000 new cases, respectively. Esophageal cancer is characterised by an extreme diversity of incidence throughout the world with rates as high as 195.3 for females and 165.3 for males in northern Gonbad in the Caspian region of Iran (Day and Muñoz, 1982) and mortality rates of 211.2 among males and 136.5 among females of Linxian county in China (Lu et al, 1985). These rates are in sharp contrast to those from Cluj county in Romania—1.9 for males and 0.4 for females. A conspicuously higher rate among males is generally observed, although rates for females may on rare occasions exceed those for males, as in parts of the Iranian Caspian littoral. In southern Ireland the incidence in females (4.2) approximates that in males (4.5).

The areas of highest risk include the so-called Asian esophageal cancer belt stretching from the Caspian littoral in northern Iran, through the southern Republics of the U.S.S.R. to eastern China (Kmet and Mahboubi, 1972). Moderately high rates are observed in southeast Africa, parts of South America, and the Caribbean (Porto Alegre, Brazil, 25.9; Bermuda blacks, 24.9; Martinique, 13.7; Asuncion, Paraguay, 11.2) and in certain areas of western Europe such as parts of France, with a rate of 26.5 among males in the department of Calvados. Rates of around 10 are observed in the Basque country, or double those elsewhere in Spain.

In India rates are in the 8 to 11 range, in Japan, from 6 to 14. Rates in St. Petersburg and Kyrgyzstan, around 11, are double those in Belarus, Estonia, and Latvia.

Striking differences have further been demonstrated, more than for any other site, over small geographic areas in northern Iran (Mahboubi et al, 1973), in the Transkei (Rose, 1973), and in Brittany, France (Tuyns and Massé, 1975).

Major variation is also seen between ethnic groups residing in the same area: the incidence rates for U.S. blacks (19.5 in Connecticut) is consistently fourfold higher than those for whites (5.3 in Connecticut), and rates for the Chinese (10.9) in Singapore are treble those for Indians and 10 times greater than those for Malays living in that republic.

Even within different dialect groups of the Chinese in Singapore, marked variations have been reported (Lee et al, 1988); the highest levels of esophageal cancer, in contrast to nasopharynx cancer, occur in Teochew males (27.0). The same pattern is seen among females, albeit at lower levels of incidence. A slow but significant decrease in incidence has been observed in that country. In Israel the relative risk of esophageal cancer fell for Jewish migrants from Asia as compared to that for the Israel-born, with increasing length of stay in Israel (Steinitz et al, 1989).

Within China (Qidong, Shanghai, and Tianjin) rates range from 13 to 17, those for Hong Kong being slightly higher.

A decline in mortality rates has recently been noted in the youngest age-groups in Linxian county, the highest incidence area of the People's Republic of China, presumably due to an improvement of nutritional standards (Lu et al, 1985). On the contrary, rates have doubled among U.S. blacks over the past 30 years (Blot and Fraumeni, 1987). A considerable increase has also been observed in the Transkei in the 1960s and 1980s, this cancer having been practically unknown before 1930 (Rose, 1973; Jaskiewicz et al, 1987). The frequency of adenocarcinoma of the lower third of the esophagus is increasing more rapidly among whites and males than among blacks and females in the U.S.; and it is also increasing in England.

Stomach (ICD–9 151)

Stomach cancer, a disease frequently more common in lower socioeconomic groups, remains numerically the most frequent malignancy in the world (Parkin et al, 1993), accounting for around 10.2% of all cancers with an estimated 775,000 new cases per year for both sexes combined (males, 473,000; females, 282,000).

Although rates for males are approximately twice those for females in high- and low-risk countries, the sex ratio is not constant by age-group: it is around unity below age 30 and rises to about 2.2 towards age 60.

The highest recorded incidence is among males in Japan, with rates of around 85 (93.3 in Yamagata prefecture and 73.6 in Osaka). Comparable levels have been reported from parts of the former Soviet Union (Napalkov et al, 1983); recent figures from St. Petersburg, Belarus, Kyrgyzstan, Estonia, and Latvia show corresponding incidence as 52.8, 46.7, 44.6, 37.0, and 34.1, respectively.

Elsewhere in eastern Europe rates are in the 20 to 30 range. There are considerable contrasts within Italy, ranging from 40.2 in Florence to 16.1 in Ragusa, Sicily—a difference confirmed in studies of southern Italian migrants who moved to the north of the country (Vigotti et al, 1988). In Villa Nueva de Gaia, Portugal, risk is high (47.8) in contrast to Spain, where rates are in the 15 to 27 range.

Fairly high rates have also been reported from parts of China (Shanghai, 51.7) and Latin America (Costa Rica, 46.9; Cali, Colombia, 36.3, Porto Alegre, 33.8). In contrast, in Cuba incidence is close to levels for U.S. whites (SEER 8.0).

In western Europe, age-standardized incidence rates are generally in the range of 15 to 25. In Africa, areas of high frequency have been reported in certain mountainous regions in Rwanda, southwest Uganda, and Tanzania around Mt. Kilimanjaro. Low levels are recorded in Gambia (3.9) and in parts of India (Ahmedabad 2.1).

As for several other sites, there are substantial differences in incidence rates between various ethnic groups living in the same country. Rates among Maoris (25.3) are double those of non-Maoris living in New Zealand; blacks covered by the U.S. SEER registries have rates 50% higher than those found among whites (8.0 and 12.4); and in Singapore Chinese incidence rates (34.7) are more than double those for Indians (15.9), which are identical to those in Madras, and over five times greater than those for Singapore Malays (6.4).

There are marked variations by socioeconomic status. Rates of stomach cancer in whites (5.9) are approximately half those for blacks (12.2) in Atlanta, and a twofold difference in cumulative mortality rates between the highest and lowest socioeconomic groups is seen in England and Wales (Logan, 1982). In Scotland, Carstairs and Morris (1991) demonstrated a 75% excess risk for the most deprived compared to the most affluent.

The risk of stomach cancer changes slowly in populations moving from high-risk to low-risk communities. Incidence rates among U.S. Japanese, although about one-third those in Japan, are nonetheless about three times greater than those among U.S. whites. In Israel the risk for Jews born in Israel (9.1) is much less than that seen in Jews born in Europe or North America (16.2). The rate for non-Jews in Israel (6.9) is close to that of Kuwaitis (4.1).

Declining risk with increasing duration of residence has been observed for some of the European populations migrating to Australia (McMichael et al, 1980).

The most remarkable feature in the epidemiology of stomach cancer is the universal declining trend in both sexes, which is somewhat more marked among females than males. Paradoxically, the decline in mortality in the high incidence area of Japan has been greater than elsewhere (Tominaga, 1987). Decreasing trends in Norway and Japan appear to be due to the disappearance of the "intestinal" type of this cancer—the variant being more subject to international variation, the "diffuse" type being more constant.

Small Intestine (ICD–9 152)

Small intestine cancer is very rare, with rates for both sexes well below unity nearly everywhere. A proportion of these cancers are malignant carcinoids. In the Middle East, attention has been drawn to a relatively high frequency of small intestinal lymphoma associated with immune deficiency, but these neoplasms would be coded to lymphomas rather than the small intestine.

Within the SEER registries, rates for whites are close to unity while they are some 50% or more for blacks. The significance of a rate of 2.3 in Basel, Switzerland and of 4.2 among Maoris is unclear.

Large Bowel (ICD–9 153–154)

For both sexes, colorectal cancer is the third ranking cancer in the world, comprising 9% of all new cancers (males, 331,000; females, 346,000). The disease is most frequent in occidental countries and particularly so in North America, Australia, New Zealand, and parts of Europe. Although some writers prefer to consider the colon and rectum together, as the boundaries between these physiologically and surgically distinct organs are not well defined, and the terms *sigmoid* (part of the colon) and *rectosigmoid* (assigned by the ICD to the rectum) tend to be used interchangeably, they are nonetheless considered separately below.

Colon (ICD–9 153)

Colon cancer is a disease of economically developed countries which frequently affects both sexes almost equally. Before 60 years of age, this disease is slightly more common among females and is more frequent among males thereafter.

High incidence rates are found in the white population of Connecticut, with age-standardized rates of 35.9 in males, and 25.4 in females. (The highest female rate 30.9 is observed in the non-Maori population of New Zealand.) In the remainder of North America rates tend to be in the 25 to 30 range. The rates of colon cancer incidence for blacks residing in the U.S. are now close to those for U.S. whites, as rates for U.S. blacks have increased more rapidly than for whites. Indeed, in Detroit, they are slightly higher for both sexes. Somewhat lower rates, in the range of 15 to 20, are observed in much of western Europe. Within Italy, the rates in Ragusa, Sicily (12.0) are about half those elsewhere. Levels in eastern Europe cluster around 10, while those in Estonia (12.1) and Finland (11.9), where populations have many similarities, are very close and have lower incidence rates than in St. Petersburg (18.4). In the developing countries of Africa, Asia, and Latin America, rates are also low, many being between 5 and 15. In Poland there are considerable differences in reported rates between urban (12.0 in Warsaw) and rural areas (4.0 in Nowy Sacz), a differential also found in Romania. Rates in India are uniformly low, around 2 to 3. The highest rate observed in China, that for Shanghai (9.2), is substantially lower than that in Hong Kong (21.7), and among Singapore Chinese (20.2) and Hawaiian Chinese (23.6).

Ethnic and racial differences in colon cancer incidence as well as studies on migrants suggest that environmental factors play a major role in the etiology of the disease. In Israel, male Jews born in Europe or North America (22.5) are at higher risk for colon cancer than those born in Africa or Asia (13.2), and a change in risk for the offspring of Japanese who migrated to the United States, as heralded by Haenszel and Kurihara (1968), has now taken place: rates for U.S.-born males are in the 25 to 35 range, compared to a rate of around 17 in Japan. Indeed, rates among Hawaiian Japanese (37.2) are higher than for any U.S. population.

In general, incidence rates of colon cancer are rising slowly, particularly in areas formerly at low risk; left-sided neoplasms usually show larger increases (Haenszel and Correa, 1971). More complex patterns are being seen in high-risk countries. In the United States, incidence among white males and females fell significantly between 1986 and 1990. While mortality rates for large bowel cancer are increasing among black men but not for black women, among whites mortality is falling in both sexes (Miller et al, 1993). Increasing rates have been observed in the Nordic countries. In England and Wales, mortality rates are declining for all age-groups of both sexes.

Rectum (ICD–9 154)

Although less frequent than colon cancer, rectal cancer shows many of the features of colon cancer in geographic distribution. In contrast to colon cancer, rectal cancer is usually more common among males, with a sex ratio of 1.5 to 2.0.

Little difference exists between the incidence rates of North America, western Europe, and Australia, with rates in the range of 15 to 20 for males and 8 to 12 for females.

Rates in eastern Europe are around 10. In Italy, incidence in Latina and Ragusa, around 9, is less than elsewhere, notably, in Trieste (20.1). A similar phenomenon is noted in Spain where incidence tends to be lower in the southern registries of Granada (6.3) and Murcia (9.5) than in those located towards the north of the country, e.g., Catalonia (11.5).

Rates in Africa, India, Latin America, and the Middle East are usually below 5. The Jewish populations of Israel have incidence rates that approximate those of the continents of origin.

Unlike colon cancer, mortality from rectal cancer did not increase much in Japanese migrants to the U.S. (Haenszel and Kurihara, 1968). However, current rectal cancer rates for U.S. Japanese (around 20) are substantially higher than in any other U.S. population. Polish migrants have shown an increased risk for both sites (Staszewski, 1972). Mortality rates for rectal cancer tend to be underestimates as a varying proportion of such deaths, about half in the U.S., are certified as cancer of the large bowel and by coding rules assigned to the colon (Chow and Devesa, 1992). Elsewhere, large bowel cancer mortality time trends are not uniform, with rising rates in Japan and Hong Kong and among Singapore Chinese, while rates in France, and England and Wales are declining.

Liver (ICD–9 155)

Liver cancer is the eighth most frequent site on a worldwide basis, accounting for 5.6% (214,000) of new cancers in males and 2.7% (101,000) in females. Around 77% of these cancers occur in developing countries; indeed, over 40% of the total is in China. In adults a large majority of liver cancers are hepatocellular carcinomas. Cholangiocarcinomas are rare except in parts of Southeast Asia and around the shore of Lake Baikal in Siberia, where the cancers are associated with liver flukes (e.g., *Clonorchis sinensis, Opisthorchis viverrini*) (Srivatanakul et al, 1988). Most liver cancers in childhood are hepatoblastomas, which are rare tumors showing little worldwide variation (Parkin et al, 1988b).

Liver cancer is more common in males than in females. The sex ratio of incidence is around 3 to 1 in the high-risk areas and 1.5 to 1 elsewhere.

This disease is most common in males of eastern and Southeast Asia and sub-Saharan Africa, while in North America only Inuit (Eskimos) and populations of Asian origin exhibit high rates. In West Africa levels of 47.9 (M) and 21.4 (F) have been reported from Bamako in Mali. Corresponding figures from Gambia are 36.0 and 12.1. As high as these rates are, they do not reach the level recorded in Lourenco Marques (Maputo) around 1960 (M, 103.8).

In China the disease has a predominantly coastal distribution with incidence rates of 89.9 (M) and 24.5 (F) recorded in Qidong. In Shanghai and Hong Kong and among Singapore Chinese, incidence is of the same order: 30.6 (M) and 10.7 (F), 39.2 (M) and 10.7 (F), and 26.8 (M) and 7.0 (F), respectively. Within Singapore, unlike other cancer sites such as nasopharynx, lung, and esophagus, the incidence in Hokkien, Teochew, Canton, Hainan, and Hakka is very similar. The incidence in Singapore-born Chinese (M, 34.5; F, 11.9) is very close to that of the foreign-born (M, 34.7; F, 7.6). In contrast, migrant Chinese in Los Angeles, California, have much lower rates, for example, 14.6 (M) and 4.6 (F), but these are substantially greater than among white populations residing in the same city (M, 2.3; F, 0.9). Koreans in Los Angeles have even higher levels of incidence (M, 20.1; F, 3.1). Incidence among Japanese residents in the United States, in the range of 4 to 6, is much lower than in Osaka (M, 41.5; F, 9.7). Rates in Miyagi and Yamagata prefectures to the east of the country are about one-third those in Osaka. Intermediate levels (M, 23.7; F, 8.0) are noted in Manila in the Philippines; those in the Malay population of Singapore are at a lower level (M, 13.2; F, 6.3). In contrast to Indians in Singapore (M, 9.4; F, 4.6), rates within India are uniformly much lower—around 3 for males and 1 for females.

The incidence of liver cancer recorded in Khon Kaen Thailand is extraordinarily high (M, 90.0; F, 38.3). A large proportion of these cancers is associated with opisthorchiasis. Rates in Chiang Mai are much lower (M, 19.8; F, 10.4).

Rates of liver cancer are low in Australia and New Zealand for whites, whereas rates for New Zealand Maoris are some five times greater (M, 11.0; F, 3.0). Rates in South America and Europe are also generally low, in the range of 1 to 3, but there is a tendency for rates in southern Europe to be higher, possibly in relation to cirrhosis following alcohol consumption. The highest rates in southern Europe are seen in Trieste (14.5), Torino (10.4), Varese (10.3), and Geneva (9.8), which are perhaps a reflection of the high autopsy rates in Geneva and Trieste (Tuyns and Obradovic, 1975; Silvestri et al, 1991).

Patterns of hepatocellular cancer are generally related to the prevalence of chronic carriers of hepatitis B surface antigen (HBsAg) in the population (Szmuness, 1978).

Mortality data are usually unreliable as they are distorted not only by unrecognized secondary neoplasms but also by change in rubric content between ICD revisions (Percy and Ries, personal communication, 1989).

Gallbladder and Extrahepatic Bile Ducts (ICD–9 156)

Over two-thirds of these rare cancers arise in the gallbladder. This disease is generally twice as frequent in females as in males. The highest rates (17.6) have been observed among the Alaskan native female population (Boss et al, 1982), in Bolivia (14.6) (Rios-Dalenz et al, 1981, in Trujillo, Peru (12.9), Cali, Colombia (9.8), and Quito, Ecuador (8.7). In the American Indian population of New Mexico rates were 13.2 for females and 10.8 for males. Elsewhere the incidence rates are in the range of 2 to 6 for females and 1 to 3 for males, Japan excepted, where rates for both sexes are in the 5 to 8 range. This disease seems to occur rarely in the absence of biliary calculi.

Mortality rates in the former Federal Republic of Germany reveal an unusual regional pattern among both sexes, with elevated rates (around 6 in females), which are much higher than elsewhere in western Europe, throughout the center of the country (Becker et al, 1984; Smans et al, 1992).

Pancreas (ICD–9 156)

Pancreatic cancer is infrequent on a worldwide basis, accounting for some 3% of all cancers in developed countries. Given the very poor survival, this site is now a major contributor to cancer mortality as it is the fourth most common cause of cancer mortality in each sex in the United States (Sondik et al, 1986). This disease is slightly more frequent in males, the sex ratio tending to increase in high-risk populations.

The highest male incidence rates, in the range of 10 and 16, are observed in the U.S. black population and in New Zealand Maoris. Pancreatic cancer is somewhat more common among U.S. black males (11.1) than among U.S. whites (8.2). While rates over 10 are seen in Bohemia, Moravia, Finland, Estonia, Latvia, and St. Petersburg, most male Caucasian populations experience incidence rates in the 5 to 9 range, or that also experienced in Japan. In Israel the disease is twice as frequent among Jews (8.4) as among non-Jews (4.0).

Increases in mortality and incidence are seen practically everywhere for both sexes which could be partly due, at least in some areas, to improvements in diagnosis. The rise has been particularly rapid among black males as compared to white males in whom incidence now seems to be falling (Miller et al, 1993). A parallel between age-specific time trends in mortality from pancreas and lung cancers has been pointed out (Moolgavkar and Stevens, 1981) in England and Wales, whereas such similarities are less obvious in the U.S. and in Scandinavia.

Nose, Nasal Cavities, Middle Ear, and Accessory Sinuses (ICD–9 160)

These cancers, mostly arising from the nasal cavities and paranasal sinuses, are rare in all countries in both sexes, with rates for males of less than unity. Rates for females are even lower, with a sex ratio of around 2.

The highest male incidence rates are observed in the department of the Somme in France (1.7), in the Miyagi prefecture, Japan (1.6), and in Martinique (1.4). Male rates in Japan are all greater than unity. Relatively high rates of the same order and high frequencies have been reported from several parts of Africa.

Maxillary sinus cancers appear to occur more frequently among males than among females, whereas the reverse is true for cancers of the nasal cavities. The rates given in Parkin et al (1992) are, however, based on small numbers.

Unlike cancers of the lung or larynx, there is a tendency for nasal sinus cancers to decrease over time or to remain stable.

Larynx (ICD–9 161)

Laryngeal cancer, strongly associated with alcohol consumption and tobacco smoking, is a relatively common cancer in males, but extremely rare in females. The highest sex ratios are observed in Latin countries (Tuyns et al, 1988). Coleman et al (1993) observed that the three- to fourfold differential between Latin and English populations has remained constant over the past 20 years.

The highest male incidence rates, in the range of 12 to 20, are reported from Brazil, Cuba, Italy, France, Spain, and parts of Hungary and Poland. Within Italy incidence is half that experienced in Latina (7.5) in the center of the country and in Ragusa, Sicily (7.4) in the south.

Rates for male U.S. blacks are frequently double those of U.S. whites: in New Orleans and Detroit the difference is less marked. Incidence rates for U.S. black females are much higher than elsewhere as they are in the 2 to 4 range. In India incidence is 10.2 in Ahmedabad, or twice that in Bangalore and Madras, whereas in Bombay and among Singapore Indians the rate was identical (8.9).

At the national level the highest mortality rates are also noted in France, Spain, Italy, Luxembourg, and Uruguay. Rates are low in the United Kingdom, or between 3 and 6, in contrast with those for lung which are among the highest in the world.

Interesting variations in the distribution of tumors at different sites within the larynx have been observed. Tumors of the glottis are predominant among Anglo-Saxon populations, whereas in France, India and in the black populations of the U.S. the numbers of glottic and supraglottic tumors are approximately equal.

Incidence and mortality rates are increasing for males in many countries in southern and eastern Europe, in Scandinavia (but not in Finland where a fall has been observed), in Australia, and among U.S. blacks.

Lung (ICD–9 162)

Lung cancer was estimated to be the second most common cancer in the world around 1980 but is now considered to be in first place, representing 896,000 new cases (males, 667,000; females, 219,000), or 12% of the world cancer burden. Large international variations occur.

These tumors are particularly common in males in North America, Europe, and Oceania. The highest male rates, in the 100 to 120 range, are seen in the U.S. black population, in the Maoris of New Zealand, and in western Scotland. Lower rates, in the range of 40–90, are seen in a large number of European countries and in the white populations of North America. In the former Soviet Union rates range from 38.4 in Kyrgyzstan to 77.6 in St. Petersburg. Rates below 40 are recorded in Norway (33.9) and Sweden (25.2) and Utah (33.8).

Low rates are seen in several centers of Latin America, ranging from 24.6 in Cali, Colombia to 8.3 in Quito, Ecuador. In Porto Alegre the rate is, however, 85.6. In Sétif, Algeria the rate is 11.7; in Bamako, Mali, 4.8. Although rates in Asian countries are generally low, from 9 to 14 for males in India and from 30 to 40 in Japan, much higher rates are seen among the male Chinese of Singapore (69.7), in Hong Kong (78.7) and Shanghai (53.0).

International differences, as well as sex and ethnic differences in lung cancer incidence, are largely attributable to different smoking patterns; the high rates in western countries reflect the increase of cigarette consumption after World War II. It will be some time before rates rise in those populations that have begun to smoke recently, but the future evolution of the burden can be assessed by looking at incidence by birth cohort. Conversely, the falls now observed among males in several populations were heralded by decreases in younger birth cohorts, even at a time when the disease was increasing in older men.

Chinese females, many of whom are non-smokers, have relatively high rates, e.g., 33.2 in Tianjin compared to 44.5 for males, and 21.9 among the Chinese of Singapore compared to 69.7 for males. Indoor air pollution through exposure to cooking oil vapors has been suspected to increase risk in Chinese women (MacLennan et al, 1977; Gao et al, 1987). Although the proportion of adenocarcinoma of lung in Japanese women, many of whom do not smoke, is high (70%), the incidence rate resembles that in northwest England, the high frequency being due to the smaller proportion of histological types more strongly associated with smoking (Hanai et al, 1987, 1988). In contrast, rates for adenocarcinoma in Chinese women are elevated.

Although lung cancer was a rare disease in the early years of this century, it has now become a leading cause of cancer mortality and morbidity. This cancer's incidence is still increasing in many developed and developing countries although, in the U.S., a decline for males below 65 and for females below 45 is now perceptible due to the decrease of total exposure to cigarette tobacco (Walker and Brin, 1988). Comparable trends have been observed among males in England and Wales, Scotland, and Finland. Nonetheless, the persistence of such trends is dependent on tobacco consumption continuing to fall. Lung cancer in females illustrates the birth cohort paradox: overall rates continue to rise while falling among younger women. The annual rate of rise for U.S. women is still on the order of 2% (Miller et al, 1993). In several countries deaths from lung cancer in women exceed those from breast cancer. In Glasgow there are now more incident cases of lung cancer than there are of breast cancer (Gillis et al, 1992).

Pleura (ICD–9 163)

The incidence of primary pleural tumors, i.e., mesothelioma, is very low, with rates on the order of 0.5 for males and 0.2 for females in most of the world. In males, incidence above 1.5 but under 2 has been recorded in the Bas-Rhin, France, and Basel, Switzerland: higher values are recorded from the ports of Genoa (3.9) and Trieste (4.7) and from Maastricht, The Netherlands (2.6), St. Gall, Switzerland (2.2), Mersey, England (2.1), the West of Scotland (2.0), and South (2.0) and Western Australia (2.9). The high rate in Western Australia is probably due to asbestos mines at Wittenoom Gorge, and raised rates have been observed in coastal areas with shipyards in several countries (See also Malker et al [1985]).

Bone (ICD–9 170)

Tumors arising in bone and cartilage are rare, accounting for about 0.5% of all malignant neoplasms. Mortality data tend to be imprecise as metastatic tumors are frequently miscoded as primary (Percy et al, 1981; Percy and Muir, 1989).

Most rates are close to or below unity. High relative frequencies, around 5% in both sexes, have been reported from the Northwest Frontier Province of Pakistan, as compared to other parts of the country (Parkin, 1986), but the nature of these tumors is not yet known.

Osteogenic sarcoma, chondrosarcoma, and Ewing's tumor are the three main clinicopathological entities grouped under this single ICD rubric. Osteosarcoma is characterised by incidence peaks around the ages 15–19 and thereafter in old age, whereas chondrosarcoma shows a gradual increase in incidence with age. Ewing's sarcoma is almost entirely confined to childhood and early adult life, and is rare among black and Asian populations. Osteosarcomas are somewhat more frequent in black than in white children. Parkin et al (1988a) report incidence rates for these cancers in many parts of the world in the age-group 0–14.

Soft Tissue (ICD–9 171)

Soft tissue sarcomas are derived from mesenchymal tissues such as muscle, fat, blood vessels, and other connective tissues—a heterogeneity of cell type concealed by the site-oriented classifications of the ICD. Further, the indexing of these cancers in the ICD is such that connective tissue malignancies are often coded to specified organs such as uterus or stomach rather than ICD–9 171 and hence "lost" unless ICD–Oncology (ICD–O) is used (WHO, 1976; Percy et al, 1990).

The *Third National Cancer Survey* and the SEER Program in the U.S. have, however, provided tabulations for these cancers both by site and cell type for 1969–1971 and 1972–77 (Cutler and Young, 1975; Young et al, 1981). Leiomyosarcoma appears to be the most common, arising mainly in the uterus in females and the gastrointestinal tract in males. Fibrosarcomas, liposarcomas and rhabdomyosarcomas all occur predominantly in males. A review of the distribution by cell type of the 20,000 such cancers histologically diagnosed and reported to the SEER Program in 1973–1987 is provided by Percy et al 1995. An increasing number of cancer registries are providing this type of information (Lee et al, 1988; Registre Genevois des Tumeurs, 1988; Mehnert et al, 1992), although numbers are much smaller.

The highest rates, around 3, are reported from Trieste, Italy, Vila Nueva de Gaia, Portugal, the Australian Capital Territory, the Maoris of New Zealand, and the Hawaiian population. Elsewhere rates tend to be around 2, rates for females being somewhat lower than for males.

Although Kaposi's sarcoma has hitherto been rare in western countries and uncommon among North American blacks, these neoplasms represent 5 to 12% of all cancers in some African countries where they arise mainly in older males and affect principally the legs and are of slow evolution. Between 1982 and 1983 in association with the AIDS epidemic, the incidence of Kaposi's sarcoma in the SEER areas doubled among men aged 20–54, increasing by another 43% in the next biennium. In San Francisco City and County, incidence in the same age-group rose from 2.0 in 1980 to 26.4 in 1982 and to 112.7 in 1985 (NCI, 1988). Under current coding rules, Kaposi's sarcoma is assigned to Other Skin (ICD–9 172) and these cancers are "lost" unless the coding classification has been based on ICD–O. A separate rubric (C 46) has been proposed for ICD–10.

Malignant Melanoma of the Skin (ICD–9 172)

In spite of the substantial increases in incidence among many fair-skinned populations, on the order of 3 to 5% per annum, cutaneous malignant melanoma remains relatively infrequent. This disease is more common among fair-skinned populations of European origin living in sunny countries. Males and females are almost equally affected. Rates are very low in dark-skinned populations, being frequently well below unity.

The highest rates, 28.9 and 25.3 for females, are reported from the Australian Capital Territory (rates in New South Wales and Western Australia being very close), and New Zealand (M, 18.6; F, 23.0), among Hawaiian whites (M, 2.2; F, 14.9), and whites in Los Angeles (M, 14.6; F, 11.6), and in other parts of the US. Moderately high levels, in the range of 7 to 10, are observed among the fair-skinned populations of Scandinavia and in Switzerland, whereas rates are low in Asia (frequently less than unity) and among U.S. blacks (M, 0.4; F, 0.6). Rates for Israel-born Jews (M, 10.6; F, 11.9) are much higher than for those born in Africa or Asia (M, 1.6; F, 2.1).

The risk of melanoma is related to latitude in Australia, the rates in Tasmania being half those for Canberra cited above. The situation is less clear-cut in Europe where rates in Scandinavia and parts of Switzerland are frequently higher than those in France or Italy, probably reflecting different skin pigmentation and the importance of intermittent or recreational sunlight exposure. There is a strong social class gradient in risk, as non-manual workers are at greater risk of developing and dying from malignant melanoma than are manual workers (Office of Population Censuses and Surveys, 1978; Lee and Strickland, 1980; Sharp et al, 1993). The affluent in Scotland were three times more likely to have a malignant melanoma than the deprived (Carstairs and Morris, 1991).

The risk of melanomas increased for northern European migrants to Australia and Israel. In both countries increasing incidence was related to duration of residence (Morshovitz and Modan, 1973; Holman and Armstrong, 1984), but for superficial spreading melanoma, migration to Australia after the age of 20 was not followed by an increased risk.

A high proportion of these tumors is found on the lower limbs of white females whereas trunk, head and neck are the most frequently affected sites in males. There is some evidence that these sex differences are diminishing. In African black populations, malignant melanoma tends to occur on the soles of the feet in relation to preexisting pigmented spots (Lewis, 1967). A subungual location is more frequent among American blacks and Asians than among whites. However, a high relative frequency of plantar melanoma may reflect a relative absence of malignant melanoma on other parts of the body surface rather than a raised incidence.

A rapid increase has been observed among both sexes almost everywhere in populations of mainly European origin. With the exception of Japan and possibly Puerto Rico, incidence rates of melanoma have remained stable in the few populations of mainly non-European origin for which reliable incidence data are available (Muir and Nectoux, 1982; Armstrong and Kricker, 1994). The greatest average annual increases are around 6% in the

Nordic countries, 7% in New Zealand, and as much as 11% in the Jewish population of Israel. Recent studies support the idea that the increase observed in cutaneous malignant melanoma over the past 60 years is real and not due to changes in diagnostic criteria (van der Esch et al, 1991). Although there has been an increase of around 3% per annum among U.S. black males, the absolute level of incidence remains low; incidence has fallen among U.S. black females.

Other Skin Cancers (ICD–9 173)

The incidence of malignant tumors of the skin, other than melanomas, shows wide variation. Given their frequency and the fact that an individual may have several basal cell carcinomas over a lifetime, many cancer registries do not record them. When registered, the true incidence is frequently difficult to assess as these tumors are often subject to underreporting. Although rarely life-threatening, these cancers nonetheless require medical attention.

The highest rates are those from Tasmania in Australia (213.2 for males and 113.1 for females) and from British Columbia in Canada (134.1 for males and 91.2 for females). In El Paso, Texas, when the cancer registry made a special effort to assess the true incidence of these cancers, rates were as high as 144.9 in Anglo males and 73.3 in Anglo females (Waterhouse et al, 1976). In Goiania, Brazil, rates of over 100 have been recorded, with a slight excess among females (M, 102.0; F, 112.5), and comparable levels are noted in several Canadian provinces. Rates in the 60 to 90 range are reported from Switzerland; rates are considerably lower in most of the British Isles. High levels (M, 71.5; F, 48.0) are noted in southern Ireland. In eastern Europe incidence levels are in the 10 to 25 range.

Non-melanoma skin cancers are much more common among whites than among dark-skinned populations and low rates in the range of 1 to 5 are reported from Africa and Asia. Cutaneous squamous cell carcinomas in blacks, however, have been recorded in relation to predisposing factors such as burns, infections, and chronic ulcers, although their frequency is believed to have declined in recent years (Samitz, 1980).

Among whites the incidence of non-melanoma skin cancers is higher in areas with more sunlight; these tumors arise mainly on the most exposed areas of the face, head and neck, contrasting with the somewhat more even distribution of malignant melanoma (Pearl and Scott, 1986). An excess of basal cell and squamous cell carcinoma among males is seen for most sites but not on the lower extremities where female rates for all forms of non-melanoma skin cancers are higher.

The reported incidence of non-melanoma skin cancer, mainly basal cell carcinoma, seems to have increased in the United States among both sexes (Fears and Scotto, 1982). Incidence is usually somewhat higher in urban than rural populations. In Scotland these tumors are more common in northern areas where a higher proportion of the population are engaged in outdoor work (Kemp et al, 1985).

Breast (ICD–9 174–175)

Globally, breast cancer is the most frequent malignancy among women with an estimated 422,000 new cases in developed countries around 1985. In developing parts of the world mammary cancer, with an estimated 298,000 new cases, ranks far behind cancer of the cervix uteri (344,000) in frequency. This disease is extremely rare in males.

The highest rates reported are those for the white population of the San Francisco Bay area (104.2), closely followed by those for Hawaiians (100.2). Rates in the range of 70 to 100 are observed in the remaining regions of the U.S. (where rates for blacks are about 70% those for whites). Rates for New Zealand Maoris (64.0) are close to those of non-Maoris (64.3); rates are substantially higher among the Pacific Polynesian Islanders (80.3) resident in that country (Cancer Incidence in Five Continents, volume V). In Canada incidence is some 20% lower than in the U.S. or in the 60 to 75 range. In Latin America incidence ranges between 25 and 40, although in Brazil the rate in Porto Alegre (78.5) is double that in Goiania (40.5).

In much of northern, western and southern Europe, rates fall into the 60 to 75 band, except for those in Spain (35 to 50, with the smaller rates observed in the south). Risk is lower in eastern European registries (25 to 40).

In Africa the rates according to volume VI of *Cancer Incidence in Five Continents* are all 10 or below. In Israel rates are high, around 75 for Jews born in Israel, North America or Europe, but are much lower (46.2) among those migrating from Africa or Asia. Incidence in the nonJewish population is low (17.0). Rates are also low among Kuwaitis (17.2) and, to a lesser extent, in China, India, Japan, and Singapore, with rates between 20 and 30. In Singapore incidence in Hokkien and Cantonese females is about 30% greater than in Teochew, Hainanese and Hakka. In the Philippines rates are between 40 and 50, whereas in Kyrgyzstan, in Central Asia, rates are just below 20.

An urban–rural gradient is observed in several European registries. This differential is still very substantial in Poland, as incidence is 22.5 in rural Nowy Sacz and 40.0 in the city of Cracow close by.

Although in a large number of Muslim countries in the developing world—Egypt, Tunisia, Sudan, Iran, Kuwait, and Pakistan—the breast, rather than the cervix uteri, is the most common female cancer site, the high relative frequencies in these countries do not necessarily mean that incidence will be high. For example, although the relative frequency among Kuwaiti females is 22%, the incidence is 17.2, whereas among Maoris a relative frequency of 20% is associated with an incidence of 64.0.

The continued rise in the age-specific incidence of female breast cancer is particularly marked in the highest incidence areas, whereas in several Asian countries a plateau or even a slight decline is observed after menopause. Intermediate age–incidence curves are seen for eastern European countries.

Muir et al (1980) drew attention to similarities of cross-sectional age-incidence curves for breast cancer at various times in the past in Iceland with current cross-sectional curves in regions of contrasting incidence, namely, Connecticut, Finland and Miyagi Prefecture, suggesting that these represented birth cohort effects that reflect differing times of entry of risk factors into the environment. Thus risk in Iceland for the periods 1911–1929, 1930–1949, and 1950–1972 was about the same as that in Japan in 1959–1960, Finland in 1959–1961, and Connecticut in 1960–1962, respectively.

The change in risk of breast cancer in migrants from low-incidence to high-incidence areas and in their descendants argues strongly for environmental influences. Incidence in Hawaii and San Francisco Bay area Japanese is now more than double that in Japan. A comparable phenomenon is observable for Chinese migrants: the incidence in Singapore and Hong Kong Chinese is about 50% higher than that in Shanghai and Tianjin, but well below that in U.S. Chinese. In Singapore the incidence among Singapore-born Chinese for the period 1968–1982 was 29.5, while that for those born elsewhere, mainly in China, was 18.2—a difference significant for all Chinese dialect groups (Lee et al, 1988).

The incidence of breast cancer is increasing slowly in most countries, the rate of increase tending to be greatest where rates were the lowest, e.g., 3.2% per annum for Singapore Chinese who have experienced an increase most noticeable in the under 50 age-group. Mortality rates have also been increasing in, for example, Japan and Hong Kong, but have had a tendency to remain stationary in western countries. In the United States mortality in white women less than 65 years of age has fallen, but among older white women and black women of all ages mortality has been increasing (Devesa et al, 1987; Miller et al, 1993).

Cervix Uteri (ICD–9 180)

Cancer of the cervix uteri is the second most common cancer among women, accounting for an estimated 437,000, or 12%, of all female malignancy on a worldwide basis. Some 80% of these cancers occur in developing countries. Under investigation are sexually transmitted agents, such as the human papillomaviruses (Muñoz et al, 1989).

Cancer of the cervix is the leading cancer among females in sub-Saharan Africa, Central and South America, and Southeast Asia. The highest recorded incidence rates in volume V of *Cancer Incidence in Five Continents* were from Recife in Brazil (83.2) and among the pacific Polynesian Islanders (64.4). In volume VI of this series, the most elevated incidence rates are those in Trujillo, Peru (54.6), Goiania, Brazil (48.9), Asuncion, Paraguay (47.1) and Madras, India (47.2). Rates in the range of 25 to 45 are seen in Cali, Colombia (42.2), in Thailand and among the Maoris (29.9). Although the rates for Bangalore fall into this range, those for Ahmedabad and Bombay are around 20. The rates are intermediate in eastern Europe (12 to 20) and are somewhat lower in North America, Australia, and in northern and western Europe, with rates between 7 and 15. In Europe, very low rates are observed in Finland, Spain, and southern Ireland (4 to 9). The lowest rates are seen in parts of China, Finland (4.4), the Netherlands and Israel, with rates of 4.2 for Jews and 2.6 for non-Jews, and among Kuwaitis (4.1).

In the U.S., large differences in incidence rates are seen between ethnic groups, with a near twofold difference between blacks (12) and whites (7). Incidence is also lower in U.S. Japanese populations (4), but is higher among Hispanics (18), Los Angeles Koreans (17), and American Indians (19.6). Differences in rates are also seen in New Zealand between the Maoris (29.9), the non-Maoris (11.8), and the Pacific Polynesian Islanders (64.4). Urban populations frequently have higher rates than rural populations (volume V, Cancer Incidence in Five Continents).

A decline in the incidence and mortality rates for cervical cancer has been observed virtually everywhere and has often occurred most rapidly in the developing countries of Latin America. Where effective national screening programs have been introduced, as in Finland, mortality has fallen substantially (Hakama et al, 1986). Rises in mortality rates for women born around 1930, however, have been observed recently in New Zealand, Australia, and Britain (Muñoz and Bosch, 1989) which suggests greater exposure to risk factors, whether new or preexisting, in the more recent birth cohorts in these countries.

Choriocarcinoma (ICD–9 181)

Choriocarcinoma is a rare disease of the trophoblast, the incidence of which seems to be much higher in Asian countries than elsewhere (Shanmugaratnam et al, 1971). Some series include chorioadenoma destruens (malignant mole) with the choriocarcinomas. The highest recorded rates (0.7) are from the Philippines and

Thailand. Elsewhere rates are very low, e.g., 0.1 in the former German Democratic Republic.

Maternal age and history of a prior hydatidiform mole are established risk factors for the disease (Bracken et al, 1984). Molar pregnancies are about 1,000 times more likely to progress to choriocarcinoma than non-molar pregnancies.

Corpus Uteri (ICD–9 182)

Globally one-third as frequent as cervical cancer and ranking 8th among cancers in females, cancer of the corpus uteri is twice as common in the developed world (92,000 cases around 1985) as in the developing world (48,000 cases).

The highest reported incidence is from La Plata, Argentina (31.1). High incidence rates in the range of 15 to 25 are found among U.S. whites, in Hawaii and in much of Canada. Within the U.S. incidence rates among blacks tend to be half those for whites; mortality, however, in blacks is double that in whites. In New Zealand incidence in Maoris (16.4), close to that of Hawaiians (18.3), is 50% greater than that in non-Maoris. In Europe rates are in the range of 10 to 15 and are somewhat lower in southern Ireland and the United Kingdom. The lowest rates, in the 3 to 6 range, are found among Asian populations, in much of Latin America, in Portugal and Romania.

In Israel incidence among Jews born in Europe or America (12.2) and in Israel (11.3) is higher than among those born in Africa or Asia (6.1).

The Chinese and Japanese in the U.S. experience rates which are at least four times those in China and Japan.

Leiomyosarcoma of the uterus accounts for 6.8% of these cancers in U.S. black women, compared to 2.2% in white women (Young et al, 1981). In Singapore in 1968–1982, the proportion was 11.6% (Lee et al, 1988) for all ethnic groups combined.

Mortality in U.S. black women from uterine corpus cancer is twice as high as that in white women (Miller et al, 1993). Although mortality rates from cancer of the corpus uteri have shown large declines in both ethnic groups, incidence trends are more variable. A substantial increase in incidence among white women, more marked in the age group 45–64 and ascribed to the use of post-menopausal estrogens, occurred in the 1970s. Many of these tumors were well differentiated. Age-specific incidence rates have now declined to, or below, previous levels after the use of these drugs ceased (Austin and Roe, 1982). Increases in Europe were minimal.

Ovary (ICD–9 183)

Ovarian cancer, ranking sixth globally (162,000 estimated cases in 1985), is a moderately frequent disease representing, however, the most frequent cause of death from gynecologic malignancies in the western world. Cystadenocarcinomas constitute the large majority of ovarian cancers. The less frequent germ cell tumors have a younger age distribution.

The range of geographic variation for this disease is rather small. The highest rate recorded in volume V was 24.9 for Polynesian Pacific Islanders residing in New Zealand. Hawaiians (11.0) have rates close to those for Maoris (9.3) whose incidence is much the same as for non-Maoris in New Zealand. The highest rates reported from Europe are 17.3 in Ardèche France (Olaya and Nectoux, 1987). Values around 15 are observed among Israeli Jews born in Europe or America, in Denmark, Iceland, Norway and Sweden; incidence in Finland is lower (10.0). In much of Europe, including parts of the former U.S.S.R. and North America, rates range between 8 and 12. Rates for U.S. blacks are about two-thirds those for whites. While women in Asia, including Kyrgyzstan, have a relatively low incidence of ovarian tumors, or in the 5 to 7 range, Chinese and Japanese who reside in the United States tend to have higher rates, although still lower than in the white population. In Latin America incidence is in the 4 to 6 range.

Little change in incidence has been observed for this disease in most registries. The rise has been slightly greater in Japan than elsewhere.

Other Female Genital (ICD–9 184)

In most countries the range of incidence is 1 to 2. Levels of 4.5 were obtained in Brazil, where about half of these cancers were stated to arise on the vulva.

Prostate (ICD–9 185)

Prostate cancer is a frequent cancer among older men; its occurrence increases exponentially with age. This disease exhibits large ethnic and international differences. It is particularly common in American blacks among whom it ranks second after lung cancer. In global terms the disease ranked fourth among males, with an estimated 291,000 new cases around 1985.

The highest rates of prostatic cancer have been recorded among the black population of the United States (SEER 82.0), with rates as high as 102.0 in Atlanta where incidence is often close to double that among whites. Only in Utah do rates (77.9) for this largely white population exceed those for a U.S. black population (Connecticut 65.0). Rates are intermediate, in the 30 to 50 range, in Canada, South America, Scandinavia, parts of Switzerland, and Oceania. More moderate rates, around 20, are seen in many European countries. In eastern Europe rates tend to be in the 10 to 15 range, and are under 10 in Japan, India, and other Asian countries, the Philippines excepted (16). In China rates are under 2. In Israel rates are around 18, with the exception, however, of the non-Jewish population (7.7).

In contrast to the pattern of distribution of overt prostatic cancers, the frequency of the smaller non-invasive lesions denoted 'latent' carcinoma does not appear to show much international variation (Breslow et al, 1977).

Japanese migrants to the U.S. have experienced a marked increase in prostatic cancer, although the rates of the Japanese in Hawaii (34.4) and in Los Angeles (32.9) are about half those of whites. Contrasts between U.S. Chinese and those elsewhere are even greater. In Singapore the risk among foreign-born Chinese was 70% that for the Singapore-born over the period 1968–1982. Polish migrants to the United States also acquired higher mortality rates upon migration (Staszewski and Haenszel, 1965), which again emphasizes the influence of the environment, possibly including dietary changes that modify hormone metabolism.

The incidence and mortality of prostatic cancer have been rising over time in many areas. While an average annual increase of 4.9% has been observed among Singapore Chinese and of 2.2% for the U.S. black population (Miller et al, 1993), a decrease in mortality in American blacks was nonetheless anticipated in the future, based on the decline in risk observed among the younger cohorts (Ernster et al, 1978). Similar observations have been made in Australia, England and Wales (Holman et al, 1981). The interpretation of time trends and incidence levels is, however, not easy, depending to a degree on local practice concerning "latent" cancer of the prostate discovered incidentally at prostatic transurethral resection or autopsy. In Malmö, Sweden, the incidence of prostate cancer was 50% higher than elsewhere in the country; at the national level, 7.6% of 298 cases were discovered at autopsy compared to 36.4% of 177 cases in Malmö (National Board of Health and Welfare, 1984). The advent of widespread screening by the estimation of prostate-specific antigen is likely to confuse the situation further.

Testis (ICD–9 186)

The incidence of testicular cancer, although uncommon, shows a fairly large geographic variation while occurring relatively frequently among young white males in the 20 to 34 age-group and rarely among Africans and Asians. Mortality rates for the highest socioeconomic classes have been shown to be twice those for the lowest (Logan, 1982).

The upper range of rates, between 6 and 9, occurs in western European countries. The highest rates occur in Switzerland (8.8 in Zurich; 8.4 in Basel) and in Denmark (8.4), and a high rate is also seen in the former German Democratic Republic (7.0). Much of Europe and Canada is in the 3 to 5 range. In Estonia, Latvia, Finland, Portugal and Spain rates are below 2. Blacks in the U.S., with rates less than 1 per 100,000 have a much lower incidence than whites, with rates in the range of 3 to 6. The reported incidence of testicular cancer is even lower for African blacks than for American blacks (McDonald et al, 1984). Despite the accessibility of this site, several of the series, e.g., Kampala in Uganda, appearing in Parkin (1986) do not contain a single case of testicular cancer (see Penis below). Most rates in Asia are around unity.

As in ovarian cancer, there are a variety of cell types with somewhat different age distributions. In most series about 50% are seminomas. International comparison of cell types (Tulinius, 1970) is influenced by differing concepts of histogenesis.

A rising incidence of testicular cancer has been observed in many countries. In the United States a dramatic decline in mortality, around 9% per annum, has been observed in the past ten years due to successful therapy, this at a time when incidence is rising at some 3% per annum. The rate of increase is greatest among the youngest birth cohorts, which suggests the introduction of a new carcinogen, perhaps prevalent at conception or during the gestational period (Brown et al, 1986).

Penis (ICD–9 187)

Although ICD–9 rubric 187 includes scrotal, epididymis, cord, seminal vesicle, and tunica tumors, these are rare compared to tumors of the penis. The rates quoted below are for the entire rubric. Cancer of the penis, a rare disease in the western world, is not uncommon in several parts of Africa, Asia, and Latin America.

Incidence rates are uniformly high in South and Central America, the highest reported being from Asunción, Paraguay (4.2), Porto Alegre, Brazil (3.9) and Puerto Rico (3.3). Although incidence is common among Indian Hindus who are not routinely circumcised, incidence rates have fallen substantially in recent years. The disease is reported to be rare among Muslims and Parsees (Reddy et al, 1977). An elevated incidence is reported from Chiang Mai in Thailand (3.1). As might be expected, rates are very low in Israel where circumcision is virtually universal, although they are greater for the Israel-born (0.9) than for those born elsewhere (0.2). Rates for U.S. blacks are slightly lower than for whites.

Caucasians in North America, Europe and Australia exhibit low penile cancer rates, around unity, in contrast to the relatively high incidence of testicular cancer in industrialized countries.

Large geographical variations are reported from Africa where incidence rates tend to reflect tribal affiliation, whereas the rates for American blacks, around unity, vary little. In Kampala, Uganda, penile cancer ranked second among males, following liver cancer (13.3%), with a relative frequency of 8.1%. However, the disease has been found to be rare in parts of the highlands of New Guinea where hygiene is poor and circumcision rare (Berg, 1974).

Cervix uteri cancer incidence rates correlate weakly with those for penile cancer. A possible common risk factor has been suggested in the human papilloma virus (Muñoz and Bosch, 1989).

Bladder (ICD–9 188)

Cancer of the bladder is common among males in many parts of the world, ranking 8th globally (an estimated 182,000 new cases in 1985). For females, bladder cancer did not figure in the first 12 ranking sites. This cancer exhibits moderate international variation, although to some extent the differences depend on whether so-called benign papillomas of the bladder are included with the overtly malignant neoplasms.

Rates are elevated in several industrialized countries, the highest being observed in Italy (34.0 in Trieste, 33.5 in Florence). For a large number of registries in the remainder of Europe and North America, and in the Jewish population of Israel, rates are around 20. Somewhat higher rates are observed in parts of Spain (26.4 in the Basque country). In much of eastern Europe rates are around 10. Rates for U.S. blacks, also around 10, are uniformly somewhat less than half those for white Americans, perhaps due in part to an underreporting of early-stage tumors (Schairer et al, 1988); mortality, however, was much the same in both groups (Miller et al, 1993). For Bermudan blacks the rate was 22.4. The lowest rates occur in Asia, notably in India, with rates between 3.6 in Bombay and 1.8 in Madras. Rates in Singapore, Thailand, Japan, and China are slightly higher, between 5 and 8 (a somewhat higher incidence is reported from Hiroshima [12.3] and Nagasaki [10.6]). Incidence among U.S. Chinese and Japanese is slightly higher than in China or Japan. Incidence in Hong Kong is substantially greater (16.1).

Females are much less affected by the disease than males, the M:F sex ratio being about 3–5 to 1, and the geographic variation in incidence is less than that for males. Smoking and occupational exposures contribute to this pattern.

Bladder cancer also occurs frequently in countries of the Middle East and Africa where urinary schistosomiasis is endemic; for example, it accounts for some 29% of all cancer in males and 11% of those in females reported to the Cairo Metropolitan Cancer Registry. In Baghdad, bladder cancer accounts for 13% of all malignant neoplasms in males (Al Fouadi and Parkin, 1984). Squamous cell carcinomas are dominant in areas where bladder cancer is related to schistosomiasis in contrast to the overwhelming preponderance of transitional cell tumors seen elsewhere. Nonetheless, the urothelial/squamous ratio varies greatly—it is 3 in Cali, Colombia; 7 in Birmingham, England; 30 in Alameda County; and 70 in Sweden—possibly due to differences in pathological interpretation and causal agent (Tulinius, 1970).

The incidence of bladder cancer is slowly increasing in many countries, with a more moderate increase in mortality.

Kidney (ICD–9 189)

Renal cell carcinoma in adults represents a large majority, around 80%, of the cancers of the kidney, renal pelvis, and ureter, which are all grouped together in this ICD rubric. In general, rates for renal pelvis and parenchymal cancers correlate well (Muir and Nectoux, 1980). In children, most of the cancers are nephroblastomas.

Worldwide variation in these tumors is moderate. The highest rates, above 10, are seen in North America (where rates are fairly close among U.S. whites [10.3] and blacks [8.9]) and in parts of Europe. The highest levels observed are in the male populations of Trieste (15.5), the Bas-Rhin department in France (15.2), in Iceland (13.0) and Sweden (11.5). Intermediate rates, around 6 to 8, are seen in most remaining areas of the western world. Rates are low, however, in India, China, the Philippines and other parts of Asia, including Kyrgyzstan, and in much of Latin America. Rates for males are generally twice those for females.

Exceptionally high levels of renal pelvis cancer are found in areas where Balkan nephropathy is endemic, such as the Vratsa area of Bulgaria (Chernozemsky et al, 1977), where incidence levels of 22.0 (M) and 28.1 (F) were found, the total incidence for renal pelvis, bladder and ureter combined being 61.7 and 62.4, respectively. In contrast, in areas with little or no nephropathy, the combined incidence was 8.4 and 7.4, respectively.

Nephroblastomas, which occur relatively frequently in children between one and three years of age, are slightly more common in blacks than whites and particularly in black females. Rates for the age-group 0–14 in the SEER registries are 7.9 and 10.0 per million white males and females and 9.9 and 12.3 for black male and female children, respectively. A differential of the same order was also noted in Los Angeles. It has been suggested that the excess risk of these tumors among blacks is the result of a higher proportion of children with a hereditary predisposition (Kramer et al, 1984). Nonetheless, even higher rates have been recorded in Finland and in the department of Bas-Rhin, France.

Eye (ICD–9 190)

Eye cancers are uniformly rare both in males and females, rates being seldom above unity. In Israel the incidence in Israel-born Jews (1.1) is double that in those born elsewhere. Surprisingly high rates were observed in the Pacific Polynesian Islanders resident in New Zealand (M, 4.4; F, 2.1 [V]).

The majority of ocular tumors in persons over 15 in western countries are melanomas. In Denmark, 80% of these tumors were located in the choroid (Osterlind, 1987). The estimated rates of ocular melanomas do not show either the geographic variations or the increase over time observed for cutaneous malignant melanomas (Hakulinen et al, 1978). The incidence of eye melanomas appears however to be higher in whites than in blacks, as is the case for malignant melanoma of the skin (Strickland and Lee, 1981).

Most ocular tumors in children are retinoblastomas which occur mainly in the first years of life, and a large proportion of these lesions appear to be transmitted through an autosomal dominant gene (Knudson, 1989). As for nephroblastoma, black populations seem to be at slightly higher risk for the disease, e.g., in Kampala, Uganda. The unilateral, generally non-genetic form seems to be responsible for the geographical variation in incidence.

Brain and Nervous System (ICD–9 191–192)

Primary tumors of the brain and nervous system are not uncommon, but their reported incidence depends to some extent on the standard of medical care which is available and the ability to exclude metastatic tumors. Further, certain registries include benign and unspecified tumors. Most of these neoplasms are intracranial, intraspinal tumors representing but 10% of the total. The highest rates for tumors of the central nervous system are reported from Sweden (10.7), Porto Alegre, Brazil (10.5), and among Israeli females born in Israel (10.0). Intermediate rates, between 5 and 9, are generally seen in most of the western world, the rates in Asian populations being lower, in the 1 to 4 range. In the U.S. incidence among blacks (3.4) is half that among whites.

Except for Israel, where female rates are marginally higher than those for males, there is a tendency for males to exhibit a slightly higher incidence. In children the highest rates, around 30 per million, are observed in Denmark and Finland.

It is misleading, however, to consider these tumors as one group since distinct epidemiological patterns have been observed for different histological types among adults (Kepes et al, 1984). Parkin et al (1988b) present information for children by cell type; the proportionate distribution seems to be much the same irrespective of level of incidence.

There is some controversy concerning time trends for these cancers (Davis et al, 1991; Muir et al, 1993), notably for older persons. The rapid changes in diagnostic methods may be responsible for at least part of the postulated increase.

Thyroid Cancer (ICD–9 193)

Thyroid cancer is relatively infrequent on a worldwide basis, representing 1–2% of all cancers, although in adolescents and young adults it is one of the most frequent neoplasms. Incidence rates are approximately three times higher for females than for males, this excess varying with age and occurring more among the young.

The highest female rates of thyroid cancer are observed among the Filipinos and Chinese residing in Hawaii (24.2 and 11.3). In the Philippines and in Los Angeles, Filipinos' rates are much lower, around 3 and 8, respectively. A comparable differential is seen for Los Angeles Chinese and other Chinese populations. High rates are also seen in Iceland (8.3) and among native Alaskan women (Lanier et al, 1976).

Incidence rates for both sexes have been increasing slightly over time among U.S. whites and blacks. In the Nordic countries, rates have tended to be stable. In contrast, a general decline in mortality rates has been observed, even in those countries, such as Austria and Switzerland, with traditionally high rates. Kerr et al (1985) suggested a decline in the proportion of tumors with poor prognosis.

Hodgkin's Disease (ICD–9 201)

Hodgkin's disease is a relatively uncommon form of malignancy with somewhat higher rates for males than for females.

The highest male rates, in the range of 3 to 4, are observed among whites from North America, in Porto Alegre, Brazil, southern Ireland, and Italy; the corresponding rates for females are between 2 and 3. In Israel rates are much the same in the Jewish (M, 2.9; F, 2.2) and non-Jewish (M, 2.6; F, 1.1) populations.

Intermediate rates, in the 2 to 3 range, are found in much of Europe and Australasia as well as for American blacks (M, 2; F, 1). The incidence is lowest in Asia, in particular in China and Japan where rates are well below unity. Mortality is decreasing in several countries following improvements in therapy.

Three main incidence peaks have been reported (Correa and O'Conor, 1971): in childhood, in young adults, and in older age-groups. Whereas the older age peak is observed early everywhere, some variation is seen in the age–incidence pattern in young age-groups. In western populations a peak between ages 25–30 is followed by a further rise after ages 40–45, whereas in developing countries the young adult peak tends to be replaced by a peak at ages 5–9. In Japan, however, Hodgkin's disease shows a unimodal increase with age. The data in Parkin et al (1988b) clearly bring out the differences in incidence for Hodgkin's disease below the age of 15 in several developing populations: rates per million in males are below 10 except for Los Angeles Hispanics, in Sao Paulo and Costa Rica, and for non-Jews in Israel and in Kuwait.

In the US, a shift in age of onset from childhood to young adulthood has been noted in successive birth cohorts, possibly in relation to changes in socioeconomic status (Gutensohn and Cole, 1977).

These epidemiological features have suggested the possible influence of infectious agents during childhood in developing countries that remain delayed until adolescence in developed countries.

Lymphosarcoma and Recticulum Cell Sarcoma (ICD–9 200)

Following changes in histopathological classification, data for this group of tumors are rather unreliable. Many neoplasms which would have been previously coded to this rubric are now found in ICD–9 202 as non-Hodgkin's lymphomas. Reticulum cell sarcomas are generally 30% more common than lymphosarcomas in most populations, irrespective of incidence. Combined rates are slightly higher for males than females. The highest rates are seen in North America, Australia, Switzerland and Israel, generally in the range of 5 to 10. In contrast, rates are in the 2 to 3 range in the British Isles and the former Federal Republic of Germany and below unity in much of eastern Europe. Low rates are seen in Japan and China and are much closer to those of the host country in migrant Chinese and Japanese populations.

Burkitt's Lymphoma (ICD–9 200.2)

Burkitt's lymphoma is a distinct pathological entity arising from B lymphocytes, occurs among children of both sexes and often involves the jaw or ovary.

The disease was first noted in Uganda where it currently represents 12% of childhood tumors. The regions of high risk are those which are affected by holoendemic malaria as in sub-Saharan Africa, with the exception, however, of the highland areas in Papua New Guinea (Evans and de Thé, 1989). Sporadic cases occur all over the world. Parkin et al (1988b) tabulated the relative frequency of Hodgkin's disease, Burkitt's lymphoma and other lymphomas in children: Burkitt's lymphoma comprised 90% in the West Nile district of Uganda, 55% in Papua New Guinea, around 30% in Baghdad, and 17% in white populations covered by the SEER program.

In endemic areas the peak incidence occurs among children from 5 to 8 years of age, whereas the disease is rare before the age of 2 as well as after 14. Incidence in males is twice that in females.

Declines in incidence were seen in the 1970s in parts of Uganda and Tanzania, although in the latter area a recent increase, possibly related to a recrudescence of malaria, has been observed (Geser et al, 1989).

Non-Hodgkin's Lymphoma (ICD–9 200, 202)

As noted above, this group of tumors has seen major differences in classification over the past decade. Many lymphomas are classified as being diffuse or nodular and recently it has proved possible to determine whether a given tumor arises from T or B lymphocytes. Unfortunately, despite attempts to create a uniform classification, there remain several schools of thought on this. The second edition of the *International Classification of Diseases-Oncology* (Percy et al, 1990) provides codes for these various descriptors.

Mycosis fungoides is a form of non-Hodgkin's lymphoma that appears to begin in the skin, the malignant cells being T lymphocytes. Sézary syndrome shares common cutaneous histopathological features. The incidence is usually well below unity.

Within Canada and in white U.S. populations, rates vary between 10 and 14 for males, but are somewhat lower, around 8, in black populations. Rates in Australia are around 10. In the British Isles, western Europe, and in the Nordic countries rates are around 8, although they are somewhat higher in Trieste (12.4) in the north of Italy and in St. Gall, Switzerland (12.7). In Israel rates are highest among the Israel-born (10.2) and are virtually double those for the non-Jewish population (5.4). In eastern Europe and the Iberian peninsula, as in much of Asia and Latin America, rates vary between 3 and 7. Rates for females, usually about three-quarters those for males, follow the same pattern.

Multiple Myeloma (ICD–9 203)

Multiple myeloma, originally classified as a bone tumor, was recognized as a separate entity in the early 1950s. It is characterized by a strong age dependence, occurring at a rather late age and predominantly among males.

This disease, common among U.S. blacks, in whom it represents the most common form of malignancy of the lympho-hematopoietic system with rates around 7, or double those for U.S. whites. Rates are generally low among blacks in Africa, perhaps on account of incomplete ascertainment, limited diagnostic facilities, and a lower number of persons reaching older ages. The incidence of multiple myeloma is intermediate, in the 2 to 4 range, in North American white populations, in western Europe, and in Israel. Rates in eastern Europe and in most Asian populations are usually lower.

Multiple myeloma seems to be increasing in most geographic regions and socioeconomic groups of both sexes, the rise being particularly marked among the elderly. Technical improvements in the diagnosis of multiple myeloma, however, may have partly contributed to this increase (Verlez et al, 1982). While the SEER cancer registries report a non-significant increase among both black and white populations, U.S. mortality figures reflect a larger significant increase (Miller et al, 1993).

Leukemia (ICD–9 204–208)

The leukemias group a variety of cancers originating in cells that arise from bone marrow and circulate in peripheral blood. Leukemias are classified by cell type in the *International Classification of Diseases*; distinction between the acute and chronic forms is made at the level of the fourth digit. Rates tend to be higher in North America and Australia (10) and in much of western and eastern Europe (7 to 9). Reported incidence is somewhat lower in Israel, Latin America, and in much of Asia (2 to 7). Similar patterns are observed for both lymphoid and myeloid leukemias. Chronic lymphoid leukemia remains relatively rare in Chinese and Japanese populations. Monocytic leukemia is uniformly rare with rates well below unity in practically all countries for both sexes.

Parkin et al (1988b) present childhood lymphoma/leukemia ratios. These are around 0.5 in most populations, rising to unity in several developing countries. The very high ratios observed in East Africa may be due to under-ascertainment of leukemia as well as the presence of Burkitt's lymphoma. Whereas chronic leukemia is rare among children, acute lymphoid leukemia is the most frequent childhood cancer in developed countries.

The incidence of and mortality from leukaemia has been virtually stable in the U.S. over the past ten years, but in children there have been substantial declines in mortality following advances in therapy.

Primary Site Uncertain

In cases where it is not always possible to determine the origin of a cancer, they are classified as *primary site uncertain*. The rates for this category range between 5 and 25 for both sexes, many values being around 10. In developing countries where the resources for extensive investigation may not exist, the proportion of such cancers is likely to be higher than elsewhere.

All Sites of Cancer (ICD–9 140–208, excluding 173)

Given that many cancer registries do not collect information on non-melanoma skin cancer (ICD–9 173), the *Cancer Incidence in Five Continents* series has included tables for all sites and all sites but 173. The comments which follow pertain to the latter. There are very large geographical and ethnic differences for the rates observed, differences which transcend possible variations in registration efficiency. The highest rates are seen in the black populations of the United States—411 in Alameda County, California, where the rates for white males are 322 (the crude rates in these populations are 389 and 398, respectively). For the combined SEER registries the ethnic differences in rates are less striking—349 and 326, respectively—but still substantial. There is always the possibility that part of the difference may be due to underenumeration of the black population by the census. However, such an effect would be seen across the board and the low levels of testis cancer, for example, among blacks as compared to whites run counter to such a hypothesis. Except for the prostate, much of the difference is due to cancers associated with alcohol, tobacco and nutritional risk factors.

In much of Europe and Japan rates are lower, or in the 250 to 300 range. Among the Chinese in Hong Kong, in Singapore, Shanghai, Qidong and the U.S., rates are in the 200 to 330 range. In much of Latin America they are less than 200, and in Africa they are below 100.

Rates for all cancers in females follow their own pattern. In Cali, Colombia, the very high levels of cervix uteri cancer result in an overall rate of 207 compared to 179 in males, a comparable differential observed in Quito, Ecuador and in the Indian cities of Bangalore and Madras. Rates are much the same for both sexes in the Philippines, but predominate among males elsewhere.

COMMENT

In selecting countries and registries for mention, the authors have become increasingly aware of the fluctuations that occur from one volume of *Cancer Incidence in Five Continents* to the next. That this should occur for infrequent tumors in small populations is of little surprise, but when sizeable populations and a five-year span are concerned, the possibility of changes in the efficiency of registration as well as a true change in incidence must be considered.

Although the data presented above are of interest, it can be difficult to visualize the global cancer map in the narrative format used, with mention of the selection of registries and wide gaps in data coverage. The patterns by sites of cancers of the developing world are different from those of the developed parts of the globe (Fig. 10–2). It is obvious that there are substantial differences between the continents and that the north, south, east, and west of Europe exhibit different cancer patterns. Hirayama proposed superimposition of incidence rates on a map of the world, but the technique permits at best some 15–20 regions per cancer site and it is difficult to portray north–south differences. Cancer atlases have become increasingly popular as a method of drawing attention to such spatial patterns as they have developed considerably in terms of sophistication and visual impact (Li et al, 1979; Kemp et al, 1985; Mehnert et al, 1992; Smans et al, 1992) since the pioneering publications by Haviland (1875), Stocks (1928), Burbank (1971) and Mason et al. (1975). Nations are much too large an administrative unit and it is now customary to use much smaller divisions, such as the county or its equivalent. The problems of data presentation in the form of a map are well described in Boyle et al (1989) who concluded that the most appropriate function to map is the age-standardized incidence or mortality rate.

The old axiom that a single picture is worth a thousand words is certainly valid for the cancer atlas. It is the pattern which is important rather than differences in the formal statistical sense, for these may be a function of population size rather than of differences in incidence. Visual distortions result from large populations residing in a relatively small area covered by a city, and from the existence of large, virtually uninhabited areas, such as in Canada, China and Australia.

For esophageal cancer in males, the excess risk in the north and northwest of France is quite outstanding; rates elsewhere in France and in the rest of Europe, other than in northern Italy, are much lower. The pattern of this cancer in females is quite different, with excesses in Scotland and Ireland, although the rates are very much lower than for males. Bearing in mind the maxim that cancer occurs in people, not in places (Kemp et al, 1985), one must ask why the excess risk for esophageal cancer ends abruptly at the Belgian border, as, at first sight, there would not appear to be great differences in tobacco/alcohol habits between northern France and southern Belgium. The difference is unlikely to be due to diagnosis or classification. The high rates for Scottish and Irish women compared to other parts of the EEC are again puzzling, unless these represent the residual influence of sideropenic dysphagia (Paterson-Brown-Kelly or Plummer-Vinson syndrome).

Unlike the substantial contrasts between and within countries in the risk of esophageal cancer, risk differentials for breast cancer seem to lie mainly at the national rather than the regional level, a finding which must have implications for the design and interpretation of etiological studies. The limited regional variation for leukemia suggests that the risk factors are likely to be widely distributed. The increasing popularity of the cancer atlas has resulted in several new portrayals of incidence patterns; for the majority of countries, however, such atlases are still confined to mortality.

UTILITY OF DESCRIPTIVE EPIDEMIOLOGY

The conspicuous geographic variations in cancer occurrence have long intrigued oncologists (see Clemmesen, 1965). Following an attempt at a general census of cancer in London in 1728, there were numerous efforts to collect better data in several countries. Yet many early writers, such as Hirsch (1864), were well aware of the problems of comparability, as reflected in his text of geographic pathology on the inadequacy of hospital and mortality statistics to portray cancer patterns. In 1915, when Hoffman published his book on cancer mortality in the world, he was well on the way to placing the subject on a sound basis, believing, like Greenwood (1928), that "it is probable that by the gradual improvement in accuracy and completeness of the medical statistics of all nations we can best prepare the way for a really illuminating survey of the cancer problem." Yet, as Medawar (1967) has pointed out, the mere compilation of raw data never gave rise to a hypothesis, a process that is outside logic and cannot be made the subject of logical rules.

While some were content to record patterns without realizing the significance of their findings, others related international differences to race or ethnicity, i.e., to genetic factors, while yet others were convinced that the environment was important. The apparent rarity of cancer in (usually) remote parts of the world was frequently uncritically accepted as reflecting the Acadian ideal, and questions of availability of medical services and relevant records were ignored (Muir, 1963).

By 1908 oral cancer in India had been ascribed to betel quid chewing, not to race, and in 1933 a case–control study—one of the first—published by Orr showed a strong dose–response effect for this habit. In 1944 Kennaway pointed out the fundamental etiologic lesson to be drawn from changes in cancer risk in migrants, a conclusion later supported by the data from the classic studies of Haenszel and Kurihara (1968) on Japanese migrants to the United States which showed that genetic factors are much less important than the environment in determining cancer risk. There are still sizeable migrant populations to be studied such as

Greeks, Italians and Yugoslavs in Australia, Indians and Pakistanis in Great Britain, Turks in Germany, and North Africans in France.

The remarkable geographic variations in cancer risk discussed here are now generally agreed to reflect the effects of environmental differences (Higginson, 1960). Such differences fall into three main groups. The first comprises well-defined personal habits such as smoking, betel quid chewing, excess alcohol consumption, and sunbathing.

The second category of environmental differences relates to the common cancers of the gastrointestinal tract and of the endocrine-dependent organs (breast, ovary, corpus uteri, prostate). Here the causes are much less well defined and those that have been identified are generally in the nature of risk factors, such as age at first full-term pregnancy or low-fiber diet. The most rational interpretation of the descriptive epidemiologic data for this second category is an association with environmental factors, using the word "environment" in its broadest sense, that is, all that impinges on the human system. Such a conclusion is based on changes in risk due to migration, whether these changes occur relatively rapidly or over one or more generations, as is the case for occurrences of colon and breast cancer, respectively, among Japanese migrants to the United States; on changes in risk over time; on sex ratios of risk; and on the differences in risk for these cancers observed in groups such as the Mormons and the Seventh-Day Adventists whose lifestyle (behavior and/or diet) departs from the norm of the country in which they live.

The third group is represented by the very much smaller number of cancers shown to be due to occupational exposures, medicaments, and radiation, or cancers that are associated with definable hereditary and congenital syndromes (Higginson and Muir, 1979).

These concepts can be regarded as simplistic and will doubtless be modified and refined as more becomes known about the role of dietary fat and calories in cancers of the endocrine-dependent organs, about genetically determined differences in the activity of metabolizing enzymes, and about the significance of endogenous nitrosation, to mention but a few factors. In fact, we are now in the position of Tanchou (1843) who, commenting on cancer deaths in Paris, arrived at the conclusion that "the cause of cancer is complex and is neither completely internal nor completely external."

It seems axiomatic that combined epidemiological and laboratory efforts should continue to be aimed at dissecting the nature and somatic effects of lifestyle factors, including diet and behavior. Such investigations are more likely to succeed if they include populations of contrasting risk (Trichopoulos et al, 1985). Further, if the proposed causes or mechanisms are not consistent with the observed distribution, taking induction period into account, they are either incomplete or incorrect (Muir, 1973). The reader who has followed the evolution of estimates of the global cancer burden and the rankings of common cancers (Parkin et al, 1984; 1988a; 1993) will not have failed to observe that not only is the world cancer burden increasing but also that some of the differences between regions are beginning to blur somewhat. Since nations are becoming increasingly homogeneous, which is likely to eventually result in a kind of globocancer pattern, the opportunities to explain differences in incidence must be seized now. Without knowledge of cause there can be no rational prevention.

REFERENCES

AL-FOUADI A, PARKIN DM. 1984. Cancer in Irak. Seven years data from the Bahgdad Tumour Registry. Int J Cancer 34:207–213.

ARMSTRONG BK, KRICKER A. 1994. Cutaneous melanoma. Cancer Surv 19/20:219–240.

AOKI K, KURIHARA M, HAYAKAWA N, SUZUKI S. 1992. Death Rates for Malignant Neoplasms for Selected Sites and Five-Year Age Group in 33 Countries 1953–57 to 1983–87. Nagoya, University of Nagoya Co-op Press.

AUSTIN DF, ROE KM. 1982. The decreasing incidence of endometrial cancer: public health implications. Am J Public Health 72:65–68.

BECKER N, FRENTZEL-BEYME R, WAGNER S. 1984. Atlas of Cancer Mortality in the Federal Republic of Germany, 2nd ed. Berlin, Springer Verlag, p. 385.

BERG D: CANCER OF THE GENITO-URINARY TRACT. *In* Atkinson L, Clezy JK, Reay-Young PS, et al (eds). 1974. The Epidemiology of Cancer in Papua New Guinea. Konedobu, Dept. of Public Health, pp. 97–103.

BLOT WJ, FRAUMENI JF. 1987. Trends in esophageal cancer mortality among US blacks and whites. Am J Public Health, 77:296–298.

BONETT A, RODER D. 1988. Epidemiology of cancer in South Australia. Incidence, mortality and survival 1977 to 1986 analysed by type, country of birth and geographical location. Adelaide, South Australia Health Commission, p. 408.

BORING CC, SQUIRES TS, TONG T, MONTGOMERY S. 1944. Cancer statistics 1994. CA Cancer J Clin 44:7–26.

BOSS LP, LANIER AP, DOHAN PH, et al. 1982. Cancers of the gallbladder and biliary tract in Alaskan natives, 1970–79. J Natl Cancer Inst 69:1005–1007.

BOYLE P, MUIR CS, GRUNDMANN E (EDS). 1989. Cancer mapping. Recent Results Cancer Res 114. New York, Springer-Verlag, p. 255.

BRACKEN MB, BRINTON LA, HAYASHI K. 1984. Epidemiology of hydatidiform mole and choriocarcinoma. Epidemiol Rev 6:52–75.

BRESLOW N, CHAN CE, DHOM G, et al. 1977. Latent carcinoma of prostate at autopsy in seven areas. Int J Cancer 20:680–688.

BROWN LM, POTTERN LM, HOOVER RN. 1986. Testicular cancer in the United States, trends in incidence and mortality. Int J Epidemiol 15:164–170.

BURBANK F. 1971. Patterns in Cancer Mortality in the US 1950–1967. Natl Cancer Inst Monograph 33. Washington, D.C., U.S. Government Printing Office.

CARSTAIRS V, MORRIS T. 1991. Deprivation and Health in Scotland. Aberdeen, Aberdeen University Press.

CHOW H-W, DEVESA SS. 1992. Death certificate reporting of colon and rectal cancers. JAMA 267:3028.

CHERNOZEMSKY IN, STOYANOV IS, PETKOVA-BOCHAROVA T, NICOLOV IG, DRAGANOV IV, STOICHEV IN, TANCHEV Y, NAIDENOV D,

KALCHEVA ND. 1977. Geographic correlation between the occurrence of endemic nephropathy and urinary tract tumours in Vratza district, Bulgaria. Int J Cancer 19:1–11.

CLEMMESEN J. 1965. Statistical Studies in the Aetiology of Malignant Neoplasms. I. Review and Results. Copenhagen, Munksgaard.

COLEMAN MP, ESTÈVE J, DAMIECKI P, ARSLAN A, RENARD H. 1993. Trends in Cancer Incidence and Mortality. IARC Sci Publ 121. Lyon, International Agency for Research on Cancer.

COOK PJ, BURKITT DP. 1971. Cancer in Africa. Br Med Bull 27:14–20.

CORREA P, O'CONOR GT. 1971. Epidemiologic patterns of Hodgkin's Disease. Int J Cancer 8:192–201.

CUTLER SJ, YOUNG J. 1975. Third National Cancer Survey: Incidence Rates. NCI Monograph, DHEW Publications NIH 75-787. Washington, D.C., U.S. Government Printing Office, p. 454.

DAVIS DL, AHLBOM A, HOEL D, PERCY C. 1991. Is brain cancer mortality increasing in industrial countries? Am J Ind Med 19:421–431.

DAVIS S, SEVERSON RK. 1987. Increasing incidence of cancer of the tongue in the United States among young adults. Lancet ii:910–911.

DAY NE. 1976. A new measure of age-standardized incidence, the cumulative rate. *In* Waterhouse J, Muir CS, Correa P, et al (eds): Cancer Incidence in Five Continents, Vol. III, IARC Sci Publ 15. Lyon, International Agency for Research on Cancer, pp. 443–452.

DAY NE, MUÑOZ N. 1982. Esophagus. *In* Schottenfeld D, Fraumeni JF (eds): Cancer Epidemiology and Prevention. W.B. Saunders Company, Philadelphia, pp. 596–622.

DEVESA SS, SILVERMAN DT, YOUNG JL, et al. 1987. Cancer incidence and mortality among whites in the United States, 1974–1984. J Natl Cancer Inst 79:701–770.

DOLL R. 1976. Comparison between registries: age-standardized rates. *In* Waterhouse J, Muir CS, Correa P et al: Cancer Incidence in Five Continents, Vol. III. IARC Sci Publ 15. Lyon, International Agency for Research on Cancer, pp. 453–459.

DOLL R, FRAUMENI JF, MUIR CS (EDS). 1994. Trends in Cancer Incidence and Mortality. Cancer Surv 19/20. New York, Cold Spring Harbor Laboratory Press.

DOLL R, PAYNE P, WATERHOUSE J (EDS). 1966. Cancer Incidence in Five Continents. A Technical Report. New York, Heidelberg, Berlin, Springer-Verlag.

DUNHAM LJ, BAILAR III JC. 1968. World maps of cancer mortality rates and frequency ratios. J Natl Cancer Inst 41:155–203.

ERNSTER VL, SELOIN S, WINKELSTEIN W. 1978. Cohort mortality for prostatic cancer among United States non-whites. Science 200:1165–1166.

ESTÈVE J, KRICKER A, FERLAY J, PARKIN DM. 1993. Facts and Figures of Cancer in the European Community. Lyon, International Agency for Research on Cancer.

EVANS AS, DE THÉ G. 1989. Burkitt's lymphoma. *In* Evans AS (ed): Viral Infections of Humans, 3rd ed. New York, Plenum Press, pp. 713–735.

FEARS TR, SCOTTO J. 1982. Changes in skin cancer morbidity between 1971–72 and 1977–78. J Natl Cancer Inst 69:365–370.

GAO YU-TANG, BLOT WJ, ZHENG W. 1987. Lung cancer among Chinese women. Int J Cancer 40:606–609.

GEDDES M, PARKIN DM, KHLAL M, BALZI D, BUIATTI C. 1993. Cancer in Italian Migrant Populations. IARC Sci Publ 123. Lyon, International Agency for Research on Cancer.

GESER A, BRUBAKER G, DRAPER CC. 1989. Effect of a malaria suppression program on the incidence of African Burkitt's lymphoma. Am J Epidemiol 129:740–752.

GILLIS CR, HOLE DJ, LAMONT DW, GRAHAM AC, RAMAGE S. 1992. The incidences of lung cancer and breast cancer in women in Glasgow. BMJ 305:1331.

GREENWOOD M. 1928. A review of recent statistical studies of cancer problems. Cancer Rev 3:97–107.

GUTENSOHN N, COLE P. 1977. Epidemiology of Hodgkin's disease in the young. Int J Cancer 19:595–604.

HAENSZEL N, CORREA P. 1971. Cancer of the colon and rectum and adenomatous polyps. A review of epidemiologic findings. Cancer 28:14–24.

HAENSZEL W, KURIHARA M. 1968. Studies of Japanese migrants I. Mortality from cancer and other diseases among Japanese in the United States. J Natl Cancer Inst 40:43–68.

HAKAMA M, HAKULINEN T, LÄÄRÄ E. 1986. Predicting cancer incidence and prevalence. *In* Health Projections in Europe: Methods and Applications. Copenhagen, WHO Regional Office for Europe.

HAKULINEN T, TEPPO L, SAXEN E. 1978. Cancer of the eye. A review of trends and differentials. World Health Stat Q 31:143–158.

HANAI A, BENN T, FUJIMOTO I, MUIR CS. 1988. Comparison of lung cancer incidence rates by histological type in high and low incidence countries, with reference to the limited role of smoking. Jpn J Cancer Res (Gann) 79:445–452.

HANAI A, WHITTAKER JS, TATEISHI R, et al. 1987. Concordance of histological classification of lung cancer with special reference to adenocarcinoma in Osaka, Japan and the north-west region of England. Int J Cancer 39:6–9.

HAVILAND A. 1875. The Geographical Distribution of Diseases in Great Britain. London, Smith, Elder & Co.

HIGGINSON J. 1960. Population studies on cancer. Acta Union Int contra Cancrum XVI: 1667–1670.

HIGGINSON J, MUIR CS. 1979. Environmental carcinogenesis: misconceptions and limitations to cancer control. A review. J Natl Cancer Inst 63:1291–1298.

HIRSCH A. 1864. Handbuch der pathologischen und historischen Pathologie. Berlin.

HOFFMAN FL. 1915. The Mortality From Cancer Throughout the World. Newark, New Jersey, The Prudential Press, p. 605.

HOLMAN CD, ARMSTRONG BK. 1984. Cutaneous malignant melanoma and indicators of total accumulated exposure to sun: An analysis separating histogenetic type. J Natl Cancer Inst 73:75–82.

HOLMAN CDH, JAMES IE, SEGAL MR, ARMSTRONG K. 1981. Recent trends in mortality from prostate cancer in male populations of Australia and England and Wales. Br J Cancer 44:340–348.

JASKIEWICZ K, MARASAS WF, VAN DER WALT FE. 1987. Oesophageal and other main cancer patterns in four districts of Transkei 1981–1984. S Afr Med J 72:27–30.

KEMP I, BOYLE P, SMANS M, MUIR CS (EDS). 1985. Atlas of Cancer in Scotland 1975–1980. Incidence and Epidemiological Perspective. IARC Sci Publ 72. Lyon, International Agency for Research on Cancer.

KENNAWAY EL. 1944. Cancer of the liver in the Negro in Africa and America. Cancer Res 4:571–577.

KEPES JJ, CHEN WY, PANG LC, et al. 1984. Tumours of the central nervous system in Taiwan, Republic of China. Surg Neurol 22:149–156.

KERR DJ, BURT AD, BREWIN TB, BOYLE P. 1985. Divergence between mortality and incidence rates of thyroid cancer in Scotland. Lancet 2:149.

KMET J, MAHBOUBI E. 1972. Esophageal cancer in the caspian littoral of Iran: initial studies. Science 175:846–853.

KNUDSON AG. 1989. Hereditary cancers disclose a class of cancer genes. *In* Fortner JG, Rhoades JE, (eds). Accomplishments in Cancer Research. Philadelphia, Lippincott, pp. 91–98.

KRAMER S, MEADOWS AT, JARRETT P. 1984. Racial variations in incidence of Wilms' tumour—relationship to congenital anomalies. Med Pediatr Oncol 12:401–405.

KURIHARA M, AOKI K, TOMINAGA S (EDS). 1984. Cancer Mortality Statistics in the World. Nagoya, University of Nagoya Press.

LANIER AP, BENDER TR, BLOT WJ, et al. 1976. Cancer incidence in Alaska natives. Int J Cancer 18:409–412.

LEE HP, DAY NE, SHANMUGARATNAM K (EDS). 1988. Trends in

Cancer Incidence in Singapore 1968–1982. IARC Sci Publ 91. Lyon, International Agency for Research on Cancer.

LEE JAH, STRICKLAND D. 1980. Malignant melanoma—social status and outdoor work. Br J Cancer 41:757–763.

LEWIS MG. 1967. Malignant melanoma in Uganda. The relationship between pigmentation and malignant melanoma on the soles of the feet. Br J Cancer 21:483–495.

LI J, LIU B, LI G, ET AL (EDS). 1979. Atlas of Cancer Mortality in the People's Republic of China. Shanghai, China Map Press.

LOGAN WPD. 1982. Cancer mortality by occupation and social class 1851–1971. IARC Scientific Publications no. 36. Studies on Medical and Population Subjects No. 44. London, Her Majesty's Stationery Office, p. 31.

LU JB, YANG WX, LIU JM, et al. 1985. Trends in morbidity and mortality for esophageal cancer in Linxian county, 1959–1983. Int J Cancer 36:643–645.

MACLENNAN R, DE COSTA J, DAY NE, et al. 1977. Risk factors for lung cancer in Singapore Chinese, a population with high female incidence rates. Int J Cancer 20:854–860.

MAHBOUBI E, KMET J, COOK PJ, et al. 1973. Oesophageal cancer studies in the Caspian Littoral of Iran—the Caspian Cancer Registry. Br J Cancer 28:197–208.

MALKER HSR, MCLAUGHLIN JK, MALDER DK, et al. 1985. Occupational risks for pleural mesothelioma in Sweden 1961–1979. J Natl Cancer Inst 74:61–66.

MASON TJ, MCKAY FW, HOOVER R, FRAUMENI JF. 1975. Atlas of cancer mortality for US counties: 1950–1969. DHEW Publication no. 75-780. Washington, D.C., U.S. Government Printing Office.

MCDONALD MW, JOHSON DE, GUINEE VF. 1984. Testicular tumors in blacks. Urology 23:543–546.

MCMICHAEL AJ, MCCALL MG, HARTSTORNE JM, WOODINGS TL. 1980. Pattern of gastro-intestinal cancer in European migrants to Australia. The role of dietary change. Int J Cancer 25:431–437.

MEDAWAR PB. 1967. Hypothesis and imagination. *In* The Art of the Soluble, London, Methuen, pp. 131–155.

MEHNERT WH, SMANS M, MUIR CS, MÖHNER M, SCHÖN D. 1992. Atlas of Cancer Incidence in the Former German Democratic Republic 1978–1982. IARC Sci Publ 106. Lyon, International Agency for Research on Cancer.

MENAKANIT W, MUIR CS, JAIN DK. 1971. Cancer in Chiang Mai, North Thailand. A relative frequency study. Br J Cancer 25:225–236.

MILLER BA, RIES LAG, HANKEY BF, KOSARY CL, HARRAS A, DEVESA SS, EDWARDS BK (EDS). 1993. SEER Cancer Statistics Review: 1973–1990. NIH Publication no. 93-2789. Bethesda, National Cancer Institute.

MOOLGAVKAR SH, STEVENS RG. 1981. Smoking and cancer of bladder and pancreas. Risks and temporal trends. J Nat Cancer Inst 67:15–23.

MORSHOVITZ M, MODAN B. 1973. Role of sun exposure in the etiology of malignant melanoma—epidemiologic inferences. J Nat Cancer Inst 51:777–779.

MUIR CS. 1963. The alleged rarity of cancer in the Far East. Cancer (Philad) 16:812–818.

MUIR CS. 1973. Geographical differences in cancer patterns. *In* Doll R, Vodopija L (eds): Host Environment Interaction in the Etiology of Cancer in Man. IARC Sci Publ 7. Lyon, International Agency for Research on Cancer.

MUIR CS, CHOI NW, SCHIFFLERS E. 1980. Time trends in cancer mortality in some countries—their possible causes and significance. *In* Proceedings of the Skandia International Symposium, Stockholm, pp. 269–309.

MUIR CS, NECTOUX J. 1980. Geographical distribution and aetiology of kidney cancer. *In* Sufrin G, Beekley SA, (eds): Renal Adenocarcinoma. UICC Tech. Rep. Series no. 49. Geneva, International Union Against Cancer, pp 135–150.

MUIR CS, NECTOUX J. 1982. Time-trends, malignant melanoma of the skin. *In* Magnus K (ed): Trends in Cancer Incidence. New York, Plenum Press, pp. 365–385.

MUIR CS, SHANMUGARATNAM K. 1967. The incidence of nasopharyngeal cancer in Singapore. *In* Muir, CS, Shanmugaratnam, K (eds): Cancer of the Nasopharynx. UICC Monograph Series no. 1. Copenhagen, Munksgaard, pp. 47–53.

MUIR CS, STORM HH, POLEDAK A. 1993. Brain and other nervous system tumours. Cancer Surv 19/20: 369–392.

MUIR CS, WATERHOUSE J, MACK T, POWELL J, WHELAN S (EDS). 1987. Cancer Incidence in Five Continents, Vol. V. IARC Sci Publ 88. Lyon, International Agency for Research on Cancer.

MUÑOZ N, BOSCH FX, JENSEN OM (EDS). 1989. Human Papillomavirus and Cervical Cancer. IARC Sci Publ 94. Lyon, International Agency for Research on Cancer.

MUÑOZ N, BOSCH FX. 1989. Epidemiology of cervical cancer. In Muñoz N, Bosch FX, Jensen OM (eds.): Human Papillomavirus and Cervical Cancer. IARC Sci Publ 94. Lyon, International Agency for Research on Cancer. pp. 9–39.

NAPALKOV NP, TSERKOVY GF, MERABISHVILI VM, PARKIN DM, SMANS M, MUIR CS (EDS). 1983. Cancer Incidence in the USSR (Supplement to Cancer Incidence in Five Continents, vol. III). IARC Sci Publ 48. Lyon, International Agency for Research on Cancer.

NATIONAL BOARD OF HEALTH AND WELFARE. 1984. The Cancer Registry. Cancer Incidence in Sweden 1981. Stockholm, Socialstyrelsen.

NATIONAL CANCER INSTITUTE. 1988. 1987 Annual Cancer Statistics Review Including Cancer Trends 1950–1985. NIH Publication no. 88-2789. Bethesda, National Cancer Institute.

OFFICE OF POPULATION CENSUSES AND SURVEYS (OPCS). 1978. Occupational Mortality. The Registrar-General's Decennial Supplement for England and Wales, 1970–1972. Series DS no 1. London, Her Majesty's Stationery Office.

OLAYA F, NECTOUX J. 1987. Le cancer en Ardèche du Nord, Incidence 1983–86. Registre des Tumeurs de l'Ardèche du Nord. Annonay.

ORR IM. 1933. Oral cancer in betel nut chewers in Travancore: its aetiology, pathology and treatment. Lancet 2:575–580.

OSTERLIND A. 1987. Trends in incidence of ocular malignant melanoma in Denmark, 1943–1982. Int J Cancer 40:161–164.

PARKIN DM (ED). 1986. Cancer Occurrence In Developing Countries. IARC Sci Publ 75. Lyon, International Agency for Research on Cancer.

PARKIN DM, LÄÄRÄ E, MUIR CS. 1988a. Estimates of the worldwide frequency of sixteen major cancers in 1980. Int J Cancer, 41:184–197.

PARKIN DM, MUIR CS, WHELAN SW, GAO Y-T, FERLAY J, POWELL J. (EDS). 1992. Cancer Incidence in Five Continents, Vol. VI. IARC Sci Publ no. 120. Lyon, International Agency for Research on Cancer.

PARKIN DM, PISANI P, FERLAY J. 1993. Estimates of the worldwide incidence of eighteen major cancers in 1985. Int J Cancer 54:594–606.

PARKIN DM, STILLER CA, BIEBER CA (EDS). 1988b. International Incidence of Childhood Cancer. IARC Sci Publ 87. Lyon, International Agency for Research on Cancer.

PARKIN DM, STJERNSWARD J, MUIR CS. 1984. Estimates of the world-wide frequency of twelve major cancers. Bull WHO 62:163–182.

PEARL DK, SCOTT EL. 1986. The anatomical distribution of skin cancers. Int J Epidemiol 15:502–506.

PERCY C, MUIR CS. 1989. The international comparability of cancer mortality data. Results of an international death certificate study. Am J Epidemiol 129:934–946.

PERCY C, STANEK E, GLOECKLER L. 1981. Accuracy of cancer death certificates and its effect on cancer mortality statistics. Am J Public Health 71:242–250.

PERCY C, VAN HOLTEN V, MUIR CS (EDS). 1990. ICD–O. International Classification of Diseases for Oncology, 2nd ed. Geneva, World Health Organization.

PERCY C, YOUNG JL, MUIR CS, RIES L, HANKEY BF, SOHIM LH, BERG JW. 1995. Histology of cancer. Incidence and prognosis. SEER population based data 1973–1987. Cancer 75:139–422.

REDDY CRRM, GOPAL RT, VENKATARATHNAM G, et al. 1977. A study of 10 patients with penile carcinoma combined with cervical biopsy study of their wives. Int Surg 62:549–553.

REGISTRE GENEVOIS DES TUMEURS. 1988. Cancer à Genève: Incidence, Mortalité et Survie 1970–1986. Geneva, Registre Genevois des Tumeurs.

RIOS-DALENZ J, CORREA P, HAENSZEL W. 1981. Morbidity from cancer in La Paz, Bolivia. Int J Cancer 28:307–314.

ROSE E. 1973. Esophageal cancer in the Transkei, 1955–1969. J Natl Cancer Inst 51:716.

SAMITZ MH. 1980. Dermatology in Tanzania—problems and solutions. Int J Dermatol 19:102–106.

SASCO AJ, HUBERT A, DE THÉ G. 1985. Diet and nasopharyngeal carcinoma: epidemiological approach to comparative dietary assessment in different populations. *In* Joosens JV, et al (eds): Diet and Human Carcinogenesis. New York, Elsevier Science Publishers (Biomedical Division).

SCHAIRER C, HARTGE P, HOOVER RN, SILVERMAN DT. 1988. Racial differences in bladder cancer risk: A case-control study. Am J Epidemiol 128:1027–1037.

SEGI INSTITUTE OF CANCER EPIDEMIOLOGY. 1964. Age-adjusted death rates for cancer for selected sites in 46 countries.

SHANMUGARATNAM K. 1982. Nasopharynx. *In* Schottenfeld D, Fraumeni JF (eds): Cancer Epidemiology and Prevention. Philadelphia, W.B. Saunders Company, pp. 536–553.

SHANMUGARATNAM K, MUIR CS, TOW SH, et al. 1971. Rates per 100,000 births and incidence of choriocarcinoma and malignant mole in Singapore Chinese and Malays. Comparison with Connecticut, Norway and Sweden. Int J Cancer 8:165–175.

SHARP L, BLACK RJ, HARKNESS EL, FINLAYSON AR, MUIR CS. 1993. Cancer Registration Statistics Scotland 1981–1990. Edinburgh, Information and Statistics Division.

SILVESTRI F, BUSSANI R, GIARELLI L. 1991. Changes in underlying causes of death during 85 years of autopsy practice in Trieste. *In* Riboli E, Delendi M (eds): Autopsy in Epidemiology and Medical Research. IACR Sci Publ 112. Lyon, International Agency for Research on Cancer, pp. 3–24.

SMANS M, MUIR CS, BOYLE P (EDS). 1992. Atlas of Cancer Mortality in the European Economic Community. IARC Sci Publ 107. Lyon, International Agency for Research on Cancer.

SONDIK E, YOUNG JL, HORM JW, RIES LAG (EDS). 1986. 1985 Annual Cancer Statistics Review. NIH Publication 86-2789. Bethesda, National Cancer Institute.

SRIVATANAKUL S, SONTIPONG P, CHOTIWAN P, PARKIN DM. 1988. Liver cancer in Thailand: Temporal and geographic variations. J Gastroenterol Hepatol 3:413–420.

STASZEWSKI J. 1972. Migrant studies in alimentary tract cancer. Recent Results Cancer Res 39:85–97.

STASZEWSKI J, HAENSZEL W. 1965. Cancer mortality among the Polish-born in the US. J Natl Cancer Inst 35:291–297.

STEINITZ R, PARKIN DM, YOUNG JL, BIEBER CA, KATZ L (EDS). 1989. Cancer Incidence in Jewish Migrants to Israel 1961–1981. IARC Sci Publ 98. Lyon, International Agency for Research on Cancer.

STOCKS P. 1928. On the evidence for a regional distribution of cancer in England and Wales. Report of the International Conference on Cancer. London, British Empire Cancer Campaign, pp. 508–519.

STRICKLAND D, LEE JAH. 1981. Melanomas of eye—stability of rates. Am J Epidemiol 113:700–702.

SZMUNESS W. 1978. Hepatocellular carcinoma and the Hepatitis B virus: evidence for a causal association. Prog Med Virl. 24:40–69.

TANCHOU S. 1843. Recherches sur la fréquence du cancer. Gaz. Hôpit. p. 313.

TOMINAGA S. 1987. Decreasing trend of stomach cancer in Japan. Jpn J Cancer Res (Gann) 78:1–10.

TRICHOPOULOS D, OURANOS G, DAY NE, et al. 1985. Diet and cancer of the stomach: a case-control study in Greece. Int J Cancer 36:291–297.

TULINIUS H. 1970. Frequency of some morphological types of neoplasm of five sites. *In* Doll R, Muir C, Waterhouse J (eds): Cancer Incidence in Five Continents, Vol. III. Berlin, Springer-Verlag, pp. 23–83.

TUYNS AJ, ESTÈVE J, RAYMOND L. 1988. Cancer of the larynx/hypopharynx, tobacco and alcohol: IARC international case-control study in Turin and Varese (Italy), Zaragoza and Navarra (Spain), Geneva (Switzerland) and Calvados (France). Int J Cancer 41:483–491.

TUYNS AJ, MASSÉ G. 1975. Cancer of the oesophagus in Brittany. An incidence study in Ille-et-Vilaine. Int J Epidemiol 4:55–59.

TUYNS AJ, OBRADOVIC M. 1975. Unexpected high incidence of primary liver cancer in Geneva, Switzerland. J Natl Cancer Inst 54:61–64.

VAN DER ESCH EP, MUIR CS, NECTOUX J, et al. 1991. Temporal change in diagnostic criteria as a cause of the increase of malignant melanoma over time is unlikely. Int J Cancer 47:483–490.

VERLEZ R, BERAL V, CUZICK J. 1982. Increasing trends of multiple myeloma mortality in England and Wales, 1950–1979. Are the changes real? J Natl Cancer Inst 69:387–392.

VIGOTTI MA, CISLAGHI C, BALZI D, GIORGI D, LA VECCHIA C, MARCHI M, DECARLI A, ZANETTI R. 1988. Cancer mortality in migrant populations within Italy. Tumori 74:107–128.

WALKER WJ, BRIN BN. 1988. US Lung cancer mortality and declining cigarette tobacco consumption. J Clin Epidemiol 41:179–185.

WATERHOUSE J, MUIR CS, CORREA P, et al. 1976. Cancer Incidence in Five Continents, Volume III. IARC Scientific Publication No. 15, Lyon, IARC.

WORLD HEALTH ORGANIZATION. 1988. World Health Statistics Annual. Geneva, World Health Organization, pp. 513.

WORLD HEALTH ORGANIZATION. 1976. ICD–O. International Classification of Diseases for Oncology. Geneva, World Health Organization.

WORLD HEALTH ORGANIZATION. 1977. International Statistical Classification of Diseases, Injuries and Causes of Death Based on the Recommendations of the 9th Revision Conference, 1975, Vol. I and II. Geneva, World Health Organization.

YOUNG JL, PERCY CL, ASIRE AJ. (eds). 1981. Surveillance, Epidemiology and End Results. Incidence and Mortality Data 1973–77. NCI Monograph 57, NIH Publication no. 81-2330. Bethesda, National Cancer Institute.

11–I Cancer incidence, mortality, and patient survival in the United States

LYNN A. GLOECKLER RIES
BENJAMIN F. HANKEY
ANGELA HARRAS
SUSAN S. DEVESA

Reliable assessment of the impact of cancer on the general population is predicated upon the availability of measurements related to cancer incidence, mortality, and patient survival. While population-based cancer mortality data have been available for nearly a century, before 1973 cancer incidence data were obtainable primarily from periodic surveys conducted in selected geographic areas of the U.S. during the periods 1937–39, 1947–48 (Dorn and Cutler, 1959) and 1969–71 (Cutler and Young, 1975). Before 1973, the National Cancer Institute (NCI) collected cancer patient survival data mainly on hospital-based cases through the End Results Program (Axtell et al, 1976).

The Surveillance, Epidemiology and End Results (SEER) Program, the successor to the End Results Program and the periodic incidence surveys, has collected population-based data on newly diagnosed cancers since 1973 for approximately ten percent of the U.S. population. The SEER Program is an ongoing contract-supported program of the NCI that funds and coordinates the collection of cancer data in population-based cancer registries located throughout the U.S. These registries, while not randomly selected, are thought to be reasonably representative of the U.S. population; a number of the registries cover diverse populations of particular epidemiologic interest. For this chapter data from nine SEER registries were used: the states of Connecticut, Iowa, Utah, New Mexico, and Hawaii; and the metropolitan areas of Atlanta, Detroit, Seattle (Puget Sound), and San Francisco-Oakland (Table 11–I–1). Incidence, mortality, and survival data are published annually by the SEER Program. The volume, *SEER Cancer Statistics Review, 1973–1991: Tables and Graphs* (CSR) (Ries et al, 1994a), contains data from 1973 to 1991 and is the primary source for much of the data in this chapter.

MATERIAL AND METHODS

The SEER Program collects information on the demographic characteristics of the patient, anatomic site of the malignancy, histologic cell type, extent (stage) of the disease at time of diagnosis, treatment, and follow-up, including survival status and cause of death.

The intent here is to provide the reader with an overview of the recent data available on cancer for all races and, in many instances, for whites and blacks sepa-

TABLE 11–I–1. *Populations by Race for Nine SEER Participants—1990 Census Data*

Area	*All Races*	*White*	*Black*
United States	248,709,874	208,704,165	30,483,281
Total SEER	23,553,609	18,972,426	2,574,897
% of U.S.	9.5	9.1	8.4
Northeast			
Connecticut	3,287,116	2,946,216	282,103
South			
Atlanta	2,177,495	1,462,579	662,495
North Central			
Detroit	3,912,679	2,901,269	939,968
Iowa	2,776,755	2,694,907	48,417
West			
Hawaii	1,108,229	379,248	27,947
New Mexico	1,515,069	1,330,645	31,651
San Francisco-Oakland	3,686,592	2,617,921	433,876
Seattle-Puget Sound	3,366,824	2,988,282	136,358
Utah	1,722,850	1,651,359	12,082

We thank Joan Hartel of IMS, Inc., for figure development and R. Scott Depuy of IMS, Inc., for data analysis and table generation.

TABLE 11–I–2. *Comparison of U.S. and SEER Cancer Mortality for Whites by Site and Sex, 1987–1991**

Site	U.S. Mortality			SEER Mortality		
	Total	Male	Female	Total	Male	Female
ALL SITES	172.8	220.2	141.1	163.3	201.6	138.7
ORAL CAVITY AND PHARYNX	3.0	4.6	1.7	2.8	4.1	1.7
Lip	0.0	0.1	0.0	0.0	0.1	0.0
Tongue	0.7	1.0	0.4	0.7	1.0	0.4
Salivary gland	0.2	0.3	0.1	0.2	0.3	0.1
Floor of mouth	0.1	0.2	0.1	0.1	0.2	0.1
Gum and other mouth	0.5	0.7	0.3	0.4	0.6	0.3
Nasopharynx	0.3	0.4	0.2	0.2	0.2	0.1
Tonsil	0.2	0.3	0.1	0.2	0.3	0.1
Oropharynx	0.2	0.3	0.1	0.2	0.3	0.1
Hypopharynx	0.2	0.3	0.1	0.2	0.3	0.1
Other buccal cavity and pharynx	0.6	0.9	0.3	0.5	0.7	0.2
DIGESTIVE SYSTEM	40.6	52.7	31.7	38.0	48.7	30.1
Esophagus	3.5	6.0	1.5	3.0	5.1	1.4
Stomach	4.8	7.0	3.1	4.3	6.5	2.8
Small intestine	0.3	0.4	0.3	0.3	0.4	0.3
Colon and rectum	19.1	23.6	16.0	18.1	22.1	15.4
Anus, anal canal, and anorectum	0.1	0.1	0.1	0.2	0.1	0.2
Liver and intrahepatic	2.8	4.1	1.8	2.4	3.4	1.6
Liver	2.4	3.5	1.5	1.9	2.9	1.2
Intrahepatic bile duct	0.4	0.5	0.4	0.5	0.5	0.4
Gallbladder	0.7	0.5	0.9	0.7	0.4	0.9
Other biliary	0.6	0.7	0.5	0.6	0.7	0.5
Pancreas	8.4	10.0	7.2	8.0	9.5	6.9
Retroperitoneum	0.1	0.1	0.1	0.1	0.1	0.1
Peritoneum, omentum, and mesentery	0.1	0.1	0.1	0.1	0.1	0.1
Other digestive organs	0.2	0.2	0.1	0.1	0.2	0.1
RESPIRATORY SYSTEM	51.1	78.2	31.3	46.1	67.2	30.9
Nose, nasal cavity, and middle ear	0.2	0.2	0.1	0.2	0.2	0.1
Larynx	1.4	2.5	0.5	1.2	2.1	0.5
Lung and bronchus	49.3	74.9	30.5	44.5	64.2	30.2
Pleura	0.2	0.3	0.1	0.2	0.4	0.1
Trachea, mediastinum, and other respiratory organs	0.1	0.2	0.1	0.1	0.2	0.1
BONES AND JOINTS	0.4	0.5	0.3	0.4	0.5	0.3
SOFT TISSUE (including heart)	1.1	1.3	1.1	1.2	1.3	1.0
SKIN (excluding basal and squamous)	2.9	4.3	1.9	3.0	4.3	2.0
Melanomas of skin	2.2	3.1	1.5	2.4	3.2	1.7
Other non-epithelial skin	0.7	1.3	0.3	0.6	1.1	0.3
BREAST	15.3	0.2	27.3	15.4	0.2	27.7
FEMALE GENITAL SYSTEM	8.4	—	14.9	8.1	—	14.5
Cervix uteri	1.6	—	3.0	1.1	—	2.1
Corpus uteri	1.0	—	1.8	1.9	—	3.3
Uterus, NOS[a]	1.0	—	1.7	0.8	—	1.5
Ovary	4.4	—	7.8	4.6	—	8.3
Vagina	0.1	—	0.2	0.1	—	0.2
Vulva	0.2	—	0.3	0.2	—	0.3
Other female genital organs	0.1	—	0.2	0.1	—	0.2
MALE GENITAL SYSTEM	9.9	26.0	—	9.4	24.8	—
Prostate	9.7	25.6	—	9.2	24.4	—
Testis	0.1	0.3	—	0.1	0.2	—
Penis	0.1	0.2	—	0.1	0.1	—
Other male genital organs	0.0	0.0	—	0.0	0.0	—

(continued)

TABLE 11–I–2. *Comparison of U.S. and SEER Cancer Mortality for Whites by Site and Sex, 1987–1991* (Continued)*

Site	U.S. Mortality			SEER Mortality		
	Total	*Male*	*Female*	*Total*	*Male*	*Female*
URINARY SYSTEM	6.8	10.8	4.1	6.7	10.7	4.0
Urinary bladder	3.2	5.7	1.7	3.2	5.7	1.6
Kidney and renal pelvis	3.4	5.0	2.3	3.3	4.7	2.3
Ureter	0.1	0.1	0.1	0.1	0.2	0.1
Other urinary organs	0.1	0.1	0.1	0.1	0.1	0.0
EYE AND ORBIT	0.1	0.1	0.1	0.1	0.1	0.1
BRAIN AND NERVOUS SYSTEM	4.2	5.1	3.5	4.6	5.5	3.8
Brain	4.1	5.0	3.4	4.5	5.4	3.7
Cranial nerves and other nervous system	0.1	0.1	0.1	0.1	0.1	0.1
ENDOCRINE SYSTEM	0.7	0.7	0.6	0.6	0.6	0.6
Thyroid	0.3	0.3	0.4	0.3	0.3	0.3
Other endocrine (including thymus)	0.3	0.4	0.3	0.3	0.3	0.2
LYMPHOMAS	6.7	8.4	5.5	7.1	8.8	5.7
Hodgkin's disease	0.6	0.7	0.4	0.6	0.8	0.4
Non-Hodgkin's lymphoma	6.2	7.6	5.0	6.5	8.0	5.2
MULTIPLE MYELOMA	2.9	3.7	2.4	2.8	3.4	2.3
LEUKEMIAS	6.3	8.3	4.9	6.4	8.3	5.0
ILL-DEFINED AND UNSPECIFIED SITES	12.2	15.2	9.9	10.7	12.9	9.1

*Mortality rates are per 100,000 person-years and are age-adjusted to the 1970 U.S. standard million population.
[a]NOS, not otherwise specified.

rately. Incidence and mortality data are based on 479,729 newly diagnosed malignancies, 213,345 cancer deaths among residents of the SEER areas, and 2,432,671 cancer deaths in the total U.S. during the period 1987–91. Trends are based on data from 1973–91. Incidence data are presented for all malignant neoplasms by primary site and are classified according to the *International Classification of Diseases for Oncology* (ICD–O) (WHO, 1976, 1986, 1988). While in situ cancers of all primary sites have been collected, they are not included in the rates except in those for bladder cancer because the distinction between in situ and early invasive bladder cancer has not been consistent, either among pathologists or over time.

Mortality data are obtained annually from the National Center for Health Statistics. The underlying cause of death is used in calculating mortality rates for both the entire U.S. and the SEER areas.

Incidence and mortality rates are presented as the number of events per 100,000 people at risk per year (person-years) and are age-adjusted by the direct method. An age-adjusted rate is a weighted average of the age-specific rates with the weights being the proportion of persons in corresponding age groups of a standard population which, in the present analysis, is the 1970 standard million population of the U.S.

Relative survival rates are presented by stage for patients diagnosed from 1983 to 1990 with follow-up through 1991. In order that a patient not be represented in multiple cohorts, survival time is computed from the time of diagnosis of the patient's first primary cancer only; all cases identified by death certificate only, autopsy only, and all cases with unknown survival time are excluded from the survival analysis. Relative survival rates estimate the likelihood that a patient will not die from causes directly related to the malignancy in question within a specific time period following diagnosis, the conventional survival interval being five years. The relative survival rate is obtained by correcting the observed survival rate for expected mortality using a procedure described by Ederer et al (1961). Survival rates are presented for all races by sex.

Trends in incidence and mortality rates from 1973 through 1991 are included in the CSR (Ries et al, 1994a) and figures are presented here only for those cancers presented where trends are noteworthy. The analysis of trends is based on two measures of change for the period 1973 to 1991: the total percent change and the estimated annual percent change (EAPC). The EAPC is obtained by fitting a straight line through the natural logarithms of the yearly rates over the period 1973 to 1991 using standard least squares procedures. The trends refer to incidence from the SEER areas and mortality for the total U.S., not just SEER areas. Mortality data for the total U.S. are used because such trends are of utmost importance in understanding the total cancer picture. These figures use the same arithmetic *x*-axis, whereas the *y*-axis is logarithmic with the maximum 20 times the minimum value, resulting in slopes that are comparable not only within but also between figures. The *y:x*–axis ratio has been chosen such that a slope of 10 degrees portrays a rate of change of 1% per year (Devesa et al, 1995). Unless otherwise specified, the incidence rates presented in the tables in this chapter are the average annual rates for 1987–91 for the SEER areas and the mortality rates are the average annual rates for 1987–91 for the U.S. Rates for each single year, 1973 to 1991, are presented in the CSR for the major cancer sites. Analysis of long-term trends may be found in the report by Devesa et al (1987) and the *1987 Annual Cancer Statistics Review* (National Cancer Institute, 1988). Estimates for the number of new cases in 1994 are provided by the American Cancer Society and are based on SEER data for 1988–90 (American Cancer Society, 1994).

Before the SEER data can be offered as a measure of cancer incidence and patient survival for the entire U.S., an assessment of how well the SEER areas represent the nation as a whole is essential. Since incidence data for the entire U.S. do not exist, SEER area mortality rates were compared with total U.S. mortality rates for specific cancers in white males and females (Table 11–I–2). There are few differences between the two sets of rates for females, whereas the total rate for males is about 8% lower in the SEER areas than in the total U.S. More than half of the difference is due to lung cancer, with several gastrointestinal sites also contributing. SEER includes Utah where abstinence from tobacco and alcohol use among the large Mormon population has resulted in low mortality rates. The close approximation of the mortality rates for SEER to the total U.S. population for most cancers provides some confidence that the experience in the SEER areas is reasonably representative of the total U.S. population and that the temporal trends are similar.

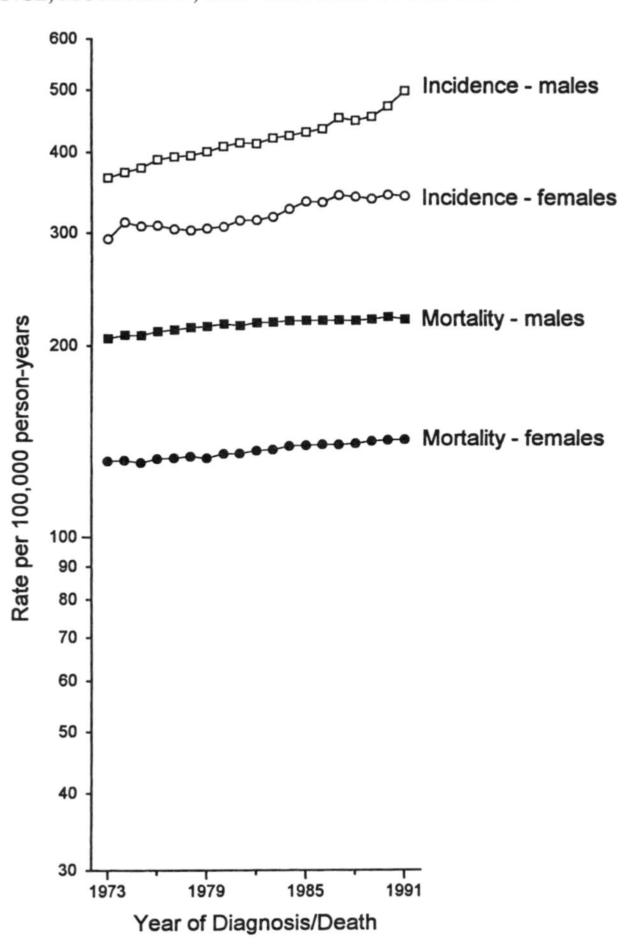

FIG. 11–I–1. All cancers combined, age-adjusted (1970 Standard) SEER incidence and United States mortality rates by sex, 1973–91.

RESULTS

During 1994, approximately 1,208,000 malignancies were diagnosed and 538,000 persons died due to cancer in the United States. From 1973 to 1991, the overall cancer mortality rates (Fig. 11–I–1) increased only slightly (between 7 and 8%) while incidence rates increased 31 and 14% among males and females, respectively. Since 1974 the five-year relative survival rate increased 5 percentage points—from 49 to 54%.

Overall cancer incidence (1987–91) was highest among black males (557.2) followed by white males (464.0), white females (348.0), and black females (331.8). Rates and trends for all cancers combined serve primarily as an indicator of the overall cancer burden on the population and by definition are the composite of many forms of cancer. Patterns of incidence, mortality, and survival for individual malignancies may vary because of differences in demographic characteristics, influences of screening programs, or lifestyle and environmental changes, and a myriad of other factors. Therefore, the remainder of this chapter will focus on individual cancers. Incidence and mortality rates by organ system are presented in Tables 11–I–3 through 11–I–11 and 11–I–13, and survival rates are presented in Tables 11–I–12, 11–I–14, and 11–I–15.

ORAL CAVITY AND PHARYNX

Cancers of the oral cavity and pharynx account for less than 3% of all cancers diagnosed in the U.S. each year; they were diagnosed in approximately 29,600 people in 1994, two-thirds of whom were males. Over the 19-year period covered by the SEER program, the incidence rate among males dropped by 7.4% while remaining stable among females. Mortality for these cancers declined 18.3% over the same time period, decreasing 22.7% in whites while rising 9.5% among blacks.

Individually, these cancers have very low incidence rates, the highest being 2.2 for cancer of the tongue; the incidence rates for the remaining subgroups are extremely low, ranging from .3 to 2.0 (Table 11–I–3). Survival for patients with cancer of the oral cavity or pharynx vary by subsite. Malignancies of the lip (excluding the skin of the lip) have a more favorable extent of disease distribution at diagnosis and a far better five-year survival rate (94%) than any of the other subsites (Table 11–I–15). While each of these cancers appears infrequently, they have had different trends with some decreasing (lip and floor of mouth) and others increasing.

Lip

Cancer of the lip is one of the more frequently diagnosed cancers of the oral cavity with an overall incidence rate of 1.2 and an associated five-year relative survival rate of 94%. From 1973 to 1991 the incidence decreased by 53.2%. Among whites the incidence was more than 6 times higher in males (2.6) than in females (0.3). The rate for blacks, however, was 0.1 for each sex.

Salivary Gland

Cancer of the salivary gland is relatively rare, occurring in less than 1 per 100,000. Nearly 50% of salivary gland cancers are diagnosed while the cancer is still confined to the salivary gland (localized stage); five-year relative survival was 91% for localized stage and 72% for all stages combined.

Nasopharynx

Cancer of the nasopharynx is a rare tumor occurring at a rate of 0.6 per 100,000 and is more frequent among

TABLE 11–I–3. *Oral Cavity and Pharynx, Average Annual Cancer Incidence and Mortality Rates per 100,000 Person-Years by Race and Sex, SEER Areas, 1987–1991**

	All Races			*Whites*			*Blacks*		
	Total	*Male*	*Female*	*Total*	*Male*	*Female*	*Total*	*Male*	*Female*
INCIDENCE									
ORAL CAVITY AND PHARYNX	10.8	16.4	6.2	10.5	15.8	6.2	14.0	23.7	6.5
Lip	1.2	2.3	0.3	1.3	2.6	0.3	0.1	0.1	0.1
Tongue	2.2	3.2	1.3	2.1	3.1	1.3	3.0	5.3	1.2
Salivary gland	0.9	1.2	0.7	0.9	1.2	0.7	0.9	1.1	0.7
Floor of mouth	1.1	1.7	0.7	1.1	1.6	0.7	1.7	2.9	0.8
Gum and other mouth	2.0	2.6	1.4	2.0	2.6	1.4	2.4	3.6	1.5
Nasopharynx	0.6	0.9	0.4	0.4	0.6	0.3	0.6	1.1	0.3
Tonsil	1.1	1.6	0.6	1.0	1.5	0.6	2.0	3.5	0.8
Oropharynx	0.3	0.5	0.2	0.3	0.5	0.2	0.6	0.9	0.3
Hypopharynx	1.1	1.8	0.4	1.0	1.7	0.4	1.9	3.7	0.4
Other buccal cavity and pharynx	0.4	0.6	0.2	0.4	0.6	0.2	0.9	1.5	0.4
MORTALITY									
ORAL CAVITY AND PHARYNX	3.0	4.6	1.7	2.7	4.2	1.6	5.2	9.2	2.3
Lip	0.0	0.1	0.0	0.0	0.1	0.0	0.0	0.0	0.0
Tongue	0.7	1.0	0.4	0.6	0.9	0.4	1.2	2.1	0.5
Salivary gland	0.2	0.3	0.1	0.2	0.3	0.1	0.2	0.3	0.1
Floor of mouth	0.1	0.2	0.1	0.1	0.2	0.1	0.2	0.4	0.1
Gum and other mouth	0.5	0.7	0.3	0.5	0.6	0.3	0.8	1.2	0.4
Nasopharynx	0.3	0.4	0.2	0.2	0.3	0.1	0.3	0.6	0.2
Tonsil	0.2	0.3	0.1	0.2	0.3	0.1	0.5	0.9	0.2
Oropharynx	0.2	0.3	0.1	0.2	0.3	0.1	0.4	0.8	0.1
Hypopharynx	0.2	0.3	0.1	0.2	0.3	0.1	0.4	0.8	0.1
Other buccal cavity and pharynx	0.6	0.9	0.3	0.5	0.8	0.3	1.2	2.2	0.4

*Incidence and mortality rates are age-adjusted to the 1970 U.S. standard million population.

males than among females, 0.9 and 0.4, respectively. Fifty-one percent of all nasopharyngeal malignancies have regional involvement at diagnosis with an associated five-year relative survival rate of 49%, which is similar to the five-year relative survival rate of 47% for all stages combined.

Tongue, Other Mouth, and Pharynx

The tongue is the most frequent primary site of oral cavity cancer. Incidence is nearly twice as high among males (3.2) as among females (1.3). The highest occurrence is among black males whose incidence rate of 5.3 is more than 4 times that for black females (1.2). The mortality rate for all races combined is 0.7. Forty percent of tongue cancers are localized and 41% have regional spread at the time of diagnosis. The five-year relative survival rate for all stages combined is 47%.

The aggregate of tongue, other mouth, and pharyngeal cancers accounts for 72–90% of all oral cavity and pharyngeal cancer cases and more than 80% of the deaths. Incidence rates for this aggregated group are highest among black males (21.4), dropping to 11.4 among white males, and lowest among females (5.4 and 4.9 among blacks and whites, respectively).

Oral cancers are diagnosed at earlier stages than pharyngeal cancers, thus resulting in better overall survival rates. Cancers of the hypopharynx, only 12% of which are diagnosed while localized, have an overall five-year survival rate of 25%. The anatomical inaccessibility and histologic complexity of certain oral and pharyngeal cancers coupled with their infrequent occurrence contribute to a relatively low rate of early diagnosis as well as poor survival. Cancer of the base of the tongue, for example, tends toward early, silent, and deep infiltration. Since the base of the tongue can only be visualized by indirect mirror examination, early asymptomatic lesions are rarely diagnosed (DeVita et al, 1989). Another factor contributing to the poor prognosis for this group of tumors is the extreme vascularity of the entire area, which promotes rapid development of lymph node involvement and metastases.

DIGESTIVE SYSTEM

Malignancies of the digestive system currently account for nearly 20% of all cancers in the U.S. Of these, 64% arise in the colon and rectum, 12% in the pancreas, and 10% in the stomach.

Five-year relative survival rates vary from 3% for pancreatic cancer to around 60% for anus and large intestine. Even when diagnosed while localized, cancers of the esophagus, liver, and pancreas have five-year relative survival rates of only 20, 15 and 9%, respectively.

Esophagus

Cancer of the esophagus is a rare malignancy with an overall incidence rate of 3.9, occurring more than three times more frequently in males than females (Table 11–I–4). The rate for white males (5.5) is less than one-third the rate for black males (17.1). Survival is poor; only 9% of patients survive five years or more.

Stomach

Stomach cancer occurs more than twice as often among males as among females (11.6 and 5.0, respectively). From 1950 to 1991 there was a 75% drop in incidence and a 77% decline in the death rate. In more recent years, 1973 to 1991, the incidence of stomach cancer decreased 26 and 25% for males and females, respectively, and mortality decreased 31 and 34% for males and females, respectively (Fig. 11–I–2). Current SEER data show an incidence rate of 7.8, a mortality rate of 4.8, and a five-year relative survival rate of 19%. Both incidence and mortality rates are nearly twice as high among blacks as among whites. For both males and females, incidence and mortality rates are higher among blacks than whites.

Colon and Rectum

Accounting for 149,000 new cases each year, cancers of the colon and rectum combined constitute the most frequently diagnosed malignancy after cancers of the lung, prostate, and breast. Colorectal cancer incidence increased until 1985 when it peaked and then subsequently decreased among both males and females (Fig. 11–I–3). The incidence trends differed by race–sex group, decreasing by 6.6% among white females while increasing by 3.0, 36.1, and 20.0% among white males, black males, and black females, respectively. Recent incidence declines have become apparent among all race–sex groups except black males. Colon cancer incidence, excluding rectum, is 34.5 per 100,000 (40.7 for males and 29.9 for females). The rate for blacks is now about 20% higher (40.6) than that for whites (34.0 per 100,000). More than half of all colon cancers occur either in the sigmoid (35%) or cecum (22%). An additional 12% occur in the ascending colon, 10% in the transverse colon, and 7% in the descending colon (National Cancer Institute, 1988). Subsite incidence patterns vary by sex, race, age, and time period (Devesa and Chow, 1993).

Colon cancer occurs at a rate two and a half times that for rectal cancer (13.8). Rectal cancer occurs less frequently among blacks than whites (11.9 compared to 13.8), and more often among males than females in

TABLE 11–I–4. *Digestive System, Average Annual Cancer Incidence and Mortality Rates per 100,000 Person-Years by Race and Sex, SEER Areas, 1987–1991**

	All Races			*Whites*			*Blacks*		
	Total	*Male*	*Female*	*Total*	*Male*	*Female*	*Total*	*Male*	*Female*
INCIDENCE									
DIGESTIVE SYSTEM	77.2	97.4	62.1	74.0	93.2	59.8	99.8	127.6	79.8
Esophagus	3.9	6.4	1.9	3.4	5.5	1.7	10.0	17.1	4.7
Stomach	7.8	11.6	5.0	6.7	10.1	4.2	12.7	19.4	7.9
Small intestine	1.2	1.5	1.0	1.2	1.5	1.0	2.2	2.9	1.8
Colon and rectum	48.2	58.9	40.4	47.8	58.7	39.9	52.4	60.9	46.7
Colon, excluding rectum	34.5	40.7	29.9	34.0	40.4	29.5	40.6	46.2	36.8
Rectum and rectosigmoid	13.8	18.2	10.4	13.8	18.3	10.4	11.9	14.7	9.9
Anus, anal canal, and anorectum	0.9	0.8	1.0	0.9	0.8	1.0	1.1	1.1	1.0
Liver and intrahepatic bile duct	3.0	4.7	1.8	2.4	3.6	1.5	4.7	7.8	2.4
Liver only	2.7	4.2	1.4	2.0	3.1	1.2	4.4	7.3	2.2
Gallbladder	1.1	0.7	1.4	1.0	0.6	1.3	1.0	0.9	1.1
Other biliary	1.1	1.4	0.9	1.1	1.3	0.9	0.9	1.1	0.8
Pancreas	9.0	10.4	7.9	8.6	10.1	7.5	13.8	15.1	12.7
Retroperitoneum	0.4	0.5	0.3	0.4	0.5	0.3	0.5	0.5	0.5
Peritoneum, omentum, and mesentery	0.2	0.2	0.2	0.2	0.2	0.3	0.2	0.2	0.2
Other digestive organs	0.2	0.3	0.2	0.2	0.3	0.2	0.3	0.5	0.2
MORTALITY									
DIGESTIVE SYSTEM	40.6	52.7	31.7	38.8	50.2	30.4	59.4	79.9	45.0
Esophagus	3.5	6.0	1.5	3.0	5.2	1.2	8.5	15.1	3.7
Stomach	4.8	7.0	3.1	4.3	6.3	2.8	8.9	13.8	5.6
Small intestine	0.3	0.4	0.3	0.3	0.4	0.2	0.5	0.6	0.4
Colon and rectum	19.1	23.6	16.0	18.8	23.3	15.6	23.5	28.0	20.6
Colon, excluding rectum	—	—	—	—	—	—	—	—	—
Rectum and rectosigmoid	—	—	—	—	—	—	—	—	—
Anus, anal canal, and anorectum	0.1	0.1	0.1	0.1	0.1	0.1	0.2	0.2	0.2
Liver and intrahepatic bile duct	2.8	4.1	1.8	2.5	3.6	1.7	4.2	6.3	2.6
Liver only	2.4	3.5	1.5	2.1	3.1	1.3	3.8	5.8	2.3
Gallbladder	0.7	0.5	0.9	0.7	0.5	0.9	0.7	0.5	0.8
Other biliary	0.6	0.7	0.5	0.6	0.7	0.5	0.5	0.6	0.4
Pancreas	8.4	10.0	7.2	8.1	9.7	6.9	11.9	14.2	10.3
Retroperitoneum	0.1	0.1	0.1	0.1	0.1	0.1	0.1	0.2	0.1
Peritoneum, omentum, and mesentery	0.1	0.1	0.1	0.1	0.1	0.1	0.1	0.1	0.1
Other digestive organs	0.2	0.2	0.1	0.1	0.2	0.1	0.3	0.3	0.2

*Incidence and mortality rates are age-adjusted to the 1970 U.S. standard million population.

both blacks (14.7 and 9.9) and whites (18.3 and 10.4 per 100,000). There has been a slight decline in the overall incidence rate since 1973.

More than one-third of colorectal cancers are diagnosed while localized and about 20% have distant disease. Patients with colorectal cancer have an overall five-year relative survival rate of about 60%, but it varies from about 90% to less than 10%, depending on the stage.

Separating mortality rates for cancer of the colon from that of the rectum is inappropriate since mortality rates for rectal cancer are underestimated; in death certification practices colon cancer is often designated as the underlying cause of death when the hospital diagnosis was rectal cancer (Percy et al, 1981). The impact of this misclassification has changed over time (Chow and Devesa, 1992). The combined colorectal mortality rates since 1973 have declined by 15.5% with an EAPC of −1.0% (Fig. 11–I–3). Mortality rates decreased for both white males (11.2%) and females (23.6%) while they increased for both black males (25.1%) and females (3.8%).

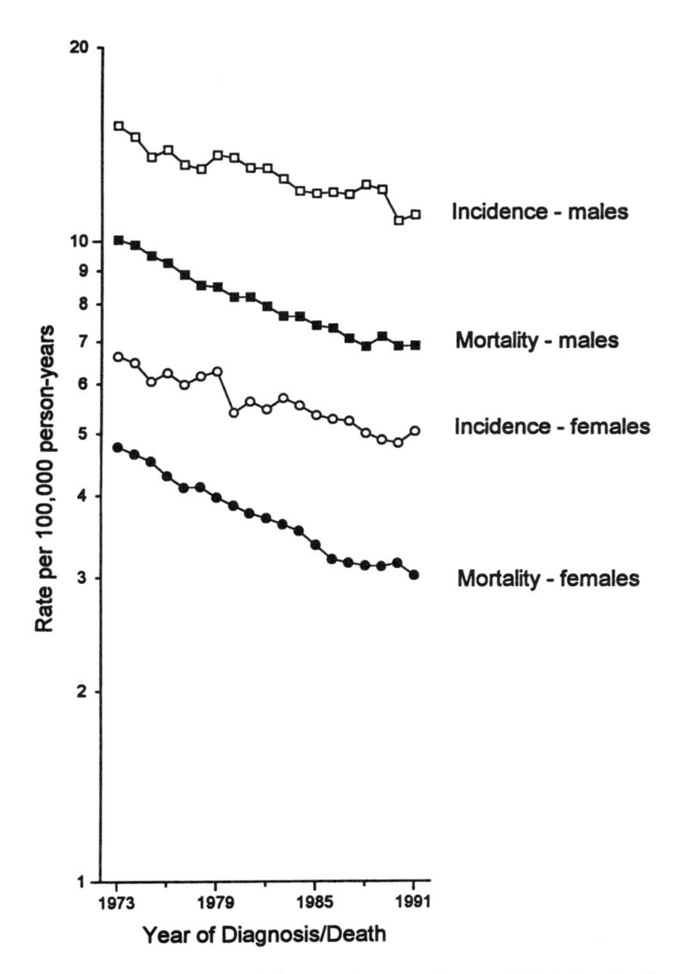

FIG. 11–I–2. Cancer of the stomach, age-adjusted (1970 Standard) SEER incidence and United States mortality rates by sex, 1973–91.

Liver

Primary cancers of the liver and intrahepatic bile duct are rare, with an overall incidence rate of only 3.0 per 100,000. The category includes hepatocellular carcinomas and to a lesser extent, intrahepatic bile duct cancers. The incidence rate for blacks (4.7) is higher than that for whites (2.4) and more than twice as high among males (4.7) as among females (1.8). The five-year relative survival rate for all stages is only 6%, but reaches 15% for localized tumors. Reported mortality rates for liver cancer overestimate the true rates because many deaths attributed to liver cancer on the death certificate may in reality be deaths due to cancers which have metastasized to the liver (Percy et al, 1990b).

Pancreas

Although incidence and mortality rates have declined slightly, cancers of the pancreas still account for about 26,000 deaths annually. The incidence rate among blacks (13.8) is more than 60% higher than that among whites (8.6). The malignancy occurs more frequently in males than in females, 10.4 and 7.9, respectively. The five-year relative survival rate of 3%, which is the poorest of any malignancy, has remained unchanged for years. Even when the disease is diagnosed while still localized, the five-year survival rate is only 9%. Due to such poor survival, the mortality rates are only slightly lower than the incidence rates; current mortality figures are 10.0 for males and 7.2 for females.

RESPIRATORY SYSTEM

Lung

In 1994 lung cancer was diagnosed in approximately 172,000 people: 100,000 males and 72,000 females.

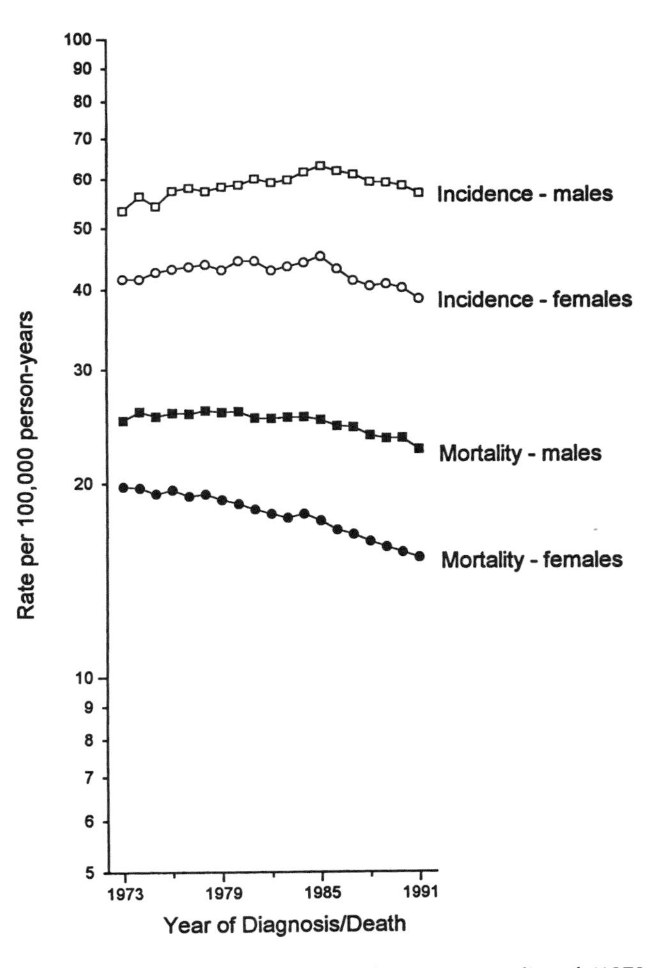

FIG. 11–I–3. Cancer of the colon and rectum, age-adjusted (1970 Standard) SEER incidence and United States mortality rates by sex, 1973–91.

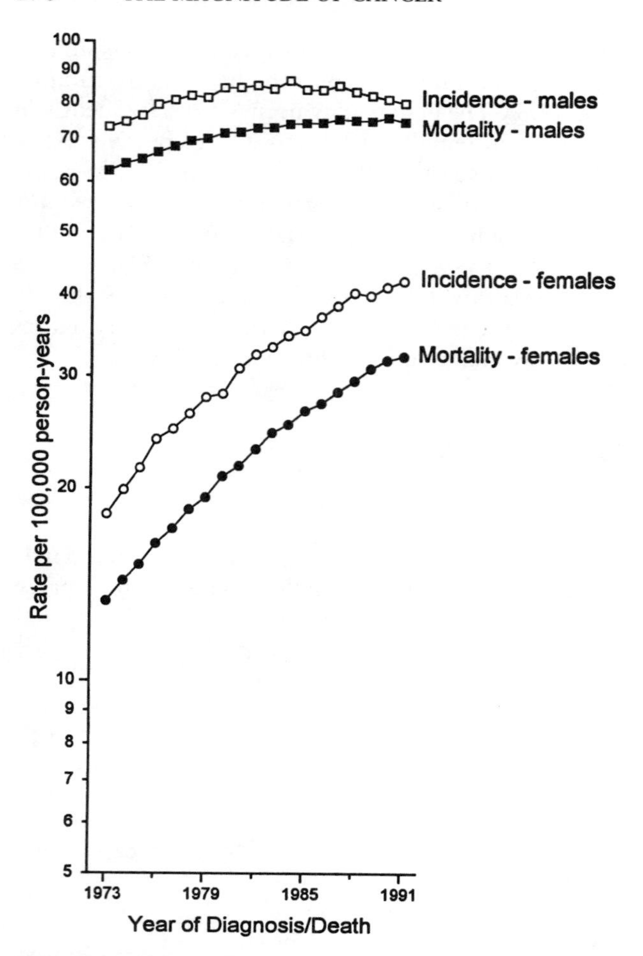

FIG. 11–I–4. Cancer of the lung, age-adjusted (1970 Standard) SEER incidence and United States mortality rates by sex, 1973–91.

For males, lung cancer incidence is second only to cancer of the prostate, and for females, it is second only to cancer of the breast.

After increasing for many years, the incidence of lung cancer among males decreased between the mid-1980s and the early 1990s (Fig. 11–I–4), apparently peaking in 1984 among both white and black males. The incidence among both white and black females increased approximately 5% per year, more than doubling between 1973 and 1991. Rates declined among the young and middle-aged, in contrast to continuing increases among the elderly (Devesa et al, 1989), with the changing trends most striking for squamous cell carcinoma (Devesa et al, 1991). Lung cancer mortality among blacks has exceeded the incidence among whites in recent years (Fig. 11–I–5).

The 1987–91 lung cancer incidence rate for white males (80.7) was almost double that for white females (41.3) (Table 11–I–5). Differences in incidence by sex were even greater among blacks; the rate for males (122.4) was more than two and a half times that for females (44.5). Even though the incidence of lung cancer among black males was more than 50% higher than white males, white and black females had similar rates.

Survival following lung cancer is generally poor—only 13% at five years. For the 15% for whom the cancer has not spread beyond the lung, i.e., the localized stage, the five-year relative survival rate is 43% for males and over 50% for females. In 1994 there were 153,000 deaths (94,000 males and 59,000 females) attributed to lung cancer, which is more than to any other cancer. The lung cancer mortality rate has increased 19% for males and 131% for females since 1973 (Fig. 11–I–4). In recent years the rate among males has levelled off at around 75 per 100,000. For females of all races combined, the lung cancer mortality rate of 28.3 in 1987 first exceeded the breast cancer mortality rate of 27.1. This first occurred in 1986 for white females but not until 1991 for black females.

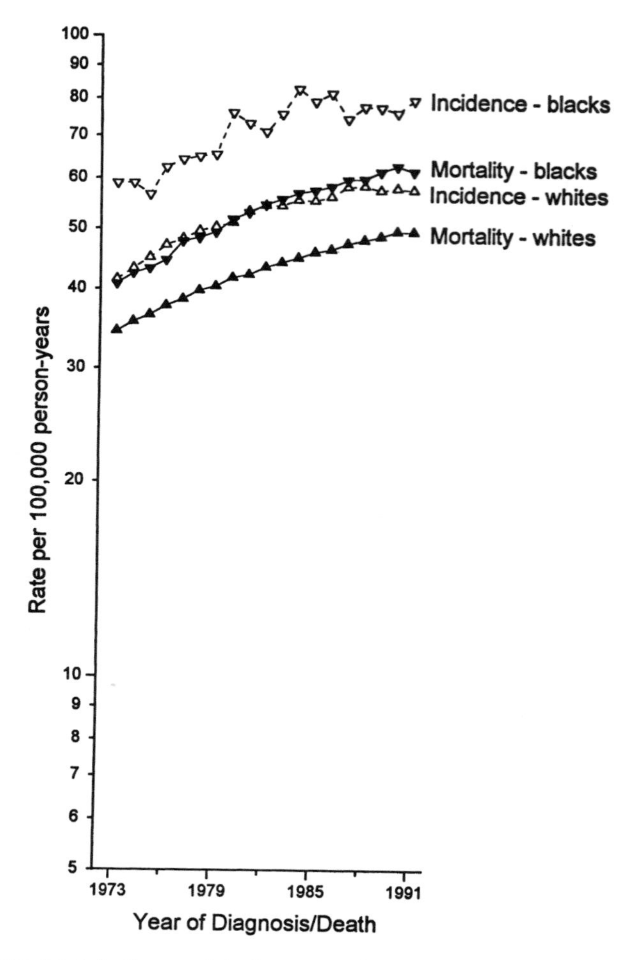

FIG. 11–I–5. Cancer of the lung, age-adjusted (1970 Standard) SEER incidence and United States mortality rates by race, 1973–91.

TABLE 11–I–5. *Respiratory System, Average Annual Cancer Incidence and Mortality Rates per 100,000 Person-Years by Race and Sex, SEER Areas, 1987–1991**

	All Races			*Whites*			*Blacks*		
	Total	*Male*	*Female*	*Total*	*Male*	*Female*	*Total*	*Male*	*Female*
INCIDENCE									
RESPIRATORY SYSTEM	64.3	92.5	43.0	64.0	91.1	43.8	85.7	137.5	48.1
Nose, nasal cavity, and middle ear	0.6	0.8	0.5	0.6	0.7	0.5	0.7	0.9	0.6
Larynx	4.5	7.9	1.7	4.4	7.8	1.7	7.1	13.0	2.7
Lung and bronchus	58.2	82.1	40.4	57.9	80.7	41.3	77.2	122.4	44.5
Pleura	0.7	1.4	0.2	0.8	1.5	0.3	0.4	0.8	0.2
Trachea, mediastinum, and other respiratory organs	0.2	0.3	0.2	0.2	0.3	0.2	0.2	0.4	0.1
MORTALITY									
RESPIRATORY SYSTEM	51.1	78.2	31.3	50.3	76.0	31.6	64.5	111.8	31.6
Nose, nasal cavity, and middle ear	0.2	0.2	0.1	0.2	0.2	0.1	0.3	0.4	0.2
Larynx	1.4	2.5	0.5	1.2	2.3	0.5	2.8	5.4	0.9
Lung and bronchus	49.3	74.9	30.5	48.6	73.0	30.9	61.2	105.5	30.4
Pleura	0.2	0.3	0.1	0.2	0.3	0.1	0.1	0.1	0.0
Trachea, mediastinum, and other respiratory organs	0.1	0.2	0.1	0.1	0.2	0.1	0.2	0.3	0.1

*Incidence and mortality rates are age-adjusted to the 1970 U.S. standard million population.

Larynx

Although less than one-tenth as frequent as lung cancer, cancer of the larynx is the second most frequently diagnosed malignancy in the respiratory system, with an overall incidence rate of 4.5 per 100,000. The incidence rate for males is more than four times that for females, 7.9 versus 1.7. The highest incidence, 13.0, is found among black males. Since 50 percent are diagnosed while localized, the five-year relative survival rate is 67 percent for all stages combined, which is considerably better than that for lung cancer.

Mesothelioma

Incidence rates for all mesotheliomas in white males nearly doubled from 1974 to 1991 (from 0.9 to 1.7 per 100,000), while the rate for white females remained at about 0.4. Rates for males aged 75–84 have more than tripled from 4.6 to 16.6 per 100,000 between 1973 and 1991. Although it is a rare malignancy, it has become the focus of intense interest because of its strong association with asbestos exposure. Rates during 1973–84 were even higher in Seattle, Hawaii, and San Francisco-Oakland, 2.1, 1.9, and 1.7, respectively, where asbestos exposures in the ship-building industry were prevalent during World War II (Connelly et al, 1987).

BONES AND JOINTS, SOFT TISSUES, AND SKIN

Bones and Joints

Cancers of the bones and joints are very rare; the incidence rate is less than one per 100,000 with slightly higher rates among whites than blacks. The current five-year relative survival rate for all stages combined is 57%.

Soft Tissues

The overall incidence rate for soft tissue malignancies is 2.1 and it is lower among females than among males (Table 11–I–6). For children, incidence increased 27% while mortality decreased 71% from 1973 to 1991. The five-year relative survival rate for all ages combined was 62 percent.

Melanoma of the Skin

Melanoma of the skin accounts for slightly less than 3% of all malignancies. It is especially common among whites (12.4) but occurs rarely among blacks (0.9). Incidence increased 94% from 1973 to 1991, or more rapidly than for any other major primary site except for female lung cancer and male prostate cancer. Incidence

TABLE 11–I–6. *Bone, Soft Tissue, and Skin, Average Annual Cancer Incidence and Mortality Rates per 100,000 Person-Years by Race and Sex, SEER Areas, 1987–1991**

	All Races			*Whites*			*Blacks*		
	Total	*Male*	*Female*	*Total*	*Male*	*Female*	*Total*	*Male*	*Female*
INCIDENCE									
BONES AND JOINTS	0.8	0.9	0.7	0.9	1.0	0.8	0.6	0.5	0.6
SOFT TISSUE (including heart)	2.1	2.6	1.8	2.1	2.5	1.7	2.6	3.0	2.2
SKIN (excluding basal and squamous)	15.0	20.1	10.6	16.5	21.9	11.8	4.3	7.1	1.9
Melanomas of skin	11.1	13.1	9.7	12.4	14.5	10.9	0.9	1.2	0.7
Other non-epithelial skin	3.9	7.0	0.9	4.0	7.3	0.8	3.3	5.9	1.2
MORTALITY									
BONES AND JOINTS	0.4	0.5	0.3	0.4	0.5	0.3	0.5	0.6	0.4
SOFT TISSUE (including heart)	1.1	1.3	1.1	1.1	1.3	1.0	1.4	1.5	1.4
SKIN (excluding basal and squamous)	2.9	4.3	1.9	3.2	4.7	2.1	1.3	2.1	0.7
Melanomas of skin	2.2	3.1	1.5	2.5	3.4	1.7	0.4	0.5	0.4
Other non-epithelial skin	0.7	1.3	0.3	0.7	1.2	0.4	0.9	1.6	0.3

*Incidence and mortality rates are age-adjusted to the 1970 U.S. standard million population.

has generally been higher among males (13.1) than among females (9.7). The overall five-year relative survival rate is 85%, ranging from a high of 93% for patients with localized disease to 15% for those with distant disease. Melanomas occurring on the skin of male and female genitalia including the vagina, vulva, scrotum, and penis are reported as cancers of the specific organ and are not included here.

Skin (Basal and Squamous Cell)

Data on basal and squamous cell carcinomas of the skin are not collected by the SEER program. While these are the most frequently diagnosed of all malignancies, they are about 99% curable and are usually diagnosed and treated in an ambulatory setting. A separate survey of non-melanoma skin cancer conducted in the 1970s estimated an incidence rate among whites of 231.3 (Scotto et al, 1983).

Kaposi's Sarcoma

Prior to the 1980s, Kaposi's sarcoma occurred mostly in specific areas of Africa where it accounted for approximately 10% of all malignancies. Infrequent occurrences in the United States were seen among older males of Jewish or Italian ancestry (DeVita et al, 1989). With the emergence of the acquired immune deficiency syndrome (AIDS), Kaposi's sarcoma became a frequent response to the compromised immune system and the incidence among high risk populations in the United States increased accordingly. Among males aged 20–54 from 1973 to 1979, the SEER Program counted a total of 18 cases (0.1/100,000). The rate in all SEER geographic areas combined increased from 0.1 in 1980 to 15.3 in 1989 for males aged 20–54. The rate appears to have decreased slightly after 1989 to 13.9 in 1991. Men in this age group in San Francisco County experienced the most dramatic increase of all SEER areas when, by 1988, the rate of Kaposi's sarcoma reached 211.6 per 100,000 compared to a rate of zero in 1973–79. In areas of the SEER Program other than San Francisco, rates among males aged 20–54 increased to 6.5 in 1989–90 (Ries et al, 1994a).

FEMALE BREAST

There were approximately 183,000 diagnoses of invasive breast cancer in 1994, only 1,000 of which were in males. Female breast cancer incidence has varied somewhat since the beginning of the SEER Program in 1973 (Fig. 11–I–6). In 1974 the incidence rate spiked when women reacted to the highly publicized breast cancer diagnoses in two nationally prominent women and sought out diagnostic testing in greater than usual numbers. The rate subsequently fell. However, since 1980, the rate has been increasing rather dramatically—from 85.2 per 100,000 to a peak of 112.4 in 1987, and subsequently levelled off. These increases have been observed in both white and black females both under 50

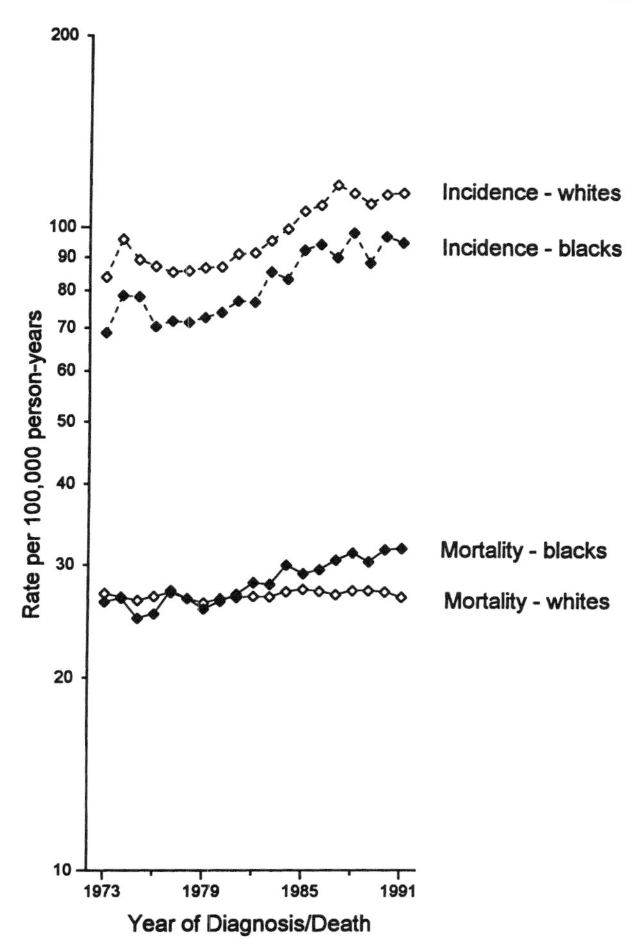

FIG. 11–I–6. Cancer of the female breast, age-adjusted (1970 Standard) SEER incidence and United States mortality rates by race, 1973–91.

and 50 years and older. The increases in incidence have been confined to women with early stage disease. Further, the increase is confined to women with small tumors, implying that the increased utilization of mammography may be partially responsible (Miller et al, 1993). The incidence rate has remained lower among blacks: 94.0 in black females versus 113.2 in white females during 1987–91.

Survival for breast cancer patients has remained relatively stable, although there was a small increase in the five-year relative rate from 75 to 77% for white females diagnosed during the periods 1974–76 and 1980–82, respectively. The survival rate for those diagnosed in 1983–90, however, jumped substantially to 82% due in part to increased screening and earlier diagnosis.

For females diagnosed during 1983–90, survival was poorer for blacks than for whites, with five-year relative rates being 66 and 82%, respectively. Blacks also had a prognostically less favorable stage distribution, with only 45% diagnosed while localized compared to 56% for whites.

Approximately 46,000 females died from breast cancer in 1994. The U.S. mortality rate for breast cancer has increased only 1.8% since 1973. For whites, breast cancer mortality only increased 0.6% while rates among blacks increased 20%. Among white females under 50 years of age, breast cancer mortality decreased 14% and increased 2% among blacks. For women aged 50 and older, mortality rates rose 4% and 26% among whites and blacks, respectively, resulting in an excess risk among blacks during the early 1980s.

FEMALE GENITAL SYSTEM

Cancers of the corpus uteri and uterus, not otherwise specified (NOS) account for over 40% of all malignancies of the female genital system. Ovarian cancer accounts for approximately 32% of such malignancies and cervical cancer, 20%. Malignancies of the vagina, vulva, and other female genital organs are rare. In situ lesions are not included in the tabulations.

Cervix Uteri

Both incidence and mortality for cervical cancer have decreased substantially over the past four decades, due at least in part to widespread use of the pap smear and advances in diagnostic techniques. From 1950 to 1991 the incidence for white females decreased 76%, while mortality decreased 74%.

Rates among blacks were about twice those for whites, or 14.0 versus 7.8 for incidence and 6.7 versus 2.6 for mortality, respectively, during 1987–91 (Table 11–I–7). Only one-half of all cases are diagnosed while the cancer is localized, i.e., still confined to the cervix uteri. Survival rates range from 90% for those women diagnosed with localized disease to 12% for distant disease, suggesting that mortality could be further reduced by improved early diagnosis.

Corpus Uteri

From 1950 to 1991 the incidence trends for cancer of the corpus uteri remained generally in the low 20s. However, shortly after the use of postmenopausal estrogens gained wide acceptance, the incidence rate increased to 32.1 in 1975. When this association was identified, the rates fell sharply as the number of prescriptions decreased and dosages were modified.

Accurate estimation of corpus uterine cancer rates is

TABLE 11–I–7. *Breast and Female Genital System, Average Annual Cancer Incidence and Mortality Rates per 100,000 Person-Years by Race and Sex, SEER Areas, 1987–1991**

	All Races		*Whites*		*Blacks*	
	Male	*Female*	*Male*	*Female*	*Male*	*Female*
INCIDENCE						
BREAST	0.9	109.5	0.9	113.2	1.4	94.0
FEMALE GENITAL SYSTEM	—	47.6	—	48.5	—	42.0
Cervix uteri	—	8.6	—	7.8	—	14.0
Corpus uteri	—	20.9	—	21.9	—	13.8
Uterus, NOS[a]	—	0.3	—	0.3	—	0.7
Ovary	—	14.8	—	15.6	—	10.3
Vagina	—	0.6	—	0.5	—	1.0
Vulva	—	1.7	—	1.8	—	1.4
Other female genital organs	—	0.7	—	0.7	—	0.8
MORTALITY						
BREAST	0.2	27.3	0.2	27.2	0.4	31.2
FEMALE GENITAL SYSTEM	—	14.9	—	14.5	—	20.1
Cervix uteri	—	3.0	—	2.6	—	6.7
Corpus uteri	—	1.8	—	1.7	—	2.7
Uterus, NOS	—	1.7	—	1.5	—	3.2
Ovary	—	7.8	—	8.0	—	6.5
Vagina	—	0.2	—	0.2	—	0.4
Vulva	—	0.3	—	0.3	—	0.3
Other female genital organs	—	0.2	—	0.2	—	0.2

*Incidence and mortality rates are age-adjusted to the 1970 U.S. standard million population.
[a]NOS, not otherwise specified.

complicated by the inclusion of women who have had hysterectomies in the population estimates. The prevalence of women with an intact uterus varies by geography, race, and time period, resulting in varying underestimations of the true risk of this cancer (Pokras and Hufnagel, 1987). This would not account, however, for the rapid changes in the incidence rates.

Patients with cancer of the corpus uteri have the most favorable prognosis of any gynecologic malignancy, with an 83% five-year relative survival rate for all stages combined. Trends in survival for this cancer seem to correspond to the increase in incidence of early lesions in the mid 1970s. The five-year relative survival rate was 88% in 1975 and 83% in 1986. The survival rate for whites is about 30 percentage points higher than that for blacks. The black–white survival differential is 12 percentage points for the under-50 age group.

Incidence is nearly 60% higher among whites (21.9) than among blacks (13.8). Cancer of the uterus, NOS is combined with that for cancer of the corpus uteri since most of these cancers probably originate in the corpus (Percy et al, 1990a). Mortality, however, is higher among blacks due to their much poorer survival rate (Fig. 11–I–7). Mortality from cancer of the corpus uteri and uterus, NOS decreased over the past 19 years by 25% for whites and 20% for blacks.

Ovary

Incidence rates for ovarian cancer increased slightly between 1973 and 1991. Since borderline lesions have only been collected in recent years, they must be excluded in order to evaluate the real trend. When borderline lesions are excluded, the incidence rate decreased among women under 65 and increased slightly for women 65 and over (Ries et al, 1994a). Incidence rates are more than 50% higher among whites, and mortality rates are more than 20% higher among whites than blacks (Fig. 11–I–8).

The silence of this disease in its early stages has impeded early detection efforts, and survival rates have remained poor. Of all ovarian cancers diagnosed from 1983 to 1990, 52% were detected in an advanced stage, with a five-year relative survival rate of only 21%. In contrast, the rate was 90% among those diagnosed with localized disease (23% of cases). The rate for all stages combined was 42%.

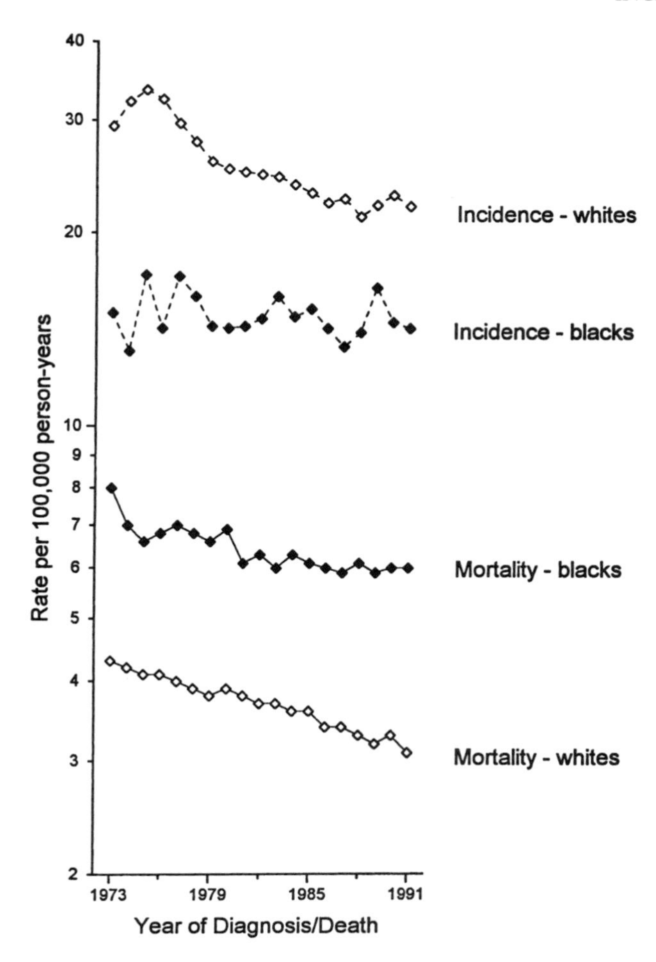

FIG. 11–I–7. Cancer of the corpus and uterus, NOS, age-adjusted (1970 Standard) SEER incidence and United States mortality rates by race, 1973–91.

MALE GENITAL SYSTEM

Genital cancers account for about 33% of all cancers diagnosed in males. Of all male genital cancers, cancer of the prostate accounts for over 95%.

Prostate

Incidence of prostate cancer is 35% higher among blacks than among whites. American blacks have the highest incidence of prostate cancer in the world (Parkin et al, 1992). Between 1973 and 1991, the incidence rates in the U.S. increased 127% among white males, while among black males the rate rose 82% (Fig. 11–I–9). There is indirect evidence that the increasing incidence over the period 1973–86 may be due to increased detection of clinically asymptomatic cases associated with increasing rates of transurethral resection of the prostate (TURP) for benign prostatic hyperplasia (Potosky et al, 1990). The increases after 1987 do not seem to be associated with TURPs. During the late 1980s, increases in incidence were seen for all stages except distant. At the same time, there were increases in the use of tests to detect prostate cancer, such as transrectal ultrasound-guided needle biopsy, and in particular, blood testing for prostate-specific antigen (PSA), which suggests that the observed increases in incidence are surveillance related (Potosky et al, 1995).

From 1973 to 1991, mortality increased less rapidly than incidence, 21% among whites and 39% among blacks. Mortality among blacks was more than twice that among whites (Table 11–I–8). Survival for patients with prostate cancer increased from 67% in 1974–76 to 80% in 1983–90. The five-year relative survival rates for 1983–90 were 66.4% among blacks and 81.3% among whites, reflecting the more favorable stage distribution at diagnosis among whites. Among cases diagnosed in 1983–90, survival was 85% for those with regional disease but fell to 29% for distant disease.

Testis

Cancer of the testis is a rare malignancy that mainly affects young adult males (median age, 32 years). Incidence rose 43% between 1973 and 1991, with the rate 6 times more common among whites (5.1) than among blacks (0.8).

Survival for patients with this malignancy is favorable and improvement in survival has been dramatic, increasing from 79% for the years 1974–76 to 93% for the years 1983–90. Survival increases were seen for both whites and blacks. As a result, the mortality rate for all races combined decreased 67% since 1973. In recent years, 63% of all cases were diagnosed while in the localized stage, with a 98% five-year relative survival rate. Even with distant metastases the survival rate has been 68%.

Penis

Cancer of the penis is rare among both blacks and whites in the United States, accounting for less than 1% of all male genital cancers. Sixty-five percent of all cases are diagnosed while localized, and the overall five-year relative survival rate is currently 69%.

URINARY SYSTEM

Cancers of the urinary tract, of which bladder cancer is the most common, are more than three times as frequent

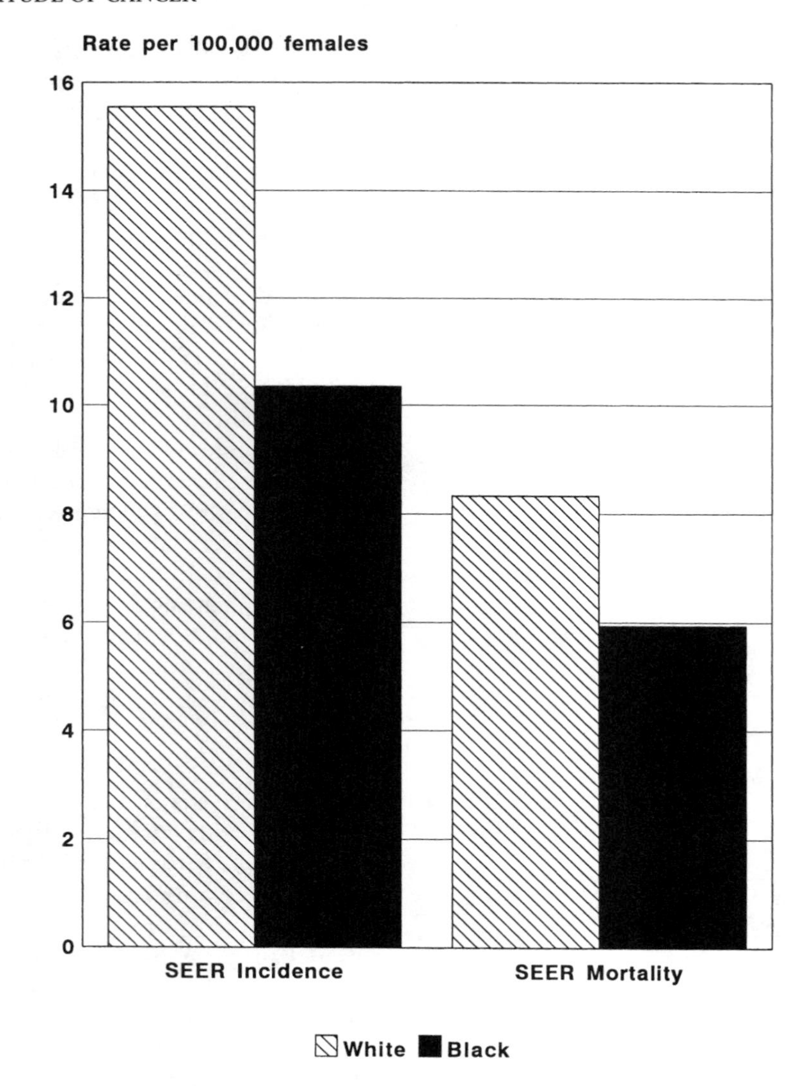

FIG. 11–I–8. Cancer of the ovary, age-adjusted (1970 Standard) SEER incidence and United States mortality, 1987–91.

in males than in females (43.2 and 13.8, respectively) and about 40% more frequent among whites than among blacks (27.7 and 19.9, respectively).

Urinary Bladder

Cancer of the bladder is predominantly a disease among white males, whose incidence rate is 32.3, more than twice that among black males (15.0), four times that among white females (7.8), and more than five times that among black females (5.9) (Table 11–I–9). Bladder cancer is a disease of later life with a median age at diagnosis of 70 years. In contrast to other cancers which only include invasive cancer, in situ cancer is combined with invasive cancer as the distinction is particularly difficult to make.

Incidence of bladder cancer increased between 1973 and 1991 for each race–sex group and increased relatively more among blacks than among whites (26 and 13%, respectively). In contrast, the mortality rates decreased. The mortality rate for both blacks and whites is 3.3. The male-to-female mortality ratio is 3.6 to 1 for whites and 2 to 1 for blacks.

The current five-year survival rate for all stages combined is 80%; for cancer diagnosed while still localized, the rate is 92%. The survival rate for whites (81%) is considerably higher than that for blacks (60%), partially reflecting the large difference in the proportion diagnosed while still localized, 74% for whites and only 57% for blacks. However, even within each stage, survival differences by race persist. In situ cancers are grouped with localized disease for bladder cancer.

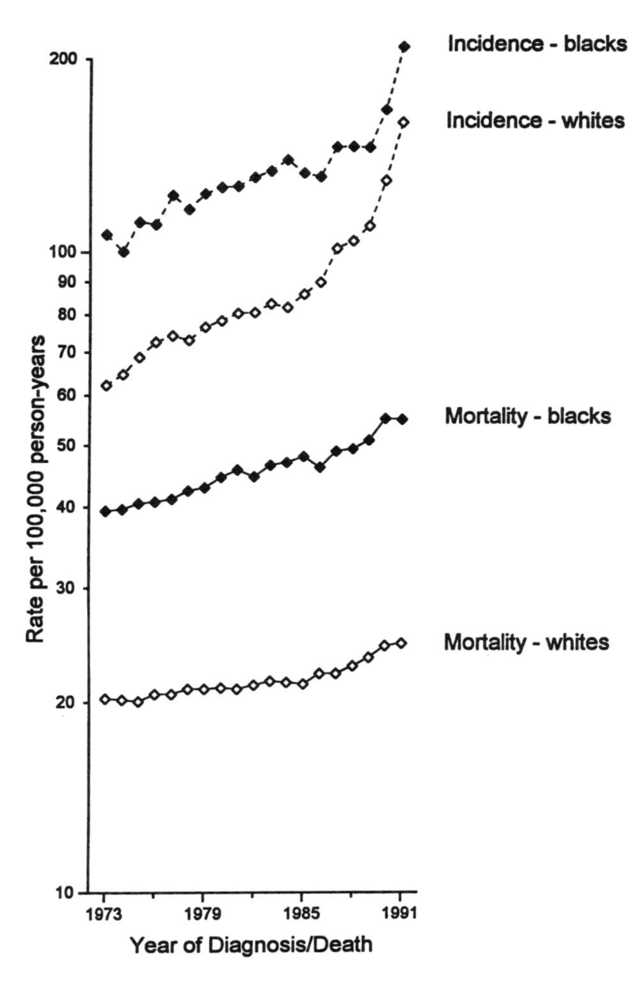

FIG. 11–I–9. Cancer of the prostate, age-adjusted (1970 Standard) SEER incidence and United States mortality rates by race, 1973–91.

Kidney and Renal Pelvis

The median age for cancer of the kidney and renal pelvis, 66 years, is less than that for bladder cancer, 70 years of age. The incidence increased 35% from 1973 to 1991, while mortality increased 17%. Risk and incidence patterns are different by site and cell type (Devesa et al, 1990). Whites and blacks experienced similar incidence rates (8.8 and 9.5, respectively) and mortality rates (3.5 and 3.3, respectively), with male-to-female ratios for both at about 2. The five-year relative survival rate for all stages is 56%; however, for localized cancer the rate is 87%.

EYE, NERVOUS SYSTEM, AND ENDOCRINE SYSTEM

This is a mixed group whose combined incidence in the general population was about 12 per 100,000 during the period 1987–91. Ocular and orbital cancer occurred at a rate of 0.7; brain and central nervous system cancer, 6.2; and endocrine cancer, 5.0 (Table 11–I–10).

Eye

Over 75% of all malignancies of the eye are melanomas; another 13% are retinoblastomas, most of which occur in childhood (DeVita et al, 1989). Although incidence rates are higher among whites than among blacks, mortality rates are similar, or less than 0.2 per 100,000 in each group. The five-year relative survival rate is 77%.

TABLE 11–I–8. *Male Genital System, Average Annual Cancer Incidence and Mortality Rates per 100,000 Person-Years by Race, SEER Areas, 1987–1991**

	All Races	*Whites*	*Blacks*
	Male	*Male*	*Male*
INCIDENCE			
MALE GENITAL SYSTEM	128.4	127.2	165.0
Prostate gland	123.0	121.2	163.1
Testis	4.5	5.1	0.8
Penis	0.7	0.7	0.9
Other male genital organs	0.3	0.3	0.3
MORTALITY			
MALE GENITAL SYSTEM	26.0	24.0	52.5
Prostate gland	25.6	23.6	52.0
Testis	0.3	0.3	0.1
Penis	0.2	0.1	0.3
Other male genital organs	0.0	0.0	0.0

*Incidence and mortality rates are age-adjusted to the 1970 U.S. standard million population.

TABLE 11–I–9. *Urinary System, Average Annual Cancer Incidence and Mortality Rates per 100,000 Person-Years by Race and Sex, SEER Areas, 1987–1991**

	All Races			*Whites*			*Blacks*		
	Total	*Male*	*Female*	*Total*	*Male*	*Female*	*Total*	*Male*	*Female*
INCIDENCE									
URINARY SYSTEM	26.4	43.2	13.8	27.7	45.8	14.3	19.9	29.6	12.9
Urinary bladder	16.9	29.9	7.4	18.2	32.3	7.8	9.7	15.0	5.9
Kidney and renal pelvis	8.6	12.1	5.9	8.8	12.2	6.1	9.5	13.7	6.5
Ureter	0.5	0.8	0.3	0.5	0.8	0.3	0.2	0.2	0.2
Other urinary organs	0.3	0.4	0.2	0.3	0.4	0.1	0.6	0.7	0.4
MORTALITY									
URINARY SYSTEM	6.8	10.8	4.1	6.9	11.0	4.1	6.9	10.0	4.8
Urinary bladder	3.2	5.7	1.7	3.3	5.8	1.6	3.3	4.8	2.4
Kidney and renal pelvis	3.4	5.0	2.3	3.5	5.0	2.3	3.3	5.0	2.2
Ureter	0.1	0.1	0.1	0.1	0.1	0.1	0.1	0.1	0.1
Other urinary organs	0.1	0.1	0.1	0.0	0.1	0.0	0.2	0.2	0.2

*Incidence and mortality rates are age-adjusted to the 1970 U.S. standard million population.

Brain and Central Nervous System

Ninety-five percent of the malignancies in this category occur in the brain. Incidence for cancer of the brain and nervous system increased 25% from 1973 to 1991. The 1987–91 incidence rate was higher for whites (6.7) than for blacks (3.9) and higher among males than among females of each race. The five-year relative survival rate for cancer of the brain is 25 percent. For cancers arising in the brain, stage at diagnosis has relatively little impact on survival. While brain cancers rarely metastasize, as space-occupying lesions they compress and damage the adjacent tissues. In contrast, patients with localized cancers arising in the cranial nerves and other parts of the

TABLE 11–I–10. *Eye, Brain, and Endocrine System, Average Annual Cancer Incidence and Mortality Rates per 100,000 Person-Years by Race and Sex, SEER Areas, 1987–1991**

	All Races			*Whites*			*Blacks*		
	Total	*Male*	*Female*	*Total*	*Male*	*Female*	*Total*	*Male*	*Female*
INCIDENCE									
EYE AND ORBIT	0.7	0.8	0.6	0.7	0.9	0.6	0.3	0.4	0.2
BRAIN AND NERVOUS SYSTEM	6.2	7.4	5.3	6.7	7.9	5.7	3.9	4.7	3.3
Brain	5.9	7.0	5.0	6.4	7.6	5.4	3.6	4.2	3.1
Cranial nerves and other nervous system	0.3	0.4	0.3	0.3	0.3	0.3	0.3	0.5	0.2
ENDOCRINE SYSTEM	5.0	3.1	6.9	5.0	3.1	6.9	3.0	1.8	4.0
Thyroid	4.5	2.5	6.4	4.5	2.5	6.4	2.5	1.2	3.4
Other endocrine (including thymus)	0.5	0.6	0.5	0.5	0.6	0.5	0.6	0.5	0.6
MORTALITY									
EYE AND ORBIT	0.1	0.1	0.1	0.1	0.1	0.1	0.0	0.1	0.0
BRAIN AND NERVOUS SYSTEM	4.2	5.1	3.5	4.5	5.4	3.7	2.6	3.2	2.1
Brain	4.1	5.0	3.4	4.3	5.3	3.6	2.4	3.0	2.0
Cranial nerves and other nervous system	0.1	0.1	0.1	0.1	0.1	0.1	0.1	0.1	0.1
ENDOCRINE SYSTEM	0.7	0.7	0.6	0.7	0.7	0.6	0.7	0.7	0.8
Thyroid	0.3	0.3	0.4	0.3	0.3	0.3	0.4	0.3	0.4
Other endocrine (including thymus)	0.3	0.4	0.3	0.3	0.4	0.3	0.4	0.4	0.3

*Incidence and mortality rates are age-adjusted to the 1970 U.S. standard million population.

TABLE 11–I–11. *Lymphomas and Myeloma, Average Annual Cancer Incidence and Mortality Rates per 100,000 Person-Years by Race and Sex, SEER Areas, 1987–1991**

	All Races			*Whites*			*Blacks*		
	Total	*Male*	*Female*	*Total*	*Male*	*Female*	*Total*	*Male*	*Female*
INCIDENCE									
LYMPHOMAS	17.3	21.2	14.0	18.2	22.2	14.7	12.3	15.2	9.9
Hodgkin's disease	2.9	3.3	2.5	3.1	3.6	2.7	2.1	2.4	1.9
Non-Hodgkin's lymphoma	14.4	17.9	11.5	15.0	18.6	12.0	10.2	12.8	8.1
MULTIPLE MYELOMA	4.4	5.5	3.6	4.1	5.1	3.3	9.1	11.1	7.7
MORTALITY									
LYMPHOMAS	6.7	8.4	5.5	7.0	8.6	5.7	4.9	6.4	3.7
Hodgkin's disease	0.6	0.7	0.4	0.6	0.8	0.5	0.6	0.7	0.4
Non-Hodgkin's lymphoma	6.2	7.6	5.0	6.4	7.9	5.2	4.3	5.7	3.3
MULTIPLE MYELOMA	2.9	3.7	2.4	2.7	3.4	2.2	5.8	7.2	4.9

*Incidence and mortality rates age-adjusted to the 1970 U.S. standard million population.

nervous system experience a survival rate of 71%, and 65% for all stages.

Endocrine System

Cancer of the thyroid accounts for about 90% of these cancers. Thyroid cancer is one of the few nongender-specific malignancies which occur more often in females than males, with incidence rates of 6.4 and 2.5, respectively. It also occurs more frequently in whites (4.5) than in blacks (2.5). The median age at diagnosis, 44 years, is relatively young. The five-year relative survival rate of 95% for all stages is the highest for any malignancy. Fifty-six percent of thyroid cancers are diagnosed while localized, and these patients experience a five-year relative survival rate close to 100%. The overall mortality rate is only 0.3 per 100,000.

LYMPHOMAS

All lymphomas arising in both lymphatic and extralymphatic sites are included in this section. For example, a lymphoma arising in the stomach is tabulated with the lymphomas and not the stomach cancers. These tumors are further subdivided into Hodgkin's disease and non-Hodgkin's lymphoma.

Hodgkin's Disease

The current incidence rate for Hodgkin's disease is 2.9 per 100,000 (Table 11–I–11). The rate has decreased 12 percent since 1973. Incidence is higher among whites (3.1) than among blacks (2.1), and is higher in males than in females. While the median age for the diagnosis of Hodgkin's disease is 33, there is a bimodal distribution with peak risks occurring in the age-groups 20 to 24 and 80 to 84 years. The five-year relative survival rate is 79%, with slightly higher rates among females than among males (Table 11–I–12). Mortality rates from Hodgkin's disease, which were fairly stable in earlier years, have been decreasing since the late 1960s, reflecting substantial improvement in survival. Since 1973 mortality decreased more than 50%.

TABLE 11–I–12. *Lymphomas and Myeloma, Five-Year Relative Survival Rates by Sex, SEER Areas, All Races, 1983–1990*

	Both Sexes		*Males*		*Females*	
Site	*Number*	*Rate*	*Number*	*Rate*	*Number*	*Rate*
LYMPHOMAS	28,109	58	15,348	56	12,761	60
Hodgkin's disease	5,307	79	2,976	77	2,331	82
Non-Hodgkin's lymphoma	22,802	52	12,372	50	10,430	55
MULTIPLE MYELOMA	7,422	28	3,888	29	3,534	27

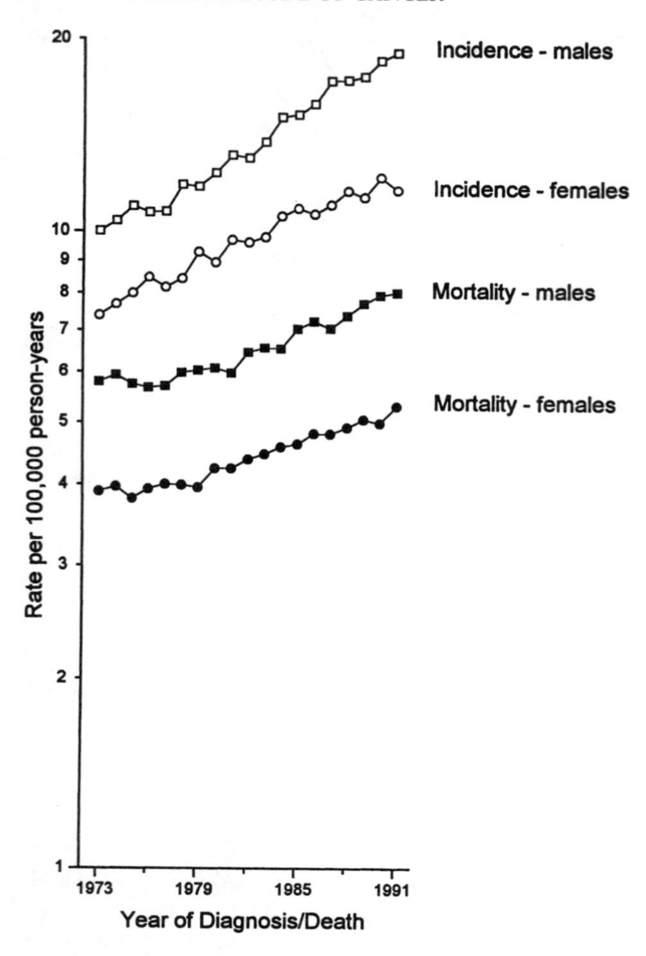

FIG. 11–I–10. Non-Hodgkin's lymphoma, age-adjusted (1970 Standard) SEER incidence and United States mortality rates by sex, 1973–91.

Non-Hodgkin's Lymphoma (NHL)

The incidence of non-Hodgkin's lymphoma is higher among whites (15.0) than among blacks (10.2). The median age at onset for non-Hodgkin's lymphoma is 65. Non-Hodgkin's lymphoma rates have been rising for many years, with acceleration in recent years, due particularly to extranodal and high-grade tumors (Devesa and Fears, 1992). Changes in diagnosis and classification can account for only a small portion of the long-term increases (Hartge and Devesa, 1992). From 1973 to 1991, NHL rose 73 percent—one of the largest increases seen in any malignancy, with more rapid increases among males than among females (Fig. 11–I–10).

Between 1973 and 1991, NHL increased most rapidly in men under 65, or by 104%. Part of the more rapid increase among men under 65 may be a reflection of the effect of more diagnoses of NHL secondary to HIV infection. Incidence rates for NHL in men aged 20–54 have been particularly high in recent years in the San Francisco-Oakland area. These dramatic increases lag by a couple of years behind the increases seen for Kaposi's sarcoma. The inclusion of San Francisco-Oakland in the incidence rates for all SEER areas combined exaggerates the overall increase in NHL incidence for men aged 20–54 (Ries et al, 1994a).

Mortality increased at a lesser rate (33% increase) than incidence. The five-year relative survival is about 52%, comprised of 55% for females and 50% for males. Survival rates improved substantially during the 1960s and 1970s, particularly among children, resulting in declining mortality rates for those under 15 years of age.

MULTIPLE MYELOMA

Multiple myeloma is a disease of later life with a median age at occurrence of 70 years. The disease occurs predominantly among black males (11.1) at a rate nearly 50% higher than for black females (7.7), more than twice that for white males (5.1), and more than three times that for white females (3.3). American blacks have among the highest multiple myeloma rates in the world (Parkin et al, 1992). Mortality rates follow a similar pattern. There has been a 16% increase in incidence since 1973, driven largely by increases among white males. The five-year relative survival is poor at only 28%.

LEUKEMIA

The leukemias are a family of malignant diseases of the blood which are subclassified into two groups—acute leukemias and chronic leukemias. These are further subdivided into categories based on cell type. The major cell types are lymphocytic and myeloid (granulocytic), and the less common forms include monocytic, basophilic, eosinophilic, plasma cell, erythro, and hairy cell leukemias. Lymphocytic leukemia occurs more frequently than does myeloid leukemia among whites, but almost equally among blacks (Table 11–I–13). From another perspective, there is little racial difference in myeloid leukemia incidence, but lymphocytic rates are higher among whites than blacks. The chronic form occurs more frequently among those with lymphocytic leukemia and the acute form more among those with myeloid leukemia. Acute lymphocytic leukemia has a bimodal distribution with peak incidence occurring in young children and again after age 80. While the incidence of total leukemia decreased by 11%, there are

TABLE 11–I–13. *Leukemia, Average Annual Cancer Incidence and Mortality Rates per 100,000 Person-Years by Race and Sex, SEER Areas, 1987–1991**

	All Races			*Whites*			*Blacks*		
	Total	*Male*	*Female*	*Total*	*Male*	*Female*	*Total*	*Male*	*Female*
INCIDENCE									
LEUKEMIAS	10.0	13.1	7.7	10.2	13.4	7.8	8.9	11.5	6.9
Lymphocytic Leukemia	4.6	6.1	3.4	4.7	6.4	3.5	3.9	4.9	3.0
Acute lymphocytic	1.6	1.8	1.3	1.6	1.9	1.4	1.0	1.0	1.0
Chronic lymphocytic	2.9	4.1	2.0	3.0	4.3	2.0	2.7	3.7	2.0
Other lymphocytic	0.1	0.1	0.1	0.1	0.1	0.1	0.1	0.2	0.1
Myeloid Leukemia	3.9	4.9	3.2	3.9	4.9	3.1	3.8	4.9	3.0
Acute myeloid	2.3	2.9	1.9	2.4	3.0	2.0	2.0	2.7	1.5
Chronic myeloid	1.3	1.7	1.0	1.3	1.7	1.0	1.5	1.9	1.2
Other myeloid	0.2	0.3	0.2	0.2	0.3	0.2	0.2	0.3	0.3
Monocytic Leukemia	0.3	0.3	0.2	0.3	0.3	0.2	0.2	0.3	0.2
Acute monocytic	0.2	0.3	0.2	0.2	0.3	0.2	0.2	0.2	0.2
Chronic monocytic	0.0	0.0	0.0	0.0	0.0	0.0	0.1	0.2	0.1
Other monocytic	0.0	0.0	0.0	0.0	0.0	0.0	0.1	0.3	0.0
Other Leukemias	1.3	1.7	0.9	1.3	1.8	1.0	1.0	1.4	0.7
Other acute	0.6	0.8	0.5	0.6	0.8	0.5	0.5	0.8	0.3
Other chronic	0.0	0.0	0.0	0.0	0.0	0.0	0.1	0.3	0.1
Aleukemic, subleukemic, and NOS[a]	0.7	0.9	0.5	0.7	1.0	0.5	0.5	0.6	0.4
MORTALITY									
LEUKEMIAS	6.3	8.3	4.9	6.4	8.5	5.0	6.0	8.0	4.7

*Incidence and mortality rates age-adjusted to the 1970 U.S. standard million population.
[a]NOS, not otherwise specified.

TABLE 11–I–14. *Leukemias, Five-Year Relative Survival Rates by Sex, SEER Areas, All Races, 1983–1990*

	Both Sexes		*Males*		*Females*	
Site	*Number*	*Rate*	*Number*	*Rate*	*Number*	*Rate*
LEUKEMIAS	17,185	38	9,845	38	7,340	38
Lymphocytic Leukemia	7,842	62	4,572	60	3,270	65
Acute lymphocytic	2,317	52	1,329	50	988	55
Chronic lymphocytic	5,343	69	3,150	67	2,193	72
Other lymphocytic	182	31[a]	93	28[b]	89	35[b]
Myeloid Leukemia	6,723	16	3,747	15	2,976	16
Acute myeloid	3,908	10	2,147	9	1,761	12
Chronic myeloid	2,360	24	1,347	23	1,013	24
Other myeloid	455	18	253	19[a]	202	17[a]
Monocytic Leukemia	430	12	218	13[a]	212	10[a]
Acute monocytic	365	11	185	13[a]	180	8
Chronic monocytic	31	20[b]	14	—[c]	17	—[c]
Other monocytic	34	12[b]	19	—[c]	15	—[c]
Other Leukemias	2,190	29	1,308	32	882	22
Other acute	1,008	9	561	9	447	10
Other chronic	44	58[b]	25	71[b]	19	—[c]
Aleukemic, subleukemic and NOS[d]	1,138	44	722	49	416	34[a]

[a]The standard error of the survival rate is between 5 and 10 percentage points.
[b]The standard error of the survival rate is greater than 10 percentage points.
[c]—, valid survival rates could not be calculated.
[d]NOS, not otherwise specified.

TABLE 11–I–15. *Historical Stage Distribution and Five-Year Relative Survival Rates by Primary Cancer Site and Stage for All Races, Males and Females, SEER Program 1983–1990*

Site	Number	Distribution (%)				5-Year Survival (%)				
		Local	Regional	Distant	Unknown	Total	Local	Regional	Distant	Unknown
ORAL CAVITY AND PHARYNX	17,457	37	43	10	10	52	79	41	19	37
Lip	2,139	83	10	1	6	94	96	82[a]	—[c]	83[b]
Tongue	3,459	40	41	9	9	47	68	37	16	36[a]
Salivary gland	1,527	49	35	8	8	72	91	58[a]	27[b]	57[b]
Floor of mouth	1,854	37	51	5	7	54	74	44	20[b]	43[b]
Gum and other mouth	3,053	32	44	7	17	54	79	50	24[a]	30[a]
Nasopharynx	1,000	15	51	18	16	47	72[b]	49[a]	24[a]	47[b]
Tonsil	1,690	17	57	18	9	40	59[a]	41	19[a]	34[a]
Oropharynx	479	13	58	18	11	24	40[b]	26[a]	12[a]	16[b]
Hypopharynx	1,703	12	64	18	7	25	50[a]	25	11	16[a]
Other buccal cavity and pharynx	553	14	53	14	19	25	46[b]	24[a]	10[a]	25[b]
DIGESTIVE SYSTEM	131,237	29	34	26	11	42	79	47	5	17
Esophagus	6,042	25	23	27	25	9	20	7	2	8
Stomach	13,630	17	33	36	14	19	59	20	2	10
Small intestine	1,596	26	35	32	7	48	70[a]	58[a]	23	38[b]
Colon and rectum	82,894	37	38	19	6	59	91	60	6	33
Colon, excluding rectum	58,693	35	39	21	5	60	93	63	7	30
Rectum and rectosigmoid	24,201	41	35	16	8	58	87	52	5	36
Anus, anal canal and anorectum	1,419	41	32	10	17	62	80[a]	58[a]	9[a]	56[a]
Liver and intrahepatic bile duct	4,349	21	23	25	32	6	15	7	3	3
Liver only	3,854	21	23	25	31	6	15	6	3	3
Gallbladder	2,074	25	32	38	4	13	43[a]	6	1	3
Other biliary	1,965	22	37	21	20	16	31[a]	18	2	8
Pancreas	15,851	9	22	49	20	3	9	4	2	4
Retroperitoneum	673	30	27	33	11	44	67[a]	52[a]	22[a]	26[b]
Peritoneum, omentum and mesentery	311	15	17	56	13	24	43[b]	40[b]	14[a]	21[b]
Other digestive organs	433	—[c]	3	68	29	4	—[c]	—[c]	2	6[a]
RESPIRATORY SYSTEM	102,558	18	29	39	14	18	55	19	2	10
Nose, nasal cavity and middle ear	1,027	28	43	20	9	54	80[a]	49[a]	25[a]	52[b]
Larynx	7,438	49	36	9	6	67	85	54	33[a]	49[a]
Lung and bronchus	92,433	15	28	41	15	13	47	15	2	8
Pleura	1,237	9	32	35	24	4	15[a]	3	7	1
Trachea and other respiratory organs	423	18	32	24	25	42[a]	73[b]	45[b]	23[a]	33[b]
BONES AND JOINTS	1,274	35	36	18	12	57	72[a]	59[a]	19[a]	62[b]
SOFT TISSUE (including heart)	3,569	55	17	16	12	62	80	58[a]	15	47[a]
SKIN (excluding basal and squamous)	23,744	65	11	5	19	69	91	46	11	27
Melanomas of skin	17,399	82	8	4	6	85	93	57	15	64
Other non-epithelial skin	6,345	19	18	10	53	28	69	33	8	14
BREAST	94,156	55	35	6	4	80	94	73	18	53
FEMALE GENITAL SYSTEM	44,077	53	19	23	6	67	92	53	22	47
Cervix uteri	8,424	50	34	9	7	67	90	51	12	58[a]
Corpus uteri	19,906	74	12	9	4	84	94	68	28	58[a]
Uterus, NOS[d]	287	9	16	39	36	29[a]	68[b]	29[b]	13[a]	35[b]
Ovary	12,865	23	19	52	5	42	90	40	21	24
Vagina	496	36	23	23	19	46[a]	61[b]	56[b]	20[a]	40[b]
Vulva	1,552	65	23	5	7	73	85	57[a]	2[a]	59[b]
Other female genital organs	547	26	16	49	10	51[a]	84[a]	41[b]	37[a]	44[b]

(continued)

TABLE 11–I–15. *(Continued)*

Site	Number	*Distribution (%)* Local	Regional	Distant	Unknown	*5-Year Survival (%)* Total	Local	Regional	Distant	Unknown
MALE GENITAL SYSTEM	77,828	58	16	16	10	81	94	86	31	75
Prostate	72,654	58	15	16	10	80	94	85	29	75
Testis	4,464	63	21	12	3	93	98	95	68	89[a]
Penis	532	65	20	4	11	69[a]	84[a]	48[b]	—[c]	47[b]
Other male genital organs	178	61	19	7	13	73[b]	86[b]	65[b]	—[c]	—[c]
URINARY SYSTEM	41,874	63	21	10	5	72	91	51	9	49
Urinary bladder	27,974	73	19	3	5	80	92	47	8	61
Kidney and renal pelvis	12,817	44	24	26	6	56	87	57	9	30
Ureter	694	45	39	8	8	62[a]	89[a]	45[a]	13[a]	30[b]
Other urinary system	389	36	22	12	30	55[a]	72[b]	33[b]	25[b]	59[b]
EYE AND ORBIT	1,103	67	15	4	13	77	85	68[b]	49[b]	59[b]
BRAIN AND NERVOUS SYSTEM	10,347	42	14	1	43	27	28	29	32[a]	26
Brain	9,817	41	13	1	45	25	25	27	23[a]	25
Cranial nerves and other nervous system	530	57	17	11	16	65[a]	71[a]	59[b]	41[b]	65[b]
ENDOCRINE SYSTEM	8,538	53	33	8	5	90	99	91	41	74[a]
Thyroid	7,645	56	34	5	4	95	100	93	49[a]	82[a]
Other endocrine and thymus	893	27	25	36	12	54	75[a]	64[a]	32[a]	48[b]

[a]The standard error of the survival rate is between 5 and 10 percentage points.
[b]The standard error of the survival rate is greater than 10 percentage points.
[c]—, valid survival rate could not be calculated.
[d]NOS, not otherwise specified.

variations by subtype: incidence of acute lymphocytic increased by 22%, chronic lymphocytic decreased by 24%, acute myeloid decreased by 2%, and chronic myeloid decreased by 17%.

Mortality rates by subtype are not presented because death certificates frequently do not specify the type of leukemia. Mortality declined for whites but increased for blacks. Childhood leukemia mortality decreased dramatically following improvements in treatment and survival.

Relative survival rates among patients with myeloid leukemia are 24% or less—considerably lower than rates of at least 50% for acute or chronic lymphocytic leukemia (Table 11–I–14). Survival rates improved over the last several decades, most notably for acute lymphocytic leukemia among children.

CANCER IN CHILDREN UNDER 15 YEARS OF AGE

Incidence rates for many childhood cancers continue to increase. Among children aged 0–14 years, increases of greater than 10% were seen for acute lymphocytic leukemia (20%), brain and nervous system (38%), bone (13%), and soft tissue (27%) over the period 1973–91. The incidence of total leukemia did not rise, implying that some of the increase in the incidence of acute lymphocytic leukemia may be an artifact due to more specificity in the diagnosis over time (Ries et al, 1993). The only childhood cancer that declined in incidence was Hodgkin's disease (−10%). During the same period, however, overall childhood cancer mortality decreased 42%, due to substantial declines in mortality for every major childhood cancer. Mortality decreased by more than 50% for Hodgkin's disease (−76%), kidney cancer (−53%), soft tissue malignancies (−70%), acute lymphocytic leukemia (−59%), and non-Hodgkin's lymphoma (−61%). These decreases in mortality in the face of rising incidence are attributable to large increases in the survival rates due to improved treatment regimens.

DISCUSSION

Males develop and die from cancer with greater frequency than females. Tobacco use and alcohol consumption as well as occupational exposures contribute to the higher rates of mouth, lung, esophagus, larynx, and bladder cancers in men. Sex differences in other malignancies, such as stomach, colon, and rectal cancers which predominate among men, and breast, gallbladder, and thyroid cancers, which predominate among women, have given rise to investigation of other factors such as biologic differences, nutrition, parity, endogenous hormones, and sex steroid receptors, in attempts to explain such differences (Fraumeni et al, 1993).

As the population continues to grow in size and shifts to an older age distribution, increasing numbers of people will be affected by cancer. Primary prevention will progress by the identification of factors influencing risk, followed by modifications in exposure. As suggested by stage-specific survival rates, substantial declines in cancer mortality could also be achieved by shifting diagnoses to earlier, less advanced, more treatable stages of disease with considerable improvements in survival.

SUMMARY

The intent of this chapter has been to show the current estimates for cancer incidence, mortality, and survival in a large subgroup of the U.S. population. Trends in cancer incidence, mortality, and survival were presented where they appeared to be important. More information on cancer trends is provided in the most recent *SEER Cancer Statistics Review*. The SEER home page on the World Wide Web (WWW-SEER.ims.nci.nih.gov) contains the most recent SEER publications and information on ordering free SEER publications. The reader is referred to other chapters in this book for additional information on changes in diagnostic procedures, diffusion of new treatments, and effects of screening programs, as well as discussion of the known and suspected risk factors.

REFERENCES

AMERICAN CANCER SOCIETY: 1994. Cancer Facts and Figures—1994. Atlanta, GA, American Cancer Society.

AXTELL LM, ASIRE AJ, MYERS MH. 1976. Cancer patient survival: report number 5. NIH Publ. No. 81-992. Bethesda, MD, National Cancer Institute.

CHOW W-H, DEVESA SS. 1992. Death certificate reporting of colon and rectal cancers. Letter to the editor. JAMA, 267:3028.

CONNELLY RR, SPIRTAS R, MYERS MH, et al. 1987. Demographic patterns for mesothelioma in the United States. J Natl Cancer Inst 78:1053–1060.

CUTLER SJ, YOUNG JL. (eds). 1975. Third National Cancer Survey: Incidence Data. National Cancer Institute Monograph 41. Washington, D.C., U.S. Government Printing Office.

DEVESA SS, BLOT WJ, FRAUMENI JF JR. 1989. Declining lung cancer rates among young men and women in the United States: a cohort analysis. J Natl Cancer Inst 81:1568–1571.

DEVESA SS, CHOW W-H. 1993. Variation in colorectal cancer incidence in the United States by subsite of origin. Cancer 71:3819–3826.

DEVESA SS, DONALDSON J, FEARS T. 1995. Graphic presentation of trends in rates. Am J Epidemiol 141:300–304.

DEVESA SS, FEARS T. 1992. Non-Hodgkin's lymphoma time trends: United States and international data. Cancer Res (Suppl.) 52:5432s–5440s.

DEVESA SS, SHAW GL, BLOT WJ. 1991. Changing patterns of lung cancer incidence by histological type. Cancer Epidemiol Biomarkers Prev 1:29–34.

DEVESA SS, SILVERMAN DT, YOUNG JL JR, et al. 1987. Cancer incidence and mortality trends among whites in the United States, 1947–84. J Natl Cancer Inst 79:701–770.

DEVESA SS, SILVERMAN DT, MCLAUGHLIN JK, BROWN CC, CONNELLY RR, FRAUMENI JF JR. 1990. Comparison of the descriptive epidemiology of urinary tract cancers. Cancer Causes Control 1:133–141.

DEVITA VT, HELLMAN S, ROSENBERG SA. 1989. Cancer: Principles and Practice of Oncology, 3rd ed. Philadelphia, J.B. Lippincott Co.

DORN HF, CUTLER SJ. 1959. Morbidity from cancer in the United States: Parts I and II. Public Health Monogr 56:1–207.

EDERER F, AXTELL LM, CUTLER SJ. 1961. The relative survival rate: a statistical methodology. *In* Cutler SJ, Ederer F (eds): End Results and Mortality Trends in Cancer. NCI Monograph No. 6. Bethesda, National Cancer Institute, pp. 101–121.

FRAUMENI JF JR, DEVESA SS, HOOVER RN, KINLEN LJ. 1993. Epidemiology of cancer. *In* DeVita VT, Hellman S, Rosenberg SA (eds): Cancer: Principles Practice of Oncology, 4th ed. Philadelphia, J.B. Lippincott Co., pp. 150–181.

HARTGE P, DEVESA SS. 1992. Quantification of the impact of known risk factors and time trends in non-Hodgkin's lymphoma incidence. Cancer Res (Suppl.) 52:5566s–5569s.

MILLER BA, FEUER EJ, HANKEY BF. 1993. Recent incidence trends for breast cancer in women and the relevance of early detection: an update. CA Cancer J Clin 43:27–41.

NATIONAL CANCER INSTITUTE. 1988. 1987 Annual Cancer Statistics Review Including Cancer Trends 1950–1985. DHHS Publication No. (NIH) 88-2789. Bethesda, National Cancer Institute.

PARKIN DM, MUIR CS, WHELAN S, GAO YT, FERLAY J, POWELL J. (eds). 1992. Cancer Incidence in Five Continents, Vol. VI. IARC Scientific Publications No. 120. Lyon, International Agency for Research on Cancer.

PERCY CL, MILLER BA, RIES LAG. 1990a. Effect of changes in cancer classification and the accuracy of cancer death certificates on trends in cancer mortality. *In* Davis DL, Hoel D (eds): Trends in Cancer Mortality in Industrial Countries. Ann N Y Acad Sci 609:87–99.

PERCY CL, RIES LAG, VAN HOLTEN VD. 1990b. The accuracy of liver cancer as the underlying cause of death on death certificates. Public Health Rep 105:361–368.

PERCY C, STANEK E III, GLOECKLER L. 1981. Accuracy of cancer death certificates and its effect on cancer mortality statistics. A J Public Health, 71:242–250.

POKRAS R, HUFNAGEL VG. 1987. Hysterectomies in the United States. DHHS Publication No. (PHS) 88-1753. Hyattsville, MD, National Center for Health Statistics.

POTOSKY AL, KESSLER L, GRIDLEY G, BROWN CC, HORM JW. 1990. Rise in prostatic cancer incidence associated with increased use of transurethral resection. J Natl Cancer Inst 82:1624–1628.

POTOSKY AL, MILLER BA, ALBERTSEN PC, KRAMER BS. 1995. The role of increasing detection in the rising incidence of prostate cancer. JAMA 273:548–552.

RIES LAG, MILLER BA, HANKEY BF, KOSARY CL, HARRAS A, EDWARDS BK. (eds). 1994a. SEER Cancer Statistics Review, 1973–1991:

Tables and Graphs. NIH Publication No. 94-2789. Bethesda, MD, National Cancer Institute.

RIES LAG, MILLER RW, SMITH MA. 1993. Cancer in children (ages 0–14 and ages 0–19). *In* Miller BA, Ries LAG, Hankey BF, Kosary CL, Harras A, Devesa SS, Edwards BK (eds): SEER Cancer Statistics Review, 1973–1990. NIH Publication No. 93-2789. Bethesda, MD, National Cancer Institute. pp. XXVII 1–15.

SCOTTO J, FEARS TR, FRAUMENI JF JR. 1983. Incidence of Nonmelanoma Skin Cancer in the United States. NIH Publication No. 83-2433. Bethesda, MD, National Cancer Institute.

WORLD HEALTH ORGANIZATION. International Classification of Diseases for Oncology, 1st ed. Geneva, World Health Organization, 1976; Field trials, 1986, 1988.

11-II

Cancer incidence, mortality, and survival among racial and ethnic minority groups in the United States

JOHN W. HORM
SUSAN S. DEVESA
LINDA BURHANSSTIPANOV

The study of cancer risk differences among racial and ethnic groups is a practical epidemiologic method for discovering important clues into the etiology of, and perhaps preventive measures for, specific cancers. Cultural differences among minority groups in personal habits, dietary practices, and environmental exposures that might be related to cancer risk deserve special attention. Rates may change over time and among migrating groups, suggesting the influence of lifestyle and other environmental factors. Although not known to affect racial and ethnic patterns generally, some marked differences in genetic susceptibility are well documented, most notably for skin cancers.

Many racial and ethnic minorities in the United States are at a disadvantage relative to the access and availability of health care, preventive services, and health education (Health Resources and Services Administration [HRSA], 1985; National Center for Health Statistics [NCHS], 1994). This is due in part to cultural and language differences and, typically, low income and education. Thus several minority groups may experience increased incidence, mortality, and survival disadvantages. Further, among low-income, low-education groups, including racial and ethnic minorities, an excess of unhealthy conditions may exist, such as employment in high-risk occupations and low usage of preventive medical services (Baquet et al, 1986; Jones, 1989; Fraumeni et al, 1993). The information presented in this chapter, in conjunction with that in other chapters focusing on specific risk factors or forms of cancer, should assist in furthering our understanding of cancer and ultimately lessening its burden on racial and ethnic minorities in the United States.

We thank Dr. Joseph F. Fraumeni, Jr., for comments on the manuscript.

METHODS

Incidence and survival data were based on the Surveillance, Epidemiology, and End Results (SEER) Program of the National Cancer Institute (NCI), and mortality data were provided by the National Center for Health Statistics (Young et al, 1981; Horm et al, 1984; Ries et al, 1994). As is described more fully elsewhere in this volume, the SEER program is a set of geographically defined, population-based tumor registries containing about 10% of the total U.S. population in diverse locations around the country. The racial and ethnic groups considered in this chapter live in discrete areas of the United States. A population of blacks sufficiently large for analysis was found in only four SEER registry areas: the metropolitan areas of San Francisco-Oakland, California; Atlanta, Georgia; Detroit, Michigan; and the state of Connecticut. Our incidence and survival data on American Indians were from the states of Arizona and New Mexico, while information on Hawaiian Natives was from the state of Hawaii. Among the SEER registries, Chinese, Japanese, and Filipinos were found in San Francisco-Oakland and Hawaii in sufficiently large numbers for analysis. Rates for Hispanics were from New Mexico only. Mortality data for most racial and ethnic groups were available on a national basis. Hispanic ethnicity, coded on death certificates on a national basis only since 1984, was not available for analysis at the time of this writing; mortality rates are therefore presented for Hispanics in New Mexico. Data were also available for the Commonwealth of Puerto Rico and for Alaska Natives.

Geographic differences among whites and nonwhites in cancer rates have been noted (Mason et al, 1975, 1976; Young et al, 1981; Pickle et al, 1987, 1990). To reduce the impact of geographic confounding on the racial comparisons, our tables use whites within the same geographic area as the study population for the comparison group. Each table is footnoted to indicate the source of the data. As an indication of the amount of geographic variation, 1977–83 incidence rates among whites for all cancers combined ranged from a low of 314.5 cases per 100,000 person-years in New Mexico (Anglos, or non-Hispanic whites) to a high of 384.9 cases per 100,000 person-years in Hawaii. Incidence and mortality rates in this report generally were based on events occurring from 1977 through 1983 and thus chosen to center on the 1980 United States Census, providing good estimates of the populations at risk. This seven-year period generally provided sufficiently large numbers of cases to permit meaningful comparisons. Exceptions were that mortality data were available only for 1977–82 for New Mexico Hispanics and for 1979–82 for Puerto Ricans; incidence and mortality data for Alaska Natives were pooled for 1969–83 to maximize numbers of events.

The incidence and mortality rates were age-adjusted by the direct method to the age distribution of the total U.S. population in 1970 and are expressed per 100,000 population per year for each specific population group.

Survival rates were based on cases diagnosed between 1975 and 1984 to provide enough cases for survival analyses, with follow-up through 1985. Survival rates were calculated by the actuarial method (Cutler et al, 1958), which does not age-adjust but corrects for the life expectancy of a normal population of similar race–sex–age distribution as the cases. This method statistically adjusts for non-cancer causes of death and permits the interpretation of the relative rate as if the only cause of death were cancer. Survival rates were available for all groups except Alaska Natives.

As compiled by NCI staff, the following table contains the July 1, 1980 population estimates by race for the total United States and for the SEER geographic areas used for each race/ethnic group analysis.

1980 Populations by Race and Registry

Geographic Area and Race	*Total United States*	*Analytic Areas*	*Percent of U.S.*
Atlanta, Connecticut, Detroit, San Francisco-Oakland			
Blacks	26,897,581	1,984,587	7.4
Whites	195,170,670	9,691,106	5.0
Hawaii, San Francisco			
Chinese	812,769	201,660	24.8
Japanese	706,503	286,000	40.5
Filipinos	781,063	236,295	30.3
Whites	195,170,670	2,786,206	1.4
New Mexico, Arizona (Indians only)			
American Indians	1,364,033	259,294	19.0
Hispanics	14,608,673	477,222	3.3
Anglos	180,256,366	691,660	0.4
Hawaii			
Hawaiian Natives	176,469	176,469	100.0
Whites	195,170,670	281,460	0.1
Puerto Rico			
Puerto Ricans	5,210,465	3,196,520	61.3
Alaska			
Alaska Natives	n/a[a]	64,357	n/a
Whites	195,170,670	17,950,952[b]	9.2

[a]n/a, not available.
[b]nine SEER areas.

The overall 1980 Census undercount rate was 5.3% but it varied from 14.9% among Puerto Ricans to 11.7% among blacks, 9.4% among Mexicans, 8.2% among other Spanish, 7.7% among native Americans, 6.7% among Asians, and 4.0% among non-Hispanic whites (Fein, 1990). The undercount rate varied inversely with education of the head of household (8.4% to 4.5%), and with 1979 household income (9.1% to 4.4%), whereas less geographic variation was evident (3.1% to 6.7%). Undercount rates were greater at younger ages and diminished with age among adults; the rates at ages 30–64 and 65+ were 4.6% and 2.9% among men, and 3.7% and 3.2% among women, respectively. Thus the cancer rates were overestimated, and differentially so. Conversely, underascertainment of cases would have lowered the rates. However, variations in cancer rates to be presented frequently exceeded those that could be explained by underenumeration or underascertainment, suggesting real differences in risk.

BLACKS

According to the 1980 Census of Population, there were almost 27 million blacks in the United States (Bureau of the Census, 1983a), constituting the largest single racial minority in the country. This population was younger than the general population, with a median age of 24.9 compared to 30.0 years. A disproportionately large number of blacks were concentrated in the lower socioeconomic status (SES) levels, as defined by education and income. In 1987 over 31% of the black population lived below the poverty level, which is significantly greater than the 13.6% for the entire population (Bureau of the Census, 1988b, 1988d). Their median family income in 1979 was $12,598, among the lowest for any population group in the nation. Thirty-six percent of the black population aged 25 years or older had less than a high school education, compared to 23% of the white population, and only 11% had completed four years of college. Blacks have a much higher unemployment rate than the majority population; for instance, 13% were unemployed in 1987 compared to 5.3%. When employed, blacks are concentrated in blue-collar occupations and service industries. On the other hand, consumption of fruits and vegetables was higher among blacks and consumption of total and saturated fat was lower than that among whites in at least three areas of the United States (Atlanta, Detroit, and New Jersey) (Swanson et al, 1993).

Cigarette smoking prevalence rates among black males were quite high; during 1987, 40.6% currently smoked, compared to 30.9% among white males (NCI, 1989). Further, smoking rates among black males have not decreased as rapidly as those for the general population (NCHS, 1988, 1994). Smoking prevalence rates among females have been more similar: 28.9% versus 26.9% among blacks and whites, respectively (NCI, 1989).

Blacks were generally less likely than the majority population to have heard of or to have availed themselves of cancer screening procedures. The National Health Interview Surveys revealed that twice as many blacks as whites had never heard of the Pap smear, and over twice as many blacks had never heard of mammography, although differences have narrowed over time (NCI, 1989; Breen and Kessler, 1994). Similar relationships held for the digital rectal exam, blood stool tests, and proctoscopy. However, increased awareness among young women has recently resulted in larger proportions of blacks than whites having had a Pap smear and/or a breast exam in the prior year (Bloom, 1986; Centers for Disease Control [CDC], 1988). A smaller proportion of the black population has been covered by private health insurers and a correspondingly larger proportion either was covered by Medicaid or had no health care coverage at all (NCHS, 1988). In 1986 over 17% of blacks were covered under Medicaid and 22.6% had no health care coverage, compared to 4% of whites covered by Medicaid and 14% with no coverage. These factors relate directly to access to and availability of medical care and to health knowledge, attitudes, and practices (Jones, 1989). Factors influencing the use of preventive and screening activities are being identified (Robinson et al, 1991; Kang and Bloom, 1993; Lacey 1993).

Based on data available from four registries (see Table 11–II–1), cancer incidence among black males exceeded that among white males for about half the forms of cancer investigated, with the rate for all sites combined being almost 20% higher. The largest relative difference was for esophageal cancer, for which the black rate of 19.7 was more than three times the white rate of 5.5; alcohol, tobacco, and dietary factors are the prime risk factors identified (Schottenfeld, 1984; Ziegler, 1986). Multiple myeloma occurred more than twice as frequently among blacks as among whites, and prostatic cancer was 71% higher; explanations are not known. Lung cancer, caused primarily by cigarette smoking (Department of Health and Human Services [DHHS], 1982; International Agency for Research on Cancer [IARC], 1986), was 36% higher among black than white males. Incidence rates were higher among black than white males for a number of other cancers, including the stomach, liver, pancreas, and oral cavity. Many studies have found strong inverse associations for such cancers as the lung (especially among males), esophagus, and stomach with several indices of socioeconomic status, including income, education, and poverty level (Williams and Horm, 1977; Devesa and Diamond, 1983; McWhorter et al, 1989; Baquet et al, 1991; Gorey and Vena, 1994). Incidence rates, however, were lower among black as compared to white males for several cancers, including those of the urinary bladder and brain, melanoma, the leukemias, and lymphomas.

Overall, cancer incidence among black females was 92% that among white females. This relationship varied, however, by cancer site. Similar to the pattern observed among males, esophageal cancer occurred about three times more frequently among black than white females, multiple myeloma was more than twice as common, and excesses were apparent for cancers of the stomach, liver, pancreas, and oral cavity. Furthermore, the relative risk for invasive cervix uteri cancer was more than two. However, many cancers were less frequent among black females. Rates for cancers of the corpus uteri and ovary were 56 and 72% those among whites, respectively. Although breast cancer incidence was higher among black women than white women under age 45, the rate among blacks for all ages combined was 81% that among whites. The increased incidence of cancer of the cervix uteri and the lower rate of postmenopausal breast cancer among black females appear related to factors associated with socioeconomic status (Williams and Horm, 1977; Devesa and Diamond, 1980; McWhorter et al, 1989; Baquet et al, 1991; Gorey and Vena, 1994). In contrast to the excess among black males, the lung cancer rate among black females was 93% that among white females.

Relative survival rates were poorer among blacks than whites for about two-thirds of the forms of cancer (Table 11–II–2), with overall five-year rates 75–81% those among whites. The largest black–white survival differences occurred for melanoma and cancers of the corpus uteri, urinary bladder, and breast. Survival rates appear to be influenced by socioeconomic status (Freeman, 1989). A larger proportion of blacks than expected presented with advanced-stage cancers (DHHS, 1986), partially explaining the survival disadvantages.

TABLE 11–II–1. *Average Annual Age-Adjusted (1970 U.S. Standard) Cancer Incidence Rates per 100,000 Population for Malignant Cases Only, Four Areas, 1977–1983**

	Both Sexes		*Male*		*Female*	
	Number	*Rate*	*Number*	*Rate*	*Number*	*Rate*
ALL SITES						
Black	39,601	382.8	21,772	502.2	17,829	298.9
White	270,460	358.5	132,983	420.3	137,477	325.6
ORAL CAVITY AND PHARYNX						
Black	1,610	15.0	1,153	24.1	457	7.6
White	8,728	11.7	5,774	17.6	2,954	7.1
Other Oral Cavity[a]						
Black	1,522	14.2	1,111	23.2	411	6.9
White	7,233	10.3	4,716	14.4	2,517	6.1
Nasopharynx						
Black	81	0.7	51	0.9	30	0.5
White	352	0.5	241	0.7	111	0.3
ESOPHAGUS						
Black	1,218	11.6	912	19.7	306	5.3
White	2,577	3.4	1,765	5.5	812	1.8
STOMACH						
Black	1,441	14.5	948	22.5	493	8.6
White	6,828	8.9	4,140	13.3	2,688	5.8
COLON AND RECTUM						
Black	4,970	50.3	2,342	56.5	2,628	46.0
White	40,492	52.8	20,056	64.5	20,436	45.0
LIVER						
Black	375	3.6	255	5.5	120	2.0
White	1,616	2.1	1,034	3.3	582	1.3
GALLBLADDER						
Black	102	1.0	34	0.8	68	1.2
White	1,025	1.3	274	0.9	751	1.6
PANCREAS						
Black	1,375	13.8	723	17.0	652	11.0
White	7,253	9.5	3,645	11.6	3,608	8.0
LUNG AND BRONCHUS						
Black	7,218	69.8	5,418	120.7	1,800	31.0
White	42,118	56.4	28,317	88.7	13,801	33.4
MELANOMA OF SKIN						
Black	81	0.8	38	0.9	43	0.7
White	7,150	9.4	3,660	10.6	3,490	8.6
BREAST						
Black	4,607	42.8	48	1.2	4,559	75.2
White	38,367	51.5	275	0.8	38,092	92.9
CERVIX UTERI						
Black	1,261	11.0	—	—	1,261	19.7
White	3,490	4.6	—	—	3,490	8.6
CORPUS UTERI						
Black	878	8.6	—	—	878	15.0
White	10,978	14.7	—	—	10,978	26.6

(continued)

TABLE 11–II–1. *Average Annual Age-Adjusted (1970 U.S. Standard) Cancer Incidence Rates per 100,000 Population for Malignant Cases Only, Four Areas, 1977–1983* (Continued)*

	Both Sexes		*Male*		*Female*	
	Number	*Rate*	*Number*	*Rate*	*Number*	*Rate*
OVARY						
Black	625	5.8	—	—	625	10.2
White	5,761	7.7	—	—	5,761	14.1
PROSTATE GLAND						
Black	4,926	51.2	4,926	125.5	—	—
White	22,020	28.6	22,020	73.2	—	—
URINARY BLADDER						
Black	948	9.6	635	15.3	313	5.5
White	13,727	18.0	10,005	31.9	3,722	8.3
KIDNEY AND RENAL PELVIS						
Black	726	6.8	452	9.7	274	4.5
White	5,302	7.2	3,420	10.7	1,882	4.5
BRAIN AND NERVOUS SYSTEM						
Black	417	3.4	236	4.2	181	2.8
White	4,500	6.3	2,460	7.5	2,040	5.3
HODGKIN'S DISEASE						
Black	250	1.8	155	2.5	95	1.3
White	2,369	3.2	1,342	3.8	1,027	2.6
NON-HODGKIN'S LYMPHOMA						
Black	782	7.2	419	8.7	363	6.0
White	8,307	11.1	4,202	13.0	4,105	8.6
MULTIPLE MYELOMA						
Black	864	8.6	440	10.3	424	7.4
White	2,814	3.7	1,403	4.5	1,411	3.1
LEUKEMIAS						
Black	988	9.1	537	11.6	451	7.4
White	7,682	10.4	4,310	13.9	3,372	8.0
Lymphocytic						
Black	386	3.7	229	5.1	157	2.6
White	3,126	4.4	1,777	5.8	1,349	3.4
Myelocytic						
Black	471	4.2	242	4.9	229	3.6
White	3,276	4.3	1,762	5.6	1,514	3.5

*The data for whites and blacks in this table are from San Francisco, Detroit, Atlanta, and Connecticut only.
[a]Other oral cavity is the total oral cavity and pharynx excluding lip and salivary glands.

Differences between blacks and whites in survival rates within individual stages were smaller than overall, but they generally persisted (DHHS, 1986; Ries et al, 1994). There were, however, a few forms of cancer for which blacks had better relative survival rates than whites, including cancer of the brain and nervous system, multiple myeloma, myelocytic leukemia, stomach cancer (male), and non-Hodgkin's lymphoma (female).

Table 11–II–5 presents age-adjusted mortality rates for various racial and ethnic groups for the entire United States. For cancers with poor survival, such as those of the esophagus, liver, or pancreas, mortality rates approximated the incidence rates. Where there was substantial racial variation in survival, mortality rates presented a pattern different from incidence. Among females, in contrast to lower overall incidence, blacks had a higher mortality rate for all cancers combined. Whereas incidence rates for lung, breast, corpus uteri, and bladder cancers were lower among black females than white females, mortality rates were similar in the two races for lung and breast cancers, and higher among blacks for corpus uteri and bladder cancers. Colorectal

TABLE 11–II–2. *Five-Year Relative Survival Rates (%) for Malignant Cases Diagnosed from 1975 to 1984 in Four Areas**

	Both Sexes		*Male*		*Female*	
	Number	*Rate*	*Number*	*Rate*	*Number*	*Rate*
ALL SITES						
Black	46,904	39.6	25,657	33.4	21,247	46.5
White	318,015	51.3	155,637	44.4	162,378	57.4
ORAL CAVITY AND PHARYNX						
Black	1,902	33.0	1,340	27.4	562	45.5
White	10,495	49.8	7,082	47.5	3,413	54.5
Other oral cavity[a]						
Black	1,820	30.1	1,313	25.6	507	41.0
White	8,796	42.9	5,875	39.3	2,921	49.7
Nasopharynx						
Black	112	36.5	74	30.8	38	46.8
White	449	37.9	305	38.7	144	36.3
ESOPHAGUS						
Black	1,416	4.2	1,061	3.4	355	6.6
White	2,884	6.1	2,002	5.7	882	7.1
STOMACH						
Black	1,716	17.5	1,131	17.3	585	17.8
White	7,922	16.6	4,995	15.1	2,927	19.1
COLON AND RECTUM						
Black	5,664	46.7	2,666	44.1	2,998	48.8
White	46,651	54.2	23,505	53.2	23,146	55.1
LIVER						
Black	362	3.1	256	2.4	106	0.0
White	1,459	3.9	950	2.2	509	7.1
GALLBLADDER						
Black	127	8.9	44	8.3	83	9.3
White	1,257	8.8	358	8.1	899	9.0
PANCREAS						
Black	1,300	3.2	682	2.4	618	4.1
White	6,853	2.3	3,585	2.4	3,268	2.1
LUNG AND BRONCHUS						
Black	8,508	11.7	6,470	10.3	2,038	15.7
White	47,013	14.2	32,039	12.5	14,974	17.5
MELANOMA OF SKIN						
Black	106	57.5	47	44.8	59	67.2
White	8,813	81.3	4,572	76.2	4,241	86.5
BREAST						
Black	5,734	63.4	60	76.5	5,674	63.2
White	47,292	75.6	331	81.0	46,961	75.5
CERVIX UTERI						
Black	1,746	61.6	—[b]	—	1,746	61.6
White	4,765	66.7	—	—	4,765	66.7
CORPUS UTERI						
Black	1,131	54.9	—	—	1,131	54.9
White	14,752	84.6	—	—	14,752	84.6

(continued)

TABLE 11–II–2. *Five-Year Relative Survival Rates (%) for Malignant Cases Diagnosed from 1975 to 1984 in Four Areas* (Continued)*

	Both Sexes		*Male*		*Female*	
	Number	*Rate*	*Number*	*Rate*	*Number*	*Rate*
OVARY						
Black	733	40.9	—	—	733	40.9
White	7,197	38.1	—	—	7,197	38.1
PROSTATE GLAND						
Black	5,937	63.4	5,937	63.4	—	—
White	25,599	70.3	25,599	70.3	—	—
URINARY BLADDER						
Black	1,120	53.4	738	59.0	382	43.1
White	16,831	75.8	12,439	76.9	4,392	72.9
KIDNEY AND RENAL PELVIS						
Black	790	56.3	486	53.3	304	60.8
White	5,788	55.2	3,741	54.4	2,047	56.4
BRAIN AND NERVOUS SYSTEM						
Black	459	28.5	268	25.2	191	33.4
White	4,977	22.6	2,830	21.4	2,147	24.1
HODGKIN'S DISEASE						
Black	349	71.0	228	70.3	121	72.5
White	3,237	73.8	1,821	71.8	1,416	76.3
NON-HODGKIN'S LYMPHOMA						
Black	964	47.9	534	42.2	430	54.4
White	10,434	49.9	5,318	49.2	5,116	50.6
MULTIPLE MYELOMA						
Black	1,020	30.1	525	28.5	495	31.5
White	3,282	24.3	1,660	23.7	1,622	24.8
LEUKEMIAS						
Black	1,246	28.0	671	26.9	575	29.2
White	9,221	32.6	5,236	32.8	3,985	32.4
Lymphocytic						
Black	484	47.5	280	46.8	204	48.3
White	3,817	58.3	2,199	57.3	1,618	59.7
Myelocytic						
Black	608	15.0	312	13.3	296	16.7
White	4,012	12.0	2,214	11.8	1,798	12.2

*The data for whites and blacks in this table are from San Francisco, Detroit, Atlanta, and Connecticut only.
[a]Other oral cavity is the total oral cavity and pharynx excluding lip and salivary glands.
[b]Dash indicates that there were too few cases for a reliable estimate of the five-year survival rate.

cancer incidence was virtually the same among females of both races, but the mortality rate was higher among blacks; among males, colorectal cancer incidence was lower among blacks but mortality rates were virtually equivalent. As expected from their high overall incidence rate, black males had a higher total cancer mortality rate than other males. Of the specific forms of cancer presented in Table 11–II–5, rates were higher among blacks than whites for 11 of the 26 forms. More recent incidence, survival, and mortality data on cancer among blacks are presented in Boring et al (1992) and Ries et al (1994).

ASIAN AMERICANS

Approximately 3.5 million members of various Asian ethnic groups resided in the United States in 1980 (Bureau of the Census, 1988a). Twelve distinct groups of Asian Americans were identified, including Chinese

(806,040), Japanese (700,794), Filipino (774,652), Korean (354,593), Vietnamese (261,729), and another 17% consisting of smaller numbers of persons of other Asian ancestries or origins. The Asian-American population is concentrated in just a few areas of the United States: the West Coast (including Hawaii), Texas, Illinois (Chicago), and the heavily populated areas of the East Coast (New York, New Jersey, and Rhode Island, with fewer found in Pennsylvania, Virginia, and Delaware). Each of these different ethnic groups has its own language and customs.

Of these 3.5 million Asian Americans, 62% were foreign-born (Bureau of the Census, 1988a), with large variations in percent foreign-born by country of origin: 77% of the Vietnamese, 63% of the Chinese, 42% of the Japanese, and 65% of the Filipinos. Cultural customs and diet probably are more like those in the country of origin among the foreign-born than the native-born. Ten percent of the foreign-born compared to 70% of U.S.-born Asian Americans speak only English at home. The language spoken at home may be related to the ability to read English and understand health-related information and literature, and thus may influence cancer control efforts.

The median family income in 1979 was $23,095 for all Asian Americans combined and $21,458 for the foreign-born (Bureau of the Census, 1988a), both of which are higher than the $20,835 comparable income for whites. This may partially reflect Asian Americans living in geographic areas of the country with higher salary levels. Only 10 to 12% of Asian Americans were below the poverty level in 1979. As a group, Asian Americans are well educated, with about 70% having graduated from high school.

Of the twelve Asian-American ethnic groups, we were able to ascertain both the numbers of cases and deaths and denominator population estimates adequately for three groups: the Chinese, the Japanese, and the Filipinos. Cancer incidence and survival experience of these groups are available from registries in the San Francisco-Oakland metropolitan area and the state of Hawaii. These two geographic areas contained 24.8% of the Chinese Americans, 40.5% of the Japanese Americans, and 30.3% of the Filipino Americans.

In San Francisco and Hawaii, stomach cancer incidence rates among the Japanese were three times those among whites, whereas an excess occurred among Chinese females but not males, and rates among Filipinos of both sexes were lower than those among whites (Table 11–II–3). Liver cancer incidence rates were high in all three Asian groups, particularly the Chinese. Nasopharynx cancer rates were markedly elevated among the Chinese, with rates about 20 times those among whites; rates were somewhat higher among the other Asian groups except for Japanese females. Excesses of esophageal cancers were apparent among all three groups of Asian males but not females. Although based on small numbers, gallbladder cancer rates showed a similar pattern. The cervix uteri cancer rate among Chinese women was 24% higher than that for whites, whereas Japanese women were at lower risk. Overall, however, these three Asian-American groups had cancer incidence rates 54–73% those among whites. For all cancers combined and both sexes, Filipinos had the lowest incidence rate (212.4), followed by the Japanese (242.5) and the Chinese (247.6), all considerably lower than the rate of 349.6 among whites. These patterns were due to lower rates of colorectal, pancreatic, and virtually all non-gastrointestinal forms of cancer.

There were smaller differences in five-year relative survival rates between Asian Americans and whites (Table 11–II–4) than between blacks and whites. In fact, survival rates for all sites combined were higher among Japanese than white females and, with the exception of the leukemias and corpus uteri cancer, at least one of the Asian-American groups had a survival rate equal to or higher than that for whites for every cancer. In several instances, it was difficult to evaluate the survival experience of the Asian-American groups because small numbers of cases gave the rates a large variability. The Chinese experienced the most favorable survival rates for cancers of the nasopharynx and other oral cavity, esophagus, cervix uteri, and non-Hodgkin's lymphomas among males. The Japanese had the highest five-year survival rates for cancers of the stomach, colorectum, breast, prostate, bladder among males, kidney and renal pelvis, and for myeloid leukemia. The best five-year survival rates occurred among Filipinos for cancers of the liver and ovary, but this group experienced relatively poor survival for a number of sites, including cancers of the colorectum, breast, corpus uteri, prostate, and bladder, and non-Hodgkin's lymphoma.

Reflecting primarily the difference in incidence rates, total cancer mortality rates for U.S. Asian Americans were 36–75% those for whites (Table 11–II–5). On a site-specific basis, the patterns of cancer mortality varied widely among these racial and ethnic groups. The Japanese had the highest mortality rates for cancer of the stomach, relatively high rates for liver cancer, and among the lowest for prostatic cancer. Filipinos had the lowest mortality rates for cancers overall and for those of the esophagus, stomach, colorectum, pancreas, lung, female breast, cervix uteri, ovary, and brain. The Chinese had high mortality rates for oral cavity cancers, the highest rates for nasopharynx and liver cancers by factors of three to fifteen, and a low mortality rate for prostatic cancer.

A number of investigators have compared the cancer risks among migrant and nonmigrant groups of Japanese, Chinese, and Filipinos (Locke and King, 1980;

TABLE 11–II–3. *Average Annual Age-Adjusted (1970 U.S. Standard) Cancer Incidence Rates per 100,000 Population for Malignant Cases Only, Two Areas, 1977–1983**

	Both Sexes		Male		Female	
	Number	*Rate*	*Number*	*Rate*	*Number*	*Rate*
ALL SITES						
Chinese	3,940	247.6	2,095	274.0	1,845	225.9
Japanese	6,139	242.5	3,255	289.2	2,884	207.4
Filipino	2,950	212.4	1,835	221.1	1,115	178.7
White	82,148	349.6	39,712	393.5	42,436	329.0
ORAL CAVITY AND PHARYNX						
Chinese	238	15.4	166	22.8	72	8.6
Japanese	121	4.8	85	7.7	36	2.5
Filipino	121	8.9	85	10.4	36	7.1
White	2,935	13.3	1,847	18.7	1,088	9.0
Other oral cavity[a]						
Chinese	229	14.8	161	22.1	68	8.0
Japanese	108	4.3	76	6.8	32	2.2
Filipino	107	7.9	76	9.2	31	6.2
White	2,382	10.8	1,435	14.5	947	8.0
Nasopharynx						
Chinese	168	11.1	112	15.4	56	7.1
Japanese	16	0.6	14	1.2	2	0.2
Filipino	30	2.1	22	2.9	8	1.1
White	116	0.5	79	0.8	37	0.3
ESOPHAGUS						
Chinese	53	3.3	45	5.9	8	0.9ep
Japanese	72	2.8	64	5.6	8	0.6
Filipino	48	3.4	38	4.5	10	1.6
White	694	2.9	423	4.3	271	2.0
STOMACH						
Chinese	165	10.5	97	13.0	68	8.4
Japanese	670	26.6	419	38.9	251	17.2
Filipino	102	7.8	73	9.3	29	5.0
White	2,130	8.7	1,285	13.0	845	5.5
COLON AND RECTUM						
Chinese	628	40.4	361	48.8	267	33.0
Japanese	1,226	48.8	709	62.3	517	37.5
Filipino	408	30.3	305	36.7	103	18.3
White	11,697	49.1	5,751	59.6	5,946	41.9
LIVER						
Chinese	182	9.6	150	17.0	32	2.8
Japanese	120	3.6	92	6.2	28	1.4
Filipino	86	5.4	69	8.0	17	2.1
White	579	2.2	383	3.5	196	1.1
GALLBLADDER						
Chinese	15	1.0	9	1.3	6	0.8
Japanese	37	1.5	16	1.5	21	1.5
Filipino	17	1.4	11	1.4	6	1.2
White	284	1.2	66	0.7	218	1.6
PANCREAS						
Chinese	126	6.3	61	6.6	65	6.1
Japanese	212	7.1	116	9.0	96	5.5
Filipino	82	4.9	61	6.1	21	3.6
White	2,318	8.0	1,138	9.7	1,180	6.8

(continued)

TABLE 11–II–3. *(Continued)*

	Both Sexes		Male		Female	
	Number	*Rate*	*Number*	*Rate*	*Number*	*Rate*
LUNG AND BRONCHUS						
Chinese	660	40.6	451	57.4	209	24.8
Japanese	715	27.1	534	45.0	181	12.6
Filipino	388	27.3	293	35.5	95	16.1
White	12,664	53.6	8,036	77.5	4,628	36.2
MELANOMA OF SKIN						
Chinese	12	0.7	4	0.6	8	0.9
Japanese	30	1.2	17	1.6	13	1.0
Filipino	13	1.0	9	1.1	4	0.5
White	2,739	11.7	1,425	13.2	1,314	10.6
BREAST						
Chinese	452	29.8	5	0.5	447	57.8
Japanese	751	30.0	4	0.4	747	55.0
Filipino	275	19.8	2	0.4	273	41.3
White	11,779	52.6	82	0.8	11,697	96.8
CERVIX UTERI						
Chinese	80	5.3	—	—	80	10.3
Japanese	79	3.2	—	—	79	5.9
Filipino	63	4.2	—	—	63	8.6
White	994	4.3	—	—	994	8.3
CORPUS UTERI						
Chinese	138	9.2	—	—	138	18.0
Japanese	246	9.5	—	—	246	17.7
Filipino	73	5.4	—	—	73	11.3
White	3,659	16.7	—	—	3,659	30.6
OVARY						
Chinese	72	4.8	—	—	72	9.2
Japanese	119	4.7	—	—	119	8.8
Filipino	60	4.5	—	—	60	9.7
White	1,666	7.3	—	—	1,666	13.5
PROSTATE GLAND						
Chinese	212	13.7	212	29.6	—	—
Japanese	450	19.0	450	43.8	—	—
Filipino	376	28.8	376	44.0	—	—
White	6,796	28.2	6,796	70.7	—	—
URINARY BLADDER						
Chinese	138	9.0	108	14.7	30	3.7
Japanese	197	8.0	133	12.0	64	4.6
Filipino	54	4.4	40	5.4	14	2.9
White	3,926	17.2	2,819	29.7	1,107	8.2
KIDNEY AND RENAL PELVIS						
Chinese	55	3.5	35	4.6	20	2.6
Japanese	96	3.6	70	5.7	26	2.0
Filipino	44	3.1	33	4.2	11	1.8
White	1,409	6.0	930	9.0	479	3.6
BRAIN AND NERVOUS SYSTEM						
Chinese	40	2.4	23	2.9	17	2.0
Japanese	53	2.4	30	2.8	23	2.1
Filipino	30	1.9	26	2.9	4	0.5
White	1,356	5.4	757	6.6	599	4.3

(continued)

TABLE 11–II–3. *Average Annual Age-Adjusted (1970 U.S. Standard) Cancer Incidence Rates per 100,000 Population for Malignant Cases Only, Two Areas, 1977–1983* (Continued)*

	Both Sexes		*Male*		*Female*	
	Number	*Rate*	*Number*	*Rate*	*Number*	*Rate*
HODGKIN'S DISEASE						
Chinese	11	0.6	6	0.6	5	0.7
Japanese	14	0.5	10	0.8	4	0.3
Filipino	20	1.2	12	1.4	8	1.2
White	644	2.9	376	3.5	268	2.4
NON-HODGKIN'S LYMPHOMA						
Chinese	125	8.5	75	10.3	50	6.8
Japanese	179	7.2	94	8.5	85	6.2
Filipino	112	8.3	75	9.3	37	7.0
White	2,518	11.1	1,293	13.0	1,225	9.5
MULTIPLE MYELOMA						
Chinese	30	1.9	17	2.4	13	1.4
Japanese	35	1.3	16	1.3	19	1.4
Filipino	44	3.2	33	3.8	11	2.0
White	834	3.4	420	4.2	414	2.9
LEUKEMIAS						
Chinese	67	4.8	41	6.3	26	3.4
Japanese	131	5.7	77	7.1	54	4.5
Filipino	95	7.1	60	8.0	35	5.8
White	2,158	9.5	1,210	12.6	948	7.3
Lymphocytic						
Chinese	19	1.7	11	2.2	8	1.2
Japanese	30	1.5	16	1.7	14	1.4
Filipino	26	1.9	14	1.9	12	2.0
White	861	4.0	480	5.2	381	3.1
Myelocytic						
Chinese	28	1.9	17	2.4	11	1.4
Japanese	84	3.5	51	4.6	33	2.6
Filipino	50	3.5	31	3.8	19	3.2
White	980	4.2	539	5.5	441	3.4

*The data in this table are from San Francisco and Hawaii only.
[a]Other oral cavity is the total oral cavity and pharynx excluding lip and salivary glands.

King et al, 1985; Kolonel, 1985, 1988; Shimizu et al, 1987; Stemmermann et al, 1991; Ziegler et al, 1993; Herrinton et al, 1994; Stellman and Wang, 1994). As persons migrate from one environment to another, it was thought that their exposures to carcinogens and hence their risk of developing cancer would change. Exceptions would be those cancers with a genetic predisposition. Perhaps among the best-known findings from these migrant studies are decreases from the high stomach cancer rates found in their homelands among those who migrate to the United States, greater decreases among those born in the U.S., and even more rapid increases in colon cancer rates. The declines in stomach cancer risk have been ascribed to westernization of the diet, eating less pickled and salted foods and more fresh vegetables and fruits (Hirayama, 1975; Namiki, 1980; Tominaga et al, 1982). Increases in colon and breast cancer rates appear to be influenced by dietary changes (Riboli, 1990), with hormonal factors probably mediating the risk of breast cancer. A sharp decrease in the high risk of liver cancer noted among migrants is most likely related to differences in the prevalence of infection with hepatitis B virus (Ho, 1979; Tu et al, 1985). Excess risks of nasopharynx cancer among the Chinese appear to be related to a combination of genetic, dietary, and viral factors (Hildesheim and Levine, 1993).

HISPANICS

Hispanic is a general term used to denote persons in the United States with Hispanic surnames or with origins

TABLE 11–II–4. *Five-Year Relative Survival Rates (%) for Malignant Cases Diagnosed from 1975 to 1984 in Two Areas**

	Both Sexes		*Male*		*Female*	
	Number	*Rate*	*Number*	*Rate*	*Number*	*Rate*
ALL SITES						
Chinese	4,702	47.5	2,475	38.9	2,227	56.2
Japanese	7,370	53.1	3,814	44.4	3,556	61.6
Filipino	3,771	46.1	2,311	38.9	1,460	56.7
White	96,220	52.9	46,366	46.1	49,854	58.7
ORAL CAVITY AND PHARYNX						
Chinese	292	55.7	199	54.3	93	58.5
Japanese	151	44.4	108	41.7	43	51.6
Filipino	161	46.6	109	40.6	52	58.4
White	3,476	50.2	2,226	49.6	1,250	51.1
Other oral cavity[a]						
Chinese	287	54.6	197	53.8	90	56.2
Japanese	138	45.1	99	42.9	39	50.5
Filipino	146	45.0	99	39.1	47	56.8
White	2,591	42.6	1,578	39.3	1,013	47.6
Nasopharynx						
Chinese	219	56.6	143	55.9	76	57.7
Japanese	26	45.1	21	—[b]	5	—
Filipino	43	47.5	28	46.3	15	—
White	146	41.1	99	43.1	47	35.5
ESOPHAGUS						
Chinese	61	11.5	51	7.0	10	—
Japanese	82	5.8	72	4.8	10	—
Filipino	63	3.4	50	6.5	13	—
White	771	5.8	486	6.3	285	4.8
STOMACH						
Chinese	204	21.6	121	17.8	83	26.6
Japanese	823	29.8	510	28.1	313	32.5
Filipino	133	18.8	96	21.2	37	0.0
White	2,455	16.3	1,554	14.8	901	18.8
COLON AND RECTUM						
Chinese	749	53.1	437	48.7	312	58.8
Japanese	1,506	61.7	899	60.8	607	62.8
Filipino	542	44.8	398	42.5	144	51.4
White	13,366	54.4	6,677	54.2	6,689	54.6
LIVER						
Chinese	184	2.0	150	1.4	34	4.1
Japanese	106	1.5	76	1.5	30	0.0
Filipino	99	6.7	82	5.0	17	—
White	528	4.2	355	3.2	173	6.1
GALLBLADDER						
Chinese	17	—	12	—	5	—
Japanese	42	16.2	14	—	28	14.9
Filipino	22	—	12	—	10	—
White	355	8.8	90	3.0	265	10.8
PANCREAS						
Chinese	118	0.0	61	0.0	57	0.0
Japanese	206	2.6	120	0.9	86	4.8
Filipino	82	5.2	57	3.8	25	0.0
White	2,212	2.1	1,140	2.2	1,072	2.1

(continued)

TABLE 11–II–4. *Five-Year Relative Survival Rates (%) for Malignant Cases Diagnosed from 1975 to 1984 in Two Areas* (Continued)*

	Both Sexes		*Male*		*Female*	
	Number	*Rate*	*Number*	*Rate*	*Number*	*Rate*
LUNG AND BRONCHUS						
Chinese	783	15.1	524	15.0	259	15.4
Japanese	830	14.3	627	13.4	203	16.8
Filipino	476	13.2	369	14.3	107	10.1
White	14,103	15.7	9,048	13.8	5,055	18.9
MELANOMA OF SKIN						
Chinese	10	—	4	—	6	—
Japanese	37	81.0	21	—	16	—
Filipino	18	—	12	—	6	—
White	3,299	83.2	1,754	78.5	1,545	88.3
BREAST						
Chinese	551	80.9	3	—	548	80.8
Japanese	979	85.4	5	—	974	85.4
Filipino	367	73.6	3	—	364	73.7
White	14,303	78.3	98	90.2	14,205	78.3
CERVIX UTERI						
Chinese	102	74.6	—	—	102	74.6
Japanese	108	70.2	—	—	108	70.2
Filipino	100	73.0	—	—	100	73.0
White	1,366	69.0	—	—	1,366	69.0
CORPUS UTERI						
Chinese	179	86.1	—	—	179	86.1
Japanese	330	84.1	—	—	330	84.1
Filipino	94	79.9	—	—	94	79.9
White	5,006	86.9	—	—	5,006	86.9
OVARY						
Chinese	98	43.3	—	—	98	43.3
Japanese	150	43.5	—	—	150	43.5
Filipino	67	44.7	—	—	67	44.7
White	2,052	37.4	—	—	2,052	37.4
PROSTATE GLAND						
Chinese	271	72.5	271	72.5	—	—
Japanese	477	80.5	477	80.5	—	—
Filipino	469	71.7	469	71.7	—	—
White	7,861	73.0	7,861	73.0	—	—
URINARY BLADDER						
Chinese	153	78.5	121	83.9	32	56.8
Japanese	254	80.8	175	85.6	79	70.1
Filipino	77	58.4	60	64.9	17	—
White	4,708	77.5	3,434	79.0	1,274	73.5
KIDNEY AND RENAL PELVIS						
Chinese	61	60.7	42	58.9	19	—
Japanese	108	63.1	74	61.4	34	66.7
Filipino	50	47.0	39	44.3	11	—
White	1,524	53.1	1,026	54.6	498	50.0
BRAIN AND NERVOUS SYSTEM						
Chinese	47	35.9	26	25.5	21	—
Japanese	64	40.6	36	26.5	28	57.4
Filipino	37	29.6	32	28.4	5	—
White	1,446	25.1	840	22.8	606	28.3

(continued)

TABLE 11–II–4. *(Continued)*

	Both Sexes		*Male*		*Female*	
	Number	*Rate*	*Number*	*Rate*	*Number*	*Rate*
HODGKIN'S DISEASE						
Chinese	15	—	8	—	7	—
Japanese	21	—	15	—	6	—
Filipino	30	43.5	18	—	12	—
White	885	73.5	519	69.7	366	78.7
NON-HODGKIN'S LYMPHOMA						
Chinese	155	50.3	92	51.4	63	48.7
Japanese	222	41.1	120	38.5	102	43.9
Filipino	154	33.8	106	32.9	48	35.1
White	3,163	49.9	1,653	47.9	1,510	52.1
MULTIPLE MYELOMA						
Chinese	38	20.5	22	—	16	—
Japanese	46	37.6	22	—	24	—
Filipino	62	17.1	45	7.8	17	—
White	975	25.4	500	26.1	475	24.6
LEUKEMIAS						
Chinese	99	19.8	61	22.1	38	16.4
Japanese	156	26.0	88	22.0	68	31.4
Filipino	128	22.3	77	21.9	51	22.5
White	2,647	32.8	1,472	33.7	1,175	31.6
Lymphocytic						
Chinese	33	36.4	20	—	13	—
Japanese	37	39.9	17	—	20	—
Filipino	35	54.3	19	—	16	—
White	1,072	62.1	607	60.8	465	63.7
Myelocytic						
Chinese	47	13.8	29	9.4	18	—
Japanese	97	18.9	61	20.1	36	16.6
Filipino	70	10.0	41	14.4	29	2.8
White	1,215	9.3	653	10.1	562	8.4

*The data in this table are from San Francisco and Hawaii only.
[a]Other oral cavity is the total oral cavity and pharynx excluding lip and salivary glands.
[b]Dash indicates that there were too few cases for a reliable estimate of the five-year survival rate.

or ancestry from any of the following: Puerto Rico, Cuba, Spain, the Spanish-speaking countries of Central and South America, or Mexico (Bureau of the Census, 1983a). Persons of Brazilian or Filipino origin or ancestry are not considered to be Hispanic. The 1980 U.S. Census of the Population counted about 14.6 million persons who identified themselves as Hispanic, of whom about 62% were Mexican American, 13% Puerto Rican, 5% Cuban-American, 12% Central or South American, and 8% other. As a group, during 1980 Hispanics living in the United States were young, with a median age of 23.2 years versus 31 for U.S. whites, were often foreign-born (ranging from 20% for Mexican Americans to 80% for Cuban Americans and Central or South Americans), and lived in an urban setting. In 1982, 15% of Hispanic Americans aged 25 and over had less than five years of schooling and only about 45% had completed high school, compared to 2.4% and over 72% of all non-Hispanics, respectively (Bureau of the Census, 1988c). Over 23% of Hispanics had incomes below the poverty level in 1981, more than double the U.S. non-Hispanic rate of 10.5%.

Hispanics were overrepresented in blue-collar jobs such as the service occupations, farming, machine operators, and laborers, and underrepresented in white-collar managerial or administrative and professional jobs (Bureau of the Census, 1988c). The cancer control supplement to the 1987 Health Interview Survey indicated that Hispanics were less likely than white non-Hispanics (Anglos) to have heard about a number of

TABLE 11–II–5. *Average Annual Age-Adjusted (1970 U.S. Standard) Cancer Mortality Rates per 100,000 Population, United States, 1977–1983**

	Both Sexes		*Male*		*Female*	
	Number	*Rate*	*Number*	*Rate*	*Number*	*Rate*
ALL SITES						
Black	312,456	209.8	180,151	288.2	132,305	154.0
American Indian	5,282	89.3	2,794	105.9	2,488	76.4
Chinese	5,547	125.0	3,420	158.0	2,127	93.5
Japanese	5,061	108.0	2,698	138.6	2,363	84.8
Filipino	2,725	72.0	1,877	84.0	848	48.2
White	2,562,285	164.2	1,376,734	209.8	1,185,551	133.5
ORAL CAVITY AND PHARYNX						
Black	8,430	5.7	6,412	9.9	2,018	2.4
American Indian	105	1.8	64	2.3	41	1.3
Chinese	268	5.4	199	8.0	69	2.7
Japanese	81	1.7	58	2.8	23	0.8
Filipino	88	2.4	69	3.0	19	1.2
White	50,326	3.3	34,093	5.2	16,233	1.8
Other oral cavity[a]						
Black	8,065	5.5	6,198	9.6	1,867	2.2
American Indian	96	1.6	60	2.1	36	1.1
Chinese	263	5.3	195	7.8	68	2.6
Japanese	75	1.6	54	2.6	21	0.7
Filipino	82	2.2	65	2.8	17	1.0
White	45,467	3.0	30,885	4.7	14,582	1.6
Nasopharynx						
Black	533	0.3	368	0.5	165	0.2
American Indian	31	0.5	20	0.6	11	0.3
Chinese	210	4.1	161	6.3	49	1.9
Japanese	18	0.4	11	0.5	7	0.2
Filipino	31	0.8	23	1.0	8	0.4
White	3,796	0.2	2,533	0.4	1,263	0.2
ESOPHAGUS						
Black	13,445	9.1	10,179	15.9	3,266	3.9
American Indian	117	2.0	91	3.4	26	0.8
Chinese	120	2.8	101	4.7	19	0.9
Japanese	97	2.1	76	3.8	21	0.8
Filipino	64	1.8	59	2.6	5	0.3
White	41,224	2.6	29,821	4.5	11,403	1.2
STOMACH						
Black	14,747	10.0	9,138	14.9	5,609	6.5
American Indian	338	5.8	198	7.5	140	4.4
Chinese	340	7.6	217	10.1	123	5.3
Japanese	812	17.9	460	24.3	352	13.2
Filipino	128	3.5	85	4.0	43	2.6
White	83,687	5.2	49,438	7.6	34,249	3.6
COLON AND RECTUM						
Black	33,090	22.4	15,515	25.3	17,575	20.4
American Indian	509	8.9	261	10.1	248	8.0
Chinese	760	17.9	487	23.8	273	12.4
Japanese	790	16.8	442	21.8	348	13.0
Filipino	288	7.9	228	9.8	60	4.2
White	343,085	21.4	167,104	25.7	175,981	18.4

(continued)

TABLE 11–II–5. *(Continued)*

	Both Sexes		Male		Female	
	Number	*Rate*	*Number*	*Rate*	*Number*	*Rate*
LIVER						
Black	5,724	3.6	3,753	5.6	1,971	2.1
American Indian	135	2.0	85	3.1	50	1.1
Chinese	482	10.1	393	16.4	89	3.8
Japanese	172	3.4	108	4.9	64	2.1
Filipino	144	3.5	119	5.3	25	1.3
White	33,059	1.9	19,222	2.7	13,837	1.3
GALLBLADDER						
Black	1,089	0.7	325	0.5	764	0.9
American Indian	148	2.6	37	1.5	111	3.6
Chinese	29	0.7	10	0.5	19	0.9
Japanese	46	1.1	17	0.9	29	1.2
Filipino	24	0.6	15	0.6	9	0.6
White	15,097	0.9	3,901	0.6	11,196	1.2
PANCREAS						
Black	16,553	11.2	8,599	13.8	7,954	9.3
American Indian	264	4.6	132	5.3	132	4.2
Chinese	277	6.4	163	7.6	114	5.3
Japanese	317	7.0	165	8.3	152	6.0
Filipino	134	3.5	102	4.5	32	2.1
White	132,131	8.4	68,304	10.4	63,827	6.8
LUNG AND BRONCHUS						
Black	76,003	51.3	58,502	92.3	17,501	20.8
American Indian	1,040	18.1	746	28.7	294	9.4
Chinese	1,372	31.7	967	45.2	405	18.6
Japanese	896	19.8	655	34.0	241	8.7
Filipino	530	14.5	430	20.0	100	6.9
White	638,827	41.6	461,377	69.6	177,450	21.0
MELANOMA OF SKIN						
Black	636	0.4	300	0.5	336	0.4
American Indian	17	0.3	13	0.5	4	0.1
Chinese	11	0.2	7	0.4	4	0.2
Japanese	10	0.2	6	0.3	4	0.1
Filipino	14	0.3	8	0.3	6	0.3
White	32,714	2.2	19,153	2.8	13,561	1.6
BREAST						
Black	23,250	15.5	241	0.4	23,009	26.9
American Indian	313	4.8	1	0.0	312	9.0
Chinese	295	6.1	4	0.2	291	12.0
Japanese	332	5.8	0	—	332	10.2
Filipino	174	3.9	3	0.2	171	7.8
White	227,823	15.0	1,580	0.2	226,243	26.8
CERVIX UTERI						
Black	7,552	5.0	—	—	7,552	8.7
American Indian	188	2.9	—	—	188	5.5
Chinese	79	1.7	—	—	79	3.3
Japanese	71	1.3	—	—	71	2.2
Filipino	43	0.9	—	—	43	1.9
White	26,088	1.7	—	—	26,088	3.2

(continued)

TABLE 11–II–5. *Average Annual Age-Adjusted (1970 U.S. Standard) Cancer Mortality Rates per 100,000 Population, United States, 1977–1983* (Continued)*

	Both Sexes		Male		Female	
	Number	*Rate*	*Number*	*Rate*	*Number*	*Rate*
CORPUS UTERI						
Black	5,586	3.8	—	—	5,586	6.5
American Indian	58	1.0	—	—	58	1.8
Chinese	59	1.3	—	—	59	2.7
Japanese	65	1.3	—	—	65	2.4
Filipino	27	0.7	—	—	27	1.7
White	25,295	2.2	—	—	25,295	3.9
OVARY						
Black	5,477	3.7	—	—	5,477	6.4
American Indian	107	1.8	—	—	107	3.2
Chinese	95	1.9	—	—	95	3.8
Japanese	143	2.5	—	—	143	4.4
Filipino	54	1.2	—	—	54	2.6
White	69,559	4.6	—	—	69,559	8.1
PROSTATE GLAND						
Black	25,400	17.5	25,400	43.9	—	—
American Indian	268	5.1	268	11.7	—	—
Chinese	134	3.5	134	7.4	—	—
Japanese	142	3.4	142	8.4	—	—
Filipino	192	6.0	192	8.7	—	—
White	133,675	8.0	133,675	21.1	—	—
URINARY BLADDER						
Black	5,527	3.8	3,238	5.4	2,289	2.6
American Indian	57	1.0	40	1.6	17	0.5
Chinese	67	1.7	48	2.6	19	0.9
Japanese	80	1.8	42	2.3	38	1.5
Filipino	42	1.4	33	1.6	9	0.7
White	62,882	3.8	43,775	6.8	19,107	1.9
KIDNEY AND RENAL PELVIS						
Black	4,023	2.7	2,491	3.8	1,532	1.8
American Indian	161	2.7	96	3.4	65	2.0
Chinese	74	1.7	51	2.4	23	1.1
Japanese	74	1.6	50	2.5	24	1.0
Filipino	29	0.8	23	1.1	6	0.5
White	48,778	3.2	30,314	4.6	18,464	2.1
BRAIN AND NERVOUS SYSTEM						
Black	3,775	2.4	2,051	2.9	1,724	1.9
American Indian	96	1.3	53	1.6	43	1.1
Chinese	67	1.3	38	1.5	29	1.1
Japanese	60	1.3	32	1.4	28	1.1
Filipino	47	1.1	31	1.3	16	0.7
White	61,061	4.2	33,689	5.0	27,372	3.4
HODGKIN'S DISEASE						
Black	1,118	0.6	661	0.9	457	0.5
American Indian	23	0.3	18	0.5	5	0.1
Chinese	14	0.3	12	0.5	2	0.1
Japanese	4	0.1	3	0.1	1	0.0
Filipino	14	0.3	10	0.3	4	0.2
White	13,158	0.9	7,539	1.1	5,619	0.7

(continued)

TABLE 11–II–5. *(Continued)*

	Both Sexes		*Male*		*Female*	
	Number	*Rate*	*Number*	*Rate*	*Number*	*Rate*
NON-HODGKIN'S LYMPHOMA						
Black	5,127	3.3	2,861	4.3	2,266	2.6
American Indian	124	2.1	66	2.4	58	1.8
Chinese	130	2.8	74	3.1	56	2.5
Japanese	163	3.5	87	4.2	76	3.0
Filipino	138	3.4	93	3.8	45	2.6
White	81,393	5.2	41,764	6.3	39,629	4.4
MULTIPLE MYELOMA						
Black	7,428	5.1	3,817	6.3	3,611	4.2
American Indian	101	1.8	51	2.1	50	1.6
Chinese	57	1.4	35	1.8	22	1.1
Japanese	59	1.3	32	1.7	27	1.0
Filipino	58	1.5	44	1.9	14	0.6
White	38,186	2.4	19,494	3.0	18,692	2.0
LEUKEMIAS						
Black	9,150	5.8	4,965	7.4	4,185	4.6
American Indian	213	2.9	129	3.6	84	2.2
Chinese	200	4.1	121	5.2	79	3.1
Japanese	165	3.5	100	4.9	65	2.4
Filipino	172	4.1	117	5.0	55	2.3
White	103,736	6.7	58,084	8.9	45,652	5.2

*The data in this table are from the total United States.
[a]Other oral cavity is the total oral cavity and pharynx excluding lip and salivary glands.

cancer screening procedures, including the Pap smear, breast exam, mammography, digital rectal exam, blood stool test, and proctoscopy (NCI, 1989). Lower proportions of Hispanics than Anglos had private health insurance coverage, and their utilization of health services was less extensive (Trevino et al, 1991).

There are very little cancer incidence, mortality, or survival data available on the different Hispanic subgroups. Although perhaps not representative of all Hispanics in the United States, data on Hispanics have been reported in two geographic areas of the SEER program: the state of New Mexico and the Commonwealth of Puerto Rico.

Hispanics in New Mexico

Many New Mexican Hispanic families have been here for many generations, descended from colonial Spaniards, while others arrived in the United States during the last two centuries, primarily from Mexico (Key, 1981). There were approximately 477,000 Hispanics in New Mexico in 1980. Anglos (non-Hispanic whites) were used as the comparison group in this section, rather than "total white." Mortality data from the state of New Mexico were used for Hispanics and Anglos because national data encoded for these ethnicities were not available from the NCHS until 1984.

Cancer incidence rates for Hispanics for all sites combined were 75 and 78% those among Anglo males and females, respectively, in spite of New Mexican Anglos having incidence rates among the lowest for whites anywhere (Table 11–II–6). The low overall rates were due to low rates, relative to Anglos, for cancers of the colorectum (65%, 70%), lung (46%, 54%), breast (63%), corpus uteri (55%), and bladder (52%, 57%). Lower daily cigarette consumption by Hispanics in spite of similar smoking prevalence appears to explain their low lung cancer rates relative to Anglos (Humble et al, 1985). However, cancers of the stomach, liver, gallbladder, pancreas, nasopharynx, and cervix uteri all occurred more frequently among Hispanics than Anglos, with the Hispanic–Anglo rate ratio for stomach cancer being 2.5 and that for gallbladder cancer among females almost seven. As among other groups, stomach cancer rates have declined, more in the past than recently (Wiggins et al, 1993). Hispanics in New Mexico experience excess gallbladder disease that is associated with their increased risk of gallbladder cancer (Samet et al, 1988).

TABLE 11–II–6. *Average Annual Age-Adjusted (1970 U.S. Standard) Cancer Incidence Rates per 100,000 Population for Malignant Cases Only, New Mexico, 1977–83**

	Both Sexes		*Male*		*Female*	
	Number	*Rate*	*Number*	*Rate*	*Number*	*Rate*
ALL SITES						
Hispanic	5,570	245.1	2,868	277.0	2,702	218.9
American Indian*	1,605	137.6	730	133.3	875	140.8
Anglo	17,004	314.5	8,800	367.9	8,204	280.8
ORAL CAVITY AND PHARYNX						
Hispanic	145	6.6	111	10.8	34	2.8
American Indian	22	2.1	16	3.0	6	1.3
Anglo	664	12.3	482	19.7	182	6.3
Other oral cavity[a]						
Hispanic	87	3.9	66	6.3	21	1.7
American Indian	17	1.7	13	2.5	4	1.0
Anglo	362	6.7	224	9.7	138	4.8
Nasopharynx						
Hispanic	13	0.5	11	0.9	2	0.2
American Indian	3	0.3	2	0.3	1	0.2
Anglo	14	0.3	11	0.4	3	0.1
ESOPHAGUS						
Hispanic	35	1.6	26	2.6	9	0.8
American Indian	10	1.0	8	1.6	2	0.4
Anglo	109	2.0	70	2.9	39	1.3
STOMACH						
Hispanic	326	15.3	209	21.1	117	10.2
American Indian	164	15.1	97	19.2	67	11.7
Anglo	310	5.8	187	7.9	123	4.0
COLON AND RECTUM						
Hispanic	573	26.2	293	28.9	280	23.9
American Indian	102	9.6	53	10.4	49	9.1
Anglo	2,091	38.6	1,042	44.2	1,049	34.2
LIVER						
Hispanic	65	3.1	45	4.6	20	1.7
American Indian	25	2.1	18	3.2	7	1.1
Anglo	102	1.9	66	2.8	36	1.2
GALLBLADDER						
Hispanic	99	4.6	12	1.2	87	7.6
American Indian	99	10.0	27	5.9	72	13.6
Anglo	52	1.0	16	0.7	36	1.1
PANCREAS						
Hispanic	237	11.0	117	11.6	120	10.5
American Indian	53	3.7	30	5.2	23	2.2
Anglo	476	8.7	258	10.7	218	7.2
LUNG AND BRONCHUS						
Hispanic	500	23.4	335	33.6	165	14.5
American Indian	67	6.3	46	9.4	21	3.6
Anglo	2,570	47.1	1,785	73.2	785	26.7
MELANOMA OF SKIN						
Hispanic	53	1.9	18	1.3	35	2.5
American Indian	20	1.9	12	2.4	8	1.6
Anglo	667	12.3	333	13.1	334	11.8

(continued)

TABLE 11–II–6. *(Continued)*

	Both Sexes		Male		Female	
	Number	*Rate*	*Number*	*Rate*	*Number*	*Rate*
BREAST						
Hispanic	655	27.6	4	0.3	651	52.1
American Indian	130	11.3	0	—	130	21.3
Anglo	2,374	44.6	23	1.0	2,351	82.3
CERVIX UTERI						
Hispanic	217	8.4	—	—	217	16.1
American Indian	120	10.5	—	—	120	19.9
Anglo	248	4.5	—	—	248	8.6
CORPUS UTERI						
Hispanic	136	6.0	—	—	136	11.3
American Indian	47	3.9	—	—	47	7.2
Anglo	597	11.0	—	—	597	20.5
OVARY						
Hispanic	147	6.0	—	—	147	11.3
American Indian	47	4.0	—	—	47	7.5
Anglo	359	6.7	—	—	359	12.5
PROSTATE GLAND						
Hispanic	737	35.2	737	76.3	—	—
American Indian	158	14.9	158	31.0	—	—
Anglo	1,874	34.0	1,874	81.5	—	—
URINARY BLADDER						
Hispanic	171	7.9	128	12.8	43	3.7
American Indian	13	1.4	11	2.8	2	0.2
Anglo	781	14.3	584	24.4	197	6.5
KIDNEY AND RENAL PELVIS						
Hispanic	141	6.4	94	9.2	47	4.1
American Indian	71	5.7	36	6.2	35	5.3
Anglo	364	6.9	238	9.9	126	4.3
BRAIN AND NERVOUS SYSTEM						
Hispanic	97	3.7	67	5.4	30	2.1
American Indian	25	1.2	16	1.6	9	0.8
Anglo	256	4.9	148	6.1	108	3.9
HODGKIN'S DISEASE						
Hispanic	75	2.6	57	4.1	18	1.2
American Indian	4	0.2	2	0.2	2	0.3
Anglo	129	2.4	73	2.8	56	2.1
NON-HODGKIN'S LYMPHOMA						
Hispanic	157	6.7	90	7.8	67	5.6
American Indian	30	2.8	14	2.6	16	3.2
Anglo	539	10.2	278	11.7	261	8.9
MULTIPLE MYELOMA						
Hispanic	57	2.7	25	2.5	32	2.8
American Indian	32	3.4	15	3.1	17	3.7
Anglo	164	3.0	86	3.6	78	2.6

(continued)

TABLE 11–II–6. *Average Annual Age-Adjusted (1970 U.S. Standard) Cancer Incidence Rates per 100,000 Population for Malignant Cases Only, New Mexico, 1977–83* (Continued)*

	Both Sexes		*Male*		*Female*	
	Number	*Rate*	*Number*	*Rate*	*Number*	*Rate*
LEUKEMIAS						
Hispanic	183	6.9	99	7.9	84	6.0
American Indian	71	4.6	40	5.2	31	4.1
Anglo	547	10.4	322	13.7	225	7.7
Lymphocytic						
Hispanic	90	3.1	49	3.6	41	2.6
American Indian	34	2.3	18	2.4	16	2.3
Anglo	263	5.1	166	7.1	97	3.4
Myelocytic						
Hispanic	72	2.9	40	3.4	32	2.6
American Indian	27	1.6	17	2.0	10	1.3
Anglo	214	4.0	113	4.9	101	3.4

*The data in this table for Hispanics and whites are from the state of New Mexico only. Data on American Indians from the state of Arizona have been added to those of New Mexico.

[a]Other oral cavity is the total oral cavity and pharynx excluding lip and salivary glands.

Notably high gallbladder cancer rates also have been reported in Cali, Colombia (Muir et al, 1987) and Chile (Nervi et al, 1988). Although based on small numbers of cases, Hispanic males, but not females, appeared to be at excess risk of Hodgkin's disease.

Five-year relative survival rates for all cancers combined among Hispanics were slightly lower than those for Anglos, 48.4 and 51.4%, respectively (Table 11–II–7). Rates for individual forms of cancer were generally very similar. In fact, the stomach cancer survival rate was somewhat higher for Hispanic than Anglo males, or 19.5% versus 8.8%. While the survival rates for males and Anglo females with cancer of the urinary bladder were about 70%, Hispanic females appeared to be at a large disadvantage, with a five-year survival rate of only 37.3%, although this rate was based on only 50 cases. Survival rates were also lower for Hispanics than for Anglos diagnosed with leukemia, especially for males, whose five-year survival rate was 23.5% versus 35.4%.

Mortality rates for Hispanics were lower than those for Anglos for virtually every cancer investigated, except cancers of the stomach, liver, gallbladder, pancreas, and cervix uteri (Table 11–II–8), reflecting the incidence experience. Differences in rates between Hispanics and Anglos in New Mexico have been diminishing over time (Wiggins et al, 1993). In other western U.S. areas, cancer patterns generally similar to those in New Mexico were seen among Hispanics relative to non-Hispanic whites, although differences may also be diminishing over time due to acculturation (Mack et al, 1985; Savitz, 1986; Muir et al, 1987).

Hispanics in Puerto Rico

The Commonwealth of Puerto Rico had 3,196,520 inhabitants according to the 1980 U.S. Census (Bureau of the Census, 1983b). The population of Puerto Rico was young, with a median age of 24.6, and 67% lived in urbanized areas. All Puerto Ricans are considered Hispanic, with 80% of the population having white or mixed blood and 20% black (Martinez et al, 1987). The cancer registry in Puerto Rico was established in 1950, and the reporting of cancer was made mandatory by public law in 1951 (Mora et al, 1987).

The overall cancer incidence rate of 202.2 (Table 11–II–9) was lower than either the Hispanic (245.1) or Anglo (314.5) rate in New Mexico, and rates were lower for many forms of cancer. However, there were several sites for which incidence rates in Puerto Rico were relatively high, including cancers of the oral cavity and pharynx, esophagus, stomach, and cervix uteri. Two of these cancers, oral cavity and pharynx, and esophagus, have strong associations with heavy alcohol and tobacco use (Schottenfeld, 1984; Schottenfeld and Bergad, 1985). A case–control study in Puerto Rico by Martinez (1969) revealed a strong association between alcohol use and esophageal cancer even after adjusting for cigarette smoking. The findings were consistent with estimates indicating an excess risk of esophageal cancer among heavy alcohol users of up to 25 times that of non-users (Wynder and Bross, 1961). Incidence rates for both stomach and cervix uteri cancers among Puerto Ricans were similar to those among Hispanics in New Mexico; they were approximately twice those among

TABLE 11–II–7. *Five-Year Relative Survival Rates (%) for Malignant Cases Diagnosed from 1975 to 1984 in New Mexico**

	Both Sexes		*Male*		*Female*	
	Number	*Rate*	*Number*	*Rate*	*Number*	*Rate*
ALL SITES						
Hispanic	6,820	48.4	3,439	45.1	3,381	51.5
American Indian	2,192	33.4	980	26.6	1,212	38.6
Anglo	21,715	51.4	11,169	46.3	10,546	56.2
ORAL CAVITY AND PHARYNX						
Hispanic	190	60.7	141	61.9	49	56.2
American Indian	34	32.5	25	25.8	9	—[b]
Anglo	789	62.9	562	66.2	227	55.6
Other oral cavity[a]						
Hispanic	116	43.8	84	40.8	32	51.6
American Indian	26	24.8	21	—	5	—
Anglo	438	43.3	268	42.6	170	44.3
Nasopharynx						
Hispanic	18	—	16	—	2	—
American Indian	7	—	6	—	1	—
Anglo	18	—	12	—	6	—
ESOPHAGUS						
Hispanic	43	0.0	30	0.0	13	—
American Indian	12	—	9	—	3	—
Anglo	142	3.8	91	1.6	51	5.8
STOMACH						
Hispanic	411	17.8	268	19.5	143	14.5
American Indian	210	8.7	125	4.9	85	14.1
Anglo	396	10.4	239	8.8	157	13.2
COLON AND RECTUM						
Hispanic	707	45.0	366	40.8	341	49.4
American Indian	136	37.8	64	34.0	72	41.0
Anglo	2,616	48.4	1,307	47.4	1,309	48.6
LIVER						
Hispanic	66	0.0	45	0.0	21	—
American Indian	37	0.0	23	—	14	—
Anglo	117	0.7	77	1.6	40	0.0
GALLBLADDER						
Hispanic	128	8.5	20	—	108	10.2
American Indian	141	3.6	39	3.2	102	3.6
Anglo	71	1.0	22	—	49	1.5
PANCREAS						
Hispanic	242	1.2	129	1.3	113	1.0
American Indian	73	0.0	40	0.0	33	—
Anglo	593	2.0	324	1.5	269	2.5
LUNG AND BRONCHUS						
Hispanic	564	10.8	372	8.7	192	14.6
American Indian	92	3.0	59	0.0	33	10.5
Anglo	3,240	11.6	2,258	10.6	982	13.6
MELANOMA OF SKIN						
Hispanic	69	82.1	25	89.3	44	78.1
American Indian	21	—	13	—	8	—
Anglo	806	80.6	398	78.5	408	82.6

(continued)

TABLE 11–II–7. *Five-Year Relative Survival Rates (%) for Malignant Cases Diagnosed from 1975 to 1984 in New Mexico* (Continued)*

	Both Sexes		*Male*		*Female*	
	Number	*Rate*	*Number*	*Rate*	*Number*	*Rate*
BREAST						
Hispanic	841	70.8	6	—	835	70.6
American Indian	183	46.5	1	—	182	46.3
Anglo	3,125	75.4	35	69.4	3,090	75.5
CERVIX UTERI						
Hispanic	328	70.5	—	—	328	70.5
American Indian	159	64.1	—	—	159	64.1
Anglo	364	69.7	—	—	364	69.7
CORPUS UTERI						
Hispanic	179	77.0	—	—	179	77.0
American Indian	65	83.9	—	—	65	83.9
Anglo	813	85.4	—	—	813	85.4
OVARY						
Hispanic	188	38.7	—	—	188	38.7
American Indian	61	45.7	—	—	61	45.7
Anglo	456	40.2	—	—	456	40.2
PROSTATE GLAND						
Hispanic	887	72.4	887	72.4	—	—
American Indian	213	50.0	213	50.0	—	—
Anglo	2,431	76.2	2,431	76.2	—	—
URINARY BLADDER						
Hispanic	210	64.6	160	72.7	50	37.3
American Indian	19	—	16	—	3	—
Anglo	972	73.9	733	74.0	239	73.7
KIDNEY AND RENAL PELVIS						
Hispanic	158	51.4	105	56.4	53	41.1
American Indian	94	38.9	55	38.6	39	38.6
Anglo	444	50.0	287	51.5	157	47.5
BRAIN AND NERVOUS SYSTEM						
Hispanic	107	32.2	74	27.3	33	42.5
American Indian	37	34.8	25	38.2	12	—
Anglo	321	24.1	188	22.3	133	26.3
HODGKIN'S DISEASE						
Hispanic	94	69.0	66	66.8	28	74.6
American Indian	5	—	3	—	2	—
Anglo	174	79.9	103	80.1	71	79.7
NON-HODGKIN'S LYMPHOMA						
Hispanic	191	41.1	103	42.6	88	39.5
American Indian	46	33.7	23	—	23	—
Anglo	702	49.9	365	48.4	337	51.4
MULTIPLE MYELOMA						
Hispanic	76	34.2	35	28.5	41	37.8
American Indian	44	25.5	20	—	24	—
Anglo	221	29.9	118	22.7	103	38.0
LEUKEMIAS						
Hispanic	243	25.7	135	23.5	108	28.1
American Indian	99	21.0	54	12.4	45	31.8
Anglo	695	35.0	408	35.4	287	34.5

(continued)

TABLE 11–II–7. *(Continued)*

	Both Sexes		*Male*		*Female*	
	Number	*Rate*	*Number*	*Rate*	*Number*	*Rate*
Lymphocytic						
Hispanic	117	40.7	65	33.7	52	48.6
American Indian	50	24.7	25	8.8	25	42.7
Anglo	331	60.4	203	57.7	128	64.6
Myelocytic						
Hispanic	98	12.6	55	14.7	43	10.0
American Indian	36	17.4	23	—	13	—
Anglo	270	9.6	148	8.9	122	10.4

*The data in this table for Hispanics and whites are from the state of New Mexico only. Data on American Indians from the state of Arizona have been added to those of New Mexico.

[a]Other oral cavity is the total oral cavity and pharynx excluding lip and salivary glands.

[b]Dash indicates that there were too few cases for a reliable estimate of the five-year survival rate.

New Mexico Anglos (Tables 11–II–6 and 11–II–9). Rates for these cancers were also relatively high in several Central and South American countries (Muir et al, 1987). Interestingly, gallbladder cancer rates did not appear to be elevated among Puerto Ricans, in contrast to those for Hispanics in New Mexico.

The five-year relative cancer survival rate of 40.2% for Puerto Rico (Table 11–II–10) was among the poorest of any racial or ethnic group in the United States. Among the racial and ethnic groups examined here, only American Indians and blacks had poorer five-year relative survival rates, 35.4 and 39.6%, respectively. Puerto Ricans had relatively poor survival rates for oral cavity, lung, cervix uteri, and prostate cancers, as well as for Hodgkin's disease and multiple myeloma. Survival rates for other forms of cancer were more comparable to those among other ethnic groups (see Tables 11–II–2, 11–II–4, 11–II–7, and 11–II–11).

Although the time period for which Puerto Rican mortality data (Table 11–II–11) were available, 1979–82, was not quite the same as for other analyses, the difference was minor and should not have a significant effect on comparisons with other mortality rates in this report. Cancer mortality rates were not as low as would be expected based on the low incidence rates, reflecting the impact of unfavorable survival rates. The total cancer mortality rate of 115.8 was higher than the Hispanic rate in New Mexico and rates for American Indians, Japanese, and Filipinos (Table 11–II–5). Mortality rates were notably high for cancers of the esophagus, stomach, and liver. However, rates were relatively low for cancers of the colorectum, lung, breast, kidney, and brain, and for non-Hodgkin's lymphomas, reflecting the incidence patterns.

Increases in cancer rates for several forms of cancer, particularly colon, have been observed among Puerto Rican–born migrants to New York and Connecticut, along with declines in stomach and cervix uteri cancers (Rosenwaike and Shai, 1986; Wolfgang et al, 1991; Polednak, 1992). Cancer mortality rates among persons born in Cuba, Mexico, or Puerto Rico were lower than among the U.S-born, with some variations among the foreign-born groups (Rosenwaike, 1987). Incidence rates among Hispanics in South Florida, who are primarily of Cuban origin, were lower than among non-Hispanics for many cancers, with some variation by race (Trapido et al, 1994a, 1994b).

AMERICAN INDIANS

The 1980 U.S. Census counted 1,364,033 American Indians, of whom about 37% resided on reservations, tribal trust lands, or historic areas and 54% lived in urbanized areas (Bureau of the Census, 1984). There are 511 federally recognized tribes, each of which has its own unique culture and history, which makes it difficult to characterize the "average American Indian." Overall, however, American Indians had a significantly lower median family income in 1979 than that for the entire country, $13,678 vs. $19,917, respectively (Bureau of the Census, 1984). More than twice as many American Indians lived at or below the poverty level as the total population, 27.5% compared to 12.4%, and unemployment rates were twice as high. In 1980, among persons aged 25 and over, 56% of American Indians were high school graduates, compared to 66% of the total U.S. population. The median age of American Indians in 1980 was 23.4, almost seven years younger than the overall U.S. figure of 30.0 years.

Cancer was not acknowledged as a major public health problem for American Indians until recently. Early researchers around the turn of the century had difficulty documenting the existence of cancer among

TABLE 11–II–8. *Average Annual Age-Adjusted (1970 U.S. Standard) Cancer Mortality Rates per 100,000 Population, New Mexico, 1977–82**

	Both Sexes		Male		Female	
	Number	*Rate*	*Number*	*Rate*	*Number*	*Rate*
ALL SITES						
Hispanic	2,455	132.0	1,296	150.1	1,159	116.5
Anglo	7,235	159.0	3,950	199.5	3,285	130.4
ORAL CAVITY AND PHARYNX						
Hispanic	35	1.9	22	2.6	13	1.3
Anglo	141	3.1	93	4.5	48	1.9
Other oral cavity[a]						
Hispanic	34	1.9	22	2.6	12	1.2
Anglo	125	2.7	82	3.9	43	1.7
Nasopharynx						
Hispanic	7	0.4	2	0.3	5	0.5
Anglo	9	0.2	7	0.3	2	0.1
ESOPHAGUS						
Hispanic	31	1.7	26	3.0	5	0.5
Anglo	95	2.1	63	3.1	32	1.3
STOMACH						
Hispanic	214	11.8	128	15.4	86	8.7
Anglo	208	4.6	116	5.8	92	3.5
COLON AND RECTUM						
Hispanic	241	13.2	131	15.4	110	11.3
Anglo	825	18.0	426	22.0	399	15.2
LIVER						
Hispanic	72	3.9	44	5.2	28	2.8
Anglo	116	2.5	78	3.9	38	1.4
GALLBLADDER						
Hispanic	57	3.2	12	1.5	45	4.6
Anglo	47	1.0	9	0.5	38	1.4
PANCREAS						
Hispanic	189	10.2	100	11.6	89	9.1
Anglo	375	8.1	207	10.2	168	6.5
LUNG AND BRONCHUS						
Hispanic	351	19.5	238	28.2	113	12.0
Anglo	1,739	38.1	1,249	61.8	490	19.9
MELANOMA OF SKIN						
Hispanic	6	0.4	2	0.2	4	0.5
Anglo	117	2.6	66	3.1	51	2.1
BREAST						
Hispanic	197	10.3	1	0.1	196	19.4
Anglo	660	14.6	21	1.0	639	25.8
CERVIX UTERI						
Hispanic	44	2.2	—	—	44	4.2
Anglo	64	1.4	—	—	64	2.6
CORPUS UTERI						
Hispanic	13	1.2	—	—	13	2.3
Anglo	100	2.2	—	—	100	3.9

(continued)

TABLE 11–II–8. *(Continued)*

OVARY						
Hispanic	60	3.1	—	—	60	5.9
Anglo	175	3.9	—	—	175	7.0
PROSTATE GLAND						
Hispanic	158	9.0	158	19.4	—	—
Anglo	440	9.5	440	23.8	—	—
URINARY BLADDER						
Hispanic	41	2.3	29	3.6	12	1.2
Anglo	175	3.8	125	6.7	50	1.9
KIDNEY AND RENAL PELVIS						
Hispanic	50	2.6	33	3.7	17	1.6
Anglo	126	2.8	82	4.2	44	1.7
BRAIN AND NERVOUS SYSTEM						
Hispanic	67	3.2	45	4.5	22	2.0
Anglo	198	4.4	113	5.5	85	3.6
HODGKIN'S DISEASE						
Hispanic	22	1.0	14	1.3	8	0.7
Anglo	32	0.7	20	0.9	12	0.5
NON-HODGKIN'S LYMPHOMA						
Hispanic	61	3.1	32	3.5	29	2.8
Anglo	212	4.7	114	5.6	98	3.9
MULTIPLE MYELOMA						
Hispanic	36	2.0	21	2.5	15	1.6
Anglo	101	2.2	53	2.8	48	1.9
LEUKEMIAS						
Hispanic	102	4.8	55	5.4	47	4.2
Anglo	329	7.4	181	9.0	148	6.0

*The data in this table for Hispanics and whites are from the state of New Mexico only.
[a]Other oral cavity is the total oral cavity and pharynx excluding lip and salivary glands.

American Indians (Hrdlicka, 1908), and some claimed that American Indians were immune to cancer (Hampton, 1989). By the end of the 1930s more cases were being reported, and it was clear that American Indians did indeed suffer from cancer and that the disease had become more prevalent (Palmer, 1938). Part of the apparent rise in cases was due to a decrease in other causes of death, resulting in increased longevity. A national analysis based on 1950–67 mortality indicated significantly lower mortality rates for most cancers among American Indians, with only gallbladder cancer rates notably higher among both males and females (Creagan and Fraumeni, 1972).

Incidence and survival analyses in this report were based on American Indians resident in the states of New Mexico and Arizona in the southwest United States. These two states contained about 19% of the American Indian population, but the data were not necessarily representative of all American Indians. The major tribes represented in these two states are the Apache, Hopi, Navajo, Papago, Pueblo, and Zuni. It is likely that cancer risk factors and the cancer experience vary significantly among different tribes and different geographic areas (DHHS, 1986; Hampton, 1989). The mortality analyses were for American Indians throughout the United States. The possibility of racial misclassification in the numerators and/or denominators should be born in mind when evaluating the observed rates (Bleed et al, 1992; Frost et al, 1992; Welty et al, 1993).

Although American Indians would be expected to be at high cancer risk on the basis of SES, they actually had very low cancer incidence rates (Table 11–II–6). Their overall incidence was far less than one-half that of whites, 137.6 compared to 314.5, and among males, it was 36% that among whites. The lower overall rates were due to notably low incidence rates for cancers of the oral cavity, colon and rectum, pancreas, lung, breast, corpus uteri, prostate, and urinary bladder, as

TABLE 11–II–9. *Average Annual Age-Adjusted (1970 U.S. Standard) Cancer Incidence Rates per 100,000 Population for Malignant Cases Only, Puerto Rico, 1977–83**

	Both Sexes		*Male*		*Female*	
	Number	*Rate*	*Number*	*Rate*	*Number*	*Rate*
ALL SITES	38,488	202.2	21,026	233.6	17,462	173.5
Oral cavity and pharynx	2,998	16.0	2,390	27.0	608	6.1
Other oral cavity[a]	2,747	14.7	2,232	25.2	515	5.2
Nasopharynx	96	0.5	73	0.8	23	0.2
Esophagus	1,734	9.3	1,288	14.5	446	4.5
Stomach	3,096	16.4	2,011	22.6	1,085	10.8
Colon and rectum	3,578	19.0	1,815	20.3	1,763	17.8
Liver	561	3.0	366	4.1	195	1.9
Gallbladder	330	1.8	87	1.0	243	2.5
Pancreas	930	4.9	528	5.9	402	4.1
Lung and bronchus	2,728	14.6	1,963	22.1	765	7.8
Breast	3,866	20.3	29	0.3	3,837	38.2
Cervix uteri	1,722	8.9	—	—	1,722	16.9
Corpus uteri	884	4.7	—	—	884	9.0
Ovary	650	3.4	—	—	650	6.5
Prostate gland	3,717	19.8	3,717	41.9	—	—
Urinary bladder	1,466	7.8	1,069	12.1	397	4.0
Kidney and renal pelvis	429	2.2	276	3.0	153	1.5
Brain and nervous system	596	2.8	347	3.5	249	2.3
Hodgkin's disease	435	2.1	254	2.5	181	1.6
Non-Hodgkin's lymphoma	1,042	5.4	564	6.0	478	4.8
Multiple myeloma	614	3.3	335	3.7	279	2.9
Leukemias	1,271	6.1	690	7.0	581	5.4
Lymphocytic	461	2.1	251	2.4	210	1.9
Myelocytic	600	3.0	311	3.2	289	2.8

*Data from Puerto Rico, SEER Program, National Cancer Institute.
[a]Other oral cavity is the total oral cavity and pharynx excluding lip and salivary glands.

well as for melanoma and most myelo- and lymphoproliferative malignancies. Lung cancer rates among American Indians were only 13% those among whites. Cigarette smoking has been uncommon among southwest American Indians, facilitating the identification of high lung cancer risk associated with uranium mining (Butler et al, 1986). Lung cancer rates are sure to rise in the future as smoking increases, unless intervention strategies are initiated (Michalek et al, 1989). In tribes where smoking was a common practice, lung cancer rates were higher than in areas of low tobacco usage (Hampton, 1989; Michalek et al, 1989). The rates for other known cancers in American Indians are likely to rise with better case ascertainment as delivery of medical care improves. Additional cancer incidence data for various American Indian populations are presented in Nutting et al (1993).

The low oral cancer rate, found both in this study and elsewhere, was of interest in light of high alcohol consumption (Heath, 1989), a strong risk factor for cancers of the oral cavity. Alcohol abuse has long been a serious problem among American Indians (Indian Health Service, 1977). While excessive alcohol consumption is a risk factor for upper aerodigestive tumors, especially in combination with smoking, it has also resulted in early alcohol-related deaths from non-cancer causes (Indian Health Service, 1989; Schinke et al, 1989), which may be moderating the apparent risk of developing cancer.

American Indians had a gallbladder cancer incidence rate ten times that among whites, however, with the excess especially prominent among females. This pattern has been noted among other groups of American Indians. Although the mechanisms are not understood, these groups also experience excess risks of gallstones, which predispose to gallbladder cancer (Weiss et al, 1984; Nervi et al, 1988). In addition, cancers of the stomach and cervix uteri occurred twice as frequently among American Indians as whites. These two cancers occur more frequently among lower socioeconomic groups (Fraumeni et al, 1993), and rates have been declining for many years among whites and blacks (Pollack and Horm, 1980; Devesa et al, 1987; NCI, 1988).

TABLE 11–II–10. *Five-Year Relative Survival Rates (%) for Malignant Cases Diagnosed from 1975 to 1984 in Puerto Rico**

	Both Sexes		*Male*		*Female*	
	Number	*Rate*	*Number*	*Rate*	*Number*	*Rate*
ALL SITES	48,137	40.2	26,140	33.5	21,997	47.6
Oral cavity and pharynx	3,863	29.9	3,038	26.6	825	42.0
Other oral cavity[a]	3,512	26.2	2,812	23.1	700	38.6
Nasopharynx	127	27.2	93	21.2	34	44.6
Esophagus	2,167	7.5	1,590	6.5	577	10.5
Stomach	3,793	14.5	2,518	13.7	1,275	16.1
Colon and rectum	4,537	44.5	2,299	41.9	2,238	47.1
Liver	559	2.3	375	2.2	184	2.3
Gallbladder	401	13.3	109	12.9	292	13.5
Pancreas	1,084	4.6	610	4.8	474	4.4
Lung and bronchus	3,161	7.8	2,308	7.4	853	8.9
Breast	5,015	66.8	39	70.2	4,976	66.8
Cervix uteri	2,376	60.2	—	—	2,376	60.2
Corpus uteri	1,132	77.5	—	—	1,132	77.5
Ovary	830	41.0	—	—	830	41.0
Prostate gland	4,628	58.8	4,628	58.8	—	—
Urinary bladder	1,816	56.7	1,353	58.3	463	52.3
Kidney and renal pelvis	554	53.5	353	49.7	201	60.3
Brain and nervous system	756	25.6	443	24.1	313	27.6
Hodgkin's disease	601	60.5	362	62.1	239	58.2
Non-Hodgkin's lymphoma	1,303	38.2	702	35.2	601	41.6
Multiple myeloma	823	19.2	458	19.1	365	19.5
Leukemias	1,650	25.3	891	24.1	759	26.7
Lymphocytic	614	39.8	329	37.5	285	42.3
Myelocytic	821	17.5	432	16.9	389	18.1

*Data from Puerto Rico, SEER Program, National Cancer Institute.
[a]Other oral cavity is the total oral cavity and pharynx excluding lip and salivary glands.

In contrast, stomach cancer rates have declined only moderately among American Indians in New Mexico (Wiggins et al, 1993).

The survival experience of American Indians once they develop cancer is generally among the poorest of any racial group studied (Table 11–II–7). The overall five-year relative survival rate was 35.4%, only two-thirds that among whites. Survival rates were notably lower for cancers of the oral cavity and breast, non-Hodgkin's lymphoma, multiple myeloma, and lymphocytic leukemia. Some of these survival differences persisted after adjustment for stage and treatment (Samet et al, 1987). However, there are several forms of cancer for which the survival rates for American Indians were equal to or greater than those of whites, including cancers of the corpus uteri, ovary, brain and nervous system, and myelocytic leukemia.

Mortality data for American Indians in the total United States are presented in Table 11–II–5. Only Filipinos had a lower overall cancer mortality rate than American Indians, among whom the rate was 54% that among whites. Similar to the incidence data, mortality rates were quite low for colorectal, lung, breast, corpus uteri, bladder, and brain cancers. Although not as striking as the excess observed in the incidence data, gallbladder cancer mortality rates were 2.5–3 times those among whites. The 70% excess of cervix uteri cancer mortality could and should be largely reduced by efficient Pap smear screening. The considerably higher incidence and poorer survival observed in New Mexico for stomach cancer among American Indian males would be consistent with high mortality rates, and indeed stomach cancer mortality rates during 1973–77 were twice as high among New Mexico American Indian males as white males in New Mexico (Young et al, 1981). The similarity in stomach cancer mortality among American Indian and white males on a national basis indicates that the excess observed in New Mexico was not uniform across the country and that stomach cancer mortality among U.S. American Indians must

TABLE 11–II–11. *Average Annual Age-Adjusted (1970 U.S. Standard) Cancer Mortality Rates per 100,000 Population, Puerto Rico, 1979–82**

	Both Sexes		*Male*		*Female*	
	Number	*Rate*	*Number*	*Rate*	*Number*	*Rate*
ALL SITES	13,006	115.8	7,732	146.0	5,274	89.3
Oral cavity and pharynx	599	6.1	483	10.6	116	2.1
Other oral cavity[a]	584	5.9	474	10.4	110	2.0
Nasopharynx	9	0.1	9	0.2	0	0.0
Esophagus	910	9.4	696	15.3	214	4.2
Stomach	1,270	12.4	848	17.5	422	7.9
Colon and rectum	930	9.3	449	9.6	481	9.0
Liver	549	5.1	309	6.1	240	4.1
Gallbladder	89	0.9	25	0.5	64	1.3
Pancreas	486	4.8	272	5.8	214	3.9
Lung and bronchus	1,372	13.4	953	19.6	419	7.9
Breast	616	5.9	5	0.0	611	11.2
Cervix uteri	162	1.8	—	—	162	3.3
Corpus uteri	271	2.7	—	—	271	5.1
Ovary	148	1.3	—	—	148	2.6
Prostate gland	981	9.3	981	20.1	—	—
Urinary bladder	317	2.2	212	3.4	105	1.2
Kidney and renal pelvis	82	0.8	48	1.1	34	0.6
Brain and nervous system	174	1.7	103	2.1	71	1.4
Hodgkin's disease	88	0.7	53	0.9	35	0.5
Non-Hodgkin's lymphoma	248	2.4	136	2.7	112	2.1
Multiple myeloma	243	2.3	119	2.4	124	2.2
Leukemias	557	4.6	300	5.3	257	4.1

*Data from the National Cancer Institute.
[a]Other oral cavity is the total oral cavity and pharynx excluding lip and salivary glands.

vary geographically. Indeed, substantial regional variation in total cancer mortality rates has been reported (Valway, 1994).

Recent unpublished mortality data for several major cancers indicate substantial variation by state of residence among American Indians in 1977–83 age-adjusted rates (Horm, unpublished data). Mortality rates per 100,000 American Indians for all cancers combined ranged from a low of 40.0 in California to a high of 223.8 in North Dakota, more than a fivefold difference. Variations were seen for individual cancers, including a tenfold difference in lung cancer mortality rates per 100,000 American Indians, which ranged from 5.4 in New Mexico to 55.0 in North Dakota. Lung and cervix cancer mortality rates among three Sioux tribes in North and South Dakota exceeded the U.S. rates (Welty et al, 1993). Mortality rates for American Indians in New Mexico and Arizona (the two states used for this incidence analysis) were similar to the national average for all cancers combined, but they were the lowest of any state for lung cancer. Incidence patterns probably were similar.

NATIVE HAWAIIANS

In 1980 more than 175,000 Native Hawaiians lived in Hawaii (unpublished data, Hawaii State Department of Health, Research and Statistics Office). Native Hawaiians were a young population, with a median age of 22.6 (Bureau of the Census, 1983c, 1988a). The entire population of Hawaii is well educated, including Native Hawaiians. Over 75% of Native Hawaiian males and 72% of females (aged 25 and over) had at least a high school education, and the median education level was 12.7 years, not much less than the 13.3 years for whites. The 1979 median family income of $22,750 among Native Hawaiians exceeded that of $20,792 among whites in Hawaii.

The overall cancer incidence rate among Native Hawaiians was only slightly lower (10%) than that among whites in Hawaii, or 346.5 versus 384.9, respectively (Table 11–II–12). It should be noted, however, that the incidence among whites in Hawaii was the highest of any racial or ethnic group in this report. The major cancers for which Native Hawaiians had lower incidence

TABLE 11–II–12. *Average Annual Age-Adjusted (1970 U.S. Standard) Cancer Incidence Rates per 100,000 Population for Malignant Cases Only, Hawaii, 1977–83**

	Both Sexes		Male		Female	
	Number	*Rate*	*Number*	*Rate*	*Number*	*Rate*
ALL SITES						
Hawaiian	2,382	346.5	1,142	372.7	1,240	329.9
White	6,196	384.9	3,364	435.2	2,832	347.2
ORAL CAVITY AND PHARYNX						
Hawaiian	61	9.0	32	10.0	29	8.0
White	303	19.1	205	25.2	98	12.6
Other oral cavity[a]						
Hawaiian	55	8.7	30	9.8	25	7.6
White	237	16.3	155	21.1	82	11.2
Nasopharynx						
Hawaiian	7	0.7	3	0.8	4	0.7
White	14	0.8	12	1.4	2	0.3
ESOPHAGUS						
Hawaiian	49	7.3	42	14.0	7	1.8
White	44	2.8	30	3.9	14	1.6
STOMACH						
Hawaiian	165	27.0	103	38.3	62	18.3
White	161	10.7	103	14.6	58	7.2
COLON AND RECTUM						
Hawaiian	199	31.7	125	42.3	74	22.4
White	705	46.7	398	55.9	307	38.4
LIVER						
Hawaiian	37	5.5	27	8.7	10	2.7
White	48	2.8	34	4.5	14	1.2
GALLBLADDER						
Hawaiian	7	1.3	4	1.5	3	1.0
White	15	1.1	4	0.6	11	1.3
PANCREAS						
Hawaiian	65	8.0	33	8.1	32	7.6
White	164	9.3	80	9.3	84	9.3
LUNG AND BRONCHUS						
Hawaiian	459	66.9	310	97.5	149	39.2
White	945	58.7	646	81.6	299	37.1
MELANOMA OF SKIN						
Hawaiian	10	1.1	5	1.4	5	0.8
White	418	22.6	237	26.3	181	19.8
BREAST						
Hawaiian	383	57.1	3	0.8	380	106.1
White	811	51.4	5	0.7	806	102.6
CERVIX UTERI						
Hawaiian	63	8.1	—	—	63	15.2
White	79	4.4	—	—	79	8.9
CORPUS UTERI						
Hawaiian	106	14.8	—	—	106	28.2
White	226	14.8	—	—	226	29.4

(continued)

TABLE 11–II–12. *Average Annual Age-Adjusted (1970 U.S. Standard) Cancer Incidence Rates per 100,000 Population for Malignant Cases Only, Hawaii, 1977–83* (Continued)*

	Both Sexes		*Male*		*Female*	
	Number	*Rate*	*Number*	*Rate*	*Number*	*Rate*
OVARY						
Hawaiian	56	7.8	—	—	56	14.4
White	106	6.5	—	—	106	13.2
PROSTATE GLAND						
Hawaiian	122	23.5	122	56.1	—	—
White	542	37.2	542	81.0	—	—
URINARY BLADDER						
Hawaiian	51	8.5	33	12.4	18	5.7
White	303	20.2	241	34.6	62	7.6
KIDNEY AND RENAL PELVIS						
Hawaiian	36	4.2	25	7.0	11	1.8
White	122	7.3	83	10.2	39	4.5
BRAIN AND NERVOUS SYSTEM						
Hawaiian	37	3.0	19	2.8	18	3.1
White	108	5.9	71	8.0	37	3.8
HODGKIN'S DISEASE						
Hawaiian	12	1.0	9	1.6	3	0.6
White	53	2.5	30	2.9	23	2.3
NON-HODGKIN'S LYMPHOMA						
Hawaiian	59	8.4	35	10.4	24	6.6
White	159	10.1	100	12.3	59	7.8
MULTIPLE MYELOMA						
Hawaiian	35	5.8	16	5.8	19	6.2
White	57	3.7	34	4.9	23	2.9
LEUKEMIAS						
Hawaiian	77	8.2	48	9.4	29	6.7
White	159	10.1	100	12.7	59	7.7
Lymphocytic						
Hawaiian	16	1.1	13	1.9	3	0.4
White	72	4.7	47	6.1	25	3.5
Myelocytic						
Hawaiian	50	5.5	31	6.4	19	4.4
White	72	4.4	43	5.1	29	3.6

*The data for Hawaiians and whites in this table are from the state of Hawaii only.
[a]Other oral cavity is the total oral cavity and pharynx excluding lip and salivary glands.

rates than whites are: cancers of the oral cavity and pharynx, colorectum, prostate, urinary bladder, and kidney, non-Hodgkin's lymphoma, and lymphocytic leukemia. However, Native Hawaiians had higher incidence rates than whites for cancers of the stomach, liver, cervix uteri, and, among males, esophagus and lung. Female breast cancer rates among both Hawaiian Natives and whites exceeded 100, considerably higher than the rates observed among whites in other SEER areas. Rates were similar among female Hawaiian Natives and whites for corpus uteri, ovarian, and lung cancers, the latter occurring notably more frequently than among mainland whites.

Native Hawaiians do not fare as well as whites once they are diagnosed with cancer (Table 11–II–13), with an overall five-year survival rate of 43.2% versus 56.9%, respectively. Survival rates for Native Hawaiians lagged behind those for whites for virtually every form of cancer investigated. Some of the largest apparent differences were 68.0% among Native Hawaiians

TABLE 11–II–13. *Five-Year Relative Survival Rates (%) for Malignant Cases Diagnosed from 1975 to 1984 in Hawaii**

	Both sexes		Male		Female	
	Number	Rate	Number	Rate	Number	Rate
ALL SITES						
Hawaiian	2,847	43.2	1,377	32.8	1,470	52.0
White	7,313	56.9	3,993	51.8	3,320	62.5
ORAL CAVITY AND PHARYNX						
Hawaiian	76	42.8	47	46.6	29	37.2
White	370	53.1	258	54.7	112	49.7
Other oral cavity[a]						
Hawaiian	70	39.8	45	45.7	25	30.5
White	280	43.4	186	43.6	94	43.1
Nasopharynx						
Hawaiian	12	—[b]	7	—	5	—
White	19	—	15	—	4	—
ESOPHAGUS						
Hawaiian	61	0.0	50	0.0	11	—
White	47	11.5	34	12.3	13	—
STOMACH						
Hawaiian	194	12.9	128	12.2	66	14.3
White	187	12.6	125	9.4	62	18.0
COLON AND RECTUM						
Hawaiian	233	58.4	147	59.3	86	57.2
White	837	59.7	465	62.1	372	56.8
LIVER						
Hawaiian	36	6.6	29	0.0	7	—
White	47	2.7	36	3.5	11	—
GALLBLADDER						
Hawaiian	9	—	4	—	5	—
White	17	—	4	—	13	—
PANCREAS						
Hawaiian	57	0.0	30	0.0	27	0.0
White	170	2.2	86	2.9	84	1.4
LUNG AND BRONCHUS						
Hawaiian	558	13.0	388	10.8	170	18.2
White	1,055	16.6	734	16.3	321	17.3
MELANOMA OF SKIN						
Hawaiian	14	—	7	—	7	—
White	492	85.0	288	82.5	204	88.6
BREAST						
Hawaiian	447	68.1	1	—	446	68.0
White	959	83.1	8	—	951	83.2
CERVIX UTERI						
Hawaiian	80	67.7	—	—	80	67.7
White	113	74.5	—	—	113	74.5
CORPUS UTERI						
Hawaiian	137	74.6	—	—	137	74.6
White	305	86.8	—	—	305	86.8

(continued)

TABLE 11–II–13. *Five-Year Relative Survival Rates (%) for Malignant Cases Diagnosed from 1975 to 1984 in Hawaii* (Continued)*

	Both sexes		*Male*		*Female*	
	Number	*Rate*	*Number*	*Rate*	*Number*	*Rate*
OVARY						
Hawaiian	64	46.8	—	—	64	46.8
White	136	41.9	—	—	136	41.9
PROSTATE GLAND						
Hawaiian	137	72.0	137	72.0	—	—
White	638	74.1	638	74.1	—	—
URINARY BLADDER						
Hawaiian	61	51.4	39	62.2	22	—
White	362	89.2	298	90.1	64	85.2
KIDNEY AND RENAL PELVIS						
Hawaiian	38	59.0	26	44.7	12	—
White	126	58.0	91	58.8	35	56.5
BRAIN AND NERVOUS SYSTEM						
Hawaiian	46	38.9	20	—	26	50.7
White	126	21.8	86	20.3	40	23.6
HODGKIN'S DISEASE						
Hawaiian	19	—	13	—	6	—
White	74	80.4	45	75.2	29	87.7
NON-HODGKIN'S LYMPHOMA						
Hawaiian	76	40.2	44	35.3	32	47.3
White	204	49.1	125	48.9	79	49.9
MULTIPLE MYELOMA						
Hawaiian	42	30.6	21	—	21	—
White	66	26.5	42	26.9	24	—
LEUKEMIAS						
Hawaiian	101	21.1	59	21.6	42	20.0
White	193	38.5	114	39.5	79	37.2
Lymphocytic						
Hawaiian	25	57.7	17	—	8	—
White	93	65.3	61	59.8	32	74.5
Myelocytic						
Hawaiian	64	4.2	37	3.6	27	4.9
White	84	7.9	44	10.9	40	4.7

*The data for Hawaiians and whites in this table are from the state of Hawaii only.
[a]Other oral cavity is the total oral cavity and pharynx excluding lip and salivary glands.
[b]Dash indicates that there were too few cases for a reliable estimate of the five-year survival rate.

versus 83.2% among whites for female breast cancer, 51.4 versus 89.2% for urinary bladder cancer, and 21.1 versus 38.5% for leukemia, respectively.

These lower survival rates resulted in overall cancer mortality rates that were higher among Native Hawaiians than among whites (207.2 versus 175.5) (Table 11–II–14), in spite of lower overall incidence rates. Native Hawaiians had death rates about double those of whites for cancers of the esophagus, cervix uteri, and corpus uteri; a stomach cancer rate almost triple that of whites; and a lung cancer rate 35% higher than that of whites. The high breast cancer incidence among white women in Hawaii may be due to screening, as they had higher incidence and better survival but the same mortality as mainland white women. In contrast, Native Hawaiian women had similar incidence to that of white women in Hawaii but poorer survival and hence higher mortality, suggesting a true increased risk among the Native women rather than a screening-related excess. One study of lung cancer revealed that Hawaiian men

TABLE 11–II–14. *Average Annual Age-Adjusted (1970 U.S. Standard) Cancer Mortality Rates per 100,000 Population, Hawaii, 1977–83**

	Both Sexes		*Male*		*Female*	
	Number	*Rate*	*Number*	*Rate*	*Number*	*Rate*
ALL SITES						
Hawaiian	1,285	207.2	699	247.3	586	174.8
White	2,604	175.5	1,449	206.9	1,155	149.6
ORAL CAVITY AND PHARYNX						
Hawaiian	25	3.9	19	5.9	6	2.1
White	94	6.1	64	8.4	30	4.0
Other oral cavity[a]						
Hawaiian	23	3.5	18	5.6	5	1.7
White	87	5.6	57	7.5	30	4.0
Nasopharynx						
Hawaiian	6	0.9	6	1.9	0	0.0
White	7	0.4	6	0.6	1	0.1
ESOPHAGUS						
Hawaiian	47	7.2	39	13.7	8	2.0
White	46	3.1	34	4.7	12	1.6
STOMACH						
Hawaiian	121	21.8	75	32.7	46	14.1
White	111	7.8	69	10.3	42	5.5
COLON AND RECTUM						
Hawaiian	86	14.6	46	17.6	40	12.5
White	286	20.0	148	21.4	138	18.2
LIVER						
Hawaiian	32	5.2	22	7.6	10	2.9
White	48	3.2	35	5.1	13	1.5
GALLBLADDER						
Hawaiian	3	0.5	2	0.8	1	0.3
White	12	0.9	3	0.6	9	1.1
PANCREAS						
Hawaiian	61	10.0	31	10.8	30	9.3
White	138	9.3	65	9.3	73	9.3
LUNG AND BRONCHUS						
Hawaiian	354	56.5	241	81.2	113	34.4
White	629	41.8	422	57.9	207	27.1
MELANOMA OF SKIN						
Hawaiian	2	0.3	1	0.2	1	0.3
White	59	3.5	37	4.7	22	2.6
BREAST						
Hawaiian	131	20.0	0	0.0	131	37.2
White	219	14.3	2	0.3	217	27.9
CERVIX UTERI						
Hawaiian	19	3.0	—	—	19	5.6
White	18	1.1	—	—	18	2.2
CORPUS UTERI						
Hawaiian	21	3.4	—	—	21	6.3
White	27	1.9	—	—	27	3.6

(continued)

TABLE 11–II–14. *Average Annual Age-Adjusted (1970 U.S. Standard) Cancer Mortality Rates per 100,000 Population, Hawaii, 1977–83* (Continued)*

	Both Sexes		*Male*		*Female*	
	Number	*Rate*	*Number*	*Rate*	*Number*	*Rate*
OVARY						
Hawaiian	26	4.5	—	—	26	8.2
White	64	4.2	—	—	64	8.2
PROSTATE GLAND						
Hawaiian	30	6.4	30	15.8	—	—
White	142	10.4	142	24.3	—	—
URINARY BLADDER						
Hawaiian	16	2.9	9	3.4	7	2.4
White	60	4.3	41	6.4	19	2.4
KIDNEY AND RENAL PELVIS						
Hawaiian	16	2.3	15	4.6	1	0.2
White	49	3.3	37	5.6	12	1.5
BRAIN AND NERVOUS SYSTEM						
Hawaiian	19	2.0	11	2.0	8	1.9
White	66	4.4	41	5.2	25	3.3
HODGKIN'S DISEASE						
Hawaiian	3	0.2	1	0.1	2	0.3
White	12	0.5	8	0.9	4	0.3
NON-HODGKIN'S LYMPHOMA						
Hawaiian	37	5.6	24	7.2	13	3.7
White	88	5.8	51	6.7	37	4.7
MULTIPLE MYELOMA						
Hawaiian	21	3.7	11	4.0	10	3.4
White	39	2.6	20	2.6	19	2.5
LEUKEMIAS						
Hawaiian	57	6.8	37	8.2	20	5.3
White	93	6.2	60	8.1	33	4.5

*The data for Hawaiians and whites in this table are from the state of Hawaii only.
[a]Other oral cavity is the total oral cavity and pharynx excluding lip and salivary glands.

were at considerably higher risk than men of other ethnic groups, even after adjusting for pack-years of smoking, occupation, education, and age, which suggests that dietary, genetic, or other risk factors should be considered (Le Marchand et al, 1992). Although Hawaiians and part-Hawaiians account for 20% of the population of Hawaii (Kolonel and Goodman, 1987), little etiologic research has focused specifically on these groups.

ALASKA NATIVES

Cancer mortality rates during 1960–69 among Alaska Natives were not significantly different from those of U.S. whites but were significantly higher than those for American Indians resident in the continental United States (Blot et al, 1975). Alaska Natives were found to have elevated mortality rates for cancers of the nasopharynx, esophagus, gallbladder among females, cervix uteri, kidneys, and salivary glands. Rates were lower than among U.S. whites for prostate, breast, corpus uteri, ovary, colorectum, and brain cancers.

The 1980 Census identified 209 Alaska Native villages and counted 64,103 Alaska Natives: 34,144 Eskimos, 8,090 Aleuts, and 21,869 American Indians (Athabascans) living in Alaska (Bureau of the Census, 1984; Indian Health Service, 1989). Similar to other Native American groups, the socioeconomic status of Alaska Natives is low. In 1980, over 18% of Alaska Natives aged 25 and older had had less than 5 years of elementary school compared to 2.6% of U.S. whites, and only 46.2% had completed high school. Over two-thirds of Alaska Natives lived in rural areas, compared to less than 30% of U.S. whites. The median age was

TABLE 11–II–15. *Average Annual Age-Adjusted (1970 U.S. Standard) Cancer Incidence Rates per 100,000 Population, Alaska, 1969–83* and Nine SEER Areas, 1974–78*

	Both Sexes		*Male*		*Female*	
	Number	*Rate*	*Number*	*Rate*	*Number*	*Rate*
ALL SITES						
Alaska Natives	1,475	314.3	756	329.7	719	300.6
SEER whites	301,900	335.4	148,662	384.9	153,238	308.9
ORAL CAVITY AND PHARYNX						
Alaska Natives	87	16.5	47	17.2	40	15.7
SEER whites	10,015	11.2	6,956	17.6	3,059	6.2
Nasopharynx						
Alaska Natives	51	9.8	35	13.1	16	6.4
SEER whites	393	0.4	267	0.6	126	0.3
Excluding nasopharynx						
Alaska Natives	36	6.7	12	4.1	24	9.3
SEER whites	9,622	10.8	6,689	16.9	2,933	6.0
ESOPHAGUS						
Alaska Natives	25	6.1	18	8.9	7	3.4
SEER whites	2,694	3.0	1,867	4.8	827	1.6
STOMACH						
Alaska Natives	71	15.5	52	22.4	19	8.4
SEER whites	7,725	8.4	4,732	12.4	2,993	5.5
COLON AND RECTUM						
Alaska Natives	261	62.6	128	61.0	133	65.2
SEER whites	44,631	49.1	21,815	57.3	22,816	43.3
LIVER						
Alaska Natives	37	6.4	31	10.8	6	2.0
SEER whites	1,682	1.9	1,055	2.7	627	1.2
GALLBLADDER						
Alaska Natives	41	10.6	12	6.7	29	14.7
SEER whites	1,289	1.4	359	1.0	930	1.7
PANCREAS						
Alaska Natives	45	9.9	24	10.1	21	9.6
SEER whites	8,366	9.2	4,441	11.6	3,925	7.4
LUNG AND BRONCHUS						
Alaska Natives	211	46.9	158	69.7	53	23.2
SEER whites	41,662	46.8	30,315	77.9	11,347	23.4
BREAST						
Alaska Natives	116	21.7	1	0.4	115	44.2
SEER whites	43,058	48.4	300	0.8	42,758	88.3
CERVIX UTERI						
Alaska Natives	83	—	—	—	83	28.0
SEER whites	5,020	—	—	—	5,020	10.5
OVARY						
Alaska Natives	25	—	—	—	25	9.5
SEER whites	6,915	—	—	—	6,915	14.4
PROSTATE GLAND						
Alaska Natives	65	—	65	34.5	—	—
SEER whites	26,001	—	26,001	70.5	—	—

(continued)

TABLE 11–II–15. *Average Annual Age-Adjusted (1970 U.S. Standard) Cancer Incidence Rates per 100,000 Population, Alaska, 1969–83* and Nine SEER Areas, 1974–78 (Continued)*

	Both Sexes		*Male*		*Female*	
	Number	*Rate*	*Number*	*Rate*	*Number*	*Rate*
URINARY BLADDER						
Alaska Natives	25	6.1	18	8.9	7	3.4
SEER whites	14,874	16.4	10,960	28.7	3,914	7.4
KIDNEY AND RENAL PELVIS						
Alaska Natives	53	11.2	26	11.4	27	11.0
SEER whites	5,894	6.6	3,760	9.6	2,134	4.4
BRAIN AND NERVOUS SYSTEM						
Alaska Natives	18	2.1	11	2.8	7	1.5
SEER whites	5,018	5.8	2,808	6.9	2,210	4.8
LYMPH NODES						
Alaska Natives	29	5.7	21	8.3	8	3.1
SEER whites	11,524	12.6	6,025	14.8	5,499	11.1
HEMATOLOGIC						
Alaska Natives	42	7.5	29	10.7	13	4.3
SEER whites	13,146	14.6	7,303	18.9	5,843	11.5
OTHER						
Alaska Natives	173	39.6	80	34.7	93	44.1
SEER whites	48,243	51.6	18,620	42.4	29,623	59.8

*Based on data from Lanier and Knutson, 1986. Data for Alaska were not available for lip, salivary gland, or corpus uteri cancers.

about 21, ten years younger than that of U.S. whites. In 1979, 25.3% of Alaska Natives lived below the poverty level versus 7.0% of U.S. whites.

As is seen in many other economically deprived groups, low-income and education status is associated with increased tobacco use. According to a 1981 smoking survey, 56% of the adult Alaska Native population smoked cigarettes as did 41% of the youth aged 12–18 (Lee, 1983), or considerably higher than U.S. rates of about 33% of adults and 12% of youths (NCHS, 1988). The same survey found that 21% of the children in grades 4–6 chewed tobacco or used snuff, over twice the corresponding U.S. figure of less than 10%. In 1986 the rate for children in grades kindergarten–12 who had ever used smokeless tobacco was 43%, and the rate of regular use was about 30% for both males and females (Schlife, 1987).

A tumor registry to collect cancer incidence data on the Native populations was begun in 1969 (Lanier and Knutson, 1986). Since there were only about 100 cancers per year, rates for the years 1969–1983 are presented separately in Table 11–II–15. Cancer incidence data on whites from all nine SEER registries for 1974–78, the mid-years of the Alaskan data, were used as the comparison group because a local comparison group was not available. A survival analysis was not possible because collecting follow-up information was not a part of the registry function.

The overall cancer incidence rate for Alaska Natives was slightly lower than that for U.S. whites, or 314.3 versus 335.2, respectively (Table 11–II–15). Rates for females were more similar (300.6 compared to 308.7) than those among males (329.7, 14% less than the U.S. white rate of 384.7). However, compared with U.S. whites, Alaska Natives had higher rates for cancers of the oral cavity and pharynx among females, nasopharynx, esophagus, stomach, colorectum, liver, gallbladder, cervix uteri, and kidney and renal pelvis. In contrast to the experience of most of the other minority groups considered in this report, colorectal cancer rates were similar for Alaska Native and white males and 50% higher among Alaska Native females than white females. The colorectal cancer incidence rate for Alaska Native females in fact exceeded that for either Alaska Native or white males.

The nasopharynx cancer rate among Alaska Natives was 9.8 compared to 0.4 among the white comparison group. Studies of Alaska Natives found the titer of antibody to the Epstein-Barr virus (EBV) among cases to be significantly greater than among controls (Lanier et al, 1980, 1983). Immunoglobulin A (IgA) antibodies to the EBV viral capsid antigen were particularly increased

TABLE 11–II–16. *Average Annual Age-Adjusted (1970 U.S. Standard) Cancer Mortality Rates per 100,000 Population, Alaska, 1969–83 and U.S. Whites, 1974–78*

	Both Sexes		*Male*		*Female*	
	Number	*Rate*	*Number*	*Rate*	*Number*	*Rate*
ALL SITES						
Alaska Natives	792	182.1	443	201.0	349	162.1
U.S. whites	1,669,286	161.4	902,146	205.8	767,140	131.1
ORAL CAVITY AND PHARYNX						
Alaska Natives	32	6.2	19	7.4	13	5.1
U.S. whites	35,500	3.4	24,701	5.6	10,799	1.8
Nasopharynx						
Alaska Natives	22	4.3	15	5.8	7	2.9
U.S. whites	2,638	0.3	1,808	0.4	830	0.2
Excluding nasopharynx						
Alaska Natives	10	1.9	4	1.6	6	2.2
U.S. whites	32,862	3.1	22,893	5.2	9,969	1.6
ESOPHAGUS						
Alaska Natives	13	3.2	10	4.9	3	1.5
U.S. whites	26,876	2.6	19,559	4.4	7,317	1.2
STOMACH						
Alaska Natives	47	10.8	34	14.8	13	6.4
U.S. whites	61,931	5.9	36,699	8.5	25,232	4.0
COLON AND RECTUM						
Alaska Natives	106	26.6	53	25.5	53	27.9
U.S. whites	231,861	22.0	111,957	25.9	119,904	19.4
LIVER						
Alaska Natives	36	6.9	27	10.0	9	3.5
U.S. whites	20,437	2.0	11,882	2.7	8,555	1.4
GALLBLADDER						
Alaska Natives	13	3.6	4	2.5	9	4.8
U.S. whites	11,172	1.1	2,875	0.7	8,297	1.3
PANCREAS						
Alaska Natives	38	8.7	21	9.1	17	8.1
U.S. whites	88,236	8.4	47,340	10.8	40,896	6.7
LUNG AND BRONCHUS						
Alaska Natives	140	32.1	112	51.5	28	12.2
U.S. whites	385,122	37.6	292,353	65.6	92,769	16.5
BREAST						
Alaska Natives	34	6.8	0	0.0	34	14.0
U.S. whites	152,143	15.0	1,225	0.3	150,918	26.8
CERVIX UTERI						
Alaska Natives	25	5.5	—	—	25	11.1
U.S. whites	21,037	2.1	—	—	21,037	3.8
CORPUS UTERI						
Alaska Natives	3	0.5	—	—	3	1.1
U.S. whites	24,475	2.3	—	—	24,475	4.1
OVARY						
Alaska Natives	8	2.0	—	—	8	4.0
U.S. whites	48,483	4.8	—	—	48,483	8.6

(continued)

TABLE 11–II–16. *Average Annual Age-Adjusted (1970 U.S. Standard) Cancer Mortality Rates per 100,000 Population, Alaska, 1969–83 and U.S. Whites, 1974–78 (Continued)*

	Both Sexes		*Male*		*Female*	
	Number	*Rate*	*Number*	*Rate*	*Number*	*Rate*
PROSTATE GLAND						
Alaska Natives	20	5.4	20	10.7	—	—
U.S. whites	85,359	7.9	85,359	20.5	—	—
URINARY BLADDER						
Alaska Natives	6	1.7	3	1.4	3	1.8
U.S. whites	44,084	4.1	31,066	7.3	13,018	2.0
KIDNEY AND RENAL PELVIS						
Alaska Natives	22	5.2	13	6.3	9	4.1
U.S. whites	31,948	3.1	19,986	4.5	11,962	2.0
BRAIN AND NERVOUS SYSTEM						
Alaska Natives	12	1.6	5	1.2	7	2.0
U.S. whites	40,495	4.1	22,544	5.0	17,951	3.4
HODGKIN'S DISEASE						
Alaska Natives	1	0.3	0	0.0	1	0.6
U.S. whites	11,043	1.1	6,415	1.4	4,628	0.8
NON-HODGKIN'S LYMPHOMA						
Alaska Natives	11	3.1	6	3.6	5	2.6
U.S. whites	50,784	4.9	26,578	6.0	24,206	4.1
MULTIPLE MYELOMA						
Alaska Natives	10	2.3	7	3.2	3	1.3
U.S. whites	23,781	2.3	12,343	2.8	11,438	1.9
LEUKEMIAS						
Alaska Natives	23	3.8	16	5.3	7	2.3
U.S. whites	68,732	6.7	38,889	8.9	29,843	5.2

in nasopharynx cancer patients and in certain high-risk populations (Hildesheim and Levine, 1993), which suggested that screening for the EBV IgA antibody could lead to early diagnosis. Other factors that contribute to the high incidence include dietary components (salted fish) and genetic susceptibility. The high oral cavity and pharynx cancer rate, excluding nasopharynx, among Alaska Native females was due almost entirely to an excess of salivary gland cancers (Lanier and Knutson, 1986).

The high incidence of primary liver cancer among Alaska Natives as compared to U.S. whites, 6.4 versus 1.9, respectively, may be related to the high proportion of the Alaska Native population that is infected with the hepatitis B virus (Heyward et al, 1981). Some success at early detection of liver cancer has been achieved by semiannual serological screening for elevated alpha-fetoprotein levels (Heyward et al, 1985). A program of immunization with hepatitis B vaccine has been undertaken with the hope that this may reduce the incidence of chronic liver disease and liver cancer among Alaska Natives.

Gallbladder cancer incidence rates were even higher among Alaska Natives than among American Indians in the southwestern United States (Table 11–II–6). A corresponding excess of benign gallbladder disease among Alaska Natives has been reported (Boss et al, 1982). Cancer incidence rates for other forms of cancer among Alaska Natives, while similar to those of U.S. whites, were over twice as high as the incidence rates for American Indians in the southwestern United States (Table 11–II–6). Those cancers for which Alaska Natives were at the greatest risk compared to southwest U.S. American Indians are: oral cavity and pharynx, eight times higher; colorectum, ten times higher; and lung and bronchus, seven times higher. Because cigarette smoking is a relatively recently acquired habit in the Native population, with over one-half of the adult Native population smoking by the early 1980s, further increases in lung cancer rates may be anticipated in the absence of intervention. Nutritional factors may be influencing patterns of several cancers. Some variations in incidence rates among the Alaska Native subgroups (Indian, Eskimo, and Aleut) have been reported (Lanier et al, 1989).

Mortality data are presented for the same years (1969–83) as the incidence data (Table 11–II–16), along with data for U.S. whites for 1974–78, the mid interval of 1969–83. The cancer mortality rate for all sites combined was slightly higher among Alaska Natives (182.1) than whites (161.4), due to a 24% excess among females but not males. Similar to the earlier mortality report and the incidence data presented here, rates were particularly high for cancers of the nasopharynx, esophagus, stomach, liver, cervix uteri, and kidney. Rates were relatively low for cancers of the lung, breast, corpus uteri, ovary, prostate, bladder, and brain. In contrast to the earlier mortality but mirroring the incidence data, colorectal cancer rates were similar among males but higher among Alaska Native females than white females; an excess of gallbladder cancer was now evident among Alaska Native males as well as females.

The cancer registry has been expanded in Alaska to assess more completely the cancer burden among the Native populations (Lanier et al, 1993). The registry collects information on cancer incidence, follow-up for survival analyses, stage at diagnosis, and treatment. The effects of low socioeconomic status on diagnosis and treatment can then be studied, as well as the effects of the vast distances that people have to travel, away from friends and families, to receive state-of-the art treatment and diagnosis. These effects could range from late diagnosis to noncompliance with treatment regimens. A comparison of incidence rates among various American Indians and Alaska natives has been reported (Nutting et al, 1993).

DISCUSSION

Of the minority groups considered, only black males had total cancer incidence and mortality rates exceeding those for geographically comparable whites. Although the overall incidence was slightly lower, total cancer mortality rates were 15% higher among black females as compared to white females. As seen in the preceding sections, however, several racial and ethnic minority groups were at a distinct disadvantage when their incidence, mortality, and relative survival rates for certain forms of cancer were compared to those among whites. Other indicators of cancer burden, such as stage distribution at diagnosis, treatment patterns, age-specific incidence, mortality, and survival rates, are useful and should be explored but are beyond the scope of this chapter. The measures presented, however, should provide an overview of variations in the distribution of cancer by race and ethnicity.

In studies primarily concerned with whites, socioeconomic status has been linked to cancer risk, with an inverse association consistently noted for cancers of the esophagus, stomach, lung among males, and cervix uteri, in contrast to positive trends for cancers of the breast and corpus uteri. Socioeconomic status, as indicated by income, education, and poverty measures, may be associated with certain lifestyle patterns, occupational risks, diet, sexual and child-bearing practices, and the use or non-use of preventive medical services. A number of the cancer patterns observed among the various racial and ethnic groups suggest the influence of socioeconomically related factors similar to those described among whites.

Higher smoking rates among black males have contributed to a 36% excess of lung cancer incidence as compared to whites. Other groups such as Hispanics do not yet have high lung cancer rates because their increased use of tobacco has been a relatively recent phenomenon. Groups experiencing high smoking prevalence rates provide a target for intervention programs designed to prevent the onset of smoking among young people and to help current smokers quit.

Both Chinese and Alaska Natives have notably high rates of nasopharyngeal cancer; excesses were suggested for some other minority groups as well, including blacks. High incidence among blacks and Puerto Ricans of oral and esophageal cancers probably are related to alcohol consumption, tobacco use, and diet, providing opportunities for etiologic research and intervention programs. Explanations for elevated rates for esophageal but not oral cancers among Japanese, Filipino, Hawaiian, and Alaska Native males are not clear. Low rates of these cancers among American Indians may be a temporary phenomenon.

Incidence rates for certain gastrointestinal cancers were elevated among several of the minority groups. Stomach cancer rates were high among all the minority groups except Chinese males and Filipinos. Liver cancer incidence rates were relatively high among virtually all the minority groups considered, with the largest excesses being among the Chinese. Gallbladder cancer was highest among American Indians, followed by Alaska Natives and Hispanics, particularly in New Mexico. Pancreatic cancer displayed a different pattern, with high rates among blacks and Hispanics in New Mexico but not in Puerto Rico, and with rates lower among most other minority groups than whites. However, relative to whites, colorectal cancer rates ranged from some excess among Alaska Natives (especially females) to similar rates among blacks, lower rates among most

Asian and Hispanic groups, and rates among American Indians only one-quarter those among whites. It is suspected that several of these patterns are related to diet, but the specific factors have remained elusive.

Excessive incidence rates for cervix uteri cancer, most notably among Alaska Natives, American Indians, blacks, and Hispanics, both in New Mexico and Puerto Rico, may be related in part to the early age of starting sexual activity or to the number of sexual partners. Having a Pap smear frequently has a strong protective effect against invasive disease, which is almost 100% curable when detected in an early stage. Improved screening of these groups could dramatically decrease their cervical cancer incidence and mortality rates. Of the population groups analyzed here, only the Japanese and Filipinos did not have excess rates for invasive cervix uteri cancer. Breast and other female genital cancer incidence rates tended to be considerably lower among most minority groups compared to whites, most likely related to reproductive, hormonal, and dietary differences. Among males, prostatic cancer was diagnosed less frequently among all minority groups except blacks, whose rates were 70% higher than among whites.

Incidence rates for most other cancers examined tended to be considerably lower among each of the minority groups, with the notable exception of the excess of multiple myeloma among blacks. Some environmental factors have been identified for several of these cancers, whereas the etiologies of others are virtually unknown. The racial and ethnic patterns of Hodgkin's disease are intriguing, with substantially lower rates among Asian groups and some suggestion of an excess among New Mexico Hispanic males. Linked to genetically influenced skin color, melanoma in all of the minority groups occurred at rates that did not exceed 20% of those among whites.

Low survival rates among certain racial and ethnic groups are, in many instances, the result of a less favorable stage distribution at diagnosis, perhaps related to delays in seeking diagnosis or difficulty in accepting treatment. English as a second language and a fatalistic attitude about the outcome following a cancer diagnosis may be significant barriers to seeking medical help.

Numerous opportunities exist for reducing the cancer burden of these population groups. Through epidemiologic and multidisciplinary approaches, high-risk and even low-risk groups can be targeted in site-specific investigations designed to clarify the causes and natural history of cancer and to identify appropriate means of prevention and control. Furthermore, programs can be designed to reduce cancer incidence by decreasing the prevalence of risk factors through prevention, cessation, and education programs. Survival of minority groups can be improved through greater emphasis on early detection and screening programs, such as mammography and self-examination for breast cancer and Pap tests for cervix cancer, and through better delivery of timely state-of-the-art therapy. Educational programs designed to combat fatalistic attitudes about cancer can help patients seek medical care promptly and adhere to recommended treatment regimens. When interventions are targeted towards specific racial and ethnic population groups, success will depend on the sensitivity and emphasis given to the distinctive cultural, socioeconomic, and language requirements of these groups. In striving to reduce cancer mortality in the United States, it is crucial that all segments of the population be reached and that differential burdens of minority groups be reduced and eventually eliminated.

REFERENCES

Baquet CR, Horm JW, Gibbs T, et al. 1991. Socioeconomic factors and cancer incidence among blacks and whites. J Natl Cancer Inst 83:551–557.

Baquet CR, Ringen K, Pollack ES, et al. 1986. Cancer Among Blacks and Other Minorities: Statistical Profiles. NIH Publ. No. 86-2785. Bethesda, MD, National Cancer Institute.

Bleed DM, Risser DR, Sperry S, et al. 1992. Cancer incidence and survival among American Indians registered for Indian health service care in Montana, 1982–1987. J Natl Cancer Inst 84:1500–1505.

Bloom B: Use of selected preventive care procedures, United States: 1982. 1986. Vital and Health Statistics, Series 10, No. 157. DHHS Publ. No. (PHS) 86-1585. Hyattsville, MD, National Center for Health Statistics.

Blot WJ, Lanier A, Fraumeni JF Jr, et al. 1975. Cancer mortality among Alaskan natives, 1960–69. J Natl Cancer Inst 55:547–554.

Boring CC, Squires TS, Heath CW Jr. 1992. Cancer statistics for African Americans. CA Cancer J Clin 42:7–17.

Boss LP, Lanier AP, Dohan PH, et al. 1982. Cancers of the gallbladder and biliary tract in Alaskan natives: 1970–79. J Natl Cancer Inst 69:1005–1007.

Breen N, Kessler L. 1994. Changes in the use of screening mammography: evidence from the 1987 and 1990 National Health Interview Surveys. Am J Public Health 84:62–67.

Bureau of the Census. 1983a. 1980 Census of the Population: General Population Characteristics, United States Summary. PC80-1-B1. Washington, D.C., U.S. Department of Commerce.

Bureau of the Census. 1983b. 1980 Census of the Population: General Population Characteristics, Puerto Rico. PC80-1-B53. Washington, D.C., U.S. Department of Commerce.

Bureau of the Census. 1983c. 1980 Census of the Population: Characteristics of the Population, General Social and Economic Characteristics, Hawaii. PC80-1-C13. Washington, D.C., U.S. Department of Commerce.

Bureau of the Census. 1984. 1980 Census of the Population: American Indian Areas and Alaska Native Villages: 1980, Supplementary Report. PC80-S1-13. Washington, D.C., U.S. Department of Commerce.

Bureau of the Census. 1988a. Asian and Pacific Islander Population in the United States: 1980. PC80-2-1E. Washington, D.C., U.S. Department of Commerce.

Bureau of the Census. 1988b. Current Population Reports, Series P-20, No. 416. Washington, D.C., U.S. Government Printing Office.

Bureau of the Census. 1988c. Current Population Reports, Series P-20, No. 422. The Hispanic Population in the United States: March 1985. Washington, D.C., U.S. Government Printing Office.

BUREAU OF THE CENSUS. 1988d. Current Population Reports, Series P-60, No. 159. Washington, D.C., U.S. Government Printing Office.

BUTLER C, SAMET JM, BLACK WC, et al. 1986. Histopathologic findings of lung cancer in Navajo men: relationship to U mining. Health Phys 51:365–368.

CENTERS FOR DISEASE CONTROL (CDC). 1988. Provisional estimates from the National Health Interview Survey Supplement on Cancer Control—United States, January–March 1987. MMWR Morb Mortal Wkly Rep 37:417–425.

CREAGAN ET, FRAUMENI JF JR. 1972. Cancer mortality among American Indians, 1950–67. J Natl Cancer Inst 49:959–967.

CUTLER SJ, EDERER F. 1958. Maximum utilization of the life table method in analyzing survival. J Chron Dis 8:699–712.

DEPARTMENT OF HEALTH AND HUMAN SERVICES (DHHS). 1982. The Health Consequences of Smoking: Cancer. A Report of the Surgeon General. DHHS Publ. No. (PHS) 82-50179. Rockville, MD, Office on Smoking and Health.

DEPARTMENT OF HEALTH AND HUMAN SERVICES (DHHS). 1986. Report of the Secretary's Task Force on Black & Minority Health, Volume III—Cancer. GPO Publ. No. 1986-621-605:00171. Washington, D.C., U.S. Government Printing Office.

DEVESA SS, DIAMOND EL. 1980. Association of breast cancer and cervical cancer incidences with income and education among whites and blacks. J Natl Cancer Inst 65:515–528.

DEVESA SS, DIAMOND EL. 1983. Socioeconomic and racial differences in lung cancer incidence. Am J Epidemiol 118:818–831.

DEVESA SS, SILVERMAN DT, YOUNG JL JR, et al. 1987. Cancer incidence and mortality trends among whites in the United States, 1947–84. J Natl Cancer Inst 79:701–770.

FEIN DJ. 1990. Racial and ethnic differences in U.S. census omission rates. Demography 27:285–302.

FRAUMENI JF JR, HOOVER RN, DEVESA SS, et al: Epidemiology of cancer. 1993. *In* DeVita VT Jr, Hellman S, Rosenberg SA (eds): Cancer—Principles and Practice of Oncology, 4th ed. Philadelphia, Lippincott, pp. 150–181.

FREEMAN HP. 1989. Cancer in the socioeconomically disadvantaged. CA Cancer J Clin 39:266–288.

FROST F, TAYLOR V, FRIES E. 1992. Racial misclassification of Native Americans in a surveillance, epidemiology, and end results cancer registry. J Natl Cancer Inst 84:957–962.

GOREY KM, VENA JE. 1994. Cancer differentials among US blacks and whites: quantitative estimates of socioeconomic-related risks. J Natl Med Assoc 86:209–215.

HAMPTON JW. 1989. The heterogeneity of cancer in Native American populations. *In* Jones LA (ed): Minorities and Cancer. New York, Springer-Verlag, pp. 45–53.

HEALTH RESOURCES AND SERVICES ADMINISTRATION (HRSA). 1985. Health Status of Minorities and Low Income Groups. DHHS Publ. No. (HRSA) HRS-P-DV 85-1. Washington, D.C., U.S. Government Printing Office.

HEATH DB. 1989. American Indians and alcohol: Epidemiological and sociocultural relevance. *In* Alcohol, Drug Abuse, and Mental Health Administration: Alcohol Use among U.S. Ethnic Minorities. DHHS Publ. No. (ADM)89-1435. Rockville, MD, National Institute on Alcohol Abuse and Alcoholism, pp. 207–222.

HERRINTON LJ, STANFORD JL, SCHWARTZ SM, et al. 1994. Ovarian cancer incidence among Asian migrants to the United States and their descendants. J Natl Cancer Inst 86:1336–1339.

HEYWARD WL, LANIER AP, BENDER TR, et al. 1981. Primary hepatocellular carcinoma in Alaskan natives, 1969–1979. Int J Cancer 28:47–50.

HEYWARD WL, LANIER AP, MCMAHON BJ, et al. 1985. Early detection of primary hepatocellular carcinoma. Screening for primary hepatocellular carcinoma among persons infected with hepatitis B virus. JAMA 254:3052–3054.

HILDESHEIM A, LEVINE PH. 1993. Etiology of nasopharyngeal carcinoma: a review. Epidemiol Rev 15:466–485.

HIRAYAMA T. 1975. Epidemiology of cancer of the stomach with special reference to its recent decrease in Japan. Cancer Res 35:3460–3463.

HO JH. 1979. Some epidemiologic observations on cancer in Hong Kong. Natl Cancer Inst Monogr 53:35–47.

HORM JW, ASIRE AJ, YOUNG JL JR, et al (eds). 1984. SEER Program: Cancer Incidence and Mortality in the United States, 1973–81. NIH Publ. No. 85-1837. Bethesda, MD, National Cancer Institute.

HRDLICKA A. 1908. Physiological and Medical Observations. Washington, D.C., U.S. Government Printing Office.

HUMBLE CG, SAMET JM, PATHAK DR, et al. 1985. Cigarette smoking and lung cancer in "Hispanic" whites and other whites in New Mexico. Am J Public Health 75:145–148.

INDIAN HEALTH SERVICE. 1977. Alcoholism: A High Priority Health Problem. DHEW Publ. No. (HSA) 77-1001. Washington, D.C., U.S. Government Printing Office.

INDIAN HEALTH SERVICE. 1989. Trends in Indian Health 1989. Washington, D.C., U.S. Department of Health and Human Services.

INTERNATIONAL AGENCY FOR RESEARCH ON CANCER (IARC). 1986. Evaluation of the Carcinogenic Risk of Chemicals to Humans, Vol. 38: Tobacco Smoking. Lyon, IARC.

JONES LA (ED). 1989. Minorities and Cancer. New York, Springer-Verlag.

KANG SH, BLOOM JR. 1993. Social support and cancer screening among older black Americans. J Natl Cancer Inst 85:737–742.

KEY CR. 1981. Cancer incidence and mortality in New Mexico, 1973–77. *In* Young JL Jr, Percy Cl, Asire AJ (eds): Surveillance, Epidemiology, and End Results: Incidence and Mortality Data, 1973–77. Natl Cancer Inst Monogr 57, pp. 489–595.

KING H, LI JY, LOCKE FB, et al. 1985. Patterns of site-specific displacement in cancer mortality among migrants: the Chinese in the United States. Am J Public Health 75:237–242.

KOLONEL L, GOODMAN MT. 1987. USA, Hawaii. *In* Muir C, Waterhouse J, Mack T, et al: Cancer Incidence in Five Continents, Vol V. IARC Scientific Publ. No. 88. Lyon, International Agency for Research on Cancer, pp. 766–785.

KOLONEL LN. 1985. Cancer incidence among Filipinos in Hawaii and the Philippines. Natl Cancer Inst Monogr 69:93–98.

KOLONEL LN. 1988. Variability in diet and its relation to risk in ethnic and migrant groups. Basic Life Sci 43:129–135.

LACEY L. 1993. Cancer prevention and early detection strategies for reaching underserved urban, low-income black women. Barriers and objectives. Cancer 72:1078–1083.

LANIER A, BENDER T, TALBOT M, et al. 1980. Nasopharyngeal carcinoma in Alaskan Eskimos, Indians, and Aleuts: a review of cases and study of Epstein-Barr virus, HLA, and environmental risk factors. Cancer 46:2100–2106.

LANIER AP, BULKOW LR, IRELAND B. 1989. Cancer in Alaskan Indians, Eskimos, and Aleuts, 1969–83: implications for etiology and control. Public Health Rep 104:658–664.

LANIER AP, HENLE W, HENLE G, et al. 1983. Epstein-Barr virus antibody patterns in Alaskan Natives at high risk for nasopharyngeal carcinoma. *In* Prasad U, Ablashi DV, Levine PH, et al (eds): Nasopharyngeal Carcinoma: Current Concepts. Kuala Lumpur, University of Malaysia, pp. 173–181.

LANIER AP, KELLY J, SMITH B, et al. 1993. Cancer in the Alaska Native Population: Eskimo, Aleut, and Indian—Incidence and Trends 1969–1988. Anchorage, AL, Alaska Area Native Health Service.

LANIER AP, KNUTSON LR. 1986. Cancer in Alaskan Natives: a 15-year summary. Alaska Med 28:37–41.

LEE JF. 1983. Smoking among Alaska Native youth: A profile of the smoking patterns in five northwest Arctic communities from surveys done for the purpose of developing and evaluating a smoking and prevention program for Alaska youth. *In* Forbes WF, Frecker RC,

Nostbakken D (eds): Proceedings of the Fifth World Conference on Smoking and Health, Winnipeg, Canada, 1983, Vol 1. Ottawa, Canadian Council on Smoking and Health, pp. 737–741.

LE MARCHAND L, WILKENS LR, KOLONEL LN. 1992. Ethnic differences in the lung cancer risk associated with smoking. Cancer Epidemiol Biomarkers Prev 1:103–107.

LOCKE FB, KING H. 1980. Cancer mortality risk among Japanese in the United States. J Natl Cancer Inst 65:1149–1156.

MACK TM, WALKER A, MACK W, et al. 1985. Cancer in Hispanics in Los Angeles County. Natl Cancer Inst Monogr 69:99–104.

MARTINEZ I. 1969. Factors associated with cancer of the esophagus, mouth, and pharynx in Puerto Rico. J Natl Cancer Inst 42:1069–1094.

MARTINEZ I, TORRES R, ECHEVARRIA L, et al. 1987. USA, Puerto Rico. *In* Muir C, Waterhouse J, Mack T, et al: Cancer Incidence in Five Continents, Vol V. IARC Scientific Publ. No. 88. Lyon, International Agency for Research on Cancer, pp. 208–211.

MASON TJ, MCKAY FW, HOOVER R, et al. 1975. Atlas of Cancer Mortality for U.S. Counties: 1950–1969. DHEW Publ. No. (NIH) 75-780. Washington, D.C., U.S. Government Printing Office.

MASON TJ, MCKAY FW, HOOVER R, et al. 1976. Atlas of Cancer Mortality among U.S. Nonwhites: 1950–1969. DHEW Publ. No. (NIH) 76-1204. Washington, D.C., U.S. Government Printing Office.

MCWHORTER WP, SCHATZKIN AG, HORM JW, et al. 1989. Contribution of socioeconomic status to black/white differences in cancer incidence. Cancer 63:982–987.

MICHALEK AM, MAHONEY MC, CUMMINGS KM, et al. 1989. Mortality patterns among a Native American population in New York State. N Y State J Med 89:557–561.

MORA LI, MARTINEZ I, TORRES LLAUGER R. 1987. Cancer en Puerto Rico 1985. Estado Libre Asociado de Puerto Rico, Departamento de Salud, Registro Central de Cancer.

MUIR C, WATERHOUSE J, MACK T, et al. 1987. Cancer Incidence in Five Continents, Vol V. IARC Scientific Publ. No. 88. Lyon, International Agency for Research on Cancer.

NAMIKI M. 1980. Westernization of eating habits and changes in stomach lesions. I To Cho 15:59–64.

NATIONAL CANCER INSTITUTE (NCI). 1988. Annual Cancer Statistics Review, Including Cancer Trends: 1950–1985. NIH Publ. No. 88-2789. Washington, D.C., U.S. Government Printing Office.

NATIONAL CANCER INSTITUTE (NCI). 1989. Cancer Statistics Review 1973–1986, Including a Report on the Status of Cancer Control. NIH Publ. No. 89-2789. Bethesda, MD, NIH.

NATIONAL CENTER FOR HEALTH STATISTICS (NCHS). 1988. Health, United States, 1987. DHHS Publ. No. (PHS)88-1232. Hyattsville, MD, PHS.

NATIONAL CENTER FOR HEALTH STATISTICS (NCHS). 1994. Health, United States, 1993. DHHS Publ. No. (PHS)94-1232. Hyattsville, MD, PHS.

NERVI F, DUARTE I, GOMEZ G, et al.1988. Frequency of gallbladder cancer in Chile, a high-risk area. Int J Cancer 41:657–660.

NUTTING PA, FREEMAN WL, RISSER DR, et al.1993. Cancer incidence among American Indians and Alaska Natives, 1980 through 1987. Am J Public Health 83:1589–1598.

PALMER EP. 1938. Cancer among the American Indians of the United States, with an analysis of cancer in Arizona. Southwestern Med 22:483–487.

PICKLE LW, MASON TJ, HOWARD N, et al. 1987. Atlas of U.S. Cancer Mortality among Whites: 1950–1980. DHHS Publ. No. (NIH) 87-2900. Washington, D.C., U.S. Government Printing Office.

PICKLE LW, MASON TJ, HOWARD N, et al. 1990. Atlas of U.S. Cancer Mortality among Nonwhites: 1950–1980. DHHS Publ. No. (NIH) 90-1582. Washington, D.C., U.S. Government Printing Office.

POLEDNAK AP. 1992. Cancer incidence in the Puerto Rican–born population of Connecticut. Cancer 70:1172–1176.

POLLACK ES, HORM JW. 1980. Trends in cancer incidence and mortality in the United States, 1969–76. J Natl Cancer Inst 64:1091–1103.

RIBOLI E. 1990. The IARC program of prospective studies on nutrition and cancer. Prog Clin Biol Res 346:189–204.

RIES LAG, MILLER BA, HANKEY BF, et al. 1994. SEER Cancer Statistics Review, 1973–1991: Tables and Graphs. NIH Publ. No. 94-2789. Bethesda, MD, National Cancer Institute.

ROBINSON RG, KESSLER LG, NAUGHTON MD. 1991. Cancer awareness among African Americans: a survey assessing race, social status, and occupation. J Natl Med Assoc 83:491–497.

ROSENWAIKE I. 1987. Mortality differentials among persons born in Cuba, Mexico, and Puerto Rico residing in the United States, 1979–1981. Am J Public Health 77:603–606.

ROSENWAIKE I, SHAI D. 1986. Trends in cancer mortality among Puerto Rican–born migrants to New York City. Int J Epidemiol 15:30–35.

SAMET JM, COULTAS DB, HOWARD CA, et al. 1988. Diabetes, gallbladder disease, obesity, and hypertension among Hispanics in New Mexico. Am J Epidemiol 128:1302–1311.

SAMET JM, KEY CR, HUNT WC, et al. 1987. Survival of American Indian and Hispanic cancer patients in New Mexico and Arizona, 1969–82. J Natl Cancer Inst 79:457–463.

SAVITZ DA. 1986. Changes in Spanish surname cancer rates relative to other whites, Denver area, 1969–71 to 1979–81. Am J Public Health 76:1210–1215.

SCHINKE SP, MONCHER MS, HOLDEN GW, et al. 1989. American Indian youth and substance abuse: Tobacco use problems, risk factors, and preventive interventions. Health Education Research, Theory and Practice 4:137–144.

SCHLIFE C. 1987. Smokeless tobacco use in rural Alaska. MMWR Morb Mortal Wkly Rep 36:140–143.

SCHOTTENFELD D. 1984. Epidemiology of cancer of the esophagus. Semin Oncol 11:92–100.

SCHOTTENFELD D, BERGAD BM. 1985. Epidemiology of cancers of the oral cavity, pharynx, and larynx. *In* Whittes RE (ed): Head and Neck Cancer. New York, Wiley, pp. 3–12.

SHIMIZU H, MACK TM, ROSS RK, et al. 1987. Cancer of the gastrointestinal tract among Japanese and white immigrants in Los Angeles County. J Natl Cancer Inst 78:223–228.

STELLMAN SD, WANG QS. 1994. Cancer mortality in Chinese migrants to New York City. Cancer 73:1270–1275.

STEMMERMANN GN, NOMURA AMY, CHYOU PH, et al. 1991. Cancer incidence in Hawaiian Japanese: migrants from Okinawa compared with those from other prefectures. Jpn J Cancer Res 82:1366–1370.

SWANSON CA, GRIDLEY G, GREENBERG RS, et al. 1993. A comparison of diets of blacks and whites in three areas of the United States. Nutr Cancer 20:153–165.

TOMINAGA S, OGAWA H, KUROISHI T. 1982. Usefulness of correlation analyses in the epidemiology of stomach cancer. Natl Cancer Inst Monogr 62:135–140.

TRAPIDO EJ, CHEN F, DAVIS K, et al. 1994a. Cancer among Hispanic males in south Florida. Arch Intern Med 154:177–185.

TRAPIDO EJ, CHEN F, DAVIS K, et al. 1994b. Cancer in south Florida Hispanic women. Arch Intern Med 154:1083–1088.

TREVINO FM, MOYER ME, VALDEZ RB, et al. 1991. Health insurance coverage and utilization of health services by Mexican Americans, mainland Puerto Ricans, and Cuban Americans. JAMA 265:233–237.

TU JT, GAO RN, ZHANG DH, et al. 1985. Hepatitis B virus and primary liver cancer on Chongming Island, People's Republic of China. Natl Cancer Inst Monogr 69:213–215.

VALWAY S. 1994. Cancer mortality in Native Americans by region. J Natl Cancer Inst 86:579.

WEISS KM, FERRELL RE, HANIS CL, et al. 1984. Genetics and epidemiology of gallbladder disease in New World native peoples. Am J Hum Genet 36:1259–1278.

WELTY TK, ZEPHIER N, SCHWEIGMAN K, et al. 1993. Cancer risk factors in three Sioux tribes. Alaska Med 35:265–272.

WIGGINS CL, BECKER TM, KEY CR, et al. 1993. Cancer mortality among New Mexico's Hispanics, American Indians, and non-Hispanic whites, 1958–1987. J Natl Cancer Inst 85:1670–1678.

WILLIAMS RR, HORM JW. 1977. Association of cancer sites with tobacco and alcohol consumption and socioeconomic status of patients: interview study from the Third National Cancer Survey. J Natl Cancer Inst 58:525–547.

WOLFGANG PE, SEMEIKS PA, BURNETT WS. 1991. Cancer incidence in New York City Hispanics, 1982 to 1985. Ethn Dis 1:263–272.

WYNDER EL, BROSS IJ. 1961. A study of etiological factors in cancer of the esophagus. Cancer 14:389–413.

YOUNG JL JR, PERCY CL, ASIRE AJ (eds). 1981. Surveillance, Epidemiology, and End Results: Incidence and mortality data, 1973–77. Natl Cancer Inst Monogr 57:1–1082.

ZIEGLER RG. 1986. Alcohol-nutrient interactions in cancer etiology. Cancer 58:1942–1948.

ZIEGLER RG, HOOVER RN, PIKE MC, et al. 1993. Migration patterns and breast cancer risk in AsianAmerican women. J Natl Cancer Inst 85:1819–1827.

12 Migrant studies

DAVID B. THOMAS
MARGARET R. KARAGAS

The incidence and mortality rates of virtually all malignancies vary among different regions of the world. When individuals move from one region to another, in time they or their descendants eventually tend to develop most cancers at rates comparable to those in the native population of their new homeland. Many studies of such changes in rates have been conducted. In addition, a variety of investigative approaches have been taken to identify factors responsible for these changes. This chapter provides a description of the types of studies that have been conducted on migrants and summarizes selected results from these efforts.

A migrant is an individual who has moved from one country and established residence in another. The country that the migrant came from is the *country of origin* (sometimes referred to as the *country of birth* or the *home country*), and the country to which the migrant moved is the *country of adoption* (sometimes referred to as the *new homeland*). Migrants are also referred to as *first generation nationals* (e.g., first generation Americans), their offspring who reside in the country of adoption are referred to as *second generation nationals*, and so forth, for subsequent generations; those who are of uncertain generation, are collectively referred to as *descendants of migrants*.

TYPES OF STUDIES IN MIGRANTS

Table 12–1 shows the types of studies that have been conducted on migrants. Studies of mortality and incidence rates are usually what are referred to as *migrant studies*. These studies serve a number of purposes, which are summarized in Table 12–2.

Observations on changes in rates for migrants and their descendants can provide etiologic clues. If rates of a cancer in migrants or their descendants tend to approach those of the country of adoption, at least part of the differences in rates among countries are presumably due to environmental and not hereditary factors. If rates in succeeding generations stabilize at a level different from the rate in the country of adoption, and if these descendants become completely acculturated to their environment, then the magnitude of this residual difference would, in theory, be a measure of the hereditary component of the difference in rates between the countries of origin and adoption.

The pattern of displacement of cancer rates in succeeding generations of migrants can also be of value in determining when exposure to a new environment is of greatest etiologic importance. If rates of a particular cancer in the migrants themselves approximate those in the country of adoption, then factors in the new environment that operate in adulthood are likely to be important determinants of risk. If rates for the second generation, but not those for the first generation, approximate those in the country of adoption, then the factors of primary etiologic importance may be largely operative early in life. Alternatively, these factors may be substances to which members of the first and second generations are differently exposed as adults. More precise estimates of the critical period and length of exposure to the new environment can be made from studies of rates in migrants by duration of residence in the country of adoption or age at immigration.

Variations among different migrant groups in the patterns of displacement of rates for a particular cancer can identify cultural environments particularly conducive to exposures to factors of etiologic or protective importance. Also, comparisons of different cancers by their patterns of displacement of rates in migrants and their descendants can provide evidence that different cancers of unknown etiology have similar or different causes.

Rates of various histologic types of cancers, or of cancers arising from different sites within the same organ, have also been compared in migrants and non-migrants. Shimizu et al (1987) compared rates of carcinomas arising from the upper colon, sigmoid region, and rectum in Hispanics and Japanese migrants in Los Angeles, natives of their respective homelands, and their U.S.-born descendants; and they compared rates of cancers in different parts of the colon in the migrants in relation to an index of age at migration (based on social security numbers). Correa and Haenszel (1978) similarly com-

TABLE 12–1. *Types of Studies in Migrants*

1. Incidence and mortality rates in migrants
   - Compared with rates in country of adoption
   - Compared with rates in country of origin
   - Compared with rates in their descendants
   - By duration of residence in country of adoption
   - By anatomic distribution and histologic type
2. Correlation studies
3. Comparisons of migrants and non-migrants
   - Exposures to known and suspected carcinogens
   - Biologic measurements
   - Prevalence of precursor lesions
4. Case–control studies
5. Cohort studies

pared rates of carcinomas arising in different regions of the colon in Japanese in Hawaii and Miyagi Prefecture, Japan, as did Kune et al (1986) in migrants to Australia. In another study, Correa et al (1973) compared rates of intestinal and diffuse types of stomach cancer among Japanese in Hawaii and Miyagi Prefecture. Studies like these can provide evidence for differing etiologies of different types of neoplasms arising from the same organ.

Another purpose served by migrant studies is to provide information on rates in the migrant's country of origin. If rates for recent migrants are similar to those in their country of origin, then this provides evidence that the reported rates in the country of origin are reasonably valid. This information is of value in interpreting differences in rates among countries. Also, with caution, rates for recent migrants can be used to estimate rates in their country of origin. This is of particular value for less developed countries where incidence or mortality rates are lacking or inadequate, and provides a way to identify areas that are likely to have unusual rates of specific neoplasms, where opportunities may exist for fruitful epidemiologic research. Examples include high observed rates of nasopharyngeal and cervical cancers in migrants from North Africa to Israel, high rates of esophageal cancer in migrants from Iran and Yemen to Israel (Katz and Steinitz, 1979) high rates of leukemia in migrants from Iraq to Israel (Halevi et al, 1971), and high rates of thyroid cancer in migrants from Ethiopia to Israel (Iscovich et al, 1993). Also, Malays in Singapore were observed to have high rates of oral cancer, and Hokkien-speaking Chinese, who are mainly from Fukien Province, were found to have high rates of esophageal cancer (Shanmugaratnam et al, 1983).

TABLE 12–2. *Purposes Served by Studies of Mortality and Incidence Rates in Migrants*

1. Provide etiologic clues
   - Distinguish effects of heredity and environment
   - Identify periods of exposure of etiologic importance
   - Identify causal or protective cultural environments
   - Provide evidence for similar or dissimilar etiologies of different cancers
2. Provide information on rates in countries of origin
   - Validate reported rates in countries of origin
   - Estimate rates in countries for which rates are unavailable
3. Identify specific health needs of migrants
4. Identify populations for further studies of individual migrants

Studies of cancer rates among migrants can also serve a public health function by identifying unusual needs that immigrants may have for preventive and medical services.

Observations of incidence and mortality rates in migrants and their descendants have logically led to more detailed studies of migrants to identify specific environmental factors of etiologic importance for various cancers. These kinds of studies are listed as items 2 through 5 in Table 12–1.

Surveys have been conducted to estimate levels of exposures to a variety of substances in migrants and native-born residents of their country of adoption. Markides et al (1987) conducted surveys of smoking habits in three generations of Mexican Americans. Drinking habits of Greek migrants to Australia have been compared to those of their siblings in Greece (Powles, et al, 1991); and smoking habits, alcohol consumption, physical activity, and other health-related practices have been compared among five racial groups in Hawaii (Chung et al, 1990). Dietary surveys have been performed among southern European migrants to Australia (McMichael and Giles, 1988), various racial groups in Hawaii (Kolonel et al, 1981a, 1981b), Mexicans in California (Bruhn and Pangborn, 1971), Koreans in Japan (Ubukata et al, 1987), and European migrants residing on a kibbutz in Israel (Rozen et al, 1981).

Results of such surveys have been used to speculate as to the possible environmental factors that have resulted in changes in rates of various cancers in migrants (Wynder and Hirayama, 1977). Some studies have taken this approach a step further by examining correlations between intakes of various substances and rates of specific cancers (correlational studies). For example, Kolonel et al (1981b) demonstrated strong correlations between incidence rates of lung cancer and cholesterol intake, stomach cancer and fish intake, breast cancer and consumption of animal protein, and cancer of the corpus uteri and intake of saturated fat, among five different ethnic groups in Hawaii (Caucasians, Japanese, Chinese, Filipino, and native Hawaiian). Also, Hinds et al (1980) assessed correlations between rates of various neoplasms and consumption of cigarettes, beer, wine, and distilled beverages among 10 ethnic–sex groups in Hawaii.

Migrants and non-migrants with different rates of cancer have also been compared with respect to biological measurements that may be of etiologic importance. For example, levels of mutagens were found to be higher in feces from Japanese in Hawaii with high risks of colon cancer, than from Japanese in Japan with low rates (Mower et al, 1982). Glober et al (1977) found stool weight to be lower for Japanese in Hawaii than for Japanese in Japan, but bowel transit time was found to be similar in individuals in these two groups. In another study, Goldin et al (1986) compared diets, plasma estrogen and androgen levels, and 24-hour urinary and fecal estrogen excretion of Caucasians and recent migrants from Vietnam and Laos to Hawaii. Compared to the Caucasians, the Oriental women had lower plasma levels of estrone and estradiol, less urinary excretion of estrogens, and more fecal estrogen excretion. These findings may provide insights into the reasons for the lower rates of endometrial, ovarian, breast, and colon cancers in Orientals than in Caucasians.

Comparisons of the prevalence of putative precursor lesions in migrants and non-migrants have helped to clarify the role of specific histologic entities in the carcinogenic process. Akazaki and Stemmermann (1973) showed that the prevalence of latent cancer of the prostate did not differ for Japanese in Japan and Hawaii, but that the prevalence of a more proliferative type was higher among the higher-risk migrants in Hawaii, suggesting that something in the new environment of the migrants exerted a promotional influence on latent prostatic carcinomas. Stemmermann and Yatani (1973) also found higher prevalence rates of adenomatous polyps of the colon for Japanese living in Hawaii than did Sato et al (1976) for Japanese in Japan.

The degree to which migrants change their lifestyles to more closely resemble that of the native-born citizens of their new country varies within migrant groups according to each member's desire and ability to adapt, by time since migration, and among succeeding generations. Exposures of interest, such as dietary intake, may thus vary more widely among migrant groups and their descendants than among members of the native population of the country of adoption. Because of this broader range of exposure, case–control and cohort studies in migrant populations may have greater power to detect associations between specific neoplasms and putative risk factors than studies of similar size in populations with more homogenous levels of exposure. In addition, the date of migration is an easily identifiable indicator of the time when changes in the exposure of interest began, and this information can be used to estimate the influence on risk of early versus late exposure and the latent period between exposure and development of the disease. Studies which include more than one migrant group, or native-born residents of the host country, can also help explain observed variations in rates among groups.

Examples of case–control studies in migrants include: a dietary study of colon cancer in Hawaiian Japanese (Haenszel et al, 1973); a study of colorectal cancer in relation to diet and physical activity in Chinese in North America and in China (Whittemore, et al, 1990); investigations in various ethnic groups in Hawaii of cancers of the breast, prostate, lung, and bladder in relation to various dietary constituents (Kolonel et al, 1983); studies in Australia of both malignant melanoma (Holman, et al, 1986) and non-melanotic skin cancers (Kricker, et al, 1991), which included assessments of risk in relation to ethnic origin and age at migration from Europe; and a study in the United States (Ziegler et al, 1993) of breast cancer among Chinese, Japanese, and Filipino migrants and their descendants in relation to various features of the place of origin and of the circumstances of immigration of the migrant generation.

A few studies have been conducted in which cohorts of migrants have been defined, their members surveyed to obtain information on exposures of interest or various biological measurements, and then followed for development of cancers and other diseases. Early attempts were made in the United States in the 1960s to conduct such cohort studies among migrants and their descendants from Norway and the United Kingdom (Reid, 1966), and among the siblings of the migrants from Norway who did not migrate (Magnus et al, 1970). Unfortunately, the effort in the United States was limited because parents' place of birth was not recorded on death certificates in many states after the 1960s. A second cohort of persons who migrated to the United States from Norway, Sweden, or Germany, or who were descendants of such individuals, or who were born in the United States of different descent, was assembled from individuals who had insurance policies with the Lutheran Brotherhood, an insurance company in Minnesota (Haenszel, 1970). Usable self-administered questionnaires were completed by 17,633 respondents. After 26 years of follow-up, reports have been published on mortality rates of cancers of the prostate (Hsing et al, 1990) and stomach (Kneller et al, 1991) in relation to nativity, smoking, alcohol use, and diet.

As part of the Honolulu Heart Study, 8,006 men of Japanese birth or ancestry in Hawaii, born between 1900 and 1919, who had been identified from World War II selective service registration records, completed a self-administered questionnaire and were clinically examined from 1965 to 1968 (Worth and Kagan, 1970; Nomura et al, 1985). From 1971 to 1975, 6860 of the men were examined again, and blood samples were obtained for measurement of serum cholesterol and for storage and future use. This cohort has been monitored for the occurrence of new cases of cancer. Studies of risk of subsequent cancers in relation to serum levels of several vitamins (Nomura et al, 1985), selenium (Nomura et al, 1987), hepatitis B surface antigen (Nomura et al, 1982), and blood lipids (Stemmermann et al, 1985) have been conducted in this cohort by measuring levels of substances of interest in the prediagnostic serum specimens from the cases and from a sample of individuals in the cohort study who have not developed cancer. Based on information from the baseline questionnaire, cancer rates in relation to various dietary constituents and other factors have also been assessed (e.g., Nomura et al, 1981b).

Also in Hawaii, between 1975 and 1980 approximately 50,000 residents were sampled and interviewed to obtain information on smoking, alcohol use, and frequency of consumption of a limited number of foods and drinks. In addition, between 1977 and 1979 a subset of 5,000 of these individuals over age 45 of Japanese, Chinese, Caucasian, Filipino, and Hawaiian descent were randomly selected and interviewed to obtain information on frequency of intake of 83 food items. Both the large cohort and the smaller subset are currently being followed for development of all cancers (Kolonel et al, 1983).

McMichael and Giles (1988) have summarized results of dietary surveys of southern European migrants to Australia. These surveyed groups may serve as the basis for the development of cohort studies of cancer in relation to diet similar to those underway in Hawaii.

The remaining portions of this chapter are devoted largely to studies of cancer incidence and mortality rates in migrants and their descendants. Other studies on migrants are more appropriately considered in the context of other etiologic investigations in the various chapters on specific neoplasms.

METHODOLOGIC CONSIDERATIONS IN THE STUDY OF INCIDENCE AND MORTALITY RATES IN MIGRANTS

Methodologic difficulties related to the identification and enumeration of migrant groups have been summarized by Staszewski et al (1970). First generation migrants from specific countries are usually readily identified from census data and from death certificates and cancer registries because country of birth is routinely recorded. In some situations, where there is considerable variation in rates of cancer within various parts of the country of origin, more refined measures of place of origin have been used. Among the Chinese in Singapore, for example, Chinese dialect has been used as an index of region of origin in China (Shanmugaratnam et al, 1983); and in Hawaii, incidence rates of cancer in migrants from Okinawa have been compared with rates in migrants from other prefectures of Japan (Stemmermann et al, 1991). Also in Hawaii, results of a survey of Japanese immigrants were used to compare rates of cancer among Japanese in Japan and Hawaii, correcting for differences in the distribution of migrants and native residents of Japan by prefecture of birth (Nomura and Hirohata, 1976). In this instance, the correction had little effect on the rates.

Unfortunately, in most countries, place of birth of parents is not routinely recorded in censuses or death certificates, so second generation immigrants cannot be directly enumerated. When race and country of origin are synonymous (e.g., Japanese or Filipinos), first generation migrants can be distinguished from their descendants and enumerated by using a combination of their race and birth place. When race is not informative as to country of origin, as with whites, rates in second generation migrants have not been readily obtainable. An exception to this is the identification of individuals in the United States with Spanish surnames. They have been assumed to be largely of Latin American descent, and their names plus place of birth have been used to distinguish first generation Mexicans from their descendants (e.g., Menck et al, 1975).

It has also been difficult to obtain information on age at migration or duration of residence in country of adoption. Armstrong et al (1983) were able to estimate person-years at risk by duration of residence in Australia, for migrants from a number of European countries, from information on duration of residence from censuses taken in 1961, 1966, and 1971. There are, however, some uncertainties in their estimates. In Los Angeles, Mack et al (1985), and Shimizu et al (1987) estimated age at migration, reasoning that individuals whose social security numbers were assigned after the usual age of entry into the work force migrated as adults, whereas those whose numbers were assigned at the usual age of initial employment most likely either migrated as children or were born locally. Unfortunately, they were able to utilize this procedure only for cases, not for individuals in the general population, and have thus only been able to directly calculate proportional incidence ratios by inferred age at migration. Utilizing data from the Israel cancer registry, Parkin et al (1990) estimated risks of various cancers in migrants from Europe and America, Asia, and Africa relative to risks in native-born Israelis, by duration of stay in Israel. A case–control approach was utilized in which each individual case group was compared with all other cases in the registry (as the controls); logistic regression techniques were used to estimate the relative risks. The same approach was used to study risk of malignant melanoma in relation to age at migration and duration of residence in Australia (Khlat, et al, 1992).

When ethnically identifiable migrants are known to have arrived in their new homeland primarily during a limited period of time, calendar year and age can be used to infer likely place of birth. In such circumstances, temporal trends in rates for such ethnic groups can be interpreted as reflecting the influences on cancer risks of longer exposures to the new environment, or exposures at earlier ages with the passage of time. Examples of studies of time trends in migrant groups include one by Savitz (1986) of Spanish surnamed whites in the Denver area of the United States, and one by Hinds et al (1981) of five ethnic groups in Hawaii.

Immigration statistics have not proven useful for estimating populations of immigrants at risk (Staszewski et al, 1970), although they have been of value in identifying migrants for inclusion in studies of individuals (Haenszel, 1970).

Another potential problem in measuring cancer rates among migrants is that the information on race and place of birth from census records may not be comparable to that from death certificates or cancer registries. This problem stems from the fact that, in many countries where studies of rates for migrants have been conducted, including the United States, information on individuals from death certificates or tumor registries cannot routinely be linked to information on the same individual from census records. Haenszel (1961) and Lilienfeld et al (1972) compared place of birth listed on an individual's death certificate with that listed in his or her 1950 and 1960 census record, respectively. Similarly, Marmot et al (1984) compared place of birth of migrants to England and Wales recorded on death certificates with that recorded in the 1971 census. Fortunately, in these instances the desired information was sufficiently comparable. The comparability of information from cancer registries and censuses has not been similarly assessed. However, since information on race and place of birth in both census and medical records usually comes from the cases themselves, it is unlikely that the numerator and denominator data would be less comparable for the components of incidence rates than for the components of mortality rates.

The problems of ensuring complete ascertainment of cases or deaths among migrant groups include all of those for native populations of various countries. In addition, there are some special problems in identifying cases and deaths among migrants. Attitudes of some migrants toward seeking medical care may influence stage of disease at diagnosis. For diseases for which screening techniques are available, such as cervical cancer, avoidance of screening could enhance rates of invasive disease in migrants. For diseases that are inoperable if not brought to medical attention at an early stage, delays in seeking care can result in underdiagnosis, due to lack of histological confirmation of tumors not treated surgically, or in inability of pathologists to identify the primary tumor site in individuals with undifferentiated disseminated neoplasms. Delay in seeking care can also adversely affect prognosis and selectively increase mortality rates. Attitudes of migrants toward autopsies can also affect observed rates of disease by influencing the proportion of cases that are histologically confirmed.

In studies of incidence and mortality rates in migrants, a variety of summary statistics have been utilized to compare rates in different populations. Using the indirect method of age standardization, standardized mortality ratios (SMR) and standardized incidence ratios (SIR) have been extensively utilized. These are of particular value when there are small numbers of cases in the migrant group. Their major disadvantage is that the age-specific ratios are assumed to be constant across all ages, and if they are not, the values for the various groups are not strictly comparable.

Alternatives are mortality rates (MR) and incidence rates (IR), adjusted for age to some standard population using the direct method, and the use of ratios of these rates, i.e., standardized incidence rate ratios (IRR) and standardized mortality rate ratios (MRR) to compare rates for various groups. These ratios have the advantage of being directly comparable if the same standard population is used to calculate the incidence or mortality rates for the various groups. Their major disadvantage is that they are subject to considerable random variation when rates are based on small numbers of cases.

When adequate denominator data have not been available, information on proportional mortality and proportional incidence have been used to calculate standardized proportional mortality ratios (PMR) and standardized proportional incidence ratios (PIR); logistic regression techniques have also been used to estimate risks among migrants relative to non-migrants by utilizing individual case groups as the cases and all other cases in a registry as controls (Parkin et al, 1990). These techniques can provide useful indications of variations in rates of various cancers among groups or within groups over time, but they must obviously be interpreted with more caution than other summary statistics since they are influenced by rates of conditions other than the one under consideration.

Another factor that must be considered in interpreting results of studies of rates in migrants is that migrants are self-selected and may not be representative of the citizens of their country of origin. Sometimes migrants tend to come from specific areas of a country with patterns of cancer occurrence that differ from those elsewhere in the same country. Migrants from China are a good example (King et al, 1985; Shanmugaratnam et al, 1983). Migrants may also be of different socioeconomic status than those who remain at home. Many Europeans who migrated to the United States did so for economic reasons and were poorer than non-migrants from the same country, whereas recent migrants from the Indian subcontinent to the United Kingdom tend to be more well off than the non-migrating population. Migrants may also differ from non-migrants by religion or ethnicity. Migrants to the United States from Russia were predominantly Jewish, and more Protestants than Catholics have moved from Ireland to England. Migrants may also, on occasion, move because of ill health, but more often they tend to be healthier than the average person from their country of origin. The infirm cannot easily move, and many countries have restrictive laws preventing immigration of individuals in ill health. This tendency for the migrant to be in good health has resulted in the observation in some instances of a "healthy migrant" effect (e.g., Marmot et al, 1984) manifested by recent migrants having lower rates of some diseases than expected from knowledge of the rates in their country of origin.

STUDIES OF MORTALITY AND INCIDENCE RATES IN SPECIFIC MIGRANT GROUPS

Table 12–3 shows the countries of origin and adoption of the subjects of the major studies of mortality and incidence rates in migrant populations that have been conducted since 1960.

Caucasian Migrants

Large numbers of migrants from a variety of European countries to the United States during the latter part of the last century and the early part of this one have provided a rich source of information on migrants. Most came from eastern Europe (Czechoslovakia, Hungary, Poland, Yugoslavia, and the Soviet Union), Scandinavia (Finland, Norway, Sweden, and Denmark), the British Isles (The United Kingdom and Ireland), Germany, Austria, and Italy. The first large investigation in which mortality rates of specific cancers were compared in migrants, their country of origin, and their country of adoption was conducted by Haenszel (1961). Standardized mortality ratios relative to U.S. whites were reported for most major cancers in migrants from 10 European countries and Canada for 1950. The reader is referred to this paper and also to the chapter on migrant studies in the first edition of this book (Haenszel, 1982) for a historical review of migrant studies prior to that investigation. The same methodology was used to compare age-specific cancer mortality rates among migrants from Poland with rates in Poland and for whites born in the United States (Staszewski and Haenszel, 1965; Staszewski, 1974). Staszewski et al (1971) also contrasted age-specific and age-adjusted mortality rates of major cancers among Polish migrants to Australia, Australians born in Australia, and Poles in Poland. More recently, mortality rates of most cancers in Polish immigrants by duration of stay in Australia have been reported (Tyczynski et al, 1994).

Lilienfeld et al (1972) updated and extended the observations of Haenszel (1961). They reported age-specific and age-adjusted mortality rates of various neoplasms in migrants to the United States from 14

TABLE 12–3. *Place of Origin and Countries of Adoption in Studies of Cancer Mortality and Incidence Rates in Migrants*

	Country of Adoption									
Place of origin	*U.S.*	*Canada*	*Australia*	*U.K.*	*Israel*	*Singapore*	*Japan*	*Argentina*	*Uruguay*	*Brazil*
Europe	X	X	X	X	X			X	X	X
Canada	X			X						
Australia				X						
New Zealand			X	X						
United States			X	X						
Japan	X									X
China	X		X			X				
Indian subcontinent			X	X		X				
Malaysia						X				
Philippines	X									
Korea							X			
Middle East			X		X			X		
Africa			X	X	X					
Mexico	X									
Puerto Rico	X									
Caribbean	X			X						
South America	X							X	X	

European countries and Canada for the years 1959–1961, and contrasted these rates with published mortality rates for their country of origin and for U.S. whites. Some of the findings from this study are presented graphically as standardized rate ratios in the next section of this chapter. Results from this study and that of Haenszel are similar, but the Lilienfeld study is based on larger numbers and provides more stable estimates of rates. Two studies of Caucasian migrants to New York City (Seidman, 1971) and New York State (Nasca et al, 1981) also yielded results comparable to those of Lilienfeld et al (1972), as did the study of Newman and Spengler (1984) of five major cancers in six European migrant groups to Ontario, Canada, and the study of Terracini et al (1990) of Italian migrants to Montreal, Canada.

A large influx of Europeans into Australia, particularly in the 1950s, has been the subject of a number of migrant studies, the largest of which is that by Armstrong et al (1983). They calculated age-adjusted mortality rates of various neoplasms for migrants from 16 European countries, New Zealand, and the United States. An important feature of this work is the estimation of rates by duration of residence in Australia. Results are presented as ratios of age-adjusted rates for migrants to those for persons born in Australia. Some of these results are shown graphically in the next section of this chapter. More recently, the incidence rates for migrants to New South Wales, Australia, from the British Isles, and various parts of Europe have been compared to rates for Australian-born individuals (McCredie et al, 1990a, 1990b).

There was a large influx of Caucasian migrants to England and Wales from Germany, Italy, Poland, and the Soviet Union after World War II. Other Caucasian groups arrived over a more prolonged period of time. Migrants from nine European countries, and also from Mediterranean islands, Australia, Canada, New Zealand, and the United States were the subjects of a study by Marmot et al (1984), with results similar to those of Lilienfeld et al (1972).

Jews began to migrate to what is now Israel early in this century, with the largest influx occurring from 1948 to 1953 (Halevi et al, 1971). The two largest groups were those from Europe after World War II, and those from Yemen and Iraq in the late 1940s and early 1950s. Age-adjusted cancer mortality (Halevi et al, 1971; Katz and Steinitz, 1979) and incidence (Steinitz and Costin, 1971; Katz and Steinitz, 1979; Parkin et al, 1990) rates for migrants by their place of origin have been reported. None of these reports contrast rates for migrants with rates in their countries of origin. Incidence rates by year of migration, but not by age at migration, have been published. As indicated above, risks relative to the risk among Israeli-born persons, by duration of residence in Israel, have also been estimated (Parkin et al, 1990).

Mortality rates for various cancers in European migrants to Argentina (Matos et al, 1991) and Uruguay (DeStefani et al, 1990) have also been reported, as have rates relative to those for persons born in the country of adoption, for both the migrants and populations in their countries of origin. Similarly, the incidence rates of various cancers in Estonian migrants to Sweden have been compared with rates in Estonia and in native-born Swedes (Nilsson et al, 1993).

A monograph on cancer incidence and mortality rates among Italian migrants to Canada, the United States, Argentina, Brazil, Uruguay, Australia, France, Switzerland, England and Wales, and Scotland was compiled under the auspices of the International Agency for Research on Cancer (Geddes et al, 1993). This is the first systematic effort to compare cancer patterns in migrants from a single country to a variety of new environments.

Japanese Migrants

Japanese laborers migrated to the United States, primarily from southwestern Japan, from the 1880s until 1924 when exclusionary legislation prohibited further immigration until 1943. Few migrated after that date. These individuals and their descendants have been the subject of a number of investigations. By using a combination of race and birthplace, first generation (Issei) and U.S.-born (Nisei) Japanese have been distinguished on death certificates and census records, and mortality rates of cancers in these two groups have been compared with those in U.S. whites (Buell and Dunn, 1965; Haenszel and Kurihara, 1968; Locke and King, 1980), and also with those for Japanese in Japan (Locke and King, 1980). Comparisons have also been published of incidence rates of specific cancers in Japanese residing in various parts of the United States, Japanese in Japan, and U.S. whites (Dunn, 1975; Thomas, 1979; Tominaga, 1985). Kolonel et al (1980) have published incidence rates separately for first and second generation Japanese (in Hawaii); and Shimizu et al (1991) estimated incidence rates of cancers of the prostate and breast separately among Japanese in Los Angeles who likely migrated as adults and who either immigrated as children or were born in the United States. Results from a study of cancer mortality in first and second generation Japanese in Sao Paulo, Brazil have also been published (Tsugane et al, 1990).

Chinese Migrants

From the 1850s until 1882, large numbers of Chinese mainly from the Guangdong area in southern China immigrated to the United States as laborers. Limited numbers of Chinese were again permitted to enter the United States after 1943, and since 1968, larger numbers were allowed to immigrate. In these latter years, migrants came primarily from the educated classes outside mainland China. King and Haenszel (1973) computed SMRs for Idai (foreign-born) and Erdai (U.S.-born) Chinese in the United States relative to U.S. whites. They also presented comparable SMRs for Chinese populations in Hong Kong, Singapore, and Taiwan. King and Locke (1980) updated these observations and also provided SMRs for Taiwanese. No rates were available for these studies from the Guangdong area of China, and since rates of many cancers vary greatly among different geographic areas of China (Atlas of Cancer Mortality in the People's Republic of China, 1979), comparisons with rates for the overseas Chinese must be interpreted with caution. King et al (1985) subsequently provided comparable SMRs for Guangdong Province in China. A small study of mortality in Chinese migrants to Australia (Zhang et al, 1984) provided limited results but generally confirmed the findings of the larger U.S. studies, as did a study of PMRs of foreign-born Chinese in New York City, Chinese in Tianjin, China, and U.S.-born white residents of New York City (Stellman and Wang, 1994).

Standardized incidence ratios relative to U.S. whites have been published for the Chinese populations of Hawaii, the San Francisco Bay Area, and Singapore (Thomas, 1979), and for Chinese in Hawaii (Kolonel, 1980), but no comparisons of incidence rates for Idai and Erdai in the United States have been published. In Singapore, Shanmugaratnam et al (1983) contrasted incidence rates of various cancers among Chinese who were born locally with those born outside the country and compared these with rates for similar years in Shanghai and the United States. They also compared rates among four groups of Chinese who were characterized by the dialect they spoke, which is an indicator of the region in China from which individuals or their ancestors originated.

Migrants from the Indian Subcontinent

Migrants from India, Pakistan, Bangladesh, and Sri Lanka have entered England and Wales continuously since the years when these countries were British colonies, but immigration was heaviest in the 1960s. The earlier migrants were predominantly white descendants of British colonists, whereas the later migrants were largely of Indian subcontinent origin. Marmot et al (1984) reported SMRs for these migrants to the United Kingdom. However, because migrants from the subcontinent who were of British origin could not be distinguished from those of subcontinent origin, except possibly by inspection of their names, only PMRs by ethnicity were calculated. More recently, Barker and Baker (1990) reported SIRs of various cancers (relative to rates in Bombay) for individuals of Indian subcontinent ethnicity in Bradford, England. Armstrong et al (1983) calculated SMRs relative to individuals born in Australia for migrants to that country from India and Pakistan (combined), and Shanmugaratnam et al (1983) computed ratios of age-adjusted incidence rates among foreign-born versus Singapore-born persons of Indian subcontinent origin. However, the interpretation of the results of all these efforts is limited for several reasons: migrants to the various destinations came from different areas of the subcontinent; accurate information on cancer incidence or mortality rates from these areas is not available; and many of the rates in migrants are based on small numbers and are hence imprecise.

Filipino Migrants

Filipinos migrated to the United States in large numbers from about 1910 to 1934. They came, mostly as laborers, from the northern provinces of Luzon. A second large influx occurred after World War II. These were mainly men who had served in the U.S. Armed Forces or were wives of servicemen. After 1968 immigration again increased; most immigrants since then have been members of the middle and upper socioeconomic classes. Kolonel (1985) reported incidence rates for Filipinos living in Hawaii for five time periods from 1962–1981. He did not distinguish Filipinos by place of birth, and since immigration continued during those years, trends in rates cannot necessarily be attributed to greater acculturation with the passage of time. He also attempted to compare rates in Hawaii with those in Manila for 1977, but case ascertainment in Manila was likely incomplete.

Other Asian Migrants

Koreans migrated to Japan up to and during World War II, and many of them and their descendants currently live in Osaka Prefecture. Ubukata et al (1987) compared incidence and mortality rates among Koreans and Japanese in Osaka. They also compared age-standardized PMRs for these groups and for Koreans in Korea, where there is a centralized hospital-based, but not a population-based, cancer registry. A major limitation of this study is that rates for many cancers were rather similar in the two countries.

Shanmugaratnam et al (1983) computed ratios of age-adjusted incidence rates in foreign-born versus Singapore-born individuals of Malay origin, but no rates for Malaysia are available.

The studies of migrants to Israel already mentioned included individuals from some Asian countries of the Middle East (Halevi et al, 1971; Steinitz and Costin, 1971; Katz and Steinitz, 1979; Parkin et al, 1990). Also, SIRs for migrants from the Middle East to Australia have been reported (McCredie et al, 1990b). No rates are available from any of these Asian countries of origin.

Matos et al (1991), De Stefani et al (1990), and McCredie et al (1990b) have also reported rates among Asians from multiple countries grouped into single categories who had migrated to Argentina, Uruguay, and Australia, respectively. Such groupings, although of limited value, were necessitated by small numbers of individual migrants from single countries.

African Migrants

Rates of cancer mortality (Halevi et al, 1971) and incidence (Steinitz and Costin, 1971; Katz and Steinitz, 1979; Iscovitch et al, 1989) in Israeli Jews from North Africa have been reported. Marmot et al (1984) calculated SMRs for migrants to the United Kingdom from the sub-Sharan African Commonwealth countries combined; and more recently, Grulich et al (1992) provided similar information separately for migrants from East and West Africa to England and Wales. Age-adjusted incidence rates of various cancers among migrants to Australia from Egypt and elsewhere in Africa relative to rates among Australian-born persons were published by Armstrong et al (1983). No rates are available for any of the countries of origin of these African migrants.

Latin American Migrants

The two major groups of migrants from Latin America that have been the subject of studies of cancer incidence and mortality in the United States are the Mexicans and the Puerto Ricans. Puerto Ricans began migrating to the United States after the Spanish American War in 1898, with large numbers of unskilled laborers migrating since the 1950s. The largest number of these migrants reside in New York City. Age-adjusted mortality rates in Puerto Rico and in the Puerto Rican–born and U.S.-born white populations of that city have been reported (Rosenwaike, 1984; Rosenwaike and Shai, 1986; Warshauer et al, 1986). Similar comparisons of incidence rates were made for colorectal and stomach cancers by Warshauer et al (1986), and for these and several other sites by Polednak (1991).

Many Mexican Americans are descendants of people who lived in what are now states that border Mexico before those areas became part of the United States in 1848. A major influx of migrants followed the Mexican revolution in 1910. Another large Mexican immigration began after World War II and continues to the present time. Many are migrant agricultural workers and unskilled laborers. Most reside in the southwestern United States.

Mortality rates among Mexican Americans were included in the studies of Haenszel (1961) and Lilienfeld et al (1972) described above. Martin and Suarez (1987) also compared mortality rates for resident Texans with and without Spanish surnames, and Savitz (1986) contrasted incidence rates in Colorado for Spanish-surnamed and other whites in two time periods. Most persons with Spanish surnames in these two studies were of Mexican origin, but their place of birth was not considered. In Los Angeles County, age-standardized incidence ratios relative to non-Hispanic whites were calculated separately for immigrant Mexicans and Mexicans born in the United States (Menck et al, 1975); Mack et al (1985) graphically presented PIRs for Mexican migrants by estimated age at migration; and Shimizu et al (1991) reported estimated incidence rates of breast and prostate cancers in Spanish-surnamed whites by estimated age at migration.

Mack et al (1985) also graphically presented PIRs for migrants to the United States from the Caribbean, Central America, and South America; and in studies of migrants to England and Wales (Marmot et al; 1984; Grulich et al, 1992), SMRs for immigrants from the Caribbean Commonwealth were calculated. Mortality rates of various cancers in migrants from several South American countries to Argentina (Matos et al, 1991) and SIRs for migrants from Argentina and Brazil to Uruguay (De Stefani et al, 1990) have also been reported.

OBSERVATIONS FROM STUDIES OF MORTALITY AND INCIDENCE RATES IN MIGRANTS

The results from the many studies of incidence and mortality rates among migrants (Table 12–3) are remarkably consistent. For virtually all cancers, with the passage of time, or in succeeding generations, rates tend to approach those of the native-born in the country of adoption. However, the patterns of displacement of rates over time vary by cancer type, and for some cancers, by migrant group. The results from selected studies of migrants are presented in Figures 12–1 through 12–8.

These figures include studies of non-white and Spanish-surnamed white migrants to the United States (collectively referred to as non-whites for brevity) from those investigations that provided information on country of origin or provided rates for second generation migrants, or both; in most instances the most recent such investigations of each ethnic group are shown because the rates from them are based on the largest numbers of second generation migrants and are hence the most stable. Unless otherwise noted, the studies included are those of Locke and King (1980) on the Japanese, King and Locke (1980) on the Chinese, Rosenwaike (1984) on the Puerto Ricans, and Lilienfeld et al (1972) and Menck et al (1975) on the Mexicans. Results from two studies of Mexicans are presented because one provides information on country of origin and the other provides information on second generation Mexicans. In all instances estimates of ratios of rates for migrants relative to rates for U.S. whites are graphed. These are SMRs as published in the original reports except those from Menck et al (1975) which provided SIRs, and those from Lilienfeld et al (1972). The latter provided age-adjusted mortality rates, and the ratios of these rates to rates for U.S. whites (MRRs) were calculated for presentation in this chapter. Some of these results have been summarized previously by Thomas and Karagas (1987).

Results from two studies of white migrants are also presented in Figures 12–1 through 12–8. Ratios of age-adjusted mortality rates (MRRs) in foreign-born whites and their country of origin relative to rates for U.S. whites were computed from the report of Lilienfeld et al (1972). Since studies of migrants between countries with large differences in rates are the most likely to be informative, for each type of cancer, results were graphed only for migrants from countries with mortality rates that were either 50% greater or 50% lower than U.S. white rates. Age-adjusted MRRs for selected white migrants, by years of residence in Australia (Armstrong et al, 1983), are also presented, but only when the 95% confidence intervals of the MRRs for the most recent migrants did not include one.

Cancers of the breast, colon, ovary, testis, endometrium, and prostate all occur more commonly in most western developed countries than in eastern or developing nations, and each has been hypothesized to have an environmentally determined hormonal or dietary component to its etiology.

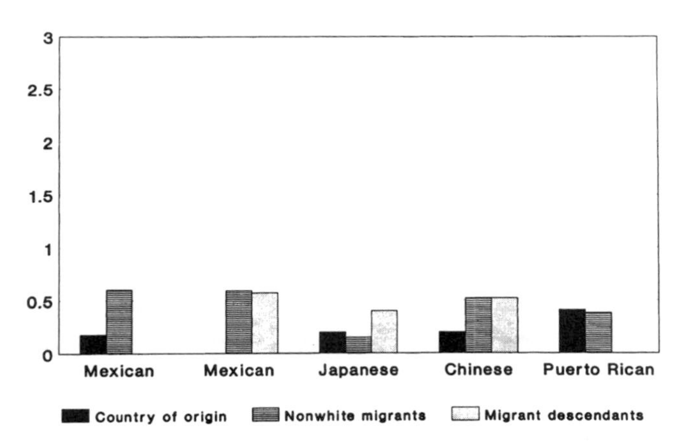

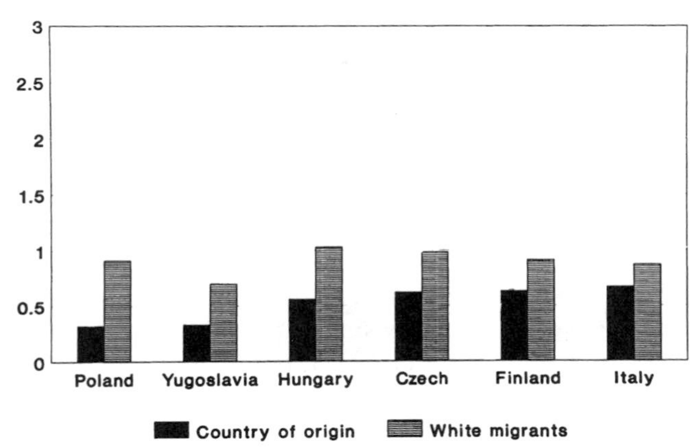

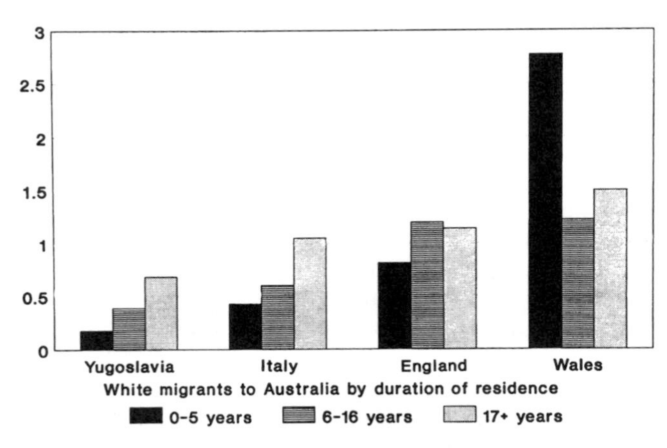

FIG. 12–1. Breast cancer in females. Standardized incidence or mortality ratios, or ratios of the age-adjusted mortality rates, using native-born whites as the standard (1.0), for selected countries.

Breast

As shown in Figure 12–1, rates of breast cancer are much lower in the countries of origin of all of the non-white migrants considered than for U.S. whites. Rates for the non-white migrants tend to be higher than the rates in their countries of origin, but even rates among the descendants of migrants are considerably lower than rates for U.S. whites. As with mortality rates, residual deficits in incidence rates have been observed among Japanese and Spanish-surnamed whites in Los Angeles (Shimizu et al, 1991), and among Asian migrants to Israel (Parkin et al, 1990). These observations are in sharp contrast to rates for white migrants, which generally approximate those of U.S. whites in the first generation (except for rates in migrants from Yugoslavia). Rates among migrants approximated those for Australian-born women after only 6 to 16 years for migrants from England and Wales, and after 17 years of residence in Australia for Italians, but remained below the rates for

Australian women in Yugoslavians even after more than 17 years since migration. These results indicate that exposures to a new environment as an adult can influence risk of breast cancer. The persistence of relatively lower rates in the more culturally distinct non-whites than in whites suggests either that the non-whites are less likely to be exposed to the environmental causes of breast cancer than white migrants, or that part of the differences in rates between whites and the non-whites considered is due to genetic differences in susceptibility to breast cancer. Measurements of rates in subsequent generations of non-whites will help determine which interpretation is correct.

Colon

Patterns of colon cancer are shown in Figure 12–2. Rates for the descendants of non-white migrants more closely approach those of U.S. whites than do rates of breast cancer but are generally not as high as rates for U.S. whites. Rates for white male migrants from most countries shown are slightly greater than rates for U.S. whites. Rates among white female migrants are more variable but are generally similar to rates for U.S. white women. Male European migrants to Australia had almost the same rates as native-born Australians after 17 years, but rates for female European migrants after 17 years in Australia tended to remain somewhat lower than rates for native-born Australians. In the aggregate, these observations suggest that the environmental causes of breast and colon cancer are different and that exposure as an adult to the causal factors for colon cancer can have a strong influence on risk of this disease. These observations also suggest that white male migrants may more readily come in contact with the environmental determinants of colon cancer than white female migrants. However, a different pattern has been observed in Israel (Parkin et al, 1990), where incidence rates increased only slightly among Asian migrants and not at all among migrants from Africa after over 30 years since migration. Rates of cancers arising from various parts of the lower bowel in migrants have been compared in Japanese in Hawaii (Nomura et al, 1981a) and Los Angeles (Shimizu et al, 1987), and in first generation European migrants in Australia (Kune et al, 1986). The findings from these studies are not consistent but do indicate that there may be different etiologic factors for neoplasms arising from different parts of the large bowel.

Ovary

The rates of ovarian cancer for second generation non-whites relative to U.S. white rates tend to be intermediate between those for breast and colon cancer. As with colon and breast cancers, rates of ovarian cancer in white migrants approach those of U.S. whites in the first generation.

Testis

Testicular cancer has occurred too infrequently in migrants for the calculation of stable rates. The pattern of

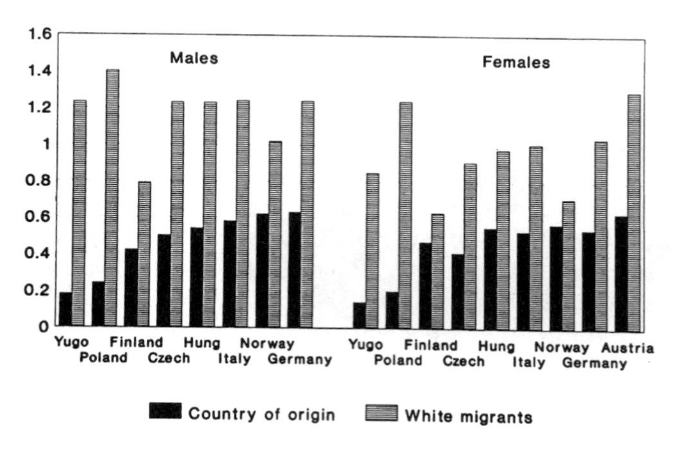

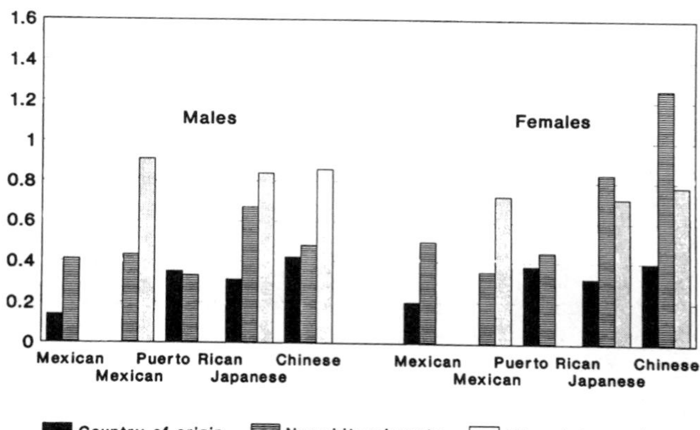

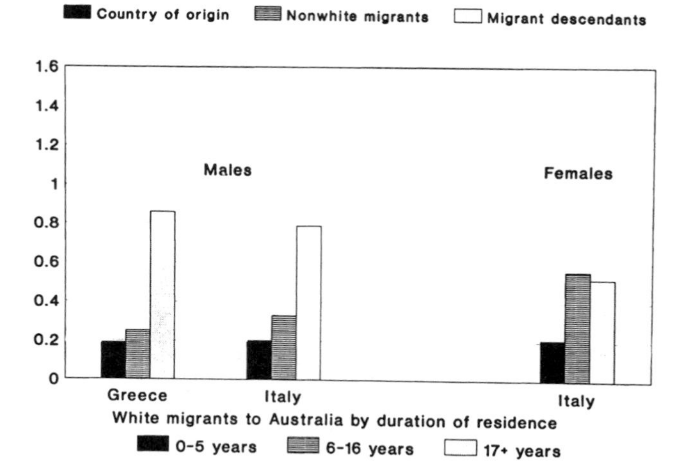

FIG. 12–2. Colon cancer in males and females. Standardized incidence or mortality ratios, or ratios of the age-adjusted mortality rates, using native-born whites as the standard (1.0), for selected countries.

displacement of rates, however, appears to be broadly similar to the patterns for ovarian, colon, and breast cancers, at least among Chinese and Mexican migrants to the United States (Thomas, 1979).

Endometrium

Endometrial carcinomas have also been poorly studied in migrants. In some studies, cancers of the corpus and cervix uteri are not distinguished, and in others, small number of cancers of the corpus precluded firm estimates of rates. However, rates of this neoplasm do appear to increase among Japanese, Chinese, and Mexican migrants to the United States (Thomas, 1979) and among Asian and African migrants to Israel (Parkin et al, 1990).

Prostate

The patterns of displacement of mortality rates of prostate cancer are not consistent among non-whites (Figure 12–3). Rates remain low among second generation Chinese and Japanese but not among second generation Mexicans, and rates for first generation Puerto Ricans are nearly as high as U.S. white rates. Similar findings, based on incidence rates, were observed in Japanese and whites with Spanish surnames in Los Angeles (Shimizu et al, 1991). Rates for white migrants almost reach those of U.S. whites in the United States. Among Italian migrants to Australia, only those who had lived for a relatively long time in Australia had rates close to those of native-born Australians. Although based on small numbers, similar observations were made in migrant populations to Australia from Greece, the Soviet Union, and Yugoslavia. With the possible exception of the findings from Australia, these results suggest that the environmental determinants of prostate cancer are operative in adult life. This interpretation is consistent with the results of the autopsy study of Akazaki and Stemmermann (1973) that showed a higher prevalence of proliferative latent carcinomas in Japanese in Hawaii than in Japanese in Japan, suggesting a promotional effect of the migrants' new environment. Migrants from Latin America may more readily come in contact with the environmental factors of etiologic importance than migrants from Japan or China.

Changes in dietary habits are a likely environmental modification responsible for the changes in rates of these neoplasms. The international rates of each of these cancers are correlated with per capita consumption of various nutrients (Armstrong and Doll, 1975); and changes in dietary practices among many migrants have been documented. These observations have led to more detailed case–control and cohort studies of some of these cancers in migrants to attempt to identify the specific nutritional factors of etiologic importance. The results to date are inconclusive. Additional studies of these cancers in relation to dietary intakes in migrants, particularly those with differing patterns of displacement of their rates, may further our understanding of the etiology of these tumors.

The next four neoplasms considered are cancers of the stomach, esophagus, liver, and uterine cervix. All

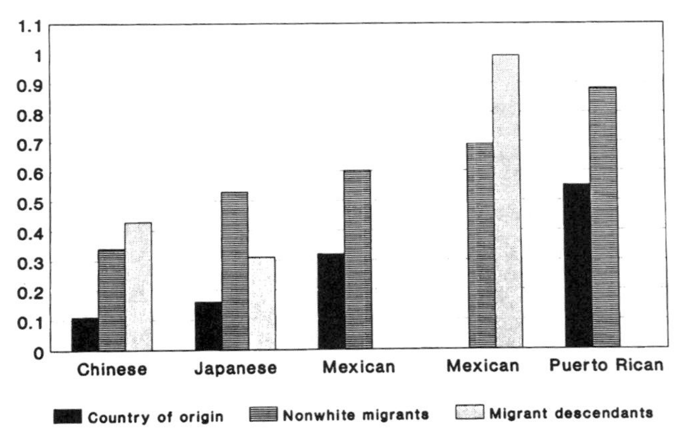

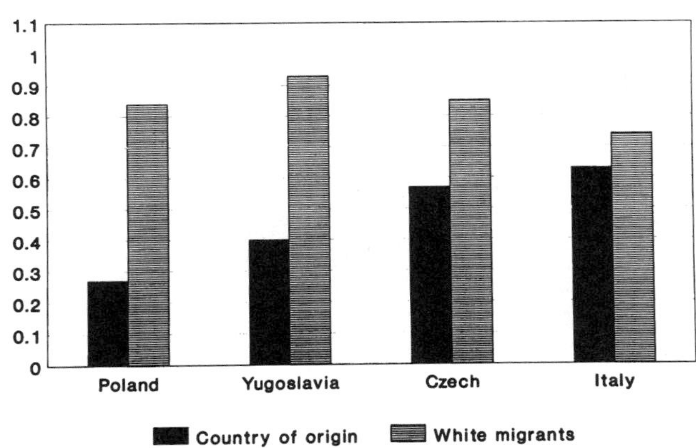

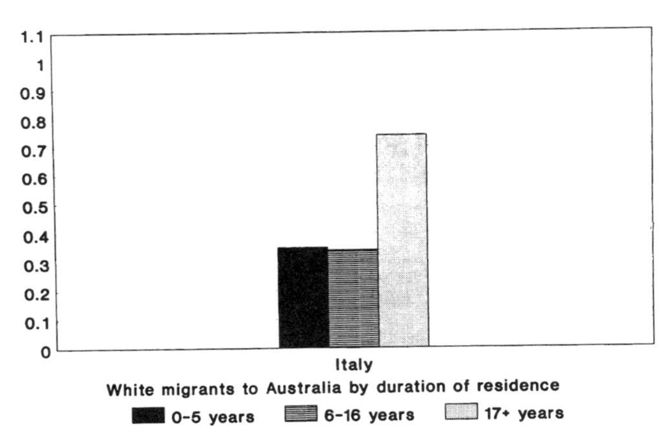

FIG. 12–3. Prostate cancer in males. Standardized incidence or mortality ratios, or ratios of the age-adjusted mortality rates, using native-born whites as the standard (1.0), for selected countries.

occur with greater frequency in many developing and Asian countries than in most developed areas of the world.

Stomach

Mortality ratios for stomach cancer in male migrants are shown in Figure 12–4. Similar ratios were observed for females. The mortality ratio for Mexicans in Mexico is probably erroneously low. In all non-white migrants, rates decline in succeeding generations, but some residual excess risk persists in the offspring of migrants, except for Chinese males. Rates for white migrants are consistently lower than rates in their country of origin, but consistently higher than rates for U.S. whites. The residual excess in the rates is not related to the level of risk in the country of origin. Rates among migrants to Australia declined with the passage of time in Australia, but a small residual excess is seen after over 17 years since immigration. A similar excess persisted among migrants to Israel after over 30 years since immigration (Parkin et al, 1990). Smoked, cured, salted or pickled products have been the most strongly implicated dietary factors of etiologic importance for stomach cancer, and constituents of fresh fruits and vegetables may be protective. The decline in rates of stomach cancer in first generation migrants provides evidence that exposures to one or more of these factors in adult life are of etiologic importance.

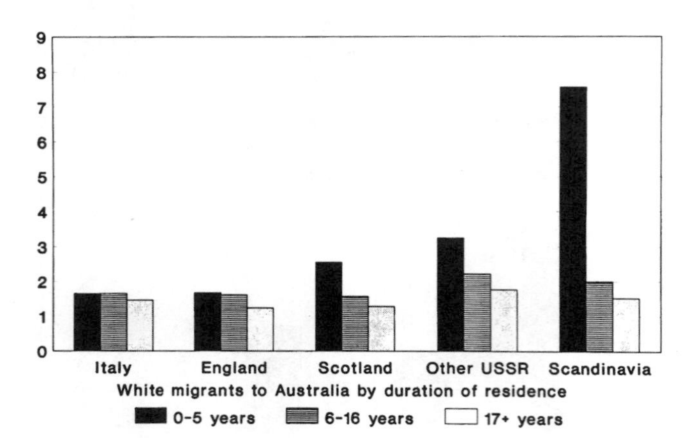

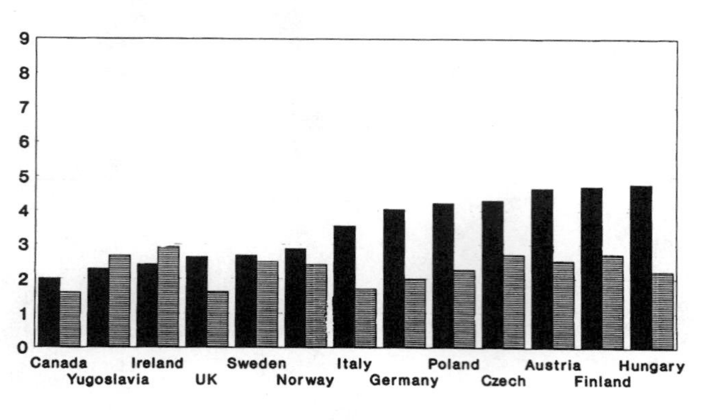

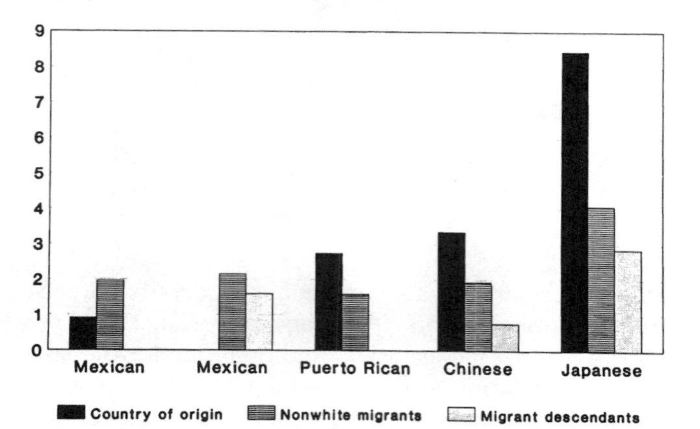

FIG. 12–4. Stomach cancer in males and females. Standardized incidence or mortality ratios, or ratios of the age-adjusted mortality rates, using native-born whites as the standard (1.0), for selected countries.

Esophagus

The patterns of displacement of rates of the esophagus in migrants are shown in Figure 12–5. In males there is little decline in rates among first generation non-white migrants, although rates for their offspring (observed in Mexicans, Chinese, and Japanese), are close to those for U.S. whites. In contrast, rates declined to levels below those of U.S. whites in first generation Japanese and Chinese females. Rates for white males who migrated to the United States tend to be higher than rates in their country of origin. This was also observed for migrants to England and Wales from Ireland but not for those from Scotland or Poland (Marmot et al, 1984). In contrast, rates for white female migrants to the U.S. were lower than rates in their country of origin, an observation also made for white migrants to England and Wales from Scotland and Ireland (Marmot et al, 1984). Rates declined with the passage of time in Australia, and this was also generally true for most migrants from the countries not shown in the figure. This was also observed among Asian migrants to Israel (Parkin et al, 1990). The esophageal cancers in most developing countries are probably not primarily related to smoking and drinking, as they are in western countries, and the decline in rates for migrants from developing countries is likely a result of diminished exposure to the unknown indigenous causes of esophageal cancer in their homeland. The same may be true for white females from at least some of the European countries considered. Perhaps the male migrants to the United States were heavier

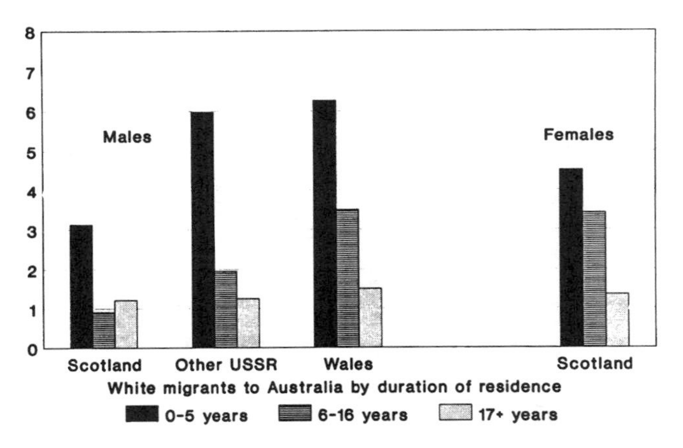

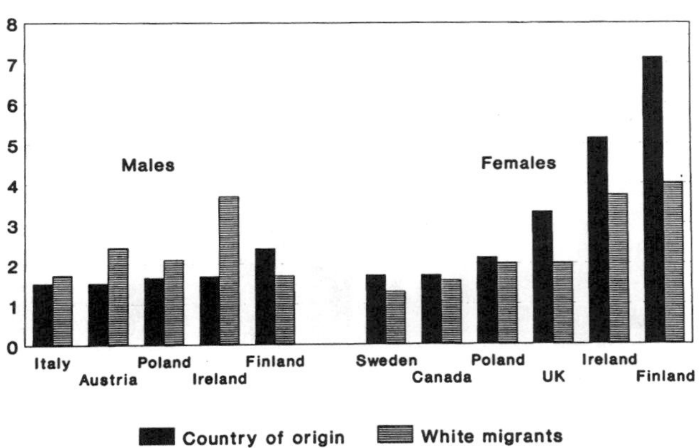

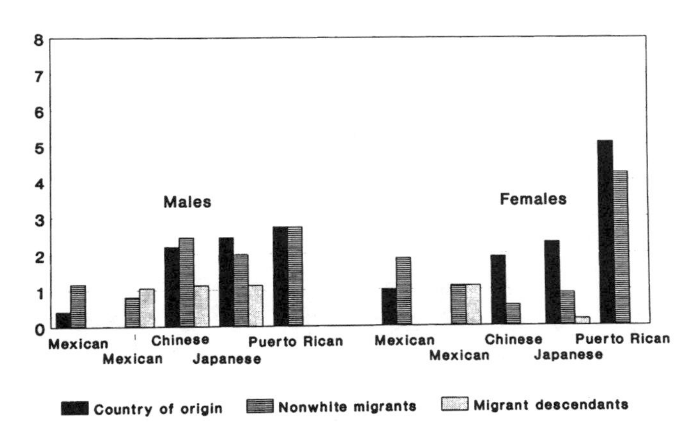

FIG. 12–5. Esophageal cancer in males and females. Standardized incidence or mortality ratios, or ratios of the age-adjusted mortality rates, using native-born whites as the standard (1.0), for selected countries.

smokers and drinkers than their countrymen who remained at home.

Liver

As shown in Figure 12–6, rates of liver cancer among Chinese migrants declined rapidly in succeeding generations. A similar pattern is apparent from an early study of Japanese (Buell and Dunn, 1965), when rates of liver cancer in Japan were relatively high. Little residual excess in rates is evident in the second generation nonwhites. If most liver cancers in their countries of origin are hepatitis B–related, then these observations are consistent with reduced exposure at an early age to this

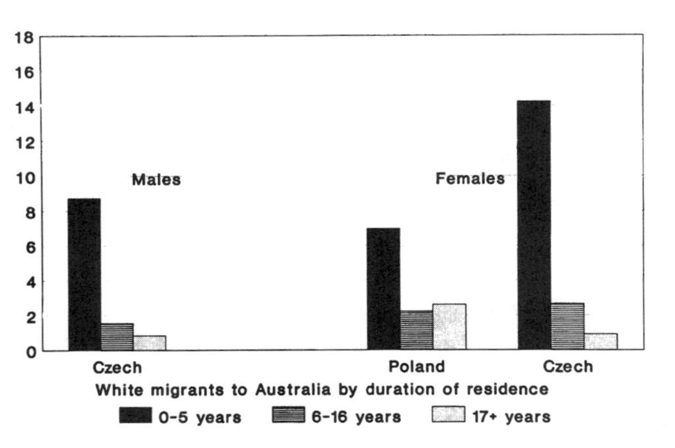

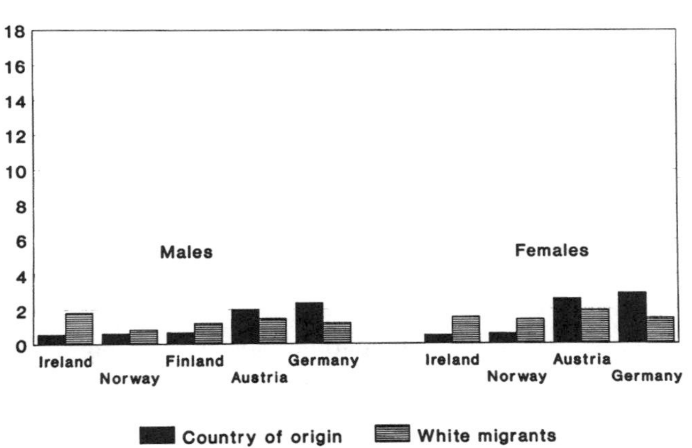

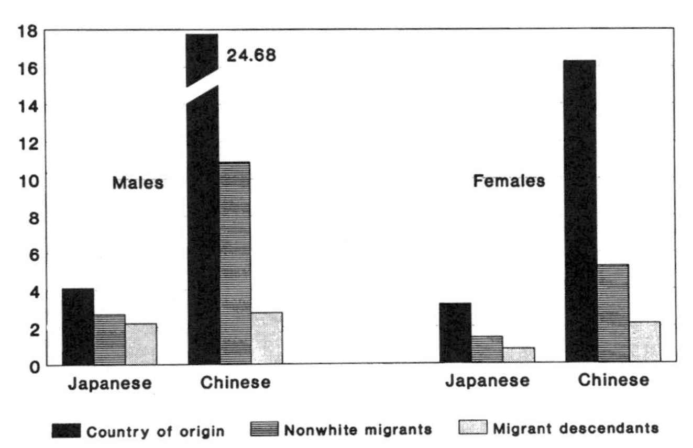

FIG. 12–6. Liver cancer in males and females. Standardized incidence or mortality ratios, or ratios of the age-adjusted mortality rates, using native-born whites as the standard (1.0), for selected countries.

virus in succeeding generations. In whites of both sexes rates decreased among migrants to the United States from high-risk countries, but remained somewhat in excess of rates for U.S. whites. In Australia, rates declined most strikingly during the period from 6 to 16 years after migration for both sexes. In Israel, however, rates declined more slowly with time among migrants from Africa and not at all for migrants from Asia (Parkin et al, 1990). Rates for most white migrants to the United States from low-risk countries tended to be slightly higher than rates for U.S. whites. Since the main determinant of liver cancer in the United States is probably alcohol use, this increase may reflect enhanced use of alcohol by these migrants, an interpretation consistent with the observations on esophageal cancer.

Cervix Uteri

A fourth cancer with higher rates in many developing countries than in developed countries is cervical carcinoma. Unfortunately, little reliable information on rates in second generation migrants is available and, in many studies, carcinomas of the cervix and corpus uteri were combined. Rates of invasive cervical cancer are higher in several Latin American countries and for Mexican-born residents of Los Angeles than for second generation Mexicans in Los Angeles and Spanish-surnamed women in New Mexico; and rates are lower among Chinese in the United States than in the Orient (Thomas, 1979). Risk of cervical cancer is related to sexual behavior of the woman or her male partner conducive to the acquisition of sexually transmitted agents. A number of viruses have been causally implicated, including certain types of human papillomaviruses. Changes in the occurrence of cervical cancer in migrants therefore probably are a reflection of changes in their sexual practices. More screening for cervical cancer in migrants than in their country of origin has possibly also contributed to their declining rates of invasive disease.

Lung

Figure 12–7 shows lung cancer rates for migrants. In non-whites (from low-risk countries) rates increase dramatically among first generation migrants, and then decline among their offspring in most groups. Rates for white migrants to the United States from both low- and high-risk countries tend to have lung cancer rates closer to those of U.S. whites than their countrymen who did not migrate. Rates for migrants to Australia are inconsistent among countries. Some show lower rates for those who lived in Australia for 0–5 years than for those who lived there from 6–16 years, possibly reflecting a healthy migrant effect. Since cigarette smoking is universally the major etiologic determinant of lung cancer,

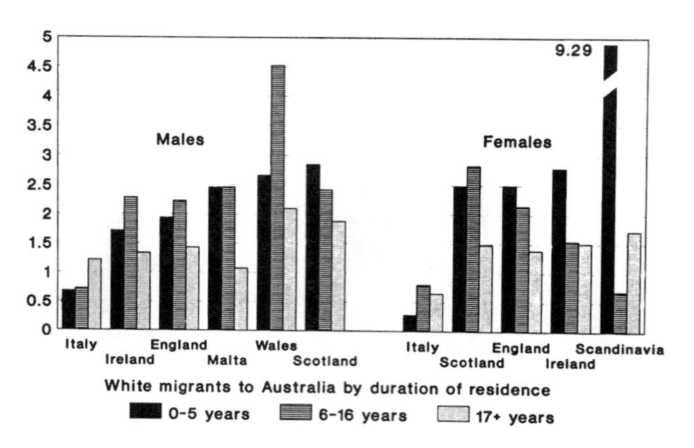

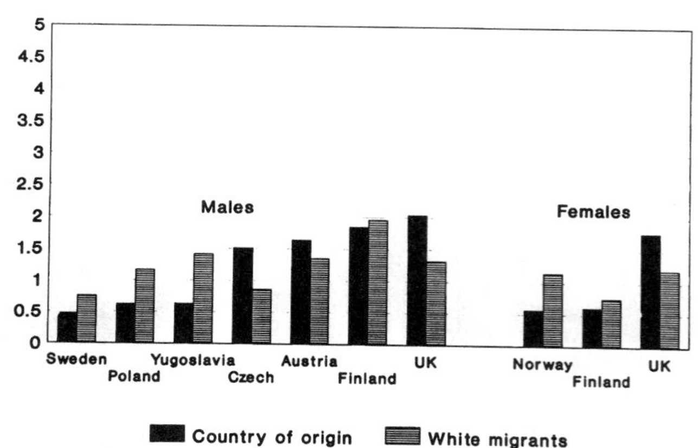

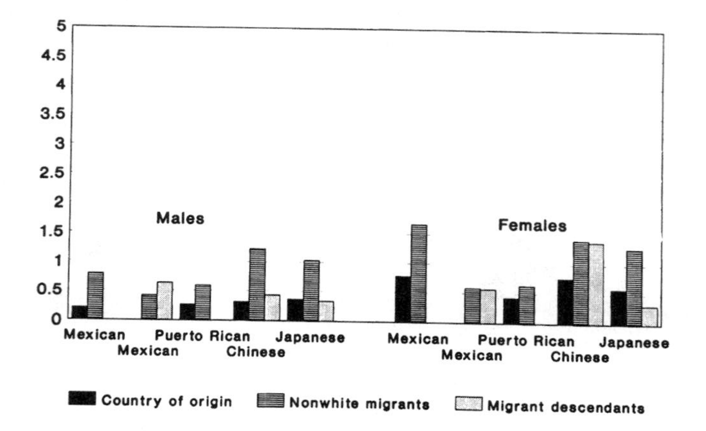

FIG. 12–7. Lung cancer in males and females. Standardized incidence or mortality ratios, or ratios of the age-adjusted mortality rates, using native-born whites as the standard (1.0), for selected countries.

these variations in rates can safely be assumed to be largely a result of differences in smoking habits.

Bladder

Patterns of rates of bladder cancer in both white and non-white migrants are similar to those for lung cancer, and probably also are determined by differences in smoking habits.

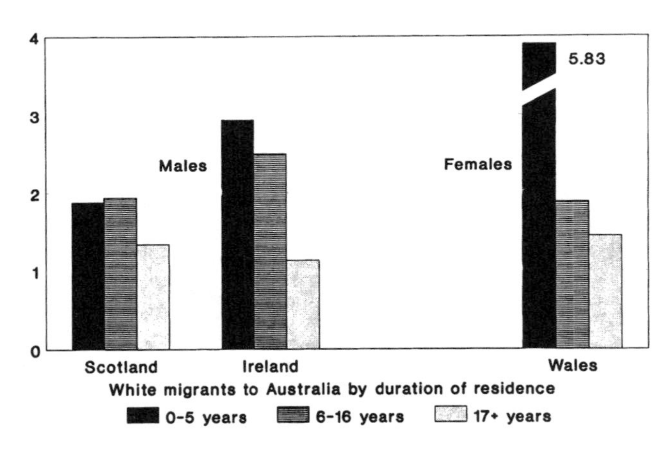

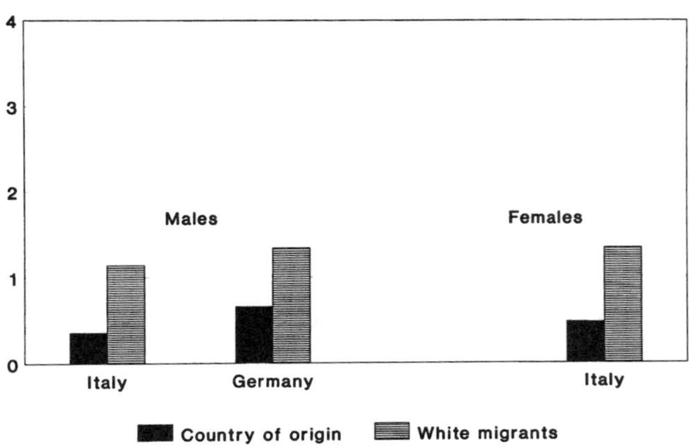

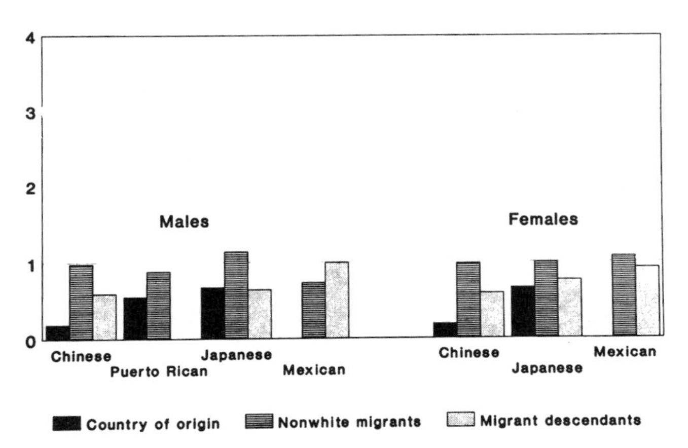

FIG. 12–8. Pancreatic cancer in males and females. Standardized incidence or mortality ratios, or ratios of the age-adjusted mortality rates, using native-born whites as the standard (1.0), for selected countries.

Pancreas

Rates of pancreatic cancer in both non-white and white male and female migrants from low-risk areas approximate the rates for U.S. whites. This is shown in Figure 12–8. In most non-whites, as with lung cancer, rates declined in the second generation, perhaps reflecting changes in smoking habits. In migrants to Australia from places with higher pancreatic cancer rates than that country, rates declined with the passage of time since migration, although some residual excess is apparent after over 17 years in the new environment. Rates for migrants to Australia from other countries not shown in the figure were unstable but generally showed the expected trends toward rates for Australian-born whites with the passage of time since migration. Rates among migrants from Europe or America, and from Asia, declined slightly with duration of residence in Israel but remained higher than for Israeli-born persons after over 30 years since immigration (Parkin et al, 1990).

Melanoma

Malignant melanoma has been most thoroughly studied in European migrants to Australia. Mortality rates have been shown by Armstrong et al (1983) and Khlat et al (1992) to increase with duration of residence in Australia, and incidence rates among migrants from Europe and Asia increased gradually with duration of residence in Israel (Parkin et al, 1990). Case–control studies, reviewed by Holman et al (1986), showed that age at migration was a more important determinant of risk than time in Australia, suggesting that exposure to sunlight at an early age is of particular etiologic importance.

Other Sites

Attempts to summarize changes in rates of other malignancies have been made by Thomas (1979) and Tominaga (1985) for Japanese migrants to the United States, and also for Chinese and Spanish-surnamed migrants to that country by Thomas (1979). These include neoplasms of the central nervous system, eye, thyroid, salivary gland, upper aerodigestive tract (oral and oropharyngeal, nasopharyngeal, sinonasal, hypopharyngeal, and laryngeal), gallbladder, small intestine, penis, the lymphatic system (lymphocytic leukemias and lymphosarcomas), and the hematopoietic system (multiple myeloma and myelogenous leukemias), as well as sarcomas of the bone, fat and connective tissue. In the aggregate, these reviews provide evidence to suggest that rates of these less common malignancies also tend to shift away from those in the country of origin and toward those of the country of adoption.

OPPORTUNITIES FOR FURTHER RESEARCH

Although studies of incidence and mortality rates in migrants have probably reached a point of diminishing returns, some additional investigations are clearly warranted. Opportunities should be taken to study migrants from areas of the world with unknown rates of cancer to provide estimates of rates in such areas and to identify regions with unusual patterns of cancer occurrence of potential for etiologic research. Most studies of second generation migrants have been based on mortality rates, and more studies of incidence rates for second generation migrants should be conducted to confirm and supplement the information from the studies based on mortality rates. In addition, studies of rates in subsequent generations, as the descendants of migrants become more acculturated, will be of value in quantifying the extent to which hereditary and environmental factors are responsible for the variability in rates of some cancers among different racial and ethnic groups. Also, additional studies of rates among migrants of different histologic types of cancers arising from the same tissue and of cancers arising from subsites of the same organ may provide evidence for etiologic heterogeneity.

More importantly, migrants offer unusual opportunities for case–control and cohort studies of cancers because they are groups in transition with larger variations in many exposures of interest than is commonly observed in indigenous populations. For example, the identification of significantly altered dietary and lifestyle practices in association with changing risks for stomach and colorectal cancer has been facilitated by conducting case-control and cohort studies in migrant populations. Similar studies in migrant groups with varying exposures to dietary and other environmental factors are likely to provide further insights into the causes of many cancers.

REFERENCES

AKAZAKI K, STEMMERMANN GN. 1973. Comparative study of latent carcinoma of the prostate among Japanese in Japan and Hawaii. J Natl Cancer Inst 50:1137–1144.

ARMSTRONG B, DOLL R. 1975. Environmental factors and cancer incidence and mortality in different countries, with special reference to dietary practices. Int J Cancer 15:617–631.

ARMSTRONG BK, WOODINGS TL, STENHOUSE NS, et al. 1983. Mortality from cancer in migrants to Australia—1962 to 1971. NH & MRC Research Unit in Epidemiology and Preventive Medicine, Raine Medical Statistics Unit—Department of Medicine, The University of Western Australia.

ATLAS OF CANCER MORTALITY IN THE PEOPLE'S REPUBLIC OF CHINA, 1979. China Map Press no. 1538, Yan An Xilu, Shanghai, China.

BARKER RM, BAKER MR. 1990. Incidence of cancer in Bradford Asians. J Epidemiol Community Health 44:125–129.

BRUHN CM, PANGBORN RM. 1971. Food habits of migrant farm workers in California. J Am Diet Assoc 59:347–355.

BUELL P, DUNN JE JR. 1965. Cancer mortality among Japanese Issei and Nisei of California. Cancer 18:656–664.

CHUNG CS, TASH E, RAYMOND J, et al. 1990. Health risk behaviours and ethnicity in Hawaii. Int J Epidemiol 19:1011–1018.

CORREA P, HAENSZEL W. 1978. The epidemiology of large bowel cancer. *In* Klein G, Weinhouse S (eds): Advances in Cancer Research, Vol 26. New York, Academic Press.

CORREA P, SASANO H, STEMMERMANN GH, et al. 1973. Pathology of gastric carcinoma in Japanese populations: Comparisons between Miyagi prefecture, Japan and Hawaii. J Natl Cancer Inst 51:1449–1459.

DE STEFANI E, PARKIN DM, KHLAT M, et al. 1990. Cancer in migrants to Uruguay. Int J Cancer 46:233–237.

DUNN JE JR. 1975. Cancer epidemiology in populations of the United States—with emphasis on Hawaii and California—and Japan. Cancer Res 35:3240–3245.

GEDDES M, PARKIN DM, KHLAT M, et al (eds). 1993. Cancer in Italian Migrant Populations. IARC Sci Publ 123. Lyon, International Agency for Research on Cancer.

GLOBER GA, KAMIYAMA S, NOMURA A, et al. 1977. Bowel transit-time and stool weight in populations with different colon-cancer risks. Lancet ii:110–111.

GOLDIN BR, ADLERCREUTZ H, GORBACH SL, et al. 1986. The relationship between estrogen levels and diets of Caucasian American and Oriental immigrant women. Am J Clin Nutr 44:945–953.

GRULICH AE, SWERDLOW AJ, HEAD J, MARMOT MG. 1992. Cancer mortality in African and Caribbean migrants to England and Wales. Br J Cancer 66:905–911.

HAENSZEL W. 1961. Cancer mortality among the foreign-born in the United States. J Natl Cancer Inst 26:37–132.

HAENSZEL W. 1970. Identification of migrants and their descendants in the United States. J Chron Dis 23:383–387.

HAENSZEL W. 1982. Migrant studies. *In* Schottenfeld D, Fraumeni JF, Jr (eds): Cancer Epidemiology and Prevention. New York, W. B. Saunders Company, pp 194–207.

HAENSZEL W, BERG JW, SEGO M, et al. 1973. Large-bowel cancer in Hawaiian Japanese. J Natl Cancer Inst 51:1765–1779.

HAENSZEL W, KURIHARA M. 1968. Studies of Japanese migrants. I. Mortality from cancer and other diseases among Japanese in the United States. J Natl Cancer Inst 40:43–68.

HALEVI HS, DREYFUSS F, PERITZ E, et al. 1971. Cancer mortality and immigration to Israel, 1950–67. Isr J Med Sci 7:1386–1404.

HINDS MW, KOLONEL LN, LEE J, et al. 1980. Associations between cancer incidence and alcohol/cigarette consumption among five ethnic groups in Hawaii. Br J Cancer 41:929–940.

HINDS MW, KOLONEL LN, NOMURA AMY, et al. 1981. 1973–77 cancer incidence in Hawaii, with special reference to trends since 1968–72 for certain sites. Cancer 40:7–11.

HOLMAN CDJ, ARMSTRONG BK, HEENAN PJ, et al. 1986. The causes of malignant melanoma: Results from the West Australian Lions Melanoma Research Project. Recent Results Cancer Res 102:18–37.

HSING AW, MCLAUGHLIN JK, SCHUMAN LM, et al. 1990. Diet, tobacco use, and fatal prostate cancer: results from the Lutheran Brotherhood Cohort Study. Cancer Res 50:6836–6840.

ISCOVICH J, STEINITZ R, ANDREEV H. 1993. Descriptive epidemiology of malignant tumors in Ethiopian jews immigrating to Israel, 1984–1989. Isr J Med Sci 29:364–367.

KATZ L, STEINITZ R. 1979. Cancer patterns in Israel: selected aspects. Isr J Med Sci 15:983–989.

KING H, HAENSZEL W. 1973. Cancer mortality among foreign- and native-born Chinese in the United States. J Chron Dis 26:623–646.

KING H, LI J-Y, LOCKW FB, et al. 1985. Patterns of site-specific displacement in cancer mortality among migrants: The Chinese in the United States. Am J Public Health 75:237–242.

KING H, LOCKE FB. 1980. Cancer mortality among Chinese in the United States. J Natl Cancer Inst 65:1141–1148.

KHLAT M, VAIL A, PARKIN M, GREEN A. 1992. Mortality from melanoma in migrants to Australia: variation by age at arrival and duration of stay. Amer J Epidemiol 135:1103–1113.

KNELLER RW, MCLAUGHLIN JK, BJELKE E, et al. 1991. A cohort study of stomach cancer in a high-risk American population. Cancer 68:672–678.

KOLONEL LN. 1985. Cancer incidence among Filipinos in Hawaii and the Philippines. Natl Cancer Inst Monogr 69:93–98.

KOLONEL LN. 1980. Cancer patterns of four ethnic groups in Hawaii. J Natl Cancer Inst 65:1127–1139.

KOLONEL LN, HANKIN JH, LEE J, et al. 1981a. Nutrient intakes in relation to cancer incidence in Hawaii. Br J Cancer 44:332–339.

KOLONEL LN, HANKIN JH, NOMURA AM, et al. 1981b. Dietary fat intake and cancer incidence among five ethnic groups in Hawaii. Cancer Res 41:3727–3728.

KOLONEL LN, HINDS MW, HANKIN JH. 1980. Cancer patterns among migrant and native-born Japanese in Hawaii in relation to smoking, drinking and dietary habits: *In* H.V. Gelboin, B. MacMahou, T. Matsushima, T. Sugimura, S. Takayama, H. Takabe (eds): Genetic and Environmental Factors in Experimental and Human Cancer. Tokyo, Japan Sci. Soc. Press, pp. 327–340.

KOLONEL LN, NOMURA AMY, HINDS MW, et al. 1983. Role of diet in cancer incidence in Hawaii. Cancer Res (Suppl) 43:2397s–2402s.

KRICKER A, ARMSTRONG BK, ENGLISH DR, HEENAN PJ. 1991. Pigmentary and cutaneous risk factors for non-melanocytic skin cancer—a case-control study. Int J Cancer 48:650–662.

KUNE S, KUNE GA, WATSON L. 1986. The Melbourne colorectal cancer study: incidence in findings by age, sex, site, migrants and religion. Int J Epidemiol 15:483–493.

LILIENFELD AM, LEVIN ML, KESSLER II. 1972. Cancer in the United States. Cambridge, Massachusetts, Harvard University Press.

LOCKE FB, KING H. 1980. Cancer mortality risk among Japanese in the United States. J Natl Cancer Inst 65:1149–1156.

MACK TM, WALKER A, MACK W, et al. 1985. Cancer in Hispanics in Los Angeles County. Natl Cancer Inst Monogr 69:99–104.

MAGNUS K, HOUGEN A, ANDERSEN A, et al. 1970. A study of disease in migrants and their siblings: development of sibling rosters. J Chron Dis 23:405–410.

MARKIDES KS, COREIL J, RAY LA. 1987. Smoking among Mexican Americans: A three-generation study. Am J Public Health 77:708–711.

MARMOT MG, ADELSTEIN AM, BULUSU L. 1984. Immigrant mortality in England and Wales 1970–78: Causes of death by country of birth. Studies on Medical and Population Subjects 47:1–144.

MARTIN J, SUAREZ L. 1987. Cancer mortality among Mexican Americans and other whites in Texas, 1969–80. Am J Public Health 77:851–853.

MATOS E, KHLAT M, LORIA DI, et al. 1991. Cancer in migrants to Argentina. Int J Cancer 49:805–811.

MCCREDIE M, COATES MS, FORD JM. 1990a. Cancer incidence in migrants to New South Wales from England, Wales, Scotland and Ireland. Br J Cancer 62:992–995.

MCCREDIE M, COATES MS, FORD JM. 1990b. Cancer incidence in migrants to New South Wales. Int J Cancer 46:228–232.

MCMICHAEL AJ, GILES GG. 1988. Cancer in migrants to Australia: extending the descriptive epidemiological data. Cancer Res 48:751–756.

MENCK HR, HENDERSON BE, PIKE MC, et al. 1975. Cancer incidence in the Mexican-American. J Natl Cancer Inst 55:531–536.

MOWER HF, ICHINOTSUBO D, WANG LW, et al. 1982. Fecal mutagens in two Japanese populations with difference colon cancer risks. Cancer Res 42:1164–1169.

NASCA PC, GREENWALD P, BURNETT WS, et al. 1981. Cancer among the foreign-born in New York State. Cancer 48:2323–2328.

NEWMAN AM, SPENGLER RF. 1984. Cancer mortality among immigrant populations in Ontario, 1969 through 1973. Can Med Assoc J 130:399–405.

NILSSON B, GUSTAVSON-KADAKA E, ROTSTEIN S, et al. 1993. Cancer incidence in Estonian migrants to Sweden. Int J Cancer 55:190–195.

NOMURA A, HEILBRUN LK, MORRIS JS, et al. 1987. Serum selenium and the risk of cancer, by specific sites: case-control analysis of prospective data. J Natl Cancer Inst 79:103–108.

NOMURA A, HIROHATA T. 1976. Cancer mortality among Japanese in Hawaii. Comparison of observed and expected rates based on Prefecture-of-Origin in Japan. Hawaii Med J 35:293–297.

NOMURA A, STEMMERMANN GN, HEILBRUN LK. 1981b. Coffee and pancreatic cancer. Lancet 2:415.

NOMURA A, STEMMERMANN GN, WASNICH RD. 1982. Presence of hepatitis B surface antigen before primary hepatocellular carcinoma. JAMA 247:2247–2249.

NOMURA AM, STEMMERMANN GN, HEILBRUN LK, et al. 1985. Serum vitamin levels and risk of cancer of specific sites in men of Japanese ancestry in Hawaii. Cancer Res 45:2369–2372.

NOMURA AMY, KOLONEL LN, HINDS MW. 1981a. Trends in the anatomical distribution of colorectal carcinoma in Hawaii, 1960–1978. Dig Dis Sci 26:1116–1120.

PARKIN DM, STEINITZ R, KHLAT M, et al. 1990. Cancer in Jewish migrants to Israel. Int J Cancer 45:614–621.

POLEDNAK AP. 1991. Cancer incidence in the Puerto Rican-born population of Long Island, New York. Amer J Public Health 81:1405–1407.

POWLES JW, MACASKILL G, HOPPER JL, KTENAS D. 1991. Differences in drinking patterns associated with migration from a Greek island to Melbourne, Australia: a study of sibships. J Stud Alcohol 52:224–231.

REID DD. 1966. Studies of disease among migrants and native populations in Great Britain, Norway, and the United States. I. Background and Design. Natl Cancer Inst Monogr 19:287–299.

ROSENWAIKE I. 1984. Cancer mortality among Puerto Rican-born residents in New York City. Am J Epidemiol 119:177–185.

ROSENWAIKE I, SHAI D. 1986. Trends in cancer mortality among Puerto Rican-born migrants to New York City. Int J Epidemiol 15:30–35.

ROZEN P, HELLERSTEIN SM, HORWITZ C. 1981. The low incidence of colorectal cancer in a "high-risk" population: its correlation with dietary habits. Cancer 48:2692–2695.

SATO E, OUCHI A, SASANO H, et al. 1976. Polyps and diverticulosis of large bowel in autopsy population of Akita prefecture, compared with Miyagi. High risk for colorectal cancer in Japan. Cancer 37:1316–1321.

SAVITZ DA. 1986. Changes in Spanish surname cancer rates relative to other whites, Denver area, 1969–71 to 1979–81. Am J Public Health 76:1210–1215.

SEIDMAN H. 1971. Cancer mortality in New York City for country-of-birth, religious, and socioeconomic groups: Environ Res 4:390–429.

SHANMUGARATNAM K, LEE HP, DAY NE, DAVIS W (ED). 1983. Cancer incidence in Singapore 1968–1977. IARC Scientific Publ 47. Lyon, International Agency for Research on Cancer.

SHIMIZU H, MACK TM, ROSS RK, et al. 1987. Cancer of the gastrointestinal tract among Japanese and white immigrants in Los Angeles County. J Natl Cancer Inst 78:223–228.

SHIMIZU H, ROSS RK, BERNSTEIN L, et al. 1991. Cancers of the prostate and breast among Japanese and white immigrants in Los Angeles County. Br J Cancer 63:963–966.

STASZEWSKI J. 1974. Cancer of the upper alimentary tract and larynx in Poland and in Polish-born Americans. Br J Cancer 29:389–399.

STASZEWSKI J, HAENSZEL W. 1965. Cancer mortality among the Polish-born in the United States. J Natl Cancer Inst 35:291–297.

STASZEWSKI J, MCCALL MG, STENHOUSE NS. 1971. Cancer mortality in 1962–66 among Polish migrants to Australia. Br J Cancer 25:599–610.

Staszewski J, Slomska J, Muir CS, et al. 1970. Sources of demographic data on migrant groups for epidemiological studies of chronic disease. J Chron Dis 23:351–373.

Steinitz R, Costin C. 1971. Cancer in Jewish immigrants. Isr J Med Sci 7:1413–1436.

Stellman SD, Wang Q-S. 1994. Cancer mortality in Chinese immigrants to New York City. Cancer 73:1270–1275.

Stemmermann G, Nomura AMY, Heilbrun LK, et al. 1985. Colorectal cancer in Hawaiian Japanese men: A progress report. Natl Cancer Inst Mongr 69:125–131.

Stemmermann GN, Nomura AMY, Chyou P-H, et al. 1991. Cancer incidence in Hawaiian Japanese: Migrants from Okinawa compared with those from other prefectures. Jpn J Cancer Res 82:1366–1370.

Stemmermann GN, Yatani R. 1973. Diverticulosis and polyps of the large bowel: Anecropsy study of Hawaiian Japanese. Cancer 31:1260–1270.

Terracini B, Siemiatycki J, Richardson L. 1990. Cancer incidence and risk factors among Montreal residents of Italian origin. Int J Epidemiol 19:491–497.

Thomas DB. 1979. Epidemiologic studies of cancer in minority groups in the western United States. Natl Cancer Inst Monogr 53:103–113.

Thomas DB, Karagas MR. 1987. Cancer in first and second generation Americans. Cancer Res 47:5771–5776.

Tominaga S. 1985. Cancer incidence in Japanese in Japan, Hawaii, and western United States. Natl Cancer Inst Monogr 69:83–92.

Tsugane S, Gotlieb SLD, Laurenti R, et al. 1990. Cancer mortality among Japanese residents of the city of Sao Paulo, Brazil. Int J Cancer 45:436–439.

Tyczynski J, Tarkowski W, Parkin DM, Zatonski W. 1994. Cancer mortality among Polish migrants to Australia. Eur J Cancer 30A:478–484.

Ubukata T, Oshima A, Morinaga K, et al. 1987. Cancer patterns among Koreans in Japan, Koreans in Korea and Japanese in Japan in relation to life style factors. Jpn J Cancer Res (Gann) 78:437–446.

Warshauer ME, Silverman DT, Schottenfeld D, et al. 1986. Stomach and colorectal cancers in Puerto Rican-born residents of New York City. J Natl Cancer Inst 76:591–595.

Waterhouse J, Muir C, Shanmugaratnam K, Powell J, Peachm D, Wheland S (eds). 1982. Cancer Incidence in Five Continents, Vol. IV. IARC Sci Publ 42. Lyon, International Agency for Research on Cancer.

Waterhouse J, Muir C, Correa P, Powell J (eds). 1976. Cancer Incidence in Five Continents, Vol. III. IARC Sci Publ 15. Lyon, International Agency for Research on Cancer.

Whittemore AS, Wu-Williams AH, Lee M, et al. 1990. Diet, physical activity, and colorectal cancer among Chinese in North America and China. J Natl Cancer Inst 82:915–926.

Worth RM, Kagan A. 1970. Ascertainment of men of Japanese ancestry in Hawaii through World War II selective service registration. J Chron Dis 23:389–397.

Wynder EL, Hirayama T. 1977. Comparative epidemiology of cancers of the United States and Japan. Prev Med 6:567–594.

Zhang YQ, MacLennan R, Berry G. 1984. Mortality of Chinese in New South Wales, 1969–1978. Int J Epidemiol 13:188–192.

Ziegler RG, Hoover RN, Pike MC, et al. 1993. Migration patterns and breast cancer risk in Asian-American women. J Natl Cancer Inst 85:1819–1827.

13 Economic impact of cancer in the United States

MARTIN L. BROWN
THOMAS A. HODGSON
DOROTHY P. RICE

There are an estimated 6.3 million Americans alive today who have a history of cancer. Of this total, 4.2 million were diagnosed five or more years ago, most of whom can be considered cured. (Unpublished National Cancer Institute estimates based on Feldman et al, 1986). Currently over 1 million people a year are diagnosed as having cancer and about half will be alive five years after diagnosis and treatment. (National Cancer Institute, 1993)

Illness and disease create a burden for the patient, family and friends, and society. The individual's burden may include pain and suffering, reduced quality of life, premature mortality, and financial loss. Family and friends suffer emotional trauma, grief, and financial loss. Society must bear the negative impact on the social conscience created by the suffering of patients, families, and acquaintances, as well as the costs of resources used for medical care and lost because of morbidity, disability, and premature mortality. The cumulative social and economic implications of disease for victims and society at large are pain, suffering, disability, and death; millions of years of life lost; vast amounts of human and economic resources devoted to detection, diagnosis, and treatment; and billions of dollars of economic output foregone annually because of lost human resources.

The costs of illness are the losses, whether pecuniary or nonpecuniary, originating in disease, with economic costs being those that can be expressed in monetary units. Three categories of costs can be identified: direct costs, resulting from the use of resources; indirect costs, resulting from the loss of resources; and psychosocial costs, resulting from intangible impacts such as pain and suffering.

Ideally, data on the economic aspects of cancer should be specific enough to make it possible to (*a*) distribute costs among diagnosis, treatment, rehabilitation, and continuing care; (*b*) estimate non-health sector costs such as those for transportation, special diets, equipment, clothing, vocational, social and family counseling, and indirect losses to family members; (*c*) relate functional health status and costs; (*d*) estimate costs according to significant attributes of disease, such as tumor site, stage of disease at diagnosis, and treatment modality; (*e*) estimate costs per person with the disease or per case. Included in this would be ascertaining the medical care used, expenditures incurred, disability, morbidity and mortality suffered from onset of a condition until death or cure. Currently available data on the cost of cancer fulfill some of these criteria and recently initiated primary data collection and modeling efforts will improve the specificity and detail of cancer-related economic data further.

DIRECT COSTS

Direct costs include resources used for medical care in the prevention, diagnosis, and treatment of illness and disease and for the continuing care, rehabilitation, and terminal care of patients. These costs include expenditures for hospitalization; outpatient clinical care; nursing home care; home health care; services of primary physicians and specialists, dentists and other health practitioners; drugs and drug sundries; and rehabilitation counseling and other rehabilitation costs, such as reconstructive surgery, prostheses, appliances, eyeglasses, wigs, hearing aids, and speech devices related to overcoming impairments resulting from illness or disease.

In addition to medical care, other direct costs borne by patients and other individuals include costs of transportation to health providers, certain household expenditures, and costs of relocating such as moving expenses. Illness can force a family to incur expenses in caring and providing for the sick member of the family. These include extra expenditures for household help for cleaning, laundering, cooking, and baby-sitting; special diets; special clothing; items for rehabilitation and comfort such as exercycles, vaporizers, humidifiers, and dehumidifiers; alterations of property, such as elevators for invalids and other special housing facilities; and vocational, social and family counseling services. Other costs originating in disease or illness are expenditures for retraining or re-education, care provided by family and friends, and certain financial costs. Financial costs include interest lost on withdrawal of savings to pay expenses, interest charges on funds borrowed to pay illness-related expenses including interest on personal loans, mortgages, and loans against the cash value of life insurance.

INDIRECT COSTS

Indirect costs are the time and output lost or foregone by the patient, family, friends, and others from employment, housekeeping, volunteer activities, and leisure. The patient suffers a cessation or reduction of activity because of morbidity, disability, or mortality associated with the illness. Family members and others may incur indirect costs in the form of time spent caring for and being with the patient, and unwanted job changes and loss of opportunities for promotion and education necessitated by the patient's illness. Additional indirect costs include the time patient and/or family spend visiting physicians, other health professionals, and hospitalized persons.

PSYCHOSOCIAL COSTS

Disease may bring about personal catastrophes that are not reflected in direct and indirect economic costs. Illness and disease are responsible for a wide variety of deteriorations in the quality of life that are frequently referred to as psychosocial costs. Victims of illness and disease; children, spouses, and siblings of victims; friends and co-workers of victims; and those who render care may all be affected. A victim may suffer a loss of a body part or speech, disfigurement, disability, impending death, pain, and grief. The patient, and those around him, or her, may be forced into economic dependence and social isolation, unwanted job changes, loss of opportunities for promotion and education, relocation of living quarters, and other undesired changes in life plans. The environment created by illness often induces anxiety, reduced self-esteem and feelings of well-being, resentment, and emotional problems that often require psychotherapy. Problems of living may develop, leading to family conflict, antisocial behavior, and suicide. The victim and others may experience marked personality changes and reduced sexual function. Disrupted development and delinquency may occur among children. The quality of life may be reduced beyond the restorative capability of current rehabilitation efforts. The combination of financial strain and psychosocial problems can be especially devastating. Assessing the quality of life ramifications of cancer and cancer treatment is currently an active area of cancer research (Nayfield and Hailey, 1991).

ESTIMATED COSTS OF CANCER

Two approaches have been developed to measure the cost of cancer (Hodgson, 1988). One approach tracks cost-generating events in the macroeconomy and attributes a monetary value to each event. This produces an estimate of the annual aggregate, or "prevalent" burden of illness measured by the value of goods and services diverted from other uses to provide medical care and lost because of idled labor. Morbidity and mortality from cancer are translated into use and expenditures for medical care, time lost from work and housekeeping, and forgone wages and salaries. Another approach tracks the longitudinal pattern of expenditures or resource use for individual cancer patients. This produces estimates for the average lifetime, "incidence" cost of cancer by cancer site. (A detailed discussion of the prevalence approach versus the incidence approach to accounting for the costs of illness is in Hodgson [1988]).

This chapter will report mainly on prevalence estimates of cost for all cancer, although some recent incidence estimates for specific cancer sites will also be discussed in Estimates of Lifetime Costs section. Direct costs other than those due to medical care and psychosocial costs will not be presented due to lack of data in these areas, although some data relevant to this question will be reviewed. The costs of illness presented are nationwide in scope and convey the aggregate burden of illness in 1985, 1990, and 1994 resulting from the prevalence of disease during these same years.

The economic costs of cancer have been estimated in the past as a major diagnostic category of the total economic costs of illness for 1963, 1972, 1975, and 1980 (Rice, 1966; Cooper and Rice, 1976; Berk et al, 1978; Rice et al, 1985) Estimates of the costs of cancer by cancer site have also been made in the past for 1976, 1977, and 1980 (Scotto and Chiazze, 1977; Rice and Hodgson, 1981; Hodgson, 1984). This chapter updates to 1985, 1990, and 1994 previous estimates by Rice and Hodgson of the economic costs of malignant neoplasms to the U.S. The methodology follows closely that originally developed by Rice (1966) to allocate expenditures among diagnoses, and is amended to include additional sources of data. This and methods used to update esti-

TABLE 13–1. *Economic Costs of All Illnesses and Cancer by Type of Cost, United States, 1985**

Type of Cost	All Illnesses: AMOUNT ($ MILLIONS)	All Illnesses: PERCENT DISTRIBUTION	Cancer: AMOUNT ($ MILLIONS)	Cancer: PERCENT DISTRIBUTION	PERCENT OF ALL ILLNESSES
Total	679,712	100.0	72,494	100.0	10.7
Direct	371,400	54.6	18,104	25.0	4.9
Indirect	308,312	45.4	54,390	75.0	17.6
Morbidity	80,850	11.9	7,170	9.9	8.9
Mortality	227,462	33.5	47,220	65.1	20.8

*Direct costs of all illnesses from Waldo, et al (1986). All other costs calculated by the authors. Mortality costs discounted at 4%.

mates to 1990 are briefly described in the Methodology section.

ECONOMIC COSTS IN 1985

In 1985 the total economic costs of all illness amounted to $680 billion, of which direct costs comprised 55% and indirect costs, 45%. Total economic costs of cancer were $72.5 billion, or 10.7% of the economic costs of all illnesses in 1985. Direct costs of cancer were 25 percent and indirect costs 75% of total cancer costs. Cancer is characterized by a higher premature mortality rate than many other diseases, resulting in higher indirect costs relative to direct costs for cancer compared to all illnesses together (Table 13–1).

DIRECT MEDICAL CARE COSTS

In 1985, medical care expenditures for cancer amounted to $18.1 billion, and comprised almost 5% of the total personal health spending in the United States (Table 13–2). Most of the cost of medical care for cancer derives from the care received in short-stay hospitals from 1.9 million patient discharges, with an average length of stay of 8.9 days, for a total of 17 million days (National Center for Health Statistics, 1987), and 20 million office visits to ambulatory care physicians for diagnosis and treatment (National Center for Health Statistics, 1988). Hospital care of cancer patients accounted for $12.1 billion, or two-thirds of total medical care expenditures. In contrast, hospital care spending for all illnesses comprised 45% of total medical spending in the United States. This relative difference is due to the higher rate of hospitalization and longer stays for cancer patients compared with many other illnesses. Physicians' services for cancer patients amounted to $4.1 billion (23% of total medical care expenditures for cancer), but considerably lesser amounts were spent for nursing home care ($919 million), drugs ($659 million), and other professional services ($326 million).

MORBIDITY COSTS

Morbidity costs are one component of indirect costs. They are the value of losses in output for people who are ill or disabled and unable to work or keep house. Illness due to cancer prevents people from leading their accustomed productive lives and keeping house. They may lose time from their activities, be forced out of the labor force, or become institutionalized. Estimated morbidity costs of cancer include losses, measured by the

TABLE 13–2. *Medical Care Expenditures for All Conditions and Cancer by Type of Medical Service, United States, 1985*

Type of Service	All Conditions: AMOUNT ($ MILLIONS)	All Conditions: PERCENT DISTRIBUTION	Cancer: AMOUNT ($ MILLIONS)	Cancer: PERCENT DISTRIBUTION
All services	371,400	100.0	18,104	100.0
Hospital care	166,700	44.9	12,118	66.9
Physicians' services	82,800	22.3	4,082	22.5
Nursing home care	35,200	9.5	919	5.1
Drugs	28,500	7.7	659	3.6
Other professional services	39,700	10.7	326	1.8
Other health services	18,500	5.0	[a]	[a]

[a]Not applicable.

TABLE 13–3. *Cancer Mortality According to Age, United States, 1985**

Age in Years	*Number of Deaths*	*Percent of All U.S. Deaths*	*Rank Order in Age-group*
Total	461,563[a]	22.2	2
1–4	543	7.4	3
5–14	1,183	13.2	2
15–24	2,142	5.6	4
25–44	20,026	17.0	2
45–64	138,829	34.4	1
65 and over	298,683	20.3	2

*From National Center for Health Statistics (1987).
[a]Includes deaths under 1 year of age and deaths with age not stated.

value of forgone earnings and the imputed value of lost housekeeping services, among the currently employed, persons not in institutions who are unable to work, persons unable to keep house because of illness or disability, and persons residing in institutions, such as nursing homes and homes for the aged, who are ill with cancer.

Morbidity and disability from cancer in the United States in 1985 resulted in $7.2 billion of lost output, representing 8.9% of the morbidity costs for all diseases (Table 13–1). Cancer is high on the list of diseases causing morbidity and concomitant economic costs (Rice et al, 1985).

MORTALITY COSTS

Mortality costs are the second component of indirect costs. If individuals had not died in 1985, they would have continued to be productive for a number of years. The present value of future output lost because of premature death constitute the mortality costs of cancer deaths in 1985.

In 1985 almost 462,000 persons died from cancer, accounting for 22% of the 2.1 million deaths in the United States and making cancer the second leading cause of death (National Center for Health Statistics, 1987). Cancer's rank as a leading cause of death varies by age. For the population aged 45–64 years, cancer was the leading cause of death and accounted for 34% of the deaths in that age group. For persons aged 15–24 years, it ranked fourth, with 6% of total deaths in that age group. The number of cancer deaths, the percent of deaths due to cancer, and the rank of cancer as a cause of death are shown in Table 13–3 for various ages.

TABLE 13–4. *Number of Deaths, Person-years Lost, and Mortality Costs by Age and Sex, United States, 1985**

	All Causes of Death				*Cancer*				
		Person-years Lost				*Person-years Lost*		*Mortality Costs[b]*	
	Number of Deaths[a]	NUMBER (THOUSANDS)	PER DEATH	*Mortality Costs[b] ($ millions)*	*Number of Deaths[a]*	NUMBER (THOUSANDS)	PER DEATH	TOTAL ($ MILLIONS)	PER DEATH (THOUSANDS)
TOTAL	2,086,440	33,253	15.9	227,462	461,563	7,210	15.6	47,220	$102
Under 25	94,237	6,149	65.2	49,172	3,982	244	61.4	2,295	576
25–44	117,667	4,772	40.6	70,758	20,026	799	39.9	10,684	533
45–64	403,114	8,843	21.9	82,197	138,829	3,084	22.2	27,296	197
65–74	482,646	6,354	13.2	18,479	142,542	1,901	13.3	5,646	40
75 and over	987,899	7,136	7.2	6,855	156,141	1,181	7.6	1,300	8
MALES	1,097,758	18,044	16.4	154,231	246,914	3,467	14.0	25,953	105
Under 25	60,846	3,756	61.7	35,092	2,333	136	58.4	1,476	632
25–44	80,848	3,150	39.0	53,693	9,344	346	37.0	5,939	636
45–64	251,031	5,067	20.2	54,697	74,883	1,486	19.8	15,570	208
65–74	283,017	3,336	11.8	8,515	81,113	962	11.9	2,489	31
75 and over	421,525	2,735	6.5	2,234	79,220	537	6.8	480	6
FEMALES	988,682	15,209	15.4	73,231	214,649	3,743	17.4	21,267	99
Under 25	33,391	2,392	71.6	14,080	1,649	108	65.6	819	497
25–44	36,819	1,623	44.1	17,065	10,682	454	42.5	4,745	444
45–64	152,083	3,776	24.8	27,501	63,946	1,598	25.0	11,726	183
65–74	199,629	3,018	15.1	9,965	61,429	939	15.3	3,157	51
75 and over	566,374	4,401	7.8	4,621	76,921	645	8.4	820	11

*Number of deaths due to all causes from National Center for Health Statistics (1987); number of cancer deaths from unpublished data from the Divisi—on of Vital Statistics, National Center for Health Statistics; person-years lost and costs calculated by the authors.
[a]Includes deaths with age not stated.
[b]Discounted at 4%.

Premature mortality from cancer is a significant drain on the productive capacity of the economy. Cancer deaths in 1985 resulted in a loss of $47 billion (at a 4% discount rate) (Table 13–4). The cost per cancer death was $102 thousand. For males who died of cancer, an estimated 3.5 million person-years were lost (14 years per death) at a cost of $26 billion. Females who died of cancer represented a loss of 3.7 million person-years (17 per death) and $21 billion. Males accounted for 53% of cancer deaths, 48% of the person-years lost, and 55% of the productivity losses, due to the higher earnings of males. Cancer was responsible for about one-fifth of all deaths, person-years lost, and mortality costs.

The number of cancer deaths, person-years lost, and mortality costs vary by age. The highest number of deaths is among the aged (65 years and older), representing almost two-thirds of the total. But this age group accounted for only 43% of years lost and 15% of mortality costs owing to a relatively short life expectancy and greatly reduced earnings. Persons 45–64 years of age accounted for only 30% of all cancer deaths, but 43% of person-years lost and 58% of mortality costs. The relatively few deaths among persons less than 45 years of age were responsible for 27% of mortality costs, due to high expected lifetime earnings remaining at the time of death.

Cancer mortality and costs also vary according to cancer site (Table 13–5). Cancers of the respiratory and intrathoracic organs accounted for 28% of cancer deaths, 27% of person-years lost, and 27% of mortality costs in 1985. Next in order of magnitude are cancers of the digestive organs and peritoneum with 25% of deaths, 22% of person-years lost, and 20% of mortality costs. Other cancer sites accounted for much smaller proportions of deaths, years lost, and costs. Although there were more deaths from cancers of the genital organs, breast cancer was responsible for the third highest number of person-years lost and mortality costs.

TOTAL INDIRECT COSTS

Morbidity and mortality from cancer in 1985 deprived the U.S. of more than 7 million person-years of productive activity at an estimated value of $54 billion. It is important to emphasize, however, that not all the person-years lost were incurred in 1985. Included in these figures are the years lost and value of productivity foregone in succeeding years as a result of premature mortality in 1985. In order to make meaningful comparisons among amounts occurring in different time periods, the stream of future money values for each individual who died in 1985 was converted to a 1985 present value. These present values were then summed over all persons to arrive at a total value of person-years lost from mortality in 1985. A discussion of the mechanics of discounting a stream of future money values into its present value can be found in Anderson and Settle (1975). A discussion of this and other issues pertinent to estimating costs of illness are in Hodgson and Meiners (1982) and Hodgson (1983).

SUMMARY OF ECONOMIC COSTS—1985

Total economic costs of neoplasms, including direct medical care expenditures and indirect losses of output, were estimated at $72.5 billion in 1985 and accounted for 10.7% of the economic costs of all illnesses in the United States. Direct costs comprised 25% of total

TABLE 13–5. *Number of Deaths, Person-years Lost, and Mortality Costs, According to Cancer Site, United States, 1985**

		Person-years Lost		*Mortality Costs*[a]	
Cancer Site	*Number of Deaths*	TOTAL (THOUSANDS)	PER DEATH	TOTAL ($ MILLIONS)	PER DEATH ($ THOUSANDS)
Total	461,563	7,210	15.6	47,220	102
Lip, oral cavity, and pharynx	8,290	136	16.4	1,045	126
Digestive organs and peritoneum	116,609	1,614	13.8	9,418	81
Respiratory and intrathoracic organs	127,311	1,951	15.3	12,869	101
Breast	40,383	793	19.6	5,165	128
Genital organs	49,690	687	13.8	3,607	73
Urinary organs	18,897	251	13.3	1,450	77
Leukemia	17,319	327	18.9	2,511	145
Lymphatic and hematopoietic tissues	25,159	416	16.5	3,097	123
Other and unspecified sites	57,905	1,035	17.9	8,057	139

*Number of deaths data from National Center for Health Statistics (1987); person-years lost and costs calculated by the authors.
[a]Discounted at 4%.

costs, morbidity costs were 10%, and mortality costs were 65%. Indirect costs were 3 times the direct costs of cancer. Chronic diseases characterized by morbidity, disability and mortality generate high indirect costs relative to medical care expenditures. Indirect losses are especially important for conditions that cause morbidity and disability and result in death, especially at younger ages. For all conditions together, total costs were more evenly distributed among direct (55% of total costs) and indirect (45% of the total) costs. This reflects the influence in the costs of all diseases of acute illnesses for which mortality is low but medical care is required when people are sick.

Large amounts of money have little meaning for most people. In order to put into perspective the $18.1 billion spent on medical care for cancer in 1985, Table 13–6 presents personal consumption expenditures for selected items in the United States during the same year (U.S. Bureau of Economic Analysis, 1986). This table shows that medical care for cancer cost 15% of the amount spent for household utilities, 20% of spending for gasoline and oil, 57% of expenditures on tobacco, and 64% of spending for legal services. On the other hand, spending for cancer was 17% higher than the nation's consumers spent on higher education, 37% more than the amount for magazines and newspapers, and 87% more than (almost double) the amount spent for admissions to a variety of spectator amusements.

TABLE 13–6. *Personal Consumption Expenditures for Selected Items, United States, 1985**

Item	*Amount ($ billions)*	*Per Capita Expenditures ($)*	*Ratio of Expenditures for Cancer to Expenditures for Item*
Household utilities[a]	121.2	508	0.15
Furniture and household equipment[b]	105.6	442	0.17
Gasoline and oil	91.9	385	0.20
Alcoholic beverages	55.5	232	0.33
Tobacco products	31.8	133	0.57
Legal services	28.1	118	0.64
Cancer medical care	18.1	76	1.00
Higher education	15.5	65	1.17
Magazines, newspapers, sheet music	13.2	55	1.37
Bank service charges[c]	11.7	49	1.55
Admissions to spectator amusements	9.7	41	1.87

*From Department of Commerce (1986).
[a]Includes electricity, gas, water and sanitary services, and fuel oil and coal.
[b]Includes furniture; kitchen and other household appliances; china, glassware, tableware, and utensils; and other durable and semidurable furnishings.
[c]Includes bank service charges, trust services, and safe deposit box rental.

TABLE 13–7. *Wages and Salaries According to Type of Activity, United States, 1985*

Activity	*Amount ($ billions)*	*Ratio of Amount for Cancer to Amount for Activity*
Construction	102.1	0.53
Transportation[a]	72.5	0.75
Cancer morbidity and mortality	54.4	1.00
Food and kindred products manufacturing	33.5	1.62
Telephone and telegraph communications	32.0	1.70
Motor vehicles and equipment	29.3	1.86
Textile mill, apparel and other textile manufacturing	25.1	2.17
Real estate	21.6	2.52
Legal services	21.5	2.53
Educational services	19.9	2.73

*From Department of Commerce (1986).
[a]Includes railroad, local, and interurban passenger transit, trucking and warehousing, water, air, pipelines (except natural gas), and other transportation services.

Indirect costs of cancer are compared in Table 13–7 to wages and salaries in selected industries. The wages and salaries given are the total dollars for all employees in that industry in the United States. The value of productive labor lost to morbidity and mortality from cancer was $54.4 billion. By comparison, the labor lost to cancer is sufficient to provide more than half the needs of the construction industry, more than twice the labor required by textile products, two-and-a-half that used to provide real estate and legal services, and almost three times the value of labor required for educational services. Indirect costs of cancer are a significant diminution in the nation's capacity to produce goods and services. Even a relatively small reduction in indirect costs of cancer would increase the value of productive labor by several billion dollars and the capacity of the economy to supply additional goods and services. Indirect costs of cancer are large, representing a significant loss of resources, and they diminish the nation's capacity to produce goods and services.

UPDATING CANCER COST ESTIMATES TO 1990 AND 1994

The methods used to update estimates to 1990 are described in the Methodology section. The estimate of the total cost of cancer in 1990 (Table 13–8) is over $96 billion; 29% of this is attributable to direct cost, 10%

TABLE 13–8. *Economic Costs of Cancer by Type of Cost, United States, 1990*

Type of Cost	*Amount ($ millions)*	*Percent Distribution*
Total	96,126	100.0
Direct	27,458	28.6
Indirect	68,668	71.4
Morbidity	9,895	10.3
Mortality	58,773	61.1

to morbidity cost, and 61% to mortality cost. Table 13–9 shows these adjustments for each component of direct cancer cost. 1990 mortality cost estimates for specific cancer sites are shown in Table 13–10. While similar methods could be applied to update costs to 1994, we applied this update only to total direct costs because the composition of direct costs has been changing significantly in recent years. This approach yields an estimate of $41.4 billion for direct costs in 1994.

With somewhat different updating methods than used here, Brown (1990) obtained the following estimates for the cost of *all* neoplasms (e.g., including non-melanoma skin cancer and in situ cancers) in 1990: direct cost = $35.3 billion; morbidity cost = $11.8 billion; mortality cost = $56.8 billion. In addition, increased screening activities for the early detection of cancer were estimated to cost between $2.98 and $3.92 billion in 1990.

ESTIMATES OF LIFETIME COSTS

The incidence approach to direct costs attempts to account for all costs which an average cancer patient incurs from the date of diagnosis until death or cure. Scotto and Chiazze (1976, 1977) ascertained the hospital care costs of a 10% sample of patients from the Third National Cancer Survey. The costs, hospital admissions, and average length of stay, of these patients—identified by cancer site and stage and diagnosed in 1969—were followed up for 24 months from the date of diagnosis. Data were also collected on the medical expenditures, in 1969, of patients diagnosed prior to 1969. Using these data, and a hospital-to-total-medical-cost ratio derived from aggregate data, Scotto and Chiazze estimated the total prevalence direct cost of cancer for 1976 to be about $6 billion. Using inflation, incidence, and prevalence adjustments to update this estimate to 1990 we obtain $28.7 billion, remarkably close to the 1990 estimate obtained above.

More recent and complete estimates of incidence cost have been obtained using Medicare records. Using the continuous Medicare history (5%) sample file (CMHSF) of patients diagnosed with cancer from 1974 through 1981, Baker et al (1989) estimated cancer site–

TABLE 13–9. *Medical Care Expenditures for Cancer by Type of Medical Service, United States, 1990**

Type of Service	*Amount ($ millions)*	*Percent Distribution*
All services	27,458	100.0
Hospital care	17,935	65.3
Physicians' services	6,613	24.1
Nursing home care	1,333	4.9
Drugs	1,068	3.9
Other professional services	509	1.9

*Updated from 1985 estimates using the fixed weight price index for personal health care expenditures (Health Care Financing Administration, 1990) to inflate costs and cancer incidence data (National Cancer Institute, 1993) to account for increased cancer cases.

TABLE 13–10. *Mortality Costs According to Cancer Site, United States, 1990**

Cancer Site	*Number of Deaths*	*Person-years Lost* TOTAL (THOUSANDS)	*Person-years Lost* PER DEATH	*Mortality Costs* TOTAL ($ MILLIONS)	*Mortality Costs* PER DEATH ($ THOUSANDS)
Total	498,698	7,309	14.6	58,711	118
Lip, oral cavity and pharynx	8,040	130	16.2	943	117
Digestive organs and peritoneum	115,633	1,396	12.1	11,249	97
Respiratory and intrathoracic organs	145,687	2,129	14.6	17,123	117
Breast	43,746	848	19.4	6,150	141
Genital organs	52,678	675	12.8	4,122	78
Urinary organs	19,297	255	13.2	1,782	92
Leukemia	17,802	327	18.4	2,990	168
Lymphatic and hematopoietic tissues	28,239	457	16.5	3,938	140
Other and unspecified sites	67,576	1,092	16.2	10,414	154

*Number of deaths from National Center for Health Statistics (1990), projected to 1990 using recent trends in cancer mortality (National Cancer Institute, 1991); mortality costs calculated by the authors.

TABLE 13–11. *Charges Made to Medicare for Treatment during the Initial, Continuing, and Terminal Phases of Cancer of 13 Sites (cases diagnosed 1974–1981, charges expressed in 1990 dollars)**

Cancer Site	*Initial (3 months)*	*Continuing (monthly)*	*Terminal (6 months)*
Colorectal	$20079	$809	$22323
Lung	18276	976	22024
Prostate	11478	792	20677
Breast	10762	683	21417
Bladder	11985	1084	26286
Leukemia	12832	957	27984
Pancreas	19822	958	20928
Stomach	20437	934	22826
Uterine corpus	13103	600	24936
Kidney	17840	948	27312
Ovary	15643	915	26389
Uterine cervix	12705	698	23225
Melanoma	9840	691	22914
All sites	14205	818	23036

*From Baker et al, 1989. Charges inflated to 1990 dollars using fixed weight price index for personal health care expenditures (Health Care Financing Administration, 1990).

specific costs for "initial" (first three months after diagnosis), "terminal" (last 6 months prior to death) and "continuing" phases of treatment. These estimates, originally published in terms of 1984 dollars, are shown in 1990 dollars in Table 13–11. The continuing care costs are almost surely an overestimate of cancer attributable costs since these data refer to any medical care costs incurred by cancer patients. Comparisons of cancer patients in the continuing care phase to non-cancer patients suggest that cancer-attributable continuing care costs are in the range of $700 to $1500 annually. From a more detailed analysis of the CMHSF data, Baker et al (1991) have estimated the average lifetime cost attributable to breast cancer at $52,249 and lung cancer at $17,701, both in 1990 dollars (1984 dollars in the original paper.)

Currently this data set is being updated and improved through a joint project of the National Cancer Institute and the Health Care Financing Administration (HCFA). The SEER/Medicare project is a linked data file between the SEER (Surveillance, Epidemiology and End Results) cancer registry system and Medicare finance records maintained by HCFA. This file will include persons diagnosed with cancer between 1973 and 1993 and detailed Medicare data on procedures and services used, reimbursements, and charges, from 1984 to 1993. This data base will make it possible, within the limitations of Medicare-based data, to construct longitudinal cost and lifetime cost estimates by cancer site and stage (Potosky, 1993).

To date, no nationally representative data on incidence-based morbidity costs for cancer have been collected. A recent study (Watson, 1990) followed the employment experience of 459 cancer survivors employed at American Telephone and Telegraph Company. These individuals, all diagnosed with cancer in 1987, were followed for two years. The average days of lost work over the two-year period was 87.2 (median = 61 days). Days lost from work due to cancer varied by sex, cancer site, employment category, salary level, geographical region, and employment at Bell Labs.

UNCOUNTED COSTS

Out-of-pocket medical costs, disease-related non-medical costs, lost wages, and unpaid family labor may represent a substantial economic burden on the families of cancer patients. There is no systematic overview of this aspect of the cost of cancer. A few studies have been done which suggest the magnitude of this component of these costs. The indirect economic impact of childhood cancer on the family has been relatively well studied. The potential for lost earnings is relatively high in these families because it is likely that parents in their prime income-earning years will become primary care givers. Two studies by Lansky and colleagues (1979, 1983) found the average weekly out-of-pocket non-medical expenditures ($62) and lost wages ($38) of the families of children with cancer to be $100, equal to 44% of family income. Including out-of-pocket medical expenditures increased this only moderately. A study of childhood cancer patients diagnosed in 1981 and followed longitudinally (Bloom et al, 1985) found that non-medical cancer-related costs and lost income amounted to 38% of family income.

Houts and colleagues (1984) studied adult cancer patients—mainly diagnosed with breast, colon, and lung cancer—who were currently receiving outpatient chemotherapy. Average non-medical expenses and lost wages for a treatment week was $73 and for a non-treatment week, $46. For half of the families surveyed, the total expenses plus loss of pay amounted to more than 25% of the weekly family income. In all of these studies median costs were substantially less than mean values, indicating that a wide variability of the economic burden was due to cancer.

In a recent study, Stommel et al (1991) estimated the value of unpaid family labor for cancer patients currently undergoing out-patient treatment. They estimated an average annual value of $14,204 in such services. They found average weekly costs due to out-of-pocket expenditures and loss of earnings to be $85, similar to the result of Houts et al.

While it is not possible to generalize from any of these studies, because they were conducted using relatively small and non-population-based samples, taken together, they suggest that the magnitude of the cancer-related costs that have not been systematically counted, is significant.

CONCLUSION

The prevalence-based costs discussed in this chapter provide an estimate of the direct and indirect economic burden incurred over a period of time (the base period) as a result of the prevalence of disease during the same base period, which is most often a year. Included are the costs of the base year manifestations or sequelae of a disease which may have had its onset in the base year or any time prior to the base year. Prevalence costs measure the value of resources used or lost during a specific period of time, regardless of the time of disease onset. These cost of illness estimates help convey the aggregate burden of illness on society, assess the relative burden of different diseases, indicate benefits to be derived from reductions in prevalence or severity of disease, and assist in setting priorities for the allocation of limited resources.

In recent years there has been an increasing demand for disease- and intervention-specific cost-benefit and cost-effectiveness analyses in health care (Russell, 1989). These types of analyses often require cancer site– or even cancer site and stage–specific incidence-based cost data. SEER/Medicare and other efforts to collect data of this kind are a response to this need.

METHODOLOGY

Details concerning the methodology for calculating the economic cost of illness may be found in previous articles on this subject (Rice, 1966; Cooper and Rice, 1976; Rice and Hodgson, 1981; Hodgson and Meiners, 1982; Hodgson, 1983; and Rice et al, 1985). What follows is a brief description of the methodology and data sources for estimating economic costs of cancer in the United States and for updating these costs to 1990 and 1994.

Direct Costs

National health expenditures, by type of expenditure, are published annually by the Health Care Financing Administration (HCFA) (Health Care Financing Administration, 1987). Total expenditures in 1985 for hospital care, physicians' services, and other direct costs of illness were distributed by diagnosis (cancer) according to utilization and cost per unit of service if available. Expenditures in community hospitals, for example, were allocated to cancer in proportion to the number of days of care attributable to cancer from the National Hospital Discharge Survey multiplied by the expense per patient day. Utilization of other medical care services, weighted by unit costs if available, determined the share of total medical care expenditures assigned to cancer.

Direct costs were updated to 1990 by making two adjustments: (1) the increase in number of cancer cases was taken into account—the number of incidence cancers increased 14% from 1985 to 1990 (National Cancer Institute, 1991); estimated prevalence increased by 18% (unpublished NCI estimates). Increased incidence was used, to be conservative, because the estimate of incidence is more reliable and total prevalence cost increase is less than proportionate to prevalence, since in many prevalent years, cancer patients incur relatively low costs. (2) The increased dollar costs of cancer related medical services was adjusted for 1990 using the appropriate components of the fixed weight price index for personal health care expenditures (Health Care Financing Administration, 1990). These price indices take all medical expenditures into account, not just out-of-pocket expenditures, as does the medical care component of the consumer price index. To update total direct cost to 1994 the medical component of the consumer price index was used because the HCFA index was not available for this year and the American Cancer Society estimates of 1994 cases was used (American Cancer Society, 1994). This method of updating is clearly approximate in that it does not take into account the changing composition of cancer incidence and prevalence, changing methods of treatment, or the changing mix of treatment setting due to the effects of reimbursement policy and other factors.

Morbidity Costs

Morbidity losses are estimated separately for those who are currently employed, housekeepers, persons unable to work because of ill health, and the institutionalized population. Days lost from work among the currently employed due to cancer are converted to years lost by age and sex and multiplied by age- and sex-specific estimates of average annual earnings to obtain lost earnings for this group. Days of bed-disability suffered by women who have cancer who usually keep house are also converted to years and multiplied by age-specific values of housewives' services to obtain morbidity costs for this group. The number of persons unable to work by age and sex is multiplied by employment rates and average annual earnings and by housekeeping rates and housekeeping values to determine indirect morbidity costs among members of this group. A similar proce-

TABLE 13–12. *Present Values of Lifetime Earnings According to Age and Sex, United States, 1985**

Age	Earnings ($ thousands) MALES	FEMALES
Under 1	$421,235	$341,574
1–4	454,561	368,388
5–9	519,459	420,790
10–14	602,092	487,557
15–19	689,576	552,141
20–24	745,680	578,481
25–29	749,695	558,019
30–34	717,630	513,796
35–39	653,498	454,897
40–44	561,016	388,555
45–49	450,452	319,279
50–54	331,478	249,422
55–59	213,719	181,151
60–64	108,880	117,333
65–69	42,879	67,346
70–74	19,176	36,593
75–79	9,383	18,847
80–84	4,698	9,164
85 and over	1,442	2,311

*Values calculated by the authors and discounted at 4%.

dure is applied to the institutionalized population to estimate morbidity costs by type of institution. These separate components of morbidity costs are aggregated to obtain a total cancer morbidity cost figure.

Morbidity costs were updated to 1990 in a fashion similar to direct costs, except that rather than using a medical expenditure inflation adjustment, the increased dollar value of average earnings was applied.

Mortality Costs

To obtain indirect costs of mortality, the numbers of deaths in 1985 by age and sex (National Center for Health Statistics, 1987) are multiplied by the present value of lifetime earnings, also by age and sex. These are shown in Table 13–12. Selected economic values used in estimating present values of lifetime earnings and housekeeping services are shown in Table 13–13. The number of person-years lost due to premature mortality is the product of number of deaths and life expectancy at the mid-year of the age group (Table 13–14). This method of estimating mortality costs accounts for life expectancy, labor force participation and housekeeping rates, future growth of earnings, imputed values of housekeeping services, and the discount rate for each age and sex group. Estimates for 1985 include imputed

TABLE 13–13. *Selected Economic Variables Used in Estimating Mortality Costs According to Age and Sex, United States, 1985**

	Percent of Population With Earnings		Mean Annual Earnings[a]		Mean Annual Value of Housekeeping Services[b] ($ thousands)			
					In Labor Force		Not in Labor Force	
Age	MALES	FEMALES	MALES	FEMALES	MALES	FEMALES	MALES	FEMALES
15–19	44.9	41.5	$6,706	$6,353	1,835	4,691	3,611	9,330
20–24	85.0	71.8	19,357	16,030	2,220	7,076	4,706	11,715
25–29	94.1	75.5	25,771	19,702	2,604	7,862	5,091	12,396
30–34	94.4	74.1	30,950	22,268	2,871	8,491	5,327	13,130
35–39	94.8	75.6	36,075	22,077	2,960	8,911	5,446	13,549
40–44	93.5	75.4	38,856	21,642	2,989	8,282	5,475	12,920
45–49	93.2	73.0	38,884	21,252	2,989	7,469	5,475	12,108
50–54	90.5	65.4	37,497	20,476	2,989	7,469	5,475	12,108
55–59	82.0	55.7	35,936	19,878	3,196	7,338	5,682	12,029
60–64	62.6	40.3	35,409	19,270	3,196	7,338	5,682	12,029
65–69	24.6	13.3	33,412	19,552	3,196	7,155	5,712	11,793
70–74	12.9	5.5	27,898	16,529	2,276	5,094	4,067	8,397
75–79	8.4	3.0	23,284	13,988	1,547	3,464	2,766	5,710
80–84	5.5	1.5	19,418	11,824	899	2,013	1,607	3,317
85 and over	3.5	1.0	16,212	9,999	509	1,139	909	1,878

*From U.S. Bureau of the Census (1987), U.S. Department of Labor (1986).

[a]Mean annual earnings for year-round full-time workers, including supplements to earnings that consist mainly of employers' contributions to social insurance.

[b]Values are imputed by multiplying hours spent in each type of domestic activity by the wages for corresponding occupations.

TABLE 13–14. *Life Expectancy According to Age and Sex, United States, 1985**

Age	*MALES*	*FEMALES*
Under 1	71.2	78.1
1–4	69.7	76.5
5–9	65.3	72.1
10–14	60.3	67.2
15–19	55.5	62.3
20–24	50.9	57.4
25–29	46.3	52.6
30–34	41.7	47.7
35–39	37.1	42.9
40–44	32.5	38.2
45–49	28.1	33.6
50–54	23.9	29.1
55–59	20.1	24.9
60–64	16.5	20.8
65–69	13.3	17.1
70–74	10.5	13.6
75–79	8.1	10.5
80–84	6.1	7.8
85 and over	5.1	6.4

*From National Center for Health Statistics (1988).

housekeeping values for women and men in the labor force who have household responsibilities.

This method of valuing the economic losses due to premature mortality is referred to as the *human capital approach* because it views an employed person as producing a stream of output over the years that is valued at the individual's earnings. The main criticism of this methodology is that it excludes intangibles, only counting earnings, and undervalues some groups relative to others because earnings may not reflect one's ability to produce. Thus men are more highly valued than women, whites more than blacks, and the middle-aged more than the young and elderly, with part of the difference being due to racial and sexual discrimination. The human capital method is still most often used because it provides valuable information based upon reliable statistics, so long as one realizes its limitations.

Mortality costs were updated to 1990 by replicating the method used for 1985. The latest year for which cancer mortality data is currently available is 1988. Age-specific cancer mortality rates for 1988 (NCHS public use tape) were applied to age-specific 1990 lifetime earnings estimates. The results were adjusted to 1990 by using cancer site–specific mortality for 1990 derived from 1984–1988 trends (separately for males and females) (National Cancer Institute, 1991) and 1990 population estimates.

REFERENCES

AMERICAN CANCER SOCIETY. 1994. Cancer Statistics, 1994. Atlanta, American Cancer Society.

ANDERSON LC, SETTLE RF. 1975. Benefit-Cost Analysis: A Practical Guide. Lexington, Massachusetts, DC Heath.

BAKER MS, KESSLER LG, SMUCKER RC. 1989. Site-specific treatment costs for cancer: an analysis of the Medicare continuous history sample file. *In* Scheffler RC, Andrews NC (eds): Cancer Care and Costs: DRGs and Beyond. Ann Arbor, Michigan, Health Administration Press.

BAKER MS, KESSLER LG, URBAN N, SMUCKER RC. 1991. Estimating the treatment costs of breast and lung cancer. Med Care 29:40–49.

BERK A, PARINGER L, MUSHKIN SJ. 1978. The economic cost of illness fiscal 1975. Med Care 16:785–790.

BLOOM BS, KNORR RS, EVANS AE. 1985. The epidemiology of disease expense, the costs of caring for children with cancer. JAMA 253:2393–2397.

BROWN ML. 1990. The national economic burden of cancer: an update. J Natl Cancer Inst 82:1811–1814.

COOPER BS, RICE DP. 1976. The economic cost of illness revisited. Soc Sec Bul 39:21–36.

FELDMAN AR, KESSLER LG, MYERS MH, et al. 1986. The prevalence of cancer. Estimates based on the Connecticut Tumor Registry. N Engl J Med 315:1394–1397.

HEALTH CARE FINANCING ADMINISTRATION. 1987. National health expenditures 1986–2000. Health Care Financing Rev 8:1–36.

HEALTH CARE FINANCING ADMINISTRATION. 1990. National health expenditures, 1988. Health Care Financing Rev 11:1–54.

HODGSON TA. 1988. Annual costs of illness versus lifetime costs of illness and implications of structural change. Drug Information J 22:323–341.

HODGSON TA. 1984. The economic burden of cancer. Proceedings of the American Cancer Society Fourth National Conference on Human Values and Cancer. New York, American Cancer Society, Inc.

HODGSON TA. 1983. The state of the art of cost of illness estimates. Adv Health Econ Health Services 4:129–164.

HODGSON TA, MEINERS MR. 1982. Cost of illness methodology—a guide to current practices and procedures. Mil Mem Fund Q 60:429–462.

HOUTS PS, LIPTON A, HARVEY HA, MARTIN B, SIMMONDS MA, DIXON RH, LONGO S, ANDREWS T, GORDON RA, MELOY J, HOFFMAN SL. 1984. Nonmedical costs to patients and their families associated with outpatient chemotherapy. Cancer 53:2388–2392.

LANSKY SB, CAIRNS NU, CLARK GM, LOWMAN J, MILLER L, TRUEWORTHY R. 1979. Childhood cancer, nonmedical costs of the illness. Cancer 43:403–408.

LANSKY SB, BLACK JL, CAIRNS NU. 1983. Childhood cancer, medical costs. Cancer 52:762–766.

NATIONAL CANCER INSTITUTE. 1993. Cancer Statistics Review, 1973–1990. Publication No. (NIH) 93-2789. Bethesda, MD, National Cancer Institute.

NATIONAL CENTER FOR HEALTH STATISTICS. 1987. Advance Report of Final Mortality Statistics, 1985. Monthly Vital Statistics Report, Vol. 36, No. 5 (Suppl.), DHHS Publication No. (PHS) 87-1120. Washington, D.C., U.S. Government Printing Office.

NATIONAL CENTER FOR HEALTH STATISTICS, GRAVES EJ. 1987. Utilization of Short-stay Hospitals, United States, 1985. Vital and Health Statistics, Series 13, No. 91, DHHS Publication No. (PHS) 87-1752. Washington, D.C., U.S. Government Printing Office.

NATIONAL CENTER FOR HEALTH STATISTICS, NELSON C, MCLEMORE T. 1988. The National Ambulatory Medical Care Survey, United States, 1975–81. Vital and Health Statistics, Series 13, No. 93, DHHS Publication No. (PHS) 88-1754. Washington, D.C., U.S. Government Printing Office.

NATIONAL CENTER FOR HEALTH STATISTICS. 1988. Vital Statistics of the United States, 1985, Vol. II, Sect. 6, Life Tables. DHHS Publication No. (PHS) 88-1104. Washington, D.C., U.S. Government Printing Office.

NAYFIELD SG, HAILEY BJ. 1991. Quality of Life Assessment in Cancer Clinical Trials. Bethesda, MD, U.S. Department of Health and Human Services.

POTOSKY AL, RILEY GF, LUBITZ JD, MENTNECH RM, KESSLER LG. 1993. Potential for cancer related health services research using a linked Medicare–tumor registry database. Med Care 31:732–748.

RICE DP. 1966. Estimating the Cost of Illness. Health Economic Series No. 6, PHS Publication No. 947-6. Washington, D.C., U.S. Government Printing Office.

RICE DP, HODGSON TA. 1981. Social and Economic Implications of Cancer in the United States. Vital and Health Statistics, Series 3, No. 20, DHHS Publication No. (PHS) 81-1404. Washington, D.C., U.S. Government Printing Office.

RICE DP, HODGSON TA, KOPSTEIN AN. 1985. The economic cost of illness—a replication and update. Health Care Financing Rev 7:61–80.

RUSSELL LB. 1989. Some of the tough decisions required by a national health plan. Science 246:892–896.

SCOTTO J, CHIAZZE L. 1976. Third National Cancer Survey: Hospitalizations and Payments to Hospitals. DHEW Publication No. (NIH) 76-1094. Bethesda, MD, U.S. Department of Health, Education and Welfare.

SCOTTO J, CHIAZZE L. 1977. Cancer prevalence and hospital payments. J Natl Cancer Inst 59:345–349.

STOMMEL M, GIVEN CW, GIVEN B. 1991. The cost of cancer care to families. Working paper, Family Care Study, Department of Family Practice, Michigan State University.

U.S. BUREAU OF THE CENSUS. 1987. Money Income of Households, Families and Persons in the United States, 1985. Current Population Reports, Series P-60, No. 156. Washington, D.C., U.S. Government Printing Office.

U.S. BUREAU OF ECONOMIC ANALYSIS. 1986. Survey of Current Business. Washington, D.C., U.S. Government Printing Office.

U.S. DEPARTMENT OF COMMERCE, BUREAU OF ECONOMIC ANALYSIS. 1986. National income and product accounts tables. Surv Curr Business 66:38,65.

U.S. DEPARTMENT OF LABOR, BUREAU OF LABOR STATISTICS. 1986. Household data annual averages. Employment and Earnings 33:154–156.

WALDO D, LEVIT K, LAZENBY H. 1986. National health expenditures, 1985. Health Care Financing Rev 8:1–21.

WATSON SD. 1990. Saving Money and Helping People: A Multimethod Analysis of the Employment Experience of Cancer Survivors. Washington, D.C., Washington Business Group on Health.

PART III | The Causes of Cancer

14 Tobacco

JOHN A. BARON
THOMAS E. ROHAN

The use of tobacco in Western societies dates from the early explorers of the New World, who discovered the practice among the American natives and carried it back to Europe. The native Americans used tobacco leaf in various ways, smoking it in pipes or cigarlike rolls, chewing it, or inhaling it into the nasal passages. In Europe, pipe smoking and the use of nasal snuff gradually became fashionable. The use of cigarettes (shreds of tobacco wrapped in paper) spread in the late nineteenth century, when the introduction of rolling machines made large-scale manufacturing of them possible. Aggressive advertising then popularized this inexpensive product and led to one of the most pervasive modern health hazards (Norman, 1982; McCusker, 1988; International Agency for Research on Cancer [IARC], 1985, 1986).

Worldwide, an estimated 1 billion people smoke cigarettes (Council on Scientific Affairs, 1990), and other practices are also widespread, including the smoking of pipes or cigars (shredded tobacco wrapped in tobacco leaf). In Asia, large numbers of people smoke tobacco hand-rolled in the dried leaf of various plants (bidis), or smoke small cigars (chuttas) with the burning end held inside the mouth, a practice called "reverse smoking" (IARC, 1986; Sankaranarayanan, 1990).

The term "smokeless tobacco" refers to the noncombustive use of various tobacco products. Chewing tobacco consists of relatively coarse shreds, wads, or twists of tobacco leaf, which are chewed and retained in the oral cavity (IARC, 1985; U.S. Department of Health and Human Services [USDHHS], 1986; Council on Scientific Affairs, 1986). Snuff is a ground or powdered product that is inhaled nasally or placed in the mouth. Flavorings or additives such as sugar, molasses, or licorice (for chewing tobacco), or mint or wintergreen (for snuff) may be added. Particularly in parts of Asia, tobacco may be mixed with betel leaf, Areca nut, lime, wood ash, or other substances to form combinations such as betel quids ("pan") or nass that are chewed and/or retained in the mouth. In the United States alone, several million people use smokeless tobacco (USDHHS, 1986; Novotny et al, 1989).

Over 2000 chemical compounds have been identified in tobacco leaf (IARC, 1986; USDHHS, 1986), and many others are formed during smoking (Dube and Green, 1982). Nicotine, which accounts for .05%–4% by weight of tobacco leaves (Schmeltz and Hoffmann, 1977), is readily absorbed after smoking or oral use; circulating nicotine levels in smokers and in smokeless tobacco users are broadly similar (Benowitz, 1988). Nicotine seems responsible for addiction to tobacco use, and withdrawal syndromes after cessation of cigarette smoking are well described (USDHHS, 1988; Benowitz, 1988). Withdrawal reactions may also occur after cessation of smokeless tobacco use (Hatsukami et al, 1987).

Most tobacco products are made from the species *Nicotiana tabacum* (IARC, 1986), but there are different tobacco strains and methods of drying the tobacco leaves ("curing"). In flue-curing, the tobacco is heated (but not allowed to come in contact with smoke); in air-curing, there is little or no use of artificial heat. The air-cured tobaccos tend to be darker and have stronger taste; until recently, these were preferred for cigarettes in some Mediterranean countries and South America. In addition to being cured, some tobaccos for use in cigars, pipes, or smokeless products are fermented before sale (Tso, 1972a; Akehurst, 1981; IARC, 1986).

The composition of tobacco smoke is studied experimentally by means of smoking machines that simulate (but by no means duplicate) human smoking (Guerin, 1980; IARC, 1986; Dube and Green, 1982). The smoke is an aerosol with a vapor phase (more than 90% of the smoke by weight) and a particulate phase. "Tar" is the material left on a glass filter through which a machine has "smoked" a cigarette, after removal of water and nicotine from the residue. The tar and nicotine yield of cigarettes can be manipulated by the use of filters and changes in the composition of the tobacco (Tso, 1972b; Gori, 1976; USDHHS, 1989). However, the manner in which a cigarette is smoked also greatly influences the delivery and retention of smoke components (Rickert et al, 1983; Hoffmann and Brunnemann, 1983; IARC, 1986). "Mainstream smoke" (MS) is generated during puffing and inhalation through the butt end of the lit cigarette (or cigar or pipe). "Sidestream smoke" (SS) is the mixture that is emitted directly into the ambient environment between puffs from the smoldering tobacco. Exhaled MS, SS, and small amounts of smoke emitted during puffing make up environmental tobacco smoke (ETS) (Committee on Passive Smoking, 1986; IARC, 1986; USDHHS, 1993).

There is only a weak relationship between the nicotine delivery of cigarettes and the smokers' circulating levels of nicotine or its metabolite, cotinine (Russell et al, 1980; Benowitz et al, 1983). This apparently is due to the tendency of smokers to self-regulate their nicotine levels. For example, after switching to lower nicotine cigarettes, smokers increase the puff volume to compensate for the decreased delivery (Herning et al, 1981; Benowitz et al, 1986). It is not clear if this compensation prevents a materially reduced exposure to nicotine (and other tobacco products) in the smokers of low tar/nicotine cigarettes (Russell et al, 1986; Wald and Froggatt, 1989).

TOBACCO USE AND CANCER: EPIDEMIOLOGICAL FINDINGS

The cancer risks of tobacco use, especially cigarette smoking, have been extensively investigated. Much relevant data can be obtained from several large cohort studies, largely of mortality (Hammond and Horn, 1958; Kahn, 1966; Hammond, 1966; Department of National Health and Welfare, 1966; Weir and Dunn, 1970; Cederlof et al, 1975; Doll and Peto, 1976; Doll et al, 1980; Garfinkel, 1980; Carstensen et al, 1987; Hirayama, 1990). While most of these studies collected detailed data on tobacco use, many did not collect information that would permit control for potentially important confounding variables such as diet, alcohol use, sexual and reproductive behavior, and body weight or body habitus. Also, the reliance of these studies on death certificate data prevented them from verifying cancer diagnoses and distinguishing the effects of smoking on cancer incidence from those on case fatality.

In many ways, the ascertainment of cigarette smoking history in epidemiological studies is relatively straightforward. Qualitative aspects of active and passive smoking can be assessed through questionnaires with relatively high repeatability, although quantitative aspects are assessed with less precision (USDHHS, 1990; Krall et al, 1989; Coultas et al, 1989). Surrogate respondents (eg, spouse, siblings) also provide qualitative information on active and passive smoking that agrees well with that obtained by self-report (USDHHS, 1990; Cummings et al, 1989). However, comparison of national sales data with survey reports suggests there may be a bias toward underreporting in interviews (Peto, 1986; USDHHS, 1990; Warner, 1978).

Concerns over the validity of questionnaire-based methods of assessment of tobacco exposure have led to the use of biochemical measures of exposure, of which the most studied have been cotinine, carbon monoxide, and thiocyanate (National Research Council, 1986; USDHHS, 1990). At present, the method of choice—by virtue of its sensitivity and specificity—is measurement of cotinine in blood, urine, or saliva. Carbon monoxide (CO) levels can be measured in exhaled alveolar air or can be estimated from blood carboxyhemoglobin levels; however, because exposure to CO can occur from sources other than cigarette smoke, this approach has relatively poor specificity. Thiocyanate testing also has lower sensitivity and specificity than other methods. One limitation of all of these methods of testing is that they relate to smoking within the last few days (for cotinine or carbon monoxide) or weeks (for thiocyanate), so that their main application is in differentiating current or recent active smokers from nonsmokers. Also, because of individual differences in metabolism of nicotine, even cotinine measurements cannot be used to quantitate the nicotine exposure of individuals (Idle, 1990; USDHHS, 1990). Adducts of tobacco smoke products with blood-based proteins such as hemoglobin are correlated with the intensity of smoking; these may both extend the period during which ex-smokers can be detected, and provide a means of quantifying the biological effect of exposure to genotoxic smoke constituents (Perera et al, 1987; Bailey et al, 1988).

Cigarette smoking poses some other unique methodological problems in epidemiological research. One difficulty derives from the fact that most smokers begin their habit over a relatively narrow age range (roughly ages 14 to 21 years). Therefore analyses of the association between duration of smoking and cancer risk among current smokers may be confounded by the close relationship between age and the duration of smoking (Morrison, et al 1984; USDHHS, 1990). Summarization of smoking history is another difficult issue. Indices produced by multiplying duration by intensity of consumption (eg, pack-years or cigarette-years) are commonly used, but these may not provide a biologically appropriate summary; separate consideration of duration and intensity of smoking may be required (Doll and Peto, 1978; Peto, 1986; Moolgavkar et al, 1989).

The Association of Cigarette Smoking with Cancer

Cancers of the Oropharynx and Respiratory Tract. Cigarette smoking has been associated with cancer over the entire respiratory tract. For cancer of the buccal cavity and pharynx, the relative risk for current smoking (after adjustment for alcohol intake) has been about 2 to 3 in most studies (IARC, 1986; Blot et al, 1988; Merletti et al, 1989; Zheng et al, 1990), but some hospital-based investigations have reported adjusted relative risks greater than 10 in heavy smokers relative to never smokers (De Stefani et al, 1988; Franceschi et al, 1990; Oreggia et al, 1991). From the limited data available regarding histological varieties of buccal/pharyngeal cancers, these associations appear to be stronger for squamous cancer than for cancers with other histological patterns (Stockwell and Lyman, 1986; Zheng et al, 1990). Bidis, like cigarettes, also confer high relative risks for cancers of the oropharynx (as well as of the larynx) (Sankaranarayanan et al, 1989b, Sankaranarayanan, 1990; Nandakumar et al, 1990).

For cancers of the larynx and lung, the risk conferred by current cigarette smoking is very high: With the strong dose-response patterns that have generally been observed, the relative risk rises to 15 or more for heavy smokers (Fig. 14–1). The relative risk also increases with duration of smoking, and consequently inversely with the age at which smoking is begun (IARC, 1986; Tuyns et al, 1988; La Vecchia et al, 1990a; Zatonski et al, 1991). For lung cancer, smoking duration seems to be a more potent risk factor than the number of cigarettes smoked (Doll and Peto, 1978; Peto, 1986) and the effects on adenocarcinoma (relative risk 3–5) are much less marked than on tumors with squamous or small-cell histology (relative risk 15 or more) (Lubin and Blot, 1984; IARC, 1986). Cigarette smoking has also been associated with preneoplastic changes in the respiratory tract (Auerbach et al, 1979).

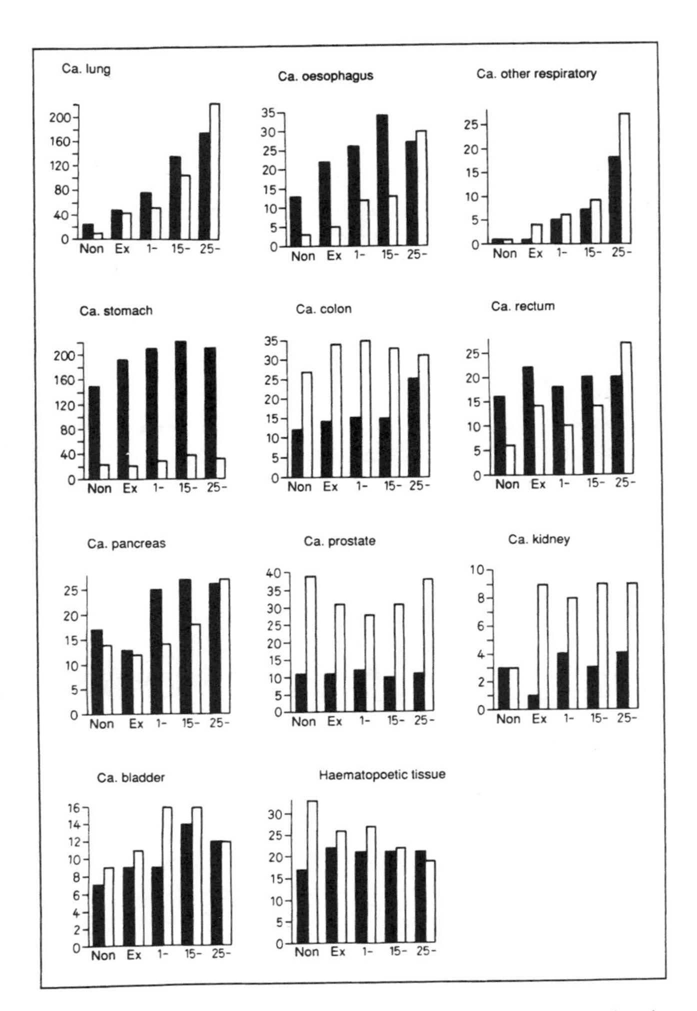

FIG. 14–1. Age-standardized mortality rates per 100,000 males, by smoking habit, in the Japanese Cohort Study (filled bars) and the UK Physicians' Study (open bars). (Adapted from Hirayama, 1990.)

Most studies of cancers of the nasal cavity and paranasal sinuses have reported an increased risk among cigarette smokers (Brinton et al, 1984; Stockwell and Lyman, 1986; Hayes et al, 1987; Fukuda and Shibata, 1990; Zheng et al, 1992). As elsewhere in the respiratory tract, the increased risk has typically been more evident for squamous cell carcinomas than for adenocarcinomas (Brinton et al, 1984; Hayes et al, 1987; Zheng et al, 1992). In contrast, studies of nasopharyngeal carcinoma have not consistently indicated a smoking-associated risk (IARC, 1986; Hildesheim and Levine, 1993; Chow et al, 1993); those of lip cancer have been inconclusive (IARC, 1986; Douglass and Gammon, 1984; Stockwell and Lyman, 1986); and those of salivary gland cancer have generally shown no association (Spitz et al, 1984; Stockwell and Lyman, 1986; Preston-Martin et al, 1988).

Cancers of the Gastrointestinal Tract. In the digestive tract, the relationship between cancer and cigarette smoking becomes weaker with progression from esophagus to rectum. For cancer of the esophagus (largely squamous carcinoma) heavy current smokers have a relative risk of about 5, which remains after control for covariates (mainly alcohol use) (IARC, 1986; Tuyns and Esteve, 1983; Li et al, 1989; Franceschi et al, 1990; DeStefani et al, 1993). However, the association of cigarette smoking with adenocarcinoma of the stomach is less clear. Most studies have reported a modest relationship (relative risk for current smokers about 1.3–1.5) (IARC, 1986; You et al, 1988; Buiatti et al, 1989; Ferraroni et al, 1989; McLaughlin et al, 1990; Hansson et al, 1994), although a few investigations have reported higher relative risks (Wu-Williams et al, 1990; Nomura et al, 1990; Kneller et al, 1991). In the positive studies, typically only a weak dose-response relationship has been found (IARC, 1986; You et al, 1988; Nomura et al, 1990; McLaughlin et al, 1990) (Fig. 14–1); few investigations have addressed possible confounding factors such as diet (You et al, 1988; Wu-Williams et al, 1990). Although several studies have suggested stronger smoking effects for adenocarcinoma of the gastric cardia than at other stomach sites, the data regarding subsite differences remains inconclusive (Wu-Williams et al, 1990; Palli et al, 1992; Jedrychowski et al, 1993; Inoue et al, 1994). Investigation of precursor lesions such as chronic atrophic gastritis and intestinal metaplasia has yielded inconsistent indications of associations with cigarette smoking (Nomura et al, 1982; Tatsuta et al, 1988; Stemmermann et al, 1990).

Cigarette smoking does not appear to substantially affect the risk of adenocarcinoma of the colon and rectum (Baron and Sandler, 1990; Kune et al, 1992) (Fig. 14–1). However, two large cohort studies have suggested that smoking may be a risk factor after a long latent interval, and several (but not all) studies of large bowel polyps suggest that cigarette smokers have an increased prevalence of adenomas (Demers et al, 1988; Kono et al, 1990; Kune et al, 1992; Giovannucci et al, 1994a,b). Cancer of the anus, a malignancy with a squamous or transitional-cell histology, has repeatedly been found to be positively associated with cigarette smoking (Holly et al, 1989; Daling et al, 1992).

Many studies of hepatocellular carcinoma have indicated a relationship with cigarette smoking (Trichopoulos et al, 1987; Hirayama, 1989; Tsukuma et al, 1990; Tsukuma et al, 1993), although few of these accounted for possible confounding (eg, by alcohol use) in detail, and other investigations found at most a weak association with smoking (Austin et al, 1986; La Vecchia et al, 1988). The relationship may be limited to hepatocellular carcinoma occurring in the absence of evident hepatitis B infection, a cancer for which an association with cigarette smoking has repeatedly been found (Lam et al, 1982; Austin et al, 1986; Trichopoulos et al, 1987; Tsukuma et al, 1990). There appears to be no substantial effect of cigarette smoking on the risk of cancer of the gallbladder or biliary tract (Williams and Horm, 1977; Garfinkel, 1980; Carstensen et al, 1987; Hirayama, 1990; Zatonski et al, 1992), although one study found evidence of an inverse association (Yen et al, 1987).

Adenocarcinoma of the pancreas is more clearly related to cigarette smoking: current smokers have a twofold or higher increase in risk in most studies (IARC, 1986; Mack et al, 1986; Bouchardy et al, 1990; Bueno de Mesquita et al, 1991) (Fig. 14–1). However, some investigators have not found a pattern of increasing risks with increasing amounts smoked (Howe et al, 1991). An increased prevalence of atypical nuclei in ductal and parenchymal cells among smokers has been noted in one autopsy survey (Auerbach and Garfinkel, 1986).

Cancers of the Urinary Tract. Cigarette smoking has been closely associated with cancers of the bladder, ureter, and pelvis of the kidney (IARC, 1986; Jensen et al, 1987, 1988; Hartge et al, 1987; Augustine et al, 1988; Burch et al, 1989; McCredie and Stewart, 1992). For transitional cell carcinoma of the bladder, the relative risks have been about 2–3 for currently smoking subjects, rising to as high as 5–6 for current heavy smokers (Fig. 14–1). Dose-response patterns have been demonstrated with the amount usually smoked and with duration of smoking. Relative risks for cancer of the renal pelvis and ureter have been at least as high as those for the bladder; two sets of studies in which both bladder and renal pelvis/ureter cancer have been investigated in one geographic area have shown the dose-response curves for smoking to be steeper for cancer of the renal pelvis/ureter (McCredie et al, 1983; Jensen et al, 1988). Smokers also have an increased prevalence of preneoplastic changes in the bladder (Auerbach and Garfinkel, 1989), but appear not to have an increased risk of adenocarcinoma of the bladder (Kantor et al, 1988).

For adenocarcinoma of the kidney the relative risks (about 2 for current smokers) are lower than those found for the squamous or transitional cell cancers lower in the urinary tract (IARC, 1986; McLaughlin et al, 1984; McLaughlin et al, 1992; McCredie and Stewart, 1992) (Fig. 14–1). Gradients in risk with increasing amounts smoked have not been large, but the association does not appear to be due to confounding by factors such as body habitus or analgesic use (McLaughlin et al, 1984; Yu et al, 1986; Talamini et al, 1990; McCredie and Stewart, 1992).

Cancers of the Reproductive Tract/Breast. Cigarette smoking has been associated with an increased risk of squamous cancer of the cervix, as well as with cervical intraepithelial neoplasia (IARC, 1986; Winkelstein, 1990; Brock et al, 1989; Herrero et al, 1989), often with trends in risk over increasing amounts or duration of smoking. Some of the studies have controlled carefully for possible confounding by factors such as sexual behavior and PAP smear testing, with retention of the effect, albeit weakened. Control for the presence of human papilloma virus (HPV) more markedly reduces the association with smoking (Herrero et al, 1989; Bosch et al, 1992; Schiffman et al, 1993), and the independent effect of smoking on risk remains unclear (Phillips and Smith, 1994). There does not appear to be an association of smoking with adenocarcinoma of the cervix (Brinton et al, 1987; Silcocks et al, 1987; Parazzini et al, 1988).

Endometrial cancer may be unique among cancers in that women who currently smoke cigarettes appear to have a *lowered* risk, even after control for relevant covariates such as body weight (Baron et al, 1990; Weiss, 1990; Brinton et al, 1993). Several (but not all) studies have reported a gradient of decreasing risks with increasing amounts smoked, and heavy smokers may have risks as low as 20% of that of never smokers. Some investigations have found that the inverse association between smoking and endometrial cancer is either confined to postmenopausal women, or is much stronger than among premenopausal women (Baron et al, 1990; Wald and Baron, 1990).

Several case-control studies have investigated the relationship of cigarette smoking with cancer of the vulva; all have found a positive association (Daling et al, 1992). However, from the very limited data available, it appears that smoking does not have an association with cancer of the vagina (Brinton et al, 1990; Daling et al, 1992).

Studies of epithelial cancer of the ovary have generally shown no substantial association with cigarette smoking (Franks et al, 1987; Beral et al, 1988; Whittemore et al, 1988). A few studies have reported higher risks in women who smoke (Doll and Peto, 1976; Cramer et al, 1984; Shu et al, 1989), but in most of these analyses the increase was not statistically significant, and there was no pattern of increasing risk with increasing amounts smoked. Moreover, other studies (Whittemore et al, 1988) have shown a weak negative association (again typically not statistically significant, and without dose-response patterns). Few of the studies have investigated separately the various histological types of epithelial ovarian cancer.

Cigarette smoking does not substantially affect the risk of breast cancer in women or in men (Wald and Baron, 1990; Palmer and Rosenberg, 1993; Mabuchi et al, 1985; Casagrande et al, 1988; Thomas et al, 1992). Moreover, separate analyses of premenopausal and postmenopausal women have not revealed an effect in either group alone, nor have investigations of estrogen-receptor positive or receptor-negative tumors (Palmer and Rosenberg, 1993). Cigarette smoking is also unrelated to "benign breast disease" among premenopausal women, although there are suggestions of an inverse relationship after menopause (Wald and Baron, 1990; Baron et al, 1990). One study suggests that cigarette smoking is not associated with the proliferative breast lesions that have been linked most strongly with breast cancer (Rohan et al, 1989).

Most investigations of adenocarcinoma of the prostate have reported no association with cigarette smoking (Cederlof et al, 1975; Doll and Peto, 1976; Garfinkel, 1980; Hirayama, 1990; Talamini et al, 1993) (Fig. 14–1), although some have noted increased risks, particularly among heavy smokers (Hammond, 1966; Honda et al, 1988; Hsing et al, 1991; Hiatt et al, 1994). Cancer of the testis has not been as extensively investigated, but seems unrelated to smoking (Schwartz et al, 1961; Henderson et al, 1979; Rogot and Murray, 1980; Coldman et al, 1982; Brown et al, 1987). Data regarding the association between cigarette smoking and cancer of the penis are conflicting (Schwartz et al, 1961; Hellberg et al, 1987; Brinton et al, 1991; Daling et al, 1992).

Other Epithelial Cancers. There are few data available regarding the effect of cigarette smoking on nonmelanoma skin cancer. Smoking appears not to increase the risk of basal cell carcinoma (Hunter et al, 1990), but it may be associated with an increased risk of squamous carcinoma (Aubry and MacGibbon, 1985; Karagas et al, 1992). Despite suggestions that cigarette smoking increases the metastatic potential of melanoma (Shaw and Milton, 1981), no consistent smoking-related effect on its incidence or mortality has been observed (Garfinkel, 1980; Rogot and Murray, 1980; Osterlind et al, 1988; Evans et al, 1988; Stryker et al, 1990). Smoking is also not related to thyroid cancer (Williams and Horm, 1977; Rogot and Murray, 1980; Garfinkel, 1980; McTiernan et al, 1984; Ron et al, 1987; Kolonel et al, 1990).

Nonepithelial Cancers. Several cohort and case-control studies have indicated that cigarette smokers have a modestly increased relative risk of leukemia (about 1.5), and especially of acute myelogenous (or acute nonlymphocytic) leukemia (Siegel, 1993). There are also reports indicating that among patients with chronic myelogenous leukemia, smokers have a shortened period to blast phase (Herr et al, 1990; Archimbaud et al, 1989).

Cigarette smoking appears unrelated to other hematological malignancies, including lymphoma in aggregate, non-Hodgkin's lymphoma, Hodgkin's disease, myeloma, mycosis fungoides, and hairy cell leukemia (Hammond and Horn, 1958; Weir and Dunn, 1970; Newell et al, 1973; Williams and Horm, 1977; Rogot and Murray, 1980; Garfinkel, 1980; Hardell et al, 1981; Oleske et al, 1985; Bernard et al, 1987; Woods et al, 1987; Tuyp et al, 1987; Franceschi et al, 1989; Brown et al, 1992). Primary neoplasms of the central nervous system are also unrelated to smoking (Cederlof et al, 1975; Garfinkel, 1980; Rogot and Murray, 1980; Burch et al, 1987; Preston-Martin et al, 1989). The data regarding soft-tissue sarcoma are mixed (Zahm et al, 1992).

Effects of Inhalation and Cessation. Investigation of the effects of inhalation of cigarette smoke is difficult because of the likelihood of confounding by the amount and pattern of smoking. Moreover, self-reports of inhalation may be unreliable (Wald et al, 1978; Stepney, 1982). Nonetheless, studies of the association between tobacco smoke inhalation and cancer risk have yielded fairly consistent results. Smokers who report inhaling have an increased risk of cancers of the larynx, bladder, and pelvis of the kidney compared to noninhalers (Tuyns et al, 1988; IARC, 1986; Jensen et al, 1988;

Clavel et al, 1989; Burch et al, 1989); for cancer of the lung, the associations are more complicated. Inhaling is associated with an increased risk among light smokers, but among heavy smokers, inhaling has been associated with *lower* risks. This may be due to the pattern of bronchial flow in heavy and light inhalers (Wald et al, 1983).

Study of the potential benefits of smoking cessation are complicated by several technical points. Smokers may quit smoking because of ill health, which would obviously tend to associate cessation with adverse events. For this reason, many studies of smoking cessation include recent quitters as current smokers. Also, former smokers may differ from current smokers with regard to important factors such as the numbers of cigarettes smoked, duration of smoking, exercise, diet, or other health-related behaviors. Finally, the benefits of cessation will be a combination of the avoidance of further tobacco exposure and the degradation (if any) of the excess risk associated with past exposure; in analyses of the reduction of risk according to time since quitting, it may be difficult or impossible to separate these effects (USDHHS, 1990).

The relative risk of cancer at most smoking-related sites is noticeably lower than that of current smokers after about 5 years' cessation (IARC, 1986; USDHHS, 1990) (Fig. 14–2). However, for cancer of the bladder, some studies have found that former smokers retain an elevated risk even after prolonged cessation (USHHS 1990; Lopez-Abente et al, 1991), and for adenocarcinoma of the kidney, it may take 10 years or more for the relative risks to decrease (McLaughlin et al, 1984; LaVecchia et al, 1990b; McCredie and Stewart, 1992). Former smokers generally have risks of cancer of the cervix intermediate between those of current and never smokers, although several studies have found no increase in risk among former smokers as a group (USDHHS, 1990).

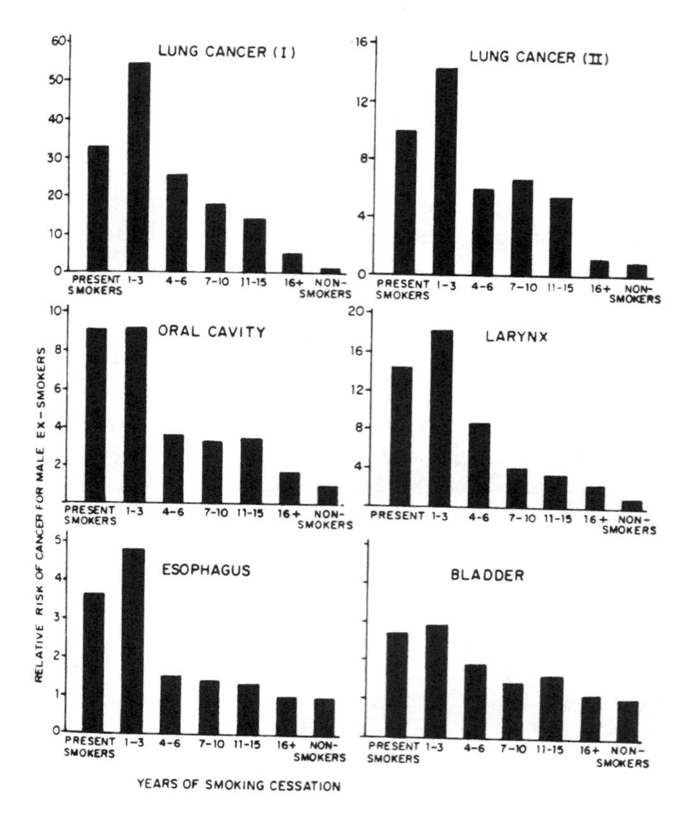

FIG. 14–2. Relative risks of cancer at selected sites in males, by years since quitting cigarette smoking. (Adapted from Wynder and Stellman, 1977.)

The Changing Cigarette and Cancer. Differences in the way in which tobacco is used will obviously influence the associated health risks, but even a particular tobacco practice may have variable effects depending on the filters used, degree of inhalation, and so on. Moreover, additives may have an impact, and the tobacco itself may vary from place to place. In some Mediterranean and South American countries there has been a recent shift from the use of dark, air-cured tobacco for cigarettes to lighter, flue-cured varieties. These changes have implications for cancer risk because there appear to be differences in the carcinogenic potential of these types of tobaccos. Smokers of dark tobacco cigarettes have repeatedly been found to have higher risks of bladder cancer than smokers of light tobacco cigarettes (D'Avanzo et al, 1990; Vineis, 1991). Similar findings have been reported for cancers of the oropharynx, larynx, esophagus, and lung as well (De Stefani et al, 1987; Merletti et al, 1989; Oreggia et al, 1991; Benhamou and Benhamou, 1993; De Stefani et al, 1993), though not for cervical cancer (Herrero et al, 1989). In contrast, mentholated cigarettes appear to be neither more, nor less, carcinogenic than nonmentholated varieties (Kabat and Hebert, 1994). However, for all these associations there remain questions of confounding by factors such as alcohol use, duration of smoking, and use of filters.

In many industrialized countries, there have been substantial changes in cigarettes since the 1950s (Norman, 1982; Ramstrom, 1986; USDHHS, 1989) (Fig. 14–3). Between the mid-1950s and the mid-1980s, the average tar delivery of American cigarettes dropped from over 35 mg to 13 mg, and nicotine yields from over 2.5 mg to 1 mg (Norman, 1982; USDHHS, 1989). Similar changes have occurred elsewhere in the industrialized world (Wald et al, 1981; Ramstrom, 1986). These changes are the result of increasing use of cigarette filters, decreases in the amount of tobacco used in each cigarette, changes in the design of the cigarettes, and changes in the preparation and characteristics of the tobacco used (Gori, 1976; USDHHS, 1981; Norman, 1982). The composition of MS and SS smoke is determined by different factors, and the decline in the nico-

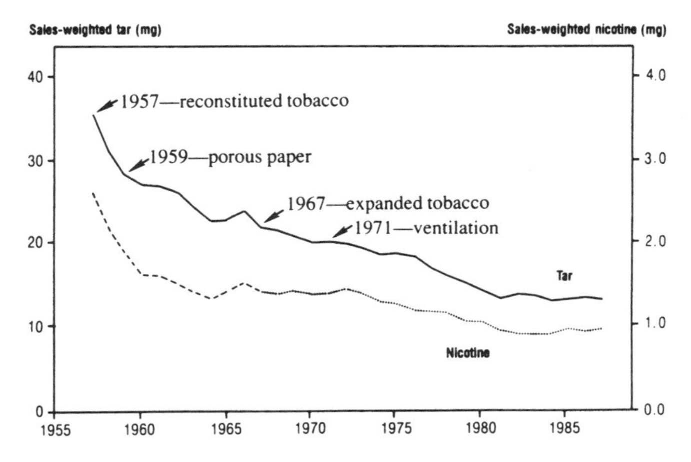

FIG. 14–3. Sales-weighted average tar and nicotine content of cigarettes sold in the United States, by years, 1957–1987. (Taken from USDHHS, 1989.)

tine and tar yields of modern cigarettes has not affected the content of SS smoke as substantially as it has changed that of MS smoke (Adams et al, 1987).

The changing cigarette has apparently had an impact on cancer risk. Smokers of filtered cigarettes have a lower risk of cancers of the lung and larynx than smokers of unfiltered brands (IARC, 1986; Stellman, 1986a; Stellman and Garfinkel, 1989; Kaufman et al 1989; La Vecchia et al, 1990a). However, even smokers of the lowest tar brands remain at substantially higher risk than those who quit smoking altogether, or who never smoked. Evidence regarding the association of low-tar cigarettes with the risk of cancer at other sites is more limited, but the patterns for cancer of the oropharynx, esophagus, and pancreas appear similar to those for cancer of the lung and larynx (Stellman, 1986a; Lee and Garfinkel, 1981; Merletti et al, 1989; La Vecchia et al, 1990a); for cancers of the bladder, the data are conflicting (IARC, 1986; Hartge et al, 1987; Wynder et al, 1988; Clavel et al, 1989; Burch et al, 1989).

Interactions with Other Exposures. Investigation of the combined effects of cigarette smoking and other exposures has largely focused on cancer sites that have strong smoking associations and on other exposures that are themselves related to cancer risk (Saracci, 1987). For cancers of the oropharynx, larynx, and esophagus, the risk models best describing the combined effect of smoking and alcohol appear to be approximately multiplicative or intermediate between additive and multiplicative (IARC, 1986; Saracci, 1987; IARC, 1988; Blot et al, 1988; Merletti et al, 1989; Franco et al, 1989; Franceschi et al, 1990; Zheng et al, 1990) (illustrated in Fig. 14–4). Similar findings have been reported for lung cancer and the joint effects of smoking and occupational exposure to radiation or asbestos (Stellman, 1986b; IARC, 1986; Saracci, 1987; Samet et al, 1989). In contrast, modeling of smoking and occupational exposure to nickel or arsenic tends to show joint lung cancer effects that are closer to additive (Saracci, 1987). For bladder cancer, the joint effect of smoking and occupational exposure to aromatic amines appears to fit a multiplicative model (Saracci, 1987; D'Avanzo et al, 1990).

Several studies have investigated whether the effects of vegetable or carotene intake on lung cancer risks differ according to smoking status, but no consistent pattern has emerged (Ziegler et al, 1986; Le Marchand et al, 1989; Steinmetz et al, 1993). A possible interaction between high intake of animal fat and smoking has been proposed, but relevant data are sparse (Xie et al, 1991). Information regarding possible interactions between smoking and diet on the risk of cervical cancer is also too scanty to permit any conclusions (Brock et al, 1988; Ziegler et al, 1990). Studies of all these topics are hampered by the difficulties of dietary assessment, and the large sample sizes required to estimate interactions reliably.

Little is known about the relationship between infectious agents and the cancer risks associated with tobacco use. The possibility that smoking may be a stronger risk factor for hepatocellular carcinoma among individuals who are not carriers of hepatitis B has been discussed above. There are data suggesting that cigarette smoking is a stronger risk factor for cervical neoplasms among women with evidence of HPV infection than among those without (Herrero et al, 1989), but there is also evidence to the contrary (Bosch et al, 1992). Investigation of these issues is greatly hampered by difficulties in measuring the presence or absence of the relevant infectious agent.

Pipe and Cigar Smoking. In assessing the risks associated with smoking pipes or cigars, cigarette smoking

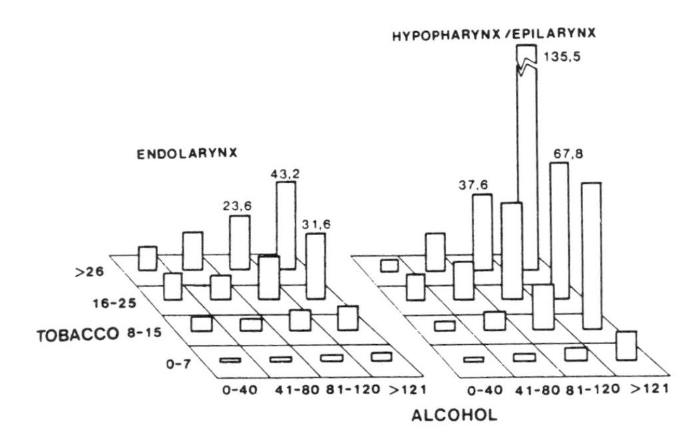

FIG. 14–4. Relative risks of cancers of the larynx and hypopharynx at combined levels of daily cigarette smoking (cigarettes per day) and alcohol consumption (grams per day). (Taken from Tuyns et al, 1988.)

must also be taken into account, either by including cigarette smoking as a covariate, or by restricting analysis to subjects who (in their lifetimes) smoked only pipes or cigars. For cancers of the oropharynx, larynx, and esophagus, cigar and/or pipe smoking is associated with relative risks similar to those for cigarette smoking (IARC, 1986; Blot et al, 1988; Merletti et al, 1989; Falk et al, 1989; Zheng et al, 1990). Smokers of pipes and/or cigars also have increased risks of lung cancer, although the relative risks are not as high as those for cigarette smokers (IARC, 1986; Higgins et al, 1988). Most studies have not shown a materially increased risk of cancer of the urinary tract associated with pipe and/or cigar smoking (Hartge et al, 1985; IARC, 1986; Jensen et al, 1987, 1988; Slattery et al, 1988; Steineck et al, 1988; Burch et al, 1989).

Passive Smoking. Epidemiological studies of the effects of environmental tobacco smoke (passive smoking) have largely focused on lung cancer. These have been complicated by several problems, including the small numbers of cases occurring among nonsmokers, possible misclassification of smokers or former smokers as never smokers, and difficulty in measuring the dose of the exposure (Committee on Passive Smoking, 1986; Lee, 1987; USDHHS, 1993). Numerous studies have considered the risk of lung cancer among nonsmoking women exposed to ETS, and several overviews have been published (eg, Committee on Passive Smoking, 1986; Spitzer et al, 1990; Fleiss and Gross, 1991; USDHHS, 1993). Relative risk estimates have varied, but have generally been less than 2 for exposed women overall; summary estimates (after adjustment for misclassification of some smokers as nonsmokers) are approximately 1.2 for studies conducted in the United States or Western Europe (USDHHS, 1993). More recent studies have reported results at least consistent with this estimate (Fontham et al, 1994), but the subject remains controversial (Lee, 1987; Fleiss and Gross, 1991). A particular impact of ETS exposure during childhood on adult lung cancer is even more uncertain (Fontham et al, 1994, Janerich et al, 1990).

Some investigators have reported increased risks of cancer at sites other than the lung among passive smokers, although the data are insufficient to permit any conclusions (Spitzer et al, 1990; Remmer, 1987; Sandler et al, 1985a; Slattery et al, 1989; Hirayama, 1990). Maternal smoking during pregnancy does not seem to be associated with childhood cancer (Pershagen et al, 1992), but investigations of its association with parental smoking during childhood have reported conflicting results (IARC, 1986; Spitzer et al, 1990; Sandler et al, 1985b; McKinney and Stiller, 1986; Buckley et al, 1986; Magnani et al, 1990).

Smokeless Tobacco

Research on smokeless tobacco is complicated by the possible confounding effects of alcohol intake and cigarette smoking, both of which are associated with all of the malignancies that may be caused by smokeless tobacco. Since there is some evidence of a *negative* correlation between the use of smokeless tobacco and cigarettes, ignoring smoking may result in conservative estimates of smokeless tobacco risks (USDHHS, 1986). However, no similar statement can be made about the confounding effects of alcohol use.

The oral use of smokeless tobacco is clearly associated with cancer of the oropharynx, often at the specific site where the tobacco is usually placed. Numerous studies have reported relative risks of 3 to 20 or more, with risk increasing with duration of use. The highest risks have been associated with cancers of the anterior tongue, buccal mucosa or gingiva, areas with the most direct contact with the tobacco (IARC, 1985; USDHHS, 1986; Stockwell and Lyman, 1986; Blot et al, 1988). The association seems stronger for oral snuff use than for chewing tobacco, possibly because of the close continued mucosal contact generated by snuff dipping (Mattson and Winn, 1989). The study by Winn and colleagues (1981, 1984) provides the most convincing epidemiological evidence for an association between smokeless tobacco use with oral cancer: there were clear dose-response effects, and the risks could not be explained by smoking, alcohol, or diet. Not surprisingly, smokeless tobacco use has also been associated with an increased incidence and prevalence of oral leukoplakia, a precancerous lesion (Mehta et al, 1981; IARC, 1985; USDHHS, 1986; Ernster et al, 1990). As with oral cancer, this association appears stronger for oral snuff use than for chewing tobacco (Ernster et al, 1990). There are few data regarding the benefits of cessation of smokeless tobacco use on cancer risk. However, for leukoplakia it appears that the relative risks decline markedly after cessation, so that former users are not at substantially increased risk (Ernster et al, 1990).

The chewing of quids containing tobacco (as well as other substances such as areca nut, betel leaf, and lime) is closely associated with oral cancer (IARC, 1985; USDHHS, 1986; Sankaranarayanan et al, 1989a,b; Sankaranarayanan, 1990; Nandakumar et al, 1990). Studies that have considered the composition of the products chewed have indicated that the users of tobacco-containing quids have higher risks of oral cancer than those who chew quids without tobacco (IARC 1985, USDHHS, 1986; Gupta et al, 1982; Nandakumar et al, 1990).

The evidence linking smokeless tobacco to cancer outside of the oropharynx is much less secure. Several investigations have reported modestly elevated risks of cancer of the esophagus among smokeless tobacco users, but none adjusted for the possible confounding effects of both smoking and alcohol intake (IARC, 1985; USDHHS, 1986; Cook-Mozaffari, 1979; Jussawalla, 1981). In Asian populations, adding tobacco to betel quids does not appear to increase the risk of esophageal cancer (Jussawalla and Deshpande, 1971; Jussawalla, 1981). This may be because tobacco chewers spit out the saliva/juice produced by chewing, whereas the chewers of quids without tobacco swallow it (Jussawalla, 1981). Data regarding the relationship between smokeless tobacco use and cancers of the larynx, nasal cavity, or sinuses are conflicting, and allow no firm conclusions to be drawn (IARC, 1985; Jussawalla and Deshpande, 1971; Wynder and Stellman, 1977; Williams and Horm, 1977; Sankaranarayanan et al, 1990; Brinton et al, 1984; Stockwell and Lyman, 1986).

THE BIOLOGY OF TOBACCO USE AND CANCER

The Carcinogenic Potential of Tobacco and Tobacco Smoke

Tobacco Leaf. While nicotine is probably not a classic tumor initiator, it may function as a promoter or cocarcinogen (Bock, 1971, 1980), and is transformed during curing and smoking to tobacco-specific nitrosamines (TSNAs), which clearly are carcinogenic (Hecht and Hoffmann, 1988). The concentration of nitrosamines in snuff far exceeds that allowed in other consumer products, and snuff dippers have high levels of hemoglobin adducts of TSNAs (Carmella et al, 1990). However, in general, animal studies have shown only weak evidence of carcinogenicity from tobacco contact, possibly because of their small size and short duration of exposure (IARC, 1985). For example, application of tobacco or snuff to the oral mucosa of rodents has generally not resulted in oral cancers except in the presence of infection with herpes simplex virus (USDHHS, 1986; Park et al, 1988). Nonetheless, extracts of cured (but not green) tobacco have tumor-promoting activity when applied topically to mouse skin (Bock, 1971). In humans, smokeless tobacco use does not appear to increase levels of DNA adducts in the oral mucosa (Dunn and Stich, 1986; Chacko and Gupta, 1988), and its effect on micronuclei in the oral mucosa has not been clearly delineated (Tolbert et al, 1991).

Tobacco Smoke. Many known carcinogens and promoters are formed during the smoking of tobacco or are transmitted to the smoke from the leaf. These include polycyclic aromatic hydrocarbons (eg, benzo[a]pyrene), aromatic amines (eg, naphthylamine), aldehydes (eg, formaldehyde), other phenolic compounds (eg, phenol, catechol), a variety of free radicals, and TSNAs (Guerin, 1980; IARC, 1986; Hoffmann and Hecht, 1990). The particulate phase of cigarette smoke is particularly rich in carcinogens (IARC, 1986; Hoffmann and Wynder, 1986), providing one rationale for the use of filters. In addition to reducing tar, the commonly used cellulose filters also reduce delivery of phenols and volatile nitrosamines (Norman, 1982; Hoffmann and Hecht, 1990).

Sidestream smoke actually contains higher concentrations of many tobacco smoke products than MS, including nicotine, carbon monoxide, benzene, and several polycyclic aromatic hydrocarbons. Of course SS and exhaled MS are diluted rapidly by ambient air under most circumstances, and so the potency of ETS as it is actually encountered is likely to be much lower than that of MS or SS in pure form. (On the other hand, it may be inhaled for prolonged periods, rather than intermittently, as is MS.) Most extrapolations indicate that persons heavily exposed to ETS absorb no more than the amount of nicotine expected from smoking one or two cigarettes per day, and probably considerably less (National Research Council, 1986; Blot and Fraumeni, 1986). For carbon monoxide and volatile nitrosamines, the "cigarette equivalents" are probably higher (Lee, 1982; Jarvis, 1989).

Cigarette smoke condensate is a classic cancer initiator when applied topically, especially the fractions containing polycyclic aromatic hydrocarbons. Animal studies confirm the carcinogenic potential of cigarette smoke in tissues having smoke contact: smoke exposure leads to laryngeal tumors and pulmonary adenomas, although pulmonary carcinomas result less often. An increased incidence of cancers outside the respiratory tree is not generally seen (IARC, 1986; Ketkar et al, 1984; Henry and Kouri, 1986). These inhalation studies are limited by the difficulties of exposing short-lived small animals to smoke for prolonged periods in a manner that resembles human smoking (IARC, 1986).

There is human evidence of genotoxicity from tobacco smoke in tissues having direct smoke contact (IARC, 1986; Gupta et al, 1989). Cigarette smokers have increased levels of DNA adducts in the lung and bronchus compared to nonsmokers (Phillips et al, 1990; van Schooten et al, 1990; Dunn et al, 1991). Data regarding the details of the actual DNA damage caused by smoking are limited; however, cigarette smoking is associated with K-*ras* mutations among patients with adenocarcinoma of the lung (Westra et al, 1993). Similar mutations are caused by TSNAs in experimental lung cancer in rats (Belinsky et al, 1989) and are found in oral cancers occurring among tobacco quid chewers (Saranath et al, 1991). Mutations in the p53 gene are also common in smoking-related cancers (Davidson et al, 1993). For cancers of the aero-digestive tract, the *ras* and p53 mutations tend to be guanine to thymine transversions, which are typical of chemical carcinogens such as benzo[a]pyrene.

Cigarette smoking is also associated with effects in organs lacking direct smoke contact, reflecting the absorption of tobacco smoke constituents into the circulation. Nicotine and cotinine are concentrated in cervical mucus as well as in ovarian follicular fluid and breast fluid (Hellberg and Nilsson, 1988; Hill and Wynder, 1979; Weiss and Eckert, 1989; McCann et al, 1992), and there are inconsistent reports that passive smokers may also have increased nicotine levels in cervical secretions (Jones et al, 1991; McCann et al, 1992). Other smoke compounds carcinogenic to visceral organs presumably also have a systemic distribution in smokers. Indeed, levels of hemoglobin adducts of several known carcinogens contained in cigarette smoke are higher in smokers than in nonsmokers and may be increased in passive smokers as well (Maclure et al, 1989; Carmella et al, 1990; Bartsch et al, 1990). Similarly, the urine, breast fluid, and amniotic fluid of cigarette smokers contain mutagens at higher levels than samples from nonsmokers (Petrakis et al, 1980; IARC, 1986; Sorsa, 1986; Rivrud et al, 1986; Rynard, 1990), although the effect of smoking on levels of mutagens in cervical mucus is uncertain (Holly et al, 1993). DNA adducts and micronuclei in the bladder, cervix, and pancreas also are more common in smokers than in nonsmokers (Vine, 1990; Cuzick et al, 1990), as is genetic damage in lymphocytes (Nordic Study Group, 1990). In experimental systems, interactions of cigarette smoke constituents with other exposures have been noted. Ethanol may increase the tissue penetration or metabolic activation of tobacco smoke carcinogens (Seitz and Simanowski, 1988; Blot, 1992), and (as noted above) infection with herpes simplex virus enhances the carcinogenicity of snuff in the hamster cheek pouch. On the other hand, dietary vitamin C supplementation may inhibit the formation or activation of TSNAs (Hoffmann et al, 1991; Tsuda and Kurashima, 1991), and antioxidant nutrients may modulate the oxidative effects of smoking (Anderson, 1991). Isothiocyanates (found in cruciferous vegetables) and indole-3-carbinol may also inhibit activation of TSNAs and polycyclic aromatic hydrocarbons (Appel, 1991; Hoffman et al, 1991). If confirmed in humans, these effects have obvious relevance for cancer prevention in smokers.

Metabolic Effects of Tobacco Use

Cigarette smoking affects the metabolism of many drugs and other exogenous compounds, in part through induction of enzymes such as those in the microsomal mixed-function oxidase system (Dawson and Vestal, 1982). This has potential relevance to cancer, since the enzyme systems affected may detoxify or activate various carcinogens, including the polycyclic aromatic hydrocarbons and nitrosamines present in the smoke itself (Guengerich, 1988). For example, aryl hydrocarbon hydroxylase (AHH) metabolizes polycyclic aromatic hydrocarbons to active moieties through cytochrome P450IA1 reactions. The inducibility of P450IA1 is under genetic control and may be related to the risk of cancer of the lung and other sites (Kouri et al, 1982; Korsgaard et al, 1984; Petruzzelli et al, 1988). Cigarette smoking induces AHH in the human lung (Petruzzelli et al, 1988; McLemore et al, 1990), and pulmonary DNA adducts correlate with the AHH activity there (Geneste et al, 1991). Similarly, smoking induces cytochrome P450IA2, which activates carcinogenic arylamines (Butler et al, 1989). The constituents of cigarette smoke that induce the relevant enzyme systems have not been identified with certainty, though they appear to be contained in the particulate phase of the smoke; the enzyme induction associated with smoking resembles that resulting from exposure to the polycyclic aromatic hydrocarbons contained in this smoke fraction (IARC, 1986). Cigarette smoking appears *not* to induce either debrisoquine metabolism (associated with cytochrome P450IID6) or *N*-acetyl transferase, both genetically determined enzyme pathways that have been linked to the risk of cancers of the lung and bladder, respectively (Steiner et al, 1985; Caporaso et al, 1990; Kaisary et al, 1987). However, smokers may have an increased rate of endogenous nitrosamine formation (Hoffmann and Brunnemann, 1983; Ladd et al, 1984; Scherer and Adlkofer, 1986). Passive smoking has some enzyme-inducing effects (Matsunga et al, 1989), but in general, these are weaker than those for active smoking (Remmer, 1987).

Cigarette smoking could also affect cancer risk through effects on immunological functioning. These include depressed activity of natural killer cells, changes in the numbers of circulating T-cell subtypes, and impaired humoral and cellular response to immune challenge (Holt, 1987; Barton et al, 1988; Tollerud et al, 1989). The disturbances that have been directly associated with an increased risk of cancer (eg, AIDS) are typically more severe. However, local immunological effects could also be pertinent for certain cancer sites (eg, lung, cervix) (USDHHS, 1990; Barton et al, 1988).

Immunological effects may be particularly relevant to the relationship between cigarette smoking and squamous carcinoma of the uterine cervix or anus, malignancies that are associated with human papillomavirus (HPV). It is not clear if infection with HPV at either site is related to smoking status (Kjaer et al, 1990; Melbye et al, 1990; Caussy et al, 1990; Ley et al, 1991; Rohan et al, 1991; Burger et al, 1993), but there are increased risks of condyloma accuminatum and cervical condyloma in smokers, both manifestations of HPV infection (Daling et al, 1986; Brisson et al, 1988).

Cigarette smokers (especially long-term smokers) have repeatedly been found to weigh less than nonsmokers, and weight gain is commonly reported after cessation of cigarette smoking (USDHHS, 1988, 1990). Smokers also have a higher waist-to-hip ratio than nonsmokers (Seidell et al, 1991; Slattery et al, 1992), which may affect the risks of malignancies associated with body weight or body habitus (eg, endometrial cancer). The metabolic basis for the effect of smoking on body fat is not clear, but appears to involve changes in diet after smoking cessation, as well as increased metabolic energy expenditure in smokers (apparently from nicotine intake) (USDHHS, 1988; USDHHS, 1990; Hofstetter et al, 1986; Perkins et al, 1989).

Cigarette smokers also have lower circulating levels of vitamin C and beta-carotene than nonsmokers, even after adjustment for reported intake (Nierenberg et al, 1989; Schectman et al, 1989; Preston, 1991). Because these vitamins may be protective against several smoking-related cancers, the lower levels may, in themselves, place smokers at a higher risk than nonsmokers (Committee on Diet and Health, 1989).

Recent laboratory and epidemiological studies have indicated that cigarette smoking has an "anti-estrogenic" effect, because women who smoke seem relatively estrogen-deficient. Thus women who smoke cigarettes have an early menopause, an increased risk of osteoporotic fractures, and apparently a reduced risk of uterine fibroids and endometriosis. This effect of smoking may explain the reduced risk observed for endometrial cancer among smokers (Baron et al, 1990).

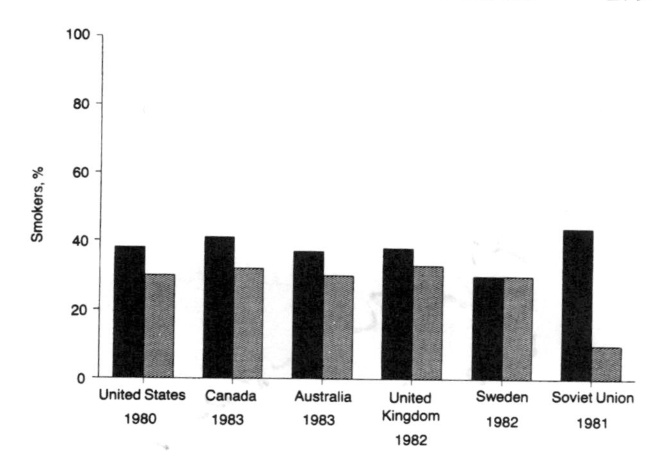

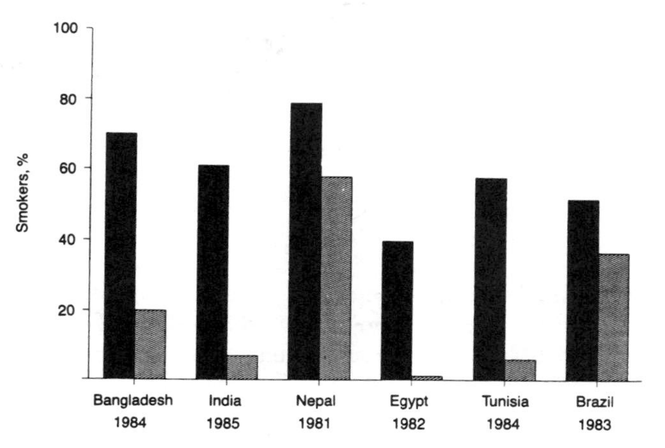

FIG. 14–5. Smoking prevalences in selected countries in selected years. (Taken from Council on Scientific Affairs, 1990.)

THE BURDEN OF TOBACCO USE

Prevalence of Tobacco Use

Cigarette sales reports and various population surveys clearly show that cigarette smoking is common in most industrialized countries (Masironi and Rothwell, 1988; Pierce, 1989; Council on Scientific Affairs, 1990), with about 30%–40% of adult males and 25%–35% of adult females currently smoking. For example, in the United States about 30%–33% of adult males and 25%–28% of adult females were currently smoking in the mid/late 1980s (USDHHS, 1989; Fiore, 1992). Smoking was more common among men than among women (except among those under 24 years old) (USDHHS, 1989; Novotny et al, 1990), and was also more prevalent among less educated individuals (USDHHS, 1989; Fiore, 1992) (Fig. 14–5).

In the United States, these patterns represent a substantial change from the 1960s, when over half of adult men and a third of adult women smoked cigarettes (USDHHS, 1989; Fiore, 1992). The reduction in the prevalence of current smoking has been observed among blacks as well as among whites, but the decreases among women have been much smaller than those for men (USDHHS, 1989; Fiore, 1992). In fact, among women under 24, the decline has been minimal or absent, and for women 65 or older, the proportion of currently smoking women actually increased slightly during the 1980s (Novotny et al, 1990).

The overall decline in the numbers of Americans smoking has been the result of two related trends. Fewer people are taking up smoking, and since the mid-1960s, an increasing proportion of smokers have quit (USDHHS, 1990; Fiore, 1992) (Fig. 14–6), to the point that more than 45% of male ever smokers and 40% of

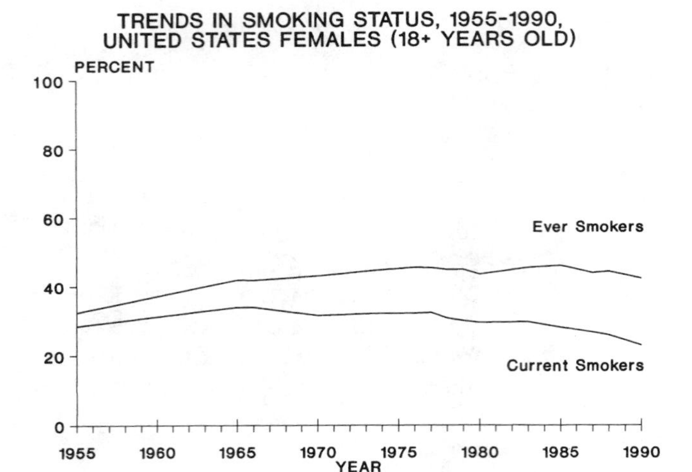

FIG. 14–6. Percentages of current and ever smokers, females and year, United States, 1955–1990. (From the 1955 Current Population Survey and 15 National Health Interview Surveys from 1965–1990; data compiled by the Office on Smoking and Health, Centers for Disease Control.)

female ever smokers no longer smoke. However, the proportion of the U.S. population that has ever smoked has not declined as sharply as that of current smokers. In other industrial countries, the trends in smoking have been roughly similar: recent declines in smoking among men and less striking decreases (or small increases) among women (Tominaga, 1986a; Masironi and Rothwell, 1988; Pierce, 1989).

In many developing countries, over 50% of adult males smoke, although often a much lower proportion of females do (IARC, 1986; Crofton, 1990). The high smoking prevalence among males is generally thought to reflect an increase in use over the past two decades (Tominaga, 1986b, IARC, 1986; Masironi and Rothwell, 1988). China produces more tobacco than any other country, between a third and a half of the total world crop. It is estimated that over 60% of adult Chinese males smoke (but less than 10% of adult Chinese females) (Council on Scientific Affairs, 1990; Yu et al, 1990).

In the United States, the prevalence of snuff and chewing tobacco use has remained stable or declined slightly between the 1960s and the 1980s. However, recently the heaviest use has been among younger males, whereas formerly it was among men over 50. In some regional surveys, as many as a quarter of males 12–18 years old use smokeless tobacco (largely oral snuff). Use among young females is rare, though in the rural southeastern parts of the country significant numbers of older women "dip snuff"—that is, use oral snuff (USDHHS, 1986; Novotny et al, 1989).

Mortality from Tobacco-Related Cancer

In the industrialized countries, cigarette smoking has been prevalent long enough to account for about a third of cancer mortality during the late twentieth century (Doll and Peto, 1981). In particular, lung cancer mortality has increased dramatically in these countries during the mid twentieth century (Tominaga, 1986a; Parkin, 1989; Davis et al, 1990). For example, in the United States, mortality rates from lung cancer among males have increased from about 10 per 100,000 population in the 1930s to about 75 per 100,000 in the 1980s. Substantial exposure to tobacco came later for women, and consequently their rates have not risen as high: from 5 per 100,000 in the 1950s to over 25 per 100,000 in the 1980s. Over 85% of lung cancer deaths can be attributed to smoking, and smokers currently face a higher excess mortality from lung cancer than from coronary heart disease (Shopland et al, 1991) (Table 14–1).

The incidence and mortality from cancer at other sites related to tobacco use is substantial, although not as high as for lung cancer (Table 14–1). In many industrialized countries, the mortality from cancers of the oral cavity, pharynx, larynx, and esophagus increased modestly during the mid twentieth century. However, the birth-cohort mortality patterns do not always reflect tobacco exposure, and the mortality for cancer of the bladder did not change substantially over the same period (Doll and Peto, 1981; Devesa et al, 1990; Davis et al, 1990). These contrasts with lung cancer may reflect the relatively strong influence of other etiologic factors on these malignancies (for example, alcohol for cancers of the upper aerodigestive tract) (Doll, 1989).

Similar data on tobacco-related cancers from developing countries are sparse. However, it is clear that lung

TABLE 14–1. *United States Mortality, Mortality Rates, and Smoking-Attributable Risks for Selected Cancers*

	Number of Deaths, 1988		*Death Rate, 1988*		*Attributable Risk (%)*	
	Male	*Female*	*Male*	*Female*	*Male*	*Female*
Lip, oral cavity, pharynx	5,497	2,702	4.6	2.1	92	61
Esophagus	6,916	2,420	5.8	1.9	78	75
Pancreas	11,722	12,126	9.8	9.6	29	34
Larynx	2,965	702	2.5	0.6	81	87
Trachea/bronchus/lung	88,059	45,225	73.5	35.9	90	79
Bladder	6,534	3,271	5.5	2.6	47	37
Kidney	5,855	3,814	4.9	3.0	48	12

*per 100,000 population
Source: From National Center for Health Statistics (NCHS), 1991; USDHHS, 1989.

cancer incidence or mortality is high or increasing in several parts of the Third World (Parkin, 1989).

Conclusions, Opportunities for Prevention

Tobacco use, especially cigarette smoking, is not only common worldwide, but also strongly associated with the risk of malignancies at several anatomic sites. There is biological evidence that tobacco and tobacco smoke products directly influence the carcinogenic process at various stages, and that cigarette smoking has other effects that may alter cancer risks. Epidemiologically, the strongest positive associations are with cancers that have a squamous histology. The evidence is overwhelming that cigarette smoking causes cancers of the oropharynx, larynx, lung, and bladder. The relationships between smoking and cancers of the esophagus and pelvis of the kidney/ureter also appear to be causal, and the association between smoking and cancer of the pancreas suggests additional carcinogenic potential. Strong evidence has also emerged linking smokeless tobacco use and oral cancer. The relationships between cigarette smoking and myelogenous leukemia and between passive smoking and lung cancer are suggestive of a causal relationship, but require further confirmation.

Although antagonism of tobacco carcinogenesis may be possible through "chemoprevention" with antioxidants, isothiocyanates, or other compounds, this is far from established. Cessation of tobacco use is associated with an attenuation of the excess cancer risks at virtually all tobacco-related sites, and this offers the best potential for a reduction in the burden of tobacco-related cancer. Indeed, the promotion of smoking cessation is probably the most cost-effective anti-cancer effort available (Eddy, 1981; Barnum and Greenberg, 1991). The declining prevalence of smoking in many of the industrialized countries suggests that the incidence and mortality from tobacco-related cancer may also decline in these areas. Because of the latent period associated with carcinogenic effects, the reductions in the prevalence of cigarette smoking and in the tar content of cigarettes have just begun to have an effect on the incidence of smoking-related cancer. In several industrialized countries (including the United States, the United Kingdom, and Finland), lung cancer mortality has been decreasing in younger males, reflecting a reduced lifetime exposure to cigarettes that are in themselves relatively low in tar (IARC, 1986; Lopez, 1990). Moreover, there are suggestions that among those under 45 years old, mortality from oral/pharyngeal and laryngeal cancers is decreasing among U.S. whites (Devesa et al, 1990) and mortality from cancers of the pharynx, larynx, and bladder is decreasing in England and Wales (Doll, 1989). Thus, in the industrialized countries, there is cause for optimism. If present tobacco-use trends continue, a decline in the burden of tobacco-related cancer can be expected to become more evident in age-adjusted statistics (Brown and Kessler, 1988).

In the developing countries the situation is unfortunately quite different. There, tobacco use seems to be becoming more popular, and the high smoking prevalence appears to be accompanied by relatively high tar delivery in cigarettes and bidis (Gray, 1985; Ramstrom, 1986). The use of cigarettes has not been widespread long enough for the full implications to be currently apparent. However, it is clear that if present smoking patterns continue, there will be an epidemic of smoking-related cancers in these countries in the early twenty-first century.

REFERENCES

ADAMS JD, O'MARA-ADAMS KJ, HOFFMANN D. 1987. Toxic and carcinogenic agents in undiluted mainstream smoke and sidestream smoke of different types of cigarettes. Carcinogenesis 8:729–731.

AKEHURST BC. 1981. *Tobacco*. London: Longman.

ANDERSON R. 1991. Assessment of the roles of vitamin C, vitamin E, and β-carotene in the modulation of oxidant stress mediatd by cigarette smoke-activated phagocytes. Am J Clin Nutr 53:358S–361S.

APPEL KE. 1991. Tobacco-specific *N*-nitrosamines: some aspects of prevention. Toxicology 21:299–304.

ARCHIMBAUD E, MAUPAS J, LECLUZE-PALAZZOLO C, et al. 1989. Influence of cigarette smoking on the presentation and course of chronic myelogenous leukemia. Cancer 63:2060–2065.

AUBRY F, MACGIBBON B. 1985. Risk factors of squamous cell carcinoma of the skin: a case-control study in the Montreal region. Cancer 55:907–911.

AUERBACH O, GARFINKEL L. 1986. Histologic changes in pancreas in relation to smoking and coffee-drinking habits. Dig Dis Sci 31:1014–1020.

AUERBACH O, GARFINKEL L. 1989. Histologic changes in the urinary bladder in relation to cigarette smoking and use of artificial sweeteners. Cancer 64:983–987.

AUERBACH O, HAMMOND EC, GARFINKEL L. 1979. Changes in bronchial epithelium in relation to cigarette smoking, 1955–1960 vs. 1970–1977. N Engl J Med 300:381–386.

AUGUSTINE A, HEBERT JR, KABAT GC, WYNDER EL. 1988. Bladder cancer in relation to cigarette smoking. Cancer Res 48:4405–4408.

AUSTIN H, DELZELL E, GRUFFERMAN S, et al. 1986. A case-control study of hepatocellular carcinoma and the hepatitis B virus, cigarette smoking, and alcohol consumption. Cancer Res 46:962–966.

BAILEY E, BROOKS AGF, DOLLERY CT, et al. 1988. Hydroxyethylvaline adduct formation in haemoglobin as a biological monitor of cigarette smoke intake. Arch Toxicol 62:247–253.

BARNUM H, GREENBERG R. 1991. *Health Sector Priorities Review*. Washington, DC: Population, Health and Nutrition Division, Population and Human Resources Department, The World Bank.

BARON JA, SANDLER RS. 1990. Cigarette smoking and cancer of the large bowel. In: *Smoking and Hormone-Related Disorders*, Wald N, Baron J (eds). Oxford: Oxford University Press, pp 167–182.

BARON JA, LA VECCHIA C, LEVI F. 1990. The antiestrogenic effect of cigarette smoking in women. Am J Obstet Gynecol 162:502–514.

BARTON SE, JENKINS D, CUZICK J, et al. 1988. Effect of cigarette smoking on cervical epithelial immunity: a mechanism for neoplastic change? Lancet 2:652–654.

BARTSCH H, CAPORASO N, CODA M, et al. 1990. Carcinogen hemoglobin adducts, urinary mutagenicity, and metabolic phenotype in active and passive cigarette smokers. J Natl Cancer Inst 82:1826–1831.

BELINSKY SA, DEVEREUX TR, MARONPOT RR, et al. 1989. Relationship between the formation of promutagenic adducts and the activation of the K-*ras* protooncogene in lung tumors from A/J mice treated with nitrosamines. Cancer Res 49:5305–5311.

BENHAMOU E, BENHAMOU S. 1993. Black (air-cured) and blond (flue-cured) tobacco and cancer risk VI: lung cancer. Eur J Cancer 29A:1778–1780.

BENOWITZ NL. 1988. Pharmacologic aspects of cigarette smoking and nicotine addiction. N Engl J Med 319:1318–1330.

BENOWITZ NL, HALL SM, HERNING RI, et al. 1983. Smokers of low-yield cigarettes do not consume less nicotine. N Engl J Med 309:139–142.

BENOWITZ NL, JACOB P III, YU L, et al. 1986. Reduced tar, nicotine, and carbon monoxide exposure while smoking ultralow- but not low-yield cigarettes. JAMA 256:241–246.

BERAL V, HANNAFORD P, KAY C. 1988. Oral contraceptive use and malignancies of the genital tract. Lancet 2:1331–1335.

BERNARD SM, CARTWRIGHT RA, DARWIN CM, et al. 1987. Hodgkin's disease: case control epidemiological study in Yorkshire. Br J Cancer 55:85–90.

BLOT WJ. 1992. Alcohol and cancer. Cancer Res 52:2119s–2123s.

BLOT WJ, FRAUMENI JF JR. 1986. Passive smoking and lung cancer. J Natl Cancer Inst 77:993–1000.

BLOT WJ, MCLAUGHLIN JK, WINN DM, et al. 1988. Smoking and drinking in relation to oral and pharyngeal cancer. Cancer Res 48:3282–3287.

BOCK FG. 1971. Tumor promoters in tobacco and cigarette-smoke condensate. J Natl Cancer Inst 48:1849–1853.

BOCK FG. 1980. Cocarcinogenic properties of nicotine. In: *Banbury Report 3—A Safe Cigarette?* Gori GB, Bock FG (eds. Cold Spring Harbor Laboratory, pp 129–139.

BOCKENSTEDT JB, LESCH CA, SQUIER CA. 1988. Smokeless tobacco, nicotine, and the pathogenesis of oral mucosal lesions. Abstract J Dent Res 67:338.

BOSCH FX, MUNOZ N, DE SANJOSE S, et al. 1992. Risk factors for cervical cancer in Colombia and Spain. Int J Cancer 52: 750–758.

BOUCHARDY C, CLAVEL F, LAVECCHIA C, et al. 1990. Alcohol, beer and cancer of the pancreas. Int J Cancer 45:842–846.

BRINTON LA, BARRETT RJ, MERMAN ML, et al. 1993. Cigarette smoking and the risk of endometrial cancer. Am J Epidemiol 137:281–291.

BRINTON LA, BLOT WJ, BECKER JA, et al. 1984. A case-control study of cancers of the nasal cavity and paranasal sinuses. Am J Epidemiol 119:896–906.

BRINTON LA, JUN-YAO L, SHOU-DE R, et al. 1991. Risk factors for penile cancer: results from a case-control study in China. Int J Cancer 47:504–509.

BRINTON LA, NASCA PC, MALLIN K, et al. 1990. Case-control study of *in situ* and invasive carcinoma of the vagina. Gynecol Oncol 38:49–54.

BRINTON LA, TASHIMA KT, LEHMAN HF, et al. 1987. Epidemiology of cervical cancer by cell type. Cancer Res 47:1706–1711.

BRISSON J, ROY M, FORTIER M, et al. 1988. Condyloma and intraepithelial neoplasia of the uterine cervix: a case-control study. Am J Epidemiol 128:337–342.

BROCK KE, BERRY G, MOCK PA, et al. 1988. Nutrients in diet and plasma and risk of in situ cervical cancer. J Natl Cancer Inst 80:580–585.

BROCK KE, MACLENNAN R, BRINTON LA, et al. 1989. Smoking and infectious agents and risk of *in situ* cervical cancer in Sydney, Australia. Cancer Res 49:4925–4928.

BROWN CC, KESSLER LG. 1988. Projections of lung cancer mortality in the United States: 1985–2025. J Natl Cancer Inst 80:43–51.

BROWN LM, POTTERN LM, HOOVER RN. 1987. Testicular cancer in young men: the search for causes of the epidemic increase in the United States. J Epidemiol Community Health 41:349–354.

BROWN LM, EVERETT GD, GIBSON R, et al. 1992. Smoking and risk of non-Hodgkin's lymphoma and multiple myeloma. Cancer Causes Control 3:49–55.

BUCKLEY JD, HOBBIE WL, RUCCIONE K, et al. 1986. Maternal smoking during pregnancy and the risk of childhood cancer. (Letter) Lancet 2:519–520.

BUENO DO MESQUITA HB, MAISONNEUVE P, MOERMAN CJ, et al. 1991. Life-time history of smoking and exocrine carcinoma of the pancreas: a population-based case-control study in the Netherlands. Int J. Cancer 49:816–122.

BUIATTI E, PALLI D, DECARLI A, et al. 1989. A case-control study of gastric cancer and diet in Italy. Int J Cancer 44:611–616.

BURCH JD, CRAIB KJP, CHOI BCK, et al. 1987. An exploratory case-control study of brain tumors in adults. J Natl Cancer Inst 78:601–609.

BURCH JD, ROHAN TE, HOWE GR, et al. 1989. Risk of bladder cancer by source and type of tobacco exposure: a case-control study. Int J Cancer 44:622–628.

BURGER MPM, HOLLEMA H, GOUW ASH, et al. 1993 Cigarette smoking and human papillomavirus in patients with reported cervical cytological abnormality. Br Med J 306:749–752.

BUTLER MA, IWASAKI M, GUENGERICH FP, KADLUBAR FF. 1989. Human cytochrome P-450_{PA} (P-450IA2, the phenacetin O-deethylase, is primarily responsible for the hepatic 3–demethylation of caffeine and N-oxidation of carcinogenic arylamines. Proc Natl Acad Sci USA 86:7696–7700.

CAPORASO NE, TUCKER MA, HOOVER RN, et al. 1990. Lung cancer and the debrisoquine metabolic phenotype. J Natl Cancer Inst 82:1264–1272.

CARMELLA SG, KAGAN SS, KAGAN M, et al. 1990. Mass spectometric analysis of tobacco-specific nitrosamine hemoglobin adducts in snuff dippers, smokers, and nonsmokers. Cancer Res 50:5438–5445.

CARSTENSEN JM, PERSHAGEN G, EKLUND G. 1987. Mortality in relation to cigarette and pipe smoking: 16 years; observation of 25,000 Swedish men. J Epidemiol Community Health 41:166–172.

CASAGRANDE JT, HANISCH R, PIKE MC, et al. 1988. A case-control study of male breast cancer. Cancer Res 48:1326–1330.

CAUSSY D, GOEDERT JJ, PALEFSKI J, et al. 1990. Interaction of human immunodeficiency and papilloma viruses: association with anal epithelial abnormality in homosexual men. Int J Cancer 46:214–219.

CEDERLOF R, FRIBERG L, HRUBEC Z, LORICH U. 1975. The relationship of smoking and some social covariables to mortality and cancer morbidity: a ten year follow-up in a probability sample of 55,000 Swedish subjects age 18 to 69. Department of Environmental Hygiene, The Karolinska Institute.

CHACKO M, GUPTA RC. 1988. Evaluation of DNA damage in the oral mucosa of tobacco users and non-users by ^{32}P-adduct assay. Carcinogenesis 9:2309–2313.

CHOW W-H MCLAUGHLIN JK, HRUBEC A, et al. 1993. Tobacco use and nasopharyngeal carcinoma in a cohort of US veterans. Int J Cancer 55:538–540.

CLAVEL J, CORDIER S, BOCCON-GIBOD L, HEMON D. 1989. Tobacco and bladder cancer in males: increased risk for inhalers and smokers of black tobacco. Int J Cancer 44:605–610.

COLDMAN AJ, ELWOOD JM, GALLAGHER RP. 1982. Sports activities and risk of testicular cancer. Br J Cancer 46:749–756.

COMMITTEE ON DIET AND HEALTH, FOOD AND NUTRITION BOARD, COMMISSION ON LIFE SCIENCES, NATIONAL RESEARCH COUNCIL. 1989. Diet and health: implications for reducing chronic disease risk. Washington, DC: National Academy Press.

Committee on Passive Smoking, National Research Council. 1986. *Environmental Tobacco Smoke: Measuring Exposures and Assessing Health Effects*. Washington, DC: National Academy Press.

Cook-Mozaffari PJ, Azordegan F, Day NE, et al. 1979. Oesophageal cancer studies in the Caspian littoral of Iran: results of a case-control study. Br J Cancer 39:293–309.

Coultas DB, Peake GT, Samet JM. 1989. Questionnaire assessment of lifetime and recent exposure to environmental tobacco smoke. Am J Epidemiol 130:338–347.

Council on Scientific Affairs. 1986. Health effects of smokeless tobacco. JAMA 255:1038–1044.

Council on Scientific Affairs. 1990. The worldwide smoking epidemic. Tobacco trade, use, and control. JAMA 263:3312–3318.

Cramer DW, Welch WR, Hutchison GB, et al. 1984. Dietary animal fat in relation to ovarian cancer risk. Obstet Gynecol 63:833–838.

Crofton J. 1990. Tobacco and the third world. Thorax 45:164–169.

Cummings KM. 1984. Changes in the smoking habits of adults in the United States and recent trends in lung cancer mortality. Cancer Detect Prev 7:125–134.

Cummings KM, Markello S, Mahoney MC, et al. 1989. Measurement of lifetime exposure to passive smoke. Am J Epidemiol 130:122–132.

Cuzick J, Routledge MN, Jenkins D, Garner RC. 1990. DNA adducts in different tissues of smokers and non-smokers. Int J Cancer 45:673–678.

Daling JR, Sherman KJ, Weiss NS. 1986. Risk factors for condyloma acuminatum in women. Sex Transm, Dis 13:16–18.

Daling JR, Sherman KJ, Hislop TG,, et al. 1992. Cigarette smoking and the risk of anogenital cancer. Am J Epidemiol 135:180–189.

D'Avanzo B, Negri E, La Vecchia C, et al. 1990. Cigarette smoking and bladder cancer. Eur J Cancer 26:714–718.

Davidson BJ, Hsu TC, Schantz SP. 1993. The genetics of tobacco-induced malignancy. Arch Otolaryngol Head Neck Surg 119:1198–1205.

Davis DL, Hoel D, Fox J, Lopez A. 1990. International trends in cancer mortality in France, West Germany, Italy, Japan, England and Wales, and the USA. Lancet 336:474–481.

Dawson GW, Vestal RE. 1982. Smoking and drug metabolism. Pharmacol Ther 15:207–221.

Demers RY, Neale AV, Demers P, et al. 1988. Serum cholesterol and colorectal polyps. J Clin Epidemiol 41:9–13.

Department of National Health and Welfare, Canada. 1966. *A Canadian Study of Smoking and Health*. Department of National Health and Welfare, Canada.

De Stefani E, Correa P, Oreggia F, et al. 1987. Risk factors for laryngeal cancer. Cancer 60:3087–3091.

De Stefani E, Correa P, Oreggia F, et al. 1988. Black tobacco, wine and mate in oropharyngeal cancer: a case-control study from Uruguay. Rev Epidem Sante Publico 36:389–394.

De Stefani E, Barrios E, Fierro L. 1993. Black (air-cured) and blond (flue-cured) tobacco and cancer risk III: Oesophageal cancer. Eur J Cancer 29A:763–766.

Devesa SS, Blot WJ, Fraumeni JF Jr. 1990. Cohort trends in mortality from oral, esophageal, and laryngeal cancers in the United States. Epidemiology 1:116–121.

Doll R. 1989. Progress against cancer: are we winning the war? Acta Oncol 28:611–621.

Doll R, Peto R. 1976. Mortality in relation to smoking: 20 years' observations on male British doctors. Br Med J 2:1525–1536.

Doll R, Peto R. 1978. Cigarette smoking and bronchial carcinoma: dose and time relationships among regular smokers and lifelong non-smokers. J Epidemiol Community Health 32:303–313.

Doll R, Peto R. 1981. Definition of the avoidability of cancer. J Natl Cancer Inst 66:1191–1308.

Doll R, Gray R, Hafner B, Peto R. 1980. Mortality in relation to smoking: 22 years' observations on female British doctors. Br Med J 5 April:967–971.

Douglass CW, Gammon MD. 1984. Reassessing the epidemiology of lip cancer. Oral Surg 57:631–642.

Dube MF, Green CR. 1982. Methods of collection of smoke for analytical purposes. In: *Formation, Analysis and Composition of Tobacco Smoke*, Recent Advances in Tobacco Science, Vol. 8. 36th Tobacco Chemists Research Conference, Raleigh, NC, pp. 42–102.

Dunn BP, Stich HF. 1986. ^{32}P-postlabelling analysis of aromatic DNA adducts in human oral mucosal cells. Carcinogenesis 7:115–120.

Dunn BP, Vedal S, San RHC, et al. 1991. DNA adducts in bronchial biopsies. Int J Cancer 48:485–492.

Eddy DM. 1981. The economics of cancer prevention and detection: getting more for less. Cancer 47:1200–1209.

Ernster VL, Grady DG, Greene JC, et al. 1990. Smokeless tobacco use and health effects among baseball players. JAMA 264:218–224.

Esteve J, Tuyns AJ, Raymond L, Vineis P. 1984. Tobacco and the risk of cancer. Importance of kinds of tobacco. IARC Publications 57:867–876.

Evans RD, Kopf AW, Lew RA et al. 1988. Risk factors for the development of malignant melanoma—I: review of case-control studies. J Dermatol Surg Oncol 14:393–408.

Falk RT, Pickle LW, Brown LM, et al. 1989. Effect of smoking and alcohol consumption on largyngeal cancer risk in coastal Texas. Cancer Res 49: 4024–4029.

Ferraroni M, Negri E, La Vecchia C, et al. 1989. Socioeconomic indicators, tobacco and alcohol in the aetiology of digestive tract neoplasms. Int J Epidemiol 18:556–562.

Fiore MC. 1992. Trends in cigarette smoking in the United States. The epidemiology of tobacco use. Med Clin North Am 65:289–303.

Fleiss JL, Gross AJ. 1991. Meta-analysis in epidemiology, with special reference to studies of the association between exposure to environmental tobacco smoke and lung cancer: a critique. J Clin Epidemiol 44:127–139.

Fontham EH, Correa P, Reynolds P, et al. 1994. Environmental tobacco smoke and lung cancer in nonsmoking women. JAMA 271:1752–1759.

Franceschi S, Serraino D, Bidoli E, et al. 1989. The epidemiology of non-Hodgkin's lymphoma in the north-east of Italy: a hospital-based case-control study. Leukemia Res 13:465–472.

Franceschi S, Talamini R, Barra S, et al. 1990. Smoking and drinking in relation to cancers of the oral cavity, pharynx, larynx and esophagus in northern Italy. Cancer Res 50:6502–6507.

Franco EL, Kowalski LP, Oliveira BV, et al. 1989. Risk factors for oral cancer in Brazil: a case-control study. Int J Cancer 43:991–1000.

Franks AL, Lee NC, Kendrick JS, et al. 1987. Cigarette smoking and the risk of epithelial ovarian cancer. Am J Epidemiol 126:112–117.

Fukuda K, Shibata A. 1990. Exposure-response relationships between woodworking, smoking or passive smoking, and squamous cell neoplasms of the maxillary sinus. Cancer Causes and Control 1:165–168.

Garfinkel L. 1980. Cancer mortality in nonsmokers: prospective study by the American Cancer Society. J Natl Cancer Inst 65:1169–1173.

Geneste O, Camus A-M, Castegnaro M, et al. 1991. Comparison of pulmonary DNA adduct levels, measured by ^{32}P-postlabelling and aryl hydrocarbon hydroxylase activity in lung parenchyma of smokers and ex-smokers. Carcinogenesis 12:1301–1305.

Giovannucci E, Rimm EB, Stampfer MJ, et al. 1994a. A prospective study of cigarette smoking and risk of colorectal adenoma and colorectal cancer in U.S. men. J Natl Cancer Inst 86:183–191.

GIOVANNUCCI E, COLDITZ GA, STAMPFER MJ, et al. 1994b. A prospective study of cigarette smoking and risk of colorectal adenoma and colorectal cancer in U.S. women. J Natl Cancer Inst 86:192–199.

GORI GB. 1976. Low-risk cigarettes: a prescription. Science 194: 1243–1246.

GRAY N. 1985. Cancer risks and cancer prevention in the Third World. In: *Cancer Risks and Prevention*, Vessey MP, Gary M (eds). Oxford: Oxford University Press, pp 269–299.

GUENGERICH FP. 1988. Roles of cytochrome P-450 enzymes in chemical carcinogenesis and cancer chemotherapy. Cancer Res 48:2946–2954.

GUERIN MR. 1980. Chemical composition of cigarette smoke. In: *Banbury Report, A Safe Cigarette*. Gori GB, Bock FG (eds). Cold Spring Harbor Laborator pp 191–205.

GUPTA PC, PINDBORG JJ, MEHTA FS. 1982. Comparison of carcinogenicity of betel quid with and without tobacco: an epidemiological review. Ecol Dis 1:213–219.

GUPTA RC, SOPORI ML, GAIROLA CG. 1989. Formation of cigarette smoke-induced DNA adducts in the rat lung and nasal mucosa. Cancer Res 49:1916–1920.

HAMMOND EC. 1966. Smoking in relation to the death rates of one million men and women. In: *Epidemiological Approaches to the Study of Cancer and Other Chronic Diseases*, Haenszel W (ed). NCI Monograph #19. Bethesda: DHEW, pp 127–204.

HAMMOND EC, HORN D. 1958. Smoking and death rates—report on forty-four months of follow-up of 187,783 men. JAMA 166:1294–1308.

HANSSON L-E, BARON J, NYREN O, et al. 1994. Tobacco, alcohol and the risk of gastric cancer: a population-based case-control study in Sweden. Int J Cancer 57:26–31.

HARDELL L, ERIKSSON M, LENNER P, LUNDGREN E. 1981. Malignant lymphoma and exposure to chemicals, especially organic solvents, chlorophenols and phenoxy acids: a case-control study. Br J Cancer 43:169–176.

HARTGE P, HOOVER R, KANTOR A. 1985. Bladder cancer risk and pipes, cigars, and smokeless tobacco. Cancer 55:901–906.

HARTGE P, SILVERMAN D, HOOVER R, et al. 1987. Changing cigarette habits and bladder cancer risk: a case-control study. J Natl Cancer Inst 78:1119–1125.

HATSUKAMI DK, GUST SW, KEENAN RM. 1987. Physiologic and subjective changes from smokeless tobacco withdrawal. Clin Pharmacol Ther 41:103–107.

HAYES RB, KARDAUN JWPF, DE BRUYN A. 1987. Tobacco use and sinonasal cancer: a case-control study. Br J Cancer 56:843–846.

HECHT SS, HOFFMANN D. 1988. Tobacco-specific nitrosamines, an important group of carcinogens in tobacco and tobacco smoke. Carcinogenesis 9:875–884.

HELLBERG D, NILSSON S. 1988. Smoking and cancer of the ovary. (Letter) N Engl J Med 318:782–783.

HELLBERG D, VALENTIN J, EKLUND T, NILSSON S. 1987. Penile cancer: is there an epidemiological role for smoking and sexual behavior? Br Med J 295:1306–1308.

HENDERSON BE, BENTON B, JING J, et al. 1979. Risk factors for cancer of the testis in young men. Int J Cancer 23:598–602.

HENRY CJ, KOURI RE. 1986. Chronic inhalation studies in mice. II. Effects of long-term exposure to 2R1 cigarette smoke on (C57BL/CumXC3H/AnfCum)F_1 mice. J Natl Cancer Inst 77:203–212.

HERNING RI, JONES RT, BACHMAN J, MINES AH. 1981. Puff volume increases when low-nicotine cigarettes are smoked. Br Med J 283:187–189.

HERR R, FERGUSON J, MYERS N, et al. 1990. Cigarette smoking, blast crisis, and survival in chronic myeloid leukemia. Am J Hematol 34:1–4.

HERRERO R, BRINTON LA, REEVES WC, et al. 1989. Invasive cervical cancer and smoking in Latin America. J Natl Cancer Inst 81:205–211.

HIATT RA, ARMSTRONG MA, KLATSKY AL, SIDNEY S. 1994. Alcohol consumption, smoking, and other risk factors and prostate cancer in a large health plan cohort in California (United States). Cancer Causes Control 5:66–72.

HIGGINS ITT, MAHAN CM, WYNDER EL. 1988. Lung cancer among cigar and pipe smokers. Prev Med 17:116–128.

HILDESHEIM A, LEVINE PH. 1993. Etiology of nasopharyngeal carcinoma: a review. Epidemiol Rev 15:466–485.

HILL P, WYNDER EL. 1979. Nicotine and cotinine in breast fluid. Cancer Lett 6:251–254.

HIRAYAMA T. 1989. A large-scale cohort study on risk factors for primary liver cancer, with special reference to the role of cigarette smoking. Cancer Chemother Pharmacol 23(suppl):S114–S117.

HIRAYAMA T. 1990. *Life-Style and Mortality. A Large-Scale Census-Based Cohort Study in Japan*. Vol. 6 in series *Contributions to Epidemiology and Biostatisics*, Wahrendorf J (series ed). Basel: Karger.

HOFFMANN D, BRUNNEMANN KD. 1983. Endogenous formation of *N*-nitrosoproline in cigarette smokers. Cancer Res 43:5570–5574.

HOFFMANN D, HECHT SS. 1990. Advances in tobacco carcinogenesis. In: *Chemical Carcinogenesis and Mutagensis I*, Cooper CS, Grover PL (eds). Berlin: Springer-Verlag.

HOFFMANN D, WYNDER EL. 1986. Chemical constituents and bioactivity of tobacco smoke. In: *Tobacco: A Major International Health Hazard*, Zaridze DG, Peto R (eds.), Lyon, France: International Agency for Research on Cancer, pp 145–165.

HOFFMANN D, RIVENSON A, CHUNG F-L, HECHT SS. 1991. Nictoine-derived N-nitrosamines (TSNA) and their relevance in tobacco carcinogenesis. Toxicology 21:305–311.

HOFSTETTER A, SCHUTZ Y, JEQUIER E, WAHREN J. 1986. Increased 24–hour energy expenditure in cigarette smokers. N Engl J Med 314:79–82.

HOLLY EA, WHITTEMORE AS, ASTON DA, et al. 1989. Anal cancer incidence: genital warts, anal fissure or fistula, hemorrhoids, and smoking. J Natl Cancer Inst 81:1726–1731.

HOLLY EA, CRESS RD, AHN DK, et al. 1993. Detection of mutagens in cervical mucus in smokers and nonsmokers. Cancer Epidemiol Biomarkers Prev 2:223–228.

HOLT PG. 1987. Immune and inflammatory function in cigarette smokers. Thorax 42:241–249.

HONDA GD, BERNSTEIN L, ROSS RK, et al. 1988. Vasectomy, cigarette smoking, and age at first sexual intercourse as risk factors for prostate cancer in middle-aged men. Br J Cancer 57:326–331.

HOWE GR, JAIN M, BURCH JD, MILLER AB. 1991. Cigarette smoking and cancer of the pancreas: evidence from a population-based case-control study in Toronto, Canada. Int J Cancer 47:323–328.

HSING AW, MCLAUGHLIN JK, HRUBEC Z, et al. 1991. Tobacco use and prostate cancer: 26–year follow-up of US veterans. Am J Epidemiol 133:437–441.

HUNTER DJ, COLDITZ GA, STAMPFER MJ, et al. 1990. Risk factors for basal cell carcinoma in a prospective cohort of women. Ann Epidemiol 1:13–23.

IDLE JR. 1990. Titrating exposure to tobacco smoke using cotinine—a minefield of misunderstandings. J Clin Epidemiol 43:313–317.

INOUE M, TAJIMA K, HIROSE K, et al. 1994. Life-style and subsite of gastric cancer—joint effect of smoking and drinking habits. Int J Cancer 56: 494–499.

INTERNATIONAL AGENCY FOR RESEARCH ON CANCER. 1985. *IARC Monographs on the Evaluation of the Carcinogenic Risk of Chemicals to Humans. Vol. 37. Tobacco Habits Other than Smoking: Betel-Quid and Areca-Nut Chewing: and Some Related Nitrosamines*. France: International Agency for Research on Cancer.

INTERNATIONAL AGENCY FOR RESEARCH ON CANCER. 1986. *IARC Monographs on the Evaluation of the Carcinogenic Risk of Chemical to Humans. Vol. 38. Tobacco Smoking*. Switzerland: International Agency for Research on Cancer.

International Agency for Research on Cancer. 1988. *IARC Monographs on the Evaluation of Carcinogenic Risks to Humans. Vol. 44. Alcohol Drinking*. France: International Agency for Research on Cancer.

Janerich DT, Thompson WD, Varela LR, et al. 1990. Lung cancer and exposure to tobacco smoke in the household. N Engl J Med 323:632–636.

Jarvis MJ. 1989. Application of biochemical intake markers to passive smoking measurement and risk estimation. Mutat Res 222:101–110.

Jedrychowski W, Boeing H, Wahrendorf J, et al. 1993. Vodka consumption, tobacco smoking and risk of gastric cancer in Poland. Int J Epidemiol 22:606–613.

Jensen OM, Wahrendorf J, Blettner M, et al. 1987. The Copenhagen case-control study of bladder cancer: role of smoking in invasive and non-invasive bladder tumours. J Epidemiol Community Health 41:30–36.

Jensen M, Knudsen JB, McLaughlin JK, Sorensen BL. 1988. The Copenhagen case-control study of renal pelvis and ureter cancer: role of smoking and occupational exposures. Int J Cancer 41:557–561.

Jones CJ, Schiffman MH, Kurman R, et al. 1991. Elevated nicotine levels in cervical lavages from passive smokers. Am J Public Health 81:378–379.

Jussawalla DJ. 1981. Oesophageal cancer in India. J Cancer Res Clin Oncol 99:29–33.

Jussawalla DJ, Deshpande VA. 1971. Evaluation of cancer risk in tobacco chewers and smokers: an epidemiologic assessment. Cancer 28:244–252.

Kabat GC, Hebert JR. 1994. Use of mentholated cigarettes and oropharyngeal cancer. Epidemiology 5:183–188.

Kahn HA. 1966. The Dorn Study of Smoking and Mortality Among U.S. Veterans: report on eight and one-half years of observation. In: *Epidemiological Approaches to the Study of Cancer and Other Chronic Diseases*, Haenszel W (ed). NCI Monograph #19. Bethesda: DHEW, pp 1–126.

Kaisary A, Smith P, Jaczq E, et al. 1987. Genetic predisposition to bladder cancer: ability to hydroxylate debrisoquine and mephenytoin as risk factors. Cancer Res 47:5488–5493.

Kantor AF, Hartge P, Hoover RN, Fraumeni JF Jr. 1988. Epidemiological characteristics of squamous cell carcinoma and adenocarcinoma of the bladder. Cancer Res 48:3853–3855.

Karagas MR, Stukel TA, Greenberg ER, et al. 1992. Risk of subsequent basal cell carcinoma and squamous cell carcinoma of the skin among patients with prior skin cancer. JAMA 267:3305–3310.

Kaufman DW, Palmer JR, Rosenberg L, et al. 1989. Tar content of cigarettes in relation to lung cancer. Am J Epidemiol 129:703–711.

Ketkar MB, Fuhst R, Mohr U. 1984. The effect of cigarette smoke exposure in European hamsters. Exp Pathol 25:103–106.

Kjaer SK, Engholm G, Teisen C, et al. 1990. Risk factors for cervical human papillomavirus and herpes simplex virus infections in Greenland and Denmark: a population-based study. Am J Epidemiol 131:669–682.

Kneller RW, McLaughlin JK, Bjelke E, et al. 1991. A cohort study of stomach cancer in a high-risk American population. Cancer 68:672–678.

Kolonel LN, Hankin JH, Wilkens LR, et al. 1990. An epidemiologic study of thyroid cancer in Hawaii. Cancer Causes Control 1:223–234.

Kono S, Ikeda N, Yanai F, et al. 1990. Serum lipids and colorectal adenoma among male self-defence officials in northern Kyushu, Japan. Int J Epidemiol 19:274–278.

Korsgaard R, Trell E, Simonsson BG, et al. 1984. Aryl hydrocarbon hydroxylase induction levels in patients with malignant tumors associated with smoking. Cancer Res Clin Oncol 108:286–289.

Kouri RE, McKinney CE, Slomiany DJ, et al. 1982. Positive correlation between high aryl hydrocarbon hydroxylase activity and primary lung cancer as analyzed in cryopreserved lymphocytes. Cancer Res 42:5030–5037.

Krall EA, Valadian I, Dwyer JT, Gardner J. 1989. Accuracy of recalled smoking data. Am J Public Health 79:200–206.

Kune GA, Kune S, Vitetta L, Watson LF. 1992. Smoking and colorectal cancer risk: data from the Melbourne Colorectal Cancer Study and brief review of literature. Int J Cancer 50:369–372.

Ladd KF, Newmark HL, Archer MC. 1984. N-nitrosation of proline in smokers and nonsmokers. J Natl Cancer Inst 73:83–87.

Lam KC, Yu MC, Leung JWC, Henderson BE. 1982. Hepatitis B virus and cigarette smoking: risk factors for hepatocellular carcinoma in Hong Kong. Cancer Res 42:5246–5248.

La Vecchia C, Negri E, Decarli A, et al. 1988. Risk factors for hepatocellular carcinoma in northern Italy. Int J Cancer 42:872–876.

La Vecchia C, Bidoli E, Barra S, et al. 1990a. Type of cigarettes and cancers of the upper digestive and respiratory tract. Cancer Causes Control 1:69–74.

La Vecchia C, Negri E, D'Avanzo B, Franceschi S. 1990b. Smoking and renal cell carcinoma. Cancer Res 50:5231–5233.

Lee PN. 1982. Passive smoking. Food Chem Toxicol 20:223–229.

Lee PN. 1987. Passive smoking and lung cancer association: a result of bias? Hum Toxicol 6:517–524.

Lee PN, Garfinkel L. 1981. Mortality and type of cigarette smoked. J Epidemiol Community Health 35:16–22.

Le Marchand L, Yoshizawa CN, Kolonel LN, et al. 1989. Vegetable consumption and lung cancer risk: a population-based case-control study in Hawaii. J Natl Cancer Inst 81:1158–1164.

Ley C, Bauer HM, Reingold A, et al. 1991. Determinants of genital human papillomavirus infection in young women. J Natl Cancer Inst 83:997–1003.

Li J-Y, Ershow AG, Chen Z-J, et al. 1989. A case-control study of cancer of the esophagus and gastric cardia in Linxian. Int J Cancer 43:755–761.

Lopez AD. 1990. Changes in tobacco consumption and lung cancer risk: evidence from national statistics. In: *Evaluating Effectiveness of Primary Prevention of Cancer*, Hakama M, Beral V, Cullen JW, Parkin DM (eds). Lyon: International Agency for Research on Cancer, pp 57–76.

Lopez-Abente G, Gonzalez CA, Errezola M, et al. 1991. Tobacco smoke inhalation pattern, tobacco type, and bladder cancer in Spain. Am J Epidemiol 134:830–839.

Lubin JH, Blot WJ. 1984. Assessment of lung cancer risk factors by histologic category. J Natl Cancer Inst 73:383–389.

Mabuchi K, Bross DS, Kessler II. 1985. Risk factors for male breast cancer. J Natl Cancer Inst 74:371–375.

Mack TM, Yu MC, Hanisch R, Henderson BE. 1986. Pancreas cancer and smoking, beverage consumption, and past medical history. J Natl Cancer Inst 76:49–60.

Maclure M, Katz RB-A, Bryant MS, et al. 1989. Elevated blood levels of carcinogens in passive smokers. Am J Public Health 79:1381–1384.

Magnani C, Pastore G, Luzzatto L, Terracini B. 1990. Parental occupation and other environmental factors in the etiology of leukemias and non-Hodgkin's lymphomas in childhood: a case-control study. Tumori 76:413–419.

Masironi R, Rothwell K. 1988. Tendances et effets du tabagisme dans le monde. World Health Statist Q 41:228–241.

Matsunga SK, Plezia PM, Karol MD, et al. 1989. Effects of passive smoking on theophylline clearance. Clin Pharmacol Ther 46:399–407.

Mattson ME, Winn DM. 1989. Smokeless tobacco: association with increased cancer risk. NCI Monogr 8:13–16.

McCann MF, Irwin DE, Walton LA. 1992. Nicotine and cotinine in the cervical mucus of smokers, passive smokers, and nonsmokers. Cancer Epidemiol, Biomarkers Prev 1:125–129.

McCredie M, Stewart JH. 1992. Risk factors for kidney cancer in New South Wales—I. Cigarette smoking. Eur J Cancer 28A:2050–2054.

McCredie M, Stewart JH, Ford JM. 1983. Analgesics and tobacco as risk factors for cancer of the ureter and renal pelvis. J Urol 130:28–30.

McCusker K. 1988. Landmarks of tobacco use in the United States. Chest 93:34S–36S.

McKinney PA, Stiller CA. 1986. Maternal smoking during pregnancy and the risk of childhood cancer. (Letter) Lancet 2:519.

McLaughlin JK, Mandel JS, Blot WJ, et al. 1984. A population-based case-control study of renal cell carcinoma. J Natl Cancer Inst 72:275–284.

McLaughlin JK, Hrubec Z, Blot WJ, Fraumeni JF Jr. 1990. Stomach cancer and cigarette smoking among U.S. veterans, 1954–1980. (Letter). Cancer Res 50:3804.

McLaughlin JK, Gao Y-T, Gao R-N, et al. 1992. Risk factors of renal cell cancer in Shanghai, China. Int J Cancer 52:562–565.

McLemore TL, Adelberg S, Liu MC, et al. 1990. Expression of CYP1A1 gene in patients with lung cancer: evidence for cigarette smoke-induced gene expression in normal lung tissue and for altered gene regulation in primary pulmonary carcinomas. J Natl Cancer Inst 82:1333–1339.

McTiernan A, Thomas DB, Johnson LK, Roseman D. 1986. Risk factors for estrogen receptor-rich and estrogen receptor-poor breast cancers. J Natl Cancer Inst 77:849–854.

McTiernan AM, Weiss NS, Daling JR. 1984. Incidence of thyroid cancer in women in relation to reproductive and hormonal factors. Am J Epidemiol 120:423–35.

Mehta FS, Gupta PC, Pindborg JJ. 1981. Chewing and smoking habits in relation to precancer and oral cancer. J Cancer Res Clin Oncol 99:35–39.

Melbye M, Palefsky J, Gonzales J, et al. 1990. Immune status as a determinant of human papillomavirus detection and its association with anal epithelial abnormalities. Int J Cancer 46:203–206.

Merletti F, Boffetta P, Ciccone G, et al. 1989. Role of tobacco and alcoholic beverages in the etiology of cancer of the oral cavity/oropharynx in Torino, Italy. Cancer Res 49:4919–4924.

Moolgavkar SH, Dewanji A, Luebeck G. 1989. Cigarette smoking and lung cancer: reanalysis of the British doctors' data. J Natl Cancer Inst 81:415–420.

Morrison AS, Buring JE, Verhoek WG, et al. 1984. An international study of smoking and bladder cancer. J Urol 131:650–654.

Nandakumar A, Thimmasetty KT, Sreeramareddy NM, et al. 1990. A population-based case-control investigation on cancers of the oral cavity in Bangalore, India. Br J Cancer 62:847–851.

National Center for Health Statistics. 1991. *Vital Statistics of the United Stats, 1988. Volume II, Mortality, Part A.* Washington: Public Health Service DHHS (PHS 91–1101.

National Research Council. 1986. *Environmental Tobacco Smoke: Measuring Exposures and Assessing Health Effects.* Washington, DC: National Academy Press.

Newell GR, Rawlings W, Kinnear BK, et al. 1973. Case-control study of Hodgkin's disease. I. Results of the interview questionnaire. J Natl Cancer Inst 51:1437–1441.

Nierenberg DW, Stukel TA, Baron JA, et al. 1989. Determinants of plasma levels of beta-carotene and retinol. Am J Epidemiol 130:511–521.

Nomura A, Yamakawa H, Ishidate T, et al. 1982. Intestinal metaplasia in Japan: association with diet. J Natl Cancer Inst 68:401–405.

Nomura A, Grove JS, Stemmermann GN, Severson RK. 1990. A prospective study of stomach cancer and its relation to diet, cigarettes and alcohol consumption. Cancer Res 50:627–631.

Nordic Study Group on the Health Risk of Chromosome Damage. 1990. A Nordic data base on somatic chromosome damage in humans. Mutat Res 241:325–337.

Norman V. 1982. Changes in smoke chemistry of modern day cigarettes. In: *Recent Advances in Tobacco Science, Vol. 8.* Formation, Analysis, and Composition of Tobacco Smoke. 36th Tobacco Chemists Research Conference, Raleigh, NC, pp 141–177.

Novotny TE, Pierce JP, Fiore MC, Davis RM. 1989. Smokeless tobacco use in the United States: the adult use of tobacco surveys. NCI Monogr 8:25–28.

Novotny TE, Fiore MC, Hatziandreu EJ, et al. 1990. Trends in smoking by age and sex, United States, 1974–1987: the implications for disease impact. Prev Med 19:552–561.

Oleske D, Golomb HM, Farber MD, Levy PS. 1985. A case-control inquiry into the etiology of hairy cell leukemia. Am J Epidemiol 121:675–683.

Oreggia F, De Stefani E, Correa P, Fierro L. 1991. Risk factors for cancer of the tongue in Uruguay. Cancer 67:180–183.

Osterlind A, Tucker MA, Stone BJ, Jensen OM. 1988. The Danish case-control study of cutaneous malignant melanoma. IV. No association with nutritional factors, alcohol, smoking or hair dyes. Int J Cancer 42:825–828.

Palli D, Bianchi S, Decarli A, et al. 1992. A case-control study of cancers of the gastric cardia in Italy. Br J Cancer 65:263–266.

Palmer JR, Rosenberg L. 1993. Cigarette smoking and the risk of breast cancer. Epidemiol Rev 15:145–156.

Parazzini F, La Vecchia C, Negri E, et al. 1988. Risk factors for adenocarcinoma of the cervix: a case-control study. Br J Cancer 57:201–204.

Park N-H, Akoto-Amanfu E, Pail DI. 1988. Smokeless tobacco carcinogenesis: the role of viral and other factors. CA—A Cancer Journal for 38:248–256.

Parkin DM. 1989. Trends in lung cancer incidence worldwide. Chest 96(suppl.):5S–8S.

Perera FP, Santella RM, Brenner D, et al. 1987. DNA adducts, protein adducts and sister chromatid exchange in cigarette smokers and nonsmokers. J Natl Cancer Inst 79:449–456.

Perkins KA, Epstein LH, Marks BL, et al. 1989. The effect of nicotine on energy expenditure during light physical activity. N Engl J Med 320:898–903.

Pershagen G, Ericson A, Otterblad-Olausson O. 1992. Maternal smoking in pregnancy: does it increase the risk of childhood cancer? Int J Epidemiol 21: 1–5.

Peto R. 1986. Influence of dose and duration of smoking on lung cancer rates. In: *Tobacco: A Major International Health Hazard*, Zaridze DG, Peto R (eds). Lyon, France: International Agency for Research on Cancer, pp. 23–33.

Petrakis NL, Maack CA, Lee RE, Lyon M. 1980. Mutagenic activity in nipple aspirates of human breast fluid. Cancer Res 40:188–189.

Petruzzelli S, Camus A-M, Carrozzi L, et al. 1988. Long-lasting effects of tobacco smoking on pulmonary drug-metabolizing enzymes: a case-control study on lung cancer patients. Cancer Res 48:4695–4700.

Phillips DH, Schoket B, Hewer A, et al. 1990. Influence of cigarette smoking on the levels of DNA adducts in human bronchial epithelium and white blood cells. Int J Cancer 46:569–575.

Phillips AN, Smith GD. 1994. Cigarette smoking as a potential cause of cervical cancer: has confounding been controlled? Int J Epidemiol 23:42–49.

Pierce JP. 1989. International comparisons of trends in cigarette smoking prevalence. Am J Public Health 79:152–157.

Preston AM. 1991. Cigarette smoking-nutritional implications. Prog Food Nutr Sci 15:183–217.

Preston-Martin S, Thomas DC, White SC, Cohen D. 1988.

Prior exposure to medical and dental x-rays related to tumors of the parotid gland. J Natl Cancer Inst 80:943–949.

Preston-Martin S, Mack W, Henderson BE. 1989. Risk factors for gliomas and meningiomas in males in Los Angeles County. Cancer Res 49:6137–6143.

Ramstrom LM. 1986. Worldwide changes and trends in cigarette brands and consumption. In: *Tobacco: A Major International Health Hazard*, Zaridze DG, Peto R (eds). Lyon, France: International Agency for Research on Cancer, pp 135–142.

Remmer H. 1987. Passively inhaled tobacco smoke: a challenge to toxicology and preventive medicine. Arch Toxicol 61:89–104.

Rickert WS, Robinson JC, Young JC, et al. 1983. A comparison of the yields of tar, nicotine, and carbon monoxide of 36 brands of Canadian cigarettes tested under three conditions. Prev Med 12:682–694.

Rivrud GN, Berge K, Anderson D, et al. 1986. Mutagenic effect of amniotic fluid from smoking women at term. Mutation Res 171:71–77.

Rogot E, Murray J. 1980. Cancer mortality among nonsmokers in an insured group of U.S. veterans. J Natl Cancer Inst 65:1163–1168.

Rohan TE, Cook MJ, Baron JA. 1989. Cigarette smoking and benign proliferative epithelial disorders of the breast in women; a case-control study. J Epidemiol Community Health 43: 362–368.

Rohan T, Mann V, McLaughlin J, et al. 1991. PCR-detected genital papillomavirus infection: prevalence and association with risk factors for cervical cancer. Int J Cancer 49:856–860.

Ron E, Kleinerman RA, Boice JD Jr, et al. 1987. A population-based case-control study of thyroid cancer. J Natl Cancer Inst 79:1–12.

Russell MAH, Jarvis M, Iyer R, Feyerabend C. 1980. Relation of nicotine yield of cigarettes to blood nicotine concentrations in smokers. Br Med J 5 i: 972–976.

Russell MAH, Jarvis MJ, Feyerabend C, Saloojee Y. 1986. Reduction of tar, nicotine and carbon monoxide intake in low tar smokers. J Epidemiol Community Health 40:80–85.

Rynard SM. 1990. Urine mutagenicity assays. In: *Biological Markers in Epidemiology*, Hulka BS, Wilcosky TC, Griffith JD (eds). New York: Oxford University Press, pp. 56–77.

Samet JM, Pathak DR, Morgan MV, et al. 1989. Radon progeny exposure and lung cancer risk in New Mexico U miners: a case-control study. Health Physics 56:415–421.

Sandler DP, Everson RB, Wilcox AJ. 1985a. Passive smoking in adulthood and cancer risk. Am J Epidemiol 121:37–48.

Sandler DP, Everson RB, Wilcox AJ, Browder JP. 1985b. Cancer risk in adulthood from early life exposure to parents' smoking. Am J Public Health 75:487–492.

Sankaranarayanan R. 1990. Oral cancer in India: an epidemiologic and clinical review. Oral Surg Oral Med Oral Pathol 69:325–330.

Sankaranarayanan R, Duffy SW, Day NE, et al. 1989a. A case-control investigation of cancer of the oral tongue and the floor of the mouth in southern India. Int J Cancer 44:617–621.

Sankaranarayanan R, Duffy SW, Padmakumary G, et al. 1989b. Tobacco chewing, alcohol and nasal snuff in cancer of the gingiva in Kerala, India. Br J Cancer 60: 638–643.

Sankaranarayanan R, Duffy SW, Nair MK, et al. 1990. Tobacco and alcohol as risk factors in cancer of the larynx in Kerala, India. Int J Cancer 45:879–882.

Saracci R. 1987. The interactions of tobacco smoking and other agents in cancer etiology. Epidemiol Rev 9:175–193.

Saranath D, Chang SE, Bhoite LT, et al. 1991. High frequency mutation in codons 12 and 61 of H-*ras* oncogene in chewing tobacco-related human oral carcinoma in India. Br J Cancer 63:573–578.

Schectman G, Byrd JC, Gruchow HW. 1989. The influence of smoking or vitamin C status in adults. Am J Public Health 79:158–162.

Scherer G, Adlkofer F. 1986. Endogenous formation of *N*-nitrosoproline in smokers and nonsmokers. In: *Mechanisms in Tobacco Carcinogenesis*, Hoffmann D, Harris CC (eds). Banbury Report #23. Cold Spring Harbor Laboratory, pp 137–148.

Schiffman MH, Bauer HM. Hoover RN, et al. 1993. Epidemiologic evidence showing that human papillomavirus infection causes most cervical intraepithelial neoplasia. J Natl Cancer Inst 85: 958–964.

Schmeltz I, Hoffmann D. 1977. Nitrogen-containing compounds in tobacco and tobacco smoke. Chem Rev 77:295–311.

Schwartz D, Flamant R, Lellough J, Denoix PF. 1961. Results of a French survey on the role of tobacco, particularly inhalation, in different cancer sites. J Natl Cancer Inst 26:1085–1108.

Seidell JC, Cigolini M, Deslypere J-P, et al. 1991. Body fat distribution in relation to physical activity and smoking habits in 38-year-old European men. Am J Epidemiol 133:257–265.

Seitz HK, Simanowski. 1988. Alcohol and carcinogenesis. Annu Rev Nutr 8:99–119.

Shaw HM, Milton GW. 1981. Smoking and the development of metastases from malignant melanoma. Int J Cancer 28:153–156.

Shopland DR, Eyre HJ, Pechacek TF. 1991. Smoking-attributable cancer mortality in 1991: is lung cancer now the leading cause of death among smokers in the United States? J Natl Cancer Inst 83:1142–1148.

Shu XO, Brinton LA, Gao YT, Yuan JM. 1989. Population-based case-control study of ovarian cancer in Shanghai. Cancer Res 49:3670–3674.

Siegel M. 1993. Smoking and leukemia: evaluation of a causal hypothesis. Am J Epidemiol 138:1–9.

Silcocks PBS, Thornton-Jones H, Murphy M. 1987. Squamous and adenocarcinoma of the uterine cervix: a comparison using routine data. Br J Cancer 55:321–325.

Slattery ML, Schumacher MC, West DW, Robison LM. 1988. Smoking and bladder cancer: the modifying effect of cigarettes on other factors. Cancer 61:402–408.

Slattery ML, Robison LM, Schuman KL, et al. 1989. Cigarette smoking and exposure to passive smoke are risk factors for cervical cancer. JAMA 261:1593–1598.

Slattery ML, McDonald A, Bild DE, et al. 1992. Associations of body fat and its distribution with dietary intake, physical activity, alcohol, and smoking in blacks and whites. Am J Clin Nutr 55:943–949.

Sorsa M. 1986. Experimental studies on the mutagenicity and related effects of low-tar and high-tar cigarettes in relation to smoker exposures. In: *Tobacco: A Major International Health Hazard*, Zaridze DG, Peto R (eds. Lyon: International Agency for Research on Cancer, pp 227–235.

Spitz MR, Tilley BC, Batsakis JG, et al. 1984. Risk factors for major salivary gland carcinoma: a case-comparison study. Cancer 54:1854–1859.

Spitzer WO, Lawrence V, Dales R, et al. 1990. Links between passive smoking and disease: a best-evidence synthesis. Clin Invest Med 13:17–42.

Steineck G, Norell SE, Feychting M. 1988. Diet, tobacco and urothelial cancer. Acta Oncol 27:323–327.

Steiner E, Iselious L, Alvan G, et al. 1985. A family study of genetic and environmental factors determining polymorphic hydroxylation of debrisoquin. Clin Pharmacol Ther 38:394–401.

Steinmetz KA, Potter JD, Folsom AR. 1993. Vegetables, fruit, and lung cancer in the Iowa Women's Health Study. Cancer Res 53:536–543.

Stellman SD. 1986a. Cigarette yield and cancer risk: evidence from case-control and prospective studies. In: *Tobacco: A Major In-*

ternational Health Hazard, Zaridge D, Peto R (eds). IARC Sci. Publ. 74. Lyon: International Agency for Research on Cancer, p 197.

STELLMAN SD. 1986b. Interactions between smoking and other exposures: occupation and diet. In: *Mechanisms in Tobacco Carcinogenesis*, Hoffmann D, Harris CC (eds). Banbury Report #23. Cold Spring Harbor Laboratory, pp 377–396.

STELLMAN SD, GARFINKEL L. 1989. Lung cancer risk is proportional to cigarette tar yield: evidence from a prospective study. Prev Med 18:518–525.

STEMMERMANN GN, NOMURA AMY, CHYOU P-H, HANKIN J. 1990. Impact of diet and smoking on risk of developing intestinal metaplasia of the stomach. Dig Dis Sci 35:433–438.

STEPNEY R. 1982. Are smokers' self-reports of inhalation a useful measure of smoke exposure? J Epidemiol Community Health 36:109–112.

STOCKWELL HG, LYMAN GH. 1986. Impact of smoking and smokeless tobacco on the risk of cancer of the head and neck. Head Neck Surg 9:104–110.

STRYKER WS, STAMPFER MJ, STEIN EA, et al. 1990. Diet, plasma levels of beta-carotene and alpha-tocopherol, and risk of malignant melanoma. Am J Epidemiol 131:597–611.

TALAMINI R, BARON AE, BARRA S, et al. 1990. A case-control study of risk factor for renal cell cancer in northern Italy. Cancer Causes Control 1:125–131.

TALAMINI R, FRANCESCHI S, LA VECCHIA C, et al. 1993. Smoking habits and prostate cancer: a case-control study in Northern Italy. Prev Med 22:400–408.

TATSUTA M, IISHI H, OKUDA S. 1988. Effect of cigarette smoking on extent of acid-secreting area and intestinal metaplasia in the stomach. Dig Dis Sci 33:23–29.

THOMAS DB, JIMENEZ LM, MCTIERNAN A, et al. 1992. Breast cancer in men: risk factors with hormonal implications. Am J Epidemiol 135:734–748.

TOLBERT PE, SHY CM, ALLEN JW. 1991. Micronuclei and other nuclear anomalies in buccal smears: a field test in snuff users. Am J Epidemiol 134:840–850.

TOLLERUD DJ, CLARK JW, BROWN LM, et al. 1989. Association of cigarette smoking with decreased numbers of circulating natural killer cells. Am Rev Respir Dis 139;194–198.

TOMINAGA S. 1986a. Smoking and cancer patterns and trends in Japan. In: *Tobacco: A Major International Health Hazard*, Zaridze DG, Peto R (eds.) Lyon, France: International Agency for Research on Cancer, pp 103–114.

TOMINAGA S. 1986b. Spread of smoking to the developing countries. In: *Tobacco: A Major International Health Hazard*, Zaridze DG, Peto R (eds). Lyon, France: International Agency for Research on Cancer, pp 125–134.

TRICHOPOULOS D, DAY NE, KAKLAMANI E, et al. 1987. Hepatitis B virus, tobacco smoking and ethanol consumption in the etiology of hepatocellular carcinoma. Int J Cancer 39:45–49.

TSO TC. 1972a. *Physiology and Biochemistry of Tobacco Plants*. Stroudsburg, PA: Dowden, Hutchinson & Ross, Inc.

TSO TC. 1972b. Manipulation of leaf characteristics through production—role of agriculture in health-related tobacco research. J Natl Cancer Inst 48:1811–1819.

TSUDA M, KURASHIMA Y. 1991. Tobacco smoking, chewing, and snuff dipping: factors contributing to the endogenous formation of N-nitroso compounds. Toxicology 21:243–253.

TSUKUMA H, HIYAMA T, OSHIMA A, et al. 1990. A case-control study of hepatocellular carcinoma in Osaka, Japan. Int J Cancer 45:231–236.

TSUKUMA H, HIYAMA T, TANAKA S, et al. 1993. Risk factors for hepatocellular carcinoma among patients with chronic liver disease. N Engl J Med 328:1797–1801.

TUYNS AJ, ESTEVE J. 1983. Pipe, commercial and hand-rolled cigarette smoking in oesophageal cancer. Int J Epidemiol 12:110–113.

TUYNS AJ, ESTEVE J, RAYMOND L, et al. 1988. Cancer of the larynx/hypopharynx, tobacco and alcohol: IARC International Case-Control Study in Turin and Varese (Italy), Zaragoza and Navarra (Spain), Geneva (Switzerland) and Calvados (France). Int J Cancer 41:483–491.

TUYP E, BURGOYNE A, AITCHISON T, MACKIE R. 1987. A case-control study of possible causative factors in mycosis fungoides. Arch Dermatol 123:196–200.

U.S. DEPARTMENT OF HEALTH AND HUMAN SERVICES. 1981. *The Health Consequences of Smoking. The Changing Cigarette. A Report of the Surgeon General.* U.S. Department of Health and Human Services, Public Health Service, Centers for Disease Control, Center for Chronic Disease Prevention and Health Promotion, Office on Smoking and Health. DHHS(PHS)81–50156.

U.S. DEPARTMENT OF HEALTH AND HUMAN SERVICES. 1986. *The Health Consequences of Using Smokeless Tobacco. A Report of the Surgeon General.* U.S. Department of Health and Human Services, Public Health Service, Centers for Disease Control, Center for Chronic Disease Prevention and Health Promotion, Office on Smoking and Health. NIH Pub. #86–2874.

U.S. DEPARTMENT OF HEALTH AND HUMAN SERVICES. 1988. *The Health Consequences of Smoking. Nicotine Addiction. A Report of the Surgeon General.* U.S. Department of Health and Human Services, Public Health Service, Centers for Disease Control, Center for Chronic Disease Prevention and Health Promotion, Office on Smoking and Health. DHHS(CDC)88–8406.

U.S. DEPARTMENT OF HEALTH AND HUMAN SERVICES. 1989. *The Health Consequences of Smoking. 25 Years of Progress. A Report of the Surgeon General.* U.S. Department of Health and Human Services, Public Health Service, Centers for Disease Control, Center for Chronic Disease Prevention and Health Promotion, Office on Smoking and Health. DHHS(PHS)89–8411.

U.S. DEPARTMENT OF HEALTH AND HUMAN SERVICES. 1990. *The Health Benefits of Smoking Cessation. A Report of the Surgeon General.* U.S. Department of Health and Human Services, Public Health Service, Centers for Disease Control, Center for Chronic Disease Prevention and Health Promotion, Office on Smoking and Health. UDHHS(PHS)90–8416.

U.S. DEPARTMENT OF HEALTH AND HUMAN SERVICES. 1993. *Respiratory Health Effects of Passive Smoking: Cancer and Other* U.S. Department of Health and Human Services, Public Health Service, National Institites of Health NIH 93–3605.

VAN SCHOOTEN FJ, HILLEBRAND MJX, VAN LEEUWEN FE, et al. 1990. Polycyclic aromatic hydrocarbon-DNA adducts in lung tissue from lung cancer patients. Carcinogenesis 11:1677–1679.

VINE MF. 1990. Micronuclei. In: *Biological Markers in Epidemiology*, Hulka BS, Wilcosky TC, Griffith JD (eds). New York: Oxford University Press, pp 125–146.

VINEIS P. 1991. Black (air-cured) and blond (flue-cured) tobacco and cancer risk, I: bladder cancer. Eur J Cancer 27:1491–1493.

WALD N, BARON J (eds). 1990. *Smoking and Hormone-Related Disorders*. Oxford: Oxford University Press.

WALD N, DOLL R, COPELAND G. 1981. Trends in tar, nicotine, and carbon monoxide yields of UK cigarettes manufactured since 1934. Br Med J 282:763–765.

WALD N, FROGGATT P. 1989. *Nicotine, Smoking and the Low Tar Programme*. Oxford: Oxford University Press.

WALD N, IDLE M, BAILEY A. 1978. Carboxyhaemoglobin levels and inhaling habits in cigarette smokers. Thorax 33:201–206.

WALD NJ, IDLE M, BOREHAM J, BAILEY A. 1983 Inhaling and lung cancer: an anomaly explained. Br Med J 287:1273–1275.

WARNER KE. 1978. Possible increases in the underreporting of cigarette consumption. J Am Statist Assoc 73:314–318.

WEIR JM, DUNN JE JR. 1970. Smoking and mortality: a prospective study. Cancer 25:105–112.

WEISS NS. 1990. Cigarette smoking and the incidence of endometrial cancer. In: *Smoking and Hormone-Related Disorders*, Wald N, Baron J (eds). Oxford: Oxford University Press, pp 145–153.

WEISS T, ECKERT A. 1989 Cotinine levels in follicular fluid and serum of IVF patients: effect on granulosa-luteal cell function *in vitro*. Hum Reprod 4:482–485.

WESTRA WH, SLEBOS RJC, OFFERHAUS GJA, et al. 1993. K-ras oncogene activiation in lung adenocarcinomas from former smokers. Cancer 72:432–438.

WHITTEMORE AS, WU ML, PAFFENBARGER RS JR, et al. 1988. Personal and environmental characteristics related to epithelial ovarian cancer. Am J Epidemiol 128:1228–1240.

WILLIAMS RR, HORM JW. 1977. Association of cancer sites with tobacco and alcohol consumption and socioeconomic status of patients: interview study from the Third National Cancer Survey. J Natl Cancer Inst 58:525–547.

WINKELSTEIN W JR. 1990. Smoking and cervical cancer—current status: a review. Am J Epidemiol 131:945–960.

WINN DM, BLOT WJ, SHY CM, et al. 1981. Snuff dipping and oral cancer among women in the southern United States. N Engl J Med 304:745–749.

WINN DM, ZIEGLER RG, PICKLE LW, et al. 1984. Diet in the etiology of oral and pharyngeal cancer among women from the southern United States. Cancer Res 44:1216–1222.

WU-WILLIAMS AH, YU MC, MACK TM. 1990. Life-style, workplace, and stomach cancer by subsite in young men of Los Angeles County. Cancer Res 50:2569–2576.

WYNDER EL, AUGUSTINE A, KABAT GC, HEBERT JR. 1988. Effect of the type of cigarette smoked on bladder cancer risk. Cancer 61:622–627.

WYNDER EL, STELLMAN SD. 1977. Comparative epidemiology of tobacco-related cancers. Cancer Res 37:4608–4622.

XIE J, LESAFFRE E, KESTELOOT H. 1991. The relationship between animal fat intake, cigarette smoking, and lung cancer. Cancer Causes Control 2:79–83.

YEN S, HSIEH C-C, MACMAHON B. 1987. Extrahepatic bile duct cancer and smoking, beverage consumption, past medical history, and oral-contraceptive use. Cancer 59:2112–2116.

YOU W-C, BLOT WJ, CHANG Y-S, et al. 1988. Diet and high risk of stomach cancer in Shandong, China. Cancer Res 48:3518–3523.

YU JJ, MATTSON ME, BOYD GM, et al. 1990. A comparison of smoking patterns in the People's Republic of China. JAMA 264:1575–1579.

YU MC, MACK TM, HANISCH R, et al. 1986. Cigarette smoking, obesity, diuretic use, and coffee consumption as risk factors for renal cell carcinoma. J Natl Cancer Inst 77:351–356.

ZAHM SH, HEINEMAN EF, VAUGHT JB. 1992. Soft tissue sarcoma and tobacco use: data from a prospective cohort study of United States veterans. Cancer Causes Control 3:371–376.

ZATONSKI W, BECHER H, LISSOWSKA J, WAHRENDORF J. 1991. Tobacco, alcohol, and diet in the etiology of laryngeal cancer: a population-based case-control study. Cancer Causes Control 2:3–10.

ZATONSKI WA, LA VECCHIA C, PRZEWOZNIAK K, et al. 1992. Risk factors for gallbladder cancer: a Polish case-control study. Int J Cancer 51:707–711.

ZHENG T, BOYLE P, HUANFANG H, et al. 1990. Tobacco smoking, alcohol consumption, and risk of oral cancer: a case-control study in Beijing, People's Republic of China. Cancer Causes Control 1:173–179.

ZHENG W, BLOT WJ, SHU X-O, et al. 1992. A population-based case-control study of cancers of the nasal cavity and paranasal sinuses in Shanghai. Int J Cancer 52:557–561.

ZIEGLER RG, MASON TJ, STEMHAGEN A, et al. 1986. Carotenoid intake, vegetables, and the risk of lung cancer among white men in New Jersey. Am J Epidemiol 123:1080–1093.

ZIEGLER RG, BRINTON LA, HAMMAN RF, et al. 1990. Diet and the risk of invasive cervical cancer among white women in the United States. Am J Epidemiol 132:432–445.

15 Alcohol

OLE MØLLER JENSEN
SALLY L. PAINE
ANTHONY J. McMICHAEL
MARIANNE EWERTZ

Humans have consumed alcoholic beverages for thousands of years. Alcohol consumption has thus come to have diverse symbolic and social functions in many cultures. Some of the world's major religions, however, have a strict prohibition against alcohol consumption. Elsewhere moderate drinking is usually socially acceptable, but the repeated excessive consumption of alcohol is regarded as a behavioral or medical disorder in most societies.

Alcohol consumption is associated with many health problems. Alcoholic liver disease ranges from the benign, reversible, fatty liver to the more severe alcoholic hepatitis and irreversible cirrhosis. Alcohol has various effects on the gastrointestinal tract and may cause acute and chronic pancreatitis. It can adversely influence the immune system and the developing fetus, and it is associated with a number of neurological and mental problems. Alcohol intoxication is a common cause of injury, accidental death and social violence. At moderate intakes, however, alcohol consumption reduces the risk of death from coronary heart disease (Doll et al., 1994) and, probably, from gallstone disease (Scragg et al., 1984).

An association between alcohol drinking and cancer has long been observed. In 1910 it was noted in Paris that some 80% of patients with cancers of the esophagus and gastric cardia were alcoholics who drank mainly absinth (Lamy, 1910). Mortality statistics in the first half of this century from various countries showed high risk for cancer of the oral cavity, pharynx, esophagus, and larynx among persons employed in the production and distribution of alcoholic beverages (Clemmesen, 1965). These early observations have been followed by many formal studies of the association between alcohol and cancer. In 1988 the International Agency for Research on Cancer (IARC) of the World Health Organization (WHO) concluded that there is sufficient evidence that alcoholic beverages are carcinogenic in humans (International Agency for Research on Cancer, 1988). While this causal relation clearly applies for cancers of certain organs, the question remains unresolved for others.

TYPES OF STUDIES

The relation between alcohol and cancer has been studied via various types of epidemiological investigations. *Correlation studies* (or ecological studies) examine the geographical, temporal, or other population-based relationship between per capita alcohol consumption and cancer rate (incidence or mortality). Whereas routine (especially registry-based) data on cancer rates are often reliable, the mean level of alcohol intake for a population or subpopulation must often be inferred from commercial sales data or from knowledge of residential location, religious affiliation, or other such characteristics. It is usually difficult to control for interpopulation differences in other risk factors for cancer, and these differences may therefore confound the observed alcohol–cancer relationship.

Better quality evidence is available from cohort and case–control studies in which information on alcohol consumption, other cancer risk factors, and cancer occurrence is obtained at an individual level. In *retrospective cohort studies* the cancer risk is typically studied in groups of persons defined as having exhibited a consumption pattern above (or below) the average pattern of the comparison population. With few exceptions, neither detailed information on the amount or type of beverage drunk, nor information on potentially confounding characteristics, notably smoking, has been available. Nevertheless, retrospective cohort studies of alcoholics, who are defined in various ways, and of oc-

Throughout this chapter, *alcohol* is used interchangeably with *alcoholic beverages*. *Ethanol* is used to denote the key component of alcoholic beverages.

cupational groups having easy access to alcohol have provided important information on the pattern of cancer related to alcohol intake. These studies are summarized in Table 15–1. More detailed information on both drinking and smoking has been available in the fewer number of *prospective cohort studies* that have been carried out, thus enabling site-specific cancer risks to be determined (also summarized in Table 15–1).

Most of the detailed information about the relationship between alcohol and cancers of individual sites has come from *case–control studies*. In these studies, as in prospective cohort studies, measurements of usual past alcohol consumption are obtained by structured interview or questionnaire. These have been found to provide satisfactory estimates of alcohol intake (Riboli et al., 1986; Willett et al., 1987).

CORRELATION STUDIES

Alcohol consumption patterns show clear spatial and temporal variations at the population level and often differ between population subgroups. Hence there have been many correlation studies of alcohol and cancer.

Strong geographic correlations have consistently been found in France between mortality from liver cirrhosis, alcoholism, and esophageal cancer; alcoholism has also been associated with cancers of the mouth, pharynx, and stomach (Lasserre et al, 1967). Similar geographic correlations have been reported between cancer mortality and per capita consumption of alcohol and tobacco in 41 of the U.S. states and in 24 countries (Breslow and Enstrom, 1974). In particular, significant tobacco-adjusted correlations were found for beer consumption in relation to stomach, colon, and rectal cancer in both men and women. In a subsequent analysis of 29 countries, this geographic correlation with colon and rectal cancer was confirmed. Changes in beer consumption over time also correlated with subsequent changes over time in occurence of rectal cancer (Potter et al, 1982).

In a similar analysis for the 46 prefectures of Japan, few consistent relationships between consumption of different types of alcoholic beverages during 1964–66 and gastrointestinal cancer mortality during 1969–71 were found (Kono and Ikeda, 1979). However, pancreatic cancer correlated significantly with the consumption of sake and whisky among both sexes after adjusting for cigarette consumption. In analysing data from 30 countries, Qiao and colleagues (1988), found that after adjustment for hepatitis B prevalence, there was a statistically significant relationship between per capita alcohol consumption and primary liver carcinoma mortality.

Time trends in per capita alcohol consumption and mortality from esophageal and laryngeal cancers have been clearly linked in France (Tuyns and Audigier, 1976), and such an association has also been described in relation to differential time trends in several other countries (McMichael, 1978; Wynder et al, 1991). Correlated time trends in alcohol consumption and colorectal cancer mortality, including trends in male–female ratios, have been confirmed in Australia, England, New Zealand, and the United States (McMichael et al, 1979).

In other correlation studies, cancer rates have been compared in subpopulations with different alcohol consumption levels. For example, in a study of the relation between cancer incidence and alcohol consumption among the five main ethnic groups in Hawaii (Hinds et al., 1980), stomach cancer incidence was strongly positively associated with beer consumption but inversely associated with wine and spirits consumption. Studies of Mormons and Seventh Day Adventists (SDA) have also contributed circumstantial evidence, since these religious groups abstain from tobacco and alcohol. Fewer cancers were observed in SDAs than were expected on the basis of general population cancer rates in studies in the U.S. (Wynder et al, 1959; Lemon et al, 1964; Phillips et al, 1980) and in Denmark (Jensen, 1983)—especially for cancers of the mouth, larynx, and esophagus. A significant deficit of colorectal cancer among SDAs has also been noted (Phillips et al, 1980; Jensen, 1983), although it is difficult to know to what extent that reduced risk might be due to vegetarianism or other dietary practices. Very low risks for cancers of the esophagus and larynx have also been found among Mormon men and women in Utah (Lyon et al, 1976). The incidence rates for cancer of the stomach, colorectum, and pancreas were about one-third lower for Mormons than for non-Mormons.

Many correlation studies have linked alcohol intake with cancers of the upper aerodigestive tract and liver cancer, and often with colon and rectal cancers. However, it has usually not been possible to infer a causal relationship because alcohol consumption is likely to be associated with other behavioral risk factors for those same cancers, especially cigarette smoking and aspects of diet. Such confounding factors can usually be adequately dealt with only in studies where individual-based measurements are made.

COHORT AND CASE–CONTROL STUDIES

Cancer of the Oral Cavity and Pharynx

The mucosa of the oral cavity and pharynx (excluding the nasopharynx) comes into close contact with alcohol upon ingestion. It is therefore biologically plausible that alcohol directly affects carcinogenesis in these sites via physiochemical or metabolic effects.

TABLE 15–1. *Summary of Results of Cohort Studies of Alcohol and Cancer*

Study Reference	Years of Enrollment	Population	Duration of Follow-up; No. of Cancer (ca) Deaths, or Incident Cases	Standardized Mortality Ratio/Relative Risk[a] (95% confidence intervals, where originally reported)								
				Oral Cavity	Pharynx	Larynx	Esophagus	Stomach	Colon	Rectum	Liver	Pancreas
RETROSPECTIVE COHORT STUDIES												
Norwegian alcoholics study Sundby (1967)	1925–1939	1,722 men	37 years; 204 ca deaths	5.0 (2.8–8.6)	4.4 (2.1–8.5)	3.1 (1.0–7.3)	4.1 (2.9–5.6)	1.3 (0.9–1.7)	1.0 (0.5–1.9)	1.9	1.9	1.6
Finnish alcohol misusers Hakulinen et al (1974)	1944–1959	Estimated 205,000 men alive in 1965–1968 (born 1881–1932)	Incidence of selected cancer sites only; 449 cases	—	—		1.7 (1.4–2.1)	—	1.0 (0.7–1.1)	—	1.5[b]	—
Finnish alcoholics study Hakulinen et al (1974)	1967–1970	Mean no. of men in registry was 4,370	4 years; 81 incident ca cases	—	5.7 (1.2–16.5)	1.4 (0.3–4.1)	4.1 (1.4–9.3)	0.8 (0.3–1.6)	1.9 (0.4–5.4)	—	2.5	1.8
U.K. alcoholics study Nicholls et al (1974); Adelstein and White (1976)	1953–1964	2,070 men and women	17 years	—	—	—	—	0.8 (0.3–1.5)	1.3 (0.6–2.5)	0.9 (0.3–2.4)	5.8 (men)[b]	1.5
Massachusetts alcoholics study Monson and Lyon (1975)	1930, 1935, 1940	1,139 men 243 women	41 years; 894 deaths, 105 ca deaths	—	3.3 (1.8–5.6)[c]	3.8 (1.4–8.2)	1.9 (0.4–5.5)	1.0 (0.6–1.7)	0.6 (0.3–1.3)	0.7 (0.2–1.8)	1.0	0.6
U.S. veterans alcoholics study Robinette et al (1979)	1944–1945	4,401 men	29 years; 166 ca deaths	—	2.2 (1.1–4.6)[c]	1.7 (0.7–4.4)	2.0 (0.9–5.1)	1.0 (0.4–2.3)	0.8 (0.3–1.9)	3.3 (0.7–22.4)	>1	0.9 (0.2–3.2)
Danish brewery workers Jensen (1979)	1939–1963	14,313 men	30 years; 951 ca deaths	1.4 (0.9–2.3)	1.9 (1.0–3.4)	2.0 (1.4–2.7)	2.1 (1.5–2.8)	0.9 (0.7–1.1)	1.0 (0.8–1.4)	1.0 (0.8–1.3)	1.5[b]	1.1
Dublin brewery workers Dean et al (1979)	1954–1973	Not stated (men; 1628 total deaths)	20 years; total ca deaths not stated	—	—	—	0.6 (0.3–1.2)	0.8 (0.6–1.1)	1.3 (0.9–1.9)	1.6 (1.1–2.3)	1.3	1.2
Canadian alcoholics study Schmidt and Popham (1981)	1951–1970	9,889 men	21 years; 240 ca deaths	—	4.2 (2.7–6.3)[c]	4.3 (1.4–4.9)	3.2 (1.8–5.2)	1.0 (0.6–1.6)	1.0 (0.6–1.6)	1.0 (0.5–1.9)	2.0	1.2
Swedish brewery workers Carstensen et al (1990)	1961–1979	6,230 men	19 years; 712 incident ca cases	—	1.2 (0.7–1.8)[c]	1.7 (0.9–2.9)	2.5 (1.5–3.8)	1.1 (0.8–1.4)	1.2 (0.9–1.5)	1.7 (1.3–2.3)	1.7 (1.0–2.8)	1.7 (1.2–2.3)
Swedish alcoholics study Adami et al (1992a,b)	1965–1983	9,353 men and women	19 years (av, 7.7 years)	—	4.1[c] (2.9–5.7)	3.3 (1.7–6.0)	6.8 (4.5–9.9)	0.9 (0.6–1.4)	1.1[d] (0.8–1.5)		3.1 (1.6–5.3)	1.5 (0.9–2.3)
Danish alcoholics study Tonnesen et al (1994)	1954–1987	18,307 men and women	av, 13 years for men; av, 9 years for women; 1623 incident cases	7.2 (5.1–9.8)	7.3 (5.4–9.5)	3.7 (2.8–4.6)	5.3 (4.0–6.8)	1.3 (1.0–1.7)	1.0 (0.7–1.3)	1.0 (0.7–1.3)	3.9 (2.8–5.40)	1.3 (1.0–1.8)

PROSPECTIVE COHORT STUDIES												
Kaiser-Permante study (I) Klatsky et al (1981)	1964–1968	8,060 men and women	10 years; 215 ca deaths	—	4.0[c] (1.7–7.9)	—	—		1.0[e]	—	—	2.1[e]
Japanese doctors study, Kono et al (1983, 1985, 1986)	1965	5,135	19 years; 381 ca deaths	—	8.6[c,e] (6.9–10.6)	—		1.2[e]	—	1.4[d,e] (0.5–4.0)	2.7[e] (1.0–6.8)	1.4
Hawaiian Japanese study. Blackwelder et al (1980); Pollack et al (1984); Stemmermann et al (1990); Nomura et al (1990); Kato et al (1992a)	1965–1968	7,572 men	24 years; 1,321 ca cases	—	+[f,b]	+[b]	+[b]	1.17[e] (0.7–1.9)	1.4[e] (1.0–2.2)	1.9[b,e]	NA[g]	NA
Framingham study Gordon and Kannel (1984)	1948	2,106 men 2,641 women	22 years; 257 ca deaths	—	—	—	—	+[b]	NA	—	—	—
Western Electric Company, Chicago Garland et al (1985)	1957	2,107 men	19 years; 235 ca cases (29 colon, 20 rectal)	—	—	—	—	—	—	NA[d]	—	—
Southern Californian retirement community Wu et al (1987); Paganini-Hill et al (1990)	1981–1982	11,888 men and women	4.5 years; 126 incident cases colorectal ca	—	—	—	—	—	2.4[d] (1.3–4.5) 1.5[d] (0.8–2.6)	— men women	—	—
Kaiser Permanente Study (II) Klatsky et al (1988)	1976–1984	106,203 men and women	1–7 years; 269 incident colorectal ca cases	—	—	—	—	—	1.7 all 1.2 men 2.6[b] women	3.2[b]	—	—
Japanese study Hirayama (1989b, 1990)	1965	265,118 men and women	17 years; 14,740 ca deaths	2.3[b,e] men	2.4[b,e] men	1.4[e] (1.0–2.1) men and women	2.3[b,e] men	0.9[b,e] men	5.4[b,e,h] men 1.9[b,e,h] women	1.4[b,e] men	1.2[b,e] men	1.0[e] (0.8–1.2) men and women
U.S. Norwegian immigrants study Kneller et al (1991); Zheng et al (1993)	1966	17,633 men and women	20 years	—	—	—	—	NA	—	—	—	3.1 (1.2–8.0)
Japanese study Kato et al (1992b)	1985	9,753 men and women	6 years; 57 stomach ca deaths	—	—	—	—	3.1 (1.4–6.9)	—	—	—	—
Netherlands study Goldbohm et al (1994)	1986	120,852 men and women	3.3 years; 217 colon ca, 113 rectal ca cases	—	—	—	—	—	NA	2.0 (1.1–3.9)	—	—
Iowa women's health study Gapstur et al (1994)	1986	41,837 postmenopausal women	5 years; 237 colon ca, 75 rectal ca cases	—	—	—	—	—	1.1 (0.6–1.9)	1.3 (0.7–2.2)	—	—

[a]Historical cohort studies present standardized mortality ratios, prospective cohort studies present relative risks. Numbers in parentheses are 95% confidence intervals except for Robinette et al (1979), where numbers in parentheses are 90% confidence intervals.
[b]Estimates are significantly different from the reference group ($P < 0.05$).
[c]Oral and pharyngeal cancers combined.
[d]Colorectal cancer.
[e]Highest vs. lowest consumption category.
[f]Positive association.
[g]NA, no association.
[h]Sigmoid colon only.

Cohort Studies. The rates of occurrence of oral cavity and/or pharyngeal cancer have been reported from nine retrospective and four prospective cohort studies (Table 15–1). The relative risk increased in all studies, particularly in the studies of alcoholics in Norway (Sundby, 1967), Canada (Schmidt and De Lint, 1972; Schmidt and Popham, 1981), Finland (Hakulinen et al, 1974), Sweden (Adami et al, 1992a), and Denmark (Tonnesen et al, 1994). Increased risks for tumor development of these sites, although not statistically significant, were also found in the studies of Danish brewery workers and Swedish brewery workers, who were not alcoholics but had an above average daily beer consumption (Jensen, 1979; Cartensen et al, 1990). A strong positive association between the level of alcohol consumption and risk of cancer of the oral cavity/pharynx was observed in all four prospective cohort studies (Klatsky et al, 1981; Kono et al, 1983, 1985, 1986; Kato et al, 1992a; Hirayama, 1989b).

Case–Control Studies. The earliest case–control studies were carried out in the U.S. (Wynder et al, 1957a) and in France (Schwartz et al, 1962). The latter study compared average smoking and drinking habits of 3,937 male patients with cancer at various sites and 1,807 control patients admitted to hospital for traffic and work accidents in Paris and certain other French towns. These initial observations linking alcohol and tobacco consumption with cancer risk have been confirmed by further studies in North and South America, Europe, Asia, and Australia.

Of the 30 studies listed in Table 15–2 comparing alcohol consumption between controls and cases with oral cancer, fourteen, ten, and eight studies showed a significant positive association between alcohol drinking and respectively, cancers of the oral cavity, pharynx, and oral cavity and pharynx combined. Six studies showed positive but non-significant associations (Hirayama, 1966; Olsen et al, 1985b; Notani, 1988; Sankaranarayanan et al, 1989, 1990b; Nandakumar et al, 1990; Zheng et al, 1992b). Four of these studies were in India where the prevalence of alcohol consumption, particularly relative to tobacco chewing and smoking, is low (see Table 15–2). Of the eleven studies providing analyses by sex, eight showed significant positive associations, two non-significant positive associations and one a non-significant negative association between drinking and oral/pharyngeal cancer in women (see Table 15–2). In only one of these studies, however, was the number of cases greater than 100 (Bross and Coombs, 1976).

In these studies, relative risk generally increases with increasing amounts of alcohol taken, and this association does not appear to be due to confounding by other known risk factors. This is particularly important for tobacco smoking since it is causally related to cancers of the oral cavity and pharynx, and personal alcohol and tobacco consumption are usually correlated.

Rothman and Keller (1972) examined further the data on both alcohol and tobacco consumption originally obtained by Keller and Terris (1965) in their study of U.S. veterans. When stratified for smoking, the relative risk for oral and pharyngeal cancer increased with increasing alcohol consumption at every level of smoking (Table 15–3). A doubling of the relative risk occurred among non-smokers who consumed 1.6 oz or more (36g+) alcohol daily. This demonstration of an independent carcinogenic effect of alcohol consumption has been confirmed in studies from Canada (Elwood et al, 1984) and southern Europe (Tuyns et al, 1988a).

The analysis by Rothman and Keller (1972) also showed a synergism between alcohol and tobacco in the development of oral cavity cancer (i.e., smoking appeared to modify the effect of alcohol); heavy drinkers who were also heavy smokers had a relative risk of 15.6 compared with persons who neither smoked nor drank. These results have been corroborated by other studies, although there is statistical inconstancy and uncertainty as to whether smoking and drinking interact in a supra-additive or supra-multiplicative fashion (Wynder et al, 1957a; Graham et al, 1977; Elwood et al, 1984; Olsen et al, 1985b; Tuyns et al, 1987; Spitz et al, 1988). More recently, Negri and colleagues (1993) have reported a case–control study of northern Italy in which alcohol and tobacco appeared to act in a supra-multiplicative way.

The increased cancer risk in the early cohort studies of alcoholics may have encouraged the view that it was strong alcoholic beverages in particular which cause an increase in cancers of the upper aerodigestive tract. Wynder et al (1957a) found the highest relative risk among whisky drinkers, but the overall trends for consumers of beer and consumers of whisky were similar. Subsequently, it emerged more clearly that the increases in the risk of oral cavity and pharyngeal cancers were similar for drinkers of different types of beverages (Keller and Terris, 1965; Williams and Horm, 1977). Overall, the results indicate that consumption of any alcoholic beverage, irrespective of its ethanol concentration, increases the risk of oral cavity and pharyngeal cancers.

Cancer of the Larynx

The several parts of the larynx must be distinguished when considering the aetiology of cancer of the larynx. The endolarynx is exposed only to inhaled agents, while the junctional area between the larynx and the pharynx is exposed to both inhaled and ingested agents.

Cohort Studies. Studies of alcoholics have consistently shown increased risks of laryngeal cancer compared with the general population, as summarized in Table

TABLE 15–2. *Summary of Results of Case–Control Studies of Oral Cavity and Pharyngeal Cancers*

	Oral Cavity		*Pharynx*		*Oral Cavity and Pharynx*		
Study Site References	*Cases, Controls*	*Relative Risk*	*Cases, Controls*	*Relative Risk*	*Cases, Controls*	*Relative Risk*	*Comments*
New York, USA Wynder et al (1957)	Men (462, 207)	5.2 (2.2–12.4)	Men (81, 207)	7.7 (1.9–31.2)	—	—	Crude RR
Buffalo, NY, USA Vincent and Marchetta (1963)	Men (33, 100)	9.7 (3.0–31.9)	Men (33, 100)	52.5 (12.7–217.0)	—	—	Crude RR
	Women (9, 50)	41.0 (3.4–495.3)	Women (7, 50)	82.0 (14.0–481.2)	—	—	—
New York, USA Keller and Terris (1965)	—	—	—	—	Men (134, 134)	3.7 (1.7–7.8)	RR based on pairs matched for smoking.
Ceylon (Sri Lanka) Hirayama (1966)	Men and Women (76, 228)	1.5 (0.9–2.8)	—	—	—	—	RR adjusted for tobacco chewing.
Puerto Rico Martinez (1969)	Men (108, 108)	2.8 (1.1–7.0)	Men (39, 39)	14.7 (2.4–89.7)	—	—	RR based on pairs matched for age and smoking.
	Women (30, 30)	0.8 (0.2–3.6)					
Buffalo, NY, USA Bross and Coombs (1976)	Women (145, 1973)	3.4 (1.7–6.6)	—	—	—	—	RR adjusted for age and smoking.
Buffalo, NY, USA Graham et al. (1977)	Men (584, 1222)	2.7 (1.9–3.7)	—	—	—	—	Crude RR
Multicenter study, USA Williams and Horm (1977)	Men (74, 1788)	1.4 (NS)[a,b]	Men (47, 1788)	6.2[c]	—	—	RR adjusted for age, race, and smoking; CI could not be calculated.
	Women (20, 3188)	9.7[b,c]	Women (18, 3188)	17.0[c]	—	—	
	Men (53, 1788)	3.7[c,d]	—	—	—	—	
	Women (25, 3188)	1.5 (NS)[d]	—	—	—	—	
New York, USA Feldman and Boxer (1979); Feldman et al (1975)	—	—	—	—	Men (96, 182)	4.5[c]	RR adjusted for age and tobacco.
British Columbia, Canada Elwood et al (1984)	Men and women (133, 133)	4.5[c]	Men and women (87, 87)	12.1[c]	—	—	RR adjusted for smoking, socioeconomic group, dental care, and risk of tuberculosis; CI could not be calculated.
Denmark Olsen et al (1985b)	—	—	Men and women (32, 1141)	1.8[e] (0.7–3.3)	—	—	RR adjusted for age, sex, and smoking.

(continued)

TABLE 15–2. *Summary of Results of Case–Control Studies of Oral Cavity and Pharyngeal Cancers (Continued)*

Study Site References	Oral Cavity		Pharynx		Oral Cavity and Pharynx		Comments
	Cases, Controls	Relative Risk	Cases, Controls	Relative Risk	Cases, Controls	Relative Risk	
Paris, France Brugere et al (1986)	Men (759, unknown)	70.3 (42.8–115.4)	Men (637, unknown)	70.3[f] (41.2–120.0)	—	—	RR adjusted for smoking.
	Men (97, unknown)	10.5[k] (4.0–27.7)	(366, unknown)	143.1[e] (61.9–330.5)			
			(217, unknown)	101.4[g] (44.0–233.9)			
Italy, Spain, Switzerland, France Tuyns et al (1988a)	—	—	Men (281, 3057)	12.5[e] (6.3–25.0)	—	—	RR adjusted for smoking, age, and area of residence.
			Men (118, 3057)	10.6[g] (4.4–25.8)			
Houston, TX, USA Spitz et al (1988)	—	—	—	—	Men (131, 131) Women (54, 54)	2.2[c]; 2.0[c,h] 0.6; 2.0[h]	RR adjusted for smoking.
Multicenter study, USA Blot et al (1988)	—	—	—	—	Men (762, 837) Women (352, 431)	8.8 (5.4–14.3) 9.1 (3.9–21.0)	RR adjusted for smoking, age, race, study location, and respondent status.
Bombay, India Notani (1988)	Men (278, 392)	1.2 (0.7–1.9)	Men (225, 392)	1.4 (0.9–2.4)	—	—	RR adjusted for age, smoking and chewing habits.
Kerala, India Sankaranarayanan et al (1989)	Men (tongue, floor of mouth) (158, 314)	NA[i]	—	—	—	—	Crude RR of 3.2, but RR no longer significant after adjustment for pan tobacco chewing, bidi smoking and bidi and cigarette smoking.
Sao Paulo, Curitiba, Goiania, Brazil Franco et al (1989)	Men and women (232, 464)	8.8[c]	—	—	—	—	RR adjusted for age, sex, and smoking.
Italy, northern region Franceschi et al (1990)	Men (157, 1272)	3.4[c]	Men (134, 1272)	3.6[c]	—	—	RR adjusted for age, area of residence, education, occupation, and smoking.
Franceschi et al (1992)	Men (tongue) (102, 726)	3.4[c]	—	—	—	—	RR adjusted for age, area of residence, occupation, and smoking status.
	(mouth) (104, 726)	3.0[c]	—	—	—	—	
Franceschi et al (1994)	—	—	—	—	Men (465, 1706) Women (81, 557)	7.8 (5.1–12.0) 4.5 (1.5–13.1)	RR adjusted for age, study center, and smoking.

Beijing, China Zheng et al (1990)	Men (248, 248)	2.3	—	—	—	—	RR adjusted for age, education, and smoking.
Bangalore, India Nandakumar et al (1990)	Men and Women (348, 348)	NA	—	—	—	—	RR not reported.
Kerala, India Sankaranarayanan et al (1990b)	Men (buccal and labial mucosa) (250, 546)	1.6 (1.0–2.6)	—	—	—	—	RR adjusted for age, smoking, betel-tobacco chewing, and snuff-taking.
Uruguay Oreggia et al (1991)	Men (57, 353)	11.6[j] (3.3–40.7)	—	—	—	—	RR adjusted for age, county, type of tobacco and smoking habits.
Seoul, Korea Choi and Kahyo (1991b)	Men (113, 339) Women (44, 132)	14.8 (5.0–43.7) 8.1 (0.3–202.7)	Men (133, 399) Women (19, 57)	11.2 (4.2–29.8) 2.0 (0.1–62.7)	—	—	RR adjusted for smoking.
Shanghai, China Zheng et al (1992a,b)	—	—	—	—	Men (115, 269) Women (89, 145)	1.7 P = 0.08 —	RR adjusted for smoking; very low prevalence of alcohol drinking in women so RR not calculated in women.
Western New York, USA Marshall et al (1992)	—	—	—	—	Men and women (290, 290)	+	?
Melbourne, Australia Kune et al (1993)	—	—	—	—	Men (41, 398)	+*	?
New Jersey, USA Mashberg et al (1993)	—	—	—	—	Men (359, 2280)	7.1 (4.1–12.2)	RR adjusted for age, race, and smoking.
Bombay, India Rao, et al (1994a,b)	Men (713, 635)	1.5 (1.1–2.1)	—	—	—	—	RR adjusted for diet, tobacco chewing, education, bidi smoking, age, and residence.
Heidelberg, Germany Maier et al (1994)	—	—	Men (105, 420)	125.2[c]	—	—	RR adjusted for smoking.

[a] NS, not significant.
[b] Lip, tongue.
[c] P < 0.05 for trend.
[d] Gum, mouth.
[e] Hypopharynx.
[f] Oropharynx.
[g] Epilarynx.
[h] Hard liquor; beer/wine. Includes larynx.
[i] NA, no association.
[j] Tongue.
[k] Lip.

TABLE 15–3. *Relative Risk of Oral Cavity and Pharynx Cancer According to Level of Exposure to Smoking and Alcohol**

	Smoking (Cigarette Equivalents per Day)			
Alcohol/Day	*0*	*<20*	*20–39*	*40+*
0	1.00	1.63	1.62	3.40
<0.4 oz (9.5g)	1.66	1.89	3.29	3.35
0.4–1.5 oz (9.5–36g)	1.88	4.85	4.84	8.20
1.6+ oz (36+ g)	2.27	4.79	9.97	15.6
Total number of cases	26	44	248	143

* Risks are expressed relative to a risk of 1.00 for persons who neither smoked nor drank. (From Rothman, 1976.)

15–1. These studies are limited by the lack of information on smoking—a well-established cause of laryngeal cancer. However, the study of Danish brewery workers (Jensen, 1979) indicates that the association can be attributed to alcohol drinking since the relative risk for laryngeal cancer was 3.7 in persons employed in beer production, while it was 0.7 in those employed in mineral water production.

Case–Control Studies. The relationship between alcohol intake and cancer of the larynx has been examined in 25 case–control studies (Table 15–4). The first study by Wynder et al (1956) showed a significantly higher alcohol consumption in cases than in control patients. In all, 22 of the 25 studies have shown a significant positive association and three show a non-significant positive association between laryngeal cancer and drinking. Adjustment for smoking, whenever feasible, has not removed this association with alcohol. Of the four studies for which separate analyses by sex were reported, three showed non-significant positive associations and one showed a non-significant negative association in women. In none of these studies, however, was the number of cases greater than 25.

The borderline areas between the larynx and pharynx (i.e., free border of epiglottis, posterior surface of suprahyoid portion, and junctional region of the folds, aryepiglottic fold, arytinoid) belong partly to the larynx and partly to the pharynx. Since these problems of anatomical definition may have exposure implications, it is important to note that Wynder and colleagues (1956) did not find any difference between the alcohol-related risk for "intrinsic" and that for "extrinsic" laryngeal cancer. In a detailed study in Italy, Spain, Switzerland, and France, Tuyns and colleagues (1988a) found significant increases in risk with increases in the daily amount of alcohol consumed, both for supraglottic tumor locations (relative risk [RR] = 2.0, 121+ gm ethanol vs. 0–120 gm ethanol per day) and for glottic and subglottic sites (RR = 3.4). These relative risks were adjusted for smoking, age, and area of residence.

The joint effect of alcohol and tobacco has been investigated in many studies (Flanders and Rothman, 1986; Burch et al, 1981; Elwood et al, 1984; Hinds et al, 1979; Herity et al, 1981, 1982; Olsen et al, 1985a; Zagraniski et al, 1986; Tuyns et al, 1988a; Brownson and Chang, 1987; De Stefani et al, 1987; Spitz et al, 1988). A synergistic effect between alcohol and tobacco in the induction of laryngeal cancer has been widely reported, and in the study by Tuyns et al. (1988a) a multiplicative model provided an adequate description of the data (Table 15–5). The association between laryngeal cancer and increasing consumption of alcohol in light smokers (Table 15–5) indicates that alcohol independently affects the risk of laryngeal cancer.

It had been previously suggested that the relative risk of laryngeal cancer was particularly high for heavy whisky consumers in the USA (Wynder et al, 1956). However, a significant relative risk was also seen for wine and beer drinkers in that study. In further studies in North America (Wynder et al, 1976; Williams and Horm, 1977; Burch et al, 1981), the relative risk was similar for consumption of comparable amounts of wine, beer, and spirits. In a large case–control study in Denmark (Olsen et al, 1985a), the only significantly increased relative risk was found for drinking beer. Although adjustment was not made for use of other beverages in any of these beverage-specific studies, the results indicate that all types of alcoholic beverages increase the risk of laryngeal cancer.

Cancer of the Esophagus

The mucosa of the esophagus comes into direct contact with alcohol upon consumption. It is therefore plausible that alcohol may influence esophageal carcinogenesis.

Cohort Studies. The relative risk of esophageal cancer has been evaluated in 11 retrospective cohort studies and two prospective cohort studies, shown in Table 15–1. With the exception of the study of Dublin brewery workers (Dean et al, 1979), all retrospective cohort studies have shown an approximately two- to seven-fold increase in risk of esophageal cancer compared with rates for the general population. No information has been available in the retrospective cohort studies on tobacco smoking or other risk factors for esophageal cancer. However, in one study of Canadian alcoholics (Schmidt and Popham, 1981), the relative risk for esophageal cancer remained doubled when the observed number of esophageal cancer deaths was compared with an expected number derived from the death rates for a group of persons with a similar average number of cigarettes smoked per day. In a large prospective cohort

TABLE 15–4. *Summary of Results of Case–Control Studies of Laryngeal Cancer*

Study Site Reference	Subjects (Cases, Controls)	Relative Risk (RR) (Highest vs. Lowest Category)	Comments
New York, USA, Wynder et al (1956)	Men (209, 209)	1.8 (1.0–2.9)	RR adjusted for smoking.
Buffalo, NY, USA Vincent and Marchetta (1963)	Men (23, 100)	5.9 (2.4–14.3)	Crude RR
Multicenter study, USA, Wynder et al (1976)	Men (224, 414)	2.3 (1.5–3.4)	RR adjusted for smoking.
France Spalajkovic (1976)	Men (200, 200)	11.2 (6.9–18.2)	Crude RR
Multicenter study, USA, Williams and Horm (1977)	Men (99, 1788)	2.3[a]	RR adjusted for smoking, age, and race.
	Women (11, 3188)	0.8 (NS)	
Washington State, USA, Hinds et al (1979)	Men (47, 47)	9.0 (2.4–34.1)	Crude RR
New York, USA, Graham et al (1981)	Men (374, 381)	1.8[a]	RR adjusted for cigarettes.
Ontario, Canada, Burch et al (1981)	Men (184, 184)	4.8 (2.3–9.9)	RR adjusted for smoking.
Dublin, Ireland, Herity et al (1981, 1982)	Men (59, 200)	3.2	Crude RR; 95% CI could not be calculated.
British Colombia, Canada, Elwood et al (1984)	Men and women (154, 154)	6.4[a,b] 2.2[a,c]	RR adjusted for smoking, socioeconomic group, marital status, dental care, and history of tuberculosis.
Denmark Olsen et al (1985a)	Men and women (326, 1134)	4.1	RR adjusted for smoking, 95% CI could not be calculated.
New Haven, CT, USA Zagraniski et al (1986)	Men (87, 153)	4.2 (1.4–12.4)	RR adjusted for smoking.
Paris, France Brugere et al (1986)	Men (224, unknown)	42.1[d] (20.5–86.4)	RR adjusted for smoking. Control group selected from national survey.
	(242, unknown)	6.1[e] (3.4–10.9)	
Missouri, USA Brownson and Chang (1987)	Men (63, 200)	4.9[a]	RR adjusted for smoking and age.
Uruguay De Stefani et al (1987)	Men (107, 290)	9.3 (3.5–24.9)	RR adjusted for smoking and age.
Italy, Spain, Switzerland, France Tuyns et al (1988a)	Men (727, 3057)	2.6[f] (1.8–3.6)	RR adjusted for smoking, age, and area of residence.
Texas, USA Falk et al (1989)	Men (151, 235)	2.1 (0.9–5.0)	RR adjusted for age, residence, fruit and vegetable consumption, occupation, and smoking.
Kerala, India Sankrayrayanan et al (1990a)	Men (191, 549)	2.6 (1.5–4.3)	RR adjusted for age, religion, and smoking.
Lower Silesia, Poland Zatonski et al (1991)	Men and women (249, 965)	10.4 (4.0–27.2)	RR adjusted for smoking, age, residence, and education; RR is for vodka drinking.
Seoul, Korea Choi and Kahyo (1991b)	Men (94, 282)	11.1 (3.8–32.4)	RR adjusted for cigarette smoking.
	Women (6, 18)	7.0 (0.2–219.0)	
Heidelberg, Germany Maier et al (1992a)	Men (164, 656)	11.7[d] (4.5–29.6) 7.9[e] (3.5–17.7)	RR adjusted for tobacco consumption.
Shanghai, China Zheng et al (1992a)	Men (177, 269)	0.8 (0.4–1.6)	RR adjusted for age, education and smoking; a small proportion of female cases and controls consumed alcohol.
	Women (24, 145)	4.8 (0.8–28.3)	
Western New York, USA Freudenheim et al (1992)	Men (250, 250)	3.5[a]	RR adjusted for cigarettes and education.
Multicenter Study, USA Muscat and Wynder (1992)	Men (194, 184)	9.6[a,d] 2.5[a,e]	RR adjusted for age, education, smoking and quetelet index; 52% of controls contacted refused interview.
Northern Italy Franceschi et al (1994) (see also LaVecchia et al, 1990; Francheschi et al, 1990)	Men (369, 1706)	2.0 (1.3–3.0)	RR adjusted for age, study area, and smoking.
	Women (19, 557)	2.6 (0.4–17.7)	

[a]$P < 0.05$; [b]Extrinsic larynx; [c]Intrinsic larynx; [d]Supraglottis; [e]Glottis and subglottis; [f]Endolarynx.

TABLE 15–5. *Combined Effect (RR) of Alcohol and Tobacco in Cancer of the Endolarynx**

Alcohol Consumption (grams Ethanol per Day)	Cigarettes per Day			
	0–7	8–15	16–25	26+
0–40	1.00	6.68	12.72	11.47
41–80	1.65	5.94	12.23	18.51
81–120	2.31	10.70	21.01	23.55
121+	3.78	12.20	31.55	43.21
Total number of cases	50	147	357	173

*From Tuyns et al (1988a) with permission. Risks are expressed relative to a risk of 1.00 in persons smoking less than 8 cigarettes per day and drinking no more than 40 g ethanol per day.

study in Japan, after adjustment for smoking, relative risks of 1.7 and 2.0 were noted for whisky and shochu drinking (Hirayama, 1989b). Similarly, in Hawaiian Japanese, the alcohol-related risk of esophageal cancer remained significantly elevated after adjustment for smoking (Kato et al, 1992a).

Case–Control Studies. The relationship between alcohol intake and esophageal cancer has been examined in 21 case–control studies, and several have evaluated the effect of various alcoholic beverages and their interactions with tobacco and nutrition. Except for two studies in South Africa (Bradshaw and Schonland, 1969, 1974) and one study in India (Notani, 1988), studies in North and South America, Europe, Singapore, and China have all found an association between esophageal cancer and alcohol. The studies are summarised in Table 15–6.

In the first study reported, Wynder and Bross (1961) investigated 150 men with squamous cell carcinoma of the esophagus and 150 hospital controls. The esophageal cancer patients consumed significantly more alcoholic drinks per day than the controls and, when the analysis was restricted to smokers of 16–34 cigarettes per day, a clear dose–response relationship was seen with increasing amounts of whisky and beer. In a large study in France (Schwartz et al, 1962), the average alcohol consumption was significantly higher among esophageal cancer patients than among controls after adjustment for tobacco.

Subsequently, two other large case–control studies were carried out in France in relation to alcohol, tobacco, and diet. Aspects of the design of these studies have been reported in detail (Pequignot and Cubeau, 1973; Tuyns et al, 1977a, 1979, 1983; Jensen et al, 1978). In the first study, alcohol and tobacco consumption were compared for 200 male cases of esophageal cancer representative of all cases in the population, and 778 controls selected randomly from the same population. After adjustment for age and smoking, a clear increase in relative risk was seen along with total amount of alcohol consumed per day derived from different types of alcoholic beverages (Tuyns et al, 1976). In the second study, of 743 cases of esophageal cancer (704 males, 39 females) and 1,976 controls chosen at random from the population of Normandy, a significant increase in relative risk accompanied the consumption of any type of alcohol (Tuyns et al, 1982). A clear dose–response relationship was also seen in that study (Tuyns et al, 1979, 1987). In these studies an association between smoking and esophageal cancer was also found, but adjustment for smoking and diet did not substantially affect the risk estimates observed for drinking. Similarly, in studies from the U.S. (Ziegler, 1986; MC Yu et al, 1988), China (Cheng et al, 1992; Gao et al, 1994), southern Brazil (Victoria et al, 1987) and northern Italy (Franceschi et al, 1994; Negri et al, 1992), the association of esophageal cancer with alcohol was independent of the association with dietary factors.

Tobacco smoking is a cause of esophageal cancer. The joint actions of alcohol and tobacco in the etiology for esophageal cancer have been investigated in several studies. In an often quoted study in the northwest of France, Tuyns and colleagues (1977b, 1979, 1987) found a combined effect which was intermediate between additive and multiplicative (Table 15–7). In a further analysis of those subjects who reported that they had never smoked, Tuyns (1983) found that the relative risk increased with increasing consumption of alcohol in both men and women (Table 15–8). Similar results were reported by LaVecchia and Negri (1989) for esophageal cancer in non-smokers from their northern Italian case–control study. In an examination of possible interaction between poor diet and alcohol consumption, Tuyns and colleagues (1987) reported a smoking-adjusted 90-fold increased risk of esophageal cancer in persons with poor nutrition and who drank more than 120 g of ethanol per day.

The risk of esophageal cancer associated with consumption of various types of drinks containing different concentrations of ethanol has been much studied. In three studies from the U.S. (Wynder and Bross, 1961; Pottern et al, 1981; MC Yu et al, 1988), an increased risk for esophageal cancer was found both among whisky drinkers and among beer and wine drinkers, but the risk seemed to be particularly pronounced for consumers of strong liquors. No difference in relative risk was found in Puerto Rico for consumers of commercial rum only, of home processed rum only, or of a mixture of beverages (Martinez, 1969). The study of the Danish brewery workers (Jensen, 1979) indicated that beer may also increase the risk for esophageal cancer.

In Europe the incidence of esophageal cancer is particularly high in the northwestern part of France (Tuyns and Massé, 1975a). While the high incidence was first assumed to be due to drinking locally produced alcoholic beverages, the case–control study indicated that esophageal cancer was associated with all types of al-

TABLE 15–6. *Summary of Results of Case–Control Studies of Esophageal Cancer*

Study Site Reference	*Subjects (Cases, Controls)*	*Relative Risk (RR) (Highest vs. Lowest Category)*	*Comments*
New York, USA Wynder and Bross (1961)	Men (150, 150)	12.5 (1.5–78.4)	Crude RR
Puerto Rico Martinez (1969)	Men (111, 111)	7.7 (3.0–20.0)	Crude RR based on pairs matched on smoking.
Minnesota, USA Bjelke (1973)	Men and women (52, 1657)	4.4[a] (2.3–8.3) 0.5[b] (0.2–1.2) 2.1[c] (1.0–4.3)	RR adjusted for sex.
Durban, South Africa Bradshaw and Schonland (1969, 1974)	Men (98, 341)	0.9 (0.4–1.9)	RR adjusted for smoking.
Johannesburg, South Africa Bradshaw and Schonland (1974)	Men (196, 1064)	1.0 (0.6–1.8)	RR adjusted for smoking.
Singapore De Jong et al (1974)	Men (95, 465)	2.9[d]	Crude RR for samsu (strong liquor) drinking.
Multicenter study, USA Williams and Horm (1977)	Men (38, 1788)	1.4	RR adjusted for age, race, and smoking.
	Women (19, 3188)	8.1[d]	
Brittany, France Tuyns et al (1977b)	Men (200, 778)	18.3	RR adjusted for smoking; 95% CI could not be calculated.
Normandy, France Tuyns et al (1979)	Men (312, 869)	11.6	RR adjusted for smoking; 95% CI could not be calculated.
Washington D.C., USA Pottern et al (1981)	Men (90, 213)	7.5 (2.5–22.0)	Crude RR remains high after adjustment for smoking; data based on proxy interviews.
Uruguay Vasallo et al (1985)	Men (185, 386)	7.6 (4.5–12.8)	RR adjusted for age and tobacco smoking.
Southern Brazil Victoria et al (1987)	Men and women (171, 342)	8.2[d,e]	Crude RR; RR remained significant after adjustment for smoking, place of residence and diet; 80% of alcohol consumed was cahaca (distilled, sugar cane spirit).
Bombay, India Notani (1988)	Men (236, 392)	1.1 (0.6–1.8)	RR adjusted for age, smoking and chewing habits.
Soweto, South Africa Segal et al (1988)	Men and women (200, 391)	18.3 (10.1–33.2)	RR adjusted for smoking; type of alcohol consumed includes beer and spirits.
Los Angeles, CA, USA MC Yu et al (1988)	Men and women (275, 275)	15.5 (5.9–41.1)	Crude RR based on pairs matched for sex, age, race and neighbourhood. Average daily intake of ethanol remained a significant risk factor after adjustment for tobacco use, diet, level of education, and exposure to metal dust.
Uruguay De Stefani et al (1990b)	Men (199, 398) Women (62, 124)	5.3 (2.7–10.2) 1.9 (0.7–4.9)	RR adjusted for age, residence, and smoking.
Kerala, India Sankaranarayanan et al (1991)	Men (207, 546) Women (60, 349)	2.3 (1.5–3.6) —	RR adjusted for daily bidi and cigarette smoking, duration of bidi smoking and pantobacco chewing. Prevalence of alcohol use in women was low and not examined.
Hong Kong Chinese Cheng et al (1992)	Men and women (400, 1598)	10.0 (5.3–18.7)	RR adjusted for age, educational attainment, place of birth, diet, and smoking.
Heilongjiang Province, China Hu et al (1994)	Men and women (196, 392)	4.2[d]	RR adjusted for smoking. RR is for hard liquor, wine was rarely consumed, and no association for beer consumption was found.
Shanghai, China Gao, et al (1994)	Men (624, 723) Women (278, 662)	4.0[d] —	RR adjusted for age, education, birthplace, tea drinking, dietary factors, and cigarette smoking; few women drank alcohol.
Northern Italy Franceschi et al (1994) (see also La Vecchia and Negri, 1989; Franceschi et al, 1990)	Men (343, 1706) Women (67, 557)	7.7 (5.1–11.5) 3.0 (0.7–12.7)	RR adjusted for age, study center, and smoking habit.

[a]Beer; [b]Wine; [c]Spirits; [d]$P < 0.05$; [e]Cachaca.

TABLE 15–7. *Relative Risks for Esophageal Cancer According to Daily Consumption of Alcohol and Tobacco**

Alcohol consumption (grams ethanol per day)	Tobacco Consumption in Grams per Day		
	0–9	10–19	20+
0–40	1.0	3.4	5.1
41–80	7.3	8.4	12.3
81+	18.0	19.9	44.4
Number of cases	78	58	308

*From Tuyns et al (1977b) with permission. Risks are expressed relative to a risk of 1.0 in persons smoking less than 10 g per day and drinking no more than 40 g ethanol per day.

coholic beverages (Tuyns et al, 1979). In an extended analysis of the same study, taking into account consumption of alcohol from other beverages, beer, cider, and wine had the strongest influence on risk, but it could not be ruled out that all types of alcoholic beverages contributed to the risk in proportion to their alcohol content (Breslow and Day, 1980). All types of alcoholic beverages thus appear to increase the risk of esophageal cancer.

Cancer of the Stomach

As with cancers of the upper aerodigestive tract, the stomach is exposed directly to ingested ethanol. Although the concentration of alcohol is diluted by gastric juices and other gastric contents, it is biologically plausible that the risk of stomach cancer could be increased by some direct carcinogenic effect of ethanol upon the mucosa.

Cohort Studies. In very few of the 17 cohort studies (Table 15–1) did the risk of stomach cancer increase in association with alcohol consumption. Only in the Framingham study (Gordon and Kannell, 1984) and the Japanese study (Kato et al, 1992b) was this increase statistically significant. In the study by Kato, daily alcohol drinkers who consumed more than 50 ml of alcohol per day had a greater risk than non-drinkers in a multivariate analysis that included smoking and cooking habits. However, only the results for males were statistically significant, while females showed similar but insignificant trends. Further, the findings from both the Framingham and Japanese studies are based on relatively few deaths from stomach cancer. A weak, but statistically significant, negative association was found in one study (Hirayama 1989a). In the subset of cohort studies of high-risk persons (i.e., categories of persons with above-average consumption of alcoholic beverages), there was a slight overall deficit in the risk of stomach cancer. However, the general absence of data on diet, a potential confounder of risk for stomach cancer, makes these cohort studies difficult to interpret.

TABLE 15–8. *Relative Risk (RR) of Esophageal Cancer in Relation to Average Daily Alcohol Consumption by Nonsmoking Males and Females in Normandy, France**

Alcohol Consumption (grams ethanol/day)	Males		Females	
	No. of cases	RR	No. of cases	RR
0–40	7	1.0	25	1.0
41–80	15	3.8	8	5.6
81–120	9	10.1	3	11.0
121+	8	101.0	—	—

*From Tuyns et al (1983) with permission.

Case–Control Studies. Of 24 case–control studies reporting on alcohol consumption and stomach cancer (see IARC, 1988, pp. 199–202; Hu et al, 1988; Lee et al, 1990; Kato et al, 1990; Wu-Williams et al, 1990; Demirer et al, 1990; De Stefani et al, 1990a; Boeing et al, 1991; Yu and Hsieh, 1991; Hoshiyama and Sasaba, 1992; Jedrychowski et al, 1993; D'Avanzo et al, 1994; Guo et al, 1994), nine have reported a positive association.

In the earliest of these positive findings (Haenszel et al, 1972), a hospital-based case–control study among Hawaiian Japanese, the risk of stomach cancer was positively associated with consumption of beer (RR = 1.2) and of sake (RR = 2.2). The association was statistically significant for persons drinking sake daily, but not beer. In two smaller hospital-based studies of men in France (Hoey et al, 1981) and Taiwan (Lee et al, 1990), the risk of stomach cancer was significantly increased among regular consumers of alcohol. In the French study, the (tobacco-adjusted) risk was greatly increased (sevenfold) for persons consuming more than 80 g of alcohol daily. A hospital-based study in Uruguay (De Stefani et al, 1990a) found a positive association with alcohol consumption for men only. In a population-based study, weekly consumption of alcohol was associated with a doubling in risk, after multivariate adjustment for other factors, including diet (Wu-Williams et al, 1990). Two separate hospital-based case–control studies in Poland found a significant positive association with vodka drinking (Jedrychowski et al, 1986, 1993). In the earlier study, this risk was particularly elevated among those who drank vodka before breakfast, while in the latter study the risk was particularly strong for cancer of the non-cardia region. In a hospital-based case–control study in northern Italy (D'Avanzo et al, 1994), a non-significant 30% increase in risk was observed among those who drank very heavily (>8 drinks/day). The authors suggested that this increase may reflect uncontrolled confounding by other risk factors (possibly related to diet and social class). In a hospital-based case–control study in Japan (Hoshiyama and Sasba, 1992), a non-significant 30% increase was observed among those who drank 50 ml or more alcohol per day.

In several other studies, no positive associations were apparent. In a population-based study (Tuyns et al, 1982) in the Calvados region of France, a non-significant inverse relationship was seen between alcohol consumption and stomach cancer. A multihospital case–control study in Germany found a positive relationship with beer consumption but statistically significant negative relationships with wine and liquor consumption (Boeing et al., 1991). In a large nested case–control study in Linxian, China of primarily gastric cancers of the cardia, no association was found with alcohol drinking (Guo et al, 1994).

In all except four of these 24 case–control studies, the controls were hospital patients with other conditions or diseases. The alcohol consumption profile of such patients may not reflect closely, and indeed may exceed, that of the non-hospitalised population of non-cases. Further, in most of these case–control studies there was no adjustment for any possible confounding effects of diet. In light of the overall lack of excess risk of stomach cancer in cohort studies and the inconsistent and mostly negative results of case–control studies, and in view of the generally inadequate control for the potential confounding effects of dietary and socioeconomic factors, there is little evidence that alcoholic beverages play a causal role in stomach cancer.

Cancer of the Large Bowel

Since ethanol is absorbed efficiently from within the stomach and upper intestine, it is unlikely that intraluminal ethanol has a direct effect upon the large bowel. Nevertheless, in view of the evidence from correlation studies of a positive relationship between alcohol consumption and large bowel cancer, many analytic studies have examined this relationship. Some studies have treated colon cancer and rectal cancer separately; in others they have been combined. A review and meta-analysis (Longnecker et al, 1990) gives the details of methods and results of 27 of these analytic studies, excluding the studies of cohorts of alcoholics and brewery workers.

Cohort Studies. From the cohort studies (Table 15–1) there is little evidence that the risk of colon cancer is associated with increased consumption of alcoholic beverages. Only two studies have shown statistically significant positive associations. In the Japanese study (Hirayama, 1989b) a significant increase in risk of sigmoid colon cancer (but not proximal) with total alcohol consumption was found for both men and women. Klatsky and colleagues (1988), however, observed a significant threefold increase in risk of colon cancer for women but not men. Six studies showed non-significant increases in risk (Hakulinen et al, 1974; Adelstein and White, 1976; Dean et al, 1979; Carstensen et al, 1990; Stemmermann et al, 1990; Gapstur et al, 1994). Two studies showed non-significant decreases in risk (Monson and Lyon, 1975; Robinette et al, 1979), and the remaining studies showed no association.

By comparison, the risk of rectal cancer has been reported to be positively associated with alcohol consumption in seven of fourteen cohort studies, with six studies showing a statistically significant increase (Table 15–1). In four of these six studies, the increased risk was with beer consumption (Dean et al, 1979; Stemmermann et al, 1990; Carstensen et al, 1990). In the other two studies the association was not specific to beer, wine, or spirits (Klatsky et al, 1988; Hirayama, 1989b; Goldbohm et al, 1994). There were no gender differences in the two studies that included both men and women (Klatsky et al, 1988; Goldbohm et al, 1994).

A dose–response relationship between alcohol and rectal cancer was observed in three of the six statistically significant studies (Klatsky et al, 1988; Hirayama, 1989b; Stemmermann et al, 1990). In two of the cohort studies of alcoholics, non-significant two- to threefold increases in the risk of rectal cancer were reported (Sundby, 1967; Robinette et al, 1979). The results of cohort studies of Danish brewery workers (Jensen, 1979) and of members of the Copenhagen Temperance Society (Jensen, 1983) enable comparison of groups with extreme differences in consumption of alcohol. The fact that neither group had a risk of rectal cancer different from that of the general population suggests that alcohol consumption is unrelated to rectal cancer.

Of four cohort studies in which colon and rectal cancers were combined, one study found a statistically significant twofold increase in risk in men only (Wu et al, 1987). In the Japanese doctors study and the Swedish alcoholics study, non-significant positive associations were found (Kono et al, 1986; Adami et al, 1992a), while no association was found in the 19-year follow-up study of men employed by the Western Electric Company in Chicago (Garland et al, 1985). The combined results from two cohort studies in the US indicate that alcohol consumption significantly increases the incidence of hyperplastic colorectal polyps, which are thought to be a dysplastic precursor of carcinoma (Kearney et al, 1995).

Case–Control Studies. A statistically significant positive relationship has been observed in 12 of 22 case–control studies of colon cancer. The association was with beer consumption in six studies (Wynder and Shigematsu, 1967; Pickle et al, 1984; Tuyns et al, 1988b; Kato et al, 1990; Longnecker, 1990), with spirits consumption in another four studies (Bjelke, 1973; Potter and McMichael, 1986; Peters et al, 1992; Newcomb et al, 1993), with total alcohol consumption in one study (Meyer and White, 1993), and with each of beer, spirits, and wine in the remaining study (Williams and Horm, 1977). However, ten other such case–control studies have shown either a non-significant increase in risk or no such association with alcohol drinking (see IARC, 1988; Ferraroni et al, 1989; Peters et al, 1989; Slattery et al, 1990; Riboli et al, 1991; Choi and Kahyo, 1991a).

Alcohol drinking was positively associated with rectal cancer in 19 of 24 case–control studies (see IARC, 1988; Graham et al, 1978; Manousos et al, 1983; Pickle et al, 1984; Tuyns et al, 1988b; Ferraroni et al, 1989; Freudenheim et al, 1990; Longnecker, 1990; Kato et al, 1990; Riboli et al, 1991). Significant associations were reported in 13 of these 19 studies, with beer consumption significant in eight of these. In five of the latter studies, beer consumption was significantly associated with rectal cancer in men only (Wynder and Shigematsu, 1967; Kabat et al, 1986; Kune et al, 1987; Freudenheim et al, 1990; Kato et al, 1990; Longnecker, 1990), and in two studies, this association was significant for men and women combined (Bjelke, 1973; Riboli et al, 1991). Beer consumption was also statistically associated with an increased risk in a study that included women only (Newcomb et al, 1993). Of the other five case–control studies with significant positive results, one study showed an association with consumption of wine in women (Potter and McMichael, 1986), one with total alcohol consumption in women only (Williams and Horm, 1977), two with total alcohol consumption in men only (Hu et al, 1991, Choi and Kahyo, 1991a) and one with total alcohol consumption in both men and women (Freudenheim et al, 1990). A case–control analysis within a cohort study of brewery workers showed a positive relationship between drinking alcohol (stout) and rectal cancer risk (Dean et al, 1979).

Of four case–control studies that combined both colon and rectal cancers, two studies (Higginson, 1966, Manousos et al., 1983) found no relationship between colorectal cancer and any alcoholic beverage for males and females combined. One of the earliest case–control studies that examined dietary factors and cancer in men only reported a non-significant association between beer consumption and cancers of the large bowel (Stocks, 1957). Slattery and colleagues (1990) found a significant dose–response in males between colorectal cancer and total alcohol consumption that disappeared after adjusting for confounding factors.

Of four case–control studies of colorectal adenomas, as found at colonoscopy, one study found a significantly increased risk associated with beer consumption only in men but not in women (Kikendall et al, 1989); one showed an increased risk with total alcohol consumption in men and women (Giovanuuci et al, 1993); while the other two studies found no association of cancer risk with any type of alcoholic beverage (Riboli et al, 1991; Olsen and Kronborg, 1993).

In over half of the case–control studies, particularly those published prior to the 1980s, there was no adjustment for the possible confounding effects of diet. This makes their interpretation difficult, especially since the size of the excess alcohol-related relative risk is usually not large. A recent comprehensive review of colon cancer epidemiology has suggested that "inconsistencies in results between alcohol and colon cancer may be a consequence of the small number of cases in some studies or the result of differences in control groups, in methods of assessing consumption and in preferred beverages across countries and between men and women" (Potter et al, 1993).

There have been recurring indications from epidemiological studies that alcohol is more strongly related to cancer of the rectum than of the colon. In view of the inconsistent findings and the probability of uncontrolled confounding by dietary factors, no firm conclusion can be drawn about the role of alcoholic beverages in the aetiology of colon cancer. Overall, the epidemiological data provide suggestive but inconclusive evidence of a causal role of alcoholic beverages, particularly beer, in the etiology of rectal cancer.

Cancer of the Liver

There have been reports over many decades of associations between chronic alcohol abuse, alcoholic liver cirrhosis, and primary liver cancer (PLC). More recently, a number of formal epidemiological studies have examined the relationship between alcohol consumption and liver cancer.

Cohort Studies. There is a strong indication from cohort studies that excessive alcohol consumption increases the risk of PLC. Of four cohort studies conducted within the general population, two showed a significantly increased risk of liver cancer among frequent drinkers of alcoholic beverages (Hirayama, 1981, 1989a; Kono et al, 1986), one study in a farming and fishing region in Japan showed an increased risk only among the subgroup of shochu drinkers (Shibata et al, 1986), and the other study showed no relationship at all (Blackwelder et al, 1980). It is of interest that these four cohort studies were all conducted within Japanese populations. In another cohort study in Italy entailing a three-year follow-up of 365 patients with liver cirrhosis, alcohol was found to be an important independent risk factor for PLC (Bargiggia et al, 1989).

Among the 12 cohort studies of high-risk persons (Table 15–1), five have shown a statistically significant association between alcohol consumption and liver cancer (Hakulinen et al, 1974; Adelstein and White, 1976; Jensen, 1979; Adami et al, 1992b; Tonnesen et al, 1994), while in another six of the twelve studies there was a non-significant positive association (Sundby, 1967; Hakulinen et al, 1974; Robinette et al, 1979; Dean et al, 1979; Schmidt and Popham, 1981; Carstensen et al, 1990). The remaining study produced null findings (Monson and Lyon, 1975). Taken together, the results of these cohort studies indicate an approximately 50% increase in risk of liver cancer in relation to alcohol consumption (see also IARC, 1988, p. 210).

In most of the cohort studies, some cases classified as having PLC probably had metastatic liver cancer. This misclassification is unlikely to have been related to level of alcohol consumption and therefore would tend to diminish the strength of the observed association between alcohol consumption and risk for PLC.

Case–Control Studies. Of 16 case–control studies of PLC and alcohol consumption (Table 15–9), nine have shown statistically significant two- to threefold increases in risk (Infante et al, 1980; Bulatao-Janme et al, 1982; Stemhagen et al, 1983; Yu et al, 1983; Hardell et al, 1984; Austin et al, 1986; HYu et al, 1988; Filipazzo et al, 1985; Tsukuma et al, 1990). In three of the other seven studies, there was some suggestion of a positive relationship (Williams and Horm, 1977; Trichopoulos et al, 1987; La Vecchia et al, 1988). One study (Lu et al, 1988) showed an inverse relationship. Two of the three case-control studies reporting results by gender have shown clearly higher alcohol-associated risks of PLC among women than among men (Stemhagen et al, 1983; Yu et al, 1983). The fact that the results have been noticeably more positive in case–control studies conducted among Western populations than in those within Asian and African populations with high PLC rates could indicate that the risk of PLC occurrence is conditioned by other risk factors (Yu et al, 1983).

A particularly strong association between the consumption of alcoholic beverages and PLC was reported in a case–control study conducted within a cohort of hepatitis B surface antigen–positive volunteer male blood donors in Japan (Oshima et al, 1984). A strong dose–dependent, statistically significant, positive association (up to eightfold relative risk) was seen between drinking habits and primary liver cancer. Evidence of a similar synergistic effect between alcohol consumption and hepatitis B seropositivity was reported by Inaba and colleagues (1984). While interactive effects between ethanol consumption and tobacco smoking have been postulated, few studies have directly addressed the issue. Data from one case–control study (Yu et al, 1983) and one cohort study (Hirayama, 1981) suggest that the risk of liver cancer is particularly high among individuals who both drink alcoholic beverages and smoke cigarettes.

Overall, the results from the cohort and case–control studies indicate that alcohol consumption is causally related to primary liver cancer. Although potential confounding due to hepatitis B virus, tobacco smoking, and aflatoxin was not explored in all studies, when it was considered it did not markedly alter the findings. The observation that there is no apparent reduction in risk of liver cancer in populations of abstainers, in comparison with the general population, suggests that the increased risk of liver cancer is largely confined to individuals with substantially above-average consumption of alcohol.

Cancer of the Pancreas

Despite strong evidence that alcohol plays a role in certain non-neoplastic chronic conditions of the pancreas (Yen et al, 1982), the evidence associating alcohol intake with increased risk of pancreatic cancer is inconsistent and generally weak. Dorken (1964) reported data on a large series of pancreatic cancer cases which suggested an increased risk associated with regular to heavy consumption of alcohol. Subsequently, a number of cohort and case–control studies have examined this relationship.

Cohort Studies. Of the six prospective cohort studies conducted within the general population, only two have reported statistically significant associations of pancreatic cancer with alcohol drinking (Table 15–1; Heuch et al, 1983). The first study, in a large Norwegian cohort (Heuch et al, 1983), found a statistically significant fivefold increase in pancreatic cancer risk among regular alcohol consumers. (However, apparent methodological irregularities have impeded interpretation of this study [IARC, 1988]). In a study of Norwegian immigrants to the U.S., a threefold increase in risk was found among those consuming ten or more drinks per month compared to non-drinkers (Zheng et al, 1993). The risks tended to increase with intake of both beer and hard liquor, although after adjustment for smoking, the trend was less pronounced and not smooth. A two- to threefold, but statistically insignificant, increase in risk was evident in the Kaiser-Permanente cohort in the U.S. (Klatsky et al, 1981) while a non-significant 50% increase was reported in the Japanese doctors study (Kono et al, 1986). The remaining two studies (Blackwelder, 1980; Hirayama, 1990) found no association between cancer of the pancreas and alcohol drinking, although

TABLE 15–9. *Summary of Case–Control Studies of Primary Liver Cancer*

Study Site Reference	*Subjects (Cases, Controls)*	*Relative Risk (Highest vs. Lowest Category)*	*Comments*
France Schwartz et al (1962)	Men (61, 61)	NA[a]	High but equal ethanol consumption among cases and controls
Multicenter study, USA, Williams and Horm (1977)	Men (18, 1770) Women (10, 3178)	2.7 (NS)[b] 5.0 (NS)	RR adjusted for age and smoking. All subjects were from national cancer survey.
Geneva, Switzerland Infante et al (1980)	Men and women (35, 433)	+[c]	Ethanol consumption in cases was twice that in controls
Phillipines Bulatao-Jayme et al (1982)	Men and women (90, 90)	3.9[d]	Hospital–based age–sex–matched design; Hepatitis B serology was not controlled for.
Hong Kong Lam et al (1982)	Men (95, 95) Women (12, 12)	NA	Alcohol consumption details were not given.
New Jersey, USA, Stemhagen et al (1983)	Men (178, 356) Women (87, 174)	2.0[d] 5.6[d]	RR adjusted for age, sex, and residence. Smoking not related to liver cancer.
Los Angeles, CA, USA, Yu et al (1983)	Men and women (78, 78)	4.2 (1.3–13.8)	RR adjusted for age, sex, and race.
Sweden Hardell et al (1984)	Men (98[e], 196)	4.3 (1.8–10.8)	Age–matched design
Italy Filippazzo et al (1985)	Men and women (120, 360)	3.2 (1.5–6.8)	Crude RR based on matching for age and sex.
Multicenter study, USA, Austin et al (1986)	Men and women (86, 161)	2.6[d]	RR adjusted for age, sex, and race.
Greece Trichopoulos et al (1987)	Men and women (194, 456)	1.2[f]	RR adjusted for age, sex, smoking, and hepatitis B serology.
New York, USA, Yu et al (1988)	Men (92, 261) Women (73, 202)	1.3 1.9	RR for age–matched design. A significant dose response relationship for liver cancer and alcohol was found in women >50 years of age.
Northern Italy La Vecchia et al (1988); Ferraroni et al (1989)	Men and women (151, 1051)	1.4 (0.8–2.5)	RR adjusted for age, sex, geographic area, education, history of hepatitis, history of cirrhosis, and smoking.
Taiwan Lu et al (1988)	Men and women (131, 207)	0.6	RR adjusted for sex and hepatitis B surface antigen.
Osaka, Japan, Tsukuma et al (1990)	Men and women (221, 266)	3.2 (2.0–5.1)	RR adjusted for hepatitis B surface antigen, history of blood transfusion, cigarette smoking, sex, age, and family history of liver cancer. RR calculated for history of heavy drinking versus no heavy drinking.
Germany Peters et al (1994)	Men and women (86, 86)	NA	Controls were patients with liver cirrhosis but not hepatocellular carcinoma. RR adjusted for hepatitis B surface antigen, antibodies to hepatitis C virus, and cigarette use.

[a]NA, no association.
[b]NS, not significant.
[c]+, positive association.
[d]$P < 0.05$
[e]Cases include 15 patients with cholangiocarcinoma
[f]For primary hepato-cellular carcinoma with cirrhosis

Hirayama found a significant threefold risk for daily whiskey drinkers.

Of twelve cohort studies of persons known to be consumers of high levels of alcohol (Table 15–1; Schmidt and de Lint, 1972), only one study (Carstensen et al, 1990) has shown a statistically significant increase in risk of pancreatic cancer. Ten studies have shown weak to moderate, but non-significant, elevated risks. In only seven of the twelve studies was the observed number of cases greater than five (Adelstein and White, 1976; Dean et al, 1979; Jensen, 1979; Schmidt and Popham, 1981; Carstenson et al, 1990; Adami et al, 1992a; Tonnesen et al, 1994). Analysis by duration of follow-up does not suggest any tendency for an increased risk after a long latency period (Velema et al, 1986).

Case–Control Studies. Of 32 case–control studies (see IARC, 1988, pp. 217–222; Mack et al, 1986; La Vecchia et al, 1987b; Raymond et al, 1987; Falk et al, 1988; Olsen et al, 1989; Cuzick and Babiker, 1989; Clavel et al, 1989; Ferraroni et al, 1989; Farrow and Davis, 1990; Jain et al, 1991; Ghadirian et al, 1991; Baghurst et al, 1991; Bueno de Mesquita et al, 1992; Lyon et al, 1992; Mizuno et al, 1992; Friedman et al, 1993; Zatonski et al, 1993; Sciallero et al, 1993), only three studies have found a statistically significant increased risk of pancreatic cancer risk among regular drinkers of alcoholic beverages (Durbec et al, 1983; Cuzick and Babiker, 1989; Sciallero et al, 1993). In one study the increased risk was with beer consumption (Cuzick and Babiker, 1989), in another it was with weekly consumption of spirits (Sciallero et al, 1993), and in the remaining study it was with total alcohol consumption (Durbec et al, 1983). Three other studies (Ferraroni et al, 1989; Olsen et al, 1989; Zatonski et al, 1993) reported a moderate but non-significant increase in risk in association with alcohol. Zatonski found a weakly positive trend in risk with life-time consumption of spirits (vodka). Interestingly, some of the case–control studies have indicated an alcohol-associated deficit in risk—particularly in relation to wine consumption—and five of these deficits were statistically significant (see IARC, 1988, pp. 221–222; Farrow and Davis, 1990; Baghurst et al, 1991).

While there are methodological reasons for suspecting some underestimation of alcohol-associated risk of pancreatic cancer in case–control studies (Velema et al, 1986; Bouchardy et al, 1990), there has nevertheless been little positive evidence from cohort studies. Overall, therefore, the evidence indicates that alcohol consumption is unlikely to be causally related to cancer of the pancreas.

Cancer of the Female Breast

Prior to 1982 little attention had been paid to the role of alcohol consumption in the etiology of female breast cancer. There was no a priori reason for expecting any biologically direct effect of alcohol on breast carcinogenesis.

Geographic correlation studies (intranational as well as international) have provided little evidence of a positive correlation of breast cancer mortality or incidence with alcohol consumption (Pochin, 1976; Kono and Ikeda, 1979; La Vecchia et al, 1982; La Vecchia and Pampallona, 1986; Schatzkin et al, 1989b), although one early study (Breslow and Enstrom, 1974) noted a positive correlation between breast cancer mortality and beer drinking. In the few follow-up studies of alcoholics that included women, most (Schmidt and de Lint, 1972; Nicholls et al, 1974; Monson and Lyon, 1975; Adelstein and White 1976; Prior, 1988; Adami, et al, 1992b) yielded too few breast cancer cases to provide any conclusive evidence. In the one study of alcoholic women where at least 40 cases of breast cancer were observed (Tonneson et al, 1994), the relative risk of breast cancer was 1.3, but this was not statistically significant.

The first study based on individual measurement of alcohol consumption that reported a positive association between alcohol and breast cancer went largely unnoticed (Williams and Horm, 1977). However, following the confirmation of this association in a case–control study (Rosenberg et al., 1982) the issue has been addressed in nine cohort studies (Table 15–10) and in at least 27 case–control studies (Table 15–11). To evaluate whether there was a dose–response relation between alcohol consumption and breast cancer risk, Longnecker (1994) performed a meta-analysis of 38 epidemiological studies available up to 1992. The analysis shows strong evidence of a dose–response relation, although the slope of the dose–response curve was modest. The risks of breast cancer associated with consumption of one, two or three drinks per day compared with non-drinkers were: 1.1 (95% confidence interval [CI] = 1.07–1.16), 1.2 (95% CI = 1.15–1.34), and 1.4 (95% CI = 1.23–1.55), respectively. An explanation for the marked variation in results between studies, however, was not apparent.

This variation in results has also been evident in the recent studies published since the meta-analysis by Longnecker (1994). In a Canadian screening study cohort, a weak positive but non-significant association was found in women drinking more than 30 g of alcohol daily (Friedenreich et al, 1993). Two case–control studies showed positive associations; one study in Spain showed a monotonic dose–response relationship (MartinMoreno et al, 1993) and one study from Greece indicated a threshold effect (Katsouyanni et al, 1994). A population-based case–control study conducted in Sweden showed a clear increase in risk for the highest quartile of alcohol intake versus that of the lowest (Holmberg et al, 1994), but no association was found when alcohol consumption was treated as a continuous variable. In the U.K., a case–control study of breast cancer in young women showed no alcohol-related risk (Smith et al, 1994).

Most of the studies in Tables 15–10 and 15–11 linking alcohol consumption with breast cancer showed the alcohol–breast cancer association to be independent of other known risk factors, such as socioeconomic status, reproductive history, obesity, benign breast diseases, and family history. In some studies, the increase in risk was greatest in women at low risk from these other fac-

TABLE 15–10. *Cohort Studies of Alcohol and Female Breast Cancer*

Reference	Location	No. of Cases/Subjects	Maximum Alcohol Intake (g/day)	Relative Risk (95% CI)[a]
Seidman et al (1982) Garfinkel et al (1988)	USA	2,933/581,321 (deaths)	≥12	1.6 (1.0–2.6)
Hiatt and Bawoll (1984)	California	838/88,477	≥39	1.5 (1.1–2.1)
Schatzkin et al (1987)	USA	121/7,188	≥5	2.0 (1.1–3.7)
Willett et al (1987)	USA	601/89,538	≥15	1.6 (1.3–2.0)
Hiatt et al (1988a)	California	303/5,835	≥78	3.3 (1.2–9.3)
Schatzkin et al (1989a)	Framingham, Massachusetts	143/2,636	≥5	0.6 (0.4–1.0)
Simon et al (1991)	Tecumseh, MI	87/1,854	≥24	1.1 (0.3–5.0)
Gapstur et al (1992)	Iowa	493/41,837	≥15	1.5 (1.0–2.0)
Friedenreich et al (1993)	Canada	519/56,837	≥30	1.2 (0.8–1.9)

[a]Relative risk for the maximum category, as shown, compared with abstainers.

TABLE 15–11. *Case–Control Studies of Alcohol and Female Breast Cancer*

Reference	Location	Study Subjects	No. of Cases, Controls	Maximum Alcohol Intake (g/day)	Relative Risk (95% CI)[a]
Rosenberg et al (1982)	Canada, Israel	Hospital	1,152, 2,694	≥7	2.5 (1.9–3.4)
Byers and Funch, (1982)	New York	Hospital	1,314, 770	≥11	1.1 (0.9–1.3)
Begg et al (1983)	USA, Canada	Hospital	997, 730	≥13	1.4 (0.9–2.0)
Paganini-Hill and Ross (1983)	California	Population	239, 239	≥26	1.0 (0.6–2.0)
Talamini et al (1984)	Italy	Hospital	368, 373	≥78	16.7 (3.1–89.7)
Lê et al (1984, 1986)	France	Hospital	500, 945	≥34	1.2 (0.7–2.0)
La Vecchia et al (1985, 1987a, 1989)	Italy	Hospital	2,402, 2,220	≥36	2.2 (1.7–2.7)
Harvey et al (1987)	USA	Population	1,524, 1,896	≥26	1.7 (1.2–2.4)
O'Connell et al (1987)	North Carolina U.S.	Population	276, 1,519	≥2	1.5 (1.0–2.1)
Rohan and McMichael (1988)	Australia	Population	451, 451	≥9	1.5 (1.0–2.5)
Harris and Wynder (1988)	USA	Hospital	1,467, 10,178	≥15	0.9 (0.8–1.1)
Adami et al (1988)	Norway and Sweden	Population	422, 527	≥15	0.5 (0.2–1.3)
Webster et al, (1983) Chu et al (1989)	USA	Population	3,217, 2,945	≥22	1.2 (0.9–1.6)
Toniolo et al (1989)	Northern Italy	Population	499	>40	1.6 (0.9–2.9)
Meara et al (1989)	UK	Hospital and screening	998, 118	≥28	1.1 (0.7–1.9)
Richardson et al (1989)	France	Hospital	349, 459	≥31	3.5 (2.0–6.1)
Young (1989)	USA	Population	277, 372	≥18	1.8 (1.3–2.6)
Van't Veer et al (1989)	Netherlands	Population	120, 164	≥30	0.9 (0.2–4.5)
Nasca et al (1990)	USA	Population	1,608, 1,609	≥15	1.4 (1.1–1.8)
Rosenberg et al (1990)	Canada	Hospital	534, 1,044	≥26	1.0 (0.7–1.5)
Ferraroni et al (1991)	Northern Italy	Hospital	214, 215	≥24	2.1 (1.1–3.9)
Ewertz (1991)	Denmark	Population	1,486, 1,336	≥12	1.3 (0.9–1.9)
Sneyd et al (1991)	New Zealand	Population	891, 1,864	≥24	1.8 (0.9–3.8)
MartinMoreno et al (1993)	Spain	Population	762, 988	>20	1.7 (1.3–2.3)[b]
Holmberg et al (1994)	Sweden	Population	265, 432	>3	1.6 (1.0–2.4)
Katsouyanni et al (1994)	Greece	Hospital	820, 1,548	≥48	3.8 (1.1–13.7)[b]
Smith et al (1994)	UK	Population	755, 755	≥15	0.8 (0.5–1.5)

[a]For the maximum category stated compared with abstainers.
[b]$P < 0.05$ for trend.

tors (Willett et al, 1987) or in lean women (Schatzkin et al, 1987). The latter finding has either been weakly supported (Harris and Wynder, 1988; Gapstur et al, 1992) or not supported at all (Garfinkel et al, 1988; La Vecchia et al, 1989b; Sneyd et al, 1991; Katsouyanni et al, 1994). In the many studies in which it was possible to adjust for dietary variables, the alcohol-related risk generally did not change much. Two studies showed a significant interaction between alcohol and dietary fat intake, with the alcohol-related risk being greatest in women with low fat intake (Richardson et al, 1989; Ewertz, 1991).

Various investigators have examined for an age-dependency of this effect of alcohol. At least four studies indicate that breast cancer risk is increased most by alcohol consumption in early adulthood (Hiatt et al, 1988; Harvey et al, 1987; Van't Veer et al, 1989; Young, 1989). However, other studies have observed no such age-related effects. Few studies have examined the effect of cumulative (lifetime) exposure to alcohol, although two studies report that the risk appears unrelated to duration of alcohol consumption (La Vecchia et al, 1989; Nasca et al, 1990).

In several studies, the risk associated with alcohol consumption was greater in premenopausal women (Schatzkin et al, 1987; Harvey et al, 1987; O'Connell et al, 1987; Rohan and McMichael, 1988; Van't Veer et al, 1989; Young, 1989; Freidenreich et al, 1993). But in others it was stronger in postmenopausal women (Hiatt et al, 1988; Ferraroni et al, 1991; MartinMoreno et al, 1994), or was unrelated to menopausal status (La Vecchia et al, 1989b; Sneyd et al, 1991; Katsouyanni et al, 1994). While several studies have suggested that the risk may be enhanced by estrogen replacement therapy (Gapstur et al, 1992; Colditz et al, 1990), others found no such relationship (Freidenreich et al, 1993; Harvey et al, 1987; Paganin-Hill and Ross, 1983; Rosenberg et al, 1990).

Each type of alcoholic beverage—beer, wine, spirits—has been implicated in at least several studies as a source of increased breast cancer risk. In particular, two studies with positive findings (Willett et al, 1987; Howe et al, 1991) made comparisons of risk estimates for each type of beverage after controlling for the intake of other types. Thus the risk of breast cancer associated with alcohol consumption appears to be independent of the source of the alcohol.

Several potential sources of bias in these studies need to be considered. In hospital-based case–control studies, women with a history of large alcohol consumption may have been less likely to be included as controls, particularly where women with alcohol-associated disorders were considered ineligible. Above-average drinkers may also be less likely to participate as controls in studies, particularly community-based studies. Such biases would cause overestimation of the strength of the association. On the other hand, random errors in the measurement of alcohol intake, especially a generalized tendency towards underreporting high consumption, would lead to underestimating the magnitude of the true association.

On balance, current evidence indicates that daily consumption of several standard glasses of alcoholic drinks per day increases the risk of female breast cancer. However, this risk elevation may be due to some as yet unrecognized confounding factor. Longnecker (1994) concluded that "the modest size of the association and variation in results across studies leave the causal role of alcohol in question." Future studies should seek more detailed exposure information (temporal and quantitative aspects) and further explore the possible interactions of alcohol with other factors (e.g., estrogen replacement therapy, menopausal status, and body size).

Cancer of Other Sites

Even though alcohol may not make direct contact with a particular tissue, it may influence biological processes that are important in the carcinogenic process. For example, it has been suggested that pituitary secretion of thyroid- and melanocyte-stimulating hormones increase in response to alcohol intake and that this increases the probabilities of thyroid cancer and malignant melanoma development (Williams, 1976).

Various cohort studies have shown increased risks of lung cancer, but this has mostly been attributed to a high consumption of tobacco by the cohorts investigated. Case–control studies indicate that the association of alcohol with lung cancer risk is secondary to that of smoking (IARC, 1988; Pierce et al, 1989). Nevertheless, there is some human and animal evidence that makes plausible a possible causal link (Potter and McMichael, 1984).

An association of melanoma of the skin with alcohol consumption was seen in the Third National Cancer Survey in the U.S. (Williams and Horm, 1977). A (nonsignificant) relative risk of 1.2 emerged from the study of Danish brewery workers (Jensen, 1979), but a detailed case–control study in Denmark found no such association (Østerlind et al, 1988).

ETIOLOGICAL MECHANISMS

Although alcohol intake has been judged to be causally related to cancer of the oral cavity, pharynx, larynx, esophagus, and liver (IARC, 1988), the carcinogenic action of alcohol is incompletely understood. There is no evidence that ethanol per se is carcinogenic in experimental animals, but most experiments have suffered from deficiencies in design (IARC, 1988). However, alcoholic beverages consumed by humans are complex mixtures which may contain small amounts of recognized carcinogens (IARC, 1988; Table 15–12). Besides, there is evidence that ethanol and its metabolite acetaldehyde influence the metabolism and DNA damaging effect of xenobiotics and endogenous compounds. Increased DNA alkylation has been observed experimentally, and long-term ingestion of alcohol increases levels of cytochrome P-450 in the liver; this in turn may lead to enhanced metabolism of a variety of xenobiotics (IARC, 1988).

While a general metabolic effect of ethanol is possible, the fact that alcohol substantially increases the risk of cancer in organs where ingested carcinogens could act directly on the mucosal cells seems to favor a local effect. Kuratsune and colleagues (1971) found that ethanol promotes the development of tumours in mice given benzo(a)pyrene, probably as a result of increased mucosal penetration. These results were reproduced in other experiments (Henefer, 1966; Elzay, 1969). However, the combined action of nitrosamines and alcohol on the esophageal epithelium has varied (IARC, 1988). One recent, isolated, finding consistent with a general metabolic effect is the observation of an increased frequency of DNA adducts in bronchial tissues in association with alcohol consumption (Dunn et al, 1991).

TABLE 15–12. *Chemical Compounds in Alcoholic Beverages Which Have Been Found To Be Carcinogenic According to IARC*[*]

	Identified in[a]			*Degree of Evidence for Carcinogenicity*[b]		
Compound	*Beer*	*Wine*	*Spirits*	*Human*	*Animal*	*Overall Evaluation*
Acetaldehyde	+	+	+	I	S	2B
Aflatoxins	+	+		S	S	1
Arsenic		+		S	L	1
Asbestos	+	+	+	S	S	1
Benz(a)anthracene			+	ND	S	2A
Benzene		+	+	S	S	1
Benzo(b)fluoranthene			+	ND	S	2B
Benzo(a)pyrene			+	ND	S	2A
Cadmium		+		L	S	2A
Chloroform		+		I	S	2B
Chromium		+		S	S	1[c]
Dichlorobenzene			+	I	S	2B
Ethylene thiourea		+		I	S	2B
Formaldehyde	+	+	+	L	S	2A
Lead		+		I	S	2B[d]
Nickel		+		S	S	1
N-Nitrosodiethylamine	+	+	+	ND	S	2A
N-Nitrosodimethylamine	+	+	+	ND	S	2A
N-Nitrosodi-n-propylamine		+	+	ND	S	2B
N-Nitrosopyrrolidine	+			ND	S	2B
Styrene	+	+	+	I	L	2B
Urethane		+	+	ND	S	2B

[a]From IARC (1988).
[b]From IARC (1987).
[*]S = sufficient; L = limited; I = inadequate; ND = no data; 1 = the agent is carcinogenic to humans; 2A = the agent is probably carcinogenic to humans; 2B = the agent is possibly carcinogenic to humans.
[c]Hexavalent chromium compounds only.
[d]Inorganic lead only.

Other mechanisms might apply more specifically to individual anatomical sites, for which a causal effect of alcohol is uncertain. For example, the stomach is exposed directly to ingested ethanol, although the concentration is quickly diluted by gastric juices and other gastric contents. Under the multi-step model of gastric carcinogenesis postulated by Correa et al (1975), concentrated alcoholic drinks might induce chronic gastritis in individuals consuming excessive amounts. Ethanol ingestion also increases the concentration of bile acids in the bile. This results from the effect of ethanol upon hepatic lipoprotein and cholesterol metabolism, and is thought to account for the reduced risk of cholesterol gallstone disease associated with alcohol consumption (Scragg et al, 1984). The profile of bile acid in the large bowel has been invoked as an etiological factor in colorectal carcinogenesis. Ethanol could also act by altering hepatic metabolism of large bowel carcinogens (Soon et al., 1986), by stimulating epithelial proliferation (Simanowski et al, 1986), or by altering folate metabolism and, hence, the methylation of mucosal-cell DNA (Kearney et al, 1995).

In the same way as the chemical carcinogenic effect of aflatoxin-B upon the liver appears to be potentiated by hepatitis (Bulatao-Jayme et al, 1982), alcoholic cirrhosis, with its associated hepatocellular hyperplasia and/or metabolic disruptions, may increase the risk of primary liver cancer. The evidence from the cohort study of hepatitis B surface antigen–positive volunteer male blood donors in Japan (Oshima et al, 1984), indicating an interactive effect between hepatitis B seropositivity and alcohol consumption in the causation of liver cancer, is compatible with such a potentiation phenomenon.

Heavy consumption of alcohol is strongly associated with pancreatitis, and chronic calcifying pancreatitis may be a potent but rare risk factor for pancreatic cancer (Velema et al, 1986). Human and animal studies have demonstrated both exocrine pancreatic hyperplasia and increased secretion of pancreatic digestive enzymes in association with alcohol consumption (Pour et al, 1983a, b). Such increases in exocrine activity could plausibly predispose one to pancreatic carcinogenesis. However, in animal experimental studies, neither alcohol nor pancreatitis have caused pancreatic cancer. On the other hand, there has been some speculation that the effects of ethanol upon blood lipoprotein concentrations, especially high-density lipoprotein, may in some way account for the repeated observations of reduced risk of pancreatic cancer in alcohol consumers (Farrow and Davis, 1990).

Ethanol might affect breast carcinogenesis via several mechanisms, including direct toxic or solvent properties of alcohol, indirect effects through stimulation of prolactin secretion (Williams, 1976), or effects upon hepatic metabolism that result in increased concentrations of bioactive estrogens in the blood (Siiteri, 1981).

CONCLUSION

The consumption of alcoholic beverages increases the risk of cancer of the oral cavity, pharynx, larynx, esophagus, and liver. Further, all types of alcoholic drinks increase the risk of those cancers, and several studies indicate that the increase in risk may reflect the total amount of ethanol consumed rather than the type of beverage.

Synergistic effects with tobacco smoking have been demonstrated for cancers of the upper aerodigestive tract, and there are indications that alcohol and hepatitis B virus infection exert a joint effect in liver carcinogenesis. While the former finding may point to a mechanism involving a local effect on the mucosa, it is currently not clear to what extent a systemic effect of ethanol influences carcinogenesis. The possible role of carcinogens present in alcoholic beverages is unknown.

For neither cancer of the rectum nor of the female breast is the relationship with alcohol clear. A consistent association with breast cancer has been shown in a large number of studies, but the lack of evidence for a biologically plausible mechanism and the continuing uncertainty about the other main causes of breast cancer make it premature to infer a cause–effect relationship. For rectal cancer the epidemiological evidence is less consistent, and there is little corroborative evidence for the several proposed mechanisms. There is little evidence that alcohol causes cancer of the colon.

Overall, the relationship between alcohol and cancer is sufficient to warrant preventive measures. Indeed, this has assumed greater public health importance as alcohol consumption has increased in many countries in recent decades along with rising affluence. Nevertheless, while personal alcohol consumption should be moderated (especially among cigarette smokers) in order to reduce cancer risk, consideration may need to be given to the balance of risks, given the apparent protective effect of moderate alcohol consumption in relation to the risk of coronary heart disease.

REFERENCES

Adami HO, Hsing AW, McLaughlin JK, et al. 1992a. Alcoholism and liver cirrhosis in the etiology of primary liver cancer. Int J Cancer 51:898–902.

Adami HO, Lund E, Bergström R, Meirik O. 1988. Cigarette smoking, alcohol consumption and risk of breast cancer in young women. Br J Cancer 58:832–837.

Adami HO, McLaughlin JK, Hsing AW, et al. 1992b. Alcoholism and cancer risk: A population-based cohort study. Cancer Causes Control 3:419–425.

Adelstein A, White G. 1976. Alcoholism and mortality. Popul Trends 6:7–13.

Austin H, Delzell E, Grufferman S, et al. 1986. A case–control study of hepatocellular carcinoma and the hepatitis B virus, cigarette smoking, and alcohol consumption. Cancer Res 46:962–966.

Baghurst PA, McMichael AJ, Slavotinek AH, et al. 1991. A case–control study of diet and cancer of the pancreas. Am J Epidemiol 134:167–179.

Bargiggia S, Piva A, Sangiovanni A, Donato F. 1989. Il carcinoma primitivo del fegato e il virus dell'epatite C in Italia. Med Firenze 9:424–426.

Begg CB, Walker AM, Wessen B, et al. 1983. Alcohol consumption and breast cancer. Lancet i:293–294.

Bjelke E. 1973. Epidemiologic studies of cancer of the stomach, colon, and rectum: with special emphasis on the role of diet. Thesis, University of Minnesota.

Blackwelder WC, Yano K, Rhoads GG, et al. 1980. Alcohol and mortality: the Honolulu heart study. Am J Cancer 68:164–169.

Blot WJ, McLaughlin JK, Winn DM, et al. 1988. Smoking and drinking in relation to oral and pharyngeal cancer. Cancer Res 48:3282–3287.

Boeing H, Frentzel-Beyme R, Berger M, et al. 1991. Case–control study on stomach cancer in Germany. Int J Cancer 47:858–864.

Bouchardy C, Clavel F, La Vecchia C, Raymond L, Boyle P. 1990. Alcohol, beer and cancer of the pancreas. Int J Cancer 45:842–846.

Bradshaw E, Schonland M. 1969. Oesophageal and lung cancers in Natal African males in relation to certain socioeconomic factors. An analysis of 484 interviews. Br J Cancer 23:275–284.

Bradshaw E, Schonland M. 1974. Smoking, drinking, and oesophageal cancer in African males of Johannesburg, South Africa. Br J Cancer 30:157–163.

Breslow NE, Day N. 1980. Statistical Methods in Cancer Epidemiology, Vol. I. IARC Scientific Publications No. 32. Lyon, International Agency for Research on Cancer.

Breslow NE, Enstrom JE. 1974. Geographic correlations between cancer mortality rates and alcohol–tobacco consumption in the United States. J Natl Cancer Inst 53:631–639.

Bross IDJ, Coombs J. 1976. Early onset of oral cancer among women who drink and smoke. Oncology 33:136–139.

Brownson RC, Chang JC. 1987. Exposure to alcohol and tobacco and the risk of laryngeal cancer. Arch Environ Health 42:192–196.

Brugere J, Guenel P, Leclerc A, Rodriguez J. 1986. Differential effects of tobacco and alcohol in cancer of the larynx, pharynx, and mouth. Cancer 57:391–395.

BUENO DE MESQUITA HB, MAISONNEUVE P, MOERMAN CJ, RUNIA S, BOYLE P. 1992. Lifetime consumption of alcoholic beverages, tea and coffee and exocrine carcinoma of the pancreas: A population-based case–control study in the Netherlands. Int J Cancer 50:514–522.

BULATAO-JAYME J, ALMERO E, CASTRO MA, et al. 1982. A case–control dietary study of primary liver cancer risk from aflatoxin exposure. Int J Epidemiol 11:112–119.

BURCH JD, HOWE GR, MILLER AB, et al. 1981. Tobacco, alcohol, asbestos, and nickel in the etiology of cancer of the larynx: a case–control study. J Natl Cancer Inst 76:1219–1224.

BYERS T, FUNCH DF. 1982. Alcohol and breast cancer. Lancet i:799–800.

CARSTENSEN JM, BYGREN LO, HATSCHEK T. 1990. Cancer incidence among Swedish brewery workers. Int J Cancer 45:393–396.

CHENG KK, DAY NE, DUFFY SW, LAM TH, FOK M, WONG J. 1992. Pickled vegetables in the aetiology of oesophageal cancer in Hong Kong Chinese. Lancet 339:1314–1318.

CHOI SY, KAHYO H. 1991a. Effect of cigarette smoking and alcohol consumption in the etiology of cancer of the digestive tract. Int J Cancer 49:381–386.

CHOI SY, KAHYO H. 1991b. Effect of cigarette smoking and alcohol consumption in the aetiology of cancer of the oral cavity, pharynx and larynx. Int J Epidemiol 20:878–885.

CHU SY, LEE NC, WINGO PA, WEBSTER LA. 1989. Alcohol consumption and the risk of breast cancer. Am J Epidemiol 130:867–877.

CLAVEL F, BENHAMOU E, AUGUIER A, TARARYRE M, FLAMANT R. 1989. Coffee, alcohol, smoking, and cancer of the pancreas: a case–control study. Int J Cancer 43:17–21.

CLEMMESEN J. 1965. Statistical studies in the aetiology of malignant neoplasms, APMIS, (Suppl) 1: 1174:86–93.

COLDITZ GA, STAMPFER MJ, WILLET WC, et al. 1990. Prospective study of estrogen replacement therapy and risk of breast cancer in postmenopausal women. JAMA 264:2648–2653.

CORREA P, HAENSZEL W, CUELLO W, et al. 1975. A model for gastric cancer epidemiology. Lancet ii:58–60.

CUZICK J, BABIKER AG. 1989. Pancreatic cancer, alcohol, diabetes mellitus and gallbladder disease. Int J Cancer 43:415–421.

D'AVANZO B, LA VECCHIA C, FRANCESCHI S. 1994. Alcohol consumption and the risk of gastric cancer. Nutr Cancer 22:57–64.

DAY GL, BLOT WJ, AUSTIN DF, et al. 1993. Racial differences in risk of oral and pharyngeal cancer: Alcohol, tobacco, and other determinants. J Natl Cancer Inst 85:465–473.

DAY GL, BLOT WJ, SHORE RE, et al. 1994. Second cancers following oral and pharyngeal cancers: Role of tobacco and alcohol. J Natl Cancer Inst 86:131–137.

DE JONG UW, BRESLOW N, GOH EH, et al. 1974. Aetiological factors in oesophageal cancer in Singapore Chinese. Int J Cancer 13:291–303.

DE STEFANI E, CORREA P, FIERRO L, et al. 1990a. Alcohol drinking and tobacco smoking in gastric cancer. A case–control study. Rev Epidemiol Sante Publique 38:297–307.

DE STEFANI E, CORREA P, OREGGIA F, et al. 1987. Risk factors for laryngeal cancer. Cancer 60:3087–3091.

DE STEFANI E, MUÑOZ N, ESTEVE J, et al. 1990b. Mate drinking, alcohol, tobacco, diet and esophageal cancer in Uruguay. Cancer Res 50:426–431.

DEAN G, MACLENNAN R, MCLOUGHLIN H, et al. 1979. Causes of death of blue-collar workers at a Dublin brewery, 1954–73. Br J Cancer 40:581–589.

DEMIRER T, ICLI F, VZUNALIMOGLU O, et al. 1990. Diet and stomach cancer incidence. A case–control study in Turkey. 65:2344–2348.

DOLL R, PETO R, HALL E, WHEATLEY K, GRAY R. 1994. Mortality in relation to consumption of alcohol: 13 years' observations on male British doctors. BMJ 309:911–918.

DORKEN J. 1964. Einige Daten bei 280 Patienten mit Pankreaskrebs. Gastroenterologia 102:47–77.

DUNN BP, VEDAL S, SAN RH, et al. 1991. DNA adducts in bronchial tissues. Int J Cancer 48:485–492.

DURBEC JP, CHEVILLOTTE G, BIDART JM, et al. 1983. Diet, alcohol, tobacco and risk of cancer of the pancreas: a case–control study. Br J Cancer 47:463–470.

ELWOOD JM, PERSON JCG, SKIPPEN DH, et al. 1984. Alcohol, smoking, and socioeconomic factors in the etiology of cancer of the oral cavity, pharynx, and larynx. Int J Cancer 34:603–612.

ELZAY RP. 1969. Effect of alcohol and cigarette smoke as promoting agents in hamster pouch carcinogenesis. J Dent Res 48:1200–1206.

EWERTZ M. 1991. Alcohol consumption and breast cancer risk in Denmark. Cancer Causes Control 2:247–252.

FALK RT, PICKLE LW, BROWN LM, et al. 1989. Effect of smoking and alcohol consumption on laryngeal cancer risk in coastal Texas. Cancer Res 49:4024–4029.

FALK RT, PICKLE LW, FONTHAM ET, et al. 1988. Lifestyle factors for pancreatic cancer in Louisiana: a case–control study. Am J Epidemiol 128:324–336.

FARROW DC, DAVIS S. 1990. Risk of pancreatic cancer in relation to medical history and the use of tobacco, alcohol and coffee. Int J Cancer 45:816–820.

FELDMAN JG, BOXER P. 1979. Relationship of drinking to head and neck cancer. Prev Med 8:507–519.

FELDMAN JG, HAZAN M, NAGARAJAN M, KISSING B. 1975. A case–control investigation of alcohol, tobacco, and diet in head and neck cancer. Prev Med 4:444–463.

FERRARONI M, DECARLI A, WILLETT WC, MARUBINI E. 1991. Alcohol and breast cancer risk: A case–control study from northern Italy. Int J Epidemiol 20:859–864.

FERRARONI M, NEGRI E, LA VECCHIA C, et al. 1989. Socioeconomic indicators, tobacco and alcohol in the aetiology of digestive tract neoplasms. Int J Epidemiol 18:556–562.

FILIPPAZZO MG, ARAGONA E, COTTONE M, et al. 1985. Assessment of some risk factors for hepatocellular carcinoma: a case–control study. Stat Med 4:345–51.

FLANDERS WD, ROTHMAN KJ. 1986. Interaction of alcohol and tobacco in laryngeal cancer. Am J Epidemiol 115:371–379.

FRANCESCHI S, BARRA S, LA VECCHIA C, et al. 1992. Risk factors for cancer of the tongue and the mouth. A case–control study from northern Italy. Cancer 70:2227–2233.

FRANCESCHI S, BIDDI E, NEGRI E, et al. 1994. Alcohol and cancers of the upper aerodigestive tract in men and women. Cancer Epidemiol Biomarkers Prev 3:299–304.

FRANCESCHI S, TALAMINI R, BARRA S, et al. 1990. Smoking and drinking in relation to cancers of the oral cavity, pharynx, larynx and esophagus in northern Italy. Cancer Res 50:6502–6507.

FRANCO EL, KOWALSKI LP, OLIVIERA BV, et al. 1989. Risk factors for oral cancer in Brazil: a case–control study. Int J Cancer 43:992–1000.

FREUDENHEIM JL, GRAHAM S, BYERS TE, et al. 1992. Diet, smoking, and alcohol in cancer of the larynx: A case–control study. Nutr Cancer 17:33–45.

FREUDENHEIM JL, GRAHAM S, MARSHALL JR, et al. 1990. Lifetime alcohol intake and risk of rectal cancer in western New York. Nutr Cancer 13:101–109.

FRIEDENREICH CM, HOWE GR, MILLER AB, JAIN MG. 1993. A cohort study of alcohol consumption and risk of breast cancer. Am J Epidemiol 137:512–520.

FRIEDMAN GD, VAN DEN EDEN SK. 1993. Risk factors for pancreatic cancer. An exploratory study. Int J Epidemiol 22:30–37.

GAO YT, MCLAUGHLIN JK, BLOT WJ, et al. 1994. Risk factors for esophageal cancer in Shanghai, China. I. Role of cigarette smoking and alcohol drinking. Int J Cancer 58:192–196.

GAPSTUR SM, POTTER JD, FOLSOM AR. 1994. Alcohol consumption and colon and rectal cancer in postmenopausal women. Int J Epidemiol 23:50–57.

GAPSTUR SM, POTTER JD, SELLERS TA, FOLSOM AR. 1992. Increased risk of breast cancer with alcohol consumption in postmenopausal women. Am J Epidemiol 136:1221–1231.

GARFINKEL L, BOFFETTA P, STELLMAN SD. 1988. Alcohol and breast cancer: a cohort study. Prev Med 17:686–693.

GARLAND C, SHEKELLE R, BARRETT-CONNOR E. 1985. Dietary vitamin D and calcium and risk of colorectal cancer: a 17-year prospective study in men. Lancet i:307–309.

GHADIRIAN P, SIMARD A, BAILLARGEON J. 1991. Tobacco, alcohol and coffee and cancer of the pancreas. Cancer 67:2664–2670.

GIOVANNUCCI E, STAMPFER MJ, COLDITZ GA, et al. 1993. Folate, methionine, and alcohol intake and risk of colorectal adenoma. J Natl Cancer Inst 85:875–884.

GOLD EB, GORDIS L, DIENER MD, et al. 1985. Diet and other risk factors for cancer of the pancreas: a case–control study. Cancer 55:460–467.

GOLDBOHM RA, VAN DEN BRANDT PA, VAN TV, DORANT E, STURMANS F, HERMUS RJJ. 1994. Prospective study on alcohol consumption and the risk of cancer of the colon and rectum in the Netherlands. Cancer Causes Control 5:95–104.

GORDON T, KANNEL WB. 1984. Drinking and mortality: The Framingham study. Am J Epidemiol 120:97–107.

GRAHAM S, DAGAL H, SWANSON M, MITTELMAN A, WILKINSON G. 1978. Diet in the epidemiology of cancer of the colon and rectum. J Natl Cancer Inst 61:709–714.

GRAHAM S, METTLIN C, MARSHALL J, et al. 1977. Dentition, diet, tobacco and alcohol in the epidemiology of oral cancer. J Natl Cancer Inst 59:1611–1618.

GRAHAM S, METTLIN C, MARSHALL J, et al. 1981. Dietary factors in the epidemiology of cancer of the larynx. Am J Epidemiol 113:675–680.

GUO W, BLOT WJ, LI JY, et al. 1994. A nested case–control study of oesophageal and stomach cancers in the Linxian nutrition intervention trial. Int J Epidemiol 23:444–450.

HAENSZEL W, KURIHARA M, SEGI M, et al. 1972. Stomach cancer among Japanese in Hawaii. J Natl Cancer Inst 49:969–988.

HAKULINEN T, LEHTIMAKI L, LEHTONEN M, et al. 1974. Cancer morbidity among two male cohorts with increased alcohol consumption in Finland. J Natl Cancer Inst 52:1711–1714.

HARDELL L, BENGTSSON NO, JONSSON U, et al. 1984. Aetiological aspects of primary liver cancer, with special regard to alcohol, organic solvents and acute intermittent porphyria—an epidemiological investigation. Br J Cancer 50:389–397.

HARRIS RE, WYNDER EL. 1988. Breast cancer and alcohol consumption. A study in weak associations. JAMA 259:2867–2871.

HARVEY EB, SCHAIRER C, BRINTON LA. 1987. Alcohol consumption and breast cancer. J Natl Cancer Inst 78:657–661.

HENEFER EP. 1966. Ethanol, 30 percent, and hamster pouch carcinogenesis. J Dent Res 45:838–845.

HERITY B, MORIARTY M, BOURKE GJ, et al. 1981. A case–control study of head and neck cancer in the Republic of Ireland. Br J Cancer 43:177–182.

HERITY B, MORIARTY M, DALY L, et al. 1982. The role of tobacco and alcohol in the aetiology of lung and larynx cancer. Br J Cancer 46:961–964.

HEUCH I, KVOLE G, JACOBSEN BK, et al. 1983. Use of alcohol, tobacco and coffee, and risk of pancreatic cancer. Br J Cancer 48:637–643.

HIATT RA, BAWOL RD. 1984. Alcoholic beverage consumption and breast cancer incidence. Am J Epidemiol 120:676–683.

HIATT RA, KLATSKY AL, ARMSTRONG MA. 1988. Alcohol consumption and the risk of breast cancer in a prepaid health plan. Cancer Res 48:2284–2287.

HIGGINSON J. 1966. Etiological factors in gastrointestinal cancer in man. J Natl Cancer Inst 37:527–545.

HINDS MW, KOLONEL LN, LEE J, et al. 1980. Associations between cancer incidence and alcohol cigarette consumption among five ethnic groups in Hawaii. Br J Cancer 41:929–940.

HINDS MW, THOMAS DB, O'REILLY HP. 1979. Asbestos, dental X-rays, tobacco, and alcohol in the epidemiology of laryngeal cancer. Cancer 44:1114–1120.

HIRAYAMA T. 1966. An epidemiological study of oral and pharyngeal cancer in Central and South-east Asia. Bull World Health Organ 34:41–69.

HIRAYAMA T. 1981. A large-scale cohort study on the relationship between diet and selected cancers of digestive organs. *In* Bruce WR, Correa P, Lipkin M, et al (eds): Gastrointestinal Cancer: Endogenous Factors (Banbury Report 7). Cold Spring Harbor, NY, Cold Spring Harbor Laboratory, pp. 409–426.

HIRAYAMA T. 1989a. A large-scale cohort study on risk factors for primary liver cancer, with special reference to the role of cigarette smoking. Cancer Chemother Pharmacol 23 (Suppl):S114–117.

HIRAYAMA T. 1989b. Association between alcohol consumption and cancer of the sigmoid colon: Observations from a Japanese cohort study. Lancet ii:725–727.

HIRAYAMA T. 1990. Contribution of a long-term prospective cohort study to the issue of nutrition and cancer, with special reference to the role of alcohol drinking. Prog Clin Biol Res 346:179–187.

HOEY J, MONTVERNAY C, LAMBERT R. 1981. Wine and tobacco: risk factors for gastric cancer in France. Am J Epidemiol 113:668–674.

HOLMBERG L, OHLANDER EM, BYERS T, et al. 1994. Diet and breast cancer risk: Results from a population-based, case–control study in Sweden. Arch Intern Med 154:1805–1811.

HOSHIYAMA Y, SASABA T. 1992. A case–control study of single and multiple stomach cancers in Saitama Prefecture, Japan. Jpn J Cancer Res 83:937–943.

HOWE G, ROHAN T, DE CARLI A, et al. 1991. The association between alcohol and breast cancer risk: evidence from the combined analysis of six dietary case–control studies. Int J Cancer 47: 707–710.

HU J, LIU Y, YU Y, et al. 1991. Diet and cancer of the colon and rectum: a case–control study in China. Int J Epidemiol 20: 362–367.

HU J, NYREN O, WOLK A, et al. 1994. Risk factors for oesophageal cancer in Northeast China. Int J Cancer 57:38–46.

HU JF, ZHANG SF, JIA EM, et al. 1988. Diet and cancer of the stomach: a case–control study in China. Int J Cancer 41:331–335.

INABA Y, MARUCHI N, MATSUDA M, et al. 1984. A case–control study on liver cancer with special emphasis on the possible aetiological role of schistosomiasis. Int J Epidemiol 13:408–412.

INFANTE T, VOIROL M, RAYMOND L, et al. 1980. Alcohol, tobacco and nutriments consumption in liver cancer and cirrhosis patients in Geneva. *In* Alcohol and the Gastrointestinal Tract (Les colloques de l'INSERM 95). Paris, Institut National de Science et de la Recherche Médicale, pp. 53–58.

INTERNATIONAL AGENCY FOR RESEARCH ON CANCER. 1988. Alcohol drinking. Monogr Eval Carcinog Risks Hum 44. Lyon, International Agency for Research on Cancer.

INTERNATIONAL AGENCY FOR RESEARCH ON CANCER. 1987. Overall evaluation of carcinogenicity: An updating of IARC Monographs Volumes 1–42. Lyon, International Agency for Research on Cancer.

JAIN M, HOWE GR, ST LOUIS P, et al. 1991. Coffee and alcohol as determinants of risk of pancreas cancer: a case–control study from Toronto. Int J Cancer 47:384–389.

JEDRYCHOWSKI W, BOEING H, WAHRENDORF J, POPIELA T, TOBIASZ ADAMCZYK TB, KULIG J. 1993. Vodka consumption, tobacco smoking and risk of gastric cancer in Poland. Int J Epidemiol 22:606–613.

JEDRYCHOWSKI W, WAHRENDORF J, POPIELA T, et al. 1986. A case–control study of dietary factors and stomach cancer risk in Poland. Int J Cancer 37:837–842.

JENSEN OM. 1979. Cancer morbidity and causes of death among Danish brewery workers. Int J Cancer 23:454–463.

JENSEN OM. 1983. Cancer risk among Danish male Seventh-Day Adventists and other temperance society members. J Natl Cancer Inst 70:1011–1014.

JENSEN OM, TUYNS AJ, PEQUIGNOT G. 1978. Usefulness of population controls in retrospective studies of alcohol consumption. Experience from a case–control study of esophageal cancer in Ille-et-Vilaine, France. Q J Stud Alcohol 39:175–182.

KABAT GC, HOWSON CP, WYNDER EL. 1986. Beer consumption and rectal cancer. Int J Epidemiol 15:494–501.

KATO I, NOMURA AMY, STEMMERMANN GN, CHYOU PH. 1992a. Prospective study of the association of alcohol with cancer of the upper aerodigestive tract and other sites. Cancer Causes Control 3:145–151.

KATO I, TOMINAGA S, IKARI A. 1990. A case–control study of male colorectal cancer in Aichi Prefecture, Japan: with special reference to occupational activity level, drinking habits and family history. Jpn J Cancer Res 81:115–121.

KATO I, TOMINAGA S, MATSUMOTO K. 1992b. A prospective study of stomach cancer among a rural Japanese population: a 6-year survey. Jpn J Cancer Res 85:568–575.

KATSOUYANNI K, TRICHOPOULOU A, STUVER S, et al. 1994. Ethanol and breast cancer: An association that may be both confounded and causal. Int J Cancer 58:356–361.

KEARNEY J, GIOVANUCCI E, RIMM EB, et al. 1995. Diet, alcohol, and smoking and the occurrence of hyperplastic polyps of the colon and rectum. Cancer Causes Control 6:45–56.

KELLER AZ, TERRIS M. 1965. The association of alcohol and tobacco with cancer of the mouth and pharynx. Am J Publ Health 55:1578–1585.

KIKENDALL JW, BOWEN PE, BURGESS MB, et al. 1989. Cigarettes and alcohol as independent risk factors for colonic adenomas. Gastroenterology 97:660–664.

KLATSKY AL, AMSTRONG MA, FRIEDMAN GD, HIATT RA. 1988. The relations of alcohol beverage use to colon and rectal cancer. Am J Epidemiol 128:1007–1015.

KLATSKY AL, FRIEDMAN GD, SIEBELAUB AB. 1981. Alcohol and mortality: a ten-year Kaiser-Permanente experience. Ann Intern Med 95:139–145.

KNELLER RW, MCLAUGHLIN JK, BJELKE E, et al. 1991. A cohort study of stomach cancer in a high-risk American population. Cancer 68:672–678.

KONO S, IKEDA M. 1979. Correlation between cancer mortality and alcoholic beverage in Japan. Br J Cancer 40:449–455.

KONO S, IKEDA M, OGATA M, et al. 1983. The relationship between alcohol and mortality among Japanese physicians. Int J Epidemiol 12:437–441.

KONO S, IKEDA M, TOKUDOME S, et al. 1985. Alcohol and cancer in male Japanese physicians. J Cancer Res Oncol 109:82–85.

KONO S, IKEDA M, TOKUDOME S, et al. 1986. Alcohol and mortality: a cohort study of male Japanese physicians. Int J Epidemiol 15:527–532.

KUNE GA, KUNE S, FIELD B, et al. 1993. Oral and pharyngeal cancer, diet, smoking, alcohol, and serum vitamin A and beta-carotene levels: A case–control study in men. Nutr Cancer 20:61–70.

KUNE S, KUNE GA, WATSON LF. 1987. Case–control study of alcoholic beverages as etiological factors: The Melbourne colorectal cancer study. Nutr Cancer 9:43–56.

KURATSUNE M, KOHCHI S, HORIE A, et al. 1971. Test of alcoholic beverages and ethanol solutions for carcinogenicity and tumour-promoting activity. Jpn J Cancer Res 62:395–405.

LA VECCHIA C, FRANCESCHI S, CUZICK J. 1982. Alcohol and breast cancer. Lancet i:621.

LA VECCHIA C, DECARLI A, FRANCHESCHI S, et al. 1985. Alcohol consumption and risk of breast cancer in women. J Natl Cancer Inst 75:61–65.

LA VECCHIA C, PAMPALLONA S. 1986. Age at first birth, dietary practices and breast cancer: mortality in various Italian regions. Oncol 43:1–6.

LA VECCHIA C, DECARLI A, FRANCESCHI S, et al. 1987a. Dietary factors and the risk of breast cancer. Nutr Cancer 10:205–14.

LA VECCHIA C, LIATI P, DECARLI A, et al. 1987b. Coffee consumption and the risk of pancreatic cancer. Int J Cancer 40:309–13.

LA VECCHIA C, NEGRI E. 1989. The role of alcohol in oesophageal cancer in nonsmokers, and of tobacco in non-drinkers. Int J Cancer 43:784–785.

LA VECCHIA C, NEGRI E, D'AVANZO B, et al. 1990. Dietary indicators of laryngeal cancer risk. Cancer Res 50:4497–4500.

LA VECCHIA C, NEGRI E, DECARLI A, et al. 1988. Risk factors for hepatocellular carcinoma in northern Italy. Int J Cancer 42:872–876.

LA VECCHIA C, NEGRI E, PARAZZINI F, et al. 1989. Alcohol and breast cancer: update from an Italian case–control study. Eur J Cancer Clin Oncol 25:1711–1117.

LAM KC, YU MC, LEUNG JWC, et al. 1982. Hepatitis B virus and cigarette smoking: risk ractors for hepatocellular carcinoma in Hong Kong. Cancer Res 42:5246–5248.

LAMY L. 1910. Etude de statistique clinique de 134 cas de cancer de l'oesophage et du cardia. Arch Mal Appar Digest 4:451–475.

LASSERRE O, FLAMANT R, LELLOUCH J, et al. 1967. Alcohol et cancer. Étude de pathologie geographique portant sur les departements francais. Bull Inserm 33:53–60.

LÉ MG, HILL C, KRAMAR A, et al. 1984. Alcoholic beverage consumption and breast cancer in a French case–control study. Am J Epidemiol 120:350–357.

LÉ MG, MOULTON LH, HILL C, et al. 1986. Consumption of dairy produce and alcohol in a case–control study of breast cancer. J Natl Cancer Inst 77:633–636.

LEE HH, WU HY, CHUANG YC, et al. 1990. Epidemiologic characteristics and multiple risk factors of stomach cancer in Taiwan. Anticancer Res 10:875–881.

LEMON FR, WALDEN RT, WOODS RH. 1964. Cancer of the lung and mouth in Seventh-Day Adventists. Preliminary report on a population study. Cancer 17:486–497.

LEVI F, LA VECCHIA C, GULIE C, NEGRI E. 1993. Dietary factors and breast cancer risk in Vaud, Switzerland. Nutr Cancer 19:327–335.

LONGNECKER MP. 1990. A case–control study of alcoholic beverages consumption in relation to risk of cancer of the right colon and rectum. Cancer Causes Control 1:5–14.

LONGNECKER MP. 1994. Alcoholic beverage consumption in relation to risk of breast cancer: Meta-analysis and review. Cancer Causes Control 5:73–82.

LONGNECKER MP, BERLIN JA, ORZA MJ, et al. 1988. A meta-analysis of alcohol consumption in relation to risk of breast cancer. JAMA 260:652–656.

LONGNECKER MP, ORZA MJ, ADAMS ME, et al. 1990. A meta-analysis of alcoholic beverage consumption in relation to risk of colorectal cancer. Cancer Causes Control 1:59–68.

LU SN, LIN TM, CHEN CJ, et al. 1988. A case-control study of primary hepatocellular carcinoma in Taiwan. Cancer 62:2051–2055.

LYON JL, KLAUBER MR, GARDNER JW, et al. 1976. Cancer incidence in Mormons and non-Mormons in Utah, 1966–1970. New Engl J Med 292:129–133.

LYON JL, MAHONEY AW, FRENCH TK, MOSER R, JR. 1992. Coffee consumption and the risk of cancer of the exocrine pancreas: A case–control study in a low-risk population. Epidemiol 3:164–170.

MACK TM, YU MC, HANISCH R, HENDERSON BE. 1986. Pancreas, smoking, beverage consumption, and past medical history. J Natl Cancer Inst 76:49–60.

MAIER H, GEWELKE U, DIETZ A, HELLER WD. 1992. Risk factors of cancer of the larynx: Results of the Heidelberg case–control study. Otolaryngol Head Neck Surg 107:577–582.

MAIER H, SENNEWALD E, WOLFDIETER-HELLER GF, WEIDAUER H. 1994. Chronic alcohol consumption—The key risk factor for pharyngeal cancer. Otolaryngol Head Neck Surg 110:168–173.

MANOUSOS O, DAY NE, TRICHOPOULOS D, et al. 1983. Diet and colorectal cancer: A case control study in Greece. Int J Cancer 32:1–5.

MARSHALL JR, GRAHAM S, HAUGHEY BP, et al. 1992. Smoking, alcohol, dentition and diet in the epidemiology of oral cancer. Eur J Cancer Part B: Oral Oncol 28:9–15.

MARTINEZ I. 1969. Factors associated with cancer of the oesophagus, mouth and pharynx in Puerto Rico. J Natl Cancer Inst 42:1069–1094.

MARTINMORENO JM, BOYLE P, GORGOJO L, et al. 1993. Alcoholic beverage consumption and risk of breast cancer in Spain. Cancer Causes Control 4:345–353.

MASHBERG A, BOFFETTA P, WINKELMAN R, GARFINKEL L. 1993. Tobacco smoking, alcohol drinking, and cancer of the oral cavity and oropharynx among U.S. Veterans. Cancer 72:1369–1375.

MCMICHAEL AJ. 1978. Recent increases in laryngeal cancer in relation to alcohol and tobacco consumption trends: Great Britain and Australia. Lancet i:1244–1247.

MCMICHAEL AJ, POTTER JD, HETZEL BS. 197?. Time trends in colorectal cancer mortality in relation to food and alcohol consumption: United States, United Kingdom, Australia and New Zealand. Int J Epidemiol 8:295–303.

MEARA J, MCPHERSON K, ROBERTS M, et al. 1989. Alcohol, cigarette smoking and breast cancer. Br J Cancer 60:70–73.

MEYER F, WHITE E. 1993. Alcohol and nutrients in relation to colon cancer in middle-aged adults. Am J Epidemiol 138:225–236.

MIZUNO S, WATANABE S, NAKAMURA K, et al. 1992. A multi-institute case–control study on the risk factors of developing pancreatic cancer. Jpn J Clin Oncol 22:286–291.

MONSON RR, LYON JL. 1975. Proportional mortality among alcoholics. Cancer 36:1077–1079.

MUSCAT JE, WYNDER EL. 1992. Tobacco, alcohol, asbestos, and occupational risk factors for laryngeal cancer. Cancer 69:2244–2251.

NANDAKUMAR A, THIMMASETTY KT, SREERAMAREDDY NM, et al. 1990. A population-based case–control investigation on cancers of the oral cavity in Bangalore, India. Br J Cancer 62:847–851.

NASCA PC, BAPTISTE MS, FIELD NA, et al. 1990. An epidemiological case–control study of breast cancer and alcohol consumption. Int J Epidemiol 19:532–538.

NEGRI E, LA VECCHIA C, FRANCESCHI S, DECARLI A, BRUZZI P. 1992. Attributable risks for oesophageal cancer in Northern Italy. Eur J Cancer Part A: General Topics 28:1167–1171.

NEGRI E, LA VECCHIA C, FRANCESCHI S, et al. 1993. Attributable risk of oral cancer in northern Italy. Cancer Epidemiol Biomarkers Prev 2:189–193.

NEWCOMB PA, STORER BE, MARCUS PM. 1993. Cancer of the large bowel in women in relation to alcohol consumption: A case–control study in Wisconsin (United States). Cancer Causes Control 4:405–411.

NICHOLLS P, EDWARDS G, KYLE E. 1974. Alcoholics admitted to four hospitals in England. II. General and cause-specific mortality. Q J Stud Alcohol 35:841–855.

NOMURA A, GROVE JS, STEMMERMANN GN, SEVERSON RK. 1990. A prospective study of stomach cancer and its relation to diet, cigarettes and alcohol consumption. Cancer Res 50:627–631.

NOTANI PN. 1988. Role of alcohol in cancers of the upper alimentary tract: use of models in risk assessment. J Epidemiol Community Health 42:187–192.

O'CONNELL DL, HULKA BS, CHAMBLESS, et al. 1987. Cigarette smoking, alcohol consumption, and breast cancer risk. J Natl Cancer Inst 78:229–324.

OLSEN GW, MANDEL JS, GIBSON RW, et al. 1989. A case–control study of pancreatic cancer and cigarettes, alcohol, coffee and diet. Am J Public Health 79:1016–1019.

OLSEN J, KRONBORG O. 1993. Coffee, tobacco and alcohol as risk factors for cancer and adenoma of the large intestine. Int J Epidemiol 22:398–402.

OLSEN J, SABROE S, FASTING U. 1985a. Interaction of alcohol and tobacco as risk factors in cancer of the laryngeal region. J Epidemiol Community Health 39:165–168.

OLSEN J, SABROE S, IPSEN J. 1985b. Effect of combined alcohol and tobacco exposure on risk of cancer of the hypopharynx. J Epidemiol Community Health 39:304–307.

OREGGIA F, DESTEFANI E, CORREA P, et al. 1991. Risk factors for cancer of the tongue in Uruguay. Cancer 67:180–183.

OSHIMA A, TSUKUMA H, HIYAMA T, et al. 1984. Follow-up study of HBsAG-positive blood donors with special reference to effect of drinking and smoking on development of liver cancer. Int J Cancer 34:775–779.

ØSTERLIND A, TUCKER MA, STONE BJ, JENSEN OM. 1988. The Danish case–control study of cutaneous malignant melanoma. IV. No association with nutritional factors, alcohol, smoking or hair dyes. Int J Cancer 42:825–828.

PAGANANI-HILL A, ROSS RK. 1983. Breast cancer and alcohol consumption. Lancet ii:626–627.

PAGANINI-HILL A, WU A, CHAO A. 1990. Re: "The relations of alcoholic beverage use to colon and rectal cancer" (Letter). Am J Epidemiol 132:394.

PEQUIGNOT G, CUBEAU J. 1973. Enquètes methodologiques comparant chez les memes sujets la consommation appreciée par interrogatoire et la consommation mesurée par pesée. Rev Epidemiol Med Soc 21:585–608.

PETERS M, WELLEK S, DIENES HP, et al. 1994. Epidemiology of hepatocellular carcinoma. Evaluation of viral and other risk factors in a low-endemic area for hepatitis B and C. Z Gastroenterol 32:146–151.

PETERS RK, GARABRANT DH, YU MC, MACK TM. 1989. A case–control study of occupational and dietary factors in colorectal cancer in young men by subsite. Cancer Res 49:5459–5468.

PETERS RK, PIKE MC, GARABRANT D, MACK TM. 1992. Diet and colon cancer in Los Angeles County, California. Cancer Causes Control 3:457–473.

PHILLIPS RL, GARFINCKEL L, KUZMA JW, ET AL. 1980. Mortality among California Seventh Day Asventists for selected cancer sites. J Natl Cancer Inst 65:1097–1107.

PICKLE LN, GREENE MH, ZIEGLER RG, et al. 1984. Colorectal cancer in Nebraska. Cancer Res 44:363–369.

PIERCE RJ, KUNE GA, KUNE S, et al. 1989. Dietary and alcohol intake, smoking pattern, occupational risk, and family history in lung cancer patients: results of a case–control study in males. Nutr Cancer 12:237–248.

POCHIN EE. 1976. Alcohol and cancer of the breast and thyroid (Letter). Lancet i:1137.

POLLACK ES, NOMURA AMY, HEIBRUN LK, et al. 1984. Prospective study of alcohol consumption and cancer. N Engl J Med 310:617–621.

POTTER JD, MCMICHAEL AJ. 1984. Alcohol, beer and lung cancer—a meaningful relationship? Int J Epidemiol 13:240–242.

POTTER JD, MCMICHAEL AJ. 1986. Diet and cancer of the colon and rectum: A case–control study. J Natl Cancer Inst 76:557–569.

POTTER JD, MCMICHAEL AJ, HARTSHORNE JM. 1982. Alcohol and

beer consumption in relation to cancers of bowel and lung: an extended correlation analysis. J Chron Dis 35:833–842.

POTTER JD, SLATTERY ML, BOSTICK RM, GAPSTUR, SM. 1993. Colon cancer: a review of the epidemiology. Epidemiol Rev 15:499–545.

POTTERN LM, MORRIS LE, BLOT WJ, et al. 1981. Esophageal cancer among black men in Washington, DC. I. Alcohol, tobacco, and other risk factors. J Natl Cancer Inst 67:777–783.

POUR PM, REBER HA, STEPON K. 1983a. Modification of pancreatic carcinogenesis in the hamster model. XII. Dose-related effect of ethanol. J Natl Cancer Inst 71:1085–1087.

POUR PM, TAHAHASHI M, DONNELLY T, et al. 1983b. Modification of pancreatic carcinogenesis in the hamster model. IX. Effect of pancreatitis. J Natl Cancer Inst 71:607–613.

PRIOR P. 1988. Long-term risk in alcoholism. Alcohol 23:163–171.

QIAO ZK, HALLIDAY ML, RANKIN JG, COATES RA. 1988. Relationship between hepatitis B surface antigen prevalence, per capita alcohol consumption and primary liver cancer death rate in 30 countries. J Clin Epidemiol 41:787–792.

RAO DN, GANESH B, DESAI PB. 1994a. Role of reproductive factors in breast cancer in a low-risk area: A case–control study. Br J Cancer 70:129–132.

RAO DN, GANESH B, RAO RS, DESAI PB. 1994b. Risk assessment of tobacco, alcohol and diet in oral cancer. A case–control study. Int J Cancer 58:469–473.

RAYMOND L, INFANTE F, TUYNS AJ, et al. 1987. Diet and pancreatic cancer (Fr.). Gastroenterol Clin Biol 11:488–492.

RIBOLI E, CAPERLE M, SABATINO C, et al. 1986. Evaluation of dietary assessment methods. Pilot phase of a case–control study on colorectal polyps. Ital J Gastroenterol 18:245–248.

RIBOLI E, CORNEE J, MACQUART-MOULIN G, KAAKS R, CASAGRANDS C, GUYADER M. 1991. Cancer and polyps of the colorectum and lifetime consumption of beer and other alcoholic beverages. Am J Epidemiol 133:157–166.

RICHARDSON S, DE VINCENZI I, PUJOL H, GERBER M. 1989. Alcohol consumption in a case–control study of breast cancer in southern France. Int J Cancer 44:84–89.

ROBINETTE CD, HRUBEC Z, FRAUMENI JF. 1979. Chronic alcoholism and subsequent mortality in World War II veterans. Am J Epidemiol 109:687–700.

ROHAN TE, MCMICHAEL AJ. 1988. Alcohol consumption and risk of breast cancer. Int J Cancer 41:695–699.

ROSENBERG L, PALMER JR, MILLER DR, CLARKE EA, SHAPIRO S. 1990. A case–control study of alcoholic beverage consumption and breast cancer. Am J Epidemiol 131:6–14.

ROSENBERG L, SLONE D, SHAPIRO S, et al. 1982. Breast cancer and alcoholic-beverage consumption. Lancet i:267–271.

ROTHMAN K, KELLER A. 1972. The effect of joint exposure to alcohol and tobacco on risk of cancer of the mouth and pharynx. J Chron Dis 25:711–716.

ROTHMAN KJ. 1976. The estimation of synergy or antagonism. Am J Epidemiol 103:506–511.

SANKARANARAYANAN R, DUFFY SW, DAY NE, NAIR MK, PADMAKUMARY G. 1989. A case–control investigation of cancer of the oral tongue and the floor of the mouth in southern India. Int J Cancer 44:617–621.

SANKARANARAYANAN R, DUFFY SW, NAIR MK, PADMAKUMARY G, DAY NE. 1990a. Tobacco and alcohol as risk factors in cancer of the larynx in Kerala. Int J Cancer 45:879–882.

SANKARANARAYANAN R, DUFFY SW, PADMAKUMARY G, DAY NE, KRISHAN NAIR M. 1990b. Risk factors for cancer of the buccal and labial mucosa in Kerala, southern India. J Epidemiol Community Health 44:286–292.

SANKARANARAYANAN R, DUFFY SW, PADMAKUMARY G, et al. 1991. Risk factors for cancer of the oesophagus in Kerala, India. Int J Cancer 49:485–489.

SCHATZKIN A, JONES DY, HOOVER RN, et al. 1987. Alcohol consumption and breast cancer in the epidemiologic follow-up study of the First National Health and Nutrition Examination Survey. N Engl J Med 316:1169–1173.

SCHATZKIN A, PIANTADOSI S, MICCOZZI M, BARTEE D. 1989b. Alcohol consumption and breast cancer: a cross-national correlation study. Int J Epidemiol 18:28–31.

SCHATZKIN A, CARTER CL, GREEN SB, KREGER BE, SPLANSKY GL, ANDERSON KM, HELSEL WE, KANNEL WB. 1989a. Is alcohol consumption related to breast cancer? Results from the Framingham heart study. J Natl Cancer Inst 81:31–35.

SCHMIDT W, DE LINT J. 1972. Causes of death of alcoholics. Q J Stud Alcohol 33:171–185.

SCHMIDT W, POPHAM RE. 1981. The role of drinking and smoking in mortality from cancer and other causes in male alcoholics. Cancer 47:1031–1041.

SCHWARTZ D, LELLOUCH J, FLAMANT R, et al. 1962. Alcool et cancer. Resultats d'une enquète retrospective. Rev Fr Clin Biol 7:590–604.

SCIALLERO S, BONELLI L, SACCOMANNO S, CONIO M, BRUZZI P, PUGLIESE V. 1993. Socioeconomic characteristics, life style, diabetes, family history of cancer and risk of pancreatic cancer. Eur J Gastroenterol Hepatol 5:367–371.

SCRAGG RKR, MCMICHAEL AJ, BAGHURST PA. 1984. Diet, alcohol and relative weight in gallstone disease: A case–control study. B M J 288:1113–1119.

SEGAL I, REINACH SG, DE BEER M. 1988. Factors associated with oesophageal cancer in Soweto, South Africa. Br J Cancer 58: 681–686.

SEIDMAN H, STELLMAN SD, MUSHINSKI MH. 1982. A different perspective on breast cancer risk factors: some implications of non-attributable risk. Cancer 32:3–15.

SHIBATA A, HIROHATA T, TOSHIMA H, et al. 1986. The role of drinking and cigarette smoking in the excess deaths from liver cancer. Jpn J Cancer 77:287–295.

SIITERI PK. 1981. Extraglandular oestrogen formation and serum binding of oestradiol: Relationship to cancer. J Endocrinol 89:119–129.

SIMANOWSKI UA, SEITZ HK, BAIER B, et al. 1986. Chronic ethanol consumption selectively stimulates rectal cell proliferation in the rat. Gut 27:278–282.

SIMON MS, CARMAN W, WOLFE R, et al. 1991. Alcohol consumption and the risk of breast cancer: a report from the Tecumseh Community Health Study. J Clin Epidemiol 44:755–761.

SLATTERY ML, WEST DN, ROBISON, LM, et al. 1990. Tobacco, alcohol, coffee and caffeine as risk factors for colon cancer in a low risk population. Epidemiol 1:141–145.

SMITH SJ, DEACON JM, CHILVERS CED, et al. 1994. Alcohol, smoking, passive smoking and caffeine in relation to breast cancer risk in young women. Br J Cancer 70:112–119.

SNEYD MJ, PAUL C, SPEARS GFS, et al. 1991. Alcohol consumption and risk of breast cancer. Int J Cancer 48:812–815.

SOON OS, FIALA ES, PUZ C, HAMILTON SR. 1986. Enhancement of azoxymethane (AOM) and methylazoxymethanol (MAM) metabolism by liver microsomes following chronic ethanol administration to rats (abstr.). Proceedings, 77th Annu Meeting Am Assoc Cancer Res 27:120.

SPALAJKOVIC M. 1976. Alcoholism and cancer of the larynx and hypopharynx. J Fr Otorhinolaryngol 25:49–50.

SPITZ MR, FUEGER JJ, GOEPFERT H, et al. 1988. Squamous cell carcinoma of the upper aerodigestive tract. A case comparison analysis. Cancer 61:203–208.

STEMHAGEN A, SLADE J, ALTMAN R, et al. 1983. Occupational risk factors and liver cancer. A retrospective case–control study of primary liver cancer in New Jersey. Am J Epidemiol 117:443–454.

STEMMERMANN GN, NOMURA AMY, CHYON P, et al. 1990. Prospective study of alcohol intake and large bowel cancer. Dig Dis Sci 35:1414–1420.

STOCKS P. 1957. Cancer incidence in North Wales and Liverpool region in relation to habits and environment. British Empire Cancer Campaign, 35th Annual Report, Suppl. to Part 2:1–127.

SUNDBY P. 1967. Alcoholism and Mortality. Oslo, Universitetsforlaget.

TALAMINI R, LA VECCHIA C, DECARLI A, et al. 1984. Social factors, diet and breast cancer in a northern Italian population. Br J Cancer 49:723–729.

TAVANI A, NEGRI E, FRANCESCHI S, LA VECCHIA C. 1993. Risk factors for esophageal cancer in women in Northern Italy. Cancer 72:2531–2536.

TONIOLO P, RIBOLI E, PROTTA F, et al. 1989. Breast cancer and alcohol consumption: a case–control study in northern Italy. Cancer Res 49:5203–5206.

TONNESEN H, MOLLER H, ANDERSEN JR, JENSEN E, JUEL K. 1994. Cancer morbidity in alcohol abusers. Br J Cancer 69:327–332.

TRICHOPOULOS D, DAY NE, KAKLAMANI E, et al. 1987. Hepatitis B virus, tobacco smoking and ethanol consumption in the etiology of hepatocellular carcinomas. Int J Cancer 39:45–49.

TSUKUMA H, HIYAMA T, OSHIMA A, et al. 1990. A case–control study of hepatocellular carcinoma in Osaka, Japan. Int J Cancer 45:231–236.

TUYNS AJ. 1983. Oesophageal cancer in non-smoking drinkers and in non-drinking smokers. Int J Cancer 32:443–444.

TUYNS AJ, MASSÉ G. 1975. Cancer of the oesophagus in Brittany: an incidence study in Ille-et-Villaine. Int J Epidemiol 13:53–57.

TUYNS AJ, AUDIGIER JC. 1976. Double wave cohort increase of oesophageal and laryngeal cancer in France in relation to reduced alcohol consumption during the Second World War. Digestion 14:197–204.

TUYNS AJ, ESTÈVE J, RAYMOND L, et al. 1988a. Cancer of the larynx/hypopharynx, tobacco and alcohol. Int J Cancer 41:483–491.

TUYNS AJ, HU MX, PEQUIGNOT G. 1983. Alcohol consumption patterns in the department of Calvados (France). Rev Epidemiol Santé Publique 31:179–197.

TUYNS AJ, JENSEN OM, PEQUIGNOT G. 1977a. Le choix difficile d'un bon groupe de témoins dans une enquête rétrospective. Rev Epidemiol Santé Publique 25:67–84.

TUYNS AJ, KAAKS R, HAELTERMAN M. 1988b. Colorectal cancer and the consumption of foods: a case–control study in Belgium. Nutr Cancer 11:189–204.

TUYNS AJ, PEQUIGNOT G, ABBATUCCI JS. 1979. Oesophageal cancer and alcohol consumption: importance of type of beverage. Int J Cancer 23:443–447.

TUYNS AJ, PEQUIGNOT G, GIGNOUX M, et al. 1982. Cancers of the digestive tract, alcohol and tobacco. Int J Cancer 30:9–11.

TUYNS AJ, PEQUIGNOT G, JENSEN OM. 1977b. Le cancer de l'oesophage en Illeet-Villaine en fonction des niveaux de comsommation d'alcool et de tabac. Des risques qui se multiplient. Bull Cancer 64:45–60.

TUYNS AJ, RIBOLI E, DOORNBOS G, et al. 1987. Diet and esophageal cancer in Calvados (France). Nutr Cancer 9:81–92.

VAN'T VEER P, KOK FJ, HERMUS RJJ, STURMANS F. 1989. Alcohol dose, frequency and age at first exposure in relation to the risk of breast cancer. Int J Epidemiol 18:511–517.

VASSALLO A, CORREA P, DE STÈFANI E, et al. 1985. Oesophageal cancer in Uruguay: a case–control study. J Natl Cancer Inst 75:1005–1009.

VELEMA JP, WALKER AM, GOLD EB. 1986. Alcohol and pancreatic cancer. Insufficient epidemiologic evidence for a causal relationship. Am J Epidemiol 124:28–41.

VICTORIA CG, MUÑOZ H, DAY NE, BARCELOS LB, PECCIN DA, BRAGA NM. 1987. Hot beverages and oesophagel cancer in southern Brazil: a case–control study. Int J Cancer 39:710–716.

VINCENT RG, MARCHETTA F. 1963. The relationship of the use of tobacco and alcohol to cancer of the oral cavity, pharynx or larynx. Am J Surg 106:501–505.

WEBSTER LA, LAYDE PM, WINGO PA, et al. 1983. Alcohol consumption and risk of breast cancer. Lancet ii:724–726.

WILLETT WC, STAMPFER MJ, COLDITZ GA, et al. 1987. Moderate alcohol consumption and the risk of breast cancer. N Engl J Med 316:1174–1180.

WILLIAMS RR. 1976. Breast and thyroid cancer and malignant melanoma promoted by alcohol-induced pituitary secretion of prolactin, TSH and MSH. Lancet i:996–999.

WILLIAMS RR, HORM JW, 1977. Association of cancer sites with tobacco and alcohol consumption and socioeconomic status of patients: Interview study from the Third National Cancer Survey. J Natl Cancer Inst 58:525–547.

WU AH, PAGANINI-HILL A, RAO RK, et al. 1987. Alcohol physical activity and other risk factors for colorectal cancer: a prospective study. Br J Cancer 55:687–694.

WU-WILLIAMS AH, YU MC, MACK TM. 1990. Life-style, workplace, and stomach cancer by subsite in young men of Los Angeles County. Cancer Res 50:2569–2576.

WYNDER EL, BROSS IJ. 1961. A study of etiological factors in cancer of the esophagus. Cancer 14:389–413.

WYNDER EL, BROSS IJ, DAY E. 1956. A study of environmental factors in cancer of the larynx. Cancer 9:86–110.

WYNDER EL, BROSS IJ, FELDMAN RM. 1957. A study of etiological factors in cancer of the mouth. Cancer 10:1300–1323.

WYNDER EL, COVEY LS, MABUCHI K, et al. 1976. Environmental factors in cancer of the larynx. A second look. Cancer 38:1591–1601.

WYNDER EL, FUJITA Y, HARRIS RE. 1991. Comparative epidemiology of cancer between the United States and Japan: a second look. Cancer 67:746–763.

WYNDER EL, LEMON FR, BROSS IJ. 1959. Cancer and coronary artery disease among Seventh-Day Adventists. Cancer 12:1016–1028.

WYNDER EL, SHIGEMATSU T. 1967. Environmental factors of cancer of the colon and rectum. Cancer 20:1520–1561.

YEN S, HSIEH CC, MACMAHON B. 1982. Consumption of alcohol and tobacco and other risk factors for pancreatitis. Am J Epidemiol 116:407–414.

YOUNG TB. 1989. A case–control study of breast cancer and alcohol consumption habits. Cancer 64:552–558.

YU GP, HSIEH CC. 1991. Risk factors for stomach cancer: a population-based case–control study in Shanghai. Cancer Causes Control 2:169–174.

YU H, HARRIS RE, KABAT GC, WYNDER EL. 1988. Cigarette smoking, alcohol consumption and primary liver cancer: a case–control study in the USA. Int J Cancer 42:325–328.

YU MC, GARABRANT DH, PETERS JM, et al. 1988. Tobacco, alcohol, diet, occupation, and carcinoma of the esophagus. Cancer Res 48:3843–3848.

YU MC, MACK T, HANISCH R, et al. 1983. Hepatitis, alcohol consumption, cigarette smoking, and hepatocellular carcinoma. Cancer Res 43:6077–6079.

ZAGRANISKI RT, KELSEY JL, WALTER SD. 1986. Occupational risk factors for laryngeal carcinoma, Connecticut, 1975–1980. Am J Epidemiol 124:67–76.

ZARIDZE D, LIFANOVA Y, MAXIMOVITCH D, DAY NE, DUFFY SW. 1991. Diet, alcohol consumption and reproductive factors in a case–control study of breast cancer in Moscow. Int J Cancer 48:493–501.

ZATONSKI W, BECHER H, LISSOWSKA J, WAHRENDORF J. 1991. Tobacco, alcohol, and diet in the etiology of laryngeal cancer: a population-based case–control study. Cancer Causes Control 2:3–10.

ZATONSKI W, BOYLE P, PRZEWOZRUAK K, et al. 1993. Cigarette

smoking, alcohol, tea and coffee consumption and pancreas cancer risk: a case–control study from Opole, Poland. Int J Cancer 53:601–607.

ZHENG TZ, BOYLE P, HU HF, et al. 1990. Tobacco smoking, alcohol consumption, and risk of oral cancer: a case–control study in Beijing, People's Republic of China. Cancer Causes Control 1:173–179.

ZHENG W, BLOT WJ, SHU X, et al. 1992a. Risk factors for laryngeal cancer in Shanghai, China. Am J Epidemiol 136:178–191.

ZHENG W, BLOT WJ, SHU X, et al. 1992b. Risk factors for oral and pharyngeal cancer in Shanghai, with emphasis on diet. Cancer Epidemiol Biomarkers Prev 1:441–448.

ZHENG W, MCLAUGHLIN JK, GRINDLEY G, et al. 1993. A cohort study of smoking, alcohol consumption, and dietary factors for pancreatic cancer (United States). Cancer Causes Control 4:477–482.

ZIEGLER RG. 1986. Alcohol-nutrient interactions in cancer etiology. Cancer 58:1942–1948.

16 Ionizing radiation

JOHN D. BOICE, JR.
CHARLES E. LAND
DALE L. PRESTON

Ionizing radiation is perhaps the most extensively studied human carcinogen. Epidemiological studies have been conducted on human populations irradiated for medical, occupational, or military reasons, and a wealth of knowledge on carcinogenic effects has been derived from experimental studies in animals and in cell culture (UNSCEAR, 1986, 1988, 1993, 1994; NAS, 1990). Many human cancers have been convincingly linked to radiation, with a few notable exceptions such as chronic lymphocytic leukemia (CLL), Hodgkin's disease, cervical cancer, and prostate cancer. The important questions, however, are not whether radiation causes cancer but how does it cause cancer? How much cancer is caused by radiation? Is risk substantially diminished when exposure is spread over time? How long does the risk last after exposure? Which organs are particularly sensitive and why do they vary in sensitivity? Although radiation can be readily detected and quantified, and precise radiation protection guidelines exist, there remains uncertainty about the shape of the dose-effect curve at low doses for sparsely ionizing radiation such as x-rays or gamma rays; the influence of physical exposure conditions such as dose rate (fractionation or protraction of dose) and type of radiation; and the influence of various biological modifiers of risk such as age and sex. Many of these issues are of current scientific, public health, and radiation protection interest.

Since our earlier review in 1982 (Boice and Land, 1982), the attention given to the health effects of ionizing radiation has intensified. The Chernobyl reactor accident in the Soviet Union in 1986 distributed radionuclides throughout the world (UNSCEAR, 1988). Indoor radon gas was recognized as a possible risk factor for lung cancer (NAS, 1988). The dosimetry for the atomic bomb survivors in Japan underwent major revisions (Fry and Sinclair, 1987). The National Institutes of Health published congressionally mandated radioepidemiological tables on the probability that a given dose of radiation may have caused a specific cancer in an individual (NIH, 1985). Living near nuclear installations (Forman et al, 1987) and preconception radiation (Gardner et al, 1990) were suggested as possible risk factors for childhood leukemia. Participants at some nuclear weapons tests appeared to be at increased risk of leukemia (Robinette et al, 1985). New studies were published of patients (Boice, 1988a) and workers (Gilbert et al, 1993a) exposed to radiation. The extent of radiation exposures associated with nuclear weapons production in the former Soviet Union was learned to be substantial (Burkhart and Kellerer, 1994). Finally, a National Academy of Sciences committee reported that estimates of lifetime cancer risk following relatively low doses may be as much as four times larger than previously thought (NAS, 1990).

In the following discussion two themes will be followed. The first will concern radiation as a carcinogen, touching on implications for public health and radiation protection. The second will involve scientific issues, stressing, whenever possible, what might be learned about carcinogenesis in general from radiation studies.

SOURCES OF EXPOSURE

The greatest population exposure to ionizing radiation comes from natural background sources, about 2.9 millisievert (mSv) (0.29 rem) per year (UNSCEAR, 1988; NCRP, 1987). These sources include cosmic rays (0.27 mSv/year), which vary by altitude; terrestrial radiations (0.28 mSv/year), which vary according to the distribution in soil of radioactive elements such as uranium; internally deposited radionuclides (0.39 mSv/year) such as potassium^{40}; and radon (2.0 mSv/year, confined mainly to lung). The greatest source of manmade radiation is from medical uses (0.53 mSv/year), with exposures increasing directly with age. Occupation, nuclear power, fallout from testing nuclear weapons, and consumer products make only a minor contribution (0.109 mSv/year). The average per capita dose from all sources of radiation, excluding radon, is thus about 1.6 mSv (0.160 rem) per year.

It was recently estimated that continuous lifetime exposure of 100,000 persons to 1 mSv (0.1 rem) of ionizing radiation per year will induce about 65 leukemias, and 495 fatal cancers of other sites (NAS, 1990). On this basis, 4%–5% of all cancers might be attributable to all sources of radiation exposure (1.6 mSv/yr), excluding indoor radon which has been suggested as an important cause of lung cancer (NAS, 1988). Previous estimates of attributable risk were lower (NAS, 1980; Jablon and Bailar, 1980; Evans et al, 1986), but all such estimates should be interpreted with caution given the substantial uncertainties in applying risks from high-dose studies to low-dose and low dose rate situations. It appears, though, that a reduction in medical x-ray exposures and possibly indoor radon are the only ways to reduce population exposure and presumed radiogenic cancer risk.

POPULATIONS STUDIED

Knowledge of radiation effects has come from medically exposed patients, occupational groups, atomic bomb survivors, and persons exposed to radioactive fallout or naturally occurring radiation such as radon (Fig. 16–1) (Boice and Fraumeni, 1984; Upton et al, 1986; UNSCEAR, 1994; NAS, 1988, 1990).

Medical Exposures

Chest Exposures

Tuberculosis. Frequent x-ray fluoroscopic examinations to monitor lung-collapse treatments for tuberculosis (TB) during 1935–1954 increased the risk of breast cancer among 2573 women in Massachusetts who received an average of 88 chest fluoroscopies, compared to 2367 nonexposed women with TB (Boice et al, 1991c). The follow-up was 97% complete. Excess breast cancers (147 observed vs 113.6 expected) were related to dose in a linear manner. The excess did not appear until 10 to 15 years after exposure and remained high throughout 50 years of observation. Exposures during the adolescent and teenage years carried the greatest risk, and exposures after age 40 the least (suggesting an important promotional role for hormonal factors). Radiation-absorbed dose to the breast per fluoroscopy was estimated as about 0.9 centigray (cGy) (rad), and the average cumulative dose as 79 cGy. The excess absolute risk was estimated as 10.7 cases per 10^4 person-years per gray (PY-Gy), and the relative risk (RR) as 1.61 at 1 Gy. A large Canadian series was gen-

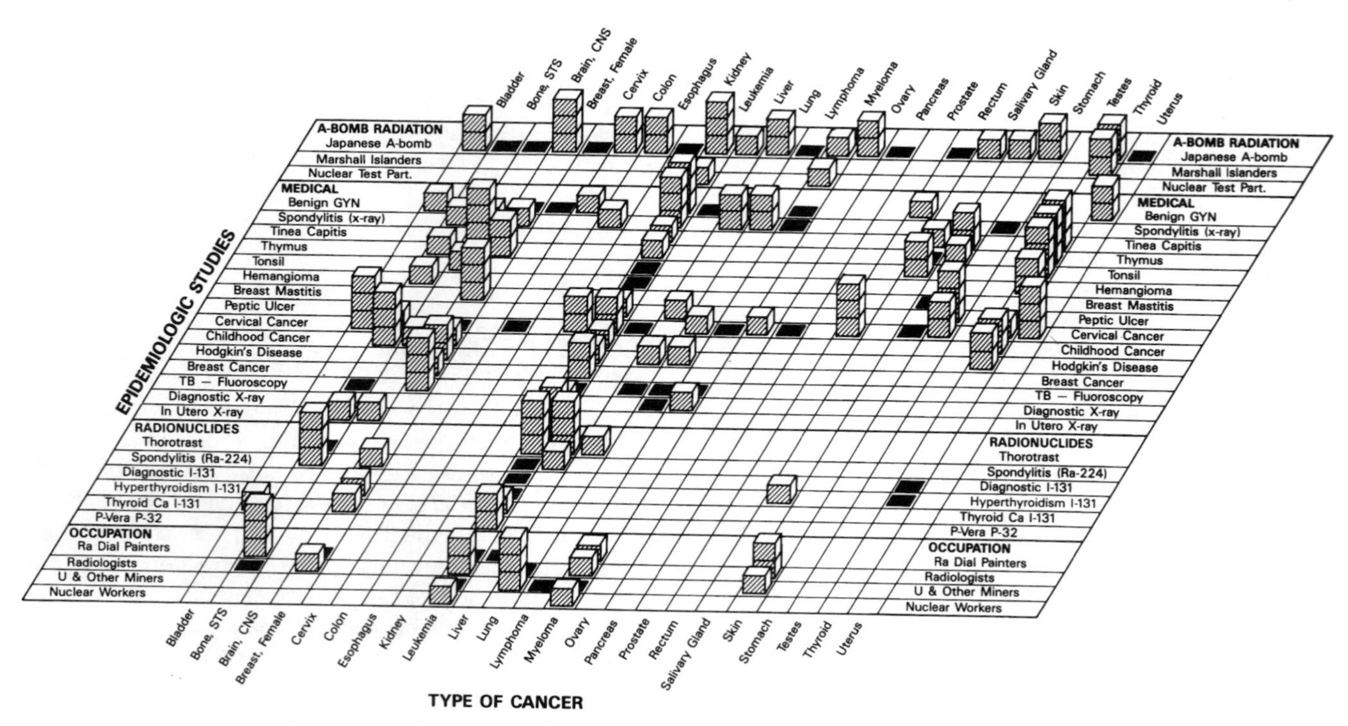

FIG. 16–1. Graphical display of various types of cancer associated with radiation in different populations. The four column sizes represent: 3 blocks = strong association; 2 blocks = meaningful association; 1 block = suggested but unconfirmed association; "flat" = no association found, although study was reasonably powerful. Blank = no or minimal data. Note that the height of a column is not related to level of risk. For example, the strong association between radiotherapy for cervical cancer and cancer of the rectum is based on very high-dose exposures and the risk coefficient is quite small (see Table 16–1).

TABLE 16–1. *Ranking of Various Tissues with Regard to the Carcinogenic Influence of Radiation**

Type of Cancer	Range of Risk Estimates: RR at 1 Gy	Range of Risk Estimates: Excess Risk × 10^4PY-Gy	Comment
Cancers Frequently Associated with Radiation with Authoritative Risk Estimates			
Leukemia	1.3–6.2	0.5–2.9	Especially myeloid leukemia
Thyroid	1.6–31	3.0–13	Low mortality
Female breast	1.1–2.7	3.5–18	Little risk if exposed >40 yr
Cancers Occasionally Associated with Radiation with Valid Risk Estimates			
Lung	1.0–1.6	0.0–1.7	Interaction with smoking uncertain
Stomach	1.0–1.7	0.0–4.7	Major A-bomb effect
Colon	1.0–1.9	0.0–3.0	Not seen after cervical cancer
Esophagus	1.3–1.6	0.3–0.5	
Bladder	1.1–2.3	0.1–1.0	Both low and high dose effect
Ovary	1.0–2.3	0.1–0.7	
Myeloma	1.0–3.3	0.0–0.3	Uncertainty if association causal
Cancers Rarely Associated with Radiation with Uncertain Risk Estimates[a]			
Brain and nervous system	1.0–5.9	0.0–1.1	Mainly after childhood exposures
Kidney	1.0–1.7	0.0–1.1	
Liver	1.0–1.5	0.0–1.6	Major Thorotrast effect
Salivary glands	1.1–1.7	0.1–0.2	Little evidence
Non-Hodgkin's lymphoma	b	b	Little evidence, possible high dose effect
Skin	1.0–2.0	0.1–2.5	Effect may be limited to high doses (or UV necessary)
Rectum	1.0–1.2	0.0–0.1	Effect may be limited to high doses
Uterus	1.0–1.01	0.0–0.5	Effect may be limited to high doses
Bone	1.0–1.1	0.0–0.1	Effect may be limited to high doses
Connective tissues	b	b	Effect may be limited to high doses
Cancers Never or Sporadically Associated with Radiation with No Risk Estimates[c]			
Chronic lymphocytic leukemia	b	b	Absent?
Pancreas	b	b	Little evidence
Hodgkin's disease	b	b	Little evidence
Prostate	b	b	Little evidence
Testis	b	b	Little evidence
Cervix	b	b	Little evidence
Certain childhood cancers[d]	b	b	Absent?
Supporting tissues of skeleton[e]	b	b	Little evidence

*Relative rankings are based on the studies summarized in this chapter, and consider the frequency that the observed cancer is reported in irradiated populations, the strength of the associations found, and the availability of reliable estimates of radiation risk per unit organ dose (cf NAS, 1980). Risk coefficients mainly from Thompson et al, 1994; Shimizu et al, 1990; NAS, 1990; UNSCEAR, 1994; Boice et al, 1988; and Darby et al, 1987b. Range of risk estimates are associated with differences in age distributions, follow-up times, and other factors among exposed populations.

[a]Association is inconsistently found and/or available estimates of risk are highly uncertain.

[b]No reliable estimate available.

[c]Sites for which radiation-induced cancers have not been reported or confirmed.

[d]Retinoblastoma, Wilms' tumor, and others of embryonic origin.

[e]Muscles, tendons, and synovial membranes of joints.

erally consistent with these findings, although based on mortality rather than incidence data (Miller et al, 1989). The breast appears to be one of the most sensitive tissues to the carcinogenic action of radiation (Table 16–1). In comparison with other studies, fractionated exposures seem similar to single exposures of the same total dose in their ability to induce breast cancer (Boice et al, 1979).

No excesses of leukemia, lymphoma, or lung cancer have been reported among TB patients repeatedly exposed to fluoroscopic x-rays (Davis et al, 1989). The mean dose to lung tissue was 84 cGy (84 rad). Similarly, the large Canadian TB fluoroscopy study included 1178 lung cancer deaths and no increase in lung cancer occurred despite an average lung dose of 1.02 Gy (102 rad) (Howe, 1995). In animal experiments, splitting dose over time also appears to reduce the risk of radiogenic lung cancer to a much greater extent than the reduction seen for radiogenic breast cancer (Ullrich et al, 1987; UNSCEAR, 1986).

Uncertainties in dosimetry limit precise quantification of radiation risks from these TB series. On the other hand, practically all environmental, occupational and nontherapeutic medical exposures involve radiation doses no greater than those received by TB patients from a single fluoroscopy, yet cumulative exposures were high enough to engender measurable excess risks. Risk estimates based on these studies of frequent low-dose exposure are thus relatively free of the problems of extrapolation to low doses that characterize studies of brief, high-dose exposures, and may be more directly relevant to public health concerns.

Mastitis. A survey of 601 women treated with radiation for acute postpartum mastitis in New York found 56 (or 9.3%) breast cancers compared with 59 (or 4.8%) in 1239 women not irradiated (Shore et al, 1986). A treatment involved 1–11 exposures (mean, 3.4), 3.8 Gy to the irradiated breast. Doses were delivered by carefully calibrated x-ray therapy units and were accurately known. Excess risk was not apparent until 10 years after treatment, and was approximately linear in dose up to 3.5 Gy, when it declined. The absolute risk was estimated as 3.5 cases/10^4 PY-Gy, and the RR at 1 Gy as 1.4. Interestingly, the age-specific absolute risk estimates obtained for mastitis patients (who were especially healthy, having just given birth) were very similar to those computed for TB fluoroscopy patients and A-bomb survivors (Boice et al, 1979; Land et al, 1980).

Other. Risk of breast cancer among women given radiation therapy (mean, 5.5 Gy) for benign breast disorders in Sweden was inversely related to age at exposure (Mattson et al, 1993). Use of a nonirradiated comparison group minimized the possibility that the underlying breast disease was the sole reason for the breast cancer excess, although the possibility that women with more serious breast disease (conceivably at higher risk for breast cancer) were selected for radiotherapy was recognized by the authors. Women with scoliosis exposed to multiple diagnostic x-rays (mean, 12 cGy) during adolescence were at increased risk of breast cancer (Hoffman et al, 1989). The numbers were small, however, and factors associated with scoliosis, such as nulliparity, could have influenced risk. Breast cancer excesses have been reported following radiotherapy for Hodgkin's disease (Bhatia et al, 1996; Hancock et al, 1993), breast cancer (Boice et al, 1992a), and during infancy for thymic enlargement (Hildreth et al, 1989). Radiation (mean, 2.8 Gy) to treat primary breast cancer appeared to result in the same age-specific RRs for secondary breast cancer as seen in other studies (Boice et al, 1992a), implying that radiation might interact with underlying host factors, for example, late parity, in a multiplicative manner. A concern over possible interaction for x-ray mammographic exposures does not appear warranted, however, because this procedure is usually recommended for women in midlife who are well past the ages of greatest breast tissue sensitivity to radiation carcinogenesis (Storm et al, 1992). It has been suggested that the ataxia-telangiectasia gene predisposes heterozygotes to radiogenic breast cancer (Swift et al, 1991), but the epidemiological and radiologic evidence to date requires confirmation (Boice and Miller, 1992b; UNSCEAR, 1994).

Spine Irradiation

Ankylosing spondylitis. The mortality experience of 14,556 persons treated between 1935 and 1954 in 87 British radiotherapy clinics for ankylosing spondylitis, a rheumatoid condition of the spine, has been carefully evaluated through 1991 with 98% follow-up (Darby et al, 1987; Weiss et al, 1994, 1995). Radiation doses, estimated for each leukemia fatality and for a 7% sample of the population, averaged about 4.4 Gy for the active bone marrow, several gray for the esophagus, stomach, upper colon, pancreas, lung, and main bronchial tree, about 2.64 Gy mean total body dose, and substantially lower doses for organs not in the treatment field (Lewis et al, 1988). Some epidemiological evaluations focused on those patients, nearly half the total, who received a single course of treatment, typically 10 exposures over a month.

Leukemia risk (60 observed vs. 21.5 expected) peaked 1–5 years after radiotherapy and gradually declined, but not to baseline levels; CLL was not significantly increased (7 observed vs 4.8 expected). The dose response for leukemia was irregular and essentially flat, possibly reflecting reduced leukemogenesis in the most heavily irradiated portions of the marrow due to cell killing or related to the fractionated nature of the exposures (Smith and Doll, 1982; Mole and Major, 1983). Compared to general population rates, the RR of leukemia can be estimated as 1.08 at 1 Gy and the absolute excess risk as 0.15/10^4 PY-Gy, although much higher estimates were suggested in a recent follow-up (Weiss et al, 1995).

Nonleukemia cancer deaths were increased by 26%, with the excess occurring in the more heavily irradiated tissue such as the lung, esophagus, central nervous system, bone, non-Hodgkin's lymphoma, and multiple myeloma. An earlier reported excess of stomach cancer was no longer apparent. For nonleukemia cancers, the estimated RR was 1.14 at 1 Gy and the absolute excess risk was 4.67 per 10^4 PY-Gy. Unlike the experience of other irradiated populations, the RR for nonleukemia cancer was as great during the first 5 years after exposure as it was later, and then declined to near normal levels after 25 years. The temporal pattern was dominated by lung cancer, which may have been affected by variations in smoking habits, as well as the influence of cigarette smoke on relatively immobile lungs. Noncancer mortality, including benign lung conditions, was increased by 51%, and was attributed to conditions associated with spondylitis and not the radiation exposure. Some of the early cancer excesses may also reflect correlates of the underlying disease (eg, ulcerative colitis is associated with both spondylitis and colon cancer), other therapies such as cytotoxic medications (Spiess et al, 1989), or possibly preexisting metastatic lesions causing pain that was misdiagnosed as ankylosing spondylitis. A study of 1201 nonirradiated patients with less severe disease, however, found no increased risk of leukemia or other cancers (Smith et al, 1977; Weiss et al, 1994).

A new follow-up through 1991 was recently completed on the entire population (Weiss et al, 1994). The mean total body dose was estimated as 2.64 Gy with the vertebrae receiving 18.6 Gy. For all cancers except leukemia the RR at 1 Gy was estimated to be between 1.11 and 1.18. Significant increases were seen for leukemia and cancer of the esophagus, pancreas, lung, bones, connective tissue, prostate, bladder, kidney, non-Hodgkin's lymphoma, and multiple myeloma. Radiation risk estimation is imprecise because of the absence of individual dosimetry on all but a sample. Organ dose could vary by several magnitudes depending on type of treatment.

Head and Neck

Thymus. In the 1930s and 1940s, newborn children often received radiation therapy to shrink enlarged thymus glands. The fifth mail survey of 2856 irradiated persons identified 30 thyroid cancers versus one in 5055 untreated siblings (Shore et al, 1985). The follow-up was 88% complete. Females were at two to three times greater absolute risk than males, and the risk among Jews seemed especially high. The data were consistent with a linear dose response (mean, 1.2 Gy), risk remained high even after 40 years, and fractionation did not appear to reduce risk. Risk estimates were 2.9 cases/10^4 PY-Gy and RR=9.90 at 1 Gy (Shore, 1992). Benign thyroid adenomas also occurred more frequently among exposed persons than among their siblings, 86 versus 11, respectively (7.0/10^4PY-Gy). The RR at 1 Gy for nodules was 6.0 (Shore et al, 1993).

The incidence of thyroid neoplasms rose abruptly during adolescence, suggesting the influence of thyroid-stimulating hormone as a promoting or secondary factor. Childhood irradiation may also be particularly damaging if rapidly proliferating cells injured by radiation are more likely to develop abnormally than cells irradiated in later life with limited growth potential. Indeed, the rapid growth of the thyroid gland, from 1–2 g at birth to 18 g at maturity, may have influenced risk. Excess breast cancers have occurred, suggesting that the immature breast is also susceptible to the carcinogenic effects of radiation (Hildreth et al, 1989). Significant excesses of leukemia and cancer of the skin have also been reported (Hempelmann et al, 1975; Hildreth et al, 1985).

Ringworm of the scalp. Among 10,834 children in Israel who received x-ray therapy to the scalp for tinea capitis, 43 thyroid cancers were observed versus 11 expected based on two comparison groups (Ron et al, 1989). Cases were ascertained from tumor registry records and from searching pathology records of all major hospitals in Israel. The dose to the thyroid was particularly low, 9 cGy (rad) on average, although alignment errors might have greatly increased the exposure for some children. The dose response was consistent with linearity up to 50 cGy. The absolute excess risk was 13 cancers/10^4PY-Gy, and the RR at 1 Gy was 31. Comparable numbers for benign tumors were 15 tumors/10^4PY-Gy and RR = 11 at 1 Gy. Risk was greatest among persons under age 5 at irradiation, and was most prominent 10 or more years later. The pattern of radiation risk over time was best described on the basis of a constant multiplication of the background rate, although few persons were followed for more than 30 years.

Evidence for a low-dose effect is tempered by the possibilities that (1) careless irradiation techniques or restless children resulted in direct thyroid exposure, (2) pituitary irradiation may have influenced thyroid cancer risk, and (3) the thyroid glands of Jewish children may be particularly sensitive to radiation (Hempelmann et al, 1975).

A dose-response relationship for brain cancer and other neural tumors was reported (Ron et al, 1988b). The brain dose was estimated as 1.5 Gy. For all neural tumors (especially meningiomas), the absolute excess risk was 1.14 tumors/10^4PY-Gy and the RR at 1 Gy was 5.9. Significant excesses of leukemia and cancers of bone and connective tissue also occurred (Ron et al, 1988a). A preliminary report suggested that breast cancer might be elevated among children exposed at ages 5–9 years; however, the data are not easily interpreted since the excess resulted from a peculiar deficit among the comparison group rather than an elevation among the exposed, and no increase was seen among children exposed at younger or older ages (Modan et al, 1989; UNSCEAR 1994). Skin cancer, other than melanoma, was significantly increased (mean, 7 Gy); the absolute excess risk was 0.31/10^4 PY-Gy and the RR at 1 Gy was 1.7 (Ron et al, 1991).

Among 2215 patients with tinea capitis treated in New York, no excess thyroid cancer was found, but thyroid adenomas, leukemia, and brain cancers were elevated (Shore et al, 1976). Radiotherapy likely contributed to excess skin cancers, especially for anatomical areas exposed to ultraviolet radiation from the sun (Shore et al, 1984). Basal cell carcinomas of the face were significantly increased among white but not black patients. Patients with psoriasis treated with 8-methoxy-psoralen and long-wave ultraviolet radiation (PUVA) also have been found to develop cancer in skin previously treated with low-energy x-rays (Stern et al, 1984).

Tonsils. Excess thyroid cancer has occurred among 5379 predominantly Jewish persons irradiated in Chicago during childhood for mostly tonsil and nasopharyngeal conditions (Favus et al, 1976; Schneider et al, 1985). The tracing was about 68% complete. Intensive clinical screening of 1922 persons included thyroid scans. About 37.5% (1,108) of the 3610 persons for whom vital status was known had nodular thyroid disease, and in 297 of these (or 8% overall) it was malignant. A large number of small tumors were apparently detected only at screening; about 80% were less than 1.5 cm. The clinical significance of these small tumors is uncertain and they may be relatively harmless (Crile et al, 1979). A recent evaluation included individual dose estimates for 3843 subjects and revealed a linear relationship between thyroid dose and cancer, radiation risk was inversely related to age at exposure, excess RR for men and women were similar, and RR decreased after 30 years of follow-up (Schneider et al, 1993). While overall rates of thyroid cancer dramatically increased after 1974 when screening programs began, the estimates of radiation risk did not vary significantly compared to those obtained prior to 1974 (Ron et al, 1992).

Interpretation of radiation risks is hindered because (1) a nonirradiated comparison group, comparably screened, was not available; (2) the significance of small, clinically silent cancers is uncertain; and (3) the follow-up was incomplete. The dose-response evaluations and consistency with other studies, however, support the reported results.

Based on clinical examinations, an excess of thyroid nodularity was reported among 1590 individuals treated with radiation for lymphoid hyperplasia compared with 1499 persons treated with surgery only (Pottern et al, 1990). There was a strong dose-response gradient (mean, 24 cGy), similar RR at 1 Gy for males and females (8.0 and 7.0, respectively), and an inverse relationship with age at exposure. Much higher risks were suggested, however, by self-reported conditions from a mailed questionnaire, apparently due to underreporting of thyroid nodularity among the surgical comparison groups.

Other. The pattern of thyroid cancer incidence in birth cohorts in Connecticut appeared to coincide with the widespread use of radiation to treat benign head and neck conditions between 1920 and 1959; rates were also lower for persons born in the 1960s when such irradiation was discouraged (Pottern et al, 1980). Prior radiotherapy in childhood may account for 9% of all thyroid cancers (Ron et al, 1987). Excess salivary gland and neural tumors can occur after childhood irradiation (Schneider et al, 1985; Land, 1986). A series of 18,030 children treated with radiation for skin hemangioma identified increased rates of thyroid cancer and soft-tissue sarcoma (Fürst et al, 1988). A smaller series linked thyroid nodularity to radiation treatments for childhood hemangiomas (deVathaire et al, 1993). Persons treated with nasopharyngeal radium applicators to shrink lymphoid tissue around the eustachian tube were not found to be at increased risk of thyroid cancer (Hazen et al, 1966; Verduijn et al, 1989), although a small excess of brain tumors was reported following treatments in childhood (Sandler et al, 1982). A comprehensive pooled analyses of studies of radiogenic thyroid cancer found that linearity best described the dose response; a downturn or leveling of risk appears at very high doses (>10 Gy); risk was greatest for childhood exposures (RR = 8.7 at 1 Gy); the attributable risk at 1 Gy was 88%; and that spreading dose over time appears to lower risk, possibly due to cellular repair processees (Ron et al, 1994a).

Pelvic/Abdominal Irradiation

Cervical cancer. In an international study involving 31 radiotherapy centers, over 30,000 women with cervical cancer were followed clinically and with blood studies for up to 10 years (mean, 5 years). Despite large radiation doses (5–15 Gy) to the pelvic bone marrow, no excess leukemia or lymphoma was observed (Boice and Hutchison, 1980). This study served as the basis for an expanded survey of more than 200,000 women from 15 countries (Boice et al, 1985a, 1987). A small but significant risk of leukemia then became apparent, together with the characteristic wavelike pattern of risk over time (Fig. 16–2). Risk was modeled to account for the inhomogeneous distribution of dose to active bone

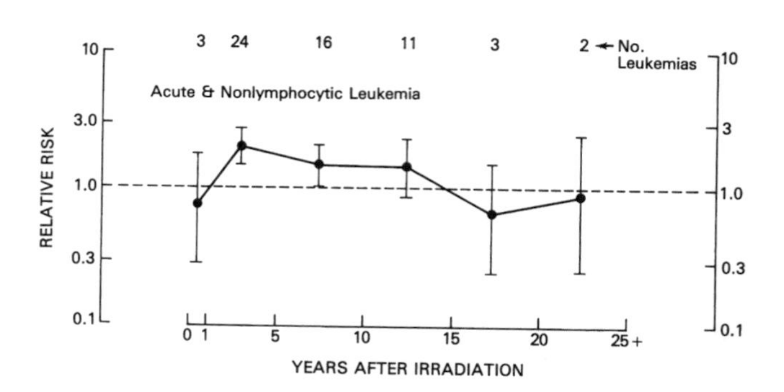

FIG. 16–2. Characteristic wavelike pattern of leukemia risk over time since exposure, seen among women with cervical cancer treated with radiation. (Reproduced from Boice et al, 1985, JNCI 74:955–975, p 966.)

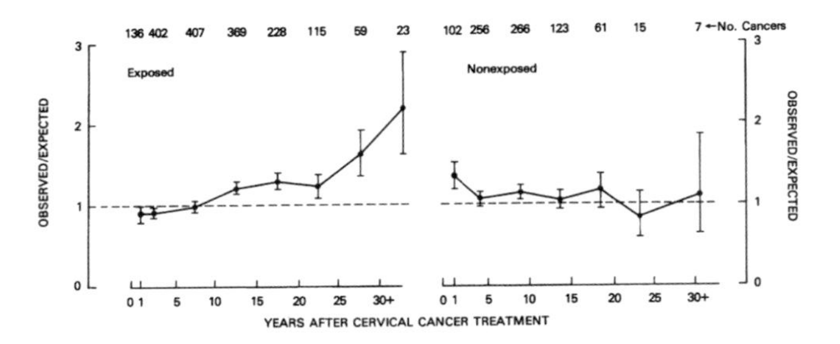

FIG. 16–3. Characteristic pattern of radiation-induced solid tumors over time since exposure, seen for heavily irradiated sites among cervical cancer patients treated with radiation. (Reproduced from Boice et al, 1985, JNCI 74:955–975, p 964.)

marrow throughout the body, and for the possibility of cell-killing at high doses. Risk increased with increasing dose up to about 4 Gy, and then decreased at the highest doses. The RR at 1 Gy was estimated to be 1.7. Evaluations of chromosome aberrations in circulating lymphocytes also revealed a dose-effect pattern similar to that seen for leukemia (Kleinerman et al, 1989). A recent international cancer registry study indicated that the risk of second primary cancers remains high for the duration of life (Kleinerman et al, 1995).

After a minimum latent interval of about 10 years, risk of second tumors following radiotherapy increased with time and reached nearly twofold among long-term survivors (Fig. 16–3). Overall, the excess RR for all second cancers was only about 10% (Boice et al, 1985a). A comprehensive dosimetry program provided organ dose estimates for individual patients based on their actual radiotherapy records. New dose-response information was provided for 18 solid tumors, including cancers of the stomach, uterus, rectum, bladder, vagina, kidney, ovary, thyroid, and breast (Boice et al, 1988b). Risk estimates for this study of incident cancers and leukemia were generally lower than those from the mortality studies of atomic bomb survivors and spondylitics (UNSCEAR, 1988). Possibly the protracted nature of the treatment for cervical cancer allowed more time for the repair of radiation damage than is possible from acute exposures; the high therapeutic doses might have resulted in substantial cell killing; or factors associated with cervical cancer might have confounded the observations.

Among women with intact ovaries, radiotherapy was linked to a significant 35% reduction in breast cancer risk, attributable in all likelihood to the cessation of ovarian function (Boice et al, 1989). Radiotherapy lowers estrogen and androgen levels, even among postmenopausal women, which may contribute to the low breast cancer risk seen among women exposed past the age of menopause (Inskip et al, 1994).

Uterine bleeding. Among 2067 women who received x-ray treatment of 5–10 Gy to their ovaries for metropathia hemorrhagica in Scotland, 12 leukemia deaths occurred (5.9 expected) following an estimated bone marrow dose of 1.3 Gy (Darby et al, 1994). Cancers of heavily irradiated pelvic sites were also significantly increased, including the colon and bladder, but not cancers of the ovary and rectum. Breast cancer occurred significantly below expectation, even among postmenopausal women, possibly related to the cessation of ovarian function after radiation castration. An incidence study of 1893 women given radiotherapy for benign gynecologic diseases in Connecticut also found significant excesses of leukemia (12 vs 5.3), uterine sarcomas, cancers of urinary organs, and lymphomas, including myeloma (Wagoner, 1984). In a new study of 9,770 women treated mainly with radium implants for bleeding disorders in New England, 64 leukemia deaths occurred and 39.6 were expected (Inskip et al, 1993). A comparison group of 3185 women was also studied. The RR at 1 Gy was estimated to be 2.9; the mean dose to bone marrow was 1.11 Gy. The lower doses used to treat benign menstrual disorders appear to have been more leukemogenic than the higher doses used to treat cervical cancer, presumably because of less cell killing (Kleinerman et al, 1994). Cancers of heavily irradiated sites were also significantly elevated, including the colon, uterus and bladder, but not the rectum or cervix, lymphomas or myeloma (Inskip et al, 1990; 1993). Only the excesses of leukemia and cancer of the bladder and uterus were consistent across these three studies. Inconsistencies might be related to different dose distributions within organs from the different radiation modalities (radium implants vs external x-rays), differences in the extent of surgical procedures or presenting conditions, differences in the comparison populations, or simply chance.

Peptic ulcer. In a new survey of 1831 patients with peptic ulcer treated with radiation (15 Gy) and 1778 nonexposed ulcer patients, significant increases were reported for cancers of the stomach, pancreas, lung and leukemia (Griem et al, 1994). The excess of pancreatic cancer was attributed to possible miscoding of stomach cancers on death certificates. Radiation combined with surgery appeared to induce carcinogenic processes that greatly enhanced the development of stomach cancer, possibly mediated by hypoacidity and bile reflux. Estimated RR at 1 Gy for stomach and lung cancers were 1.15 and 1.66, respectively. Corresponding excess risks were 0.25 and $2.33/10^4$ PY-Gy. A substantial difference in absolute (but not relative) risk estimates for stomach cancer between ulcer patients and A-bomb survivors points to the difficulty in generalizing from one population to another when baseline disease rates differ appreciably.

Infertility. Another new series evaluated mortality among 816 women treated for infertility (Ron et al,

1994b). Doses were, on average, 0.9, 0.6, 0.5, and 0.3 Gy to the ovary, brain, colon, and bone marrow, respectively. No unusual cancer patterns were observed, in all likelihood due to the small study size.

Prenatal Irradiation. Most, but not all, studies are consistent with a 40% increased risk of childhood leukemia associated with low-dose intrauterine exposure to diagnostic radiation of between 1 and 10 cGy just before birth (Stewart et al, 1958; MacMahon, 1962; Bithell and Stewart, 1975; Monson and MacMahon, 1984). These studies have been extensively reviewed (UNSCEAR, 1972, 1986, 1994; NAS, 1972, 1980; Miller and Boice, 1986). It has been postulated, however, that selection factors, related to the medical reasons why women receive prenatal x-rays, were responsible for the increased leukemia risk and not the x-ray exposures themselves. The absence of any childhood leukemia (and only one childhood cancer) in atomic bomb survivors exposed in utero (Jablon and Kato, 1970) supported the selection hypothesis, as did Miller's observation (1969) that it was peculiar that diagnostic x-rays would increase all childhood malignancies by about the same percentage (50%) when there is such a remarkable degree of variability between tissues in their response to radiation at other ages. Further, childhood cancers are primarily embryonal and developmental neoplasms which are not known to be induced by radiation (Miller, 1995). Animal experiments do not suggest an enhanced sensitivity to leukemia induction following irradiation during fetal stages (UNSCEAR, 1986).

The indication of a leukemia risk for preconception irradiation in one study (Graham et al, 1966), when no genetic effects were noted in the much larger A-bomb survivor study (Neel and Schull, 1991), and the finding of an excess risk in white, but not black, children prenatally exposed (Diamond et al, 1973), further suggested that fetal x-rays might just be an indicator of a poor future health experience.

A small prospective study in Chicago evaluated about 1000 unselected children whose mothers received x-ray pelvimetry as a matter of hospital policy, and not medical indications, and no excess cancers were found (Oppenheim et al, 1974). Court Brown and coworkers (1960) studied nearly 40,000 children irradiated in utero and observed nine cases of leukemia versus an expected number of 10.5. The sample sizes of the prospective studies, however, were such that an increased risk of 40–50% could not be excluded. Several large cohort studies of twins, however, also fail to find childhood leukemia to be increased.

A New England study was extended to include 1342 childhood cancers among 1,429,499 births (Monson and MacMahon, 1984). The RR associated with prenatal x-ray was 1.52 for leukemia and 1.27 for other cancers, and there was no evidence that the associations were due to confounding. A reanalysis of the large Oxford Survey of childhood cancer in England concluded that x-raying 1000 fetuses with 1 cGy (1 rad) would yield about two or three extra cases of childhood cancer in the first 15 years of life (Bithell and Stiller, 1988). An early report of increased adult cancer following fetal irradiation of A-bomb survivors was apparently not substantiated with further follow-up (Yoshimoto et al, 1994).

Evidence against the selection hypothesis comes from the demonstration of a dose-response relationship for childhood leukemia based on number of x-ray films taken (Stewart and Kneale, 1970); and from the observation that the excess risk was as great among twins for whom x-ray pelvimetry was far more frequent (55%) than among singletons (15%) simply because of a greater likelihood to determine fetal positioning before delivery (Mole, 1974). This observation was confirmed in a case-control study of twins born in Connecticut (Harvey et al, 1985). Nonetheless, it is argued that number of x-rays is not necessarily equivalent to fetal dose, and that twin studies are somewhat difficult to interpret. For example, despite substantial exposure to prenatal x-rays, cohort studies consistently find twins to be at significantly low risk of childhood cancer compared to single births (UNSCEAR, 1986, 1994; Inskip et al, 1991). Further, while there is no reason to believe that the fetus should be immune to the leukemogenic effects of ionizing radiation, there is also little reason to believe that the risk should be substantially greater for exposures just prior to birth than for exposures in early childhood. Thus, while it is established that prenatal x-ray is associated with an increased risk of childhood leukemia, the magnitude of the hazard, and even the causal nature of the cancer association, remain uncertain (UNSCEAR, 1986, 1994; MacMahon, 1989).

General Diagnostic Radiation. Studies linking diagnostic radiation with adult leukemia are inconsistent. The first report from England was later retracted when the author attributed the concentration of x-rays within 5 years of the leukemia diagnosis to symptoms related to preclinical disease, including an increased susceptibility to infection (Stewart, 1973). Excesses of chronic myelogenous leukemia (CML) in some studies appeared restricted to those who received extremely large numbers of x-rays (Gibson et al, 1972). A study at the Mayo Clinic, which included accurate estimates of bone marrow doses, found no link between leukemia and diagnostic x-rays but the numbers were small (Linos et al, 1980). A recent report from California found an association between diagnostic radiography, particularly low-back x-rays, and CML based on personal interviews of 136 cases and 136 neighborhood controls (Preston-Martin et al, 1989). Based on x-ray records with two prepaid health plans, another recent study concluded that persons with leukemia and lymphoma are x-rayed frequently just prior to diagnosis for conditions related to the development or natural history of their disease (Boice et al, 1991b). However, the possibility of small increases in myeloma could not be discounted among persons who received rather extensive x-ray exposures. Diagnostic x-rays, however, were not linked to multiple myeloma in an interview study of 399 cases and 399 controls in the United Kingdom (Cuzick and DeStavola, 1988). An evaluation of medical x-ray records among 484 persons with thyroid cancer and matched controls revealed no association between x-rays to the head and neck and thyroid cancer (Inskip et al, 1995).

Past exposures to dental or medical radiography of the head and neck have been correlated with meningiomas, gliomas, and salivary gland tumors in some case-control interview studies (Preston-Martin et al, 1980, 1982, 1988) but not in others (Kuijten et al, 1990). Radiation doses were not known, but might have been substantial. In one investigation, an association between skull x-rays and brain cancer was thought to be due to early symptoms of brain cancer prompting the radiographic examinations (Howe et al, 1989). Multiple fluoroscopic chest x-rays appear to increase the risk of breast cancer, but not lung cancer or leukemia among tuberculosis patients (Davis et al, 1989; Howe, 1995), and not cancer or leukemia among children undergoing heart catheterization (McLaughlin et al, 1993a).

Limitations of many of these studies include the potential for response bias in interview surveys; incomplete verification of the actual numbers of x-rays; limited dosimetry; and study sizes too small to detect risks on the order of currently accepted estimates (cf Boice and Land, 1979). The possible contribution of diagnostic radiology to the cancer burden appears small in comparison with other causes (Evans et al, 1986).

Radiotherapy for Cancer

Adult treatments. The most serious consequences of curative therapies for cancer is the heightened risk of developing a new cancer (Boice et al, 1985b; Boice, 1993a). Leukemia has been linked to high-dose radiotherapy, but to a lesser extent than seen in patients treated with lower doses for nonmalignant diseases (Curtis et al, 1985; Boivin et al, 1986). Large international studies have revealed twofold leukemia risks following radiotherapy for cervical and uterine cancer, whereas much higher risks were predicted based on simple linear risk extrapolation (Boice et al, 1987; Curtis et al, 1994; Kleinerman et al, 1995). When such high doses are delivered to small volumes of tissue, cell killing likely predominates over cell transformation and overall leukemia risk is reduced. A variety of risk coefficients per Gy has been observed among medical studies of partial-body exposures (Fig. 16–4). Systemic chemotherapy and radiotherapy together, however, appeared to enhance the risk of leukemia over 17-fold among patients with breast cancer (Curtis et al, 1992). Increased leukemia risks have also been reported after radiotherapy for Hodgkin's (Tucker et al, 1988; Kaldor et al, 1990) and non-Hodgkin's lymphoma (Travis et al, 1991, 1994). Total or hemibody irradiation for non-Hodgkin's lymphoma (NHL), a unique treatment that exposes large volumes of bone marrow to relatively low therapeutic doses, was seen to increase leukemia risk (Greene et al, 1983; Travis et al, 1996).

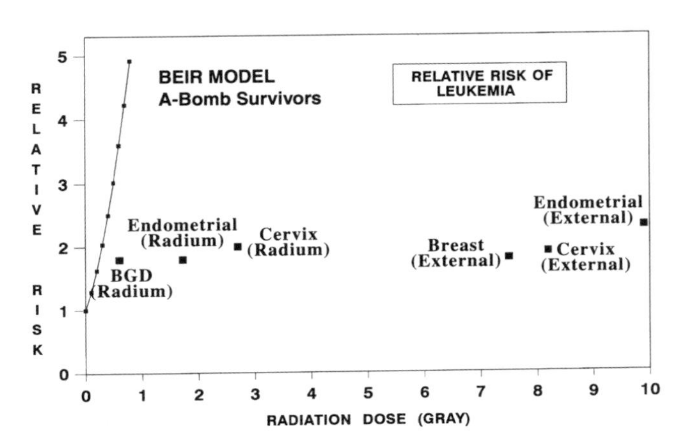

FIG. 16–4. Relative risk of leukemia by bone marrow dose for A-bomb survivors (NAS, 1990), and women treated for menstrual bleeding (Inskip et al, 1993), and cancers of the cervix (Boice et al, 1987), endometrium (Curtis et al, 1994), and breast (Curtis et al, 1992).

Cancers of the lung and breast are elevated after radiotherapy for Hodgkin's disease (Tucker et al, 1988; van Leeuwen et al, 1989, 1995; Swerdlow et al 1992; Hancock et al 1993; Travis et al, 1995a). Non-Hodgkin's lymphoma is increased after Hodgkin's disease (Travis et al, 1991) and cervical cancer (Boice et al, 1988b), but it is possibly related to immune deficiencies. Only very high doses of radiation seem to elevate the risk of cancers of the rectum and uterus (Boice et al, 1988b) and osteogenic sarcomas of the bone and soft tissues (NAS, 1990). Excess bladder cancer has been reported after 10 Gy, but not colon or liver cancer (Boice et al, 1988b). Second breast cancer has been linked to radiotherapy for primary breast cancer, but only among women under age 45 at exposure (Boice et al, 1992a). Lung cancer has recently been recognized as a late effect following radiotherapy for breast cancer (Inskip et al,

1994a; Inskip and Boice, 1994; Travis et al, 1995; Neugut et al, 1994). Significantly low rates of breast cancer can follow ovarian doses greater than 6 Gy (Boice et al, 1989).

Many studies, however, used general population rates for comparison, which may not be appropriate if the underlying disease predisposes to second cancers. Other treatments, such as alkylating agents or other drugs of high toxicity, might also influence subsequent cancer risk. Only a few studies attempted to quantify risk in terms of radiation-absorbed dose to organs (Boice et al, 1988b). It appears that radiotherapy may account for only 5%–10% of second cancers among cancer patients, with cigarette smoking, alcohol, hormonal factors, chemotherapy, and other cofactors playing more important roles (Boice et al, 1985a, 1985b).

Childhood Treatments. Children treated for cancer are at high risk for developing new cancers (Miké et al, 1982; Tucker et al, 1984; Hawkins et al, 1987; Breslow et al, 1988; de Vathaire et al, 1989). Only a few series, however, have estimated radiation doses to specific organs, or evaluated dose-response relationships. Radiotherapy was not found to increase the risk of leukemia in one study (Tucker et al, 1987b), possibly because of the predominance of cell-killing effects over oncogenic transformation at such high levels. A more recent study reported a leukemia risk following radiotherapy (Hawkins et al, 1992), possibly because of interactive effects with chemotherapeutic agents. Radiogenic thyroid cancer has been reported at 30 Gy (de Vathaire et al, 1988; Tucker et al, 1991).

A dose response over the range of 10–60 Gy has been seen for bone cancer (Tucker et al, 1987a). Interestingly, the RR for radiogenic bone cancer in children with retinoblastoma (who possess an underlying predisposition to develop osteosarcoma) was similar to that among children irradiated for other cancers; cumulative and absolute risks, however, were much greater among children with retinoblastoma. Children with familial retinoblastoma have a deletion in chromosome 13 that predisposes to osteosarcoma, and radiation appears to cause a second mutation in an osteoblast that leads to a high rate of osteosarcoma development (NAS, 1990). A survey of 1602 children with retinoblastoma revealed significant increases in cancers of the bone, connective tissue, brain and skin melanoma for which radiotherapy appeared to further enhance the inborn susceptibility to cancer development (Eng et al, 1993). Radiogenic bone cancers have been reported after childhood cancer in other series (Draper et al, 1986; Hawkins et al, 1996), and among children treated for Ewing's sarcoma (Strong et al, 1979). Children treated for medulloblastoma who have basal cell nevus syndrome develop multiple basal cell carcinomas in irradiated skin (Strong, 1977). Children with leukemia treated with cranial irradiation also are at high risk for developing brain malignancies (Neglia et al, 1991).

Military Exposures from Atomic and Thermonuclear Weapons

Japanese Atomic Bomb Survivors. The Life Span Study (LSS) of the Radiation Effects Research Foundation (RERF) includes about 93,000 atomic bomb survivors and 27,000 nonexposed comparison subjects. Recent analyses of cancer mortality cover 1950–1985 (Shimizu et al, 1990). The first comprehensive report on cancer incidence was recently completed based on data from the Hiroshima and Nagasaki Tumor Registries during the period 1958–1987 (Thompson et al, 1994). These and other recent studies of cancer risk among A-bomb survivors, reflect increases in numbers of cancer cases associated with the natural aging of the population, notably among the youngest survivors, who appear to be at greatest relative risk of radiation-associated cancer. The findings also reflect modifications in dosimetry, and advances in statistical methods for the analysis of cohort survival data that facilitate modeling of age, sex, time since exposure, and other cofactors as modifiers of radiation dose-response relationships (NAS, 1990; Pierce and Vaeth, 1991, Pierce et al, 1991).

The new atomic bomb dosimetry. In the early 1980s, the accuracy of the Tentative 1965 Dosimetry (T65D), used to estimate doses for individuals, was questioned. A new dosimetry, called Dosimetry System 1986 or DS86 was developed, and revised estimates were computed for 86,000 of the 93,000 exposed survivors in the LSS, called the DS86 subcohort. Under reasonable assumptions about the relative biological effectiveness (RBE) of neutrons, risk estimates based upon the new dosimetry are 1.5 to 2 times greater than those under the old dosimetry (Preston and Pierce, 1988; Shimizu et al, 1989). Recent neutron activation measurements of metal and other minerals in Hiroshima, however, suggest that the DS86 dosimetry may have underestimated the neutron exposure (Straume et al, 1992, 1994). If true, then the risks for low-linear energy transfer (LET) radiations have been overestimated.

Leukemia, multiple myeloma, and malignant lymphoma. Leukemia was the first radiation-induced cancer reported among A-bomb survivors, with the risk peaking within 10 years of exposure (Ichimaru et al, 1986; Preston et al, 1994). The dose response for leukemia appeared to follow a linear-quadratic relationship with some flattening at doses over 3–4 Gy (Fig. 16–5) (Shimizu et al, 1990; NAS, 1990). Differences between Hiroshima and Nagasaki were no longer significant (Preston and Pierce, 1988). Based on mortality data, the overall RR at 1 Gy was 6.21, and the absolute excess per 10^4 PY-Gy was 2.94 (Shimizu et al, 1990). Multiple

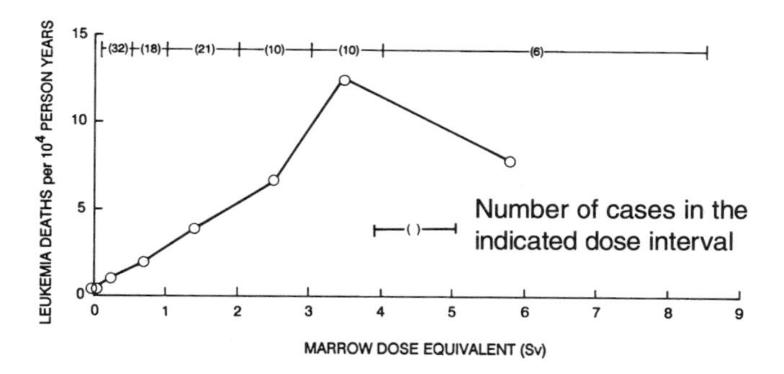

FIG. 16–5. Dose-response relationship for radiation-induced leukemia among atomic bomb survivors. (Reproduced from NAS, 1990, p 243.)

myeloma was significantly increased based on mortality (Shimizu et al, 1990) but not incidence data (Preston et al, 1994). Malignant lymphoma was not related to radiation exposure.

Radiation-related risks were seen for acute lymphocytic and myelogenous leukemias, and chronic myelocytic leukemia (CML), but not CLL or adult T-cell leukemia (Ichimaru et al, 1986; Preston et al, 1994). A sharp peak in CML occurred within 5 years of exposure, notably among children under 15 at time of bombings (ATB), but also at older ages (Ishimaru, 1979). Excess risks have declined since this early peak. In absolute terms, CML risks in Hiroshima are much larger than those in Nagasaki. Based on these differences, it was suggested that CML may be a neutron-dependent cancer (Ishimaru, 1979; Mole, 1975). However, CML was much less common among unexposed survivors in Nagasaki than in Hiroshima, and, in relative terms, there was no difference in CML risk. The CML dose response was well described by a linear model.

For acute leukemias, primarily myelogenous, the temporal pattern of the excess risk depended on age at exposure. Among survivors under 20 when exposed, absolute excess risks peaked within 10 years and then fell rapidly. For ages 20–35, the peak was less pronounced and the fall less rapid. For older survivors, the excess varied little over time. For all leukemias combined, males had almost twice the absolute excess risk as females, but similar RR.

Breast. Female breast cancer has been comprehensively studied (Tokunaga et al, 1994). The dose response was linear in both cities, and age at exposure strongly influenced risk. The risk among women irradiated before age 10 (RR=4.2 at 1 Sv) was comparable with that seen for ages 10–20 (RR = 3.2). A lesser risk was observed among survivors aged 20–40 (RR=2.3) in 1945 with an even lower risk in women exposed after age 40. Excess risk did not appear until 10 years after exposure and not before about age 30. Measures of RR remained roughly constant over time after exposure, within age cohorts, with the notable exception of early-onset breast cancer before age 35 among women exposed before age 20 whose risk (RR = 14.5 at 1 Sv) was sufficiently high to suggest a possible genetically susceptible subgroup (Land et al, 1993a). Estimates of risk at 1 Gy are roughly 2.6 for the RR, and 6.7 excess cancers/10^4 PY-Gy (Thompson et al, 1994). Interestingly, an early age at first birth appeared to protect against both baseline and radiation-induced breast cancer in roughly equal proportions (Land et al, 1994).

Lung. Excess lung cancers of all major types have been reported, including adenocarcinoma, squamous cell carcinoma, and small-cell carcinoma (Yamamoto et al, 1987; Thompson et al, 1994). Among A-bomb survivors and uranium miners, it appears that the typical radiogenic lung cancer is small cell and the atypical is adenocarcinoma (Land et al, 1993b). Except for the absence of effect among those exposed under 10, age at exposure had little influence on the level of risk. Females had higher RR than males; however, this difference was substantially reduced when adjusted for smoking history (Prentice et al, 1983; Kopecky et al, 1986). The interaction between smoking history and radiation remains unclear, having been reported as approximately additive (Blot et al, 1984; Kopecky et al, 1986) and intermediate between additive and multiplicative (Prentice et al, 1983). The RR at 1 Gy was 1.63, and the absolute excess was 1.68/10^4 PY-Gy (Shimizu et al, 1990).

Thyroid. Thyroid cancer was the first solid tumor reported to be increased among A-bomb survivors. Subsequent surveys found higher background rates among those who receive biennial clinical examinations, high prevalences of occult cancer less than 1.5 cm in size at autopsy, significant excesses of papillary and follicular carcinoma, and no significant elevations for medullary or anaplastic cancer (Prentice et al, 1982; Sampson et al, 1969; Ezaki et al, 1986). The dose response was consistent with linearity; RRs were similar for males and females and highest among survivors less than age 20 at exposure (Thompson et al, 1994). Since women are about three times more likely to develop thyroid cancer than men, equality of the RRs implies higher absolute risks among women. For persons younger than 10, between 10 and 20, and 20 and older ATB, the RRs at 1 Gy were 10.5, 4.02, and 1.10, respectively (2.25 overall). Corresponding absolute excess risks were 4.4, 2.7 and 0.21/10^4 PY-Gy (1.61 overall), indicating only a small risk following adult exposures.

Other Cancers. Significant excess risks were found for both mortality and incidence of cancers of the stomach, colon, lung, breast, ovary, and urinary bladder (Shimizu et al, 1990; Thompson et al, 1994; Ron et al, 1994c). There was a suggested increase for mortality from tumors of the esophagus and central nervous system, excluding the brain. The incidence data also provided new

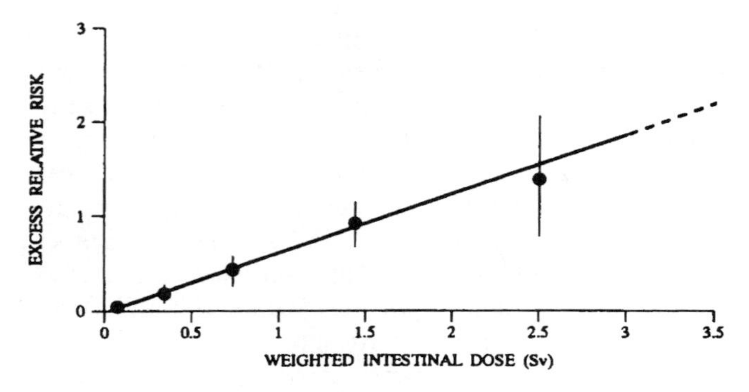

FIG. 16–6. Dose-response relationship for all cancers excluding leukemia among atomic bomb survivors (Thompson et al, 1994).

evidence for excess risks of liver (RR = 1.45 at 1 Gy) and nonmelanoma skin cancers (RR = 2.0 at 1 Gy). For all cancers, excluding leukemia, the dose-response relationship was consistent with linearity down to about 0.2 Gy (Fig. 16–6). No significant risks were seen for cancers of the rectum, gallbladder, pancreas, uterus, bone, oral cavity and pharynx, or nasal passages and larynx.

For radiogenic cancers other than leukemia, the minimal latent period was at least 10 years, and subsequent excess risks were roughly proportional to the background rates. The RR for all cancers as a group, except leukemia, and for specific tumors did not vary significantly over time. On the other hand, relative and absolute risks differed significantly by age at exposure, with younger survivors having higher risks. Among those under age 10 when exposed, excess absolute risks continued to increase but RR have decreased with time. For nonleukemia deaths, the dose-response gradient appeared to be linear. Among the 41,791 survivors exposed to more than 1 cGy and followed through 1985, 55.4% of the leukemias (112 of 202) and 10.2% of the nonleukemia deaths (585 of 5734) have been attributed to the atomic radiation in 1945 (Shimizu et al, 1990). About 1% of deaths from all causes could be attributable to the atomic bomb radiations. The RR for mortality at 1 Gy was 1.41 and the absolute excess was $10.1/10^4$ PY-Gy for the period from 1950–1985. The estimated average RR at 1 Gy based on the solid tumor incidence data was 1.63 while the average excess absolute risk was $29.7/10^4$ PY-Gy (Thompson et al, 1994).

General comments. The atomic bomb survivor studies provide an important human experience from which estimates of radiation risk can be derived. The population is large and not selected because of disease or occupation. Estimates of doses are based upon a comprehensive program that included interviews with virtually all proximal survivors. Despite its strengths, the study is not large enough to provide direct evidence of the effects of low doses (less than about 0.2 Gy); inferences about low-dose risk therefore depend upon dose-response models fitted to data obtained at a wide range of doses. The statistically important high-dose data are surprisingly few; there were only about 3000 survivors who received over 1 Gy. Because the exposures were acute and the dose rate was high, the data provide no direct information on the effects of protracted, low dose rate exposures. Additional factors which might affect interpretations include (1) the relative absence of healthy men of military age in the cities in 1945; (2) restricting the study population to 5-year survivors; (3) possible effects of thermal or mechanical injury on those close to the hypocenter; (4) possible effects of poor nutrition or health problems on subsequent cancer risks; and (5) inaccuracies in dose assessment and death certificate diagnoses of cancer. Increasingly sophisticated techniques are being incorporated to adjust for biases in dose estimates. With regard to possible biases introduced by selection factors, various studies suggest that some such effects, if present initially, tend to disappear over time (Howe et al, 1988).

Exposure to Radionuclides

Radium (^{224}Ra). In a study of 900 German patients repeatedly injected with ^{224}Ra to treat bone tuberculosis and ankylosing spondylitis, 56 osteosarcomas developed versus 0.3 expected (Mays and Speiss, 1984; Chmelevsky et al, 1988; Spiess et al, 1989; van Kaick et al, 1995). Similar to the pattern seen for radiogenic leukemia in other studies, risk peaked at 6 to 8 years, and decreased to normal level after about 33 years. Children and adults were at similar risk, as were males and females. The dose response was best described by a linear-quadratic-exponential equation. Average dose to the bone volume was estimated as 4.2 Gy, the excess risk as 0.8 cancers/10^4PY-Gy, and the lifetime risk as 2.0% per person per gray (NAS, 1972, 1988).

Risk per unit dose was 10 times greater than that seen in radium dial painters who ingested ^{226}Ra and ^{228}Ra (Rowland et al, 1978), reflecting, perhaps, different dose distributions in bone. Radium 224 has a short half-life (3.62 days) and releases its energy on bone surfaces where the "critical" cells for osteosarcoma induction, the endosteal cells, are located. In contrast, ^{226}Ra is a bone-volume seeker with a very long half-life (1600 years), and distributes its energy more uniformly throughout the bone, the dose to the bone matrix being essentially irrelevant to risk. For the same average bone dose, the risk from ^{224}Ra will always be greater than that from ^{226}Ra because more radiation will reach the endosteal cells. Precise quantification of risk in the study of German patients is limited, however, because of (1) the nonuniform distribution of ^{224}Ra in bone, and

(2) the possible effects of the underlying disease or other medications on cancer risk.

Protracted exposure to radium alpha particles appeared more carcinogenic than acute exposures (Mays and Spiess, 1984). This "protraction-enhancement" from alpha-emitting radiation might be related to (1) less killing of premalignant cells, (2) exposing more cells, (3) increasing the stimulus for cell division, and/or (4) preventing repair of local damage. In contrast, for x-rays and gamma rays, a decrease in the carcinogenic effectiveness of a given dose generally occurs when dose rates are decreased or protraction times are increased (NCRP, 1980).

Small excesses of leukemia and cancers of the liver, kidney, and breast were reported (Spiess et al, 1989). The authors point out that phenylbutazone taken to relieve pain associated with spondylitis has been linked to acute forms of leukemia. Among 1473 German patients with spondylitis given ^{224}Ra, but in smaller doses (0.65 Gy), three skeletal tumors (but no osteosarcomas) and six leukemias occurred (Wick and Gössner, 1989). In contrast, one skeletal tumor and four leukemias developed in 1338 nonexposed spondylitics.

Iodine 131

Thyrotoxicosis. In a cooperative study of over 30,000 patients with thyrotoxicosis, leukemia was not linked to radioiodine treatments (Saenger et al, 1968). Among 18,400 patients treated with ^{131}I, 17 leukemias developed, contrasted with 16 in 10,700 patients who received surgery only. The value of a nonexposed comparison group was underscored in that an excess of leukemia was suggested when general population rates were used for comparison. The dose to the whole body was low (7–13 cGy). Other studies of patients treated for hyperthyroidism have also failed to link ^{131}I with leukemia (Holm et al, 1991; Hall et al, 1992a, 1992b).

Thyroid cancer has not been correlated with ^{131}I therapy (Holm et al, 1991), possibly because of the cellular destruction and loss of thyroid function that follows a dose of 10–100 Gy to the thyroid. No cancer has been convincingly linked to ^{131}I treatments for hyperthyroidism. Excess cancers of organs such as the bladder that concentrate iodine (Hoffman, 1984) and of the breast (Goldman et al, 1988) have been suggested in some studies, but were not confirmed in a large incidence series of 10,552 patients followed for up to 30 years (Holm et al, 1991).

Thyroid Cancer. In a study of 258 persons treated with high-dose ^{131}I for inoperable thyroid cancer, four leukemias were observed versus 0.08 expected based on general population rates (Edmonds and Smith, 1986). Small excesses of bladder cancer and breast cancer were also noted. A slight excess of leukemia (4 vs 1.6) was reported among 834 patients treated with ^{131}I for thyroid cancer in Sweden, but cancers of the bladder and breast were not excessive (Hall et al, 1991). The doses to the bone marrow and other organs in these series were large and likely between 0.5 and 1.0 Gy.

Diagnostic ^{131}I. A study of 35,074 Swedish patients failed to link the incidence of any cancer with diagnostic doses of ^{131}I (Holm et al, 1988, 1989; Hall et al, 1996). The dose to the thyroid was 1.1 Gy (110 rad) and a substantial excess of thyroid cancer was anticipated. The absence of an effect supports the notion that internal ^{131}I beta particles may be less carcinogenic than external x-rays or gamma rays, perhaps due to the protracted nature of the exposure (half-life = 8 days) or to the distribution of dose within the gland from ^{131}I. However, if age at exposure significantly modifies the effectiveness of radiation to cause thyroid cancer (Thompson et al, 1994), then the absence of an increased risk in the Swedish series might merely reflect the small number of exposed children and adolescents. Patients examined because of a suspicion of a thyroid tumor were found to be at risk of thyroid cancer independent of ^{131}I exposure. It is also possible that thyroid cancer risks were affected by subsequent surgery or hormonal medications. A series of nearly 14,000 patients in Germany given ^{131}I also failed to identify a thyroid cancer risk (Glöbel et al, 1984). Overall, ^{131}I appears to be less carcinogenic than x-rays by at least a factor of four.

Phosphorus 32. Among 1222 patients treated for polycythemia vera (PV), a blood disease characterized by overproduction of red cells, leukemia developed in 11% of 228 patients treated with ^{32}P, 9% of 79 treated with x-rays, and 16% of 72 treated with both x-rays and ^{32}P, in contrast to 1% of 133 nonirradiated patients (Modan and Lilienfeld, 1965). It is possible that the bone marrow of patients with PV may be unusually sensitive to radiation. However, the causal nature of the association with ^{32}P was not entirely clear because (1) the incidence of leukemia was also associated with spleen size at the time of treatment, suggesting that biological factors determining treatment, rather than the treatment itself, could be associated with leukemia (UNSCEAR, 1972); (2) the underlying myeloproliferative disease may predispose to leukemia; (3) biases in the selection of patients being treated could not be discounted; that is, patients treated with "additional radiation" had to be removed from either the nonexposed, ^{32}P only, or x-ray only groups; and (4) PV patients are exposed to other medications, including powerful cytotoxic drugs, that could increase leukemia risk. A randomized clinical trial found that 9 of 156 (6%) patients treated with ^{32}P developed leukemia in contrast to 1 of 134 (1%) treated by phlebotomy (Berk et al, 1981). Patients treated with chlorambucil were at highest risk (16 of 141, 11%).

Thorotrast. A colloidal solution of thorium dioxide (Thorotrast) was used between 1928 and 1955 as a contrast agent during radiographic procedures (van Kaick et al, 1995). The thorium, however, remained in body tissue for life and resulted in continuous alpha particle exposure at a low dose rate. The annual dose from a typical injection of 25 ml of Thorotrast was 25 cGy to liver and 16 cGy to bone marrow. Surveys in Denmark, Germany, Japan, and Portugal show substantial excesses of liver cancer, including angiosarcoma and cholangiocarcinoma, and acute myeloid leukemia (NAS, 1988; Taylor et al, 1989; Andersson and Storm, 1992, Andersson et al, 1993, 1994). Hemangioendothelioma of the liver appears uniquely related to Thorotrast. Among 2326 exposed persons in the German Thorotrast study, 396 (17%) have died from liver cancer in contrast to only 2 (0.1%) among 1,890 controls (van Kaick et al, 1989; NAS, 1988). Excess lung cancer has been reported in some series, suggesting a possible effect of exhaled Thoron (^{220}Rn) (Andersson and Storm, 1992; Andersson et al, 1995). Small increases in bone cancer have also been noted, possibly due to translocating ^{224}Ra from Thorotrast deposits (NAS, 1988). The relative effectiveness of alpha particles to cause leukemia appears very similar to that expected from external irradiation at doses to bone marrow of the order of 1.3 Gy (Boice, 1993b).

The nonuniform deposition of thorium in the liver and bone marrow likely resulted in very high local doses, which may be the important determinant of cancer risk (Guilmette and Mays, 1992). If so, the convention of averaging dose over the entire organ would be misleading. Risk estimation is also hindered because (1) the chemical nature of thorium, a heavy metal, may be related to risk; (2) the average dose to the liver was about 5 Gy, and a portion of this radiant energy, expended in necrotic tissue, was probably not essential for carcinogenesis; (3) the completeness of patient follow-up was generally poor; and (4) the combination of necrosis and liver regeneration might influence risk. Further, Thorotrast was often administered to diagnose and evaluate liver diseases that may intrinsically have contributed to the development of subsequent cancer, although such patients were excluded from the German study. Nonetheless, Thorotrast appears to be one of the most carcinogenic exposures known to man, with cumulative lifetime incidences of cancer estimated to be as high as 86% (Andersson and Storm, 1992).

Occupational Exposure

Radium Dial and Clock Painters. Among 1474 women employed in the U.S. radium dial industry before 1930, 61 bone sarcomas and 21 head carcinomas have occurred (Rowland et al, 1978; Stebbings et al, 1984). The habit of licking paint brushes to make fine tips resulted in the ingestion of large quantities of bone-seeking ^{226}Ra (mean to bone, 17 Gy) and some quantities of ^{228}Ra. Cancers in mastoid air cells or paranasal sinuses (head carcinomas) likely were caused by radon gas emitted as a decay product of radium. The "latency period" for osteosarcoma was not related to dose (Polednak, 1978). Age at first exposure did not influence risk. Risk was estimated as 0.1 bone cancers/10^4PY-Gy (NAS, 1972).

No excess of leukemia was observed (10 vs 9.24 expected) among U.S. dial painters (Spiers et al, 1983) or among 1100 English radium luminisers (Baverstock and Papworth, 1989). Early reports linking breast cancer with radium or external gamma ray exposures were not confirmed (Stebbings et al, 1984; Baverstock and Papworth, 1989). Multiple myeloma was increased in the U.S. study, but correlated with duration of employment (a surrogate for gamma ray exposure), rather than radium intake. Liver cancer was not increased. The British study reported only one osteosarcoma, but the systemic intake of radium was much lower than for the United States. Other than for radiogenic cancer, there was no general life-shortening effect (Stehney et al, 1978).

An equation of the form $I = (c + bD^2)e^{-aD}$ fits the osteosarcoma data, whereas a linear form, $I = c+bD$, fits the head carcinoma data. Marshall and coworkers (1977, 1978) developed an elaborate two-target model proposing that two successive initiating events and a later promoting event are required for osteosarcoma induction. The initiation events remove the ability of a cell to stop dividing; the promotion event is a signal to divide associated with natural remodeling of bone. The model also allowed for the competitive effects of cell killing.

The actual dose-incidence curve determined for radium dial painters must be considered tentative for the following reasons: (1) the estimation of dose was made many years after the ingestion of radium; (2) the nonuniform distribution of radium in bone likely resulted in "hot spots" that caused extensive cell killing; (3) the dose responsible for tumor induction cannot be distinguished from the "irrelevant" or "wasted" dose received after initiation; (4) the relative effectiveness and contribution of the alpha particle emissions cannot easily be separated from the other radiations accompanying radium decay; and (5) the fraction of the total dose to the endosteal cells cannot be specified precisely.

Radiologists. The first cancer attributed to ionizing radiation occurred on the hand of a radiologist in 1902 (NAS, 1990), and leukemia was first associated with chronic exposure in studies of radiologists (March, 1944). Leukemia, aplastic anemia, and skin cancer were excessive among radiologists who practiced during the early part of this century before radiation protection guidelines were in use, but these risks appear to have disappeared among more recent radiologists (Matanoski et al, 1975; Smith and Doll, 1981; Wang et al, 1990a).

Multiple myeloma was increased among U.S. radiologists practicing in later years (Lewis, 1963; Matanoski et al, 1975), but not among English or Chinese radiologists. Cancers of the pancreas and lung were increased among the pioneering radiologists in the United Kingdom, but not in the United States or China. Suggested increases of breast, thyroid, and bone cancers were correlated with radiation work in China only (Wang et al, 1990a). Neither leukemia nor cancer was reported to be in excess among U.S. Army x-ray technologists, who likely received much lower total doses (Jablon and Miller, 1978). A new survey of 145,000 radiologic technologists in the United States may be able to evaluate risks more precisely (Boice et al, 1992c). Recent evaluation of 600 breast cancers reported on mail questionnaires was not able, however, to convincingly link years worked with breast cancer (Boice et al, 1995).

A generally higher mortality rate among U.S. radiologists from all causes was originally interpreted as evidence of an acceleration of the aging process by radiation. Other than the loss of life due to cancer deaths, however, nonspecific life-shortening has not been demonstrated in animal experiments or seen in British radiologists, or radium dial painters (UNSCEAR, 1982). Recent mortality analyses among A-bomb survivors, however, leave open the possibility that excess non-cancer deaths may have occurred following high doses over 2–3 Gy (Shimizu et al, 1992).

The absence of accurate estimates of radiation dose is a serious limitation of these studies. Cumulative doses were likely between 1 and 8 Gy during the early part of this century, and it is possible that radiologists who developed cancer were those who scorned safety measures and received even greater doses. It was not uncommon for x-ray workers to be given time off from work because of severe depression of white blood cell counts. Radiologists also receive more personal (non-occupational) exposures to diagnostic and therapeutic radiation than other specialists (Jessup and Silverman, 1981). Nonetheless, these studies indicate that leukemia and skin cancer can result from repeated, presumably small, radiation exposures received over a period of many years.

Workers at Nuclear Shipyards. A proportional mortality study of naval shipyard workers suggested an increased risk of cancer and leukemia among nuclear workers in Portsmouth, New Hampshire (Najarian and Colton, 1978), which was not borne out in a subsequent cohort study (Rinsky et al, 1981). Radiation exposure histories, ascertained from next-of-kin by newspaper reporters, did not correlate with employment records. Further, relatives of workers who died from cancer were more likely to be located and interviewed, which, in combination with a lower all-cause mortality among nuclear workers, contributed to the spurious result (Greenberg et al, 1985). Case-control studies of leukemia and lung cancer also found no association with radiation work (Rinsky et al, 1988; Stern et al, 1986). A comprehensive evaluation of workers at eight nuclear shipyards found no increase in any cancer except mesothelioma, attributable in all likelihood to asbestos exposures (Matanoski, 1993).

Workers at Nuclear Installations. The mortality experience of nearly 31,500 male and 12,600 female workers employed between 1944 and 1978 at the Hanford nuclear installation in Richland, Washington, has been reported by several investigators. An early proportional mortality analysis on 3520 certified deaths (Mancuso et al, 1977) was widely criticized and discounted (Hutchison et al, 1979; NCRP, 1980; NAS, 1980). Conclusions were inconsistent with subsequent follow-up studies (Gilbert et al, 1993a,b). The most recent analyses revealed a strong "healthy worker" effect, a significant deficit of cancer mortality, including leukemia, and no evidence for increasing risk with increasing film badge exposure for any cancer. A previously reported excess of multiple myeloma was no longer significant.

Results from studies of workers at nuclear installations are generally inconsistent. Leukemia was not in excess among U.K. Sellafield workers, although a dose response was suggested when exposure was lagged 15 years (Smith and Douglas, 1986). Leukemia was elevated at the Oak Ridge National Laboratory (ORNL), but risk was inversely related to dose (Checkoway et al, 1985; Gilbert et al, 1993b). Multiple myeloma was excessive at Sellafield, although based on only two cases receiving over 50 cGy (Smith and Douglas, 1986). Prostate cancer was increased at the U.K. Atomic Energy Authority and the U.K. Atomic Weapons Establishment (Beral et al, 1988; Rooney et al, 1993), and bladder cancer at Sellafield (Smith and Douglas, 1986). Lung cancer is often found to be significantly low in nuclear workers (Gilbert et al, 1993b). Prostate cancer was negatively linked to radiation among U.S. workers (Gilbert et al 1993b).

A recent analysis of data on workers at the ORNL has received considerable criticism (Wing et al, 1991). An excess of leukemia, including CLL, was emphasized, although risk decreased with increasing levels of exposure. Confounding by smoking likely contributed to the correlations reported, making the data difficult to interpret since lung cancer dominated the analysis (Gilbert, 1992, 1993b). Compared to the general population, the ORNL workers were at a 28% significantly reduced risk of dying from lung cancer. Interestingly, Oak Ridge workers hired during WWII were previously reported to be at high risk of lung cancer unrelated to radiation exposure (Frome et al, 1990). This "unhealthy worker effect" appeared due to the selection out of the workforce of physically fit individuals to serve in the armed forces.

Another recent study from a large registry of 95,000 radiation workers in the United Kingdom reported significant increased risks due to leukemia, excluding CLL (Kendall et al, 1992). Other cancers were elevated but not significantly. Risk estimates were consistent with A-bomb survivor data but not with U.S. worker studies. This first report should be interpreted with some caution because the leukemia risk seemed apparent only at one facility, Sellafield, where cumulative exposures over 40 cGy have occurred and where potential exposure to leukemogenic chemicals during fuel reprocessing activities were possible.

A new report from Canada exemplifies the difficulties in detecting risks following low-dose radiation exposures (Gribbin et al, 1993). A careful study of nearly 9000 workers revealed a significant deficit of cancer (SMR=0.87), and there were no significant correlations with radiation for any site or combination of sites. Less than 1% of workers received greater than 5 cGy. Risk estimates were computed and stated to be consistent with extrapolations from A-bomb survivor data; that is, RR = 1.0036 at 1 cGy. Although true, the data were equally consistent with no effect at all, and reflect the extremely small excess risk expected at such low exposure levels and the associated low power to detect such risk.

The first comprehensive effort to combine series of nuclear workers involved four U.S. studies (Gilbert et al, 1993b). Excess relative risk estimates per sievert were 0.0 for all cancer and −1.0 for leukemia. The authors concluded that data extrapolations from higher dose studies are unlikely to underestimate risks at lower doses. A new analysis combines data from 75,006 employees in three nuclear establishments in the United Kingdom (Carpenter et al, 1994). Excess RR estimates per Sv were −0.02 for all cancers and 4.2 for leukemia. Leukemia was elevated only in one of the three nuclear establishments. Significant increases in cancer of the pleura suggest that employees were exposed to other hazardous agents such as asbestos. Recently, 95,673 nuclear industry workers in three countries were analyzed (Cardis et al, 1995). Leukemia was increased, but not other cancers. Interpretations are limited because, overall, only about 9 of the 3976 cancer deaths could be attributable to radiation. Even combinations of larger studies may have difficulty in providing risk estimates of useful precision, because the sample sizes and ranges of exposures appear small for acceptable power at the most likely effect level (Land, 1980; Cook-Mozaffari et al, 1987). The average cumulative doses for workers employed in research and development or weapons production range between about 1–3 cGy, with only about 5%–15% over 5 cGy (Gilbert et al, 1993a,b; Beral et al, 1988). Higher doses occur during nuclear fuel processing; for example, badged employees at Sellafield have accumulated 13 cGy on average (Carpenter et al, 1994). Studies of nuclear utility workers may eventually provide useful information on radiation risks because of relatively higher exposures and larger numbers (Jablon and Boice, 1993).

Occupational studies of radiation workers must be interpreted carefully because (1) film badge or thermoluminescent dosimeter (TLD) exposures are imperfect measures of organ doses; (2) the dose from natural background radiation (about 7 cGy in 70 years) is often greater than the occupational dose; (3) other occupational and nonoccupational carcinogens are usually not considered; and (4) ascertainment bias is possible if the working population receives better medical care and more accurate cancer diagnoses recorded on death certificates than the general population. This surveillance bias was suggested as a possible explanation for the excess of multiple myeloma (in the absence of a leukemia excess) seen among Hanford workers (NIH, 1985). However, chance might have been responsible for the early excess, which was no longer significant in the latest follow-up (Gilbert et al, 1993a).

Workers Exposed to Plutonium. At one time, plutonium was thought to be one of the most toxic elements known to man. Animal experiments clearly indicate that excessive exposure to plutonium can cause cancers of the lung, bone and liver; however, the evidence in man is sketchy (NAS, 1988). Twenty-six heavily exposed individuals who worked on the Manhattan Project in Los Alamos, New Mexico, and who received extensive clinical examinations over the last 40 years, have not died at a higher rate than expected (Voelz and Lawrence, 1991). However, three lung cancers developed in long-term smokers, and the occurrence of one osteosarcoma is noteworthy. In 224 males with plutonium body burdens of 10 nanocuries or more, a lower than expected cancer mortality was reported, and lung cancer and osteosarcoma were not excessive (Voelz, 1991). Lung cancer has been reported to be excessive among 2346 workers at the Mayak radiochemical plant in Russia (Hohryakov and Romanov, 1994). Studies of large populations of workers exposed to lower levels of plutonium find no correlation between plutonium intake and cancer mortality (Wilkinson et al, 1987; Beral et al, 1988; Gilbert et al, 1993a).

Underground Miners. Among 3366 white and 780 nonwhite U.S. uranium miners who worked at least one month underground, a substantial excess of respiratory cancer was observed: 155 deaths versus 30.4 expected based on general population rates (Hornung and Meinhardt, 1987). Lung irradiation was from inhaled radon gas, and the mean dose was about 4.7 Gy (NAS, 1972). Most lung cancers developed in cigarette smokers, but an excess risk was also seen among 516 nonsmoking miners exposed to very high radon levels (Roscoe et al, 1989). Radiation and smoking appear to interact in a way that enhances risk, though somewhat less than multiplicative (NAS, 1988).

Dose-response data for lung cancer in the U.S. miners are difficult to interpret because of (1) uncertainties in lung doses for individual miners, which had to be estimated based on infrequent measurements in over 2500 mines; (2) the relationship between exposure (the concentration of radioactive materials in mine atmospheres) and actual dose to respiratory tissue; (3) the dose to individual cells, which could vary depending on cell type, the thickness of the epithelial and overlapping mucous layers, and the clearance rate of absorbed radioactive particles; (4) the doses received in non-uranium mines; and (5) the contribution to risk of cigarette smoking and of pollutants, like diesel exhaust, in mine atmospheres (NAS, 1991).

Many of the above concerns were addressed in underground miner studies in Sweden (Radford et al, 1984), Canada (Howe et al, 1987; Morrison et al, 1988), China (Xuan et al, 1993), Czechoslovakia (Sevc et al, 1988) and other countries (NAS, 1988) where radon exposures were lower and better characterized than in Colorado mines. An analysis of four major studies concluded that the dose-response relationship between cumulative radon exposure and lung cancer was linear, that the increase in RR per working level month (WLM) was approximately 1.5%, that age at first exposure had little influence on risk, and that relative (but not absolute) risk declined with both time since exposure stopped and attained age (NAS, 1988).

The most recent analysis of underground miner data sets combines 11 individual studies (Lubin et al, 1994a; 1995a). The linearity of the dose response across all studies was remarkable, although individual risk estimates differed somewhat. Age at exposure did not influence subsequent risk, even among children exposed under age 10. Excess RR per WLM decreased with time since exposure and with age at observation. Mine contaminants such as arsenic were important lung carcinogens and adjustment resulted in lower radon risks. The overall excess RR per WLM was 0.49% (Fig. 16–7). Risk coefficients for nonsmoking miners were higher than for smokers as might be anticipated from a submultiplicative relationship between radon and smoking. The temporal relationships between radon exposure and cigarette smoking appears important (Thomas et al, 1994; Yao et al, 1994; van Leeuwen et al, 1995). An "inverse dose rate" effect was apparent at the highest cumulative exposures but appeared to level off at cumulative exposure of the order of 100 WLM (Lubin et al, 1995b), as might be expected based on biophysical principles (Brenner et al, 1993, Brenner, 1994).

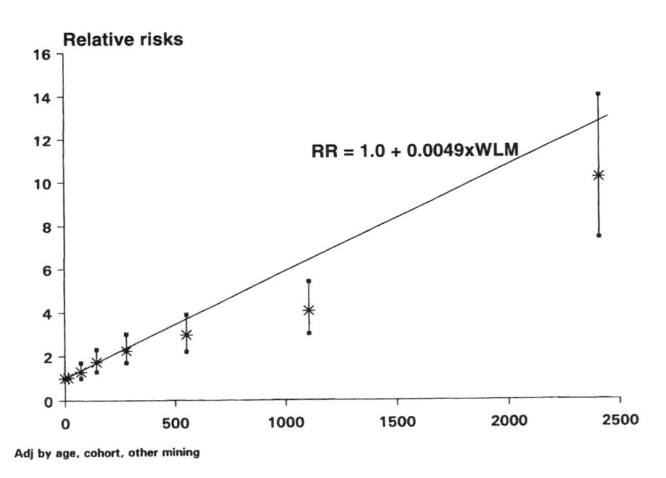

FIG. 16–7. Relative risk of lung cancer by cumulative radon concentrations for 11 cohort studies, combined, of underground miners (Lubin et al, 1994a).

Several studies suggest that exposure at a low rate may be more harmful than at a high rate for the same total dose (Hornung and Meinhardt, 1987; Howe et al, 1987; Lubin et al, 1990a, 1994a, 1995b). For very high doses, a lower rate of exposure (or equivalently, a longer duration of exposure) might result in less cell killing and thus higher risk. At very low doses, such as experienced in domestic situations, no dose-rate effect would be expected because multiple alpha particle traversals of single cell nuclei would be rare (Brenner et al, 1993, Brenner, 1994). No excess leukemia or lymphoma has been reported, although miners were heavily exposed to uranium, radon, and their decay products (Tomaser et al, 1993). Much lower levels of exposure associated with environmental contamination from uranium mill tailings also have not been linked to increased cancer risks (Mason et al, 1972). The evidence that radon causes lung cancer comes mainly from miners exposed to over 100 WLM (about 0.5 Gy), and significant risks below about 50 WLM have not been observed (NAS, 1988). In contrast, average levels of indoor radon are estimated as 0.2 WLM per year (NAS, 1991).

Indoor Radon

Although it has long been recognized that radon causes lung cancer among underground miners (NAS, 1988; Samet, 1989), the possible hazard to homeowners exposed to much lower levels was not appreciated until recently. Indoor radon accounts for over half of all radiation exposures received by the general population, and, based on extrapolations from high-dose miner studies, may cause between 6600 and 24,000 lung cancer deaths per year in the United States (Lubin and Boice, 1989; Lubin et al, 1994a, 1995a).

In 1979, lung cancer was linked to living in stone houses compared to wood houses (Axelson et al, 1979). Subsequent case-control studies in Sweden showed positive associations between lung cancer and living in structures where radon levels were measured to be high, although the associations were appreciably weakened when adjustment for occupancy was made (Pershagen et al, 1992). A new national study finds a positive association between radon and lung cancer based on comprehensive measurements and large numbers (Pershagen et al, 1994). In New Jersey, lung cancer risk was increased more than twofold among women living in homes with radon levels greater than 4 picoCuries (pCi) per liter, but there were only six cases and two controls with such exposure (Schoenberg et al, 1990). A comprehensive case-control study of 308 women recently diagnosed with lung cancer in China found no association between lung cancer and increasing radon exposure (Blot et al, 1990). Year-long measurements of radon were made in current residences, and 20% of the readings exceeded 4 pCi/liter, the level above which remedial action is suggested in the United States. It was concluded that projections from surveys of miners exposed to high radon levels may overestimate the risks of lung cancer associated with levels typically seen in homes. Similar findings and conclusions were reached in a large study in Canada of over 750 lung cancer cases (Létourneau et al, 1994).

Combined analyses of radon data sets have been conducted to help clarify apparent discrepancies. A recent pooling of data from three studies in Sweden, New Jersey, and China involved nearly 1000 lung cancer cases among women (Lubin et al, 1994b). No association with cumulative radon measures were found. Another recent study of 600 lung cancer cases in Missouri among nonsmoking women also found no overall association with radon, and the estimated population attributable risk to radon was at most 2% (Alavanja et al, 1994, 1995). The later study had several methodological advantages, such as being an incident survey with exposure measurements made close in time to the lung cancer diagnosis, nonsmokers would enhance the probability of detecting an effect given that their risk coefficient would be high, direct smoking was not a meaningful confounder, there was relatively little migration of residents, and a comprehensive dosimetry program was in place. Nevertheless, when all the studies to date are considered together, they are not powerful enough to either accept or reject the possibility that residential radon contributes to the lung cancer burden in a manner expected based on extrapolations from studies on underground miners (Fig. 16–8) (Lubin, 1994).

Circumstances associated with underground mines have led some to question whether extrapolations from miner studies have direct relevance to residential situations (Abelson, 1991). The role of concomitant exposures such as silica, arsenic, and diesel and blasting fumes has not been clearly elucidated. Conceivably, exposures that damage or irritate lung tissue and promote cell proliferation might potentiate the carcinogenic effect of radon (NAS, 1991). One ecological study has suggested an inverse relationship between county measures of radon and lung cancer mortality (Cohen, 1995), but such studies are inherently weak and susceptible to many biases, especially the inability to adjust for smoking habits in individuals (Greenland and Robins, 1994; Stidley and Samet, 1993).

Studies of indoor radon have to be interpreted with caution because of inherent difficulties in accurately estimating exposures that occurred many years ago based on current measurements (Lubin et al, 1990b, 1995c). The expected risk associated with average residential exposures is accordingly low (RR <1.2), which necessitates accurate adjustment for the effect of smoking, including involuntary exposures. Exposure reconstruction is complicated further because of mobility (persons

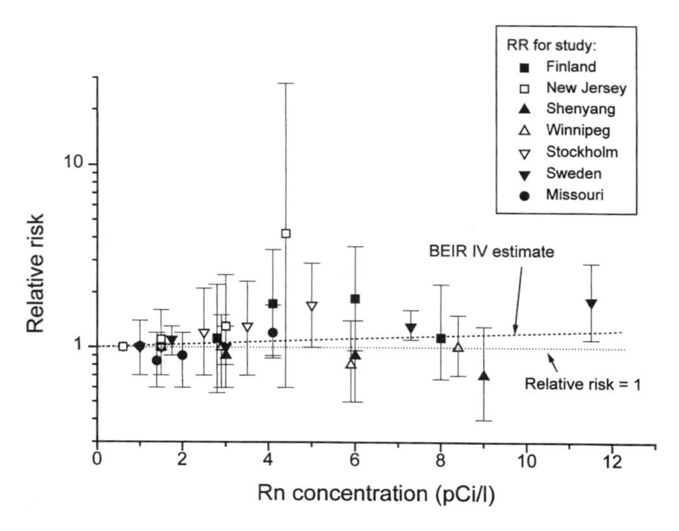

FIG. 16–8. Relative risk of lung cancer by residential radon concentrations for seven case-control studies (Lubin, 1994; Blot et al, 1990; Schoenberg et al, 1990; Pershagen et al, 1992, 1994; Létourneau et al, 1994; Alavanja et al, 1994).

reside in many homes throughout life), home modifications, and uncertain estimates of time actually spent in the home. While pooling data sets might help to define the possible level of risk associated with indoor radon, current data suggest that even these results may be equivocal.

Natural Background Radiation

Correlation studies attempting to link cancer mortality with natural background radiation have generally been negative (Mason and Miller, 1974; NAS, 1990), but are fraught with uncertainties of dose levels, migration patterns, selection factors for place of residence, and geographic variations in the accuracy of cancer diagnoses (Pochin, 1976). In England, childhood cancer has been correlated with maternal irradiation from background sources (Knox et al, 1988), and leukemia (but not lung cancer) to radon (Henshaw et al, 1990), but the interpretations remain clouded by the serious limitations of ecological correlation analyses (NAS, 1990; Muirhead et al, 1991). The most extensive investigation on the possible health effects of naturally occurring radiation was conducted in China on a stable population of 73,000 persons who received three times the amount of background radiation as 77,000 inhabitants of a comparison region (Wei, 1980, 1990). Cancer was not increased among residents of the high background area. Thyroid nodularity, a sensitive indicator of low-dose radiation effects, was also found to be similar among female residents of the high (14 cGy) and low (5 cGy) radiation areas based on clinical screenings of 2000 elderly women (Wang et al, 1990b). Differences in chromosome aberrations in circulating lymphocytes indicated that the background radiation levels were meaningfully different. A dose of 9 cGy accumulated gradually over a lifetime apparently produced many fewer thyroid tumors than seen following a similar dose of x-rays received briefly in childhood (Ron et al, 1989).

Fallout

Marshall Islands. Over 200 native residents of four inhabited atolls east of Bikini Island were accidentally exposed to nuclear fallout from the BRAVO weapons test in 1954 (Conard, 1984; Robbins and Adams, 1989). Whole-body gamma ray doses were estimated as 0.11 Gy, 1.1 Gy, and 1.9 Gy to the Marshallese on three atolls. Mean thyroid dose, from gamma radiation plus radioiodines, was estimated as 3–52 Gy to children, depending upon age, and 1.6–12 Gy to adults. During 32 years of observation, 60 (or 24%) of 253 subjects developed thyroid nodules and cancer, excluding seven occult papillary carcinomas found incidentally during surgery. Thyroid cancers appeared in 7 of 130 women and 2 of 113 men; and in 6 of 127 children under age 19 at exposure and in 3 of 126 older natives. The offspring of 2 of 12 women pregnant at the time of the test developed thyroid nodules. The earliest thyroid lesion appeared 9 years after exposure. Impairment of thyroid function and some clinically evident hypothyroidism occurred at doses between 3.9 and 21 Gy. Growth retardation was apparent in some children. One leukemia occurred in each group of exposed and nonexposed (135) islanders. Two pituitary tumors developed in women exposed as young children, suggesting a possible link with thyroid injury.

Calculated risk coefficients were $8.3/10^4$ PY-Gy and $1.5/10^4$ PY-Gy for nodules and cancer, respectively. Risk estimates are uncertain, however, because (1) the large thyroid doses may have caused lethal cellular damage that decreased the number of cells at risk for malignant transformation; (2) frequent surgery for benign tumors and nodules might have removed tissue destined to develop into cancer; (3) increased levels of TSH, secondary to thyroid hypofunction, and prophylactic thyroid hormone treatments might have influenced risk; and (4) the effects of gamma ray exposures could not be distinguished from those of internal radioiodines. Further, dosimetry for the radioiodines is complex. Most beta particle energy from ^{131}I is supposedly deposited in the colloid of the large follicles without reaching the critical follicular cells, and the low dose rate would tend to minimize risk. In contrast, the shorter-lived and more energetic isotopes (^{132}I, ^{133}I, and ^{135}I) contributed two to three times the dose of ^{131}I and exposed the thyroid more uniformly and at a higher dose rate. Thus, while the study clearly shows that short-lived iodines are carcinogenic, the contribution of ^{131}I could not be distinguished.

A study of 7000 Marshall Islanders from 14 atolls, including several not previously studied, revealed a linear relationship between thyroid nodules and proximity to Bikini (Hamilton et al, 1987). An estimate of 11 nodules/10^4PY-Gy was based on clinical examinations.

Utah

Thyroid. Clinical examinations of 2945 children in the sixth to twelfth grades from 1965–1971 were conducted in two counties in Utah and Nevada that received fallout from nuclear weapons tests in the 1950s, and also on 2271 children in Arizona exposed to negligible fallout (Rallison et al, 1975). No cancers and 18 nodules (1.3%) were detected in 1378 children living in the exposed counties at the time of the weapons tests. In contrast, two thyroid cancers and 19 thyroid nodules (1.4%) occurred in 1313 nonexposed children who moved into the area after the time of fallout; and no cancers and 20 nodules (0.9%) were found in 2140 nonexposed Arizona children. Nearly 75% of the original cohort of children were reexamined in 1985–1986 and the authors concluded that radioiodines from fallout were responsible for a small excess of thyroid neoplasms (Kerber et al, 1993). The study is remarkable for the comprehensive dose reconstruction based on milk and green vegetable consumption, radionuclide deposition, and milk production and deposition. Estimates of individual thyroid doses ranged from 0 to 4.6 Gy and averaged 0.17 Gy in Utah. A significant association with dose was found for period prevalence of neoplasms (n = 19), but not for benign (n = 11) or malignant (n = 8) neoplasms separately. No excess of nonneoplastic thyroid nodules (n = 34) was found. Although the estimated radiation risks were roughly consistent with those reported in studies of children exposed to external x-rays or gamma rays, the small number of cases limit the conclusions that can be drawn.

In addition to the small sample size, other concerns include (1) the apparent lack of a correlation between thyroid neoplasms and proximity to the Nevada test site (NTS) (Rallison et al, 1990); (2) the dosimetry relied on recall of dietary habits of 30 years ago, which must be uncertain; (3) recall bias was possible because the dietary questionnaire was administered after the thyroid examination; (4) observation bias was possible in that nurse practitioners referred nearly twice as many subjects for clinical thyroid examination from the high fallout areas—32% from Utah and 17% from Arizona; and (5) the absence of a clear association between dose and the larger number of nonneoplastic thyroid nodules is unusual because nodules have been related to fallout radiation among residents of the Marshall Islands (Conard, 1984) and among children exposed to cranial irradiation (Ron et al, 1989).

Leukemia. A geographical study of childhood cancer mortality within Utah suggested an increase of leukemia in "high-fallout" counties near the NTS (Lyon et al, 1979). However, there was a significantly low risk of other childhood cancers in the high-exposure counties, and no overall association with total childhood cancers (Land, 1979; NCRP, 1980). Attempts to duplicate the leukemia findings using county mortality statistics from the National Center for Health Statistics (NCHS) also failed (Land et al, 1984). It appeared that the earlier finding reflected an anomalously low rate of childhood leukemia rates in southern Utah during 1944–1949, and not an association with fallout.

A telephone survey of Mormon church members of certain communities in the southwest claimed that fallout had caused exceptionally high risks of leukemia and cancer (Johnson, 1984). Self-reported cancers, obtained by volunteer interviewers, were not verified. Some purported risks were far greater than seen among A-bomb survivors exposed to near-lethal doses of over 4 Gy, and suggested biases in the study methodology (Cook-Mozaffari et al, 1987; MacMahon, 1989). A geographical analysis of NCHS mortality data for counties in Utah covered by the telephone survey found a significant deficit of cancer, although leukemia was increased (Machado et al, 1987).

A recent case-control study of over 1000 individuals who died of leukemia in southwestern Utah identified a weak association between estimated bone marrow dose and all leukemia, though the trend was not significant (Stevens et al, 1990). Significant risks, however, were observed for acute leukemia among those under age 20 when exposed to fallout, consistent with that expected based on other studies of exposed populations. The increasing trends seen for CLL, a tumor not known to be elevated after irradiation, and the difficulty in estimating doses retrospectively add caution to causal interpretations.

Nordic Countries. Trends in childhood leukemia within Nordic countries were evaluated for possible changes that might be related to fallout from atmospheric nuclear weapons testing in the 1950s and 1960s (Darby et al, 1992). Estimates of fetal bone marrow exposure, primarily from cesium 137 (^{137}Cs), were low and about 0.14 mSv, and no increase in leukemia incidence could be tied to such levels. A 7-year cumulative exposure was estimated to be 1.5 mSv, and although no correlation with exposure was found, small increases were not inconsistent with a possible radiation effect. There was no evidence for a preconception effect based on estimated parental testicular dose. These data suffer from the same uncertainties of all ecological surveys in that dose to individuals is unknown. Further, there have been a great many new exposures in childhood occurring after World War II, other than low-level radioactive fallout, that might influence the incidence, diagnosis, and reporting of leukemia over time.

Nuclear Weapons Test Participants

Nevada. No excess in total cancer mortality (112 vs 117.5) was found among 3017 of 3217 participants in military maneuvers during the 1957 nuclear test "SMOKY" (Caldwell et al, 1983). Leukemia, however, was significantly elevated; 10 cases were observed, including the index case that prompted the investigation and one case that developed after radiation therapy for lymphoma, versus 4.0 expected. Lower cancer frequencies were generally noted among the military units with the highest exposures based on film badge doses (mean, 0.46 cGy). A survey of 46,186 military participants in two test series conducted at the NTS and three in the Pacific also found no excess of nonleukemia deaths (990 vs. 1187) (Robinette et al, 1985). Excluding SMOKY, 46 leukemia deaths occurred versus 52.4 expected, suggesting that the leukemia excess among SMOKY participants was either due to chance or to circumstances peculiar to that shot (or its participants).

United Kingdom. Cancer mortality and incidence among 21,358 participants in the United Kingdoms' atmospheric nuclear weapons tests in Australia and the Pacific Ocean between 1952 and 1967 and in 22,333 matched controls were recently evaluated (Darby et al, 1993). Mortality from all causes Standardized Mortality Ratio (SMR) (SMR = 0.86 and 0.99), and from all cancers (SMR = 0.85 and 0.96) were comparable, but lower among participants. Leukemia and bladder cancer risks were significantly higher among participants than controls, whereas controls had significantly higher levels of lung and oral cancer. Mortality from leukemia among participants, however, was equal to that predicted from national rates (SMR = 1.0, based on 29 deaths), but was extremely low among controls (SMR = 0.56 based on 17 deaths). Thus the possible increased risks of leukemia was related more to a significant deficit among the controls than to an excess among the exposed.

Cancer Around Nuclear Installations

Systematic Surveys. Reports of small clusters of childhood leukemia around nuclear installations in the United Kingdom in the 1980s prompted several large-scale systematic surveys. Lymphoid leukemia among persons under age 25 was found to be generally increased in populations living near nuclear fuel reprocessing or weapons production facilities in the United Kingdom, but not plants that generated electricity (Cook-Mozaffari et al, 1987; Forman et al, 1987). Mortality from Hodgkin's disease at ages 0–24 was also increased, whereas mortality from lymphoid leukemia at ages 25–64 was significantly reduced. Overall, there was no general increase in cancer deaths in the vicinity of nuclear installations.

Interestingly, a study from Britain evaluated residents of areas where construction of nuclear power stations had only been considered, or just recently completed. Excesses of childhood leukemia and Hodgkin's disease, and deficits of adult leukemia, were reported that were similar to those previously identified in areas with operating nuclear facilities (Cook-Mozaffari et al, 1989). The authors concluded that the unexpected increases in some childhood cancers around nuclear installations are unlikely to be due to environmental radiation pollution, but rather to other risk factors yet to be identified. An infective agent associated with large migrations of people into these areas, for example, has been proposed as one possible explanation (Kinlen et al, 1991, 1993a).

In the largest survey to date, over 900,000 cancer deaths in 113 counties in the United States containing or adjacent to 62 nuclear facilities were compared to 1,800,000 cancer deaths in control counties with similar population and socioeconomic characteristics (Jablon et al, 1991). Overall, and for specific groups of nuclear installations, there was no evidence that mortality for any cancer, including childhood leukemia, was higher in counties with nuclear reactors than in the control counties. For childhood leukemia, the RR in the study counties versus their controls after plant start-up was 1.03; before start-up it was 1.08. For all leukemia, the RRs were 0.98 after start-up and 1.02 before. Systematic studies in France, Germany, and Canada also failed to identify clusters of childhood cancer around nuclear facilities (Hill and Laplanche, 1990; Michaelis et al, 1992; McLaughlin et al, 1993b). Small area data were recently analyzed in England and Wales and, except for Sellafield, there was little evidence that childhood leukemia was related to proximity to nuclear installations (Bithell et al, 1994).

The ecological correlation analyses are not without problems because (1) radiation dose to the population is unknown, although likely much below natural background (Darby and Doll, 1987; UNSCEAR, 1988); (2) mortality is not the best indicator of cancer hazard due to inaccuracies of death certificates, and cancer registration may also be incomplete and variable between areas; (3) other important risk factors often cannot be identified; (4) the county or district may be too large an administrative unit to detect localized increases in cancer rates; and (5) the many comparisons made with regard to individual cancers, ages, and time frames increase the likelihood that chance plays a role in highlighting areas with seemingly high, or low, cancer rates.

Clusters. In 1983, a team of investigative television reporters from Yorkshire set out to evaluate the risk of cancer in workers at the Sellafield (Windscale) nuclear fuel reprocessing complex in West Cumbria, U.K. Learning that neither cancer nor leukemia was excessive in these workers (Smith and Douglas, 1986), the reporters focused on an apparent cluster of seven young people who developed leukemia between 1950 and 1983 in Seascale, a village about 3 kilometers south of Sellafield. A government report confirmed that childhood leukemia (4 vs 0.25) was elevated in the region near Sellafield (Black, 1984). An assessment of total radiation exposure of the population revealed that natural background contributed the greatest amount (66%), with Sellafield discharges contributing only 16%. Thus, environmental pollution from radioactive releases seemed an unlikely culprit. Additional studies found that the excess of leukemia occurred entirely among individuals born in Seascale (5 vs 0.53) and not among children born elsewhere (0 vs 0.54), suggesting that factors present in early life or before birth might be important (Gardner et al, 1987). A subsequent case-control study, discussed below, raised the possibility that parental exposure among Sellafield workers might explain the cluster (Gardner et al, 1990).

Other studies around nuclear facilities have failed to provide clear insights into the reasons, other than chance or gerrymandering, for apparent clusterings of childhood cancer (Boice, 1991; MacMahon, 1992; Draper et al, 1993). In some investigations, findings were entirely dependent upon the selection of particular geographic and calendar time groupings. Even the Seascale cluster might be considered suspect, because it was the *occurrence of the cases* that determined both the geographic boundary and the age definition of the cluster. Recall that the TV reporters first went to Sellafield, not Seascale, and were seeking excesses of cancer among adult workers, not leukemia among young people in the general population.

Preconception. The most provocative (and controversial) finding from the Seascale studies was the association between leukemia and preconception irradiation of the fathers working at Sellafield (Gardner et al, 1990). If true, the apparent cluster might be explained in terms of occupational rather than environmental radiation exposure. The numbers were small, however, and the association relied on only four high-exposed fathers. Other correlates of occupation, such as chemical exposures, were not evaluated. Most of the nine fathers who worked at Sellafield were chemists or were involved with chemical processing; parental exposure to chemicals has been suggested as a possible risk factor for leukemia in offspring (Buckley et al, 1989). The leukemia and lymphoma diagnoses evaluated occurred over a 35-year period and included "children" up to age 25. Conceivably, medical care, cancer diagnoses, and cancer registration might be slightly better among skilled workers at a nuclear facility, resulting in spurious associations between parental exposure and childhood cancer.

The study was also at odds with the prospective investigation of children of the atomic bomb survivors where no excess of cancer, chromosome aberrations, or genetic mutations in blood proteins were observed (UNSCEAR, 1988; Neel and Schull, 1991). Childhood cancer also has not been increased among offspring of long-term survivors of cancer treated with radiation (Mulvihill et al, 1987). Experimental studies indicate that chronic exposures, such as experienced among Sellafield workers, produce fewer mutations than equivalent acute doses (UNSCEAR, 1988). One experimental study, however, has suggested that preconception x-rays might induce heritable tumors (mainly of the lung) in mice (Nomura, 1982). On the other hand, if radiation were acting to cause heritable mutations, then an epidemic of known heritable diseases and congenital malformations, and not leukemia, might be expected in the Sellafield area whereas none was noted (Evans, 1990).

A similar but small study at the Dounreay nuclear facility failed to replicate the Sellafield preconception findings (Urquhart et al, 1991). Another recent report purports to corroborate the preconception effect found at Sellafield (McKinney et al, 1991). Unfortunately, radiation exposures were not verified or quantified, and, perhaps more importantly, the study included many of the same fathers previously evaluated in the investigation by Gardner and coworkers (1990) that raised the hypothesis (Smith, 1991). Excluding these overlapping individuals, as would be appropriate for an independent assessment, meaningfully reduced the evidence for an association. Still another study around other U.K. nuclear facilities failed to link childhood leukemia with external exposures to occupational radiation, although an association was suggested with being "monitored" for such exposures (Roman et al, 1993).

Two recent surveys in Scotland (Kinlen et al, 1993b) and Canada (McLaughlin et al, 1993c) also failed to confirm the Gardner hypothesis. Further, a recent study of 10,363 children who were born to fathers who worked at Sellafield evaluated the geographical distribution in Cumbria of the paternal dose received prior to conception (Parker et al, 1993). Paternal doses were consistently higher among fathers of children born outside Seascale. Since childhood leukemia was not increased in these areas of West Cumbria despite the higher preconception exposures, the authors concluded that paternal exposure to radiation before conception is unlikely to be a causal factor for childhood leukemia.

An explanation of the Seascale cluster in terms of preconception radiation of the fathers appears now to have been a provocative hypothesis that was unsubstantiated by further studies (Doll et al, 1994). Other than chance, one hypothesis being pursued is the possibility that childhood leukemia may occur as a rare response to an unidentified infection whose transmission is facilitated when large numbers of people come together, such as might occur when large industrial complexes are built in rural areas (Kinlen et al, 1991, 1993a).

Nuclear Reactor Accidents

The nuclear reactor accident at Three Mile Island released little radioactivity into the environment and resulted in population exposure that was much less than what was received from natural background. Any presumed increase in cancer at these levels would be negligible and undetectable (Upton, 1981). An ecological survey did not link increased cancer rates with estimated patterns of radiation releases (Hatch et al, 1990), nor were any peculiar mortality patterns noted (Jablon et al, 1991). In contrast, the accident at Chernobyl resulted in a massive release of radioactivity (UNSCEAR, 1988; Karaoglov et al, 1996). Initial studies did not link increases in childhood leukemia (Parkin et al, 1993; Auvinen et al, 1994; Hjalmars et al, 1994; Ivanov et al, 1993; Boice and Linet, 1994), or thyroid cancer (Mettler et al, 1992) with the Chernobyl accident but the follow-up may not be sufficient. An abrupt increase in childhood thyroid cancer in Belarus and the Ukraine (Kazakov et al, 1992) may have been partially due to increased medical surveillance and reporting (Ron et al, 1992). While it is becoming clear that an unusual increase of thyroid cancer in children hs occurred (Williams et al, 1993, 1994; Stsjazhko et al, 1995), the absence of radiation dose estimates, the possibility of surveillance bias, the absence of a similar excess in Russia, and the very short latency adds caution to a causal interpretation in terms of radiation. Over 600,000 workers were sent to Chernobyl after the accident to clean up the environment and entomb the reactor. Allowable occupational exposures were 0.35 Gy, suggesting that future health studies might be informative. Studies of thyroid cancer and modularity among cleanup workers from the Baltic countries, however, have failed to find associations with radiation exposure (Inskip et al, 1996; Bigbee et al, 1996). Recently, it was revealed that an explosion in 1957 in a storage tank at the Chelyabinsk nuclear facility (the Kyshtym accident) in the former Soviet Union released large amounts of radioactive waste. High-level radioactive effluents also had been dumped into the Techa river prior to the accident between 1949 and 1956 (Kossenko and Degteva, 1994). Population doses among 28,000 residents were as high as 4 Gy and leukemia was reported to be significantly increased.

BASIC CONCEPTS

Radiation

Radiation generally refers to energy emitted from a source, such as heat or light from the sun, radio waves from a broadcast antenna, microwaves from a radar unit or cellular phone, x-rays from an x-ray tube, or gamma rays from radioactive elements. Radiation that can remove electrons from atoms is called *ionizing* and includes electromagnetic rays such as x-rays and gamma rays and energetic particles such as protons, fission nuclei, and alpha and beta particles. Neutrons, unlike these other particles, have no charge and cannot ionize directly. Instead they impart energy to protons through elastic collisions, and the protons then cause the subsequent ionizations. The amount of energy absorbed in matter as a result of radiation interactions is called the dose, which is measured in gray (Gy): 1 Gy = 1 joule per kilogram. Until recently the standard unit for dose was the rad (1 rad = 100 ergs per gram), but the conversion is simple: 1 Gy = 100 rad. An acute whole-body dose of about 5 Gy (500 rad) is lethal about half the time in humans; yet this dose ionizes only about 1 of every 40 million molecules. Permanent damage thus can be produced after a relatively small amount of energy is absorbed.

Nonionizing radiations, such as radiowaves, do not possess enough energy to strip electrons from atoms. Microwaves, such as used in ovens (2450 MHz) or cellular telephones (850 MHz), and extremely low frequency electromagnetic fields (60 Hz) from household appliances or electrical power transmission lines also are nonionizing. While generating great public concern, exposures to nonionizing electromagnetic fields have not been convincingly linked to cancer in humans or animals, and the evidence to date is sufficient only to formulate hypotheses for testing in further studies (NRPB, 1992a).

Ionizing radiation is absorbed randomly by atoms and molecules in cells and can alter molecular structure. These alterations can be amplified by biological processes to result in observable effects. The biological effects, however, depend not only on the total absorbed dose but also on the linear energy transfer (LET), or ionization density, of the type of radiation. LET is a measure of the energy loss per unit distance traveled and depends on the velocity, charge, and mass of a particle or on x-ray or gamma-ray energy. High-LET radiations such as alpha particles (helium nuclei) release energy in short tracks of dense ionizations. Low-LET, or sparsely ionizing, radiations such as x-rays produce ionizing events that are not close together. Depending on the biological end point, the effect per Gy may differ widely as a function of LET but is usually greater for high-LET radiation.

The relative biological effectiveness (RBE) of radiation characterizes its ability to produce a specific disorder (eg, cell death, chromosome aberration, or cancer) compared to a standard, usually x-rays or gamma rays. A RBE of 20 for neutrons at 0.1 Gy (10 rad), for example, would imply that the biological effect from 0.1 Gy of neutrons is the same as that from 2.0 Gy (200 rad) of gamma rays. The unit of biological dose equivalence used in radiologic protection is the sievert (Sv), which has replaced the rem (1 Sv = 100 rem). The sievert represents the absorbed dose in grays multiplied by an appropriate weighting factor (specific to the type of radiation) and other possible modifying factors (ICRP, 1991). The sievert has also been applied to assess the effects of mixed-field exposures. For example, the dose equivalence of an exposure to 0.1 Gy of gamma ray and

0.1 Gy of neutrons, with gamma rays as the standard and an RBE of 20 for neutrons, would be 2.1 Sv (210 rem). Another unit, the "effective dose equivalent," expresses the dose equivalent to a particular tissue in terms of whole-body risk. For example, indoor radon results in an annual dose equivalent of 24 mSv to lung tissue, which converts to an effective dose equivalent of 2 mSv (NAS, 1990).

Mechanisms of Cellular Damage

Cellular damage depends on the type of radiation, the amount of energy deposited per volume of tissue, the rate at which the energy is deposited, the way in which the energy is distributed throughout the tissue of interest, and the time over which a given dose is accumulated.

The physical properties of radiation have been used (Kellerer and Rossi, 1978) to describe how the transfer of energy at the cellular level might induce malignant transformation (NAS, 1990; UNSCEAR, 1993). Essentially, it is postulated that sublesions (eg, single-strand break in DNA helix) are produced within cells at a rate proportional to the energy deposited, and a biological effect results if two sublesions occur close enough in both time and space. The double-strand DNA molecule, essential for cellular replication, is thought to be the critical target for radiation-induced damage. For high-LET radiation, such as neutrons or alpha particles, the concentration of transferred energy is such that both sublesions are usually produced by one track or "hit," implying a biological response proportional to dose; that is, a linear response.

For sparsely ionizing low-LET radiation, ionizations and any consequent sublesions will usually be distributed uniformly throughout the cell. The occurrence of two sublesions close together would be rare, with probability approximately proportional to the square of the dose, D^2; that is, two "hits" are required and a quadratic response would be expected. Low-LET radiation, however, is thought to have a high-LET component at the end of each track whose biologic effect should be proportional to dose.

For low-LET radiation, a general equation for biological effect is

$$I = c + a\mathrm{D} + b\mathrm{D}^2$$

where I is the incidence of the effect, c is the spontaneous rate, D is the radiation dose, and a and b are positive constants. This model appears to fit a wide range of studies on the induction of chromosome aberrations, point mutations, and other radiation effects on single cells, and some carcinogenic studies in animals (NCRP, 1980; UNSCEAR, 1986). Experimental studies with low-energy x-rays, however, do not conform to this biophysical model in that biological effects can be produced from single tracks that are too short to break separate strands on two independent chromosomes (NRPB, 1992b). Nonetheless, the linear-quadratic model has been applied to derive risk estimates from human studies (NAS, 1980; NIH, 1985). Recent analyses of atomic bomb survivor data found little reason to reject linearity for most cancers, except leukemia (NAS, 1990).

A further modification can be made to account for the possible competing effects of cell killing or inactivation, which prevents a cell from developing into a cancer (Mole, 1975; Major and Mole, 1978; UNSCEAR, 1986; NAS, 1990):

$$I = (c + a\mathrm{D} + b\mathrm{D}^2)\exp(-p\mathrm{D} - q\mathrm{D}^2)$$

where the exponential term, which predominates at high doses, corresponds to a decrease in incidence after some maximal value is reached. For low-LET radiation, the linear term predominates at very low doses, the quadratic at higher doses, and the exponential at very high doses.

Dose Rate. When exposures are protracted or separated in time, the contributions of D^2 become less and less important for both cancer induction and cell killing. It is generally found in experimental settings (Fig. 16–9) that lengthening the time over which a dose is delivered reduces the amount of cellular damage and cancer induction from low-LET radiations, related in part to the repair of damage (Upton et al, 1970; Han et al, 1980; Mole and Major, 1983; NCRP, 1980; Ullrich and Storer, 1979b; UNSCEAR, 1986, 1993). To estimate risks for persons exposed at low dose rates, various committees have recommended that a dose-rate effectiveness

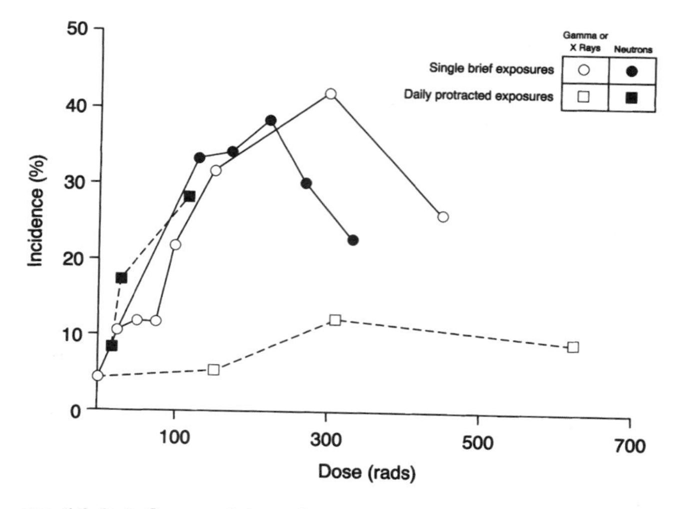

FIG. 16–9. Influence of dose, dose rate, and type of radiation on the cumulative incidence of myeloid leukemia in male RF mice. (Modified from Upton AC, et al, 1970, Radiat Res 41:467–491, p 476.)

factor (DREF) of between 2 and 10 should be used to scale down risk coefficients obtained from studies of brief exposure, such as among A-bomb survivors (NCRP, 1980; UNSCEAR, 1988). A DREF of 2.5 was used in the probability of causation tables (NIH, 1985), estimating cancer risks associated with space travel (NCRP, 1989), and estimating risks from continuous exposures to low doses (NAS, 1980). Except for leukemia, a DREF was not incorporated in risk models employed by the BEIR V committee, although a preference for a value of about 2 was expressed (NAS, 1990). Other committees have assumed a DREF of 2 for radiation protection purposes (ICRP, 1991; NRPB, 1992b). There is no reason to believe, however, that a single DREF value is appropriate for every human cancer.

In experimental studies the induction of cancer by high-LET radiations has generally followed a linear dose response. Moreover, protraction and fractionation of dose tend not to decrease cancer risk but rather, especially at high total doses, to increase risk because of a reduction in the competing effect of cell killing and perhaps other factors (NCRP, 1980; UNSCEAR, 1986, 1993). An inverse dose-rate effect has also been suggested among underground miners exposed to radon (Lubin et al, 1990a), although such an effect would not be expected at domestic levels (Brenner et al, 1993). Recently, α-particle irradiation of mouse stem cells was linked to chromosome aberrations in progeny cells that were not apparent until after 10 to 13 cell divisions, suggesting a form of "transmissible genetic instability" not seen after x-ray irradiation (Kadhim et al, 1992). Similar studies of human bone marrow cells indicate that α-particles can induce transmissible genetic instability (Kadhim et al, 1994). The implications of such observations are not clear but add an additional complexity to risk predictions following low-dose high-LET exposures.

There is no reason to believe that only one type of dose-response curve is appropriate to describe the induction of all human cancers. Experiments in mice demonstrate, for example, the diversity of dose-response relationships possible for even the same class of tumors: linear for myeloid leukemia; curvilinear for thymic lymphoma; and a negative (or protective) response for reticulum cell sarcoma (Ullrich and Storer, 1979a). The influence of carcinogenic modifiers, including genetic susceptibility, is likely reflected in the wide range of dose-response relationships seen for different cancers and for different species with respect to both low-LET and high-LET radiation (NCRP, 1980; UNSCEAR, 1986; 1993).

Modifiers. Initiation following radiation exposure appears to be a common cellular event (NAS, 1990), and secondary factors that facilitate transformation might offer a way to control carcinogenesis (Little, 1981, 1993). After initiation, at least one other event seems necessary for irradiated cells to become malignant; this second event may occur randomly during cellular growth (Kennedy and Little, 1984). Nutritional and environmental factors, hormones, and cigarette smoking, among others, have been shown to markedly influence the process of radiation carcinogenesis. The phorbol ester tumor promoter TPA, for example, can greatly enhance and change the shape of the dose-response curve for radiation-induced cellular transformation (Kennedy et al, 1978). Other agents, such as selenium or the retinoids (or vitamin A analogues), suppress radiogenic transformation (NAS, 1990). Hormonal stimulation appears necessary for mammary tumor development in rats after an initiating event has occurred (Sukumar et al, 1991). It is interesting, in this respect, that excess breast cancer risk among A-bomb survivors exposed after age 40 has been relatively low (Tokunaga et al, 1994), and that a dose-related excess of preneoplastic lesions was observed in autopsy tissue from women exposed during their 40s; that is, shortly before menopause (Tokunaga et al, 1993). Terminal differentiation following exposure may limit the capacity of radiation-initiated breast cells to progress to cancer, as demonstrated experimentally (Clifton and Crowley, 1978) and as suggested by the observation that A-bomb survivors exposed during childhood or adolescence were at significantly less risk of radiation-related breast cancer if they subsequently experienced a full-term pregnancy (Land et al, 1994).

Oncogenes. Advances in molecular biology have uncovered oncogenes and tumor-suppressor genes in human cells that, when mutated or deleted, can result in cancer through a multi-step process (Weinberg, 1989). Oncogenes are thought to arise from activated proto-oncogenes, that is, normal genes that help a cell divide. Tumor-suppressor genes are believed, when inactivated, to lose their normal function of regulating cell growth. Conceivably, radiation could cause the genetic changes that activate or inactivate these genes (Guerrero et al, 1984; Weichselbaum et al, 1989). The breakage and repair of chromosomes, including the insertion or translocation of genetic material, might be one mechanism for radiation to modify the function of these genes. Interestingly, unique "molecular signatures" such as radiation-induced deletions in the *p53* tumor-suppressor gene have been implicated in the etiology of radon (Vahakangas et al, 1992; Taylor et al, 1994) and x-ray (de Benedetti et al, 1996) related lung cancers. Similarly, certain *p53* mutations appear more common in UV-associated skin cancer (Brash et al, 1991). Deletion or mutation of the *Rb* gene in patients with retinoblastoma likely contributes to the enormous risk of osteosarcoma of the orbit seen after radiotherapy (Eng et al, 1993). Inactivation of the *Rb* and *p53* tumor suppressor genes may contribute to other types of radiation-induced sarcomas (Brachman et al, 1991). Patients with the Li-Fraumeni syndrome who inherit a mutated *p53* allele also appear to be at high risk for radiation-induced cancers (Li et al, 1988).

Repair. Mammalian cells are capable of repairing potentially lethal damage caused by radiation, and the risk of cancer induction also may be influenced by an effective repair mechanism (Elkind and Han, 1979; Han et al, 1980). A genetic defect in patients with xeroderma pigmentosum, for example, reduces cellular capability to repair UV-related DNA damage, and skin cancers can result (NAS, 1990). Recently it was reported that the *p53* tumor-suppressor gene plays an important role in G_1 arrest—the delay phase before a cell divides when the cell checks for and repairs DNA damage (Kastan et al, 1992). Following DNA damage from x-rays, normal cells enter G_1 arrest only after the production of *p53* protein is increased. Cells incapable of producing *p53* proteins, such as cells from patients with ataxia telangiectasia, are extremely sensitive to the impact of radiation and chemotherapy; genetic damage is not repaired, and either the cell dies or flawed genetic information is passed on to subsequent cell generations. Since mutation of the *p53* gene is the most common known genetic defect in human cancer, it is conceivable that radiation damage to *p53* genes, or to other genes that affect *p53* protein production, contributes to the carcinogenic process by limiting the time a cell stays in G_1 to repair mutations.

While physical models reasonably describe the occurrence of some biological effects following radiation exposure, they are nonetheless simplifications of a complex carcinogenic process. Cancer develops as a sequence of cellular events, and it is clear that initiation, promotion, and progression are all important components of this process (Upton, 1987). Inactivation of tumor-suppressor and/or other genes by radiation likely contributes to cancer development, but may represent only one of several steps necessary for a cell to become transformed. The number of steps required appears to vary, probably just two mutational lesions for childhood cancers such as retinoblastoma and probably five to 10 for adult tumors such as colorectal cancer. Radiation likely acts as an early stage initiator but perhaps not in all circumstances. Tissue proliferation, promoting factors, and misrepair of genetic damage also play important roles in the carcinogenic process. More sophisticated understanding of carcinogenesis through molecular biology should result in more precise estimates of risk at low doses and low dose rates.

Modeling Risk: Age, Time, and Population

Age at exposure is a strong determinant of future cancer risk, but the reasons appear complex. The growing child is at highest risk for many cancers, perhaps because tissue proliferation somehow converts (or fixes) the initial lesion into genetic alterations that are transmitted to daughter cells, or proliferation somehow promotes the progression of altered cells into cancer cells. Breast cancer, for which risk is greatest following exposure during childhood or adolescence and least for exposure after age 40, suggests an age-dependent opportunity for promotion of radiation-initiated cells by hormonal stimulation (Tokunaga et al, 1994). For the most part, however, modeling of risk by age at exposure is done on an ad hoc basis (NIH, 1985; NAS, 1990).

Modeling of risk as a function of *time* following exposure is often done to estimate lifetime risk based on limited periods of observation. Relevant questions concern how soon after exposure excess risk begins and whether it persists until the end of life. Estimated lifetime risks differ according to whether radiation is assumed to add to or multiply the baseline risk, since for most cancers the baseline risk increases with increasing age. Recent studies have tended to support constancy of relative measures of risk and to reject constancy of absolute measures of risk over time after exposure, for fixed ages at exposure (NAS, 1990). There are, however, notable exceptions. British spondylitics show a marked diminution of risk 25 years after exposure, particularly for lung cancer (Darby et al, 1987b; Weiss et al, 1994). Lung cancer RR among underground miners declines after cessation of work, and a step function was recently used to model risk over time (NAS, 1988). The RR of breast cancer decreased with time in one large series of tuberculosis patients (Miller et al, 1989). RRs for lung and breast cancer mortality were accordingly modeled by the NAS BEIR V committee to decrease with time after reaching some maximal value (NAS, 1990). Lifetime risk projections based on limited periods of observation must be interpreted with caution, however, especially when applying the relatively high RRs seen following childhood exposures to older ages.

Modeling for the purpose of transporting estimated excess risk from one *population* to another is even less developed than that for projecting risk forward in time. There is a tendency to assume that either absolute or relative measures of risk are the same in the two populations, but this is not always straightforward (NAS, 1990). For example, absolute measures of breast cancer risk appear similar for Japanese A-bomb survivors and irradiated Western women (Land et al, 1980), whereas relative measures of stomach cancer risk appear similar (Griem et al, 1994). These models are simplifications of a complex process in which other causes and modifying factors, that vary by age and among populations, influence the expression of radiogenic cancer.

Estimation of Cancer Risks: Epidemiological Studies

Epidemiological studies have conclusively linked high-dose radiation to increased cancer risks. Estimates of risk for low-level exposures, however, are based on uncertain extrapolations and require assumptions about the shape of the dose-effect relationship and about the mechanisms of radiation carcinogenesis. These assumptions are often guided by experimental investigations and radiobiology theory. Similar to other epidemiological investigations, however, studies of radiogenic cancers are also susceptible to the problems of inappropriate comparison groups; biases of selection, observation and response; multiple comparisons; cluster analyses; inadequate control of confounding factors; inadequate measures of dose and cancer outcome; and low statistical power due to small numbers of excess cancers at low doses (Land, 1980; Beebe, 1984; UNSCEAR, 1988, 1994; MacMahon, 1989; NAS, 1990).

An appropriate comparison group is important. Comparisons with general population rates could be misleading when the irradiated population is ill, because the disease itself could be related to the occurrence of cancer, and other competing risks or treatments could influence subsequent cancer incidence (such as chemotherapy among cancer patients). Many employed populations are also self-selected, with different expectations of disease than the general population. Interpretation should be made cautiously, however, when an elevated "risk" is related more to a decreased incidence in the comparison group than an increased incidence among the exposed.

More thorough case-finding among an irradiated population than among the general population used to compute expected numbers could bias study results in a positive direction (ascertainment bias). Special screening of exposed but not nonexposed persons is an extreme but not uncommon example of observational bias. It could, for example, account for many of the excess benign tumors seen in persons with histories of head and neck irradiation during childhood. In case-control studies of cancer and diagnostic x-rays, a respondent might be a more reliable witness if he or she recently developed a cancer (response bias).

Radiation dose should be accurately estimated, and dose-response gradients add meaningfully to causal interpretations. If doses are not known for individuals, an excess in a presumably low-dose group could be concentrated in those few individuals who received high doses. When the radiogenic response is low, chance events are also more likely to be misinterpreted, and the influence of confounding factors more worrisome (Beebe, 1984). Care should be exercised in performing statistical tests on investigations generated because of an apparent cluster of disease in the study population that prompted the investigation. The statistical problems of cluster analysis are complex, especially in light of possible gerrymandered time and geographic groupings. When multiple comparisons are made, investigators should be careful not to over-interpret unexpected findings.

The confounding influence of other carcinogenic exposures should be evaluated. Estimates of lung cancer risks obtained without adjusting for smoking or estimates of occupational risks obtained without controlling for toxic chemical exposures may be misleading. Other radiation exposures, such as excessive medical x-rays or environmental background radiation, are not often considered in low-dose studies, despite the possibility that their contribution to the total radiation burden may be greater than the exposure under study (Spiers, 1979).

It is important that exposed populations be followed for substantial periods of time to detect excesses of solid tumors. If the A-bomb survivor studies had been terminated after about 15 years, the leukemia effect would have been observed but not the solid tumor effect. Evidence that the exposure precedes the disease is obviously important. In the case of diagnostic radiation and adult leukemia, however, it was likely that many x-rays occurred during the early stages of cancer when symptoms were being evaluated but before any diagnosis was actually made or onset recognized. Findings should be consistent with other studies. Excesses in sites not frequently seen after radiation, such as prostate cancer or Hodgkin's disease, in the absence of elevations in leukemia or other sensitive sites, should be interpreted cautiously.

There are substantial difficulties in studying directly the carcinogenic effects of very small radiation doses, such as impracticably large study size requirements and the inability to control for other factors that influence cancer incidence (Beebe, 1984). An unfortunate consequence of small study sizes (and in studies of cancer and low radiation dose, one million persons may be a small study size) is that when a positive result is obtained (and reported), it is likely to be mainly the result of random variation and, if so, must yield an overestimate of risk (Land, 1980). Further, because positive studies appear more likely to be written up and published than negative studies, such reporting bias might operate in studies of low-dose radiation, as seems to be the case for nonionizing radiation (NRPB, 1992a).

Epidemiological methods may be capable of directly

detecting RRs perhaps as low as 1.3–1.4 (ie, 30%–40% relative excesses). However, the RRs of interest following low doses of radiation (1–10 cGy) are on the order of 1.01 to 1.05. Thus not much should be anticipated from direct observations at 1 cGy (1 rad), and indirect approaches must be used to estimate low-dose effects. Such approaches include studies of populations exposed to a wide range of doses, both low and high, and the development of models to interpolate the effects at high and moderate doses to those at low doses.

FUTURE RESEARCH

Epidemiological studies of irradiated human populations should focus on producing refined estimates of cancer risk due to low-level exposure. Studies of populations receiving a distribution of doses, both low level and high level, should receive highest priority because (1) such populations are rare and it is important that they be thoroughly studied while there is an opportunity to do so; (2) estimates of risks are obtainable with reasonable expenditures of resources; and (3) the possibility for confounding by factors other than radiation is minimized.

Studies of populations exposed to high doses are also valuable because many questions about age effects, tissue sensitivity, time response, and the interaction of radiation with other factors can be addressed. Populations exposed to fractionated or protracted radiation over long periods should be pursued, especially if cumulative levels of more than 25 cGy (rad) are reached. Separation of ionizing events in time likely simulates spatial separation of events at low doses, and any resulting dose response should be linear and directly applicable to estimation of low-level effects.

Current issues or opportunities include clarification of the level of risk from residential radon; comprehensive evaluations of populations exposed to radiation from Chernobyl and Chelyabinsk; pooling data of worker and patient studies; creation of national registries of radiation workers, especially in the utility industry; clarification of the role genetic susceptibility might play; and identification of any radiation fingerprints or signatures in tumor tissue.

Because of the multifactorial nature of carcinogenesis, studies should be encouraged that integrate biochemical and molecular measures of response (Langlois et al, 1987; Elkind et al, 1991). Such studies are needed to provide insights into the mechanisms of carcinogenesis, and to help in the setting of guidelines for occupational, medical, and environmental exposures to radiation.

REFERENCES

ABELSON PH. 1991. Mineral dusts and radon in uranium mines. Science 254:777.

ALAVANJA MCR, BROWNSON RC, LUBIN JH. et al. 1994. Residential radon exposure and lung cancer among nonsmoking women. J Natl Cancer Inst 86:1829–1837.

ALAVANJA MCR, BROWNSON RC, BENICHOU J, et al. 1995. Attributable risk of lung cancer in lifetime nonsmokers and long-term ex-smokers (Missouri, United States). Cancer Causes Control 6:209–216.

ANDERSSON M, STORM HH. 1992. Cancer incidence among Danish Thorotrast-exposed patients. J Natl Cancer Inst 84:1318–1325.

ANDERSSON M, CARTENSEN B, VISFELDT J. 1993. Leukemia and other related hematological disorders among Danish patients exposed to Thorotrast. Radiat Res 134:224–233.

ANDERSSON M, VYBERG M, VISFELDT J, et al. 1994. Primary liver tumors among Danish patients exposed to Thorotrast. Radiat Res 137:262–273.

ANDERSSON M, WALLIN H, JONSSON M, et al. 1995. Lung carcinoma and malignant mesothelioma in patients exposed to Thorotrast: incidence, histology and p53 status, Int J Cancer 63:1–7.

AUVINEN A, HAKAMA M, ARVELA H, et al. 1994. Fallout from Chernobyl and incidence of childhood leukaemia in Finland, 1976–92. Br Med J 309:151–154.

AXELSON O, EDLING C, KLING H. 1979. Lung cancer and residency—a case-referent study on the possible impact of exposure to radon and its daughters in dwellings. Scand J Work Environ Health 5:10–15.

BAVERSTOCK KF, PAPWORTH DG. 1989. The UK radium luminiser survey. *In*: Risks from Radium and Thorotrast. Taylor DM, Mays CW, Gerber GB, Thomas RG (eds). BIR Report 21. London, Br Inst Radiol, pp 72–76.

BEEBE GW. 1984. A methologic assessment of radiation epidemiology studies. Health Phys 46:745–762.

BERAL V, FRASER P, CARPENTER L, et al. 1988. Mortality of employees of the Atomic Weapons Establishment. Br Med J 297:757–770.

BERK PD, GOLDBERG JD, SILVERSTEIN MN, et al. 1981. Increased incidence of acute leukemia in polycythemia vera associated with chlorambucil therapy. N Engl J Med 304:441–447.

BHATIA S, ROBISON LL, OBERLIN O, et al. 1996. Breast cancer and other second neoplasms after childhood Hodgkin's disease. N Engl J Med 334:745–751.

BIGBEE WL, JENSEN RH, RAHU M, et al. 1996. Glycophorin A biodosimetry of Chernobyl cleanup workers from the Baltic countries. Br Med J 312:1078–1079.

BITHELL JF, STEWART AM. 1975. Pre-natal irradiation and childhood malignancy: a review of the British data from the Oxford Survey. Br J Cancer 31:271–287.

BITHELL JF, STILLER CA. 1988. A new calculation of the carcinogenic risk of obstetric X-raying. Stat Med 7:857–864.

BITHELL JF, DUTTON SJ, NEARY NM. 1994. Distribution of childhood leukaemias and non-Hodgkin's lymphomas near nuclear installations in England and Wales. Br Med J 309:501–505.

BLACK D. 1984. Investigation of the possible increased incidence of cancer in West Cumbria. Report of the Independent Advisory Group. London, Her Majesty's Stationery Office.

BLOT WJ, AKIBA S, KATO H. 1984. Ionizing radiation and lung cancer: a review including preliminary results from a case-control study among A-bomb survivors. *In*: *Atomic Bomb Survivor Data: Utilization and Analysis*, Prentice RL, Thompson DJ (eds). Philadelphia, SIAM, pp 235–248.

BLOT WJ, XU Z-Y, BOICE JD JR, et al. 1990. Indoor radon and lung cancer in China. J Natl Cancer Inst 82:1025–1030.

BOICE JD JR. 1991. Epidemiologic studies of radioactively contaminated environments and cancer clusters. NCRP Proc 12:94–116.

BOICE JD JR. 1993a. Second cancer after Hodgkin's disease—the price of success? J Natl Cancer Inst 85:4–5.

BOICE JD JR. 1993b. Leukemia risk in Thorotrast patients (letter) Radiat Res 136:301–302.

BOICE JD JR, FRAUMENI JF JR (EDS). 1984. *Radiation Carcinogenesis: Epidemiology and Biological Significance*. New York: Raven Press, pp 1–473.

BOICE JD, HUTCHISON GB. 1980. Leukemia in women following radiotherapy for cervical cancer: Ten-year follow-up of an international study. J Natl Cancer Inst 65:115–129.

BOICE JD, LAND CE. 1979. Adult leukemia following diagnostic X-rays? Am J Public Health 69:137–145.

BOICE JD JR, LAND CE. 1982. Ionizing radiation. *In: Cancer Epidemiology and Prevention*, Schottenfeld D, Fraumeni JF Jr (eds). New York, Saunders, pp 231–253.

BOICE JD JR, LAND CE, SHORE RE, et al. 1979. Risk of breast cancer following low-dose radiation exposure. Radiology 131:589–597.

BOICE JD JR, DAY NE, ANDERSEN A, et al. 1985a. Second cancers following radiation treatment for cervical cancer: an international collaboration among cancer registries. J Natl Cancer Inst 74:955–975.

BOICE JD JR, STORM HH, CURTIS RE, et al (eds). 1985b. Multiple primary cancers in Connecticut and Denmark. Natl Cancer Inst Monogr 68. Washington D.C., U.S. Govt Print Off, pp 1–437.

BOICE JD JR, BLETTNER M, KLEINERMAN RA, et al. 1987. Radiation dose and leukemia risk in patients treated for cancer of the cervix. J Natl Cancer Inst 79:1295–1311.

BOICE JD JR. 1988a. Carcinogenesis—a synopsis of human experience with external exposure in medicine. Health Phys 55:621–630.

BOICE JD JR, ENGHOLM G, KLEINERMAN RA, et al. 1988b. Radiation dose and second cancer risk in patients treated for cancer of the cervix. Radiat Res 116:3–55.

BOICE JD JR, BLETTNER M, KLEINERMAN RA, et al. 1989. Radiation dose and breast cancer risk in patients treated for cancer of the cervix. Int J Cancer 44:7–16.

BOICE JD JR, MORIN MM, GLASS AG, et al. 1991b. Diagnostic X-ray procedures and risk of leukemia, lymphoma and multiple myeloma. JAMA 265:1290–1294.

BOICE JD JR, PRESTON D, DAVIS FG, et al. 1991c. Frequent chest X-ray fluoroscopy and breast cancer incidence among tuberculosis patients in Massachusetts. Radiat Res 125:214–222.

BOICE JD JR, HARVEY E, BLETTNER M, et al. 1992a. Cancer in the contralateral breast after radiotherapy for breast cancer. N Engl J Med 326:781–785.

BOICE JD JR, MILLER RW. 1992b. Risk of breast cancer in ataxia-telangiectasia. (Letter). N Engl J Med 326:1357–1358.

BOICE JD JR, MANDEL JS, DOODY MM, et al. 1992c. A health survey of radiologic technologists. Cancer 69:586–598.

BOICE JD JR, MANDEL JS, DOODY MM. 1995. Breast cancer among radiological technologists. JAMA 274:394–401.

BOICE JD JR, LINET M. 1994. Chernobyl, childhood cancer and chromosome 21. (Editorial) Br Med J 309:139–140.

BOIVIN J-F, HUTCHISON GB, EVANS FB, et al. 1986. Leukemia after radiotherapy for first primary cancers of various anatomic sites. Am J Epidemiol 123:993–1003.

BRACHMAN DG, HALLAHAN DE, BECKETT MA, et al. 1991. *p53* gene mutations and abnormal retinoblastoma protein in radiation-induced human sarcomas. Cancer Res 51:6393–6396.

BRASH DE, RUDOLPH JA, SIMON JA, et al. 1991. A role for sunlight in skin cancer: UV-induced *p53* mutations in squamous cell carcinoma. Proc Natl Acad Sci USA 88:10124–10128.

BRENNER DJ, HALL EJ, RANDERS-PEHRSON G, et al. 1993. Mechanistic considerations on the dose-rate/LET dependence of oncogenic transformation by ionizing radiations. Radiat Res 133:365–369.

BRENNER DJ. 1994. The significance of dose rate in assessing the hazards of domestic radon exposure. Radiat Res 67:76–79.

BRESLOW NE, NORKOOL PA, OLSHAN A, et al. 1988. Second malignant neoplasms in survivors of Wilms' tumor: a report from the National Wilms' Tumor Study. J Natl Cancer Inst 80:592–595.

BUCKLEY JD, ROBISON LL, SWOTINSKY R, et al. 1989. Occupational exposures of parents of children with acute nonlymphocytic leukemia: a report from the Children Cancer Study Group. Cancer Res 49:4030–4037.

BURKHART W, KELLERER AM (EDS). 1994. Radiation exposure in the Southern Urals. Sci Total Environ 142:1–125.

CALDWELL GG, KELLEY D, ZACK M, et al. 1983. Mortality and cancer frequency among military nuclear test (SMOKY) participants, 1957 through 1979. JAMA 250:620–624.

CARDIS E, GILBERT ES, CARPENTER L, et al. 1995. Effects of low doses and low dose rates of external ionizing radiation: cancer mortality among nuclear industry workers in three countries. Radial Res 142:117–132.

CARPENTER L, HIGGINS C, DOUGLAS A, et al. 1994. Combined analysis of mortality in three United Kingdom nuclear industry workforces, 1946–1988. Radiat Res 138:224–238.

CHECKOWAY H, MATHEW RM, SHY CM, et al. 1985. Radiation, work experience, and cause specific mortality among workers at an energy research laboratory. Br J Ind Med 42:525–533.

CHMELEVSKY D, KELLERER AM, LAND CE, et al. 1988. Time and dose dependency of bone-sarcomas in patients injected with radium-224. Radiat Environ Biophys 27:103–114.

CLIFTON KH, CROWLEY J. 1978. Effects of radiation type and role of glucocorticoids, gonadectomy and thyroidectomy in mammary tumor induction in MLT-grafted rats. Cancer Res 38:1507–1513.

CONARD RA. 1984. Late radiation effects in Marshall Islanders exposed to fallout twenty-eight years ago. *In: Radiation Carcinogenesis: Epidemiology and Biological Significance*. Boice JD Jr, Fraumeni JF Jr (eds). New York, Raven Press, pp 57–71.

COOK-MOZAFFARI PJ, ASHWOOD FL, VINCENT T, et al. 1987. Cancer incidence and mortality in the vicinity of nuclear installations, England and Wales, 1959–1980. OPCS Studies on Medical and Population Subjects 51. London, Her Majesty's Stationery Office.

COOK-MOZAFFARI P, DARBY S, DOLL R. 1989. Cancer near potential sites of nuclear installations. Lancet 2:1145–1147.

COURT BROWN WM, DOLL R, HILL AB. 1960. Incidence of leukemia after exposure to diagnostic radiation in utero. Br Med J 2:1539–1545.

CRILE G JR, ESSELSTYN CB JR, HAWK WA. 1979. Needle biopsy in the diagnosis of thyroid nodules appearing after radiation. N Engl J Med 301:997–999.

CURTIS RE, BOICE JD JR, KLEINERMAN RA, et al. 1985. Summary: multiple primary cancers in Connecticut, 1935–82. Natl Cancer Inst Monogr 68:219–242.

CURTIS RE, BOICE JD JR, STOVALL M, et al. 1992. Risk of leukemia after chemotherapy and radiation treatment for breast cancer. N Engl J Med 326:1745–1751.

CURTIS RE, BOICE JD JR, STOVALL M, et al. 1994. Relation of leukemia risk to radiation dose after cancer of the uterine corpus. J Natl Cancer Inst 86:1315–1324.

CUZICK J, DESTAVOLA B. 1988. Multiple myeloma—a case-control study. Br J Cancer 57:516–520.

DARBY SC, DOLL R. 1987. Fallout, radiation doses near Dounreay, and childhood leukaemia. Br Med J 294:603–607.

DARBY SC, DOLL R, GILL SK, et al. 1987. Long term mortality after a single treatment course with X-rays in patients treated for ankylosing spondylitis. Br J Cancer 55:179–190.

DARBY SC, OLSEN JH, DOLL R, et al. 1992. Trends in childhood leukaemia in the Nordic countries in relation to fallout from atmospheric nuclear weapons testing. Br Med J 304:1005–1009.

DARBY SC, KENDALL GM, FELL TP, et al. 1993. Further follow-up of mortality and incidence of cancer in man from the United Kingdom who participated in the United Kingdom's atmospheric nuclear weapon tests and experimental programmes. Br Med J 307:1530–1535.

DARBY SC, REEVES G, KEY T, et al. 1994. Mortality in a cohort of women given x-ray therapy for metropathia haemorrhagica. Int J Cancer 56:793–801.

DAVIS FG, BOICE JD JR, HRUBEC Z, et al. 1989. Cancer mortality in a radiation-exposed cohort of Massachusetts tuberculosis patients. Cancer Res 49:6130–6136.

DE BENEDETTI VMG, TRAVIS LB, WELSH JA, et al. 1996. *p53* mutations in lung cancer following radiation therapy for Hodgkin's disease. Cancer Epidemiol Biomarkers Prev 5:93–98.

DE VATHAIRE F, FRANÇOIS P, SCHWEISGUTH O, et al. 1988. Irradiated neuroblastoma in childhood as potential risk factor for subsequent thyroid tumor. Lancet 2:455.

DE VATHAIRE F, FRANÇOIS P, HILL C, et al. 1989. Role of radiotherapy and chemotherapy in the risk of second malignant neoplasms after cancer in childhood. Br J Cancer 59:792–796.

DE VATHAIRE F, FRAGU P, FRANÇOIS P, et al. 1993. Long-term effects on the thyroid of irradiation for skin angiomas in childhood. Radiat Res 133:381–386.

DIAMOND EL, SCHMERLER H, LILIENFELD AM. 1973. The relationship of intrauterine radiation to subsequent mortality and development of leukemia in children. Am J Epidemiol 97:283–313.

DOLL R, EVANS HJ, DARBY SC. 1994. Paternal exposure not to blame. Nature 367:678–680.

DRAPER GJ, SANDERS BM, KINGSTON JE. 1986. Second primary neoplasms in patients with retinoblastoma. Br J Cancer 53:661–671.

DRAPER GJ, STILLER CA, CARTWRIGHT RA, et al. 1993. Cancer in Cumbria and in the vicinity of the Sellafield nuclear installation, 1963–90. Br Med J 306:89–94.

EDMONDS CJ, SMITH T. 1986. The long-term hazards of the treatment of thyroid cancer with radioiodine. Br J Radiol 59:45–51.

ELKIND MM, HAN A. 1979. Neoplastic transformation and dose fractionation: does repair of damage play a role? Radiat Res 79:233–240.

ELKIND MM, BENJAMIN SA, SINCLAIR WK, et al. 1991. Oncogenic mechanisms in radiation-induced cancer. Cancer Res 51:2740–2747.

ENG C, LI FP, ABRAMSON DH, et al. 1993. Mortality from second tumors among long-term survivors of retinoblastoma. J Natl Cancer Inst 85:1121–1128.

EVANS HJ. 1990. Gardner report. Leukaemia and radiation. Nature 345:16–17.

EVANS JS, WENNBERG JE, MCNEIL BJ. 1986. The influence of diagnostic radiography on the incidence of breast cancer and leukemia. N Engl J Med 315:810–815.

EZAKI H, ISHIMARU T, HAYASHI Y, et al. 1986. Cancer of the thyroid and salivary glands. In: *Cancer in Atomic Bomb Survivors*, Shigematsu I, Kagan A (eds). GANN Monograph on Cancer Research No. 32. Tokyo, Plemun Press, pp 129–142.

FAVUS MJ, SCHNEIDER AB, STACHURA ME, et al. 1976. Thyroid cancer occurring as a late consequence of head-and-neck irradiation: evaluation of 1056 patients. N Engl J Med 294:1019–1025.

FORMAN D, COOK-MOZAFFARI P, DARBY S, et al. 1987. Cancer near nuclear installations. Nature 329:499–505.

FROME EL, CRAGLE DL, MCLAIN RW. 1990. Poisson regression analysis of the mortality among a cohort of World War II nuclear industry workers. Radiat Res 123:138–152.

FRY RJM, SINCLAIR WK. 1987. New dosimetry of atomic bomb radiations. Lancet 2:845–848.

FÜRST CJ, LUNDELL M, HOLM L-E, et al. 1988. Cancer incidence after radiotherapy for skin hemangioma: a retrospective cohort study in Sweden. J Natl Cancer Inst 80:1387–1392.

GARDNER MJ, HALL AJ, DOWNES S, et al. 1987. Follow-up study of children born to mothers resident in Seascale, West Cumbria (birth cohort). Br Med J 295:822–827.

GARDNER MJ, SNEE MP, HALL AJ, et al. 1990. Results of case-control study of leukaemia and lymphoma among young people near Sellafield nuclear plant in West Cumbria. Br Med J 300:423–429.

GIBSON R, GRAHAM S, LILIENFELD A, et al. 1972. Irradiation in the epidemiology of leukemia among adults. J Natl Cancer Inst 48:301–311.

GILBERT ES. 1992. Mortality of workers at the Oak Ridge National Laboratory. Health Phys 62:260–261.

GILBERT ES, CRAGLE DL, WIGGS LD, et al. 1993a. Updated analyses of combined mortality data for workers at the Hanford Site, Oak Ridge National Laboratory, and Rocky Flats Weapons Plant. Radiat Res 136:408–421.

GILBERT ES, OMOHUNDRO JA, BUCHANAN JA, et al. 1993b. Mortality of workers at the Hanford site: 1945–1986. Health Phys 64:577–590.

GLÖBEL B, GLÖBEL H, OBERHAUSEN E. 1984. Epidemiologic studies on patients with iodine-131 diagnostic and therapy. In: Radiation-risk-protection, vol II, Kaul A, Neider R, Pensko J, et al (eds). IRPA. Köln: Fachverband für Strahlenschutz eV., pp 565–568.

GOLDMAN MB, MALOOF F, MONSON RR, et al. 1988. Radioactive iodine therapy and breast cancer. A follow-up study of hyperthyroid women. Am J Epidemiol 127:969–980.

GRAHAM S, LEVIN ML, LILIENFELD AM, et al. 1966. Preconception, intrauterine and postnatal irradiation as related to leukemia. Natl Cancer Inst Monogr 19:347–371.

GREENBERG ER, ROSNER B, HENNEKENS C, et al. 1985. An investigation of bias in a study of nuclear shipyard workers. Am J Epidemiol 121:301–308.

GREENE MH, YOUNG RC, MERRILL JM, et al. 1983. Evidence of a treatment dose response in acute nonlymphocytic leukemias which occur after therapy of non-Hodgkin's lymphoma. Cancer Res 43:1891–1898.

GREENLAND S, ROBINS J. 1994. Invited commentary; ecologic studies—biases, misconceptions, and counterexamples. Am J Epidemiol 139:747–760.

GRIBBIN MA, WEEKS JL, HOWE GR. 1993. Cancer mortality (1956–1985) among male employees of Atomic Energy Canada Limited with respect to occupational exposure to external low-linear-energy-transfer ionizing radiation. Radiat Res 133:375–380.

GRIEM ML, KLEINERMAN RA, BOICE JD JR, et al. 1994. Cancer following radiotherapy for peptic ulcer. J Natl Cancer Inst 86:842–849.

GUERRERO I, VILLASANTE A, CORCES V, et al. 1984. Activation of a c-K-ras oncogene by somatic mutation in mouse lymphomas induced by gamma radiation. Science 225:1159–1162.

GUILMETTE RA, MAYS DM, EDS. 1992. Total body evaluation of a Thorotrast patient. Health Phys 63:1–100.

HALL P, HOLM L-E, LUNDELL G, et al. 1991. Cancer risks in thyroid cancer patients. Br J Cancer 64:159–163.

HALL P, BERG G, BJELKENGREN G, et al. 1992a. Cancer mortality after iodine-131 therapy for hyperthyroidism. Int J Cancer 50:886–890.

HALL P, BOICE JD JR, BERG G, et al. 1992b. Leukaemia incidence after iodine-131 exposure. Lancet 340:1–4.

HALL P, MATTSON A, BIOCE JD JR, et al. 1996. Thyroid cancer following diagnostic iodine-131 exposure. Radiat Res 145:86–92.

HAMILTON TE, VAN BELLE G, LOGERFO JP. 1987. Thyroid neoplasia in Marshall Islanders exposed to nuclear fallout. JAMA 258:629–635.

HAN A, HILL CK, ELKIND MM. 1980. Repair of cell killing and neoplastic transformation at reduced dose rates of ^{60}Co γ-rays. Cancer Res 40:3328–3332, 1980.

HANCOCK SL, TUCKER MA, HOPPE RT. 1993. Breast cancer after treatment of Hodgkin's disease. J Natl Cancer Inst 85:25–31.

HARVEY EB, BOICE JD JR, HONEYMAN M, et al. 1985. Prenatal X-ray exposure and childhood cancer in twins. N Engl J Med 312:541–545.

HATCH MC, BEYEA J, NIEVES JW, et al. 1990. Cancer near the Three Mile Island nuclear plant: radiation emissions. Am J Epidemiol 132:397–412.

HAWKINS MM, DRAPER GJ, KINGSTON JE: 1987. Incidence of second primary tumours among childhood cancer survivors. Br J Cancer 56:339–347.

HAWKINS MM, KINNIER-WILSON LM, STOVALL MA, et al. 1992. Epipodophyllotoxins, alkylating agents, and radiation and risk of secondary leukaemia after childhood cancer. Br Med J 304:951–958.

HAWKINS MM, KINNIER WILSON LM, BURTON HS, et al. 1996. Radiotherapy, alkylating agents, and risk of bone cancer after childhood cancer. J Natl Cancer Inst 88:270–278.

HAZEN RW, PIFER JW, TAYOOKA ET, et al. 1966. Neoplasms following irradiation of the head. Cancer Res 26:305–311.

HEMPELMANN LH, HALL WJ, PHILLIPS M, et al. 1975. Neoplasms in persons treated with X-rays in infancy: fourth survey in 20 years. J Natl Cancer Inst 55:519–530.

HENSHAW DL, EATOUGH JP, RICHARDSON RB. 1990. Radon as a causative factor in induction of myeloid leukaemia and other cancers. Lancet 335:1008–1012.

HILDRETH NG, SHORE RE, HEMPELMANN LH, et al. 1985. Risk of extrathyroid tumors following radiation treatment in infancy for thymic enlargement. Radiat Res 102:378–391.

HILDRETH NG, SHORE RE, DVORETSKY PM. 1989. The risk of breast cancer after irradiation of the thymus in infancy. N Engl J Med 321:1281–1284.

HILL C, LAPLANCHE A. 1990. Overall mortality and cancer mortality around French nuclear sites. Nature 347:755–757.

HJALMARS U, KULLDORFF M, GUSTAFSSON G. 1994. For the Swedish Child Leukaemia Group. Fallout from the Chernobyl accident and risk of acute leukaemia in Sweden. Br Med J 309:154–157.

HOFFMAN D. 1984. Effects of I-131 therapy in the United States. *In: Radiation Carcinogenesis: Epidemiology and Biological Significance*, Boice JD Jr, Fraumeni JF Jr (eds). New York: Raven Press, pp 273–280.

HOFFMAN DA, LONSTEIN JE, MORIN MM, et al. 1989. Breast cancer in women with scoliosis exposed to multiple diagnostic X-rays. J Natl Cancer Inst 81:1307–1312.

HOHRYAKOV VF, ROMANOV SA. 1994. Lung cancer in radiochemical industry workers. Sci Total Environ 142:25–28.

HOLM L-E, WIKLUND KE, LUNDELL GE, et al. 1988. Thyroid cancer after diagnostic doses of iodine-131: a retrospective cohort study. J Natl Cancer Inst 80:1132–1138.

HOLM L-E, WIKLUND KE, LUNDELL GE, et al. 1989. Cancer risk in population examined with diagnostic doses of 131–I. J Natl Cancer Inst 81:302–306.

HOLM L-E, HALL P, WIKLUND KE, et al. 1991. Cancer risk after iodine-131 therapy for hyperthyroidism. J Natl Cancer Inst 83:1072–1077.

HORNUNG RW, MEINHARDT TJ. 1987. Quantitative risk assessment of lung cancer in U.S. uranium miners. Health Phys 52:417–430.

HOWE GR. 1995. Lung cancer mortality between 1950 and 1987 after exposure to fractionated moderate-dose–rate ionizing radiation in the Canadian fluocoscopy chart study and a comparison with lung cancer mortality in the atomic bomb survivor study. Radiat Res 142:295–304.

HOWE GR, NAIR RC, NEWCOMBE HB, et al. 1987. Lung cancer mortality (1950–80) in relation to radon daughter exposure in a cohort of workers at the Eldorado Port Radium uranium mine: possible modification of risk by exposure rate. J Natl Cancer Inst 79:1255–1260.

HOWE GR, CHIARELLI AM, LINDSAY JP. 1988. Components and modifiers of the healthy worker effect: evidence from three occupational cohorts and implications for industrial compensation. Am J Epidemiol 128:1364–1375.

HOWE GR, BURCH JD, CHIARELLI AM, et al. 1989. An exploratory case-control study of brain tumors in children. Cancer Res 49:4349–4352.

HUTCHISON GB, MACMAHON B, JABLON S, et al. 1979. Review of report by Mancuso, Stewart and Kneale of radiation exposure of Hanford workers. Health Phys 37:207–220.

ICHIMARU M, OHKITA T, ISHIMARU T. 1986. Leukemia, multiple myeloma, and malignant lymphoma. In: *Cancer in Atomic Bomb Survivors*, Shigematsu I, Kagan A (eds). GANN Monograph on Cancer Research No. 32. Tokyo, Plemun Press, pp 113–128.

ICRP (International Commission on Radiological Protection). 1991. 1990 Recommendation of the International Commission on Radiological Protection. Oxford: Pergamon Press.

INSKIP PD, BOICE JD JR. 1994. Radiotherapy-induced lung cancer among women who smoke (Editorial) Cancer 73:1541–1543.

INSKIP PD, EBY NL, COOKFAIR D, et al. 1994a. Serum estrogen and androgen levels following treatment for cervical cancer. Cancer Epidemiol Biomarkers Prev 3:37–45.

INSKIP PD, EKBOM A, GALANTI MR, et al. 1995. Medical diagnostic x-rays and thyroid cancer. J Natl Cancer Inst 87:1613–1621.

INSKIP PD, TEKKEL M, RAHU M, et al. 1996. Studies of leukemia and thyroid disease among Chernobyl clean-up workers from the Baltics. National Council on Radiation Protection Proceedings. In Press.

INSKIP PD, KLEINERMAN RA, STOVALL, et al. 1993. Leukemia, lymphoma, and multiple myeloma following pelvic radiotherapy for benign disease. Radiat Res 135:108–124.

INSKIP PD, MONSON RR, WAGONER JK, et al. 1990. Cancer mortality following radium treatment for uterine bleeding. Radiat Res 123:331–344.

INSKIP PD, HARVEY EB, BOICE JD JR, et al. 1991. Incidence of childhood cancer in twins. Cancer Causes Control 2:315–324.

INSKIP PD, STOVALL M, FLANNERY JT. 1994. Lung cancer risk and radiation dose among women treated for breast cancer. J Natl Cancer Inst 86:983–988.

ISHIMARU T, OTAKE M, ICHIMARU M. 1979. Dose-response relationship of neutrons and gamma rays to leukemia incidence among atomic bomb survivors in Hiroshima and Nagasaki by type of leukemia, 1950–1971. Radiat Res 77:377–394.

IVANOV EP, TOLOCHKO G, LAZAREV VS, et al. 1993. Childhood leukaemia after Chernobyl. Nature 365:702.

JABLON S, KATO H. 1970. Childhood cancer in relation to prenatal exposure to atomic-bomb radiation. Lancet 2:1000–1003.

JABLON S, MILLER RW. 1978. Army technologists: 29–year follow-up for cause of death. Radiology 126:677–679.

JABLON S, BAILAR JC III. 1980. The contribution of ionizing radiation to cancer mortality in the United States. Prev Med 9:219–226.

JABLON S, HRUBEC Z, BOICE JD JR. 1991. Cancer in populations living near nuclear facilities: a survey of mortality nationwide and incidence in two states. JAMA 265:1403–1408.

JABLON S, BOICE JD JR. 1993. Mortality among workers at a nuclear power plant in the United States. Cancer Causes Control 4:427–430.

JESSUP GL, SILVERMAN C. 1981. Personal usage of medical radiological procedures by radiologists, pathologists, and their families. Am J Epidemiol 114:53–62.

JOHNSON CJ. 1984. Cancer incidence in an area of radioactive fallout downwind from the Nevada Test Site. JAMA 251:230–236.

KADHIM MA, MACDONALD DA, GOODHEAD DT, et al. 1992. Transmission of chromosomal instability after plutonium α-particle irradiation. Nature 355:738–740.

KADHIM MA, LORIMORE SA, HEPBURN MD, et al. 1994. α-particle-induced chromosomal instability in human bone marrow cells. Lancet 344:987–988.

KALDOR JM, DAY NE, CLARKE EA, et al. 1990. Leukemia following Hodgkin's disease. N Engl J Med 322:7–13.

KARAOGLOV A, DESMET G, KELLY GN, et al (eds) 1996. The Radiological consequences of the Chernobyl accident. EUR 16544 Brussels: European Community.

KASTAN MB, ZHAN Q, EL-DEIRY WS, et al. 1992. A mammalian cell cycle checkpoint pathway utilizing *p53* and *GADD45* is defective in ataxia-telangiectasia. Cell 71: 587–597.

KAZAKOV VS, DEMIDCHIK EP, ASTAKHOVA LN. 1992. Thyroid cancer after Chernobyl. Nature 359:21.

KELLERER AM, ROSSI HH. 1978. A generalized formulation of dual radiation action. Radiat Res 75:471–488.

KENDALL GM, MUIRHEAD CM, MACGIBBON BH, et al. 1992. Mortality and occupational exposure to radiation: first analysis of the National Registry for Radiation Workers. Br Med J 304:220–225.

KENNEDY AR, MONDAL S, HEIDELBERGER C, et al. 1978. Enhancement of X-ray transformation by 12–0–tetradecanoyl-phorbol-13–acetate in a cloned line of C3H mouse embryo cells. Cancer Res 38:439–443.

KENNEDY AR, LITTLE JB. 1984. Evidence that a second event in X-ray-induced oncogenic transformation *in vitro* occurs during cellular proliferation. Radiat Res 99:228–248.

KERBER RA, TILL JE, SIMON SL, et al. 1993. A cohort study of thyroid disease in relation to fallout from nuclear weapons testing. JAMA 270:2076–2082.

KINLEN LJ, HUDSON CM, STILLER CA. 1991. Contacts between adults as evidence for an infective origin of childhood leukaemia: an explanation for the excess near nuclear establishments in West Berkshire. Br J Cancer 64:549–554.

KINLEN LJ, O'BRIEN F, CLARKE K, et al. 1993a. Rural population mixing and childhood leukaemia: effects of the North Sea oil industry in Scotland, including the area near Dounreay nuclear site. Br Med J 306:743–748.

KINLEN LJ, CLARKE K, BALKWILL A. 1993b. Paternal preconceptional radiation exposure in the nuclear industry and leukaemia and non-Hodgkin's lymphoma in young people in Scotland. Br Med J 6:1153–1158.

KLEINERMAN RA, LITTLEFIELD LG, TARONE RE, et al. 1989. Chromosome aberrations in peripheral lymphocytes and radiation dose to active bone marrow in patients treated for cancer of the cervix. Radiat Res 119:176–190.

KLEINERMAN RA, LITTLEFIELD LG, TARONE RE, et al. 1994. Chromosome aberrations in lymphocytes from women irradiated for benign and malignant gynecological disease. Radiat Res 139:40–46.

KLEINERMAN RA, BOICE JD JR, STORM HH, et al. 1995. Second primary cancer after treatment for cervical cancer. An international cancer registry study. Cancer 76:442–452.

KNOX EG, STEWART AM, GILMAN EA, et al. 1988. Background radiation and childhood cancers. J Radiol Prot 8:9–18.

KOPECKY KJ, NAKASHIMA E, YAMAMOTO T, et al. 1986. Lung cancer radiation and smoking among A-bomb survivors, Hiroshima and Nagasaki. RERF TR 13–86. Hiroshima, RERF.

KOSSENKO MM, DEGTEVA MO. 1994. Cancer mortality and radiation risk for the Techa river population. Sci Total Environ 142:73–89.

KUIJTEN RR, BUNIN GR, NASS CC, et al. 1990. Gestational and familial risk factors for childhood astrocytoma: results of a case-control study. Cancer Res 50:2608–2612.

LAND CE. 1979. The hazards of fallout or of epidemiologic research? (Editorial) N Engl J Med 300:431–432.

LAND CE. 1980. Estimating cancer risks from low doses of ionizing radiation. Science 209:1197–1203.

LAND CE, BOICE JD JR, SHORE RE, et al. 1980. Breast cancer risk from low-dose exposures to ionizing radiation: results of parallel analysis of three exposed populations of women. J Natl Cancer Inst 65:353–376.

LAND CE, MCKAY FW, MACHADO SG. 1984. Childhood leukemia and fallout from the Nevada nuclear tests. Science 223:139–144.

LAND CE. 1986. Carcinogenic effects of radiation on the human digestive tract and other organs. *In*: *Radiation Carcinogenesis*. Upton AC, et al (eds). New York: Elsevier, pp 347–378.

LAND CE, TOKUNAGA M, NAKAMURA N. 1993a. Early-onset breast cancer among Japanese A-bomb survivors: evidence of a radiation susceptible subgroup? *Lancet* 342:237.

LAND CE, SHIMOSATO Y, SACCOMANNO G, et al. 1993b. Radiation-associated lung cancer: a comparison of the pathology of lung cancers in uranium miners and survivors of the atomic bombings of Hiroshima and Nagasaki. Radiat Res 134:234–243.

LAND CE, HAYAKAWA N, MACHADO SG, et al. 1994. A case-control interview study of breast cancer among Japanese A-bomb survivors. II. Interactions with radiation dose. Cancer Causes Control 5:167–176.

LANGLOIS RG, BIGBEE WL, KYOIZUMI S, et al. 1987. Evidence for increased somatic cell mutations at the glycophorin A locus in atomic bomb survivors. Science 236:445–448.

LÉTOURNEAU EG, KREWSKI D, CHOI NW, et al. 1994. Case-control study of residential radon and lung cancer in Winnipeg, Manitoba, Canada. Am J Epidemiol 140:310–322.

LEWIS EB. 1963. Leukemia, multiple myeloma, and aplastic anemia in American radiologists. Science 142:1492–1494.

LEWIS CA, SMITH PG, STRATTON IM, et al. 1988. Estimated radiation doses to different organs among patients treated for ankylosing spondylitis with a single course of X rays. Br J Radiol 61:212–220.

LI FP, FRAUMENI JF JR, MULVIHILL JJ, et al. 1988. A cancer family syndrome in twenty-four kindreds. Cancer Res 48:5358–5362.

LINOS A, GRAY JE, ORVIS AL, et al. 1980. Low-dose radiation and leukemia. N Engl J Med 302:1101–1105.

LITTLE JB. 1981. Influence of noncarcinogenic secondary factors on radiation carcinogenesis. Radiat Res 87:240–250.

LITTLE JB. 1993. Cellular, molecular, and carcinogenic effects of radiation. Hematol Oncol Clin N Am 7:337–352.

LUBIN JH, BOICE JD JR. 1989. Estimating Rn-induced lung cancer in the United States. Health Phys 57:417–427.

LUBIN JH, QIAO Y-L, TAYLOR PR, et al. 1990a. Quantitative evaluation of the radon and lung cancer association in a case control study of Chinese tin miners. Cancer Res 50:174–180.

LUBIN JH, SAMET JM, WEINBERG C. 1990b. Design issues in epidemiologic studies of indoor exposure to Rn and risk of lung cancer. Health Phys 59:807–817.

LUBIN JH, BOICE JD JR, EDLING C et al. 1994a. Lung cancer following radon exposure among underground miners: a joint analysis of 11 studies. NIH Publ No. 94–3644. Washington, DC: US Govt Print Office.

LUBIN JH, LIANG Z, HRUBEC Z, et al. 1994b. Radon exposure in residences and lung cancer among women: combined analysis of three studies. Cancer Causes Control 5:114–128.

LUBIN JH. 1994. Lung cancer and exposure to residential radon. Am J Epidemiol 140:323–332.

LUBIN JH, BOICE JD JR, EDLING C, et al. 1995a. Lung cancer in radon-exposed miners and estimation of risk from indoor exposure. J Natl Cancer Inst 87:817–827.

LUBIN JH, BOICE JD JR, EDLING C, et al. 1995b. Radon-exposed underground miners and the inverse dose-rate (protraction enhancement) effects. Health Phys 69:494–500.

LUBIN JH, BOICE JD JR, SAMET JM. 1995c. Errors in radon dosimetry might explain mixed results for indoor studies. Radiat Res 144:329–341.

LYON JL, KLAUBER MR, GARDNER JW, et al. 1979. Childhood leukemias associated with fallout from nuclear testing. N Engl J Med 300:397–402.

MACHADO SG, LAND CE, MCKAY FW. 1987. Cancer mortality and radioactive fallout in southwestern Utah. Am J Epidemiol 125:44–61.

MACMAHON B. 1962. Prenatal X-ray exposure and childhood cancer. J Natl Cancer Inst 28:1173–1191.

MACMAHON B. 1989. Some recent issues in low-exposure radiation epidemiology. Environ Health Perspect 81:131–135.

MACMAHON B. 1992. Leukemia clusters around nuclear facilities in Britain. Cancer Causes Control 3:283–288.

MAJOR IR, MOLE RH. 1978. Myeloid leukemia in X-ray irradiated CBA mice. Nature 272:455–456.

MANCUSO TF, STEWART A, KNEALE G. 1977. Radiation exposures of Hanford workers dying from cancer and other causes. Health Phys 33:369–385.

MARCH HC. 1944. Leukemia in radiologists. Radiology 43:275–278.

MARSHALL JH, GROER PG. 1977. A theory of the induction of bone cancer by alpha radiation. Radiat Res 71:149–192.

MARSHALL JH, GROER PG, SCHLENKER RA. 1978. Dose to endosteal cells and relative distribution factors for radium-224 and plutonium-239 compared to radium-226. Health Phys 35:91–101.

MASON TJ, FRAUMENI JF JR, MCKAY FW JR. 1972. Uranium mill tailings and cancer mortality in Colorado. J Natl Cancer Inst 49:661–664.

MASON TJ, MILLER RW. 1974. Cosmic radiation at high altitudes and U.S. cancer mortality, 1950–1969. Radiat Res 60:302–306.

MATANOSKI GM, SELTSER R, SARTWELL PE, et al. 1975. The current mortality rates of radiologists and other physician specialists: specific causes of death. Am J Epidemiol 101:199–210.

MATANOSKI G. 1993. Nuclear shipyard workers study. Radiat Res 133:126–127.

MATTSON A, RUDEN B, HALL R, et al. 1993. Radiation-induced breast cancer and long term follow-up of radiotherapy for benign breast disease. J Natl Cancer Inst 85:1679–1685.

MAYS CW, SPIESS H. 1984. Bone sarcomas in patients given radium-224. In: *Radiation Carcinogenesis: Epidemiology and Biological Significance*. Boice JD Jr, Fraumeni JF Jr (eds): New York: Raven Press, pp 241–252.

MCKINNEY PA, ALEXANDER FE, CARTWRIGHT RA, et al. 1991. Parental occupations of children with leukaemia in West Cumbria, North Humerside, and Gateshend. Br Med J 302:681–687.

MCLAUGHLIN JR, KREIGER N, SLOAN MP, et al. 1993a. An historical cohort study of cardiac catherization during childhood and the risk of cancer. Int J Epidemiol 22:584–591.

MCLAUGHLIN JR, CLARKE EA, NISHRI D, et al. 1993b. Childhood leukaemia in the vicinity of Canadian nuclear facilities. Cancer Causes Control 4:51–58.

MCLAUGHLIN JR, KING WD, ANDERSON TW, et al. 1993c. Paternal radiation exposure and leukaemia in offspring: the Ontario case-control study. Br Med J 307:959–966.

METTLER FA, WILLIAMSON MR, ROYAL HD, et al. 1992. Thyroid nodules in the population living around Chernobyl. JAMA 268:616–619.

MICHAELIS J, KELLER B, HAAF G, et al. 1992. Incidence of childhood malignancies in the vicinity of West German nuclear power plants. Cancer Causes Control 3:255–263.

MIKÉ V, MEADOWS AT, D'ANGIO GJ. 1982. Incidence of second malignant neoplasms in children: results of an international study. Lancet 2:1326–1331.

MILLER AB, HOWE GR, SHERMAN GJ, et al. 1989. Mortality from breast cancer after irradiation during fluoroscopic examinations in patients being treated for tuberculosis. N Engl J Med 321:1285–1289.

MILLER RW. 1969. Delayed radiation effects in atomic-bomb survivors. Science 166:569–574.

MILLER RW, BOICE JD JR. 1986. Radiogenic cancer after prenatal or childhood exposure. In: *Radiation Carcinogenesis*, Upton AC, et al (eds). New York, Elsevier, pp 379–386.

MILLER RW. 1995. Delayed effects of external radiation exposure: a brief history. Radiat Res 144:160–169.

MODAN B, LILIENFELD AM. 1965. Polycythemia vera and leukemia—the role of radiation treatment: a study of 1222 patients. Medicine 44:305–344.

MODAN B, CHETRIT A, ALFANDARY E, et al. 1989. Increased risk of breast cancer after low-dose irradiation. Lancet 1:629–631.

MOLE RH. 1974. Antenatal irradiation and childhood cancer: causation or coincidence? Br J Cancer 30:199–208.

MOLE RH. 1975. Ionizing radiation as a carcinogen: practical questions and academic pursuits. Br J Radiol 48:157–169.

MOLE RH, MAJOR IR. 1983. Myeloid leukaemia frequency after protracted exposure to ionizing radiation: experimental confirmation of the flat dose-response found in ankylosing spondylitis after a single treatment course with X-rays. Leuk Res 7:295–300.

MONSON RR, MACMAHON B. 1984. Prenatal X-ray exposure and cancer in children. In: *Radiation Carcinogenesis: Epidemiology and Biological Significance*, Boice JD Jr, Fraumeni JF Jr (eds). New York: Raven Press, pp 97–105.

MORRISON HI, SEMENCIW RM, MAO Y, et al. 1988. Cancer mortality among a group of fluorspar miners exposed to radon progeny. Am J Epidemiol 128:1266–1275.

MUIRHEAD CR, BUTLAND BK, GREEN BM, et al. 1991. Childhood leukaemia and natural radiation. Lancet 337:503–504.

MULVIHILL JJ, MYERS MH, CONNELLY RR, et al. 1987. Cancer in offspring of long-term survivors of childhood and adolescent cancer. Lancet 2:813–817.

NAJARIAN T, COLTON T. 1978. Mortality from leukemia and cancer in shipyard nuclear workers. Lancet 1:1018–1020.

NAS (NATIONAL ACADEMY OF SCIENCES) 1972. Advisory Committee on the Biological Effects of Ionizing Radiations (The BEIR Report): The Effects on Populations of Exposure to Low Levels of Ionizing Radiation. Washington D.C., U.S. Government Printing Office.

NAS. 1980. Committee on the Biological Effects of Ionizing Radiations (BEIR III). The Effects on Populations of Exposure to Low Levels of Ionizing Radiation: 1980. Washington, DC: Natl Acad Press.

NAS. 1988. Health Risks of Radon and Other Internally Deposited Alpha-Emitters (BEIR IV Report). Washington, DC, Natl Acad Press.

NAS. 1990. Health Effects of Exposure to Low Levels of Ionizing Radiation (BEIR V). Washington, DC: Natl Acad Press.

NAS. 1991. Comparative Dosimetry of Radon in Mines and Homes. Washington, DC: Natl Acad Press.

NCRP (NATIONAL COUNCIL ON RADIATION PROTECTION AND MEASUREMENTS). 1980. Report No. 64. Influence of Dose and Its Distribution in Time on Dose-Response Relationships for Low-LET Radiations. Washington, DC: NCRP.

NCRP. 1987. Report No. 93. Ionizing Radiation Exposure of the Population of the United States. Bethesda, Md: NCRP.

NCRP. 1989. Report No. 98. Guidance on Radiation Received in Space Activities. Bethesda, Md: NCRP.

NEEL JV, SCHULL WJ, (EDS). 1991. *The Children of Atomic Bomb Survivors. A Genetic Study*. Washington, DC: Natl Acad Press, pp 1–518.

NEGLIA JP, MEADOWS AT, ROBISON LL, et al. 1991. Second neoplasms after acute lymphoblastic leukemia in childhood. N Engl J Med 325:1330–1336.

NEUGUT AI, ROBINSON E, LEE WC, et al. 1994. Lung cancer after radiotherapy for breast cancer. Cancer 71:3054–3057.

NIH (NATIONAL INSTITUTES OF HEALTH). 1985. Report of the National Institutes of Health Ad Hoc Working Group to Develop Radioepidemiological Tables, NIH Publ No 85–2748, U.S. DHHS, Public Health Service, NIH, Washington, DC.

NOMURA T. 1982. Prenatal exposure to X-rays and chemicals induces heritable tumours and anomalies in mice. Nature 296:575–577.

NRPB (NATIONAL RADIOLOGICAL PROTECTION BOARD). 1992a. *Electromagnetic Fields and the Risk of Cancer*. London: HMSO.

NRBP. 1992b. Estimates of late radiation risks to the UK population. NRPB-R226(rev). Oxon, NRPB.

OPPENHEIM BE, GRIEM ML, MEIER P. 1974. Effects of low-dose prenatal irradiation in humans: analysis of Chicago lying-in data and comparison with other studies. Radiat Res 57:508–544.

PARKIN DM, CARDIS E, MASUYER E, 1993. et al. Childhood leukaemia following the Chernobyl accident: the European Childhood Leukaemia-Lymphoma Incidence Study (ECLIS). Eur J Cancer 29A:87–95.

PARKER L, CRAFT AW, SMITH J, et al. 1993. Geographical distribution of preconceptional radiation doses to fathers employed at the Sellafield nuclear installation, West Cumbria. Br Med J 307:966–971.

PERSHAGEN G, LIANG Z-H, HRUBEC Z, et al. 1992. Residential radon exposure and lung cancer in Swedish women. Health Phys 63:179–186.

PERSHAGEN G, AKERBLOM G, AXELSON O, et al. 1994. Residential radon exposure and lung cancer in Sweden. N Engl J Med 330:159–164.

PIERCE DA, VAETH M. 1991. The shape of the cancer mortality dose-response curve for A-bomb survivors. Radiat Res 126:36–42.

PIERCE DA, VAETH M, PRESTON DL. 1991. Analysis of time and age patterns in cancer risk for A-bomb survivors. Radiat Res 126:171–186.

POCHIN EE. 1976. Problems involved in detecting increased malignancy rates in areas of high natural radiation background. Health Phys 31:148–151.

POLEDNAK AP. 1978. Bone cancer among female radium dial workers: latency periods and incidence rates by time after exposure: brief communication. J Natl Cancer Inst 60:77–82.

POTTERN LM, STONE BJ, DAY NE, et al. 1980. Thyroid cancer in Connecticut, 1935–1975: an analysis by cell type. Am J Epidemiol 112:764–774.

POTTERN LM, KAPLAN MM, LARSEN PR, et al. 1990. Thyroid nodularity after childhood irradiation for lymphoid hyperplasia: a comparison of questionnaire and clinical findings. J Clin Epidemiol 43:449–460.

PRENTICE RL, KATO H, YOSHIMOTO K, et al. 1982. Radiation exposure and thyroid cancer incidence among Hiroshima and Nagasaki residents. Natl Cancer Inst Monogr 62:207–212.

PRENTICE RL, YOSHIMOTO Y, MASON MW. 1983. Relationship of cigarette smoking and radiation exposure to cancer mortality in Hiroshima and Nagasaki. J Natl Cancer Inst 70:611–622.

PRESTON DL, PIERCE DA. 1988. The effect of changes in dosimetry on cancer mortality risk estimates in the atomic bomb survivors. Radiat Res 114:437–466.

PRESTON D, KUSUMI S, TOMONAGA M, et al. 1994. Cancer incidence in atomic bomb survivors. Part III: leukemia, lymphoma, and multiple myeloma, 1950–87. Radiat Res 137:S68–S97.

PRESTON-MARTIN S, PAGANINI-HILL A, HENDERSON BE, et al. 1980. Case-control study of intracranial meningiomas in women in Los Angeles County, California. J Natl Cancer Inst 65:67–73.

PRESTON-MARTIN S, YU MC, BENTON B, et al. 1982. *N*-nitroso compounds and childhood brain tumors: a case-control study. Cancer Res 42:5240–5245.

PRESTON-MARTIN S, THOMAS DC, WHITE SC, et al. 1988. Prior exposure to medical and dental X-rays related to tumors of the parotid gland. J Natl Cancer Inst 80:943–949.

PRESTON-MARTIN S, THOMAS DC, YU MC, et al. 1989. Diagnostic radiography as a risk factor for chronic myeloid and monocytic leukaemia (CML). Br J Cancer 59:639–644.

RADFORD EP, RENARD KG. 1984. Lung cancer in Swedish iron miners exposed to low doses of radon daughters. N Engl J Med 310:1485–1494.

RALLISON ML, DOBYNS BM, KEATING FR, et al. 1975. Thyroid nodularity in children. JAMA 233:1069–1072.

RALLISON ML, LOTZ TM, BISHOP M, et al. 1990. Cohort study of thyroid disease near the Nevada Test Site: a preliminary report. Health Phys 59:739–746.

RINSKY RA, ZUMWALDE RD, WAXWEILER RJ, et al. 1981. Cancer mortality at a naval nuclear shipyard. Lancet 1:231–235.

RINSKY RA, MELIUS JM, HORNUNG RW, et al. 1988. Case-control study of lung cancer in civilian employees at the Portsmouth Naval Shipyard, Kittery, Maine. Am J Epidemiol 127:55–64.

ROBBINS J, ADAMS WH. 1989. Radiation effects in the Marshall Islands. In: *Radiation and the Thyroid*, Nagataki S (ed): Tokyo: Excerpta Medica, pp 11–24.

ROBINETTE CD, JABLON S, PRESTON TL. 1985. *Mortality of Nuclear Weapons Test Participants*. Washington, DC: Natl Acad Press.

ROMAN E, WATSON A, BERAL V, et al. 1993. Case-control study of leukaemia and non-Hodgkin's lymphoma among children aged 0–4 years living in West Berkshire and North Hampshire health districts. Br Med J 306:615–621.

RON E, KLEINERMAN RA, BOICE JD JR, et al. 1987. A population-based case-control study of thyroid cancer. J Natl Cancer Inst 79:1–12.

RON E, LUBIN J, SCHNEIDER AB. 1992. Thyroid cancer incidence. Nature 360:113.

RON E, MODAN B, BOICE JD JR. 1988a. Mortality after radiotherapy for ringworm of the scalp. Am J Epidemiol 127:713–725.

RON E, MODAN B, BOICE JD JR, et al. 1988b. Tumors of the brain and nervous system after radiotherapy in childhood. N Engl J Med 319:1033–1039.

RON E, MODAN B, PRESTON D, et al. 1989. Thyroid neoplasia following low-dose radiation in childhood. Radiat Res 120:516–531.

RON E, MODAN B, PRESTON D, et al. 1991. Radiation-induced skin carcinoma of the head and neck. Radiat Res 125:318–325.

RON E, LUBIN JH, SHORE RE, et al. 1995. Thyroid cancer after exposure to external radiation: a pooled analysis of seven studies. Radiat Res 141:259–277.

RON E, BOICE JD JR, HAMBURGER S, et al. 1994. Mortality following radiation treatment for infertility of hormonal origin or amenorrhoea. Int J Epidemiol 23:1165–1173.

RON E, PRESTON DL, MABUCHI K, et al. 1994c. Cancer incidence in atomic bomb survivors. Part IV: Comparison of cancer incidence and mortality. Radiat Res 137:S98–S112.

ROONEY C, BERAL V, MACONOCHIE N, et al. 1993. Case-control study of prostate cancer in the United Kingdom Atomic Energy Authority employees. Br Med J 307:1391–1397.

ROSCOE, RJ, STEENLAND K, HALPERIN, WE, et al. 1989. Lung cancer mortality among nonsmoking uranium miners exposed to radon daughters. JAMA 262:629–633.

ROWLAND RE, STEHNEY AF, LUCAS HF JR. 1978. Dose-response relationships for female radium dial workers. Radiat Res 76:368–383.

SAENGER EL, THOMA GE, TOMPKINS EA. 1968. Incidence of leukemia following treatment of hyperthyroidism: preliminary report of the Cooperative Thyrotoxicosis Therapy Follow-up Study. JAMA 205:855–862.

SAMET JM. 1989. Radon and lung cancer. J Natl Cancer Inst 81:745–757.

SAMPSON RJ, KEY CR, BUNCHER CR, et al. 1969. Thyroid carcinoma in Hiroshima and Nagasaki. I. Prevalence of thyroid carcinoma at autopsy. JAMA 209:65–70.

SANDLER DP, COMSTOCK GW, MATANOWSKI GM. 1982. Neoplasms following childhood radium irradiation of the nasopharynx. J Natl Cancer Inst 68:3–8.

SCHNEIDER AB, SHORE-FREEDMAN E, RYO UY, et al. 1985. Radiation-induced tumors of the head and neck following childhood irradiation. Prospective studies. Medicine 64:1–15.

SCHNEIDER AB, RON E, LUBIN J, et al. 1993. Dose-response relationships for radiation-induced thyroid cancer and thyroid nodules: evidence for the prolonged effects of radiation on the thyroid. J Clin Endocrinol Metab 77:362–364.

SCHOENBERG JB, KLOTZ JB, WILCOX HB, et al. 1990. Case-control study of residential radon and lung cancer among New Jersey women. Cancer Res 50:6520–6524.

SEVC J, KUNZ E, TOMASEK L, et al. 1988. Cancer in man after exposure to Rn daughters. Health Phys 54:27–46.

SHIMIZU Y, KATO H, SCHULL WJ, et al. 1989. Studies of the mortality of A-bomb survivors. 9. Mortality, 1950–1985: Part 1. Comparison of risk coefficients for site-specific cancer mortality based on the DS86 and T65DR shielded kerma and organ doses. Radiat Res 118:502–524.

SHIMIZU Y, KATO H, SCHULL WJ. 1990. Studies of the mortality of A-bomb survivors. 9. Mortality, 1950–1985. Part 2. Cancer mortality based on the recently revised doses (DS86). Radiat Res 121:120–141.

SHIMIZU Y, KATO H, SCHULL WJ, et al. 1992. Studies of the mortality of A-bomb survivors. 9. Mortality, 1950–1985. Part 3. Noncancer mortality based on the revised doses (DS86). Radiat Res 130:249–266.

SHORE RE. 1990. Overview of radiation-induced skin cancer in humans. Int J Radiat Biol 57:809–827.

SHORE RE. 1992. Issues and epidemiological evidence regarding radiation-induced thyroid cancer. Radiat Res 131:98–111.

SHORE RE, ALBERT RE, PASTERNACK BS. 1976. Follow-up study of patients treated by X-ray epilation for tinea capitis: resurvey of post-treatment illness and mortality experience. Arch Environ Health 31:21–28.

SHORE RE, ALBERT RE, REED M, et al. 1984. Skin cancer incidence among children irradiated for ringworm of the scalp. Radiat Res 100:192–204.

SHORE RE, WOODWARD E, HILDRETH N, et al. 1985. Thyroid tumors following thymus irradiation. J Natl Cancer Inst 74:1177–1184.

SHORE RE, HILDRETH N, WOODARD E, et al. 1986. Breast cancer among women given X-ray therapy for acute postpartum mastitis. J Natl Cancer Inst 77:689–696.

SHORE RE, HILDRETH N, DVORETSKY P, et al. 1993. Benign thyroid adenomas among persons x-irradiated in infancy for enlarged thymus gland. Radiat Res 134:217–223.

SMITH PG, DOLL R, RADFORD EP. 1977. Cancer mortality among patients with ankylosing spondylitis not given X-ray therapy. Br J Radiol 50:728–734.

SMITH PG, DOLL R. 1981. Mortality from cancer and all causes among British radiologists. Br J Radiol 54:187–194.

SMITH PG, DOLL R. 1982. Mortality among patients with ankylosing spondylitis after a single treatment course with X-rays. Br Med J 284:449–460.

SMITH PG, DOUGLAS AJ. 1986. Mortality of workers at the Sellafield plant of British Nuclear Fuels. Br Med J 293:845–854.

SMITH PG. 1991. Case-control studies of leukaemia clusters. Br Med J 302:672–673.

SPIERS FW. 1979. Background radiation and estimated risks from low-dose irradiation. Health Phys 37:784–789.

SPIERS FW, LUCAS HF, RUNDO J, et al. 1983. Leukaemia incidence in the U.S. dial workers. Health Phys 44(Suppl 1):65–72.

SPIESS H, MAYS CW, CHMELEVSKY D. 1989. Malignancies in patients injected with radium 224. In: *Risks from Radium and Thorotrast*, Taylor DM, Mays CW, Gerber GB (eds). BIR Report 21. London: Brit Inst Radiol, pp 7–12.

STEBBINGS JH, LUCAS HF, STEHNEY AF. 1984. Mortality from cancers of major sites in female radium dial workers. Am J Ind Med 5:435–459.

STEHNEY AF, LUCAS HF JR, ROWLAND RE. 1978. Survival times of women radium dial workers first exposed before 1930. In: *Late Biological Effects of Ionizing Radiation*, Vol 1. Vienna: International Atomic Energy Agency, pp 333–351.

STERN RS, LAIRD N, MELSKI J, et al. 1984. Cutaneous squamous-cell carcinoma in patients treated with PUVA. N Engl J Med 310:1156–1161.

STERN FB, WAXWEILER RA, BEAUMONT JJ, et al. 1986. A case-control study of leukemia at a naval nuclear shipyard. Am J Epidemiol 123:980–992.

STEVENS W, THOMAS DC, LYON JL, et al. 1990. Leukemia in Utah and radioactive fallout from the Nevada test site: a case-control study. JAMA 264:585–591.

STEWART A, WEBB J, HEWITT D. 1958. A survey of childhood malignancies. Br Med J 1:1495–1508.

STEWART A, KNEALE GW. 1970. Radiation dose effects in relation to obstetric X-rays and childhood cancers. Lancet 1:1185–1188.

STEWART A. 1973. The carcinogenic effects of low level radiation: a re-appraisal of epidemiologists methods and observations. Health Phys 24:223–240.

STIDLEY CA, SAMET JM. 1993. A review of ecologic studies of lung cancer and indoor radon. Health Phys 65:234–251.

STORM HH, ANDERSSON M, BOICE JD JR, et al. 1992. Adjuvant radiotherapy and risk of contralateral breast cancer. J Natl Cancer Inst 84:1245–1250.

STRAUME T, EGBERT SD, WOOLSON WA, et al. 1992. Neutron discrepancies in the DS86 Hiroshima dosimetry system. Health Phys 63:421–426.

STRAUME T, HARRIS LJ, MARCHETTI AA, EGBERT SD. 1994. Neutrons confirmed in Nagasaki and at one Army Pulsed Radiation Facility: Implications for Hiroshima. Radiat Res 138:193–200.

STRONG LC. 1977. Genetic and environmental interactions. Cancer 40:1861–1866.

STRONG LC, HERSON J, OSBORNE BM, et al. 1979. Risk of radiation-related subsequent malignant tumors in survivors of Ewing's sarcoma. J Natl Cancer Inst 62:1401–1406.

STSJAZHKO VA, TSYB AF, TRONKO ND, et al. 1995. Childhood thyroid cancer since accident at Chernobyl. Br Med J 310:801.

SUKUMAR S, UPADHYAY A, YANG X. 1991. Activation of *ras* oncogenes precedes the onset of mammary neoplasia induced by N-nitroso N[1]-methylurea. In: *Origins of Human Cancer*, Brugge J, Curran T, Harlow E, et al (eds). New York: Cold Spring Harbor Laboratory Press, pp 153–161.

SWERDLOW AJ, DOUGLAS AJ, HUDSON GV, et al. 1992. Risk of second primary cancers after Hodgkin's disease by type of treatment: analysis of 2846 patients in the British National Lymphoma Investigation. Br Med J 304:1137–1143.

SWIFT M, MORRELL D, MASSEY RB, et al. 1991. Incidence of cancer in 161 families affected by ataxia-telangiectasia. N Engl J Med 325:1831–1836.

TAYLOR DM, MAYS CW, GERBER GB, ET AL, (EDS). 1989. *Risks from Radium and Thorotrast*, BIR Report 21. London: Br Inst Radiol.

TAYLOR JA, WATSON MA, DEVERUX TR, et al. 1994. p53 mutation hotspot in radon-associated lung cancer. Lancet 343:86–87.

THOMAS D, POGODA J, LANGHOLZ B, et al. 1994. Temporal modifiers of radon-smoking interaction. Health Phys 66:257–262. [erratum, Health Phys 1994; 67:675.]

THOMPSON DE, MABUCHI K, RON E, et al. 1994. Cancer incidence in atomic bomb survivors. Part II: solid tumors, 1958–1987. Radiat Res 137:S17–S67.

TOKUNAGA M, LAND CE, AOKI Y, et al. 1993. Proliferative and non-proliferative breast disease in relation to radiation dose from the atomic bombings of Hiroshima and Nagasaki. Results of a histopathology review of autopsy tissue. Cancer 72:1657–1665.

TOKUNAGA M, LAND CE, TOKUOKA S, et al. 1994. Incidence of female breast cancer among atomic bomb survivors, 1950–1985. Radiat Res 138:209–223.

TOMASEK L, DARBY SC, SWERDLOW AJ, et al. 1993. Radon exposure and cancer other than lung cancer among uranium miners in West Bohemia. Lancet 341:919–923.

TRAVIS LB, CURTIS RE, BOICE JD JR, et al. 1991. Second cancers following non-Hodgkin's lymphoma. Cancer 67:2002–2009.

TRAVIS LB, CURTIS RE, STOVALL M, et al. 1994. Risk of leukemia following treatment for non-Hodgkin's lumphoma. J Natl Cancer Inst 86:1450–1457.

TRAVIS LB, CURTIS RE, BENNETT WP, et al. 1995a. Lung cancer after Hodgkin's disease. J Natl Cancer Inst 87:1324–1327.

TRAVIS LB, CURTIS RE, INSKIP PD, et al. 1995b. Re: Lung cancer risk and radiation dose among women treated for breast cancer. J Natl Cancer Inst 87:60–61.

TRAVIS LB, WEEKS J, CURTIS RE, et al. 1996. Leukemia following total body irradiation and chemo-therapy for non-Hodgkin's lymphoma. J Clin Oncol, in press.

TUCKER MA, MEADOWS AT, BOICE JD JR, et al. 1984. Cancer risk following treatment of childhood cancer. In: *Radiation Carcinogenesis: Epidemiology and Biological Significance*, Boice JD Jr, Fraumeni JF Jr (eds). New York: Raven Press, pp 211–224.

TUCKER MA, D'ANGIO GJ, BOICE JD JR, et al. 1987a. Bone sarcomas linked to radiotherapy and chemotherapy in children. N Engl J Med 317:588–593.

TUCKER MA, MEADOWS AT, BOICE JD JR, et al. 1987b. Leukemia after therapy with alkylating agents for childhood cancer. J Natl Cancer Inst 78:459–464.

TUCKER MA, COLEMAN CN, COX RS, et al. 1988. Risk of second cancers after treatment for Hodgkin's disease. N Engl J Med 318:76–81.

TUCKER MA, MORRIS JONES PH, BOICE JD JR, et al. 1991. Therapeutic radiation at a young age is linked to secondary thyroid cancer. Cancer Res 51:2885–2888.

ULLRICH RL, STORER JB. 1979a. Influence of γ irradiation on the development of neoplastic disease in mice. I. Reticular tissue tumors. Radiat Res 80:303–316.

ULLRICH RL, STORER JB. 1979b. Influence of γ irradiation on the development of neoplastic disease in mice. III. Dose-rate effects. Radiat Res 80:325–342.

ULLRICH RL, JERNIGAN MC, SATTERFIELD LC, et al. 1987. Radiation carcinogenesis: time-dose relationships. Radiat Res 111:179–184.

UNSCEAR (UNITED NATIONS SCIENTIFIC COMMITTEE ON THE EFFECTS OF ATOMIC RADIATION). 1972. Ionizing Radiation Levels and Effects, Vol 2: Effects. Publ E.72.IX.18. New York; United Nations.

UNSCEAR. 1982. Ionizing Radiation: Sources and Biological Effects. Publ E.82.IX.8. New York: United Nations.

UNSCEAR. 1986. Genetic and Somatic Effects of Ionizing Radiation. Publ E.86.IX.9. New York: United Nations.

UNSCEAR. 1988. Sources, Effects, and Risks of Ionizing Radiation. Publ E.88.IX.7. New York: United Nations.

UNSCEAR. 1993. Sources and Effects of Ionizing Radiation. Publ E.94.IX.2. New York: United Nations.

UNSCEAR. 1994. Sources and Effects of Ionizing Radiation. E.94.IX.11. New York: United Nations.

UPTON AC, RANDOLPH ML, CONKLIN JW, et al. 1970. Late effects of fast neutrons and gamma-rays in mice as influenced by the dose rate of irradiation: induction of neoplasia. Radiat Res 41:467–491.

UPTON AC. 1981. Health impact of the Three Mile Island accident. Ann NY Acad Sci 365:63–75.

UPTON AC. 1987. Biological basis of radiological protection and its application to risk assessment. Br J Radiol 60:1–16.

UPTON AC, ALBERT RE, BURNS FJ, ET AL, EDS. 1986. *Radiation Carcinogenesis*. New York, Elsevier, pp 1–459.

URQUHART JD, BLACK RJ, MUIRHEAD MJ, et al. 1991. Case-control study of leukaemia and non-Hodgkin's lymphoma in children in Caithness near the Dounreay nuclear installation. Br Med J 302:687–692.

VAHAKANGAS KH, SAMET JM, METCALF RA, et al. 1992. Mutations of p53 and ras genes in radon-associated lung cancer from uranium miners. Lancet 339:576–580.

VAN KAICK G, WESCH H, LÜHRS H, et al. 1989. The German Thorotrast Study—report on 20 years follow-up. In: *Risks from Radium and Thorotrast*, Taylor DM, Mays CW, Gerber GB, Thomas RG (eds). BIR Report 21. London: Br Inst Radiol, pp 98–104.

VAN KAICK G, KARAOGLOU A, KELLERER AM (eds.). 1995. Health effects of Internally Deposited Radionuclides: Emphasis on Radium and Thorium, Singapore: World Scientific.

VAN LEEUWEN FE, SOMERS R, TAAL BG, et al. 1989. Increased risk of lung cancer, non-Hodgkin's lymphoma, and leukemia following Hodgkin's disease. J Clin Oncol 7:1046–1058.

VAN LEEUWEN FE, KLOKMAN WJ, STOVALL M, et al. 1995. Roles of radiotherapy and smoking in lung cancer following Hodgkin's disease. J Natl Cancer Inst 87:1530–1537.

VERDUIJN PG, HAYES RB, LOOMAN C, et al. 1989. Mortality after nasopharyngeal radium irradiation for eustachian tube dysfunction. Ann Otol Rhinol Laryngol 98:839–844.

VOELZ GL. 1991. Health considerations for workers exposed to plutonium. Occup Med 6:681–694.

VOELZ GL, LAWRENCE JNP. 1991. A 42–year medical follow-up of Manhattan Project plutonium workers. Health Phys 61:181–190.

WAGONER JK. 1984. Leukemia and other malignancies following radiation therapy for gynecological disorders. In: *Radiation Carcinogenesis: Epidemiology and Biological Significance*, Boice JD Jr, Fraumeni JF Jr (eds). New York: Raven Press, pp 153–159.

WANG JX, INSKIP PD, BOICE JD JR, et al. 1990a. Cancer incidence among medical diagnostic X-ray workers in China, 1950 to 1985. Int J Cancer 45:889–895.

WANG ZY, BOICE JD JR, WEI LX, et al. 1990b. Thyroid nodularity and chromosome aberrations among women in areas of high background radiation in China. J Natl Cancer Inst 82:478–485.

WEI L. 1980. Health survey in high background radiation areas in China. Science 209:877–880.

WEI L, ZHA Y, TAO Z, et al. 1990. Epidemiological investigation of radiological effects in high background radiation areas of Yangjiang, China. J Radiat Res 31:119–136.

WEICHSELBAUM RR, BECKETT MA, DIAMOND AA. 1989. An important step in radiation carcinogenesis may be inactivation of cellular genes. Int J Radiat Oncol Biol Phys 16:277–282.

WEINBERG RA. 1989. Oncogenes, antioncogenes, and the molecular bases of multistep carcinogenesis. Cancer Res 49:3713–3721.

WEISS HA, DARBY SC, DOLL R. 1994. Cancer mortality following x-ray treatment for ankylosing spondylitis. Int J Cancer 59:327–338.

WEISS HA, DARBY SC, FEARN T, et al. 1995. Leukemia mortality after x-ray treatment for ankylosing spondylitis. Radiat Res 142: 1–11.

WICK RR, GÖSSNER W. 1989. Recent results of the follow-up of radium-224–treated ankylosing spondylitis patients. In: *Risks from Radium and Thorotrast*, Taylor DM, Mays CW, Gerber GB, et al (eds). BIR Report 21. London: Br Inst Radiol, pp 25–28.

WILKINSON GS, TIETJEN GL, WIGGS LD, et al. 1987. Mortality among plutonium and other radiation workers at a plutonium weapons facility. Am J Epidemiol 125:231–250.

WILLIAMS D, PINCHERA A, KARAOGLOU A, CHADWICK KH, EDS. 1993. Thyroid cancer in children living near Chernobyl. Luxembourg: Commission of the European Communities, (Report EUR 15248).

WILLIAMS D. 1994. Chernobyl, eight years on. Nature 371:556.

WING S, SHY CM, WOOD JL, et al. 1991. Mortality among workers at Oak Ridge National Laboratory. Evidence of radiation effects in follow-up through 1984. JAMA 265:1397–1402.

XUAN X-Z, LUBIN JH, LI J-Y, et al. 1993. A cohort study in southern China of tin miners exposed to radon and radon decay products. Health Phys 64:120–131.

YAMAMOTO T, KOPECKY KJ, FUJIKURA T, et al. 1987. Lung cancer incidence among Japanese A-bomb survivors, 1950–80. J Radiat Res 28:156–171.

YAO SX, LUBIN JH, QIAO YL, et al. 1994. Exposure to radon progeny, tobacco use and lung cancer in a case-control study in southern China. Radiat Res 138:326–336.

YOSHIMOTO Y, DELONGCHAMP R, MABUCHI K. 1994. *In-utero* exposed atomic bomb survivors: cancer risk update. Lancet 344:345–346.

17 Solar radiation

JOSEPH SCOTTO
THOMAS R. FEARS
JOSEPH F. FRAUMENI, JR.

The sun emits electromagnetic radiation, which makes life as we know it possible on earth. Solar radiation is characterized by its wavelength, the distance from one crest of the wave to the next. The shorter the wavelength, the more energetic the radiation, and the greater the capacity to produce chemical and biologic reactions. Visible sunlight, which we perceive as the colors—violet, blue, green, yellow, orange, and red (in order of decreasing energy)—varies in wavelength from about 400 nanometers (nm) to over 700 nm. (A nanometer is one-billionth of a meter and is equal to 10A [Angstrom units]). The electromagnetic spectrum of sunlight is illustrated in Figure 17–1 (Environmental Studies Board, 1973).

In 1801 J.W. Ritter discovered radiation beyond the short end of the visible spectrum, which has since been known as *ultraviolet (UV) radiation* (Jagger, 1967). Earlier, in 1800, Sir William Herschel detected invisible radiation at the long end of the spectrum, known as *infrared radiation*. UV radiation in the wavelengths ranging from about 100 to 400 nm is invisible to the naked eye and is shorter in wavelength than the violet light, thus its name; it provides more energetic radiation than the visible light. Radiation of even shorter wavelengths, i.e., X rays and gamma rays, is so energetic it can cause atoms and molecules to ionize (add or remove electrons) and is thus referred to as ionizing radiation.

Non-ionizing UV radiation has been subdivided into three wavelength groups according to photobiologic effects, with each group showing carcinogenic activity in laboratory animals. UVC radiations are less than 280 nm, and they are referred to as *far-UV* or germicidal radiation because of their effectiveness in killing various microbes. UVA radiations, or *near-UV*, range from about 330 nm to 400 nm. Electromagnetic energy at these wavelengths can produce skin erythema (sunburn) and pigmentation (tanning) in humans, as well as skin tumors in experimental animals, especially at the shorter wavelengths of UVA (International Agency for Research on Cancer [IARC], 1992). Although large quantities are usually required for biologic effects, UVA predominates in the solar radiation reaching the earth's surface and may contribute to the carcinogenic effects of sunlight (Gange and Rosen, 1986).

Of major concern are the UVB radiations (280 nm to about 330 nm), also called *middle-UV*. While solar radiation below 290 nm virtually never reaches the earth's surface since it is absorbed by the earth's atmosphere, a small quantity of UVB, less than 1% of the sun's total energy, does. Under experimental conditions UVB is three to four times more effective than UVA in producing skin erythema in humans and skin cancer in animals (IARC, 1992). Epidemiologic studies have conclusively linked UVB exposure from sunlight and from artificial sources (Morison, 1988) to the major forms of skin cancer, including the nonmelanoma types (basal cell and squamous cell carcinomas) and malignant melanoma (National Institutes of Health [NIH], 1991). Among young people with xeroderma pigmentosum, whose DNA repair mechanisms are defective, the risk of developing skin cancer is about 5,000 times that of the general population under 20 years of age (Kraemer et al, 1984). Cumulative exposure to UVB is also considered at least partly responsible for the "aging" process of the skin in humans (Wei et al, 1993). In addition, there is mounting evidence that UVB radiation causes immune alterations that inhibit rejection of transformed epidermal cells and promote the growth of skin cancer (Kripke, 1994). At the molecular level, Brash et al (1991) have reported that most squamous cell carcinomas of the skin have mutations of the tumor-suppressor gene, *p53*, with the mutations being located at dipyrimidine sites and involving specific double-base changes characteristic of UVB-induced mutations in model systems.

On the other hand, it is well known that UVB helps to prevent vitamin D deficiency rickets, which is now confined to underdeveloped parts of the world with inadequate nutrition. In recent years, the latitudinal gradients for colon, breast, and prostate cancers have led to suggestions that solar radiation may protect against these common tumors, perhaps by increasing vitamin D

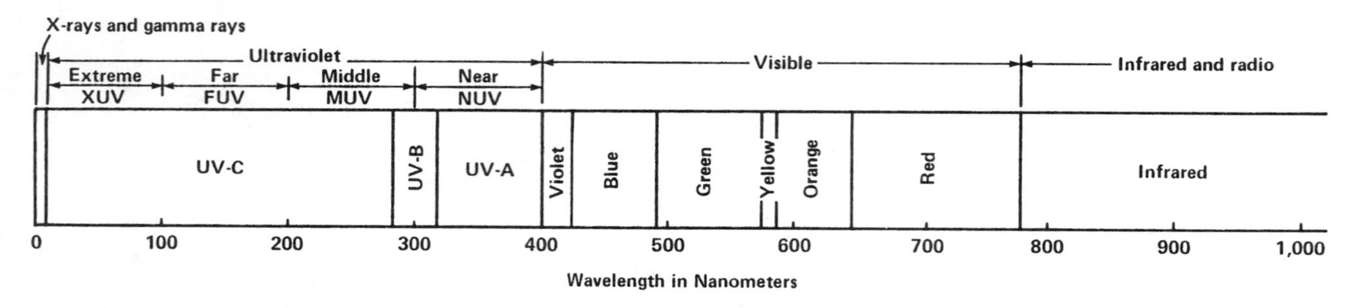

FIG. 17–1. The electromagnetic spectrum. [Adapted from Environmental Studies Board, 1973, with permission.]

and calcium levels (Garland et al, 1990; Emerson and Weiss, 1992), although other factors may account for the geographic patterns observed.

THE OZONE LAYER

One of the principal components of the earth's atmosphere that protects us from excessive radiation is ozone (O_3), which is both formed and destroyed by the action of solar UV radiation on oxygen molecules (Armstrong, 1994). Ozone gases absorb most UV light in the stratosphere (at heights of between 10 and 50 kilometers), where about 90% of the total column ozone is distributed, and allow only small amounts of UVB to penetrate to the earth's surface. Disturbances in the stratospheric ozone layer may increase the amount of UVB reaching the earth and cause changes in temperature, wind patterns, precipitation, and other weather elements. The greenhouse effect, crop failures, soil erosions and decreasing shorelines, and disturbances of marine life are among the environmental consequences of sustained stratospheric ozone depletion (Titus and Seidel, 1986). Thus, maintaining the proper balance of ozone levels in the biosphere is an ecologic necessity.

Over the past two decades, there have been widespread concern and publicity that the protective "ozone shield" may be damaged or depleted by various human activities (Roan, 1990; Armstrong, 1994). Initial alerts from the U.S. Department of Transportation raised concern about the use of supersonic transport aircraft (the SSTs), nitrogen fertilizers, and nuclear weapons, all of which result in ozone-depleting nitrogen oxide gases at high altitudes (Environmental Studies Board, 1973; Cutchis, 1974). Soon thereafter it was discovered that chlorine atoms contained in man-made chlorofluorocarbon (CFC) compounds have an even greater potential for absorbing ozone (Rowland and Molina, 1975). The lifetime of halocarbons that reach stratospheric heights may exceed 75 years and during that time a single reprocessed chlorine atom may destroy as many as 100,000 ozone molecules (Moran and Morgan, 1991).

While the Climatic Impact Committee (1975) of the National Academy of Sciences (NAS) suggested that large fleets of early model SSTs would eventually reduce ozone levels, Rowland and Molina (1975) urged that the use of CFCs, particularly F-11 and F-12, which travel as inert gases into the upper stratosphere, be discontinued. These compounds, generally known as *freons*, are used as propellants in aerosol spray cans and as refrigerants in cooling and air conditioning units. Their trade names are listed in Table 17–1. In 1975 a Federal Task Force on the Inadvertent Modification of the Stratosphere (IMOS) concluded that

> ". . . any release to the atmosphere of man-made chemicals that reach the stratosphere and react to destroy ozone would create additional decreases in the stratospheric ozone content over and above those caused naturally. . ."

and that

> ". . . current model calculations predict that if release of fluorocarbons were to continue at the 1972 rate, a maximum reduction of about 7 percent in the equilibrium ozone concentration would be expected after several decades."

The IMOS report also found that

> "[a]n approximately 1.4% to 2.5% (median of 2%) increase in UV-B radiation at the earth's surface at mid-latitudes would occur for each 1% reduction in stratospheric ozone concentration. This relationship holds true for small percentage changes in ozone concentration. For larger reductions in ozone, it is expected that the associated increase in UV-B radiation reaching the earth's surface would be disproportionately greater."

The relative change in UVB dose due to the relative change in ozone value is referred to as the *physical amplification factor*. In 1976 the Committee on Impacts of Stratospheric Change (CISC) of the NAS further recommended steps to "(a) regulate the uses of CFCs selectively, and (b) regulate the handling of CFCs on the basis of threats to plants and animals important to human life."

In 1977, an amendment to the Clean Air Act (Public Law 95-95) provided for an "ozone protection policy." It acknowledged that stratospheric ozone reductions resulting from halocarbon compounds introduced into the environment would cause harmful biologic effects, and called for continued and detailed investigations by federal agencies to estimate the magnitude of the problem and the potential threat to food crops as well as human suffering. An updated report from the CISC

TABLE 17–1. *List of Trade Names of Chlorofluorocarbons by Country and Manufacturer, 1974*

Country	Company	Trade Name
Argentina	Fluoder S.A.	Algeon
	I.R.A., S.A.	Frateon
Czechoslovakia	Slovek Pro Chemickov A Hutni Vyobu, Ustianad Cabem	Ledon
England	Imperial Chemical Industries, Ltd.	Arcton
	Imperial Smelting Corp., Ltd.	Isceon
France	Products Chimiques Penchiney-Saint-Gobain	Flugene
	Societe d'Electro-Chimie d'Electro-Metallurgie et des Acieres Electrique d'Ugine	Forane
East Germany	V.E.B. Alcid Fluorwerk Dohna	Frigedohn
West Germany	Chemische Fabrik von Heyden AG	Heydogen
	Farbwerke Hoechst AG	Frigen
	Kali-Chemie AG	Kaltron
India	Everest Refrigerants, Ltd.	Everkalt
	Navin Fluorine Industries	Mafron
Italy	Montecatini-Edison	Algofrene
		Edifren
Japan	Daikin Kigyl Co., Ltd.	Daiflon
	Asahi Glass Co., Ltd.	Asahiflon
Netherlands	Uniechemie N.V.	Fresane
	Noury van Der Lande N.V.	FCC
U.S.S.R.		Eskimon
United States	E.I. du Pont de Nemours and Co.	Freon
	Allied Chemical and Dye Corp.	Genetron
	Kaiser Chemicals	Kaiser
	Pennwalt Chemical Co.	Isotron
	Racon, Inc.	Racon
	Union Carbide Corp.	Ucon

*From Rowland and Molina (1975). The chlorofluoromethanes are frequently described by trademark names plus identifying number, such as Freon-11 for $CFCl_3$ and Freon-12 for CF_2Cl_2 for these compounds when manufactured by E.I. du Pont de Nemours and Company.

(1979) estimated that "the eventual ozone depletion due to continued release of CFCs at the 1977 level is 16.5 percent." The relative increase in UVB reaching the earth's surface then would be about twice as much ($16.5 \times 2 = 33\%$). Questions were asked about health consequences, especially with respect to the risk of skin cancer, and steps were taken to collect appropriate physical and epidemiologic information. Several federal agencies have responsibilities for research programs to study and monitor the atmospheric and biospheric consequences of ozone depletion. Since nonmelanoma skin cancers are not routinely included in population-based registries that measure cancer incidence, the National Cancer Institute (NCI) began studies to measure the incidence of skin cancer in various parts of the United States and to evaluate the effects of UVB and other risk factors. In collaboration with the National Oceanic and Atmospheric Administration (NOAA) and Temple University, the NCI started to monitor the counts of UVB reaching the earth's surface (Scotto et al, 1976).

By the end of 1978, the United States and many European countries banned the production of CFCs as propellants in nonessential products, especially aerosol-spray cans. In the following years the estimates of projected ozone depletion by the NAS were revised downward to 7.6% in 1980, and then to 2–4% in 1982 (CISC, 1982, 1984). Concerns were raised that the relatively small changes in ozone, projected over many years into the 21st century, would be very difficult to monitor, and measurements would be confounded by variations in other atmospheric pollutants capable of absorbing UVB. However, by the mid-1980s, it became apparent that the global production and use of CFCs were increasing due to the lack of restrictions in many countries, as well as the continued use of CFCs in air conditioners, styrofoam containers, and as solvents in the manufacture of computer chips (Hoffman, 1987). In the fall (i.e., austral spring) of 1985 the dramatic finding of a "hole," amounting to 40% depletion in the ozone layer over Antarctica, renewed worldwide interest in developing environmental safeguards (Farman et al, 1985).

THE MONTREAL PROTOCOL AND THE OZONE HOLE

In 1987 a consortium of 43 nations met in Montreal, Canada to assess the scientific evidence regarding ozone depletion and its causes and to recommend protective measures. About the same time, studies of the Antarctic ozone hole suggested a strong correlation with the presence of highly reactive chlorinated and brominated compounds aided by the polar vortex, a natural circulation of wind occurring each winter (Solomon, 1988; World Meterological Organization [WMO], 1990). It was suggested that the halogen molecules crystalize and remain on the surface of stratospheric clouds during the winter and then react with ozone when sunlight returns in the austral spring. This condition is temporary, as warm air masses dissipate the polar vortex and replenish the ozone layer over the Antarctic. Similar observations have been made over the Arctic polar vortex, although the ozone depletion appears less pronounced due to wind and cloud patterns. By 1990 the United States and over 60 other countries agreed to ratify the so-called Montreal protocol, which recommended the limitation and eventual ban of the use and production of CFCs by the year 2000.

RECENT OZONE AND UVB TRENDS

Based on risk assessment models, it has been predicted that a 6% depletion of the global ozone layer may occur by the middle of the 21st century and a 40% depletion by the year 2075 if CFC consumption continues unabated (Hoffman, 1987). Statistical analyses combining ozone measurements at various geographic sites at first revealed no significant decreasing trends during the 1960s and 1970s (Reinsel and Tiao, 1987). However, recent updates and re-analyses of the ozone data obtained from satellites indicate that, on a worldwide basis, stratospheric ozone was depleted by 3% between 1969 and 1987 (Watson et al, 1988; Stolarski et al, 1992). As a result, the U.S. Environmental Protection Agency (EPA) (1988) has predicted that by the middle of the 21st century, cumulative excesses in skin cancer incidence may reach several hundred thousand cases. Some workers have suggested that recent increases in skin cancer rates could be related to ozone depletion, particularly in view of the increases in UVB levels reported in Toronto, Canada (Kerr and McElroy, 1993) and in a mountainous region of Switzerland (Blumthaler and Ambach, 1990). However, surface levels of solar UVB have not shown increases at various urban locations of the United States (Scotto et al, 1988) or in other countries such as Norway (Moan and Dahlback, 1992). Although variations in UVB exposure may be influenced by meterological conditions such as cloud cover, sulfur dioxide, nitrogen oxides, tropospheric ozone, and UVB-absorbing particulates (Frederick et al, 1991), it is important to continue the monitoring of the ozone layer and surface levels of UV radiation as well as incidence trends for nonmelanoma skin cancer and melanoma. At present the steady increases reported in the incidence of melanoma, squamous cell carcinoma, and basal cell carcinoma appear largely due to increased sun exposures from changing leisure-time activities and clothing habits (Glass and Hoover, 1989; Gallagher et al, 1990; Miller and Weinstock, 1994).

CARCINOGENIC EFFECTS OF SUNLIGHT

There is abundant evidence in humans and laboratory animals that solar radiation causes both melanoma and nonmelanoma skin cancer. Urbach (1987) reports that in 1820 Sir Everard Home, by exposing one hand to the sun and covering the other with a black cloth, was the first to observe that sunlight other than heat "scorches" the skin. In the late 19th century Thiersch (1875) and Unna (1894) described the high frequency of skin changes, which terminated in cancer, among sailors exposed to the sun (*Seemanshaut*). In the early 20th century, Dubreuilh (1907) and Bellini (1909) recognized an excess risk of skin cancer among people in rural communities, notably vineyard workers and farmers. Hyde (1906) linked sunlight exposure to the exceptional risk of skin cancer in children with the inherited condition xeroderma pigmentosum. He also noted that pigmented races are relatively protected from skin cancer, while Caucasians with fair complexions and outdoor occupations are more susceptible. An excellent historical review of events linking solar radiation to skin cancer was provided by Blum (1959), while more recent evidence has been reviewed by a working group of the International Agency for Research on Cancer (IARC, 1992).

As is often the case, clinical and epidemiologic observations relating environmental exposure to disease preceded the laboratory evidence. Findlay (1928) is credited with first detecting the carcinogenic action of UV radiation on the skin of experimental mice. These observations were soon verified (Roffo, 1934; Rusch et al, 1941). Findlay's source of ultraviolet light was a quartz mercury vapor lamp, while Roffo induced tumors in rats by exposure to direct sunlight. In subsequent animal studies, broad-spectrum UV radiation from sunlight or from sunlamps emitting mostly UVB produced a variety of benign and malignant skin tumors, most notably squamous cell carcinomas. Basal cell carcinomas were seen occasionally in athymic nude mice and rats exposed to UV radiation, while melanocytic tumors were reported following exposure of opossums and hybrid fish (IARC, 1992).

The evidence linking skin cancer to solar radiation, as reviewed by the IARC (1992) and by others (Koh, 1991; Preston and Stern, 1992; Marks, 1995), may be summarized as follows:

1. Skin cancer (melanoma and nonmelanoma types) occurs predominantly in white populations. It is uncommon in blacks, Asians, Hispanics, and other populations with protective melanin pigmentation of the skin.
2. It is especially common in fair-complexioned individuals who freckle and sunburn easily, notably those of Celtic ancestry having Irish, Scottish, or Welsh background.
3. It occurs primarily on parts of the body most often exposed to sunlight, with the anatomic pattern being more pronounced for squamous cell carcinoma than for basal cell carcinoma and being least evident for melanoma.
4. The incidence of skin cancer is inversely correlated with latitude and shows a positive relation to estimated or measured levels of UV radiation.
5. Outdoor workers with chronic sun exposure are at greater risk than indoor workers for nonmelanoma skin cancer, while indoor workers with intermittent sun-intensive exposure appear more prone to melanoma.
6. The risk of skin cancer is associated with various measures of solar skin damage, including actinic keratoses and solar elastosis.
7. Individuals with certain genetic skin diseases, such as xeroderma pigmentosum and albinism, are prone to skin cancer by virtue of their exceptional sensitivity to UV radiation.
8. Experimental animals develop skin cancer with repeated doses of UV radiation, especially in the UVB

spectral range that produces delayed erythema in human skin, i.e., 290–320 nm.

9. Most squamous cell skin cancers have highly specific mutations of the tumor-suppressor gene, *p53*, that are characteristic of UV-induced changes in model systems (Brash et al, 1991).

Lip cancer is also related to sunlight exposure based on the following factors: a latitudinal gradient, predilection for the more exposed lower lip, association with labial actinic keratoses, greater risk among outdoor workers including farmers and fisherman, and predisposition of individuals who are fair complexioned or have sun-sensitive genetic diseases (Lindqvist and Teppo, 1978; Wiklund and Holm, 1986). The lip tumors are predominantly squamous cell carcinomas. Tobacco smoking is also a risk factor, most notably in outdoor workers, suggesting an interaction with solar radiation (Lindqvist, 1979).

Although a latitudinal gradient has not been reported, ocular melanoma has been related to UV radiation based on risk factors resembling those for skin melanoma, including exposure and sensitivity to sunlight (Tucker et al, 1985; Holly et al, 1990). Some epidemiologic and experimental similarities to skin cancer have been noted recently for non-Hodgkin's lymphoma (Cartwright et al, 1994), raising speculation that UV radiation may be a risk factor.

ACTION SPECTRUMS AND UVB METERS

The sun's angle in relation to the earth (which is 0° at zenith when the sun lies directly overhead and 90° when the sun sets at the horizon), and the distance through the atmosphere which the sun's rays must travel (which is shortest, or one *airmass* at solar noon near the equator when the zenith angle is 0°) vary with season and time of day as well as latitude and altitude. Although zenith angle and airmass (except for large zenith angles, airmass equals the secant of the zenith angle) dictate for the most part how much solar UV radiation may reach the earth's surface, other meterological factors, such as sky cover, make it difficult to estimate the amounts of biologically effective UV radiation reaching specific locations. Meters specifically designed to measure the UVB irradiance were developed by Donald Robertson (1968) in Australia, and were refined, manufactured, and implemented by Dan Berger (1975) of Temple University. These photosensitive Robertson-Berger (R-B) meters were installed at a network of various National Weather Service stations (usually airports) and have been used to measure the solar UVB intensities around the United States and in other countries since 1974 (Scotto et al, 1988). Each meter is calibrated to the action spectrum which parallels that for human skin erythema and provides a single reading by weighting the UVB wavelengths according to the relative erythema response.

The wavelength most effective in producing erythema on the "average untanned" Caucasian skin is 297 nm in length (Robertson, 1982). Figure 17–2A shows the classical action spectrum which depicts the relative biologic response for erythema at various UVB wavelengths compared to the effects of radiation at 297 nm (set at 1.00). The biological effectiveness of UVB decreases logarithmically within the UVB range; at about 325 nm it is .001% as effective as at 297 nm. In terms of energy units, about 250,000 ergs per cm^2 at 297 nm are required to produce a minimum perceptible erythema. This is equivalent to 0.025 w-s per cm^2 or 25,000 μw-s per cm^2. The R-B meter, with a response about 2–3 nm toward the longer wavelengths, integrates the weighted amounts of UVB and provides counts in sunburn units (SU). McKinley and Diffey (1987) have recently developed a human erythema action spectrum that includes wavelengths longer than 330 nm. In do-

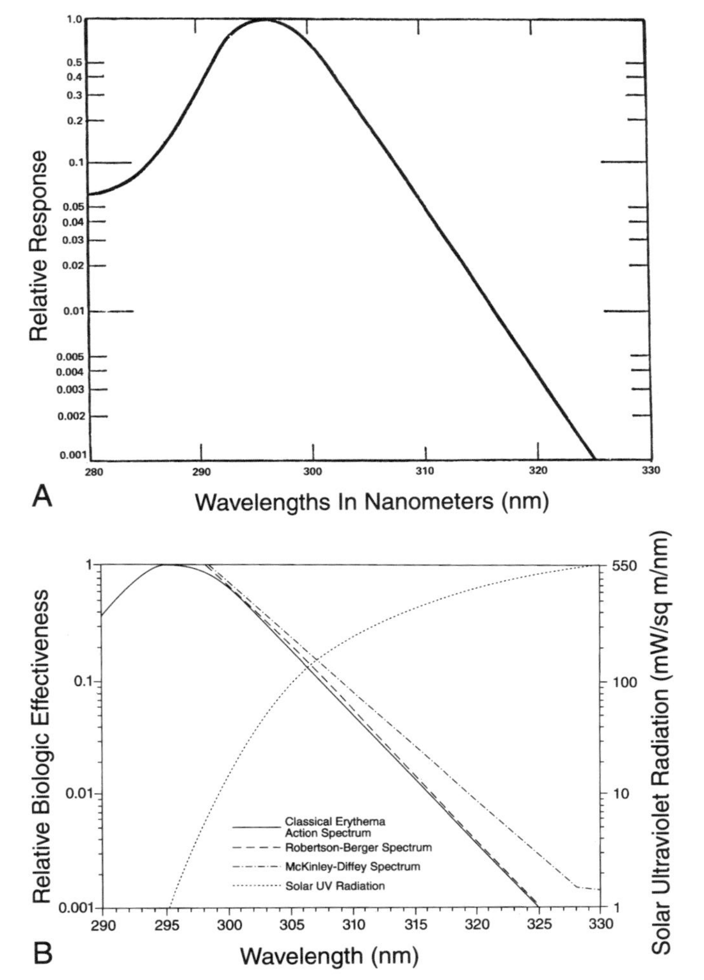

FIG. 17–2. *A*: Erythema action spectrum. *B*: Comparison of classical erythema, Robertson-Berger, and McKinley-Diffey action spectrums, with solar UV measurements at ground level.

simetry studies, the R-B meter has shown a high degree of correlation with measurements of solar radiation from other spectroradiometric instruments (Diffey, 1987). Figure 17–2B indicates how the R-B action spectrum compares with the McKinley-Diffey and classical action spectrums, along with measures of solar UV radiation reaching the earth's surface. It has been estimated (Koller, 1965) that an exposure of about 20 minutes to midsummer noonday sunlight may produce a perceptible sunburn or minimal erythemal response in nontanned Caucasian skin. In R-B meter units this amounts to a count of about 440, and is equivalent to about 25–35 mJ/cm² (DeLuisi and Harris, 1983).

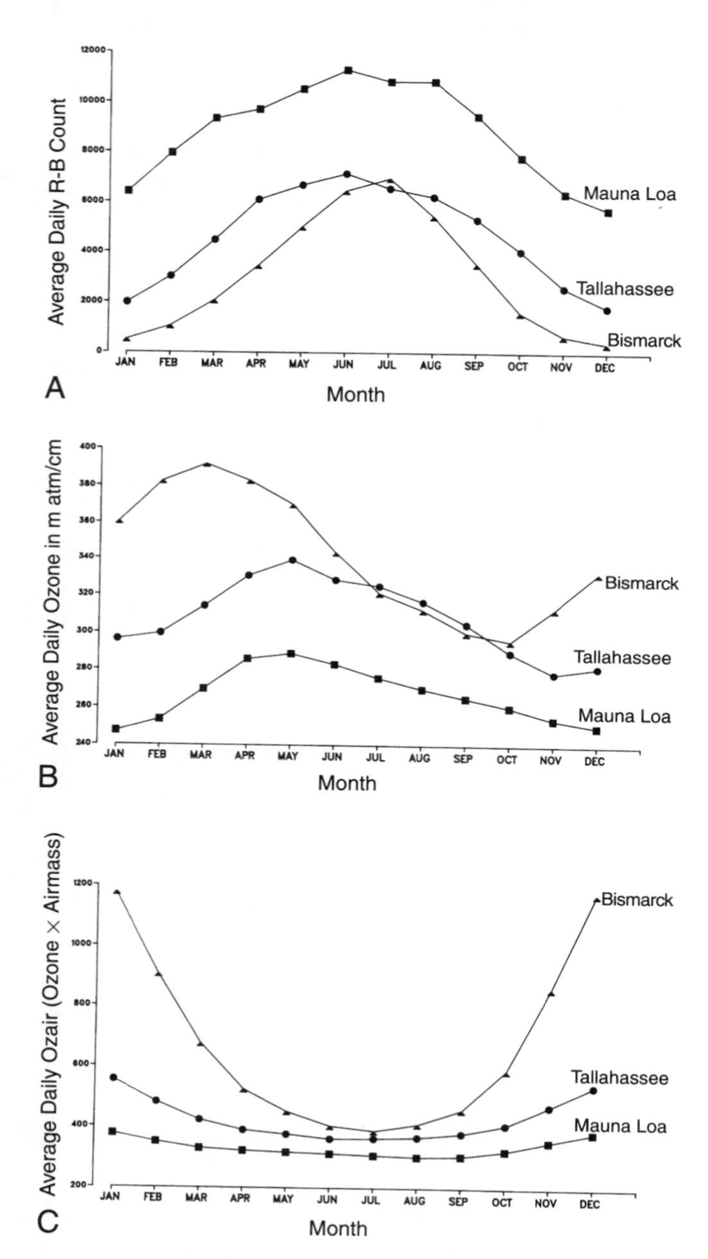

FIG. 17–3. *A*: Average daily UVB counts (Robertson-Berger meter units) by month for selected locations. *B*: Average daily ozone (Dobson units) by month for selected locations. C: Average daily ozair (ozone × airmass) by month for selected locations.

There is good evidence that skin cancer may arise from UV-induced changes in DNA, and Setlow (1974) has shown that the action spectrum for DNA damage parallels that for skin erythema over the UVB portion of the spectrum between 295 and 320 nm. Setlow also noted that estimates of the biologic amplification factor (BAF) based on the classical erythema action spectrum may be about 20–40% less than those observed for a DNA action spectrum (CISC, 1982). Compared to the DNA reference, which has an estimated BAF of 2.0 (CISC, 1979), BAFs based on the R-B and McKinley-Diffey action spectrums would be even further reduced (Frederick and Lubin, 1988; Urbach, 1989).

MEASUREMENTS OF ULTRAVIOLET RADIATION AND OZONE

It has been possible to link UVB measurements at various locations (Scotto et al, 1988; Elwood and Diffey, 1993) with ozone data from the Dobson meter network assembled by the World Meterological Organization (1990). Figures 17–3A and 17–3B show patterns in average monthly UVB and ozone levels at three U.S. locations of widely varying latitude, altitude, and sky cover: Mauna Loa, Hawaii (low latitude, high altitude, and relatively clear skies); Tallahassee, Florida (low latitude, low altitude, and very cloudy skies); and Bismarck, North Dakota (high latitude, moderate altitude, and relatively cloudy skies except for the summer months). Ozone levels peak during the spring months and drop during the fall season, and the levels rise with increasing latitude. In contrast, UVB levels decrease as latitude increases; but their peaks (in summer) and troughs (in winter) do not appear synchronized with the seasons of low and high ozone values. However, when the effects of ozone and airmass are combined, it is evident that the seasonally high levels of UVB are associated with the path of least resistance for solar radiation (Figure 17–3C). While ozone is the main factor associated with surface measurements of UVB, Frederick et al (1989) showed that cloud cover and atmospheric particulates and gases (usually associated with urban pollution) can offset the effects of small changes in the ozone layer. Thus we see that the amount of UVB reaching Bismarck in July is actually greater than that for Tallahassee, which is almost 17° latitude closer to the equator. The difference is mainly due to the effect of heavy cloud cover at the southern location, as the ozone values varied by only 4 Dobson units.

As shown in Figure 17–4, annual levels of surface-based UVB readings decrease as latitude increases. In a statistical analysis of UVB exposure at various locations in the United States, latitude alone explained 68% of the variation; altitude and latitude, 91%; and sky cover,

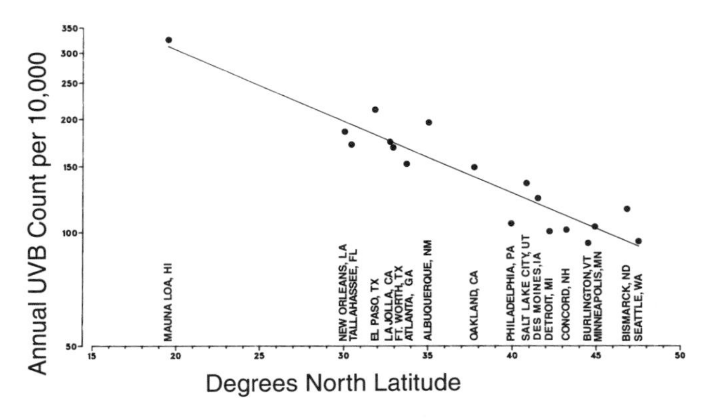

FIG. 17–4. Average annual UVB measurements (Robertson-Berger meter units) by latitude for selected locations, 1974–1990.

altitude and latitude, as much as 97% (Scotto et al, 1982). It is estimated that a one-degree decrease in latitude will increase the annual amount of UVB radiation by 4%. Also, for each mile in altitude above sea level, UVB radiation may increase by 17%. An estimate of the annual amount of UVB reaching the earth's surface at a particular location, when only latitude and altitude are known, may be obtained by using the following formula:

$$\text{Ln(UVB)} = 15.545 - 0.039(L) + .0001038(A)$$

where, L is the latitude in degrees north and A is the altitude or sea elevation in meters. Table 17–2 shows

TABLE 17–2. *Estimated Annual Solar Ultraviolet (UVB) Radiation in the Coterminous United States in Robertson-Berger (R-B) Units According to State of Residence**

State	*Annual R-B Count* $\times 10^{-4}$	*State*	*Annual R-B Count* $\times 10^{-4}$
Alabama	154	Nebraska	125
Arizona	196	Nevada	160
Arkansas	145	New Hampshire	105
California (North)	145	New Mexico	195
California (South)	164	New York	104
Colorado	158	North Carolina	142
Connecticut	108	North Dakota	105
Florida	175	Ohio	113
Georgia	152	Oklahoma	144
Idaho	129	Oregon	93
Illinois	117	Pennsylvania	113
Indiana	120	Rhode Island	110
Iowa	117	South Carolina	148
Kansas	138	South Dakota	115
Kentucky	124	Tennessee	141
Louisiana	172	Texas	180
Maine	103	Utah	133
Maryland	117	Vermont	96
Massachusetts	109	Virginia	129
Michigan	100	Washington	98
Minnesota	100	Wisconsin	105
Missouri	133	Wyoming	137
Montana	109		

*A count of about 440 R-B units = 1 minimal erythema dose (MED) for an "average" Caucasian skin. Estimation model for each state includes latitude, altitude and cloud cover.

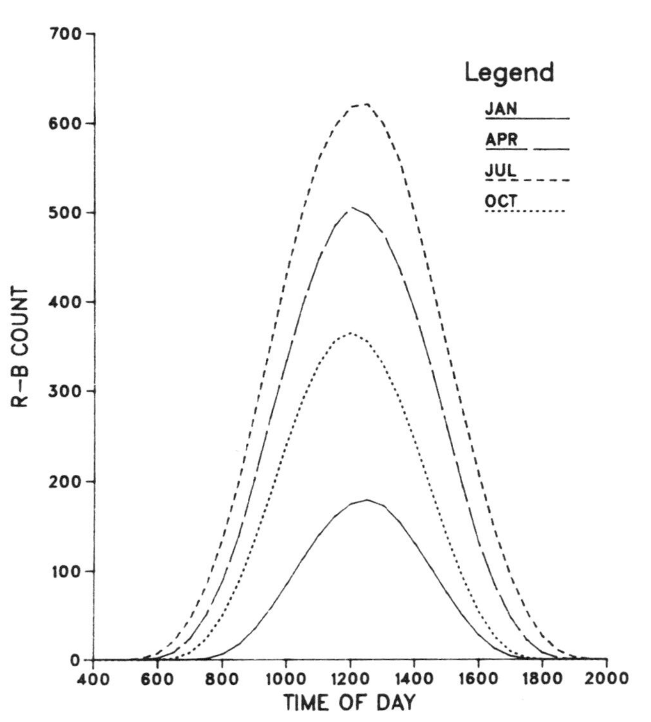

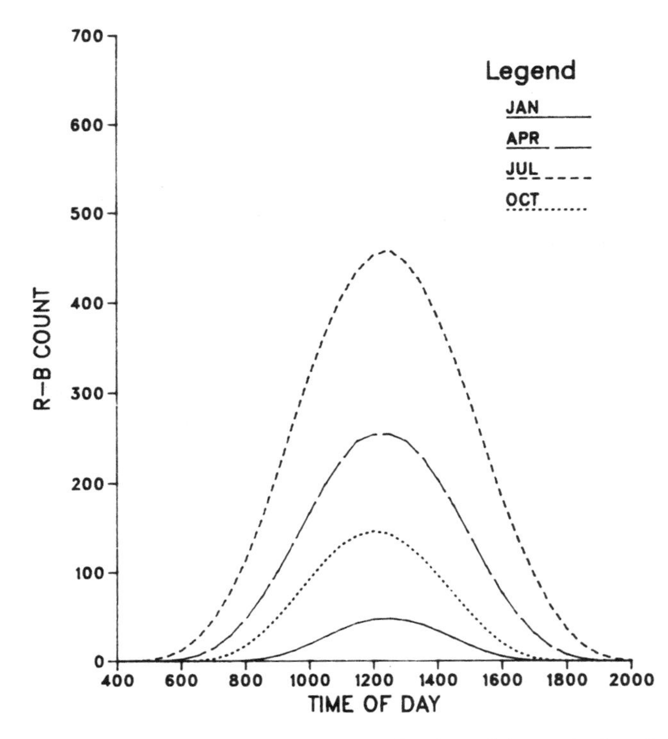

FIG. 17–5. Average UVB measurements by time of day and selected months for southern and northern regions of the United States.

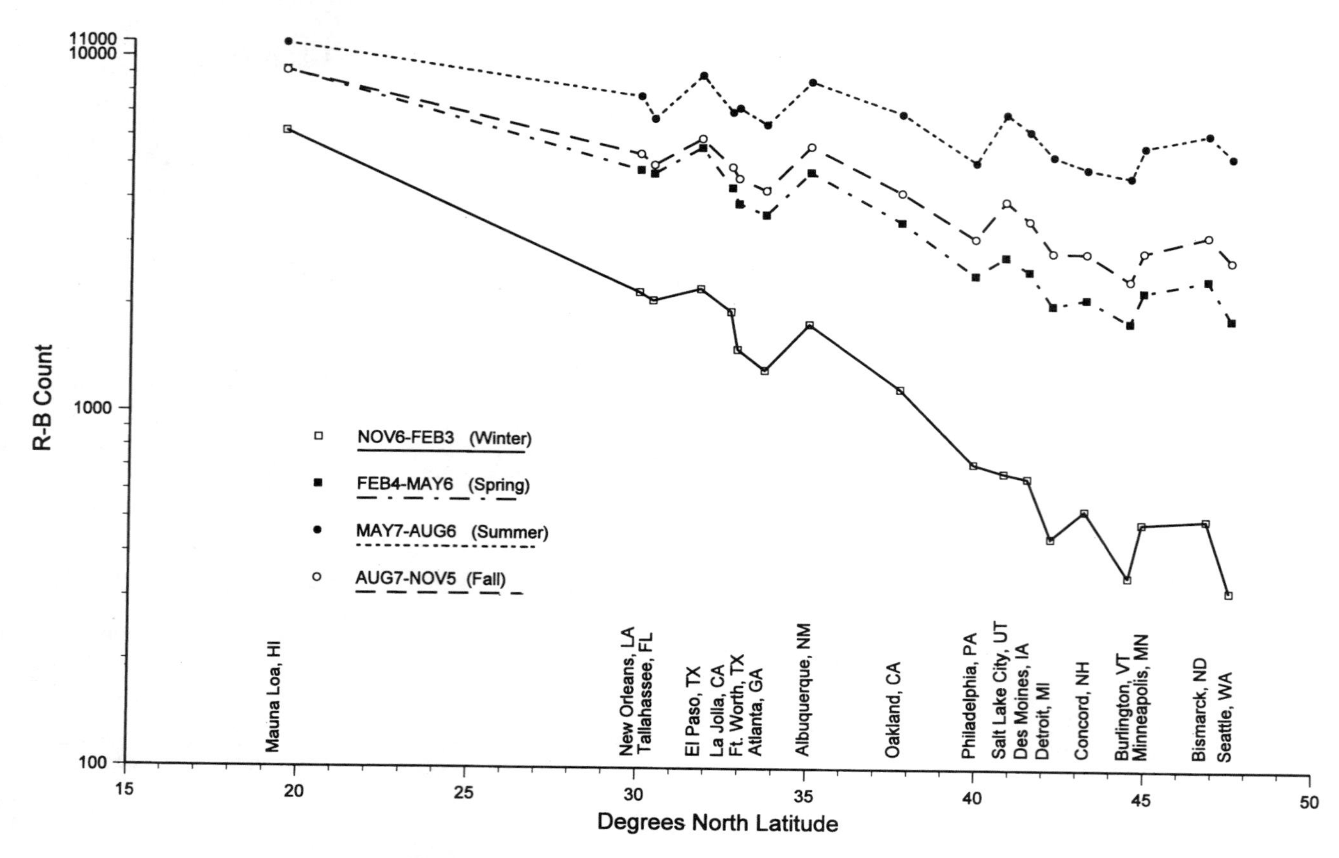

FIG. 17–6. Average daily UVB counts (Robertson-Berger meter units) by latitude and solar quarter.

our estimates in R-B units of the ambient annual levels of solar UVB radiation (averaged from 1974 to 1987, for available data) for each state where monthly UVB levels were estimated using latitude, altitude, and monthly cloud cover data in the models.

Solar UV intensity varies by the time of day and season of the year (Smith et al, 1993). Figure 17–5 illustrates the UVB exposure patterns for selected months of each season at southern (30° to 40° N. latitude) and northern (40° to 50° N. latitude) locations. The daily peak for each month and region centers around noontime, and the amplitudes are greatest in July and lowest in January. On average about one-sixth of the total daily UVB count occurs during the 1-hour period from 11:30 a.m. to 12:30 p.m. local time. Over 60% occurs between the 4-hour span of 10:00 a.m. and 2:00 p.m., with the percentage increasing as latitude increases. Figure 17–6 shows the huge differences in average daily intensity between solar quarters centered around the winter solstice (about December 21, the shortest day) and the summer solstice (about June 21, the longest day) at each location. Division by solar quarters is a more precise way of adjusting for zenith angle changes than the classical method of using three calendar months for each season. It can be seen that the solar quarter centered around the fall equinox (about September 21, when the number of hours of daylight and darkness are equal) receives greater amounts of UVB than that centered around the spring equinox (about March 21), mainly because the ozone is at its annual nadir between August and November.

SKIN CANCER AND UV MEASUREMENTS

Since nonmelanoma skin cancer is not routinely reported by population-based cancer registries in the United States, special incidence surveys have been conducted by the NCI at various areas that participated in the Third National Cancer Survey (TNCS), and the Surveillance, Epidemiology and End Results (SEER) program. In 1971–72, as an adjunct to the TNCS, a 6-month survey of nonmelanoma skin cancer was conducted in 1971–1972 in four areas: Dallas-Fort Worth, San Francisco-Oakland, Iowa, and Minneapolis-St. Paul (Scotto et al, 1974). The NAS Climatic Impact Committee (1975) utilized the TNCS data for nonmelanoma skin cancer and melanoma, along with prevalence data from the National Health and Nutrition Examination Survey (NHANES) (Figure 17–7). As expected from earlier U.S. surveys (Haenszel, 1963; MacDonald, 1978), the incidence and prevalence rates for

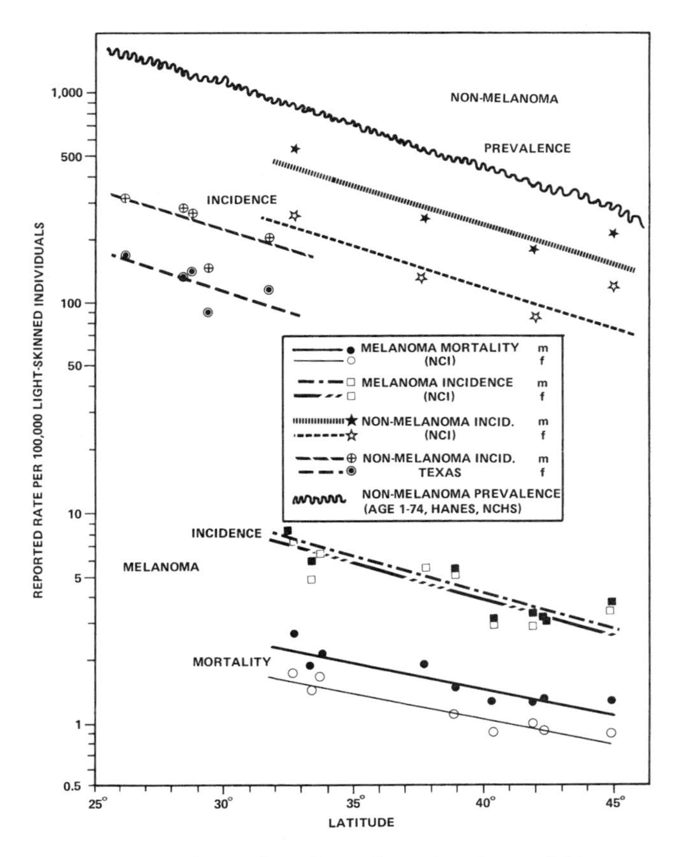

FIG. 17–7. Annual age-adjusted rates for various forms of skin cancer by latitude. [Adapted from Climatic Impact Committee, 1975, with permission.]

nonmelanoma skin cancer, as well as the incidence and mortality rates for melanoma showed an inverse correlation with latitude. In addition, measures of the maximum cumulative lifetime UVB exposure, obtained by multiplying average age by the total annual R-B counts at the four locations, showed a positive correlation with the age-specific incidence rates for nonmelanoma skin cancer (Scotto et al, 1982). When applying mathematical models to the age-specific data for nonmelanoma skin cancer and melanoma, it appeared that these tumors are related to UV exposure in different ways (Fears et al, 1977). The incidence patterns of nonmelanoma skin cancer seemed associated with cumulative UV exposure, and the melanoma patterns with intermittent exposure to high-intensity UV radiation.

To obtain more reliable dose–response estimates, the NCI carried out in 1977–78 a 1-year incidence survey of nonmelanoma skin cancer in eight geographic areas: Atlanta standard metropolitan statistical area (SMSA), Detroit (SMSA), Minneapolis-St. Paul (SMSA), New Mexico (State), New Orleans (SMSA), San Francisco-Oakland (SMSA), Seattle (King County), and Utah (Scotto et al, 1983). All except Minneapolis-St. Paul were part of the SEER program and were included in the UVB monitoring network. To further enhance the dose–response estimates, the survey was extended in 1979–80 to cover New Hampshire-Vermont and San Diego, areas with relatively low and high levels of insolation, respectively (Scotto, 1986; Serrano et al, 1991). UVB data from the R-B meters surface measurements were averaged by location over the calender years 1977–80.

Figure 17–8 shows the latitudinal gradient of age-adjusted incidence rates for nonmelanoma skin cancer among white males and females for the survey conducted in 1977–80. The male-to-female ratios were about two and were higher in the southern than the northern locations. Figure 17–9 shows the regional variation in age-specific incidence patterns of nonmelanoma skin cancer for the ten areas. In the southern locations, the male rates appear to diverge from the female rates and show increased risk as early as age 30. In the northern and central regions, the male rates do not exceed the female rates until about age 45, presumably because of lower cumulative exposures to UVB. Tables 17–3a and 17–3b show the age-adjusted incidence rates by anatomic site and geographic location for white males and females. Over 80% of all patients had at least one skin cancer on the face, head or neck. Among females, the nose was the most common site, while among males, tumors of the nose, cheek and scalp were equally high. Tumors of the ear occurred more frequently among men compared to women by a factor of 10 or more, especially in the southern areas, whereas tumors of the leg were more common among females. A similar anatomic pattern has been described for melanoma (Lee and Yongchaiyudha, 1971). In both sexes, tumors were much more common in the skin affecting the lower lip than the upper lip.

Figure 17–10 compares the area-specific incidence

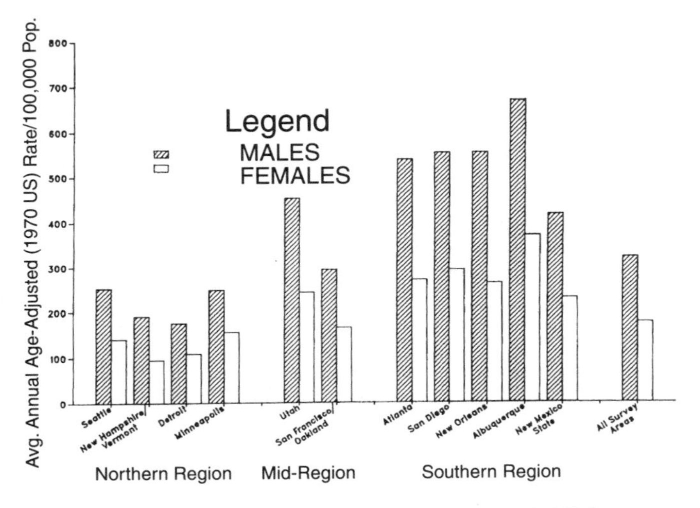

FIG. 17–8. Annual age-adjusted incidence rates (1977–80) for nonmelanoma skin cancer among white males and females according to geographic areas of the United States.

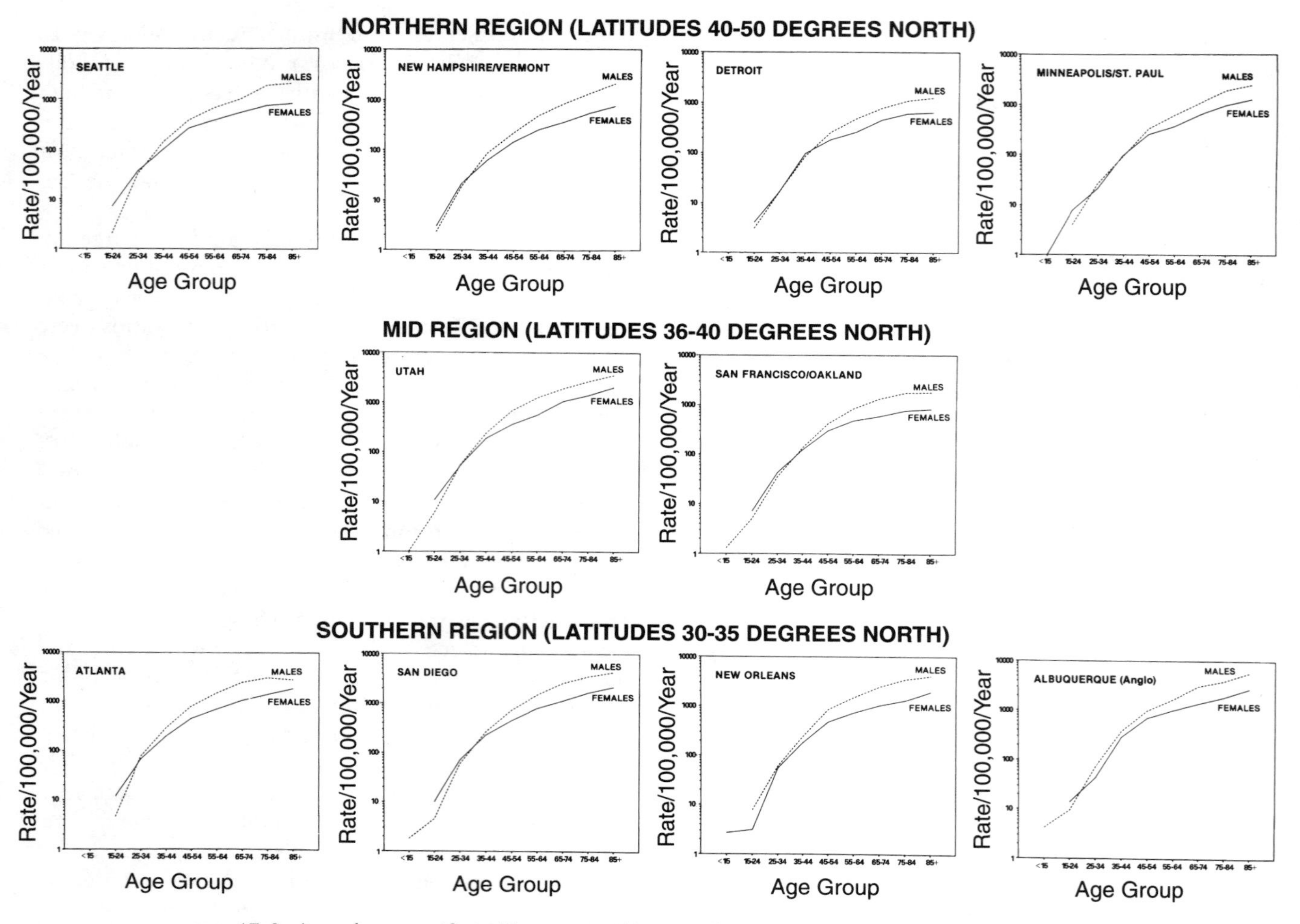

FIG. 17–9. Annual age-specific incidence rates (1977–80) for nonmelanoma skin cancer among white males and females in selected regions of the United States.

rates for nonmelanoma skin cancer with the rates for total cancer reported by the SEER program (Ries et al, 1991). The strong latitudinal gradient for skin cancer contrasts with the lack of any trend for other cancers combined. In the southern areas, the incidence of skin cancer surpassed that for all other cancers, while in the northern areas, skin cancer rates were about 40% those of other sites. Based on data from the two surveys, incidence appeared to increase by 15–20% over the 6-year period in the 1970s, consistent with the upward trend reported for nonmelanoma skin cancer and melanoma in other surveys. When rates from various surveys of nonmelanoma skin cancer are projected to 1994, the annual incidence is estimated to be 900,000 to 1.2 million cases, which is similar to the magnitude of all noncutaneous malignancies (Miller and Weinstock, 1994).

Figure 17–11 displays for white males and females the annual UVB levels and age-adjusted incidence rates for nonmelanoma skin cancer in the two surveys. The incidence data are plotted on a log scale so that a straight line with a positive slope represents a constant percentage increase in incidence. Mathematical models are used to describe dose–response relationships, and do not reflect the mechanism by which UV causes skin cancer. Using an exponential model previously applied to the 1971–72 data (Fears et al, 1976), estimates of the biologic amplification factor (i.e., the relative change in skin cancer incidence due to a relative change in UVB radiation) are derived. Assuming a common slope, the exponential model for each time period may be written as a logarithmic expression:

$$\mathrm{Ln}(R_{ij}) = a_i + b(UV_j) + \epsilon_{ij}$$

where

i = 1,2 denotes the two surveys
j = 1,2 . . . 10 denotes the location
R_{ij} = the age-adjusted incidence rate
UV_j = the annual UV-B count $\times 10^4$
a_1, a_2, b = constants

and the ϵ_{ij}'s are normally and independently distributed with mean zero.

TABLE 17–3a. *Annual Age-Adjusted (1970 U.S. Standard) Incidence Rates (per 100,000) for Nonmelanoma Skin Cancer among White Males by Anatomic Site and Geographic Area, 1977–80, with UVB Index and Latitude*

	Seattle (King Co.)	*New Hampshire Vermont*[a] *(States)*	*Detroit (SMSA)*	*Minneapolis-St. Paul (SMSA)*	*Utah*[a] *(State)*	*San Francisco-Oakland (SMSA)*	*Atlanta (SMSA)*	*San Diego (SMSA)*	*New Orleans (Metro)*[b]	*Albuquerque*[a] *(Anglos)*	*All Survey Areas*
UVB RADIATION INDEX[c]	95	94–102	101	104	136	150	153	175	186	197	94–197
DEGREES IN LATITUDE	47.5	45.0–42.7	42.2	44.9	40.7	37.8	33.7	32.9	30.0	35.1	47.5–30.0
SURVEY PERIOD	1977–78	1979–80	1977–78	1977–78	1977–78	1977–78	1977–78	1979–80	1977–78	1977–78	1977–80
All anatomic sites	253.0	190.6	175.2	250.4	455.4	297.0	542.3	557.7	558.7	673.0	326.0
Face, head or neck (FHN)	189.7	134.3	127.5	186.2	340.7	204.0	374.0	356.5	379.8	481.0	227.8
Scalp or forehead	43.0	35.1	28.7	40.6	80.7	43.3	84.6	93.1	83.4	122.6	53.2
Eyelid	13.2	8.1	7.2	11.7	20.0	11.4	11.0	19.3	20.6	26.0	12.5
Ear	23.8	16.5	13.2	18.2	38.5	25.8	51.6	42.6	51.9	50.1	27.1
Nose	39.8	28.5	29.8	37.8	68.9	41.1	80.3	68.9	84.6	111.3	47.7
Cheek, chin or jaw	38.5	32.0	29.4	50.3	73.9	50.2	93.0	85.6	87.2	110.8	54.0
Neck-supraclavicular	13.7	7.3	12.4	13.3	29.5	17.1	26.1	27.5	27.3	31.0	17.8
Lip	12.5	5.9	6.2	13.1	25.3	12.9	19.4	19.3	22.1	25.2	13.3
Head or neck, NOS	5.3	0.9	0.5	1.2	4.0	2.2	8.0	0.1	2.8	4.0	2.1
Trunk	29.7	22.4	14.0	25.3	26.4	29.5	51.3	50.7	34.6	48.7	29.2
Trunk, front	10.1	6.9	4.8	7.1	10.6	12.1	24.7	18.4	14.4	23.0	11.1
Trunk, back	16.4	15.3	8.6	18.2	14.7	15.9	26.2	32.2	20.2	24.6	17.3
Trunk, NOS	3.3	0.2	0.5	—	1.1	1.5	0.3	—	—	1.0	0.7
Upper extremities (UE)	8.6	9.2	9.9	9.3	31.4	22.0	41.6	51.5	67.9	35.1	23.2
Arm	4.5	5.0	5.7	4.8	14.3	13.9	19.9	34.6	38.4	12.3	13.4
Hand	3.6	4.2	3.9	4.5	17.0	7.2	21.6	16.9	27.3	21.0	9.4
Arm or hand, NOS	0.5	—	0.3	—	—	0.8	0.2	—	2.2	1.8	0.4
Lower extremities (LE)	2.0	4.0	2.3	3.0	2.5	4.2	6.2	5.7	5.1	11.2	3.8
Leg	1.9	3.6	1.9	2.4	2.1	3.8	5.7	5.3	5.1	11.2	3.4
Foot	0.1	0.2	0.4	0.4	0.4	0.3	0.5	0.4	—	—	0.3
Leg or foot, NOS	—	0.2	—	0.2	—	0.2	—	—	—	—	0.1
Other sites	2.8	1.4	1.3	1.9	1.6	4.0	1.7	1.8	6.8	—	2.3
Genitals	0.4	0.5	0.5	1.9	1.4	1.2	—	0.1	0.6	—	0.8
Skin, NOS	2.4	0.9	0.8	—	0.2	2.8	1.7	1.6	6.2	—	1.6
Multiple sites	20.2	19.4	20.3	24.7	52.9	33.3	67.5	91.6	64.4	97.0	39.7
FHN only	10.4	12.7	12.6	15.8	44.6	18.5	39.9	47.8	40.3	68.7	24.0
FHN and trunk	4.7	2.9	4.9	5.0	3.0	5.6	11.1	14.3	8.3	13.7	6.5
FHN and UE	1.6	0.9	1.5	1.1	3.3	3.0	7.3	14.6	11.1	8.1	4.2
FHN and LE	0.4	0.6	0.3	—	0.9	0.5	2.0	1.8	0.3	1.0	0.7
FHN and other	—	—	—	—	—	—	—	—	—	—	—
Other multiples	3.1	2.3	1.0	2.8	1.1	5.7	7.1	13.1	4.5	5.5	4.4

[a]UVB counts and latitudes are for Salt Lake City, Utah; Albuquerque, New Mexico; Burlington, Vermont; and Concord, New Hampshire, respectively.
[b]Includes three parishes: Jefferson, Orleans, and St. Bernard.
[c]Index = estimated UVB counts per 10,000 per annum.

TABLE 17–3b. *Annual Age-Adjusted (1970 U.S. Standard) Incidence Rates (per 100,000) for Nonmelanoma Skin Cancer among White Females by Anatomic Site and Geographic Area, 1977–80, with UVB Index and Latitude*

	Seattle (King Co.)	*New Hampshire-Vermont*[a] *(States)*	*Detroit (SMSA)*	*Minneapolis-St Paul (SMSA)*	*Utah*[a] *(State)*	*San Francisco-Oakland (SMSA)*	*Atlanta (SMSA)*	*San Diego (SMSA)*	*New Orleans (Metro)*[b]	*Albuquerque*[a] *(Anglos)*	*All Survey Areas*
UVB RADIATION INDEX[c]	95	94–102	101	104	136	150	153	175	186	197	94–197
DEGREES IN LATITUDE	47.5	45.0–42.7	42.2	44.9	40.7	37.8	33.7	32.9	30.0	35.1	47.5–30.0
SURVEY PERIOD	1977–78	1979–80	1977–78	1977–78	1977–78	1977–78	1977–78	1979–80	1977–78	1977–78	1977–80
All anatomic sites	140.3	94.9	108.7	155.9	245.5	166.1	274.1	297.5	267.2	374.2	178.7
Face, head or neck (FHN)	102.3	69.8	83.3	120.6	187.8	121.3	192.3	210.7	198.0	266.0	131.4
Scalp or forehead	24.3	15.2	18.9	29.3	46.9	22.1	43.5	45.4	37.2	43.4	28.4
Eyelid	8.4	4.4	6.0	7.9	12.3	9.3	9.9	12.9	18.6	15.4	9.1
Ear	2.4	0.9	1.5	1.5	3.6	1.9	4.0	2.9	5.0	4.6	2.3
Nose	29.0	22.9	24.5	32.4	61.9	38.1	64.3	62.8	64.2	107.5	40.7
Cheek, chin or jaw	21.6	16.8	18.8	30.6	33.0	31.3	43.4	53.0	46.3	48.2	30.6
Neck-supraclavicular	5.8	5.1	6.7	7.8	15.4	7.8	12.3	14.3	10.9	21.0	9.0
Lip	7.0	4.1	6.7	10.7	13.4	9.7	12.0	19.3	14.6	24.5	10.3
Head or neck, NOS	3.8	0.4	0.2	0.5	1.3	1.1	2.9	0.1	1.2	1.5	1.0
Trunk	18.0	8.5	7.4	13.0	13.3	12.3	23.8	22.7	10.1	34.0	13.6
Trunk, front	6.1	3.2	2.7	3.8	4.8	5.1	11.2	11.6	4.4	15.9	5.6
Trunk, back	10.5	5.2	4.4	9.1	7.3	7.0	12.3	11.1	5.7	18.1	7.7
Trunk, NOS	1.3	0.2	0.3	0.1	1.2	0.3	0.3	—	—	—	0.3
Upper extremities (UE)	6.1	4.0	4.0	6.0	15.8	10.5	19.8	20.9	24.4	29.1	10.6
Arm	2.7	3.0	2.0	2.7	7.2	6.5	11.7	14.3	14.3	15.9	6.2
Hand	3.2	1.0	1.9	3.1	8.5	3.5	8.1	6.6	10.2	11.6	4.3
Arm or hand, NOS	0.2	—	0.1	0.1	0.2	0.5	—	—	—	1.6	0.2
Lower extremities (LE)	3.7	3.1	3.4	3.3	4.7	7.1	10.0	11.5	6.1	8.8	5.7
Leg	3.3	2.8	3.3	3.0	4.5	6.4	9.8	11.0	6.1	8.8	5.4
Foot	0.2	0.1	0.1	0.3	—	0.4	0.2	0.5	—	—	0.2
Leg or foot, NOS	0.2	0.1	—	—	0.2	0.3	—	—	—	—	0.1
Other sites	1.3	1.2	0.7	1.6	2.0	3.2	2.1	0.9	4.9	1.6	1.8
Genitals	0.8	0.5	0.6	1.6	1.4	1.8	1.0	0.6	0.4	1.6	1.0
Skin, NOS	0.6	0.7	0.1	—	0.5	1.4	1.1	0.3	4.5	—	0.8
Multiple sites	9.0	8.3	10.0	11.5	21.8	11.8	26.2	30.8	23.7	34.8	15.5
FHN only	6.1	5.0	6.7	8.3	14.3	7.4	14.8	17.1	15.8	24.9	9.7
FHN and trunk	1.0	1.7	1.7	1.9	4.2	1.8	5.8	4.0	3.2	5.4	2.5
FHN and UE	0.7	0.6	0.5	0.3	1.2	0.6	1.7	3.5	2.2	1.5	1.0
FHN and LE	0.3	0.1	0.5	0.2	0.8	0.4	1.3	1.8	0.5	—	0.6
FHN and other	—	—	—	0.1	0.2	—	0.1	—	—	—	0.0
Other multiples	0.9	0.9	0.6	0.6	1.1	1.6	2.4	4.3	1.9	3.0	1.5

[a]UVB counts and latitudes are for Salt Lake City, Utah; Albuquerque, New Mexico; Burlington, Vermont; and Concord, New Hampshire, respectively.

[b]Includes three parishes: Jefferson, Orleans, and St. Bernard.

[c]Index = estimated UVB counts per 10,000 per annum.

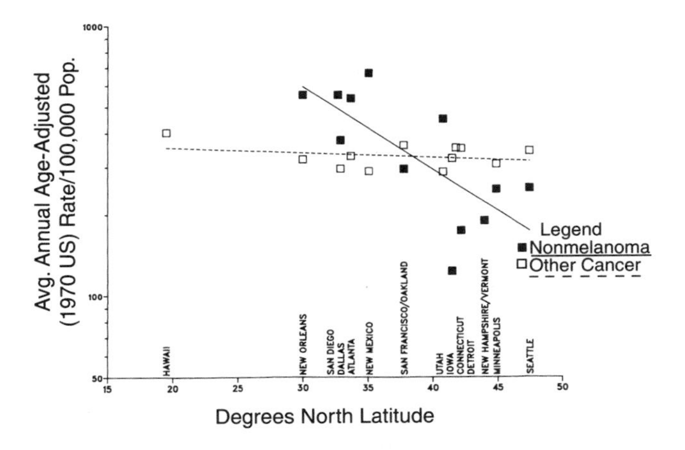

FIG. 17–10. Annual age-adjusted incidence rates for nonmelanoma skin cancer (1977–80) and all other cancers by latitude in the white population of the United States.

In the regression analyses, the logarithms of the age-adjusted incidence rates are weighted by the inverse of their estimated variances. Assuming that the annual UVB counts were to increase by 1% at each location, the relative effects on skin cancer incidence are found to vary from a low of 1.03% to a high of 2.49% (Table 17–4). The estimates are lowest for females residing in areas of low UVB exposure levels. Overall, the biologic amplification factors appear consistent with earlier estimates based on the 1971–72 data (Fears et al, 1977; Rundel and Nachtwey, 1978), and with recent estimates using other models and action spectrums, skin cancer incidence data from other countries, and UVB data imputed from satellite measurements of the ozone layer (Table 17–5). These estimates may be conservative if the skin cancer action spectrum differs from the erythema action spectrum as measured by the R-B meters (CISC, 1984; Moan et al, 1989).

HOST AND ENVIRONMENTAL CO-FACTORS

The effects of solar UV radiation on the development of skin cancer, including melanoma, vary according to a number of host and environmental factors (Kricker et al, 1991, 1994; Preston and Stern, 1992; Marks, 1995). The risks of skin cancer of all types are generally reported to be greater among persons with fair skin complexion, red or blond hair, blue or light eyes, tendency to freckle and sunburn, inability to tan, Celtic ancestry, pre-existing skin tumors, and solar skin damage as measured by actinic keratoses or solar elastosis. In addition, the combination of sun exposure and fair complexion has been linked to actinic keratoses, a common precursor of squamous cell carcinoma (Sober and Burstein, 1995). The risk of melanoma is increased not only by sun exposure and light skin complexion but also by the presence of multiple nevi, especially atypical or dysplastic nevi that may evolve into melanoma (Tucker, 1988). No known precursor lesion exists for basal cell carcinoma.

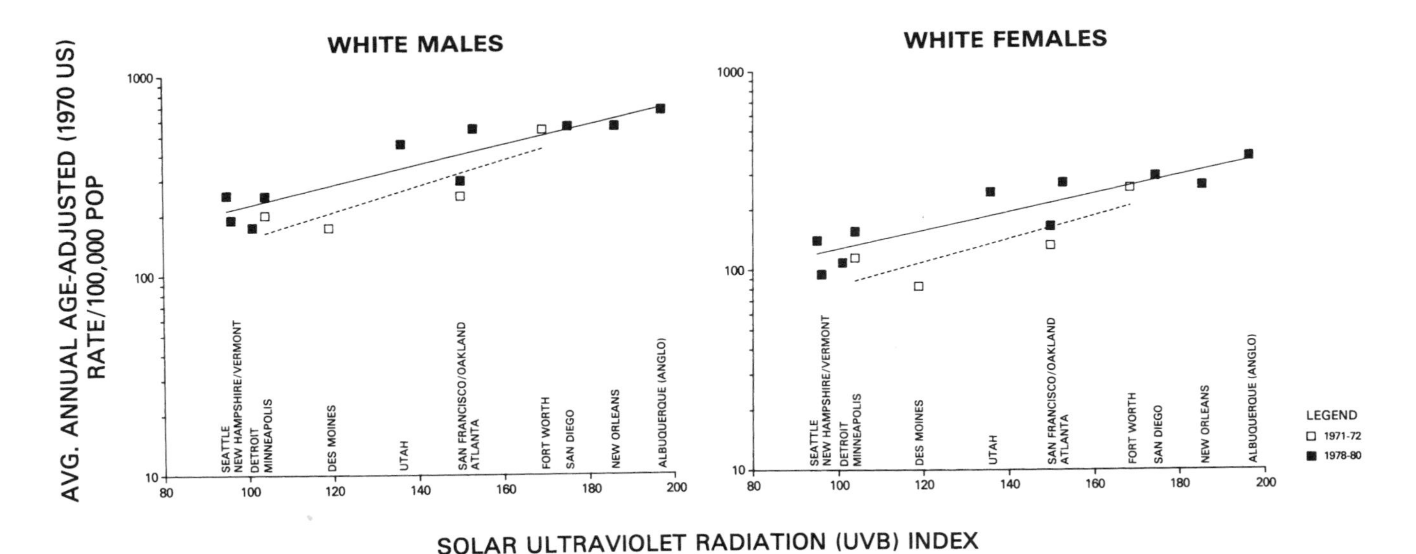

FIG. 17–11. Annual age-adjusted incidence rates (1971–72 and 1977–80) for nonmelanoma skin cancer among white males and females according to UVB index in selected areas of the United States, with regression lines based on exponential model.

TABLE 17–4. *Estimated Relative Increase (Biological Amplification Factor) in Age-Adjusted Incidence Rates for Nonmelanoma Skin Cancer among White Males and Females, Associated with a 1% Increase in UVB Exposures in Specific Areas of the United States**

Location	UVB Index	White Males	White Females
Seattle	95	1.19	1.03
New Hampshire-Vermont	96	1.20	1.04
Detroit	101	1.27	1.10
Minneapolis-St. Paul	104	1.31	1.13
Utah	136	1.71	1.48
San Francisco-Oakland	150	1.89	1.64
Atlanta	153	1.93	1.67
San Diego	175	2.21	1.91
New Orleans	186	2.35	2.03
Albuquerque (Anglo)	197	2.49	2.15

*Exponential model: Ln Rate (AAR) = a+b (UV).

Logistic regression analyses (Vitaliano, 1978) have shown that the effects of sunlight exposure, adjusting for constitutional factors, are greater for patients with squamous cell carcinoma than those with basal cell carcinoma. The finding is consistent with demographic data showing that the latitudinal gradient with UVB levels and the age curves are steeper for squamous cell carcinoma than for basal cell carcinoma and melanoma (Scotto and Fears, 1987). In addition, the available evidence from analytical studies suggests that chronic repeated exposures to sunlight are important in the development of nonmelanoma skin cancer, notably the squamous cell type, whereas intermittent exposures with sunburning tend to be associated with melanoma (Marks, 1995). Risk of melanoma has been linked especially to history of sunburns during childhood, which is consistent with migration studies indicating elevated rates among those moving to sunny climates, particularly when the migration occurs during childhood (Koh, 1991). It has been suggested that intermittent types of exposure may be involved also in basal cell carcinoma based on its anatomic patterns (Gallagher et al, 1990) and the absence of dose dependence at high exposure levels (Strickland et al, 1989).

In conjunction with the 1977–80 survey of nonmelanoma skin cancer in the United States, the NCI conducted a telephone interview study of patients and general population controls at nine locations (Scotto and Fears, 1978) to obtain information on several host and environmental risk factors. Our primary objective was to depict the UVB dose–skin cancer relationship for individuals with and without certain host characteristics (Scotto et al, 1982; Scotto, 1986). Despite sizable variations in the prevalence of risk factors across geographic locations, overall dose–response relationships remained consistent for skin complexion, eye and hair color, and ancestry. As shown in Table 17–6 and Figure 17–12 (for males), patients with nonmelanoma skin cancer are more likely to be light-colored or fair-complexioned than the general population, as expected from earlier studies (IARC, 1992). Although women tended to be more often fair-skinned than men, the responses to this question are sometimes criticized as being too subjective, but in our survey an objective measure of determining skin color was provided. Attached to the bottom of the questionnaire was a series of ten colors ranging from dark to light (1–10), which were replicas of skin swatches used to match skin types for artificial limbs. At each location women were "lighter" than men, so they may indeed be the "fairer sex."

Our study also showed that individuals with blue or green eyes and red or blond hair color were at elevated

TABLE 17–5. *Recent Results from Dose–Response Models**

Year	Authors	Model	Results
1990	Henriksen et al	Quadratic	2% increase in skin cancer for each 1% decrease in ozone.
1990	Dahlbach and Moan	Exponential	BAFs for either BCC or SCC range from 1.5–2.72.
1990	Kelfkens et al	Various	Including UVA wavelengths, BAF = 1.56; 1% decrease in ozone results in 2.7% increase in skin cancer (BAF = 1.7).
1990	United Nations Environment Programme	Exponential-Quadratic	10% ozone reduction yields 30% and 50% increases in BCC and SCC.
1992	Moan and Dahlbach	Exponential	10% ozone depletion results in 16–18% increase in SCC incidence.
1993	Ambach and Blumthaler	Exponential-Power	BAF varies between 1.1 and 1.7, depending on tumor type; 10% ozone reduction increases nonmelanoma skin cancer by 26%.
1992	Diffey	Various	Continued ozone depletion may result in an additional lifetime skin cancer risk of 5% for adults and 10–15% for children.
1993	Madronich and de Gruijl	Exponential-Other	BAFs of 1.4 for BCC and 2.5 for SCC are applied to erythema and DNA dose increases for various estimates of ozone depletion by latitude. Ozone depletion and resultant increases in erythema dose are relatively greater at higher latitude, yielding relatively greater increases in BCC and SCC.

*Abbreviations: BAF = Biological amplification factor; BCC = Basal cell carcinoma; SCC = Squamous cell carcinoma.

TABLE 17–6. *Estimates of Annual Age-Adjusted (1970 U.S. Standard) Incidence Rates (per 100,000 Population) for Nonmelanoma Skin Cancer According to Selected Host Factors, and Relative Risks (Compared to Individuals without Factor) among White Males and Females*

	White Males		*White Females*	
Host Factors	*Rate*	*RR*	*Rate*	*RR*
Fair complexion	533	2.6	236	1.6
Skin color test >8	451	1.8	234	1.9
Blue/green eye color	418	1.5	227	1.4
Blond/red hair color	497	1.5	224	1.3
Scottish ancestry	534	1.6	308	1.8
Irish ancestry	494	1.7	234	1.6

risk, although these pigmentary associations appear to be secondary to the sun-sensitive skin type (Kricker et al, 1991). In addition, individuals with Scottish and Irish ancestry were prone to skin cancers, consistent with the predisposition reported for Celtic ancestry in some (Carey and Hogan, 1990) but not all studies (Kricker et al, 1994). Since we found no clear excess risk among those of Scandinavian ancestry, it would appear that the degree of skin pigmentation is not the sole determinant of sun sensitivity. It is noteworthy that a UVB dose–response gradient was seen among individuals without fair complexion or Celtic ancestry, indicating the importance of solar radiation dose as well as individual susceptibility to sunlight in the development of skin cancer. Another risk factor in our study was exposure to ionizing radiation, in accord with several studies linking radiotherapy to skin cancer (Fragu et al, 1991). Further work is needed to clarify the influence of other host and environmental factors, including cigarette smoking, photosensitizing chemicals, immunosuppressive states, dietary factors, human papilloma viruses, and genetic susceptibility, which may enhance the carcinogenicity of UVB radiation (Hunter et al, 1992; Karagas et al, 1992; Kune et al, 1992; Preston and Stern, 1992; Black et al, 1994; Leigh and Glover, 1995). The importance of genetic predisposition is further indicated by the recent finding of impaired DNA repair in patients with basal cell carcinoma (Wei et al, 1994) and by the discovery of susceptibility genes for familial occurrences of melanoma and dysplastic nevi (Goldstein et al, 1994).

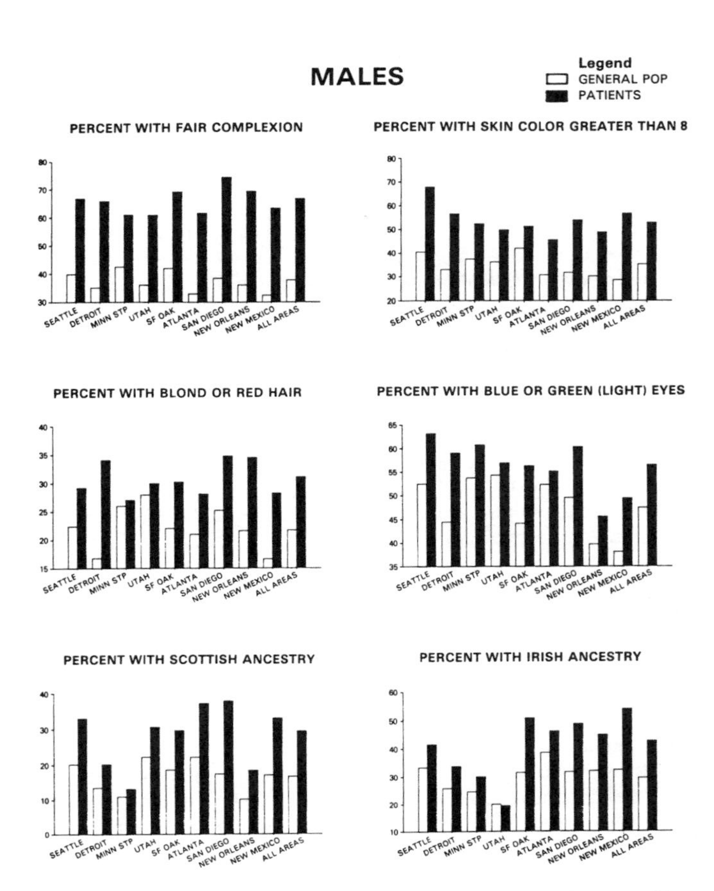

FIG. 17–12. Proportion of white male patients (nonmelanoma skin cancer) and general population controls with selected host characteristics in selected areas of the United States.

CONCLUSIONS

Recent investigations into the hazards of solar radiation have focused on the inadvertent modifications of the biosphere that may result from extensive use of man-made products, including supersonic aircraft exhausts and chlorofluorocarbons (Lloyd, 1993). Epidemiologic and physical data underscore concerns about the potentially harmful effects to humans if reduction of the stratospheric ozone layer permits greater amounts of solar UV radiation to reach the earth's surface. The current and projected magnitude of the skin cancer problem, particularly in light-skinned populations, should be heeded in spite of the generally favorable prognosis of nonmelanoma skin cancers and the decreases reported in mortality rates (Weinstock, 1993). In the United States, newly diagnosed skin cancers may have affected up to 1.2 million individuals in 1994 (Miller and Weinstock, 1994). The upward trends reported in the incidence rates for nonmelanoma skin cancer and melanoma (Kaldor et al, 1993) are worrisome, although the increases so far appear related mainly to changing clothing habits and outdoor recreational activities. However, continued surveys are needed that simultaneously monitor stratospheric ozone depletion, UVB exposures, and skin cancer incidence trends, along with epidemiologic and laboratory studies to further define the impact of solar radiation and its interactions with other environmental and susceptibility factors. Based on the available information, a 2–4% or greater increase in nonmelanoma skin cancer may be expected for each 1% reduction in stratospheric ozone, with the increase being greater for squamous cell than basal cell carcinomas. Although stratospheric ozone levels have declined during the 1980s (World Meterological Organization, 1990), especially at the poles and during winter months (Bojkov et al, 1990), the UVB network in the United States has not yet detected increases in surface measurements of UVB radiation at various locations, including areas showing increases in skin cancer (Scotto et al, 1988).

As more is learned about the exact UV wavelengths and amounts of solar energy that may be carcinogenic (de Gruijl et al, 1993), and the precise chemical actions and biologic processes that result in the transformation and proliferation of cutaneous cells, educational campaigns are urgently needed to reduce exposure to sunlight, especially around the noontime period when a large proportion of UVB reaches the earth's surface. Sensible sun-exposure behaviors need to be encouraged, particularly in high-risk individuals with fair complexions who burn readily, and in those with precursor lesions such as dysplastic nevi or actinic keratoses. The added hazard of artificial UV sources, including sunlamps for recreational tanning, needs to be publicized. Preventive measures, including protective clothing and sunscreen lotions, should be disseminated to physicians and the general public before sunlight-induced skin cancers become an even greater public health burden than they are today (Thompson et al, 1993; Rhodes, 1995). Stern et al (1986) have estimated that the risk of developing skin cancer could be reduced by as much as 50% if sunscreening and other preventive measures were taken to reduce the amount of sunlight exposure sustained during childhood, when UVB exposures are common and may pose unusual risks, especially for melanoma. Greater emphasis should also be given to routine screening of the skin by health professionals and to self-examinations aimed at early detection and prompt treatment of skin cancer (Kopf et al, 1995). It is very important to intensify surveillance among highly susceptible individuals, such as those with an exceptional risk of melanoma associated with dysplastic nevi and a positive family history (Tucker et al, 1993).

REFERENCES

AMBACH W, BLUMTHALER M. 1993. Biological effectiveness of solar UV radiation in humans. Experientia 49:747–753.

ARMSTRONG BK. 1994. Stratospheric ozone and health. Int J Epidemiol 23:873–885.

BELLINI A. 1909. Dell' influenza degli agenti fisci e piu particolaramente della luce nella etiologia dell epithielioma cutaneo. Gior Ital di Mal Ven e Pelle 50:732.

BERGER D, ROBERTSON DF, et al. 1975. Field measurements of biologically effective UV radiation. *In* Impacts of Climatic Change of the Biosphere. CIAP Monograph 5, Department of Transportation DOT-TST-75-55. Springfield, VA, NTIS, pp. 2-235–2-263.

BLACK HS, HERD JA, GOLDBERG LH, et al. 1994. Effect of a low-fat diet on the incidence of actinic keratosis. N Engl J Med 330:1272–1275.

BLUM H. 1959. Carcinogenesis by Ultraviolet Light. Princeton, NJ, Princeton University Press.

BLUMTHALER M, AMBACH W. 1990. Indications of increasing solar ultraviolet radiation flux in alpine regions. Science 248:206–208.

BOJKOV RL, BISHOP WJ, HILL GC, et al. 1990. A statistical trend analysis of revised Dobson total ozone data over the northern hemisphere. J Geophys Res 95:9785–9807.

BRASH DE, RUDOLPH JA, SIMON JA, et al. 1991. A role for sunlight in skin cancer: UV-induced p53 mutations in squamous cell carcinoma. Proc Natl Acad Sci USA 88:10124–10128.

CAREY FA, HOGAN JM. 1990. The relationship of sun exposure and solar elastosis to skin cancer in a high risk population. Ir J Med Sci 159:44–47.

CARTWRIGHT R, MCNALLY R, STAINES A. 1994. The increasing incidence of non-Hodgkin's lymphoma (NHL): the possible role of sunlight. Leuk Lymphoma 14:387–394.

CLIMATIC IMPACT COMMITTEE. 1975. Environmental Impact of Stratospheric Flight. Washington, D.C., National Academy of Sciences.

COMMITTEE ON IMPACTS OF STRATOSPHERIC CHANGE (CISC). 1979. Protection Against Depletion of Stratospheric Ozone by Chlorofluorocarbons. Washington, D.C., National Academy of Sciences.

COMMITTEE ON IMPACTS OF STRATOSPHERIC CHANGE. 1982. Cause and Effects of Stratospheric Ozone Reduction—An Update. Washington D.C., National Academy of Sciences.

COMMITTEE ON IMPACTS OF STRATOSPHERIC CHANGE. 1976. Halocarbons: Effects on Stratospheric Ozone. Washington, D.C., National Academy of Sciences.

COMMITTEE ON IMPACTS OF STRATOSPHERIC CHANGE. 1984. Causes and Effects of Changes in Stratospheric Ozone—Update 1983. Washington, D.C., National Academy of Sciences.

CUTCHIS P. 1974. Stratospheric ozone depletion and solar ultraviolet radiation on earth. Science 184:13–19.

DAHLBACK A, MOAN J. 1990. Annual exposures to carcinogenic radiation from the sun at different latitudes and amplification factors related to ozone depletion: The use of different geometrical representations of the skin surface receiving the ultraviolet radiation. Photochem Photobiol 52:1025–1028.

DE GRUIJL FR, STERENBORG HJ, FORBES PD, et al. 1993. Wavelength dependence of skin cancer induction by ultraviolet irradiation of albino hairless mice. Cancer Res 53:53–60.

DELUISI JJ, HARRIS JM. 1983. A determination of the absolute radiant energy of a Robertson-Berger meter sunburn unit. Atmos Environ 17:751–758.

DIFFEY BL. 1987. A comparison of dosimeters used for solar ultraviolet radiometry. Photochem Photobiol 46:55–60.

DIFFEY BL. 1992. Stratospheric ozone depletion and the risk of non-melanoma skin cancer in a British population. Phys Med Biol 37:2267–2279.

DUBREUILH W. 1907. Des hyperketoses circonscribes. Ann Dermatol Syphil (Paris) 8:387.

ELWOOD JM, DIFFEY L. 1993. A consideration of ambient solar ultraviolet radiation in the interpretation of studies of the aetiology of melanoma. Melanoma Res 3:113–122.

EMERSON JC, WEISS NS. 1992. Colorectal cancer and solar radiation. Cancer Causes Control 3:95–99.

ENVIRONMENTAL STUDIES BOARD. AD HOC PANEL ON THE BIOLOGICAL IMPACTS OF ULTRAVIOLET RADIATION. 1973. Biological Impacts of Increased Intensities of Solar Ultraviolet Radiation. Washington, D.C., National Academy of Sciences.

FARMAN JC, GARDINER BG, SHANKLIN JD. 1985. Large losses of

total ozone in Antarctica reveal seasonal ClO/NO interaction. Nature 315:207–210.

Fears TR, Scotto J, Schneiderman MA. 1976. Skin cancer, melanoma and sunlight. Am J Public Health 66:461–464.

Fears TR, Scotto J, Schneiderman MA. 1977. Mathematical models of age and ultraviolet effects on the incidence of skin cancer among whites in the United States. Am J Epidemiol 105:420–427.

Federal Task Force on Inadvertent Modification of the Stratosphere (IMOS). Fluorocarbons and the Environment. 1975. Council on Environmental Quality, and Federal Council for Science and Technology.

Findlay GM. 1928. Ultraviolet light and skin cancer. Lancet 2:1070–1073.

Fragu P, Lemarchand-Venencie F, Benhamou S, et al. 1991. Long-term effects in skin and thyroid after radiotherapy for skin angiomas: A French retrospective cohort study. Eur J Cancer 27:1215–1222.

Frederick JE, Lubin D. 1988. The budget of biologically active ultraviolet radiation in the earth–atmosphere system. J Geophys Res 93:3825–3832.

Frederick JE, Snell HE, Haywood EK. 1989. Solar ultraviolet radiation at the earth's surface. Photochem Photobiol 50:443–450.

Frederick JE, Weatherhead EC, Haywood EK. 1991. Long-term variations in ultraviolet sunlight reaching the biosphere: Calculations for the past three decades. Photochem Photobiol 54:781–788.

Gallagher RP, Ma B, McLean DI, et al. 1990. Trends in basal cell carcinoma, squamous cell carcinoma, and melanoma of the skin from 1973 through 1987. J Am Acad Dermatol 23:413–421.

Gange RW, Rosen CF. 1986. UVA effects on mammalian skin and cells. Photochem Photobiol 43:701–705.

Garland FC, Garland CF, Gorham ED, Young JF. 1990. Geographic variation in breast cancer mortality in the United States: A hypothesis involving exposure to solar radiation. Prev Med 19:614–622.

Glass AG, Hoover RN. 1989. The emerging epidemic of melanoma and squamous cell skin cancer. JAMA 262:2097–2100.

Goldstein AM, Dracopoli NC, Engelstein M, et al. 1994. Linkage of cutaneous malignant melanoma/dysplastic nevi to chromosome 9p, and evidence for genetic heterogeneity. Am J Hum Genet 54:489–496.

Haenszel W. 1963. Variations in skin cancer incidence within the United States. Natl Cancer Inst Monogr 10:225–243.

Henriksen T, Dahlback A, Larsen SH, et al. 1990. Ultraviolet-radiation and skin cancer: Effect of an ozone layer depletion. Photochem Photobiol 51:579–582.

Hoffman JS. 1987. Assessing the Risks of Trace Gases that Can Modify the Stratosphere. Vol. 1: Executive Summary. Washington, D.C., Office of Air and Radiation, EPA 400/1-87/001A. pp. ES 1–64.

Holly EA, Aston DA, Char DH, et al. 1990. Uveal melanoma in relation to ultraviolet light exposure and host factors. Cancer Res 50:5773–5777.

Hunter DJ, Colditz GA, Stampfer MJ, et al. 1992. Diet and risk of basal cell carcinoma of the skin in a prospective cohort of women. Ann Epidemiol 2:231–239.

Hyde JN. 1906. On the influence of light in the production of cancer of the skin. Am J Med Sci 131:1–22.

International Agency for Research on Cancer. 1992. Solar and Ultraviolet Radiation. IARC Monogr Eval Carcinog Risks Hum 55. Lyon, IARC.

Jagger J. 1967. Introduction to Research in Ultraviolet Photobiology. Englewood Cliffs, NJ, Prentice Hall.

Kaldor J, Shugg D, Young B, et al. 1993. Non-melanoma skin cancer: ten years of cancer-registry-based surveillance. Int J Cancer 53:886–891.

Karagas MR, Stukel TA, Greenberg ER, et al. 1992. Risk of subsequent basal cell carcinoma and squamous cell carcinoma of the skin among patients with prior skin cancer. JAMA 267:3305–3310.

Kelfkens G, de Gruijl FR, van der Leun JC. 1990. Ozone depletion and increase in annual ultraviolet radiation dose. Photochem Photobiol 52:819–823.

Kerr JB, McElroy CT. 1993. Evidence for large upward trends of ultraviolet-B radiation linked to ozone depletion. Science 262:1032–1034.

Koh HK. 1991. Cutaneous melanoma. N Eng J Med 325:171–182.

Koller LR. 1965. Ultraviolet Radiation, 2nd ed. New York, John Wiley and Sons, Inc.

Kopf AW, Salopek TG, Slade J, et al. 1995. Techniques of cutaneous examination for the detection of skin cancer. Cancer 75:684–690.

Kraemer KH, Lee MM, Scotto J. 1984. DNA repair protects against cutaneous and internal neoplasia: Evidence from xeroderma pigmentosum. Carcinogenesis 5:511–514.

Kricker A, Armstrong BK, English DR. 1994. Sun exposure and non-melanocytic skin cancer. Cancer Causes Control 5:367–392.

Kricker A, Armstrong BK, English DR, Heenan PJ. 1991. Pigmentary and cutaneous risk factors for non-melanocytic skin cancer: A case–control study. Int J Cancer 48:650–662.

Kripke ML. 1994. Ultraviolet radiation and immunology: Something new under the sun—Presidential address. Cancer Res 54:6102–6105.

Kune GA, Bannerman S, Field B, et al. 1992. Diet, alcohol, smoking, serum β-carotene, and vitamin A in male nonmelanocytic skin cancer patients and controls. Nutr Cancer 18:237–244.

Lee JA, Yongchaiyudha S. 1971. Incidence of and mortality from malignant melanoma by anatomical site. J Natl Cancer Inst 47:253–263.

Leigh IM, Glover MT. 1995. Cutaneous warts and tumours in immunosuppressed patients. J R Soc Med 88:61–62.

Lindqvist C. 1979. Risk factors in lip cancer: A questionnaire survey. Am J Epidemiol 109:521–530.

Lindqvist C, Teppo L. 1978. Epidemiological evaluation of sunlight as a risk factor of lip cancer. Br J Cancer 37:983–989.

Lloyd SA. 1993. Stratospheric ozone depletion. Lancet 342:1156–1158.

MacDonald EJ, Heinze EB. 1978. Epidemiology of cancer in Texas: Incidence analysed by type, ethnic group and geographic location. New York, Raven Press.

Madronich S, de Gruijl FR. 1994. Stratospheric ozone depletion between 1979 and 1992: Implications for biologically active ultraviolet-B radiation and non-melanoma skin cancer incidence. Photochem Photobiol 59:541–546.

Marks R. 1995. An overview of skin cancers: Incidence and causation. Cancer 75:607–612.

McKinley AF, Diffey BL. 1987. A reference action spectrum for ultraviolet induced erythema in human skin. *In* Passchier WF, Bosnjakovic BFM (eds): Human Exposure to Ultraviolet Radiation—Risks and Regulations. Amsterdam, Elsevier Science Publishers, pp. 83–87.

Miller DL, Weinstock MA. 1994. Nonmelanoma skin cancer in the United States: Incidence. J Am Acad Dermatol 30:774–778.

Moan J, Dahlback A. 1992. The relationship between skin cancers, solar radiation and ozone depletion. Br J Cancer 65:916–921.

Moan J, Dahlback A, Henriksen T, Magnus K. 1989. Biological amplification factor for sunlight-induced nonmelanoma skin cancer at high latitudes. Cancer Res 49:5207–5212.

Moran JM, Morgan MD. 1991. Meterology: The Atmosphere and the Science of Weather: The Ozone Shield. New York, MacMillan Publishing Company, pp. 459–463.

Morison WL. 1988. Skin cancer and artificial sources of UV radiation. J Dermatol Surg Oncol 14:893–896.

National Institutes of Health. 1991. Summary of the Consensus Development Conference on Sunlight, Ultraviolet Radiation, and the Skin. J Am Acad Dermatol 24:608–612.

PRESTON DS, STERN RS. 1992. Nonmelanoma cancers of the skin. N Engl J Med 327:1649–1662.

REINSEL GC, TIAO GC. 1987. Impact of chlorofluoromethanes on stratospheric ozone. J Am Stat Assoc 82:20–30.

RHODES AR. 1995. Public education and cancer of the skin: What do people need to know about melanoma and nonmelanoma skin cancer? Cancer 75:613–636.

RIES LAG, HANKEY BF, MILLER BA, et al. 1991. Cancer Statistics Review, 1973–1988. National Cancer Institute. NIH Publ. No. 91-2789. Bethesda, National Cancer Institute.

ROAN S. 1990. Ozone Crisis: The 15-year Evolution of a Sudden Global Emergency. New York, John Wiley & Sons, Inc.

ROBERTSON DF. 1968. Solar ultraviolet radiation in relation to sunburn and skin cancer. Med J Aust 2:1123–1132.

ROBERTSON DF. 1982. Ultraviolet effects and prevention. *In* Emmett AJ et al (eds): Malignant Skin Tumors. New York, Churchill and Livingstone Inc., pp. 12–22.

ROFFO AH. 1934. Cancer et soleil: Carcinomes et sarcomes provoquees par l'action du soleil in toto. Bull Cancer (Paris) 23:590–616.

ROWLAND FS, MOLINA MJ. 1975. Chlorofluoromethanes in the environment. Rev Geophys Space Physics 13:1–35.

RUNDEL RD, NACHTWEY DS. 1978. Skin cancer and ultraviolet radiation. Photochem Photobiol 28:345–356.

RUSCH HP, KLINE BE, BAUMANN CA. 1941. Carcinogenesis by ultraviolet rays with reference to wavelength and energy. Arch Pathol 31:135–146.

SCOTTO J. 1986. Nonmelanoma skin cancer—UVB effects. *In* Titus JG (ed): Effects of Changes in Stratospheric Ozone and Global Climate, Vol. 2: Stratospheric Ozone. Washington, D.C., U.S. Environmental Protection Agency, pp. 33–61.

SCOTTO J, COTTON G, URBACH F, et al. 1988. Biologically effective ultraviolet radiation: Surface measurements in the United States, 1974 to 1985. Science 239:762–764.

SCOTTO J, FEARS TR. 1978. Skin cancer epidemiology: Research needs. Natl Cancer Inst Monogr 50:169–177.

SCOTTO J, FEARS TR. 1987. The association of solar ultraviolet and skin melanoma incidence among Caucasians in the United States. Ca Invest 5:275–283.

SCOTTO J, FEARS TR, FRAUMENI JF JR. 1982. Solar radiation. *In* Schottenfeld D, Fraumeni JF Jr (eds): Cancer Epidemiology and Prevention. Philadelphia, WB Saunders Company, pp. 254–276.

SCOTTO J, FEARS TR, FRAUMENI JF JR. 1983. Incidence of Nonmelanoma Skin Cancer in the United States. DHEW Publ. No. (NIH) 83-2433. Washington, D.C., U.S. Government Printing Office.

SCOTTO J, FEARS TR, GORI GB. 1976. Measurements of Ultraviolet Radiation in the United States and Comparisons with Skin Cancer Data. DHEW (NIH) 76-1029. Bethesda, National Cancer Institute.

SCOTTO J, KOPF A, URBACH F. 1974. Nonmelanoma skin cancer among Caucasians in four areas of the United States. Cancer 34:1333–1338.

SERRANO H, SCOTTO J, SHORNICK G, et al. 1991. Incidence of nonmelanoma skin cancer in New Hampshire and Vermont. J Am Acad Dermatol 23:574–579.

SETLOW RB. 1974. The wavelength in sunlight effective in producing skin cancer: A theoretical analysis. Proc Natl Acad Sci USA 71:3363–3366.

SMITH GJ, WHITE MG, RYAN KG. 1993. Seasonal trends in erythemal and carcinogenic ultraviolet radiation at mid-southern latitudes, 1989–1991. Photochem Photobiol 57:513–517.

SOBER AJ, BURSTEIN JM. 1995. Precursors to skin cancer. Cancer 75:645–650.

SOLOMON S. 1988. The mystery of the Antarctic ozone "hole." Rev Geophys 26:131–148.

STERN RS, WEINSTEIN MC, BAKER SG. 1986. Risk reduction for nonmelanoma skin cancer with childhood sunscreen use. Arch Dermatol 122:537–545.

STOLARSKI R, BOJKOV R, BISHOP L, et al. 1992. Measured trends in stratospheric ozone. Science 256:342–349.

STRICKLAND PT, VITASA BC, WEST SK, et al. 1989. Quantitative carcinogenesis in man: Solar ultraviolet B dose dependence of skin cancer in Maryland watermen. J Natl Cancer Inst 81:1910–1913.

THIERSCH K. 1875. Der Epithelialkrebs, namentlich der äusseren Haut. Leipzig, Germany.

THOMPSON SC, JOLLEY D, MARKS R. 1993. Reduction of solar keratoses by regular sunscreen use. N Engl J Med 329:1147–1151.

TITUS JG, SEIDEL SR. 1986. Effects of changes in stratospheric ozone and global climate, Vol 1: Overview. Washington, D.C., U.S. Environmental Protection Agency, pp. 3–19.

TUCKER MA. 1988. Individuals at high risk of melanoma. *In* Mackie RM (ed): Pigment Cell. Basel, Karger, pp. 254–276.

TUCKER MA, FRASER MC, GOLDSTEIN AM, et al. 1993. Risk of melanoma and other cancers in melanoma-prone families. J Invest Dermatol 100:350S–355S.

TUCKER MA, SHIELDS JA, HARTGE P, et al. 1985. Sunlight exposure as risk factor for intraocular malignant melanoma. N Engl J Med 313:789–792.

UNITED NATIONS ENVIRONMENT PROGRAMME ENVIRONMENTAL EFFECTS PANEL. 1990. Environmental Effects of Ozone Depletion. Nairobi, United Nations Environment Programme.

UNNA PG. 1894. Die Histopathologie der Hautkrankheiten. Berlin, August Hirschwald.

URBACH F. 1987. Man and ultraviolet radiation. *In* Passchier WF, Bosnjakovic BFM (eds): Human Exposure to Ultraviolet Radiation—Risks and Regulations. Amsterdam, Elsevier Science Publishers, pp. 3–20.

URBACH F. 1989. Potential effects of altered solar ultraviolet radiation on human skin cancer. Photochem Photobiol 501:507–513.

U.S. ENVIRONMENTAL PROTECTION AGENCY. 1988. Regulatory Impact Analysis: Protection of Stratospheric Ozone. Washington, D.C., U.S. Government Printing Office.

VITALIANO PP. 1978. The use of logistic regression for modelling risk factors: With application to non-melanoma skin cancer. Am J Epidemiol 108:402–414.

WATSON RT, PRATHER MJ, KURYLO MJ. 1988. Present State of Knowledge of the Upper Atmosphere: An Assessment Report. NASA Reference Publication 1208. Washington, D.C., U.S. Government Printing Office.

WEI Q, MATANOSKI GM, FARMER ER, et al. 1993. DNA repair and aging in basal cell carcinoma: A molecular epidemiology study. Proc Natl Acad Sci USA 90:1614–1618.

WEI Q, MATANOSKI GM, FARMER ER, et al. 1994. DNA repair and susceptibility to basal cell carcinoma: A case–control study. Am J Epidemiol 140:598–607.

WEINSTOCK MA. 1993. Nonmelanoma skin cancer mortality in the United States, 1969 through 1988. Arch Dermatol 129:1286–1290.

WIKLUND K, HOLM LE. 1986. Trends in cancer risks among Swedish agricultural workers. J Natl Cancer Inst 77:657–664.

WORLD METEROLOGICAL ORGANIZATION. 1990. Global Ozone Research and Monitoring Project, Report No. 20: Scientific Assessment of Stratospheric Ozone. Geneva, WMO.

18 Occupation

RICHARD R. MONSON

Exposures that occur in the workplace may cause cancer. This fact has been known for over two hundred years (Pott, 1775). Conversely, no workplace exposure has been shown conclusively not to be associated with an increased risk of cancer (IARC, 1987). Either this means that many workplace exposures cause cancer or that sufficient information has not been assembled to demonstrate a lack of an excess of cancer. The role of the occupational epidemiologist is to collect data that will permit judgment to be made about whether a substance at some defined level of exposure does or does not present a risk for cancer and other diseases.

Historically, occupational cancers have been initially detected by clinical means. Most carcinogens in the workplace about which we have definitive knowledge were present at high levels, had strong associations with one or more types of cancer, and occurred among sufficiently exposed workers to present a clear causal picture to the alert clinician. From Pott's recognition of scrotal cancer among chimney sweeps in 1775 to Creech and Johnson's identification of angiosarcoma of the liver among vinyl chloride workers in 1974, unusual cancers among persons with unusual occupations were sufficient evidence to judge that the occupation caused the cancer. Prevention of scrotal cancer or of angiosarcoma of the liver could readily be accomplished by reduction of exposure to soot or to vinyl chloride.

The observations of Pott and of Creech and Johnson were made possible because the causal exposure and the disease caused were present at the same time in the same individual. Pott was a physician who treated chimney sweeps, and Creech was a physician who treated vinyl chloride workers. When a rare cancer occurred among several members of each group, a clear causal relation to occupation could be inferred. However, had excess lung cancer occurred following retirement from the chimney sweep business, or had vinyl chloride caused prostate cancer rather than angiosarcoma of the liver, it is uncertain whether clinical observations would have been sufficient to identify the causal relation between occupation and cancer.

The era of initial identification of occupational cancer by a clinician has extended into the last quarter of the twentieth century. This illustrates the inadequacy that still exists in our ability to control exposure to hazardous substances in the workplace. Also, it illustrates the inadequacy of scientific observation to identify some occupational hazards before exposure sufficient to cause cancer has taken place.

The Kennaways were among the first to use quantitative methods to assess the occurrence of occupational cancer (Kennaway, 1925; Kennaway and Kennaway, 1936, 1947). However, the era of formal epidemiological assessment of the occurrence of cancer and other diseases in relation to workplace exposures did not begin until after World War II. In a proportional mortality analysis of deaths in a British arsenical factory, Hill and Faning (1948) noted an excess of lung and of skin cancers. In a retrospective cohort study of British gas workers, Doll (1952) also noted excess lung cancer. And Case and his colleagues started a retrospective cohort study of workers in the British dyestuffs industry (Case et al, 1954).

In the United States lung cancer among chromate workers was one of the first occupational cancers to be studied using epidemiological methods. In a retrospective cohort study Machle and Gregorius (1948) used both death proportions and death rates to demonstrate an excess occurrence of lung cancer among chromate workers relative to Metropolitan Life Insurance Company industrial policyholders. In a case-control study of lung cancer among patients in two Baltimore hospitals, Baetjer (1950b) identified a higher percentage of chromate-exposed workers among persons with lung cancer than among controls.

The many retrospective cohort and case-control studies that have been done during the last half of the twentieth century reflect the second stage of identification of occupational cancer. Through the use of historical records, persons in defined occupational groups can be evaluated for the excess occurrence of cancer or persons with cancer can be described as to past occupations. It is not necessary that the cancer develop while the person is employed in the exposed occupation. However, both retrospective cohort studies and case-control studies have a major limitation—the assessment of exposure must be done retrospectively. Usually this means that exposure to specific substances can only be approximated; often no information at all is available on level of exposure; occasionally even fact of exposure to specific substances is a matter of guesswork. The result of this imprecision in assessment of exposure is that weak causal relationships between occupational exposure and cancer may not be identifiable. While the epidemiologist of today can identify causal relative risks that are much lower than those identified by the clinician of yesterday, weak relative risks, say those less than two, may not be detected and interpreted with any degree of confidence. Further, because of the imprecision in measurement of exposure, the powerful information that comes from an assessment of dose-response relationships frequently is not available.

Therefore, the pressing need that faces today's occupational epidemiologist is to establish prospective cohort studies. Actual measurement of level and type of exposure to specific substances in the workplace must be made. This measurement must continue prospectively so that an exposure profile may be developed for each worker. Persons in the workplace must be followed from initial employment through job changes through retirement to development of disease and death. The goal of the occupational epidemiologist must be to become less a seeker of causes of occupational cancer and more a describer of patterns of morbidity and mortality according to level of exposure to one or more substances in the workplace. The ideal is to develop convincing information that may be interpreted as showing that a defined level of exposure of a chemical, in the presence of defined levels of exposure to other chemicals, is not associated with an increase in morbidity or mortality.

HISTORY

As suggested above, alert clinicians have historically been the first to identify occupational cancers. The observation by Pott in 1775 that chimney sweeps in London developed excess cancer of the scrotum was followed by a report of scrotal cancer among Cornish smelter workers, presumably due to arsenic (Paris, 1822). Other clinicians reported excess skin cancer following occupational exposure to a variety of coal tar products (Volkman, 1875; Manouvriez, 1876; Lueke, 1907). Also, excess skin cancer was noted among workers involved in a variety of mineral oils: "paraffin pressmen" in the Scottish shale oil industry (Bell, 1876), "mule spinners" in the English cotton industry (Southam and Wilson, 1922), and workers exposed to cutting oils in the English machine tooling industry (Cruickshank and Squire, 1950).

For centuries, metal miners in central Europe were known to suffer from "Bergkrankheit" or "miner's phthisis" (Hueper, 1966; Frank, 1987). In 1879, Haerting and Hesse identified the disease as cancer of the lung. Over the subsequent decades, the cause was thought to be due to arsenic, pneumoconiosis, silicosis, and eventually radioactivity (Peller, 1939). During the first half of the twentieth century, other substances were recognized to be causes of lung cancer: arsenic in English factory workers (Hill and Faning, 1948); asbestos in an American mill weaver (Lynch and Smith, 1935); chromium compounds among American chromate producers (Machle and Gregorius, 1948); coal carbonization in Japanese gas workers (Kuroda and Kawahata, 1936); and nickel refining in Wales (Annual Report, 1933). In general the recognition proceeded from clinical case report to quantitative epidemiological studies. Prior to 1950, cigarette-induced lung cancer was not common, so it was possible for a relative excess among an occupational group to be detected by clinical observation. Currently, over 90% of lung cancer is estimated to be caused by cigarette smoking (Doll and Peto, 1981). The detection of occupationally induced lung cancers against this high background is difficult. Nevertheless, in 1973 Figueroa and coworkers identified a causal excess of lung cancer among chloromethyl methyl ether workers.

Other occupational cancers recognized before 1950 were bladder cancer among German dyestuffs workers (Rehn, 1895), bone cancer among American radium dial painters (Martland, 1931), leukemia among Italian workers exposed to benzene (see Vigliani and Saita, 1964), and cancer of the nasal sinuses among Welsh nickel refiners (Annual Report, 1933). The wide geographic dispersion of these largely clinical identifications indicates the widespread nature of dangerous industrial environments as well as the recognition by physicians that work can be harmful to one's health.

Nevertheless, before 1950 the identification of occupational cancer was largely reactive rather than proactive. The only routine surveillance system to estimate the occurrence of occupationally induced cancers was that of the Registrar General in England and Wales (1958, 1978). After World War II, the increasing recognition that occupational cancer was not uncommon led to proportional mortality analyses of death certificates (Hill and Faning, 1948; Machle and Gregorius, 1948), to retrospective follow-up studies among exposed workers (Machle and Gregorius, 1948; Doll, 1952), and to case-control studies (Baetjer, 1950b). It is of interest that what essentially were prospective follow-up studies among occupational cohorts were started by at least two investigators before 1950. In 1948 Meigs initiated a comprehensive monitoring, control, and research program at a Connecticut plant that manufactured benzidine (Meigs et al, 1986). In 1949, Archer started a follow-up study of uranium miners that extended the information available on the association between exposure to radon and lung cancer (Archer et al, 1962, 1976). Finally, occupation has been evaluated in many of the case-control studies that have been conducted since 1950 (Lilienfeld and Lilienfeld, 1979).

CURRENT STATUS OF EPIDEMIOLOGICAL FINDINGS

The International Agency for Research on Cancer categorizes chemicals according to four levels (Tomatis et al, 1978; IARC, 1987):

Group 1: There is sufficient evidence of carcinogenicity in humans
Group 2: There is limited evidence of carcinogenicity in humans
Group 3: There is insufficient evidence of carcinogenicity
Group 4: There is evidence suggesting lack of carcinogenicity

Group 2 is subdivided into 2A—probably carcinogenic—and 2B—possibly carcinogenic, depending primarily upon the strength of evidence in experimental animals.

The agents or industrial processes listed in Table 18–1 are in general those that are categorized by IARC as Group 1—the agent is carcinogenic to humans. Where groups of chemicals are listed, not all chemicals in the group are necessarily carcinogenic. Where industrial processes are listed, insufficient information currently exists to specify the substance (or substances) that is the carcinogen. While it is unlikely that the classification of a specific Group 1 chemical would change, it is possible that other groups of chemicals or industrial processes could be reclassified as more specific information becomes available.

In the discussion of Tables 18–1 and 18–2, general reference is made to the IARC (1987) citation for information on carcinogenicity among humans and among animals. The only specific agent for which there is sufficient evidence of carcinogenicity in humans and limited evidence in animals is arsenic and arsenic compounds. In 1981, benzene was considered to be carcinogenic to humans but to have only limited evidence of carcinogenicity among animals (IARC, 1982a; Decouflé, 1982). Since then, additional experimental studies have demonstrated a variety of benzene-induced cancers in animals (IARC, 1987).

Among the bladder carcinogens listed in Table 18–1, 2-naphthylamine is likely to be the substance that accounted for the excess bladder cancer in the rubber industry. It seems likely that this agent was not used extensively in the American rubber industry, therefore an excess bladder cancer was noted mainly in Europe. In Great Britain, the use of antioxidants containing 2-naphthylamine was discontinued in 1949 (IARC, 1982b). It is likely that polynuclear aromatic compounds were responsible for the excess bladder cancer among workers at gas retorts (coal carbonization) and in the aluminum reduction industries (coal tar pitch volatiles).

As noted above, benzene has only recently been demonstrated to be carcinogenic in animals. In humans, also, the judgment that benzene causes leukemia has been arrived at recently. In the early part of this century, exposure to high levels (hundreds of parts per million [ppm]) were recognized to cause aplastic anemia, and there were a number of case reports of leukemia among workers exposed to benzene (Vigliani and Saita, 1964). However, when Infante et al in 1977 reported an excess of leukemia among "Pliofilm" workers who were exposed to less than 100 ppm, there was considerable controversy as to the generalizability of this finding (IARC, 1982b). Subsequently, the new and updated studies cited provide persuasive evidence that moderate exposure to benzene in the workplace has caused leukemia.

Among radiologists, excess leukemia was observed among early radiologists, who were exposed to high levels of radiation. No excess has been seen among persons who became radiologists after 1939 (Matanoski, 1981). It is of interest that excess leukemia has not been observed among the radium dial painters, in whom there was a high excess of bone cancer (Stebbings et al, 1984).

Sulfuric acid has recently been judged by IARC (1992) to be a cause of cancer of the larynx and of the lung.

As can be seen from Table 18–1, a number of chemicals or processes have been identified as causes of lung cancer in humans. For most of the categories listed, there are several specific chemical elements or compounds that may be the causal agent. However, in most studies not only is there exposure to a number of compounds of the likely causal agent, there also is exposure to a number of other substances that may interact with the primary causal agent. Thus, prevention through reduction of exposure must be aimed at the general working environment rather than at the specific causal agent.

Most of the information on the association between arsenic and lung cancer comes from workers in mines

TABLE 18–1. *Cancer Sites for Which Relationships with Occupational Exposures Are Well-Established in Human Studies**

Site	Agent or Industrial Process	References
Bladder	Benzidine, 2-naphthylamine; 4-Aminobiphenyl (xenylamine)	Rehn, 1895; Scott, 1952; Case et al, 1954; Melick et al, 1955; Goldwater et al, 1965; Mancuso and El-Attar, 1967; Melick et al, 1971; Zavon et al, 1973; Tsuchiya et al, 1975; Zack and Gaffey, 1983; Meigs et al, 1986; Vineis and Simonato, 1986
	Manufacture of certain dyes (e.g., auramine and magenta)	Case and Pearson, 1954; Gardiner et al, 1982; (Ott and Langner, 1983;) Boyko et al, 1985
	Gas retorts	Doll, 1952; Doll et al, 1972; Vineis and Simonato, 1986; Gustavsson and Reuterwall, 1990
	Rubber and cable making industries	Case and Hosker, 1954; Davies, 1965; Baxter and Werner, 1980; Parkes et al, 1982; Sorahan et al, 1986; Vineis and Simonato, 1986; Sorahan et al, 1989
	Coal tar pitch volatiles (aluminum reduction plants, chimney sweeps)	Andersen et al, 1982; Rockette and Arena, 1983; Thériault et al, 1984; Gibbs, 1985; Gustavsson et al, 1988; Rönneberg and Langmark, 1992
Blood (leukemia)	Benzene	Vigliani and Saita, 1964; Girard et al, 1971; Aksoy et al, 1974; Vigliani, 1976; Infante et al, 1977; Decouflé et al, 1983; Yin et al, 1987; Rinsky et al, 1987; Wong, 1987a; Wong, 1987b; Austin et al, 1988; Paci et al, 1989
	X-radiation	March, 1944; Seltser and Sartwell, 1965; Warren and Lombard, 1966; Matanoski, 1981; Logue et al, 1986; (Matanoski et al, 1987); Wang et al, 1990; Wing et al, 1991
Bone	Radium, mesothorium	Martland and Humphries, 1929; Martland, 1931; Polednak et al, 1978; Stebbings et al, 1984
Larynx	Mustard gas	Wada et al, 1968; Manning et al, 1981
	Sulfuric acid mist	Weil et al, 1952; Lynch et al, 1979; Soskolne et al, 1984; Forastiere et al, 1987; Steenland et al, 1988; IARC, 1992
Liver (angiosarcoma)	Arsenic (inorganic compounds)	Roth, 1958
	Vinyl chloride	Creech and Johnson, 1974; Monson et al, 1974; Waxweiler et al, 1976; Fox and Collier, 1977; Spirtas and Kaminski, 1978; Cooper, 1981; Jones et al, 1988; Doll, 1988; Simonato et al, 1991a
Lung, bronchus	Arsenic (inorganic compounds)	Henry, 1934; Hill and Faning, 1948; Roth, 1958; Lee and Fraumeni, 1969; Milham and Strong, 1974; Tokudome and Kuratsune, 1976; Pinto et al, 1978; Axelson et al, 1978; Wall, 1980; Mabuchi et al, 1980; Buiatti et al, 1985; Lee-Feldstein 1986; Enterline et al, 1987b; Enterline et al, 1987c; Sobel et al, 1988; Järup et al, 1989; Simonato et al, 1994
	Asbestos	Lynch and Smith, 1936; Merewether, 1949; Doll, 1955; Mancuso and Coulter, 1963; Selikoff et al, 1964; Enterline and Kendrick, 1967; Selikoff et al, 1968; Knox et al, 1968; Newhouse, 1969; Fletcher, 1972; Newhouse et al, 1972; Selikoff et al, 1979; McDonald et al, 1980; Dement et al, 1983; McDonald et al, 1983; Finkelstein, 1984; Peto et al, 1985; Seidman et al, 1986; Hughes et al, 1987; Enterline et al, 1987a; Talcott et al, 1989
	Beryllium and beryllium compounds	Mancuso, 1980; Wagoner et al, 1980; Saracci, 1987; Ward et al, 1992; IARC, 1993b; (MacMahon, 1994)
	Bis(chloromethyl) ether, chloromethyl methyl ether	Figueroa et al, 1973; DeFonso and Kelton, 1976; McCallum et al, 1983; Maher and DeFonso, 1987; Collingwood et al, 1987
	Cadmium and cadmium compounds	Sorahan and Waterhouse, 1983; Elinder et al, 1985; Thun et al, 1985; Oberdörster, 1986; Ades and Kazantzis, 1988; Sullivan and Waterman, 1988; Stayner et al, 1992; Kazantzis et al, 1992; IARC, 1993b
	Chromium compounds	Machle and Gregorius, 1948; Baetjer, 1950a; Baetjer, 1950b; Mancuso and Hueper, 1951; Bidstrup and Case, 1956; Enterline, 1974; Långard and Norseth, 1975; Michel-Briand and Simonin, 1977; Davies, 1978; Hayes et al, 1979; Dalager et al, 1980; Långard et al, 1980; Sheffet et al, 1982; Sjögren et al, 1987; Sorahan et al, 1987; Långard, 1990; IARC, 1990b; Davies et al, 1991; Lees, 1991

(*continued*)

TABLE 18–1. *(Continued)*

Site	Agent or Industrial Process	References
	Coal carbonization processes (coke ovens, gas retorts, producer gas)	Kuroda and Kawahata, 1936; Kennaway and Kennaway, 1947; Doll, 1952; Christian, 1962; Kawai et al, 1967; Lloyd, 1971; Redmond et al, 1972; Doll et al, 1972; Mazumdar et al, 1975; Rockette and Redmond, 1985; Bertrand et al, 1987; Gustavsson and Reuterwall, 1990; Swaen et al, 1991
	Coal tar pitch volatiles (roofing materials, aluminum reduction plants, chimney sweeps)	Hammond et al, 1976; Milham, 1979; Hansen et al, 1982; Andersen et al, 1982; (Rockette and Arena, 1983); Gibbs, 1985; Kjuus et al, 1986b; Gustavsson et al, 1988; Hansen, 1991; Rönneberg and Langmark, 1992; Armstrong et al, 1994
	Foundry workers	Turner and Grace, 1938; Koskela et al, 1976; Decouflé and Wood, 1979; Tola et al, 1979, Egan-Baum et al, 1981; Gibson et al, 1983; Fletcher and Ades, 1984; Silverstein et al, 1986; Sorahan and Cooke, 1989; Moulin et al, 1990; Sherson et al, 1991; Moulin et al, 1993; Delzell et al, 1993
	Iron ore (hematite) mining	Faulds and Stewart, 1956; Boyd et al, 1970; (Lawler et al, 1985); Chen et al, 1990
	Mustard gas	Case and Lea, 1955; Wada et al, 1968; Easton et al, 1988
	Nickel and nickel compounds	Annual report, 1933; Doll, 1958; Mastromatteo, 1967; Pedersen et al, 1973; Enterline and Marsh, 1982; Kaldor et al, 1986; Grandjean et al, 1988; Roberts et al, 1989; Doll et al, 1990; IARC, 1990b
	Painters	IARC, 1989c
	Radiation (radioactive ores or radon)	Haerting and Hesse, 1879; Peller, 1939; Lorenz, 1944; Archer et al, 1962; DeVilliers and Windish, 1964; Wagoner et al, 1965; Archer et al, 1976; Fox et al, 1981; Radford and Renard, 1984; Samet et al, 1984; Solli et al, 1985; Howe et al, 1986; Howe et al, 1987; Hornung and Meinhardt, 1987; Battista et al, 1988; Morrison et al, 1988; Hodgson and Jones, 1990; Woodward et al, 1991
	Sulfuric acid mist	Beaumont et al, 1987; Siemiatycki, 1991; IARC, 1992
Nasal cavity, sinuses	Isopropanol manufacture by strong acid process	Weil et al, 1952
	Mustard gas	Wada et al, 1968
	Nickel and nickel compounds	Annual Report, 1933; Doll, 1958; Mastromatteo, 1967; Pedersen et al, 1973; Kaldor et al, 1986; Grandjean et al, 1988; Roberts et al, 1989; Doll et al, 1990
	Radium, mesothorium	Hasterlik et al, 1964
	Shoe manufacturing (leather dust?)	Acheson, 1976; Acheson et al, 1981; Merler et al, 1986
	Woodworking (wood dust?)	Acheson, 1976; Brinton et al, 1977; Roush et al 1980; Acheson et al 1981; Wills, 1982; Acheson et al 1984b; Gerhardsson et al 1985; Finkelstein, 1989; (Viren and Imbus, 1989)
Peritoneum (mesothelioma)	Asbestos	Selikoff et al, 1965; Newhouse and Thompson, 1965; Selikoff et al, 1972; Greenberg and Lloyd Davies, 1974; Peto et al, 1982; Finkelstein, 1984; Hughes et al, 1987; Enterline et al, 1987a
Pharynx	Mustard gas	Wada et al, 1968
Pleura (mesothelioma)	Asbestos	Wagner et al, 1960; Selikoff et al, 1965; Newhouse and Thompson, 1965; Selikoff et al, 1972; Greenberg and Lloyd Davies, 1974; Peto et al, 1982; Berry and Newhouse, 1983; Finkelstein, 1984; Peto et al, 1985; Hughes et al, 1987; Enterline et al, 1987a
Skin (including scrotum)	Arsenic (inorganic compounds)	Paris, 1822; Kennaway, 1925; Roth, 1958; Mabuchi et al, 1980
	Coal tar products (mainly coal tar, creosote, pitch, soot)	Pott, 1775; Volkmann, 1875; Manouvriez, 1876; Lueke, 1907; Kennaway, 1925; Henry, 1946; Doll et al, 1972; Kipling and Waldron, 1976
	Coal hydrogenation	Sexton, 1960
	Mineral oils (from coal, petroleum, shale)	Volkmann, 1875; Bell, 1876; Scott, 1922; Southam and Wilson, 1922; Kennaway, 1925; Henry, 1946; Cruickshank and Square, 1950; Cruickshank and Gourevitch, 1952; Hendricks et al, 1959; Kipling, 1968; Kipling and Waldron, 1976; Roush et al, 1982; Waldron et al, 1984; Järvholm and Lavenius, 1987
	Ultraviolet light	Spitzer et al, 1975; Burmeister, 1981; Wiklund, 1983; Hagmar et al, 1992
	X-radiation	Court Brown and Doll, 1958; Matanoski, 1981

*References in parentheses are consistent with no excess of occupationally caused cancer.

or in smelters. Inorganic arsenic compounds are the likely causal factors. All commercial forms of asbestos tested by inhalation are carcinogenic in laboratory animals. In humans, an increased risk of lung cancer has been observed following occupational exposure to chrysotile, amosite, and anthophyllite asbestos and to mixtures containing crocidolite. While in some studies, little or no excess lung cancer has been reported among workers exposed to asbestos, there is no known safe level of exposure.

The data on beryllium and on cadmium constitute a hazard for epidemiologists, as noted by Sir Richard Doll (1985). These substances have recently been judged by IARC (1993b) as being causes of lung cancer in humans. However, the judgment with respect to beryllium has been criticized on the basis of a lack of unambiguous data (MacMahon, 1994).

Not infrequently, persons are exposed concurrently to chromium compounds and to nickel compounds. Thus, uncertainty may exist as to the specific compounds that are associated with excess lung cancer. Excess lung and nasal cancers among nickel refiners were not related to concurrent chromium exposure, and nickel subsulfide and nickel oxide were considered to be the most likely causal compounds. Nickel subsulfide is also carcinogenic to animals via inhalation. There is little evidence for excess lung cancer among workers in nickel alloy plants. Hexavalent chromium is clearly carcinogenic both to humans and to animals.

As is the case with bladder cancer, polynuclear aromatic compounds (PACs) are judged to be responsible for the excess lung cancer observed among persons exposed to coal-related compounds. Polynuclear aromatic compounds are also likely to be involved in causing the excess lung cancer among foundry workers. In addition, other compounds such as silica, metal fumes (eg, chromium or nickel), and formaldehyde may be present in the atmosphere of a foundry and may be related to excess lung cancer.

It is likely that the excess lung cancer observed among certain groups of hematite miners is caused by exposure to radon gas, just as miners are the main group affected by radioactive ores. Other substances present in some mining environments are silica and arsenic, which either are carcinogenic themselves or interact with other compounds. In animals, there is evidence that ferric oxide is not carcinogenic.

Some substances that cause lung cancer are also associated with excess cancers of the nasal sinuses, the pharynx, the pleura, or the peritoneum. Workers in two industries that produce a complex dust, shoe manufacturing and woodworking, have greatly increased rates of nasal adenocarcinoma. No greater degree of specificity other than leather dust and wood dust is available. Leather workers also are reported to have excess bladder cancer, and woodworkers are reported to have excess Hodgkin's disease (see Table 18–3).

There are four categories of documented causes of occupational skin cancer: ultraviolet light, ionizing radiation, polycyclic hydrocarbons, and arsenic (Emmett, 1987; Shmunes, 1987). Working in the sunlight is the likely cause of excess lip cancer among fishermen (Spitzer et al, 1975) and in farmers (Burmeister, 1981; Wiklund, 1983). A variety of polycyclic aromatic compounds are contained in coal products and in mineral oils.

Most of the materials listed in Table 18–2 are judged by IARC to be Group 2—the agent is probably or possibly carcinogenic to humans. Also included are some substances that have not been reviewed by IARC (abrasives), that are definitely causal to other sites (asbestos, coke oven emissions, radium, vinyl chloride), or for which there is recent information (polypropylene manufacture). In addition, cutting oils may be composed of mineral oils, some of which are known to be carcinogenic, or may be synthetic or semi-synthetic compounds.

Over 50 years ago, synthetic abrasives replaced sandstone as a grinding material (Wegman and Eisen, 1981). In the past, coal tar pitches were used as polishing materials (Wang et al, 1983). In addition, workers with abrasives may be exposed to metal oxides, silicon carbide, and cutting oils. Stomach cancer and/or colorectal cancers have most consistently been reported to be in excess. Also, a slight excess of lung cancer has been reported among a group of bearing manufacturers (Park et al, 1988).

There is a lack of consistency in the reporting of excess laryngeal or gastrointestinal cancers among persons exposed to asbestos. Since there is a strong causal association between asbestos and lung cancer, any misclassification of lung (or pleural) cancer may lead to an apparent excess of cancer of the larynx or of the gastrointestinal tract. Different forms of asbestos may have different associations with different tissues. The relative risk of the association between asbestos and nonrespiratory cancers likely is closer to 2 than to 10, so that it is not surprising that some inconsistency is seen across studies.

The judgment as to the potential of cadmium to cause cancer of the prostate is inconsistent (Doll, 1985; Elinder et al, 1985; Oberdörster, 1986; Ades and Kazantzis, 1988). Early case reports were followed by formal epidemiological studies that included the early cases. Later compilations of all available data suggested that little if any excess prostate cancer has occurred in some of the groups with continued follow-up. Yet within group, there is a tendency for excess cancer among the more heavily exposed workers.

TABLE 18–2. *Industrial Materials for Which Epidemiological Studies Suggest (or Do Not Suggest) Carcinogenicity**

Material	*Site(s)*	*References*
Abrasives	Digestive organs	Sparks and Wegman, 1980; Wegman and Eisen, 1981; Järvholm et al, 1982; Wang et al, 1983; (Edling et al, 1987); Park et al, 1988; Svensson et al, 1989
Acrylonitrile	Lung	O'Berg, 1980; (Werner and Carter, 1981); Delzell and Monson, 1982b; Koerselman and van der Graaf, 1984; (Chen et al, 1987); (Collins et al, 1989b)
Asbestos	Gastrointestinal	Selikoff et al, 1979; Seidman et al, 1986; Frumkin and Berlin, 1988
	Kidney	Smith et al, 1989
	Larynx	Stell and McGill, 1973; Shettigara and Morgan, 1975; Burch et al, 1981; Olsen and Sabroe, 1984; (Hughes et al, 1987); (Enterline et al, 1987a); Smith et al, 1990
	Ovary	Wignall and Fox, 1982
1,3-Butadiene	Lymphatic and hematopoietic	Meinhardt et al, 1982; Divine, 1990; Matanoski et al, 1990; IARC, 1992; (Cole et al, 1993); (Cowles et al, 1994)
Cadmium	Prostate	Potts, 1965; Kipling and Waterhouse, 1967; Lemen et al, 1976; (Armstrong and Kazantzis, 1983); Elinder et al, 1985; (Thun et al, 1985); Sorahan and Waterhouse, 1985; (Sullivan and Waterman, 1988); (Kazantzis et al, 1992); (IARC, 1993b)
Chlorophenoxy herbicides	Soft-tissue sarcoma	Hardell, 1977; Hardell and Sandstrom, 1979; Eriksson et al, 1981; Lynge, 1985; (Hoar et al, 1986); Wiklund and Holm, 1986); (Coggon et al, 1986); (Kang et al, 1987); (Ott et al, 1987); (Woods et al, 1987); Hardell and Eriksson, 1988; Kogan and Clapp, 1988; Zahm et al, 1988; Bond et al, 1989a; Fingerhut et al, 1991; Saracci et al, 1991; (Green, 1991); (Kogevinas et al, 1993); Lynge, 1993
	Non-Hodgkin's lymphoma	Hardell et al, 1981; (Lynge, 1985); Hoar et al, 1986; (Pearce et al, 1986); Ott et al, 1987; (Woods et al, 1987); (Wiklund et al, 1988); (Zahm et al, 1988); (Bond et al, 1989a); Zahm et al, 1990; (Fingerhut et al, 1991); (Saracci et al, 1991); (Green, 1991); (Kogevinas et al, 1993)
	Reviews	Sterling and Arundel, 1986; Lynge et al, 1987; Lilienfeld and Gallo, 1989; Bond et al, 1989a; Johnson, 1990; Ibrahim et al, 1991
Coke oven emissions	Kidney, prostate	Redmond et al, 1972
Cutting oils	Digestive organs	Waterhouse, 1972; Vena et al, 1985; (Järvholm and Lavenius, 1987); Park et al, 1988; Silverstein et al, 1988; Tolbert et al, 1992; (Acquavella et al, 1993)
	Lung	Waterhouse 1972; Decouflé, 1978; Vena et al, 1985; (Järvholm and Lavenius, 1987); Park et al, 1988; (Silverstein et al, 1988); (Tolbert et al, 1992); Acquavella et al, 1993
	Skin	Waterhouse 1972; Järvholm and Lavenius, 1987; (Eisen et al, 1992)
Dimethyl formamide	Testis	Ducatman et al, 1986; Levin et al, 1987; (Chen and Kennedy, 1988)
	Buccal cavity and pharynx	Chen et al, 1988
Diesel fumes	Lung	Howe et al, 1983; Wong et al, 1985; Garshick et al, 1988; Boffetta et al, 1988; NIOSH, 1988; IARC, 1989b; Boffetta et al, 1990; Emmelin et al, 1993; (Van Den Eeden and Friedman, 1993)
Dust	Stomach	Wright et al, 1988; Coggon et al, 1990
Ethylene oxide	Blood (leukemia)	(Morgan et al, 1981a); Hogstedt et al, 1986; (Gardner et al, 1989); (Greenberg et al, 1991); (Steenland et al, 1991a); (Hagmar et al, 1991); (Wong and Trent, 1993); Bisanti et al, 1993
	Stomach	Hogstedt et al, 1986; (Gardner et al, 1989); (Greenberg et al, 1990); (Steenland et al, 1991a); (Hagmar et al, 1991)
Formaldehyde	Lung	(Jensen and Andersen, 1982); (Walrath and Fraumeni, 1983); (Acheson et al, 1984a); Bertazzi et al, 1986; Blair et al, 1986; Sterling and Weinkam, 1988; (Partanen et al, 1990); (Marsh et al, 1994)
	Nasopharyngeal	(Vaughn et al, 1986); Olsen and Asnaes, 1986; Blair et al, 1986; Roush et al, 1987
	Sinonasal	Olsen et al, 1984; (Acheson et al, 1984a); (Vaughan et al, 1986); (Blair et al, 1986); (Roush et al, 1987)
	Reviews	Gough et al, 1984; Levine et al, 1984; Blair et al, 1990

(*continued*)

TABLE 18–2. *Industrial Materials for Which Epidemiological Studies Suggest (or Do Not Suggest) Carcinogenicity* (Continued)*

Material	Site(s)	References
Ionizing radiation	Prostate	Beral et al, 1985; Beral et al, 1988
Man-made mineral fibers	Lung	Saracci R, 1986; Simonato et al, 1987; Enterline et al, 1987d; Doll, 1987; (Gardner et al, 1988); March et al, 1990
Methylmethacrylate/ethyl acrylate	Colon/rectum	(Collins et al, 1989a); Walker et al, 1991
Polychlorinated biphenyls	Various sites	Bahn et al, 1976; Ikeda et al, 1986; Bertazzi et al, 1987; Brown, 1987; Yassi et al, 1994
Polypropylene manufacture	Colorectal	Acquavella et al, 1988; (Acquavella and Owen, 1990); Lewis et al, 1994
Radium	Lung, Multiple myeloma	Stebbings et al, 1984
	Thyroid	Polednak, 1986
Silica (crystalline)	Lung	Forastiere et al, 1986; (Kjuus et al, 1986b); Lynge et al, 1986; Koskela et al, 1987; Finkelstein et al, 1987; Thomas and Stewart, 1987; Guenel et al, 1989; Ng et al, 1990; Simonato et al, 1990; Amandus, 1991; (Hnizdo and Sluis-Cremer, 1991); (Carta et al, 1994)
	Stomach	Finkelstein et al, 1987
Talc	Lung	Lamm et al, 1988
	Ovary	Cramer et al, 1982; Whittemore et al, 1988
Vinyl chloride	Brain	Monson et al, 1974; Cooper, 1981; (Jones et al, 1988); (Simonato et al, 1991a)
	Lung	Monson et al, 1974; (Cooper, 1981); Heldaas et al, 1987; Smulevich et al, 1988; (Jones et al, 1988); (Simonato et al, 1991a)
	Lymphatic and hematopoietic	Monson et al, 1974; Smulevich et al, 1988; (Simonato et al, 1991a)

*References in parentheses are not consistent with a suggestion of carcinogenicity.

The data on the possible health effects of exposure to chlorophenoxy herbicides are also subject to controversy. Two of the most used of these herbicides were 2,4-dichlorophenoxyacetic acid (2,4-D) and 2,4,5-trichlorophenoxyacetic acid (2,4,5-T). Dioxin (2,3,7,8-tetrachlorodibenzo-para-dioxin or TCDD) is a contaminant in 2,4,5-T but not in 2,4-D. Agent Orange, a common herbicide used in the Vietnam war, is a 50:50 mixture of 2,4-D and 2,4,5-T (Sterling and Arundel, 1986). In addition to the scientific uncertainty about the interpretation of epidemiological data on the chlorophenoxyacetic acids, there is substantial political criticism of the conduct of these studies as well as the interpretation of data deriving from them (Gough, 1986).

In general, but not consistently, positive associations between occupational exposure to chlorophenoxy herbicides and soft-tissue sarcoma or Hodgkin's disease have been seen in case-control studies. Data from follow-up studies, while not consistently showing no association, are less indicative of an association. Because of reliance in case-control studies on the assessment of exposure via interview, there is concern about biased reporting of exposure as well as about biased inclusion of exposed cases. Retrospective follow-up studies in which no association between exposure and disease are seen may be criticized because of inclusion of many persons with low exposure or because of inadequate length of time elapsed between exposure and end of follow-up. Thus, the current uncertainty about the health effects of exposure to chlorophenoxy herbicides serves as a paradigm for the criticism of epidemiological methods.

Early studies from Sweden suggested that leukemia and stomach cancer occurred in excess among workers exposed to ethylene oxide (Hogstedt et al, 1986). However, more recent studies show no excess of these cancers. Ethylene oxide has been judged by IARC to be an animal carcinogen.

The data on formaldehyde are quite inconsistent. The largest studies were done in Great Britain by Acheson and colleagues (1984a) and in the United States by Blair and colleagues (1986). An apparent lack of any dose-response relationship may be due to imprecise measurement of past exposures. Also, interpretation of internal analyses differs somewhat from interpretation of anal-

TABLE 18–3. *Occupational Groups Associated (or Not Associated) with Excess Risks for Cancer, with No Specific Agents Identified**

Occupational Group	*Site(s)*	*References*
Agricultural workers	Leukemia	Blair and Thomas, 1979; (Linos et al, 1980); Burmeister, 1981; Blair and White, 1981; Delzell and Grufferman, 1985; (Stark et al, 1987)
	Lip (sun?)	Burmeister, 1981; Wiklund, 1983; Fincham et al, 1992
	Liver	Alavanja et al, 1987
	Lung	Rothschild and Mulvey, 1982; (McDuffie et al, 1990); (Fincham et al, 1992)
	Non-Hodgkin's lymphoma	Burmeister, 1981; Cantor, 1982; Schumacher, 1985; Hoar et al, 1986; (Stark et al, 1987); Dubrow et al, 1988; Wigle et al, 1990
	Testis	(Wiklund, 1983); Mills et al, 1984
	Reviews	Blair et al, 1985; Council, 1988; Blair et al, 1992
Architects	Kidney	Lowrey et al, 1991
Artists	Various sites	Miller et al, 1985; Miller et al, 1986
Bakers	Lung	Tuchsen and Nordholm, 1986
Benzoyl chloride manufacture	Lung	Sakabe et al, 1976
Brewery workers	Various sites	Dean et al, 1979; Jensen, 1979; Carstensen et al, 1990
Calcium carbide manufacture	Colon, prostate	Kjuus et al, 1986a
Cement workers	Lung (chromium?)	(McDowell, 1984); Rafnsson and Johannesdottir, 1986
	Stomach	McDowell, 1984; (Rafnsson and Johannesdottir, 1986); (Amandus, 1986)
Chemists or chemical workers	Brain	Olin and Ahlbom, 1980
	Breast	Walrath et al, 1985
	Cervix	O'Berg et al, 1987
	Genitourinary	Marsh, 1983
	Large intestine	Hoar and Pell, 1981
	Lung	Bond et al, 1985b; Wolf et al, 1987
	Lymphatic and hematopoietic	Li et al, 1969; Walrath et al, 1985
	Ovary	Walrath et al, 1985
	Skin	O'Berg, et al, 1987
	Testis	Bond et al, 1987a
	"Other and unspecified"	Bond et al, 1985a; Bond et al, 1987a
	None	Ott et al, 1985; Guberand and Raymond, 1985; Harrington and Goldblatt, 1986; Maher and Defonso, 1986; Chiazze et al, 1986; Bond et al, 1987b; Thomas, 1987
Coal miners	Stomach	Rockette, 1977; Ames, 1983; (Swaen et al, 1985)
	Leukemia	Gilman et al, 1985
	Lung	(Ames et al, 1983); (Meijers et al, 1988)
Coke by-product plant workers	Colon, pancreas	Redmond et al, 1976
Dry cleaning solvent–exposed workers	Bladder	(Blair et al, 1979); Katz and Jowett, 1981; (Duh and Asal, 1984); Smith et al, 1985; Brown and Kaplan, 1987
	Cervix	Blair et al, 1979; Katz and Jowett, 1981; Brown and Kaplan, 1987
	Kidney	Katz and Jowett, 1981; Duh and Asal, 1984
	Liver	Lynge and Thygesen, 1990
	Lung	Blair et al, 1979; (Katz and Jowett, 1981); Duh and Asal, 1984
Firefighters	Various sites	(Musk et al, 1978); Heyer et al, 1990; Hanson, 1990; Sama et al, 1990; Beaumont et al, 1991; Demers et al, 1994; Tornling et al, 1994; Aronson et al, 1994
	Review	Howe and Burch, 1990
Glass manufacturers	Review	IARC, 1993b
Hairdressers and barbers	Review	IARC, 1993a

(*continued*)

TABLE 18–3. *Occupational Groups Associated (or Not Associated) with Excess Risks for Cancer, with No Specific Agents Identified* (Continued)*

Occupational Group	*Site(s)*	*References*
Lead workers	Various sites	Malcolm and Barnett, 1982; Cooper et al, 1985; Selevan et al, 1985; (Fanning, 1988)
Leather workers	Bladder	Wynder et al, 1963; Cole et al, 1972; Decouflé, 1979; (Decouflé and Walrath, 1983); Garabrant and Wegman, 1984; Morrison et al, 1985; Marrett et al, 1986; (Walrath, et al, 1987); Costantini et al, 1989
Meat workers	Hodgkin's disease	Johnson et al, 1986a
	Lung	Johnson et al, 1986b; Coggon et al, 1989; Johnson 1989; Reif et al, 1989; Guberand et al, 1993
Nonionizing radiation–exposed workers	Blood (leukemia)	Milham, 1982; Savitz and Calle, 1987; Coleman and Beral, 1988; Christie et al, 1991; Tynes et al, 1992; Floderus et al, 1993; Guenel et al, 1993; (Tynes et al, 1994); Thériault et al, 1994
	Brain	Lin et al, 1985; (Milham, 1985); (Tornquist et al, 1986); Thomas et al, 1987; Loomis and Savitz, 1990; (Tynes et al, 1992); Floderus et al, 1993; (Guenel et al, 1993); (Tynes et al, 1994); Thériault et al, 1994
Oil refinery/petro-worker	Blood (leukemia)	McCraw et al, 1985; Divine and Barron, 1986; Wongsrichanalai et al, 1989
	Bone	Wen et al, 1983
	Brain[a]	Thériault and Goulet, 1979; Thomas et al, 1982; Austin and Schnatter, 1983; Waxweiler et al, 1983; (Thomas et al, 1986); Magnani et al, 1987; Teta et al, 1991
	Kidney	Shallenberger et al, 1992
	Lymphatic	Divine and Barron, 1986; Wong et al, 1986; Marsh et al, 1991; Christie et al, 1991
	Pancreas	Hanis et al, 1985; Divine and Barron, 1986
	Skin	Rushton and Alderson, 1981; Nelson et al, 1987; Magnani et al, 1987
	None	(Kaplan, 1986); (Divine and Barron, 1987)
	Reviews	Savitz and Moure, 1984; Harrington, 1987; Wong and Raabe, 1989; IARC, 1989a
Paint manufacturers	Liver	(Chiazze et al, 1980); Englund, 1980; Matanoski et al, 1986; (Bethwaite et al, 1990)
	Lung	Chiazze et al, 1980; Englund, 1980; (Morgan et al, 1981b); (Matanoski et al, 1986); Olsen and Jensen, 1987; (Bethwaite et al, 1990)
	Bladder, kidney, myeloma	Bethwaite et al, 1990
	Review	IARC, 1989c
Pattern makers	Colon	Robinson et al, 1980; Swanson et al, 1985; Tilley et al, 1990
Pesticide-exposed workers	Lung	(Morgan et al, 1980); Blair et al, 1983; (Shindell et al, 1986); MacMahon et al, 1988; (Wiklund et al, 1989); Pesatori et al, 1994
	Lymphatic, skin	Corrao et al, 1989; Hansen et al, 1992
	Reviews	Council, 1988; IARC, 1991
Plumbers	Lung	Kaminski et al, 1980; Englund, 1980; Cantor et al, 1986
	Lymphatic and hematopoietic	Kaminski et al, 1980; Cantor et al, 1986
Printing workers	Lung	Moss et al, 1972; (Greene et al, 1979); Bertazzi and Zocchetti, 1980; Paganini-Hill et al, 1980; Malker and Gemne, 1987; Leon, 1994
	Skin	Greene et al, 1979; Dubrow, 1986
Pulp and paper workers	Various sites	Milham and Demers, 1984; Robinson et al, 1986; Jappinen et al, 1987; Schwartz, 1988; Henneberger et al, 1989; Solet et al, 1989; Hogstedt, 1990; Jappinen and Pukkala, 1991
Rubber industry work areas	Bladder	McMichael et al, 1976; Monson and Fine, 1978; Delzell and Monson, 1981; Checkoway et al, 1981; Negri et al, 1989
	Blood (leukemia)	McMichael et al, 1976; Andjelkovich et al, 1977; Monson and Fine, 1978; Delzell and Monson, 1981; Checkoway et al, 1984
	Lung	McMichael et al, 1976; Andjelkovich et al, 1977; Monson and Fine, 1978; Baxter and Werner, 1980; Delzell and Monson, 1985; Sorahan et al, 1986; Andjelkovich et al, 1988; Sorahan et al, 1989

(*continued*)

TABLE 18–3. (*Continued*)

Occupational Group	*Site(s)*	*References*
	Skin	Monson and Fine, 1978
	Stomach	McMichael et al, 1976; Andjelkovich et al, 1977; Monson and Fine, 1978; Baxter and Werner, 1980; Delzell and Monson, 1982a; Sorahan et al, 1986
Steelmakers	Lung	Finkelstein and Wilk, 1990; Finkelstein et al, 1991
Textile workers	Several sites	Delzell and Grufferman, 1983; O'Brien and Decouflé, 1988; IARC, 1990a
Truck drivers	Bladder	Silverman et al, 1983; Hoar and Hoover, 1985
Veterinarians	Various sites	Blair and Hayes, 1980; Blair and Hayes, 1982; Kinlen, 1983
Waitpersons	Lung	Kjaerheim and Andersen, 1993; Kjaerheim and Andersen, 1994
Welders	Lung	(Blot et al, 1978); Beaumont and Weiss, 1981; Polednak, 1981; Stern, 1983; Lerchen et al, 1987; Sjögren et al, 1987; Tola et al, 1988; Hull et al, 1989; Simonato et al, 1991b; (Steenland et al, 1991b); Danielsen et al, 1993
	Reviews	IARC, 1990b; Sjögren et al, 1994
Woodworkers	Lymphatic tissue (Hodgkin's disease)	Milham and Hesser, 1967; Petersen and Milham, 1974; Grufferman et al, 1976; Greene et al, 1978; (Acheson et al, 1984b); (Miller et al, 1994;
	Review	Nylander and Dement, 1993

*References in parentheses are not consistent with a suggestion of carcinogenicity.
[a]Austin, Waxweiler, and Teta references describe the same study population.

yses based on external (general) population comparison groups. In a reanalysis of the U.S. data, a dose-response association was reported (Sterling and Weinkam, 1988).

Similar difficulties are present in the interpretation of data from studies of workers exposed to man-made mineral fibers (MMMF), mainly fiberglass or rock wool. Coincidentally, formaldehyde is a potentially confounding exposure in some of the MMMF studies.

Exposure to silica is common in miners, foundry workers, ceramic workers, and persons exposed to abrasives. However, persons exposed to silica are also exposed to a number of substances known or suspected to cause lung cancer—arsenic, mineral oils, polycyclic aromatic hydrocarbons, radon. The most persuasive information for a causal association comes from the excess of lung cancers seen in many of the studies of persons with silicosis.

A wide variety of occupations are listed in Table 18–3, and the likelihood that any of the associations listed is causal is quite uncertain. The common element in all of the occupation-cancer associations in this table is the general nature of the occupation. A task before today's occupational epidemiologist is to define with greater specificity the exposures of workers in these occupations and to follow these exposed groups to assess the likelihood of dose-response relationships.

In Tables 18–4 and 18–5 a number of materials from Tables 18–1 and 18–2, respectively, have arbitrarily been selected for inclusion. For each substance an assessment is made of early clinical, early epidemiological, and recent epidemiological reports. An indication is made as to when the association was described, when an early epidemiological study took place, what was the approximate size of the relative risk in these early studies, and how a more precise measure of exposure and of any dose-response relationship evolved. It is a tenet in the interpretation of epidemiological data that strong causal associations do not need an epidemiologist to point them out, and that even epidemiologists may not be able to provide a definitive evaluation of weak associations of uncertain causal nature.

Arsenic (Table 18–4) is unusual in that the early case reports linking arsenic and lung cancer apparently occurred in an environment where the relative risk may only have been about two. (Alternatively, there may have been considerable misclassification in the data used by Hill and Faning [1948]). In the early reports by Lee and Fraumeni (1969) and by Pinto and colleagues (1978) on smelter workers, clear dose-response relationships were present, even though the measure of exposure was quite imprecise. However, in the most recent reports of these two groups of authors (Lee-Feldstein, 1986; Enterline et al, 1987b), a much weaker dose-response relationship is seen in spite of greater precision in the measure of dose. It is likely that this apparent paradox relates to a reduction in exposure with the passage of time coupled with a greater percentage of per-

TABLE 18–4. *Examples of the Development of Information in Humans on Well-Established Occupational Cancers*

Material/Cancer	Study Type[a]	Years of Occurrence	Study Population	Measure of Exposure[b]	Exposed Cases (n)	Risk[c]	Location	Reference
Arsenic/Respiratory	Clin	1933	Sheep-dip makers	—	2	?	England	Henry, 1934
	PMR	1900–43	Arsenical packers	—	7	2.0	England	Hill and Faning, 1948
	RC	1938–63	Smelter workers	Light	45	2.4	Montana	Lee and Fraumeni, 1969
				Medium	44	4.8		
				Heavy	18	6.7		
	RC,PC	1938–67	Smelter workers				Montana	Lee-Feldstein, 1986
			1st employment, <1925	<100 mgm	6	2.2 (1)		
				100–499 mgm	64	3.8 (2.2)		
				500+ mgm	50	5.3 (4.8)		
			1st employment, 1948–55	<100 mgm	61	1.9 (1.3)		
				100–499 mgm	40	3.0 (2.1)		
				500+ mgm	30	1.1 (0.5)		
	RC	1949–73	Smelter workers (urine index)	<3000	5	1.6	Washington	Pinto et al, 1978
				3000–8999	18	2.9		
				9000+	9	6.9		
	RC,PC	1941–76	Smelter workers (air index)	<2000 μgy	24	1.6	Washington	Enterline et al, 1987b
				2000–7999 μgy	40	1.9		
				8000+ μgy	40	2.3		
Asbestos/Lung	Clin	1934	Case report	—	1	?	South Carolina	Lynch and Smith, 1935
	RC	1935–53	Asbestos workers	—	11	14	England	Doll, 1955
	RC	1943–62	Insulation workers	—	45	6.8	USA	Selikoff et al, 1964
	RC	1940–75	Chrysotile workers	<1000 fcd	5	1.4	USA	Dement et al, 1983
				1000–40,000 fcd	16	3.1		
				40,000+ fcd	12	11.8		
	RC		Amosite workers	2200 fcd	14	2.6	USA	Seidman et al, 1986
				2200–36,500 fcd	56	4.9		
				36,500+ fcd	32	8.5		
Benzene/Leukemia	Clin	1928–63	Case reports	—	6	?	Italy	Vigliana and Saita, 1964
	Clin	1967–73	Shoemakers	—	26	?	Turkey	Aksoy et al, 1974
	RC	1950–75	Pliofilm makers	—	7	4.7	Ohio	Infante et al, 1977
	RC,PR	1950–81	Pliofilm makers	<40 pmy	2	1.1	Ohio	Rinsky et al, 1987
				40–400 pmy	4	5.1		
				400+ pmy	3	66		
	RC	1972–81	Benzene producers	—	25	7.0	China	Yin et al, 1987
Benzidine/Bladder	Clin	1895	Dye workers	Many chem's	4	?	Germany	Rehn, 1895
	Clin	1935–51	Dye workers	Benzidine	23	?	England	Scott, 1952
	PMR	1921–52	Dye workers	Benzidine	10	14	Great Britain	Case et al, 1954
	PC	1945–78	Benzidine makers	<2 yr	2	1.1	Connecticut	Meigs et al, 1986
				2+ yr	6	13		

Chloroethers/Lung	Clin	1962–71	Chem. wkrs	Open kettles	14	(8)	Phila.	Figueroa et al, 1973
	(RC)	1954–71	Chem. wkrs	Scale of 0–6	19	3.8	Phila.	DeFonso and Kelton, 1976
	RC	1948–80	Chloroether makers	Low risk	2	1	Great Britain	McCallum et al, 1983
				Medium risk	3	9		
				High risk	6	27		
Nickel and nickel compounds/ Nasal	Clin	?	Nickel refineries	—	10	10	Wales	Annual Report, 1933
	PMR	1938–56	Nickel refineries	—	29	196	Wales	Doll, 1958
	RC	1934–81	Nickel refineries	<1 yr	5	1	Wales	Kaldor et al, 1986
				1–4 yr	18	4.7		
				5–9 yr	9	4.0		
				10–14 yr	16	12.7		
				15+ yr	8	20.5		
Radium, mesothorium/ Bone	Clin	1924–27	Dial painters	Brush licking	2	?	New Jersey	Martland and Humphries, 1929
	(PMR)	1924–31	Dial painters	Brush licking	5	(7000)	New Jersey	Martland, 1931
	(RC)	1930–76	Dial painters	Brush licking	22	82	USA	Polednak et al, 1978
Radon/Lung	Clin	1869–77	Miners	Schneeberg	150	?	Germany	Haerting and Hesse, 1879
	RC	1929–38	Miners	Joachimsthal	43	29	Czechoslov.	Peller, 1939
	PC	1950–59	Uranium miners	3 yr	1	1.1	USA	Archer et al, 1962
				3+ yrs	5	4.5		
	(PC)	1950–74	Uranium miners	1800 wlm,			USA	Archer et al, 1976
				<20 cig	12	1		
				20+ cig	63	3.5		
				1800+ wlm,				
				<20 cig	8	4.2		
				20+ cig	45	12.5		
	RC	1950–80	Uranium miners	<100 wlm	20	1.3	Canada	Howe et al, 1987
				100–399 wlm	11	3.1		
				400–1599 wlm	9	2.9		
				1600+ wlm	8	7.7		
Vinyl chloride/ Liver	Clin	1971–73	PVC makers	—	3	?	Kentucky	Creech and Johnson, 1974
	(PMR)	1947–73	PVC makers	—	8	11	Kentucky	Monson et al, 1974
	(RC)	1942–73	PVC makers	—	7	12	USA	Waxweiler et al, 1976
	RC	1940–74	PVC makers	—	3	3.2	Great Britain	Fox and Collier, 1977

[a]Study type: Clin = clinical report; PMR = proportional mortality ratio; CC = case-control; RC = retrospective cohort; PC = prospective cohort. (Studies in parentheses include data from previous listed study.)

[b]mgm = mg/m^3-months; gy = g/m^3-yr; fcd = fibers/cc-days; pmy = parts/million-years; yr = years exposed; wlm = working level month; cig = cigarettes/day.

[c]Risk is mortality ratio or relative risk. Exp = expected number. (Risks in parentheses are approximate.)

TABLE 18–5. *Examples of the Development of Information in Humans on Suspected Occupational Cancers*

Material/Cancer	*Study Type*[a]	*Years of Occurrence*	*Study Population*[b]	*Measure of Exposure*[b]	*Exposed Cases (n)*	*Risk*[c]	*Location*	*Reference*
Acrylonitrile/ Lung	RC	1956–76	AN users	—	8	1.9	South Carolina	O'Berg, 1980
	RC	1950–78	AN makers	—	9	1.2	Great Britain	Werner and Carter, 1981
	RC	1940–78	AN users	—	9	1.5	Ohio	Delzell and Monson, 1982b
	RC	1956–83	AN users	—	5	0.7	Virginia	Chen et al, 1987
Cadmium/ Prostate	Clin	1920–64	Battery makers	—	3	?	England	Potts, 1965
	(RC)	19??–66	Battery makers	—	4	6.7	England	Kipling and Waterhouse, 1967
	(RC)	1946–81	Battery makers, mortality	—	8	1.2	England	Sorahan and Waterhouse, 1983
	(RC)	1950–80	Battery makers, incidence	High Low	8 7	4.0 0.8	England	Sorahan and Waterhouse, 1985
	RC	1940–69	Cadmium smelters	—	4	3.5	USA	Lemen et al, 1976
	(RC)	1940–78	Cadmium smelters	—	3	1.3	USA	Thun et al, 1985
Ethylene oxide/ Leukemia	Clin	1972–77	Cluster	Sterilizers	3	(15)	Sweden	Hogstedt et al, 1979a
	RC	1961–77	ETO producers	—	3	11	Sweden	Hogstedt et al, 1979b
	RC,PC	1961–82	ETO producers	—	8	10	Sweden	Hogstedt et al, 1986
	RC	1955–77	ETO producers	—	0	(Exp = 0.7)	USA	Morgan et al, 1981
Formaldehyde/ Lung	CC	1943–76	Physicians	Pathologist, anatomist	8	0.9	Denmark	Jensen and Andersen, 1982
	RC	1941–81	Makers/users	Nil Low Moderate High	37 39 14 109	0.9 0.9 0.7 1.1	Great Britain	Acheson et al, 1984a

	RC	1930–80	Makers/users	0 pmy	14	0.6	USA	Blair et al, 1986
				0.5 pmy	88	1.1		
				0.51–5.5 pmy	86	0.9		
				5.5+ pmy	62	1.0		
Man-made mineral fibers/Lung	RC	1945–72	Glasswool	—	5	0.8	USA	Enterline and Henderson, 1975
	RC	1945–73	Mineral wool	<20 yrl	6	1.4	USA	Enterline and Marsh, 1980
				20+ yrl	8	1.0		
			Fibrous glass	<20 yrl	23	0.7		
				20+ yrl	17	1.0		
	(RC,PC)	1946–82	Mineral wool, 20+ yrl	0–9 yrs	23	1.6	USA	Enterline et al, 1987d
				10–19 yr	6	1.1		
				20+ yr	16	1.1		
			Glass wool, 20+ yrl	0–9 yr	132	1.2		
				10–19 yr	36	1.0		
				20+ yr	88	1.4		
	RC	1942–79	MMMF producers	Rockwool	50	1.1	Europe	Saracci et al, 1984
				Glasswool	44	0.9		
	(RC,PC)	1942–82	Rockwool, 20+ yrl	Early production phases	21	2.2	Europe	Simonato et al, 1987
				Late production phases	13	0.9		
			Glasswool, 20+ yrl	Early production phases	46	1.1		
				Late production phases	0	(exp = 0.1)		

[a]Study type: Clin = clinical report; PMR = proportional mortality ratio; CC = case-control; RC = retrospective cohort; PC = prospective cohort. (Studies in parentheses include data from previous listed study.)
[b]pmy = parts/million-years; yrl = years of latency; yr = years exposed.
[c]Risk is mortality ratio or relative risk. Exp = expected number. (Risks in parentheses are approximate.)

son-years of follow-up (and deaths) occurring among workers with lower exposure. Any absolute uncertainty in the measurement of exposure has a greater relative effect on low relative risks than on higher relative risks.

The first case report on lung cancer and asbestos occurred in a person with asbesto-silicosis (Lynch and Smith, 1935). The subsequent evolution of information on the certainty of asbestos and the uncertainty of silica as a cause of lung cancer underlines the caution that must be attached to the interpretation of case reports. In many of the early epidemiological reports on asbestos and lung cancer, fact of exposure to asbestos was the only measure of exposure. It is of interest that the recent dose-response data from Dement and colleagues (1983) and from Seidman and colleagues (1986) show quite similar patterns in the dose-response relationship based on the relative risk. In contrast to many industrial materials, the societal reaction to asbestos is to eliminate its use rather than to reduce exposure to an apparently safe level. This phenomenon may relate to the availability of alternative materials (man-made mineral fibers) as well as to the widespread presence of asbestos in homes and schools. Nevertheless, as time passes, a goal of research on the health effects of exposure to asbestos must be to evaluate whether or not a safe level of exposure can be recommended.

To date, little information exists on the dose-response relationship between exposure to benzene and the development of leukemia. The Rinsky study (1987) is an extension of the Infante study (1977), and only two additional cases of leukemia have been noted. An industry-wide study is currently following 4600 male workers with some history of benzene exposure (Wong 1987a,b). While to date there is not sufficient information collected to evaluate any dose-response relationship between benzene and type of leukemia, an extensive estimation of past exposure has been conducted. It is essential that this study and other studies with accurate exposure estimates continue for the indefinite future.

The data on the relation between benzidine and bladder cancer illustrate a gradual evolution from general to specific; yet the final step of an exposure-based dose-response assessment is yet to be done. Rehn (1895) noted clinically an excess of bladder cancer among workers exposed to many chemicals in the manufacture of dyestuffs. Scott (1952) reported on persons exposed only to benzidine. In 1948, based on the potential health risks of benzidine, a control and monitoring program was established that evolved into an epidemiological follow-up study (Meigs, 1986). This was not a prototypical prospective cohort study, in that continuous exposure measurement and disease assessment was not set in place. When a later follow-up was done, persons who had been exposed to benzidine for more than 2 years were found to have excess bladder cancer. Yet the process of risk evaluation and the establishment of control of exposure should precede rather than follow the setting up of an epidemiological study. That the best efforts based on current information in 1948 were not sufficient to prevent excess occurrence of bladder cancer illustrates the need for continuous evaluation and refinement of exposure standards.

The data on the chloroethers and on vinyl chloride are similar in that clinical observations in the early 1970s were sufficient to enable a causal judgment to be made as to cancer caused by an occupational exposure. These observations were not made earlier because sufficient time had not passed since initial exposure. These observations were not made by epidemiologists because exposure assessment and disease measurement systems were not in place. In the case of chloroether exposure, excess lung cancer in one area of the plant was suggested on the basis of periodic chest x-rays (Figueroa et al, 1973). Yet it took 11 years and 14 cases of lung cancer before the link with chloromethyl methyl ether could be established. In contrast, the report of the association between vinyl chloride exposure and angiosarcoma of the liver was available after 6 years and three cases. The unusual nature of angiosarcoma and the very high relative risk were the likely reasons for the timely clinical association to be noted.

The lesson of benzidine must not be forgotten in considering current exposure to the chloroethers or to vinyl chloride. Manufacturing processes were changed, exposures were reduced, and follow-up studies were started (Collingwood et al, 1987; Cooper, 1981). Yet these studies have been able to do little more than quantify the original clinical observations. Long-term prospective follow-up with characterization of current exposure and confounding factors is needed to establish within a reasonable degree of certainty that current exposure is not harmful.

Whereas there is no doubt that excess nasal and lung cancers have occurred among workers at nickel refineries, there is considerable uncertainty as to the agent(s) responsible. Prevention at the refinery has largely been accomplished by a general reduction in environmental exposures (Grandjean et al, 1988). Studies of workers exposed to nickel and nickel compounds in other settings have yielded inconsistent results, in part because of likely confounding by other chemicals (IARC, 1987). The current need is to measure concurrent exposure to specific nickel compounds, asbestos, chromium, and cigarettes and to follow exposed persons forward in time.

Finally, radium and radon provide an interesting contrast as factors in the development of occupational cancer. Radium caused a fairly specific type of cancer (osteosarcoma), and exposure was controlled by elimination of the occupation. Radon causes lung cancer in general, cannot be eliminated from the air in an essential industry (mining), and must be controlled by some form of ventilation. Thus, a thorough knowledge of the dose-response relationship between radon exposure and lung cancer is needed in order to establish a safe working environment in mines. One of the first epidemiological studies to be conducted of miners was a prospective cohort study in which potential confounding by cigarette smoking could be controlled (Archer, 1976). Yet in most recent studies, investigators have had to rely on retrospective follow-up with no control of confounding by cigarettes or other supected causal agents such as arsenic or silica (Howe et al, 1987). As noted in the data from the Canadian study of workers at the Eldorado Port Radium mine, exposure of around 100 working level months has not been demonstrated to be a level with no excess cancer.

In contrast to the exposure-cancer associations listed in Table 18–4, those in Table 18–5 have relatively weak relative risks and show little consistency across studies. Not all have been reported in clinical series, and retrospective epidemiological studies provide a mixed picture. Yet each of the chemicals listed could on grounds of biological plausibility be considered a potential cause of human cancer in that each is, or contains contaminants that are, carcinogenic to animals (IARC 1987, 1988). Further, many of these and other chemicals are present in the general living environment (herbicides, formaldehyde, man-made mineral fibers), and a small increase in risk could have profound adverse public health consequences.

The first report on lung cancer among workers exposed to acrylonitrile came from the Du Pont Company (O'Berg, 1980) as did a recent report (Chen et al, 1987). A contrasting picture is presented among two independent groups of Du Pont employees. As noted above, the epidemiological picture on cadmium is inconsistent. The data on ethylene oxide are not consistent. Given the widespread nature of ethylene oxide as a sterilant in the health care industry, there is a pressing need to establish and document a safe level of exposure. Finally, formaldehyde and man-made mineral fibers have become widespread in the construction of houses. Formaldehyde has well-known irritant effects, and some forms of man-made mineral fibers have been suggested to carry risks similar to those of asbestos (Stanton and Wrench, 1972; McDonald, 1984). Clearly, prospective cohort studies are needed to characterize recent and current exposure and to quantify morbidity as well as mortality.

PRIORITIES FOR RESEARCH ON OCCUPATIONAL CANCER

A number of suggestions have been made as to the priorities to be followed in future research relating to occupational cancer (Dubrow and Wegman, 1983; Cole and Merletti, 1983; IARC, 1986). These are summarized below.

Dubrow and Wegman focus on large occupational groups in the United States or Great Britain with known or apparent excesses of occupational cancer. Identification and elimination of an occupational cause of cancer would potentially have a major positive public health impact. On the basis of twelve surveillance studies, five groups are recommended for study:

1. *Asbestos workers.* While the adverse health effects of asbestos are well-known, additional work is needed to characterize level of exposure in a number of occupations and to establish safe working environments.
2. *Motor vehicle drivers.* Lung and other cancers are reported to be in excess among this group of over 3.5 million workers. The role of cigarette smoking and diesel exhaust must be evaluated.
3. *Machinists and related occupations.* Over 1.5 million workers may be exposed to abrasives and cutting oils.
4. *Electrical workers.* An exposure of uncertain carcinogenic potential is non-ionizing radiation.
5. *Metal molders.* Exposures of concern include polycyclic aromatic hydrocarbons, metal dusts, and oxides.

Cole and Merletti (1983) suggest how improved epidemiological methodology would contribute to the prevention of occupational cancer. Their recommendations relate to the development of long-term institutional programs that would enable continuous and standardized collection of information on occupational exposures and illnesses:

1. *A list of known and suspected animal carcinogens should be maintained.* Such a list is contained in a recent publication from the International Agency for Research on Cancer (IARC, 1987). Human exposure to animal carcinogens calls for long-term epidemiological assessment.
2. *An exposure-based classification scheme for occupations should be developed.* While work on such a scheme has been proceeding for over a decade (Hoar et al, 1980), results to date suggest that retrospective characterization of exposure leads to insensitivity (Hinds et al, 1985; Magnani et al, 1988). It seems likely that concurrent assessment of exposure will be needed to develop a sensitive and specific scheme.

3. *The National Death Index should be extended back in time.* While a number of countries have for years had national systems of identifying deaths and causes of death, a National Death Index (NDI) has existed in the United States only since 1979 (Wentworth, 1983). This index is proving to be of great value in following occupational cohorts, in that a death search need be done through only the NDI rather than through the 50 states.

4. *Registries of exposed workers should be established.* The establishment of exposure registries to complement disease registries is a logical way to pool data from more than one organization. An essential component of an exposure registry is that past, current, and future exposure to occupational substances must be documented and maintained.

5. *Medical and occupational information should be linked.* In essence, this recommendation would establish ongoing prospective cohort studies of occupational groups who are potentially exposed to toxic substances. Such a linkage system should become a national priority.

6. *Research on improved epidemiological methodology should be encouraged.* As large amounts of specific data on exposure and disease in individual workers are collected, sensitive and efficient methods must be developed to deal with data where both the measure of exposure and the measure of disease change with time.

Finally, a Panel from IARC (1986) developed ten criteria to assist in selecting occupational exposures for epidemiological study. These criteria relate to issues of potential public health importance as well as to interpretation of epidemiological data.

1. *Number of workers exposed.* The evaluation of substances to which many workers are exposed should take priority.
2. *Level of exposure to workers.* Measure of level of exposure is essential to assess priority as well as to relate exposure to disease.
3. *Quality of exposure data.* Dose-response relationships can be evaluated only if exposure (and disease) are measured accurately.
4. *Carcinogenic potential.* Human exposure to animal carcinogens calls for long-term epidemiological assessment.
5. *Evidence of human carcinogenicity.* Clinical case reports should be followed by epidemiological studies. Studies of established human carcinogens should focus on dose-response relationships or mechanisms of action.
6. *Ongoing exposure to known carcinogens at permissible levels of exposure.* Regulations of exposure must be established and reevaluated continuously. The safe standard of yesterday may not be the safe standard of tomorrow.
7. *Trends in exposure.* Suspect carcinogens whose use is increasing must receive a high priority for study.
8. *Control of confounding factors.* Identification and evaluation of potential confounding factors is necessary to establish valid conclusions.
9. *Cases potentially attributable to exposure.* The absolute number of cases of cancer that may result from an occupational exposure is a function of the number of persons exposed, the level and duration of exposure, and the relative risk. The eventual public impact of any disease-causing exposure is the number of cases of disease caused.
10. *Time since first exposure.* Sufficient time must pass before the effects of exposure to a carcinogen can occur. Thus, studies that result in data showing no association between exposure and disease must take into account time since first exposure. The past may not be predictive of the future.

A common thread runs through these three sets of recommendations with respect to occupational cancer: measure exposure, measure confounding factors, measure disease, relate exposure to disease, set standards of exposure, and control exposure. Historically, this has been more a retrospective than a prospective process. Disease has occurred among employed persons, clinicians have noticed an apparent excess, epidemiologists have quantified the excess, and exposure has been controlled. The need now and in the future is to link the measure of exposure with the measure of disease in the prospective collection of data among employed persons.

OPTIONS FOR THE FUTURE

In 1987 a Workshop on Needs and Resources for Occupational Mortality Data was held to evaluate how data relating to occupational safety and health could be improved (National Center for Health Statistics, 1988). Ten options were reviewed to improve the collection of data on occupational mortality in ongoing vital statistics programs in the United States. An example of an innovative study in this context has been conducted in Canada, where a 10% sample of the Canadian Labor Force was linked to the Canadian mortality data base (Howe and Lindsay, 1983). Within the context of ongoing surveillance programs or the conduct of ad hoc studies, collection of data on occupational cancer can be considered to be disease-based or exposure-based. After the collection of these data, there are issues that relate to data analysis, setting of standards to exposure, and control of exposure.

Disease-based Data Collection

A clinical case-report on the occurrence of cancer in a person with a specified occupation is disease-based. While the co-occurrence of exposure and disease is the phenomenon of interest, the development of the disease is the factor that leads to further investigation. Historically, case reports have led to the prevention of occupational cancer, but better and earlier methods are needed. A formalization and generalization of case reports is the Sentinal Health Event (Rutstein et al, 1983). The occurrence of diseases known to be induced by occupational exposures can lead to identification of currently uncontrolled exposures and the prevention of future occupational disease, including cancer. Sentinal Health Events, however, are of limited use in identifying previously unrecognized occupational carcinogens.

Evaluation of occupation in routinely collected data on persons with cancer may lead to the identification of unrecognized occupational hazards (Williams et al, 1977; Dubrow and Wegman, 1983; Whorton et al, 1983). While such screening programs usually have little information on specific exposures, they serve to focus attention on occupational groups that may be at risk of excess cancer.

The next level of disease-based study is the conduct of formal case-control studies (Siemiatycki et al, 1981; Coggan et al, 1984; Gerin et al, 1985; Goldberg et al, 1986). These studies are useful in evaluating past and present occupational exposures in persons with cancer. The goal in case-control studies is to identify occupational exposures that may be factors in causing cancer.

The advantages of disease-based studies of potential occupational cancer are that specific cancers can be targeted for evaluation and that a wide variety of occupations can be related to the occurrence of cancer. The disadvantages are that there may be a small number of persons with any single occupation and that quantitative assessment of past occupational exposures usually is not possible. Thus, case-control studies are most useful in finding new occupational causes of cancer or for evaluating whether known causes are present in a general population.

Exposure-based Data Collection

Cohort or follow-up studies are exposure-based. Persons with an occupation of concern are identified and followed in order to measure the rate of occurrence of cancer. If follow-up is retrospective, exposure assessment will be difficult and approximate; if follow-up is prospective, exposure can be measured with greater accuracy. The goal in follow-up studies is to quantify past, current, and future exposure to specific chemicals (Ballantyne, 1985; Hoar et al, 1985; Smith, 1987). A logical extension is to measure biological markers of exposure in human tissues (Perera, 1987).

In considering which new retrospective cohort studies of occupational groups to conduct, there are issues of what to study, who to study, whether to study, and how to study. An extensive source of what has been studied is the Publications Catalogue of the National Institute for Occupational Safety and Health (Maloney and Grooms, 1987). Levine and Eisenbud (1988) have identified over 20 industrial populations that potentially could be studied retrospectively. Among these populations are persons with exposure to known human carcinogens (benzene, chromates), suspected human carcinogens (beryllium, dioxins), and chemicals for which little information exists (flour, nitroglycerine). Steenland and colleagues (1987) have discussed issues about whether or not sufficient information exists to warrant the setting up of a retrospective follow-up study. In the context of ethylene oxide, they address sample size, levels of exposure, and adequacy of records. Marsh (1987) has described methods that may be used to collect and combine data from industrywide studies.

While the goal in retrospective cohort studies is to quantify exposure and to relate exposure to disease, obvious limitations exist. If industrial hygiene measurements of past exposure do not exist, exposure assessment must be more qualitative than quantitative. If the relation between exposure and disease is weak, this imprecision in measurement of exposure may prevent an accurate assessment of the relative risk. The establishment of safe standards of exposure and of control of exposure will be approximate at best.

Thus, consideration must be given to setting up long-term prospective cohort studies of occupational groups. Exposure can be quantified with precision, and persons can be followed with relative ease. The obvious disadvantage is that decades may have to pass before an accurate dose-response assessment can be made. But now is the time to start.

Analysis of Data on Occupational Cancer

There is nothing unique about data relating occupational exposures to cancer. As with all epidemiological data, there are concerns about presence and control of confounding, appropriateness of comparisons, accurate relating of exposure to disease, and cost. A number of publications address these and other issues (Monson, 1974, 1986, 1990; Breslow and Day, 1980, 1987; Prentice, 1986; Wacholder and Boivin, 1987; Whittemore, 1987; Stewart and Hunting, 1988; Siemiatycki et al, 1988). An issue of increasing concern as time-related data accumulate is the dynamic interrelation between measure of exposure and measure of disease (Pearce et al, 1988). Not only may an occupational exposure cause a change in the rate of disease, the occurrence of disease may change the degree to which one is exposed (Robins 1985, 1987).

Exposure Standards and Control

The ultimate aim of epidemiology is the prevention of disease. Disease is not prevented by the conduct of an epidemiological study, but by the maintenance of safe levels of exposure to toxic substances. Epidemiological information is of value in the establishment of standards that approximate safe levels of exposure. But the main actions that prevent disease are those that minimize exposures to harmful substances.

In the occupational setting, exposure standards have been established that aim to provide a safe working environment (Holmberg and Winell, 1977; Corn, 1983; ACGIH, 1987). Historically, these standards were developed based on considerations of acute toxicity; as experience accumulated it was recognized that prevention of chronic diseases such as cancer was also essential (Hatch, 1973). While these standards are intended to have a wide margin of safety, perhaps 10-fold, it has become apparent that for many substances, for example, asbestos or vinyl chloride, long-term exposure at the prevailing standard may lead to the development of cancer. The ultimate prevention of occupational cancer will come to pass only when epidemiologists, industrial hygienists, and occupational physicians work together to provide accurate guidelines to be followed in control of the occupational environment. (Burgess, 1981; Levy and Wegman, 1988; Zenz, 1988; Monson, 1990; Rom, 1992).

EPILOGUE

Mortality studies have been conducted among chimney sweeps in Copenhagen and in Sweden (Hansen et al, 1982; Gustavsson et al, 1988). Excess skin cancer was not observed, but there was excess lung cancer. The control of one form of occupational cancer does not necessarily prevent all forms. "The condition upon which God hath given liberty to man is eternal vigilance" (Curran, 1790).

REFERENCES

ACGIH. 1987. Threshold Limit Values and Biological Exposure Indices for 1986–87. Cincinnati, American Conference of Governmental Industrial Hygienists Inc.

ACHESON ED. 1976. Nasal cancer in the furniture and boot and shoe manufacturing industries. Prev Med 5:295–315.

ACHESON ED, BARNES HR, GARDNER MJ, et al. 1984a. Formaldehyde in the British chemical industry: an occupational cohort study. Lancet 1:611–616.

ACHESON ED, COWDELL RH, RANG EH. 1981. Nasal cancer in England and Wales: an occupational survey. Br J Ind Med 38:218–224.

ACHESON ED, PIPPARD EC, WINTER PD. 1984b. Mortality of English furniture makers. Scand J Work Environ Health 10:211–217.

ACQUAVELLA JF, DOUGLASS TS, PHILLIPS SC. 1988. Evaluation of excess colorectal cancer incidence among workers involved in the manufacture of polypropylene. J Occup Med 30:439–442.

ACQUAVELLA JF, OWEN CV. 1990. Assessment of colorectal cancer incidence among polypropylene pilot plant employees. J Occup Med 32:127–130.

ACQUAVELLA J, LEET T, JOHNSON G. 1993. Occupational experience and mortality among a cohort of metal components manufacturing workers. Epidemiology 4:428– 434.

ADES AE, KAZANTZIS G. 1988. Lung cancer in a non-ferrous smelter: the role of cadmium. Br J Ind Med 45:435–442.

AHLBORG G, HOGSTEDT C, SUNDELL L, et al. 1981. Laryngeal cancer and pickling house vapors. Scand J Work Environ Health 7:239–240.

AKSOY M, ERDEM S, DINCOL G. 1974. Leukemia in shoeworkers exposed chronically to benzene. Blood 44:837–841.

ALAVANJA MCR, MALKER H, HAYES RB. 1987. Occupational cancer risk associated with the storage and bulk handling of agricultural foodstuffs. J Toxicol Environ Health 22:247–254.

AMANDUS HE. 1986. Mortality from stomach cancer in United States cement plant and quarry workers, 1950–80. Br J Ind Med 43:520–528.

AMANDUS HE, SHY C, WING C, et al. 1991. Silicosis and lung cancer in North Carolina dusty trades workers. Am J Ind Med 20:57–70.

AMES RG. 1983. Gastric cancer and coal mine dust exposures: a case-control study. Cancer 52:1346–1350.

AMES RG, AMANDUS H, ATTFIELD M, et al. 1983. Does coal mine dust present a risk for lung cancer? A case-control study of U.S. coal miners. Arch Environ Health 38:331–333.

ANDERSEN A, DAHLBERG BE, MAGNUS K, et al. 1982. Risk of cancer in the Norwegian aluminium industry. Int J Cancer 29:295–298.

ANDJELKOVICH D, ABDELGHANY N, MATHEW RM, et al. 1988. Lung cancer case-control study in a rubber manufacturing plant. Am J Ind Med 14:559–574.

ANDJELKOVICH D, TAULBEE J, SYMONS M, et al. 1977. Mortality of rubber workers with reference to work experience. J Occup Med 19:397–405.

ANNUAL REPORT OF THE CHIEF INSPECTOR OF FACTORIES AND WORKSHOPS FOR THE YEAR 1932. 1933, London: Her Majesty's Stationery Office pp 103–104.

ARCHER VE, GILLAM JD, WAGONER JK. 1976. Respiratory disease mortality among uranium miners. Ann NY Acad Sci 271:280–293.

ARCHER VE, MAGNUSON JH, HOLADAY DA, et al. 1962. Hazards to health in uranium mining and milling. J Occup Med 4:55–60.

ARMSTRONG B, TREMBLAY C, BARIS D et al. 1994. Lung cancer mortality and polynuclear aromatic hydrocarbons. a case-control study of aluminum production workers in Arvida, Quebec, Canada. Am J Epidemiol 139:250–262.

ARMSTRONG BG, KAZANTZIS G. 1983. The mortality of cadmium workers. Lancet 1:1425–1427.

ARONSON KJ, TOMLINSON GA, SMITH L. 1994. Mortality among fire fighters in metropolitan Toronto. Am J Ind Med 26:89–101.

AUSTIN H, DELZELL E, COLE P. 1988. Benzene and leukemia: a review of the literature. Am J Epidemiol 127:419–439.

AUSTIN SG, SCHNATTER AR. 1983. A cohort mortality study of petrochemical workers. J Occup Med 25:304–312.

AXELSON O, DAHLGREN E, JANSSON CD, et al. 1978. Arsenic exposure and mortality: a case-referent study from a Swedish copper smelter. Br J Ind Med 35:8–15.

BAETJER AM. 1950a. Pulmonary carcinoma in chromate workers. I. A review of the literature and report of cases. AMA Arch Ind Hyg Occup Med 2:487–504.

BAETJER AM. 1950b. Pulmonary carcinoma in chromate workers. II. Incidence on basis of hospital records. AMA Arch Ind Hyg Occup Med 2:505–516.

BAHN AK, ROSENWAIKE I, HERRMANN N, et al. 1976. Melanoma after exposure to PCB's.N Engl J Med 295:450.

BALLANTYNE B. 1985. Evaluation of hazards from mixtures of chemicals in the occupational environment. J Occup Med 27:85–94.

BATTISTA G, BELLI S, CARBONCINI F, et al. 1988. Mortality among pyrite miners with low-level exposure to radon daughters. Scand J Work Environ Health 14:280–285.

BAXTER PJ, WERNER JB. 1980. Mortality in the British rubber industries 1967–76. London. Her Majesty's Stationery Office.

BEAUMONT JJ, CHU GST, JONES JR, et al. 1991. An epidemiologic study of cancer and other causes of mortality in San Francisco firefighters. Am J Ind Med 19:357–372.

BEAUMONT JJ, LEVETON J, KNOX K, et al. 1987. Lung cancer mortality in workers exposed to sulfuric acid mist and other acid mists. J Natl Cancer Inst 79:911–921.

BEAUMONT JJ, WEISS NJ. 1981. Lung cancer among welders. J Occup Med 23:839–844.

BELL J. 1876. Paraffin epithelioma of the scrotum. Edinburgh Med J 22:135–137.

BERAL V, FRASER P, CARPENTER L, et al. 1988. Mortality of employees of the Atomic Weapons Establishment. Br Med J 297:757–770.

BERAL V, INSKIP H, FRASER P, et al. 1985. Mortality of employees of the United Kingdom Atomic Energy Authority, 1946–79. Br Med J 291:440–447.

BERRY G, NEWHOUSE ML. 1983. Mortality of workers manufacturing friction materials using asbestos. Br J Ind Med 40:1–7.

BERTAZZI PA, PESATORI AC, RADICE L, et al. 1986. Exposure to formaldehyde and cancer mortality in a cohort of workers producing resins. Scand J Work Environ Health 12:461–468.

BERTAZZI PA, RIBOLDI L, PESATORI A, 1987. et al. Cancer mortality of capacitor manufacturing workers. Am J Ind Med 11:165–176.

BERTAZZI PA, ZOCCHETTI C. 1980. A mortality study of newspaper printing workers. Am J Ind Med 1:85–97.

BERTRAND JP, CHAU N, PATRIS A. 1987. Mortality due to respiratory cancers in the coke oven plants of the Lorraine coal mining industry (Houilleres du Bassin de Lorraine). Br J Ind Med 44:559–565.

BETHWAITE PB, PEARCE N, FRASER J. 1990. Cancer risks in painters: study based on the New Zealand Cancer Registry. Br J Ind Med 47:742–746.

BIDSTRUP PL, CASE RAM. 1956. Carcinoma of the lung in workmen in the bichromates-producing industry in Great Britain. Br J Ind Med 13:260–264.

BISANTI L, MAGGINI M, RASCHETTI R, et al. 1993. Cancer mortality in ethylene oxide workers. Br J Ind Med 50:317–324.

BLAIR A, DECOUFLÉ P, GRAUMAN D. 1979. Causes of death among laundry and dry cleaning workers. Am J Public Health 69:508–511.

BLAIR A, GRAUMAN DJ, LUBIN JH, et al. 1983. Lung cancer and other causes of death among licensed pesticide applicators. J Natl Cancer Inst 71:31–37.

BLAIR A, HAYES HM JR. 1980. Cancer and other causes of death among U.S. veterinarians, 1966–1977. Int J Cancer 25:181–185.

BLAIR A, HAYES HM JR. 1982. Mortality patterns among U.S. veterinarians 1947–1972: an expanded study. Int J Epidemiol 11:391–397.

BLAIR A, MALKER H, CANTOR KP, et al. 1985. Cancer among farmers: a review. Scand J Work Environ Health 11:397–407.

BLAIR A, SARACCI R, STEWART PA, et al. 1990. Epidemiologic evidence on the relationship between formaldehyde exposure and cancer. Scand J Work Environ Health 16:381–393.

BLAIR A, STEWART P, O'BERG M, et al. 1986. Mortality among industrial workers exposed to formaldehyde. J Natl Cancer Inst 76:1071–1084.

BLAIR A, THOMAS TL. 1979. Leukemia among Nebraska farmers. a death certificate study. Am J Epidemiol 110:264–273.

BLAIR A, WHITE DW. 1981. Death certificate study of leukemia among farmers from Wisconsin. J Natl Cancer Inst 66:1027–1030.

BLAIR A, ZAHM SH, PEARCE NE, et al. 1992. Clues to cancer etiology from studies of farmers. Scand J Work Environ Health 18:209–216.

BLOT WJ, HARRINGTON JM, TOLEDO A, et al. 1978. Lung cancer after employment in shipyards during World War II. N Engl J Med 299:620–624.

BOFFETTA P, HARRIS RE, WYNDER EL. 1990. Case-control study on occupational exposure to diesel exhaust and lung cancer risk. Am J Ind Med 17:577–592.

BOFFETTA P, STELLMAN SC, GARFINKEL L. 1988. Diesel exhaust exposure and mortality among males in the American Cancer Society prospective study. Am J Epidemiol 14:403–415.

BOND GG, BODNER KM, COOK RR. 1989a. Phenoxy herbicides and cancer: insufficient epidemiologic evidence for a causal relationship. Fund Appl Toxicol 12:172–188.

BOND GG, MCLAREN EA, CARTMILL JB, et al. 1987a. Cause-specific mortality among male chemical workers. Am J Ind Med 12:353–383.

BOND GG, MCLAREN EA, CARTMILL JB, et al. 1987b. Mortality among female employees of a chemical company. Am J Ind Med 12:563–578.

BOND GG, MCLAREN EA, LIPPS TE, et al. 1989b. Update of mortality among chemical workers with the potential exposure to the higher chlorinated dioxins. J Occup Med 31:121–123.

BOND GG, REEVE GR, OTT MG, et al. 1985b. Mortality among a sample of chemical company employees. Am J Ind Med 7:109–121.

BOND GG, SHELLENBERGER RJ, FISHBECK WA, et al. 1985a. Mortality among a large cohort of chemical manufacturing employees. J Natl Cancer Inst 75:859–869.

BOYD JT, DOLL R, FAULDS JS, et al. 1970. Cancer of the lung in iron ore (haematite) miners. Br J Ind Med 27:97–105.

BOYKO RW, CARTWRIGHT RA, GLASHAN RW. 1985. Bladder cancer in dye manufacturing workers. J Occup Med 27:799–803.

BRESLOW NE, DAY NE. 1980. Statistical Methods in Cancer Research. Vol. 1—The Analysis of Case-Control Studies. Lyon, IARC.

BRESLOW NE, DAY NE. 1987. Statistical Methods in Cancer Research. Vol. 2—The Design and Analysis of Cohort Studies. Lyon, IARC.

BRINTON LA, BLOT WJ, STONE BJ, et al. 1977. A death certificate analysis of nasal cancer among furniture workers in North Carolina. Cancer Res 37:3473–3474.

BROWN DP. 1987. Mortality of workers exposed to polychlorinated biphenyls—an update. Arch Environ Health 42:333–339.

BROWN DP, KAPLAN SD. 1987. Retrospective cohort mortality study of dry cleaner workers using perchlorethylene. J Occup Med 29:535–541.

BUIATTI E, GEDDES M, SANTUCCI M, et al. 1985. A case control study of lung cancer in Florence, Italy: I. Some occupational risk factors. J Epidemiol Community Health 39:244–250.

BURCH JD, HOWE GR, MILLER AB, et al. 1981. Tobacco, alcohol, asbestos, and nickel in the etiology of cancer of the larynx: a case-control study. J Natl Cancer Inst 67:1219–1224.

BURGESS WA. 1981. *Recognition of Health Hazards in Industry: a Review of Materials and Processes.* New York: Wiley.

BURMEISTER LF. 1981. Cancer mortality in Iowa farmers, 1971–78. J Natl Cancer Inst 66:461–464.

CANTOR KP. 1982. Farming and mortality from non-Hodgkin's lymphoma: a case-control study. Int J Cancer 29:239–247.

CANTOR KP, SONTAG JM, HEID MF. 1986. Patterns of mortality among plumbers and pipefitters. Am J Ind Med 10:73–89.

CARSTENSEN JM, BYGREN LO, HATSCHEK T. 1990. Cancer incidence among Swedish brewery workers. Int J Cancer 45:393–396.

CARTA P, COCCO P, PICCHIRI G. 1994. Lung cancer mortality and airways obstruction among metal miners exposed to silica and low levels of radon daughters. Am J Ind Med 25:489–506.

CASE RAM, HOSKER ME. 1954. Tumour of the urinary bladder as an occupational disease in the rubber industry in England and Wales. Br J Prev Soc Med 8:39–50.

CASE RAM, HOSKER ME, MCDONALD DB, et al. 1954. Tumours of the urinary bladder in workmen engaged in the manufacture and use of certain dyestuff intermediates in the British chemical industry. Part I. The role of aniline, benzidine, alpha-naphthylamine and beta-naphthylamine. Br J Ind Med 11:75–104.

CASE RAM, LEA AJ. 1955. Mustard gas poisoning, chronic bronchitis and lung cancer. Br J Prev Soc Med 9:62–72.

CASE RAM, PEARSON JT. 1954. Tumours of the urinary bladder in workmen engaged in the manufacture and use of certain dyestuff intermediates in the British chemical industry. Part II. Further consideration of the role of aniline and of the manufacture of auramine and magenta (fuchsine) as possible causative agents. Br J Ind Med 11:213–216.

CHECKOWAY H, SMITH AH, MCMICHAEL AJ, et al. 1981. A case-control study of bladder cancer in the United States rubber and tyre industry. Br J Ind Med 38:240–246.

CHECKOWAY H, WILCOSKY T, WOLF P, et al. 1984. An evaluation of the associations of leukemia and rubber industry solvent exposures. Am J Ind Med 5:239–249.

CHEN JL, FAYERWEATHER WE, PELL S. 1988. Cancer incidence of workers exposed to dimethylformamide and/or acrylonitrile. J Occup Med 30:813–818.

CHEN JL, KENNEDY GL. 1988. Dimethylformamide and testicular cancer. Lancet 1:55.

CHEN JL, WALRATH J, O'BERG MT, et al. 1987. Cancer incidence and mortality among workers exposed to acrylonitrile. Am J Ind Med 11:157–163.

CHEN SY, HAYES RB, LIANG SR, et al. 1990. Mortality experience of haematite mine workers in China. Br J Ind Med 47:175–181.

CHIAZZE L JR, FERENCE LD, WOLF PH. 1980. Mortality among automobile assembly workers. I. Spray painters. J Occup Med 22:520–526.

CHIAZZE L JR, WOLF P, FERENCE LD. 1986. An historical cohort study of mortality among salaried research and development workers of the Allied Corporation. J Occup Med 28:1185–1188.

CHRISTIAN HA. 1962. Cancer of the lung in employees of a public utility. J Occup Med 4:133–139.

CHRISTIE D, ROBINSON K, GORDON I, et al. 1991. A prospective study in the Australian petroleum industry. II. Incidence of cancer. Br J Ind Med 48:511–514.

COGGON D, BARKER DJP, COLE RB. 1990. Stomach cancer and work in dusty industries. Br J Ind Med 47:298–301.

COGGON D, PANNETT B, ACHESON ED. 1984. Screening for new occupational hazards of cancer in young persons. Ann Occup Hyg 28:145–150.

COGGON D, PANNETT B, PIPPARD ED, et al. 1989. Lung cancer in the meat industry. Br J Ind Med 46:188–191.

COGGON D, PANNETT B, WINTER PD. 1986. Mortality of workers exposed to 2 methyl-4 chlorophenoxyacetic acid. Scand J Work Environ Health 12:448–454.

COLE P, HOOVER R, FRIEDELL GH. 1972. Occupation and cancer of the lower urinary tract. Cancer 29:1250–1260.

COLE P, MERLETTI F. 1983. Occupational cancer. In: *The Epidemiology of Cancer*, Bourke G (ed). London: Croom Helm, pp 260–291.

COLE P, DELZELL E, ACQUAVELLA J. 1993. Exposure to butadiene and lymphatic and hematopoietic cancer. Epidemiology 4:96–103.

COLEMAN M, BERAL V. 1988. A review of epidemiological studies of the health effects of living near or working with electricity generation and transmission equipment. Int J Epidemiol 17:1-13.

COLLINGWOOD KW, PASTERNAK BS, SHORE RE. 1987. An industry-wide study of respiratory cancer in chemical workers exposed to chloromethyl ethers. J Natl Cancer Inst 78:1127–1136.

COLLINS JJ, PAGE LC, CAPOROSSI JC, et al. 1989a. Mortality patterns among men exposed to methyl methacrylate. J Occup Med 31:41–46.

COLLINS JJ, PAGE LC, CAPOROSSI JC, et al. 1989b. Mortality patterns among employees exposed to acrylonitrite. J Occup Med 31:368–371.

COOPER WC. 1981. Epidemiologic study of vinyl chloride workers: mortality through December 31, 1972. Environ Health Perspect 41:101–106.

COOPER WC, WONG O, KHEIFETS L. 1985. Mortality among employees of lead battery plants and lead producing plants, 1947–1980. Scand J Work Environ Health 11:331–345.

CORN M. 1983. Regulations, standards and occupational hygiene within the U.S.A. in the 1980s. Ann Occup Hyg 27:91–105.

CORRAO G, CALLERI M, CARLE F, et al. 1989. Cancer risks in a cohort of licensed pesticide users. Scand J Work Environ Health 15:203–209.

COSTANTINI AS, PACI E, MILIGI L. 1989. Cancer mortality among workers in the Tuscan tanning industry. Br J Ind Med 46:384–388.

COUNCIL ON SCIENTIFIC AFFAIRS (AMA). 1988. Cancer risk of pesticides in agricultural workers. JAMA 260:959–966.

COURT BROWN WM, DOLL R. 1958. Expectation of life and mortality from cancer among British radiologists. Br Med J ii:181–187.

COWLES SR, TSAI SP, SNYDER PJ, et al. 1994. Mortality, morbidity, and haematological results from a cohort of long term workers involved in 1,3–butadiene monomer production. Occup Environ Med 51:323–329.

CRAMER DW, WELCH WR, SCULLY RE, et al. 1982. Ovarian cancer and talc. Cancer 50:372–376.

CREECH JL JR, JOHNSON MN. 1974. Angiosarcoma of liver in the manufacture of polyvinyl chloride. J Occup Med 16:150–151.

CRUICKSHANK CND, GOUREVITCH A. 1952. Skin cancer of the hand and forearm. Br J Ind Med 9:74–79.

CRUICKSHANK CND, SQUIRE JR. 1950. Skin cancer in the engineering industry from the use of mineral oil. Br J Ind Med 7:1–11.

CURRAN JP. (1790) Speech upon the Right of Election. In: *Bartlett's Familiar Quotations*, Morley C, Everett LD (eds). Boston, Little, Brown and Company, 1951, p 277.

DALAGER NA, MASON TJ, FRAUMENI JF JR, et al. 1980. Cancer mortality among workers exposed to zinc chromate paints. J Occup Med 22:25–29.

DANIELSEN TE, LANGARD S, ANDERSEN A, et al. 1993. Incidence of cancer among welders of mild steel and other shipyard workers. Br J Ind Med 50:1097–1103.

DAVIES JM. 1965. Bladder tumours in the electric-cable industry. Lancet 2:143–146.

DAVIES JM. 1978. Lung cancer mortality of workers making chrome pigments. Lancet 1:384.

DAVIES JM, EASTON DF, BIDSTRUP PL. 1991. Mortality from respiratory cancer and other causes in United Kingdom chromate production workers. Br J Ind Med 48:299–313.

DEAN G, MACLENNAN R, MCLOUGHLIN H, et al. 1979. Causes of death of blue-collar workers at a Dublin brewery, 1954–73. Br J Cancer 40:581–589.

DECOUFLÉ P. 1978. Further analysis of cancer mortality patterns among workers exposed to cutting oil mists. J Natl Cancer Inst 61:1025–1030.

DECOUFLÉ P. 1979. Cancer risks associated with employment in the leather and leather products industry. Arch Environ Health 34:33–37.

DECOUFLÉ P. 1982. Occupation. In. *Cancer Epidemiology and Prevention*, Schottenfeld D, Fraumeni JF Jr (eds). Philadelphia: WB Saunders Company, pp 318–335.

DECOUFLÉ P, BLATTNER WA, BLAIR A. 1983. Mortality among chemical workers exposed to benzene and other agents. Environ Res 30:16–25.

DECOUFLÉ P, WALRATH J. 1983. Proportionate mortality among US shoeworkers, 1966–1977. Am J Ind Med 4:523–532.

DECOUFLÉ P, WOOD DJ. 1979. Mortality patterns among workers in a gray iron foundry. Am J Epidemiol 109:667–675.

DEFONSO LR, KELTON SC SR. 1976. Lung cancer following exposure to chloromethyl methyl ether. Arch Environ Health 31:125–130.

DELZELL E, GRUFFERMAN S. 1983. Cancer and other causes of death among female textile workers, 1976–78. J Natl Cancer Inst 71:735–740.

DELZELL E, GRUFFERMAN S. 1985. Mortality among white and nonwhite farmers in North Carolina, 1976–78. Am J Epidemiol 121:391–402.

DELZELL E, MONSON RR. 1981. Mortality among rubber workers. III. Cause-specific mortality, 1940–1978. J Occup Med 23:677–684.

DELZELL E, MONSON RR. 1982a. Mortality among rubber workers: V. Processing workers. J Occup Med 24:539–545.

DELZELL E, MONSON RR. 1982b. Mortality among rubber workers. VI. Men with potential exposure to acrylonitrile. J Occup Med 24:767–769.

DELZELL E, MONSON RR. 1985. Mortality among rubber workers: IX. Curing workers. Am J Ind Med 8:537–544.

DELZELL E, MACALUSO M, HONDA Y, et al. 1993. Mortality patterns among men in the motor vehicle manufacturing industry. Am J Ind Med 24:471–484.

DEMENT JM, HARRIS RL JR, SYMONS MJ, et al. 1983. Exposures and mortality among chrysotile asbestos workers. Part II: Mortality. Am J Ind Med 4:421–433.

DEMERS PA, CHECKOWAY H, VAUGHAN TL, et al. 1994. Cancer incidence among firefighters in Seattle and Tacoma, Washington. Cancer Causes Control 5:129–135.

DEVILLIERS AJ, WINDISH JP. 1964. Lung cancer in a fluorspar mining community. I. Radiation, dust and mortality experience. Br J Ind Med 21:94–109.

DIVINE BJ, BARRON V. 1986. Texas mortality study. II. Patterns of mortality among white males by specific job groups. Am J Ind Med 10:371–381.

DIVINE BJ, BARRON V. 1987. Texas mortality study: III. A cohort study of producing and pipeline workers. Am J Ind Med 11:189–202.

DIVINE BJ. 1990. An update on mortality among workers at a 1,3- butadiene facility—preliminary results. Environ Health Perspect 86:119–128.

DOLL R. 1952. The causes of death among gasworkers with special reference to cancer of the lung. Br J Ind Med 9:180–185.

DOLL R. 1955. Mortality from lung cancer in asbestos workers. Br J Ind Med 12:81–86.

DOLL R. 1958. Cancer of the lung and nose in nickel workers. Br J Ind Med 15:217–223.

DOLL R. 1985. Occupational cancer: a hazard for epidemiologists. Int J Epidemiol 14:22–31.

DOLL R. 1987. Symposium on MMMF, Copenhagen, October 1986: overview and conclusions. Ann Occup Hyg 31:805–819.

DOLL R. 1988. Effects of exposure to vinyl chloride: an assessment of the evidence. Scand J Work Environ Health 14:61–78.

DOLL R, ANDERSEN A, COOPER WC, et al. 1990. Report of the International Committee on Nickel Carcinogenesis in Man. Scand J Work Environ Health 16:1–82.

DOLL R, PETO R. 1981. The causes of cancer: quantitative estimates of avoidable risks of cancer in the United States today. J Natl Cancer Inst 66:1191–1308.

DOLL R, VESSEY MP, BEASLEY RWR, et al. 1972. Mortality of gasworkers—final report of a prospective study. Br J Ind Med 29:394–406.

DUBROW R. 1986. Malignant melanoma in the printing industry. Am J Ind Med 10:119–126.

DUBROW R, PAULSON JO, INDIAN RW. 1988. Farming and malignant lymphoma in Hancock County, Ohio. Br J Ind Med 45:25–28.

DUBROW R, WEGMAN DH. 1983. Setting priorities for occupational cancer research and control: synthesis of the results of occupational disease surveillance studies. J Natl Cancer Inst 71:1123–1142.

DUCATMAN AM, CONWILL DE, CRAWL J. 1986. Germ cell tumors of the testicle among aircraft repairmen. J Urol 136:834–836.

DUH R-W, ASAL NR. 1984. Mortality among laundry and dry cleaning workers in Oklahoma. Am J Public Health 74:1278–1280.

EASTON DF, PETO J, DOLL R. 1988. Cancers of the respiratory tract in mustard gas workers. Br J Ind Med 45:652–699.

EDLING C, JÄRVHOLM B, ANDERSSON L, 1987. et al. Mortality and cancer incidence among workers in an abrasive manufacturing factory. Br J Ind Med 44:57–59.

EGAN-BAUM E, MILLER BA, WAXWEILER RJ. 1981. Lung cancer and other mortality patterns among foundrymen. Scand J Work Environ Health 7(suppl 4):147–155.

EISEN EA, TOLBERT PE, MONSON RR, et al. 1992. Mortality studies of machining fluid exposure in the automobile industry I: A standardized mortality ratio analysis. Am J Ind Med 22:809–824.

ELINDER C-G, KJELLSTROM T, HOGSTEDT C, et al. 1985. Cancer mortality of cadmium workers. Br J Ind Med 42:651–655.

EMMELIN A, NYSTRÖM L, WALL S. 1993. Diesel exhaust exposure and smoking: A case-control study of lung cancer among Swedish dock workers. Epidemiology 4:237–244.

EMMETT EA. 1987. Occupational skin cancers. In: *Occupational Medicine: State of the Art Reviews.* Vol 2—Number 1. *Occupational Cancer and Carcinogenesis*, Brandt-Rauf PW (ed): Philadelphia: Hanley & Belfus, pp 165–177.

ENGLUND A. 1980. Cancer incidence among painters and some allied trades. J Toxicol Environ Health 6:1267–1273.

ENTERLINE PE. 1974. Respiratory cancer among chromate workers. J Occup Med 16:523–526.

ENTERLINE PE, HARTLEY J, HENDERSON V. 1987a. Asbestos and cancer: a cohort followed up to death. Br J Ind Med 44:396–401.

ENTERLINE PE, HENDERSON V. 1975. The health of retired fibrous glass workers. Arch Environ Health 30:113–116.

ENTERLINE PE, HENDERSON VL, MARSH GM. 1987b. Exposure to arsenic and respiratory cancer: a reanalysis. Am J Epidemiol 125:929–938.

ENTERLINE PE, KENDRICK MA. 1967. Asbestos-dust exposures at various levels and mortality. Arch Environ Health 15:181–186.

ENTERLINE PE, MARSH GM. 1980. Mortality of workers in the man-made mineral fibre industry. In: *Biological Effects of Mineral Fibres*, Vol. 1, Wagner JC (ed). Lyon, IARC, pp 965–972.

ENTERLINE PE, MARSH GM. 1982. Mortality among workers in a nickel refinery and alloy manufacturing plant in West Virginia. J Natl Cancer Inst 68:925–933.

ENTERLINE PE, MARSH GM, ESMEN NA, et al. 1987c. Some effects of cigarette smoking, arsenic, and SO_2 on mortality among US copper smelter workers. J Occup Med 29:831–838.

ENTERLINE PE, MARSH GM, HENDERSON V, et al. 1987d. Mortality update of a cohort of U.S. man-made mineral fibre workers. Ann Occup Hyg 31:625–656.

ERIKSSON M, HARDELL L, BERG NO, et al. 1981. Soft tissue sarcomas and exposure to chemical substances: a case-referent study. Br J Ind Med 38:27–33.

FANNING D. 1988. A mortality study of lead workers, 1926–1985. Arch Environ Health 43:247–251.

FAULDS JS, STEWART MJ. 1956. Carcinoma of the lung in haematite miners. J Pathol Bacteriol 72:353–366.

FIGUEROA WG, RASZKOWSKI R, WEISS W. 1973. Lung cancer in chloromethyl methyl ether workers. N Engl J Med 288:1096–1097.

FINCHAM SM, HANSON J, BERKEL J. 1992. Patterns and risks of cancer in farmers in Alberta. Cancer 69:1276–1285.

FINGERHUT MA, HALPERIN WE, MARLOW DA, et al. 1991. Cancer mortality in workers exposed to 2,3,7,8–tetrachlorodibenzo-p-dioxin. N Engl J Med 324:212–218.

FINKELSTEIN MM. 1984. Mortality among employees of an Ontario asbestos-cement factory. Am Rev Respir Dis 219:754–761.

FINKELSTEIN MM. 1989. Nasal cancer among North American woodworkers: another look. J Occup Med 31:899–901.

FINKELSTEIN MM, BOULARD M, WILK N. 1991. Increased risk of lung cancer in the melting department of a second Ontario steel manufacturer. Am J Ind Med 19:183–194.

FINKELSTEIN M, LISS GM, KRAMMER F, et al. 1987. Mortality among workers receiving compensation awards for silicosis in Ontario 1940–85. Br J Ind Med 44:588–594.

FINKELSTEIN M, WILK N. 1990. Investigation of a lung cancer cluster in the melt shop of an Ontario steel producer. Am J Ind Med 17:483–491.

FLETCHER AC, ADES A. 1984. Lung cancer mortality in a cohort of English foundry workers. Scand J Work Environ Health 10:7–16.

FLETCHER DE. 1972. A mortality study of shipyard workers with pleural plaques. Br J Ind Med 29:142–145.

FLODERUS B, PERSSON T, STENLUND C, et al. 1993. Occupational exposure to electromagnetic fields in relation to leukemia and brain tumors: a case-control study in Sweden. Cancer Causes Control 4:465–476.

FORASTIERE F, LAGORIO S, MICHELOZZI P, et al. 1986. Silica, silicosis and lung cancer among ceramic workers: a case-referent study. Am J Ind Med 10:363–370.

FORASTIERE F, VALESINI S, SALIMEI E, et al. 1987. Respiratory cancer among soap production workers. Scand J Work Environ Health 31:258–260.

FOX AJ, COLLIER PF. 1977. Mortality experience of workers exposed to vinyl chloride monomer in the manufacture of polyvinyl chloride in Great Britain. Br J Ind Med 34:1–10.

FOX AJ, GOLDBLATT P, KINLEN LJ. 1981. A study of mortality of Cornish tin miners. Br J Ind Med 38:378–380.

FRANK A. 1987. Occupational cancers of the respiratory system. Semin Occup Med 2:257–266.

FRUMKIN H, BERLIN J. 1988. Asbestos exposure and gastrointestinal malignancy. Review and meta-analysis. Am J Ind Med 14:79–95.

GARABRANT DH, WEGMAN DH. 1984. Cancer mortality among shoe and leather workers in Massachusetts. Am J Ind Med 5:303–314.

GARDINER JS, WALKER JA, MACLEAN AJ. 1982. A retrospective mortality study of substituted anthraquinone dyestuffs workers. Br J Ind Med 39:355–360.

GARDNER MJ, COGGON D, PANNETT B, et al. 1989. Workers exposed to ethylene oxide: a follow-up study. Br J Ind Med 46:860–865.

GARDNER MJ, MAGNANI C, PANNETT B, et al. 1988. Lung cancer among glass fibre production workers. a case-control study. Br J Ind Med 45:631–618, 1988.

GARSHICK E, SCHENKER MB, MUNOZ A, et al. 1988. A retrospective cohort study of lung cancer and diesel exhaust exposure in railroad workers. Am Rev Respir Dis 137:820–825.

GERHARDSSON MR, NORELL SE, KIVIRANTA HJ, et al. 1985. Respiratory cancers in furniture workers. Br J Ind Med 42:403–405.

GERIN M, SIEMIATYCKI J, KEMPER H, et al. 1985. Obtaining occupational exposure histories in epidemiologic case-control studies. J Occup Med 27:420–426.

GIBBS GW. 1985. Mortality of aluminum reduction plant workers, 1950 through 1977. J Occup Med 27:761–770.

GIBSON ES, MCCALLA DR, KAISER-FARRELL C, et al. 1983. Lung cancer in a steel foundry: a search for causation. J Occup Med 25:573–578.

GILMAN PA, AMES RG, MCCAWLEY MA. 1985. Leukemia risk among U.S. white male coal miners. J Occup Med 27:669–671.

GIRARD R, TOLOT F, BOURRET J. 1971. Emopatie maligne e benzolismo. Med Lav 62:71–76.

GOLDBERG MS, SIEMIATYCKI J, GERIN M. 1986. Inter-rater agreement in assessing occupational exposure in a case-control study. Br J Ind Med 43:667–676.

GOLDWATER LJ, ROSSO AJ, KLEINFELD M. 1965. Bladder tumors in a coal tar dye plant. Arch Environ Health 11:814–817.

GOUGH M. 1986. *Dioxin, Agent Orange: the Facts.* London: Plenum Publishing.

GOUGH M, HART R, KARRH BW, et al. 1984. Report on the consensus workshop on formaldehyde. Environ Health Perspect 58:323–381.

GRANDJEAN P, ANDERSEN O, NIELSEN GD. 1988. Carcinogenicity of occupational nickel exposures: an evaluation of the epidemiological evidence. Am J Ind Med 13:193–209.

GREEN LM. 1991. A cohort mortality study of forestry workers exposed to phenoxy and herbicides. Br J Ind Med 48:234–238.

GREENBERG HL, OTT MG, STONE RE. 1990. Men assigned to ethylene oxide production or other ethylene oxide related chemical manufacturing: a mortality study. Br J Ind Med 47:221–230.

GREENBERG M, LLOYD DAVIES TA. 1974. Mesothelioma register 1967–68. Br J Ind Med 31:91–104.

GREENE MH, BRINTON LA, FRAUMENI JF JR, et al. 1978. Familial and sporadic Hodgkin's disease associated with occupational wood exposure. Lancet 2:626–627.

GREENE MH, HOOVER RN, ECK RL, et al. 1979. Cancer mortality among printing plant workers. Environ Research 20:66–73.

GRUFFERMAN S, DUONG T, COLE P. 1976. Occupation and Hodgkin's disease. J Natl Cancer Inst 57:1193–1195.

GUBERAND E, RAYMOND L. 1985. Mortality and cancer incidence in the perfumery and flavour industry of Geneva. Br J Ind Med 42:240–245.

GUBERAND E, USEL M, RAYMOND L, et al. 1993. Mortality and incidence of cancer among a cohort of self employed butchers from Geneva and their wives. Br J Ind Med 50:1008–1016.

GUENEL P, HOJBERG G, LYNGE E. 1989. Cancer incidence among Danish stone workers. Scand J Work Environ Health 15:265–270.

GUENEL P, RASKMARK P, ANDERSEN JB, et al. 1993. Incidence of cancer in persons with occupational exposure to electromagnetic fields in Denmark. Br J Ind Med 50:758–764.

GUSTAVSSON P, GUSTAVSSON A, HOGSTEDT C. 1988. Excess of cancer in Swedish chimney sweeps. Br J Ind Med 45:777–781.

GUSTAVSSON P, REUTERWALL C. 1990. Mortality and incidence of cancer among Swedish gas workers. Br J Ind Med 47:169–174.

HAERTING FH, HESSE W. 1879. Der Lungenkrebs, die Bergkrankheit in den Schneeberger Gruben. Vrtljhrssch Gerichtl Med 30:296–309; 31:102–132, 313–337.

HAGMAR L, LINDÉN K, NILSSON A, et al. 1992. Cancer incidence and mortality among Swedish Baltic Sea fishermen. Scand J Work Environ Health 18:217–224.

HAGMAR L, WELINDER H, LINDEN K, et al. 1991. An epidemiological study of cancer risk among workers exposed to ethylene oxide using hemoglobin adducts to validate environmental exposure assessments. Int Arch Occup Environ Health 63:271–277.

HAMMOND EC, SELIKOFF IJ, LAWTHER PL, et al. 1976. Inhalation of benzpyrene and cancer in man. Ann NY Acad Sci 271:116–124.

HANIS NM, SHALLENBERGER LG, DONALESKI DL, et al. 1985. A

retrospective mortality study of workers in three major U.S. refineries and chemical plants. J Occup Med 27:283–292.

HANSEN ES. 1990. A cohort study on the mortality of firefighters. Br J Ind Med 47:805–809.

HANSEN ES. 1991. Mortality of mastic asphalt workers. Scand J Work Environ Health 17:20–24.

HANSEN ES, OLSEN JH, TILT B. 1982. Cancer and non-cancer mortality of chimney sweeps in Copenhagen. Int J Epidemiol 11:356–361.

HANSEN ES, HASLE H, LANDER F. 1992. A cohort study on cancer incidence among Danish gardeners. Am J Ind Med 21:651–660.

HARDELL L. 1977. Soft tissue sarcomas and exposure to phenoxyacetic acids—a clinical observation. Lakartidningen 74:2753–2754.

HARDELL L, ERIKSSON M. 1988. The association between soft tissue sarcoma and exposure to phenoxyacetic acids. Cancer 62:652–656.

HARDELL L, ERIKSSON M, LENNER P, et al. 1981. Malignant lymphoma and exposure to chemicals especially organic solvents, chlorophenols and phenoxy acids: a case-control study. Br J Cancer 43:169–176.

HARDELL L, SANDSTROM A. 1979. Case-control study: soft-tissue sarcoma and exposure to phenoxyacetic acids or chlorophenols. Br J Cancer 39:711–717.

HARRINGTON JM. 1987. Health experience of workers in the petroleum manufacturing and distribution industry: a review of the literature. Am J Ind Med 21:475–497.

HARRINGTON JM, GOLDBLATT P. 1986. Census based mortality study of pharmaceutical workers. Br J Ind Med 43:206–211.

HASTERLIK RJ, FINKEL AJ, MILLER CE. 1964. The cancer hazards of industrial and accidental exposure to radioactive isotopes. Ann NY Acad Sci 114:832–837.

HATCH TF. 1973. Criteria for hazardous exposure limits. Arch Environ Health 27:231–235.

HAYES RB, LILIENFELD AM, SNELL LM. 1979. Mortality in chromium chemical production workers: a prospective study. Int J Epidemiol 8:365–374.

HELDAAS SS, ANDERSON AA, LANGARD S. 1987. Incidence of cancer among vinyl chloride and polyvinyl chloride workers: further evidence for an association with malignant melanoma. Br J Ind Med 44:278–280.

HENDRICKS NV, BERRY CM, LIONE JG, et al. 1959. Cancer of the scrotum in wax pressmen; I: Epidemiology. AMA Arch Ind Health 19:524–529.

HENNEBERGER PK, FERRIS BG JR, MONSON RR. 1989. Mortality among pulp and paper workers. Br J Ind Med 46:658–664.

HENRY SA. 1934. *Industrial Maladies*. London: Legge, pp 83–84.

HENRY SA. 1946. *Cancer of the Scrotum in Relation to Occupation*. London: Oxford University Press.

HEYER N, WEISS NS, DEMERS P, et al. 1990. Cohort mortality study of Seattle fire fighters: 1945–1983. Am J Ind Med 17:493–504.

HILL AB, FANING EL. 1948. Studies in the incidence of cancer in a factory handling inorganic compounds of arsenic. I. Mortality experience in the factory. Br J Ind Med 5:1–6.

HINDS MW, KOLONEL LN, LEE J. 1985. Application of a job-exposure matrix to a case-control study of lung cancer. J Natl Cancer Inst 75:193–197.

HNIZDO E, SLUIS-CREME GK. 1991. Silica exposure, silicosis, and lung cancer: a mortality study of South Africa gold mines. Br J Ind Med 48:53–60.

HOAR SK, BLAIR A, HOLMES FF, et al. 1986. Agricultural herbicide use and risk of lymphoma and soft-tissue sarcoma. JAMA 256:1141–1147.

HOAR SK, HOOVER R. 1985. Truck driving and bladder cancer mortality in rural New England. J Natl Cancer Inst 74:771–774.

HOAR SK, MORRISON AS, COLE P, et al. 1980. An occupation and exposure linkage system for the study of occupational carcinogenesis. J Occup Med 22:722–726.

HOAR SK, PELL S. 1981. A retrospective cohort study of mortality and cancer incidence among chemists. J Occup Med 23:485–494.

HOAR SK, SANTODONATO J, CAMERON TP, et al. 1985. Monographs on human exposures to chemicals in the workplace. J Occup Med 27:585–586.

HODGSON JT, JONES RR. 1990. Mortality of a cohort of tin miners 1941–86. Br J Ind Med 47:665–676.

HOGSTEDT C, MALMQVIST N, WADMAN B 1979a. Leukemia in workers exposed to ethylene oxide. JAMA 241:1132–1133.

HOGSTEDT C, ROHLEN O, BERNDTSSON BS, et al. 1979b. A cohort study of mortality and cancer incidence in ethylene oxide production workers. Br J Ind Med 36:276–280.

HOGSTEDT C, ARINGER L, GUSTAVSSON A. 1986. Epidemiologic support for ethylene oxide as a cancer causing agent. JAMA 255:1575–1578.

HOGSTEDT C. 1990. Cancer epidemiology in the paper and pulp industry. IARC Scientific Publications. 104:382–389.

HOLMBERG B, WINELL M. 1977. Occupational health standards: an international comparison. Scand J Work Environ Health 3:1–15.

HORNUNG RW, MEINHARDT TJ. 1987. Quantitative risk assessment of lung cancer in U.S. uranium miners. Health Phys 52:417–430.

HOWE GR, BURCH JD. 1990. Firefighters and cancer: an assessment and overview of the epidemiologic evidence. Am J Epidemiol 132:1039–1050.

HOWE GR, FRASER D, LINDSAY J, et al. 1983. Cancer mortality (1965–77) in relation to diesel fume and coal exposure in a cohort of retired railway workers. J Natl Cancer Inst 70:1015–1019.

HOWE GR, LINDSAY JP. 1983. A follow-up of a ten-percent sample of the Canadian labor force; I: Cancer mortality in males, 1965–73. J Natl Cancer Inst 70:37–44, 1983.

HOWE GR, NAIR RC, NEWCOMBE HB, et al. 1986. Lung cancer mortality (1950–1980) in relation to radon daughter exposure in a cohort of workers at the Eldorado Beaverlodge uranium mine. J Natl Cancer Inst 77:357–362.

HOWE GR, NAIR RC, NEWCOMBE HB, et al. 1987. Lung cancer mortality in a cohort of workers at the Eldorado Port Radium uranium mine: possible modification of risk by exposure rate. J Natl Cancer Inst 79:2155–2160.

HUEPER WC. 1966. *Occupational and Environmental Cancers of the Respiratory System*. New York: Springer-Verlag, p 127.

HUGHES JM, WEILL H, HAMMAD YY. 1987. Mortality of workers employed in two asbestos cement manufacturing plants. Br J Ind Med 44:161–174.

HULL CJ, DOYLE E, PETERS JM, et al. 1989. Case-control study of lung cancer in Los Angeles County welders. Am J Ind Med 16:103–112.

IARC MONOGRAPHS ON THE EVALUATION OF CARCINOGENIC RISK OF CHEMICALS TO HUMANS. 1982a. *The Rubber Industry*, Vol. 28. Lyon, IARC, p 160, 227–229.

IARC MONOGRAPHS ON THE EVALUATION OF CARCINOGENIC RISK OF CHEMICALS TO HUMANS. 1982b. *Some Industrial Chemicals and Dyestuffs*, Vol. 29. Lyon, IARC, p 127.

IARC. 1987. Overall Evaluations of Carcinogenicity: An Updating of IARC Monographs Volumes 1 to 42. IARC Monographs Supplement 7. Lyon, France, IARC.

IARC MONOGRAPHS ON THE EVALUATION OF CARCINOGENIC RISKS TO HUMANS. 1988. *Man-made Mineral Fibres and Radon*, Vol. 43. Lyon, IARC, p 152.

IARC MONOGRAPHS ON THE EVALUATION OF CARCINOGENIC RISK OF CHEMICALS TO HUMANS. 1989a. Occupational Exposures in Petroleum Refining; Crude Oil and Major Petroleum Fuels. Vol. 45. Lyon, IARC.

IARC MONOGRAPHS ON THE EVALUATION OF CARCINOGENIC RISK OF CHEMICALS TO HUMANS. 1989b. Diesel and Gasoline Engine Exhausts and some Nitroarenes. Vol. 46. Lyon, IARC.

IARC Monographs on the Evaluation of Carcinogenic Risk of Chemicals to Humans. 1989c. Some Organic Solvents, Resin Monomers and Related Compounds, Pigments and Occupational Exposures in Paint Manufacture and Painting. Vol. 47. Lyon, IARC.

IARC Monographs on the Evaluation of Carcinogenic Risk of Chemicals to Humans. 1990a. Some Flame Retardants and Textile Chemicals, and Exposures in the Textile Manufacturing Industry. Vol. 48. Lyon, IARC.

IARC Monographs on the Evaluation of Carcinogenic Risk of Chemicals to Humans. 1990b. Chromium, Nickel and Welding. Vol. 49. Lyon, IARC.

IARC Monographs on the Evaluation of Carcinogenic Risk of Chemicals to Humans. 1991. Occupational Exposures in Insecticide Application, and Some Pesticides. Vol. 53. Lyon, IARC.

IARC Monographs on the Evaluation of Carcinogenic Risk of Chemicals to Humans. 1992. Occupational Exposures to Mists and Vapours from Strong Inorganic Acids; and Other Industrial Chemicals. Vol. 54. Lyon, IARC.

IARC Monographs on the Evaluation of Carcinogenic Risk of Chemicals to Humans. 1993a. Occupational Exposure of Hairdressers and Barbers and Personal Use of Hair Colourants; Some Hair Dyes, Cosmetic Colourants, Industrial Dyestuffs and Aromatic Amines. Vol 57. Lyon, IARC.

IARC Monographs on the Evaluation of Carcinogenic Risk of Chemicals to Humans. 1993b. Beryllium, Cadmium, Mercury, and Exposures in the Glass Manufacturing Industry. Vol. 58. Lyon, IARC.

IARC. 1986. Priorities in Occupational Cancer Epidemiology. IARC Internal Technical Report No 86/004. Lyon, France, IARC.

Ibrahim MA, Bond GG, Burke TA, et al. 1991. Weight of the evidence on the human carcinogenicity of 2,4-D. Environ Health Perspect 96:213–222.

Ikeda M, Kuratsune M, Nakamura Y, et al. 1986. A cohort study on mortality of Yusho patients. Fukuoka Acta Med 78:297–300.

Infante PF, Wagoner JK, Rinsky RA, et al. 1977. Leukemia in benzene workers. Lancet 2:76–78.

Jappinen P, Hakulinen T, Pukkala E, et al. 1987. Cancer incidence of workers in the Finnish pulp and paper industry. Scand J Work Environ Health 31:197–202.

Jappinen P, Pukkala E. 1991. Cancer incidence among pulp and paper workers exposed to organic chlorinated compounds formed during chlorine pulp bleaching. Scand J Work Environ Health 17:356–359.

Järup L, Pershagen G, Wall S. 1989. Cumulative arsenic exposure and lung cancer in smelter workers: a dose-response study. Am J Ind Med 15:31–41.

Järvholm B, Lavenius B. 1987. Mortality and cancer morbidity in workers exposed to cutting fluids. Arch Environ Health 42:361–366.

Järvholm B, Thiringer G, Axelson O. 1982. Cancer morbidity among polishers. Br J Ind Med 39:196–197.

Jensen OM, Andersen SK. 1982. Lung cancer risk from formaldehyde. Lancet 1:913.

Jensen OM. 1979. Cancer morbidity and causes of death among Danish brewery workers. Int J Cancer 23:454–463.

Johnson ES. 1989. Mortality among nonwhite men in the meat industry. J Occup Med 31:270–272.

Johnson ES. 1990. Association between soft tissue sarcomas, malignant lymphomas, and phenoxy herbicides/chlorophenols: evidence from occupational cohort studies. Fund Appl Toxicol 14:219–234.

Johnson ES, Fischman HR, Matanoski GM, et al. 1986a. Cancer mortality among white males in the meat industry. J Occup Med 28:23–32.

Johnson ES, Fischman HR, Matanoski GM, et al. 1986b. Occurrence of cancer in women in the meat industry. Br J Ind Med 43:597–604.

Jones RD, Smith DM, Thomas PG. 1988. A mortality study of vinyl chloride monomer workers employed in the United Kingdom in 1940–1974. Scand J Work Environ Health 14:153–160.

Kaldor J, Peto J, Easton D, et al. 1986. Models for respiratory cancer in nickel refinery workers. J Natl Cancer Inst 77:841–848.

Kaminski R, Geissert KS, Dacey E. 1980. Mortality analysis of plumbers and pipefitters. J Occup Med 22:183–188.

Kang H, Enziger F, Breslin P. 1987. Soft tissue sarcoma and military service in Vietnam: a case-control study. J Natl Cancer Inst 79:693–699.

Kaplan SD. 1986. Update of a mortality study of workers in petroleum refineries. J Occup Med 28:514–516.

Katz RM, Jowett D. 1981. Female laundry and dry cleaning workers in Wisconsin: a mortality analysis. Am J Public Health 71:305–307.

Kawai M, Amamoto H, Harada K. 1967. Epidemiologic study of occupational lung cancer. Arch Environ Health 14:859–864.

Kazantzis G, Blanks RG, Sullivan KR. 1992. Is cadmium a human carcinogen? In: *Cadmium in the Human Environment; Toxicity and Carcinogenicity*, Nordberg GF, Herber RFM, Alessio L, (eds). IARC Scientific Publication No. 118. Lyon, IARC, pp. 435–446.

Kennaway EL. 1925. The anatomical distribution of the occupational cancers. J Ind Hyg 7:69–93.

Kennaway EL, Kennaway NM. 1947. A further study of the incidence of cancer of the lung and larynx. Br J Cancer 1:260–298.

Kennaway NM, Kennaway EL. 1936. A study of the incidence of cancer of the lung and larynx. J Hyg (Cambridge) 36:236–267.

Kinlen LJ. 1983. Mortality among British veterinary surgeons. Br Med J 287:1017–1019.

Kipling MD. 1968. Oil and the skin. In: *Annual Report of HM Chief Inspector of Factories, 1967.* London: Her Majesty's Stationery Office, pp 105–119.

Kipling MD, Waldron HA. 1976. Polycyclic aromatic hydrocarbons in mineral oil, tar, and pitch, excluding petroleum pitch. Prev Med 5:262–278.

Kipling MD, Waterhouse JAH. 1967. Cadmium and prostatic carcinoma. Lancet 1:730–731.

Kjærheim K, Andersen A. 1993. Cancer incidence among male waiters and cooks: two Norwegian cohorts. Cancer Causes Control 4:419–426.

Kjærheim K, Andersen A. 1994. Cancer incidence among waitresses in Norway. Cancer Causes Control 5:31–37.

Kjuus H, Andersen A, Langård S. 1986a. Incidence of cancer among workers producing calcium carbide. Br J Ind Med 43:237–242.

Kjuus H, Andersen A, Langård S, et al. 1986b. Cancer incidence among workers in the Norwegian ferroalloy industry. Br J Ind Med 43:227–236.

Knox JF, Holmes S, Doll R, et al. 1968. Mortality from lung cancer and other causes among workers in an asbestos textile factory. Br J Ind Med 25:293–303.

Koerselman W, van der Graaf M. 1984. Acrylonitrile: a suspected human carcinogen. Int Arch Occup Environ Health 54:317–324.

Kogan MD, Clapp RW. 1988. Soft tissue sarcoma mortality among Vietnam veterans in Massachusetts, 1972 to 1983. Int J Epidemiol 17:39–43.

Kogevinas M, Saracci R, Winkelmann R, et al. 1993. Cancer incidence and mortality in women occupationally exposed to chlorophenoxy herbicides, chlorophenols, and dioxins. Cancer Causes Control 4:547–553.

Koskela RS, Hernberg S, Karava R, et al. 1976. A mortality study of foundry workers. Scand J Work Environ Health 2 (Suppl 1): 73–89.

KOSKELA RS, KLOCKARS M, JÄRVINEN E, et al. 1987. Cancer mortality of granite workers. Scand J Work Environ Health 13: 26–31.

KURODA S, KAWAHATA K. 1936. Uber die gewerbliche Entstehung des Lungenkrebses bei Generatorgasarbeitern. Z Krebsforsch 45:36–39.

LAMM SH, LEVINE, MS, STARR JA, et al. 1988. Analysis of excess lung cancer risk in short-term employees. Am J Epidemiol 217:2102–2109.

LANGÅRD S. 1990. One hundred years of chromium and cancer: a review of epidemiological evidence and selected case reports. Am J Ind Med 17:189–215.

LANGÅRD S, ANDERSEN A, GLYSETH B. 1980. Incidence of cancer among ferrochromium and ferrosilicon workers. Br J Ind Med 37:l14–120.

LANGÅRD S, NORSETH T. 1975. A cohort study of bronchial carcinomas in workers producing chromate pigments. Br J Ind Med 32:62–65.

LAWLER AB, MANDEL JS, SCHUMAN LM, et al. 1985. A retrospective cohort mortality study of iron ore (hematite) miners in Minnesota. J Occup Med 27:507–517.

LEE AM, FRAUMENI JF JR. 1969. Arsenic and respiratory cancer in man: an occupational study. J Natl Cancer Inst 42:1045–1052.

LEE-FELDSTEIN A. 1986. Cumulative exposure to arsenic and its relationship to respiratory cancer among copper smelter employees. J Occup Med 28:296–302.

LEES PS. 1991. Chromium and disease: review of epidemiologic studies with particular reference to etiologic information provided by measures of exposure. Environ Health Perspect 92:93–104.

LEMEN RA, LEE JS, WAGONER JK, et al. 1976. Cancer mortality among cadmium production workers. Ann NY Acad Sci 271:273–279.

LEON DA. 1994. Mortality in the British printing industry: a historical cohort study of trade union members in Manchester. Occup Environ Med 51:79–86.

LERCHEN ML, WIGGINS CL, SAMET JM. 1987. Lung cancer and occupation in New Mexico. J Natl Cancer Inst 79:639–645.

LEVIN SM, BAKER DB, LANDRIGAN PJ, et al. 1987. Testicular cancer in leather workers exposed to dimethylformamide. Lancet 1:1153.

LEVINE RJ, ANDJELKOVICH DA, SHAW LK. 1984. The mortality of Ontario undertakers and a review of formaldehyde-related mortality studies. J Occup Med 26:740–746.

LEVINE RJ, EISENBUD M. 1988. Have we overlooked important cohorts for follow-up studies? Report of the Chemical Industry Institute of Toxicology conference of World War II-era industrial health specialists. J Occup Med 30:655–660.

LEVY BS, WEGMAN DH, EDS. 1988. *Occupational Health*, 2nd Ed. Boston: Little, Brown and Company.

LEWIS RJ, LERMAN SE, SCHNATTER AR, et al. 1994. Colorectal polyp incidence among polypropylene manufacturing workers. J Occup Med 36:174–181.

LI FP, FRAUMENI JF JR, MANTEL N, et al. 1969. Cancer mortality among chemists. J Natl Cancer Inst 43:1159–1164.

LILIENFELD DE, GALLO MA. 1989. 2,4-D, 2,4,5-T, and 2,3,7,8-TCDD: an overview. Epidemiol Rev 11:28–58.

LILIENFELD AM, LILIENFELD DE. 1979. A century of case-control studies: progress? J Chronic Dis 32:5–13.

LIN RS, DISCHINGER PC, CONDE J, et al. 1985. Occupational exposure to electromagnetic fields and the occurrence of brain tumors. J Occup Med 27:413–419.

LINOS A, KYLE RA, O'FALLON WM, et al. 1980. A case-control study of occupational exposures and leukemia. Int J Epidemiol 9:131–135.

LLOYD JW. 1971. Long-term mortality study of steelworkers. V. Respiratory cancer in coke plant workers. J Occup Med 13:53–68.

LOGUE JN, BARRICK MK, JESSUP GL JR. 1986. Mortality of radiologists and pathologists in the radiation registry of physicians. J Occup Med 28:91–97.

LOOMIS DP, SAVITZ DA. 1990. Mortality from brain cancer and leukemia among electrical workers. Br J Ind Med 47:633–638.

LORENZ E. 1944. Radioactivity and lung cancer: a critical review of lung cancer in the miners of Schneeberg and Joachimsthal. J Natl Cancer Inst 5:1–15.

LOWREY JT, PETERS JM, DEAPEN D, et al. 1991. Renal cell carcinoma among architects. Am J Ind Med 10:123–125.

LUEKE AW. 1907. Epithelioma in carbon workers. Cleveland Med J 6:199–202.

LYNCH J, HANIS NM, BIRD MG, et al. 1979. An association of upper respiratory cancer with exposure to diethyl sulfate. J Occup Med 21:333–341.

LYNCH KM, SMITH WA. 1935. Pulmonary asbestosis III: Carcinoma of lung in asbesto-silicosis. Am J Cancer 24:56–64.

LYNGE E. 1985. A follow-up study of cancer incidence among workers in manufacture of phenoxy herbicides in Denmark. Br J Cancer 52:259–270.

LYNGE E, KURPPA K, KRISTOFERSEN L, et al. 1986. Silica dust and lung cancer: Results from the Nordic occupational and cancer incidence registers. J Natl Cancer Inst 77:883–889.

LYNGE E, STORM HH, JENSEN OM. 1987. The evaluation of trends in soft tissue sarcoma according to diagnostic criteria and consumption of phenoxy herbicides. Cancer 60:1896–1901.

LYNGE E, THYGESEN L. 1990. Primary liver cancer among women in laundry and dry-cleaning work in Denmark. Scand J Work Environ Health 16:108–112.

LYNGE E. 1993. Cancer in phenoxy herbicide manufacturing workers in Denmark, 1947–87—an update. Cancer Causes Control 4:261–272.

MABUCHI K, LILIENFELD AM, SNELL LM. 1980. Cancer and occupational exposure to arsenic: a study of pesticide workers. Prev Med 9:51–77.

MACHLE W, GREGORIUS F. 1948. Cancer of the respiratory system in the United States chromate-producing industry. Public Health Rep 63:1114–1127.

MACMAHON B, MONSON RR, WANG HH, et al. 1988. A second follow-up of mortality in a cohort of pesticide applicators. J Occup Med 30:429–432.

MACMAHON B. 1994. The epidemiological evidence on the carcinogenicity of beryllium in humans. J Occup Med 36:15–24.

MAGNANI C, COGGON D, OSMOND C, et al. 1987. Occupation and five cancers: a case-control study using death certificates. Br J Ind Med 44:769–776.

MAGNANI C, PANNETT B, WINTER PD, et al. 1988. Application of a job-exposure matrix to national mortality statistics for lung cancer. Br J Ind Med 45:70–72.

MAHER KV, DEFONSO LR. 1986. A historical cohort study of mortality among chemical researchers. Arch Environ Health 41:109–116.

MAHER KV, DEFONSO LR. 1987. Respiratory cancer among chloromethyl ether workers. J Natl Cancer Inst 78:839–843.

MALCOLM D, BARNETT HAR. 1982. A mortality study of lead workers 1925–76. Br J Ind Med 39:404–410.

MALKER HSR, GEMNE G. 1987. A register-epidemiology study on cancer among Swedish printing industry workers. Arch Environ Health 42:73–82.

MALONEY CB, GROOMS GA, EDS. 1987. NIOSH Publications Catalogue. 7th Ed. Cincinnati, NIOSH.

MANCUSO TF. 1980. Mortality study of beryllium workers' occupational lung cancer. Environ Res 21:48–55.

MANCUSO TF, COULTER EJ. 1963. Methodology in industrial health studies. The cohort approach, with special reference to an asbestos company. Arch Environ Health 6:210–226.

MANCUSO TF, EL-ATTAR AA. 1967. Cohort study of workers exposed to beta-naphthylamine and benzidine. J Occup Med 9:277–285.

MANCUSO TF, HUEPER WC. 1951. Occupational cancer and other health hazards in a chromate plant: a medical appraisal; I: Lung cancers in chromate workers. Ind Med Surg 20:358–363.

MANNING KP, SKEGG DCG, STELL PM, et al. 1981. Cancer of the larynx and other occupational hazards of mustard gas workers. Clin Otolaryngol 6:165–170.

MANOUVRIEZ A. 1876. Maladies et hygiene des ouvriers, travaillant a la fabrication des agglomeres de houille et de brai. Ann Hyg Public Med Leg 45:459–482.

MARCH HC. 1944. Leukemia in radiologists. Radiology 43:275–278.

MARRETT LD, HARTGE P, MEIGS JW. 1986. Bladder cancer and occupational exposure to leather. Br J Ind Med 43:96–100.

MARSH GM. 1983. Mortality among workers from a plastics producing plant: a matched case-control study nested in a retrospective cohort study. J Occup Med 25:219–230.

MARSH GM. 1987. A strategy for merging and analyzing work history data in industry-wide occupational epidemiology studies. Am Ind Hyg Assoc J 48:414–419.

MARSH GM, ENTERLINE PE, MCGRAW D. 1991. Mortality patterns among petroleum refining and chemical plant workers. Am J Ind Med 19:29–42.

MARSH GM, ENTERLINE PE, STONE RA, et al. 1990. Mortality among a cohort of US man-made mineral fiber workers: 1985 follow-up. J Occup Med 32:594–604.

MARSH GM, STONE RA, ESMEN NA, et al. 1994. Mortality patterns among chemical plant workers exposed to formaldehyde and other substances. J Natl Cancer Inst 86:384–386.

MARTLAND HS. 1931. The occurrence of malignancy in radioactive persons. Am J Cancer 15:2435–2516.

MARTLAND HS, HUMPHRIES RE. 1929. Osteogenic sarcoma in dial painters using luminous paint. Arch Pathol 7:406–417.

MASTROMATTEO E. 1967. Nickel: a review of its occupational health aspects. J Occup Med 9:127–136.

MATANOSKI GM. 1981. Risk of cancer associated with occupational exposure in radiologists and other radiation workers. In: *Cancer: Achievements, Challenges and Prospects for the 1980s*, Burchenal JH, Oettgen HF (eds). New York: Grune and Stratton, pp 241–254.

MATANOSKI GM, STERNBERG A, ELLIOTT EA. 1987. Does radiation exposure produce a protective effect among radiologists? Health Phys 52:637–643.

MATANOSKI GM, STOCKWELL HG, DIAMOND EL, et al. 1986. A cohort mortality study of painters and allied tradesmen. Scand J Work Environ Health 12:16–21.

MATANOSKI GM, SANTOS-BURGOA C, SCHWARTZ L. 1990. Mortality of a cohort of workers in the styrene-butadiene polymer manufacturing industry (1943–1982). Environ Health Perspect 86:107–117.

MAZUMDAR S, REDMOND C, SOLLECITO W, et al. 1975. An epidemiologic study of exposure to coal tar pitch volatiles among coke oven workers. J Air Pollut Control Assoc 25:382–389.

MCCALLUM RI, WOOLLEY V, PETRIE A. 1983. Lung cancer associated with chloromethyl methyl ether manufacture: an investigation at two factories in the United Kingdom. Br J Ind Med 40:384–389.

MCCRAW DS, JOYNER RE, COLE P. 1985. Excess leukemia in a refinery population. J Occup Med 27:220–222.

MCDONALD AD, FRY JS, WOLLEY AJ, et al. 1983. Dust exposure and mortality in an American chrysotile textile plant. Br J Ind Med 40:361–367.

MCDONALD JC. 1984. Mortality of workers exposed to MMMF—current evidence and future research. In: *Biological Effects of Man-made Mineral Fibers*, Vol. 1. Copenhagen, WHO, pp 369–380.

MCDONALD JC, LIDDELL FDK, GIBBS GW, et al. 1980. Dust exposure and mortality in chrysotile mining, 1910–75. Br J Ind Med 37:11–24.

MCDOWELL ME. 1984. A mortality study of cement workers. Br J Ind Med 41:179–182.

MCDUFFIE HH, KLAASSEN DJ, DOSMAN JA. 1990. Is pesticide use related to the risk of primary lung cancer in Saskatchewan? J Occup Med 32:996–1002.

MCMICHAEL AJ, SPIRTAS R, GAMBLE JF, et al. 1976. Mortality among rubber workers: relationship to specific jobs. J Occup Med 18:178–185.

MEIGS JW, MARRETT LD, ULRICH FU, et al. 1986. Bladder tumor incidence among workers exposed to benzidine: a thirty-year follow-up. J Natl Cancer Inst 76:1–8.

MEIJERS JMM, SWAEN GMH, SLANGEN JJM, et al. 1988. Lung cancer among Dutch coal miners: a case-control study. Am J Ind Med 14:597–604.

MEINHARDT TJ, LEMEN RA, CRANDALL MS, et al. 1982. Environmental epidemiologic investigation of the styrene-butadiene rubber industry: mortality patterns with discussion of the hematopoietic and lymphatic malignancies. Scand J Work Environ Health 8:250–259.

MELICK WF, ESCUE HM, NARYKA JJ, et al. 1955. The first reported cases of human bladder tumors due to a new carcinogen—xenylamine. J Urol 74:760–766.

MELICK WF, NARYKA JJ, KELLY RE. 1971. Bladder cancer due to exposure to paraaminobiphenyl: a 17–year followup. J Urol 106:220–226.

MEREWETHER ERA. 1949. Asbestosis and carcinoma of the lung. In: Annual Report of the Chief Inspector of Factories for the Year 1947. London: Her Majesty's Stationery Office, pp 79–81.

MERLER E, BALDASSERONI A, LARIA R, et al. 1986. On the causal association between exposure to leather dust and nasal cancer: further evidence from a case-control study. Br J Ind Med 43:91–95.

MICHEL-BRIAND C, SIMONIN M. 1977. Cancers broncho-pulmonaires survenus chez deux salariés occupés à un poste de travail dans le meme atelier de chromage électrolytique. Arch Mal Prof 38:1001–1013.

MILHAM S JR. 1976. Occupational Mortality in Washington State, 1950–1971. DHEW (NIOSH) Pub Nos. 76-175-A,B,C. Washington, DC: USGPO.

MILHAM S JR. 1979. Mortality in aluminum reduction plant workers. J Occup Med 21:475–480.

MILHAM S JR. 1982. Mortality from leukemia in workers exposed to electrical and magnetic fields. N Engl J Med 307:249.

MILHAM S JR. 1985. Mortality in workers exposed to electromagnetic fields. Environ Health Perspect 62:297–300.

MILHAM S JR, DEMERS RY. 1984. Mortality among pulp and paper workers. J Occup Med 26:844–846.

MILHAM S JR, HESSER JE. 1967. Hodgkin's disease in woodworkers. Lancet 2:136–137.

MILHAM S JR, STRONG T. 1974. Human arsenic exposure in relation to a copper smelter. Environ Res 7:176–182.

MILLER BA, BLAIR A, MCCANN M. 1985. Mortality patterns among professional artists: a preliminary report. J Environ Pathol Toxicol Oncol 6:303–313.

MILLER BA, SILVERMAN DT, HOOVER RN, et al. 1986. Cancer risk among artistic painters. Am J Ind Med 9:281–287.

MILLER BA, BLAIR A, REED EJ. 1994. Extended mortality follow-up among men and women in a U.S. furniture workers union. Am J Ind Med 25:537–549.

MILLS PK, NEWELL GR, JOHNSON DE. 1984. Testicular cancer associated with employment in agriculture and oil and natural gas extraction. Lancet 1:207–209.

MONSON RR. 1974. Analysis of relative survival and proportional mortality. Computers Biomed Res 7:325–332.

MONSON RR. 1990. *Occupational Epidemiology*, 2nd ed. Boca Raton, Florida: CRC Press.

MONSON RR. 1986. Observations on the healthy worker effect. J Occup Med 28:425–433.

MONSON RR, FINE LJ. 1978. Cancer mortality and morbidity among rubber workers. J Natl Cancer Inst 61:1047–1053.

MONSON RR, PETERS JM, JOHNSON MN. 1974. Proportional mortality among vinyl-chloride workers. Lancet 2:397–398.

MORGAN DP, LIN LI, SAIKALY HH. 1980. Morbidity and mortality in workers occupationally exposed to pesticides. Arch Environ Contam Toxicol 9:349–382.

MORGAN RW, CLAXTON KW, DIVINE BJ, et al. 1981a. Mortality among ethylene oxide workers. J Occup Med 23:767–770.

MORGAN RW, KAPLAN SD, GAFFEY WR. 1981b. A general mortality study of production workers in the paint and coating manufacturing industry. J Occup Med 23:13–21.

MORRISON AS, AHLBOM A, VERHOEK WG, et al. 1985. Occupation and bladder cancer in Boston, USA, Manchester, UK, and Nagoya, Japan. J Epidemiol Community Health 39:294–300.

MORRISON HI, SEMENCIW RM, MAO Y, et al. 1988. Cancer mortality among a group of Fluorspar miners exposed to radon progeny. Am J Epidemiol 128:1266.

MOSS E, SCOTT TS, ATHERLEY GRC. 1972. Mortality of newspaper workers from lung cancer and bronchitis 1952–66. Br J Ind Med 29:1–14.

MOULIN JJ, PORTEFAIX P, WILD P, et al. 1990. Mortality study among workers producing ferroalloys and stainless steel in France. Br J Ind Med 47:537–543.

MOULIN JJ, WILD P, MANTOUT B, et al. 1993. Mortality from lung cancer and cardiovascular disease among stainless-steel producing workers. Cancer Causes Control 4:75–81.

MUSK AW, MONSON RR, PETERS JM, et al. 1978. Mortality among Boston firefighters, 1915–1975. Br J Ind Med 35:104–108.

NATIONAL CENTER FOR HEALTH STATISTICS. 1988. Proceedings of the Workshop on Needs and Resources for Occupational Mortality Data. Vital and Health Statistics. Series 4, No. 26. DHHS Pub. No. (PHS) 88-1463. Hyattsville, MD, DHHS.

NEGRI E, PIOLATTO G, PIRA E. 1989. Cancer mortality in a northern Italian cohort of rubber workers. Br J Ind Med 46:624–628.

NELSON NA, VAN PEENEN PFD, BLANCHARD AG. 1987. Mortality in a recent oil refinery cohort. J Occup Med 29:610–612.

NEWHOUSE ML. 1969. A study of the mortality of workers in an asbestos factory. Br J Ind Med 26:294–301.

NEWHOUSE ML, BERRY G, WAGNER JC, et al. 1972. A study of the mortality of female asbestos workers. Br J Ind Med 29:134–141.

NEWHOUSE ML, THOMPSON H. 1965. Mesothelioma of pleura and peritoneum following exposure to asbestos in the London area. Br J Ind Med 22:261–269.

NG TP, CHAN SL, LEE J. 1990. Mortality of a cohort of men in a silicosis register: further evidence of an association with lung cancer. Am J Ind Med 17:163–171.

NIOSH. 1988. Carcinogenic Effects of Exposure to Diesel Exhaust. Current Intelligence Bulletin No. 50, DHHS (NIOSH) Publication No. 88-116. Atlanta, NIOSH.

NYLANDER LA, DEMENT JM. 1993. Carcinogenic effects of wood dust. review and discussion. Am J Ind Med 24:619–647.

O'BERG MT. 1980. Epidemiologic study of workers exposed to acrylonitrile. J Occup Med 22:245–252.

O'BERG MT, BURKE CA, CHEN JL, et al. 1987. Cancer incidence and mortality in the Du Pont Company: an update. J Occup Med 29:245–252.

O'BRIEN TR, DECOUFLÉ P. 1988. Cancer mortality among northern Georgia carpet and textile workers. Am J Ind Med 14:15–24.

OBERDÖRSTER G. 1986. Airborne cadmium and carcinogenesis of the respiratory tract. Scand J Work Environ Health 12:523–537.

OLIN GR, AHLBOM A. 1980. The cancer mortality among Swedish chemists graduated during three decades. Environ Res 22:154–161.

OLSEN J, SABROE S. 1984. Occupational causes of laryngeal cancer. J Epidemiol Community Health 38:l17–121.

OLSEN JH, ASNAES S. 1986. Formaldehyde and the risk of squamous cell carcinoma of the sinonasal cavities. Br J Ind Med 43:769–774.

OLSEN JH, JENSEN SP, HINK M, et al. 1984. Occupational formaldehyde exposure and increased nasal cancer risk in man. Int J Cancer 34:639–644.

OLSEN JH, JENSEN OM. 1987. Occupation and risk of cancer in Denmark: an analysis of 93,810 cancer cases, 1970–79. Scand J Work Environ Health 13, Suppl 1:1–91.

OTT MG, CARLO GL, STEINBERG S, et al. 1985. Mortality among employees engaged in chemical manufacturing and related activities. Am J Epidemiol 122:311–322.

OTT MG, LANGNER RR. 1983. A mortality survey of men engaged in the manufacture of organic dyes. J Occup Med 25:763–768.

OTT MG, OLSON RA, COOK RR, et al. 1987. Cohort mortality study of chemical workers with potential exposure to the higher chlorinated dioxins. J Occup Med 29:422–429.

PACI E, BUIATTI E, COSTANTINI AS, et al. 1989. Aplastic anemia, leukemia and other cancer mortality in a cohort of shoe workers exposed to benzene. Scand J Work Environ Health 15:313–318.

PAGANINI-HILL A, GLAZER E, HENDERSON BE. 1980. Cause-specific mortality among newspaper web pressman. J Occup Med 22:542–544.

PARIS JA. 1822. *Pharmacologia*, vol 2. Fifth edition. London: W. Phillips, pp 88–89.

PARK RM, WEGMAN DM, SILVERSTEIN MA, et al. 1988. Causes of death among workers in a bearing manufacturing plant. Am J Ind Med 13:569–580.

PARKES HG, VEYS CA, WATERHOUSE JAH, et al. 1982. Cancer mortality in the British rubber industry. Br J Ind Med 39:209–220.

PARTANEN T, KAUPPINEN T, HERNBERG S, et al. 1990. Formaldehyde exposure and respiratory cancer among woodworkers—an update. Scand J Work Environ Health 16:394–400.

PEARCE N, CHECKOWAY H, DEMENT J. 1988. Exponential models for analysis of time-related factors, illustrated with asbestos textile worker mortality data. J Occup Med 30:517–522.

PEARCE NE, SMITH AH, HOWARD JK, et al. 1986. Non-Hodgkin's lymphoma and exposure to phenoxyherbicides, chlorophenols, fencing work, and meat works employment: a case-control study. Br J Ind Med 43:75–83.

PEDERSEN E, HOGETVEIT AC, ANDERSEN A. 1973. Cancer of respiratory organs among workers at a nickel refinery in Norway. Int J Cancer 12:32–41.

PELLER S. 1939. Lung cancer among mine workers in Joachimsthal. Hum Biol 11:130–143.

PERERA FP. 1987. Molecular cancer epidemiology: a new tool in cancer prevention. J Natl Cancer Inst 78:887–898.

PESATORI AC, SONTAG JM, LUBIN JH, et al. 1994. Cohort mortality and nested case-control study of lung cancer among structural pest control workers in Florida (United States). Cancer Causes Control 5:310–318.

PETERSEN GR, MILHAM S JR. 1974. Hodgkin's disease mortality and occupational exposure to wood. J Natl Cancer Inst 53:957–958.

PETO J, DOLL R, HERMON C, et al. 1985. Relationship of mortality to measures of environmental asbestos pollution in an asbestos textile factory. Ann Occup Hyg 29:305–355.

PETO J, SEIDMAN H, SELIKOFF IJ. 1982. Mesothelioma mortality in asbestos workers: implications for models of carcinogenesis and risk assessment. Br J Cancer 45:124–135.

PINTO SS, HENDERSON V, ENTERLINE PE. 1978. Mortality experience of arsenic-exposed workers. Arch Environ Health 33:325–331.

POLEDNAK AP. 1981. Mortality among welders, including a group exposed to nickel oxides. Arch Environ Health 36:235–242.

POLEDNAK AP. 1986. Thyroid tumors and thyroid function in women exposed to internal and external radiation. J Environ Pathol Toxicol Oncol 7:53–64.

POLEDNAK AP, STEHNEY AF, ROWLAND RE. 1978. Mortality

among women first employed before 1930 in the U.S. radium dial-painting industry. Am J Epidemiol 107:179–195.

POTT P. 1775. Cancer scroti. In *Chirurgical Observations*. London: Hawes, Clarke, and Collins, pp 63–68.

POTTS CL. 1965. Cadmium proteinuria: the health of battery workers exposed to cadmium oxide dust. Ann Occup Hyg 8:55–61.

PRENTICE RL. 1986. A case-cohort design for epidemiologic cohort studies and disease prevention trials. Biometrika 73:1–11.

RADFORD EP, RENARD KGSC. 1984. Lung cancer in Swedish iron miners exposed to low doses of radon daughters. N Engl J Med 310:1485–1494.

RAFNSSON V, JOHANNESDOTTIR SG. 1986. Mortality among masons in Iceland. Br J Ind Med 43:522–525.

REDMOND CK, CIOCCO A, LLOYD JW, et al. 1972. Long-term mortality study of steelworkers VI. Mortality from malignant neoplasms among coke oven workers. J Occup Med 14:621–629.

REDMOND CK, STROBINO BR, CYPESS RH. 1976. Cancer experience among coke by-product workers. Ann NY Acad Sci 271:102–115.

THE REGISTRAR GENERAL'S DECENNIAL SUPPLEMENT, ENGLAND AND WALES, 1951. 1958. Part II, Vol. 2. Occupational Mortality Tables. London: Her Majesty's Stationery Office.

THE REGISTRAR GENERAL'S DECENNIAL SUPPLEMENT, ENGLAND AND WALES, 1970–72. 1978. Occupational Mortality Series DS No. 1, London: HMSO.

REHN L. 1895. Blasengeschwulste bei Fuchsin-Arbeitern. Arch Klin Chir 50:588–600.

REIF JS, PEARCE NE, FRAZER J. 1989. Cancer risks among New Zealand meat workers. Scand J Work Environ Health 15:24–29.

RINSKY RA, SMITH AB, HORNUNG R, et al. 1987. Benzene and leukemia: an epidemiologic risk assessment. N Engl J Med 316:1044–1050.

ROBERTS RS, JULIAN JA, MUIR DCF, et al. 1989. A study of mortality in workers engaged in the mining, smelting, and refining of nickel. Toxicol Ind Health 5:957–992.

ROBINS J. 1985. A new theory of causality in observational survival studies—application to the healthy worker effect. Biometrics 41: 331.

ROBINS J. 1987. A graphical approach to the identification and estimation of causal parameters in mortality studies with sustained exposure periods. J Chron Dis 40, suppl. 2:1395–1615.

ROBINSON CV, WAXWEILER RJ, FOWLER DP. 1986. Mortality among production workers in pulp and paper mills. Scand J Work Environ Health 12:552–560.

ROBINSON C, WAXWEILER RJ, MCCAMMON CS. 1980. Pattern and model makers, proportionate mortality 1972–1978. Am J Ind Med 1:159–165.

ROCKETTE HE. 1977. Cause-specific mortality of coal miners. J Occup Med 19:795–801.

ROCKETTE HE, ARENA VC. 1983. Mortality studies of aluminum reduction plant workers: Potroom and carbon department. J Occup Med 25:549–557.

ROCKETTE HE, REDMOND CK. 1985. Selection, follow-up, and analysis in the coke oven study. Natl Cancer Inst Monogr 67:89–94.

ROM WN, Ed. 1992. *Environmental and Occupational Medicine*. 2nd ed. Boston, Little, Brown and Company.

RÖNNEBERG A, LANGMARK F. 1992. Epidemiologic evidence of cancer in aluminum reduction plant workers. Am J Ind Med 22:573–590.

ROTH F. 1958. Uber den Bronchialkrebs arsengeschadigter Winzer. Virchows Arch 331:119–137.

ROTHSCHILD H, MULVEY JJ. 1982. An increased risk for lung cancer mortality associated with sugarcane farming. J Natl Cancer Inst 68:755–760.

ROUSH GC, KELLY JA, MEIGS JW, et al. 1982. Scrotal carcinoma in Connecticut metal workers: sequel to a study of sinonasal cancer. Am J Epidemiol 116:76–85.

ROUSH GC, MEIGS JW, KELLY J, et al. 1980. Sinonasal cancer and occupation: a case-control study. Am J Epidemiol 111:183–193.

ROUSH GC, WALRATH J, STAYNER LT, et al. 1987. Nasopharyngeal cancer, sinonasal cancer, and occupations related to formaldehyde: a case-control study. J Natl Cancer Inst 79:1221–1224.

RUSHTON L, ALDERSON MR. 1981. An epidemiological survey of eight oil refineries in Britain. Br J Ind Med 38:225–234.

RUTSTEIN DD, MULLAN RJ, FRAZIER TM, et al. 1983. Sentinel health events (occupational): a basis for physician recognition and public health surveillance. Am J Public Health 73:1054–1062.

SAKABE H, MATSUSHITA H, KOSHI S. 1976. Cancer among benzoyl chloride manufacturing workers. Ann NY Acad Sci 271:67–70.

SAMA SR, MARTIN TR, DAVIS LK, et al. 1990. Cancer incidence among Massachusetts firefighters, 1982–1986. Am J Ind Med 18:47–54.

SAMET JM, KUTVIRT DM, WAXWEILER RJ, et al. 1984. Uranium mining and lung cancer in Navajo men. N Engl J Med 310:1481–1484.

SARACCI R. 1986. Ten years of epidemiologic investigations on man-made mineral fibers and health. Scand J Work Environ Health 12. suppl 1, 5–11.

SARACCI R: BERYLLIUM: epidemiological evidence. In: *Interpretation of Negative Epidemiological Evidence for Carginogenicity*, Wald NJ, Doll R (Eds). IARC Scientific Publications No. 65. Lyon, France, IARC, 1987, pp 203–219.

SARACCI R, SIMONATO L, ACHESON ED, et al. 1984. Mortality and incidence of cancer of workers in the man-made vitreous fibres producing industry. an international investigation at 13 European plants. Br J Ind Med 41:425–436.

SARACCI R, KOGEVINAS M, BERTAZZI PA, et al. 1991. Cancer mortality in workers exposed to chlorophenoxy herbicides and chlorophenols. Lancet 338:1027–1032.

SAVITZ DA, CALLE EE. 1987. Leukemia and occupational exposure to electromagnetic fields: review of epidemiologic surveys. J Occup Med 29:47–51.

SAVITZ DA, MOURE R. 1984. Cancer risk among oil refinery workers. A review of epidemiologic studies. J Occup Med 26:662–620.

SCHUMACHER MC. 1985. Farming occupations and mortality from non-Hodgkin's lymphoma in Utah. J Occup Med 27:580–584.

SCHWARTZ E. 1988. A proportionate mortality ratio analysis of pulp and paper mill workers in New Hampshire. Br J Ind Med 45:234–238.

SCOTT A. 1922. On the occupation cancer of the paraffin and oil workers of the Scottish shale oil industry. Br Med J 2:1108–1109.

SCOTT TS. 1952. The incidence of bladder tumours in a dyestuffs factory. Br J Ind Med 9:127–132.

SEIDMAN H, SELIKOFF IJ, GELBS K. 1986. Mortality experience of amosite asbestos factory workers: dose-response relationships 5 to 40 years after onset of short-term work exposure. Am J Ind Med 10:497–514.

SELEVAN SG, LANDRIGAN PJ, STERN FB, et al. 1985. Mortality of lead smelter workers. Am J Epidemiol 122:673–783.

SELIKOFF IJ, CHURG J, HAMMOND EC. 1964. Asbestos exposure and neoplasia. JAMA 118:22–26.

SELIKOFF IJ, CHURG J, HAMMOND EC. 1965. Relation between exposure to asbestos and mesothelioma. N Engl J Med 272:560–565.

SELIKOFF IJ, HAMMOND EC, CHURG J. 1968. Asbestos exposure, smoking, and neoplasia. JAMA 204:106–112.

SELIKOFF IJ, HAMMOND EC, CHURG J. 1972. Carcinogenicity of amosite asbestos. Arch Environ Health 25:183–186.

SELIKOFF IJ, HAMMOND EC, SEIDMAN H. 1979. Mortality experience of insulation workers in the United States and Canada, 1943–1976. Ann NY Acad Sci 330:91–116.

SELTSER R, SARTWELL PE. 1965. The influence of occupational exposure to radiation on the mortality of American radiologists and other medical specialists. Am J Epidemiol 81:1–22.

SEXTON RJ. 1960. The hazards to health in the hydrogenation of coal. IV. The control program and the clinical effects. Arch Environ Health 1:208–231.

SHALLENBERGER LG, ACQUAVELLA JF, DONALESKI D. 1992. An updated mortality study of workers in three major United States refineries and chemical plants. Br J Ind Med 49:345–354.

SHEFFET A, THIND I, MILLER AM, et al. 1982. Cancer mortality in a pigment plant utilizing lead and zinc chromates. Arch Environ Health 37:44–52.

SHERSON D, SVANE O, LYNGE E. 1991. Cancer incidence among foundry workers in Denmark. Arch Environ Health 46:75–81.

SHETTIGARA PT, MORGAN RW. 1975. Asbestos, smoking and laryngeal carcinoma. Arch Environ Health 30:517–519.

SHINDELL S, ULRICH S. 1986. Mortality of workers employed in the manufacture of chlordane: an update. J Occup Med 28:497–501.

SHMUNES F. 1987. Occupational skin cancer. Seminars Occup Med 2:267–274.

SIEMIATYCKI J, DAY NE, FABRY J, et al. 1981. Discovering carcinogens in the occupational environment: a novel epidemiologic approach. J Natl Cancer Inst 66:217–225.

SIEMIATYCKI J, WACHOLDER S, DEWAR R, et al. 1988. Degree of confounding bias related to smoking, ethnic group, and socio-economic status in estimates of the associations between occupation and cancer. J Occup Med 30:617–625.

SIEMIATYCKI J, ED. 1991. Risk Factors for Cancer in the Workplace. Boca Raton, Fla: CRC Press.

SILVERMAN DT, HOOVER RN, ALBERT S, et al. 1983. Occupation and cancer of the lower urinary tract in Detroit. J Natl Cancer Inst 70:237–245.

SILVERSTEIN M, MAIZLISH N, PARK R, et al. 1986. Mortality among ferrous foundry workers. Am J Ind Med 10:27–43.

SILVERSTEIN M, PARK R, MARMOR R, et al. 1988. Mortality among bearing plant workers exposed to metal working fluids and abrasives. J Occup Med 30:706–714.

SIMONATO L, FLETCHER AC, CHERRIE JW, et al. 1987. The International Agency for Research on Cancer historical cohort study of MMMF production workers in seven European countries: extension of the follow-up. Ann Occup Hyg 31:603–623.

SIMONATO L, L'ABBÉ KA, ANDERSEN A, et al. 1991a. A collaborative study of cancer incidence and mortality among vinyl chloride workers. Scand J Work Environ Health 17:159–169.

SIMONATO L, FLETCHER AC, ANDERSEN A, et al. 1991b. A historical prospective cohort study of European stainless steel, mild steel, and shipyard welding. Br J Ind Med 48:145–154.

SIMONATO L, FLETCHER AC, SARACCI R, ET AL, EDS. 1990. Occupational exposure to silica and cancer risk. IARC Scientific Publications No. 97, Lyon, IARC.

SIMONATO L, MOULIN JJ, JAVELAUD B, et al. 1994. A retrospective mortality study of workers exposed to arsenic in a gold mine and refinery in France. Am J Ind Med 25:625–633.

SJÖGREN B, GUSTAVSSON A, HEDSTROM L. 1987. Mortality in two cohorts of welders exposed to high- and low-levels of hexavalent chromium. Scand J Work Environ Health 13:247–251.

SJÖGREN B, HANSEN KS, KJUUS H, et al. 1994. Exposure to stainless steel welding fumes and lung cancer: a meta-analysis. Occup Environ Med 51:335–336.

SMITH AH, HANDLEY MA, WOOD R. 1990. Epidemiological evidence indicates asbestos causes laryngeal cancer. J Occup Med 32:499–507.

SMITH AH, SHEARN VI, WOOD R. 1989. Asbestos and kidney cancer: the evidence supports a causal association. Am J Ind Med 16:159–166.

SMITH EM, MILLER ER, WOOLSON RF, et al. 1985. Bladder cancer risk among laundry workers, dry cleaners, and others in chemically-related occupations. J Occup Med 27:295–297.

SMITH TJ. 1987. Exposure assessment for occupational epidemiology. Am J Ind Med 12:249–268.

SMULEVICH VB, FEDOTOVA IV, FILATOVA VS. 1988. Increasing evidence of the rise of cancer in workers exposed to vinyl chloride. Br J Ind Med 45:93–97.

SOBEL W, BOND GG, BALDWIN CL, et al. 1988. An update of respiratory cancer and occupational exposure to arsenicals. Am J Ind Med 13:263–270.

SOLET D, ZOLOTH SR, SULLIVAN C, et al. 1989. Patterns of mortality in pulp and paper workers. J Occup Med 31:627–630.

SOLLI HM, ANDERSEN A, STRANDEN E, et al. 1985. Cancer incidence among workers exposed to radon and thoron daughters at a niobium mine. Scand J Work Environ Health 11:7–13.

SORAHAN T, BURGES DCL, WATERHOUSE JAH. 1987. A mortality study of nickel/chromium platers. Br J Ind Med 44:250–258.

SORAHAN T, COOKE MA. 1989. Cancer mortality in a cohort of United Kingdom steel foundry workers. 1946–85. Br J Ind Med 46:74–81.

SORAHAN T, PARKES HG, VEYS CA, et al. 1986. Cancer mortality in the British rubber industry. 1946–80. Br J Ind Med 43:363–373.

SORAHAN T, PARKES HG, VEYS CA, et al. 1989. Mortality in the British rubber industry 1946–85. Br J Ind Med 46:1–11.

SORAHAN T, WATERHOUSE JAH. 1983. Mortality study of nickel-cadmium battery workers by the method of regression models in life tables. Br J Ind Med 40:293–300.

SORAHAN T, WATERHOUSE JAH. 1985. Cancer of prostate among nickel-cadmium battery workers. Lancet 1:459.

SOSKOLNE CL, ZEIGHAMI EA, HANIS NM, et al. 1984. Laryngeal cancer and occupational exposure to sulfuric acid. Am J Epidemiol 120:358–369.

SOUTHAM AH, WILSON SR. 1922. Cancer of the scrotum: the etiology, clinical features, and treatment of the disease. Br Med J 2:971–973.

SPARKS P, WEGMAN DH. 1980. Cause of death among jewelry workers. J Occup Med 22:733–736.

SPIRTAS R, KAMINSKI R. 1978. Angiosarcoma of the liver in vinyl chloride/polyvinyl chloride workers: 1977 update of the NIOSH register. J Occup Med 20:427–429.

SPITZER WO, HILL GB, CHAMBERS LW, et al. 1975. The occupation of fishing as a risk factor in cancer of the lip. N Engl J Med 293:419–424.

STANTON MF, WRENCH C. 1972. Mechanisms of mesothelioma induction with asbestos and fibrous glass. J Natl Cancer Inst 48:797–821.

STARK AD, CHANG H-G, FITZGERALD EF, et al. 1987. A retrospective cohort study of mortality among New York State Farm Bureau members. Arch Environ Health 42:204–212.

STAYNER L, SMITH R, THUN M, et al. 1992. A dose-response analysis and quantitative assessment of lung cancer risk and occupational cadmium exposure. Ann Epidemiol 2:177–194.

STEBBINGS JH, LUCAS HF, STEHNEY AF. 1984. Mortality from cancers of major sites in female radium dial workers. Am J Ind Med 5:435–459.

STEENLAND K, BEAUMONT J, ELLIOT L. 1991b. Lung cancer in mild steel welders. Am J Epidemiol 133:220–229.

STEENLAND K, SCHNORR T, BEAUMONT J, et al. 1988. Incidence of laryngeal cancer and exposure to acid mists. Br J Ind Med 45:766–776.

STEENLAND K, STAYNER L, GRIEFE A. 1987. Assessing the feasibility of retrospective cohort studies. Am J Ind Med 12:419–430.

STEENLAND K, STAYNER L, GREIFE A, et al. 1991a. Mortality

among workers exposed to ethylene oxide. N Engl J Med 324:1402–1407.

STELL PM, MCGILL T. 1973. Asbestos and laryngeal carcinoma. Lancet 2:416–417.

STERLING TD, ARUNDEL AV. 1986. Health effects of phenoxy herbicides: a review. Scand J Work Environ Health 12:161–173.

STERLING TD, WEINKAM JJ. 1988. Reanalysis of lung cancer mortality in a National Cancer Institute study on mortality among industrial workers exposed to formaldehyde. J Occup Med 30:895–901.

STERN RM. 1983. Assessment of risk of lung cancer for welders. Arch Environ Health 38:148–155.

STEWART W, HUNTING K. 1988. Mortality odds ratio, proportionate mortality ratio, and healthy worker effect. Am J Ind Med 14:345–353.

SULLIVAN K, WATERMAN L. 1988. Cadmium and cancer: the current position. Report of an international meeting in London, September, 1988. Ann Occup Hyg 32:557–560.

SVENNSON BG, ENGLANDER V, AKKESSON B, et al. 1989. Deaths and tumors among workers grinding stainless steel. Am J Ind Med 15:51—59.

SWAEN GMH, AERDTS CWHM, STURMANS F, et al. 1985. Gastric cancer in coal miners: a case-control study in a coal mining area. Br J Ind Med 42:627–630.

SWAEN GMH, SLANGEN JJM, VOLOVICS A, et al. 1991. Mortality of coke plant workers in The Netherlands. Br J Ind Med 48:130–135.

SWANSON GM, BELLE SH, BURROWS RW. 1985. Colon cancer incidence among model makers and pattern makers in the automobile industry: a continuing dilemma. J Occup Med 27:567–569.

TALCOTT JA, THURBER WA, KANTOR AF, et al. 1989. Asbestos-associated diseases in a cohort of cigarette-filter workers. N Engl J Med 321:1220–1223.

TETA MJ, OTT MG, SCHNATTER AR. 1991. An update of mortality due to brain neoplasms and other causes among employees of a petrochemical facility. J Occup Med 33:45–51.

THÉRIAULT G, GOULET L. 1979. A mortality study of oil refinery workers. J Occup Med 21:367–370.

THÉRIAULT G, TREMBLAY C, CORDIER S, et al. 1984. Bladder cancer in the aluminium industry. Lancet 1:947–950.

THÉRIAULT G, GOLDBERG M, MILLER AB, et al. 1994. Cancer risks associated with occupational exposure to magnetic fields among electric utility workers in Ontario and Quebec, Canada, and France: 1970–1989. Ann J Epidemiol 139:550–572.

THOMAS TL. 1987. Mortality among flavour and fragrance chemical plant workers in the United States. Br J Ind Med 44:733–737.

THOMAS TL, FONTHAM ETH, NORMAN SA, et al. 1986. Occupational risk factors for brain tumors: a case-referent death certificate analysis. Scand J Work Environ Health 12:121–127.

THOMAS TL, STEWART PA. 1987. Mortality from lung cancer and respiratory disease among pottery workers exposed to silica and talc. Am J Epidemiol 125:35–43.

THOMAS TL, STOLLEY PD, STEMHAGEN A, et al. 1987. Brain tumor mortality risk among men with electrical and electronics jobs: a case-control study. J Natl Cancer Inst 79:233–238.

THOMAS TL, WAXWEILER RJ, MOURE-ERASO R, et al. 1982. Mortality patterns among workers in three Texas oil refineries. J Occup Med 24:135–141.

THUN MJ, SCHNORR TM, SMITH AB, et al. 1985. Mortality among a cohort of US cadmium production workers—an update. J Natl Cancer Inst 74:325–33.

TILLEY BC, JOHNSON CC, SCHULTZ LR, ET AL. 1990. Risk of colorectal cancer among automotive pattern and model makers. J Occup Med 32:541–546.

TOKUDOME S, KURATSUNE M. 1976. A cohort study on mortality from cancer and other causes among workers at a metal refinery. Int J Cancer 17:310–317.

TOLA S, KALLIOMAKI P-L, PUKKALA E. 1988. Incidence of cancer among welders, platers, machinists, and pipe fitters in shipyards and machine shops. Br J Ind Med 45:209–218.

TOLA S, KOSKELA RS, HERNBERG S, et al. 1979. Lung cancer mortality among iron foundry workers. J Occup Med 21:753–760.

TOLBERT PE, EISEN EA, POTHIER LJ, et al. 1992. Mortality studies of machining-fluid exposure in the automobile industry II. Risks associated with specific fluid types. Scand J Work Environ Health 18:351–360.

TOMATIS L, AGTHE C, BARTSCH H, et al. 1978. Evaluation of the carcinogenicity of chemicals: a review of the monograph program of the International Agency for Research on Cancer (1971–1977). Cancer Res 38:877–885.

TORNLING G, GUSTAVSSON P, HOGSTEDT C. 1994. Mortality and cancer incidence in Stockholm fire fighters. Am J Ind Med 25:219–228.

TORNQUIST S, NORELL S, AHLBOM A, et al. 1986. Cancer in the electric power industry. Br J Ind Med 43:212–213.

TSUCHIYA K, OKUBO T, ISHIZU S. 1975. An epidemiological study of occupational bladder tumours in the dye industry of Japan. Br J Ind Med 32:203–209.

TUCHSEN F, NORDHOLM L. 1986. Respiratory cancer in Danish bakers: a 10–year cohort study. Br J Ind Med 43:516–521.

TURNER HM, GRACE HG. 1938. An investigation into cancer mortality among males in certain Sheffield trades. J Hyg (London) 38:90–103.

TYNES T, ANDERSEN A, LANGMARK F. 1992. Incidence of cancer in Norwegian workers potentially exposed to electromagnetic fields. Am J Epidemiol 136:81–88.

TYNES T, JYNGE H, VISTNES AI. 1994. Leukemia and brain tumors in Norwegian railway workers, a nested case-control study. Am J Epidemiol 139:645–653.

VAN DEN EEDEN SK, FRIEDMAN GD. 1993. Exposure to engine exhaust and risk of subsequent cancer. J Occup Med 35:307–311.

VAUGHAN TL, STRADER C, DAVIS S, et al. 1986. Formaldehyde and cancers of the pharynx, sinus and nasal cavities: I. Occupational exposures. Int J Cancer 38:677–683.

VENA JE, SULTZ HA, FIEDLER RC, et al. 1985. Mortality of workers in an automobile engine and parts manufacturing complex. Br J Ind Med 42:85–93.

VIGLIANI EC. 1976. Leukemia associated with benzene exposure. Ann NY Acad Sci 271:143–151.

VIGLIANI EC, SAITA G. 1964. Benzene and leukemia. N Engl J Med 271:872–876.

VINEIS P, SIMONATO L. 1986. Estimates of the proportion of bladder cancers attributable to occupation. Scand J Work Environ Health 12:55–60.

VIREN JR, IMBUS HR. 1989. Case-control study of nasal cancer in workers employed in wood-related industries. J Occup Med 31:35–40.

VOLKMANN R. 1875. Über Theer-, Paraffin und Russkrebs (Schornsteinfegerkrebs). In: *Beitrage zur Chirurgie*. Leipzig: Druck and Verlag von Breitkopf und Hartel, pp 370–381.

WACHOLDER S, BOIVIN J-F. 1987. External comparisons with the case-control design. Am J Epidemiol 126:1198–1209.

WADA S, MIYANISHI M, NISHIMOTO Y, et al. 1968. Mustard gas as a cause of respiratory neoplasia in man. Lancet 1:1161–1163.

WAGNER JC, SLEGGS CA, MARCHAND P. 1960. Diffuse pleural mesothelioma and asbestos exposure in North Western Cape Province. Br J Ind Med 17:260–271.

WAGONER JK, ARCHER VE, LUNDIN FE JR, et al. 1965. Radiation as the cause of lung cancer among uranium miners. N Engl J Med 273:181–188.

WAGONER JK, INFANTE PF, BAYLISS DL. 1980. Beryllium: an etiologic agent in the induction of lung cancer, non-neoplastic respiratory disease and heart disease among industrially exposed workers. Environ Res 21:15–34.

WALDRON HA, WATERHOUSE JAH, TESSEMA N. 1984. Scrotal cancer in the West Midlands, 1936–1976. Br J Ind Med 41:437–444.

WALKER AM, COHEN AJ, LOUGHLIN JE, et al. 1991. Mortality from cancer of the colon or rectum among workers exposed to ethyl acrylate and methyl methacrylate. Scand J Work Environ Health 17:7–19.

WALL S. 1980. Survival and mortality patterns among Swedish smelter workers. Int J Epidemiol 9:73–87.

WALRATH J, DECOUFLE P, THOMAS TL. 1987. Mortality among workers in a shoe manufacturing company. Am J Ind Med 12:615–623.

WALRATH J, FRAUMENI JF JR. 1983. Mortality patterns among embalmers. Int J Cancer 31:407–411.

WALRATH J, LI FP, HOAR SK, et al. 1985. Causes of death among female chemists. Am J Public Health 75:883–885.

WANG J-D, WEGMAN DH, SMITH TJ. 1983. Cancer risks in the optical manufacturing industry. Br J Ind Med 40:177–181.

WANG JX, INSKIP P, BOICE JD JR, et al. 1990. Cancer incidence among medical diagnostic X-ray workers in China, 1950 to 1985. Int J Cancer 45:889–895.

WARD E, OKUN A, RUDER A, et al. 1992. A mortality study of workers at seven beryllium processing plants. Am J Ind Med 22:885–904.

WARREN S, LOMBARD OM. 1966. New data on the effects of ionizing radiation on radiologists. Arch Environ Health 13:415–421.

WATERHOUSE JAH. 1972. Lung cancer and gastro-intestinal cancer in mineral oil workers. Ann Occup Hyg 15:43–44.

WAXWEILER RJ, ALEXANDER V, LEFFINGWELL SS, et al. 1983. Mortality from brain tumor and other causes in a cohort of petrochemical workers. J Natl Cancer Inst 70:75–81.

WAXWEILER RJ, STRINGER W, WAGONER JK, et al. 1976. Neoplastic risk among workers exposed to vinyl chloride. Ann NY Acad Sci 271:40–48.

WEGMAN DH, EISEN E. 1981. Causes of death among employees of a synthetic abrasive product manufacturing plant. J Occup Med 24:748–754.

WEIL CS, SMYTH HF JR, NALE TW. 1952. Quest for a suspected industrial carcinogen. AMA Arch Ind Hyg Occup Med 5:535–547.

WEN CP, TSAI SP, MCCLELLAN WA, et al. 1983. Long-term mortality study of oil refinery workers; I: Mortality of hourly and salaried workers. Am J Epidemiol l18:526–542.

WENTWORTH DN, NEATON JD, RASMUSSEN WL. 1983. An evaluation of the Social Security Administration master beneficiary record file and the National Death Index in the ascertainment of vital status. Am J Public Health 73:1270–1274.

WERNER JB, CARTER JT. 1981. Mortality of United Kingdom acrylonitrile polymerisation workers. Br J Ind Med 38:247–253.

WHITTEMORE AS. 1987. Methods old and new for analyzing occupational cohort data. Am J Ind Med 12:233–248.

WHITTEMORE AS, WU ML, PAFFENBARGER RS JR, et al. 1988. Personal and environmental characteristics related to epithelial ovarian cancer, II: Exposure to talcum powder, tobacco, alcohol, and coffee. Am J Epidemiol 128:1228–1240.

WHORTON MD, SCHULMAN J, LARSON SR, et al. 1983. Feasibility of identifying high-risk occupations through tumor registries. J Occup Med 25:657–660.

WIGLE DT, SEMENCIW RM, WILKINS K, et al. 1990. Mortality study of Canadian male farm operators. non-Hodgkin's lymphoma mortality and agricultural practices in Saskatchewan. J Natl Cancer Inst 82:575–582.

WIGNALL BK, FOX AJ. 1982. Mortality of female gas mask assemblers. Br J Ind Med 39:34–38.

WIKLUND K. 1983. Swedish agricultural workers: a group with a decreased risk of cancer. Cancer 51:566–568.

WIKLUND K, DICH J, HOLM L-E, ET AL. 1989. Risk of cancer in pesticide oeprators in Swedish agriculture. Br J Ind Med 46:809–814.

WIKLUND K, HOLM L-E. 1986. Soft tissue sarcoma risk in Swedish agricultural workers. J Natl Cancer Inst 76:229–234.

WIKLUND K, LINDEFORS B-M, HOLM L-E. 1988. Risk of malignant lymphoma in Swedish agricultural and forestry workers. Br J Ind Med 45:19–24.

WILLIAMS RR, STEGENS NL, GOLDSMITH JR. 1977. Associations of cancer site and type with occupation and industry from the Third National Cancer Survey Interview. J Natl Cancer Inst 59:1147–1185.

WILLS JH. 1982. Nasal carcinoma in woodworkers: a review. J Occup Med 24:526–530.

WING S, SHY CM, WOOD JL, et al. 1991. Mortality among workers at Oak Ridge National Laboratory. JAMA 265:1397–1402.

WOLF P, CHIAZZE L, JR, FERRENCE L. 1987. An historical cohort study of mortality among salaried research and development pensioners of the Allied Corporation. J Occup Med 29:613–615.

WONG O. 1987a. An industry-wide mortality study of chemical workers occupationally exposed to benzene; I: General results. Br J Ind Med 44:365–381.

WONG O. 1987b. II: Dose response analysis. Br J Ind Med 44:382–395.

WONG O, MORGAN RW, BAILEY WJ, et al. 1986. An epidemiological study of petroleum refinery employees. Br J Ind Med 43:6–17.

WONG O, MORGAN RW, KHEIFETS L. 1985. Mortality among members of a heavy construction equipment operators union with potential exposure to diesel exhaust emissions. Br J Ind Med 42:435–448.

WONG O, RAABE GK. 1989. Critical review of cancer epidemiology in petroleum industry employees, with a quantitative meta-analysis by cancer site. Am J Ind Med 15:283–310.

WONG O, TRENT LS. 1993. An epidemiological study of workers potentially exposed to ethylene oxide. Br J Ind Med 50:308–316.

WONGSRICHANALAI C, DELZELL E, COLE P. 1989. Mortality from leukemia and other diseases among workers at a petroleum refinery. J Occup Med 31:106–111.

WOODS JS, POLISSAR L, SEVERSON RK, et al. 1987. Soft tissue sarcoma and non-Hodgkin's lymphoma in relation to phenoxy herbicide and chlorinated phenol exposure in western Washington. J Natl Cancer Inst 78:899–910.

WOODWARD A, RODER D, MCMICHAEL AJ, et al. 1991. Radon daughter exposures at the Radium Hill uranium mine and lung cancer rates among former workers, 1952–87. Cancer Causes Control 2:213–220.

WRIGHT WE, BERNSTEIN L, PETERS JM, et al. 1988. Adenocarcinoma of the stomach and exposure to occupational dust. Am J Epidemiol 128:64–73.

WYNDER EL, ONDERDONK J, MANTEL N. 1963. An epidemiological investigation of cancer of the bladder. Cancer 16:1388–1407.

YASSI A, TATE R, FISH D. 1994. Cancer mortality in workers employed at a transformer manufacturing plant. Am J Ind Med 25:425–437.

YIN S-N, LI G-L, TAIN F-D, et al. 1987. Leukaemia in benzene workers: a retrospective cohort study. Br J Ind Med 44:124–128.

ZACK JA, GAFFEY WR. 1983. A mortality study of workers employed at the Monsanto Company plant in Nitro, West Virginia. Environ Sci Res 26:575–591.

ZAHM SH, BLAIR A, HOLMES FF, et al. 1988. A case-referent study of soft-tissue sarcoma and Hodgkin's disease. Scand J Work Environ Health 14:224–230.

ZAHM SH, WEISENBURGER DD, BABBITT PA, et al. 1990. A case-control study of non-Hodgkin's lymphoma and the herbicide 2,4-dichlorophenoxyacetic acid (2,4-D) in Eastern Nebraska. Epidemiology 1:349–356.

ZAVON MR, HOEGG U, BINGHAM E. 1973. Benzidine exposure as a cause of bladder tumors. Arch Environ Health 27:1–7.

ZENZ C. 1988. *Occupational Medicine: Principles and Practical Applications*. Chicago: Year Book Medical Publishers.

19 Air pollution

CARL M. SHY

The relationship of acute and chronic nonmalignant respiratory disease with ambient air pollution is well established, but the evidence for an effect of community air quality on cancer risk is far less conclusive. Three major obstacles lie in the path of establishing a causal connection between ambient air and cancer risk: the latency between exposure and cancer occurrence, combined with pronounced temporal changes in air quality; the difficulty of estimating cumulative personal exposure to ambient air pollution; and confounding of cancer risk by other personal exposures, especially active smoking and environmental tobacco smoke. These obstacles have not been adequately addressed in the body of epidemiological literature on cancer and air pollution. As a consequence, the magnitude of the ambient air pollution effect on cancer risk is uncertain. At the same time, there is sufficient convergence of evidence from many population-based studies that ambient air pollution has contributed to the human cancer burden. These converging lines of evidence are as follows:

1. Known and probable human carcinogens are present in the ambient air environment. Prominent examples are organic products of incomplete combustion, arsenic, chromium, and asbestos.
2. Urban residents show a consistent lung cancer excess in comparison with rural inhabitants, even when risk estimates are appropriately adjusted for tobacco smoking and occupational exposures.
3. Among urban residents, gradients of community air pollution levels correspond with area differences in lung cancer risk.
4. Communities adjacent to certain large point sources of carcinogenic air pollutants, such as arsenic smelters, show an excess of lung cancer, adjusted for tobacco and occupational exposures, in proportion to the nearness of the household to the point source.

In this chapter, the literature that bears on these four lines of evidence will be discussed. Since several literature reviews on this subject have been recently published (Tomatis, 1990; Pershagen, 1990; Speizer, 1986; and several following articles in Volume 70 of *Environmental Health Perspectives*, 1986), this work will not review all relevant articles but rather will attempt to identify the missing links that limit our ability to quantify the attributable risk of air pollution–induced cancer. The focus of concern in this chapter is ambient air pollution, that is air pollution in the outdoor environment of a community, as opposed to indoor sources of air pollution or occupational exposures.

KNOWN AND PROBABLE HUMAN CARCINOGENS IN AMBIENT AIR

In 1990, the U.S. Environmental Protection Agency (U.S. EPA, 1990a) published a report estimating cancer risks from outdoor exposure to airborne toxic pollutants in the United States. Ninety toxic air pollutants from sixty-five source categories were evaluated. Information on the sources, ambient levels and distribution of these pollutants was obtained from twenty-two previously published national and regional studies. Cancer risks attributable to individual air pollutants were estimated by multiplying the unit risk factor for a pollutant by the average ambient concentration of that pollutant in a given region. The unit risk factor is a numerical estimate of the probability of developing cancer as a result of lifetime exposure to 1 $\mu g/m^3$. For example, if the unit risk factor for a specific pollutant has a value of $3 \times 10^{-5}/\mu g/m^3$, that is, a risk of three cancers per 100,000 persons exposed for a lifetime to 1 $\mu g/m^3$, and if the average pollutant concentration in the region is 5 $\mu g/m^3$, the estimated lifetime cancer risk attributable to exposure is 3×10^{-5} $\mu g/m^3 \times 5$ $\mu g/m^3$ or 15 cancers per 100,000 exposed persons. By applying these results to the estimated pollutant distribution in the total population of the United States (240 million in 1986) and dividing the result by 70 years (ie, the approximate life expectancy) the total annual number of cancer cases attributable to each pollutant was derived. Table 19–1 presents EPA's summary of estimated nationwide annual cancer cases by pollutant. The total is a simple sum of annual cancer cases attributed to individual pollutants. Of the listed pollutants, five—products of incomplete combustion, 1,3-butadiene, chromium, benzene,

TABLE 19–1. *Estimated Contribution of Individual Air Pollutants to U.S. Nationwide Cancer Cases*

Pollutant	*EPA Classification*[a]	*Cases Attributable to Pollutant*	
		Annual Cases	*Percent Distribution*
PIC[b]	—	780	35.2
1,3-Butadiene	B2	266	12.0
Chromium	A	206	9.3
Benzene	A	181	8.2
Formaldehyde	B1	124	5.6
Chloroform	B2	115	5.2
Asbestos	A	88	4.0
Arsenic	A	68	3.1
Ethylene dibromide	B2	68	3.1
Dioxin	B2	64	2.9
Gasoline vapors	B2	46	2.1
Ethylene dichloride	B2	45	2.0
Carbon tetrachloride	B2	41	1.9
Vinyl chloride	A	25	1.1
Acrylonitrile	B1	13	0.6
Cadmium	B1	10	0.5
Vinylidene chloride	C	10	0.5
Hexachlorobutadiene	C	9	0.4
Trichloroethylene	B2	7	0.3
Coke oven emissions	A	7	0.3
Perchloroethylene	B2	6	0.3
Hydrazine	B2	6	0.3
Ethylene oxide	B1–B2	6	0.3
Methylene chloride	B2	5	0.2
Radionuclides (outdoor)	A	3	0.1
Radon (outdoor)	A	2	0.1
Miscellaneous	—	15	0.7
Totals		2216	100.0

Source: U.S. Environmental Protection Agency. Cancer Risk from Outdoor Exposure to Air Toxics. Vol. I. Final Report. EPA-450/1-90-004a.Research Triangle Park, N.C.: Office of Air Quality Planning and Standards. September 1990.

[a]The EPA classification of carcinogens is as follows: A = proven human carcinogen; B1 = probable human carcinogen, limited evidence from human studies and sufficient evidence from animal studies; B2 = probable human carcinogen, inadequate evidence from human studies and sufficient evidence from animal studies; C = possible human carcinogen.

[b]PIC = Products of incomplete combustion, an ill-defined group composed of benzo(a)pyrene for which EPA has developed a carcinogenic classification (B2) and a mixture of other hydrocarbons that have not been classified.

and formaldehyde—account for 70% of the total estimated annual cancer cases attributable to air pollution; the products of incomplete combustion alone account for 35% of the total. By partitioning individual pollutants into the 65 source categories covered in the studies, the relative contribution of major sources of air pollution to total estimated nationwide cancer cases was estimated, as shown in Figure 19–1.

The estimates given in Table 19–1 and Figure 19–1 should be viewed with considerable skepticism, given the many assumptions and uncertainties incorporated into the estimation process. There are some major limitations.

1. The majority of toxic air pollutants listed in Table 19–1 are not established human carcinogens. Pollutants classified as B1 have limited human evidence for carcinogenicity, and those classified as B2 have inadequate human evidence. The evidence for carcinogenicity of the B class of pollutants is primarily based on animal studies.

2. Unit risk factors for individual pollutants were derived mostly by EPA's Carcinogenic Assessment Group and have undergone periodic review by the Carcinogen Risk Assessment Verification Endeavor, a working group of EPA. However, all unit risk factors have not received EPA verification. Unit risk factors for each pollutant were generated by applying linear multistage models to extrapolate from high doses observed in occupational studies or in animal bioassays to considerably lower ambient concentrations. The uncertainty in these extrapolations ranges from one to five orders of magnitude, with estimates based on animal bioassays being at the high end of the uncertainty range.

3. The unit risk factor for products of incomplete combustion (PICs), the largest single estimated contributor to total cancer risk, had to be derived from representative surrogate compounds because PICs refer to a large and variable number of organic particulates that result from incomplete combustion. Products of incomplete combustion consist primarily of polycyclic organic matter, a generic term that covers hundreds of chemical substances containing two or more ring structures containing carbon and hydrogen, sometimes with a ring nitrogen, and sometimes nitrated or chlorinated as in the case of dioxins. Depending on the source of PICs, different unit risk factors were applied. Some estimates were based on the assumption that all of the risk from PICs could be adequately represented by benzo(a)pyrene (BaP), in which case the estimated BaP concentration from that source would be multiplied by the BaP unit risk. For other sources, a category-specific PIC unit risk factor was derived from published studies of that category. The EPA report (U.S. EPA, 1990b) noted that "the unit risk factors for specific PIC mixtures have not received the same level of scrutiny as other pollutants and that all cancer risk estimates for PICs remain highly uncertain." Emissions of PICs vary as a function of combustion efficiency, which changes over time depending on the maintenance and age of the combusting unit, be it a power plant or an automobile. Likewise, the chemical constituents of PICs vary as a function of temperature, input fuels, and other factors. Therefore any ge-

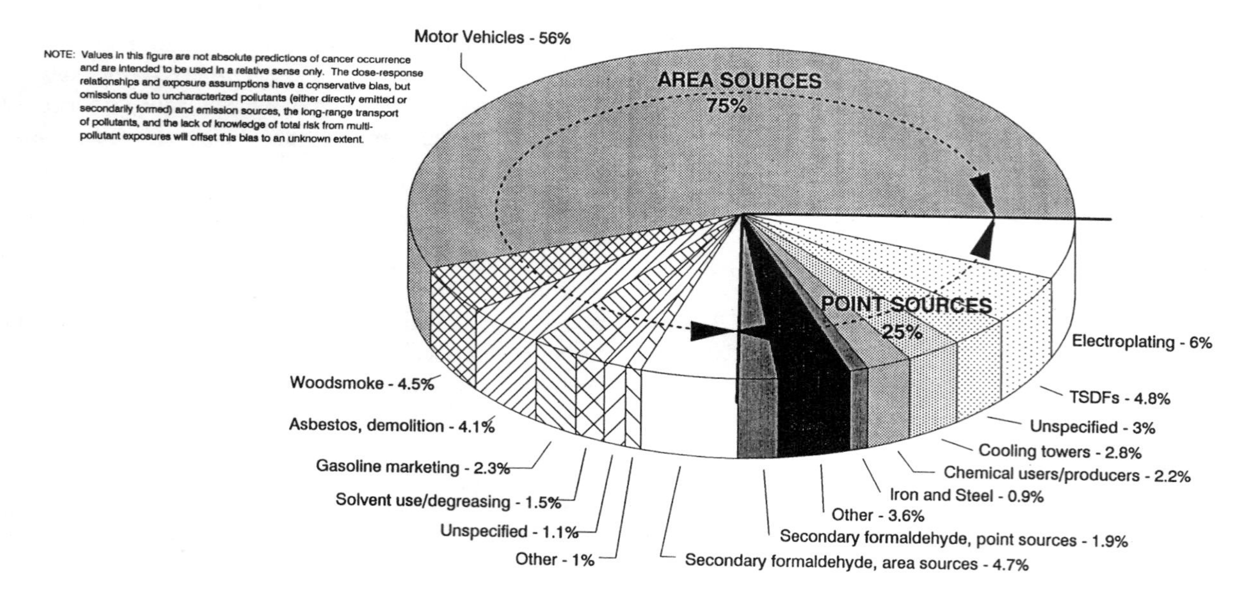

FIG. 19–1. Relative contribution by source categories to total estimated nationwide cancer cases per year. Source: U.S. EPA, 1990a.

neric unit risk factor for PICs must be viewed with considerable caution.

4. The application of a single unit risk factor to express the carcinogenic potency of a pollutant in the entire population over a lifetime assumes constant linear dose-response relationships and the absence of any important modifiers of carcinogenic exposures by factors such as age at first exposure, rate of exposure, or interaction with other exposures such as tobacco smoke. These assumptions are not valid, but the consequence of making alternative assumptions was not evaluated in the EPA report.

The utility of the estimates given in Table 19–1 and Figure 19–1 lies less in the absolute numbers of cancer cases attributable to air pollutants and more in providing a basis for evaluating the relative contribution from different air pollutants and from source categories. The estimates take into account not only the potency of the carcinogen but magnitude and distribution of population exposure to each pollutant. On a national scale, motor vehicles appear to be the dominant source of cancer risk from ambient air pollutants (Fig. 19–1), and products of incomplete combustion appear to be the primary class of pollutants contributing to risk. In specific localities, certain point sources of pollution such as an electroplating plant (emitting hexavalent chromium), a smelter of arsenic-bearing ores, or a producer of 1,3-butadiene may be the dominant source of risk.

The potential carcinogenic effect of secondary pollutants, that is, air pollutants formed in the atmosphere by chemical transformation of primary pollutants emitted from a source, are not understood and are not represented in Table 19–1 or Figure 19–1, with the exception of secondary formaldehyde (the human carcinogenicity of which has not been determined). For example tropospheric ozone is produced through a series of photochemical reactions involving hydrocarbons and nitrogen oxides. Ozone is known to cause free radical formation in exposed biological tissue, but thus far ozone is not known to increase the risk of cancer in humans. On the other hand, the degradation of chlorofluorocarbons in the atmosphere causes depletion of ozone in the stratosphere (McElroy and Salawitch, 1989), the consequence of which will probably be an increase in skin cancers from greater amounts of ultraviolet radiation and possibly in other UV-related adverse health effects.

The total annual number of cancers (n = 2216) estimated to be attributable to the 90 toxic air pollutants evaluated in the EPA report represents 0.2% of the annual incidence of cancers in the United States. (The 0.2% figure is obtained from the ratio of 2216 attributable cancers to 190,000 incident cancers estimated to have occurred in the United States ([Silberg and Lubera, 1986] in the year 1986, the year for which the attributable cancers were derived in the EPA report.) The figure of 2216 cancers would underestimate the true cancer burden to the extent that unidentified pollutants, uncharacterized sources of air pollution, or pollutants undergoing atmospheric transformation to an active carcinogen have not been incorporated in the estimation process. The 2216 figure would overestimate the attributable risk if some of the pollutants are not carcinogenic to humans, if the unit risk estimates are too large, or if the extent of population exposure has been overstated. It is likely that over- and underestimating factors are both present. The figure of 0.2% attributable risk is at the low end of the series of risk estimates made by various authors, as will be discussed later (cf Table 19–4). One frequently cited issue that probably does not affect these figures is that of additive or multiplicative interaction between combinations of these pollutants. Smith (1988) has shown that the magnitude of risk from the joint action of two risk factors, each of which has a relative risk (RR) less than 2.0, is quite similar whether an additive or multiplicative model is assumed. To illustrate, if factor 1 has a relative risk of 1.1 and factor 2 has a relative risk of 1.2, addition of the two factors yields a relative risk of 1.30 and multiplication a risk of 1.32. Given the small number of cancers estimated for each pollutant in Table 19–1, none of the relative risks are as large as 1.1 or 1.2.

Any estimate of total cancer burden generated by summing effects attributable to individual known carcinogens will inevitably miss some pollutant-induced cancers, assuming that we have not identified all carcinogens likely to be in the atmosphere. Epidemiological studies contrasting cancer risks in populations more exposed and populations less exposed to a suspect carcinogenic air environment are more likely to generate the appropriate data for estimating populationwide estimates of cancer burden. In states where regionwide cancer registries exist, a reasonably complete count of cancers can be made. Subgroups living in different air environments can also be identified, and these environments can be sufficiently characterized to describe the contrast in exposure in general terms sufficient to see whether findings can be replicated in similar environments. Thus, without measuring individual carcinogens specifically, it is possible to obtain quite comprehensive assessments of cancer risks from population-based studies, and these assessments will not be biased downwards by failing to include some carcinogens in the exposure measurement scheme, since, the carcinogens, if present will exert their effect whether measured or not. Nationwide estimates of cancer burden attributable to so complex a risk factor as community air pollution require data from direct observations of exposed populations.

URBAN-RURAL LUNG CANCER RATIOS

Pershagen and Simonato (1990) provide a recent review of ecological or aggregate studies of lung cancer mortality in urban versus rural areas; the average urban/rural lung cancer mortality ratio in these studies ranges from 1.3 to 2.0. As pointed out by these authors, ecological studies are of limited use for evaluating an ambient air pollution effect because they generally lack information on important confounders such as active smoking, environmental tobacco smoke, and occupational exposures. These lung cancer risk factors occur in greater proportions among urban residents. Thus, Doll (1978) alludes to evidence that cigarette smoking became common first in large cities of the United Kingdom; he cites data from the Tobacco Research Council (1972) showing that even in 1970 men and women in large metropolitan areas smoked twice as many cigarettes as men in rural parts of the United Kingdom. The average cigarette consumption was 12, 11, 10, and 9 per adult per day in conurbations, county districts, other urban districts, and rural districts, respectively. Even if aggregate data on cigarette consumption were available in comparisons of urban and rural residents, the incidence of lung cancer would still be strongly affected by age at starting to smoke and other aspects of the smoking habit, so that adjustments of observed lung cancer rates for aggregate measures of smoking could still be significantly biased by residual confounding. Therefore, in the absence of information on individual smoking habits, descriptive observations on urban/rural risk ratios are not informative in regard to an ambient air pollution effect.

A number of analytical cohort and case-control studies, described in Table 19–2, have provided estimates of lung cancer risk among urban and rural residents, controlling for smoking habits of study participants. The primary objective of many of these studies was to quantify the risk of tobacco smoking rather than to evaluate effects of air pollution. Exposures to air pollution were crudely estimated from aggregate measures such as urban versus rural residence or residence stratified by size of city. Urban/rural lung cancer mortality risk ratios were generally on the order of 1.2 to 1.5. None of these studies considered personal exposure to environmental tobacco smoke, and few took into account lifetime residence. These two factors exert opposite effects on air pollution–lung cancer risk estimates. Environmental tobacco smoke exerts a lung cancer risk of approximately 1.2 to 1.4 (National Research Council, 1986), equal in magnitude to the above risk estimates for urban residence. Since exposure to environmental tobacco smoke is likely to be more prevalent in urban areas, given the higher prevalence of active smokers, some of the excess risk in urban residents is likely to be attributable to environmental tobacco smoke. In the above studies, adjustments for active cigarette smokers were made for individuals, not households. Therefore, a smoking-adjusted risk estimate of urban-rural differences does not control for the positive confounding effect of environmental tobacco smoke. The consequence is an upward bias if the urban excess is attributed to ambient air pollution. On the other hand, failure to account for lifetime residence will exert a downward bias, because exposure estimates based on current residence will nondifferentially misclassify lifetime exposures, which results in underestimation of risks.

The excess urban relative risk for lung cancer re-

TABLE 19–2. *Summary of Cohort and Case-Control Studies on Lung Cancer in Urban and Rural Areas, Controlling for Smoking*

Study Population	Findings on Lung Cancer	References
I. COHORT STUDIES		
United States, 187,783 white males followed 1952–55; 69,868 followed 1958–62	Urban/rural mortality ratio of 1.33 for cities over 50,000	Hammond and Horn (1958)
California: 69,868 men followed 1958–62	Relative mortality ratio of 130 in densely populated urban counties (Los Angeles, San Francisco, San Diego) compared with other California counties	Buell et al (1967)
Sweden, 25,444 men and 26,467 women followed 1958–62	Relative mortality ratio of 1.6 and 1.2 in male smokers of cities and towns respectively, compared with rural smokers. Similar trend in women	Cederlof et al (1975)
United Kingdom, 34,440 physicians followed 1951–71	No increase in relative death rate in conurbations, large towns, or small towns in comparison with rural areas	Doll and Peto (1981)
Sweden, 7.5 million men and women followed 1961–73	About 40% and 20% of male and female lung cancer explainable by urban factors other than smoking	Ehrenberg et al (1985)
Finland, 4475 men in 3 urban and 3 rural areas, followed 1964–80	Increased risk (RR = 1.2) in "urbanized" but not in urban married smokers in relation to rural married smokers	Tenkanen and Teppo (1987)
II. CASE CONTROL STUDIES		
United Kingdom, 725 male lung cancers, 12,000 hospital controls	Relative risks of 1.1 to 3.4 in different groups of urban vs. rural smokers	Stocks and Campbell (1955)
United States, 2381 white male lung cancer deaths, 31,516 population controls	1.43 urban/rural ratio, with positive trend for duration of urban residence. Joint effects of urban residence and smoking exceed additivity	Haenszel et al (1962)
United States, 749 white female lung cancer deaths, 34,339 population controls	1.27 urban/rural ratio, with positive trend for duration of urban residence. Joint effects of urban residence and smoking exceed additivity	Haenszel and Taeuber (1964)
Northern Ireland, 2873 male and 167 female lung cancer deaths, equal number of deceased controls with non-respiratory illness	1.5 to 5.0 urban/rural ratios in men and women of different smoking groups. Joint effects of urban residence and smoking exceed additivity	Dean (1966)

Source: Table adapted from Pershagen, 1990.

ported in case-control studies (Table 19–2) was of similar magnitude to estimates in cohort studies. In several of these studies, the joint effect of air pollution and smoking appeared to be greater than the addition of individual risks.

The major limitations of urban-rural comparisons are the absence of quantitative measures of exposure to ambient air pollution, and the urban-rural difference in indoor environments caused by environmental tobacco smoke exposures. If these studies were the only sources of evidence, it would be difficult to determine whether the "urban effect" is due to indoor or outdoor exposures, neither of which were directly evaluated.

GRADIENTS OF EXPOSURE AND RISK WITHIN URBAN AREAS

The potential confounding effect of differences in urban-rural indoor exposures should be diminished in studies comparing two or more similarly urbanized areas, if appropriate care is given to the consideration of sociodemographic and occupational variables. Several such studies have been reported. Hitosugi (1968) conducted such a study in the metropolitan area of Osaka, Japan, in the 1960s. Lung cancer cases (n = 216) occurring over 7 years and a random sample of the same area population (n = 4443) were interviewed; smoking habits and place of residence were determined. The population was divided into three areas according to measured concentrations of several air pollutants including suspended particulates, trace elements, and aromatic hydrocarbons. Pollutant ratios of highest to lowest exposure areas ranged from 2 to 3 for the different pollutants. Among nonsmokers (7 males and 33 female cases) there was no correspondence between risk and air pollution levels. Among smokers, risk increased slightly among males only in the highest air pollution area, where the risk was 1.6 times that of the low and middle exposure areas; among female smokers the risk was unrelated to the air pollution gradient but the number of smokers (n = 34) in the total female case group was small. In this study, it is likely that the assignment of individual exposures to the air pollution level of each place of residence will misclassify exposure status, because commuting to different parts of the same metropolitan area is common, and these movements will cause a regression toward the mean exposure of the population. Given random misclassification of air pollution exposure status, an air pollution effect would be biased downwards in any such intraregional study unless cumulative individual exposures over the past 20–40 years could be estimated.

Jedrychowski and coworkers (1990) conducted a similar but larger intra-urban case-control study in Cracow, Poland. Lung cancer deaths (901 males, 198 females) were compared with age and sex frequency matched deaths from causes other than respiratory (875 males, 198 females); all deaths occurred between 1980 and 1985, a period of time during and after an interval of relatively high levels of air pollution in eastern Europe. Questionnaires were sent to next of kin, and data were collected concerning demographics, residency, occupation, and smoking habits, with a response rate of 64%–74%, similar for cases and controls and similar across pollution levels. Total suspended particulate levels, averaged over the years 1973–1980, were less than 120, 120–150, and greater than 150 $\mu g/m^3$ in the three areas, representing a concentration gradient of 1.5 to 2.0 from the lowest to highest exposure area. When lung cancer risk estimates were simultaneously controlled for smoking intensity, age at start and years since stopped smoking, and occupational exposures, the adjusted relative risk was 1.0, 1.0 and 1.46 in the low, middle, and high air pollution areas among males, and 1.0 and 1.17 in the low and medium + high areas among females.

The joint action of smoking, occupational exposure and air pollution was found to fit a multiplicative model, although at these low relative risks, the difference between an additive and multiplicative effect is slight, and it is unlikely that a study of this size could distinguish between the two models of interaction.

Vena (1982) limited his analysis of lung cancer cases (n = 417 white males) and controls (n = 752 white male hospital controls without cancer, or infectious or respiratory diseases) to lifetime residents of Erie County, New York. All study subjects were admitted to a cancer research hospital between 1957 and 1965. Lifetime cigarette use, residential, and occupational histories were obtained by interview during the first hospital admission, prior to diagnosis. A network of 21 air-sampling stations during the early 1960s in Erie County provided 2 years of data for stratifying all residential areas into a grid of total suspended particulate concentrations, and these data were combined with historical information on major point sources of air pollution between 1880 and 1960 to develop concentration isopleths for the entire county. A surrogate measure of lifetime exposure was constructed for each case and control by summing years of exposure to high or medium levels of air pollution. However, high or medium levels are not specifically defined in the report. When exposure was defined as either 50 or more years of residence in a high or medium concentration isopleth, or lifetime residence in a high or medium isopleth for persons contracting lung cancer before age 50, the age-adjusted lung cancer odds ratio for air pollution alone was 0.93, for combined occupation and cigarette smoking 5.81, and for the combination of all three factors 5.91. Thus air pollution as defined did not increase the risk of lung cancer, nor did it appreciably alter the lung cancer risk from the combination of smoking and occupation, although the author concludes that the air pollution effect was greater than additive to the effect of the other two factors. Since the lower concentration isopleths were generally in the more rural parts of Erie County, the air pollution estimates are likely to be confounded by urban-rural differences in exposure to environmental tobacco smoke. Hence any apparent small effect of ambient air pollution in this study must be viewed with reservation. Also, as in the two previously described intraregional studies, normal travel of residents within the same county would produce nondifferential misclassification of air pollution exposure and a consequent bias towards finding no effect.

Archer (1990) took advantage of the low prevalence of smoking in the predominantly nonsmoking Mormon population of Utah to compare lung cancer mortality and air pollution exposures in two counties of that state; in one, a steel mill was constructed in the early 1940s while the other had no major point source of air pollution. The prevalence of active smokers, determined by a telephone survey conducted in 1986, was 6% in the steel mill county and 10% in the comparison county. The average total suspended particulate level in the steel mill county between 1962 and 1979 (80 $\mu g/m^3$) was twice that of the comparison county. This difference was probably greater in the 1940s and 1950s, prior to the development of national air quality standards. Whereas the age-adjusted respiratory cancer mortality rates were nearly equal in the two counties in the 1950–1959 period, the rate in the steel mill county increased steadily between 1960 and 1987 to an average of 15 deaths per 100,000 (approximately double the 1950–1959 rates), while rates in the comparison county averaged 9.3 deaths per 100,000 during the same time period and showed little increase. This mortality rate ratio is 1.6. Mortality rates for all other cancers were nearly the same in the two counties between 1950 and 1979 and showed no time trend. If the excess respiratory cancer mortality rate of 5.7 deaths per 100,000 (1.5 − 9.3) observed in the steel mill county was caused by community air pollution during the years 1960–1987, 38% of respiratory cancer mortality in this county would be attributable to air pollution exposure. However, this estimate is likely to be biased upwards due to the nature of the aggregate data used in this analysis. No information on smoking habits or occupation was obtained from individuals. While Mormons constituted 90% of the population in both counties, differences in smoking prevalence among the remaining 10% are likely because the steel mill county was more urbanized in 1950 (79% urban) than the comparison county (50% urban). Furthermore, a higher proportion of residents in the steel mill county were likely to be employed in jobs having occupational exposures associated with increased lung cancer risk. The absence of any control for tobacco and occupational exposures is likely to bias relative risk estimates upwards, while the dilution of exposure estimates, resulting from the lack of individual exposure measures, are likely to bias relative risk estimates downwards. The consequence of these two opposing vectors cannot be evaluated in the absence of individual risk factor data; such data were incorporated in a subsequent analysis by Blindauer and colleagues (1993) of incident lung cancer rates from the same steel mill county and comparison county as in Archer's publication, and from all other urban and rural counties in the entire state of Utah. The proportion of cigarette smokers in each county was estimated from data obtained by interviews with statewide controls selected for inclusion in an ongoing (from 1991–1994) case-control study of lung cancer and radon. Controls less than 65 years of age were identified by random-digit dialing, while controls 65 years and older were selected randomly from Medicare records. Cases of lung cancer were enumerated from the Utah Cancer Registry for the years 1970 through 1988, and age- and sex-specific lung cancer incidence rates were calculated for each county and were directly adjusted to the 1970 population distribution of the United States. The number of smokers among cases was estimated from the reported proportion among lung cancer cases in the lung cancer and radon study, and the number of smokers in the population of each county was estimated from the age- and sex-specific proportion of smokers in the controls from that same study. Among males who ever smoked cigarettes, the resultant lung cancer incidence rates per 100,000 were 196 in the steel mill county (which is urban in population density), 197 in the comparison county (which is rural), 230 in all urban counties, and 194 in all rural counties. Among females who ever smoked, corresponding incidence rates were 179 in the steel mill county, 78 in the comparison county, 138 in all urban counties, and 140 in all rural counties. Among nonsmokers, lung cancer incidence rates were 20 to 50 times lower than those of smokers, and rates in the steel mill county were somewhat lower than those of all urban and of all rural counties among both men and women. These results fail to find an independent effect of residence in the steel mill county or in urban areas on lung cancer incidence. There is a suggestion of a combined smoking and urban residence effect on lung cancer risk among males, and of a combined smoking and steel mill residence effect among females, but these estimates are based on ecological estimates of exposure to tobacco smoke and air pollution and thus suffer from the limitations of data that are not linked at the individual level. The authors conclude that the finding from the Archer (1990) study of a 38% attributable risk for air pollution exposure is largely explained by the differences in smoking rates between the county with the steel mill and the comparison county.

Several studies of nonsmokers have failed to show any difference in lung cancer risk stratified by population density or by urban/rural residence. Doll (1953) estimated lung cancer mortality rates for nonsmokers in Greater London, other urban areas, and rural districts of England for the year 1950. These rates were, respectively, 8.5, 8.7, and 7.0 per 100,000 in the 45–64 year age group, and 28.3, 15.7, and 27.3 per 100,000 in the 65–74 year age group. Lyon and coworkers (1980) studied lung cancer incidence during 1967–1975 in the Mormon population of Utah, among whom use of tobacco is proscribed by church rules. The age-adjusted lung cancer incidence rates among urban and rural Mormons were respectively 27.1 and 27.3 per 100,000 among males, and 4.8 and 4.4 per 100,000 among females. The urban population consisted of four metropolitan counties containing 78% of the Utah population; the other 25 counties constituted the rural area. By contrast, the non-Mormon population showed an urban/rural lung cancer incidence rate ratio of 1.9 for males (urban = $75.7/10^5$; rural $40.3/10^5$) and 1.2 for females (urban = $11.2/10^5$; rural = $9.4/10^5$). In the absence of smoking data, these latter urban/rural ratios are evidently confounded by the usual urban excess of tobacco use.

The cohort of 8111 adults selected for participation in the Harvard Six Cities Study on the health effects of air pollution provides one of the most complete characterizations of air pollution exposures among all studies reported to date. Dockery and colleagues (1993) reported on the 14–16 year mortality follow-up of this cohort through 1989. Ambient concentrations of particulate matter and gases were monitored in each of the six cities at a centrally located site from the late 1970s through the follow-up period. At enrollment, all members of the cohort were queried regarding smoking history, occupational exposure, and medical history. Mortality rate ratios for air pollution were estimated by simultaneously adjusting for other risk factors in Cox proportional hazards regression models; other risk factors included in the model were age, sex, smoking status, number of pack-years of smoking, education, and body-mass index. Increased total mortality was most strongly associated with smoking and also with having less than a high school education and with an increased body-mass index. After simultaneous adjustment for all other variables, city-specific mortality rates were associated with the average levels of air pollutants, strongly so with levels of fine and inhalable particulates (ie, particles less than 2.5 μm and 10μm diameter, respectively) and sulfate particles, less so with total suspended particulates, sulfur dioxide, nitrogen dioxide, and the acidity of the aerosol. Positive associations between mortality and air pollution were observed in all subgroups defined by occupational exposure and sex, and differences between subgroups were not significant. For a difference in the air pollution level equal to that between the most polluted and least polluted city, whether measured in terms of fine particulates (range, 11.0 to 29.6 $\mu m/m^3$), inhalable particulates (range, 18.2 to 46.5 $\mu m/m^3$), or sulfate particles (range, 4.8 to 12.8 $\mu m/m^3$), the adjusted mortality rate ratios were nearly equal at 1.27, 1.26, and 1.26, respectively, with the lower bound of all confidence intervals (CI) at 1.08. When the air pollution effect on cause-specific mortality was estimated, the authors found a positive association only with deaths from lung cancer and cardiopulmonary diseases, not with all other causes. For lung cancer, the adjusted mortality rate ratio, comparing the most polluted with the least polluted city, was 1.37 (95% confidence interval, 0.81–2.31), based on 120 lung cancers. Although not statistically significant, this rate ratio was equal to that for cardiopulmonary disease (1.37, 95% CI, 1.11–1.68), based on 759 deaths from that cause. These results, which are individually adjusted for all known important population risk factors for lung cancer, suggest a 14%–20% increase in lung cancer mortality for every 10 $\mu g/m^3$ increase in long-term exposure to fine particulate or inhalable particulate air pollution, a finding that exceeds most other estimates but which is also derived from a study that has more accurate measurements of long-term air pollution exposure as well as detailed information on confounding factors.

Of the above studies, three (Hitosugi, 1968; Doll, 1953; Lyon et al., 1980) failed to find excess risk of lung cancer among nonsmokers in urban versus rural areas or in nonsmokers living in more polluted communities of a metropolis. Vena (1982) failed to find any increased risk attributable to air pollution alone. In the Cracow study (Jedrychowski et al, 1990) nonsmokers in the high pollution area had 1.14 times the lung cancer risk of nonsmokers in the low and medium areas. Results from Archer (1990) were biased by residual confounding from smoking among the more exposed population. However, the more recent results obtained from the Harvard Six Cities Study, as reported by Dockery and colleagues (1993), suggest a larger lung cancer effect of particulate air pollution than was observed in most other studies. It is possible that nondifferential misclassification of exposure, which is a major source of bias towards the null in most epidemiological studies of the chronic effects of air pollution, was greatly reduced in the study by Dockery and colleagues because ambient air concentrations were monitored throughout the period of mortality follow-up, unlike most analyses of the lung cancer–air pollution relationship. However, the magnitude of the lung cancer effect per unit of particulate air pollution may have been biased upward by the convergence of two factors: first, if particulate air pollution exerts its carcinogenic effect relatively early in the multistage process, resulting in a lag of 20 or more years between effective exposure and manifestation of lung cancer; and second, if differences in the concentrations of particulate air pollution between the most and least polluted cities of the Six Cities Study were greater in the 1950s and 1960s than during the follow-up period when air monitoring data were being generated for this study. Dockery and colleagues (1993) observed declining annual concentrations of total suspended particulates in the more polluted cities over the course of their follow-up period from 1975 through 1986, but annual average concentrations of fine particulates and sulfate particles showed little trend over time, so it is difficult to judge whether intercity differences in carcinogenic air pollution were greater during the two or three decades prior to the period of observation. But even if exposure differences were as much as twofold greater in the past, the observed lung cancer rate ratios would still result in an estimate of 7%–10% excess lung cancer per 10 $\mu g/m^3$ particulate air pollution, which is a sizable effect given that differences of 30 to 50 $\mu g/m^3$ are not uncommon even today between relatively clean and polluted cities in the United States.

CANCER RISK IN COMMUNITIES NEAR LARGE POINT SOURCES OF CARCINOGENIC AIR POLLUTION

Populations living near industries emitting large quantities of certain pollutants into the community air environment have been studied to determine whether excess cancers occur, in comparison with national cancer rates or with less exposed communities. At an aggregate level of analysis, Blot and Fraumeni (1976) reported higher lung cancer mortality, adjusted for age, population density and indicators of socioeconomic level, in U.S. counties with higher proportions of persons employed in petroleum, chemical, paper and pulp industries, and in counties having smelters that release substantial amounts of arsenic (Blot and Fraumeni, 1975). Although part of the excess mortality in males may be attributed to employment in these industries, the estimated number of such workers is generally only a small fraction of the total population (less than 1% for the most counties with these industries), whereas the excess mortality is in the range of 10%–15%. If occupational exposures alone accounted for these excesses, the hypothetical relative risk due to occupation would have to be 10- to 15-fold in a county where only 1% of the population is occupationally exposed. These hypothetical relative risks are considerably larger than those actually observed in occupational cohort studies, in which risks of three- to five-fold are observed.

Case-control studies performed on residents of areas near arsenic-emitting smelters are more persuasive of a community air pollution effect on lung cancer risk. Brown and colleagues (1984) studied a three-county area of eastern Pennsylvania where a primary zinc smelter and a large steel manufacturing plant were located. They obtained lifetime residential, occupational, and smoking histories from the next of kin of 335 white males who died of lung cancer and 332 randomly selected white males who died of causes other than respiratory diseases or suicide. Soil samples were collected from the study area and were analyzed for arsenic, copper, lead, manganese, zinc, and cadmium. Residence near the zinc smelter, but not near the steel plant, and residence in areas with high soil levels of arsenic and cadmium were associated with a 1.6-fold risk for lung cancer, controlling for smoking and occupation; this risk increased slightly to 1.9-fold when residential exposures 25 years prior to the death of cases were considered. Pershagen (1985) reported very similar results from a lung cancer case-control study conducted in a county in northern Sweden where an arsenic-emitting smelter was located. A relative risk of 2.0 for lung cancer, controlling for smoking and occupation, was observed among men who lived within 20 km of the smelter. Smelter workers and miners had relative risks of 3.0 and 4.1, respectively. Frost and colleagues (1987) conducted a lung cancer death certificate case-control study among female residents of Tacoma and Ruston, Washington, for the years 1935 through 1969. A copper smelter had operated in the town of Ruston since 1905, and an arsenic refinery was added in 1922–1923. Thirty percent of the area population lived within 3 miles of the smelter, and elevated air arsenic levels had been measured within 7 miles. Few women were employed at the smelter, and the prevalence of smoking in older cohorts of women was low. Cases and controls were stratified into quintiles of exposure scaled according to year of residence in the study area, distance from the smelter, and a weighting factor that accounted for temporal changes in arsenic emissions. The odds ratios for lung cancer across the five quintiles were 1.0, 0.97, 1.07, 1.17, and 1.58 (p value for trend = 0.07). The index of exposure for the fifth quintile was more than 10 times higher than the fourth quintile, whereas exposure differences between the other quintiles were much smaller. Despite the absence of data on cigarette smoking, the results are consistent with other individual risk studies of arsenic-exposed communities in suggesting a 1.5- to 2.0-fold increased risk of lung cancer among persons living close to arsenic-emitting smelters.

In an earlier case-control study, Lyon and colleagues (1977) failed to demonstrate any association between residence in an arsenic-emitting smelter area and lung cancer. Given the relatively small excess risk noted in the above positive studies, it is conceivable that even well-conducted population studies may fail to find excess risks, especially if the proportion of the population sufficiently exposed to the pollutant of interest is quite small and if their risk is diluted by the admixture of considerable numbers of minimally exposed persons.

Overall, there are sufficient numbers of point source studies to conclude that excess lung cancer risk was very likely caused by large, relatively uncontrolled point sources of community air pollution, particularly arsenic-emitting smelters. Based on strong evidence for human carcinogenicity from occupational studies, large point sources of chromium, nickel, and possibly of cadmium should also be considered as potential contributors to lung cancer risk in adjacent communities. However, the risks from community exposure are likely to be quite small, between 1.5 and 2.0, and will require substantial study populations and careful assessment of other known lung cancer risk factors.

THE MAGNITUDE OF THE AMBIENT AIR POLLUTION–INDUCED CANCER RISK; RESEARCH DESIGN ISSUES

Two parameters must be estimated to calculate the proportion of cancers in a population attributable to ambient air pollution: the average relative risk associated with exposure to air pollution, and the proportion of the population exposed. For lung cancer, relative risk estimates have ranged from 1.0 among nonsmokers (Doll, 1953; Lyon et al, 1980) to 1.4 (studies cited in Table 19–2 and the more recent Six Cities Study) based on smoking- and occupation-adjusted estimates in several well-conducted cohort and case-control studies. By applying this range of relative risks to alternative assumptions regarding the proportion of the population exposed to "sufficient" concentrations of air pollution to induce an excess risk, a theoretical range of population-attributable risks can be calculated. For illustrative purposes, three figures for the proportion exposed were chosen: 25%, 10%, and 1%. An exposure proportion of 25% might apply in a circumscribed region having a major point source of air pollution. The 10% figure might apply to a more regional or national population exposed to a highly prevalent category of pollutants such as fine particulates or products of incomplete combustion from motor vehicles, and the 1% figure would apply if effective exposures were relatively uncommon. The resulting theoretical proportion of cancers attributable to air pollution is shown in Table 19–3. For these calculations, it seems reasonable to consider only lung cancers as attributable to air pollution, because evidence for an air pollution effect on any other cancer site is lacking or otherwise inconclusive (Pershagen and Simonato, 1990).

Several authors have attempted to estimate the risk of lung cancer attributable to air pollution; these estimates were summarized by Speizer (1986) and are reiterated in modified form in Table 19–4. Speizer (1986) notes that each of these estimates is flawed by lack of sufficient data on exposure, latency, and potential confounders. As previously discussed, some epidemiological studies of air pollution and lung cancer risk had a high likelihood of residual confounding by tobacco smoking, especially due to variations in aspects of active smoking other than intensity of smoking, and also due to inadequate attention to exposures from environmental tobacco smoke.

These sources of flawed estimates should be addressed in any future studies of cancer risk and community air pollution. The first of these issues—exposure—is the most difficult to cope with in epidemiological studies of cancer risk. Exposure to air pollution begins at birth and continues for a lifetime. In present day industrialized countries, most people spend 90% of their time indoors, where exposures to particulate and volatile organic air pollution can often exceed ambient concentrations. It is not feasible to obtain direct measures of lifetime exposure, but studies can be designed to identify relative differences in lifetime exposures in subgroups of the population. The important known determinants of personal exposure to various sources of air pollution can be enumerated and queried retrospectively. These determinants include information on all places of residence; presence and number of regular cigarette smokers in the home in childhood and early adult life; years of participation in a hobby that entails use of volatile organics indoors; if ever a cigarette smoker, age at start, intensity and duration of smoking; use of a wood-burning stove or of any unvented space heaters; years of work involving exposure to dusts, fumes, or gases; proportion of time usually spent outdoors during daylight hours and any occupational or recreational activities that would regularly involve strenuous activity outdoors. It is unreasonable to expect a high degree of accuracy in responses to all of these questions, but the

TABLE 19–3. *Theoretical Proportion of Respiratory Cancer in the Total Population Attributable to Ambient Air Pollution*

	Proportion of Respiratory Cancers Attributable to Air Pollution (PAR%)[a]		
	Proportion of Population "Effectively" Exposed (%)		
Relative Risk of Air Pollution	*0.25*	*0.10*	*0.01*
1.0	0	0	0
1.1	2	1	0.1
1.2	5	2	0.2
1.4	9	4	0.4
1.6	13	6	0.6

[a] $PAR\% = \dfrac{RR - 1\ (P_E)}{1 + [(RR - 1)\ (P_E)]}$

where P_E = proportion of population exposed, expressed as a fraction

point of seeking such information is to reduce the gross exposure misclassification produced by using place of residence and adjacent stationary outdoor air monitors as the only marker of air pollution exposure. Recall of lifetime dietary habits regarding a hundred or so food items is far more challenging than attempting to obtain qualitative information on personal sources of air pollution, as described above. Yet dietary studies have provided consistent evidence for a protective effect against cancer from certain categories of food. Some of the personal exposure data would be used to construct an index of cumulative exposure, and other data from this

TABLE 19–4. *Estimates by Various Authors of Risk of Lung Cancer Attributable to Air Pollution*

Reference	*Attributable Risk*
Stocks and Campbell (1955)	Urban air adds approximately 100 deaths/100,000
National Research Council (1972)	5% of all lung cancers
Carnow and Meier (1973)	5% increase in lung cancer per ng/m^3 of benzo(a)pyrene (BaP)
Higgins (1976)	Possibly 1/10 of the effect of cigarette smoking
Pike et al (1975)	0.4 deaths/10^5/ng/m^3 of BaP in nonsmokers 1.4 deaths/10^5/ng/m^3 of BaP in smokers
Report of the Task Group (1978)	5–10 cases/10^5, in combination with cigarette smoking
Doll and Peto (1981)	1–2% of lung cancer; less than 1% of all cancers in the future
Speizer (1983)	Less than 2% but more than 0% of lung cancer
U.S. EPA (1990a)	2216 cancer cases in the 1986 U.S. population, representing 0.2% of all cancer cases

Source: Modified from Speizer 1986.

list would provide the means to control for potentially important confounders of an ambient air pollution effect. The most important confounders are active smoking, environmental tobacco smoke, and occupational respiratory exposures. However the potential for confounding by these factors can be reduced by control for occupation and socioeconomic level, which are common correlates of those confounders.

The more ambient air pollution exerts a carcinogenic effect at an early stage in the multistage process, the greater the importance of latency. In that case, cumulative exposures through childhood and early adult years will be very important to estimate carefully. This is a difficult task for a study population currently between ages 50 and 75 years of age (the age at which excess cancers can be more readily detected), because childhood exposures for this cohort would have occurred in the 1910s to 1940s at a time when inefficient combustion of coal was the dominant source of residential heating and virtually no air pollution controls were in use on automobiles or on major point sources of air pollution. However, there are ample historical records to document the existence and location of major point sources, and a few historical records of air pollution measurements exist to provide "ballpark" estimates of the magnitude of change in air pollution concentrations over time. On the other hand, if air pollution exerts a carcinogenic effect at a late stage of the multistage process, more recent exposures will be the important determinants of risk. Considerably more measurements of air pollution have been made during the past 15–20 years in many geographical areas of the United States and other industrialized countries than previously, so that more quantitative data are available to estimate cumulative ambient exposures of the last decade or two.

There are some special populations that could be studied epidemiologically to estimate the magnitude of cancer risks attributable to community air pollution. The combination of a relatively stable population, a nonsmoking culture, and changes in industrialization introduced in some but not in other segments of this population would greatly reduce the most important confounders of lung cancer risk, while allowing observation of the effect of a contrast in ambient air exposure both over time in the same exposed subgroup (that is, in the population before and after the introduction of a major air pollution source) and over space in the nonexposed versus exposed subgroups. Since many of the less developed areas of the world are undergoing industrialization (sometimes with far less control of pollutant emissions than in industrialized countries) and since cultural or religious proscriptions against smoking exist in some of these areas, new opportunities are being presented for the less confounded studies of air pollution–induced cancers.

In some populations of the world, high levels of personal exposure to indoor or outdoor sources exist, and allow the investigator to detect risks of greater magnitude (thus less likely to be strongly biased by active and passive smoking) than in most population groups. For example Xu and colleagues (1989) conducted a lung cancer case-control study in an industrial city in northeastern China, where bedroom spaces were frequently heated by brick beds heated by the unvented combustion of coal or wood. Lung cancer risk among women, adjusted for age, education, and smoking, increased in proportion to the number of years this method of heating was used in the home, and the risk was 3.4-fold greater in women exposed to this type of heating for 50 or more years compared with unexposed women. This risk was larger than the risk associated with active tobacco smoking (RR = 2.6) in the women. Heating with vented coal stoves was associated with a small increase in risk (RR = 1.5 in the longest exposed group), while central gas heating showed no association with risk.

As previously discussed, the isolated effect of ambient air pollution on lung cancer risk appears to be in the relative risk range of 1.05 to 1.4. It is also likely that between 1% and 10% of the population are exposed to sufficient amounts of air pollution to have a detectable effect on risk. If these assumptions are correct, the population attributable risk (ie, the proportion of lung cancers attributable to exposure in the total population) is somewhere between 0.1% and 4.0% (cf Table 19–3). This estimate accords with Doll (1978) and Speizer (1986), who estimate (cf Table 19–4) attributable risks of 1%–2% for past exposures and less than 1% of all cancers in the future. The U.S. EPA (1990a) estimates cited in Table 19–1 also fall within this range.

These attributable risk estimates are too low if more than 10% of the population is exposed to cancer-inducing levels of air pollution or if the relative risk from exposure is larger than 1.05 to 1.4. What proportion of the population is exposed can be addressed more easily than the question of the magnitude of the relative risk from air pollution. New information is being obtained on population exposures to volatile organics, metals and products of incomplete combustion, sometimes from direct measurements and otherwise from implementation plans for achieving air quality goals. However, to generate a credible estimate of relative risk will require new epidemiological studies that account for, or otherwise control for, important indoor sources of exposure to carcinogens. In a mixed environment of smokers and nonsmokers, environmental tobacco smoke must be assessed. If a study area is known to have elevated radon within homes, this exposure becomes very important. Special environments should be sought, especially stable populations living in a nonsmoking culture but undergoing industrialization. If such studies continue to find relative risks of 1.1 to 1.4, we can have greater confidence that air pollution plays a minor role in the lung cancer burden of the population living in the air environment that has been achieved in the United States and western Europe. At the same time, epidemiological evidence from areas adjacent to major point source emitters are sufficient to argue that high levels of air pollution pose a substantial lung cancer risk, similar to that of environmental tobacco smoke.

REFERENCES

ARCHER VE. 1990. Air pollution and fatal lung disease in three Utah counties. Arch Environ Health 45:325–334.

BLINDAUER KM, ERICKSON L, MCELWEE N, SORENSON G, GREN LH, LYON JL. 1993. Age and smoking-adjusted lung cancer incidence in a Utah County with a steel mill. Arch Environ Health 48:84–190.

BLOT WJ, FRAUMENI JF. 1975. Arsenical air pollution and lung cancer. Lancet 2:142–144.

BLOT WJ, FRAUMENI JF. 1976. Geographic patterns of lung cancer: industrial correlations. Am J Epidemiol 103:539–550.

BROWN LM, POTTERN LM, BLOT WJ. 1984. Lung cancer in relation to environmental pollutants emitted from industrial sources. Environ Res 34:250–261.

BUELL P, DUNN JE, BRESLOW L. 1967. Cancer of the lung and Los Angeles type air pollution. Cancer 20:2139–2147.

CARNOW BW, MEIER P. 1973. Air pollution and pulmonary cancer. Arch Environ Health 27:207–218.

DEAN G. 1966. Lung cancer and bronchitis in Northern Ireland. Br Med J 1:1506–1514.

DOCKERY DW, POPE CA, XIPING X, SPENGLER JD, WARE JH, FAY ME, FERRIS BG JR AND SPEIZER FE. 1993. An association between air pollution and mortality in six U.S. cities. N Engl J Med 329:1753–1759.

DOLL R. 1953. Mortality from lung cancer among non-smokers. Br J Cancer 7:303–312.

DOLL R. 1978. Atmospheric pollution and lung cancer. Environ Health Perspect 22:23–31.

DOLL R, PETO R. 1981. The causes of cancer: quantitative estimates of avoidable risks of cancer in the United States today. J Natl Cancer Inst 66:1191–1308.

EHRENBERG L, VON BAHR B, EKMAN G. 1985. Register analysis of measures of urbanization and cancer incidence in Sweden. Environ Int 11:393–399.

FROST F, HARTER L, MILHAM S, ROYCE R, SMITH AH, HARTLEY J, ENTERLINE P. 1987. Lung cancer among women residing close to an arsenic emitting copper smelter. Arch Environ Health 42:148–152.

HAENSZEL W, LOVELAND DB, SIRKEN MG. 1962. Lung cancer mortality as related to residence and smoking histories: white males. J Natl Cancer Inst 28:947–1001.

HAENSZEL W, TAEUBER KE. 1964. Lung-cancer mortality as related to residence and smoking histories: white females. J Natl Cancer Inst 32:803–838.

HAMMOND EC, HORN D. 1958. Smoking and death rates—report on forty-four months of follow-up of 187,783 men. JAMA 166:1294–1308.

HIGGINS ITT. 1976. Epidemiologic evidence on the carcinogenic risk of air pollution. INSER 52:41–52.

HITOSUGI M. 1968. Epidemiological study of lung cancer with special reference to the effect of air pollution and smoking habit. Bull Inst Public Health 17:237–256.

JEDRYCHOWSKI W, BECHER H, WAHRENDORF J, BASA-CIERPIALEK Z. 1990. A case-control study of lung cancer with special reference to the effect of air pollution in Poland. J Epidemiol Community Health 44:114–120.

LYON JL, FILMORE JL, KLAUBER MR. 1977. Arsenical air pollution and lung cancer. Lancet 2:869.

LYON JL, GARDNER JW, WEST DW. 1980. Cancer risk and life style: cancer among Mormons from 1967–1975. In: *Cancer Incidence in Defined Populations*, Cairns J, Lyon JL, Skolnik M (eds). Banbury Report No. 4 Cold Spring Harbor, NY: CSH Press, pp. 3–30.

MCELROY MB, SALAWITCH RJ. 1989. Changing composition of the global stratosphere. Science 243:763–770.

NATIONAL RESEARCH COUNCIL. 1972. Particulate polycyclic organic matter. National Academy of Sciences, Washington, DC.

NATIONAL RESEARCH COUNCIL COMMITTEE ON PASSIVE SMOKING, BOARD ON ENVIRONMENTAL STUDIES AND TOXICOLOGY. 1986. Environmental tobacco smoke: measuring exposures and assessing health effects. Washington, DC: National Academy Press.

PERSHAGEN G. 1985. Lung cancer mortality among men living near an arsenic-emitting smelter. Am J Epidemiol 122:684–694.

PERSHAGEN G. 1990. Air pollution and cancer. In: *Complex Mixtures and Cancer Risk*, Vainio H, Sorsa M, McMichael AJ (eds). IARC Scientific Publication No. 104, Lyon, International Agency for Research on Cancer, pp 240–251.

PERSHAGEN G, SIMONATO L. 1990. Epidemiological evidence on air pollution and cancer. In: *Air Pollution and Human Cancer*. Tomatis L (ed). Berlin: Springer-Verlag, pp 65–74.

PIKE MC, GORDON RJ, HENDERSON BE, MENCK HR, SOO HOO J. 1975. Air pollution. In: *Persons at High Risk of Cancer*, Fraumeni JF (ed) New York: Academic Press, pp 225–239.

REPORT OF THE TASK GROUP. 1978. Air pollution and cancer: risk assessment methodology and epidemiologic evidence. Environ Health Perspect 22:1–12.

SELBERG E, LUBERA J. 1986. Cancer statistics, 1986. CA 36:9–15.

SMITH AH. 1988. Epidemiologic input to environmental risk assessment. Arch Environ Health 43:124–127.

SPEIZER FE. 1983. Assessment of the epidemiological data relating lung cancer to air pollutants. Environ Health Perspect 47:33–42.

SPEIZER FE. 1986. Overview of the risk of respiratory cancer from airborne contaminants. Environ Health Perspect 70:9–15.

STOCKS P, CAMPBELL JM. 1955. Lung cancer death rates among non-smokers and pipe and cigarette smokers: an evaluation in relation to air pollution by benzpyrene and other substances. Br Med J 2:923–939.

TENKANEN L, TEPPO L. 1987. Migration, marital status and smoking as risk determinants of cancer. Scand J Soc Med 15:67–72.

TOBACCO RESEARCH COUNCIL. 1972. *Statistics of Smoking in the United Kingdom*. 6th ed, Todd GF, ed. Tobacco Research Council, London.

TOMATIS L. 1990. Air pollution and human cancer. Berlin: Springer-Verlag, 86 pp.

U.S. ENVIRONMENTAL PROTECTION AGENCY. September, 1990a. Cancer risk from outdoor exposure to air toxics. Vol. 1. Office of Air Quality Planning and Standards, Research Triangle Park, NC, 27711, EPA-450/1-90-004a.

U.S. ENVIRONMENTAL PROTECTION AGENCY. September, 1990b. Cancer risk from outdoor exposure to air toxics. Vol. II: Appendices. Office of Air Quality Planning and Standards, Research Triangle Park, NC 27711, EPA-450/1-90-004b.

VENA JE. 1982. Air pollution as a risk factor in lung cancer. Am J Epidemiol 116:42–56.

XU ZY, BLOT WJ, X HP, WU A, FEND YP, STONE BJ, SUN J, ERSHOW AG, HENDERSON B, FRAUMENI JF. 1989. Smoking, air pollution, and the high rates of lung cancer in Shenyang, China. J Natl Cancer Inst 81:1800–1806.

20 Water pollution

KENNETH P. CANTOR
CARL M. SHY
CLAIR CHILVERS

Although quality of drinking water in industrialized nations is considered the finest in the world, there is growing concern that various waterborne contaminants may contribute to the overall burden of environmental carcinogenesis. This idea is not new. In a classic report published three decades ago, W.C. Hueper (1960) warned of the potential carcinogenic dangers of the increasing use of drinking water contaminated with various natural and man-made pollutants. This concern has been fueled by more recent reports of the widespread distribution of many proven or suspected carcinogens in drinking water, mostly at trace levels. Further evidence has come from epidemiological studies indicating that contaminated water may be associated with an elevated risk of cancer. To determine whether water contaminants contribute to the human cancer burden, and if so, what the potential for prevention is, we will review the epidemiological evidence regarding a variety of contaminants and will include relevant information on their levels and environmental distribution. We will also discuss future research priorities and mention strategies for prevention.

Other approaches to assessing the impact of drinking water quality in environmental carcinogenesis, such as extrapolation of dose-response data from animal studies, will not be discussed here. These have been covered in a series of publications from the National Research Council (1977a,1986,1987,1989).

CATEGORIES OF POTENTIAL EXPOSURE

Drinking water contaminants that may be carcinogenic can be grouped into five general categories: (1) organic chemicals; (2) inorganic solutes; (3) radionuclides; (4) solid particulates; and (5) microbiological agents. Although these groups are discussed separately below, drinking water is a complex mixture of agents that may interact in various ways. This interaction often has a direct bearing on their carcinogenic potential, on their ability to enter and be removed from drinking water, and on the difficulty and validity of an epidemiological investigation.

Table 20–1 displays the salient features of the epidemiological studies of drinking water quality, most of which were published since the first edition of this volume. In separate sections, the table covers organic chemicals, including (1) industrial, commercial, and agricultural chemicals and (2) chlorination by-products; inorganic solutes (arsenic, metals, and nitrates); radionuclides; and solid particulates (asbestos). Within each of these sections, studies are grouped by type of study design and then listed alphabetically by senior author. Site-specific results are reported as such whenever possible, along with the direction of the association, plus or minus (+ or −). For several multivariate analyses from studies in which a number of sites were examined, only major significant results are listed. All other sites examined are marked as "no association" (NA), a conclusion that generally agrees with that of the original authors. Unless otherwise indicated, all statistical tests are two-tailed, with 0.05 being the level of significance used. Microbiological agents (primarily *Schistosoma haematobium*) are covered in the text.

ORGANIC CHEMICALS

Among potential waterborne carcinogens, synthetic organic chemicals are a major focus of concern (Wilkins et al, 1979; National Research Council, 1980; Ram et al, 1990; Valema, 1987). Synthetic organics in drinking water can be divided into two major groupings: man-made chemicals from industrial, agricultural, commercial, or domestic sources; and chemical by-products that arise during the disinfection process from the interaction of chlorine or other disinfectants with organic chemical precursors in the untreated water. Both have been the subject of epidemiological evaluation. The widespread use of chlorine to disinfect drinking water,

TABLE 20–1. *Summary of Epidemiological Studies of Drinking Water*

Senior Author (year) Country	Study Design Incidence or Mortality Regional Description	Sex Race	Age Years Covered	Exposure Description	Cancer Sites Included	Summary of Findings
				ORGANICS: INDUSTRIAL, COMMERCIAL, AND AGRICULTURAL CHEMICALS		
Aschengrau (1993) United States	Case-control Incidence Massachusetts	M F	? 1983–86	Estimated exposure to PCE	Leukemia Bladder Kidney	Leuk: OR=1.9 (CI=0.7-5.0) Blad: OR=1.9 (CI=0.9-3.7) Kidney: OR=1.2 (CI=0.4-3.0)
Budnick (1984) United States	Ecological/cluster investigation Mortality Clinton County, PA	M F	All 1950–79	Drake Superfund site, with β-naphthylamine, benzidine, benzene, and other compounds	All Site-specific	+ Bladder (M), "Other" lymphomas (M,F), several other sites
DeKraay (1978) United States	Ecological Lymphoma incidence Iowa counties	M F	All 1969–71	Chlorinated hydrocarbon pesticides in drinking water	Non-Hodgkin's lymphoma Hodgkin's disease	+ Non-Hodgkin's lymphoma incidence in communities served by rivers with detectable pesticide levels
Delong (1979) China (PRC)	Ecological (geog. and time trend) Mortality 4 counties of Jiangsu Province	M F	All 1973,1978	Stagnant ditch water polluted with agricultural chemicals	Liver cell cancer	+ Liver cancer mortality with use of polluted water. Rates decreased after a change in water supply
Fagliano (1990) United States	Ecological Incidence New Jersey towns	M F W N	All 1979–84	14 non-THM volatile organic carbon (VOC) compounds (tetrachloroethylene, trichloroethylene, etc.) in public drinking water supplies	Leukemia	+ (F) NA (M)
Griffith (1989) United States	Ecological Mortality Counties with hazardous waste sites	M F W	All 1970–79	339 U.S. counties with hazardous waste sites (compared with other U.S. counties)	All Site-specific	+ Lung, bladder, stomach, large intestine, rectum (M,F); + Esophagus (M); breast (F)
Hoff (1992) Norway	Cross-sectional screening Prevalence Telemark, Norway	M F	50–59 Early 1980s	Residents of Telemark exposed to drinking water from four sources.	Colorectal adenomas	+ for water with high organic content compared with low organic content
Janerich (1981) United States	Ecological Incidence Love Canal area of Niagara Falls, New York State	M F	All 1955–77	80+ chemicals deposited in a toxic waste site between the 1920s and 1953	All Site-specific	+ for respiratory cancer (M+F), but not consistent by age, and similar to city of Niagara Falls rates
Lagakos (1986) United States	Ecological/cluster investigation Childhood leukemia incidence Woburn, Massachusetts	M F	<20 1964–83	Halogenated organic compounds in drinking water wells, and 48 EPA priority pollutants and 22 metals in nearby test wells	Leukemia	+ for location of contaminated wells and residences of affected children
Lampi (1992) Finland	Ecological Non-Hodgkin's lymphoma, soft-tissue sarcoma, others.	M F	All 1953–86	Drinking water contaminated with chlorophenol from a sawmill	Lymphomas, leukemia, bladder, soft tissue, others	+ Soft tissue sarcoma, non-Hodgkin's lymphoma
Mallin (1990) United States	Cluster investigation Incidence Northern Illinois counties	M F W N	All 1978–85	Wells contaminated with halogentated organic solvents near a 22-acre municipal and industrial landfill	Bladder	+ SIR=1.7 (M) + SIR=2.6 (F) in town with contaminated wells
Najem (1985) United States	Ecological Mortality 194 municipalities in New Jersey	M F W N	All 1968–77	Municipalities with chemical toxic waste disposal sites	13 major sites	+ For 8 cancers in locations with toxic waste disposal sites

(continued)

TABLE 20–1. *Summary of Epidemiological Studies of Drinking Water (Continued)*

Senior Author (year) Country	*Study Design Incidence or Mortality Regional Description*	*Sex Race*	*Age Years Covered*	*Exposure Description*	*Cancer Sites Included*	*Summary of Findings*
				ORGANICS: CHLORINATION BY-PRODUCTS		
Bean (1982b) United States	Ecological Incidence Iowa (Municipalities)	M F W	All 1969–78	Water source Well depth	7 specific sites	+ Lung, p=0.0088 (M), p=0.0128 (F) + Rectum, p=0.0005 (M), p=0.0001 (F)
Beresford (1983) United States	Ecological Incidence S. London area (14 boroughs)	M F	25–74 1968–74	Percent reused water	GI and urinary tract sites	NA after adjustment for social factors
Brenniman (1980) United States	Case-control Mortality Illinois (communities with ground water)	M F W	All 1973–76	Chlorinated vs. nonchlorinated well water	9 specific sites	+ Colorectal (F), OR=1.19
Cantor (1987) United States	Case-control interview Incidence 5 states, 5 metropolitan areas	M F W	21–84 1978	(1) Years chlorinated surface source (2) Tapwater consumption	Bladder	+ Gradient for tapwater consumption among long-term chl. surface water users. OR=1.8 for highest vs. lowest consumption quintile
Cragle (1985) United States	Case-control interview Incidence North Carolina (all places)	M F W M	All 1978–80	Water source and chlorination status	Colon	Age-dependent result: NA, OR=0.94, Age 50 NA, OR=2.15, Age 70
Flaten (1992) Norway	Ecological Incidence and mortality Counties and municipalities (two analyses)	M F	All 1975–84 (incid.) 1974–83 (mort.)	Chlorination practice of municipalities	16 specific sites/all combined	+ Colon + Rectum (both after adjustment for other risk factors)
Gottlieb (1981) United States	Case-control Mortality Louisiana (20 parishes in southern Louisiana)	M F W N	All 1960–75	(1) Water source in parish of residence at death and birth (2) Chlorination level	Colon Rectum	NA Colon, OR=0.96 NA Rectum, OR=2.07 for mostly surface vs. least surface over lifetime
Koivusalo (1994) Finland	Ecological Incidence 56 cities	M F	All 1967–86	Estimated mutagenicity of drinking water in the past	Urinary and GI tract cancers	+ Bladder + Kidney
Lawrence (1984) United States	Case-control Mortality New York State	F W	28–94 1962–78	(1) Water source (2) 20-year cumulative $CHCl_3$	Colorectal	NA, OR=1.07, exposed to $CHCl_3$ vs. not exposed NA for cumulative $CHCl_3$
Lynch (1989) United States	Case-control interview Incidence Iowa	M F W	21–84 1978	Type of water source	Bladder	+ Higher OR with greater exposure specificity (methodologic study—see Cantor (1987))
McGeehin (1993) United States	Case-control interview Incidence Colorado	M F	21–84 1990–91	Chlorinated surface water	Bladder	+ 30+ years chlorinated surface: RR=1.8
Wilkins (1981) United States	Retrospective cohort Incidence Maryland (Washington County)	M F W	25+ 1963–75	Surface (chlorinated) vs. ground source	All sites Site-specific	+ Bladder (M) for 12+ yrs chlorinated surface; RR=6.5 + Breast (F), RR=2.3
Young (1981) United States	Case-control Mortality Wisconsin (28 counties)	F W	21–84 1972–77	(1) Chlorine dose (2) Rural runoff contaminants	GI sites Urinary tract sites, brain, lung, breast	+ Colon, OR=1.6, high vs. no chlorine

Young (1987) United States	Case-control interview Incidence Wisconsin	F W	35–90 1980–82	(1) Water source (2) Cumulative THM	Colon	NA, OR=0.73 (High vs. low THM, life) NA, OR=0.92 (1971, surf vs. gnd source) + , OR=1.66 (1971, mun gnd vs. pvt gnd)
Zierler (1988) United States	Case-control (proxy interviews) Mortality Massachusetts communities	M F W N	45+ 1978–84	Chlorinated vs. chloraminated	Bladder	+ OR=1.6 for lifetime exposure
				INORGANICS: ARSENIC AND METALS		
Bates (1995) United States	Case-control interview Incidence Utah	M F	21–84 1978	Arsenic in municipal water supplies (level and timing of exposure)	Bladder	+ Association among male smokers, esp. in time period 30–39 yrs before diagnosis
Cebrian (1983) Mexico	Cross-sectional Cutaneous abnormalities Central North Mexico	M F	All Unknown	Arsenic in well water Town 1: 0.41 mg/liter avg. Town 2: 0.005 mg/liter avg.	Various cutaneous lesions	+ RR=13.6, Papular keratoses + RR=3.6, Ulcerative zones (both considered as basal cell carcinomas)
Chen (1985) Taiwan	Ecological Mortality SW Taiwan region with high water arsenic levels and endemic blackfoot disease	M F	All 1968–82	Water sources with high and low arsenic content	13 specific sites	+ bladder, kidney, skin, lung, liver, colon
Chen (1986) Taiwan	Case control Mortality SW Taiwan	M F	Unknown 1980–82	Artesian well water (median As=0.78 ppm) vs. shallow well water (median As=0.04 ppm)	Bladder Lung Liver	+ Dose-response with no. yrs. exposed for each cancer site
Chen (1990) Taiwan	Ecological Mortality Countrywide precincts and townships (N=314)	M F	All 1972–83	Arsenic in water from 83,656 wells nationwide: 18.7% >0.05ppm; 2.7% >0.35 ppm	21 specific sites	+ Liver, nasal cavity, lung, skin, bladder, kidney (M,F) + Prostate
Flaten (1991) Norway	Ecological Incidence 97 Municipalities	M F	All 1975–84	NA for most cancer site/ contaminant combinations + for some	16 cancer sites	NA for most site/contaminant combinations + For a few
Harrington (1978b) United States	Cross-sectional Cutaneous abnormalities/other signs/symptoms Fairbanks, Alaska	M F	Unknown Unknown	Arsenic in well water Range: 1.0-2450 μg/liter Mean : 224 μg/liter	Various cutaneous lesions	NA
Isacson (1985) United States	Ecological Incidence Iowa towns of population 1,000–10,000	M F	All 1969–71	Selected volatile organics Trace elements and metals	5 cancer sites in both sexes, F. breast, prostate	+ Bladder, nickel exposure + Lung, nickel exposure + Colon, dichlorethane exposure + Rectum, dichloroethane exposure
Morton (1976) United States	Ecological Incidence Lane County, OR census tracts	M F	All 1958–71	Arsenic in municipal well water 5% of samples >100 μg/liter	Basal and squamous cell carcinoma	NA
Wu (1989) Taiwan	Ecological Mortality SW Taiwan (42 villages)	M F	All 1973–86	Arsenic in well water Low: <0.30 ppm Intermediate: 0.30–0.59 ppm High: 60+ ppm	12 specific sites	+ Bladder, kidney, skin, lung (M,F) + Liver, prostate (M)
				INORGANICS: NITRATE		
Armijo (1975) Chile	Ecological Mortality All 25 provinces	M F	All 1957–71	Nitrogen fertilizer use in kg/capita, by province	Stomach	+

(continued)

TABLE 20–1. *Summary of Epidemiological Studies of Drinking Water (Continued)*

Senior Author (year) Country	*Study Design Incidence or Mortality Regional Description*	*Sex Race*	*Age Years Covered*	*Exposure Description*	*Cancer Sites Included*	*Summary of Findings*
Armijo (1981) Chile	Ecological Incidence High- and low-risk areas	M F	11–13 1977–80	Salivary nitrate in high- and low-risk stomach cancer areas	Salivary nitrate	− Nitrate levels in urine and salivary nitrite with stomach cancer rates
Beresford (1985) United Kingdom	Ecological Mortality 253 urban areas	M F	25–74 1969–73	Nitrate in community drinking water	All cancer Stomach	NA, All cancer − stomach (M,F)
Boeing (1991) Germany	Case-control Incidence Hospitals from 2 regions	M F	<80 yrs 1985–88	Public water supply or other (mostly private well)	Stomach	+ For well water use, not nitrate specifically
Cuello (1976) Colombia	Case-control/Ecological Incidence High- and low-risk areas	M F	All 1968–72	Nitrate in drinking water (173 samples)	Stomach cancer and precursor lesions	+ With stomach cancer or precursors
Dutt (1987) Singapore	Ecological Incidence Ethnic group rates	M F	All Unknown	Total dietary nitrate intake	Stomach	+ Chinese, with more dietary nitrate, have higher rates than Malays or Indians
Forman (1985) Great Britain	Ecological Levels of nitrate in saliva High- and low-risk areas for gastric cancer	M F	15–75 Unknown	Salivary nitrate/nitrite measurements	Saliva nitrate	− Association for salivary nitrate and residence in a low or high stomach cancer risk area
Fraser (1981) United Kingdom	Ecological Mortality Rural districts in E. England	M F	All 1969–73	(1) Cumulative fertilizer use, 1938–72 (2) Nitrate in drinking water from 32 rural districts	Stomach	− For fertilizer use + Stomach (M) − Stomach (F), both with no social class correction
Gilli (1984) Italy	Ecological Incidence 1199 communities of Piemonte Region	M F	All 1976–79	Drinking water nitrate > 20 mg/liter vs. <20 mg/liter	Stomach	+ For nitrate above 20 mg/liter
Haenszel (1976) Japan	Case-control Incidence Two prefectures	M F	All 1962–64	Well water vs. other water used between 1950 and diagnosis	Stomach	+ For well water use. Implications for nitrate not clear
Hartman (1983) International	Ecological Mortality 12-country comparison	M F	All 1974–75	Dietary nitrate intake	Stomach	+ Correlation coefficient (r) = 0.88
Jensen (1982) Denmark	Ecological Incidence Two towns in Jutland	M F	All 1943–72	Mean nitrate level in drinking water of two towns (30 mg/liter and 0.2 mg/liter)	Stomach	+ RR=1.25(1.15-1.35)(M) + RR=1.20(1.10-1.32)(F)
Juhasz (1980) Hungary	Ecological Incidence High- and low-nitrate areas of a county	M F	All 1960–79	Nitrate in drinking water, also soil type	Stomach	NA for nitrate alone + For soil type/nitrate combination
Rademacher (1992) United States	Ecological Mortality Nitrate levels in Wisconsin drinking water	M F	All 1982–85	Nitrate levels in municipal supplies and private wells	Stomach	No association observed

Steindorf (1994) Germany	Case-control Incidence Estimated past exposure to nitrate from community drinking water	M F	Adults 1987–88	Nitrate levels in municipal supplies after 1970	Brain	No association with mean nitrate concentration in drinking water
Morales Suarez-Varela (1993) Spain	Ecological Mortality Time trends in Valencia Province compared to oth. Spain; Communities in Valencia with high and low nitrate in water	M F	All 1975–88	Nitrate levels in municipal water supplies	Bladder	+ (1) Bladder cancer mortality increased more rapidly in Valencia than other Spanish provinces + (2) OR=1.4 (CI=0.7-2.8) for communities with high (above std.) vs. low nitrate in water
Takacs (1981) Hungary	Ecological Incidence of 6 cancer sites 12 towns with different drinking water nitrate levels	M F	All 1953–80	Nitrate in drinking water, ranging to > 100 mg/liter	Esophagus, stomach, bladder, others	+ (?) Elevated proportion of gastric cancer patients with NO_3 >100mg/liter
Vincent (1983) France	Ecological Mortality 753 communities in Northern France	M F	All 1968–75	Average nitrate in drinking water of each community	5 digestive tract and urinary sites	NA
Ward (1994) United States	Case-control interview Incidence Eastern Nebraska	M	21+ 1983–86	Nitrate level in community water supplies, back to 1946	Non-Hodgkin's lymphoma	+ Significant risk for cumulative exposure; highest vs. lowest quintile, OR=2.3
Weisenburger (1991) United States	Ecological Incidence Eastern Nebraska counties (N=66)	M F	All 1984	"Exposed": More than 20% of wells with nitrate exceeding the standard; "Unexposed": Less than 10% of wells exceed the standard	Non-Hodgkin's lymphoma	+ "Exposed" counties rate = $21.0/10^5$; "Unexposed" rate = $11.6/10^5$
				RADIONUCLIDES		
Bean (1982a) United States	Ecological Incidence 28 Iowa towns with deep wells	M F	All	Radium level in municipal well water	Lung, colon, bladder, rectum, fem. breast, prostate	+ Lung (M,F), bladder (M), and breast (F) in towns with radium-226 >5.0 pCi/liter
Collman (1991) United States	Ecological Mortality All North Carolina counties	M F	<15 yrs 1950–79	Radon level in public water supplies	Major sites of childhood cancer	+ Leukemia
Fuortes (1990) United States	Ecological Incidence 59 Iowa towns	M F	All 1969–84	Radium level in municipal well water	All leukemia, AML	+ Total leukemia NA Granulocytic leukemia (weak associations)
Hess (1983) United States	Ecological Mortality All 16 Maine counties	M F	All	Average radon level in water by county (from 2000 sampled public and private wells)	All sites, Lung	+ All cancer, lung with waterborne radon (F) NA (M)
Lyman (1985) United States	Ecological Incidence 27 counties in Florida	M F	All	Radium from 50 wells in each county	Leukemia, AML	+ Leukemia and AML with mean county radium
				PARTICULATES: ASBESTOS		
Andersen (1993) Norway	Cohort Incidence Norwegian lighthouse keepers	M	All 1960–91	Drinking water from cisterns contaminated with runoff from asbestos-cement roof tiles	All	+ Stomach for latency >20 yr.

(continued)

TABLE 20–1. *Summary of Epidemiological Studies of Drinking Water (Continued)*

Senior Author (year) Country	*Study Design Incidence or Mortality Regional Description*	*Sex Race*	*Age Years Covered*	*Exposure Description*	*Cancer Sites Included*	*Summary of Findings*
Conforti (1981) United States	Ecological Incidence Census tracts of San Francisco Bay Area, California	M F	All 1969–74	Estimated asbestos levels in public water supplies in 722 census tracts, and 410 "super" tracts sharing demographic and asbestos exposure levels (natural source)	All Site-specific	+ All sites, all digestive, esophagus, stomach, pancreas (M,F) + Colon, respiratory, prostate (M) retroperitoneum, pleura (F)
Harrington (1978a) United States	Ecological Incidence Connecticut townships	M F	All 1935–73	Towns using asbestos cement pipe vs. other towns	Colon, rectum, stomach	NA
Howe (1989) United States	Ecological Incidence Census block groups of the Woodstock, New York, region	M F	All 1973–83	Asbestos levels in municipal water from asbestos-cement pipes	All Site-specific	+ Buccal, kidney, prostate (M) − NA colon, lung (M)
Millette (1983b) United States	Ecological Mortality Census tracts of Escambia County, Florida	M F	All 1963–76	Asbestos levels in public water supplies from asbestos-cement pipes	Bladder, kidney, GI, pancreas, liver, lung, other	NA
Polissar (1982) United States	Ecological Incidence, Mortality Puget Sound Region, WA	M F	All 1974–77 (incid.) 1955–75 (mort.)	Asbestos in local water supplies (natural source)	All Site-specific	NA (Nonsignificant elevation of small intestine [M,F])
Polissar (1984) United States	Case-control Incidence Everett, Washington, area	M F	40–79 11/1977–12/1980	Cumulative lifetime imbibed asbestos (natural source)	Buccal cavity, pharynx, resp. system, diges. system, kidney, bladder	NA
Sadler (1984) United States	Ecological Incidence 41 Utah communities	M F W	All 1967–76	Communities using asbestos cement pipe vs. other communities	11 sites Site-specific	+ Kidney (M) + Leukemia (F)
Sigurdson (1981) United States	Ecological Incidence Duluth, MN	M F	All 1969–71	Comparison of rates in a city using tailings-contaminated lake water with rates of other nearby cities	Lung and site-specific digestive system tumors	+ Pancreas (F)

and our ability to characterize past exposures to chlorination by-products, using available historical records of water source and treatment, have facilitated epidemiological study of these contaminants. The study of the more sporadic contamination of drinking water with anthropogenic chemicals has been more challenging.

Enormous advances in the capabilities of analytical chemistry over the past 20 years to detect low levels of contaminants have both vastly increased our knowledge of organics in drinking water, and greatly complicated the questions of risk assessment, since detectable levels of compounds are often quite low, beneath the concentrations at which it may be possible to detect health effects by epidemiological methods. Hundreds of organic chemicals have been found in U.S. drinking waters, but most occur infrequently and at low concentration (in the part per trillion or part per billion [ppb] range). It is likely that many remain to be detected. Of the detected chemicals, at least 40 are known or suspected carcinogens, three of which are associated with human cancer induction: vinyl chloride, benzene, and chloromethyl ether (International Agency for Research on Cancer, 1987).

Organic Chemicals from Human Commerce

Contamination of underground and surface water with organic chemicals from industrial, agricultural, commercial, and domestic sources, as well as from hazardous waste disposal sites, is increasingly found. Usually, the contamination is geographically restricted, but some materials such as agricultural pesticides and organic solvents used for cleaning cesspools may affect extensive aquifers (U.S. EPA, 1988). There are relatively few epidemiological assessments of the health impact of such drinking water contaminants. This is due to the difficulty in estimating the levels, timing, and specific chemicals involved in past exposures; the relatively small populations usually exposed to high contaminant levels; and the problem of deciding which health end points, or intermediate biological markers, to examine. When effects are observed, it is often impossible to sort out the specific exposures involved. Of special concern are studies of hazardous waste sites, because the route of exposure from such sources often involves contamination of groundwater used for drinking.

County and local cancer mortality and incidence rates, calculated from routinely collected information, have been examined in places with hazardous waste sites, or with municipal water supplies with documented contamination. An early study from Iowa described elevated county lymphoma rates in places served by rivers with measurable levels of dieldrin (DeKraay, 1978). A bladder cancer cluster was noted in a Northwestern llinois community with exposure to several contaminants in the community drinking water supply, including trichloroethylene, tetrachlorethylene, and 1,1-dichloroethane (Mallin, 1990). The contamination source was a 22-acre industrial and municipal landfill that leached into local aquifers. In a nationwide study, age-adjusted cancer mortality rates from 339 U.S. counties with 593 hazardous waste sites listed by EPA were compared with rates from 2726 other counties (Griffith et al, 1989). Significant associations were found for lung, bladder, stomach, colon, and rectal cancers in white males and females, esophageal cancer in white males, and breast cancer in white females. In New Jersey, significant positive associations between chemical toxic waste disposal sites and eight cancer sites, especially stomach and lung, were found in one or more subpopulations living in 194 municipalities with over 10,000 population, after adjustment for sociodemographic characteristics (Najem et al, 1985). In another New Jersey study, female leukemia incidence rates in 27 towns were associated with an index of volatile organic chemicals in municipal drinking water, but no association was observed in males (Fagliano et al, 1990). In Clinton County, Pa., the location of the Drake Superfund Site, bladder cancer mortality among white males was significantly elevated (Budnick et al, 1984).

Several studies have evaluated populations near specific toxic waste sites. Love Canal in Niagara Falls, N.Y., served as a toxic waste disposal site from 1947 to 1952, and residential housing was later built adjacent to the area. Most exposure to residents likely was via inhalation, as volatile chemicals outgassed from the groundwater and contaminated the air in neighborhood houses. An assessment of cancer incidence rates for the period 1955–1977 revealed elevated lung cancer that was not consistent across age groups (Janerich et al, 1981). Other cancers did not appear to be elevated, but the statistical power to detect elevated rates of less common sites was limited. Rates of chromosomal aberrations and sister chromatid exchange frequencies were as expected (Heath et al, 1984). An elevated incidence of low birth weight was found for the period when chemicals were being dumped (Vianna and Polan, 1984). A household survey and review of medical and vital statistics records in communities near the Stringfellow Hazardous Waste Site in Riverside County, Calif., (Baker et al, 1988) did not reveal excesses of cancer or adverse birth outcomes, but increases of several other conditions were reported. The authors noted that these findings may be explained by differential reporting from neighboring residents. A Finnish community with drinking water contaminated with chlorophenols, probably from sawmills, had an elevated incidence of soft-tissue sarcoma and non-Hodgkin's lymphoma (Lampi et al, 1992). These findings are of concern because these tumors have been linked with exposure to the closely related chlorinated phenoxy-acetic acids and/or their dioxin contaminants (Lilienfeld and Gallo, 1989). Furthermore, primary liver cancer in China was strongly linked to consuming drinking water from ditches highly polluted with agricultural runoff that presumably contained a variety of organic and other chemicals (Delong, 1979).

A cluster of childhood leukemia cases associated with contaminated community drinking water in Woburn, Mass., has been the subject of scientific, legal, and political controversy (Lagakos et al, 1986; MacMahon et al, 1986; Cutler et al, 1986; Byers et al, 1988). Woburn, with a population of 37,000, has been an industrial site for more than 130 years. Two of eight drinking water wells were discovered in 1979 to be contaminated with trichloroethylene (267 ppb), tetrachloroethylene (21 ppb), trichlorotrifluoroethane (23 ppb), and dichloroethylene (28 ppb). Forty-eight EPA priority pollutants and elevated levels of 22 metals were found in 61 additional test wells drilled to sample the groundwater (Lagakos et al, 1986). An elevated rate of childhood leukemia was found and statistically linked in space and time to the contamination. Associations were also observed for two of five categories of congenital anomalies, and two of nine categories of childhood disorders. In addition, lymphocyte abnormalities were noted among family members of cases (Byers et al, 1988).

A population-based case-control study from upper Cape Cod, Mass., evaluated associations of bladder cancer (N=61), kidney cancer (N=35) and leukemia (N=34) with exposure to tetrachloroethylene in public drinking water, which had leached from the plastic lining of improperly cured vinyl lined water distribution pipes (Aschengrau et al, 1993). Elevated risk for leukemia was found, especially among subjects with exposure levels over the 90th percentile, as well as nonsignificant elevations in bladder cancer risk.

A health survey in Hardeman County, Tenn., where leachate from a pesticide waste dump contaminated the drinking water, found significant differences in hepatic profiles of exposed and unexposed members of the population that included alkaline phosphatase, albumin, total bilirubin, and SGOT (Clark et al, 1982). This may be of relevance to cancer induction, because detoxification of potentially carcinogenic compounds or conversion of procarcinogens to direct-acting carcinogens may be linked to enzyme profiles. The most frequently detected contaminants in the air of exposed homes were carbon tetrachloride and tetrachloroethylene. Continued health surveillance of potentially exposed populations in the vicinity of toxic waste disposal sites should continue to be of high priority.

Organic Chemicals: Chlorination By-Products

Chlorination byproducts are found in almost every chlorinated drinking water in the United States. Chloroform and other trihalomethanes (THM) are found at the highest concentration in this chemical mixture. The concentration of total THM ranges from less than one ppb (in treated water from deep wells low in organics) to several hundred ppb (certain chlorinated surface waters). Among the chlorination byproducts, the THMs account for 20%–80% of the covalently bound halogen (mostly chlorine and bromine), with the remaining halogen bound to a large number (typically > 200) of higher molecular weight, nonvolatile compounds, such as a variety of carboxylic acids, aldehydes, ketones, and ethers (Stevens et al, 1989; Singer and Chang, 1989). The organically bound bromine originates as naturally occurring bromide ion, which is oxidized by chlorine to highly reactive Br^0.

The observation of elevated chlorination by-products in treated surface water, as contrasted to well water, has served as the basis for epidemiological evaluation of these exposures. Studies of chlorination by-products may be placed in one of three groups that describe the methodological approach, and roughly correspond to the time period during which they were conducted. A detailed review is available (International Agency for Research on Cancer, 1991).

The first studies were ecological; both the exposure and outcome measures (cancer mortality or incidence) were estimated for populations, not individuals. In most of these studies, the county was the geographic unit of observation. Age-adjusted, site-, sex-, and race-specific county cancer mortality rates were used as outcomes, and characteristics (chlorinated vs nonchlorinated, surface vs ground, THM level) of the predominant county drinking water source as the exposure variable (Cantor et al, 1978; Hogan et al, 1979; Kuzma et al, 1977; Page et al, 1976; Salg, 1977). Incidence rates were used as outcomes in studies of water quality and cancer in Iowa towns (Bean et al, 1982b; Isacson et al, 1983), Norwegian municipalities (Flaten, 1992), and Finnish cities (Koivusalo et al, 1994). In these ecological studies, bladder, colon, and rectum were the sites of cancer most commonly associated with surface water, with chlorination, with THM level (Wilkins et al, 1979; National Research Council, 1980), or, in the case of the Finnish study (Koivusalo et al, 1994), with estimates of water mutagenicity.

The second group of studies were of case-comparison design, and used mortality records as the sources of case and comparison subjects. In the earliest studies (Alavanja et al, 1978; Brenniman et al, 1980; Young et al, 1981; Gottlieb and Carr, 1982; Crump and Guess, 1982), the exposure variable was a characteristic of the water supply (surface/ground, chlorinated/nonchlorinated, Mississippi River/other source) that served the decedent's residence town at the time of death, abstracted from mortality records. In later studies, attempts were made to gather information about previous residences and their sources of drinking water. These data were either inferred from the place of birth listed on the death certificate (Gottlieb et al, 1981), obtained from available records (Lawrence et al, 1984), or collected in interviews with next of kin (Zierler et al, 1988). Most of these studies focused on cancers of the bladder, colon, or rectum. Their results were largely supportive of the findings from the earlier ecological studies. A notable exception is the study of Lawrence and colleagues (1984), which found no association for colorectal cancer with type of water source or imputed past THM level.

The third group of investigations were disaggregate studies in which past exposures were estimated through linking historical community water supply records with residential history information gathered in personal interviews. One community cohort follow-up study and five case-comparison studies used this approach (Wilkins and Comstock, 1981; Cantor et al, 1987; Young et al, 1987; Cragle et al, 1985; IJsselmuiden et al, 1992; McGeehin et al, 1993). Three of the case-comparison studies also gathered information about the tap water consumption of individuals.

In a population of nearly 31,000 persons in Washington County, Maryland, Wilkins and Comstock (1981) found elevated (but not statistically significant) bladder cancer incidence among men, and cancer of the liver among women, in the drinking water subcohort supplied with chlorinated surface water at home. The low exposure comparison was the subcohort with a history of unchlorinated ground water consumption. The male bladder cancer excess increased with duration of residence with a chlorinated surface water source. A subsequent nested case-comparison study of cancer of the pancreas (IJsselmuiden et al, 1992) found a significantly elevated odds ratio of 2.2 (confidence interval of 1.2–4.1) for "chlorinated municipal water" as contrasted with users of nonmunicipal, nonchlorinated water.

Colon cancer was the subject of case-comparison interview studies in North Carolina (Cragle et al, 1985) and Wisconsin (Young et al, 1987). In the former, an association was observed with use of chlorinated surface water, but only among cases more than 60 years old. In Wisconsin, where the authors estimated trihalomethane ingestion at various times in the past, no associations with colon cancer were noted. In Telemark, Norway, where some residents were served with chlorinated water high in organic content, the prevalence of colorectal adenomas was higher than among residents using water with lower levels of organics (Hoff et al, 1992). However, there were no differences in the chloroform content of these waters, challenging an interpretation of a link with chlorination by-products. Bladder cancer risk as related to water source and tap water consumption was evaluated in a case-comparison interview study conducted in ten areas of the United States (Cantor et al, 1987). Approximately 3000 cases and 6000 comparison subjects were personally interviewed regarding known and suspected bladder cancer risk factors. A lifetime profile of home drinking water source and treatment was developed for each respondent by merging individual residential histories with water utility information. Bladder cancer risk increased with the amount of tap water consumed, and this increase was strongly influenced by the duration of living at residences served by chlorinated surface water. Among respondents who resided for 60+ years at places served by surface water, a risk of 2.0 was found for persons in the highest tap water consumption quintile relative to those in the lowest quintile. There was no increase of risk with tap water consumption among persons who had lived at places served by nonchlorinated ground water for most of their lives. Similar findings were reported from a smaller case-comparison study of bladder cancer and disinfection methods (327 cases, 261 controls) in Colorado (McGeehin et al, 1993).

Results of these studies and that of Wilkens and Comstock (1981) support a link between bladder cancer risk and elevated levels of chlorination by-products in drinking water. The findings for cancer of the rectum are weaker, since most studies are death certificate based, with little detailed exposure information, while the results for colon cancer are inconclusive. For the bladder cancer findings, the two disaggregate studies meet sample size and other criteria, and the relative risks are small, mostly in the range below 2.0. A formal meta-analysis of the epidemiological data was conducted with the purpose of better quantifying cancer risk linked to chlorinated by-products (Morris et al, 1992). The meta-analysis may have been premature, because most available studies were methodologically weak, especially with regard to incomplete exposure assessment and inadequate control for confounding (Cantor, 1994). Thus it will be necessary to develop information in additional disaggregate studies in other settings before risks can be quantified with confidence.

INORGANIC SOLUTES

A wide variety of inorganic solutes are found in drinking waters, and several are suspected to increase cancer risk in exposed populations. Certain metals and transition elements, notably arsenic, and nitrates are of particular concern. Also of interest is fluoride because of broad population exposure and equivocal evidence from animal studies suggesting a carcinogenic risk.

Metals and Transition Elements

Several metals and transition elements are considered to be carcinogenic in man (arsenic, chromium, and nickel) and others are known carcinogens in animals (Berg and Burbank, 1972). These are present in a wide range of concentrations in U.S. drinking waters (usually under 100 μg/liter) and can increase or decrease during water treatment. The sources include leaching from soil or distribution systems, industrial or mining activities, or water treatment itself.

Other than arsenic, there has been relatively little study of trace metals in water and cancer risk. An early correlational study (Berg and Burbank, 1972) found several significant links between site-specific cancer mortality in U.S. sites and drinking water concentrations of eight trace metals in 16 major water basins. The most frequent associations were with beryllium, cadmium, and lead. An Iowa study observed geographic correlations between town-level cancer incidence of lung and bladder cancers and levels of nickel in drinking water (Isacson et al, 1985). The authors suggested that nickel was not directly implicated, but an indicator of other contamination. A Norwegian study in 97 municipalities evaluated the correlation of 17 inorganic ions in drinking water with 16 groups of cancer morbidity (Flaten and Bolviken, 1991). Several significant associations were found, many of which could have been due to chance.

The strongest evidence comes from studies of inorganic arsenic. Initial investigations reported elevated prevalence of non-melanoma skin cancer in areas of chronic arsenicism from contaminated water supplies in Mexico (Cebrian et al, 1983), Argentina (Bergoglio, 1964), Chile (Borgoño and Grieber, 1971), and Taiwan (Tseng et al, 1968; Tseng, 1977). A study by Tseng and colleagues (1968) in Taiwan utilized a cross-sectional design and detected a dose-response association between sampled arsenic concentrations (ca. 0.5 ppm) in wells and the prevalence of skin cancer. These results were substantiated by further studies in Taiwan (Tseng, 1977). Skin cancer prevalence and/or incidence has not been found elevated in U.S. locations where populations are exposed to elevated arsenic levels in drinking water (Morton et al, 1976; Harrington et al, 1978b), suggesting that higher doses of arsenic or etiological cofactors (eg, other water pollutants, sunlight) are important in endemic areas like Taiwan.

Recent studies in Taiwan have revealed geographic associations of inorganic arsenic in drinking water with risk of mortality from several other cancers, notably cancers of the bladder, kidney, lung, nasal cavity, liver, and prostate (Wu et al, 1989; Chen et al, 1985; Chen and Wang, 1990). The most extensive study (Chen and Wang, 1990) extended the correlations to the whole of Taiwan (excepting Taipei City and 30 townships that had surface water or small populations), using data from 314 precincts and townships. Arsenic levels came from a nationwide survey of more than 83,000 wells conducted in 1974–76. The strongest correlations were found for bladder and kidney cancers, with the multivariate-adjusted regression coefficients indicating an increase in age-adjusted mortality per 100,000 person-years of 3.9 and 4.2 (bladder) for every 0.1 ppm increase in arsenic level of well water, and 1.1 and 1.7 (kidney) among males and females, respectively. Chen and colleagues (1986) conducted a case-comparison study of bladder, lung, and liver cancers in an area of Taiwan with arsenic-contaminated artesian wells. They found a positive dose-response relationship for each of these cancer sites, with odds ratios of 3.9 for bladder cancer, 3.4 for lung cancer, and 2.7 for liver cancer among those who drank contaminated water for 40 years or longer, as compared with never users. In a case-control study, an association between bladder cancer and arsenic in drinking water was found among male smokers, especially among those exposed in the time period 30–39 years before diagnosis (Bates et al, 1994). An excess of bladder cancer has been reported in a cohort of patients treated with Fowler's solution (potassium arsenite) (Cuzick et al, 1992).

The Taiwanese studies suggest that arsenic causes not only skin cancer, but also certain other cancers by ingestion of ambient trace amounts (Bates et al, 1992; Smith et al, 1992). The broad distribution of these metals in drinking water indicates a need for further study. In particular, additional disaggregate studies that exploit situations of high exposures or high disease rates should receive top priority.

Nitrate

Nitrate ion occurs in surface and ground waters in concentrations ranging from less than 1.0 mg/liter to over 100 mg/liter. The U.S. Environmental Protection Agency (EPA) has established a maximum contaminant level for nitrate in drinking water of 45 mg/l (10 mg/l nitrate-nitrogen), primarily to protect against methemoglobinemia in young infants. Nitrate in drinking water comes from numerous natural and man-made sources, including waste waters and agricultural and urban runoff. Nitrate is seldom removed during treatment. Nitrogen fertilizers have been implicated as an ever more important source of drinking water nitrate in rural areas, and more than 20% of wells may have nitrate levels above the EPA limit (Johnson and Kross, 1990; McDonald and Splinter, 1982; Hallberg, 1985), especially if their depth is less than 30 m. When drinking water nitrate is well below 10 mg/liter, most ingested nitrate comes from dietary sources, and average intake is about 100 mg/day. However, when water levels are near or exceed the EPA limit, water may increase nitrate intake to 200 mg/day or more. At levels near the EPA limit, about 30% of ingested nitrate comes from water, rising to almost 70% at levels between 50 and 100 mg/liter (Chilvers et al, 1984).

The main concern is that nitrate can act as a procarcinogen, interacting with secondary amines and amides to form a variety of *N*-nitroso compounds, after reduction in the saliva of nitrate to nitrite (Eisenbrand et al, 1980; Walters and Smith, 1981; Walters, 1980; Hart and Walters, 1983; Moller et al, 1989). Many *N*-nitroso compounds are potent carcinogens in multiple species (International Agency for Research on Cancer, 1978). The potential for forming N-nitroso compounds in humans has been demonstrated by exposing people orally to l-proline and nitrate, and then measuring the resulting levels of *N*-nitrosoproline (a noncarcinogenic *N*-nitrosamine) in the urine. For example, the urinary concentration of *N*-nitrosoproline was significantly associated with well water nitrate levels among Nebraskan men given oral doses of 500 mg *l*-proline (Mirvish et al, 1992). *N*-nitrosoproline formation can be inhibited by vitamin C (Mirvish, 1994). *N*-nitrosoproline in *l*-proline-exposed Italians (Knight et al, 1991) and Costa Rican children (Sierra et al, 1993) was elevated in areas with an elevated incidence of stomach cancer. In southern China, the same test showed excess *N*-nitrosoproline excretion in high-risk areas for nasopharyngeal carcinoma (Zeng et al, 1993). In a high-risk area for gastric cancer in China, premalignant histological changes in the gastric mucosa were related to nitrate content of the drinking water, which ranged above 100 mg/l (Xu et al, 1992).

Despite the data indicating the carcinogenic potential of nitrate in drinking water, direct epidemiological evidence is equivocal. Several studies, most of ecological design, have shown associations between nitrate concentrations in drinking water and gastric cancer. Brain cancer, bladder cancer, and non-Hodgkin's lymphoma are also of interest, although there is less evidence. As shown in Table 20–1, positive geographic associations of nitrate with gastric cancer have been found in Chile, Hungary, England, Colombia, Italy, and Denmark (Armijo and Coulson, 1975; Juhasz et al, 1980; Takacs and Gomori, 1981; Fraser and Chilvers, 1981; Cuello et al, 1976; Gilli et al, 1984; Jensen, 1982). However, several other studies have not demonstrated a positive association for gastric cancer. A positive association with bladder cancer incidence was found in Spain (Morales Suarez-Varela et al, 1993). Incidence rates of non-Hodgkin's lymphoma in eastern Nebraska counties were associated with the proportion of wells high in nitrate (Weisenburger, 1991). Geographic correlations of this type may be subject to "publication bias," whereby positive associations may be more likely to find their way into print than null findings. Retrospective cohort studies of fertilizer workers who are presumably exposed to nitrate dusts have not shown excess cancer risk (Rafnsson and Gunnarsdottir, 1990; Al-Dabbagh et al, 1986; Fraser et al, 1989). Among the few disaggregate studies is a case-control study of gastric cancer deaths from Wisconsin that did not show a link with nitrate level of the water source at the last residence of decedents (Rademacher et al, 1992). A population-based case-control study from Germany of incident primary brain tumors, which estimated exposures for the 18-year period prior to diagnosis, showed no association with drinking water nitrate (Steindorf et al, 1994). A case-control study of incident non-Hodgkin's lymphoma in eastern Nebraska found a link with estimates of cumulative nitrate ingestion from community sources of drinking water, going back almost 40 years (Ward et al, in press). Until more information is available from drinking water studies of nitrate conducted on the individual level, where diet and other risk factors can be taken into account, the epidemiological evidence must be considered as being weak. However, in view of the widespread and increasing contamination of water supplies with nitrate, especially in agricultural regions, and the established potential for forming N-nitroso compounds, this area of research should have a high priority.

Fluoride

Fluoride is present in most natural waters at concentrations that rarely exceed 5.0 mg/liter and are usually less than 1.0 mg/liter. Its natural source is mainly the dissolution of fluoride ion from minerals, such as apatite, amphibole, and fluorite. In the United States, the principal source in an increasing number of communities over the past four decades has been the successful prophylactic addition of fluoride to prevent dental caries. The usual dosage is approximately 1.0 mg/liter.

Fluoride in drinking water came under suspicion as a human carcinogen with the release of data showing that the overall cancer mortality rates of the ten largest U.S. cities that practiced water fluoridation were significantly higher than those of the ten largest that did not (Burk and Yiamouyiannis, 1975). Site-specific differences were found for cancers of the urinary and gastrointestinal tracts, female breast, and ovary. Subsequent analyses of the same data showed that the differences initially observed disappeared when relevant sociodemographic variables were taken into account (Hoover et al, 1976; Chilvers, 1983). Additional studies, almost all of ecological design, provided no supporting evidence. Given the important public health implications of this question, the epidemiological findings on fluoridation and cancer risk were independently reviewed by an international panel (International Agency for Research on Cancer, 1982) and by three separate expert committees convened in the United States (National Research Council, 1977a; U.S. Public Health Service; 1991) and Great Britain (Knox, 1985). All groups concluded that the available evidence does not support the hypothesis that fluoride in drinking water influences cancer risk.

However, concern was again fueled by a finding of "equivocal evidence" of carcinogenicity from a lifetime sodium fluoride rodent feeding study (Bucher et al, 1991). Three of 50 male rats in the highest dose category (79 ppm) and 1 of 50 in the next-to-highest group (45 ppm) had a rare bone tumor (osteosarcoma), while no osteosarcomas were found in the lower dose groups, nor in female rats, or male or female mice. In the brief period since, epidemiological assessments have found no time trend nor geographic pattern of bone cancer or osteosarcoma consistent with a causal role for fluoride in drinking water (McGuire et al, 1991; Hoover et al, 1991; Hrudey et al, 1990; Mahoney et al, 1991). This continues to be an area of active research interest.

RADIONUCLIDES

Traces of natural and man-made radioactivity from radionuclides are found in drinking water supplies throughout the United States. Levels vary geographically with local soil and rock conditions and may be increased by industrial and other point discharges, such as activities associated with radiopharmaceutical production and use, radionuclide production, and nuclear power generation. The principal naturally occurring species include radium 226, radium 228, uranium, radon 222, lead 210, polonium 210, thorium 230, and thorium 232 (Cothern et al, 1986).

In 1976, the U.S. Environmental Protection Agency promulgated regulations setting standards for maximum allowed levels of radionuclides in drinking water. Among other requirements, the regulations mandated monitoring of the almost 60,000 U.S. public water supplies (Federal Register, Vol. 41, No.133, pp 28404–9, 9 July, 1976). Data from this monitoring program and other surveys have been used to estimate the occurrence of uranium (Cothern and Lappenbusch, 1983), radon 222 (Cross et al, 1985), radium (Mays et al, 1985), and total radioactivity (Hess et al, 1985), and the contribution of drinking water to total natural background radiation (Cross et al, 1985; Cothern et al, 1986; Nazaroff et al, 1987).

Most of the population dose of alpha radiation derived from drinking water is from airborne radon released from water in dish and clothes washers, showers, baths, toilets, and cooking, drinking, and cleaning (Nazaroff et al, 1987). The primary exposure is to the lungs. Ingested radon or other radionuclides are not thought to be important as environmental determinants of cancer (National Research Council, 1977b). Although the predominant source of indoor radon 222 in most U.S. houses is the soil underlying and adjacent to the foundation, in some circumstances groundwater constitutes the predominant source (Hess et al, 1983). On the average, water contributes less than 2% of airborne household radon. Radon 222 concentrations in water vary over an extremely large range, from nearly zero to more than 10^6 becquerel (Bq)/m^3. Surface waters, serving about half the U.S. population, have the lowest concentrations (0.1 Bq/m^3 average), followed by public groundwater supplies (1.3 Bq/m^3) and private wells (24 Bq/m^3).

Most epidemiological studies of cancer and radon in dwellings have evaluated lung cancer as related to airborne radon, without regard to the primary sources of the measured radon. The few investigations of cancer and radioactivity in drinking water are ecological in design. A study of county leukemia incidence rates in Florida found a relative risk of 1.5 for total leukemia and 2.0 for acute myeloid leukemia in high groundwater radium versus low radium counties (Lyman et al, 1985). In Maine, a study of county cancer mortality found an association between female lung cancer for 1950–1969 and average county radon concentrations in water (Hess et al, 1983). In Iowa, the incidence rates for cancers of the lung and bladder among males and cancers of the lung and breast among females were elevated in towns with a radium 226 level in the water supply exceeding 5.0 pCi/liter (Bean et al, 1982a). The associations in Iowa could not be explained by smoking patterns, water treatment factors, or sociodemographic factors. A subsequent study of leukemia incidence in 59 Iowa towns revealed a small, increasing trend for total leukemia incidence with radium content in drinking water, consistent with either no or a small effect (Fuortes et al, 1990). Although several case-control studies have examined the association of airborne radon in homes with lung cancer risk, the contribution of drinking water to total household radon has not been considered.

SOLID PARTICULATES

Drinking water always contains small amounts of solid particles that vary in size from approximately 0.005 to

100 μm, a range of over four orders of magnitude. These particles may be inorganic or organic (eg, detritus). Solid particulates can occur naturally as derivatives of rocks, soils, or decaying organic matter, or they may be man-made, and they can be present in raw water or introduced during water treatment. Solid particulates can be classified in three general groups: clays, asbestos particles, and organic particulates, although asbestos is sometimes grouped together with the clays.

Particulates are relevant to the issue of drinking water and cancer in several ways. First, although most waterborne particulates are not known to be directly associated with cancer, asbestos fibers have been implicated. Second, many of these substances, especially the clays, can adsorb and bind a number of potentially carcinogenic agents, rendering them biologically unavailable. Finally, they can also be important in enhancing chemical and biological activity. Only asbestos fibers will be discussed here because of their direct relevance to cancer.

The term asbestos refers to a large group of "naturally occurring hydrated silicate minerals possessing fibrous morphology and commercial utility" (National Research Council, 1977b). However, practically all of commercially produced asbestos consists of chrysotile (95%) and amosite and crocidolite (remaining 5%). Almost 90% of asbestos is used in the production of cement and other construction products; the remainder is used in transportation, textiles, and plastics. Asbestos fibers are widely distributed in the aqueous environment, with higher concentrations usually found near cities and industrial centers.

Asbestos fibers reach drinking water primarily through weathering from natural deposits such as serpentine, by release from asbestos-cement pipes, and from processes associated with mining and production of certain types of iron ore (Millette et al, 1983a; Langer et al, 1979). Concentrations vary enormously, ranging from a barely detectable background level of 10^4 fibers/liter, to over 10^{11} fibers/liter (Millette et al, 1983a). For human carcinogenesis, the size, shape, and crystalline structure of these fibers (particularly the ratio of length to diameter) is as important as concentration, and these characteristics are modified by physicochemical processes resulting from exposure to water or gastric fluid (Seshan, 1983).

There is considerable epidemiological evidence, primarily from occupational settings, that asbestos is a human carcinogen of the respiratory tract and possibly, because of lung clearance and subsequent swallowing, the gastrointestinal tract. Despite this evidence, epidemiological studies of populations served by water containing high concentrations of asbestos have failed to yield conclusive results.

All but two studies (Polissar et al, 1984; Andersen et al, 1993) involving asbestos in drinking water are ecological, comparing the geographic distribution of asbestos levels in drinking water with cancer incidence or mortality rates. Related studies in census tracts of the San Francisco Bay area (Kanarek et al, 1980; Conforti et al, 1981) found associations between measured (naturally occurring) asbestos in drinking water and incidence rates for cancers of the esophagus, stomach, pancreas in both sexes (Conforti et al, 1981), of the lung in males, and of the gallbladder and peritoneum in females (Kanarek et al, 1980). However, potentially confounding factors such as diet, smoking, and occupation could not be adequately controlled. Mortality in Quebec communities was associated with asbestos in drinking water for cancers of the stomach (males), pancreas (females), and lung (males) (Wigle, 1977). An ecological study (Polissar et al, 1982) and a case-control study (Polissar et al, 1984) in the Puget Sound region, based on incident cancer, evaluated the risk of imbibing water from a river with high levels of naturally occurring asbestos. Neither found overall patterns consistent with an asbestos effect. However, positive associations for male stomach cancer, based on small numbers, were observed in the case-control study. A cohort study of incident cancer among Norwegian lighthouse keepers exposed to asbestos in their drinking water also reported an excess of stomach cancer (Andersen et al, 1993). The excess was 2.4-fold and statistically significant among persons first exposed at least 20 years prior to diagnosis.

Duluth, Minn., had high levels of asbestos in its drinking water from 1955 to 1973, due to contamination of Lake Superior with tailings from an iron ore (taconite) processing facility about 60 miles away. Cancer mortality (Mason et al, 1974) and incidence (Levy et al, 1976; Sigurdson et al, 1981) in Duluth or its county were compared with rates in other Minnesota cities (or their respective counties). Some excesses of gastrointestinal mortality and morbidity were observed, but with inconsistent patterns. The variability of these results may be related to a limited time period between first exposure and the observation period of cancer mortality and incidence.

Cancer incidence as related to drinking water distributed by asbestos-cement water mains has been evaluated in Connecticut (Meigs et al, 1980; Harrington et al, 1978a), Utah (Sadler et al, 1984), and Woodstock, N.Y. (Howe et al, 1989), and mortality studied in Escambria County, Florida (Millette et al, 1983b), with inconsistent findings. In Utah, an association was found for kidney cancer (males) and leukemia (females), and in Woodstock for cancer of the oral cavity.

Laboratory studies cannot provide conclusive evidence, principally because of methodological problems and the absence of suitable animal model systems (National Research Council, 1977b). Epidemiological and experimental research on this topic should nevertheless continue, since none of the available data can rule out adverse health effects of carcinogens present in water. Furthermore, these substances are widespread in the aqueous environment, and a period of 20 to 40 years may be required before their effects in humans are seen. In particular, the approaches of Mason and colleagues (1974), Levy and colleagues (1976), and Sigurdson and colleagues (1981) on changes in cancer rates over time in high-exposure areas should be given priority. In addition, asbestos in drinking water should be considered a risk factor whenever large case-control studies of stomach, kidney, pancreas, or other cancers are conducted in regions with sources of asbestos-contaminated water.

MICROBIOLOGICAL AGENTS

Viruses, bacteria, and protozoa are the principal microbes in drinking water that can be transmitted to man by ingestion. Their concentrations and sources vary greatly in different raw water sources, but the dramatic decreases and the continued low incidence of waterborne infectious disease during this century underscore the effectiveness and importance of disinfection in maintaining acceptable low levels of these agents in finished water. An important characteristic of these organisms is that they exist in water primarily as aggregates, either with other microorganisms or with solid particulates; this has an important bearing on their effectiveness as pathogens and on methods for their removal.

These pathogens are generally not thought to be important as water-borne carcinogens, and they are discussed as noncarcinogens in a National Research Council (1977a) review of this subject. Mounting evidence suggests that several viruses (principally hepatitis B, human papilloma virus, Epstein-Barr virus, and human immunodeficiency virus 1 (HIV-1)) are associated with human cancer, but there has been no evidence of waterborne transmission. However, at least one waterborne microorganism, *Schistosoma haematobium*, has been associated with elevated bladder cancer rates in many tropical and subtropical countries where schistosomiasis is endemic (Cheever, 1978), such as Egypt (Mustacchi and Shimkin, 1958) and Zimbabwe (Thomas et al, 1990). Schistosomiasis-related bladder cancer is usually of squamous-cell origin, whereas most other bladder carcinomas have transitional cell type. In endemic areas, infections with *S. haematobium* start at an early age, persist for many years, and are related to bladder cancers of early onset. In a series of Egyptian bladder cancer patients, the average age of those found with schistosome eggs at cystoscopy was 46.7 years (El-Bolkainy et al, 1981). In places where schistosomal infection is not endemic, the median age of bladder cancer patients is 69 years (1992). It is not yet known whether the carcinogenic effects of *S. haematobium* infections are due to chronic inflammation of the bladder epithelium or the release of chemical carcinogens from the eggs, such as *N*-nitroso compounds (Cheever, 1978; Tricker et al, 1991; Badawi et al, 1992). Infections with *S. mansoni* and *S. japonicum*, which primarily affect the liver and intestines, may increase hepatocellular carcinoma and colon cancer in developing countries. *Helicobacter pylori* infection, identified in many studies as a risk factor for gastric cancer (The Eurogast Study Group, 1993; Parsonnet, 1993), is associated in industrialized countries with low socio-economic status and crowded living conditions. In some developing countries, drinking water may be important as a source of infection. In Peru, *H. pylori* infection among children from Lima was associated with source of water (Klein et al, 1991).

RESEARCH PRIORITIES AND PREVENTION STRATEGIES

On the basis of existing evidence, it is clear that the water we drink contains a complex mixture of known or suspected carcinogenic substances, usually found at trace level concentrations (<10 ppb). The substances that are regularly present in nearly all water supplies form a small minority; for example, the THMs and, in particular, chloroform. Many epidemiological studies to date have relied mainly on differences in surrogate exposure variables; for example, the higher levels of synthetic organic chemicals in surface versus ground water, or chlorinated versus nonchlorinated waters. Based on these and other investigations, the following relationships have been suggested:

1. Inorganic arsenic (and possibly other trace metals) with cancer of several sites, including non-melanoma skin cancer, bladder, kidney, and lung
2. Synthetic organic chemicals (especially chlorination byproducts) with cancers of the urinary bladder and gastrointestinal tract, especially the rectum
3. Radon in water, by contributing to airborne levels in homes, with lung cancer
4. Asbestos or nitrates with cancers of the gastrointestinal tract, especially the stomach

For these waterborne substances, hypothesis-generating work, as represented by the large number of aggregate (ecological) studies, has already been adequately carried out. To improve our understanding of the important relationships, further case-comparison or cohort studies based on individual information are indispensable, especially using refined chemical measures of exposure and appropriate biomarkers whenever possible. However, in the absence of precise data on exposures that occurred twenty years or more in the past, three paths of epidemiological investigation are possible: (1) estimating past exposures to contaminants through the use of models that apply our current understanding of water chemistry to knowledge of historical sources and treatment modalities; (2) refinement and continued use of surrogate exposure data; and (3) studies of persons occupationally exposed to elevated concentrations of specific waterborne substances of concern, such as chloroform or arsenic. Although the last option is necessary to determine the carcinogenic potential of specific substances, and to quantify risk for standard setting, it cannot be the only approach taken. Certain types of drinking water expose some populations to a number of suspected carcinogens. Risk estimates based on exposure to individual compounds may not tell us much about the interactive effects with other aqueous chemicals or with other exposures. Only disaggregate studies of populations exposed to complex mixtures can help to determine whether the combined effects of these substances are additive, synergistic, antagonistic, or nonexistent.

Future epidemiological investigations should profit from a recognition of limitations of previous work. Specific areas include the following. (1) Studies relating individual exposure to individual risk of cancer are generally preferred to ecological studies. Except in selected circumstances, aggregate studies have already met their goals. (2) It is important to estimate continuous exposure for many decades in the past to account for latency of adult cancers. (3) Large sample sizes adequate to detect the putative small differences in risk are necessary. (4) Since the carcinogenic risk conferred by drinking water contaminants is likely to be relatively small, it is of utmost importance that studies be controlled for potentially confounding factors, such as occupation, diet, smoking, physical activity, and other risk factors contributing to the cancer site under consideration. (5) Better estimates of past exposure are needed, including more information on groundwater, types of treatment practices, presence and type of upstream discharges for surface sources, and surveillance of major chemical contaminants in water supplies. (6) Future investigations should collect and validate information on individual consumption of tap water and other fluids, including water used in cooking and in beverages such as coffee and tea. (7) Understanding of carcinogenic risks and mechanisms of action will be enhanced by analysis of body fluids to test for differences in levels of major water contaminants and their associated biomarkers among populations using water of differing quality.

Strategies to minimize exposure to water contaminants include various watershed protection programs and water treatment options, some of which are expensive and technologically complex. Pollution control and watershed management can limit sources of industrial, domestic, and agricultural pollution and should be a part of any strategy to minimize contamination of water sources. The use of alternate, unpolluted source waters can reduce exposures. However, this may not be an option because these sources are often unavailable or not economically feasible. Therefore, options to reduce chemical exposures are generally limited to the following: (1) Reduction of disinfectant by-products through application of alternate disinfection procedures or more selective use of existing disinfection methods; and (2) Removal of organic, inorganic, and particulate contaminants through use of more advanced water treatment technologies.

Chlorine has generally served us well and continues to be the most cost-effective disinfectant to prevent transmission of waterborne disease. The use of alternate disinfectants such as ozone, chlorine dioxide, and chloramine will reduce chlorinated by-products. However, their use may result in other potentially toxic by-products and may not be feasible or effective for all communities. Before alternative disinfectants are considered, their effectiveness and potential by-products must be fully evaluated. Changing the location of chlorination from the beginning of the water treatment process to the end, and reducing the amount of chlorine used, can lower the concentration of chlorinated by-products. However, caution is required to ensure this process does not increase microbial risk.

Concerns about cancer risks that may be associated with long-term exposure to disinfected water must be tempered with considerations of the benefits provided by water disinfection, especially for developing countries where infectious disease risks are great. Disinfection is the final barrier against transmission of waterborne pathogens, but it must not be the sole barrier. Source protection is required, and water filtration is necessary for all surface sources except those of unusually high quality. Properly designed and operated filtration plants make disinfection more effective by reducing microbiological contamination, turbidity, and other substances that exert chlorine demand and may interfere with the efficacy of the process. The amount of disinfectant required is also reduced, thereby lowering disinfection by-products. In general, the water treatment strategy for disinfection by-products is to either remove the precursor compounds before they react with the disinfectant or remove the by-products after they are formed.

Advanced water treatment processes, such as activated carbon adsorption, ion exchange, desalinization, and membrane microfiltration can be used to remove contaminants not usually removed during conventional water filtration/disinfection. These processes are usually designed for specific contaminants or classes of contaminants, but some processes also reduce or remove a wide range of organic and microbial contaminants. They are often expensive and complex to operate. Advanced treatment may therefore be an option only for wealthy, more technologically advanced communities. Where advanced treatment is feasible, chemical exposures from drinking water can be reduced. However, it is not possible at present to quantify the reduction in carcinogenic risks. Further epidemiological studies can help quantify the relative benefits of different levels of water treatment, but some communities may prefer not to wait for this information before reducing exposures to at least some of these contaminants.

REFERENCES

AL-DABBAGH S, FORMAN D, BRYSON D, et al. 1986. Mortality of nitrate fertiliser workers. Br J Ind Med 43:507–515.

ALAVANJA M, GOLDSTEIN I, SUSSER M. 1978. A case control study of gastrointestinal and urinary tract cancer mortality and drinking water chlorination. In: *Water Chlorination: Environmental Impact and Health Effects*, Jolley RL, Gorchev H, Hamilton DH,Jr. (eds). Vol 2. Ann Arbor, Mich: Ann Arbor Science, pp 395–409.

ANDERSEN A, GLATTRE E, JOHANSEN BV. 1993. Incidence of cancer among lighthouse keepers exposed to asbestos in drinking water. Am J Epidemiol 138:682–687.

ARMIJO R, COULSON AH. 1975. Epidemiology of stomach cancer in Chile—The role of nitrogen fertilizers. Int J Epidemiol 4:301–309.

ARMIJO R, GONZALEZ A, ORELLANA M, et al. 1981. Epidemiology of gastric cancer in Chile: II—Nitrate exposures and stomach cancer frequency. Int J Epidemiol 10:57–62.

ASCHENGRAU A, OZONOFF D, PAULU C, et al. 1993. Cancer risk and tetrachloroethylene (PCE) contaminated drinking water in Massachusetts. Arch Environ Health 48:284–292.

BADAWI AF, MOSTAFA MH, O'CONNOR PJ. 1992. Involvement of alkylating agents in schistosome-associated bladder cancer: the possible basic mechanisms of induction. Cancer Lett 63:171-188.

BAKER DB, GREENLAND S, MENDLEIN J, et al. 1988. A health study of two communities near the Stringfellow waste disposal site. Arch Environ Health 43:325–334.

BATES MN, SMITH AH, HOPENHAYN-RICH C. 1992. Arsenic ingestion and internal cancers: a review. Am J Epidemiol 135:462–476.

BATES MN, SMITH AH, CANTOR KP. 1995. Case-control study of bladder cancer and arsenic in drinking water. Am J Epidemiol 141:523–530.

BEAN JA, ISACSON P, HAHNE RMA, et al. 1982a. Drinking water and cancer incidence in Iowa: II. Radioactivity in drinking water. Am J Epidemiol 116:924–932.

BEAN JA, ISACSON P, HAUSLER WJ, et al. 1982b. Drinking water and cancer incidence in Iowa: I. Trends and incidence by source of drinking water and size of municipality. Am J Epidemiol 116:912–923.

BERESFORD SAA. 1983. Cancer incidence and reuse of drinking water. Am J Epidemiol 117:258–268.

BERESFORD SAA. 1985. Is nitrate in the drinking water associated with the risk of cancer in the urban UK? Int J Epidemoil 14:57–63.

BERG JW, BURBANK F. 1972. Correlations between carcinogenic trace metals in water supplies and cancer mortality. Ann NY Acad Sci 199:249–264.

BERGOGLIO RM. 1964. Mortalidad por cancer en zonas de aguas arsenicales de la Provincia de Cordoba, Republica Argentina. Pren Med Argent 51:994–998.

BOEING H, FRENTZEL-BEYME R, BERGER M, et al. 1991. Case-control study on stomach cancer in Germany. Int J Cancer 47:858–864.

BORGOÑO JM, GRIEBER R. 1971. Estudio epidemiologico del arsenicismo en la ciudad de Antofagasta. Rev Med Chil 99:702–707.

BRENNIMAN GR, VASILOMANOLAKIS-LAGOS J, AMSEL J, et al. 1980. Case-control study of cancer deaths in Illinois communities served by chlorinated or nonchlorinated water. In: *Water Chlorination: Environmental Impact and Health Effects*, vol. 3, Jolley RL, Brungs WA, Cumming RB (eds). Ann Arbor, Mich: Ann Arbor Science, pp 1043–1057.

BUCHER JR, HEJTMANCIK MR, TOFT JD,II, et al. 1991. Results and conclusions of the National Toxicology Program's rodent carcinogenicity studies with sodium fluoride. Int J Cancer 48:733–737.

BUDNICK LD, SOKAL DC, FALK H, et al. 1984. Cancer and birth defects near the Drake superfund site, Pennsylvania. Arch Environ Health 39:409–413.

BURK D, YIAMOUYIANNIS J. July 21, 1975. Fluoridation and cancer. Congressional Record.

BYERS VS, LEVIN AS, OZONOFF DM, et al. 1988. Association between clinical symptoms and lymphocyte abnormalities in a population with chronic domestic exposure to industrial solvent-contaminated domestic water supply and a high incidence of leukaemia. Cancer Immunol Immunother 27:77–81.

CANTOR KP. 1994. Water chlorination, mutagenicity, and cancer epidemiology. (Editorial) Am J Public Health 84:1211–1212.

CANTOR KP, HOOVER R, MASON TJ, et al. 1978. Associations of cancer mortality with halomethanes in drinking water. J Natl Cancer Inst 61:979–985.

CANTOR KP, HOOVER R, HARTGE P, et al. 1987. Bladder cancer, drinking water source, and tap water consumption: a case-control study. J Natl Cancer Inst 79:1269–1279.

CEBRIAN ME, ALBORES A, AGUILAR M, et al. 1983. Chronic arsenic poisoning in the north of Mexico. Hum Toxicol 2:121–133.

CHEEVER AW 1978. Schistosomiasis and neoplasia. (Guest editorial) J Natl Cancer Inst 61:13–18.

CHEN C-J, CHUANG Y-C, LIN T-M, et al. 1985. Malignant neoplasms among residents of a blackfoot disease-endemic area in Taiwan: high-arsenic artesian well water and cancers. Cancer Res 45:5895–5899.

CHEN C-J, CHUANG Y-C, YOU S-L, et al. 1986. A retrospective study on malignant neoplasms of bladder, lung, and liver in blackfoot disease endemic area in Taiwan. Br J Cancer 53:399–405.

CHEN C-J, WANG C-J. 1990. Ecological correlation between arsenic level in well water and age-adjusted mortality from malignant neoplasms. Cancer Res 50:5470–5474.

CHILVERS C. 1983. Cancer mortality and fluoridation of water supplies in 35 US cities. Int J Epidemiol 12:397–404.

CHILVERS C, INSKIP H, CAYGILL C, et al. 1984. A survey of dietary nitrate in well-water users. Int J Epidemiol 13:324–331.

CLARK CS, MEYER CR, GARTSIDE PS, et al. 1982. An environmental health survey of drinking water contamination by leachate from a pesticide waste dump in Hardeman County, Tennessee. Arch Environ Health 37:9–18.

COLLMAN GW, LOOMIS DP, SANDLER DP. 1991. Childhood cancer mortality and radon concentration in drinking water in North Carolina. Br. J Cancer 63:626–629.

CONFORTI PM, KANAREK MS, JACKSON LA, et al. 1981. Asbestos in drinking water and cancer in the San Francisco Bay area: 1969–1974 incidence. J Chronic Dis 34:211–224.

COTHERN CR, LAPPENBUSCH WL, MICHEL J. 1986. Drinking-water contribution to natural background radiation. Health Physics 50:33–47.

COTHERN DR, LAPPENBUSCH WL. 1983. Occurrence of uranium in drinking water in the U.S. Health Physics 45:89–99.

CRAGLE DL, SHY CM, STRUBA RJ, et al. A case-control study of colon cancer and water chlorination in North Carolina. In: *Water*

Chlorination: Chemistry, Environmental Impact and Health Effects, Vol 5, Jolley RL, Bull RJ, Davis WP, et al (eds). Chelsea, Mich: Lewis Publishers, Inc., pp 153–160.

CROSS FT, HARLEY NH, HOFMANN W. 1985. Health effects and risks from radon-222 in drinking water. Health Physics 48:649–670.

CRUMP KS, GUESS HA. 1982. Drinking water and cancer: review of recent epidemiological findings and assessment of risks. Annu Rev Public Health 3:339–357.

CUELLO C, CORREA P, HAENSZEL W, et al. 1976. Gastric cancer in Colombia, I: Cancer risk and suspect environmental agents. J Natl Cancer Inst 57:1015–1020.

CUTLER JJ, PARKER GS, ROSEN S, et al. 1986. Childhood leukemia in Woburn, Massachusetts. Public Health Rep 101:201–205.

CUZICK J, SASIENI P, EVANS S. 1992. Ingested arsenic, keratoses, and bladder cancer. Am J Epidemiol 136:417–421.

DEKRAAY WH. 1978. Pesticides and lymphoma in Iowa. J Iowa Med Soc 1978:50–53.

DELONG S. 1979. Drinking water and liver cell cancer. Chinese Med J 92:748–756.

DUTT MC, LIM HY, CHEW RKH. 1987. Nitrate consumption and the incidence of gastric cancer in Singapore. J Chem Toxicol 25:515–520.

EISENBRAND G, SPEIGELHALDER B, PREUSSMANN R. 1980 Nitrate and nitrite in saliva. Oncology 37:227–231.

EL-BOLKAINY MN, MOKHTAR NM, GHONEIM MA, et al. 1981. The impact of Schistosomiasis on the pathology of bladder carcinoma. Cancer 48:2643–2648.

THE EUROGAST STUDY GROUP. 1993. An international association between Helicobacter pylori infection and gastric cancer. Lancet 341:1359–1362.

FAGLIANO J, BERRY M, BOVE F, et al. 1990. Drinking water contamination and the incidence of leukemia: an ecologic study. Am J Public Health 80:1209–1212.

FLATEN TP. 1992. Chlorination of drinking water and cancer incidence in Norway. Int J Epidemiol 21:6–15.

FLATEN TP, BOLVIKEN B. 1991. Geographical associations between drinking water chemistry and the mortality and morbidity of cancer and some other diseases in Norway. Sci Total Environ 102:75–100.

FORMAN D, AL-DABBAGH S, DOLL R. 1985. Nitrates, nitrites and gastric cancer in Great Britain. Nature 313:620–625.

FRASER P, CHILVERS C. 1981. Health aspects of nitrate in drinking water. Sci Total Environ 18:103–116.

FRASER P, CHILVERS C, DAY M, et al. 1989. Further results from a census based mortality study of fertiliser manufacturers. Br J Ind Med 46:38–42.

FUORTES L, MCNUTT LA, LYNCH C. 1990. Leukemia incidence and radioactivity in drinking water in 59 Iowa towns. Am J Public Health 80:1261–1262.

GILLI G, CORRAO G, FAVILLI S. 1984. Concentrations of nitrates in drinking water and incidence of gastric carcinomas: first descriptive study of the Piemonte region, Italy. Sci Total Environ 34:35–48.

GOTTLIEB MS, CARR JK. 1982. Case-control cancer mortality study and chlorination of drinking water in Louisiana. Environ Health Perspect 46:169–177.

GOTTLIEB MS, CARR JK, MORRIS DT. 1981. Cancer and drinking water in Louisiana: colon and rectum. Int J Epidemiol 10:117–125.

GRIFFITH J, DUNCAN RC, RIGGAN WB, et al. 1989. Cancer mortality in U.S. counties with hazardous waste sites and ground water pollution. Arch Environ Health 44:69–74.

HAENSZEL W, KURIHARA M, LOCKE FB, et al. 1976. Stomach cancer in Japan. J Natl Cancer Inst 56:265–274.

HALLBERG GR. 1985. Agricultural chemicals and groundwater quality in Iowa: status report 1985. Cooperative Extension Service, Iowa State University.

HARRINGTON JM, CRAUN GF, MEIGS JW, et al. 1978a. An investigation of the use of asbestos cement pipe for public water supply and the incidence of gastrointestinal cancer in Connecticut, 1935–1973. Am J Epidemiol 107:96–103.

HARRINGTON JM, MIDDAUGH JP, MORSE DI, et al. 1978b. A survey of a population exposed to high concentrations of arsenic in well water in Fairbanks, Alaska. Am J Epidemiol 108:377–385.

HART RJ, WALTERS CL. 1983. The formation of nitrite and *N*-nitroso compounds in salivas in vitro and in vivo. Food Cosmet Toxicol 21:749–753.

HARTMAN PE. 1983. Nitrate/nitrite ingestion and gastric cancer mortality. Environ Mutagen 5:111–121.

HEATH CW, NADEL MR, ZACK MM, et al. 1984. Cytogenetic findings in persons living near the Love Canal. JAMA 251:1437–1440.

HESS CT, MICHEL J, HORTON TR, et al. 1985. The occurrence of radioactivity in public water supplies in the United States. Health Physics 48:553–586.

HESS CT, WEIFFENBACH CV, NORTON SA. 1983. Environmental radon and cancer correlations in Maine. Health Physics 45:339–348.

HOFF G, MOEN IE, MOWINCKEL P, et al. 1992. Drinking water and the prevalence of colorectal adenomas: an epidemiologic study in Telemark, Norway. Eur J Cancer Prev 1:423–428.

HOGAN MD, CHI P-Y, HOEL DG. 1979. Association between chloroform levels in finished drinking water supplies and various site-specific cancer mortality rates. J Environ Pathol Toxicol 2:873–887.

HOOVER RN, DEVESA S, CANTOR K, et al. 1991. Appendix F: Time trends for bone and joint cancers and osteosarcomas in the Surveillance, Epidemiology and End Results (SEER) Program, National Cancer Institute. In: *Review of Fluoride: Benefits and Risks.* Report of the Ad Hoc Subcommittee on Fluoride of the Committee to Coordinate Environmental Health and Related Programs, Washington, DC, Public Health Service, DHHS.

HOOVER RN, MCKAY FW, FRAUMENI JF. 1976. Fluoridated drinking water and the occurrence of cancer. J Natl Cancer Inst 57:757–768.

HOWE HL, WOLFGANG PE, BURNETT WS, et al. 1989. Cancer incidence following exposure to drinking water with asbestos leachate. Public Health Rep 104:251–256.

HRUDEY SE, SOSKOLNE CL, BERKEL J, et al. 1990. Drinking water fluoridation and osteosarcoma. Can J Public Health 81:415–416.

HUEPER WC. 1960. Cancer hazards from natural and artificial water pollutants. In: Faber HA, Bryson LJ (eds): Proceedings, Physiological Aspects of Water Quality, Washington, D.C., U.S. Public Health Service, pp 181–193.

IJSSELMUIDEN CB, GAYDOS C, FEIGHNER B, et al. 1992. Cancer of the pancreas and drinking water: a population-based case-control study in Washington County, Maryland. Am J Epidemiol 136:836–842.

INTERNATIONAL AGENCY FOR RESEARCH ON CANCER. 1978. IARC Monographs on the Evaluation of the Carcinogenic Risk of Chemicals to Humans, Volume 17: Some *N*-Nitroso Compounds, Lyon: IARC.

INTERNATIONAL AGENCY FOR RESEARCH ON CANCER. 1982. Inorganic fluorides. In: IARC Monographs on the Evaluation of Carcinogenic Risk of Chemicals to Humans, Volume 27: Some Aromatic Amines, Anthraquinones and Nitroso Compounds, and Inorganic Fluorides, Lyon, IARC, pp 235–303.

INTERNATIONAL AGENCY FOR RESEARCH ON CANCER. 1987. Overall Evaluations of Carcinogenicity: An Updating of IARC Monographs Volumes 1 to 42, Lyon, France: IARC.

INTERNATIONAL AGENCY FOR RESEARCH ON CANCER. 1991. IARC Monographs on the Evaluation of Carcinogenic Risks to Humans, Volume 52: Chlorinated Drinking-Water; Chlorination By-Products; Some Other Halogenated Compounds; Cobalt and Cobalt Compounds, Lyon: IARC.

ISACSON P, BEAN JA, LYNCH C. 1983. Relationship of cancer incidence rates in Iowa municipalities to chlorination status of drinking water. In: *Water Chlorination: Environmental Impact and Health Ef-*

fects, vol 4, Jolley RL, Brungs WA, Cotruvo JA, et al (eds). Ann Arbor, Mich.: Ann Arbor Science, pp 1353–1363.

ISACSON P, BEAN JA, SPLINTER R, et al. 1985. Drinking water and cancer incidence in Iowa: III, Association of cancer with indices of contamination. Am J Epidemiol 121:856–869.

JANERICH DT, BURNETT WS, FECK G, et al. 1981. Cancer incidence in the Love Canal area. Science 212:1404–1407.

JENSEN OM. 1982. Nitrate in drinking water and cancer in northern Jutland, Denmark, with special reference to stomach cancer. Ecotoxicol Environ Safety 6:258–267.

JOHNSON CJ, KROSS BC. 1990. Continuing importance of nitrate contamination of groundwater and wells in rural areas. Am J Ind Med 18:449–456.

JUHASZ L, HILL MJ, NAGY G. 1980. Possible relationship between nitrate in drinking water and incidence of stomach cancer. IARC Sci Publ 31:619–623.

KANAREK MS, CONFORTI PM, JACKSON LA, et al. 1980. Asbestos in drinking water and cancer incidence in the San Francisco Bay area. Am J Epidemiol 112:54–72.

KLEIN P, GRAHAM DY, GAILLOUR A, et al. 1991. Water source as risk factor for Helicobacter pylori infection in Peruvian children. Lancet 337:1503–1506.

KNIGHT T, FORMAN D, LEACH SA, et al. 1991. The N-nitrosoproline test as a measure of cancer risk in geographical comparison studies: results from Italy and an overall comparison. In: *Relevance to Human Cancer of N-Nitroso Compounds, Tobacco Smoke and Mycotoxins*, O'Neill IK, Chen J, Bartsch H (eds). Lyon, IARC, pp 146–151.

KNOX EG. 1985. Fluoridation of water and cancer: a review of the epidemiological evidence. Report of the Working Party on Fluoridation of Water and Cancer in London: Her Majesty's Stationery Office.

KOIVUSALO M, JAAKKOLA JJK, VARTIAINEN T, et al. 1994. Drinking water mutagenicity and gastrointestinal and urinary tract cancers: an ecological study in Finland. Am J Public Health 84:1223–1228.

KUZMA RJ, KUZMA CM, BUNCHER CR. 1977. Ohio drinking water source and cancer rates. Am J Public Health 67:725–729.

LAGAKOS SW, WESSEN BJ, ZELEN M. 1986. An analysis of contaminated well water and health effects in Woburn, Massachusetts. J Am Statist Assoc 81:583–596.

LAMPI P, HAKULINEN T, LUOSTARINEN T, et al. 1992. Cancer incidence following chlorophenol exposure in a community in southern Finland. Arch Environ Health 47:167–175.

LANGER AM, MAGGIORE CM, NICHOLSON WJ, et al. 1979. The contamination of Lake Superior with amphibole gangue minerals. Ann NY Acad Sci 330:549–572.

LAWRENCE CE, TAYLOR PR, TROCK BJ, et al. 1984. Trihalomethanes in drinking water and human colorectal cancer. J Natl Cancer Inst 72:563–568.

LEVY BS, SIGURDSON E, MANDEL J, et al. 1976. Investigating possible effects of asbestos in city water: surveillance of gastrointestinal cancer incidence in Duluth, Minnesota. Am J Epidemiol 103:362–368.

LILIENFELD DE, GALLO MA. 2,4-D, 2,4,5-T, and 2,3,7,8-TCDD. 1989. An overview. In: *Epidemiologic Reviews*, vol 11, Armenian HK, Gordis L, Gregg MB, et al (eds). Baltimore, Am J Epidemiol 28–58.

LYMAN GH, LYMAN CG, JOHNSON W. 1985. Association of leukemia with radium groundwater contamination. JAMA 254:621–626.

LYNCH CF, WOOLSON RF, O'GORMAN T, et al. 1989. Chlorinated drinking water and bladder cancer: Effect of misclassification on risk estimation. Arch Environ Health 44:252–259.

MACMAHON B, PRENTICE RL, ROGAN WJ, et al. 1986. Comments and rejoinder on Lagakos, Wessen, and Zelen article on contaminated well water and health effects in Woburn, Massachusetts. J Am Statist Assoc 81:597–614.

MAHONEY MC, NASCA PC, BURNETT WS, et al. 1991. Bone cancer incidence rates in New York State: Time trends and fluoridated drinking water. Am J Public Health 81:475–479.

MALLIN K. 1990. Investigation of a bladder cancer cluster in Northwestern Illinois. Am J Epidemiol 132, Suppl.1:S96–S106.

MASON TJ, MCKAY FW, MILLER RW. 1974. Asbestos-like fibers in Duluth water supply. JAMA 228:1019–1020.

MAYS CW, ROWLAND RE, STEHNEY AF. 1985. Cancer risk from the lifetime intake of Ra and U isotopes. Health Physics 48:635–648.

MCDONALD DB, SPLINTER RC. 1982. Long-term trends in nitrate concentration in Iowa water supplies. J Am Water Works Assoc 74:437–440.

MCGEEHIN MA, REIF JS, BECKER J, et al. 1993. A case-control study of bladder cancer and water disinfection methods in Colorado. Am J Epidemiol 138:492–501.

MCGUIRE SM, VANABLE ED, MCGUIRE MH, et al. 1991. Is there a link between fluoridated water and osteosarcoma? J Am Dent Assoc 122:38–45.

MEIGS JW, WALTER SD, HESTON JF, et al. 1980. Asbestos cement pipe and cancer in Connecticut 1955–1974. J Environ Health 42:187–191.

MILLETTE JR, CLARK PJ, STOBER J, et al. 1983a. Asbestos in water supplies of the United States. Environ Health Perspect 53:45–48.

MILLETTE JR, CRAUN GF, STOBER JA, et al. 1983b. Epidemiology study of the use of asbestos-cement pipe for the distribution of drinking water in Escambia County, Florida. Environ Health Perspect 53:91–98.

MIRVISH SS. 1994. Experimental evidence for inhibition of N-nitroso compound formation as a factor in the negative correlation between vitamin C consumption and the incidence of certain cancers. Cancer Res (Suppl) 54:1948s–1951s.

MIRVISH SS, GRANDJEAN AC, MOLLER H, et al.1992. N-Nitrosoproline excretion by rural Nebraskans drinking water of varied nitrate content. Cancer Epidemiol Biomark Prev 1:455–461.

MOLLER H, LANDT J, PEDERSEN E, et al. 1989. Endogenous nitrosation in relation to nitrate exposure from drinking water and diet in a Danish rural population. Cancer Res 49:3117–3121.

MORALES SUAREZ-VARELA M, LLOPIS GONZALEZ A, TEJERIZO PEREZ ML, et al. 1993. Concentration of nitrates in drinking water and its relationship with bladder cancer. J Environ Pathol Toxicol Oncol 12:229–236.

MORRIS RD, AUDET A-M, ANGELILLO IF, et al. 1992. Chlorination, chlorination by-products, and cancer: a meta-analysis. Am J Public Health 82:955–963.

MORTON W, STARR G, POHL D, et al. 1976. Skin cancer and water arsenic in Lane County, Oregon. Cancer 37:2523–2532.

MUSTACCHI P, SHIMKIN MB. 1958. Cancer of the bladder and infestation with Schistosoma hematobium. J Natl Cancer Inst 20:825–842.

NAJEM GR, LOURIA DB, LAVENHAR MA, et al. 1985. Clusters of cancer mortality in New Jersey municipalities; with special reference to chemical toxic waste disposal sites and per capita income. Int J Epidemiol 14:528–537.

NATIONAL INSTITUTES OF HEALTH. 1992. Cancer Statistics Review: 1973–1989, Bethesda, MD: National Cancer Institute. NIH Pub. No.92-2789.

NATIONAL RESEARCH COUNCIL. 1977a. Drinking Water and Health, vol 1. Washington, DC: National Academy of Sciences.

NATIONAL RESEARCH COUNCIL. 1977b. Inorganic solutes. In: Drinking Water and Health, vol 1. Washington, DC: National Academy of Sciences, pp 369–400.

NATIONAL RESEARCH COUNCIL. 1980. Epidemiological Studies. In: Drinking Water and Health, vol 3, Safe Drinking Water Committee (ed). Washington, DC: National Academy Press, pp 5–24.

NATIONAL RESEARCH COUNCIL. 1986. Drinking Water and Health, vol 6. Washington, DC: National Academy Press.

NATIONAL RESEARCH COUNCIL. 1987. Chemistry and toxicity of disinfection. In: Drinking Water and Health, vol 7, Safe Drinking Water Committee National Research Council (ed). Washington, DC: National Academy Press, pp 27–79.

NATIONAL RESEARCH COUNCIL. 1989. Selected issues in risk assessment. In: Drinking Water and Health, vol 9. Washington, DC: National Academy Press.

NAZAROFF WW, DOYLE SM, NERO AV, et al. 1987. Potable water as a source of airborne ^{222}Rn in U.S. dwellings: a review and assessment. Health Physics 52:281–295.

PAGE T, HARRIS RH, EPSTEIN SS. 1976. Drinking water and cancer mortality in Louisiana. Science 193:55–57.

PARSONNET J. 1993. Helicobacter pylori and gastric cancer. Gastroenterol Clin North Am 22:89–104.

POLISSAR L, SEVERSON RK, BOATMAN ES, et al. 1982. Cancer incidence in relation to asbestos in drinking water in the Puget Sound region. Am J Epidemiol 116:314–328.

POLISSAR L, SEVERSON RK, BOATMAN ES. 1984. A case-control study of asbestos in drinking water and cancer risk. Am J Epidemiol 119:456–471.

RADEMACHER JJ, YOUNG TB, KANAREK MS. 1992. Gastric cancer mortality and nitrate levels in Wisconsin drinking water. Arch Environ Health 47:292–297.

RAFNSSON V, GUNNARSDOTTIR H. 1990. Mortality study of fertiliser manufacturers in Iceland. Br J Ind Med 47:721–725.

RAM NM, CHRISTMAN RF, CANTOR KP. 1990. Significance and Treatment of Volatile Organic Compounds in Water Supplies. Chelsea, Mich.: Lewis Publishers.

SADLER TD, ROM WN, LYON JL, et al. 1984. The use of asbestos-cement pipe for public water supply and the incidence of cancer in selected communities in Utah. J Community Health 9:285–293.

SALG J. 1977. Cancer Mortality Rates and Drinking Water in 346 Counties of the Ohio River Valley Basin, University of North Carolina, Chapel Hill: Ph.D. Thesis.

SESHAN K. 1983. How are the physical and chemical properties of chrysotile asbestos altered by a 10-year residence in water and up to 5 days in simulated stomach acid? Environ Health Perspect 53:143–148.

SIERRA R, CHINNOCK A, OHSHIMA H, et al. 1993. In vivo nitrosoproline formation and other risk factors in Costa Rican children from high- and low-risk areas for gastric cancer. Cancer Epidemiol Biomark Prev 2:563–568.

SIGURDSON EE, LEVY BS, MANDEL J, et al. 1981. Cancer morbidity investigations: lessons from the Duluth study of possible effects of asbestos in drinking water. Environ Res 25:50–61.

SINGER PC, CHANG SD. 1989. Correlations between trihalomethanes and total organic halides formed during water treatment. J Am Water Works Assoc 81;8:61–65.

SMITH AH, HOPENHAYN-RICH C, BATES MN, et al. 1992. Cancer risks from arsenic in drinking water. Environ Health Perspect 97:259–267.

STEINDORF K, SCHLEHOFER B, BECHER H, et al. 1994. Nitrate in drinking water: a case-control study on primary brain tumours with an embedded drinking water survey in Germany. Int J Epidemiol 23:451–457.

STEVENS AA, MOORE LA, MILTNER RJ. 1989. Formation and control of non-trihalomethane disinfection by-products. J Am Water Works Assoc 81;8:54–60.

TAKACS S, GOMORI A. 1981. Nitrate content of drinking water and malignant tumors of the digestive organs and urinary bladder. Egeszsegrudomany 25:235–247.

THOMAS JE, BASSETT MT, SIGOLA LB, et al. 1990. Relationship between bladder cancer incidence, Schistosoma haematobium infection, and geographical region in Zimbabwe. Trans R Soc Trop Med Hyg 84:551–553.

TRICKER AR, MOSTAFA MH, SPIEGELHALDER B, et al. 1991. Urinary nitrate, nitrite and N-nitroso compounds in bladder cancer patients with schistosomiasis (bilharzia). In: *Relevance to Human Cancer of N-Nitroso Compounds, Tobacco Smoke and Mycotoxins*, O'Neill IK, Bartsch H (eds). IARC Sci Publ no. 105. Lyon: IARC. 178–181.

TSENG W-P. 1977. Effects and dose-response relationships of skin cancer and blackfoot disease with arsenic. Environ Health Perspect 19:109–119.

TSENG WP, CHU HM, HOW SW. 1968. Prevalence of skin cancer in an endemic area of chronic arsenicism in Taiwan. J Natl Cancer Inst 40:453–463.

U.S. ENVIRONMENTAL PROTECTION AGENCY. OFFICE OF PESTICIDE PROGRAMS. 1988. Pesticides in ground water data base: 1988 interim report. Washington, DC.

U.S. PUBLIC HEALTH SERVICE. COMMITTEE TO COORDINATE ENVIRONMENTAL HEALTH AND RELATED PROGRAMS SUBCOMMITTEE ON FLUORIDE. 1991. Review of Fluoride: Benefits and Risks, Washington, DC: Department of Health and Human Services.

VALEMA JP. 1987. Contaminated drinking water as a potential cause of cancer in humans. J Environ Sci Health [C] C5:1–28.

VIANNA NJ, POLAN AK. 1984. Incidence of low birth weight among Love Canal residents. Science 226:1217–1219.

VINCENT P, DUBOIS G, LECLERC H. 1983. Nitrates dans l'eau de boisson et mortalité par cancer. Rev Epidemiol Santé Publique 31:199–207.

WALTERS CL. 1980. The exposure of humans to nitrite. Oncology 37:289–296.

WALTERS CL, SMITH PLR. 1981. The effect of water-borne nitrate on salivary nitrite. Food Cosmet Toxicol 19:297–302.

WARD MH, MARK SD, CANTOR KP, et al. Drinking water nitrate and risk of non-Hodgkin's lymphoma. Epidemiology (in press).

WEISENBURGER DD. 1991. Potential health consequences of ground-water contamination by nitrates in Nebraska. In: *Nitrate Contamination*, Bogardi I, Kuzelka RD (eds). Berlin: Springer-Verlag, pp 309–315.

WIGLE DT. 1977. Cancer mortality in relation to asbestos in municipal water supplies. Arch Environ Health 32:185–189.

WILKINS JR III, COMSTOCK GW. 1981. Source of drinking water at home and site-specific cancer incidence in Washington County, Maryland. Am J Epidemiol 114:178–190.

WILKINS JR III, REICHES NA, KRUSE CW. 1979. Organic chemical contaminants in drinking water and cancer. Am J Epidemiol 110:420–447.

WU M-M, KUO T-L, HWANG Y-H, et al. 1989. Dose-response relation between arsenic concentration in well water and mortality from cancers and vascular diseases. Am J Epidemiol 130:1123–1132.

XU G, SONG P, REED PI. 1992. The relationship between gastric mucosal changes and nitrate intake via drinking water in a high-risk population for gastric cancer in Moping county, China. Eur J Cancer Prev 1:437–443.

YOUNG TB, KANAREK MS, TSIATIS AA. 1981. Epidemiologic study of drinking water chlorination and Wisconsin female cancer mortality. J Natl Cancer Inst 67:1191–1198.

YOUNG TB, WOLF DA, KANAREK MS. 1987. Case-control study of colon cancer and drinking water trihalomethanes in Wisconsin. Int J Epidemiol 16:190–197.

ZENG Y, OHSHIMA H, BOUVIER G, et al. 1993. Urinary excretion of nitrosamino acids and nitrate by inhabitants of high- and low-risk areas for nasopharyngeal carcinoma in southern China. Cancer Epidemiol Biomark Prev 2:195–200.

ZIERLER S, FEINGOLD L, DANLEY RA, et al. 1988. Bladder cancer in Massachusetts related to chlorinated and chloraminated drinking water: a case-control study. Arch Environ Health 43:195–200.

21 Diet and nutrition

WALTER C. WILLETT

The possibility that diet may be important in the cause and prevention of cancer in humans has received major attention only recently, despite longstanding knowledge that tumor incidence in animals can be influenced by nutritional manipulation (Tannenbaum, 1942). In an extensive review of causes of cancer, Doll and Peto (1981) suggested that 35% of cancers in the United States might be due to dietary factors. However, this estimate was highly uncertain, as they believed that the effect of diet could actually be as low as 10% or as high as 70%. The specific dietary factors that may cause or prevent cancer are also uncertain (Willett, 1994).

Possible relationships of diet with specific cancer sites are discussed within the appropriate chapters of this book. For this reason and because information on diet and cancer is rapidly evolving at present, this chapter will be devoted primarily to a review of approaches and methods that are used to study relationships of diet and cancer, including considerations of their strengths and limitations. Issues involved in epidemiological studies of diets are discussed in more detail elsewhere (Willett, 1987, 1989). This chapter will conclude by briefly noting some dietary factors that have received particular attention as being possibly related to risk of certain cancers.

GENERAL APPROACHES TO THE STUDY OF DIET AND CANCER

Hypotheses and supporting evidence relating dietary factors to cancer can be obtained from a variety of sources including in vitro studies, animal experiments, metabolic studies, epidemiological observations, and randomized trials.

In Vitro Studies and Animal Experiments

Many substances that cause mutations among microorganisms also cause cancer in animals and humans. This observation underlies the usefulness of microbial mutagenicity tests (such as the Ames test), which have been widely used to study components of human diets. These tests are attractive because results are available in only days and at a relatively low cost. Although these tests are helpful in directing human research and elucidating mechanisms of action, they cannot by themselves provide information that is directly relevant to humans (Ames et al, 1987). For example, many substances, such as asbestos, that influence the risk of cancer are not mutagenic. They may act, for example, by affecting the permeability of host tissues to carcinogens, by altering hormonal balances that inhibit or promote tumor growth, by changing the immune response of the host, or by affecting the rate of cell division, which in turn influences the likelihood that a mutation is reproduced. Because these functions are not all replicated in bacterial testing systems, false-negative and false-positive results will appear.

Experimental exposure of laboratory animals to substances that may influence cancer incidence is more likely to simulate the effect of a chemical or food on the incidence of cancer in humans. However, high doses of potential carcinogens that do not reflect human experience are generally used, and species often differ in the way their enzymatic systems activate or deactivate potentially carcinogenic substances. Such factors preclude direct extrapolation of findings from animal experiments to humans, even though they may provide critical direction for research and aid in the interpretation of epidemiological studies.

Metabolic and Biochemical Studies

Another approach to the study of diet and cancer involves metabolic or biochemical studies in humans. For example, Goldin and coworkers (1981) have studied the effect of diet on estrogen profiles, which in turn are thought to be related to the risk of breast cancer. These studies do not address the relations between dietary intake and the occurrence of cancer directly, but they can also be invaluable in the interpretation of other forms of evidence.

Epidemiological Studies

Epidemiological studies of diet and cancer constitute a relatively new area of research. Until recently, many nutritionists and epidemiologists have thought that the difficulties of assessing the diets of free-living human beings over extended periods of time made large-scale studies impossible. However, a number of useful approaches for assessing dietary intake have been developed. These include standardized questionnaires to assess intakes of foods from which nutrient intakes can be calculated, biochemical determinations of body tissues, and anthropometric measurements. Because the measurement of dietary intake is a central issue, these methods will be discussed in more detail later.

Correlation Studies. Until recently, epidemiological investigations of diet and cancer consisted largely of "ecological" or "correlational" studies—comparisons of disease rates in populations with the population per capita consumption of specific dietary factors. Usually the dietary information in such studies is based on "disappearance" data, meaning the national figures for food produced and imported minus the food that is exported, fed to animals, or otherwise not available for humans. Many of the correlations based on such information are remarkably strong; for example, the correlation between meat intake and incidence of colon cancer is 0.85 for men and 0.89 for women (Armstrong and Doll, 1975).

The use of international correlational studies to evaluate the relationships between diet and cancer has several strengths. Most importantly, the contrasts in dietary intake are typically very large. For example, within the United States, most individuals consume between 30% and 45% of their calories from fat (Willett et al, 1987), whereas the *mean* fat intake for populations in different countries varies from approximately 15% to 42% of calories (Goodwin and Boyd, 1987). Second, the average of diets for persons residing in a country are likely to be more stable over time than are the diets of individual persons within the country; for most countries the changes in per capita dietary intakes over a decade or two are relatively small. Finally, the cancer rates on which international studies are based are usually derived from relatively large populations and are therefore subject to only small random errors.

The primary problem of such correlational studies is that many potential determinants of cancer other than the dietary factor under consideration may vary between areas with a high and low incidence of disease. Such confounding factors can include genetic predisposition; other dietary factors, including the availability of total energy intake; and other environmental or lifestyle practices. For example, with few exceptions, such as Japan, countries with a low incidence of colon cancer tend to be economically undeveloped. Therefore, any variable related to industrialization will be similarly correlated with incidence of colon cancer. Indeed, the correlation between gross national product and colon cancer mortality rate is 0.77 for men and 0.69 for women (Armstrong and Doll, 1975). More complex analyses can be conducted of such ecological data that control for some of the potentially confounding factors. For example, McKeown-Eyssen and Bright-See (1985) have found that an inverse association of per capita dietary fiber intake and national colon cancer mortality rates persisted after adjustment for fat intake.

Most correlational studies are also limited by the use of disappearance data that are only indirectly related to intake and are likely to be of variable quality. For example, the higher "disappearance" of calories per capita for the United States compared with most countries is probably related in part to wasted food in addition to higher actual intake. In addition, aggregate data for a geographical unit as a whole may be only weakly related to the diets of those individuals at risk of disease. As an extreme example, the interpretation of correlational data regarding alcohol intake and breast cancer is complicated because, in some cultures, most of the alcohol is consumed by men, but it is the women who develop breast cancer. These issues of data quality can potentially be addressed by collecting information on actual dietary intake in a uniform manner from the population subgroups of interest. This has been done in a study conducted in 65 geographical areas within China that are characterized by an unusually large variation in rates of many cancers (Junshi et al, 1990).

Another serious limitation of the international correlational studies is that they cannot be independently reproduced, which is an important part of the scientific process. Although the dietary information can be improved and the analyses can be refined, the data will not really be independent even as more information becomes available over time; the populations, their diets, and the confounding variables will be the same. Thus, it is not likely that many new insights will be obtained from further ecological studies among countries.

The role of correlational studies in nutritional epidemiology is controversial. Clearly these analyses have stimulated much of the current research on diet and cancer and in particular they have emphasized the major differences in cancer rates among countries. Traditionally, such studies have been considered the weakest form of evidence, primarily due to the potential for confounding by factors that are difficult to measure and control (Kinlen, 1983). More recently, some have felt that such studies provide the strongest form of evidence for evaluating hypotheses relating diet to cancer (Hebert and Miller, 1988; Prentice et al, 1988). On balance, ecological studies have unquestionably been useful, but are far from conclusive regarding the relationships between dietary factors and disease and may sometimes be highly misleading.

Special Exposure Groups. Subgroups within a population that consume unusual diets provide an additional opportunity to learn about the relation of dietary factors and disease. These groups are often defined by religious or ethnic characteristics and provide many of the same strengths as ecological studies. In addition, the special populations often live in the same general environment as the comparison group, which may somewhat reduce the number of alternative explanations for any differences that might be observed. For example, the observation that colon cancer mortality in the largely vegetarian Seventh-Day Adventists is only about half that expected (Phillips et al, 1980) has been used to support the hypothesis that meat consumption is a cause of colon cancer.

Findings based on special exposure groups are subject to many of the same limitations as ecological studies. Many factors, both dietary and nondietary, are likely to distinguish these special groups from the comparison population. Thus, another possible explanation for the lower colon cancer incidence and mortality among the Seventh-Day Adventist population is that differences in rates are attributable to a lower intake of alcohol or higher vegetable consumption. Given the many possible alternative explanations, such studies may be particularly useful when a hypothesized association is *not* observed. For example, the finding that the breast cancer mortality rate among the Seventh-Day Adventists is not appreciably different from the rate among the general U.S. population provides fairly strong evidence that eating meat does not cause a major increase in the risk of breast cancer.

Migrant Studies and Secular Trends. Migrant studies have been particularly useful in addressing the possibility that the correlations observed in the ecological studies are due to genetic factors. For most cancers, populations migrating from an area with its own pattern of cancer incidence rates acquire rates characteristic of their new location (Staszewski and Haenszel, 1965; Adelstein et al, 1979; McMichael and Giles, 1988) although, for a few tumor sites, this change occurs only in later generations (Haenszel et al, 1972; Buell, 1973). Therefore, genetic factors cannot be primarily responsible for the large differences in cancer rates among these countries. Migrant studies may also be useful for examining the latency or relevant time of exposure.

Major changes in the rates of a disease within a population over time provide evidence that nongenetic factors play an important role in the etiology of that disease. In Iceland, for example, rates of breast cancer rose dramatically over the first half of this century (Bjarnason et al, 1974). These secular changes clearly demonstrate that environmental factors, possibly including diet, are primary causes of this disease, even though genetic factors may still influence who becomes affected given an adverse environment.

Case-Control and Cohort Studies. Many of the weaknesses of correlational studies are potentially avoidable in case-control studies (in which information about previous diet is obtained from diseased patients and compared to that of subjects without the disease) or cohort investigations (in which information on diet is obtained from disease-free subjects who are then followed to determine disease rates according to levels of dietary factors). In such studies, the confounding effects of other factors can be controlled either in the design (by matching subjects to be compared on the basis of known risk factors, or by restriction) or in the analysis (by any of a variety of multivariate methods) if information has been collected on the confounding variables. Furthermore, dietary information can be obtained for the individuals actually affected by disease, rather than using the average intake of the population as a whole.

Case-control studies generally provide information more efficiently and rapidly than cohort studies because the number of subjects is typically far smaller and no follow-up is necessary. However, it remains unclear whether consistently valid results can be obtained from case-control studies of dietary factors and disease because of the inherent potential for methodological bias. This potential for bias is not unique for diet but is likely to be unusually serious for several reasons. Due to the limited range of variation in diet within most populations and some inevitable error in measuring intake, realistic relative risks in most studies of diet and disease are likely to be modest, say on the order of 0.5 to 2.0. These relative risks may seem small, but would be quite important because the prevalence of exposure is high. Given typical distributions of dietary intake, these relative risks are usually based on differences in means for cases and controls (or those who become cases and those who remain non-cases in prospective studies) of only about 5%. Thus, a systematic error of even 3% or 4% can seriously distort such a relationship. In case-control studies it is easy to imagine that biases (due to selection or recall) of this magnitude could often occur, and it is extremely difficult to exclude the possibility that this degree of bias has occurred in any specific study. Hence, it would not be surprising if case-control studies of dietary factors provide inconsistent findings.

The selection of an appropriate control group for a study of diet and cancer is also usually problematic. One common practice is to use patients with another disease for comparison, with the assumption that the exposure under study is unrelated to the condition of this control group. However, because diet may influence the incidence of many diseases, it is often difficult to identify disease groups that are, with confidence, unrelated to the aspect of diet under investigation. A common alternative is to use a sample of persons from the general population as the control group. In many areas, particularly large cities, participation rates are low; it is now common for only 60% or 70% of eligible population controls to complete an interview (Hartge et al, 1984). Because diet is particularly associated with the level of general health consciousness, the diets of those who participate are likely to differ substantially from those who do not; unfortunately little information is available that directly bears on this issue.

The many potential opportunities for methodological bias in case-control studies of diet raise a concern that incorrect associations may frequently occur. So far, empirical evidence regarding the magnitude of these biases is limited. In two large prospective studies of diet and cancer, diet of patients with breast cancer and a sample of control patients were also assessed retrospectively. In one study, no evidence of recall bias was observed (Friedenreich et al, 1991), but in the other the combination of recall and selection bias did seriously distort associations with fat intake (Giovannucci, 1991). Even if many studies arrive at correct conclusions, distortion of true associations in a substantial percentage would produce an inconsistent body of published data, making a coherent synthesis difficult or impossible for a specific diet and cancer relationship. Methodological sources of inconsistency may be particularly troublesome in nutritional epidemiology becuase of the inherent biological complexity resulting from nutrient-nutrient interactions. Since the effect of one nutrient may depend on the level of another (which can differ between studies and may not have been measured), such interactions may result in apparently inconsistent findings in epidemiological studies. Thus, compounding biological complexity with methodological inconsistency may result in an uninterpretable literature. Existing data do not provide a clear answer as to whether consistent findings can be expected to accrue from case-control studies of diet. In studies of green and yellow vegetable intake in relation to lung cancer, remarkably consistent inverse associations have been found (Willett, 1990a). On the other hand, findings from case-control studies of fat intake in relation to breast cancer have been inconsistent (Howe et al, 1990).

Prospective cohort studies avoid most of the potential sources of methodological bias associated with case-control investigations. Because the dietary information is collected before the diagnosis of disease, illness cannot affect the recall of diet. Although losses to follow-up that vary by level of dietary factors can result in distorted associations in a cohort study, follow-up rates tend to be rather high because participants have already provided evidence of willingness to participate and they may also be followed passively by means of disease registries and vital record listings (Stampfer et al, 1984). In addition to being less susceptible to bias, prospective cohort studies provide the opportunity to obtain repeated assessments of diet over time and to examine the effects of diet on a wide variety of diseases, including total mortality, simultaneously.

The primary constraints on prospective studies of diet are practical. Even for common cancers such as those of the lung, breast, or colon, it is necessary to enroll tens of thousands of subjects. The use of structured, self-administered questionnaires has made studies of this size possible, although still expensive. For diseases of somewhat lower frequency, however, even very large cohorts will not accumulate a sufficient number of cases within a reasonable amount of time. Therefore, case-control studies will continue to play an important role in nutritional epidemiology. Given current uncertainty about measuring diets early in life, it is possible that neither study design will be able to address the influence of childhood diet on disease occurring decades later.

Controlled Trials

The most rigorous evaluation of a dietary hypothesis is the randomized trial, optimally conducted as a double-blind experiment. The principal strength of a randomized trial is that potentially distorting variables should be distributed at random between the treatment and control groups, thus minimizing the possibility of confounding by these extraneous factors. In addition, it is sometimes possible to create a larger contrast between the groups being compared by use of an active intervention. Such experiments among humans, however, are best justified after considerable nonexperimental data have been collected to ensure that benefit is reasonably probable and that an adverse outcome is unlikely. Experimental studies are particularly practical for evaluating hypotheses that minor components of the diet, such as trace elements or vitamins, can prevent cancer as these nutrients can be formulated into pills or capsules.

Even if feasible, randomized trials of dietary factors and disease are likely to encounter several limitations. The time between change in the level of a dietary factor and any expected change in the incidence of disease is typically uncertain. Therefore, trials must be of long duration, and usually one cannot eliminate the possibility that any lack of difference between treatment groups may be due to insufficient duration. Compliance with the treatment diet is likely to decrease during an extended trial, particularly if treatment involves a real change in food intake, and the control group may well adopt the dietary behavior of the treatment group if the treatment diet is thought to be beneficial. Such trends, which were found in the Multiple Risk Factor Intervention Trial of coronary disease prevention (Multiple Risk Factor Intervention Trial Research Group, 1982), may obscure a real benefit of the treatment.

A related potential limitation of trials is that participants who enroll in such studies tend to be highly selected on the basis of health consciousness and motivation. Therefore, it is possible that the subjects at highest potential risk on the basis of their dietary intake, and thus susceptible to intervention, are seriously underrepresented. For example, if low beta-carotene intake is thought to be a risk factor for lung cancer and a trial of beta-carotene supplementation is conducted among a health-conscious population that includes few individuals with low beta-carotene intake, one might see no effect simply because most members of the study population were already receiving the maximal benefit of this nutrient through their usual diet. In such an instance, it would be useful to measure dietary intake of beta-carotene before starting the trial. Because the effect of supplementation is likely to be greatest among those with low dietary intakes, it would be possible to exclude those with high intakes (the potentially nonsusceptibles) either before randomization or in sub-analyses at the conclusion of the study. This requires, of course, a reasonable measurement of dietary intake.

It is sometimes said that trials provide a better quantitative measurement of the effect of an exposure or treatment because the difference in exposure between groups is better measured than in an observational study. Although this contrast may at times be better defined in a trial (it is usually clouded by some degree of noncompliance), trials still usually produce an imprecise measure of the effect of exposure because of marginally adequate sample sizes and ethical considerations that require stopping soon after a statistically significant effect is seen. For example, with a *P*-value close to 0.05, the 95% confidence interval will extend from no effect to a strong effect that is usually implausible. In an observational study an ethical imperative to stop does not exist when statistical significance occurs; continued accumulation of data can provide increasing precision regarding the relation between exposure and disease. A trial can provide unique information on the latent period between change in an exposure and change in diet; since spontaneous changes in diet are typically not clearly demarcated in time, the estimation of latent periods for dietary effects will usually be difficult in observational studies.

Although all hypotheses would ideally be evaluated in randomized trials, this will sometimes be impossible for practical or ethical reasons. For example, our knowledge of the effects of cigarette smoking on risk of lung cancer is based on observational studies, and it is similarly unlikely that randomized trials could be conducted to examine the effect of alcohol use on human breast cancer risk. It remains unclear whether trials of sufficient size, duration, and degree of compliance can be conducted to evaluate many hypotheses that involve major behavioral changes in eating patterns, such as a reduction in fat intake (Michels and Willett, 1992).

MEASUREMENT OF DIET IN EPIDEMIOLOGICAL STUDIES

The complexity of the human diet represents a daunting challenge to anyone contemplating a study of its relation to cancer. The foods we consume each day contain literally thousands of specific chemicals, some known and well quantified, some characterized only poorly, and others completely undescribed and presently unmeasurable. In human diets, intakes of various components tend to be intercorrelated. With few exceptions, all individuals are exposed; for example, everyone eats fat, fiber, and vitamin A. Thus, dietary exposures can rarely be characterized as present or absent; rather they are continuous variables, often with rather limited range of variation between persons. Furthermore, individuals are generally not aware of the content of the foods that they eat; hence, the consumption of nutrients is usually determined indirectly. The chemicals that constitute our food can be described by the non-mutually exclusive categories given in Table 21–1.

TABLE 21–1. *Aspects of Diet Related to Cancer*

Category	*Examples*
Essential nutrients	Vitamins, specific fatty acids, amino acids, and minerals
Major energy sources	Proteins, carbohydrates, fats, and alcohol
Additives	Preservatives (nitrates, BHT, salt) and coloring and flavoring agents
Agricultural chemical contaminants	Pesticides, herbicides, fungicides, growth hormones
Microbial toxin contaminants	Aflatoxin
Inorganic contaminants	Cadmium, lead, polychlorinated biphenyls
Chemicals formed in cooking or processing of food	Heterocyclic amines from cooked meat
Natural toxins	Safrole (in natural root beer), pyrrolizidine alkaloid (in comfrey tea), hydrazines (in mushrooms)
Other natural compounds	Protease inhibitors, indoles, cholesterol

Nutrients versus Foods

Throughout nutrition in general and in much of the existing cancer literature, diet has usually been described in terms of its nutrient content. Alternatively, diet can be described in terms of foods or food groups. The primary advantage of representing diets as specific compounds, such as nutrients, is that such information can be directly related to our fundamental knowledge of biology. From a practical perspective, the exact structure of a compound must usually be known if it is to be synthesized and used for supplementation. In epidemiological studies, measurement of total intake of a nutrient (as opposed to using the contribution of only one food at a time) provides the most powerful test of a hypothesis, particularly if a number of foods each contribute only modestly to intake of that nutrient. For example, in a particular study it is quite possible that total fat intake could be clearly associated with risk of disease, whereas none of the contributions to fat intake by individual foods would be significantly related to disease on its own.

The use of foods to represent diet has several practical advantages when examining relationships with disease. Particularly when suspicion exists that some aspect of diet is associated with risk but a specific hypothesis has not been formulated, an examination of the relations of foods and food groups with risk of disease will provide a means to explore the data. Associations observed with specific foods may lead to a hypothesis relating to a defined chemical substance. For example, observations that higher intakes of green and yellow vegetables were associated with reduced rates of lung cancer led to the hypothesis that beta-carotene might protect DNA from damage caused by free radicals and singlet oxygen (Peto et al, 1981). The finding by Graham and coworkers (1978) that intake of cruciferous vegetables was inversely related to risk of colon cancer supported the suggestion that indole compounds contained in these vegetables may be protective (Wattenberg and Loub, 1978).

Even more seriously than the lack of a well-formulated hypothesis, the premature focus on a specific nutrient that turns out to have no relation with disease may lead to the erroneous conclusion that diet has no effect. Mertz (1984) has pointed out that foods are not fully represented by their nutrient composition, noting as an example that milk and yogurt produce different physiologic effects despite a similar nutrient content. Furthermore, the valid calculation of a nutrient intake from data on food consumption requires that reasonably accurate food composition information is available, which markedly constrains the scope of dietary chemicals that may be investigated because such information exists for only several dozen commonly studied nutrients.

Epidemiological analyses based on foods, as opposed to nutrients, are generally most directly related to dietary recommendations because individuals and institutions ultimately manipulate nutrient intake largely by their choice of foods. Even if the intake of a specific nutrient is convincingly shown to be related to risk of cancer, this is not sufficient information on which to make dietary recommendations. Because foods are an extremely complex mixture of different chemicals that may compete with, antagonize, or alter the bioavailability of any single nutrient contained in that food, it is not possible to predict with certainty the health effects of any food solely on the basis of its content of one specific factor. For example, there is concern that high intake of nitrates may be deleterious, particularly with respect to gastrointestinal cancer. However, the primary sources of nitrates in our diets are green, leafy vegetables, which, if anything, appear to be associated with reduced risk of cancer at several sites. Similarly, because of the high cholesterol content of eggs, their avoidance has received particular attention in diets aimed at reducing the risk of coronary heart disease; per capita consumption of eggs declined by 25% in the United States between 1948 and 1980 (Welsh and Marston, 1982). However, eggs are more than cholesterol capsules; they provide a rich source of essential animo acids and micronutrients and are relatively low in saturated fat. It is thus difficult to predict the net effect of egg consumption on risk of coronary heart disease, much less the effect on overall health without empirical evidence.

Given the strengths and weaknesses of using nutrients or foods to represent diet, it appears that an optimal approach to epidemiological analyses will employ both. In this way, a potentially important finding is least likely to be missed. Moreover, the case for causality is strengthened when an association is observed with overall intake of a nutrient and also with more than one food source of that nutrient, particularly when the food sources are otherwise different. This provides, in some sense, multiple assessments of the potential for confounding by other nutrients; if an association was observed for only one food source of the nutrient, other factors contained in that food would tend to be similarly associated with disease. As an example, the hypothesis that alcohol intake causes breast cancer was strengthened by observing not only an overall association between alcohol intake and breast cancer risk, but also by independent associations with both beer and liquor intake, thus making it less likely that some factor other than alcohol in these beverages was responsible for the increased risk.

One practical drawback of using foods to represent

diet is their large number and complex, often reciprocal, interrelationships that are largely due to individual behavioral patterns. Many reciprocal relationships emerge upon perusal of typical data sets; for example, eaters of dark bread tend not to eat white bread, margarine users tend not to eat butter, and skim milk users tend not to use whole milk. This complexity is, of course, one of the reasons to compute nutrient intakes that summarize the contributions of all foods.

An intermediate solution to the problem posed by the complex interrelationships among foods is to utilize food groups or to compute the contribution of nutrient intake from various food groups. For example, Manousos and coworkers (1983) combined the intakes of foods from several predefined groups to study the relation of diet with risk of colon cancer; they observed increased risk among subjects with high meat intake and with low consumption of vegetables. The computation of nutrient intakes from different food groups is illustrated by a prospective study among British bank clerks conducted by Morris and coworkers (1977), who observed an inverse relation between overall fiber intake and risk of coronary heart disease. It is well recognized that fiber is an extremely heterogeneous collection of substances and that the available food composition data for specific types of fiber is quite incomplete. Therefore, these authors computed fiber intake separately from various food groups and found that the entire protective effect was attributable to fiber from grains; fiber from fruits or vegetables was not associated with risk of disease. This analysis both circumvents the inadequacy of food composition databases, and provides information in a form that is directly useful to individuals faced with decisions regarding choices of foods.

In general, maximal information will be obtained when analyses are conducted at the levels of nutrients, foods, and food groups.

The Dimension of Time

The assessment of diet in studies of cancer incidence is further complicated by the dimension of time. Because our understanding of the pathogenesis of most cancers is limited, considerable uncertainty exists about the period in time before diagnosis for which diet might be relevant. For some cancers, aspects of diet may be important during childhood even though the disease occurs decades later. For other cancers, it has been suggested that diet may act as a promoting or inhibiting factor; thus intake over a continuous period up to just prior to diagnosis may be important. Ideally, data on dietary intake at different points prior to diagnosis could help to resolve these issues. However, individuals rarely make clear changes in their diet at identifiable points in time; more typically, eating patterns evolve over periods of years. Thus, epidemiologists are usually forced to direct questions about diet to a period several years before diagnosis of cancer with the hope that diet at this point in time will represent, or at least be correlated with, diet during the critical period in cancer development. Fortunately, diets of individuals do tend to be correlated from year to year, so that some imprecision in identification of critical periods of exposure may not be serious. For most nutrients, correlations for repeated assessments of diet at intervals from one to about 10 years tend to be on the order of 0.6 to 0.7 (Willett et al, 1985; Rohan and Potter, 1984; Byers et al, 1987), with decreasing correlations over longer intervals (Byers et al, 1983). For scientists accustomed to measurements made under highly controlled conditions in a laboratory, this may seem like a low degree of reproducibility. However, these correlations are similar to other biological measurements made in free-living populations, such as serum cholesterol (Shekelle et al, 1981) and blood pressure (Rosner et al, 1977).

Even though diets of individuals tend to have a strong element of consistency over intervals of years, they are characterized by marked variation from day to day (Beaton et al, 1979). This variation differs from nutrient to nutrient, being moderate for total energy intake, but extreme for cholesterol and vitamin A. For this reason, even perfect information about diet on any single day or the average of a small number of days will poorly represent long-term average intake, which is likely to be more relevant to cancer etiology.

General Methods of Dietary Assessment

Three general approaches have been used to assess dietary intake: information about intake of foods that can be used directly or to calculate intake of nutrients, biochemical measurements of blood or other body tissues that provide indicators of diet, and measures of body dimensions or composition that reflect the long-term effects of diet. Since the interpretation of data on diet and cancer is heavily influenced by the methods used to assess diet, features of these methods and their limitations will be considered.

Methods Based on Food Intake

Short-term recall and diet records. The 24-hour recall, in which subjects are asked to report their food intake during the previous day, has been the most widely used dietary assessment method. It has been the basis of most national surveys, including NHANES, and numerous prospective studies of coronary heart disease. Interviews are conducted by nutritionists or trained interviewers, usually using visual aids such as food models or shapes to obtain data on quantities of foods. The 24-hour recall requires about 10 to 20 minutes for an experienced interviewer; although usually conducted in person, it has also been done by telephone using a two-dimensional chart that is mailed beforehand to assist in the estimation of portion sizes (Posner et al, 1982). This method has the advantages of requiring no training or literacy and minimal effort on the part of the participant.

Dietary records or food diaries are detailed meal-by-meal recordings of types and quantities of foods and beverages consumed during a specified period, typically 3 to 7 days. Ideally, subjects weigh each portion of food before eating, although this is frequently impossible for all meals. Alternatively, household measures can be used to estimate portion sizes. The method places a considerable burden upon the subject, thus limiting its application to those who are literate and highly motivated. In addition, the effort involved in keeping diet records may increase awareness of food intake and induce an alteration in diet. However, diet recording has the distinct advantages of not depending on memory and allowing direct measurements of portion sizes.

The validity of 24-hour recalls has been assessed by observing the actual intake of subjects in a controlled environment and interviewing them the next day. In such a study, Karvetti and Knuts (1985) observed that subjects both erroneously recalled foods that were not actually eaten and omitted foods that were eaten; correlations between nutrients calculated from observed intakes with calculations from the recalled information ranged from 0.58 to 0.74. In a similar study among elderly persons, Madden and coworkers (1976) found correlations ranging from 0.28 to 0.87. Relatively few validation studies have been conducted of diet recordings. In a recent comparison of nitrogen intake calculated from diet records, with intake based on analyses of replicate meals, Bingham and Cummings (1985) found a correlation of 0.97.

The most serious limitation of the 24-hour recall method is that dietary intake is highly variable from day to day. Diet records reduce the problem of day-to-day variation because the average of a number of days is used. For nutrients that vary substantially, however, even a week of recording will still not provide an accurate estimate of an individual's intake (Beaton et al, 1979). The variability in intake of specific foods is even greater than for nutrients (Salvini et al, 1989), so that only very commonly eaten foods can be studied by this method. The problem of day-to-day variation is not an issue if the objective of a study is to estimate a mean intake for a population, as might be the goal in a correlational study. However, in case-control or cohort investigations, accurate estimation of individual intakes is necessary.

Practical considerations and issues of study design further limit the application of short-term recall and diet record methods in epidemiological studies. Because they provide information on current diet, their use will typically be inappropriate in case-control studies because the relevant exposure will have occurred earlier and diet may have changed as a result of the cancer or its treatment. A few exceptions may occur, such as in the case of very early tumors or premalignant lesions. While the average of multiple days of 24-hour recalls or diet recording could theoretically be used in prospective studies of diet and cancer, the costs are prohibitive because of the large numbers of subjects required and substantial expense involved in collecting this information and processing it. These methods, however, can play an important role in the validation or calibration of other methods of dietary assessment that are more practical for epidemiological studies.

Food frequency questionnaire. Because short-term recall and diet record methods are generally expensive, unrepresentative of usual intake, and inappropriate for assessment of past diet, investigators have sought alternative methods for measuring long-term dietary intake. Burke developed a detailed dietary history interview that attempted to assess an individual's usual diet; this included a 24-hour recall, a menu recorded for 3 days, and a checklist of foods consumed over the preceding month. This method was time-consuming and expensive because a highly skilled professional was needed for both the interview and processing of information. The checklist, however, was the forerunner of the more structured dietary questionnaires in use today. During the 1950s, Stephanik and Trulson (1962), Heady, (1961), Wiehl and Reed (1960), and Marr (1971) developed food frequency questionnaires and evaluated their role in dietary assessment. Heady, using diet records collected by British bank clerks, demonstrated that the *frequencies* with which foods were used correlated highly with the total *weights* of the same foods consumed over a several-day period, thus providing the theoretical basis for the food frequency method. Multiple investigators have converged toward the use of food frequency questionnaires as the method of dietary assessment best suited for most epidemiological studies of diet and cancer. During recent years substantial refinement, modification, and evaluation of food frequency questionnaires have occurred, so that data derived from their use has become considerably more interpretable.

The basic food frequency questionnaire consists of two components: a food list and a frequency response section for subjects to report how often each food was eaten. Questions related to further details of quantity and composition may be appended. A basic decision in designing a questionnaire is whether the objective is to measure intake of a few specific foods or nutrients, or whether a comprehensive assessment of dietary intake is desired. A comprehensive assessment is generally desirable whenever possible. It is often impossible to anticipate at the beginning all the questions regarding diet that will appear important at the end of a study; a highly restricted food list may not have included an item that is, in retrospect, important. Furthermore, total food intake, represented by energy consumption, may be related to disease outcome and thus confound the effects of specific nutrients or foods. Even if total energy intake is not related to a disease outcome, adjustment for total intake may increase the accuracy of specific nutrient measurements (Willett and Stampfer, 1986). Nevertheless, epidemiological practice is usually a compromise between the ideal and reality, and it may simply not be possible to include a comprehensive diet assessment in a particular interview or questionnaire, especially if diet is not the primary focus of the study.

Since diets tend to be reasonably correlated from year to year, most investigators have asked subjects to describe their frequency of using foods in reference to the preceding year. This provides a full cycle of seasons so that, in theory, the responses should be independent of the time of year. In case-control studies, the time frame could be in reference to a period or a specified number of years previously.

Typically, investigators have provided a multiple-choice response format, with the number of options usually ranging from five to ten. Another approach is to use an open-ended format and provide subjects the option of answering in terms of frequency per day, week, or month (Block et al, 1986). In theory, an open-ended frequency response format might provide for some enhanced precision in reporting because the frequency of use is truly a continuous rather than a categorical variable. However, it is unlikely that the overall increment in precision is large, because the estimation of the frequency a food is used is inherently an approximation.

Several options exist for collecting additional data on serving sizes. The first is to collect no additional information on portion sizes at all; that is, to use a simple frequency questionnaire. A second possibility is to specify a portion size as part of the question on frequency; for example, to ask how often a *glass* of milk is consumed rather than only how often milk is consumed, which has been termed a semiquantitative food frequency questionnaire. A third alternative is to include an additional question for each food to describe the usual portion size, in words (Block et al, 1986), using food models (Morgan et al, 1978), or pictures of different portion sizes (Hankin et al, 1983). Because most of the variation in intake of a food is explained by frequency of use rather than differences in serving sizes, several investigators have found that portion size data are relatively unimportant (Samet et al, 1984; Pickle and Hartman, 1985; Block et al, 1990). Cummings and coworkers (1987) found that adding questions on portion sizes to a simple frequency questionnaire only slightly improved estimation of calcium intake; others have found that the use of food models in an in-person interview did not increase the validity of a self-administered, semi-quantitative food frequency questionnaire (Hernandez-Avila et al, 1988). These findings have practical implications because the cost of data collection by mail or telephone is far less than the cost of personal interviews, which are necessary if food models are to be used for assessing portion sizes. Cohen and coworkers (1990) also found that the portion size information included in the Block questionnaire added only slightly to validity assessed by comparison with diet records (average correlation 0.41 without portion sizes and 0.43 with portion sizes).

Food frequency questionnaires are extremely practical in epidemiological applications because they are easy for subjects to complete, often as a self-administered form. Processing is readily computerized and inexpensive, so that even prospective studies involving tens of thousands of subjects are feasible.

Validity of Dietary Assessment Methods

The interpretation of epidemiological data on diet and cancer depends directly on the validity of the methods used to measure dietary intake. This is particularly true when no association is found because one possible explanation could be that the method used to measure diet was not able to discriminate among persons. During the past 10 years a substantial body of evidence has accumulated regarding the validity of food frequency questionnaires, which has been the method most commonly used in epidemiological studies.

In evaluating the validity of a dietary assessment method, the choice of a standard for comparison is a critical issue. As for all variables, no perfect standard exists. Thus, a desirable feature for the comparison method is that its errors be independent from the method being evaluated so that an artificial correlation will not be observed. For this reason, biochemical indicators of diet are probably the optimal standard. Their greatest limitation is that markers of diet do not exist for most of the nutrients of current interest, such as total fat, fiber, and sucrose intake. Moreover, the available biochemical indicators of diet are likely to be quite imprecise measures of diet because they are influenced by many factors such as differences in absorption and metabolism, short-term biological variation, and laboratory measurement error. However, the capacity to demonstrate a correlation between a questionnaire estimate of nutrient intake and a biochemical indicator provides useful qualitative evidence of validity. Such correlations have been reported for questionnaire estimates of dietary carotene, vitamin E, vitamin B-6, and omega-3 fatty acids (see Table 21–2).

Validation studies of dietary questionnaires have also been conducted by comparing computed intakes with those based on other dietary assessment methods. Among the possible comparison methods, diet records are particularly attractive because they do not depend on memory and, when scales are used to assess portion sizes, do not depend on perception of amounts of foods eaten. Several of the most comprehensive validation studies involving comparisons of questionnaires completed at about a 1-year interval, before and after multiple diet records collected during the intervening months, are summarized in Table 21–3 (Willett et al, 1985; Pietinen et al, 1988a,b; Block et al, 1990; Rimm et al, 1992; Goldbohm et al, 1995). Similar degrees of misclassification were seen in these studies; for questionnaires completed at the end of the 1-year recording of diet (which corresponds to the time frame of the questionnaires), correlations adjusted for total energy intake tended to be mainly between 0.5 and 0.7.

Although, the degree of measurement error associated with nutrient estimates calculated from food frequency questionnaires appears to be similar to that for many epidemiological measures, these errors will lead to important underestimates of relative risks. Less commonly appreciated, the errors will also result in observed confidence intervals that are inappropriately narrow; this is of particular concern when no association is seen because the entire interest is then in the range of possible relative risks that are reasonably excluded by the data. In part generated by the interest in diet and cancer and the recognized issue of measurement error in assessing dietary intake, considerable effort has been directed to the development of methods that provide corrected estimates of relative risks and confidence intervals based on quantitative assessments of measurement error (Byars and Gail, 1989; Willett, 1989a; Rosner et al, 1992). Thus, validation studies of dietary questionnaires can provide important estimates of error that can be used to quantitatively interpret the influence of error on observed associations. Based on such analyses, it can be shown that important associations will generally not be missed by typical dietary questionnaires (Rosner et al, 1989), although sample sizes for studies will need to be several times larger than those estimated assuming that measurement error did not exist (Walker and Blettner, 1985).

Caution is necessary when interpreting validation studies when the standard method is based on calculated nutrient intakes, such as diet records. For nutrients that vary substantially from one specimen of a food to another, the calculated values may be highly correlated

TABLE 21–2. *Comparison of Food Frequency Questionnaires with Biochemical Indicators of Diet*

	Subjects	*r*
Dietary carotene vs plasma total carotenoid, plasma beta-carotene		
Willett et al, 1983	59 men and women	0.35[a]
Russell-Briefel et al, 1985	187 men	0.25
Stryker et al, 1988	137 men/193 women	0.53/0.51[a]
Coates et al, 1991	50 nonsmoking/41 smoking women	0.43/0.23[b]
Ascherio et al, 1992	121 men/186 women	0.34/0.30[ac]
Jacques et al, 1993[d]	57 men/82 women	0.37[e]
Dietary vitamin A vs Plasma retinol		
Ascherio et al, 1992	121 men/186 women	0.25/0.08[b,c]
Dietary vitamin E vs Plasma alpha-tocopherol		
Willett et al, 1983	59 men and women	0.34[a]
Stryker et al, 1988[d]	137 men/186 women	0.53/0.51[a]
Ascherio et al, 1992[d]	121 men/186 women	0.51/0.41[b,c]
Dietary vitamin D vs Plasma vitamin D		
Jacques et al, 1993[d]	57 men/82 women	0.35[f]
Vitamin B_6 intake vs Plasma pyridoxal phosphate		
Willett et al, 1985	94 men/25 women	0.37/0.39
Selhub et al, 1993[d]	457 men/703 women	0.51
Vitamin B_{12} intake vs Plasma vitamin B_{12}		
Jacques et al, 1993	57 men/82 women	0.35[e]
Folate intake vs Plasma folate		
Jacques et al, 1993	57 men/82 women	0.63[e]
Selhub et al, 1993	457 men/703 women	0.56
Vitamin C intake vs Plasma total vitamin C		
Jacques et al, 1993	57 men/82 women	0.43[e]
Saturated fat intake vs Serum cholesterol		
Sacks et al, 1986	19 men and women	0.54
Trans fatty acid intake vs Adipose saturated fat		
London et al, 1991	115 women	0.51[h]
Hunter et al, 1992	118 men	0.0.34[h]
Dietary N-3 fatty acids from marine sources vs Plasma phospholipid eicosapentaenoic acid, adipose N-3 fatty acid		
Silverman et al, 1990	42 men	0.54
London et al, 1991	115 women	0.48[h]
Hunter et al, 1992	118 men	0.0.49[h]
Dietary linoleic acid vs Serum cholesterol, subcutaneous fat aspirate		
Sacks et al, 1986[g]	19 men and women	−0.51
London et al, 1991	115 women	0.35[h]
Hunter et al, 1992	118 men	0.37[h]

[a]Adjusted for caloric intake and plasma lipids.

[b]Adjusted for caloric and alcoholic intake, age, body mass index, plasma lipids, use of medications, supplementary vitamin A intake, and number of cigarettes smoked per day for smokers.

[c]Includes nonsmokers only (110 men/162 women).

[d]Includes supplements.

[e]Adjusted for caloric intake, sex, age.

[f]Adjusted for caloric intake, sex, age, plasma cholesterol concentration.

[g]Subjects were participants in a dietary intervention trial: change in diet was correlated with change in serum cholesterol.

[h]Percentage of fat.

TABLE 21–3. *Comparison of Food Frequency Questionnaires with other Dietary Assessment Methods*

Source	*Population*	*Comparison Methods*	*Interval between Methods*	*Reference Period*	*Range of Correlations*	*Comments*
Willett et al (1985)	Registered nurses (n = 194)	Diet record	1 month–1 year	Previous year	0.36 Vitamin A without supplements to 0.75 vitamin C	
Pietinen et al (1988b)	Finnish men (n = 189)	Twelve 2-day diet records (vs 273-item questionnaire)	1–6 months	1 year	0.51 vitamin A to 0.73 polyunsaturated fat	Adjustment for energy had little effect on correlations
Block et al (1990)	260	Three 4-day diet records	1–12 months	6 months	0.37 vitamin A to 0.74 vitamin C, with supplements average = 0.55	Correlations were similar in low fat and usual diet group. Variable portion sizes added little to correlations
Rimm et al (1992)	127 U.S. health professionals	Two 1-week diet records	1–12 months	1 year	0.28 for iron to 0.86 for vitamin C with supplements, average = 0.59	Mean correlation increased to 0.65 with adjustment for variation in diet records
Goldbohm et al (1995)	59 men 48 women	Three 3-day diet records	3–15 months	1 year	0.33 for B-1 to 0.75 for polyunsaturated fat, average = 0.64	Adjustment for sex and energy intake had little effect except for fat intake, changing from 0.72 to 0.52

Source: From Willett, 1989.

because each of the foods is measured well by methods, but neither method is actually measuring the nutrient well. This can occur when the nutrient contents of the food vary greatly with the soil on which it was grown or raised, as is true for selenium, or when the nutrient is sensitive to degradation during processing or storage.

BIOCHEMICAL INDICATORS OF DIET

The use of biochemical measurements made on blood or other tissues to indicate intake of a nutrient is attractive because it does not depend on the memory or knowledge of the subject. Furthermore, such measurements can be made in retrospect; for example, using blood specimens that have been collected and stored for other purposes.

Choice of Tissues for Analysis

Most commonly, serum or plasma has been used in epidemiological studies to measure biochemical indicators of diet. However, consideration should also be given to red blood cells, subcutaneous fat, hair, and nails. The choices should be governed by the ability of the tissue to reflect dietary intake of the factor of interest, the time-integrating characteristics of the tissue, practical considerations in collecting, transporting and storing the specimen, and cost. These considerations are examined in detail elsewhere for a number of dietary factors (Hunter, 1989); some general comments are provided here.

Red Blood Cells. For a number of dietary factors, red cells are less sensitive to short-term fluctuations in diet than plasma or serum and may thus provide a better index of long-term exposure. Nutrients that can be usefully measured in red cells include fatty acids, folic acid, and selenium.

Subcutaneous Fat. Composed primarily of fatty acids, the adipose tissue turns over slowly among individuals with relatively stable weight. For at least some fatty acids, the half-life is on the order of 600 days, which makes this an ideal indicator of long-term diet in epidemiological studies. Fat-soluble vitamins such as retinol, vitamin E, and carotenoids are also measurable in subcutaneous fat, although their relations to diet are yet to be clearly established.

Hair and Nails. Hair and nails incorporate many elements into their matrix during formation and for many heavy metals these may be the tissues of choice because these elements tend to be rapidly cleared from the blood. Nails appear to be the optimal tissue for the assessment of long-term selenium intake because of their capacity to integrate exposure over time (Morris et al, 1983). Because the hair and nails can be cut at various times after formation (a few weeks for hair close to the scalp and approximately one year for the great toe), an index of exposure can be obtained that may be little affected by recent experiences. This can be a particular advantage in the context of a case-control study of diet and cancer. Contamination poses the greatest problem for measurements in hair due to its intense exposure to the environment and great surface area; these problems are generally much less for nails but still need to be considered.

Limitations of Biochemical Indicators

Although the use of biochemical indicators for assessing diet is attractive, no practical indicators exist for many of the dietary factors implicated in the etiology of cancer. Even when tissue levels of a nutrient can be measured, these levels are often highly regulated and thus reflect dietary intake poorly; blood retinol and cholesterol are good examples. Just as with dietary intake, the blood levels of some nutrients fluctuate substantially over time, so that one measurement may not provide a good reflection of long-term intake. Furthermore, experience has provided sobering evidence that the tissue levels of many nutrients can be affected by the presence of cancer, even several years prior to diagnosis (Wald et al, 1986), rendering the use of many biochemical indicators treacherous in most case-control studies. Despite these limitations, careful application of biochemical indicators can provide unique information about dietary intake, particularly for nutrients that cannot be accurately calculated from data on food intake.

ANTHROPOMETRY AND MEASURES OF BODY COMPOSITION

The influence of energy balance at various times in life is likely to have important effects on the incidence of some cancers. Energy balance is better reflected by measurements of body dimensions and composition than by assessments based on the difference between energy intake and expenditure (largely physical activity) because both of these variables are measured with considerable error (Willett, 1990).

The most common use of anthropometric measurements is in the calculation of obesity using either indices such as Quetelet Index or Body Mass Index (weight divided by the second power of height), or relative weight (weight standardized for height). Remarkably valid estimates of weight and height can be obtained even by questioning (Stunkard and Albaun, 1981), including their recall for several decades earlier (Rhoads and Kagan, 1979). Thus, estimates of obesity can be obtained easily for large prospective investigations or retrospectively in the context of case-control studies. The major limitation of obesity estimates based on height and weight is that an assessment of weight cannot differentiate between fat and lean body mass, most importantly muscle and bone. For this reason, these are imperfect measures of obesity. Until recently, studies of the validity of Body Mass Index (BMI) as a measure of obesity have used as a "gold standard" body fat expressed as a percent of total weight, usually determined by underwater weighing. However, BMI is actually a measure of fat mass adjusted for height rather than a measure of percent body fat. When fat mass, determined from densitometry, is adjusted for height and used as the standard, the correlation with BMI is approximately 0.90, indicating a substantially higher degree of validity than has generally been appreciated (Spiegelman et al, 1992). Moreover, in the same study, fat mass adjusted for height correlated more strongly with biologically relevant variables such as blood pressure and fasting blood glucose than did percent body fat. Using the simple measure of BMI, much has been learned about the relation of positive energy balance with cancer as well as with coronary heart disease. Newer methods that are also practical in epidemiological studies may provide improved measurements of obesity. In particular, the electrical impedance method (Hodgdon and Fitzgerald, 1987) can provide an estimate that is likely to be more accurate than those based on weight and height, although this needs further evaluation.

The use of one or a small number of skin fold thicknesses does not appear to be appreciably more accurate than weight and height in the estimation of overall adiposity, but can provide additional information on the distribution of body fat. The ratio of waist to hip circumferences has received considerable attention in relation to cardiovascular disease, diabetes, and blood pressure (Hartz et al, 1984; Bjorntrop, 1987). This ratio has also been of interest with respect to hormonally sensitive cancers as it has been suggested that central fat functions differently than peripheral fat with respect to estrogen metabolism (Vague, 1956).

Height has often been ignored as a variable of potential interest in epidemiological studies. However, it can provide unique information on energy balance during the years before adulthood, a time period that may be important in the development of some tumors that occur many years later. For example, in a number of studies, height has been positively associated with risk of breast cancer (Swanson et al, 1988). Furthermore, this information can be valid even in the context of case-control studies because height will usually be unaffected even if illness has caused recent weight loss. Caution is indicated, however, if associations are not found with height because it is possible that, in some populations, few individuals will have been sufficiently deprived of energy intake during development to reduce their longitudinal growth. In such populations, height will primarily reflect genetic factors. Further information on the measurement and interpretation of body dimensions and composition is provided elsewhere (Lohman et al, 1988; Willett, 1990).

METHODOLOGICAL ISSUES IN NUTRITIONAL EPIDEMIOLOGY

Between-Person Variation in Dietary Intake

In addition to the availability of a sufficiently precise method for measuring dietary intake, an adequate degree of variation in diet is necessary to conduct observational studies within populations; if no variation in diet exists among persons, no associations can be observed. Some have argued that the diets within populations such as the United States are too homogeneous to study relationships with diet (Goodwin and Boyd, 1987; Hebert and Miller, 1988; Prentice et al, 1988). The true between-person variation in diet is difficult to measure directly, but it cannot be measured by the questionnaires used by epidemiologists because the observed variation will combine true differences with those due to measurement error; more quantitative methods must be used for this purpose. The fat content of the diet varies less among persons than does any other specific nutrient (Beaton et al, 1979); for women in our prospective study (Willett et al, 1987) the mean fat intake assessed by the mean of four 1-week diet records for those in the top quintile as 44% of calories while for those in the bottom quintile, 32% of calories were derived from fat. Although this is not a large range of fat intake and is certainly smaller than the variation among countries, it is of considerable interest because it corresponds closely to the changes (from about the present average intake of 40% of energy to about 30% of energy) recommended by the National Research Council (Committee on Diet, Nutrition, and Cancer, 1982) and other organizations. Other nutrients vary much more among persons than does total fat intake (Beaton, 1979; Willett, 1990).

Evidence that measurable and informative variation in diet exists within the U.S. population is provided by several sources. First, the correlations between food frequency questionnaires and independent assessments of diet found in the validation studies noted above could not have been observed if variation in diet did not exist. For the same reason, the correlations between questionnaire estimates of nutrient intakes and biochemical indicators of intake provide solid evidence of variation. In addition, the ability to find associations between dietary factors and incidence of disease (particularly when based on prospective data) indicates that measurable and biologically relevant variation exists. Reproducible relationships have been demonstrated between dietary fats and cardiovascular disease (Shekelle et al, 1981; Kushi et al, 1985), fat or meat intake and colon cancer (Willett, 1989b; Giovannucci et al, 1994), dietary carotenoids and lung cancer (Willett, 1990a), and alcohol and multiple cancer sites (IARC Working Group, 1988).

Although accumulated evidence has indicated that informative variation in diets exists within the U.S. population and that these differences can be measured, it is important that findings be interpreted in the context of that variation. For example, a lack of association with fat intake within the range of 32% to 44% of energy should not be interpreted to mean that fat intake has no relation with risk of disease under any circumstances. It is possible that the relation is nonlinear and that risk changes at lower levels of fat intake—for example, at 20% of total energy.

Implications of Total Energy Intake

Energy balance is likely to have important associations with some cancers; however, this cannot be studied directly by examining the relation of energy intake with risk of cancer because energy intake largely reflects factors other than over- or undereating in relation to requirements (Willett and Stampfer, 1986). The implications of total energy intake can be appreciated by realizing that variation among persons is to a large degree secondary to differences in body size and in physical activity. Persons also appear to differ somewhat in metabolic efficiency, inefficient persons requiring higher energy intake for the same level of function; however, these differences in metabolic efficiency are not practically measurable in epidemiological studies. Because virtually all nutrient intakes tend to be correlated with total energy intake, much of the variation in intake of specific nutrients is secondary to factors that may be unrelated to risk of disease. The effect of extraneous variation is, of course, to increase misclassification of diet and attenuate associations. Although the interrelations of diet and factors that determine variation in total energy intake are complex and beyond the scope of this discussion, failure to adjust for total energy intake may result in lack of significant associations.

When total energy intake is related to risk of disease—for example, when physical activity is protective—failure to consider total energy intake in the analysis can be particularly serious because it will confound associations with specific nutrients. The example of coronary heart disease is instructive: Because of the inverse relation with total energy intake, specific nutrients such as saturated fat will also tend to be inversely related to risk. Adjustment for total energy intake is necessary to avoid misleading conclusions; a number of statistical methods can be used (Willett, 1989a; Willett, 1990). However, the most commonly employed method, division by total energy, which is also called a nutrient density, is not an adequate solution, because the inverse of energy intake can then be confounding; this may or may not be a serious problem in any particular study. Appropriate adjustment for energy intake can be a nontrivial issue in some studies; the direction of association can be reversed, such as in the relation between saturated fat intake and myocardial infarction (Gordon et al, 1981) and between fiber intake and risk of colon cancer (Lyon, 1987). Unfortunately, total energy intake has been either not measured or, when associated with disease, not appropriately accounted for in many of the published studies on diet and cancer, thus rendering the interpretation of many studies unclear.

Nutrient intakes adjusted for total energy can be viewed conceptually as measures of nutrient composition rather than as measures of absolute intake. Measures of nutrient composition are most relevant to personal decisions and public health policy because individuals must alter nutrient intakes primarily by manipulating the composition of their diets rather than their total energy intake. This reasoning underlies, for example, the use of fat as a percent of calories in expressing a dietary objective (Committee on Diet, Nutrition, and Cancer, 1982).

ASSOCIATIONS OF DIET WITH SPECIFIC CANCERS

In this section several aspects of diet that have been considered in relation to cancer etiology will be noted. It is intended to provide a sense of the scope of the issues and direction to other sources of information, including the chapters in this book relating to specific cancers. This is not a comprehensive or critical review, which would require a volume in itself.

Total Energy Intake

In animal studies, restriction of energy intake sufficient to reduce growth consistently and substantially reduces the occurrence of many tumors (Ross and Bras, 1971; Weindruch and Walford, 1982). In humans, total energy intake, as assessed by indices of obesity, is strongly related to risk of endometrial cancer and cancer of the biliary system (Lew and Garfinkel, 1979) and a modest association may exist with renal cell cancer (Goodman et al, 1986) and cancer of the colon in men, but probably not women (Lew and Garfinkel, 1979). Weak and inconsistent associations have been observed between obesity and breast cancer incidence among postmenopausal women (Wynder et al, 1978; Paffenbarger et al, 1980; Lubin et al, 1985; Helmrich et al, 1983; Le Marchand et al, 1988; Swanson et al, 1988; Tretli, 1989). A modest association between obesity and mortality due to breast cancer was seen in the large American Cancer Society cohort (Lew and Garfinkel, 1979); this is probably, at least in part, related to delayed diagnosis and poorer prognosis among obese women. Among premenopausal women, obesity appears to be protective for breast cancer (Willett et al, 1985; Le Marchand et al, 1988), perhaps because heavier women have more anovulatory menstrual cycles.

Height, which in part reflects energy balance during development, has been positively related to risk of breast cancer in a number of studies (Valaoras et al, 1969; Swanson et al, 1988; Tretli, 1989). This has not been observed in some studies, particularly those in affluent countries, which may be due to a paucity of women in these populations who were sufficiently restricted so as to stunt their growth. Moderate restriction of energy intake during adult life may not be adequate to reduce breast cancer incidence since the relatively least obese at age 18 years of age appear to be at highest risk of breast cancer during the premenopausal years (Willett et al, 1985).

Dietary Fat

Fat intake has been singled out (Committee on Diet, Nutrition, and Cancer, 1982) as the aspect of diet most clearly related to risk of cancer. The most important sites for which associations have been suggested are cancers of breast, colon, and prostate. Much of the support for these relationships is based on the striking international correlations between per capita fat intake and rates of these malignancies (Armstrong and Doll, 1975; Prentice et al, 1988). For breast cancer, other data are much less clear (Willett, 1989); only weak or no association with fat intake has been found in most case-control (Graham et al, 1982; Hirohata et al, 1985; Hirohata et al, 1987; Katsouyanni et al, 1988; Miller et al, 1978; Rohan et al, 1988) and cohort studies (Willett et al, 1987; Jones et al, 1987; Howe et al, 1991; Kushi et al, 1992; Willett et al, 1992; van den Brandt, 1993; Graham, 1992). For colon cancer, associations with fat or meat intake have been seen more frequently (Willett, 1989a; Willett et al, 1990; Giovannucci et al, 1994); whether this represents a specific effect of fat intake or other factors in red meat is less clear. Associations have also been reported between animal fat intake and risk of prostate cancer (Kolonel et al, 1988; Graham et al, 1983; Heshmat et al, 1985; Giovannucci, 1993; Le Marchand, 1994) and ovarian cancer (Cramer et al, 1984; LaVecchia et al, 1987), but the literature is far from conclusive.

Fiber

Interest in the relation between fiber intake and colon cancer is largely the result of Burkitt's observation of low rates of colon cancer in areas of Africa where fiber consumption and stool bulk were high (Burkitt, 1971). Fiber has been hypothesized to dilute potential carcinogens and speed their transit through the colon. Inverse associations with total fiber intake have been seen in most case-control studies (Trock, 1990). When specific sources of fiber have been examined, fiber intake from fruits or vegetables have been most consistently associated with lower incidence whereas fiber from cereals has either been related to an increased risk or not associated with colon cancer (Potter and McMichael, 1986; Macquart-Moulin et al, 1986; Slattery et al, 1988; Modan et al, 1975; Miller et al, 1983; LaVecchia et al, 1988; Manousos et al, 1983; Martinez et al, 1979; Haenszel et al, 1980; Graham et al, 1978). The inverse associations with vegetable or fruit intake may be due to specific forms of fiber, or to other components of plants such as vitamin C, protease inhibitors (Troll et al, 1987), or indoles (Wattenberg and Loub, 1978). However, this relation has not been so clear in prospective studies (Willett, 1990; Giovannucci, 1994; Steinmetz, 1994).

Preformed Vitamin A and Carotenoids

Because vitamin A plays a central role in regulating cell differentiation, ample reason exists to suspect that it may be related to cancer incidence. In a number of animal models, preformed vitamin A or chemical analogues can inhibit tumor development, even when administered well after the carcinogen (Lippman and Meyskens, 1989), which has major potential epidemiological and public health importance. Vegetable precursors of vitamin A, the carotenoids, have been less studied in animals but have reduced tumor incidence in some models, particularly skin cancers (Mathews-Roth, 1989). Whether carotenoids act by virtue of conversion to retinol, the main circulating form of vitamin A with physiologic activity, or by other mechanisms, such as being an antioxidant or quencher of singlet oxygen (Peto et al, 1981), remains uncertain.

Epidemiological studies of preformed vitamin A or carotenoids in relation to cancer incidence have used either questionnaire assessments of diet or blood measurements. The distinction between these two forms of vitamin A has important practical implications because preformed vitamin A is obtained only from foods derived from animal sources or vitamin supplements, whereas carotenoid precursors of vitamin A are obtained almost entirely from plant sources. The initial reports of an inverse relation between total vitamin A intake and risk of lung cancer (Bjelke, 1975; Mettlin et al, 1979) did not clearly distinguish between these sources. In a subsequent prospective study by Shekelle and coworkers (1981), the protective effect of total vitamin A for lung cancer was found to be entirely attributable to carotenoid sources; preformed vitamin A was unrelated to risk of this disease. Subsequent studies, based both on dietary intake (Gregor et al, 1980; Hinds et al, 1984; Ziegler et al, 1984; Samet et al, 1985; Wu et al, 1985) and beta-carotene measurements in prospectively collected blood (Nomura et al, 1985; Menkes et al, 1986; Stahelin et al., 1984), have provided remarkably consistent evidence for a protective relationship between carotenoid intake and risk of lung cancer after controlling for cigarette smoking, but little support for any relationship with preformed vitamin A (Willett, 1990b; Hunter, 1994).

The relation of preformed vitamin A and carotenoid intake with risk of cancers other than lung is unclear at this time because only a few studies have been conducted for any single cancer site. Total vitamin A or carotenoid intake has been inversely related to risk of cancers of the bladder (Mettlin and Graham, 1979), oral cavity (Marshall, 1982), larynx (Graham et al, 1981), esophagus (Mettlin et al, 1980), and breast (Graham et al, 1982). In two additional case-control studies (Howe et al, 1990; Katsouyanni, 1988), and two large prospective studies (Hunter et al, 1991; Rohan et al, 1993) total vitamin A intake was related to lower risk of breast cancer, but in another case-control study neither intake nor blood levels of preformed vitamin A or beta-carotene were associated with reduced risk of this disease (Marubini et al, 1988). Total vitamin A intake was positively related to risk of prostatic cancer in three case-control studies (Kolonel et al, 1988; Graham et al, 1983; Heshmat et al, 1985), but an inverse association was seen with carotenoid intake in a Japanese study (Ohno et al, 1988). Beta-carotene intake has been associated with reduced risk of gastric neoplasia (Haenszel et al, 1985), and some evidence suggests that an inverse relation may exist with cervical cancer (Brock et al, 1988). Neither preformed vitamin A nor carotenoid intake has been consistently associated with risk of colon cancer, although these relationships have been examined in several studies.

Although existing data strongly support an association between intake of carotenoid precursors of vitamin A and risk of lung cancer, uncertainty exists as to whether this relationship is confounded by other components of fruits and vegetables or by nondietary factors and whether this apparent protective effect extends to cancers at other sites. Randomized trials conducted to determine whether supplements of beta-carotene will reduce the risk of cancer have not been promising up to this point. In a randomized study among patients with previous skin cancer, beta-carotene did not prevent the development of new skin cancer (Greenberg et al, 1990). Similarly, beta-carotene—as well as vitamins C and E—did not influence the recurrences of adenomatous colon polyps (Greenberg et al, 1994). The most surprising finding has been from the large Finnish Trial among men at high risk of lung cancer (Heinonen et al, 1994); a statistically significant 18% increase in incidence of this malignancy was seen in those randomized to beta-carotene. Although these trials do not support the hypothesis that beta-carotene specifically reduces risk of these cancers, they do not necessarily refute the many epidemiological observations that higher consumption of vegetables and fruits is associated with lower risk, as these foods contain many other carotenoids as well as other nutrients and phytochemicals that may be the active agents. Moreover, a 6-year study may be of insufficient duration to observe a protective effect that operates at an early stage of carcinogenesis.

Vitamin C

Vitamin C has been hypothesized to reduce cancer risk by its antioxidant properties, by blocking the conversion of nitrates and nitrogen-containing compounds to carcinogens under conditions found in the stomach (Mirvish et al, 1972) and in food (Raineri and Weisburger, 1975), and by other mechanisms (Cameron et al, 1979). In case-control studies, evidence for a protective effect of vitamin C has been seen for laryngeal cancer (Graham et al, 1981), oral cancer (Winn et al, 1984), esophageal cancer (Mettlin et al, 1981; Ziegler et al, 1981), stomach cancer (Correa et al, 1985), and cervical dysplasia (Romney et al, 1985; Wassertheil-Smoller et al, 1981). As discussed elsewhere (Block and Menkes, 1989; Willett and MacMahon, 1984), the interpretation of these data, while supporting a preventive effect of vitamin C, are also compatible with the possibility that other factors in fruits and vegetables are the primary cause of reduced cancer risk.

Vitamin E

The concept that vitamin E might reduce risk of human cancer derives from its role as a potent intracellular antioxidant and from suggestive animal studies (Mergens and Bhagavan, 1989; Bieri et al, 1983). Wald reported an extremely strong inverse relation between prediagnostic blood levels of vitamin E and risk of breast cancer (Wald et al, 1984); however, this was later found to be an artifact of differential handling of case and control specimens (Wald et al, 1988). In a separate study population, Wald reported a protective association between prediagnostic blood vitamin E levels and cancer at all sites combined, but provided evidence that this was likely due to an effect of preclinical disease on vitamin E levels rather than a preventive effect of this micronutrient (Wald et al, 1987). Also using blood collected from a large cohort, Menkes and coworkers (1986) reported an inverse association with lung cancer; this was not confirmed in a similar study by Nomura and coworkers (1985). Although associations have generally not been seen for other cancer sites (Nomura et al, 1985), an inverse association was reported in a Finnish cohort between prediagnostic serum vitamin E levels and cancers at all sites combined, which was particularly strong for non–smoking-related cancers (Knekt et al, 1988). In the recent Finnish Trial (Heinonen, 1994), vitamin E supplementation did not influence risk of lung cancer but was associated with a somewhat lower risk of prostate cancer. The overall data thus remain unclear at this time; this may be the result of only modest numbers of specific cancers in the studies that have been reported, but a large beneficial effect of vitamin E against cancer seems unlikey.

Selenium

That higher intake of selenium might reduce the risk of some human cancers has been suggested by numerous animal experiments (Combs and Combs, 1986) and ecological studies in which indices of selenium intake have been inversely related to risk of cancer, both internationally (Schrauzer et al, 1977) and within the United States (Shamberger et al, 1976). The correlational data have been particularly strong for cancers of the colon and breast. Inverse associations have been seen between serum selenium levels and subsequent risk of all cancers combined in several large prospective studies (Willett et al, 1983; Salonen et al, 1984; Salonen et al, 1985; Kok et al, 1987), but no evidence of a protective effect has been found in other similar investigations (Virtamo et al, 1987; Peleg et al, 1985; Menkes et al, 1986; Nomura et al, 1987; Coates et al, 1988). In two prospective studies that together included a large number of breast cancer cases, no relation was found between selenium in nails and subsequent risk of this malignancy (Van Noord et al, 1987; Hunter et al, 1990). A strong inverse association between nail selenium levels and risk of lung cancer was seen in a prospective study from Holland (van den Brandt et al, 1993). Other than for breast and lung, studies have not included a sufficiently large number of specific cancers to clearly confirm or exclude a modest association, thus the data for human cancer remain inconclusive (Willett and Stampfer, 1988).

Salt

Ecological associations have led to the suggestion that high salt intake, which has been traditionally used in many societies for the preservation of food, might increase the risk of gastric cancer (Joossens and Geboers, 1987; Howson et al, 1986). Salt is hypothesized to act as a local irritant that may compromise the gastric mucosal barrier and thus facilitate the action of local carcinogens. Positive associations of salt intake with risk of gastric cancer have been seen in several case-control studies (Haenszel et al, 1972; You et al, 1988; Fontham et al, 1986). This hypothesis is compatible with the striking decline in gastric cancer in most industrialized countries over this century as refrigeration reduced the need of salt for preservation. However, economic improvements also enhanced the supply of fresh fruits and vegetables on a year-round basis and improved hygiene, which may have reduced the transmission of helicobacter infection. A strong association between salted fish intake during childhood and risk of nasopharyngeal cancer has been noted among several Chinese populations (You et al, 1988).

Natural Carcinogens and Products of Food Preparation

Ames (1987) has reviewed the large number of naturally occurring compounds in foods that are known to be mutagenic or carcinogenic in laboratory settings. Many of these toxic compounds have probably been developed by plants during evolution as a form of protection. In addition, a wide variety of mutagens and carcinogens are formed during the process of cooking meat and other foods, even under conditions that do not involve charring (Sugimura, 1986). With few exceptions—such as the bracken fern, which may cause bladder cancer when used regularly as a tea (Pamukcu et al, 1970)—little evidence exists that these compounds contribute substantially to human cancer. On the contrary, vegetable intake has generally been found to be protective for many human cancers. However, the role of carcinogens that occur naturally or that are formed during cooking has not been studied thoroughly with respect to human cancer and may be rather difficult to investigate.

PREVENTION OF CANCER BY DIETARY MEANS

Intense interest in the possible prevention of cancer by dietary manipulations has generated a series of recommendations from numerous private and governmental bodies, worldwide and within the United States (Committee on Diet, Nutrition, and Cancer, 1982; Greenwald and Sondick, 1986; Committee on Diet and Health, 1989). Those of the National Academy of Sciences (Committee on Diet, Nutrition, and Cancer, 1982) are typical:

1. The consumption of both saturated and unsaturated fats should be reduced, from an average of approximately 40% of total calories to 30%.
2. The intake of fruits, vegetables, and whole grain cereal products in the diet should be emphasized.
3. The consumption of food preserved by salt-curing (including salt-pickling) or smoking should be minimized.
4. Efforts should continue to be made to minimize contamination of foods with carcinogens from any source, including those that are natural or occurring inadvertently during production, processing, and storage.
5. Further efforts should be made to identify mutagens in food and to expedite testing for their carcinogenicity. Where feasible and prudent, mutagens should be removed or minimized.
6. If alcoholic beverages are consumed, it should be done in moderation.

The potential impact of these changes in diet is extremely difficult to quantify. Based on similar recommendations, the U.S. National Cancer Institute suggests that, within 10 years, cancer of the colon and rectum would be reduced by 50%, cancer of the breast by 25%, cancers of the prostate, endometrium, and gallbladder by 15%, and the cancers of the stomach, esophagus, pancreas, ovaries, liver, lung, and bladder by a possible but not precisely quantifiable amount (Greenwald and Sondick, 1986). In this same publication, the large uncertainty of these estimates was noted, including the possibility that no reductions for some of these cancers might occur.

Dietary recommendations for the United States and other Western countries have primarily focused on ways to reduce cancers of the breast, large bowel, and prostate and to a lesser extent pancreas and ovary because these are the most important cancers not caused by smoking or alcohol that are plausibly related to diet. In other parts of the world, different cancer sites, such as stomach and esophagus, are dominant. These upper gastrointestinal cancers in particular are almost surely influenced by dietary factors; although uncertainty exists about the specific alterations of diet that will be effective, a change toward the contemporary U.S. diet is likely to be beneficial. However, a more precise understanding of etiologic factors is needed to avoid exchanging one pattern of cancer for another that includes high rates of breast and colon cancer.

The actual benefit in cancer reduction that might be realized by dietary change is, of course, a function of both the biological relationships and the success of an intervention. Probably the most certain associations of diet and cancer are those with total energy balance, especially with cancers of the endometrium and gallbladder. The effects of weight control on breast cancer incidence are unclear and include the possibility that a reduced prevalence of obesity might actually increase the incidence of this disease during the premenopausal years. A modest reduction in breast cancer mortality might occur with weight loss in postmenopausal women as a result of a lower case-fatality rate. However, barring an effective pharmacological treatment of obesity, the prospects for any substantial influence on cancer incidence in the general population by control of weight during the near future is remote because the cancers for which the association is strong do not contribute greatly to cancer incidence or mortality. Moreover, efforts to attain long-term reductions in weight in population groups have been disappointing, and the overall trend in the United States appears to be toward greater obesity (Van Itallie, 1978) despite widespread desire for slim body builds and solid evidence that obesity is associated with a large increased risk of cardiovascular disease.

After energy balance, epidemiological data provide the strongest evidence for a potential impact of dietary change on cancer incidence by increasing the intake of fruits and vegetables. Increasing these foods is likely to be a more attainable goal than altering energy balance or making major shifts in macronutrient intake. Whether the apparent protective effect of fruits and vegetables is mediated by beta-carotene, vitamin C, dietary fiber, or any other specific substance remains uncertain. Despite uncertainty regarding the active component, intake of these plant products has been inversely related to cancers of the lung, colon, breast, and many other sites. Unfortunately, the advice to eat more fruits and vegetables is rather vague; epidemiologists could provide further practical guidance by giving more detail about relations of cancers with specific foods and food groups in their analyses.

The primary focus of most dietary recommendations thus far has been on intake of dietary fat; it has been suggested that intake should be reduced to an average of about 30% of energy (Committee on Diet, Nutrition, and Cancer, 1982). Anticipated benefits have related primarily to cancers of breast and colon and possibly prostate, endometrium, and ovary. While most would agree that the evidence of benefit for cancer is not conclusive, the recommendation to reduce fat intake has been in part justified on the basis of being harmless and also being likely to result in a reduced risk of coronary heart disease. However, this recommendation appears overly simplistic and not without potential harm. Polyunsaturated fats, contained primarily in vegetable oils, are likely to reduce risk of coronary heart disease (Shekelle et al, 1981) whereas saturated fats, primarily from animal sources, are likely to increase the risk. The relation of type of fat with risk of human cancer remains unclear; what evidence there is suggests that any positive association pertains mainly to fat from animal sources. Without a careful selective reduction in the type of fat, it is quite conceivable that some individuals might primarily reduce their intake of vegetable fat and thereby increase their risk of cardiovascular disease. Rather than focusing on fat intake, a reduction in meat consumption is better supported; associations have been seen with cancers of the colon and prostate in multiple studies. Whether these relationships are due to the fat content of meat is uncertain, and some data for colon cancer suggest other components contribute to risk.

The level of scientific certainty that is appropriate for launching public health interventions aimed at changing diets to prevent cancer is an issue of legitimate debate. As has been pointed out elsewhere (Greenwald and Sondick, 1986), waiting to change dietary behavior until the scientific evidence is almost certain could mean the loss of thousands of lives. On the other hand, promulgating policies that turn out to be wrong has costs in terms of diverting attention and resources from interventions that are effective, such as smoking cessation and mammography, and in the loss of credibility, which is essential for any public health program. Fortunately, the dietary recommendations noted above, with the qualification regarding type of fat, are generally consistent with those designed to reduce the incidence of coronary heart disease (Consensus Conference, 1985), and for which the evidence is more compelling.

Specific actions for implementing dietary recommendations have been developed by the U.S. National Cancer Institute (Greenwald and Sondick, 1986). These include encouraging federal agencies and industries to include cancer prevention dietary recommendations in federal food production, marketing, and distribution policies; encouraging the production of leaner meat products and lower fat content of dairy products; informing the public about the relationship between diet and cancer; expanding nutrition labeling to cover the full range of mass-marketed foods so consumers can be better informed and make wiser shopping decisions; and developing diet and cancer programs that make use of the mass media and other high-technology communication approaches. State and local agencies are also encouraged to review school curricula to reflect newer knowledge of diet and cancer risks and strategies for risk reduction; to review school menus in relation to the cancer control objectives; to promote diet and cancer information programs; to encourage restaurants to provide sufficient information to allow patrons to choose nutritious foods; to coordinate governmental planning activities to ensure that attention is given to reducing dietary risk factors for cancer; to promote dissemination of information about proper food selection to protect against cancer risk; and to include information on diet and cancer in existing food, nutrition, and health programs with the use of innovative approaches to reach high-risk groups.

SUMMARY

A wide variety of evidence based on comparisons of cancer rates in different geographic areas, migrating populations, and religious orders strongly suggests that the high rates of breast, colon, and other important cancers in the affluent countries are due to environmental rather than genetic factors. Furthermore, aspects of diet are likely to be important etiological factors for some of these cancers. Similarly, the incidence rates of many cancers that are still of great importance in other parts of the world, such as those of the oral cavity, esophagus, and stomach, are also likely to be strongly influenced by dietary factors. Despite the substantial evidence that dietary factors are likely to be important, the specific aspects of food and nutrient intake that are either causative or preventive remain inconclusively defined for most of these cancers. The most consistent evidence is that higher intake of fruits and vegetables reduces the risk of many of these cancers; however, the specific components of these plant-derived foods responsible for the protective effects are not clearly established. Evidence, although not entirely consistent, is accumulating that meat or animal fat intake is associated with risks of colon and prostate cancers; the hypothesized relationship of these factors with breast cancer is less well supported. Evidence relating the fat composition of the diet to other cancer sites remains sporadic. Individual and policy decisions regarding dietary changes should consider not only the possible benefits for cancer reduction but also the effects on coronary heart disease because this remains the dominant cause of mortality in the United States and its relation with diet is better established.

REFERENCES

ABRAMSON JH, SLOME C, KOSOVSKY C. 1963. Food frequency interview as an epidemiological tool. Am J Public Health 53:1093–1101.

ADELSTEIN AM, STASZEWSKI J, MUIR CS. 1979. Cancer mortality in 1970–1972 among Polish-born migrants to England and Wales. Br J Cancer 40:464–475.

AMES BN. 1983. Dietary carcinogens and anticarcinogens. Science 221:1256–1264.

AMES BN, MAGAW R, GOLD LS. 1987. Ranking possible carcinogenic hazards. Science 236:271–280.

ARMSTRONG B, DOLL R. 1975. Environmental factors and cancer incidence and mortality in different countries, with special reference to dietary practices. Int J Cancer 15:617–631.

ASCHERIO A, STAMPFER MJ, COLDITZ GA, RIMM EB, LITIN L, WILLETT WC. 1992. Correlations of vitamin A and E intakes with the plasma concentrations of carotenoids and tocopherols among American men and women. J Nutr 122:1792–1801.

BALOGH M, MEDALIE, JH, SMITH H, GROEN. 1968. The development of a dietary questionnaire for an ischemic heart disease survey. Isr J Med Sci 4:195–203.

BEATON GH, MILNER J, COREY P, et al. 1979. Sources of variance in 24-hour dietary recall data: implications for nutrition study design and interpretation. Am J Clin Nutr 32:2546–2549.

BIERI JG, CORASH L, HUBBARD VS. 1983. Medical uses of vitamin E. N Engl J Med 308:1063–1071.

BINGHAM SA, CUMMINGS JH. 1985. Urine nitrogen as an independent validatory measure of dietary intake: a study of nitrogen balance in individuals consuming their normal diet. Am J Clin Nutr 42:1276–1289.

BJARNASON O, DAY N, SNAEDAL G, TULINIUS H. 1974. The effect of year of birth on the breast cancer age-incidence curve in Iceland. Int J Cancer 13:689–696.

BJELKE E. 1975. Dietary vitamin A and human lung cancer. Int J Cancer 15:561–565.

BJORNTROP P. 1987. Classification of obese patients and complications related to the distribution of surplus fat. Am J Clin Nutr 45(s):1120–1125.

BLOCK G, HARTMAN AM, DRESSER CM, et al. 1986. A data-based approach to diet questionnaire design and testing. Am J Epidemiol 3:453–469.

BLOCK G, MENKES M. 1989. Ascorbic acid in cancer prevention. In: *Nutrition and Cancer Prevention*, Moon TE and Micozzi MS (eds). New York: Marcel Dekker, pp 341–388.

BLOCK G, WOODS M, POTOSKY A, CLIFFORD C. 1990. Validation of a self-administered diet questionnaire using multiple diet records. J Clin Epidemiol 43:1327–1335.

BROCK KE, BERRY G, MOCK PA, MACLENNAN R, TRUSWELL AS, BRINTON LA. 1988. Nutrients in diet and plasma and risk of in situ cervical cancer. J Natl Cancer Inst 80:580–585.

BROWE JH, GOFSTEIN RM, MORLLEY DM, MCCARTHY MC. 1966. Diet and heart disease study in the Cardiovascular Health Center. J Am Diet Assoc 48:95–100.

BUELL P. 1973. Changing incidence of breast cancer in Japanese-American women. J Natl Cancer Inst 51:1479–1483.

BURKITT DP. 1971. Epidemiology of cancer of the colon and rectum. Cancer 28:3–13.

BYARS D, GAIL M. 1989. Errors-in-variables workshop. Stat Med 8:1027–1029.

BYERS T, MARSHALL J, ANTHONY E, FIEDLER R, ZIELEZNY M. 1987. The reliability of dietary history from the distant past. Am J Epidemiol 125:999–1011.

BYERS TE, ROSENTHAL RI, MARSHALL JR et al. 1983. Dietary history from the distant past: a methodological study. Nutr Cancer 5:69–77.

CAMERON E, PAULING L, LEIBOVITZ B. 1979. Ascorbic acid and cancer: a review. Cancer Res 39:663–681.

COATES RJ, ELEY JW, BLOCK G, GUNTER EW, SOWELL AL, GROSSMAN C, GREENBERG RS. 1991. An evaluation of a food frequency questionnaire for assessing dietary intake of specific carotenoids and vitamin E among low-income black women. Am J Epidemiol 134:658–671.

COATES RJ, WEISS NS, DALING JR, MORRIS JS, LABBE RF. 1988. Serum levels of selenium and retinol and the subsequent risk of cancer. Am J Epidemiol 128:515–523.

COHEN NL, LAUS MJ, FERRIS AM et al. 1990. The contributions of portion data to estimating nutrient intake by food frequency. Research Bulletin Number 730/Dec 1990. Amherst, Mars Agricultural Experiment Station, University of Massachusetts.

COMBS GJ JR, COMBS SB. 1986. Selenium and cancer. In: *The Role of Selenium in Nutrition*, Combs GJ Jr, Combs SB (eds). New York: Academic Press, pp 413.

COMMITTEE ON DIET AND HEALTH. 1989. Diet and health: implications for reducing chronic disease risk. Food and Nutrition Board. National Research Council. Washington, DC: National Academy Press.

COMMITTEE ON DIET, NUTRITION AND CANCER, NATIONAL RESEARCH COUNCIL. 1982. Diet, nutrition, and cancer. Washington, DC: National Academy Press.

CONSENSUS CONFERENCE. 1985. Lowering blood cholesterol to prevent heart disease. JAMA 253:2080–2090.

CORREA P, FONTHAM E, PICKLE LW, et al. 1985. Dietary determinants of gastric cancer in south Louisiana inhabitants. J Natl Cancer Inst 75:645–654.

CRAMER DW, WELCH WR, HUTCHISON GB, WILLETT WC, SCULLY RE. 1984. Dietary animal fat in relation to ovarian cancer risk. Obstet Gynecol 63:833–838.

CUMMINGS SR, BLOCK G, MCHENRY K, BARON RB. 1987. Evaluation of two food frequency methods of measuring dietary calcium intake. Am J Epidemiol 126:796–802.

DOLL R, PETO R. 1981. The causes of cancer: quantitative estimates of avoidable risks of cancer in the United States today. J Natl Cancer Inst 66:1191–1308.

EPSTEIN LM, RESHEF A, ABRAMSON JH, BIALIK O. 1970. Validity of a short dietary questionnaire. Isr J Med Sci 6:589–597.

FEX G, PETTERSSON B, AKESSON B. 1987. Low plasma selenium as a risk factor for cancer death in middle-aged men. Nutr Cancer 10:221–229.

FONTHAM E, ZAVALA D, CORREA P, RODRIGUEZ E, HUNTER F, HAENSZEL W, TANNENBAUM SR. 1986. Diet and chronic atrophic gastritis: a case-control study. J Natl Cancer Inst 76:621–627.

FRIEDENREICH CM, HOWE GR, MILLER AB. 1991. An investigation of recall bias in the reporting of past food intake among breast cancer cases and controls. Ann Epidemiol 1:439–453.

GIOVANNUCCI E, RIMM EB, STAMPFER MJ, COLDITZ GA, ASCHERIO A, CHUTE CC, WILLETT WC. 1993. A prospective study of dietary fat and risk of prostate cancer. J Natl Cancer Inst 85:1571–1579.

GIOVANNUCCI E, RIMM EB, STAMPFER MJ, COLDITZ GA, ASCHERIO A, WILLETT WC. 1994. Intake of fat, meat, and fiber in relation to risk of colon cancer in men. Cancer Res 54:2390–2397.

GIOVANNUCCI E, STAMPFER MJ, COLDITZ GA, MANSON J, ROSNER B, LONGNECKER M, SPEIZER F. 1991. A comparison of prospective and retrospective assessments of diet in the study of breast cancer. (Abstract) Am J Epidemiol 134:714.

GOLDBOHM RA, VAN DEN BRANDT PA, BRANTS HAM, et al. 1995. Validation of a dietary questionnaire used in a large-scale prospective cohort study on diet and cancer. Eur J Clin Nutr 49:420–429.

GOLDIN B, ADLERCREUTZ H, DWYER JT SWENSON L, WARRAM JH, GORBACH SL. 1981. Effect of diet on excretion of estrogens in pre- and postmenopausal women. Cancer Res 41:3771–3773.

GOODMAN MT, MORGENSTERN H, WYNDER EL. 1986. A case-control study of factors affecting the development of renal cell cancer. Am J Epidemiol 124:926–941.

GOODWIN PJ, BOYD NF. 1987. Critical appraisal of the evidence that dietary fat intake is related to breast cancer risk in humans. J Natl Cancer Inst 79:473–485.

GORDON TA, KAGAN A, GARCIA-PALMIERI MR, et al. 1981. Diet and its relationship to coronary heart disease and death in three populations. Circulation 63:500–515.

GRAHAM S, HAUGHEY B, MARSHALL J, PRIORE R, BYERS T, RZEPKA T, METTLIN C, PONTES JE. 1983. Diet in the epidemiology of carcinoma of the prostate gland. J Natl Cancer Inst 70:687–692.

GRAHAM S, METTLIN C, MARSHALL J, PRIORE R, RZEPKA T, SHEDD D. 1981. Dietary factors in the epidemiology of cancer of the larynx. Am J Epidemiol 113:675–680.

GRAHAM S, DAYAL H, SWANSON M, MITTELMAN A, WILKINSON G. 1978. Diet in the epidemiology of cancer of the colon and rectum. J Natl Cancer Inst 61:709–714.

GRAHAM S, DAYAL H, ROHRER T, et al. 1977. Dentition, diet, tobacco, and alcohol in the epidemiology of oral cancer. J Natl Cancer Inst 59:1611–1618.

GRAHAM S, MARSHALL J, METTLIN C, RZEPKA T, NEMOTO T, BYERS T. 1982. Diet in the epidemiology of breast cancer. Am J Epidemiol 116:68–75.

GRAHAM S, ZIELEZNY M, MARSHALL J, et al. 1992. Diet in the epidemiology of postmenopausal breast cancer in a New York State cohort. Am J Epidemiol 136:1327.

GRAY GE, PAGANINI-HILL A, ROSS RK, HENDERSON BE. 1984. Assessment of three brief methods of estimation of vitamin A and C intakes for a prospective study of cancer: comparison with dietary history. Am J Epidemiol 119:581–590.

GREENBERG ER, BARON JA, STUKEL TA, STEVENS MM, MANDEL JS, SPENCER SK, ELIAS PM, LOWE N, NIERENBERG DW, BAYRD G, et al. 1990. A clinical trial of beta carotene to prevent basal-cell and squamous-cell cancers of the skin. The Skin Cancer Prevention Study Group. N Engl J Med 323:789–795.

GREENBERG ER, BARON JA, TOSTESON TD, et al. 1994. A clinical trial of antioxidant vitamins to prevent colorectal adenoma. N Engl J Med 331:141–147.

GREENWALD P, SONDICK EJ, eds. 1986. Cancer Control Objectives for the Nation: 1985–2000. Bethesda, MD, National Cancer Institute Monograph, U. S. Dept. Health and Human Services, National Institutes of Health Pub. No. 86-2880 No. 2.

GREGOR A, LEE PN, ROE FJC, et al. 1980. Comparison of dietary histories in lung cancer cases and controls with special reference to vitamin A. Nutr Cancer 2:93–97.

HAENSZEL W, CORREA P, LOPEZ A, et al. 1985. Serum micronutrient levels in relation to gastric pathology. Int J Cancer 36:43–48.

HAENSZEL W, KURIHARA M, SEGI M, LEE RK. 1972. Stomach cancer among Japanese in Hawaii. J Natl Cancer Inst 49:969–988.

HAENSZEL W, LOCKE FB, SEGI M. 1980. A case-control study of large bowel cancer in Japan. J Natl Cancer Inst 64:17–22.

HANKIN JH, RHOADS GG, GLOBER GA. 1975. A dietary method for an epidemiologic study of gastrointestinal cancer. Am J Clin Nutr 28:1055–1061.

HANKIN JH, NOMURA, AM, LEE J, HIROHATA T, KOLONEL LN. 1983. Reproducibility of a dietary history questionnaire in a case-control study of breast cancer. Am J Clin Nutr 37:981–985.

HARTGE, P BRINTON LA, ROSENTHAL JF, CAHILL JI, HOOVER RN, WAKSBERG J. 1984. Random digit dialing in selecting a population-based control group. Am J Epidemiol 120:825–833.

HARTZ AJ, RUPLEY DC, RIMM AA. 1984. The association of girth measurements with disease in 32,856 women. Am J Epidemiol 119:71–80.

HEADY JA. 1961. Diets of bank clerks: development of a method of classifying the diets of individuals for use in epidemiologic studies. J R Stat Soc (A) 124:336–361.

HEBERT JR, MILLER DR. 1988. Methodologic considerations for investigating the diet-cancer link. Am J Clin Nutr 47:1068–1077.

HEINONEN OP, et al. 1994. Effect of vitamin E and beta-carotene on the incidence of lung cancer and other cancers in male smokers. N Engl J Med 330:1029–1035.

HELMRICH SP, SHAPIRO S, ROSENBERG L, et al. 1983. Risk factors for breast cancer. Am J Epidemiol 117:35–45.

HENNEKENS CH, PHYSICIANS HEALTH STUDY RESEARCH GROUP. 1983. Strategies for a primary prevention trial of cancer and cardiovascular disease among U. S. physicians. (Abstract). Am J Epidemiol 118:453–454.

HERNANDEZ-AVILA M, MARTEZ C, HUNTER DJ, et al. 1988. Influence of additional portion size data on the validity of a semi-quantitative food frequency questionnaire. Am J Epidemiol 128:891.

HESHMAT MY, KAUL L, KOVI J, et al. 1985. Nutrition and prostate cancer: a case-control study. Prostate 6:7–17.

HINDS MW, KOLONEL LN, HANKIN JH, LEE J. 1984. Dietary vitamin A, carotene, vitamin C, and risk of lung cancer in Hawaii. Am J Epidemiol 119:227–237.

HIROHATA TA, NOMURA AM, HANKIN JH, KOLONEL LN, LEE J. 1987. An epidemiologic study on the association between diet and breast cancer. J Natl Cancer Inst 78:595–600.

HIROHATA T, SHIGEMATSU T, NOMURA AM, et al. 1985. Occurrence of breast cancer in relation to diet and reproductive history: a case-control study in Fukuoka, Japan. NCI Monogr 69:187–190.

HODGDON JA, FITZGERALD PI. 1987. Validity of impedance predictions at various levels of fatness. Hum Biol 59:281–298.

HOWE GR, HIROHATA T, HISLOP TG, et al. 1990. Dietary factors and risk of breast cancer: combined analysis of 12 case-control studies. J Natl Cancer Inst 82:561–569.

HOWE GR, FRIEDENREICH CM, JAIN M, MILLE AB. 1991. A cohort study of fat intake and risk of breast cancer. J Natl Cancer Inst 83:336–340.

HOWSON CP, HIYAMA T, WYNDER EL. 1986. The decline in gastric cancer: epidemiology of an unplanned triumph. Epidemiol Rev 8:1–27.

HUNT IF, LIKE LS, MURPHY NJ, CLARK VA, COULSON AH. 1979. Nutrient estimates for computerized questionnaires vs. 24-hr. recall interviews. J Am Diet Assoc 74:656–659.

HUNTER D, WILLETT WC. 1994. Vitamin A and cancer: epidemiological evidence in humans. In: *Vitamin A in Health and Disease*, Blomhoff R (ed). New York: Marcel Dekker, pp 561–584.

HUNTER DC. 1989. Biochemical indicators of dietary intake. In: *Nutritional Epidemiology*, Willett WC (ed). New York: Oxford University Press, pp 143–216.

HUNTER, DJ MORRIS JS, STAMPFER MJ, COLDITZ GA, SPEIZER FE, WILLETT WC. 1990. A prospective study of selenium status and breast cancer risk. JAMA 264:1128–1131.

HUNTER DJ, RIMM EB, SACKS FM, STAMPFER MJ, COLDITZ GA, LITIN LB, WILLETT WC. 1992. Comparison of measures of fatty acid intake by subcutaneous fat aspirate, food frequency questionnaire, and diet records in a free-living population of US men. Am J Epidemiol 135:418–427.

HUNTER DJ, STAMPFER MJ, COLDITZ GA, et al. 1991. A prospective study of consumption of vitamins A, C, and E and breast cancer risk. (Abstract). Am J Epidemiol 134:715.

IARC WORKING GROUP. 1988. Alcohol drinking, International Agency for Cancer Research Monograph on the Evaluation of Carcinogenic Risks to Humans, Vol. 44. Lyon, France, IARC.

JACQUES PF, SULSKY SI, SADOWSKI, PHILLIPS, JCC, RUSH D, WILLETT WC. 1993. Comparison of micronutrient intake measured by a dietary questionnaire and biochemical indicators of micronutrient status. Am J Clin Nutr 57:182–189.

JAIN MG, HARRISON L, HOWE GR, MILLER AB. 1982. Evaluation of a self-administered dietary questionnaire for use in a cohort study. Am J Clin Nutr 36:931–935.

JENSEN OM, WAHRENDORF J, ROSENQVIST A, et al. 1984. The reliability of questionnaire-derived historical dietary information and temporal stability of food habits in individuals. Am J Epidemiol 120:281–290.

JONES DY, SCHATZKIN A, GREEN SB, et al. 1987. Dietary fat and breast cancer in the National Health and Nutrition Examination Survey I Epidemiologic Follow-up Study. J Natl Cancer Inst 79:465–471.

JOOSSENS JV, GEBOERS J. 1987. Dietary salt and risks to health. Am J Clin Nutr 45 (suppl):1277–1288.

JUNSHI C, et al. 1990. Diet, lifestyle, and mortality, a study of the characteristics of 65 Chinese counties. Oxford: Oxford University Press.

KARVETTI RL, KNUTS LR. 1985. Validity of the 24-hour recall. J Am Diet Assoc 85: 1437–1442.

KATSOUYANNI K, WILLETT WC, BOYLE P, et al. 1988. Risk of breast cancer among Greek women in relation to nutrient intake. Cancer 61:181–185.

KINLEN LJ. 1983. Fat and cancer. Br Med J 286:1081–1082.

KNEKT P, AROMAA A, MAATELA J, et al. 1988. Serum vitamin E and risk of cancer among Finnish men during a 10-year follow-up. Am J Epidemiol 127:28–41.

KOK FJ, DE BRUIJN AM, HOFMAN A, VERMEEREN R, VALKENBURG HA. 1987. Is serum selenium a risk factor for cancer in men only? Am J Epidemiol 125:12–16.

KOLONEL LN, YOSHIZAWA CN, HANKIN JH. 1988. Diet and prostatic cancer: a case-control study in Hawaii. Am J Epidemiol 127:999–1012.

KUSHI LH, LEW RA, STARE FJ. 1985. Diet and 20-year mortality from coronary heart disease: the Ireland-Boston Diet-Heart study. N Engl J Med 312:811–818.

KUSHI LH, SELLERS TA, POTTER JD, et al. 1992. Dietary fat and postmenopausal breast cancer. J Natl Cancer Inst 84:1092–1099.

LAVECCHIA C, DECARLI A, NEGRI E, et al. 1987. Dietary factors and the risk of epithelial ovarian cancer. J Natl Cancer Inst 79:663–669.

LAVECCHIA C, NEGRI E, DECARLI A, et al. 1988. A case-control study of diet and colo-rectal cancer in northern Italy. Int J Cancer 41:492–498.

LE MARCHAND L, KOLONEL LN, EARLE ME, MI MP. 1988. Body size at different periods of life and breast cancer risk. Am J Epidemiol 128:137–152.

LE MARCHAND L, KOLONEL LN, WILKENS LR, MYERS BC, HIROHATA T. 1994. Animal fat consumption and prostate cancer: a prospective study in Hawaii. Epidemiology 5:276–282.

LEW EA, GARFINKEL L. 1979. Variations in mortality by weight among 750,000 men and women. J Chronic Dis 32:563–576.

LIPPMAN SM, MEYSKENS FL. 1989. Retinoids for the prevention of cancer. In: *Micronutrients and Cancer Prevention*, Moon TE, Micozzi MS (eds). New York: Marcel Dekker, Inc., pp 243–272.

LOHMAN TG, ROCHE AF, MARTORELL R. 1988. Anthropometric Standardization Reference Manual. Champaign, IL: Human Kinetics Books.

LONDON SJ, SACKS FM, CAESAR J, STAMPFER MJ, SIGUEL E, WILLETT WC. 1991. Fatty acid composition of subcutaneous adipose tissue and diet in postmenopausal US women. Am J Clin Nutr 54:340–345.

LUBIN F, RUDER AM, WAX Y, MODAN G. 1985. Overweight and changes in weight throughout adult life in breast cancer etiology: a case-control study. Am J Epidemiol 122:579–588.

LYON AW, MAHONEY JL, WEST DW, et al. 1987. Energy intake: its relation to colon cancer risk. J Natl Cancer Inst 78:853–861.

MACQUART-MOULIN GE, RIBOLI E, CORNEE J. 1986. Case-control study on colorectal cancer and diet in Marseilles. Int J Cancer 38:183–191.

MADDEN JP, GOODMAN SJ, GUTHRIE HA. 1976. Validity of the 24-hour recall: analysis of data obtained from elderly subjects. J Am Diet Assoc 68:143–147.

MANOUSOS O, DAY NE, TRICHOPOULOS D. 1983. Diet and colorectal cancer: a case-control study in Greece. Int J Cancer 32:1–5.

MARR JW. 1971. Individual dietary surveys: purposes and methods. World Rev Nutr Diet 13:105–164.

MARSHALL J, GRAHAM S, METTLIN C, et al. 1982. Diet in the epidemiology of oral cancer. Nutr and Cancer 3:145–149.

MARTINEZ I, TORRES R, FRIAS Z, COLON JR, FERNANDEZ N. 1979. Factors associated with adenocarcinomas of the large bowel in Puerto

Rico. In: *Adv Med Oncol Res Education 3*, Birch JM (ed). New York: Pergamon Press, pp 45–52.

MARUBINI E, DECARLI A, COSTA A, et al. 1988. The relationship of dietary intake and serum levels of retinol and beta-carotene with breast cancer: results of a case-control study. Cancer 61:173–180.

MATHEWS-ROTH MM. 1989. Beta-carotene, canthaxanthin, and phytoene. In: *Micronutrients and Cancer Prevention*, Moon TE, Micozzi MS (eds). New York: Marcel Dekker, Inc., pp 273–290.

MCKEOWN-EYSSEN GE, BRIGHT-SEE E. 1985. Dietary factors in colon cancer: international relationships: an update. Nutr Cancer 7:251–253.

MCMICHAEL AJ, GILES GG. 1988. Cancer in migrants to Australia: extending the descriptive epidemiological data. Cancer Res 48:751–756.

MENKES MS, COMSTOCK GW, VAULLEUMIER JP, HELSING KJ, RIDER AA, BROOKMEYER R. 1986. Serum beta-carotene, vitamins A and E, selenium, and the risk of lung cancer. N Engl J Med 315:1250–1254.

MERGENS WJ, BHAGAVAN HN. 1989. a-Tocopherols (vitamin E). In *Nutrition and Cancer Prevention*, Moon TE, Micozzi MS (eds). New York: Marcel Dekker, Inc., pp 341–388.

MERTZ W. 1984. Foods and nutrients. J Am Diet Assoc 84:769–770.

METTLIN C, GRAHAM S, SWANSON M. 1979. Vitamin A and lung cancer. J Natl Cancer Inst 62:1435–1438.

METTLIN C, GRAHAM S. 1979. Dietary risk factors in human bladder cancer. Am J Epidemiol 110:255–263.

METTLIN C, GRAHAM S, PRIORE R, et al. 1981. Diet and cancer of the esophagus. Nutr and Cancer 2:143–147.

MICHELS KB, WILLETT WC. 1992. The women's health initiative: daughter of politics or science? In *Cancer Prevention*, DeVita VT, Hellman S, Rosenberg SA (eds). Philadelphia: JB Lippincott Company, pp 1–11.

MILLER AB, KELLY A, CHOI, NW et al. 1978. A study of diet and breast cancer. Am J Epidemiol 107:499–509.

MILLER AB, HOWE GR, JAIN M, CRAIB KJ, HARRISON L. 1983. Food items and food groups as risk factors in a case-control study of diet and colo-rectal cancer. Int J Cancer 32:155–161.

MIRVISH SS, WALLCAVE L, EAGEN M, SHUBIK P. 1972. Ascorbate-nitrite reaction: possible means of blocking the formation of carcinogenic N-nitroso compounds. Science 177:65–68.

MODAN B, BARELL V, LUBIN F, MODAN M, GREENBERG RA, GRAHAM S. 1975. Low fiber intake as an etiologic factor in cancer of the colon. J Natl Cancer Inst 55:15–18.

MORGAN RW, JAIN M, MILLER AB, et al. 1978. A comparison of dietary methods in epidemiologic studies. Am J Epidemiol 107:488–498.

MORRIS JN, MARR JW, CLAYTON DG. 1977. Diet and heart: a postscript. Br Med J 2: 1307–1314.

MORRIS JS, STAMPFER MJ, WILLETT WC. 1983. Toenails as an indicator of dietary selenium. Biol Trace Element Res 5:529–537.

MULTIPLE RISK FACTOR INTERVENTION TRIAL RESEARCH GROUP. 1982. Risk factor changes and mortality results. J Am Med Assoc 248:1465–1477.

NOMURA AM, STEMMERMANN GN, HEILBRUN LK, et al. 1985. Serum vitamin levels and the risk of cancer of specific sites in men of Japanese ancestry in Hawaii. Cancer Res 45:2369–2372.

NOMURA A, HEILBRUN LK, MORRIS JS, STEMMERMANN GN. 1987. Serum selenium and risk of cancer by specific sites: case-control analysis of prospective data. J Natl Cancer Inst 79:103–108.

OHNO Y, YOSHIDA O, OISHI K, OKADA K, YAMABE H, SCHROEDER FH. 1988. Dietary beta-carotene and cancer of the prostate; a case-control study in Kyoto, Japan. Cancer Res 48:1331–1336.

PAFFENBARGER RS JR, KAMPERT JB, CHANG HG. 1980. Characteristics that predict risk of breast cancer before and after the menopause. Am J Epidemiol 112:258–268.

PAMUKCU AM, PRICE JM, BRYAN GT. 1970. Assay of fractions of bracken fern (Pteris aquilina) for carcinogenic activity. Cancer Res 30:902–905.

PELEG I, MORRIS S, HAMES CG. 1985. Is serum selenium a risk factor for cancer? Med Oncol Tumor Pharmacother 2:157–163.

PETO R, DOLL R, BUCKLEY JD, SPORN MD. 1981. Can dietary beta-carotene materially reduce human cancer rates? Nature 290:201–208.

PHILLIPS RL, GARFINKEL L, KUZMA JW, BEESON WL, LOTZ T, BRIN B. 1980. Mortality among California Seventh-Day Adventists for selected cancer sites. J Natl Cancer Inst 65:1097–1107.

PICKLE LW, HARTMAN AM. 1985. Indicator foods for vitamin A assessment. Nutr Cancer 7:3–23.

PIETINEN P, HARTMAN AM, HAAPA E, et al. 1988a. Reproducibility and validity of dietary assessment instruments: II. A qualitative food frequency questionnaire. Am J Epidemiol 128:667–676.

PIETINEN P, HARTMAN AM, HAAPA E, et al. 1988b. Reproducibility and validity of dietary assessment instruments: I. A self-administered food use questionnaire with a portion size picture booklet. Am J Epidemiol 128:655–666.

POSNER BM, BORMAN CL, MORGAN JL, BORDEN WS, OHLS JC. 1982. The validity of a telephone-administered 24-hour dietary recall methodology. Am J Clin Nutr 36:546–553.

POTTER JD, MCMICHAEL AJ. 1986. Diet and cancer of the colon and rectum: a case-control study. J Natl Cancer Inst 76:557–569.

PRENTICE RL, KAKAR F, HURSTING S, SHEPPARD L, KLEIN R, KUSHI LH. 1988. Aspects of the rationale for the Women's Health Trial. J Natl Cancer Inst 80:802–814.

RAINERI R, WEISBURGER JH. 1975. Reduction of gastric carcinogens with ascorbic acid. Ann NY Acad Sci 258:181–189.

REVICKI DA, ISRAEL RG. 1986. Relationship between body mass indices and measures of body adiposity. Am J Public Health 76:992–994.

RHOADS GG, KAGAN A. 1983. The relation of coronary disease, stroke, and mortality to weight in youth and in middle age. Lancet 1:492–495.

RIMM EB, GIOVANNUCCI E, STAMPFER MJ, COLDITZ GA, LITIN L, WILLETT WC. 1992. Reproducibility and validity of an expanded self-administered semiquantitative food frequency questionnaire among male health professionals. Am J Epidemiol 135:1114–1126.

ROHAN TE, HOWE GR, FRIEDENREICH CM, et al. 1993. Dietary fiber, vitamins A, C, and E, and risk of breast cancer: a cohort study. Cancer Causes Control 4:29–37.

ROHAN TE, MCMICHAEL AJ, BAGHURST PA. 1988. A population-based case-control study of diet and breast cancer in Australia. Am J Epidemiol 128:478–489.

ROHAN TE, POTTER JD. 1984. Retrospective assessment of dietary intake. Am J Epidemiol 120:876–887.

ROMNEY SL, DUTTAGUPTA C, BASU J, et al. 1985. Plasma vitamin C and uterine cervical dysplasia. Am J Obstet Gynecol 151:976–980.

ROSNER B, HENNEKENS CH, KASS EH, MIALL WE. 1977. Age-specific correlation analysis of longitudinal blood pressure data. Am J Epidemiol 106:306–313.

ROSNER B, SPIEGELMAN D, WILLETT WC. 1992. Correction of logistic regression relative risk estimates and confidence intervals for random within-person measurement error. Am J Epidemiol 136:1400–1413.

ROSNER B, WILLETT WC, SPIEGELMAN D. 1989. Correction of logistic regression relative risk estimates and confidence intervals for systematic within-person measurement error. Stat Med 8:1051–1069.

ROSS MH, BRAS G. 1971. Lasting influence of early caloric restriction on prevalence of neoplasms in the rat. J Natl Cancer Inst 47:1095–1113.

RUSSELL-BRIEFEL R, BATES MW, KULLER LH. 1985. The relationship of plasma carotenoids to health and biochemical factors in middle-aged men. Am J Epidemiol 122:741–749.

SACKS FM, HANDYSIDES GH, MARIAS GE, ROSNER B, KASS EH. 1986. Effects of a low-fat diet on plasma lipoprotein levels. Arch Intern Med 146:1573–1577.

SALONEN JT, ALFTHAN G, HUTTUNEN JK, PUSKA P. 1984. Association between serum selenium and the risk of cancer. Am J Epidemiol 120:342–349.

SALONEN JT, SALONEN R, LAPPETLAINEN R, MEAENPAA PH, ALFTHAN G, PUSKA P. 1985. Risk of cancer in relation to serum concentrations of selenium and vitamins A and E: matched case-control analysis of prospective data. Br Med J 290:417–420.

SALVINI S, HUNTER DJ, SAMPSON L, STAMPFER MJ, COLDITZ GA, ROSNER B, WILLETT WC. 1989. Food-based validation of a dietary questionnaire: the effect of week-to-week variation in food consumption. Int J Epidemiol 18:858–867.

SAMET JM, HUMBLE CG, SKIPPER BE. 1984. Alternatives in the collection and analysis of food frequency interview data. Am J Epidemiol 120:572–581.

SAMET JM, SHIPPER BJ, HUMBLE CG, PATHAK DR. 1985. Lung cancer risk and vitamin A consumption in New Mexico. Am Rev Respir Dis 131:198–200.

SCHRAUZER GN, WHITE DA, SCHNEIDER CJ. 1977. Cancer mortality correlation studies—III: Statistical associations with dietary selenium intakes. Bioinorgan Chem 7:23–31.

SELHUB J, JACQUES PF, WILSON PWF, RUSH D, ROSENBERG IH. 1993. Vitamin status and intake as primary determinants of homocysteinemia in an elderly population. JAMA 270:2693–2698.

SHAMBERGER RJ, TYTKO SA, WILLIS CE. 1976. Antioxidants and cancer, Part VI: Selenium and age-adjusted human cancer mortality. Arch Environ Health 31:231–235.

SHEKELLE RB, SHRYOCK AM, PAUL O, et al. 1981. Diet, serum cholesterol, and death from coronary heart disease: the Western Electric study. N Engl J Med 304:64–70.

SHEKELLE RB, LEPPER M, LIU S, et al. 1981. Dietary vitamin A and risk of cancer in the Western Electric study. Lancet 2:1186–1190.

SILVERMAN I, REIS GJ, SACKS FM, et al. 1990. Usefulness of plasma phospholipid n-3 fatty acids in predicting dietary fish intake in patients with coronary heart disease. Am J Cardiol 66:680–682.

SLATTERY ML, SCHUMACHER MC, SMITH KR, WEST DW, ABDEIGHANY N. 1988. Physical activity, diet, and risk of colon cancer in Utah. Am J Epidemiol 128:989–999.

SPIEGELMAN D, ISRAEL RG, BOUCHARD C, WILLETT WC. 1992. Absolute fat mass, percent body, and body fat distribution: which is the real risk factor for diabetes and hypertension? Am J Clin Nutr 55:1033–1044.

STAHELIN HB, ROSEL F, BUESS E, et al. 1984. Cancer, vitamins, and plasma lipids: prospective Basel study. J Natl Cancer Inst 73:1463–1468.

STAMPFER MJ, WILLETT WC, SPEIZER FE, et al. 1984. Test of the National Death Index. Am J Epidemiol 119: 837–839.

STAMPFER MJ, WILLETT WC, HENNEKENS CH. 1989. Choice of populations for cancer prevention trials. In *Nutrition and Cancer Prevention*, Moon TE, Micozzi MS (eds). New York: Marcel Dekker, Inc., pp 473–482.

STASZEWSKI J, HAENSZEL W. 1965. Cancer mortality among the Polish-born in the United States. J Natl Cancer Inst 35:291–297.

STEINMETZ KA, KUSHI LH, BOSTICK RM, FOLSOM AR, POTTER JD. 1994. Vegetables, fruit, and colon cancer in the Iowa Women's Health Study. Am J Epidemiol 139:1–15.

STEPHANIK PA, TRULSON MF. 1962. Determining the frequency of foods in large group studies. Am J Clin Nutr 2:335–343.

STRYKER WS, KAPLAN LA, STEIN EA, et al. 1988. The relation of diet, cigarette smoking, and alcohol consumption to plasma beta-carotene and alpha-tocopherol levels. Am J Epidemiol 127:283–296.

STUFF JE, GARZA C, SMITH EO, NICHOLS BL, MONTANDON CM. 1983. A comparison of dietary methods in nutritional studies. Am J Clin Nutr 37:300–306.

STUNKARD AJ, ALBAUM JM. 1981. The accuracy of self-reported weights. Am J Clin Nutr 34:1593–1599.

SUGIMURA T. 1986. Studies on environmental chemical carcinogenesis in Japan. Science 233:312–318.

SWANSON CA, JONES DY, SCHATZKIN A, et al. 1988. Breast cancer risk assessed by anthropometry in the NHANES I epidemiological follow-up study. Cancer Res 48:5363–5367.

TANNENBAUM A. 1942. The genesis and growth of tumors, III: Effects of a high fat diet. Cancer Res 2:468–475.

TRETLI S. 1989. Height and weight in relation to breast cancer morbidity and mortality: a prospective study of 570,000 women in Norway. Int J Cancer 44:23–30.

TROCK B, LANZA E, GREENWALD P. 1990. Dietary fiber, vegetables, and colon cancer: critical review and meta-analyses of the epidemiologic evidence. J Natl Cancer Inst 82:650–661.

TROLL W, WIESNER R, FRENKEL K. 1987. Anticarcinogenic action of protease inhibitors. Adv Cancer Res 49:265–283.

VAGUE J. 1956. The degree of masculine differentiation of obesity: a factor determining predisposition to diabetes, atherosclerosis, gout and uric-calculous disease. Am J Clin Nutr 4:20–34.

VALAORAS VG, MACMAHON B, TRICHOPOULOS D, POLYCHRONOPOULOU A. 1969. Lactation and reproductive histories of breast cancer patients in greater Athens, 1965–67. Int J Cancer 4:350–363.

VAN DEN BRANDT PA, GOLDBOHM RA, VAN'T VEER P, DORANT E, HERMUS RJ, STURMANS F. 1993. A prospective cohort study on selenium status and the risk of lung cancer. Cancer Res 53:4860–4865.

VAN DEN BRANDT PA, VAN'T VEER P, GOLDBOHM RR, et al. 1993. A prospective cohort study on dietary fat and the risk of postmenopausal breast cancer. Cancer Res 53:75–82.

VAN ITALLIE TB. 1978. Dietary fiber and obesity. Am J Clin Nutr 31 (suppl):543–552.

VAN NOORD PA, COLLETTE HJ, MAAS MJ, DE WAARD F. 1987. Selenium levels in nails of premenopausal breast cancer patients assessed prediagnostically in a cohort-nested case-referent study among women screened in the DOM project. Int J Epidemiol 16:318–322.

VIRTAMO J, VALKEILA E, ALFTHAN G, PUNSAR S, HUTTUNEN JK, KARVONEN MJ. 1987. Serum selenium and risk of cancer: a prospective follow-up of nine years. Cancer 60:145–148.

WALD N, BOREHAM J, BAILEY A. 1986. Serum retinol and subsequent risk of cancer. Br J Cancer 54:957–961.

WALD NJ, NICOLAIDES-BOUMAN A, HUDSON GA. 1988. Plasma retinol, beta-carotene and vitamin E levels in relation to the future risk of breast cancer. (Letter) Br J Cancer 57:235.

WALD NJ, BOREHAM J, HAYWARD JL, BULBROOK RD. 1984. Plasma retinol, beta-carotene, and vitamin E levels in relation to the future risk of breast cancer. Br J Cancer 49:321–324.

WALD NJ, THOMPSON SG, DENSEM JW, BOREHAM J, BAILEY A. 1987. Serum vitamin E and subsequent risk of cancer. Br J Cancer 56:69–72.

WALKER AM, BLETTNER M. 1985. Comparing imperfect measures of exposure. Am J Epidemiol 121:783–790.

WASSERTHEIL-SMOLLER S, ROMNEY SL, WYLIE-ROSETT J, et al. 1981. Dietary vitamin C and uterine cervical dysplasia. Am J Epidemiol 114: 714–724.

WATTENBERG LW, LOUB WD. 1978. Inhibition of polycyclic aromatic hydrocarbon-induced neoplasia by naturally occurring indoles. Cancer Res 38:1410–1413.

WEINDRUCH R, WALFORD RL. 1982. Dietary restriction in mice beginning at 1 year of age: effect on life-span and spontaneous cancer incidence. Science 215:1415–1418.

WELSH SO, MARSTON RM. 1982. Review of trends in food use in the United States, 1909 to 1980. J Am Diet Assoc 81:120–128.

WIEHL DG, REED R. 1960. Development of new or improved dietary methods for epidemiological investigation. Am J Public Health 50:824.

WILLETT WC. 1987. Nutritional epidemiology: issues and challenges. Int J Epidemiol 16:312–317.

WILLETT WC. 1989a. An overview of issues related to the correction of non-differential exposure measurement error in epidemiologic studies. Stat Med 8:1031–1040.

WILLETT WC. 1989b. The search for the causes of breast and colon cancer. Nature 338: 389–394.

WILLETT WC. 1990. Nutritional Epidemiology. New York: Oxford University Press.

WILLETT WC. 1990a. Total energy intake and nutrient composition: dietary recommendations for epidemiologists. Int J Cancer 46:770–771.

WILLETT WC. 1990b. Vitamin A and lung cancer. Nutr Rev 48:201–211.

WILLETT WC. 1994. Diet and health: what should we eat? Science 264:532–537.

WILLETT WC, HUNTER DJ, STAMPFER MJ. 1992. Dietary fat and fiber in relation to risk of breast cancer: an eight-year follow-up. JAMA 268:2037–2044.

WILLETT WC, MACMAHON B. 1984. Diet and cancer: an overview. N Engl J Med 310:633–638.

WILLETT WC, REYNOLDS RD, COTTRELL-HOEHNER S, SAMPSON L, BROWN ML. 1987. Validation of a semi-quantitative food frequency questionnaire: comparison with a one-year diet record. J Am Diet Assoc 87:43–47.

WILLETT WC, SAMPSON LS, STAMPFER MJ, et al. 1985. Reproducibility and validity of a semiquantitative food frequency questionnaire. Am J Epidemiol 122:51–65.

WILLETT WC, STAMPFER MJ. 1986. Total energy intake: implications for epidemiologic analyses. Am J Epidemiol 124:17–27.

WILLETT WC, STAMPFER MJ. 1988. Selenium and cancer. (Editorial) Br Med J 297:573–574.

WILLETT WC, STAMPFER MJ, COLDITZ GA, ROSNER BA, HENNEKENS CH, SPEIZER FE. 1987. Dietary fat and the risk of breast cancer. N Engl J Med 316:22–28.

WILLETT WC, STAMPFER MJ, COLDITZ GA, ROSNER BA, SPEIZER FE. 1990. Relation of meat, fat, and fiber intake to the risk of colon cancer in a prospective study among women. N Engl J Med 323:1664–1672.

WILLETT WC, STAMPFER MJ, UNDERWOOD BA, SPEIZER FE, ROSNER B, HENNEKENS CH. 1983. Validation of a dietary questionnaire with plasma carotenoid and α-tocopherol levels. Am J Clin Nutr 38:631–639.

WINN DM, ZIEGLER RG, PICKLE LW, et al. 1984. Diet in the etiology of oral and pharyngeal cancer among women from the southern United States. Cancer Res 44:1216–1222.

WOMERSLEY J. 1977. A comparison of the skinfold method with extent of "overweight" and various weight-height relationships in the assessment of obesity. Br J Nutr 38:271–284.

WU AH, HENDERSON BE, PIKE MC, YU MD. 1985. Smoking and other risk factors for lung cancer in women. J Natl Cancer Inst 74:747–751.

WYNDER EL, MACCORNACK FA, STELLMAN SD. 1978. The epidemiology of breast cancer in 785 United States Caucasian women. Cancer 41:2341–2354.

YOU WC, BLOT WJ, CHANG YS, et al. 1988. Diet and high risk of stomach cancer in Shandong, China. Cancer Res 48:3518–3523.

YOU MC, MO CC, CHONG WX, YEH FS, HENDERSON BE. 1988. Preserved foods and nasopharyngeal carcinoma: a case-control study in Guangxi, China. Cancer Res 48:1954–1959.

ZIEGLER RG, MORRIS LE, BLOT WJ, et al. 1981. Esophageal cancer among black men in Washington, DC, II: Role of nutrition. J Natl Cancer Inst 67:1199–1206.

ZIEGLER RG, MASON TJ, STEMHAGEN A, et al. 1984. Dietary carotene and vitamin A and risk of lung cancer among white men in New Jersey. J Natl Cancer Inst 73:1429–1435.

22 Exogenous hormones

LESLIE BERNSTEIN
BRIAN E. HENDERSON

A substantial body of experimental, clinical, and epidemiological evidence indicates that hormones play a major role in the etiology of several human cancers. Based on experimental studies of estrogens and mammary cancer in mice, Bittner (1947) first proposed that hormones can cause, that is, increase the incidence of, neoplasia. This concept has been refined into epidemiological hypotheses related to cancers of the breast, endometrium, prostate, ovary, and testis (Henderson et al, 1982; Henderson et al, 1988a). A key element of these hypotheses is that neoplasia is the consequence of excessive hormonal stimulation of the particular target organ, the normal growth and function of which is under the control of one or more steroid or polypeptide hormones. In this model, hormones exert an effect that is independent of outside initiators such as chemicals or ionizing radiation.

The evidence for an association of endogenous hormones with risk for each of the hormone-related cancers mentioned above is reviewed in the chapters on those cancer sites. Taken together, these sites currently account for more than 20% of all newly diagnosed male and more than 40% of all newly diagnosed female cancers in the United States. Because of the evidence that endogenous hormones affect the risk of these cancers and the importance of these cancers in absolute frequency, there is reason for concern about the effects on cancer risk if the same or closely related hormones are administered for therapeutic purposes, for example, as contraceptives, as hormone replacement therapy, or for the prevention of miscarriages. This chapter briefly reviews the vast amount of epidemiological information regarding the effects of therapeutic hormones on the risk of cancer. Where results of specific case-control and cohort studies are reported, the terminology relative risk (RR) has been used to represent odds ratios as well as rate ratios.

ORAL CONTRACEPTIVES

Because of the widespread use of oral contraceptives as a birth control method, the assessment of the possible relationship between oral contraceptive use and cancer continues to be of great public health importance. A substantial body of literature exists on the relationship between oral contraceptive use and subsequent risk of cancers of the endometrium, ovary, breast, cervix, and liver. Reports have also been published assessing whether oral contraceptive use affects the risk of malignant melanoma or thyroid cancer.

When evaluating the results of epidemiological studies on the possible effects of oral contraceptives on cancer risk, the following factors must be considered: latent period, temporal changes in pill formulation, timing of exposure (both in terms of the woman's age and in terms of her reproductive history), a woman's baseline risk for the particular cancer, and differences in study design.

The period of time between first exposure to a carcinogen and the development of overt malignant disease (the latent period) is generally long and considered to be on the order of 15 to 30 years (Doll and Peto, 1981). In order to detect the effect of an exposure in epidemiological studies, a sufficient number of cases must arise as a result of the exposure. In addition to time since first exposure, exposure intensity and exposure duration are important factors. Since widespread use of oral contraceptives began in the middle 1960s, results of early epidemiological studies may have been premature, as few women would have had both prolonged exposure and extended follow-up. Rates of acceptance of oral contraceptives as a birth control method have varied geographically and by subgroups of women, so that these factors must be considered in the critical evaluation of epidemiological studies of cancer risks. There have been marked changes in pill composition over time. Sequential oral contraceptives, which administered a constant, relatively high dose of estrogen for 14 to 16 days and an estrogen-progestogen combination for 5 to 6 days, were removed from sale in the United States in 1976 because of reports of increased endometrial cancer risk associated with their use (see below) and because they were less efficacious than combination oral contraceptives. Combination oral contraceptives, the most popular pill type, commonly contain a fixed amount of estrogen and progestogen and are taken for 20 to 21 days in each 28-day cycle. Progestogen-only pills, which contain a considerably lower dose of progestogen than other pill types and no estrogen, were introduced in the United States in 1973 but have never been widely used (Piper and Kennedy, 1987). Biphasic and triphasic oral contraceptives, introduced in 1983, generally deliver a fixed, relatively low estrogen dose over 21 days, and alter the dosage of progestogen given in each phase.

Over time, combination oral contraceptives have evolved from pills with a high steroidal content to lower dose combinations (Piper and Kennedy, 1987). The more recently introduced multiphasic pills deliver the low doses of estrogen that are characteristic of newer combination formulations. Data on prescription sales in the United States indicate that pills with less than 50μg of estrogen (including multiphasics) made up 78.6% of the market share, with 50μg products constituting 19% of the market (IMS America, 1987). Only 2.4% of the prescriptions filled were for oral contraceptives with more than 50μg of estrogen. Multiphasic pills have continued to grow in popularity, constituting 32% of prescriptions (IMS America, 1987).

Exposure to contraceptive steroids at particular ages or reproductive times of life, such as during adolescence, prior to first pregnancy or in the perimenopausal period, may be especially important. Initially, the majority of oral contraceptive users were married women who used this method of contraception for spacing births after the first full-term pregnancy. The results of studies of cancer risk in such women may not be relevant to women who begin oral contraceptive use during adolescence. Age at first use has declined substantially, and by the early 1980s, oral contraceptives were the contraceptive method of choice for sexually active teenaged girls (Tyrer, 1984; Russel-Briefel et al, 1985).

Some women are at higher risk for a particular cancer than others. It is possible that oral contraceptives may have no effect on cancer risk for the general population of women, but may have a striking effect on the risk for women with certain predisposing factors (e.g., for breast cancer, women with a positive family history of breast cancer, or those with a history of benign breast disease).

In addition to the timing of the study in relation to the availability of and prolonged use of different preparations, the study design, methods of data collection and relevant characteristics of study subjects are important. Results are reviewed here for both cohort studies and case-control studies. Since these studies are observational, potential sources of bias must be considered before interpreting the results and the study population must be considered in drawing generalizations.

Endometrial Cancer

Estrogen stimulates endometrial cell division, but only in the absence of progestogen; that is, "unopposed" estrogen stimulates endometrial cell division. In a normal menstrual cycle endometrial cell mitotic activity peaks during the early follicular phase when unopposed serum estradiol levels are approximately 50 pg/ml; further increases in estradiol do not appear to increase the mitotic rate (Ferenczy et al, 1979; Goebelsmann and Mishell, 1979). Following ovulation, serum progesterone rises and endometrial cell proliferation ceases despite continued elevated estradiol levels. Thus, it is not surprising that during the time that the association of prolonged use of estrogen replacement therapy and endometrial cancer was being established, case-series reports suggested a similar association between sequential oral contraceptives and endometrial cancer (Silverberg and Makowski, 1975). Sequential pills would be expected to have this effect on the endometrium because these formulations result in a menstrual cycle that begins with a 14- to 16-day unopposed estrogen phase followed by a short, 7-day secretory phase (estrogen-progestogen combination) and ends with a 5- to 7-day period with low unopposed estrogen. Three case-control studies with sufficient data on the use of sequential oral contraceptives show a twofold increased risk of endometrial cancer following use of these preparations (Weiss and Sayvetz, 1980; Centers for Disease Control [CDC], 1983c; Henderson et al, 1983a).

In contrast to the adverse effects on the endometrium of sequential oral contraceptives, use of combination oral contraceptives would be predicted to lower risk. Since combination oral contraceptives contain both estrogen and progestogen, endometrial cells are exposed to unopposed estrogen only during the 7 days in 28 when the combination pill is not taken; endogenous estrogen levels during these 7 days remain quite low. Use of combination oral contraceptives has been reported consistently in case-control studies to decrease the risk of endometrial cancer by about 50% (Table 22–1). The Walnut Creek Contraceptive Drug Study (Ramcharan et al, 1981) and Royal College of General Practitioners' Oral Contraception Study (Beral et al, 1988), prospective cohort studies, have demonstrated similar decreases in risk.

In the large, multicenter Cancer and Steroid Hormone (CASH) study sponsored by the CDC and the National Institute of Child Health and Human Development, there was no apparent difference in risk for short-term use of combination oral contraceptives (< 5 years) compared with longer use (CDC, 1983c), although very short term users (< 1 year) were not protected (CDC, 1987a). In contrast, Henderson and colleagues (1983a) and Stanford and colleagues (1993) observed clear de-

TABLE 22–1. *Case-Control Studies of Combination Oral Contraceptives and Endometrial Cancer*

First Author and Reference	*Age Range*	*Relative Risk*[a]	*Number of Cases Using Oral Contraceptives*
Kaufman (1980)	≤59	0.5	16
Weiss (1980)	35–54	0.5	17
Hulka (1982b)	≤59	0.4	5
Kelsey (1982)	45–74	0.6	6
Centers for Disease Control (CASH) (1983c, 1987a)	20–54	0.6	70
Henderson (1983a)	≤45	0.5	43
WHO Collaborative Study (1988)	25–59	0.6	12
Stanford (1993)	20–74	0.4	78

[a]Ever vs never users of oral contraceptives.

clines in risk with increasing duration of use. In both studies, the relative risk for the category of longest use (≥ 6 years in Henderson et al and ≥ 10 years in Stanford et al) was less than 0.2.

Whether the protective effect persists with increasing duration of time since last use is an important question, and study results are mixed. In both the CASH study (CDC, 1983c) and the study of Stanford and colleagues (1993), the protective effect of pill use persisted for women who discontinued using oral contraceptives 15–20 years prior to participation in the study.

Voigt and colleagues (1994) combined data from two case-controls studies conducted in western Washington. In their analysis, the protective effect of oral contraceptives was observed only among women who had never used unopposed postmenopausal estrogen replacement therapy or who had used such therapy for less than 3 years.

No consistent differential effect on endometrial cancer risk was demonstrated by specific formulation of combination oral contraceptive used in the CASH study (CDC, 1987a) or by dichotomizing the ratio of estrogen to progestogen into high and low potency in the study by Henderson and colleagues (1983a). Voigt and colleagues (1994) assessed endometrial cancer risk according to progestin potency and found the reduction in endometrial cancer risk of women who had used low progestin content pills was similar to that of women using high progestin content pills. These results contrast with those of two other studies. Hulka and associates (1982b) ranked products by their progestogen content and found the greatest reduction in risk occurred among women using products with the highest progestogen dose. A similar result has been reported by the WHO Collaborative study (Rosenblatt et al, 1991).

In the studies of Henderson and colleagues (1983a) and Stanford and colleagues (1993), no protective effect of combination oral contraceptive use on endometrial cancer risk was observed in women in the highest weight category. When not taking oral contraceptives, obese premenopausal women may experience increased frequency of anovulatory menstrual cycles (ie, unopposed estrogen exposure) and lower progesterone levels during ovulatory menstrual cycles (Shoup, 1991), both of which would contribute to their greater endometrial cancer risk. Because combination oral contraceptives provide progestins throughout the 21-day treatment cycle, an explanation for the lack of an oral contraceptive effect in obese women is not obvious.

Ovarian Cancer

A number of case-control studies have examined the association between prior use of oral contraceptives and ovarian cancer (primarily epithelial cancers). Results from 13 of these studies are presented in Table 22–2. Except for a small series of women in Utah reported by Risch and associates (1983), each of these studies has shown a decreased risk among oral contraceptive users, averaging about 40%. Reports from major cohort studies of oral contraceptive use are consistent with these results (Ramcharan et al, 1981; Vessey et al, 1987; Beral

TABLE 22–2. *Case-Control Studies of Oral Contraceptives and Epithelial Carcinoma of the Ovary*

First Author and Reference	*Age Range*	*Relative Risk*[a]	*Number of Cases Using Oral Contraceptives*
Newhouse (1977)	All ages	0.6	19
Casagrande (1979)	25–49	0.8	41
McGowan (1979)	Mean, 52	0.7	NP
Hildreth (1981)	45–74	0.5	3
Willett (1981)	30–55	0.8	13
Cramer (1982)	≤59	0.4	34
Franceschi (1982)	≤69	0.7	17
Rosenberg (1982)	≤59	0.6	29
Centers for Disease Control (CASH) (1983b)	20–54	0.6	90
Risch (1983)			
Washington	34–74	0.4[b]	NP[c]
Utah	20–74	1.1[b]	NP[c]
La Vecchia (1984)	≤59	0.6	18
Wu (1988)	18–85	0.7	111
Booth (1989)	≤64	0.5	35

Abbreviation: NP = not provided.
[a]Ever vs never users of oral contraceptives.
[b]Estimated.
[c]Study provides percentage of cases exposed to oral contraceptives adjusted to age distribution of controls: 10.6% of 216 Washington cases and 10.9% of 68 Utah cases exposed to oral contraceptives.

et al, 1988). Oral contraceptives also appear to protect against borderline ovarian tumors (tumors of low malignant potential) (Harlow et al, 1988).

Because epithelial ovarian tumors are more common in less fertile women, this factor must be considered in interpreting the results of these studies as it could lead to a spurious, protective effect of pill use. Recent studies indicate that this explanation is unlikely to account for the lower risk among oral contraceptive users. The risk of ovarian cancer clearly decreases with increasing duration of oral contraceptive use (Casagrande et al, 1979; CDC, 1983b; Wu et al, 1988; Booth et al, 1989) and this dose-response effect appears to be independent of parity (Wu et al, 1988; Booth et al, 1989). The protection appears to be long-lasting (Rosenberg et al, 1982; CDC, 1983b; Wu et al, 1988; Booth et al, 1989). In the CASH study (CDC, 1983b), women who first used oral contraceptives 10 or more years before participating in the study had about one-half the risk of non-users. This study also examined risk associated with several specific oral contraceptive formulations and found similar protective effects for each (CDC, 1987b).

The Collaborative Ovarian Cancer Group combined data from 12 case-control studies conducted in the United States between 1956 and 1986 (Whittemore et al, 1992). For white women, the six hospital-based studies provided data on oral contraceptive use for 704 cases and 2901 controls; the six population-based studies provided data for 1283 cases and 5520 controls. Compared with nonusers of oral contraceptives, the ovarian cancer risk of women who had used oral contraceptives for 6 or more years was 0.30 in the combined population-based studies and 0.55 in the combined hospital-based studies. Women who had stopped using oral contraceptives at least 15 years prior to the studies' reference dates were more protected against ovarian cancer than were more recent pill users. This may reflect the usage of lower potency formulations by women whose use was more recent. Among black women in these studies (110 cases and 365 controls), a reduction in ovarian cancer risk was associated with oral contraceptive use, but risk did not decline linearly with increasing duration of use (John et al, 1993).

The risk of ovarian cancer is decreased by any pregnancy, whether complete or incomplete. Casagrande and coworkers (1979) suggested that this protection, as well as that provided by oral contraceptive use, resulted from the suppression of ovulation. They combined periods of pregnancy and oral contraceptive use into a single measure of "protected time" in the analysis of their case-control study and demonstrated that risk of ovarian cancer decreased as protected time increased.

It has been suggested that oral contraceptives containing only progestogens may enhance the formation of ovarian cysts (Moghiss, 1972; Aref et al, 1973; Tayob et al, 1985; Vessey et al, 1987). Tayob and colleagues (1985) reported higher frequency of functional ovarian cysts in women taking progestogen-only oral contraceptives compared with women using other birth control methods. Although findings were based on small numbers, Vessey and coworkers (1987) also noted higher rates of functional cysts in current users of progestogen-only pills.

Breast Cancer

The relationship of oral contraceptives to breast cancer risk has been the topic of many review articles (see, for example, Malone et al, 1993). Not all agree. Although numerous epidemiological studies have examined the relationship between oral contraceptives and the risk of breast cancer, this possible relationship continues to be a major source of controversy (Editorial, 1985; McPherson and Coope, 1986; Meirik, 1986a; Stadel et al, 1986; Drife, 1989; Peto, 1989; Pike and Bernstein, 1989). A number of studies were begun in the late 1960s, only a few years after oral contraceptives became available for clinical use. Unlike the consistent protective effects of combination oral contraceptives on the risk of endometrial and ovarian cancer, no clear trend is evident across breast cancer studies. If one can draw any conclusion from these studies, it is that oral contraceptives *do not protect* against breast cancer. In fact, one might argue that use at two particular times during the reproductive years, the postmenarcheal period and the perimenopausal period, would increase breast cancer risk if oral contraceptives provided greater hormonal exposure to estrogens and progestogens than would have occurred naturally during these time periods. Furthermore, certain subgroups of women may have increased risk of breast cancer following use of oral contraceptives, particularly women with benign breast disease, women with a positive family history of breast cancer, and nulliparous women.

Perimenopausal Period. Few studies have assessed the effects on breast cancer risk of oral contraceptive use around the time of menopause. Four that have either presented results for oral contraceptive use after age 40 or 45 years or presented results for current users aged 45 years or older have reported an elevated risk, although the range of risk estimates is wide (Vessey et al, 1979; Jick et al, 1980a; Brinton et al, 1982; Lipnick et al, 1986). These findings have not been confirmed in other studies (Rosenberg et al, 1984; Stanford et al, 1989; Thomas et al, 1991). Pike and colleagues (1993) summarized the results of six population-based studies that assessed total oral contraceptive use (use at any age) and the risk of breast cancer in women older than 45 years of age. Although three of these showed a positive

TABLE 22–3. *Design Aspects of Case-Control Studies of Oral Contraceptives and Breast Cancer*

Study and Reference	Dates of Diagnoses	Number of young women (Cases/Controls), Age	Source of Cases/Controls	Age Matched	Type of Interview
CASH (CDC 1983a, Stadel 1985 and 1989)	1980–1982	2088/2065 <45	Population-based/Random digit dial	No	In-person
Drug Epidemiology Unit I (Rosenberg 1984, Miller 1986)	1976–1983	521/521 <45	Hospital/Hospital	Yes[a]	In-person
Drug Epidemiology Unit II (Miller 1989)	1983–1986	407/424 25–44	Hospital/Hospital	No	In-person
London/Oxford Phases 1–4 (Vessey 1982 and 1983a)	1968–1980	1176/1176 ≤50	Hospital/Hospital	Yes	In-person
London/Oxford Phase 5 (McPherson 1987)	1980–1984	351/351 <45	Hospital/Hospital	Yes	In-person
Los Angeles (Pike 1981 and 1983, Bernstein 1990)	1972–1983	439/439 <38	Population-based/Neighborhood	Yes	Telephone
New Zealand (Paul 1986)	1983–1985	433/897 <45	Population-based/Electoral rolls	No	Telephone
Sweden/Norway (Meirik 1986b)	1984–1985	422/722[b] <45	Population-based/Population register	Yes	In-person
United Kingdom (UKNCCSG 1989)	1980–1985	755/755 <36	Population-based/General Practitioner rolls	Yes	In-person
Western Washington State (White 1994)	1983–1990	747/961 21–45	Population-based/Random digit dial	No	In-person

[a]Subgroup analysis presented in Miller et al (1986) is aged matched.
[b]Sweden only: 195 cases, 195 controls under age 40.

association, none was statistically significant. Overall, the studies provided no evidence that oral contraceptive use increases the risk of breast cancer among these older women; however, no firm conclusions can yet be drawn as women with access to oral contraceptives for most of their reproductive lives are only now entering the perimenopausal and postmenopausal ages. Several large-scale studies currently in the field should provide more complete assessment of this risk in the near future.

Postmenarcheal Period. Women who use oral contraceptives for long periods of time early in menstrual life, particularly before their first full-term pregnancy, may be at increased risk of breast cancer. Because prolonged use by very young women is a recent phenomenon, only the more recently conducted studies may have been able to measure such an effect. The results of 10 major case-control studies completed in the 1980s that have either specifically examined breast cancer risk associated with early oral contraceptive use in young women (under age 45), or that have provided subgroup results for young women, are reviewed here (Tables 22–3 through 22–5). [Note: The major cohort studies are not reviewed here, as few subjects had relevant exposure, ie, had used oral contraceptives in early reproductive life (Kay and Hanaford, 1988; Romieu et al, 1989; Vessey et al, 1989).]

TABLE 22–4. *"Negative" Case-Control Studies of the Relationship between Oral Contraceptive Use and Risk of Breast Cancer (Results presented for total duration of use by young women)*

Study and Reference	Age Range	Duration of Use	Relative Risk[a]
CASH (Stadel 1989)	20–54	1–47 mo	1.1
		48–95 mo	1.2
		96–143 mo	1.2
		≥144 mo	0.9
Drug Epidemiology Unit (Miller 1986)	20–45	1–11 mo	0.7[b]
		1–2 yr	1.4
		3–4 yr	0.8
		5–6 yr	1.5
		≥7 yr	1.4
London/Oxford Phases 1–4 (Vessey, 1982, 1983a)	16–35	1–12 mo	0.8
		13–48 mo	0.8
		49–96 mo	1.6
		≥97 mo	1.0
New Zealand (Paul 1986)	25–34	1–23 mo	2.8
		2–5 yr	1.6
		6–9 yr	1.8
		≥10 yr	4.6
	35–44	1–23 mo	0.9
		2–9 yr	0.9
		≥10 yr	0.8

[a]Risk relative to that of non-users.
[b]Use before first birth.

TABLE 22–5. *"Positive" Case-Control Studies of the Relationship between Oral Contraceptive Use and Risk of Breast Cancer (Results presented for total duration of use by young women)*

Study and Reference	*Age Range*	*Duration of Use*	*Relative Risk*[a]
Drug Epidemiology Unit II (Miller 1989)	25–44	<3 mo	2.5
		3–11 mo	1.8
		1–4 yr	1.8
		5–9 yr	1.9
		≥10 yr	4.1
London/Oxford Phase 5 (McPherson 1987)	16–44	1–48 mo	1.1
		4–12 yr	1.2
		≥12 yr	1.8
Sweden/Norway (Meirik 1986b)	<45	1–47 mo	1.1
		4–7 yr	1.2
		8–11 yr	1.4
		≥12 yr	2.2
Sweden (Meirik 1986b)	<40	1–47 mo	0.9
		4–7 yr	1.4
		8–11 yr	2.2
		≥12 yr	2.1
Los Angeles (Bernstein 1990)	<38	1–48 mo	0.9
		49–96 mo	1.1
		≥97 mo	1.7
United Kingdom (UKNCCSG 1989)	<36	1–48 mo	1.0
		49–96 mo	1.4
		≥97 mo	1.7
Western Washington[b] (White 1994)	36–45	1–2 yr	0.9
		3–5 yr	0.9
		6–9 yr	1.0
		≥10 yr	1.2
	21–35	1–2 yr	0.8
		3–5 yr	1.2
		6–9 yr	1.2
		≥10 yr	1.7

[a]Risk relative to that of non-users.
[b]Baseline comparison group includes women who had used oral contraceptives for less than 1 year as well as women who had never used oral contraceptives.

Overall, case-control studies (as well as cohort studies) have produced conflicting results. However, greater consensus appears in the latest reports from European studies (Meirik et al, 1986b; McPherson et al, 1987; UK National Case-Control Study Group [UKNCCSG], 1989), a recent United States hospital-based study (Miller et al, 1989), as well as more current analyses of the CASH Study (Stadel et al, 1988; Peto 1989; Pike and Bernstein 1989) and two population-based case-control studies, one conducted in Los Angeles (Bernstein et al, 1990) and the other in western Washington State (White et al, 1994) (Table 22–4).

Variations in design aspects of these studies may account for some of the early discrepant results that were reported and the resulting controversy regarding oral contraceptives and breast cancer risk. Studies have varied in terms of the source of cases and controls (population-based vs hospital-based), matching criteria used in selecting controls (none vs age, socioeconomic status, parity) and method of interview (in-person vs telephone) (Table 22–3). Using patients with diseases and conditions considered to be unrelated to oral contraceptive use as controls in the early hospital-based studies may have produced biased estimates of relative risk. A survey conducted in the United States during the early 1970s showed that oral contraceptive users were 20%–40% more likely to be hospitalized for non–life-threatening conditions than were nonusers (Hoover et al, 1978). If present, this bias would have resulted in underestimates of the true strength of the association between oral contraceptive use and breast cancer. No similar data on oral contraceptive use by women admitted to hospitals have been published for the 1980s.

The degree of age-matching in these studies also has varied widely, from matching on individual year of birth (Meirik et al, 1986b; UKNCCSG, 1989) to not matching on age at all (CDC 1983a; Rosenberg et al, 1984; Paul et al, 1986; White et al, 1994). Close age-matching may be critical because cohort trends in oral contraceptive use at young ages (before age 25 and before first full-term pregnancy) have been reported (Le et al, 1985). In-person interviews with subjects are preferable to telephone interviews because in-person interviews allow the use of photographs of oral contraceptives and a calendar to facilitate accurate recall of dates of use as well as formulations used.

Differential recall or reporting of oral contraceptive use by cases and controls must also be considered when examining the various study results. The results of some studies have been highly publicized so that, conceivably, subjects participating in some later studies may have been aware of the study hypotheses at the time of interview. Early studies that validated women's reported oral contraceptive use by examining their medical records found that cases had more accurate recall than controls and that controls were more likely to overestimate use than to underestimate it (Stolley et al, 1974; Rosenberg et al, 1983; Coulter et al, 1986). In the UK National Case-Control Study (1989), the comparison of subjects' self-reported use of oral contraceptives to general practitioners' notes revealed that cases more accurately reported their prescribed oral contraceptive use than controls with cases over-reporting at most 2% of their use.

Case selection bias must also be considered. If women who use oral contraceptives are more likely to practice breast self-examination or to have routine medical examinations, thereby resulting in earlier detection of breast cancer, a positive association with oral contraceptive use could result. The results of studies that examined pill use in association with breast tumor stage or size at diagnosis are not consistent. Mant and associates (1982) reported less advanced tumors at diagnosis in oral contraceptive users than in nonusers in Britain. However, in a United States series of breast cancer patients aged 35 and younger, Rosner and colleagues (1985) found no differences between oral contraceptive users and nonusers in clinical stage, histologic features of the primary tumor, or axillary node involvement. Among women with breast cancer who participated in the CASH study, oral contraceptive users had tumors that were slightly smaller and less likely to be late-stage (TNM stage III or IV) (Schlesselman et al, 1992). The net effect of such a diagnostic bias would be to advance the date of cancer diagnosis less than 8 weeks, which would correspond to, at most, a 2.4% increase in the risk of breast cancer associated with oral contraceptive use.

Control selection bias may also be an issue if, due to the selection process, controls do not represent the population from which the cases originated, or if the oral contraceptive usage of responders and nonresponders differs. Not only has concern been expressed regarding the appropriateness of hospital controls, but the use of random digit dial controls has been criticized because of a possibly high nonresponse rate during the first phase of contact (Editorial, 1986).

Response rates for cases may reflect an underlying survival bias associated with oral contraceptive use. Although longer survival of oral contraceptive users may be an explanation for positive study findings (Vessey et al, 1982), two studies of breast cancer survival among young women provide evidence against this potential source of bias. Rosner and colleagues (1985, 1986) reported no differences between oral contraceptive users and nonusers in terms of breast cancer disease-free interval, metastatic period, or survival. Furthermore, Swedish investigators (Olsson et al, 1988) found that premenopausal breast cancer patients who first used oral contraceptives before age 20 had significantly poorer survival than women who had never used oral contraceptives or who were older at time of first use. A detailed analysis of breast cancer survival in the Swedish and Norwegian case-control study (described below) found short-term (< 4 years) oral contraceptive users to be at significantly lower risk of dying than nonusers but found no difference between longer-term users and nonusers (Holmberg et al, 1994).

The largest of the "negative" studies (ie, studies that, overall, have reported no increased risk of breast cancer in young women associated with oral contraceptive use) is the CASH study (CDC, 1983a; Stadel et al, 1985), which was conducted simultaneously in eight areas of the United States (the metropolitan areas of Atlanta, Detroit, San Francisco, and Seattle; the states of Connecticut, Iowa, and New Mexico; and four urban areas of Utah). For women under age 45, no increased risk was found for any duration of oral contraceptive use category or for oral contraceptive use prior to first full-term pregnancy (Stadel et al, 1985). In a later publication, an excess risk associated with oral contraceptive use was reported among the small subgroup of premenopausal nulliparous women under age 45 who had menarche before age 13 (Stadel et al, 1988). Using the relative risks published in this paper, Peto (1989) noted an apparent contradiction with the earlier publication, calculating that, overall, premenopausal women with at least 4 years of oral contraceptive use had a significantly elevated relative risk of 1.5 (compared to the previously reported estimate of 1.2). These discrepancies in reporting appear to be due to differences in stratification and the methods of statistical adjustment for other variables (Peto, 1989; Pike and Bernstein, 1989). Analyses of the specific pill formulations (restricted to women aged 20–44 who used only one formulation) found no appreciable variation in overall relative risks associated with the estrogen component of the pill (Schlesselman et al, 1987). Although nulliparous women who used mestranol exclusively appeared to be at increased risk, no trend in risk with increasing duration of use, time since first use, or time since last use was observed.

The initial Boston University Drug (Slone) Epidemiology Unit study (Rosenberg et al, 1984) also is considered "negative," although one subgroup of women (aged 30–39 with 5 or more years of oral contraceptive use that began or ended many years prior to diagnosis) had a significantly elevated risk of breast cancer. A later report considered women younger than 45 years of age, with controls selected from the larger control group and individually matched to cases by age, year of interview, and geographic area (Miller et al, 1986). In this subgroup, no increased risk of breast cancer associated with oral contraceptive use was found among all women or among nulliparous women. However, women with long-term use before first full-term pregnancy had nonstatistically significant, elevated relative risks of 1.5 for 5 to 6 years of use and 1.4 for 7 or more years of use.

Using the same design methodology, the results of a second study by these investigators indicated a statistically significant, twofold increased risk of breast cancer associated with any use of oral contraceptives (Miller et al, 1989). No variation in risk was evident for durations of use of less than 10 years including short-term use (< 3 mos); the relative risks were approximately 2 in all categories of duration. For at least 10 years of use, the relative risk was 4.1. The elevated risk in short-term users could reflect recall bias, but it is unlikely that this explanation would account for the increased risk in women with long durations of use. Risk did not vary appreciably by age at first use of oral contraceptives or with respect to duration of use before first pregnancy. Results for individual pill formulations were inconclusive; based on the authors' presentation of 95% confidence intervals for the relative risk, estimates of the relative risk for each formulation studied were consistent with the study's overall relative risk of 2.

Results have been reported for five phases of the London/Oxford study of breast cancer and oral contraceptive use, a study restricted to married women. Control patients were individually matched to breast cancer case patients for age, hospital, and, in Phases I–IV, parity. No increased risk of breast cancer associated with oral contraceptive use was observed in the first four phases of the study (Vessey et al, 1982; 1983a). Results for Phase 5 indicate a statistically significant trend of increasing breast cancer risk with increasing duration of oral contraceptive use prior to first full-term pregnancy and elevated risk for long-term users overall (McPherson et al, 1987). These authors noted that publicity related to pill use and risk of breast cancer that followed publication of the paper of Pike and associates (1983) in the *Lancet* did not affect Phase 5 subjects' responses, as the majority of subjects were interviewed prior to this publication; the distributions of reported oral contraceptive use for cases and controls did not change after this publication. Analyses of risk related to pill formulation suggest that pills containing ethinylestradiol made a larger contribution to the increased risk of breast cancer prior to first full-term pregnancy than did pills containing mestranol (McPherson et al, 1987).

The results of a study conducted in New Zealand by Paul and associates (1986) are also considered "negative." Analyses of breast cancer risk by total duration of oral contraceptive use, age at first use and time since first use showed no increased risk, although one subgroup of women aged 25–34 at diagnosis did show an elevated relative risk of 2.2 for any use of oral contraceptives. In this age group, women with at least 10 years of use had a relative risk of breast cancer of 4.6. According to Stadel and colleagues (1988), no increased risk of breast cancer associated with oral contraceptive use was observed for nulliparous women in this study.

For women under age 33 living in Los Angeles County, California, Pike and coworkers (1981) reported that the risk of breast cancer increased with increasing duration of oral contraceptive use before the first full-term pregnancy; a relative risk of 3.5 was observed for 8 or more years of use compared with no use. Later, Pike and coworkers (1983) updated their ongoing study to include 317 breast cancer patients under age 37. Patients used oral contraceptives for an average of 49 months compared to 39 months for the control group; a majority (60%) of this difference in average duration of use was for use before age 23. For oral contraceptive use before age 25, the relative risk was 2.5 for 4 or more years of use and the trend of increasing risk with increasing duration of use was statistically significant. Pike and colleagues suggested that use of oral contraceptives with a high "progestogen potency" conferred especially high risk of breast cancer. Of three studies that subsequently evaluated this issue (Stadel et al, 1985; McPherson et al, 1987; White et al, 1994), only one has confirmed this observation (White et al, 1994). In the final report of the Los Angeles study, based on 439 case-control pairs, total oral contraceptive use and use before age 25 were significantly associated with increased risks of breast cancer, with relative risks of 1.68 for 97 or more months of total use and 3.15 for 73 or more months of use before age 25. A statistically significant distinction between parous and nulliparous women could not be drawn concerning these effects of oral contraceptive use, although the increased risks were greater for parous women (Bernstein et al, 1990).

A study conducted in Sweden and Norway included Swedish patients under age 45 and Norwegian patients under age 40 at diagnosis (Meirik et al, 1986b). Controls were individually matched to case patients on exact year of birth. For Swedish case patients under age 40, a second control was individually matched on exact year of birth and exact age at first full-term pregnancy; separate analyses were presented for these women. A statistically significant trend of increasing breast cancer risk with increasing duration of oral contraceptive use was observed for all women as well as for the subgroup of younger Swedish women. For the younger Swedish women, a statistically significant trend in risk associated with increasing duration of oral contraceptive use prior to first full-term pregnancy was observed. In subgroup analyses by parity status, Meirik and colleagues (1989) showed that the increased risk of breast cancer before age 45 associated with long-term oral contraceptive use was more pronounced in nulliparous women than in parous women.

In the most recent British study (UKNCCSG, 1989), which studied women under age 36 at breast cancer diagnosis and controls matched exactly on age, a highly significant trend in risk of breast cancer was associated with increasing total duration of oral contraceptive use (relative risk, RR=1.74 for more than 8 years of use). Use before and after first full-term pregnancy showed similar significant trends in risk with increasing duration of use. Although few women had substantial long-term use of oral contraceptives containing less than 50 μg of estrogen, the results suggest that the risk associated with use of these low-dose pills was lower than that associated with use of pills with greater estrogen content.

A western Washington State study of women aged 21 to 45 years is considered "positive" as White and colleagues (1994) found a statistically significant trend in the risk of breast cancer with increasing duration of oral contraceptive use; the elevation in risk in the longest use category was modest, however ($\geq$ 10 years use,

RR=1.3). Analyses by age group indicated that among women 36 to 45 years of age the relative risk for long-term users was 1.2. It was among women aged 35 years or younger that the effect for long-term users was substantially elevated (≥ 10 years use, RR=1.7). This greater risk among younger women is consistent with the findings of the studies in Britain (UKNCCSG, 1989) and Los Angeles (Bernstein et al, 1990), which were restricted to younger women, and with the subgroup results for women under age 35 years in the New Zealand study (Paul et al, 1986). Also consistent with these results is a subgroup analysis of the CASH study, which was restricted to black women aged 20 to 39 years (Mayberry, 1994). Among these women, breast cancer risk was nearly three times greater for those who used oral contraceptives for more than 10 years than for women who had never used oral contraceptives (RR=2.8). Risk was also elevated 50%–70% among shorter term users. No increase in risk was observed among women 40 to 54 years of age.

The results of these recent studies of the effect of oral contraceptives on the risk of breast cancer in young women confirm that oral contraceptives do not protect them against breast cancer. A meta-analysis of population-based case-control and cohort studies of women younger than age 45 years at diagnosis estimates that breast cancer risk increases, on average, 3.1% per year of oral contraceptive use (Pike et al, 1993).

High-Risk Women. No clear picture emerges when breast cancer risk associated with oral contraceptive use is examined in young women who have a mother or sister diagnosed with breast cancer or in those with benign breast disease who subsequently take oral contraceptives. In the second Drug (Slone) Epidemiology Unit study (Miller et al, 1989), oral contraceptive use was significantly associated with risk of breast cancer in women with a positive family history (RR=3.6) and this risk was greater than that of women with no family history (RR=2.1). Brinton and coworkers (1982) reported that, among women whose sisters had been diagnosed with breast cancer, oral contraceptive users had a greater risk of breast cancer than nonusers; however, no increased risk was found among oral contraceptive users whose mothers had been diagnosed with breast cancer. In other studies, no increased risk associated with oral contraceptive use was found for women with such a family history (Rosenberg et al, 1984; Lipnick et al, 1986; Murray et al, 1989).

Results of studies that have examined the risk of breast cancer associated with oral contraceptive use in women with benign breast disease are also inconsistent (Pike et al, 1981; Brinton et al, 1982; Vessey et al, 1983a; Rosenberg et al, 1984; Miller et al, 1989). In interpreting these findings, it is important to consider the sequence of "exposures" to determine whether the diagnosis of benign breast disease precedes the onset of oral contraceptive use (Stadel and Schlesselman, 1986).

Progestin-only Pills. Few case-control studies have examined breast cancer risk in relation to use of progestin-only pills (minipills). Those that have looked at this exposure have reported relatively few users (Stanford and Thomas, 1993). Two studies had sufficient usage to examine duration of use in relation to breast cancer risk (UKNCCSG 1989; Ewertz, 1992). Both suggest that breast cancer risk is moderately lower among long-term users of these pills. Because of the paucity of data, however, it is not possible to draw any firm conclusions regarding minipills. As noted previously, these pills have not become widely used in the United States.

Cervical Cancer

Although the relation between oral contraceptives and cervical neoplasia has also received considerable attention, several factors complicate the interpretation of results of these studies. Sexual factors such as age at first sexual intercourse and number of sexual partners are risk factors for cervical cancer that may also be associated with the use of oral contraceptives, with oral contraceptive users more likely to have been younger at first sexual intercourse or to have had more sexual partners than nonusers (see, for example, Swan and Brown, 1981, and Ebeling et al, 1987). Smoking and exposure to sexually transmitted agents, especially human papilloma virus, are other possible confounders of the cervical cancer–oral contraceptive association (zur Hausen, 1982). Barrier methods of contraception are protective against cervical neoplasia (Boyce et al, 1977; Vessey et al, 1983b; Brinton et al, 1986b; Peters et al, 1986b) and this further complicates the analysis of risk associated with oral contraceptive use, as women who use these methods will be less likely to have used oral contraceptives. Thus, one must carefully control for such factors in the statistical analyses.

Invasive cervical cancer is the end result of a series of changes in the cervical epithelium (progressing from normal to dysplasia to carcinoma in situ to invasive cancer), and oral contraceptives may act at one or more of these stages. Stern and colleagues (1977) suggested that oral contraceptives altered the progression rates of preinvasive lesions to neoplastic states, although Zarcovic (1985) detected no significant differences in patterns of cytological alterations between oral contraceptive users and controls who were followed by periodic Pap screening over an 8-year period. A number of analytic epidemiological studies of oral contraceptive use and cervical neoplasia have focused on preinvasive abnormalities that are prone to pathological classification difficulties (Editorial, 1975) and that may, in fact, be easier to detect among oral contraceptive users (Editorial, 1977).

The frequency of Pap screening may also confound the association of cervical cancer and oral contraceptive use. Oral contraceptive users may have more frequent Pap tests (Swan and Brown, 1981; Hellberg et al, 1985; La Vecchia et al, 1986a; Irwin et al, 1988). As a result of frequent Pap screening, earlier stages of the disease process have been diagnosed and invasive cervical cancer incidence rates have declined (Brinton et al, 1986b; Ebeling et al, 1987). If women using oral contraceptives are under more intensive medical surveillance, and are tested more frequently than other women, one would expect to observe an increased risk of cervical dysplasia and in situ cervical cancer in oral contraceptive users, with fewer oral contraceptive users progressing to invasive cervical cancer.

The majority of early studies of the possible relation between oral contraceptive use and cervical cancer dealt with a mixture of preinvasive lesions, dysplasia, and carcinoma in situ (CIS) and did not control for sexual behavior as well as for other important sources of confounding (Swan and Pettiti, 1982). Characteristics of the design and statistical analysis of more recent studies of cervical dysplasia, CIS, and invasive disease that have attempted to deal with possible bias and confounding are presented in Table 22–6, with relevant results presented in Table 22–7. However, with perhaps one ex-

TABLE 22–6. *Design Aspects of Analytic Studies of Oral Contraceptives and Cervical Neoplasia*

Study and Reference	*Type of Study/Source of Subjects*	*Dates of Diagnoses*	*Number of Cases*	*Age Range*	*Handling of Potential Biases*[a]
Harris (1980)	Case-control/Hospital-based	1974–1979	Dysplasia: Mild 44, Severe 81; CIS: 65	Most <40	Analysis of combined abnormalities adjusted for factors A, B, C
Swan (1981)	Case-control/HMO patients	1969–1976	CIS: 67; Invasive: 2	18–54	Analysis of combined abnormalities adjusted for factors A, D. Matching on factor E.
Vessey (1983b)	Cohort/Family planning clinics Follow-up: 10 yrs	Formed: 1968–1974	Dysplasia: 64; CIS: 59; Invasive: 13	25–39 at entry	Oral contraceptive users compared to IUD users.
Hellberg (1985)	Case-control/Maternity clinic (all subjects pregnant)	1977–1981	CIN: 140	16–41	Excluded users of barrier methods from controls; analysis adjusted for factors A, C
Clarke (1985)	Case-control/Cases: Hospital clinic; Controls: Neighborhood	1979–1981	Dysplasia: 250	20–59	Analysis adjusted for factors A, C, D
WHO (1985)	Case-control/Hospital-based	1979–1983	Invasive: 726	<58	Analysis adjusted for factors A, D, E, F
La Vecchia (1986a)	Case-control/Hospital and clinic	1979–1985	CIN: 202	<60	Analysis adjusted for factors A, D, E, G, H
Brinton (1986b)	Case-control/Cases: hospital; Controls: RDD	1982–1985	Invasive: 479	20–69	Analysis adjusted for factors A, D, G, I. No confounding by factor C.
Ebeling (1987)	Case-control/Hospital-based	1983–1985	Invasive: 129	20–54	Analysis adjusted for factors A, C, D, H, G
Irwin (1988)	Case-control/Population-based	1982–1984	CIS: 583; Invasive: 293	25–59	Analysis adjusted for factors A, D, E, J. No confounding by factor B.
Beral (1988)	Cohort/GPs' patients	Formed: 1968–1969	CIS: 207; Invasive: 65		Analysis adjusted for factors C (at entry), E and J.
Brinton (1990)	Case-control/Cases: hospital; Controls: hospital and community	1986–1987	Invasive: 759	<70	Analysis adjusted for factors A, D, G. Assessment of effects of nonconfounding factors B, C, J (HPV 16/18 detection status).
Jones (1990)	Case-control/Cases: hospital; Controls: RDD	1982–1984	CIS: 293	20–74	Analyses adjusted for factors A, B, C, E, G, I. No confounding by D, J.
Parazzini (1990)	Case-control/Hospital-based	1981–1987	Invasive: 367	20–59	Analyses adjusted for factors A, B, C, D, E. No confounding by factor G.
Kjær (1993)	Case-control/Population-based	1987–1988	CIS: 586; Invasive: 59		Analyses adjusted for A, B, C, H, I, any Pap smear

Abbreviations: CIS=carcinoma in situ, CIN=cervical intraepithelial neoplasia, RDD=random digit dial, HPV=human papilloma virus.
[a]Factors: A=number of sexual partners; B=use of barrier methods of contraception; C=smoking; D=age at first or regular intercourse; E=number of Pap tests; F=history of vaginal discharge; G=time since last Pap test; H=other contraceptive practices; I=history of nonspecific genital infection or sore; J=history of sexually transmitted disease or pelvic inflammatory disease.

TABLE 22–7. *Cervical Neoplasia Risk and Oral Contraceptive Use*

Pathologic Classification	Study and Reference	Adjusted[a] Relative Risk Estimate: Any Use	Long-Term Use		Significant Dose-Response
Dysplasia	Vessey (1983b)	1.5	>8 yr	4.0	NP
	Hellberg (1985)	NA	NP		No
	Clarke (1985)	1.7[b]	NP		No
	LaVecchia (1986a)	0.7	>2 yr	0.9	No
CIS	Harris[c] (1980)	NP	≥10 yr	2.1	Yes
	Swan[d] (1981)	1.7	>6 yr	1.5	No
	Vessey (1983b)	1.6	>8 yr	2.0	NP
	Irwin (1988)	1.6	≥10 yr	2.0	Yes
	Beral (1988)	2.9	≥10 yr	4.8	Yes
	Jones (1990)	1.8[e] 1.4[f]	≥10 yr	1.4	Yes
	Kjær (1993)	1.4	≥10 yr	1.7	Yes
Invasive	Vessey (1983b)	13 exposed cases (9 with >6 yrs), 0 unexposed cases			
	WHO (1985)	1.2	>8 yr	1.6	Borderline
	Brinton (1986b)	1.5	≥10 yr	1.8	Yes
	Ebeling (1987)	1.5	≥7 yr	1.8	No
	Irwin (1988)	0.8	NP		No
	Beral (1988)	1.8	≥10 yr	4.4	Yes
	Parazzini (1990)	1.8	>2 yr	2.5	Yes
	Brinton (1990)	1.2	≥10 yr	1.2	No
	Kjær (1993)	1.3	≥6 yr	1.3	No

Abbreviations: NA=no association, adjusted relative risk estimate not provided; NP=not provided; CIS=carcinoma in situ.

[a]Adjusted for factors indicated in last column of Table 21–6; risk relative to that of non-users.

[b]Adjusted only for number of sexual partners.

[c]Combines dysplasia and CIS.

[d]Restricted to incident cases.

[e]Current users.

[f]Former users.

ception (Brinton et al, 1990), no study fully accounts for all factors that might influence the comparison.

Dysplasia. No consistent picture regarding the relationship of oral contraceptive use and the risk of cervical dysplasia emerges upon examination of the data presented in Table 22–7. Cohort data from the Oxford–Family Planning Association Contraceptive Study (Vessey et al, 1983b,c) suggest a positive effect, but this effect is not confirmed in case-control studies (Clarke et al, 1985; Hellberg et al, 1985; La Vecchia et al, 1986a). Although the risk estimate for any use of oral contraceptives was elevated in the study by Clarke and associates (1985), they were unable to demonstrate an effect of duration of use in spite of substantial numbers of long-term users (8 or more years).

Carcinoma in situ (CIS). The results of studies of CIS are more consistent than those of cervical dysplasia. The overall pattern suggests a moderate increase in risk of CIS associated with oral contraceptive use, with long-term users having about double the risk of nonusers. Irwin and colleagues (1988) attributed the increased risk observed in their study to detection bias because no increased risk was observed when analyses were restricted to subgroups of subjects for whom no association between Pap screening and oral contraceptive use existed. Yet, in the study conducted by Kjær and colleagues (1993), the risk of CIS was increased in both groups of women, those who had never had a previous Pap screening test and those who had been screened previously.

Invasive Cervical Cancer. As noted above, if oral contraceptive users receive more frequent Pap screening, one would expect to detect an association with preinvasive cervical lesions, but not an association with invasive disease. With the exception of the study by Irwin and colleagues (1988), positive associations with oral contraceptive use were observed in the studies presented in Tables 22–6 and 22–7, with long-term use associated with approximately a 1.5-fold to 2-fold increase in risk. Again, one must consider possible confounding and bias when interpreting these results.

Two cohort studies conducted in England have at least 10 years of follow-up (Vessey et al, 1983b, Beral et al, 1988). In the Oxford study (Vessey et al, 1983b), all 13 cases of invasive cervical cancer that were identified occurred in women who were oral contraceptive users; nine of these women had used oral contraceptives for more than 6 years. Women participating in the Royal College of General Practitioners' study had significantly increased risk with increasing durations of oral contraceptive use (Beral et al, 1988).

The preliminary report of the World Health Organization (WHO) study on cervical cancer showed a relative risk of 1.2 for users of oral contraceptives that was of borderline statistical significance (WHO, 1985). Risk increased with longer duration of use, with 8 or more years of use associated with a relative risk of 1.6. In this study, the majority of cases had diagnoses of squamous cell carcinoma; only 8% had been diagnosed with adenocarcinomas.

Brinton and associates (1986b) reported a relative risk of 1.5 overall for invasive cervical cancer associated with oral contraceptive use. In this study, long-term users (5 or more years) had approximately a twofold higher risk than nonusers. The association held for both squamous cell carcinoma and adenocarcinoma of the cervix. Risk declined with interval since last use; for women who had used oral contraceptives within one year of study, the relative risk was 2.0, whereas the relative risk was 1.4 for women who had terminated use more than one year earlier. Overall risks were highest for women who used pills containing high estrogen content.

Ebeling and coworkers (1987) found both long-term use (7 or more years) and early age at first use (24 years of age or younger) significantly associated with increased risk of invasive cervical cancer (RR=1.8 and RR=3.0 respectively). The relative risk for current users was 2.0.

In a multicenter case-control study conducted in Mexico, Costa Rica, Panama, and Colombia, Brinton and colleagues (1990) reported a modest 21% nonsignificant elevation in invasive cervical cancer risk associated with any oral contraceptive use, with recent long-term users (≥ 5 years use) at highest risk (RR=1.7). Careful evaluation ruled against any detection bias associated with a history of recent Pap smear; other risk factors, including smoking and detection of human papilloma viruses, had little effect on risk associated with oral contraceptive use.

Analytic studies involving oral contraceptive use and invasive cervical cancer have focused almost entirely on squamous cell malignancies or have not provided analyses by cell type (with the exception of Brinton and colleagues 1986b and 1990); however, the influence of oral contraceptives may well be greater on adenocarcinomas that originate from progesterone-responsive endocervical glandular cells. An increasing incidence of adenocarcinoma of the cervix has been reported among women under 35 years of age in Los Angeles County, California (Peters et al, 1986a) and in areas served by population-based cancer registries participating in the Surveillance, Epidemiology and End Results Program (Schwartz and Weiss, 1986). In these areas incidence has remained essentially constant over the same period among older women. Peters and coworkers (1986a) hypothesized that the use of oral contraceptives during the teenage years might account for this trend as oral contraceptives produce morphologic changes in the endocervix, characterized by stromal edema, excessive mucus production, and glandular hyperplasia (Minteot and Fievez, 1974). The extent of these histologic changes increases as continuous use of the contraceptive agents increases (Gall et al, 1969). In the study by Brinton and colleagues (1990), the invasive cervical cancer risk associated with oral contraceptive use was significantly increased for adenocarcinomas (RR=2.2) compared with a nonsignificant minimal effect for squamous cell tumors (RR=1.1). A population-based case-control study conducted in Los Angeles County, California, that was limited to young women (born after 1935) diagnosed with adenocarcinoma of the cervix has recently been completed (Ursin et al, 1994). Based on personal interviews of 195 cases and 386 age-, race-, and neighborhood-of-residence–matched controls, the risk of adenocarcinoma of the cervix was statistically significantly greater among women who had used oral contraceptives than among those who had not (RR=2.1). The highest risk was observed for oral contraceptive use that exceeded 12 years (RR=4.4). No further increased risk was suggested for early age at first use, long-term use beginning at an early age, long time since first use, recent use, or particular formulations of oral contraceptives.

Liver Cancer

A causal association between the use of oral contraceptives and benign liver tumors, variously described as adenomas or focal nodular hyperplasia, is well documented (Edmondson et al, 1976, Rooks et al, 1979). Experimental animal studies have shown that oral contraceptives can cause hepatocellular carcinomas in mice and are effective promoters of hepatocarcinogenesis in diethylnitrosamine-primed rats (Yager and Yager, 1980).

At least 10 case reports of hepatocellular carcinoma arising in women taking oral contraceptives have been published. Because of the rarity of primary liver cancer, few analytic studies investigating the risk associated with oral contraceptive use have been conducted. Liver cancer is usually rapidly fatal, so population-based epidemiological studies are particularly difficult to conduct; studies therefore have either had to be hospital-based or to rely, in large part, on proxy interviews (or incomplete medical records) to obtain information on the oral contraceptive use of cases.

Henderson and associates (1983b) compared the oral contraceptive use of 11 young women diagnosed with hepatocellular carcinoma to that of 22 age-matched neighborhood control women. Ten case patients had used oral contraceptives for periods ranging from 6 to 168 months. The other patient had received multiple "hormone" shots of undetermined type for regulation of menstrual periods during the 9 months preceding diagnosis. Six of the 11 patients were taking hormones at the time of diagnosis. On average, they had used oral contraceptives significantly longer than had control patients (65 months vs 27 months).

Results of more recent case-control studies are all consistent with an increased risk of hepatocellular carcinoma in long-term oral contraceptive users. In one British study (Neuberger et al, 1986), oral contraceptive use by a series of 26 women under age 50 diagnosed with hepatocellular carcinoma was compared to the use of controls from the London/Oxford breast cancer case-control study described earlier (Vessey et al, 1983a; McPherson et al, 1987). Although short-term oral contraceptive use was not associated with increased liver cancer risk, use for 8 or more years was associated with a significantly elevated relative risk of 4.4. When the case group was restricted to women without markers of hepatitis B infection, the relative risk remained significantly elevated in long-term users (RR=7.2). A study of young British women (aged 20 to 44 years) who died of liver cancer showed that oral contraceptive use for 8 or more years was associated with a significantly increased relative risk of 20.1 (Forman et al, 1986). No increased risk for cholangiocarcinoma associated with oral contraceptive use was found in this study. Yu and colleagues (1991) also found a significant association of oral contraceptive use and hepatocellular carcinoma risk among women in Los Angeles County, California (any use: RR=3.0, >5 years use: RR=5.5); exclusion of women with serologically determined viral hepatitis from the analysis increased the magnitude of the association.

Two hospital-based case-control studies also found positive associations between oral contraceptives and liver cancer. Tavani and colleagues (1993) reported a statistically significant trend in the risk of hepatocellular carcinoma with increasing years of oral contraceptive use (≤5 years use: RR=1.5; > 5 years use: RR=3.9). Similarly, Palmer and coworkers (1989) found a greater proportion of the 12 liver cancer cases they studied had used oral contraceptives than controls. No data were available on the hepatitis B status of subjects in these latter two studies.

Only one study has provided results for geographic areas where hepatitis B virus is prevalent and background liver cancer incidence rates are relatively high. This study conducted by the World Health Organization (WHO) found no evidence that short-term use of oral contraceptives increased liver cancer risk; no data were available for long-term users (WHO, 1989).

Other Cancers

Thyroid Cancer. Several case-control studies have reported on the association of oral contraceptive use and risk of thyroid cancer in young women; all have shown some evidence of an increase in risk. In a study conducted in Washington State, the risk for all histologic types of thyroid cancer (papillary, follicular, and mixed tumors) was increased with oral contraceptive use (RR=1.6), but the finding was significant only for follicular carcinoma (RR=3.6) (McTiernan et al, 1984). In Los Angeles County, California, a statistically significant overall increased risk for thyroid cancer of 2.4 was observed in oral contraceptive users compared to nonusers (Preston-Martin et al, 1987). Similarly, in Shanghai, oral contraceptive use was associated with a statistically significant elevation in female thyroid cancer risk (RR=1.7) (Preston-Martin et al, 1993). For Connecticut women under age 35, oral contraceptive use was associated with an elevated relative risk of 1.8 that was not statistically significant (Ron et al, 1987). The Washington and Los Angeles studies examined duration of use and observed the greatest risk in short-term users (McTiernan et al, 1984; Preston-Martin et al, 1987). This finding was explained to some extent in the Los Angeles study by the fact that control patients had fewer pregnancies, possibly due to their greater duration of oral contraceptive use, and by the fact that more case patients than controls (and particularly short-term users) had stopped taking oral contraceptives because they wanted to become pregnant.

Malignant Melanoma. Because the anatomic distribution of cutaneous malignant melanoma differs for men and women, and because women apparently have a survival advantage, the effects of femal hormones, including oral contraceptives, on melanoma risk are of interest (Franceschi et al, 1990). The majority of studies that have evaluated the association of oral contraceptive use and risk of malignant melanoma have reported either a weak association or no association with any use, with relative risk estimates ranging from 0.7 to 1.2 (Adams et al, 1981; Kay, 1981; Bain et al, 1982; Holly et al, 1983; Beral et al, 1984; Helmrich et al, 1984; Holman et al, 1984; Gallagher et al, 1985; Green and Bain, 1985; Osterlind et al, 1988; Zanetti et al, 1990; Palmer et al, 1992). One small case-control study (39 cases/69 controls) that was based on the medical records of a health plan found an elevated risk (RR=1.8) of malignant melanoma among oral contraceptive users (Beral et al, 1977). A statistically significant relative risk of 3.5 associated with use of oral contraceptives was reported in the Walnut Creek Contraceptive Drug Study (Ramcharan et al, 1981), although two British cohort studies found no association (Hannaford et al, 1991).

Overall, the case-control study data on duration of oral contraceptive use are not convincing of an association with risk of malignant melanoma. Although in three studies, long-term oral contraceptive users had elevated risks (Adams et al, 1981: ≥ 5 years use, RR=1.6; Holly et al, 1983: > 10 years use, RR=2.1; Beral et al, 1984: ≥ 10 years use, RR=1.6), none of the dose-response effects was statistically significant.

The stage at which melanoma is diagnosed varies considerably; this may be due to differences among individuals in awareness of the disease, access to health care, and educational level, factors that may also be related to oral contraceptive use. In a hospital-based case-control study, Palmer and colleagues (1992) investigated this possibility by examining the effects of oral contraceptive use on risk of severe and non-severe malignant melanoma where severity was defined by the depth of invasion of the malignant lesion. Among severe cases, oral contraceptive use was not related to the risk of melanoma (RR=1.1); however, among non-severe cases, oral contraceptive use was significantly associated with melanoma risk (OR=1.5) although risk did not increase substantially with increasing duration of use. These results point out the need to consider surveillance bias when interpreting associations between melanoma and oral contraceptive use.

INJECTABLE CONTRACEPTIVES

Depot-medroxyprogesterone acetate (DMPA), a progestogen, is a long-acting injectable contraceptive that has been used worldwide since the mid-1960s. It was not licensed for use in the United States until 1992 because of a concern about effects on breast cancer risk. This concern stems, in part, from the results of animal studies of DMPA that have found increased numbers of malignant breast nodules in female beagle dogs (Finkel and Berlinger, 1973; Geil and Lamar, 1977), high incidence of mammary tumors in female BALB/c mice (Lanari et al, 1986), and endometrial carcinoma in rhesus monkeys (Fraser and Weisberg, 1981).

Epidemiological data related to cancer risk associated with use of DMPA are limited. Early studies of these associations are difficult to interpret because of design limitations; studies were based on small samples, limited DMPA exposure, or inadequate comparison groups. For example, one record linkage study conducted in Atlanta, Georgia, matched family planning clinic records of approximately 5000 women who had used DMPA with hospital admission records to ascertain cancer incidence (Liang et al, 1983). Most women in this study received DMPA for less than 1 year; less than 13% had used DMPA for more than 3 years. One further problem with this study was an estimated 45% underascertainment of cancer in the cohort; although an attempt was made to adjust for this problem in the statistical analyses, it casts doubt on the results of the study.

Endometrial Cancer

One would expect that DMPA use would protect against endometrial cancer. The addition of a cyclic progestogen to estrogen replacement therapy in perimenopausal and postmenopausal women reduces the increased risk of endometrial cancer associated with estrogen replacement therapy. Furthermore, combination oral contraceptives, which deliver progestogens continuously over the cycle, are protective against endometrial cancer. Data on DMPA use and endometrial cancer are limited. Only one case of endometrial cancer was identified in the Atlanta study compared with an expected number, adjusted for underascertainment, of 0.83 (Liang et al, 1983). The WHO Collaborative Study of Neoplasia and Steroid Contraceptives, a hospital-based case-control study, which included 122 endometrial cancer case patients (three of whom had used DMPA as a contraceptive) and 939 controls (84 exposed to DMPA), found a statistically significant protective effect of DMPA on endometrial cancer risk (RR=0.2) which appears to persist for at least 8 years after cessation of DMPA use (WHO, 1991a). Of note, however, data on duration of DMPA use are limited in this study.

Ovarian Cancer

Because DMPA is thought to reduce gonadotropin levels and inhibit ovulation, it is conceivable that it would be associated with a reduced risk of ovarian cancer. One woman was diagnosed with ovarian cancer in the Atlanta DMPA cohort compared with 1.2 expected after adjustment for underascertainment (Liang et al, 1983). In the WHO study, 22 of the 224 case patients with ovarian cancer had used DMPA compared to 229 of 1781 controls exposed, resulting in a nonsignificant relative risk estimate of 1.1 controlling for the confounding effects of number of live births and oral contraceptive use (WHO, 1991b). Thus, the limited data currently available suggest that the risk of epithelial ovarian cancer is not altered by the use of DMPA.

Breast Cancer

Seven cases of breast cancer were identified in the Atlanta study compared with 10.1 expected after adjustment for lack of complete follow-up (Liang et al, 1983). Lee and associates (1987) reported a statistically significant increased risk of breast cancer associated with DMPA use (RR=2.6) in a study conducted in Costa Rica. Risk was elevated for all durations of use evaluated up to 6 years (less than 12 months, RR=2.3; 12 to 23 months, RR=4.4; 24 to 71 months RR=3.4). The results of this study have been questioned because the case response rate was only 66%, raising concern that selection bias may have produced spurious results.

Two recent studies, the WHO study that was conducted at five centers in three developing countries (WHO, 1991c) and a population-based case-control study conducted in New Zealand (Paul et al, 1989) show no overall association between DMPA use and breast cancer; however, they do find some evidence of an increased risk among women diagnosed before age 35, among recent users of DMPA, and among women who had used DMPA before age 25. Both studies had similar prevalences of DMPA use among controls (just under 14%). The WHO study reported on 869 breast cancer patients and 11,890 control patients (WHO, 1991c). Overall, the risk of breast cancer did not increase with increasing duration of DMPA use, nor did it increase among women who began using DMPA more than 5 years previously. Among women under age 35, however, breast cancer risk was elevated (RR=1.5), particularly among those who began DMPA use within the previous 4 years (RR=2.2). Paul and coworkers (1989) reported results for 891 case patients and 1864 controls aged 25 to 54 years. A twofold increased risk of breast cancer associated with DMPA use was observed in the youngest age group of women (25 to 34 years of age). Among women who had 2 to 5 years of DMPA use before age 25, risk was significantly elevated (RR=4.6). The 25-to-34-year-old age group also had a significantly elevated risk of breast cancer associated with oral contraceptive use (Paul et al, 1986), but adjustment for oral contraceptive use did not affect the DMPA results.

If estrogens alone are a cause of breast cancer, then one would expect that DMPA would decrease breast cancer risk because the regimen prevents ovulation and does not include any exposure to exogenous estrogen. After the administration of DMPA, estradiol levels vary between 20 and 50 pg/ml; these levels are slightly lower than normal early follicular phase estradiol levels (Jeppsson et al, 1977; Mishell, 1991). The results of the epidemiological studies described above suggest that DMPA offers no protection against breast cancer; one explanation for these observations is that progesterone (or progestins) play some role in stimulating breast cell growth.

Cervical Cancer

In the WHO study, the risk for invasive squamous cell cancer of the cervix associated with use of DMPA was not significantly elevated (2009 cases/9583 controls; RR=1.1) (WHO, 1992). There were no trends in risk with increasing duration of use, nor with recency of use or age at first use. Oberle and coworkers (1988) found no effect of DMPA on risk of cervical CIS or invasive cervical cancer in a case-control study conducted in Costa Rica; however, this study was limited in that few women had used DMPA for more than 2 years.

Risk of cervical cancer associated with use of monthly injectable estrogen-progestogen contraceptives has also been evaluated within the WHO study (Thomas et al, 1989). Although preliminary results from Chile suggested a strong association of these products with invasive cervical cancer, further data collection failed to confirm the association.

Liver Cancer

There is concern that DMPA may increase the risk of liver cancer because progestins are a component of oral contraceptives that are associated with higher liver cancer risk. Based on interviews with subjects from Kenya and Thailand, where hepatitis B is endemic, there is no apparent effect of DMPA use on the risk of liver cancer, although the results for Kenya (RR=1.6) differ from those of Thailand (RR=0.3) (WHO, 1991d). These results are based on 8 DMPA users among the 63 case patients and 77 DMPA users among the 453 controls.

HORMONE REPLACEMENT THERAPY

Currently, more than 30 million postmenopausal women live in the United States. By the mid-1970s, over 28 million prescriptions of noncontraceptive estrogens were being filled annually in the United States. Because of concerns about the carcinogenic potential of estrogen replacement therapy on endometrium, the number of estrogen prescriptions declined 50% by 1980. Later, a cyclic estrogen-progestogen regimen became widely recommended and prescribed. By 1983, prescriptions of estrogen had increased to 18 million and, compared to 1981, progestogen prescriptions, exclusive of oral contraceptives, had increased more than 50% (Kennedy et al, 1985). By the mid-1980s, nearly 30% of all noncontraceptive estrogen prescriptions were combined with a progestogen prescription (Hemminki et al, 1988).

The advisability of long-term use of estrogen replacement therapy for postmenopausal women remains controversial. This controversy centers on three issues: the potential benefits to be derived from such therapy compared with the potential risks, the most favorable dose to maximize the benefit to risk ratio, and the benefits and risks to be derived by adding a progestogen to the estrogen regimen.

Endometrial Cancer

Case reports of endometrial cancer occurring in women following the use of estrogens have appeared in the medical literature for more than 30 years, but only since 1975 have there been serious, controlled efforts to study this relationship. Within 5 years of the initial studies, more than 20 studies appeared in the literature which examined this association. Nearly all studies demonstrated a strong association between estrogen use and disease risk that was related to both dose and duration of use (see, for example, Smith et al, 1975; Ziel and Finkle, 1975; Mack et al, 1976; Antunes et al, 1979). Chapter 49 presents a full discussion of the relationship of estrogen replacement therapy to endometrial cancer risk and the reversal of effects obtained by combined estrogen-progestogen therapy. The benefit of adding a progestogen to estrogen replacement therapy to reduce estrogen-induced endometrial mitotic activity has been clearly established in clinical practice (Studd et al, 1980; Gambrell, 1982; Gal et al, 1983); however, the preferred dose should be the lowest possible to achieve the desired histologic changes in the endometrium because of the potential for adverse effects on risk of heart disease risk and breast cancer (Henderson et al, 1988b). Whitehead and coworkers (1982) have shown that the duration of progestogen therapy is more important than the dose of progestogen given; however, the optimal type, dose, and duration of progestogen have not been established.

Ovarian Cancer

Data on ovarian cancer risk associated with estrogen replacement therapy are sparse, as most studies have been based on relatively few cases. Results that are available generally have indicated that menopausal estrogens do not alter risk (Kelsey and Hildreth, 1983). However, several studies have identified subgroups of women with possible increased risk.

Hoover and associates (1977) conducted a follow-up study of women with at least 6 months of exposure to conjugated equine estrogens (Premarin), and found an excess risk among women who had also taken diethylstilbestrol (DES). Weiss and coworkers (1982), however, found no increased risk of ovarian cancer associated with DES use in their case-control study.

Among Greek women, Tzonou and colleagues (1984) observed a moderately elevated, although not statistically significant, relative risk of ovarian cancer associated with use of replacement estrogens (RR=1.6). Weiss and coworkers (1982) and Cramer and associates (1983) observed similar modest elevations in ovarian cancer risk associated with postmenopausal estrogen use (RR=1.3 and RR=1.6, respectively). Long duration of use had no significant effect on risk in either study, although Cramer and associates (1983) observed a relative risk of 2.8 associated with 5 or more years of use that approached statistical significance. Other recent case-control studies have found no elevation in risk with estrogen therapy (Hildreth et al, 1981; LaVecchia et al, 1982; Kaufman et al, 1989).

Weiss and colleagues (1982) and LaVecchia and colleagues (1982) examined risk by histologic type of tumor and observed elevated risks (RRs of 3.1 and 2.3, respectively) associated with noncontraceptive estrogen use for endometrioid carcinoma of the ovary, which resembles adenocarcinoma of the endometrium histologically. Cramer and associates (1983) also found a higher proportion of estrogen users among women with endometrioid tumors. Kaufman and coworkers (1989), however, did not find such an effect in their hospital-based study.

No data are available regarding the effect of combined estrogen-progestogen replacement therapy on risk of cancer of the ovary. If any possible increase in risk due to estrogen therapy is restricted to endometrioid tumors, then it is likely that the addition of a progestogen might counteract the effects of estrogen.

Breast Cancer

Most early studies of the possible effects of estrogen replacement therapy on risk of breast cancer were uncontrolled follow-up studies. The most credible of these studies was conducted by Hoover and colleagues (1976). These investigators reported a 25% excess of breast cancer in their cohort of menopausal estrogen users compared to the number expected based on general population rates (49 observed versus 39 expected) and a more substantial excess risk among women using high doses for a long time.

Early case-control studies that reported findings on menopausal estrogens and breast cancer were often limited by small numbers, by insufficient data on dose and duration of use, and by the definite possibility of bias. A new round of carefully conducted case-control studies using healthy population controls has recently been published (Ross et al, 1980; Hoover et al, 1981; Hulka et al 1982a; Hiatt et al, 1984; Brinton et al, 1986a; McDonald et al, 1986; Nomura et al, 1986; Wingo et al, 1987) (Table 22–8). Overall, these studies have found small to moderate increases in the risk of breast cancer after long-term use, but substantial inconsistencies exist with regard to the effect of estrogen replacement therapy use on the breast cancer risk of women with or without a family history of breast cancer, with or without a personal history of benign breast disease, or with respect to ovarian status (intact ovaries vs ovaries removed) or hysterectomy status (surgical vs natural menopause).

In women with intact ovaries, Ross and coworkers (1980) found that those with a total cumulative dose in excess of 1500 mg Premarin had a 2.5-fold increased risk relative to nonusers. No such increase was observed for oophorectomized women. In the CASH study (Wingo et al, 1987), risk with long-term use was elevated only for women who reported surgical menopause. The age range of women included in this study (ages 20 to 54 years) was lower than that of the other studies, resulting in a higher percentage of women with surgical menopause (hysterectomy with or without bilateral oophorectomy). Hiatt and associates (1984), who studied only women who had undergone bilateral

TABLE 22–8. *Recent Case-Control Studies of Breast Cancer after Estrogen Replacement Therapy (ERT) Using Population Controls*

Study and Reference	Source of Cases	No. Cases/Controls (% controls exposed)		Relative Risk[a] Any Use	Long-Term Use		Comments
Ross (1980)	Retirement communities	101/187	(45%)	1.4	TMD	2.5	Results for NM
		26/66	(56%)	0.8	TMD	0.7	Results for BSO
							High in NM with BBD
Hoover (1981)	Prepaid health plan	345/611	(29%)	1.4	5+yr	1.7	High in FH
Hulka (1982a)	Hospitals	152/620	(18%)	1.8	10+yr	1.7	Results for NM
		21/117	(50%)	1.3	NP		Results for H
							High in NM with FH, users of INJ
Hiatt (1984)	Prepaid health plan	119/119	(90%)	0.7	3+yr	1.8	All subjects had BSO
Nomura (1986)	Population						
	Japanese	181/181	(50%)	1.1	6+yr	1.9	Both results include
	Caucasian	160/159	(62%)	0.9	6+yr	1.3	21% premenopausal
							women. High in FH, BBD
Brinton (1986a)	Nationwide screening program	1127/1308	(41%)	1.1	15+yr	1.7	Results for NM
		485/517	(59%)	1.0	15+yr	1.3	Results for H, no BSO
		320/393	(77%)	1.1	15+yr	1.4	Results for BSO
							Overall, high in BBD with 10+ yrs estrogen use
McDonald (1986)[b]	Population	96/307	(40%)	1.3	6+yr	1.2	Results for BSO
		43/120	(67%)	0.5	6+yr	0.5	Results for H, no BSO
		35/89	(79%)	0.8	6+yr	0.7	Results for NM
Wingo (1987)	Population	295/401	(67%)	1.3	15+yr	1.7	Results for BSO
		564/652	(25%)	1.1	15+yr	2.0	Results for H, no BSO
		510/592	(16%)	0.8	5+yr	0.7	Results for NM
							High in BSO with FH

Abbreviations: NP=not provided, NM=women with natural menopause, H=women with hysterectomy, BSO=women with bilateral salpingo-oophorectomy, BBD=benign breast disease, FH=family history, INJ=injectable estrogens, TMD=total milligram accumulated dose greater than 1500.

[a]Risk relative to that of non-users.

[b]Ever users are women who have used estrogens for at least 1 year; ever users and long-term users are compared with women with either less than 1 year or no estrogen use.

oophorectomy, also reported increased risk of breast cancer with long-term estrogen replacement therapy use. No elevated risk was observed by McDonald and colleagues (1986) in their study conducted in Washington State. However, in this study, interviews were completed for only 54% of eligible cases.

Risk of breast cancer associated with the use of replacement estrogens was elevated for women with and without intact ovaries in two studies (Hoover et al, 1981; Brinton et al, 1986a). In one of the largest case-control studies conducted to date, Brinton and colleagues (1986a) observed a significant trend in risk with increasing duration of estrogen use. Estrogen users with 15 or more years of exposure had a 50% elevation in risk, which would be sufficient to produce approximately a 2% cumulative absolute excess risk in women aged 65 to 79 years.

Studies using hospital patients as their comparison group generally found no evidence to suggest that breast cancer risk was increased either overall or with long duration of estrogen replacement therapy use (Table 22–9) (Kelsey et al, 1981; Sherman et al, 1983; Kaufman et al, 1984; Nomura et al, 1986); however, two studies reported significantly elevated risks associated with use by women who had natural menopause (Jick et al, 1980b; LaVecchia et al, 1986b). Hulka and coworkers (1982a) reported comparable risks using hospital-based and community-based control patients. One possible explanation for the lack of an effect of long-term use in most of these hospital-based studies is that these hospital control patients have more contact with the health care system and are therefore more likely to have greater use of elective drugs than the population as a whole.

In a recent meta-analysis, based on 15 population-based or hospital-based case-control studies, Steinberg and colleagues (1991) quantified the effect of estrogen replacement therapy on breast cancer risk. They concluded that for women who experienced any type of menopause, risk of breast cancer did not increase until after 5 years of estrogen use. These investigators estimated that breast cancer risk is increased 30% after 15 years of use, although this estimate is influenced in large part by studies that included premenopausal women or

TABLE 22–9. *Recent Case-Control Studies of Breast Cancer after Estrogen Replacement Therapy (ERT) Using Hospital Controls*

Study and Reference	Source of Cases	No. Cases/Controls (% controls exposed)	Relative Risk: Any Use	Relative Risk: Long-term Use	Comments
Jick (1980b)	Prepaid health plan	60/78 (44%)	1.1	NP	Results for H
		37/61 (70%)	3.4	NP	Results for NM
Kelsey (1981)	Hospital-based	41/219 (44%)	0.9	50+mgM 1.0	Results for BSO
		286/1089 (76%)	0.9	50+mgM 0.6	Results for at least 1 ovary
					Analyses include premenopausal women
Hulka (1982a)	Hospitals	152/309 (18%)	1.7	10+yr 0.7	Results for NM
		21/63 (52%)	1.2	NP	Results for H
					High in NM with FH, users of INJ
Sherman (1983)	Hospital-based	113/113 (45%)	0.6	NP	High in OW
Kaufman (1984)	Hospital-based	1610/1606 (30%)	1.0		Overall
		NP	0.9	10+yr 1.3	Results for NM
		NP	0.9	10+yr 0.3	Results for H
		NP	0.5	10+yr 0.5	Results for BSO
Nomura (1986)	Hospital-based				
	Japanese	181/183 (53%)	1.0	6+yr 1.2	Both results include premenopausal women
	Caucasian	160/161 (66%)	0.7	6+yr 0.8	
LaVecchia (1986b)	Hospital-based	1108/1281 (4%)	1.8	2+yr 2.0	Combines NM, H, but risk with 2+yrs elevated only in NM

Abbreviations: NP=not provided, NM=women with natural menopause, H=women with hysterectomy, BSO=bilateral salpingoophorectomy, mgM=milligram months, FH=family history, INJ=injectable estrogens, OW=overweight.

women using estradiol (see discussion of Bergkvist et al, 1989a, below) rather than conjugated equine estrogens (the most popular replacement estrogen in the United States).

Certain subgroups of women may be relatively more susceptible to the carcinogenic effects of estrogens than others. Use of estrogen replacement therapy by postmenopausal women with a positive family history of breast cancer was associated with a much elevated breast cancer risk in several studies (Hoover et al, 1981; Hulka et al, 1982a; Nomura et al, 1986; Wingo et al, 1987). Several studies found elevated breast cancer risk following estrogen use in women with surgically proven benign breast disease (Hoover et al, 1976; Ross et al, 1980; Brinton et al, 1986a), particularly when estrogen use followed the diagnosis of benign breast disease (Thomas et al, 1982).

Results that have been published regarding the risk of breast cancer associated with postmenopausal hormone use among a cohort of nurses who are being followed prospectively indicate a statistically significant elevation in risk among current users, but no apparent increase in the risk of past users (Colditz et al, 1990). In the extended follow-up of participants in the Nurses' Health Study, the risk of breast cancer was significantly increased in women who were currently using estrogen alone (relative risk, 1.32; 95% CI 1.14 to 1.54); estrogen plus progestin (relative risk, 1.41; 95% CI 1.15 to 1.74); but was not increased in past users after two or more years of stopping (Colditz et al, 1995). In the 6-year follow-up of a cohort of Seventh-Day Adventist women, any use of hormone replacement therapy (in 1976 and thus, almost totally estrogen therapy) was associated with a statistically significant 69% increase in breast cancer risk (Mills et al, 1989); no strong dose-response effect with increasing duration of use was evident, however.

The breast cancer risk of a cohort of Swedish women 35 years of age or older who had been prescribed noncontraceptive hormones was compared to that of other women from the same geographic area (Bergkvist et al, 1989a). Although risk overall was increased only 10%, there was a 70% elevation in risk with long-term use (more than 9 years). This increased risk was attributable to estradiol compounds, which were the most commonly used formulations in this study, but which are not generally used in the United States. There were few women who had used conjugated estrogens in this cohort and those who had generally had received low-dose regimens. The greater effect of estradiol compounds than conjugated estrogens on breast cancer risk is consistent with the published data on the biological effects of these different compounds (Roy, 1987). Although both conjugated estrogens and estradiol compounds increase plasma estradiol levels, the percentage increase in sex-hormone-binding globulin (SHBG) is more than twice as large for conjugated estrogen compounds. The amount of SHBG is believed to be a crucial factor as it binds estradiol and reduces the estrogen activity on target cells such as those in the breast. Transdermal administration of replacement estrogens by subcutaneous estradiol pellets or transdermal patches results in similar average increases in plasma estradiol levels, but does not alter SHBG levels.

Little information is available on the relationship between combination hormone replacement therapy and breast cancer. The best known data on this issue come from the Swedish cohort (Bergkvist et al, 1989a; Persson et al, 1992). For women with 6 or fewer years of follow-up, the relative risk for the combined regimen was 1.2; and for those with 7 to 11 years of follow-up, the relative risk was 1.6 (Persson et al, 1992). Hunt and colleagues (1987) studied a cohort of 4544 British women attending specialist menopause clinics. The average duration of hormone replacement therapy use was 67 months with use roughly equally divided between estrogen only and combination replacement therapy. The overall incidence of breast cancer was increased 60% compared to that expected based on national data, but no detailed breakdown was given for combined therapy use alone.

In a population-based case-control study conducted in western Washington state among women 50 to 64 years of age, the use of estrogen alone (usually conjugated estrogens) or combined with progestin (usually medroxyprogesterone acetate), for intervals of 8 years or longer, was not associated with an increased risk of breast cancer. A significantly positive association with breast cancer was observed, however, in the subset of users of combined hormone replacement therapy following bilateral oophorectomy (Stanford et al, 1995).

In combination hormone replacement therapy, progestogens may enhance the carcinogenic effect of estrogen therapy on the breast. Unlike the endometrium, for which maximal mitotic activity occurs during the follicular phase of the menstrual cycle, cell replication in breast epithelium peaks in the luteal phase (Ferguson and Anderson, 1981). This phenomenon suggests that progesterone in conjunction with the luteal phase estradiol peak could stimulate breast tissue mitotic activity and increase breast cancer risk. If estrogen-progestogen hormone replacement therapy is given during the perimenopausal period, a woman's hormonal exposure to both estrogens and progestogens would be greater than that which occurs naturally at this time. Finally, the Swedish results on combined therapy are consistent with the hypothesis that estrogen plus progestogen is more carcinogenic to the breast than estrogen alone (Bergkvist et al, 1989a; Persson et al, 1992).

There are also relatively few data available on the relationship between hormone replacement therapy and breast cancer mortality. Survival analyses comparing breast cancer patients within the Swedish cohort of estrogen-treated women to breast cancer patients with no recorded estrogen treatment have suggested a relative survival advantage for estrogen-treated women (Bergkvist et al, 1989b). However, this advantage was restricted to women who were diagnosed with breast cancer while actually on estrogen therapy or who had stopped therapy in the previous 12 months. The 5-year relative survival among "current" estrogen replacement therapy users was 85% compared with 74% for women who had discontinued such therapy more than a year before diagnosis. Although these investigators provided no specific data on breast cancer mortality rates in current estrogen users versus past users, these survival data clearly suggest that the breast cancer mortality experience among women using replacement therapy is more favorable than their morbidity experience (Bergkvist et al, 1989a). Several other investigators have reported a reduction in mortality from breast cancer among estrogen replacement therapy users overall (Henderson et al, 1991; Hunt et al, 1987); as yet, there are no reports on the breast cancer mortality experience among women using combination therapy for extended periods of time.

One possible explanation for the apparent anomaly between the effects of estrogen replacement therapy on breast cancer incidence and breast cancer mortality, consistent with what has been proposed to explain a similar phenomenon that occurs with endometrial cancer (Chu et al, 1982), is that estrogen replacement therapy users are diagnosed with breast (or endometrial) cancer at an earlier stage, on average, because as a group such women are under closer medical surveillance than nonusers. Alternative explanations are possible. It is also feasible that replacement therapy leads to a detection bias, although currently no data exist to suggest that screening by mammography or other means detects breast tumors that would otherwise not come to medical attention. There could also exist a fundamental difference in the biological behavior of or in the response to therapy of breast cancers diagnosed among women taking replacement therapy.

Substantial epidemiological and clinical evidence indicate that estrogens prevent osteoporosis (Lindsay et al, 1984; Savras et al, 1988) and its most serious medical consequence, hip fracture (Paganini-Hill et al, 1981; Kiel et al, 1987). Women using estrogens for 5 years in the postmenopausal period reduce their risk of sustaining a nontraumatic osteoporotic hip fracture approximately 50% to 60%. Recent case-control studies have provided compelling evidence that estrogens lower risk of coronary heart disease (eg, Henderson et al, 1986). This effect is most likely mediated through raised high-density and reduced low-density lipoprotein cholesterol levels in estrogen users (Bush and Barrett-Connor, 1985). Since death rates from coronary heart disease among United States women are four times those of breast and endometrial cancer combined, this benefit alone could far outweigh any carcinogenic potential.

TAMOXIFEN

Tamoxifen is a synthetic, nonsteroidal antiestrogen in the breast that has proven effective in the treatment of breast cancer (Early Breast Cancer Trialists' Collaborative Group, 1988). It blocks estrogen receptors at the level of the tumor by competitively inhibiting estradiol binding (Lerner and Jordan, 1990; Jordan 1990a) and it has been labeled an "antiestrogen" on that basis. Tamoxifen also may act as an antitumor agent on the hypothalamic-pituitary axis, where it affects the release of growth hormone, thereby reducing the amount of insulin-like growth factor, a stimulatory growth factor for breast tissue (Pollack et al, 1990). Thus, tamoxifen may provide a model of direct (by interference with estrogen binding to receptors) and indirect (by its effects on the hypothalamic-pituitary axis) endocrine control of estrogen-regulated breast tumor growth. As a result of its efficacy in preventing or delaying breast cancer recurrence, tamoxifen chemoprevention trials have begun in healthy "high risk" women (ie, those with approximately the breast cancer risk of a 60-year-old woman). The most compelling argument for using tamoxifen as a breast cancer chemoprevention agent is the lower risk of contralateral primary breast cancer observed among women receiving adjuvant tamoxifen therapy for breast cancer. A summary of data from eight randomized trials of tamoxifen-treated versus control breast cancer patients (Nayfield et al, 1991) shows approximately a 35% reduction in the risk of contralateral breast cancer after an average treatment duration of 2 years.

Ongoing concerns that have subdued the optimism about the probable efficacy of such a regimen in primary breast cancer prevention are the possible adverse effects of tamoxifen on other organ systems (Jordan, 1990b). Reports of increased incidence of endometrial cancer among breast cancer patients treated with tamoxifen (Nayfield et al, 1991; Fisher et al, 1994; van Leeuwen et al, 1994) have generated the most concern. The magnitude of this increased endometrial cancer risk is estimated to be comparable to that associated with unopposed estrogen replacement therapy.

Experimental evidence and biochemical effects of tamoxifen treatment support a causal relationship between tamoxifen and endometrial cancer. Tamoxifen acts directly on the ovaries to stimulate estrogen biosynthesis, and in premenopausal women, plasma estrogen levels are increased after tamoxifen treatment (Groom et al, 1976). Tamoxifen causes estrogen-like changes in the vaginal epithelium (Boccardo et al, 1981) and endometrium (Boccardo et al, 1984) of some women. In the British Pilot Breast Cancer Prevention Trial, women taking tamoxifen had a significantly larger uterus and lower impedance to blood flow in the uterine arteries compared with control women (Kedar et al, 1994). In addition, a substantially larger proportion of women taking tamoxifen had histologic evidence of an abnormal endometrium compared to the control group (39% vs 10%). Gottardis and colleagues (1988) have reported that while tamoxifen inhibits the growth of breast tumors implanted in athymic mice, it stimulates the growth of implanted endometrial tumors; and Anzai and coworkers (1989) have shown that tamoxifen stimulates the division of endometrial cancer cells in culture.

Another concern is that tamoxifen may have estrogen-like effects on the liver. In rats, estrogens act as promoters of liver carcinogenesis (Yager and Yager, 1980). Liver tumors have been produced in rats that have been treated with large doses of tamoxifen over an extended period (Jordan, 1990b). However, no increase in primary liver tumor incidence has been reported among tamoxifen-treated patients in any clinical trial to date, although Fornander and coworkers (1989) have reported two cases of hepatocellular carcinoma among their patients receiving tamoxifen.

HORMONES DURING PREGNANCY

Diethylstilbestrol (DES), a nonsteroidal estrogen, was promoted during the 1940s as a useful drug for the treatment of habitual miscarriage and threatened miscarriage (Smith, 1948; Smith and Smith, 1949). It has been estimated that during the next 20 years, 2 to 3 million women were given DES during pregnancy. In 1971, Herbst and coworkers reported a strong association between such maternal exposure and the occurrence of clear cell adenocarcinoma of the vagina in female offspring. The peak incidence occurred during the daughters' late teenage years, with risk declining once these young women reached their 20s (Herbst et al, 1979; Herbst, 1981). It has been estimated that approximately one in 1000 exposed women will develop clear cell adenocarcinoma by the age of 34 (Melnick et al, 1987). It is noteworthy that the highest risk occurred among the offspring of mothers initially exposed to DES during the first trimester of the index pregnancy. Based on an evaluation of the scientific data on DES and clear cell adenocarcinoma, the International Agency for Research on Cancer has concluded that sufficient evidence exists for DES to be classified as a human carcinogen (International Agency for Research on Cancer, 1987).

Squamous cell cervical abnormalities have been identified in a follow-up study of a cohort of DES-exposed daughters, although the association may be spurious (Robboy et al, 1984). In this study, a subset of 744 DES-exposed daughters identified from reviews of obstetrical records was matched with an unexposed group of women and both groups were screened over a 7-year period. The overall incidence rate of dysplasia and carcinoma in situ of the uterine cervix was substantially higher in the exposed women than in unexposed women (respectively, 15.7 vs 7.9 cases per 1000 person-years of follow-up). The investigators noted that exposed women with an abnormal cytologic smear may have been more likely to have had a biopsy than unexposed women and that more exposed women had a history of genital herpes.

Until recently little information was available on the cancer risk of male offspring exposed in utero to DES. The relationship between exogenous sex steroids in pregnancy (DES, hormonal pregnancy tests, or inadvertent use of oral contraceptives after conception) and the risk of testis cancer in male offspring has been examined in four case-control studies (Henderson et al, 1979; Schottenfeld et al, 1980; Depue et al, 1983; Moss et al, 1986). Three of these studies (Henderson et al, 1979; Schottenfeld et al, 1980; Depue et al, 1983) found an increased risk in the male offspring of women exposed to any of these hormone preparations. The relative risks ranged from 2.8 to 5.3. In the study of Depue and coworkers (1983), all hormone use began in the first 2 months of the pregnancy. Of the nine exposed women, five had only a single exposure as a result of the pregnancy test.

The effect of DES exposure during pregnancy on the risk of cancer in the mother has been the subject of several reports (Bibbo et al, 1978; Beral and Cowell, 1980; Brian et al, 1980; Hubby et al, 1981; Hadjimichael et al, 1984; Meara et al, 1989, Colton et al, 1993). Three are based on the long-term follow-up of women who were subjects in randomized clinical trials (Bibbo et al, 1978; Beral and Cowell, 1980; Meara et al, 1989). Taken together these reports demonstrated a 30% excess of breast cancer cases in treated women (48 treated women compared to 37 women in the placebo control groups). Although this excess is not statistically significant, it is consistent with the magnitude of risk that might be expected for exposure to an estrogenic drug over a relatively short duration. A comparable, statistically significant elevation in risk was observed for a historical cohort of women treated with DES between 1940 and 1960 after an average follow-up of more than 36 years (overall RR=1.35) (Colton et al, 1993). By decade of follow-up, no increase in risk was observed during the first two decades following exposure in this cohort, but during the subsequent two decades risk was increased 33%–36%. The authors noted that detection bias was an unlikely explanation for the increased risk because DES-exposed women had excesses of both large and small tumors and the breast cancer detection practices of the DES-exposed women were similar to those of the unexposed, comparison cohort.

REFERENCES

ADAMS SA, SHEAVES JK, WRIGHT NH, et al. 1981. A case control study of the possible association between oral contraceptives and malignant melanoma. Br J Cancer 44:45–50.

ANTUNES CMF, STOLLEY PD, ROSENSHEIN NB, et al. 1979. Endometrial cancer and estrogen use. N Engl J Med 300:9–13.

ANZAI Y, HOLINKA CF, KURAMOTO H, et al. 1989. Stimulatory effects of 4-hydroxytamoxifen on proliferation of human endometrial adenocarcinoma cells (Ishikawa line). Cancer Res 49:2362–2365.

AREF I, HEFNAWI F, KANDEL O. 1973. Changes in human ovaries after long-term administration of microdose progestogens. Contraception 7:503–513.

BAIN C, HENNEKENS CH, SPEIZER FE, et al. 1982. Oral contraceptive use and malignant melanoma. J Natl Cancer Inst 68:537–539.

BERAL V, COWELL L. 1980. Randomized trial of high doses of stilboestrol and thisterone in pregnancy: long-term follow-up of mothers. Br Med J 281:1098–1101.

BERAL V, EVANS S, SHAW H, MILTON G. 1984. Oral contraceptive use and malignant melanoma in Australia. Br J Cancer 50:681–685.

BERAL V, HANNAFORD P, KAY C. 1988. Oral contraceptive use and malignancies of the genital tract. Lancet 2:1331–1335.

BERAL V, RAMCHARAN S, FARIS R. 1977. Malignant melanoma and oral contraceptive use among women in California. Br J Cancer 36:804–809.

BERGKVIST L, ADAMI HO, PERSSON I, et al. 1989a. The risk of breast cancer after estrogen and estrogen-progestin replacement. N Engl J Med 321:293–297.

BERGKVIST L, ADAMI HO, PERSSON I, et al. 1989b. Prognosis after breast cancer diagnosis in women exposed to estrogen and estrogen-progestogen replacement therapy. Am J Epidemiol 130:221–228.

BERNSTEIN L, PIKE MC, KRAILO M, HENDERSON BE. 1990. Update of the Los Angeles Study of oral contraceptives and breast cancer: 1981 and 1983. In *Oral Contraceptives and Breast Cancer,* Mann R (ed). London: Parthenon Publishing Group, pp 169–180.

BIBBO M, GILL WB, AZIZI F, et al. 1978. A 25-year follow-up study of women exposed to diethylstilbestrol during pregnancy. N Engl J Med 2998:763–767.

BITTNER JJ. 1947. The causes and control of mammary cancer in mice. Harvey Lect 42:221–246.

BOCCARDO F, BRUZZI P, RUBAGOTTI A, et al. 1981. Estrogen-like action of tamoxifen on vaginal epithelium in breast cancer patients. Oncology 38:281–285.

BOCCARDO F, GUARNIERI D, RUBAGOTTI A, et al. 1984. Endocrine effects of tamoxifen in postmenopausal breast cancer patients. Tumori 70:61–68.

BOOTH M, BERAL V, SMITH P. 1989. Risk factors for ovarian cancer: a case-control study. Br J Cancer 60:592–598.

BOYCE JG, LU T, NELSON JH, FRUCHTER RG. 1977. Oral contraceptives and cervical carcinoma. Am J Obstet Gynecol 128:761–766.

BRIAN DD, TILLEY BC, LABARTHE DR, et al. 1980. Breast cancer in DES-exposed mothers: absence of association. Mayo Clin Proc 55:89–93.

BRINTON LA, HOOVER R, FRAUMENI JF. 1986a. Menopausal oestrogens and breast cancer risk: an expanded case-control study. Br J Cancer 54:825–832.

BRINTON LA, HOOVER R, SZKLO M, FRAUMENI JF. 1982. Oral contraceptives and breast cancer. Int J Epidemiol 11:316–322.

BRINTON LA, HUGGINS GR, LEHMAN HF, et al. 1986b. Long-term use of oral contraceptives and risk of invasive cervical cancer. Int J Cancer 38:339–344.

BRINTON LA, REEVES WC, BRENES MM, et al. 1990. Oral contraceptive use and risk of invasive cervical cancer. Int J Epidemiol 19:4–11.

BUSH TL, BARRETT-CONNOR E. 1985. Non-contraceptive estrogen use and cardiovascular disease. Epidemiol Rev 7:80–104.

CASAGRANDE JT, LOUIE EW, PIKE MC, et al. 1979. "Incessant ovulation" and ovarian cancer. Lancet 2:170–173.

CENTERS FOR DISEASE CONTROL. 1983a. Long-term oral contraceptive use and the risk of breast cancer. JAMA 249:1591–1595.

CENTERS FOR DISEASE CONTROL. 1983b. Oral contraceptive use and the risk of ovarian cancer. JAMA 249:1596–1599.

CENTERS FOR DISEASE CONTROL. 1983c. Oral contraceptive use and the risk of endometrial cancer. JAMA 249:1600–1604.

CENTERS FOR DISEASE CONTROL. 1987a. Combination oral contraceptive use and the risk of endometrial cancer. JAMA 257:796–800.

CENTERS FOR DISEASE CONTROL. 1987b. The reduction in risk of ovarian cancer associated with oral-contraceptive use. N Engl J Med 316:650–655.

CHU J, SCHWEID A, WEISS NS. 1982. Survival among women with endometrial cancer: a comparison of estrogen users and non-users. Am J Obstet Gynecol 143:569–573.

CLARKE EA, HATCHER J, MCKEOWN-EYSSEN GE, LICKRISH GM. 1985. Cervical dysplasia: association with sexual behavior, smoking and oral contraceptive use? Am J Obstet Gynecol 151:612–616.

COLDITZ GA, STAMPFER MJ, WILLETT WC, et al. 1990. Prospective study of estrogen replacement therapy and risk of breast cancer in postmenopausal women. JAMA 264:2648–2653.

COLDITZ GA, HANKINSON SE, HUNTER DJ, et al. (1995). The use of estrogens and progestins and the risk of breast cancer in postmenopausal women. N Engl J Med 332:1589–1593.

COLTON T, GREENBERG R, NOLLER K, et al. 1993. Breast cancer in mothers prescribed diethylstilbestrol in pregnancy: further follow-up. JAMA 269:2096–2100.

COULTER A, VESSEY M, MCPHERSON K. 1986. The ability of women to recall their oral contraceptive histories. Contraception 33:127–137.

CRAMER DW, HUTCHINSON GB, WELCH WR, et al. 1982. Factors affecting the association of oral contraceptives and ovarian cancer. N Engl J Med 307:1047–1051.

CRAMER DW, HUTCHINSON GB, WELCH WR. 1983. Determinants of ovarian cancer risk, I: Reproductive experiences and family history. J Natl Cancer Inst 71:711–716.

DEPUE RH, PIKE MC, HENDERSON BE. 1983. Estrogen exposure during gestation and risk of testicular cancer. J Natl Cancer Inst 71:1151–1155.

DOLL R, PETO R. 1981. The Causes of Cancer: Quantitative Estimates of Avoidable Risks of Cancer in the United States Today. New York: Oxford University Press.

DRIFE JO. 1989. The contraceptive pill and breast cancer in young women. Br Med J 298:1269–1270.

EARLY BREAST CANCER TRIALISTS' COLLABORATIVE GROUP. 1988. Effects of adjuvant tamoxifen and of cytotoxic therapy on mortality in early breast cancer. N Engl J Med 319:1681–1692.

EBELING K, NISCHAN P, SCHINDLER C. 1987. Use of oral contraceptives and risk of invasive cervical cancer in previously screened women. Int J Cancer 39:427–430.

EDITORIAL. 1975. Cervical epithelial dysplasia. Br Med J 1:294.

EDITORIAL. 1977. Cervical neoplasia and the pill. Lancet 2:644.

EDITORIAL. 1986. Oral contraceptives and breast cancer. Lancet 2:665–666.

EDITORIAL. 1985. Another look at the pill and breast cancer. Lancet 2:985–987.

EDMONDSON HA, HENDERSON B, BENTON B. 1976. Liver cell adenomas associated with use of oral contraceptives. N Engl J Med 294:470–472.

EWERTZ M. 1992. Oral contraceptives and breast cancer risk in Denmark. Eur J Cancer 28a:1176–1181.

FERENCZY A, BERTRAND G, GELFAND MM. 1979. Proliferation kinetics of human endometrium during the normal menstrual cycle. Am J Obstet Gynecol 133:859–867.

FERGUSON DJP, ANDERSON TJ. 1981. Morphological evaluation of cell turnover in relation to the menstrual cycle in the 'resting' human breast. Br J Cancer 44:177–181.

FINKEL MC, BERLINGER VR. 1973. The extrapolation of experimental findings (animal to man): the dilemma of systematically administered contraceptives. Bull Soc Pharmacol Environ Pathol 4:13–18.

FISHER B, COSTANTINO JP, REDMOND CK, et al. 1994. Endometrial cancer in tamoxifen-treated breast cancer patients: findings from the National Surgical Adjuvant Breast and Bowel Project (NSABP) B-14. J Natl Cancer Inst 86:527–537.

FORMAN D, VINCENT TJ, DOLL R. 1986. Cancer of the liver and the use of oral contraceptives. Br Med J 292:1357–1361.

FORNANDER T, RUTQVIST LE, CEDERMARK B, et al. 1989. Adjuvant tamoxifen in early breast cancer: occurrence of new primary cancers. Lancet 1:117–120.

FRANCESCHI S, BARON AE, LAVECCHIA C. 1990. The influence of female hormones on malignant melanoma. Tumori 76:439–449.

FRANCESCHI S, LAVECCHIA C, HELMRICH SP, et al. 1982. Risk factors for epithelial ovarian cancer in Italy. Am J Epidemiol 115:714–719.

FRASER IS, WEISBERG E. 1981. A comprehensive review of injectable contraception with special emphasis on depot medroxyprogesterone. Med J Aust 1(Suppl):1–19.

GAL D, EDMAN CD, VELLIOS F, FORNEY JP. 1983. Long-term effect of megestrol acetate in the treatment of endometrial hyperplasia. Am J Obstet Gynecol 146:316–321.

GALL SA, BOURGEOIS CH, MAGUIRE R. 1969. The morphologic effects of oral contraceptive agents on the cervix. JAMA 202:2243–2247.

GALLAGHER RP, ELWOOD JM, HILL GB, et al. 1985. Reproductive factors, oral contraceptives and risk of malignant melanoma: Western Canada melanoma study. Br J Cancer 52:901–907.

GAMBRELL RD. 1982. Clinical use of progestins in the menopausal patient: dosage and duration. J Reprod Med 27:531–538.

GEIL RG, LAMAR K. 1977. FDA studies of oestrogen, progestogen and oestrogen-progestogen combinations. J Toxicol Environ Health 3:179–193.

GOEBELSMANN U, MISHELL DR. 1979. The menstrual cycle. In *Reproductive Endocrinology, Infertility and Contraception*, Mishell DR, Davajan V (eds). Philadelphia: F. A. Davis Co., pp 67–89.

GOTTARDIS MM, ROBINSON SP, SATYASWAROOP PS, et al. 1988. Contrasting actions of tamoxifen on endometrial and breast tumor growth in the athymic mouse. Cancer Res 48:812–815.

GREEN A, BAIN C. 1985. Hormonal factors and melanoma in women. Med J Aust 142:446–448.

GROOM GV, GRIFFITHS K. 1976. Effect of the anti-oestrogen tamoxifen on plasma levels of luteinizing hormone, follicle-stimulating hormone, prolactin, oestradiol and progesterone in normal premenopausal women. J Endocrinol 70:421–428.

HADJIMICHAEL OC, MEIGS JW, FALCIER FW, et al. 1984. Cancer risk among women exposed to exogenous estrogens during pregnancy. J Natl Cancer Inst 73:831–834.

HANNAFORD PC, VILLARD-MACKINTOSH L, VESSEY MP, KAY CR. 1991. Oral contraceptives and malignant melanoma. Br J Cancer 63:430–433.

HARLOW BL, WEISS NS, ROTH GJ, et al. 1988. Case-control study of borderline ovarian tumors: reproductive history and exposure to exogenous female hormones. Cancer Res 48:5849–5852.

HARRIS RWC, BRINTON LA, COWDELL RH, et al. 1980. Characteristics of women with dysplasia or carcinoma-in-situ of the cervix uteri. Br J Cancer 42:359–369.

HELLBERG D, VALENTIN J, NILSSON S. 1985. Long-term use of oral contraceptives and cervical neoplasia: an association confounded by other risk factors? Contraception 32:337–346.

HELMRICH SP, ROSENBERG L, KAUFMAN DW, et al. 1984. Lack of

an elevated risk of malignant melanoma in relation to oral contraceptive use. J Natl Cancer Inst 72:617–620.

HEMMINKI E, KENNEDY DL, BAUM C, MCKINLAY SM. 1988. Prescribing non-contraceptive estrogens and progestogens in the United States, 1974–1986. Am J Public Health 78:1479–1481.

HENDERSON BE, BENTON B, JING J, et al. 1979. Risk factors for cancer of the testis in young men. Int J Cancer 23:598–602.

HENDERSON BE, CASAGRANDE JT, PIKE MC, et al. 1983a. The epidemiology of endometrial cancer in young women. Br J Cancer 47:749–756.

HENDERSON BE, PAGANINI-HILL A, ROSS RK. 1991. Decreased mortality in users of estrogen replacement therapy. Arch Intern Med 151:75–78.

HENDERSON BE, PRESTON-MARTIN S, EDMONDSON HA, et al. 1983b. Hepatocellular carcinoma and oral contraceptives. Br J Cancer 48:437–440.

HENDERSON BE, ROSS RK, BERNSTEIN L. 1988a. Estrogens as a cause of human cancer: The Richard and Hinda Rosenthal Foundation Award Lecture. Cancer Res 48:246–253.

HENDERSON BE, ROSS RK, LOBO RA, et al. 1988b. Re-evaluating the role of progestogen therapy after the menopause. Fertil Steril 49(Suppl):9S–15S.

HENDERSON BE, ROSS RK, PAGANINI-HILL A, MACK TM. 1986. Estrogen use and cardiovascular disease. Am J Obstet Gynecol 154:1181–1186.

HENDERSON BE, ROSS RK, PIKE MC, CASAGRANDE JT. 1982. Endogenous hormones as a major factor in human cancer. Cancer Res 43:3232–3239.

HERBST AL. 1981. The epidemiology of vaginal and cervical clear cell adenocarcinoma. In *Developmental Effects of Diethylstilbestrol (DES) in Pregnancy*, Herbst AL, Bern HA (eds). New York: Thieme Stratton, pp 63–70.

HERBST AL, COLE P, NORUSIS MJ, et al. 1979. Epidemiologic aspects and factors related to survival in 384 registry cases of clear cell adenocarcinoma of the vagina and cervix. Am J Obstet Gynecol 135:876–886.

HERBST AL, ULFELDER H, POSKANZER DC. 1971. Association of maternal stilbestrol therapy with tumor appearance in young women. N Engl J Med 248:878–881.

HIATT RA, BAWOL R, FRIEDMAN GW, HOOVER R. 1984. Exogenous estrogens and breast cancer after oophorectomy. Cancer 54:139–144.

HILDRETH NG, KELSEY JL, LIVOLSI VA, et al. 1981. An epidemiological study of epithelial carcinoma of the ovary. Am J Epidemiol 14:398–405.

HOLLY EA, WEISS NS, LIFF JM. 1983. Cutaneous melanoma in relation to exogenous hormones and reproductive factors. J Natl Cancer Inst 70:827–831.

HOLMAN CDJ, ARMSTRONG BK, HEENAN PJ. 1984. Cutaneous malignant melanoma in women: exogenous sex hormones and reproductive factors. Br J Cancer 50:673–680.

HOLMBERG L, LUND E, BERGSTROM R, et al. 1994. Oral contraceptives and prognosis in breast cancer: effects of duration, latency, recency, age at first use and relation to parity and body mass index in young women with breast cancer. Eur J Cancer 30A:351–354.

HOOVER R, BAIN C, COLE P, MACMAHON B. 1978. Oral contraceptive use: association with frequency of hospitalization and chronic disease risk indicators. Am J Public Health 68:335–341.

HOOVER R, GLASS A, FINKLE WD, et al. 1981. Conjugated estrogens and breast cancer risk in women. J Natl Cancer Inst 67:815–820.

HOOVER R, GRAY LA, COLE P, MACMAHON B. 1976. Menopausal estrogens and breast cancer. N Engl J Med 295:401–405.

HOOVER R, GRAY LA, FRAUMENI JF. 1977. Stilboestrol (diethylstilbestrol) and the risk of ovarian cancer. Lancet 2:533–534.

HUBBY MM, HAENSZEL WM, HERBST AL. 1981. Effects on the mother following exposure to diethylstilbestrol in pregnancy. In *Developmental Effects of Diethylstilbestrol (DES) in Pregnancy*, Herbst AL, Bern JA (eds). New York: Thieme Stratton, pp 120–128.

HULKA BS, CHAMBLESS LE, DEUBNER DC, WILKINSON WE. 1982a. Breast cancer and estrogen replacement therapy. Am J Obstet Gynecol 143:638–644.

HULKA BS, CHAMBLESS LE, KAUFMAN DG, et al. 1982b. Protection against endometrial carcinoma by combination-product oral contraceptives. JAMA 247:475–477.

HUNT K, VESSEY M, MACPHERSON K, COLEMAN M. 1987. Long-term surveillance of mortality and cancer incidence in women receiving hormone replacement therapy. Br J Obstet Gynaecol 94:620–635.

IMS AMERICA. 1987. National Prescription Audit. Ambler PA, IMS America.

INTERNATIONAL AGENCY FOR RESEARCH ON CANCER. 1987. IARC Monographs on the Evaluation of Carcinogenic Risk of Chemicals to Man, Supplement 7, Overall Evaluations of Carcinogenicity: An Updating of IARC Monographs, Vols 1–42. Lyon, IARC, pp 273–278.

IRWIN KL, ROSERO-BIXBY L, OBERLE MW, et al. 1988. Oral contraceptives and cervical cancer risk in Costa Rica: detection bias or causal association? JAMA 259:59–64.

JEPPSSON J, JOHANSSON EDB, LJUNGBERG O, et al. 1977. Endometrial histology and circulating levels of medroxyprogesterone acetate (MPA): estradiol, FSH and LH in women with MPA induced amenorrhoea compared with women with secondary amenorrhoea. Acta Obstet Gynecol Scand 56:43–48.

JICK H, WALKER AM, WATKINS RN, et al. 1980a. Oral contraceptives and breast cancer. Am J Epidemiol 112:577–585.

JICK H, WALKER AM, WATKINS RN, et al. 1980b. Replacement estrogens and breast cancer. Am J Epidemiol 112:586–594.

JOHN EM, WHITTEMORE AS, HARRIS R, et al. 1993. Characteristics relating to ovarian cancer risk: collaborative analysis of seven U.S. case-control studies. Epithelial ovarian cancer in black women. J Natl Cancer Inst 85:142–147.

JONES CJ, BRINTON LA, HAMMAN RF, et al. 1990. Risk factors for in situ cervical cancer: results from a case-control study. Cancer Res 50:3657–3662.

JORDAN VC. 1990a. Estrogen receptor-mediated direct and indirect antitumor effects of tamoxifen. J Natl Cancer Inst 82:1662–1663.

JORDAN VC. 1990b. Tamoxifen for the prevention of breast cancer. In *Cancer Prevention*, DeVita VT, Hellman S, Rosenberg SA (eds). Philadelphia: JB Lippincott Company, pp 1–12.

KAUFMAN DW, KELLY JP, WELCH WR, et al. 1989. Noncontraceptive estrogen use and epithelial ovarian cancer. Am J Epidemiol 130:1142–51.

KAUFMAN DW, MILLER DR, ROSENBERG L, et al. 1984. Noncontraceptive estrogen use and risk of breast cancer. JAMA 252:63–67.

KAUFMAN DW, SHAPIRO S, SLONE D, et al. 1980. Decreased risk of endometrial cancer among oral contraceptive users. N Engl J Med 303:1045–1047.

KAY CR. 1981. Malignant melanoma and oral contraceptives. (Letter) Br J Cancer 44:479.

KAY CR, HANNAFORD PC. 1988. Breast cancer and the pill—a further report from the Royal College of General Practitioners' oral contraception study. Br J Cancer 58:675–680.

KEDAR RP, BOURNE TH, POWLES TJ, et al. 1994. Effects of tamoxifen on uterus and ovaries of postmenopausal women in a randomised breast cancer prevention trial. Lancet 343:1318–1321.

KELSEY JL, FISCHER DB, HOLFORD JR, et al. 1981. Exogenous estrogens and other factors in the epidemiology of breast cancer. J Natl Cancer Inst 67:327–333.

KELSEY JL, HILDRETH NG. 1983. Breast and Gynecologic Cancer Epidemiology. Boca Raton, Fla: CRC Press.

KELSEY JL, LIVOLSI VA, HOLFORD TR, et al. 1982. A case-control study of cancer of the endometrium. Am J Epidemiol 116:333–342.

KENNEDY LD, BAUM C, FORBES MD. 1985. Noncontraceptive estrogens and progestins: use patterns over time. Obstet Gynecol 65:441–446.

KIEL DP, FELSON DT, ANDERSON JJ, et al. 1987. Hip fracture and the use of estrogens in postmenopausal women. The Framingham Study. N Engl J Med 317:1169–1174.

KJÆR SK, ENGHOLM G, DAHL C, et al. 1993. Case-control study of risk factors for cervical squamous-cell neoplasia in Denmark, III: Role of oral contraceptive use. Cancer Causes Control 4:513–519.

LANARI C, MOLINOLO AA, PASQUALINI CD. 1986. Induction of mammary adenocarcinomas by medroxyprogesterone acetate in BALB/c female mice. Cancer Lett 33:215–223.

LAVECCHIA C, DECARLI A, FASOLI M, et al. 1986a. Oral contraceptives and cancers of the breast and female genital tract: interim results from a case-control study. Br J Cancer 54:311–317.

LAVECCHIA C, DECARLI A, PARAZZINI F, et al. 1986b. Non-contraceptive oestrogens and the risk of breast cancer in women. Int J Cancer 38:853–858.

LAVECCHIA C, FRANCESCHI S, DECARLI A. 1984. Oral contraceptive use and the risk of epithelial ovarian cancer. Br J Cancer 50:31–34.

LAVECCHIA C, LIBERATI A, FRANCESCHI S. 1982. Noncontraceptive estrogen use and the occurrence of ovarian cancer. (Letter) J Natl Cancer Inst 69:1207.

LE MG, HILL C, KRAMAR A, MOULTON LH. 1985. Possible cohort effects in studies of oral contraceptive use and breast cancer. (Letter) Br J Cancer 52:805.

LEE NC, ROSERO-BIXBY L, OBERLE MW, et al. 1987. A case-control study of breast cancer and hormonal contraception in Costa Rica. J Natl Cancer Inst 79:1247–1254.

LERNER LJ, JORDAN VC. 1990. Development of antiestrogens and their use in breast cancer: Eighth Cain Memorial Award Lecture. Cancer Res 50:4177–4189.

LIANG AP, LEVENSON AG, LAYDE PM, et al. 1983. Risk of breast, uterine corpus and ovarian cancer in women receiving medroxyprogesterone injections. JAMA 249:2909–2912.

LINDSAY R, HART DM, CLARK DM. 1984. The minimum effective dose of estrogen for the prevention of post-menopausal bone loss. Obstet Gynecol 63:759–763.

LIPNICK RJ, BURING JE, HENNEKENS CH, et al. 1986. Oral contraceptives and breast cancer: a prospective cohort study. JAMA 255:58–61.

MACK TM, PIKE MC, HENDERSON BE, et al. 1976. Estrogens and endometrial cancer in a retirement community. N Engl J Med 294:1262–1267.

MALONE KE, DALING JR, WEISS NS. 1993. Oral contraceptives and breast cancer risk. Epidemiol Rev 15:80–97.

MANT D, VESSEY MP, NEIL A, et al. 1982. Breast self-examination and breast stage at diagnosis. Br J Cancer 55:207–211.

MAYBERRY RM. 1994. Age-specific patterns of association between breast cancer risk factors in black women, ages 20 to 39 and 40 to 54. Ann Epidemiol 4:205–213.

MCDONALD JA, WEISS NS, DALING JR, et al. 1986. Menopausal estrogen use and the risk of breast cancer. Breast Cancer Res Treat 7:193–199.

MCGOWAN L, PARENT L, LEDNAR W, NORRIS HJ. 1979. The woman at risk for developing ovarian cancer. Gynecol Oncol 7:325–344.

MCPHERSON K, COOPE PA. 1986. Early oral contraceptive use and breast cancer risk. (Letter) Lancet 1:685–686.

MCPHERSON K, VESSEY MP, NEIL A, et al. 1987. Early oral contraceptive use and breast cancer: results of another case-control study. Br J Cancer 56:653–660.

MCTIERNAN AM, WEISS NS, DALING JR. 1984. Incidence of thyroid cancer in women in relation to reproductive and hormonal factors. Am J Epidemiol 120:423–435.

MEARA J, VESSEY M, FAIRWEATHER DV. 1989. A randomized double-blind controlled trial of the value of diethylstilboestrol therapy in pregnancy: 35-year follow-up of mothers and their offspring. Br J Obstet Gynaecol 96:620–622.

MEIRIK O. 1986a. Oral contraceptives and breast cancer in young women: some notes on a current controversy. Acta Obstet Gynecol Scand 134(Suppl):5–7.

MEIRIK O, FARLEY TMM, LUND E, et al. 1989. Breast cancer and oral contraceptives: patterns of risk among parous and nulliparous women—further analyses of the Swedish-Norwegian material. Contraception 39:471–475.

MEIRIK O, LUND E, ADAMI HO, et al. 1986b. Oral contraceptive use and breast cancer in young women. Lancet 2:650–653.

MELNICK S, COLE P, ANDERSON D, HERBST A. 1987. Rates and risks of diethylstilbestrol-related clear-cell adenocarcinoma of the vagina and cervix: an update. N Engl J Med 316:514–516.

MILLER DR, ROSENBERG L, KAUFMAN DW, et al. 1986. Breast cancer risk in relation to early oral contraceptive use. Obstet Gynecol 68:863–868.

MILLER DR, ROSENBERG L, KAUFMAN DW, et al. 1989. Breast cancer before age 45 and oral contraceptive use: new findings. Am J Epidemiol 129:269–280.

MILLS PK, BEESON WL, PHILLIPS RL, FRASER GE. 1989. Prospective study of exogenous hormone use and breast cancer in Seventh-day Adventists. Cancer 64:591–597.

MINTEOT R, FIEVEZ CL. 1974. Endocervical changes with the use of synthetic steroids. Obstet Gynecol 44:53–59.

MISHELL DR. 1991. Long-acting contraceptive steroids: postcoital contraceptives and antiprogestins. In *Infertility, Contraception and Reproductive Endocrinology*. Mishell DR, Davajan V, Lobo RA (eds). Boston: Blackwell Scientific, pp 872–894.

MOGHISS K. 1972. Morphologic changes in the ovaries of women treated with microdose progestogens. Fertil Steril 23:739–744.

MOSS AR, OSMOND D, DACCHETTI P, et al. 1986. Hormonal risk factors in testicular cancer: a case-control study. Am J Epidemiol 124:39–52.

MURRAY PP, STADEL BV, SCHLESSELMAN JJ. 1989. Oral contraceptive use in women with a family history of breast cancer. Obstet Gynecol 73:977–983.

NAYFIELD SG, KARP JE, FORD LG, et al. 1991. Potential role of tamoxifen in prevention of breast cancer. J Natl Cancer Inst 83:1450–1459.

NEUBERGER J, FORMAN D, DOLL R, WILLIAMS R. 1986. Oral contraceptives and hepatocellular carcinoma. Br Med J 292:1355–1357.

NEWHOUSE ML, PEARSON RM, FULLERTON JM, et al. 1977. A case control study of carcinoma of the ovary. Br J Prev Soc Med 31:148–153.

NOMURA AMY, KOLONEL LN, HIROHATA T, LEE J. 1986. The association of replacement estrogens with breast cancer. Int J Cancer 37:49–53.

OBERLE MW, ROSERO-BIXBY L, IRWIN KL, et al. 1988. Cervical cancer risk and use of depot-medroxyprogesterone acetate in Costa Rica. Int J Epidemiol 17:718–723.

OLSSON H, MOLLER TR, RANSTAM J, et al. 1988. Early oral contraceptive use as a prognostic factor in breast cancer. Anticancer Res 8:29–32.

OSTERLIND A, TUCKER MA, STONE BJ, JENSEN OM. 1988. The Danish case-control study of cutaneous malignant melanoma, III: Hormonal and reproductive factors in women. Int J Cancer 42:821–824.

PAGANINI-HILL A, ROSS RK, GERKINS VR, et al. 1981. Menopausal estrogen therapy and hip fractures. Ann Intern Med 95:28–31.

PALMER JR, ROSENBERG L, KAUFMAN D, et al. 1989. Oral contraceptive use and liver cancer. Am J Epidemiol 130:878–882.

PALMER JR, ROSENBERG L, STROM BL, et al. 1992. Oral contraceptive use and risk of cutaneous malignant melanoma. Cancer Causes Control 3:547–554.

PARAZZINI F, LAVECCHIA C, NEGRI E, MAGGI R. 1990. Oral contraceptive use and invasive cervical cancer. Int J Epidemiol 19:259–263.

PAUL C, SKEGG, DCG, SPEARS GFS. 1989. Depot medroxyprogesterone (Depo-Provera) and risk of breast cancer. Br Med J 299:759–762.

PAUL C, SKEGG DCG, SPEARS GFS, KALDOR JM. 1986. Oral contraceptives and breast cancer: a national study. Br Med J 293:723–726.

PERSSON I, YUEN J, BERGKVIST L, et al. 1992. Combined oestrogen-progestogen replacement and breast cancer risk. (Letter) Lancet 340:1044.

PETERS RK, CHAO A, MACK TM, et al. 1986a. Increased frequency of adenocarcinomas of the uterine cervix in young women in Los Angeles County. J Natl Cancer Inst 76:423–428.

PETERS RK, THOMAS DC, HAGAN DG, et al. 1986b. Risk factors for invasive cervical cancer among Latinas and non-Latinas in Los Angeles County. J Natl Cancer Inst. 77:1063–1077.

PETO J. 1989. Oral contraceptives and breast cancer: is the CASH study really negative? (Letter) Lancet 1:552.

PIKE MC, BERNSTEIN L. 1989. Oral contraceptives and breast cancer. (Letter) Lancet 1:615–616.

PIKE MC, BERNSTEIN L, SPICER D. 1993. Exogenous hormones and breast cancer risk. In Current Therapy in Oncology, Neiderhuber JE (ed). St. Louis: BC Decker, pp 292–303.

PIKE MC, HENDERSON BE, CASAGRANDE JT, et al. 1981. Oral contraceptive use and early abortion as risk factors for breast cancer in young women. Br J Cancer 43:72–76.

PIKE MC, HENDERSON BE, KRAILO MD, et al. 1983. Breast cancer in young women and use of oral contraceptives: possible modifying effect of formulation and age at use. Lancet 2:926–930.

PIPER JM, KENNEDY DL. 1987. Oral contraceptives in the United States: trends in content and potency. Int J Epidemiol 16:215–221.

POLLACK M, CONSTANTINO J, POLYCHRONAKOS C, et al. 1990. Effect of tamoxifen on serum insulinlike growth factor I levels in stage I breast cancer patients. J Natl Cancer Inst 82:1693–1697.

PRESTON-MARTIN S, BERNSTEIN L, PIKE MC, et al. 1987. Thyroid cancer among young women related to prior thyroid disease and pregnancy history. Br J Cancer 55:191–195.

PRESTON-MARTIN S, JIN F, DUDA MJ, et al. 1993. A case-control study of thyroid cancer in women under age 55 in Shanghai (People's Republic of China). Cancer Causes Control 4:431–440.

RAMCHARAN S, PELLEGRIN FA, RAY R, HSU JP. 1981. A prospective study of the side effects of oral contraceptive use. In: The Walnut Creek Contraceptive Drug Study, NIH Publ. 81-564, Vol. 3. Washington, DC: US Government Printing Office.

RISCH HA, WEISS NS, LYON JL, et al. 1983. Events of reproductive life and the incidence of epithelial ovarian cancer. Am J Epidemiol 177:128–139.

ROBBOY SJ, NOLLER KL, O'BRIEN P, et al. 1984. Increased incidence of cervical and vaginal dysplasia in 3,980 diethylstilbestrol-exposed young women: experience of the National Collaborative Diethylstilbestrol Adenosis Project. JAMA 252:2979–2983.

ROMIEU I, WILLET WC, COLDITZ GA, et al. 1989. Prospective study of oral contraceptive use and risk of breast cancer in women. J Natl Cancer Inst 81:1313–1321.

RON E, KLEINERMAN RA, BOICE JD, et al. 1987. A population-based case-control study of thyroid cancer. J Natl Cancer Inst 79:1–12.

ROOKS JB, ORY HW, ISHAK KG, et al. 1979. Epidemiology of hepatocellular adenoma: the role of oral contraceptive use. JAMA 242:644–648.

ROSENBERG L, MILLER DR, KAUFMAN DW, et al. 1984. Breast cancer and oral contraceptive use. Am J Epidemiol 119:167–176.

ROSENBERG L, SHAPIRO S, SLONE D, et al. 1982. Epithelial ovarian cancer and combination oral contraceptives. JAMA 247:3210–3212.

ROSENBERG MJ, LAYDE PM, ORY HW, et al. 1983. Agreement between women's histories of oral contraceptive use and physician records. Int J Epidemiol 12:84–87.

ROSENBLATT KA, THOMAS DB AND THE WHO COLLABORATIVE STUDY OF NEOPLASIA AND STEROID CONTRACEPTIVES. 1991. Hormonal content of combined oral contraceptives in relation to the reduced risk of endometrial cancer. Int J Cancer 49:870–874.

ROSNER D, LANE WW, BRETT RP. 1985. Influence of oral contraceptives on the prognosis of breast cancer in young women. Cancer 55:1556–1562.

ROSNER D, LANE WW. 1986. Oral contraceptive use has no adverse effect on the prognosis of breast cancer. Cancer 57:591–596.

ROSS RK, PAGANINI-HILL A, GERKINS VR, et al. 1980. A case-control study of menopausal estrogen therapy and breast cancer. JAMA 243:1635–1639.

ROY S. 1987. Hepatic effects of hormone therapy. Postgrad Med (Special Report, September 14, 1987):39–47.

RUSSELL-BRIEFEL R, EZZATI T, PERLMAN J. 1985. Prevalence and trends in oral contraceptive use in premenopausal females aged 12–54 years, United States 1971–1980. Am J Public Health 75:1173–1176.

SAVRAS M, STUDD JWW, FOGELMAN I, et al. 1988. Skeletal effects of oral oestrogen compared with subcutaneous oestrogen and testosterone in postmenopausal women. Br Med J 297:331–333.

SCHLESSELMAN JJ, STADEL BV, KORPER M, et al. 1992. Breast cancer detection in relation to oral contraception. J Clin Epidemiol 45:449–459.

SCHLESSELMAN JJ, STADEL BV, MURRAY P, LAI S. 1987. Breast cancer risk in relation to type of estrogen contained in oral contraceptives. Contraception 36:595–613.

SCHOTTENFELD D, WARSHAUER ME, SHERLOCK S, et al. 1980. The epidemiology oftesticular cancer in young adults. Am J Epidemiol 112:232–246.

SCHWARTZ SM, WEISS NS. 1986. Increased incidence of adenocarcinoma of the cervix in young women in the United States. Am J Epidemiol 124:1045–1047.

SHERMAN B, WALLACE R, BEAN J. 1983. Estrogen use and breast cancer: interaction with body mass. Cancer 51:1527–1531.

SHOUP D. 1991. Effect of body weight and reproductive function. In *Infertility, Contraception and Reproductive Endocrinology*, Mishell DR, Davajan V, Lobo RA (eds). Boston: Blackwell Scientific Publications, pp 288–313.

SILVERBERG SG, MAKOWSKI EL. 1975. Endometrial carcinoma in young women taking oral contraceptive agents. Obstet Gynecol 46:503–506.

SMITH DC, PRENTICE R, THOMPSON DJ, HERRMANN W. 1975. Association of exogenous estrogen and endometrial cancer. N Engl J Med 293:1164–1167.

SMITH OW. 1948. Diethylstilbestrol in the prevention and treatment of complications of pregnancy. Am J Obstet Gynecol 56:821–834.

SMITH OW, SMITH G VAN S. 1949. The influence of diethylstilbestrol on the progress and outcome of pregnancy as based on a comparison of treated with untreated primigravidas. Am J Obstet Gynecol 58:994–1009.

STADEL BV, LAI S, SCHLESSELMAN JJ, MURRAY P. 1988. Oral contraceptives and premenopausal breast cancer in nulliparous women. Contraception 38:287–299.

STADEL BV, RUBIN GL, WINGO PA, SCHLESSELMAN JJ. 1986. Oral contraceptives and breast cancer in young women. (Letter) Lancet 1:436.

STADEL BV, SCHLESSELMAN JJ. 1986. Oral contraceptive use and the risk of breast cancer in women with a "prior" history of benign breast disease. Am J Epidemiol 123:373–382.

STADEL BV, SCHLESSELMAN JJ, MURRAY PA. 1989. Oral contraceptives and breast cancer. (Letter) Lancet 1:1257–1258.

STADEL BV, WEBSTER LA, RUBIN GL, et al. 1985. Oral contraceptives and breast cancer in young women. Lancet 2:970–973.

STANFORD JL, BRINTON LA, BERMAN ML, et al. 1993. Oral contraceptives and endometrial cancer: do other risk factors modify the association? Int J Cancer 54:243–248.

STANFORD JL, BRINTON LA, HOOVER RN. 1989. Oral contraceptives and breast cancer: results from an expanded case-control study. Br J Cancer 60:375–381.

STANFORD JL, THOMAS DB. 1993. Exogenous progestins and breast cancer. Epidemiol Rev 15:98–107.

STANFORD JL, WEISS NS, VOIGT LF, et al. 1995. Combined estrogen and progestin hormone replacement therapy in relation to risk of breast cancer in middle-aged women. JAMA 274:137–142.

STEINBERG KK, THACKER SR, SMITH SJ, et al. 1991. A meta-analysis of the effect of estrogen replacement therapy on the risk of breast cancer. JAMA 265:1985–1990.

STERN E, FORSYTHE AB, YOUKELES L, COFFELT CF. 1977. Steroid contraceptive use and cervical dysplasia: increased risk of progression. Science 196:1460–1462.

STOLLEY PD, TONASCIA JA, SARTWELL PE, et al. 1974. Agreement rates between oral contraceptive users and prescribers in relation to drug use histories. Am J Epidemiol 107:226–235.

STUDD JWW, THOM MH, PATERSON MEL. 1980. The prevention and treatment of endometrial pathology in postmenopausal women receiving exogenous oestrogens. In: *The Menopause and Postmenopause*. Pasetto W, Pavletti R, Lambrus J (eds). Lancaster, England: MTP Press, p 127.

SWAN SH, BROWN WL. 1981. Oral contraceptive use, sexual activity and cervical carcinoma. Am J Obstet Gynecol 139:52–57.

SWAN SH, PETITTI DB. 1982. A review of problems of bias and confounding in epidemiologic studies of cervical neoplasia and oral contraceptive use. Am J Epidemiol 115:10–18.

TAVANI A, NEGRI E, PARAZZINI F, et al. 1993. Female hormone utilisation and risk of hepatocellular carcinoma. Br J Cancer 67:635–637.

TAYOB Y, ADAMS J, JACOBS HS, GUILLEBAUD J. 1985. Ultrasound demonstration of increased frequency of functional ovarian cysts in women using progestogen-only oral contraceptives. Br J Obstet Gynaecol 92:1003–1009.

THOMAS DB, MOLINA R, CUEVAS HR, et al. 1989. Monthly injectable steroid contraceptives and cervical carcinoma. Am J Epidemiol 130:237–247.

THOMAS DB, NOONAN EA. 1991. Risk of breast cancer in relation to use of combined oral contraceptives near the age of menopause: WHO Collaborative Study of Neoplasia and Steroid Contraceptives. Cancer Causes Control 2:389–394.

THOMAS DB, PERSING JP, HUTCHINSON WG. 1982. Exogenous estrogens and other risk factors for breast cancer in women with benign breast diseases. J Natl Cancer Inst 69:1017–1025.

TYRER LB. 1984. Oral contraception for the adolescent. J Reprod Med 29:551–559.

TZONOU A, DAY NE, TRICHOPOULOS D, et al. 1984. The epidemiology of ovarian cancer in Greece: a case-control study. Eur J Cancer Clin Oncol 20:1045–1052.

UK NATIONAL CASE-CONTROL STUDY GROUP. 1989. Oral contraceptive use and breast cancer risk in young women. Lancet 1:973–982.

URSIN G, PETERS RK, HENDERSON BE, et al. 1994. Oral contraceptive use and adenocarcinoma of the cervix. Lancet 344:1390–1394.

VAN LEEUWEN FE, BENRAADT J, COEBERGH JW, et al. 1994. Risk of endometrial cancer after tamoxifen treatment of breast cancer. Lancet 343:448–452.

VESSEY M, BARON J, DOLL R, et al. 1983a. Oral contraceptives and breast cancer: final report of an epidemiological study. Br J Cancer 47:455–462.

VESSEY M, METCALFE A, WELLS C, et al. 1987. Ovarian neoplasms, functional ovarian cysts, and oral contraceptives. Br Med J 294:1518–1520.

VESSEY MP, DOLL R, JONES K, et al. 1979. An epidemiological study of oral contraceptives and breast cancer. Br Med J 1:1755–1758.

VESSEY MP, LAWLESS M, MCPHERSON K, YEATES D. 1983b. Neoplasia of the cervix uteri and contraception—a possible adverse effect of the pill. Lancet 2:930–934.

VESSEY MP, LAWLESS M, MCPHERSON K, YEATES D. 1983c. Oral contraceptives and cervical cancer. Lancet 2:1358–1359.

VESSEY MP, MCPHERSON K, VILLARD-MACKINTOSH L, YEATES D. 1989. Oral contraceptives and breast cancer: latest findings in a large cohort study. Br J Cancer 59:613–617.

VESSEY MP, MCPHERSON K, YEATES D, DOLL R. 1982. Oral contraceptive use and abortion before first term pregnancy in relation to breast cancer risk. Br J Cancer 45:327–331.

VOIGT LF, DENG Q, WEISS NS. 1994. Recency, duration and progestin content of oral contraceptives in relation to the incidence of endometrial cancer (Washington, USA). Cancer Causes Control 5:227–233.

WEISS NS, LYON JL, KRISHNAMURTHY S, et al. 1982. Noncontraceptive estrogen use and the occurrence of ovarian cancer. J Natl Cancer Inst 68:95–98.

WEISS NS, SAYVETZ TA. 1980. Incidence of endometrial cancer in relation to the use of oral contraceptives. N Engl J Med 302:551–554.

WHITE E, MALONE KE, WEISS NS, et al. 1994. Breast cancer among young U.S. women in relation to oral contraceptive use. J Natl Cancer Inst 86:505–514.

WHITEHEAD MI, TOWNSEND PT, PRYSE-DAVIES J, et al. 1982. Effects of various types and dosages of progestogens on the postmenopausal endometrium. J Reprod Med 27:539–547.

WHITTEMORE AS, HARRIS R, ITNYRE J, et al. 1992. Characteristics relating to ovarian cancer risk: collaborative analysis of 12 US case-control studies, II: Invasive epithelial ovarian cancers in white women. Am J Epidemiol 136:1184–1203.

WHO COLLABORATIVE STUDY OF NEOPLASIA AND STEROID CONTRACEPTIVES. 1985. Invasive cervical cancer and combined oral contraceptives. Br Med J 290:961–965.

WHO COLLABORATIVE STUDY OF NEOPLASIA AND STEROID CONTRACEPTIVES. 1988. Endometrial cancer and combined oral contraceptives. Int J Epidemiol 17:263–269.

WHO COLLABORATIVE STUDY OF NEOPLASIA AND STEROID CONTRACEPTIVES. 1989. Combined oral contraceptives and liver cancer. Int J Cancer 43:254–259.

WHO COLLABORATIVE STUDY OF NEOPLASIA AND STEROID CONTRACEPTIVES. 1991a. Depot-medroxyprogesterone acetate (DMPA) and risk of endometrial cancer. Int J Cancer 49:186–190.

WHO COLLABORATIVE STUDY OF NEOPLASIA AND STEROID CONTRACEPTIVES. 1991b. Depot-medroxyprogesterone acetate (DMPA) and risk of epithelial ovarian cancer. Int J Cancer 49:191–195.

WHO COLLABORATIVE STUDY OF NEOPLASIA AND STEROID CONTRACEPTIVES. 1991c. Breast cancer and depot-medroxyprogesterone acetate: a multinational study. Lancet 338:833–838.

WHO COLLABORATIVE STUDY OF NEOPLASIA AND STEROID CONTRACEPTIVES. 1991d. Depot-medroxyprogesterone acetate (DMPA) and risk of liver cancer. Int J Cancer 49:182–185.

WHO COLLABORATIVE STUDY OF NEOPLASIA AND STEROID CONTRACEPTIVES. 1992. Depot-medroxyprogesterone acetate (DMPA) and risk of invasive squamous cell cervical cancer. Contraception 45:299–312.

WILLETT WC, BAIN C, HENNEKENS CH, et al. 1981. Oral contraceptives and risk of ovarian cancer. Cancer 48:1684–1687.

WINGO PA, LAYDE PM, LEE NC, et al. 1987. The risk of breast cancer in postmenopausal women who have used estrogen replacement therapy. JAMA 257:209–215.

WU ML, WHITTEMORE AS, PAFFENBARGER RS, et al. 1988. Personal and environmental characteristics related to epithelial ovarian cancer, I: Reproductive and menstrual events and oral contraceptive use. Am J Epidemiol 128:1216–1227.

YAGER JD, YAGER R. 1980. Oral contraceptive steroids as promoters of hepatocarcinogenesis in female Sprague-Dawley rats. Cancer Res 40:3680–3685.

YU MC, TONG MJ, GOVINDARAJAN S, et al. 1991. Nonviral risk factors for hepatocellular carcinoma in a low-risk population, the non-Asians of Los Angeles County, California. J Natl Cancer Inst 83:1820–1826.

ZANETTI R, FRANCESCHI S, ROSSO S, et al. 1990. Cutaneous malignant melanoma in females: the role of hormonal and reproductive factors. Int J Epidemiol 19:522–526.

ZARCOVIC G. 1985. Alterations of cervical cytology and steroid contraceptive use. Int J Epidemiol 14:369–377.

ZIEL HK, FINKLE WD. 1975. Increased risk of endometrial carcinoma among users of conjugated estrogens. N Engl J Med 293:1167–1170.

ZUR HAUSEN H. 1982. Human genital cancer: synergism between two virus infections or synergism between a virus infection and initiating events? Lancet 2:1370–1372.

23 Pharmaceuticals other than hormones

JOSEPH V. SELBY
GARY D. FRIEDMAN
LISA J. HERRINTON

Among the substances in the environment that are of concern as possible carcinogens are therapeutic drugs. Drugs are deliberately ingested by, or injected into, people in amounts often much greater than other chemicals in the environment that are suspected to be carcinogenic. A few drugs have been demonstrated to cause or promote the development of cancer in humans. Some others have these effects in experimental animals, but their status as carcinogens in humans remains unclear.

This chapter is concerned with the carcinogenic effects of drugs other than hormones. Those both known and suspected to cause cancer are discussed.

SURVEILLANCE: DISCOVERY AND VERIFICATION OF DRUG–CANCER ASSOCIATIONS

Current understanding of chemical carcinogenesis suggests that chemicals act at one or more stages in a process that includes initiation of previously normal cells and promotion of these cells toward malignancy. The process may require 20 years or more to produce clinically detectable cancer (Farber, 1987). For both initiation and promotion, prolonged exposure is considered important, although in some cases a single exposure may be sufficient to initiate cells. One implication of this theory is that drugs taken for long intervals may be more suspect as possible carcinogens than those used only briefly. Another is that prolonged observation following initial exposure may be needed to detect a carcinogenic effect and will always be necessary before such an effect can be ruled out.

Surveillance for adverse effects of drugs has frequently been divided into "first-alert" or "hypothesis-generating" activities and subsequent verification or "hypothesis-testing" analyses (Venning, 1983). For many adverse effects, individual case reports by astute clinicians provide the first suspicion of an increase in risk. For drug-induced cancer, only very rare cancers or those occurring in unusual circumstances (eg, an unusual anatomic site or age of onset) would be likely to be detected in this manner. The long interval between drug exposure and diagnosis of most cancers and the occurrence of the cancer in the absence as well as the presence of drug exposure make it less likely that suspicion will be raised by an individual case, and underscore the importance of epidemiological surveillance.

Initial suspicion of drug–cancer associations often results from theoretical considerations of the chemical and pharmacokinetic properties of the compound, from results of in vivo or in vitro tests for mutagenicity or other genetic effects, or from reports of experiments in animals. The International Agency for Research on Cancer (IARC) conducts systematic evaluations of the evidence of carcinogenicity of hundreds of chemicals, including many agents used primarily for medicinal purposes. The evaluations to date have been published in a series of monographs, which have been summarized (IARC, 1987) and recently updated concerning certain drugs (IARC, 1990).

Computerized databases that link drug prescription data with subsequent medical records in large populations have been proposed as a nearly ideal drug surveillance system. The advantages of this approach are that unbiased drug exposure information is obtained prior to occurrence of the adverse effect and that ascertainment of cases is complete, avoiding possible selection biases. Given the rarity of many cancers and the low prevalence of usage for most drugs, these databases must be very large, covering populations of one million persons or more, to have sufficient power for surveillance of more than the most frequently used drugs. Several automated systems of this size are now being developed in the United States and Canada (Edlavitch, 1988).

Systematic testing of drug-cancer associations in these

We gratefully acknowledge the editorial assistance of Lyn Wender, and support for our studies of drug carcinogenesis by Public Health Service grants R37-CA19939 and R35-CA49761 from the National Cancer Institute.

databases, using either longitudinal or case-control methods, could provide a powerful method for identifying previously unsuspected adverse drug effects. Of course, many spurious findings would also be found in testing the large number of hypotheses (Friedman, 1972; Thomas et al, 1985), and more detailed case-control studies would be essential to test these hypotheses further. These same databases could provide an unbiased group of cases and objective drug exposure information for the subsequent case-control studies. Additional information on possible confounding factors could then be gathered on the cases and an appropriate control group from the same cohort.

Once such a system is in place, 20 or more years of data collection will be necessary before negative findings can be considered definitive. Until that time, ad hoc case-control studies offer the most feasible method of testing hypotheses regarding drug carcinogenicity. For these, prior drug use by cases and controls is ascertained by interview or, preferably for prescription drugs, by review of medical records if they are available. For rarely used drugs, the only practical approach is to assemble cohorts of users of the drug and compare subsequent cancer incidence with that of appropriate nonuser groups.

Presented below are summaries of available information for nonhormonal medications that are known or suspected to be carcinogenic to man. Table 23-1 summarizes IARC evaluations through 1990 (IARC, 1987, IARC, 1990) for nonhormonal drugs judged to be at least possibly carcinogenic in humans and for which at least some epidemiological evidence in humans is available. The term *carcinogenic*, as used here, includes any effect, either initiating or promoting, that ultimately increases the incidence of cancer.

TABLE 23–1. *Nonhormonal Drugs Considered to Be Definitely, Probably, or Possibly Carcinogenic to Humans**

	Data Source		
Drug	*Human*[a]	*Animal*[a]	*Overall Evaluation*[b]
Adriamycin	I	S	2A
Arsenic and arsenic compounds	S	S	1
Azathioprine	S	L	1
Bleomycins	I	L	2B
Chlorambucil	S	S	1
Chloramphenicol	L	I	2A
Cisplatin	I	S	2A
Cyclophosphamide	S	S	1
Cyclosporine	S	L	1
Dacarbazine	I	S	2B
Diphenylhydantoin (Phenytoin)	L	L	2B
Iron dextran	I	S	2B
Melphalan	S	S	1
Methoxsalen	S	S	2A
Metronidazole	I	S	2B
Nitrogen mustard	L	S	2A
Phenacetin-containing analgesic mixtures	S	S	1
Phenazopyridine	I	S	2B
Phenobarbital	I	L	2B
Procarbazine hydrochloride	I	S	2A
Propylthiouracil	I	S	2B
Thiotepa	S	S	1

*IARC summary findings (IARC, 1987) for all drugs judged to be at least possibly carcinogenic to humans and for which there exist at least some epidemiological data in humans.

[a]S, L, and I signify sufficient, limited, and inadequate (or conflicting) evidence of carcinogenicity, respectively.

[b]Overall evaluation: 1 = agent is carcinogenic to humans; 2A = agent is probably carcinogenic to humans; 2B = agent is possibly carcinogenic to humans.

ARSENICALS

Arsenic and compounds containing it have been associated with increased cancer risk in humans exposed in three different ways—occupationally, in drinking water, and in drugs (IARC, 1987). Arsenic may also be ingested in foods, where it may occur as pesticide residues on fruits and vegetables, or be derived from feed additives for livestock or poultry. It is also concentrated from environmental sources in some species of fish and shellfish (Klaasen, 1980).

Medicinal arsenic was formerly given orally for psoriasis, asthma, and a variety of other conditions in the form of inorganic trivalent compounds such as Fowler's solution (potassium arsenite). As such, it has been shown to cause skin cancer (Cuzick et al, 1982). Suspected associations of other types of cancer with these drugs, based on case reports, have not been confirmed epidemiologically. These compounds are now rarely used.

At present, medicinal arsenic is commonly administered only in the form of organic compounds for therapy of advanced stages of African trypanosomiasis, a tropical parasitic disease (American Medical Association, 1986). These arsenicals have not been studied in relation to risk of subsequent cancer.

CHLORAMPHENICOL

Because the antibiotic chloramphenicol can cause aplastic anemia, its use has been greatly restricted in the United States. However, in developing countries it is still commonly employed to treat infections. Because some patients with chloramphenicol-induced aplastic anemia go on to develop leukemia (IARC, 1987), this drug has for many years been suspected of being a cause of leukemia. Adding to the suspicion, acute nonlymphocytic leukemia and aplastic anemia have other causal factors in common such as ionizing radiation and benzene exposure. Only recently, however, has there been a large, population-based epidemiological study supporting the chloramphenicol–leukemia link.

In a case-control study of 309 children with leukemia and 618 matched controls in Shanghai, chloramphenicol users showed a statistically significant 2.3-fold increased risk of leukemia. Supporting a causal interpretation was a dose-response relationship—the relative risk reaching 9.7 for all leukemias, 11.0 for acute lymphocytic leukemia, and 12.0 for acute nonlymphocytic leukemia when the duration of chloramphenicol use was over 10 days. Also, a closely related drug, syntomycin, was associated with subsequent leukemia, whereas other drugs, including many antibiotics, were not. The greater prior use of chloramphenicol in the leukemia patients persisted when attention was restricted to the period at least 2 years before diagnosis, suggesting that the association was not attributable to treatment of leukemia- or preleukemia-induced infections with chloramphenicol (Shu et al, 1987).

Based on present evidence, chloramphenicol is probably leukemogenic. It should only be administered when no appropriate alternatives are available, and its duration of use should be as short as possible. It is still not clear whether topical application of chloramphenicol, particularly to the eyes, results in sufficient exposure to be of concern (Besamusca and Bastiaensen, 1986; Stevens and Mission, 1987).

COAL TAR

Occupational exposure to coal tar has been shown to cause cancer of the skin, including the scrotum, and lungs, and possibly of the urinary and digestive tracts as well (IARC, 1987). Coal tar in ointments has been applied to the skin in the treatment of psoriasis and eczematous dermatitis. Thus, concern has been raised about its possible carcinogenicity when used medicinally in this way. Sometimes its use is combined with ultraviolet radiation in what is known as the Goeckerman regimen (Pittelkow, 1981).

Epidemiological data regarding cancer risk after coal tar ointment application have been inconclusive. In one case-control study, the risk of skin cancer after the Goeckerman regimen was increased 4.7-fold over that in matched psoriasis patients (Stern et al, 1980). However, in two 25-year follow-up studies, the observed increase in risk was much smaller, and not apparently greater than that in age-sex-matched residents of the Dallas–Fort Worth, Texas, area (Pittelkow et al, 1981; Maughan et al, 1980). Another follow-up study found a similar attack rate of skin cancer before and after the Goeckerman regimen was used (Menter and Cram, 1983).

In weighing the advantages and disadvantages of topical coal tar versus other dermatologic preparations, the possible small added risk of skin cancer should be considered and appropriate follow-up instituted if coal tar is selected.

CYTOTOXIC DRUGS

Cytotoxic drugs comprise a variety of agents used mostly to treat cancer, but used for some other conditions as well. Major categories include alkylating agents, antimetabolites, antitumor antibiotics, and several other types of compounds. Evaluation of the carcinogenic effects of each of these agents is difficult because the cancer or other condition being treated may itself be associated with subsequent new malignancies and because of the administration to a patient of more than one such drug plus, in many cases, radiation therapy as well.

The complexity of the problem is illustrated by so-called MOPP therapy for Hodgkin's disease. MOPP is a combination of (1) nitrogen mustard, an alkylating agent that damages DNA and prevents cell replication, (2) vincristine, a plant alkaloid that inhibits mitosis, (3) prednisone, an adrenal corticosteroid that damages lymphoid cells and interferes with their proliferation, and (4) procarbazine, a synthetic drug that inhibits DNA, RNA, and subsequent protein synthesis. Both nitrogen mustard and procarbazine have been shown to be carcinogenic in experimental animals, but neither has been studied epidemiologically as a single agent (IARC, 1987). MOPP therapy was introduced in 1967 and was found, along with radiation therapy alone and MOPP plus radiation, to cure 70% of all cases of Hodgkin's disease. This resulted in many long-term survivors of a disease that had usually been fatal within a few years (Blayney et al, 1987). Several studies have shown a markedly increased risk of acute nonlymphocytic leukemia (ANLL) in persons treated with MOPP with or without radiation therapy and a lesser and possibly nonelevated risk after radiation therapy alone (IARC, 1987). In a recent study of long-term survivors there appeared to be a window of increased ANLL risk with peak incidence between 3 and 9 years after MOPP; those who survived at least 11 years appeared to be at no increased risk (Blayney et al, 1987). At present, it is not known whether one or more components or MOPP as a whole is responsible for the heightened risk of ANLL or how much is attributable to radiation therapy and, perhaps, other factors associated with Hodgkin's disease itself. Also observed has been an excess of solid tumors among Hodgkin's disease survivors, but the causes of this are obscure. Complicating the interpretation of the many studies that have been done are differences in the patients investigated, the methods and timing of MOPP administration, and the study criteria and methods, all of which could have contributed to the wide variation in the reported risks of ANLL and other cancers (IARC, 1987).

Other cytotoxic agents with substantial evidence for carcinogenic effects in humans include the alkylating agents busulfan, chlorambucil, melphalan, thiotepa, and cyclophosphamide, all of which can cause ANLL, and the last of which can also cause bladder cancer; chlornaphazine, which can cause bladder cancer and is no longer used; and one of the nitrosureas, methyl-CCNU, which can cause ANLL (IARC, 1987). Because of the relation of alkylating-agent therapy with secondary ANLL, etoposide (epipodophyllotoxin) has been favored over alkylating-agent therapy in recent years. Unfortunately, reports of ANLL following treatment with etoposide are mounting, and a monitoring plan recently was initiated so that the risks and benefits of etoposide relative to alkylating agents can be compared (Smith et al, 1993). Still other cytotoxic agents with sufficient evidence of carcinogenicity only in animals may be found in the table.

In addition to the demonstrated risks of cytotoxic drugs to patients, there has also been concern about occupational exposures to oncologists, nurses, pharmacists, and other health care workers who handle them (Fishbein, 1987). The risks for these personnel are not well quantitated, but prudence dictates that exposure be minimized.

DIPHENYLHYDANTOIN (PHENYTOIN)

Diphenylhydantoin, an anticonvulsant drug, can cause immune dysfunction in animals and humans (Sorrell and Forbes, 1975), and the development of pseudolymphoma (Saltzstein and Ackerman, 1959; Gams et al, 1968), a hypersensitivity reaction that includes generalized lymphadenopathy and usually regresses on discontinuation of the medication. Numerous cases of Hodgkin's and non-Hodgkin's lymphoma have been reported in persons taking diphenylhydantoin (Hyman and Sommers, 1966; Rubinstein et al, 1985), sometimes preceded by, and arising in, pseudolymphoma. Occasional cases of leukemia (Gyte, 1985) and multiple myeloma (Matzner and Polliack, 1978) have also been noted. Two case-control studies (Charlton and Lunsford, 1971; Li et al, 1975) found increased frequencies of prior exposure to diphenylhydantoin in cases of Hodgkin's or non-Hodgkin's lymphoma, but each study was based on a very small number of exposed cases.

Longitudinal studies have been inconclusive. In three cohorts of persons with epilepsy (White et al, 1979; Shirts et al, 1986; Olsen et al, 1989), incidence or mortality from lymphoma after 13 to 30 years of follow-up was slightly increased compared to general population rates. These studies could not distinguish phenytoin users from the small proportion of subjects who did not take the drug. In the Kaiser Permanente study of carcinogenicity of prescription drugs (Selby et al, 1989), incidence of non-Hodgkin's lymphoma after 11 to 15 years of follow-up was increased among the 954 users of diphenylhydantoin (two observed cases, 0.64 expected). However, for all hematologic malignancies, a slight deficit was noted (four observed versus 4.56 expected). Neither difference was statistically significant.

Excesses of central nervous system neoplasms are frequently noted in follow-up studies of persons with epilepsy (Clemmesen et al, 1974; Shirts et al, 1986; White et al, 1979) and of diphenylhydantoin users (Friedman and Ury, 1980). These associations are most likely due to inclusion of persons whose seizures are an early manifestation of slow-growing tumors such as low-grade astrocytomas (Mathieson, 1975) rather than to carcinogenic effects of either seizures or anticonvulsants. Other confounding factors in these studies are greater surveillance (detection bias) and more frequent exposure to diagnostic radiation (or, in earlier studies, to Thorotrast) in persons with epilepsy, and concomitant use of phenobarbital, which has itself been associated with subsequent occurrence of brain tumors (see below).

Of some concern are recent case reports of neuroblastoma and lymphoma in children exposed to diphenylhydantoin in utero who display the constellation of congenital anomalies known as fetal hydantoin syndrome (Cohen, 1981). No epidemiological assessment of cancer risk in this group has yet been reported.

All in all, there is suggestive evidence that use of diphenylhydantoin may increase risk for non-Hodgkin's lymphoma slightly, but the link is by no means well established.

DIURETICS

Two cohort (Fraser et al, 1990; Lindblad et al, 1993) and five case-control (Finkle et al, 1993; Hiatt et al, 1994; Krieger et al, 1993; McLaughlin et al, 1988; Yu et al, 1986) studies have observed a link between diuretic or antihypertensive use and subsequent risk of renal cell carcinoma in women, with ever users being at two- to four-fold increased risk. The relation exists both in hypertensives and in women who use diuretics for weight control. Hiatt and coworkers (1994) specifically examined thiazides, noting an odds ratio of 4.0 (95% confidence interval [CI], 1.5–11). Finkle and coworkers (1993) excluded women who had been diagnosed with the cancer within the 10 years following first use of diuretics, observing an odds ratio of 3.5 (95% CI, 1.7–7.4). There is also evidence that risk increases with increasing cumulative dose (Finkle et al, 1993; Hiatt et al, 1994). The association has not consistently been found in men, and the possible biological basis for the relationship has not been elucidated. Further investigation of the role of diuretics in the etiology of renal cell carcinoma is needed.

HISTAMINE H_2-RECEPTOR ANTAGONISTS

The histamine H_2-receptor antagonists were introduced beginning in the mid-1970s for treatment and secondary prevention of peptic ulcer disease. These agents suppress gastric production of hydrochloric acid and are now widely used for a variety of conditions related to gastric acidity. As early as 1979 (Elder et al, 1979) theoretical concern was raised that H_2-receptor blockade could cause gastric cancer. Inhibition of gastric acid secretion raises intragastric pH, which may allow bacterial colonization of the normally sterile stomach with increased production of carcinogenic nitrates, nitrites, and N-nitroso compounds. Certain H_2-receptor antagonists may also act directly as carcinogens (Wormsley, 1984).

Early reports of gastric cancer developing shortly after use of cimetidine (Taylor et al, 1981) were apparently explained by use of the medication for preexistent but undiagnosed cancer (Piper, 1981). Animal studies (Poynter, 1985) reportedly find an increase in gastric carcinoid tumors in rats and mice following lifetime achlorhydria induced by potent experimental H_2-receptor antagonists, but not after exposure to currently marketed agents (cimetidine, ranitidine, famotidine). Postmarketing follow-up studies (summarized in IARC, 1990) to date have detected no increased risk of cancer in humans that is not compatible with use of the drug for preexisting cancer. On balance, available evidence suggests no increased cancer risk with usual doses of the H_2-receptor antagonists in current use (Penston and Wormsley, 1985). However, continued observation is needed to establish the long-term safety of these widely used drugs.

IMMUNOSUPPRESSIVE AGENTS

Immunosuppressive agents are administered routinely to prevent graft rejection in organ transplantation and are also used frequently, although in smaller doses, to treat rheumatoid arthritis, systemic lupus erythematosus, and other autoimmune disorders. Commonly used agents include azathioprine (an antimetabolite), cyclophosphamide and chlorambucil (alkylating agents), and, more recently, cyclosporine A.

Earlier studies of organ transplant recipients, most of whom received either azathioprine, cyclophosphamide, or both (Penn, 1977; Fraumeni and Hoover, 1977; Kinlen, 1979) have consistently found large increases in risk for certain cancers, including lymphoma (particularly non-Hodgkin's or B-cell lymphoma), Kaposi's sarcoma, squamous cell skin cancer, malignant melanoma, and hepatocellular carcinoma. Slightly elevated risks, on the order of two- to four-fold, are also suggested for lung and bladder cancer (Fraumeni and Hoover, 1977). The incidence of lymphoma and Kaposi's sarcoma is increased within months after treatment is begun. An unusual predilection has been noted for the central nervous system as the primary or only site of occurrence of the lymphomas.

Cancer risk following cyclosporine therapy is similar in magnitude to that following earlier immunosuppressive regimens (Penn and Brunson, 1988; Penn, 1988), but lymphomas, Kaposi's sarcomas, and renal cell carcinomas constitute a greater proportion of all resulting tumors and skin cancers are correspondingly less frequent. The average interval between treatment and diagnosis of lymphoma or Kaposi's sarcoma is even shorter after cyclosporine treatment than earlier therapies. Most patients treated with cyclosporine also receive other immunosuppressive agents. There have been reports of spontaneous regression of both lymphomas and Kaposi's sarcoma upon cessation of cyclosporine therapy (Starzl et al, 1984; Bencini et al, 1987).

Increased risk for both non-Hodgkin's lymphoma and squamous cell skin cancer has also been reported in patients receiving immunosuppressive therapy for other conditions such as rheumatoid arthritis (Kinlen, 1985), although the excess risk was considerably lower than that following transplantation. Both azathioprine and cyclophosphamide appeared to increase risk for these two cancers. A potential confounder is the condition being treated, since an increased occurrence of non-Hodgkin's lymphoma has been reported in rheumatoid arthritis patients even in the absence of immunosuppressive therapy (Isomaki et al, 1978). Chronic lymphoid stimulation from an autoimmune process such as rheumatoid arthritis could cause the increased occurrence of lymphoma. However, the increase in risk for lymphoma due to rheumatoid arthritis itself appears to be much less than the 13-fold increase (Kinlen, 1985) seen after immunosuppressive therapy.

Several mechanisms by which immunosuppression could increase cancer risk have been proposed (Penn, 1977). The brief latent period between treatment and increased cancer incidence, particularly for lymphomas, suggests that classic chemical carcinogenesis is not involved. The specificity for certain cancer types and sites following immunosuppression, whether drug-induced, congenital, or acquired (as in acquired immune deficiency syndrome) has been interpreted to support the hypothesis of impaired immunosurveillance (Kripke, 1988). Immunosurveillance, the recognition and destruction of tumor cells by the immune system, is most effective for tumors with easily recognized foreign antigens. Tumors induced by oncogenic viruses (non-Hodgkin's lymphomas, Kaposi's sarcoma, and hepatocellular carcinoma) and those induced by ultraviolet irradiation (squamous cell skin cancer and melanoma) are highly antigenic. Impaired immunosurveillance would thus be expected to result in excesses of these tumors, but not of chemically induced and "spontaneous" tumors, which are less antigenic and not, in fact, increased by immunosuppression.

IRON

Iron is a dietary element essential for the synthesis and function of hemoglobin, myoglobin, and intracellular enzymes such as cytochromes and other oxidases. Iron deficiency, as a result of dietary deficiency, excessive menstrual blood loss, or acute or chronic bleeding, is a frequently seen medical condition. Medicinal iron, in the form of iron dextran injections, or more frequently as orally administered ferrous salts, is commonly used to treat this condition.

Reports of soft tissue tumors developing at the site of iron dextran injections appeared as early as 1960 (Robinson et al, 1960). However, no epidemiological studies of this association have appeared to date and the observations may well represent coincidence given the widespread use of this drug. Repeated injections of doses of iron dextran much larger than those used clinically have also induced formation of fibrosarcomas in some animal species, but not in others (Richmond et al, 1959).

Concern that excessive body iron stores could lead to increased risk of both infection and cancer has been raised on the basis of biological considerations (Weinberg, 1984). Both tumor cells and bacteria require iron for cell growth. Pathogenic bacteria and neoplastic cells are specifically adapted to enhance iron acquisition from the host (Nielands, 1980; Weinberg, 1984). The hypoferremia and iron sequestration by the reticuloendothelial system, which are components of the host response to both infection and neoplasia, may be a defense that withholds iron from invading cells (Roeser, 1980; Weinberg, 1984).

Five recent epidemiologic studies (Stevens et al, 1986; Selby and Friedman, 1988; Stevens et al, 1994; Knekt et al, 1994; Herrinton et al, 1995) have examined the association of iron stores with risk of cancer. Although there have been inconsistent associations observed with cancer of several particular sites (lung, stomach, colon and rectum, and hematologic malignancies), it is not clear that there is a general relation with cancer per se.

ISONIAZID

Isoniazid, a drug commonly used to treat and prevent tuberculosis, is a derivative of hydrazine, a potent mutagen and carcinogen in animals (Balo, 1979). Hydrazine is released during metabolism of isoniazid in humans and can be detected in the plasma and urine of subjects taking the drug (Blair et al, 1985), particularly in patients who metabolize the drug slowly (slow acetylator phenotype). Isoniazid induces lung tumors in mice after both intraperitoneal and oral administration (Balo, 1979). Two large follow-up studies in humans treated for tuberculosis (Stott et al, 1976; Clemmesen and Hjalgrim-Jensen, 1979) found increased cancer mortality, particularly from lung cancer, in isoniazid users compared to the general population. In general, these studies did not control for cigarette smoking, which may have been more frequent among persons with tuberculosis than in the general population, nor for the known association of lung cancer with tuberculosis that is independent of isoniazid use (Zheng et al, 1987). An association of isoniazid with bladder cancer has also been reported (Miller et al, 1978).

A large randomized trial of isoniazid chemoprophylaxis for household contacts of tuberculosis patients conducted by the U.S. Public Health Service in the late 1950s provides the best evaluation of possible isoniazid carcinogenicity. This study avoids confounding by the presence of tuberculosis among isoniazid users and, by randomization, minimizes differences in smoking between groups. Follow-up of 14 years for cancer mortality (Glassroth et al, 1977a) and 19 years for cancer incidence (Costello and Snider, 1980) have failed to show increased risks for lung, bladder, or all cancer. No association of isoniazid with bladder cancer was found in two recent case-control studies (Glassroth et al, 1977b; Kantor et al, 1985). Although these findings are reassuring, the animal studies and the biological considerations noted above dictate longer-term follow-up before a delayed carcinogenic effect of isoniazid can be ruled out.

METRONIDAZOLE

Metronidazole is an antiprotozoal and antibacterial drug that is used to treat a variety of infections, most often vaginal or intestinal. Because of its apparent carcinogenicity in rats and mice (IARC, 1987) there has been concern that it might also have this effect in humans.

Follow-up studies have been performed in three cohorts. In one study, 771 women treated at the Mayo Clinic with metronidazole for vaginal trichomoniasis showed statistically significant elevations in the incidence of lung cancer and, more recently, of all cancers combined after 15 to 25 years of follow-up (Beard et al, 1979, 1988). In another study of 2236 female and 224 male patients who received metronidazole from a Kaiser Permanente Medical Care Program pharmacy, there was no significant increase in either total cancer or lung cancer incidence after 11 to 15 years of follow-up. An increase in cervical cancer was believed to be due to sexual behavior that led also to vaginitis treated with metronidazole (Friedman, 1980; Friedman and Selby, 1989). A third study group of 12,280 patients who received the drug at the Group Health Cooperative of Puget Sound were followed for up to 2 ½ years and showed no increase over expected cancer incidence (Danielson et al, 1982b). Another study in the same setting, which focused on breast cancer, showed a nonsignificantly elevated risk ratio of 1.1 (Danielson et al, 1982a).

There is still insufficient evidence to demonstrate that metronidazole is carcinogenic in humans or to be sure that it is safe in this regard. If there is an added risk, it is probably small. Longer follow-up and more studies are both needed.

NONSTEROIDAL ANTI-INFLAMMATORY DRUGS

Three case-control studies have indicated that the use of nonsteroidal anti-inflammatory drugs (NSAIDs), including aspirin, may help prevent colon cancer (Kune et al, 1988; Rosenberg et al, 1991; Suh et al, 1993). In the study of Rosenberg and coworkers (1991), use for 4 or more days a week for 3 months or longer was associated with a 50% reduction in risk. A similar relation with fatal colon cancer was noted in the American Cancer Society cohort (Thun et al, 1991). Analysis of the National Health and Nutrition Examination Survey (Schreinemachers and Everson, 1994) also gave evidence for a protective effect, although information on prior aspirin use was quite limited. A prospective study of the residents of a California retirement community did not find evidence for the relationship (Paganini-Hill et al, 1991). Animal and in vitro studies suggest that NSAIDs inhibit cyclooxygenase, an enzyme important in converting arachidonic acid to prostaglandins and other molecules that influence cellular proliferation (Ernest et al, 1992). Analysis of existing randomized trials of aspirin prophylaxis will provide important information about this hypothesis.

PHENACETIN

Phenacetin is an aniline derivative closely related to acetaminophen. It was widely used during the 1940s and 1950s as an ingredient in many nonprescription, combination analgesic, antipyretic preparations. These preparations were often used to excess because of mild, subjective stimulation or euphoria induced by phenacetin. Phenacetin is principally metabolized by the liver to *N*-acetyl-*p*-aminophenol (acetaminophen), conjugated, and excreted in the urine (Flower et al, 1980). However, a small proportion is metabolized in the kidney to *p*-aminophenol and other known urinary tract carcinogens (Carpenter, 1981). Phenacetin has been shown to be a potent promotor of tumor formation in previously initiated rat bladder tissue (Ito et al, 1984).

An association between chronic abuse of combination analgesic, antipyretic preparations and a distinctive form of interstitial nephropathy with renal papillary necrosis was first described in the 1950s (Hultengren, 1961). Because phenacetin was included in nearly all preparations associated with the nephropathy, this agent has been most frequently implicated. However, phenacetin was rarely used as a single agent and other analgesics may also produce papillary necrosis (Prescott, 1982).

Increased occurrence of transitional cell cancers of the renal pelvis and urinary bladder in persons with analgesic nephropathy was subsequently reported (Hultengren et al, 1968; Bengtsson et al, 1968; Johansson et al, 1974). Case-control studies have confirmed associations of chronic or excessive use of phenacetin-containing analgesics with both of these urinary cancers (Fokkens, 1979; McCredie et al, 1982; McCredie et al, 1983; Piper et al, 1985; McCredie and Stewart, 1988; McLaughlin et al, 1992; Krieger et al, 1993; McCredie et al, 1993). A weaker association with renal cell carcinoma has also been observed (McLaughlin et al, 1984; McCredie et al, 1988). The level of exposure at which risk begins to increase cannot be specified from these studies, but Fokkens (1979) found no increase in risk for bladder cancer if lifetime consumption was below 2.0 kg. Associations of nonphenacetin analgesics, acetaminophen, or aspirin with urothelial cancers have not been found in the three studies that could address this question (McCredie et al, 1983; Piper et al, 1985; McCredie and Stewart, 1988; McCredie et al, 1988).

Although it is highly probable that abuse of phenacetin-containing analgesics increases risk for urothelial cancers, it is not clear that occasional use of such products in appropriate doses conveys any increase in risk. Likewise, it has not been established whether other analgesics, alone or in combination with phenacetin, can also increase cancer risk.

PHENAZOPYRIDINE

Oral administration of phenazopyridine, an orange-red azo dye used as a urinary tract analgesic alone or in combination with sulfonamide preparations, has been shown to increase the incidence of hepatic carcinomas in mice and to induce colon and rectum tumors in rats (National Cancer Institute, 1978). The only epidemiological data in humans comes from the Kaiser Permanente study of prescription drugs. Among 2214 recipients of the drug, no significant excess was noted for cancer at any site after 3 to 7 years of follow-up (Friedman and Ury, 1980). Eight additional years of follow-up have now been reported (Selby et al, 1989), again with no excess of cancer for any site or for all sites combined. Thus, the limited epidemiological data available provide no evidence for carcinogenicity of phenazopyridine in humans.

PHENOBARBITAL

Barbiturates such as phenobarbital, secobarbital, and pentobarbital have been widely used since 1920 as sedatives and hypnotics, and for treatment of epilepsy. Barbiturates are potent inducers of hepatic microsomal enzymes known as mixed-function oxidases, which are responsible for the metabolic activation as well as detoxification of many chemical carcinogens (Mayer et al, 1980). Phenobarbital is also a known promoter of liver tumors following exposure to initiating carcinogens in rats (Peraino et al, 1971).

An increased occurrence of hepatic cancer (11 observed cases versus 2.8 expected) was noted in one large follow-up study of persons treated with phenobarbital for epilepsy (Olsen et al, 1989). However, eight of the 11 cases had also been exposed to Thorotrast (a diagnostic radiopharmaceutical known to be carcinogenic) in the workup of their epilepsy. Other follow-up studies of persons with epilepsy (White et al, 1979; Shirts et al, 1986) found no excess of hepatic cancer.

A greater than expected occurrence of brain tumors in these follow-up studies (White et al, 1979; Shirts et al, 1986; Olsen et al, 1989) is most likely due to use of anticonvulsants for early symptoms of preexistent brain tumors. The incidence of the tumors was increased mainly during the early years of treatment, reverting toward normal after 10 years of use. As pointed out by Olsen and coworkers (1989) and Shirts and coworkers (1986), this is the opposite of what would be expected if exposure to phenobarbital were causally related to brain tumor. No increase in risk of brain tumors was observed among 5834 recipients of phenobarbital prescriptions in the Kaiser Permanente study of prescription drugs (Selby et al, 1989), most of whom received phenobarbital as a sedative rather than an anticonvulsant.

Gold and coworkers (1978) reported an association of brain tumors in children with prenatal exposure to barbiturates in a case-control study (odds ratio = 1.5, $P=0.03$). However, the association was based on only six discordant case-control pairs, and was noted only when cases were compared to other cancer controls, not when compared with ordinary controls. Heinonen and coworkers (1977) found no excess of all cancer among 1415 children exposed to phenobarbital in utero, nor was the association confirmed in a larger case-control study (Goldhaber et al, 1990).

A 1.7-fold increase in the incidence of lung cancer was observed among users of three barbiturate preparations in the Kaiser Permanente study of prescription drugs (Friedman and Ury, 1980; Friedman and Ury, 1983). The association persisted after adjustment for cigarette smoking (Friedman, 1981) and was seen among nonsmokers as well as smokers, although the association in nonsmokers was based on only four observed cases (versus 2.7 expected). No effect of duration of use on risk could be demonstrated, nor did the distribution of histologic types for barbiturate-related cancers differ from that of other lung cancers. Increases of similar size in the incidence of lung cancer were noted in the three follow-up studies of persons treated for epilepsy (White et al, 1979; Shirts et al, 1986; Olsen et al, 1989). One of these cohorts formed the basis for a nested case-control study in which more detailed information about drug use, smoking history, and exposure to Thorotrast was obtained (Olsen et al, 1993). The earlier-observed association with lung cancer was appreciably lower after adjustment for smoking (odds ratio [OR] = 1.2, 95% CI, 0.7–2.2). The association of a history of use of barbiturates with lung cancer risk merits further investigation.

Increasing doses of phenobarbital have also been associated with increasing protection against the occurrence of bladder cancer, such that persons whose cumulative dose was 720 g or greater were at one-fifth the risk of nonusers (95% CI, 0.0–0.9) (Olsen et al, 1989, 1993). The authors hypothesized that phenobarbital induces liver enzymes that deactivate bladder carcinogens.

Thus, although there are biological links that could explain a carcinogenic effect of phenobarbital and other barbiturates, the data from humans are inconclusive.

PHENYLBUTAZONE

Phenylbutazone is a potent anti-inflammatory drug. It was commonly used in the past to treat rheumatic conditions, but it is now used less because of concern about side effects and because several other potent nonsteroidal anti-inflammatory agents have become available.

One of its feared although infrequent side effects is bone marrow depression with resulting leukopenia, agranulocytosis, or aplastic anemia (American Medical Association, 1986). There have been a sizeable number of case reports of leukemia following phenylbutazone administration, but such occurrences are difficult to ascribe to anything but coincidence, particularly since phenylbutazone was so commonly prescribed when they were reported (IARC, 1987). A follow-up study of 489 patients with rheumatoid arthritis revealed an incidence of non-Hodgkin's lymphoma far greater than expected. Sixty percent of the hospital charts of those who developed this and other lymphohematopoietic malignancies showed evidence of phenylbutazone use, but there were reasons to doubt that phenylbutazone was the cause (Symmons, 1985; IARC, 1987). Two Kaiser Permanente studies found no significant excess risk of leukemia attributable to phenylbutazone (Friedman, 1982; Friedman and Ury, 1980). An association of musculoskeletal disease with leukemia was noted; this could underlie an apparent phenylbutazone-leukemia association.

Evidence to date is limited but it does not indicate that phenylbutazone is carcinogenic. Leukemia is probably not one of the blood dyscrasias that phenylbutazone can cause.

PROPYLTHIOURACIL

Propylthiouracil is an antithyroid drug that interferes with synthesis of thyroid hormone. It is used for the temporary control of and sometimes as definitive therapy for hyperthyroidism. An unspecified excess of thyroid cancer was reported in a follow-up study of 331 patients treated with propylthiouracil and subsequent thyroidectomy (Dobyns et al, 1974). Propylthiouracil produces thyroid tumors in several animal species after oral administration (summarized in IARC, 1974). There were 107 recipients of this drug in the Kaiser Permanente study of prescription drugs, with subjects averaging more than four prescriptions each. After 11 to 15 years' follow-up, no significant excess of cancer has been noted for any site (Selby et al, 1989). One thyroid cancer was observed (compared to 0.07 expected), but this cancer was diagnosed less than 1 year after the first prescription of propylthiouracil, and may have been present before treatment began. Further study of the possible carcinogenicity of this drug is needed.

PSORALENS

Methoxsalen (8-methoxypsoralen or 8-MOP) is a photosensitizing agent that is sometimes used with long-wave ultraviolet radiation in the treatment of severe psoriasis, vitiligo, and mycosis fungoides. It may be applied topically or given orally if large areas of skin are to be treated.

While methoxsalen alone has not been shown to cause cancer in humans or animals, the combination of the drug plus long-wave ultraviolet light (often abbreviated as PUVA) is carcinogenic for human and mouse skin (IARC, 1987). In three follow-up studies of psoriatic patients treated with PUVA, the incidence of squamous cell carcinoma of the skin was increased over general population rates, with persons exposed to high doses having as much as a 60-fold higher risk (Stern et al, 1984; Bruynzeel et al, 1991; Lindelhof et al, 1991). There was a much smaller increase in the incidence of basal cell carcinoma (Bruynzeel et al, 1991; Stern et al, 1984). Other studies, which did not find increased risk of skin cancer after PUVA therapy, may have been affected by lower doses of PUVA, a lower baseline skin cancer risk in Europe than in the United States, and low statistical power (IARC, 1987; Henseler et al, 1987). The evidence to date thus dictates both caution in the use of PUVA and careful follow-up after it is used.

A related compound, 5-methoxypsoralen (5-MOP), is used in some sunscreens, with the objective of increasing tanning by admitting longer ultraviolet waves while protecting against radiation-induced skin damage by blocking shorter ultraviolet waves (Cartwright and Walter, 1983). Limited experimental evidence suggests that the combination of ultraviolet radiation and 5-methoxypsoralen increases risk of skin cancer in mice (IARC, 1986). The degree to which use of sunscreens containing 5-methoxypsoralen augments the known link between sun exposure and skin cancer in humans is unknown.

RESERPINE

There has been considerable interest in the possibility that reserpine (or rauwolfia), a commonly used antihypertensive drug, can cause breast cancer in women. About 20 epidemiological studies have yielded conflicting results, with relative risk estimates ranging from 0.6 to over 3 (IARC, 1987; Danielson et al, 1982a; Shapiro et al, 1984; Stanford et al, 1986). Although the studies that are methodologically most sound tend to show little if any increased risk (IARC, 1987), there is recent evidence that a larger risk may be found among women using the drug for long durations. One study suggested that previous contradictory findings could be explained by the hypothesis that reserpine use for at least 5 years causes breast cancer occurring after age 50 (Williams et al, 1978), but another study aimed at this specific hypothesis (Friedman, 1983) did not confirm it. More recently, a large case-control study found evidence for a moderately strong association of reserpine with breast cancer only for women who had taken the drug for at least 10 years, or where there had been a latency interval from first use to diagnosis of cancer of 10 years or more (Stanford et al, 1986). Animal experiments have given mixed results with limited evidence for carcinogenicity in rats and mice (IARC, 1987).

The proposed mechanism linking reserpine to breast cancer is the drug's stimulation of prolactin secretion. The degree of elevation of prolactin levels in women taking reserpine was found to be consistent with only small increases in breast cancer risk as judged by a postulated statistical model of breast cancer incidence (Ross et al, 1984).

The overall body of evidence to date suggests that reserpine may be used to treat hypertension for several years with little if any added risk of breast cancer. Caution is still appropriate with regard to long-term use, pending additional studies.

MAGNITUDE OF THE PROBLEM OF CARCINOGENESIS DUE TO DRUGS

What does the authors' experience to date in large-scale monitoring for carcinogenic effects (Friedman and Ury, 1980; Friedman and Ury, 1983; Selby et al, 1989) suggest about the relative importance of drugs as causes of cancer in our society? With the well-known exceptions described here and in the chapter on hormones, it appears that most drugs, as they are ordinarily used in clinical practice, do not pose a problem. This general observation must be tempered with the proviso that more follow-up (than our present maximum of 15 years) is needed to rule out longer-term effects, and that our power to detect relatively weak effects is low for many drugs, given the low incidence of most cancers.

REFERENCES

American Medical Association, Department of Drugs, Division of Drugs and Technology. 1986. Drug Evaluations. 6th ed. Chicago: American Medical Association, 1579–1580.

Balo J. 1979. Role of hydrazine in carcinogenesis. Adv Cancer Res 30:151–163.

Beard CM, Noller KL, O'Fallon WM, et al. 1979. Lack of evidence for cancer due to use of metronidazole. N Engl J Med 301:519–522.

Beard CM, Noller KL, O'Fallon WM, et al. 1988. Cancer after exposure to metronidazole. Mayo Clinic Proc 63:147–153.

Bencini PL, Marchesi L, Cainelli T, et al. 1987. Kaposi's sarcoma in kidney transplant recipients treated with cyclosporin. Br J Dermatol 118:709–714.

Bengtsson U, Angervall L, Ekman H, et al. 1968. Transitional cell tumours of the renal pelvis in analgesic abusers. Scand J Urol Nephrol 2:145–150.

Besamusca FW, Bastiaensen LA. 1986. Blood dyscrasias and topically applied chloramphenicol in ophthalmology. Doc Ophthalmol 64:87–95.

Blair IA, Tinoco RM, Brodie MJ, et al. 1985. Plasma hydrazine concentrations in man after isoniazid and hydralazine administration. Hum Toxicol 4:195–202.

Blayney DW, Longo DL, Young RC, et al. 1987. Decreasing risk of leukemia with prolonged follow-up after chemotherapy and radiotherapy for Hodgkin's disease. N Engl J Med 316:710–714.

Bruynzeel I, Bergman W, Hartevelt HM, et al. 1991. 'High single-dose' European PUVA regimen also causes an excess of nonmelanoma skin cancer. Br J Dermatol 124:49–55.

Carpenter HM, Mudge GH. 1981. Acetaminophen nephrotoxicity: studies on renal acetylation and deacetylation. J Pharmacol Exp Ther 218:161–167.

Cartwright LE, Walter JF. 1983. Psoralen-containing sunscreen is tumorigenic in hairless mice. J Am Acad Dermatol 8:830–836.

Charlton MH, Lunsford D. 1971. Le sostanze di idantoina come possibili cause del linfoma maligno. Minerva Med 62:2185.

Clemmesen J, Frederiksen VF, Plum CM. 1974. Are anticonvulsants oncogenic? Lancet 1:705–707.

Clemmesen J, Hjalgrim-Jensen S. 1979. Is isonicotinic acid hydrazide (INH) carcinogenic to man? A 24-year follow-up of 3,371 tuberculosis cases. Ecotoxicol Environ Safety 3:439–450.

Clissold SP. 1986. Paracetamol and phenacetin. Drugs 32(Suppl 4):46–59.

Cohen MM. 1981. Neoplasia and the fetal alcohol and hydantoin syndromes. Neurobehav Toxicol Teratol 3:161–162.

Colin-Jones DG, Langman MJS, Lawson DH, et al. 1985. Postmarketing surveillance of the safety of cimetidine: mortality during second, third, and fourth years of follow-up. Br Med J 291:1084–1088.

Costello HD, Snider DE. 1980. The incidence of cancer among participants in a controlled, randomized isoniazid prevention therapy trial. Am J Epidemiol 111:67–74.

Cuzick J, Evans S, Gillman M, et al. 1982. Medicinal arsenic and internal malignancies. Br J Cancer 45:904–911.

Danielson DA, Jick H, Hunter, et al. 1982a. Nonestrogenic drugs and breast cancer. Am J Epidemiol 116:329–332.

Danielson DA, Hannan MT, Jick H. 1982b. Metronidazole and cancer. (Letter) JAMA 247:2498–2499.

Dobyns BM, Sheline GE, Workman JB, et al. 1974. Malignant and benign neoplasms of the thyroid in patients treated for hyperthyroidism: a report of the cooperative thyrotoxicosis therapy follow-up study. J Clin Endocrinol Metab 38:976–998.

Edlavitch SA. 1988. Postmarketing surveillance methodologies. Drug Intell Clin Pharm 22:68–78.

Elder JB, Ganguli PC, Gillespie I. 1979. Cimetidine and gastric cancer. Lancet 1:1005–1006.

Ernst DL, Hixson LJ, Alberts DS. 1992. Piroxicam and other cyclooxygenase inhibitors: potential for cancer chemoprevention. J Cell Biochem (Suppl) 16I:156–166.

Farber E. 1987. Possible etiologic mechanisms in chemical carcinogenesis. Environ Health Perspect 75:65–70.

Finkle WD, McLaughlin JK, Rasgon SA, et al. 1993. Increased

risk of renal cell cancer among women using diuretics in the United States. Cancer Causes Control 4:555–558.

FISHBEIN L. 1987. Perspectives on occupational exposure to antineoplastic drugs. Arch Geschwulstforsch 57:219–248.

FLOWER RJ, MONCADA S, VANE JR. 1980. Analgesic-antipyretics and anti-inflammatory agents; drugs employed in the treatment of gout. In: The Pharmacological Basis of Therapeutics, 6th ed, Gilman AG, Goodman LS, Gilman A (eds). New York: Macmillan, pp 701–704.

FOKKENS W. 1979. Phenacetin abuse related to bladder cancer. Environ Res 20:192–198.

FRASER GE, PHILLIPS RL, BEESON WL. 1990. Hypertension, antihypertensive medication and risk of renal carcinoma in California Seventh Day Adventists. Int J Epidemiol 19:832–838.

FRAUMENI JF JR, HOOVER R. 1977. Immunosurveillance and cancer: epidemiologic observations. Natl Cancer Inst Monogr 47:121–126.

FRIEDMAN GD. 1972. Screening criteria for drug monitoring: the Kaiser Permanente drug reaction monitoring system. J Chron Dis 25:11–20.

FRIEDMAN GD. 1980. Cancer after metronidazole. (Letter) N Engl J Med 302:519.

FRIEDMAN GD. 1981. Barbiturates and lung cancer in humans. J Natl Cancer Inst 67:291–295.

FRIEDMAN GD. 1982. Phenylbutazone, musculoskeletal disease, and leukemia. J Chronic Dis 35:233–243.

FRIEDMAN GD. 1983. Rauwolfia and breast cancer: no relation found in long term users age fifty and over. J Chronic Dis 36:367–370.

FRIEDMAN GD, URY HK. 1983. Screening for possible drug carcinogenicity: Second report of findings. J Natl Cancer Inst 71:1165–1175.

FRIEDMAN GD, SELBY JV. 1989. Metronidazole and cancer. (Letter) JAMA 261:866.

FRIEDMAN GD, URY HK. 1980. Initial screening for carcinogenicity of commonly used drugs. J Natl Cancer Inst 65:723–733.

GAMS RA, NEAL JA, CONRAD FG. 1968. Hydantoin-induced pseudo-pseudolymphoma. Ann Intern Med 69:557–568.

GLASSROTH JL, WHITE MC, SNIDER DE. 1977a. An assessment of the possible association of isoniazid with human cancer deaths. Am Rev Respir Dis 116:1065–1074.

GLASSROTH JL, SNIDER DE, COMSTOCK GW. 1977b. Urinary tract cancer and isoniazid. Am Rev Respir Dis 116:331–333.

GOLD E, GORDIS L, TONASCIA J, et al. 1978. Increased risk of brain tumors in children exposed to barbiturates. J Natl Cancer Inst 61:1031–1034.

GOLDHABER MK, SELBY JV, HIATT RA, et al. 1990. Exposure to barbiturates *in utero* and during childhood and risk of intracranial and spinal cord tumors. Cancer Res 50:4600–4603.

GYTE GML, RICHMOND JE, WILLIAMS JRB, et al. 1985. Hairy cell leukemia occurring during phenytoin (diphenylhydantoin) treatment. Scand J Hematol 35:358–362.

HEINONEN OP, SLONE D, SHAPIRO S. 1977. Birth Defects and Drugs in Pregnancy. Littleton, Mass: PSG Publishing Co.

HENSELER T, CHRISTOPHERS E, HONIGSMANN H, et al. 1987. Skin tumors in the European PUVA study. J Am Acad Dermatol 16:108–116.

HERRINTON LJ, FRIEDMAN GD, BAER D, et al. 1995. Transferrin saturation and risk of cancer. Am J Epidemiol (In press)

HIATT RA, TOLAN K, QUESENBERRY CP JR. 1994. Renal cell carcinoma and thiazide use: a historical, case-control study (California, USA). Cancer Causes Control 5:319–325.

HOWE GR. 1985. Use of computerized record linkage in follow-up studies of cancer epidemiology in Canada. Natl Cancer Inst Monogr 67:117–121.

HULTENGREN N. 1961. Renal papillary necrosis, a clinical study of 103 cases. Acta Chir Scand (suppl 277).

HULTENGREN N, LAGERGREN C, LJUNGQVIST A. 1968. Carcinoma of the renal pelvis in renal papillary necrosis. Acta Chir Scand 130:314–320.

HYMAN GA, SOMMERS SC. 1966. The development of Hodgkin's disease and lymphoma during anticonvulsant therapy. Blood 28:416–427.

INTERNATIONAL AGENCY FOR RESEARCH ON CANCER. 1974. Some anti-thyroid and related substances, nitrofurans and industrial chemicals. In: IARC Monographs on the evaluation of carcinogenic risk of chemicals to man; vol 7. Lyon, France: IARC.

INTERNATIONAL AGENCY FOR RESEARCH ON CANCER. 1986. Some naturally occurring and synthetic food components, furocoumarins and ultraviolet radiation. In: IARC Monographs on the evaluation of the carcinogenic risk of chemicals to humans; vol. 40. Lyon, France: IARC.

INTERNATIONAL AGENCY FOR RESEARCH ON CANCER. 1987. Overall evaluations of carcinogenicity: an updating of IARC Monographs Volumes 1 to 42. In: IARC Monographs on the evaluation of the carcinogenic risk of chemicals to humans (Suppl 7). Lyon, France: IARC.

INTERNATIONAL AGENCY FOR RESEARCH ON CANCER. 1990. Pharmaceutical drugs. In: IARC Monographs on the evaluation of carcinogenic risks to humans; vol. 50. Lyon, France: IARC.

ISOMAKI HA, HAKULINEN T, JOUTSENLAHTI U. 1978. Excess risk of lymphomas, leukemia and myeloma in patients with rheumatoid arthritis. J Chronic Dis 31:691–696.

ITO N, FUKUSHIMA S, SHIRA T, et al. 1984. Drugs, food additives and natural products as promoters in rat urinary bladder carcinogenesis. IARC Sci Publ 56:399–407.

JOHANSSON S, ANGERVALL L, BENGTSSON U, et al. 1974. Uroepithelial tumors of the renal pelvis associated with abuse of phenacetin-containing analgesics. Cancer 33:743–753.

KANTOR AF, HARTGE P, HOOVER RN, et al. 1985. Tuberculosis chemotherapy and risk for bladder cancer. Int J Epidemiol 14:182–184.

KINLEN LJ. 1985. Incidence of cancer in rheumatoid arthritis and other disorders after immunosuppressive treatment. Am J Med 78(Suppl 1A):44–49.

KINLEN LJ, SHEIL AGR, PETO J, et al. 1979. Collaborative United Kingdom-Australasian study of cancer in patients treated with immunosuppressive drugs. Br Med J 2:1461–1466.

KLAASEN CD. 1980. Heavy metal and heavy-metal antagonists. In: The Pharmacological Basis of Therapeutics, 6th ed, Gilman AC, Goodman LS, Gilman A (eds). New York: Macmillan pp 1615–1637.

KNEKT P, REUNANEN TAKKUNEN H, et al. 1994. Body iron stores and risk of cancer. Int J Cancer 56:379–382.

KRIEGER N, MARRETT LD, DODDS L, et al. 1993. Risk factors for renal cell carcinoma: results of a population-based case-control study. Cancer Causes Control 4:101–110.

KRIPKE ML. 1988. Immunoregulation of carcinogenesis: past, present and future. J Natl Cancer Inst 80:722–727.

KUNE GA, KUNE S, WATSON LF. 1988. Colorectal cancer risk, chronic illnesses, operations, and medications: case control results from the Melbourne Colorectal Cancer Study. Cancer Res 48:4399–4404.

LI EP, WILLARD DR, GOODMAN R, et al. 1975. Malignant lymphoma after diphenylhydantoin (Dilantin) therapy. Cancer 36:1359–1362.

LINDBLAD P, MCLAUGHLIN JK, MELLEMGAARD A, et al. 1993. Risk of kidney cancer among patients using analgesics and diuretics: a population-based cohort study. Int J Cancer 55:5–9.

LINDELHOF B, SIGURGEIRSSON B, TEGNER E, et al. 1991. PUVA and cancer: a large-scale epidemiological study. Lancet 338:91–93.

Mathieson G. 1975. Pathologic aspects of epilepsy with special reference to the surgical pathology of focal cerebral seizures. Adv Neurol 8:107–138.

Matzner Y, Polliack A. 1978. Myelomatosis after phenytoin therapy: a chance association? Scand J Hematol 21:309–312.

Maughan WZ, Muller SA, Perry HO, et al. 1980. Incidence of skin cancers in patients with atopic dermatitis treated with coal tar. J Am Acad Dermatol 3:612–615.

Mayer SE, Melmon KL, Gilman AG. 1980. Introduction: the dynamics of drug absorption, distribution, and elimination. In: The Pharmacological Basis of Therapeutics, 6th ed, Gilman AG, Goodman LS, Gilman A (eds). New York: Macmillan, pp 1–27.

McCredie M, Ford JM, Taylor JS, et al. 1982. Analgesics and cancer of the renal pelvis in New South Wales. Cancer 49:2617–2625.

McCredie M, Steward JH, Ford JM, et al. 1983. Phenacetin-containing analgesics and cancer of the bladder or renal pelvis in women. Br J Urol 55:220–224.

McCredie M, Stewart JH. 1988. Does paracetamol cause urothelial cancer or renal papillary necrosis? Nephron 49:296–300.

McCredie M, Ford JM, Stewart JH. 1988. Risk factors for cancer of the renal parenchyma. Int J Cancer 42:13–16.

McCredie M, Stewart JH, Day NE. 1993. Different roles for phenacetin and paracetamol in cancer of the kidney and renal pelvis. Int J Cancer 53:245–249.

McLaughlin JK, Blot WJ, Mandel JS, et al. 1983. Etiology of cancer of the renal pelvis. J Natl Cancer Inst 71:287–291.

McLaughlin JK, Mandel JS, Blot WJ, Schuman LM, et al. 1984. A population-based case-control study of renal cell carcinoma. J Natl Cancer Inst 72:275–284.

McLaughlin JK, Blot WJ, Fraumeni JF Jr. 1988. Diuretics and renal cell cancer. J Natl Cancer Inst 80:378.

McLaughlin JK, Gao YT, Gao RN, et al. 1992. Risk factors for renal-cell cancer in Shanghai, China. Int J Cancer 52:562–565.

Menter A, Cram DL. 1983. The Goeckerman regimen in two psoriasis day care centers. J Am Acad Dermatol 9:59–65.

Miller CT. 1974. Isoniazid and cancer risks. JAMA 230:1254.

Miller CT, Neutel CI, Nair RC, et al. 1978. Relative importance of risk factors in bladder carcinogenesis. J Chronic Dis 31:51–56.

National Cancer Institute. 1978. Bioassay of phenazopyridine hydrochloride for possible carcinogenicity (Tech. Rep. Ser. No. 99), Department of HEW, Publ. No. (NIH) 78-1349, Washington, DC, U.S. Government Printing Office.

Nielands JB. 1980. Microbial metabolism of iron. In: Iron in Biochemistry and Medicine, II, Jacobs A, Worwood M, (eds). London: Academic Press, pp. 529–572.

Olsen JH, Boice JD, Jensen JPA, et al. 1989. Cancer among epileptic patients exposed to anticonvulsant drugs. J Natl Cancer Inst 81:803–808.

Olsen JH, Wallin H, Boice JD Jr, et al. 1993. Phenobarbital, drug metabolism, and human cancer. Cancer Epidemiol Biomarkers Prev 2:449–452.

Paganini-Hill A, Chao A, Ross RK, et al. 1991. Aspirin use and incidence of large-bowel cancer in a California retirement community. J Natl Cancer Inst 183:1182–1183.

Penn I. 1977. Development of cancer as a complication of clinical transplantation. Transplant Proc 9:1121–1127.

Penn I, Brunson ME. 1988. Cancers after cyclosporine therapy. Transplant Proc 20(Suppl 3):885–892.

Penston J, Wormsley KG. 1985. H_2-receptor antagonists and gastric cancer. Med Toxicol 1:163–168.

Peraino C, Fry RJM, Staffeldt E. 1971. Reduction and enhancement by phenobarbital of hepatocarcinogenesis induced in the rat by 2-acetylaminofluorene. Cancer Res 31:1506–1512.

Piper JM, Tonascia J, Matanoski GM. 1985. Heavy phenacetin use and bladder cancer in women aged 20 to 49 years. N Engl J Med 313:292–295.

Piper DW. 1981. Cimetidine and cancer. Med J Aust 1:327.

Pittelkow MR, Perry HO, Muller SA, et al. 1981. Skin cancer in patients with psoriasis treated with coal tar. Arch Dermatol 117:465–468.

Porter JB, Janeway CM, Hunter JR, et al. 1984. Absence of a causal association between cimetidine and gastric cancer. Gastroenterology 87:987–988.

Poynter D. 1985. Long-term effects of reduced gastric acidity in laboratory animals. Digestion 31:174.

Prescott LF. 1982. Analgesic nephropathy: a reassessment of the role of phenacetin and other analgesics. Drugs 23:75–149.

Richmond HG. 1959. Induction of sarcoma in the rat by iron-dextran complex. Br Med J 1:947–949.

Robinson CEG, Bell DN, Sturdy JH. 1960. Possible association of malignant neoplasm with non-dextran injection. Br Med J 2:648.

Roeser HP. 1980. Iron metabolism in inflammation and malignant disease. In: Iron in Biochemistry and Medicine, II, Jacobs A, Worwood M (eds). London: Academic Press, pp 605–640.

Rosenberg L, Palmer JR, Zauber AG, et al. 1991. A hypothesis: nonsteroidal anti-inflammatory drugs reduce the incidence of large-bowel cancer. J Natl Cancer Inst 83:355–358.

Ross RK, Paganini-Hill A, Krailo MD, et al. 1984. Effects of reserpine on prolactin levels and incidence of breast cancer in postmenopausal women. Cancer Res 44:3106–3108.

Rubinstein I, Langevitz P, Shibi G. 1985. Isolated malignant lymphoma of the jejunum and long-term diphenylhydantoin therapy. Oncology 42:104–106.

Saltzstein SL, Ackerman LV. 1959. Lymphadenopathy induced by anticonvulsant drugs and mimicking clinically and pathologically malignant lymphomas. Cancer 12:164–182.

Schreinemachers DM, Everson RB. 1994. Aspirin use and lung, colon, and breast cancer incidence in a prospective study. Epidemiology 5:138–146.

Selby JV, Friedman GD, Fireman BH. 1989. Screening prescription drugs for possible carcinogenicity: eleven to fifteen years of follow-up. Cancer Res 49:5736–5747.

Selby JV, Friedman GD. 1988. Epidemiologic evidence of an association between body iron stores and risk of cancer. Int J Cancer 41:677–682.

Shapiro S, Parsells JL, Rosenberg JL, et al. 1984. Risk of breast cancer in relation to the use of rauwolfia alkaloids. Eur J Clin Pharmacol 26:143–146.

Shirts SB, Annegers JF, Hauser WA, et al. 1986. Cancer incidence in a cohort of patients with seizure disorders. J Natl Cancer Inst 77:83–87.

Shu XO, Gao YT, Linet MS, et al. 1987. Chloramphenicol use and childhood leukaemia in Shanghai. Lancet 2:934–937.

Smith MA, Rubinstein L, Cazenave L, et al. 1993. Report of the Cancer Therapy Evaluation Program Monitoring Plan for Secondary Acute Myeloid Leukemia Following Treatment with Epipodophyllotoxins. J Natl Cancer Inst 85:554–558.

Sorrell TC, Forbes IJ. 1975. Depression of immune competence by phenytoin and carbamazepine. Clin Exp Immunol 20:273–285.

Stanford JL, Martin EJ, Brinton LA, et al. 1986. Rauwolfia use and breast cancer: a case-control study. J Natl Cancer Inst 76:817–822.

Starzl TE, Nalesnik MA, Porter KA, et al. 1984. Reversibility of lymphomas and lymphoproliferative lesions developing under cyclosporin-steroid therapy. Lancet 1:583–587.

Stern RS, Laird N, Melski J, et al. 1984. Cutaneous squamous-cell carcinoma in patients treated with PUVA. N Engl J Med 310:1156–1161.

Stern RS, Zierler S, Parrish JA. 1980. Skin carcinoma in patients with psoriasis treated with topical tar and artificial ultraviolet radiation. Lancet:731–735.

STEVENS JD, MISSION GP. 1987. Ophthalmic use of chloramphenicol (Letter). Lancet:1456.

STEVENS RG, BEASLEY RP, BLUMBERG BS. 1986. Iron-binding proteins and risk of cancer in Taiwan. J Natl Cancer Inst 76:605–610.

STEVENS RG, GRAUBARD BI, MICOZZI MS, et al. 1994. Moderate elevation of body iron level and increased risk of cancer occurrence and death. Int J Cancer 56:364–369.

STOTT H, PETO J, STEPHENS R. 1976. An assessment of the carcinogenicity of isoniazid in patients with pulmonary tuberculosis. Tubercle 57:1–15.

SUH O, METTLIN C, PETRELLI NJ. 1993. Aspirin use, cancer, and polyps of the large bowel. Cancer 72:1171–1177.

SYMMONS DPM. 1985. Neoplasms of the immune system in rheumatoid arthritis. Am J Med 78(suppl 1A):22–28.

TAKKUNEN H, REUNANEN A, KNEKT P, et al. 1989. Body iron stores and risk of cancer. N Engl J Med 320:1013–1014.

TAYLOR TV, LEE D, HOWATSON AG, et al. 1981. Gastric cancer and cimetidine. J R Coll Surg Edinb 26:34–35.

THOMAS DB, SIEMIATYCKI J, DEWAR R, et al. 1985. The problem of multiple inference in studies designed to generate hypotheses. Am J Epidemiol 122:1080–1095.

THUN MJ, NAMBOODIRI MM, HEATH CW. 1991. Aspirin use and reduced risk of fatal colon cancer. N Engl J Med 325:1593–1596.

VENNING GR. 1983. Identification of adverse reactions to new drugs. II-How were 18 important adverse reactions discovered and with what delays. Br Med J 286:289–292.

WEINBERG ED. 1984. Iron withholding: a defense against infection and neoplasia. Physiol Rev 64:65–102.

WHITE SJ, MCLEAN AEM, HOWLAND C. 1979. Anticonvulsant drugs and cancer: a cohort study in patients with severe epilepsy. Lancet 2:458–460.

WILLIAMS RR, FEINLEIB M, CONNOR RJ, et al. 1978. Case-control study of antihypertensive and diuretic use by women with malignant and benign breast lesions detected in a mammography screening program. J Natl Cancer Inst 61:327–335.

WORMSLEY KG. 1984. Assessing the safety of drugs for the long-term treatment of peptic ulcers. Gut 25:1416–1423.

YU MC, MACK TM, HANISCH R, et al. 1986. Cigarette smoking, obesity, diuretic use, and coffee consumption as risk factors for renal cell carcinoma. J Natl Cancer Inst 77:351–356.

ZHENG W, BLOT WJ, LIAO ML, et al. 1987. Lung cancer and prior tuberculosis infection in Shanghai. Br J Cancer 40:501–504.

24 Viruses

NANCY E. MUELLER
ALFRED S. EVANS
W. THOMAS LONDON

The oncogenic potential of several types of viruses has been recognized for some time. Early in this century, Ellerman, Bang, and Rous observed that an apparently infectious agent was responsible for transmitting malignancy among chickens. Shope later determined that some tumors in rabbits were caused by papillomavirus infection (Shope and Hurst, 1933). Around 1950, the identification of a family of murine retroviruses that caused leukemia and other malignancies provided researchers with animal systems suitable for laboratory experiments. The study of these systems fostered understanding of the molecular biology of transformation, culminating in the identification of oncogenes (Wold and Green, 1979; Dulbecco, 1987). However, these systems provided only limited insight into the role of viruses in naturally occurring malignancies because they were based both on laboratory isolates of viruses, selected for their high level of oncogenicity, and on inbred hosts, selected for susceptibility to tumor induction. Further, the routes and doses used for virus exposure were quite artificial. Thus the laboratory observations bore little resemblance to what happened in nature.

Beginning in the 1970s, many researchers became interested in virally induced cancer occurring naturally in animal populations. Studies at this time established that under some circumstances, horizontally transmitted infection with certain "wild type" viruses endemic in animal populations can lead to the induction of malignancy. The major animal systems used in these investigations are listed in Table 24–1.

These animal models have provided a window on the natural history of oncogenic viruses, and in the case of Marek's disease and feline leukemia, preventive vaccination programs have been implemented. Of these models of animal viruses, the feline leukemia model has been the most amenable to observation. As such, it provides a paradigm for the epidemiologist concerned with the role of viruses in human malignancy (Onions, 1985).

The feline leukemia virus (FeLV) is a typical retrovirus, a class of RNA virus distinguished by a replicatory cycle which involves reverse transcription into DNA. In infected hosts, this double-stranded DNA provirus is integrated into the host genome, establishing latency. In cats the virus causes a range of disease, including lymphoma and leukemia, aplastic anemia, glomerulonephritis, abortion and fetal resorption, and opportunistic infections (Essex, 1982).

The initial immune response to the viral infection is strongly related to the risk of subsequent disease outcome. Most cats exposed to the virus under natural conditions develop protective immunity as indexed by the development of antibodies against viral proteins and against the so-called FOCMA, a tumor-associated antigen (Essex, 1982). However, in some circumstances a chronic viremia occurs and this normal serologic response is not seen. Certain conditions foster persistent viremia, including early age at infection (Hoover et al, 1976) and high virus dose to a mature cat (Essex et al, 1977). A simple assay for the presence of FeLV antigens on peripheral blood lymphocytes, commonly used in veterinary practice, can determine whether a cat is chronically viremic (Hardy et al, 1973).

The natural history of FeLV infection was described by Francis et al (1979, 1981b), who noted its similarities to that of hepatitis B virus (HBV) infection. As shown in Figure 24–1, about 10% of domestic cats become infected with the FeLV annually. Of these, the great majority will have a subclinical or mild infection, develop antibody to FOCMA and other viral antigens, and become immune to further infection. The role of cell-mediated immunity in controlling FeLV infection is unclear.

However, an estimated 2% will not gain immunologic control of the infection and will become chroni-

Dr. Mueller was a recipient of an American Cancer Society Faculty Research Award; her work is supported by NIH grant R37 CA 38450. Dr. London's work is supported by NIH grants CA 40737, CA 57577, CA 06927, and by an appropriation from the Commonwealth of Pennsylvania. The authors are indebted to Ms. Sara Vargas and Ms. Sandra Chinn for editorial assistance.

TABLE 24–1. *Characteristics of Major Animal Models for Naturally Occurring, Viral-Induced Malignancy**

Host Species	*Malignancy*	*Virus*	*Note*
Chicken	Marek's disease (lymphoma)	Marek's disease (herpesvirus)	Preventive vaccination
Cotton-tail rabbit	Lymphoma	Herpesvirus sylvilagus	Mononucleosis-like syndrome can occur in primary infection
Cat	Leukemia/ lymphoma	Feline leukemia virus (retrovirus)	Associated with immunosuppression
Ox	Leukemia	Bovine leukemia virus (retrovirus)	Prolonged preleukemia state
Ox	Alimentary carcinoma	Bovine alimentary papilloma virus	Co-factor: bracken fern ingestion
Woodchuck	Hepatocellular carcinoma	Woodchuck hepatitis virus (hepadna virus)	Risk associated with chronic infection following early infection

*From Essex et al (1980b).

cally viremic. These cats will remain asymptomatic for an extended latency period. Serologically, they will have low or absent anti-FOCMA antibodies and positive blood smears. Eventually, all will develop a virally induced disease. About one in three or four will develop a leukemia/lymphoma in which the malignant cells express both FOCMA and FeLV antigens. The rest will

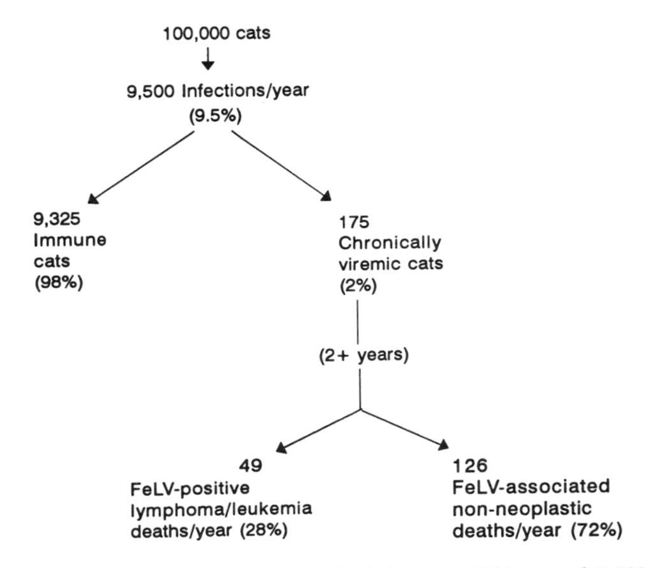

FIG. 24–1 An epidemiologic model of the natural history of FeLV infection in a steady-state of cats population [From Francis et al (1979) with permission.]

develop opportunistic infections or other serious complications of immune suppression (Essex, 1982).

The mechanism by which malignancy arises in conjunction with chronic viremia is unknown. Although wild type FeLV contains no oncogene, evidence of defective FeLV containing the *myc* gene in FeLV-positive malignancy in pet cats has been found (Hardy, 1984) and integration of the provirus in specific domains of the host DNA may be involved (Levesque et al, 1990; Tsujimoto et al, 1993). It may be that with chronic virus replication the probability of in vivo genetic recombination is enhanced, leading to the production of acutely transforming virus comparable to the laboratory isolates. In addition, among immune (non-viremic) older cats, FOCMA-positive but FeLV-negative leukemia occurs (Francis et al, 1981a). Rojko et al (1982) have found that such immune cats harbor latent FeLV which can be reactivated by immune suppression. This suggests that an alternate route of oncogenesis could occur by endogenous immune suppression and reactivation of latent FeLV (Essex, 1982).

The following characteristics of the feline leukemia model are generally representative for the natural animal models of viral oncogenesis which have been studied:

1. The virus is a common infection within the host population.
2. The virus has the capacity to persist (a latent or persistent infection).
3. Virus-associated malignancies occur in a small proportion of infected individuals after a protracted period of latency.
4. The probability of developing malignancy is associated with factors which influence immune response at primary infection. (It is likely that factors influencing reactivation of latent infections are also involved.)
5. The latent period preceding disease is marked by serologically detectable chronic viremia or altered antibody response.

These same principles generally hold true for the role of viruses in human malignancies. The types of viruses that have been determined to cause malignancy in the animal models are the same as those associated with human cancer. Table 24–2 lists the major virus-associated human malignancies for which there is substantial evidence for a causal relationship (Evans and Mueller, 1990). These are listed in order of the strength of evidence, from strongest to weakest and are reviewed in detail below.

Before turning to a discussion of each of the classes of human oncogenic viruses and the major related malignancies, two observations are important to note. These regard the contribution of viruses to the public health burden of cancer incidence and mortality. First, viral-associated malignancies have an age–incidence curve which generally peaks before middle age (Doll, 1978). This shape is quite different from that characterizing most other malignancies, such as stomach cancer, which have an exponential increase with age, with incidence peaking among the elderly (Fig. 24–2). Thus these virus-related malignancies occur in relatively young people. As such, they impose a greater cost in years of life lost than other cancers. Second, it has been estimated that a relatively small proportion of cancer mortality in the United States (10%) is "attributable" to infection (Doll and Peto, 1981). However, among people in economically developing populations, these malignancies are generally more common. Thus the identification of strategies for preventing these malignancies could have a substantial impact on public health in the developing world (Essex and Gutensohn, 1981).

TABLE 24–2. *Major Human Virus-Associated Malignancies**

Malignancy	*Virus (Family)*
Adult T-cell leukemia/lymphoma	HTLV-I (retrovirus)
Hepatocellular carcinoma	HBV (hepadna) HCV (? flaviviridae)
Burkitt's lymphoma	EBV (herpes)
Nasopharyngeal carcinoma	EBV (herpes)
Hodgkin's disease	EBV (herpes)
Cervical carcinoma	HPV 16/18 (papilloma)

*Abbreviations: HTLV-I, human T-cell lymphotropic virus type I; HBV, hepatitis B virus; EBV, Epstein-Barr virus; HPV, human papillomavirus

HERPESVIRUSES

The human herpesviruses are all potentially oncogenic. These viruses consist of an icosahedral capsid and a core containing DNA, both enclosed in an envelope of host cell and viral components. Most herpesviruses persist in their infected hosts as latent infections. As such, these viruses can be periodically activated into replication. Human herpesviruses include the Epstein-Barr virus (EBV), cytomegalovirus (CMV), herpes simplex I and II, varicella, and the more recently identified human herpesvirus types 6 and 7. Of these, there is convincing evidence of a role in oncogenesis for only the EBV.

EPSTEIN-BARR VIRUS

The EBV is a double-stranded DNA virus containing over 100 genes which have been identified by DNA recombinant technology (Miller, 1990). Like all herpesviruses, EBV consists of an outer envelope, a viral capsid, and a DNA core. The DNA exists in a circular form in the latent stage and in a linear form in the replicative stage.

The virus is complex, consisting of many antigens, some expressed early in the replicative cycle and some expressed late. The early antigens (EA) consist of two complexes, the restricted (R) and the diffuse (D), which are distinguishable by immunofluorescence staining patterns. The late antigens include the viral capsid antigen (VCA) and the EB nuclear antigen (EBNA), which has six components. The presence and level of antibodies to these various antigens as well as the time of their appearance in primary infections vary in the diverse clinical conditions associated with EBV infection. EBNA-1, for example, is important in maintaining the virus's

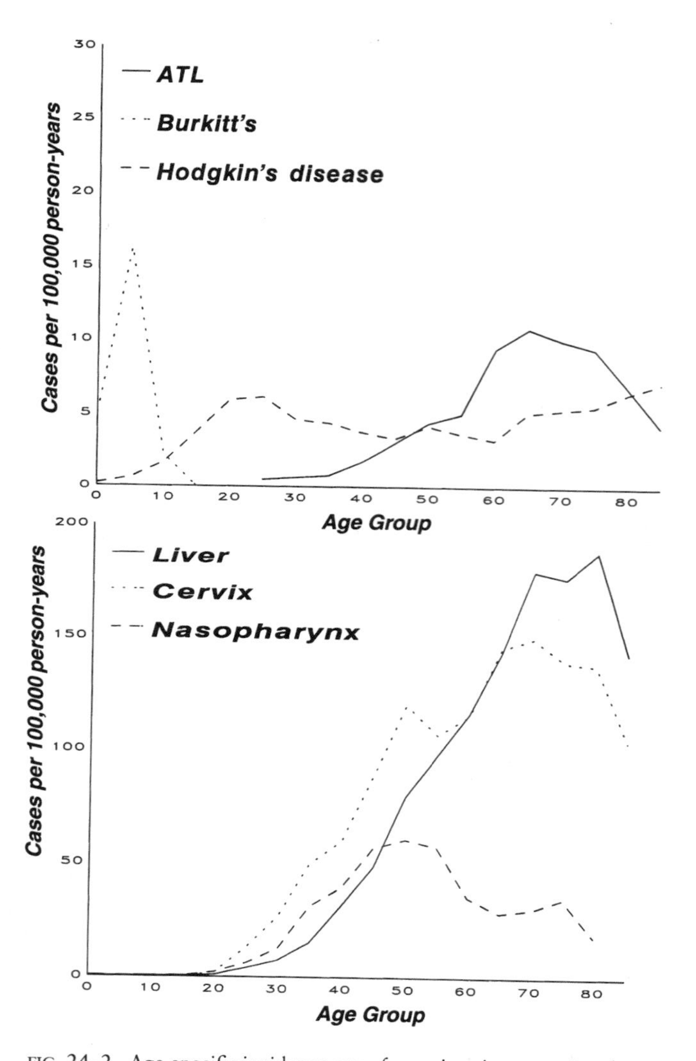

FIG. 24–2. Age-specific incidence rates for major virus-associated malignancies. Adult T-cell leukemia/lymphoma (ATL): males, 1986–87, Kyushu (Japan); Burkitt's lymphoma: males, 1961–75, West Nile District (Uganda); Hodgkin's disease: males, 1986–90, SEER Program; liver, males, 1983–87, Shanghai (China); cervix: 1982–86, Cali (Colombia); nasopharynx: males, 1983–87, Chinese (Singapore). (Parkin et al, 1992).

latent state. Antibody to EBNA-1 is normally present in infected individuals but is absent in some 30% of patients with chronic fatigue syndrome as well as in children with human immunodeficiency virus type I (HIV) infection who develop chronic lymphocytic interstitial pneumonitis (Miller, 1990).

Molecular studies indicate that the EBNA-2 gene is involved in the transformation of B lymphocytes, and that this process appears to involve the replication of other viral and cellular genes including the latent membrane protein (LMP) genes. This process requires that another gene termed ZEBRA is not expressed, as its activation is necessary for the virus to switch from latent to replicative states (Marx, 1989).

EBV enters and multiplies in primate B lymphocytes via a receptor identical to the C3 complement receptor. It can also multiply in epithelial cells of the oropharynx, parotid gland, and uterine cervix (Miller, 1990). B lymphocytes infected with EBV become "immortalized," meaning that they are capable of continual growth in vitro. In this process they enlarge into blastoid forms, lose their contact inhibition, and develop new antigens on their surface. In vivo, such EBV-infected cells (although not malignant) may undergo polyclonal proliferation, which, if uncontrolled, may progress to the infiltration of various organs. This may lead to death, in both children (Robinson et al, 1980) and adults (Snydmann et al, 1982). In experiments EBV has been used to immortalize nonhuman lymphocytes. A malignant lymphoma can be induced in vivo in cotton-top marmosets and owl monkeys by the injection of EBV or EBV-infected lymphocytes (Epstein et al, 1973; Miller, 1974; Miller et al, 1977).

There are two major EBV strains (A and B) that have been identified, and there are some differences in their geographic distribution (Sixbey et al, 1989). Genotypic variants have been identified from patients with infectious mononucleosis (IM) following primary EBV infection (Miller et al, 1987). The same variant is usually isolated from several sites in the same patient, but different patients show different genotypes. An instance of two EBV genotypes in an HIV-infected mother and her baby has been described (Miller et al, 1987). These genotypic variants may be useful in epidemiologic studies examining person-to-person transmission, reinfection versus reactivation, and clustering of cases. However, it is not known whether they result in different clinical or oncogenic expressions of EBV (Evans, 1987).

The host response to primary EBV infection varies with age at the time of infection. When infection occurs early in life, it is usually subclinical. This is common in most underdeveloped countries, and in developed populations, among people with poorer socioeconomic living conditions. When infection with the virus is delayed until older childhood or young adult life, IM occurs in about half of those infected (Evans and Niederman, 1989). A primary infection in an adult is marked by the initial appearance of IgM antibodies to VCA. These disappear with the emergence of IgG antibodies against VCA. Transient IgA antibody may also be seen at this point. Within a few weeks, antibodies against the EA-D are detectable and persist for several months. These tend to be replaced by antibodies to EA-R. Heterophile antibodies are also detectable during acute primary infection (Evans and Niederman, 1989). Antibodies against EBNA develop after a delay of several months to a year (de Thé, 1979). When the infection is accompanied clinically with IM, most of the symptoms reflect the vigorous cytotoxic T-cell response to EBNA positive–infected B lymphocytes. Children differ from adults in their antibody response to primary infection as they rarely develop clinical IM, anti-EA-D, or heterophil antibodies. The serologic mark of an established, latent EBV infection for all ages is that of IgG antibodies against VCA and against EBNA. The level (or titer) of these antibodies tends to remain constant for a patient's lifetime once the primary infection is resolved. For those with more severe infection, such as with IM, these levels are established at a relatively high level (Niederman et al 1970; Evans and Niederman, 1989). This is also true among children who are infected as infants (Melbye et al, 1984). Failure to develop anti-EBNA following seroconversion results in chronic viremia and lymphoproliferative disease (Purtilo et al, 1982).

Following a primary EBV infection, the virus remains latent in a non-productive form in a small percentage of B lymphocytes. It is also excreted intermittently from lytic infections of oropharyngeal epithelial cells. At any time, some 15%–20% of EBV antibody–positive persons excrete EBV in the oropharynx. Changes in immune competence may result in reactivation of EBV in B lymphocytes; this is usually asymptomatic, but if sufficiently vigorous it may lead to lymphoproliferative disease and B-cell lymphomas, as has been observed in HIV-infected patients, renal-transplant patients, and other severely immune-depressed individuals.

The serology of EBV reactivation has been evaluated prospectively in therapeutically immunosuppressed populations. In general, reactivation is marked by an increase in IgG titers against VCA and EA-R. The presence of IgM against VCA has also been noted (Ho et al, 1985). We have also observed a low prevalence of IgM against VCA in a normal population with established EBV infection (Evans and Mueller, unpublished results). In addition, there is a decrease or loss of antibody against EBNA (List et al, 1987; Riddler et al, 1994).

Quantitation of antibody levels against the various EBV antigens can provide insight into the virus–host interaction. (Because cell lines used in the traditional EBV immunofluorescence assays may differ in amount of antigen, titer levels from different laboratories may not be comparable but should be internally consistent, as evidenced in de Thé et al, 1978.) It has been proposed by Nilsson and Klein (1982) that anti-VCA titer levels reflect the relative proportion of B cells carrying latent virus. Such a relationship has been demonstrated for antibody titers against latent human T-cell lymphotropic virus type I (HTLV-I) infection which are positively correlated with proviral level (Ishihara et al, 1994). Kusunoki et al (1993) have shown that the number of precursor cytotoxic T lymphocytes to autologous EBV-transformed B cells is positively correlated with anti-EBNA titer and negatively correlated with anti-EA titer. Thus the level of anti-EBNA is a marker of cellular immune control of latent EBV infection while that for anti-EA reflects viral replication.

Epidemiology of Infection

The factors that determine *infection* with EBV differ from those affecting *clinical disease* among the infected (Evans and Niederman, 1989). EBV infection is related to factors influencing exposure to the virus, and may occur at different ages. EBV infection is prevalent throughout the world, even in the most remote tribes along the Amazon (Black et al, 1974).

Transmission presumably occurs via contact with the saliva of asymptomatic virus excretors. In developing countries, the infection of young children may be due to mothers' prechewing of their babies' food or to the transfer of EBV from inanimate objects in settings of poor hygiene. In such circumstances, infection generally occurs early in life. In Ghana, for example, about 80% of the children are infected by the time they reach 18 months of age (Biggar et al, 1978).

Infection generally occurs later in life in developed countries, where transmission is less frequent because of less dense housing, smaller families, and better hygiene. For example, about half of entering American college students in the early 1970s lacked EBV antibody (Evans and Niederman, 1989). In this age group, transmission is thought to occur largely during intimate oral kissing with salivary exchange. The presence of the virus in cervical secretions (Sixbey et al, 1986) suggests the possibility of sexual transmission. Transfusion-transmitted EBV infections also occur, but rarely result in any clinical disease.

There is substantial evidence that EBV infection is a causal factor in a substantial proportion of Burkitt's lymphoma (BL), undifferentiated nasopharyngeal carcinoma (NPC), and Hodgkin's disease (HD) (Evans and Mueller, 1990; Neri et al, 1991). For each of these, there is conclusive evidence of clonal EBV genome in tissue of restricted latent protein expression, and a consistent pattern of altered EBV antibody response in patients as shown in Table 24–3. (Some evidence of EBV involvement has been reported for a variety of other malignancies as diverse as T-cell non-Hodgkin's lymphoma and gastric cancer; however, these findings will not be discussed in this chapter.)

BURKITT'S LYMPHOMA

BL is a malignancy that occurs endemically, primarily among children in central Africa and New Guinea, and sporadically among all ages in other parts of the world. Endemic areas correlate strongly with the presence of holoendemic malaria. The risk of BL is thought to result from the enhanced proliferation of B lymphocytes by early infection with EBV interacting with the repeated mitogenic effect of malaria. In these areas, mainly chil-

TABLE 24–3. *Pattern of EBV Biomarkers in Associated Malignancies*

Marker	*Burkitt's Lymphoma*	*Nasopharyngeal Carcinoma*	*Hodgkin's Disease*
Antibody			
VCA			
IgG	↑↑	↑	↑
IgA	—	↑↑	↑
IgM	—	—	↓
EBNA	—	↑↑	↑↑
Early Antigen			
Diffuse	—	↑ (IgA)	↑
Restricted	↑[a]	—	±
Molecular			
Clonality	Yes	Yes	Yes
Latent Phenotype	EBNA1 only	EBNA1+, EBNA2−, LMP1+	EBNA1?, EBNA2−, LMP1+

[a]Predictive of recurrence following treatment

dren are affected, with a peak incidence at about 8 years of age. The jaw and abdominal organs are the most frequent sites of the malignancy (Evans and Mueller, in press).

Endemic BL is limited mostly to central Africa, in settings lying lower than 3,000 feet above sea level and having an annual rainfall of more than 40 inches (Burkitt, 1962; Burkitt and Wright, 1966). In these hot, wet rural lowlands, the clustering of cases both in space and time has been observed. This phenomenon may be related to the varying malarial infection rate (Morrow, 1985; Morrow et al, 1977). In these areas, BL is the most common childhood cancer, with the incidence rate in focal areas reaching as high as 4–5/100,000 person-years among children of age 15 or less. The range of incidence of all non-Hodgkin's lymphoma per 100,000 person-years in the age-group 4–14 years, and the percent contributed by BL (shown in parentheses) in different geographic areas extends from 9 to 15 (95%) in Uganda in East Africa, 2 to 4 (47%) in Algeria in North Africa, and 1 to 2 (30%) in industrialized countries, such as France and the United States (de Thé, 1985).

In the United States, a registry for BL has been established, with 256 confirmed cases reported from 1971 to 1985. Data from the Surveillance, Epidemiology and End Results (SEER) study of the National Cancer Institute show an overall annual incidence of 1.4 per million among white males and 0.4 per million among white females between 1973 and 1981 (Levine et al, 1985). The cases span a broad age-group; only half are children. The malignancy occurs predominantly in white males, with a few cases occurring among non-whites.

Of 128 cases in the American BL registry tested for EBV VCA IgG antibody, 34% had elevated titers, 45% had levels within normal range, and 20% lacked antibody entirely. Less than 30% had demonstrable EBV genome in tumor tissue. Thus only one-third or less of American BL had an association with EBV similar to African BL, and 20% apparently had never even been infected with EBV. (Evans and Mueller, in press). Similar data were also reported earlier for non-endemic cases by Ziegler (1981).

Thus the risk factors for BL in the industrialized countries are quite different from those seen in endemic areas. The more recent observation of the occurrence of BL in conjunction with infection with HIV, of which about 35%–40% are EBV positive (Hamilton-Dutoit et al, 1993), provides the opportunity to gain more insight into this disease (Ziegler et al, 1984).

Independent of geographic origin, essentially all BL shows one of the three following reciprocal chromosomal shifts involving the long arm of chromosome 8 q. These include a translocation either with 14q (75% of the cases), or with the short arm of chromosome 2p (9%) or with the long arm of chromosome 22q (16%). These translocations have been found consistently in over 100 established BL cell lines, irrespective of EBV positivity. The translated portion of chromosome 8 includes the c-*myc* oncogene, which, when translocated adjacent to the heavy chain genes on 14q, the K light chain gene on 2p, or the D light chain gene on 22q, becomes activated (derepressed) during antibody generation. Alteration of c-*myc* activity appears to be an essential event in the development of the malignant cell clone whose replication leads to BL (Leder, 1985a, b).

Viral-Specific Data

EBV is closely associated with the pathogenesis of almost all cases of BL occurring in highly endemic areas such as Africa but with only a minority of cases occurring in industrialized nations. This association is defined by the demonstration of clonal episomal EBV in tumors, characteristically expressing only EBNA-1 (Klein, 1994). In terms of antibody patterns, while there is no significantly higher frequency of the *prevalence* of these antibodies between cases and controls, a significantly higher *level* of IgG antibodies to the VCA, EBNA, and to a lesser extent, to EA-R, occurs than in age- and sex-matched controls from the same area. For example, Henle et al (1969) found titers to VCA-IgG antibody levels of 1:160 or higher in 81% of 139 patients with African BL, as compared with only 14% of 489 controls. The geometric mean of the antibody titers was 1:275 and 1:37, respectively.

Under the auspices of the International Agency for Research on Cancer (IARC), a prospective study was done involving samples from a cohort of 42,000 children ages 0–8 in the West Nile district of Uganda (de Thé et al, 1978). Baseline blood specimens were obtained and stored. Fourteen BL cases occurred in the first 5 years of follow-up, and two additional cases were later identified (Geser et al, 1982). All patients with BL had EBV antibody present in the initial serum sample, taken between 7 and 54 months prior to diagnosis, and 12 of 13 EBV-associated BL cases had pre-tumor VCA antibody titers as high or higher than any control bled at the same time. The risk for development of BL in children with titers two dilutions or more above the geometric mean titer (standardized for age, sex, and area) of the controls was estimated to be 30 times higher than those with normal levels. In addition, nine of the ten confirmed cases from whom biopsies had been obtained at the time of diagnosis had detectable EBNA or EBV DNA in the tumor tissue, including one case in whom the pre-tumor antibody level was normal. Antibodies to other herpesviruses as well as to measles virus were not elevated in the baseline bleeding, indicating a specificity of the virus association.

Other Factors

The major cofactor in endemic areas appears to be holoendemic malaria. Malaria acts as a B-cell mitogen, stimulating polyclonal expansion and providing greatly increased opportunity for chromosomal translocation to occur. It also interferes with the action of cytotoxic T cells that regulate B-cell replication. Nearly all of the epidemiological characteristics of African BL can be explained on the basis of the intensity of the exposure to *Plasmodium falciparum* malaria. These include the geographic distribution, the young age-group affected, time–space clustering, the occurrence of BL among older migrants from areas of non-holoendemic malaria to holoendemic areas, and the decreasing incidence of the tumor in areas where death rates from malaria are declining (Morrow, 1985). In a series of elegant studies, Magrath et al have shown that the specific site of chromosomal breakpoint varies substantially between geographic areas (Shiramizu et al, 1991; Magrath et al, 1993). The proportion of EBV-positive BL in a given area correlates with that of tumors in which the breakpoint on chromosome 8 is distant from c-*myc*. These proportions are highest in endemic areas, lowest in North American tumors, and intermediate in those from South America, pointing to more than one causal pathway leading to common molecular lesions, these pathways being influenced by environmental factors.

The current view of the natural history of endemic BL was first suggested by Klein (1982). EBV infection usually occurs very early in African children, resulting in transformation and rapid replication of a relatively large subset of B lymphocytes. This process is augmented by repeated malarial infection, which acts as a secondary B-cell mitogen and interferes with normal control mechanisms for T-cell regulation of B-cell replication. During this process of amplified replication of immunoglobulin genes on chromosomes 14, 2, and 22, a chromosomal translocation may occur, involving chromosome 8 which carries the normally repressed c-*myc*. This translocation apparently results in the inappropriate expression of c-*myc*, setting off less-regulated cell replication. The activation of a second oncogene, B-*lym*, may then be necessary to gain independent monoclonal proliferation (Leder et al, 1983; Leder, 1985b; Magrath et al, 1993).

The evidence indicting the EBV in endemic BL has led to the call for an EBV vaccine to be given to susceptible infants in endemic areas (Epstein, 1976, 1986; Epstein and Morgan, 1985). However, the testing of a vaccine will be difficult in Africa because of the decreasing incidence of BL, corresponding with the decrease in malaria in many areas, and the logistical difficulties related to intervention in infancy. However, trials now underway in this age-group for the prevention of primary hepatocellular carcinoma (HCC) by a vaccine against HBV may lead to solutions for these problems.

NASOPHARYNGEAL CARCINOMA

NPC occurs worldwide. Most commonly these carcinomas are classified histologically as poorly differentiated or undifferentiated. The highest incidence is in the Far East, primarily in persons of Chinese descent and in related populations, wherever they may migrate (de Thé et al, 1989). Rates differ among various Chinese populations in the same area, and are highest among those from the South. The disease appears to be relatively common among Eskimos and native Greenlanders (an Eskimo group of Caucasian heritage). The age-adjusted incidence rates (world standard) for males in high incidence areas range from 6 to 28 per 100,000 person-years and 3 to 11 for females. This rate falls to less than 1 per 100,000 person-years for males in the UK, USA, and New Zealand (Parkin et al, 1992).

The age-specific incidence among Chinese in Hong Kong and Singapore shows a peak rising from ages 20–24 to about age 50, then drops off thereafter (Fig. 24–2). This type of age curve suggests an infectious etiology with exposure occuring early in life (Doll, 1978). In Sweden by contrast, the rise occurs some two decades later and continues until over age 70 (Parkin et al, 1992). In the United States, a trimodal distribution has been noted by Green et al (1977), who suggest that this may reflect varying etiologies operating in different age-groups in a racially mixed population. The epidemiology of NPC is described in detail in Chapter 29.

Viral-Specific Data

As in the case of BL, high antibody titers to VCA-IgG mark an association with EBV in NPC (Henle et al, 1970, 1973). Such high titers are found in over 80% of NPC patients. Antibody to EA is also elevated, but usually it is the diffuse form (EA-D) rather than EA-R, which is elevated in BL. The level of these antibodies increases as the stages of disease progress (Henle et al, 1977). A unique feature of NPC cases is the presence of VCA-IgA antibody in both serum and saliva (Henle and Henle, 1976). Mathew et al (1994) found that of 100 NPC patients with anti-VCA IgA, 75% had IgG antibodies against ZEBRA, indicative of viral replication. NPC patients also have high antibody levels against EBNA (de Thé et al, 1989). Chatani et al (1991) have reported that cases have high titers against both EBNA-1 and EBNA-2. Frech et al (1993) have reported that 38% of 83 NPC cases had antibodies against the latent infection terminal proteins, but none of 19 EBV-positive BL patients nor of 62 HD patients had such antibodies.

The presence of IgA against the EBV has served as the basis for a screening test for NPC in massive population studies in China (Zeng et al, 1980). There investigators have found that anti-VCA IgA can be present for years prior to clinical evidence of the disease and, in the presence of a positive computerized axial tomographic scan, is a very strong indicator of the presence of NPC (Prasad, 1988). However, the presence of VCA-IgA antibody on stored serum samples was not predictive of subsequent NPC in a small study among Alaskan Eskimos (Lanier et al, 1980) nor for seven cases from California (Chan et al, 1991).

Evidence of EBV "fingerprints" in NPC tissue has also been found regularly in biopsies (including carcinoma in situ) by several molecular techniques and occur predominantly in epithelial cells, not in the infiltrating lymphocytes (Wolf et al, 1973; Klein et al, 1974; Pagano et al, 1975; Yeung et al, 1993). The viral genome is clonal (Raab-Traub and Flynn, 1986); clonal EBV has also been found in preinvasive lesions (Pathmanathan et al, 1995). It has been shown that the integrated viral genome expresses a restricted pattern of viral latent proteins, with only EBNA-1 and LMP detected (Fåhraeus et al, 1988). This restricted phenotype is similar to that seen in EBV-positive HD (Table 24–3).

Other Factors

Major risk factors for NPC include genetic susceptibility and related environmental exposures, especially dietary factors (de Thé et al, 1989; Hildesheim and Levine, 1993). Genetic influences are evident because of the familial aggregation of NPC patients in areas of high risk and its high occurrence in persons of southern Chinese descent, irrespective of where they live. There is an associated human leukocyte antigen (HLA) profile among Chinese patients which is characterized by an increased frequency of the first-locus antigen (HLA-A2) and by a deficit at the second locus, which has been demonstrated to represent Bw46. However, not all data from Chinese populations are consistent. Furthermore, it has recently been reported that among American Caucasians A2 was associated with a significantly protective effect for NPC (Burt et al, 1994). Linkage analysis based on affected sib pairs suggests that a gene closely linked to the HLA locus confers a greatly increased risk (Lu et al, 1990).

The epidemiological importance of environmental factors, primarily dietary, are now being recognized (Yu, 1991). The ingestion of smoked and dried fish, especially during infancy, has been suspected as a risk factor for some time (Ho, 1971). Recent dietary surveys focusing on the presence of nitrosamines in the high-risk countries of China, Tunisia, and Greenland have supported this association. Representative food samples were analyzed for the presence of volatile nitrosamines which were detected in salted and dried fish from southern China, in radish roots and Chinese cabbage in brine, in some preserved food in Tunisia, and in dry but not salted fish in Greenland (Poirier et al, 1987; de Thé et al, 1989). The disease is also associated with the reduced ingestion of fresh fruits and vegetables (Anderson et al, 1978).

Other environmental factors found in some case–control studies include a history of repeated acute respiratory infections, use of traditional Chinese medicines for the nose and throat, and exposure to smoke from coils of mosquito repellant (Shanmugaratnam and Higginson, 1967). Henderson et al (1976) evaluated exposures associated with occupation in a case–control study of 156 NPC patients and 267 controls in California. They found risk associated with exposure to fumes (relative risk [RR] = 2.0), smoke exposure (RR = 3.0), and chemicals (RR = 2.4). The results were the same for both Chinese and white subjects. Tobacco use has also been implicated (Nam et al, 1992).

Synthesis of Present Knowledge

Very little is clear about the natural history of NPC. In most settings where NPC is endemic, infection with EBV is presumed to occur early in life. In a recent study in the Republic of China, EBV antibody was present in 80% of children under 5 years old. However, among the Chinese in Singapore, only 20% were EBV antibody–positive by age 3, while in Hong Kong, infection appears to occur earlier (Wang and Evans, 1986). Whether the level of oropharyngeal EBV infection is influenced by age of infection is not known, but it is likely to be heavier.

During the next 20 years or more before a tumor is evident, a variety of factors may contribute to enhancing oropharyngeal replication. These include genetic susceptibility, exposure to dietary nitrosamines and smoke, and perhaps repeated respiratory infections. There is some evidence that enhanced replication of EBV plays a role because of the increased EBV-IgA level prior to diagnosis and the presence of anti-ZEBRA. At some point a malignant clone arises, apparently without a demonstrable chromosomal translocation as in BL. Once the tumor is in situ, EBV can be found consistently in malignant epithelial cells of biopsy specimens.

NPC appears to be the result of a chronically reactivated EBV infection rather than a primary EBV infection, since the tumor does not occur until adult life. An EBV vaccine might not be protective, even if it were feasible to administer one prior to infection, unless it is very early EBV infection that is crucial to the development of NPC. It should also be noted that EBV has also been implicated in other tumors of epithelial tissues such as salivary gland, palatine tonsil, and thymic carcinoma (Evans, 1988).

HODGKIN'S DISEASE

The relationship of EBV to HD is suggested by the epidemiological similarities between HD among young adults and infectious mononucleosis (IM) in economically advantaged populations. For both diseases, risk is associated with higher social class and small family size (Gutensohn and Cole, 1977, 1981). These similarities suggest that exposure to the causative agent is delayed until young adult life. It has been consistently found that people with a history of IM have about a threefold increase in their risk of developing HD. In addition, a larger proportion of HD cases have elevated antibody titers to several EBV antigens, primarily VCA-IgG and EA-D, as compared to controls. Generally, some 30%–40% of HD cases are found to have elevated titers. This has been a consistent finding in many studies over different geographic areas (Mueller, 1987). It has also been found that these titer elevations precede the immunosuppressive therapy given for this disease, but the question of whether they are the consequence of the immunosuppression of HD itself, or precede it as a risk factor, can only be answered by prospective studies. A pilot study based on two cases of HD occurring prospectively among 25,802 persons for whom serum samples had been banked showed that in comparison to matched controls, EBV antibodies were significantly elevated *prior* to diagnosis, in contrast to three other herpesviruses whose antibody titers were not elevated (Evans and Comstock, 1981). This study was then extended to include sera from over 240,000 persons based on five serum banks. In this study, 43 persons who developed HD between 1 and 13 years following blood collection were identified and matched with 96 controls (Mueller et al, 1989). EBV antibody analysis of these sera confirmed the findings of the pilot study in that the proportion of patients with elevated antibody against VCA-IgG and IgA, and EBNA, was significantly higher than that of the controls, and this was associated with a three- to sevenfold increased risk of HD. It is of interest that the cases had significantly decreased levels of IgM against the VCA as compared to controls. These findings were stronger in sera collected at least 3 years prior to diagnosis than in sera collected within 3 years of diagnosis (Mueller et al, 1989). More than half (56%) of the sera from pre-HD cases had elevated titers of one or more EBV antibody compared to 35% of controls. This pattern of anti-EBV was quite different from that seen in prediagnosis serum samples from non-Hodgkin lymphoma patients obtained from the same serum banks (Mueller et al, 1991); no significant differences were found for antibody titers against CMV.

Recently, more direct evidence of EBV involvement in the etiology of HD has been gained by the application of molecular hybridization assays as first reported by Weiss et al (1987); these studies are summarized in detail in Chapter 41 of this book and in Evans and Mueller (in press). In brief, the findings for the almost 2,000 HD cases studied through 1993 suggest that about half of HD cases are EBV positive as defined by the presence of monoclonal EBV genome or of viral gene products. The presence of these viral fingerprints is isolated in the great majority of cases to the Reed-Sternberg cells (RSC). As first reported by Pallesen et al (1991a), it has further been demonstrated that the EBV-positive RSC express the restricted latent infection phenotype of only LMP-1+/EBNA2−, which it shares with NPC. However, although it has been found that NPC tissues express EBNA1, there are conflicting data on whether this is true for RSC in HD (Grässer et al, 1994; Khan and Naase, 1995). These two malignancies share similar transcriptional programs (Deacon et al, 1993) and similar serologic patterns of elevated anti-EA-D and IgA antibodies against the VCA and elevated anti-EBNA (Evans and Mueller, 1990).

In HD, EBV-genome status appears to be stable over time based on follow-up biopsies (Delsol et al, 1992; Coates et al, 1991). The presence of both LMP-1 and the abundant EBV-encoded small RNAs, namely EBERs, indicate that the episomal viral genome is not silent but that the latent state is actively maintained. Pallesen et al (1991b) evaluated whether the BZLF1 gene product ZEBRA was expressed in 47 LMP-1+ HD biopsies. This product induces the switch from latency to the lytic cycle and virus replication. They found that it was rarely expressed—only 3 were positive—and no structural viral proteins were detected. This observation suggested to these investigators that the latent state of the episomal EBV genome in HD is not severely impaired; rather, that the infrequent activation of replication is impaired, resulting in an abortive viral productive cycle. Thus the maintenance of the malignant state appears not to be related to EB viral replication *per se*; it may rather involve the transforming properties of LMP-1 which inhibits terminal differentiation by upregulation of *bcl-2* protein expression (Knecht et al, 1993).

EBV positivity is more strongly associated with the

histologic subtypes which connote more advanced disease and is higher in HD among children and somewhat lower among young adults. These findings imply that there are two types of HD: EBV-genome positive and EBV-genome negative, which may reflect differing causal pathways. Alternatively, EBV may be involved in early events in both types of HD, but the genome is lost under certain conditions. Future research should focus on the integration of both risk factor and serologic data to gain insight into these questions.

RETROVIRUSES: HTLV-I

HTLV-I is the first identified retrovirus that naturally infects humans. In 1980 Poiesz et al made the original isolation from an African-American with a cutaneous lymphoma. The same virus was isolated independently by Yoshida, Miyoshi and Hinuma from a cell line established from a Japanese patient with T-cell leukemia (Yoshida et al, 1982). The subsequent evidence that the virus is a causal factor in the etiology of adult T-cell leukemia/lymphoma (ATL) is so compelling that it has been unchallenged. Yet, little is known about the natural history of the infection and the role of other factors which affect oncogenesis.

A closely related retrovirus, HTLV-II, has also been isolated (Kalyanaraman et al, 1982). Although early serologic assays could not distinguish between the two, new assays are now able to do so (Wiktor et al, 1990; Chen et al, 1990). The oncogenicity of HTLV-II is currently under investigation (Mueller and Blattner, in press).

The HTLV-I, an RNA-containing C-type virus, has a general structure similar to that of the known animal retroviruses, with coding areas for the "gag" internal proteins, the "pol" polymerase proteins, and the "env" envelope proteins (Seiki et al, 1983; Cann et al, 1990). The pol gene codes for an RNA-dependent DNA polymerase which allows the virus to integrate into the host DNA, thus establishing latency. The HTLV-I genome has long terminal repeats at each end which code for transcription initiation signals. There is an additional open reading frame (ORF) called the "X region" which codes for regulatory proteins as well as several alternatively spliced novel m-RNAs. The first regulatory protein called "tax" (p40 or p42) is responsible for the transactivation of transcription of the virus, as well as for the host genes for interleukin 2 (IL-2) and the IL-2 receptor α (ILRα, or CD25) component of the high-affinity receptor on T cells (Lee et al, 1984; Sodrowski et al, 1984). It also transactivates the gene for granulocyte-macrophage colony-stimulating factor (Nimer et al, 1989), but transrepresses the β-polymerase gene, which is involved in host cell DNA repair among other host genes (Jeang et al, 1990). A second negative regulatory protein, *rex* (p27), has been shown to modulate RNA processing in balance with tax activity (Yoshida and Fujisawa, 1992).

Host Response

Following primary infection with HTLV-I, a latent infection is established. Unlike other retroviruses such as FeLV or HIV-1, HTLV-I is a highly cell-associated infection, with no circulating virus products detectable. This property accounts for its extremely low level of infectivity. As reviewed by Rosenblatt et al (1988), the apparent reservoir of latent infection is in peripheral blood T lymphocytes. These cells can be immortalized by HTLV-I in vitro, where they continue to grow in the absence of extraneous IL-2. The immortalized cells are generally of an activated T-helper cell phenotype (CD4+, CD25), the phenotype of essentially all cases of ATL.

As is generally true for the other latent infections, it is likely that periodic virus reactivation occurs. Although there is no direct evidence of this, Okayama et al (1987) has observed that among HTLV-I carriers in Miyazaki, Japan, antibody titers tend to increase with age, which may reflect a cumulative response to viral antigen expression.

Epidemiology of Infection

A unique feature of the epidemiology of HTLV-I infection is its highly restricted geographic distribution as summarized in Table 24–4 (Mueller and Blattner, in press). The highest prevalence occurs in Japan, primarily among the residents of the southern islands of Kyushu, Shikoku, and Okinawa. There the rates among broad population samples range from 10 to 20% (Kohakura et al, 1986; Tajima et al, 1987; Stuver et al, 1992). Within highly endemic populations, there is still striking variability between adjacent communities (Tajima et al, 1987; Stuver et al, 1992). In the northern part of Japan, most of the carriers are migrants from the endemic areas (Tajima et al, 1986), with the exception of the isolated Ainu aboriginal population in northern Hokkaido, among whom the prevalence is 18% (Ishida et al, 1985). However, there is very little infection evident in the rest of Asia (Levine et al, 1988), other than among the aboriginal Aeta people in the Philippines (Ishida et al, 1988).

A second focus of infection has been identified in the Caribbean area where the prevalence is lower (Clark et al, 1985; Levine et al, 1988; Murphy et al, 1989). Here

TABLE 24–4. *Patterns of HTLV-I Seroprevalence Among Population Groups by Apparent Level of Endemicity*

Geographic Region	*Population Group*
HIGHLY ENDEMIC (≥15%)[a]	
Japan	Kyushu, Shikoku, Okinawa, Ainu Aborigines
South Pacific	Papua New Guinea, Solomon Islands, Australian Aborigines
South America	Brazil (Bahia)
INTERMEDIATELY ENDEMIC (5–14%)	
Caribbean	Jamaica, Trinidad, Martinique, French Guiana
West Africa	Gabon, Cameroon, Equatorial Guinea, Ivory Coast
South America	Andes Mountain highland Indians
LOW SEROPREVALENCE (1–<5%)	
Caribbean	Barbados
West Africa	Southern Chad, Nigeria
America	Native Alaskans
Philippines	Aeta Aborigines

[a]Among adults ≥ 40 years of age in the general population.

the infection was likely carried by the slave trade from West Africa. In West Africa there is a scattering of low-to-moderate prevalence of infection ranging from about 1% to as high as 15% (de Thé and Gessain, 1988; Levine et al, 1988; Delaport et al, 1989; Verdier et al; 1989). Of interest, the infection has been found among a Pygmy population in the Central African Republic (Gessain et al, 1993). The infection is also present among several Amerindian tribes in South America (Zaninovic et al, 1994) and native Alaskans (Kaplan et

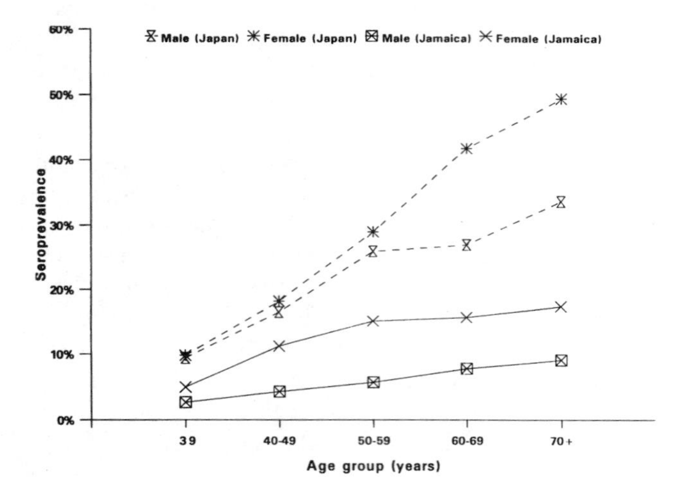

FIG. 24–3. Age-specific incidence of HTLV-I by sex in Miyazaki Cohort (Japan) and Jamaican food handlers. Jamaican data adapted from Murphy et al, 1991.

al, 1991). A third focus has been characterized in Aboriginal peoples in the South Pacific (Madeleine et al, 1993; Yanagihara, 1992).

The explanation for this unique geographic pattern appears to come from phylogenetic analysis on viral isolates from the scattered populations. Given the high level of transcription fidelity of HTLV-I, it appears that the present geographic endemicity reflects the ancient migration patterns of initially infected populations. These data also suggest that the origin of the infection is likely in the Indo-Malay region (Gessain et al, 1992; Saksena et al, 1992).

In the endemic populations, infection rates are quite low and stable among children, reflecting perinatal infection (Kusuhara et al, 1987). There is a slow increase with advancing age, which plateaus among men at about age 50. Among older women rates continue to increase with age (Tajima et al, 1987; Mueller et al, 1990) (Fig. 24–3). Infection in adults appears to be due primarily to sexual exposure (Murphy et al, 1989; Stuver et al, 1993) and, to a much lesser extent, through transfusion of infected blood cells. The divergence of seroprevalence curves after age 50 likely reflects the greater probability of heterosexual transmission from men than vice versa (Stuver et al, 1993).

ADULT T-CELL LEUKEMIA/LYMPHOMA

ATL, an aggressive malignancy of mature T lymphocytes, was first recognized as a distinct entity by Japanese clinicians in the 1970s (Uchiyama et al, 1977). The syndrome is characterized by hypercalcemia, cutaneous involvement, and depressed cellular immunity (T- and B-cell Malignancy Study Group, 1981). Although the malignant cells are of an activated T-helper cell phenotype, they function as suppressor cells in cell culture (Yamada, 1983).

A spectrum of premalignant states have been described. All are distinguishable by the detection on peripheral blood smears of abnormal ("flower-like") lymphocytes which are characteristic of ATL (Kim and Durack, 1988). These cells are also phenotypically CD4+ and CD25+, and are thought to contain the HTLV-I genome (Matutes et al, 1986). The premalignant states can be distinguished by the clonality of viral integration (polyclonal versus monoclonal) and by the presence or absence of symptoms.

Yamaguchi et al (1988) have described 15 individuals with polyclonal integration of HTLV-I and a low level of circulating abnormal lymphocytes (≤2%). Fourteen of these were patients who were seen for a variety of complaints suggestive of immune dysfunction. Of these, one case showed a subsequent loss of circulating detectable abnormal lymphocytes and one progressed to ATL during up to 3 years of follow-up. In an earlier report, five persons with low levels of circulating abnormal lymphocytes (≤2%) were detected due to presentation with either skin or infectious problems, and were followed for extended periods of time. Of these, two developed ATL (Yamaguchi et al, 1983). Clonality was not determined. Kinoshita et al (1985) have described and followed 18 cases with 10 to 40% circulating abnormal lymphocytes. Of these, 14 had monoclonally integrated HTLV-I genome. Ten of the 18 presented with a rash or infectious complications. Of 13 followed for more than 1 year, three developed ATL (mean follow-up, 4.1 years), three had persistent lymphocytosis (4.4 years), and seven had regression of abnormalities (2.8 years).

Virus-Specific Data

Antibodies against HTLV-I have been consistently detected in sera from nearly all ATL patients in endemic areas (Hinuma et al, 1981; Robert-Guroff et al, 1982). All show monoclonal integration of HTLV-I provirus in their malignant cells (Yoshida et al, 1985). The integration sites differ between patients, and no oncogene has been identified, suggesting that another mechanism of oncogenesis is involved, probably involving transactivation (Seiki et al, 1983, 1984). We have found that ATL patients have a significantly lower prevalence of antibodies to p40 by radioimmunoprecipitation assay, in comparison to healthy carriers. However, whether this is true prior to disease manifestation is unknown (Yokota et al, 1989).

Cofactors

It was initially proposed that risk of ATL was associated with undernutrition and with repeated exposure to filariasis in childhood, as both of these conditions were common in the past in endemic areas of Japan (Tajima and Hinuma, 1984). However, in view of the evidence of immunosuppression in premalignant disease, it is likely that the association of disseminated filariasis with ATL is not a primary event (Nakada et al, 1987). In addition, Neva et al (1989) have reported no difference in the prevalence of antibody against *S. stercoralis* between HTLV-I carriers and controls in Jamaica. We have reported that asymptomatic carriers have significantly reduced response to PPD antigen challenge. This reduction is strongest among carriers over age 60 years, suggesting that immune suppression is a late correlate of the disease process (Tachibana et al, 1988; Murai et al, 1990).

Tajima and Hinuma (1984) also proposed that early age at infection may be another modifier of risk, since the sex ratio among ATL cases is essentially equal (with some male predominance), similar to the ratio of seroprevalence among children following perinatal infection, and quite different from the sex ratio among older persons (Fig. 24–4). Further, the age–incidence curve of ATL is unimodal, peaking at about age 50 and decreasing thereafter (Kondo et al, 1987; Murphy et al, 1989). This distribution suggests that the cases share a very early etiologic exposure (Doll, 1978).

Genetic susceptibility to HTLV-I–induced malignancy has been considered. Several investigations have evaluated the HLA phenotype of ATL patients; however, the findings have been inconsistent (Tajima et al, 1984; Tanaka et al, 1984; Usuku et al, 1988; T- and B-Cell Malignancy Study Group, 1988; Uno et al, 1988). Usuku et al (1988) and Sonoda et al (1993) have found what appears to be two subgroups as identified by HLA phenotype in Kagoshima who differ in their cellular immune response to HTLV-I in vitro. *High responders* appear to be associated with risk of HTLV-I–associated myelopathy, an autoimmune type disorder observed in <1% of carriers. *Low responders* are associated with the occurrence of ATL.

Based on these observations, a potential model for the pathogenesis of ATL would include several steps: early infection, development of detectable circulating polyclonally transformed T cells, increasing immunosuppression, expansion of a monoclonal pool of cells, and progression to malignancy. In this process, a central role for tax, the transactivating gene product, has been postulated by several leading scientists (Yoshida et al, 1984; Haseltine et al, 1985).

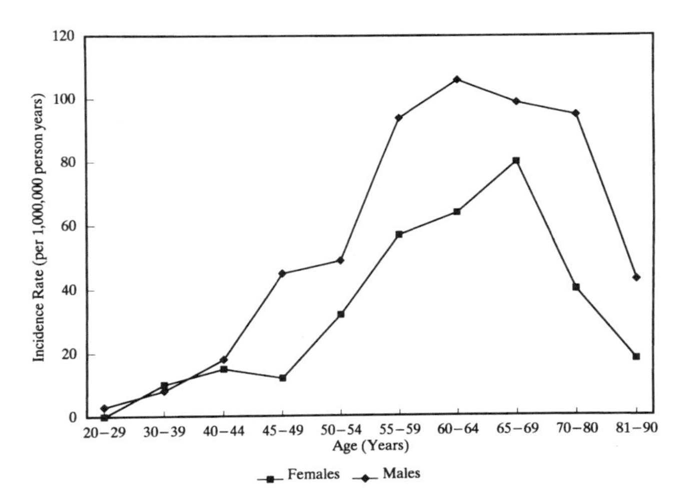

FIG. 24–4. Age-specific incidence of ATL in Kyushu Prefecture, Japan, 1986–87, by sex. (Adapted from Tajima et al, 1990).

Unresolved Issues and Prevention

It is clear that infection with HTLV-I results in the occurrence of malignancy in a subset of carriers. However, the actual risk is not established. Based on age-specific incidence estimated for Tsushima Island, the cumulative lifetime incidence among all carriers is about 5% (Tajima et al, 1987). Based on data from the Miyazaki Cohort Study the estimate is 2–3%. However, if risk of ATL is limited to only those who are infected perinatally, the cumulative risk in that group would be substantially higher. Murphy et al (1989) have modelled the risk for those infected prior to age 20 using population data in Jamaica; their estimate for lifetime risk of ATL for that group alone is about 4%. Reconciliation of these discrepant estimates will depend on the accrual of longitudinal population-based data; standardization for life expectancy differences between these populations is also necessary.

Based on the observational evidence that perinatal transmission occurs primarily through breast milk, there is now an uncontrolled intervention trial in Nagasaki Prefecture, in which carrier mothers are advised not to breast-feed, which finds a substantial reduction in the rate of infant infection (Hino et al, 1987, 1994). If it is true that risk is related to very early infection, then with time, the incidence of ATL in this area should approach zero. However, the generalizability of this intervention to populations with poor nutrition is questionable. Of note are findings from several observational studies in Japan that suggest that breast-feeding for less than 6 months is not associated with increased transmission (Takahashi et al, 1991; Hirata et al, 1992; Wiktor et al, 1993). In addition, several investigators have found that perinatal transmission is associated with high maternal antibody titer against the HTLV-I—especially to the tax protein (Hino et al, 1987; Sawada et al, 1989). These indices of viral status could be used to identify those mothers most likely to transmit in intervention programs.

Of more immediate public health value is the identification of clinically relevant markers of premalignant status. With the identification of the subset of carriers who are at high risk of developing ATL, potential therapeutic interventions can be considered.

HEPATITIS B VIRUS

HBV is a double-stranded virus that contains a single-stranded region of variable length (Summers et al, 1975). It is a member of a family of hepatotrophic DNA viruses called hepadnaviruses, which have similar genomic structures and replicate by similar mechanisms (Robinson et al, 1982).

Hepadnaviruses are unique among DNA viruses because they all replicate through an RNA intermediate by reverse transcription (Summers and Mason, 1982). The virion, or "Dane particle," is a spherical particle 42 nm in diameter. It contains an outer protein coat, hepatitis B surface antigen (HBsAg), and an inner core protein hepatitis B core antigen (HBcAg) (Dane et al, 1970). Located within the core are the viral genome and a DNA polymerase (Tiollais et al, 1988). Excess HBsAg is synthesized during viral replication, resulting in the production of 22 nm spherical particles and rod-shaped particles which are 22 nm in width and variable in length. All morphologic forms are found in the peripheral blood (Fig. 24–5).

The HBV genome contains four genes: "S," "C," "pol," and "X." The products of these genes are expressed during HBV infection and have been identified in human serum and/or in infected hepatocytes (Tiollais et al, 1988). S encodes the envelope protein, HBsAg; C, the core protein, HBcAg; pol, the polymerase; and X, a protein of uncertain function, probably located in replication complexes (core-like particles) in hepatocyte cytoplasm. Two pre-S regions are present which are expressed with S to yield proteins larger than HBsAg. There is evidence that the pre-S regions are involved in binding the virus to the hepatocyte membrane (Pontisso et al, 1987). The amino terminal region of the C gene encodes the hepatitis B e antigen (HBeAg). Its production is regulated by a short pre-C DNA sequence. The X protein may bind or interact with the p-53 protein (Feitelson et al, 1993) and thereby deregulate the cell cycle.

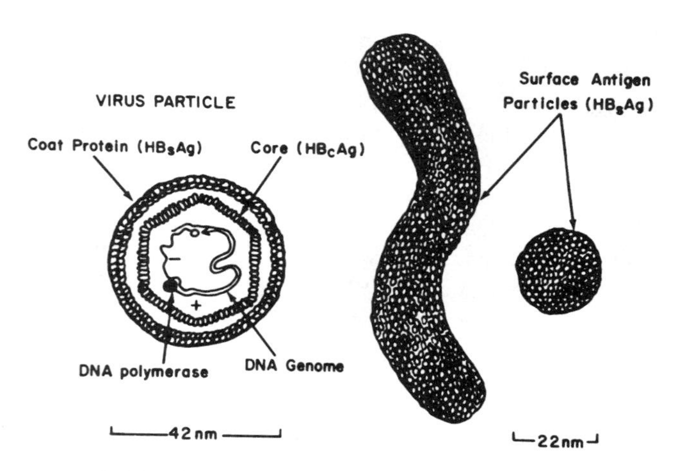

FIG. 24–5. Morphologic forms of hepatitis B virus. The non-infectious surface antigen particles are always produced in great excess over the complete virus particles (virions, Dane particles).

Host Response

Hepadnaviruses primarily infect the liver, but they can also infect certain other cells and tissues, including the pancreas, lymphocytes, and monocytes. After exposure to HBV, the time until the first appearance of virus (HBsAg) in the blood may be as short as 2 weeks or as long as 6 months, depending mainly on the dose of virus. Infections can be transient or chronic and can result in subclinical, mild, severe, or fulminant hepatitis. In general, the course of infection is determined by the age at infection. In infants HBV infection carries a high risk of chronicity and is usually subclinical, whereas in adults infection is likely to be transient and accompanied by clinical signs and symptoms of hepatitis. Seventy to 90% of infants exposed to HBV at birth via an infected mother will develop a chronic infection. By contrast, only 5%–10% of adults will develop a chronic infection (Hoofnagle et al, 1978).

The serologic profiles of response in acute and chronic infections are quite different. HBsAg is usually the first marker detected in both types of infection. In transient infections HBsAg may be present for a few days or up to several months. HBeAg appears in the circulation at about the same time as HBsAg (Werner and Blumberg, 1978). As its presence correlates with viremia, HBeAg is a good marker of infectivity and of active viral replication in the liver (Werner et al, 1977). In acute infection, e antigen is generally present for a few days to a few weeks.

If HBsAg persists in the blood for more than 6 months, there is a greater than 90% probability that the patient will remain HBsAg+ indefinitely, meaning that the patient will be a chronic carrier (London et al, 1977). In chronic infections, HBeAg may be present for years, but it disappears more quickly than HBsAg. Only 1% of HBsAg+ persons will become HBsAg− each year, whereas 10%–12% of HBeAg+ persons will become HBeAg− every year (Alward et al, 1985). The persistent presence of HBeAg is associated with an increased risk of developing severe forms of chronic liver disease, including chronic active hepatitis, cirrhosis, and HCC. IgM antibody to HBcAg also appears in the early phase of infection. IgG anti-HBc antibodies tend to persist for the lifetime of the individual, whether or not a chronic infection is established.

In acute hepatitis essentially all hepatocytes become infected with HBV (Jilbert et al, 1992; Kajino et al, 1994). Until recently it was thought that in transient infections all infected hepatocytes were eliminated by cytotoxic T lymphocytes (Eddleston et al, 1982). Now it appears that cell killing by cytotoxic T cells accounts for only a small portion of hepadnavirus clearance from the liver. Other mechanisms that may be involved include an increase in cell turnover by increased programmed cell death (apoptosis) with replacement of infected hepatocytes with uninfected liver stem cells (Jilbert et al, 1992), inhibition of HBV gene expression in infected hepatocytes by cytokines released by T lymphocytes (Guidotti et al, 1994a), loss or inhibition of virus by cell division (Guidotti et al, 1994b), and spontaneous clearance of virus from non-dividing hepatocytes (Kajino et al, 1994). Whatever the mechanisms, over time, damaged hepatocytes are replaced, inflammatory cells disappear, neutralizing antibody develops, and the liver returns to a morphologically normal appearance.

In chronic hepatitis, for reasons that are poorly understood, some virus-infected hepatocytes escape elimination by the immune system and other clearance mechanisms. As infected cells die and new liver cells regenerate, they become infected with HBV which is produced by persisting cells that are still replicating the virus. These newly infected cells, in turn, become targets for the immune system.

There is also a second process which affects chronicity of infection and the immune response. HBV DNA may integrate into the host cell DNA of some hepatocytes. Such cells often express HBsAg, but rarely, if ever, express HBcAg. Cells with integrated viral sequences are also unlikely to replicate HBV, and therefore, they are resistant to immune responses directed at HBcAg in hepatocyte membranes. Over time, HBcAg+ cells gradually disappear from the liver, leaving only HBsAg+ cells. By this process inflammation is reduced but not entirely eliminated (Eddleston et al, 1982).

Epidemiology of Infection

In the United States and other low prevalence areas, HBV is spread mainly by exposure to contaminated blood through intravenous drug use and sexual contact with an HBV carrier. Since 1982 the Centers for Disease Control have monitored four sentinel counties in the United States for new cases of hepatitis B and have interviewed these patients to identify the probable mode of acquisition (Table 24–5) (Centers for Disease Control, 1988a). Sexual contact with a person infected with HBV accounted for about 30% of the cases. Intravenous drug use was associated with 25 to 28% of the cases. All other known risk factors, including health care exposures, blood transfusions, hemodialysis therapy, and exposure within institutions for the developmentally disabled accounted for less than 10% of the cases. In about a third of the cases, no source of infection was identified. Many of these "unknowns" were probably either sexual exposures or inapparent blood exposures such as sharing a toothbrush or razor with an HBV carrier.

In the highly endemic areas of Asia, including China, Taiwan, Vietnam, and Korea, about half of all chronic infections result from perinatal transmission by exposure of babies during birth to maternal blood containing HBV (Beasley, 1988). Usually such babies are born HBsAg− and become positive at the age of 6 weeks to 3 months (Beasley et al, 1977). There is both direct and indirect evidence that fetuses may be exposed to the virus in utero (Li et al, 1986; Stevens et al, 1985), and in some series, up to 10% of babies born to carrier mothers are viremic by the time of their birth (Stevens et al, 1988). Whether the virus found in the venous blood of some newborn babies is produced by the fetal liver or is maternal in origin is unknown.

In endemic areas outside of Asia, perinatal transmission is much less common. For example, among Alaska Eskimos, who have a carrier prevalence of 5%–10%, less than 5% of all chronic infections are the result of perinatal transmission (Estroff et al, 1985). In Alaska the phenomenon is explained by a much lower prevalence of HBeAg positivity among Eskimo women of reproductive age than among Asian women. In Africa there is also a low rate of HBeAg positivity with an additional, unidentified factor contributing to the low rate of perinatal transmission. African babies are very rarely infected in the first 6 months of life, even by HBeAg+ mothers (Marinier et al, 1985).

TABLE 24–5. *Risk Factors Associated with Reported Cases of Clinical Hepatitis B in four Sentinel Counties in the United States**

Risk Factor	Percentage of Cases with Risk Factor 1982 $n = 326^a$	1987 $n = 295^a$
Homosexuality	20	9
Intravenous drug abuse	15	28
Heterosexual activity[b]	15	22
Health care worker (frequent blood contact)	3	2
Household contact	<1	3
Blood transfusion	4	2
Dialysis	<1	<1
Resident of institution for developmentally disabled	1	1
No known source	42	32

*From Centers for Disease Control (1988[a])

[a]Number of cases interviewed within six months after onset of symptoms for risk factors that occurred within six months before onset of symptoms.

[b]Sexual contact with a known hepatitis B patient, an HBV carrier, or with multiple partners.

HEPATOCELLULAR CARCINOMA

Current evidence strongly supports the hypothesis that chronic infection with HBV is the most significant etiologic factor in HCC and is associated with about 80% of HCC incidence worldwide. There is a direct correlation between the prevalence of HBV carriers in a country and the incidence of HCC. Case–control studies in all areas of the world have consistently shown a prevalence of HBsAg higher in cases with HCC than in appropriate controls (London, 1981). The strongest evidence for an etiologic association has come from prospective studies. The largest and most convincing of these have been those by Beasley and his colleagues in Taiwan (Beasley et al, 1981; Beasley, 1988). In these studies, chronic carriers have a relative risk of HCC of about 100 compared with non-carriers. Among chronic adult male carriers in Taiwan, China, Japan, and Alaska, the annual incidence of HCC is about four to five cases per thousand men (Beasley, 1988). The incidence of HCC among carrier women is much lower, but, because prospective studies have been limited to carrier men, with the exception of studies in Alaska, no precise estimates are available.

Virus-Specific Data

HBV is closely associated with HCC at the cellular level. In studies using immunohistologic methods, HBsAg has been found in non-tumor cells surrounding primary liver cancers in 50% to 90% of patients with HCC. In cancer cells, HBsAg was detected much less frequently (Nayak et al, 1977; Nazarewicz et al, 1977). Extracts of the DNA of HCC tissues have revealed integrated HBV DNA sequences in virtually all cases that have HBsAg in the serum, as well as in 10% to 20% of HBsAg−, anti-HBs+ cases (Shafritz et al, 1981; Brechot et al, 1982). No preferred integration site in the hepatocyte genome has been identified. Usually the integrated HBV DNA sequences are considerably rearranged and contain deletions. This is thought to be the reason that viral proteins are not commonly expressed in HCC cells.

Cofactors

In humans there are probably cofactors which interact with chronic HBV infection to produce HCC. As noted above, male chronic carriers are much more likely to develop HCC than female carriers. Androgens, male-associated behaviors, and high iron stores in men have been proposed as explanations for this difference in risk (Blumburg, 1986; Beasley, 1988). Mycotoxins such as aflatoxin-B are carcinogenic in their own right, and ingestion of these compounds in all likelihood accelerates the development of HCC and increases the likelihood that HCC will develop in an HBV carrier (Wogan, 1976). Similarly, the consumption of alcohol, which is hepatotoxic, probably has a promotional effect on an HBV-infected liver by increasing cell death and hepatocyte regeneration (Lieber et al, 1986). A further discussion of these cofactors is presented in Chapter 36.

Synthesis of Present Knowledge

Although many theories have been proposed, the precise role of HBV in hepatocarcinogenesis is unknown (London and Buetow, 1988). Histopathologic studies have demonstrated that in most cases HCC arises in an already abnormal liver. Eighty percent of the cases have cirrhosis and 10%–15% have chronic active or chronic persistent hepatitis. Since most HBV infections that lead to HCC are initiated in the perinatal period or in early childhood and most cases do not occur until the fifth decade of life, the events in the process of carcinogenesis must take place during this long latent period. It is unknown whether chronic hepatitis and cirrhosis are precipitating events in the progress to cancer or are merely correlated disease processes which also take place over a prolonged time period.

All available sources of evidence, including epidemiology, pathology, molecular biology, and experimental induction, indicate that HBV can cause HCC and is the probable cause of HCC in at least 80% of the cases worldwide. A working group of the IARC has stated that "chronic infection with hepatitis B virus is carcinogenic to humans" and thus is classified as a Group 1 carcinogen (IARC, 1994). However, there are two missing pieces of information which would provide the final links in the chain. First, the prevention of HBV infection should also prevent HCC in those populations in which HCC has been endemic. Second, the elimination of HBV infection in already chronically infected persons should greatly reduce their risk of HCC.

Treatment

Interferon-α is the only currently available, effective therapy for chronic hepatitis B. A meta-analysis of 15 randomized controlled studies that included 837 adult subjects, published between 1986 and 1992, showed a demonstrable benefit in selected patients (Wong et al, 1993). The main outcome variable was the frequency of conversion from HBeAg+ (a surrogate marker of viral replication) to HBeAg−. Following 6 to 12 months of interferon-α therapy, HBeAg loss was 33% compared with 12% among the untreated patients; similarly, loss of HBV DNA was 37% vs. 17% and loss of HBsAg was 7.8% vs. 1.8%. It is unknown whether the risk of cirrhosis or HCC is reduced in patients who respond favorably to this treatment. There is no information regarding whether there are long-term adverse effects on the two-thirds of patients who fail to respond to interferon-α. Furthermore, interferon therapy is very expensive, requires parenteral administration 3 or more times a week for 6 months, and is often accompanied by significant side effects.

Prevention

The United States Food and Drug Administration approved the license for commercial distribution of the plasma-based hepatitis B vaccine in 1982 and in 1987 approved a yeast-based recombinant vaccine. Both vaccines have been shown in clinical trials to be safe and effective. Over 50 million doses of the plasma-based vaccine have been administered with no serious side effects. Neither HBV infection itself nor HIV has ever been transmitted by the vaccine.

A large-scale prospective study is in progress in Gambia to determine whether vaccination against HBV will prevent the development of HCC (Gambia Hepatitis Study Group, 1987). Although it may take 40 years to complete the study, in 10 to 15 years sufficient information may be available to adequately test this hypothesis. In the meantime, nationwide programs for the vaccination of all newborns are being introduced in many countries in Asia and to a lesser extent in Africa. In the United States and Europe, the testing for HBsAg of all pregnant women has been recommended (Centers for Disease Control, 1988b). Babies born to positive women are currently immunized at birth with hyperimmune globulin and hepatitis B vaccine. The Immunization Practices Advisory Committee (ACIP) of the Centers for Disease Control and Prevention now recommends that all babies in the United States be vaccinated against HBV at birth or in the first few months of life (ACIP, 1991). If the hypothesis that chronic HBV infection is the major cause of HCC is correct, then these measures should result in a drop in the incidence of HCC to very low levels within the first generation.

HEPATITIS C VIRUS (HCV)

HCV is a single positive-stranded RNA virus of about 9,400 nucleotides (Houghton et al, 1991) that is similar in molecular structure to Flaviviruses (yellow fever virus, Dengue virus) and even more closely related to Pestiviruses like hog cholera virus and bovine diarrhea virus (Miller et al, 1990). Both of these groups of viruses belong to the Flaviviradae family (Collett et al, 1988). Therefore, HCV has been tentatively classified as a genus among the Flaviviradae (Bradley et al, 1993). The HCV genome consists of a single open reading frame which apparently codes for one large polyprotein of 3,010 amino acids. This large polyprotein is processed into seven proteins which, by analogy with the flaviviruses, have been labelled C (core), E1 (envelope 1, a glycoprotein), E2/NS1 (non-structural 1), NS2, NS3, NS4, and NS5. The functions of these proteins are poorly understood. A replicase function for NS5 and helicase and protease functions for NS3 have been postulated (Okamoto et al, 1991). The genomic HCV RNA positive strand is transcribed into a minus strand RNA. There are no DNA intermediate forms and HCV does not integrate into the host cell genome (Choo et al, 1989). The lack of tissue culture and laboratory animal models has limited the investigation of HCV replication. In fact, the molecular characterization of HCV has proceeded much more rapidly than has understanding of its virology, immunology, or biology (Houghton et al, 1991).

History

HCV was discovered as a result of investigations of the cause of non-A, non-B hepatitis. Until very recently, the diagnosis of non-A, non-B hepatitis was one of exclusion. It was reserved for cases of acute or chronic hepatitis that, according to serologic tests, were not caused by hepatitis A or B viruses or other viruses that can cause liver damage, such as the EBV or CMV. Two types of non-A, non-B disease had been recognized: (1) an epidemic, acute hepatitis probably spread by contaminated water; and (2) a sporadic hepatitis that frequently became chronic and was blood transmitted. The agent which causes the enterically transmitted hepatitis has been identified as a single-stranded RNA virus that appears to differ significantly from other mammalian RNA virus families (Tam et al, 1991). It has been named hepatitis E virus (HEV). Because it does not cause chronic infections and has not been associated with chronic liver disease or liver cancer, HEV will not be discussed further here.

Although many aspects of the blood-transmitted non-A, non-B virus remain elusive, serum assays have been developed that are reasonably specific for detection of antibodies to the agent (Kuo et al, 1989) and its nucleic acid (Weiner et al, 1990; Kaneko et al, 1990). These assays have permitted initial epidemiologic studies and preliminary characterization of the virus now termed HCV.

The existence of a blood-borne non-A, non-B virus was proposed shortly after blood banks began routine testing of donors for HBV (Prince et al, 1974). A series of studies in the following 15 years provided clear epidemiologic, experimental, and pathological evidence of a blood-transmitted virus, different from the known hepatitis viruses, which could cause chronic hepatitis, cirrhosis, and possibly HCC (Feinstone et al, 1975; Knodell et al, 1977; H. Alter et al, 1978, 1982; Tabor et al, 1978; Aach et al, 1981). Attempts to identify the virus or specific host antibodies were futile until molecular biological techniques were applied to the problem.

It is beyond the scope of this chapter to review in depth the experiments that led to the present state of knowledge of HCV. The story is remarkable, however, and reading the original reports of Houghton and his colleagues is recommended (Choo et al, 1989; Kuo et al, 1989). Briefly, they extracted and cloned the nucleic acids from a large pool of infectious plasma (from an experimentally infected chimpanzee) into an expression vector and screened the proteins produced by the resulting DNA library for binding with antibodies in a serum sample from a patient with chronic non-A, non-B hepatitis. Among a million clones, only five tested positive; and of these five, only one appeared on subsequent testing to be specifically associated with non-A, non-B hepatitis. This clone was then used to both produce polypeptides for serological tests and to recover the cDNA insert for hybridization studies. The candidate nucleic acid sequence was not encoded in the human or chimpanzee genome, nor was it derived from a DNA intermediate. Eventually, the investigators were able to clone and sequence a single-stranded, approximately 9,400 nucleotide RNA virus.

Experiments in chimpanzees have documented that HCV infects the liver (Shimizu et al, 1990; Jacob et al, 1991), but it is likely that it also infects other tissues including macrophages and lymphocytes (Qian et al, 1992; Hsieh et al, 1992) in the peripheral blood and possibly the kidney and pancreas. The amount of virus circulating in the blood and the quantity in the liver is very low. It is detected by polymerase chain reaction (PCR) amplification methods in serum (Kaneko et al, 1990; Garson et al, 1990; Weiner et al, 1990) and by immunohistochemistry (Hiramatsu et al, 1992; Krawczynski et al, 1992) and molecular methods (Fong et al, 1991; Akyol et al, 1992) in liver tissue. No animal, other than the chimpanzee, has been found susceptible to HCV infection and no naturally occurring HCV-related animal virus has been identified.

Host Response

Many studies have demonstrated that antibodies to HCV are found in 50 to 80% of transfusion recipients who acquired non-A, non-B hepatitis (H. Alter et al,

1989; Van der Poel et al, 1990; Roggendorf et al, 1990; Mosley et al, 1990). These studies also showed that one or more of the blood donors of these patients had detectable antibodies to HCV. Usually the antibody response to HCV infection was delayed. In one study, the mean time for appearance of antibodies to HCV nonstructural proteins following transfusion was almost 22 weeks; this was 15 weeks after the onset of clinical symptoms (H. Alter et al, 1989). Second generation and immunoblot assays have shown that antibodies to the core and envelope proteins appear earlier, about 2 weeks after infection (Mattson et al, 1992). The development of antibodies to either structural or non-structural HCV proteins is unrelated to resolution of infection. It is likely that the cellular immune response to HCV is responsible for the liver damage that usually accompanies acute and chronic infection. Because so little is known about the virology and biology of HCV, the cellular immune response has also not been adequately characterized as yet.

Studies in chimpanzees have shown that the antibodies generated during the course of infection do not protect against subsequent exposure to either the infecting strain or heterologous strains of HCV (Farci et al, 1992; Prince et al, 1992). Neutralizing antibodies have been detected in humans, but they fail to prevent the emergence of viral mutants that escape neutralization (Shimizu et al, 1994).

Epidemiology of Infection

HCV is transmitted by the parenteral route. Other routes of transmission probably occur, but have been difficult to document. Forty percent of patients with acute hepatitis C in the United States have no identifiable risk factor for infection (M. Alter et al, 1990). Persons at greatest risk of infection are intravenous drug users (M. Alter et al, 1990; van den Hoek et al, 1990), hemodialysis patients (Schlipkoter et al, 1990; Yamaguchi et al, 1990), blood transfusion recipients (whole blood, cellular components, or plasma) (H. Alter et al, 1989; van der Poel et al, 1990), and health care workers exposed to blood (M. Alter et al, 1990). Unlike HIV and HBV, transmission of HCV from health care workers to patients has not been observed (Centers for Disease Control, 1991).

Several studies of patients with chronic renal failure undergoing hemodialysis have found a prevalence of HCV infection of greater than 20% (Hayashi et al, 1991; Evans et al, 1990; Kuhns et al, 1994). These high rates cannot be ascribed to exposure to blood transfusions alone, because in the absence of any blood transfusions high prevalence was still observed (Hayashi et al, 1991; Fabrizi et al, 1993). In one study, patients with renal insufficiency who had not been dialyzed had anti-HCV antibodies at about the same frequency as the dialysis patients (Evans et al, 1990). What the routes of transmission in these instances may be is unknown. No evidence has been reported of HCV transmission through common environmental exposures such as sharing meals or eating utensils, sneezing, coughing, or causal person-to-person contact (Centers for Disease Control, 1991), but transmission by these routes has not been thoroughly investigated in hemodialysis units or among the general population.

Sexual transmission of HCV is less common than such transmissions of HBV and HIV, but probably does occur. Case–control studies of HCV-infected persons (M. Alter et al, 1989) showed that persons with non-A, non-B hepatitis with no history of parenteral exposures were more likely to have had sexual contacts with persons who had a past history of hepatitis. Among patients attending sexually transmitted disease clinics, both heterosexual men and women and homosexual men had significantly higher prevalence of anti-HCV antibodies (5%–15%) than those found in control populations (1% or less) (Hess et al, 1989; Esteban et al, 1989; Stevens and Taylor, 1991; Thomas et al, 1994). Studies of the sexual partners of hepatitis C viremic individuals have revealed very low levels of transmission (Bresters et al, 1993; Brackmann et al, 1993). Men who carry both HIV and HCV are more likely to transmit HCV to their sex partners than men infected with HCV alone (Eyster et al, 1991), but the rate of such transmissions is still very low (<3%).

Stevens and Taylor (1991) concluded from seroepidemiologic evidence that perinatal transmission, which is also common with HBV and HIV, rarely occurs with HCV. In those instances in which maternal transmission has been documented, the mothers have had high titers of viremia (Lin et al, 1994; Ohto et al, 1994). When the mother is infected with HCV and HIV, however, transmission to the neonate may be more likely. In one study, 44% of 25 babies born to such women became infected with HCV (and with HIV) (Giovannini et al, 1990). Other studies have not confirmed an increased maternal transmission rate with HIV coinfection (Marcellin et al, 1993).

Many of the flavi- and pestiviruses are transmitted by insects. It is not known whether insect vectors are involved in the transmission of HCV, but at our current stage of knowledge the possibility of arthropod transmission should not be dismissed.

Liver Disease and Hepatocellular Carcinoma

What is most important about HCV infections is that they usually become chronic and have the potential to cause severe forms of chronic liver disease. Longitudinal studies of community-acquired HCV, identified among patients with acute hepatitis, suggest such infections become chronic in almost all patients who develop antibodies to HCV (M. Alter et al, 1992). Initial case reports and case series implied that of the individuals who became chronically infected, 20%–50% developed chronic active hepatitis and cirrhosis, and 25%–50% of the patients with serious liver disease after 15 to 30 years developed HCC (Kiyosawa et al, 1990; Tremolada et al, 1990). More recent studies indicate that two-thirds of chronically infected individuals develop some form of chronic liver disease (M. Alter, 1994) and 20% of all patients with chronic hepatitis C progress to cirrhosis over a period of 20 years (Mendenhall et al, 1991, Mondelli and Colombo, 1991). The route of infection does not appear to affect this risk.

Soon after the development of the first generation tests for detecting anti-HCV antibodies, several groups reported cross-sectional studies of the prevalence of HCV antibodies in various forms of chronic liver diseases (Table 24–6). Although concerns were raised about the specificity of the first generation assays, it is likely that most of these cases were truly associated with chronic HCV infection. In areas where HBV is endemic, dual infections with HBV and HCV have been reported (Colombo et al, 1989; Chen, 1991). Although dual infections may increase the risk of serious liver disease over that imparted by chronic infection with either virus alone, critical studies to test this hypothesis have not been done.

Several studies have shown associations of HCV with HCC in both HBsAg+ and HBsAg− cases. In a population-based case–control study of 50 cases of HCC from Los Angeles County, Yu et al (1990) reported a synergistic effect of infection with HBV and HCV on HCC. The RR for anti-HCV alone was 4.8, for HBV markers alone was 4.4, and for both markers together was significantly higher than either alone (>14). There were 10 HCC cases, but no controls, with dual infections. The source of HCV infection in these HCC patients was not apparent; 10 of 15 had no history of blood transfusion. Kaklamani et al (1991), reported similar observations from a hospital-based case–control study of HCC in Greece; anti-HCV positivity alone was associated with a RR of 4.8; anti-HCV with HBsAg positivity had a RR of 20. More recent case–control studies, using second generation assays, have uniformly shown high RRs, ranging from 10 to 75 (Tanaka et al, 1991; Stroffolini et al, 1992; Zavitsanos et al, 1992). These studies also appear to support a higher risk of HCC associated with dual HCV and HBV infections, but the numbers of coinfected individuals in such studies are too few to draw firm conclusions.

Recent studies using molecular methods to examine histopathological specimens of liver and tumor from patients with HCV associated HCC have demonstrated HCV RNA plus and minus strands in tumor and adjacent non-tumor tissue (Haruna et al, 1994; Kobayashi et al, 1994). Such studies suggest that HCV may replicate in HCC cells and participate directly in the carcinogenesis process.

Mechanism of Carcinogenesis

Based on current evidence, HCV is an RNA virus that does not replicate through DNA intermediates and therefore cannot integrate into the host cell genome. If this statement is correct, then other models of oncogenesis must be considered (London and Buetow, 1988). HCV-associated chronic hepatitis and cirrhosis are likely mediated by immunologic response to the infection. The increased death rate of hepatocytes in these diseases results in increased cell division and hence, increased opportunities for mutational events. As proposed by London and Blumberg (1982) with respect to chronic HBV infection, the cellular immune response to HCV may be directed against mature hepatocytes, thereby selectively promoting the division of immature

TABLE 24–6. *Prevalence of Antibodies to Hepatitis C Virus in HBsAg Negative Cases of Chronic Liver Disease and Primary Hepatocellular Carcinoma*

Country	*Controls*	*Chronic Hepatitis*	*Cirrhosis*	*PHC*	*Reference*
Italy	—	86/132 (65%)	—	64/91 (70%)	Colombo et al (1990)
Spain	13/177 (7%)	—	59/106 (56%)	72/96 (75%)	Bruix et al (1990)
France	—	—	14/70 (20%)	21/74 (28%)	Ducreux et al (1990)
	12/1296 (1%)	92/120 (77%)	—	—	Ouzan et al (1990)
Taiwan	40/420 (10%)	28/43 (65%)	11/25 (44%)	15/24 (63%)	Chen (1991)
Japan	—	210/305 (69%)	147/201 (73%)	144/201 (72%)	Mitamura et al (1990)
U.S.	5/115 (4%)	—	—	5/29 (17%)	Yu et al (1990)

hepatocytes or liver stem cells. Such cells have a greater capacity for cell division than mature hepatocytes, and mutations in immature cells would carry a greater risk of oncogenesis than mutations in mature liver cells. In a test of this hypothesis, Tarao et al (1994) performed liver biopsies on 28 patients with early (Child's stage A) cirrhosis and antibodies to HCV. Using bromodeoxyuridine labelling of the liver tissues as a measure of cell proliferation, they categorized the patients as having high DNA synthesis activity (above the median) or low or lower DNA synthesis activity. After 3 years of follow-up, 9 of the 14 patients with high DNA synthesis activity developed HCC compared with 2 of the 14 patients with low or lower DNA synthesis activity.

Other observations related to HCV infection may be relevant to the virus's oncogenic potential, but at the current stage of knowledge it is difficult to fit these into a model. Defective, subgenomic virus particles appear to be present in some HCV-infected hepatocytes (Houghton et al, 1991). Such particles may have a role in promoting chronicity. In experiments like those of Choo et al (1989), Mishiro et al (1990) isolated a cDNA clone from the plasma of a chimpanzee experimentally infected with a human non-A, non-B hepatitis agent. This clone had unusual characteristics. It was not similar to any HCV sequences, but was present in a single copy in the human genome. It coded for a protein designated GOR by the investigators. Antibodies to GOR were found in most patients with HCV-associated hepatitis, cirrhosis, and HCC but rarely in the general population, in HBV carriers, or in cases of HBV-associated HCC. Takahashi et al (1990) also described a host-encoded protein associated with HCV infection, which was involved in microtubule assembly. Expression of these proteins during HCV infection may reflect effects of site-specific binding of HCV proteins to host DNA.

Examination of HCV isolates has revealed significant nucleotide and amino acid sequence heterogeneity. At least four virus genotypes have been recognized and two or more other genotypes have been provisionally identified (Okamato et al, 1992; Simmonds et al, 1994). Genotypes differ in their geographic distribution; dual infections with more than one virus genotype can occur (Houghton et al, 1991). In one study, type II (1b) HCV was associated with more severe liver disease than type I (1a) (Pozzato et al, 1991), but more recent studies have not found an association of genotype with type or severity of liver disease (Yamada et al, 1994).

Within an infected individual several different but related genotypes, called *quasispecies*, may co-exist (Weiner et al, 1992; Murakami et al, 1992). How these quasispecies might affect the pathogenesis of HCV is under investigation.

Treatment

About 50% of both acute and chronic HCV infections respond well to treatment with natural (Omata et al, 1991) or recombinant interferons (Hoofnagle and Di Bisceglie, 1989). In responding patients, HCV RNA disappears from the circulation, transaminase levels fall, and histologically the liver is improved. The recurrence rate after discontinuing interferon therapy, however, is high (50%–60%), and the long-term risks and benefits of interferon therapy are unknown.

Summary

HCV is a newly identified viral agent that is readily transmitted by parenteral inoculation. It appears to be etiologically associated with a majority of the cases of HCC in Europe, Japan, and the United States. Much will be learned in the next few years about the biology, epidemiology, and pathogenicity of this virus. Efforts are under way to develop an HCV vaccine. The failure of infected individuals to develop protective antibodies and the heterogeneity of viral strains, however, limit optimism that an effective vaccine will be developed in the near future.

PAPILLOMAVIRUSES

Biology and Epidemiology

Relatively little is known about the natural history of infection by human papillomaviruses (HPV). This is due to the fact that these viruses replicate only in highly differentiated epithelia and that an in vitro cultivation system has not been available. Much of our understanding of HPV is quite recent and comes from studies using recombinant DNA technology. As extensively reviewed by Koutsky et al (1988), Schneider and Koutsky (1992), and Schiffman (1994), it is now known that many different genotypes of HPV exist. Each is generally specific to a site of infection and a type of clinical manifestation; typically infections produce benign warts.

There are at least 19 types of HPV known to infect the genital tract and anus. Of these, types 16 and 18 are most closely associated with malignancy. The oncogenic potential of these two strains is underlined by the ability of specific encoded proteins to bind to tumor suppressor genes. This includes the E6 proteins from types 16 and 18 which bind to p53, and the E7 protein of strain 16 which binds to the retinoblastoma gene, RB1. In these cases, the genes' functions in regulating cell growth are compromised (Dyson et al, 1989; Werness et al, 1990).

The HPVs are non-enveloped icosahedral capsids containing double-stranded, circular DNA. These are exquisitely controlled, cell-associated viruses, whose life cycle is "intimately tied to the growth and differentiation of the host epithelial cell" (Koutsky et al, 1988). Transmission occurs by direct contact, such as genital-to-genital exposure, and it is likely facilitated by local abrasion (Oriel, 1971). There is evidence of perinatal infection but this needs to be evaluated further (Schneider and Koutsky, 1992).

Like all the other oncogenic viruses, HPV infections can persist as latent infections. However, it appears that at least in the cervix, many HPV infections are transient, with loss of detectable viral shedding. Thus on cross-sectional analysis, the peak occurrence of viral detection occurs among young women aged 15–35 years and then drops with age. This does not appear to represent a cohort effect (Schiffman, 1992, 1994). Whether the virus remains in a silent, undetectable latent state or is actually eliminated is unknown.

Cellular immunity clearly plays a role in the control of HPV infections since with immunosuppression, as from organ transplantation (Barr et al, 1989) or from pregnancy (Kistner and Hertig, 1955), the frequency and size of lesions increase. Furthermore, regressions are frequent, particularly with trauma, suggesting cytolytic immune reaction. The role of humoral response is unknown at present (Koutsky et al, 1988; Schiffman, 1994).

Because of the lack of a serologic assay suitable for seroepidemiologic studies, relatively little had been known about the epidemiology of genital HPV infection. Koutsky et al (1988) had noted that the incidence of clinically apparent genital warts, *condyloma acuminatum*, is common in the United States and the United Kingdom and appears to have been increasing recently, in parallel with the increased occurrence of genital herpes. However, there were no firm estimates of the prevalence of inapparent genital HPV infections.

Recently, antibody assays have been developed based on recombinant viral proteins which are now beginning to address these questions. However, the validity and performance of these assays need to be established, as does the identification of which antigens are important (Galloway, 1992). In general, cases who are virus positive also have higher antibodies against viral antigens than do controls (Köchel et al, 1991; Dillner et al, 1994; Kirnbauer et al, 1994).

Cancer of the Cervix

There is evidence that HPV infections are involved in a variety of malignancies. These include esophageal carcinoma (Chang et al, 1990), anal cancer (Daling et al, 1987), penile cancer (Maden et al, 1993), and oral cancer (Maden et al, 1992), as discussed elsewhere in this text. However, most of the research has focused on the association of HPV with carcinoma of the cervix.

The epidemiology of cervical cancer is similar to that of a venereally transmitted disease. Risk is associated with early age at first sexual intercourse and with the number of sexual partners of a woman and her partner (Nahmias et al, 1982; Buckley et al, 1981; Brinton, 1992). This epidemiology suggests that a venereally transmitted oncogenic infection plays a causal role.

The association between HPV and cervical cancer is now clearly established, based on the detection of viral genetic material in tumor tissue. As summarized by Koutsky et al (1988), case–control studies have been consistent in yielding a positive association between the detection of the DNA of HPV types 16 and 18 and cervical cancer risk, with relative risks ranging from two to infinity. The prevalence of detection among case series ranges from 45% to 92%. This variation may reflect the sensitivity of different assays (Caussy et al, 1988). Furthermore, it is also established that HPV infection directly precedes the occurrence of cervical intraepithelial neoplasia (Koutsky et al, 1992).

HPV infection may be much more prevalent than currently recognized (Tidy et al, 1989). If so, what may be most relevant are the factors associated with the establishment of persistence and the frequency of viral expression. Cofactors which influence the initial host response and viral dose are likely to be important. Such factors may include age at first sexual intercourse, frequency and type of other venereally transmitted infection, parity, smoking, and oral contraceptive use (Brinton et al, 1987).

Synthesis of Present Knowledge

zur Hausen (1986) has proposed a model by which HPV infection leads to the development of cervical cancer and other HPV-associated malignancies. This model proposes a sequential process of structural genetic changes in HPV-infected cells that lead to a malignant phenotype. These changes result from the failure of host cells to control persisting viral genes by the modification of controlling cellular genes that result from toxic exposures, such as smoking and other viral infections. Clearly, factors which selectively induce the turnover of HPV-infected differentiated epithelial cells could promote this process.

Resolution of the role of HPV in cervical cancer may come from large, well-designed case–control studies which obtain data on immunosuppressed high-risk women, with appropriate biologic sampling of early lesions. The presence of a substantial number of women infected with HIV provides such an opportunity (Bradbier, 1987). In addition, elucidation of the natural history of HPV-associated cervical cancer could serve as a paradigm for understanding the role of HPV in the pathogenesis of other associated malignancies. It is quite possible that HPV infections may prove to play a role in a wide range of malignancies.

CONCLUDING COMMENTS

It is encouraging to find that the naturally occurring animal models of virus-associated malignancy are a useful prototype for their human counterparts. The biologic processes involved also fit with our general concepts of carcinogenesis derived from experimental systems. The development of cancer appears to require at least two kinds of mechanisms, one which alters the genetic makeup of the target cell (initiation) and a second chronic exposure which induces cell division (promotion). All of the potentially latent human infections discussed above are capable of producing both effects. Perhaps the clearest example is that of HBV in HCC, where through integration of viral sequences in the cellular genome, chronic HBV infection can add new genetic information and can also cause rearrangements and deletions of cellular genes. The host response to chronic HBV infection leads to repeated cycles of cell death and cell division. This effect is strongly modified by age at infection and the premalignant state is serologically detectable. In terms of cancer control, it is unlikely that humans can be protected from all of these oncogenic infections. However, control may come from reducing the risk of chronic viremia—as in HBV—or less likely, from developing therapeutic interventions for those at high risk of malignancy.

REFERENCES

AACH RD, SZMUNESS W, MOSLEY JW, et al. 1981. Serum alanine aminotransferase of donors in relation to the risk of non-A, non-B hepatitis in recipients. N Engl J Med 304:989–994.

AKYOL G, DASH S, SHIEH YSC, et al. 1992. Detection of hepatitis C RNA sequences by polymerase chain reaction in fixed liver tissue. Mod Pathol 5:501–504.

ALTER HJ, PURCELL RH, FEINSTONE FM, TEGTMEIER GE. 1982. Non-A, non-B hepatitis: Its relationship to cytomegalovirus, chronic hepatitis and to direct and indirect test methods. *In* Szmuness W, Alter JH, Maynard JE (eds): Viral Hepatitis. 1981 International Symposium. Philadelphia, Franklin Institute Press, pp. 279–294.

ALTER HJ, PURCELL RH, HOLLAND PV, et al. 1978. Transmissible agent in non-A, non-B hepatitis. Lancet i:459–463.

ALTER HJ, PURCELL RH, SHIH JW, et al. 1989. Detection of antibody to hepatitis C virus in prospectively followed transfusion recipients with acute and chronic non-A and non-B hepatitis. N Engl J Med 321:494–500.

ALTER MJ. 1994. Review of serologic testing for hepatitis C virus infection and risk of posttransfusion hepatitis C. Arch Pathol Lab Med 118:342–345.

ALTER MJ, COLEMAN PJ, ALEXANDER WJ, et al. 1989. Importance of heterosexual activity in the transmission of hepatitis B and non-A, non-B hepatitis. JAMA 262:1201–1205.

ALTER MJ, HADLER SC, JUDSON FN, et al. 1990. Risk factors for acute non-A, non-B hepatitis in the United States and association with hepatitis C virus infection. JAMA 264:2231–2235.

ALTER MJ, MARGOLIS HS, KRAWCZYNSKI K, et al. 1992. The natural history of community-acquired hepatitis C in the United States. N Engl J Med 327:1899–1905.

ALWARD WLM, MCMAHON BJ, HALL DB, et al. 1985. The long-term serologic course of asymptomatic hepatitis B virus carriers and the development of primary hepatocellular carcinoma. J Infect Dis 151:604–609.

ANDERSON EN JR, ANDERSON ML, HO JHC. 1978. A study of the environmental backgrounds of young Chinese nasopharyngeal carcinoma patients. *In* de Thé G, Ito Y (eds): Nasopharyngeal Carcinoma: Etiology and Control. Lyon, France, International Agency for Research on Cancer, pp. 231–239.

BARR BB, MCLAREN K, SMITH IW, et al. 1989. Human papillomavirus infection and skin cancer in renal allograft recipients. Lancet 1:124–129.

BEASLEY RP. 1988. Hepatitis B virus: the major etiology of hepatocellular carcinoma. Cancer 61:1942–1956.

BEASLEY RP, HWANG L-Y, LIN C-C, et al. 1981. Hepatocellular carcinoma and hepatitis B virus: a prospectice study of 22,707 men in Taiwan. Lancet 2:1129–1133.

BEASLEY RP, TREPO C, STEVENS CE, et al. 1977. The e antigen and vertical transmission of hepatitis B surface antigen. Am J Epidemiol 105:94–98.

BIGGAR RJ, HENLE W, FLEISHER G, et al. 1978. Primary Epstein-Barr virus infections in African infants. I. Decline of maternal antibodies and time of infection. Int J Cancer 22:239–243.

BLACK FL, HIERHOLZER WJ, PINHEIRO DP, et al. 1974. Evidence for persistence of infectious agents in isolated human populations. Am J Epidemiol 100:230–250.

BLUMBERG BS. 1986. Hepatitis B virus, iron and iron binding proteins. *In* Szentivanyi A, Friedman H (eds): Viruses, Immunity, and Immunodeficiency. New York, Plenum Press, pp. 81–99.

BRACKMANN SA, GERRITZEN A, OLDENBURG J, et al. 1993. Search for intrafamilial transmission of hepatitis C virus in hemophilia patients. Blood 81:1077–1082.

BRADBIER C. 1987. Is infection with HIV a risk factor for cervical intraepithelial neoplasm? Lancet ii:1277–1278.

BRADLEY DW, BEACH MJ, PURDY MA. 1993. Molecular characterization of hepatitis C and E viruses. Arch Virol (Suppl.) 7:1–14.

BRECHOT C, POURCEL C, HADCHOUEL M, et al. 1982. State of hepatitis B virus DNA in liver diseases. Hepatology 2:27S–34S.

BRESTERS D, MAUSER-BUNSCHOTEN EP, REESINK HW, et al. 1993. Sexual transmission of hepatitis C virus. Lancet 342:210–211.

BRINTON LA. 1992. Epidemiology of cervical cancer—overview. IARC Scientific Publication No. 119, Lyon, International Agency for Research on Cancer, pp. 3–22.

BRINTON LA, TASHIMA KT, LEHMAN HF, et al. 1987. Epidemiology of cervical cancer by cell type. Cancer Res 47:1706–1711.

BRUIX J, BARRERA JM, CALVET X, et al. 1990. Prevalence of antibodies to hepatitis C virus in Spanish patients with hepatocellular carcinoma and hepatic cirrhosis. Lancet ii:1004–1006.

BUCKLEY JD, DOLL R, HARRIS RWC, et al. 1981. Case–control study of the husbands of women with dysplasia or carcinoma of the cervix uteri. Lancet ii:1010–1014.

BURKITT D. 1962. A children's cancer dependent on climate factors. Nature (London) 194:232–234.

BURKITT D, WRIGHT DH. 1966. Geographical and tribal distribution of the African lymphoma in Uganda. BMJ 5487:569–573.

BURT RD, VAUGHAN TL, NISPEROS B, et al. 1994. A prospective association between the HLA-A2 antigen and nasopharyngeal carcinoma in US Caucasians. Int J Cancer 56:465–467.

CANN AJ, CHEN ISY. 1990. Human T-cell leukemia viruses type I and II. *In* Fields BN, Knipe DM, Chanock RM, Hirsch MS, Melnick JL, Monath TP, Roizman B, (eds): Field Virology, 2nd ed. New York, Raven Press, pp. 1437–1500.

CAUSSY D, ORR W, DAYA AD, et al. 1988. Evaluation of methods for detecting human papillomavirus deoxyribonucleotide sequences in clinical specimens. J Clin Microbiol 26:236–243.

CENTERS FOR DISEASE CONTROL. 1988a. Changing patterns of groups at high risk for hepatitis B in the United States. MMWR 37:429–432,437.

CENTERS FOR DISEASE CONTROL. 1988b. Prevention of perinatal transmission of hepatitis B virus: prenatal screening of all pregnant women for hepatitis B surface antigen. MMWR 37:341–346.

CENTERS FOR DISEASE CONTROL. 1991. Screening donors of blood, plasma, organs, tissue and semen for evidence of hepatitis B and hepatitis C. Public Health Service inter-agency guidelines. MMWR 40:1–17.

CHAN CK, MUELLER N, EVANS A, et al. 1991. Epstein-Barr virus antibody patterns preceding the diagnosis of nasopharyngeal carcinoma. Cancer Causes and Control 2:125–131.

CHANG F, SYRJÄNEN S, SHEN Q, et al. 1990. Human papillomavirus (HPV) DNA in esophageal precancer lesions and squamous cell carcinomas from China. Int J Cancer 45:21–25.

CHATANI M, TESHIMA T, INOUE T, et al. 1991. Antibody response against the Epstein-Barr virus-coded nuclear antigen2 (EBNA2) in nasopharyngeal carcinoma. Laryngoscope 101:626–629.

CHEN DS. 1991. Control of hepatitis B in Asia: Mass immunization program in Taiwan. *In* Hollinger FB, Lemon SM, Margolis HS (eds): Viral Hepatitis and Liver Disease. Baltimore, Williams and Wilkins, pp. 716–719.

CHEN Y-MA, LEE T-H, WIKTOR SZ, et al. 1990. Type-specific antigens for serological discrimination of HTLV-I and HTLV-II infection. Lancet 336:1153–1155.

CHOO QL, KUO G, WEINER AJ, et al. 1989. Isolation of a cDNA clone derived from a blood-borne non-A, non-B viral hepatitis genome. Science 244:359–362.

CLARK J, SAXINGER C, GIBBS WN, et al. 1985. Seroepidemiologic studies of human T-cell leukemia/lymphoma virus type I in Jamaica. Int J Cancer 36:37–41.

COATES PJ, SLAVIN G, D'ARDENNE AJ. 1991. Persistence of Epstein-Barr virus in Reed-Sternberg cells throughout the course of Hodgkin's disease. J Pathol 164:291–297.

COLLETT MS, ANDERSON DK, RETZEL E. 1988. Comparisons of the pestivirus bovine viral diarrhea virus and members of the Flaviviridae. J Gen Virol 69:2637–2643.

COLOMBO M, KUO G, CHOO QL, et al. 1990. Prevalence of antibodies to hepatitis C virus in Italian patients with hepatocellular carcinoma. Lancet ii:1006–1008.

DALING JR, WEISS NS, HISLOP TG, et al. 1987. Sexual practices, sexually transmitted diseases and the incidence of anal cancer. N Engl J Med 317:973–977.

DAMBAUGH T, NKRUMAH FK, BIGGAR RJ, KIEFF E. 1979. Epstein-Barr virus RNA in Burkitt tumor tissue. Cell 16:313–322.

DANE DS, CAMERON CH, BRISS M. 1970. Virus-like particles in serum of patients with Australia-antigen associated hepatitis. Lancet 1:695–698.

DEACON EM, PALLESEN G, NIEDOBITEK G, et al. 1993. Epstein-Barr virus and Hodgkin's disease: transcriptional analysis of virus latency in the malignant cells. J Exp Med 177:339–349.

DELAPORTE E, PEETERS M, DURAND J-P, et al. 1989. Seroepidemiological survey of HTLV-I infection among randomized populations of western central African countries. J Aquir Immune Defic Syndr 2:410–413.

DELSOL G, BROUSSET P, CHITTAL S, et al. 1992. Correlation of the expression of Epstein-Barr virus latent membrane protein and *in Situ* hybridization with biotinylated *Bam* HI-W probes in Hodgkin's disease. Am J Pathol 140:247–253.

DE THÉ G, GESER A, DAY NE, et al. 1978. Epidemiological evidence for evidence for causal relationship between Epstein-Barr virus and Burkitt's lymphoma from Ugandan prospective study. Nature (London) 274:756–761.

DE THÉ G, GESSAIN A. 1988. HTLV-I and associated diseases in Europe and Africa: a sero-epidemiological survey. Working paper, scientific group on HTLV-I and its associated diseases. World Health Organization, Regional Office for the Western Pacific, Kagoshima, Japan, December, 1988.

DE THÉ G, HO JHC, MUIR CS. 1989. Nasopharyngeal cancer. *In* Evans AS (ed): Viral Infections of Humans: Epidemiology and Control, 3rd ed. New York, Plenum Press, pp. 737–767.

DE THÉ G. 1985. Epstein-Barr virus and Burkitt's lymphoma worldwide: The causal relationship revisited. *In* Lenoir GM, O'Conor GT, Olweny CLM (eds): Burkitt's Lymphoma: A Human Cancer Model. New York, Oxford University Press, pp. 165–176.

DE THÉ G. 1979. The epidemiology of Burkitt's lymphoma: evidence for causal association with Epstein-Barr virus. Epidemiol Rev 1:32–54.

DILLNER J, LENNER P, LEHTINEN M, et al. 1994. A population-based seroepidemiological study of cervical cancer. Cancer Res 54:134–141.

DOLL R. 1978. An epidemiologic perspective of the biology of cancer. Cancer Res 38:3573–3583.

DOLL R, PETO R. 1981. The causes of cancer: quantitative estimate of avoidable rises of cancer in the United States today. J Natl Cancer Inst 66:1196–1308.

DUCREUX M, BUFFET C, DUSSAIX E, et al. 1990. Antibody to hepatitis C virus in hepatocellular carcinoma. Lancet 335:301.

DULBECCO R. 1987. A turning point in cancer research: sequencing the human genome. *In* Gallo RC, Haseltine W, Klein G, zur Hausen H (eds): Viruses and Human Cancer. New York, Alan R. Liss, Inc., pp. 1–14.

DYSON N, HOWLEY PM, MÜNGER, et al. 1989. The human papilloma virus-16 E7 oncoprotein is able to bind to the retinoblastoma gene product. Science 243:934–936.

EPSTEIN MA. 1976. Epstein-Barr virus issues—Is it time to develop a vaccine program? J Natl Cancer Inst 56:697–700.

EPSTEIN MA. 1986. Vaccination against Epstein-Barr virus: current progress and future strategies. Lancet 1:1425–1427.

EPSTEIN MA, HUNT RD, RABIN H. 1973. Pilot experiments with EB virus in owl monkeys (Aotus Tririgotus): reticuloproliferative disease in an inoculated animal. Int J Cancer 12:309–318.

EPSTEIN MA, MORGAN AJ. 1985. Prevention of endemic Burkitt's lymphoma. *In* Lenoir GM, O'Conor GT, Olweny CLM (eds): Burkitt's Lymphoma: A Human Cancer Model. Lyon, France, International Agency for Research on Cancer, pp. 197–204.

ESSEX M, COTTER SM, SLISKI AH, et al. 1977. Horizontal transmission of feline leukemia virus under natural conditions in a feline leukemia cluster household. Int J Cancer 19:90–96.

ESSEX M, GUTENSOHN (MUELLER) N. 1981. A comparison of the pathobiology and epidemiology of cancers associated with viruses in humans and animals. Prog Med Virol 27:114–126.

ESSEX M, SLISKI AH, WORLEY M, et al. 1980a. Significance of the feline oncornavirus-associated cell-membrane antigen (FOCMA) in the natural history of feline leukemia. *In* Essex M, Todaro G, zur Hausen H (eds): Viruses in Naturally Occurring Cancers. Cold Spring Harbor, New York, Cold Spring Harbor Laboratory, pp. 589–602.

ESSEX M, TODARO G, ZUR HAUSEN H. (eds). 1980b. Viruses in Naturally Occurring Cancers. Cold Spring Harbor, Cold Spring Harbor Laboratory.

ESSEX ME. 1982. Feline leukemia: A naturally occurring cancer of infectious origin. Epidemiol Rev 4:189–201.

ESTEBAN JI, ESTEBAN R, VILADOMIU L, et al. 1989. Hepatitis C virus antibodies among risk groups in Spain. Lancet 2:294–296.

ESTROFF DT, GREENMAN JH, HEYWARD WL, et al. 1985. Increased prevalence of hepatitis B surface antigen in pregnant Alaska Eskimos. *In* Fortune R (ed): Circumpolar Health 84. Seattle, University of Washington Press, pp. 206–208.

EVANS AA, WERNER BG, HEINZ-LACEY B, et al. 1990. Antibody to hepatitis C virus (HCV) in patients with chronic renal failure. Hepatology 12:845.

EVANS AS. 1987. Discussion of some recent developments in the molecular epidemiology of Epstein-Barr virus infections. Yale J Biol Mol 60:317–319.

EVANS AS. 1985. Epidemiology of Burkitt's lymphoma: other factors. *In* Lenoir GM, O'Conor GT, Olweny CLM (eds): Burkitt's Lymphoma: A Human Cancer Model. Lyon, France, International Agency for Research on Cancer, pp. 197–201.

EVANS AS. 1988. Epstein-Barr virus: An organism for all seasons. *In* de la Maga M, Peterson EM (eds): Medical Virology VII. New York, Elseira, pp. 57–97.

EVANS AS, COMSTOCK GW. 1981. Presence of elevated antibody titers to Epstein-Barr virus before Hodgkin's disease. Lancet 1:1183–1186.

EVANS AS, MUELLER NE. Malignant lymphomas. *In* Evans AS, Kaslow R (eds): Viral Infections of Humans: Epidemiology and Control, 4th ed. New York, Plenum, (in press).

EVANS AS, MUELLER NE. 1990. Viruses and cancer: causal associations. Ann Epidemiol 1:71–92.

EVANS AS, NIEDERMAN JC. 1989. Epstein-Barr virus. *In* Evans AS (ed): Viral Infections of Humans: Epidemiology and Control, 3rd ed. New York, Plenum Press, pp. 265–292.

EYSTER ME, ALTER HJ, ALEDORT LM. 1991. Heterosexual co-transmission of hepatitis C virus (HCV) and human immunodeficiency virus (HIV). Ann Intern Med 115:764–768.

FABRIZI F, RAFFAELE L, BACCHINI G, et al. 1993. Antibodies to hepatitis C virus (HCV) and transaminase concentration in chronic haemodialysis patients: a study with second-generation assays. Nephrol Dial Transplant 8:744–747.

FÅHRAEUS R, FU HL, ERNBERG I, et al. 1988. Expression of Epstein-Barr virus-encoded proteins in nasopharyngeal carcinoma. Int J Cancer 42:329–338.

FARCI P, ALTER HJ, GOVINDARAJAN S, et al. 1992. Lack of protective immunity against reinfection with hepatitis C virus. Science 258:135–140.

FEINSTONE SM, KAPIKIAN AZ, PURCELL RH, et al. 1975. Transfusion-associated hepatitis not due to viral hepatitis type A or B. N Engl J Med 292:767–770.

FEITELSON MA, ZHU M, DUAN LX, LONDON WT. 1993. Hepatitis B x antigen and p53 are associated *in vitro* and in liver tissues from patients with primary hepatocellular carcinoma. Oncogene 8:1109–1117.

FONG TL, SHINDO M, FEINSTONE SM, et al. 1991. Detection of replication intermediates of hepatitis C viral RNA in liver and serum of patients with chronic hepatitis C. J Clin Invest 88:1058–1060.

FRANCIS DP, ESSEX M, COTTER S, et al. 1981a. Epidemiologic association between virus-negative feline leukemia and the horizontally transmitted feline leukemia virus. Cancer Lett 12:37–42.

FRANCIS DP, ESSEX M, COTTER S, et al. 1979. Feline leukemia virus infections: the significance of chronic viremia. Leuk Res 3:435–441.

FRANCIS DP, ESSEX M, MAYNARD JE. 1981b. Feline leukemia virus and hepatitis B virus: A comparison of late manifestations. Prog Med Virol 27:127–132.

FRECH B, ZIMBER-STROBL U, YIP TT, et al. 1993. Characterization of the antibody response to the latent infection terminal proteins of Epstein-Barr virus in patients with nasopharyngeal carcinoma. J Gen Virol 74:811–818.

GALLOWAY D. 1992. Serological assays for the detection of HPV antibodies. *In* Muñoz N, Bosch FX, Shah KV, and Meheus A (eds): The Epidemiology of Human Papillomavirus and Cervical Cancer. IARC Scientific Publication No. 119, Lyon, International Agency for Research on Cancer, pp. 147–162.

GAMBIA HEPATITIS STUDY GROUP. 1987. The Gambia hepatitis intervention study. Cancer Res 47:5782–5787.

GARSON JA, TUKE PW, MAKRIS M, et al. 1990. Demonstration of viremia patterns in haemophiliacs treated with hepatitis C virus contaminated factor VIII concentrates. Lancet 336:1022–1025.

GESER A, DE THÉ G, LENOIR G, et al. 1982. Final case reporting from the Ugandan prospective study of the relationship between EBV and Burkitt's lymphoma. Int J Cancer 29:397–400.

GESSAIN A, GALLO RC, FRANCHINI G. 1992. Low degree of human T-cell leukemia/lymphoma virus type I genetic drift in vivo as a means of monitoring viral transmission and movement of ancient human populations, J Virol 66:2288–2295.

GESSAIN A, HERVÉ V, JEANNEL D, et al. 1993. HTLV-1 but not HTLV-2 found in Pygmies from Central African Republic. J Acquired Immunedefic Syndr 6:1373–1375.

GIOVANNINI M, TAGGER A, RIBERO ML, et al. 1990. Maternal-infant transmission of hepatitis C virus and HIV infections: a possible interaction. Lancet 335:1166.

GRÄSSER FA, MURRAY PG, KREMMER E et al. 1994. Monoclonal antibodies directed against the Epstein-Barr virus-encoded nuclear antigen 1 (EBNA1): Immunohistologic detection of EBNA1 in the malignant cells of Hodgkin's disease. Blood 84:3792–3798.

GREEN MH, FRAUMENI JF JR, HOOVER R. 1977. Nasopharyngeal cancer among adults in United States: racial variations by cell type. J Natl Cancer Inst 58:1267–1270.

GUIDOTTI LG, GUILHOT S, CHISARI FV. 1994a. Interleukin-2 and alpha/beta interferon down regulate hepatitis B virus gene expression in vivo by tumor necrosis factor-dependent and -independent pathways. J Virol 68:1265–1270.

GUIDOTTI LG, MARTINEZ V, LOH YT, et al. 1994b. Hepatitis B virus nucleocapsids particles do not cross the hepatocyte nuclear membrane in transgenic mice. J Virol 68:5469–5475.

GUTENSOHN (MUELLER) N, COLE P. 1981. Childhood social environment and Hodgkin's disease. N Engl J Med 304:135–140.

GUTENSOHN (MUELLER) N, COLE P. 1977. Epidemiology of Hodgkin's disease in the young. Int J Cancer 19:595–604.

HAMILTON-DUTOIT SJ, RAPHAEL M, AUDOUIN J, et al. 1993. In situ demonstration of Epstein-Barr virus small RNAs (EBER1) in acquired immunodeficiency syndrome induced lymphomas: correlation with tumor morphology and primary site. Blood 82:619–624.

HARDY WD JR. 1984. A new package for an old oncogene. Nature 308:775.

HARDY WD JR, HIRSHAUT Y, HESS P. 1973. Detection of the feline leukemia virus and other mammalian oncornaviruses by immunofluorescence. *In* Dutcher RM, Chieco-Bianchi L (eds): Unifying Concepts of Leukemia. Basil, Karger, pp. 778–799.

HARUNA Y, HAYASHI N, KAMADA T, et al. 1994. Expression of hepatitis C virus in hepatocellular carcinoma. Cancer 73:2253–2258.

HASELTINE WA, SODROSKI J, ROSEN C. 1985. Structure and function of Human Leukemia and AIDS Viruses. *In* Miwa M, Sugano H, Sugimura T (eds): Retroviruses in Human Lymphoma/Leukemia. Tokyo, Japan Sci Soc Press, pp. 93–108.

HAYASHI J, NAKASHIMA K, KAJIYAMA W, et al. 1991. Prevalence of hepatitis C antibody in hemodialysis patients. Am J Epidemiol 124:651–657.

HENDERSON BE, LOUIE E, JING JSH, et al. 1976. Risk factors associated with nasopharyngeal carcinoma. N Engl J Med 295:1101–1106.

HENLE G, HENLE W. 1976. Epstein-Barr virus-specific IgA serum antibodies as an outstanding feature of nasopharyngeal carcinoma. Int J Cancer 17:1–7.

HENLE G, HENLE W, CLIFFORD P, et al. 1969. Antibodies to the Epstein-Barr virus in Burkitt's lymphoma and control groups. J Natl Cancer Inst 43:147–159.

HENLE W, HENLE G, HO H-C, et al. 1970. Antibodies to Epstein-Barr virus in nasopharyngeal carcinoma, other head and neck neoplasms, and control groups. J Nat Cancer Inst 44:225–231.

HENLE W, HO HC, KWAN HC. 1973. Antibodies to the Epstein-Barr related antigens in nasopharyngeal carcinoma: comparison of active cases with long term survivors. J Natl Cancer Inst 51:361–369.

HENLE W, HO JHC, HENLE G, et al. 1977. Nasopharyngeal carcinoma: significance of changes in Epstein-Barr virus-related antibody patterns following therapy. Int J Cancer 20:663–672.

HESS G, MASSING A, ROSSOL S, et al. 1989. Hepatitis C virus and sexual transmission. Lancet 2:987.

HILDESHEIM A, LEVINE PH. 1993. Etiology of nasopharyngeal carcinoma: a review. Epidemiol Rev 15:466–485.

HINO S, DOI H, YOSHIKUNI H, et al. 1987. HTLV-I carrier mothers with high titer antibody are at high risk as a source of infection. Jpn J Cancer Res 78:1156–1158.

HINO S, KATAMINE S, KAWASE K, et al. 1994. Intervention of maternal transmission of HTLV-I in Nagasaki, Japan. Leukemia 8 (Supplement 1) 68s–70s.

HINUMA Y, NAGATA K, HANAOKA M, et al. 1981. Adult T-cell leukemia: antigen in an ATL cell line and detection of antibodies to the antigen in human sera. Proc Nat Acad Sci USA 78:6476–6480.

HIRAMATSU N, HAYASHI N, HARUNA Y, et al. 1992. Immunohistochemical detection of hepatitis C virus-infected hepatocytes in chronic liver disease with monoclonal antibodies to core, envelope, and NS3 regions of the hepatitis C virus genome. Hepatology 15:777–781.

HIRATA M, HAYASHI J, NOGUCHI A, et al. 1992. The effects of breast feeding and presence of antibody to $p40^{tax}$ protein of human T-cell lymphotropic virus type-1 on mother-to-child transmission. Int J Epidemiol 21:989–994.

HO JHC. 1971. Genetic and environmental factors in nasopharyngeal carcinoma. *In* Nakahara W, Nishioka K, Hirayama T, et al (eds): Recent Advances in Human Tumor Virology and Immunology. Tokyo, University of Tokyo Press, pp. 275–295.

HO M, MILLER G, ATCHINSON RW, et al. 1985. Epstein-Barr virus infections and DNA hybridization studies in posttransplantation lymphoma and lymphoproliferative lesions: the role of primary infection. J Infec Dis 152:876–886.

HOOFNAGLE JH, DIBISCEGLIE AM. 1989. Treatment of chronic type C hepatitis with alpha interferon. Semin Liver Dis 9:259–263.

HOOFNAGLE JH, SEEF LB, BATES ZB, et al. 1978. Serologic responses in hepatitis B. *In* Vyas G, Cohen SN, Schmid R (eds): Viral Hepatitis. Philadelphia, Franklin Institute Press, pp. 219–244.

HOOVER EA, OLSEN RG, HARDY WD JR, et al. 1976. Feline leukemia virus infection: age-related variation in response of cats to experimental infection. J Natl Cancer Inst 57:365–369.

HOUGHTON M, WEINER A, HAN J, et al. 1991. Molecular biology of the hepatitis C viruses: implications for diagnosis, development and control of viral disease. Hepatology 14:381–388.

HSIEH TT, YAO DS, SHEEN IS, et al. 1992. Hepatitis C virus in peripheral blood mononuclear cells. Am J Clin Pathol 98:392–396.

INTERNATIONAL AGENCY FOR RESEARCH ON CANCER (IARC). 1994. Hepatitis Viruses. IARC Monogr Eval Carcinog Risks Hum 59:129.

ISHIDA T, YAMAMOTO K, OMOTO K, et al. 1985. Prevalence of a human retrovirus in native Japanese: evidence for a possible ancient origin. J Infect 11:153–157.

ISHIDA T, YAMAMOTO K, OMOTO K. 1988. A seroprevalence survey of HTLV-I in the Philippines. Int J Epidemiol 17:625–628.

ISHIHARA S, OKAYAMA A, STUVER S, et al. 1994. Association of HTLV-I antibody profile of asymptomatic carriers with proviral DNA levels of peripheral blood mononuclear cells. J Aquir Immune Defic Syndr 7:199–203.

IMMUNIZATION PRACTICES ADVISORY COMMITTEE (ACIP). 1991. Hepatitis B virus: a comprehensive strategy for eliminating transmission in the United States through universal childhood vaccination-recommendations of the Immunization Practices Advisory Committee (ACIP). MMWR 40:RR 13:11–14.

JACOB JR, SUREAU C, BURK KH. 1991. *In vitro* replication of non-A, non-B hepatitis virus. *In* Hollinger FB, Lemon SM, Margolis HS (eds): Viral Hepatitis and Liver Disease. Baltimore, Williams and Wilkins, pp. 387–392.

JEANG K-T, WIDDEN SG, SEMMES OJ IV, WILSON SH. 1990. HTLV-I trans-activator protein, tax, is a transrepressor of the human 3-β polymerase gene. Science 247:1082–1084.

JILBERT AR, WU TT, ENGLAND JM, et al. 1992. Rapid resolution of duck hepatitis B virus infections occurs after massive hepatocellular involvement. J Virol 66:1377–1388.

KAJINO K, JILBERT AR, SAPUTELLI J, et al. 1994. Woodchuck hepatitis virus infections: very rapid recovery after a prolonged viremia and infection of virtually every hepatocyte. J Virol 5792–5803.

KAKLAMANI E, TRICHOPOULOS D, TZONOU A, et al. 1991. Hepatitis B and C viruses and their interaction in the origin of hepatocellular carcinoma. JAMA 265:1974–1976.

KALYANARAMAN VS, SARNGADHARAN MG, ROBERT-GUROFF M, et al. 1982. A new subtype of human T-cell leukemia virus (HTLV-II) associated with a T-cell variant of hairy cell leukemia. Science 218:571–573.

KANEKO S, UNOURA M, KOBAYASHI K, et al. 1990. Detection of serum hepatitis C virus RNA. Lancet 335–976.

KAPLAN MH, HALL WW, SUSIN M, et al. 1991. Syndrome of severe skin disease, eosinophilia and dermatopathic lymphadenopathy in patients with HTLV-II complicating human immunodeficiency virus infection, Am J Med 91:300–309.

KHAN G, NAASE MA. 1995. Down-regulation of Epstein-Barr virus nuclear antigen 1 in Reed Sternberg cells of Hodgkin's disease. J Clin Pathol 48:845–848.

KIM JH, DURACK DT. 1988. Manifestations of human T-lymphotropic virus type I infection. Am J Med 84:919–928.

KINOSHITA K, AMAGASAKI T, IKEDA S, et al. 1985. Preleukemic state of adult T-cell leukemia: abnormal T lymphocytosis induced by human adult T-cell leukemia-lymphoma virus. Blood 56:120–127.

KIRNBAUER R, HUBBERT NL, WHEELER CM, et al. 1994. A virus-like particle enzyme-linked immunosorbent assay detects serum antibodies in a majority of women infected with human papillomavirus type 16. J Natl Cancer Inst 86:494–499.

KISTNER RW, HERTIG AT. 1955. Papillomas of the uterine cervix: their malignant potentiality. Obstet Gynecol 6:147–161.

KIYOSAWA K, SODEYAMA T, TANAKA E, et al. 1990. Interrelationship of blood transfusion, non-A, non-B hepatitis and hepatocellular carcinoma: analysis by detection of antibody to hepatitis C virus. Hepatology 12:671–675.

KLEIN G. 1982. Epstein-Barr virus, malaria, and Burkitt's lymphoma. Scand J Infect Dis (Suppl.) 36:15–23.

KLEIN G. 1994. The paradoxical coexistence of EBV and the human species. Epstein-Barr Virus Report 1:5–9.

KLEIN G, GIOVANELLA BC, LINDAHL T, et al. 1974. Direct evidence for the presence of Epstein-Barr virus DNA and nuclear antigen in malignanct epithelial cells from patients with poorly differentiated carcinoma of the nasopharynx. Proc Nat Acad Sci USA 71:4737–4741.

KNECHT H, BROUSSET P, BACHMANN E, et al. 1993. Latent membrane protein 1: A key oncogene in EBV-related carcinogenesis? Acta Haematol 90:167–171.

KNODELL RG, CONRAD ME, ISHAK KG. 1977. Development of chronic liver disease after acute non-A, non-B post-transfusion hepatitis. Role of gamma globulin prophylaxis in its prevention. Gastroenterology 72:902–909.

KOBAYASHI S, HAYASHI H, ITOH Y, et al. 1994. Detection of minus-strand hepatitis C virus RNA in tumor tissues of hepatocellular carcinoma. Cancer 73:48–52.

KÖCHEL HG, SIEVERT K, MONAZAHAIN M, et al. 1991. Antibodies to human papillomavirus type-16 in human sera as revealed by the use of prokaryotically expressed viral gene products. Virology 182:644–654.

KOHAKURA M, NAKADA K, YONAHARA M, et al. 1986. Seroepidemiology of the human retrovirus (HTLV/ATLV) in Okinawa where adult T-cell leukemia is highly endemic. Jpn J Cancer Res 77:21–23.

KONDO T, KONDO H, NORAKA, et al. 1987. Risk of adult T-cell leukemia/lymphoma in HTLV-I carriers. Lancet ii:159.

KOUTSKY LA, GALLOWAY DA, HOLMES KK. 1988. Epidemiology of genital human papilloma virus infection. Epidemiol Rev 10:122–163.

KOUTSKY LA, HOLMES KK, CRITCHLOW CW, et al. 1992. A cohort study of the risk of cervical intraepithelial neoplasia grade 2 or 3 in relation to papilloma virus infection. N Engl J Med 327:1272–1278.

KRAWCZYNSKI K, BEACH MJ, BRADLEY DW, et al. 1992. Hepatitis C virus antigen in hepatocytes: immunomorphologic detection and identification. Gastroenterology 103:622–629.

KUHNS M, DE MEDINA M, MCNAMARA A, et al. 1994. Detection of hepatitis C virus RNA in hemodialysis patients. J Am Soc Nephrol 4:1491–1497.

KUO G, CHOO QL, ALTER HJ, et al. 1989. An assay for circulating antibodies to a major etiologic virus of human non-A, non-B hepatitis. Science 244:362–364.

KUSUHARA K, SONODA S, TAKAHASHI K, et al. 1987. Mother-to-child transmission of human T-cell leukemia virus type I (HTLV-I): a fifteen year follow-up study in Okinawa, Japan. Int J Cancer 40:755–757.

KUSUNOKI Y, HUANG H, FUKUDA Y, et al. 1993. A positive correlation between the precursor frequency of cytotoxic lymphocytes to autologous Epstein-Barr virus-transformed B cells and antibody titer level against Epstein-Barr virus-associated nuclear antigen in healthy seropositive individuals. Microbiol Immunol 37:461–469.

LANIER AP, HENLE W, BENDER TR, et al. 1980. Epstein-Barr virus-specific antibody titers in seven Alaskan natives before and after diagnosis of nasopharyngeal carcinoma. Int J Cancer 26:133–138.

LEDER P. 1985a. Chromosomal dislocations among antibody genes in human cancer. *In* Lenoir GM, O'Conor GM, Olweny CLM (eds): Burkitt's Lymphoma: A Human Cancer Model. Lyon, International Agency for Research on Cancer, pp. 341–358.

LEDER P. 1985b. The state and prospect for molecular genetics in Burkitt's lymphoma. *In* Lenoir GM, O'Conor GM, Olweny CLM (eds): Burkitt's Lymphoma: A Human Cancer Model. Lyon, International Agency for Research on Cancer, pp. 465–468.

LEDER P, BATTEY J, LENOIR G, et al. 1983. Translocations among antibody genes in human cancer. Science 222:765–771.

LEE TH, COLIGAN JE, SODROWSKI JG, et al. 1984. Antigens encoded by the 3′-terminal region of human T-cell leukemia virus: evidence for a functional gene. Science 226:57–61.

LEVESQUE KS, BONHAM L, LEVY LS. 1990. Flvi-1, a common integration domain of feline leukemia virus in naturally occurring lymphomas of a particular type. J Virol 64:3455–3462.

LEVINE P, BLATTNER WA, CLARK J, et al. 1988. Geographic distribution of HTLV-I and identification of a new high risk population. Int J Cancer 42:7–12.

LEVINE P, CONNELLY RR, MCKAY FW. 1985. Burkitt's lymphoma cases reported to the American Burkitt's Lymphoma Registry compared with population-based incidence and mortality data. *In* Lenoir GM, O'Conor GT, Olweny CLM (eds): Burkitt's Lymphoma: A Human Cancer Model. Lyon, International Agency for Research on Cancer, pp. 217–224.

LI L, SHEN MH, LI YQ, et al. 1986. A study of mother-child transmission of hepatitis B virus. *In* Proc. Update of the 1986 Shanghai International Symposium on Liver Cancer and Hepatitis, January 15–17, 1986.

LIEBER CS, GARRO A, LEO MA, et al. 1986. Alcohol and cancer. Hepatology 6:1005–1019.

LIN HH, KAO JH, HSU HY, et al. 1994. Possible role of high-titer maternal viremia in perinatal transmission of hepatitis C virus. J Infect Dis 169:638–641.

LIST AF, GRECO FA, VOGLER LB. 1987. Lymphoproliferative diseases in immunocompromised hosts: the role of Epstein-Barr virus. J Clin Oncol 5:1673–1689.

LONDON WT. 1981. Primary hepatocellular carcinoma: etiology, pathogenesis and prevention. Human Pathol 12:1085–1097.

LONDON WT, BLUMBERG BS. 1982. A cellular model of the role of hepatitis B virus in the pathogenesis of primary hepatocellular carcinoma. Hepatology 2:10S–14S.

LONDON WT, BUETOW K. 1988. Controversies in basic science: hepatitis B virus and primary hepatocellular carcinoma. Cancer Invest 6:317–326.

LONDON WT, DREW JS, LUSTBADER ED, et al. 1977. Host responses to hepatitis B infection in patients in a chronic hemodialysis unit. Kidney Int 12:51–58.

LU S, DAY NE, DEGOS L, et al. 1990. Linkage of a nasopharyngeal carcinoma susceptibility locus to the HLA region. Nature 346:470–471.

MADDEN C, BECKMANN AM, THOMAS DB, et al. 1992. Human papillomaviruses, herpes simplex viruses, and the risk of oral cancer in men. Am J Epidemiol 135:1093–1102.

MADDEN C, SHERMAN KJ, BECKMANN AM, et al. 1993. History of circumcision, medical conditions, and sexual activity and risk of penile cancer. J Natl Cancer Inst 85:19–24.

MADELEINE MM, WIKTOV SZ, GOEDERT JJ, MANNS A, LEVINE PH, BIGGAR RJ, BLATTNER WA. 1993. HTLV-I and HTLV-II world-wide distribution: Reanalysis of 4,832 immunoblot results. Int J Cancer 54:255–260.

MAGRATH I, JAIN V, BHATIA K. 1993. Molecular epidemiology of Burkitt's lymphoma. *In* Tursz T, Pagano JS, Ablashi DV, de The G, Lenoir G, Pearson GR (eds): The Epstein-Barr Virus and Associated Diseases. Colloque INSERM/John Libbey Eurotext 225:377–396.

MARCELLIN P, BERNUAU J, MARTINOT-PEIGNOUX M, et al. 1993. Prevalence of hepatitis C virus infection in asymptomatic anti-HIV1 negative pregnant women and their children. Dig Dis Sci 38:2151–2155.

MARINIER E, BARROIS V, LAROUZE B, et al. 1985. Lack of perinatal transmission of hepatitis B infection in Senegal, West Africa. J Pediatr 106:843–849.

MARX JL. 1989. How DNA viruses may cause cancer. Science 243:1012–1013.

MATHEW A, CHENG H-M, SAM C-K, et al. 1994. A high incidence of serum IgG antibodies to the Epstein-Barr virus replication activator protein in nasopharyngeal carcinoma. Cancer Immunol Immunother 38:68–70.

MATTSON L, GRILLNER L, WEILAND O. 1992. Seroconversion to hepatitis C antibodies in patients with acute post-transfusion non-A, non-B hepatitis in Sweden with a second generation test. Scand J Infect Dis 24:15–20.

MATUTES E, DALGLEISH AG, WEISS RA, et al. 1986. Studies in healthy human T-cell leukemia lymphoma virus (HTLV-I) carriers from the Caribbean. Int J Cancer 38:41–45.

MELBYE M, EBBESON P, LEVINE PH, BENNIKE T. 1984. Early primary infection and high Epstein-Barr virus antibody titers in Greenland Eskimos at high risk for nasopharyngeal carcinoma. Int J Cancer 34:619.

MENDENHALL CL, SEEF L, DIEHL AM, et al. 1991. Antibodies to hepatitis B virus and hepatitis C virus in alcoholic hepatitis and cirrhosis: their prevalence and clinical relevance. Hepatology 14:581–589.

MILLER G. 1990. Epstein-Barr virus: Biology, pathogenesis and medical aspects. *In* Fields B, Knipe DM (eds): Virology, 2nd ed. New York, Raven Press, pp. 1921–1958.

MILLER G. 1974. Oncogenicity of Epstein-Barr virus. J Infect Dis 130:187–205.

MILLER G, SHOPE T, COOPER D, et al. 1977. Lymphoma in cotton top marmosets after inoculation with Epstein-Barr virus: tumor incidence, histologic spectrum, antibody responses, demonstration of viral DNA, and characterization of virus. J Exp Med 145:948–967.

MILLER G, KATZ BZ, NIEDERMAN JC. 1987. Some recent developments in the molecular epidemiology of Epstein-Barr virus infections. Yale J Biol Med 60:307–316.

MILLER RH, PURCELL RH. 1990. Hepatitis C virus shares amino acid sequence similarity with pestiviruses and flaviviruses as well as members of two plant family virus supergroups. Proc Natl Acad Sci USA 87:2057–2061.

MISHIRO S, HOSHI Y, TAKEDA K, et al. 1990. Non-A, non-B hepatitis specific antibodies directed at host-derived epitope: implication for an autoimmune process. Lancet 336:1400–1403.

MITAMURA K, TANAKA N, AIKAWA T, et al. 1990. Detection of antibodies to hepatitis C virus in patients with various liver diseases in Japan. 1990 International Symposium on Viral Hepatitis and Liver Disease, Houston, April 4–8, 1990.

MONDELLI MU, COLOMBO M. 1991. The emerging picture of hepatitis C. Dig Dis 9:245–252.

MONDELLI M, VERGANI GM, ALBERTI A, et al. 1982. Specificity of T lymphocyte cytotoxicity to autologous hepatocytes in chronic hepatitis B virus infection: evidence that T cells are directed against HBV core antigen expressed on hepatocytes. J Immunol 129:2273–2278.

MORROW RH, PIKE MC, SMITH PG. 1977. Further studies of time-space clustering in Uganda. Br Cancer J 35:668–673.

MORROW RW. 1985. Epidemiological evidence for a role of falciparum malaria in the pathogenesis of Burkitt's lymphoma. *In* Lenoir GM, O'Conor GT, Olweny CLM (eds): Burkitt's Lymphoma: A Human Cancer Model. Lyon, France, International Agency for Research on Cancer, pp. 177–186.

MOSLEY JW, AACH RD, HOLLINGER FB, et al. 1990. Non-A, non-B hepatitis and antibody to hepatitis C virus. JAMA 263:77–78.

MUARAKAMI K, ESUMI M, KATO T, et al. 1992. Heterogeneity within the nonstructural protein 5-encoding region of hepatitis C viruses from a single patient. Gene 117:229–232.

MUELLER N. 1987. Epidemiological studies assessing the role of Epstein-Barr virus in Hodgkin's disease. Yale J Biol Med 60:321–327.

MUELLER N, BLATTNER WA. Retroviruses: HTLV. *In*: Evans AS, Kaslow R (eds): Viral Infections of Humans: Epidemiology and Control, 4th ed., New York, Plenum Press, (in press).

MUELLER N, EVANS A, HARRIS NL, et al. 1989. Hodgkin's disease and Epstein-Barr virus: Altered antibody pattern before diagnosis. New Engl J Med 320:696–701.

MUELLER N, MOHAR A, EVANS A, et al. 1991. Epstein-Barr virus antibody patterns preceeding the diagnosis of non-Hodgkin's lymphoma. Int J Cancer 49:387–393.

MUELLER N, TACHIBANA N, STUVER S, et al. 1990. Epidemiologic perspectives of HTLV-I. *In* Blattner WA, (ed): Human Retrovirology: HTLV. New York, Raven Press, pp. 281–293.

MURAI K, TACHIBANA N, SHIOIRI S, et al. 1990. Suppression of delayed-type hypersensitivity to PPD and PHA in elderly HTLV-I carriers. J Acquir Immune Defic Syndr 3:1006–1009.

MURPHY EL, FIGUEROA JP, GIBBS WN, et al. 1989a. Sexual transmission of human T-lymphotropic virus. Ann Intern Med 111:555–560.

MURPHY EL, FIGUEROA JP, GIBBS WN, et al. 1991. Human T-lymphotropic virus type I (HTLV-I) seroprevalence in Jamaica. I. Demographic determinants. Am J Epidemiol 133:1114–1124.

MURPHY EL, HANCHARD B, FIGUEROA JP, et al. 1989b. Modelling the risk of adult T-cell leukemia/lymphoma virus type I. Int J Cancer 43:250–253.

NAHMIAS AJ, JOSEY WE, OLESKE JM. 1982. Cervical cancer. *In* Evans AS (ed): Viral Infections of Humans: Epidemiology and Control, 2nd ed. New York, Plenum, pp. 653–673.

NAKADA K, YAMAGUCHI K, FURUGEN S, et al. 1987. Monoclonal integration of HTLV-I proviral DNA in patients with strongyloidiasis. Int J Cancer 40:145–148.

NAM JM, MCLAUGHLIN JK, BLOT WJ. 1992. Cigarette smoking, alcohol, and nasopharyngeal carcinoma: a case–control study among U.S. whites. J Nat Cancer Inst 84:619–622.

NAYAK NC, DHARK A, SACHDEVA R, et al. 1977. Association of human hepatocellular carcinoma and cirrhosis with hepatitis B virus surface and core antigens in the liver. Int J Cancer 20:643–654.

NAZAREWICZ T, KRAWCYNSKI K, SLUSARCZYK J, et al. 1977. Cellular localization of hepatitis B virus antigen in patients with hepatocellular carcinoma coexisting with liver cirrhosis. J Infect Dis 135:298–302.

NERI A, BARRIGA F, INGHIRAMI G, et al. 1991. Epstein-Barr virus infection precedes clonal expansion in Burkitt's and acquired immunodeficiency syndrome-associated lymphomas. Blood 77:1092–1095.

NEVA FA, MURPHY EL, GAM A, et al. 1989. Antibodies to *Strongyloides Stercoralis* in healthy Jamaican carriers of HTLV-I. N Engl J Med 320:252–253.

NIEDERMAN JC, EVANS AS, SUBRAHMANJAN L, MCCOLLUM RV. 1970. Prevalence, incidence, and persistence of EBV antibody in young adults. N Engl J Med 282:361–365.

NILSSON K, KLEIN G. 1982. B-cell lines and etiology of Burkitt's lymphoma. Adv Cancer Res 37:319–380.

NIMER SD, GASSON JC, HU K, et al. 1989. Activation of the GM-CSF promoter by HTLV-I and -II tax proteins. Oncogene 4:671–676.

OHTO H, TERAZAWA S, SASAKI N, et al. 1994. Transmission of hepatitis C virus from mothers to infants. The Vertical Transmission of Hepatitis C Virus Collaborative Study Group. N Engl J Med 330:744–750.

OKAMOTO H, KURAI K, OKADA S, et al. 1992. Full length sequence of a hepatitis C genome having poor homology to reported isolates: comparative study of four distinct genotypes. Virology 188:331–341.

OKAMOTO H, OKADA S, SUGIYAMA Y, et al. 1991. Nucleotide sequence of the genomic RNA of hepatitis C virus isolated from a human carrier: comparison with reported isolates for conserved and divergent regions. J Gen Virol 72:2697–2704.

OKAYAMA A, TACHIBANA N, ISHIZAKI J, et al. 1987. An immunological study of human T-cell leukemia virus type I (HTLV-I) infection (I): detection of low-titer anti-HTLV-I antibodies by HTLV-I associated membrane antigen (HTLV-MA) method. J Jap Assoc Infect Dis 61:1363–1368.

OMATA M, YOKOSUKA O, TAKANO S, et al. 1991. Resolution of acute hepatitis C after therapy with natural beta interferon. Lancet 338:914–915.

ONIONS D. 1985. Animal models: lessons from feline and bovine leukemia virus infections. Leuk Res 9:709–711.

ORIEL JD. 1971. Natural history of genital warts. Br J Vener Dis 47:1–13.

OUZAN D, TIRTAINE C, FOLLANA R, et al. 1990. Prevalence of anti-HCV in chronic liver diseases and in blood donors in southern France. 1990 International Symposium on Viral Hepatitis and Liver Disease, Houston, April 4–8, 1990. Abstract 383.

PAGANO JS, HUANG CH, KLEIN G, et al. 1975. Homology of Epstein-Barr viral DNA in nasopharyngeal carcinoma from Kenya, Taiwan, Singapore and Tunis. *In* de Thé G, Epstein MA, zur Hausen (eds): Oncogenesis and Herpesviruses II. Lyon, International Agency for Research on Cancer, pp. 191–193.

Pallesen G, Hamilton-Dutoit SJ, Rowe M, et al. 1991a. Expression of Epstein-Barr virus latent gene products in tumour cells of Hodgkin's disease. Lancet 337:320–322.

Pallesen G, Sandvej K, Hamilton-Dutoit SJ, et al. 1991b. Activation of Epstein-Barr virus replication in Hodgkin and Reed-Sternberg cells. Blood 78:1162–1165.

Parkin DM, Muir CS, Whelan SL, et al. (eds). 1992. Cancer Incidence in Five Continents, Vol. VI. IARC Sci Publ 120, pp 205, 438, 532.

Pathmanathan R, Prasad U, Sadler R, et al. 1995. Clonal proliferation of cells infected with Epstein-Barr virus in preinvasive lesions related to nasopharyngeal carcinoma. N Engl J Med 333:693–698.

Poiesz BJ, Ruscetti FW, Gazdar AF, et al. 1980. Detection and isolation of type C retrovirus particles from fresh and cultured lymphocytes of a patient with cutaneous T-cell lymphoma. Proc Natl Acad Sci USA 77:7415–7419.

Poirier S, Oshima H, de Thé G, et al. 1987. Volatile nitrosamine levels in common foods from Tunisia, South China and Greenland, high risk areas for nasopharyngeal carcinoma. (NPC). Int J Cancer 39:293–296.

Pontisso P, Bankowski M, Petit M-A, et al. 1987. Recombinant HBsAg particles containing pre-S proteins bind to human liver plasma membranes. *In* Robinson W, Koika K, Will H (eds): Hepadna Viruses. New York, Alan R. Liss, pp. 205–222.

Pozzato G, Moretti M, Franzin F, et al. 1991. Severity of liver disease with different hepatitis C viral clones. Lancet 338: 509.

Prasad U. 1988. Early diagnosis of nasopharyngeal carcinoma: A multipronged approach. (Poster) Presented at 3rd International Symposium on Epstein-Barr Virus and Associated Malignant Diseases, Rome, October 3–7, 1988.

Prince AM, Brotman B, Grady GF, et al. 1974. Long-incubation post transfusion hepatitis without serological evidence of exposure to hepatitis B virus. Lancet ii:241–246.

Prince AM, Brotman B, Huima T, et al. 1992. Immunity to hepatitis C infection. J Infect Dis 165:438–443.

Purtilo DT, Sakamotok K, Barnabei V, et al. 1982. Epstein-Barr virus-induced diseases in boys with the X-linked lymphoproliferation syndrome (XLP). Am J Med 73:49–56.

Qian C, Camps J, Maluenda MD, et al. 1992. Replication of hepatitis C virus in peripheral blood mononuclear cells. Effect of interferon therapy. J Hepatol 16:380–383.

Raab-Traub N, Flynn K. 1986. The structure of the termini of Epstein-Barr virus as a marker of clonal cellular proliferation. Cell 47:883–889.

Riddler SA, Breinig MC, McKnight JLC. 1994. Increased levels of circulating Epstein-Barr virus (EBV)-infected lymphocytes and decreased EBV nuclear antigen antibody responses are associated with the development of posttransplant lymphoproliferative disease in solid-organ transplant recipients. Blood 84:972–984.

Robert-Guroff M, Nakao Y, Notake K, et al. 1982. National antibodies to human retrovirus HTLV in a cluster of Japanese patients with adult T-cell leukemia. Science 215:975–978.

Robinson JE, Brown N, Andiman W, et al. 1980. Diffuse polyclonal B-cell lymphoma with Epstein-Barr virus. N Engl J Med 320:1293–1296.

Robinson WS, Marion PL, Feitelson M, et al. 1982. The hepadnavirus group: Hepatitis B and related viruses. *In* Szmuness W, Alter HJ, Maynard JE (eds): Viral Hepatitis: 1981 International Symposium. Philadelphia, Franklin Institute Press, pp. 57–68.

Roggendorf M, Deinhardt F, Rasshofer R, et al. 1989. Antibodies to hepatitis C virus. Lancet 2:324–325.

Rojko JL, Hoover EA, Quackenbush SL, et al. 1982. Reactivation of latent feline leukemia virus infection. Nature 298:385–388.

Rosenblatt JD, Chen ISY, Wachsman W. 1988. Infection with HTLV-I and HTLV-II: evolving concepts. Semin Hematol 25:230–246.

Saksena NK, Sherman MP, Yanagihara R, Dube DK, Poiesz BP. 1992. LTR sequence and phylogenetic analyses of a newly discovered variant of HTLV-I isolated from the Hagahai of Papua New Guinea. Virology 189:1–9.

Sawada T, Tohmatsu J, Obara T, et al. 1989. High risk of mother-to-child transmission of HTLV-I in [p40^{tax}] antibody-positive mothers. Jpn J Cancer Res 80:506–508.

Schiffman MH. 1994. Epidemiology of cervical human papilloma infections. Curr Top Microbiol Immunol 186:56–81.

Schiffman MH. 1992. Recent progress in defining the epidemiology of human papillomavirus infection and cervical neoplasia. J Natl Cancer Inst 84:394–398.

Schlipkoter U, Roggendorf M, Ernst G, et al. 1990. Hepatitis C virus antibodies in hemodialysis patients. Lancet 335:1409.

Schneider A, Koutsky L. 1992. Natural history and epidemiological features of genital HPV infection. *In* Muñoz N, Bosch FX, Shah KV, and Meheus A (eds): The Epidemiology of Human Papillomavirus and Cervical Cancer. IARC Sci Publ 119:23–52.

Seiki M, Eddy R, Shows TB, et al. 1984. Non-specific integration of the HTLV provirus genome into adult T-cell leukemia cells. Nature 309:640–642.

Seiki M, Hattori S, Hirayama V, et al. 1983. Human adult T-cell leukemia virus: complete nucleotide sequence of the provirus genome integrated in leukemia cell DNA. Proc Natl Acad Sci USA 80:3618–3622.

Shafritz D, Shouval D, Sherman HI, et al. 1981. Integration of hepatitis B virus DNA into the genome of liver cells in chronic liver disease and hepatocellular carcinoma: studies in percutaneous liver biopsies and post-mortem tissue specimens. N Engl J Med 305:1067–1073.

Shanmugaratnam K, Higginson J. 1967. Aetology of nasopharyngeal carcinoma: report on a retrospective survey in Singapore. *In* Muir CS, Shanmugaratnam (eds): Cancer of the Nasopharynx. UICC Monograph Series I. Copenhagen, Munksgaard, pp. 130–137.

Shimizu YH, Weiner AJ, Rosenblatt J. 1990. Early events in hepatitis C virus infection of chimpanzees. Proc Natl Acad Sci USA 87:6441–6444.

Shimizu YK, Hijikata M, Iwamoto A, et al. 1994. Neutralizing antibodies against hepatitis C virus and the emergence of neutralization escape mutant viruses. J Virol 68:1494–1500.

Shiramizu B, Barriga F, Neequaye J, et al. 1991. Patterns of chromosomal breakpoints location in Burkitt's lymphoma: relevance of geography and Epstein-Barr virus association. Blood 77:1516–1526.

Shope RE, Hurst EW. 1933. Infectious papillomatosis of rabbits with a note on histopathology. J Exp Med 58:607–624.

Simmonds P, Alberti A, Alter HJ, et al. 1994. A proposed system for the nomenclature of hepatitis C viral genotypes. Hepatology 19:1321–1324.

Sixbey JW, Chesney PJ, Shirley P, et al. 1989. Detection of a second widespread strain of Epstein-Barr virus. Lancet ii:761–765.

Sixbey JW, Lemon SN, Pagano JS. 1986. A second site for Epstein-Barr shedding: the uterine cervix. Lancet 2:1122–1124.

Snydmann DR, Rudders RA, Baoust P, et al. 1982. Infectious mononucleosis in an adult progressing to fatal immunoblastic lymphoma. Ann Intern Med 96:737–742.

Sodrowski JG, Rosen CA, Haseltine WA. 1984. Trans-acting transcriptional activation of the long terminal repeat of human T-lymphotropic viruses in infected cells. Science 225:381–385.

Sonoda S, Yashiki S, Fujiyoshi T, Arima N, Tanaka H, Izumo S, Osame M. 1993. Ethnically defined immunogenetic factors involved in the pathogenesis of HTLV-I associated diseases. Bio Bulletin 5:79–88.

STEVENS CE, TAYLOR PE, TONG MJ, et al. 1988. Prevention of perinatal hepatitis B virus infection with hepatitis B immune globulin and hepatitis B vaccine. *In* Zuckerman AJ (ed): Viral Hepatitis and Liver Disease. New York, Alan R. Liss, pp. 982–988.

STEVENS CE, TAYLOR PE. 1991. Perinatal and sexual transmission of HCV, a preliminary report. *In* Hollinger FB, Lemon SM, Margolis HS (eds): Viral Hepatitis and Liver Disease. Baltimore, Williams and Wilkins, pp. 407–409.

STEVENS CT, TOY PT, TONG MJ, et al. 1985. Perinatal hepatitis B virus transmission in the United States: prevention by passive-active immunization. JAMA 253:1740–1745.

STROFFOLINI T, CHIARAMONTE M, TIRIBELLI C, et al. 1992. Hepatitis C virus infection, HBsAg carrier state and hepatocellular carcinoma: relative risk and population attributable risk from a case–control study in Italy. J Hepatol 16:360–363.

STUVER SO, TACHIBANA N, OKAYAMA A, ROMANO F, YOKOTA T, MUELLER N. 1992. Determinants of HTLV-I seroprevalence in Miyazaki Prefecture, Japan: A cross-sectional study, J Acquir Immune Def Syndr 5:12–18.

STUVER SO, TACHIBANA N, OKAYAMA A, SHIOIRI S, TSUNETOSHI Y, TSUDA K, MUELLER N. 1993. Heterosexual transmission of human T-cell leukemia/lymphoma virus type I among married couples in South-western Japan: An initial report from the Miyazaki Cohort Study. J Infect Dis 167:57–65.

SUGDEN B. 1977. Comparison of Epstein-Barr viral DNA's in Burkitt lymphoma biopsy cells and in cells clonally transformed *in vitro*. Proc Natl Acad Sci USA 74:4651–4655.

SUMMERS J, MASON WS. 1982. Replication of a hepatitis B-like virus by reverse transcription of an RNA intermediate. Cell 29:403–415.

SUMMERS J, O'CONNELL A, MILLMAN I. 1975. Genome of hepatitis B virus: restriction enzyme cleavage and structure of DNA extracted from Dane particles. Proc Natl Acad Sci, USA 72:4597–4601.

TABOR E, GERETY RJ, DRUCKER JA, et al. 1978. Transmission of non-A, non-B hepatitis from man to chimpanzee. Lancet i:463–466.

TACHIBANA N, OKAYAMA A, ISHIZAKI J, et al. 1988. Suppression of tuberculin skin reaction in healthy HTLV-I carriers from Japan. Int J Cancer 42:829–831.

TAJIMA K. (T- AND B-CELL MALIGNANCY STUDY GROUP). 1990. The 4th nation-wide study of adult T-cell leukemia/lymphoma (ATL) in Japan: Estimates of risk of ATL and its geographical and clinical features. Int J Cancer 45:237–243.

TAJIMA K, AKAZA T, KOIKE K, et al. 1984a. HLA antigens and adult T-cell leukemia virus infection: a community-based study in the Goto Islands, Japan. Jpn J Clin Oncol 14:347–352.

TAJIMA K, HINUMA Y. 1984b. Epidemiological features of adult T-cell leukemia virus. *In* Mathe G, Reizenstein P (eds): Pathophysiological Aspects of Cancer Epidemiology. Oxford, Pergamon Press, pp. 75–87.

TAJIMA K, KAMURA S, ITO S, et al. 1987. Epidemiological features of HTLV-I carriers and incidence of ATL in an ATL-endemic island: a report of the community-based co-operative study in Tsuschima, Japan. Int J Cancer 40:741–746.

TAJIMA K, TOMINAGA S, SUCHI T, et al. 1986. HTLV-I carriers among migrants from an ATL-endemic area to ATL non-endemic metropolitan areas in Japan. Int J Cancer 37:383–387.

TAKAHASHI K, KITAMURA N, SHIBUI T, et al. 1990. Cloning, sequencing, and expression in *Escherichia coli* of cDNA for a non-A, non-B hepatitis-associated microtubular aggregates protein. J Gen Virol 71:2005–2011.

TAKAHASHI K, TAKEZAKI T, OKI T, et al. 1991. Inhibitory effect of maternal antibody on mother-to-child transmission of human T-lymphotropic virus type I. Int J Cancer 49:673–677.

TAM AW, SMITH MM, GUERRA ME, et al. 1991. Hepatitis E virus: cDNA isolation and sequencing. *In* Hollinger FB, Lemon SM, Margolis HS (eds): Viral Hepatitis and Liver Disease. Baltimore, Williams and Wilkins, pp. 521–526.

TANAKA K, HIROHATA T, KOGA S, et al. 1991. Hepatitis C and hepatitis B in the etiology of hepatocellular carcinoma in the Japanese population. Cancer Res 51:2842–2847.

TANAKA K, SATO H, OKOCHI K. 1984. HLA antigens in patients with adult T-cell leukemia. Tissue Antigens 23:81–83.

T- AND B-CELL MALIGNANCY STUDY GROUP. 1981. Statistical analysis of immunologic, clinical and histopathologic data in lymphoid malignancies in Japan. Jpn J Clin Oncol 11:15–38.

T- AND B-CELL MALIGNANCY STUDY GROUP. 1988. The third nation-wide study of adult T-cell leukemia/lymphoma (ATL) in Japan: characteristic patterns of HLA antigen and HTLV-I infection in ATL patients and their relatives. Int J Cancer 41:505–512.

TARAO K, OHKAWA S, SHIMIZU A, et al. 1994. Significance of hepatocellular proliferation in the development of hepatocellular carcinoma from anti-hepatitis C virus-positive cirrhotic patients. Cancer 73:1149–1154.

THOMAS DL, CANNON RO, SHAPIRO CN, et al. 1994. Hepatitis C, hepatitis B, and human immunodeficiency virus infections among non-intravenous drug-using patients attending clinics for sexually transmitted diseases. J Infect Dis 169:990–995.

TIDY JA, PARRY GNC, WARD P, et al. 1989. High rate of human papillomavirus type 16 infection in cytologically normal cervices. Lancet i:434.

TIOLLAIS P, BUENDIA M-A, BRECHOT C, et al. 1988. Structure, genetic organization and transcription of hepadna viruses. *In* Zuckerman AJ (ed): Viral Hepatitis and Liver Disease. New York, Alan R. Liss, pp. 295–300.

TREMOLADA F, BENVEGNU L, CASARIN C, et al. 1990. Antibody to hepatitis C virus in hepatocellular carcinoma. Lancet 335:300–301.

TSUJIMOTO H, FULTON R, NISHIGAKI K, et al. 1993. A common proviral integration region, fit-1, in T-cell tumors induced by myc-containing feline leukemia viruses. Virology 196:845–848.

UCHIYAMA T, YODOI J, SAGAWA K, et al. 1977. Adult T-cell leukemia: clinical and hematological features of 16 cases. Blood 50:481–492.

UNO H, KAWANO K, MATSUOKA H, et al. 1988. HLA and adult T cell leukemia: HLA genes controlling susceptibility to human T cell leukemia virus type I. Clin Exp Immunol 71:211–216.

USUKU W, SONODA S, OSAME M, et al. 1988. HLA haplotype-linked high immune responsiveness against HTLV-I in HTLV-I-associated myelopathy: comparison with adult T-cell leukemia/lymphoma. Ann Neurol 23:S143–S150.

VAN DEN HOEK JAR, VAN HAASTRECHT HJA, GOUDSMIT J, et al. 1990. Prevalence, incidence and risk factors of hepatitis C virus infection among drug users in Amsterdam. J Infect Dis 162:823–826.

VAN DER POEL CL, REESINK HW, SCHAASBERG W, et al. 1990. Infectivity of blood seropositive for hepatitis C virus antibodies. Lancet 335:558–560.

VERDIER M, DENIS F, SANGARE' A, et al. 1989. Prevalence of antibody to human T cell leukemia virus type I (HTLV-I) in populations of Ivory Coast, West Africa. J Infect Dis 160:363–370.

WANG PS, EVANS AS. 1986. Prevalence of antibodies to Epstein-Barr virus and cytomegalovirus in sera from a group of children in the Peoples Republic of China. J Infect Dis 153:150–152.

WEINER AJ, GEYSEN HM, CHRISTOPHERSON C, et al. 1992. Evidence for immune selection of hepatitis C virus (HCV) putative envelope glycoprotein variants: putative role in chronic HCV infections. Proc Natl Acad Sci USA 89:3468–3472.

WEINER AJ, KUO G, BRADLEY DW, et al. 1990. Detection of hepatitis C viral sequences in non-A, non-B hepatitis. Lancet 335:1–3.

WEISS LM, STRICKLER JG, WARNKE RA, et al. 1987. Epstein-Barr viral DNA in tissue of Hodgkin's disease. Am J Pathol 129:86–91.

WERNER BG, BLUMBERG BS. 1978. E Antigen in hepatitis B virus infected dialysis patients: Assessment of its prognostic value. Ann Intern Med 89:310–314.

WERNER BG, O'CONNELL AP, SUMMERS J. 1977. Association of e antigen with Dane particle DNA in sera from asymptomatic carriers of hepatitis B surface antigen. Proc Natl Acad Sci USA 74:2149–2151.

WERNESS BA, LEVINE AJ, HOWLEY PM. 1990. Association of human papillomavirus types 16 and 18 E6 proteins with p53. Science 248:76–79.

WIKTOR SZ, ALEXANDER SS, SHAW GM, et al. 1990. Distinguishing between HTLV-I and HTLV-II by western blot. Lancet 335:1533.

WIKTOR SZ, PATE EJ, MURPHY EL, et al. 1993. Mother-to-child transmission of human T-cell lymphotropic virus type I (HTLV-I) in Jamaica: association with antibodies to envelope glycoprotein (gp46) epitopes. JAIDS 6:1162–1167.

WOGAN, GN. 1976. Aflatoxins and their relationship to hepatocellular carcinoma *In* Okuda K, Peters RL (eds): Hepatocellular Carcinoma. New York, Wiley, pp. 25–42.

WOLD WSM, GREEN M. 1979. Historic milestones in cancer virology. Semin Oncology 6:461–478.

WOLF H, ZUR HAUSEN H, BECKER V. 1973. EB viral genomes in epithelial nasopharyngeal carcinoma cells. Nature (London) New Biol 244:245–257.

WONG DK, CHEUNG AM, O'ROURKE K, et al. 1993. Effect of alpha-interferon treatment in patients with hepatitis B e antigen-positive chronic hepatitis B. A meta-analysis. Ann Intern Med 119:312–323.

YAMADA M, KAKUMU S, YOSHIOKA K, et al. 1994. Hepatitis C virus genotypes are not responsible for development of serious liver disease. Dig Dis Sci 39:234–239.

YAMADA Y. 1983. Phenotypic and functional analysis of leukemia cells from 16 patients with Adult T-cell leukemia/lymphoma. Blood 61:192–199.

YAMAGUCHI K, KIYOKAWA T, NAKADA K, et al. 1988. Polyclonal integration of HTLV-I proviral DNA in lymphocytes from HTLV-I seropositive individuals: an intermediate state between the healthy carrier state and smouldering ATL. Br J Haematol 68:169–174.

YAMAGUCHI K, NISHIMA H, KOHROGI H, et al. 1983. A proposal for smoldering adult T-cell leukemia: A clinicopathologic study of five cases. Blood 62:758–766.

YAMAGUCHI K, NISHIMURA Y, FUKUOKA N, et al. 1990. Hepatitis C virus antibodies in hemodialysis patients. Lancet 335:1409–1410.

YANAGIHARA R. 1992. Human T-cell lymphotropic virus type I infection and disease in the Pacific basin. Hum Biol 64:843–854.

YEUNG WM, ZONG YS, CHIU CT, et al. 1993. Epstein-Barr virus carriage by nasopharyngeal carcinoma *in situ*. Int J Cancer 53:746–750.

YOKOTA T, CHO M-J, TACHIBANA N, et al. 1989. The prevalence of antibody to p42 of HTLV-I among ATLL patients in comparison to healthy carriers in Japan. Int J Cancer 43:970–974.

YOSHIDA M, FUJISAWA T-I. 1992. Positive and negative regulation of HTLV-I gene expression and their roles in leukemogenesis in ATL. *In* Takatsuki K, Hinuma Y, Yoshida M, (Eds): Advances in Adult T-cell Leukemia and HTLV-I Research. Tokyo, Gann Monograph on Cancer Research No. 39, Japan Scientific Societies Press and Boca Raton, CRC Press, pp. 217–235.

YOSHIDA M, HATTORI S, SEIKI M. 1985. Molecular biology of human T-cell leukemia. *In* Voigt P (ed): Current Topics in Microbiology and Immunology, Vol. 5, No. 115. Berlin, Springer-Verlag, pp. 157–175.

YOSHIDA M, MIYOSHI I, HINUMA Y. 1982. Isolation and characterization of retrovirus from cell lines of human T-cell leukemia and its implication in the disease. Proc Natl Acad Sci USA 79:2031–2035.

YOSHIDA M, SEIKI M, YAMAGUCHI K, et al. 1984. Monoclonal integration of human T-cell leukemia suggests causative role of human T-cell leukemia virus in the disease. Proc Natl Acad Sci USA 81:2534–2537.

YU MC. 1991. Nasopharyngeal carcinoma: epidemiology and dietary factors. IARC Publ 105:39–47.

YU MC, TONG MJ, COURSAGET P, et al. 1990. Prevalence of hepatitis B and C viral markers in black and white patients with hepatocellular carcinoma in the United States. J Natl Cancer Inst 82:1038–1041.

ZANINOVIC V, SANZON F, LOPEZ F, VELANDIA G, BLANK A, BLANK M, FUJIYAMA C, YASHIKI S, MATSUMOTO D, KATAHIRA Y, MIYASHITA H, FUJIYOSHI T, CHAN L, SAWADA T, MIURA T, HATAMI M, TAJIMA K, SONODA S. 1994. Geographic independence of HTLV-I and HTLV-II foci in the Andes Highland, the Atlantic coast, and the Orinoco of Colombia. AIDS Res Hum Retroviruses 10:97–101.

ZAVITSANOS X, HATZAKIS A, KAKLAMANI E, et al. 1992. Association between hepatitis C virus and hepatocellular carcinoma using assays based on structural and nonstructural hepatitis C virus peptides. Cancer Res 52:5364–5367.

ZENG Y, LIU Y, LIU CR, ET AL. 1980. Application of immunozymatic method and immunoantoradiographic method of the mass survey of nasopharyngeal carcinoma. Intervology 133:166–168.

ZIEGLER JL. 1981. Burkitt lymphoma. N Engl J Med 305:735–745.

ZIEGLER JL, BECKSTEAD MD, VOLBERDING, et al. 1984. Non-Hodgkin's lymphoma in 90 homosexual men: Relation to generalized lymphadenopathy and the Acquired Immunodeficiency Syndrome. N Engl J Med 311:565–570.

ZUR HAUSEN H. 1986. Intracellular surveillance of persisting viral infections: Human genital cancer results from deficient cellular control of papillomavirus gene expression. Lancet ii:489–491.

25 Immunologic factors, including AIDS

LEO J. KINLEN

Recent interest in immunologic factors in cancer etiology was greatly stimulated by the concept of immunosurveillance put forward by Thomas (1959) and developed by Burnet (1965). This postulated that cancer originates in aberrant and antigenically distinctive cells produced in the course of cell replication. Whereas such cells would normally be eliminated by a healthy immune system, the hypothesis implies that failure of this process may allow progression to cancer to occur. Intensive experimental work over the past 30 years has greatly increased our knowledge of the immune system. Its application to the study of human cancer etiology is, however, far from straightforward. For cancer itself affects the immune system so that laboratory tests are unreliable in case-control studies. In prospective studies, on the other hand, immunologic tests are too complex and time consuming to be applied to the necessarily large populations that have to be followed. Epidemiologists have therefore concentrated on determining the incidence of cancer among individuals with clear evidence of immune impairment whether by disease or immunosuppressive treatment. More recently, the worldwide epidemic of the acquired immunodeficiency syndrome (AIDS), with certain malignancies among its manifestations, has underlined the relevance of the immune function to malignancy.

TRANSPLANT RECIPIENTS

The development of organ transplantation provided an important opportunity for testing the immunosurveillance concept. If cancer does develop from the aberrant cells that are normally eliminated by a healthy immune system, then the immunosuppressive treatment associated with transplantation should increase the incidence of malignancy. Reports of de novo cancer in renal transplant recipients first appeared in the literature in the 1960s. As the number of reports mounted, some workers saw them as indicating a generalized increase of cancers, consistent with the simplest interpretation of impaired immunosurveillance. Unfortunately, data of this sort can mostly not be evaluated because no means exists for estimating the numbers that would be "expected" if transplant patients had the same incidence of cancer as the general population. But one early exception was striking, for even by 1970 it could be deduced that the total number of published case reports of non-Hodgkin's lymphoma among transplant patients must represent a real excess, even after making generous assumptions about the numbers and survival of such patients around the world (Doll and Kinlen, 1970).

For reliable information a cohort study was required and the first to be reported was an analysis of data held by the (now discontinued) international registry of transplant patients of the American College of Surgeons (Hoover and Fraumeni, 1973; Hoover, 1977). The second study and the first specifically set up to investigate the subject involved transplant centers in Britain, Australia, and New Zealand (Kinlen et al, 1979). Both these studies found an increased incidence of cancer of about threefold, mainly due to marked increases of a few malignancies, including non-Hodgkin's lymphoma and skin cancer. However it was striking that the excesses observed in these early studies involved none of the fatal cancers that are characteristically common in Western societies. The modest excess of cancers other than those mentioned above included several that might reasonably be expected to be detected more readily in this carefully supervised group of patients than in the general population, while others were related to the underlying renal disease (such as renal pelvis tumors associated with analgesic nephropathy). With larger numbers of transplant recipients under study and longer periods of follow-up, it has become evident, however, that such cancers do not explain all the excess in this group (Sheil, 1991; Birkeland et al, 1995).

Lymphomas

The excess of non-Hodgkin's lymphoma (NHL) in transplant patients is remarkable for its magnitude, the predilection shown for the brain, and the very short induction period. The early cohort studies recorded increases of 27- and 49-fold, respectively (Hoover and Fraumeni, 1973; Kinlen et al, 1979) but the excess in the latest studies have been lower, at about 10-fold (see Table 25–1).The induction period of these lymphomas can be extremely short, even within 6 months of transplantation, less than in any other human malignancy. Cerebral involvement is unusually frequent, in more than a third of the cases associated with azathioprine. This is in marked contrast to the corresponding (very small) proportion of the lymphomas in the general population. An excess of lymphomas and of other lymphoproliferative lesions occurs not only after renal but also cardiac (Anderson et al, 1978), liver (Polson et al, 1988), and bone marrow (Forman et al, 1987; Shapiro et al, 1988) transplants, and is associated with both azathioprine and cyclosporine. Most of the lymphomas in transplant recipients are of B-cell type and of host origin (Penn, 1979). There has been no suggestion of an increase of Hodgkin's disease in any study.

Intensity of immunosuppression is an important determinant of the level of lymphoma risk. Early indications of this came from the unusually high incidence among transplant patients who received a particularly intensive immunosuppressive regimen (Anderson et al, 1978; Calne et al, 1979). Similarly the occurrence of a lymphoma in more than one transplant patient at the injection site of anti-lymphocytic globulin (Cotton et al, 1973) suggests a local dose-related effect. A decline in the incidence of post-transplant lymphomas in successive calender periods in both the early cohort studies before the advent of cyclosporine probably reflected reductions in the intensity of immunosuppressive therapy with the growth of medical experience (Kinlen, 1982). The incidence of lymphoproliferative disorder among cardiac transplant recipients increased markedly when a new and potent immunosuppressive agent was introduced, the monoclonal antibody OKT3 (Swinnen et al, 1990). A recent multicenter study of 45,141 kidney and 7634 heart transplant recipients over the period 1983–1991 found that the risk of NHL after intensive immunosuppressive therapy was 15 times greater than after a less aggressive regimen (Opelz et al, 1993). This was reflected in a higher incidence among cardiac than renal transplant patients, in the first year after the graft than subsequently and in those who received combinations of immunosuppressive agents.

No consistent relationship has been found between the risk of lymphoma in renal transplant recipients and the underlying renal disease. However, the risk was higher following cardiac transplantation for idiopathic cardiomyopathy than it was after coronary artery disease, possibly reflecting the additional immune impairment that has been reported in the former disorder (Anderson et al, 1978).

The very short induction period indicated by lymphomas developing within a few months of renal transplantation is so unlike that associated with chemical carcinogens that a quite different category of causation seemed to be implied. This, and the predisposition of transplant patients to virus infections, raised the possibility that these lymphomas might also be viral in origin. Furthermore, if the virus was already present in cells of the host, malignant transformation might occur within a short period. Since this was suggested in the first edition of this work, strong evidence has emerged for the Epstein-Barr virus (EBV) as the cause. The EBV genome has been detected in the malignant cells of all cases examined (Crawford et al, 1981; Hanto et al, 1981). Immunosuppressive therapy has been shown to permit EBV reactivation and sometimes polyclonal B-cell proliferation (Frizzara et al, 1981). Some of the lymphoproliferative disorders in transplant patients are of doubtful malignancy, but many others are true lymphomas of multiclonal or oligoclonal B-cell origin (Cleary and Sklar, 1984).

TABLE 25–1. *Cancer in Renal Transplant Recipients: Observed to Expected Ratios (Observed Numbers)*

Malignancy	*Hoover 1977 Many Countries*	*Kinlen et al 1979 UK, Aust, NZ*[a]	*Sheil et al 1991 Aust, NZ*[a]	*Birkeland et al 1995 Nordic Countries*
Non-Hodgkin's lymphoma	32.0 (52)	49.4 (42)	10.4 (50)	10.4 (25)
Skin cancer				
Melanoma	3.9 (6)	8.7 (2)	4.0 (40)	1.7 (7)
Other	b	8.9[c] (19)	b	24.9 (127)
Vulval cancer	d	d	35.5 (18)	31.0 (11)
Cervical cancer	b	b	4.5 (11)	8.6 (28)
Liver cancer	d	37.5 (3)	8.3 (d)	0.7 (1)
Kaposi's sarcoma	1000+ (1)	1000+ (1)	1000+ (14)	500+ (2)
Other	1.6 (82)	1.4 (41)	2.8 (320)	3.0 (309)
Total	2.6 (140)	3.3 (108)	3.3 (424)	4.6 (471)

[a]Aust = Australia, NZ = New Zealand.
[b]Details not presented and excluded from total.
[c]Squamous cell skin cancer: 27.6(8).
[d]Not presented.

Skin Cancer

Skin cancer has long figured prominently among malignancies in transplant recipients, an early observation being the predominance of the squamous cell type (Walder et al, 1971) in contrast to the general population in which the basal cell type is commonest. Increases of skin cancer are most marked for squamous cell skin cancer (27-fold), but basal cell cancers and melanomas are also increased (Kinlen et al, 1979). Further observations are required to clarify whether the excess of rodent ulcers is real or due to the combined effects of chance, better diagnosis of skin lesions in transplant patients, and under-registration in cancer registries thereby producing falsely low expected numbers. All the main cohort studies have found excesses of melanoma and all cases investigated in one study were found to have originated in precursor nevi (Greene et al, 1981).

These cancers, which are often multiple, mainly involve light-exposed surfaces. It is of interest that in a recent follow-up study of 56 long-term survivors of bone marrow transplants, two developed squamous cell skin cancer and another a melanoma, all in sites involved by chronic graft-versus-host disease (Lishner et al, 1990). Human papillomavirus (HPV) type 5/8 DNA has been identified in skin cancers in transplant recipients (Lutzner et al, 1983; Barr et al, 1989) suggesting a similar etiological role to that in the squamous cell skin cancers that often complicate the rare disorder epidermodysplasia verruciformis (Ostrow et al, 1982). Excesses of other HPV types have been found in other studies, but the significance of these virologic findings overall is at present unclear (IARC, 1995).

Vulval and Anal Cancers

The main cohort studies have recorded a marked excess of squamous cell cancer of the vulva (see Table 25–1). More recently evidence has emerged for their causation in transplant recipients by human papillomavirus infection, as in epidermodysplasia verruciformis (Caterson et al, 1984; Alloub et al, 1989). The many anal cancers that have been recorded in transplant recipients suggest a marked excess though this is usually unquantified because of the convention of including them with rectal cancer. A 40-fold increase has been recorded in a cohort study (Fairley et al, 1994).

Cervical Cancer

Evaluation of the cases of cervical cancer (mainly in situ) in the early cohort studies was hindered by the difficulty of making appropriate allowance for the frequency of cervical smears in these closely supervised patients. The larger and more recent studies, however, have found significant increases of invasive cervical cancer (Table 25–1). In addition, screened female transplant recipients have shown a significantly greater prevalence of cervical neoplasia than have screened control patients (Halpert et al, 1986) as well as a greater prevalence of human papillomavirus type 16/18 (Alloub et al, 1989; IARC, 1995).

Kaposi's Sarcoma

Penn (1982) was able to trace no less than 47 cases of Kaposi's sarcoma among a total of 1438 malignancies in transplant patients. The lack of any denominator prevents calculation of a precise expected value but for the pre-AIDS era, this number points to a very large increase in risk that must amount at least to several hundred fold. All the cohort studies have found excesses, amounting to about 1000-fold in one large study based on 14 cases, though data on the HIV status of the individuals concerned were not presented (Sheil, 1991).

Other Cancers

In the early cohort studies, most of the excess of cancers other than NHL and skin cancers could be explained by malignancies that are either related to the disorder that led to transplantation, or more likely than the average to be detected in a closely monitored hospital population. Most of the cohort studies have recorded increases of primary liver cancer (see Table 25–1). It has become clear, however, that malignancies other than those mentioned above are also increased in this group, including colon and lung cancers (Sheil, 1991; Birkeland et al, 1995). It is noteworthy, however, that the magnitude of these increases is much lower than in the case of lymphomas and squamous cell skin cancer. Furthermore, there is still no evidence that *all* the major malignancies are increased; for example, there is no appreciable excess of breast or stomach cancers (Sheil, 1991; Birkeland et al, 1995).

Significance of the Cancer Excesses

It seems noteworthy that most of the cancers that show marked excesses in transplant recipients, such as NHL, cervical cancer, and Kaposi's sarcoma, are well known for the evidence that exists for their being infective in origin. Furthermore, the viral causation of squamous cell skin cancers in epidermodysplasia verruciformis may be relevant to their increased incidence after transplantation, though an alternative or additional factor is suggested by the unusual antigenicity of skin cancers in mice. Indeed these ultraviolet light–induced skin tumors have been shown to be the most highly antigenic of all neoplasms (Kripke, 1974; Daynes et al, 1979). Overall, the epidemiological evidence accords with the principal findings from animal work indicating that immunosurveillance mainly operates against tumors of viral origin (Klein, 1991). The less marked increases of lung and other cancers recently recorded in the largest cohort studies may reflect impaired immunosurveillance of cancers of noninfective origin as found in certain animal studies (Trainin et al, 1967; Daynes et al, 1979; Shinozuka et al, 1988; Johnson et al, 1968).

The Behavior of Cancer

Early encouragement for the view that immunologic factors are important in cancer came from two remarkable case reports of cancers inadvertently transplanted with a kidney graft and which later regressed on withdrawal of immunosuppressive therapy (Wilson et al, 1968). In the best-documented example, a kidney from a donor who had died with a bronchial carcinoma was successfully transplanted to a 34-year-old patient with chronic glomerulonephritis. An abdominal mass developed in the recipient about 17 months later, which was found to be metastatic carcinoma indistinguishable from the original bronchial cancer of the donor. When immunosuppressive therapy was discontinued, the grafted kidney was promptly rejected, but at laparotomy only partial removal of the cancer was possible. Nine months later, however, when the patient received a second renal graft, the residual tumor had disappeared. No recurrence of cancer occurred following renewal of immunosuppressive treatment (Wilson et al, 1968). Despite such suggestions that immunosuppression can influence the behavior of transplanted cancer, transplantation in patients with a previous cancer is often successful without reactivation of the malignancy (Evans and Calne, 1974).

Clinical observations suggest that the skin cancers in transplant recipients are unusually aggressive. Further evidence of the influence of immune factors on the behavior or course of malignancy has come from regression both of non-Hodgkin's lymphoma and Kaposi's sarcoma reported after reduction of the immunosuppressive therapy in organ transplant recipients (Starzl et al, 1984; Penn, 1991). Of 214 Kaposi's sarcomas after transplantation, no less than 26 regressed after such modification (Penn, 1991).

IMMUNOSUPPRESSIVE THERAPY WITHOUT TRANSPLANTATION

The incidence of cancer in relation to immunosuppressive therapy in the absence of organ transplantation has obvious relevance because this controls for the possible effects of the graft and its foreign antigens. Despite this, it has received relatively little attention and the largest prospective study involved only 1634 patients treated mainly with azathioprine (1109 patients) or cyclophosphamide (461), and followed for up to 10 years (Kinlen, 1982, 1985; Kinlen et al, 1979). The numbers of tumors observed are shown in Table 25–2, together with the numbers that would be expected if the cancer incidence rates in the general population had applied. Despite the relatively small numbers, it is noteworthy that the tumors that are increased are mainly those that show marked excesses in the transplant group, namely non-Hodgkin's lymphomas, squamous cell cancer of the skin, primary liver cancer, and mesenchymal tumors. The lymphomas in these patients do not show the same predilection for the brain as those in transplant recipients. Nevertheless some excess is implied by the number of case reports of cerebral lymphomas in patients without transplants treated with immunosuppressive drugs, for these seem unlikely merely to reflect biased reporting, so rare are such tumors in the general population (Lipsmeyer, 1972; Uhl et al, 1974; Ulrich and Wuthrich, 1974; Moser et al, 1972; Jellinger et al, 1979; Neuhas et al, 1976; Varadachari et al, 1978; Lindeman et al, 1976). Indeed not many more cases were ascertained by the US Third National Cancer Survey among 21 million people observed over 3 years (Cutler and Young, 1975).

Prior to the AIDS epidemic, at least 18 cases of Kaposi's sarcoma had been reported in patients without transplants who had received immunosuppressive drugs, including steroids (Gange and Jones, 1978; Klepp et al, 1978; Ilie et al, 1981; Hoshaw and Schwartz, 1980). For such a rare neoplasm, these case reports suggest an increased incidence, a conclusion supported by the finding that more than 10% of all (53) cases of Kaposi's sarcoma recorded in Norway over a 5-year period

TABLE 25–2. *Observed (Obs) and Expected (Exp) Numbers of Cancer in Patients without Transplants after Immunosuppressive Therapy*

Type of Cancer	*Obs*	*Exp*	*Relative Risk*
Non-Hodgkin's lymphoma	6	0.55	10.9
Skin			
Basal cell	2	2.66	0.8
Squamous cell	3	0.60	5.0
Melanoma	0	0.29	—
Bladder cancer	6	1.64	3.7
Primary liver cancer	1	0.11	9.1
Other cancers	47	34.44	1.4
Total	65	40.29	1.6

Excluding cervical carcinoma in situ.

had previously received such treatment (Klepp et al, 1978).

The only cancer in Table 25–2 that showed an appreciable excess in this group but not among transplant patients is bladder cancer. This was restricted to the subgroup that received cyclophosphamide, of which it appears to be a specific effect, as with hemorrhagic cystitis. A similar excess was found in another prospective study (Plotz et al, 1979). The moderate excess of cancers of other sites shown in Table 25–2 needs to be interpreted with caution (47 observed, 34.4 expected). Cancers are likely to be detected more promptly and more completely in such a carefully supervised group than in the general population, but some of the excess is also due to the inclusion of four mesenchymal tumors and a vulval cancer, all of which also show an excess in transplant patients. Exclusion of these cases and cancers likely to be related to the underlying disorder reduces the relative risk to 1.2 (based on 40 observed).

A substantial proportion of the patients in the above study had rheumatoid arthritis, a disorder in which there is evidence of an increase of lymphomas in the absence of immunosuppressive therapy of about 2.5-fold in a pooled analysis (Kinlen, 1992; Gridley et al, 1993). However, studies of rheumatoid patients treated with azathioprine or cyclophosphamide have found a greater increase of lymphomas, amounting overall to about 10-fold, (see Table 25–3; Kinlen, 1985; Silman et al, 1988; Baker et al, 1987; Renier et al, 1978; Pinals, 1976; Love and Sowa, 1975; Baltus et al, 1983). Details of other malignancies after such therapy are sparse, but include an excess of cervical cancer based on two cases (expected 0.5) noted in a recent study of ulcerative colitis and Crohn's disease treated with azathioprine (Connell et al, 1994). An excess of anal cancer was also observed (two compared to 0.03 expected) but cannot be evaluated because an excess (of uncertain magnitude) has been recorded in Crohn's disease in the absence of azathioprine.

TABLE 25–3. *Relative Risk of Non-Hodgkin's Lymphoma in Cohort Studies in Rheumatoid Arthritis*

			Non-Hodgkin's Lymphoma		
Azathioprine or Cyclophosphamide	*No. of Patients*	*Total Cancers*	*Obs*	*Exp*[a]	*Relative Risk*
With[b] (7 studies)	1609+	136	20	2.0	9.7
Without[b,c] (14 studies)	67429	2439	92	41.82	2.2

[a]Conservatively estimated from total cancers, when not given in the original paper.
[b]Kinlen, 1992.
[c]Gridley et al, 1993.

GENETICALLY DETERMINED IMMUNODEFICIENCY DISEASES

Knowledge has greatly increased in recent decades about rare genetically determined disorders of the immune system, such as ataxia telangiectasia, the Wiskott-Aldrich syndrome, severe combined immunodeficiency, and common variable immunodeficiency. In these disorders the frequency of case reports of malignancy, often in children, have suggested an increased incidence of malignancy.

Of 491 malignancies in patients with immunodeficiency disorders notified to an international registry, no less than 51% were non-Hodgkins lymphoma (Filipovich et al, 1987). Details are not available of the populations of the immunodeficient patients from which these malignancies are drawn, so precise evaluation is impossible. Nevertheless this high proportion of non-Hodgkin's lymphoma is striking, being higher than any cancer registry has recorded in any age group.

Attempts have recently been made to quantify the risk of malignancy associated with certain of these immunodeficiency disorders. A prospective study of 377 patients with primary hypogammaglobulinemia, mainly common variable immunodeficiency (CVID), found a five-fold increase of cancer due mainly to large increases of stomach cancer (47-fold) and lymphomas (30-fold) (Kinlen et al, 1985). The excess of stomach cancer is probably related to the achlorhydria that is a frequent feature of CVID. Among 98 patients with this disorder who were followed for up to 13 years in New York, no fewer than 11 developed cancer (seven non-Hodgkin's lymphomas). It was estimated that this amounted to an eight- to 13-fold increase of cancer and a more than 100-fold increased risk of lymphomas (Cunningham-Rundles et al, 1987).

In a follow-up study of 301 individuals with the Wiskott-Aldrich syndrome, 23 non-Hodgkin's lymphomas were observed, estimated to represent a more than 100-fold increased risk (Perry et al, 1980). The lymphomas in this disorder often involve the brain. In ataxia telangiectasia major chromosomal changes and immunologic defects coexist, though their relative roles in the associated increased incidence of malignancy are unclear. The increase in malignancy involves not only lymphomas and leukemia, but apparently also ovarian dysgerminomas and stomach and liver cancers. Of some interest is the fact that most cases of lymphoid leukemia in this disorder have been of T-cell type (Spector et al, 1982).

In the very rare X-linked lymphoproliferative syndrome, affected males are vulnerable to fatal Epstein-Barr virus (EBV) infection. T-cell defects allow uncontrolled B-cell proliferation, and there is also a greatly increased incidence of malignant lymphoma (Purtilo et al, 1977). The evidence for a causative role for EBV in the lymphomas complicating this syndrome extends to the lymphoproliferative disorders in ataxia telangiectasia (Saemundsen et al, 1982), severe combined immunodeficiency (Reece et al, 1981), and common variable immunodeficiency (Purtilo et al, 1981).

THE ACQUIRED IMMUNODEFICIENCY SYNDROME

Kaposi's Sarcoma

Kaposi's sarcoma has figured prominently in the acquired immunodeficiency syndrome (AIDS) from the outset of the epidemic (Centers for Disease Control, 1981a,b). In San Francisco, where AIDS is unusually prevalent, the incidence of Kaposi's sarcoma in 1984 was found to be 2000 times greater than that in 1973–1978 among 20–49-year-old never-married men, the closest surrogate group in cancer registry data to homosexual males (Biggar et al, 1987). More recently by cross-matching registries of cancer and AIDS it has been estimated that in AIDS patients in this area, the risk of this malignancy is increased by more than 50,000 relative to a pre-AIDS population (Reynolds et al, 1993).

There are striking differences in the frequency of Kaposi's sarcoma among the different subgroups of AIDS patients, being highest in homosexual or bisexual men (21%), but less than 3% in patients with hemophilia-associated AIDS (Beral et al, 1990). The lower frequency with parenterally than with sexually transmitted HIV infection suggests that Kaposi's sarcoma is due to a sexually transmitted infection. It has long been clear that the relevant agent is not the human immune deficiency virus itself, and recently strong evidence has been found that the causative agent is a virus of the gamma herpes family (Chang et al, 1994). This would explain the cases in homosexual men without HIV infection (Friedman-Kien et al, 1990), a group with immune impairment as a result of the infections to which they are prone. The extraordinarily high incidence of Kaposi's sarcoma in homosexual men with AIDS may therefore reflect the combination of heavy exposure to the causative virus and the severe immune impairment that facilitates its expression as a malignancy. The declining proportion of this malignancy among AIDS (particularly homosexual) patients since 1983 may reflect reduced exposure to the causal agent as a result of altered sexual behavior.

Non-Hodgkin's Lymphomas

Recognition of AIDS was followed within a few years by revision of its clinical definition to include high-grade B-cell lymphomas, which were clearly increased in affected patients (Ziegler et al, 1984). Their histological pattern shows a wide variety, including immunoblastic and Burkitt-like subtypes (Ziegler et al, 1982). Up to a quarter of AIDS-associated lymphomas have been reported as affecting the brain (Lowenthal et al, 1988). A greater frequency of rectal involvement in AIDS-associated lymphomas has been reported in homosexual men than among intravenous drug users (Freter, 1990). The lymphomas in AIDS patients tend to be of high-grade histological type and extranodal (Rabkin et al, 1991).

Appreciable increases of non-Hodgkin's lymphomas and Burkitt-like lymphomas were seen in San Francisco in 1984 of 4.2- and 11.2-fold respectively, relative to 1973–1978, among never-married men aged 20–49 (Biggar et al, 1987). Compared to the general population, a relative risk of 141 for NHL was found in men with AIDS in Illinois in 1986–1987 (Cote et al, 1991). A lower risk of 71 found in such men in the San Francisco Bay area (Reynolds et al, 1993) may reflect a greater prevalence of AIDS in the reference population of that study compared to that in Illinois.

The lack of integration of the HIV genome in host cells of affected patients indicates that this virus is not the direct cause. As in other states of immune impairment, there is evidence that EBV is the cause of many AIDS-associated lymphomas (Baumgartner et al, 1989; Rosenburg et al, 1986; Uccini et al, 1989) though not all (Kaplan et al, 1989; Subar et al, 1988).

Hodgkin's Disease

In contrast to transplant recipients, Hodgkin's disease has often been recorded in AIDS patients, among whom nervous system involvement appears to be more frequent than in the general population (Knowles et al, 1988). Recently evidence of an increased incidence has been reported from a linkage of the San Francisco registries for cancer and for AIDS, with a relative risk of 8.8 in men with AIDS based on a total of 16 cases (Reynolds et al, 1993). The possibility of some misclassification of non-Hodgkins lymphoma remains to be clarified in future analyses of this and similar studies (Cote et al, 1991).

Anal Cancer

A relative risk of 2.6 was found for anorectal cancer among single men in San Francisco County in the period 1985–1987 relative to the pre-AIDS era (Rabkin et al, 1991). Furthermore a cancer-AIDS linkage study in the San Francisco area found a relative risk of 3.5 for anorectal cancers in men with AIDS in the period 1980–1987 (Reynolds et al, 1993). For anal cancer itself, a relative risk of 63.4 was found in a study based on AIDS registries in seven U.S. health departments (Melbye et al, 1994).

It is not possible to assess the contribution by HIV infection itself to the increases mentioned above because an increased incidence of anal cancer was recorded in homosexual men even before the AIDS epidemic (Austin, 1982; Li et al, 1982; Daling et al, 1987; Frisch et al, 1993).

Among active homosexuals, immune impairment is common as a result of the immunosuppressive effects of repeated infections and of seminal fluid itself, and these influences may in turn play a role in the excess incidence of anal cancers even before the AIDS epidemic (Austin, 1982; Li et al, 1982; Daling et al, 1987). The high prevalence of HPV 16 and 18 in HIV-positive patients (Caussy et al, 1990) together with certain characteristics shared by anal and cervical cancers (Melbye et al, 1991; Rabkin et al, 1992) points to HPV in the etiology of this cancer.

Other Tumors

Increases of squamous cell carcinomas of the conjunctiva in AIDS patients have been recorded, particularly in Africa (Ateeyni-Agaba, 1995; Goedert and Cote, 1995; Kestelyn et al, 1990). Other malignancies that have been reported as showing excesses include non-melanoma skin cancers (10-fold) and nasal and middle ear cancers (18-fold), though based on two and three cases, respectively (Reynolds et al, 1993). The lack of appreciable information on skin cancer in this disorder is striking.

IMMUNOSTIMULATION

In animals immunostimulation by bacille Calmette-Guérin (BCG) vaccination reduces the yield, or even causes regression, of tumors in certain experimental models. Inevitably, therefore, the report that BCG vaccination in infancy in Canada halved the leukemia death rate below age 5 (Davignon et al, 1971) aroused much interest. This claim was based on matching death certificates of children with leukemia against central BCG records. Misspelling and changes of names and migration would interfere with the matching process and result in the inappropriate allocation of deaths to the non-vaccinated group (Stewart and Draper, 1971; Hoover, 1976). Such biases and the use of an inappropriate denominator (Hoover, 1976) may also have contributed to the observation of an 80% reduction in deaths from leukemia and other malignancies among black children in Chicago vaccinated in the neonatal period (Rosenthal et al, 1961; Crispen, 1974). In Quebec and Glasgow, where BCG vaccination of the newborn has been routine, mortality from childhood leukemia was not appreciably lower than in the areas of Canada and Scotland without such a policy (Kinlen and Pike, 1971). Furthermore the proportion of children receiving BCG in England and Wales at about age 13 has risen to more than 70% without any decline in leukemia mortality in the relevant cohorts at ages 15–29 (Sutherland 1982). Age-specific leukemia mortality rates are remarkably similar in Denmark, Sweden, and Norway, though BCG vaccination is given at markedly different ages (Waaler 1971); they also remained similar in the north and south islands of New Zealand after BCG vaccination was discontinued in the south (Skegg, 1978).

Given the contradictions mentioned above, the evidence of the three randomized controlled trials of BCG are of particular interest. These have been carried out, all outside the neonatal period, in Puerto Rico (at 1–18 years), Georgia and Alabama (at 5 years or more), and England (at 14 or 15 years) and these have shown no significant reduction in leukemia cases or deaths (Snider et al, 1978; Kendrick and Comstock, 1981; Sutherland, 1982).

Unexpectedly, one of the studies that looked for evidence of leukemia protection found instead a four-fold increase of non-Hodgkin's lymphoma in the vaccinated group in the Puerto Rico BCG trial (Comstock et al, 1975). A significant excess of deaths from non-Hodgkin's lymphoma (though not of cases) was also found in the BCG-vaccinated part of New Zealand relative to the unvaccinated part (Skegg, 1978). In summary, there is overall no good evidence that BCG vaccination provides any protection against childhood leukemia.

Multiple myeloma has been associated in several case reports with previous exposure to unusual antigenic challenge from chronic infections, multiple immunizations, or desensitization injections for allergy. In some cases the M-component protein has shown antibody activity against the relevant antigen (Seligmann et al, 1968, 1973; Osterland and Espinoza, 1975; Kalliomaki et al, 1978). However, case-control studies of myeloma have provided little or no support for the immunostimulation hypothesis (Gallagher et al, 1983; Koepsell et al; 1987; Linet et al, 1987; Cohen et al, 1987). Similar findings were obtained in studies of non-Hodgkin's lymphoma (Tielsch et al, 1987) and mycosis fungoides (Whittemore et al, 1989).

HYPERSENSITIVITY STATES (ATOPY)

The immunologic basis of allergy gives it relevance to the present subject. Several studies have reported an unusually low incidence of cancer among affected individuals, suggesting that an unusually active immune system may be correspondingly efficient in eliminating early malignancies. Unfortunately this attractively simple hypothesis has not found overall support in relevant studies. Whereas several studies have supported the hypothesis (Fisherman, 1960; MacKay, 1966; Ure, 1969; Gabriel et al, 1972; Meers, 1973; Alderson, 1974; Vena et al, 1985; Mack et al, 1986), others have not (Dworwin et al, 1955; Shapiro et al, 1971; Logan and Saker, 1953; Robinette and Fraumeni, 1978; Chilvers et al, 1986; McWhorter, 1988), and one study found a significant decreased risk among females, but the reverse, namely a significant excess of cancers, among males (Mills et al, 1992).

The marked difference in frequency of allergic disorders between case patients and control patients in certain of these interview studies raises the possibility of recall or interviewer bias. Questions about trivial disorders are likely to be asked differently of ill and dying patients than of less severely ill control patients. Interviewer bias was specifically suggested by the difference in reported allergies between cases and controls in one particular pilot study (Chilvers et al, 1986): When this potential source of bias was minimized by keeping the interviewer in ignorance of the hypothesis, the previous difference did not persist. Similarly, no support was found in one of the largest case-control studies, in which the data were collected routinely by interviewers ignorant both of the hypothesis and the case or control status of the patient (Shapiro et al, 1971). Given the inconsistencies mentioned above, prospective studies have particular importance. However neither of those that have covered several different types of allergy found any evidence overall for a protective effect against cancer (McWhorter, 1988; Mills et al, 1992).

The evidence that individuals with allergies have a lower than average incidence of a variety of cancers is therefore weak. Indeed, certain studies have even suggested a positive relation with certain malignancies. Among prospective studies of individuals with asthma, two found a significant excess of lung cancer (Robinette and Fraumeni, 1978; Reynolds and Kaplan, 1987), and another a nonsignificant deficit (Alderson, 1974). Among patients with leukemia, lymphoma, and myeloma a positive association with allergy was found both in a case-control (Linet et al, 1987) and in two prospective studies (McWhorter, 1988; Mills et al, 1992).

THYMECTOMY, TONSILLECTOMY, AND SPLENECTOMY

Neonatal thymectomy in mice is a potent immunosuppressive influence that increases the incidence of malignancy in several experimental systems. In humans, however, this operation is seldom carried out in the neonatal period so that corresponding observations are not available. However a follow-up study of 383 older children and adults after thymectomy found no evidence of an increase in extrathymic cancer (Vessey et al, 1979).

The many studies of Hodgkin's disease in relation to previous tonsillectomy have produced conflicting results (Vianna et al, 1971, 1974; Ruuskanene et al, 1971; Johnson and Johnson, 1972; Cole et al, 1973; Teillet et al, 1973; Newell et al, 1973; Shimaoka et al, 1973; Gutensohn (Mueller) et al, 1975; Paffenbarger et al, 1977; Abramson et al, 1978; Andersen and Isager, 1978; Mueller et al, 1987; Bonelli, et al 1990). Studies that use siblings as controls lose some statistical power but gain in that they control for the social factors that are known to influence both Hodgkin's disease and tonsillectomy. A recent review concluded that tonsillectomy is unlikely to be a risk factor for this malignancy in young and middle life, though the evidence for the disease as it occurs late in life was unclear (Mueller et al, 1987).

No excess of cancer was detected among men followed up after splenectomy (Robinette and Fraumeni, 1977), while an increase reported after appendectomy was based on inappropriate comparisons (McVay, 1964; Bierman, 1968) and was not confirmed by a prospective study (Moertel et al, 1974).

CHRONIC RENAL FAILURE

Chronic renal failure impairs cellular immunity while its treatment by hemodialysis may produce additional impairment (Newbury and Sanford, 1971; Miyakoshi et al, 1974; Nelson and Penrose, 1975; Holdsworth et al, 1978). Certain reports have suggested that a variety of cancers are increased in dialysis patients, though only one of these studies formally compared the number of cancers observed (11) with that expected (less than two) (Matas et al, 1975). In this case the difference was made more impressive by the inclusion of tumors diagnosed before dialysis or of doubtful malignancy. Three studies of dialysis patients have found an appreciable excess of non-Hodgkin's lymphoma but not of other cancers (Kinlen et al, 1980; Slifkin et al, 1977; Herr et al, 1979). The largest and most recent study, however, found no significant increase (relative risk 1.2) of this malignancy (Kantor et al, 1987), conceivably because of changes over time, or differences between the United States and Britain in the management of dialysis patients.

In acquired cystic disease, which affects the native kidneys of long-term dialysis patients, a number of renal cell carcinomas have been reported, but their significance is uncertain (Dunnill et al, 1977; Hughson et al, 1986, MacDougall et al, 1987).

OTHER IMMUNOLOGIC DISORDERS

Laboratory tests have revealed some degree of immune impairment in a variety of disorders, but in rheumatoid arthritis these are more marked. These may be relevant to the increased incidence of non-Hodgkin's lymphomas recorded among rheumatoid patients (Table 25–3). A greater increase of this malignancy exists among patients with Sjögren's syndrome (Talal and Bunim, 1964) estimated at about 40-fold. This is particularly marked in association with parotid enlargement, splenomegaly, and lymphadenopathy (Kassan et al, 1978). The increases of this and other hematopoietic malignancies in individuals with thyroid diseases may be related to their autoimmune basis (Holm et al, 1985; Fukuda et al, 1987; Goldman et al, 1990). Similarly, the increases recorded after intensive treatment of Hodgkin's disease, both of NHL (Krikorian et al, 1979; Jacquillet et al, 1984) and melanoma (Tucker et al, 1985; Kaldor et al, 1987), may reflect the effects of immune impairment.

It is possible that the immunologic abnormalities in gluten enteropathy are relevant to the increases of lymphomas and of adenocarcinoma of the small intestine associated with that disorder (Harris et al, 1967; Holmes et al, 1976; Swinson et al, 1983). Similarly, the immunodeficiency of patients with chronic lymphatic leukemia may play a role in the associated increases of second cancers. These include lung cancer, melanoma, and soft tissue sarcomas and perhaps skin cancer, though here the greater opportunity for detection by physicians than in the general population make this association less certain (Greene et al, 1978; Davis et al, 1987).

Malaria, which can both stimulate and depress immune responses, appears to be involved with the Epstein-Barr virus in the etiology of Burkitt's lymphoma (Kafuko and Burkitt, 1970; Morrow et al, 1976. Dilantin (diphenylhydantoin) alters certain immune responses, and can cause a transient syndrome of lymphoid hyperplasia and, less consistently, an excess of lymphomas (including Hodgkin's disease) (IARC, 1987).

AGING

It has sometimes been suggested that the steep rise in cancer incidence with increasing age is due to a decline in the ability of the immune system to eliminate malignant cells. However, the cancers that show the greatest increases with age are not those that show the most marked excesses among individuals with immune impairment. Furthermore, there has for some decades been much circumstantial evidence for more plausible explanations involving the multistage model of carcinogenesis. These include the importance of duration of exposure to carcinogens and interval from first exposure as well as the greater opportunities with increasing age for partial transformation of cells to occur. Recently, more direct support for the multistage model has emerged from laboratory studies of mutations, oncogenes, and gene expression. In epidemiological studies it is usually difficult to separate any effects of age itself from those of duration of exposure to carcinogens. It is noteworthy, however, that a large and well-controlled animal experiment found that the incidence of skin tumors in mice was directly related to duration of exposure to painting with benzo(a)pyrene, but not to age at first exposure per se (Peto et al, 1975).

Data on the role of duration of smoking in relation to lung cancer risk are confounded by differences in cigarette consumption, tar content, and inhaling. Nevertheless the marked difference in risk between those who started to smoke before age 16 and those after age 25 strongly suggests that duration is important (Kahn, 1966; Doll, 1978). Mesothelioma is notable in that age at first exposure to asbestos is not correlated with risk, which depends on time since first exposure (Peto et al, 1982).

In other malignancies, the evidence of age-related effects is more readily explained by the multistage model of carcinogenesis than by declining efficiency of the immune system in older people. Thus observations on ex-smokers strongly suggest that cigarette smoke acts both early and late in the production of lung cancer. Whereas asbestos appears to initiate mesothelioma, as a cause of lung cancer it seems to act at a later stage (Peto et al, 1982). Studies of the early nickel refinery workers in south Wales suggest an early effect for lung cancer but a late effect for nasal sinus cancer (Peto et al, 1984). A greater sensitivity of the fetus to the carcinogenic effects of radiation may be due to the large numbers of actively dividing cells at that stage of life.

CONCLUSION

Epidemiological evidence suggests that the immune system does not play a major and equal role in all cancers, though it is undoubtedly important in certain malignancies. Non-Hodgkin's lymphoma stands out in showing increases in a variety of different immunological disturbances. It is striking that the malignancies that show the most marked excesses in immune impairment are those for which there is evidence of an infective origin. This also accords with experimental work that suggests that immunosurveillance primarily operates against oncogenic viruses. It is probable that immunosurveillance is also important in relation to cancers that are highly antigenic, as demonstrated in skin cancers in mice. However, this does not exclude some additional functions of the immune system in relation to malignancy. Thus renal transplant recipients have shown in recent studies limited but significant increases of certain cancers usually associated with chemical causation, such as cancers of the lung and colon. It may be relevant, therefore, that certain animal studies have shown that chemical carcinogenesis can be influenced by impaired immunosurveillance. However, it remains the case that transplant patients have so far *not* shown increases of every major malignancy, as implied by the crudest interpretation of the immunosurveillance theory.

The real or apparent inconsistencies in the malignancies that have shown excesses in different states of immune impairment is not necessarily remarkable. These may reflect differences in the severity and type of the immune impairment, as well as the power of particular studies. A delicate balance is exercised over the many different and complex elements of the immune system so that it is easy to envisage how defects acting at different points might differ in their effects. In some cases what is regarded as immune impairment may in effect be immunostimulation through the release of elements that are normally checked, as in the B-cell proliferation following T-cell inhibition.

Overall, the evidence on cancer and immune impairment suggests that immunosurveillance in humans operates primarily against malignancies that are either viral in origin or possibly highly antigenic in nature. In this respect there is a striking similarity between the human and animal evidence.

REFERENCES

ABRAMSON JH, PRIDAN H, SACKS MI, et al. 1978. A case-control study of Hodgkin's disease in Israel. J Natl Cancer Inst 61:307–314.

ALDERSON M. 1974. Mortality from malignant disease in patients with asthma. Lancet 2:1475–1477.

ALLOUB MI, BARR BBB, MCLAREN KM, et al. 1989. Human papillomavirus infection and cervical intraepithelial neoplasia in women with renal allografts. Br Med J 298:153–156.

ANDERSEN E, ISAGER H. 1978. Pre-morbid factors in Hodgkin's disease, II: BCG vaccination status, tuberculosis, infectious diseases, tonsillectomy and appendectomy. Scand J Haematol 21:273–277.

ANDERSON JL, BIEBER CP, FOWLES RE, et al. 1978. Idiopathic cardiomyopathy, age and suppressor-cell dysfunction at risk determinant of lymphoma after cardiac transplantation. Lancet 2:1174–1177.

ATEEYNI-AGABA C. 1995. Conjunctival squamous cell carcinoma associated with HIV infection in Kampala, Uganda. Lancet 345:695–696.

AUSTIN DF. 1982. Etiological clues from descriptive epidemiology: squamous carcinoma of the rectum or anus. Natl Cancer Inst Monogr 62:89–90.

BAKER GL, KAHL LE, ZEE BC, STOLZER BL, AGARIVAL AK, MEDSGER TA. 1987. Malignancy following treatment of rheumatoid arthritis with cyclophosphamide. Am J Med 83:1–9.

BALTUS JAM, BOERSMA JW, HARTMAN AP, VANDENBROUCKE JP. 1983. The occurrence of malignancies in patients with rheumatoid arthritis treated with cyclophosphamide: a controlled retrospective follow-up. Ann Rheum Dis 42:368–373.

BARR BBB, BENTON EC, MCLAREN K. 1989. Human papilloma virus infections and skin cancer in renal allograft recipients. Lancet 1:124–129.

BAUMGARTNER J, RACHLIN J, ROSENBLUM M, et al. 1990. (1989) quoted in Freter CE. J Natl Cancer Inst Monogr 10:45–54.

BERAL V, PETERMAN TA, BERKELMAN RL, JAFFE HW. 1990. Kaposi's sarcoma among persons with AIDS: a sexually transmitted infection? Lancet 335:123–128.

BIERMAN HR. 1968. Human appendix and neoplasia. Cancer 21:109–118.

BIGGAR RJ, HORM J, GOEDERT JJ, MELBYE M. 1987. Cancer in a group at risk of acquired immunodeficiency syndrome (AIDS) through 1984. Am J Epidemiol 126:578–586.

BIRKELAND SA, STORM HH, LAMM LU, BARLOW L, BLOHME I, FORSBERG B, EDLUND B, FJELDBORG O, FRIEDBERG M, FRODIN L, GLATTRE E, HALVORSEN S, HOLM NV, JAKOBSEN A, JORGENSEN HE, LADEFOGED J, LINDHOLM T, LUNDGREN G, PUKKALA E. 1995. Cancer risk after renal transplantation in the Nordic Countries 1964–1986. Int Cancer 60:183–189.

BONELLI L, VITALE V, BISTOLFI F, LANDUCCI M, BRUZZI P. 1990. Hodgkin's disease in adults: association with social factors and age at tonsillectomy: a case-control study. Int J Cancer 45:423–427.

BURNET FM. 1965. Somatic mutation and chronic disease. Br Med J 1:338–342.

CALNE RF, ROLLES K, WHITE DJG, et al. 1979. Cyclosporin A initially as the only immunosuppressant in 34 recipients of cadaveric organs: 32 kidneys, 2 pancreases and 2 livers. Lancet 2:1033–1036.

CATERSON RJ, FURBER J, MURRAY J, et al. 1984. Carcinoma of the vulva in two young renal allograft recipients. Transplant Proc XVI; 559–561.

CAUSSY D, GOEDERT JJ, PALEFSKY J, et al. 1990. Interaction of human immunodeficiency virus and papillomaviruses: association with anal epithelial abnormality in homosexual men. Int J Cancer 46:214–219.

CENTERS FOR DISEASE CONTROL. 1981. Kaposi's sarcoma and pneumocystis pneumonia among homosexual men—New York City and California. MMWR 30(25):305–308.

CENTERS FOR DISEASE CONTROL. 1981b. Follow up on Kaposi's sarcoma and pneumocystis pneumonia. MMWR 30(33):409–410.

CHANG Y, CESARMAN E, PESSIN MS, LEE F, CULPEPPER J, KNOWLES DM, MOORE PS. 1994. Identification of Herpes-like DNA sequences in AIDS-associated Kaposi's sarcoma. Science 266:1865–1869.

CHILVERS C, JOHNSON B, LEACH S, TAYLOR C, VIGAR E. 1986. The common cold, allergy, and cancer. Br J Cancer 54:123–126.

CLEARY ML, SKLAR J. 1984. Lymphoproliferative disorders in cardiac transplant recipients are multiclonal lymphomas. Lancet 2:489–493.

COHEN HJ, BERNSTEIN RJ, GRUFFERMAN S. 1987. Role of immune stimulation in the etiology of multiple myeloma: a case control study. Am J Hematol 24:119–126.

COLE P, MACK T, ROTHMAN K, et al. 1973. Tonsillectomy and Hodgkin's disease. N Engl J Med 288:63.

COMSTOCK GW, MARTINEZ I, LIVESAY BT. 1975. Efficacy of BCG vaccination in prevention of cancer. J Natl Cancer Inst 54:834–839.

CONNELL WR, KAMM MA, DICKSON M, BALKWILL AM, RITCHIE JK, LENNARD-JONES JE. 1994. Long-term neoplasia risk after azathioprine treatment in inflammatory bowel disease. Lancet 343:1249–1252.

COTE TR, HOWE HL, ANDERSON SP, MARTIN RJ, EVANS B, FRANCIS BJ. 1991. A systematic consideration of the neoplastic spectrum of AIDs: registry linkage to Illinois. AIDS 5:49–53.

COTTON JR, SARLES HE, REMMERS AR JR, et al. 1973. The appearance of reticulum cell sarcoma at the site of A.L.G. injection. Transplantation 16:154–157.

CRAWFORD DH, EDWARDS JMB, SWENY P, et al. 1981. Studies on long-term cell-mediated immunity to Epstein-Barr virus in immunosuppressed renal allograft recipients. Int J Cancer 28:705–709.

CRISPEN RG. 1974. Immunoprophylaxis with BCG. Neoplasm Immunity: 69–75.

CUNNINGHAM-RUNDLES C, SIEGAL FP, CUNNINGHAM-RUNDLES S, LIEBERMAN P. 1987. Incidence of cancer in 98 patients with common varied immunodeficiency. J Clin Immunol 7:294–299.

CUTLER SJ, YOUNG JL. 1975. In: Third National Cancer Survey: Incidence data: National Cancer Institute Monograph 41: US Department of Health and Welfare.

DALING JR, WEISS NS, HISLOP TG, et al. 1987. Sexual practices, sexually transmitted diseases, and the incidence of anal cancer. N Engl J Med 317:973–77.

DAVIGNON L, LEMONDE P, ST-PIERRE J, et al. 1971. BCG vaccination and leukaemia mortality. Lancet 1:80–81.

DAVIS JW, WEISS NS, ARMSTRONG BK. 1987. Second cancers in patients with chronic lymphocytic leukaemia. J Natl Cancer Inst 78:91–94.

DAYNES RA, HARRIS CC, CONNOR RJ, et al. 1979. Skin cancer development in mice exposed chronically to immunosuppressive agents. J Natl Cancer Inst 62:1075–1081.

DOLL R. 1978. An epidemiological perspective of the biology of cancer. Cancer Res 38:3573–3583.

DOLL R, KINLEN L. 1970. Immunosurveillance and cancer: epidemiological evidence. Br Med J 4:420–422.

DUNNILL MS, MILLARD PR, OLIVER D. 1977. Acquired cystic disease of the kidneys, a hazard of long-term intermittent maintenance haemodialysis. J Clin Pathol 30:868–877.

DWORWIN M, DIAMOND HD, CRAVER LF. 1955. Hodgkin's disease and allergy. Cancer 8:128–131.

EVANS DB, CALNE RY. 1974. Renal transplantation in patients with carcinoma. Br Med J 4:134–136.

FAIRLEY CK, SHEIL AGR, MCNEIL J-J, UGONI AM, DISNEY APS, GILES GG, AMIS N. 1994 The risk of ano-genital malignancies in dialysis and transplant patients. Clin. Nephrol. 41:101–105.

FILIPOVICH AH, HEINITZ KJ, ROBISON LL, FRIZZERA G. 1987. The immunodeficiency cancer registry: a research resource. Am J Pediatr Hematol Oncol 9(2):183–184.

FISHERMAN EW. 1960. Does the allergic diathesis influence malignancy? J Allergy 31:74–78.

FORMAN SJ, SULLIVAN JL, WRIGHT C, et al. 1987. Epstein-Barr-virus-related malignant B cell lymphoplasmacytic lymphoma following allogeneic bone marrow transplantation for aplastic anemia. Transplantation 44:244–249.

FRETER CE. 1990. Acquired immunodeficiency syndrome-associated lymphomas. NCI Monogr 10:45–54.

FRIEDMAN-KIEN AE, SALTZMAN BR, CAO Y, et al. 1990. Kaposi's sarcoma in HIV-negative homosexual men. Lancet 335:168–169.

FRISCH M, MELBYE M, MØLLER H. 1993. Trends in incidence of anal cancer in Denmark. Br Med J 306:419–422.

FRIZZERA G, HANTO DW, GAJL-PECZALSKA, et al. 1981. Polymorphic diffuse B-cell hyperplasias and lymphomas in renal transplant recipients. Cancer Research 41:4262–4279.

FUKUDA A, HIROHATA T, NOGUCHI S, et al. 1987. Risks for malignancies in patients with chronic thyroiditis: a long-term follow-up study. Jpn J Cancer Res 8:1329–1334.

GABRIEL R, DUDLEY DM, ALEXANDER WD. 1972. Lung cancer and allergy. Br J Clin Pract 26:202–204.

GALLAGHER RP, SPINELLI JT, ELLWOOD JM, SKIPPEN DH. 1983. Allergies and agricultural exposure as risk factors for multiple myeloma. Br J Cancer 48:853–857.

GANGE RW, JONES EW. 1978. Kaposi's sarcoma and immunosuppressive therapy: an appraisal. Clin Exp Dermatol 3:135–146.

GOEDERT JJ, COTE TR. 1995. Conjunctival malignant disease with AIDS in USA. Lancet 345:257–258.

GOLDMAN MB, MONSON RR, MALOOF F. 1990. Cancer mortality in women with thyroid disease. Cancer Res 50:2283–2289.

GREAVES MF. 1986. Annotation: Is spontaneous mutation the major 'cause' of childhood acute lymphoblastic leukaemia? Br J Haematol 64:1–13.

GREENE MH, HOOVER RN, FRAUMENI JF JR. 1978. Subsequent cancer in patients with chronic lymphocytic leukemia—a possible immunologic mechanism. J Natl Cancer Inst 61:337–340.

GRIDLEY G, MCLOUGHLIN JK, EKBOM A, KLARKESKOG L, ADAMI H-O, HACKER DG, HOOVER R, FRAUMENI JF. 1993 Incidence of cancer among patients with rheumatoid arthritis. J Natl Cancer Inst 85:307–311.

GREENE MH, YOUNG TI, CLARK WH JR. 1981. Malignant melanoma in renal transplant recipients. Lancet 1:1196–1199.

GUTENSOHN (MUELLER) N, LI FP, JOHNSON RE, et al. 1975. Hodgkin's disease, tonsillectomy and family size. N Engl J Med 292:22–25.

HALPERT R, FRUCHTER RG, SEDLIS A, et al. 1986. Human papillomavirus and lower genital neoplasia in renal transplant patients. Obstet Gynecol 68:251–258.

HANTO DW, FRIZZERA G, PURTILO DT, et al. 1981. Clinical spectrum of lymphoproliferative disorders in renal transplant recipients and evidence for the role of Epstein-Barr virus. Cancer Res 41:4253–4261.

HARRIS OD, COOKE WT, THOMPSON H, et al. 1967. Malignancy in adult coeliac disease and idiopathic steatorrhoea. Am J Med 42:899–912.

HERR HW, ENGEN DE, HOSTETLER J. 1979. Malignancy in uremia: dialysis versus transplantation. J Urol 121:584–586.

HOLDSWORTH SR, FITZGERALD MG, HOSKING CS, et al. 1978. The effect of maintenance dialysis on lymphocyte function, I: Haemodialysis. Clin Exp Immunol 33:95–101.

HOLM L-E, BLOMGREN H, LOWHAGEN T. 1985. Cancer risks in patients with chronic lymphocytic thyroiditis. N Engl J Med 312(10):601–604.

HOLMES GKT, STOKES PL, SOREHAN TM, et al. 1976. Coeliac disease, gluten-free diet and malignancy. Gut 17:612–619.

HOOVER R, FRAUMENI JF JR. 1973. Risk of cancer in renal transplant recipients. Lancet 2:55–57.

HOOVER RN. 1976. BCG vaccination and cancer prevention: a critical review of the human experience. Cancer Res 36:352–354.

HOOVER R. 1977. Effects of drugs—immunosuppression. In: *Origins of Human Cancer*, Hiatt, Watson JD, Winsten JA (eds). Cold Spring Harbor Laboratory, pp 369–379.

HOWSHAW RA, SCHWARTZ RA. 1980. Kaposi's sarcoma after immunosuppressive therapy with prednisone. Arch Dermatopathol 16:1280–1282.

HUGHSON MD, BUCHWALD D, FOX M. 1986. Renal neoplasia and acquired cystic kidney disease in patients receiving long-term dialysis. Arch Pathol Lab Med 110:592–601.

ILIE B, BREMNER S, LIPITZ R, et al. 1981. Kaposi's sarcoma after steroid therapy for pemphigus foliaceus. Dermatologica 163:455–459.

INTERNATIONAL AGENCY FOR RESEARCH ON CANCER. 1995. IARC monographs on the evaluation of carcinogenic risks to humans. Vol 64. Human Papillomaviruses. Lyon, France, IARC.

JACQUILLAT C, KHAYAT D, DESPREZ-CURELY JP, et al. 1984. Non-Hodgkin's lymphoma occurring after Hodgkin's disease. Cancer 53:459–462.

JELLINGER K, KOTHBAUER P, WEISS R, et al. 1979. Primary malignant lymphoma of the CNS and polyneuropathy in a patient with necrotizing vasculitis treated with immunosuppression. J Neurol 220:259.

JOHNSON SK, JOHNSON RE. 1972. Tonsillectomy history in Hodgkin's disease. N Engl J Med 287:1122–1125.

JOHNSON S. 1968. Effect of thymectomy on the induction of skin tumours by DBA and of breast tumours by DMBA in mice of the IF strain. Br J Cancer 22:755–761.

KAFUKO GW, BURKITT DP. 1970. Burkitt's lymphoma and malaria. Int J Cancer 6:1–9.

KAHN HA. 1966. The Dorn study of smoking mortality among U.S. veterans: report on eight and one half years of observation. In: Epidemiological Study of Cancer and Other Chronic Disease. NCI Monogr 19:1.

KALDOR JM, DAY NE, BLANK P, et al. 1987. Recent malignancies followingtesticular cancer, ovarian cancer and Hodgkin's disease: an international collaborative study among cancer registries. Int J Cancer 39:571–585.

KALLIOMAKI JL, GRANFERS K, TARVANEN A. 1978. An immunoglobulin G myeloma with anti-streptolysis activity and a lifelong history of intravenous streptococcal infection. Clin Immunol Immunopathol 9:22–27.

KANTOR AF, HOOVER RN, KINLEN LJ, et al. 1987. Cancer in patients receiving long-term dialysis treatment. Am J Epidemiol 126:370–376.

KAPLAN LD, ABRAMS DI, FEIGAL L, et al. 1989. AIDS-associated non-Hodgkins lymphoma in San Francisco. JAMA 261:719–724.

KASSAN SS, THOMAS TL, MOUTSOPOULOS HM, et al. 1978. Increased risk of lymphoma in sicca syndrome. Ann Intern Med 89:888–892.

KENDRICK MA, COMSTOCK GW. 1981. BCG vaccination and the subsequent development of cancer in humans. J Natl Cancer Inst 66:431–437.

KESTELYN P, STEVENS AM, NDAYAMBAJE A, HANSSENS M, VAN DE PERRE P. 1990. HIV and conjunctival malignancies. Lancet 336:51–52.

KINLEN LJ. 1982. Immunosuppressive therapy and cancer. Cancer Surv 1:565–583.

KINLEN LJ. 1985. Incidence of cancer in rheumatoid arthritis and other disorders after immunosuppressive treatment. Am J Med 78 (Suppl 1A):44–49.

KINLEN LJ. 1992. Malignancy in autoimmune diseases. J Autoimmun 5 (Suppl A):363–371.

KINLEN LJ, DOLL R, PETO J. 1983. The incidence of tumors in human transplant recipients. Transplant Proc 15:1039–1042.

KINLEN LJ, SHEIL AGR, PETO J, et al. 1979. A collaborative U.K.-Australasian study of cancer in patients treated with immunosuppressive drugs. Br Med J 2:1461–1466.

KINLEN LJ, PIKE MC. 1971. BCG vaccination and leukaemia: evidence of vital statistics. Lancet 2:398–402.

KINLEN LJ, EASTWOOD JB, KERR DNS, et al. 1980. A study of cancer in dialysis patients. Br Med J 280:1401–1403.

KINLEN LJ, PETO J, DOLL R, SHEIL AGR. 1981. Cancer in patients treated with immunosuppressive drugs. Br Med J 1:474.

KINLEN LJ, WEBSTER ADB, BIRD AG, HAILE R, PETO J, SOOTHILL JF, THOMPSON RA. 1985. Prospective study of cancer in patients with hypogammaglobulinaemia. Lancet 1:263–265.

KLEIN G. 1991. Immunovirology of transforming viruses. Curr Opin Immunol 3:665–673.

KLEPP O, DAHL O, STENWIG JT. 1978. Association of Kaposi's sarcoma and prior immunosuppressive therapy. Cancer 42:2626–2630.

KNOWLES DM, CHAMULAK GA, SUBAR M, et al. 1988. Lymphoid neoplasia associated with the acquired immunodeficiency syndrome (AIDS). Ann Intern Med 108:744–753.

KOEPSELL TD, DALING JR, WEISS NS, TAYLOR JW, OLSHAM AF, LYON JL, SWANSON GM, CHILD M. 1987. Antigenic stimulation and the occurrence of multiple myeloma. Am J Epidemiol 126:1051–1062.

KRIKORIAN JG, BURKE JS, ROSENBERG SA, et al. 1979. Occurrence of non-Hodgkin's lymphoma after therapy for Hodgkin's disease. N Engl J Med 300:452–458.

KRIPKE ML. 1981. Immunologic mechanisms in UV radiation carcinogenesis. Adv Cancer Res 34:69–106.

KRIPKE ML. 1990. Effects of UV radiation on tumor immunity. J Natl Cancer Inst 82:1392–1395.

KRIPKE ML. 1974. Antigenicity of murine skin tumors induced by ultraviolet light. J Natl Cancer Inst 53:1333–1336.

LI FP, OSBORN D, CRONIN CM. 1982. Anorectal squamous carcinoma in two homosexual men. Lancet 2:391.

LINDEMAN RD, PETERSON JA, MATTER BJ. 1976. Long-term azathioprine-corticosteroid therapy in lupus nephritis and idiopathic nephrotic syndrome. J Chronic Dis 29:189–204.

LINET MS, HARBOUR SD, MCLOUGHLIN JK. 1987. A case-control study of multiple myeloma in whites: chronic antigenic stimulation, occupation and drugs use. Cancer Res 47:2978–2981.

LIPSMEYER EA. 1972. Development of malignant cerebral lymphoma in a patient with systemic lupus erythematosus treated with immunosuppression. Arthritis Rheum 15:183.

LIPSMEYER EA. 1972. Development of malignant cerebral lymphoma in a patient with systemic lupus erythematosus treated with immunosuppression. Arthritis Rheum 15:183–186.

LISHNER M, PATTERSON B, KANDEL R, et al. 1990. Cutaneous and mucosal neoplasms in bone marrow transplant recipients. Cancer 65:473–476.

LOGAN J, SAKER D. 1953. The incidence of allergic disorders in cancer. NZ Med J 52:210–212.

LOVE RR, SOWA JM. 1975. Myelomonocytic leukemia following cyclophosphamide therapy of rheumatoid disease. Ann Rheum Dis 34:534–535.

LOWENTHAL DA, STRAUS DJ, CAMPBELL SW, et al. 1988. AIDS-related lymphoid neoplasia: the Memorial Hospital experience. Cancer 61:2325–2337.

LUTZNER MA, ORTH G, DUTRONQUAY V, et al. 1983. Detection of human papillomavirus type 5DNA in skin cancers of an immunosuppressed renal allograft recipient. Lancet 2:422–424.

MACDOUGALL ML, WELLING LW, WIEGMANN TB. 1987. Renal adenocarcinoma and acquired cystic disease in chronic hemodialysis patients. Am J Kidney Dis 9:166–171.

MACK TM, YU MC, HANISCH R, HENDERSON BE. 1986. Pancreas cancer and smoking, beverage consumption, and past medical history. J Natl Cancer Inst 76(1):49–60.

MACKAY WD. 1966. The incidence of allergic disorders and cancer. Br J Cancer 20:434–437.

MATAS AJ, SIMMONS RL, KJELLSTRAND CM, et al. 1975. Increased incidence of malignancy during chronic renal failure. Lancet 1:883–886.

MCDONNELL JM, MAYR AJ, MARTIN WJ. 1989. DNA of human papillomavirus type 16 in dysplastic and malignant lesions of the conjunctiva and cornea. N Engl J Med 320:1442–1446.

MCVAY JR, JR. 1964. The appendix in relation to neoplastic disease. Cancer 17:929–937.

MCWHORTER WP. 1988. Allergy and risk of cancer. Cancer 62:451–455.

MEERS PD. 1973. Allergy and cancer. Lancet 1:884–885.

MELBYE M, SPROGEL P. 1991. Aetiological parallel between anal cancer and cervical cancer. Lancet 338:657–659.

MELBYE M, COTE TR, KESSLER L, GAIL M, BIGGAR RJ, AND THE AIDS/CANCER WORKING GROUP. 1994. High incidence of anal cancer among AIDS patients. Lancet 343:636–639.

MILLS PK, LAWRENCE BEESON W, FRASER GE, PHILIPS RL. 1992. Allergy and cancer: organ site-specific results from the Adventist Health Study. Am J Epidemiol 136(3):287–295.

MIYAKOSHI H, AOKI T, HIRASAWA Y. 1974. Effects of serum and plasma from hemodialysis patients on the lymphoproliferative response. Clin Nephol 12(6).

MOERTEL CG, NOBREGA FT, ELVEBACK LR, WENTZ JR. 1974. A prospective study of appendectomy and predisposition to cancer. Surg Gynecol Obstet 138:549–553.

MORROW RH, KISUULE A, PIKE MC, et al. 1976. Burkitt's lymphoma in the Mengo districts of Uganda: epidemiologic features and their relationship to malaria. J Natl Cancer Inst 56:479–485.

Moser KD, Araoz CA, Smith PL. 1972. Immunosuppressive therapy and reticulum cell sarcomas of the brain. Panminerva Med 34:1–2:436.

Mueller N, Swanson GM, Hsieh CC, Cole P. 1987. Tonsillectomy and Hodgkin's disease: results from comparison population-based studies. J Natl Cancer Inst 78:1–5.

Nelson DS, Penrose JM. 1975. Brief report: effect of hemodialysis and transplantation on inhibition of lymphocyte transformation by sera from uremic patients. Clin Immunol Immunopathol 4:143–146.

Neuhas K, Thorhurst J, Bertol O, Speck B. 1976. Multiple neoplasms in a case of rheumatoid arthritis treated with azathioprine. Praxis 10:2131.

Newberry WM, Sanford JP. 1971. Defective cellular immunity in renal failure: depression of reactivity of lymphocytes to photohemagglutinin by renal failure serum. J Clin Invest 50:1262–1271.

Newell GR, Rawlings W, Kinnear BK, et al. 1973. Case-control study of Hodgkin's disease: results of the interview questionnaire. J Natl Cancer Inst 51:1437–1441.

Opelz G, Henderson R. 1993. Incidence of non-Hodgkins lymphoma in kidney and heart transplant recipients. Lancet 342:1514–1516.

Osterland CK, Espinoza LR. 1975. Biological properties of myeloma proteins. Arch Intern Med 135:32–36.

Ostrow RS, Bender M, Nimura M, et al. 1982. Human papillomavirus DNA in cutaneous primary and metastasized squamous cell carcinomas from patients with epidermodysplasia verruciformis. Proc Natl Acad Sci (USA) 79:1634–1638.

Paffenbarger RS Jr, Wing AL, Hyde RT. 1977. Brief communication: characteristics in youth indicative of adult-onset Hodgkin's disease. J Natl Cancer Inst 58:1489–1491.

Penn I. 1982. The occurrence of cancer in immune deficiencies. Curr Probl Cancer 6:1–64.

Penn I. 1979. Host origin of lymphomas in organ transplant recipients. Transplantation 27:214.

Penn I, Halgrimson CG, Starzl TE, et al. 1971. Malignant tumors in organ transplant recipients. Transplant Proc 3:773–778.

Perry GS, Spector BD, Shuman LM, Mandel JS, Anderson VE, McHugh RB, Hanson MR, Fahlstrom SM, Krivit W, Kersey JH. 1980. The Wiscott-Aldrich syndrome in the United States and Canada (1892–1979). J Pediatr 97:72–78.

Peto J, Seidman H, Soli Koff IJ. 1982. Mesothelioma mortality inasbestos workers: implications for models of carcinogenesis and risk assessment. Br J Cancer 45:124–135.

Peto R, Row FJC, Lee PN, et al. 1975. Cancer and ageing in mice and men. Br J Cancer 32:411–426.

Peto J. 1984. Early and late-stage carcinogenesis in mouse skin and in man. In: *Models, Mechanisms and Etiology of Tumor Promotion*, Borzsonyi M, Day NE, Lampis K, Yamasaki H (eds). IARC Scientific Publications No. 56, International Agency for Research on Cancer, Lyon.

Pinals RS. 1976. Azathioprine in the treatment of chronic polyarthritis: long-term results and adverse effects in 25 patients. J Rheumatol 3(2):140–144.

Plotz PH, Klippel JH, Decker JL, et al. 1979. Bladder complications in patients receiving cyclophosphamide for systemic lupus erythematosus or rheumatoid arthritis. Ann Intern Med 91:221–223.

Polson RJ, Neuberger J, Forman D, et al. 1988. De novo malignancies after liver transplantation. Transplant Proc XX:94–97.

Purtilo DT, De Florio D, Young PS, et al. 1977. Variable phenotypic expressions of an X-linked recessive lymphoproliferative syndrome. N Engl J Med 297:1077–1081.

Purtilo DT, Sakamoto K, Saemundsen, et al. 1981. Documentation of Epstein-Barr virus infection in immunodeficiency patients with life-threatening lymphoproliferative diseases of clinical, immunological and pathological studies. Cancer Res 41:4226–4236.

Rabkin CS, Blattner WA. 1991. HIV infection and cancers other than non-Hodgkin lymphoma and Kaposi's sarcoma. Cancer Surv 10:151–160.

Rabkin CS, Biggar RJ, Melbye M, Curtis RE. 1992. Second primary cancers following anal and cervical carcinoma: evidence of shared etiologic factors. Am J Epidemiol 136(1):54–59.

Reece ER, Gartner JG, Seemayer TA, et al. 1981. Epstein-Barr virus in a malignant lymphoproliferative disorder of B-cells occurring after thymic epithelial transplantation for cerebral immunodeficiency. Cancer Res 41:4243–4247.

Renier JC, Bregeon C, Bonnette C, Boasson M, Bernat M, Basle M, Besson J, Wellinger C, Bourgeois B, Teisseire N. 1978. Le deviner des sujets atteints de polyarthrite rhumatoide et traites par les immunodepresseurs entre 1965 et 1973 inclus. Rev Rhum Mal Osteoartic 45(7–9):453–461.

Reynolds P, Saunders LD, Layefsky ME, Lemp GF. 1993. The spectrum of acquired immunodeficiency syndrome (AIDS)-associated malignancies in San Francisco, 1980–87. Am J Epidemiol 137(1):19–31.

Robinette CD, Fraumeni JF, Jr. 1978. Asthma and subsequent mortality in World War II veterans. J Chron Dis 31:619–624.

Robinette CD, Fraumeni JF. 1977. Splenectomy and subsequent mortality in veterans of the 1939–45 war. Lancet 2:127–129.

Rosenburg NL, Hochberg FH, Miller G, et al. 1986. Primary central nervous system lymphoma related to Epstein-Barr virus in a patient with acquired immunodeficiency syndrome. Ann Neurol 20:98–102.

Rosenthal SR, Loewinsohn E, Graham ML, et al. 1961. BCG vaccination against tuberculosis in Chicago: a 20 year study statistically analysed. Paed 28:622–641.

Ruuskanen O, Vanha-Perttula T, Kouvalainen K. 1971. Tonsillectomy, appendectomy and Hodgkin's disease. Lancet 1:1127–1128.

Saemundsen AK, Purtilo DT, Sakamoto K, et al. 1981. Documentation of Epstein-Barr virus infection in immunodeficient patients with life threatening lymphoproliferative diseases by DNA-DNA hybridisation. Cancer Res 41:4237–4242.

Seligmann M, Danon F, Basch A, Bernard J. 1968. IgM myeloma cryoglobulin with antistrepsolysin activity. Nature (London) 220:711.

Seligmann M, Brouet JC. 1973. Antibody activity of human myeloma globulin. Semin Hematol 10:163.

Shapiro S, Heinonen OP, Siskind V. 1971. Cancer and allergy. Cancer 28:396–400.

Shapiro RS, McClain K, Frizzera G, et al. 1988. Epstein-Barr virus associated B cell lymphoproliferative disorders following bone marrow transplantation. Blood 71:1234–1243.

Sheil AGR. 1991. Cancer survey. In: 14th Report of the Australia and New Zealand Dialysis and Transplants Registry, Disney, APS (ed). The Queen Elizabeth Hospital, Woodville, South Australia.

Shimaoka K, Bross ID, Tiding J. 1973. Tonsillectomy and Hodgkins disease. N Engl J Med 288:634–635.

Shinozuka H, et al. 1988. Experimental models of malignancies after cyclosporine therapy. Transplant Proc 20:893–899.

Silman AJ, Petrie J, Hazleman B, Evans SJW. 1988. Lymphoproliferative cancer and other malignancy in patients with rheumatoid arthritis treated with azathioprine: a 20 year follow up study. Ann Rheum Dis 47:988–992.

Skegg DCG. 1978. BCG vaccination and the incidence of lymphoma and leukaemia. Int J Cancer 21:18–21.

Slifkin RF, Goldberg J, Neff MS, et al. 1977. Malignancy in end-stage renal disease. Trans Am Soc Intern Organs 23:34–39.

Snider DE, Comstock GW, Martinez I, Caras GJ. 1978. Efficacy of BCG vaccination in prevention of cancer: an update: brief communication. J Natl Cancer Inst 60:785–788.

SPECTOR BD, FILIPOVICH AH, PERRY GS III, KERSEY JH. 1982. Epidemiology of cancer in ataxia-telangiectasia. In: *Ataxia-telangiectasia*, Bridges BA, Harnden DG (eds.), pp 103–123.

STARZL TE, NALESNIK MA, PORTER KA, et al. 1984. Reversibility of lymphomas and lymphoproliferative lesions developing under cyclosporin-steroid therapy. Lancet 1:583–587.

STEWART A, DRAPER G. 1971. BCG vaccination and leukaemia mortality. Lancet 1:799.

SUBAR M, NERI A, INGHIRAMI G, et al. 1988. Frequent c-myc oncogene activation and infrequent presence of Epstein-Barr virus genome in AIDS-associated lymphoma. Blood 72:667–671.

SUTHERLAND I. 1982. BCG and vole Bacillus vaccination in adolescence and mortality from leukaemia. Stat Med 1:329–335.

SWINNEN LJ, COSTANZO-NORDIN MR, FISHER SG, O'SULLIVAN EJ, JOHNSON MR, HEROUX AL, DIZIKES GJ, PIFARRE R, FISHER RI. 1990. Increased incidence of lymphoproliferative disorder after immunosuppression with the monoclonal antibody OKT3 in cardiac transplant recipients. N Engl J Med 323(25):1723–1728.

SWINSON CM, SLAVIN G, COLES EC, BOOTH CC. 1983. Coeliac disease and malignancy. Lancet 1:111–115.

TALAL N, BUNIM JJ. 1964. The development of malignant lymphoma in the course of Sjogren's syndrome. Am J Med 36:529–540.

TEILLET F, WEISGERBER C, FEINGOLD N. 1973. Maladie de Hodgkin: essai d'evaluation du role joue par l'appendicectomie et l'amygdalectomie. Nouv Presse Med 2:2097–2099.

THOMAS L, LAWRENCE HS (ED). 1959. In: *Cellular and Humoral Aspects of the Hypersensitive States,* London: Cassel, p 259.

TIELSCH JM, LINET MS, SEKLO M. 1987. Acquired disorders affecting the immune system and non-Hodgkin's lymphoma. Prev Med 16:96–106.

TRAININ N, et al. 1967. The enhancement of lung adenoma formation by neonatal thymectomy in mice treated with 7, 12-DMBA or urethan. Int J Cancer 2:326–336.

TUCKER MA, MISFELDT D, COLEMAN N, CLARK WH, ROSENBERG SA. 1985. Cutaneous malignant melanoma after Hodgkin's disease. Ann Intern Med 102:37–41.

UCCINI S, MONARDO F, RUCO LP, BARONI CD, FAGGIONI A, AGLIANO AM, et al. 1989. High frequency of Epstein-Barr virus genome in HIV-positive patients with Hodgkins disease. Lancet 1:1458.

UHL GS, WILLIAMS JE, ARNETT FC. 1974. Intracerebral lymphoma in a patient with central nervous system lupus on cyclophosphamide. J Rheumatol 1:282–286.

ULRICH J, WUTHRICH R. 1974. Multiple sclerosis: reticular cell sarcoma of the nervous system in a patient treated with immunosuppressive drugs. Eur Neurol 12:65–78.

URE DMJ. 1969. Negative association between allergy and cancer. Scot Medical Journal 14:51–54.

VARADACHARI C, PALUTHE M, CLIMIE ARW, et al. 1978. Immunoblastic sarcoma (histiocytic lymphoma) of the brain with B cell markers. J Neurosurg 49:887.

VENA JE, BONA JR, BYERS TE, MIDDLETON E, SWANSON MK, GRAHAM S. 1985. Allergy-related diseases and cancer: an inverse association. Am J Epidemiol 122 (1):66–74.

VESSEY MP, DOLL R, NORMAN-SMITH B, et al. 1979. Thymectomy and cancer: a further report. Br J Cancer 39:193–195.

VIANNA NJ, GREENWALD P, POLAN A, et al. 1974. Tonsillectomy and Hodgkin's disease. Lancet 2:168–169.

VIANNA NJ, GREENWALD P, DAVIES JN. 1971. Tonsillectomy and Hodgkin's disease: the lymphoid tissue barrier. Lancet 1:431–432.

WAALER HT. 1971: BCG and mortality Lancet 2:1314.

WALDER BK, ROBERTSON MR, JEREMY D. 1971. Skin cancer and immunosuppression. Lancet 2:1282–1283.

WHITTEMORE AS, HOLLY EA, LEE IM, ABEL EA, ADAMS RM, NICKELOFF BJ, BLEY L, PETERS JM, GIBNEY C. 1989. Mycosis fungoides in relation to environmental exposures and immune response: a case-control study. J Natl Cancer Inst 81:1560–1567.

WILSON RE, HAGER EB, HAMPERS CL, et al. 1968. Immunologic rejection of human cancer transplanted with a renal allograft. N Engl J Med 278:479–483.

ZIEGLER JL, BECKSTEAD JA, VOLBERDING PA, et al. 1984. Non-Hodgkin's lymphoma in 90 homosexual men: relation to generalized lymphadenopathy and the acquired immunodeficiency syndrome. N Engl J Med 311:565–570.

ZIEGLER JL, DREW WL, MINER RC, et al. 1982. Outbreak of Burkitt's-like lymphoma in homosexual men. Lancet 2:631–633.

26 Familial aggregation

FREDERICK P. LI

The present era of molecular biology has revolutionized the study of cancer in families. Powerful new tools can now be applied to identify genotypic alterations in hereditary cancers and neoplasms in general (White and Caskey, 1988; Bishop, 1987). This chapter summarizes the patterns of cancer in families, and knowledge of human carcinogenesis gained from studies of these kindreds (Knudson, 1985; Friend et al, 1988).

Epidemiological studies show that most cancers manifest a tendency to aggregate in families. Close relatives of a cancer patient can be considered to have increased risk of that neoplasm, but not all forms of cancer. The excess site-specific cancer risk is usually in the order of two- to threefold above the baseline rate (Muller and Weber, 1985; Mulvihill et al, 1977). However, some inherited cancer genes increase the relative risk of a specific cancer by hundreds-fold, and absolute risk to nearly 100% (Li, 1988). These potent cancer genes are rare in the population, but serve as important models for studies of carcinogenesis. Inherited cancer genes are the most potent oncogenic influence in humans, exceeding the effects of such environmental agents as ionizing radiation, tobacco, and occupational carcinogens (Li, 1987).

ONCOGENES IN FAMILIAL AND SPORADIC CANCERS

Until recently, little was known about the molecular basis of cancer in humans. Viruses were shown to produce cancers in experimental animals, and neoplastic features (transformation) in cultured cells (Bishop, 1985). However, the role of oncogenic virus in human cancers was uncertain, and biological mechanisms of viral carcinogenesis were poorly understood. Oncogenic viruses were thought to possess transforming genes (virogenes), but the structure and protein products of these genes were unknown.

In the last decade, much has been learned about the fundamental molecular and cellular changes that convert a normal cell into a cancer cell. The basic lesion in cancer appears to be an alteration in the genetic control of cellular processes; that is, cancer at the molecular level is a genetic disease. Among the estimated 100,000 genes in the human genome, only a small fraction seems to be critically involved in cancer development. These genes can be classified into two major groups: dominant oncogenes and tumor suppressor genes (Knudson, 1985; Friend et al, 1988). Several dozen oncogenes have been discerned, and more will be found in the future. Multiple alterations of these genes appear to be required to produce cancer, in accordance with evidence that carcinogenesis is a multistage process.

Knowledge of the dominant oncogenes stems largely from studies of the oncogenic RNA viruses (Bishop, 1985; Friend et al, 1988). The transforming genes of these viruses were found, unexpectedly, to be cellular genes acquired during the intracellular phase of the viral life cycle. These cellular genes (proto-oncogenes) gained tumorigenic potential when incorporated into the viral genome. Additional studies showed that proto-oncogenes have been strictly conserved through evolution; their DNA sequences bear a high degree of structural homology in humans and lower species such as drosophila and mouse. Gene conservation through the millennia strongly suggests production of proteins vital to the function and survival of the organism. Indeed, several proto-oncogenes have been shown to encode proteins that are growth factors, growth factor receptors, signal transducers and transcription activators (Aaronson, 1991). Qualitative or quantitative changes in these genes can confer certain behavioral characteristics of neoplasia. Dominant oncogenes appear to be involved in a high proportion of cancers in humans, but they have not been shown to be the inherited defect in familial cancers. An exception is the RET oncogene, which produces multiple endocrine neoplasia (MEN) type 2 when the RET mutation exists in the germ line cells (Mulligan et al, 1994).

Unlike the dominant oncogenes, tumor suppressor genes were discovered through clinical and epidemiological observations of cancer families. Knudson's two-mutation hypothesis provides the conceptual framework for studying these rare families to gain new understanding of human carcinogenesis (Knudson, 1983, 1985). He proposed that at least two mutations are required to transform a normal cell into a cancer cell. At the molecular level, familial and sporadic (non-familial) forms of a cancer involve the same gene(s). In the sporadic cancer, no mutation is inherited and two somatic mutations must occur within one cell. Hereditary cancer is due to a germinal mutation that has been inherited from a parent and propagated in all somatic cells of susceptible family members; a second mutation transforms the cell. The hypothesis implies that any somatic cell of cancer gene carriers can be examined for the first mutation, and a comparison of their tumor and somatic cells can reveal the second mutation. Thus the complex carcinogenic process in the sporadic form of a cancer can be dissected into two components in the familial form. Laboratory studies reveal that in certain cancers the two mutations result in loss or inactivation of both alleles of specific genes. Generally, these genes act as tumor suppressors, of which the prototype is hereditary retinoblastoma (Knudson, 1978, 1971). The next section describes the discovery that loss of recessive tumor suppressor genes is the underlying defect in certain hereditary and familial cancers.

RETINOBLASTOMA: THE MODEL OF FAMILIAL CANCERS

Retinoblastoma is a rare childhood cancer (annual incidence rate, 3.3 per million white children in the United States). Approximately 200 children are affected nationally each year, most within the first 5 years of life. Despite its rarity, retinoblastoma has been studied as the model of hereditary cancers in humans. The heritable form accounts for nearly 40% of retinoblastomas, but only a small fraction of most other cancers (Knudson, 1971). Retinoblastoma is inherited in an autosomal dominant pattern with high penetrance. All retinoblastoma patients with a family history of the tumor or with bilateral lesions have the hereditary form of the neoplasm. Approximately 10% of those with a unilateral tumor and an unaffected family also have the hereditary neoplasm on the basis of a new germinal mutation. The high cure rate of retinoblastoma in recent decades has yielded living members of multiple affected generations for genetic studies.

The retinoblastoma gene has been isolated through a series of clinical, cytogenetic, and molecular studies that spanned the past two decades (Cowell et al, 1992). In 1971, review of hospital records of more than 1600 children with retinoblastoma showed an excess frequency of concurrent mental retardation (Jensen and Miller, 1971). There were 15 children with severe mental retardation (expected, 4.7 cases), some with other anomalies such as short stature, microcephaly, colobomas of the eye, and hypertelorism; chromosome studies showed a constitutional chromosome D deletion (Francke, 1983). When chromosome banding was developed, the deletion was localized to chromosome 13. In particular, the deleted segment consistently spanned band 14 on the long arm (chromosome 13q14). Mental retardation correlated with the finding of a large deletion, suggesting that association of the two disorders is due to loss of physically linked genes on this chromosome band. Additional studies showed that a few families with hereditary retinoblastoma had constitutional rearrangements that resulted in loss or derangement of chromosome 13q14 (Strong et al, 1981). Subsequent biochemical studies revealed loss of esterase D, a co-dominant gene mapped to 13q14, in a high proportion of retinoblastoma specimens with acquired chromosome 13q14 deletions (Dryja et al, 1983).

Detailed mapping and isolation of the retinoblastoma gene were made possible through the use of recombinant DNA techniques (Cavenee et al, 1991). Friend and coworkers (1986) isolated the retinoblastoma gene RBI from chromosome 13q14. Loss of this gene was associated with tumor development; the gene functions as a tumor suppressor. Analysis of its DNA sequence showed no homology to that of any dominant oncogene. Highly polymorphic segments of the gene have been identified and used in linkage analysis of families with retinoblastoma. In 18 of 19 evaluable kindreds, coinheritance of marker DNA fragments with retinoblastoma was demonstrated to be useful in identifying gene carriers; uncertainty regarding phenotype complicated data interpretation in the remaining family (Wiggs et al, 1988).

Recent studies have expanded the spectrum of human cancers associated with loss of the retinoblastoma gene. The gene is deleted in a proportion of sporadic soft tissue sarcomas and osteogenic sarcoma, the most common second neoplasms among survivors of hereditary retinoblastoma (Dryja et al, 1986; Friend et al, 1987). Loss of the retinoblastoma gene has also been reported in two common forms of cancer, carcinoma of the breast and lung, and other sites (Harbour et al, 1988; Lee et al, 1988; Cowell et al, 1992). The gene, therefore, appears to be important in the genesis of diverse forms of human cancer. Insights into the pathogenic role of the retinoblastoma gene have been gleaned from the finding that it encodes a DNA-binding nuclear protein (Lee et al, 1987). In particular, this protein binds the transforming T antigen of SV-40 virus and E1A protein of adenovirus, which immortalizes cells (De Caprio et al, 1988; Whyte et al, 1988). These viral proteins inactivate the retinoblastoma protein and lead to development of the transformed phenotype. These observations suggest the retinoblastoma gene is central to the suppression of unregulated growth in a range of tissues. Other studies show that the Rb gene is involved in control of the cell cycle. The Rb protein associates with the transcription factor, E2F, and cell cycle-regulated cyclin complexes that control progression through the G1 phase (Nevins, 1992).

Evidence to date suggests that all families with hereditary retinoblastoma have an inherited defect of the candidate gene on chromosome 13q14. However, additional chromosomal and molecular changes, such as abnormalities of chromosomes 1 and 17, have been found in retinoblastoma cells (Gardner et al, 1982). These defects may also be involved in the multistage process of retinoblastoma development.

From the study of a rare familial and hereditary cancer, new information is being generated about the fundamental biology of human carcinogenesis.

EXTENSIONS OF THE RETINOBLASTOMA MODEL

The retinoblastoma model has been applied to other cancers, notably childhood cancers such as Wilms' tumor. A major epidemiological feature of Wilms' tumor is its association with sporadic aniridia or the Beckwith-Wiedemann syndrome (Miller et al, 1964). The aniridia–Wilms' tumor syndrome is caused by a constitutional deletion involving chromosome 11p13; a gene associated with Beckwith-Wiedemann syndrome has been mapped to a distal portion of chromosome 11p (band 15) (Koufos et al, 1985). Deletions of chromosome 11p have also been found in the Wilms' tumor cells of patients with neither malformations nor constitutional chromosomal deletions. When a normal chromosome 11 was inserted into a Wilms' tumor cell line, tumorigenicity in nude mice was lost (Weissman et al, 1987). These observations suggest that loss of a tumor suppressor gene on chromosome 11p is involved in Wilms' tumor development (Koufos et al, 1985). The Wilms' tumor gene on 11p13 has been isolated and work on the 11p15 locus is in progress (Pritchard-Jones et al, 1990). The gene on 11p13, called WT1, is deleted or altered in all patients with associated aniridia. Inherited mutations in WT1 have also been found in a few patients who have associated genitourinary defects but not aniridia. This finding and several experimental studies suggest that the gene is involved in the embryologic development of the genitourinary tract. In rare instances, WT1 mutation is transmissible through the germline (Pelletier et al, 1991). WT1 protein appears to have a role in activation of transcription (Rauscher et al, 1990). However, genes at sites other than chromosome 11p have been implicated in development of most of the familial form of Wilms' tumor. Fewer than 100 kindreds with Wilms' tumor have been reported and many have only two affected relatives. In 1979, a large kindred was reported with Wilms' tumor in five cousins in the third and fourth generations of the family (Cordero et al, 1980). Subsequently, two more children in generation four developed Wilms' tumor. Forty-eight family members have been examined for linkage with molecular probes for chromosome 11p13 and 11p15. Unexpectedly, highly negative LOD (logarithm of the odds) scores were obtained that excluded linkage between these chromosome 11 markers and Wilms' tumor in the family (Grundy et al, 1988). The same results emerged from linkage studies of several other Wilms' tumor families. In aggregate, the findings raise the prospect of one or more "Wilms' tumor gene(s)" on chromosome 11 and yet another elsewhere in the genome. It is unclear whether these genes are involved in alternative pathways in the pathogenesis of Wilms' tumor, or represent different steps in its multistage development. In any case, the genetic alterations appear more complex for Wilms' tumor than for retinoblastoma. Mutations in the common forms of carcinoma in adults also appear to involve multiple genes (Steenman et al, 1994).

Patients with dominantly inherited familial adenomatous polyposis (FAP) and variants such as Gardner's syndrome have an exceptionally high risk of adenocarcinomas of the colon and rectum in early adulthood (Bodmer et al, 1987). In 1986, Herrera and coworkers reported a patient with polyposis, multiple malformations, mental retardation, and a constitutional deletion of chromosome 5q 13-22 region. This single case raised the possibility that the constellation of diseases, including colonic polyposis and carcinoma, resulted from loss of linked genes on chromosome 5q.Tests of this hypothesis by linkage analysis of affected families showed that a gene for FAP (and Gardner's syndrome) is on chromosome 5q (Bodmer et al, 1987; Leppert et al, 1987). Genetic heterogeneity of FAP and its variants has not been found. The gene, called APC, was isolated in 1991, and appears to account for virtually all polyposis families. Like the Rb and WT1 genes, APC is a tumor suppressor gene (Kinzler et al, 1991). Another gene on chromosome 5q, the MCC gene (missing in colon cancer) may also be involved in the pathogenesis of colonic cancer. However, this locus does not seem to be the inherited defect in familial colon cancer without antecedent polyposis, raising the specter of several hereditary "colon cancer genes." Analyses of colon tumor tissue from unselected cases have revealed that chromosome 5q sequences are lost in many carcinomas and adenomas (Okamoto et al, 1988; Vogelstein et al, 1988). Deletions on chromosome 17 involving the p53 tumor suppressor gene and on chromosome 18 involving the DCC (deleted in colon cancer) gene are common in colon neoplasms (Kinzler, 1991; Weinberg, 1991). Additionally, losses in other chromosomes and the activation of *ras* oncogene have been found in colon cancers (Vogelstein et al, 1988; Law et al, 1988). The number of changes increase in the progression from early adenomas to invasive carcinoma. Thus, a cascade of alterations of oncogenes and tumor suppressor genes may be involved in the multistep transformation of the normal colonic mucosa to cancer. Similar findings are emerging from studies of other cancers, including carcinomas of the breast and lung (Yokota et al, 1987; Ali et al, 1987).

ANALYSIS OF CANCER FAMILIES

Family aggregation of cancer may be due to hereditary influences, shared exposure to environmental carcinogens, chance association, or a combination of these factors (Li, 1987). The distinction between inherited susceptibility and chance association can be particularly difficult in families with common forms of cancer, such as carcinomas of the breast and colon. One person in three in the United States develops an internal malignant neoplasm within the course of a lifetime (Li, 1987). The lifetime cancer risk is one in two when carcinomas of the skin are included in the analysis. A family history of cancer is, therefore, the rule and not the exception. The 240 million persons nationwide form many striking family aggregates of cancer by chance. Family clusters of rare cancers are less likely to be due to chance association unless ascertainment procedures involve extreme selection.

An important step in the analysis of a cancer family is confirmation of the family history, a lengthy and often neglected process. A study of accuracy of family history data shows that the primary site of cancer was correctly identified for 180 of 216 first-degree relatives (83%) of patients attending a cancer genetics clinic (Love et al, 1985). The corresponding rate for more distant relatives was only 60%. Patients at a genetics clinic are probably more knowledgeable about their family history than cancer patients in general.

Segregation analysis and linkage analysis are classical approaches to the study of the distribution of a trait within kindreds (Schneider et al, 1986). Segregation analysis of cancer families examines the pattern of neoplasia for evidence of Mendelian transmission of a predisposing gene. Available computer programs can now evaluate the contribution of multiple factors, both genetic (including polygenic) and environmental. Appropriate use of segregation analysis requires attention to avoid bias in ascertainment of families for study. Ideally, probands are identified through a random sampling of the population. The family history should only include defined relatives without regard for their history of cancer. However, much of the literature is composed of small series and individual families selected through multiple probands with the cancer(s) of interest. Attempts to correct for ascertainment bias are often inadequate (Williams and Anderson, 1984). Portions of these study families and other kindreds not conforming to the suspected Mendelian pattern may have been systematically excluded from analysis.

Linkage analysis is based on the tendency for genes in close proximity to be inherited together (Cavenee et al, 1983). A cancer gene can be localized and eventually isolated by finding polymorphic markers that are coinherited with the predisposition to cancer. Linkage studies have been limited in the past by the small number of available genetic markers, mostly blood groups and serum proteins. These markers have been replaced by restriction fragment length polymorphisms (RFLPs), and more recently short repeat nucleotide sequences such as Variation in the Number of short Tandem Repeats (VNTRs) and oligonucleotide (CA)n repeats, that are widely distributed throughout the genome (Vogelstein et al, 1985; White, 1984). Restriction endonucleases cleave DNA at specific sequences, and the resulting fragments can be sorted by electrophoretic techniques. Molecular weight of these fragments are inherited traits that may differ within the normal human population. The location of a specific RFLP can be identified by molecular hybridization techniques. By selecting the appropriate polymorphic markers, linkage can be sought in virtually any region of the genome. Linkage analysis with these markers has been particularly fruitful when cytogenetic and clinical data have localized the disease of interest to a specific region of the genome, such as chromosome 13q14 in retinoblastoma. An untargeted search of the entire genome is becoming less of a laborious and costly effort.

Case series can be studied for the familial tendency of cancers. The frequency of neoplasia among relatives of case patients with cancer is compared with corresponding figures for relatives of cancer-free control patients, or with population rates. However, bias arises when selected cancer families that prompted the study are included in the analysis, or when the control group is inappropriate. Within study families, demographic data are seldom complete, and historical data for cancers in family members may be inaccurate unless confirmation has been obtained.

Inherited susceptibility to certain cancers can be recognized by the presence of a predisposing syndrome. More than 200 single-gene traits are known to be associated with the development of neoplasia (Mulvihill et al, 1977). The frequency of neoplastic manifestations differ markedly among these inherited disorders. Benign and malignant tumors are the sole manifestation of some disorders but are rarely featured in others. In general, twin studies have made only limited contributions to the knowledge of familial cancers.

Several clinical features have been described in hereditary cancers (Li, 1987). These include specificity of the cancers by organ site or tissue of origin; earlier age of occurrence than is usual for that neoplasm; multifocal cancers of polyclonal origin within the susceptible organ; and development of multiple primary cancers in individual patients. These findings are most informative when found together in a family, but are not specific to hereditary neoplasms. Family cancer syndromes have been reported with diverse neoplasms of seemingly unrelated anatomic sites and histology. With improved cancer survival due to better treatments, more patients in general are developing multiple primary cancers. Furthermore, early age of diagnosis of cancer may not be a very reliable indicator of genetic predisposition (Schneider et al, 1983).

MULTIPLE CANCER SYNDROMES

Families have been reported with cancers at multiple anatomic sites. Some of them have well-recognized hereditary neoplastic disorders such as multiple endocrine neoplasia, types I and II; these dominantly inherited disorders have been mapped to chromosomes 11 and 10, respectively (Larsson et al, 1988; Simpson et al, 1987). Other syndromes have been identified on the basis of statistical association. The diagnosis of these syndromes can be difficult in individual families encountered in the clinic. Aggregation of diverse cancers in a family may be due to shared exposure to environmental risk factors (Li, 1987). Familial clusters of lung, bladder, and oral cancers can result from cigarette smoking; familial cancers of diverse sites have occurred after radiotherapy for benign conditions (Smith and Levitt, 1974). Breast, ovary, and endometrial cancer in a family may be due to shared reproductive and dietary risk factors. These and other environmental influences might also account for the association of breast cancer with neoplasms of the salivary glands, thyroid, and colon.

A syndrome of multiple primary adenocarcinomas has been described, but remains poorly defined. It occurred in a large family with an autosomal dominant pattern of cancers of the colon, endometrium, and other sites that was described initially by Warthin in 1895, and Hauser and Weller in 1936. Lynch showed that this family continued to develop cancers at an excess frequency, and collected additional families with the same constellation of tumors (Lynch and Krush, 1971; Lynch and Lynch, 1980). He and others have gradually expanded the tumor phenotype to encompass "adenocarcinomas of all varieties," predominantly of the colon, rectum, breast, pancreas, stomach, ovary, and endometrium (Lynch and Lynch, 1980). Leukemia and tumors of the brain and urinary tract have also occurred in multiple members of some of these families (Love, 1985; Lynch et al, 1988). As described below, many families with a predominance of colon cancers (hereditary nonpolyposis colon cancer) have been found to have inherited mutations in the mismatch repair genes (Peltomaki et al, 1993; Bronner et al, 1994). However, adenocarcinomas alone account for approximately one-half of all cancers among males in the United States; one male in six will eventually develop an adenocarcinoma (Young et al, 1977). Adenocarcinomas are even more common among women. Innumerable families have a history of multiple adenocarcinomas on the basis of chance. Presently, no simple means are available to distinguish these phenocopies from the phenotype of the familial adenocarcinoma syndrome. The syndrome should be diagnosed with caution unless, as in the family of Warthin, excess adenocarcinomas have been found on unbiased prospective observation. Chance association has not been excluded in some families reported in the literature to have the syndrome. Clinical features such as early age at diagnosis, consistency of tumor type, and multiple primary cancers are nonspecific, as noted previously. Additional uncertainty arises in studies that employ novel and unproven tests of cancer susceptibility to support the diagnosis of this syndrome.

Family cancer syndromes involving rare neoplasms are less likely to be due to chance. One of these is the family cancer syndrome of breast cancer in young women and childhood sarcomas and other neoplasms (Li-Fraumeni syndrome) that has been examined by several groups of investigators (Li et al, 1988). After this constellation of tumors was identified in one family, a medical records review uncovered three other affected kindreds, when less than 0.1 was expected. Segregation analysis of the four families was inappropriate but prospective study of these families showed an excess of the component neoplasms during follow-up observation. In two other studies, mothers of children with sarcoma in a population-based series were shown to have an excess of breast cancers (Hartley et al, 1986; Birch et al, 1984). Also, a study of 159 families of survivors of childhood soft-tissue sarcoma at one institution found at least nine kindreds with features of the syndrome (Strong et al, 1987). Segregation analysis of these kindreds showed evidence for transmission of a dominant cancer susceptibility gene. Other childhood neoplasms, including childhood acute leukemia, brain tumors, gonadal germ cell tumors and adrenocortical carcinoma, have been identified. The possibility exists of other component neoplasms that tend to occur at early ages. Observations of an unusual constellation of tumors in these few families have enabled recognition of a dominantly transmitted gene that predisposes to an unexpectedly wide spectrum of cancers. Searches for this inherited cancer-predisposing gene have found inherited mutations in the p53 tumor suppressor gene in several Li-Fraumeni families (Malkin et al, 1990). Somatic mutations in the p53 gene are found in nearly one half of a wide range of human cancers, and studies of families with Li-Fraumeni syndrome provided evidence that germline mutations in the p53 gene are also strongly associated with cancer development in families. It remains uncertain whether germline p53 mutations account for some or all Li-Fraumeni families (Barnes et al, 1992; Birch et al, 1994). However, recently developed transgenic mouse lines, including "knockout" mice, show that animals with germline mutations in both p53 alleles die of cancer before 1 year of age. Most of these mice develop T-cell lymphomas. Mice with one normal and one mutant p53 allele develop cancer later in life. Most of these heterozygous animals develop sarcomas, but other tumor types also occur (Lowe et al, 1993; Donehower et al, 1992).

Reports of unusual constellations of cancer in one or a few families can be useful to generate new hypotheses. Unless these hypotheses are properly tested, chance association remains to be excluded.

SITE-SPECIFIC CANCERS IN FAMILIES

In recent years, studies of the molecular genetics of familial cancers have overshadowed the purely descriptive reports of family clusters. This section summarizes the major reports of site-specific familial cancers in recent decades.

Gastrointestinal Tract

Esophageal cancer shows marked variations in rates worldwide. Rates of the neoplasm are highest in parts of China, Russia, Iran, and Africa where diet is suspected to be the major etiologic factor (Kmet et al, 1972; Li, 1982). Striking family aggregates of the tumor have been described in the high-risk regions, particularly in north China (Li and He, 1986). Studies are in progress to exclude chance association. Familial esophageal cancer is rare in low-risk areas such as the United States, and may be associated with dominantly inherited keratosis of the palmar and plantar surfaces (tylosis) (Ritter and Petersen, 1976).

A major review by Graham and Lilienfeld summarized and critiqued the literature on familial gastric carcinoma. All six case-control studies examined showed a higher frequency of gastric cancer (relative risks, 1.7–5.9) among relatives of patients with the neoplasm (Graham and Lilienfeld, 1958). The finding may be due in part to an association between gastric cancer and blood type A. Among reports of individual families with gastric cancer, constitutional IgA deficiency and other immunologic deficits have been found in several instances (Creagan and Fraumeni, 1973). Atrophic gastritis and intestinal metaplasia occur in families, are associated with the "intestinal" form of gastric carcinoma, and might account for some familial clusters of the tumor (Correa et al, 1975).

Most reports of familial aggregation of pancreatic cancers concern familial endocrine adenomatoses involving the islet cells (Larsson et al, 1988). Individual families have been reported with pancreatic adenocarcinoma, some in association with familial pancreatitis (Reimer et al, 1977; Riccardi et al, 1975). A recent case-control study suggested a five-fold excess risk when the cancer was reported in close relatives (Falk et al, 1988). Studies of familial pancreatic adenocarcinoma are hampered by difficulties in diagnosis, particularly in patients with extensive abdominal adenocarcinomatosis.

A few families with primary hepatocellular carcinoma have been reported (Hagstrom and Baker, 1968). The role of inherited susceptibility in these families is uncertain because hepatitis B virus, a major etiological factor, can be transmitted both vertically and horizontally within families (Joske et al, 1972). In children, hereditary tyrosinemia is associated with hepatoma, and hepatoblastoma occurs in families with dominantly inherited adenomatous polyposis (Weinberg et al, 1976; Li et al, 1987).

Much attention has been given to familial aggregation involving cancer of the colon and rectum, the commonest internal neoplasm in the United States and many parts of Europe. Colorectal carcinoma develops in nearly all patients with dominantly inherited adenomatous polyposis coli (APC) and Gardner's syndrome (polyposis of the colon and stomach associated with osseous tumors of the jaw, skull and other sites, fibromas of the mesentery and skin, and in rare instances, sarcoma and carcinoma of the ampulla of Vater) (Cannon-Albright et al, 1988; Herrera et al, 1986). The frequency of the APC mutant in the general population is in the order one per 10,000 persons. Colon cancers in polyposis gene carriers tend to arise at early ages, occasionally in teenagers, and at multiple foci in the bowel. Nearly all patients with dominantly inherited familial adenomatous polyposis and Gardner's syndrome develop colon cancer by 60 years of age (Bodmer et al, 1987). Identification of the APC gene on chromosome 5q should facilitate identification of gene carriers among children in affected families (Kinzler et al, 1991). Prophylactic colectomy is currently recommended when multiple polyposis is detected. Some patients are subjected to a total proctocolectomy with permanent ileostomy, whereas the lower rectum is spared in others. The latter procedure requires periodic proctoscopic examinations to remove new polyps that may arise. Excluding patients with adenomatous polyposis, the data suggest that close relatives of colon cancer cases have a threefold excess risk of colorectal cancer when compared with control groups or population incidence rates (Neel, 1971). Striking clusters of colon cancers have been reported in some families. The affected relatives tend to have carcinoma arising in the right (proximal) colon, often at early ages. Pedigree analysis of series of families has shown significant clustering of colon cancer in blood relatives. Whether the degree of aggregation detected in these reports applies to randomly selected families is unknown; population-based samples are difficult to collect (Bale et al, 1984). Inherited susceptibility may have a major role in colon cancers in the general population (Cannon-Albright et al, 1988). The investigators examined by proctosigmoidoscopy 670 persons in 34 families with either a "colon cancer cluster" or a proband with at least one adenomatous polyp. Results showed that susceptibility to colonic adenomas and cancer was dominantly inherited; the gene frequency was 19%. These findings, if confirmed, would strengthen both the link between adenomas and carcinomas and the role of hereditary influences in colonic neoplasia. A range of abnormalities have been described within somatic cells of families with colon cancer, but additional studies are needed (Lipkin et al, 1980).

In contrast to rare APC families, families with hereditary nonpolyposis colon cancer (HNPCC) including Lynch syndrome appear to account for approximately 4% of all colorectal cancer cases in industrialized nations (Lynch and Lynch, 1993). A series of important discoveries in 1993 led to cloning two HNPCC genes. The first set of studies demonstrated linkage of HNPCC to chromosome 2 (Peltomaki et al, 1993). Tumor specimens from these patients showed DNA instability in short repeat sequences called microsatellites. The finding raised the possibility that the DNA instability is due to a DNA mismatch repair gene on chromosome 2. Using two different approaches, positional cloning and functional cloning, investigators found the first mismatch repair gene, MSH2, within several months (Fishel, 1993). Soon thereafter, additional mismatch repair genes (MLH1, PMS1 and PMS2) were identified (Bronner et al, 1994). Together, these genes appear to account for the large majority of HNPCC families, as well as other familial and sporadic colon cases that have yet to develop strong family histories of the neoplasm.

Cancers of the Breast and Reproductive Organs

Epidemiological studies show that a family history of breast cancer is a dominant risk factor for the neoplasm (Sattin et al, 1985). In affected families, the risk may be transmitted through either parent, and males have been affected in some kindreds (Kozak et al, 1986). The relative risk of breast cancer is approximately two- to threefold among close relatives of case patients. In some studies, hereditary influences are more prominent in premenopausal breast cancer and may result in an autosomal dominant pattern of the cancer. Patients at highest risk tend to have a family history of breast cancer affecting both mother and maternal grandmother, or mother and sister (Anderson and Badzioch, 1985). However, analyses of the genetic epidemiology of breast cancer have been complicated by several factors, including sex-dependent susceptibility, variable age at onset of disease, and genetic heterogeneity among affected families. Pedigree analyses of larger series of families have yielded discordant interpretation of the same data set (Bailey-Wilson et al, 1986). Linkage studies suggesting association with the glutamate pyruvate transaminase locus on chromosome 10 have not been substantiated, but genetic heterogeneity might be the explanation (King et al, 1980). Cytogenetic analyses show that breast cancer cells are highly aneuploid and karyotypes are difficult to interpret. Several chromosome regions show nonrandom losses, and several oncogenes have been shown to be activated by point mutation (ras) or gene amplification (Her-2/neu). Recent data have identified several inherited single-gene defects that predispose to breast cancer. One of these may be the ataxia-telangiectasia (ATM) gene on chromosome 11q (Swift et al, 1991). In a follow-up study of obligate carriers of the ATM gene, a fivefold excess of breast cancer was found when compared with controls. However, germline ATM mutations appear to be uncommon among breast cancer cases (Vořechovský et al, 1996). Germline mutations in the p53 tumor suppressor gene has been detected in some families with Li-Fraumeni syndrome, which features early-onset breast cancer (Li et al, 1992). Isolated breast cancer families without the syndrome can also have inherited p53 mutations, but the frequency is probably less than 1%. A third gene on chromosome 17q was identified by linkage analysis of families with breast cancer of early onset (Hall et al, 1990; Narod et al, 1991). This major gene, called BRCA1, has now been isolated and may account for up to one-half of familial breast cancers in young women (Miki et al, 1994). Another gene for breast cancer in females and males, BRCA2, was recently found to be on chromosome 13q (Wooster et al, 1995).

The major gene for familial ovarian cancer also appears to be BRCA-1, particularly when the family history includes breast cancer (Narod et al, 1991). Cancers of the uterine corpus and ovary share several risk factors in common with breast cancer (Lingeman, 1974). The neoplasms occur excessively as multiple primary tumors and as component tumors in cancer families. They develop with high frequency in the industrialized nations of North America and Europe in association with nulliparity. The similarities may be due to shared genetically determined hormonal influences. A recent study suggests that close relatives of women with ovarian carcinoma have a three-fold excess risk of ovarian cancer (Schildkraut and Thompson, 1988). Ovarian germ cell tumors also occur in families, and in association with gonadal dysgenesis featuring a Y chromosome (Verp and Simpson, 1987).

Familial testicular cancer has been reported in numerous case studies, despite the relative rarity of the neoplasm in the population (Anderson et al, 1984). Siblings have been affected in some kindreds and multiple generations in others. Cryptorchidism is a risk factor for testis cancer, and has been found in families with testis cancer. In addition, Klinefelter's syndrome (XXY) has been reported in association with germ cell neoplasms, particularly primaries of the mediastinum (McNeil et al, 1981).

Urinary Tract

A family has been identified with renal cell carcinoma, 10 members which have a constitutional translocation involving chromosomes 3 and 8 (Cohen et al, 1979). The finding raises the possibility that a "renal carcinoma gene" is at one of these breakpoints. Subsequent studies show that nearly all renal cell carcinomas bear translocations or deletions of chromosome 3, often involving bands 14 and 21 on the short arm (Zbar et al, 1987; Kovacs et al, 1988; Li et al, 1993). The gene spanning the chromosome 3 breakpoint FHIT, was recently cloned. FHIT and the von Hippel-Lindau gene on distal 3p are involved in the genesis of renal and other cancers (Ohta et al, 1996).

In the lower urinary tract, both bladder and ureteral cancers have been reported in the same kindred (Marchetto et al, 1983). A close relative of patients with bladder cancer appears to be at increased risk of this neoplasm, often in association with cigarette smoking within the family (Kantor et al, 1985). Abnormal tryptophan metabolism, which may elevate the levels of carcinogens in the urine, has been evaluated in familial bladder cancer (Fraumeni and Thomas, 1967). In addition, slow acetylation of carcinogenic aromatic amines is in part an inherited trait that may be associated with an increased risk of bladder cancer (Evans et al, 1983).

Cancer of the prostate, though one of the commonest cancers in men, remains a disease of unknown etiology. Prostatic cancer has been reported to have a familial tendency, but the importance of family history is only beginning to be quantified (Carter, 1992). A recent hospital-based study of male relatives of 691 consecutive prostate cancer patients showed an odds ratio of 2 for men with an affected first-degree relative or second-degree relative (Steinberg, 1990). However, the odds ratio was 8.8 for those with both an affected first- and second-degree relative. The risk increases with the total number of affected family members. Familial prostate cancer tends to occur at early ages and accounts for a substantial fraction of the disease in younger men. The study represents the most complete analysis of familial prostate cancer to date. The findings suggest that familial prostate cancer occurs in patterns similar to other familial cancers, including dominant inheritance and early age of onset.

Respiratory Tract

Tobacco smoking is the dominant cause of cancers of the upper and lower respiratory system. The few studies of familial factors show that lung cancer in a blood relative constitutes a risk factor for the neoplasm after adjustment for the effect of cigarette smoking (Ooi et al, 1986). However, lung cancer was often diagnosed in relatives on the basis of death certificate data or reports by surviving family members, which may be unreliable. In addition, the effect of passive smoking on family members may not have been fully taken into account in the analysis (Blot and Fraumeni, 1986). Linkage studies of familial clusters of lung cancers have not been possible because of the high mortality from the tumor (Goffman et al, 1982). Recent reports of the use of polymerase chain reaction to recover specific DNA sequences from paraffin-fixed tissues may permit examination of these families in future studies (Lench et al, 1988). Chromosomes 3p21 and 13q14, which are deleted in many lung cancer specimens, are regions of particular interest (Yokota et al, 1987). Familial occurrence of lung cancer has been associated with genetically determined metabolism of carcinogens in cigarette smoke. Many carcinogens in tobacco smoke require metabolic activation within the target tissues, particularly through pathways of the cytochrome P450 gene family. Early studies focused on aryl hydrocarbon hydroxylase (AHH), but its association with increased lung cancer risk remains tenuous. Current studies are examining the pathway within the P450 gene system that is measured by the metabolism of debrisoquine, a medication for hypertension (Caporaso et al, 1990). Available data suggest that lung and bladder cancers occur with higher frequency among smokers who are active metabolizers of debrisoquine, and additional studies are in progress. Although genetic influences have a role in lung cancer etiology, the observation does not alter the fact that smoking cessation is the most effective solution to the lung cancer epidemic (Shilling, 1992).

Hematologic System

Familial clustering has been reported for all the major forms of acute and chronic leukemia (Gunz et al, 1975; Heath and Moloney, 1965). Some aggregates are due to predisposing Mendelian disorders such as Fanconi's anemia and ataxia-telangiectasia (Li and Bader, 1987). Other families have antecedent hematologic conditions such as constitutional thrombocytopenia or bone marrow hypoplasia (Dowton et al, 1985; Li et al, 1979). Studies of leukemia concordance in twins show a greater frequency in monozygotic (or like-sex) twins as compared with dizygotic twins; concordance rate is highest in children under 1 year of age (MacMahon and Levy, 1964; Miller, 1971). However, leukemia in identical twins could be due to spread of the disease through an interconnected fetal circulation, rather than inherited susceptibility (Chaganti et al, 1979).

Familial lymphoma can be histology-specific or involve several subtypes (Anderson et al, 1986; Johnson and Peters, 1957; Blattner et al, 1979, 1980). Inherited immunological defects such as X-linked lymphoproliferative syndrome have been identified in some kindreds (Purtilo et al, 1977). Certain human leukocyte antigen (HLA) patterns may be associated with familial Hodgkin's disease (Greene et al, 1979). Hodgkin's disease in sibships tends to occur at young ages and in like-sex siblings; brothers of a male Hodgkin's disease patient appear to be at higher risk than sisters (Grufferman et al, 1977). The finding raises the possibility that some of these aggregates are due to environmental influences shared by like-sex siblings. Familial occurrence of another B-lymphocyte neoplasm, multiple myeloma, appears to be rare (Shoenfeld et al, 1982). Most reported aggregates consist of only two affected relatives. The age and sex patterns of familial myeloma are not atypical, and the monoclonal immunoglobulins produced by the tumors in family members are often dissimilar.

Neuroendocrine and Neurocutaneous Systems

Neuroendocrine neoplasms constitute only a small proportion of all human neoplastic diseases, but they contribute to a substantial number of hereditary syndromes (Mulvihill et al, 1977). Benign and malignant tumors in hereditary disorders such as neurofibromatosis (NF) types 1 and 2 arise primarily in the central and peripheral nervous system. Both the NF1 and NF2 genes have recently been cloned (Trofatter et al, 1993). In the multiple endocrine neoplasia (MEN) syndromes types I and II, tumors develop primarily in the endocrine organs. The gene for MEN type 2 was recently found to be a known gene, RET, which has properties of an oncogene. RET appears to be the first example of an oncogene transmitted through the germline in its mutant form (Mulligan et al, 1994). Recent studies have also identified germline mutations in the p16 and CDK4 genes in familial melanoma (Goldstein et al, 1995; Zuo et al, 1996). These syndromes may also affect non-neuroendocrine tissues, such as the occurrence of renal cell carcinoma in von Hippel-Lindau disease, pancreatic cancer in p16 carriers (Goldstein et al, 1995), and acute leukemia and Wilms' tumor in von Recklinghausen's neurofibromatosis type I (Li, 1987). Familial brain tumors have also been reported in the absence of an identifiable hereditary predisposition (Challa et al, 1983; Farwell and Flannery, 1984).

CANCER PREVENTION IN FAMILIES

A family history of cancer is a consistent risk factor for nearly all forms of neoplasia in humans. The knowledge can be applied to primary and secondary prevention of cancer (Parry et al, 1987). In families with a known predisposing gene, the risk of cancer can often be estimated and used in genetic counseling. Advances in molecular genetics have broadened the use of linkage analysis in prenatal diagnosis of carriers of hereditary cancers such as retinoblastoma. In addition, fetal tissues can be assayed for biological abnormalities such as chromosomal breakage in families with Fanconi's anemia (Auerbach et al, 1986). Early cancer detection in families should focus on cancers of the breast, colon, stomach and other sites that are associated with better prognosis when diagnosed early. With the isolation of increasing numbers of inherited tumor suppressor genes, the possibility arises for testing healthy members of cancer families. Predictive testing for cancer susceptibility genes is new, and careful considerations of the risks and benefits are needed (National Advisory Council, 1994). A few model testing programs for rare inherited susceptibility genes such as p53 have been initiated to measure the impact of predictive testing. With the cloning of MSH2 and MLH1 for colon cancer and BRCA1 for breast and ovarian cancers, predictive testing of larger segments of the population can be expected in the near future. In this manner, the new information can be better used to care for cancer families.

Inherited susceptibility is only one of multiple steps in the carcinogenic process (Sugimura, 1992). Additional mutations, often due to environmental carcinogens, occur to fully transform a normal cell. Cancer prevention in high-risk families can be achieved through avoidance of carcinogens in the environment such as ultraviolet light in patients with xeroderma pigmentosum or dysplastic nevus syndrome, and cigarette smoking in families prone to lung or bladder cancers. Precancerous lesions should be removed to prevent progression. The procedure is often simple, as in removal of dysplastic nevi in familial melanoma, and polypectomy in certain colon cancer families. Long-term surveillance of these families can be an effective means of reducing morbidity and mortality of cancer. In addition, the possibility of chemoprevention, such as the use of tamoxifen for breast cancer prevention, should be examined in controlled clinical trials (Love et al, 1992; Benner et al, 1994).

REFERENCES

AARONSON SA. 1991. Growth factors and cancer. Science 254:1146–1153.

ALI IU, LINDEREAU R, THEILLET C, et al. 1987. Reduction to homozygosity of genes on chromosome 11 in human breast neoplasia. Science 238:185–188.

ANDERSON DE, BADZIOCH MD. 1985. Risk of familial breast cancer. Cancer 56:383–387.

ANDERSON KC, LI FP, MARCHETTO DJ. 1984. Dizygotic twinning, cryptorchism, and seminoma in a sibship. Cancer 53:374–376.

ANDERSON KC, JAMISON DS, PETERS WP. 1986. Familial Burkitt's lymphoma: association with altered lymphocyte subsets in family members. Am J Med 81:158–162.

AUERBACH AD, MIN Z, GHOSH R, et al. 1986. Clastogen-induced chromosomal breakage as a marker for first trimester prenatal diagnosis of Fanconi anemia. Hum Genet 73:86–88.

BAILEY-WILSON JE, CANNON LA, KING MC. 1986. Genetic analysis of human breast cancer: a synthesis of contributions to GAW IV. Genet Epidemiol 1:15–35.

BALE SJ, CHAKRAVARTI A, STRONG LC. 1984. Aggregation of colon cancer in family data. Genet Epidemiology 1:53–61.

BARNES DM, HANBY AM, GILLETT CE. 1992. Abnormal expression of wild type p53 protein in normal cells of a cancer family patient. Lancet 340:259–263.

BENNER SE, PASTORINO U, LIPPMAN SM, HONG WK. 1994. Second International Cancer Chemoprevention Conference. Cancer Res 54:854–856.

BIRCH JM, HARTLEY AL, MARSDEN HB, et al. 1984. Excess risk of breast cancer in the mothers of children with soft tissue sarcomas. Br J Cancer 49:325–331.

BIRCH JM, HARTLEY AL, TRICKER KJ, et al. 1994. Prevalence and diversity of constitutional mutations in the p53 gene among 21 Li-Fraumeni families. Cancer Res 54:1298–1304.

BISHOP JM. 1987. The molecular genetics of cancer. Science 235:305–311.

BISHOP JM. 1985. Viral oncogenes. Cell 42:23–38.

BLATTNER WA, DEAN JH, FRAUMENI JF JR. 1979. Familial lymphoproliferative malignancy: clinical and laboratory follow-up. Ann Intern Med 90:943–944.

BLATTNER WA, GARBER JE, MANN DL, et al. 1980. Waldenstrom's macroglobulinemia and autoimmune disease in a family. Ann Intern Med 93:830–832.

BLOT WJ, FRAUMENI JF JR. 1986. Passive smoking and lung cancer. J Natl Cancer Inst 77:993–1000.

BODMER WF, BAILEY CJ, BODMER J, et al. 1987. Localization of the gene for familial adenomatous polyposis on chromosome 5. Nature 328:614–616.

BOONE CW, KELLOFF GJ, MALONE WE. 1990. Identification of candidate cancer chemopreventive agents and their evaluation in animal models and human clinical trials: a review. Cancer Res 50:2–9.

BRONNER CE, BAKER SM, MORRISON PT, et al. 1994. Mutation in the DNA mismatch repair gene homologue hMLH1 is associated with hereditary nonpolyposis colon cancer. Nature 368:258–261.

CANNON-ALBRIGHT LA, SKOLNICK MH, BISHOP T, et al. 1988. Common inheritance of susceptibility to colonic adenomatous polyps and associated colorectal cancers. N Engl J Med 319:533–537.

CAPORASO NE, TUCKER MA, HOOVER RN, et al. 1990. Lung cancer and the debrisoquine metabolic phenotype. J Natl Cancer Inst 82:1264–1272.

CARTER BS, BEATY TH, STEINBERG GD, et al. 1992. Mendelian inheritance of familial prostate cancer. Proc Natl Acad Sci USA 89:3367–3371.

CAVENEE WK, DRYJA TP, PHILLIPS RA, et al. 1983. Expression of recessive alleles by chromosomal mechanisms in retinoblastoma. Nature 305:779–784.

CAVENEE WK. 1991. Recessive mutations in the causation of human cancer. Mutat Hum Cancer 67:2431–2435.

CHAGANTI RSK, MILLER DR, MEYERS PA, et al. 1979. Cytogenetic evidence of the intrauterine origin of acute leukemia in monozygotic twins. N Engl J Med 300:1032–1034.

CHALLA VR, GOODMAN HO, DAVIS CH. 1983. Familial brain tumors: studies of two families and review of recent literature. Neurosurgery 12:18–23.

CHANG EH, PIROLLO KF, QIANG ZOU Z, et al. 1987. Oncogenes in radioresistant, noncancerous skin fibroblasts from a cancer-prone family. Science 237:1036–1039.

COHEN AJ, LI FP, BERG S, et al. 1979. Hereditary renal-cell carcinoma associated with a chromosomal translocation. N Engl J Med 301:592–595.

COPPES MJ, LIEFERS GJ, HIGUCHI M, et al. 1992. Inherited WT1 mutation in Denys-Drash syndrome. Cancer Res 52:6125–6128.

CORDERO JF, LI FP, HOLMES LB, et al. 1980. Wilms' tumor in five cousins. Pediatr 66:716–719.

CORREA P, HAENSZEL W, CUELLO C, et al. 1975. A model for gastric cancer epidemiology. Lancet 2:58–59.

COWELL JK, HOGG A. 1992. Genetics and cytogenetics of retinoblastoma. Cancer Genet Cytogenet 64:1–11.

CREAGAN ET, FRAUMENI JF, JR. 1973. Familial gastric cancer and immunologic abnormalities. Cancer 32:1325–1331.

DECAPRIO JA, LUDLOW JW, FIGGE J, et al. 1988. SV40 large tumor antigen forms a specific complex with the product of the retinoblastoma susceptibility gene. Cell 54:275–283.

DONEHOWER LA, HARVEY M, SLAGLE BL, et al. 1992. Mice deficient for p53 are developmentally normal but susceptible to spontaneous tumours. Nature 356:215–221.

DOWTON SB, BEARDSLEY D, JAMISON D, et al. 1985. Studies of a familial platelet disorder. Blood 65:557–563.

DRYJA TP, BRUNS GAP, GALLIE B, et al. 1983. Low incidence of deletion of the esterase D locus in retinoblastoma patients. Hum Genet 64:151–155.

DRYJA TP, RAPAPORT JM, EPSTEIN J, et al. 1986. Chromosome 13 homozygosity in osteosarcoma without retinoblastoma. Am J Hum Genet 38:59–66.

EVANS DAP, EZE LC, WHIBLEY EJ. 1983. The association of the slow acetylator phenotype with bladder cancer. J Med Genet 20:330–333.

FALK RT, PICKLE LW, FONTHAM ET, et al. 1988. Life-style risk factors for pancreatic cancer in Louisiana: a case control study. Am J Epidemiol 128:324–336.

FARWELL J, FLANNERY JT. 1984. Cancer in relatives of children with central-nervous-system neoplasms. N Engl J Med 311:749–753.

FISHEL R, LESCOE MK, RAO RS, et al. 1993. The human mutator gene homolog MSH2 and its association with hereditary nonpolyposis colon cancer. Cell 75:1027–1038.

FRANCKE U. 1983. Specific chromosome changes in the human heritable tumors retinoblastoma and nephroblastoma. In: *Chromosomes and Cancer*, Rowley J, Ultmann JE (eds). Academic Press, Inc, pp 99–115.

FRAUMENI JF JR, THOMAS LB. 1967. Malignant bladder tumors in a man and his three sons. JAMA 201:507–509.

FRIEND SH, DRYJA TP, WEINBERG RA. 1988. Oncogenes and tumor-suppressing genes. N Engl J Med 318:618–622.

FRIEND SH, BERNARDS R, ROGELJ S, et al. 1986. Identification of a human DNA segment having properties of the gene that predisposes to retinoblastoma and osteosarcoma. Nature 323:643–646.

FRIEND SH, HOROWITZ JM, GERBER MR, et al. 1987. Deletions of a DNA sequence in retinoblastomas and mesenchymal tumors: organization of the sequence and its encoded protein. Proc Natl Acad Sci U S A 84:9059–9063.

GARDNER HA, GALLIE BL, KNIGHT LA, et al. 1982. Multiple karyotypic changes in retinoblastoma tumor cells: presence of normal chromosome No. 13 in most tumors. Cancer Genet Cytogenet 6:201–211.

GOFFMAN TE, HASSINGER DD, MULVIHILL JJ. 1982. Familial respiratory tract cancer. JAMA 247:1020–1023.

GOLDSTEIN AM, FRASER MC, STRUEWING JP, et al. 1995. Increased risk of pancreatic cancer in melanoma-prone kindreds with $p16^{INK4}$ mutations. N Engl J Med 333:970–974.

GRAHAM S, LILIENFELD AM. 1958. Genetic studies of gastric cancer in humans: an appraisal. Cancer 11:945–958.

GREENE MH, MCKEEN EA, LI FP, et al. 1979. HLA antigens in familial Hodgkin's disease. Int J Cancer 23:777–780.

GRUFFERMAN S, COLE P, SMITH PG, et al. 1977. Hodgkin's disease in siblings. N Engl J Med 296:248–250.

GRUNDY P, KOUFOS A, MORGAN K, et al. 1988. Familial predisposition to Wilms' tumor does not map to the short arm of chromosome 11. Nature 366:374–376.

GUNZ FW, FUNZ JP, VEALE AMO, et al. 1975. Familial leukaemia: a study of 909 families. Scand J Haematol 15:117–131.

HAGSTROM RM, BAKER TD. 1968. Primary hepatocellular carcinoma in three male siblings. Cancer 22:142–150.

HALL JM, LEE MK, NEWMAN B, et al. 1990. Linkage of early-onset familial breast cancer to chromosome 17q21. Science 250:1684–1689.

HARBOUR JW, LAI SL, WHANG-PENG J, et al. 1988. Abnormalities in structure and expression of the human retinoblastoma gene in SCLC. Science 24:353–357.

HARTLEY AL, BIRCH JM, MARSDEN HB, et al. 1986. Breast cancer risk in mothers of children with osteosarcoma and chrondrosarcoma. Br J Cancer 54:819–823.

HEATH CW JR, MOLONEY WC. 1965. Familial leukemia: five cases of acute leukemia in three generations. N Engl J Med 272: 882–887.

HERRERA L, KAKATI S, GIBAS L, et al. 1986. Gardner syndrome in a man with an interstitial deletion of 5q. Am J Med Genet 25:473–476.

JENSEN RD, MILLER RW. 1971. Retinoblastoma: epidemiologic characteristics. N Engl J Med 285:307–311.

JOHNSON MJE, PETERS CH. 1957. Lymphomas in four siblings. JAMA 163:20–25.

JOSKE RA, LAURENCE BH, MATZ LR. 1972. Familial active chronic hepatitis with hepatocellular carcinoma. Gastroenterology 62:441–444.

KANTOR AF, HARTGE P, HOOVER RN, et al. 1985. Familial and environmental interactions in bladder cancer risk. Int J Cancer 35:703–706.

KING MC, GO RCP, ELSTON RC, et al. 1980. Allele increasing susceptibility to human breast cancer may be linked to the glutamate-pyruvate transaminase locus. Science 208:406–408.

KINZLER KW, NILBERT MC, SU LK, et al. 1991. Identification of FAP locus genes from chromosome 5q21. Science 253:661–665.

KLEIN LA. 1979. Prostatic carcinoma. N Engl J Med 300:824–833.

KMET J, MAHBOUBI E. 1972. Esophageal cancer in the Caspian Littoral of Iran: initial studies. Science 175:846–853.

KNUDSON AG JR. 1985. Hereditary cancer, oncogenes, and antioncogenes. Cancer Res 45:1437–1443.

KNUDSON AG JR. 1983. Hereditary cancers of man. Cancer Invest 1:187–193.

KNUDSON AG JR. 1978. Retinoblastoma: a prototypic hereditary neoplasm. Semin Oncol 5:57–60.

KNUDSON AG JR. 1971. Mutation and cancer: statistical study of retinoblastoma. Proc Natl Acad Sci U S A 68:820–823.

KOUFOS A, HANSEN MF, COPELAND NG, et al. 1985. Loss of heterozygosity in three embryonal tumours suggests a common pathogenetic mechanism. Nature 316:330–334.

KOVACS G, ERLANDSSON R, BOLDOG F, et al. 1988. Consistent chromosome 3p deletion and loss of heterozygosity in renal cell carcinoma. Proc Natl Acad Sci U S A 85:1571–1575.

KOZAK FK, HALL JG, BAIRD PA. 1986. Familial breast cancer in males. Cancer 58:2736–2739.

LARSSON C, SKOGSEID B, OBERG K, et al. 1988. Multiple endocrine neoplasia type 1 gene maps to chromosome 11 and is lost in insulinoma. Nature 332:85–87.

LAW DJ, OLSCHWANG S, MONPEZAT JP, et al. 1988. Concerted nonsyntenic allelic loss in human colorectal carcinoma. Science 241:961–966.

LEACH FS, NICOLAIDES N, PAPADOPOULOS N, et al. 1993. Mutations of a mutS homolog in hereditary nonpolyposis colorectal cancer. Cell 75:1215–1216.

LEE EY, TO H, SHEW JY, et al. 1988. Inactivation of the retinoblastoma susceptibility gene in human breast cancers. Science 241:218–221.

LEE WH, SHEW JY, HONG FD, et al. 1987. The retinoblastoma susceptibility gene encodes a nuclear phosphoprotein associated with DNA binding activity. Nature 329:642–645.

LENCH N, STANIER P, WILLIAMSON R. 1988. Simple non-invasive method to obtain DNA for gene analysis. Lancet 1:1356–1358.

LEPPERT M, DOBBS M, SCAMBLER P, et al. 1987. The gene for familial polyposis coli maps to the long arm of chromosome 5. Science 238:1411–1413.

LI FP. 1988. Cancer families: human models of susceptibility to cancer. Cancer Res 48:5381–5386.

LI FP. 1993. Molecular epidemiology studies of cancer in families. Br J Cancer 68:217–219.

LI FP, DECKER HJH, ZBAR B, et al. 1993. Clinical and genetic studies of renal cell carcinomas in a family with a constitutional chromosome 3;8 translocation. Ann Intern Med 118:106–111.

LI FP, GARBER JE, FRIEND SH, et al. 1992. Recommendations on predictive testing for germ line p53 mutations among cancer-prone individuals. J Natl Cancer Inst 84:1156–1160.

LI FP. 1987. Cancer epidemiology and prevention. In: Rubenstein E, Federman DD (eds). Sci Am Med, 10:12:I:28.

LI FP, FRAUMENI JF JR, MULVIHILL JJ, et al. 1988. A cancer family syndrome in twenty-four kindreds. Cancer Res 48:5358–5362.

LI FP, THURBER WA, SEDDON J, et al. 1987. Hepatoblastoma in families with polyposis coli. JAMA 257:2475–2477.

LI FP, BADER JL. 1987. Epidemiology of cancer in childhood. In: *Hematology of Infancy and Childhood*, Nathan DG, Oski FA (eds). Philadelphia: W.B. Saunders, pp 918–941.

LI FP, MARCHETTO DJ, VAWTER GF. 1979. Acute leukemia and preleukemia in eight males in a family: an X-linked disorder? Am J Hematol 6:61–69.

LI GH, HE LJ. 1986. A survey on the familial aggregation of esophageal cancer in Yangcheng county, Shanxi province. In: *Genes and Disease*, Wu M, Nebert DW, (eds). Beijing: Science Press.

LI JY. 1982. Epidemiology of esophageal cancer in China. In: Third Symposium on Epidemiology and Cancer Registries in the Pacific Basin, 1981, Henderson B (ed). NCI Monogr 62:113–120. Washington DC: United States Government Printing Office.

LINGEMAN CH. 1974. Etiology of cancer of the human ovary. J Natl Cancer Inst 53:1603–1618.

LIPKIN M, SHERLOCK P, WINAWER SJ. 1980. Early diagnosis and detection of colorectal cancer in high-risk population groups. In: *Gastrointestinal Tract Cancer*, Lipkin M, Good RA (eds). New York: Plenum Medical Book Company, pp 421–436.

LITTLE JB, NOVE J, DALBERG WK, et al. 1987. Normal cytotoxic response of skin fibroblasts from patients with Li-Fraumeni familial cancer syndrome to DNA-damaging agents in vitro. Cancer Res 47:4229–4234.

LOVE RR, MAZESS RB, BARDEN HS, et al. 1992. Effects of tamoxifen on bone mineral density in postmenopausal women with breast cancer. N Engl J Med 326:852–856.

LOVE RR, EVANS AM, JOSTEN DM. 1985. The accuracy of patient reports of a family history of cancer. J Chron Dis 38:289–293.

LOVE RR. 1985. Small bowel cancers, B-cell lymphatic leukemia, and six primary cancers with metastases and prolonged survival in the cancer family syndrome of Lynch. Cancer 55:499–502.

LOWE SW, SCHMITT EM, SMITH SW, et al. 1993. P53 is required for radiation-induced apoptosis in mouse thymocytes. Nature 362:847–849.

LYNCH HT, KRUSH AJ. 1971. Cancer family "G" revisited: 1895–1970. Cancer 27:1505–1511.

LYNCH HT, LYNCH JF. 1993. Familial predisposition and cancer management. Contemp Oncol 12–25.

LYNCH HT, LYNCH PM. 1980. Hereditary and gastrointestinal tract cancer. In: *Gastrointestinal Tract Cancer*, Lipkin M, Good RA (eds). New York: Plenum Medical Book Company, pp 259–260.

LYNCH HT, ENS J, LYNCH JF, et al. 1988. Tumor variation in three extended Lynch syndrome II kindreds. Am J Gastroenterol 83:741–747.

MACMAHON B, LEVY MA. 1964. Prenatal origin of childhood leukemia. N Engl J Med 21:1082–1085.

MALKIN D, LI FP, STRONG LC, et al. 1990. Germline p53 mutations in a familial syndrome of breast cancer, sarcomas, and other neoplasms. Science 250:1233–1238.

MARCHETTO D, LI FP, HENSON DE. 1983. Familial carcinoma of ureters and other genitourinary organs. J Urol 130:772–773.

MCNEIL MM, LEONG AS-Y, SAGE RE. 1981. Primary mediastinal embryonal carcinoma in association with Klinefelter's syndrome. Cancer 47:343–345.

MIKI Y, SWENSEN J, SHATTUCK-EIDENS D, et al. 1994. A strong candidate for the breast and ovarian cancer susceptibility gene BRCA1. Science 266:66–71.

MILLER RW, FRAUMENI JF JR, MANNING MD. 1964. Association of Wilms' tumor with aniridia, hemihypertrophy and other congenital malformations. N Engl J Med 270:922–927.

MILLER RW. 1971. Deaths from childhood leukemia and solid tumors among twins and other sibs in the United States, 1960–67. J Natl Cancer Inst 46:203–209.

MULLER H, WEBER W, eds. 1985. Familial Cancer. Basel: Karger.

MULLIGAN LM, ENG C, HEALEY CS, et al. 1994. Specific mutations of the RET proto-oncogene are related to disease phenotype in MEN 2A and FMTC. Nature Genet 6:70–74.

MULVIHILL JJ, MILLER RW, FRAUMENI JF, JR, eds. 1977. Genetics of Human Cancer. New York: Raven Press.

NAROD SA, LYNCH HT, CONWAY T, et al. 1991. Familial breast-ovarian cancer locus on chromosome 17q12-q23. Lancet 338: 82–83.

NATIONAL ADVISORY COUNCIL OF THE HUMAN GENOME PROGRAM. 1994. Statement on use of DNA testing for presymptomatic identification of cancer risk. JAMA 271:785.

NEEDLEMAN SW, YUASA Y, SRIVASTAVA S, et al. 1983. Normal cells of patients with high cancer risk syndromes lack transforming activity in the NIH/3T3 transfection assay. Science 222:173–174.

NEEL JV. 1971. Familial factors in adenocarcinoma of the colon. Cancer 28:46–50.

NEVINS JR. 1992. E2F: a link between the Rb tumor suppressor protein and viral oncoproteins. Science 258:424–429.

OHTA M, INOVE H, COTTICELLI MG, et al. 1996. The FHIT gene, spanning the chromosome 3p14.2 fragile site and renal carcinoma-associated t(3;8) breakpoint, is abnormal in digestive tract cancers. Cell 84:587–597.

OKAMOTO M, SASAKI M, SUGIO K, et al. 1988. Loss of constitutional heterozygosity in colon carcinoma from patients with familial polyposis coli. Nature 331:273–277.

OOI WL, ELSTON RC, CHEN VW, et al. 1986. Increased familial risk for lung cancer. J Natl Cancer Inst 76:217–222.

PARRY DM, MULVIHILL JJ, MILLER RW, et al. 1987. Strategies for controlling cancer through genetics. Cancer Res 47:6814–6817.

PELLETIER J, BRUENING W, LI FP, et al. 1991. WT1 mutations contribute to abnormal genital system development and hereditary Wilms' tumour. Nature 353:431–434.

PELTOMAKI P, AALTONEN LA, SISTONEN P, PYLKKANEN L. 1993. Genetic mapping of a locus predisposing to human colorectal cancer. Science 260:751–752, 810–819.

PRITCHARD-JONES C, FLEMING S, DAVIDSON A, et al. 1990. The candidate Wilms' tumor gene is involved in genitourinary development. Nature 346:194–197.

PURTILO DT, DEFLORIO D, HUTT LM, et al. 1977. Variable phenotypic expression of an X-linked recessive lymphoproliferative syndrome. N Engl J Med 297:1077–1081.

RAUSCHER FJ, MORRIS JF, TOURNAY OE, et al. 1990. Binding of the Wilms' tumor locus zinc finger protein to the EGR-1 consensus sequence. Science 250:1259–1262.

REIMER RR, FRAUMENI JF JR, OZOLS RF, et al. 1977. Pancreatic cancer in father and son. Lancet 1:911.

RICCARDI VM, SHIH VE, HOLMES LB, et al. 1975. Hereditary pancreatitis. Arch Intern Med 135:822–825.

RITTER SB, PETERSEN G. 1976. Esophageal cancer, hyperkeratosis and oral leukoplakia: occurrence in a 25-year-old woman. JAMA 235:1723–1724.

SATTIN RW, RUBIN GL, WEBSTER LA, et al. 1985. Family history and the risk of breast cancer. JAMA 253:1908–1913.

SCHILDKRAUT JM, THOMPSON WD. 1988. Familial ovarian cancer: a population-based case-control study. Am J Epidemiol 128: 456–466.

SCHNEIDER NR, WILLIAMS WR, CHAGANTI RSK. 1986. Genetic epidemiology of familial aggregation of cancer. Adv Cancer Res 47:1–35.

SCHNEIDER NR, CHAGANTI SR, GERMAN J, et al. 1983. Familial predisposition to cancer and age at onset of disease in randomly selected cancer patients. Am J Hum Genet 35:454–467.

SHILLING TC. 1992. Addictive drugs: the cigarette experience. Science 255:430–433.

SHOENFELD Y, BERLINER S, SHAKLAI M, et al. 1982. Familial multiple myeloma: a review of thirty-seven families. Postgrad Med J 58:12–16.

SIMPSON NE, KIDD KK, GOODFELLOW PJ, et al. 1987. Assignment of multiple endocrine neoplasia type 2A to chromosome 10 by linkage. Nature 328:528–530.

SMITH DG, LEVITT SH. 1974. Radiation carcinogenesis: an unusual familial occurrence of neoplasia following irradiation in childhood for benign disease. Cancer 34:2069–2071.

STEENMAN MJC, RAINIER S, DOBRY CJ, et al. 1994. Loss of imprinting of IGF2 is linked to reduced expression and abnormal methylation of H19 in Wilms' tumour. Nature Genet 7:433–439.

STEINBERG GD, CARTER BS, BEATTY TH, et al. 1990. Family history and risk of prostate cancer. Prostate 17:337–347.

STRONG LC, RICCARDI VM, FERRELL RE, et al. 1981. Familial retinoblastoma and chromosome 13 deletion transmitted via an insertional translocation. Science 213:1501–1503.

STRONG LC, STINE M, NORSTED TL. 1987. Cancer in survivors of childhood soft tissue sarcoma and their relatives. J Natl Cancer Inst 79:1213–1220.

SUGIMURA T. 1992. Multistep carcinogenesis: a 1992 perspective. Science 258:603–607.

SWIFT M, MORRELL D, MASSEY RB, et al. 1991. Incidence of cancer in 161 families affected by ataxia-telangiectasia. N Engl J Med 325:1831–1836.

T'ANG A, VARLEY JM, CHAKRABORTY S, et al. 1988. Structural rearrangement of the retinoblastoma gene in human breast carcinoma. Science 242:263–266.

TROFATTER JA, MACCOLLIN MM, RUTTER JL, et al. 1993. A novel moesin-, ezrin-, radixin-like gene is a candidate for neurofibromatosis 2 tumor suppressor. Cell 72:791–800.

VERP MS, SIMPSON JE. 1987. Abnormal sexual differentiation and neoplasia. Cancer Genet Cytogenet 25:191–218.

VOGELSTEIN B, FEARON ER, HAMILTON SR, et al. 1988. Genetic alterations during colorectal-tumor development. N Engl J Med 319:525–532.

VOGELSTEIN B, FEARON ER, HAMILTON SR, et al. 1985. Use of restriction fragment length polymorphisms to determine the clonal origin of human tumors. Science 227:642–645.

VOŘECHOVSKÝ I, RASIO D, LUO L, et al. 1996. The ATM gene and susceptibility to breast cancer: analysis of 38 breast tumors reveals no evidence for mutation. Cancer Res 56:2726–2732.

WEINBERG AG, MIZE CE, WORTHEN HG. 1976. The occurrence of hepatoma in the chronic form of hereditary tyrosinemia. Pediatrics 88:434–438.

WEINBERG AG. 1991. Tumor suppressor genes. Science 254:1138–1146.

WEISSMAN BE, SAXON PJ, PASQUALE SR, et al. 1987. Introduction of a normal human chromosome 11 into a Wilms' tumor cell line controls its tumorigenic expression. Science 236:175–180.

WHITE R, CASKEY T. 1988. The human as an experimental system in molecular genetics. Science 240:1483–1488.

WHITE RL. 1984. Human genetics. Lancet 2:1257–1262.

WHYTE P, BUCHKOVICH KJ, HOROWITZ JM, et al. 1988. Association between an oncogene and an antioncogene: the adenovirus E1A proteins bind to the retinoblastoma gene product. Nature 334:124–129.

WIGGS J, NORDENSKJOLD M, YANDELL D, et al. 1988. Prediction of the risk of hereditary retinoblastoma, using DNA polymorphisms within the retinoblastoma gene. N Engl J Med 318:151–157.

WILLIAMS WR, ANDERSON DE. 1984. Genetic epidemiology of breast cancer: segregation analysis of 200 Danish pedigrees. Genet Epidemiology 1:7–20.

WOOSTER R, BIGNELL G, LANCASTER J, et al. 1995. Identification of the breast cancer susceptibility gene BRCA2. Nature 378:789–792.

YOKOTA J, WADA M, SHIMMOSATO Y, et al. 1987. Loss of heterozygosity on chromosomes 3, 13, and 17 in small-cell carcinoma and on chromosome 3 in adenocarcinoma of the lung. Proc Natl Acad Sci U S A 84:9252–9256.

YOUNG JL, PERRY CL, ASIRE AJ, eds. 1977. Surveillance, Epidemiology and End Results: Incidence and Mortality Data, 1973–1977, NCI Monogr 57:70–73. Washington, DC: United States Government Printing Office.

ZBAR B, BRAUCH H, TALMADGE C, et al. 1987. Loss of alleles of loci on the short arm of chromosome 3 in renal cell carcinoma. Nature 327:721–724.

ZUO L, WESER J, YANG Q, et al. 1996. Germline mutations in the $p16^{INK4a}$ binding domain of CDK4 in familial melanoma. Nature Genetics 12:97–99.

27 Inherited susceptibility

LOUISE C. STRONG
CHRISTOPHER I. AMOS

Population-based studies reveal some excess familial cancer aggregation for most cancer sites (Cannon-Albright et al, 1994; Goldgar et al, 1994b), but a clear genetic susceptibility has been identified for only a few cancer sites. Easton and Peto (1990) demonstrated that the overall percentage of cancer cases caused by the rare, highly penetrant Mendelian syndromes with associated stigmata might account for less than 0.1% of all cancer in the United Kingdom. Although the survey did not include the cancer cases caused by the more recently identified or localized breast or colon cancer genes, it still underlines the rarity of what are often considered the paradigms for hereditary cancer syndromes. The rationale for studying genetic susceptibility to cancer is not primarily its direct impact on the public health burden, however. Studies of the relatively rare paradigm familial cancers have led to the identification of specific genes and mechanisms of tumor development relevant to the common nonheritable cancers.

The concept of cancer as a genetic disease at the cellular level, resulting from an accumulation of specific mutations, is discussed in more detail in other chapters but underlies the presentation here as well. The simplest mechanism of genetic predisposition might be the case in which an individual is rendered susceptible by inheriting a mutation in one of the genes on the critical pathway. Retinoblastoma is an example where there may be as few as two rate-limiting genetic events. Other tumors may require additional mutational changes. An alternative mechanism of inherited susceptibility consistent with a multi-hit model would be inheritance of mutations in genes involved in DNA replication or repair, which then permit the accumulation of mutations. In either model, the genetically susceptible tissues would achieve the critical mutant genotype more rapidly than those requiring more mutations or more time to accrue mutations, and hence the susceptible individuals would manifest the phenotype of a younger age at onset and a high frequency of multiple primary tumors. The effect of cancer susceptibility genes that are highly penetrant at young ages may be the elimination of susceptible individuals with advancing age.

In this chapter we will review methods of detecting genetic susceptibility to cancer, paradigms for Mendelian-inherited tumor susceptibility and the mechanisms of tumor susceptibility involved, and evidence for genetic-environmental interactions in some common cancers. Evidence for genetic susceptibility by tumor type is provided in the chapters on those tumors.

METHODS TO IDENTIFY GENETIC EFFECTS IN THE ETIOLOGY OF CANCER

Various methods are available to identify genetic factors influencing cancer risk and to evaluate gene-environment interactions in cancer etiology. A general paradigm for genetic epidemiological studies that can be applied for identifying genetic predisposition to cancer is depicted in Figure 27–1. According to this schema, a preliminary step consists of case-series and clinical observations that suggest aggregation of cancer in families. These clinical observations are followed by epidemiological studies that evaluate evidence that increased cancer risk at a particular site is associated with a family history of cancer, either at the site of interest or at other sites. To identify the most likely genetic mechanism underlying susceptibility to disease, segregation analysis is performed. Provided there is evidence for a genetic effect, genetic linkage studies are then undertaken. For these studies, a genetic model based on prior segregation analysis or population studies is needed. Finally, if a genetic factor that influences susceptibility for disease has been identified, then molecular epidemiological studies may be undertaken. We now describe some aspects of these designs.

Terms specific to genetic epidemiological studies are essential to understanding these study designs. For example, a genetic locus is a particular position on a chro-

This investigation was supported by Retina Research Foundation and by grants PO1 CA-34936 and RO1 CA-38929 awarded by the National Cancer Institute. We acknowledge Dr. Margaret Spitz and Jan Bressler for their helpful discussions and Tess Derryberry and Beverly Connaly for their clerical assistance.

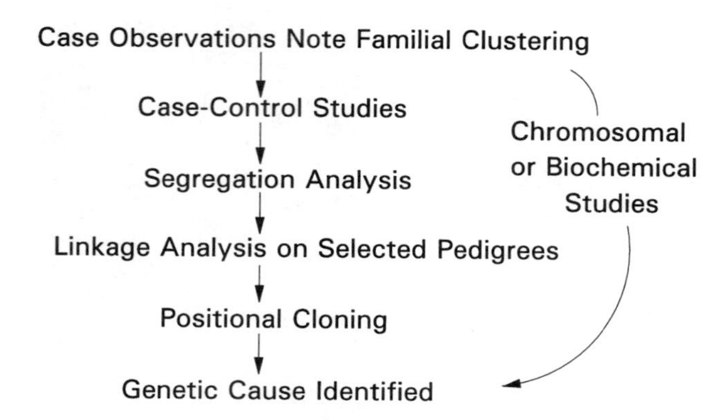

FIG. 27–1. Paradigm for epidemiological studies for identifying genetic predisposition to cancer.

mosome that may be occupied by DNA that can be transcribed, in which case a gene occupies the locus. If a locus shows variation, the variant forms are called alleles. The genotype of an individual is composed of the alleles carried by that individual. For an autosomal locus, if there are k alleles at a locus, then each individual can have one of $k(k+1)/2$ distinct genotypes for this locus. Observations about an individual, such as his or her disease status, are called the phenotype. The penetrance is the probability that an individual with a particular genotype becomes diseased.

Epidemiological Designs

Twin studies or case-control studies can be used to document evidence for familial factors, which may include inherited susceptibility. The contrast between monozygous (who are genetically identical) and dizygous (who share, on average, half their genes) twin pairs, can be exploited to partition interindividual variability into components reflecting genetic and environmental exposures (Neale and Cardon, 1993). Population-based twin studies are difficult to apply to the study of cancer because of its late onset, and the rarity of any particular cancer site or histology in most populations, but have nevertheless been applied to the study of some common cancers (Thomas et al, 1990). Twin studies are more generally useful for studying quantitative risk factors for cancers, such as aryl-hydrocarbon hydroxylase inducibility (Atlas et al, 1976), and debrisoquine phenotype (Evans et al, 1983b). Methods to analyze twin data and allow for the late age at onset of cancers have only recently become available (Thomas et al, 1990; Prentice, 1988).

Case-Control Studies

Case-control studies are more practical than twin studies for the study of uncommon diseases such as cancers. Two designs are typically employed to assess familial risk of cancer. Often all that is requested is the family history of cancer for case and control subjects in some defined constellation of relatives such as all those of first degree (full siblings, parents, and offspring). The odds ratio is then used to summarize the association between case or control status and family history of disease, with the possibility of adjusting for environmental or lifestyle-related risk factors in the case or control subject. For this approach to provide acceptable information about the familial risk of disease, at least the total number of relatives (including affected and unaffected individuals) as well as the period at risk (ie, current age, age at onset of cancer, or death from competing causes) should be collected to ensure the comparability of the control subjects to the patients. In addition, the validity of self-reported family history from the index case and control subjects can be questionable, especially for abdominal cancer sites (Love et al, 1985), though some sites, such as breast cancer, are well reported in first-degree relatives.

An alternative, and perhaps more appealing, approach for analysis uses the cases and controls to define historical cohorts that include the relatives of the case and control subjects. From this type of data, the absolute risk of disease can be estimated, and relative risks of disease among first-degree relatives of case and control subjects can be compared. More importantly, characteristics of the relatives that may influence their risk of cancer can be evaluated. For instance, for most cancer sites, increased risk of cancer among relatives of patients tends to occur mainly at earlier ages. Identifying the age-related distribution of cancer occurrence among relatives of case and control subjects provides valuable information for risk assessment. Similarly, construction of historical cohorts can provide evidence for family history–environment interactions that are difficult to assess in usual case-control studies. The standard errors of risk estimates from familial cohort studies are usually downwardly biased, but frailty (Mack et al, 1990) and quasilikelihood (Qaqish and Liang, 1992; Zhao and Le Marchand, 1992) modeling procedures have recently been adapted to allow for familial correlations in risk.

Segregation and Linkage Analysis

The usual epidemiological designs are not appropriate in evaluating specific genetic hypotheses, but these can be assessed by segregation and linkage analysis. Segregation analytic approaches have been developed specifically to permit modeling of environmental and genetic effects on disease etiology, including effects from a major gene (monogenic) as well as effects from many genes each having small effects (polygenic effects). The purpose of segregation analysis is to identify (a) how monogenic factors are expressed, (b) the gene frequencies of any monogenic factor, and (c) the relative importance of Mendelian, polygenic, and nongenetic factors in disease etiology. The selection of families through an affected individual introduces biases in the estimators of the penetrances and gene frequencies that require statistical correction (Sawyer, 1990). Provided well-established criteria are followed in the collection of families (Cannings and Thompson, 1977; Elston and Sobel, 1979), relatively simple ascertainment corrections are available. Alternatively, if the selection process is unclear, ascertainment-free methods to construct estimates of the penetrance and gene frequency parameters are available, but these provide relatively inefficient estimators (Shute and Ewens, 1988). Modeling the inheritance of polygenic factors has been computationally difficult in extended pedigrees, and a number of approaches have been taken. The mixed model, which includes both polygenic and monogenic factors, is implemented either by treating the nuclear family as the unit of analysis (Lalouel and Morton, 1981), or through an approximation that permits full pedigree analysis (Hasstedt, 1991). A third approach focuses on estimating Mendelian and nongenetic factors, with any possible polygenic effects represented by residual familial risk factors for disease. These regressive models (Bonney, 1986; Demenais, 1991) have been developed to model the logit transform of risk of disease as a function of inferred genetic susceptibility, as well as measured genotypic and environmental effects, if these are available. Regressive models sequentially condition pedigree data, beginning with the founders and proceeding through the pedigree, so that: (a) all of the dependence among pedigree members can be captured in the analysis and (b) subject to some mild assumptions, efficient algorithms to evaluate the data can be developed (Demenais et al, 1990). Gene-environment interactions can be included in the modeling process, but in the analysis of a dichotomous disorder little statistical information is likely to remain after the other parameters have been estimated. Segregation analysis nonetheless suggests that genetic susceptibility is a more important factor in the etiology of lung cancer among young patients (ie, less than age 50), whereas smoking plays the predominant role at older ages, when lung cancer most commonly occurs (Sellers et al, 1990).

Classic linkage studies (Ott, 1991) are conducted to identify coinheritance of a disease with a genetic marker: the penetrance and other parameters of the genetic model are usually derived prior to the linkage analyses. Because no mechanism other than inheritance of a susceptibility locus would result in the cosegregation of disease with genetic markers in families, linkage designs can provide conclusive evidence in favor of genetic factors in disease etiology (Williamson and Amos, 1990). Linkage analytic studies usually estimate only the recombination fraction and the LOD score, which measures support for genetic linkage. The recombination fraction measures the probability that the alleles at two distinct loci are not coinherited. A recombination fraction of zero indicates complete coinheritance of alleles at the loci; 0.5 indicates independent inheritance. A LOD score of 3.0 or greater is generally taken as definitive evidence for genetic linkage, provided sex-averaged recombination fractions are being reported and only a single genetic model was evaluated in the analysis (Weeks et al, 1990). Maximum likelihood linkage approaches in which the disease-related parameters are fixed prior to analysis have been successful in identifying many cancer-susceptibility loci, including the multiple endocrine neoplasias MEN1 and MEN2, von Hippel-Lindau syndrome, retinoblastoma, hereditary nonpolyposis colon cancer, and familial breast and ovarian cancers.

When the inheritance pattern of a disease is uncertain, linkage analysis can still be employed, but the power to detect linkage may be reduced and the recombination fraction poorly estimated (Clerget-Darpoux et al, 1986). Modeling strategies that can accommodate the complex etiology of most common cancers, including effects from environmental and monogenic factors as well as their interactions, are being developed. Conjoint segregation and linkage analysis is numerically difficult to implement, and these methods have only rarely been applied in the study of cancer aggregation in families (Demenais et al, 1992), despite theoretical support that this approach improves estimates of the penetrance (Amos and Rubin, 1995). Alternatively, similarity among affected individuals within pedigrees with respect to allelic markers can be evaluated for departure from that expected under independent segregation of the marker and disease-related locus (Weeks and Lange, 1988; Whittemore and Halpern, 1994). This approach provides a genetic model-free method of analysis. However, the power to detect genetic linkage can be low if, for example, there is heterogeneity in the major genes influencing disease risk.

In large families, identifying genetically susceptible individuals because of cosegregation of closely linked markers is possible. In these families, environmental and demographic effects on cancer risk can be directly assessed among genetically susceptible individuals, even when the specific genetic factor has not been identified. For example, results from a consortium study of breast cancer families, in which a suceptibility locus has been identified at chromosome 17q21 (the BRCA1 locus), show the median age at onset for breast cancer among genetically susceptible women to be about 50 years of age (Easton et al, 1993), much younger than the median age at onset among breast cancer patients in the United States.

Molecular Epidemiology and Association Studies

Molecular biology provides myriad tools for characterizing interindividual variability and, ultimately, for teasing apart the separate and joint genetic and environmental effects on cancer risk. As specific genetic factors are identified in the etiology of common cancers, these genetic markers and biomarkers can be used in classic case-control and hybrid designs such as the nested case-control study (Wacholder, 1991). For case-control designs, care must be taken to ensure that the controls are drawn from the same ethnic population as the cases, to allow for the considerable variation in gene frequencies among ethnic groups. In U.S. urban populations matching on ethnicity is often problematic. One approach to circumvent the difficulty in matching on ethnicity is to use unaffected sibling controls and to construct the set of control alleles from those inherited by the unaffected sibling(s) but not the case subjects (Falk and Rubenstein, 1987). Alternatively, alleles transmitted to an affected offspring can be compared with those not transmitted to provide an approach that matches on the ethnic background of the parents and thus provides protection against spurious associations that might arise because of population stratification (Schaid and Sommers,1994; Ewens et al, 1995).

The detection of DNA mutations by molecular biological techniques has minimal error. However, identifying all of the alleles that are implicated in disease etiology is often difficult because numerous different mutations often can produce altered gene expression. Rothman and coworkers (1993) provide examples showing that large bias in the estimated odds ratio can accrue even when the sensitivity in defining individuals who would have altered gene expression by a DNA-based genotyping assay is 95% or better. Moreover, the bias in the odds ratio depends upon the gene frequency of the alleles conferring at-risk status, and ethnic risk comparisons should allow for the effect of different allelic frequencies on attenuation of the odds ratio when not all genotypic variants can be detected. Direct measures of enzymatic activity or protein levels are available for a variety of products that affect genetic risk and progression of cancers. These assays are often preferable to DNA-based assays because of the direct relationship between protein level and disease risk (Khouri et al, 1993). For gene products that are inducible or show diurnal variation, however, care must be exercised to quantify modifying factors. Finally, to assist in the required confirmation of association studies, the measurement error of phenotypic assays or diagnostic criteria must be carefully documented.

Comparison Between Association and Genetic Linkage Studies

To evaluate causal relationships in the etiology of genetically influenced diseases, both association and linkage studies provide valuable information. The alternate hypothesis in genetic linkage studies postulates a genetic effect from a locus in a region of the genome. Provided there is evidence from segregation analysis for major gene effects in the etiology of a disease, the generality of the linkage hypothesis provides protection against spurious false-positive results because the number of independent genetic linkage tests that could be constructed is finite (Ott, 1991) and the critical LOD score value of 3.0 required to document evidence for genetic linkage provides a posterior probability of linkage of 5%. On the other hand, families and materials for genetic linkage studies are difficult to assemble, and large numbers of families are typically needed to document linkage. Molecular epidemiological association studies are much simpler to perform, and more usual epidemiological designs can often be employed. The alternate hypothesis in an association study—that some particular allele is associated with increased disease risk—ensures greater power in an association than in a linkage study to detect an effect, provided a specific genetic test is available for the susceptibility allele(s). Unless strong biological hypotheses can be invoked to reduce the number of alleles that need to be evaluated in an association study, the number of hypotheses to be considered for association studies is essentially infinite, and the probability of a false-positive result is high (ie, approaches 1). In addition, associations can result from population stratification and for other noncausal reasons. Therefore, to suggest causality, any association study must be confirmed by a subsequent study, and stratified analyses are needed to allow for potential confounders such as ethnicity and, possibly, gender. Further support for a causal relationship in disease etiology from association studies is provided if linkage studies (allowing for the association) document the coinheritance of susceptibility with the implicated allele, by comparative studies showing associations in different populations, and/or by the study of model systems such as animal and in vitro assays. For alleles that confer only a modest increase in susceptibility, linkage studies may be impractical because huge sample sizes may be required (Greenberg, 1993). One reason for finding a consistent association in one population but not in any other is linkage disequilibrium (Thomson and Bodmer, 1977). Even for closely linked loci, detection of disequilibrium is difficult unless the rarer alleles of both loci are in disequilibrium (Thompson et al, 1988). Exceptionally, populations that have recently been admixed and have subsequently engaged in random mating for a few generations can provide data in which association studies could identify genetic factors through linkage disequilibrium (Chakraborty and Weiss, 1988).

CLASSES OF GENES THAT PREDISPOSE TO CANCER

The recent revolution in molecular genetic technology and the progress in mapping of the human genome has provided rapidly increasing numbers of highly polymorphic markers throughout the genome available for study of genes segregating in families as well as in tumors. The advances have permitted identification and characterization of many hereditary and acquired genetic changes in cancer, with some limited characterization of the mechanism of genetic susceptibility. The major classes of genes conferring genetic susceptibility recognized to date are listed in Table 27–1.

Tumor Suppressor Genes

The best-characterized cancer susceptibility genes to date are the tumor suppressor genes. Tumor suppressor genes are negative regulators of cell growth, such that loss of the negative growth control may be permissive for neoplasia. Loss of tumor suppressor function may be associated with hyperproliferation of benign or malignant tumors, as described below. Interestingly, the concept of tumor suppressor genes arose from two independent approaches. The initial experimental data came from the demonstration that fusion of normal and malignant cell lines led to hybrids with a normal but unstable phenotype. Reversion to a malignant phenotype correlated with loss of a specific chromosome from the normal parental line (Harris et al, 1969; Stanbridge, 1976). More recently, this functional approach to identification of tumor suppressor genes has been refined by use of microcell-mediated transfer of single chromosomes or chromosome fragments into malignant cell lines, or by other mechanisms of transfer and expression of specific genes into tumor cell lines, with demonstration of morphologic change or loss of tumorigenicity (Sanchez et al, 1994).

TABLE 27–1. *Classes of Heritable Tumor Susceptibility Genes*

Class of Genes	*Mode of Inheritance*	*Tumor Genotype*
Tumor suppressor genes	AD	AR
DNA mismatch repair genes	AD	AR
Genomic instability syndromes	AR	AR
Dominant transforming genes	AD	AD
Carcinogen metabolizing genes	AD, AR	AD, AR

AD = autosomal dominant
AR = autosomal recessive

The Two-Hit Model: Retinoblastoma. The other approach that eventually led to the identification of the first human tumor suppressor gene, the retinoblastoma gene (Rb1), evolved from clinical observations and statistical, cytogenetic, and molecular genetic analyses. The approaches that led to the identification of Rb1 as a tumor suppressor still serve as a model for the study of genetic susceptibility in human cancer. The relative rarity of retinoblastoma in general (roughly 1/20,000 live births) (Vogel, 1979) permitted easy recognition of familial cases as unusual. Follow-up of survivors of retinoblastoma demonstated that the risks to offspring of bilateral retinoblastoma patients approached the 50% risk consistent with a Mendelian dominant gene (Schappert-Kimmijser et al, 1966). To explain a common genetic pathway for a tumor that could be heritable or nonheritable, unilateral or bilateral, Knudson (1971) suggested that the same genetic events at the cell level might underlie both the heritable and nonheritable tumors. His analysis of the mean number of tumors and age of onset in bilateral and unilateral cases suggested that the pattern could be explained by two genetic events if, in heritable cases, one of those events was a germ line mutation and one a somatic mutation. In the nonheritable cases, both events would occur as somatic mutations.

Localizing the predisposing mutation was facilitated by the cytogenetic observations of rare retinoblastoma patients with congenital anomalies or failure to thrive and constitutional chromosomal deletion at 13q14 (Knudson et al, 1976). The finding of rare cases with a consistent chromosome deletion was significant in the development of the tumor suppressor model not only because it provided a region of the genome on which to focus for linkage analysis and eventual positional cloning of the gene, but also because it provided the first clinical evidence that cancer susceptibility might be associated with loss of genetic material and possibly loss of function.

With the 13q14 region providing a focus, cytogenetic studies of tumors demonstrated frequent deletion of 13q14 in sporadic tumors (Balaban et al, 1982), consistent with the idea of a common genetic region being altered in both heritable and nonheritable tumors. Linkage analysis in familial retinoblastoma demonstrated the inherited cancer susceptibility gene in the absence of gross cytogenetic deletion also involved this same chromosomal 13q14 region (Sparkes et al, 1983).

Localization of the inherited region of a cancer predisposition gene provided no new information with respect to the relationship of the first and second mutations that might occur in tumor development. However, a simple hypothesis was that the second mutation might involve the second allele at the same genetic locus, rendering the cell without a normal copy of the retinoblastoma gene. If that second event involved a gross chromosomal alteration, then contrast of tumor and normal tissue from the same individual using polymorphic DNA markers from flanking regions on chromosome 13 might provide evidence for tumor-specific alteration. Cavenee and coworkers (1983) tested that hypothesis in a series of retinoblastoma tumors and demonstrated a high frequency of loss of heterozygosity for the chromosome 13 markers in tumors. They further confirmed the "loss of function" model by demonstrating that the alleles lost in the tumor were consistently those from the unaffected parent, whereas the alleles retained in the tumor were those linked to the retinoblastoma mutant based on inheritance from an affected parent (Cavenee et al, 1985). These findings suggested that inherited mutation and tumor-specific loss of the other Rb1 (or functional gene product) were associated with tumor development, a finding that facilitated the positional cloning of the gene (Friend et al, 1986). Functional evidence for Rb1 as a tumor suppressor gene—that introduction of the normal gene product could reverse the malignant phenotype in cultured tumor cells lacking a normal Rb1—was demonstrated by a series of studies beginning with those of Huang and coworkers (1988).

The hypothesis of the two-hit model and the later demonstration of Rb1 as a tumor suppressor were based on data using the tumor retinoblastoma as the indication of the affected phenotype; that is, a tissue-specific cancer phenotype. However, follow-up of patients with successfully treated hereditary retinoblastoma revealed increased cancer risk at other sites. Initially the second tumors were attributed to radiation therapy (Forrest, 1961; Sagerman et al, 1969); however, further observations demonstrated an increased risk of additional tumors, particularly osteosarcoma, even in the absence of the radiation exposure (Kitchin and Ellsworth, 1974). These findings suggested that the cancer susceptibility conferred by mutations at the Rb1 locus might involve a broad spectrum of tumors. Although no other tumors occur with the same high penetrance or predictability as retinoblastoma, the risk of nonocular cancer for a mutation carrier during the first 40 years of life appears to be highly elevated even in the absence of radiotherapy (Eng et al, 1993).

Study of various sporadic tumors has demonstated a high frequency of somatic mutations at the Rb1 locus. For some tumors, mutations at the Rb1 locus may correlate with prognosis (Cance et al, 1990; Logothetis et al, 1992), or staging (Cryns et al, 1994).

Genetic Susceptibility to Diverse Tumor Types: p53 and Li-Fraumeni Syndrome. The observations that the retinoblastoma gene might predispose to many other cancer types, none with extraordinarily high penetrance, raised the possibility that there might be inherited cancer susceptibility genes with a broad tissue specificity but without one consistent or predictable tumor type. The phenotype might be nonrandom aggregation of diverse cancers in families. The best-defined general cancer susceptibility gene is the p53 tumor suppressor gene. In contrast to Rb1, p53 was identified as a tumor-specific alteration before its role in inherited susceptibility was recognized (Finlay et al, 1989). The initial concept of a familial cancer syndrome involving a diversity of tumor types came from a clinical observation/family report followed by a systematic survey of medical records and death certificates of children with soft tissue sarcomas by Li and Fraumeni in 1969 (a, b). The remarkable findings of childhood sarcomas, young-onset breast cancer, and other diverse cancers in one family were reproduced in a few families ascertained through the systematic series. Follow-up of these families over more than 20 years demonstrated a cancer-prone pattern of new tumors in the individuals initially affected, as well as new cancers developing in previously unaffected family members (Li and Fraumeni, 1975; Li et al, 1988;). Anecdotal case reports of similar clusters of childhood sarcomas, young-onset breast cancers, brain tumors, and other neoplasms appeared in the literature from a variety of different populations (for review see Strong et al, 1992). Formal genetic analysis of a systematically ascertained series of kindreds through probands with childhood soft tissue sarcoma suggested that the most likely explanation for the tumor distribution in the families was a rare autosomal dominant gene, with high penetrance for cancer of varied types. The age-specific penetrance for this statistically defined gene suggested a 50% risk of cancer by the age of 45 years, rising to 90% by age 65. Most of the evidence for a dominant gene came from 5% to 10% of the families. In those families, an excess of cancer was observed for a wide range of sites, including the expected sarcomas, breast cancers, brain tumors, and leukemias, but in addition cancer of the lung, prostate, uterine-cervix, and others (Lustbader et al, 1992).

p53 was considered a candidate gene based on observations that it was altered somatically in a wide variety of human cancers, including sarcomas and other tumors characteristic of the Li-Fraumeni syndrome (Hollstein et al, 1991). Other supportive evidence came from observations of cultured fibroblasts as a model system. Experimental studies had demonstrated cooperation in cellular transformation by cotransfection of rat embryo fibroblasts with mutant p53 and mutant *ras* oncogene (Parada et al, 1984). Study of cultured human fibroblasts revealed that those from patients with Li-Fraumeni syndrome underwent spontaneous immortalization in culture (Bischoff et al, 1990). The immortalized but nontumorigenic fibroblasts became tumorigenic when transfected with mutant *ras*, suggesting that the immortalized human fibroblasts might be analogous to the mutant p53 rat embryo fibroblasts (Bischoff et al, 1991).

To test the hypothesis that the cancer family syndrome might be attributable to p53 germ line mutation, normal tissue DNAs were amplified and sequenced at the p53 conserved exons 5–8, and mutations were detected in five of five families with a clinical phenotype of Li-Fraumeni syndrome (Malkin et al, 1990). As for retinoblastoma, the normal but cancer-prone tissues were heterozygous for the p53 mutations, whereas most of the tumors had undergone loss of heterozygosity at the p53 locus, with loss of the normal or wild-type allele, rendering the tumor cells homozygous for mutant p53. In vitro studies of tumors with mutant p53 reveal that transfection of a wild-type p53 can alter the morphology and tumorigenicity (Diller et al, 1990), confirming the functional "tumor suppressor" model.

As for other genetic syndromes, the clinical phenotype used in the initial syndrome description may not correlate exactly with that associated with the mutant genotype. As more data on mutation carriers accrue, it seems likely that the "syndrome" will need to be redefined with respect to age- and cancer site–specific risk. Further, not all kindreds with the clinical phenotype of Li-Fraumeni syndrome have been found to have p53 germ line mutations, suggesting there may be other genes that produce a similar phenotype (Birch et al, 1994). Lack of information then poses significant problems for recommendations in genetic testing and counseling, and programs in early detection and prevention. Further study of host and environmental factors that might affect cancer outcome in the genetically susceptible are difficult because of the diversity of outcomes encountered within a given family. Given that mice heterozygous for p53 mutations have been developed, they likely will serve as unique models to determine the role of other host and environmental factors in tumor development and tumor response to therapy, as well as the potential for intervention or prevention (Donehower et al, 1992; Harvey et al, 1993a, b; Hursting et al, 1994, 1995). Such experimental systems have already provided provocative findings with respect to lack of tumor response to chemotherapy and radiation based on the tumor mutant p53 genotype (Lowe et al, 1994).

Retinoblastoma and Li-Fraumeni syndrome have been presented as paradigms for cancer susceptibility due to tumor suppressor genes. Germ line mutations in these genes are rare, with retinoblastoma occurring in about one in 20,000 live births, of which 25% to 30% of cases may be heritable (Vogel, 1979). Li-Fraumeni syndrome or germ line p53 mutation accounts for only a few percent of childhood sarcomas or young-onset breast cancer and is rare in common cancers but perhaps more frequent in exceptionally rare cancers such as adrenocortial carcinoma or choroid plexus tumors (Borresen et al, 1992; Wagner et al, 1994; Diller et al, 1995; Garber et al, 1990). Yet these genes are very frequently somatically altered in many common cancers, demonstrating their important role in cellular growth control. Interestingly, the phenotype of the germ line mutation carrier is primarily cancer, and rarely benign neoplasia, a further observation that may ultimately provide clues to cellular growth controls.

Genetic Susceptibility Associated with Hyperproliferation and Cancer Precursor States: Familial Polyposis Coli and the *apc* Gene. The same tools used to identify the tumor suppressor gene Rb1 were informative in study of the syndrome of familial adenomatous polyposis (FAP), associated with increased risk primarily of colon cancer. The initial clinical observations from the 1800s (for review see Veale, 1965) were of a rare familial syndrome characterized by hundreds of adenomatous polyps of the colon in adolescence or young adulthood, almost inevitably leading to colon cancer by 40 years of age. The phenotype was expanded by Gardner in 1951, who noted the association of mandibular and other osteomas, epidermoid cysts, and benign but often life-threatening desmoid tumors with the colon polyposis in some families (Gardner, 1951). Others later described additional tumors occurring much less frequently with the polyposis syndrome(s), including other gastrointestinal tumors of the small intestine, stomach, biliary tract, and pancreas (Rustgi, 1994); brain tumors (often referrred to as Turcot's syndrome) (Turcot et al, 1959); hepatoblastoma (Garber et al, 1988); endocrine tumors of the adrenal cortex, pituitary, and thyroid (Schneider et al, 1983); and congenital hypertrophy of the retinal pigment epithelium (Lyons et al, 1988).

The first clue to the localization of the gene came from the observation of a mentally retarded patient with developmental anomalies and colonic polyposis, and a constitutional chromosome deletion on 5q (Herrera et al, 1986). Rapidly thereafter linkage analysis confirmed the localization of the FAP gene to 5q (Bodmer et al, 1987), and demonstrated tumor-specific loss of heterozygosity for 5q in sporadic colon tumors (Solomon et al, 1987). The *apc* gene was eventually identified by positional cloning (Groden et al, 1991). Its protein product has been localized to the cytoplasm and is thought to function in cell-cell interactions by association with the microtubule cytoskeleton (Smith et al, 1994).

Vogelstein and colleagues (Fearon and Vogelstein 1990; Vogelstein et al, 1988) have studied the molecular changes associated with various stages in colon neoplasia, and demonstrated that most colon adenomatous polyps, hereditary or acquired, show alterations at the *apc* locus. Microdissection of adenomatous polyps from FAP patients and from mice with germ line mutations at the homologous mouse locus have shown early loss of the wild-type allele (Ichii et al, 1992; Oshima et al, 1995). Other investigators have shown that the additional tumors associated with FAP, including gastrointestinal adenomas and carcinomas, and desmoid tumors, also show *apc* mutations with loss of heterozygosity (Toyooka et al, 1995; Okamoto et al, 1990). Although the *apc* gene is involved early in the neoplastic process, in vitro addition of the wild-type allele to malignant colonic tumors alters the morphology and tumorigenicity (Groden et al, 1995).

In contrast to Rb1 and p53, for which the primary mutant phenotype is cancer, not necessarily preceded by premalignant lesions, mutations at the *apc* locus are associated with an increase in *premalignant* lesions. *Apc* mutations, then, are not sufficient for malignant transformation. However, for carriers with hundreds of premalignant lesions in the colon, the risk of one or more proceeding to cancer is essentially 100%, and the cancer risk for the gene carrier is increased 700-fold by 45 years of age (Moolgavkar and Luebeck, 1992). The mechanism by which *apc* mutations increase cancer risk may be related to the increased cellular proliferation, perhaps increasing the proliferative compartment and hence the number of cells at risk, resulting in a high probability of at least one cell sustaining additional critical mutations. Germ line *apc* mutations occur at a frequency of one in 5000 to one in 7500 and may account for no more than 1% of colon cancer (Rustgi, 1994); somatic mutations at *apc*, however, may define a pathway common for the colon adenoma-carcinoma sequence. Therefore, FAP patients should be ideal subjects for trials of intervention, as have been initiated with wheat fiber and nonsteroidal anti-inflammatory drugs (DeCosse et al, 1989 and Labayle et al, 1991).

Clinical data had never resolved the question of genetic heterogeneity in the polyposis syndromes including "simple" familial polyposis, Gardner's syndrome, and Turcot's syndrome. Following cloning of the *apc* gene it became possible to examine genotype-phenotype correlations. Current data suggest that most *apc* mutations produce a truncated or disabled protein, but that not all mutations are equally severe. Mutations at the most 5′ region of the gene are associated with a consistent "attentuated" or more mild phenotype (Spirio et al, 1993), possibly due to alternate splice sites in the *apc* gene (Samowitz et al, 1995). Mutations distal to exon 9 are associated with congenital hypertrophy of the retinal pigment epithelium (Olschwang et al, 1993). No unique *apc* mutation has been identified with Turcot's syndrome, but mutations both in *apc* and the hereditary nonpolyposis colon cancer syndrome genes (see below) have been identified in patients, demonstrating genetic heterogeneity in the syndrome (Hamilton et al, 1995). In addition to variation in risk associated with allelic heterogeneity, at least in the mouse model, with mutation at the *min* locus homologous to *apc*, there is also evidence for modifier genes that can dramatically reduce

TABLE 27–2. *Autosomal Dominant Tumor Susceptibility Syndromes with Tumor Suppressor Genes*

Hereditary Condition	*Chromosomal Localization/Gene*	*Tumor Type(s)*	*References*
Bilateral acoustic neurofibromatosis	22q11-q12/Merlin	Meningioma, schwannoma, neurofibroma, glioma, acoustic neurofibroma	Trofatter et al, 1993 Rouleau et al, 1993 Lutchman and Rouleau, 1995
Familial polyposis coli (Gardner's syndrome)	5q21/APC	Colon adenoma and adenocarcinoma, brain tumor, desmoid, other GI, sarcoma, adrenocortical, thyroid, pituitary, other endocrine tumor, hepatoblastoma	Groden et al, 1995
Li-Fraumeni syndrome	17p13/p53	Sarcoma, breast, brain, leukemia, adrenocortical, lung, prostate, other	Malkin et al, 1990
Melanoma, hereditary	9p21/p16	Melanoma, pancreas	Cannon-Albright et al, 1992 Kamb et al, 1994 Goldstein et al, 1995 Whelan et al, 1995 Arap et al, 1995
von Hippel-Lindau disease	3p25/VHL	Renal cell carcinoma, hemangioblastoma of central nervous system and retina, pheochromocytoma	Duan et al, 1995 Iliopoulos et al, 1995 Latif et al, 1993 Neumann et al, 1993
von Recklinghausen's neurofibromatosis	17q11.2/NF-1	Optic neuroma, brain tumor, neurogenic and non-neurogenic sarcoma, neuroblastoma, Wilms' tumor, nonlymphocytic leukemia, melanoma, hepatoma	Xu et al, 1990 Clausen et al, 1989 Shannon et al, 1994
Wilms' tumor WAGR, Drash syndrome	11p13/WT1	Wilms' tumor, genitourinary anomalies, mesangial sclerosis	Huff and Saunders, 1993 Haber et al, 1993

TABLE 27–3. *Autosomal Dominant Tumor Susceptibility Syndromes, Likely Tumor Suppressor Genes by Linkage and Tumor-Specific Loss of Heterozygosity*

Hereditary Condition	*Chromosomal Localization/Gene*	*Tumor Type(s)*	*References*
Beckwith-Wiedemann syndrome (imprinted)	11p15.5	Wilms' tumor, adrenocortical adenocarcinoma, hepatoblastoma, brain tumor, rhabdomyosarcoma	Koufos et al, 1985
Breast, breast/ovarian cancer susceptibility	17q21/BRCA1	Breast, ovary, ? colon, prostate	Miki et al, 1994 Ford et al, 1994
	13q14/BRCA2	Breast (male, female), ovary	Wooster et al, 1994 Thorlacius et al, 1995 Collins et al, 1995
Hereditary multiple exostoses	8q24/EXT1	Exostosis, osteosarcoma	Hecht et al, 1995
	11 Pericentric	Exostosis, osteosarcoma	Ahn et al, 1995
Multiple endocrine adenomatosis I	11q13	Parathyroid, pituitary, pancreatic islet cell	Thakker, 1993 Larsson et al, 1992
Nevoid basal cell carcinoma syndrome	9q22.3-q31	Basal cell carcinoma, medulloblastoma, ovarian fibroma	Gailani et al, 1992 Farndon et al, 1992
Tuberous sclerosis	16p13.3(TSC2)	Brain tumor, renal cell carcinoma, renal angiomyolipoma, cardiac rhabdomyoma	Green et al, 1994
	9q34	Brain tumor, renal cell carcinoma, renal angiomyolipoma, cardiac rhabdomyoma	Fryer et al, 1987

the risk of gastrointestinal neoplasia (Dietrich et al, 1993).

Other Tumor Suppressor Genes or Candidate Tumor Suppressor Genes. The approaches that led to the localization, cloning, and characterization of the tumor suppressor genes *Rb1*, *p53* and *apc* have been applied to other tumor types and familial aggregates. Other tumor suppressor genes, and possible tumor suppressor genes involved in inherited tumor susceptibility are listed in Tables 27–2 and 27–3, with additional autosomal dominantly inherited tumor susceptibility syndromes of unknown mechanism listed in Table 27–4. The most valuable tools to localize cancer susceptibility genes have been demonstration of familial aggregation, constitutional and tumor-specific cytogenetics, genetic linkage, tumor-specific loss of heterozygosity, and functional tumor suppression. For several cancer susceptibility syndromes, genes have been localized by linkage, and tumor specific loss of heterozygosity has been observed, suggesting that loss of gene function is important for tumor development. As described below, not all loss of function mutations represent tumor suppressor loci.

It should be noted that analysis of tumor and normal DNA has been useful in identifying loss of function mutations that may be heritable or sporadic. However, in nonheritable tumor development, loss of function may occur not only due to alterations in the DNA but as well by mechanisms that involve loss of gene expression or functional inactivation of the protein at the cell level. One mechanism of somatic loss of tumor suppressor function with normal DNA sequence involves aberrant DNA methylation and silencing of the *p16* gene (Merlo et al, 1995). Another involves sequestration of the normal tumor suppressor protein by binding to other proteins. Examples of such protein sequestration include (a) binding to oncoproteins of DNA tumor viruses, including the human papilloma viruses, (b) binding to genes overexpressed in tumors as the MDM2 protein with p53 or Rb1 (Vogelstein and Kinzler, 1992; Xiao et al, 1995), and (c) even binding to a mutant tumor suppressor protein, as for p53 or the WT1 Wilms' tumor gene (Milner et al, 1991; Haber et al, 1992). In the latter case, at the DNA level the tumor would have one mutant and one normal gene sequence for the given tumor suppressor locus, but there could be complete loss of normal protein function. Because the mutant protein could functionally inactive the normal protein, the mu-

TABLE 27–4. *Autosomal Dominant Tumor Susceptibility Syndromes of Unknown Type*

Hereditary Condition	*Chromosomal Localization/Gene*	*Tumor Type(s)*	*References*
Paraganglioma, hereditary (imprinted)	11q14-qter	Non-chromaffin paraganglioma	Heutink et al, 1992 Mariman et al, 1993
Tylosis	17q23-qter	Carcinoma of esophagus	Risk et al, 1994 Marger and Marger, 1993
Wilms' tumor (familial)	??	Wilms' tumor	Huff and Saunders, 1993

tation would confer a new or "gain of function" to the mutant protein. Other mechanisms that interfere with gene transcription or translation, or protein localization in the nucleus or cytoplasm, could lead to functional inactivation as well.

Mismatch Repair Genes and the "Mutator Phenotype"

Given the successful approach to identification of autosomal dominant cancer susceptibility genes using the above approaches of genetic linkage in familial cancer aggregates and loss of heterozygosity in the tumors, it was natural to assume that the approaches would be successful for other autosomal dominant cancer susceptibility syndromes. For colon cancer, in addition to the relatively rare FAP described above, familial aggregates of colon and other gastrointestinal cancers have been noted from the time of Warthin in the early 1900s. Follow-up of Warthin's original kindreds and others led to a clinically defined syndrome of hereditary nonpolyposis colon cancer (HNPCC) (reviewed by Marra and Boland, 1995), a familial aggregation of colon, endometrial, and other gastrointestinal and urothelial cancers at relatively young ages in a pattern consistent with autosomal dominant inheritance. Tumors in affected patients had the distinct characteristics of early age of onset (often occurring in the late forties), a high frequency of right colon location, and multiple primary lesions. Discrete polyps were occasionally observed, but the carpeting of the colon with polyps, characteristic of FAP, was not present.

Linkage analysis using microsatellite markers throughout the genome in a few large kindreds demonstrated evidence for a cancer susceptibility gene on chromosome 2p, as well as evidence for genetic heterogeneity (Peltomaki et al, 1993). However, analysis of polymorphic microsatellite markers in tumor DNA from family members failed to reveal the expected loss of heterozygosity at chromosome 2p; in contrast it unexpectedly revealed a distinct phenotype of microsatellite instability at loci throughout the tumor genome (Aaltonen et al, 1993). Ionov and coworkers (1993) and Thibodeau and colleagues (1993) also observed the microsatellite instability in sporadic colon tumors of individuals with a relatively young age of disease onset and a relative prevalence of tumors of the right colon, characteristics that had also been observed in HNPCC patients.

The microsatellite instability phenotype was recognized by microbial geneticists as resembling the phenomenon associated with errors in mismatch repair, a pathway well defined in bacteria and yeast (Strand et al, 1993). The hypothesis that the HNPCC syndrome might be attributed to mutations in the human homologues of the mismatch repair genes was confirmed as the human homologues to the microbial *MutS* and *MutL* genes were identified, localized to regions of the genome showing linkage to HNPCC, including the original observation at 2p as well as another at 3p, and shown to harbor mutations (Fishel et al, 1993; Leach et al, 1993; Lindblom et al, 1993; Bronner et al, 1994; Papadopoulos et al, 1994). Additional *MutL* homologues—PMS1 and PMS2—have been identified and shown to be involved at least occasionally in HNPCC (Nicolaides et al, 1994), and another that may bind to MSH2 in recognition of the mismatch and be involved at least in some sporadic colon cancer (Papadopoulos et al, 1995; Palombo et al, 1995; Drummond et al, 1995). It is estimated from linkage analysis that mutations in the MSH2 and MLH1 genes account for 90% of HNPCC cases, with most mutations predicted to disrupt the protein (Nystrom-Lahti et al, 1994). The microsatellite instability phenotype in tumors and germ line mutations at the MSH2 locus have also been observed in the related Muir-Torre syndrome as noted in Table 27–5 (Honchel et al, 1994; Kolodner et al, 1994).

The HNPCC syndrome as been estimated to account for 4% to 13% of colon cancer; however, the Finland registry suggests the frequency may be more in the range of 1% to 2% of colon cancer (Aaltonen et al, 1994). Penetrance has not been estimated based on gene carrier status but is thought to be high (Marra and Boland, 1995).

The finding of microsatellite instability in hereditary and sporadic colon cancers has prompted investigators

TABLE 27–5. *Autosomal Dominant Tumor Susceptibility Syndromes with Mismatch Repair Defects and "Mutator" Phenotype*

Hereditary Condition	*Chromosomal Localization/Gene*	*Tumor Type(s)*	*References*
Hereditary nonpolyposis colon cancer (HNPCC)	2p16/MSH2 3p21/MLH1 2q31-33/PMS1 7p22/PMS2	Colon, endometrial, other GI, ovarian, genitourinary, ? breast carcinoma	Fishel et al, 1993 Leach et al, 1993 Bronner et al, 1994 Papadopoulos et al, 1994 Nicolaides et al, 1994
Muir-Torre syndrome	2p16/MSH2 3p21/MLH1	Same as HNPCC plus sebaceous adenoma	Kolodner et al, 1994

TABLE 27–6. *Autosomal Recessive Tumor Susceptibility Syndromes with Genomic Instability*

Hereditary Condition	*Chromosomal Localization/Gene*	*Tumor Type(s)*	*References*
Ataxia-telangiectasia	11q22-23/ATM	Lymphoma, leukemia, Hodgkin's disease, brain, gastric, ovarian, or other epithelial tumors; possibly increased risk to heterozygote for breast cancer	Savitsky et al, 1995 Swift et al, 1991
Bloom's syndrome	15q26.1/BLM	Leukemia, lymphoma, gastrointestinal, skin, other epithelial tumors	Ellis et al, 1995 German, 1993
Fanconi's anemia	9q22.3(FACC) 20q?	Leukemia, hepatoma, post–androgen therapy brain tumors, gynecologic, GI	Mann et al, 1991 Strathdee et al, 1992 Alter, 1993 Giampietro et al, 1993
Xeroderma pigmentosum multiple complementation groups	Multiple	Basal and squamous cell carcinoma of skin, melanoma, squamous cell carcinoma of tongue	Robbins et al, 1974 Hoeijmakers, 1993

to examine other tumor types for the phenotype; although microsatellite instability has not been rigorously defined, such alterations have been observed in most tumor types associated with HNPCC and many different sporadic cancer types (Eshleman and Markowitz, 1995).

Although loss of heterozygosity was not observed in tumors from the HNPCC patients initially studied (Aaltonen et al, 1993), the microsatellite instability appeared restricted to tumor and not heterozygous normal tissue from HNPCC patients (Parsons et al, 1993). Further analysis of HNPCC tumors with additional markers revealed that most often tumors have undergone loss or somatic mutation of the original wild-type allele, rendering the tumor with loss of wild-type repair function (Hemminki et al, 1994). Tumor cell lines with microsatellite instability have been shown to have a greater than 100-fold increased mutation rate as compared with tumor cell lines without microsatellite instability (Eshleman et al, 1995), confirming the concept of a "mutator phenotype." Presumably the mechanism of cancer susceptibility is through the increased risk of sustaining mutations in cancer-related genes, including the common pathway of *apc*, *ras,* and *p53*. In addition, a high frequency of inactivating mutations has been observed for the tumor suppressor transforming growth factor–β (TGF-β) receptor type 2 locus in colon cancer cell lines with microsatellite instability (Markowitz et al, 1995). The relative specificity for the association of gastrointestinal and urothelial tumors with this mutator phenotype remains unexplained, however.

Autosomal Recessive Syndromes of Genomic Instability and Cancer Susceptibility

The above-cited genes that predispose to cancer are inherited in an autosomal dominant manner, but function in tumor development by loss of function or in a cellular recessive manner. In addition, there are disorders associated with cancer susceptibility and loss of gene function but inherited in an autosomal recessive manner. These disorders are often generically referred to as DNA repair disorders or disorders of genomic instability (Table 27–6). Individually and collectively these disorders are extraordinarily rare, but have been important models for the initial concept of mutation as important in cancer development, and in providing insights into mechanisms of mutation and DNA replication and repair. From the population perspective, an interesting but unresolved question is whether these syndromes that are extremely rare in their recessive syndromic phenotype might have an effect on cancer susceptibility in the much more common heterozygous state. Swift and coworkers (1991) have suggested that at least for ataxia-telangiectasia (AT), the heterozygotes, who may make up 1% of the population, might have a significant fivefold increased risk of breast cancer and be uniquely sensitive to very low doses of ionizing radiation. Study of kindreds at high risk for breast cancer by linkage analysis, however, has not demonstrated involvement of the AT locus (Wooster et al, 1993; Cortessis et al, 1993). The recent cloning of the ataxia-telangiectasia gene (Savitsky et al, 1995) will permit direct testing of that hypothesis.

Dominant Transforming Cancer Susceptibility Genes

From study of tumor-specific genetic alterations, gain of function mutations in proto- oncogenes are well known and common events in tumor development. However, in terms of cancer susceptibility, gain of function mutations to date have only rarely been encountered. There are selected examples of possible gain of function mutations that may occur in classic tumor suppressor genes, in which the mutations may not only knock out or disrupt the wild-type function but may as well permit addition of function (Haber et al, 1992; Harvey et al, 1995b). However, the only examples to date of consistent gain of function mutations that predictably predispose to cancer are those observed in familial medullary thyroid carcinoma and multiple endocrine neoplasia (MEN) 2A and B, associated with germ line mutations in the *ret* proto-oncogene. The syndromes have in common an autosomal dominant pattern of inheritance of medullary thyroid carcinoma; clinical penetrance is approximately 60% by age 70 years, but by screening for the earliest manifestation using pentagastrin stimulation, penetrance is found to be nearly 95% by age 30 (Easton et al, 1989). The syndromes differ in their association with other abnormalities, with MEN2A being characterized by a high risk of pheochromocytoma and hyperparathyroidism, and MEN2B being more severe, including in addition skeletal anomalies, gastrointestinal ganglioneuromas, and mucosal neuromas (Mulligan et al, 1993). Each syndrome breeds true. The clinical phenotype of high penetrance for early onset and multiple primary tumors of specific endocrine sites, with thyroid C-cell hyperplasia preceding overt malignant neoplasia (Easton et al, 1989), suggested similarity to FAP and other loss of function or tumor suppressor gene disorders. However when the gene was localized by linkage analysis to the centromeric region of chromosome 10, the expected tumor-specific loss of heterozygosity was not observed for chromosome 10, but instead for chromosome 22 (Takai et al, 1987). Germ line mutations were identified in the proto-oncogene *ret*, specifically in the extracellular membrane cysteine-rich region in patients with multiple endocrine neoplasia type 2A and familial medullary thyroid carcinoma (Mulligan et al, 1993), and in the intracellular tyrosine kinase region (Hofstra et al, 1994) in patients with the distinct MEN2B phenotype. Sporadic medullary thyroid carcinomas frequently have somatic mutations in the tyrosine kinase region (Santoro et al, 1995). To date neither the normal nor mutant function of the *ret* gene have been clarified; however, the protein is a member of the receptor tyrosine kinase family, spans the cell membrane, and presumably is involved in signal transduction. Mutations appear to lead to a constitutively active tyrosine kinase (Santoro et al, 1995). Hereditary and sporadic medullary thyroid carcinomas are heterozygous for *ret* mutations and express both the normal and mutant alleles.

The tumor specificity of the MEN2 syndromes, and the unique association with a dominant acting transforming gene *ret*, might suggest a pathway to malignancy different from that of tumor suppressor gene mutations. Curiously, however, in mice heterozygous for germ line inactivation at the Rb1 and p53 loci, the most common tumors seen were of endocrine origin and included medullary thyroid carcinoma, a tumor not observed in mice deficient either in Rb1 or p53 singly. Most tumors showed loss of heterozygosity for both Rb1 and p53, typical of tumor suppressor genes (Harvey et al, 1995a). Such unexpected observations demonstrate the commonality of the tumor suppressor gene p53 and Rb1 pathways in tumor development.

GENE-ENVIRONMENT INTERACTION

Although Mendelian disorders that confer increased risk of cancer have been described, these account for only a small proportion of cancers on a population basis. However, logical arguments suggest that potentially 80% of common cancers can be attributed to gene-environment interactions (Taylor, 1990). Results from animal and pharmacogenetic studies demonstrate dramatic variation among individuals in their ability to metabolize endogenous and exogenous carcinogens. In addition, some variation in cancer risk may be attributed to variation in the susceptibility of particular DNA sequences to damage and variability in control of transcription of DNA repair and tumor suppressor loci following exposure to DNA-damaging agents. Mechanisms that confer increased cancer risk through gene-environment interactions have been established for several common cancer sites including skin, lung, bladder, and colon cancers. The constituents of tobacco smoke are among the best characterized chemical carcinogens, and examples of gene-environment interaction are drawn from studies of these relatively well characterized systems. We first provide as an example a description of gene-environment interactions in the etiology of skin cancers. We then discuss variation in cancer risk for several common cancer sites with emphasis on lung cancer and its relationship to various metabolic phenotypes.

Gene-Environment Interaction in the Etiology of Skin Cancers

Exposure to ultraviolet B light is generally necessary for the development of basal and squamous skin cancers, the most common of all cancers, but the genetic background of individuals exposed to sunlight determines their risk. It has been recognized since the late nineteenth century that individuals of fair complexion are at much greater risk from this exposure than those having darker skin (Fitzpatrick et al, 1987). The genetic basis of skin type and color has not been well characterized but it is multigenic in origin. Some rare syndromes also confer greatly increased risk of skin cancer following sun exposure. Oculocutaneous albinism results from mutations in any of a number of genes that regulate melanin production (Witkop et al, 1989). Compared with noncarriers, individuals with these single gene defects have an increased risk of skin cancers because more UV radiation reaches the basal epithelium.

Xeroderma pigmentosum (XP) results from a lack of excision-repair mechanisms. In XP, the pyrimidine dimers that result from UV-B radiation (Cleaver and Kraemer, 1989) cannot be repaired, and the accumulation of DNA damage increases the risk of cancer. Three different genetic conditions (fair skin, occulocutaneous albinism, XP) confer increased risk of skin cancer by generally modulating the extent of permanent DNA damage to the basal epithelium.

In contrast, several syndromes have been described that confer increased risk for only a single histologic type of skin cancer. Generally, for these conditions, sun exposure plays an important but perhaps less critical role in tumorigenesis. Nevoid basal cell carcinoma (NBCC) syndrome is a single gene disorder recently localized to chromosome 9q (Gailani et al, 1992) that confers greatly increased risk of basal cell cancers, along with various developmental anomalies and increased risk of medulloblastoma. Loss-of-heterozygosity studies among basal cell carcinomas from NBCC carriers as well as in nonfamilial basal cell cancers suggests a tumor suppressor role for this gene (Gailani et al, 1992; van der Riet et al, 1994). No effect of sun exposure on risk of basal cell cancers was found in a survey (Goldstein et al, 1993a), but the low risk of basal cell cancers among black NBCC carriers suggests that UV-induced DNA damage encourages the progression to skin cancer among NBCC carriers (Goldstein et al, 1994). Ferguson-Smith syndrome has also been localized to the same region of chromsome 9q (Goudie et al, 1993). In contrast to NBCC carriers, individuals with this rare syndrome are at increased risk only for keratoacanthomas and squamous carcinomas (Ferguson-Smith et al, 1971). Finally, genetic loci that predispose for increased melanoma risk have been localized to chromosomes 9p and 1p. Genetic linkage studies from independent groups have confirmed the existence of a melanoma susceptibility locus on 9p (Cannon-Albright et al, 1992), apparently attributable to the locus for p21, a cell cycle protein. (Kamb et al, 1994). In contrast, conclusive evidence for a 1p-linked factor is currently provided by a single research group (Goldstein et al, 1993b; Bale et al, 1989). A reluctance to agree upon standardized definitions for dysplastic nevi and melanoma in situ has hampered comparative studies among research groups (Greene, 1991) . For both chromosomal regions, tumor suppressor activity has been suggested by loss of heterozygosity in nonfamilial melanoma (Ranade et al, 1995; Kamb et al, 1994).

In summary, the majority of skin cancers result from an environmental exposure among individuals who are at risk because of a fair skin type, which usually results from the multigenic effects of many separate loci. However, a few rare single-gene syndromes have been described that confer greatly increased risk of skin cancers, although sun exposure appears to be relevant as well. These syndromes result in (a) extremely fair complexion, (b) poor DNA repair of UV-induced damage, or (c) induction of mutations at a critical putative tumor suppressor locus. Genetic linkage studies have identified chromosomal regions that are critical for development of skin cancers among the rare individuals who inherit a susceptible genotype. However, loss-of-heterozygosity studies among individuals without family history of disease also show that these same loci are likely to be important in the etiology of skin cancers among normative individuals.

Evidence for Genetic Variation in Tobacco-Related Risk of Lung Cancer

Case-Control Studies. Familiality of lung cancer has been studied in case-control studies by comparing the recurrence risk among close (first-degree) relatives in case families with that observed in control families. In a landmark study, Tokuhata and Lillienfeld (1963) demonstrated excess lung cancer mortality among the relatives of lung cancer patients. A primary observation from this study was a synergism between smoking behavior and the occurrence of lung cancer in the relatives of the patients. In men the effect from smoking appeared to be stronger than that which could be attributed to familial factors, but in women the familial effect dominated. Using as referent group the control subjects who did not smoke, the risks associated with smoking and familial factors were a fourfold increase in mortality among case relatives who did not smoke, a fivefold increase in mortality among control relatives who smoked, and a 14-fold increase in mortality among case relatives who smoked. These findings are supported by more recent studies (Ooi et al, 1986; Sellers et al, 1988). Subsequent segregation analyses (Sellers et al, 1990) of the data collected by Ooi and coworkers (1986) were consistent with Mendelian segregation of a single codominant locus segregating in the case families when a model was fitted that allowed for a genetic component that could affect the age of onset of lung cancer.

Biological Processes in Lung Carcinogenesis, and Molecular Epidemiology. A variety of metabolic systems help to protect against chemically induced genotoxic damage and provide hypotheses that can be tested for identifying specific genetic loci that might be critical in lung cancer etiology. Exogenous genotoxic compounds such as polycyclic aromatic hydrocarbons (PAHs) are modified in phase I oxidative processes. The phase I reactions almost exclusively involve P450 cytochromes and often result in metabolites that are more chemically reactive than the parent compounds. These derivative compounds may in turn covalently bind to DNA and form carcinogen-macromolecular adducts. Provided adduct formation does not occur, conjugation, mediated through phase II metabolic processes, eliminates genotoxic compounds. Alternative and competing routes of phase II metabolism may lead to inactivation of carcinogens (eg, PAHs) through the formation of conjugates (glutathiones, glucuronides, and sulphate esthers) that are more hydrophilic and are excreted by the cell. The balance between metabolic activation and metabolic detoxification, as well as efficiency of DNA-repair mechanisms, may define cancer risk for an individual exposed to PAHs, arylamines, or other chemical carcinogens. Thus, individual-specific susceptibility to chemical carcinogenesis results from a delicate balance between the rate of cellular phase I and phase II reactions, with individuals who have rapid phase I and slow phase II metabolism presumably being at the highest risk.

Cytochrome P450s. The P450 cytochromes (CYP) consist of a super-multigene family important in steroidogenesis and detoxification (Nebert, 1991). In this section we describe risk conferred from CYP1A1, CYP1A2, CYP2D6, and CYP3A4, but, as shown in Table 27–7, many other cytochrome P450s are involved in oxidation and detoxification of xenobiotic compounds. In addition, cytochromes involved in steroidogenesis may play some role in regulating individual-specific risk of cancers.

The related genes CYP1A1 and CYP1A2 are contiguously located on chromosome 15q22-qter and catabolize PAHs and arylamines. CYP1A1 is expressed in parenchymal lung, is induced by interaction with an aryl-hydrocarbon (Ah) receptor-ligand complex, and has high affinity for PAHs. In contrast, CYP1A2 is not expressed in lung tissue but is active in liver and, to a small extent, in duodenum and brain; has a higher affinity for arylamines than for PAHs; and is constitutively expressed, though expression is further inducible by the Ah receptor. The Ah receptor is multimeric (Swanson and Bradfield, 1993), being composed of a nuclear receptor translocator protein (Reyes et al, 1992; Johnson et al, 1993), a ligand-binding subunit (Burbach et al, 1992), and heat-shock protein 90 (Wilhelmsson et al, 1990). The receptor-ligand complex is transported to the nucleus, where it binds to promotor regions upstream of the structural CYP1A1 or CYP1A2 genes.

Although animal studies (Nebert et al, 1991a,b)

TABLE 27–7. *Polymorphic Enzymes That Have Been Correlated with Interindividual Variation in Cancer Risk*

Genetic Locus	*Chromosome Location*	*Inheritance Pattern*	*Carcinogenic Exposures*[a]	*Cancer Sites*[b]	*References*
Cytochrome P450s					
CYP1A1	15q22-qter	D	B[a]P, PAHs	Lu	Guengerich et al, 1992 Nebert and Gonzalez, 1987
CYP1A2	15q22-qter	D	Aflatoxins, arylamines, heterocyclic amines	Li	Guengerich et al, 1992 Nebert and Gonzalez, 1987
CYP2A6	19q13.1-13.2	D	Nitrosoamines		Pelkonen and Raunio, 1995
CYP2D6	22q11.2-qter	D	N-nitrosoamines	Lu	Guengerich et al, 1992 Nebert and Gonzalez, 1987
CYP2E1	10	D	Steroids, PAHs, nitrosamines		Guengerich et al, 1992 Nebert and Gonzalez, 1987
CYP3A4	7p	D	Aflatoxins, pyrrolizidine alkaloids, arylamines, heterocyclic amines	Li, Bl, Co	Guengerich et al, 1992 Nebert and Gonzalez, 1987
Glutathione-S-transferases			Electrophiles		
GST-μ	1	R	TSO, BPO	Lu, Bl, Ae	Heckbert et al, 1992 Siedegard et al, 1990 Nazar-Stewart et al, 1993 Lafuente et al, 1993
GST-π	11q12	R	BPDE	Lu	Heckbert et al, 1992
Epoxide hydratase			PAH-epoxides	Lu?, Bl?	Heckbert et al, 1992
UDP-Glucuronosyl transferases			Glucuronidation of phenols, arylamines, steroids, bilirubin	Lu?	Kadlubar et al, 1992 Daly et al, 1993
Sulfotransferase			N-hydryoxylated arylamines	Li?, Bl?	Kadlubar et al, 1992 Daly et al, 1993
N-acetyl transferase-2	8pter-q11	R	Arylamines	Bl, Br?, Co?	Hein, 1988 Blum et al, 1990

[a]B[a]P = benzo[a]pyrene, PAHs = polycyclic aromatic hydrocarbons, TSO = *trans*-stilbene-oxide, BPDE = (+*anti*-benzo[a]pyrene-7,8-diol-9,10-epoxide, BPO = benzo[a]pyrene-4,5-oxide
[b]Li = liver, Lu = lung, Bl = bladder, Co = colorectal, Ae = aerodigestive, Br = breast

clearly implicate CYP1A1 expression in mediating risk from chemical carcinogens found in tobacco smoke (notably benzo[a]pyrene), establishing the importance of this enzyme in mediating lung cancer risk in humans has been difficult. Because CYP1A1 levels are strongly inducible, and lung cancer patients often change their smoking behavior after lung cancer diagnosis, direct measurements of CYP1A1 expression are not very informative in quantifying lung cancer risk. Instead, measurements have often been made in lymphocytes from peripheral blood, which have been activated by exposure to benzo[a]pyrene. Using this approach, early studies by Kellerman and colleagues (1973) and others showed CYP1A1 inducibility was predictive of case-control status, but these studies were not validated by others (Paigen et al, 1977). Recent studies have attempted to quantitate lung cancer risk from CYP1A1 by searching for polymorphic variants in the vicinity of the structural CYP1A1 locus on chromosome 15. An isoleucine to valine mutation in the CYP1A1 locus was associated with increased risk of lung cancer among Japanese (Kawajiri et al, 1990). The frequency of this allele varies among populations and a relation between high CYP1A1 inducibility and the valine change has also been noted in a very small study of Caucasians (Cosma et al, 1993b). A restriction site downstream of the CYP1A1 locus, digested by Msp1, is associated with lung cancer risk among Japanese smokers (Hayashi et al, 1991), but no association is noted in other populations (Kirvonen et al, 1992; Cosma et al, 1993a). The Msp1 site was inherited along with high CYP1A1 levels in a Caucasian family (Petersen et al, 1991). The variation among populations at risk from having the Msp1 site and coinheritance of the alleles with CYP1A1 levels suggests that the restriction site does not directly affect lung cancer risk, but that other nearby allelic variants, such as the isoleucine to valine mutation, in the structural gene may affect CYP1A1 expression.

The cytochrome CYP2D6 is important in the metabolism of a variety of drugs including neuroleptics, beta blockers, antidepressants, dextromethorphan, and notably debrisoquine, an antihypertensive agent. Although a major role in catabolism of genotoxic substances has not been established, CYP2D6 has been noted to activate 4-(methylnitrosoamino)-1-(3-pyridyl)-1-butanone, a nitroso ketone in tobacco smoke. Unlike CYP1A1, CYP2D6 is not inducible, but individuals vary greatly in their metabolic capacity, which is usually expressed as the metabolic ratio of debrisoquine metabolites to debrisoquine in urine. The poor metabolizer phenotype occurs in 5% to 10% of the population, and occurs among individuals who have two mutant alleles, neither of which expresses functional copies of CYP2D6. Heterozygotes for mutant alleles are intermediate metabolizers and these cannot be well separated from homozygous wild-type individuals on the basis of debrisoquine phenotype. A summary analysis of seven independent studies provided an aggregate odds ratio estimate of 2.3 comparing lung cancer risk among extensive or intermediate metabolizer versus risk among poor metabolizers (Amos et al, 1992). Phenotyping is awkward, requiring a loading with a drug such as dextromethorphan or debrisoquine, followed by a standardized protocol for urine collection and the subsequent assay through relatively expensive HPLC. Attention has therefore focused on trying to develop inexpensive DNA-based assays for CYP2D6 allelic variants that do not express a functional CYP2D6 enzyme. Currently, about 95% of CYP2D6 variants can be detected by DNA analyses.

Mixed function oxidase, CYP3A4, plays a major role in the catabolism of a variety of drugs, dietary procarcinogens such as aflatoxin B_1 and senecionine, and arylamines. CYP3A4 activity varies among individuals (Kirby et al, 1993). CYP3A4 is expressed at a high level in human liver and plays a major role in the catabolism of aflatoxin B_1. Aflatoxin B^1 can be oxidized to its 8,9-oxide by the action of CYP3A4, which subsequently forms DNA adducts at the N7 positive guanine residues. Alternatively, glutathione-S-transferases (GSH) can act to eliminate this metabolite. In animals, the Â and μ isoforms of GSH have been shown to participate primarily in this reaction, and high levels of these enzymes may confer protection to rodents from aflatoxin toxicity (Guengerich et al, 1992). Catabolism of aflatoxins is complex, and the cytochrome P450 enzymes CYP1A2, CYP2A3, CYP2B7, CYP3A3, CYP3A4, and CYP3A5 have all been shown to participate (Aoyama et al, 1990).

Glutathione-S-Transferases. The glutathione-S-transferases (GST) comprise five related gene families, of which four are cytosolic (α, μ, π, θ) and one is microsomal (Ketterer et al, 1992). The cytosolic forms assemble as dimers. Generally, expression of GSTs varies by tissue and is also inducible. Affinity for activated carcinogens varies greatly among the classes; with GSTM1 (also denoted GST-μ) has been shown to have high affinity for transtilbene-oxide and activated forms of B[a]P, and GSTP1 (also denoted GST-π) shows high affinity for (+)anti-benzo[a]pyrene-7,8-diol-9,10-oxide of B[a]P, but not for other catabolites. Notably, nearly 50% of Caucasians do not carry a functional copy of the GSTM1 gene, and do not express this enzyme. The enzyme is ordinarily expressed in all tissues, though the level of expression varies by tissue site and by level of induction. As shown in Table 27–7, studies of numerous cancer sites have indicated that individuals who are exposed to chemical carcinogens and who lack a functional GSTM1 gene are at increased risk for cancers. In addition, among smokers, the formation of DNA adducts is higher among GSTM1-null individuals than among those carrying a functional copy of this gene (Shields et al, 1993).

N-Acetyl Transferases. N-Acetylation detoxifies a wide range of drugs including isoniazid, sulfamethazine, hydralazine, and caffeine and other xenobiotics that have aromatic amine or hydrazine groups such as benzidine and -naphthylamine (Hein, 1988). The N-acetyl transferase 2 (NAT2) locus catabolizes each of these compounds. Common allelic variants of this gene have been characterized and have been demonstrated to be responsible for slow metabolic rates for these compounds (Vatsis et al, 1991). The slow, intermediate, and fast phenotypes can be distinguished on the basis of drug metabolism determinations, but clinically relevant slow metabolism of drugs such as isoniazid is inherited as a recessive condition, and most studies combine intermediate and fast acetylators. Metabolites of caffeine generated by N-acetylation can be simply identified in urine, providing an easy means for phenotyping individuals at the NAT2 locus (Butler et al, 1986).

Many of the activated xenobiotic substrates for NAT2 are carcinogenic, and in particular 4-aminobiphenyl and β-naphthylamine are tumorigenic to the bladder. As a result, many studies have evaluated the association between NAT2 phenotype and bladder cancer. Summary analyses (Hein, 1988) from case-control studies provide a significant association between bladder cancer and slow acetylator phenotype, with a pooled odds ratio of 1.24.Although arylamines are a constituent of cigarette smoke, slow acetylators who smoked were not at higher risk for bladder cancer than nonsmoking slow acetylators (Evans et al, 1983a). Among studies in which the patients had documented occupational exposure to arylamines the odds ratio for bladder cancer associated with being a slow acetylator was greater (Cartwright et al, 1982), with an aggregate odds ratio over five studies of 2.24 (Hein, 1988). Associations between NAT2 phenotype and other cancer sites have been more complex (Hein, 1988).

Harvey-Ras Polymorphisms. Many case-control studies (Devlin et al, 1993) have documented an association between rare alleles of microsatellite polymorphism about 1000 base pairs downstream of the Harvey-ras proto-oncogene. The aggregate odds ratio across studies for carrying a single rare allele was 1.85; for carrying two rare alleles the odds ratio was 4.62, but because of the rarity of homozygous carriers of rare alleles these odds ratios are not significantly different. Some variation in the strength of association is noted across sites; bladder and colorectal cancer are most strongly associated, followed by leukemia, breast, and lung. A possible confounder in any molecular epidemiological studies is population stratification. However, carefully conducted population genetic studies (Devlin et al, 1993) document relatively little variation among Caucasian populations in the frequency of rare mutations. Thus the observed associations between rare Harvey-ras alleles and risk of cancer cannot be attributed to unobserved population stratification. No mechanism for the association between rare variants of Harvey-ras and cancer risk has been documented, although microsatellite regions in the proximity of other loci have been shown to affect transcription (Takeda et al, 1989).

In a case-control study, rare alleles of a variable number of tandem repeats (VNTR) polymorphism located 5′ to the Harvey-ras oncogene were significantly ($P<0.05$) more common among black lung cancer patients than among black controls (Sugimura et al, 1990). Among whites, the frequencies of all rare alleles were similarly higher among lung cancer patients than among controls, but no significant differences were observed.

GENETIC HETEROGENEITY: BREAST CANCER AS THE PARADIGM

Familial studies of breast cancer have an ancient tradition, with literature extending back into the Roman era. Attempts to characterize the familial occurrence of breast cancer have identified several distinct familial forms of breast and other cancers. Segregation analyses of families selected through breast cancer–affected women showed evidence for a rare autosomal dominant factor with a lifetime penetrance of about 80% (Go et al, 1983; Newman et al, 1988; Claus et al, 1991). Segregation analyses and population-based family studies suggest that about 5% to 10% of early-onset breast cancer can be attributed to this dominant factor (Claus et al, 1991; Newman et al, 1988), and also document coaggregation of breast and ovarian cancers in some families (Go et al, 1983). Clinical observation also led to the definition of the much rarer Li-Fraumeni or SBLA syndrome, which is the coaggregation of sarcoma, brain, breast, lymphoma, leukemia, lung, and adrenocortical tumors (Li et al, 1988). Clinical observation also has suggested that breast cancer is more common among families that include several colon cancer or endometrial cancer affected individuals, and this syndrome has been called Lynch syndrome II, or more recently hereditary nonpolyposis colon cancer (Lynch et al, 1988). The coaggregation of breast cancer with colon cancer and endometrial cancers has remained controversial, and coaggregation of breast with endometrial cancers was not supported by population studies (Schildkraut et al, 1989).

These results led several groups to search for a genetic

etiology for breast cancer. After an exhaustive search of the genome, a group led by Mary-Claire King (Hall et al, 1990) finally identified, through genetic linkage studies, a major locus, BRCA1, for breast cancer at 17q21-22 that is particularly important in the etiology of early-onset breast cancer. This observation was quickly confirmed by a group led by Gilbert Lenoir and Steve Narod (Narod et al, 1991) using extended families collected by Henry Lynch and colleagues on the basis of breast and ovarian cancers. Because of the high prevalence of breast cancer, results from a single group were insufficient to refine the location of the BRCA1 and a consortium was formed (Easton et al, 1993). Results from the consortium's study led to a refined localization of BRCA1 on chromosome 17, and the observation that only about 40% of families that included multiple breast cancer cases could be linked to BRCA1, whereas nearly 100% of breast-ovarian cancer families could be linked to BRCA1.

In 1994, the BRCA1 locus was identified by a consortium of investigators headed by Mark Skolnick (Miki et al, 1994). More than 100 kilobases of DNA and 22 coding exons constitute BRCA1, whose 1,823–amino acid protein product is projected to contain a zinc finger motif potentiating DNA-binding capabilities and transcriptional influences. Risk estimates from evaluation of BRCA1 mutations in relatives of breast cancer probands show 80% risk for breast cancer to age 75, 60% risk for ovarian cancer, and possibly a threefold increased risk of prostate cancer and fourfold risk of colon cancer (Ford et al, 1994). The gene frequency of BRCA1 has been estimated to be six per 10,000 alleles (ie, 12 per 10,000 women are carriers) and mutations account for about 5% of breast cancer cases in women under 40 years of age, 2% in women between 40 and 49, and 1% in women between 50 and 70 (Ford et al, 1995). Several groups have published initial efforts to identify BRCA1 mutations relative to familial disease characteristics including numbers of breast and ovarian cancers and average ages of onset (Futreal et al, 1994; Friedman et al, 1994; Simard et al, 1994; Castilla et al, 1994; Friedman et al, 1995). A deletion of an AG dinucleotide pair at position 185 has been noted to occur in 0.9% of Ashkenazi Jews screened for other conditions (Struewing et al, 1995) and appears to represent a founder effect for this allele (Friedman et al, 1995) based upon haplo-identity among supposedly unrelated families for closely linked markers in the region. Expression of the BRCA1 gene has been shown to be indirectly regulated by estrogen levels (Gudas et al, 1995), and cytoplasmic localization of BRCA1 may be associated with the invasive phenotype in sporadic breast cancers (Chen et al, 1995).

A second susceptibility gene (Wooster et al, 1994), BRCA2 on chromosome 13q12-13, was identified through genetic linkage analysis of the families that did not segregate BRCA1. BRCA2 confers a 90% lifetime risk of breast cancer in women and an elevated, but not currently quantified risk in male breast cancer. It is likely to account for approximately 40% to 70% of the site-specific breast cancer families not linked to BRCA1. Discovery of additional families with high incidence of early-onset breast cancers that show no linkage to either BRCA1 or BRCA2 implies the existence of one or possibly more additional susceptibility genes (Friedman et al, 1995). Families that have been studied to date are strongly selected to contain many affected individuals and often selected for early onset. It is, therefore, difficult to generalize findings from this highly selected set of patients to the more general population of familial cases who report only a single first-degree relative, and who typically present during the postmenopausal period.

In addition to these loci identified through breast cancer probands, study of Li-Fraumeni families identified p53 as a causative agent (Malkin et al, 1990) in the majority of cases. For women younger than 45 years of age, a 17.9-fold increased risk of breast cancer was observed among women who were unaffected at the time of family ascertainment but who were inferred to be carriers of Li-Fraumeni syndrome and followed up for a median of 14.1 years (Garber et al, 1991). However, case-series of familial and nonfamilial breast cancer patients showed that p53 mutations are rare in this group (Børresen et al, 1992). Although p53 mutations are rare in the population, carriers of p53 mutations are at considerable breast cancer risk. Chemopreventive agents have been shown to protect p53 knockout mice from the development of cancers (Hursting et al, 1995), and carriers of p53 mutations may be a particularly appropriate group of women for chemopreventive clinical trials. Mutations in the DNA repair genes hMLH1, hMSH2, PMS1, and PMS2 have been identified among individuals from HNPCC families, with the microsatellite instability phenotype in the tumors. The significance of mutations in these loci in determining breast cancer risk has not been determined. Finally, heterozygotes for mutations in the ataxia-telangiectasia gene(s) may be at increased risk for breast cancer (Swift et al, 1991).

With the identification of several genetic loci that play a critical role in determining inherited risk of breast cancer, the elucidation of the interplay of genetic and environmental factors that cause breast cancer can be greatly refined. For instance, although gravidity and early first full-term pregnancy are protective factors for breast cancer in the general population, women carrying BRCA1 may not be afforded protection by pregnancy-related outcomes. Currently, a single publication has addressed the relationship between usual epidemiological risk factors and risk of breast cancer among women identified as having BRCA1 mutations (Goldgar et al, 1994a). Mean parity among unaffected gene carriers was less than among affected carriers, and the age at menarche for unaffected carriers was less than that of affected carriers. However, this study was much too small to draw definitive conclusions regarding the possible role of lifestyle-related factors in mediating breast cancer risk among BRCA1 carriers. Comparisons of disease parameters between carriers of mutated susceptibility genes and appropriately biomatched control populations will provide valuable information regarding interactions of genetics and the environment in the etiology of these cancers.

SUMMARY

We have described a variety of cancer susceptibility genes, syndromes, and mechanisms of tumor susceptibility. Undoubtedly many others await definition. To date the most common theme among the different cancer susceptibility genes may be the disruption of genomic stability. Maintenance of the integrity of the genome seems essential to normal cell function; disruption of this normally well regulated process can lead to cell death or neoplasia. Cell cycle regulation is intimately tied to DNA replication and repair to permit orderly cell division. It was initially suggested by Boveri (1929) that cancer might arise following aberrant cell division. The notion that genetic susceptibility to cancer was related to genomic instability was initially supported primarily by the rare autosomal recessive disorders associated with in vivo and in vitro chromosomal instability and increased cancer risk. The notion that the autosomal dominant cancer susceptibility genes, including tumor suppressor genes, might be involved in maintaining the integrity of the genome has only recently evolved, in part as the relationship of cell cycle genes to DNA repair and replication was recognized. The identification of the role of DNA mismatch repair genes, initially characterized in bacteria and yeast, in hereditary nonpolyposis colon cancer, and the growing list of tumors showing that mismatch repair phenotype, further demonstrate that errors in DNA repair are involved in susceptibility to common cancers in individuals without associated stigmatizing anomalies. The relationship of cancer susceptibility to DNA repair was further strengthened by the demonstration of genomic instability associated with mutations in p53, and the concept of p53 as the "guardian of the genome" (Lane, 1992; Yin et al, 1992; Livingstone et al, 1992). Recent data even suggest that p53 may be directly involved in recognition of, and binding to, insertion/deletion lesions in DNA, with recruitment of repair proteins to the site (Lee et al, 1995).

Many familial cancers demonstrate an earlier-than-average age of onset and in some cases a high frequency of multiple primary tumors. In some instances the specific genes involved have been localized or cloned, and the tumors examined for loss of heterozygosity. In many cases, as shown in Tables 27–2 and 27–3, the mechanism of tumor development seems to involve loss of function, although the MEN2 syndromes are a notable exception. While tumor-specific loss of function may suggest a tumor suppressor gene, recent findings in the HNPCC syndromes demonstrate an alternative mechanism of cancer susceptibility that permits the accumulation of mutations, including tumor suppressor genes (Markowitz et al, 1995). As described above, occasionally tumor suppressor gene mutations confer gain of function properties to the mutant protein, so that mutation at the homologous locus is not necessary to inactive the protein. At present, the phenotype of the autosomal dominant cancer susceptibility syndromes in terms of site specificity, occurrence of precursor lesions, age of onset, and distribution in the family provide little ability to discriminate among possible mechanisms of tumor predisposition.

The identification of the cancer susceptibility genes described above has provided major new biological insights into the regulation of cell growth and maintenance of orderly cell division that should eventually provide new approaches to cancer detection and prevention. For the immediate future the ability to identify genetically susceptible individuals creates not only opportunity for detection and prevention research, but obligation to use the power to detect genetic susceptibility wisely and ethically. The legal and ethical issues arising with the opportunities for genetic testing suggest the need for new partnerships in research in genetic susceptibility and its implications.

REFERENCES

AALTONEN LA, SANKILA R, MECKLIN J-P, JÄRVINEN H, PUKKALA E, PELTOMÄKI P, DE LA CHAPELLE A. 1994. A novel approach to estimate the proportion of hereditary nonpolyposis colorectal cancer of total colorectal cancer burden. Cancer Detect Prev 18:57–63.

AALTONEN LA, PELTOMÄKI P, LEACH FS, SISTONEN P, PYLKKÄNEN L, MECKLIN JP, JÄRVINEN H, POWELL SM, JEN J, HAMILTON SR, PETERSEN GM, KINZLER KW, VOGELSTEIN B, DE LA CHAPELLE A. 1993. Clues to the pathogenesis of familial colorectal cancer. Science 260 812–816.

AHN J, LUDECKE HJ, LINDOW S, HORTON WA, LEE B, WAGNER MJ, HORSTHEMKE B, WELLS DE. 1995. Cloning of the putative tumour suppressor gene for hereditary multiple exostoses (EXT1). Nature Genet 11:137–143.

ALTER BP. 1993. Fanconi's anaemia and its variability. Br J Haematol 85:9–14.

AMOS CI, CAPORASO NE, WESTON A. 1992. Host factors in lung cancer risk: A review of interdisciplinary studies. Cancer Epidemiol Biomarkers Prev 1:505–513.

AMOS CI, RUBIN LA. 1995. Major gene analysis for disease and disorders of complex etiology. Exp Clin Immunogenet 12:141–155.

ARAP W, NISHIKAWA R, FURNARI FB, CAVENEE WK, HUANG HJS. 1995. Replacement of the p16/CDKN2 gene suppresses human glioma cell growth1. Cancer Res 55:1351–1354, 1995.

ATLAS SA, VESELL ES, NEBERT DW. 1976. Genetic control of interindividual variations in the inducibility of aryl hydrocarbon hydroxylase in cultured human lymphocytes. Cancer Res 36:4619–4630, 1976.

AOYAMA T, YAMANO S, GUZELIAN PS, GELBOIN HU, GONZALEZ FJ. 1990. Five of 12 forms of vaccinia virus-expressed human hepatic cytochrome P450s metabollically activate aflatoxin B. Proc Natl Acad Sci USA 87:4790–4793.

BALABAN G, GILBERT F, NICHOLS W, MEADOWS AT, SHIELDS J. 1982. Abnormalities of chromosome #13 in retinoblastoma from individuals with normal constitutional karyotypes. Cancer Genet Cytogenet 6:213–221.

BALE SJ, DRACOPOLI NC, TUCKER MA, CLARK WH JR, FRASER MC, STANGER BZ, GREEN P, DONIS-KELLER H, HOUSMAN DE, GREEN MH. 1989. Mapping the gene for hereditary cutaneous malignant melanoma-dysplastic nevus to chromosome 1p. N Engl J Med 320:l367–1372.

BIRCH JM, HARTLEY AL, TRICKER KJ, PROSSER J, CONDIE A, KELSEY AM, HARRIS M, JONES PHM, BINCHY A, CROWTHER D, CRAFT AW, EDEN OB, EVANS GR, THOMPSON E, MANN JR, MARTIN J, MITCHELL ELD, SANTIBÁÑEZ-KOREF MF. 1994. Prevalence and diversity of constitutional mutations in the *p53* gene among 21 Li-Fraumeni families. Cancer Res 54:1298–1304.

BISCHOFF FZ, STRONG, LC, YIM SO, PRATT DR, SICILIANO MJ, GIOVANELLA BC, TAINSKY MA. 1991. Tumorigenic transformation of spontaneously immortalized fibroblasts from patients with a familial cancer syndrome. Oncogene 6:183–186.

BISCHOFF FZ, YIM SO, PATHAK S, GRANT G, SICILIANO MJ, GIOVANELLA BC, STRONG LC, TAINSKY MA. 1990. Spontaneous abnormalities in normal fibroblasts from patients with Li-Fraumeni cancer syndrome: Aneuploidy and immortalization. Cancer Res 50:7979–7984.

BLUM M, GRANT DM, MCBRIDE W, HEIM M, MEYER UA. 1990. Human arylamine N-acetyltransferase genes: isolation, chromosomal localization, and functional expression. DNA Cell Biol 9:193–203.

BODMER WF, BAILEY CJ, BODMER J, BUSSEY HJR, ELLIS A, GORMAN P, LUCIBELLO FC, MURDAY VA, RIDER SH, SCAMBLER P, SHEER D, SOLOMON E, SPURR NK. 1987. Localization of the gene for familial adenomatous polyposis on chromosome 5. Nature 328:614–616.

BONNEY GE. 1986. Regressive logistic models for familial disease and other binary traits. Biometrics 42:611–625.

BØRRESEN A-L, ANDERSEN TI, GARBER J, BARBIER-PIRAUX N, THORLACIUS S, EYFJÖRD J, OTTESTAD L, SMITH-SØRENSEN B, HOVIG E, MALKIN D, FRIEND SH. 1992. Screening for germ line TP53 mutations in breast cancer patients. Cancer Res 52:3234–3236.

BOVERI T. 1929. The Origin of Malignant Tumors. Baltimore; Williams & Wilkins, 119 pp.

BRONNER CE, BAKER SM, MORRISON PT, WARREN G, SMITH LG, LESCOE MK, KANE M, EARABINO C, LIPFORD J, LINDBLOM A, TANNERGÅRD P, BOLLAG RJ, GODWIN AR, WARD DC, NORDENSKJØLD M, FISHEL R, KOLODNER R, LISKAY RM. 1994. Mutation in the DNA mismatch repair gene homologue *hMLH 1* is associated with hereditary non-polyposis colon cancer. Nature 368:258–261.

BURBACH KM, POLAND A, BRADFIELD CA. 1992. Cloning of the Ah-receptor cDNA reveals a distinctive ligand-activated transcription factor. Proc Natl Acad Sci USA 9:8185–8189.

BUTLER MA, IWASAKI M, GUENGERICH P, KADLUBAR FF. 1986. Human cytochrome P-450 PA (P450IA2), the phenacetin-deethylase, is primarily responsible for the hepatic 3-demethylation of caffeine and the N-oxidation of carcinogenic arylamines. Proc Natl Acad Sci USA 86:7696–7700.

CANCE WG, BRENNAN MF, DUDAS ME, HUANG C-M, CORDON-CARDO C. 1990. Altered expression of the retinoblastoma gene product in human sarcomas. N Engl J Med 323:1457–1462.

CANNINGS C, THOMPSON EA. 1977. Ascertainment in the sequential sampling of pedigrees. Clin Gen 12:208–212.

CANNON-ALBRIGHT LA, GOLDGAR DE, MEYER LJ, LEWIS CM, ANDERSON DE, FOUNTAIN JW, HEGI ME, WISEMAN RW, PETTY EM, BALE AE, OLOPADE OI, DIAZ MO, KWIATKOWSKI DJ, PIEPKORN MW, ZONE JJ, SKOLNICK MH. 1992. Assignment of a locus for familial melanoma, MLM, to chromosome 9p13-p22. Science 258:1148–1152.

CARTWRIGHT RA, GLASHAN RW, ROGERS HJ, AHMAD RA, HALL DB, HIGGNS E, KAHN MA. 1982. Role of N-acetyltransferase phenotypes in bladder carcinogenesis: a pharmacogenetic epidemiological approach to bladder cancer. Lancet 2: 842–846.

CASTILLA LH, COUCH FJ, ERDOS MR, HOSKINS KF, CALZONE K, GARBER JE, BOYD J, LUBIN MB, DESHANO ML, BRODY LC, COLLINS FS, WEBER B. 1994. Mutations in the BRCA1 gene in families with early-onset breast and ovarian cancer. Nature Genet 8:387–391.

CAVENEE WK, DRYJA TP, PHILLIPS RA, BENEDICT WF, GODBOUT R, GALLIE BL, MURPHREE AL, STRONG LC, WHITE RL. 1983. Expression of recessive alleles by chromosomal mechanisms in retinoblastoma. Nature 305:779–784.

CAVENEE WK, HANSEN MF, NORDENSKJOLD M, KOCK E, MAUMENEE I, SQUIRE JA, PHILLIPS RA, GALLIE BL. 1985. Genetic origin of mutations predisposing to retinoblastoma. Science 228: 501–503.

CHAKRABORTY R, WEISS K. 1988. Admixture as a tool for finding linked genes and detecting that difference from allelic association between loci. Proc Natl Acad Sci USA 85:9119–9123.

CHEN Y, CHEN C-F, RILEY DJ, ET AL. 1995. Aberrant subcellular localization of BRCA1 in breast cancer. Science 270:789–791.

CLAUS EB, RISCH N, THOMPSON WD. 1991. Genetic analysis of breast cancer in the Cancer and Steroid Hormone Study. Am J Hum Genet 48: 232–241.

CLAUSEN N, ANDERSSON P, TOMMERUP N. 1989. Familial occurrence of neuroblastoma, von Recklinghausen's neurofibromatosis, Hirschsprung's agangliosis and jaw-winking syndrome. ACTA Paediatr Scand 78:736–741.

CLEAVER JE, KRAEMER KH. 1989. Xeroderma pigmentosum. In: *The Metabolic Basis of Inherited Disease, 6th ed*, CL Scriver, AL Beaudet, WS Sly, D Valle (eds). McGraw Hill, pp 2905–2948.

CLERGET-DARPOUX FM, BONAÏTI-PELLIÉ C, HOCHEZ J. 1986. Effects of misspecifying genetic parameters in lod score analysis. Biometrics 42:393–399.

COLLINS N, MCMANUS R, WOOSTER R, ET AL. 1995. Consistent loss of wild type allele in breast cancers from a family linked to the BRCA2 gene on chromosome 13q12-13. Oncogene 10:1673–1675.

CORTESSIS V, INGLES S, MILLIKAN R, DIEP A, GATTI RA, RICHARDSON L, THOMPSON WD, PAGANINI-HILL A, SPARKES RS, HAILE RW. 1993. Linkage analysis of *DRD2*, a marker linked to the ataxia-telangiectasia gene, in 64 families with premenopausal bilateral breast cancer. Cancer Res 53:5083–5086, 1993.

COSMA GN, CROFTS F, CURRIE D, WIRGIN I, TONIOLO P, GARTE SJ. 1993a. Racial differences in restriction fragment length polymorphisms and mRNA inducibility of the human CYP1A1 gene. Cancer Epidemiol Biomarkers Prev 2:53–57.

COSMA G, CROFTS F, TAIOLI E, TONIOLO P, GARTE S. 1993b. Relationship between genotype and function of the human CYP1A1 gene. J Toxicol Environ Health 40:309–316.

CRYNS VL, THOR A, XU H-J, HU S-X, WIERMAN ME, VICKERY AL, BENEDICT WF, ARNOLD A. 1994. Loss of the retinoblastoma tumor-suppressor gene in parathyroid carcinoma. N Engl J Med 330:757–761.

DALY AK, CHOLERTON S, GREGORY W, IDLE JR. 1993. Metabolic polymorphisms. Pharmacol Ther 57:129–160.

DECOSSE JJ, MILLER HH, LESSER ML. 1989. Effect of wheat fiber and vitamins C and E on rectal polyps in patients with familial adenomatous polyposis. J Natl Cancer Inst 81:1290–1297.

DEMENAIS FM. 1991. Regressive logistic models for familial diseases: a formulation assuming an underlying liability model. Am J Hum Genet 49:773–785.

DEMENAIS FM, MARTINEZ MM, LAING AE. 1992. Regressive logistic models in linkage analysis of the cutaneous malignant melanoma-dysplastic nevus syndrome. Cytogenet Cell Genet 59:191–193.

DEMENAIS FM, MURIGANDE C, BONNEY GE. 1990. Search for faster methods of fitting the regressive models to quantitative traits. Genet Epidemiol 7:319–334.

DEVLIN B, KRONTIRIS T, RISCH N. 1993. Population genetics of the HRAS1 minisatellite locus. Am J Hum Genet 53:1298–1305.

DIETRICH WF, LANDER ES, SMITH JS, MOSER AR, GOULD KA, LUONGO C, BORENSTEIN N, DOVE W. 1993. Genetic identification of mom-1, a major modifier locus affecting min-induced intestinal neoplasia in the mouse. Cell 75:631–639.

DILLER L, KASSEL J, NELSON CE, GRYKA MA, LITWAK G, GEBHARDT M, BRESSAC B, OZTURK M, BAKER SJ, VOGELSTEIN B, FRIEND SH. 1990. p53 functions as a cell cycle control protein in osteosarcomas. Mol Cell Biol 10:5772–5781.

DILLER L, SEXSMITH E, GOTTLIEB A, LI FP, MALKIN D. 1995. Germline p53 mutations are frequently detected in young children with rhabdomyosarcoma. J Clin Invest 95:1606–1611.

DONEHOWER LA, HARVEY M, SLAGLE BL, MCARTHUR MJ, MONTGOMERY CA JR, BUTEL JS, BRADLEY A. 1992. Mice deficient for p53 are developmentally normal but susceptible to spontaneous tumours. Nature 356:215–221.

DRUMMOND JT, LI GM, LONGLEY MJ, MODRICH P. 1995. Isolation of an hMSH2-p160 heterodimer that restores DNA mismatch repair to tumor cells. Science 268:1909–1912.

DUAN DR, PAUSE A, BURGESS WH, ET AL. 1995. Inhibition of transcription elongation by the VHL tumor suppressor protein. Science 269:1402–1406.

EASTON DF, BISHOP DT, FORD D, CROCKFORD GP, AND BREAST CANCER LINKAGE CONSORTIUM. 1993. Genetic linkage analysis in familial breast and ovarian cancer: results from 214 families. Am J Hum Genet 52:678–701.

EASTON D, PETO J. 1990. The contribution of inherited predisposition to cancer incidence. Cancer Surv 9:395–416.

EASTON DF, PONDER MA, CUMMINGS T, GAGEL RF, HANSEN HH, REICHLIN S, TASHJIAN AH JR, TELENIUS-BERG M, PONDER BAJ, AND THE CANCER RESEARCH CAMPAIGN MEDULLARY THYROID GROUP. 1989. The clinical and screening age-at-onset distribution for the MEN-2 syndrome. Am J Hum Genet 44:208–215.

ELLIS NA, GRODEN J, YE TZ, STRAUGHEN J, LENNON DJ, CIOCCI S, PROYTCHEVA M, GERMAN J. 1995. The Bloom's syndrome gene product is homologous to RecQ helicases. Cell 83:655–666.

ELSTON RC, SOBEL E. 1979. Sampling considerations in the analysis of human pedigree data. Am J Hum Genet 31:62–69.

ESHLEMAN JR, LANG EZ, BOWERFIND GK, PARSONS R, VOGELSTEIN B, WILLSON JKV, VEIGL ML, SEDWICK WD, MARKOWITZ SD. 1995. Increased mutation rate at the hprt locus accompanies microsatellite instability in colon cancer. Oncogene 10:33–37.

ESHLEMAN JR, MARKOWITZ SD. 1995. Microsatellite instability in inherited and sporadic neoplasms. Oncology 7:83–89.

EVANS DAP, EZE LC, WHIBLEY EJ. 1983a. The association of the slow acetylator phenotype with bladder cancer. J Med Genet 20: 330–333.

EVANS DAP, HARMER D, DOWNHAM DY, WHIBLEY EJ, IDLE JR, RITCHIE J, SMITH RL. 1983b. The genetic control of sparteine and debrisoquine metabolism in man with new methods of analyzing bimodal distributions. J Med Genet 20:321–329.

EWENS WJ, SPIELMAN RS, MCGINNIS RE. 1995. Transmission test for linkage disequilibrium: the insulin gene region and insulin-dependent diabetes mellitus (IDDM). Am J Human Genet 52:506–516.

FALK CT, RUBINSTEIN P. 1987. Haplotype relative risks: An easy reliable way to construct a proper control sample for risk calculations. Ann Hum Genet 51:227–233.

FARNDON PA, DEL MASTRO RG, EVANS DGR, ET AL. 1992. Location of gene for Gorlin syndrome. Lancet 339:581–582.

FEARON ER, VOGELSTEIN B. 1990. A genetic model for colorectal tumorigenesis. Cell 61:759–767.

FERGUSON-SMITH MA, WALLACE DC, JAMES ZH, RENWICK JH. 1971. Multiple self-healing squamous epithelioma. Birth Defects (8):157–163.

FINLAY CA, HINDS PW, LEVINE AJ. 1989. The p53 proto-oncogene can act as a suppressor of transformation. Cell 57:1083–1093.

FISHEL R, LESCOE MK, RAO MRS, COPELAND NG, JENKINS NA, GARBER J, KANE M, KOLODNER R. 1993. The human mutator gene homolog *MSH2* and its association with hereditary nonpolyposis colon cancer. Cell 75:1027–1038.

FITZPATRICK T, EISEN AA, WOLFF K, FREEDBERG IM, AUSTEN KF. 1987. Dermatology in General Medicine, 3rd ed. New York: McGraw Hill.

FORD D, EASTON DF, BISHOP DT, ET AL. 1994. Risks of cancer in BRCA1-mutation carriers. Lancet 343:692–695.

FORD D, EASTON DF, PETO J. 1995. Estimates of the gene frequency of BRCA1 and its contribution to breast and ovarian cancer incidence. Am J Hum Genet 57:1457–1462.

FORREST AW. 1961. Tumors following radiation about the eye. Trans Am Acad Ophthal Otolaryn 65:694–717.

FRIEDMAN LS, OSTERMEYER EA, SZABO CI, DOWD P, LYNCH ED, ROWELL SE, KING MC. 1994. Confirmation of BRCA1 by analysis of germline mutations linked to breast and ovarian cancer in ten families. Nat Genet 8:399–404.

FRIEDMAN LS, SZABO CI, OSTERMEYER EA, DOWD P, BUTLER L, PARK T, LEE MK, GOODE EL, ROWELL SE, KING MC. 1995. Novel inherited mutations and variable expressivity of BRCA1 alleles, including the founder mutation 185delAG in Ashkenazi Jewish families. Am J Hum Genet 57: 1284–1297.

FRIEND SH, BERNARDS R, ROGELJ S, WEINBERG RA, RAPAPORT JM, ALBERT DM, DRYJA TP. 1986. A human DNA segment with properties of the gene that predisposes to retinoblastoma and osteosarcoma. Nature 323:643–646.

FRYER AE, CHALMERS A, CONNOR JM, ET AL. 1987. Evidence that the gene for tuberous sclerosis is on chromosome 9. Lancet 1:659–661.

FUTREAL PA, LIU Q, SHATTUCK-EIDENS D, COCHRAN C, HARSHMAN K, TAVTIGIAN S, BENNETT LM, HAUGEN-STRANO A, SWENSEN J, MIKI Y, EDDINGTON K, MCCLURE M, FRYE C, WEAVER-FELDHAUS J, DING W, GHOLAMI Z, SODERKVIST P, TERRY L, JHANWAR S, BERCHUCK A, IGLEHART JD, MARKS J, BALLINGER DG, BARRET JC, SKOLNICK MH, KAMB A, WISEMAN R. 1994. BRCA1 mutations in primary breast and ovarian carcinomas. Science 266:120–122.

GAILANI MR, BALE SJ, LEFFELL DJ, DIGIOVANNA JJ, PECK GL, POLIAK S, DRUM MA, PASTAKIA B, MCBRIDE OW, KASE R, GREENE M, MULVIHILL JJ, BALE AE. 1992. Developmental defects in Gorlin syndrome related to a putative tumor suppressor gene on chromosome 9. Cell 69:111–117.

GARBER JE, BURKE EM, LAVALLY BL, BILLETT AL, SALLAN SE, SCOTT RM, KUPSKY W, LI FP. 1990. Choroid plexus tumors in the breast cancer-sarcoma syndrome. Cancer 66:2658–2660.

GARBER JE, GOLDSTEIN AM, KANTOR AF, DREYFUS MG, FRAUMENI JF JR, LI FP. 1991. Follow-up study of twenty-four families with Li-Fraumeni syndrome. Cancer Res 51:6094–6097.

GARBER JE, LI FP, KINGSTON JE, KRUSH AJ, STRONG LC, FINEGOLD MJ, BERTARIO L, BULOW S, FILIPPONE A JR, GEDDE-DAHL T JR, JARVINEN HJ. 1988. Hepatoblastoma and familial adenomatous polyposis. J Natl Cancer Inst 80:1626–1628.

GARDNER EJ. 1951. A genetic and clinical study of intestinal polyposis, a predisposing factor for carcinoma of the colon and rectum. Am J Hum Genet 3:167–176.

German J. 1993. Bloom syndrome: A Mendelian prototype of somatic mutational disease. Medicine 72:393–406.

Giampietro PF, Adler-Brecher B, Verlander PC, et al. 1993. The need for more accurate and timely diagnosis in Fanconi anemia: A report from the International Fanconi Anemia Registry. Pediatrics 91:1116–1120.

Go RCP, King M-C, Bailey-Wilson J, Elston RC, Lynch H. 1983. Genetic epidemiology of breast cancer and associated cancers in high-risk families. I. Segregation analysis. J Natl Cancer Inst 71:455–461.

Goldgar DE, Fields P, Lewis CM, Tran TD, Cannon-Albright LA, Ward JH, Swensen J, Skolnick MH. 1994a. A large kindred with 17q-linked breast and ovarian cancer: genetic, phenotypic, and genealogical analysis. J Natl Cancer Inst 86:200–209.

Goldgar DE, Easton DF, Cannon-Albright LA, Skolnick MH. 1994b. Systematic population-based assessment of cancer risk in first-degree relatives of cancer probands. J Natl Cancer Inst 86:1600–1608.

Goldstein AM, Bale SJ, Peck GL, DiGiovanna JJ. 1993a. Sun exposure and basal cell carcinomas in the nevoid basal cell carcinoma syndrome. J Am Acad Dermatol 29:34–41.

Goldstein AM, Dracopoli NC, Ho EC, Fraser MC, Kearns KS, Bale SJ, McBride OW, Clark WH Jr, Tucker MA. 1993b. Further evidence for a locus for cutaneous malignant melanoma-dysplastic nevus (CMM/DN) on chromosome 1p, and evidence for genetic heterogeneity. Am J Hum Genet 52:537–550.

Goldstein AM, Fraser MC, Struewing JP, Hussussian CJ, Ranade K, Zametkin DP, Fontaine LS, Organic SM, Dracopoli NC, Clark WH Jr, Tucker MA. 1995. Increased risk of pancreatic cancer in melanoma-prone kindreds with $p16^{INK4}$ mutations. N Engl J Med 333:970–974.

Goldstein AM, Pastakia B, DiGiovanna JJ, Poliak S, Santucci S, Kase R, Bale AE, Bale SJ. 1994. Clinical findings in two African-American families with the nevoid basal cell carcinoma syndrome (NBCC). Am J Med Genet 50:272–281.

Goudie DR, Yuille MAR, Leversha MA, Furlong RA, Carter NP, Lush MJ, Affara NA, Ferguson-Smith MA. 1993. Multiple self-healing squamous epitheliomata (ESS1) mapped to chromosome 9q22-q31 in families with common ancestry. Nat Genet 3:165–169.

Green AJ, Smith M, Yates JRW. 1994. Loss of heterozygosity on chromosome 16p13.3 in hamartomas from tuberous sclerosis patients. Nature Genet 6:193–196.

Greenberg DA. 1993. Linkage analysis of "necessary" disease loci versus "susceptibility" loci. Am J Hum Genet 52:135–143.

Greene MH. 1991. Rashomon and the Procrustean bed: A tale of dysplastic nevi. J Natl Cancer Inst 83:1720–1724.

Groden J, Joslyn G, Samowitz W, Jones D, Bhattacharyya N, Spirio L, Thliveris A, Robertson M, Egan S, Meuth M, White R. 1995. Response of colon cancer cell lines to the introduction of APC, a colon-specific tumor suppressor gene. Cancer Res 55:1531–1539.

Groden J, Thliveris A, Samowitz W, Carlson M, Gelbert L, Albertsen H, Joslyn G, Stevens J, Spirio L, Robertson M, Sargeant L, Krapcho K, Wolff E, Burt R, Hughes JP, Warrington J, McPherson J, Wasmuth J, Le Paslier D, Abderrahim H, Cohen D, Leppert M, White R. 1991. Identification and characterization of the familial adenomatous polyposis coli gene. Cell 66:589–600.

Gudas J, Nguyen H, Li T, Cowan KH. 1995. Hormone-dependent regulation of BRCA1 in human breast cancer cells. Cancer Res 55:4561–4565.

Guengerich FP, Shimada T, Raney KD, Yun C-H, Meyer DJ, Ketterer B, Harris TM, Groopman JD, Kadlubar FF. 1992. Elucidation of catalytic specificities of human cytochrome P450 and glutathione S-transferase enzymes and relevance to molecular epidemiology. Environ Health Perspect 98:75–80.

Haber DA, Park S, Maheswaran S, et al. 1993. WT1-mediated growth suppression of Wilms' tumor cells expressing a WT1 splicing variant. Science 262:2057–2059.

Haber DA, Timmers H Th M, Pelletier J, Sharp PA, Housman DE. 1992. A dominant mutation in the Wilms tumor gene *WT1* cooperates with the viral oncogene *E1A* in transformation of primary kidney cells. Proc Natl Acad Sci USA 89:6010–6014.

Hall JM, Lee MK, Newman B, Morrow JE, Anderson LA, Huey B, King MC. 1990. Linkage of early-onset familial breast cancer to chromosome 17q21. Science 250:1684–1689.

Hamilton SR, Liu B, Parsons RE, Papadopoulos N, Jen J, Powell SM, Krush AJ, Berk T, Cohen Z, Tetu B, Burger PC, Wood PA, Taqi F, Booker SV, Petersen GM, Offerhaus GJA, Tersmette AC, Giardiello FM, Vogelstein B, Kinzler KW. 1995. The molecular basis of Turcot's syndrome. N Engl J Med 332:839–847.

Harris H, Miller OJ, Klein G, Worst P, Tachibana T. 1969. Suppression of malignancy by cell fusion. Nature 223:363–368.

Harvey M, McArthur MJ, Montgomery CA Jr, Bradley A, Donehower LA. 1993b. Genetic background alters the spectrum of tumors that develop in p53-deficient mice. FASEB J 7:938–943.

Harvey M, McArthur MJ, Montgomery CA Jr, Butel JS, Bradley A, Donehower LA. 1993a. Spontaneous and carcinogen-induced tumorigenesis in p53-deficient mice. Nat Genet 5:225–229.

Harvey M, Vogel H, Lee E Y-H P, Bradley A, Donehower LA. 1995a. Mice deficient in both p53 and Rb develop tumors primarily of endocrine origin. Cancer Res 55:1146–1151.

Harvey M, Vogel H, Morris D, Bradley A, Bernstein A, Donehower LA. 1995b. A mutant p53 transgene accelerates tumour development in heterozygous but not nullizygous p53-deficient mice. Nat Genet 9:305–311.

Hasstedt SJ. 1991. A variance components/major locus likelihood approximation on quantitative data. Genet Epidemiol 8:113–125.

Hayashi S, Watanabe J, Nakachi K, Kawajiri K. 1991. Genetic linkage of lung cancer-associated *Msp*-1 polymorphisms with amino acid replacement in the heme binding region of the human cytochrome p450IaI gene. J Biochem 110:407–410.

Hecht JT, Hogue D, Strong LC, et al. 1995. Hereditary multiple exostosis and chondrosarcoma: linkage to chromosome 11 and loss of heterozygosity for EXT-linked markers on chromosomes 11 and 8. Am J Hum Genet 56:1125–1131.

Heckbert SR, Weiss NS, Hornung SK, Eaton DL, Motulsky AG. 1992. Glutathione S-transferase and epoxide hydrolase activity in human leukocytes in relation to risk of lung cancer and other smoking-related cancers. J Natl Cancer Inst 84:414–422.

Hein DW. 1988. Acetylator genotype and arylamine-induced carcinogenesis. Biochim Biophys Acta 948:37–66.

Hemminki A, Peltomaki P, Mecklin J-P, Jarvinen H, Salovaara R, Nystrom-Lahti M, de la Chapelle A, Aaltonen LA. 1994. Loss of the wild type MLH1 gene is a feature of hereditary nonpolyposis colorectal cancer. Nat Genet 8:405–410.

Herrera L, Kakati S, Gibas L, Pietrzak E, Sandberg AA. 1986. Brief clinical report: Gardner syndrome in a man with an interstitial deletion of 5q. Am J Med Genet 25:473–476.

Heutnik P, van der Mey AGL, Sandkuijl LA, et al. 1992. A gene subject to genomic imprinting and responsible for hereditary paragangliomas maps to chromosome 11q23-qter. Hum Mol Genet 1:7–10.

Hoeijmakers JHJ. Nucleotide excision repair II: from yeast to mammals 1993. Trends Genet 9:211–217.

Hofstra RMW, Landsvater RM, Ceccherini I, Stulp RP, Stelwagen T, Luo Y, Pasini B, Höppener JWM, van Amstel HKP, Romeo G, Lips CJM, Buys CHCM. 1994. A mutation in the *RET* proto-oncogene associated with multiple endocrine neoplasia type 2B and sporadic medullary thyroid carcinoma. Nature 367:375–376.

HONCHEL R, HALLING KC, SCHAID DJ, ET AL. 1994. Microsatellite instability in Muir-Torre syndreome. Cancer Res 54:1159–1163.

HOLLSTEIN M, SIDRANSKY D, VOGELSTEIN B, ET AL. 1991. p53 mutations in human cancers. Science 253:49–53.

HUANG H-JS, YEE J-K, SHEW J-Y, CHEN P-L, BOOKSTEIN R, FRIEDMANN T, LEE EY-HP, LEE W-H. 1988. Suppression of the neoplastic phenotype by replacement of the RB gene in human cancer cells. Science 242:1563–1566.

HUFF V, SAUNDERS GF. 1993. Wilms' tumor genes. Biochem Biophys ACTA 1155:295—306.

HURSTING SD, PERKINS SN, HAINES DC, WARD JM, PHANG JM. 1995. Chemoprevention of spontaneous tumorigenesis in p53-knockout mice. Cancer Res 55:3949–3953.

HURSTING SD, PERKINS SN, PHANG JM. 1994. Calorie restriction delays spontaneous tumorigenesis in p53-knockout transgenic mice. Proc Natl Acad Sci USA 91:7036–7040.

ICHII S, HORII A, NAKATSURU S, FURUYAMA J, UTSUNOMIYA J, NAKAMURA Y. 1992. Inactivation of both APC alleles in an early stage of colon adenomas in a patient with familial adenomatous polyposis (FAP). Hum Mol Genet 1:387–390.

ILIOPOULOS O, KIBEL A, GRAY S, ET AL. 1995. Tumor suppression by the human von Hippel-Lindau gene. Nature Med 1:822–826.

IONOV Y, PEINADO MA, MALKHOSYAN S, SHIBATA D, PERUCHO M. 1993. Ubiquitous somatic mutations in simple repeated sequences reveal a new mechanism for colonic carcinogenesis. Nature 363:558–561.

JOHNSON B, BROOKS BA, HEINZMANN C, DIEP A, MOHANDES T, SPARKES RT, REYES H, HOFFMAN E, LANGE E, GATTI R, XIA Y-R, LUSIS AJ, HANKINSON O. 1993. The Ah receptor nuclear translocation gene (ARNT) is located on q21 of human chromosome 1 and on mouse chromosome 3 near Cf-3. Genomics 17:592–598.

KADLUBAR FF, BUTLER MA, KADERLIK KR, CHOU H-C, LANG NP. 1992. Polymorphisms for aromatic amine metabolism in humans: relevance for human carcinogenesis. Environ Health Perspect 98:69–74.

KAMB A, GRUIS NA, WEAVER-FELDHAUS J, LIU Q, HARSHMAN K, TAVTIGIAN SV, STOCKERT E, DAY RS, JOHNSON BE, SKOLNICK MH. 1994. A cell cycle regulator potentially involved in genesis of many tumor types. Science 264:436–439.

KAWAJIRI K, NAKACHI K, IMAI K, YOSHII A, SHINODA N, WATANABE J. 1990. Identification of genetically high risk individuals to lung cancer by DNA polymorphisms of the cytochrome P4501A1 gene. FEBS Lett 260:131–133.

KELLERMAN G, SHAW CR, LUYTEN-KELLERMAN M. 1973. Aryl hydrocarbon hydroxylase inducibility and bronchogenic carcinoma. N Engl J Med 289:934–937.

KETTERER B, HARRIS JM, TALASKA G, MEYER DJ, PEMBLE SE, TAYLOR JB, LANG NP, KADLUBAR FF. 1992. The human glutathione S-transferase supergene family, its polymorphism, and its effects on susceptibility to lung cancer. Environ Health Perspect 98:87–94.

KHOURI MJ, BEATY TH, COHEN BH. 1993. Fundamentals of Genetic Epidemiology. Baltimore: Johns Hopkins Press.

KIRBY GM, WOLF CR, NEAL GE, JUDAH DJ, HENDERSON CJ, SRIVATANAKUL P, WILD CP. 1993. In vitro metabolism of aflatoxin B by normal and tumorous in vivo tissues from Thailand. Carcinogenesis 14:2613–2620.

KIRVONEN A, HUSGAFVEL-PURSAINEN K, KARJALAINEN A, ANTTILA S, VAINIO H. 1992. Point-mutational *MSP*1 and *Ile-Val* polymorphisms closely linked in the CYP1A1 gene: lack of an association with susceptibility to lung cancer in a Finnish study population. Cancer Epidemiol Biomarkers Prev 1:485–489.

KITCHIN FD, ELLSWORTH RM. 1974. Pleiotropic effects of the gene for retinoblastoma. J Med Genet 11:244–246.

KNUDSON AG JR. 1971. Mutation and cancer: a statistical study of retinoblastoma. Proc Natl Acad Sci USA 68:820–823.

KNUDSON AG JR, MEADOWS AT, NICHOLS WW, HILL R. 1976. Chromosomal deletion and retinoblastoma. N Engl J Med 295:1120–1123.

KOLODNER RD, HALL NR, LIPFORD J, ET AL. 1994. Structure of the human MSH-2 locus and analysis of two Muir-Torre kindreds for msh2 mutations. Genomics 24:516–526.

KOUFOS A, HANSEN MF, COPELAND NG, ET AL. 1985. Loss of heterozygosity in three embryonal tumours suggests a common pathogenetic mechanism. Nature 316:330–334.

LABAYLE D, FISCHER D, VIELH P, DROUHIN F, PARIENTE A, BORIES C, DUHAMEL O, TROUSSET M, ATTALI P. 1991. Sulindac causes regression of rectal polyps in familial adenomatous polyposis. Gastroenterology 101:635–639.

LAFUENTE A, PUJOL F, CARRETERO P, VILLA JP, CUCI A. 1993. Human glutathione S-transferase mu deficiency as a marker for the susceptibility to bladder and larynx cancer among smokers. Cancer Lett 68:49–54.

LALOUEL JM, MORTON NE. 1981. Complex segregation analysis with pointers. Hum Hered 31:312–321.

LANE DP. 1992. p53, guardian of the genome. Nature 358:15–16.

LARSSON C, WEBER G, NORDENSKJÖLD M, ET AL. 1992. Genetic aspects of tumor development in multiple endocrine neoplasia type 1 Diagnost Oncol 2:342–345.

LATIF F, TORY K, GNARRA J, ET AL. 1993. Identification of the von Hippel-Lindau disease tumor suppressor gene. Science 260:1317–1320.

LEACH FS, NICOLAIDES NC, PAPADOPOULOS N, LIU B, JEN J, PARSONS R, PELTOMÄKI, P, SISTONEN P, AALTONEN LA, NYSTRÖM-LAHTI M, GUAN X-Y, ZHANG J, MELTZER PS, YU J-W, KAO F-T, CHEN DJ, CEROSALETTI KM, FOURNIER REK, TODD S, LEWIS T, LEACH RJ, NAYLOR SL, WEISSENBACH J, MECKLIN J-P, JÄRVINEN H, PETERSEN GM, HAMILTON SR, GREEN J, JASS J, WATSON P, LYNCH HT, TRENT JM, DE LA CHAPELLE A, KINZLER KW, VOGELSTEIN B. 1993. Mutations of a *mutS* homolog in hereditary nonpolyposis colorectal cancer. Cell 75:1215–1225.

LEE S, ELENBAAS B, LEVINE A, GRIFFITH J. 1995. p53 and its 14 kDa C-Terminal domain recognize primary DNA damage in the form of insertion/deletion mismatches. Cell 81:1013–1020.

LI FP, FRAUMENI JF JR. 1975. Familial breast cancer, soft-tissue sarcomas and other neoplasms. Ann Intern Med 83:833–834.

LI FP, FRAUMENI JF JR. 1969a. Soft-tissue sarcomas, breast cancer, and other neoplasms: a familial syndrome? Ann Intern Med 71:747–752.

LI FP, FRAUMENI JF JR. 1969b. Rhabdomyosarcoma in children: epidemiologic study and identification of a familial cancer syndrome. J Natl Cancer Inst 43:1365–1373.

LI FP, FRAUMENI JF JR, MULVIHILL JJ, BLATTNER WA, DREYFUS MG, TUCKER MA, MILLER RW. 1988. A cancer family syndrome in twenty-four kindreds. Cancer Res 48:5358–5362.

LINDBLOM A, TANNERGÅRD P, WERELIUS B, NORDENSKJÖLD M. 1993. Genetic mapping of a second locus predisposing to hereditary non-polyposis colon cancer. Nature Genet 5:279–282.

LIVINGSTONE LR, WHITE A, SPROUSE J, ET AL. 1992. Altered cell cycle arrest and gene amplification potential accompany loss of wild-type p53. Cell 70:923–935.

LOGOTHETIS CJ, XU H-J, RO JY, HU S-X, SAHIN A, ORDONEZ N, BENEDICT WF. 1992. Altered expression of retinoblastoma protein and known prognostic variables in locally advanced bladder cancer. J Natl Cancer Inst 84:1256–1260.

LOWE SW, BODIS S, MCCLATCHEY A, REMINGTON L, RULEY HE, FISHER DE, HOUSMAN DE, JACKS T. 1994. p53 status and the efficacy of cancer therapy in vivo. Science 266:807–810.

LOVE RR, EVANS AM, JOSTEN DM. 1985. The accuracy of patient reports of a family history of cancer. J Chron Dis 3:289–293.

LUSTBADER ED, WILLIAMS WR, STROM SS, BONDY ML, STRONG LC. 1992. Segregation analysis of cancer in families of childhood soft tissue sarcoma patients. Am J Hum Genet 51:344–356.

LUTCHMAN M, ROULEAU GA. 1995. The neurofibromatosis type 2 gene product, schwannomin, suppresses growth of NIH 3T3 cells. Cancer Res 55:2270–2274.

LYNCH HT, WATSON P, KRIEGLER M, LYNCH JF, LANSPA SJ, MARCUS J, SMYRK T, FITZGIBBONS RJ JR, CRISTOFARO G. 1988. Differential diagnosis of hereditary nonpolyposis colon cancer (Lynch syndrome I and Lynch syndrome II). Dis Colon Rectum 31:372–377.

LYONS LA, LEWIS RA, STRONG, LC, ZUCKERBROD S, FERRELL RE. 1988. A genetic study of Gardner syndrome and congenital hypertrophy of the retinal pigment epithelium. Am J Hum Genet 42:290–296.

MACK W, LANHOLZ B, THOMAS DC. 1990. Survival models for familial aggregation of cancer. Environ Health Perspect 87:27–35.

MALKIN D, LI FP, STRONG LC, FRAUMENI JF JR, NELSON CE, KIM DH, KASSEL J, GRYKA MA, BISCHOFF JZ, TAINSKY MA, FRIEND SH. 1990. Germ line p53 mutations in a familial syndrome of breast cancer, sarcomas, and other neoplasms. Science 250:1233–1238.

MANN WR, VENKATRAJ VS, ALLEN RG, ET AL. 1991. Fanconi anemia: Evidence for linkage heterogeneity on chromosome 20q. Genomics 9:329–337.

MARIMAN ECM, VAN BEERSUM SEC, CREMERS CWRJ, ET AL. 1993. Analysis of a second family with hereditary non-chromaffin paragangliomas locates the underlying gene at the proximal region of chromosome 11q. Hum Genet 91:357–361.

MARGER RS, MARGER D. 1993. Carcinoma of the esophagus and tylosis. A lethal genetic combination. Cancer 72:17–19.

MARKOWITZ S, WANG J, MYEROFF L, PARSONS R, SUN L, LUTTERBAUGH J, FAN RS, ZBOROWSKA E, KINZLER KW, VOGELSTEIN B, BRATTAIN M, WILLSON JKV. 1995. Inactivation of the type II TGF-β receptor in colon cancer cells with microsatellite instability. Science 268:1336–1338.

MARRA G, BOLAND CR. 1995. Hereditary nonpolyposis colorectal cancer: the syndrome, the genes, and historical perspectives. J Natl Cancer Inst 87:1114–1125.

MERLO A, HERMA JG, MAO L, LEE DJ, GABRIELSON E, BURGER PC, BAYLIN SB, SIDRANSKY D. 1995. 5′ CpG island methylation is associated with transcriptional silencing of the tumour suppressor p16/CDKN2/MTS1 in human cancers. Nature Med 1:686–692.

MIKI Y, SWENSEN J, SHATTUCK-EIDENS D, FUTREAL PA, HARSHMAN K, TAVTIGIAN S, LIU Q, COCHRAN C, BENNETT LM, DING W, BELL R, ROSENTHAL J, HUSSEY C, TRAN T, MCCLURE M, FRYE C, HATTIER T, PHELPS R, HAUGEN-STRANO A, KATCHER H, YAKUMO K, GHOLAMI Z, SHAFFER D, STONE S, BAYER S, WRAY C, BOGDEN R, DAYANANTH P, WARD J, TONIN P, NAROD S, BRISTOW PK, NORRIS FH, HELVERING L, MORRISON P, ROSTECK P, LAI M, BARRETT JC, LEWIS C, NEUHAUSEN S, CANNON-ALBRIGHT L, GOLDGAR D, WISEMAN R, KAMB A, SKOLNICK MH. 1994. A strong candidate for the breast and ovarian cancer susceptibility gene BRCA1. Science 266:66–71.

MILNER J, MEDCALF EA, COOK AC. 1991. Tumor suppressor p53: analysis of wild-type and mutant p53 complexes. Mol Cell Biol 11:12–19.

MOOLGAVKAR SH, LUEBECK EG. 1992. Multistage carcinogenesis: population-based model for colon cancer. J Natl Cancer Inst 84:610–618.

MULLIGAN LM, KWOK JBJ, HEALEY CS, ELSDON MJ, ENG C, GARDNER E, LOVE DR, MOLE SE, MOORE JK, PAPI L, PONDER MA, TELENIUS H, TUNNACLIFFE A, PONDER BAJ. 1993. Germ-line mutations of the *RET* proto-oncogene in multiple endocrine neoplasia type 2A. Nature 363:458–460.

NAROD S, FEUNTEUN J, LYNCH HT, WATSON P, CONWAY T, LYNCH J, LENOIR GM. 1991. Familial breast-ovarian cancer locus on chromosome 17q21-q23. Lancet 338:82–83.

NAZAR-STEWART V, MOTULSKY AG, EATON DL, WHITE E, HORNUNG SK, LENG Z-T, STAPLETON P, WEISS NS. 1993. The glutathione S-transferase m polymorphism as a marker for susceptibility to lung carcinoma. Cancer Res 53:2313–2318.

NEALE MC, CARDON LR. 1993. *Methodology for Genetic Studies of Twins and Families.* Dordrecht, Netherlands: Kluwer Academic Publishers, Vol 67.

NEBERT DW. 1991. Role of genetics and drug metabolism in human cancer risk. Mutat Res, 247:267–281.

NEBERT DW, NELSON DR, COON MJ, ESTABROOK RW, FEYEREISEN R, FUJII-KURIYAMA Y, GONZALEZ FJ, GUENGERICH FP, GUNSALUS IC, JOHNSON EF, ET AL. 1991a. The p450 superfamily: update on new sequences gene mapping, and recommended nomenclature. DNA Cell Biol 10:1–14.

NEBERT DW, PETERSEN DD, PUGA A. 1991b. Human AH locus polymorphism and cancer: inducibility of CYP1A1 and other genes by combustion products and dioxin. Pharmacogenetics 1:68–78.

NEBERT DW, GONZALEZ FJ. 1987. P450 Genes: Structure, evolution, and regulation. Ann Rev Biochem 56:945–993.

NEUMANN HPH, BERGER DP, SIGMUND G, ET AL. 1993. Pheochromocytomas, multiple endocrine neoplasia type 2, and von Hippel-Lindau disease. N Engl J Med 329:1531–1538.

NEWMAN B, AUSTIN MA, LEE M, KING M-C. 1988. Inheritance of human breast cancer: Evidence for autosomal dominant transmission in high-risk families. Proc Natl Acad Sci USA 85:3044–3048.

NICOLAIDES NC, PAPADOPOULOS N, LIU B, WEI YF, CARTER KC, RUBEN SM, ROSEN CA, HASELTINE WA, FLEISCHMANN RD, FRASER CM, ADAMS MD, VENTER JC, DUNLOP MG, HAMILTON SR, PETERSEN GM, DE LA CHAPELLE A, VOGELSTEIN B, KINZLER KW. 1994. Mutations of two PMS homologues in hereditary nonpolyposis colon cancer. Nature 371:75–80.

NYSTROM-LAHTI M, PARSONS R, SISTONEN P, ET AL. 1994. Mismatch repair genes on chromosomes 2p and 3p account for a major share of hereditary nonpolyposis colorectal cancer families evaluable by linkage. Am J. Hum Genet 55:659–665.

OKAMOTO M, SATO C, KOHNO Y, MORI T, IWAMA T, TONOMURA A, MIKI Y, UTSUNOMIYA J, NAKAMURA Y, WHITE R, MIYAKI M. 1990. Molecular nature of chromosome 5q loss in colorectal tumors and desmoids from patients with familial adenomatous polyposis. Hum Genet 85:595–599.

OLSCHWANG S, TIRET A, LAURENT-PUIG P, MULERIS M, PARC R, THOMAS G. 1993. Restriction of ocular fundus lesions to a specific subgroup of *APC* mutations in adenomatous polyposis coli patients. Cell 75:959–968.

OOI WL, ELSTON RC, CHEN VW, BAILEY-WILSON JE, ROTHSCHILD H. 1986. Increased familial risk for lung cancer. J Natl Cancer Inst 76:217–222.

OSHIMA M, OSHIMA H, KITAGAWA K, KOBAYASHI M, ITAKURA C, TAKETO M. 1995. Loss of Apc heterozygosity and abnormal tissue building in nascent intestinal polyps in mice carrying a truncated Apc gene. Proc Natl Acad Sci USA 92:4482–4486.

OTT J. 1991. Analysis of Human Genetic Linkage. Baltimore: Johns Hopkins University Press, pp 54–81.

PAIGEN B, GURTOO HL, MINOWADA J, HOUTEN L, BINCENT R, PAIGEN K, PARKER NB, WARD E, HAYNER NT. 1977. Questionable relation of aryl hydrocarbon hydroxylase to lung-cancer risk. N Engl J Med 297:346–350.

PALOMBO F, GALLINARI P, IACCARINO I, LETTIERI T, HUGHES M, D'ARRIGO A, TRUONG O, HSUAN JJ, JIRICNY J. 1995. GTBP, a 160-kilodalton protein essential for mismatch-binding activity in human cells. Science 268:1912–1914.

PAPADOPOULOS N, NICOLAIDES NC, LIU B, PARSONS R, LENGAUER C, PALOMBO F, D'ARRIGO A, MARKOWITZ S, WILLSON JKV, KINZLER KW, JIRICNY J, VOGELSTEIN B. 1995. Mutations of GTBP in genetically unstable cells. Science 268:1915–1917.

PAPADOPOULOS N, NICOLAIDES NC, WEI Y-F, RUBEN SM, CARTER KC, ROSEN CA, HASELTINE WA, FLEISCHMANN RD, FRASER CM, ADAMS MD, VENTER JC, HAMILTON SR, PETERSEN GM, WATSON P, LYNCH HT, PELTOMÄKI P, MECKLIN J-P, DE LA CHAPELLE A, KINZLER

KW, VOGELSTEIN B. 1994. Mutation of a *mutL* homolog in hereditary colon cancer. Science 263:1625–1629.

PARADA LF, LAND H, WEINBERG RA, WOLF D, ROTTER V. 1984. Cooperation between gene encoding p53 tumour antigen and ras in cellular transformation. Nature 312:649–651.

PARSONS R, LI G-M, LONGLEY MJ, FANG W-H, PAPADOPOULOS N, JEN J, DE LA CHAPELLE A, KINZLER KW, VOGELSTEIN B, MODRICH P. 1993. Hypermutability and mismatch repair deficiency in RER+ tumor cells. Cell 75:1227–1236.

PELKONEN O, RAUNIO H. 1995. Individual expression of carcinogen-metabolizing enzymes: cytochrome P4502A. J Occup Environ Health 37:19–24.

PELTOMÄKI P, LOTHE RA, AALTONEN LA, PYLKKÄNEN L, NYSTRÖM-LAHTI M, SERUCA R, DAVID L, HOLM R, RYBERG D, HAUGEN A, BRØGGER A, Børresen A-L, de la Chapelle A. 1993. Microsatellite instability is associated with tumors that characterize the hereditary non-polyposis colorectal carcinoma syndrome. Cancer Res 53:5853–5855.

PETERSEN DD, MCKINNEY CE, IKEYA K, SMITH HH, BALE AE, MCBRIDE OW, NEBERT DW. 1991. Human CP1A1 gene: cosegregation of the enzyme inducibility phenotype and an RFLP. Am J Hum Genet 48:720–725.

PRENTICE RL. 1988. Correlated binary regression with covariates specific to each binary observation. Biometrics 44:1033–1048.

QAQISH BF, LIANG KY. 1992. Marginal models for correlated binary responses with multiple classes and multiple levels of nesting. Biometrics 48:939–950.

RANADE K, HUSSUSSIAN CJ, SIKORSKI RS, VARMUS HE, GOLDSTEIN AM, TUCKER MA, SERRANO M, HANNON GJ, BEACH D, DRACOPOLI NC. 1995. Mutations associated with familial melanoma impair $p16^{ink4}$ function. Nat Genet 10:114–116.

REYES H, REISZ-PORSZASZ S, HANKINSON O. 1992. Identification of the Ah receptor nuclear translocator protein (Arnt) as a component of the DNA binding form of the Ah receptor.

RISK JM, FIELD EA, FIELD JK, WHITTAKER J, FRYER A, ELLIS A, SHAW JM, FRIEDMANN PS, BISHOP DT, BODMER J, LEIGH IM. 1994. Tylosis oesophageal cancer mapped. Nat Genet 8:319–321.

ROBBINS JH, KRAEMER KH, LUTZNER MA, ET AL. 1974. Xeroderma pigmentosum: An inherited disease with sun sensitivity, multiple cutaneous neoplasms, and abnormal DNA repair. Ann Intern Med 80:221–248.

ROTHMAN N, STEWART W, CAPORASO NE, HAYES RB. 1993. Misclassification of genetic susceptibility biomarkers: Implications for case-control studies and cross-population comparisons. Cancer Epidemiol Biomarkers Prev 2:299–303.

ROULEAU GA, MEREL P, LUTCHMAN M, SANSON M, ZUCMAN J, MARINEAU C, HOANG-XUAN K, DEMCZUK S, DESMAZE C, PLOUGASTEL B, PULST SM, LENOIR G, BIJLSMA E, FASHOLD R, DUMANSKI J, DE JONG P, PARRY D, ELDRIDGE R, AURIAS A, DELATTRE O, THOMAS G. 1993. Alteration in a new gene encoding a putative membrane-organizing protein causes neuro-fibromatosis type 2. Nature 363:515–521.

RUSTGI AK. 1994. Hereditary gastrointestinal polyposis and non-polyposis syndromes. N Engl J Med 331:1694–1702.

SAGERMAN RH, CASSADY JR, TRETTER P, ELLSWORTH RM. 1969. Radiation induced neoplasia following external beam therapy for children with retinoblastoma. Am J Roentgenol Radium Ther Nucl Med 105:529–535.

SAMOWITZ WS, THLIVERIS A, SPIRIO LN, WHITE R. 1995. Alternatively spliced adenomatous polyposis coli (APC) gene transcripts that delete exons mutated in attenuated APC. Cancer Res 3732–3734.

SANCHEZ Y, EL-NAGGAR A, PATHAK S, KILLARY AM. 1994. A tumor suppressor locus within 3p14-p12 mediates rapid cell death of renal cell carcinoma in vivo. Proc Natl Acad Sci USA 91:3383–3387.

SANTORO M, CARLOMAGNO F, ROMANO A, BOTTARO DP, DATHAN NA, GRIECO M, FUSCO A, VECCHIO G, MATOSKOVA B, KRAUS MH, DI FIORE PP. 1995. Activation of *RET* as a dominant transforming gene by germline mutations of MEN2A and MEN2B. Science 267:381–383.

SAVITSKY K, BAR-SHIRA A, GILAD S, ROTMAN G, ZIV Y, VANAGAITE L, TAGLE DA, SMITH S, UZIEL T, SFEZ S, ASHKENAZI M, PECKER I, FRYDMAN M, HARNIK R, PATANJALI SR, SIMMONS A, CLINES GA, SARTIEL A, GATTI RA, CHESSA L, SANAL O, LAVIN MF, JASPERS NGJ, TAYLOR AMR, ARLETT CF, MIKI T, WEISSMAN SM, LOVETT M, COLLINS FS, SHILOH Y. 1995. A single ataxia telangiectasia gene with a product similar to P1-3 kinase. Science 268:1749–1753.

SAWYER S. 1990. Maximum likelihood estimators for incorrect models, with an application to ascertainment bias for continuous characters. Theor Popul Biol 38:351–366.

SCHAID DJ, SOMMERS SS. 1994. Comparison of statistics for candidate-gene association studies using cases and parents. Am J Hum Genet 55:402–409.

SCHAPPERT-KIMMIJSER J, HEMMES GD, NIJLAND R. 1966. The heredity of retinoblastoma. Ophthalmologica 151:197–213.

SCHILDKRAUT J, RISCH N, THOMPSON WD. 1989. Evaluating genetic association among ovarian, breast, and endometrial cancer: evidence for a breast-ovarian cancer relationship. Am J Hum Genet 45:521–529.

SCHNEIDER NR, CUBILLA AL, CHAGANTI RSK. 1983. Association of endocrine neoplasia with multiple polyposis of the colon. Cancer 51:1171–1175.

SELLERS TA, BAILEY-WILSON JE, ELSTON RC, WILSON AE, ROTHSCHILD H. 1990. Evidence for Mendelian inheritance in the pathogenesis of lung cancer. J Natl Cancer Inst 82:1272–1279.

SELLERS TA, ELSTON RC, STEWART C, ROTHSCHILD H. 1988. Familial risk of cancer among randomly selected cancer probands. Genet Epidemiol 5:381–392.

SHANNON KM, O'CONNELL P, MARTIN GA, ET AL. 1994. Loss of the normal NF1 allele from the bohe marrow of children with type I neurofibromatosis and malignant myeloid disorders. New Engl J Med 330:597–601.

SHIELDS PG, BOWMAN ED, HARRINGTON AM, DOAN VT, WESTON A. 1993. Polycyclic aromatic hydrocarbon-DNA adducts in human lung and susceptibility genes. Cancer Res 53:3486–3492.

SHUTE N, EWENS W. 1988. A resolution of the ascertainment sampling problem, III. Pedigrees. Am J Hum Genet 43:387–395.

SIEDEGARD J, PERO RW, MARKOWITZ MM, ROUSH G, MILLER DG, BEATTIE EJ. 1990. Isoenzyme(s) of glutathione transferase (class mu) as a marker for the susceptibility to lung cancer: a follow up study. Carcinogenesis 11:33–36.

SIMARD J, TONIN P, DUROCHER F, MORGAN K, ROMMENS J, GINGRAS S, SAMSON C, LEBLANC J-F, BELANGER C, DION F, LIU Q, SKOLNICK M, GOLDGAR D, SHATTUCK-EIDENS D, LABRIE F, NAROD SA. 1994. Common origins of BRCA1 mutations in Canadian breast and ovarian cancer families. Nat Genet 8:392–398.

SOLOMAN E, VOSS R, HALL V, BODMER WF, JASS JR, JEFFREYS AJ, LUCIBELLO FC, PATEL I, RIDER SH. 1987. Chromosome 5 allele loss in human colorectal carcinomas. Nature 328:616–619.

SPARKES RS, MURPHREE AL, LINGUA RW, SPARKES MC, FIELD LL, FUNDERBURK SJ, BENEDICT WF. 1983. Gene for hereditary retinoblastoma assigned to human chromosome 13 by linkage to esterase D. Science 219:971–973.

SPIRIO L, OLSCHWANG S, GRODEN J, ROBERTSON M, SAMOWITZ W, JOSLYN G, GELBERT L, THLIVERIS A, CARLSON M, OTTERUD B, LYNCH H, WATSON P, LYNCH P, LAURENT-PUIG P, BURT R, HUGHES JP, THOMAS G, LEPPERT M, WHITE R. 1993. Alleles of the *APC* gene: an attenuated form of familial polyposis. Cell 75:951–957.

STANBRIDGE EJ. 1976. Suppression of malignancy in human cells. Nature 260:17–20.

STRAND M, PROLLA TA, LISKAY RM, PETES TD. 1993. Destabilization of tracts of simple repetitive DNA in yeast by mutations affecting DNA mismatch repair. Nature 365:274–276.

STRATHDEE CA, BUCHWALD M. 1992. Molecular and cellular biology of Fanconi anemia. Am J Pediat Hematol Oncol 14:177–185.

STRONG LC, WILLIAMS WR, TAINSKY MA. 1992. The Li-Fraumeni syndrome: from clinical epidemiology to molecular genetics. Am J Epidemiol 135:190–199.

STRUEWING JP, ABELIOVICH D, PERETZ T, AVISHAI N, KABACK MM, COLLINS FS, BRODY LC. 1995. The carrier frequency of the BRCA1 mutation 185delAG mutation is approximately 1 percent in Ashkenazi Jewish individuals. Nat Genet 11:198–200.

SUGIMURA H, CAPORASO NE, HOOVER RN, MODALI RV, RESAU JH, TRUMP BF, LONERGAN JA, KRONTIRIS TG, MANN DL, WESTON A, HARRIS CC. 1990. Association of rare alleles of the Harvey *ras* proto-oncogene locus with lung cancer. Cancer Res 50:1857–1862.

SWANSON HI, BRADFIELD CA. 1993. The Ah receptor: genetics, structure and function. Pharmacogenetics 3:203–230.

SWIFT M, MORRELL D, MASSEY RB, CHASE CL. 1991. Incidence of cancer in 161 families affected by ataxia-telangiectasia. N Engl J Med 325:1831–1836.

TAKAI S, TATEISHI H, NISHISHO I, MIKI T, MOTOMURA K, MIYAUCHI A, KATO M, IKEUCHI T, YAMAMOTO K, OKAZAKI M, YAMAMOTO M, HONJO T, KUMAHARA Y, MORI T. 1987. Loss of genes on chromosome 22 in medullary thyroid carcinoma and pheochromocytoma. Jpn J Cancer Res 78:894–898.

TAKEDA J, ISHII S, SEINO Y, IMAMOTO F, IMURA H. 1989. Negative regulation of human insulin gene expression by the 5′ flanking region in non-pancreatic cells. FEBS Lett 247:41–45.

TAYLOR JA. 1990. Epidemiologic evidence of genetic susceptibility to cancer. In: Spatz L, Bloom AD, Paul NW, eds. Detection of Cancer Predisposition: Laboratory Approaches. White Plains, NY: March of Dimes Foundation; 113–127, Monograph 3.

THAKKER RV. 1993. The molecular genetics of the multiple endocrine neoplasia syndromes. Clin Endocrinol 38:1–14.

THIBODEAU SN, BREN G, SCHAID D. 1993. Microsatellite instability in cancer of the proximal colon. Science 260:816–819.

THOMAS DC, LANGHOLZ B, MACK W, FLODERUS B. 1990. Bivariate survival models for analysis of genetic and environmental effects in twins. Genet Epidemiol 7:121–135.

THOMPSON EA, DEEB S, WALKER D, MOTULSKY AG. 1988. The detection of linkage disequilibrium between closely linked markers: RFLPs at the AI-CIII apolipoprotein genes. Am J Hum Genet 42:113–124.

THOMSON G, BODMER WF. 1977. The genetics analysis of HLA and disease associations. In: Dausset J, Svejgaard A (eds), HLA and Disease. Munksgard, Copenhagen, pp 84–93.

THORLACIUS S, TRYGGVADOTTIR L, OLAFSDOTTIR GH, ET AL. 1995. Linkage to BRCA2 region in hereditary male breast cancer. Lancet 346:544–545.

TOKUHATA GK, LILLIENFELD AM. 1963. Familial aggregation of lung cancer in humans. J Natl Cancer Inst 30:289–312.

TOYOOKA M, KONISHI M, KIKUCHI-YANOSHITA R, IWAMA T, MIYAKI M. 1995. Somatic mutations of the adenomatous polyposis coli gene in gastroduodenal tumors from patients with familial adenomatous polyposis. Cancer Res 55:3165–3170.

TROFATTER JA, MACCOLLIN MM, RUTTER JL, ET AL. 1993. A novel moesin-, ezrin-, radixin-like gene is a candidate for the neurofibromatosis 2 tumor suppressor cell 72:791–800.

TURCOT J, DEPRES JP, ST. PIERRE F. 1959. Malignant tumors of the central nervous system associated with familial polyposis of the colon: report of two cases. Dis Colon Rectum 2:465–468.

VAN DER RIET P, KARP D, FARMER E, WEI Q, GROSSMAN L, TOKINO K, RUPPERT JM, SIDRANSKY D. 1994. Progression of basal cell carcinoma through loss of chromosome 9q and inactivation of a single p53 allele. Cancer Res 54: 25–27.

VATSIS KP, MARTELL KJ, WEBER WW. 1991. Diverse point mutations in the human gene for polymorphic N-acetyltransferase. Proc Natl Acad Sci USA 88:6333–6337.

VEALE AMO. 1965. Intestinal polyposis. Eugenics Laboratory Memoirs No. 90, Cambridge: Cambridge University Press.

VOGELSTEIN B, FEARON ER, HAMILTON SR, KERN SE, PREISINGER AN, LEPPERT M, NAKAMURA Y, WHITE R, SMITS AMM, BOS JL. 1988. Genetic alterations during colorectal-tumor development. N Engl J Med 319:525–532.

VOGELSTEIN B, KINZLER KW. 1992. p53 Function and dysfunction. Cell 70:523–526.

VOGEL F. 1979. Genetics of retinoblastoma. Hum Genet 52:1–54.

WACHOLDER S. 1991. Practical considerations in choosing between the case-cohort and nested case-control designs. Epidemiology 2:155–158.

WAGNER J, PORTWINE C, RABIN K, LECLERC JM, NAROD SA, MALKIN D. 1994. High frequency of germline p53 mutations in childhood adrenocortical cancer. J Natl Cancer Inst 86:1707–1710.

WEEKS DE, LANGE K. 1988. The affected-pedigree-member method of linkage analysis. Am J Hum Genet 42:315–326.

WEEKS DE, LEHNER T, SQUIRES-WHEELER E, KAUFMANN C, OTT J. 1990. Measuring the inflation of the LOD score due to its maximization over model parameter values in human linkage analysis. Genet Epidemiol 7:237–243.

WHELAN AJ, BARTSCH D, GOODFELLOW PJ. 1995. Brief report: a familial syndrome of pancreatic cancer and melanoma with a mutation in the CDKN2 tumor-suppressor gene. N Engl J Med 333:975–977.

WHITTEMORE AS, HALPERN J. 1994. A class of tests for linkage using affected pedigree members. Biometrics 50:118–128.

WILHELMSSON A, CATHILL S, DENIS M, WILHELMSSON AC, GUSTUFFSON JA, POELLINGER L. 1990. The specific DNA binding activity of the dioxin receptor is modulated by the 90 kd heat shock protein. EMBO J 9:69–76.

WILLIAMSON JA, AMOS CI. 1990. On the asymptotic behavior of the estimate of the recombination fraction under the null hypothesis of no linkage when the model is misspecified. Genet Epidemiol 7: 309–318.

WITKOP CJ, QUEVEDO WC, FITZPATRICK TB, KING RA. 1989. Albinism. In: *The Metabolic Basis of Inherited Disease,* 6th ed, Scriver CL, Beaudet AL, Sly WS, Valle D (eds). New York: McGraw Hill, pp 2905–2948.

WOOSTER R, NEUHAUSEN SL, MANGION J, QUIRK Y, FORD D, COLLINS N, NGUYEN K, SEAL S, TRAN T, AVERILL D, FIELDS P, MARSHALL G, NAROD S, LENOIR GM, LYNCH H, FEUNTEUN J, DEVILEE P, CORNELISSE CJ, MENKO FH, DALY PA, ORMISTON W, MCMANUS R, PYE C, LEWIS CM, CANNON-ALBRIGHT LA, PETO J, PONDER BAJ, SKOLNICK MH, EASTON DF, GOLDGAR DE, STRATTON MR. 1994. Localization of a breast cancer susceptibility gene, BRCA2, to chromosome 13q12-13. Science 265:2088–2090.

WOOSTER R, FORD D, MANGION J, PONDER BAJ, PETO J, EASTON DF, STRATTON MR. 1993. Absence of linkage to the ataxia telangiectasia locus in familial breast cancer. Hum Genet 92:91–94.

XIAO Z-X, CHEN J, LEVINE AJ, MODJTAHEDI N, XING J, SELLERS WR, LIVINGSTON DM. 1995. Interaction between the retinoblastoma protein and the oncoprotein MDM2. Nature 375:691–698.

XU H-J, XU K, ZHOU Y, LI J, BENEDICT WF, HU S-X. 1994. Enhanced tumor cell growth suppression by an N-terminal truncated retinoblastoma protein. Proc Natl Acad Sci USA 91:9837–9841.

YIN Y, TAINSKY MA, BISCHOFF FZ, STRONG LC, WAHL GM. 1992. Wild-type p53 restores cell cycle control and inhibits gene amplification in cells with mutant p53 alleles. Cell 70:937–948.

ZHAO LP, LE MARCHAND L. 1992. An analytical method for assessing patterns of familial aggregation in case-control studies. Genet Epidemiol 9:141–154.

PART IV | Cancer by Tissue of Origin

28 Cancers of the nasal cavity and paranasal sinuses

GEORGE C. ROUSH

Cancer of the nose and paranasal sinuses (sinonasal cancer, or SNC) affects fewer than one in a thousand persons in their lifetime. This low absolute risk in the general population has been accompanied by high relative risks for specific chemical exposures and occupational settings, such as nickel refining and woodworking. The histologic, preneoplastic, and etiologic features of SNC are distinct from those head and neck cancers arising in contiguous sites. For these reasons, SNC has been designated a "sentinel cancer" that may permit the identification of environmental cancer risk factors (Rutstein et al, 1983; Olsen, 1988).

New data have accumulated on dysplasia in relation to putative carcinogenic agents and on rhinitis and nasal polyps as potential markers of risk for this cancer. Also, the age distribution of SNC and other types of data suggest that estrogens may play a role in the etiology of this nongynecologic cancer (Roush et al, 1987a; Roush et al, 1987a).

DEMOGRAPHIC PATTERNS

Histopathology and Anatomic Distribution

The anatomic boundaries of the sinonasal region are described in a standardized staging manual for this and other cancers (American Joint Committee on Cancer, 1983). Anteriorly, the nasal cavity borders on the skin of the nose. Posteriorly, the nasal cavity joins the nasopharynx; the two regions can be demarcated by a line from the posterior portion of the hard palate to the base of the skull. The inferior portion of the maxillary sinus is to be distinguished from the oropharynx.

Misclassification of SNC with cancers of surrounding anatomic sites may affect observed population-based incidence and mortality rates and may also affect reported etiologic correlates. The designation "nasal cancer" might conceivably be given to a cancer of the skin of the nose (ICDO 173.3), cancer of the nasopharynx (NPC, ICDO 147), or cancer of the internal nares (ICDO 160.0). Since 1950, more than 85% of sinonasal cancers in the Connecticut Tumor Registry have been confirmed microscopically (Roush, 1987a).

For many cancers of the head and neck, key etiologic differences depend on distinguishing cancers that arise only a few millimeters away. Table 28-1 places SNC anatomically and histologically in the context of tumors arising in these adjacent areas. The normal epithelium of most of the sinonasal region is characterized by ciliated, pseudostratified columnar epithelium, which includes a substantial number of goblet cells that permit mucus secretion (Guerkink, 1983). The sinonasal respiratory epithelium creates a mucociliary blanket that allows clearance of particulate matter. Benign and premalignant lesions of the sinonasal region include nasal polyps, which are extremely common, and the inverted papilloma (Osborn, 1970, 1982). In most regions of the world, the most common histology of SNC is squamous cell carcinoma, with a fraction occurring as adenocarcinoma.

The predominant histopathology of SNC in the U.S. SEER Program is represented by squamous and undifferentiated carcinomas (Table 28-2). An interesting observation in condensing the data in Table 28-2 is the relative deficit of squamous and undifferentiated carcinomas in women (121/255, or 47%, in women versus 64% in men). The sex differences are particularly striking for melanomas and esthesioneurocytomas.

The most common subsites for SNC are the nasal cavity (ICDO 160.0) and the maxillary sinus (ICDO 160.2), which together constitute roughly fourth-fifths of all SNC (Roush, 1978; Muir and Nectoux, 1980) (Table 28-3). The ethmoid sinus (ICDO 160.3) is generally the next most common subsite, while cancers of the internal and middle ear, frontal sinus, and sphenoid sinus (ICDO 160.1, 160.4, and 160.5, respectively) are extremely rare. In most industrialized populations, the distribution is typical of that described above. Some geographic deviations from these patterns are noted in

TABLE 28–1. *Differences in Histopathologic Features between the Sinonasal Region and Adjacent Anatomic Sites**

Anatomic Site (ICDO)	Histopathologic Feature: Characteristic Normal Epithelium	Examples of Benign Neoplasms or Putative Precursors	Histology of Malignant Neoplasms	Prominent Etiologic Correlates
1. Skin of nose and cheek (contained in ICDO 173.3)	Keratinized stratified squamous	Actinic keratosis; lentigo malignant	Basal cell; keratinized squamous cell; lentigo malignant melanoma	Chronic sun exposure
2. Sinonasal region; (nasal cavity; maxillary sinus; ethmoids; and other sinuses (160)	Pseudostratified ciliated columnar; goblet cells; stratified squamous	Nasal polyps; inverted papilloma	Squamous cell; adenocarcinoma; melanoma; ethesioneurocytoma	Nickel refining; woodworking; other occupational chemical exposures
3. Nasopharynx (147)	Stratified squamous; pseudostratified ciliated columnar; "transitional"	Epithelial dysplasia	Squamous cell; lymphoepithelioma; transitional cell carcinoma	Epstein-Barr virus; salted fish
4. Oropharynx (141–145)	Stratified squamous epithelium	Oral leukoplakia	Squamous cell	Tobacco and alcohol

*General references: Ash (1964); American Joint Committee on Cancer (1983); Schottenfeld and Fraumeni (1982); Young et al (1981). Specific references corresponding to number: 1. Osborn (1970); Snyder and Perzin (1972); 2. Ashley (1978); 3. Yu et al (1986); Armstrong et al (1983); 4. WHO Collaborating Centre for Oral Precancer Lesions (1978).

TABLE 28–2. *Histology of Sinonasal Cancer, U.S. SEER Program, All Areas, Excluding Puerto Rico, 1973–1977**

Histology	Total	Men	Women
Squamous and undifferentiated carcinomas	344	223	121
Transitional cell carcinomas	27	16	11
Adenocarcinomas	94	47	47
Melanoma	19	5	14
Esthesioneurocytoma and neuroblastoma	17	5	12
Sarcomas	27	14	13
Other	6	4	2
Carcinoma, NOS	69	34	35
Total	603	348	255

*Data from Young et al (1981).

Table 28-4. In the High Wycomb area of Bucks, England (Hadfield, 1970), the distribution is characterized by the predominance of adenocarcinoma of the ethmoid sinus, presumably as a result of occupational wood dust exposure; in Japan and in Nigeria, cancers of the paranasal sinuses are diagnosed far more commonly than cancers of the nasal cavity. In Africa, the predominance of cancer of the maxillary sinus may be due to the occurrence of Burkitt's lymphoma, an aggressive form of non-Hodgkin's lymphoma.

Incidence, Mortality, Survival, and Second Primary Cancers

The age-adjusted incidence rates for SNC in the United States are 0.5 to 0.7 per 100,000 annually, occurring

TABLE 28–3. *Incident Cases of SNC by Anatomic Site in the U.S. SEER Program, 1973–1977 (All Areas Excluding Puerto Rico)**

		All Races			White			Black			Other		
	%	Total	Men	Women	Total	Men	Women	Total	Men	Women	Total	Men	Women
Nasal cavity (160.0)	37.6	233	140	93	197	118	79	13	8	5	23	14	9
Middle ear (160.1)	4.5	28	12	16	26	12	14	1	0	1	1	0	1
Maxillary sinus (160.2)	41.4	256	144	112	193	106	87	34	25	9	29	13	16
Ethmoid sinus (160.3)	7.8	48	28	20	44	26	18	0	0	0	4	2	2
Frontal sinus (160.4)	1.5	9	4	5	7	3	4	1	1	0	1	0	1
Sphenoid sinus (160.5)	2.1	13	11	2	13	11	2	0	0	0	0	0	0
Other (160.8)	2.7	17	8	9	15	7	8	0	0	0	2	1	1
Accessory sinus, NOS (160.9)	2.4	15	8	7	13	6	7	1	1	0	1	1	0
Total	100.0	619	355	264	508	289	219	50	35	15	61	31	30

*From Young et al (1981).

TABLE 28–4. *Percentage of Cancers across Subsites of the Sinonasal Region in Selected Population-based Incidence Registries**

	Geographic Region									
	TNCS, USA		*Birmingham, UK*		*Oxford, UK*		*Ibadan, Nigeria*		*Osaka, Japan*	
Anatomic Subsite of SNC	*Men*	*Women*	*Men*	*Women*	*Men*	*Women*	*Men*	*Women*	*Men*	*Women*
Nasal cavity	41.6%	54.0%	26.2%	23.9%	12.3%	18.5%	0.0%	0.0%	2.8%	2.7%
Maxillary sinus	40.2%	29.3%	53.0%	47.8%	59.7%	48.2%	56.3%	63.6%	92.2%	96.6%
Ethmoids and other sinuses	13.0%	12.0%	11.6%	13.6%	26.3%	22.2%	37.5%	36.4%	3.1%	0.0%
Eustachian tube	5.2%	4.7%	9.2%	14.7%	1.7%	11.1%	6.2%	0.0%	1.9%	0.7%
Total:	100.0%	100.0%	100.0%	100.0%	100.0%	100.0%	100.0%	100.0%	100.0%	100.0%

*Data extracted from Muir and Nectoux (1980).

more commonly among men than among women (Table 28-5). From these data and from trends in incidence and mortality (Roush et al, 1987a, 1987c; McKay et al, 1982; Young et al, 1981), estimates for the entire U.S. for the year 1990 can be computed as approximately 550 deaths from this cancer and 1,600 new cases. In the absence of competing causes of death, the lifetime cumulative probability of contracting SNC can be estimated from these same sources as 0.1% for men and 0.07% for women.

TABLE 28–5. *Descriptive Epidemiology of Sinonasal Cancer**

Males			*Females*	
HIGH INCIDENCE				
Hong Kong		3.2	India, Poona	1.5
France, Doubs		2.7	Switzerland, Neuchatel	1.4
India, Poona		2.2	New Mexico, Amerind	1.4
Shanghai		2.2	Shanghai	1.3
Brazil, Sao Paulo		2.2	Colombia, Cali	1.3
Hawaii, Chinese		2.1	Hong Kong	1.2
Japan, Miyagi		2.1	Bay Area, Chinese	1.2
Japan, Nagasaki		2.0	Japan, Nagasaki	1.1
Japan, Osaka		1.8	Poland, Cieszyn	1.1
Switzerland, Geneva		1.7	Japan, Osaka	1.0
LOW INCIDENCE				
Alameda County, White		0.4	Israel, born Europe	0.2
Romania, County Cluj		0.3	Canada, Saskatchawan	0.2
Hungary, Szabol		0.3	Singapore, Malay	0.1
Canada, Saskatchewan		0.3	UK, no Scotland	0.1
Canada, Maritime Provinces		0.3	Spain, Zaragoza	0.1
Senegal, Dakar		0.3	Atlanta, Black	0.1
Bay Area, Chinese		0.2	Hawaii, White	0.0
Atlanta, Black		0.0	Spain, Navarra	0.0
Bay Area, Japanese		0.0	Israel, born Israel	0.0
Canada, Yukon		0.0	Canada, Yukon	0.0
U.S. SEER incidence rates[a] per 100,000 per year, 1986–90	Whites	0.7		0.5
	Blacks	0.9		0.6
U.S. mortality rates per 1000,000 per year, 1986–90[a]	Whites	0.2		0.1
	Blacks	0.4		0.1
U.S. SEER relative 5-year survival rates (%), 1983–89[a]	Whites	57.7		54.7
	Blacks	23.3		30.5

*World variation, 1973–1977, incidence rate per 100,000 age-adjusted to 1970 world population. Data from Waterhouse et al (1982).
[a]Data from Miller et al (1993); incidence and mortality rates are age-adjusted to 1970 U.S. standard population.

TABLE 28–6. *Percentage in Each Stage and 5-Year Relative Survival Rates in the U.S. SEER Program, 1979**

Stage	Stage Distribution (%)	5-Year Relative Survival (%)
Localized	31.0	70.0[a]
Regional	40.0	45.0
Remote	22.0	26.0
Unknown	7.0	64.0[a]
All categories	(100%, n = 714)	50.0%

*All persons, cancer of the nose and paranasal sinuses (NCI, Division of Cancer Prevention and Control, 1988).
[a]Standard error of the survival rate was 5% to 10%.

The highest incidence rates have been reported among men in Hong Kong (3.2 per 100,000 annually). In the United States, American Indian women have rates around 1.4 per 100,000 annually, although this rate may be unstable.

Nasal congestion is a typical presenting symptom, and when the tumor involves the maxillary sinus, an Xray may show evidence of fluid and of bony erosion. Chemotherapy and radiation are primarily palliative. The relative 5-year survival rate for persons diagnosed in the SEER Program is 50% (Table 28-6). Although numbers are limited for study of survival rates, the available data suggest poorer survival among blacks than whites in the United States (National Cancer Institute, Division of Cancer Prevention and Control, 1988); these results are consistent with the somewhat less favorable incidence-to-mortality ratio among blacks as compared to whites.

Studies of second primary cancers following a diagnosis of SNC suggest associations with other respiratory cancers but little association with cancers of the mouth and pharynx (Boice and Fraumeni, 1985; Olsen, 1985). In women, cancer of the breast occurs more frequently following a diagnosis of SNC, as found in studies of second primaries in Connecticut and in Denmark, as summarized in Table 28-7.

Population studies of broad occupational categories indicate higher rates among laborers; although cancers of the mouth and pharynx are also relatively more common among lower socioeconomic groups, the pattern for cancers of the mouth and pharynx may differ from that for SNC (see Fig. 28-1).

Time Trends

SNC has shown little change in population-based long-term incidence rates since the 1940s, as shown in Figures 28-2a and 28-2b. In contrast to incidence rates, population-based mortality rates in the United States have shown declines by year of birth, as shown in Figure 28-2b. Similar overall patterns have been observed in Canada and in Denmark (Ayiomayitis et al, 1988; Olsen, 1987).

Age Trends

The median age of diagnosis is 63 in men and 65 in women in the U.S. SEER program in 1986–1990 (Hiller, 1993). Population-based rates for SNC increase with age (Waterhouse, 1974; Roush, 1978; Redmond et al, 1982). Population-based Connecticut incidence and U.S. mortality rates have since been modeled to account for changes by year of birth (Roush, 1987a, 1987c). As with other adult epithelial nongynecologic cancers, this approach shows a roughly linear increase of the incidence rate with age on the log-log scale, particularly among males (Fig. 28-3). Rates for females also show an increase with age, but there is a pause in this increase for women around the age of 50 (Fig. 28-3). The pause in this increase occurs in both Connecticut incidence and U.S. mortality data (Fig. 28-3), and the difference in male and female age trends is statistically significant

TABLE 28–7. *Second Primary Cancers after a Diagnosis of SNC*

Site of Second Primary Cancer	Connecticut, 1935–1982			Denmark, 1943–1980		
	Observed	Expected	Ratio	Observed	Expected	Ratio
All sites	43	32.18	1.3	58	47.38	1.2
Buccal cavity and pharynx	2	1.27	1.6	0	1.17	0.0
Gastrointestinal	7	10.22	0.7	19	16.85	1.1
Respiratory	10	4.98	2.0[a]	12	7.37	1.6[a]
Female breast	6	2.66	2.3[a]	6	3.57	1.7
Female genital tract	2	1.61	1.2	2	3.14	0.6
Lymphopoietic and hematopoietic	5	2.11	2.4[a]	4	2.94	1.4[a]
Other sites	6	7.76	0.8	14	10.82	1.3

[a]The authors noted the elevations for these cancers in presenting the results (Boice and Fraumeni, 1985; Olsen, 1985).

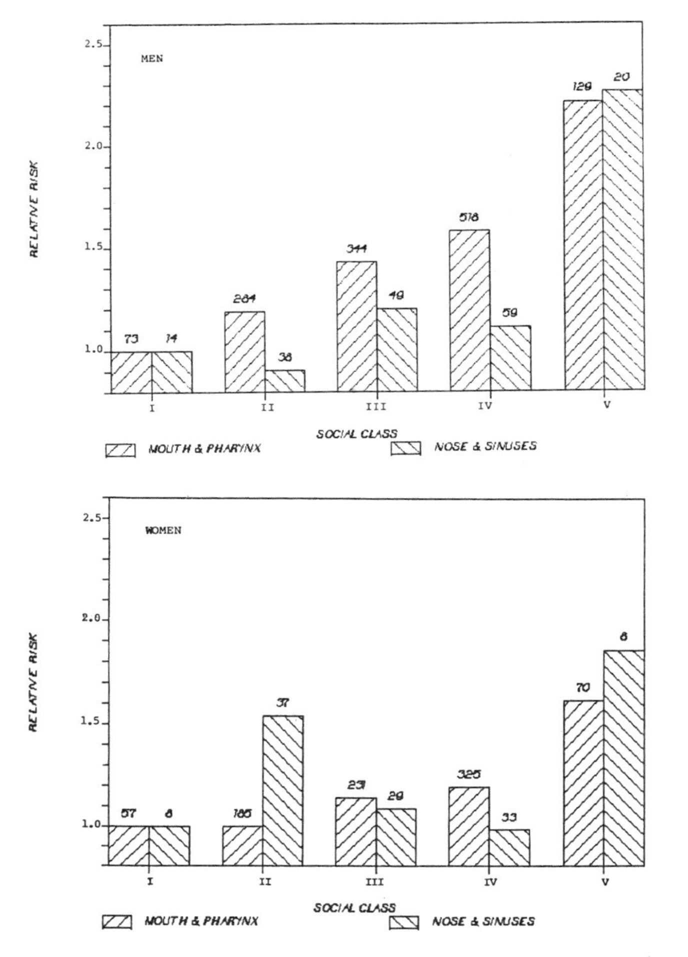

FIG. 28–1. Social class and relative risks of mouth and pharynx and sinonasal cancers, Los Angeles County, California, 1972–1978, whites only (from Preston-Martin et al, 1982).

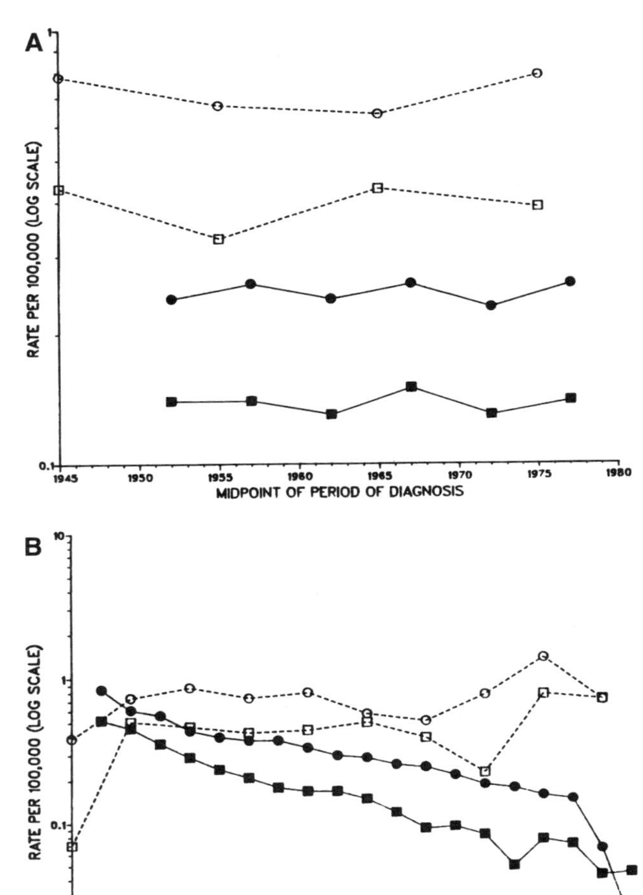

FIG. 28–2(A). Age-adjusted incidence rates (Connecticut) and mortality (United States) for sinonasal cancer by time period based on an age-period-cohort model. Linear effect of period is assumed to equal zero. ● Male mortality, US whites; ■ female mortality, US whites; ○ male incidence; □ female incidence. (B) Age-adjusted rates for sinonasal cancer by birth cohort for Connecticut incidence and US mortality based on age-period-cohort model. ● Male mortality, US whites; ■ female mortality, US whites; ○ male incidence, Connecticut; □ female incidence, Connecticut.

(Roush et al, 1987a). Review of other previously published descriptive studies reveals an apparent deficit in risk among women after age 50 in the U.S. Third National Cancer Survey (Redmond et al, 1982), and in data from England (Waterhouse, 1974) and from Japan (Hiyama et al, 1983). This change in risk may be compared to the menopausal hook in female breast cancer (Roush et al, 1987a, 1987b) and is discussed in this chapter under "Host Factors."

EXOGENOUS FACTORS

For most human cancers, tobacco and dietary agents are the most important known etiologic factors (Doll and Peto, 1981; Roush et al, 1987a) and occupational agents are responsible for less than 6%. For SNC, however, cigarette smoking is less important, dietary factors have not been identified, and occupational agents are particularly prominent. Table 28-8 summarizes studies of specific exposures, primarily in the occupational setting and usually of the retrospective cohort type. Since the early 1980s, there have been at least 10 case-control studies adding knowledge of occupational factors and cigarette smoking, as seen in Table 28-9.

Tobacco

Most information regarding the role of tobacco in the etiology of SNC is derived from descriptive epidemiol-

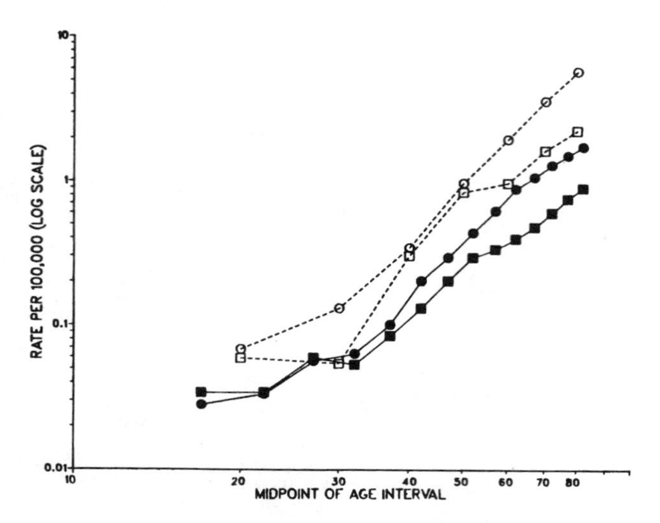

FIG. 28–3. Time-adjusted rates for sinonasal cancer by age for Connecticut (incidence) and the United States (mortality), based on an age-period-cohort model. ● Male mortality, US whites; ■ female mortality, US whites; ○ male incidence, Connecticut; □ female incidence, Connecticut.

ogy and from case-control studies. The socioeconomic pattern of SNC does not consistently follow the pattern of a smoking-related tumor, such as cancer of the mouth and pharynx. Second, tobacco-related cancers of the upper aerodigestive tract, including cancers of the pharynx and larynx, have increased over the decades. For example, for cohorts from 1875 through 1925, lung cancer has increased 5- to 20-fold, while cancers of the larynx, pharynx, and esophagus have increased 1.5- to 5-fold (Roush et al, 1987c). In contrast, incidence rates for SNC have shown no change over the same 50 years of birth cohorts (Fig. 28-2b). Studies of second primary tumors fail to support correlations of smoking-related tumors in the same way that cancers of the pharynx, larynx, esophagus, and lung are intercorrelated, as shown in Table 28-7 (Boice and Fraumeni, 1985; Olsen, 1985). Finally, the case-control studies show either no associations (as in the large detailed study of Hernberg et al (1983) in three Nordic countries) or only a moderate elevation in risk, and usually limited to the squamous or undifferentiated carcinomas (see Table 28-9). When showing an association, odds ratios have ranged from 1.4 to 3.3 (Ng, 1986; Shimizu et al, 1989; Zheng et al, 1993; Fukuda and Shibata, 1988; Leclerc et al, 1994).

Two other exposures include a possible relationship of SNC to passive smoking (Hirayama, 1984) and to intranasal snuff use (Harrison, 1967; Keen, 1974). There are very few controlled data available on either of these two types of exposures.

Nickel

The earlier studies of specific industrial cohorts in Norway, England, and Canada suggested that the risk for SNC associated with nickel exposure arose in the course of the nickel-refining process. Studies of nickel in the manufacturing setting have failed to yield risks that begin to approach those found in nickel refining (see Table 28-9; Hernberg et al, 1983; Roush et al, 1980; Brinton et al, 1984). Four workers in the United States who processed nickel matte imported from the Canadian nickel-smelting operation appeared to have developed SNC (Enterline and Marsh, 1982). In Norway, the risk for lung cancer from nickel refining appears to have been sustained, while that for SNC has declined dramatically (Magnus et al, 1982). An effect of nickel refining in combination with cigarette smoking has been postulated (Magnus et al, 1982).

Chromium

SNC has been associated with hexavalent chromate in pigment manufacturing but not with uses of chromium such as in plating processes. Case-control studies of SNC have not uncovered risks for SNC due to this exposure, though the prevalence of the occupational exposure index in any one of the studies may be low or correlated with other occupational factors.

Polyaromatic Hydrocarbons

Polyaromatic hydrocarbons are common to four different occupational processes associated with SNC, namely, petroleum-producing counties (Blot et al, 1977), furnace oven workers and coke production (Bruusgaard, 1959; Acheson et al, 1981), and mineral oil in metal-cutting occupations (Roush et al, 1980, 1982). These risks appear to have been reduced (Roush et al, 1980). Associations between SNC and metal industries have been noted in Denmark (Olsen, 1988). Although four- and five-ring aromatic hydrocarbons are causally linked in cancers of the skin and respiratory tract, current exposures may be relatively uncommon so as to prevent detection of elevations in risk for SNC in epidemiologic studies.

Formaldehyde

Formaldehyde produces nasal cancers in rodents exposed to formaldehyde vapor (Albert et al, 1982). The widespread ambient exposures (e.g., via particleboard and insulation) have led to substantial interest in risk

TABLE 28–8. *Studies of Specific Agents Suspected of Causing SNC**

Occupational Setting[a]	Suspect Carcinogen	Cases of SNC	Relative Risk	Anatomic Site	Histology	Mean Latent Period[b]	Other Cancers Associated with the Exposure
OCCUPATIONAL AGENTS CORRELATED WITH SINONASAL CANCER, ALSO HAVING LABORATORY CONFIRMATION							
1. Nickel refining	Metallic nickel, nickel subsulfide oxide or carbonyl	143	Up to 800	Nose, ethmoids	Squamous, Anaplastic	24 years (5–40)	Lung, larynx
2. Chrome pigment manufacturing	Calcium chromate zinc potassium chromate	9	21	Sinuses, nose	Adenocarcinoma and not specified	—[c]	Lung
3. Dial painting	Radium	4	—	Antrum	Squamous	23 years (18–27)	Osteosarcoma Mastoid carcinoma
4. Mustard gas manufacturing	BB-dichlorethyl sulfide	3	30+	Sphenoid	Squamous	25 years (23–28)	Tongue, pharynx, larynx, lung
5. Isopropyl alcohol manufacturing	Isopropyl oil diisopropyl sulfate	6	21+	Ethmoid	Adenocarcinoma and not specified	<20 years	Larynx
6. Gas manufacture	Hydrocarbons	3		Paranasal sinuses	—	—	Lung, larynx, pharynx, bladder, Esophagus
OCCUPATIONAL AGENTS CORRELATED WITH SINONASAL CANCER IN EPIDEMIOLOGIC STUDIES, WITHOUT LABORATORY CONFIRMATION							
7. Furniture and other woodworking	Wood dust (hard woods) (beech, oak)	100+	3–80+	Ethmoids, nasal cavity	Adenocarcinoma	43 years (27–69)	None
8. Boot and shoe manufacturing and repair	Leather or wood constituents	88+	2–87	Ethmoids, nasal cavity	Adenocarcinoma Squamous	55 years 42 years	None
9. Textile and clothing manufacturing	Wool dust constituents	40+	2–8	—	Adenocarcinoma and melanoma	—	Tongue, mouth, pharynx
10. Chemical and petroleum manufacturing	Nitrosamines dioxane, PAH, Ni catalysts	—	Up to 3	—	—	—	Lung, larynx, skin, bladder, liver, bone
NONOCCUPATIONAL AGENTS SUSPECTED OF CAUSING SINONASAL CANCER							
11. Thorium dioxide for X-ray diagnosis	Mesothorium alpha, beta	14	—	Antrum	Squamous mucoepidermoid	17 (10–21)	Liver, kidney, pancreas, bone

*Updated from Roush (1979) and Redmond et al (1982)

[a]References from which data were obtained:

1. Chief Inspector of Factories Bridge (1933), Committee on Medical and Biological Effects of Environment Pollution (1975), Doll (1958), Doll et al (1970a), Hill (1939), Hueper (1966, 1979), Morgan (1958), NIOSH (1977), Ottolengi et al (1975), Grenfell (1932), Pedersen et al (1973), Sunderman (1963, 1968, 1973, 1976, 1977), Sunderman and Donnelly (1965), Sunderman and Sunderman (1963), Magnus et al (1982), Enterline & Marsh (1982), Andrews (1983).
2. Enterline (1974), Hueper (1966), Langard and Forseth (1975), Levy (1975), Newman (1890), Schoental (1975), Davies (1991).
3. Aub et al (1952), Brues and Kirsh (1977), Rowland (1975), Polednak et al (1978).
4. Heston and Levillian (1953), Wada et al (1968).
5. Eckardt (1974), IARC Working Group (1976), NIOSH (1976), Weil et al (1952).
6. Bruusgaard (1959), Hueper (1966).
7. Acheson et al (1967, 1968, 1972), Anderson et al (1977), Brinton et al (1977), Curtes et al (1977), Debois (1969), Fombeur (1972), Gignoux and Bernard (1969), Hadfield (1970), Haguenauer et al (1977), Ironside and Matthews (1975), and see Table 28.9 for recent case-control studies of woodworking.
8. Acheson et al (1976), Acheson et al (1975), Hadfield (1972), and see Table 28.9 for case-control studies. Boot and shoe industries are not strongly related to SNC in the United States (DeCoufle and Walrath, 1987).
9. Acheson et al (1972) and see Table 28.9 for case-control studies.
10. Blot et al (1977), Hoover and Fraumeni (1975), and see Table 28.9 for case-control studies.
11. Baserga et al (1960), Hasterlik et al (1964), Hofer (1952), Rankow et al (1974), Rubin (1972).

[b]Mean latent period: time of first exposure to time of cancer incidence (range given in parentheses).

[c]A dash (—) indicates that data were not available.

TABLE 28–9. *Case-control Studies of SNC**

Methods	*Wood Dust*	*Formaldehyde*	*Cigarette Smoking*	*Other*
Denmark, Sweden, Finland, 1977–1980. SNC cases: 66% men, 11% adenocarcinoma. Controls: 167 colorectal cancer. Personal interview. (Hernberg et al, 1983)	All SNC: 4.5 Aenoca: >9 Hardwood was key exposure adenoca	Exposure to wood dust hindered evaluation	Any: 0.7 (.5, 1.1). 1+ PPD: 0.8 (.4, 1.6)	Lacquers and paints: 14+ Welding etc: 2.8 Chromium: 2.7 Nickel: 2.4
Denmark, 1970–1982. SNC cases: 67% men. Controls: Cancer of colorectum, prostate, breast. Record linkage for occupational information. (Olsen et al, 1984)	All SNC: 2.5. No important effects by adjustment for formaldehyde index	All SNC: 2.8, reduced to 1.6 after adjustment for wood dust	No information	Paint, etc: 1.6–2.1 Leather: 1.7 Chlorphenols: Men: 1.4/Wom: 0.5 Textiles: Men: 0.7/Wom: 1.3 Asbestos: 1.5 Metal work: 1.4 Plastics manufacturing: Men: 1.1/Wom: 2.8
Sweden, 1970–1979. SNC: N = 44, all men, 11% adenocarcinoma. Controls: Sarcoma and lymphoma patients. Mail questionnaire. (Hardell et al, 1982)	2.0 (1.1–3.6)	Not studied	1.0 (0.6–2.0)	Phenoxy acids and chlorpenols: 2.2 (1.0–4.8) Asbestos: 1.7(0.6–4.7)
Netherlands, 1978–1981. SNC, N = 91, 100% men, 25% adenocarcinoma. Controls, N = 259. Home interview. (Hayes et al, 1986a, 1986b)	All SNC: 2.5 (1.4–4.6) Adenocarcinoma: All wood: 17.6 (6.9–49.2) Furniture and cabinet makers: 139.8 (31.6–999.4)	Two independent classifiers: A & B. Any exposure: A: 2.5 (1.2–5.0) B: 1.6 (0.9–2.8) Results suggested dose-response effect	"Moderate elevation in risk . . ." (alcohol not related)	Adenocarcinoma: Leather: 2.5 (0.4–11.7) Textiles: 1.8 (0.5–5.4) Squamous cell: Chemicals: 1.7 (0.4–11.7)
England and Wales, 1963–67. SNC, N = 1,602, 58% men, 8% adenocarcinoma. Controls: general population. Mail questionnaire to cases. Census for general population.[a] (Acheson et al, 1981)	All SNC:[a] 2.8 Adenocarcinoma: 4.5	Not reported here (see text)	Not reported	(These are SIRs) Leather: 4.4 Clothing: 2.1 Gas, coke and chemicals: 8.7 Furnace, forge, and rolling mills: 2.5 Furnacemen: >3.0 Rolling tube mill: 2.7 Printers: 5.3 Miners: 1.7
Sienna, Italy, 1963–1981. SNC cases, N = 36, all men, 25% adenocarcinoma. Controls, N = 164, from same medical clinic. Postal questionnaire. (Battista et al, 1983)	All SNC: 5.4 (1.7–17.2) Adenocarcinoma: 89.7 (19.8–407.3)	No information given	No information given	No information given
Lombardy, Italy, 1968–1982. SNC, N = 37. Controls, N = 74, from general population. Exposures from interview. (Merler et al, 1986)	Not reported	Not reported	Not reported	Exposure to leather dust: Men: 47.1 Women: 3.5. For low exposures, OR = 7.5. Higher for adenocarcinoma
British Columbia, Canada; Y: 1939–77. SNC, N = 121, all men. Controls from same clinics with cancer[b]. Exposures from chart review. (Elwood, 1981)	All SNC: Adjusted OR = 2.3	Not examined	Matched comparison: Classifying as nonsmokers those with no information on smoking: Includes sun-related controls: Smoking: Ex-, Light: Heavy:	Y N N N Y Y Y N N N N Y 3.5 2.1 2.3 1.9 5.3 2.1 2.3 1.7

(*continued*)

TABLE 28–9. *(Continued)*

Methods	*Wood Dust*	*Formaldehyde*	*Cigarette Smoking*	*Other*
British Columbia, Canada, 2.5-year period, SNC, N = 25, controls from same clinics, age-sex matched. Exposures from interview (Elwood, 1981)	Not reported	Not reported	"... No tionship with alcohol or tobacco ..."	Not reported
USA, North Carolina and Virginia, 1970–1980. SNC, N = 160, 58% men, 15% adenocarcinoma. Controls, N = 290, from same 4 hospitals as cases. Personal interview. (Brinton et al, 1977, 1984, 1985)	All SNC: Estimates vary by industry: 0.6 to 1.5. Adenocarcinoma: All industries: 3.7. Furniture: 5.7 (1.7–18.5)	1.4 (0.5–4.1)	All SNC: 1.2 (0.8–1.9) Adenocarcinoma: 0.6 Squamous: 1.8 For squamous, years smoked was associated with increasing risk from 1.7 to 3.0. (Alcohol not related)	Self-report of ENT conditions 10 years prior to diagnosis: Nasal polyps: 7.8 (2.0–30.0) Sinus trouble: 2.2 (1.3–3.7) Nosebleeds: 1.9 (1.1–3.2)
				Chemical manufacturing: 3.0 (1.0 .0) Mineral oils: 1.4 (0.5–4.1) Asbestos: 0.7 (0.3–1.8) Leather: 0.7 (0.2–2.0) Insecticides and herbicides: 1.3 (0.7–2.2)
Connecticut, 1935–1977. SNC, N = 198, dying of any cause, all men, 13% adenocarcinoma. Controls: non–lung cancer decedents. Death certificates and city directories gave job and industry. (Roush et al, 1980, 1987a)	4.0 (1.5–10.8)	No overall association to SNC; risk increased from 0.8 to 1.5 (0.6–3.9) increase in estimated level and latency	Not studied	Nickel: 0.7 (0.4–1.5) Cutters in rubber and paper: >4 Construction workers: >7
USA, Western Washington, 1979–1983. SNC, N = 53. >50% men, 11% adenocarcinoma. Controls: population-based. Personal interview. (Vaughan et al, 1986a, 1986b)	Not reported in detail in these reports	Overall occupational classification: no relationship, upper 95% confidence limits 1.3 to 2.9. Particleboard and plywood: 1.8 (0.9–3.8). Mobile home residence: 0.6 (0.2–1.7)	Not reported in detail in these reports	Not reported in detail in these reports
Tohoku, Univ. hosp., 10-year period, SNC, N = 107. Controls from same hospital. (Takasaka, 1987)	"No evidence"	Not reported	Not reported	Not reported
Hong Kong, 1974–1978. SNC, N = 225, 70% men, 2% adenocarcinoma. Controls, N = 225, were other cancers. Exposure based on medical record review. (Ng, 1986)	2 of 225 SNC versus 1 of 225 controls	Not evaluated	1.4 (0.9–2.3)	Textiles: 2.9 (1.1–7.9), higher among weavers (4.7) and among those with more than 15+ years employment
				Fisherman: 3.4 (1.3–8.9) Farmers: 1.9 (1.0–3.7) Construction: 1.9 (1.0–3.7)

(continued)

TABLE 28–9. *Case-control Studies of SNC* (Continued)*

Methods	*Wood Dust*	*Formaldehyde*	*Cigarette Smoking*	*Other*
Shanghai, China, 1988–1990. Population-based, 60 cases, 414 controls. In-person interview. (Zheng et al, 1992)	Wood dust exposure: 1.9 (0.7–5.0)	No increased risk	30+ years of cigarette smoking: 1.8 (0.7–4.9) for squamous cell cancer	Chronic nasal disease, onset 10+ years prior to diagnosis: 4.0 (2.1–7.4)
				Orange and tangerine intake, highest tertile: 0.4 (0.2–0.7) Salted food intake, highest tertile: 4.8 (2.2–10.5)
Northeast Japan, 1983–1985, Tohoku University. Squamous cell cancer of maxillary sinus, N = 66. 132 controls, sex-age-residence matched. Self-administered interview. (Shimizu et al, 1989)	In men, sanding or lathe work: 7.5 (1.5–38.5)	—	In men: 2.0 (0.6–6.2)	Chronic sinusitis 2.3 (1.0–5.5)
Hokkaido Island, Japan, 1982–1984. 116 maxillary sinus cancer (89% squamous cell), 232 controls, mathced on sex-age-residence. Self-administered interview. (Fukuda and Shibata, 1988)	In men, carpenter, furniture maker, or other woodworker: 2.9 (1.5–5.6)	—	In men, past or current cigarette smoking: 3.3 (1.3–8.1)	In men, for chronic sinusitis: 3.1 (1.4–6.7); for nasal polyps: 5.7 (1.7–18.6)
Verona and Vicenza provinces, Sienna, Italy, 1982–1987. 78 cases 254 controls, matched on sex-age-residence and date of admission. Personal interview. (Comba et al, 1992)	Wood industry: 5.8 (2.2–16)	—	—	Leather industry: 6.8 (1.9–25)
U.S., National Mortality Survey, 1% sample of U.S. deaths, 1985–86. N = 147 white men, controls = 449 dying from non-tobacco-related causes. Mail questionnaire to next of kin. (Zheng et al, 1993)	Carpenters and other wood-related occupations: 1.7 (0.6–4.3)	—	Cigarettes 35+ per day for 25+ years: 2.0 (1.0–4.0)	Daily alcohol use: 1.8 (1.0–3.3); Maxillary sinus cancer and vegetable intake: 0.5 (0.3–0.8); Maxillary sinus cancer and salted or smoked food: 2.7 (1.2–6.0)
France, 1986–1988, 27 hospitals. SNC: 207 (81% men). Controls: 409 (323 hospital controls, 86 friend controls). In-person interview. Exposure classified by an industrial hygienist (Luce, 1992; Lareo et al, 1992; Luce et al, 1993; Leclerc et al, 1994)	All results are for men.	*Adenocarcinomas*: in men exposed >20 years, after adjusting for age, wood dust, and glues: 6.9 (1.7–27.8)	—	*Adenocarcinomas*, in men with medium-heavy exposure to glues: 51.2 (19.0–138.0)
	Adenocarcinomas: Cabinetmakers: 35.4 (18.1–69.3) Carpenters: 25.2 (14.6–43.6) Woodworking machine operators: 7.4 (3.4–15.8); Exposed >35 years to hardwoods: 303 (64–1,427)			*Squamous carcinomas*: In men: A 10+ year history of sinusitis, bleeding from the nose, and nasal trauma gave a relative risk of 3-fold. Bakers: 3.9 (1.2–12.8) Construction workers: 3.7 (1.7–8.0) Farm workers: 2.2 (1.1–4.4)

(*continued*)

TABLE 28–9. *(Continued)*

Methods	*Wood Dust*	*Formaldehyde*	*Cigarette Smoking*	*Other*
	Squamous carcinomas: 15+ years as carpenters 8.1 (1.3–50.3) 16+ years exposed to hardwoods: 1.5 (0.6–3.5)			
				In Women: Textile workers: 9.5 (1.7–54.1) Farm workers: 4.9 (1.0–24.9)

*Numbers in the body of the table represent odds ratios unless otherwise indicated.

[a]The authors computed the SIR, the standardized incidence ratio; for consistency, these observed-to-expected ratios have been given as relative risk estimates in this table.

[b]Three comparison groups: Tumors related to neither smoking nor outdoor exposures (N = 121); tumors related to smoking or but not to outdoors (N = 119); tumors related to outdoors (N = 118).

assessment (Acheson, 1985). Epidemiologic studies have suggested associations most commonly with NPC (nasopharyngeal cancer) rather than with SNC (Vaughan et al, 1986a, 1986b; Blair et al, 1986; Blair et al, 1987). In the occupational setting, the study of Blair and colleagues obtained prior selected occupational exposures in different occupational settings (Blair et al, 1986). In residential exposures, Vaughan and colleagues (1986b) have conducted a study of SNC, nasopharyngeal cancer, and oropharyngeal cancer.

In a large case-control study in France, exposures to formaldehyde were determined after an hour-long in-person interview and classification by an industrial hygienist without knowledge of case-control status (Luce et al, 1993). Independent risks were determined for exposure to wood dust from hardwoods, exposures to glues, and exposures to formaldehyde. After adjustment for the former risk factors, exposure to formaldehyde for more than 20 years persisted as an independent risk factor for adenocarcinoma of the nasal cavity and sinuses: odds ratio 6.9 (95% confidence limits 1.7–27.8). Cigarette smoking was said to have little effect on the association. This comprehensive study is summarized in Table 20-9. The authors note the possibility, however, of residual confounding effects (Luce et al, 1993).

Wood Dust

SNC has now been associated with woodworking in many reports, including England, France, Denmark, Sweden, Finland, Norway, the Netherlands, Italy, the United States, Canada and Australia (references cited in Tables 28-8 and 28-9 and Demers et al, 1995). In three North American studies (Roush et al, 1980; Brinton et al, 1977, 1984; Elwood, 1981; Vaughan and Davies, 1991; Vaughan, 1989), the relative risks for SNC due to woodworking were 3- to 7-fold, considerably lower than the 8- to 40-fold or greater observed in the European studies.

However, the qualitative features of all of the studies, including those in North America, are similar: Wood dust exposure is associated with adenocarcinomas of the paranasal sinuses, particularly the ethmoid sinuses, and the highest risk appears to be among furniture and cabinet makers, as distinguished from general carpenters. Exposures to hardwoods, alone or in combination with softwoods, appear to be the most relevant (Hernberg, 1983; Leclerc et al, 1994). In France, exposure to hardwoods for more than 35 years was associated with adenocarcinomas, odds ratio 303, with lower 95% confidence limit of 64, whereas exposures to softwoods alone had no association with this cancer (Leclerc et al, 1994). The median latent period appears to be more than 40 years where length of exposure was considered (Acheson et al, 1982; Hayes et al, 1986b), and following termination of exposure, the risk for SNC may persist for many years. These observations imply that wood dust operates at an early stage of carcinogenesis.

Leather Dust and the Shoe Industry

Both Tables 28-8 and 28-9 suggest a strong association of SNC to occupations involving boot and shoe manufacture. Some of the exposures found in these industries (such as formaldehyde and tannins) may overlap with those found in woodworking, and it is interesting that the adenocarcinomas appear to be more strongly related to this type of exposure. Occupations in this industry have been strongly associated with SNC in the United States (DeCoufle and Walrath, 1987).

Radiation Exposure

Radiation exposure has been associated with SNC in radium dial painting and the medical instillation of thorotrast (Table 28-8). Licking brushes to moisten the tips for painting of watch dials apparently led to the absorption of radium particles via the lymphatics with uptake by the facial bones, followed by long-term radiation of the surrounding epithelium, including the epithelium of the paranasal sinuses. In the instance of thorotrast (thorium dioxide), the substance was used as a radio contrast agent and was injected intravenously, but was also instilled directly into the paranasal sinuses. Therapeutic radiation continues to be used in oncology, and represents another potential form of exposure to the sinonasal region.

Infectious Agent

A *viral etiology* for SNC has been suggested. Epstein-Barr virus may play a causal role in Burkitt's lymphoma, which involves the jaw and often the maxillary sinus. Epstein-Barr virus has also been associated with nasopharyngeal carcinoma, and the undifferentiated histology of this tumor has led to such an hypothesis for the undifferentiated carcinomas of SNC in Kenya, where this histology appears to be more common (Bjerregaard et al, 1992). AIDS-related Kaposi's sarcoma occurs in the head and neck region, including the sinonasal region (Fliss et al, 1992).

CONSTITUTIONAL FACTORS

Benign Nasal Conditions as Possible Markers of Increased Risk

It has been suspected for many years that there is a relationship of SNC to recurrent nasal polyps, and particularly to inverted papillomas, which tend to recur and which appear to undergo malignant transformation (Osborn, 1970; Osborn and Friedman, 1982). Epidemiologic studies in the last several years have provided some support for this observation (Fukuda and Shibata, 1988; Lareo et al, 1992). These recent studies have attempted to address the possibility that occult undiagnosed SNC is a cause of the benign sinusitis or in some fashion stimulates polyp recurrence. In a case-control interview study, Brinton et al (1984) found a 2- to 7-fold increase in risk for SNC in those with long-standing (10+ years) history of polyps, sinusitis, and nosebleeds. In Japan, Hiyama et al (1983) have conducted both case-control and prospective studies. In the case-control investigation, risk for SNC from chronic sinusitis was estimated as at least 3-fold, with documentation of chronic sinusitis by three methods: medical records, physical exam, and Xray. In prospective data, patients with recurrent polyps have developed SNC years following removal of benign polyps (Hiyama et al, 1983).

Estrogenic Hormones

Estrogenic hormones have been hypothesized to alter risk for SNC with possible reduction in risk postmenopausally (Roush et al, 1987a, 1987b). This hypothesis is consistent with five different types of observation: (1) the observed deficit in risk for SNC among women in their 50s as noted earlier in Figure 28-3 (i.e., similar to the Clemmesen's hook in breast cancer associated with menopause); (2) the association of first primary SNC with second primary cancer of the breast in the two comprehensive studies in Connecticut and Denmark (see Table 28-5, as obtained from Boice and Fraumeni, 1985; and from Olsen, 1985); (3) changes in the respiratory epithelium of the head and neck with pregnancy and with menopause (Walker, 1976; Utiani, 1980), squamous metaplasia of the nasal epithelium and vasomotor rhinitis following prolonged estrogen administration in men (Harrison, 1957; Taylor, 1961), and the apparent existence of sex-hormone receptors on epithelial cells of the head and neck (Saez and Sakai, 1975; Molteni et al, 1981); (4) reduced risk for nasal cancer in ovariectomized rodents with induction of nasal cancer via intravenous nitrosamine injection (Pour and Goutz, 1983; Pour and Stepan, 1988); and (5) decreased serum dehydroepiandrosterone-sulfate in Kenyans with nasopharyngeal carcinoma as compared with controls (cited by Clifford, 1970, and see Wang et al, 1968). To our knowledge, an hypothesis involving estrogens in the etiology of SNC has not been evaluated in case-control or cohort studies.

CONCEPTS OF PATHOGENESIS

Any attempt to arrive at a unified concept of pathogenesis for SNC must account for substantial variability in clinical and etiologic features. For example, risk for the predominantly squamous and anaplastic carcinomas of the nasal cavities follows nickel-refining exposures with a median latent period of about 25 years and has dropped sharply following alteration of the sintering (heating agglomeration) process (Magnus et al, 1982), whereas the adenocarcinomas of the sinuses following wood dust and boot and shoe occupations have a median latent period of at least 40 years (Table 28-8).

Airborne exposures from particulates and vapors characterize several of the risk factors in Tables 28-8 and 28-9. The occurrence of cancers of the lung for five of these exposures suggests some deposition of carcinogen in the lower respiratory tract, whereas exposures in the wood industry and boot and shoe industry are unassociated with these lower respiratory tract cancers. Particles more than 5 mm in diameter tend to be trapped by the respiratory epithelium of the upper airways (Stokinger, 1977), and these physiologic features may explain the relative lack of lower respiratory cancers in dusty occupations such as woodworking.

Metaplasia of the pseudostratified ciliated columnar epithelium and subsequent dysplasia may occur (Boysen and Solberg, 1982; Edling et al, 1987) and predispose to SNC. Histopathologically, such a stage would bear some similarity to the metaplasia and dysplasia that occurs in cigarette smokers. Both respiratory routes of exposure and indirect systemic effects require consideration. Regarding systemic effects, there is the organ-specific carcinogenic effect of peripherally injected nitrosamines in rodents (Pour and Goutz, 1983; Pour and Stepan, 1988), and there is the possibility that estrogenic effects could lead to rhinitis, squamous metaplasia, and ciliary paralysis (Clifford, 1970). Because of the presence of the mucus-producing goblet cells and subsequent congestion, development of recurring polyps could also compromise the integrity of the epithelium.

Although concepts on the etiology of SNC stress the effects of particulates (regardless of chemical composition) and the morphologic alterations, it is important to recognize the specificity of effects. Wood dust is more effective than comparably sized plastic dust in slowing the mucociliary transport in nasal epithelium (Anderson et al, 1977). In a recent study involving rodents exposed to a variety of carcinogens, the irritant effects of the agent had little detectable correlation with its ability to induce cancer (Gardner et al, 1985). Finally, in animals, there is an organ-specific effect that is poorly understood (e.g., N-nitrosobis(2-oxopropyl)amine), and this effect may in some way depend on systemic endocrine factors (Pour and Goutz, 1983; Pour and Stepan, 1988).

PREVENTIVE MEASURES

Morbidity and mortality from SNC may be avoided in a high percentage of cases because in a number of populations, most of SNC has been attributable to a single occupational agent, such as woodworking. This concept of "avoidable risk" is worth noting (Doll and Peto, 1981). Perhaps the major obstacle to prevention of SNC is its overall rarity, even among those at high relative risk. In many occupational settings, relative risks for SNC tend to be much higher than for the more common cancers, such as cancers of lung, whereas lung cancers are far more important in absolute numbers. Better understanding of precursor conditions such as dysplasias and inverted papillomas might assist in identifying the subgroup of exposed persons at highest risk for SNC.

FUTURE RESEARCH

Two of the most important areas of research have to do with constitutional factors. It would be useful to obtain validation of the estimates of the risk for SNC in association with polyps and chronic sinusitis. Also, a thorough test of the hypothesis regarding effects of estrogens on risk for nasal cancer would be of interest. The latter problem could be evaluated by reproductive history and gynecologic history, as well as by more direct biochemical endocrine measures. As noted above, the development of squamous metaplasia and polyp formation might be related to endocrine status.

REFERENCES

ACHESON ED. 1976. Nasal cancer in the furniture and boot and shoe manufacturing industries. Prev Med 5:295–315.

ACHESON ED. 1985. Formaldehyde: epidemiological evidence. IARC Sci Publ (65):91–95.

ACHESON ED, COWDELL RH, HADFIELD E, et al. 1968. Nasal cancer in woodworkers in the furniture industry. Br Med J 2:587–596.

ACHESON ED, COWDELL RH, JOLLES B. 1975. Nasal cancer in the Northamptonshire boot and shoe industry. Br Med J 1:385–393.

ACHESON ED, COWDELL RH, RANG E. 1972. Adenocarcinoma of the nasal cavity and sinuses in England and Wales. Br J Ind Med 29:21–03.

ACHESON ED, COWDELL RH, RANG EH. 1981. Nasal cancer in England and Wales: an occupational survey. Br J Ind Med 38:218–224.

ACHESON ED, GARDNER MJ, PENNETT B, BARNES HR, OSMOND C, TAYLOR CP. 1984. Formaldehyde in the British chemical industry: an occupational cohort study. Lancet 1:611–616.

ACHESON ED, HADFIELD EH, MACBETH RG. 1967. Carcinoma of the nasal cavity and accessory sinuses in woodworkers. Lancet 1:311–312.

ACHESON ED, PIPPARD EC, WINTER PD. 1982. Nasal cancer in the Northamptonshire boot and shoe industry: Is it declining? Br J Cancer 46:940–946.

ALBERT RE, SELLAKUMAR AR, LASKIN S, et al. 1982. Gaseous formaldehyde and hydrogen chloride induction of nasal cancer in the rat. J Natl Cancer Inst 68(4):597–603.

AMERICAN JOINT COMMITTEE ON CANCER. 1983. Manual for Staging of Cancer. Philadelphia: Lippincott.

ANDERSON HC, ANDERSON I, SOLGAARD J. 1977. Nasal cancers, symptoms and upper airway function in woodworkers. Br J Ind Med 34:201–207.

ANDREWS P. 1983. Carcinomas of the nose and paranasal sinuses in former employees of a sinter plant at Copper Cliff, Ontario. J Otolaryngol 12(4):255–256.

ARMSTRONG RW, ARMSTRONG MJ, YU MC, et al. 1983. Salted fish and inhalants as risk factors for nasopharyngeal carcinoma in Malaysian Chinese. Cancer Res 43:2967–2970.

ASH JE, BECK MR, WOLKES JD. 1964. Tumors of the Upper Respiratory Tract and Ear. Washington, D.C.: Armed Forces Institute of Pathology.

ASHLEY DJB. 1978. Evans' Histologic Appearances of Tumors. Edinburgh: Churchill Livingstone.

AUB JC, EVANS RD, HEMPELMANN LH, et al. 1952. The late effects of internally deposited radioactive materials in man. Medicine 31:221–329.

AYIOMAMITIS A, PARKER L, HAVAS T. 1988. The epidemiology of malignant neoplasms of the nasal cavities, the paranasal sinuses and the middle ear in Canada. Arch Otorhinolaryngol 244(6):367–371.

BASERGA R, YOKOO H, HENEGAR GC. 1960. Thorotrast-induced cancer in man. Cancer 13:1021–1051.

BATTISTA G, CAVALLUCCI F, COMBA P, QUERCIA A, et al. 1983. A case-referent study on nasal cancer and exposure to wood dust in the province of Siena, Italy. Scand J Work Environ Health 9(1): 25–29.

BJERREGAARD B, OKOTH-OLENDA CA, GATEI D, et al. 1992. Tumours of the nose and maxillary sinus. Ten year survey from Kenya. J Laryngol Otol 106:337–341.

BLAIR A, STEWART P, O'BERG M, et al. 1986. Mortality among industrial workers exposed to formaldehyde. J Natl Cancer Inst 76:1071–1084.

BLAIR A, STEWART P, HOOVER RN, et al. 1987. Letter to the Editor: Cancers of the nasopharynx and oropharynx and exposure to formaldehyde. J Natl Cancer Inst 78:191–193.

BLOT WJ, BRINTON LA, FRAUMENI JF, et al. 1977. Cancer mortality in US countries with petroleum industries. Science 198:51–53.

BOICE JB, FRAUMENI JF, JR. 1985. Second cancer following cancers of the respiratory system in Connecticut, 1935–1982. NCI Monogr 68: NIH Pub. No. 85-2714, 68:83–98.

BOYSEN M, SOLBERG LA. 1982. Changes in the nasal mucosa of furniture workers. Scand J Work Environ Health 8:273–282.

BRIDGE JC. 1933. Annual Report of the Chief Inspector of Factories and Workshops for the Year 1932. London: Her Majesty's Stationery Office, pp. 103–104.

BRINTON L, BECKER J, BLOT WJ, HOOVER R, FRAUMENI J, JR. 1983. A case-control study of cancer of the nasal cavity and sinuses. Am J Epidemiol 118:436–437.

BRINTON LA, BLOT WJ, STONE BJ, et al. 1977. A death certificate analysis of nasal cancer among furniture workers in North Carolina. Cancer Res 37:3474.

BRINTON LA, BLOT WJ, BECKER JA, WINN DM, et al. 1984. A case-control study and cancers of the nasal cavity and paranasal sinuses. Am J Epidemiol 119(6):896–906.

BRINTON LA, BLOT WJ, FRAUMENI JF, JR. 1985. Nasal cancer in the textile and clothing industries. Br J Ind Med 42(7):469–474.

BRUES AM, KIRSH IE. 1977. The fate of individuals containing radium. Trans Am Clin Climatol Assoc 88:211–218.

BRUUSGAARD A. 1959. Occurrence of certain forms of cancer in gas workers. Tidsskr Nor Laegeioren 79:755–756.

CECCHI F, BUIATTI E, KRIEBEL D, et al. 1980. Adenocarcinoma of the nose and paranasal sinuses in shoemakers and woodworkers in the province of Florence, Italy (1963–1977). Br J Ind Med 37:4–14.

CLIFFORD P. 1970. On the epidemiology of nasopharyngeal carcinoma. Int J Cancer 5:287–309.

COMBA P, BATTISTA G, BELLI S, et al. 1992. A case-control study of cancer of the nose and paranasal sinuses and occupational exposures. Am J Ind Med 22:511–520.

COMMITTEE ON MEDICAL AND BIOLOGICAL EFFECTS OF ENVIRONMENTAL POLLUTANTS, PANEL ON NICKEL. SUNDERMAN FW (CHAIRMAN). 1975. Nickel, Washington, D.C.: National Academy of Sciences.

CURTES JP, TROTEL E, BOURDINIERE J. 1977. Les adenocarcinomas de l'ethmoide chez les travailleurs du bois. Arch Mal Prof 38:773–786.

DAVIES JM, EASTON DF, BIDSTRUP PI. 1991. Mortality from respiratory cancer and other causes in United Kingdom chromato production workers. Br J Ind Med 48:299–313.

DEBOIS JM. 1969. Tumoren van de neusholte by houtbewerkers. Tijdschr Geneeskol 25:92–93.

DECOUFLE P, WALRATH J. 1987. Nasal cancer in the U.S. shoe industry: does it exist? Am J Ind Med 12(5):605–613.

DEMERS PA, KOGEVINAS M, BOFFETTA P, et al. 1995. Wood dust and sino-nasal cancer: pooled reanalysis of twelve case-control studies. Am J Indust Med 28:151–166.

DOLL R. 1958. Cancer of the lung and nose in nickel workers. Br J Ind Med 15:217–223.

DOLL R, MORGAN LG, SPEIZER FE. 1970. Cancer of the lung and nasal sinuses in nickel workers. Br J Cancer 24:623–632.

DOLL R, PETO R. 1981. The Causes of Cancer: Quantitative Estimates of Avoidable Risks of Cancer in the United States Today. London, Oxford University Press.

ECKARDT RD. 1974. Annals of industry noncasualties of the workplace. J Occup Med 16:472–477.

EDLING C, HELLQUIST H, ODKVIST L. 1987. Occupational formaldehyde exposure and the nasal mucosa. Rhinology 25(3):181–187.

ELWOOD JM. 1981. Wood exposure and smoking: Association with cancer of the nasal cavity and paranasal sinuses in British Columbia. Can Med Assoc J 124:1573–1577.

ENTERLINE PE. 1974. Respiratory cancer among chromate workers. J Occup Med 16:523–526.

ENTERLINE PE, MARSH GM. 1982. Mortality among workers in a nickel refinery and alloy manufacturing plant in West Virginia. J Natl Cancer Inst 68(6):925–933.

FLISS DM, PARIKH J, FREEMAN JL. 1992. AIDS-related Kaposi's sarcoma of the sphenoid sinus. J Otolaryngol 21:235–237.

FOMBEUR JP. 1972. A propos de cas recents de tumeurs ethmoido-maxillaires chez les travailles de bois. Arch Mal Prof 33:453–455.

FUKUDA K, SHIBATA A. 1988. A case-control study of past history of nasal diseases and maxillary sinus cancer in Hokkaida, Japan. Cancer Res 48:1651–1652.

GARDNER RJ, BURGESS BA, KENNEDY GL, JR. 1985. Sensory irritant potential of selected nasal tumorigens in the rat. Food Chem Toxicol 23:87–92.

GIGNOUX M, BERNARD P. 1969. Tumeurs malignes de l'ethmoide chez les travaileurs du bois. J Med Lyon 50:731–736.

GRENFELL DM, SAMUEL H. 1932. Cancer among Welsh nickel workers. Lancet 1:375.

GUERKINK N. 1983. Nasal anatomy, physiology, and function. J Allergy Clin Immunol 72:123–128.

HADFIELD EH. 1970. A study of adenocarcinoma of the paranasal sinuses in woodworkers in the furniture industry. Ann R Coll Surg Engl 46:301–319.

HADFIELD EH. 1972. Cancer hazard from wood dust and in the boot and shoe industry. Ann Occup Hyg 15:39–41.

HAGUENAUER JP, ROMANET P, DUCLOS JC, et al. 1977. Les cancers professionels de l'ethmoide. Arch Mal Prof 38:819–823.

HARDELL L, JOHANSSON B, AXELSON O. 1982. Epidemiologic study of nasal and nasopharyngeal cancer and their relation to phenoxy acid or chlorphenol exposure. Am J Ind Med 3:247–257.

HARRISON DFN. 1957. Familial haemorrhagic telangiectases: a survey of cases treated by oestrogen therapy. J Laryngol 71:577–596.

HARRISON DFN. 1967. Snuff—its use and abuse: An essay on nasal physiology. In Muir CS, Shanmugaratnam K (eds): Cancer of the Nasopharynx. UICC Monogr 1. Copenhagen: Munksgaard, pp. 119–123.

HASTERLIK RJ, FINKEL AJ, MILLER CE. 1964. The cancer hazards of industrial and accidental exposure to radioactive isotopes. Ann NY Acad Sci 14:832–837.

HAYES RB, GERIN M, RAATGEVER JW, DE BRUYN A. 1986a. Wood-related occupations, wood dust exposure, and sinonasal cancer. Am J Epidemiol 124(4):569–577.

HAYES RB, RAATGEVER JW, DE BRUYN A, GERIN M. 1986b. Cancer of the nasal cavity and paranasal sinuses, and formaldehyde exposure. Int J Cancer 37(4):487–492.

HERNBERG S, WESTERHOLM P, SCHULTZ-LARSEN K, et al. 1983.

Nasal and sinonasal cancer: connection with occupational exposures in Denmark, Finland and Sweden. Scand J Work Environ Health 9(4):315–326.

HESTON WE, LEVILLIAN WD. 1953. Pulmonary tumors in strain A mice exposed to mustard gas. Proc Soc Exp Biol Med 82:457–460.

HILL AB. 1939. Statistical report to the Mond Nickel company relating to the incidence of carcinoma of the respiratory system at the Clydach Works. Wales: Mond Nickel Company.

HIRAYAMA T. 1984. Lung cancer in Japan: Effects of nutrition and passive smoking. In Mizell M, Correa P (eds): Lung Cancer: Causes and Prevention, p. 179.

HIYAMA T, OSHIMA A, HANAI A, et al. 1983. Chronic maxillary sinusitis and the epidemiology of cancer of the maxillary sinusus. In Reznik G, Stinson, SF (eds): Nasal Tumors in Animals and Man. Boca Raton, CRC Press, Inc., Vol. I, Anatomy, Physiology and Epidemiology, pp. 137–149.

HOFER O. 1952. Kiefer Lohlenkarzinom durch radium haltiges Kontrastmittel Hervogerufen. Dtsch Zahnaertzl Z 7:736.

HOOVER R, FRAUMENI JF. 1975. Cancer mortality in US counties with chemical industries. Environ Res 9:196–207.

HUEPER WC. 1966. Occupational and environmental cancers of the respiratory system. In Rentchnick P (ed): Recent Results in Cancer Research 3. New York: Springer-Verlag.

HUEPER WC. 1979. Some comments on the history and experimental explorations of metal carcinogens and cancers. J Natl Cancer Inst 62(4):723–725.

IARC (INTERNATIONAL AGENCY FOR RESEARCH ON CANCER) WORKING GROUP. 1975. Nickel. In: Evaluation of the Carcinogenic Risk of Chemicals to Man. Geneva: WHO, pp. 75–112.

IARC (INTERNATIONAL AGENCY FOR RESEARCH ON CANCER) WORKING GROUP. 1976. Isopropyl alcohol and isopropyl oils. In: Evaluation of the Carcinogenic Risk of Chemicals to Man, Vol. 15. Geneva: WHO pp. 223–243.

IRONSIDE P, MATTHEWS J. 1975. Carcinoma of the nose and paranasal sinuses in woodworkers in the state of Victoria, Australia. Cancer 36:1115–1121.

KEEN P. 1974. Trace elements in plants and soil in relation to cancer. S Afr Med J 48:2363–2364.

LANGARD S, FORSETH T. 1975. A cohort study of bronchial carcinomas in workers producing chromate pigments. Br J Ind Med 32:62–65.

LAREO AC, LUCE D, LECLERC A, et al. 1992. History of previous nasal diseases and sinonasal cancer: A case-control disease. Laryngoscope 102:439–442.

LECLERC A, CORTES MM, GERIN M, et al. 1994. Sinonasal cancer and wood dust exposure: results from a case-control study. Am J Epidol 140:340–349.

LEVY LS, VERRITT S. 1975. Carcinogenic and mutagenic activities of chromium-containing materials. Br J Cancer 32:262–263.

LUCE D, GERIN M, LECLERC A, et al. 1993. Sinonasal cancer and occupational exposure to formaldehyde and other substances. Int J Cancer 53:224–231.

MAGNUS K, ANDERSEN A, HGETVEIT AC. 1982. Cancer of respiratory organs among workers at a nickel refinery in Norway. Int J Cancer 30(6):681–685.

MCKAY WF, HANSON MR, MILLER RW. 1982. Cancer mortality in the United States, 1950–1977. NCI Monograph No. 59. Washington: US GPO.

MERLER E, BALDASSERONI A, LARIA R, FARAVELLI P, et al. 1986. On the causal association between exposure to leather dust and nasal cancer: further evidence from a case-control study. Br J Ind Med Feb; 43(2):91–95.

MILLER BA, RIES LAG, HANKEL BF, et al (eds). 1993. SEER Cancer Statistics Review: 1973–1990, National Cancer Institute; NIH Pub. No. 93-2789.

MOLTENI A, WARPEHA RL, BRIZIO-MOLTENI L, FORS EM. 1981. Estradiol receptor-binding protein in head and neck neoplastic and normal tissue. Arch Surg 116:207–210.

MUIR CS, NECTOUX J. 1980. Descriptive epidemiology of malignant neoplasms of nose, nasal cavities, middle ear and accessory sinuses. J Clin Otolaryngol (UK) 5:195–211.

NIOSH (NATIONAL INSTITUTE OF OCCUPATIONAL SAFETY AND HEALTH). 1976. Criteria for a Recommended Standard Occupational Exposure to Isopropyl Alcohol. Washington, D.C.: DHEW (NIOSH) Publ. No. 76-142.

NIOSH (NATIONAL INSTITUTE OF OCCUPATIONAL SAFETY AND HEALTH). 1977. Criteria for a Recommended Standard Occupational Exposure to Inorganic Nickel. Washington, D.C.: DHEW (NIOSH) Publ. No. 77-164.

NATIONAL CANCER INSTITUTE, DIVISION OF CANCER PREVENTION AND CONTROL. 1988. 1987 Annual Cancer Statistics Review, NIH Publ. No. 88-2789.

NATIONAL RESEARCH COUNCIL, COMMITTEE ON MEDICAL AND BIOLOGICAL EFFECTS OF ENVIRONMENTAL POLLUTANTS. 1975. Nickel. Washington, D.C.: National Academy of Sciences.

NEWMAN D. 1890. A case of adenocarcinoma of the left turbinate body and perforation of the nasal septum in the person of a worker in chrome pigments. Glasgow Med J 33:469–470.

NG TP. 1986. A case-referent study of the nasal cavity and sinuses in Hong Kong. Int J Epidemiol 15(2):171–175.

OLSEN J, JENSEN S, HINDS M, et al. 1984. Occupational formaldehyde exposure and increased nasal cancer risks in man. Int J Cancer 34:639–644.

OLSEN JH. 1985. Second cancer following cancer of the respiratory system in Denmark, 1943–1980. Natl Cancer Inst Monogr 68:309–324.

OLSEN JH. 1987. The epidemiology of sinonasal cancer in Denmark, 1943–1982. Acta Pathol Microbiol Immunol Scand 95:171–175.

OLSEN JH. 1988. Occupational risks of sinonasal cancer in Denmark. Br J Ind Med 45:329–335.

OSBORN DA. 1970. Nature and behavior of transitional tumors in the upper respiratory tract. Cancer 25:50–60.

OSBORN DA, FRIEDMANN I. 1982. Pathology of Granulomas and Neoplasms of the Nose and Paranasal Sinuses. Edinburgh, London, Melbourne, New York: Churchill Livingstone, pp. 103–117, 1–35.

OTTOLENGHI AD, HASEMAN JK, PAYNE WW, et al. 1975. Inhalation studies of nickel subsulfide in pulmonary carcinogenesis of rats. J Natl Cancer Inst 54:1165–1172.

PEDERSEN E, HOGETVEIT AC, ANDERSEN A. 1973. Cancer of the respiratory organs among workers at a nickel refinery in Norway. Int J Cancer 12:32–41.

POLEDNAK AP, STEHNEY F, ROWLAND RE. 1978. Mortality among women first employed before 1930 in the US radium dial-painting industry: A group ascertained from employment lists. Am J Epidemiol 107:179–195.

POUR PM, GOUTZ U. 1983. Prevention of N-nitrosobis (2-oxopropyl) amine-induced nasal cavity tumors in rats by orchietomy. J Natl Cancer Inst 700:353–357.

POUR PM, STEPAN KR. 1988. The role of testosterone in the nasal cavity tumors induced by N-nitrosobis(2-oxopropyl)amine in rats. Carcinogenesis 9(8):1417–1420.

PRESTON-MARTIN S, HENDERSON BE, PIKE MC. 1982. Descriptive epidemiology of cancers of the upper respiratory tract in Los Angeles. Cancer 49:2201–2207.

RANKOW RM, CONLEY J, FODOR P. 1974. Carcinoma of the maxillary sinus following thorotrast instillation. J Maxillofacial Surg 2:119–126.

REDMOND CK, SASS RE, ROUSH GC. 1982. Nasal Cavity and Paranasal Sinuses. In Schottenfeld D, Fraumeni JF, Jr (eds): Cancer Epidemiology and Prevention. Philadelphia: W.B. Saunders.

ROUSH GC. 1978. Sinonasal Cancer and Occupation in Connecticut. Masters Thesis. New Haven: Yale University.

ROUSH GC. 1979. Epidemiology of cancer of the nose and paranasal sinuses: Current concepts. Head and Neck Surgery 2:3–11.

ROUSH GC, KELLY JA, MEIGS FLANNERY JT. 1982. Scrotal carcinoma in Connecticut metal-workers: sequel to a study of sinonasal cancer. Am J Epidemiol 116:76–85.

ROUSH GC, MEIGS JW, KELLY J, et al. 1980. Sinonasal cancer and occupation: A case-control study. Am J Epidemiol 111:183–193.

ROUSH GC, HOLFORD TR, SCHYMURA MJ, WHITE C. 1987a. Cancer Risk and Incidence Trends. Washington, D.C.: Hemisphere.

ROUSH GC, SCHYMURA MJ, STEVENSON JM, HOLFORD TR. 1987b. Time and age trends for sinonasal cancer in Connecticut incidence and US mortality rates. Cancer 60:422–428.

ROUSH GC, WALRATH J, STAYNER LT, et al. 1987c. Nasopharyngeal cancer, sinonasal cancer and occupations related to formaldehyde: A case-control study. J Natl Cancer Inst 79:1221–1224.

ROWLAND RE. The risk of malignancy from internally deposited radioisotopes. In Nygaard OF, Adler HI, Sinclair WK (eds). Radiation Research: Biomedical, Chemical, and Physical Perspectives. New York, Academic Press, pp. 146–155.

RUTSTEIN DD, MULLAN RJ, FRAZIER TM, et al. 1983. Sentinel health events (occupational): a basis for physician recognition and public health surveillance. Am J Public Health 73:1054–1062.

RUBIN P. 1972. Radionuclide carcinogenesis and sinus carcinoma. JAMA 219:354–355.

SAEZ S, SAKAI F. 1975. Androgen receptors in human pharyngeolaryngeal mucosa and pharyngeal-laryngeal epithelioma. J Steroid Biochem 7:919–921.

SCHOENTAL R. 1975. Chromium carcinogenesis, formation of expoxaldehydes and tanning (letter). Br J Cancer 32:403–404.

SCHOTTENFELD D, FRAUMENI JF, JR. 1982. Cancer Epidemiology and Prevention. Philadelphia: W.B. Saunders.

SHIMIZU H, HOZAWA J, SAITO H, et al. 1989. Chronic sinusitis and woodworking as risk for cancer of the maxillary sinus in Northeast Japan. Laryngoscope 99:58–61.

SNYDER RN, PERZIN KH. 1972. Papillomatosis of the nasal cavity and paranasal sinuses (inverted papilloma, squamous papilloma) Cancer 30:668–690.

STOKINGER HE. 1977. Routes of entry and modes of action. In Key MM, Henschel AF, Butler J, et al (eds): Occupational Diseases: A Guide to Their Recognition. Washington D.C.: DHEW, pp. 11–21.

SUNDERMAN FW. 1963. Studies of nickel carcinogenesis: Alterations of ribonucleic acid following inhalation of nickel carbonyl. Am J Clin Pathol 39:549–561.

SUNDERMAN FW. 1968. Epidemiology of respiratory cancer among nickel workers. Dis Chest 54–41.

SUNDERMAN FW. 1973. The current status of nickel carcinogenesis. Ann Clin Lab Sci 3:156–180.

SUNDERMAN FW. 1976. A review of the carcinogenicities of nickel, chromium and arsenic compounds in man and animals. Prev Med 5:279–295.

SUNDERMAN FW. 1977. A review of the metabolism and toxicology of nickel. Ann Clin Lab Sci 7:377–398.

SUNDERMAN FW, DONNELLY AJ. 1965. Studies of nickel carcinogenesis: Metastasizing pulmonary tumors in rats induced by the inhalation of nickel carbonyl. Am J Pathol 46:1027–1041.

SUNDERMAN FW, SUNDERMAN FW, JR. 1963. Studies of nickel carcinogenesis: The subcellular partition of nickel in lung following inhalation of nickel carbonyl. Am J Clin Pathol 40:563–575.

TAKASAKA T, KAWAMOTO K, NAKAMURA K. 1987. A case-control study of nasal cancers. An occupational survey. Acta Otolaryngol Suppl (Stockh) 435:136–142.

TAYLOR M. 1961. Histopathological and histochemical studies on atropic rhinitis. J Laryngol 75:574–590.

UTIAN WH. 1980. Menopause in Modern Perspective: A Guide to Clinical Practice. New York: Appleton-Century-Crofts, p. 57.

VAUGHAN TL, STRADER C, DAVIS S, DALING JR. 1986a. Formaldehyde and cancers of the pharynx, sinus and nasal cavity: I. Occupational exposures. Int J Cancer 38(5):677–83.

VAUGHAN TL, STRADER C, DAVIS S, DALING JR. 1986b. Formaldehyde and cancers of the pharynx, sinus and nasal cavity: II. Residential exposures. Int J Cancer 38(5):685–688.

VAUGHAN TL. 1989. Occupation and squamous cell cancers of the pharynx and sinonasal cavity. Am J Ind Med 16:493–510.

VAUGHAN TL, DAVIES S. 1991. Wood dust exposure and squamous cell cancers of the upper respiratory tract. Am J Epidemiol 133:560–564.

WADA S, MIYANISHI M, NISHIMOTO Y, et al. 1968. Mustard gas as a cause of neoplasia in man. Lancet 1:1161–1163.

WALKER J, MACGILLIVRAY I, MACNAUGHTON MC. 1976. Combined Textbook of Gynecology and Obstetrics. Edinburgh: Churchill Livingston, p. 293.

WANG DY, BULBROOK RD, CLIFFORD P. 1968. Plasma levels of sulphate esters of dehydroepiandrosterone and androsterone in Kenyan men and their relation to cancer of the nasopharynx. Lancet i:1003–1005.

WATERHOUSE JAH. 1974. Cancer Handbook of Epidemiology and Prognosis. London: Churchill Livingstone.

WATERHOUSE JAH, MUIR C, SHANMUGARATNAM K, POWELL J (eds). 1982. Cancer Incidence in Five Continents. Lyon: IARC.

WEIL CS, SMITH HF, JR., NALE TW. 1952. Quest for a suspected industrial carcinogen. AMA Arch Industr Hyg Occup Med 5:535–547.

WHO COLLABORATING CENTER FOR ORAL PRECANCEROUS LESIONS. 1978. Definition of leukoplakia and related lesions: An aid to studies on oral precancer. Oral Surg 46:518–539.

YOUNG J, PERCY CL, ASIRE AJ. 1981. Cancer incidence and mortality in the United States, 1973–1977. Natl Cancer Inst Monogr No. 57.

YU MC, HO JH, LAI S-H, et al. 1986. Cantonese-style salted fish as a cause of nasopharyngeal carcinoma: Report of a case-control study in Hong Kong. Cancer Res 46:956–961.

ZHENG W, BLOT WJ, SHU X-O, et al. 1992. A population-based case-control study of cancers of the nasal cavity and paranasal sinuses in Shanghai. Int J Cancer 52:557–561.

ZHENG W, MCLAUGHLIN JK, CHOW W-H, et al. 1993. Risk factors for cancers of the nasal cavity and paranasal sinuses among white men in the United States. Am J Epidemiol 138:965–972.

29 Nasopharyngeal cancer

MIMI C. YU
BRIAN E. HENDERSON

Cancer of the nasopharynx is a disease with a remarkable racial and geographical distribution. It is very rare (incidence of less than 1 per 100,000 person-years) in most parts of the world, and only a handful of populations deviate from this low-risk profile. Regardless of race and geography, the commonest form of nasopharyngeal cancers is that which arises from the epithelial cells lining the nasopharynx. These carcinomas (commonly referred to as NPCs) constitute 75%–95% of nasopharyngeal cancers in low-risk populations and virtually all nasopharyngeal cancers in high-risk populations (Ho, 1971; Sugano et al, 1978; Levine and Connelly, 1985). In this chapter, we shall discuss primarily the epidemiology of NPC.

DEMOGRAPHIC PATTERNS

Histopathology

On the basis of light microscopic studies, the World Health Organization classified NPC into two histological types, namely, squamous cell carcinoma and nonkeratinizing carcinoma. Nonkeratinizing carcinomas are further subdivided into two subtypes, namely, differentiated nonkeratinizing carcinoma and undifferentiated carcinoma (Shanmugaratnam and Sobin, 1991):

1. Squamous cell carcinoma (keratinizing squamous cell carcinoma)—which shows squamous differentiation with the presence of intercellular bridges and/or keratinization over most of its extent.

2. Nonkeratinizing carcinoma—this group comprises a differentiated type of nonkeratinizing carcinoma and an undifferentiated type.

2a. Differentiated nonkeratinizing carcinoma—the tumor cells show differentiation with a maturation sequence that results in cells in which squamous differentiation is not evident on light microscopy. The cells have fairly well-defined cell margins and show an arrangement that is stratified or pavemented and not syncytial. A plexiform pattern is common.

2b. Undifferentiated carcinoma—the tumor cells generally have vesicular nuclei and prominent nucleoli. The cell margins are indistinct and the tumor exhibits a syncytial appearance. Spindle-shaped tumor cells, some with hyperchromatic nuclei, may be present. The tumor cells are arranged in irregular and moderately well-defined masses and/or strands of loosely connected cells in a lymphoid stroma.

Shanmugaratnam et al (1979) compared the distributions of NPC cases in Singapore by age, sex, HLA antigen profile, cell-mediated immune status, and antibodies against various Epstein-Barr virus (EBV)–related antigens across the histological types and concluded that they are variants of a homogeneous group of neoplasms.

Besides NPC, cancer of the nasopharynx can be any one of the following pathological types (Shanmugaratnam and Sobin, 1991):

1. Malignant tumors of glandular epithelium—adenocarcinoma, adenoid cystic carcinoma, others.
2. Malignant tumors of soft tissues—fibrosarcoma, rhabdomyosarcoma, others.
3. Malignant tumors of bone and cartilage—chondrosarcoma, osteosarcoma.
4. Malignant lymphomas of various types.
5. Miscellaneous malignant tumors—malignant melanoma, chordoma, malignant germ cell tumors.

Anatomic Distribution

The majority of NPCs arise in the lateral walls of the nasopharynx, especially from the pharyngeal recesses (fossae of Rosenmuller) and eustachian cushions. NPC may also arise in the superoposterior wall, in particular the roof of the nasopharynx, but only rarely in the anterior and inferior walls of the nasopharynx (Simons and Shanmugaratnam, 1982).

International Patterns

NPC is a rare malignancy in most parts of the world where the age-standardized incidence rate for either sex is generally less than 1 per 100,000 persons per year (Parkin et al, 1992). Table 29-1 lists the handful of populations that are known to deviate from this low-risk pattern together with their age-standardized (world population) incidence rates of nasopharyngeal cancer for men and women separately. Overall incidence of NPC is elevated in China, with substantial variation between regions. In general, incidence increases as one travels from north to south China. Whereas rates in Chinese men in the northernmost provinces are about 2–3/100,000 person-years, those residing in the southernmost province of Guangdong exhibit rates of 25–40/100,000 person-years (National Cancer Control Office, 1979; Yu et al, 1981; Parkin et al, 1992). High rates approaching those observed in southern China are seen in Eskimos and other natives of the Arctic region (Albeck et al, 1992; Nutting et al, 1993). Intermediate rates of NPC (3–6/100,000 person-years) are observed among many indigenous people of southeast Asia, including Thais (Parkin et al, 1992), Vietnamese (Anh et al, 1993), Malays (Parkin et al, 1992), and Filipinos (Parkin et al, 1992). In Sabah, Malaysia, rates similar to those observed among the Eskimos have been reported for the native Kadazans (Rothwell, 1979). Modestly raised rates of NPC are observed among the people of Kuwait, both local-born Arabs and immigrants from neighboring Arab countries (Parkin et al, 1992). Based on reviews of hospital series, it is believed that rates of NPC are also raised in the mainly Arab populations of Algeria, Tunisia, Morocco, Sudan, and Saudi Arabia (Muir, 1971; Cammoun et al, 1974; Hidayatalla et al, 1983; Al-Idrissi, 1990). The intermediate rates of NPC among Israeli Jews born in Morocco, Algeria, or Tunisia tend to support this view (Steinitz et al, 1989).

TABLE 29–1. *Populations at Increased Risk for Nasopharyngeal Cancer*

Population	Age-standardized (World) Incidence[a]		Reference
	Male	Female	
Chinese (Hong Kong)	28.5	11.2	Parkin et al, 1992
Chinese (Taipei)	8.1	3.2	Chen et al, 1988a
Chinese (Shanghai)	4.0	1.9	Parkin et al, 1992
Chinese (Tianjin)	1.8	0.6	Parkin et al, 1992
Eskimos (Greenland)	12.7	9.2	Albeck et al, 1992
Eskimos, Athabascan, Aleuts (Alaska)	11.9	5.6	Nutting et al, 1993
Thais (Chiang Mai)	4.1	1.6	Parkin et al, 1992
Vietnamese (Hanoi)	4.8	2.4	Anh et al, 1993
Malays (Singapore)	4.3	1.5	Parkin et al, 1992
Filipinos (Rizal)	6.3	3.0	Parkin et al, 1992
Kadazans (Sabah)	15.9	8.7	Rothwell, 1979
Kuwaitis (Kuwait)	1.3	0.8	Parkin et al, 1992
Non-Kuwaitis (Kuwait)	1.5	1.2	Parkin et al, 1992
Israeli Jews born in Morocco, Algeria, and Tunisia	2.8	1.3	Steinitz et al, 1989

[a]Per 100,000 person-years.

Migration

Most Chinese living outside of China originate from the provinces of Guangdong and Fujian in southeastern China (Ho, 1959), a region of high NPC incidence (National Cancer Control Office, 1979). Southern Chinese migrants, irrespective of their country of migration, continue to demonstrate a high rate of NPC (Worth and Valentine, 1967; King and Haenszel, 1973; Armstrong et al, 1979; Gallagher and Elwood, 1979; Lee et al, 1988; Parkin et al, 1992) although succeeding generations of these immigrants in Occidental countries such as the United States (King and Haenszel, 1973; Buell, 1974; Yu et al, 1981) and Australia (Worth and Valentine, 1967) show continually declining rates. In contrast, Singapore-born Chinese do not experience decreased rates of NPC relative to China-born Chinese (Lee et al, 1988). It is interesting to note that Chinese in southeast Asia generally adhere to their traditional culture and customs, while those in Western countries gradually adopt the Occidental way of life.

There have been reports of low-risk racial groups born and raised in high-risk areas experiencing elevated risk of NPC. Buell (1973) in a review of deaths due to NPC in California, observed that white males born in the Philippine Islands or China had increased risk of NPC relative to other white males. Among Jews in Israel, those born in North Africa had raised rates of NPC relative to other Jews (Steinitz et al, 1989). Males of French origin who were born in North Africa exhibited a significantly higher rate of NPC than French males born in France (Jeannel et al, 1993). These migrant studies thus suggest that environmental factors play an important role in the etiology of NPC.

Sex and Age

In virtually all populations studied, rates are higher in males than in females. For most populations, the male:female ratio is about 2–3:1 (Parkin et al, 1992). The age distribution, on the other hand, shows interesting differences between different populations. In high-risk southern Chinese, the incidence in both sexes increases steadily with age, reaching a peak between ages 45 and 54, and shows a definite decline at older ages (Armstrong et al, 1979; Yu et al, 1981; Parkin et al, 1992). However, the rates in China as a whole show no such decline after age 55 years; the increase with age continues to at least age 70–74 years (National Cancer Control Office, 1979). The rates in low-risk populations studied, at least after age 20 years, show a distribution similar to the overall rates in China (Balakrishnan, 1975; Burt et al, 1992; Parkin et al, 1992).

An adolescent age peak in incidence has been observed in a number of populations of low to moderately high risk for NPC. In the U.S., a minor peak in the ages 10–19 years is evident in blacks of both sexes (Burt et al, 1992). In Sabah, Malaysia, Kadazan men demonstrate a secondary peak between ages 15 and 24 years; no data are available on Kadazan women (Rothwell, 1979). In India, the age distribution of 666 consecutive cases of NPC showed a peak in the age group 13–22 years regardless of sex (Balakishnan, 1975). When Balakrishnan (1975) pooled the incidence data on nasopharyngeal cancer from 48 population groups published in Doll et al (1970), he demonstrated a definite mode between ages 10 and 19 years for either sex, which is absent when similarly pooled data for cancers of the nose and nasal sinuses were plotted against age.

Race and Ethnicity

High risk to NPC among Chinese is mainly confined to those residing in the southern provinces of Guangdong, Guangxi, Hunan, and Fujian (Fig. 29-1, National Cancer Control Office, 1979). Several distinct racial-ethnic groups reside in this high-risk region, and these groups possess different rates of NPC. Highest rates are observed among the Tankas, a subethnic group of the Cantonese, who inhabit the Pearl River Delta Basin in central Guangdong. One distinguishing feature of the Tankas from the other Cantonese is that they are seafaring people (either fishermen or sea transporters) who live on houseboats parked along the banks of the many branches of the Pearl River. The rates of NPC among the Tankas are two times those in the land-dwelling Cantonese (Ho, 1978; Li et al, 1985). In turn, the land-dwelling Cantonese (who comprise 98%–99% of Cantonese) have a 2-fold rate of NPC relative to the Hakka and Chiu Chau dialect groups who reside in northeast Guangdong (Yu et al, 1981; Li et al, 1985). The people of Fujian Province are culturally similar to the Chiu Chau people in Guangdong Province, and so are their rates of NPC (Summary data of the Cancer Mortality Survey in the People's Republic of China, 1980). It is interesting to note that the Hakkas (who rarely intermarry with other dialect groups) originated from northern China more than 500 years ago (Ho, 1959), but their rates resemble those of their Chiu Chau neighbors instead of their low-risk ancestors in the north. Even after migration to southeast Asia, the Cantonese continue to exhibit a 2-fold risk of NPC relative to the Hakkas, Chiu Chaus, and Fujianese (Armstrong et al, 1979; Lee et al, 1988).

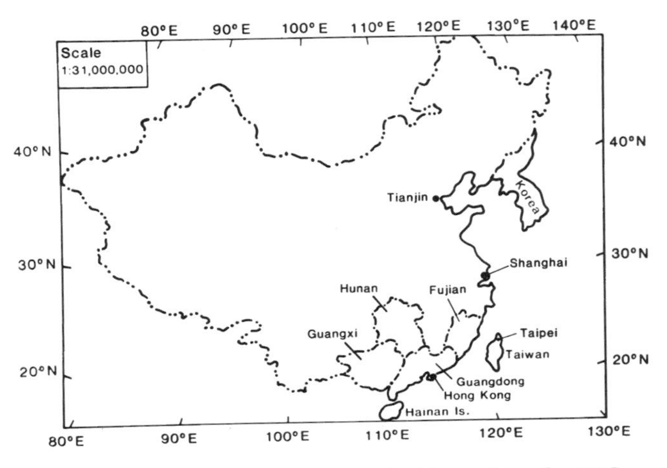

FIG. 29–1. Map of China showing high-risk provinces for NPC.

Two distinct racial groups inhabit the Autonomous Region of Guangxi. While the Zhuang people in western Guangxi possess one-fifth the NPC rate in Cantonese, the Han (the predominant race in China) people of eastern Guangxi, who are ethnically close to the Cantonese in Guangdong, show similar rates. Hunan Province borders both Guangxi and Guangdong to the north, and not surprisingly areas that border Guangdong and Guangxi have high NPC rates. In addition, the Tujia and Miao tribes (minority races in China), who inhabit the mountainous region of western Hunan, are found to possess NPC rates approaching those in the Cantonese (Summary data of the Cancer Mortality Survey in the People's Republic of China, 1980).

In summary, the geographic variation of NPC incidence within southern China closely parallels the distribution of racial-ethnic groups inhabiting the region. The relatively high NPC rates observed among the Hakkas who originated from low-risk northern China argues against genetic predisposition as a major cause of the varying risk patterns among these population groups. On the other hand, these ethnic groups are distinct in their customs and food habits, and it is possible that environmental factors inherent in their traditional cultures are responsible for their varying susceptibility to NPC.

Ethnic variation in NPC risk also has been noted in the African countries of Uganda and Sudan, which possess low (Uganda) to intermediate (Sudan) frequencies of NPC. Of the four major tribes in Uganda, rates are similar between the Nilotic and the Para-Nilotic people, but both are considerably higher than the Bantu and Sudanic groups, which have comparable rates (Schmauz and Templeton, 1972). In the Sudan, Hidayatalla et al (1983) reported the highest frequencies of NPC in the African tribes, intermediate frequencies in the Arab/African mixed tribes, and lowest frequencies in the Arab tribes.

In Malaysia and Singapore, large numbers of ethnic Chinese and Indians live alongside the native Malays. We have mentioned earlier that rates are raised among the Chinese and the Malays. In contrast, Indians in Southeast Asia show very low rates of NPC, comparable to those seen in whites in the U.S. (Armstrong et al, 1979; Parkin et al, 1992).

Socioeconomic Status

Among high-risk southern Chinese, individuals in the lower social strata experience a higher rate of NPC relative to those in the higher social strata (Geser et al, 1978; Armstrong et al, 1978; Yu et al, 1981). Information on low-risk populations is scanty. In the U.S., white males residing in rural or semirural counties demonstrate an inverse association between years of schooling and NPC mortality rate, while no clear trend is apparent among those residing in predominantly urban counties (Hoover et al, 1975).

Urbanization

Among high-risk southern Chinese, there is no observable difference in risk of NPC between urban and rural residents. In the Malaysian state of Selangor, Chinese urban and rural residents have comparable rates of NPC (Armstrong et al, 1979). In metropolitan Hong Kong, local-born Cantonese exhibited rates similar to those born and raised in the rural regions of Guangdong Province (Yu et al, 1981). On the other hand, urban residents in some low-risk populations seem to have higher rates of NPC relative to their rural counterparts. In the U.S., counties that are 100% urban have about 2 times the NPC mortality rate of counties that are 100% rural (Hoover et al, 1975). In Muir et al (1987), rates between urban and rural residents in 11 populations in Japan, Australia, the United Kingdom, and Europe are compared. Seven populations show similar rates between urban and rural areas, while urban rates are higher than rural rates (1.4–2-fold) in four populations.

Time Trends

Early records showed that NPC was a common cancer among southern Chinese well over 50 years ago (Ho, 1978). Examinations of cancer registry data over time in Hong Kong (1961–79), Malaysia (1968–77), and Singapore (1968–82) showed little change in NPC incidence in these southern Chinese populations (Armstrong et al, 1979; Ho et al, 1982; Lee et al, 1988). In the U.S., data from the Connecticut Tumor Registry between 1935 and 1974 showed relatively stable rates over the 40-year period (Levine et al, 1980). Similarly, an analysis of data collected from the nationwide Surveillance, Epidemiology and End Results program in the U.S. during 1973–1986 showed no evidence of change in incidence rates during the 14-year study period (Burt et al, 1992). Among Canadian Eskimos, review of data over a 25-year period (1950–74) also indicate no appreciable variation in rates over time (Schaefer et al, 1975). In contrast, rates in Chinese Americans have been declining steadily since 1950 such that nasopharyngeal mortality rate in men was halved between 1950–54 and 1970–79 (12 vs. 6/100,000 person-years) (Fraumeni and Mason, 1974; Levine et al, 1987). This trend is likely to be the result of (1) increased representation of local-born Chinese in the age groups at high risk to NPC as this lower-risk population ages, and (2) increased migration from Taiwan and other intermediate- to low-risk regions in China since the 1950s (prior to that time, virtually all Chinese Americans originated from the Cantonese region of Guangdong Province (Chinn et al, 1969; Lai, 1988)).

Survival

In the U.S., overall 5-year relative survival rate of NPC is about 25%, with prognosis favoring earlier stage of disease, less differentiated tumors, younger ages, the Chinese race (as opposed to whites and blacks), and the female gender (Burt et al, 1992). In Hong Kong, Ho (1978, 1985) reported an overall 5-year actuarial survival rate of about 45% posttreatment, with better results in females and in younger patients. In Taiwan, Hsu et al (1987) reported an overall 5-year survival rate of 44%, with prognosis favoring histological types of nonkeratinizing and undifferentiated carcinomas as compared to keratinizing squamous cell carcinoma.

U.S. Incidence and Mortality

The age-standardized (world population) incidence of NPC in white, black, Filipino, and Chinese American males during 1973–1986 were 0.5, 0.8, 3.1, and 13.9 per 100,000 person-years, respectively. For females, the comparable rates were 0.2, 0.3, 1.8, and 6.6 per 100,000 person-years. Among Filipino, black, and white Americans, incidence increased with age after age 20 years until at least age 70 years. Incidence in Chinese Americans, on the other hand, plateaued around age 50–54 years and declined thereafter, resembling the age pattern in southern China from where most of them originated. There was a minor peak in incidence in the ages 10–19 in blacks that was absent in the other ethnic groups (Burt et al, 1992).

The age-adjusted (1960 U.S. standard population) mortality of nasopharyngeal cancer in white, black, and

Chinese American males during 1970–79 were 0.4, 0.5, and 6.1 per 100,000 person-years, respectively. For females, the corresponding figures were 0.1, 0.2, and 2.2 per 100,000 person-years. The patterns of age-specific mortality in these three groups of Americans resemble their patterns of age-specific incidence described above (Levine et al, 1987).

ENVIRONMENTAL FACTORS

The Epstein-Barr Virus (EBV)

Ever since Old et al (1966) first noticed that a high proportion of the sera from NPC patients in Africa and the U.S. reacted with antigen prepared from cultured Burkitt's lymphoma cells, a large body of literature on the association between EBV and NPC has accumulated. NPC patients of all races and geographical locales consistently show significantly higher antibody titers to various EBV-associated antigens (viral capsid antigen, early antigen, nuclear antigen, complement-fixing antigen) compared to controls (Henle et al, 1970; Lin et al, 1973b; Sawaki et al, 1976; Henderson et al, 1977; Lanier et al, 1981; Saemundsen et al, 1982; Zeng, 1985; Bogger-Goren et al, 1987). These antibody levels increase with advancing stages of the disease and decrease to the range of control values among long-term survivors who remain disease-free (Henle et al, 1973; de Schryver et al, 1974; Naegele et al, 1982; Tamada et al, 1984). EBV DNA is present in epithelial cells of NPC tumor tissues irrespective of their degrees of differentiation (zur Hausen et al, 1970; Wolf et al, 1975; Lanier et al, 1981; Saemundsen et al, 1982; Raab-Traub, 1987; Dickens et al, 1992), and these epithelial tumor cells express EBV nuclear antigens (Huang et al, 1974; Klein et al, 1974; Lanier et al, 1981). Recently, integrated EBV was detected in several NPC biopsy samples (Kripalani-Joshi and Law, 1994). These observations have led many investigators to conclude that EBV is etiologically related to NPC, although there is as yet no conclusive evidence that virus reactivation precedes and contributes to the neoplastic disease process instead of being triggered by it.

Whether or not EBV plays an etiologic role in NPC development, it is unlikely that the virus is capable of inducing the disease by itself. Throughout China, there is little variation in the prevalence of infection and the age at primary infection with EBV (Zeng, 1985) although a greater than 20-fold difference in NPC risk exists within the country (National Cancer Control Office, 1979). Virtually all Chinese children are infected by ages 3–5 years (Zeng, 1985). Compared to the Singapore Chinese, age at primary infection by EBV is generally earlier in Ugandan and Singapore Indian and later in French Caucasian (de-The et al, 1975), and yet high risk to NPC is unique to Singapore Chinese (Parkin et al, 1992). In all of the four populations studied (Singapore Chinese and Indian, Ugandan, and French Caucasian), virtually every young adult after age 20 years is infected (de-The et al, 1975).

Chinese Salted Fish

The higher rates of NPC among the boat-dwelling Tankas as compared to the land-dwelling Cantonese was first noted by Ho of Hong Kong, who further observed that these boat people had little exposure to domestic inhalants as they "live all their lives in open boats and cook their food in the open air . . ." (Ho, 1967). Ho then turned his attention to dietary factors, especially the traditional foods of southern China. He observed that salted fish is dominant in the diet of the boat people, being the principal source of supplementary food in a diet consisting mainly of rice. Often spending long periods at sea, southern Chinese fishermen salt most of their catch as a means of preservation. These fishermen and their families prefer to consume salted instead of fresh fish, since the latter can command a much higher price. In 1971, Ho suggested that Chinese salted fish, "a common and favorite item of food among most (Cantonese) in and outside China" be investigated as a "possible etiological factor" for NPC (Ho, 1971). Ho made two additional observations crucial to his salted fish hypothesis. The salting process actually was inefficient and the product, aged several days to weeks, became partially putrefied, liberating a pungent odor offensive to those who were not raised in the southern Chinese culture, including most Chinese from the northern provinces (Ho, 1972b). Later, in an attempt to explain the early onset of NPC and its peak incidence during the fifth and sixth decades of life in southern Chinese, Ho recognized that salted fish mixed with soft rice is a popular weaning food in southern China (Ho, 1976). Thus, the final formulation of the hypothesis dictates early and repeated exposure to chemicals formed in decayed fish as a result of inadequate salting and drying, which is in part deliberate to produce the special flavor relished by those who enjoy the food.

Eight case-control studies were conducted among various Chinese populations with distinct risks for NPC to investigate this possible exposure-disease association (Table 29-2). Four were conducted in populations that are predominantly Cantonese (Chinese in California, Hong Kong, and Guangzhou). While the two earlier studies among Cantonese (Henderson et al, 1978; Geser et al, 1978) examined exposure at a single time point, the latter two studies conducted in this ethnic group (Yu et al, 1986, 1989a) investigated exposures during mul-

TABLE 29–2. *Case-control Studies of NPC That Examine Exposure to Chinese Salted Fish*

Chinese Population Studied*	*Years of Diagnosis of Cases*	*Number of Cases/Controls*	*Period of Exposure to Salted Fish*	*Estimate of Risk Relative to No/Rare Consumption*	*Reference*
California, USA	1971–74	74/109	Current	1/wk, 2.1	Henderson and Louie, 1978
				2+/wk, 3.1	
Hong Kong	1973–74	108/103	During weaning	Ever, 2.6	Geser et al, 1978
Selangor, Malaysia	1973–80	100/100	During childhood	Weekly, 3.1	Armstrong et al, 1983
				Daily, 17.4	
			During adolescence	Weekly, 1.3	
				Daily, 3.5	
Hong Kong	1981–83	250/250	During weaning	Ever 7.5	Yu et al, 1986
			At age 10	Weekly/daily[a] 37.7	
			3 yr before	Weekly, 3.2	
				Daily, 7.5	
Guangzhou, China	1983–85	306/306	During weaning	Ever, 2.1	Yu et al, 1989a
			At age 10	Weekly, 1.1	
				Daily, 2.4	
			3 yr before	Weekly, 1.4	
				Daily, 1.8	
Yulin, China	1984–86	128/174	During weaning	Ever, 2.6	Yu et al, 1988
			At age 10	Weekly[b], 1.5	
Taipei, Taiwan	Not stated	205/205	Before age 20	1–9/month, 0.8	Chen et al, 1988b
				10+/month, 1.5	
Tianjin, China	1985–86	100/300	At age 10	Weekly/Daily, 6.7	Ning et al, 1990
			3 yr before	Monthly/Weekly[b], 1.2	
Zangwu, China	1986	88/176	During weaning	Ever, 2.4	Zheng et al, 1994b
			Between ages 2–10	Monthly/Weekly, 3.2	
Northeast Thailand (Mainly Thai Population)	1987–90	120/120	Current	Less than weekly, 1.5	Sriamporn et al, 1992
				Weekly, 2.5	

*Unless otherwise specified.
[a]At least once a week is the highest frequency category.
[b]No subject reported daily consumption.

tiple time periods throughout the subjects' lifetime. All four studies demonstrated a significant and positive association between salted-fish intake and NPC risk. Moreover, in the two studies that investigated exposures at various time points, both found childhood exposure, especially during infancy (at weaning), to be more strongly related to risk than adulthood exposure (Yu et al, 1986, 1989a). Yu et al (1989a) pointed out that the apparent disparity in the magnitude of relative risks observed among the Cantonese in Guangzhou compared to those in Hong Kong was an artifact related to the influence of exposure prevalence on the diminution of the observed relative risk toward unity through random misclassification of subjects' exposure status. Indeed, a study in Hong Kong a decade earlier and examining older patients (Geser et al, 1978) reported an exposure prevalence at weaning almost identical to that noted in Guangzhou (Yu et al, 1989a), and consequently the two studies reported comparable relative risks.

Three case-control studies examining consumption of salted fish in non-Cantonese populations of southern China also showed a significant association between NPC risk and early exposure to this food. Armstrong et al (1983) studied 100 cases of NPC in Malaysian Chinese, of whom approximately one-third were Cantonese, another one-third were Hakka, and the remaining one-third were Chiu Chau/Fujianese. Childhood or adolescent exposure to salted fish was both positively associated with NPC risk in all three ethnic groups, with exposure during childhood exhibiting a stronger association with NPC than exposure during adolescence. Yu et al (1988) and Zheng et al (1994b) investigated salted-fish intake in two non-Cantonese populations in eastern Guangxi where consumption level is relatively low and again found exposure during infancy to be most strongly associated with risk. In Taiwan, Chen et al (1988b) compared salted-fish intake before age 20 years between NPC cases and controls and observed a non-significant positive association between intake frequency and risk of NPC. Childhood exposure to salted fish was not investigated in the Taiwan study.

A case-control study in Tianjin, a coastal city in northern China where NPC is relatively rare (incidence of 2/100,000 in men), confirmed the association between salted fish and NPC previously observed in southern Chinese populations (Ning et al, 1990). Four characteristics of exposure to salted fish were shown to independently contribute to the increased risk for NPC: (1) earlier age at first exposure, (2) increasing duration of consumption, (3) increasing frequency of consumption, and (4) cooking the fish by steaming it as opposed to frying, grilling, or boiling it. It is estimated that 40% of NPC cases occurring in this low-risk region can be attributed to consumption of salted fish (Ning et al, 1990).

In Northeast Thailand, two types of salted fish are consumed by the local Thai population. The home-prepared Thai-style salted fish are freshwater fish that are preserved in salty water until consumption. The local residents also consumed Chinese salted fish, which are available in the markets. A recent case-control study examined the possible association between current intake of either type of salted fish and NPC risk. Interestingly, consumption of Chinese salted fish showed a clear and statistically significant dose-response relationship with NPC, while no association was observed with exposure to Thai-style salted fish (Sriamporn et al, 1992).

In summary, all case-control studies to date have produced remarkably consistent findings in support of exposure to Chinese salted fish as a cause of NPC. Data derived from Cantonese populations (Yu et al, 1986, 1989a) indicate that 90% of NPC cases occurring in people of this ethnic group are related to early exposure to this food.

Chinese salted fish as an etiologic agent of NPC with early age at exposure being an important codeterminant of risk is compatible with the epidemiological profile of NPC in southern China. The peak incidence of NPC in southern Chinese are between the ages 45 and 54 with a definite decline at subsequent ages, suggesting that exposure occurs early and that exposure either declines or the target tissue is less susceptible (or both) at later ages. Exposure to salted fish can also explain the inverse association between NPC risk and socioeconomic status in these high-risk people. In Hong Kong (Yu et al, 1986), 38% of controls with primary school or less education were weaned on salted fish, compared with 21% of controls with higher levels of education. In Malaysia (Armstrong and Eng, 1983), 25% of controls belonging to the low-income group consumed salted fish at least once a week, compared to 15% of controls in the higher income groups. Finally, the 2-fold higher risk of NPC in the Cantonese relative to the Hakka and Chiu Chau dialect groups in Guangdong is compatible with the varying prevalence of salted-fish consumption between the three ethnic groups. Whereas 50% of mothers of controls in Guangzhou (Cantonese population) indicated that the subjects were exposed at weaning (Yu et al, 1989a), only 10 (20%) of 50 mothers of healthy subjects in Shantou Prefecture (Chiu Chau population) and 7 (14%) of 50 similar mothers in Meixian Prefecture (Hakka population) indicated likewise exposure (Yu, unpublished data).

Data from whole-animal experiments have further strengthened the hypothesis that Chinese salted fish is a human nasopharyngeal carcinogen. Huang et al (1978) successfully induced cancers of the nasal cavity in Wistar rats fed cooked Chinese salted fish, which otherwise rarely occurs in this animal species. Yu et al (1989b) confirmed those findings in a larger study, which demonstrated a dose-response relationship between level of intake and rate of tumor occurrence. Furthermore, the amounts of salted fish (in terms of percent of total diet) fed to the Wistar rats in Yu et al (1989b) were within the range of potential human (Cantonese) consumption, and the tumor (nasal cavity) rate observed in those rats was in general agreement with the rate of NPC occurrence in Cantonese. Recently, Zheng et al (1994a) demonstrated dose-dependent induction of nasal tumors in Sprague-Dawley rats fed cooked Chinese salted fish.

Low-levels (subparts per million) of several volatile nitrosamines, including N-nitrosodimethylamine, N-nitrosodiethylamine, N-nitrosodi-n-propylamine, N-nitrosodi-n-butylamine and N-nitrosomorpholine, have been detected in samples of Chinese salted fish (Huang et al, 1981; Tannenbaum et al, 1985). Most of these volatile nitrosamines can induce nasal and paranasal cavity tumors in animals (Haas et al, 1973; Pour et al, 1973; Althoff et al, 1974; Lijinsky and Taylor, 1978). In addition to these preformed nitrosamines, bacterial mutagens have been detected in Chinese salted fish that had been exposed to a nitrosating agent under simulated gastric conditions (Tannenbaum et al, 1985; Weng et al, 1992). Directly acting genotoxic substances have also been found in extracts of this food (Poirier et al, 1989). At present, it is not clear whether the volatile nitrosamines, bacterial mutagens, or genotoxic substances present in Chinese salted fish are the putative carcinogens for NPC; the food may contain other types of carcinogenic substances that have not been identified. In addition, samples of Chinese salted fish were found to contain substance(s) capable of activating EBV in latently infected Raji cells (Shao et al, 1988).

Other Dietary Factors

There is some preliminary evidence that early exposure to other types of salted fish may explain at least some of the raised rates of NPC in the native peoples of southeast Asia and the arctic region. In a small case-control study (13 cases, 50 controls) of NPC among Malays in Selangor, Malaysia, Armstrong and Armstrong (1983) found 5 (38%) cases versus 4 (8%) controls to be daily eaters of salted fish during childhood. In the Philippines, West et al (1993) observed a nonsignificant 30% excess risk among subjects belonging to the highest tertile of usual adult intake of salted fish relative to those in the lowest tertile. In Alaska, interviews on 13 NPC patient-control pairs revealed more cases than controls to be frequent users of salted fish during childhood (case yes/control no vs. control yes/case no = 4 vs. 1) (Lanier et al, 1980).

Besides salted fish, early exposure to other preserved food products has been shown to be related to NPC risk. In Yulin Prefecture in southern China, exposures before age two years to chung choi (a kind of salted root), salted duck eggs, salted mustard green, dried fish, and fermented soybean paste were independent risk factors for NPC (Yu et al, 1988). In Guangzhou, exposures at age 10 years to fermented fish sauce, moldy bean curd, salted shrimp paste, and *chan pai mui* and *gar ink gee* (two kinds of preserved plum) were independently related to NPC risk (Yu et al, 1989a). In Taiwan, exposures before age 20 years to fermented bean products and smoked meat increased risk of NPC independently (Chen et al, 1988b). In Tianjin, exposure to salted shrimp paste at age 10 years was related to NPC risk independent of salted-fish intake (Ning et al, 1990). While childhood exposure levels to most of these foods were low in the case series studied, chung choi was a weaning food for 60% of cases in Yulin, salted shrimp paste was consumed at age 10 years by 48% of cases in Tianjin, and 63% of cases in Taiwan consumed fermented bean products before age 20 years. Thus, preserved foods other than salted fish may account for a substantial proportion of NPC cases in certain Chinese populations.

Intake of preserved foods early in life was also shown to be associated with NPC risk among the Arabs of north Africa, who are believed to possess raised rates of NPC. In Tunisia, Jeannel et al (1990) observed significant associations between NPC risk and childhood exposure to three preserved foods in the local diet: Quaddid (dried mutton preserved in olive oil); Touklia (stewing mixture of red and black peppers, paprika, caraway seed and/or coriander seed, salt, and olive or soya oil); and Harissa (mixture of red pepper, garlic, caraway seed, salt, and olive oil).

Low levels (parts per billion) of several volatile nitrosamines have been detected in samples of Chinese mustard green, chung choi and fermented soybean pastes, and Tunisian Quaddid and Touklia (Poirier et al, 1987). N-nitrosodimethylamine was detected in Quaddid, Touklia, salted mustard green, and chung choi; N-nitrosopiperidine in Touklia and salted mustard green; and N-nitrosopyrrolidine in Quaddid, Touklia, salted mustard green, chung choi, and fermented soybean pastes. In addition, directly acting genotoxic substances have been found in samples of Chinese salted shrimp and fermented soybean pastes; and Tunisian Quaddid, Touklia, and Harissa (Poirier et al, 1989). As in the case of salted fish, it is not clear yet whether any of the volatile nitrosamines or genotoxic substances detected in these preserved foods are directly involved in the carcinogenic process.

In an uncontrolled study of very young (under age 25 years) NPC patients in Hong Kong, Anderson et al (1978) reported that "all families felt that vegetables and fruits were bad for babies, and the children had been fed accordingly." These observations were later confirmed in case-control studies. In both Hong Kong and Guangzhou, cases ingested significantly less fresh vegetables and fruits than controls, especially during childhood. Whereas in Hong Kong the protective effects of fresh vegetables and fruits were no longer significant after adjustment for salted fish intake, in Guangzhou such effects were not explained by the differing consumption pattern of salted fish and other preserved foods between cases and controls (Yu et al, 1989a). In Tianjin (Ning et al, 1990), although general consumption of "fresh fruit" or "fresh vegetables" was not associated with a reduction in NPC risk, a significant protective effect with carrot intake at age 10 years was evident, and garlic, the only other fresh vegetable item on the questionnaire, also showed declining risks with increasing frequency of consumption, although the effect was not statistically significant. Fruits and vegetables are rich in an array of chemical compounds that have been suggested to be protective against cancer (Wattenberg, 1978). It is interesting to note that African NPC patients showed significantly lower levels of serum carotene compared to controls (Clifford, 1972). The hypothesis that substance(s) present in certain fresh vegetables and fruits exert a modifying and beneficial effect on risk of NPC deserves further investigation.

Inhalants

Dobson (1924), in an attempt to explain the high risk of NPC in southern Chinese, first proposed that exposure to smoke from wood fires inside chimneyless houses may be a cause of NPC in these people. Later in Kenya, Clifford (1972) also noted the presence of wood fires in chimneyless houses among tribal groups at moderately elevated rates of NPC. However, there is little support from case-control studies that domestic smoke exposure is a risk factor for NPC. Five of the six studies that investigated this potential risk factor in southern Chinese found no evidence of an association (Shanmugaratnam and Higginson, 1967; Geser et al, 1978; Yu et al, 1986, 1988, 1990; Zheng et al, 1994b). Furthermore, it was observed that in China chimneyless houses were not confined to the southern region, and that the highlanders of Papua New Guinea who also lived in poorly ventilated houses and were heavily exposed to smoke from wood fires had low rates of NPC (Ho, 1972a). Exposures to burning incense and anti-mosquito coils have also been suggested as risk factors for NPC; overall, there is little evidence that such exposures are related to NPC risk (Yu et al, 1986, 1988, 1990; Chen et al, 1988b; West et al, 1993).

In a case-control study involving 156 NPC patients and 267 controls in California, Henderson et al (1976) found occupational exposure to fumes, smoke, and chemicals to be significantly related to NPC risk. Later, Armstrong et al (1983) reported occupational exposure to smoke or dust as a risk factor for NPC in Malaysian Chinese, independent of salted-fish intake. The authors pointed out that airborne particles associated with the types of smoke and dusts their cases were exposed to were of the size and weight that would be deposited mostly in the nasopharynx. In Taiwan, occupational exposure to smoke was significantly related to NPC risk (Chen et al, 1988b). In Guangzhou, Yu et al (1990) observed significant, duration-dependent increased risks of NPC associated with occupational exposures to smoke and chemical fumes. In the Philippines, West et al (1993) reported significant associations between NPC risk and exposure to dusts and exhaust fumes. A number of studies have also reported an increased risk for nasopharyngeal cancer among wood workers who are potentially exposed to wood dust and various chemicals that are applied to the wood, including pesticides, phenols, chlorophenols, asbestos, etc. (Mould and Bakowski, 1976; Hardell et al, 1982; Lam and Tan, 1984; Ng, 1986; Kawachi et al, 1989; Vaughan and Davis, 1991). These results suggest that inhalation of carcinogen-containing fumes, smoke, or dust in the more intensely exposed occupational environment may be a risk factor for NPC.

A number of rodent experiments that demonstrated the induction of squamous cell carcinomas of the nasal cavity in rats and mice exposed to formaldehyde vapors (Swenberg et al, 1980; Albert et al, 1982; Kerns et al, 1983) have led to a suspicion that the chemical, with annual commercial production in the U.S. exceeding 9 billion pounds (Chemical Information Services, 1979), may be a human carcinogen. Humans are nose and mouth breathers, and so the affected sites are likely to include the buccal-pharyngeal cavity, which would come into direct contact with gaseous formaldehyde (Blair et al, 1987). In a historical cohort study involving more than 26,000 industrial workers employed in 10 formaldehyde-producing or -using facilities, a significant excess of nasopharyngeal cancer deaths relative to the general U.S. population was noted (Blair et al, 1986). It was further found that risk increased with increasing cumulative exposure to formaldehyde among those who were also exposed to particulates, although the trend was not statistically significant (Blair et al, 1987). Four case-control studies also have examined the possible association between nasopharyngeal cancer and formaldehyde exposure. In Denmark, the occupational experiences of 266 cases of nasopharyngeal cancer were compared with those of 2,465 cancer controls, and no association with probable formaldehyde exposure was detected (Olsen et al, 1984). On the other hand, when 27 cases of nasopharyngeal cancer in western Washington were compared to 552 population controls in terms of prior probable exposure to formaldehyde in an occupational setting, a 2-fold risk was observed in individuals belonging to the highest exposure category relative to those without any known occupational exposure (Vaughan et al, 1986a). Among these same individuals, a history of living in a mobile home (which is in general associated with higher residential exposures to formaldehyde) carried a RR of 3.0 and risk increased with increasing years of mobile home residence; in the presence of both high occupational and high residential exposures, the risk of nasopharyngeal cancer was increased 7-fold (Vaughan et al, 1986b). In Connecticut, 173 cases of nasopharyngeal cancer and 605 controls were compared in terms of their occupational histories, and probable exposure to high levels of formaldehyde 20 or more years before was associated with a 2-fold risk (Roush et al, 1987). West et al (1993) investigated occupational exposure to formaldehyde in 104 NPC cases and 205 hospital and community controls in the Philippines, and observed a 4-fold excess risk of NPC among subjects who were first exposed to formaldehyde 25 or more years ago relative to unexposed subjects. In Sweden, Malker et al (1990) linked nasopharyngeal cancer incidence (1961–79) and census data (1960) on industry and occupation for all employed men and found a significant 4-fold increased risk associated with fiberboard manufacturing, a process that uses formaldehyde-based urea resins. An examination of the causes of mortality among 4,046 male embalmers and funeral directors (who would be exposed to formaldehyde in their jobs) in the U.S. revealed a nonsignificant 2-fold excess for nasopharyngeal cancer (Hayes et al, 1990). Thus, the available data, although relatively sparse, tend to support the hypothesis that formaldehyde is a nasopharyngeal carcinogen.

In Guangzhou, China, exposure to cotton dust was found to be significantly associated with a decreased risk for NPC (relative risk = 0.3) (Yu et al, 1990). The degree of protection was proportional to the duration of exposure and the occupations of exposed subjects were all consistent with their claims of exposure. The authors suggested that the putative protective effect might be related to the high concentrations of bacterial endotoxins, which are capable of eliciting various antitumor responses in the host (Enterline et al, 1985), that are contained in cotton dust. However, this novel finding was not supported by a later study in Shanghai, China, which compared employment information at the time of cancer diagnosis in 996 incident NPC cases diagnosed during 1980–1984 with occupational data for the Shanghai general population obtained from the 1982 census. In this occupation-cancer linkage study, female textile weavers and knitters actually displayed significantly elevated risks for NPC (Zheng et al, 1992).

Tobacco and Alcohol

A number of case-control studies have examined the relationship between tobacco use and NPC among Chinese in Southeast Asia, Hong Kong, Taiwan, and China; whites in the U.S.; and natives of the Philippine Islands (Shanmugaratnam and Higginson, 1967; Lin et al, 1973a; Henderson et al, 1976; Armstrong et al, 1978, 1983; Shanmugaratnam et al, 1978; Li et al, 1985; Mabuchi et al, 1985; Yu et al, 1986, 1990; Chen et al, 1988b; Nam et al, 1992; Chow et al, 1993; West et al, 1993). Although earlier data are equivocal, more recent data from well-designed studies are consistent in supporting cigarette smoking as a risk factor for NPC regardless of race. Increased risks of 3–5-fold were observed among the heaviest smokers in the U.S., China, or the Philippines (Nam et al, 1992; Chow et al, 1993; Yu et al, 1990; West et al, 1993).

A case-control study in Guangxi, China (Yu et al, 1988), found living with a smoker during childhood to be a significant and independent risk factor for NPC, with a positive trend in risk by increasing number of cigarettes smoked per day by the father. This novel finding, however, was not confirmed in a subsequent case-control study in Guangzhou, China (Yu et al, 1990).

The possible association between alcohol intake and NPC development have been investigated in a number of case-control studies among Chinese in and outside of China, and among U.S. whites (Shanmugaratnam and Higginson, 1967; Lin et al, 1973a; Henderson et al, 1976; Shanmugaratnam et al, 1978; Geser et al, 1978; Armstrong et al, 1983; Mabuchi et al, 1985; Chen et al, 1988b; Nam et al, 1992). All studies except Nam et al (1992) found no association between alcohol consumption and NPC risk. Nam et al (1992) relied on surrogate interviews for exposure information (all cases and controls were identified from death certificates). The 80% excess risk noted in that study after controlling for level of cigarette smoking could have been the result of residual confounding.

Other Factors

A number of Chinese herbal plants have been shown to induce EBV antigens in EBV-genome carrying human lymphoblastoid cell lines (Hirayama and Ito, 1981; Zeng et al, 1983; Zeng, 1987), raising the possibility that exposure to these products may influence one's risk of NPC. It was pointed out that one of these EBV-inducer plants, croton tiglium, whose seeds are used in Chinese herbs, possesses a geographical distribution that loosely parallels NPC incidence within China (Hirayama and Ito, 1981). Actually, due to their extreme potency, croton seeds are rarely used in herbal mixtures. None of the study subjects in Yu et al (1986, 1988, 1990) claimed prior exposure to croton seeds. Yu et al (1990) also examined usage of *Phyllanthus emblica* and *Croton crassifolius,* two EBV-inducing herbs that are commonly prescribed in Guangzhou (according to government sales figures); no relationship with NPC was observed. General use of herbal drugs had been reported to be associated with NPC in three case-control studies (Lin et al, 1973a; Hildesheim et al, 1992; Zheng et al, 1994b). However, other case-control studies in southern China did not find any residual (after adjustment for salted-fish consumption) association with intake of "cooling soup," the most popular herbal drink in southern China (Yu et al, 1986, 1988, 1989a).

Chinese investigators in Guangdong Province compared the contents of trace elements in rice and drinking water and in the hairs of normal subjects from two counties with varying NPC incidence (7–8-fold difference in male rates), and found the levels of nickel to be 1.7–2.7 times higher in the high-incidence compared to the low-incidence county. Moreover, NPC cases from the high-incidence county had significantly higher nickel contents in their hairs than normal subjects (Li et al, 1983). In Hunan Province, the nickel content in drinking water from an area with higher NPC incidence also was significantly raised relative to a lower-incidence area (Xia et al, 1988). These interesting observations deserve further and more extensive studies to establish the pattern of oral exposure to nickel throughout China and its relationship to NPC incidence.

The use of Chinese nasal oil, of which the main ingredients are camphor and menthol, has been postulated as a risk factor for NPC. The overall evidence does not suggest a causal role for nasal oil in NPC development. Yu et al (1986, 1990) noted higher recent (3 years before) use among cases compared to controls, which was related to clinical symptoms of NPC. The more relevant exposure during childhood was examined in three case-control studies (Yu et al, 1986, 1988, 1990). Although in two studies (Yu et al, 1988, 1990) more case- than control-mothers reported use by subjects during childhood, most of the exposures were infrequent and/or unsubstantiated by a medical condition that could suggest a more intense and sustained use.

Seven case-control studies have examined the possible role of prior ear or nose conditions in the development of NPC, and six have observed an association (Lin et al, 1973a; Henderson et al, 1976; Shanmugaratnam et al, 1978; Geser et al, 1978; Yu et al, 1988, 1990). In Yu et al (1990), the statistically significant excess risk persisted after recent conditions (those diagnosed within the last 10 years) and conditions that did not require medical treatment were excluded. The NPC-associated conditions include rhinitis or allergic rhinitis, sinusitis, nasal polyp, and otitis media (Yu et al, 1988, 1990). The overall evidence, therefore, suggests that inflammatory and certain other benign conditions of the ear and nose predispose the nasopharyngeal mucosa to transformation by environmental carcinogens.

HOST FACTORS

HLA Genes

Case-control studies have established several associations between HLA-locus A and B antigens and NPC risk in southern Chinese. A joint occurrence of A2-BW46 antigens was associated with a 2-fold increased risk of NPC among Chinese in Singapore, Malaysia, Hong Kong, and Guangzhou (Simons et al, 1976, 1977, 1978, 1981; Chan et al, 1983a). Interestingly, the frequency of the A2-BW46 phenotype is 2 times more common in Cantonese relative to the Chiu Chau/Fujianese dialect group, in parallel to the 2-fold difference in NPC incidence between these two ethnic groups (Simons et al, 1976). Other HLA antigens showing an association with NPC risk in southern Chinese are B16 (RR = 6.0), B17 (RR = 2.1) especially the co-occurrence of AW19-B17 (RR = 2.5), A11 (RR = 0.5), and B13 (RR = 0.5) (Simons et al, 1978; Chan et al, 1981, 1983a; Wu et al, 1989). In addition, preliminary work on HLA-locus DR typing in this high-risk population has shown significant differences in antigen frequencies between NPC cases and controls (Simons et al, 1981; Chan et al, 1981, 1983b; Wu et al, 1989). Recently, a linkage study based on affected sib pairs among southern Chinese suggests that a gene (or genes) closely linked to the HLA locus is associated with a 20-fold increased risk of NPC (Lu et al, 1990).

An association between HLA profile and NPC risk also has been reported in non-Chinese populations. Antigen B17 has been found to be positively associated with NPC risk in Malays (Chan et al, 1985) and Australian whites (Simons and Shanmugaratnam, 1982). Other antigens that exhibited an association with NPC in selected populations were: A29 in Kenyans and Tanzanians, B18 in Malays, A3 in Australian whites, B5 in Germans, and A2 in U.S. whites (Kruger et al, 1981; Hall et al, 1982; Simons and Shanmugaratnam, 1982; Chan et al, 1985; Burt et al, 1994). In contrast to southern Chinese, BW46 is an uncommon antigen in U.S. whites, Europeans, Tunisians, and Malays, and no association with NPC was evident in these populations (Betuel et al, 1975; Chan et al, 1979, 1985; Beigel et al, 1983; Moore et al, 1983).

Other Genetic Markers

Kirk et al (1978) studied 25 red-cell enzyme and 5 serum protein systems in 229 Singapore-Chinese NPC patients and 240 controls, and found the gene frequencies between the two groups to differ significantly in two systems. In Tunisia, several immunoglobulin allotypic markers were tested in 80 NPC patients and 404 controls. The frequencies of the Km (1) allotype and two uncommon Gm phenotypes, Gm (1,17; 11,15,21) and Gm (1,3; 5,11), were significantly increased in NPC patients relative to controls (Chaabani and Ellouz, 1986). The distributions of Gm and Km allotypes were also examined among 50 Chinese NPC cases and 140 Chinese controls, and 50 Malay cases and 79 Malay controls in Malaysia (Tarone et al, 1990), but no significant differences between cases and controls were found. In the U.S., Danes (1986) examined the incidence of hyperdiploidy exclusive of tetraploidy (IVH) in cultures derived from skin biopsies of members of an NPC-prone family (a history of NPC in three consecutive generations). Two of 2 NPC patients, 4 of 16 first-degree relatives of NPC patients, and none of 6 spouse controls showed IVH. Later, Danes (1987) assayed for IVH in 39 NPC patients and 29 clinically normal subjects without a family history of cancer. No controls but 19 (49%) NPC patients showed IVH; the mean age of IVH-positive patients was 52 years, while that of IVH-negative patients was 67 years. The possible association between ABO blood groups and NPC risk was investigated in Chinese, and no relationship was seen (Ho, 1972a). On the other hand, Clifford (1970) compared ABO blood group distributions in 233 NPC patients and historical controls in Kenya, and noted a significant deficit of A/O among NPC patients.

Familial Aggregation

Multiple cases of NPC occurring in first-degree relatives have been documented in diverse populations, ranging from high-risk southern Chinese and Alaskan and Greenland natives, low- to intermediate-risk Africans, to low-risk Caucasians (Stinson, 1940; Bell and Maguda, 1970; Nevo et al, 1971; Ho, 1972a; Williams and de-The, 1974; Brown et al, 1976; Jonas et al, 1976; Lanier et al, 1979; Gajwani et al, 1980; Fischer et al, 1984; Yu et al, 1986, 1990; Schimke et al, 1987; Albeck et al, 1993). Familial aggregation can be the result of shared genes, shared environments, or both. Among the high-risk southern Chinese, a potent environmental factor that correlates highly within families (dietary exposures at weaning) has been identified, and consistent associations with certain HLA antigens implicate the presence of disease-susceptibility genes. Genetic studies in non-Chinese populations also suggest the involvement of hereditary factors in the development of NPC, and analytic studies have implicated environmental factors. Familial clusterings of NPC, therefore, is likely to be a product of genetic constitution and environmental exposures.

PREVENTIVE MEASURES

There is strong evidence implicating dietary factors (exposure to preserved foods, especially during childhood) as a major cause of NPC in the handful of populations with raised incidence of this disease (southern Chinese, natives of the Arctic region and Southeast Asia, Arabs of north Africa). These at-risk populations, therefore, should be educated about the carcinogenic potential of those local foods, and mothers especially should be discouraged from feeding those foods to their young children.

FUTURE RESEARCH

1. Although a number of potentially carcinogenic substances have been identified in Chinese salted fish and other NPC-associated foods, it is presently unclear whether any of them are involved as nasopharyngeal carcinogens. Laboratory work to systematically search for the compound(s) contained in Chinese salted fish and other NPC-associated foods that give rise to NPC in humans should receive a high priority.
2. Analytic data relating diet to NPC risk are sparse in non-Chinese populations. Detailed diet studies with adequate sample sizes are needed to investigate NPC development among the indigenous people of Southeast Asia and the Arctic region, and in North Africans.
3. There is some suggestion that ingestion of certain fruits and vegetables may have a modifying and beneficial effect on NPC development in high-risk populations. More and better data are needed to confirm these preliminary observations. One should consider incorporating biochemical measurements into the new studies.
4. Results of rodent experiments first led to a suspicion that gaseous formaldehyde may be a human carcinogen. Epidemiological data on the possible formaldehyde-cancer association, albeit relatively sparse, tend to support the hypothesis that formaldehyde is a nasopharyngeal carcinogen. More analytical studies with improved exposure assessments are needed to better quantify the exposure-disease relationship.
5. Although there is evidence that genetic susceptibility plays a role in NPC development, we are far from identifying such disease-susceptibility genes. Genetic studies examining HLA and other systems in Chinese as well as other populations should continue.

REFERENCES

ALBECK H, BENTZEN J, OCKELMANN HH, et al. 1993. Familial clusters of nasopharyngeal carcinoma and salivary gland carcinomas in Greenland Natives. Cancer 72:196–200.

ALBECK H, NIELSEN NH, HANSEN HE, et al. 1992. Epidemiology of nasopharyngeal and salivary gland carcinoma in Greenland. Arctic Med Res 51:189–195.

ALBERT RE, SELLAKUMAR AR, LASKIN S, et al. 1982. Gaseous formaldehyde and hydrogen chloride induction of nasal cancer in the rat. J Natl Cancer Inst 68:597–603.

AL-IDRISSI HY. 1990. Head and neck cancer in Saudi Arabia: retrospective analysis of 65 patients. J Int Med Res 18:515–519.

ALTHOFF J, MOHR U, PAGE N, et al. 1974. Carcinogenic effect of dibutylnitrosamine in European hamsters (*Cricetus cricetus*). J Natl Cancer Inst 53:795–800.

ANDERSON EN, ANDERSON ML, HO HC. 1978. Environmental backgrounds of young Chinese nasopharyngeal carcinoma patients. IARC Sci Publ 20:231–239.

ANH PTH, PARKIN DM, HANH NT, et al. 1993. Cancer in the population of Hanoi, Vietnam, 1988–1990. Br J Cancer 68:1236–1242.

ARMSTRONG RW, ARMSTRONG MJ. 1983. Environmental risk factors and nasopharyngeal carcinoma in Selangor, Malaysia: a cross-ethnic perspective. Ecol Disease 2:185–198.

ARMSTRONG RW, ARMSTRONG MJ, YU MC, et al. 1983. Salted fish and inhalants as risk factors for nasopharyngeal carcinoma in Malaysian Chinese. Cancer Res 43:2967–2970.

ARMSTRONG RW, ENG ACS. 1983. Salted fish and nasopharyngeal carcinoma in Malaysia. Soc Sci Med 17:1559–1567.

ARMSTRONG RW, KANNAN KUTTY M, ARMSTRONG MJ. 1978. Self-specific environments associated with nasopharyngeal carcinoma in Selangor, Malaysia. Soc Sci Med 12D:149–156.

ARMSTRONG RW, KANNAN KUTTY M, DHARMALINGAM SK, et al. 1979. Incidence of nasopharyngeal carcinoma in Malaysia, 1968–1977. Br J Cancer 40:557–567.

BALAKRISHNAN V. 1975. An additional younger-age peak for cancer of the nasopharynx. Int J Cancer 15:651–657.

BEIGEL A, PEULEN JF, WESTPHAL E. 1983. The spectrum of histocompatibility antigens (HLA) in tumors of the nasopharynx. Arch Otorhinolaryngol 237:285–288.

BELL RB, MAGUDA TA. 1970. Nasopharyngeal carcinoma in Caucasian siblings: report of two cases. J Tenn Med Assoc 63:753–754.

BETUEL H, CAMMOUN M, COLOMBANI J, et al. 1975. The relationship between nasopharyngeal carcinoma and the HL-A system among Tunisians. Int J Cancer 16:249–254.

BLAIR A, STEWART PA, O'BERG M, et al. 1986. Mortality among industrial workers exposed to formaldehyde. J Natl Cancer Inst 76:1071–1084.

BLAIR A, STEWART PA, HOOVER RN, et al. 1987. Cancers of the nasopharynx and oropharynx and formaldehyde exposure. J Natl Cancer Inst 78:191–192.

BOGGER-GOREN S, GOTLIEB-STEMATSKY T, RACHIMA M, et al. 1987. Nasopharyngeal carcinoma in Israel: Epidemiology and Epstein-Barr virus–related serology. Eur J Cancer Clin Oncol 23:1277–1281.

BROWN TM, HEATH CW, LANG RM, et al. 1976. Nasopharyngeal cancer in Bermuda. Cancer 37:1464–1468.

BUELL P. 1973. Race and place in the etiology of nasopharyngeal cancer: a study based on California death certificates. Int J Cancer 11:268–272.

BUELL P. 1974. The effect of migration on the risk of nasopharyngeal cancer among Chinese. Cancer Res 34:1189–1191.

BURT RD, VAUGHAN TL, MCKNIGHT B. 1992. Descriptive epidemiology and survival analysis of nasopharyngeal carcinoma in the United States. Int J Cancer 52:549–556.

BURT RD, VAUGHAN TL, NISPEROS B, et al. 1994. A protective association between the HLA-A2 antigen and nasopharyngeal carcinoma in US Caucasians. Int J Cancer 56:465–467.

CAMMOUN M, HOERNER GV, MOURALI N. 1974. Tumors of the nasopharynx in Tunisia. An anatomic and clinical study based on 143 cases. Cancer 33:184–192.

CHAABANI H, ELLOUZ R. 1986. Immunoglobulin allotypes in patients with nasopharyngeal carcinoma. Hum Hered 36:402–404.

CHAN SH, CHEW CT, PRASAD U, et al. 1985. HLA and nasopharyngeal carcinoma in Malays. Br J Cancer 51:389–392.

CHAN SH, DAY NE, KHOR TH, et al. 1981. HLA markers in the development and prognosis of NPC in Chinese. In Grundmann E, Krueger GRF, Ablashi DV (eds): Cancer Campaign, Vol. 5, Nasopharyngeal Carcinoma. Stuttgart: Gustav Fischer Verlag, pp. 205–211.

CHAN SH, DAY NE, KUNARATNAM N, et al. 1983a. HLA and nasopharyngeal carcinoma in Chinese—a further study. Int J Cancer 32:171–176.

CHAN SH, WEE GB, KUNARATNAM N, et al. 1983b. HLA locus B and DR antigen associations in Chinese NPC patients and controls. In Prasad U, Ablashi DV, Levine PH, et al (eds): Nasopharyngeal Carcinoma: Current Concepts. Kuala Lumpur: University of Malaya Press, pp. 307–312.

CHAN SH, WEE GB, SRINIVASAN N, et al. 1979. HLA antigens in three common populations in South East Asia—Chinese, Malay and Filipino. Tissue Antigens 13:361–368.

CHEMICAL INFORMATION SERVICES. 1979. Directory of Chemical Producers, United States of America. Menlo Park: SRI International, pp. 637–638.

CHEN C-J, CHEN J-Y, HSU M-M, et al. 1988a. Epidemiological characteristics and early detection of nasopharyngeal carcinoma in Taiwan. In Wolf GT, Carey TE (eds): Head and Neck Oncology Research. Amsterdam-Berkeley: Kugler Publications, pp. 505–513.

CHEN C-J, WANG Y-F, SHIEH T, et al. 1988b. Multifactorial etiology of nasopharyngeal carcinoma. Epstein-Barr virus, familial tendency and environmental cofactors. In Wolf GT, Carey TE (eds): Head and Neck Oncology Research. Amsterdam-Berkeley: Kugler Publications, pp. 469–476.

CHINN TW, LAI HM, CHOY PP (EDS). 1969. A History of the Chinese in California. A Syllabus. San Francisco: Chinese Historical Society of America, pp. 2–4, 20.

CHOW W-H, MCLAUGHLIN JK, HRUBEC Z, et al. 1993. Tobacco use and nasopharyngeal carcinoma in a cohort of US veterans. Int J Cancer 55:538–540.

CLIFFORD P. 1970. Blood-groups and nasopharyngeal carcinoma. Lancet 2:48–49.

CLIFFORD P. 1972. Carcinogens in the nose and throat: nasopharyngeal carcinoma in Kenya. Proc Roy Soc Med 65:682–686.

DANES BS. 1986. *In vitro* hyperdiploidy in a family with nasopharyngeal cancer. Cancer Genet Cytogenet 21:107–115.

DANES BS, BOYLE PD, TRAGANOS F, et al. 1987. Evidence for genetic predisposition for some nasopharyngeal cancers by *in vitro* hyperdiploidy in human dermal fibroblasts. Cancer Genet Cytogenet 26:261–270.

DE SCHRYVER A, KLEIN G, HENLE W, et al. 1974. EB virus-associated antibodies in Caucasian patients with carcinoma of the nasopharynx and in long-term survivors after treatment. Int J Cancer 13:319–325.

DE-THE G, DAY NE, GESER A, et al. 1975. Sero-epidemiology of the Epstein-Barr virus: Preliminary analysis of an international study—a review. IARC Sci Publ 11(2):3–16.

DICKENS P, SRIVASTAVA G, LOKE SL, et al. 1992. Epstein-Barr virus DNA in nasopharyngeal carcinoma from Chinese patients in Hong Kong. J Clin Pathol 45:396–397.

DOBSON WH. 1924. Cervical lympho-sarcoma. Chin Med J (Engl) 38:786–787.

DOLL R, MUIR CS, WATERHOUSE JAH. 1970. Cancer Incidence in Five Continents, Vol. 2. UICC, Geneva.

ENTERLINE PE, SYKORA JL, KELETI G, et al. 1985. Endotoxins, cotton dust, and cancer. Lancet 2:934–935.

FISCHER A, FISCHER GO, COOPER E. 1984. Familial nasopharyngeal carcinoma. Pathology 16:23–24.

FRAUMENI JF, MASON TJ. 1974. Cancer mortality among Chinese Americans, 1950–69. J Natl Cancer Inst 52:659–665.

GAJWANI BW, DEVEREAUX JM, BEG JA. 1980. Familial clustering of nasopharyngeal carcinoma. Cancer 46:2325–2327.

GALLAGHER RP, ELWOOD JM. 1979. Cancer mortality among Chinese, Japanese, and Indians in British Columbia, 1964–73. Natl Cancer Inst Monogr 53:89–94.

GESER A, CHARNEY N, DAY NE, et al. 1978. Environmental factors in the etiology of nasopharyngeal carcinoma: report on a case-control study in Hong Kong. IARC Sci Publ 20:213–229.

HAAS H, MOHR U, KRUGER FW. 1973. Comparative studies with different doses of N-nitrosomorpholine, N-nitrosopiperidine, N-nitrosomethylurea, and dimethylnitrosamine in Syrian golden hamsters. J Natl Cancer Inst 51:1295–1301.

HALL PJ, LEVIN AG, ENTWISTLE CC, et al. 1982. HLA antigens in East African Black patients with Burkitt's lymphoma or nasopharyngeal carcinoma and in controls: a pilot study. Hum Immunol 5:91–105.

HARDELL L, JOHANSSON B, AXELSON O. 1982. Epidemiological study of nasal and nasopharyngeal cancer and their relation to phenoxy acid or chlorophenol exposures. Am J Ind Med 3:247–257.

HAYES RB, BLAIR A, STEWART PA, et al. 1990. Mortality of U.S. embalmers and funeral directors. Am J Ind Med 18:641–652.

HENDERSON BE, LOUIE E. 1978. Discussion of risk factors for nasopharyngeal carcinoma. IARC Sci Publ 20:251–260.

HENDERSON BE, LOUIE E, JING JS, et al. 1976. Risk factors associated with nasopharyngeal carcinoma. N Engl J Med 295:1101–1106.

HENDERSON BE, LOUIE EW, JING JS, et al. 1977. Epstein-Barr virus and nasopharyngeal carcinoma: is there an etiologic relationship? J Natl Cancer Inst 59:1393–1395.

HENLE W, HENLE G, HO H-C. 1970. Antibodies to Epstein-Barr virus in nasopharyngeal carcinoma, other head and neck neoplasms, and control groups. J Natl Cancer Inst 44:225–231.

HENLE W, HO H-C, HENLE G, et al. 1973. Antibodies to Epstein-Barr virus–related antigens in nasopharyngeal carcinoma. Comparison of active cases with long-term survivors. J Natl Cancer Inst 51:361–369.

HIDAYATALLA A, MALIK MOA, EL HADI AE, et al. 1983. Studies on nasopharyngeal carcinoma in the Sudan. I. Epidemiology and aetiology. Eur J Cancer Clin Oncol 19:705–710.

HILDESHEIM A, WEST S, DE VEYRA E, et al. 1992. Herbal medicine use, Epstein-Barr virus, and risk of nasopharyngeal carcinoma. Cancer Res 52:3048–3051.

HIRAYAMA T, ITO Y. 1981. A new view of the etiology of nasopharyngeal carcinoma. Prev Med 10:614–622.

HO HC. 1967. Nasopharyngeal carcinoma in Hong Kong. UICC Monogr Ser 1:58–63.

HO HC. 1972b. Current knowledge of the epidemiology of nasopharyngeal carcinoma—a review. IARC Sci Publ 2:357–366.

HO HC. 1976. Epidemiology of nasopharyngeal carcinoma. Gann Monogr Cancer Res 18:49–61.

HO JH. 1978. An epidemiologic and clinical study of nasopharyngeal carcinoma. Int J Radiat Oncol Biol Phys 4:183–198.

HO JHC. 1971. Genetic and environmental factors in nasopharyngeal carcinoma. Nakahara W, Nishioka K, Hirayama T, Ito Y (eds): Recent Advances in Human Tumor Virology and Immunology. Tokyo: University of Tokyo Press, pp. 275–295.

HO JHC. 1972a. Nasopharyngeal carcinoma (NPC). Adv Cancer Res 15:57–92.

HO JHC. 1985. Nasopharyngeal carcinoma. West J Med 143:70–73.

HO JHC, CHAN CL, LAU WH, et al. 1982. Cancer in Hong Kong: some epidemiological observations. Natl Cancer Inst Monogr 62:47–55.

HO P-T. 1959. Studies on the Population of China, 1368–1953. Cambridge: Harvard University Press, pp. 166–168.

HOOVER R, MASON TJ, MCKAY FW, et al. 1975. Geographic patterns of cancer mortality in the United States. In Fraumeni JF (ed): Persons at High Risk of Cancer. New York: Academic Press, pp. 343–360.

HSU H-C, CHEN C-L, HSU M-M, et al. 1987. Pathology of nasopharyngeal carcinoma. Proposal of a new histological classification correlated with prognosis. Cancer 59: 945–951.

HUANG DP, HO JHC, HENLE W, HENLE G. 1974. Demonstration of Epstein-Barr Virus-associated nuclear antigen in nasopharyngeal carcinoma cells from fresh biopsies. Int J Cancer 14:580–588.

HUANG DP, HO JHC, WEBB KS, et al. 1981. Volatile nitrosamines in salt-preserved fish before and after cooking. Food Cosmet Toxicol 19:167–171.

HUANG DP, SAW D, TEOH TB, et al. 1978. Carcinoma of the nasal and paranasal regions in rats fed Cantonese salted marine fish. IARC Sci Publ 20:315–328.

JEANNEL D, GHNASSIA M, HUBERT A, et al. 1993. Increased risk of nasopharyngeal carcinoma among males of French origin born in Maghreb (North Africa). Int J Cancer 54:536–539.

JEANNEL D, HUBERT A, DE VATHAIRE F, et al. 1990. Diet, living conditions and nasopharyngeal carcinoma in Tunisia—a case-control study. Int J Cancer 46:421–425.

JONAS JH, RIOUX E, ROBITAILLE R, et al. 1976. Multiple cases of lymphoepithelioma and Burkitt's lymphoma in a Canadian family. In Clemmesen J, Yohn DS (eds): Comparative Leukemia Research 1975. Basel, Karger, pp. 224–226.

KAWACHI I, PEARCE N, FRASER J. 1989. A New Zealand cancer registry–based study of cancer in wood workers. Cancer 64:2609–2613.

KERNS WD, PAVKOV KL, DONOFRIO DJ, et al. 1983. Carcinogenicity of formaldehyde in rats and mice after long-term inhalation exposure. Cancer Res 43:4382–4392.

KING H, HAENSZEL W. 1973. Cancer mortality among foreign- and native-born Chinese in the United States. J Chron Dis 26:623–646.

KIRK RL, BLAKE NM, SERJEANTSON S, et al. 1978. Genetic components in susceptibility to nasopharyngeal carcinoma. IARC Sci Publ 20:283–297.

KLEIN G, GIOVANELLA BC, LINDAHL T, et al. 1974. Direct evidence for the presence of Epstein-Barr virus DNA and nuclear antigen in malignant epithelial cells from patients with poorly differentiated carcinoma of the nasopharynx. Proc Natl Acad Sci USA 71:4737–4741.

KRIPALANI-JOSHI S, LAW HY. 1994. Identification of integrated Epstein-Barr virus in nasopharyngeal carcinoma using pulse field gel electrophoresis. Int J Cancer 56:187–192.

KRUGER J, IEROMNIMON V, DAHR W. 1981. Frequencies of HLA antigens in patients with NPC. In Grundmann E, Krueger GRF, Ablashi DV (eds): Cancer Campaign, Vol. 5, Nasopharyngeal Carcinoma. Stuttgart: Gustav Fischer Verlag, pp. 201–203.

LAI HM. 1988. On Chinese Americans: state of the art or challenge to the future? Amerasia Journal 14(2):xi–xiii.

LAM YM, TAN TC. 1984. Mortality from nasopharyngeal carcinoma and occupation in men in Hong Kong from 1976–1981. Ann Acad Med Singapore 13:361–365.

LANIER AP, BENDER TR, TSCHOPP CF, et al. 1979. Nasopharyngeal carcinoma in an Alaskan Eskimo family: report of three cases. J Natl Cancer Inst 62:1121–1124.

LANIER A, BENDER T, TALBOT M, et al. 1980. Nasopharyngeal carcinoma in Alaskan Eskimos, Indians, and Aleuts: a review of cases and study of Epstein-Barr virus, HLA, and environmental risk factors. Cancer 46:2100–2106.

LANIER AP, BORNKAMM GW, HENLE W, et al. 1981. Association of Epstein-Barr virus with nasopharyngeal carcinoma in Alaskan native patients: serum antibodies and tissue EBNA and DNA. Int J Cancer 28:301–305.

LEE HP, DUFFY SW, DAY NE, et al. 1988. Recent trends in cancer incidence among Singapore Chinese. Int J Cancer 42:159–166.

LEVINE PH, CONNELLY RR, EASTON JM. 1980. Demographic patterns for nasopharyngeal carcinoma in the United States. Int J Cancer 26:741–748.

LEVINE PH, CONNELLY RR. 1985. Epidemiology of nasopharyngeal cancer. In Wittes RE (ed): Head and Neck Cancer. New York: John Wiley & Sons, pp. 13–34.

LEVINE PH, MCKAY FW, CONNELLY RR. 1987. Patterns of nasopharyngeal cancer mortality in the United States. Int J Cancer 39:133–137.

LI C-C, PAN Q-C, CHEN J-J, et al (eds). 1983. Nasopharyngeal Carcinoma. Clinical and Laboratory Research. Guangzhou: Guangdong Scientific Publishing Co., pp. 129–130 (in Chinese).

LI C-C, YU MC, HENDERSON BE. 1985. Some epidemiologic observations of nasopharyngeal carcinoma in Guangdong, People's Republic of China. Natl Cancer Inst Monogr 69:49–52.

LIJINSKY W, TAYLOR HW. 1978. Relative carcinogenic effectiveness of derivatives of nitrosodiethylamine in rats. Cancer Res 38:2391–2394.

LIN TM, CHEN KP, LIN CC, et al. 1973a. Retrospective study on nasopharyngeal carcinoma. J Natl Cancer Inst 51:1403–1408.

LIN TM, YANG CS, CHIOU JF, et al. 1973b. Sero-epidemiological studies on carcinoma of the nasopharynx. Cancer Res 33:2603–2608.

LU S-J, DAY NE, DEGOS L, et al. 1990. Linkage of a nasopharyngeal carcinoma susceptibility locus to the HLA region. Nature 346:470–471.

MABUCHI K, BROSS DS, KESSLER II. 1985. Cigarette smoking and nasopharyngeal carcinoma. Cancer 55:2874–2876.

MALKER HSR, MCLAUGHLIN JK, WEINER JA, et al. 1990. Occupational risk factors for nasopharyngeal cancer in Sweden. Br J Ind Med 47:213–214.

MOORE SB, PEARSON GR, NEEL HB, et al. 1983. HLA and nasopharyngeal carcinoma in North American Caucasoids. Tissue Antigens 22:72–75.

MOULD RF, BAKOWSKI MT. 1976. Adenocarcinoma of nasopharynx. Lancet 2:1134–1135.

MUIR CS. 1971. Nasopharyngeal carcinoma in non-Chinese populations with special reference to south-east Asia and Africa. Int J Cancer 8:351–363.

MUIR C, WATERHOUSE J, MACK T, et al (eds). 1987. Cancer Incidence in Five Continents, Vol. 5. IARC Scientific Publications, No. 88. Lyon: International Agency for Research on Cancer.

NAEGELE RF, CHAMPION J, MURPHY S, et al. 1982. Nasopharyngeal carcinoma in American children: Epstein-Barr virus-specific antibody titers and prognosis. Int J Cancer 29:209–212.

NAM J-M, MCLAUGHLIN JK, BLOT WJ. 1992. Cigarette smoking, alcohol, and nasopharyngeal carcinoma: a case-control study among U.S. whites. J Natl Cancer Inst 84:619–622.

NATIONAL CANCER CONTROL OFFICE, NANJING INSTITUTE OF GEOGRAPHY. 1979. Atlas of Cancer Mortality in the People's Republic of China. Shanghai: China Map Press.

NEVO S, MEYER W, ALTMAN M. 1971. Carcinoma of nasopharynx in twins. Cancer 28:807–809.

NG TP. 1986. A case-referent study of cancer of the nasal cavity and sinuses in Hong Kong. Int J Epidemiol 15:171–175.

NING J-P, YU MC, WANG Q-S, et al. 1990. Consumption of salted fish and other risk factors for nasopharyngeal carcinoma (NPC) in Tianjin, a low-risk region for NPC in the People's Republic of China. J Natl Cancer Inst 82:291–296.

NUTTING PA, FREEMAN WL, RISSER DR, et al. 1993. Cancer incidence among American Indians and Alaska Natives, 1980 through 1987. Am J Public Health 83:1589–1598.

OLD LJ, BOYSE EA, OETTGEN HF, et al. 1966. Precipitating antibody in human serum to an antigen present in cultured Burkitt's lymphoma cells. Proc Natl Acad Sci 56:1699–1704.

OLSEN JH, JENSEN SP, HINK M, et al. 1984. Occupational formaldehyde exposure and increased nasal cancer risk in man. Int J Cancer 34:639–644.

PARKIN DM, MUIR CS, WHELAN SL, et al (eds). 1992. Cancer Incidence in Five Continents, Volume 6. IARC Scientific Publications, No. 120. Lyon: International Agency for Research on Cancer.

POIRIER S, OHSHIMA H, DE-THE G, et al. 1987. Volatile nitrosamine levels in common foods from Tunisia, south China and Greenland, high-risk areas for nasopharyngeal carcinoma (NPC). Int J Cancer 39:293–296.

POIRIER S, BOUVIER G, MALAVEILLE C, et al. 1989. Volatile nitrosamine levels and genotoxicity of food samples from high-risk areas for nasopharyngeal carcinoma before and after nitrosation. Int J Cancer 44:1088–1094.

POUR P, KRUGER FW, CARDESA A, et al. 1973. Carcinogenic effect of di-n-Propylnitrosamine in Syrian golden hamsters. J Natl Cancer Inst 51:1019–1027.

RAAB-TRAUB N, FLYNN K, PEASON G, et al. 1987. The differentiated form of nasopharyngeal carcinoma contains Epstein-Barr virus DNA. Int J Cancer 39:25–29.

ROTHWELL RI. 1979. Juvenile nasopharyngeal carcinoma in Sabah (Malaysia). Clin Oncol 5:353–358.

ROUSH GC, WALRATH J, STAYNER LT, et al. 1987. Nasopharyngeal cancer, sinonasal cancer, and occupations related to formaldehyde: a case-control study. J Natl Cancer Inst 79:1221–1224.

SAEMUNDSEN AK, ALBECK H, HANSEN JPH, et al. 1982. Epstein-Barr virus in nasopharyngeal and salivary gland carcinomas of Greenland Eskimos. Br J Cancer 46:721–728.

SAWAKI S, HIRAYAMA T, SUGANO H. 1976. Studies on nasopharyngeal carcinoma in Japan. Gann Monograph on Cancer Research 18:63–74.

SCHAEFER O, HILDES JA, MEDD LM, et al. 1975. The changing pattern of neoplastic disease in Canadian Eskimos. Can Med Assoc J 112:1399–1404.

SCHIMKE RN, COLLINS D, CROSS D. 1987. Nasopharyngeal carcinoma, aplastic anemia, and various malignancies in a family: possible role of Epstein-Barr virus. Am J Med Genet 27:195–202.

SCHMAUZ R, TEMPLETON AC. 1972. Nasopharyngeal carcinoma in Uganda. Cancer 29:610–621.

SHANMUGARATNAM K, CHAN SH, DE-THE G, et al. 1979. Histopathology of nasopharyngeal carcinoma. Correlations with epidemiology, survival rates and other biological characteristics. Cancer 44:1029–1044.

SHANMUGARATNAM K, HIGGINSON J. 1967. Aetiology of nasopharyngeal carcinoma. Report on a retrospective survey in Singapore. UICC Monogr Ser 1:130–137.

SHANMUGARATNAM K, SOBIN LH. 1991. Histological Typing of Tumours of the Upper Respiratory Tract and Ear, 2nd Edition. Berlin: Springer-Verlag.

SHANMUGARATNAM K, TYE CY, GOH EH, et al. 1978. Etiological factors in nasopharyngeal carcinoma: a hospital-based, retrospective, case-control, questionnaire study. IARC Sci Publ 20:199–212.

SHAO YM, POIRIER S, OHSHIMA H, et al. 1988. Epstein-Barr virus activation in Raji cells by extracts of preserved food from high risk areas for nasopharyngeal carcinoma. Carcinogenesis 9:1455–1457.

SIMONS MJ, CHAN SH, OU BX. 1981. Nasopharyngeal carcinoma (NPC), including analysis of HLA gene patterns in Chinese patients with cervical and hepatocellular carcinoma. In Simons MJ, Tait BD (eds): Proceedings of the Second Asia and Oceania Histocompatibility Workshop Conference. Victoria (Australia): Immunopublishing, pp. 369–378.

SIMONS MJ, CHAN SH, WEE GB, et al. 1978. Nasopharyngeal carcinoma and histocompatibility antigens. IARC Sci Publ 20:271–282.

SIMONS MJ, SHANMUGARATNAM K (EDS). 1982. The Biology of Nasopharyngeal Carcinoma. UICC Technical Report Series, Volume 71. Geneva: International Union Against Cancer, pp. 46–54.

SIMONS MJ, WEE GB, GOH EH, et al. 1976. Immunogenetic aspects of nasopharyngeal carcinoma. IV. Increased risk in Chinese of nasopharyngeal carcinoma associated with a Chinese-related HLA profile (A2, Singapore 2). J Natl Cancer Inst 57:977–980.

SIMONS MJ, WEE GB, SINGH D, et al. 1977. Immunogenetic aspects of nasopharyngeal carcinoma. V. Confirmation of a Chinese-related HLA profile (A2, Singapore 2) associated with an increased risk in Chinese for nasopharyngeal carcinoma. Natl Cancer Inst Monogr 47:147–151.

SRIAMPORN S, VATANASAPT V, PISANI P, et al. 1992. Environmental risk factors for nasopharyngeal carcinoma: a case-control study in Northeastern Thailand. Cancer Epidemiol Biomarkers Prev 1:345–348.

STEINITZ R, PARKIN DM, YOUNG JL, et al. 1989. Cancer Incidence in Jewish Migrants to Israel, 1961–1981. IARC Scientific Publications, No. 98. Lyon: International Agency for Research on Cancer.

STINSON WD. 1940. Epidermoid carcinoma of the nasopharynx occurring in two young brothers. Ann Otol Rhinol Laryngol 49:536–539.

SUGANO H, SAKAMOTO G, SAWAKI S, et al. 1978. Histopathological types of nasopharyngeal carcinoma in a low-risk area: Japan. IARC Sci Publ 20:27–39.

SUMMARY DATA OF THE CANCER MORTALITY SURVEY IN THE PEOPLE'S REPUBLIC OF CHINA. 1980. Beijing: National Cancer Control Office, Ministry of Public Health (in Chinese).

SWENBERG JA, KERNS WD, MITCHELL RI, et al. 1980. Induction of squamous cell carcinomas of the rat nasal cavity by inhalation exposure to formaldehyde vapor. Cancer Res 40:3398–3402.

TAMADA A, MAKIMOTO K, YAMABE H, et al. 1984. Titers of Epstein-Barr virus–related antibodies in nasopharyngeal carcinoma in Japan. Cancer 53:430–440.

TANNENBAUM SR, BISHOP W, YU MC, et al. 1985. Attempts to isolate N-nitroso compounds from Chinese-style salted fish. Natl Cancer Inst Monogr 69:209–211.

TARONE RE, LEVINE PH, YADAV M, et al. 1990. Relationship between immunoglobulin allotypes and susceptibility to nasopharyngeal carcinoma in Malaysia. Cancer Res 50:3186–3188.

VAUGHAN TL, DAVIS S. 1991. Wood dust exposure and squamous cell cancers of the upper respiratory tract. Am J Epidemiol 133:560–564.

VAUGHAN TL, STRADER C, DAVIS S, et al. 1986a. Formaldehyde and cancers of the pharynx, sinus and nasal cavity: I. Occupational exposures. Int J Cancer 38:677–683.

VAUGHAN TL, STRADER C, DAVIS S, et al. 1986b. Formaldehyde and cancers of the pharynx, sinus and nasal cavity: II. Residential exposures. Int J Cancer 38:685–688.

WATTENBERG LW. 1978. Inhibitors of chemical carcinogenesis. Adv Cancer Res 26:197–226.

WENG YM, HOTCHKISS JH, BABISH JG. 1992. N-nitrosamine and mutagenicity formation in Chinese salted fish after digestion. Food Addit Contam 9:29–37.

WEST S, HILDESHEIM A, DOSEMECI M. 1993. Non-viral risk factors for nasopharyngeal carcinoma in the Philippines: results from a case-control study. Int J Cancer 55:722–727.

WILLIAMS EH, DE-THE G. 1974. Familial aggregation in nasopharyngeal carcinoma. Lancet 2:295–296.

WOLF H, ZUR HAUSEN H, KLEIN G, et al. 1975. Attempts to detect virus-specific DNA sequences in human tumors. III. Epstein-Barr viral DNA in non-lymphoid nasopharyngeal carcinoma cells. Med Microbiol Immunol 161:15–21.

WORTH RM, VALENTINE R. 1967. Nasopharyngeal carcinoma in New South Wales, Australia. UICC Monogr Ser 1:73–76.

WU S-B, HWANG S-J, CHANG A-S, et al. 1989. Human leukocyte antigen (HLA) frequency among patients with nasopharyngeal carcinoma in Taiwan. Anticancer Res 9:1649–1654.

XIA L-W, LIANG S-X, JIANG J-W, et al. 1988. Trace element content in drinking water of nasopharyngeal carcinoma patients. Cancer Lett 41:91–97.

YU MC, GARABRANT DH, HUANG T-B, et al. 1990. Occupational and other non-dietary risk factors for nasopharyngeal carcinoma in Guangzhou, China. Int J Cancer 45:1033–1039.

YU MC, HO JHC, LAI S-H, et al. 1986. Cantonese-style salted fish as a cause of nasopharyngeal carcinoma: report of a case-control study in Hong King. Cancer Res 46:956–961.

YU MC, HO JHC, ROSS RK, et al. 1981. Nasopharyngeal carcinoma in Chinese—salted fish or inhaled smoke? Prev Med 10:15–24.

YU MC, HUANG T-B, HENDERSON BE. 1989a. Diet and nasopharyngeal carcinoma: a case-control study in Guangzhou, China. Int J Cancer 43:1077–1082.

YU MC, MO C-C, CHONG W-X, et al. 1988. Preserved foods and nasopharyngeal carcinoma: a case-control study in Guangxi, China. Cancer Res 48:1954–1959.

YU MC, NICHOLS PW, ZOU X-N, et al. 1989b. Induction of malignant nasal cavity tumours in Wistar rats fed Chinese salted fish. Br J Cancer 60:198–201.

ZENG Y. 1985. Sero-epidemiological studies on nasopharyngeal carcinoma in China. Adv Cancer Res 44:121–138.

ZENG Y. 1987. Prospective studies on nasopharyngeal carcinoma and Epstein-Barr virus inducers. In Wagner G, Zhang YH (eds): Cancer of the Liver, Esophagus, and Nasopharynx. New York: Springer-Verlag, pp. 164–169.

ZENG Y, ZHONG JM, MO YK, et al. 1983. Epstein-Barr virus early antigen induction in Raji cells by Chinese medicinal herbs. Intervirology 19:201–204.

ZHENG W, MCLAUGHLIN JK, GAO YT, et al. 1992. Occupational risks for nasopharyngeal cancer in Shanghai. J Occup Med 34:1004–1007.

ZHENG X, LUO Y, CHRISTENSSON B, et al. 1994a. Induction of nasal and nasopharyngeal tumors in Sprague-Dawley rats fed with Chinese salted fish. Acta Otolaryngol (Stockh) 114:98–104.

ZHENG YM, TUPPIN P, HUBERT, et al. 1994b. Environmental and dietary risk factors for nasopharyngeal carcinoma: a case-control study in Zangwu County, Guangxi, China. Br J Cancer 69:508–514.

ZUR HAUSEN H, SCHULTE-HOLTHAUSEN H, KLEIN G, et al. 1970. EBV DNA in biopsies of Burkitt tumours and anaplastic carcinomas of the nasopharynx. Nature 228:1056–1058.

30 Laryngeal cancer

DONALD F. AUSTIN
PEGGY REYNOLDS

Cancer of the larynx was rarely diagnosed until about 1860, after the invention of the laryngoscope by Garcia and the development of histopathology by Virchow. The first total laryngectomy was performed on a 36-year-old teacher of theology by Billroth, in 1873, for cancer (epithelioma), and by 1887 a total of 103 laryngectomies for cancer had been reported in the world's literature. Nine of these patients had their life extended by over 12 months, the longest by over 5 years (Weir, 1973; Stell, 1975).

HISTOPATHOLOGY

Although the larynx may be the site for primary neoplasms such as sarcomas, adenocarcinomas, cylindromas, lymphomas, or histiocytomas, these are rare, and "laryngeal cancer" refers almost exclusively to squamous carcinomas of varying degrees of histologic differentiation. Of the 17,098 invasive neoplasms of the larynx reported in the population-based SEER Program from 1973 to 1990, 94.4% were classified as squamous cell carcinoma (SEER, 1993). Another 3.6% were classified as "carcinoma" (mostly not otherwise specified) and 1.0% as verrucous carcinoma. Only 0.4% were classified as some type of adenocarcinoma, 0.1% as some type of sarcoma, and the remaining 1.5% were a variety of less frequent classifications, including 10 lymphomas of several types. In this chapter, the term *laryngeal* cancer refers to squamous cell carcinoma.

ANATOMIC DISTRIBUTION

The TNM classification system divides the larynx into three anatomic regions: supraglottis (extrinsic larynx), glottis (true or intrinsic larynx), and subglottis (Speissl et al, 1989). Tumors arising in any of the three regions are further classified into four subgroups, depending on the degree of tumor involvement and vocal cord mobility. Supraglottic tumors are superior to the true vocal cord and include tumors of the epiglottis, false cords, and laryngeal ventricles. These tumors arise from columnar ciliated epithelium, similar to that of the trachea. Glottic tumors are those of the true vocal cord, including the anterior and posterior commissures, and generally arise from the stratified squamous epithelium of the true cord. Subglottic or infraglottic tumors arise below the true vocal cord down to the level of the cricoid cartilage. The current subsite classification system of the International Classification of Disease: Oncology (ICD-0) used by the SEER Program, also recognizes laryngeal cartilage as a separate subsite, and of 16,237 laryngeal cancers classified by subsite, this accounts for 0.7% while two or more autochthonous subsites account for 3.4%. In the remaining 95.9% of SEER laryngeal cancers, supraglottic, glottic, and subglottic subsites occur in a ratio of 30:53:1, respectively.

Significant differences in subsite distribution occur between sexes and among races, however, for reasons that have not been established (Yang et al, 1989; Stephensen et al, 1991; Silvestri et al, 1992). These are illustrated in Table 30–1.

STAGE AT DIAGNOSIS

In the United States, approximately 56% of all patients with staged laryngeal cancer are diagnosed with the tumor still localized to the larynx (SEER, 1993). This is illustrated in Table 30–2. Another 37% are not diagnosed until the cancer has progressed to involve nearby tissues or lymph nodes (regional stage). For the remaining 7%, the cancer has spread to remote parts of the body at the time of diagnosis.

The supraglottic region is richly supplied with lymphatics, and cancers arising there are characterized by a high rate of metastasis to cervical lymph nodes. Hoarseness seldom occurs until late in the course of supraglottic cancer, which is frequently heralded by vague pain or by a lump in the neck. Only about a third of patients with supraglottic cancer have localized disease at the time of diagnosis.

Cancer of the glottis has the most favorable prognosis. This is most likely because hoarseness is frequently an early symptom and because glottic cancer has a small

TABLE 30–1. *Percent Distribution of Subsites for Invasive Laryngeal Cancer, by Sex and Ethnic Group (SEER 1973–1989, excluding Puerto Rico)*

			Subsite distribution (%)				
Group	*N (inc. NOS)*	*Percent NOS*	*Supraglottis*	*Glottis*	*Subglottis*	*Cartilage*	*Two or More Subsites*
Total	17,098	10.4	35.0	59.5	1.2	0.8	3.6
All males	14,062	10.3	30.9	63.7	1.1	0.7	3.7
All females	3,036	10.9	54.1	39.9	1.6	1.3	3.0
Total non-Hispanic whites	14,395	10.2	34.5	60.2	1.2	0.7	3.4
Non-Hispanic white males	11,845	10.0	30.4	64.4	1.1	0.6	3.6
Non-Hispanic white females	2,550	11.1	53.5	40.9	1.6	1.4	2.6
Total blacks	1,865	12.6	41.2	51.6	1.3	0.9	5.0
Black males	1,511	13.0	36.1	57.0	1.1	0.8	4.8
Black females	354	10.7	62.3	29.1	1.9	1.0	5.7
Total Hispanics	341	10.0	32.9	60.3	2.3	1.0	3.6
Hispanic males	279	10.0	29.1	64.1	2.4	0.8	3.6
Hispanic females	62	9.7	50.0	42.9	1.8	1.8	3.6
Total other	497	8.1	28.2	65.4	0.9	1.5	3.9
Other males	427	8.2	26.3	66.8	1.0	1.8	4.1
Other females	70	7.1	40.0	56.9	0.0	0.0	3.1

Source: SEER Public Use Tape, 1/93.

probability of metastasis until it has extended into tissues with more lymphatics. Approximately 70% of patients with glottic cancer have localized disease at the time of diagnosis.

Subglottic cancer rarely causes hoarseness but may cause dyspnea from partial obstruction of the airway. The subglottis is also well supplied with lymphatics and, like supraglottic cancers, about two-thirds of the neoplasms of this region are found to be metastatic at the time of diagnosis. A study of clinical characteristics of patients in the high-incidence region of Torino, Italy, by Merletti et al (1990) documented a male:female ratio of 13:1, with a subsite distribution in males of approximately 57:36:1 for the supraglottis:glottis:subglottis ratio. Among males, 94% of the supraglottic tumors had invaded two or more subsites at diagnosis, while only 53% of the glottic tumors had done so. Nearly 99% of the patients with cancer of the glottis acknowledged dysphonia at the time of diagnosis. No other symptoms exceeded 4% for patients with cancer of the glottis. In contrast, 80% of patients with cancer of the supraglottis reported dysphonia, followed by dysphagia (27%).

TABLE 30–2. *Percent of Invasive Laryngeal Cancers Diagnosed at a Localized Stage, by Sex and Subsite (SEER 1973–1989, excluding Puerto Rico)*

	Males		Females		Total	
	N	*% Localized*	*N*	*% Localized*	*N*	*% Localized*
Glottis	6,592	70.5	844	70.4	7,436	70.5
Supraglottis	3,216	34.0	1,181	37.5	4,397	34.9
Subglottis	118	28.0	28	17.9	146	26.0
Cartilage	60	43.3	31	54.8	91	47.3
Two or more subsites	377	44.6	66	37.9	443	43.6
NOS	972	49.7	217	43.8	1,189	48.6
All	11,335	56.9	2,367	49.8	13,703	55.7

Source: SEER Public Use Tape. 1/93.

Approximately 5% of laryngeal neoplasms were diagnosed in an in situ stage during the Third National Cancer Survey in 1969–1971 (Cutler and Young, 1975) and approximately 6% of such neoplasms reported to the SEER Program, 1973–1989, were in situ (SEER, 1993). Miller and Fisher (1971) followed a clinical series of over 250 patients with carcinoma in situ, and about 16% of these lesions progressed to invasive cancer in spite of treatment, suggesting that preinvasive lesions are candidates for aggressive therapy. This view is supported by Hojslet and coworkers (1989), who followed patients with biopsy-proven dysplastic changes of the larynx and described a high risk of invasive malignancy in this group, most of whom were active (84%) or former (9%) smokers and 24% of whom were excessive drinkers. Of those with mild dysplasia, 5% developed invasive carcinoma after an average of 65 months, while of 9 with moderate dysplasia, 4 developed carcinoma after a mean of 17 months. Of 10 patients with severe dysplasia or carcinoma in situ, 7 were treated; 2 of these developed invasive disease while two of three untreated patients did likewise.

SURVIVAL

The prognosis for all patients with laryngeal cancer has remained unchanged since the mid-1970s, with a relative survival rate of 66%. In the late 1960s, there was a significant improvement in the five-year survival of patients with laryngeal neoplasms, mostly due to improvements in the prognosis of patients with regional disease (SEER, 1992). Robbins (1988) conducted a study of disease-free survival among males and females with laryngeal cancer, matched (2:1) for age, subsite, T-stage, N-stage, and treatment. He reported no significant survival differences between males and females, although females had about 10% higher survival at 84 months than males. Within the U.S., five-year relative survival rates do not differ much by sex; however, the rates for whites are more favorable than those for Hispanics, blacks, and Filipinos, and less favorable than for Japanese and Hawaiians. Notable survival differences exist by major subsite, even within stage. These are presented in Table 30–3.

DEMOGRAPHIC PATTERNS

Yang et al (1989) have described sex ratio differences in larynx cancer incidence rates by subsite in the United States. The subsite sex ratios in European countries are close to unity, however, a fact noted by Levi and LaVecchia (1990).

Incidence and Mortality

Cancer of the larynx is more common in men than women, with an overall sex ratio in the U.S. of roughly 5:1. For the years 1987–88 the SEER Program reported an average incidence rate for males of 8.2 per 100,000 population, and for females of 1.7 per 100,000 population (Reis et al, 1991). In the U.S., incidence rates also tend to be 50% higher among black than among white males, and twice as high among whites (male and female) than among Hispanics and Asians (USDHHS, 1986a). There is little variation in incidence rates between SEER areas in the United States, except for Utah, from which reported rates among both white males and females are roughly half those reported elsewhere (USDHHS, 1984).

The age-adjusted mortality rate (1985–1986) for U.S. males of all races is 2.5 (per 100,000), 5 times higher than that for females (0.5). Unlike the case for incidence, black males during this time period experienced a disproportionately higher mortality rate, roughly twice that of white males in the U.S. (4.9 vs. 2.3). Similar to the case for incidence, mortality rates among whites were twice those among Asian ethnicities (USDHHS, 1986a).

Time Trends

There is some evidence that over the last several decades incidence and mortality rates have experienced an overall increase both worldwide and in the United States

TABLE 30–3. *Relative 5-year and 10-year Survival Rates* and Observed Median Survival for Laryngeal Cancer for Two Major Subsites, by Stage and Sex (SEER 1973–1986, excluding Puerto Rico)*

	Males				*Females*			
Stage	*Localized*	*Regional*	*Distant*	*Unstaged*	*Localized*	*Regional*	*Distant*	*Unstaged*
GLOTTIS								
(n)	(3,939)	(1,492)	(164)	(248)	(483)	(176)	(15)	(40)
Yr. 5	89.8	67.4	41.5	72.4	91.4	68.0	36.8	66.3
Yr. 10	79.9	59.2	39.1	60.5	79.7	50.0	32.0	51.7
Obs. median	> 10.00	6.49	2.07	6.86	> 10.00	9.03	1.25	5.81
SUPRAGLOTTIS								
(n)	(897)	(1,453)	(330)	(128)	(364)	(496)	(77)	(35)
Yr. 5	63.8	41.5	23.4	45.1	70.7	51.4	27.7	44.1
Yr. 10	46.2	31.7	14.3	36.2	55.2	34.7	21.6	40.7
Obs. median	5.79	2.83	1.30	2.67	8.51	4.29	1.87	2.77

*Relative survival is the observed survival for those with disease, divided by the survival for those without the disease, expressed as a percent.
Source: SEER Public Use Tape, 9/92

(Rothman et al, 1980; DeRienzo et al, 1991). In Connecticut, during the 45-year time period 1935–1979, age-adjusted incidence rates (per 100,000) in males went from 4.2 (1935–1939) to 9.9 (1975–1979) and in females went from 0.4 to 1.6 (USDHHS, 1986b). These increases could, in part, reflect improvements in diagnostic accuracy. During the same 45-year time period in Connecticut, the proportion of laryngeal cancer cases with microscopic confirmation went from slightly over half to nearly 100% of all cases. Review of the long-term U.S. morbidity patterns by Devesa el al (1990) suggests that there are strong cohort effects for laryngeal cancer among women, peaking with cohorts born in 1895 to 1920, and similar but less pronounced cohort effects among white men. Among nonwhite men, there appear to be continued increases among successive birth cohorts.

In Canada, Ayiomamitis (1989) has reported an increase in laryngeal cancer incidence during the 1970s for both sexes, with cohort effects identified for both sexes, especially for males born in the period 1895–1905. Age-adjusted incidence rates among males increased over 50%, to 7.61 per 100,000 (World Standard Population), while that for females doubled, to 1.19 per 100,000. Among males only, a modest increase in laryngeal cancer mortality occurred over that decade.

Incidence rates for laryngeal cancer in the U.S. have remained relatively unchanged since the mid-1970s (Harras et al, 1993), with the age-adjusted annual incidence rates for males varying around 8.5 per 100,000, and those for females averaging about 1.4 in the 1970s and 1.6 in the 1980s. Mortality rates have evidenced only slight changes since 1973, with those for males decreasing from about 2.8 in the 1970s to 2.5 in the 1980s and those for females increasing from 0.4 to 0.5 over the same period. Trend data from the 1950s highlight longer-term increases among women and nonwhite men, in contrast to stable rates among white men (Devesa et al, 1990).

International Patterns

Although the male : female ratio is reasonably consistent worldwide, there is considerable international variation in the incidence of laryngeal cancer. Age-adjusted incidence rates (per 100,000 population) for men in areas of Brazil (Porto Alegre, 16.0), Spain (Basque country, 20.4), Italy (Torino, 14.7), and France (Somme, 17.5) are more than double those for white men in California (Los Angeles, 6.1; San Francisco–Oakland MSA, 6.9). Incidence rates for men in areas of China (Shanghai, 2.8), Japan (Miyagi, 3.5), and several northern European countries (Norway, 3.5; Sweden, 2.6; the Southern Region of England, 3.3) are roughly half those for California males (Parkin et al, 1992). In the more recent editions of Cancer Incidence in Five Continents (Muir et al, 1987, Parkin et al, 1992), the very high incidence rate previously reported for Bombay, India (Waterhouse et al, 1982), now appears to be in line with other mid-high areas.

Similar international patterns exist for mortality rates. During 1978–79, U.S. males experienced an intermediate age-adjusted (to the World Standard) mortality rate (2.05 per 100,000 population) compared to substantially higher rates in France (11.24) and Italy (6.51) and lower rates in Japan (1.24), Norway (0.88), and Sweden (0.92) (Kurihara et al, 1984). These same contrasts are not evident for women. Among 40 population groups ranked by rates by Kurihara et al (1984) for larynx cancer mortality, only 3 of the top 10 for males are also in the top 10 for females (Cuba, Hungary, and Yugoslavia). Overall, there is little relationship between ranking of male rates and female rates.

ENVIRONMENTAL FACTORS

Tobacco and Alcohol

The best established environmental risk factors for cancer of the larynx are tobacco and alcohol. Both factors demonstrate consistent and compelling independent dose-response associations with incidence, and a synergistic combined effect.

The tobacco relationship has been known since the epidemiologic studies of the effects of smoking in the 1950s. Careful analyses of several sources of epidemiologic information on the overall smoking and larynx cancer association, validating a strong dose-response association, is available in the review by Rothman and associates (1980). Wynder et al (1956) reported that cigarette smoking was the principal risk factor for both glottic and supraglottic cancer. In 1970, Auerbach et al published the results of histologic examinations of the larynxes of 942 men who died of causes other than cancer of the larynx. Some degree of epithelial atypia was found in 99% of cigarette smokers, 16% of whom had carcinoma in situ at the time of death. In contrast, only 25% of those never having smoked had abnormal cells. In 1971, Jussawalla and Deshpande reported that the relative risk of laryngeal cancer in nondrinking Indian males was 7.7 for cigarette smokers, 4.6 for tobacco chewers, and 20.1 for those who had both habits. No risk distinction between glottic and supraglottic tumors was reported for any of these studies.

Although both retrospective and prospective studies have identified smoking as a risk factor for laryngeal cancer, several curious anomalies in epidemiologic descriptive data exist. Stell, in 1972, reported that although the incidence of lung cancer in Britain increased 500% from 1900 to 1970 and generally paralleled the increase in tobacco consumption, the incidence of laryngeal cancer remained constant. Similarly, the mortality from lung cancer in Australia between 1950 and 1970 increased 300%, while the mortality rate for laryngeal cancer remained stationary (Anon., 1976; Atkinson, 1975). Striking differences in birth cohort trends in the United States among white males, females, and nonwhite males appear to coincide with some, but clearly not with all, secular trends in the consumption of tobacco, alcohol, and fresh fruit and vegetables (Devesa et al, 1990). Wynder et al (1991), in examining trends of cancer mortality in the United States and Japan over a 30-year period (1955–1985), found the laryngeal cancer mortality pattern in Japan to be discrepant when considering the established risk factors of per capita tobacco and alcohol use, whereas lung and oropharyngeal cancer patterns were found to be consistent with past alcohol and tobacco utilization. A 50% reduction in laryngeal cancer mortality among Japanese males and females over the period studied is at variance with increasing tobacco and alcohol use over that period. The authors, who also examined per capita food supply and specific nutrient consumption trends in the two countries, offered no hypotheses for this anomalous trend. However, a study by Guenel et al (1988a) of per capita alcohol and tobacco use in Denmark from 1920 to 1980 and laryngeal cancer incidence from 1943 to 1982 concluded that the rates are most consistent with the concept that a minority of smokers and drinkers, those with heavy consumption, is responsible for the majority of the consumption, and accordingly, contribute disproportionately to laryngeal cancer risk.

Like other aerodigestive cancer sites, the rate of larynx cancer among blacks is significantly higher than among whites. Several cancer studies of sites anatomically close to the larynx (oral cavity and pharynx by Day et al, 1993; esophagus by Brown et al, 1994) have found higher risk among blacks even after controlling for exposures to the major risk factors (alcohol and tobacco). Brown et al suggest a greater susceptibility among blacks to these factors.

Few studies have addressed alcohol alone with respect to laryngeal cancer, although alcoholics are noted to have elevated risks (Rothman et al, 1980). Hedberg et al (1994) found that persons scoring higher on the Michigan alcohol screening test (MAST) have a higher risk (1.9) for laryngeal cancer even after adjusting for alcohol and tobacco use. In a population-based study in the Uppsala Medical Care Region of Sweden, Adami et al (1992) found a 3.3-fold increase in laryngeal cancer among those discharged from care facilities with a diagnosis of alcoholism, although no adjustment for tobacco use was possible. Jensen (1979) followed a large group of Danish brewery workers who had a consumption of beer estimated to be 4 times higher than that of the general male population in Denmark. An excess of cancer mortality and morbidity was mainly limited to cancers of the esophagus and larynx. Among those workers affiliated with the Brewery Workers Union who had worked in the production of mineral and soda water, no such excess was found. Tuyns (1990) has demonstrated the correspondence of laryngeal cancer rates (as well as oral, hypopharyngeal, and esophageal cancer rates) with alcohol consumption in Mediterranean countries. Unfortunately, smoking habits of subjects reported in these alcohol studies are unknown.

A case-control study conducted in six United States cities and reported by Wynder et al (1976) found patients with glottic or supraglottic laryngeal cancer to have heavier cigarette smoking and alcohol consumption. Although the investigators reported a dose-response effect for both tobacco and alcohol use, and demonstrated a multiplicative interaction between these factors, the control group systematically excluded persons with a "current diagnosis of tobacco or alcohol-related disease," thus creating an overestimate of the contribution to risk of these two factors, which would be greatest in those groups with the greatest consumption. The investigators also reported that, while in a similar 1956 study the male-to-female ratio of cases was approximately 15 : 1, they found a ratio of less than 5 : 1, which they attributed to an increase in cigarette smoking among females. A French study by Luce et al (1988) compared female patients with cancers of the mouth, pharynx, and larynx to male patients with the same cancers and provided the opportunity to evaluate presenting differences for abstainers from tobacco and/or alcohol (over 35% for each in the female series, less than 5% each among the males). Abstainers presented at much later ages than consumers of these products, hence reinforcing the etiologic importance of alcohol and tobacco for either their influence on age at onset or cohort effects.

Rothman et al (1989) evaluated the relative carcinogenicity of "dark" vs. "light" distilled liquors on cancer risk and concluded that while dark spirits constituted a 4-fold greater risk than light spirits for cancer of the hypopharynx, for the glottic and supraglottic laryngeal cancers the distinction was slight. The investigators suggested that for laryngeal tumors the carcinogenic effect of alcoholic beverages is through topical exposure to ethanol.

The interaction of alcohol and tobacco as risk factors for laryngeal cancer, without distinguishing between glottic and supraglottic tumors, has been reported by Bridges and Reay-Young (1976), Wynder and Stellman (1977), Brownson and Chang (1987), Cann and Fried (1984) in a summary article, and Choi and Kahyo

(1991), all of whom also emphasize the dose-response effects in addition to interactive effects. Spitz et al (1988) and Franceschi et al (1990) also reported progressively reduced risk of laryngeal cancer with increasing length of smoking cessation. Zatonski et al (1990) found the same relationship and also reported lower risk among intermittent smokers.

The effect of both tobacco and alcohol on laryngeal cancer mortality was uniquely documented by Tuyns and Audigier (1976), who conducted an analysis of mortality rates of birth cohorts in France. They found that cancer of the lung, larynx, and esophagus were all elevated in birth cohorts of French males who were young adults prior to World War II. During World War II, alcohol availability and consumption were reduced markedly, but this was not the case with tobacco. Lung cancer continued its rise in those birth cohorts who were young adults during and after World War II, but both cancer of the larynx and esophagus fell in the cohorts who were young adults during World War II. Both these latter neoplasms again continued their rise in cohorts who were young adults after World War II, when alcohol was again more heavily consumed.

In 1978, McMichael analyzed mortality data from England and Australia for cancers of the larynx and esophagus and related the trends to both alcohol and tobacco use. He noted an upturn in mortality from both types of cancer in both countries, especially in younger females, and related this to an increase in alcohol consumption. He attributed the relatively stable incidence of laryngeal cancer until that period to the fact that the use of chewing tobacco and distilled alcoholic beverages both decreased, also until that period, along with an increase in cigarette smoking. Yet another study, tracing English mortality data (Ramadan et al, 1982) from 1911 to 1978, also noted that the changes in trend follow patterns of alcohol rather than tobacco consumption. In fact, these findings were similar to those reported in France by Tuyns and Audigier (1976). Although McMichael and Ramadan both suggested that alcohol was a stronger risk factor for laryngeal cancer than cigarette smoking, their assessments were based on mortality data. Because the case-fatality rate for supraglottic cancer is higher than for glottic cancer, mortality data should be more representative of supraglottic cancer. Given that caveat, their suggestion is probably accurate. At any rate, this study and that of Tuyns and Audigier may explain the peculiar lack of laryngeal cancer increases in some countries having experienced increases in lung cancer.

Several European studies have addressed alcohol and tobacco risks for cancer of the two major larynx subsites. In a Danish study, Olsen et al (1985) found both substances to be major risk factors for each subsite and that their combined effect appeared multiplicative. A later study in France (LeClerc et al, 1987; Guenel, 1988b) produced similar results. The French study, which compared male cases from a Paris treatment center to a national population sample of French males, and which excluded ex-smokers, found that certain alcoholic beverages seemed to elevate the risks for one subsite disproportionately. It also produced an estimate that in the highest-consumption category of alcohol and tobacco, approximately 90% of the cases could be attributed to the interactive effect. Further, the relative risks from tobacco were substantially greater than those from alcohol for both subsites, and for each substance the risks rose, with increasing exposure, to a greater degree in the supraglottis than in the glottis. This finding of a greater effect from tobacco than alcohol is somewhat different from conclusions drawn from mortality data in England and Australia or from American studies (McMichael, 1978; Ramadan et al, 1982; Schottenfeld, 1979; Rothman et al, 1980). Another difference with the Paris study is that, among males, supraglottic cancers slightly outnumbered glottic cancers, rather than the 1:2 ratio seen in U.S. males.

Tuyns et al (1988) have also reported finding separate and multiplicative effects of tobacco smoke and alcohol. Most important, although they combined glottic and subglottic tumors, they also reported separate risks and interactions for this combined group compared to supraglottic tumors. This study, another of the few rare attempts to study laryngeal cancer risks by subsite, was a multinational case-control interview study conducted in the "Latin" countries of southwest Europe (Turin and Varese in Italy, Zaragosa and Navarra in Spain, Geneva in Switzerland, and Calvados in France). In all of these regions, the consumption of a large amount of alcohol, primarily wine, is a common feature and the tobacco commonly used is "black" tobacco, richer in aromatic amines and tobacco-specific nitrosamines and "stronger" than "blond" or flue-cured tobaccos commonly used in the United States. The influence of dark tobacco, with striking interactions with alcohol consumption, has also been implicated in a case-control study from Ecuador (DeStefani et al, 1987). Sancho-Garnier and Theobald (1993) examined the relative effect of black and blond tobacco on the risk of cancer of the pharynx and of the larynx. After taking into account a number of smoking-related factors (age at starting, duration, etc.), they concluded that black tobacco imparted a risk twice that of blond tobacco.

From studies of the effects of smoking cessation and from other studies, it also appears that smoking is a risk factor for both supraglottic and glottic cancer, but that smoking interacts with different cofactors in the two locations. For example, in smokers, alcoholism increases the risk of supraglottic tumors (Wynder et al, 1956), as it does for cancer of the oral cavity, pharynx, and esophagus. In 1974, Schottenfeld and associates reported that the relative risk of a second primary tumor after the diagnosis of supraglottic cancer was about 30 for cancer of the oral cavity and pharynx, about 18 for the esophagus, and about 5 for the lung. On the other hand, the relative risk of a second primary after a diagnosis of glottic cancer was only about 3 for all of the preceding sites. This suggests that in this country supraglottic cancer is more likely to arise from the interaction of several risk factors, such as alcohol and tobacco, as in cancer of the oral cavity, pharynx, and esophagus, while glottic cancer may be less affected by alcohol. This conclusion has also been reached by Schottenfeld (1979). Elwood et al (1984) found, in a case-control study of oral cavity, pharynx, and larynx cancers, that supraglottic tumors, like oral and pharyngeal tumors, were significantly associated with alcohol consumption, while glottic tumors were associated with smoking.

Dietary Factors

An increasing number of studies suggest that there are dietary constituents also influencing larynx cancer risk. Middleton et al (1986) used food frequency history to study dietary vitamin A intake in the year prior to the first onset of symptoms among cancer cases admitted to Roswell Park Memorial Institute and hospital controls. Among males, a highly significant protective effect for laryngeal cancer was noted among the middle and highest tertile of vitamin A consumers, as compared to the lowest third, even when controlling for age, smoking, and alcohol (RR = 0.61, 0.54, respectively). No such relationship was detected among women. A subsequent study in males by Freudenheim et al (1992), from the same institution, found that dietary carotenoids were associated with lower risk, especially among lighter smokers, while retinol, total calories, protein, and dietary fat were associated with elevated risk, the latter especially among heaviest smokers. They found no effect of vitamins C or E, dietary carbohydrate, or fiber. Esteve and associates also noted a relative risk of 2.7 associated with low consumption of fruits and vegetables, a finding consistent with as yet unpublished dietary results from the European collaborative study that show a clear dose-response relationship for beta-carotene, vitamins C and E, and polyunsaturated to saturated fatty acid ratios for risk of larynx and hypopharynx cancers (summarized in the 1988–1989 IARC Biennial Report). Case-control research from the Gulf Coast of Texas (Mackerras et al, 1988) found an odds ratio of 2.1 associated with low beta-carotene intake, and no association with total vitamin A or retinol, a result also found by McLaughlin et al (1988) with oral and pharyngeal cancer. Mackerras et al also noted that this inverse association was strongest for former smokers (OR = 5.9). LaVecchia et al (1990) identified three protective dietary factors using a food frequency questionnaire in a case-control study of laryngeal cancers in northern Italy. In the highest tertile of consumption, fish (RR = 0.6), green vegetables (RR = 0.4), and fresh fruit (RR = 0.3) were independent protective factors, a finding paralleled by that for oral and pharyngeal cancer risk by McLaughlin et al (1988).

Some dietary factors also seem to elevate the risk for laryngeal cancer. Several case-control studies have identified the South American custom of drinking maté tea as a risk factor for oropharyngeal and esophageal cancers. DeStefani et al (1987) and Pintos et al (1994) identify the practice of drinking maté to be associated with an elevated risk of laryngeal cancer of over 2-fold. A case-control study of laryngeal cancer in Yugoslavia (Sokic et al, 1994) found that a diet consisting predominantly of tinned food and meat products was an independent risk factor.

Enough epidemiologic and animal studies have yielded consistent findings to provide a scientific rationale for the apparent protective effects of various micronutrients and chemopreventive agents (Boone et al, 1990; Meyskens, 1990). Hong and coworkers (1990) have even demonstrated a significant protective effect of oral isotretinoin (13-cis-retinoic acid) against second primary head and neck cancers in a controlled clinical trial of patients previously treated for primary squamous cell cancers of the oral cavity, pharynx, or larynx. Schottenfeld (1991) has summarized the relationship of antioxidant micronutrients to the risk of laryngeal cancer, in a review of etiology and prevention of aerodigestive cancers.

Occupational Factors

Exposure to asbestos has been proposed as a risk factor for cancer of the larynx, as it is for lung cancer (Doll and Peto, 1987). The evidence for this is somewhat mixed. Stell and McGill (1973) reported in a retrospective study that a significant excess of patients with laryngeal cancer had asbestos exposure, as compared to controls. Newhouse and Berry (1973) then reported that in a cohort of asbestos workers, two cases of laryngeal cancer occurred, whereas 0.37 were expected. The possibility of a causal link between asbestos and laryngeal cancer has also been suggested on clinical grounds by Libshitz et al (1974), who reported on three patients with pulmonary asbestosis and laryngeal cancer of the glottic type. All three patients were also smokers. More recently, Hillerdal and Lindholm (1980) reviewed chest X-rays from a series of 156 Swedish patients with laryngeal cancer, and found typical pleural plaques in 14, significantly more than would be expected from the general population.

Shettigara and Morgan (1975) investigated 43 male laryngeal cancer patients and matched controls and found that asbestos was more strongly associated with the disease than was smoking or alcohol. Brown et al (1988) conducted a case-control interview study on the Gulf Coast of Texas and identified an odds ratio of 1.5 for occupational exposure to asbestos, controlling for smoking and alcohol. They also identified a clear dose-response gradient. Other studies have noted elevations in self-reported or putative asbestos exposure (Morgan, 1976; Zheng et al, 1992; Muscat and Wynder, 1992; Wortley et al, 1992; Stell and McGill, 1973). These findings are at odds with those of Hinds et al (1979) and of Blot et al (1980), who saw no evidence for an asbestos association independent of smoking and alcohol. For a plethora of studies the findings for asbestos are simply equivocal (Wynder et al, 1956; Hillerdal and Lindholm, 1980; Burch et al, 1981; Flanders and Rothman, 1982; Flanders et al, 1984; Elwood et al, 1984; Olsen and Sabroe 1984; Zagraniski et al, 1986; Brownson and Chang, 1987; Ahrens et al, 1991). Chan and Gee (1988) reviewed the evidence from 9 case-control and 12 cohort studies, and concluded that asbestos has a negligible association with laryngeal cancer after adjusting for the effects of tobacco and alcohol consumption, a conclusion also reached in reviews by Edelman (1989) and by Liddell (1990). Smith et al (1990), in their review of epidemiological evidence, reached a contrary conclusion.

The relationship of laryngeal cancer to occupations that do not involve asbestos handling is even less well substantiated, although a number of possibilities have been explored. Adelstein (1972) reviewed cancer statistics of occupational mortality based on the 1961 census in Britain. He reported a higher proportional mortality from larynx cancer for brewers, wine makers, publicans, innkeepers, stevedores, dock laborers, barmen, and barmaids. Except for stevedores and dock laborers, the contribution by alcohol to the larynx cancer mortality is likely the explanation for the excess in these occupational groups. Peterson and Milham (1980) analyzed death certificates from California (1959–1961) and from Washington (1950–1971) and calculated the proportional mortality ratio (PMR) for various occupations. An elevated PMR was observed for cancer of the larynx in both states for bartenders, sailors, deck hands and seamen, meat cutters, and salesclerks. California also evidenced excess PMRs among operative and kindred workers. Flanders and Rothman (1982) used interview data from the Third National Cancer Survey (1969–1971) to assess industrial and occupational groups at enhanced risk, adjusted for tobacco and alcohol consumption, and identified ratio estimates above 3.0 for members of the railroad industry and lumber industry, as well as sheet-metal workers, grinding wheel operators, and automobile mechanics. Guenel et al (1990) linked all persons in the Denmark 1970 census to the Danish Cancer Registry, accounting for those who died or emigrated, and determining laryngeal cancer risk by occupation and other sociodemographic variables. In addition to identifying risks associated with marital state (reduced for single, elevated for widowed or divorced), they computed relative risks for a variety of occupations. Among males those occupations with relative risks over 6 were waiters and caterers; over 5 were firemen and shop assistants in department stores; over 4 were actors and boatbuilders; and over 3 were brewery workers and shipyard mechanics.

Elwood et al (1984) found no association with specific occupational exposures in their case-control study of oropharyngeal and laryngeal cancer in Vancouver, Canada. Flanders et al (1984) examined the employment histories of 42 newly diagnosed laryngeal cancer patients in Richmond County, Georgia, and 85 individually matched (by age, sex, area of residence, and smoking and alcohol-drinking history) hospital controls, and identified rate ratios above 3.0 for farmers, textile processors, and laborers or maintenance personnel. In somewhat larger hospital-based studies (Flanders et al, 1984; Ahrens et al, 1991) significantly elevated risks were also observed for textile workers. Zagraniski et al (1986) used a similar design to recruit 92 cases and 181 general surgery controls from hospitals in New Haven, Connecticut, and found only machinists to have a statistically significant elevated odds ratio. Brownson and Chang (1987), in a case-control study conducted through the Missouri Cancer Registry, found an elevated laryngeal cancer risk (OR = 3.8) among nonconstruction laborers after controlling for tobacco and alcohol use. Spinelli et al (1990) examined occupation at diagnosis for male British Columbia cancer patients and found that among laryngeal cancer patients, as compared to all other male cancer patients, air transport workers were overrepresented (OR = 12.1, 2.2–65.9), with small excesses also noted for rail transport workers (OR = 2.6), janitors (OR = 2.2), and food preparation workers (OR = 1.7). Bravo et al (1990) examined occupational factors among larynx cancer cases and hospital controls in Madrid, Spain, and found that 48 of 85 cases, as compared to 60 of 170 controls, were categorized as service industry personnel (civil servants, office workers, etc.) (crude OR = 2.4, $p < 0.01$), while only small (1.1–2.6) and insignificant odds ratios were associated with various industrial exposures. No tobacco or alcohol exposures were assessed.

An analysis of the average annual mortality rate from laryngeal cancer, by county, for 1950–1969 in the United States was conducted by Blot et al (1978). They found an increased mortality from laryngeal cancer correlated with several factors, including the presence of chemical and printing industries, the presence of shipyards during World War II, and the per capita tax revenue on alcoholic beverage sales. In addition, the distribution correlated with that of other cancer sites, most notably with lung cancer, followed closely by esophageal and oral cancers. In 1976, Segnan and Tanturri reported the geographic distribution of bladder and laryngeal cancers among males in Italy. Laryngeal cancer was elevated in an area of chrysotile asbestos mining and in an area where a chemical factory had used 2-naphthylamine and benzidine. In the latter area, bladder cancer was also excessively high. Follow-up of a "cluster" of laryngeal cancers near an incinerator of waste solvents and oil in Great Britian (Elliott et al, 1992) found no evidence for an increased disease rate.

Wada et al (1968) reported greatly elevated mortality from respiratory tract cancer, including laryngeal cancer, among Japanese workers manufacturing mustard gas during the period 1929–45. Easton et al (1988) also reported an excess of larynx cancer among mustard gas workers employed longer than 10 years. Mustard gas has also produced respiratory neoplasms in laboratory animals (Heston, 1950). Holmes et al (1970) reported that males with scrotal epithelioma, most likely induced by cutting oil, had subsequent malignancies of the skin, digestive tract, and respiratory tract at rates significantly higher than expected. The observed respiratory tumors were of the lung (7) and larynx (1), where approximately 2.5 were expected ($p = 0.004$). Waldron (1975) subsequently found a significant excess of larynx and lung cancers among 288 cases of scrotal cancer. The excess was limited to workers with oil exposure. This suggests that the carcinogen responsible for scrotal epithelioma may also be responsible for respiratory tumors, including those of the larynx.

Wynder et al (1976) noted in their case-control interview study that laryngeal cancer cases were more likely to report having worked in a woodworking occupation than were matched controls. This is somewhat contrary to a case-control study by Brownson and Chang (1987) that found elevated risks only among nonconstruction laborers, as well as to studies by Vaughan and Davis (1991) and Bravo et al (1990) that found no association with exposure to wood dust. Although based on very small numbers, a Finnish nested case-control study found an elevation of upper respiratory tract tumors in formaldehyde-exposed woodworkers (Partanen et al, 1990). A larger German case-control study found significantly elevated larynx cancer risk associated with pinewood dust exposure for glottic, but not for supraglottic, tumors (Maier et al 1992).

Pederson et al (1973) reported nearly 6 times the expected deaths from respiratory cancer among men employed at a nickel refinery in Norway, including 5 deaths from laryngeal cancer, whereas only 1.4 were expected. Four of the 5 deaths from laryngeal cancer occurred among the employees roasting and smelting ore, whereas 24% of all employees and 28% of all deaths were from that group. No distinction between glottic and supraglottic neoplasms was made. Nickel exposure has also been implicated in an Italian study (Forastiere et al, 1987).

Moulin and coworkers (1986), investigating potential work-related cancer risks for the French National Institute for Research in Safety and Occupational Health, reported an elevated incidence of larynx cancer (SIR = 2.3), along with elevated rates of buccal cavity and pharynx but not lung cancer, among workers of a fiberglass insulation production factory. Moulin et al (1989), in a cohort mortality study of workers presumably exposed to polycyclic aromatic hydrocarbons, in two plants in southwestern France manufacturing graphite industrial electrodes from coal tar, found no elevated risk of larynx, pharynx, and buccal cavity cancers (combined). A nested case-referent study in which past smoking habits was a matching variable also produced negative findings. Exposure to silica and insecticides were the strongest occupational risk factors for larynx cancer in a Spanish study by Bravo et al (1990).

Lynch et al (1979) found a significant excess of laryngeal cancer among workers in an alcohol manufacturing plant who were exposed to a "strong acid" process of ethanol production using high concentrations of diethyl sulfate. Their methods of calculating the expected occurrence of laryngeal cancer were faulty in several instances, but the striking proportion of laryngeal cancer among all cancer cases (4/17) was supportive evidence for the elevated risk among that group. Diethyl sulfate was also indirectly implicated in a study by Soskolne et al (1984) of workers on an ethanol unit using strong concentrations of sulfuric acid at a large refinery and chemical plant in Baton Rouge, Louisiana. Of the 50 cases of upper respiratory cancer identified, 34 were of the larynx, which represented a 4-fold excess. These results are also consistent with those of Steenland et al (1988), who noted 9 cases of laryngeal cancer in a cohort of male steelworkers exposed to sulfuric acid mist, compared to a smoking-adjusted expected estimate of 3.9, and Forastiere et al (1987), who noted 5 cases of larynx cancer among Italian soap production workers exposed to sulfuric acid, when only 0.7 to 1.4 might have been expected. Zemla et al (1987) also reported, from a case-control study of larynx cancers in Poland, that risk was higher in workers exposed to acid vapors.

Other

A case-control study of 47 male laryngeal cancer patients conducted by Hinds et al (1979) suggested a possible association with exposure to dental X-rays, particularly among heavy smokers. Evidence consistent with dental X-ray exposure comes from the study of French female laryngeal cancer patients, in which abstainers from both alcohol and tobacco were significantly more likely than cases consuming one or both of these products to be edentulous or have dental prostheses (Luce et al, 1988). It is a commonly held belief among otolaryngologists that irradiation of symptomatic laryngeal papillomata dramatically increases the risk of malignant degeneration (Quick et al, 1978).

As a further note on environmental influences, an increased mortality rate from laryngeal cancer with increased urbanization in Oklahoma was reported by Cucchiara and Asal (1976), but an attempt by Caston et al (1972) to correlate current levels of air pollution in three urban counties in South Carolina to mortality rates for cancer of the lung and larynx combined was unsuccessful. Likewise, Elliott et al (1992) were unable to identify any excess of laryngeal or lung cancers in populations living near incinerators of waste solvents and oils in Great Britain.

Summary

Most epidemiological studies linking environmental agents to laryngeal cancer risk are of males only or of males and females combined, representing primarily males, and therefore largely glottic cancer risk. The separate and combined effects of tobacco and alcohol as major risk factors are well established for males and females. In addition, there is much evidence to suggest that the influence of these agents on subsites of the larynx may differ considerably. Low dietary vitamin A is a consistently reported risk factor among males, independent of smoking and alcohol. Much of the occupational risk evidence must be interpreted with caution since only a few of these studies evaluate occupational exposure in the context of the rather powerful contribution of alcohol and tobacco exposure. Even so, exposure to sulfuric acid mist and mustard gas appear to be risk factors, and cutting oil mist, nickel smelting, and asbestos exposures may also elevate risk. Evidence for radiation as a risk factor is weak and suggestive at most.

HOST FACTORS

Little evidence exists to link laryngeal cancer to heritable factors, but familial cases have been reported. Gencik et al (1986) described a Swiss family in which a father and both sons developed cancer of the larynx. They collected an additional 21 reports of similar families in the literature and noted that the familial cases had an unusually early onset and an alteration of the usual sex ratio.

Attempts to characterize genetic susceptibility by some laboratory measurement have been unsuccessful using HLA histocompatibility antigens (Tarpley et al, 1975) and ABO blood groups (Sokolowski and Woszczyk, 1980), but several studies (among them Korsgaard et al, 1984; Andreasson et al, 1987) suggest that individual susceptibility may be related to inducibility of the enzyme arylhydrocarbon hydroxylase (AHH). It is believed that the chief carcinogens of tobacco smoke are metabolically activated in the cell by AHH, which is subject to genetic control. In the general population, there appear to be three subgroups—low, intermediate, and high—for levels of AHH inducibility, corresponding to the homozygous (low), heterozygous, and homozygous (high) gene states (Kellermann et al, 1973). In 1978, Brandenburg and Kellermann reported that patients with laryngeal cancer were more likely to have intermediate and high AHH inducibility than controls, and Trell et al (1976) found a frequency of high AHH inducibility among laryngeal cancer cases of nearly 40%, whereas only about 9% was expected.

More recently, Lafuente et al (1993) reported a 2-fold risk for laryngeal cancer and bladder cancer among smokers deficient in the enzyme glutathione S-transferase [μ]. Similar findings for the same enzyme also have been found in relation to lung cancer (Seidgard et al, 1990), adding plausibility to the findings. It is of interest that Flagg and associates (1994) have identified increased dietary glutathione to be associated with reduced risk of oropharyngeal cancer.

Trell et al (1980) have also demonstrated a significant overrepresentation of AHH inducibility among patients with chronic laryngitis and laryngeal leukoplakia, but not with polyploid degeneration of the larynx (Reinke's edema), corresponding well with the malignant potential of the first two clinical conditions but not the latter.

The possibility of individual susceptibility to the carcinogenic effects of cigarette smoking was suggested by Hiranandani (1975). He examined the oro-respiratory tract of 1,000 smokers selected "at random" and found that 30% showed no leukoplakial change in the oral cavity or larynx, despite having smoked heavily for prolonged periods. These individuals were characterized as nonsusceptible. Another 10% had marked leukoplakial changes, but were relatively light smokers of short duration. These were called highly susceptible. The remaining 60% fell between the extremes, showing varying degrees of leukoplakia and tobacco use.

The two extreme groups were followed for three years. Among the 100 "highly susceptible" individuals, 20 developed laryngeal cancer, whereas among the 300 "nonsusceptible" individuals, only 2 developed laryngeal cancer. The leukoplakia may represent a highly individualized host reaction to the carcinogenic effects of smoking, but this susceptibility might stem from interactions with environmental cofactors.

There is evidence that patients with head and neck squamous cell cancer, about half of which are laryngeal neoplasms, also have immunologic abnormalities (Chretien, 1985). Weiss and Chretien (1985) summarized these abnormalities and their relationship to cigarette smoking. Whether or not the abnormalities are etiologically related to the malignancy, it does illustrate an apparent altered state of host resistance. This same state may be observed epidemiologically as multiple tumors involving the larynx and others of the oral cavity and respiratory tract, reported in this country (Moore, 1971; Wynder and Stellman, 1977), Denmark (Christensen et al, 1987), Sweden (Lundgren and Olofsson, 1986), Japan (Hiyama and Fujimoto, 1984; Miyahara et al, 1985), Israel (Deviri et al, 1982), and the Netherlands (Karim et al, 1983). Also from the Netherlands, deVries et al (1986) reported multiple primary tumors (primarily lung) in patients with laryngeal squamous cell hyperplasia.

Fechner (1985) summarized a number of histologic, antigenic, and biologic changes in premalignant and malignant squamous cell cancers of the head and neck. He cites the study of Lin et al (1977) in which the A, B, and H isoantigens, normally present in laryngeal epithelial cells, evidenced a gradual loss with transition from morphologically normal to dysplasia to neoplasia. Ten cases had morphologically normal epithelium devoid of antigens adjacent to laryngeal cancers. An additional four patients, in whom an initial biopsy was benign but who had a complete loss of the ABH antigens in the biopsy tissue, all developed subsequent carcinoma.

DeVries et al (1986) also reported on an immunoglobin allotype, Km(1), which seemed to be associated with elevated risk for developing multiple primary tumors of the head and neck and respiratory tract.

Schantz et al (1990) have investigated the sensitivity of patients to mutagen-induced chromosome breaks from bleomycin by dichotomizing the sensitivity of lymphocytes from patients with squamous cell carcinoma of the head and neck (a third of which were laryngeal in origin). They found that those patients with greater sensitivity were 4.4 times as likely to develop multiple primary tumors, independent of previous exposures. They hypothesize this finding to be evidence of genetic susceptibility.

The reported association between laryngocele and laryngeal cancer may be due to the fact that laryngoceles arise as a result of conditions that raise intralaryngeal pressure—for example, occupations such as glassblowing—or from obstructive lesions, including tumors (Lindell et al, 1978; Micheau et al, 1978; Close et al, 1987). There is no evidence that laryngoceles predispose to carcinoma.

Clinical evidence suggests that gastroesophageal reflux may increase the risk of laryngeal cancer. Morrison (1988) reported 6 cases of glottic carcinoma in lifetime nonsmokers and users of no or minimal alcohol, but all of whom had clinical gastroesophageal reflux. A subsequent record review was conducted of the 21 nonsmoker cases (4.6%) from all glottic cancer patients presenting to the Cancer Control Agency of British Columbia 1970–1980 and of the 52 cases (11.4%) who had stopped smoking 10 or more years previously at diagnosis. Among the never smokers, definite or probable recorded evidence of reflux existed in 33%, while for former smokers only 7% had such chart evidence. A similar clinical study by Ward and Hanson (1988) reviewed charts and 16-mm pictures or videotapes of patients seen in a clinical practice in Los Angeles where cinematic or video evaluation of the larynx was routinely included in the patient evaluation, of whom 138 initially or subsequently were diagnosed with laryngeal cancer. Of these, 19 patients who had never smoked, including 16 who were nonusers of alcohol and 3 with "social use only," were identified. On a clinical scale of 1–4+, 12 patients evidenced 4+ gastroesophageal reflux, 6 evidenced 3+, and one 2+. The three "social drinkers" were either 2+ or 3+. Of the 19 malignancies, 14 were glottic, all of which involved the posterior glottis. The prevalence of reflux in patients without laryngeal disease was not determined, and until well-designed epidemiologic evaluations of the effect of reflux are conducted, the clinical information must serve to define an interesting hypothesis.

Concepts of Pathogenesis

Little work on the pathogenesis of cancer has been focused on the larynx, no doubt because of its relative rarity among cancers. However, an epidemiologic study of the incidence of laryngeal keratosis (leukoplakia), carcinoma in situ, and carcinoma in Rochester County, Minnesota, by Bouquot et al (1991) found a male preponderance in all three. A 3-fold increase in incidence of keratosis and carcinoma occurred over a 50-year period, but the in situ incidence remained relatively stable. They also noted that the age of peak incidence of keratosis occurred 20 years prior to the peak of invasive carcinoma.

It is apparent that concepts of tobacco carcinogenesis apply generally to the larynx. Alcohol appears to be both an independent risk factor and a potent cocarcinogen with tobacco. It appears, however, that the relative contribution of tobacco and alcohol in the pathogenesis of cancer is different for the two major subsites of the larynx, although there is no evidence that the interaction of these two are different in males than females.

The causal role of viruses in laryngeal cancer is not conclusive, although substantial evidence exists to support the biologic plausibility of that hypothesis, at least for some proportion of cases. The hypothetical pathway is infection with a human papillomavirus (HPV) of the type that causes condyloma acuminata, acquired perhaps during parturition from a maternal infection. The HPV results in laryngeal papilloma development early (juvenile laryngeal papillomatosis) or later in life (adult laryngeal papillomas), which may undergo malignant degeneration depending upon host factors and environmental stimulation, such as radiation.

The etiology of laryngeal papillomas is usually accepted as being viral. In 1973, Cook et al reported that 7 of 9 children with laryngeal papilloma were delivered of mothers with a history of condyloma acuminata. All 5 of those who developed papillomas during the first 6 months of life were delivered of mothers with genital warts. In 1978, Quick et al reported that 60% of their series of children with laryngeal papillomatosis had a positive history of maternal genital warts during pregnancy and parturition. They also established that the viral agent involved was not the same as that causing cutaneous papillomas and postulated a strain of HPV as the etiological agent. The etiologic roles of HPV types 6 and 11 were reported by Mounts et al (1982) and Steinberg et al (1983) for laryngeal papillomata of both juvenile and adult onset. Terry et al (1987) and Wright et al (1990) identified HPV types 6 and 11 in cases of juvenile papillomatosis examined using in situ hybridization. The relationship of juvenile papillomatosis to HPV, especially strains 6 and 11, is summarized by Bennet and Powell (1987), who propose obstetrical methods to prevent parturitional transmission by infected mothers. Hallmo and Naess (1991) describe a unique clinical anecdote of the development of laryngeal papillomatosis, positive for both HPV types 6 and 11, in a laser surgeon who had treated five patients with anogenital condyloma acuminata without a laser smoke evacuator system. They comment that the surgeon's wife had no history of anogenital condylomas.

Mullooly et al (1988) have described a strong correlation between dosage of alpha-interferon as a treatment for HPV-positive laryngeal papillomas (both adult and juvenile) and clinical response. Levinthal and others in the Papilloma Study Group (1991) report a high rate of remission of recurrent respiratory papillomatosis using an alpha-interferon from lymphoblasts. Steinberg et al (1983, 1988) have also established the persistence of HPV in laryngeal tissues during periods of papilloma remission and in surrounding histologically normal tissue in patients with active papillomata.

Ibrahim et al (1985) have demonstrated the apparent identity of two of three tumor-associated antigens between squamous cell carcinoma of the cervix and squamous cell carcinoma of the larynx, strongly suggesting the antigenic identity of these two malignancies. These investigators took the results to suggest a possible common virus etiology. Spitz and her associates (1992) reported that the odds ratio of laryngeal cancer after diagnosis of cervical cancer, or the reverse, was about 5.5. Other factors, such as tobacco use and diet, could also contribute to this finding. Aurelian (1985) described an apparent association between seropositivity to herpes simplex virus (HSV) type 1 and head and neck squamous cancers. This finding must be interpreted with caution, since a similar association exists between HSV-2 and cervical cancer, although the virus now thought to be etiologically linked is the papilloma virus (deVilliers et al, 1987). Human papillomavirus has also been detected in malignancies of the mouth (Demetrick et al, 1990), conjunctiva (McDonnell et al, 1989), and esophagus (Williamson et al, 1991).

An epidemiological study of both juvenile and adult laryngeal papillomatosis in the Copenhagen region (Bomholt, 1988a, 1988b) revealed that there is no epidemiologic basis for considering the adult and juvenile conditions to be separate syndromes, that regression of the condition in childhood may still result in recurrence in later life (up to 22 years later), that the condition carries with it a higher risk of laryngeal cancer with or without radiation of the benign condition, and that a variable clinical course is seen in different individuals. In extremely aggressive cases, multiple papillomata extending into the bronchial tree may be seen, which is also an indicator of high risk for pulmonary malignancy, a finding also reported by Alberti and Dykun (1981).

Quiney et al (1989) reviewed records of 113 patients with laryngeal papillomatosis treated at the Royal National Throat Nose and Ear Hospital in London and noted similar male:female ratios under age 25 but a marked male preponderance among older ages. They also report two in situ and four invasive laryngeal carcinomas occurring in this group during follow-up, half of which they suggest were the result of prior irradiation treatment of the papillomatosis.

Lindeberg and Elbrond (1990) discuss the epidemiology of laryngeal papillomas in a subpopulation of Denmark and their relationship to laryngeal cancer risk. They point out that if papilloma virus infection was acquired during childbirth, one would expect a 1:1 male:female ratio. That ratio is, in fact, found among juveniles but not among adults, suggesting an additional route of transmission among adults. They suggest orogenital sexual contact as a possible route but offer no gender-specific data on sexual practices in Denmark in support of this suggestion. Jenison et al (1990) found approximately equal prevalences (about 20%) of HPV 6b and HPV 16 in oral scrapings from Seattle preschoolers and adults.

Lie et al (1994) report the development of squamous cell carcinoma of the larynx among 7 of 102 patients followed for laryngeal papillomatosis, producing a risk ratio of 88. An additional case of bronchial carcinoma was also noted. Two of the cases had received radiation and two had received bleomycin for treatment of the papillomas. Brandwein et al (1993) cite studies in which the range of HPV prevalence in laryngeal cancers ranged from 0% to 54%, depending upon the technique. Using consensus primers to "hot-start" the polymerase chain reaction, a technique that is sensitive and that minimizes contamination, they found a prevalence of 8% of 40 laryngeal cancers and detectable HPV, suggesting that the fraction of cases associated with HPV is small. Hagen et al (1993) argues that the uncommon verrucous carcinoma of the larynx (about 1% of all laryngeal cancers), which is well differentiated but persistently recurrent, which is noted for anaplastic transformation following radiation, and in which HPV type 16 have been isolated (Brandsma et al, 1986), should be treated surgically but not with radiation. They cite a surgical cure rate of over 90% but a radiation cure rate of less than 50%.

PREVENTIVE MEASURES

The two most important approaches for primary prevention of laryngeal cancer are avoidance of tobacco and alcohol. Singly and in combination, these two factors must account for the majority of laryngeal cancer in any society. Thomas (1985) estimates that three-quarters of all carcinomas of the larynx in the United States are due to the use of tobacco and alcohol. In Auerbach et al's (1970) meticulous studies demonstrating 16% in situ carcinoma and 99% atypia in an autopsy series, it is notable that no ex–cigarette smokers had carcinoma in situ and only 25% had mild atypia, similar to nonsmokers. In a later electron microscopy study of ultrastructural abnormalities in upper airway and digestive tract epithelial tissues, Incze et al (1982) found that smokers with cancers had an average of 6.3 abnormalities per cell, smokers without cancer had 2.3 abnormalities, but nonsmokers and ex-smokers each had an average of 1.2. One of the ex-smokers had morphologic abnormalities before quitting smoking.

These two pathologic studies reinforce the epidemiologic observation that the well-established risk for multiple oral and respiratory tract cancers among smokers is reduced among patients who stop smoking after the first diagnosis (Moore, 1971; Wynder and Stellman, 1977).

Evidence is mounting that beta-carotene, but not retinol, and perhaps glutathione or other micronutrients found in fresh or lightly cooked fruits and vegetables, can reduce the risk of a variety of upper aerodigestive tract epithelial cancers. This effect is observed in the presence of other major risk factors and may reduce risk by 50%–80% in the high-consumption group as compared to the lowest-consumption group.

Presumptive evidence is sufficient to warrant protection against occupational exposure to sulfuric acid mist, cutting oil mist, nickel-smelting fumes, mustard gas, and asbestos or similar fibers, although protection from exposure to these substances is warranted on other grounds also.

Early Detection

Glottic cancer tends to cause symptoms, especially hoarseness, early in the course of disease, so examination of all patients with hoarseness of more than a few days duration is a useful means of detecting this malignancy at a curable stage. Not only does glottic cancer cause symptoms early, it has a low rate of metastasis and a high survival rate. Because glottic cancer is the most common laryngeal subsite (especially among males, who have the higher incidence), the use of hoarseness has been used in a mass screening trial (Ono, 1982) in Japan. Patients over 50 years of age with hoarseness, at 53 cooperating institutions, were selected to undergo laryngeal cancer screening. Of 941 so screened, 16 laryngeal cancers and 7 lower pharyngeal cancers were detected, a yield that compares favorably with many other types of cancer screening.

Laryngeal cytopathology screening has been advocated, but primarily as a means of following previously irradiated laryngeal cancers (Osborn and Sunderman, 1971; Glennie et al, 1976) or as an adjunct to histologic examination (Lundgren et al, 1981; Gaafar et al, 1989).

The potential of detecting a possible laryngeal neoplasm by an alteration in the tonal quality of the voice has intrigued investigators. Earlier work (Rontal et al, 1975; Kitajima and Gould, 1976; Murry, 1978) in this country did not produce a procedure for laryngeal screening, but a later Japanese attempt (Mashima et al, 1987) produced optimism in the investigators that an acoustic screening system could be built for mass screening.

Likewise, earlier hopes for developing a serologic method of detecting laryngeal cancer have not been realized, although investigators are still pursuing promising leads (Ibrahim et al, 1985; Aurelian, 1985). So far, the only accepted procedure for routine detection of laryngeal cancer is direct or indirect laryngoscopy, and biopsy of suspicious lesions.

FUTURE RESEARCH

Even though the major etiologic factors for laryngeal cancer apparently have been fairly well established, their relationship to incidence and mortality rates is not clear. It is not clear why males are much more likely than females to develop glottic cancer, which has a better prognosis. If the proportion of glottic cancers were a function of the incidence rate, one would expect lower proportions of glottic cancer among males in areas with lower incidence, but this seems not to be the case. Perhaps hormonal factors influence the risk in different larynx subsites. Perhaps tobacco type and alcohol type are important to characterize for each subsite. Perhaps a different combination of alcohol use, dietary factors, and tobacco use accounts for the different subsite risks by sex. Additional epidemiological research is necessary to elucidate the role of risk factors on larynx subsites.

Occupational risk factors are in need of better characterization, and attention to subsite is important, since it appears that the two major subsites may respond quite differently to exposures.

The viral etiology of laryngeal cancer is becoming better characterized, and the current perspective appears to be that HPV infection may be etiologically related to a small portion of the total number of cases. However, the relationship of laryngeal cancer to other viral agents, such as HSV-2 infection, and the interaction of viral infection with other factors, including tobacco products, alcohol, irradiation, and vitamin A deficiency, is largely unknown.

A means of identifying individuals at high risk for developing laryngeal cancer is needed. Seropositivity to a particular viral antigen, an immunoglobin allotype, a DNA adduct, a specific genetic marker, or the demonstration of the presence of a particular inducible enzyme might be developed into a possible test. However, regarding the identification of high-risk individuals, age and hoarseness currently offer the only accepted improvements over a history of alcohol and tobacco use. Future research may determine whether gastroesophageal reflux is also clinically useful in identifying individuals at elevated risk. Although several imaging techniques, cytopathology, and other laboratory techniques show promise for improving the amount of information obtained from a diagnostic evaluation, no procedure other than laryngoscopy has yet been shown to be effective for mass screening.

REFERENCES

ADAMI H-O, MCLAUGHLIN JK, HSING AW, et al. 1992. Alcoholism and cancer risk: a population-based cohort study. Cancer Causes Control 3:419–425.

ADELSTEIN AM. 1972. Occupational mortality: cancer. Ann Occup Hyg 15:53–57.

AHRENS W, KARL-HEINZ J, PATZACK W, ELSNER G. 1991. Alcohol, smoking, and occupational factors in cancer of the larynx: A case-control study. Am J Ind Med 20:477–493.

ALBERTI PW, DYKUN R. 1981. Adult laryngeal papillomata. J Otolaryngol 10(6):463–470.

ANDREASSON L, BJORLIN G, HOCHERMAN M, et al. 1987. Laryngeal cancer, aryl hydrocarbon hydroxylase inducibility and smoking. A follow-up study. ORL 49:187–192.

ANON. 1976. (Editorial): Smoking and laryngeal cancer. Med J Aust ii:284.

ATKINSON L. 1975. Some features of the epidemiology of cancer of the larynx in Australia and Papua, New Guinea. Laryngoscope 85:1173–1184.

AUERBACH O, HAMMOND EC, GARFINKEL L. 1970. Histologic changes in relation to smoking habits. Cancer 25:92–104.

AURELIAN L. 1985. HSV antigens as diagnostic and/or therapeutic markers in squamous cancer of the cervix and head and neck: In Chretien PB, Johns ME, Shedd DP, et al (eds): Head and Neck Cancer, Vol. 1. Philadelphia/Toronto: B.C. Decker Inc. pp. 573–580.

AYIOMAMITIS A. 1989. The epidemiology of malignant neoplasia of the larynx in Canada: 1931–1984. Clin Otolaryngol 14:349–355.

BENNETT RS, POWELL KR. 1987. Human papillomaviruses: associations between laryngeal papillomas and genital warts. Pediatr Infect Dis J 6:(3)229–232.

BLOT WJ, MORRIS LE, STROUBE R, et al. 1980. Lung and laryngeal cancers in relation to shipyard employment in coastal Virginia. J Natl Cancer Inst 65(3):571–575.

BLOT WJ, FRAUMENI JF JR, MORRIS LE. 1978. Patterns of laryngeal cancer in the United States. Lancet ii:674–675.

BOMHOLT A. 1988a. Juvenile laryngeal papillomatosis. An epidemiological study from the Copenhagen region. Acta Otolaryngol 105(3-4):367–371.

BOMHOLT A. 1988b. Laryngeal papillomas with adult onset. An epidemiological study from the Copenhagen region. Acta Otolaryngol (Stockh) (106) (1–2):240–14.

BRANDENBURG JH, KELLERMAN G. 1978. Aryl hydrocarbon hydroxylase inducibility in laryngeal carcinoma. Arch Otolaryngol 104:(3)151–152.

BOONE CW, KELLOFF GJ, MALONE WE. 1990. Identification of candidate cancer chemopreventive agents and their evaluation in animal models and human clinical trials: a review. Cancer Res 50:2–9.

BOUQUET JE, KURLAND LT, WEILAND LH. 1991. Laryngeal keratosis and carcinoma in the Rochester, MN, population, 1935–1984. Cancer Detect Prev 15(2):83–91.

BRANDSMA JL, STEINBERG BM, et al. 1986. Presence of human papillomavirus type 16 sequences in verrucous carcinoma of the larynx. Cancer Res 46:2185–2188.

BRANDWEIN MS, NUOVO GJ, BILLER H. 1993. Analysis of prevalence of human papilloma virus in laryngeal carcinomas: study of 40 cases using polymerase chain reaction and consensus primers. Ann Otol Rhinol Laryngol 102:309–313.

BRAVO MP, ESPINOSA J, et al. 1990. Occupational risk factors for cancer of the larynx in Spain. Neoplasma 37:477–481.

BRIDGES GP, REAY-YOUNG P. 1976. Laryngeal cancer and smoking. Med J. Aust ii:293–294.

BROWN LM, MASON TJ, PICKLE LW, et al. 1988. Occupational risk factors for laryngeal cancer on the Texas Gulf Coast. Cancer Res 48:1960–1964.

BROWN LM, HOOVER RN, GREENBERG RS, et al. 1994. Are racial differences in squamous cell esophageal cancer explained by alcohol and tobacco use? J Natl Cancer Inst 86:1340–1345.

BROWNSON RC, CHANG JC. 1987. Exposure to alcohol and tobacco and the risk of laryngeal cancer. Arch Environ Health 42:192–196.

BURCH JD, HOWE GR, MILLER AB, et al. 1981. Tobacco, alcohol, asbestos, and nickel in the etiology of cancer of the larynx: a case controlled study. J Natl Cancer Inst 67:1219–1224.

CANN CI, FRIED MP. 1984. Determinants and prognosis of laryngeal cancer. Otolaryngol Clin North Am 17:139–150.

CASTON JC, FINKLEA JF, SANDIFER SH. 1972. Cancer of the larynx and lung in three urban counties in South Carolina. South Med J 65:753–756.

CHAN CK, GEE JB. 1988. Asbestos exposure and laryngeal cancer: an analysis of the epidemiologic evidence. J Occup Med 30(1): 23–27.

CHOI SY, KAHYO H. 1991. Effect of cigarette smoking and alcohol consumption in the aetiology of cancer of the oral cavity, pharynx and larynx. Int J Epidemiol 20(4):878–885.

CHRETIEN PB. 1985. Immunology and Immunotherapy. In Chretien PB, Johns ME, Shedd DP, et al (eds.). Head and Neck Cancer, Vol. 1. Philadelphia/Toronto: B.C. Decker Inc., pp. 557–559.

CHRISTENSEN PH, JOERGENSEN K, MUNK J, et al. 1987. Hyperfrequency of pulmonary cancer in a population of 415 patients treated for laryngeal cancer. Laryngoscope 97(5):612–614.

CLOSE LG, MERKEL M, BURNS DK, et al. 1987. Asymptomatic laryngocele: incidence and association with laryngeal cancer. Ann Otol Rhinol Laryngol 96(4):393–399.

COOK TA, COHN AM, BRUNSCHWIG JP, et al. 1973. Laryngeal papilloma: etiologic and therapeutic considerations. Ann Otol 82:649–655.

CUCCHIARA AJ, ASAL NR. 1976. Laryngeal neoplasm mortality in Oklahoma: 1950–1970. South Med J 69:908–910.

CUTLER SJ, YOUNG JL. 1975. Third National Cancer Survey: Incidence Data. Natl Cancer Inst Monogr 41:1–454.

DAY GL, BLOT WJ, AUSTIN DF, et al. 1993. Racial differences in risk of oral and pharyngeal cancer: alcohol, tobacco, and other determinants. J Natl Cancer Inst 85:465–473.

DEMETRICK DJ, INOUE M, et al. 1990. Human papillomavirus type 16 associated with oral squamous carcinoma in a cardiac transplant recipient. Cancer 6:1726–1731.

DERIENZO DP, GREENBERG D, FRAIRE A. 1991. Carcinoma of the larynx: changing incidence in women. Arch Otolaryngol Head Neck Surg 117:681–684.

DESTEFANI E, CORREA P, OREGGIA F, et al. 1987. Risk factors for laryngeal cancer. Cancer 60(12):3087–3091.

DEVESA SS, BLOT WJ, FRAUMENI JF. 1990. Cohort trends in mortality from oral, esophageal, and laryngeal cancers in the United States. Epidemiology 1:116–121.

DEVILLIERS EM, SCHNEIDER A, et al. 1987. Human papillomavirus infection in women with and without abnormal cervical cytology. Lancet 703–706.

DEVIRI E, ELIACHAR I, BARTAL A, et al. 1982. Occurrence of additional primary neoplasms in patients with laryngeal carcinoma in Israel. Ann Otol Rhinol Laryngol 91(3):261–265.

DEVRIES N, OLDE KALTER P, SNOW GB. 1986. Multiple primary tumors in patients with laryngeal squamous cell hyperplasia. Arch Otorhinolaryngol 243(2):143–145.

DOLL R, PETO J. 1987. Other asbestos-related neoplasms. In Antman K, Aisner J, eds Asbestos-Related Malignancy. London, Grume G Stratton, Inc, pp. 81–96.

DOLL R, PETO J, EASTON DF, PETO J, DOLL R. 1988. Cancer of the respiratory tract in mustard gas workers. Br J Ind Med 45:652–659.

EASTON DF, PETO J, DOLL R. 1988. Cancer of the respiratory tract in mustard gas workers. Br J Ind Med 45:652–659.

EDELMAN DA. 1989. Laryngeal cancer and occupational exposure to asbestos. Int Arch Occup Environ Health 61:223–227.

ELLIOTT P, HILLS M, BERESFORD J, et al. 1992. Incidence of cancers of the larynx and lung near incinerators of waste solvents and oils in Great Britain. Lancet 339:854–858.

ELWOOD JM, PEARSON JCG, SKIPPEN DH, et al. 1984. Alcohol, smoking, social and occupational factors in the aetiology of cancer of the oral cavity, pharynx and larynx. Int J Cancer 34:603–612.

ESTEVE J, RIBOLI E, TUYNS AJ. 1988–89. Laryngeal and pharyngeal cancer: case-control study in southwestern Europe. IARC Biennial Report. Lyon: Int'l Agency for Research Against Cancer, p. 54.

FECHNER RE. 1985. New and innovative aspects of pathology: In Chretien PB, Johns ME, Shedd DP, et al (eds): Head and Neck Cancer, Vol. 1. Philadelphia/Toronto: B.C. Decker Inc., pp 18–26.

FLAGG EW, COATES RJ, JONES DP, et al. 1994. Dietary glutathione intake and the risk of oral and pharyngeal cancer. Am J Epidemiol 139:453–65.

FLANDERS WD, ROTHMAN KJ. 1982. Occupational risk for laryngeal cancer. Am J Public Health 72(4):369–372.

FLANDERS WD, CANN CI, ROTHMAN KJ, et al. 1984. Work-related risk factors for laryngeal cancer. Am J Epidemiol 119(1):23–32.

FORASTIERE F, VALESINI S, SALIMEI E, et al. 1987. Respiratory cancer among soap production workers. Scand J Work Environ Health 13:258–260.

FRANCESCHI S, TALAMINI R, SALVATORE B, et al. 1990. Smoking and drinking in relation to cancers of the oral cavity, pharynx, larynx, and esophagus in northern Italy. Cancer Res 50:6502–6507.

FREUDENHEIM JL, GRAHAM S, BYERS TE, et al. 1992. Diet, smoking, and alcohol in cancer of the larynx: a case-control study. Nutr Cancer 17:33–45.

GAAFAR H, HUSSEIN M, EL-ASSI H. 1989. Cytopathology in cancer of larynx. Otorhinolaryngol 51:216–220.

GENCIK A, WEY W, MULLER H. 1986. High incidence of laryngeal carcinoma in a Swiss family. J Otorhinolaryngol Relat Spec 48(3):162–166.

GLENNIE HRR, GILBERT JG, MELCHER DH, et al. 1976. The place of cytology in laryngeal diagnosis. Clin Otolaryngol 1:134–136.

GOLDSMITH JR. 1980. The "urban factor" in cancer: smoking, industrial exposures and air pollution as possible explanations. J Environ Pathol Toxicol 3:205–217.

GUENEL P, MOLLER H, LYNGE E. 1988a. Incidence of the upper respiratory and digestive tract cancers and consumption of alcohol and tobacco in Denmark. Scand J Soc Med 16:257–263.

GUENEL P, CHASTANG JF, LUCE D, et al. 1988b. A study of the interaction of alcohol drinking and tobacco smoking among French cases of laryngeal cancer. J Epidemiol Community Health 42:350–354.

GUENEL P, ENGHOLM G, LYNGE E. 1990. Laryngeal cancer in Denmark: a nationwide longitudinal study based on register linkage data. Br J Ind Med 47:473–479.

HAGEN P, LYONS GD, HAINDEL C. 1993. Verrucous carcinoma of the larynx: role of human papillomavirus, radiation, and surgery. Laryngoscope 103:253–257.

HALLMO P, NAESS O. 1991. Laryngeal papillomatosis with human papillomavirus DNA contracted by a laser surgeon. Eur Arch Otorhinolaryngol 248:425–427.

HARRAS A, LUBIN J, FEIGAL E. 1993. Larynx. In Miller BA, Reis

LAG, Hankey B, et al. eds, Cancer Statistics Review 1973–1990. US Department of Health and Human Services, NIH Publication No. 93-2789, Bethesda, Maryland.

HEDBERG K, VAUGHN TL, WHITE E, et al. 1994. Alcoholism and cancer of the larynx: a case-control study in western Washington. Cancer Causes Control 5(1):3–8.

HESTON WE. 1950. Carcinogenic action of the mustards. J Natl Cancer Inst 11:415–423.

HILLERDAL G, LINDHOLM CE. 1980. Laryngeal cancer and asbestos. Otorhinolaryngol 42(4):233–241.

HINDS MW, THOMAS DB, O'REILLY HP. 1979. Asbestos, dental x-rays, tobacco, and alcohol in the epidemiology of laryngeal cancer. Cancer 44:1114–1120.

HIRANANDANI LH. 1975. Panel on epidemiology and etiology of laryngeal carcinoma. Laryngoscope 85:1197–1207.

HIYAMA T, FUJIMOTO I. 1984. Epidemiological studies on multiple primary cancers—observations on the second primary cancers among cervical and laryngeal cancer cases. Gan No Rinsho 30(12 Suppl.):1459–1506.

HOJSLET P-E, NIELSON VM, PALVIO D. 1989. Premalignant lesions of the larynx. Acta Otolaryngol 107:150–155.

HOLMES JG, KIPLING MD, WATERHOUSE JAH. 1970. Subsequent malignancies in men with scrotal epithelioma. Lancet ii:214–215.

HONG WK, LIPPMAN SM, ITRI LM, et al. 1990. Prevention of second tumors with isotretinoin in squamous-cell carcinoma of the head and neck. N Engl J Med 323:795–801.

IBRAHIM AN, TUCKER RA, MARR L, et al. 1985. Tumor-associated antigens in head and neck cancer tissues and in sera of tumor-bearing patients; In Chretien PB, Johns ME, Shedd DP, et al (eds.): Head and Neck Cancer, Vol. 1. Philadelphia/Toronto: B.C. Decker Inc., pp. 568–573.

INCZE J, VAUGHAN CW JR, LUI P, et al. 1982. Premalignant changes in normal appearing epithelium in patients with squamous cell carcinoma of the upper aerodigestive tract. Am J Surg 144:401–405.

JENISON SA, XIU-PING Y, et al. 1990. Evidence of prevalent genital-type human papillomavirus infections in adults and children. J Inf Dis 162:61–69.

JENSEN OM. 1979. Cancer morbidity and causes of death among Danish brewery workers. Int J Cancer 23:454–463.

JUSSAWALLA DJ, DESHPANDE VA. 1971. Evaluation of cancer risk in tobacco chewers and smokers: an epidemiologic assessment. Cancer 28:244–252.

KARIM AB, SNOW GB, SIEK HT, et al. 1983. The quality of voice in patients irradiated for laryngeal carcinoma. Cancer 51(1):47–49.

KELLERMANN G, LUYTEN-KELLERMANN M, SHAW CR. 1973. Genetic variation of aryl hydrocarbon hydroxylase in human lymphocytes. Am J Hum Genet 25:327–331.

KITAJIMA K, GOULD WJ. 1976. Vocal shimmer in sustained phonation of normal and pathologic voice. Ann Otol Rhinol Laryngol 85:377–381.

KORSGAARD R, TRELL E, KITZING P, et al. 1984. Arylhydrocarbon-hydroxylase inducibility and smoking habits in patients with laryngeal carcinomas. Acta Otolaryngol (Stockh) 98:368–373.

KURIHARA M, AOKI J, TOMINAGA S. (EDS.). 1984. Cancer Mortality Statistics in the World. Nagoya, Japan: University of Nagoya Press.

LAFUENTE A, PUJOL F, CARRETERO P, et al. 1993. Human glutathione S-transferase (μ) (GSTμ) deficiency as a marker for the susceptibility to bladder and larynx cancer among smokers. Cancer Lett 68:49–54.

LAVECCHIA C, NEGRI E, et al. 1990. Dietary indicators of laryngeal cancer risk. Cancer Res 50:4497–4500.

LECLERC A, BRUGERE J, LUCE D, et al. 1987. Type of alcoholic beverage and cancer of the upper respiratory and digestive tract. Eur J Cancer Clin Oncol 23(5):529–534.

LEVI F, LAVECCHIA C. 1990. Sex ratio of laryngeal cancer by anatomic subsite (letters). J Clin Epidemiol 43(7):729–730.

LEVINTHAL BG, KASHIMA HK, et al. 1991. Long-term response of recurrent respiratory papillomatosis to treatment with lymphoblastoid interferon Alfa-n1. N Engl J Med 325(9):613–617.

LIBSHITZ HI, WERSHBA MS, ATKINSON GW, et al. 1974. Asbestosis and carcinoma of the larynx. JAMA 228:1571–1572.

LIDDELL FDK. 1990. Laryngeal cancer and asbestos. Br J Ind Med 47:289–291.

LIE ES, ENGH V, et al. 1994. Squamous cell carcinoma of the respiratory tract following laryngeal papillomatosis. Acta Otolaryngol (Stockh) 114:209–212.

LIN F, LIU PI, MCGREGOR DH. 1977. Isoantigens A, B, and H in morphologically normal mucosa and in carcinoma of the larynx. Am J Clin Pathol 68:372–376.

LINDEBERG H, ELBROND O. 1990. Laryngeal papillomas: the epidemiology in a Danish subpopulation 1965–1984. Clin Otolaryngol 15:125–131.

LINDELL MM JR, JING B, FISCHER EP, et al. 1978. Laryngocoele. Am J Roentgenol 131:259–262.

LUCE D, GUENEL P, BRUGERE J, et al. 1988. Alcohol and tobacco consumption in cancer of the mouth, pharynx and larynx: A study of 316 female patients. Laryngoscope 98:313–316.

LUNDGREN J, OLOFFSON J, HELLQUIST HB, et al. 1981. Exfoliative cytology in laryngology: Comparison of cytologic and histologic diagnosis in 350 microlaryngoscopic examinations—A prospective study. Cancer 47:1336–1343.

LUNDGREN J, OLOFSSON J. 1986. Multiple primary malignancies in patients treated for laryngeal carcinoma. J Otolaryngol 15(3):145–150.

LYNCH J, HANIS NM, BIRD MG, et al. 1979. An association of upper respiratory cancer with exposure to diethyl sulfate. J Occup Med 21:333–341.

MACKERRAS D, BUFFLER PA, RANDALL DE, et al. 1988. Carotene intake and the risk of laryngeal cancer in coastal Texas. Am J Epidemiol 128(5):980–988.

MAIER H, GEWELKE U, DIETZ, HELLER W. 1992. Risk factors of cancer of the larynx: results of the Heidelberg case-control study. Otolaryngol Head Neck Surg 107:577–582.

MASHIMA K, EBIHARA S, KASUYA H. 1987. Acoustic screening for laryngeal cancer. Jpn J Clin Oncol 17(1):41–47.

MCDONNELL JM, MAYR AJ, et al. 1989. DNA of human papillomavirus type 16 in dysplastic and malignant lesions of the conjunctiva and cornea. N Engl J Med 320(22):1442–1445.

MCLAUGHLIN JK, GRIDLEY G, BLOCK G, et al. 1988. Dietary factors in oral and pharyngeal cancer. J Natl Cancer Inst 80:1237–1243.

MCMICHAEL AJ. 1978. Increases in laryngeal cancer in Britain and Australia in relation to alcohol and tobacco consumption trends. Lancet i:1244–1247.

MERLETTI F, FAGGIANO F, et al. 1990. Topographic classification, clinical characteristics, and diagnostic delay of cancer of the larynx/hypopharynx in Torino, Italy. Cancer 66:1711–1716.

MEYSKENS FL. 1990. Coming of age—the chemoprevention of cancer. N Engl J Med 323:825–827.

MICHEAU C, LUBOINSKI B, LANCHI P, et al. 1978. Relationship between laryngoceles and laryngeal carcinomas. Laryngoscope 88:680–688.

MIDDLETON B, BYERS T, MARSHALL J, et al. 1986. Dietary vitamin A and cancer—a multisite case-control study. Nutr Cancer 8(2):107–116.

MILLER AH, FISHER HR. 1971. Clues to the life history of carcinoma in situ of the larynx. Laryngoscope 81(9):1475–1480.

MIYAHARA H, YOSHINO K, UMATANI J, et al. 1985. Multiple primary tumors in laryngeal cancer. J Laryngol Otol 99(10):999–1004.

MOORE C. 1971. Cigarette smoking and cancer of the mouth, pharynx, and larynx (a continuing study). JAMA 218:553–558.

MORGAN RW, SHETTIGARA PT. 1976. Occupational asbestos exposure, smoking and laryngeal carcinoma. Ann NY Acad Sci 271:308–310.

MORRISON MD. 1988. Is chronic gastroesophageal reflux a causative factor in glottic carcinoma? Otolaryngol Head Neck Surg 99(4):370–373.

MOULIN JJ, MUR JM, WILD P, et al. 1986. Oral cavity and laryngeal cancers and man-made mineral fiber production workers. Scand J Work Environ Health 12:27–31.

MOULIN JJ, WILD P, et al. 1989. Risk of lung, larynx, pharynx and buccal cavity cancers among carbon electrode manufacturing workers. Scand J Work Environ Health 15:30–37.

MOUNTS P, SHAH KV, KASHIMA H. 1982. Viral etiology of juvenile and adult onset squamous papilloma of the larynx. Proc Natl Acad Sci USA 79:5425–5429.

MUIR C, WATERHOUSE J, MACK T, POWELL J, WHELAN S (EDS). 1987. Cancer Incidence on Five Continents, Vol. V. Lyon: International Agency for Research on Cancer (IARC Scientific Publication Number 88).

MULLOOLY VM, ABRAMSON AL, STEINBERG BM, et al. 1988. Clinical effects of alpha-interferon dose variation on laryngeal papillomas. Laryngoscope 98(12):1324–1329.

MURRY J. 1978. Speaking fundamental frequency characteristics associated with voice pathologies. J Speech Hear Disord 43:374–379.

MUSCAT JE, WYNDER EL. 1992. Tobacco, alcohol, asbestos, and occupational risk factors for laryngeal cancer. Cancer 69:2244–2851.

NEWHOUSE ML, BERRY G. 1973. Asbestos and laryngeal carcinoma. Lancet ii:615.

OLSEN J, SABROE S. 1984. Occupational causes of laryngeal cancer. J Epidemiol and Community Health 38:117–121.

OLSEN J, SABREO S, FASTING U. 1985. Interaction of alcohol and tobacco as risk factors in cancer of the laryngeal region. J Epidemiol Community Health 39:165–168.

ONO I. 1982. Mass screening for laryngeal cancer. Second Report: Incidence of Laryngeal Cancer in High Risk Groups. Nippon Jibiinkoka Gakkai Kaiho 85(11):1494–1497.

OSBORN GR, SUNDERMAN J. 1971. Laryngeal cytology: histological basis and clinical applications. Med J Aust 2:756–762.

PARKIN DM, MUIR CS, WHELAN SL, GAO WY, FERLAY J, POWELL J (EDS). 1992. Cancer Incidence in Five Continents, Vol. VI. Lyon: International Agency for Research on Cancer (IARC Scientific Publication No. 120).

PARTANEN T, KAUPPINEN T, et al. 1990. Formaldehyde exposure and respiratory cancer among woodworkers—an update. Scand J Work Environ Health 16:394–400.

PEDERSON E, HOGETVEIT AC, ANDERSON A. 1973. Cancer of respiratory organs at a nickel refinery in Norway. Int J Cancer 12:32–41.

PETERSON GR, MILHAM S, JR. 1980. Occupational mortality in the State of California 1959–61. NIOSH Research Report DHEW (NIOSH) Publ. No. 80-104.

PINTOS J, FRANCO EL, et al. 1994. Maté, coffee, and tea consumption and risk of cancers of the upper aerodigestive tract in Southern Brazil. Epidemiology 5:583–590.

QUICK CA, FARAS A, KRZYSEK R. 1978. The etiology of laryngeal papillomatosis. Laryngoscope 88(11):1789–1795.

QUINEY RE, HALL D, CROFT B. 1989. Laryngeal papillomatosis: analysis of 113 patients. Clin Otolaryngol 14:217–225.

RAMADAN MF, MORTON RP, STELL PM, et al. 1982. Epidemiology of laryngeal cancer. Clin Otolaryngol 7(6):417–428.

ROACH M III, ALEXANDER M, COLEMAN JL. 1992. The prognostic significance of race and survival from laryngeal carcinoma. J Natl Med Assoc 84(8):668–674.

ROBBINS KT. 1988. Prognostic and therapeutic implications of gender and menopausal status in laryngeal cancer. J Otolaryngol 17(2):81–85.

RONTAL E, RONTAL M, TOLNICK MI. 1975. Objective evaluation of vocal pathology using voice spectrography. Ann Otol 84:662–671.

ROTHMAN KJ, CANN CI, FLANDERS D, et al. 1980. Epidemiology of laryngeal cancer. Epidemiol Rev 2:195–209.

ROTHMAN KJ, CANN CI, FRIED MP. 1989. Carcinogenicity of dark liquor. Am J Public Health 79(11):1516–1520.

SANCHO-GARNIER H, THEOBALD S. 1993. Black (air-cured) and blond (flue-cured) tobacco and cancer risk II: pharynx and larynx cancer. Eur J Cancer 29A(2):273–276.

SCHANTZ SP, SPITZ MR, HSU TC. 1990. Mutagen sensitivity in patients with head and neck cancers: A biologic marker for risk of multiple primary malignancies. J Natl Cancer Inst 82(22):1773–1775.

SCHOTTENFELD D, GANTT RC, WYNDER EL. 1974. The role of alcohol and tobacco in multiple primary cancers of the upper digestive system, larynx and lung: a prospective study. Prev Med 3:277–293.

SCHOTTENFELD D. 1979. Alcohol as a co-factor in the etiology of cancer. Cancer 43:1962–1966.

SCHOTTENFELD D. 1991. Etiology and prevention of aerodigestive tract cancers. In Newell GR, Hong WK (eds): Biology and Prevention of Aerodigestive Cancers. New York: Plenum Publ. Co. pp 1–19.

SEER. 1992. Public Use Tape, September.

SEER. 1993. Public Use Tape, January.

SEGNAN N, TANTURRI G. 1976. Study of the geographical pathology of laryngeal, bladder and childhood tumors in the Province of Turin. Tumori 62:377–385.

SELDGARD J, PETO RW, MARKOWITZ MM, ROUSH G, MILLER DG, BEATTIE EJ. 1990. Isoenzymes of glutathione transferase (class μ) as a marker for the susceptibility to lung cancer: a follow-up study. Carcinogenesis (Lond.), 11:33–36.

SHETTIGARA PT, MORGAN RW. 1975. Asbestos, smoking and laryngeal carcinoma. Arch Environ Health 30:517–519.

SILVESTRI F, BUSSANI R, et al. 1992. Supraglottic versus glottic laryngeal cancer: epidermiological and pathological aspects. ORL 54:43–48.

SMITH AH, HANDLEY MA, WOOD R. 1990. Epidemiological evidence indicates asbestos causes laryngeal cancer. J Occup Med 32(6):499–507.

SOKIC SI, ADANJA BJ, MARINKOVIC JP, et al. 1994. Case-control study of risk factors in laryngeal cancer. Neoplasma 41(1):43–47.

SOKOLOWSKI Z, WOSYCZYK J. 1980. Relative incidence of laryngeal carcinoma and ABO blood groups. Wiad Lek 33(23):1869–1873.

SOSKOLNE CL, ZEIGHAMI EA, HANIS NM, et al. 1984. Laryngeal cancer and occupational exposure to sulfuric acid. Am J Epidemiol 120(3):358–369.

SPEISSL B, BEAHRS OH, HERMANEK P, et al. (eds.) 1989. TNM Atlas: Illustrated guide to the TNM/pTNM Classification of Malignant Tumors, 3rd Ed. New York: Springer-Verlag.

SPINELLI JJ, GALLAGHER RP, BAND PR, et al. 1990. Occupational associations among British Columbia male cancer patients. Canadian Journal of Public Health. Revue Canadian de Sante Publique. 81:254–258.

SPITZ MR, FUEGER JJ, GEOPFERT H, et al. 1988. Squamous cell carcinoma of the upper aerodigestive tract: a case comparison analysis. Cancer 61:203–280.

SPITZ MR, SIDER JG, et al. 1992. Association between malignancies of the upper aerodigestive tract and uterine cervix. Head Neck 14:347–351.

STEENLAND K, SCHNORR T, BEAUMONT J, et al. 1988. Incidence of laryngeal cancer and exposure to acid mists. Br J Ind Med 45:766–776.

STEINBERG BM, TOPP WC, SCHNEIDER PS, et al. 1983. Laryngeal papillomavirus infection during clinical remission. N Engl J Med 308:1261–1264.

STEINBERG BM, GALLAGHER T, STOLER M, et al. 1988. Persistence and expression of human papillomavirus during interferon therapy. Arch Otolaryngol 114:27–32.

STELL PM. 1972. Smoking and laryngeal cancer. Lancet i:617–618.

STELL PM, MCGILL T. 1973. Asbestos and laryngeal cancer. Lancet ii:416–417.

STELL PM. 1975. The first laryngectomy. J Laryngol Otol 89:353–358.

STEPHENSON WT, BARNES DE, HOLMES FF, et al. 1991. Gender influences subsite of origin of laryngeal carcinoma. Arch Otolaryngol Head Neck Surg 117:774–778.

TARPLEY JL, CHRETIEN P, ROGENTINE GH, JR. 1975. Histocompatibility antigens and solid malignant neoplasms. Arch Surg 110:269–271.

TERRY RM, LEWIS GA, et al. 1987. Demonstration of human papillomavirus types 6 and 11 in juvenile laryngeal papillomatosis by insity DNA probes. J Pathol 153:245–248.

THOMAS DB. 1985. Sinonasal, nasopharyngeal, oral, pharyngeal, laryngeal and esophageal cancers: epidemiology opportunities for primary prevention. In Chretien PB, Johns ME, Shedd DP, et al. (eds.): Head and Neck Cancer. Philadelphia/Toronto: B.C. Decker Inc., pp. 585–591.

TRELL E, KOSGAARD R, HOOD B, et al. 1976. Letter: Aryl hydrocarbon hydroxylase inducibility and laryngeal carcinomas. Lancet ii:140.

TRELL E, MATTIASSON I, KITZING P, et al. 1980. Smoking, arylhydrocarbon hydroxylase inducibility and laryngeal precancerous lesions. IRCS Med Sci. Cancer 8(5):339.

TUYNS AJ, AUDIGIER JC. 1976. Double wave cohort increase for oesophageal and laryngeal cancer in France in relation to reduced alcohol consumption during the second world war. Digestion 14(3):197–208.

TUYNS AJ, ESTEVE J, RIBOLI E, et al. 1984. Laryngeal and pharyngal cancer in south-western Europe: IARC Annual Report. Lyon: International Agency for Research on Cancer, pp. 66–68.

TUYNS AJ, ESTEVE J, RAYMOND L, et al. 1988. Cancer of the larynx/hypopharynx, tobacco and alcohol: IARC international case-control study in Turin and Varese (Italy), Zaragosa and Navarra (Spain), Geneva (Switzerland) and Calvados (France). Int J Cancer 41:483–491.

TUYNS AJ. 1990. Alcohol-related cancers in Mediterranean countries. Tumori 76:315–320.

U.S. DEPARTMENT OF HEALTH AND HUMAN SERVICES, SEER PROGRAM. 1984. Cancer incidence and mortality in the United States, 1973–1981. Bethesda, MD: NIH Publ. No. 85-1837.

U.S. DEPARTMENT OF HEALTH AND HUMAN SERVICES, NATIONAL INSTITUTES OF HEALTH. 1986a. Cancer among blacks and other minorities: statistical profiles. Bethesda, MD: NIH Publ. No. 86-2785.

U.S. DEPARTMENT OF HEALTH AND HUMAN SERVICES, NATIONAL INSTITUTES OF HEALTH. 1986b. Forty-five years of cancer incidence in Connecticut 1935-79. Bethesda, MD: NCI Monograph 70.

VAUGHAN TL, DAVIS S. 1991. Wood dust exposure and squamous cell cancers of the upper respiratory tract. Am J Epidemiol 133:560–564.

WADA S, MIYA NISHI M, NISHIMOTO Y, et al. 1968. Mustard gas as a cause of respiratory neoplasia in a man. Lancet 1:1161–1163.

WALDRON HA. 1975. The carcinogenicity of oil mist. Br J Cancer 32:256–257.

WARD PH, HANSON DG. 1988. Reflux as an etiological factor of carcinoma of the laryngopharynx. Laryngoscope 98:1195–1199.

WATERHOUSE J, MUIR C, SHANMUGARTANAM K, POWELL J (EDS). 1982. Cancer Incidence in Five Continents, Volume IV. Lyon: International Agency for Research on Cancer (IARC Scientific Publication No. 42).

WEIR NF. 1973. Theodore Billroth. The first laryngectomy for cancer. J Laryngol Otol 87:1161–1169.

WEISS JF, CHRETIEN PB. 1985. Interrelationship of immune response, circulating proteins, and etiologic factors for head and neck cancer. In Chretien PB, Johns ME, Shedd DP, et al. (eds.): Head and Neck Cancer, Vol. 1. Philadelphia/Toronto: B.C. Decker Inc., pp. 559–563.

WILLIAMSON AL, JASKIESICZ K, GUNNING A. 1991. Anticancer Res II 263–266.

WORTLEY P, VAUGHAN TL, DAVIS S, MORGAN MS, THOMAS DB. 1992. A case-control study of occupational factors for laryngeal cancer. Br J Ind Med 49:837–844.

WRIGHT RG, MURTHY DP, ET AL. 1990. Comparative in situ hybridisation study of juvenile laryngeal papillomatosis, in Papua, New Guinea and Australia. J Clin Pathol 43:1023–1025.

WYNDER EL, BROSS IJ, DAY E. 1956. Epidemiological approach to etiology of cancer of the larynx. JAMA 160:1384–1391.

WYNDER EL, COVEY LS, MARUCHI K, et al. 1976. Environmental factors in cancer of the larynx: a second look. Cancer 38:1591–1601.

WYNDER EL, STELLMAN SD. 1977. Comparative epidemiology of tobacco-related cancers. Cancer Res 37:4608–4622.

WYNDER EL, FUJITA Y, HARRIS RE, et al. 1991. Comparative epidemiology of cancer between the United States and Japan: A second look. Cancer 67:746–763.

YANG PC, THOMAS DB, DALING JR, et al. 1989. Differences in the sex ratio of laryngeal cancer incidence rates by anatomic subsite. J Clin Epidemiol 42:755–758.

ZAGRANISKI RT, KELSEY JL, WALTER SD. 1986. Occupational risk factors for laryngeal carcinoma: Connecticut, 1975–1980. Am J Epidemiol 124(1):67–76.

ZATONSKI W, BECKER H, LISSOWSKA J. 1990. Smoking cessation: Intermediate non-smoking periods and reduction of laryngeal cancer risk. J Natl Cancer Inst 82:1427–1428.

ZEMLA B, DAY N, et al. 1987. Larynx cancer risk factors. Neoplasma 34(2)223–233.

ZHENG W, BLOT WJ, XIAO-OU S, et al. 1992. Diet and other risk factors for laryngeal cancer in Shanghai, China. Am J Epidemiol 136:178–191.

31 Cancers of the lung and pleura

WILLIAM J. BLOT
JOSEPH F. FRAUMENI, JR.

This chapter provides an update of the epidemiology of lung and pleural cancer (Fraumeni and Blot, 1982), with emphasis on recent research into the distribution and causes of these cancers. Highlighted are their changing patterns of occurrence and clarification of the effects associated with active and passive smoking, indoor radon and other pollutants, occupational hazards, and dietary factors. Also reviewed are markers of host susceptibility and means of prevention of these cancers.

LUNG CANCER

Demographic Factors

Geographic Variation. Lung cancer continues to be the leading cause of cancer death in most countries (Kurihara et al, 1989). In several areas, the annual age-adjusted (world standard) incidence rates among males exceed 100 per 100,000 (Table 31–1), some of the highest reported for any malignancy (Parkin et al, 1992). The international variations are striking. Especially low rates (<6 per 100,000) have been reported among Fiji islanders, even though many smoke cigarettes (Henderson et al, 1985), while the highest rates are now reported among urban American black men.

Geographic variation has also been described by cancer mapping within countries, although differences are usually less striking than between nations. The first cancer maps from the United States showed elevated rates in the 1950s and 1960s in urban areas of the north and in southern coastal counties (Mason et al, 1975). As shown in Figure 31–1, lung cancer mortality rates among males in the 1980s were higher in southern rural areas than in northern cities, largely reflecting changes in smoking practices: by the mid-1980s the prevalence of smoking was higher in the south than in any other region of the country (Marcus et al, 1989). High rates of lung cancer in the 1960s and 1970s were seen in areas along the Atlantic and Gulf coasts in the United States, at least partly due to shipyard exposures to asbestos, particularly during World War II (Blot et al, 1978, 1980). Similar patterns have been described in Japan and Poland (Minowa et al, 1988; Zatonski and Becker, 1988). In most parts of the world, rates are higher in urban than rural areas, with smoking being more responsible than air pollution for the urban excess (Doll and Peto, 1981).

Gender and Age. Throughout the world the incidence of lung cancer among men exceeds, usually by 2-fold or more, that among women, among whom annual age-adjusted rates are generally below 40 per 100,000 population. The sex difference, primarily due to a lower prevalence of smoking by females than males, is shrinking, however, as gender differences in cigarette consumption have become less pronounced. The male/female ratio is lowest in parts of China, where some of the world's highest rates of female lung cancer, especially adenocarcinoma, occur (Gao et al, 1987; Mumford et al, 1987). Rates of lung cancer rise progressively with age until the oldest age groups (Fig. 31–2). The plateau and fall after age 80 in men and age 70 in women is mostly attributable to lower smoking prevalences in earlier-born cohorts.

Time Trends. Incidence and mortality rates for lung cancer have risen dramatically since the turn of the century. Figure 31–3 shows trends in age-adjusted lung cancer mortality in the United States during the period 1950–1989 according to sex and race. The rates have risen in all four groups, particularly among females and among black males, whose death rates surpassed those for white males in the late 1960s. However, the upward trend has slowed and the end of the epidemic appears near in several countries, including the United States. Figure 31–4 shows trends in age-specific mortality among white males in the United States by cohort year of birth (Devesa et al, 1989). Rates at ages above 55 rose throughout the 35-year period, although the curves have begun to flatten. At ages below 55 there have been actual declines in lung cancer mortality. Indeed, between the mid-1970s and mid-1980s, lung cancer death rates among white males under age 45 declined nearly

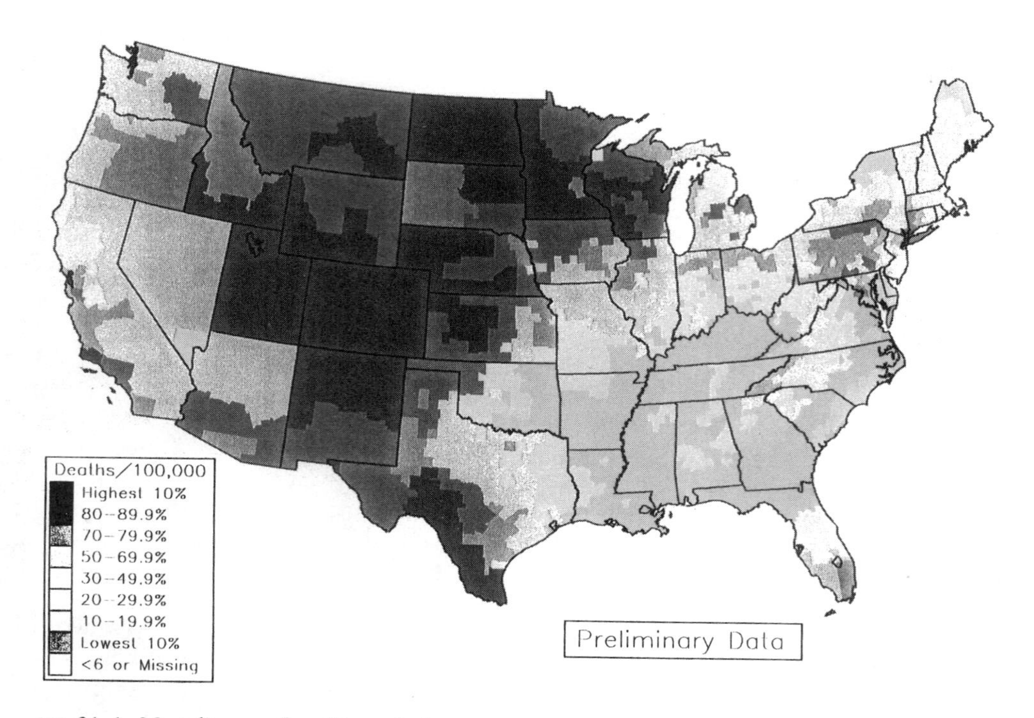

FIG. 31–1. Mortality rates for white males by state economic area, 1980–1989, from cancer of the trachea, bronchus, lung, and pleura.

30%. It the trends continue, rates will begin to decrease at successively older ages, and the overall age-adjusted rates among American men will decline in the 1990s. Among American women, lung cancer mortality also has decreased recently at young ages, although the declines lag behind those for men by about 10 years. Thus, overall rates among females will not level off and drop until after the year 2000 (Brown and Kessler, 1988). These patterns reflect strong cohort effects, with males born during the late 1920s and women born during the late 1930s showing the highest risks of lung cancer. These same cohorts demonstrate the highest prevalence of cigarette smoking (Harris, 1983). Lung cancer mortality is abating in several other countries as well. In-

TABLE 31–1. *Lung Cancer Incidence among Males in Selected Countries, 1980s**

Annual Age-Adjusted Rate (World Standard) per 100,000				
<25	*26–50*	*51–75*	*76–100*	*100+*
Fiji	U.S. (Utah)	Canada	U.S. (South)	U.S. (blacks)
India	U.S. (Hispanic)	U.S. (White)	U.K.	New Zealand (Maori)
Puerto Rico	Israel	France	Netherlands	
Sweden	Japan	Poland		
Norway (rural)	Spain	Finland		
	Ireland	Australia		
		Hong Kong		

*From Cancer Incidence in Five Continents, Vol. VI (Parkin et al, 1992). The time periods covered differed by country, but typically centered about the mid-1980s. Rates are age-adjusted to standard world population.

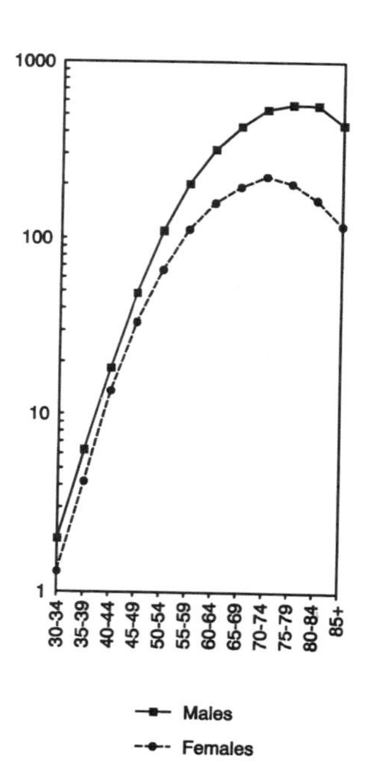

FIG. 31–2. Annual age-specific lung cancer incidence rates in the United States, 1985–1989, by sex.

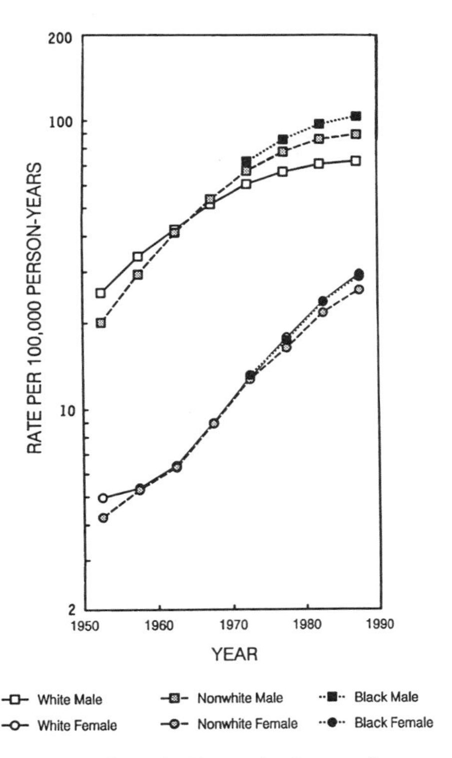

FIG. 31–3. U.S. age-adjusted (70 standard) mortality rates for lung cancer by year of death, 1950–54 to 1985–89.

deed, in England and Wales, Scotland, and Finland, age-adjusted lung cancer mortality rates began to decline in the 1980s (Kurihara et al, 1989).

Socioeconomic and Religious Patterns. An inverse association between lung cancer and socioeconomic status, particularly among males, has been observed in several studies. A 2-fold difference in mortality between low and high social class, as measured primarily by occupation, is seen in British mortality data (Registrar General, 1978), with similar results in other surveys measuring income or education (Fraumeni and Blot, 1982). Smoking habits account for at least part of the socioeconomic differentials, with rates of smoking considerably higher among blue- than white-collar workers and among those with lower levels of education (Novotny et al, 1989; Pierce et al, 1989).

In surveys in New York, Pittsburgh, and Montreal, a 20% to 50% lowered rate of lung cancer was found among Jewish males, although some excess risk has been noted among Jewish females (Horowitz and Enterline, 1970). The deficit in males has been attributed mostly to lower cigarette consumption, but the excess in females remains unexplained. In Israel, incidence among males is low by western standards (Muir et al, 1987), but not among females whose tumors are mostly adenocarcinomas (Modan, 1978). At even lower risk are Mormons and Seventh-Day Adventists, whose religious dictates proscribe the use of tobacco products (Lyon et al, 1976; Phillips et al, 1980).

Ethnicity. Incidence data from the Surveillance, Epidemiology, and End Results (SEER) program of the National Cancer Institute permit a breakdown for several ethnic and racial groups within the United States (Table 31–2). Low rates are seen for some groups, notably Hispanic males, American Indians, and Japanese, related in part to low tobacco consumption. The highest rates are seen in blacks and native Hawaiians. Hispanic American females were once reported to have increased rates for lung cancer, but current data suggest that the excess no longer exists. The lower rates in Hispanic males seem to be due to lower smoking prevalences, since the effects of smoking upon risks of lung cancer appear to be the same in Hispanics and whites (Pathak et al, 1986). Rates for females used to be highest among Chinese (Fraumeni and Mason, 1974), consistent with the high rates of lung adenocarcinoma reported among Chinese females in China and elsewhere in Southeast Asia even though few smoked cigarettes (Gao et al, 1987). Rates among Chinese Americans have now been surpassed by rates among whites and blacks, among whom lung cancer incidence has risen rapidly as a consequence of cigarette smoking.

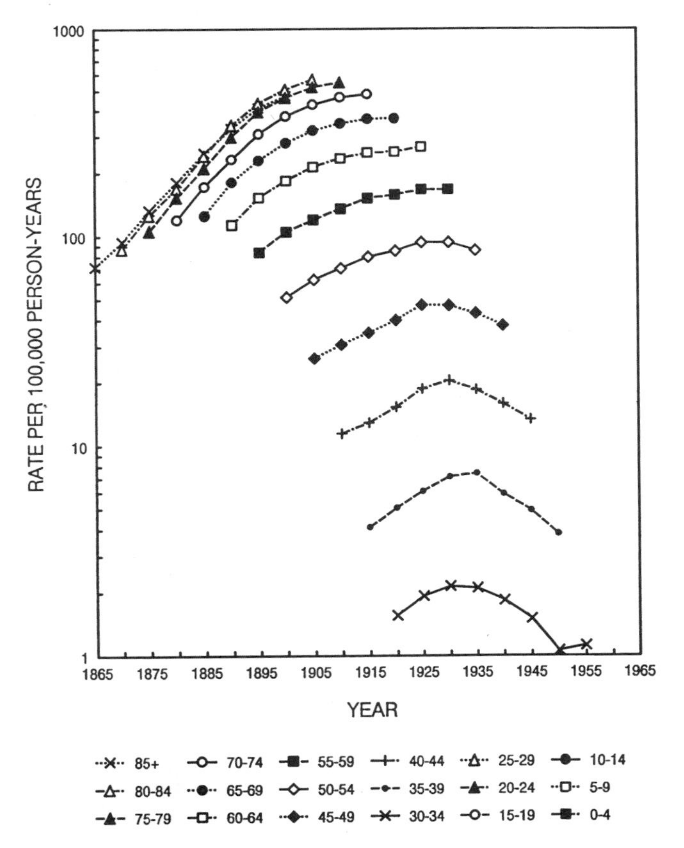

FIG. 31–4. U.S. age-specific mortality rates for white male lung cancer by cohort year of birth: 1865–1965.

TABLE 31–2. *Average Annual Age-Adjusted (1970 U.S. Standard) Lung Cancer Incidence, 1977–83, in SEER Registry Areas and Alaska According to Sex, Racial, and Ethnic Groups*

	Incidence (Cases/yr/100,000)	
Racial or Ethnic Group	*Male*	*Female*
White	80.0	30.8
Hispanic (New Mexico)	33.6	13.7
Black	110.8	28.3
Chinese (San Francisco, Hawaii)	57.4	24.8
Japanese (San Francisco, Hawaii)	45.0	12.6
Hawaiian	97.5	39.2
American Indian (New Mexico)	9.4	3.6
Alaskan Natives	69.7	23.2

Histology. Virtually all lung cancers arise from epithelial tissue. There are several histologic types, the most common being squamous cell carcinomas, adenocarcinomas, and small (oat) cell carcinomas. Squamous and small cell carcinomas are more closely linked to smoking than are adenocarcinomas. Squamous cell carcinomas until recently were by far the most frequent, paricularly among men. In 1973–77 data from the SEER program, there were more than twice as many squamous cell carcinomas than adenocarcinomas among males, whereas adenocarcinomas were slightly more common among females (Young et al, 1981). By the mid–1980s, however, the excess of squamous cell cancer was only about 40% among males, while adenocarcinomas outnumbered squamous cell cancers by about 50% among females (Devesa et al, 1991). The incidence of small cell carcinomas has also risen faster than squamous cell cancer. Cohort analyses suggest that the epidemic rise of squamous cell cancer has already ended, while the increases of adenocarcinoma and small cell cancers have yet to peak. Among the other histologic types, the most frequent is large cell carcinoma. Its rising incidence, with large cell carcinomas now accounting for about 9% of all lung cancers, is probably due in part to improved diagnostic techniques.

Survival. Most people who develop lung cancer succumb to the disease. Five-year relative survival rates have remained low, being 12% for white males and 16% for white females in the latest statistics evaluating survival through the late-1980s among SEER participants (Miller et al, 1993). The corresponding percentages for blacks are slightly lower. Variation in survival by cell type is limited, with the poorest survival (about 5%) for small cell carcinomas. Five-year survival rates reach 46% for localized tumors, but these account for only 16% of all lung cancers (Miller et al, 1993).

Risk Factors

Tobacco. In the 1920s and 1930s, an alarming increase in lung cancer incidence along with clinical observations raised suspicion that smoking might be a causal factor. By the early 1950s, case-control studies in the United States and Great Britain supported the link (Doll and Hill, 1952; Levin et al, 1950; Wynder and Graham, 1950), and the evidence became conclusive through surveys of large cohorts of smokers. In 1964 the first Surgeon General's report on smoking summarized existing evidence and declared cigarette smoking to be the major cause of lung cancer among American men. In the ensuing 30+ years, further evidence has accumulated to clarify the relationship between lung cancer incidence and the timing, duration, intensity, and other characteristics of smoking. Table 31–3 shows relative risks (RR) of lung cancer according to number of cigarettes smoked per day among male current smokers in three of the largest cohort studies: the American Cancer Society (ACS) follow-up over 6 years of nearly one-half million men (Hammond, 1966); the 40-year assessment of mortality among 34,000 British physicians (Doll et al, 1994); and the 26-year follow-up of 290,000 U.S. veterans (McLaughlin et al, 1995). All 3 studies showed a steady rise in lung cancer death rates with increasing amount smoked, so that the risk for smokers of 2 or more packs per day was about 20 times that of nonsmokers.

The first reports of lung cancer and smoking usually concerned men, who in almost all countries began smoking earlier and consumed greater quantities of tobacco than women. When the association was examined by sex, therefore, the relative risks were considerably higher for men. Recently, however, the prevalence of smoking in many countries, including the United States, has increased greatly among females (Harris, 1983; Fiore et al, 1989; Pierce, 1989). As female smoking habits have begun to resemble those of men, so have their

TABLE 31–3. *Relative Risks of Death from Lung Cancer among Male Smokers According to Number of Cigarettes Smoked*

Number of Cigarettes Smoked per Day	*American Cancer Society (ACS) Volunteers*	*United States Veterans*	*British Physicians*
Nonsmokers[a]	1.0	1.0	1.0
Current cigarette smokers[b]	9.2	11.6	14.9
1–9	4.6	3.7	7.5
10–19	8.6	9.9	14.9
20–39	14.7	16.9	25.4
40+	18.8	22.9	

[a]Did not smoke any form of tobacco.

[b]Classification refers to ACS study. The categories for United States veterans were 1–9, 10–20, 21–39, and 40+, and for British physicians were 1–14, 15–24, and 25+ per day. Only current smokers included.

lung cancer risks. In a 4-year follow-up during 1982–86 of approximately 600,000 American women by the ACS, the RR of lung cancer among current smokers was 12.7, with 20-fold excesses for those smoking more than 30 cigarettes per day (Garfinkel and Stellman, 1988). Similarly, in Great Britain, the smoking habits of female doctors born after 1920 were similar to those of their male counterparts, and nearly a 30-fold increase in risk in lung cancer has been observed among women smoking 25 or more cigarettes per day (Doll et al, 1980).

While lung cancer risks have risen sharply with increasing numbers of cigarettes smoked per day, the trends have been reported to be even stronger with duration of smoking. Doll and Peto (1978), using data from the follow-up of British doctors, reported that excess risks of lung cancer rose in proportion to the square of the number of cigarettes smoked per day, but to the 4th or 5th power of the duration of smoking. The interrelationships of intensity (number smoked per day) and duration of smoking on lung cancer risk are complicated, however, and in some mathematical models it has been shown that intensity may be nearly as important as duration of smoking in influencing lung cancer risk (Moolgavkar et al, 1989). In most studies the small numbers of lung cancers among nonsmokers and within various age-intensity-duration categories have made it difficult to separate the effects of intensity vs. duration of smoking. Table 31–4 shows the RRs from a large population-based case-control study of lung cancer in China, with approximately 1,400 lung cancer patients and 1,500 controls. This investigation (Gao et al, 1988) revealed clear independent effects of intensity and duration. Doubling either intensity (from 1–19 to 30+ cigarettes per day) or duration (from 1–29 to 40+ years) approximately quadrupled the risk of lung cancer. Similar results were reported in an even larger multicenter hospital-based case-control study in western Europe (Lubin et al, 1984a).

Epidemiologic investigations have not shown consistent associations between depth of inhalation of tobacco smoke and lung cancer, although risks were higher among moderate/deep vs. none/slight inhalers in the largest cohort (Garfinkel and Stellman, 1988) and case-control studies (Lubin et al, 1984a).

The risk of lung cancer is related to the type of tobacco smoked. The effect of smoking low-tar and nicotine cigarettes is still not well quantified, but reductions in risk for users of filter or low-tar brands have been found in both case-control and cohort studies. In the western European study, lifelong filter cigarette smokers experienced significantly lower risks (40% lower for males, 20% for females) than lifelong nonfilter smokers after adjusting for differing amounts smoked (Lubin et al, 1984a). Qualitatively similar results have been seen in several other case-control studies (Sidney et al, 1993).

TABLE 31–4. *Relative Risks of Lung Cancer among Chinese Men Associated with Intensity and Duration of Cigarette Smoking*[a]

Number of Cigarettes per Day	*Duration of Smoking (years)*		
	1–29	*30–39*	*40+*
1–19	0.9	3.2	3.8
20–29	2.1	7.1	7.2
30+	3.0	10.8	15.4

[a]All risks relative to lifelong nonsmokers. Data from Gao et al (1988).

In the recent ACS cohort (Garfinkel and Stellman, 1988), women who smoked only filters experienced about 70% of the risk of those who smoked mostly nonfilters, as did smokers of cigarettes containing 10 mg compared to 20 mg tar (the median tar intake in the early 1980s declined to about 12 mg). In one hospital-based survey in North America, smokers of "low-tar" (<22 mg) cigarettes had one-fourth the risk of lung cancer than smokers of "high-tar" (>29 mg) cigarettes (Kaufman et al, 1989), while in another population-based case-control study risk was 40% lower among smokers of <14 mg vs. 21–28 mg tar cigarettes (Wilcox et al, 1988). Not all studies have found such tar effects, with little or no reduced risk in one prospective study in the 1980s of smokers in a California health plan, although long-term use of filter cigarettes was linked to lowered risk of lung cancer (Sidney et al, 1993). While these findings suggest that switching from nonfilter to filter, or high- to low-tar, cigarettes may reduce the risk of lung cancer, the greatest reduction in risk comes from cessation of smoking. As shown in Table 31–5, RR steadily decline (compared to continued smoking) with increasing duration from cessation, with risks among long-term ex-smokers approaching those of nonsmokers. It has been suggested that ex-smokers will never completely achieve the low baseline risk of lifelong nonsmokers, always maintaining a nearly constant arithmetic excess (IARC, 1986), although a dwindling excess

TABLE 31–5. *Relative Risks of Lung Cancer According to Years Since Quitting Smoking among Males in Three Cohort Studies of Smokers*[a]

Cohort	*Years Since Quitting Smoking*					
	0	*1–4*	*5–9*	*10–14*	*15–19*	*20+*
British physicians	15.8	16.0	5.9	5.3	2.0	2.0
U.S. veterans	11.3	18.8	7.5	5.0	5.0	2.1
American Cancer Society[b]	13.7	12.0	7.2	1.1	1.1	1.1

[a]All risks relative to lifelong nonsmokers. Data from IARC (1986).
[b]Excludes those who smoked less than one pack of cigarettes per day.

with time since quitting has been noted (Freedman and Navidi, 1990). The percentage reduction in risk after quitting depends on the duration of time smoked, with larger relative decreases in risk among shorter-term and younger smokers (Lubin et al, 1984a; Halpern et al, 1993).

Pipe and cigar smoking are linked to lung cancer, but the risks are smaller than those seen with either filter or nonfilter cigarettes (e.g., RR ~ 2 in the ACS and U.S. veterans studies, and RR ~ 7 among British physicians). It has been suggested that cigarette smoke is less irritating and thus more easily inhaled than pipe or cigar smoke. In one study that classified cigar smokers according to extent of inhalation, those who inhaled deeply experienced nearly 10 times the risk of lung cancer than noninhalers (Lubin et al, 1984b). Furthermore, in some Scandinavian countries where pipe and cigar smoking is nearly as common as cigarette smoking, risks from pipes/cigars have been almost as high as for cigarettes (Carstensen et al, 1987).

Risks of lung cancer may also vary with the type of tobacco used in cigarettes. In Cuba, dark tobaccos have been associated with a somewhat greater risk than light tobaccos (Joly et al, 1983), and in Italy the levels of hemoglobin adducts to the cigarette-smoke carcinogen 4-aminobiphenyl were higher in smokers of black than blond tobaccos (Bryant et al, 1988). Cigarettes manufactured in China were once thought to be less harmful, but recent studies indicate that risks of lung cancer among Chinese smokers are comparable to those in Western societies once the amounts smoked are standardized (Gao et al, 1988). In the United States use of mentholated cigarettes is common, especially among blacks, but risks of lung cancer have been reported to be similar in smokers who did vs. did not use this type of cigarettes (Kabat and Hebert, 1991).

Smoking induces lung cancers of all the major histologic types. The strongest associations are for squamous cell and small cell carcinomas, but dose–response relationships for adenocarcinomas and other cell types have also been reported. Based on the western European study, Table 31–6 presents risk estimates for squamous cell carcinoma, small cell carcinoma, and adenocarcinoma according to amount smoked, with the increases generally 2–4 times greater for squamous cell cancers (Lubin and Blot, 1984).

It has been estimated that in the United States in 1985 cigarette smoking accounted for 90 percent of lung cancer in males and 79% in females (Surgeon General, 1989). The attributable risk for women likely will eventually reach that for men, because of increasing similarities in both the RRs and the prevalences of smoking. Smoking will continue to be the dominant risk factor for lung cancer in the years to come, but its relative importance may decline if recent trends toward reduced

TABLE 31–6. *Relative Risks of Squamous Cell Carcinoma, Small Cell Carcinoma, and Adenocarcinoma of the Lung According to Intensity of Cigarette Smoking*

Sex	*Number Cigarettes Smoked per Day*	*Squamous Cell Carcinoma*	*Small Cell Carcinoma*	*Adenocarcinoma*
Males	Nonsmoker	1.0	1.0	1.0
	1–9	8.1	3.1	1.4
	10–19	12.2	5.6	2.7
	20–29	17.0	7.8	3.5
	30+	25.1	9.9	4.9
Females	Nonsmoker	1.0	1.0	1.0
	1–9	2.8	2.3	1.0
	10–19	6.7	5.5	2.0
	20–29	14.8	14.9	1.1
	30+	11.8	12.9	2.3

[a]Adapted from Lubin and Blot (1984).

cigarette consumption are maintained (Devesa et al, 1989; Wynder 1989; Pierce 1989). Although the evidence that smoking causes lung cancer is indisputable, more remains to be learned about the changing risk of various diseases following alterations in smoking habits and product modification, and the extent to which smoking interacts with other environmental and host determinants of lung cancer.

Passive Smoking. In 1981 two nearly simultaneous publications indicated that lung cancer risks were increased among nonsmoking women married to smokers (Hirayama, 1981; Trichopoulos et al, 1981). Since then nearly 30 epidemiologic studies have evaluated passive smoking as a risk factor, with the consensus of data from around the world indicating that risk of lung cancer was elevated by about 30% among female nonsmokers whose husbands smoked (Surgeon General, 1986; National Research Council, 1980; Environmental Protection Agency, 1992). Table 31–7 lists the RRs from several studies around the world which evaluated dose–response trends. Typically, risks rose with amounts smoked by the husbands, with about a 70% excess on average among those most heavily exposed. Although it is not clear that passive smoking is entirely responsible for these associations, an etiologic role is likely since environmental tobacco smoke contains various mutagens, carcinogens, and other toxic agents, sometimes in higher concentrations (e.g., nitrosamines) than in inhaled mainstream smoke (Table 31–8). Furthermore, elevated levels of cotinine, the major metabolite of nicotine, have been consistently detected in body fluids of passive smokers (Surgeon General, 1986; National Research Council, 1986; Riboli et al, 1990; Environmental Protection Agency, 1992). Hemoglobin ad-

TABLE 31–7. *Relative Risks of Lung Cancer among Nonsmoking Women from Epidemiologic Studies Evaluating Trends in Risk According to Level of Husband's Smoking*

Reference	Number of Lung Cancers	Husband's Smoking Status		
		Nonsmoker	Light	Heavy[a]
Hirayama, 1981	201	1.0	1.4	1.9
Trichopolous et al, 1983, 1984	77	1.0	1.9	2.5
Garfinkel, 1981	153	1.0	1.3	1.1
Correa et al, 1983	22	1.0	1.2	3.5
Koo et al, 1984	88	1.0	1.9	1.2
Wu et al, 1985	28	1.0	1.2	2.0
Garfinkel et al, 1985	134	1.0	1.1	2.0
Akiba et al, 1986	94	1.0	1.4	2.1
Pershagen et al, 1987	67	1.0	1.0	3.2
Lam et al, 1987	199	1.0	1.9	2.1
Gao et al, 1987	406	1.0	1.2	1.7
Janerich et al, 1990	191	1.0	0.8	1.1
Brownson et al, 1992	432	1.0	0.9	1.3
Stockwell et al, 1992	210	1.0	1.5	2.4
Fontham et al, 1994	653	1.0	1.1	1.8

[a]Definitions of heavy smokers vary by study, but typically include those who smoked ≥20 cigarettes per day.

ducts of 4-aminobiphenyl, a carcinogen in tobacco smoke, have been detected in passive smokers, including fetuses whose mothers smoked (MacLure et al, 1989; Coghlin et al, 1991; Hammond et al, 1993). Comparison of cotinine concentrations suggests that passive smokers may smoke the equivalent of about one-half cigarette a day, although this figure is not precise (estimates usually range from 0.1 to 1.0, occasionally up to 3). Direct estimates of risk associated with this low level of smoking are unavailable, but linear interpolation between the nearly 5-fold excess risk among smokers of 1–9 cigarettes per day and the baseline risk of 1.0 among all nonsmokers (Table 31–2) predicts increased risks among passive smokers resembling those actually observed. Public awareness of the potential harmful effect of environmental tobacco smoke has already led to expanding restrictions on smoking in public places and at work, and should facilitate reductions in the prevalence of smoking as the attitudes and motivations of current and potential smokers change.

TABLE 31–8. *Selected Constituents of Tobacco Smoke and Their Approximate Ratio in Sidestream to Mainstream Smoke*

Constituent	Ratio in Sidestream to Mainstream Smoke
VAPOR PHASE	
Benzene	5–10
1,3-Butadiene	3–6
Carbon monoxide	2–5
Formaldehyde	0.1–50
Hydrogen cyanide	0.1–0.25
N-nitrosodimethylamine	20–100
PARTICULATE PHASE	
4-Aminobiphenyl	30
Benzo(a)pyrene	2–4
Cadmium	7
NNK	1–4

[a]From Environmental Protection Agency, 1992.

Occupational Factors. *Arsenic.* Although experimentalists have not succeeded in producing tumors in laboratory animals with arsenic, there is little question that occupational lung cancer may result from inorganic arsenic compounds (Blot and Fraumeni, 1994). Hill and Fanning (1948) reported a relative excess of deaths from lung and skin cancers among heavily exposed workers involved in the manufacture of sheep dip containing inorganic arsenicals. Lee and Fraumeni (1969) found a 3-fold increase in mortality from lung cancer among 8,047 copper smelter workers in the United States. Updated follow-up showed that the excess persisted into the 1970s, with a 4-fold gradient in risk according to estimated level of arsenic exposure (Lubin et al, 1981; Lee-Feldstein, 1986). Similar dose-response relationships have been observed at other copper smelters in the United States, Japan, and Sweden (Enterline et al, 1987; Jarup et al, 1989), with an even stronger effect reported among arsenic-exposed tin miners in China (Taylor et al, 1989). Examination of risks according to the timing of exposure suggests that arsenic may be primarily a late-stage promoting agent (Brown and Chu, 1983). Although few studies have evaluated the smoking habits of smelter workers, limited data suggest that the two exposures exert independent additive, or between additive and multiplicative, effects (Welsch et al, 1982; Pershagen et al, 1981; Taylor et al, 1989; Jarup and Pershagen, 1991). The risk of lung cancer is elevated also among vineyard workers in Germany and France who were heavily exposed to arsenical insecticides, and among American workers who handled arsenic in the manufacture of pesticides and herbicides (Mabuchi et al, 1980; Ott et al, 1974). Elevated mortality from lung cancer has been described in some mining groups heavily exposed to arsenic, notably Rhodesian gold miners (Osburn, 1969). Thus, despite the negative results from experimental studies, the epidemiologic evidence from several occupational settings indicates that inhaled arsenicals are carcinogenic to the lung. Inorganic arsenic also has the capacity to induce characteristic dermatologic changes, including skin cancer, when ingested in the form of drugs (Fowler's solution) or contaminated drinking water (Cuzik et al, 1992; Chen et al, 1986). In Taiwan, excess risks of lung and urinary cancer have been linked to long-term consumption of arsenic-contaminated well water (Chen et al, 1986), but no increased risks of lung cancer have been reported in a follow-up of British patients treated with medicinal arsenic solutions (Cuzik et al, 1992).

Asbestos. Over the past 40 years epidemiologic evidence has accumulated indicating that the risk of lung cancer, mesothelioma, and asbestosis is increased in various asbestos industries, including miners, millers, textile, gas mask, friction product, insulation, shipyard, and cement workers (McDonald and McDonald, 1987). Asbestos was first quantitatively associated with lung cancer risk among British textile workers in the 1950s: 11 cases were observed among men who had worked at least 20 years vs. 0.8 expected based on natural rates—all 11 had preexisting asbestosis (Doll, 1955). Since then, lung cancer has become recognized as an asbestos-related disease, resulting in about 20% of all deaths in some exposed cohorts with the highest intensity and duration of exposure (Selikoff et al, 1979; Newhouse et al, 1985). In a review of 47 cohort studies of male asbestos-exposed workers, Morgan (1992) noted that mortality from lung cancer was increased in 40. The overall weighted-average SMR for these cohorts, among whom over 4,000 lung cancer deaths were reported, was 1.65. Most were studies of heavily exposed long-term workers, but the length of exposure required to induce lung cancer is not necessarily long, as indicated by the doubling of risk 20 years after working for less than 9 months in a U.S. amosite factor (Seidman et al, 1979), and by the 60% excess risk among American men who worked temporarily in shipyards during World War II (Blot et al, 1978; Blot and Fraumeni, 1981). Because of its carcinogenic potential and widespread distribution in many industries, asbestos is the agent generally considered to have posed the largest carcinogenic threat in the workplace, although uncertainties about the extent of exposure hinder estimation of the numbers of asbestos-related lung cancers in the United States or abroad (Walker et al, 1983).

Occupational exposures are usually to mixed forms of asbestos, so that distinguishing effects of fiber types (amosite, anthophyllite, chrysotile, crocidolite) is difficult. All types seem capable of inducing cancer in experimental animals (Doll and Peto, 1985). Chrysotile, the most common type of commercial asbestos, however, is reported to be much less hazardous than other types (McDonald and McDonald, 1987; Mossman et al, 1990). Risks of lung cancer among chrysotile-exposed workers, including miners and millers in Canada, are increased only about 20% (Hughes and Weill, 1994), and no excess of lung cancer was detected up to 47 years following exposure to generally controlled levels of chrysotile asbestos in one group of British workers manufacturing friction materials (Newhouse and Sullivan, 1989). However, lung cancer has been linked to chrysotile in some other groups, including textile workers in South Carolina (Sebastian et al, 1989). In contrast, risks of lung cancer are increased more than 2-fold in insulation and several other workers exposed to amphibole fibers (Hughes and Weill, 1994).

Asbestos-induced lung cancer is generally characterized by a latent period of 15 to 20 years or longer between start of exposure and onset of the disease. In a mortality follow-up of 17,800 U.S. and Canadian asbestos insulation workers, there was a 2-fold increase of lung cancer during the period 10 to 14 years after initial employment, reaching nearly 6-fold 30 to 34 years after employment, and declining at longer intervals (Selikoff et al, 1979). Risk rises as amount of exposure to asbestos increases, but whether the dose-response relationship is linear, exponential, or some other form is difficult to ascertain epidemiologically because of the absence of detailed or precise exposure data. Whereas duration of employment typically was known in most studies, level or intensity of asbestos exposure generally was not. In 9 cohorts, however, amount of exposure could be classified in asbestos concentration-years. Assuming a linear dose-response yields an increase in the relative risk of lung cancer ranging from .0003 to .01 per fiber/ml-year, reflecting the wide variability across studies and the concomitant uncertainty in risk assessment (Hughes and Weill, 1994).

A characteristic of asbestos-related lung cancer is its synergistic relation with cigarette smoking. In a combined analysis of 6 occupational groups, increased risks were found among asbestos-exposed workers who did not smoke, while among smokers asbestos was shown to interact with smoking in a more-than-additive, and probably multiplicative, fashion (Berry et al, 1985; Saracci, 1987). Small numbers of lung cancers among nonsmokers, however, result in imprecise estimation of the magnitude of the risk among nonsmokers. Because the bulk of the excess lung cancer results from the combined effect of smoking and asbestos, programs aimed at smoking cessation would significantly lower the occupational risk.

Besides its enhancement of the effect of cigarette smoking, the mechanisms by which asbestos induces lung cancer are not clear. Relative risk of lung cancer appears to fall following cessation of exposure (Seidman and Selikoff, 1990; Sanden et al, 1992), suggesting that asbestos may affect later stages of the carcinogenic process. The decline is a hopeful sign for the future, since occupational exposures to asbestos generally were curtailed by the 1970s. The lower risk associated with chrysotile seems consistent with its reported easier clearance from the lung, whereas the longer, straighter amphiboles appear to have greater penetration and lung retention times (Wagner et al, 1988). A primary role of asbestos's fibrogenic action is supported by observations in a number of occupational groups, including U.S. and Canadian insulation workers, that lung cancers developed mainly (in some groups, only) in those with asbestosis (Kipen et al, 1987; Sluis-Cremer and Bezuidenhout, 1989; Hughes and Weill, 1991). A fibrogenesis-carcinogenesis link is plausible, especially since asbestos is not a mutagen, and its carcinogenicity is closely related to its physical dimensions—long thin fibers being the most hazardous (Davis, 1986; Barrett et al, 1989; Browne, 1991). The link to fibrogenesis has implications regarding dose-response trends, because asbestosis is generally thought to occur only following sufficiently high levels of asbestos exposure (perhaps 25 fibers/cc-years) (Doll and Peto, 1985). Thus, if asbestos-induced lung cancer occurs primarily or only among those with asbestosis, then it too occurs primarily or only when exposures are above a minimal level. The asbestos-related tumors tend to arise more often peripherally and in the lower lobes, but all histologic types of lung cancer seem to be affected.

An increased risk of respiratory cancer has recently been reported among large cohorts of American and European workers handling man-made mineral fibers (Enterline, 1990; Boffetta et al, 1992). The 30%–40% excess 20 years after initial exposure was most prominent among those who produced fibrous wool from rock or slag. Some of the 40,000 man-made mineral fiber workers in these studies may have also been exposed to asbestos, polycyclic hydrocarbons, or arsenic, so the extent of the effect due to man-made fibers per se is not clear (IARC, 1988a). Experimental studies have reported mixed results, although several have found increased risks of lung tumors (and mesotheliomas) among exposed rats and hamsters (Infante et al, 1994).

Chloromethyl Ethers. One of the few carcinogens detected in laboratory animals before human studies is bis(chloromethyl)ether (BCME). Following positive bioassay reports of this haloether in the late 1960s, a high risk of lung cancer was reported among American, Japanese, German, and French chemical workers exposed to BCME and chloromethyl methyl ether (CMME) during the manufacture of ion exchange resins (Pasternack et al, 1977; Gowers et al, 1993). The tumors were primarily small cell anaplastic carcinomas. Dose-response relationships were evident, with a high proportion of tumors in young men and nonsmokers (Weiss, 1980; Collingwood et al, 1987). Risk appears to decrease following cessation of exposure, suggesting that the chemical may affect late as well as early stages of carcinogenesis. It is not possible to distinguish on epidemiologic grounds between the effects of CMME and BCME. Commercial-grade CMME is nearly always contaminated by BCME, which is highly carcinogenic in rodents by inhalation, skin application, or subcutaneous injection. The carcinogenicity of commercial-grade CMME is of a lower order of magnitude (Laskin et al, 1975).

Chromium. Since the initial observation in 1948 of an elevated risk of lung cancer in the U.S. chromate-producing industry (Machle and Gregorius, 1948), several studies have reported similar results. In the largest study, Alderson et al (1981) reported 116 deaths from respiratory cancer in a follow-up survey of British chromate workers, 2.4 times that expected from national death rates. Elevated risks have been observed also among U.S., Japanese, German, and Italian chromate workers, chrome pigment industry workers, chromium platers, and workers producing ferrochromium alloys (Langard, 1990; IARC, 1990). In a review of 19 published reports of lung cancer among workers occupationally exposed to chromates, increased SMRs were found in all (Coultas, 1994). Although it is not entirely clear which chromium compounds are carcinogenic in humans, both epidemiologic and experimental data implicate the hexavalent but not trivalent forms.

Mustard Gas. Wada et al (1968) summarized the cancer mortality experience of Japanese workers in a factory that manufactured mustard gas in the period 1929–45. There were 33 deaths after 1950 from respiratory tract cancer, compared to 0.9 expected. Tumors tended to develop centrally along the upper respiratory tract and major bronchus, and were squamous or undifferentiated carcinomas. An excess of lung cancer was also reported among factory workers in Germany and in England (IARC, 1987a; Easton et al, 1988). In the British study, the relative excesses in a follow-up until 1984 of World War II mustard gas workers were greater for oral, pharyngeal, and laryngeal cancers, but nevertheless 200 lung cancers were observed vs. 138 expected. The findings are consistent with the capacity of mustard gas to produce lung tumors in laboratory animals (IARC, 1987a). Sporadic military exposures during World War I were apparently insufficient to raise the incidence of lung cancer (Norman, 1975).

Nickel Refining. In 1958, epidemiologic studies documented an excess risk of lung and nasal sinus cancers among workers in a nickel refinery in South Wales. In an updated follow-up of 967 workers at that refinery, Doll et al (1977) found that the increased risk was limited to men employed before 1930, indicating that changes in the refining process have eliminated the hazard. Studies of refinery workers in other countries, notably Norway and Canada, confirmed that the risk was confined to the earliest stage of refining involving heavy exposure to dust from relatively crude ore (IARC, 1990). The hazard was in operations such as smelting, roasting, and electrolysis, involving especially the calcination of impure nickel sulfide. In some nickel refineries, the high levels of PAHs, arsenic, or other agents may have influenced cancer risk. The view that nickel in some form is responsible is consistent with animal studies indicating that certain nickel compounds can produce local sarcomas by injection and pulmonary tumors by inhalation and intratracheal instillation (IARC, 1990). In a recent combination of data from 10 cohort studies, it was concluded that several forms of nickel may contribute to occupational lung cancer, with the evidence strongest for oxidic, sulfitic, and soluble nickel, but not metallic nickel in nonrefining processes (Doll, 1990).

Polycyclic Hydrocarbons. An elevated risk of lung cancer has been reported in several occupational groups heavily exposed to polycyclic aromatic hydrocarbons (PAHs) (IARC, 1983). Early results came from Great Britain (Doll et al, 1972), where coal carbonization products were implicated in the high rates of lung cancer among gas workers. In the United States, Lloyd (1971) reported the mortality experience of 58,828 steelworkers, and found that men in the coke plant had a risk of lung cancer $2\frac{1}{2}$ times greater than other steelworkers. The excess mortality was mainly among men working at coke ovens, reaching 10-fold among those employed 5 or more years at the top of the ovens. Further analyses indicated that the risks rise in proportion to estimated cumulative exposure to coke oven emissions (Redmond, 1983). Modeling taking into account age, duration, and intensity of exposure yields predictions that the lifetime probability of developing lung cancer among the most heavily exposed coke oven workers could reach 40% (Dong et al, 1988). PAHs seem responsible for at least part of the excess risk of lung cancer, especially since benzo(a)pyrene-DNA adducts, markers of biologically effective PAH doses that correlate with exposure measurements, have been detected in blood samples of coke oven workers in the United States (Harris et al, 1985) and foundry workers in Finland (Perera et al, 1988). A case-control study in eastern Pennsylvania found an 80% smoking-adjusted increased risk of lung cancer among long-term (15+ years) steelworkers, only a few of whom were coke oven workers, suggesting that PAHs or other exposures across the steel industry may be associated with increased risk (Blot et al, 1983). The excess was greatest for men who worked in foundries, consistent with reports of elevated lung cancer mortality among iron and steel foundry workers elsewhere in North America and Europe (IARC, 1983; Sorahan and Cooke, 1989).

PAHs appear to be involved in the excess risk of lung cancer among workers exposed to tars in the aluminum-smelting industry and among roofers exposed to asphalt and pitch (IARC, 1983). Lung cancer is also excessive among asphalt workers exposed to bitumen fumes, although other factors may be involved since the PAH content of the bitumens is low (Hansen, 1989). There have been a few reports of increased lung cancer among petroleum workers exposed to PAHs, but in an analysis combining data from over 20 industry-wide and company studies, the overall SMR for lung cancer was 0.77, significantly less than the comparison population mortality rates (Wong and Raabe, 1989; IARC, 1989a).

Diesel exhausts, to which PAHs may be adsorbed, have been associated with increased risks of lung cancer in truck drivers, railroad workers, and other occupational groups (IARC, 1989b; Steenland et al, 1990), but causal relationships are not clearly defined. Cohort studies of nearly 100,000 railroad workers in the United States and Canada report about a 40% higher risk of lung cancer among subgroups with the longest duration in jobs likely to involve diesel exposure (Howe et al, 1983; Garshick et al, 1988). In addition, PAHs have been a long-recognized cause of occupational skin and scrotal cancers, and a follow-up of men with scrotal tumors associated with exposure to mineral oil revealed an excess risk of lung cancer (Kipling and Waldron, 1976).

Radon. Increased risks of lung cancer have been observed among underground miners in North America, Europe, and Asia and quantitatively related to the inhalation of radon daughter products (Samet, 1989). Among miners with the highest exposures, the smoking-adjusted relative risk of lung cancer is about 20. The early studies among Colorado uranium miners indicated that most of the radon-induced lung cancers were small cell anaplastic tumors (Archer et al, 1973). Although a predilection for small cell cancers remains, more recent data indicate that all cell types are affected (Saccomanno, 1982; Samet, 1989). Radon appears to combine with cigarette smoking to increase the risk of lung cancer in a more-than-additive and nearly multiplicative fashion (National Research Council, 1988; Lubin et al, 1990). Nevertheless, radon in the absence of smoking still exerts a strong effect. In a 34-year follow-up of nonsmoking Colorado uranium miners, a 13-fold increased risk of lung cancer was observed (Roscoe et al, 1989), and significant excess risks have been observed among nonsmoking miners elsewhere in the United States and in Europe (Samet et al, 1984; Radford and Renard, 1984; Svec et al, 1988). Declines in risk after cessation of underground mining suggest that radon may act at a late stage in the carcinogenic process, and for the same cumulative dose, prolonged exposure at low dose rates seems more hazardous than shorter exposures at higher doses (Hornung and Meinhardt, 1987; Lubin et al, 1990). Interest in dose-response relationships in these occupational cohorts has increased recently with heightened concern over the potential hazards of household radon. A linear dose-response relation for lung cancer risk seems to hold over the exposure range seen in the miner studies, generally 100 to 3,000 working level months (WLM), with one Swedish and one Canadian investigation suggesting that risk may be nearly doubled following exposures as low as 50 WLM (Radford and Renard, 1984; Howe et al, 1986). An excess risk of lung cancer has been described among phosphate workers, whose exposure levels to radon appear to be lower than among underground miners (Checkoway et al, 1985; Block et al, 1988).

Silica. Exposures to crystalline silica have induced lung cancers and histiocytic lymphomas in experimental animals (IARC, 1987b). The epidemiologic evidence is less clear, although increased risks of lung cancer have been observed among silicotics in Europe, North America, and Asia, as well as among foundry workers, miners, and other groups heavily exposed to silica dusts (Goldsmith et al, 1986; Infante-Rivard et al, 1989; Forastiere et al, 1989; Ng et al, 1990; Amandus and Costello, 1991; Sherson et al, 1991). Silica's etiologic role remains in doubt because several studies have not found positive associations (Goldsmith et al, 1986; Hessel et al, 1990; Carta et al, 1991); those exposed to silica are often exposed to PAHs, radon, asbestos, or other workplace carcinogens; and smoking typically was not controlled for in the studies reported to date. In a recent survey in Montreal, silica was among several inorganic dusts associated with significantly increased risks of lung cancer after adjusting for exposure to other potential carcinogens (Siemiatycki et al, 1989). In a nested case-control study of lung cancer among a large cohort of silica-exposed miners and pottery workers in China, however, only small increases in smoking-adjusted risks of lung cancer were detected among silicotics, and trends in risk with increasing cumulative silica exposure were slight and varied by factory (McLaughlin et al, 1992). Pottery workers exposed to talc dusts have been reported to experience an increased risk of lung cancer (Thomas and Stewart, 1987), as have rubber workers handling talc during tire curing (Zhang et al, 1989).

Other Exposures. Several industrial exposures are suspected as causes of lung cancer, although epidemiologic evidence is preliminary. Initial surveys of chemical workers exposed to acrylonitrile suggested an excess lung cancer risk (O'Berg, 1980; Thiess et al, 1980; Delzell and Monson, 1982), consistent with inhalation studies in rats, but no increased risks have been noted in other groups of American workers (Chen et al, 1987; Collins et al, 1989). Some surveys of the vinyl chloride industry have indicated an association with lung cancer, in addition to liver angiosarcoma (Buffler et al, 1979). An increased risk has also been reported among rubber workers, especially those involved in tire curing and in fuel cells and deicers (Monson and Fine, 1978).

Excess mortality from lung cancer has been reported among workers exposed to beryllium (Steenland and Ward, 1991). Although a causal relationship is uncertain, beryllium compounds have induced lung tumors in rats and monkeys following inhalation. An increase of lung cancer has been reported in some, but not other, studies of metalworkers exposed to ferric oxide dust (Axelson and Sjoberg, 1979). One investigation found elevated lung cancer mortality in ferrochromium but not ferrosilicon workers (Langard et al, 1980). Follow-up surveys of workers in lead and cadmium smelters have reported an increased mortality from certain cancers, including those of the lung, although the responsible agents are uncertain (Doll, 1982). Several investigations in the United States and Europe have reported increased risks of lung cancer among welders in shipyards and other settings (IARC, 1990). Fumes from stainless steel (chromium) welding may contribute, although the occurrence of mesothelioma in some studies suggests that asbestos may be involved, and no increase in lung cancer was detected among welders in three U.S. plants where concomitant exposure to asbestos and stainless steel fumes could be ruled out (Steenland et al, 1991). In a European survey, no excess risk of lung cancer was found for stainless steel welders, although a nonsignificant increase was detected among mild steel welders (Moulin et al, 1993). Elevated risks of respiratory cancer have been reported in steel pickling and other operations where exposure to sulfuric and other acid mists is high. The excesses have been most pronounced for laryngeal cancer, but the acid mists have been reported to affect lung cancer as well, and an international panel has judged the evidence as sufficient to declare these agents as carcinogenic to humans (IARC, 1992).

Formaldehyde has been evaluated as a respiratory carcinogen, but no clear associations were detected in large-scale cohort and case-control studies of exposed workers (Blair et al, 1986; Gerin et al, 1989 IARC, 1995). Several surveys of workers exposed to chlorinated toluenes, including the animal carcinogen benzotrichloride, have found about a 3-fold increased risk of respiratory cancer, but the results are based on small numbers (IARC, 1982; Sorahan and Cathcart, 1989; Wong, 1989). Epichlorohydrin, an alkylating agent used in producing epoxy resins and synthetic glycerin that has induced respiratory cancer in laboratory animals, and isopropyl alcohol were linked to lung cancer in a small group of U.S. chemical factory workers (Enterline, 1982). A 2-fold increase in lung cancer was reported among workers exposed to inorganic mercury, but prior exposure to asbestos may have taken place (Barregard et al, 1990). Elevated rates of lung cancer have been detected among pesticide applicators in the United States and Germany (Blair et al, 1983), but no specific exposures could be implicated. Some increase in lung cancer risk has been reported among workers involved in the manufacture of DDT, and a nonsignificant excess was found among South Carolina residents with antecedent high serum DDT levels, but evidence linking DDT or other specific pesticides and lung cancer was considered inadequate in one international review (IARC, 1991).

Paper and pulp industry workers have been reported at increased risk of lung cancer in some surveys (Solet et al, 1989), but not others (Milham and Demers, 1984; Blot et al, 1978; Robinson et al, 1986; Schwartz, 1988). Carpenters and other groups exposed to wood dust have also been reported to be at increased risk of lung cancer in some surveys (Blot et al, 1982b; Siemiatycki et al, 1989), with one (Zahm et al, 1989) suggesting that adenocarcinomas may be most affected, an interesting finding in view of the clear excess of nasal adenocarcinomas reported among furniture workers in several areas of the world exposed to wood dusts (IARC, 1981). A recent international review, however, noted that evidence linking wood dust exposure and lung cancer was inconsistent (IARC, 1995). Increased risks of lung cancer have been observed among butchers and meat packers in Europe and the United States (Coggon et al, 1989), but the responsible agents have not been identified. Lung cancer risks have also been reported to occur excessively among cooks and bakers (Tuchsen and Nordholm, 1986; Carstensen et al, 1988).

Some reports have pointed to decreased risks of lung cancer among certain occupational groups. Most notable is the 20%–40% lowered risk reported among cotton textile workers in the United States, Great Britain, and China (Levin et al, 1987). This pattern could not be attributed to lowered levels of smoking or competing risks from byssinosis, raising the possibility of a protective effect of bacterial endotoxins found in cotton and other agricultural dusts (Enterline et al, 1985).

Radiation. *Medical and Atomic Radiation.* Lung cancer is one of the major effects of exposure to high doses of ionizing radiation. In addition to the increased risks among miners exposed to radon and its daughter products, significant excesses of lung cancer have been observed among patients receiving radiation therapy for ankylosing spondylitis in Great Britain and among atomic bomb survivors in Japan (National Research Council, 1980). The relative risks associated with high (100+ rad) exposures in the British and Japanese data were only moderately elevated, on the order of 1.5 to 2, but the excess absolute risk per rad for lung cancer in each series is estimated to exceed that for all other neoplasms (National Research Council, 1980). These studies have not clarified the interactive roles of radiation and smoking, although there was little evidence of synergism in autopsy and case-control studies of lung cancer in Japan (Blot et al, 1984; National Research Council, 1988). Among atomic bomb survivors, the radiation dose gradient for lung cancer was more pronounced for small cell carcinomas, which is also the cell type predominant among uranium miners.

Indoor Radon. Indoor radon has been estimated to account for about one-half of all radiation exposures received by the general population (Clarke and Southwood, 1989). Thus, there is much concern that household exposures might induce lung cancer. Some estimates suggest that in the United States between 6,000 and 24,000 lung cancers annually are related to indoor radon (Lubin and Boice, 1989). The uncertainty arises since projections are generally based on dose-response curves derived from data on lung cancer risks among underground miners exposed to high levels of radon.

Only a relatively small number of investigations have directly assessed risks associated with household radon exposure (Samet, 1989). The first report of an association came in 1979, when Axelson et al (1979) noted an increased lung cancer risk among persons living in stone compared to wood houses in Sweden. Subsequent case-control studies in Sweden have generally (Axelson et al, 1988; Svensson et al, 1989), but not always (Damber and Larsson, 1987), found higher smoking-adjusted risks associated with living in structures where radon levels were thought to be high. Data are more limited from outside Sweden. No appreciable differences in lung cancer risk according to housing type were found in Maryland (Simpson and Comstock, 1983), but 2-fold elevations (based on only 6 cases and 2 controls) have been reported among New Jersey residents in homes with radon levels exceeding 4 picocuries per liter (Schoenberg et al, 1989), the level above which the U.S. Environmental Protection Agency recommends remedial action. In Canada, a 2-fold increase of lung cancer was found among residents of homes built with radioactive materials, but the result is based on small numbers of cases (Lees et al, 1987). In a large-scale study in China, there was no evidence of a rising trend in risk of lung cancer among female residents as radon levels rose from <2, 2–3.9, 4–7.9 to 8.0 picocuries per liter, although a slight excess was seen for small cell carcinomas (Blot et al, 1990). The epidemiologic findings thus are mixed with respect to the effects of home exposures. Furthermore, there is uncertainty in extrapolations from higher-level mine exposures (Toohey et al, 1987). Hence, although radon is a known lung carcinogen, further epidemiologic studies in different populations are needed, with pooled analyses when possible, to clarify the impact of indoor radon upon lung cancer risk.

Air Pollution. While there has been recent concern about indoor air pollution from radon and environmental tobacco smoke, pollutants in the urban air have long been suspected in the etiology of lung cancer. Epidemiologic evaluation has been confounded by difficulties in defining and measuring air pollution, and in evaluating the effects of low-level exposures in the general population (National Research Council, 1979). Of special concern are products from the combustion of fossil fuels, notably PAHs. The major sources of pollution are motor vehicle exhausts (including diesel engines), residential and commercial space heating, oil- and coal-fired power plants, and industrial emissions. In several studies the rates for lung cancer have shown geographic correlations with measurements of benzo(a)pyrene in the ambient air, yet the available evidence suggests that the urban excess of lung cancer is mainly due to cigarette smoking, with some effect from occupational hazards. In the large-scale follow-up study of the American Cancer Society, age- and smoking-standardized rates for lung cancer were computed according to residence among men not occupationally exposed to dust, fumes, or vapors (Hammond and Garfinkel, 1980). Only small differences in mortality were seen between urban and rural areas, and between cities categorized by indices of pollution. Another approach has been to extrapolate from studies of workers heavily exposed to PAHs. Based on these data, Doll (1978) has suggested that the effect of urban air pollutants is small but may cause as many as 10 cases of lung cancer per year per 100,000 men with average smoking habits. Some studies suggest that the effect of smoking a particular amount is greater in urban than in rural areas, indicating that tobacco smoke may interact with carcinogens in the ambient atmosphere (Friberg and Cederlof, 1978).

Recent investigations in areas of China with exceptionally high rates of lung cancer provide some of the strongest evidence to date that specific air pollutants may increase cancer risk. In a rural county in Yunnan province, the excess risk among men and women was attributed almost entirely to living in chimneyless houses heated by a local soft, smoky coal (Mumford et al, 1987). In urban Shenyang and Harbin in northeastern China, indoor pollution from the use of "kang" and other coal-burning heating devices contributes to the area's high rates of lung cancer (Xu et al, 1989; Wu-Williams et al, 1990). In both instances, detection of the hazard was aided by extremely high pollutant levels, with indoor and outdoor levels of benzo(a)pyrene in Shenyang exceeding recommended standards for U.S. cities by over 60-fold. Air pollution has also been associated with a significant (50%) increase in lung cancer among men in Cracow, Poland, where airborne particulate levels are also high, with a smaller (20%) excess among women (Jedrychowski et al, 1990).

PAHs are not the only components of air pollution that are carcinogenic. In Shanghai, increased risks of lung cancer have been associated with prolonged exposure to oil vapors, particularly from unrefined rapeseed oil used in high-temperature wok cooking (Gao et al, 1987). This may contribute to the high rates of lung adenocarcinoma described in Chinese women worldwide. In addition, it has been shown that lung cancer occurs excessively in neighborhoods adjacent to arsenic-emitting smelters in the United States, Sweden, and China (Brown et al, 1984; Pershagen, 1986; Xu et al, 1989). Asbestos bodies and calcified pleural plaques have been reported in large segments of the urban population (Churg and Warnock, 1979). The nearly linear dose-response relation observed in some occupational settings has led to concern about airborne exposures to asbestos in consumer products, schools, office buildings, and other public places, although it has not been established that lung cancer occurs excessively following low-dose nonoccupational exposures to asbestos (Mossman et al, 1990).

Diet and Nutrition. Epidemiologic studies over the past decade have provided evidence that dietary and nutritional factors influence lung cancer risk. The most consistent association is a lowered risk associated with consumption of fresh vegetables and fruits, a pattern seen in multiple case-control and cohort studies (Colditz et al, 1987). Risks among subjects in the upper quantile (usually tertile, quartile, or quintile) of consumption tend to be about one-half those in the lowest intake categories. Several ingredients in vegetables may contribute to the reduced risks, but much attention has focused on carotenoids, particularly beta-carotene. Table 31–9 lists investigations that have evaluated dietary intakes of carotene (or total vitamin A), and shows that protective effects associated with consumption of foods high in carotenoids have been replicated across different populations in the United States, Europe, and Asia. Although beta-carotene is one of the few carotenoids converted to retinol in vivo, it may act as a cancer inhibitor through different mechanisms, perhaps by quenching free radicals, since those epidemiologic studies distinguishing dietary beta-carotene from retinol intake have tended to find protective effects only for beta-carotene (Ziegler, 1989). Several biochemical studies (Stahelin et al, 1984; Nomura et al, 1985; Menkes et al, 1986; Knekt et al, 1991), but not all (Willet et al, 1984), have shown reduced levels of beta-carotene in stored sera from persons who subsequently developed lung cancer, whereas serum retinol levels were lower only when serum was collected shortly before the diagnosis of cancer

TABLE 31–9. *Epidemiologic Investigations Reporting Risks of Lung Cancer Associated with Dietary Carotene Intake*

Reference	*Approximate Study Location*	*Dietary Variable*	*No. of Lung Cancers*	*RR in High vs. Low Consumers*[a]
Bjelke, 1975	Norway	Vitamin A	19	0.4
MacLennan et al, 1977	Singapore	Green vegetables	233	0.7
Mettlin et al, 1979	New York	Vitamin A	292	0.4
Hirayama, 1979	Japan	Green-yellow vegetables	807	0.6
Gregor et al, 1980	England	Vitamin A	100	0.7
Shekelle et al, 1981	Chicago	Beta-carotene	33	0.2
Kvale et al, 1983	Norway	Vitamin A	70	0.6
Hinds et al, 1984	Hawaii	Carotene	364	0.5
Samet et al, 1985	New Mexico	Vitamin A	447	0.8
Wang and Hammond, 1985	U.S.	Green salad	2952	0.8
Wu et al, 1985	Los Angeles	Beta-carotene	220	0.4
Pisani et al, 1986	Italy	Carrots	417	0.5
Ziegler et al, 1986	New Jersey	Beta-carotene	763	0.8
Byers et al, 1987	New York	Carotene	450	0.6
Paginini-Hill et al, 1987	Los Angeles	Beta-carotene	56	0.7
Bond et al, 1987	Texas	Carotene	308	0.5
Pastorino et al, 1987	Italy	Carotene	47	0.3
Gao et al, 1987	Shanghai	Carotene	672	2.0
Koo, 1988	Hong Kong	Green vegetables, carrots, fruit	88	0.5
Fontham et al, 1988	Louisiana	Carotene	1253	0.9
Mettlin, 1989	New York	Carrots, broccoli, spinach	569	0.4
LeMarchand et al, 1989	Hawaii	Beta-carotene	332	0.5
Wu-Williams et al, 1990	China	Vegetables high in carotene	965	0.9
Dartigues et al, 1990	France	Beta-carotene	106	0.2
Fraser et al, 1991	California	Cooked green vegetables, tomatoes	61	1.1
Kalandidi et al, 1990	Greece	Beta-carotene	154	1.0
Jain et al, 1990	Toronto	Beta-carotene	839	0.9
Knekt et al, 1991	Finland	carotenoids	117	0.4
Shibata et al, 1992	Los Angeles	Beta-carotene	94	1.1
Candelora et al, 1992	Florida	Beta-carotene	124	0.4
Steinmetz et al, 1993	Iowa	Beta-carotene	138	0.9

[a]Definitions vary from study to study, but high consumers were often those in the upper quartile of intake.

(Friedman et al, 1986; Wald et al, 1986; Comstock et al, 1992). Carotenoid intake and serum beta-carotene concentrations tend to be lower in smokers (Stryker et al, 1988), but smoking was often controlled for in the studies reported. There have been some reports that the protective effects of carotenoids may be greater among current and recent smokers (Ziegler et al, 1986; LeMarchand et al, 1989), but the interactive roles of dietary factors and smoking are not clear. A stronger effect of carotene upon squamous and small cell lung cancers has also been noted in some studies, but all cell types seem to be affected.

Given the strong observational data suggesting that dietary intake of beta-carotene may protect against lung cancer, the recent finding of an increased risk following up to 8 years of supplementation with 20 mg per day of beta-carotene capsules in a randomized intervention trial among male smokers in Finland and an average of 4 years of daily supplementation with 30 mg of beta carotene plus 25,000 IU of retinol among heavy smokers and asbestos workers in the United States was completely unexpected (ATBC Study Group, 1994; Omenn et al, 1996). An 18% higher incidence of lung cancer ($p = .01$) was found among the supplemented group in Finland; a 28% increase in the United States. The findings raise the possibility that correlates of beta-carotene have been responsible for the protective effect of foods high in carotene seen in epidemiologic studies. In a randomized trial in Linxian, China, nonsignificantly lowered risks of lung cancer were seen among those who received daily supplementation with beta-carotene, vitamin E, and selenium, but the numbers of lung cancers were small (Blot et al, 1994). A small (7%) reduction in lung cancer was also observed in a trial of 22,000 male American physicians at low risk for lung cancer (Hennekens et al, 1996). A 14-week regimen of 20 mg of beta-carotene daily was shown to result in a significant reduction in micronuclei in the sputum of smokers (Van Poppel et al, 1992).

In addition to carotenoids, fresh fruits and vegetables contain other micronutrients, including vitamin C, which can inhibit the formation of carcinogenic nitrosamines (Mirvish, 1983), as well as phenols, flavones, isothiocyanates, and other compounds which may influence cancer risk. In studies in Louisiana (Fontham et al, 1988) and California (Fraser et al, 1991), stronger protective effects were observed for dietary vitamin C than for carotene intake. Dietary vitamin E from vegetable oils and other foods may play a role, since prediagnostic serum levels appear to be inversely related to lung cancer risk (Menkes et al, 1986; Knekt et al, 1991). One survey reported 33% lower serum vitamin E levels in lung cancer patients than hospital controls, the most marked reduction among the several nutrients examined (LeGardeur et al, 1991). Although selenium has been postulated as a tumor inhibitor (Coombs, 1989), blood levels have not been reported to be related to risk of lung cancer (Menkes et al, 1986; Nomura et al, 1987), except in Finland, where selenium intake is exceptionally low and 3-fold or greater increases in risk have been found among those with the lowest levels (Knekt et al, 1990). In the randomized clinical trial in Finland, no significant reduction in lung cancer incidence occurred within the 8-year study period among those supplemented with 50 mg daily of alpha tocopherol (ATBC Study Group, 1994).

An excess of lung cancer has been reported among persons with high dietary intake of foods rich in fat and cholesterol, including whole milk and eggs (Hinds et al, 1987; Byers et al, 1987; Goodman et al, 1989; Mettlin, 1989; Jain et al, 1990; Shekelle et al, 1991). In one case-control study, there was a greater than 6-fold increase in risk associated with high saturated fat intake (Alavanja et al, 1993), although this is almost surely an overestimate (Kolonel, 1993). However, cohort studies generally have not found increases of lung cancer among persons with elevated serum cholesterol (Schatzkin et al, 1988). Despite the positive association with dietary fat, lung cancer risk tends to be inversely related to body mass. Data from a large case-control study enrolling patients in hospitals in several American cities and from a cohort study in Finland showed that risks were nearly twice as high among both males and females in the lowest compared to highest quantiles of body mass index (Knekt et al, 1991; Kabat and Wynder, 1992). In one study, however, the association was primarily with body size 5 years prior to diagnosis rather than at age 20–29, calling into question the etiologic significance of the finding (Goodman and Wilkens, 1993). In the study by Drinkard et al (1995), the inverse association between risk of lung caner and body mass index was substantially reduced after controlling for cigarette smoking.

Recent case-control studies in North and South America have suggested that consumption of alcoholic beverages, particularly beer, may be associated with increased risk of lung cancer (Potter et al, 1992; Bandera et al, 1992; DeStefani et al, 1993). These studies reported smoking-adjusted RRs of 1.6 to about 3 among beer drinkers, although the association was limited to heavy smokers in one study (Bandera et al, 1992). An association between lung cancer and alcohol was noted in some earlier case-control cohort studies, but the relationship was usually attributed to confounding by smoking, and lung cancer has not generally been considered an alcohol-related cancer (IARC, 1988b).

Prior Lung Disease. Lung cancer risk has been reported to be increased among persons with a history of certain nonmalignant lung diseases, including asbestosis, silicosis, tuberculosis (TB), chronic bronchitis/emphysema, and pneumonia (Skillrud et al, 1986; Zheng et al, 1987; Wu et al, 1985, 1989; Browne, 1991; Alavanja et al, 1992). As noted earlier in this review, lung cancers in asbestos-exposed workers are most prominent among those with asbestosis. Similarly, excess risks of lung cancer associated with silica exposure seem to occur mainly among those with silicosis (McLaughlin et al, 1992). There have been several clinical series of lung cancer, particularly adenocarcinomas, arising from scar tissue (Auerbach et al, 1979a; Bakris et al, 1983), but scarring can also occur during tumor growth, so the etiologic implications of the relationship are not clear. An increased risk of lung cancer among TB patients has been seen in some recent cohort as well as case-control studies (Zheng et al, 1987; Wu et al, 1989). Isoniazid, a mainstay in TB therapy, was suspected for a while because of its capacity to induce lung cancer in experimental animals, but the drug has been exonerated in epidemiologic studies (Boice and Fraumeni, 1980). Perhaps the strongest evidence for an association with TB comes from a case-control study in Shanghai (Zheng et al, 1987), where TB has affected a sizable percentage of the population (20% of adult males). Risk of lung cancer was increased by 50% among survivors of TB, with a more than 2-fold increase among those diagnosed with TB within the past 20 years. The risks were more apparent for adenocarcinoma than squamous cell cancer, with the location of the TB lesions and lung cancers highly correlated. Other preexistent respiratory diseases have been associated with lung cancer risk, with the link to chronic bronchitis/emphysema generally stronger for squamous and small cell cancers, even after adjusting for smoking habits (Gao et al, 1987; Wu et al, 1989). A link between asthma and increased risk of lung cancer has been reported in some studies (Vena et al, 1985; Reynolds and Kaplan, 1987; Alavanja et al, 1992), but not others (Osann, 1991). The association has been said to be stronger for males, but the potential etiologic significance of these mixed findings is not clear. Risk of lung cancer has been reported in several studies to be elevated among owners of pet birds, perhaps as a result of pulmonary interstitial fibrosis from bird dander, but further evaluation of this intriguing finding is needed (Holst et al, 1988; Kohlmeier et al, 1992; Gardiner et al, 1992).

Host Factors

The role of genetic factors is easily obscured by the potent environmental determinants of lung cancer, notably smoking. There have been several clinical reports of familial lung cancer, often of adenocarcinoma and alveolar cell carcinoma, the cell types less closely related to smoking (Mulvihill, 1976). Tokuhata and Lilienfeld (1963) reported a case-control study showing a significant tendency for lung cancer to aggregate in families. Since then, other investigators have reported 2- to 4-fold increased risks of lung cancer among close relatives of patients (Ooi et al, 1986a, 1986b; Horwitz et al, 1988; Wu et al, 1989; Shaw et al, 1991), as well as excesses of certain other cancers (Sellers et al, 1988; McDuffie, 1991). A segregation analysis involving 337 families with lung cancer suggested a codominant inheritance pattern, with tumors tending to arise at an early age among affected members (Sellers et al, 1990). In addition, a familial tendency to chronic obstructive pulmonary disease (COPD) among patients with lung cancer has been reported (Cohen et al, 1977; Samet et al, 1986). The available evidence suggests that, in addition to smoking and shared environmental exposures, heritable factors may contribute to the familial aggregation of lung cancer, along with other cancers and COPD.

In the search for genetic markers of susceptibility, Kellermann et al (1973) reported increased levels of inducible aryl hydrocarbon hydroxylase activity in cultured lymphocytes of lung cancer patients. This suggested a genetically regulated enzyme defect altering the metabolism of PAHs, but subsequent studies have failed to uphold the promise of the initial observations (Kakri et al, 1987; Law, 1989). More recently, DNA polymorphisms in the cytochrome P450 gene (CYP1A1) responsible for the metabolic activation of benzo(a)pyrene have been associated in some studies with lung cancer; and among those with susceptible genotypes, the amount of exposure to cigarettes required to induce squamous cell carcinomas of the lung may be reduced (Nakachi et al, 1991). Findings are mixed, however, with no association between lung cancer and CYP1A1 polymorphisms found in Finland and Norway (Hirvonen et al, 1992). The genetically controlled ability to metabolize the antihypertensive agent debrisoquine also has been linked to risk of lung cancer. The P450 gene (CYP2D6) regulating debrisoquine metabolism may also influence the metabolism of NNK, a tobacco-specific nitrosamine that is a potent lung carcinogen in experimental animals (Hoffmann and Hecht, 1985). Sixfold or greater increases in risk have been reported among extensive metabolizers of debrisoquine, a trait affecting 73% of controls in one study in the United States (Caporaso et al, 1990), but other studies have found the association to be more modest, with combined data indicating about a doubling in risk among extensive metabolizers (Amos et al, 1992). A recent survey enrolling over 300 patients found no evidence that the risk of lung cancer was related to the debrisoquine metabolic phenotype (Shaw et al, 1995). It has also been reported that susceptibility may be influenced by individual variability in the detoxification of carcinogens. Reduced activity of glutathione S-transferase (GST) enzymes that catalyze the conjugation of PAHs has been linked to increased risk of lung cancer (Siedegard et al, 1986). Little difference was seen, however, in GST activity in lung vs. non-smoking-related cancers, although levels were somewhat lower for lung cancer patients than healthy controls in a population-based survey in Washington (Heckbert et al, 1992). In an analysis combining data from 12 case-control studies with 1,593 lung cancer patients, GSTM1 deficiency was associated with a summary relative risk of 1.4 for lung cancer (McWilliams et al, 1995). Another potential marker of susceptibility is slow acetylator phenotype, which has been related to the frequency of 4-aminobiphenyl (a constituent of cigarette smoke) hemoglobin adducts and linked to risk of bladder cancer (Vineis et al, 1990), but no differences in acetylator phenotype or in adduct levels were found in recent comparisons of lung cancer cases vs. controls (Philip et al, 1988; Weston et al, 1991).

Genetic determinants are further suggested by molecular studies showing that a DNA sequence is deleted at the chromosome locus 3p14–23 in all major forms of lung cancer, particularly small cell carcinomas (Birrer and Minna, 1988). It is not clear whether these alterations are a consequence or a cause of the lung cancers, but the natural history of lung cancer may involve a sequence of gene mutations. Mutations in the p53 tumor suppressor gene and in *ras* oncogenes are common in lung tumor tissue, although *ras* mutations appear limited to non–small cell lung cancers (Takahashi et al, 1989; Lehman et al, 1991; Mitsudomi et al, 1991). Activation of *myc* oncogenes has been reported in small cell carcinomas and chromosome alterations may be frequent on *5q* (Kok et al, 1989; Miura et al, 1992). The frequency of mutations in lung tumor tissue is still uncertain, but the majority of cancers may express mutated p53 genes, and 20%–35% *ras* genes. Furthermore, p53 and *ras* mutations tend to be seen in the same tumor specimens, indicating that one may enhance activities of the other in the process of lung carcinogenesis. In one survey of 54 lung adenocarcinomas, K-*ras* mutations occurred significantly more often in patients who were cigarette smokers than in nonsmokers (Slebos et al, 1991).

Some fragmentary evidence exists that immunosuppressive states may predispose to lung cancer. Hoover and Fraumeni (1973) reported an increased risk of lung cancer, primarily adenocarcinoma, among kidney transplant recipients receiving immunosuppressive drugs, although the risk was not nearly as high as for lymphoma. The risk of lung cancer is also increased among patients with various lymphoproliferative diseases, perhaps due to the accompanying immunodeficiency state along with radiotherapy and smoking (Greene et al, 1978; Tucker et al, 1988). Also noteworthy is the finding of subclinical immune defects found in a family with multiple cases of lymphoproliferative neoplasms and lung adenocarcinoma (Fraumeni et al, 1975). However, the risk of lung cancer does not appear elevated in all immunodeficiency disorders or in autoimmune diseases, except for scleroderma, which predisposes to adenocarcinoma and alveolar cell carcinoma of the lung (Tomkin, 1969).

Hormonal risk factors have been suggested by the observation that among nonsmokers adenocarcinoma affects proportionately more females than males (Lubin and Blot, 1984), by the possible role of menstrual variables, particularly menstrual cycle length (Gao et al, 1987), and by the finding of sex steroid receptors in lung cancer (Beattie et al, 1985).

Preventive Measures

Autopsy studies have uncovered a spectrum of pathologic lesions (hyperplasia, metaplasia, carcinoma in situ, and invasive cancer) throughout the tracheobronchial tree whose prevalences vary in relation to the duration and amoung of cigarette smoking (Auerbach et al, 1979b). The premalignant lesions have shown some evidence of reversibility among ex-smokers. Although the relationship of these lesions to atypical cells released into the sputum has not been clearly defined, it has seemed reasonable to assume that periodic surveillance of high-risk groups by sputum cytology may detect early-stage cancers that are curable. However, controlled clinical trials of asymptomatic individuals (including heavy smokers) screened by chest Xray and sputum cytology have not as yet shown significant reductions in mortality from lung cancer (Fontana, 1986). Further studies are needed to clarify the relation of atypical metaplasia in sputum cytology to lung cancer risk (Vine et al, 1990).

It is obvious that the major hope in controlling lung cancer is through primary prevention (Wynder, 1989). Although smoking cigarettes with low tar and nicotine appears less dangerous than the use of unfiltered cigarettes, clearly the most effective approach to reducing mortality is through strategies aimed at smoking cessation and avoidance in large segments of the population, including targeting young people for prevention programs. Major reductions in lung cancer and other smoking-related diseases should ensue (Devesa et al, 1989). Recent sharp declines in smoking prevalence following imposition of taxes on cigarettes in California (Pierce et al, 1991) and Canada (Kaiserman and Rogers, 1991) indicate that governmental policies can have a marked impact in hastening the reduction in cigarette use. An important impact should also result from antismoking measures in the workplace and public places, now increasing in frequency as the potential effects of environmental tobacco smoke have become clearer (Environmental Protection Agency, 1992). In addition, the role of nutritional deficiencies in lung cancer suggests that chemoprevention studies deserve further emphasis. Further work is needed to clarify the interaction of smoking with occupational and other environmental hazards, and with various susceptibility states based on genetic, nutritional, immunologic, and hormonal factors. By better understanding the interplay of multiple risk factors and multistage mechanisms, it should be possible to augment the development of sound programs aimed at the prevention of lung cancer.

PLEURAL CANCER

Mesotheliomas of the pleural and peritoneal lining were rarely noted until Wagner et al (1960) reported a large case series among South African crocidolite miners and neighborhood residents. Since then, the incidence of mesothelioma has been increasing, with most tumors arising from the pleura as a result of occupational asbestos exposure.

Demographic Factors

Worldwide Occurrence. Statistics on the incidence and mortality of mesothelioma are not routinely reported because of problems in the diagnosis and classification of this uncommon tumor. Recent data are available, however, from the SEER program of population-based cancer registries covering about 10% of the total U.S. population. The annual age-adjusted incidence of mesothelioma from 1985 to 1989 was 1.6 per 100,000 among white males, and 0.4 per 100,000 among white females. The rates in nonwhites were lower, but based on small numbers. In total, 78% of all mesotheliomas occurred among males, 22% among females. Pleural outnumbered peritoneal mesotheliomas by a 9-to-1 margin among males, but by less than 3 to 1 among women, a pattern resembling that seen in other nations (Theriault and Grand-bois, 1978; Zwi et al, 1989). The tumors arise rarely in other sites, such as the pericardium.

There is considerable international variation in rates, related partly to differences in the completeness of case ascertainment (McDonald and McDonald, 1977). Although underdiagnosis and underreporting of mesothelioma are serious problems, particularly in death certificate surveys, there is some tendency in the opposite direction, since tumors initially called mesothelioma (especially of the peritoneum) may actually be other malignancies after review by expert pathologists (Greenberg and Lloyd Davies, 1974; McDonald, 1979; Spirtas et al, 1986b). Nevertheless, there are well-documented pockets of elevated incidence of mesothelioma, particularly where shipbuilding has been a major industry. Along coastal areas in the states of Virginia and Washington, annual incidence rates exceed 2.5 per 100,000 among males (Tagnon et al, 1980; Connelly et al, 1987). In England and Wales, elevated rates among men tend to cluster in shipbuilding centers, while among women the highest mortality occurs in areas where gas masks (with asbestos filters) were manufactured (Gardner et al, 1982). Mesotheliomas are rare in Japan except in shipbuilding centers (Kishimoto et al, 1989). In South Africa, excess mesothelioma is largely concentrated in mining districts (Botha et al, 1986).

Time Trends and Age Curves. In Connecticut, where cancer has been a reportable disease since 1935, rates of mesothelioma have continued to increase since the 1950s. In SEER areas of the United States over the period 1973–84, pleural mesothelioma incidence rose by nearly 12% per year among males, vs. 1% per year among females, with the increase among males primarily for diagnoses at ages over 55 years (Spirtas et al, 1986a; Connelly et al, 1987). The latest SEER data through the end of the 1980s show that age-adjusted rates among males continued to increase, but at a slower pace. Indeed, rates of mesothelioma appear to have peaked among those born around 1910 and declined among later-born cohorts. Rates at ages below 55 years were already declining in the 1980s. If the SEER data are representative of the total population and the trends continue, over 2,000 Americans annually will be diagnosed with mesothelioma in the 1990s. Histopathologic review of cases from New York and Los Angeles suggests that the increase in incidence is not simply due to changing diagnostic procedures. Rising rates also have been seen in Canada, Great Britain, France, and other nations (Bignon et al, 1979; Gardner et al, 1982; Morrison et al, 1984; Zwi et al, 1989). At least part of the increase may result from asbestos exposures in shipbuilding, the major manufacturing industry in the United States and several other countries during World War II. It has been estimated that occupational exposures to asbestos may account for about 20,000 mesothelioma deaths in the United States between the 1980s and the first decade of the next century (Peto et al, 1981; Walker et al, 1983; Lilienfeld et al, 1988).

Figure 31–5 shows the age-specific incidence rates of pleural mesothelioma among white males based on the data from the SEER program for 1975–79, 1980–84, and 1985–89. Incidence rises almost linearly (on a semi-log scale) with age before reaching a plateau or falling around age 80. The deviations at these older ages seem at least partly due to cohort effects, with earlier-born cohorts less likely to receive asbestos exposures as young adults.

Survival. Based on follow-up of nearly 1,500 mesothelioma patients diagnosed during 1973–84 in the United States, the median survival was 7 months (Spirtas et al, 1988), a figure somewhat lower than that reported in most other (and smaller) case series (Pisani et al, 1988). Five-year survival rates were about 5% among males,

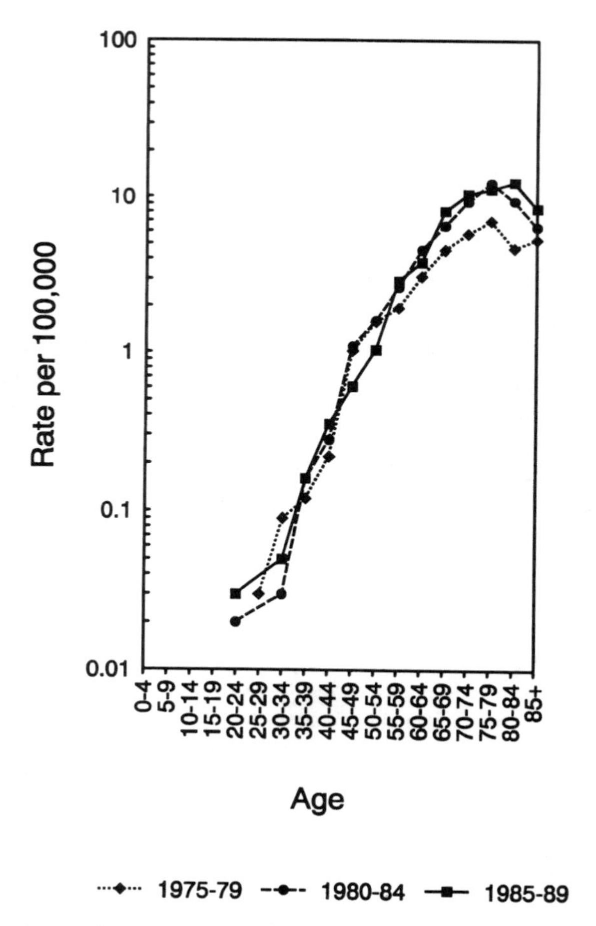

FIG. 31–5. Pleural mesothelioma incidence in the 9 SEER white males.

but were higher among females, exceeding 30% among women diagnosed before age 50. It has been suggested that survival may be longer for mesotheliomas without asbestos exposure (Law et al, 1984), but confirmatory evidence is still awaited.

Risk Factors

Occupational Asbestos. The principal cause of mesothelioma is asbestos, primarily through occupational exposure. An increased risk has been documented among workers in asbestos mines, asbestos mills and factories, insulation manufacture and installation, gas mask manufacture, shipbuilding, railroad machinery, and other occupations involving inhalation of asbestos dust (IARC, 1977; McDonald and McDonald, 1986). In the only national survey linking pleural mesothelioma and occupation, which covered all incident cases diagnosed in Sweden between 1961 and 1979, increased risks were linked to work in a number of industries, particularly the manufacture of transportation equipment (both shipbuilding and railroad equipment), paper and wood products, and machinery and electronic equipment, as well as in construction and sugar processing (Malker et al, 1985).

All types of asbestos seem capable of causing pleural mesotheliomas in both experimental animals and in human populations, although the risks in humans are greater for crocidolite, amosite, and other amphibole fibers. Peritoneal mesotheliomas have generally been reported only among amphibole- (and not chrysotile-) exposed workers (Doll and Peto, 1985). The mechanisms of induction are unknown, but appear closely related to the physical properties of fiber size and dimension (Stanton et al, 1981). The greatest carcinogenicity has been reported for fibers with higher length-to-width ratios, particularly those greater than 8 μm long and less than 0.25 μm in diameter. Especially hazardous are the amphiboles, straight rodlike fibers that can most easily penetrate to peripheral segments of the lung.

The rate of mesothelioma appears proportional to the amount of asbestos exposure. A gradient in risk according to intensity of exposure was seen among male and female London factory workers, with mesotheliomas accounting for 7% and 9% of all deaths in men and women, respectively (Newhouse et al, 1985). Rising risks with increasing duration of employment have been found in other groups, including insulation and amosite manufacturing workers (Selikoff, 1977). Among long-term shipyard workers in Virginia, pleural mesotheliomas were especially common in jobs with intense asbestos exposure, notably pipecovers and pipefitters, whereas the elevated risk of lung cancer could not be related to particular shipyard duties or length of employment (Blot et al, 1980; Tagnon et al, 1980).

It has been suggested that high levels of asbestos exposure are related more closely to peritoneal than to pleural mesotheliomas (IARC, 1977), since the peritoneal tumors prevail in heavily exposed groups, including workers in the U.S. and Canadian insulation industries and in some U.S. and British asbestos factories (Newhouse et al, 1985; Selikoff et al, 1979). The issue is in some doubt, however, since exposures in shipyards, railroads and certain other industries produce pleural tumors almost exclusively (Tagnon et al, 1980; Mancuso, 1988).

Perhaps the most prominent feature of mesothelioma is the long duration between initial exposure to asbestos and onset of the disease. Indeed, incidence of mesothelioma is primarily related to time since first exposure. Peto et al (1982) showed that mesothelioma death rates rise in proportion to about the 3rd power of duration since initial exposure to asbestos, with the cancers rarely occurring within 20 years of first exposure. Table 31-10 shows the numbers of deaths attributed to pleural and peritoneal mesotheliomas among asbestos insulation workers (Seidman and Selikoff, 1990). For both pleural and peritoneal tumors, the peak mortality was 45 years after first employment. Surveys of shipyard-related mesotheliomas of the pleura indicate latency periods of the same order. The median duration between initial employment and tumor onset was 34 to 39 years in Norfolk and Newport News, Walcheren Island, Nantes, and Plymouth (Tagnon et al, 1980; Blot and Fraumeni, 1981). In these series, very few cancers developed within 20 years of first exposure. The long latent period suggests that the current increase in mesothelioma incidence is not likely to end until the late 1990s or after the year 2000, when the effects of asbes-

TABLE 31–10. *Numbers of Deaths and Death Rates during 1967–86 from Pleural and Peritoneal Mesotheliomas**

Time from Initial Employment (years)	*Pleural*		*Peritoneal*	
	Number[a]	*Rate*[b]	*Number*[a]	*Rate*[b]
<15	0	0.0	0	0.0
15–19	2	3.8	3	5.7
20–24	10	17.4	8	13.9
25–29	33	65.3	40	79.2
30–34	40	107.6	65	174.9
35–39	33	162.2	58	285.2
40–44	17	166.7	42	411.7
45+	38	332.9	69	604.4

*According to duration from onset of employment among United States and Canadian asbestos insulation workers. Data from Siedman and Selikoff (1990).

[a]Numbers based on "best evidence" diagnosis.

[b]Number of deaths per 10^5 person-years observation.

tos controls introduced in the 1960s and 1970s become apparent and cases linked to asbestos exposures around World War II and shortly thereafter have subsided.

Nonoccupational Asbestos Exposure. In the early South African report (Wagner et al, 1960), one-third of the mesothelioma cases were exposed as residents living near asbestos mines and mills. Mesotheliomas may result from neighborhood exposures to various asbestos industries and from household contact with asbestos dust, primarily through the laundering of work clothing (Newhouse, 1977; Browne and Goffe, 1984; Kane et al, 1990; Otte et al, 1990). Concern has arisen that asbestos in homes, schools, and buildings may pose a significant health threat, but the levels of exposure are generally very low and to date mesothelioma occurrence has not been clearly linked to low-dose exposure from such sources (Mossman et al, 1990; Gaensler, 1992).

Other Factors. In virtually all surveys of mesothelioma, a fraction of cases have no documented exposure to asbestos (Peterson et al, 1984). One review of published material lists the percentage of cases without reported exposure at 38% (McDonald and McDonald, 1977), another at 46% (Walker et al, 1983), but contact with asbestos may be unrecognized by the patient or unreported by the next of kin, so that the actual percentage of exposure-free cases may be less. In some occupational groups the asbestos-related fraction approaches 100%, as seen when intensive interviews found evidence of exposure in 69 of 70 patients with mesothelioma in South Africa (Cochrane and Webster, 1978), and when combined occupational history/autopsy information implicated asbestos in 160 of 170 mesotheliomas occurring during the period 1968–87 among Italian shipyard workers (Giarelli et al, 1992). Nevertheless, there is little doubt that there is a baseline incidence of mesothelioma around the world that is not attributable to asbestos exposure. This is particularly true for mesothelioma among women, with the majority of patients appearing not to have had asbestos exposure. One population-based survey in Los Angeles indicated that 76% of female mesothelioma patients had no known asbestos exposure (Peto et al, 1981), and a hospital-based survey in New York found 84% unexposed (Muscat and Wynder, 1991). A background, non-asbestos-related occurrence of mesothelioma has also been reported in several studies of experimental animals (Ilgren and Wagner, 1990; Cicala et al, 1993). Mesothelioma is rarely reported in children: of 13 verified mesotheliomas identified by screening all childhood cancer deaths in the United States during the period 1960–69, 11 were of pleural origin (Grundy and Miller, 1972).

In rural villages in Turkey, a high rate of pleural mesothelioma has been traced to naturally occurring zeolite (erionite) fibers (Artvinli and Baris, 1979). This is the only exposure other than asbestos that has been clearly linked to mesothelioma in humans, although other man-made mineral fibers, notably fibrous glass, have induced mesotheliomas in experimental animals (IARC, 1988). It is noteworthy that smoking does not enhance the risk for mesothelioma as it does for asbestos-related lung cancer (Muscat and Wynder, 1991). Case reports of mesothelioma have been reported among sugarcane workers in the United States and sugar beet processors in Sweden, but concomitant asbestos exposures could not be ruled out (Brooks et al, 1992; Malker et al, 1985). Clues to dietary factors come from a case-control study in Louisiana involving 37 pleural mesothelioma patients (Schiffman et al, 1988). Risks were elevated by 2- to 3-fold among subjects with a low intake of vegetables in general and carotene-containing foods in particular. Exposure to high doses of ionizing radiation, usually as cancer treatment, has been linked to some cases of mesothelioma (Peterson et al, 1984; Hofmann et al, 1994)). Simian virus 40 has recently been shown to induce mesothelioma in hamsters, providing an experimental model for mesothelioma and raising the possibility that viruses may be involved in human pleural tumors (Cicala et al, 1993).

Genetic factors may predispose to some familial aggregations of mesothelioma (Hammar et al, 1989), and the role of tumor suppressor genes has been suggested by chromosome loss involving 1p, 3p, and 22p in mesothelioma tissue (Flejter et al, 1989). Although mutations in the p53 tumor-suppressor gene were reported to be common in human mesothelioma cell lines (Cote et al, 1991), a larger series did not confirm this finding or show activation of the K-*ras* oncogene (Metcalf et al, 1992). In view of the variable fractions of mesotheliomas unrelated to asbestos, and the multiple agents that can induce mesotheliomas in animal models, further epidemiologic research on non-asbestos causes of this tumor is warranted.

Preventive Measures

The key to prevention of mesothelioma is control of asbestos exposures in industry and other settings where asbestos products are used. This approach is vital, since to date mesothelioma has been virtually resistant to therapy, even when detected at an early stage during surveillance of high-risk groups (Selikoff, 1977).

REFERENCES

AKIBA S, KATO H, BLOT WJ. 1986. Passive smoking and lung cancer among Japanese women. Cancer Res 46:4806–4807.

ALAVANJA M, BROWNSON R, BOICE J, et al. 1992. Preexisting lung disease and lung cancer among nonsmoking women. Am J Epidemiol 136:623–632.

ALAVANJA M, BROWN L, SWANSON C, et al. 1963. Saturated fat-intake and lung cancer risk among nonsmoking women in Missouri. J Natl Cancer Inst 85:1906–1916.

ALDERSON MR, RATTAN NS, BIDSTRUP L. 1981. Health of workmen in the chromate producing industry in Britain. Br J Ind Med 38:117–124.

AMANDUS H, COSTELLO J. 1991. Silicosis and lung cancer in U.S. metal miners. Arch Environ Health 46:82–89.

AMOS CT, CAPORASO N, WESTON A. 1992. Host Factors in lung cancer risk: a review of interdisciplinary studies. Cancer Epidemiol Biomarkers Prev 1:505–513.

ARCHER VE, WAGONER JK, LUNDIN FE. 1973. Lung cancer among uranium miners in the United States. Health Phys 25:351–371.

ARTVINLI M, BARIS YI. 1979. Malignant mesotheliomas in a small village in the Anatolian region of Turkey: An epidemiologic study. J Natl Cancer Inst 63:17–22.

ATBC STUDY GROUP. 1994. The effect of vitamin E and beta carotene on the incidence of lung cancer and other cancers in male smokers. N Engl J Med 330:1029–1035.

AUERBACH O, GARFINKEL L, PARKS VR. 1979a. Scar cancer of the lung. Cancer 43:636–642.

AUERBACH O, HAMMOND EC, GARFINKEL L. 1979b. Changes in bronchial epithelium in relation to cigarette smoking, 1955–1960 vs. 1970–1977. N Engl J Med 300:381–386.

AXELSON O, SJOBERG A. 1979. Cancer incidence and exposure to iron oxide dust. J Occup Med 21:419–422.

AXELSON O, EDLING C, KLING H. 1979. Lung cancer and residency—a case-referent study on the possible impact of exposure to radon and its daughters in dwellings. Scand J Work Environ Health 5:10–15.

AXELSON O, ANDERSON K, DESAI G, et al. 1988. Indoor radon exposure and active and passive smoking in relation to the occurrence of lung cancer. Scand J Work Environ Health 14:286–292.

BAKRIS GL, MULOPULOS GP, KARCHIK R, et al. 1983. Pulmonary scar cancer: a clinicopathologic analysis. Cancer 52:493–497.

BANDERA E, FREUDENHEIM J, GRAHAM S, et al. 1992. Alcohol consumption and lung cancer in white males. Cancer Causes Control 3:361–369.

BARREGARD L, SALLSTEN G, JARVHOLM B. 1990. Mortality and cancer incidence in chloralkali workers exposed to inorganic mercury. Br J Ind Med 47:99–104.

BARRETT JC, LAMB PW, WISEMAN RW. 1989. Multiple mechanisms for the carcinogenic effects of asbestos and other mineral fibers. Env Health Perspect 81:81–89.

BEATTIE CW, HANSEN NW, THOMAS PA. 1985. Steroid receptors in human lung cancer. Cancer Res 45:4206–4214.

BERRY G, NEWHOUSE ML, ANTONIS P. 1985. Combined effects of asbestos and smoking on mortality from lung cancer and mesothelioma in factory workers. Br J Ind Med 42:12–18.

BIGNON J, SEBASTIEN P, DI MENZA L, et al. 1979. French mesothelioma register. Ann NY Acad Sci 330:455–466.

BIRRER MJ, MINNA JD. 1988. Molecular genetics of lung cancer. Semin Oncol 15:226–232.

BJELKE EA. 1975. Dietary vitamin A and human lung cancer. Int J Cancer 15:561–565.

BLAIR A, GRAUMAN D, LUBIN J, et al. 1983. Lung cancer and other causes of death among licensed pesticide applicators. J Natl Cancer Inst 71:31–37.

BLAIR A, STEWART P, O'BERG M, et al. 1986. Mortality among industrial workers exposed to formaldehyde. J Natl Cancer Ins 76:1071–1084.

BLOCK G, MATANOSKI G, SELTZER R, et al. 1988. Cancer morbidity and mortality in phosphate workers. Cancer Res 48:7298–7303.

BLOT WJ, HARRINGTON JM, TOLEDO A, et al. 1978. Lung cancer after employment in shipyards during World War II. N Engl J Med 299:620–624.

BLOT WJ, MORRIS LE, STROUBE R, et al. 1980. Lung and laryngeal cancers in relation to shipyard employment in coastal Virginia. J Natl Cancer Inst 65:571–575.

BLOT WJ, FRAUMENI JF. 1981. Cancer among shipyard workers. Banbury Rpt 9:37–46.

BLOT WJ, FRAUMENI JF. 1982. Changing patterns of lung cancer in the United States. Am J Epidemiol 115:664–673.

BLOT WJ, DAVIES JE, BROWN LM, et al. 1982b. Occupation and the high risk of lung cancer in northeast Florida. Cancer 50:364–371.

BLOT WJ, BROWN LM, POTTERN LM, et al. 1983. Lung cancer among long-term steel workers. Am J Epidemiol 117:706–716.

BLOT WJ, AKIBA S, KATO H. 1984. Ionizing radiation and lung cancer: a review including preliminary results from a case-control study among A-bomb survivors. In Prentice R, Thampson D (eds): Atomic Bomb Survivor Data. Philadelphia: SIAM, pp. 235–248.

BLOT WJ, ZU ZY, BOICE JD, et al. 1990. Indoor radon and lung cancer in China. J Natl Cancer Inst 82:1025–1030.

BLOT WJ, FRAUMENI JF, JR. 1994. Arsenic and lung cancer. In Samet J (ed): The Epidemiology of Lung Cancer. New York: Marcell Dekker, pp. 207–218.

BLOT WJ, LI JY, TAYLOR PR, et al. 1994. Lung cancer and vitamin supplementation. N Engl J Med 331:614.

BOFFETTA P, SARACEI R, ANDERSEN A, et al. 1992. Lung cancer mortality among workers in the European production of man made mineral fibers—a Poisson regression analysis. Scand J Work Environ Health 18:279–284.

BOICE JD, FRAUMENI JF. 1980. Late effects following isoniazid therapy. Am J Public Health 70:987.

BOND GC, THOMPSON FE, COOK RR. 1987. Dietary vitamin A and lung cancer: Results of a case-control study among chemical workers. Nutr Cancer 9:109–121.

BOTHA JL, IRWIG LM, STREBEL PM. 1986. Excess mortality from stomach cancer, lung cancer, and asbestosis and/or mesothelioma in crocidolite mining districts in South Africa. Am J Epidemiol 123:30–40.

BROOKS SM, STOCKWELL HG, PINKHAM PA. 1992. Sugarcane exposure and risk of lung cancer and mesothelioma. Environ Res 58:195–203.

BROWN CC, CHU KS. 1983. Implications of the multistage theory of carcinogenesis applied to occupational arsenic exposure. J Natl Cancer Inst 70:455–462.

BROWN CC, KESSLER LG. 1988. Projections of lung cancer mortality in the United States: 1985–2025. J Natl Cancer Inst 80:45–51.

BROWN LM, POTTERN LM, BLOT WJ. 1984. Lung cancer in relation to environmental pollutants emitted from industrial sources. Environ Res 34:250–261.

BROWNE K, GOFFE T. 1984. Mesothelioma due to domestic exposure to asbestos. Br Med J 289:110.

BROWNE K. 1991. Asbestos related malignancy and the Cairns hypothesis. Br J Ind Med 48:73–76.

BROWNSON RC, ALVANJA MC, HOOK ET, et al. 1992. Passive smoking and lung cancer in nonsmoking women. Am J Public Health 82:1525–1530.

BRYANT MS, VINEIS P, SKIPPER P, et al. 1988. Hemoglobin adducts of aromatic amines: associations with smoking status and type of tobacco. Proc Natl Acad Sci USA 85:9788–9791.

BUFFLER PA, WOOD S, EIFLER C, et al. 1979. Mortality experience of workers in a vinyl chloride monomer production plant. J Occup Med 21:195–203.

BYERS TE, GRAHAM S, HAUGHEY BP, et al. 1987. Diet and lung cancer risk: Findings from the Western New York Diet Study. Am J Epidemiol 125:351–363.

CANDELORA EC, STOCKWELL HG, ARMSTRONG AW, et al. 1992. Dietary intake and risk of lung cancer in women who never smoked. Nutr Cancer 17:263–270.

CAPORASO NE, TUCKER MA, HOOVER RN, et al. 1990. Lung cancer and the debrisoquine metabolic phenotype. J Natl Cancer Inst 82:1264–1272.

CARSTENSEN JM, WICKSELL L, EKLUND G, et al. 1988. Lung cancer incidence among Swedish bakers and pastry cooks: temporal variation. Scand J Soc Med 16:81–85.

CARSTENSEN JHM, PERSHAGEN G, EKLUND G. 1987. Mortality in relation to cigarette and pipe smoking: 16 years observation in 25,000 Swedish men. J Epidemiol Community Health 41:166–172.

CARTA P, COCCO PL, CASULA D. 1991. Mortality from lung cancer among Sardinian patients with silicosis. Br J Ind Med 48:122–129.

CHECKOWAY H, MATHEW RM, HICKEY J, et al. 1985. Mortality among workers in the Florida phosphate industry. J Occup Med 27:855–896.

CHEN JL, WALRATH J, O'BERG MT, et al. 1987. Cancer incidence and mortality among workers exposed to acrylonitrile. Am J Ind Med 11:157–163.

CHEN C, CHUANG Y, YOU S, et al. 1986. A retrospective study on malignant neoplasm of bladder, lung, and liver in blackfoot disease endemic area in Taiwan. Br J Cancer 53:399–405.

CHURG AM, WARNOCK ML. 1979. Numbers of asbestos bodies in urban patients with lung cancer and gastrointestinal cancer and in matched controls. Chest 76:143–149.

CICALA C, POMPETTI F, CARBONE M. 1993. SV40 induces mesotheliomas in hamsters. Am J Pathol. 142:1524–1533.

CLARKE RH, SOUTHWOOD TRE. 1989. Risks from ionizing radiation. Nature 338:197–198.

COCHRANE JC, WEBSTER I. 1978. Mesothelioma in relation to asbestos fibre exposure: A review of 70 serial cases. S Afr Med J 54:279–281.

COGHLIN J, GANN PH, HAMMOND SK, et al. 1991. 4-aminobiphenyl hemoglobin adducts in fetuses exposed to tobacco smoke carcinogen in utero. J Natl Cancer Inst 83:274–280.

COGGON D, PANNETT B, PIPPARD EC, et al. 1989. Lung cancer in the meat industry. Br J Ind Med 46:188–191.

COHEN BH, DIAMOND EL, GRAVES CG, et al. 1977. A common familial component in lung cancer and chronic obstructive pulmonary disease. Lancet 2:523–526.

COLDITZ GA, STAMPFER MJ, WILLET WC. 1987. Diet and lung cancer: a review of the epidemiologic evidence in humans. Arch Intern Med 147:157–160.

COLLINGWOOD KW, PASTERNACK BS, SHORE RE. 1987. An industry-wide study of respiratory cancer in chemical workers exposed to chloromethyl ethers. J Natl Cancer Inst 78:1127–1131.

COLLINS JC, PAGE LC, CAPOROSSI JC, et al. 1989. Mortality patterns among employees exposed to acrylonitrile. J Occup Med 31:368–371.

COMSTOCK G, BUSH T, HELZLSOUER K. 1992. Serum retinol, beta-carotene, vitamin E, and selenium as related to subsequent cancer of specific sites. Am J Epidemiol 135:115–121.

CONNELLY RR, SPIRTAS R, MYERS MH, et al. 1987. Demographic patterns for mesothelioma in the United States. J Natl Cancer Inst 78:1053–1060.

COOMBS GF. 1989. Selenium. In Moon TE, Micozi MS (eds): Nutrition and Cancer Prevention. New York: Marcell Dekker, pp. 389–420.

COOPER WC. 1976. Cancer mortality patterns in the lead industry. Ann NY Acad Sci 271:250–259.

CORREA P, PICKLE LW, FONTHAM E, et al. 1983. Passive smoking and lung cancer. Lancet 2:595–597.

COTE RJ, JHANWAR SC, NOVICK S, et al. 1991. Genetic alterations of the p53 gene are a feature of malignant mesotheliomas. Cancer Res 51:5410–5416.

COULTAS DB. 1994. Other occupational carcinogens. In Samet JM (ed): Epidemiology of lung cancer. New York: Marce I Dekker, pp. 299–333.

CUZIK J, SASIENI D, EVANS S. 1992. Ingested arsenic, keratoses and bladder cancer. Am J Epidemiol 136:417–421.

DAMBER LA, LARSSON LG. 1987. Lung cancer in males and type of dwelling: and epidemiologic pilot study. Acta Oncol 20:211–215.

DARTIGUES JF, DABIS F, GROS N, et al. 1990. Dietary vitamin A, beta carotene and risk of epidermoid lung cancer in southern western France. Eur J Epidemiol 6:261–265.

DAVIS JM. 1986. The pathogenicity of long versus short fibre samples of amosite. Br J Exp Pathol 67:415–430.

DELZELL E, MONSON RR. 1982. Mortality among rubber workers: VI. Men with potential exposure to acrylonitrile. J Occup Med 24:767–769.

DESTEFANI E, CORREA P, FIERRO L, et al. 1993. The effect of alcohol on the risk of lung cancer in Uruguay. Cancer Epidemiol Biomarkers Prev 2:21–26.

DEVESA SS, BLOT WJ, FRAUMENI JF. 1989. Declining lung cancer among young men and women in the United States: a cohort analysis. J Natl Cancer Inst 81:1568–1571.

DEVESA SS, SHAW GL, BLOT JW. 1991. Changing patterns of lung cancer incidence by histologic type. Cancer Epidemiol Biomarkers Prev 1:29–34.

DOLL R, HILL AB. 1952. A study of the aetiology of carcinoma of the lung. Br Med J 2:1271–1286.

DOLL R. 1955. Mortality from lung cancer in asbestos workers. Br J Ind Med 12:81–86.

DOLL R, VESSEY MP, BEASLEY RW, et al. 1972. Mortality of gas workers—final report of a prospective study. Br J Ind Med 29:394–406.

DOLL R, PETO R, WHEATLEY K, et al. 1994. Mortality in relation to smoking: 40 years' observations on male British doctors. Br Med J 309:901–911.

DOLL R, MATHEWS JD, MORGAN LG. 1977. Cancers of the lung and nasal sinuses in nickel workers: A reassessment of the period of risk. Br J Ind Med 34:102–105.

DOLL R. 1978. Atmospheric pollution and lung cancer. Environ Health Perspect 22:23–31.

DOLL R, PETO R. 1978. Cigarette smoking and bronchial carcinoma: dose and time relationships among regular smokers and lifelong nonsmokers. J Epidemiol Community Health 32:303–313.

DOLL R, GRAY R, HAFNER B, et al. 1980. Mortality in relation to smoking: 22 years' observations on female British doctors. Br Med J 1:967–971.

DOLL R, PETO R. 1981. The causes of cancer: quantitative estimates of avoidable risks of cancer in the United States today. J Natl Cancer Inst.

DOLL R, PETO J. 1985. Asbestos. Effects on health of exposure to asbestos. Merseyside: HMSO.

DOLL R. 1990. Report of the International Committee on Nickel Carcinogenesis in Man. Scand J Work Environ Health 16:1–82.

DOLL R. 1982. Cadmium in the human environment. In Nordberg GF, Hesber R, Alessio L (eds): Cadmium in the Human Environment: Toxicity and Carcinogenicity. Lyon: IARC, pp. 459–464.

DONG MH, REDMOND CK, MAZUMDAR S, et al. 1988. A multistage approach to the cohort analysis of lifetime lung cancer risk among steelworkers exposed to coke oven emissions. Am J Epidemiol 128:860–873.

DRINKARD CK, SELLERS TA, POTTER JD, et al. 1995. Association of body mass index and body fat distribution with risk of lung cancer in older women. Am J Epidemiol 142:600–607.

EASTON DF, PETO J, DOLL R. 1988. Cancers of the respiratory tract in mustard gas workers. Br J Ind Med 45:652–659.

ENTERLINE PE. 1982. Importance of sequential exposure in the production of epichlorhydrin and isopropanol. Ann NY Acad Sci 381:344–349.

ENTERLINE PE, SYKORA JL, KELETI G, et al. 1985. Endotoxins, cotton dust, and cancer. Lancet 2:934–935.

ENTERLINE PE, MARSH GM, ESMEN NA, et al. 1987. Some effects of cigarette smoking, arsenic and SO^2 on mortality among US copper smelter workers. J Occup Med 29:831–838.

ENTERLINE PE. 1990. Role of manmade mineral fibers in the causation of cancer. Br J Ind Med 47:145–146.

ENVIRONMENTAL PROTECTION AGENCY. 1992. Respiratory health effects of passive smoking: lung cancer and other disorders. Washington: EPA.

FIORE MC, NOVOTNY TE, PIERCE JP, et al. 1989. Trends in cigarette smoking in the United States: The changing influence of gender and race. JAMA 261:49–55.

FLEJTER WL, LI FP, ANTMAN KH, et al. 1989. Recurring loss involving chromosomes 1, 3, and 22 in malignant mesothelioma. Genes Chromosom Cancer 1:148–154.

FONTANA RS. 1986. Screening for lung cancer: recent experience in the United States. In Hansen H (ed): Lung Cancer: Basic and Clinical Aspects. Boston: Martinus Nijhoff Pub, pp. 91–111.

FONTHAM ET, PICKLE LW, HAENSZEL W, et al. 1988. Dietary vitamins A and C and lung cancer risk in Louisiana. Cancer 62:2267–2273.

FONTHAM ET, CORREA P, REYNOLDS P, et al. 1994. Environmental tobacco smoke and lung cancer in nonsmoking women: a multicenter study. JAMA 271:1752–1759.

FORASTIERE F, LAGORIO S, MICHELOZZI P, et al. 1989. Mortality pattern of silicotic subjects in the Latium region, Italy. Br J Ind Med 46:877–880.

FRAUMENI JF, MASON TJ. 1974. Cancer mortality among Chinese Americans, 1950–69. J Natl Cancer Inst 52:659–665.

FRAUMENI JF, WERTELECKI W, BLATTNER WA, et al. 1975. Varied manifestations of a familial lymphoproliferative disorder. Am J Med 59:45–151.

FRAUMENI JF, BLOT WJ. 1982. Lung and Pleura. In Schottenfeld D, Fraumeni JF (eds): Cancer Epidemiology and prevention. Philadelphia: Saunders, pp. 564–582.

FRASER GE, BEESON WL, PHILLIPS RL. 1991. Diet and lung cancer in California Seventh Day Adventists. Am J Epidemiol 133:683–693.

FREEDMAN DA, NAVIDI WC. 1990. Ex-smokers and the multistage model for lung cancer. Epidemiol 1:21–29.

FRIBERG L, CEDERLOF R. 1978. Late effects of air pollution with special reference to lung cancer. Environ Health Perspect 22:45–66.

FRIEDMAN G, BLANER W, GOODMAN D, et al. 1986. Serum retinol and retinol-binding protein do not predict subsequent lung cancer. Am J Epidemiol 123:781–789.

GAENSLER EA. 1992. Asbestos exposure in buildings. Clin Chest Med 13:231–242.

GAO YT, BLOT WJ, ZHENG W, et al. 1987. Lung cancer among Chinese women. Int J Cancer 40:604–609.

GAO YT, BLOT WJ, ZHENG W, et al. 1988. Lung cancer and smoking in Shanghai. Int J Epidemiol 17:277–280.

GARDINER A, FOREY Z, LEE P. 1992. Avian exposure and bronchogenic carcinoma. Br Med J 305:989–992.

GARDNER MJ, ACHESON ED, WINTER RD. 1982. Mortality from mesothelioma of the pleura during 1968–1978 in England and Wales. Br J Cancer 46:81–88.

GARFINKEL L. 1981. Time trends in lung cancer mortality among non-smokers and a note on passive smoking. J Natl Cancer Inst 66:1061–1066.

GARFINKEL L, AUERBACH O, JOUBERT I. 1985. Involuntary smoking and lung cancer: A case-control study. J Natl Cancer Inst 79:463–469.

GARFINKEL L, STELLMAN SD. 1988. Smoking and lung cancer in women: findings in a prospective study. Cancer Res 48:6951–6955.

GARSHICK E, SCHENKER M, MUNOZ A, et al. 1988. A retrospective cohort study of lung cancer and diesel exhaust exposure in railroad workers. Am Rev Respir Dis 137:820–825.

GERIN M, SIEMIATYEKI J, NADON L, et al. 1989. Cancer risks due to occupational exposure to formaldehyde: results of a multi-site case-control study in Montreal. Int J Cancer 44:53–58.

GIARELLI L, BIANCHI C, GRANDI G. 1992. Malignant mesothelioma of the pleura in Trieste, Italy. Am J Ind Med 22:521–530.

GOLDSMITH DF, WINN DM, SHY CM (EDS). 1986. Silica, Silicosis, and Cancer: Controversy in Occupational Medicine. New York: Praeger.

GOODMAN MT, KOLONEL LN, YOSHIZAWA CN, et al. 1989. The effect of dietary cholesterol and fat on the risk of lung cancer in Hawaii. Am J Epidemiol 128:1241–1255.

GOODMAN MT, WILKENS LR. 1993. Relation of body size and risk of lung cancer. Nutr Cancer 20:179–186.

GOWERS DS, DEFONSO LR, SCHAFFER P, et al. 1993. Incidence of respiratory cancer among workers exposed to chloromethyl-ethers. Am J Epidemiol 137:31–42.

GREENBERG M, LLOYD DAVIES TA. 1974. Mesothelioma register 1967–68. Br J Ind Med 31:91–104.

GREENE MH, HOOVER RN, FRAUMENI JF, JR. 1978. Subsequent cancer in patients with chronic lymphocytic leukemia. A possible immunologic mechanism. J Natl Cancer Inst 61:337–340.

GREGOR A, LEE PN, ROE FJ, et al. 1980. Comparison of dietary histories in lung cancer cases and controls with special reference to vitamin A. Nutr Cancer 2:93–97.

GRUNDY GW, MILLER RW. 1972. Malignant mesothelioma in childhood: Report of 13 cases. Cancer 30:1216–1218.

HALPERN MT, GILLESPIE BW, WARNER KE. 1993. Patterns of absolute risk of lung cancer mortality in former smokers. J Natl Cancer Inst 85:457–464.

HAMMAR ST, BROCKUS D, REMINGTON F, et al. 1989. Familial mesothelioma: a report of two families. Hum Pathol 20:107–112.

HAMMOND EC. 1966. Smoking in relation to the death rates of one million men and women. Natl Cancer Inst Monogr 19:127–204.

HAMMOND EC, GARFINKEL L. 1980. General air pollution and cancer in the United States. Prev Med 9:206–211.

HAMMOND SK, COGHLIN J, GANN P, et al. 1993. Relationship between environmental tobacco smoke exposure and carcinogen-hemoglobin adduct levels in nonsmokers. J Natl Cancer Inst 85:474–478.

HANSEN ES. 1989. Cancer incidence in an occupational cohort exposed to bitumen fumes. Scand J Work Environ Health 15:101–105.

HARRIS CC, VAHAKANGAS K, NEWMAN M, et al. 1985. Detection of benzoapryene diol epoxide-DNA adducts in peripheral blood lymphocytes and antibodies to the adducts in serum from coke oven workers. Proc Natl Acad Sci 82:6672–6876.

HARRIS JE. 1983. Cigarette smoking among successive birth cohorts of men and women in the United States during 1900–1980. J Natl Cancer Inst 71:473–479.

HECKBERT SR, WEISS NS, HORNUNG SK, et al. 1992. Glutathione S-transferase and epoxide hydrolase activity in human leukocytes in relation to the risk of lung and other smoking-related cancers. J Natl Cancer Inst 84:414–422.

HENDERSON BE, KOLONEL LN, DWORSKY R, et al. 1985. Cancer incidence in the islands of the Pacific. Natl Cancer Inst Monogr 69:78–82.

HENNEKENS CH, BURING JE, MANSON JE, et al. 1996. Lack of effect of long-term supplementation with beta carotene on the incidence of malignant neoplasms and cardiovascular disease. N Engl J Med 334:1145–1149.

HESSEL PA, SLUIS-CREMER GK, HNIZDO E. 1990. Silica exposure, silicosis, and lung cancer: a necropsy study. Br J Ind Med 49:4–9.

HILL AB, FANNING EL. 1948. Studies in the incidence of cancer in a factory handling inorganic compounds of arsenic. I. Mortality experience in the factory. Br J Ind Med 5:1–15.

HINDS MW, KOLONEL LN, HANKIN JH, et al. 1984. Dietary vitamin A, carotene, vitamin C and risk of lung cancer in Hawaii. Am J Epidemiol 119:227–237.

HINDS MW, KOLONEL LN, LEE J, et al. 1987. Dietary cholesterol and lung cancer risk among men in Hawaii. Am J Clin Nutr 37:192–193.

HIRAYAMA T. 1979. Diet and cancer. Nutr Cancer 1:67–81.

HIRAYAMA T. 1981. Non-smoking wives of heavy smokers have a higher risk of lung cancer: A study from Japan. Br Med J 282:183–185.

HIRVONEN K, HUSGAFVEL-PURSIANEN K, KARJALAINEN A, et al. 1992. Point mutational Msp1 and 11e-Vallpolymophisms closely linked to the CYP 1A1 gene: lack of association with susceptibility to lung cancer in a Finnish study population. Cancer Epidemiol Biomarkers Prev 1:485–489.

HOFMANN J, MINTZER D, WARHOL M, et al. 1994. Malignant mesothelioma following radiation therapy. Am J Med 97:379–382.

HOFFMANN D, HECHT S. 1985. Nicotine-derived N-nitrosamines and tobacco-related cancer: current status and future directions. Cancer Res 45:935–944.

HOLST PA, KROMHOUT D, BRAND R. 1988. Pet birds as an independent risk factor for lung cancer. Br Med J 297:1319–1321.

HOOVER R, FRAUMENI JF, JR. 1973. Risk of cancer in renal-transplant recipients. Lancet 2:55–57.

HORNUNG RW, MEINHARDT TJ. 1987. Quantitative risk assessment of lung cancer in U.S. uranium miners. Health Phys 52:417–430.

HOROWITZ I, ENTERLINE PE. 1970. Lung cancer among the Jews. Am J Public Health 60:275–282.

HORWITZ RI, SMALDONE LF, VISCOLI CM. 1988. An ecogenetic hypothesis for lung cancer in women. Arch Intern Med 148:2609–2612.

HOWE GR, FRASER D, LINDSAY J, et al. 1983. Cancer mortality (1965–1967) in relation to diesel fume and coal exposure in a cohort of retired railway workers. J Natl Cancer Inst 70:1015–1019.

HOWE GR, NAIR RC, NEWCOMBE HB, et al. 1986. Lung cancer mortality (1950–80) in relation to radon daughter exposure in a cohort of workers at the Eldorado Beaverlodge uranium mine. J Natl Cancer Inst 77:357–362.

HUGHES JM, WEILL H. 1991. Asbestosis as a precursor of asbestos related lung cancer: results of a prospective mortality study. Br J Ind Med 48:229–233.

HUGHES JM, WEILL H. 1994. Asbestos and man-made fibers. In Samet JM (ed): Epidemiology of Lung Cancer. New York: Marcell Dekker, pp. 185–205.

IARC. 1977. Asbestos. Monographs on the Evaluation of Carcinogenic Risk of Chemicals to Man, Vol. 14. Lyon: International Agency for Research on Cancer.

IARC. 1981. Wood, leather, and some associated industries. Monographs on the Evaluation of Carcinogenic Risk of Chemicals to Man, Vol. 55. Lyon: International Agency for Research on Cancer.

IARC. 1982. Some industrial chemicals and dye stuffs. Monographs on the Evaluation of Carcinogenic Risk of Chemicals to Man, Vol. 29. Lyon: International Agency for Research on Cancer.

IARC. 1983. Polynuclear aromatic hydrocarbons. Monographs on the Evaluation of Carcinogenic Risk of Chemicals to Man, Vol. 34. Lyon: International Agency for Research on Cancer.

IARC. 1986. Tobacco smoking: Monographs on the Evaluation of Carcinogenic Risk of Chemicals to Man, Vol. 38. Lyon: International Agency for Research on Cancer.

IARC. 1987a. Overall evaluations of carcinogenicity: Monographs for Research to Man, Supplement 7. Lyon: International Agency for Research on Cancer.

IARC. 1987b. Silica and some silicates. Monographs on the Evaluation of Carcinogenic Risk of Chemicals to Man, Vol. 42. Lyon: International Agency for Research on Cancer.

IARC. 1988a. Man-made mineral fibres and radon. Monographs on the Evaluation of Carcinogenic Risk of Chemicals to Man, Vol. 43. Lyon: International Agency for Research on Cancer.

IARC. 1988b. Alcohol drinking. Monographs on the Evaluation of Carcinogenic Risk of Chemicals to Man, Vol. 43. Lyon: International Agency for Research on Cancer.

IARC. 1989a. Occupational exposures in petroleum refining; crude oil and major petroleum fuels. Monographs on the Evaluation of Carcinogenic Risk of Chemicals to Man, Vol. 45. Lyon: International Agency for Research on Cancer.

IARC. 1989b. Diesel and gasoline exhausts and some nitroarenes. Monographs on the Evaluation of Carcinogenic Risk of Chemicals to Man, Vol. 46. Lyon: International Agency for Research on Cancer.

IARC. 1990. Chromium, nickel and molding. Monographs on the Evaluation of Carcinogenic Risk of Chemicals to Man, Vol. 49. Lyon: International Agency for Research on Cancer.

IARC. 1991. Occupational exposure in insecticide application and same pesticides. Monographs on the Evaluation of Carcinogenic Risk of Chemicals to Man, Vol. 53. Lyon: International Agency for Research on Cancer.

IARC. 1992. Occupational exposures to mists and vapors from strong inorganic acids. Monographs on the Evaluation of Carcinogenic Risk of Chemicals to Man, Vol. 54. Lyon: International Agency for Research on Cancer.

IARC. 1995. Wood Dust and Formaldehyde. Evaluation of Carcinogenic Risk of Chemicals to Humans, vol 62, Lyon, International Agency for Research on Cancer.

ILGREN EB, WAGNER JC. 1990. Background incidence of mesothelioma: animal and human evidence. Regul Toxicol Pharmocol 13:133–149.

INFANTE-RIVARD C, ARMSTRONG B, PETITCLERC M, et al. 1989. Lung cancer mortality and silicosis in Quebec, 1938–85. Lancet 2:1504–1507.

INFANTE PC, SCHUMAN L, DEMENT J, et al. 1994. Fibrous glass and cancer. Am J Ind Med 26:559–584.

JAIN M, BURCH J, HOWE G, et al. 1990. Dietary factors and risk of lung cancer: results from a case-control study, Toronto, 1982–1985. Int J Cancer 45:287–293.

JANERICH DT, THOMPSON WD, VARELA LR, et al. 1990. Lung cancer and exposure to tobacco smoke in the household. N Engl J Med 323:632–636.

JARUP L, PERSHAGEN G, WALL G. 1989. Cumulative arsenic exposure and lung cancer in smelter workers: a dose-response study. Am J Ind Med 15:31–41.

JARUP L, PERSHAGEN G. 1991. Arsenic exposure, smoking, and lung cancer in smelter workers: a case-control study. Am J Epidemiol 134:545–551.

JEDRYCHOWSKI W, BEECHER H, WAHRENDORF J, et al. 1990. A case-control study of lung cancer with special reference to the effect of air pollution in Poland. J Epidemiol Community Health 44:114–120.

JOLY OG, LUBIN JH, CARABALLOSO M. 1983. Dark tobacco and lung cancer in Cuba. J Natl Cancer Inst 70:1033–1039.

KABAT GC, HEBERT JR. 1991. Use of mentholated cigarettes and lung cancer risk. Cancer Res 51:6510–6514.

KABAT GC, WYNDER EL. 1992. Body mass index and lung cancer risk. Am J Epidemiol 135:769–774.

KAISERMAN M, ROGERS B. 1991. Tobacco consumption declining faster in Canada than in the U.S.: Am J Public Health 81:902–904.

KAKRI NT, POKELA R, NUUTINEN L, et al. 1987. Aryl hydrocarbon hydroxylase in lymphocytes and lung tissue from lung cancer patients and controls. Int J Cancer 39:565–570.

KALANDIDI A, KATSOUYANNI K, VOROPOULOU N, ET AL. 1990. Passive smoking and diet in the etiology of lung cancer among non-smokers. Cancer Causes Control 1:15–21.

KANE MJ, CHAHINIAN AP, HOLLAND JF. 1990. Malignant mesothelioma in young adults. Cancer 65:1449–1455.

KAUFMAN DW, PALMER JR, ROSENBERG L, et al. 1989. Tar content of cigarettes in relation to lung cancer. Am J Epidemiol 129:703–711.

KELLERMANN G, SHAW CR, LUYTEN-KELLERMANN M. 1973. Aryl hydrocarbon hydroxylase inducibility and bronchogenic carcinoma. N Engl J Med 289:934–937.

KIPEN HM, LILIS R, SUZUKI Y, et al. 1987. Pulmonary fibrosis in asbestos insulation workers with lung cancer: a radiological histopathological evaluation. Br J Ind Med 44:96–100.

KIPLING MD, WALDRON HA. 1976. Polycyclic aromatic hydrocarbons in mineral oil, tar, and pitch, excluding petroleum pitch. Prev Med 5:262–278.

KISHIMOTO T, SATO T, ONO T, et al. 1989. Malignant mesothelioma in Kure City, Japan: The relationship to asbestos exposure. Cancer Invest 7:407–410.

KOLONEL L. 1993. Lung cancer: another consequence of a high-fat diet? J Natl Cancer Inst 85:1886–1887.

KNEKT P, AROMAA A, MAATELA JS, et al. 1990. Serum selenium and subsequent risk of cancer among Finnish men and women. J Natl Cancer Inst 82:864–868.

KNEKT P, JARVINEN R, SEPPANEN R, et al. 1991. Dietary antioxidants and risk of lung cancer. Am J Epidemiol 134:471–479.

KOHLMEIER L, ARMINGER B, BARTOLOMEYCIK S, et al. 1992. Pet birds as an independent risk factor for lung cancer: case-control study. Br Med J 305:988–989.

KOK K, OSINGA J, SCHOTANUS DC, et al. 1989. Amplification and expression of different myc-family genes in a tumor specimen and 3 cell lines derived from one small-cell lung cancer patient during longitudinal follow-up. Int J Cancer 44:75–78.

KOO LC, HO JH, SAW D. 1984. Is passive smoking an added risk factor for lung cancer in Chinese women? J Exp Clin Cancer Res 3:277–283.

KOO LC. 1988. Dietary habits and lung cancer risk among Chinese females in Hong Kong who never smoked. Nutr Cancer 11:155–173.

KURIHARA M, AOKI K, HISAMICHI S. 1989. Cancer Mortality Statistics in the World, 1950–1985. Nagoya: Nagoya University Press.

KVALE G, BJELKE E, GART JJ. 1983. Dietary habits and lung cancer risk. Int J Cancer 31:397–405.

LAM TH, KUNG IT, WONG EM, et al. 1987. Smoking passive smoking and histological types of lung cancer in Hong Kong chinese women. Br J Cancer 56:673–679.

LANGARD S, ANDERSEN A, GYLSETH B. 1980. Incidence of cancer among ferrochromium and ferrosilicon workers. Br J Ind Med 37:114–120.

LANGARD S. 1990. One hundred years of chromium and cancer: a review of epidemiological evidence and selected case reports. Am J Ind Med 17:189–315.

LASKIN S, DREW RT, CAPPIELLO V, et al. 1975. Inhalation carcinogenicity of alpha halo ethers. Arch Environ Health 30:70–72.

LAW MR, GREGOR A, HODSON ME, et al. 1984. Malignant mesothelioma of the pleura: a study of 52 treated and 64 untreated patients. Thorax 39:255–259.

LAW MR. 1989. Genetic predisposition to lung cancer. Br Med J.

LEE AM, FRAUMENI JF, JR. 1969. Arsenic and respiratory cancer in man: An occupational study. J Natl Cancer Inst 42:1045–1052.

LEE-FELDSTEIN A. 1986. Cumulative exposure to arsenic and its relationship to respiratory cancer among copper smelter employees. J Occup Med 28:296–302.

LEES RE, STEELE R, ROBERTS JH. 1987. A case-control study of lung cancer relative to domestic radon exposure. Int J Epidemiol 16:7–12.

LEGARDEUR BY, LOPEZ A, JOHNSON WD. 1991. A case-control study of serum vitamin A, E, and C in lung cancer patients. Nutr Cancer 14:133–140.

LEHMAN TA, BENNETT WP, METCALF RA, et al. 1991. p53 mutations, ras mutations, and p53-heat shock to protein complexes in human lung carcinoma cell lines. Cancer Res 51:4090–4096.

LEMARCHAND L, YOSHIZAWA CN, KOLONEL LN, et al. 1989. Vegetable consumption and lung cancer risk: a population-based case-control study in Hawaii. J Natl Cancer Inst 81:1158–1164.

LEVIN ML, GOLDSTEIN H, GERHARDT PR. 1950. Cancer and tobacco smoking: A preliminary report. JAMA 143:336–338.

LEVIN LI, GAO YT, BLOT WJ, et al. 1987. Decreased risk of lung cancer in the cotton textile industry of Shanghai. Cancer Res 47:5777–5781.

LILIENFELD DE, MANDEL JS, COIN P, et al. 1988. Projection of asbestos related diseases in the United States, 1985–2009. Br J Med 45:283–291.

LLOYD JW. 1971. Long-term mortality study of steelworkers. V. Respiratory cancer in coke plant workers. J Morphol 13:53–68.

LUBIN JH, POTTERN LM, BLOT WJ, et al. 1981. Respiratory cancer among copper smelter workers: recent mortality statistics. J Occup Med 23:779–784.

LUBIN JH, BLOT WJ. 1984. Assessment of lung cancer risk factors by histologic category. J Natl Cancer Inst 73:383–389.

LUBIN JH, BLOT WJ, BERRINO F, et al. 1984a. Patterns of lung cancer risk according to type of cigarette smoked. Int J Cancer 33:569–576.

LUBIN JH, RICHTER BS, BLOT WJ. 1984b. Lung cancer risk with cigar and pipe use. J Natl Cancer Inst 73:377–381.

LUBIN JH, BOICE JD. 1989. Estimating Rn-induced lung cancer in the United States. Health Phys 57:417–427.

LUBIN JH, QIAO TL, TAYLOR PR, et al. 1990. Quantitative evaluation of the radon and lung cancer association in a case-control study of Chinese tin miners. Cancer Res 50:174–180.

LYON JL, KLAUBER MR, GARDNER JW, et al. 1976. Cancer incidence in Mormons and non-Mormons in Utah, 1966–1970. N Engl J Med 294:129–133.

MABUCHI K, LILIENFELD AM, SNELL LM. 1980. Cancer and occupational exposure to arsenic: A study of pesticide workers. Prev Med 9:51–77.

MACHLE W, GREGORIUS F. 1948. Cancer of the respiratory system in the United States chromate-producing industry. Public Health Rep 63:1114–1127.

MACLENNAN R, DA COSTA J, DAY NE, et al. 1977. Risk factors for lung cancer in Singapore Chinese, a population with high female incidence rates. Int J Cancer 20:854–860.

MACLURE M, KATZ RB, BRYANT MS, et al. 1989. Elevated blood levels of carcinogens in passive smokers. Am J Public Health 79:1381–1384.

MALKER H, MCLAUGHLIN JK, MALKER B, et al. 1985. Occupational risks for pleural mesothelioma in Sweden, 1961–79. J Natl Cancer Inst 74:61–66.

MANCUSO T. 1988. Relative risk of mesotheliomas among railroad workers exposed to chrysotile. Am J Ind Med 15:353–356.

MARCUS AC, SHOPLAND DR, CRANE LA, et al. 1989. Prevalence of cigarette smoking in the United States: estimates from the 1985 Current Population Survey. J Natl Cancer Inst 81:409–414.

MASON TJ, MCKAY FW, HOOVER RN, et al. 1975. Atlas of cancer mortality for U.S. counties: 1950–1969. Washington, D.C.: USHDEW.

MCDONALD JC, MCDONALD AD. 1977. Epidemiology of mesothelioma from estimated incidence. Prev Med 6:426–446.

MCDONALD AD. 1979. Mesothelioma registries in identifying asbestos hazards. Ann NY Acad Sci 330:441–454.

MCDONALD AD, MCDONALD JC. 1987. Epidemiology of malignant mesothelioma. In Antman K, Aisner T (eds): Asbestos-related Malignancy. Orlando: Grune and Straton, pp. 31–55.

MCDONALD JC, MCDONALD AD. 1987. Epidemiology of asbestos-related lung cancer. In Antman K, Aisner J (eds): Asbestos-related Malignancy. Orlando: Grune & Straton, pp. 57–79.

MCDUFFIE HH. 1991. Clustering of cancer in families of patients with primary lung cancer. J Clin Epidemiol 44:69–76.

MCLAUGHLIN JK, CHEN JC, DOSEMECI M, et al. 1992. A nested

case-control study of lung cancer among silica exposed workers in China. Br J Ind Med 49:167–171.

McLaughlin JK, Hrubec Z, Blot WJ, et al. 1995. Smoking and cancer mortality among US veterans: a 26-year followup. Int J Cancer 60:190–193.

McWilliams JE, Sanderson BS, Harris EL, et al. 1995. Glutathione S-Transferase M1 (GSTM1) deficiency and lung cancer risk. Cancer Epidemiol Biomarkers Prevention 4:589–594.

Menkes MS, Comstock GW, Vuilleumier JP, et al. 1986. Serum beta-carotene, vitamins A and E, selenium, and the risk of lung cancer. N Engl J Med 315:1250–1254.

Metcalf RA, Welsh JA, Bennett WP, et al. 1992. p53 and Kirsten-ras mutations in human mesothelioma cell lines. Cancer Res 52:2610–2615.

Mettlin C, Graham S, Swanson M. 1979. Vitamin A and lung cancer. J Natl Cancer Inst 62:1435–1438.

Mettlin C. 1989. Milk drinking, other beverage habits, and lung cancer risk. Int J Cancer 43:608–612.

Milham S, Demers R. 1984. Mortality among pulp and paper workers. J Occup Med 26:844–846.

Miller BA, Ries LAG, Hankey BF, et al. 1993. SEER Cancer Statistics Review 1973–1990. Bethesda, MD: NIH Pub. No. 93-2789.

Minowa M, Stone BJ, Blot WJ. 1988. Geographic patterns of lung cancer in Japan and its environmental correlations. Jpn J Cancer Res 79:1017–1023.

Mirvish S. 1983. The etiology of gastric cancer: intragastric nitrosamine formation and other theories. J Natl Cancer Inst 71:629–647.

Mitsudomi T, Steinberg SM, Okie HK, et al. 1991. Ras gene mutations in non small cell lung cancers are associated with shortened survival irrespective of treatment intent. Cancer Res 51:4999–5002.

Miura I, Graziano W, Cheng J, et al. 1992. Chromosome alterations in human small cell lung cancer: frequent involvement of 5q. Cancer Res 52:1322–1324.

Modan B. 1978. Population distribution of histological types of lung cancer: Epidemiologic aspects in Israel and review of the literature. Isr J Med Sci 14:771–784.

Monson RR, Fine LJ. 1978. Cancer mortality and morbidity among rubber workers. J Natl Cancer Inst 61:1047–1053.

Moolgavkar SH, Dewanji A, Luekbeck G. 1989. Cigarette smoking and lung cancer: reanalysis of the British doctors' data. J Natl Cancer Inst 81:415–420.

Morgan RW. 1992. Attitudes about asbestos and lung cancer. Am J Ind Med 22:437–441.

Morrison HI, Brand PR, Gallagher R, et al. 1984. Recent trends in incidence rates of pleural mesothelioma in British Columbia. Can Med Assoc J 131:1069–1071.

Mossman BT, Bignon J, Corn M, et al. 1990. Asbestos: scientific developments and implications for public policy. Science 247:294–301.

Moulin J, Wild P, Haguenoer J, et al. 1993. A mortality study among mild steel and stainless steel welders. Br J Ind Med 50:234–243.

Muir C, Waterhouse J, Mack T, et al. 1987. Cancer Incidence in Five Continents, Vol. V. Lyon: IARC.

Mulvihill JJ. 1976. Host factors in human lung tumors: An example of ecogenetics in oncology. J Natl Cancer Inst 57:3–7.

Mumford JL, He XZ, Chapman RS, et al. 1987. Lung cancer and indoor air pollution in Xuan Wei, China. Science 235:217–220.

Muscat J, Wynder EL. 1991. Cigarette smoking, asbestos exposure and malignant mesothelioma. Cancer Res 51:2263–2267.

Nakachi N, Imai K, Hayashi S, et al. 1991. Genetic susceptibility to squamous cell carcinoma of the lung in relation to cigarette smoking dose. Cancer Res 51:5177–5180.

National Cancer Institute. 1992. Cancer Statistics Review 1973–1989. Bethesda, MD: NCI.

National Research Council. 1979. Committee on Medical and Biologic Effects of Environmental Pollutants: Airborne Particles. Baltimore: University Park Press.

National Research Council. 1980. Committee on the Biological Effects of Ionizing Radiations: The effects on populations of exposure to low levels of radiation. Washington D.C.: National Academy of Science.

National Research Council. 1986. Environmental Tobacco Smoke. Washington, D.C.: National Academy Press.

National Research Council. 1988. Committee on the Biological Effects of Ionizing Radiations: Health risks of radon and other internally deposited alpha-emitters. Washington, D.C.: National Academy of Sciences.

Newhouse ML. 1977. The geographic pathology of mesothelial tumors. J Morphol 19:480–482.

Newhouse ML, Berry G, Wagner JC. 1985. Mortality of factory workers in east London, 1933–1980. Br J Ind Med 42:4–11.

Newhouse ML, Sullivan KR. 1989. A mortality study of workers manufacturing friction materials: 1941–86. Br J Ind Med 46:176–179.

Nomura A, Heilbrum L, Morris S, et al. 1987. Serum selenium and risk of cancer by specific cites: Case-control analysis of prospective data. J Natl Cancer Inst 79:103–108.

Nomura AMY, Stemmerman GN, Heilbrun LK, et al. 1985. Serum vitamin levels and the risk of cancer of specific sites in men of Japanese ancestry in Hawaii. Cancer Res 45:2369–2372.

Ng TP, Chan SL, Lee J. 1990. Mortality of a cohort of men in a silicosis register: further evidence of an association with lung cancer. Am J Ind Med 17:163–171.

Norman JE, Jr. 1975. Lung cancer mortality in World War I veterans with mustard-gas injury: 1919–1965. J Natl Cancer Inst 54:311–317.

Novotny TE, Warner KE, Kendrick JS, et al. 1989. Smoking by blacks and whites: socioeconomic and demographic differences. Am J Public Health 78:1187–1189.

O'Berg MT. 1980. Epidemiologic study of workers exposed to acrylonitrile. J Morphol 22:245–252.

Omenn GS, Goodman GE, Thornquist MD et al. 1996. Effects of a combination of beta carotene and vitamin A on lung cancer and cardiovascular disease. N Engl J Med 334:1150–1155.

Ooi WL, Elston RC, Chen VW, et al. 1986a. Increased familial risk for lung cancer. J Natl Cancer Inst 76:217–222.

Ooi WL, Elston RC, Chen VW, et al. 1986b. Familial lung cancer-correcting an error in calculation. J Natl Cancer Inst 77:990.

Osann KE. 1991. Lung cancer in women: importance of smoking, family history of cancer, and medical history of respiratory disease. Cancer Res 51:4893–4897.

Osburn HS. 1969. Lung cancer in a mining district in Rhodesia. S Afr Med J 43:1307–1312.

Ott MG, Holder BB, Gordon HL. 1974. Respiratory cancer and occupational exposure to arsenicals. Arch Environ Health 29:250–255.

Otte KE, Sigsgaard TI, Kjaerulff J. 1990. Malignant mesotheliomas clustering in a family producing asbestos cement in their home. Br J Ind Med 47:10–13.

Paganini-Hill A, Chao A, Ross RK, et al. 1987. Vitamin A, beta-carotene, and the risk of cancer: A prospective study. J Natl Cancer Inst 79:443–448.

Parkin DM, Muir CS, Whelon SL, et al. 1992. Cancer Incidence in Five Continents, Vol. VI. Lyon: IARC Sci Publ 120.

Pasternack BS, Shore RE, Albert RE. 1977. Occupational exposure to chloromethyl ethers. J Morphol 19:741–746.

Pastorino U, Pisani P, Berrino F, et al. 1987. Vitamin A and female lung cancer: A case-control study on plasma and diet. Nutr Cancer 10:171–179.

Pathak DR, Samet JM, Humble CG, et al. 1986. Determinants of lung cancer risk in cigarette smokers in New Mexico. J Natl Cancer Inst 76:597–604.

PERERA FP, HEMMINKI K, YOUNG TL, et al. 1988. Detection of polycyclic aromatic hydrocarbon-DNA adducts in white blood cells of foundry workers. Cancer Res 48:2288–2291.

PERSHAGEN G, WALL S, TAUBE A, et al. 1981. On the interaction between occupational arsenic exposure and smoking and its relation to lung cancer. Scand J Work Environ Health 7:302–309.

PERSHAGEN G. 1986. Lung cancer mortality among men living near an arsenic-emitting smelter. Am J Epidemiol 122:654–694.

PERSHAGEN G, HRUBEC Z, SVENSON C. 1987. Passive smoking and lung cancer in Swedish women. Am J Epidemiol 125:17–24.

PETERSON JT, GREENBERG SD, BUFFLER PA. 1984. Non-asbestos-related malignant mesothelioma. Cancer 54:951–960.

PETO J, HENDERSON BE, PIKE MC. 1981. Trends in mesothelioma incidence in the United States and the forecast epidemic due to asbestos exposure during World War II. Banbury Rpts 9:51–69.

PETO J, SEIDMAN H, SELIKOFF IJ. 1982. Mesothelioma mortality in asbestos workers: implications for models of carcinogenesis and risk assessment. Br J Cancer 45:124–135.

PHILLIPS RL, KUZMA JW, BEESON WL, et al. 1980. Influence of selection versus lifestyle on risk of fatal cancer and cardiovascular disease among Seventh-day Adventists. Am J Epidemiol 112:296–314.

PHILIP P, FITZGERALD D, CARTWRIGHT R, et al. 1988. Polymorphic N-acetylation capacity in lung cancer. Carcinogenesis 4:491–493.

PIERCE JP, FIORE MC, NOVOTNY TE, et al. 1989. Trends in cigarette smoking in the United States: Educational differences are increasing. JAMA 261:56–60.

PIERCE JP. 1989. International comparisons of trends in cigarette smoking prevalence. Am J Public Health 79:152–157.

PIERCE JP, BURNS DM, BERRY C, et al. 1991. Reducing tobacco consumption in California: Proposition 99 seems to work. JAMA 265:1257–1258.

PISANI P, BERRINO F, MACALUSO M, PASTORINO U, CROSIGNANI P, BALDASSERONI A. 1986. Carrots, green vegetables, and lung cancer: A case-control study. Int J Epidemiol 15:463–468.

PISANI RJ, COLBY TV, WILLIAMS DE. 1988. Malignant mesothelioma of the pleura. Mayo Clin Proc 63:1234–1244.

POTTER JD, SELLERS TA, FOLSON AR, et al. 1992. Alcohol, beer and lung cancer in postmenopausal women: The Iowa Women's Health study. Ann Epidemiol 2:557–595.

RADFORD EP, RENARD K. 1984. Lung cancer in Swedish iron miners exposed to low doses of radon daughters. N Engl J Med 310:1485–1494.

REDMOND CK. 1983. Cancer mortality among coke oven workers. Environ Health Perspect 52:67–73.

REGISTRAR GENERAL. 1978. Occupational Mortality. Decennial Supplement for England and Wales, 1970–1972. London: HMSO.

REYNOLDS P, KAPLAN G. 1987. Asthma and cancer. Am J Epidemiol 125:539–540.

RIBOLI E, PRESTON-MARTIN S, SARACCI R, et al. 1990. Exposure of nonsmoking women to environmental tobacco smoke: a 10-country collaborative study. Cancer Causes Control 1:243–252.

RIMINGTON J. 1971. Smoking, chronic bronchitis, and lung cancer. Br Med J 2:373–375.

ROBINSON C, WAXWEILER R, FOWLER D. 1986. Mortality among production workers in pulp and paper mills. Scand J Work Environ Health 12:522–560.

ROSCOE RJ, STEENLAND K, HALPERIN W, et al. 1989. Lung cancer mortality among non smoking uranium miners exposed to radon daughters. JAMA 262:629–633.

SACCOMANNO G. 1982. The contribution of uranium miners to lung cancer histogenesis. Recent Results Cancer Res 82:43–52.

SAKABE TT, MATSUSHITA H, KOSHI S. 1976. Cancer among benzol chloride manufacturing workers. Ann NY Acad Sci 271:67–70.

SAMET JM, KUTVIRT DM, WAXWEILER RJ, et al. 1984. Uranium mining and lung cancer in Navajo men. N Engl J Med 310:1481–1484.

SAMET JM, SKIPPER BJ, HUMBLE CG, et al. 1985. Lung cancer risk and vitamin A consumption in New Mexico. Am Rev Respir Dis 131:198–202.

SAMET JM, HUMBLE CG, PATHAK DR. 1986. Personal and family history of respiratory disease and lung cancer risk. Am Rev Respir Dis 134:466–470.

SAMET JM. 1989. Radon and lung cancer. J Natl Cancer Inst 81:745–757.

SANDEN A, JARVHOLM B, LARSSON S, et al. 1992. The risk of lung cancer and mesothelioma after cessation of asbestos exposure: a prospective study of shipyard workers. Eur Respir J 5:281–285.

SARACCI R. 1987. The interactions of tobacco smoking and other agents in cancer etiology. Epidemiol Rev 9:175–193.

SCHATZKIN A, HOOVER RN, TAYLOR PR, et al. 1988. Site-specific analysis of total serum cholesterol and incident cancer in the National Nutrition Examination Survey I Epidemiologic follow-up study. Cancer Res 48:452–458.

SCHIFFMAN MH, PICKLE LW, FONTHAM E, et al. 1988. Case-control study of diet and mesothelioma in Louisiana. Cancer Res 48:2911–2915.

SCHOENBERG JB, KLOTZ JB, WILCOX HB, et al. 1989. Lung cancer and exposure to radon in women in New Jersey. MMWR 42:715–718.

SCHWARTZ E. 1988. A proportionate mortality ratio analysis of pulp and paper workers in New Hampshire. Br J Ind Med 45:234–238.

SEBASTIAN P, MCDONALD JC, MCDONALS AC, et al. 1989. Respiratory cancer in chrysotile textile and mining industries: exposure inferences from lung analysis. Br J Ind Med 46:180–187.

SEIDMAN H, SELIKOFF IJ, HAMMOND EC. 1979. Short-term asbestos work exposure and long-term observation. Ann NY Acad Sci 330:61–90.

SEIDMAN H, SELIKOFF IJ. 1990. Decline in death rates among asbestos insulation workers 1967–86 associated with diminution of work exposure to asbestos. Ann NY Acad Sci 609:300–317.

SELIKOFF IJ. 1977. Cancer risk of asbestos exposure. In Hiatt HH, Watson JD, Winsten JA (eds): Origins of Human Cancer. Cold Spring Harbor, NY: Cold Spring Harbor Laboratory, pp. 1765–1784.

SELIKOFF IJ, HAMMOND EC, SEIDMAN H. 1979. Mortality experience of insulation workers in the United States and Canada, 1943–1976. Ann NY Acad Sci 330:91–116.

SELLERS TA, ELSTON RC, STEWART C, et al. 1988. Familial risk of cancer among randomly selected cancer probands. Genet Epidemiol 5:381–391.

SELLERS TA, BAILEY-WILSON J, ELSTON RC, et al. 1990. Evidence for Mendelian inherticance in the pathogenesis of lung cancer. J Natl Cancer Inst 82:1272–1279.

SHAW GL, FALK R, PICKLE LW, et al. 1991. Lung cancer risk associated with cancer in relatives. J Clin Epidemiol 44:429–437.

SHAW GL, FALK RT, DESLAURIERS J, et al. 1995. Debrisoquine metabolism and lung cancer risk. Cancer Epidemiol Biomarkers Prev 4:41–48.

SHEKELLE RB, LEPPER M, LIU S, et al. 1981. Dietary vitamin A and risk of cancer in the Western Electric Study. Lancet 2:1185–1190.

SHEKELLE RB, ROSSOF A, STAMLER J. 1991. Dietary cholesterol and incidence of lung cancer: the Western Electric Study. Am J Epidemiol 134:480–484.

SHERSON D, SVANE O, LYNGE E. 1991. Cancer incidence among foundry workers in Denmark. Arch Environ Health 46:75–81.

SHIBATA A, PAGANINI-HILL A, ROSS R, et al. 1992. Intake of vegetable, fruits, beta-carotene, vitamin C and supplements and cancer incidence among the elderly: a prospective study. Br J Cancer 68:673–679.

SIDNEY S, TEKAWN I, FRIEDMAN G. 1993. A prospective study of cigarette tar yield and lung cancer. Cancer Causes Control 4:3–10.

SIEDEGARD J, PERO PW, MILLER DG, et al. 1986. A glutathione

transferase in human leukocytes as a marker for the susceptibility to lung cancer. Carcinogenesis 7:751–753.

SIEMIATYCKI J, DEWAR R, LAKHANI R, et al. 1989. Cancer risks associated with 10 organic dusts: results from a case-control study in Montreal. Am J Ind Med 16:547–567.

SIMPSON SG, COMSTOCK GW. 1983. Lung cancer and housing characteristics. Arch Environ Health 38:248–251.

SKILLRUD DM, OFFORD KP, MILLER RD. 1986. Higher risk of lung cancer in chronic obstructive pulmonary disease: a prospective matched controlled study. Ann Intern Med 105:503–507.

SLEBOS RJ, HRUBAN RH, DALESIO O, et al. 1991. Relationship between k-ras oncogene activation and smoking in adenocarcinoma of the human lung: J Natl Cancer Inst 83:1024–1027.

SLUIS-CREMER GK, BEZUIDENHOUT BN. 1989. Relation between asbestosis and bronchial cancer in amphibole asbestos miners. Br J Ind Med 46:537–540.

SOLET D, ZOLOTH SR, SULLIVAN C, et al. 1989. Patterns of mortality in pulp and paper workers. J Occup Med 31:627–630.

SORAHAN T, COOKE MA. 1989. Cancer mortality in a cohort of United Kingdom steel foundry workers: 1946–85. Br J Ind Med 46:74–81.

SORAHAN T, CATHCART M. 1989. Lung cancer mortality among workers in a factory manufacturing chlorinated toluene: 1961–84. Br J Ind Med 46:425–427.

SPIRTAS R, BEEBE GU, CONNELLY RR, et al. 1986a. Recent trends in mesothelioma incidence in the United States. Am J Ind Med 9:397–407.

SPIRTAS R, KEEHN RJ, BEEBE GU, et al. 1986b. Results of pathology reviews of recent US mesothelioma cases. Accomp Oncol 1:144–152.

SPIRTAS R, CONNELLY RR, TUCKER MA. 1988. Survival patterns for malignant mesothelioma: The SEER experience. Int J Cancer 41:525–530.

STAHELIN HB, ROSEL F, BUESS E, et al. 1984. Cancer, vitamins, and plasma lipids: Prospective Basel Study. J Natl Cancer Inst 73:1463–1468.

STANTON MF, LAYARD M, TEGERIS A, et al. 1981. Relation of particle dimension to carcinogenicity of amphibole asbestos and other fibrous minerals. J Natl Cancer Inst 67:965–975.

STEENLAND NK, SILVERMAN DT, HORNUUG RW. 1990. Case-control study of lung cancer and truck driving in the Teamsters Union. Am J Public Health 80:670–674.

STEENLAND NK, BEAUMONT J, ELLIOT L. 1991. Lung Cancer in mild steel welders. Am J Epidemiol 133:220–229.

STEENLAND K, WARD E. 1991. Lung cancer incidence among patients with beryllium disease: a cohort mortality study. J Natl Cancer Inst 83:1380–1385.

STEINMETZ KA, POTTER JD, FOLSON AR. 1993. Vegetables, fruit, and lung cancer in the Iowa Women's Health Study. Cancer Res 53:536–543.

STOCKWELL HG, GOLDMAN AL, LYMAN GH, et al. 1992. Environmental tobacco smoke and lung cancer risk in nonsmoking women. J Natl Cancer Inst 84:1417–1422.

STRYKER WS, KAPLAN LA, STEIN EA, et al. 1988. The relation of diet, cigarette smoking, and alcohol consumption to plasma beta-carotene and alpha-tocopherol levels. Am J Epidemiol 127:282–296.

SURGEON GENERAL. 1986. The health consequences of involuntary smoking. Washington, D.C.: U.S. Government Printing Office.

SURGEON GENERAL. 1989. Reducing the health consequences of smoking: 25 years of progress. Washington, D.C.: U.S. Government Printing Office.

SVEC J, KUNZ E, TOMASEK L, et al. 1988. Cancer in man after exposure to Rn daughters. Health Phys 54:27–46.

SVENSSON C, PERSHAGEN G, KLOMINEK J. 1989. Lung cancer in women and type of dwelling in relation to radon exposure. Cancer Res 49:1861–1865.

TAGNON I, BLOT WJ, STROUBE RB, et al. 1980. Mesothelioma associated with the shipbuilding industry in coastal Virginia. Cancer Res 40:3875–3879.

TAKAHASHI T, NAU MM, CHIBA I, et al. 1989. p53, a frequent target for genetic abnormalities in lung cancer. Science 246:491–494.

TAYLOR PR, QIAO YL, SCHATZKIN A, et al. 1989. Relation of arsenic exposure to lung cancer among tin miners Yunnan Province, China. Br J Ind Med 46:881–886.

THERIAULT GP, GRAND-BOIS L. 1978. Mesothelioma and asbestos in the Province of Quebec, 1969–1972. Arch Environ Health 33:15–19.

THIESS AM, FRENTZEL-BEYME R, LINK R, et al. 1980. Mortality study on skilled chemical workers employed in various production plants with exposure to acrylonitrile. Zentralbl Arbeitsmed 30 (Suppl. 7):259–267.

THOMAS TL, STEWART PA. 1987. Mortality from lung cancer and respiratory disease among pottery workers exposed to silica and talc. Am J Epidemiol 125:35–43.

TOKUHATA GK, LILIENFELD AM. 1963. Familial aggregation of lung cancer in humans. J Natl Cancer Inst 30:289–312.

TOMKIN GH. 1969. Systemic sclerosis associated with carcinoma of the lung. Br J Dermatol 81:213–216.

TOOHEY RE, ESSLING MA, RUNDO J, et al. 1987. Some measurements of the equilibrium factor for ^{2}22Rn daughters in houses. Health Phys 53:87–91.

TUCHSEN F, NORDHOLM L. 1986. Respiratory cancer in Danish bakers: a 10-year cohort study. Br J Ind Med 43:516–521.

TUCKER MA, COLEMAN CN, COX RS, et al. 1988. Risk of second cancers after treatment for Hodgkin's disease. N Engl J Med 38:76–81.

TRICHOPOLOUS D, KALANDIDI A, SPARROS L, et al. 1981. Lung cancer and passive smoking. Int J Cancer 27:1–4.

TRICHOPOLOUS D, KALANDIDI A, SPARROS L. 1983. Lung cancer and passive smoking: Conclusion of Greek study. Lancet 2:677–678.

TRICHOPOLOUS D, KALANDIDI A, SPARROS L. 1984. Passive smoking and lung cancer. Lancet 1:684.

VAN POPPEL G, KOK F, HERMUS R. 1992. Beta-carotene supplementation in smokers reduces the frequency of micronuclei in sputum. Br J Cancer 66:1164–1168.

VENA JE, BONA JR, BYERS TE, et al. 1985. Allergy-related diseases and cancer: an inverse association. Am J Epidemiol 122:66–74.

VINE MF, SCHOENBACH VJ, HULKA BS, et al. 1990. Atypical metaplasia and incidence of bronchogenic carcinoma. Am J Epidemiol 131:781–793.

VINEIS P, CAPORASO N, TANNEBAUM SR, et al. 1990. Acetylation phenotype, carcinogen-hemoglobin adducts and cigarette smoking. Cancer Res 50:2002–3004.

WADA S, MIYANISHI M, NISHIMOTO Y, et al. 1968. Mustard gas as a cause of respiratory neoplasia in man. Lancet 1:1161–1163.

WAGNER JC, STEGGS CA, MARCHAND P. 1960. Diffuse pleural mesothelioma and asbestos exposure in the north western Cape Province. Br J Ind Med 17:260–271.

WAGNER JC, NEWHOUSE M, CORRIN B, et al. 1988. Correlation between fibre content of the lung and disease in east London asbestos factory workers. Br J Ind Med 45:305–308.

WALD NJ, BOREHAM J, BAILEY A. 1986. Serum retinol and subsequent risk of cancer. Br J Cancer 54:597–961.

WALKER AM, LOUGHLIN J, FRIEDLANDER E, et al. 1983. Projections of asbestos-related disease 1980–2009. J Occup Med 25:405–425.

WANG L, HAMMOND EC. 1985. Lung cancer, fruit, green salad and vitamin pills. Chin Med J 98:206–210.

WEISS W. 1980. The cigarette factor in lung cancer due to chloromethyl ethers. J Morphol 22:527–529.

WELSCH K, HIGGINS I, OH M, et al. 1982. Arsenic exposure, smoking and respiratory cancers in copper smelter workers. Arch Environ Health 37:325–335.

WESTON A, CAPORASO N, TAGHIZADEH K, et al. 1991. Measurement of 4-aminobiphenyl hemoglobin adducts in lung cancer cases and controls. Cancer Res 51:5219–5223.

WILCOX H, SCHOENBERG J, MASON T, et al. 1988. Smoking and lung cancer: risk as a function of cigarette tar content. Prev Med 17:263–272.

WILLETT WC, POLK VF, UNDERWOOD BA, et al. 1984. Relation of serum vitamins A and E and carotenoids to the risk of cancer. N Engl J Med 310:430–434.

WONG O, RAABE GK. 1989. Critical review of cancer epidemiology in petroleum industry employees with a quantitative meta analysis by cancer site. Am J Ind Med 15:283–310.

WONG O. 1989. A cohort mortality study of employees exposed to chlorinated chemicals. Am J Ind Med 14:417–431.

WU AH, HENDERSON BE, PIKE MC, et al. 1985. Smoking and other risk factors for lung cancer in women. J Natl Cancer Inst 74:747–751.

WU AH, YU MC, THOMAS DC, et al. 1989. Personal and family history of lung disease as risk factors for adenocarcinoma of the lung. Cancer Res 49:7279–7284.

WU-WILLIAMS AH, DAI XD, BLOT WJ, et al. 1990. Lung cancer among women in northeast China. Br J Cancer 62:982–987.

WYNDER EL. 1989. Lung cancer and smoking: The science of applying prevention strategies. J Natl Cancer Inst 81:388–389.

ZHENG W, BLOT WJ, LIAO ML, et al. 1987. Lung cancer and prior tuberculosis infection in Shanghai. Br J Cancer 56:501–504.

ZIEGLER RG, MASON TJ, STEMHAGEN A, et al. 1986. Carotenoid intake, vegetables, and the risk of lung cancer among white men in New Jersey. Am J Epidemiol 123:1080–1093.

ZIEGLER RG. 1989. A review of the epidemiologic evidence that carotenoids reduce the risk of cancer. J Nutr 119:116–122.

ZWI AB, REID G, LANDAU SP, et al. 1989. Mesothelioma in South Africa, 1976–84: Incidence and case characteristics. Int J Epidemiol 18:320–329.

32 Cancers of the oral cavity and pharynx

WILLIAM J. BLOT
JOSEPH K. McLAUGHLIN
SUSAN S. DEVESA
JOSEPH F. FRAUMENI, JR.

This chapter reviews the epidemiology of cancers of the oral cavity and pharynx, describing their marked variation in occurrence in different populations, the factors known and suspected to cause the tumors, and prospects for prevention. Cancers of the tongue (ICD 141), the gum, floor and other parts of the mouth (ICD 143–145), and the pharynx (ICD 146, 148–149) are included. These will be treated as a single entity and often referred to simply as oral cancer, although the occasional differences in epidemiologic patterns according to anatomic site will be noted. Almost all of these tumors are squamous cell carcinomas. The epidemiologic characteristics of cancers of the lip (ICD 140) and salivary glands (ICD 142), which differ markedly from those of other oral cancers, are described separately at the end of the chapter, while nasopharyngeal tumors (ICD 146), which present yet different features, are considered elsewhere in this volume.

ORAL CANCER

Descriptive Patterns

Geographic Variation. Oral cancer varies strikingly around the world. In parts of India and Southeast Asia it is the most common cancer, owing to the use of chews containing betel and tobacco, while it ranks 7th among blacks and 12th among whites in cancer incidence in the United States (Ries et al, 1991; Parkin et al, 1992; Blot et al, 1994). Figure 32-1 portrays age-adjusted incidence rates of oral cancer in several areas of the world. The variation exceeds 20-fold. The highest incidence among males is reported in France, with annual rates of more than 40 per 100,000 in the east-central part of the country along the German border (Bas-Rhin) and on the Brittany coast (Calvados), while the highest rates among females occur in India. In most parts of the world oral cancer occurs more frequently in males, with the sex ratio usually between 2 and 6. Higher rates for females, however, have been reported among Filipinos, among Indians in Singapore and Bangalore, India, and in Iceland (Muir et al, 1987).

Figure 32–1 also shows geographic variation in the anatomic distribution of tumors within the oral cavity and pharynx. Among males in many areas of the world, cancers arise more frequently in the pharynx than other oral sites. Among French males, for example, the majority (about 60% in Calvados) of the tumors are pharyngeal in origin. In the United States, the most common site among black males is the pharynx, accounting for about 50% of oral tumors, whereas among white males the mouth (usually gum or floor) and pharynx each account for about 35%. Mouth cancers predominate among females in Bangalore, India, where the highest oral cancer rates are reported, accounting for about 80% of the tumors. Tongue cancers typically are less frequent than other mouth and pharyngeal cancers, except in Japan, where overall rates are low. High tongue cancer rates among males and females are reported in parts of France and India.

Geographic variation also exists within countries, with one of the most striking patterns seen in the United States. The mapping of cancer mortality from 1950 to 1969 revealed elevated rates of oral cancer among males in the north, particularly in large urban centers (Mason et al, 1975; Blot and Fraumeni, 1977). This pattern is consistent with the distribution of the major risk factors: cigarette smoking and alcohol drinking. Among females, however, mortality was highest in the south, especially in rural areas where the long-standing use of smokeless tobacco products is commonplace (Winn et al, 1981a). A recent update of the oral cancer maps among women for the period 1970–89 revealed some diminution in the high-risk southeast and several new

We thank Mr. Vladimir Dragunsky, Mr. James Abbott, Ms. Joan Hertel, Mr. Gray Williams, Mr. Jie Sun, and Ms. Ruth Parsons for computer programming and graphics preparation, and Mr. Dan Grauman for mapping.

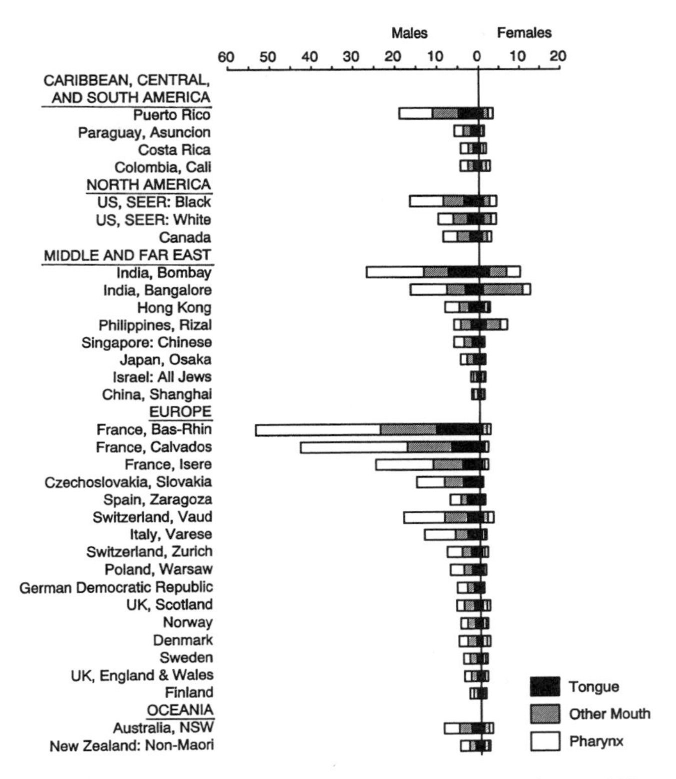

FIG. 32–1. International oral and pharyngeal cancer incidence, 1983–1987. Age-adjusted (world standard) annual rates per 100,000 for tongue, other mouth, and pharyngeal cancers. (From Blot et al., 1994.)

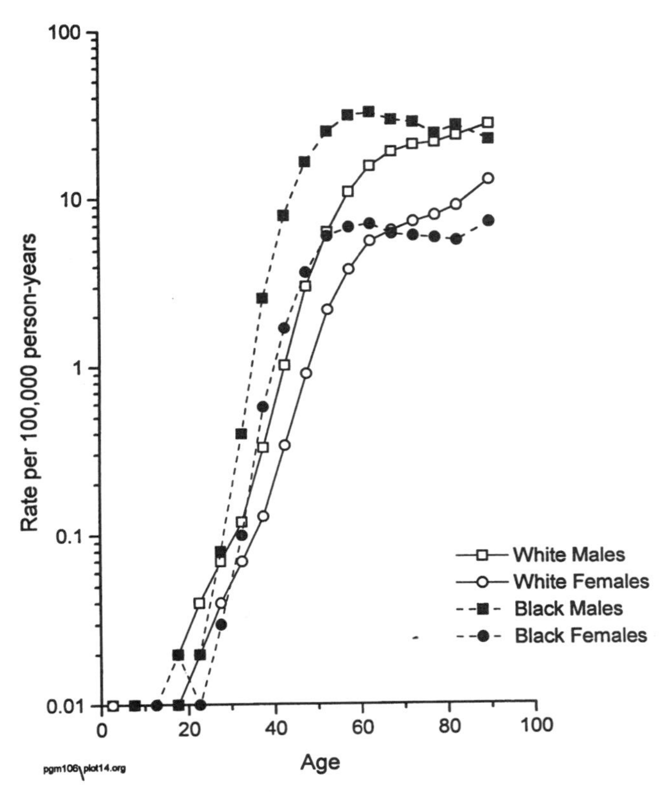

FIG. 32–2. Age-specific oral and pharyngeal cancer mortality rates by race and sex in the United States, 1975–1990 (excludes cancers of the lip, salivary gland, and nasopharynx). (Based on data from the National Center for Health Statistics.)

high-rate areas appearing along the Pacific and Florida coasts (Blot et al, 1994). This emergent pattern resembles that for lung cancer among females, suggesting the influence of cigarette smoking on both cancers (Pickle et al, 1987).

Demographic Patterns. Around the world, oral cancer displays the age pattern typical of many epithelial cancers, with rates rising progressively with advancing age. The median age at diagnosis of oral cancer in the United States is 63 years, and the median age at death is 65 years (Young et al, 1981). Figure 32-2 shows age-specific oral cancer mortality rates in the United States from 1975 to 1990. Death rates among whites increase to about age 60 in a nearly linear fashion when log mortality is plotted against age, after which the rate of increase declines. Mortality rates among blacks plateau at younger ages, reflecting sizable cohort effects. The figure also shows the substantial excess in rates among blacks compared to whites up to age 60–70, a disparity that is also seen in oral cancer incidence data for this period from the Surveillance, Epidemiology and End Results (SEER) program of cancer registration covering slightly more than 10% of the U.S. population (not shown) (Miller et al, 1993; Weller et al, 1993).

Between 1950–54 and 1985–89, the age-adjusted oral cancer mortality rates were relatively stable for white males until they began to decline in recent years, while those for nonwhite males doubled, surpassing those for whites in the early 1960s (Blot et al, 1994) (Fig. 32-3). Rates increased among females of both racial groups during the 1950s to 1970s, with declines suggested during the 1980s. Cohort analyses revealed peak mortality among white males born around 1910–15 and white females born around 1915–20 (Devesa et al, 1990). The recent decline in mortality among white males is apparent across all age groups and is probably a reflection of reductions in smoking. The nonwhite excess of oral cancer reflects elevated rates among blacks, with mortality figures among American Indians, Chinese, and Japanese Americans at or below levels for whites (Mason et al, 1976). In contrast to the overall declines in rates, rising tongue cancer mortality (Depue, 1986) and incidence (Davis and Severson, 1987) in the United States have been reported at young ages and postulated to be due to increasing use of snuff by teenage and young adult males. Figure 32-4 displays the rising tongue cancer death rates among white males below age 45 (Blot et al, 1994). However, no concomitant in-

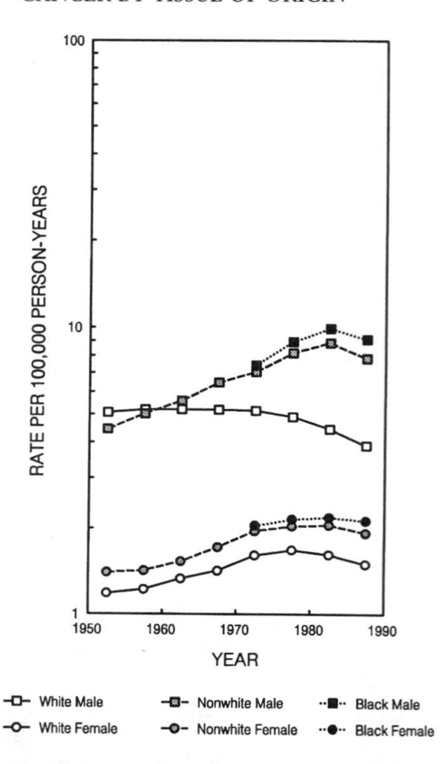

FIG. 32–3. Trends in age-adjusted (1970 U.S. standard) oral and pharyngeal cancer mortality rates in the United States by race and sex, 1950–1989. (From Blot et al., 1994.)

creases have been seen in the rates for cheek, gum, and other mouth cancers, which are more closely linked to smokeless tobacco use (Surgeon General, 1986). Furthermore, increases in tongue cancer mortality have occurred also in the United Kingdom, where oral snuff and

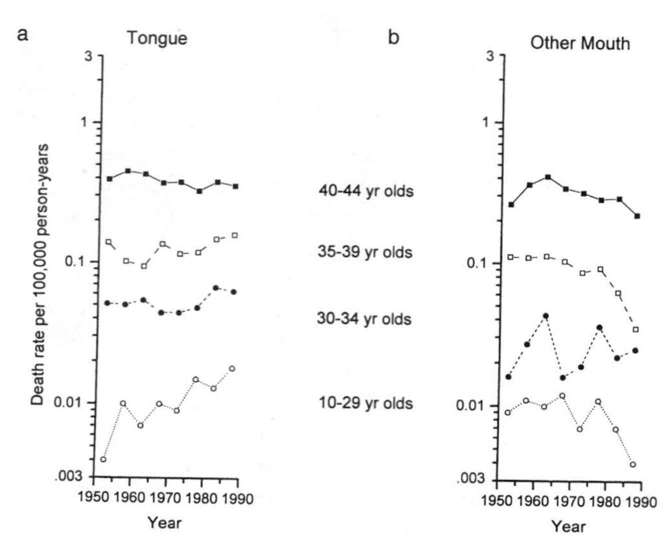

FIG. 32–4. Trends in age-specific mortality from (*a*) tongue cancer and (*b*) other mouth cancer among young American white males, 1950–1989. (From Blot et al., 1994.)

chewing tobacco are seldom used (MacFarlane et al, 1987).

Mortality trends in other countries over the past 35 years have generally been fairly stable or rising (Kurihara et al, 1989). Sizable increases have been seen recently in France and other western European countries, the German Democratic Republic, where rates of oral cancer rose faster than those for any other tumor during the period 1968–81 (Haas et al, 1986), and eastern and central Europe (Blot et al, 1994). A decrease in the exceptionally high rates of oral cancer in parts of India has recently been reported, as incidence has declined in later-born cohorts in Bombay (Jayant and Yeole, 1987).

The urban-rural gradient for oral cancer is one of the strongest seen for any malignant neoplasm (Blot and Fraumeni, 1982). Death rates for oral cancer are nearly twice as high in urban compared to rural counties of the United States. There are also strong social class differences, with rates higher in persons with lower income and education. In the United Kingdom, for example, mortality in both sexes was 60% higher among those in the lowest category of social class as defined by the British Office of Census and Population Surveys. The urban/rural and socioeconomic differences, as well as the sex and racial variations, are consistent with patterns of smoking and drinking in the population.

Survival Patterns. As shown in Table 32-1, 5-year relative survival rates, 1975-89, range from 18% to 62% depending on sex, race, and anatomic site, being lowest for pharyngeal tumors. For each anatomic site, survival rates are lower among males than females, and among blacks than whites. Survival trends have shown little change in recent decades. Survival percentages are higher if the tumor is localized (reaching nearly 80% for mouth cancer among white females) at the time of diagnosis than if regional or distant spread has occurred.

Oral cancer is characterized by a high incidence of second primary cancers of the oral cavity and adjacent sites. In a follow-up of nearly 8,000 patients with oral cancers diagnosed in Connecticut during the period

TABLE 32–1. *Five-year Relative Survival Rates among U.S. White and Black Males and Females with Oral Cancer, According to Anatomic Location of the Tumor, 1975–1989**

Anatomic Location	*Whites*		*Blacks*	
	Males	*Females*	*Males*	*Females*
Tongue	43%	49%	24%	35%
Other mouth	52%	62%	36%	47%
Pharynx	30%	36%	18%	28%

*Data from 9 SEER Registries.

1935–82, 11% developed a second primary cancer despite an average follow-up time of only 3.4 years (Winn and Blot, 1985). The number of new cancers was more than twice that expected, based on general population rates, with excesses most prominent for second oral and esophageal tumors, but rates of second primaries were also increased for other digestive and respiratory organs. Among those who survived 10 or more years, 24% developed a second primary cancer. Similar patterns were seen in a recent follow-up of over 20,000 oral cancer cases reported to SEER, with increases documented among both men and women and blacks and whites, especially among those below age 60 (Day and Blot, 1992). In this large survey, second tumors developed at a constant rate of 3.7% per year. In Japan, excessive rates of multiple oral cancers have been reported among patients with tongue cancer and associated leukoplakia (Shibuya et al, 1986).

Risk Factors

Tobacco. A major risk factor for oral cancer is tobacco smoking, affecting cancers of the tongue, mouth, and pharynx (IARC, 1986). In some populations, most tumors of the cheek and gum are induced by smokeless tobacco products. The elevated risks associated with tobacco consumption are typically large. Table 32-2 shows the relative risks of oral cancer from cohort studies of cigarette smokers conducted in several areas of the world. The relative risks have ranged from 2.9 to 13. Similar risks among smokers were observed in the case-control studies of oral cancer reported in the 1950s (Sanghvi and Rao, 1955; Wynder et al, 1957a) as well as recently (Elwood et al, 1984; Tuyns et al, 1988; Blot et al, 1988; Franco et al, 1989; Merletti et al, 1989; Kabat et al, 1989; Sankaranarayanan et al, 1989; Franceschi et al, 1990; Zheng et al, 1990; Oreggia et al, 1991). When dose-response relationships were examined, the risks tended to rise with increasing amounts of tobacco smoked. This pattern is evident from a recent case-control study of oral cancer conducted in four areas of the United States (Blot et al, 1988). In total, 1,104 oral cancer patients and 1,268 population-based controls participated in this study, with the large numbers permitting more precise estimates of relative risk than were possible in previous studies. Table 32-3 shows the positive trends in relative risk according to number of cigarettes smoked, rising to more than 4 among males and 10 among females who are heavy smokers, after adjusting for the effects of alcohol intake. In addition, men who smoked pipes and/or cigars exclusively showed a 2-fold increased risk of oral cancer. Also seen was an upward trend in risk with increasing pipe and cigar consumption, with the effects stronger for mouth than for tongue or pharyngeal cancers. This study also showed that risk was lower among lifelong male filter smokers than among nonfilter smokers, but a concomitant reduction in risk was not observed among females. Exclusive use of filtered cigarettes was linked to a lowered (compared to use of nonfiltered cigarettes) risk in a multicenter study of hypopharyngeal cancer in Europe (Tuyns et al, 1988), with a similar but less pronounced pattern in Italy (Merletti et al, 1989). In another case-control study in Italy, risks of oral cancer were higher for users of high- vs. low-tar cigarettes (LaVecchia et al, 1990). In Italy, risks associated with smoking black vs. blond tobaccos were similar (Merletti et al, 1989), but in Uraguay the risk was 4 times higher among black tobacco smokers (Oreggia et al, 1991). Use of mentholated cigarettes, more common among blacks than whites in the United States, was not associated with higher risks than use of nonmentholated cigarettes (Kabat and Hebert, 1994).

Further evidence of the role of smoking, and an important clue for prevention, comes from observations of reduced risk of oral cancer following cessation of smoking (Wynder and Stellman, 1977; Blot et al, 1988; Franco et al, 1989; Merletti et al, 1989; Franceschi et al, 1990; Oreggia et al, 1991). The decline in risk, now reported from three continents, appears to be rapid, with no detectable elevation in oral cancer risk among

TABLE 32–2. *Relative Risks of Oral Cancer from Cohort Studies of Male Cigarette Smokers**

Cohort	*RR (Smokers vs. Nonsmokers)*
U.S. veterans	6.1
American Cancer Society	6.5
British physicians	13.0
Japanese population	2.9

*Data from Surgeon General (1982).

TABLE 32–3. *Relative Risks of Oral Cancer According to Amount of Tobacco Smoked*

	Males		*Females*	
Smoking Status	*RR*[a]	*95% CI*	*RR*[a]	*95% CI*
Nonsmokers	1.0	—	1.0	—
Short duration or former[b]	1.1	0.7–1.7	1.0	0.5–1.8
Light[c]	1.6	0.9–2.7	3.0	1.9–5.2
Moderate[d]	2.8	1.8–4.3	4.4	2.7–7.2
Heavy[e]	4.4	2.7–7.2	10.2	5.2–20.4
Pipe/cigar only	1.9	1.1–3.4	—	—

[a]All risks relative to nonsmokers of any tobacco product and adjusted for alcoholic beverage intake. Data from Blot et al (1988).

[b]Quit smoking at least 10 years earlier or smoked for less than 20 years.

[c]Smoked 1–19 cigarettes per day for 20 or more years.

[d]Smoked 20–39 cigarettes per day for 20 or more years.

[e]Smoked 40 or more cigarettes per day for 20 or more years.

those who quit smoking at least 10 years before. This elimination of excess risk shortly after cessation suggests that smoking operates primarily at a late stage in oral carcinogenesis and that its effects may be reversible.

Smokeless tobacco is a well-documented cause of oral cancer (Surgeon General, 1986). The chewing of products containing tobacco, betel, and other substances, such as "pan" and "nass," has long been thought to contribute to the elevated rates of oral cancer in India and other parts of Central Asia (Orr, 1937; Sanghvi, 1974; Jayant and Deo, 1986; Sankaranarayanan et al, 1989). A review of relevant epidemiologic data indicates that the excess risk of oral cancer is associated mainly with tobacco-containing chews, suggesting that tobacco is the key ingredient, although other components of the quid mixtures may enhance the risk (Gupta et al, 1982). In the United States, a link between smokeless tobacco and oral cancer has been suspected for many years. In 1915, Abbe noted that several patients with oral cancer were tobacco chewers and commented upon a possible etiologic relation. By the 1950s smokeless tobacco was implicated in several clinical reports from southern medical centers describing verrucous carcinomas of the oral cavity among snuff users, and the term "snuff-dipper's cancer" was coined (Wilkins and Vogler, 1957; Vogler et al, 1962; Rosenfeld and Callaway, 1963). This association was not confirmed, however, until the 1980s, when a case-control study in North Carolina showed that nonsmoking white women who used snuff experienced a significant increased risk of oral cancer, 4.2 times that of nonusers of tobacco (Winn et al, 1981a). Among long-term users, the relative risk reached nearly 50 for tumors arising in the cheek and gum, tissues in contact with the snuff powder.

Cultural variations in the use of tobacco products also underlie regional and anatomic patterns of oral cancer in other populations. For example, in parts of India, oral (lip) tumors arising in users of smokeless tobacco have been named "Khaini" cancers, after the Khaini tobacco used in the quids, and cancers of the palate among women smoking Chutta cigars with the lighted ends inside their mouths have been called "Chutta" cancers (Sanghvi, 1974; Gupta et al, 1982).

It is not clear which of the many compounds in tobacco smoke or tobacco itself are carcinogenic to oral tissue. While combustion products from smoked tobacco probably are involved, tobacco-specific nitrosamines have been isolated from commercially available smokeless tobacco products as well as from cigarettes (Hoffmann and Hecht, 1985). Some of these substances, such as N-nitrosonornicotine (NNN) and 4-methylnitrosamino-l-3-pyridyl-l-butanone (NNK), occur in smokeless tobacco at levels an order of magnitude higher than allowable levels of nitrosamines in food in the United States. These agents are potent animal carcinogens at doses that approach those consumed by long-term users of smokeless tobacco (Hoffmann and Hecht, 1985). Smokeless tobacco itself did not appear to produce cancers in experimental animals until recently, when snuff was shown to induce oral tumors in rats when surgically implanted in the oral cavity (Hecht et al, 1986; Johansson et al, 1989).

Alcohol. Epidemiologic investigations over the past few decades have provided conclusive evidence that consumption of alcoholic beverages can increase risk of oral cancer (Martinez, 1969; Tuyns, 1982; Elwood et al, 1984; Mashberg et al, 1981; Tuyns et al, 1988; IARC, 1988; Blot et al, 1988; Kabat and Wynder, 1989; Franco et al, 1989; Merletti et al, 1989; Franceschi et al, 1990; Zheng et al, 1990; Oreggia et al, 1991). Table 32-4 shows the relative risks of oral cancer according to amount of alcoholic beverages usually consumed per week, using data from an American case-control study (Blot et al, 1988). The smoking-adjusted risks increased steadily with amount consumed, with relative risks of 9 among both males and females who were heavy drinkers.

Only limited data are available to distinguish differences in risk of oral cancer according to type of alcoholic beverage. Intake of all types of alcohol, however, appears to increase risk (IARC, 1988). In the large American study referred to earlier (Blot et al, 1988), the risks associated with individual types of alcoholic beverages were adjusted for other types of alcoholic beverages and smoking. Strong trends were found for hard liquor and for beer intake, with elevated risks for heavy, but not light or moderate, wine drinkers. In a hospital-based case-control study in the United States (Kabat and Wynder, 1989), increased risks also were observed among those who drank mainly hard liquor and those who drank mainly beer. In Torino, Italy, the strongest effects were found for beer consumption (Merletti et al, 1989). Specific alcoholic beverages have been linked to clustering of elevated cancer rates in some areas of the world. In Brittany, France, apple brandies have been implicated in the elevated rates of hypopharyngeal cancer (Tuyns et al, 1988), while cachaca, a spirit derived

TABLE 32–4. *Relative Risks of Oral Cancer According to Number of Alcoholic Beverages Consumed*

	Males		*Females*	
Number of Drinks per Week	*RR*[a]	*95% CI*	*RR*[a]	*95% CI*
<1	1.0	—	1.0	—
1–4	1.2	0.7–2.0	1.2	0.7–1.9
5–14	1.7	1.0–2.7	1.3	0.8–2.1
15–29	3.3	2.0–5.4	2.3	1.2–4.5
30+	8.8	5.4–14.3	9.1	3.9–21.0

[a]All risks adjusted for smoking and relative to those who drank less than 1 alcoholic drink per week. Data from Blot et al (1988).

from sugarcane, contributes to the high rates of oral cancer in Brazil (Franco et al, 1989).

Several studies have established the joint effects of tobacco and alcohol on oral cancer. The exact form of the interrelationship has been difficult to quantify because intake of the two substances is so highly correlated, but the consensus is that drinking and smoking multiply the effects of each other (Rothman and Keller, 1972; Elwood et al, 1984; Olsen et al, 1985; Blot et al, 1988; Franco et al, 1989). Table 32-5 lists relative risks following joint exposure to alcohol and tobacco, using data from the U.S. Those who were both heavy drinkers and heavy smokers had 38 times the risk of oral cancer for abstainers from both products. Furthermore, the risk increased with amount of alcohol consumed among lifelong nonsmokers, indicating that tobacco is not a prerequisite cofactor for alcohol-induced cancer. Since ethanol is not carcinogenic in laboratory animals, the mechanism by which alcohol promotes oral carcinogenesis is not clear. Under suspicion are nutritional deficiencies associated with heavy drinking, the effects of congeners or contaminants (e.g., nitrosamines, hydrocarbons) in alcoholic beverages, the capacity of alcohol to solubilize carcinogens or enhance their penetration into oral tissues, alcohol-induced P450 enzyme activities that can affect the metabolic activation of some compounds into carcinogens, alcohol-induced liver damage that inhibits the detoxication of carcinogenic compounds, and an increase in cellular exposure to oxidants (Ziegler, 1986; IARC, 1988; Blot, 1992).

It is estimated that smoking and drinking account for 75% of all oral cancers in the United States (Blot et al, 1988). Differences in the prevalence of use and levels of risk of tobacco and particularly alcohol appear almost completely responsible for the higher rates of oral cancer among American men than women, and among blacks than whites (Day et al, 1993). The attributable fractions in other countries are uncertain, but it seems that one or both of these exposures contribute to most cases in high-risk areas of the world. In France, alcohol intake of the general population is high by world standards and higher still among oral cancer patients. The median consumption among 1,759 oral cancer patients treated at the Institute Curie in Paris during the period 1975–82 was approximately 80 drinks per week (with a typical drink being 6 ounces of wine), rising to nearly 100 drinks for patients with cancers of the hypopharynx and floor of the mouth (Brugere et al, 1986). Alcohol may also contribute to the high rates reported in Ireland (Herrity et al, 1981). In India, tobacco is the dominant factor, with smoking of bidi and other cigarettes and chewing of quids containing tobacco and betel contributing to the majority of cases (Sanghvi, 1974; Jayant et al, 1977). Although changes in risk following cessation or reduction of alcohol consumption are not well documented, it seems that preventive strategies should focus on reducing exposure to both alcohol and tobacco. If both affect primarily later stages in the carcinogenic process, as is believed, substantial reductions in oral cancer risk may quickly follow.

Diet and Nutrition. In the 1950s, nutritional deficiencies of iron, riboflavin, and other vitamins were implicated in the Plummer-Vinson (or Paterson-Kelly) Syndrome. This condition was seen particularly among Swedish women, and it predisposed mainly to hypopharyngeal or postcricoid cancer (Wynder et al, 1957b). With the advent of programs to supplement iron and vitamins in the population, the incidence of oral cancer has declined in Sweden. Recently, several case-control studies (Marshall et al, 1982; Winn et al, 1984; Notani and Jayant, 1987; McLaughlin et al, 1988; Franco et al, 1989; Gridley et al, 1992a; LaVecchia et al, 1991; Oreggia et al, 1991; Zheng et al, 1992) have consistently found that oral cancer patients have histories of diets low in fruits and vegetables, even after accounting for their high alcohol intake. As shown in Table 32-6, relative risks of oral cancer among American men and women declined as the consumption of fruit rose, even when controlling for smoking and drinking patterns. Protective effects of vegetable intake were not as strong, except for vegetables likely to be eaten uncooked. Similar findings were seen in North Carolina (Winn et al, 1984), Brazil (Franco et al, 1989), and Italy (LaVecchia et al, 1991).

TABLE 32–5. *Relative Risks of Oral Cancer among Males According to Magnitude of Consumption of Alcoholic Beverages and Cigarettes**

	Number of Cigarettes/Day			
Number of Drinks per Week	*None*[a]	*1–19*[b]	*20–39*[b]	*40+*[b]
<1	1.0	1.7	1.9	7.4
1–4	1.3	1.5	2.4	0.7
5–14	1.6	2.7	4.4	4.4
15–29	1.4	5.4	7.2	20.2
30+	5.8	7.9	23.8	37.7

*Data from Blot et al (1988).
[a]These persons never smoked any tobacco product.
[b]These persons all smoked cigarettes for 20 or more years.

TABLE 32–6. *Relative Risks of Oral Cancer According to Adult Consumption of Fruit**

Quartile of Fruit Intake	*Males*	*Females*
I (low)	1.0	1.0
II	0.6	0.9
III	0.4	0.8
IV (high)	0.4	0.5

*All risks adjusted for smoking and alcohol consumption. Data from McLaughlin et al (1988).

Although the role of micronutrients is difficult to distinguish from that of other constituents of fruits and vegetables that may lower the risk of oral cancer, some epidemiologic studies of oral cancer point to beta-carotene, the precursor of vitamin A derived from plant sources. This nutrient has shown cancer-inhibitory effects in some animal experiments, including inhibition and regression of dimethylbenzanthracene-induced oral carcinomas in hamsters (Suda et al, 1986; Schwartz and Shklar, 1988), and it has been linked through epidemiologic studies to a lowered risk of other squamous cell cancers, notably cancers of the lung (Willett and MacMahon, 1984). In a U.S. survey using stored serum, serum levels of beta-carotene were lower in persons who subsequently developed oral cancer than in controls (Zheng et al, 1993). Twice-weekly supplementation with beta-carotene and retinol reduced the frequency of micronuclear aberrations in buccal cells of betel/tobacco quid chewers in the Philippines (Stich et al, 1984). Beta-carotene concentrations were also lower in exfoliated oral mucosal cells of heavy drinkers than in persons at low risk for oral cancer (Stich et al, 1986). Although the epidemiologic evidence favors carotene, a protective role of vitamin A itself is suggested by the lower risk of oral cancer among users of retinol supplements in one case-control study (Rossing et al, 1989). In addition, regression of oral leukoplakia was seen in a controlled clinical trial of 13-cis-retinoic acid (Hong et al, 1986), as well as following weekly administration of 200,000 IU of vitamin A (Stich et al, 1988a). Vitamin A combined with beta-carotene was more effective than beta-carotene alone in reducing micronucleated cells and leukoplakia among tobacco chewers in India (Stich et al, 1988b, 1991). The synthetic retinoid 13-cis-retinoic acid has also been shown in an American clinical trial to lower the incidence of second primary cancers among patients with head and neck cancers (Hong et al, 1990). The link between dietary retinol and oral cancer is not clear, however, and some case-control studies have found increased rather than decreased risks among those with high levels of intake of retinol-rich foods (McLaughlin et al, 1988).

The protective effects of fruit intake in some studies have suggested that vitamin C (ascorbic acid) may play a role. Experimental studies have shown mixed results with regard to cancer inhibition (Birt, 1986), but vitamin C is known to block the formation of nitrosamines, potent animal carcinogens (Mirvish, 1983). In an investigation of pharyngeal cancer in Seattle, Washington, dietary intake of vitamin C was associated with reduced risk, whereas there was little or no effect with consumption of carotenoids or retinol (Rossing et al, 1989). In the national U.S. study, protective effects were seen with increasing consumption of fruits with and without high vitamin C or carotene content, suggesting that components other than these nutrients may be involved (McLaughlin et al, 1988). These include non-nutritive organic compounds such as phenols, flavones, and aromatic isothiocyanates that can inhibit carcinogenesis (Wattenberg, 1985). In laboratory animals, vitamin E has inhibited and iron deficiency has promoted oral carcinogenesis (Trickler and Shklar, 1987; Shklar et al, 1990). A sharply reduced risk of oral cancer recently has been seen among users of vitamin E supplements in two case-control studies in the United States (Gridley et al, 1992b; Barone et al, 1992). In each, the risk of oral cancer was only 50% as high among users compared to nonusers of the supplements. In clinical trials, vitamin E has proven effective in reversing oral leukoplakia (Benner et al, 1993; Zaridze et al, 1993). The high rate of oral cancer in patients with pernicious anemia suggests that deficiencies of vitamin B_{12} or other nutrients may be involved (McLaughlin et al, 1988; Brinton et al, 1989).

No relationship has been found between oral cancer and nonalcoholic beverages, except for a type of tea (maté) that is heavily consumed, typically at high temperatures, in areas of southern Brazil (Franco et al, 1989; Oreggia et al, 1991).

Precancerous Lesions. Oral leukoplakia is defined as a white patch or plaque occurring on the oral mucosal surface that cannot be characterized clinically or pathologically as any other disease (WHO, 1978). The condition is not uncommon; leukoplakia prevalence rates among Americans over age 35 have been estimated to be 43 per 1,000 for males and 21 per 1,000 for females (Bouquot and Gourlin, 1986), while in Sweden the prevalence of "snuff dipper's lesion" reached 80 per 1,000 (Axell, 1987). Leukoplakias have been considered as precancerous lesions, since some may progress to dysplasia, carcinoma in situ, and invasive cancer. Most of the information available on oral premalignant lesions pertains to this entity (Vogler et al, 1962; Pindborg et al, 1968; Shklar, 1986; Gupta et al, 1989). Some studies have reported transformation rates from leukoplakia to oral cancer as high as 17% (Silverman et al, 1984), although the rates are much lower in most studies (Surgeon General, 1986; Lind, 1987). Leukoplakia can be induced by tobacco, both smoked and unsmoked, and can disappear following cessation of tobacco use, so the association of leukoplakia with oral cancer is conditional in part on tobacco use (Gianta and Connolly, 1986). In a prospective follow-up of 12,000 tobacco users in Kerela, India, 79% of the newly detected oral cancers arose from preexisting lesions, usually the nodular type of leukoplakia (Gupta et al, 1989). To a lesser extent, oral submucosal fibrosis, seen mainly in India and Indian immigrants, appears to increase the risk of oral cancer.

Oral erythroplasia refers to red patches on the oral surface, and indicates epithelial atrophy and inflammation. These lesions have been reported to have an even higher risk of malignant transformation than leukoplakia (Mashberg, 1977). Oral epithelial dysplasias are more advanced lesions, although their rates of transformation to cancer are unknown. The lesions occur throughout the oral cavity but tend to cluster in the buccal mucosa among smokeless tobacco users (64% of dysplasias among snuff dippers or tobacco chewers appeared in the buccal mucosa/vestibule vs. 19% in nonusers, in a recently reported series of 1,651 biopsy-proven oral dysplasias in Richmond, Virginia) (Kaugars et al, 1989). In early studies, syphilitic lesions seemed to contribute to the development of tongue cancers, but the decline in late-stage infections has virtually eliminated syphilis as the source of a possible premalignant lesion. In a linkage of cancer and syphilis registry data in the state of Washington, however, significantly increased risks of oral and pharyngeal cancer were found among persons testing positive for syphilis, although the numbers of cancers were small (Daling et al, 1982). Chronic candidiasis, lichen planus, pemphigus vulgaris, and verrucous hyperplasia have also been reported to predispose to oral cancer, but the evidence linking these conditions to subsequent malignancy is incomplete (Fowler et al, 1987; Gupta et al, 1989).

Other Risk Factors. Poor oral hygiene has been postulated as a risk factor in some studies. Ill-fitting dentures have been linked to oral cancer risk, and poor dentition was shown to enhance the risks associated with tobacco and alcohol (Wynder et al, 1957a; Graham et al, 1977; Young et al, 1986). Winn et al (1981b) observed 2- to 3-fold increased risks associated with loss of 10 or more teeth among women who wore dentures as well as those who did not, and no association with denture-wearing was seen in Brazil, where most cases and controls wore dentures (Franco et al, 1989), suggesting that underlying oral hygiene may be a more important factor than the wearing of dentures.

Mouthwash use has been associated with oral cancer in some case-control studies, with effects seen mainly after long-term use among women and nonsmokers/nondrinkers (Weaver et al, 1979; Wynder et al, 1983; Blot et al, 1983; Mashberg et al, 1985; Kabat et al, 1989). The largest investigation into the role of mouthwash revealed that the association may be limited to mouthwashes high in alcohol content (Winn et al, 1991). Some brands contain over 25% alcohol. Although biologically plausible, because alcohol drinking is a strong oral carcinogen whose effect may be via topical exposure, the findings regarding mouthwash use are not yet considered conclusive. Further study is important, since mouthwash has been used regularly by over 40% of American adults (Winn et al, 1991).

Viruses may play an etiologic role in oral cancer, but information is limited. Human papillomavirus (HPV) antigens have been detected in oral papillomas and leukoplakias, with HPV type 16 found especially among patients with oral cancer (De Villiers et al, 1985; Ostrow et al, 1987; Greer et al, 1990; Watts et al, 1991). In Taiwan, HPV 16 was detected in tumor tissue of 13 of 17 oral cancer patients, most of whom were tobacco smokers or chewers (Chang et al, 1989). Prototypes of HPV 16, however, appear to be common in normal oral tissue as well (Maitland et al, 1987, 1989; Scully et al, 1987; Greer et al, 1990), and the etiologic role between HPV exposure and oral cancer is unclear. Recent technologic advances using polymerase chain reaction methods have permitted the enhanced detection and identification of HPV, which should help in assessing the virus role in oral cancer. Herpes simplex virus has been suspected as a risk factor in clinical and laboratory studies, but confirmatory evidence is lacking (Shillitoe, 1987). It is noteworthy, however, that in one study experimental animals exposed to smokeless tobacco developed oral tumors only when also infected with herpes simplex type l virus (Park et al, 1986). The Epstein-Barr virus (EBV) has been suggested as a risk factor by the presence of EBV DNA in some oral cancers (Brichacek et al, 1984), and EBV, along with papilloma, herpes simplex type l, and other viruses, has been found in the oral "hairy" leukoplakia lesions associated with the acquired immunodeficiency syndrome (Greenspan et al, 1984, 1985).

Occupational factors may play a limited role in oral cancer (Huebner et al, 1992). Jobs involving opportunities for heavy alcohol consumption, such as bartending or working in a brewery, are associated with increased oral cancer risk (Wynder et al, 1957a; Dean et al, 1979; Jensen, 1979; Herrity et al, 1981). Insulation workers exposed to asbestos and workers producing man-made mineral fibers in France have experienced 2-fold excesses of oral cancer, although the numbers of affected individuals were small (Selikoff et al, 1979; Moulin et al, 1986). In three small surveys of oral cancer (OPCS, 1978; Vagero and Olin, 1983; Winn et al, 1982), increased risk was associated with work in the electronics manufacturing industry. Workers in the textile industry were reported at increased risk of oral cancer (Moss and Lee, 1974), but subsequent studies have shown no association or decreased risks (Moss, 1976; Winn et al, 1982; Huebner et al, 1992). A possible effect of indoor air pollution has been reported in Brazil by an association of oral cancer with the use of woodstoves for cooking and heating (Franco et al, 1989).

Familial and genetic susceptibility appear to play little role in oral cancer, although few studies have evaluated this issue. Oral and pharyngeal cancer patients have been reported to have increased sensitivity to chromosome damage, independent of their tobacco and alcohol habits (Spitz et al, 1993). In some rare inherited genodermatoses, the predisposition to skin cancer extends to the oral mucous membranes, as seen with xeroderma pigmentosum, dyskeratosis congenital, and polydysplastic epidermolysis bullosa (Fraumeni, 1982). In Bloom's syndrome, which features chromosomal breakage, there is an exceptional risk of leukemia and several other neoplasms, including oral cancer (German and Passage, 1989). Multiple-case families have been reported occasionally (Hara et al, 1988), including occurrences in identical twins (Bhaskar et al, 1988), but it has not been possible to distinguish genetic factors from environmental or chance events.

LIP CANCER

Cancers of the lip are mainly squamous cell carcinomas. They are uncommon in most parts of the world, with age-adjusted incidence rates generally in the range of 0.1 to 5 per 100,000 population per year (Fig. 32-5), but occasionally exceeding 10 per 100,000 per year, as in parts of Canada and Australia (Parkin et al, 1992; Blot et al, 1994). The highest rates have been observed in Newfoundland fishermen, with the annual incidence reported to exceed 50 per 100,000 (Spitzer et al, 1975). However, geographic differences may be complicated by variations in distinguishing lip cancers from cancers arising from the adjacent skin and oral mucosa. Nevertheless, the incidence of lip cancer appears to be declining in many areas. For example, decreases of at least 50% in age-adjusted rates have reported among men in England and Wales, and in parts of Canada and the United States, from the 1960s to 1980s (Morton et al, 1983; Blot et al, 1994). Table 32-7, which shows incidence rates for lip cancer in the United States, illustrates the substantial excesses (nearly 10- to 40-fold) among white males as compared to black males and to females of both races. Nearly all lip cancers occur on the lower lip, often associated with labial solar keratoses. Among more than 3,700 microscopically confirmed cancers of the lip included in the U.S. SEER program, 1975–85, when the site was specified, 92% occurred on the lower lip. Prognosis for patients with lip cancer is good, with a 5-year relative survival of 90% (National Cancer Institute, 1989), and mortality rates even in high-risk areas do not exceed 0.2 deaths per 100,000 per year (Young et al, 1981).

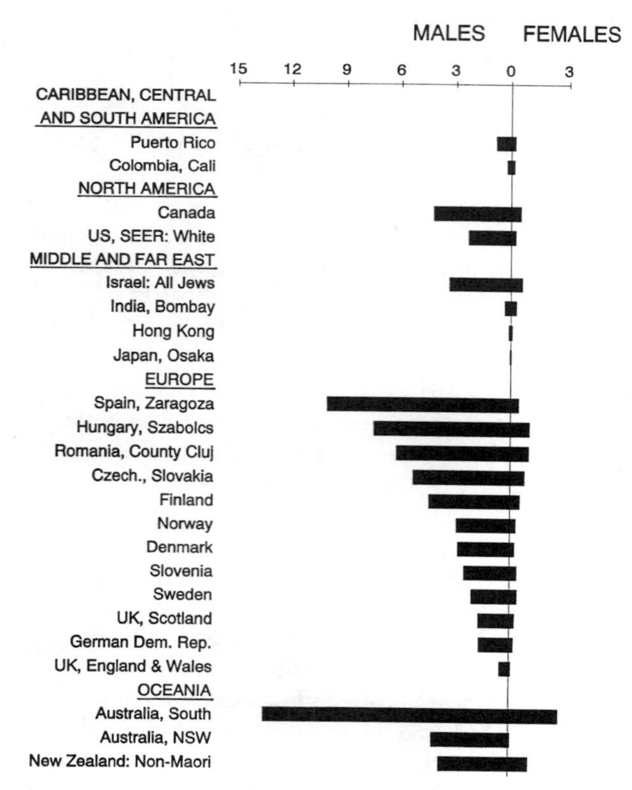

FIG. 32–5. International variation in lip cancer incidence 1983–1987. Age-adjusted (world standard) annual rates per 100,000. (From Blot et al., 1994.)

The primary causes of lip cancer are exposures to sunlight, as with cancers of facial skin, and to tobacco products (Keller, 1970; Lindquist, 1979). Although the latitudinal gradient is less pronounced than with skin cancer, an association with sunlight is consistent with the concentration of tumors on the more exposed lower lip, the male predominance, and association with outdoor occupations, such as farming and fishing, and the predisposition of those with fair complexions or with sun-sensitive genodermatoses such as xeroderma pigmentosum (Spitzer et al, 1975; Lindquist, 1979; Preston-Martin et al, 1982; Dardanoni et al, 1984; Wiklund and Holm, 1986). Patients with lip cancer have an excess risk of skin cancers and intraoral cancers (Winn and Blot, 1985), also consistent with the role of sunlight and tobacco use.

Reports from the 1950s and earlier emphasized the relation of lip cancer to pipe smoking, but more recent data indicate that as smoking habits have changed, the excess risk is mainly among cigarette smokers (Spitzer et al, 1975; Lindquist, 1979; Dardanoni et al, 1984). Still, the thermal and mechanical irritation from pipe smoking appears to exert a further risk. In one case-control study (Lindquist, 1979), tobacco smoking and outdoor occupations seemed to combine to greatly enhance risk. Little is known about other potential risk factors, although a viral origin is suggested by an excess of labial herpes infections in lip cancer patients (Lindquist, 1979).

SALIVARY GLAND CANCER

Cancers of the salivary glands are relatively rare, accounting for 8% of newly diagnosed cancers of the oral cavity and pharynx (Young et al, 1981). The tumors are mainly adenocarcinomas. Geographic comparisons may be distorted by inclusion of benign (mixed) tumors of the salivary glands in some registries. In Western countries, the majority of cancers arise in the parotid gland, but the proportion appears to be lower in certain underdeveloped areas. Among the 100 incidence rates listed for registries reporting to Cancer Incidence in Five Continents (Parkin et al, 1992), in only two instances—males in Canada's Yukon and Northwest Territories and both sexes in northeast Scotland—were the age-adjusted incidence rates as high as 2 per 100,000 per year, although higher rates have been reported among Alaskan natives (Lanier et al, 1976). International variation, as shown in Figure 32-6, is thus very limited (Blot et al, 1994). In most areas of the world, the frequency is greater in men than women (see Table 32-7 for U.S. data), but the sex ratio is generally less than two. In the United States, a recent increase in the incidence of salivary gland cancer has been noted among men residing in the San Francisco–Oakland area, although the reason for this trend is unclear (Horn-Ross et al, 1991). Five-year relative survival is 65% for men and 80% for women (National Cancer Institute, 1989). During the period 1975–90, mortality rates for salivary gland cancer in the United States were 0.3 per 100,000 per year among males and 0.2 among females, showing only a slight decline since the 1950s (National Cancer Institute, unpublished data; McKay et al, 1982; Blot et al, 1994). As with other oral tumors, salivary gland cancer rates increase steadily with advancing age, although rates for black males increase more rapidly at young ages before plateauing (Fig. 32-7).

TABLE 32–7. *Incidence of Lip and Salivary Gland Cancer in the United States by Sex and Race, 1975–1990**

		Lip		*Salivary Glands*	
Sex	*Race*	*No.*	*Rate*	*No.*	*Rate*
Male	White	4972	3.6	1641	1.2
	Black	17	0.2	112	0.9
Female	White	688	0.4	1363	0.8
	Black	12	0.1	118	0.7

*Data from 9 SEER Registries.

The causes of salivary gland cancers are largely unknown, although high levels of ionizing radiation from the atomic bombs of Hiroshima and Nagasaki and repeated medical and dental X-irradiation have been reported to increase risk (Belsky et al, 1975; Spitz et al, 1984, 1990; Preston-Martin et al, 1988; Preston-Martin and White, 1990). Case-control studies have not shown a relationship to tobacco or alcohol use, except possibly in women (Preston-Martin et al, 1988; Spitz et al, 1990). Associations with use of hair dyes and mouthwash have been suggested (Spitz et al, 1990). Although

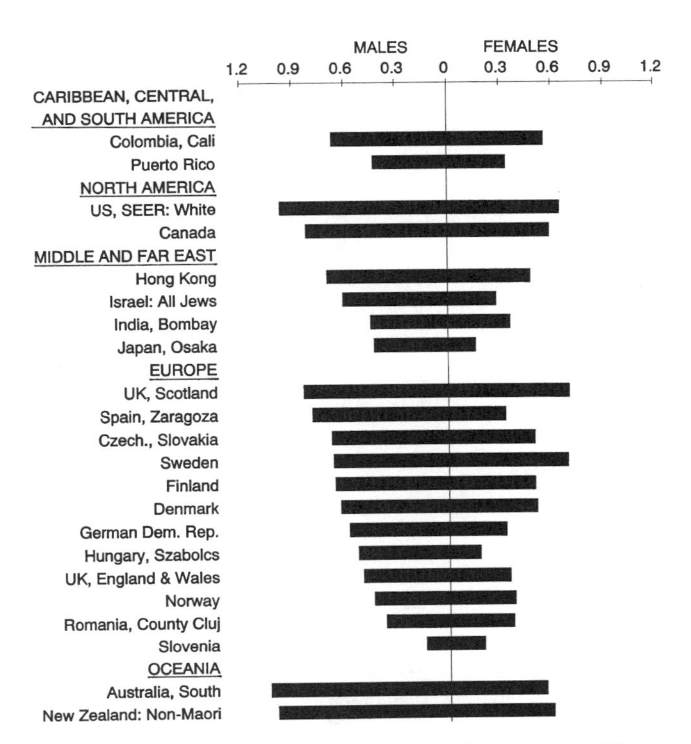

FIG. 32–6. International variation in salivary gland cancer incidence, 1983–1987. Age-adjusted (world standard) annual rates per 100,000. (From Blot et al., 1994.)

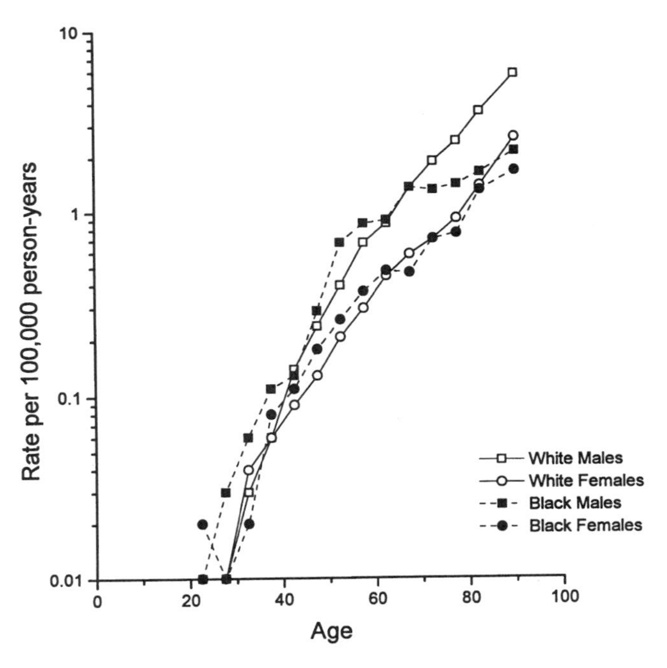

FIG. 32–7. Age-specific mortality rates for salivary gland cancer in the United States by race and sex, 1975–1990. (Based on data from the National Center for Health Statistics.)

experimental studies suggest that vitamin A deficiency may enhance salivary gland carcinogenesis (Rowe et al, 1970), supplementation with retinol palmitate, beta-carotene, or canthaxanthin did not inhibit DMBA-induced salivary tumors in rats (Alam et al, 1988), and the limited epidemiologic data have not identified dietary risk factors (Spitz, 1984). Occupational factors may be involved in some cases, with reports of excessive rates of salivary gland cancers among rubber workers, automotive industry woodworkers, and farmers (Mancuso and Brennan, 1970; Swanson and Belle, 1982). Hormonal risk factors have been suggested by reports that salivary and breast cancers occur excessively together as multiple primaries (Abbey et al, 1984; Harvey et al, 1985), although these findings are not always observed (Winn and Blot, 1985). In case reports of parotid gland cancers among Eskimos, EBV genome equivalents in biopsy material suggest a role for viruses (Saemundsen et al, 1982). Familial clustering of these tumors has also been reported among Eskimos (Merrick et al, 1986).

PREVENTIVE MEASURES

Most cancers of the oral cavity and pharynx are preventable. The single most effective measure to lower the incidence and mortality of these cancers is to reduce exposure to tobacco and alcohol. This requires continued educational efforts to encourage smokers to quit smoking and young people to avoid the tobacco habit. Antismoking campaigns should be directed also toward minority groups, blue-collar workers, and other segments of the population with excessive exposures and risks. The prevalence of smoking among adult males in the United States has been declining over the past 25 years, but still approximately 30% of American men and nearly as many women smoke cigarettes (Marcus et al, 1989). Since smoking reduction results in a lower risk of oral cancer relatively soon after quitting, programs to maintain and accelerate these downward trends in smoking should be emphasized. The effects may already be occurring, as national age-adjusted oral cancer mortality rates among white males declined over 15% in the past 15 years, with decreases affecting nearly all age groups. There is concern that the recent upturn in smokeless tobacco use by teenage boys (Orlandi and Boyd, 1989) may eventually increase oral cancer rates in the United States. Not only is there a risk of oral cancer associated with long-term use of smokeless tobacco, but adolescent users can become addicted to nicotine and convert to smoking later in life (Surgeon General, 1986). Recent labels mandated for snuff and chewing tobacco packages warning of cancer risk, and educational campaigns indicating that smokeless tobacco is not a safe alternative to smoking (Blot and Boyd, 1986), should help stem the rising prevalence of smokeless tobacco use. Educational campaigns to reduce intake of smokeless tobacco and smoking have been conducted successfully in parts of India, with a subsequent 4- to 5-fold reduction in oral leukoplakia (Gupta et al, 1986).

Prevention activities should emphasize reduction in alcohol consumption along with tobacco intake. Alcohol abstention appears to convey the greatest protection, but since most oral cancers arise in heavy drinkers, campaigns that encourage limiting intake to light drinking should also be effective in lowering oral cancer risk.

There is considerable promise that dietary modification may help reduce oral cancer risk. Increasing intake of fresh fruits and salad vegetables appears to be protective, but further research is needed to clarify the dietary associations with oral cancer and determine the specific nutrients (e.g., carotene or vitamin C) or other dietary constituents that are responsible. Although it is perhaps too early to make definitive recommendations, the inclusion of fruit and fresh vegetables in the daily diet seems prudent, and strategies for chemoprevention should be considered in high-risk groups with clinical or subclinical markers of precancerous states.

Because the prognosis for oral cancer is not good, and because curative surgery can lead to facial disfigurement, major emphasis should be placed on strategies for prevention and early diagnosis, with special efforts to encourage avoidance of tobacco and alcohol. Since the likelihood of a second cancer among long-term survivors of oral cancer is substantial, continued surveillance of patients with these cancers is required. Screening of oral cancer patients as well as those belonging to high-risk groups is feasible and may help identify new cancers at a stage when posttreatment morbidity is low and survival relatively high (Mashberg and Barsa, 1984; Silverman, 1988; Mashberg and Samit, 1989).

Further research into the origins and natural history of oral cancer will help develop and target additional measures for primary and secondary prevention, but the current need is urgent to undertake more ambitious programs aimed at reducing intake of the major risk factors, tobacco and alcohol.

REFERENCES

ABBE R. 1915. Cancer of the mouth. NY Med J 102:1–2.

ABBEY LM, SCHWAB BH, LANDAU GC, et al. 1984. Incidence of second primary breast cancer among patients with a first primary salivary gland tumor. Cancer 54:1439–1442.

ALAM BS, ALAM SQ, WEIR SC. 1988. Effects of excess vitamin A and canthaxanthin on salivary gland tumors. Nutr Cancer 11:233–241.

AXELL T. 1987. Occurrence of leukoplakia and some other oral white lesions among 20,333 adult Swedish people. Community Dent Oral Epidemiol 15:46–51.

BARONE J, TAIOLI E, HEBERT J, et al. 1992. Vitamin supplement use and risk of oral and esophageal cancer. Nutr Cancer 18:31–41.

BELSKY JL, TAKEICHI N, YAMAMOTO T, et al. 1975. Salivary gland neoplasms following atomic irradiation. Cancer 35:555–559.

BENNER SE, WINN RJ, LIPPMAN SM, et al. 1993. Regression of oral leukoplakia with α-tocopherol: a community clinical oncology program chemoprevention study. J Natl Cancer Inst 85:44–47.

BHASKAR PB, SMITH RG, BAUGHMAN RA. 1988. Oral squamous cell carcinoma in identical twins: report of a case. J Oral Maxillofac Surg 46:1096–1098.

BIRT D. 1986. Update on effects of vitamins A, C, and E and selenium on carcinogenesis. Proc Soc Exp Biol Med 183:311–320.

BLOT WJ, FRAUMENI JF, JR. 1977. Geographic patterns of oral cancer in the United States: Etiologic implications. J Chron Dis 30:745–757.

BLOT WJ, FRAUMENI JF, JR. 1982. Geographic epidemiology of cancer in the United States. In Schottenfeld D, Fraumeni, JF, Jr (eds): Cancer Epidemiology and Prevention. Philadelphia: Saunders, pp. 179–193.

BLOT WJ, WINN DM, FRAUMENI JF, JR. 1983. Oral cancer and mouthwash. J Natl Cancer Inst 70:251–253.

BLOT WJ, BOYD G. 1986. Health implications of smokeless tobacco use. Public Health Rep 101:349–354.

BLOT WJ, MCLAUGHLIN JK, WINN DM, et al. 1988. Smoking and drinking in relation to oral and pharyngeal cancer. Cancer Res 48:3282–3287.

BLOT WJ. 1992. Alcohol and cancer. Cancer Res 52 (Suppl.): 2119s–2123s.

BLOT WJ, DEVESA SS, MCLAUGHLIN JK, et al. 1994. Oral and pharyngeal cancer. Cancer Surv 19:23–42.

BOUQOUT JE, GOURLIN RJ. 1986. Leukoplakia, lichen planus and other oral keratoses in 23,616 white Americans over the age of 35 years. Oral Surg Oral Med Oral Pathol 61:373–381.

BRICHACEK B, HIRSCH I, SIBL O, et al. 1984. Presence of Epstein-Barr virus DNA in carcinomas of the palatine tonsil. J Natl Cancer Inst 72:809–811.

BRINTON LA, GRIDLEY G, HRUBEC Z, et al. 1989. Cancer risk following pernicious anemia. Br J Cancer 59:810–813.

BRUGERE J, GUENEL P, LECLERC A, et al. 1986. Differential effects of tobacco and alcohol in cancer of the larynx, pharynx, and mouth. Cancer 57:391–395.

CHANG KW, CHANG CS, LAI KS, et al. 1989. High prevalence of human papilloma virus infection and possible association with betel quid chewing and smoking in oral epidermoid carcinomas in Taiwan. J Med Virol 28:57–61.

DALING JR, WEISS NS, KLOPFENSTEIN LL, et al. 1982. Correlates of homosexual behavior and the incidence of anal cancer. JAMA 247:1988–1990.

DARDANONI L, GAFA L, PATERNO R, et al. 1984. G: A case-control study on lip cancer risk factors in Ragusa (Sicily). Int J Cancer 34:335–337.

DAVIS S, SEVERSON RK. 1987. Increasing incidence of cancer of the tongue in the United States among young adults. Lancet 2:910–911.

DAY GL, BLOT WJ. 1992. Second primary malignancies in patients with oral cancer. Cancer 70:14–19.

DAY GL, BLOT WJ, AUSTIN D, et al. 1993. Racial differences in risk of oral and pharyngeal cancer. J Natl Cancer Inst 85:465–473.

DEAN G, MACLENNAN R, MCLOUGHLIN H, et al. 1979. Causes of death of blue-collar workers at a Dublin brewery, 1954–73. Br J Cancer 40:581–589.

DEPUE R. 1986. Rising mortality from cancer of the tongue in young white males. N Engl J Med 315:647.

DEVESA SS, BLOT WJ, FRAUMENI JF, JR. 1990. Cohort trends in mortality from oral, esophageal, and laryngeal cancers in the United States. Epidemiology 1:116–121.

DEVILLIERS E, WEIDAUER H, OTTO H, et al. 1985. Papillomavirus DNA in human tongue carcinomas. Int J Cancer 36:575–578.

ELWOOD JM, PEARSON JCG, SKIPPEN DH, et al. 1984. Alcohol, smoking, social and occupational factors in the etiology of cancer of the oral cavity, pharynx, and larynx. Int J Cancer 34:603–612.

FOWLER CB, REES TD, SMITH BK. 1987. Squamous cell carcinoma of the tongue arising in a long-standing lesion of erosive lichen planus. J Am Dent Assoc 115:707–710.

FRANCESCHI S, TALAMINI R, BARRA S, et al. 1990. Smoking and drinking in relation to cancers of the oral cavity, pharynx, larynx and esophagus in northern Italy. Cancer Res 50:6502–6507.

FRANCO EL, KOWALSKI LP, OLIVEIRA BV, et al. 1989. Risk factors for oral cancer in Brazil: A case-control study. Int J Cancer 43:992–1000.

FRAUMENI JF, JR. 1982. Genetic factors. In Holland JF, Frei E III (eds): Cancer Medicine, 2nd ed. Philadelphia: Lea and Febiger.

GERMAN J, PASSAGE E. 1989. Bloom's syndrome-XII. Report from the registry for 1987. Clin Genet 35:57–69.

GIANTA JL, CONNOLLY G. 1986. The reversibility of leukoplakia caused by smokeless tobacco. J Am Dent Assoc 113:50–52.

GRAHAM S, DAYAL H, ROHRER J, et al. 1977. Dentition, diet, tobacco, and alcohol in the epidemiology of oral cancer. J Natl Cancer Inst 59:1611–1617.

GREENSPAN D, GREENSPAN JS, CONANT M, et al. 1984. Oral "hairy" leukoplakia in male homosexuals: evidence of association with both papilloma virus and a herpes-group virus. Lancet 2:831–834.

GREENSPAN JS, GREENSPAN D, LENNETTE ET, et al. 1985. Replication of Epstein-Bear virus within the epithelial cells of oral "hairy" leukoplakia, an AIDS-associated lesion. N Engl J Med 313:1564–1571.

GREER RO, EVERSOLA LR, CROSBY LK. 1990. Detection of human papilloma virus genomic DNA in oral epithelial dysplasias, oral smokeless tobacco-associated leukoplakias, and epithelial malignancies. J Oral Maxillofac Surg 48:1201–1205.

GRIDLEY G, MCLAUGHLIN JK, BLOCK G, et al. 1992a. Diet and oral and pharyngeal cancer among blacks. Nutr Cancer 14:212–225.

GRIDLEY G, MCLAUGHLIN JK, BLOCK G, et al. 1992b. Vitamin supplement use and reduced risk of oral and pharyngeal cancer. Am J Epidemiol 135:1083–1092.

GUPTA PC, PINDBORG JJ, MEHTA FS. 1982. Comparison of carcinogenicity of betal quid with and without tobacco: an epidemiological review. Ecol Dis 1:213–219.

GUPTA PC, MEHTA FS, PINDBORG JJ, et al. 1986. Intervention study for primary prevention of oral cancer among 36000 Indian tobacco users. Lancet 1:1235–1239.

GUPTA PC, BHOUSLE RB, MURTI PR, et al. 1989. An epidemiologic assessment of cancer risk in oral and precancerous lesions in India with special reference to nodular leukoplakia. Cancer 63:2249–2252.

HAAS JF, RAHU M, STANECZEK W. 1986. Time trends in cancer incidence in the German Democratic Republic, 1968–81. Neoplasma 33:129–139.

HARA H, OZEKI S, SHIRATSUCHI Y, et al. 1988. Familial occurrence of oral cancer: report of cases. J Oral Maxillofac Surg 46:1098–1102.

HARVEY EB, BRINTON LA. 1985. Second cancer following cancer of the breast in Connecticut, 1935–82. Natl Cancer Inst Monogr 68:99–112.

HECHT S, RIVENSON A, BRALEY J, et al. 1986. Induction of oral cavity tumors in F344 rats by tobacco-specific nitrosamines and snuff. Cancer Res 46:4162–4166.

HERRITY B, MORIARTY M, BOURKE G, et al. 1981. A case-control study of head and neck cancer in the Republic of Ireland. Br J Cancer 43:177–182.

HOFFMANN D, HECHT S. 1985. Nicotine-derived N-nitrosamines

and tobacco-related cancer. Current status and future directions. Cancer Res 45:935–944.

HONG WK, ENDICOTT J, ITRI L, et al. 1986. 13-cis-retinoic acid in the treatment of oral leukoplakia. N Engl J Med 315:1801–1505.

HONG WK, LIPPMAN SM, ITRI L, et al. 1990. Prevention of second primary tumors with isotretinonin in squamous cell carcinoma of the head and neck. N Engl J Med 323:795–801.

HORN-ROSS PL, WEST DW, BROWN SR. 1991. Recent trends in the incidence of salivary gland cancer. Int J Epidemiol 20:628–633.

HUEBNER W, SCHOENBERG J, KELSEY J, et al. 1992. Oral and pharyngeal cancer and occupation: a case-control study. Epidemiol 3:300–309.

INTERNATIONAL AGENCY FOR RESEARCH ON CANCER. 1986. Tobacco smoking. IARC Monogr 38:1–421.

INTERNATIONAL AGENCY FOR RESEARCH ON CANCER. 1988. Alcohol drinking. IARC Monogr 44:1–416.

JAYANT K, BALAKRISHNAN V, SANGHVI LD, et al. 1977. Quantification of the role of smoking and chewing tobacco in oral, pharyngeal, and esophageal cancer. Br J Cancer 35:232–235.

JAYANT K, DEO MG. 1986. Oral cancer and cultural practices in relation to betel quid and tobacco chewing and smoking. Cancer Detect Prev 9:207–213.

JAYANT K, YEOLE BB. 1987. Cancers of the upper alimentary and respiratory tracts in Bombay, India: A study of incidence over two decades. Br J Cancer 56:847–852.

JENSEN O. 1979. Cancer morbidity and causes of death among Danish brewery workers. Int J Cancer 23:459–463.

JOHANSSON SL, HIRSCH JM, LARSSON PA, et al. 1989. Snuff-induced carcinogensis: effect of snuff in rats initiated with 4-Nitroquinidine N-oxide. Cancer Res 49:3063–3069.

KABAT GC, HEBERT JR, WYNDER EL. 1989. Risk factors for oral cancer in women. Cancer Res 49:2803–2806.

KABAT GC, WYNDER EL. 1989. Type of alcoholic beverage and oral cancer. Int J Cancer 43:190–194.

KABAT GC, HEBERT JR. 1994. Use of mentholated cigarettes and oropharyngeal cancer. Epidemiology 5:183–184.

KAUGARS GE, MEHAILESCU WL, GUNSOLLEY JC. 1989. Smokeless tobacco use and oral epithelial dysplasia. Cancer 64:1527–1530.

KELLER AZ. 1970. Cellular types, survival, race, nativity, occupations, habits and associated diseases in the pathogenesis of lip cancer. Am J Epidemiol 91:486–499.

KURIHARA M, AOKI K, HISAMACHI S. 1989. Cancer Mortality Statistics in the World 1950–85. Nagoya: Nagoya University Press.

LANIER AP, BENDER TR, BLOT WJ, et al. 1976. Cancer incidence in Alaskan natives. Int J Cancer 18:409–412.

LAVECCHIA C, BIDOLI E, BARRA S, et al. 1990. Type of cigarettes and cancers of the upper digestive and respiratory tract. Cancer Causes Control 1:69–74.

LAVECCHIA C, NEGRI E, DAVANZO B, et al. 1991. Dietary indications of oral and pharyngeal cancer. Int J Epidemiol 20:39–44.

LIND PO. 1987. Malignant transformation in oral leukoplakia. Scand J Dent Res 95:449–455.

LINDQUIST C. 1979. Risk factors in lip cancer. Am J Epidemiol 109:521–530.

MACFARLANE GJ, BOYLE P, SCULLY C. 1987. Rising mortality from cancer of the tongue in young Scottish males. Lancet 2:912.

MAITLAND NJ, COX MF, LYNAS C, et al. 1987. Detection of human papillomavirus DNA in biopsies of human oral tissue. Br J Cancer 51:245–250.

MAITLAND NJ, BROMIDGE T, COX MF, et al. 1989. Detection of human papillomavirus genes in human oral tissue biopsies and cultures by polymerase chain reaction. Br J Cancer 59:698–703.

MANCUSO TF, BRENNAN MJ. 1970. Epidemiological considerations of cancer of the gallbladder, bile ducts and salivary glands in the rubber industry. J Occup Med 12:333–341.

MARCUS AC, SHOPLAND DR, CRANE LA, et al. 1989. Prevalence of cigarette smoking in the United States: estimates from the 1985 current population survey. J Natl Cancer Inst 81:409–414.

MARSHALL J, GRAHAM S, METTLIN C, et al. 1982. Diet in the epidemiology of oral cancer. Nutr Cancer 3:145–149.

MARTINEZ I. 1969. Factors associated with cancer of the esophagus, mouth, and pharynx in Puerto Rico. J Natl Cancer Inst 42:1069–1094.

MASHBERG A. 1977. Erythroplasia vs leukoplakia in the diagnosis of early aymptomatic oral squamous carcinoma. N Engl J Med 297:101–110.

MASHBERG A, GARFINKEL L, HARRIS S. 1981. Alcohol as a primary risk factor in oral squamous carcinoma. CA Cancer J Clin 31:146–156.

MASHBERG A, BARSA P. 1984. Screening for oral and oropharyngeal squamous carcinomas. CA Cancer J Clin 34:262–268.

MASHBERG A, BARSA P, GROSSMAN M. 1985. A study of the relationship between mouthwash use and oral and pharyngeal cancer. JADA 110:731–734.

MASHBERG A, SAMIT AM. 1989. Early detection, diagnosis, and management of oral and oropharyngeal cancer. CA Cancer J Clin 39:67–88.

MASON TJ, MCKAY FW, HOOVER RN, et al. 1975. Atlas of Cancer Mortality for U.S. Counties: 1950–1969. Washington, D.C.: U.S. Govt. Printing Office, DHEW Publ. No. (NIH) 75-780.

MASON TJ, MCKAY FW, HOOVER RN, et al. 1976. Atlas of Cancer Mortality among U.S. Nonwhites: 1950–1969. Washington, D.C.: U.S. Govt. Printing Office, DHEW Publ. No. (NIH) 76-1204.

MCKAY FW, HANSEN MR, MILLER RW. 1982. Cancer Mortality in the United States: 1950–1977. Natl Cancer Inst Monogr 59:1–475.

MCLAUGHLIN JK, GRIDLEY G, BLOCK G, et al. 1988. Dietary factors in oral and pharyngeal cancer. J Natl Cancer Inst 80:1237–1243.

MERLETTI F, BOFFETTA P, CICCONE G, et al. 1989. Role of tobacco and alcoholic beverages in the etiology of cancer of the oral cavity and oropharynx in Torino, Italy. Cancer Res 49:4919–4924.

MERRICK Y, ALBECK H, NIELSEN NH, et al. 1986. Familial clustering of salivary gland carcinoma in Greenland. Cancer 57:2097–2102.

MILLER BA, RIES LA, HANKEY BF, et al. 1993. SEER Cancer Statistics Review 1973–1990 Bethesda, MD: National Cancer Institute, NIH Publ. No. 93-2789.

MIRVISH SS. 1983. The etiology of gastric cancer. J Natl Cancer Inst 71:629–647.

MORTON RP, MISSOTTEN FE, PHAROAH OP. 1983. Classifying cancer of the lip: an epidemiological perspective. Eur J Cancer Clin Oncol 19:875–877.

MOSS E, LEE WR. 1974. Occurrence of oral and pharyngeal cancers in textile workers. Br J Ind Med 31:224–232.

MOSS E. 1976. Oral and pharyngeal cancer in textile workers. Ann NY Acad Sci 271:301–307.

MOULIN JJ, MUR JM, WILD P, et al. 1986. Oral cavity and laryngeal cancers among man-made mineral fiber production workers. Scand J Work Environ Health 12:27–31.

MUIR C, WATERHOUSE J, MACK T, et al. 1987. Cancer Incidence in Five Continents, Vol. V. Lyon: International Agency for Research on Cancer, IARC Publ. No. 88.

NATIONAL CANCER INSTITUTE. 1989. Annual Cancer Statistics Review, 1973–1986, Including a Report on the Status of Cancer Control. Bethesda, MD: National Cancer Inst., NIH Publ. No. 89-2789.

NOTANI PN, JAYANT K. 1987. Role of diet in upper aerodigestive tract cancers. Nutr Cancer 10:103–113.

OFFICE OF POPULATION CENSUSES AND SURVEYS. 1978. Occupational Mortality 1970–1972. London: Her Majesty's Stationery Office, p. 115.

OLSEN J, SABROE S, IPSEN J. 1985. Effect of combined alcohol and tobacco exposure on risk of cancer of the hypopharynx. J Epidemiol Community Health 39:304–307.

OREGGIA F, DE STEFANI E, CORREA P, et al. 1991. Risk factors for cancer of the tongue in Uruguay. Cancer 67:180–183.

ORLANDI MA, BOYD G. 1989. Smokeless tobacco use among adolescents: Theoretical overview. Natl Cancer Inst Monogr 89:5–12.

ORR IM. 1937. Oral cancer in betel nut chewers in Travancore. Lancet 2:575–580.

OSTROW RS, MANIAS D, FONG W, et al. 1987. A survey of human cancers for human papillomavirus DNA by filter hybridization. Cancer 59:429–434.

PARK NW, HERBOSA E, SAPP J. 1986. Herpes simplex infection and simulated snuff dipping. Oral Surg, Oral Med, Oral Pathol 62:164–168.

PARKIN DM, MUIR CS, WHELAN SL, et al. 1992. Cancer Incidence in Five Continents, Vol. VI. 1992 IARC Sci. Publ. No. 120, Lyon: International Agency for Research on Cancer.

PICKLE LW, MASON TJ, HOWARD N, et al. 1987. Atlas of U.S. Cancer Mortality among Whites: 1950–1980. Washington, D.C.: U.S. Government Printing Office, DHHS Publ. No. (NIH) 87-2900.

PINDBORG J, JOLST O, RENSTRUP G, et al. 1968. Studies in oral leukoplakia: a preliminary report on the period prevalence of malignant transformation in leukoplakia based on follow-up study of 248 patients. J Am Dent Assoc 78:767–771.

PRESTON-MARTIN S, HENDERSON BE, PIKE MC. 1982. Descriptive epidemiology of cancer of the upper respiratory tract in Los Angeles. Cancer 49:2201–2207.

PRESTON-MARTIN S, THOMAS DC, WHITE SC, et al. 1988. Prior exposure to medical and dental x-rays related to tumors of the salivary gland. J Natl Cancer Inst 80:943–949.

PRESTON-MARTIN S, WHITE SC. 1990. Brain and salivary gland tumors related to prior dental radiography: implications for correct practice. JADA 120:151–158.

RIES LG, HANKEY BF, MILLER BA, et al. 1991. Cancer Statistics Review 1973–88. Bethesda, MD: National Cancer Institute, NIH Publ. No. 91-2789.

ROSENFELD L, CALLAWAY J. 1963. Snuff dipper's cancer. Am J Surg 106:840–844.

ROSSING MA, VAUGHAN TL, MCKNIGHT B. 1989. Diet and pharyngeal cancer. Int J Cancer 44:593–597.

ROTHMAN K, KELLER A. 1992. The effect of joint exposure to alcohol and tobacco on risk of cancer of the mouth and pharynx. J Chronic Dis 25:711–716.

ROWE N, GRAMMAR F, WATSON F, et al. 1970. A study of environmental influence upon salivary gland neoplasia in rats. Cancer 26:436–444.

SAEMUNDSEN AK, ALBECK H, HANSEN JP, et al. 1982. Epstein-Barr virus in nasopharyngeal and salivary gland carcinomas of Greenland Eskimos. Br J Cancer 46:721–728.

SANGHVI LD, RAO KC. 1955. Smoking and chewing of tobacco in relation to cancer of the upper alimentary tract. Br Med J 1:1111–1114.

SANGHVI LD. 1974. Cancer epidemiology in India: a critique. Indian J Med Res 62:1950–1870.

SANKARANARAYANAN R, DUFFY SW, DAY NE, et al. 1989. A case-control investigation of cancer of the oral tongue and the floor of the mouth in southern India. Int J Cancer 44:617–621.

SCHWARTZ J, SHKLAR G. 1988. Regression of experimental oral carcinomas by local injection of b-carotene and canthaxanthin. Nutr Cancer 11:35–40.

SCULLY C, MAITLAND N, COX M, et al. 1987. Human papillomavirus DNA and oral mucosa. Lancet 8:336.

SELIKOFF IJ, HAMMOND EC, SEIDMAN H. 1979. Mortality experience of insulation workers in the United States and Canada 1943–1976. Ann NY Acad Sci 330:91–116.

SHIBUYA H, AMAGASA T, SETO K, et al. 1986. Leukoplakia-associated multiple carcinomas in patients with tongue carcinoma. Cancer 57:843–846.

SHILLITOE EJ. 1987. Viruses in the etiology of head and neck cancer. Cancer Bull 39:82–88.

SHKLAR G. 1986. Oral leukoplakia. N Engl J Med 315:24–26.

SHKLAR G, SCHWARTZ JL, TRICKLER DP, et al. 1990. Prevention of experimental cancer and immunostimulation by vitamin E. J Oral Pathol Med 19:60–64.

SILVERMAN S, JR, GORSKY M, LOZADA F. 1984. Oral leukoplakia and malignant transformation. Cancer 53:563–568.

SILVERMAN S, JR. 1988. Early diagnosis of oral cancer. Cancer 62:1796–1799.

SPITZ MR. 1984. Risk factors for salivary gland cancer—a review. Cancer Bull 36:115–117.

SPITZ MR, FUEGER JJ, GOEPFERT H, et al. 1990. Salivary gland cancer: a case-control investigation of risk factors. Arch Otolaryngol Head Neck Surg 116:1163–1166.

SPITZ MR, FUEGER JJ, HALAB S, et al. 1993. Mutagen sensitivity in upper aerodigestive tract cancer: a case-control analysis. Cancer Epidemiol, Biomarkers, Prev 2:329–333.

SPITZER WO, HILL GB, CHAMBERS LV, et al. 1975. The occupation of fishing as a risk factor in cancer of the lip. N Engl J Med 293:419–423.

STICH HF, ROSIN MP, VALLAJERA MO. 1984. Reduction with vitamin A and beta-carotene administration of proportion of micronucleated buccal mucosal cells in Asian betel nut and tobacco chewers. Lancet 1:1204–1206.

STICH HF, HORNBY AP, DUNN BP. 1986. Beta-carotene levels in exfoliated mucosal cells of population groups at low and elevated risk for oral cancer. Int J Cancer 37:389–393.

STICH HF, HORNBY AP, MATHEW B, et al. 1988a. Response of oral leukoplakia to the administration of vitamin A. Cancer Lett 40:93–101.

STICH HF, ROSIN MP, HORNBY AP, et al. 1988b. Remission of oral leukoplakias and micronuclei in tobacco betel quid chewers treated with beta-carotene and with beta-carotene plus vitamin A. Int J Cancer 42:195–199.

STICH HF, MATHEW B, SANKARANARYANAN R, et al. 1991. Remission of oral precancerous lesions of tobacco areca nut chewers following administration of B-carotene or vitamin A and maintenance of the protective effect. Cancer Detect Prev 15:93–95.

SUDA D, SCHWARTZ J, SHKLAR G. 1986. Inhibition of experimental oral carcinogenesis by topical beta-carotene. Carcinogenesis 7:711–715.

SURGEON GENERAL. 1982. The Health Consequences of Smoking: Cancer. Rockville, MD: Department of Health and Human Services, DHHS (PHS) 82-50179.

SURGEON GENERAL. 1986. The Health Consequences of Using Smokeless Tobacco. Bethesda, MD: Department of Health and Human Services, NIH Publ. No. 86–2874.

SWANSON GM, BELLE SH. 1982. Cancer morbidity among woodworkers in the U.S. automobile industry. J Occup Med 24:315–319.

TRICKLER D, SHKLAR G. 1987. Prevention by vitamin E of experimental oral carcinogenesis. J Natl Cancer Inst 78:165–169.

TUYNS AJ. 1982. Alcohol. In Schottenfeld D, Fraumeni JF, Jr (eds): Cancer Epidemiology and Prevention. Philadelphia: Saunders, pp. 293–303.

TUYNS AJ, ESTEVE J, RAYMOND L, et al. 1988. Cancer of the larynx/hypopharynx, tobacco, and alcohol. Int J Cancer 41:483–491.

VAGERO D, OLIN R. 1983. Cancer incidence in the electronics industry using the new Swedish Cancer Environment Registry as a screening instrument. Br J Ind Med 40:188–192.

VOGLER WR, LLOYD JW, MILMORE BK. 1962. A retrospective study of etiological factors in cancer of the mouth, pharynx, and larynx. Science 15:246–258.

WATTENBERG LW. 1985. Chemoprevention of cancer. Cancer Res 45:1–8.

WATTS SL, BREWER EE, FRY TL. 1991. Human papillomavirus DNA types in squamous cell carcinomas of the head and neck. Oral Surg Oral Med Oral Pathol 71:701–707.

WEAVER A, FLEMING SM, SMITH DB. 1979. Mouthwash and oral cancer: carcinogen or coincidence? J Oral Surg 37:250–253.

WELLER EA, BLOT WJ, FEIGAL E. 1993. Oral cavity and pharynx. In Miller BA, Ries LAG, Hankey BF, et al (eds): SEER Cancer Statistics Review: 1973–1990. NIH Publ. No. 93-2789, Bethesda, MD: Natl Cancer Inst, pp. XIX.1–15.

WHITAKER CJ, MOSS E, LEE WR, et al. 1979. Oral and pharyngeal cancer in the Northwest and West Yorkshire regions of England, and occupation. Br J Ind Med 36:292–298.

WIKLUND K, HOLM LE. 1986. Trends in cancer risks among Swedish agricultural workers. J Natl Cancer Inst 77:657–664.

WILKINS SA, VOGLER WR. 1957. Cancer of the gingiva. Surg Gynecol Obstet 105:145–152.

WILLETT WG, MACMAHON B. 1984. Diet and cancer: an overview. N Engl J Med 310:633–638.

WINN DM, BLOT WJ, SHY CM, et al. 1981a. Snuff dipping and oral cancer among women in the southern United States. N Engl J Med 304:745–749.

WINN DM, BLOT WJ, FRAUMENI JF, JR. 1981b. Snuff dipping and oral cancer. N Engl J Med 305:230–231.

WINN DM, BLOT WJ, SHY CM, et al. 1982. Occupation and oral cancer among women in the south. Am J Ind Med 3:161–167.

WINN DM, ZIEGLER RG, PICKLE LW, et al. 1984. Diet in the etiology of oral and pharyngeal cancer among women from the southern United States. Cancer Res 44:1216–1223.

WINN DM, BLOT WJ. 1985. Second cancer following cancers of the buccal cavity and pharynx in Connecticut, 1935–1981. Natl Cancer Inst Monogr 68:23–48.

WINN DM, BLOT WJ, MCLAUGHLIN JK, et al. 1991. Mouthwash use and oral conditions in the risk of oral and pharyngeal cancer. Cancer Res 51:3044–3047.

WORLD HEALTH ORGANIZATION. 1978. Definition of leukoplakia and related lesions: an aid to studies of oral precancer. Oral Surg 46:318–339.

WYNDER EL, BROSS IJ, FELDMAN RM. 1957a. A study of the etiological factors in cancer of the mouth. Cancer 19:1300–1323.

WYNDER EL, HULTBERG S, JACOBSON F, et al. 1957b. Environmental factors in cancer of the upper alimentary tract: Swedish study with special reference to Plummer-Vinson (Paterson-Kelly) syndrome. Cancer 10:470–487.

WYNDER EL, STELLMAN SD. 1977. Comparative epidemiology of tobacco related cancers. Cancer Res 37:4608–4622.

WYNDER EL, KABAT G, ROSENBERG S, et al. 1983. Oral cancer and mouthwash use. J Natl Cancer Inst 70:255–260.

YOUNG JL, JR, PERCY CL, ASIRE AJ. 1981. Surveillance, epidemiology and end results: incidence and mortality data 1973–77. Natl Cancer Inst Monogr 57:54–55.

YOUNG TB, FORD CN, BRANDENBURG JH. 1986. An epidemiological study of oral cancer in a statewide network. Am J Otolaryngol 7:200–208.

ZARIDZE D, EVSTIFEEVA T, BOYLE P. 1993. Chemoprevention of oral leukoplakia and chronic esophagitis in an area of high incidence of oral and esophageal cancer. Ann Epidemiol 3:225–234.

ZHENG T, BOYLE P, HU H, et al. 1990. Tobacco smoking, alcohol consumption, and risk of oral cancer: a case-control study in Beijing, People's Republic of China. Cancer Causes Control 1:173–179.

ZHENG W, BLOT WJ, SHU X, et al. 1992. Risk factors for oral and pharyngeal cancer in Shanghai, with emphasis on diet. Cancer Epidemiol Biomarkers Prev 1:441–448.

ZHENG W, BLOT WJ, DIAMOND EL, et al. 1993. Serum micronutrients and subsequent risk of oral and pharyngeal cancer. Cancer Res 53:795–798.

ZIEGLER RG. 1986. Alcohol-nutrient interactions in cancer etiology. Cancer 58:1942–1948.

ZUR HAUSEN H. 1987. Papillomavirus in human cancer. In Fortner JG, Rhoads JE (eds): Accomplishments in Cancer Research, 1986. Philadelphia: Lippincott, pp. 74–81.

33 Esophageal cancer

NUBIA MUÑOZ
NICHOLAS E. DAY

Cancer of the esophagus is the ninth-most common cancer in the world, with about 300,000 cases diagnosed every year; in developing countries it ranks fifth (Parkin et al, 1993). The disease is rapidly fatal for most of those whom it strikes even where medical care meets the highest standards, and the prospect of reducing this toll through earlier diagnosis or improvements in treatment appears poor. Its epidemiological behavior, marked by large differences in incidence within small geographic confines and sharp changes in incidence over time, suggests a predominant role for external environmental factors. Among some populations, major risk factors have already been identified by epidemiologic methods, and there is now a potential for primary prevention. In other areas of the world, primary causes have not been unequivocally identified, but the prospects are encouraging.

Cancer of the esophagus, like cancer of the lung, appears to be a disease whose control will come about by primary prevention utilizing the findings of epidemiologic studies. In addition to a potentially major contribution to public health, the epidemiology of esophageal cancer has yielded insights into factors—genetic, nutritional, or otherwise environmentally determined—that may modify the susceptibility of the esophageal epithelium for neoplastic development and that are running ahead of experimental work in suggesting the parameters of importance in the mechanism involved.

In this chapter, we shall outline the broad features of the occurrence of esophageal cancer in the world, and then discuss the factors related, or hypothesized as being related, to the disease, and their role in determining its geographic and temporal patterns. We conclude by examining the possibilities of prevention, including the nature and distribution of possibly precancerous lesions.

Most published studies reviewed in this chapter do not distinguish between various histological types of esophageal cancer. Consequently, their results are mainly applicable to squamous cell carcinomas, which represent over 90% of esophageal cancer in most populations. When available, data is given separately for squamous cell carcinomas and adenocarcinomas.

DESCRIPTIVE EPIDEMIOLOGY

Worldwide Distribution

Survival from cancer of the esophagus is poor, so that mortality and incidence rates should be comparable. Table 33-1 gives a brief résumé of available mortality and incidence rates, indicating the main features of intercountry variation, with some indication of within-country differences.

Salient features of the table are: (1) very low rates in north and west Africa and among females in many of the populations; (2) high or very high rates among male blacks in both South Africa and North America; (3) intermediate or high rates in some areas in the Caribbean and southeastern Latin America; (4) intermediate rates in the Indian subcontinent; (5) very high rates for China, and in some migrant Chinese populations.

These figures give an indication of the magnitude of the public health problem posed by the disease, but are of limited value for considering the etiological implications. For the latter, finer detail is required.

China

About half the cases of esophageal cancer occurring in the world each year are estimated to occur in China, where it is the second most common cancer after stomach cancer. The national annual mortality rates for the two cancers are in fact very close (for stomach cancer, 32.3 per 100,000 males and 15.9 in females, as compared to 31.7 per 100,000 and 15.9, respectively, for the esophagus). The distribution of the two diseases over the country, however, are very markedly different. Stomach cancer is more common in the north and less common in the south, the changes in incidence are smooth, and in few counties is the disease rare. Esophageal cancer, by contrast, is rare over large tracts of the country, the disease occurring mainly in a few sharply demarcated areas, in which the incidence rises to levels considerably higher than seen anywhere for stomach cancer (see Fig. 33–1).

TABLE 33–1. *Incidence Rates of Esophageal Cancer per Year per 10^5 (standardized to the world population)*

Region—Population	*Male*	*Female*	*Reference*
Africa			
Zimbabwe—Bulawayo-African	58.6	8.1	Parkin et al, 1994
Uganda—Kyadondo	13.0	7.2	Wabinga et al, 1993
Swaziland	11.5	2.4	Parkin, 1986
Nigeria—Ibadan	1.5	1.1	Waterhouse et al, 1976
Algeria—Setif	1.4	0.5	Parkin et al, 1992
Mali—Bamako	1.3	0.7	" "
The Gambia	0.9	0.6	" "
Caribbean			
Bermuda—Black	24.9	0.9	Parkin et al, 1992
White and other	2.7	1.7	" "
Martinique	13.7	2.5	" "
Puerto Rico	9.8	2.1	" "
Cuba	5.2	1.7	" "
Latin America			
Brazil—Puerto Alegre	25.9	6.9	" "
Goiania	9.8	2.6	" "
Paraguay—Asuncion	11.2	1.7	" "
Ecuador—Quito	4.4	0.5	" "
Colombia—Cali	3.6	1.6	" "
Costa Rica	3.8	1.2	" "
Peru—Trujillo	1.0	0.6	" "
North America			
USA, SEER—Black	14.2	3.6	" "
White	4.0	1.3	" "
Canada	4.2	1.3	" "
Asia			
Iran—North Gonbad	165.5	195.5	Mahboubi et al, 1973
China—Linxian	161.0[a]	103.0[a]	National Cancer Control Office, 1980
Shanghai	14.9	6.4	Parkin et al, 1992
Hong Kong	18.1	3.6	" "
Japan—Miyagi	14.1	2.4	" "
Osaka	8.4	1.8	" "
Kyrgyzstan	11.8	5.5	" "
India—Bombay	11.4	8.4	" "
Madras	7.6	6.3	" "
Singapore—Chinese	10.9	2.7	" "
Indian	3.2	3.4	" "
Malay	1.2	0.9	" "
Thailand—Chiang Mai	4.1	2.7	" "
Philippines—Manila	3.1	2.3	" "
Israel—all Jews	1.4	1.1	" "
Europe			
France—Calvados	26.5	1.7	Parkin et al, 1992
Somme	9.5	0.8	" "
Russia—St. Petersburg	11.1	3.7	" "
Spain—Basque country	10.3	0.7	" "
Granada	4.4	0.3	" "
UK, North Scotland	9.4	4.7	" "

(continued)

TABLE 33–1. (*Continued*)

Region—Population	*Male*	*Female*	*Reference*
UK, England & Wales	6.5	3.2	" "
Slovenia	7.7	0.6	" "
Italy—Varese	7.6	0.8	" "
Ragusa	1.6	0.2	" "
Switzerland—Geneva	7.5	1.5	" "
Zurich	3.5	0.8	" "
Germany—Saarland	6.1	0.8	" "
Czechoslovakia—Slovakia	5.6	0.5	" "
Poland—Warsaw City	5.2	0.9	" "
Estonia	5.0	0.7	" "
Ireland—Southern	4.5	4.2	" "
Belarus	4.4	0.5	" "
Iceland	4.0	2.2	" "
Denmark	3.9	1.3	" "
Finland	3.3	2.2	" "
Netherlands—Eindhoven	3.2	1.0	" "
Sweden	3.2	0.9	" "
Norway	2.6	0.8	" "
Australia—Victoria	5.0	2.3	" "
Western	3.9	1.7	" "
New Zealand—Maori	7.0	1.0	" "
Non Maori	5.3	2.4	" "

[a]Mortality rates.

The Central Asian Esophageal Cancer Belt

Westward from the high-incidence area in northern Sinkiang, areas of extremely high incidence are seen in the Republics of Kazakhstan, Uzbekistan, and Turkmenistan, in the northeast of Iran and northern Afghanistan. These regions, together with western Sinkiang, form the center of the old Turkic Kingdom of Uleg Beg and Timur, with Samarkand as capital. In all four countries, high rates of the disease are seen almost exclusively in the groups of Turkic origin—Turkoman, Uzbek, and Kazakh—and not in the groups of Indo-European origin—Persian, Pathan, and Russian. Rates are also high among both sexes in northern and eastern Siberia, the affected populations being also of Mongol origin (Yakuts, Chakchi, Eskimos, Evenki, and Yukagir). The rates for males for the whole central Asian region are displayed in Figure 33–2. One can see, as in Figure 33–1, not only the areas of very high incidence, but also the remarkably rapid fall-off to areas with low or moderate rates (the corresponding map displaying female rates is almost identical).

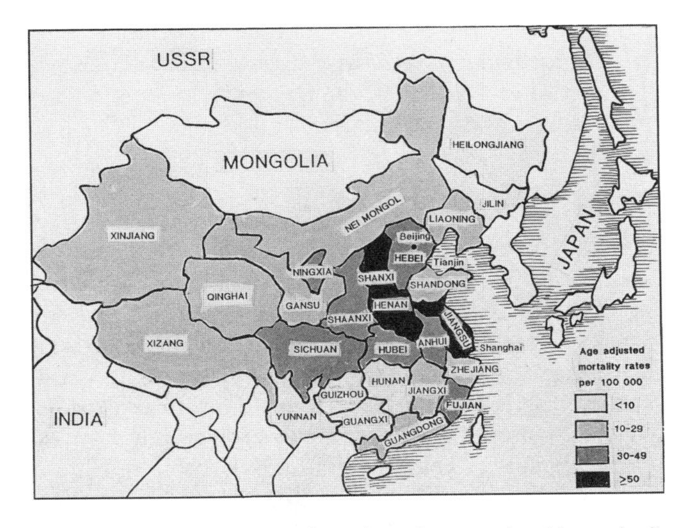

FIG. 33–1. Mortality rates of esophageal cancer (world standard) among males in China.

The area of this region that has been most extensively studied is northern Iran; Figure 33–3 displays the incidence rates as recorded by the Caspian Cancer Registry. Studies undertaken to exploit the range of incidences are described in a later section.

A noteworthy feature of the incidence pattern seen in China and central Asia is the parallelism between male and female rates. When the rates are high they are equally high in both sexes, with the highest rates sometimes seen in females. When the rates are low, there is typically a 2- or 3-fold male excess. There is little evidence that rates are changing over time among the indigenous population of these areas.

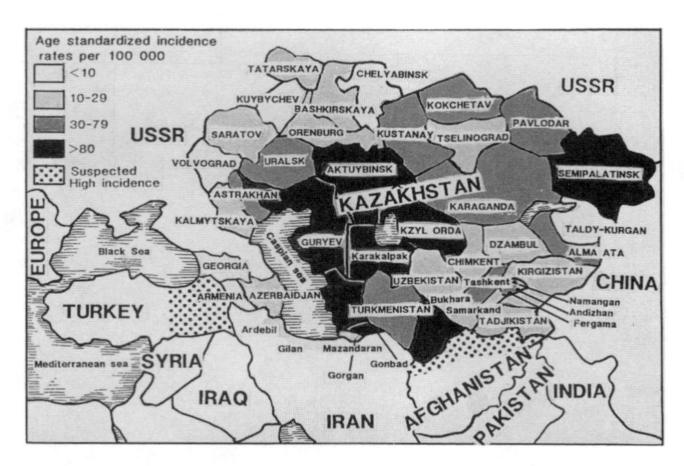

FIG. 33–2. Incidence rates (world standard) of esophageal cancer among males in Central Asia.

TABLE 33–2. *Esophageal Cancer among Chinese in Singapore: Age-Standardized Annual Incidence Rates, 1968–77**

	Male	*Female*
By dialect group		
Cantonese	4.5	2.2
Teochew	30.7	7.8
Hokkien	27.5	6.7
By place of birth		
China	22.8	6.1
Singapore	7.0	2.2
Annual decrease in incidence over the period 1968–82	3.4%	6.1%
Age-adjusted incidence, 1968–72	20.1	6.4
Age-adjusted incidence, 1978–82	13.5	3.7

*From Shanmugaratnam et al (1983); Lee et al (1988).

Chinese Migrant Population: Singapore

Given the variation in rates in China (Fig. 33–1), incidence or mortality figures for Chinese living outside China can be used to assess the effect of migration only if their place of origin in China is known. For many Chinese populations outside China, such information is not fully available. An exception is Singapore, where the cancer registry has information both on place of origin of the family in China (that is, dialect group) and on whether the person was born in China or Singapore. Most Chinese in Singapore come either from the south of Kwantung province (Cantonese speakers), from Fukkien province (Hokkien speakers), or from the neighborhood of Swatow in northeast Kwantung province (Teochew speakers). The last two groups come from one of the areas shown in Figure 33–1 as having exceptionally high incidence. The rates in Table 33-2 reflect these differences. Table 33-2 indicates also the first-generation effect in esophageal cancer incidence. Unlike cancer of the stomach, where the difference is minimal, Singapore-born Chinese have only 40% of the risk of China-born. The esophagus, in fact, is the only site where the China-born have a substantially higher risk.

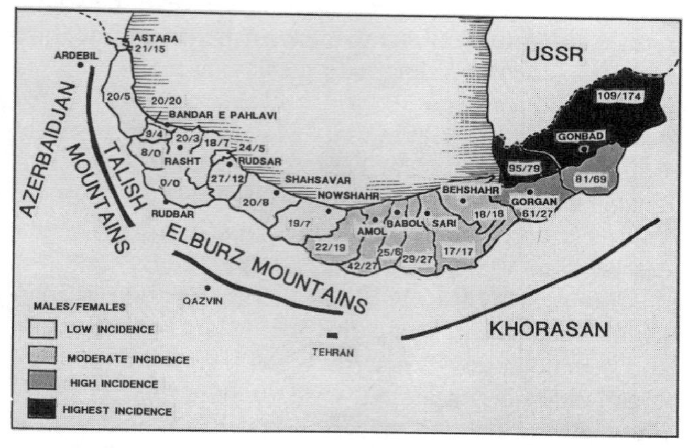

FIG. 33–3. Incidence of esophageal cancer (world standard) among males and females in the Caspian littoral of Iran. (From Mahboubi et al, 1973.)

Africa

The epidemiology of esophageal cancer in the African continent has been frequently reviewed (Van Rensburg et al, 1983). Throughout north, west, and central Africa, the disease is rare. In east and southern Africa, areas of high and low incidence are intermingled, with sharp gradients of incidences. Unlike China and Central Asia, however, in some of the areas of high interest mainly males are affected, as in Bulawayo (see Table 33-1) or some regions around Lake Victoria. In South Africa, particularly in the associated rural regions of the Transkei and the Ciskei, the incidence in females rises in parallel with that in males.

Europe

Males. The major patterns of variation in Europe are seen for males, the incidence among females being low or very low in most of Europe except in Ireland and Scotland (see Table 33-1). Even in Europe, a striking feature of the epidemiology of the disease is the large variation, greater in relative terms than for most other cancers. Brittany and Normandy provide the most extreme examples. The distribution by canton in Brittany is shown in Figure 33–4. Data by canton have not yet been published for the other two departments with high rates, Manche and Mayenne, which would round out

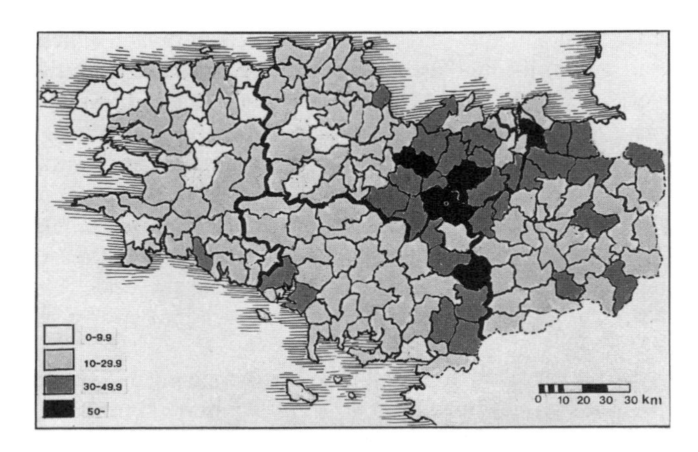

FIG. 33–4. Age-standardized mortality rates per 100,000 for cancer of the esophagus among males in Brittany, 1958–1966. (From Tuyns and Vernhes, 1981.)

the picture. The rates in western Brittany and in the southeast of Orne are similar to the average rates in France. In the foci of high incidence, the rates are 5 to 10 times higher.

In Italy, the European country with the highest alcohol consumption after France, esophageal cancer rates nowhere reach the levels seen in Brittany, but of the commoner cancers, the rates show the greatest variation. Between the northeast and south, there is more than a 6-fold difference (see Fig. 33–5), compared to differences of only 3-fold for cancers of the stomach, colon, or lung.

Within Scotland the highest rates are seen in the main whisky-distilling areas (Kemp et al, 1992).

Females. Among females in Europe, the picture is completely different. Throughout the Mediterranean region, including France and Italy, and central and eastern Europe, the disease is very rare (see Table 33–1). Only in Scandinavia, particularly in the north, in St. Petersburg, and in the British Isles is the disease seen with any frequency.

The Americas

High rates are seen, particularly among men, in Uruguay, southeast Brazil (Puerto Alegre in Table 33–1), and northeast Argentina. This is the maté-drinking area, discussed later. Moderately high rates are seen in much of the Caribbean. In North America, high rates are observed among United States blacks, particularly urban blacks, among whom the disease is now one of the more common types of cancer (Muir et al, 1988). Among counties on the southeastern Atlantic coast, high rates are also seen, especially among blacks (Fraumeni and Blot, 1977). In Alaska and Greenland, Eskimos and

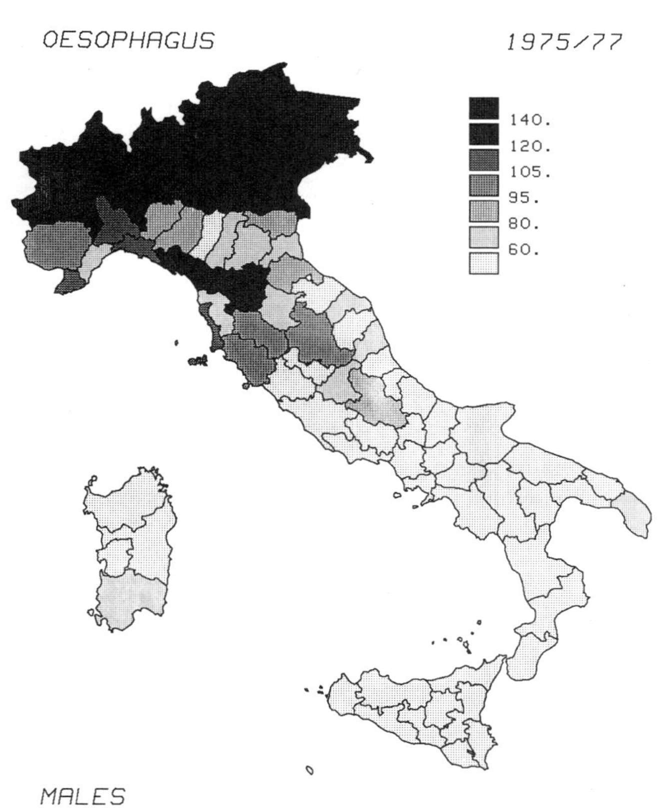

FIG. 33–5. Mortality rates per 100,000 for cancer of the esophagus in Italy. (From Cislaghi et al, 1986.)

Aleuts formerly suffered a high frequency of the disease, particularly in women, which has declined in recent years (Lanier et al, 1980). The similarity with northern and eastern Siberia is noteworthy.

TIME TRENDS

Asia and Oceania

In the areas covered by the "Asian esophageal cancer belt" this cancer appears to have been common for many centuries. Changes have been reported recently in some of these areas. In Linxian, China, for example, where the incidence and mortality rates have been high, a slight recent decrease has been reported among younger age groups (Lu et al, 1985), but in Shanghai the rates have decreased more than 50% from 1972 to 1989 (Zheng et al, 1993). In the Central Asian Republic of Karakalpakstan, with rates reaching 126 per 100,000 in males and 151 in females in the northern region, a substantial reduction in both sexes over the last 20 years has been reported (Zaridze et al, 1992). Time trends using incidence data from selected populations included in the six volumes of Cancer Incidence in Five Continents and mortality rates for the period 1955–1985 from the World Health Organization database have been reported (Coleman and Estève, 1993). These data show stable rates among males in Japan and Hong Kong and among females in New Zealand and Australia; recent increasing trends are seen among males in New Zealand and Australia and decreasing rates in Singapore, in Bombay, India, and among females in Japan and Hong Kong.

Strong correlations have been shown in Australia between the time trends in sex-specific mortality from cancers of the esophagus and of the larynx and alcohol consumption (McMichael, 1978).

The most dramatic changes have occurred among Chinese in Singapore, where the incidence is falling rapidly, especially among females (Table 33–2). Among Singapore-born females, the disease has now become rare. The fall in both sexes is more rapid than for any of the other cancers common in mainland China. The causes of this decline remain to be determined.

Africa

There is also some evidence that the disease is of recent origin and has been increasing. Patterns of contrasting incidence in the Transkei have been extensively documented, but it seems that in the areas formerly of low incidence in northern Transkei, the incidence has risen rapidly in the last 15 years (Table 33–3).

Europe

A recent analysis of the time trend from 1951 to 1985 of the mortality from esophageal cancer in 17 European countries shows that, except among the younger age group in men, esophageal cancer had either decreased or increased only slightly in most countries. The increase was more than 100% only in the youngest age group in men (50–59 years) in four of these 17 countries: Northern Ireland, Czechoslovakia, Spain, and Denmark. This trend differed from that of mortality from lung cancer and cirrhosis and that of alcohol consumption, which had generally increased substantially during the study period (Cheng et al, 1992a). Among females the rates have been decreasing in most countries, with slight increases (20%–37%) only in four countries: Scotland, Ireland, England and Wales, and Spain. More than 100% increase was observed only in Norway in women 50–59 years of age (Cheng et al, 1992a). The decrease has been more marked in Finland, where the once relatively high rates have largely disappeared, as shown in Table 33-4.

Møller et al (1990) attributed the increasing mortality in male cohorts born after 1910 in Denmark, Hungary, Germany, and Czechoslovakia to rising alcohol consumption. In addition, it has been suggested that the decrease in esophageal cancer mortality observed in some European countries is unlikely to be due to an improvement in treatment and that these decreases and the slight increases observed in most countries are probably the result of population-wide changes in certain undetermined risk/protective factor(s), one of which is possibly the consumption of fruit that had partially overridden the effect of tobacco and alcohol (Cheng et al, 1992a).

In relation to histologic types, since the early 1970s increases in the incidence of adenocarcinoma of the esophagus and of the gastric cardia have been reported in the West Midlands Region of the United Kingdom (Powell and McConkey, 1990) and in Denmark (Møller, 1992). In the Oxford region of the United Kingdom, a significant increase over time in the incidence of adenocarcinoma of the cardia but no appreciable change in the incidence of esophageal cancer was reported (Harrison et al, 1992). In some cancer registries in France and Switzerland a trend toward an increasing proportion of adenocarcinomas has been observed (Tuyns, 1992).

It is not clear how much of the increase in adenocarcinoma might be explained by shifts in classification, diagnostic practices, or in the proportion of unspecified tumors.

TABLE 33–3. *Changing Patterns of Esophageal Cancer Incidence in the Transkei**

	Annual Rates per 100,000 Population					
	Males			*Females*		
	1955–59	*1965–69*	*1981*	*1955–59*	*1965–69*	*1981*
Northern Transkei	13	14	51	8	5	33
Southern Transkei	93	68	63	48	33	65

*From Van Rensburg et al (1983).

TABLE 33–4. *Decreasing Rates (per 10^5) per Year of Esophageal Cancer among Females in Finland**

Year	*Age-Standardized Rate*	*Age Group*						
		45–49	*50–54*	*55–59*	*60–64*	*65–69*	*70–74*	*75–79*
1954	6.4	2.9	7.6	12.1	25.9	41.6	62.1	91.2
1964	4.9	1.5	5.5	6.6	19.8	34.9	54.8	72.8
1974	3.3	0	4.2	7.8	12.7	20.3	32.0	47.4
1984	2.1	0	1.5	5.0	4.4	14.7	17.7	31.5

*From the Finnish Cancer Registry (1982).

The Americas

During the period 1950–80, a dramatic increase in the incidence and mortality rates of esophageal cancer occurred among blacks in the United States, while the rates for whites remained nearly unchanged (Blot and Fraumeni, 1987; Bang et al, 1988).

That rising mortality among blacks is due to poorer medical care seems unlikely, since survival rates for esophageal cancer are very low regardless of race. In addition, similar trends are observed in the incidence data (Bang et al, 1988). Therefore, the observed black/white differences are probably real and not the result of artifacts of diagnosis or reporting. Race-specific trends in smoking and alcohol consumption suggest that these two factors, the major determinants of esophageal cancer in the U.S., are small contributors to the increasing trend in blacks (Blot and Fraumeni, 1987). It is thus possible that racial differences in nutritional status may also underlie the racial differences in the time trends of esophageal cancer in the United States.

An analysis of cancer incidence data from nine areas of the United States by histological type revealed stable trends for squamous cell carcinoma from 1976 to 1987 for both blacks and whites and steadily rising rates of adenocarcinoma of the esophagus and of the gastric cardia. The increases among men ranged from 4% to 10% per year and thus exceeded those of any other types of cancer (Blot et al, 1991). Improved specification of diagnosis and changes in classification and diagnostic practices over time might explain part of this increase. The causes of the real increase remaining after these factors have been taken into account are unknown.

In most Latin American countries stable or slightly decreasing trends are observed. One exception is São Paulo, Brazil, where the incidence rates have been increasing both in males and females (Coleman and Estève, 1993). In Uruguay, where the highest rates are reported in Latin America, a recent decline has been observed (de Stefani et al, 1994).

EXOGENOUS CAUSATIVE FACTORS

Tobacco, Alcohol, Betel, Opium

Heavy consumption of alcohol and tobacco have long been suspected of increasing risk for the disease (Young and Russel, 1926; Craver, 1932). Case-control studies in Denmark (Mosbech and Videback, 1955), France (Schwartz et al, 1962), and the United States (Steiner, 1956) gave more formal support to the association. The degree of risk and the interaction between the two factors were first studied in some detail by Wynder and Bross (1961). Table 33-5 gives the risk associated with different levels of smoking and drinking separately, showing a well-defined dose response and substantial levels of risk for heavy consumers of either. Tobacco chewing also significantly increased risk, although the numbers were small.

A study performed in the Department of Ille-et-Vilaine (Tuyns et al, 1977) further quantified the association between alcohol, tobacco, and esophageal cancer. Table 33-6 gives the associated risks over a wide range of levels of both factors. A multiplicative model for the combined risk fits the data well. The very high risk suffered by those who both drink and smoke heavily is striking.

The risk associated with varying degrees of consumption of alcohol and tobacco can be described by a simple parametric function, given by

$$\text{Relative risk} = \text{Exp}\ (0.025 \times \text{ALC})\ (\text{TOB} + 1)^{0.54}$$

where ALC is the average daily consumption of ethanol, in grams, and TOB is the average daily quantity of tobacco smoked, in grams (Breslow and Day, 1980). The exponential increase in risk associated with increasing alcohol consumption is interesting and contrasts with the less than linear increase in risk associated with increased tobacco smoking.

An extension of the study in the department of Calvados has provided risk estimates for alcohol in the ab-

TABLE 33–5. *Relative Risk of Esophageal Cancer Associated with Differing Levels of Tobacco and Alcohol Consumption in North American Males**

Smoking				*Alcohol*			
Cigarette Equivalents per Day	*Percentages*			*Alcohol Consumption*	*Percentages*		
	Case	*Controls*	*RR*		*Case*	*Controls*	*RR*
None	5	15	1.00	Never or rarely	12	48	1.00
1–9	7	9	2.33	1–2 drinks a day	17	26	2.62
10–20	39	43	2.72	≥3 drinks a day	71	26	10.92
21–34	22	16	4.13				
≥35	26	17	4.59				

*Adapted from Wynder and Bross (1961).

TABLE 33–6. *Relative Risk of Esophageal Cancer Associated with Varying Levels of Consumption of Alcohol and Tobacco, in Brittany Males**

Alcohol	*Tobacco*			
	Grams Smoked per Day			
Grams of Ethanol Consumed per Day	*0–9*	*10–19*	*20–29*	*≥30*
0–40	1.0	3.4	3.2	7.8
41–80	7.3	8.4	8.8	35.0
81–120	11.8	13.6	12.6	83.0
≥121	49.6	65.9	137.6	155.6

*Adapted from Tuyns et al (1977).

sence of smoking, and for smoking in the absence of alcohol. The effect of each factor in the absence of the other is clear (Table 33-7).

The role of alcohol and tobacco has been demonstrated in many areas of the world, including Puerto Rico (Martinez, 1969), Southern Brazil (Victoria et al, 1987), Uruguay (Vassallo et al, 1985; de Stefani et al, 1990), South Africa (Segal et al, 1988; McGlashan et al, 1982), Italy (La Vecchia et al, 1986; Decarli et al, 1987), Japan (Hirayama, 1979), and the black population of the United States (Pottern et al, 1981). In the high-incidence areas of China and Central Asia, however, where the majority of cases worldwide occur, and also in Singapore, tobacco and alcohol play a negligible role in the etiology (de Jong et al, 1974; Cook-Mozaffari et al, 1979; Crespi et al, 1984; Li et al, 1989; Yu et al, 1993). However, in a recent case-control study in Heilongjiang province, a low-risk area in China, alcohol and tobacco were identified as the major risk factors (Hu et al, 1994).

Although many studies have examined the issue, little evidence has been forthcoming to show that different types of alcoholic drinks affect risk differently. The main effect relates to the total consumption of ethanol (IARC, 1988). However, accurate information on the relative quantities of different drinks consumed is difficult to obtain, and most of the proposed mechanisms of action of alcoholic drinks would suggest that higher alcohol concentration should convey higher risk (e.g., as a solvent, as a transport sector to the basal layer of the esophageal mucosa, or as an irritant). The issue must be regarded as unresolved. There is some evidence that high-tar, hand-rolled, black tobacco cigarettes (La Vecchia et al, 1986; de Stefani et al, 1990, 1993) and pipe smoking (Tuyns and Estève, 1983) may increase risk per gram of tobacco more than other forms of smoking.

TABLE 33–7. *Relative Risk among Males for Esophageal Cancer (number of cases in parentheses)**

Alcohol (gm) per Day	*Alcohol among Nonsmokers*	*Tobacco (gm) per Day*	*Smoking among Nondrinkers*
0–40	1.0 (7)		
>40–80	3.8 (15)	0–15	1.0 (4)
>80–120	10.2 (9)	>15	5.2 (7)
>120	101.0 (8)		

*Adapted from Tuyns (1983).

In Western Europe and North America, 90% or more of the risk of esophageal cancer can be attributed to alcohol and tobacco. Even in these areas, however, low socioeconomic status and poor nutrition status are of importance. In other regions of the world, dietary factors and other exogenous agents assume a larger role; tobacco is also used in different ways.

Jussawalla (1971) gives a comprehensive review of the role of smoking, chewing (both betel and tobacco), and drinking habits in Bombay, where esophageal cancer is about equally common in males and females. A summary of the findings is given in Table 33-8. Alcohol on its own is not significant. In conjunction with smoking, drinking local brews containing a high proportion of raw spirits is associated with particularly high risk, as is smoking the local type of cigarette, the bidi. The seemingly paradoxical finding that the betel quid without tobacco engenders greater risk than the quid with

TABLE 33–8. *Relative Risk of Esophageal Cancer Associated with Combinations of Smoking, Chewing, and Drinking, in Bombay**

	Males	*Females*
Smoking		
Bidi	8.0	7.4
With cigarettes	2.8	—[a]
Both types	37.5	—[a]
Chewing		
Betel with tobacco	2.9	1.8
Betel without tobacco	15.9	6.3
Alcohol		
Foreign brew	2.4	—[a]
Local brew	12.0	—[a]
Smoking and chewing		
With tobacco	24.4	4.9
Without tobacco	94.2	—[a]
Smoking and alcohol use	18.1	—[a]
Chewing and alcohol use	12.0	—[a]
Smoking alone	4.2	17.8
Chewing alone	3.5	2.3
Alcohol use alone	0.4	—[a]

*Based on Jussawalla (1971).
[a]Insufficient numbers for a relative risk estimate.

tobacco is explained by Jussawalla on the grounds that tobacco chewers usually spit the liquid extract produced by chewing, whereas betel chewers habitually swallow most of the liquid. Exposure to the esophagus will differ accordingly. As can be seen, combined exposures lead to particularly high risks. Betel quid chewing with tobacco (pan tobacco) was not found to be a significant risk factor for cancer of the esophagus in both sexes in the southern Indian state of Kerala (Sankaranarayanan et al, 1991). Tobacco smoking in the form of bidi smoking and bidi plus cigarette smoking and alcohol emerged as independent risk factors in males on multivariate analysis. Significant interaction between alcohol and tobacco smoking was observed in this study. Of great interest is the inability of any researcher to attribute more than a small fraction of the incidence in males to chewing, smoking, or drinking. Few women indulge in more than one of the three different habits, and few drink alcohol. In contrast to the oral cavity, for which 70% of tumors are attributable to chewing and smoking, the figure for the esophagus is only 50%, both sexes combined (Jayant et al, 1977).

Chewing tobacco (nass) is also widespread in central Asia. In areas of very high incidence, however, it does not make an appreciable contribution to the overall risk (Cook-Mozaffari et al, 1979). The use of opium, in contrast, appears of major importance, at least in northern Iran. Among adults in the high-incidence areas, use is widespread in both sexes, almost 50% of the population having levels of morphine metabolites in the urine, suggestive of addictive intake (Ghadirian et al, 1985). Use takes two main forms, smoking and eating, but the residues formed in the pipe when opium is smoked are recycled to retrieve the morphine (opium dross contains some 3% to 5% morphine). This residue, known as sukhteh, is either extracted with boiling water and evaporated to dryness (known as shireh) or simply eaten or smoked in its crude form. Of particular significance is the widespread use of sukhteh addictively and medicinally for headaches and gastrointestinal complaints. Sukhteh is strongly active in the Ames test (Hewer et al, 1978), is an initiator on mouse skin in a two-stage carcinogenesis model, and displays a range of other genotoxic activities (Friesen et al, 1985, 1987). The active components of sukhteh, substituted hydroxyphenanthrenes, represent a new class of carcinogenic compounds, and are related structurally to benzo[c]phenanthrene, the metabolic products of which display intense tumorigenic activity in rodents (Levin et al, 1980). The frequency of opium use, and hence the availability of sukhteh, parallels the incidence of esophageal cancer in northern Iran, and is also higher in households of esophageal cancer patients (Ghadirian et al, 1985). Opium use is also frequent in parts of Afghanistan (Gobar, 1976). The role of opium in the Soviet central Asia and China is unclear; its use was certainly frequent in both areas formerly. The extent to which the habit, or the initiating effect of earlier use, may have continued to the present is unclear. Of possible relevance is the reported decline in the disease in Lin Xiang in China among those born after 1940 or so—i.e., those who reached adolescence after the revolution (Lu et al, 1987).

Unusual practices associated with pipe smoking have been described in the areas of the Transkei where the disease is common (Rose, 1978). The residue in the stem (injonga) is sucked out through a straw and swallowed, and the residues in the bowl of the pipe (isixaxa) are scraped out and then chewed. These residues have demonstrated mutagenic activity in the Ames test (Hewer et al, 1978), at a considerably higher level on a weight-for-weight basis than cigarette smoke condensates. The association of high incidence and the chewing of highly mutagenic pyrolyzed residues in both Iran and the Transkei deserves further study.

The Effect of Reducing Alcohol or Tobacco Consumption. There appear to be no data in the literature on the combined smoking and drinking history of those who have given up either habit. Data are available on ex-smokers from the prospective study of United States veterans (Rogot, 1979), as shown in Table 33-9. However, ex-smokers may well have drunk less alcohol than continuing smokers, and to examine this possibility the corresponding relative risks for cirrhosis (a surrogate measure of alcohol consumption) from the study of veterans are given (Rogot, 1979). The lower risk in ex-smokers appears to be at least partially due to their lower alcohol consumption. One might speculate that

TABLE 33–9. *Relative Risks for Esophageal Cancer and for Cirrhosis among Smokers and Ex-smokers*

A. Current Smokers (cigarettes only)			
Number Smokers/Day	*Esophageal Cancer*[a]	*Cirrhosis*[a]	*Esophageal Cancer*[b]
<10	3.06	2.01	
10–20	4.34	2.26	
21–39	12.42	3.49	
≥40	9.20	4.69	
All smokers	6.43	2.69	6.1
B. Ex-smokers			
Interval since Quitting	*Esophageal Cancer*[a]	*Cirrhosis*[a]	*Esophageal Cancer*[b]
<5 years	4.77	0.0	2.9 (<5 and 5–9 years)
5–9 years	2.50	1.58	
10–14 years	2.06	1.60	
15–19 years	1.21	1.06	1.2
≥20 years	2.48	1.57	

[a]From Rogot (1979).
[b]From Doll and Peto (1976).

tobacco pyrolysates affect early stages in the induction of esophageal tumors, implying a long delay between elimination of exposure and appreciable reduction of risk (Day and Brown, 1980), whereas alcoholic beverages accelerate later stages in the process. The excess relative risk would then fall relatively rapidly after cessation of alcohol consumption. The results from Puerto Rico (Martinez, 1969) suggest a large reduction in risk 10 years or more after giving up alcohol, but neither the level of former alcohol consumption nor that of tobacco consumption is given, rendering the interpretation unclear.

Ingestion of Hot Food and Drink. Hot drinks have regularly been proposed as augmenting the risk for esophageal cancer, but convincing evidence is difficult to obtain. Both the quantity of liquid consumed and the temperature to which the esophagus is exposed are not easy to measure (de Jong et al, 1972). In the high-incidence region of southern Brazil, Uruguay, and northeast Argentina, the habit of maté drinking presents an unusual opportunity for assessing the role of hot drinks. It has long been suggested that the intake of maté, a hot infusion of *Ilex paraguariensis,* may be responsible for this high incidence. This tea is drunk through a metal tube that brings the hot liquid onto the posterior part of the tongue, whence it is promptly swallowed. This habit is very common in the high-incidence area and not elsewhere, and large quantities of maté (often more than one liter) may be drunk each day. In addition, unlike other high-incidence areas, South America has a well-defined unexposed group, since approximately 10%–20% of the adult population do not drink maté at all. Studies in these areas (Vasallo et al, 1985; Victoria et al, 1987; de Stefani et al, 1990; Castelletto et al, 1994) demonstrate a clear effect of alcohol and tobacco and a moderate independent effect of hot maté drinking. A clear and independent increase in risk was observed in Uruguay with both amount and duration of hot maté drinking (Vasallo et al, 1985; de Stefani et al, 1990). In Brazil, a nonsignificant increase in risk was observed among daily drinkers of maté after adjustment for confounding variables (Victora et al, 1987), but in Argentina a moderate increase in risk was observed only among those who reported drinking maté hot or very hot versus those drinking it warm (Castelletto et al, 1994). Alcohol, mainly spirits, and tobacco, together with low fruit consumption, increased risk independently. Quantitatively, the risk associated with maté drinking appeared sufficient to explain the high rates in the area. A complementary study has demonstrated that maté drinking is also associated with histologically confirmed esophagitis (Muñoz et al, 1987). Based on the above studies, hot maté drinking has been classified as probably carcinogenic to humans (IARC, 1991). The effect could be due to components of maté themselves being carcinogenic or promoting, or to the temperature. No relevant in vitro activity has been demonstrated. On the other hand, studies in other parts of the world have associated different types of hot food and drink with increased risk. The evidence for each study is less clear than from the South American studies, but together they point strongly in the same direction.

Ecological studies from Japan (Segi, 1975), the Soviet Union (Kolicheva, 1980), and northern Iran (IARC/Iran Study Group, 1977; Ghadirian, 1987) have suggested that inhabitants from high-risk areas drink larger quantities of hot tea than do those from low-risk areas. Also from Iran, a case-control study indicated similar differences (Cook-Mozaffari et al, 1979). De Jong et al (1974) found that esophageal cancer cases in Singapore were more likely than controls to report drinking "burning-hot" beverages. The same association was found in another case-control study in Puerto Rico investigating the intake of hot coffee (Martinez, 1969). A prospective study carried out by Hirayama (1971) in Japan also showed a higher risk among those drinking hot green tea.

A study among young adults in a high-risk area of China revealed that the habit of drinking "burning-hot" beverages was the strongest risk factor for esophagitis (Wahrendorf et al, 1989), and it was a strong risk indicator in a low-risk area for esophageal cancer in northeast China (Hu et al, 1994). In Hong Kong, preference for consuming drinks or soups at high temperatures was reported to account for 14% of esophageal cancer (Cheng et al, 1992b).

OTHER EXOGENOUS FACTORS

Pickled Vegetables

Consumption of pickled vegetables was held to be one of the major determinants of the high risk of esophageal cancer in Henan province, China. This was not confirmed in the large-scale case-control study conducted in Linxian (Li et al, 1989), but in a recent case-control study of chronic esophagitis carried out in the same area, consumption of pickled vegetables during adolescence was associated with an increased risk (Chang-Claude et al, 1990). In addition, a strong association with pickled vegetables was detected in a large case-control study of esophageal cancer conducted recently in Hong Kong, with an attributable risk of about 30% (Cheng et al, 1992b). On the other hand, pickled vegetables and moldy food consumption were not associated with esophageal cancer in a recent retrospective cohort study in Linxian, China (Yu et al, 1993). In an international evaluation of the carcinogenic potential of pickled vegetables, it was concluded that pickled vegetables as prepared traditionally in Asia are possibly carcinogenic to humans (IARC, 1993). N-nitroso compounds and mycotoxins from fungi present in the pickled vegetables have been postulated as the responsible carcinogenic agents, but final proof of their role needs to be established.

Nitrosamines

Nitrosamines were thought, some years ago, to be the key to the etiology of esophageal cancer, in view of the specificity of action of some nitrosamines for the esophagus of several animal species. However, studies generated by these hypotheses, hypotheses that may have considerable theoretical attraction, have not provided conclusive data. The diet in northern Iran and alcoholic drinks from Brittany and Normandy have been extensively analyzed for nitrosamine levels (Walker et al, 1979) and for the levels of nitrate and nitrite from which nitrosamines may be formed in vivo. The results have been negative, and for alcoholic drinks particularly would suggest that nitrosamines are not involved, since beer contained the greatest quantities and is less strongly associated with the disease. In China, nitrosamines and their precursors have been found in food consumed in the high-risk areas, particularly in fungus-infected samples, including moldy cornbread and pickled vegetables. Feeding of these moldy foods and pickled vegetables to rodents induced precancerous changes in the esophagus and stomach (Yang, 1980). However, no association with these moldy foods or pickled vegetables was found in a large recent case-control study in this population (Li et al, 1989) nor in a retrospective cohort study (Yu et al, 1993). Higher amounts of O^6-methyldeoxyguanosine, a DNA alkylation adduct resulting from exposure to nitrosamines among other alkylating agents, have been found in the esophageal mucosa of subjects from China than in subjects from Europe (Wild et al, 1987), but the application of these assays to large-scale epidemiological studies is not yet possible. Endogenous formation of N-nitroso compounds assessed by the N-nitrosoproline test in subjects from high- and low-risk areas in China have provided suggestive results (Chen et al, 1987; Wu et al, 1993). Chronic exposure to dietary amines and nitrates has been documented in a population at high risk for esophageal cancer in Kashmir, India (Siddiqi et al, 1992).

Infectious Agents

Human papillomavirus (HPV) has been considered as a potential etiological agent in esophageal cancer, but the evidence is largely inconclusive. Some investigators have been able to detect HPV DNA in 20% to 70% of biopsies from esophageal cancers (Chang et al, 1993; Williamson et al, 1991; Benamouzig et al, 1992), but others have failed to do so (Loke et al, 1990; Ashworth et al, 1993). The association has not been evaluated in any formal epidemiological study.

The suggestion that syphilis is associated with esophageal cancer was not confirmed by case-control studies (Mosbech and Videback, 1955; Wynder and Bross, 1961).

Contamination of wheat and maize with *Fusariarum moniliformis*, a fungus characteristic of hot dry climates that produces carcinogenic toxins called fumonisins, has been suspected to be associated with esophageal cancer in South Africa and China (Sydenham et al, 1990), but formal studies to assess this association are lacking.

A significant positive relation has been reported between mortality from esophageal cancer in Shanxi, China, and the consumption of dietary corn and wheat flour (Chen et al, 1993). Fumonisin B1 and other mycotoxins have been detected in moldy corn collected from high-risk areas for esophageal cancer in China (Chu and Li, 1994).

Physical and Chemical Chronic Injury

Like most tissues, the esophagus is susceptible to the carcinogenic effects of ionizing radiation. Data from A-bomb survivors (Beebe et al, 1977) and from the cohort treated by radiation for ankylosing spondylitis (Smith and Doll, 1978) demonstrate the effect.

The follow-up of 17,800 insulation workers in North America (Selikoff and Hammond, 1978) suggests that asbestos exposure increases risk for the disease, with 18 cases observed when only 7.01 were expected.

Silica fibers and fragments are common contaminants of coarse bread eaten by the high-risk populations of Iran, Transkei, and China. Silica has also been found in the esophageal mucosa surrounding tumors in patients from Henan, China, in amounts 10 times higher than those found in tissue for a control group from London. It has been postulated that these silica fragments produce trauma and may stimulate proliferation of epithelial cells (O'Neill et al, 1986).

Cicatricial strictures of the esophagus due to the ingestion of lye occasionally give rise to malignant tumors. Vinson (1940), writing fifty years ago, stated that malignancy is rarely, if ever, observed in benign strictures arising from other causes. Lye, however, was formerly responsible for some 60% of strictures, which may also have been more severe. A specific effect for lye is not established.

Bracken Fern

The eating of bracken fern has been associated with increased risk of esophageal cancer in Japan (Hirayama,

1979). Daily consumption increases risk 2-fold or more compared to less frequent consumption. There has been speculation that the relatively high incidence of the disease in North Wales is in part related to local use of bracken fern.

Occupation

Two studies from Sweden have identified occupational groups at high risk of esophageal cancer—vulcanization workers (Norell et al, 1983) and chimney sweeps. For neither would excessive smoking or drinking be likely contributors. The former also had a high rate of laryngeal cancer. The chimney sweeps would have been heavily exposed to soot from wood-burning stoves, i.e. pyrolyzed vegetable matter. A 3-fold increase in mortality from esophageal cancer has been reported among Swedish workers exposed to combustion products—i.e., chimney sweeps, waste incinerator workers, gas workers, and bus garage workers exposed to diesel exhausts. Tobacco smoking and alcohol consumption did not contribute greatly to this excess in risk (Gustavsson et al, 1993). Long-term occupational exposure to metal dust, especially beryllium, has been found to increase the risk of tumors of the lower third of the esophagus, after adjustment for alcohol, tobacco, and other risk factors (Yu et al, 1988).

Various other occupations have slightly higher risks for the disease, most of which one can assume to have high alcohol consumption (Clemmesen, 1965). Thus, the risk of esophageal cancer has been found to be reduced among Danish male farmers and increased among Italian farmers, probably reflecting differences in alcohol consumption between farmers of the two countries compared to the general population (Ronco et al, 1992). Clemmesen also mentions as being at elevated risk a group of occupations involving various types of metal work—plumbers, brass and bronze workers, and electrical-apparatus makers. However, the overall occupational component to the causation of esophageal cancer is probably small.

SOCIOECONOMIC STATUS

Esophageal cancer is a disease of the poor in most areas of the world. Not all impoverished populations have a high rate for the disease, but where the disease is common the population is frequently deprived in some manner (Day, 1975). Furthermore, case-control studies have frequently shown that within a population risk is higher among the lower socioeconomic strata.

In the United States, the ten-city survey of 1947 showed a smooth decrease in risk with income, the poorest group having some two and a half times the incidence of the richest group. The case-control study reported by Wynder and Bross (1961) found lower educational status among the cases, as well as a poorer dietary history. Duration of schooling was also found to be inversely related to risk of esophageal cancer in a case-control study in Singapore (de Jong et al, 1974). In Puerto Rico, Martinez (1969) showed, in addition to the effects of alcohol and tobacco, that the disease was more common in the lower income groups. Farmers and agricultural workers had twice the risk of managerial and professional workers (Martinez, 1964). In the former Soviet Union, Kolicheva (1980) refers to the poor diet among the native groups in northern and eastern Siberia, with vitamin C deficiency and few fruits or vegetables.

Among blacks in Washington, D.C., risk was highest among the poorest (Pottern et al, 1981), and even in the deprived township of Soweto, cases were more common among the lowest socioeconomic stratum (Segal et al, 1988). A clear gradient with social class has been observed in a review including case-control and cohort studies from 13 countries in Europe, North America, South America, and Asia (Faggiano et al, 1994).

In Soviet Central Asia the situation is perhaps similar to that in neighboring regions of Iran, where studies have shown a restricted diet among high-incidence groups. We refer later to the specific nutritional deficiencies that have been observed. In addition to population studies, a case-control study (Cook-Mozaffari et al, 1979), in which controls were individually matched to cases for village of residence, age, and sex, showed a strong socioeconomic effect. Other tumors were included in the study to exclude the possibility that any socioeconomic effect demonstrated was simply a reflection of being sick. Although low socioeconomic status increased risk for other tumors (particularly of the stomach), the effect was greatest for the esophagus. As in other studies relating level of education to esophageal cancer risk, the Iranian study showed that indicators of socioeconomic status in childhood and early adult life were as strongly associated with risk as were markers of socioeconomic status just before the onset of disease. The significance of this finding is that the observed low economic level among cases is not the result of a debilitating condition, such as alcoholism or opium addiction, but may itself be the cause of the disease. The low economic level precedes the possible onset of such conditions.

RISK FACTORS FOR ADENOCARCINOMA

The most common site of adenocarcinoma is the lower third of the esophagus, and its incidence is higher in whites, males, and higher socioeconomic groups. Longstanding reflux esophagitis has been suspected of leading to Barrett's esophagus (columnar metaplasia of the squamous cell epithelium of the lower esophagus), and an increased risk of adenocarcinoma has been reported in patients with Barrett's esophagus (Bonelli, 1993; Moghissi et al, 1993; Spechler, 1994). However, the magnitude of the risk remains to be determined (Spechler and Goyal, 1986). Experimental studies in rats suggest that reflux of duodenal contents rather than gastric contents are important in the development of esophageal adenocarcinoma (Mirvish et al, 1993).

Few epidemiological studies have investigated the environmental factors linked to adenocarcinoma, in part owing to the rarity of these tumors. In China, where cardia cancer is common, a large case-control study including 214 adenocarcinomas of the cardia and of the esophagus did not reveal strong risk factors. A slight increase in risk was observed with tobacco smoking, but only in the communes at lower risk for esophageal cancer. Alcohol consumption in this population was too low to allow a proper evaluation (Li et al, 1989). Other studies in Japan and the United States are consistent with weak associations of tobacco and alcohol with cardia cancer (Unakami et al, 1989; Wu-Williams et al, 1990). A case-control study conducted in Italy including cancers of the cardia and of the stomach revealed no association with tobacco smoking and a weak effect with total alcohol intake (Palli et al, 1992). In a comparison of 30 cases of adenocarcinoma of the cardia with 140 cases of uncomplicated Barrett's esophagus, no significant association with tobacco or alcohol was detected (Levi et al, 1990), suggesting that these two factors do not increase the risk of progression from Barrett's to cancer, but their effects in the induction of Barrett's esophagus remain to be determined. Independent associations between adenocarcinoma of the distal esophagus/cardia and tobacco smoking and alcohol consumption have been reported in a multicenter case-control study in the U.S. In addition, total fat and vitamin A were positively associated with the risk of adenocarcinoma, while fiber intake was inversely associated with it (Kabat et al, 1993). The weak associations between adenocarcinoma and tobacco and alcohol consumption contrast with the strong effects shown earlier for the squamous cell carcinoma of the esophagus.

Concerning dietary factors, no clear associations were detected in China (Li et al, 1989), but in Italy remarkably similar associations were observed for cancers of the cardia and of the stomach. Protective effects were found for high intake of raw vegetables and fruits or vitamin C, and increased risk was associated with the consumption of traditional soups and meat and a preference for salty foods (Palli et al, 1992).

A positive family history of esophageal or cardia cancer was a significant risk factor for cancer of the cardia both in China and Italy (Li et al, 1989; Palli et al, 1992). This association could be the result of sharing environmental or genetic factors. The possibility of a genetic component is suggested by the higher risk associated with having a parent or sibling than a spouse with cancer in the Chinese study, but the importance of exposures early in life cannot be excluded.

A family with six cases of Barrett's esophagus, three of which were associated with adenocarcinoma, suggests an autosomal dominant pattern of transmission (Jochem et al, 1992).

SUMMARY OF EXOGENOUS CAUSATIVE FACTORS

The theme common to the exposures that augment risk for cancer of the esophagus appears to be intimate contact between the agent and the esophageal mucosa, and the increased ability of the agent to penetrate through the mucosa to the basal layer, presumably where the target cells are to be found (Cairns, 1975). Tobacco smoke condensates in the saliva; pipe scrapings, whether opium or tobacco, chewed in the mouth, and the exudate from a betel quid will pass slowly down the esophagus by peristaltic action. The contact will be close. Alcohol and hot drinks may well act both as solvents and transport media for these carcinogens. Kuratsune et al (1965) have shown, for example, that benzo[a]pyrene penetrates more into the mucosa of a rat's esophagus when in a strong ethanol solution than when in a weak ethanol solution. Benzo[a]pyrene is also known to be greatly more soluble in coffee than in water. The compounds in coffee that solubilize benzo[a]pyrene are also present in tea; so one might speculate that one role for hot tea or coffee or hot tea gruel might be to increase the solubility of the carcinogens in the esophagus, thereby increasing their penetration into the mucosa. In addition, both strong alcohol and hot drinks will act as direct irritants to the esophagus, which, increasing cell turnover, will increase the contact between carcinogen and dividing target cells.

Thus, the three components that seem to lead to high risk are intimate contact between a carcinogenic agent and the esophageal wall, transport through the mucosa to the basal layer, and esophageal irritants that lead to increased cell turnover. In short, external factors so far identified as risk factors are those that favor contact between carcinogen and a dividing target cell. In the next section we consider how systemic factors, whether nutritional or genetic, may modify risk.

HOST SUSCEPTIBILITY

The striking features of the epidemiology of esophageal cancer are the great variation in incidence, even within short distances; the tendency for the male excess to disappear in many areas of high incidence; and the higher incidence in lower socioeconomic groups.

If tumor incidence is considered to be related both to the increased susceptibility and to the action of an exogenous carcinogen, then this variation in incidence could be explained by variation in either or both of these factors. Most research efforts in this field have been directed toward the identification of environmental esophageal carcinogens. However, poor diet and low socioeconomic status seem to be important features of the high-risk profile in many areas of the world, even though the environmental agents vary. It is, then, unlikely that the variations in incidence of this cancer are due solely to variations in the exposure to environmental carcinogens. Variation in susceptibility may well be responsible for much of the great variation in incidence of esophageal cancer. Individual or tissue susceptibility may be genetically or environmentally induced, or both.

Genetic Susceptibility

A striking example of genetic susceptibility is provided by the joint segregation of esophageal cancer and keratosis palmaris et plantaris (tylosis) observed in some families. The two conditions appear to be due to a single autosomal gene with dominant effect. This association was originally described in 18 patients with esophageal cancer belonging to two Liverpool families (Howel-Evans et al, 1958). The tylosis in these cases was of the late-onset form, appearing after one year of age. The esophageal cancers were squamous cell carcinomas arising mostly in the middle and lower thirds of the esophagus. The mean age at onset of cancer was 45 years, and the youngest patient was 20 years old. Two additional families with tylosis, in each of which one member has developed esophageal carcinoma, have been reported from Liverpool, in addition to six new cases of esophageal cancer in one of the original families (Harper et al, 1970). In one of them an association between oral leukoplakia and esophageal cancer was also reported (Tyldesley, 1974), which has also been described in a 26-year-old patient with esophageal cancer, oral leukoplakia, and hyperkeratosis (Ritter and Petersen, 1976). In another family, tylosis has been associated with a congenital esophageal stricture and the subsequent development of esophageal carcinoma (Shine and Allison, 1966). In an Indian family tylosis has been associated with an increased risk of squamous cell carcinoma of the tylotic skin and of the esophagus (Yesudian et al, 1980).

A further report on a member of one of the Liverpool families describes the association of esophageal cancer with tylosis and diffuse follicular hyperkeratosis and raises the interesting possibility of an inherited abnormal vitamin A metabolism as the cause of this syndrome (O'Mahony et al, 1984). HPV DNA has not been detected in the squamous carcinomas arising in a large Liverpool family (Ashworth et al, 1993).

In epidemiological surveys carried out in the high-risk populations of Iran and China no clear tylosis was detected in over 1,600 individuals examined, although it would be difficult to differentiate it from plantar or palmar hyperkeratosis due to walking barefoot or performing manual labor (Crespi et al, 1979; Muñoz et al, 1982, 1985a). This type of genetic susceptibility accounts for only a minimal proportion of esophageal cancers, since only a small number of tylosis-associated cancers have been reported.

Family studies have been inconclusive. One of these studies, involving 877 relatives of 101 esophageal cancer patients and 2,572 relatives of control patients, failed to show any influence by hereditary factors, but showed a clear association of this cancer with alcohol abuse (Mosbech and Videback, 1955). Another study, from the Soviet Union, showed an increased risk for esophageal cancer among spouses of patients with this cancer, suggesting exposure to common environmental factors rather than a hereditary component (Nasipov, 1977). In a village in northern Iran, an aggregation of esophageal cancer in one family has been described; the occurrence of 13 cases of esophageal cancer among 19 relatives from 3 generations is striking (Pour and Ghadirian, 1974). An unusual proportion of these cases were under age 40, some even being under age 30. Two cousin marriages, plus the remoteness of the village, indicate a high degree of inbreeding in the family. In a subsequent report on this population, a positive family history of esophageal cancer was reported in 47% of Turkoman patients with this disease compared to only 2% in non-Turkoman patients (Ghadirian, 1985). Familial aggregation of esophageal cancer has also been reported in some areas of China (Li and He, 1985). How much of this familial aggregation is the result of genetic susceptibility and how much is due to shared environment remains to be elucidated.

Case-control studies among the population of northeast Iran, using various genetic markers such as red blood cell enzymes (Kirk et al, 1977) and HLA antigens (Hashemi et al, 1979) have, however, yielded negative results. In a recent case-control study carried out in Linxian, China, a significant increase in risk of 1.7-fold was associated with the fact of having had one or both parents affected with esophageal and stomach cancer (Li et al, 1989).

A segregation analysis on 221 high-risk families from the same area indicated an autosomal recessive Medelian inheritance with a recessive gene present at a frequency of 19%, causing 4% of this population to be predisposed to esophageal cancer (Carter et al, 1992).

As discussed in an earlier section, the populations at high risk in central Asia and eastern and northern Siberia are of Turkic or Mongol origin. Populations of Caucasian origin in the same region do not suffer the same high rates. The role of genetic factors in this area is in need of further study.

Nutritional Deficiency

Environmental susceptibility and the role of nutritional deficiencies in this susceptibility is illustrated by the increased frequency of cancer of the upper esophagus and hypopharynx in patients with sideropenic dysphagia (Ahlbom, 1936; Beveridge et al, 1965; Jacobsson, 1948; Simpson, 1939; Wynder, 1971). This syndrome was described by Plummer and Vinson in the United States (Vinson, 1922) and earlier by Paterson (1919) and Kelly (1919) in the United Kingdom. The condition is now rare, but it used to be common in some northern parts of the world—for example, certain rural areas of northern Sweden (Waldenstrom, 1946). Relatively high rates for esophageal cancer in females are still seen in northern areas of Norway (Norwegian Cancer Society, 1978) and rural Wales (United Kingdom). These high rates may be the remnants of a high prevalence of Plummer-Vinson syndrome 40 to 50 years ago.

There is some disagreement over the definition of the syndrome. The term Plummer-Vinson, or Paterson-Kelly, syndrome is sometimes used to group all epithelial lesions (atrophic changes of nails, mouth, tongue, hypopharynx, esophagus, and stomach) that may accompany hypochromic anemia, but in a more restricted sense it is reserved for cases with postcricoid dysphagia and the typical radiologic changes observed in the hypopharynx and upper esophagus. Although hypochromic anemia has been reported to occur frequently in patients with this syndrome (Beveridge et al, 1965; Lundholm, 1939; Waldenstrom, 1938; Waldenstrom and Kjellberg, 1939; Wynder et al, 1957), dysphagia has been reported to be uncommon in populations with a high prevalence of severe iron deficiency (Jacobs, 1963).

At present, therefore, the pathogenesis of this syndrome is not clear. Even though iron deficiency may be of prime importance, other nutritional deficiencies, specifically of riboflavin, thiamine, pyridoxine, vitamin C, and animal protein, are likely to be involved (Jacobs and Cavill, 1968; Wynder et al, 1957).

Apart from the Plummer-Vinson syndrome, a more general role for nutritional deficiencies in cancer of the upper alimentary tract has long been suspected. The evidence for this is derived from three types of studies:

1. Ecological studies in the Caspian littoral of Iran have shown strong geographical correlations between esophageal cancer risk and low intakes of animal protein, fresh fruits, and vegetables, which resulted in low intake of vitamins A, C, and riboflavin (IARC/Iran Study Group, 1977). In subsequent correlation studies in African and Asian populations, it was noted that in populations at high risk for esophageal cancer the dietary staple was wheat or corn with low content of riboflavin, nicotinic acid, magnesium, and zinc, whereas in the low-risk populations the staples (sorghum, millet, and cassava) were rich in these micronutrients (Van Rensburg, 1981). In Japan, correlation between data from a nationwide nutrition survey and mortality of esophageal cancer yielded positive correlations with wheat, pork, and dried or salted fish (Nagai et al, 1982). In an international correlation study involving data from 59 countries a protective effect of fruits and total caloric intake and an increased risk with consumption of meat and vegetable oil were reported (Hebert et al, 1993).

2. Case-control studies in various populations have confirmed some of the associations detected in ecological studies: in general in most studies, patients with esophageal cancer reported a history of lower intake of fresh vegetables and fruits than control patients (Wynder and Bross, 1961; Martinez, 1969; Cook-Mozaffari et al, 1979; Ziegler et al, 1981; Victoria et al, 1987; Decarli et al, 1987; Tuyns et al, 1987; Yu et al, 1988; Hu et al, 1994). Associations with other foods, such as meat, dairy products, eggs, and cereals, are controversial: in some studies a reduction in risk has been associated with a high intake of fresh meat and fish (Ziegler et al, 1981; Decarli et al, 1987; Tuyns et al, 1987), but not in others (Victora et al, 1987; Notani and Jayant, 1987; Yu et al, 1988; Li et al, 1989). On the other hand, an increased risk associated with frequent consumption of barbecued meat has been reported in some populations (Victora et al, 1987; Yu et al, 1988; de Stefani et al, 1990). As regards cereals, a case-control study among Zulu men in South Africa identified the consumption of commercial maize meal as one of the main risk factors in this population (Van Rensburg et al, 1983); a strong trend of increasing risk with rising wheat consumption was recently reported in a high-risk population of China (Li et al, 1989), and an increased risk among those who preferred white to whole-grain bread was found in a study in the U.S. (Yu et al, 1988). In two case-control studies an attempt has been made to estimate the combined effect of the food groups affecting the esophageal cancer risk. In the study among black males in Washington, D.C., a nutrition index was constructed taking into account the degree of consumption of the three food groups inversely associated with esophageal cancer—i.e., fresh meat and fish, fruits and vegetables, and dairy products and eggs. The RRs for combinations of high, moderate, and low consumption

TABLE 33–10. *Ethanol-adjusted Risk of Esophageal Cancer by an Overall Measure of Food Consumption Patterns**

Food Consumption Pattern[a]	*Number of Cases*	*Number of Controls*	*Relative Risk*
HHH	2	20	1.0
HHM, HMM	24	65	3.8
HHL, MMM, HML, HLL	32	68	4.5
MML, MLL	36	46	6.7
LLL	11	8	15.0

*From Ziegler (1986).
[a]Concurrent level of consumption of fresh or frozen meat and fish, fruits and vegetables, and dairy products and eggs, each rated as high (H), moderate (M), or low (L). For example, HML indicates high consumption of one of the three food groups, moderate consumption of a second, and low consumption of a third.

of the three food groups were estimated adjusting for alcohol intake. Compared to those who consumed high quantities of all three food groups (HHH), those who consumed low quantities of all three (LLL) had a 15 times higher risk (Table 33–10) (Ziegler, 1986). A similar approach was used in a case-control study in France. A nutritional index was calculated based on the degree of consumption of three food groups associated with a protective effect: fresh meat, citrus fruits, and oil, after adjustment for age and tobacco and alcohol consumption. Compared to those with a low consumption of the three food groups, those with a high consumption of these food groups had one-tenth of the risk (Tuyns et al, 1987).

3. Data from a large-scale cohort study in Japan have shown a reduction in the risk for cancer of the esophagus and of other sites in those who ate green-yellow vegetables daily, even when smoking and drinking habits were maintained (Hirayama, 1986). The interaction of nutritional status with alcohol intake has been examined in two studies which show that these two factors appear to act in a multiplicative way (Ziegler et al, 1981; Tuyns et al, 1987). Table 33–11 summarizes data from the French study.

Concerning the effect of specific nutrients, several studies indicate that subpopulations at high risk for esophageal cancer in Iran, South Africa, and China have low intake and/or low plasma levels of vitamins A, C, beta-carotene, riboflavin, and other micronutrients (IARC/Iran Study Group, 1977; Van Rensburg et al, 1983; Yang et al, 1984). Case-control studies have also reported a history of lower intake of vitamins A, C, and riboflavin among cases than among controls (Martinez, 1969; Cook-Mozaffari et al, 1979; Ziegler et al, 1981; Mettlin et al, 1981). The associations with these micronutrients were, however, in general less strong than those observed for the food groups providing them, raising the possibility that other unidentified constituents of these foods might contribute to their protective effect. A further source of difficulty in the assessment of the effect of specific nutrients is the high degree of correlation among them. In the case-control study in France strong correlations were found between nutrients, while between foods the correlations were weak (Tuyns et al, 1987). Intervention studies might help in elucidating the role of certain micronutrients in the development of esophageal cancer. One such study has been carried out in Huixian, a high-risk area for esophageal cancer in China. It was a double-blind randomized trial involving 610 randomly selected individuals and using the regression of precancerous lesions and micronuclei formation as endpoints. Although no reduction in the prevalence of histologically diagnosed precancerous lesions was observed, a significantly lower prevalence of esophageal micronucleated cells was found in the group receiving a combined treatment of riboflavin, retinol, and zinc during one year as compared to the control group receiving a placebo (Table 33–12) (Muñoz et al, 1985b; 1987). One difficulty in the final interpretation of this trial arises from the fact that at the end of the trial an increase in blood retinol levels occurred in 47% of subjects in the placebo group and in 76% of those receiving the treatment. The corresponding figures for riboflavin were 17% and 66%. These changes in blood levels of the vitamins were probably the result of dietary changes

TABLE 33–11. *Relative Risks of Esophageal Cancer for Combined Levels of Dietary Score and Alcohol Consumption**

Dietary Score[a]	*Alcohol Consumption, g/day of Ethanol*			
	0–40[b]	*40–80*	*80–120*	*120+*
HHH, HHM, HMM	1	3.7 (1.1–12.6)	15.8 (4.3–58.1)	33.6 (8.3–136.6)
HHL, HML, MML	4.1 (1.1–15.4)	10.2 (2.9–35.6)	32.0 (0.1–111.9)	147.0 (39.1–557.2)
HLL, MLL, LLL	16.3 (4.5–58.4)	38.8 (11.2–135.1)	41.6 (11.8–147.1)	89.3 (25.0–320.5)

*From Tuyns et al (1987). Adjusted for age, area of residence, and tobacco smoking.
[a]Combination of high (H), moderate (M), or low (L) consumption of fresh meat, citrus fruits, and oils.
[b]40 g equals approximately 1.4 oz; 1 ml alcohol weighs 0.8 g.

TABLE 33–12. *Effect of Riboflavin, Retinol, and Zinc Treatment on the Prevalence of Micronuclei and of Histologically Diagnosed Precancerous Lesions of the Esophagus**

	Placebo	Vitamins
Micronuclei (mean ± SD)	0.31 (±0.29)	0.19 (±0.15)
Histological diagnosis		
Normal esophagus	53.6%	49.6%
Chronic esophagitis	30.4%	34.1%
Epithelial atrophy	12.7%	12.3%
Dysplasia	2.2%	2.5%
Squamous cancer	0.7%	1.5%
Adenocarcinoma	0.4%	0.0%
Number of subjects	276	276

*Adapted from Muñoz et al (1985b); Muñoz et al (1987).

that occurred during the study period (Thurnham et al, 1988). To account for these changes a multivariate analysis was made and a reduction in the prevalence of precancerous lesions was seen in those whose blood levels of retinol, riboflavin, and zinc improved or remained unchanged as compared to those whose levels got worse during the study period (Table 33–13) (Wahrendorf et al, 1988). The overall results of this trial underline the difficulty of carrying out intervention studies in populations undergoing rapid changes in dietary habits and suggest a beneficial effect of retinol, riboflavin, and zinc on the prevalence of precancerous lesions. Further data on the effect of these micronutrients on the occurrence of esophageal cancer have emerged from the results of two large-scale intervention studies being conducted in the same high-risk population in China in which the endpoints are changes in incidence and mortality of esophageal cancer (Li et al, 1985).

In the first of these trials about 30,000 adults from Linxian were randomized to one of the 8 vitamin/mineral supplement combinations. No significant reduction in the incidence or mortality from esophageal cancer was observed after 5 years of treatment. A moderate reduction of cancer risk was observed only for those receiving beta-carotene, vitamin E, and selenium, and this reduction was mainly due to lower rates of stomach cancer (RR = 0.79; 95% CI = 0.64–0.99) (Blot et al, 1993). The second trial included 3,300 with cytological diagnosis of esophageal dysplasia randomized to receive either a multivitamin preparation (14 vitamins and 12 minerals) or a placebo during 6 years. Cumulative esophageal/gastric cardia death rates were 8% lower (RR = 0.92; 95% CI = 0.67–1.28) among subjects receiving supplements rather than placebo, but the difference was nonsignificant ($p > 0.10$). In addition, the incidence rate for esophageal/gastric cancer was similar in the treatment and placebo groups (RR = 0.98; 95% CI = 0.81–1.19) and the incidence of stomach cancer was significantly increased in the subjects receiving supplements (RR = 3.54; 95% CI = 1.17–10.76) (Li et al, 1993).

TABLE 33–13. *Effect of Blood Level Changes of Riboflavin, Retinol, and Zinc on the Prevalence of Precancerous Lesions of the Esophagus**

	Odds Ratio for Precancerous Lesions		
Vitamin Change	Retinol	Riboflavin	Zinc
Worse	1.00	1.00	1.00
Unchanged	0.56	0.76	0.14
Improved	0.41	0.61	0.11
p for linear trend	0.04	0.13	0.001

*Adapted from Wahrendorf et al (1988).

The informativeness of the first trial in which improvements in nutritional status of the untreated arms of the study population took place during the intervention period has been questioned (Day et al, 1994).

Some minerals and trace elements (i.e., iron, zinc, calcium, cobalt) have been suspected to be associated with esophageal cancer risk (Rogers et al, 1993), but firm evidence of this association is lacking.

A further example of the role of individual susceptibility is provided by the association between esophageal cancer and idiopathic steatorrhea or celiac disease (Harris et al, 1967; Holmes et al, 1976). This association may be either a genetic or an environmental susceptibility. Celiac disease is an absorption disorder of the small intestine and is characterized by a flat jejunal mucosa whose histologic abnormalities and clinical features can be reversed by gluten withdrawal. The main symptoms are diarrhea, anemia, weight loss, lassitude, and some skeletal disorders (Cooke and Asquith, 1974). Since the upper small intestine is the most seriously involved portion of the intestine, deficiencies of iron, folic acid, B_{12}, pyridoxine, and vitamins A, C, and K have been observed, as well as disturbances of carbohydrate, protein, and calcium metabolism (Hoffbrand, 1974). It is of interest to note that severe zinc deficiency has been observed in patients with celiac disease who do not respond to gluten-free diets (Love et al, 1978).

Celiac disease is a familial condition, with approximately 10% of first-degree relatives affected (Stokes et al, 1973). The mode of inheritance remains to be established, but studies of histocompatibility antigens have shown that HLA-B8 and HLA-DW3 are important risk factors for the disease (Falchuk et al, 1972; Kenning et al, 1976). Malignant lymphoma of the jejunum has been the most common complication of celiac disease (Harris et al, 1967; Holmes et al, 1976), but an excess of esophageal cancer has been observed. The patients who developed esophageal cancer had a long history of celiac disease (mean age 50 years), and the most frequent location of the tumor was the middle or lower third (Harris et al, 1967). An increased incidence of esophageal cancer has also been reported in male relatives of patients with celiac disease, but no excess of cancer deaths due to lymphoma was observed in relatives of either sex (Stokes et al, 1976).

The increased susceptibility to esophageal cancer in these patients may be the result of both genetic factors and nutritional deficiencies. The long latent period between the onset of celiac disease and the development of esophageal cancer may favor the nutritional hypothesis.

Precancerous Lesions

Little is known about the precursor lesions of esophageal cancer in man. The limited number of studies reported are based on postmortem or surgical specimens in the presence of unequivocal cancers, and the changes in the mucosa surrounding this cancer have been assumed to be the only changes that can denote a precancerous condition (Postlethwait and Wendell Musser, 1974; Ushigome et al, 1967). Thus, epithelial dysplasia has been proposed as a precancerous condition (Ushigome et al, 1967; Mukada et al, 1976; Coordinating Group, 1974), but no information on the lesions preceding the dysplasia was available until recently.

Mass surveys using esophageal cytology have been carried out in the high-incidence regions of China. Cytology using an abrasive balloon was obtained in 7,212 subjects over 30 years of age in Linxian, Henan Province. In the northern part of the country, where the incidence of esophageal cancer is high, the prevalence rates for mild and severe dysplasia were 26% and 2%, respectively, and in the south, with a lower incidence of esophageal cancer, these rates were 18% and 0.7%, respectively (Coordinating Group, 1974). In other regions of Henan Province, 21,581 subjects over 30 years of age were examined, and the prevalence rates of mild and severe dysplasia were 13% and 1.2%. The prevalence rate of esophageal carcinoma was 0.9%. It was also observed that the frequency of dysplasia increased progressively with age, especially in the case of severe dysplasia. Follow-up studies of over 500 individuals with severe esophageal dysplasia revealed that 40% regressed to mild dysplasia or normal, 20% remained unchanged, 20% fluctuated between severe and mild dysplasia, and 20% progressed to carcinoma. In comparison, only 0.12% of 11,011 individuals with normal epithelium developed cancer during the 5–8-year follow-up period (Xia, 1984).

During the intervention trials carried out in Linxian, China, by the NCI more than 12,000 subjects underwent esophageal balloon cytology in 1983, with the following results: normal esophagus, 31%; hyperplasia, 44%; dysplasia 1, 16%; dysplasia 2, 4%; near cancer, 2%; and cancer, 3%. It was of interest that the prevalence of dysplasia was higher than in earlier surveys in the same population, probably reflecting changes in cytological classification (Shen et al, 1993). In 1987, esophageal biopsies were evaluated from 750 subjects from the dysplasia trial after 30 months of intervention, with the following results: normal mucosa, 56.5%; esophagitis, 4.6%; dysplasia, 22.7%; and cancer, 4.6%. However, it should be noted that the histological criterion of esophagitis was different from the one we have used in our surveys (Dawsey et al, 1994a). The same investigators estimated the subsequent risk of esophageal cancer in more than 12,000 persons from Linxian in whom esophageal balloon cytology was carried out in 1974. After adjusting for confounding factors, the risk for esophageal cancer by cytological diagnosis was: esophagitis, 1.5 (95% CI 1.1–2.1); hyperplasia, 1.2 (1.1–1.3); dysplasia 1, 1.5 (1.1–2.1); dysplasia 2, 1.9 (1.5–2.4); suspicious for cancer, 5.8 (3.8–8.8) (Dawsey et al, 1994b).

In comparing the results reported from China with those reported from other populations, it should be borne in mind that the cytological criteria used in China and the histological criteria of esophagitis used in recent studies are different from those used in other parts of the world.

The low prevalence of esophageal dysplasia (0.2% observed) in the postmortem study in the United States (Postlethwait and Wendell Musser, 1974) is not surprising considering the low incidence of esophageal cancer in this population, but the high prevalence (37%) observed in Japan and the lack of correlation with the risk for esophageal cancer are puzzling (Mukada et al, 1976). Possible explanations for these inconsistencies are: (1) there is no clear definition for esophageal dysplasia; (2) irradiation and chemotherapy can produce changes in the esophageal mucosa that resemble dysplastic lesions, and patients having received these treatments must therefore be excluded from postmortem studies (Mandard et al, 1978); (3) lysis postmortem and poor fixation can also mimic dysplasia.

Although esophageal leukoplakia has been considered a precancerous lesion (Sharp, 1931; Etienne et al, 1969), it is not possible to establish a clear-cut correlation between this lesion and cancer, as there is no agreement in the literature as to its precise definition (WHO Collaborating Centre for Oral Precancerous Lesions, 1978). It has been suggested that the term leukoplakia should be used only when lichen planus, candidiasis, white sponge nevus, and other specific entities can be excluded (WHO Collaborating Centre for Oral

Precancerous Lesions, 1978). Therefore, this term must be used exclusively in a clinically descriptive sense.

In an attempt to characterize the premalignant lesions of the esophagus and in particular those preceding dysplasia, endoscopic surveys involving over 1,700 subjects have been carried out in high- and low-risk areas for esophageal cancer in Iran and China, and in intermediate-risk areas of France and Argentina. The main histological findings are summarized in Table 33–14. In Iran, the study population were volunteers from three Turkoman villages, while in China random samples of the population of the selected communes from Linxian and Jiaoxian were examined. Study subjects in Argentina were symptomatic patients attending gastroenterological clinics, and in France they were volunteers. The prevalence of chronic esophagitis, epithelial atrophy, and dysplasia correlated well with the risk of esophageal cancer. The endoscopic characteristics of the chronic esophagitis observed in these populations was different from the reflux esophagitis seen in the low-risk populations of America and Europe. It was a diffuse lesion involving more frequently the middle and lower thirds of the esophagus and characterized by an irregular, swollen, friable, and hyperemic mucosa with scattered or confluent patches of leukoplakia but without the erosions and ulcerations that characterize the reflux esophagitis. Histologically, this esophagitis was characterized by infiltration of the mucosa and submucosa by chronic inflammatory cells and occasionally by acute cells, elongation of the vascular papillae, and proliferation and dilatation of blood vessels. According to the severity of the changes, three degrees of chronic esophagitis were considered. Lesions were slightly more severe in males than in females and in older age groups than in young age groups (Crepsi et al, 1979; Muñoz et al, 1982; Crespi et al, 1984; Castelleto et al, 1992; Jacob et al, 1993). Studies on the pattern of cell proliferation of epithelial esophageal cells using tritiated thymidine were conducted in a subsample of subjects from the high- and low-risk areas in China. A clear difference was observed between the two groups; the high-risk one showed abnormal cell proliferation in the upper layers of the epithelium more often than the low-risk group, in which 90% of the labeled cells were located in the first two layers of cells from the basal membrane (Muñoz et al, 1985a). The presence of cell proliferation in the superficial layers of the epithelium could be the result of chronic injury to the esophagus.

Concerning the prevalence of possible risk factors for these precancerous lesions, the prevalence of tobacco smoking and alcohol drinking was higher in Jiaoxian (low-risk area) than in Linxian (high-risk area). History of esophageal cancer in a close relative was reported in 61% of the subjects in Linxian and only in 1% in Jiaoxian. Oral leukoplakia and angular stomatitis (lesion suggesting riboflavin deficiency) were observed in 2% of the subjects in Jiaoxian, while in the high-risk population of Linxian, oral leukoplakia was observed in 20% and angular stomatitis in 6%. As regards blood levels of vitamins, no significant difference was observed in the mean values of retinol, beta-carotene, and zinc for the two communities, and only the riboflavin status was significantly different in the two populations: although riboflavin deficiency was highly prevalent in both populations, it was more severe in Linxian than in Jiaoxian (Muñoz et al, 1982; Crespi et al, 1984). To study further

TABLE 33–14. *Histologic Findings on Precursor Lesions of Esophageal Cancer in High- and Low-Risk Populations*

	Men					*Women*			
	High Risk[a]		*Intermediate*[b,c]		*Low Risk*[d]	*High Risk*[a]		*Intermediate*[b]	*Low Risk*[d]
Number of Subjects	*Iran—Turkoman 213%*	*China—Linxian 292%*	*Argentina—La Plata 210%*	*France—Calvados 134%*	*China 152%*	*Iran—Turkoman 205%*	*China—Linxian 235%*	*Argentina—La Plata 196%*	*China—Turkoman 100%*
Esophagitis									
Mild	58.7	55.8	38.1	54.0	33.5	57.6	56.2	35.7	18.0
Moderate	21.6	7.5	3.4	3.2	0.7	17.6	6.4	0.5	0.0
Severe	2.8	1.7	0.5	1.6	0.0	1.0	0.9	0.0	0.0
Total	83.1	65.0	41.9	62.9	34.2	76.2	63.5	36.2	18.0
Clear-cell acanthosis	66.2	80.8	27.6		82.9	64.9	72.4	29.0	85.0
Atrophy	12.7	11.6	3.8	1.6	0.7	8.3	9.8	2.5	0.0
Dysplasia	4.7	7.9	2.4	4.8	0.0	2.9	8.1	0.0	0.0

[a]Crespi et al (1979); Muñoz et al (1982).
[b]Castelleto et al (1992).
[c]Jacob et al (1993).
[d]Crespi et al (1984).

the role of these vitamins in the human esophageal carcinogenesis, an intervention study was carried out in Huixian, a high-risk population of China. The overall results described in the previous section suggested a beneficial effect of retinol, riboflavin, and zinc on the prevalence of esophageal micronucleated cells and of the precursor lesions of esophageal cancer (Muñoz et al, 1985; Muñoz et al, 1987; Wahrendorf et al, 1988).

A case-control study of esophagitis was conducted in the same area. One-third of the subjects were selected from households with a case of esophageal cancer in the past 6 years, and two-thirds came from control households. The prevalence of histologically diagnosed chronic esophagitis was 44% in males and 36% in females. In a case-control analysis of the data, the consumption of burning-hot beverages, a family history of esophageal cancer, and an infrequent consumption of fresh fruit were identified as the main risk factors for chronic esophagitis as shown in Table 33–15 (Wahrendorf et al, 1989). These results support the findings of an earlier study carried out in southern Brazil showing that thermal injury resulting from maté drinking is associated with an increased risk of histologically diagnosed esophagitis (Muñoz et al, 1987).

Tobacco and alcohol drinking have been associated with an increased risk of chronic esophagitis in Argentina and France (Castelletto et al, 1992; Jacob et al, 1993).

Although final proof of the precancerous nature of these lesions can only come from long-term follow-up studies, there is indirect evidence in favor of their precancerous nature: the good correlation between the prevalence of these lesions and the incidence of esophageal cancer, the similar location in the esophagus of these lesions and of the cancer, the results of a small follow-up study showing a high progression rate of these lesions to cancer (Muñoz et al, 1982), the similar risk factors for chronic esophagitis and for esophageal cancer, and the similarity between these lesions and those induced in nonhuman primates treated with a nitrosamine (Adamson et al, 1977). Based on these observations, we have suggested that the natural history of esophageal cancer is as follows:

$$\text{Chronic esophagitis} \rightleftarrows \text{atrophy} \rightleftarrows \text{dysplasia} \rightarrow \text{cancer.}$$

Since chronic esophagitis was present even below 20 years of age, exposure to the various risk factors (thermal injury, dietary insufficiencies, etc.) probably commences early in life.

TABLE 33–15. *Risk Factors for Chronic Esophagitis in Huixian, China**

Risk Factor	*Odds Ratio (95% CI)*
Consumption of fresh fruits > 1/week	0.29 (0.15–0.56)
Drinking of burning-hot beverages	4.39 (1.72–11.25)
Family history of esophageal cancer	2.69 (1.44–5.02)
Consumption of wheat flour products > 2/day	0.41 (0.22–0.75)

*From Wahrendorf et al (1989).

CONCLUSIONS

We have almost ignored in our review a number of topics that on occasion have been stressed by others. There is considerable literature on the possible role of tannins (Morton, 1968, 1979). "Cancer gardens" in the Transkei (Burrell et al, 1966) and the role of mineral deficiencies, especially molybdenum, in the soil were widely discussed at one time.

We have not stressed the role of genetics, which is probably fundamental to understanding the disease process. However, there is little evidence that genetic aspects have much influence on the epidemiology of the disease, and they are unlikely to be helpful for control. The association of esophageal cancer with Turkic or Mongol origin in central and northeastern Asia has now led to the identification of specific high-risk genotypes, but the recessive genes involved predispose only 4% of the population (Carter et al, 1992). Alterations of various oncogenes associated with human neoplasia are being looked for in esophageal tumors. No mutations in the *ras* gene family have been found in esophageal tumors from China, France, Transkei, and Uruguay, while P53 point mutations were found in almost half of the tumors (Hollstein et al, 1991). The etiological implications of these genetic alterations remain to be established.

The large number of studies reviewed here indicate that the sharp changes in incidence characteristics of this disease are probably a reflection of multifactor causation. Chronic injury to the esophagus, resulting from drinking very hot beverages, eating hot and coarse food, and nutritional deficiencies or imbalances, is probably the common denominator. In America, Europe, and parts of Africa and Asia, alcohol and tobacco have been identified as the main exogenous etiological factors. In northern Iran, opium residues appear to be the main directly acting carcinogens. Although opium use was widespread throughout Central Asia and much of China, its role in these high-risk populations is unclear. In the high-risk populations of China, N-nitroso compounds ingested as such or formed in vivo, and fungal contamination have been proposed as etiological candidates, but clear evidence of their involvement is still lacking.

Esophageal cancer thus appears to provide an excellent model of multifactorial action, where, although not all the components have been unambiguously identified, one can perhaps suggest how different factors take their place in a multistage process of carcinogenesis. One might propose that early stages in carcinogenesis consist of genetic (heritable) damage to the relevant cell, which take place with greater frequency the greater the access that agents with DNA-damaging capability have to the genetic material of these cells, and that later stages are associated with some form of promoting action. Given the presence of tobacco or opium residues with their mutagenic potential, one can then consider the role of modifying agents such as alcohol, thermal irritation, or dietary deficiency. Alcohol might act in a number of ways. First, as a transport agent in the manner described by Kuratsune (1965): Alcohol will facilitate the transfer of active agents through the esophageal mucosa to the cells of the basal layer. Second, as an irritant: It will lead to an increased turnover of the esophageal epithelium, thereby both increasing the rate at which genetic damage is fixed and perhaps accelerating the progression through later stages. Third, by inducing nutritional imbalance, since for a number of micronutrients (riboflavin, thiamin, zinc, for example) high alcohol intake will lead to physiological deficiency even though dietary intake appears adequate. The role of these deficiencies has been discussed earlier. Excessively hot food and drink might act, like alcohol, both as a transport agent and as an irritant. Dietary deficiency, acting through dietary-dependent enzyme systems, might alter the rate of activation (or deactivation) of precarcinogens and thus accelerate the early stages; or, as Wynder and Chan (1970) showed for riboflavin, their effect on the relevant tissue may be to increase the rate of later stages. The mechanism by which the different factors act is not simply of scientific interest; understanding their nature may lead to practical and effective ways of intervention and primary prevention.

The possibilities for early detection and secondary prevention do not appear encouraging. The early-detection program in China seems to have had little effect on mortality, and we are not aware of any other genuine mass-screening program in existence or planned. Further work is needed to evaluate screening tests.

By contrast, there is now a mass of evidence that exogenous factors and poor nutrition are involved, and that control of these factors would lead to a great reduction in the disease. The exogenous factors so far identified, or under suspicion, appear to act directly on the esophagus, and not systemically. The critical parameters are the rate at which carcinogens can be transported through the mucosa to the target basal cells, and the susceptibility of these cells to carcinogenic action. Research should now concentrate on how these factors interact to augment risk, so that aspects of the overall mechanism that are amenable to control can be identified. A particularly promising area for future research is the relationship between early esophageal lesions and nutritional status, and attempts should be made to modify these lesions, or induce them to regress, by means of diet supplements.

A further area that needs elucidation is the role that alcoholic drinks play in the process. The differential effect of different drinks needs clarifying. For both smoking and drinking, one needs to know the effect on subsequent risk of stopping exposure. How quickly does risk decrease? There seems little information on the role of different types of cigarettes. The role of hot drinks needs further clarifying, particularly the effect of thermal irritation. The extent to which tea, coffee, and strong alcoholic drinks act as transport mechanism for other carcinogens needs elaboration, and in general there has been a neglect of the physical properties of the esophagus. The hydrodynamics of the passage of fluid down the esophagus would probably prove worthy of study. One would like to investigate, probably using in vitro tissue systems, the degree of DNA damage suffered by basal cells of the esophageal mucosa when various combinations of liquid and carcinogens are applied at the mucosal surface.

For many cancer sites, the notion that 80% or 90% of tumors are of environmental origin is academic, and the possibilities of primary prevention still theoretical. For cancer of the esophagus, the issues are not theoretical. Primary prevention is largely possible; epidemiologists must determine how to achieve it.

REFERENCES

ADAMSON RH, KROLIKOWSKI, CORREA P, et al. 1977. Carcinogenicity of 1-methyl-1-nitrosourea in non-human primates. J Natl Cancer Inst, 59:415–422.

AHLBOM HE. 1936. Simple achlorhydric anaemia. Plummer-Vinson syndrome and carcinoma of the mouth, pharynx and oesophagus in women. Br Med J, 2:331–333.

ASHWORTH MT, MCDICKEN IW, SOUTHERN SA, NASH JRG. 1993. Human papillomavirus in squamous cell carcinoma of the oesophagus associated with tylosis. J Clin Pathol, 46(6):573–575.

BANG KM, WHITE JE, GAUSE BL, LEFFALL LD. 1988. Evaluation of recent trends in cancer mortality and incidence among blacks. Cancer, 61:1255–1261.

BEEBE GW, KATO H, LAND CE. 1978. Studies of the mortality of A-bomb survivors: 6. Mortality and radiation dose, 1950–1974. Radiation Res 75(1):138–201.

BENAMOUZIG R, PIGOT F, QUIROGA G, et al. 1992. Human papillomavirus infection in esophageal squamous-cell carcinoma in western countries. Int J Cancer 50:549–542.

Beveridge BR, Bannerman RM, Evanson JM, et al. 1965. Hypochromic anaemia. A retrospective study and follow-up of 378 inpatients. Quart J Med, 34:145–161.

Blot WJ, Fraumeni JF. 1987. Trends in esophageal cancer mortality among US blacks and whites. Am J Public Health 77:296–298.

Blot WJ, Devesa SS, Kneller RW, Fraumeni JF. 1991. Rising incidence of adenocarcinoma of the esophagus and gastric cardia. JAMA 265:1287–1289.

Blot WJ, Devesa SS, Fraumeni JF, Jr. 1993. Continuing climb in rates of esophageal adenocarcinoma: an update. JAMA 270:1320.

Bonnelli L. 1993. Barrett's esophagus: results of a multicentric survey. G.O.S.P.E. (Gruppo Operativo per lo Studio delle Precancerosi Esofagee). Endoscopy, 25:652–654.

Breslow NE, Day NE. 1980. Statistical methods in cancer research. The analysis of case-control studies (IARC Scientific Publications No. 32). Lyon: International Agency for Research on Cancer.

Burrell RJW, Roach WA, Shadwell A. 1966. Esophageal cancer in the Bantu of the Transkei associated with mineral deficiency in garden plants. J Natl Cancer Inst, 36:201–209.

Cairns J. 1975. Mutation, selection and the natural history of cancer. Nature 255:197–200.

Carter CL, Hu N, Wu M, Lin PZ, Murigande C, Bonney GE. 1992. Segregation analysis of esophageal cancer in 221 high-risk Chinese families. J Natl Cancer Inst, 84:771–776.

Castelletto R, Muñoz N, Landoni N, Jmelnitzky A, Crespi M, Belloni P, Chopita N, Teuchmann S. 1992. Pre-cancerous lesions of the oesophagus in Argentina: prevalence and association with tobacco and alcohol. Int J Cancer 51:34–37.

Castelletto R, Castellsague X, Muñoz N, Iscovich J, Chopita N, Jmelnitsky A. 1994. Alcohol, tobacco, diet, maté drinking and oesophageal cancer in Argentina. Cancer Epidemiol Biomarkers Prev (In Press). 3:557–564.

Chang F, Syrjanen S, Shen Q, Wang L, Syrjanen K. 1993. Screening for human papillomavirus infections in esophageal squamous cell carcinomas by in situ hybridization. Cancer 72:2525–2530.

Chang-Claude J, Wahrendorf J, Qui SL, Yang GR, Muñoz N, Crespi M, et al. 1990. An epidemiologic study of precursor lesions of esophageal cancer among young persons in a high-risk population in Huixian, China. Cancer Res 50:2268–2274.

Chen J, Ohshima H, Yang H, Li J, Campbell TC, Peto R, Bartsch H. 1987. A correlation on urinary excretion of N-nitroso compounds and cancer mortality in China: interim results. In Bartsch H, O'Neill IK, Schulte-Hermann R (eds): The Relevance of N-nitroso Compounds to Human Cancer: Exposures and Mechanisms (IARC Scientific Publications No. 84). Lyon: International Agency for Research on Cancer, pp. 503–506.

Chen F, Cole P, Mi Z, Xing LY. 1993. Corn and wheat-flour consumption and mortality from esophageal cancer in Shanxi, China. Int J Cancer 53:902–906.

Cheng KK, Day NE, Davies TW. 1992a. Esophageal cancer mortality in Europe: paradoxical time trend in relation to smoking and drinking. Br J Cancer 65:613–617.

Cheng KK, Day NE, Duffy SW, Lam TH, Fok M, Wong J. 1992b. Pickled vegetables in the aetiology of esophageal cancer in Hong Kong Chinese. Lancet 339:1314–1318.

Chu FS, Li GY. 1994. Simultaneous occurrence of fumonisin B1 and other mycotoxins in moldy corn collected from the People's Republic of China in regions with high incidences of esophageal cancer. Appl Environ Microbiol 60:847–852.

Cislaghi C, DeCarli A, La Vecchia C, Laverda N, Mezzanotte G, Smans M. 1986. Data, Statistics and Maps on Cancer Mortality, Italy 1975/1977. Bologna: Pitagora.

Clemmesen J. 1965. Statistical studies in malignant neoplasms. I. Review and results. Copenhagen: Munksgaard.

Coleman M, Estève J, Damiecki P, Arslan A, Renard H. 1993. Time trends in cancer incidence and mortality (IARC Scientific Publications No. 121). Lyon: International Agency for Research on Cancer.

Cooke WT, Asquith P. 1974. Introduction and definition. Clinics Gastroenterol 3:3–11.

Cook-Mozaffari PJ, Azordegan F, Day NE, et al. 1979. Esophageal cancer studies in the Caspian littoral of Iran: results of a case-control study. Br J Cancer 39:293–309.

Coordinating Group for the Research of Esophageal Carcinoma. 1974. Studies in the relationship between epithelial dysplasia and carcinoma of the esophagus. Peking: Chinese Academy of Medical Sciences.

Craver LF. 1932. Clinical study of etiology of gastric and esophageal cancer. Am J Cancer 16:68–102.

Crespi M, Muñoz N, Grassi A, et al. 1979. Esophageal lesions in northern Iran: A premalignant condition? Lancet ii:217–221.

Crespi M, Muñoz N, Grassi A, Shen Q, Wang KJ, Lin JJ. 1984. Precursor lesions of esophageal cancer in a low-risk population in China: comparison with high-risk populations. Int J Cancer 34:599–602.

Dawsey SM, Yu T, Taylor PR, Li JY, Shen Q, Shu YJ, Liu SF, Zhao HZ, Cao SG, Wang GQ, et al. 1994a. Esophageal cytology and subsequent risk of esophageal cancer. A prospective follow-up study from Linxian, China. Acta Cytol 38:183–192.

Dawsey SM, Lewin KJ, Liu FS, Wang GQ, Shen Q. 1994b. Esophageal morphology from Linxian, China. Cancer 73:2027–2037.

Day NE, Bingham SA. 1994. Nutrition intervention trials in Linxian, China: supplementation with specific vitamin/mineral combinations, cancer incidence, and disease-specific mortality in the general population [letter]. Natl Cancer Inst 86(21):1645–1648.

Day NE. 1975. Some aspects of the epidemiology of esophageal cancer. Cancer Res 35:3304–3307.

Day NE, Brown CC. 1980. Multistage models and the primary prevention of cancer. J Natl Cancer Inst 64:977–989.

Day NE. 1994. Personal communication.

Decarli A, Liati P, Negri E, Franceschi S, La Vecchia C. 1987. Vitamin A and other dietary factors in the etiology of esophageal cancer. Nutr Cancer 10:29–37.

de Jong UW, Day NE, Mounier-Kuhn PL, et al. 1972. The relationship between the ingestion of hot coffee and intra-esophageal temperature. Gut 13:24–30.

de Jong UW, Breslow NE, Goh Ewe Hong J, et al. 1974. Aetiological factors in esophageal cancer in Singapore Chinese. Int J Cancer 13:291–303.

de Stefani E, Muñoz N, Estève J, Vasallo A, Victora CG, Teuchmann S. 1990. Maté drinking, alcohol, tobacco, diet and esophageal cancer in Uruguay. Cancer Res, 50:426–431.

de Stefani E, Barrios E, Fierro L. 1993. Black (air-cured) and blond (flue-cured) tobacco and cancer risk. III: Esophageal cancer. Eur J Cancer 29A:763–766.

de Stefani E, Fierro L, Barrios E, Ronco A. 1994. Cancer mortality trends in Uruguay 1953–1991. Int J Cancer, 56:634–639.

Doll R, Peto R. 1976. Mortality in relation to smoking: 20 years' observations in male British doctors. Br Med J, 2:1525–1536.

Etienne JP, Delavierre PH, Petite JP, et al. 1969. Les leucoplasies esophagiennes au cours des cirrhoses. Sem Hôp Paris 45:1589–1598.

Faggiano F, Partenen T, Kogevinas M, Boffetta P. 1995. Evidence of social inequities in cancer mortality and incidence. In Kogevinas M, Boffetta P, Pearce N, Susser M (eds): Socio-Economic Factors and Cancer. Lyon: IARC Scientific Publication, International Agency for Research on Cancer (In Press).

Falchuk ZM, Rogentine GN, Strober W. 1972. Predominance of histocompatibility antigen HL-A8 in patients with gluten sensitive enteropathy. J Clin Invest 51:1602–1605.

Finnish Cancer Registry. 1982. Development of cancer morbidity in Finland up to the Year 2002. Predictions on incidence rates and numbers of new cases for some common cancers in Finland based on analysis by age, period and cohort. Helsinki: National Board of Health.

FRAUMENI JF, BLOT WJ. 1977. Geographic variation in esophageal cancer mortality in the United States. J Chron Dis 30:759–767.

FRIESEN M, O'NEILL IK, MALAVEILLE C, GARREN L, HAUTEFEUILLE A, CABRAL JRP, GALENDO D, LASNE C, SALA M, CHOUROULINKOV I, MOHR U, TURUSOV V, DAY NE, BARTSCH H. 1985. Characterization and identification of 6 mutagens in opium pyrolysates implicated in esophageal cancer in Iran. Mutat Res 150:177–191.

FRIESEN M, O'NEILL IK, MALAVEILLE C, GARREN L, HAUTEFEUILLE A, BARTSCH H. 1987. Substituted hydroxyphenanthrenes in opium pyrolysates implicated in esophageal cancer in Iran: structures and in vitro metabolic activation of a novel class of mutagens. Carcinogenesis 8:1423–1432.

GHADIRIAN P. 1985. Familial history of esophageal cancer. Cancer 56:2112–2116.

GHADIRIAN P. 1987. Thermal irritation and esophageal cancer in northern Iran. Cancer 60:1909–1914.

GHADIRIAN P, STEIN GF, GORODITZKY A, ROBERFROID MB, MAHON GAT, BARTOCH H, DAY N. 1985. Esophageal cancer studies in the Caspian littoral of Iran: some residual results, including opium use as a risk factor. Int J Cancer 35:593–597.

GOBAR AH. 1976. L'abus des drogues en Afghanistan. Bull Stupéfiants, 28:1–12.

GUSTAVSSON P, EVANOFF B, HOGSTEDT C. 1993. Increased risk of esophageal cancer among workers exposed to combustion products. Arch Environ Health, 48:243–245.

HARPER PS, HARPER RMJ, HOWEL-EVANS AW. 1970. Carcinoma of the esophagus with tylosis. Q J Med, 155:317–333.

HARRIS OD, COOKE WT, THOMPSON H, et al. 1967. Malignancy in adult coeliac disease and idiopathic steatorrhoea. Am J Med, 42:899–912.

HARRISON SL, GOLDACRE MJ, SEAGROATT V. 1992. Trends in registered incidence of esophageal and stomach cancer in the Oxford region, 1974–88. Eur J Cancer Prev, 1:271–274.

HASHEMI S, DOWLATSHAHI K, MOHAGHEGHPOUR N, et al. 1979. Esophageal cancer studies in the Caspian littoral of Iran: introductory assessment of the HLA profile in patients and controls. Tissue Antigens 14:422–425.

HEBERT JR, LANDON J, MILLER DR. 1993. Consumption of meat and fruit in relation to oral and esophageal cancer: a cross-national study. Nutr Cancer 19:169–179.

HEWER T, ROSE E, GHADIRIAN P, et al. 1978. Ingested mutagens from opium and tobacco pyrolysis products and cancer of the oesophagus. Lancet ii:494–496.

HIRAYAMA T. 1971. An epidemiological study of cancer of the oesophagus in Japan, with special reference to the combined effect of selected environmental factors. In Monograph No. 1. Int Seminar on Epidemiology of Oesophageal Cancer, Bangalore, India, 4 November 1971, pp 45–60.

HIRAYAMA T. 1979. Diet and cancer. Nutr Cancer, 1:67–81.

HIRAYAMA T. 1986. Nutritional intervention as a means of cancer prevention. In Khogali M, Omar YT, Gjorgov A, Ismail AS (eds): Cancer Prevention in Developing Countries. Oxford: Pergamon Press, pp 287–289.

HOFFBRAND AV. 1974. Anaemia in adult coeliac disease. In: Clinics Gastroenterol 3:71–89.

HOLLSTEIN MC, PERI L, MANDARD AM, WELSH JA, MONTESANO R, METCALF A, BAK M, HARRIS CC. 1991. Genetic analysis of human esophageal tumors from two high incidence geographic areas: frequent p53 base substitutions and absence of ras mutations. Cancer Res 51:4102–4106.

HOLMES GKT, STOKES PL, SORAHAN TM, et al. 1976. Coeliac disease, gluten-free diet, and malignancy. Gut 17:612–619.

HOWEL-EVANS AW, MCCONNELL RB, CLARKE CA, et al. 1958. Carcinoma of the oesophagus with keratosis palmaris et plantaris (tylosis): a study of two families. Qu J Med 27:413–429.

HU J, NYREN O, WOLK A, BERGSTROM R, YUEN J, ADAMI HO, GUO L, LI H, HUANG G, XU X, et al. 1994. Risk factors for oesophageal cancer in northeast China. Int J Cancer 57:38–46.

IARC/IRAN STUDY GROUP. 1977. Esophageal cancer studies in the Caspian littoral of Iran: results of population studies. A prodrome. J Natl Cancer Inst 59:1127–1138.

IARC. 1988. Monographs on the Evaluation of the Carcinogenic Risk of Chemicals to Humans, Vol. 44, Alcohol and alcoholic beverages. Lyon: International Agency for Research on Cancer.

IARC. 1991. Monographs on the Evaluation of the Carcinogenic Risk of Chemicals to Humans, Vol. 51, Coffee, Tea, Maté, Methylxanthines and Methylglyoxal. Lyon: International Agency for Research on Cancer.

IARC. 1993. Monographs on the Evaluation of the Carcinogenic Risk of Chemicals to Humans, Vol. 56, Pickled Vegetables. Lyon: International Agency for Research on Cancer.

JACOB JH, RIVIERE A, MANDARD AM, MUÑOZ N, CRESPI M, ETIENNE Y, CASTELLSAGUE X, MARNAY J, LEBIGOT G, QIU SF. 1993. Prevalence survey of precancerous lesions of the oesophagus in a high-risk population for esophageal cancer in France. Eur J Cancer Prev 2:53–59.

JACOBS A. 1963. Epithelial changes in anaemic East Africans. Br Med J 5347:1711–1712.

JACOBS A, CAVILL IAJ. 1968. Pyridoxine and riboflavin status in the Paterson-Kelly syndrome. Br J Haematol 14:153–160.

JACOBSSON F. 1948. Carcinoma of the tongue. A clinical study of 227 cases treated at Radiumhemmet, 1931–1942. Acta Radiol 68:1–184.

JAYANT K, BALAKRISHNAN V, SANGHVI LD, et al. 1977. Quantification of the role of smoking and chewing tobacco in oral, pharyngeal and oesophageal cancers. Br J Cancer 35:232–235.

JOCHEM VJ, FUERST PA, FROMKES JJ. 1992. Familial Barrett's esophagus associated with adenocarcinoma. Gastroenterol 102:1400–1402.

JUSSAWALLA DJ. 1971. Epidemiological assessment of aetiology of oesophageal cancer in greater Bombay. Monograph No. 1, Int. Seminar on Epidemiology of Oesophageal Cancer, Bangalore, India, 4 November 1971, pp 20–30.

KABAT GC, NG SK, WYNDER EL. 1993. Tobacco, alcohol intake, and diet in relation to adenocarcinoma of the esophagus and gastric cardia. Cancer Causes Control 4:123–132.

KELLY AB. 1919. Spasm at the entrance of the oesophagus. J Laryngol Otol 34:285–289.

KEMP IW, CLARKE K, KINLEN J. 1992. Oesophageal cancer and distilleries in Scotland. Br Med J 304:1543–1544.

KENNING JJ, PENA AS, VAN LEUWEN A, et al. 1976. HLA-DW3 associated with coeliac disease. Lancet i:606–608.

KIRK RL, KEATS B, BLAKE NM, et al. 1977. Genes and people in the Caspian littoral. Am J Phys Anthropol 46:377–390.

KOLICHEVA NI. 1974. Data on the epidemiology and morphology of precancerous changes and of cancer of the oesophagus in Kazakhstan, USSR. Thesis, Alma Ata.

KOLICHEVA NI. 1980. Epidemiology of esophagus cancer in the USSR. In Levin D (ed): Joint USA/USSR Monograph on Cancer Epidemiology in the USA and USSR.

KURATSUNE M, KOHCHI S, HORIE A. 1965. Carcinogenesis in the esophagus. I. Penetration of benzo(a)pyrene and other hydrocarbons into the esophageal mucosa. Gann 56:177–187.

LANIER AP, BLOT WJ, BENDER TR, FRAUMENI JF JR. 1980. Cancer in Alaska Indians, Eskimos and Aleuts. J Natl Cancer Inst 65:1157–1159.

LA VECCHIA C, LIATI P, DECARLI A, NEGRELLO I, FRANCESCHI S. 1986. Tar yields of cigarettes and the risk of oesophageal cancer. Int J Cancer 38:381–385.

LEE HP, DAY NE, SHANMUGARATNAM K. 1988. Trends in cancer incidence in Singapore 1968–1982 (IARC Scientific Publications No. 91). Lyon: International Agency for Research on Cancer.

LEVI F, OLLYO JP, LA VECCHIA C, BOYLE P, MONNIER P, SAVARY M. 1990. Int J Cancer 45:852–854.

LEVIN W, WOOD AW, CHANG RG, ITTAH Y, CROISY-DELCEY M, YOGI H, JERINA DM, CONNEY AH. 1980. Exceptionally high tumour initiating activity of benzo(c)phenanthrene bay-region diol-epoxides on mouse skin. Cancer Res 40:3910–3914.

LI GH, HE LJ. 1985. A survey of the familial aggregation of esophageal cancer in Yangcheng County. Chin Med J (Engl.), 98:749–752.

LI JY, LI GY, ZHENG SF, et al. 1985. A pilot vitamin intervention trial in Linxian, People's Republic of China. Natl Cancer Inst Monogr 69:19–22.

LI JY, ERSHOW AG, CHEN ZJ, WACHOLDER S, LI GY, GUO W, LI B, BLOT WJ. 1989. A case-control study of cancer of the esophagus and gastric cardia in Linxian. Int J Cancer 43:755–761.

LI JY, TAYLOR PR, LI B, DAWSEY S, WANG GY, ERSHOW AG, GUO W, LIU SF, YANG CS, SHEN Q, WANG W, MARK SD, ZOU XN, GREENWALD P, WU YP, BLOT WJ. 1993. Nutrition intervention trials in Linxian, China: Multiple/mineral supplementation, cancer incidence, and disease-specific mortality among adults with esophageal dysplasia. J Natl Cancer Inst 85:1492–1498.

LOKE SL, MA L, WONG M, et al. 1990. Human papillomavirus in oesophageal squamous cell carcinoma. J Clin Pathol 43:909–912.

LOVE AGG, ELMES M, GOLDEN NK, et al. 1978. Zinc deficiency and coeliac disease. In McNichol B, McCarthy CF, Fottrell PF (eds). Perspectives in Coeliac Disease. MTP Press Limited, Kluwer Acad Publ, Lancaster, UK, pp 335–342.

LU JB, YANG WX, LIU JM, LI YS, QIN YM. 1985. Trends in morbidity and mortality for oesophageal cancer in Linxian County. Int J Cancer 36:643–645.

LU SH, YANG WX, GUO LP, LI FM, WANG GJ, ZHANG JS, LI PZ. 1987. Determination of N-nitrosamines in gastric juice and urine and a comparison of endogenous formation of N-nitrosoproline and its inhibition in subjects from high- and low-risk areas for oesophageal cancer. In Bartsch H, O'Neill I, Schulte-Hermann R (eds): The relevance of N-nitroso compounds to human cancer: Exposure and mechanisms (IARC Scientific Publications No. 84). Lyon: International Agency for Research on Cancer.

LUNDHOLM I. 1939. Hereditary hypochromic anaemia. A clinical-statistical study. Acad Med Scand 102:1–237.

MAHBOUBI E, KMET J, COOK PJ, et al. 1973. Oesophageal cancer studies in the Caspian littoral of Iran: The Caspian cancer registry. Br J Cancer 28:197–214.

MANDARD AM, CHASLE J, MARNAY J. 1978. Cancer of the oesophagus and dysplasias (preliminary results). Eur J Cancer (Suppl.):15–26.

MARTINEZ I. 1964. Cancer of the esophagus in Puerto Rico. Mortality and incidence analysis, 1950–1964. Cancer 17:1279–1288.

MARTINEZ I. 1969. Factors associated with cancer of the esophagus, mouth and pharynx in Puerto Rico. J Natl Cancer Inst 42:1069–1094.

MCGLASHAN ND, BRADSHAW E, HARRINGTON JS. 1982. Cancer of the oesophagus and the use of tobacco and alcoholic beverages in Transkei, 1975–6. Int J Cancer 29:249–256.

MCMICHAEL AJ. 1978. Increases in laryngeal cancer in Britain and Australia in relation to alcohol and tobacco consumption trends. Lancet i:1244–1247.

METTLIN C, GRAHAM S, PRIORE S, MARSHALL J, SWANSON M. 1981. Diet and cancer of the esophagus. Nutr Cancer 2:143–147.

MIRVISH SS, HUANG Q, CHEN SC, BIRT DF, CLARK GW, HINDER RA, SMYRK TC, DEMEESTER TR. 1993. Metabolism of carcinogenic nitrosamines in the rat and human esophagus and induction of esophageal adenocarcinoma in rats. Endoscopy 25:627–631.

MOGHISSI K, SHARPE DA, PENDER D. 1993. Adenocarcinoma and Barrett's oesophagus. A clinico-pathological study. Eur J Cardiothorac Surg 7:126–131.

MØLLER H, BOYLE P, MAISONNEUVE P, LA VECCHIA C, JENSEN OM. 1990. Changing mortality from esophageal cancer in males in Denmark and other European countries, in relation to changing levels of alcohol consumption. Cancer Causes Control 1:181–188.

MØLLER H. 1992. Incidence of cancer of the oesophagus, cardia and stomach in Denmark. Eur J Cancer Prev 1:159–164.

MORTON JF. 1968. Plants associated with oesophageal cancer cases in Curacao. Cancer Res 28:2268–2271.

MORTON JF. 1979. Plant tannins and esophageal cancer. In Deichmann WB Amsterdam (ed): Toxicology and Occupational Medicine. Elsevier North Holland, Inc, pp 129–137.

MOSBECH L, VIDEBACK A. 1955. On the etiology of esophageal carcinoma. J Natl Cancer Inst 15:1665–1673.

MUIR CS, WATERHOUSE J, MACK T, POWELL J, WHELAN S. 1988. Cancer Incidence in Five Continents, Vol. V (IARC Scientific Publications No. 88). Lyon: International Agency for Research on Cancer.

MUKADA T, SATO E, SASANO N. 1976. Comparative studies on dysplasia of esophageal epithelium in four prefectures of Japan (Miyagi, Nara, Wakayama and Aomori) with reference to risk of carcinoma. Tohoku J Exp Med 119:51–63.

MUÑOZ N, CRESPI M, GRASSI A, WANG GUO QING, SHEN QIONG, LI ZHANG CAI. 1982. Precursor lesions of oesophageal cancer in high-risk populations in Iran and China. Lancet i:876–879.

MUÑOZ N, LIPKIN M, CRESPI M, WAHRENDORF J, GRASSI A, LU SH. 1985a. Proliferative abnormalities of the esophageal epithelium of Chinese populations at high and low risk for esophageal cancer. Int J Cancer 36:187–189.

MUÑOZ N, WAHRENDORF J, LU JIAN BANG, CRESPI M, THURNHAM DI, DAY NE, ZHENG HONG JI, GRASSI A, LI WEN YAN, LIU GUI LIN, LANG YU QUAN, ZHANG CAI YUN, ZHENG SU FANG, LI JUN YAO, CORREA P, O'CONOR GT, BOSCH X. 1985b. No effect of riboflavine, retinol and zinc on prevalence of precancerous lesions of esophagus: a randomized double-blind intervention study in a high-risk population of China. Lancet ii:111–114.

MUÑOZ N, HAYASHI M, LU JB, WAHRENDORF J, CRESPI M, BOSCH FX. 1987. Effect of riboflavin, retinol and zinc on micronuclei of buccal mucosa and of esophagus: a randomized double-blind intervention study in China. J Natl Cancer Inst 79:687–691.

NAGAI M, HASHIMOTO T, YANAGAWA H, YOKOYAMA H, MINOVA M. 1982. Relationship of diet to the incidence of esophageal and stomach cancer in Japan. Nutr Cancer 3:257–268.

NASIPOV SN. 1977. Esophageal cancer morbidity as evidenced by the genealogy of patients registered in the Gur'ev province. Vop Onkol 23:81–85.

NATIONAL CANCER CONTROL OFFICE. 1980. Atlas of Cancer Mortality in the People's Republic of China.

NORELL S, AHLBOM A, LIPPING H, ÖSTERBLOM L. 1983. Esophageal cancer and vulcanisation work. Lancet i:462–463.

NORWEGIAN CANCER SOCIETY. 1978. Geographical variations in cancer incidence in Norway, 1966–1975. Oslo: Norwegian Cancer Society.

NOTANI PN, JAYANT K. 1987. Role of diet in upper aerodigestive tract cancers. Nutr Cancer 10:103–113.

O'MAHONY MY, ELLIS JP, HELLIER M, MANN R, HUDDY P. 1984. Familial tylosis and carcinoma of the esophagus. J R Soc Med 77:515–516.

O'NEILL C, JORDAN P, BHATT T, NEWMAN R. 1986. Silica and esophageal cancer. Ciba Found Symp 121:214–230.

PALLI D, BIANCHI S, DECARLI A, CIPRIANI F, AVELLINI C, COCCO P, FALCINI F, PUNTONI R, RUSSO A, VINDIGNI C, FRAUMENI JF JR, BLOT WJ, BUIATTI E. 1992. A case-control study of cancers of the gastric cardia in Italy. Br J Cancer 65:263–266.

PARKIN DM. 1986. Cancer Occurrence in Developing Countries

(IARC Scientific Publications No. 75). Lyon: International Agency for Research on Cancer.

PARKIN DM, MUIR CS, WHELAN SL, GAO YT, FERLAY J, POWELL J. (eds). 1992. Cancer Incidence in Five Continents, Volume VI (IARC Scientific Publications No. 120). Lyon: International Agency for Research on Cancer.

PARKIN DM, PISANI P, FERLAY J. 1993. Estimates of the worldwide incidence of eighteen major cancers in 1985. Int J Cancer 54:594–606.

PARKIN DM, VIZCAINO AP, SKINNER MEG, NDHLOVU A. 1994. Cancer patterns and risk factors in the African population of Southwestern Zimbabwe, 1969–1977. Cancer Epidemiol Biomarkers Prev 3:537–547.

PATERSON DR. 1919. A clinical type of dysphagia. J Laryngol Otol 34:289–291.

POSTLETHWAIT RW, WENDELL MUSSER A. 1974. Changes in the esophagus in 1000 autopsy specimens. Thorac Cardiovasc Surg 68:953–956.

POTTERN LM, MORRIS LE, BLOT WJ, ZIEGLER RG, FRAUMENI JF. 1981. Esophageal cancer among black men in Washington, D.C. I. Alcohol, tobacco and other risk factors. J Natl Cancer Inst 67:777–783.

POUR P, GHADIRIAN P. 1974. Familial cancer of the esophagus in Iran. Cancer 33:1649–1652.

POWELL J, MCCONKEY CC. 1990. Increasing incidence of adenocarcinoma of the gastric cardia and adjacent sites. Br J Cancer 62:440–443.

RITTER SB, PETERSEN G. 1976. Esophageal cancer, hyperkeratosis and oral leukoplakia: occurrence in a 25-year-old woman. JAMA 235:1723.

ROGERS MA, THOMAS DB, DAVIS S, VAUGHAN TL, NEVISSI AE. 1993. A case-control study of element levels and cancer of the upper aerodigestive tract. Cancer Epidemiol Biomarkers Prev 2:305–312.

ROGOT E. 1979. Personal communication.

RONCO G, COSTA G, LYNGE E. 1992. Cancer risk among Danish and Italian farmers. Br J Ind Med 49:220–225.

ROSE E. 1978. Environmental factors associated with cancer of the esophagus in Transkei. In Silber W. (ed): Carcinoma of the Esophagus. Rotterdam: Balkema, pp. 91–98.

SANKARANARAYANAN R, DUFFY SW, PADMAKUMARY G, NAIR SM, DAY NE, PADMANABHAN TK. 1991. Risk factors for cancer of the esophagus in Kerala, India. Int J Cancer 49:485–489.

SCHWARTZ D, FLAMANT R, LELLOUCH J, et al. 1962. Alcool et cancer. Résultats d'une étude rétrospective. Rev Fr Etudes Clin Biol 7:590–604.

SEGAL I, REINACH SG, DE BEER M. 1988. Factors associated with esophageal cancer in Soweto, South Africa. Br J Cancer 58:681–686.

SEGI M. 1975. Tea-gruel as a possible factor for cancer of the esophagus. Gann 66:199–202.

SELIKOFF IO, HAMMOND EC. 1978. Asbestos-associated disease in United States shipyards. CA Cancer J Clin 28:87–99.

SHANMUGARATNAM K, LEE HP, DAY NE. 1982. Cancer incidence in Singapore 1968–1977 (IARC Scientific Publications No. 47). Lyon: International Agency for Research on Cancer.

SHARP GS. 1931. Leukoplakia of the esophagus. Am J Cancer 15:2029–2043.

SHEN O, LIU SF, DAWSEY SM, CAO J, ZHOU B, WANG DY, CAO SG, ZHAO HZ, LI GY, TAYLOR PR, et al. 1993. Cytologic screening for esophageal cancer: results from 12,877 subjects from a high risk population in China. Int J Cancer 54:185–188.

SHINE I, ALLISON PR. 1966. Carcinoma of the esophagus with tylosis (keratosis palmaris et plantaris). Lancet i:951–953.

SIDDIQI M, KUMAR R, FAZILI Z, SPIEGELHALDER B, PREUSSMAN R. 1992. Increased exposure to dietary amines and nitrate in a population at high risk of esophageal and gastric cancer in Kashmir (India). Carcinogenesis 13:1331–1335.

SIMPSON RR. 1939. Anaemia with dysphagia: a precancerous condition? Proc Roy Soc Med 32:1447–1474.

SMITH P, DOLL R. 1978. Age- and time-dependent changes in the rates of radiation-induced cancers in patients with ankylosing spondylitis following a single course of x-ray treatment. In: Late Biological Effects of Ionizing Radiation. Vol. I. Vienna, International Atomic Energy Agency, pp. 205–218.

SPECHLER SJ, GOYAL RK. 1986. Barrett's esophagus. N Engl J Med 315:362–371.

SPECHLER SJ. 1994. Pathogenesis and epidemiology of Barrett esophagus. Chirurg 65:84–87.

STEINER P. 1956. Etiology and histogenesis of carcinoma of esophagus. Cancer 9:436–452.

STOKES PL, ASQUITH P, COOKE WT. 1973. Genetics of coeliac disease. In: Clinics Gastroenterol. London: W.B. Saunders, p. 547.

STOKES PL, PRIOR P, SORAHAN TM, et al. 1976. Malignancy in relatives of patients with coeliac disease. Br J Prev Soc Med 30:17–21.

SYDENHAM E, THIEL PG, MARASAS WFO, SHEPHARD GS, VAN SCHALKWYK DJ, KOCH KR. 1990. Natural occurrence of some fusarium mycotoxins in corn from low and high esophageal cancer prevalence areas of the Transkei, Southern Africa. J Agric Food Chem 38:1900–1903.

THURNHAM DI, MUÑOZ N, LU JB, WAHRENDORF J, ZHENG SF, HAMBIDGE KM, CRESPI M. 1988. Nutritional and haematological status of Chinese farmers: the influence of 13.5 months treatment with riboflavin, retinol and zinc. Eur J Clin Nutrition 42:647–660.

TUYNS AJ. 1983. Oesophageal cancer in non-smoking drinkers and in non-drinking smokers. Int J Cancer 32:443–444.

TUYNS AJ. 1992. Oesophageal cancer in France and Switzerland: recent time trends. Eur J Cancer Prev 1:275–278.

TUYNS AJ, ESTÈVE J. 1983. Pipe, commercial and hand-rolled cigarette smoking in oesophageal cancer. Int J Epidemiol 12:110–113.

TUYNS AJ, VERNHES JC. 1981. La mortalité par cancer de l'oesophage dans les départements du Calvados et de l'Orne. Gastroenterol Clin Biol 5: 257–265.

TUYNS AJ, PÉQUIGNOT G, JENSEN OM. 1977. Le cancer de l'oesophage en Ille-et-Vilaine en fonction des niveaux de consommation d'alcool et de tabac. Des risques qui se multiplient. Bull Cancer 64:45–60.

TUYNS AJ, RIBOLI E, DOORNBOS G, PÉQUIGNOT G. 1987. Diet and esophageal cancer in Calvados (France). Nutr Cancer 9:81–92.

TYLDESLEY WR. 1974. Oral leukoplakia associated with tylosis and oesophageal carcinoma. J Oral Pathol 3:62–70.

UNAKAMI M, HARA M, FUKUCHI S, AKIYAMA H. 1989. Cancer of the gastric cardia and the habit of smoking. Acta Pathol Jpn 39:420.

USHIGOME S, SPJUT HJ, NOON GP. 1967. Extensive dysplasia and carcinoma in situ of esophageal epithelium. Cancer 20:1023–1034.

VAN RENSBURG SJ. 1981. Epidemiologic and dietary evidence for a specific nutritional predisposition to esophageal cancer. J Natl Cancer Inst 67:243–251.

VAN RENSBURG SJ, BENADE AS, ROSE EF, DU PLESSIS JP. 1983. Nutritional status of African populations predisposed to esophageal cancer. Nutr Cancer 4:206–216.

VASSALLO A, CORREA P, DE STEFANI E, CENDAN M, ZAVALA D, CHEN V, CARZOGLIO J, DENEO-PELLEGRINI H. 1985. Esophageal cancer in Uruguay: A case-control study. J Natl Cancer Inst 75:1005–1009.

VICTORIA CG, MUÑOZ N, DAY NE, BARCELOS LB, PECCIN DA, BRAGA NM. 1987. Hot beverages and oesophageal cancer in southern Brazil: a case-control study. Int J Cancer 39:710–716.

VINSON PP. 1922. Hysterical dysphagia. Minn Med 5:107–108.

VINSON PP. 1940. Diagnosis and Treatment of Diseases of the Esophagus. London: Baillière, Tindall and Cox.

WABINGA HR, PARKIN DM, WBWIRE-MANGEN F, MUGERWA JW.

1993. Cancer in Kampala, Uganda, in 1989–1991: changes in incidence in the era of AIDS. Int J Cancer 54:26–36.

WAHRENDORF J, MUÑOZ N, LU JB, THURNHAM DI, CRESPI M, BOSCH FX. 1988. Blood, retinol and zinc riboflavin status in relation to precancerous lesions of the esophagus: findings from a vitamin intervention trial in the People's Republic of China. Cancer Res 48:2280–2283.

WAHRENDORF J, CHANG-CLAUDE J, QUI SL, YANG GR, MUÑOZ N, CRESPI M, RAEDSCH R, THURNHAM D, CORREA P. 1989. Precursor lesions of oesophageal cancer in adolescents in a high-risk population in China. Lancet ii:1239–1241.

WALDENSTROM J. 1938. Iron and epithelium. Some clinical observations. Part I. Regeneration of the epithelium. Acta Med Scand 90:380–397.

WALDENSTROM J. 1946. Incidence of "iron deficiency" (sideropenia) in some rural and urban populations. Acta Med Scand 70:252–279.

WALDENSTROM J, KJELLBERG SR. 1939. The roentgenological diagnosis of sideropenic dysphagia (Plummer-Vinson's syndrome). Acta Radiol 20:618–638.

WALKER EA, CASTEGNARO M, GARREN L, TOUSSAINT G, KOWALSKI B. 1979. Intake of volatile nitrosamines from consumption of alcohols. J Natl Cancer Inst 63:947–951.

WATERHOUSE J, MUIR C, CORREA P, POWELL J. 1976. Cancer Incidence in Five Continents, Volume III (IARC Scientific Publications No. 15). Lyon: International Agency for Research on Cancer.

WHO COLLABORATING CENTRE FOR ORAL PRECANCEROUS LESIONS. 1978. Definition of leukoplakia and related lesions: an aid to studies on oral precancers. Oral Surg 46:518–539.

WILD CP, LU SH, MONTESANO R. 1987. Radioimmunoassay used to detect DNA alkylation adducts in tissues from populations at high risk for oesophageal and stomach cancer. In Bartsch H, O'Neill I, Schulte-Hermann R (eds). The Relevance of N-nitrosocompounds to Human Cancer. Exposure and Mechanisms (IARC Scientific Publications No. 84), pp 534–537.

WILLIAMSON AL, JASKIEWICZ K, GUNNING A. 1991. The detection of human papillomavirus in oesophageal lesions. Anticancer Res 11:263–265.

WU Y, CHEN J, OHSHIMA H, PIGNATELLI B, BOREHAM J, LI J, CAMPBELL TC, PETO R, BARTSCH H. 1993. Geographic association between urinary excretion of N-nitroso compounds and oesophageal cancer mortality in China. Int J Cancer 54:713–719.

WU-WILLIAMS AH, YU MC, MACK TM. 1990. Life-style, workplace, and stomach cancer by sub-site in young men of Los Angeles County. Cancer Res 50:2569.

WYNDER EL. 1971. Etiological aspects of squamous cancers of the head and neck. JAMA 215:452–453.

WYNDER EL, BROSS IJ. 1961. A study of etiological factors in cancers of the esophagus. Cancer 14:389–413.

WYNDER EL, CHAN PC. 1970. The possible role of riboflavin deficiency in epithelial neoplasia. II. Effect on skin tumor development. Cancer 26:1221–1224.

WYNDER EL, HULTBERT S, JACOBSSON F, et al. 1957. Environmental factors in cancer of the upper alimentary tract: Swedish study with special reference to Plummer-Vinson (Paterson-Kelly syndrome). Cancer 10:470–487.

XIA QJ. 1984. Carcinogenesis in the esophagus. In Huang GJ, Wu Ku (eds): Carcinoma of the Esophagus and Gastric Cardia. New York: Springer-Verlag, pp 53–76.

YANG CS. 1980. Research on esophageal cancer in China: a review. Cancer Res 40:2633–2644.

YANG CS, SUN Y, YANG QU, MILLER KW, LI GY, ZHENG SF, ERSHOW AG, BLOT WJ, LI JY. 1984. Vitamin A and other deficiencies in Linxian, a high esophageal cancer incidence area in northern China. J Natl Cancer Inst 73:1449–1453.

YESUDIAN P, PREMALATHA S, THAMBIAH AS. 1980. Genetic tylosis with malignancy: a study of a South Indian pedigree. Br J Dermatol 102:597–600.

YOUNG M, RUSSEL WT. 1926. An investigation into the statistics of cancer in different trades and professions. Medical Research Council, Special Report Series No. 99. London, England: His Majesty's Stationery Office.

YU MC, GARABRANT DH, PETERS JM, MACK TM. 1988. Tobacco, alcohol, diet, occupation, and carcinoma of the esophagus. Cancer Res 48:3843–3848.

YU Y, TAYLOR PR, LI JY, DAWSEY SM, WANG GQ, GUO WD, WANG W, LIU BQ, BLOT WJ, SHEN Q, et al. 1993. Retrospective cohort study of risk factors for esophageal cancer in Linxian, People's Republic of China. Cancer Causes Control 4:195–202.

ZARIDZE DG, BASIEVA T, KABULOV M, DAY NE, DUFFY SW. 1992. Esophageal cancer in the Republic of Karakalpakstan. Int J Epidemiol 21:643–648.

ZHENG W, JIN F, DEVESA SS, BLOT WJ, FRAUMENI JF JR, GAO YT. 1993. Declining incidence is greater for esophageal than gastric cancer in Shanghai, People's Republic of China. Br J Cancer 68:978–982.

ZIEGLER RG. 1986. Alcohol-nutrient interactions in cancer etiology. Cancer 58:1942–1948.

ZIEGLER RG, MORRIS LE, BLOT WJ, POTTERN LM, HOOVER R, FRAUMENI JF. 1981. Esophageal cancer among black men in Washington, D.C. II. Role of nutrition. J Natl Cancer Inst 67:1199–1206.

34 Stomach cancer

ABRAHAM NOMURA

One outstanding feature of stomach cancer has been the remarkable decline in its mortality rate, worldwide, over the past 50 years or so (Haenszel, 1958; Kurihara et al, 1984). In 1930 it was the leading cause of death due to cancer in the United States (American Cancer Society, 1995). Since then, the U. S. mortality rate for stomach cancer has decreased to about one-fifth of its earlier rate. These data provide encouragement that a similar reduction is achievable for other cancers and support the view that environmental causes play a major role in the occurrence of gastric cancer.

In spite of its decline, stomach cancer is still a disease of significant impact. Internationally, it appears to be the second leading cause of death due to cancer (Kurihara et al, 1984). In the United States, stomach cancer is the seventh leading cause of cancer deaths. It is estimated that for 1995 there will be 22,800 new cases diagnosed and 14,700 stomach cancer deaths in the country (American Cancer Society, 1995).

Although there has been some improvement in the 5-year relative survival rates of gastric cancer over the past 25 years, the disease has a high case-fatality rate of over 80% (Miller et al, 1993). This emphasizes the importance of isolating its causes so that preventive measures can be taken to reduce further its occurrence. In this chapter, the histopathology of stomach cancer related to its epidemiology is reviewed. The observed patterns in mortality, incidence, time trends, and survival are presented and interpreted. The demography of stomach cancer with regard to age, sex, race, and socioeconomic status is also discussed in detail. This is followed by a listing of antecedent conditions studied in association with gastric cancer and a review of environmental factors suspected in the causation of stomach cancer. Emphasis is on studies related to diet. Then the role of host factors is briefly covered, followed by a discussion of possible pathogenetic mechanisms. Finally, there is a section on preventive measures, and recommendations are made for future research.

This work was supported in part by grants RO1 CA 33644 and P01 CA 33619 from the National Cancer Institute.

DEMOGRAPHIC PATTERNS

Histopathology

Adenocarcinoma of the stomach constitutes 95% of all cancers of the stomach in the United States. Of the remaining 5%, more than one-half are non-Hodgkin's lymphomas, and the rest are often leiomyosarcomas (Schein and Levin, 1985).

In 1951, Jarvi and Lauren noted that the histological structure of gastric carcinomas often displayed features characteristic of intestinal mucosa. Later, Lauren divided gastric cancer into two histologic types, intestinal and diffuse (Lauren, 1965). The intestinal type had large, irregular nuclei in large, distinct cells arranged in a well-polarized, columnar fashion, giving a glandular appearance. There was usually a pronounced inflammatory cell infiltration, but a sparse amount of connective tissue. Intestinal metaplasia or atrophic gastritis was often found in surrounding regions.

In contrast to the intestinal type, diffuse stomach cancer has been characterized by small cells scattered either as solitary cells or as clusters of cells, arranged in a non-polarized pattern and rarely with glandular lamina. Inflammatory cell reaction is minimal and the connective tissue has a more scirrhous pattern. Intestinal metaplasia or atrophic gastritis has been less frequently found in neighboring regions.

Munoz and colleagues used the Jarvi-Lauren classification of stomach cancer to study the pattern of stomach cancer occurrence by sex, age, and country. They observed that the intestinal type predominated in high-risk areas, especially in men and in older age groups (Munoz et al, 1968; Munoz and Connelly, 1971; Munoz and Steinitz, 1971; Munoz and Matko, 1972). In low-risk areas, the diffuse type was more frequent at younger ages, and its sex ratio was close to one. These studies were done in Colombia, Mexico, Israel, Poland, Yugoslavia, and the United States.

In Norway, time-trend patterns showed that the decrease in stomach cancer mortality from 1940 to 1966 was primarily due to diminished numbers of intestinal cancers, although the occurrence of diffuse cancer also decreased over that time period (Munoz and Asvall, 1971). A separate study comparing stomach cancer in Japanese people living in Miyagi, Japan, and in Hawaii showed that the decrease in gastric cancer among the Hawaii Japanese was chiefly due to fewer cases of the intestinal type (Correa et al, 1973).

Although Munoz and Matko (1972) hypothesized that the two types of stomach cancer may have different causes, differences in host susceptibility and response and in the level of exposure to cancer-causing agents could produce the observations that have been made with regard to the occurrence of intestinal and diffuse stomach cancer.

Time Trends and Mortality Patterns

In 1930, there was little difference in the stomach cancer mortality rates between the United States and England and Wales. Their rates were much lower than those of Japan and the Netherlands. Over the next 20 years, the rate of decrease in the United States was greater than that of the other three countries (Haenszel, 1958).

From 1950 to 1979, the rate of decline among men was still greater in the United States, as shown in Figure 34–1 (Kurihara et al, 1984). Countries with a high stomach cancer mortality rate, such as Japan and Chile, were also experiencing a decrease in their rates, beginning around 1962–63. Although there is a certain degree of inaccuracy in the use of death certificates and mortality data (Moriyama et al, 1958; Steer et al, 1976), the information in Figure 34–1 is probably not misleading with respect to time trends in gastric cancer occurrence.

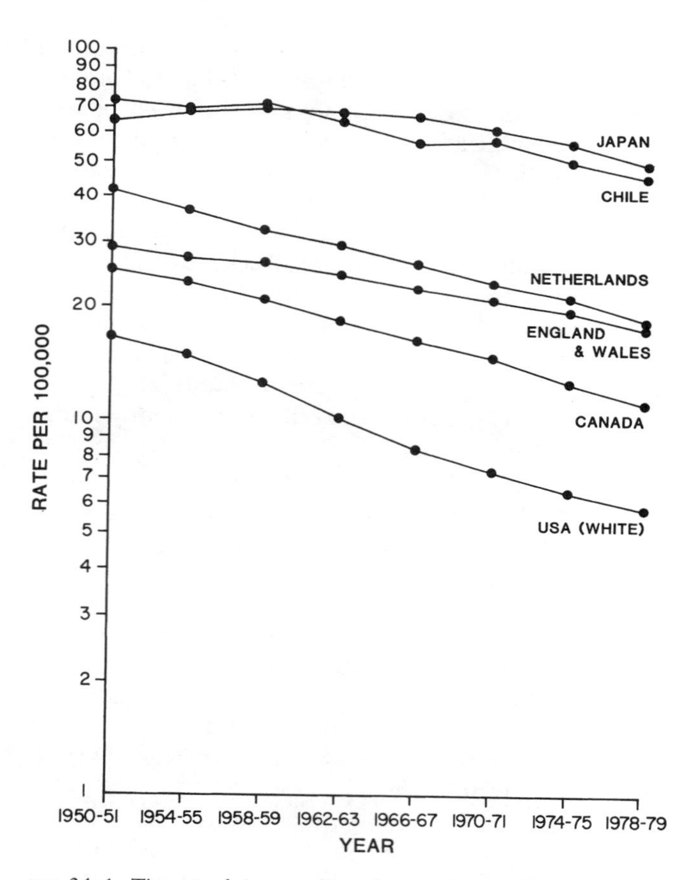

FIG. 34–1. Time trends in age-adjusted stomach cancer mortality rates per 100,000 men in six countries. (Kurihara et al., 1984.)

Within the United States, there are still regional differences among whites in stomach cancer mortality rates. The patterns for both men and women have shown clusters of excessive mortality in the north central regions of the country, with elevated rates in counties with many residents of foreign stock (Hoover, 1975). This cluster has persisted but was less apparent in the 1970s (Pickle et al, 1987). High rates were also present in urban areas of the northeastern region of the United States.

International Patterns in Incidence

Stomach cancer incidence rates by countries present several noteworthy patterns, as shown in Table 34–1 (Parkin et al, 1992). First, there is about a 20-fold difference in stomach cancer rates in comparing the high-risk Japanese in Miyagi with the low-risk Filipinos in Los Angeles, California. Second, there is obvious heterogeneity in the ethnicity of people who have high and low rates of gastric cancer. People in Japan, Russia, China, and Costa Rica have high rates, while residents of Thailand and Kuwait, and American Filipinos have low rates. Third, Japanese and Chinese migrants to Hawaii and their offspring have lower rates than the Japanese in Japan and the Chinese in China or Singapore. Conversely, Indians in Singapore have higher rates than Indians in India. Although it is recognized that cancer rates vary geographically within a country of origin, there is a general pattern in which migrants tend to gravitate toward the cancer risk of their adopted country. Fourth, Polynesians (Maoris and Hawaiians) in New Zealand and Hawaii have higher rates than their white neighbors. Fifth, whites in English-speaking countries (United Kingdom, New Zealand, Australia, United States, and Canada) have relatively low rates.

Factors related to the causation of stomach cancer should be reconciled with the incidence patterns in different countries. However, there is a caveat. Caution should be exercised in comparing stomach cancer incidence rates from different countries, because of possible differences in diagnostic methods, criteria for determining malignancy, and other medical care practices. Where these differences are minimal between countries,

TABLE 34–1. *Average Annual Age-Adjusted* Stomach Cancer Incidence per 100,000 from Selected Registries†*

Country	Locale	Race/Ethnicity	Men	Women
Japan	Miyagi		85.4	36.7
Russia	St. Petersburg		52.8	25.3
China	Shanghai		51.7	21.9
Costa Rica			46.9	21.3
United States	Los Angeles	Korean	41.5	22.9
Italy	Parma		38.4	17.9
Colombia	Cali		36.3	19.9
Singapore		Chinese	34.7	15.6
United States	Los Angeles	Japanese	29.7	13.8
Iceland			28.8	9.9
Yugoslavia	Slovenia		27.9	12.8
Romania	County Cluj		26.1	10.7
New Zealand		Maori	25.3	20.4
United States	Hawaii	Hawaiian	24.3	11.8
United States	Hawaii	Japanese	24.3	11.1
Hong Kong			22.1	11.2
Germany	Saarland		20.4	11.5
Finland			20.3	11.2
United Kingdom	Oxford		17.5	6.8
Singapore		Indian	15.9	7.5
Norway			15.7	8.0
France	Doubs		15.1	5.5
United States	Connecticut	Black	15.0	4.1
United States	Los Angeles	Black	14.8	6.0
Puerto Rico			14.5	6.7
Philippines	Manila		13.5	8.1
United States	Los Angeles	Chinese	13.0	7.9
Australia	South		12.8	4.3
Sweden			12.7	6.5
United States	Los Angeles	Hispanic	12.6	8.0
Denmark			12.5	5.7
New Zealand		Non-Maori	12.3	5.2
Canada	Alberta		11.3	5.2
United States	Hawaii	White	10.2	3.9
United States	Connecticut	White	9.0	3.9
United States	Hawaii	Filipino	8.6	5.3
United States	Hawaii	Chinese	8.5	6.1
United States	Los Angeles	White	7.4	3.3
India	Bombay		7.3	4.3
Singapore		Malay	6.4	5.4
Thailand	Khon Kaen		5.0	2.5
Kuwait		Kuwaiti	4.1	2.0
United States	Los Angeles	Filipino	4.0	3.7

*Based on world standard population.
†From Parkin et al (1992).

and where there is a high degree of completeness in case ascertainment, the rates should be reliable for comparative purposes.

Survival

Among the different types of cancer, stomach cancer has the fifth poorest 5-year relative survival rate, following cancers of the pancreas, liver, esophagus, and lung (Miller et al, 1993). From 1960 to 1989, the 5-year relative survival rate among white males and females improved from 11% to 17%. The rate among blacks also improved from 8% to 18%. Figure 34–2 presents the 5-year relative survival rates by stage for whites and blacks, both sexes combined. Obviously, the key to improving survival is early diagnosis. Among black men and women, 18% were diagnosed with local disease, 31% with regional disease, 37% with distant disease, and 14% unstaged. Among whites, the percentages were 16, 34, 36, and 14, respectively.

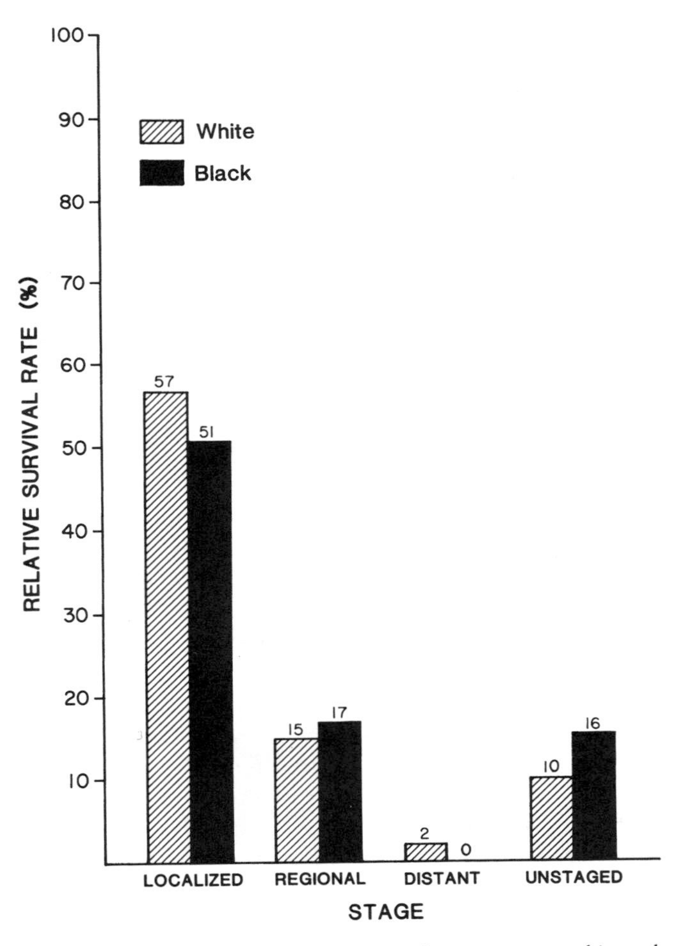

FIG. 34–2. Five-year relative survival rates by stage among white and black males and females, 1983–1987. (Miller et al., 1993.)

Migration

Migrant studies have presented a strong argument that environmental factors assume a dominant role over genetic factors in the occurrence of stomach cancer. Haenszel (1961) first observed that migrants to the United States had lower stomach cancer mortality rates than their peers in the country of origin. This applied to migrants from Germany,Italy, Norway, Sweden, Canada, Ireland, England, and Wales. The standard mortality ratios (SMR=100 for residents of country of origin) for 1950 ranged from 50 to 88 among men and 52 to 100 among women. Similar results were observed in a study by Gregorio et al (1992). This suggested that a change in environmental exposures could reduce stomach cancer mortality by at least 50%. Incidence rates in Table 34–1 for the Japanese in Hawaii, Los Angeles, and Miyagi and the Chinese in Hawaii, Los Angeles, Singapore, and Shanghai indicate that the stomach cancer incidence in migrant populations can be reduced even more than 50%. These migrant studies, along with the marked decrease in stomach cancer mortality over the past 50 years, provide a convincing case that environmental exposures mainly account for the differences in stomach cancer rates. These comparisons make the assumption that selection factors that lead to migration do not affect the occurrence of stomach cancer. Even if they do, it is unlikely they would cause such a remarkable change in rates.

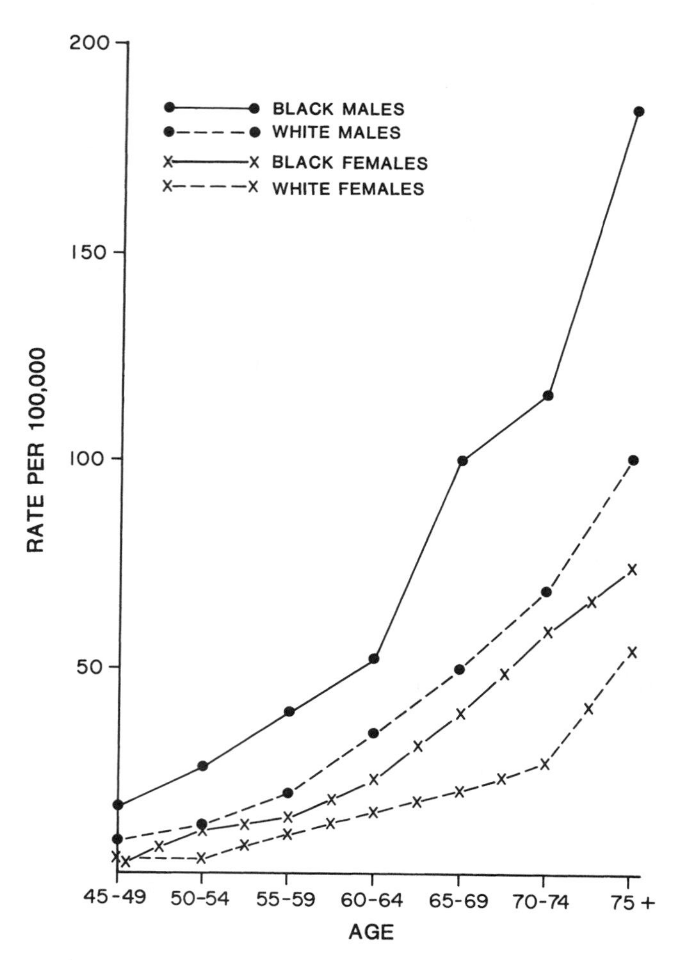

FIG. 34–3. Average annual age-specific incidence rates per 100,000 population by race and sex, 1983–1987, Los Angeles County, California, USA. (Parkin et al., 1992.)

Age and Sex

Like many other diseases, the incidence rate of stomach cancer increases markedly with age. Figure 34–3 shows the increase in rates among black and white residents in Los Angeles County, California (Parkin et al, 1992). This age pattern is typical of many ethnic groups in the United States and elsewhere.

An interesting feature of stomach cancer is that the male:female sex ratio of population-based incidence rates is usually in the range of 1.5–2.5. There is some tendency for the high-risk populations to have higher ratios than the low-risk populations, although many exceptions exist (Table 34–1). The pattern is not surprising in view of the male predominance in the intestinal type of stomach cancer in high-risk areas, while the sex ratio for the diffuse type is closer to one in low-risk areas.

The location of the cancer also affects the sex ratio. It has been reported that adenocarcinomas arising in the cardia have a male:female ratio of 7.0 compared with a ratio of 2.2 for cancers in the distal stomach (Yang and Davis, 1988). However, cancers occurred in the distal region three and a half times more frequently than in the cardia in the same report.

Race and Ethnicity

In many areas of the United States, blacks consistently have higher stomach cancer incidence rates than whites. This pattern has been observed in Alameda, Los Angeles, and the San Francisco Bay area, as well as in Atlanta, New Orleans, and Detroit (Parkin et al, 1992). The incidence rates are about two times greater among blacks in most of these locales. Blacks are also more likely to develop cancers in the distal stomach than whites, but are less likely to be diagnosed with tumors in the cardia than whites (Yang and Davis, 1988).

When the other ethnic groups are included, there is a greater diversity of rates. For example, in Los Angeles, the annual stomach cancer incidence rates per 100,000 men from 1983 to 1987 were 41.5 for Koreans, 29.7 for Japanese, 14.8 for blacks, 13.0 for Chinese, and 12.6 for Spanish-surnamed whites, 7.4 for other whites, and 4.0 for Filipinos. In Hawaii, the rates were 24.3 for Hawaiians, 24.3 for Japanese, 10.2 for whites, 8.6 for

Filipinos, and 8.5 for Chinese during the same period of time. Ethnic differences in susceptibility to stomach cancer need to be considered, but it is unlikely that they are mainly due to inherited biological or ethnic traits. Differences in environmental, dietary, and other personal exposures between the ethnic groups could account for much of the variation in rates of stomach cancer.

Social Class and Occupation

Gastric cancer has typically been a disease of the poor. Studies have consistently shown an association of stomach cancer with low socioeconomic status, based either on census tract information (Torgersen and Petersen, 1956), education (Tajima and Tominaga, 1985; Jedrychowski et al, 1993), family income (You et al, 1988), or occupation (Sigurjonsson, 1967; Haenszel et al, 1972). Most such studies have found that the gastric cancer risk of the lower social class was up to two times greater than that of the upper social class. Studies have been conducted in Norway, Japan, Poland, China, Iceland, and the United States, which attests to the universality of the finding.

Although social class is related to occupation, available evidence indicates that occupational exposures do not play a major role in the incidence of gastric cancer. It is suspected that coal miners (Ames, 1983) and asbestos workers (Selikoff et al, 1968; Enterline et al, 1972) have an increased risk for stomach cancer, but studies are not conclusive (Davies, 1980; Creagan et al, 1974). Other occupations associated with gastric cancer include employment in the chemical (Viadana et al, 1976), rubber (McMichael et al, 1976; Monson and Fine, 1978), oil refinery (Thomas et al, 1982; Rushton and Alderson, 1981), metal-products industries (Wu-Williams et al, 1990; Kraus et al, 1957), and other industries involving mineral dust exposure (Wright et al, 1988). Since exposures in these occupations have been related to stomach cancer in some studies, a number of carcinogenic agents have been suspected, including asbestos, polycyclic aromatic hydrocarbons, and N-nitroso compounds (Mirvish, 1983). However, relatively few people in the general population have had heavy industrial exposures, so such exposures would not contribute significantly to the overall risk for stomach cancer.

ANTECEDENT CONDITIONS

Gastric Polyps

There have been few epidemiological studies on the association of gastric cancer with gastric polyps, which are relatively uncommon (Lawrence, 1936). Pathologically, the most frequent types are hyperplastic polyps and adenomatous polyps. The former are small, seldom over 2 cm in diameter, and have revealed no evidence of malignant potential (Tomasulo, 1971; Ming and Goldman, 1965). On the other hand, adenomatous polyps have shown carcinomatous changes in 25% to 72% of studied lesions, and over 80% are 2 cm in diameter or larger (Ming, 1973).

In three pathology series of polyp cases, an accompanying gastric carcinoma was present in 12% to 35% of the cases (Ming and Goldman, 1965; Berg, 1958; Tomasulo, 1971). In a fourth study, 28% of patients with gastric polyps had an associated carcinoma, and in 5% of patients with gastric carcinomas there were associated polyps (Stewart, 1929). These observations suggest that conditions fostering the growth of polyps could also promote the development of carcinoma. It is not known whether polyp patients without carcinoma are at increased risk for stomach cancer after polypectomy or partial gastrectomy.

Gastric Ulcer

The relationship between gastric ulcer and gastric cancer has been the subject of much controversy. Studies in Western countries tend to support the view that gastric ulcers are not a significant source of gastric carcinoma. In 1962, Thunold and Wetteland found only 19 (2.5%) cases of ulcer-carcinoma in 726 stomachs resected for gastric ulcer. The diagnosis of ulcer-carcinoma was based upon the criteria first described by Hauser (1926): (1) the histological picture of a peptic ulcer with typical reactive changes at the base and edge of the ulcer; (2) tumor infiltration at ulcer edge but not in its base. In two other series, only 1.1% (5 of 473) and 3.6% (10 of 278) of cases with gastric ulcer were found with ulcer-carcinoma (Ihre et al, 1964; Rønnov-Jessen et al, 1965). Others have further argued against a close relationship of gastric ulcer to gastric carcinoma (Flood, 1961; Eisenberg and Woodward, 1963). In a follow-up study of 1038 patients in Massachusetts with medically treated gastric ulcer, only 4 subsequently died with gastric cancer 5 or more years after entry into the study, as compared to 3 expected deaths. One of the 4 patients may have had a true ulcer-cancer (Hirohata, 1968).

Reports from Japan appear to support both sides of the question. Several researchers in Japan have claimed that ulcer-cancer can arise from shallow ulcers as well as deep ones, which were described by Hauser and others. On this basis the frequency of ulcer-cancer in Japan is higher, ranging from about 40% to 70% (Nakamura et al, 1967). Sakita et al (1971) have proposed that a life cycle of ulceration, healing, and recurrent ulceration can take place in malignant ulcers. In 1967, Majima et al succeeded in producing ulcer-carcinoma in rats by implanting 4-nitroquinoline 1-oxide in beeswax into the gastric wall. The ulcer developed first and carcinoma appeared after the ulcer became chronic. However, two unique studies that investigated the pathology of a total of 91 stomach carcinomas less than 5 mm in diameter concluded that the majority of early gastric cancers are not preceded by gastric ulcers or polyps (Nakamura et al, 1968; Nagayo, 1975). They believed that either "chronic gastritis" or epithelium of the metaplastic type played a more important role.

Gastroenterostomy

Past studies support the view that patients who have had a gastroenterostomy for benign disease are at increased risk for developing gastric cancer many years (usually 20 or more) after surgery. In a prospective study of 4466 patients who had partial gastrectomy, the gastric cancer risk increased after surgery (Caygill et al, 1986). For gastric ulcer patients after their operation, there was a 2.7-fold increase in risk for the first 20 years, which rose to 5.5-fold thereafter. For duodenal ulcer patients, the risk was lower than expected for the first 20 years after surgery, but it increased 3.6-fold thereafter. Patients who had undergone the Billroth II procedure, which results in a duodenal stump with a gastrojejunal anastomosis, had a greater risk than patients who had had the Billroth I procedure, which resulted in a gastroduodenal anastomosis. Similar findings were observed in another large follow-up study with 6459 gastrectomy patients (Lundegardh et al, 1988), except there was no increase in risk less than 20 years after gastrectomy. The increase in gastric cancer risk after surgery has also been supported in other investigations (Fisher et al, 1993; Tersmette et al, 1991; Viste et al, 1986; Stalsberg and Taksdal, 1971). Studies that have not found this association usually either had fewer patients or had an insufficient number followed for more than 20 years to detect the increased risk (Ross et al, 1982; Schafer et al, 1985; Tokudome et al, 1984).

There is supporting evidence that the observed association is real. Studies have noted that gastric carcinomas or polyps occurred within or close to the stomal opening in patients with gastroenterostomy (Domellof et al, 1977) and that there was more cellular atrophy of the mucosa of the gastric stump after gastrojejunostomy (Billroth II) than after gastroduodenostomy (Billroth I) (Jones and Williams, 1963). It is believed that the regurgitation of alkaline bile and pancreatic juice through the gastrojejunostomy contributes to postoperative gastritis, whereas regurgitation of duodenal contents seldom occurs after the gastroduodenostomy (Kobayashi et al, 1970). In most series, the percentage of gastric cancer patients who had previous gastric surgery ranged from 2.6% to 8.7% (Liavaag, 1962; Saegesser and James, 1972; Eberlein et al, 1978; Stalsberg and Taksdal, 1971).

Chronic Atrophic Gastritis

Correa and colleagues (1976) have conducted detailed studies of chronic atrophic gastritis, defined as the loss of gastric glands, either antral or corporal. They have found that the prevalence of this type of gastritis is increased in subjects at high stomach cancer risk. Others have made a similar observation (Imai et al, 1971; Siurala et al, 1966). Correa (1985) further categorized chronic atrophic gastritis into three types: environmental, autoimmune, and hypersecretory. Environmental chronic gastritis, which starts as multiple small foci in the corpus-antrum junction, is most closely linked to stomach cancer. Autoimmune chronic gastritis is synonymous with proximal atrophic gastritis, which involves mainly the corpus of the stomach (Strickland and Mackey, 1973). It is found in association with pernicious anemia, which has been identified with an increase in gastric cancer risk in the past (Brinton et al, 1989; Shearman et al, 1966; Zamcheck et al, 1955; Mosbech and Videback, 1950). The hypersecretory type of chronic gastritis is associated with duodenal or antral ulcers. Histologically, it is characterized by regenerating epithelium and lymphocytic infiltration. This type of gastritis is not associated with gastric cancer.

Intestinal Metaplasia

Intestinal metaplasia, which may be defined as the replacement of antral and oxyntic gastric mucosa by glands which have the histological, histochemical, and physiological characteristics of the small intestine (Stemmermann et al, 1978), has been strongly associated with stomach cancer. In pathological-epidemiological studies, the prevalence of intestinal metaplasia was correlated more with intestinal cancer than with diffuse stomach cancer (Correa et al, 1970, 1973). Intestinal metaplasia and the intestinal type of stomach cancer are more commonly found in the pyloric antrum, with intestinal metaplasia usually first appearing at the junction of the corpus and the pyloric antrum along or adjacent to the lesser curvature (Stemmermann et al, 1978). Minute carcinomas of the intestinal type have arisen in areas surrounded by intestinal metaplasia (Matsukura et al, 1980).

Two types of intestinalized gastric mucosa, complete and incomplete, have been identified, based on differences in enzyme production, mucus content, and presence of Paneth cells (Matsukura et al, 1980). It has been suggested that intestinal gastric cancer may arise from the incomplete type of intestinal metaplasia, but this is still not certain (Stemmermann, 1988).

ENVIRONMENTAL FACTORS

Cigarette Smoking

Table 34–2 presents a list of environmental factors that have been studied in relation to stomach cancer. Although cigarette smoking has been related to several different cancers, its association with stomach cancer is equivocal. Several studies have found that smokers have an increased gastric cancer risk, especially with heavy usage (Risch et al, 1985; Hu et al, 1988; You et al, 1988; McLaughlin et al, 1990; Wu-Williams et al, 1990). Other investigators have also found a positive association with cigarette smoking, but a dose-response effect was not observed or reported (Hammond, 1966; Haenszel et al, 1972; Correa et al, 1985; Nomura et al, 1990; Kato et al, 1992; Hoshiyama and Sasaba, 1992). Furthermore, there was no relation between cigarette smoking and stomach cancer in other studies (Wynder et al, 1963; Jedrychowski et al, 1986; La Vecchia et al, 1987; Buiatti et al, 1989). Because mainstream and sidestream tobacco smoke are known to contain *N*-nitroso compounds (Hoffman and Hecht, 1985), which are suspected carcinogens for gastric cancer (Mirvish, 1983), and because it has been reported that smokers who routinely swallowed cigarette smoke had a heightened risk (Saha, 1991), more work is needed to clarify this issue.

Alcohol

The data supporting an association of alcoholic beverages with stomach cancer are weak. Several studies have observed that alcohol drinkers have a greater risk for stomach cancer (Segi et al, 1957; Haenszel et al, 1972; Correa et al, 1985; Jedrychowski et al, 1986; Hu et al, 1988; Kato et al, 1992), but others have not supported this observation (Wynder et al, 1963; Hirayama, 1971; Pollack et al, 1984; Trichopoulos et al, 1985; La Vecchia et al, 1987; You et al, 1988; Nomura et al, 1990). The studies that found an association implicated beer (Haenszel et al, 1972), hard liquor (Correa et al, 1985), sake (Japanese rice wine) (Segi et al, 1957), or the combined sources of alcohol (Jedrychowski et al, 1986; Hu et al, 1988), but a dose-response was either not found or reported. Overall, the results are not convincing that alcohol intake is related to stomach cancer risk.

TABLE 34–2. *Environmental Factors Studied in Relation to Stomach Cancer*

Cigarette smoking
Alcohol
Radiation
Nitrate and related compounds
Salted foods
Carbohydrates
Fruits and vegetables
Serum markers

Radiation

Ionizing radiation increases the risk for gastric cancer. Among the atomic bomb survivors in Japan, Nakamura (1977) observed that in Hiroshima the standardized mortality ratio for stomach cancer rose steadily with increasing dosage up to 200 rad and over. In Nagasaki, the same pattern was not found, but in the very high dose range (500 rad and over) 10 deaths were observed while 2.6 deaths were expected. Court Brown and Doll (1965) reported that patients treated by x-ray for ankylosing spondylitis had an increased mortality from stomach cancer, with 28 deaths observed and 16 expected. It has further been shown that persons exposed to radiation at younger ages tend to have a greater risk for stomach cancer than those exposed at later ages (Kohn and Fry, 1984).

Nitrate and Related Compounds

A series of studies have linked the intake of nitrates and related compounds to stomach cancer. Excellent reviews of this subject have been written by Mirvish (1983) and Forman (1987). Nitrate is readily available in the human diet and is found in drinking water, green vegetables, cured meats, some cheeses, and other foods. When combined with oral bacteria, nitrate is reduced to nitrite. The reduction of salivary nitrate provides 80% of the nitrite entering the stomach, while 20% comes from dietary nitrite sources (Mirvish, 1986) such as cured meats, cereals, baked goods, and vegetables. Nitrite can combine with secondary amines and alkylamides from many types of fish, pork-based products, tea, cereals, beer, and certain spices to form *N*-nitroso compounds. This nitrosation reaction is catalyzed by thiocyanate from the saliva or takes place in the presence of bacteria at a neutral pH in the stomach. *N*-nitroso compounds, which can be found in smoked or salt-dried fish, bacon, sausages, other cured meats, beer, pickled vegetables, and mushrooms, are potent carcinogens, as shown in many experiments with laboratory animals (Bogovski and Bogovski, 1981). These compounds have produced tumors at a number of different sites in 39 different animal species. Concern about nitrite and related compounds has led to a reduction in their concentrations in the processing of certain foods (Engel, 1977).

In a number of studies, subjects at high risk for gastric cancer have had high concentrations of nitrite or *N*-nitroso compounds in their gastric juice. This has been found in pernicious anemia patients (Ruddell et al, 1978), Billroth II gastrectomy patients (Schlag et al, 1980), and other patients with pernicious anemia, gastrectomy, or gastric cancer (Reed et al, 1981). The increased concentrations were linked to the presence of high levels of nitrate-reducing bacteria and elevated pH levels in the gastric juice. The presence of gastric juice with an alkaline pH is associated with the presence of chronic atrophic gastritis (Tannenbaum et al, 1981; Reed et al, 1981), which is considered a precursor lesion for stomach cancer. These results indirectly support a role for *N*-nitroso compounds in gastric carcinogenesis.

A number of case-control studies on diet and gastric cancer have been done and are summarized in Table 34–3. Some of these studies have observed a positive association with consumption of foods likely to contain preformed *N*-nitroso compounds (Kawabata et al, 1984; Ishidate et al, 1972). These include bacon (Higginson, 1966), salty foods (Hirayama, 1971; Graham et al, 1990; Nazario et al, 1993), dried salted fish and pickled vegetables (Haenszel et al, 1972; Tajima and Tominaga, 1985), salted fish (Bjelke, 1974; Buiatti et al, 1989), smoked/pickled foods (Ramon et al, 1993), home-cured meats (Correa et al, 1985), nitrite-rich foods (Risch et al, 1985; Buiatti et al, 1990), ham (La Vecchia et al, 1987), sour pancakes (You et al, 1988), and processed meats (Boeing et al, 1991). Other studies have not supported these findings (Graham et al, 1967; Modan et al, 1974; Trichopoulos et al, 1985; Stehr et al, 1985; Kono et al, 1988; Hoshiyama and Sasaba, 1992; Hansson et al, 1993), but variations in the dietary patterns of population groups may have contributed to the different results.

A case has been made that nitrosamides, which are volatile *N*-nitroso compounds, may be involved in the etiology of gastric cancer (Mirvish, 1983). They are potent carcinogens in laboratory animals and could be produced in the stomach from nitrite and amides. Because of their instability, nitrosamides are difficult to detect in the stomach. Furthermore, it is unlikely that they need enzyme activation, so they are less susceptible to inhibitors of carcinogenesis.

Salted Foods

Evidence has accumulated that salt or salted foods contribute to gastric cancer risk. There has been a decrease in salt intake in the United States since the early 1900s (Hartman, 1983), which has accompanied the decrease in stomach cancer mortality rates. In Japan, urinary salt excretion and the consumption of salted fish and vegetables have been correlated with stomach cancer rates in different regions (Tsugane et al, 1991; Sato et al, 1959). In experimental studies, Mirvish (1983) has noted that a high salt concentration can injure the gastric mucosa and also can be a promoting factor for gastric cancer. Furthermore, salt may also facilitate gastric absorption of known carcinogens in laboratory animals.

Supporting but less convincing evidence has been gathered from dietary case-control studies. Investigators in Japan (Hirayama, 1971; Tajima and Tominaga, 1985), Norway (Bjelke, 1974), China (Hu et al, 1988), Italy (La Vecchia et al, 1987; Buiatti et al, 1989), Spain (Ramon et al, 1993), Puerto Rico (Nazario et al, 1993), and the United States (Haenszel et al, 1972; Correa et al, 1985; Graham et al, 1990) have found that salted foods or cured meats increase the risk for stomach cancer. Other dietary studies, as shown in Table 34–3, have not reported similar results. It is possible that the difficulties in measuring the intake of salt or salted foods in the diet can limit the effectiveness of interview studies (Negri et al, 1990). Nonetheless, there is still a high index of suspicion that salted foods with their accompanying products are related to stomach cancer risk. Furthermore, salted foods may contain *N*-nitroso compounds, which have been implicated as causative agents for gastric cancer (Kawabata et al, 1984).

The availability of refrigeration since 1900 has lessened the need to preserve foods by various means such as salting, smoking, or pickling (Howson et al, 1986). Home refrigeration has also promoted the availability and consumption of fruits and vegetables, as well as other foods. It is possible that the use of refrigeration to keep foods fresh has contributed to the reduction of stomach cancer, as has been observed recently by several investigators (Boeing et al, 1991; Graham et al, 1990; Buiatti et al, 1989; Risch et al, 1985; Hansson et al, 1993).

Carbohydrates

Along with the decline of stomach cancer, there has been a 50% reduction in starch consumption in the United States from 1889 to 1974 (Hartman, 1983). Earlier case-control studies reported that a high starch intake was associated with an increased risk of stomach cancer (Graham et al, 1967; Modan et al 1974; Bjelke, 1974). These studies were conducted in New York, Israel, Minnesota, and Norway, as shown in Table 34–3. Subsequent investigations in Canada (Risch et al, 1985), Greece (Trichopoulos et al, 1985),Italy (La Vecchia et al, 1987), China (Hu et al, 1988), and Belgium (Tuyns

TABLE 34–3. *Dietary Findings from Case-Control Studies of Stomach Cancer*

Authors and Year	*Location*	*Positive Association*	*Inverse Association*
Higginson, 1966	Kansas, United States	Cooked fat Animal fat Fried foods Bacon	Fruits Dairy products
Graham et al, 1967	New York, United States	Cabbage Potatoes	Lettuce
Hirayama, 1971	Japan	Salty foods	Milk, meat Green and yellow vegetables
Haenszel et al, 1972	Hawaii, United States	Dried/salted fish Pickled vegetables	Many vegetables
Modan et al, 1974	Israel	Starchy foods	Squash Eggplant
Bjelke, 1974	Norway	Cooked cereals Salted fish	Many vegetables Many fruits
	Minnesota, United States	Cooked cereals Smoked fish Canned fruits	Lettuce Tomatoes
Haenszel et al, 1976	Japan	—	Celery, lettuce Fruits
Correa et al, 1985	Louisiana, United States	Smoked foods Home-cured meats	Fruits Vitamin C
Risch et al, 1985	Canada	Nitrite foods Chocolate Carbohydrates	Citrus fruits Dietary fiber
Trichopoulos et al, 1985	Greece	Pasta, beans Nuts	Oranges, lemons Raw vegetables Brown bread
Tajima and Tominaga, 1985	Japan	Dried/salted fish Pickled vegetables	—
Jedrychowski et al, 1986	Poland	Protein foods	Fruits, salads Vegetables
La Vecchia et al, 1987	Italy	Pasta, rice Ham Corn porridge	Green vegetables Fresh fruits Citrus fruits
Hu et al, 1988	China	Potatoes Salted/fermented soya paste	Vegetables
Stehr et al, 1988	Pennsylvania, United States	—	Vitamin A foods
You et al, 1988	China	Sour pancakes	Fresh fruits Fresh vegetables Carotene Vitamin C
Kono et al, 1988	Japan	—	Fruits
Buiatti et al, 1989	Italy	Traditional soups Meats Salted/dried fish	Raw vegetables Fresh fruits Citrus fruits Spices, garlic
You et al, 1989	China	—	Garlic, onions Allium vegetables
Buiatti et al, 1990	Italy	Nitrites Protein	Ascorbic acid Beta-carotene Alpha-tocopherol Vegetable fat
Graham et al, 1990	New York, United States	Sodium Fat Retinol	Carotene Raw vegetables
Chyou et al, 1990	Hawaii, United States	—	Vegetables Fruits
Boeing et al, 1991	Germany	Smoked meat Processed meat	Vitamin C Raw vegetables Citrus fruits

(continued)

TABLE 34–3. *Dietary Findings from Case-Control Studies of Stomach Cancer (Continued)*

Authors and Year	*Location*	*Positive Association*	*Inverse Association*
Tuyns et al, 1992	Belgium	Flour products	Many vegetables Fresh fruits
Hoshiyama and Sasaba, 1992	Japan	—	Fresh vegetables
Ramon et al, 1992	Spain	Smoked/pickled foods Salt	Citrus fruits Green vegetables
Nazario et al, 1993	Puerto Rico	Salted foods	—
Hansson et al, 1993	Sweden	—	Fruits Vegetables
Lopez-Carrillo et al, 1994	Mexico	Chili pepper	—
Gonzalez et al, 1994	Spain	Exogenous nitrosamines	Vitamin C Fiber Folate Nitrate

et al, 1992) have made similar observations. The starchy food categories in these studies have included potatoes, bread, rice, pasta, and carbohydrates in general.

If a high carbohydrate diet contributes to the occurrence of stomach cancer, several mechanisms have been proposed (Mirvish, 1983). Physical irritation of the gastric mucosa may result from the consumption of rough, whole-grain cereals. A high carbohydrate/low protein diet could lead to a reduction of gastric mucus production, thus facilitating carcinogen absorption. Lastly, a high carbohydrate/low protein diet might decrease the availability of compounds that remove nitrite and inhibit nitrosation in the gastric juice. Low socioeconomic groups, which have a high stomach cancer risk, historically consume more carbohydrates, but it is still uncertain whether or not starchy foods are involved in promoting stomach cancer.

Fruits and Vegetables

The most consistent dietary finding in studies of stomach cancer has been the inverse association with intake of fresh fruits and vegetables (Table 34–3). This consistency is remarkable in view of the limited precision of past questionnaire instruments used in the collection of dietary data. It is difficult to collect data representative of a person's early and typical dietary experience, particularly in view of the long incubation period suspected for stomach cancer. Consequently, the similar results of many studies are noteworthy.

Some of the fruits and vegetables listed in Table 34–3 are rich in vitamin C or ascorbic acid. They include oranges, lemons, citrus fruits, tomatoes, lettuce, and green vegetables. Vitamin C can prevent the formation of *N*-nitroso compounds in vitro or in vivo (Mirvish et al, 1972; Rainieri and Weisburger, 1975). On this basis, these sources of vitamin C may be helpful against gastric cancer. Some of these vegetables are also sources of nitrate, but the potential harmful effects of nitrate may be offset by the antinitrosating properties of the vegetables (Mirvish, 1983).

Beta-carotene, or provitamin A, may also be protective against stomach cancer. It is a potent singlet oxygen scavenger and has antioxidant properties (Burton and Ingold, 1984). Beta-carotene can also inhibit carcinogenesis in laboratory animals (Matthews-Roth, 1983; Alam et al, 1984). Recent dietary studies (You et al, 1988; Stehr et al, 1985; Buiatti et al, 1990) gave results that suggest that vitamin A foods may protect against stomach cancer.

Alpha-tocopherol, or vitamin E, is another vitamin that has been inversely associated with gastric cancer (Buiatti et al, 1990). More studies are needed to verify this association. Vitamin E is widely distributed in foods (viz., vegetable oils, whole grain cereals, wheat germ, and margarines), but is difficult to quantify (Bertram et al, 1987). It has antioxidant properties (Bieri et al, 1983) and can inhibit endogenous nitrosation reactions (Bartsch et al, 1983).

In addition to vitamins, allium vegetables, including garlic and onions, may also be protective against gastric cancer (Buiatti et al, 1989; You et al, 1989). Allium vegetables have been used for centuries in folk medicine and as a flavor enhancer in foods. Allium compounds have anticarcinogenic properties in laboratory animals (Belman, 1983; Niukian et al, 1987), but little information is available on their effects in humans.

Serum Markers

It would be useful if serum or other biochemical markers could be found to identify subjects at increased risk for developing gastric cancer. In a prospective study of survivors at Hiroshima, subjects with a low serum pepsin level or an abnormal Diagnex Blue test indicating achlorhydria had a greater risk for stomach cancer (Pastore et al, 1972). A separate study was then done measuring serum pepsinogen I, which is a precursor of pepsin (Samloff and Liebman, 1973), a proteolytic enzyme. It was observed that persons with low levels had an increased risk for the intestinal type of stomach cancer (Nomura et al, 1980). However, these patients usually had an advanced stage of cancer when diagnosed. Consequently, a low serum pepsinogen I level does not appear to be a useful marker for identifying subjects with early gastric cancer.

Haenszel et al (1985) found that patients with gastric dysplasia had low levels of serum beta-carotene and vitamin E. Zhang et al (1994) also reported that subjects with intestinal metaplasia had low levels of serum beta-carotene and vitamin C. However, in nested case-control studies using stored prediagnostic serum, there were no significant differences in serum beta-carotene and vitamin E levels between stomach cancer cases and controls (Stahelin et al, 1984; Nomura et al, 1985). Vitamin C could not be adequately measured in the stored serum samples.

Helicobacter pylori are gram-negative spiral bacteria that have only been identified and cultured in the past decade (Warren and Marshall, 1983). They have been strongly associated with antral gastritis (Blaser, 1990) and peptic ulcer disease (Nomura et al, 1994). Because of their association with conditions related to gastric cancer, researchers have suggested that *H. pylori* be studied in populations at high risk for this cancer (Dooley et al, 1989).

Three nested case-control studies were conducted in 1991 (Forman et al, 1991; Parsonnet et al, 1991; Nomura et al, 1991). In these studies stored sera collected years prior to the diagnosis of gastric cancer were tested. They found that subjects with IgG antibody to *H. pylori* had an increased risk or odds ratio for gastric carcinoma which ranged from 2.8 to 6.0. Both the intestinal and diffuse histological types of gastric carcinoma were related to *H. pylori*. Anywhere from 47% to 76% of the controls in these studies were also infected with *H. pylori*. Because it is unlikely that most of these infected subjects will eventually be diagnosed with gastric carcinoma, this suggests that other factors must also play an important role in the pathogenesis of this disease. There was no association between a prior *H. pylori* infection and cancers of the cardia and gastro-esophageal junction (Parsonnet et al, 1991; Nomura et al, 1991).

HOST FACTORS

Studies of the genetic aspects of stomach cancer have used several different approaches: (1) family pedigree reports; (2) twin studies; (3) familial aggregation studies; and (4) blood typing studies. A perceptive review of genetic studies of gastric cancer was published by Graham and Lilienfeld in 1958. In the pedigree approach, investigators have reported the aggregation of gastric cancer over several generations (Maimon and Zinninger, 1953; Woolf and Gardner, 1950) and have suggested that immunogenetic mechanisms may explain familial susceptibility (Creagan and Fraumeni, 1973). Although these pedigree studies are important in proposing a role for genetic predisposition, it should be recognized that such families are selected because of their high frequency of stomach cancer. An assumption is often made that the degree of familial association present in selected families is unusual and more than one would expect in the general population. To show that this assumption is true, the pedigree study should be based on an adequate sample of families in the general population.

The standard approach in twin studies is to separate the pairs into monozygotic or dizygotic twins and to compute the percentage of twins in each group in which both members have the disease. If the percentage is higher for the monozygotic twins, it is believed that a genetic factor is operating. Using this approach, Harvald and Hauge (1956) investigated 1900 out of 9360 twins born in Denmark from 1870 to 1910. They found no evidence of a difference between monozygotic and dizygotic twins in the frequency of stomach cancer in both twins, but only 35 cases of stomach cancer were in the study. Until more extensive studies are done using this design, our knowledge of the contribution of twin studies in gastric cancer is very limited.

Familial aggregation studies typically compare the occurrence of gastric cancer in relatives of a case or proband with the occurrence of the same cancer in relatives of suitable controls. These studies have usually shown that family members of gastric cancer cases have two to three times the risk of developing this cancer compared to the family members of controls (Graham and Lilienfeld, 1958; La Vecchia et al, 1992; Palli et al, 1994). However, these studies do not separate out genetic from environmental factors, because family members tend to share the same environment as well.

Blood type A has been consistently associated with stomach cancer. A number of studies done in Switzerland (Aird et al, 1953), Great Britain (Aird et al, 1953), Denmark (Køster et al, 1955), Australia (Billington, 1956), and the United States (Buckwalter et al, 1957; Hogg and Pack, 1957; Eisenberg et al, 1958) have shown that there is 2% to 8% excess of blood type A among stomach cancer patients compared to the general population. A separate study divided stomach cancer patients into the intestinal and diffuse types and found an association of blood type A with only the diffuse type

(Correa et al, 1973). Forty-nine percent of 164 diffuse cases had type A compared to 39% of 326 intestinal type cases and 38.3% of the general population. These findings suggest there is a genetic factor in blood type A subjects that increases their risk for diffuse stomach cancer.

More recently, researchers have identified a variety of oncogenes found to be activated in stomach cancer. Oncogenes are a class of genes which are capable of inducing neoplastic changes in cells. They include *c-myc*, *c-erbB-2*, *sam*, and *c-erbA*, which have been amplified and overexpressed in gastric cancer (Tsuchiya et al, 1989). Amplification of *c-erbB-2* has been reported for the well-differentiated, tubular type of gastric carcinoma, suggesting a relation between this type of oncogenes and the histological type of cancer (Yokota et al, 1987). However, *c-erbB-2* has also been found in poorly differentiated adenocarcinomas as well (Tsuchiya et al, 1989). Although much work still needs to be done to identify and determine the mechanisms by which genetic defects lead to cancer, the discovery of oncogenes enhances the opportunity to learn more about the genetics of gastric cancer in humans.

EXPERIMENTAL CARCINOGENESIS

The most widely used experimental model for the study of stomach cancer was developed by Sugimura and Fujimura in 1967, when they produced adenocarcinomas in the glandular stomach of rats by adding *N*-methyl-*N'*-nitro-*N*-nitrosoguanidine (MNNG) to the drinking water. Since then, MNNG or related *N*-nitroso compounds have been used repeatedly in laboratory studies to study the pathogenesis of stomach cancer. For example, the short-term administration of MNNG has led to the development of intestinal metaplasia (Matsukura et al, 1978). In a similar fashion, Watanabe (1978) was able to produce intestinal metaplasia in Wistar rats by localized x-irradiation at doses less than necessary for cancer induction. It was suggested that in humans a small dose of carcinogen might cause only intestinal metaplasia, whereas increasing the dose level would result in carcinoma associated with metaplasia.

Dietary treatment in rats with the addition of sodium chloride increased glandular stomach tumors produced by MNNG, suggesting that a high salt concentration can enhance the induction of stomach cancer (Takahashi et al, 1983; Tatematsu et al, 1975). Vitamin C, on the other hand, can inhibit the biological activity of MNNG (Mirvish, 1986) and can block the formation of *N*-nitroso compounds (Mirvish et al, 1972).

MNNG and ENNG (*N*-ethyl-*N'*-nitro-*N*-nitrosoguanidine) have produced adenocarcinomas of the stomach in dogs (Sugimura et al, 1971; Kurihara et al, 1974), as well as in rats. Researchers have also been successful in producing gastric carcinomas in nonhuman primates with ENNG (Ohgaki et al, 1986). Although reported, spontaneous stomach tumors in nonhuman primates have been very rare. This supports the possibility that human gastric carcinomas could be caused by *N*-nitroso compounds.

CONCEPTS OF PATHOGENESIS

The identification of the causes of stomach cancer has proven to be a very challenging task. In 1975, Correa et al proposed a hypothesis for the etiology of gastric cancer of the intestinal type. The hypothesis, which has been subsequently refined (Correa, 1992), postulates that gastric cancer results from a series of changes that appear sequentially in the precancerous process, namely, superficial gastritis, chronic atrophic gastritis, small intestinal metaplasia, colonic metaplasia, and dysplasia. The carcinogenic agent could be *N*-nitroso compounds that are found in the stomach after nitrosation. Normally, these compounds would not harm gastric mucosal cells because of their inability to pass the mucous barrier or because their synthesis would be inhibited by vitamin C and antioxidants. Infection with *H. pylori* leads to active inflammation resulting in chronic diffuse superficial gastritis (Blaser, 1992). High concentrations of salted foods or other gastric irritants or abrasives could lead to further mucosal injury and facilitate the progression to atrophic gastritis. The low intake of vitamins and proteins and the postgastrectomy state could foster the spread of atrophic gastritis and the replacement of gastric glands by intestinal-type epithelium. In this environment, the gastric pH becomes elevated and nitrate-reducing bacteria multiply. This leads to an increase of *N*-nitroso compounds in the stomach. If this process persists over time, metaplasia is followed by mild to severe dysplasia and then carcinoma. This model, as developed by Correa and colleagues and presented here in a simplified manner, provides a useful framework in attempting to identify the causes of stomach cancer.

The leading candidate as a carcinogenic agent continues to be *N*-nitroso compounds, which are potent carcinogens in bioassay studies (Bogovski and Bogovski, 1981). The difficulty arises in proving that their actions lead to gastric cancer. Many people have frequent exposure to nitrate, nitrite, or *N*-nitroso compounds because of their ubiquitous nature. Certain *N*-nitroso compounds, such as nitrosamides, are very volatile and have not been measured in the stomach. As a result, it is difficult to evaluate their role in the etiology of gastric cancer.

Little is known about the pathogenesis of the diffuse histopathological type of stomach cancer. Persons with this disease may have a genetic susceptibility, as suggested by its association with blood type A (Correa et al, 1973). The earlier age of diagnosis with diffuse cancer in comparison to intestinal cancer also supports this impression (Munoz and Steinitz, 1971; Munoz et al, 1968). However, because diffuse gastric cancer has not been associated with distinctive precancerous lesions (Lauren, 1965), it is more difficult to propose an etiological model for this disease.

PREVENTIVE MEASURES

Low socioeconomic status seems to be a common characteristic of stomach cancer cases, but this is an indirect indicator of a shared experience that places subjects at higher risk. Cigarette smokers may be more susceptible, but a clear dose-response effect is lacking. This suggests that cigarette smokers, as a group, may be at an increased risk, possibly due to confounding factors. Exposure to high doses of radiation or a past history of gastrectomy appears to increase the risk for gastric cancer, but relatively few people have these characteristics.

The main focus of the primary prevention of gastric cancer will most likely center on the diet. A nutritious diet with at least 12% of caloric intake from protein to balance the intake from carbohydrates would be advisable (Select Committee on Nutrition and Human Needs, 1977). Studies to date suggest that avoidance or diminished intake of foods altered by salting, pickling, or other means of chemical preservation may be helpful. Also, the decreased use of foods rich in nitrate or related compounds may be a prudent course to follow. The National Academy of Sciences (1981) has recommended that nitrite be eliminated from all cured meats except for certain slow-cured products. Agricultural methods have been recommended to reduce the nitrate content of vegetables (Maynard, 1978). Greater consumption within reasonable limits of fresh vegetables, citrus fruits, and other foods rich in vitamin C and other antioxidants could be helpful in reducing the risk of stomach cancer and possibly other cancers as well. Indeed, there has been about a 400% increase in the consumption of citrus fruits in the United States between 1909 and 1961 (Antar et al, 1964).

Screening and the early detection of stomach cancer have been practiced primarily in Japan, where more deaths have been due to gastric cancer than all other cancers combined (Segi and Kurihara, 1972). With the use of x-ray photofluorography to identify suspicious lesions, followed by gastroscopy, the Japanese have detected more cases with the cancer limited to the submucosa among screenees, compared to patients diagnosed without mass screenings. In one series, 43% of the stomach cancer cases detected by screening techniques had early carcinoma compared to 23% of other patients (Kaneko et al, 1977). The 5-year relative survival rates were 96% for the patients with early carcinoma, so that the overall 5-year relative survival rate among the screenees was 63%, which is very impressive. These data suggest that patients are being saved with mass screening, even though there has not been a well-controlled randomized study to evaluate fully the effectiveness of the mass screening survey in Japan. It has been observed that screening by photofluorography with an image intensifier is equivalent to that of screening with direct radiography and both are superior to that of screening by photofluorography with a mirror camera (Murakami et al, 1990).

It is obvious that screening and early detection would be more cost-effective if such efforts were directed to high-risk groups. The characteristics of persons susceptible to gastric cancer are as follows: (1) male; (2) age 60 or older; (3) low socioeconomic status; (4) a family history of gastric cancer; (5) a history of pernicious anemia, gastric polyp, gastroenterostomy, intestinal metaplasia, chronic atrophic gastritis, or possibly gastric ulcer; and (6) high radiation exposure to the gastric region. Because stomach cancer is not as great a problem in the United States as it is in Japan, the cost-effectiveness of screening and early detection is less apparent.

FUTURE RESEARCH

The significant decline in the incidence of stomach cancer in many countries of the world is very encouraging. It is hoped that the trend will continue, but any possibility of relegating stomach cancer to the category of rare diseases requires a better understanding of its causative factors and the multistage mechanisms involved in gastric carcinogenesis. Only then will primary prevention, early detection and therapeutic measures be sufficiently effective in combatting this disease.

To improve our understanding of the nature of stomach cancer, the following should be pursued:

1. The continued search for biochemical markers in serum or other biological material to help identify subjects at high or low risk for stomach cancer. Attempts have been made to identify markers (Pastore et al, 1972; Stahelin et al, 1984; Nomura et al, 1985), such as the *H. pylori* IgG antibody (Forman et al, 1991; Parsonnet et al, 1991; Nomura et al, 1991), but more are needed

to improve our understanding of the pathogenesis of stomach cancer.

2. Improvement in the methods of reliably measuring the amounts and types of *N*-nitroso compounds in the gastric juice and other specimens (Bartsch and O'Neill, 1988). Improved biochemical methods should enhance our knowledge of relationship between *N*-nitroso compounds and gastric cancer.

3. Studies with improved dietary methodologies. Reasonably comprehensive dietary histories should be taken to assess further the association of nitrate-containing foods, salted foods, carbohydrates, and vitamins A, C, and E with stomach cancer. If possible, the studies should separate intestinal from diffuse types of stomach cancer, which has been done infrequently in past diet studies (Haenszel et al, 1976, 1972). With improved and more precise dietary information, well-designed prospective studies are also needed.

4. Further testing of suspected food items or their extracts for the presence of mutagenic, carcinogenic, or protective properties. Fava beans, which are commonly consumed in high-risk Colombian populations, were found to have mutagenic properties (Montes et al, 1984). Nitrosated fava beans appear to contain *N*-nitroso indoles (Yang et al, 1984), as do Chinese cabbage and soy sauce (Wakabayashi et al, 1987), which are frequently consumed in Japan. Similar studies should be done to identify potential carcinogenic agents in other suspected high-risk foods.

5. More studies regarding the epidemiology and pathogenesis of diffuse stomach cancer. A useful model has been proposed for the etiology of intestinal gastric cancer (Correa et al, 1975), but diffuse cancer is also a major problem and is more fatal than intestinal cancer (Stemmermann and Brown, 1974).

6. The identification of genetic markers, which may be associated with stomach cancer by histological type. For example, are HL-A or other immunogenetic markers related to diffuse or intestinal stomach cancer? Additional studies are required to confirm the association of blood type A with diffuse stomach cancer, as noted by Correa et al (1973). New studies are needed to determine the association of oncogenes and tumor suppressor genes with stomach cancer.

7. Studies have indicated that intestinal metaplasia is associated more with intestinal than diffuse cancer (Lauren, 1965; Munoz and Steinitz, 1971; Correa et al, 1973). More information is needed about factors responsible for the progression of metaplasia to dysplasia and cancer.

8. Studies which reflect the collaborative efforts of pathologists, epidemiologists, and biochemists to delineate further the relationship between nitrates, *N*-nitroso compounds and gastric cancer. Correa and coworkers (1975, 1976, 1985) have been very effective with their multidisciplinary team approach, and it should be pursued further.

REFERENCES

AIRD I, BENTALL HH, FRASER ROBERTS JA. 1953. A relationship between cancer of stomach and the ABO blood groups. Br Med J 1:799–801.

ALAM BS, ALAM SQ, WEIR JC JR, GIBSON WA. 1984. Chemopreventive effects of beta-carotene and 13-cis-retinoic acid on salivary bland tumors. Nutr Cancer 6:4–12.

AMERICAN CANCER SOCIETY. 1995. Cancer Facts and Figures—1995. Atlanta, pp. 4, 6.

AMES RG. 1983. Gastric cancer and coal mine dust exposure: A case-control study. Cancer 52:1346–1350.

ANTAR MA, OHISON MA, HODGES RE. 1964. Changes in retail market food supplies in the United States in the last seventy years in relation to the incidence of coronary heart disease, with special reference to dietary carbohydrates and essential fatty acids. Am J Clin Nutr 14:169–178.

BARTSCH H, OHSHIMA H, MUNOZ N, CRESPI N, LU SH. 1983. Measurement of endogenous nitrosation in humans: Potential application of a new method and initial results. *In* Harris CC, Autrup HN (eds): Human Carcinogenesis New York, Academic Press, pp. 833–856.

BARTSCH H, O'NEILL IK. 1988. Ninth International Meeting on N-nitroso compounds: Exposures, mechanisms, and relevance to human cancer. Cancer Res 48:4711–4714.

BELMAN S. 1983. Onion and garlic oils inhibit tumor promotion. Carcinogenesis 4:1063–1065.

BERG J. 1958. Histological aspects of the relation between gastric adenomatous polyps and gastric cancer. Cancer 11:1149–1155.

BERTRAM JS, KOLONEAL LN, MEYSKENS FL JR. 1987. Rationale and strategies for chemoprevention of cancer in humans. CancerRes 47:3012–3031.

BIERI JG, CORASH L, HUBBARD VS. 1983. Medical uses of vitamin E. N Engl J Med 308:1063–1071.

BILLINGTON BP. 1956. Gastric cancer. Relationships between ABO blood groups, site, and epidemiology. Lancet 2:859–862.

BJELKE E. 1974. Epidemiologic studies of cancer of the stomach, colon, and rectum; with special emphasis on the role of diet. Scand J Gastroenterol 9:Suppl 31:42–53.

BLASER MJ. 1990. Helicobacter pylori and the pathogenesis of gastroduodenal inflammation. J Infect Dis 161:626–633.

BLASER MJ. 1992. Hypothesis of the pathogenesis and natural history of *Helicobacter pylori*-induced inflammation. Gastroenterology 102:720–272.

BOEING H, FRENTZEL-BEYME R, BERGER M, et al. 1991. Case-control study on stomach cancer in Germany. Int J Cancer 47:858–864.

BOGOVSKI P, BOGOVSKI S. 1981. Animal species in which N-nitroso compounds induce cancer. Int J Cancer 27:471–474.

BRINTON LA, GRIDLEY G, HRUBEC Z, HOOVER R, FRAUMENI JF JR. 1989. Cancer risk following pernicious anaemia. Br J Cancer 59:810–813.

BUCKWALTER JA, WOHLWEND CB, COLTER DC, et al. 1957. The association of the ABO blood groups to gastric carcinoma. Surg Gynecol Obstet 104:176–179.

BUIATTI E, PALLI D, DECARLI A, et al. 1989. A case-control study of gastric cancer and diet in Italy. Int J Cancer 44:611–616.

BUIATTI E, PALLI D, DECARLI A, et al. 1990. A case-control study of gastric cancer and diet in Italy. II. Association with nutrients. Int J Cancer 45:896–901.

BURTON GW, UNGOLD KU. 1984. B-carotene: An unusual type of lipid antioxidant. Science 224:569–573.

CAYGILL CPJ, HILL MJ, KIRKHAM JS, NORTHFIELD TC. 1986. Mortality from gastric cancer following gastric surgery for peptic ulcer. Lancet 1:929–931.

CHYOU P-H, NOMURA AMY, HANKIN JH, STEMMERMANN GN. 1990. A case-cohort study of diet and stomach cancer. Cancer Res 50:7501–7504.

CORREA P. 1985. Clinical implications of recent developments in gastric cancer pathology and epidemiology. Semin Oncol 12:2–10.

CORREA P. 1992. Human gastric carcinogenesis. A multistep and multifactorial process—first American Cancer Society award lecture on cancer epidemiology and prevention. Cancer Res 52:6735–6740.

CORREA P, CUELLO C, DUQUE E. 1970. Carcinoma and intestinal metaplasia of the stomach in Colombian migrants. J Natl Cancer Inst 44:297–306.

CORREA P, CUELLO C, DUQUE E, et al. 1976. Gastric cancer in Colombia. III. Natural history of precursor lesions. J Natl Cancer Inst 57:1027–1035.

CORREA P, FONTHAM E, PICKLE LW, CHEN V, LIN Y, HAENSZEL W. 1985. Dietary determinants of gastric cancer in south Louisiana inhabitants. J Natl Cancer Inst 75:645–654.

CORREA P, HAENSZEL W, CUELLO W, et al. 1975. A model for gastric cancer epidemiology. Lancet 2:58–59.

CORREA P, SASANO N, STEMMERMANN GN, et al. 1973. Pathology of gastric carcinoma in Japanese populations: Comparisons between Miyagi Prefecture, Japan, and Hawaii. J Natl Cancer Inst 51:1449–1459.

COURT BROWN WM, DOLL R. 1965. Mortality from cancer and other causes after radiotherapy for ankylosing spondylitis. Br Med J 2:1327–1332.

CREAGAN ET, FRAUMENI JF JR. 1973. Familial gastric cancer and immunologic abnormalities. Cancer 32:1325–1331.

CREAGAN ET, HOOVER RN, FRAUMENI JF JR. 1974. Mortality from stomach cancer in coal mining regions. Arch Environ Health 28:28–30.

DAVIES JM. 1980. Stomach cancer mortality in worksop and other Nottinghamshire mining towns. Br J Cancer 41:438–445.

DOMELLOF L, ERICKSON S, JANUNGER KG. 1977. Carcinoma and possible precancerous changes of the gastric stump after Billroth II resection. Gastroenterology 73:462–468.

DOOLEY CP, COHEN H, FITZGIBBONS PL, et al. 1989. Prevalence of helicobacter pylori infection and histologic gastritis in asymptomatic persons. N Engl J Med 321:1562–1566.

EBERLEIN TJ, LORENZO FV, WEBSTER MW. 1978. Gastric carcinoma following operation for peptic ulcer disease. Ann Surg 187:251–256.

EISENBERG H, GREENBERG RA, YESNER R. 1958. ABO blood group and gastric cancer. J Chronic Dis 8:342–348.

EISENBERG H, WOODWARD ER. 1963. Gastric cancer: A midcentury look. Arch Surg 87:810–824.

ENGEL RE. 1977. Nitrites, nitrosamines, and meat. J Am Vet Med Assoc 171:1157–1160.

ENTERLINE P, DECOUFLE P, HENDERSON V. 1972. Mortality in relation to occupational exposure in the asbestos industry. J Occup Med 14:897–903.

FISHER SG, DAVIS F, NELSON R, WEBER L, GOLDBERG J, HAENSZEL W. 1993. A cohort study of stomach cancer risk in men after gastric surgery for benign disease. J Natl Cancer Inst 85:1303–1310.

FLOOD CA. 1961. Precancerous disease of the gastrointestinal tract. Am J Dig Dis 6:555–569.

FORMAN D. 1987. Dietary exposure to *N*-nitroso compounds and the risk of human cancer. Cancer Surv 6:719–738.

FORMAN D, NEWELL DG, FULLERTON F, et al. 1991. Association between infection with Helicobacter pylori and risk of gastric cancer: Evidence from a prospective investigation. Br Med J 302:1302–1305.

GONZALEZ CA, RIBOLI E, BADOSA J, et al. 1994. Nutritional factors and gastric cancer in Spain. Am J Epidemiol 139:466–473.

GRAHAM S, HAUGHEY B, MARSHALL J, et al. 1990. Diet in the epidemiology of gastric cancer. Nutr Cancer 13:19–34.

GRAHAM S, LILIENFELD AM. 1958. Genetic studies of gastric cancer in humans: An appraisal. Cancer 11:945–958.

GRAHAM S, LILIENFELD AM, TIDINGS JE. 1967. Dietary and purgation factors in the epidemiology of gastric cancer. Cancer 20:2224–2234.

GREGORIO DI, FLANNERY JT, HANSEN H. 1992. Stomach cancer patterns in European immigrants to Connecticut, United States. Cancer Causes Control 3:215–221.

HAENSZEL W. 1961. Cancer mortality among the foreign born in the United States. J Natl Cancer Inst 26:37–132.

HAENSZEL W. 1958. Variation in incidence of and mortality from stomach cancer, with particular reference to the UnitedStates. J Natl Cancer Inst 21:213–262.

HAENSZEL W, CORREA P, LOPEZ A, et al. 1985. Serum micronutrient levels in relation to gastric pathology. Int J Cancer 36:43–48.

HAENSZEL W, KURIHARA M, LOCKE FB, et al. 1976. Stomach cancer in Japan. J Natl Cancer Inst 56:265–278.

HAENSZEL W, KURIHARA M, SEGI M, et al. 1972. Stomach cancer among Japanese in Hawaii. J Natl Cancer Inst 49:969–988.

HAMMOND EC. 1966. Smoking in relation to the death rates of 1 million men and women. *In* Haenszel W (ed): Epidemiological Approaches to the Study of Cancer and Other Chronic Diseases. National Cancer Institute Monograph, No. 19, Bethesda, MD, U.S. Public Health Service, pp. 127–204.

HANSSON L-E, NYREN O, BERGSTROM R, et al. 1993. Diet and risk of gastric cancer. A population-based case-control study in Sweden. Int J Cancer 55:181–189.

HARTMAN PE. 1983. Putative mutagens and carcinogens in foods. I. Nitrate/nitrite ingestion and gastric cancer mortality. Environ Mutagen 5:111–121.

HARVALD B, HAUGE M. 1956. Catamnestic investigation of Danish twins; Preliminary Report. Dan Med Bull 3:150–158.

HAUSER G. 1926. *In* Henke F, Lubarsch O: Handb. d. spez. path. Anat. u. Histol. Vol. IV. Berlin, Julius Springer, p. 497.

HIGGINSON J. 1966. Etiological factors in gastrointestinal cancer in man. J Natl Cancer Inst 37:527–545.

HIRAYAMA T. 1971. Epidemiology of stomach cancer. Gann 11:3–19.

HIROHATA T. 1968. Mortality from gastric cancer and other causes after medical or surgical treatment for gastric ulcer. J Natl Cancer Inst 41:895–908.

HOFFMANN D, HECHT SS. 1985. Nicotine-derived N-nitrosamines and tobacco-related cancer: Current status and future directions. Cancer Res 45:935–944.

HOGG L, PACK GT. 1957. The controversial relationship between blood group A and gastric cancer. Gastroenterology 32:797–806.

HOOVER R, MASON TJ, MCKAY FW, et al. 1975. Cancer by country: New resource for etiologic clues. Science 189:1005–1007.

HOSHIYAMA Y, SASABA T. 1992. A case-control study of stomach cancer and its relation to diet, cigarettes, and alcohol consumption in Saitama Prefecture, Japan. Cancer Causes Control 3:441–448.

HOWSON CP, HIYAMA T, WYNDER EL. 1986. The decline in gastric cancer: Epidemiology of an unplanned triumph. Epidemiol Rev 8:1–27.

HU J, ZHANG S, JIA E, et al. 1988. Diet and cancer of the stomach: A case-control study in China. Int J Cancer 41:331–335.

IHRE BJ, BARR H, HAVERMARK G. 1964. Ulcer-cancer of the stomach. A follow-up of 473 cases of gastric ulcer. Gastroenterologica 102:78–91.

IMAI T, KUBO T, WATANABE H. 1971. Chronic gastritis in Japanese with reference to high incidence of gastric carcinoma. J Natl Cancer Inst 47:179–195.

ISHIDATE M, TANIMURA A, ITO Y, et al. 1972. Secondary amines, nitrites and nitrosamines in Japanese foods. *In* Topics in Chemical Carcinogenesis—Proceedings of the 2nd International Symposium of the Princess Takamatsu CancerResearch Fund. Baltimore, University Park Press, pp. 313–322.

JARVI O, LAUREN P. 1951. On the role of heterotopias of the intestinal epithelium in the pathogenesis of gastric cancer. Acta Pathol Microbiol Scand 29:26–44.

JEDRYCHOWSKI W, BOEING H, WAHRENDORF J, POPIELA T, TOBIASZ-ADAMCZYK B, KULIG J. 1993. Vodka consumption, tobacco smoking and risk of gastric cancer in Poland. Int J Epidemiol 22:606–613.

JEDRYCHOWSKI W, WAHRENDORF J, POPIELA T, RACHTAN J. 1986. A case-control study of dietary factors and stomach cancer risk in Poland. Int J Cancer 37:837–842.

JONES CT, WILLIAMS JA. 1963. The Effects of Gastric Operations on the Gastric Mucosa in Partial Gastrectomy. London, Butterworth and Company, pp. 132.

KANEKO E, NAKAMURA T, UMEDA N, et al. 1977. Outcome of gastric carcinoma detected by gastric mass survey in Japan. Gut 18:626–630.

KATO I, TOMINAGA S, MATSUMOTO K. 1992. A prospective study of stomach cancer among a rural Japanese population: a 6-year survey. Jpn J Cancer Res 83:568–575.

KAWABATA T, MATSUI M, ISHIBASHI T, HAMANO M. 1984. Analysis and occurrence of total N-nitroso compounds in the Japanese diet. *In* O'Neill JK, von Borstel RC, Miller CT, Long J, Bartsch H (eds): N-Nitroso Compounds: Occurrence, Biological Effects, and Relevance to Human Cancer. Lyon, International Agency for Research on Cancer, pp. 25–31.

KOBAYASHI S, PROLLA JC, KIRSNER JB. 1970. Late gastric carcinoma developing after surgery for benign conditions. Am J Dig Dis 15:905–912.

KOHN HI, FRY RJM. 1984. Radiation carcinogenesis. N Engl J Med 310:504–509.

KONO S, IKEDA M, TOKUDOME S, KURATSUNE M. 1988. A case-control study of gastric cancer and diet in Northern Kyushu, Japan. Jpn J Cancer Res (Gann) 79:1067–1074.

KØSTER KH, SINDRUP E, SEELE V. 1955. ABO blood groups and gastric acidity. Lancet 2:52–55.

KRAUS AS, LEVIN ML, GERHARDT PR. 1957. A study of occupational associations with gastric cancer. Am J Public Health 47:961–970.

KURIHARA M, AOKI K, TOMINAGA S (EDS). 1984. Cancer Mortality Statistics in the World. Nagoya, University of Nagoya Press, pp. 8–9.

KURIHARA M, SHIRAKABE H, MURAKAMI T, et al. 1974. A new method for producing adenocarcinomas in the stomach of dogs with *N*-ethyl-*N'*-nitro-*N*-nitrosoguanidine. Gann 65:163–177.

LAUREN P. 1965. The two histological main types of gastric carcinoma. Diffuse and so-called intestinal-type. Acta Pathol Microbiol Scand 64:31–49.

LA VECCHIA C, NEGRI E, DECARLI A, D'AVANZO B, FRANCESCHI S. 1987. A case-control study of diet and gastric cancer in northernItaly. Int J Cancer 40:484–489.

LA VECCHIA C, NEGRI E, FRANCESCHI S, GENTILE A. 1992. Family history and the risk of stomach and colorectal cancer. Cancer 70:50–55.

LAWRENCE JC. 1936. Gastrointestinal polyps: A statistical study of malignancy incidence. Am J Surg 31:499–500.

LIAVAAG K. 1962. Cancer development in gastric stump after partial gastrectomy for peptic ulcer. Ann Surg 155:103–106.

LOPEZ-CARRILLO L, AVILA MH, DUBROW R. 1994. Chili pepper consumption and gastric cancer in Mexico: A case-control study. Am J Epidemiol 139:263–271.

LUNDEGARDH G, ADAMI H-O, HELMICK C, ZACK M, MEIRIK O. 1988. Stomach cancer after partial gastrectomy for benign ulcer disease. N Engl J Med 319:195–200.

MAIMON SN, ZINNINGER MM. 1953. Familial gastric cancer. Gastroenterology 25:139–152.

MAJIMA S, TAKAHASHI T, YOSHIDA K, et al. 1967. A typical epithelial proliferation in the course of experimental production of ulcer-carcinoma of the stomach. Tohoku J Exp Med 93:363–376.

MATSUKURA N, KAWACHI T, SASAJIMA K, et al. 1978. Induction of intestinal metaplasia in the stomachs of rats by N-methyl-N'-nitroso-N-nitrosoguanidine. J Natl Cancer Inst 61:141–144.

MATSUKURA N, SUZUKI K, KAWACHI T, et al. 1980. Distribution of marker enzymes and mucin in intestinal metaplasia in human stomach and relation of complete and incomplete types of intestinal metaplasia to minute gastric carcinomas. J Natl Cancer Inst 65:231–240.

MATTHEWS-ROTH MM. 1983. Carotenoid pigment administration and delay in development of UV-B-induced tumors. Photochem Photobiol 37:509–511.

MAYNARD DN. 1978. Potential nitrate levels in edible plant parts. *In* Nielsen DR, MacDonald JG (eds): Nitrogen in the Environment, Vol. 2. New York, Academic Press, pp. 221–233.

MCLAUGHLIN JK, HRUBEC Z, BLOT WJ, FRAUMENI JF JR. 1990. Stomach cancer and cigarette smoking among U.S. veterans, 1954–1980. Cancer Res 50:3804.

MCMICHAEL AJ, ANDJELKOVIC DA, TYROLER HA. 1976. Cancer mortality among rubber workers. Ann NY Acad Sci 271:125–142.

MILLER BA, GLOOCKLER RIES LA, HANKIN BF, KOSARY CL, HARRAS A, DEVESA SS, EDWARDS BK (EDS). 1993. SEER Cancer Statistics Review: 1973–1990, Bethesda, MD. NIH Publication No. 93–2789.

MING SC. 1973. Tumors of the Esophagus and Stomach. 2nd ser, fasc 7. Firminger HI (ed): Atlas of Tumor Pathology. Washington, D.C., Armed Forces Institute of Pathology, pp. 124–143.

MING SC, GOLDMAN H. 1965. Gastric polyps. A histogenetic classification and its relation to carcinoma. Cancer 18:721–726.

MIRVISH SS. 1983. The etiology of gastric cancer. Intragastric nitrosamide formation and other theories. J Natl Cancer Inst 71:629–647.

MIRVISH SS. 1986. Effects of vitamins C and E on N-nitroso compound formation, carcinogenesis, and cancer. Cancer 58:1842–1850.

MIRVISH S, WALLCAVE L, EAGEN M, et al. 1972. Ascorbate-nitrite reaction: Possible means of blocking the formation of carcinogenic N-nitroso compounds. Science 177:65–68.

MODAN B, LUBIN F, BARELL V, et al. 1974. The role of starches in the etiology of gastric cancer. Cancer 34:2087–2092.

MONSON RR, FINE LJ. 1978. Cancer mortality and morbidity among rubber workers. J Natl Cancer Inst 61:1047–1053.

MONTES G, CUELLO C, CORREA P, HAENSZEL W, ZARAMA G, GORDILLO G. 1984. Mutagenic activity of nitrosated foods in an area with a high risk for stomach cancer. Nutr Cancer 6:171–175.

MORIYAMA IM, BAUM WS, HAENSZEL W, et al. 1958. Inquiry into diagnostic evidence supporting medical certification of death. Am J Publ Health 48:1376–1387.

MOSBECH J, VIDEBACK A. 1950. Mortality from and risk of gastric carcinoma among patients with pernicious anemia. Br Med J 2:390–394.

MUNOZ N, ASVALL J. 1971. Time trends of intestinal and diffuse types of gastric cancer in Norway. Int J Cancer 8:144–157.

MUNOZ N, CONNELLY R. 1971. Time trends of intestinal and diffuse types of gastric cancer in the United States. Int J Cancer 8:158–164.

MUNOZ N, CORREA P, CUELLO C, et al. 1968. Histologic types of gastric carcinoma in high and low risk areas. Int J Cancer 3:809–818.

Munoz N, Matko I. 1972. Histological types of gastric cancer and its relationship with intestinal metaplasia. Cancer Res 39:99–105.

Munoz N, Steinitz R. 1971. Comparative histology of gastric cancer in migrant groups in Israel. Israel J Med Sci 7:1479–1487.

Murakami R, Tsukuma H, Ubukata T, et al. 1990. Estimation of validity of mass screening program for gastric cancer in Osaka, Japan. Cancer 65:1255–1260.

Nagayo T. 1975. Microscopical cancer of the stomach—A study on histogenesis of gastric carcinoma. Int J Cancer 16:52–60.

Nakamura K. 1977. Stomach cancer in atomic-bomb survivors. Lancet 2:866–867.

Nakamura K, Sugano H, Takagi K. 1968. Carcinoma of the stomach in incipient phase: Its histogenesis and histological appearances. Gann 59:251–258.

Nakamura K, Sugano H, Takagi K. 1967. Histopathological study on early carcinoma of the stomach: Some considerations on the ulcer-cancer by analysis of 144 foci of the superficial spreading carcinomas. Gann 58:377–387.

National Academy of Sciences. 1981. The Health Effects of Nitrate, Nitrite, and N-Nitroso Compounds. Washington, National Academy Press, pp. 1–544.

Nazario CM, Szklo M, Diamond E, et al. 1993. Salt and gastric cancer: A case-control study in Puerto Rico. Int J Epidemiol 22:790–797.

Negri E, La Vecchia C, D'Avanzo B, Gentile A, Boyle P, Franceschi S. 1990. Salt preference and the risk of gastrointestinal cancers. Nutr Cancer 14:227–232.

Niukian K, Schwartz J, Shklar G. 1987. Effects of onion extract on the development of hamster buccal pouch carcinomas as expressed in tumor burden. Nutr Cancer 9:171–176.

Nomura A, Grove JS, Stemmermann GN, Severson RK. 1990. A prospective study of stomach cancer and its relation to diet, cigarettes, and alcohol consumption. Cancer Res 50:627–631.

Nomura A, Stemmermann GN, Chyou P-H, Kato I, Perez-Perez GI, Blaser MJ. 1991. Helicobacter pylori infection and gastric carcinoma in a population of Japanese-Americans in Hawaii. N Engl J Med 325:1132–1136.

Nomura A, Stemmermann GN, Chyou P-H, Perez-Perez GI, Blaser MJ. 1994. Helicobacter pylori infection and the risk for duodenal and gastric ulceration. Ann Intern Med 120:977–981.

Nomura AMY, Stemmermann GN, Heilbrun LK, Salkeld RM, Vuilleumier JP. 1985. Serum vitamin levels and the risk of cancer of specific sites in men of Japanese ancestry in Hawaii. Cancer Res 45:2369–2372.

Nomura AMY, Stemmermann GN, Samloff IM. 1980. Serum pepsinogen I as a predictor of stomach cancer. Ann Intern Med 93:537–540.

Ohgaki H, Hasegawa H, Kusama K, et al. 1986. Induction of gastric carcinomas in nonhuman primates by *N*-ethyl-*N*'-nitro-N-nitrosoguanidine. J Natl Cancer Inst 77:179–186.

Palli D, Galli M, Caporaso NE, et al. 1994. Family history and risk of stomach cancer in Italy. Cancer Epidemiol Biomarkers Prev 3:15–18.

Parkin DM, Muir C, Whelan SL, Ga OYT, Ferlay J, Powell J. (eds). 1992. Cancer Incidence in Five Continents, Vol. VI Lyon, IARC Scientific Publications No. 120.

Parsonnet J, Friedman GD, Vandersteen DP, et al. 1991. Helicobacter pylori infection and the risk of gastric carcinoma. N Engl J Med 325:1127–1131.

Pastore JO, Kato H, Belsky JL. 1972. Serum pepsin and tubeless gastric analysis as predictors of stomach cancer. N Engl J Med 286:279–284.

Pickle LW, Mason TJ, Howard N, Hoover R, Fraumeni JF Jr. 1987. Atlas of U.S. Cancer Mortality Among Whites: 1950–1980. DHHS Publication No. (NIH) 87-2900, Washington, D.C., U.S. Government Printing Office.

Pollack ES, Nomura AMY, Heilbrun LK, Stemmermann GN, Green SB. 1984. Prospective study of alcohol consumption and cancer. N Engl J Med 310:617–621.

Raineri R, Weisburger JH. 1975. Reduction of gastric carcinogens with ascorbic acid. Ann NY Acad Sci 258:181–189.

Ramon JM, Serra L, Cerdo C, Oromi J. 1993. Dietary factors and gastric cancer risk. A case-control study in Spain. Cancer 71:1731–1735.

Reed PI, Smith PLR, Haines K, House FR, Walters CL. 1981. Gastric juice N-nitrosamines in health and gastroduodenal disease. Lancet 2:550–552.

Risch HA, Jain M, Won Choi N, et al. 1985. Dietary factors and the incidence of cancer of the stomach. Am J Epidemiol 122:947–959.

Rønnov-Jessen V, Ahlgren P, Qvist CF. 1965. Incidence of gastric cancer in medically treated patients with gastric cancer. Acta Med Sci 178:141–153.

Ross AHM, Smith MA, Anderson JR, Small WP. 1982. Late mortality after surgery for peptic ulcer. N Engl J Med 307:519–522.

Ruddell WSJ, Bone ES, Hill MJ, Walters CL. 1978. Pathogenesis of gastric cancer in pernicious anemia. Lancet 1:521–523.

Rushton I, Alderson MR. 1981. An epidemiological survey of eight oil refineries in Britain. Br J Ind Med 38:225–234.

Saegesser F, James D. 1972. Cancer of the gastric stump after partial gastrectomy (Billroth II principle) for ulcer. Cancer 29:1150–1159.

Saha SK. 1991. Smoking habits and carcinoma of the stomach: A case-control study. Jpn J Cancer Res 82:497–502.

Sakita T, Oguro Y, Takasu S, et al. 1971. Observations on the healing of ulcerations in early gastric cancer. Gastroenterology 60:835–844.

Samloff IM, Liebman WM. 1973. Cellular localization of the group II pepsinogens in human stomach and duodenum by immunofluorescence. Gastroenterology 65:36–42.

Sato T, Fukuyama T, Suzuki T, et al. 1959. Studies of the causation of gastric cancer. 2. The relation between gastric cancer mortality rate and salted food intake in several places in Japan. Bull Inst Publ Health (Japan) 8:187–198.

Schafer LW, Larson DE, Melton LJ III, Higgins JA, Zinsmeister AR. 1985. Risk of development of gastric carcinoma in patients with pernicious anemia: A population-based study in Rochester, Minnesota. Mayo Clin Proc 60:444–448.

Schein PS, Levin B. 1985. Neoplasms of stomach. *In* Calabresi P, Schein PS, Rosenberg SA (eds): Medical Oncology. New York, Macmillan Publishing Co, pp. 806–827.

Schlag P, Bockler R, Ulrich H, Peter M, Merkle P, Herfarth C. 1980. Are nitrite and N-nitroso compounds in gastric juice risk factors for carcinoma in the operated stomach? Lancet 1:727–729.

Segi M, Fukushima I, Fujisaku S, et al. 1957. An epidemiological study of cancer in Japan. Gann 48:1–63.

Segi M, Kurihara M. 1972. Cancer Mortality for Selected Sites in 24 Countries, No. 6 (1966–1967). Japan Cancer Society, p. 98.

Select Committee on Nutrition and Human Needs, U.S. Senate. 1977. Dietary Goals for the United States. Washington, D.C., U.S. Government Printing Office.

Selikoff IJ, Hammond EL, Churg J. 1968. Asbestos exposure, smoking, and neoplasia. JAMA 204:104–110.

Shearman DJC, Finlayson MDC, Wilson R, et al. 1966. Carcinoma of the stomach and early pernicious anemia. Lancet 2:403–405.

Sigurjonsson J. 1967. Occupational variations in mortality from gastric cancer in relation to dietary differences. Br J Cancer 21:651–656.

SIURALA M, VARIS K, WILJASALO M. 1966. Studies of patients with atrophic gastritis: A 10–15 year follow-up. Scand J Gastroenterol 1:40–48.

STAHELIN HB, ROSEL F, BUESS E, BRUBACHER G. 1984. Cancer, vitamins, and plasma lipids: Prospective Basel study. J Natl Cancer Inst 73:1463–1468.

STALSBERG H, TAKSDAL S. 1971. Stomach cancer following gastric surgery for benign conditions. Lancet 2:1175–1177.

STEER A, LAND CE, MORIYAMA IM, et al. 1976. Accuracy of diagnosis of cancer among autopsy cases: JNIH-ABCC population for Hiroshima and Nagasaki. Gann 7:625–632.

STEHR PA, GLONINGER MF, KULLER LH, MARSH GM, RADFORD EP, WEINBERG GB. 1985. Dietary vitamin A deficiencies and stomach cancer. Am J Epidemiol 121:65–70.

STEMMERMANN GN. 1988. Gastric cancer and its precursors: Clinical implications to be drawn from morphological changes. *In* Gastrointestinal Cancer: Current Approaches to Diagnosis and Treatment, Annual Clinical Conference on Cancer, Vol. 30. University of Texas System Cancer Center, pp. 353–363.

STEMMERMANN GN, BROWN C. 1974. A survival study of intestinal and diffuse types of gastric carcinoma. Cancer 33:1190–1195.

STEMMERMANN GN, ISHIDATE T, SAMLOFF IM, et al. 1978. Intestinal metaplasia of the stomach in Hawaii and Japan. A study of its relation to serum pepsinogen I, gastrin, and parietal cell antibodies. Am J Dig Dis 23:815–820.

STEWART MJ. 1929. Observations on the relation of malignant disease to benign tumors of the gastrointestinal tract. Br Med J 2:567–569.

STRICKLAND RG, MACKAY IR. 1973. A reappraisal of the nature and significance of chronic atrophic gastritis. Am J Dig Dis 18:426–440.

SUGIMURA T, FUJIMURA S. 1967. Tumor production in glandular stomach of rat by *N*-methyl-*N'*nitro-*N*-nitrosoguanidine. Nature 216:943–944.

SUGIMURA T, TANAKA N, KAWACHI T, et al. 1971. Production of stomach cancer in dogs by *N*-methyl-*N'*-nitro-*N*-nitrosoguanidine. Gann 62:67–68.

TAJIMA K, TOMINAGA S. 1985. Dietary habits and gastro-intestinal cancers: A comparative case-control study of stomach and large intestinal cancers in Nagoya, Japan. Jpn J Cancer Res (Gann) 76:705–716.

TAKAHASHI M, KOKUBO T, FURUKAWA F, KUROKAWA Y, TATEMATSU M, HAYASHI Y. 1983. Effect of high salt diet on rat gastric carcinogenesis induced by *N*-methyl-*N'*-nitro-*N*-nitrosoguanidine. Gann 74:28–34.

TANNENBAUM SR, MORAN D, FALCHUK KR, CORREA P, CUELLO C. 1981. Nitrite stability and nitrosation potential in human gastric juice. Cancer Lett 14:131–136.

TATEMATSU M, TAKAHASHI M, FUKUSHIMA S, HANANOUCHI M, SHIRAI T. 1975. Effects in rats of sodium chloride on experimental gastric cancers induced by *N*-methyl-*N'*-nitro-*N*-nitrosoguanidine or 4-nitroquinoline-1-oxide. J Natl Cancer Inst 55:101–106.

TERSMETTE AC, GOODMAN SN, OFFERHAUS GJA, et al. 1991. Multivariate analysis of the risk of stomach cancer after ulcer surgery in an Amsterdam cohort of postgastrectomy patients. Am J Epidemiol 134:14–21.

THOMAS TL, WAXWEILER RJ, MOURE-ERASO R, ITAYA S, FRAUMENI JF JR. 1982. Mortality patterns among workers in three Texas oil refineries. J Occup Med 24:135–141.

THUNOLD S, WETTELAND P. 1962. Ulcer-carcinoma of the stomach in a 10-year biopy series. Acta Pathol Microbiol Scand 56: 155–165.

TOKUDOME S, KONO S, IKEDA M, et al. 1984. A prospective study on primary gastric stump cancer following partial gastrectomy for benign gastroduodenal diseases. Cancer Res 44:2208–2212.

TOMASULO J. 1971. Gastric polyps. Histologic types and their relationship to gastric carcinoma. Cancer 27:1346–1355.

TORGERSEN O, PETERSON M. 1956. The epidemiology of gastric cancer in Oslo: Cartographic analysis of census tracts and mortality rates of sub-standard housing areas. Br J Cancer 10:299–306.

TRICHOPOULOS D, OURANOS G, DAY NE, et al. 1985. Diet and cancer of the stomach. A case-control study in Greece. Int J Cancer 36:291–297.

TSUCHIYA T, UEYAMA Y, TAMAOKI N, YAMAGUCHI S, SHIBUYA M. 1989. Co-amplification of c-myc and c-erB-2 oncogenes in a poorly differentiated human gastric cancer. Jpn J Cancer Res 80:920–923.

TSUGANE S, AKABANE M, INAMI T, et al. 1991. Urinary salt excretion and stomach cancer mortality among four Japanese populations. Cancer Causes Control 2:165–168.

TUYNS AJ, KAAKS R, HAELTERMAN M, RIBOLI E. 1992. Diet and gastric cancer. A case-control study in Belgium. Int J Cancer 51:1–6.

VIADANA E, BROSS ID, HOUTEN L. 1976. Cancer experience of men exposed to inhalation of chemicals or to combustion products. J Occup Med 18:787–792.

VISTE A, BJORNESTAD E, OPHEIM P, et al. 1986. Risk of carcinoma following gastric operations for benign disease. Lancet 2:502–505.

WAKABAYASHI K, NAGAO M, OCHIAI M, et al. 1987. Recently identified nitrite-reactive compounds in food: Occurrence and biological properties of the nitrosated products. *In* Bartsch H, O'Neill I, Schulte-Hermann R (eds): Relevance of N-Nitroso Compounds to Human Cancer: Exposures and Mechanisms, Vol. 84. Oxford, United Kingdom, Oxford University Press, pp 287–291.

WARREN JR, MARSHALL B. 1983. Unidentified curved bacilli on gastric epithelium in active chronic gastritis. Lancet 1:1273–1275.

WATANABE H. 1978. Experimentally induced intestinal metaplasia in Wistar rats by X-ray irradiation. Gastroenterology 75:796–799.

WOOLF CM, GARDNER EJ. 1950. Carcinoma of gastrointestinal tract in Utah family. J Hered 41:273–276.

WRIGHT WE, BERNSTEIN L, PETERS JM, GARABRANT DH, MACK TM. 1988. Adenocarcinoma of the stomach and exposure to occupational dust. Am J Epidemiol 128:64–73.

WU-WILLIAMS AH, YU MC, MACK TM. 1990. Life-style, workplace, and stomach cancer by subsite in young men of Los Angeles County. Cancer Res 50:2569–2576.

WYNDER EL, KMET J, DUNGAL N, et al. 1963. An epidemiological investigation of gastric cancer. Cancer 16:1461–1496.

YANG D, TANNENBAUM SR, BUCHI G, LEE GCM. 1984. 4-Chloro-6-methoxyindole is the precursor of a potent mutagen that forms during nitrosation of the fava bean (Vicia faba). Carcinogenesis (Lond.) 5:1219–1224.

YANG PC, DAVIS S. 1988. Epidemiological characteristics of adenocarcinoma of the gastric cardia and distal stomach in the United States, 1973–1982. Int J Epidemiol 17:293–297.

YOKOTA J, YAMAMOTO T, MIYAJIMA N, et al. 1987. Genetic alterations of the c-erB-2 oncogene occur frequently in tubular adenocarcinoma of the stomach and are often accompanied by amplification of the v-erbA homologue. Oncogene 2:283–288.

YOU W-C, BLOT WJ, CHANG Y-S, et al. 1988. Diet and high risk of stomach cancer in Shandong, China. Cancer Res 48:3518–3523.

YOU W-C, BLOT WJ, CHANG Y-S, et al. 1989. Allium vegetables and reduced risk of stomach cancer. J Natl Cancer Inst 81:162–164.

ZAMCHECK N, GRABLE E, LEY A, et al. 1955. Occurrence of gastric cancer among patients with pernicious anemia at the Boston City Hospital. N Engl J Med 252:1103–1110.

ZHANG L, BLOT WJ, YOU W-C, et al. 1994. Serum micronutrients in relation to pre-cancerous gastric lesions. Int J Cancer 56:650–654.

35 Pancreatic cancer

KRISTIN E. ANDERSON
JOHN D. POTTER
THOMAS M. MACK

Cancer of the pancreas is one of the most rapidly fatal cancers and its presentation and course are usually marked by severe pain. The pain may be insidious in onset, it may be difficult for either patient or physician to localize, and it may become severe as the tumor spreads, even before the pathophysiologic effects of specific organ malfunction occur (Richard and Cohn, 1969). Presumably because of this unhappy combination of characteristics, the pain may result not only in ordinary anxiety but also in serious emotional disturbances. There are currently no safe and effective means of early diagnosis. The disease progresses more or less relentlessly. There is less than one chance in five of surviving a year and hardly any chance of surviving more than a few years (American Cancer Society, 1993; U.S. DHSS, 1990); long-term survival may even constitute evidence against the accuracy of the original diagnosis. Available treatments are not known to be effective and, despite their focus on palliation and pain relief, are themselves responsible for serious morbidity. (Carter, 1990).

While there are neoplasms that kill people by virtue of being more common, the inevitability of death from cancer of the pancreas ensures that this relatively uncommon disease is a major source of mortality. Some 28,000 Americans are killed by it annually, accounting for approximately 5% of all cancer deaths (American Cancer Society, 1993). To complete the dismal outline, there are just a few leads on etiology and therefore only a little hope of disease prevention in the foreseeable future (recent reviews of various aspects of the epidemiology and etiology include Boyle et al, 1989; Fontham and Correa, 1989; Potter, 1990; Haddock and Carter, 1990; Raymond and Bouchardy, 1990; Poston et al, 1991; Pietri and Clavel, 1991; Warshaw and Fernández-Del Castillo, 1992; Bueno de Mesquita, 1992).

This discussion of pancreas cancer epidemiology begins by reviewing the imperfections in the available system of disease classification and the impact of that on the quality of information. The descriptive epidemiology of cancer of the pancreas is summarized, followed by a critical review of evidence pertinent to specific etiologic hypotheses.

HISTOPATHOLOGY

Classification

The pancreas consists of two separate functional entities—an endocrine portion that produces, most importantly, insulin and glucagon, and an exocrine organ that is an integral part of the digestive system, producing enzymes such as trypsin, chymotrypsin, amylase, and lipase. In addition, ductal cells excrete bicarbonate, electrolytes, and water into the duodenum to maintain the luminal pH at the optimum for the function of pancreatic enzymes. For a review of the evolutionary and embryologic relatedness of the two pancreatic organs, see Pictet et al (1972), Rutter (1980), Cubilla and Fitzgerald (1984), and Lebenthal and Leung (1991). For a review of the physiology of endocrine and exocrine pancreas, see Go et al (1986) and Cubilla and Fitzgerald (1984). For purposes of this discussion, cancer of the pancreas will be considered synonymous with exocrine adenocarcinoma of the pancreas. The islet tumors of the endocrine pancreas present a different clinical appearance, have a more favorable prognosis, are difficult to classify in relation to degree of malignancy, and occur in a different pattern in the population (Mack and Paganini-Hill, 1981; Sindelar et al, 1985). While many analyses of epidemiologic data do not distinguish between exocrine and endocrine neoplasms, the latter are quite rare and their rigid exclusion would have altered few conclusions from studies in which they were included. The same can be said of those rare sarcomas and lymphomas that arise within the pancreas and that also have been inadvertently included in some studies. None of these less common tumors of the pancreas will be given further attention here.

Given adequate material of unambiguous origin, pathologists do not find the diagnosis of exocrine carcinoma of the pancreas to be difficult. Benign neoplasms, endocrine neoplasms, and cysts are uncommon and usually are not difficult to identify. Most exocrine lesions are quickly recognized because they are first perceived after having grown to macroscopic proportions (Frantz, 1959; Sindelar et al, 1985; Klöppel and Maillet, 1991).

The large majority of exocrine adenocarcinomas are believed to arise in the cells that line the pancreatic ductules, but this is somewhat controversial (Cubilla and Fitzgerald, 1984; Klöppel, 1984). The proportion thought to be of acinar origin is variously estimated at from 1% to 15% (Cubilla and Fitzgerald, 1984; Robbins and Cotran, 1979; Klöppel, 1984), and, as the breadth of that range suggests, the criteria used for classification are subject to local variation. Indeed, few community pathologists appear to concern themselves greatly with distinctions between cells of origin, reporting the histology simply as pancreatic adenocarcinoma. While the criteria for identifying the cell of origin include the presence or absence of zymogen granules characteristic of acinar cells and, with less reliability, the presence or absence of the mucin characteristic of ductal cells, the characterization of individual tumors is often based solely on such features as shape and growth pattern. In fact, some tumors in animals (Pour, 1980; Longnecker et al, 1984) and humans have been reported to contain both types of cells, and even islet cells, all of which have a common embryologic origin (Cubilla and Fitzgerald, 1984; Klöppel and Maillet, 1991). It has been argued (Jamieson, 1975) that the apparent distinction between cells of ductal and acinar origin is, in reality, a difference in degree of differentiation, since the cuboidal, granule-free ductal cells closely resemble the progenitor cells of both lines. Evidence from experimental pancreatic cancers supports the view that some ductlike carcinomas may arise from acinar cells (Flaks, 1984; Bockman, 1981). Recent evidence demonstrating acinar to ductal transdifferentiation in human cultured cells and in transgenic mice support the same view, i.e., that acinar cells may be the target for carcinogenic events that lead to tumors with ductal phenotype (Hall and Lemoine, 1992; Sandgren et al, 1990; Jhappen et al, 1990).

Anatomic Distribution

One subclassification that has been thought useful, at least clinically, is that of subsite within the pancreas. The distinction between cancer of the head of the pancreas and that arising in the remainder (body or tail) is not based on histologic differences, because there appear to be none (except for the occasional inadvertent assignment of improperly diagnosed ampullary carcinoma to the head of the pancreas) (Williams et al, 1979; Cubilla and Fitzgerald, 1980). Rather, it is thought to result from the tendency for tumors of the head of the pancreas to produce symptoms while still at a comparatively small size, because the growing tumor mass is adjacent to, and impinges upon, the flexible wall of the common bile duct or the duodenum itself. In those cases of cancer of the pancreas occurring in the mid 1970s among the residents of Los Angeles County, subsite was indicated for about half of the total. Of those, over two-thirds occurred in the head (Mack and Paganini-Hill, 1981). This figure is consistent with other series (Cubilla and Fitzgerald, 1978b; Howard and Jordan 1977; Sener et al, 1991).

The epidemiologic pattern of tumors in the head of the pancreas differs somewhat from those in the body and tail, but these differences are consistent with those expected on the basis of mode and timing of presentation. Designation of the body or tail as the subsite of origin usually requires that the lesions be localized by direct or indirect observation, whereas designation of the head is often based on the symptoms of patients in whom, for whatever reason, surgery or other technical means of localization are not employed. One might expect, therefore, that the body or tail would be specified more often in younger and more intensively studied patients, and this does seem to be the case in Los Angeles (Mack and Paganini-Hill, 1981).

Diagnosis

The foregoing suggests that the observed pattern of occurrence of cancer in such a well-hidden organ might itself depend somewhat on the quality and conventions of medical care. Unfortunately, this is likely to be true, and it is an important obstacle to our understanding of the epidemiology of the disease.

Most patients with pancreatic cancer are identified on the basis of their presenting symptoms. Commonly, these include weight loss, pain, and jaundice (Warshaw and Fernández-Del Castillo, 1992; Bakkevold et al, 1992). The current diagnostic imaging techniques include ultrasound imaging (US), computed tomography (CT), and endoscopic retrograde cholangiopancreatography (ERCP) (Niederau and Grendell, 1992; Sindelar et al, 1985). Considerable effort has been made to identify serum tumor markers, but none has proven to be both sufficiently sensitive and specific for use in routine diagnosis or screening (Livingston and Reber, 1992; Niederau and Grendell, 1992; Appert, 1990). Percutaneous fine-needle aspiration (FNA) is increasingly being used to obtain a biopsy for cytologic diagnosis (Rösch et al, 1992). Overall, these techniques have improved the ability of physicians to diagnose and to stage the disease and have reduced the number of diagnostic laparotomies performed, but early detection is still rare. At diagnosis, less than 10% of patients have tumors confined to the pancreas and more than 50% have visceral metastatic disease (Sindelar et al, 1985).

Because the diagnosis of pancreas cancer is so often made at a time when nothing can be offered the patient, because the organ is inconveniently located, and because of the morbidity associated with biopsy, pancreatic cancer continues to have the lowest proportion of histologically verified cases of any major cancer. This, too, has important implications for epidemiologic studies.

For comparable recent years, the average proportion of incident male cases that have been verified histopathologically prior to notification to various registries is given in Table 35–1 (Parkin et al, 1992). These figures suggest, indeed, that for pancreas cancer, more than for other neoplasms, estimates of incidence depend heavily on accurate enumeration of cases with and without microscopic examination.

There is certainly an extraordinary geographic variation in the frequency of histologic confirmation (Parkin et al, 1992), and the level of this indicator does not correlate well with the presumed quality of diagnosis. Even within regions with relatively homogeneous medical services, such as Europe, there is great variation. Therefore, the international variation in the specificity and sensitivity of the diagnosis is likely to be large, and its impact should be presumed to be even larger in areas where histologic confirmation is less frequent than in Europe, North America, and Oceania (Kurihara, 1979; Parkin et al, 1992).

TABLE 35–1. *Percentages of Incident Cancer of the Pancreas Confirmed Histopathologically* in Males, All Ages*

Area	*Number of Registry Entries*	*Mean (%)*	*Range (%)*
Poland	6	20.8	11–31
Africa	3	29	14–40
United Kingdom	13	37.9	24–64
Latin America	9	38.6	13–73
Japan	6	44.3	28–56
Canada	12	51	33–65
Scandinavia	5	74	55–86
United States[a]	14	76.9	63–85

From Parkin et al, 1992.
*Means and ranges include date from registries where cytologic verification was excluded. For details, see Parkin et al (1992), Chapter 6, pp. 45–173.
[a]Where percentages were provided by race, the data for "white" or "other white" were used.

There is evidence that some of the variation in both mortality and incidence may be due to variation in methods and completeness of case ascertainment. The proportion of deaths that went to autopsy in the province of Trieste has been approximately 60% since 1978 (Riboli et al, 1991); during 1970–1984, pancreatic cases ascertained through autopsy accounted for 45% of the pancreatic cancers (Riboli et al, 1991). It may be that, in regions with relatively high percentages of autopsied deaths, cases ascertained by autopsy may account, in part, for correspondingly high incidence and mortality rates. This is illustrated for some cancer sites, though, perversely, not for pancreas, in Malmö. Malmö has the highest autopsy rate in Sweden, and twice as many cancer cases (12.4%) were found incidentally than in Sweden as a whole (Sternby, 1991).

Histologically confirmed cases fall into two categories—those diagnosed at postmortem examination and those diagnosed before death. Among the latter are not only those where specimens of pancreas were taken under full visualization, but also those where a specimen of lymph node, liver, or other nonpancreatic site was believed to contain pancreas cancer, and those where a specimen taken under conditions of indirect or imperfect localization was believed to derive from the pancreas.

The cases with diagnoses that are unconfirmed histologically include those in which a mass was identified and localized at operation and either not biopsied or biopsied, but in which a tumor was not demonstrated. This group also includes those who refused unpromising surgery, and those who, for a variety of reasons, received only symptomatic care. Many such clinical diagnoses come to registration only through the screening of death certificates or, for hospital cases, through the enumeration of discharge diagnoses. The completeness and the consistency of enumeration are therefore highly dependent upon the accuracy of clinical records for both the most probable diagnosis and the probable site of origin. Unlike pathology records, neither death certificates nor discharge records are primarily maintained for purposes of nosology, and their quality reflects the variable need for documenting clinical decisions (Levin and Connelly, 1973). Enumeration depends as well upon the motivation and training of the persons who code the records and those who screen them for evidence of cancer diagnosis; neither group is usually paid by, or directly responsible to, the relevant cancer registry.

These effects of transcription upon enumeration also pertain to one class of microscopically verified case. When suspect cases come to autopsy and receive a definitive diagnosis from the pathologist, this final diagnosis may not be reflected in either the clinical records or the death certificate. Such cases may not be ascertained, or properly stricken from the record, unless the registry seeks out the autopsy records, which often become available only after a long delay (Engel et al, 1980).

These factors suggest that the enumeration of accurate diagnoses may be incomplete and variable. Additional variation and inaccuracy derive from the process of diagnosis itself.

Because of the late appearance and nonspecific nature of symptoms and signs, preoperative clinical diagnostic criteria have resulted simultaneously in both overdiagnosis, which produces false-positive diagnoses, and underdiagnosis, which produces missed, false-negative cases. The differential diagnosis of prolonged abdominal pain in an extremely ill patient includes not only other conditions of the pancreas and malignancies at other intra-abdominal sites, but also a wide range of nonmalignant, intra-abdominal, retroperitoneal, and systemic illnesses (Malagelada, 1979; Sindelar et al, 1985). Even with localizing symptoms, a variety of diseases of the liver, biliary tree, duodenum, and pancreas may be clinically indistinguishable from pancreatic cancer. Over the past decade, the use of computed tomography (CT), ultrasound imaging (US), endoscopic retrograde cholangiopancreatography (ERCP), and percutaneous fine-needle aspiration (FNA) has helped improve physicians' ability to diagnose correctly, and to stage, the disease thereby avoiding inappropriate surgery for patients with advanced disease and increasing resectability rates from 5% to 22% for patients who ultimately undergo laparotomy (Niederau and Grendell, 1992; Beazley et al, 1991).

Finally, factors similar to those that result in erroneous diagnosis sometimes lead to an inaccurate designation of primary site of origin (Cassiere et al, 1980; Riboli et al, 1991). Review of cases routinely designated as pancreas cancer is more likely to turn up sizable numbers of tumors of the ampulla (Cubilla and Fitzgerald, 1980), the stomach (Lazar et al, 1960), the biliary tree, the small intestine, the ovary, or, often, those of unknown origin (Gudjonsson et al, 1978).

While it is difficult to quantify such errors in diagnosis, their frequency, even in the recent past, appears to have been high. Some idea of the sensitivity of the clinical diagnosis can be obtained from the proportion of autopsy-verified cases that have been correctly diagnosed prior to death. In Boston from 1955 to 1965, 47.5% of 139 cases had been diagnosed accurately (Bauer and Robbins, 1972). Of 100 cases that were histologically verified by either biopsy or necropsy in Cleveland between 1962 and 1967, 59% had been previously diagnosed correctly (Rastogi and Brown, 1967). In a prospective study of hospital autopsies, Cameron and McGoogan (1981) found agreement on clinical and autopsy diagnoses of cancer in only 7 of 26 cases of pancreas cancer.

Riboli and colleagues (1991) compared causes of death from cancers of the digestive tract as reported on death certificates and as determined by autopsy. The data covered the period 1970–84 in Trieste and included 30,895 autopsies of which 688 were cases of pancreatic cancer and over 3800 were cases of other cancers of the digestive tract reported by death certificate and/or autopsy. The study was an indirect comparison of the accuracy of clinical diagnoses, since nearly all of the death certificates were completed in the same hospitals in which patients were treated, and a parallel study revealed that about 80% of the death certificates that listed a cancer of the digestive tract agreed with clinical records. An assessment of all 688 reported pancreatic cancers yielded a 37% agreement on primary cancer site (concordance on the 3-digit ICD code) between death certificate and autopsy report. There were 14% (n = 96) false-positive (for pancreas cancer) death certificates; the autopsy data revealed cancer at a different site for about 88% (n = 85) of these false-positives and no cancer in the remainder.

The specificity of the diagnosis is more difficult to assess. When autopsy data from the Trieste study (Riboli et al, 1991) were used to correct death certificate diagnoses, a net gain of 45% was found in pancreas cancers. Of these false-negatives, a different cancer was found at autopsy in 45% to 55% of the individuals. Of 197 patients given a discharge diagnosis of pancreas cancer in a major Connecticut teaching hospital from 1960 to 1971 (Gudjonsson et al, 1978), only 100 had histologically verified disease, 70 had no histologic proof of cancer, and 27 were seen on review to have disease that originated at a different site. Over 65% of those diagnosed without histologic verification had undergone laparotomy. In a community hospital reporting to the Connecticut Tumor Registry (Suguitan et al, 1973), only 15 out of 40 patients diagnosed from 1969 to 1973 had been histologically verified, and over half of these were by biopsy of a metastatic site, with assignment of primary site based on palpation at time of surgery. In 10 of the remainder, the diagnosis was based solely on clinical criteria, and in none of the clinical diagnoses had there been confirmation of the primary site by autopsy or surgery at the end of a 4-year follow-up period. Another estimate of the specificity of the diagnosis comes from a review of all deaths from cancer reported to the province of Saskatchewan from 1950 to 1956 (Barclay and Phillips, 1962). Of the 375 deaths alleged to have been due to pancreas cancer, 231 had been seen in provincial clinics and were presumed to be accurately diagnosed. Of the 124 reported by private physicians, only 39 (31.5%) could be confirmed by a review of records using conventional criteria (not demanding histologic verification). Eight cases of pancreas cancer were found on review among the 1547 nonclinic diagnoses of cancer of other sites similarly reviewed. Thus 23% of the reported cases were believed to be in error after reviewing only 38.4% of the total. Although improved techniques will have altered the picture somewhat, for many centers diagnostic accuracy remains problematic.

The errors in specificity and sensitivity are large, and false-positives and false-negatives do not consistently balance each other. Further, although certain clinical conventions might involve consistent errors, these must account for a small proportion of the total errors and will have been quantitatively inconsistent over time and place.

One must conclude that errors in the diagnosis of carcinoma of the pancreas may be quantitatively more important, perhaps by an order of magnitude, than errors in the diagnosis of other common cancers. Moreover, whereas the consequences of errors in incidence data can often be overcome by scrutiny of the relatively insensitive, but more specific, mortality tabulations, that is not possible for pancreas cancer; measures of incidence and mortality are quite interdependent, more so than those for other sites. Clinically unambiguous diagnoses that are recorded in death certificates for want of an alternative constitute a substantial number of the reported incident cases. Therefore, major differences between mortality and incidence are more likely to reflect errors due to the process of registration rather than errors in the diagnosis itself.

Random misclassification merely tends to obscure differences rather than produce them; therefore, none of the preceding errors would seriously restrict positive interpretation of descriptive information were it not for a systematic component to many of them. Substantial variation over place and time must be presumed to exist in the clinical acumen of the average practitioner, the customary level of diagnostic technology, the risks of surgery, the perceived dangers of biopsy, the confidence of frightened patients in their proposed treatment, the spectrum of differential diagnosis, and even the perceived likelihood of each of these diseases in the demographic subgroup represented by the patient.

As noted, variation in the quality of diagnosis must be assumed to be a function of time at least as much as of geography. The dramatic trends in the technology of surgical support systems, and in access to early medical care as well as the falling rates of autopsy in many places ensure that changes in the frequency of histologic confirmation over the decades within any given country are great, with, however, not all trends being in the same direction. The specificity and sensitivity of clinical diagnoses are likely to have changed greatly, even in recent years. To a certain extent, the clinical diagnosis of pancreatic carcinoma has been a diagnosis of exclusion. On the other hand, because of the increasing rarity of alternative diagnoses of exclusion, and because of the proliferation of methods for the treatment of other occult possibilities, the diagnosis of pancreatic carcinoma has remained relatively available for use in labeling a moribund patient with ambiguous localizing signs who cannot be subjected to highly invasive diagnostic or therapeutic measures. Such a trend is likely to have worked in the opposite direction to increase the nonspecificity of the diagnosis.

Summary of Diagnostic Issues. For the time being, we may be on relatively safe ground if we compare rates from within populations living at the same time and place; if we accept only substantial differences as meaningful; and if we can presume that the groups being compared have received a comparable standard of health care. This last condition may be questionable when the comparison is among socioeconomically diverse groups, extreme age groups, etc. When comparing chronologically or geographically disparate populations, there is no safe ground; extreme caution must be used in interpretation. Superficial measures of the quality of data or the quality of medical care cannot ensure comparability in the assigning and reporting of diagnoses. This should be borne in mind while considering the descriptive epidemiology below.

DESCRIPTIVE EPIDEMIOLOGY

Incidence

Pancreatic cancer is the ninth most common cause of cancer in the United States with a similar ranking in the United Kingdom and Sweden (Parkin et al, 1992). The American Cancer Society (1993) estimated that there would be 27,700 new cases in the United States in 1993, accounting for approximately 2.5% of cancer diagnoses. The age-adjusted (U.S. 1970 standard population) incidence rates per 100,000 people for pancreatic cancer among males and females (SEER, all races) in the United States in 1989 were 9.9 and 7.6 respectively; for both sexes, the rate was 8.7 (Miller et al, 1992).

Mortality

Carcinoma of the pancreas is the fifth leading cause of cancer death in the United States. It was estimated that there would be 25,000 deaths from this disease in 1993, or about 5% of all cancer deaths (American Cancer Society, 1993). The 1989 age-adjusted (U.S. 1970 standard population) annual mortality rates (SEER) per 100,000 people for pancreatic cancer in the United States were 9.7 for white males, 7.2 for white females, 12.5 for black males, and 11.1 for black females (Miller et al, 1992).

Survival

Survival rates for pancreatic cancer are among the worst for any cancer. Median survival is about 3 months (Axtell et al, 1976; Riela et al, 1992). Fewer than 3% of newly diagnosed cases are expected to live beyond 5 years (American Cancer Society, 1993); 1-year survival is around 16% (U.S. DHSS, 1990). In that minority of patients for whom surgery is an option, the 5-year survival rate is better than the rate for all stages, but is still less than 10% (Livingston et al, 1991). The majority of cases (perhaps 75% to 85%) present with relatively advanced disease and unresectable tumors and none of the standard treatment options—surgery, radiation therapy, and chemotherapy—have been shown to influence significantly their high mortality rate; palliation is the most common therapy (Beazley et al, 1991; Livingston and Reber, 1992).

Time Trends in the U.S.

Pancreatic cancer incidence and mortality rates have increased in the United States over this century; between 1920 and 1965, the age-adjusted mortality rate increased from 2.9 to 8.2 per 100,000 people (Krain, 1970). Both mortality and incidence rates have been relatively stable since about 1970, with slight decreases that reflect decreases in rates for white males (American Cancer Society, 1993; Miller et al, 1992; Devesa et al, 1987). From 1973 to 1989, there has been little change in either the incidence or mortality rates among black males and white females and a slight increase in these same rates in black females. The current age-adjusted (U.S. 1970 standard population) mortality rate (SEER) for both sexes and all races is 8.4/100,000 people (Miller et al, 1992).

Reasons for the increase earlier in this century are not known, but it is believed to be due, in part, to improvements in diagnostic procedures (IARC, 1986). Another possible explanation comes from the observation of a lagged correlation between the prevalence rates of cigarette use and cancer mortality rates for men and women in the United States (Weiss and Bernarde, 1983). Given the strong epidemiologic data that implicate cigarettes as a risk factor for pancreatic cancer (see below), trends in cigarette use might explain both the increase seen until about 1970 (Fontham and Correa, 1989) and the recent decrease in white males.

Race, Ethnicity, and International Patterns

There is an approximately 30-fold variation in pancreas cancer incidence around the world (Parkin et al, 1992). In a comparison of age-standardized annual incidence rates per 100,000 people, the highest rates are found among U. S. black populations in Alameda County of California (13.7, males; 11.9, females) and the San Francisco Bay Area (13.5, males; 11.6, females). In general, the incidence rates in blacks are 1.5 to 1.9 times those of whites throughout the United States. Rates are also very high among the Polynesians of Hawaii (10.5, males; 7.8, females) and New Zealand (11.0, males; 9.8, females). Among the lowest incidence rates reported are those from regional population-based registries of India, for example, Ahmedabad (0.7, males; 0.1, females). Low rates are also found in Thailand, Kuwait (Kuwaitis), and Algeria.

The highest mortality rates (Aoki et al, 1992) occur in northern Europe, including Britain, and in countries populated by migration from those areas. The corresponding rates in central and southern Europe are generally lower. The age-adjusted (world population) mortality rates per 100,000 people for the period 1983–87 are 9.8 for males and 6.3 for females in Finland; 8.6 and 6.6 in Sweden; 8.0 and 5.4 in Norway; 7.7 and 5.1 in England and Wales; 7.4 and 5.1 in the United States (whites); 7.1 and 3.5 in France; 7.0 and 4.1 in Italy; and 5.0 and 2.8 in Spain (Aoki et al, 1992).

Mortality rates are lowest in Asia (Aoki et al, 1992); for example, in Hong Kong the rates per 100,000 people are 4.1 for males and 2.8 for females, and in Singapore (5.1 and 3.3). Though relatively low in the past (Segi and Kurihara, 1972), mortality rates in Japan are now similar to rates in Western countries at 8.0 and 4.5 (Aoki et al, 1992).

Incidence patterns (Parkin et al, 1992) are similar to those seen for mortality; for example, incidence rates per 100,000 people in Finland are 10.1 for males and 6.7 for females; in Sweden 8.4 and 6.3; in England and Wales 7.4 and 4.9; in the white population of the United States (SEER) 8.2 and 6.0; in the white population (non-Maori) of New Zealand 7.2 and 4.8. Although lower incidence rates are generally found in central and southern Europe, there are numerous exceptions. For example, relatively low rates are reported in Granada, Spain (3.3 and 2.4); in Tarn, France (3.7 and 1.4); and Latina, Italy (3.9 and 2.7), but rates similar to those in the United States, New Zealand, or Britain have been reported in Genoa, Italy (7.7 and 4.8), Somme, France (7.4 and 2.8), and Vaud, Switzerland (8.5 and 5.7). High rates can be found in Trieste (10.4 and 6.7) and Parma, Italy (10.1 and 4.5).

The incidence rates are relatively low in Asia, for example, among the Malay of Singapore (4.1 and 2.0). Again, Japan is an exception where the rates are not very different from those in U. S. whites (8.9 and 5.0, in Osaka). While incidence rates in Americans of Asian descent have generally, but not always, appeared to fall between those of Asians in Asia and those of Americans of European origin (Young et al, 1978; Mack and Paganini-Hill, 1981; Parkin et al, 1992), mortality rates have been consistently comparable to those for the European Americans (Smith, 1956; Buell and Dunn, 1965; Haenszel and Kurihara, 1968; King and Haenszel, 1973; Fraumeni and Mason, 1974).

In South America, Cuba, and Puerto Rico (Parkin et al, 1992), incidence appears low. Hispanic populations in the United States have been variously reported to have rates that are somewhat lower (Waterhouse et al, 1976), somewhat higher (Young et al, 1978; New Mexico Tumor Registry, personal communication, 1993); and quite comparable (Menck et al, 1975; Mack and Paganini-Hill, 1981) to those of non-Hispanic white Americans. The New Mexico Tumor Registry, a participant in the SEER program, covers a population that is 38% Hispanic (based on 1990 census figures). The average annual age-adjusted (1970 U.S. standard population) incidence rates per 100,000 people for the Hispanic population were 10.8 and 7.4 in 1988–91. The corresponding rates in the non-Hispanic white population for the same period were 10.1 and 6.7 (New Mexico Tumor Registry, personal communication). Since "Hispanic" is not a well-defined category, one must use caution in interpreting incidence and mortality rates for this heterogeneous group.

Although based on very limited data, the incidence rates in Africa are low, in contrast to the high rates in African Americans (Parkin et al, 1992; Walker et al, 1993).

Available estimates of incidence for American Indians are based on small numbers. Studies of mortality for both American Indians (Creagan and Fraumeni, 1972) and Alaskan natives (Blot et al, 1975; Lanier et al, 1976) in the past have shown no consistent or extreme variation from the patterns among whites. For the period 1988–91, average annual age-adjusted incidence rates per 100,000 people for Native Americans in New Mexico and Arizona were 12.0 and 10.2. These rates were somewhat higher than the comparable rates for the non-Hispanic white population of New Mexico (10.1, 6.7), but the rates for Native Americans are based on a total of only 33 cases (New Mexico Tumor Registry, personal communication).

It is important to bear in mind that some, perhaps much, of the variation in both mortality and incidence patterns may be due to variation in methods and completeness of case ascertainment.

Migration

Examination of morbidity and mortality in relation to place of birth has not produced information that is easily interpreted. In the late 1950s and early 1960s, U. S. mortality rates were 2- to 3-fold higher than those in Japan, but the rates in those of Japanese origin in the United States at this time were actually higher than those in U. S. whites (Haenszel and Kurihara, 1968). A similar observation has been made in Australia for the 1960s and 1970s, when migrants from lower risk southern Europe and Poland, after a duration of 16 or more years, experienced a higher risk of pancreas cancer than native-born Australians (McMichael et al, 1980). Mortality in European immigrants to the United States has been reported to be somewhat higher than in the members of second or subsequent generations as well (Haenszel, 1961); mortality has also been reported to be higher in United States counties populated by a high percentage of residents of northern European descent (Blot et al, 1978). Israelis born in Europe or America experience higher rates than those born in Africa or Asia (Parkin et al, 1992).

These differences are not as great as racial differences, however, and the association with place of birth has not been a consistent finding. Mortality from pancreas cancer in New York City has been shown to be related to European nativity as well as to Judaism (MacMahon, 1960; Newill, 1961), but there was no consistent relation with nativity among Jews in either study. Mortality from pancreas cancer in Chinese in the United States does not appear to be related to nativity (King and Haenszel, 1973).

Age

The most reliable and important known predictor of pancreas cancer incidence is age. In the first three decades of life, this cancer is extremely uncommon, although it can occur even in childhood (Moynan et al, 1964; Tsukimoto et al, 1973; Taxy, 1976; Grosfeld et al, 1990). After the age of 30, as in most epithelial cancers, rates increase with age in approximately log-linear fashion. The slopes of these curves are remarkably similar from population to population, regardless of race, environment, or absolute level of age-adjusted incidence (Figs. 35–1 and 35–2). Those in the eighth decade of life experience a risk approximately 40 times that of those in the fourth decade. The median age at diagnosis in the United States is 71 years (Miller et al, 1992), and the majority of cases occur between age 65 and 79.

The age-specific incidence curves in white United States females and males (SEER) increase continuously, even through the last age category (85+), as do the most recent curves from England and Wales, Sweden, and Nagasaki, Japan (Parkin et al, 1992). In Granada, Spain, rates decline in the last age category in males, but not in females, the reverse is true in Zaragoza, Spain, and in the Miyagi Prefecture, Japan. A decline in incidence rates is evident after age 85 in the curves for black

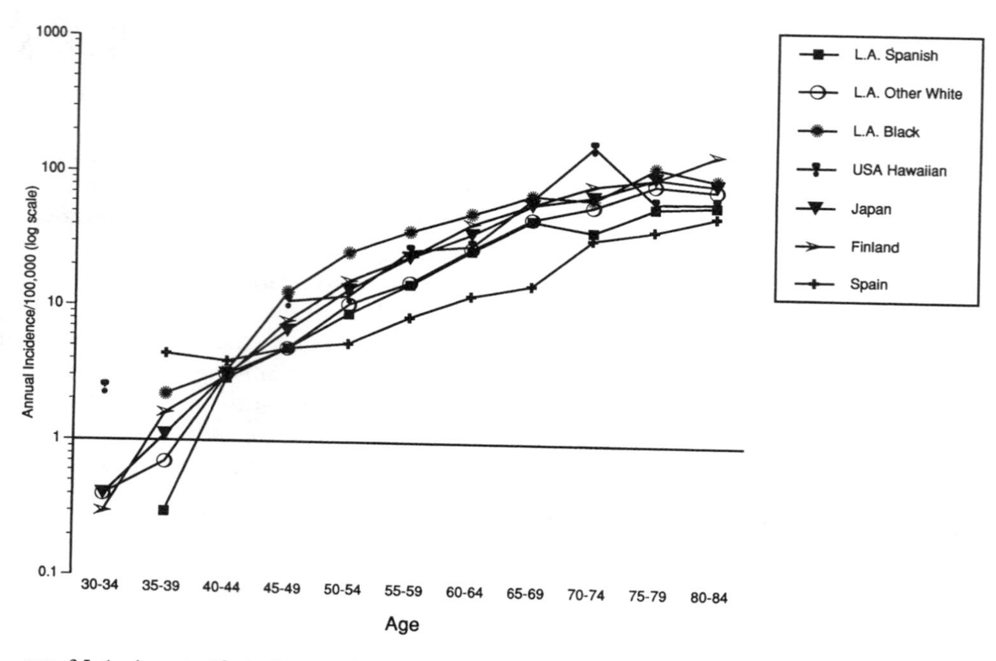

FIG. 35–1. Age-specific incidence of cancer of the pancreas per 10^5 per year for different racial groups in males. Data from Parkin et al, 1992.

males and females in the United States (SEER) and for Spanish-surnamed (Los Angeles) females. In contrast, incidence rates for Spanish-surnamed males (Los Angeles) show a sharp increase in the last age category. Since some of these patterns are different from those reported for a half-decade earlier in Muir et al (1987), the oldest-age-related phenomena are quite consistent with an artifact of diagnosis, ascertainment, or demography. Alternatively, of course, there could be a genuine elimination of susceptibles or a higher proportion of unexposed (particularly, for example, fewer smokers) in this oldest age group in some of these populations.

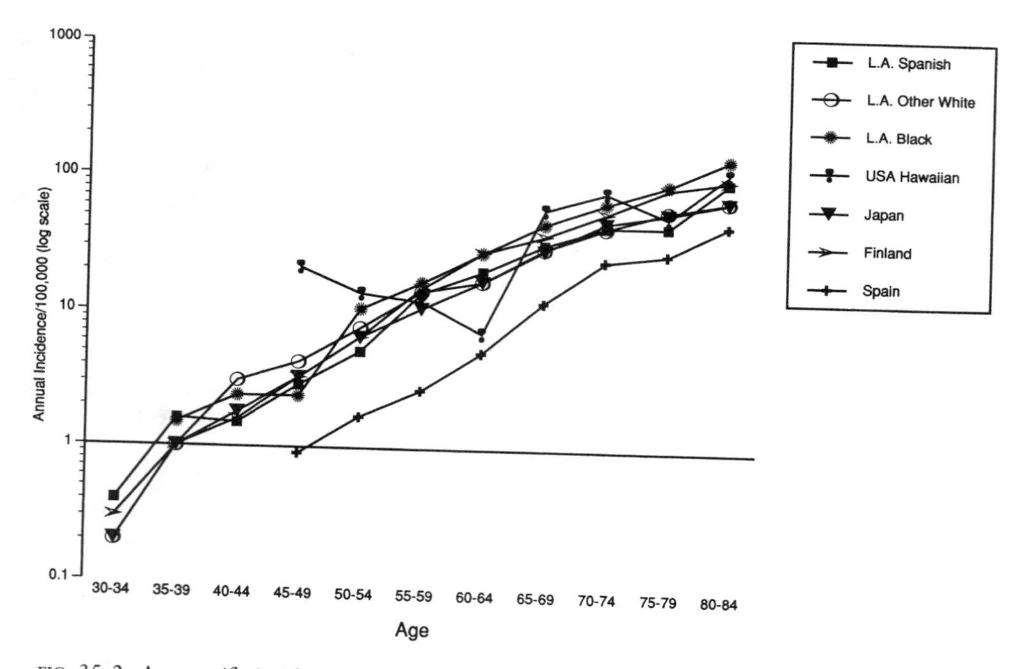

FIG. 35–2. Age-specific incidence of cancer of the pancreas per 10^5 per year for different racial groups in females. Data from Parkin et al, 1992.

Sex

Pancreas cancer is about 50% more common in men than in women, varying somewhat by race, geographical location, and histological type. This ratio is remarkably constant as long as comparisons are made using data from relatively complete population-based registries (Muir et al, 1987, Parkin et al, 1992). In the United States, the current male : female ratio ranges from 1.7 : 1.0 for ages 40–59 to 1.3 : 1.0 for ages 70 and over (Miller et al, 1992). Among U. S. whites, the sex ratios for both incidence and mortality peaked about 1970 at more than a 60% male excess and have declined continuously since (Devesa et al, 1987; Muir et al, 1987; Parkin et al, 1992). A similar decrease was observed by Riela et al (1992) in Olmsted County, Minnesota, where the male : female incidence ratio declined from 2 : 1 for 1940 through 1949 to 1.5 : 1 for 1980 through 1988. These changes over time are consistent both with changes in exposure (particularly increased smoking among women) and with possible differences between the sexes in the changes that have occurred in diagnostic work-up, cancer treatment, and reporting of the disease over time.

Socioeconomic Status

The relation between pancreas cancer and socioeconomic status seems to have changed over the years. In England and Wales in the early 1930s, mortality from the disease, at least in women, was somewhat more common in lower socioeconomic status households (Registrar General, 1938). In the next report of the Registrar General (1954), the trends were inconsistent, but mortality tended to be higher for persons in the upper social classes. In the most recent report (Logan, 1982), no trends were discernible. Similarly in the United States, observations from earlier periods suggested either no social class association (Cohart and Muller, 1955; Graham et al, 1960) or higher rates in the lower socioeconomic categories (Dorn and Cutler, 1958; Seidman, 1970; Krain, 1971a, b; Young et al, 1975). In more recent periods, some have observed no association (Moldow and Connelly, 1968; Wynder et al, 1973a, 1983; Williams and Horm, 1977; Blot et al, 1978), while others have observed an inconsistent association with higher social class (Levin et al, 1981; Levin and Connelly, 1973; Lin and Kessler, 1981; Mack and Paganini-Hill, 1981; Falk et al, 1988; Ferraroni et al, 1989). Whether the observed trends have been judged positive, inverse, or absent, however, the magnitude of any effect is usually small, and risk in both the lowest and highest categories has usually been elevated in comparison with intermediate categories.

Urbanization

The evidence concerning the relative frequency of pancreas cancer in rural and urban areas is more or less consistent, but not striking. Rates in the urban areas of Denmark (Clemmesen, 1974), Norway (Waterhouse et al, 1976), and Finland (Klintrup, 1966) have been reported to be consistently higher than in rural areas. Urban versus rural cancer rates were available for 11 regions of the world in Muir et al (1987). In all of the regions, rates among rural males were never higher than the rates among urban males. The rate ratios (urban: rural) ranged from 1.0, for both New South Wales, Australia, and Szabolcs, Hungary, to 1.5 for Calvados, France. A similar pattern is observed among females with the exceptions of a higher rural versus urban rate for females of Vaud, Switzerland, and the Szabolcs region of Hungary. The urban : rural rate ratios for females in these regions were 0.8 and 0.9, respectively, while the largest ratio, 1.8, was observed for females in Doubs, France. There are no comparable data in Cancer Incidence in Five Continents, vol VI (Parkin et al, 1992).

A clear trend in incidence with several levels of population density was observed in New York State (Nasca et al, 1980). For men, the incidence of pancreas cancer was higher in urban than in rural Olmsted County, Minnesota (Maruchi et al, 1979). There was also a correlation, for men, between United States county mortality rates from pancreas cancer and an index of county urbanization (Blot et al, 1978). None of these associations suggests that urban risks are more than twice those in rural areas. In Utah, there appears to be no clear relation to urbanization, but the situation is complicated by some uncertainty about the distribution of the lower risk members of the Church of Jesus Christ of the Latter Day Saints (LDS), often called Mormons (Lyon et al, 1976, 1980). Falk et al (1988) found residents in rural Louisiana at higher risk than urban residents. Finally, no relation to urbanization was found in Iowa and Colorado in data from the Third National Cancer Survey (Levin et al, 1981).

Religion

Both higher and lower than average susceptibility to develop pancreatic cancer have been observed in one or other religious groups. An increased mortality from pancreas cancer in New York Jews could not be explained by age, nativity (MacMahon, 1960; Newill, 1961; King et al, 1965), or socioeconomic status based on place of residence (Seidman, 1970). Such an excess among Jewish men, but not women, was also reported in a multicenter case-control study (Wynder, 1973a) and is evident in data from New York (Greenwald et al, 1975).

Cohort studies of Seventh-Day Adventists have shown a considerable deficit of deaths from pancreas cancer (Phillips, 1975; Phillips et al, 1980; Mills et al, 1988), and studies of both incidence (Lyon et al, 1976, 1980) and mortality (Enstrom, 1978, 1980) in LDS have indicated a deficit of pancreas cancer of similar magnitude. In Los Angeles (Mack and Paganini-Hill, 1981), a slight deficit of incident cases among LDS and a slight excess among Jews are evident.

Summary of Descriptive Epidemiology. Risk from exocrine pancreas cancer increases dramatically with age and is higher in men and in certain racial groups. Seemingly consistent differences by religion and population density could be explained by differences in diagnostic criteria, and such differences may have completely obscured the true international and chronological trends. More interesting, these differences could be explained by behavioral differences, particularly differences in smoking; this explanation is especially likely for the patterns seen in Adventists and LDS. Socioeconomic effects are weak and inconsistent, and probably explain few cases. Although migration effects are also weak, the patterns may hold some clues regarding etiology, particularly for identifying early versus late exposures.

INDIVIDUAL-LEVEL RISK FACTORS

Smoking

The most consistent risk factor for pancreatic cancer is cigarette smoking. In 1986, an IARC working group evaluating the carcinogenic risk of tobacco concluded that cigarette smoking is an important cause of pancreatic cancer (IARC, 1986, p. 313). The conclusion was based on the evaluation of findings from nine cohort studies (Doll and Peto, 1976; Kahn, 1966; Lossing et al, 1966; Hammond and Horn, 1958; Hammond, 1966; Cederlöf et al, 1975; Weir and Dunn, 1970; Hirayama, 1981; Heuch et al, 1983) and eight case-control studies (Wynder et al, 1973, 1983; Lin and Kessler, 1981; MacMahon et al, 1981; Whittemore et al, 1983; Durbec et al, 1983; Kinlen and McPherson, 1984; Polissar et al, 1984). All of the cohort studies and all but one of the case-control studies showed increased risks for smokers and most had evidence of a positive dose-response. Relative risk estimates are around 2-fold, with some as high as 6-fold in association with high exposure. In the one case-control study (hospital-based) (Lin and Kessler, 1981) that did not show a positive association between smoking and pancreatic cancer, a design flaw was cited in the IARC report—the control group contained smoking-related diseases. Studies subsequent to the IARC report support its conclusions, including three cohort studies (Hirayama 1988; Hiatt et al, 1988; Mills et al, 1988) and seventeen case-control studies (Mack et al, 1986; Norell et al, 1986a; Hsieh et al, 1986; Wynder et al, 1986; La Vecchia et al, 1987, Falk et al, 1988, Olsen et al, 1989; Cuzick and Babiker, 1989; Farrow and Davis, 1990a; Baghurst et al, 1991; Bueno de Mesquita et al, 1991a; Howe et al, 1991; Ghadirian et al, 1991b; Lyon et al, 1992b; Mizuno et al, 1992; Friedman and van den Eeden, 1993; Zatonski et al, 1993). A recent hospital-based case-control study reported finding no association (Clavel et al, 1989); although, the odds ratios (ORs) reported are consistent with an increased risk with cigarette smoking.

Howe et al (1991) reported a rapid decrease in risk with time since quitting. Many studies report a relative risk estimate in former smokers that is lower than in current smokers; indeed, in some studies the difference in risk between never smokers and ex-smokers is not statistically significant (Falk et al, 1988; Farrow and Davis, 1990a; Bueno de Mesquita, 1991a; Howe et al, 1991; Ghadirian et al, 1991b; Friedman and van den Eeden, 1993).

Wynder et al (1983) reported a 2-fold increased risk associated with pipe and cigar smoking, but this has not been found by others (Kahn, 1966; Williams and Horm, 1977; Mack et al, 1986; Falk et al, 1988; Farrow and Davis, 1990a; Bueno de Mesquita, 1991a; Howe et al, 1991).

Diet

The pancreas is, of course, intimately related to digestion and absorption and since diet is implicated in the cause and modulation of cancer at other gastrointestinal sites, it is reasonable to place diet high among the possible causal elements for pancreatic carcinoma (Longnecker, 1990; Willett and MacMahon, 1984a, b). In considering the relation with dietary constituents, however, it is worth bearing in mind that, unlike every other part of the gastrointestinal tract, the pancreas is never exposed either directly (mouth to anus) or indirectly (liver) to ingested foods or their modified, digested, and absorbed products. Accordingly, the effects of diet on pancreatic carcinogenesis must be via changes in the internal metabolic environment of that organ, exposure to blood-borne agents, or (more likely) both. The empirical approach, via ecologic studies, to the question of the relation between diet and pancreas cancer has raised interest in fat (Lea, 1967; Segi and Kurihara, 1972; Ghadirian et al, 1991d), eggs (Lea, 1967; Armstrong and Doll, 1975; Ghadirian et al, 1991d), animal protein (Lea, 1967; Armstrong and Doll, 1975; Ghadirian et al, 1991d), milk (Lea, 1967; Ghadirian et al, 1991d), and sugar (Yanai et al, 1979).

A number of individual-level studies have examined dietary habits in relation to pancreatic cancer risk and although the dietary data are not quite as consistent as the data on smoking, investigators have generally found increased risks associated with animal protein and fat consumption and decreased risks associated with vegetable and fruit intake.

Animal Products. The risk factors—meats, grilled meat, and fat—are closely correlated in the diet and can be regarded either as risk factors in their own right or as markers for a specific common exposure. Positive associations in individual-level studies have been described with fat intake (Durbec et al, 1983); beef and bacon (Mack et al, 1986); fried and grilled meat (Norell et al, 1986a); pork, beef, and dairy foods (Falk et al, 1988) (Table 35–2). Other studies have reported elevated risks associated with intake of beef, pork, and dairy products (Olsen et al, 1989); eggs, pork, and fish, but not beef (Bueno de Mesquita et al, 1991b); beef, chicken, and pork (Farrow and Davis, 1990b). Hirayama's study (1981, 1989) of diet and pancreas cancer in a Japanese cohort indicated an increased risk for daily meat consumption. La Vecchia et al (1990) reported inconsistent findings with respect to meat, animal protein, and fat intake, with elevated risks for ham and eggs, a marginally increased risk for meat, and decreased risks associated with fish and dairy products. Mills et al (1988) reported an increased risk with consumption of meat and eggs that disappeared after controlling for smoking while Gold and colleagues (1985) reported an increased risk associated with butter, but not eggs or meat. Baghurst found that cases reported a higher consumption of boiled eggs and omelettes, but no consistent findings among men and women were reported for meat intake (Baghurst et al, 1991). Raymond et al (1987) found that meat intake did not alter the risk except for lean pork, which was associated with a decreased risk. In the same study, the authors found an excess risk associated with increased consumption of butter, but margarine was associated with a decreased risk. Mizuno et al (1992) found no elevated risks associated with meat consumption in a case-control study in Japan, but found that daily fish and milk consumption were both inversely associated with the disease.

Vegetables and Fruits. In a recent review of the epidemiological literature on vegetables, fruit, and cancer, Steinmetz and Potter (1991a) cite seven studies that examined the association between vegetable and fruit consumption and pancreatic cancer (Norell et al, 1986a; Gold et al, 1985; Mack et al, 1986; Voirol et al, 1987; Falk et al, 1988; Olsen et al, 1989; Farrow and Davis, 1990b); five of the seven reported statistically significant inverse associations between cancer of the pancreas and one or more fruits or vegetables (see Table 35–2). In six studies, each OR presented suggested an inverse association between vegetable and fruit consumption and pancreatic cancer, although the associations were not found consistently with particular items. Three case-control studies published subsequent to the above review have also analyzed food groups (Baghurst et al, 1991; La Vecchia et al, 1990; Bueno de Mesquita et al, 1991b). Baghurst et al (1991) reported on a general pattern of lower fruit juice and vegetable consumption among the cases compared with controls, but ORs were not provided. Bueno de Mesquita et al (1991b) reported significant inverse associations for daily intake of vegetables and several subgroups of vegetables, while La Vecchia et al (1990) reported a decreasing trend in risk associated with higher intakes of both vegetables and fresh fruit, statistically significant for the latter.

Of the above studies that examined the relations with subgroups of vegetables and fruit, Norell et al (1986a) found the most extreme OR for carrots (0.3); Olsen et al (1989) for cruciferous vegetables (0.6); Voirol et al (1987) for both vegetables (0.5) and fruit (0.5); Falk et al (1988) for fruit (0.6); La Vecchia et al (1990) for fruit (0.7); and Bueno de Mesquita et al (1991b) for low-fiber vegetables (0.3). Farrow and Davis (1990b) found a slightly and nonsignificantly *higher* consumption of green and yellow vegetables by cases than controls, but no association for any other vegetable or fruit subgroup.

Mills et al (1988) analyzed mortality data in a cohort study of Seventh-Day Adventists and reported a reduced risk in association with higher consumption of vegetable protein products, for pulses (beans, lentils, and peas), and for dried fruit.

Our overall interpretation of these data is that there is indeed a lower risk associated with a lifestyle that includes a higher intake of plant foods, that this is probably a causal association, but that it is not confined to a specific group or groups of plant food although the association with cereals is ambiguous at best (see below).

Cereals and Sugar. Some authors have reported *increased* risks associated with carbohydrate food groups, for example, rice, breads and cereals (Falk et al, 1988), white bread (Gold et al, 1985), breads and cereals (Olsen et al, 1989), pasta (Raymond et al, 1987), and refined sugar (Baghurst et al, 1991). On the other hand, Mack et al (1986) reported a decreased risk associated with whole grain-breads.

Nutrients. Howe et al (1991) reported on the nutrient data gathered on 802 cases from five simultaneous case-control studies of pancreatic cancer and diet conducted

TABLE 35–2. *Studies of Diet and Pancreas Cancer*

Authors (year)	*Study Type and Size*[a]	*Comparison*[b]	*Relative Risk Estimate by Control Category*	
VEGETABLES AND FRUIT				
Gold et al (1985)	Hospital-based case-control 201/402	*Raw fruits & vegetables*	*Hospital*	*Population*
		Ever vs never	0.5	0.2[c]
		≥ vs <2/week	0.5[c]	0.7
		≥ vs <5/week	0.6[c]	0.6[c]
Mack et al (1986)	Population-based case control 490/490	*Fresh fruits or vegetables*	*Direct Interview*	*All*
		≤5/week	1.0	1.0
		≥5/week	0.8	0.7[c]
Norell et al (1986a)	Population-based case control 99/301	*Vegetables*	*Hospital*	*Population*
		<1/week	1.0	1.0
		Every week	1.0	1.0
		Almost daily	0.5	0.8
		Raw vegetables		
		<1/week	1.0	1.0
		Every week	0.5[d]	0.7
		Almost daily	0.5	0.6
		Citrus fruits		
		<1/week	1.0	1.0
		Every week	0.6	1.0
		Almost daily	0.3[d]	0.5[d]
		Fruit juices		
		<1/week	1.0	1.0
		Every week	0.9	0.6
		Almost daily	0.6	0.6
Voirol et al (1987), Raymond (1987)	Population-based control 88/336	*Vegetables*		*Population*
		<1110 g/week		1.0
		1110–1609 g/week		0.87
		≥1610 g/week		0.47[d]
		Fruits		
		<280 g/week		1.0
		280–619 g/week		1.1
		≥620 g/week		0.56
Falk et al (1988)	Hospital-based case control 363/1,234	*Fruits & juices*	*Male*	*Female*
		<25/month	1.0	1.0
		25-63/month	0.6[c]	0.6
		≥64/month	0.4[c]	0.5[c]
Mills et al (1988)	Cohort 40/193,483	*Beans, lentils, peas*	*Noncases*	
		<1/week	1.0	
		≥3/week	0.4	
		Dried fruits (quintiles)		
		<1/month	1.0	
		≥3/week	0.4[c]	
		Vegetarian protein products		
		<1/week	1.0	
		≥3/week	0.4[c]	
		Green salad	<1.0	
		Cooked green vegetables	<1.0	
Hirayama (1989)	Cohort 679/265,118[e] × 17y follow-up	*Green yellow vegetables*	No difference between cases and noncases	
Olsen (1989)	Mortality-based case-control 212/220	*Cruciferous vegetables*	*Population*[f]	
		≤2/month	1.0	
		≥9/month	0.6	
		Noncruciferous vegetables		
		≤16/month		1.0
		17–31/month		0.55[c]
		≥32/month		0.95
		Fruit & juices		
		≤21/month		1.0
		≥53/month		0.88

(continued)

TABLE 35–2. *(Continued)*

Authors (year)	*Study Type and Size*[a]	*Comparison*[b]	*Relative Risk Estimate by Control Category*	
Farrow & Davis (1990b)	Population-based case-control 148/188	*Vegetables*	*Population*	
		U vs L quartile	No association	
		Raw vegetables		
		U vs L quartile		No association
		Green & yellow vegetables		
		U vs L quartile		No association
		Fruit		
		U vs L quartile		No association
		Citrus fruit		
		U vs L quartile		No association
La Vecchia (1990)	Hospital-based case-control 247/1,089	*Fresh fruit* (tertiles)		*Population*
		1		1.0
		3		0.68[c]
		Green vegetables (tertiles)		
		1	1.0	
		3	0.84	
Bueno de Mesquita (1991b)	Population-based case-control 164/480	*Vegetables* (quintiles)	*Direct Interview*	All
		1	1.0	1.0
		5	0.22[g]	0.34[g]
		Cooked vegetables (quintiles)		
		1	1.0	1.0
		5	0.32[g]	0.35[g]
		Raw vegetables (quintiles)		
		1	1.0	1.0
		5	0.30[g]	0.42[g]
		Fruits total (quintiles)		
		1	-	1.0
		5	-	1.1
		Fruit juices (quintiles)		
		1	-	1.0
		5	-	0.77
Baghurst et al (1991)	Population-based case-control 104/253	**Cases consuming less than controls**	*Male*	*Female*
		Tomato	$0.01<p<0.05$	$0.01<p<0.05$
		Dried grapes	$p<0.01$	$p<0.01$
Mizuno et al (1992)	Hospital-based case-control 124/124	*Green, yellow vegetables*	*Hospital*	
		Daily vs less often	1.2	
		Other vegetables		
		Daily vs less often	0.71	
		Fruit		
		Daily vs less often	0.62	
MEAT, EGGS, AND DAIRY PRODUCTS				
Gold et al (1985)	Hospital-based case-control 201/402	*Butter*	*Hospital*	*Population*
		<2 vs >2/week	2.4[c]	1.1
		Deep fried foods	<1.0	
		Beef	<1.0	
Mack et al (1986)	Population-based case-control 490/490	*Beef*	*Direct Interview*	*All*
		<5/week	1.0	1.0
		≥5/week	2.1[c]	1.2
		Eggs		
		<5/week	1.0	1.0
		≥5/week	0.7	0.8
		Fried bacon/ham		
		<5/week	1.0	1.0
		≥5/week	1.4	0.9

(continued)

TABLE 35–2. *Studies of Diet and Pancreas Cancer (Continued)*

Authors (year)	*Study Type and Size*[a]	*Comparison*[b]	*Relative Risk Estimate by Control Category*	
Norell et al (1986a)	Population-based case-control 99/301	*Fried/grilled meat*	*Hospital*	*Population*
		<1/week	1.0	1.0
		Every week	1.5	1.7[d]
		Almost daily	4.6[d]	13.4[d]
Voirol et al (1987), Raymond (1987)	Population-based case-control 88/336	*Red meat*		*Population*
		<480 g/week		1.0
		≥480 g/week		0.77
		Poultry		
		<18 g/week		1.0
		18–59 g/week		1.6
		≥60 g/week		1.1
		Lean pork		
		0 g/week		1.0
		<150 g/week		0.44
		>150 g/week		0.62
		Butter		
		<108 g/week		1.0
		108–194 g/week		1.4
		≥195 g/week		2.0[d]
		Margarine		
		any vs none		0.35[d]
		Whole milk		
		0 ml/week		1.0
		<630 ml/week		1.2
		≥630 ml/week		
Falk et al (1988)	Hospital-based case-control 363/1,234	*Beef*	*Male*	*Female*
		<6/month	1.0	1.0
		6–15 month	1.2	0.8
		≥16/month	1.1	0.7
		Pork		
		<9/month	1.0	1.0
		9–30/month	1.4	1.6
		≥31/month	1.7[c]	1.3
		Dairy		
		<34/month	1.0	1.0
		34–67/month	1.6	1.6
		≥68/month	2.2[c]	1.0
		Seafood		
		<2/month	1.0	1.0
		2–7/month	1.0	1.2
		≥8/month	1.0	1.9
Mills et al (1988)	Cohort 40/193,483	*Current use of meat, poultry, fish* </week 1–2/week ≥/week	*Noncases*	
			1.0	
			0.8	
			2.2	
		Current use of eggs <1/week 1–2/week ≥3/week	1.0	
			1.5	
			2.5[c]	
		Butter	~1.0	
		Milk	~1.0	
Hirayama (1989)	Cohort 679/265,118[e] × 17y follow-up	*Meat*[h] Never Occasionally Daily	1.0	
			1.4	
			1.8	
Olsen et al (1989)	Mortality-based case-control 212/220	*Beef* ≤8/month≥18/month		*Population*
				1.0
				11.8

(continued)

TABLE 35–2. *(Continued)*

Authors (year)	*Study Type and Size*[a]	*Comparison*[b]	*Relative Risk Estimate by Control Category*	
		Pork≤2/month ≥9/month		
				1.0
				1.9
		Poultry ≤2/month ≥6/month		
				1.0
				0.95
Farrow & Davis (1990b)	Population-based case-control 148/188	*Beef* <1.6/week 2.5–4.0/ week>4.0/week	*Population*	
			1.0	
			2.4[c]	
			2.8[c]	
		Chicken <0.71/week 1.1–2.0/week >2.0/week		
			1.0	
			1.8	
			2.5[c]	
		Pork <0.21/week 0.51–1.0/week >1.0/week		
			1.0	
			1.3	
			1.7	
La Vecchia et al (1990)	Hospital-based case-control 247/1,089	*Meat* (tertiles) 1 3	*Hospital*	
			1.0	
			1.1	
		Ham (tertiles) 1 3		
			1.0	
			1.4	
		Fish (tertiles) 1 3		
			1.0	
			0.74	
		Eggs (tertiles) 1 3		
			1.0	
			1.4	
		Milk (tertiles) 1 3		
			1.0	
			0.67	
Bueno de Mesquita (1991b)	Population-based case-control 164/480	*Pork* (quintiles)	*Direct Interview*	All
		1	—	1.0
		5	—	1.4
		Beef (quintiles)		
		1	—	1.0
		5	—	0.51
		Fish (quintiles)		
		1	1.0	1.0
		5	2.5[g]	1.8
		Cheese (quintiles)		
		1	1.0	1.0
		5	0.44	1.81
		Eggs (quintiles)		
		1	1.0	1.0
		5	1.6	2.2[g]
		Milk & milk products (quintiles)		
		1	—	1.0
		5	—	0.78
		Oil & fats (quintiles)		
		1	1.0	1.0
		5	—	1.1
Baghurst et al (1991)	Population-based case-control 104/254	**Cases consuming more than controls**	*Male*	*Female*
		Omelette	$0.01<p<0.05$	$p<0.01$
		Boiled egg	$p<0.01$	$p<0.01$
		Cases consuming less than controls	$0.01<p<0.05$	No association
		Fried fish		

(continued)

TABLE 35–2. *Studies of Diet and Pancreas Cancer (Continued)*

Authors (year)	*Study Type and Size*[a]	*Comparison*[b]	*Relative Risk Estimate by Control Category*
Mizuno et al (1992)	Hospital-based case-control 124/124	*Meat*	*Hospital*
		Every day vs less often	1.18
		Fish	
		Every day vs less often	0.56[c]
		Milk	
		Every day vs less often	0.41[c]

[a]Study size as cases/controls or cases/person-years.
[b]Frequency of consumption or quantiles.
[c]95% CI excludes 1.0.
[d]90% CI excludes 1.0.
[e]Initial cohort size.
[f]All interviews were indirect.
[g]p for trends <0.05.
[h]Also shows there is an interaction with smoking.
g = grams; U = uppermost; L = lowermost.

under the auspices of the International Agency for Research on Cancer (IARC). Individual groups that contributed to the IARC study have also published their study-specific findings on some of the same factors (Baghurst et al, 1991; Zatonski et al, 1991, 1993; Ghadirian et al, 1991b, c; Bueno de Mesquita et al, 1990, 1991b, 1992a, b; Howe et al, 1990; Jain et al, 1991). When relative risks were estimated with highest versus lowest quintiles of consumption in the combined analysis, inverse associations were found with dietary fiber (OR = 0.5, 95% CI, 0.3–0.6) and vitamin C (OR = 0.5, 95% CI, 0.4–0.8); and increased risks were observed for higher intake of carbohydrate (OR = 2.57, 95% CI, 1.6–4.0) and cholesterol (OR = 2.7, 95% CI, 1.7–4.2), but not fat. The estimates were derived using a model that adjusted for energy by the calorie-partition method of Howe (1989). The authors examined the relation of disease risk with total energy intake and reported that the strong positive association was almost entirely due to the positive association with total carbohydrate intake—both simple and complex. They also noted that the relations were generally consistent among all five studies.

Four other case-control studies have reported on associations between pancreatic cancer and nutrients (Durbec et al, 1983; Falk et al, 1988; Farrow and Davis, 1990b; Olsen et al, 1991). Falk et al (1988) found a significant inverse trend for vitamin C in both men and women. Durbec et al (1983) found a positive association for fat intake and an inverse association for carbohydrates—both were statistically significant. Farrow and Davis (1990b) analyzed data from their study, using the residual method of Willett and Stampfer (1986) (see also Willett, 1990). They found no associations for fats, cholesterol, or vitamins A and C; they reported a positive association for total protein consumption that appeared to be largely due to meat consumption (their findings in relation to meat are described above), and they reported an unexpected finding of an inverse association between calcium intake and disease risk. Olsen et al (1991) also reported risk estimates for energy-adjusted nutrient intake [residual method of Willett and Stampfer (1986)]; inverse trends were observed for polyunsaturated fat, linoleic acid, vitamin C, and beta-carotene. Positive trends were associated with retinol and riboflavin. No significant associations were found for carbohydrates or calcium. In contrast to findings in studies by Durbec et al (1983) and Farrow and Davis (1990b), Olsen et al (1991) found that caloric intake was 10% higher in cases than controls.

In a nested case-control analysis of data from a longitudinal study conducted in Washington County, Maryland, Burney et al (1989) compared prediagnostic serum micronutrient levels in individuals who subsequently developed cancer of the pancreas and their matched controls. The samples were assayed for several carotenoids, vitamin E, and selenium. The authors reported statistically significant lower levels of the carotenoid, lycopene (a major source is tomatoes), and, in men only, selenium, in cases than controls.

Overall, the nutrient data do not appear to provide much more information than the food analyses. In general, meat, animal protein, and fat seem associated with increased risk and vegetables and fruit and the micronutrients of which they are significant sources are associated with decreased risk. Only cereals and carbohydrates present unclear associations.

Coffee. The possibility that coffee consumption might be related to pancreatic cancer was first suggested by a study (Stocks, 1970) of correlations between cigarette and beverage consumption and cancer mortality. The author found an inconsistent correlation between coffee consumption and mortality from pancreas cancer, based largely on the coincidence of the two in northern Europe. No correlation was found with use of cigarettes or tea.

In 1981, a 2- to 3-fold increased risk was reported for coffee drinkers of three cups per day in a case-control study; the effect was not explained by the observed effect of smoking (MacMahon et al, 1981). This report generated a great deal of publicity and controversy. The findings were criticized on methodologic grounds (Feinstein et al, 1981). Important among these was the exclusion of potential controls with gastrointestinal disease or cancer without having assessed the possible effect these conditions might have had on coffee-drinking habits. A second flaw was the exclusion of possible controls with diseases known to be associated with smoking or alcohol without knowledge of the effect that exclusion might have on the distribution of coffee-drinking among the remaining controls. Gordis (1990) reviewed 30 epidemiologic studies addressing the relation between coffee and pancreatic cancer. He concluded that the current epidemiologic evidence does not support the hypothesis that coffee consumption increases the risk of pancreatic cancer. He argued that, despite certain ecologic and case-control studies that suggest an association, 14 of 17 case-control studies and six of six prospective studies show no statistically significant increased risk.

An IARC working group on the evaluation of carcinogenic risks to humans also assessed the epidemiologic evidence for the association with coffee (IARC, 1991). Evaluating 21 case-control studies and six cohort studies [a largely overlapping subset of that examined by Gordis et al (1990)], the authors concluded that the data as a whole were suggestive of a weak relation between high levels of coffee consumption and pancreatic cancer, but that bias or confounding might account for the association. They also reported that, although the results with decaffeinated coffee were less comprehensive, they were generally null. The same working group examined the evidence on the relation between tea consumption and pancreatic cancer; three of four cohort studies found no association and one reported a small inverse association. Only one of six case-control studies designed to evaluate the relation found an increased risk.

Of the subsequent case-control studies, most have been null for coffee consumption (Farrow and Davis, 1990a; Jain et al, 1991; Baghurst et al, 1991; Bueno de Mesquita, 1992a; Mizuno et al, 1992; Friedman and van den Eeden, 1993; Zatonski et al, 1993); at least one has been positive (Lyon et al, 1992b), and one, (Ghadirian et al, 1991b) reported a statistically nonsignificant lower risk among coffee drinkers than among nondrinkers. In a Japanese cohort, Hirayama (1989) reported a positive association. The possibility that coffee is associated with a small, but real, increased risk of pancreatic cancer remains; however, it appears likely that the increased risk associated with coffee results from residual confounding with cigarette smoking or, possibly, from other sources of confounding or bias.

Alcohol. It was first suggested by Dörken (1964), in discussing the findings of a case-series, that alcohol abuse may increase the risk of pancreatic adenocarcinoma. In an ecologic study, Hinds et al (1980), in Hawaii, found an association with beer consumption that is largely explainable by a single value. In several other ecologic studies, alcohol consumption is not correlated with pancreatic cancer incidence in the United States (Blot et al, 1978), Japan (Kono and Ikeda, 1979), or internationally (Sarles, 1973).

Among the first individual-level studies, case-control studies using hospital controls showed positive associations (Burch and Ansari, 1968; Ishii et al, 1968; Lin and Kessler, 1981), but the lack of detail about control selection in each instance reduces confidence in the findings. One similarly designed study was null (Wynder, 1973a). A case-control study using consenting cases from the Third National Cancer Survey, and other cancer patients as a comparison, found a small excess risk of pancreas cancer in male drinkers, but the effect disappeared after controlling for smoking (Williams and Horm, 1977). Durbec et al (1983) reported an increased risk associated with beer and wine, but not spirits.

In the first cohort studies, results were generally null, although in some studies the results were inconclusive because of small numbers. Of 4370 Finnish alcoholics observed for less than 4 years (Hakulinen et al, 1974), four cases of pancreatic cancer were observed compared with two expected. A proportional mortality analysis of the 909 deaths identified among 1382 known alcoholics revealed 3 deaths compared with 5.2 expected (Monson and Lyon, 1975). Klatsky et al (1981) found 6 deaths among individuals with reported consumption of six or more alcoholic drinks per day compared with 2 among matched nondrinkers in a follow-up study of members of a health plan (RR = 3.0 [95% CI, 1.1–6.5]).

In a cohort study of nearly 17,000 Norwegians, Heuch et al (1983) found a relative risk of 2.7 [95% CI, 1.2–6.4—calculated by Velema et al (1986)] among those who drank at least 14 times per month compared to those who did not drink or who drank infrequently.

In a cohort study of over 14,000 Danish brewery workers (Jensen, 1979), the observed number of cases did not differ significantly from the number expected.

In 1986, Velema et al reviewed the literature and argued that evidence for a causal association was weak and that neither total alcohol consumption nor any specific type of alcohol showed a strong and consistent relation. They pointed out that there is a degree of selection bias in case identification in case-control studies and that this could possibly be associated with alcohol consumption. However, cohort studies do not produce consistently stronger or more consistent evidence for a casual association than case-control studies. There remains a suggestion that chronic high intake may increase the risk.

A number of subsequent studies have reported no consistent associations. In Japan, 265,118 adults (a population-based sample) were followed for 17 years. Data were analyzed using the 679 incident cases that occurred during the follow-up (Hirayama, 1989). While an association was found (risk ratio 2.8 [95% CI, 1.2–6.2]) among a small group of Japanese whiskey drinkers), there was no overall association with alcohol consumption in the cohort. Using a pooled analysis of three case-control studies from Italy, France, and Switzerland (La Vecchia et al, 1987; Raymond et al, 1987; Clavel et al, 1989), Bouchardy et al (1990) reported on 494 cases and 1704 controls. The authors found no consistent association with consumption of wine, beer, or spirits, nor any evidence of a dose-response. Other case-control studies with generally null findings for alcohol include those of Mack et al (1986), Norell et al (1986a), Falk et al (1988), Farrow and Davis (1990a), Jain et al (1991), Ghadirian et al (1991b), Bueno de Mesquita et al (1992a), Lyon et al (1992b), Mizuno et al (1992), Friedman and van den Eeden (1993). On the other hand, Olsen et al (1989) found positive associations with heavy consumption of beer, hard liquor, and total alcohol, but the elevations in risks were not statistically significant. Cuzick and Babiker (1989) also found elevated risks associated with alcohol consumption, particularly beer; the authors speculated that any role of alcohol in the etiology of pancreatic cancer is likely to be among heavy drinkers and of importance only in smokers; this view is close to the current consensus.

Occupation and Industry

Descriptive information about occupation and industry is especially difficult to interpret because of the hundreds of categories, the uncertainty of the significance—from a toxicological or carcinogenic exposure viewpoint—of job titles, the variety of ways in which they can be classified, and the low frequency of observations in each. It is inevitable that many associations between single occupations and single outcomes will be observed, and that many of these will be the result of chance. Nonetheless, attempts to quantify the risk from the workplace have proceeded in one of several ways. Links between the workplace and disease have been screened by analyzing the employment described on the death certificates of all decedents in a defined population, or on the hospital charts of all cancer cases diagnosed in a population or in a large hospital. The members of many cohorts defined by occupation, employment in a company or industry, insured status, or union membership have been followed until death, or, in some cases, by recording all cancer diagnoses among the members. In general, it has not been possible to analyze the available information on an individual basis or to consider alternative explanations for the associations found. There have also been a few individual-level case-control studies in which occupation has been examined; again, the number of cases with any single occupational exposure is usually small.

Population-based mortality or morbidity studies of occupation and cancer, including pancreas cancer, have been conducted in the United States (Guralnick, 1963; Williams et al, 1977), the United Kingdom (Registrar General, 1978; Logan, 1982), Denmark (Olsen and Jensen, 1987), Norway (Central Bureau of Statistics, 1976), Washington State (Milham, 1976), California (Petersen and Milham, 1980), Illinois (Mallin et al, 1989), three English counties (Magnani et al, 1987), New Orleans (Pickle and Gottlieb, 1980), Los Angeles (Mack and Paganini-Hill, 1981), and Tokyo (Ishii, 1968). Information about pancreas cancer has come from similar studies of multiple outcomes using hospital patients in New York City (Cubilla and Fitzgerald, 1978a), Buffalo, New York (DeCouflé et al, 1977a), and Rochester, New York (Maruchi et al, 1979), and in representative groups defined in other ways in Canada (Best et al, 1966) and Japan (Hirayama, 1975, 1978). Occupational results have been reported from population-based case-control studies in New York City (Wynder, 1973a), Baltimore (Lin and Kessler, 1981), Los Angeles (Mack et al, 1985), Stockholm (Norell et al, 1986c), Paris (Pietri et al, 1990), and Louisiana (Falk et al, 1990). Positive results from at least 18 occupational cohorts have been reported; in a few of these a superimposed case-control analysis did permit the occupational findings to be adjusted individually for other exposures (Hanis et al, 1982; Garabrant, 1992).

The positive results of the published inquiries are shown in Table 35–3; many comparisons were part of almost every study, and while many of the differences found were statistically significant, the tests of significance are hard to interpret and have not been presented. The following summarizes the most interesting findings.

Asbestos. One observation suggestive of an increased risk for pancreas cancer among workers exposed to crocidolite has been reported (Newhouse et al, 1988). More cases than controls reported past asbestos expo-

TABLE 35–3. *Occupations Reported to be at High Risk of Pancreas Cancer*

Occupation/Exposure	Place	Reported by	Year
	Risk Ratio >OR = 2.0		
>10 UNEXPECTED CASES			
Engineers	Sheffield, U.K.	Turner and Grace	1938
Professionals and technicians	Japan	Hirayama	1978
Acetylene production (crocidolite)	Bilston, U.K.	Newhouse et al[b]	1988
Assemblers	Illinois	Mallin et al	1989
Sales/Commodities	Illinois	Mallin et al	1989
Clerks/administrative staff	Illinois	Mallin et al	1989
Asbestos	South Louisiana	Falk et al[a]	1990
Cotton dust	South Louisiana	Falk et al[a]	1990
4–9 UNEXPECTED CASES			
Stationary engineers	Washington	Milham	1976
Aluminum mill workers	Washington	Milham	1976
Nurserymen	Washington	Milham	1976
Motion picture projectionists	Washington	Milham	1976
Stone cutters	Washington	Milham	1976
Mechanics and repairmen	Buffalo, NY	Viadana et al[b]	1976
Metal craftsmen	Olmsted Co, MN	Maruchi et al	1979
Cement finishers	California	Peterson & Milham	1980
Airplane mechanics	California	Peterson & Milham	1980
Oil refinery workers	New Orleans, LA	Pickle & Gottlieb	1980
Managers and administrators	Baltimore, MD	Lin & Kessler[a]	1981
Dry cleaners, service station workers, garagemen	Baltimore, MD	Lin & Kessler[a]	1981
Coke oven workers	Allegheny Co, PA	Redmond[bc]	1983
Thorium-processing workers	Illinois	Polednak et al[b]	1983
Dyestuffs	Los Angeles, CA	Mack et al[a]	1985
Chemical company workers	U.S.A.	Bond et al[b]	1985
Tire-curing	U.S.A.	Delzell & Monson[b]	1985
Auto engine/parts mfg workers	New York	Vena et al[bc]	1985
Welding materials	Stockholm, Sweden	Norell et al[a]	1986c
Cleaning agents	Stockholm, Sweden	Norell et al[a]	1986c
Methylene chloride in film mfg	Rochester, NY	Hearne et al[b]	1987
Metal/cutting oil workers	Connecticut	Silverstein et al[bc]	1988
Auto mechanics	Denmark	Hansen[b]	1989
Sales/business services	Illinois	Mallin et al	1989
Photoengravers/lithographers	Illinois	Mallin et al	1989
Brickmasons/stonemasons	Illinois	Mallin et al	1989
Misc moving equipment operators	Illinois	Mallin et al	1989
Sheet metal workers	Illinois	Mallin et al	1989
Plant, system operators	Illinois	Mallin et al	1989
Crane and tower operators	Illinois	Mallin et al	1989
Precision metal workers	Illinois	Mallin et al	1989
Moving equipment operators	Illinois	Mallin et al	1989
Mechanic/machine operators	South Louisiana	Falk et al[a]	1990
Chlorhydrins	Connecticut	Greenberg et al	1990
DDT/Related compound mfg	Philadelphia, PA	Garabrant et al[ac]	1992

(continued)

TABLE 35–3. *Occupations Reported to be at High Risk of Pancreas Cancer (Continued)*

Occupation/Exposure	*Place*	*Reported by*	*Year*
2–3 UNEXPECTED CASES			
Bus, taxi, truck drivers	Buffalo, NY	Viadana et al	1967
Beta-naphthylamine/benzidine	Pittsburgh, PA	Mancuso & El-Attar[b]	1967
Managers	Tokyo, Japan	Ishii et al	1968
Service workers	Tokyo, Japan	Ishii et al	1968
Chemists	Washington	Milham	1976
Stationary engineers	Buffalo, NY	Decouflé et al	1977
Primary metal workers	Buffalo, NY	Decouflé et al	1977
Machine operators, miscellaneous	United States	Williams et al	1977
Printing workers	United States	Williams et al	1977
Construction workers	United States	Williams et al	1977
Hairdressers	New York, NY	Cubilla & Fitzgerald	1978
Telegraph operators	California	Peterson & Milham	1980
Stationary engineers	California	Peterson & Milham	1980
Tanners	Linkoping, Sweden	Edling et al[b]	1986
Butchers	3 English counties	Magnani et al	1987
Fish filleters, fish shops	3 English counties	Magnani et al	1987
Traffic, shipping, receiving clerks	Illinois	Mallin et al	1989
	Risk Ratio 1.4–1.9		
>10 UNEXPECTED CASES			
Electric fitters	United Kingdom	Registrar General	1954
Mine workers	United States	Guralnick	1963
Metal workers	United States	Guralnick	1963
Chemists	United States	Li et al[b]	1969
Civil servants	Washington	Milham	1976
Sawmill workers	Washington	Milham	1976
Insurance agents	Washington	Milham	1976
Electrical machinery manufacture	Los Angeles, CA	Mack & Paganini-Hill	1981
Professionals/managers	Southern Louisiana	Falk et al[a]	1990
Paint sprays	Southern Louisiana	Falk et al[a]	1990
Supervisors, precision production	Illinois	Mallin et al	1989
4–9 UNEXPECTED CASES			
Fishermen	United Kingdom	Registrar General	1954
Coal, gas, coke workers	United Kingdom	Registrar General	1954
Merchant seamen	Sweden	Otterland[b]	1967
Produce buyers, shippers	Washington	Milham	1976
Dentists	Washington	Milham	1976
Furniture store workers	Washington	Milham	1976
Civil servants	Washington	Milham	1976
Managers and administrators	Washington	Milham	1976
Cranemen and derrickmen	Washington	Milham	1976
Canning and food processing	Washington	Milham	1976
Delivery men	Washington	Milham	1976
Fruit warehousemen	Washington	Milham	1976
Sheetmetal workers	Washington	Milham	1976
Managers and administrators	Washington	Milham	1976
Farmers	United States	Williams et al	1977
Paper mill workers	United States	Williams et al	1977
Produce buyers, shippers	New Orleans, LA	Pickle & Gottlieb	1980
Civil servants	California	Peterson & Milham	1980
	California	Peterson & Milham	1980

(continued)

TABLE 35–3. (*Continued*)

Occupation/Exposure	*Place*	*Reported by*	*Year*
4–9 UNEXPECTED CASES (continued)			
Managers and administrators	California	Peterson & Milham	1980
Jewelers	Attleboro, MA	Sparks & Wegman[b]	1980
Petroleum refining/petrochemicals	Texas	Thomas et al[b]	1980
Refinery/chemical plant workers	Baton Rouge, LA	Hanis et al[b]	1982
Petrol stations	Stockholm, Sweden	Norell et al[a]	1986c
Textile manufacturing workers	Denmark	Olsen & Jensen	1987
Textile spinning, weaving, finishing	Denmark	Olsen & Jensen	1987
Baking	Denmark	Olsen & Jensen	1987
Textile mfg	Paris, France	Pietri et al[a]	1990
Hairdressers	Finland	Pukkala et al[b]	1992

[a]Analytic case-control study of individuals, adjusted for other determinants.
[b]Cohort study of individuals, not adjusted.
[c] Evidence of dose/response relation.

sure in one case-control study (Falk et al, 1990), and high risk has also been reported among auto mechanics, who also experience significant asbestos exposure (Hansen, 1989). However, in asbestos workers, the cohort most intensively exposed to asbestos, no excess of pancreas cancer was found (Selikoff and Seidman, 1981).

Ionizing Radiation. Initial analyses of the occurrence of pancreatic cancer among British radiologists indicated a possible excess, but the study of U. S. radiologists (Matanoski, 1975) and a more complete follow-up of the British cohort (Smith and Doll, 1981) have suggested otherwise. Similarly, when atomic workers at the Hanford plant in Washington State were initially examined (Mancuso et al, 1977) and re-examined (Hutchison et al, 1979; Gilbert and Marks, 1979), it was concluded that an excess risk had occurred in the highest of six radiation dose categories, but subsequent follow-up has failed to confirm the excess (Tolley et al, 1983). Other than a study showing increased risk in workers exposed to thorium processing (Polednak et al, 1983), there is currently no evidence of a link between pancreas cancer and occupational exposure to radiation (Committee BEIR V, 1990).

Fossil Fuel Products. Knowledge of the link between cigarette smoking and pancreas cancer suggests the possibility that pancreas cancer might also be caused by other organic materials, especially if these have been subjected to incomplete combustion. Consistent with such a suggestion are the observed increases in risk that have been recorded among workers exposed to various forms of petroleum products (Registrar General, 1954; Pickle and Gottlieb, 1980; Thomas et al, 1980; Lin and Kessler, 1981; Hanis et al, 1982; Norell et al, 1986c), as well as stationary engineers (Milham, 1976; Peterson and Milham, 1980), coke oven workers (Redmond et al, 1976), aluminum mill workers (Milham, 1976), printers and lithographers (Williams et al, 1977; Mallin et al, 1989), vehicle drivers (Viadana et al, 1976; Mallin et al, 1989), various metal workers with possible exposure to metalworking fluids (Guralnick, 1963; Milham, 1976; Maruchi et al, 1979; DeCouflé et al, 1977a; Mallin et al, 1989; Silverstein et al, 1988; Vena et al, 1985), and mechanics of various kinds (Viadana et al, 1976; Peterson and Milham, 1980; Falk et al, 1990; Hansen, 1989). Subsequent investigations of workers exposed to organic particles from coke ovens (Redmond, 1983) and aluminum reduction plants (Rockette and Arena, 1983) have produced some corroborating evidence: in the former study, some evidence of a relation between length of exposure and risk was found, and, in the latter, the increased risk was consistent in all exposure circumstances. Risk also has been observed to increase after longer exposure to metalworking fluids and abrasives (Silverstein et al, 1988), and similar exposures in the manufacture of auto parts (Vena et al, 1985); however, in the largest such cohort study (Eisen et al, 1992), the increased risk was restricted to African-American workers.

No excess risk was found among British gas workers (Doll et al, 1972), and observations of refinery workers have shown generally minor elevations; under detailed analysis, those subgroups with higher risk have no special exposure to petroleum products, and no relation between length of exposure and risk (Thomas et al, 1980, 1982; Hanis et al, 1985; Divine et al, 1985, Divine and Barron, 1986; Kaplan, 1986; Nelson et al, 1987; Theriault and Provencher, 1987; Schottenfeld et al, 1981; Rushton and Alderson, 1981; Wen et al, 1983; Wong et al, 1986).

Pressworkers have also been studied with inconsistent results; a minor increase in risk has been found among commercial pressmen (Zoloth et al, 1986) and among a group of printing pressmen (Lloyd et al, 1977) where the increase was found only in the youngest age group.

No risk was found among the members of the American Cancer Society cohort who had been exposed to diesel exhaust (Boffetta et al, 1988), nor was any observed among a cohort of stationary engineers and firemen (DeCouflé et al, 1977b), a group that has been singled out several times in screening studies.

Rubber Manufacture. Early studies of rubber workers produced evidence of both decreased (McMichael et al, 1974) and increased (Monson and Fine, 1978) risk; more recent results from the latter study (Delzell et al, 1981; Delzell and Monson, 1985) show a consistent low-level elevation in risk, still based on small numbers of observed cases.

Tanning. Studies of cohorts of workers in the tanning industries of both Tuscany, Italy (Costantini et al, 1989) and Sweden (Edling et al, 1986) revealed increases in risk of pancreas cancer. Population-based screening of industrial categories has not consistently identified leather manufacturing as a high-risk industry, but a study of chromate pigment workers (chrome being one exposure in the tanning process) found a few excess cases (Sheffet et al, 1982).

Chemicals. Early studies of cohorts of chemists (Li et al, 1969) and chemical company employees (Mancuso and El-Attar, 1967) found excess risk based on a small number of cases; while a similar small excess among the workers of one chemical company has subsequently been reported (Bond et al, 1985), only a few cases had occurred among the young workers studied in a second company (Hoar and Pell, 1981), and a study of British chemists (Searle et al, 1981) showed no increased risk. Among a cohort of film manufacturing workers with daily exposure to methylene chloride (Hearne et al, 1987), more than twice the expected number of cases was observed, but without a dose-response relation.

Pesticides. Workers in companies engaged in the manufacture of phenoxy acid herbicides (Coggon et al, 1986) and brominated chemical pesticides, including DCBP, TRIS, and brominated organic and inorganic compounds (Wong et al, 1984), have been followed without finding any excess risk of pancreas cancer. However, a study of workers in a chemical plant where there was a known excess of pancreas cancer unexpectedly found substantial excess among those workers with exposure to DDT (Garabrant et al, 1992): higher risk was associated with longer exposure; DDT derivatives were independently shown linked to risk; and adjustment for individual exposure to other risk factors failed to alter the findings. No similar excess was found among workers exposed to DDT production elsewhere (Wong et al, 1984). No increased risk or dose-response relation was found among Swedish agricultural workers (Wiklund and Holm, 1986) or Swedish pesticide applicators (Wiklund et al, 1989), and only two unexpected pancreas cancer cases were observed among the 1153 deaths occurring in U. S. pesticide applicators and flight instructors (Cantor and Booze, 1991). No excess has been found among farmers in Iowa (Burmeister, 1990) or Wisconsin (Saftlas et al, 1987), nor has a consistent excess been found using international observations on the mortality of farmers (Blair et al, 1985; Franceschi et al, 1993). Falk et al (1990) have reported no excess risk associated with farming as an occupation but did find an excess risk in association with cotton dust exposure. It is of interest that as production of DDT in the United States diminished around 1970, most of that produced was used in cotton fields (IARC, 1991). In a nested case-control study of 450 cases, performed in a prepaid care setting in California, Friedman and van den Eeden (1993) found an elevation in risk associated with exposure to "insect or plant sprays." An interesting anecdote (Rubio and Rodriguez, 1989) concerns a chlorinated insecticide manufacturing worker and his wife, each of whom developed pancreas cancer after (in her case 18 years after) residing many years on the grounds of the insecticide factory.

No truly common element in the list of occupations in Table 35–3 is obvious, and the breadth of workplace experience represented is broad. Several of the categories are such that the most distinctive job exposures that can be imagined occur during refreshment breaks, and some of the most credible associations represent very rare occupational experiences. Thus, there are no common occupations that can be considered, on the available evidence, as certifiable causes of pancreas cancer. There are suggestive findings in relation to the products of incomplete combustion, to certain pesticides, and to other chemicals or chemical processes.

It is important to emphasize, for balance, that, in addition to the above-mentioned published results from studies that have failed to find any association between the workplace and pancreas cancer, there are an unknown, but very large, number of cohorts that have been examined but for which negative results have gone unpublished; for reasons of apathy or economics, such findings are often not disseminated except as adjuncts to other, positive, results. Moreover, few extreme results have emanated from the studies of occupational mortality and morbidity that are based on very large populations. Even with rather detailed occupational categorizations, such as those used by the British, Danish, and U. S. mortality and Los Angeles incidence studies, few occupations at high risk are singled out. Indeed, in the most recent examination of occupational mortality in Britain (Logan, 1982), no occupations at all met the rather liberal criteria for inclusion. This should serve to emphasize, again, that even many of the positive observations are likely to be due to chance.

Finally, other observations emphasize the probable unimportance of occupational causality in the broad pattern of pancreas cancer occurrence. As already described above, the pattern of occurrence in relation to social class is generally flat or inconsistent (Logan, 1982; Williams and Horm, 1977; Mack and Paganini-Hill, 1981; Ferraroni et al, 1989), even in poorer countries. Again, as noted above, there is currently little difference between rates in rural and in urban environments. In Los Angeles (Mack and Paganini-Hill, 1981) and in Olmsted County, Minnesota (Riela et al, 1992), there has been no increase or decrease in the rate in men of working age over 20 years. In Scandinavia, where diagnostic and treatment facilities are uniformly of good quality and access to care is universal, age-adjusted rates of pancreas cancer in the larger industrialized countries are identical to those in Iceland (Arnar et al, 1991) and the Faroe Islands (Jacobsen et al, 1985), which, especially in the case of the latter, are almost completely nonindustrialized.

Host Factors

Familiality. Endocrine tumors of the pancreas are known to occur in families; familial occurrence of exocrine pancreas cancer, though rare, has also been reported (Mulvihill, 1985). Further, adenocarcinoma of the pancreas has been reported to occur in "cancer families" (Li and Fraumeni, 1969; Lynch, 1967) and in hereditary nonpolyposis colon cancer (Lynch et al, 1985). A class of inherited conditions known as hereditary pancreatitis, which involve pancreatic enzyme deficiencies, has been described. Affected family members seem to be at high risk of pancreatic adenocarcinoma (Castleman et al, 1972; Kattwinkel et al, 1973; Davidson et al, 1983).

Among the reports of familial clusterings of pancreas cancer itself are two sibships in which four members died from pancreas adenocarcinoma (MacDermott and Kramer, 1973; Friedman and Fialkow, 1976). In neither family was there evidence of hereditary pancreatitis. Pancreas cancer has also been reported in three women of consecutive generations: a 29-year-old woman, her 42-year-old mother and 76-year-old maternal grandmother (Ehrenthal et al, 1987). Lynch et al (1992) reported on a family in which pancreatic cancer was documented in the proband's brother, father, and grandfather, and in the grandfather's daughter by another marriage.

Eight of 71 (8.9%) unselected cases of pancreas cancer in a case series, without controls, proved to have first-degree relatives with pancreas cancer (Anderson, 1978). Ghadirian et al (1991a) found that 7.8% of the cases in a population-based case-control study of pancreatic cancer had a positive family history of the disease, compared to 0.6% of the controls.

Associated Medical Conditions

Diabetes Mellitus. Diabetes has repeatedly been seen in connection with pancreas cancer. In the United States, geographic correlations have been reported between pancreas cancer and diabetes, notably in women (Blot et al, 1978). Review of the charts of patients with diabetes has always resulted in an excess of cases with pancreas carcinoma (Marble, 1934; Ellinger and Landsman, 1944; Bell, 1957). While pancreas cancer appearing in persons with a long history of diabetes has been documented (Cohen, 1965), it does seem clear that a large majority of pancreas cancer patients diagnosed with diabetes mellitus received that diagnosis during the course of their cancer or in the period immediately preceding it (Green et al, 1958; Clark and Mitchell, 1961; Karmody and Kyle, 1969). The question therefore must be phrased in terms of whether established diabetics are really at higher subsequent risk of pancreas cancer or whether the risks of cancer and diabetes are related in some other way.

Kessler followed 21,000 diabetics seen at a large Boston clinic between 1930 and 1956 for evidence of cancer on death certificates through 1959 (Kessler, 1970). Eligibility criteria included survival for at least 1 year after diagnosis of diabetes, and a large number of pancreas cancer cases (20% of all deaths) were ineligible by this criterion, reaffirming that the diagnosis of cancer coincident with the diagnosis of diabetes is commonplace. An additional 11 of the 78 observed cases were diagnosed but did not die within 1 year following the diagnosis of diabetes. Based on overall mortality in Massachusetts, the standard mortality ratios for males and females were 1.5 and 2.1, and these fell to 1.3 and 1.8 after excluding the 11 cases diagnosed within a year after diagnosis of diabetes. A potential bias in this study exists because the physicians at the diabetes clinic had a strong interest in diseases of the pancreas and may have determined pancreas cancer as a cause of death more often than other Massachusetts physicians.

In Olmsted County, Minnesota (Maruchi et al, 1979), no excess of pancreas cancer in diabetics was observed after cases diagnosed more than 2 years after the initial diagnosis of diabetes were excluded.

Ragozzino et al (1982) followed a population-based cohort of 1135 diabetics in Minnesota diagnosed between 1945 and 1969. There were 9 observed pancreatic cancers and 2.1 expected. When 5 cancer cases that were diagnosed in the first year following the onset of diabetes were excluded, the SMR was 2.6 (95% CI, 0.9–6.1) with similar findings for both sexes.

Green and Jensen (1985) followed a cohort of 1499 insulin-dependent diabetics in Denmark. Based on age- and sex-specific Danish cancer incidence rates, 2.4 pancreas cancer cases were expected among the cohort during the 8.5 years of follow-up. Two cases in whom cancer was diagnosed less than 5 years from the onset of diabetes were excluded from the analysis, four other cases of pancreatic cancer were observed (O/E = 1.69, p = 0.29); the four included in the analysis were diagnosed with cancer 6, 7, 8, and 37 years after the onset of diabetes.

The association between pre-existing diabetes and pancreatic cancer has been examined in other prospective studies. Whittemore et al (1983) found a statistically significant increased risk of approximately 5-fold for the development of pancreas cancer among diabetics in a large prospective study of college men. Mills et al (1988) reported a relative risk of 3.4 (95% CI, 1.7–8.3) for pancreatic cancer among self-reported diabetics in a cohort of Seventh-Day Adventists; the analysis was restricted to individuals who survived at least 1 year after entry into the study.

An association with pre-existing diabetes was observed in two prospective studies of members of a prepaid health plan in the San Francisco Bay area; Hiatt et al (1988) reported a relative risk of 2.1 for subjects with a history of diabetes among a cohort of 122,894 individuals; all of the cancer cases were diagnosed with diabetes at a minimum of 5.7 years prior to the diagnosis of cancer. A recent prospective study (nested case-control study) conducted within this same health plan found a 2-fold increase in risk of pancreatic cancer among subjects who had previously responded "yes" to questions on diabetes history during their first multiphasic health checkup (Friedman and van den Eeden, 1993). The relative risk was virtually unchanged when cases whose cancer developed within 5 years of the first checkup were excluded.

Among the case-control studies that have examined pre-existing diabetes as an independent variable, several have included other hospital patients as controls (Wynder, 1973a; Lin and Kessler, 1981; MacMahon et al, 1981; Gold et al, 1985; La Vecchia et al, 1990). Only two of these studies (Wynder, 1973a; La Vecchia et al, 1990) found an association between diabetes and pancreas carcinoma: one noted the association with longstanding diabetes and then only in women (Wynder, 1973a); the other found an increased risk, but the authors did not indicate if recently diagnosed diabetics were excluded from the analysis. A simple interpretation of these various results is difficult because of the inclusion of hospital patients in the control series: such a series may contain an excess of subjects with diabetes-related conditions relative to the general population.

Cuzick and Babiker (1989) addressed this issue in their report of results from a case-control study which included both hospital and general practice controls. The authors noted that there were no material differences in their results when only one of the two control groups was used. After excluding patients diagnosed with diabetes less than a year prior to diagnosis of cancer, they reported a 4-fold risk ratio associated with diabetes which did not change with the further exclusion of diabetics diagnosed within 2–5 years of their cancer.

Among five other population-based case-control studies that have examined this issue, at least three reported positive associations. Norell et al (1986b) reported an OR of 2.4 (90% CI, 0.6–9.7); Farrow and Davis (1990a) found an OR of 6.7 (95% CI, 1.8–24.9). In both studies, subjects diagnosed with cancer less than 5 or 3 years, respectively, after the onset of diabetes, were excluded from analysis. Jain et al (1991) found an OR of 2.1 (95% CI, 0.7–6.2) for subjects diagnosed with diabetes between 5 to 10 years prior to their cancer. Two other studies have relevant data: Mack et al (1986) found a relative risk estimate of 1.3, which was compatible with chance as well as a modest increase in risk; Bueno de Mesquita et al (1992b) found an elevated risk associated with diabetes in both women and men, but that was statistically significant only in men.

Pancreatitis. Pathologists have observed that pancreatitis occurs in a large proportion of autopsied cases of pancreatic carcinoma (Mikal and Campbell, 1950), and clinical signs of pancreatitis have been observed in many patients with pancreatic cancer (Gambill, 1971). A hereditary form of pancreatitis has been described in which affected family members appear at high risk of pancreatic adenocarcinoma (Castleman et al, 1972; Kattwinkel et al, 1973). It has been demonstrated that, in some instances, chronic pancreatitis clearly precedes the diagnosis of carcinoma of the pancreas (Bartholomew et al, 1958; Robinson et al, 1970; Lundh and Nordenstam, 1970; Ammann et al, 1984; Lowenfels, 1984; Ammann and Schueler, 1984), as well as other carcinomas (Ammann et al, 1980).

The hypothesis that chronic pancreatitis conveys a higher risk of pancreas cancer has been examined in a number of case-control studies, and evidence for a positive association (Lin and Kessler, 1981; Mack et al, 1986; Farrow and Davis, 1990a; La Vecchia et al, 1990; Jain et al, 1991) and for no association (Wynder et al, 1973a; Gold et al, 1985; Bueno de Mesquita, 1992b) has been reported. However, the data from such studies are based on relatively few individuals with evidence of prior pancreatitis.

A multicenter historical cohort study of 2015 patients with chronic pancreatitis was reported by Lowenfels et al in 1993. The risk of pancreatic cancer was significantly elevated. Even after excluding individuals with only 2 or 5 years of follow-up, the standardized incidence ratios were 16.5 (95% CI, 11.1–23.7) and 14.4 (95% CI, 8.5–22.8), respectively. These ratios were derived from the observed number of cases and the expected number based on country-specific incidence data. The increased risk was observed in men and women; was associated with both alcoholic and nonalcoholic pancreatitis; and was observed in the individual cohorts from all six participating countries. The center-specific relative risks were all statistically significant and ranged from 9.7 to 19.9 for the analysis restricted to individuals with 2 or more years of follow-up; all but one of the relative risk estimates were statistically significant when the analysis was restricted to individuals with 5 or more years of follow-up, with a range of 3.6 to 24.3.

Gastric Surgery. A number of studies have shown higher risks for pancreas cancer following gastrectomy or "peptic ulcer surgery." McLean-Ross and colleagues (1982) observed 11 cases of pancreatic cancer (3.9 expected) when they followed-up nearly 780 members of a Scottish gastrectomy cohort. Caygill et al (1985) reported a 3.2-fold excess of pancreatic cancers among approximately 4200 gastrectomy patients after a 20-year latency period. Increased risks for other cancers were also reported in the cohort, including tumors of the large bowel, bronchus, biliary tract, and other sites. In contrast to these findings, Maringhini et al (1987) followed 336 gastrectomy patients in a cohort study in Olmsted County, Minnesota, and found 1 pancreatic cancer where 1.6 were expected. In 2633 gastrectomy patients followed for more than 5 years after surgery, Tersmette et al (1990) found O/E ratios of 1.7 (95% CI, 1.1–2.4) in males and 1.7 (95% CI, 0.4–5.0) in females. In a similar study, Eide et al (1991) reported O/E ratios of 1.7 for males (95% CI, 1.2–2.4) and 0.2 (95% CI, 0.1–1.4) for females in a cohort of 4224 patients. A marginally increased risk for pancreatic cancer, though not statistically significant, was also observed in another cohort of over 4000 gastrectomy patients (Møller and Toftgaard, 1991).

Offerhaus et al (1987) conducted a case-control autopsy study and included three control groups, each with a high prevalence of cigarette smoking, in order to adjust indirectly for the possible confounding effect of smoking. Increased risks for pancreatic cancer were found in comparisons with each control group. When all controls were included in the analysis, an OR of 3.1 (95% CI, 1.2–8.0) was found. Mack et al (1986) also adjusted for smoking and reported a positive association for pancreatic cancer and gastrectomy (OR = 5.3, 95% CI, 1.6–21.5), as did Farrow and Davis (1990a) (OR = 2.3, 95% CI, 0.4–12.7), and Mills et al (1988) for peptic ulcer surgery (OR = 2.6, 95% CI, 1.0–6.9). Studies reporting no strong association include those of Wynder et al (1973a), La Vecchia et al (1990), and Bueno de Mesquita et al (1992b).

Cholecystitis. Cholecystitis has been thought by clinicians (Berk, 1941) and pathologists (Mikal and Campbell, 1950) to be commonly present in patients with pancreas carcinoma, but the findings for an association between pancreatic cancer and cholecystectomy are inconsistent. Although Wynder (1973b) found no increased frequency of antecedent cholecystectomy in males, there was an excess among female cases, which may be explained by diagnostic bias. A modest increase was also observed among Olmsted County residents (Maruchi et al, 1979), although it was also recognized that more clinical attention had probably been focused upon the biliary organs of the cases. Lin and Kessler (1981) found evidence for an increased risk associated with a history of gallstones; Mack et al (1986) found an inverse association with cholecystectomy (OR = 0.8); Farrow and Davis (1990a) reported an OR of 1.1 for cholecystectomy and 1.2 for gallstones. Cuzick and Babiker (1989) reported a 2-fold risk associated with a history of gallstones and the same value for prior cholecystectomy; risk estimates were similar for men and women. La Vecchia et al (1990) reported a modestly increased risk of 1.3, which was not statistically significant. Norell et al (1986b), using population controls, found an OR of 2.9 (90% CI, 1.5–5.6) for pancreatic cancer for subjects reporting a history of gallstone disease 5 years prior to diagnosis of cancer.

Allergies. The association of prior allergies with pancreatic cancer has been examined in a number of studies (Lin and Kessler, 1981; Gold et al, 1985; Mack et al, 1986; Mills et al, 1988; Jain et al, 1991; Farrow and Davis, 1990a; La Vecchia et al, 1990; Bueno de Mesquita, 1992b). Although the data are somewhat equivocal, the preponderance of evidence suggests that a history of allergies may be inversely associated with the risk of subsequently developing pancreas cancer.

A cohort of asthmatic veterans was followed for 25 to 30 years and their cause-specific mortality compared to national expectations and to the mortality occurring in a cohort of similar size and age but with an initial diagnosis of acute nasopharyngitis (Robinette and Fraumeni, 1978). In relation to both the expected deaths from all digestive system cancers (based on national mortality) and the observed pancreas cancer deaths in the comparison cohort, a substantial excess of pancreas cancer mortality occurred among the asthmatics. The authors expressed concern that this effect might have been related to aminophylline therapy for asthma, on the basis of an effect upon the DNA binding of carcinogens that has been observed in cultured cells (Huberman and Sachs, 1977). Others have examined the relation between these conditions and found no increase in pancreas cancer (Farrow and Davis, 1990a); most have observed an overall reduced risk of cancer in asthmatics (Shapiro et al, 1971; Meers, 1973; Alderson, 1974; Mack et al, 1986; Jain et al, 1991), which is consistent with the findings for a history of allergies noted above.

Other Conditions. Lin and Kessler (1981), Gold et al (1985), and Farrow and Davis (1990a) have all reported finding prior tonsillectomy associated with a significantly reduced risk of pancreatic cancer. Mills et al (1988) reported a slight, though nonsignificant inverse association, as did Mack et al (1986). Bueno de Mesquita et al (1992b) found no association.

No increased risk was found in a large cohort of patients with rheumatoid arthritis studied in Finland (Isomaki et al, 1978); nor was an excess found in patients with celiac disease (Holmes et al, 1976). An increased incidence of pancreatic neoplasia (O/E = 3.8, $p<0.02$) in pernicious anemia patients versus the general population of Sweden has been reported (Borch et al, 1988).

CONCEPTS OF PATHOGENESIS

Animal Models

Spontaneous Tumors. Spontaneous exocrine adenocarcinomas of the pancreas have been reported in a wide range of species, including camels, cattle, horses, jackals, dogs, cats, marmots, bears, rats, mice, and Syrian hamsters (Rowlatt, 1967; Slye et al, 1935). In dogs, at least, the frequency and prognosis of the disease warrant about the same attention as in humans (Priester, 1974). The histology is as similarly varied as that in humans, and most tumors also seem to be of ductal origin (Kirchner and Nielsen, 1976). The incidence in animals is strongly associated with increasing age, but there is no male preponderance in either dogs or cats.

Experimental Carcinogenesis. Pancreatic carcinogenesis in experimental animals has been extensively reviewed (Longnecker et al, 1984; Longnecker, 1986, 1990; Pour, 1989; Watanapa and Williamson, 1993). Two well-characterized and extensively used models are the Syrian hamster, where intraperitoneal injection with any of several nitrosamines results in ductlike adenocarcinoma of the pancreas (Pour et al, 1975a, b; Levitt et al, 1977; Pour, 1980, 1989), and various strains of rats, especially Wistar and Lewis, where injection of azaserine produces adenocarcinomas of acinar cell origin (Longnecker and Curphey, 1975; Longnecker, 1984). Similarly invasive tumors, also with features suggesting acinar cell origin, are produced by feeding methylnitrosourea or related compounds to guinea pigs (Reddy and Rao, 1977) and the tobacco-specific *N*-nitrosamine, NNK, to rats (Rivenson et al, 1988). Pancreatic neoplasms can also be induced by other chemical carcinogens. Adenocarcinomas that metastasize and have ductal morphology can be induced by direct implantation of dimethylbenzanthracene (DMBA) (Dissin et al, 1975). The heterocyclic aromatic amine, 2-amino-3-methylimidazo[4,5-*f*]quinoline (IQ), has been shown to produce benign tumors in rats (Tanaka et al, 1985). The *N*-hydroxy heterocyclic arylamine, 4-hydroxyaminoquinoline 1-oxide (4-HAQO), has been shown to induce both benign (Hayashi et al, 1972) and malignant (Konishi et al, 1976) pancreatic tumors in rats.

A new model of exocrine pancreatic carcinoma has been developed with transgenic mice (Ornitz et al, 1987; Longnecker et al, 1990). A fusion gene was constructed which contains the transforming gene (the T-antigen) from simian virus 40 under the control of the regulatory elements of a rat elastase gene which is pancreas-specific. Homozygous strains of the transgenic mice can dominantly transmit the oncogene construct in their germ cell line. In the mice possessing the oncogenes, all offspring develop exocrine pancreatic carcinomas spontaneously.

As mentioned above, the cellular origin of tumors with ductlike morphology is not established. Evidence from experimental pancreatic cancers supports the view that some ductlike carcinomas may arise from acinar cells (Flaks, 1984; Bockman, 1981; Longnecker et al, 1984). Acinar to ductal transdifferentiation in human cultured cells and in transgenic mice supports the same view, i.e., that acinar cells may be the target for carcinogenic events which lead to tumors with ductal phenotype (Hall and Lemoine, 1992; Sandgren et al, 1990; Jhappen et al, 1990).

ras **in Animal Models.** Mutations in c-Kirsten-*ras* (K-*ras*) genes occur in some but not all experimental pancreatic cancers. In reports from at least three laboratories, a high proportion of the pancreatic adenocarcinomas induced in the hamster by *N*-nitroso-bis-(2-oxypropyl)amine (BOP) were found to have activated K-*ras* genes due to mutations in codon 12 (Cerny et al, 1990, 1992; Fujii et al, 1990; van Kranen et al, 1991). Activation of *c*-K-*ras* has not been found in pancreatic acinar-cell neoplasms arising in azaserine-treated rats (Schaeffer et al, 1990; van Kranen et al, 1991). As noted below, mutations in *ras* may be an important similarity between the disease in animals and humans.

Dietary Modulation of Experimental Carcinogenesis. Dietary factors have both inhibitory and enhancing effects on pancreatic growth and carcinogenesis depending upon the experimental model used. Many studies have been conducted in this area; for further references see Longnecker et al (1984); Longnecker (1990); Watanapa and Williamson (1993); and Poston et al (1991).

Caloric restriction has been shown to decrease tumor incidence in a variety of tissues and animal models (Tannenbaum, 1959; Pariza, 1987). More specifically, reduced caloric intake protects against pancreatic carcinogenesis in rats initiated with azaserine (Roebuck et al, 1981a, 1993). The mechanism is not known but may involve reduced trophic stimuli to the pancreas, reduced levels of carcinogen-activating enzymes within the pancreas, or other physiologic differences (Longnecker, 1990; Pariza, 1987).

Dietary protein has been shown to modulate carcinogenesis in animals but not in a consistent fashion. Incidence of pancreatic carcinomas was increased in BOP-treated hamsters when dietary protein was increased during the postinitiation phase of carcinogenesis (Pour and Birt, 1983). The enhancing effect of high protein on carcinogenesis did not occur when the fat content was low, suggesting a possible interaction between the two components (Birt et al, 1983b). In contrast, azaserine-treated rats on a high protein diet (50% casein by weight) had a lower incidence of adenomas and carcinomas than did rats fed a similar diet with 20% protein by weight (Roebuck et al, 1981a).

Some of the dietary effects on pancreatic carcinogenesis in animal systems, possibly including the inconsistently enhancing effects of high dietary protein (Longnecker, 1990), are thought to be mediated by cholecystokinin (CCK), the gastrointestinal peptide hormone that is a potent stimulator of pancreatic function and cell growth (Axelson et al, 1992). Exogenous administration of CCK has been shown to cause pancreatic hypertrophy and hyperplasia, and to enhance tumorigenesis (Mainz et al, 1973; Barrowman and Mayston, 1974; Howatson and Carter, 1985). Furthermore, Bell et al (1992) have demonstrated the overexpression of a high affinity CCK receptor in both premalignant and malignant foci in azaserine-induced tumors in rats.

Diets that contain trypsin inhibitor—both natural, from raw soya flour (McGuiness et al, 1982; Liener and Hasdi, 1986), or synthetic (Göke et al, 1986; Lhoste et al, 1988; Gumbmann et al, 1989; Douglas et al, 1990)—have been shown to stimulate pancreatic growth and the formation of preneoplastic and neoplastic lesions in some, but not all, animal models. The stimulatory effects of trypsin inhibitors may work through the release of CCK; administration of these compounds leads to increased circulating levels of CCK (Fölsch et al, 1984; Lu et al, 1989).

Certain dietary fats have been shown to increase susceptibility to pancreatic cancer in animals (Roebuck, 1992). Post-initiation enhancement of tumor incidence and multiplicity has been shown in azaserine-treated rats fed a high proportion (20% by weight) of unsaturated, but not saturated, fat in the diet (Roebuck et al, 1981a, b). In addition, Roebuck et al (1985) have shown that a minimum proportion of the diet (4%–8% by weight) must be linoleic acid, an essential polyunsaturated fatty acid, to produce the enhancing effects of dietary unsaturated fat in the azaserine/rat model. Hoffmann et al (1993) reported enhanced nitrosamine-induced pancreatic tumor development in rats fed a high unsaturated fat (20% corn oil by weight) vs low fat (5% corn oil by weight) diet. Similar findings with unsaturated fat have been reported for BOP-treated hamsters (Birt et al, 1981a). In more recent studies, Birt et al (1990) compared tumor incidence in BOP-treated hamsters receiving diets with corn oil or beef tallow; animals on beef tallow had a higher incidence of both adenomas and adenocarcinomas compared to those fed corn oil at a similar proportion of calories. Woutersen and van Garderen-Hoetmer (1988a, b) have reported enhancement of "(pre)neoplastic" lesions by a diet high in saturated fat (20% lard by weight) in both BOP-treated hamsters and azaserine-treated rats.

In contrast to the enhancing effects on carcinogenesis by some dietary fats, dietary fish oil (which is rich in omega-3 fatty acids), at 20% of the diet by weight, has been shown to produce a significantly smaller size and number of preneoplastic lesions in azaserine-treated rats compared with those on a diet containing 20% corn oil by weight (O'Connor et al, 1989).

Certain retinoids have been shown to modulate carcinogenesis in animals (Longnecker et al, 1983, 1986; Roebuck et al, 1984a; Birt et al, 1981b, 1983a; Woutersen and van Garderen-Hoetmer, 1988a, b; Appel et al, 1991). A number have inhibited carcinogen-induced pancreatic tumors in rats, but they have a variety of effects—depending on the model used—including an increase in tumor yield in hamsters (Birt et al, 1983a).

Other dietary components that have modulated pancreatic neoplasia in experimental systems include vitamin C (Woutersen and van Garderen-Hoetmer, 1988a; Appel et al, 1991), selenium (Birt et al, 1986; Woutersen and van Garderen-Hoetmer, 1988b; Appel et al, 1991), and the phenolic antioxidants, BHA and BHT (Roebuck et al, 1984b).

There are a number of key parallels between the animal and human data: in general, pancreatic cancer is more common in males than females in both animal models and humans; humans are exposed—through cigarette smoke and diet—to chemical carcinogens that induce pancreas cancer in animals, for example, polycyclic aromatic hydrocarbons, nitrosamines, and aromatic amines; K-*ras* mutations are common in both BOP-treated hamsters and humans (Cerny et al, 1992; Shibata et al, 1990b); and abnormalities in the structure and function of other oncogenes, growth factors, and hormones have been observed in both the animal and human disease (Lemoine and Hall, 1990; Longnecker, 1991; Andren-Sandberg and Johansson, 1990). There are also parallels between animals and humans in the dietary data. For example, fat intake has been associated with an increased risk in carcinogen-induced animal models and in humans. Certain carotenoids and vitamin C have been shown to inhibit some phases of carcinogenesis in some animal models, and these compounds are present in fruits and vegetables, which have been consistently associated with reduced risk in humans. However, the species specificity of both carcinogenicity and pancreatic physiology demand that special caution be exercised in the interpretation of results from animal models (Hegsted, 1975; Longnecker et al, 1984). This is particularly true for diet where the findings—in both animals and man—are not consistent, the potential exposures are complex, and the measurement techniques problematic.

Humans

As with many other human neoplasms, for pancreas cancer there are now extensive data on the epidemiologic risk factors, relevant animal data, and a steadily accumulating body of knowledge regarding the molecular events involved in carcinogenesis. Also, as with many other cancers, there is a lack of a clear and coherent account of how these data are to be reconciled. What we know at present includes evidence of relevant somatic mutations that are a plausible consequence of specific chemical carcinogens; evidence of various factors that may be important in modifying the mutagenic process—either positively or negatively; evidence of host-environment interactions particularly those involving metabolic activation of carcinogens; and the possible importance of genetic differences between individuals in this activation.

Molecular Events—Oncogenes and Tumor Suppressor Genes. There is now a large body of evidence to support the view that mutations in cellular proto-oncogenes and tumor suppressor genes are important events in pancreatic carcinogenesis. The *ras* gene family encodes proteins involved in cell growth and differentiation. These proto-oncogenes encode membrane-bound proteins thought to be involved in GTP-mediated signal transduction across the cell membrane (Barbacid, 1987). Point mutations in *ras* genes can render the protein constitutively activated, and the association of such mutations with several human tumors including pancreas, colon, myeloid leukemia, breast, and bladder (Bos, 1989, 1990; Marshall et al, 1989; Fearon and Vogelstein, 1990) has led to the view that they probably play an important role early in carcinogenesis.

The highest frequency of *ras* mutations has been found in case series of adenocarcinomas of the pancreas (over 95% in some series) with the great majority of these mutations being found in codon 12 of c-Kirsten-*ras* (K-*ras*) (Bos, 1989, 1990; Shibata et al, 1990b; Almoquera et al, 1988; Tada et al, 1990; Nagata et al, 1990). Numerous lines of evidence suggest that K-*ras* mutations are an early and important event in the pathogenesis of pancreatic cancer; for example, the high proportion of malignant tumors with mutations in K-*ras*; the presence of the mutation in some preinvasive lesions; the presence of the mutation in both primary and metastatic foci; and the reported amplification of the oncogene in some malignant tumors (Lemoine et al, 1992b; Yamada et al, 1986; Parsa et al, 1988) and cell lines (Hirai et al, 1985). Because of the high proportion of exocrine tumors with this mutation, analysis for mutations in K-*ras* in tumor cells recovered from peripheral blood, pancreatic juice, and fine needle aspirates shows promise as a diagnostic tool (Tada et al, 1991, 1993; Shibata et al, 1990a).

It is possible that human pancreatic carcinogens from cigarettes, diet, and occupational or environmental exposures cause mutations in the *ras* gene. It has been argued that, although carcinogens can cause reproducible mutations at defined positions, the heterogeneity of mutations in codon 12 of K-*ras* in pancreas cancer is not consistent with the interpretation that mutations might be caused by a specific carcinogen and that they are more likely to be caused by multiple carcinogens (Shibata et al, 1990b). That multiple carcinogens may cause pancreatic cancer is plausible; however, one could argue that there is a degree of consistency in the mutations. Transversions and transitions of nucleotides from G to T or G to A in codon 12 of K-*ras* accounted for the majority of K-*ras* mutations in at least five studies of pancreatic tumors (Smit et al, 1988; Grunewald et al, 1989; Mariyama et al, 1989; Nagata et al, 1990; Shibata et al, 1990b; Höhne et al, 1992) and have been seen in other tumors as well. It is noteworthy in that regard, that arylamine-modified DNA can lead to transversion and transition mutations and that the specific mutations cited above are consistent with the predicted genetic consequences of arylamine-DNA adducts (Beland and Kadlubar, 1985). In fact, Beland and Kadlubar (1985) have suggested that aromatic amines may activate *ras* genes via this mechanism. It should be noted that G to A transitions are also consistent with mutations caused by some alkylating agents. For example, in two studies using BOP-induced pancreatic adenocarcinomas in the hamster, the point mutations in codon 12 of the K-*ras* gene were exclusively G to A transitions (Fujii et al, 1990; Cerny et al, 1992); and the nitrosamine *N*-nitrosomethylurea has been associated with G to A transitions in codon 12 of the Ha-*ras* oncogene in a rat mammary tumor model (Tricker and Preussmann, 1991).

The possible role of some other oncogenes in pancreatic cancer has also been examined. For example, c-*myc* has been reported to be amplified in one pancreatic carcinoma (Yamada et al, 1986). Further, in a case-series of pancreatic tumors, Hall and coworkers (1990) examined the expression of the c-*erbB*-2 proto-oncogene, a probable growth factor receptor that is closely related to the epidermal growth factor receptor; abnormal expression of the c-*erbB*-2 protein was observed in 19% of the 87 tumors examined. Overexpression of a related receptor, the *erbB*-3 protein, has recently been found in a majority of pancreatic carcinomas investigated (Lemoine et al, 1992c).

Alterations in tumor suppressor genes (*apc,* p53) associated with familial cancer syndromes that include colon and breast cancers have been reported in some human pancreas cancers. Using probes close to the gene associated with familial adenomatous polyposis coli (the *apc* gene), Neuman et al (1991) reported chromosome 5 allele loss in two of six pancreatic tumors. Subsequently, Horii et al (1992) found somatic mutations within the *apc* coding region that would result in a truncated *apc* product in four of ten pancreatic cancers. A mutant form of the p53 tumor suppressor gene was reported in 28 of 124 (23%) of pancreatic adenocarcinomas (Barton et al, 1991b, 1992). The loss of expression of another potential tumor suppressor gene, *dcc,* has also been observed in pancreatic tumors. The *dcc* gene product is a probable cell-adhesion molecule, and mutations in *dcc* are found in a high proportion of colon cancers (Fearon et al, 1990; Fearon and Vogelstein, 1990). Höhne et al (1992), reported a loss of *dcc* gene expression in four of eight pancreatic tumors and in eight of eleven human pancreatic cell lines.

Clearly, an understanding of the function and the causes of mutations in K-*ras, myc, erbB*-2, *apc,* p53, *dcc,* and perhaps other oncogenes and tumor suppressor genes will reveal more about the etiology and the pathogenesis of pancreatic cancer. The overlap with colon cancer genes is striking, but may as plausibly be a consequence of the particular genes that are being examined as of shared biology.

Genetic Predisposition. Although shared environmental exposure (or coincidence) may explain some familial clusters of pancreatic cancer, it appears likely—particularly because of the young cases reported—that genetic predisposition to pancreatic cancer can occur. However, the evidence described previously suggests that only a small proportion of cases is likely to be explained by familiality. Nonetheless, information on genes that may predispose to this cancer, as with other cancers with larger familial components, may be very useful in increasing understanding of etiology and therefore relevant to the sporadic cases as well.

The evidence suggesting associations between pancreatic cancer and the tumor suppressor (and probable tumor suppressor) genes p53, *apc,* and *dcc* is based on somatic mutations found in pancreatic carcinomas. Altered p53 and *apc* genes have been found as germline mutations in families with elevated risk for breast, colon, and other cancers. It is important to establish if the rare individuals with a family history of pancreatic cancer harbor such mutations.

There may be genetic differences between individuals in their ability to activate and inactivate pancreatic carcinogens. Of current interest are differences in the ability to activate aromatic amines—via acetyltransferase and cytochrome P-4501A2 (Probst et al, 1992; Anderson et al, 1992; Kadlubar et al, 1992, 1993)—and the nitrosamines NNK and NNN (Carmella et al, 1990; Hecht et al, 1993; SS Hecht, personal communication).

Carcinogens

Smoking. Despite the strong evidence that smoking is a cause of pancreatic cancer, to date there has been no unequivocal biological mechanism demonstrated to explain this finding. There are numerous chemical carcinogens in cigarette smoke that could play a role. Wynder proposed that carcinogens absorbed from tobacco smoke may reach the pancreas through the blood, or alternatively, through refluxed bile (Wynder et al, 1973b). It has been argued that there may be both early- and late-stage effects of smoking (Mack et al, 1986). Cigarette smoking has been associated with histologic changes in the pancreas (Auerbach and Garfinkel, 1986). Several studies have reported carcinogen-DNA-adduct levels to be higher in the pancreas of smokers compared to nonsmokers (Cuzick et al, 1990; Kaderlik et al, 1993).

Nitrosamines have been suggested as human pancreatic carcinogens. These compounds are present at high levels in cigarettes (Hecht and Hoffmann, 1991). The Surgeon General's report of 1989 (U.S. DHHS, 1989) suggested the *N*-nitrosamine, NNK, as a putative human pancreatic carcinogen in cigarette smoke; other *N*-nitroso compounds have also been suggested (Hecht and Hoffmann, 1991). As described earlier, nitrosamines induce pancreatic cancers in several animal models.

Aromatic amines may also play a role in pancreas cancer (Mancuso and El-Attar, 1967; Weisburger, 1991; Anderson et al, 1992; Kaderlik et al, 1993; Kadlubar et al, 1993). About 30 arylamines are present in nanogram quantities in mainstream cigarette smoke and in even higher levels in sidestream smoke, including 2-naphthylamine (2-NA) and 4-aminobiphenyl (ABP) (Patrianakos, 1979). These two compounds are known human bladder carcinogens and are the components of tobacco smoke that are the likely causative agents of bladder cancer (Surgeon General's Report, U.S. DHHS, 1989).

Diet. Genotoxic chemical carcinogens, such as *N*-nitroso compounds and heterocyclic amines are present in food as a result of cooking, curing, smoking, pickling, or salting; as mentioned above, both of these classes of carcinogens have been suggested as human pancreatic carcinogens. *N*-nitroso compounds are present in the human diet, particularly in cured and smoked meat and fish, and in pickled and salt-preserved foods such as vegetables; they are also found in beer and some cheeses (Tricker and Preussmann, 1991; IARC, 1984). Nitrosamines and nitrosamides can be formed endogenously via the combination of nitrosating compounds (such as nitrite) with amines or amides, respectively; these are all found in human diets. The hypothesis that dietary *N*-nitroso compounds, activated in the liver and blood-borne to the pancreas, play a role in human pancreatic cancer, as in animals, is plausible.

The associations between meat consumption and pancreatic cancer are intriguing in the light of the presence of a variety of carcinogenic and mutagenic heterocyclic aromatic amines—particularly in cooked fish and meats, but also in eggs—that are formed as pyrolysis products of amino acids and proteins (Sugimura and Sato, 1983; Sugimura, 1985; Turesky et al, 1991; Grivas et al, 1986; Bjeldanes et al, 1982). Mutagenic activities of heterocyclic amines are high, especially those of IQ, MeIQ, MeIQx, Trp-P-1, Trp-P-2, and Glu-P-1, when assayed by the bacterial strain commonly used in the Ames test, *S. typhimurium* TA98 (Sugimura and Sato, 1983). Furthermore, these compounds exhibit appreciable rates of DNA-binding when activated by human liver and colon enzymes (Turesky et al, 1991). Arylamines are receiving considerable attention as possible carcinogens for the human colon (Turesky et al, 1991; Lang et al, 1986; Kadlubar et al, 1988; Schiffman and Felton, 1990) and other organs (Weisburger, 1993) and have been suggested as possible human pancreatic carcinogens (Mancuso and El-Attar, 1967; Weisburger 1991; Anderson et al, 1992).

There are differences in the levels of heterocyclic aromatic compounds formed in meat and fish, depending upon the method of cooking and time and temperature employed (Felton and Knize, 1991). Frying and broiling cause formation of mutagenic compounds; boiling also produces mutagens, but far more slowly (Spingarn and Weisburger, 1979). In contrast, Nader et al (1981) found no mutagenic activity was produced by microwaving beef—even at three times the normal cooking period—while high levels of mutagens were formed by pan-broiling. If heterocyclic amines are carcinogenic for the human pancreas, then differences in cooking methods might explain some of the inconsistencies reported in the literature for meat consumption and risk of pancreatic cancer. Attention to method of cooking meat and fish, as well as overall consumption, may be essential in future studies in order to clarify risks (Steineck et al, 1993).

Coffee. Interest in coffee as a causal agent for pancreatic cancer has biologic plausibility stemming from the fact that caffeine and other xanthines are mutagenic (Kuhlmann et al, 1968). The plasma clearance of xanthines is reduced by constituents of tobacco smoke (Welch et al, 1977), and xanthines produce hyperglycemia and mobilize fatty acids (MacCornack, 1977). In addition, coffee is an extremely complex chemical mixture, with phenolics derived from chlorogenic acid, products of pyrolyzed proteins and carbohydrates, volatile aldehydes and ketones (MacCornack, 1977), and other substances that might enhance the carcinogenicity of other etiologic agents. However, as stated earlier, the current epidemiologic evidence does not provide strong support for the hypothesis that coffee (or tea) consumption increases the risk for pancreatic cancer (Gordis, 1990; IARC, 1991), so plausible mechanisms are largely irrelevant. Of course, given the complexity of the mixture of compounds, the likely variability of that mixture from coffee to coffee, and the possible mixed enhancing and inhibiting effects that compounds like polyphenolics have on carcinogenesis, it may be that specific kinds or preparations of coffee actually do vary in their cancer-related potential.

Metabolism of Carcinogens. The agents that have been suggested as human pancreatic carcinogens, for example, *N*-nitroso compounds and aromatic amines, both require metabolic activation to bind to DNA and cause mutations. Procarcinogens for the pancreas may be fully or partially activated in the pancreas or liver (Braganza, 1983). Enzymes that activate these compounds include cytochrome P-450s for nitrosamines and arylamines (Hecht et al, 1993; Hecht and Hoffmann, 1991; Kadlubar and Hammons, 1987) and *O*-acetyltransferase for arylamines (Hein, 1988). Partially or fully activated carcinogens may reach the pancreas via bile reflux, although both theoretical and empirical considerations support the notion of access via the blood. Organotropism also appears to be a factor.

Available evidence in humans suggests that the pancreas lacks sufficient quantities of the cytochrome P-450s needed to activate nitrosamines (Anderson et al, 1992; SS Hecht, personal communication). Therefore for these possible pancreatic carcinogens, a plausible mechanism is activation of procarcinogens to ultimate carcinogens in the liver followed by blood-borne transport to the pancreas, where binding to DNA takes place.

Recent studies have shown that in animal models where NNK (and other nitrosamines) cause tumors, there is a strong correlation between adduct levels of NNK in hemoglobin and the adduct levels in DNA of tissues where tumors arise (Hecht et al, 1993). In humans, it has been shown that smokers and snuff dippers have higher average levels of hemoglobin-adducts of NNK than nonsmokers; similarly, higher levels of these DNA-adducts are found in the lung and trachea of smokers as compared to nonsmokers (Carmella et al, 1990; Hecht et al, 1993). It is plausible that such DNA-adducts may be formed in the pancreata of smokers as well.

For arylamines, cytochrome P-4501A2, which completes the first step in a multistage activation of these compounds, is apparently not present in human pancreas (Anderson et al, 1992). Yet, the presence of arylamine-DNA adducts in the pancreas of smokers together with evidence of *O*-acetyltransferase activity in this tissue suggests that the first step in activation, conversion to an *N*-hydroxy arylamine, may take place in the liver with subsequent transport to the pancreas for further activation to the *N*-acetoxy compound, the highly reactive species that binds to DNA (Kadlubar et al, 1992, 1993).

Animal studies have suggested a pathway that may be important for the food-borne heterocyclic amines. In the rat and dog, oral administration of radiolabeled PhIP results in high levels of radioactivity bound to DNA in many organs, with the levels of DNA-adducts highest in the pancreas in both species. Moreover, intravenous injection of radiolabeled *N*-acetoxy PhIP, the putative ultimate carcinogenic form of PhIP, into rats similarly results in high levels of DNA-PhIP adducts in the pancreas (FF Kadlubar, personal communication). It appears, therefore, that *N*-acetoxy heterocyclic amines are relatively stable (the analogous metabolites of the aromatic amines such as 4-aminobiphenyl or 2-naphthylamine are not). The data suggest that activation of the food-borne heterocyclic amines by the liver may be sufficient to lead to formation of DNA-adducts in the pancreas. Further, these data and evidence on compounds including nitrosamines (Pour, 1980), other nitroso compounds (Reddy and Rao, 1975), 4-hydroxyaminoquinoline-1-oxide (Hayashi and Hasegawa, 1971), and other various compounds (Hayashi and Hasegawa, 1971; Scarpelli, 1975; Rao et al, 1974; Longnecker, 1970) support the notion that organotropism for the pancreas may govern, to some degree, the susceptibility of this organ to carcinogenic agents.

Finally, there are metabolic capacities in the pancreas that could directly activate some carcinogens. Hall et al (1989), using immunochemical techniques, showed that human pancreatic ductal cells contain NADPH-cytochrome P-450 reductase, and metabolic studies have shown the human pancreas has 4-nitrobiphenyl reductase activity, which would be consistent with the presence of the P-450 reductase as well as some other enzymes (Anderson et al, 1992). Such activity could reduce airborne nitroaromatic hydrocarbons (nitro-PAHs) to aromatic amines and their *N*-hydroxy derivatives (Kadlubar et al, 1988; Poirier and Weisburger, 1974; Djuric et al, 1985); these in turn could be further activated by pancreatic *O*-acetyltransferase to their ultimate carcinogenic form. There is no strong epidemiologic evidence consistent with such a mechanism; however, humans can be exposed to nitro-PAHs in industrial settings and such a mechanism may underlie some of the elevated risks associated with some occupations.

Modulators of Carcinogenesis

Diet. 1. *Vegetables and fruit.* Steinmetz and Potter (1991b) have reviewed evidence on mechanisms by which vegetables and fruit might be protective against cancer in general. They discuss numerous agents in fruits and vegetables with anticarcinogenic potential including carotenoids, vitamins C and E, isoflavones, phenols, protease inhibitors, isothiocyanates, flavonoids, dithiolthiones, indoles, glucosinolates, selenium, plant sterols, allium compounds, and limonene.

A variety of protective mechanisms—many complex—have been postulated by which vegetables and fruit may lower the risk of cancer (Wattenberg, 1985; Adlercreutz, 1990; for other references in this area see Steinmetz and Potter, 1991b). They include, among others, the induction of detoxification enzymes, inhibition of nitrosamine formation, dilution and binding of carcinogens in the digestive tract, antioxidant effects, alterations in hormone metabolism, and provision of substrates for the formation of endogenous anticarcinogens. Several mechanisms of possible importance to pancreatic cancer will be discussed briefly.

A number of compounds present in plants can induce glutathione *S*-transferase and increase levels of glutathione (GSH). These include isothiocyanates and dithiolthiones, which are present in cruciferous vegetables, and limonene, the majority component of citrus oil. There is some evidence that GSH can inhibit the mutagenic activation of the food-borne heterocyclic amine Trp-P-2 in vitro (Saito et al, 1983); it is therefore plausible that nutrients from fruits and vegetables exert a protective effect against pancreatic cancer through GSH- or GSH *S*-transferase-mediated inhibition of arylamine activation.

Ascorbic acid, alpha-tocopherol, and certain polyphenols can interfere with the process of nitrosamine formation by inhibiting the conversion of dietary nitrate to nitrite by bacteria in the saliva and stomach (Steinmetz and Potter, 1991b; IARC, 1984; Mirvish, 1986). Isothiocyanates have been found to be inhibitors of experimental tumorigenesis induced by the tobacco-specific nitrosamine NNK; the mechanism is thought to involve inhibition of DNA-adduct formation (Morse et al, 1989). If nitrosamines are human pancreatic carcinogens, then vegetables and fruits may exert a protective effect, indirectly, via inhibition of nitrosamine formation or, directly, by blocking formation of DNA-adducts.

Dietary fiber, derived in part from vegetables and fruits, may dilute or bind carcinogens in the digestive tract and thereby decrease their absorption (Steinmetz and Potter, 1991b; Adlercreutz, 1990). Such action may explain the inverse association observed by Howe et al (1991) for fiber, although this may be merely the measured marker for a variety of unmeasured plant anticarcinogens.

Steinmetz and Potter (1991b) have argued that the number of potentially anticarcinogenic agents in vegetables and fruits, some of which have complementary and overlapping mechanisms of action, make it extremely unlikely that any one substance is responsible for all of the associations observed with these foods and cancer risk. Furthermore, they suggest that humans are adapted to a high intake of plant foods containing substances upon which their metabolism is dependent—only some of which are currently identified as "essential nutrients"—and that cancer may result from reducing the level of intake of foods that are metabolically essential [see also Potter (1992)].

2. *Fat.* The association between high fat foods and pancreas cancer is well established in both the epidemiologic and experimental animal literature. In this regard, pancreas cancer is like colon cancer. Unlike colon cancer, however, where at least one plausible mechanism has been described (invoking the effects of fat on both hepatic and bacterial bile acid metabolism) no clear mode of action presents itself as an explanation for fat per se in pancreatic carcinogenesis. Nonetheless, there are both general and specific consequences of a high fat diet, as well as other quite specific dietary exposures for which a high fat diet may be a general marker, that could provide explanations for the association.

It has been known since the 1920s that calorie restriction lowers the incidence of many tumors in mice, rats, fish, and other species. While the mechanism of calorie restriction remains to be fully explicated, there are clear and important differences in the metabolic profile of ad lib fed (who might be better regarded as obese rather than normal) rodents and their calorie-restricted (who might be better regarded as normal) littermates particularly in levels and response-rates of a variety of hormones and enzymes (e.g., glucocorticoids, prolactin, cholecystokinin, gastrin, and ornithine decarboxylase) that are important in energy metabolism and cell proliferation.

Pariza (1987) has pointed out that these data on calorie intake bear on the fat-cancer relation in two ways: high fat/high calorie diets are more likely to contain "adequate" levels of essential fatty acids to provide for the growth requirements of tumors as well as an overall excess of fat which is used more efficiently than other sources of energy.

The mechanism by which dietary fat enhances (or in the case of fish oil, inhibits) carcinogenesis in animals is not known, but several mechanisms have been proposed (Roebuck et al, 1987). One hypothesis is that corn oil may enhance and fish oil inhibit carcinogenesis through opposite effects on prostaglandin synthesis (O'Connor et al, 1989). Corn oil is rich in omega-6 fatty acids, the precursors of prostaglandins, and therefore, a high corn oil diet may lead to higher prostaglandin levels. Fish oil, on the other hand, contains omega-3 fatty acids, which are competitive inhibitors of cyclooxygenase—a key enzyme in prostaglandin synthesis. O'Connor et al (1989) demonstrated that increasing the ratio of omega-3 to omega-6 fatty acids in the diets of rats resulted in a statistically significant lowering of several serum prostaglandin levels.

Other suggested mechanisms for enhancement of carcinogenesis by dietary fat include altered cell membrane or receptor function, or even less well specified mechanisms involving energy intake and retention (Roebuck et al, 1987, 1989; Longnecker, 1990; Pariza, 1987, 1988).

These considerations are not specific to pancreas cancer. A more important observation may be that human diets that are high in fat and calories are also higher in meat and, therefore, in known carcinogens with direct effects upon the pancreas. These include nitrosamines and heterocyclic arylamines and are discussed in more detail above.

3. *Alcohol.* The epidemiologic evidence of a role for alcohol in the genesis of pancreatic cancer is, as noted above, quite weak. Together with a high fat diet, it is an important determinant of chronic calcifying pancreatitis (Johnson and Zintel, 1963; Ishii et al, 1973; Sarles and Tiscornia, 1974; Sarles et al, 1980), the form of pancreatitis most strongly suspected of constituting a risk factor for pancreatic carcinoma (Paulino-Netto et al, 1960; Ishii et al, 1973). The mechanism whereby alcohol increases the risk for pancreatic cancer, should this prove not to be a spurious association, could be via pancreatitis. However, in several studies where pancreatitis was associated with an increased risk for pancreatic cancer, the increase was not specific to alcohol-induced pancreatitis (Amman et al, 1984; Amman and Schueler, 1984; Lowenfels, 1984; Lowenfels et al, 1985, 1993). In some animal models, alcohol has been shown to promote carcinogenesis (Kuratsune et al, 1971), but other studies do not support a role for alco-

hol (Pour et al, 1983a), or pancreatitis (Pour, et al, 1983b).

Steroid Hormones. Pancreatic cancer is more common among males than females, in both humans and in several experimental models. The differences stimulated interest in the role sex hormones might play in the development of this disease. Steroid hormones play a role in normal pancreatic function; it is plausible, therefore, that they may modify pancreatic carcinogenesis (Andren-Sandberg and Johansson, 1990; Longnecker, 1991; Poston et al, 1991; Bueno de Mesquita, 1992c).

Pancreatic tissue has been examined for receptors for hormones that influence normal cell growth. The presence of estrogen and androgen receptors have been demonstrated in normal human pancreas and in some carcinomas (Greenway et al, 1981; Corbishley et al, 1986). The effects of hormones on pancreas cells, however, are unclear. The growth of human pancreas carcinoma in cell cultures has been shown to be stimulated, impaired, and unaffected by estradiol (Benz et al, 1986). Testosterone has stimulated the growth of some human pancreas cancer xenografts in nude mice and had no effect on others (Greenway et al, 1982; Klöppel et al, 1986). Serum concentrations of testosterone have been shown to be significantly lower in pancreatic cancer patients than controls (Greenway et al, 1983; Militello et al, 1984; Tulassay et al, 1988), but whether this is a precursor or a consequence of the disease is not clear. The low serum levels of the hormone in these patients may be explained by the presence of aromatase and 5-alpha-reductase, two enzymes that metabolize testosterone, in pancreatic cancer tissue (Greenway et al, 1983).

Both the experimental data on hormones and the presence of steroid receptors in human pancreatic tissue provided the rationale for clinical trials with tamoxifen, an antiestrogen, and other drugs which alter sex hormone levels. These agents, however, have not had appreciable effects on pancreatic cancer patient survival (Bakkevold et al, 1990; Keating et al, 1989; Theve et al, 1983).

At present, the conservative interpretation of the sex differences in human populations is that smoking rates, intakes of meat and fat, and exposure to carcinogens through occupation are higher in men than women, and that intake of plant foods is lower. There is little need to invoke a biologic (sex-hormone) mechanism.

Gastrointestinal Hormones. Cholecystokinin-pancreozymin (CCK), secretin, gastrin, and other gastrointestinal hormones originating in the cells of the stomach and small intestine have trophic and hyperplastic effects on the exocrine pancreas (Lemoine and Hall, 1990). Hormonal function is regulated by mechanisms that respond to various characteristics of the small intestine, including pH, the concentration of various nutrients, the presence of various drugs, and the intraluminal contents of proteolytic enzymes, such as trypsin and enterokinase. Function at the cellular level is probably regulated by the dynamics of the calcium ion and cyclic AMP (Poston et al, 1991; Williams and Hootman, 1986; Williams, 1987).

CCK and gastrin are two potent hormones that are structurally related: they are 33 and 17 amino acids long, respectively, and they share the same four C-terminal amino acids. For gastrin, the terminal tetrapeptide is as active as the whole molecule. When CCK or its analogue, cerulein, are administered chronically to rats they cause pancreatic growth; in a similar manner, the gastrin analogue, pentagastrin, promotes pancreatic growth in rats (Peterson et al, 1978). CCK has been shown to stimulate growth in cultures of human pancreatic carcinoma cells (Smith et al, 1987). In addition, using nude mice, it has been shown that a CCK receptor antagonist blocks the growth of human pancreatic carcinoma xenografts, and blocks the tumor-promoting effects of a high fat diet (Maani et al, 1988; Smith et al, 1990). It appears that insulin also has a role in maintaining normal function of the exocrine pancreas (Lebenthal and Leung, 1991). Among the other peptide hormones that promote pancreatic growth are secretin, neurotensin, and bombesin (Poston et al, 1991). In contrast, treatment with somatostatin inhibits the growth of pancreatic tumors in animals (Redding and Schally, 1984), and a somatostatin analogue inhibits the growth of human pancreatic cell lines grown as xenografts (Upp, 1988).

The modulating role of peptide hormones in experimental carcinogenesis has been established (Longnecker, 1991). There is evidence to support the notion that these hormones modulate human carcinogenesis (Axelson et al, 1992) and it has been suggested that they may serve as mediators of known or suspected dietary (and other) risk factors (McMichael, 1981; Poston et al, 1991), but this remains to be established.

Growth Factors. There is considerable evidence for a role of growth factors in normal pancreatic growth and function as well as in the pathogenesis of pancreatic cancer (Lemoine and Hall, 1990; Poston et al, 1991). This area was reviewed by Lemoine and Hall (1990) and is only briefly discussed here. Overexpression of epidermal growth factor receptor (EGF-R) and/or its ligands, transforming growth factor alpha (TGF-alpha) and epidermal growth factor (EGF), may be involved in the genesis of pancreatic cancer through an autocrine stimulatory loop (Korc, 1990; Barton et al, 1991a). EGF and TGF-alpha bind to the EGF-R and cause trophic and other effects in the normal pancreas. Normal pancreas tissue expresses TGF-alpha, but not EGF (Barton et al, 1991a). Overexpression of TGF-alpha was observed in 80 of 84 (95%) pancreatic tumors examined, while 12% overexpressed EGF. Furthermore, overexpression of the EGF-R was found in 95% of these same tumors (Lemoine et al, 1992c), and in other pancreatic tumors (Korc et al, 1986; Klöppel et al, 1989). This overexpression is believed to be due to increased transcription of the normal gene. Thus, various lines of evidence support the hypothesis that TGF-alpha may stimulate the growth of pancreatic cells via an autocrine loop in which TGF-alpha binds to EGF-R expressed by those same cells that produce the TGF-alpha. Thus a growth advantage may be provided to cells which concomitantly produce—or overproduce—TGF-alpha and overexpress EGF-R to bind it (Barton et al, 1991a). Although such loops—autocrine as here, paracrine in other tissues—are plausible mechanisms for growth promotion of tumors, there are no data that currently allow such mechanisms to be related to epidemiologic risk factors or known metabolism.

Medical Conditions. 1. *Diabetes.* It has been argued that the association between diabetes and pancreatic cancer is artifactual—due to increased medical surveillance of diabetics or that undiagnosed cancer causes diabetes via destruction of islets by invading tumor. Ragozzino et al (1982) found little evidence for this first possibility in their follow-up of a cohort of diabetics, citing the fact that relative risk estimates for other cancers, both those "easily observed," such as breast cancer, and "occult" tumors (other than pancreas) such as bladder or ovary, were not substantially different from expected. Regarding the second possibility, it has long been known that glucosuria and hyperglycemia may appear after the nutritional deprivation associated with carcinomatosis (Glicksman et al, 1956), and it is reasonable to suppose that islet cell function is sometimes interrupted after invasion by exocrine carcinoma (Frantz, 1959). However, many studies that have addressed this question have excluded cancer cases diagnosed within 1 year of the onset of diabetes (a number have excluded cases diagnosed within 5 years) and still have found increased risks associated with long-standing diabetes. Given what is known about the behavior of pancreas cancer in general, it does not seem reasonable to suppose that islet cell function is interrupted by tumor invasion in individuals who have had diabetes for 5 years or more. An alternative hypothesis is that the two diseases are associated because of a common susceptibility to toxic stimuli shared by the embryologically related exocrine and endocrine cells (Rutter, 1980).

It is this last argument that served, in part, as a rationale for Walker's conclusions in a 1988 review of the literature on the association between pancreatic cancer and diabetes (Walker, 1990). Several salient arguments regarding the nature of the relation will be paraphrased here. First, the manifestation of diabetes often precedes that of the cancer by a period sufficient to make it unlikely that the association is due to a simple process of islet cell compression by the tumor. Second, the interval between diabetes and cancer onset is sufficiently short as to make it unlikely that the tumor results from a process that begins de novo with the appearance of diabetes. Third, the clinical appearance of the tumor is often accompanied by widespread abnormalities suggesting a more general chemical or metabolic disorder. These arguments, together with the anatomic, metabolic, and pathophysiologic links between endocrine and exocrine organ, support the view that neither condition causes the other, but, to paraphrase Walker, diabetes mellitus is a sign of the breakdown of islet cell function under stress from metabolic by-products that have been toxic to the islet cells and carcinogenic to the ductal cells.

Pursuing this argument further, one could argue that the collapse of the islet cells means that an interaction between endocrine and exocrine pancreas, which is necessary for maintaining or controlling normal growth and function in the exocrine pancreas, is lost; the result is a promoting effect—perhaps a late-stage promoting effect—upon initiated cells in the exocrine tissue. The relation of insulin or glucagon to the initial development of the autocrine loops described above may be important.

2. *Pancreatitis.* There is increasing evidence to support the hypothesis that patients with chronic pancreatitis, independent of the factors that caused the pancreatitis, are at increased risk for pancreatic cancer. It is also true, however, that even if chronic pancreatitis is a risk factor for pancreatic cancer, it could explain only a small fraction of pancreatic cancers (Gold and Cameron, 1993). The significance of such a link is that it may provide clues about the etiology of this enigmatic cancer.

The underlying biology that may predispose patients with pancreatitis to pancreas cancer is not known, but it is interesting to note that there are a number of alterations at the genetic level that have been associated with pancreatic cancer and to a lesser extent with pancreatitis. For example, overexpression of epidermal growth factor receptor—which has been associated with enhanced metastatic potential and tumor invasiveness (Korc, 1990), and overexpression of *erbB*-3 protein, with growth-factor-receptor-like characteristics, has been observed in biopsied samples of chronic pancreatitis as well as in a majority of pancreatic cancers examined by Lemoine et al (1992a, 1992c).

3. *Cholecystectomy and gall stones.* An explanation for a possible predisposition for cancer among subjects with cholelithiasis is discussed by Haddock and Carter (1990). The authors point out that cholecystectomy in hamsters can lead to an increase in circulating CCK levels and to hypertrophy and hyperplasia in the pancreas. Receptors for CCK have been found in human pancre-

atic cancer cells and CCK stimulates the growth of some human pancreatic cancer cell lines (Axelson et al, 1992). Thus, a role for cholecystectomy as a promoting factor for pancreatic cancer, mediated by the trophic effects of CCK, is plausible, though not established.

4. *Gastrectomy and allergies.* Several plausible mechanisms for an increased risk of pancreatic cancer among gastrectomy patients have been described (Mack et al, 1986). Both hormonal and neurologic regulation of pancreas are mediated by gastric secretion, and gastrectomy could alter homeostatic regulation of hormones that are trophic for the pancreas. Detoxification of endogenous and exogenous substances in the small intestine might be less efficient after gastrectomy. Finally, gastrectomy can increase the endogenous production of *N*-nitroso compounds (Schlag et al, 1980), possibly as a result of pH-induced changes in bacterial growth and is a plausible mechanism to explain the observed increased risk of pancreas cancer in gastrectomy patients (Caygill et al, 1985; Mack et al, 1986). Increased endogenous production of *N*-nitroso compounds has also been suggested as a possible mechanism to explain the increased incidence of pancreas cancer observed in pernicious anemia patients (Borch et al, 1988). Trophic hormones may mediate the observed associations of pancreatic cancer with both tobacco smoke and gastric surgery and the possible protective effect of allergies (Mack et al, 1986). The argument is as follows: it has been shown that both gastrectomy and nicotine suppress pancreatic secretion. IgE-linked allergy, on the other hand, indirectly stimulates pancreatic secretion via histamine-mediated stimulation of gastric acid secretion. Thus the effects of tobacco and gastrectomy, on the one hand, and allergy, on the other, are opposite both in their effects on pancreatic secretion and in their association with risk of pancreatic cancer.

PREVENTIVE MEASURES

Screening and early detection for pancreatic cancer are not feasible at this time, and, aside from surgery for a small minority of patients, there is no effective treatment for this formidable disease; therefore, in the future, our only hope is prevention.

The most significant step that could be taken to prevent pancreas cancer would be to eliminate cigarette smoking. The major argument for the reduction of cigarette consumption, however, clearly arises from its relation with heart disease and lung cancer. Nonetheless, a reduction in pancreatic cancer would be an excellent bonus.

Evidence suggests that some of the dietary recommendations proposed by the National Research Council's "Committee on Diet and Health" to decrease the risk of chronic disease overall may function to prevent pancreatic cancer; i.e., individuals should strive to reduce total fat consumption to 30% or less of calories; consume five or more servings of fruits and vegetables per day; and maintain protein intake at moderate levels, which, in general, means lowering meat consumption (National Research Council, 1989).

It may also be prudent to limit the consumption of burned or charred animal-protein-containing foods and pickled and preserved foods in order to limit intake of carcinogenic compounds.

FUTURE RESEARCH

The growing use of molecularly defined subgroups of cancer in epidemiology may help us to discover more about the etiology of pancreatic cancer. The use of biomarkers may allow us to better determine and measure dietary and environmental exposures (Potter et al, 1993). Epidemiology, in combination with genetics, may elucidate differences in carcinogen metabolism that influence risk.

It would be useful to have a better understanding of mechanisms of action of dietary factors in order to learn more about their possible role in pancreatic physiology and carcinogenesis. For example, what are the effects of dietary habits and dietary change on gastrointestinal hormone levels? What effect does dietary intervention, for example, increased fruit and vegetable consumption, have on serum and pancreatic levels of compounds that may be protective against this cancer? What are the effects of meat consumption on the induction of carcinogen-activating enzymes? Can fruit, vegetable, or fiber intake alter blood-borne nitrosamine and heterocyclic amine levels in smokers and individuals with high meat intake?

Molecular genetic research has pinpointed genes that are frequently mutated in this cancer. Further studies to elucidate the normal function and the consequences of mutation in *ras, myc, erbB*-2, *apc,* p53, *dcc,* and other genes may teach us a great deal about the pathogenesis of pancreatic cancer and may provide strategies for prevention and possible targets for growth inhibition of neoplasia (Weinberg, 1991; Aaronson, 1991).

Finally, there are methodologic issues. The accuracy of diagnosis remains a significant factor for epidemiologists. Many case-control studies have used proxy respondents, which increase the chance of misclassifying exposures (Lyon et al, 1992a). Hospital-based studies have the advantage of a higher proportion of direct versus surrogate interviews, yet are burdened with other problems related to the selection of the control series. More population-based studies, attempting direct interview with patients (and thus requiring interviews with cases as early as possible), may help to clarify some risk factors associated with the disease, particularly diet. To establish clearly the gene-environment interactions that characterize most cancers, large cohort studies with baseline bloods and access to tumor tissue will ultimately prove to be crucial.

REFERENCES

AARONSON SA. 1991. Growth factors and cancer. Science 254:1146–1153.

ADLERCREUTZ H. 1990. Western diet and western diseases: Some hormonal and biochemical mechanisms and associations. Scand J Clin Lab Invest 50 (Suppl 201):3–23.

ALDERSON M. 1974. Mortality from malignant disease in patients with asthma. Lancet 2:1475–1477.

ALOMOQUERA C, SHIBATA D, FORRESTER K, et al. 1988. Most human carcinomas of the exocrine pancreas contain mutant *c*-K-*ras* genes. Cell 53:549–554.

AMERICAN CANCER SOCIETY. 1993. Cancer Facts and Figures—1993. New York, American Cancer Society.

AMMANN RW, AKOVBIAMTZ A, LARGIADER F, et al. 1984. Course and outcome of chronic pancreatitis: Longitudinal study of a mixed medical-surgical series of 245 patients. Gastroenterology 86:820–828.

AMMANN RW, KNOBLAUCH M, MÖHR P, et al. 1980. High incidence of extrapancreatic carcinoma in chronic pancreatitis. Scand J Gastroenterol 15:395–399.

AMMANN RW, SCHUELER G. 1984. Chronic pancreatitis, pancreatic cancer, alcohol, and smoking. (Letter). Gastroenterology 87:744–745.

ANDERSON DE. 1978. Familial cancer and cancer families. Semin Oncol 5:11–16.

ANDERSON KE, POTTER JD, HAMMONS GJ, et al. 1992. Metabolic activation of aromatic amines by human pancreas. (Abstract). Proc Am Assoc Cancer Res 33:152.

ANDREN-SANDBERG A, JOHANSSON J. 1990. Influence of sex hormones on pancreatic cancer. Int J Pancreatol 7:167–176.

AOKI K, HAYAKAWA N, KURIHARA M, et al (eds). 1992. Death Rates for Malignant Neoplasms for Selected Sites by Sex and Five-year Age Group in 33 Countries 1953–57 to 1983–87. Nagoya, Japan, The University of Nagoya Coop Press.

APPEL MJ, ROVERTS G, WOUTERSEN RA. 1991. Inhibitory effects of micronutrients on pancreatic carcinogenesis in azaserine-treated rats. Carcinogenesis 12:2157–2161.

APPERT HE. 1990. Composition and production of pancreatic tumor related antigens. Int J Pancreatol 7:13–24.

ARMSTRONG B, DOLL R. 1975. Environmental factors and cancer incidence and mortality in different countries with special reference to dietary practices. Int J Cancer 15:617–631.

ARNAR DO, THEODORS A, ISAKSSON HJ, et al. 1991. Cancer of the pancreas in Iceland: An epidemiologic and clinical study, 1974–85. Scand J Gastroenterol 26:724–730.

AUERBACH O, GARFINKEL L. 1986. Histologic changes in pancreas in relation to smoking and coffee-drinking habits. Dig Dis Sci 31:1014–1020.

AXELSON J, IHSE I, HÅKANSON R. 1992. Pancreatic cancer: The role of cholecystokinin? Scand J Gastroenterol 27:993–998.

AXTELL LM, ASIRE AJ, MYERS MH. 1976. Cancer patient survival, Report No. 5. Bethesda, U.S. Department of Health, Education, and Welfare.

BAGHURST PA, MCMICHAEL AJ, SLAVOTINEK AH, et al. 1991. A case-control study of diet and cancer of the pancreas. Am J Epidemiol 134:167–179.

BAKKEVOLD KE, ARNESJØ B, KAMBESTAD B. 1992. Carcinoma of the pancreas and papilla of Vater: Presenting symptoms, signs and diagnosis related to stage and tumour site. Scand J Gastroenterol 27:317–325.

BAKKEVOLD KE, PETTERSEN A, ARNESJØ B, et al. 1990. Tamoxifen therapy in unresectable adenocarcinoma of the pancreas and the papilla of Vater. Br J Surg 77:725–730.

BARBACID M. 1987. *ras* Genes: Annu Rev Biochem 56:779–827.

BARCLAY THC, PHILLIPS AJ. 1962. The accuracy of cancer diagnosis on death certificates. Cancer 15:5–9.

BARROWMAN JA, MAYSTON PD. 1974. The trophic influence of cholecystokinin in the rat pancreas. J Physiol 238:73P–75P.

BARTHOLOMEW LG, et al. 1958. Carcinoma of the pancreas associated with chronic relapsing pancreatitis. Gastroenterology 35:473–477.

BARTON CM, HALL PA, HUGHES CM, et al. 1991a. Transforming growth factor alpha and epidermal growth factor in human pancreatic cancer. J Pathol 163:111–116.

BARTON CM, STADDON SL, HUGHES CM, et al. 1991b. Abnormalities of the p53 tumor suppressor gene in human pancreatic cancer. Br J Cancer 64:1076–1082.

BARTON CM, STADDON SL, HUGHES CM, et al. 1992. Abnormalities of the p53 tumour suppressor gene in human pancreatic cancer. (Corrigendum.) Br J Cancer 65:485.

BARTON CM, HALL PA, HUGHES CM, et al. 1991b. Transforming growth factor alpha and epidermal growth factor in human pancreatic cancer. J Pathol 163:111–116.

BAUER FW, ROBBINS SL. 1972. An autopsy study of cancer patients. JAMA 221:1471–1474.

BEAZLEY RM, MCANENY DB, COHN I JR. 1991. Progress in pancreatic cancer. American Cancer Society.

BELAND FA, KADLUBAR FF. 1985. Formation and persistence of arylamine DNA adducts *in vivo*. Environ Health Perspect 62:19–30.

BELL ET. 1957. Carcinoma of the pancreas. Am J Pathol 33:499–523.

BELL RH JR, KUHLMANN ET, JENSEN RT, et al. 1992. Overexpression of cholecystokinin receptors in azaserine-induced neoplasms of the rat pancreas. Cancer Res 52:3295–3299.

BENZ C, HOLLANDER C, MILLER B. 1986. Endocrine-responsive pancreatic carcinoma: Steroid binding and cytotoxicity studies in human tumor cell lines. Cancer Res 46:2276–2281.

BERK JE. 1941. Diagnosis of carcinoma of the pancreas. Arch Intern Med 68:525–559.

BEST EWR, et al. 1966. A Canadian Study of Smoking and Health. Ottawa, Canada. Dept Natl Health and Welfare.

BIRT DF, DAVIES MH, POUR PM, et al. 1983a. Lack of inhibition by retinoids of bis (2-oxypropyl) nitrosamine-induced carcinogenesis in Syrian hamsters. Carcinogenesis 4:1215–1220.

BIRT DF, JULIUS AD, DWORK E, et al. 1990. Comparison of the effects of dietary beef tallow and corn oil on pancreatic carcinogenesis in the hamster model. Carcinogenesis 11:745–748.

BIRT DF, JULIUS AD, RUNICE CE, et al. 1986. Effects of dietary selenium on bis (2-oxypropyl) nitrosamine-induced carcinogenesis in Syrian golden hamsters. J Natl Cancer Inst 77:1281–1286.

BIRT DF, SALMASI S, POUR PM. 1981a. Enhancement of experimental pancreatic cancer in Syrian golden hamsters by dietary fat. J Natl Cancer Inst 67:1327–1332.

BIRT DF, SAYED S, DAVIES MH, et al. 1981b. Sex differences in the effects of retinoids on carcinogenesis by *N*-nitrosobis(2-oxypropyl)amine in Syrian hamsters. Cancer Lett 14:13–21.

BIRT DF, STEPAN KR, POUR PM. 1983b. Interaction of dietary fat and protein on pancreatic carcinogenesis in Syrian golden hamsters. J Natl Cancer Inst 71:355–360.

BJELDANES LF, MORRIS MM, FELTON JS, et al. 1982. Mutagens from the cooking of food. II. Survey by Ames/Salmonella test of mutagen formation in the major protein-rich foods of the American diet. Food Chem Toxicol 20:357–363.

BLAIR A, MALKER H, CANTOR KP, et al. 1985. Cancer among farmers: A review. Scand J Work Environ Health 11:397–407.

BLOT WJ, FRAUMENI JF JR, STONE BJ. 1978. Geographic correlates of pancreas cancer in the United States. Cancer 42:373–380.

BLOT WJ, LANIER A, FRAUMENI JF JR, et al. 1975. Cancer mortality among Alaskan natives, 1960–69. J Natl Cancer Inst 55:547–554.

BOCKMAN DE. 1981. Cells of origin of pancreatic cancer: Experimental animal tumors related to human pancreas. Cancer 47:1528–1534.

BOFFETTA P, STELLMAN SD, GARFINKEL L. 1988. Diesel exhaust exposure and mortality among males in the American Cancer Society prospective study. Am J Ind Med 14:403–415.

BOND GG, RECYE GR, OTT MG, et al. 1985. Mortality among a sample of chemical company employees. Am J Ind Med 7:109–20.

BORCH K, KULLMAN E, HALLHAGEN S, et al. 1988. Increased incidence of pancreatic neoplasia in pernicious anaemia. World J Surg 12:866–870.

BOS JL. 1989. *ras* Oncogenes in human cancer: A review. Cancer Res 49:4682–4689.

BOS JL. 1990. *ras* Oncogenes in human cancer: A review. (Erratum.) Cancer Res 50:1352.

BOUCHARDY C, CLAVEL F, LA VECCHIA C, et al. 1990. Alcohol, beer and cancer of the pancreas. Int J Cancer 45:842–846.

BOYLE P, HSIEH C-C, MAISONNEUVE P, et al. 1989. Epidemiology of pancreas cancer (1988). Int J Pancreatol 5:327–346.

BRAGANZA JM. 1983. Pancreatic disease: A casualty of hepatic "detoxification"? Lancet 2:1000–1003.

BUELL P, DUNN JE. 1965. Cancer mortality among Japanese Issei and Nisei of California. Cancer 18:656–664.

BUENO DE MESQUITA HB, MAISONNEUVE P, MOERMAN CJ, et al. 1991a. Life-time history of smoking and exocrine carcinoma of the pancreas: A population-based case-control study in The Netherlands. Int J Cancer 49:816–822.

BUENO DE MESQUITA HB, MAISONNEUVE P, MOERMAN CJ, et al. 1991b. Intake of foods and nutrients and exocrine carcinoma of the pancreas: A population-based case-control study in The Netherlands. Int J Cancer 48:540–549.

BUENO DE MESQUITA HB. 1992. On the causation of cancer of the exocrine pancreas. (Thesis.) Utrecht, The Netherlands, University of Utrecht.

BUENO DE MESQUITA HB, MAISONNEUVE P, MOERMAN CJ, et al. 1992a. Lifetime consumption of alcoholic beverages, tea and coffee and exocrine carcinoma of the pancreas: A population-based case-control study in The Netherlands. Int J Cancer 50:514–522.

BUENO DE MESQUITA HB, MAISONNEUVE P, MOERMAN CJ, et al. 1992b. Aspects of medical history and exocrine carcinoma of the pancreas: A population-based case-control study in The Netherlands. Int J Cancer 52:17–23.

BUENO DE MESQUITA HB, MAISONNEUVE P, MOERMAN CJ, et al. 1992c. Anthropometric and reproductive variables and exocrine carcinoma of the pancreas: A population-based case-control study in The Netherlands. Int J Cancer 53:24–29.

BUENO DE MESQUITA HB, MOERMAN CJ, RUNIA S, et al. 1990. Are energy and energy-providing nutrients related to exocrine carcinoma of the pancreas. Int J Cancer 46:435–444.

BURCH GE, ANSARI A. 1968. Chronic alcoholism and carcinoma of the pancreas. Arch Intern Med 122:273–275.

BURMEISTER LF. 1990. Cancer in Iowa farmers: Recent results. Am J Ind Med 18:295–301.

BURNEY PGJ, COMSTOCK GW, MORRIS JS. 1989. Serologic precursors of cancer: Serum micronutrients and the subsequent risk of pancreatic cancer. Am J Clin Nutr 49:895–900.

CAMERON HM, MCGOOGAN E. 1981. A prospective study of 1152 hospital autopsies. II. Analysis of inaccuracies in clinical diagnoses and their significance. J Pathol 133:285–300.

CANTOR KP, BOOZE CF JR. 1991. Mortality among aerial applicators and flight instructors: A reprint. Arch Environ Health 46:110–116.

CARMELLA SG, KAGAN SS, KAGAN M, et al. 1990. Mass spectrometric analysis of tobacco-specific nitrosamine hemoglobin adducts in snuff dippers, smokers, and nonsmokers. Cancer Res 50:5438–5445.

CARTER DC. 1990. Cancer of the pancreas. Gut 31:494–496.

CASSIERE SG, MCLAIN DA, BROOKS EMORY W, et al. 1980. Metastatic carcinoma of the pancreas simulating primary bronchogenic carcinoma. Cancer 46:2319–2321.

CASTLEMAN B, SCULLY RE, MCNEELY BU (EDS). 1972. Case records of the Massachusetts General Hospital. N Engl J Med 286:1353–1359.

CAYGILL CPG, HILL MJ, HALL N, et al. 1985. Gastric surgery as a risk factor in human carcinogenesis. (Abstract). Gastroenterology 88:1344.

CEDERLÖF R, FRIBERG L, HRUBEC Z, et al. 1975. The Relationship of Smoking and Some Social Covariables to Mortality and Cancer Morbidity. Stockholm, The Karolinska Institute.

CENTRAL BUREAU OF STATISTICS, NORWAY. 1976. Yrke og dodelighed 1970–73. Statistiske Analyser, No. 21, Oslo.

CERNY WL, MANGOLD KA, SCARPELLI DG. 1990. Activation of K-*ras* in transplantable pancreatic ductal adenocarcinomas of Syrian golden hamsters. Carcinogenesis 11:2075–2079.

CERNY WL, MANGOLD KA, SCARPELLI DG. 1992. K-*ras* mutation is an early event in pancreatic duct carcinogenesis in the Syrian golden hamster. Cancer Res 52:4507–4513.

CLARK CG, MITCHELL PEG. 1961. Diabetes mellitus and primary carcinoma of the pancreas. Br Med J 2:1259–1262.

CLAVEL F, BENHAMOU D, AUQUIER A, et al. 1989. Coffee, alcohol, smoking and cancer of the pancreas: A case-control study. Int J Cancer 43:17–21.

CLEMMESEN J. 1974. Statistical studies in the aetiology of malignant neoplasms. IV. Lung/bladder ratio for Denmark 1943–67. Acta Pathol Microbiol Scand 247:7–266.

COGGON D, PANNETT B, WINTER PD, et al. 1986. Mortality of workers exposed to 2-methyl-4-chlorophenoxyacetic acid. Scand J Work Environ Health 12:448–454.

COHART EM, MULLER C. 1955. Socioeconomic distribution of cancer of the gastrointestinal tract in New Haven. Cancer 8:1126–1129.

COHEN GF. 1965. Early diagnosis of pancreatic neoplasms in diabetics. Lancet 2:267–269.

COMMITTEE ON THE BIOLOGICAL EFFECTS OF IONIZING RADIATIONS. 1990. Health effects of exposure to low levels of ionizing radiation: BEIR V. Washington, D.C. National Academy Press.

CORBISHLEY TP, IQBAL MJ, WILKINSON ML, et al. 1986. Androgen receptors in human normal and malignant pancreatic tissue and cell lines. Cancer 57:1992–1995.

COSTANTINI A, PACI E, MILIGI L, et al. 1989. Cancer mortality among workers in the Tuscan tanning industry. Br J Ind Med 46:384–388.

COURT-BROWN WM, DOLL R. 1958. Expectation of life and mortality from cancer among British radiologists. Br Med J 2:181–187.

CREAGAN ET, FRAUMENI JF JR. 1972. Cancer mortality among American Indians, 1950–67. J Natl Cancer Inst 49:959–967.

CUBILLA AL, FITZGERALD PJ. 1978a. Pancreas cancer (non-endocrine): A review. Part II. Clin Bull 8:143–155.

CUBILLA AL, FITZGERALD PJ. 1978b. Pancreas cancer. I. Duct adenocarcinoma, a clinical-pathologic study of 380 patients. *In* Pathology Annual, Part 1. New York, Appleton-Century-Crofts, pp. 241–287.

CUBILLA AL, FITZGERALD PJ. 1980. Surgical pathology aspects of cancer of the ampulla-head-of-pancreas region. *In* Fitzgerald PJ, Morrison AB (eds): The Pancreas. Baltimore, Williams & Wilkins, pp. 67–81.

CUBILLA AL, FITZGERALD PJ. 1984. Tumors of the exocrine pancreas. *In* Hartmann WH, Sobin LH (eds): Atlas of Tumor Pathology. Second series, fasc. 19. Washington, Armed Forces Institute of Pathology.

CUZICK J, BABIKER AG. 1989. Pancreatic cancer, alcohol, diabetes mellitus and gallbladder disease. Int J Cancer 43:415–421.

CUZICK J, ROUTLEDGE MN, JENKINS D, et al. 1990. DNA adducts in different tissues of smokers and non-smokers. Int J Cancer 45:673–678.

DAVIDSON P, COSTANZA D, SWIECONER JA, et al. 1983. Hereditary pancreatitis: A kindred without gross aminoaciduria. Ann Intern Med 68:88–96.

DECOUFLÉ P, et al. 1977a. A retrospective survey of cancer in relation to occupation. Washington, DC, U.S. Government Printing Office, NIOSH Pub No, 77-178.

DECOUFLÉ P, LLOYD JW, SALVIN LG. 1977b. Mortality by cause among stationary engineers and stationary firemen. J Occup Med 19:679–682.

DELZELL E, LOUIK C, LEWIS J, et al. 1981. Mortality and cancer morbidity among workers in the rubber tire industry. Am J Ind Med 2:209–216.

DELZELL E, MONSON RR. 1985. Mortality among rubber workers. IX. Curing workers. Am J Ind Med 8:537–544.

DEVESA SS, SILVERMAN DT, YOUNG JL JR, et al. 1987. Cancer incidence and mortality trends among whites in the United States, 1947–1984. J Natl Cancer Inst 79:701–770.

DISSIN J, MILLS LR, MAINS DL, et al. 1975. Experimental induction of pancreatic adenocarcinoma in rats. J Natl Cancer Inst 55:4.

DIVINE BJ, BARRON V. 1986. Texaco mortality study. II. Patterns of mortality among white males by specific job group. Am J Ind Med 10:371–381.

DIVINE BJ, BARRON V, KAPLAN SD. 1985. Texaco mortality study. I. Mortality among refinery petrochemical, and research workers. J Occup Med 27:445–447.

DJURIC Z, FIFER EK, BELAND FA. 1985. Acetyl coenzyme A-dependent binding of carcinogenic and mutagenic dinitropyrenes to DNA. Carcinogenesis 6:941–944.

DOLL R, PETO R. 1976. Mortality in relation to smoking: 20 years' observation on male British doctors. Br Med J 2:1525–1536.

DOLL R, VESSEY MP, BEASLEY RW, et al. 1972. Mortality of gasworkers—Final report of a prospective study. Br J Ind Med 29:394–406.

DÖRKEN VH. 1964. Einige daten bei 280 Patienten mit Pankreaskrebs. Gastroenterologia 102:47–77.

DORN HF, CUTLER SJ. 1958. Morbidity from cancer in the United States. Part II. Trend in morbidity association with income and stage at diagnosis. Public Health Monogr 56.

DOUGLAS BR, WOUTERSEN RA, JANSEN JBMJ, et al. 1990. Comparison of the effect of lorglumide on pancreatic growth stimulated by camostate in rat and hamsters. Life Sci 46:281–286.

DURBEC JP, CHEVILLOTTE G, BIDART JM, et al. 1983. Diet, alcohol, tobacco and risk of cancer of the pancreas: A case-control study. Br J Cancer 47:467–470.

EDLING C, KLING H, FLODIN U, et al. 1986. Cancer mortality among leather tanners. Br J Ind Med 43:494–496.

EHRENTHAL D, HAEGER L, GRIFFIN T, et al. 1987. Familial pancreatic adenocarcinoma in three generations: A case report and a review of the literature. Cancer 59:1661–1664.

EIDE TJ, VISTE A, ANDERSEN A, et al. 1991. The risk of cancer at all sites following gastric operation for benign disease. A cohort study of 4,224 patients. Int J Cancer 48:333–339.

EISEN EA, TOLBERT PE, MONSON RR, et al. 1992. Mortality studies of machining fluid exposure in the automobile industry. I. A standardized mortality ratio analysis. Am J Ind Med 22:809–824.

ELLINGER F, LANDSMAN H. 1944. Frequency and course of cancer in diabetics. New York State J Med 44:259–265.

ENGEL LW, STRAUCHEN JA, CHIAZZE L JR, et al. 1980. Accuracy of death certification in an autopsied population with specific attention to malignant neoplasms and vascular diseases. Am J Epidemiol, 111:99–112.

ENSTROM JE. 1978. Cancer and total mortality among active Mormons. Cancer 42:1943–1951.

ENSTROM JE. 1980. Health and dietary practices and cancer mortality among California Mormons. *In* Cairns J, et al (eds): Banbury Report 4. Cancer Incidence in Defined Populations. Cold Spring Harbor, NY, Cold Spring Harbor Laboratory, pp. 69–92.

FALK RT, PICKLE LW, FONTHAM ET, et al. 1988. Life-style risk factors for pancreatic cancer in Louisiana: A case-control study. Am J Epidemiol 128:324–336.

FALK RT, PICKLE LW, FONTHAM ET, et al. 1990. Occupation and pancreatic cancer risk in Louisiana. Am J Ind Med 18:565–576.

FARROW DC, DAVIS S. 1990a. Risk of pancreatic cancer in relation to medical history and the use of tobacco, alcohol and coffee. Int J Cancer 45:816–820.

FARROW DC, DAVIS S. 1990b. Diet and risk of pancreatic cancer in men. Am J Epidemiol 132:423–431.

FEARON ER, CHO K, NIGRO J, et al. 1990. Identification of a chromosome 18q gene that is altered in colorectal cancers. Science 247:49–56.

FEARON ER, VOGELSTEIN B. 1990. A genetic model for colorectal tumorigenesis. Cell 61:759–767.

FEINSTEIN AR, HORWITZ RI, SPITZER WO, et al. 1981. Coffee and pancreatic cancer: The problems of etiologic science and epidemiologic case-control research. JAMA 246:957–961.

FELTON JS, KNIZE MG. 1991. Occurrence, identification and bacterial mutagenicity of heterocyclic amines in cooked food. Mutat Res 259:205–217.

FERRARONI M, NEGRI E, LA VECCHIA C, et al. 1989. Socioeconomic indicators, tobacco and alcohol in the aetiology of digestive tract neoplasms. Int J Epidemiol 18:556–562.

FLAKS B. 1984. Histogenesis of pancreatic carcinogenesis in the hamster: Ultrastructural evidence. Environ Health Perspect 56:187–203.

FÖLSCH UR, MUSTROPH D, SCHAFMAYER A, et al. 1984. Elevated CCK plasma concentrations during acute and chronic feeding of soybean flour. Digestion 30:88.

FONTHAM ETH, CORREA P. 1989. Epidemiology of pancreatic cancer. Surg Clin North Am 69:551–567.

FRANCESCHI S, BARBONE F, BIDOLI E, et al. 1993. Cancer risk in farmers: Results from a multi-site case-(hospital) control study in North-eastern Italy. Int J Cancer 53:740–745.

FRANTZ VK. 1959. Atlas of tumor pathology, Section VII, Fascicles 27–28, *In* Tumors of the Pancreas. Washington, DC, AFIP, pp. 5–78.

FRAUMENI JF JR, MASON TJ. 1974. Cancer mortality among Chinese Americans, 1950–69. J Natl Cancer Inst 52:659–665.

FRIEDMAN GD, VAN DEN EEDEN SK. 1993. Risk factors for pancreatic cancer: An exploratory study. Int J Epidemiol 22:30–37.

FRIEDMAN JM, FIALKOW PJ. 1976. Familial carcinoma of the pancreas. Clin Genet 9:463–469.

FUJII H, EGAMI H, CHANEY W, et al. 1990. Pancreatic ductal adenocarcinomas induced in Syrian hamsters by *N*-nitrobis(2-oxopropyl)amine contain a c-Ki-*ras* oncogene with a point-mutated codon 12. Mol Carcinog 3:296–301.

GAMBILL EE. 1971. Pancreatitis associated with pancreatic carcinoma: A study of 26 cases. Mayo Clin Proc 46:174–177.

GARABRANT DH, HELD J, LANGHOLZ B, et al. 1992. DDT and related compounds and risk of pancreatic cancer. J Natl Cancer Inst 84:764–771.

GHADIRIAN P, BOYLE P, SIMARD A, et al. 1991a. Reported family aggregation of pancreatic cancer within a population-based case-control study in the Francophone community in Montreal, Canada. Int J Pancreatol 10:183–196.

GHADIRIAN P, SIMARD A, BAILLARGEON J. 1991b. Tobacco, alcohol, and coffee and cancer of the pancreas. Cancer 67:2664–2670.

GHADIRIAN P, SIMARD A, BAILLARGEON J, et al. 1991c. Nutritional factors and pancreatic cancer in the Francophone community in Montreal, Canada. Int J Cancer 47:1–6.

GHADIRIAN P, THOUEZ J-P, PETITCLERC C. 1991d. International comparisons of nutrition and mortality from pancreatic cancer. Cancer Detect Prev 15:357–362.

GILBERT ES, MARKS S. 1979. An analysis of the mortality of workers in a nuclear facility. Radiat Res 79:122–128.

GLICKSMAN AS, MYERS WPL, RAWSON R. 1956. Diabetes mellitus and carbohydrate metabolism in patients with cancer. Med Clin North Am 40:887–900.

GO VLW, GARDERNER JD, BROOKS FP, et al (eds). 1986. The Exocrine Pancreas: Biology, Pathobiology and Diseases. New York, Raven Press.

GÖKE B, PRINTZ H, KOOP I, et al. 1986. Endogenous CCK release and pancreatic growth after feeding a proteinase inhibitor (camostate). Pancreas 1:509–515.

GOLD EB, CAMERON JL. 1993. Chronic pancreatitis and pancreatic cancer. (Editorial). N Engl J Med 328:1485–1486.

GOLD EB, GORDIS L, DIENER MD, et al. 1985. Diet and other risk factors for cancer of the pancreas. Cancer 55:460–467.

GORDIS L. 1990. Consumption of methylxanthine-containing beverages and risk of pancreatic cancer. Cancer Lett 52:1–12.

GRAHAM S, LEVIN M, LILIENFELD AM. 1960. The socioeconomic distribution of cancer of various sites in Buffalo, NY: 1948–1952. Cancer 13:180–190.

GREEN A, JENSEN OM. 1985. Frequency of cancer among insulin-treated diabetic patients in Denmark. Diabetologia 28:128–130.

GREEN RC, BAGGENSTOSS AH, SPRAGUE RG. 1958. Diabetes mellitus in association with primary carcinoma of the pancreas. Diabetes 7:308–311.

GREENBERG HL, OTT MG, SHORE RE. 1990. Men assigned to ethylene oxide production or other ethylene oxide related chemical manufacturing: a mortality study. Br J Ind Med 47:221–230.

GREENWALD P, KORNS RF, NASCA PL, et al. 1975. Cancer in United States Jews. Cancer Res 35:3507–3512.

GREENWAY B, DUKE D, PYM B, et al. 1982. The control of human pancreatic adenocarcinoma xenografts in nude mice by hormone therapy. Br J Surg 69:595–597.

GREENWAY B, IQBAL MJ, JOHNSON PJ, et al. 1981. Oestrogen receptor proteins in malignant and fetal pancreas. Br Med J 283:751–753.

GREENWAY B, IQBAL MJ, JOHNSON PJ, et al. 1983. Low serum testosterone concentration in patients with carcinoma of the pancreas. Br Med J 286:93–95.

GRIVAS S, NYHAMMAR T, OLSSON K, et al. 1986. Isolation and identification of the food mutagens IQ and MEIQx from heated model system of creatine, glycine and fructose. Food Chem 20:127–136.

GROSFELD JL, VANE DW, RESCORLA FJ, et al. 1990. Pancreatic tumors in childhood: Analysis of 13 cases. J Pediatr Surg 25:1057–1062.

GRUNEWALD K, LYONS J, FROHLICH A, et al. 1989. High frequency of Ki-*ras* codon 12 mutations in pancreatic adenocarcinomas. Int J Cancer 43:1037–1041.

GUDJONSSON B, LIVSTONE EM, SPIRO HM. 1978. Cancer of the pancreas, diagnostic accuracy and survival statistics. Cancer 42:2494–2506.

GUMBMANN MR, DUGAN GM, SPANGLER WL, et al. 1989. Pancreatic response in rats and mice to trypsin inhibitors from soy and potato after short- and long-term dietary exposure. J Nutr 119:1598–1609.

GURALNICK L. 1963. Mortality by Occupation Level and Cause of Death Among Men 20 to 64 Years of Age: U.S., 1950. Vital Statistics Special Report 53. Washington, DC, U.S. Government Printing Office, DHEW Pub, pp. 439–446.

HADDOCK G, CARTER DC. 1990. Aetiology of pancreatic cancer. Br J Surg 77:1159–1166.

HAENSZEL W. 1961. Cancer mortality among the foreign-born in the United States. J Natl Cancer Inst 26:37–132.

HAENSZEL W, KURIHARA M. 1968. Studies of Japanese migrants. I. Mortality from cancer and other diseases among Japanese in the United States. J Natl Cancer Inst 40:43–68.

HAKULINEN T, LEHTINAKI L, LEHTONEN M, et al. 1974. Cancer morbidity among two male cohorts with increased alcohol consumption in Finland. J Natl Cancer Inst 52:1711–1713.

HALL PA, HUGHES CM, STADDON SL, et al. 1990. The *c-erbB*-2 proto-oncogene in human pancreatic cancer. J Pathol 161:195–200.

HALL PA, LEMOINE NR. 1992. Rapid acinar to ductal transdifferentiation in cultured human exocrine pancreas. J Pathol 166:97–103.

HALL PM, STUPANS I, BURGESS W, et al. 1989. Immunohistochemical localization of NADPH-cytochrome P450 reductase in human tissues. Carcinogenesis 10:521–530.

HAMMOND EC. 1966. Smoking in relation to the death rates of one million men and women. Natl Cancer Inst Monogr 19:127–204.

HAMMOND EC, HORN D. 1958. Smoking and death rates—report on fourty-four months of follow-up of 187,783 men. II. Death rates by cause. JAMA 166:1294–1308.

HANIS NM, HOLMES TM, SHALLENBERGER LG, et al. 1982. Epidemiologic study of refinery and chemical plant workers. J Occup Med 24:203–212.

HANIS NM, SHALLENBERGER LG, DONALESKI DL, et al. 1985. A retrospective mortality study of workers in three major U.S. refineries and chemical plants. Part I. J Occup Med 27:283–292.

HANSEN ES. 1989. Mortality of auto mechanics. A ten-year follow-up. Scand J Work Environ Health 15:43–46.

HAYASHI Y, FURUKAWA H, HASEGAWA T. 1972. *In* Nakahara W, Takayma S, Sugimura T, et al (eds): Topics in Chemical Carcinogenesis. Baltimore, University Park Press, pp. 53–61.

HAYASHI Y, HASEGAWA T. 1971. Experimental pancreatic tumor in rats after intravenous injection of 4-hydroxyaminoquinoline I-oxide. Gann 62:329–330.

HEARNE FT, GROSE F, PIFER JW, et al. 1987. Methylene chloride mortality study: Dose-response characterization and animal model comparison. J Occup Med 29:217–228.

HECHT SS, CARMELLA SG, FOILES PG, et al. 1993. Tobacco-specific nitrosamine adducts: Studies in laboratory animals and humans. Environ Health Perspect 99:57–63.

HECHT SS, HOFFMANN D. 1991. *N*-nitroso compounds and tobacco-induced cancers in man. *In* O'Neill IK, Chen J, Bartsch H (eds): Relevance to Human Cancer of *N*-Nitroso Compounds, Tobacco Smoke and Mycotoxins. IARC Sci Pub No. 105. Lyon, France, International Agency for Research on Cancer. pp. 54–61.

HEGSTED DM. 1975. Relevance of animal studies to human disease. Cancer Res 35:3537–3539.

HEIN DW. 1988. Acetylator genotype and arylamine-induced carcinogenesis. Biochim Biophys Acta 948:37–66.

HEUCH I, KVALE G, JACOBSEN BK, et al. 1983. Use of alcohol, tobacco and coffee and risk of pancreatic cancer. Br J Cancer 48:637–643.

HIATT RA, KLATSKY AL, ARMSTRONG MA. 1988. Pancreatic cancer, blood glucose and beverage consumption. Int J Cancer 41:794–797.

HINDS MW, KOLONEL IN, LEE J, et al. 1980. Association between cancer incidence and alcohol/cigarette consumption among five ethnic groups in Hawaii. Br J Cancer 41:929–940.

HIRAI H, OKABE T, ANRUKA Y, et al. 1985. Activation of the *c*-K-

ras oncogene in a human pancreas carcinoma. Biochem Biophys Res Commun 127:168–174.

HIRAYAMA T. 1975. Prospective studies on cancer epidemiology based on census population in Japan. Proceedings of XI International Cancer Congress, Vol 3. Cancer Epidemiology, Environmental Factors. Florence, Italy, pp. 26–35.

HIRAYAMA T. 1978. Prospective studies on cancer epidemiology based on census population in Japan. *In* Nieburgs HE (ed): Prevention and Detection of Cancer. Vol 1, Etiology. New York, Marcel Dekker, pp. 1139–1148.

HIRAYAMA T. 1981. A large-scale cohort study on the relationship between diet and selected cancers of digestive organs. *In* Bruce WR, Correa P, Lipkin M, et al (eds): Banbury Report 7. Gastrointestinal Cancer: Endogenous Factors. Cold Spring Harbor, NY, Cold Spring Harbor Laboratory, pp. 409–426.

HIRAYAMA T. 1988. Epidemiology of pancreatic cancer in Japan. Int J Pancreatol 3:S203–204.

HIRAYAMA T. 1989. Epidemiology of pancreatic cancer in Japan. Jpn J Clin Oncol 19:208–215.

HOAR SK, PELL SA. 1981. A retrospective cohort study of mortality and cancer incidence among chemists. J Occup Med 23:485–494.

HOFFMANN D, RIVENSON A, ABBI R, et al. 1993. A study of tobacco carcinogenesis: Effect of the fat content of the diet on the carcinogenic activity of 4-(methylnitrosamino)-1-(3-pyridyl)-1-butanone in F344 rats. Cancer Res 53:2758–2761.

HÖHNE MW, HALATSCH M-E, KAHL GF, et al. 1992. Frequent loss of expression of the potential tumor suppressor gene *DCC* in ductal pancreatic adenocarcinoma. Cancer Res 52:2616–2619.

HOLMES GKT, STOKES PL, SORAHAN TM, et al. 1976. Coeliac disease, gluten free diet, and malignancy. Gut 17:612–619.

HORII A, NAKATSURU S, MIYOSHI Y, et al. 1992. Frequent somatic mutations of the *APC* gene in human pancreatic cancer. Cancer Res 52:6696–6698.

HOWARD JM, JORDAN GL. 1977. Cancer of the pancreas. Curr Probl Cancer 2:1–52.

HOWATSON AG, CARTER DC. 1985. Pancreatic carcinogenesis—enhancement by cholecystokinin in the hamster-nitrosamine model. Br J Cancer 51:107–114.

HOWE GR. 1989. Re: Total energy intake: implications for epidemiologic analyses. (Letter). Am J Epidemiol 129:1314–1315.

HOWE GR, JAIN M, BURCH JD, et al. 1991. Cigarette smoking and cancer of the pancreas: Evidence from a population-based case-control study in Toronto, Canada. Int J Cancer 47:323–328.

HOWE GR, JAIN M, MILLER AB. 1990. Dietary factors and risk of pancreatic cancer: Results of a Canadian population-based case-control study. Int J Cancer 45:604–608.

HSIEH C-C, MACMAHON B, YEN S, et al. 1986. Coffee and pancreatic cancer. (Letter). N Engl J Med 315:587–589.

HUBERMAN E, SACHS L. 1977. DNA binding and its relationship to carcinogenesis by different polycyclic hydrocarbons. Int J Cancer 19:122–127.

HUTCHISON GB, MACMAHON B, JABLON S, et al. 1979. Review of report by Mancusco, Stewart and Kneale of radiation exposure of Hanford workers. Health Physics 37:207–220.

IARC. 1984. *N*-Nitroso Compounds: Occurrence, Biological Effects and Relevance to Human Cancer. IARC Sci Pub No. 57. O'Neill IK, von Borstel RC, Miller CT, et al (eds): Lyon, International Agency for Research on Cancer.

IARC. 1986. IARC Monographs on the Evaluation of the Carcinogenic Risk of Chemicals to Humans. Vol. 38, Tobacco Smoking. Lyon, International Agency for Research on Cancer.

IARC. 1991. IARC Monographs on the Evaluation of the Carcinogenic Risk of Chemicals to Humans. Vol. 51, Coffee, Tea, Mate, Methylxanthines and Methylglyoxal. Lyon, International Agency for Research on Cancer.

IARC. 1991. IARC Monographs on the Evaluation of the Carcinogenic Risk of Chemicals to Humans. Vol. 53, DDT and Associated Compounds. Lyon, International Agency for Research on Cancer.

ISHII K, NAKAMURA K, OZAKI H, et al. 1968. Epidemiological problems of pancreas cancer. Jpn J Clin Med 26:1839–1842.

ISHII K, NAKAMURA K, TAKEUCHI T, et al. 1973. Chronic calcifying pancreatitis and pancreatic carcinoma in Japan. Digestion 9:429–437.

ISOMAKI HA, HAKULINEN T, JOUTSENLAHTI V. 1978. Excess risk of lymphomas, leukemia and myeloma in patients with rheumatoid arthritis. J Chronic Dis 31:691–696.

JACOBSEN O, WINTHER OLSEN S, NIELSEN NA. 1985. Pancreatic cancer in the Faroe Islands. Scand J Gastroenterol 20:1142–1146.

JAIN M, HOWE GR, ST LOUIS P, et al. 1991. Coffee and alcohol as determinants of risk of pancreas cancer: A case-control study from Toronto. Int J Cancer 47:384–389.

JAMIESON JD. 1975. Prospectives for cell and organ culture systems in the study of pancreatic carcinoma. J Surg Oncol 7:139–141.

JENSEN OM. 1979. Cancer morbidity and causes of death among Danish brewery workers. Int J Cancer 23:454–463.

JHAPPEN C, STAHLE C, HARKINS RN, et al. 1990. TGF-alpha overexpression in transgenic mice induces liver neoplasia and abnormal development of the mammary gland and pancreas. Cell 61:1137–1146.

JOHNSON JR, ZINTEL HA. 1963. Pancreatic calcification and cancer of the pancreas. Surg Gynecol Obstet 117:585–588.

KADERLIK KR, LIN D-X, FRIESEN MD, et al. 1993. Human biomonitoring of arylamine-DNA adducts in colon and pancreas tissues. (Abstract). Proc Am Assoc Cancer Res 34:152.

KADLUBAR FF, BUTLER MA, KADERLIK KR, et al. 1992. Polymorphisms for aromatic amine metabolism in humans: Relevance for human carcinogenesis. Environ Health Perspect 98:69–74.

KADLUBAR FF, HAMMONS GJ. 1987. The role of cytochrome P-450 in the metabolism of chemical carcinogens. *In* Guengerich FP (ed): Mammalian Cytochromes P-450, vol 2. Boca Raton, FL, CRC Press, pp. 81–130.

KADLUBAR FF, KADERLIK KR, LIN D-X, et al. 1993. Detection of aromatic amine-DNA adducts in human populations. (Abstract). Proc Am Assoc Cancer Res 34:606.

KADLUBAR FF, TALASKA G, LANG NP, et al. 1988. Assessment of exposure and susceptibility to aromatic amine carcinogens. *In* Bartsch H, Hemminki K, O'Neill IK (eds): Methods for Detecting DNA Damaging Agents in Humans: Applications in Cancer Epidemiology and Prevention. IARC Sci Pub No. 89. Lyon, International Agency for Research on Cancer, pp. 166–174.

KAHN HA. 1966. The Dorn study of smoking and mortality among U.S. veterans: Report on eight and one-half years of observation. Natl Cancer Inst Monogr 19:1–125.

KAPLAN SD. 1986. Update of a mortality study of workers in petroleum refineries. J Occup Med 28:514–516.

KARMODY AJ, KYLE J. 1969. The association between carcinoma of the pancreas and diabetes mellitus. Br J Sur 56:362–364.

KATTWINKEL J, LOPEY A, DISANT'AGNESE PA, et al. 1973. Hereditary pancreatitis: Three new kindreds and a critical review of the literature. Pediatrics 51:55–69.

KEATING JJ, JOHNSON PJ, COCHRANE AMG, et al. 1989. A prospective randomised controlled trial of tamoxifen and cyproterone acetate in pancreatic carcinoma. Br J Cancer 60:789–792.

KESSLER II. 1970. Cancer mortality among diabetics. J Natl Cancer Inst 44:673–686.

KING H, DIAMOND E, BAILAR JC III. 1965. Cancer mortality and religious preference: A suggested method in research. Milbank Mem Fund Q 43:349–357.

KING H, HAENSZEL W. 1973. Cancer mortality among foreign and native-born Chinese in the United States. J Chronic Dis 26:623–646.

KINLEN LJ, MCPHERSON K. 1984. Pancreas cancer and coffee and tea consumption: A case-control study. Br J Cancer 49:93–96.

KIRCHNER CH, NIELSEN SW. 1976. Tumors of the pancreas. Bull WHO 53:195–202.

KLATSKY AL, FRIEDMAN GD, SIEGELAUB AB. 1981. Alcohol and mortality: A ten-year Kaiser-Permanente experience. Ann Intern Med 95:139–145.

KLINTRUP HE. 1966. Carcinoma of the pancreas. Acta Chir Scand 362:1–96.

KLÖPPEL G. 1984. Pancreatic, non-endocrine tumors. *In* Klöppel G, Heitz PU (eds): Pancreatic Pathology. New York, Churchill Livingstone, pp. 79–113.

KLÖPPEL G, LOHR M, MÖESTA M, et al. 1986. The effects of sex steroid hormones on pancreatic carcinoma grown in nude mice and tissue culture. (Abstract). Dig Dis Sci 31:1137.

KLÖPPEL G, MAILLET B. 1991. Histological typing of pancreatic and periampullary carcinoma. Eur J Surg Oncol 17:139–152.

KLÖPPEL G, MAILLET B, SCHEWE K, et al. 1989. Immunocytochemical detection of epidermal growth factor receptors (EGRF) and transferrin receptor (TR) on normal, inflamed and neoplastic tissue. (Abstract). Pancreas 4:649.

KONISHI Y, DENADA A, INUI S, et al. 1976. Pancreatic carcinoma induced by 4-Hydroxyaminoquinoline 1-oxide after partial pancreatectomy and splenectomy in rats. Gann 67:919–920.

KONO S, IKEDA M. 1979. Correlation between cancer mortality and alcoholic beverage in Japan. Br J Cancer 40:449–455.

KORC M. 1990. Potential role of the epidermal growth factor receptor in human pancreatic cancer. Int J Pancreatol 7:71–81.

KORC M, MELTZER P, TRENT J. 1986. Enhanced expression of epidermal growth factor receptor correlates with alterations of chromosome 7 in human pancreatic cancer. Proc Natl Acad Sci USA 83:5141–5144.

KRAIN LS. 1970. The rising incidence of carcinoma of the pancreas—real or apparent? J Surg Oncol 2:115–124.

KRAIN LS. 1971a. The rising incidence of cancer of the pancreas. Further epidemiologic studies. J Chronic Dis 23:685–690.

KRAIN LS. 1971b. Cancer of the pancreas in California, 1942–1967. Calif Med 115:38–41.

KUHLMANN W, FROMME H-G, HEEGE E-M, et al. 1968. The mutagenic action of caffeine in higher organisms. Cancer Res 28:2375–2389.

KURATSUNE M, KOCHI S, HORIE A, et al. 1971. Test of alcoholic beverages and ethanol solutions for carcinogenicity and tumor promoting activity. Gann 62:395.

KURIHARA M. 1979. National cancer mortality and incidence in Japan. Environ Health Perspect 32:59–74.

LANG NP, CHU DZT, HUNTER CF, et al. 1986. Role of aromatic amine acetyltransferase in human colorectal cancer. Arch Surg 121:1259–1261.

LANIER AP, BENDER TR, BLOT WJ, et al. 1976. Cancer incidence in Alaska natives. Int J Cancer 18:409–412.

LA VECCHIA C, LIATI P, DECARLI A, et al. 1987. Coffee consumption and risk of pancreatic cancer. Int J Cancer 40:309–313.

LA VECCHIA C, NEGRI E, D'AVANZO B, et al. 1990. Medical history, diet and pancreatic cancer. Oncology 47:463–466.

LAZAR HP, SPELLBERG MA, FOX RE. 1960. The increasing incidence of carcinoma of the pancreas. Am J Gastroenterol 34:235–347.

LEA AJ. 1967. Neoplasms and environmental factors. Ann R Coll Surg Engl 41:432–438.

LEBENTHAL E, LEUNG Y-K. 1991. Fetal and neonatal development of the exocrine pancreas. *In* Morrisset J, Solomon TE (eds): Growth of the Gastrointestinal Tract: Gastrointestinal Hormones and Growth Factors. Boca Raton, FL, CRC Press, pp. 73–88.

LEMOINE NR, HALL PA. 1990. Growth factors and oncogenes in pancreatic cancer. Baillières Clin Gastroenterol 4:815–832.

LEMOINE NR, HUGHES CM, BARTON CM, et al. 1992a. The epidermal growth factor receptor in human pancreatic cancer. J Pathol 166:7–12.

LEMOINE NR, JAIN S, HUGHES CM, et al. 1992b. Ki-*ras* oncogene activation in preinvasive pancreatic cancer. Gastroenterology 102:230–236.

LEMOINE NR, LOBRESCO M, LEUNG H, et al. 1992c. The *c-erbB*-3 gene in human pancreatic cancer. J Pathol 168:269–273.

LEVIN DL, CONNELLY RR. 1973. Cancer of the pancreas. Cancer 31:1231–1236.

LEVIN DL, CONNELLY RR, DEVESA SS. 1981. Demographic characteristics of cancer of the pancreas: Mortality, incidence, and survival. Cancer 47:1456–1468.

LEVITT MH, HARRIS CC, SQUIRE R, et al. 1977. Experimental pancreatic carcinogenesis. I. Morphogenesis of pancreatic adenocarcinoma in the Syrian golden hamster induced by *N*-nitroso-bis(2-hydroxypropyl)amine. Am J Pathol 88:5–28.

LHOSTE EF, ROEBUCK BD, LONGNECKER DS. 1988. Stimulation of the growth of azaserine-induced nodules in the rat pancreas by dietary camostate (FOY-305). Carcinogenesis 9:901–906.

LI FP, FRAUMENI JF JR. 1969. Soft-tissue sarcomas, breast cancer, and other neoplasms: A familial syndrome? Ann Intern Med 71:747–752.

LI FP, FRAUMENI JF JR, MANTEL N, et al. 1969. Cancer mortality among chemists. J Natl Cancer Inst 43:1159–1164.

LIENER IE, HASDI A. 1986. The effect of long-term feeding of raw soyflour on the pancreas of the mouse and hamster. Adv Exp Med Biol 199:189–197.

LIN RS, KESSLER II. 1981. A multifactorial model for pancreatic cancer in man. JAMA 245:147–152.

LIVINGSTON EH, REBER HA. 1992. Cancer of the pancreas. Current Opinion in Gastroenterology 8:844–851.

LIVINGSTON EH, WELTON ML, REBER HA. 1991. Surgical treatment of pancreatic cancer: The United States experience. Int J Pancreatol 9:153–157.

LLOYD JW, DECOUFLE P, SALVIN LG. 1977. Unusual mortality experience of printing pressmen. J Occup Med 19:543–550.

LOGAN WPD. 1982. Cancer Mortality by Occupation and Social Class 1851–1971. OPCS, Studies on Medical and Population Subjects No. 44./IARC Sci Pub No. 36. London/Lyon, HM Stat Off, International Agency for Research on Cancer.

LONGNECKER DS. 1970. Organ distribution of puromycin in rats, a possible basis for selective cytoxicity. Lab Invest 22:400–403.

LONGNECKER DS. 1984. Lesions induced in rodent pancreas by azaserine and other pancreatic carcinogens. Environ Health Perspect 56:245–251.

LONGNECKER DS. 1986. Experimental models of exocrine pancreatic tumors. *In* Go VLW, Garderner JD, Brooks FP, et al (eds): The Exocrine Pancreas: Biology, Pathobiology and Diseases. New York, Raven Press, pp. 443–458.

LONGNECKER D. 1990. Experimental pancreatic cancer: Role of species, sex and diet. Bull Cancer 77:27–37.

LONGNECKER DS. 1991. Hormones and pancreatic cancer. Int J Pancreatol 9:81–86.

LONGNECKER DS, CURPHEY TJ. 1975. Adenocarcinoma of the pancreas in azaserine-treated rats. Cancer Res 35:2249–2258.

LONGNECKER DS, CURPHEY TJ, KUHLMANN ET, et al. 1986. Effects of retinoids in *N*-nitrosobis(2-oxypropyl)amine-treated hamsters. Pancreas 1:224–231.

LONGNECKER DS, KUHLMANN ET, CURPHEY TJ. 1983. Divergent effects of retinoids on pancreatic and liver carcinogenesis in azaserine-treated rats. Cancer Res 43:3219–3225.

LONGNECKER DS, KUHLMANN ET, FREEMAN DH JR. 1990. Characterization of the elastase 1-simian virus 40 T-antigen mouse model of pancreatic carcinoma: Effects of sex and diet. Cancer Res 50:7552–7554.

LONGNECKER DS, WIEBKIN P, SCHAEFFER BK, et al. 1984. Experimental carcinogenesis in the pancreas. Int Rev Exp Pathol 26:177–229.

LOSSING EH, BEST EWT, MCGREGOR JT, et al. 1966. A Canadian study of smoking and Health. Ottawa, Department of National Health and Welfare.

LOWENFELS AB. 1984. Chronic pancreatitis, pancreatic cancer, alcohol, and smoking. (Letter). Gastroenterology 87:744.

LOWENFELS AB, MAISONNEUVE P, CAVALLINI G, et al. 1993. Pancreatitis and the risk of pancreatic cancer. N Engl J Med 328:1433–1437.

LOWENFELS AB, PATEL VP, PITCHUMONI CS. 1985. Chronic calcific pancreatitis and pancreatic cancer. (Abstract). Dig Dis Sci 30:982.

LU L, LOUIE D, OWYANG C. 1989. A cholecystokinin releasing peptide mediates feedback regulation of pancreatic secretion. Am J Physiol 256:G430–G435.

LUNDH G, NORDENSTAM H. 1970. Pancreas calcification and pancreas cancer. Acta Chir Scand 136:493–496.

LYNCH HT. 1967. Hereditary factors in cancer. *In* Lynch HT (ed): Recent Results in Cancer Research, vol 12. New York, Springer-Verlag, pp. 125–142.

LYNCH HT, FUSARO L, LYNCH JF. 1992. Familial pancreatic cancer: A family study. Pancreas 7:511–515.

LYNCH HT, VOORHEES GH, LANSPA SJ, et al. 1985. Pancreatic carcinoma and hereditary nonpolyposis colorectal cancer: A family study. Br J Cancer 52:271–273.

LYON JL, MAHONEY AW, FRENCH TK, et al. 1992a. Coffee consumption and the risk of cancer of the exocrine pancreas: A case-control study in a low-risk population. Epidemiology 3:164–170.

LYON JL, EGGER MF, ROBISON LM, et al. 1992b. Misclassification of exposure in a case-control study: The effects of different types of exposure and different proxy respondents in a study of pancreatic cancer. Epidemiology 3:223–231.

LYON JL, GARDENER JW, WEST DW. 1980. Cancer risk and lifestyle: Cancer among Mormons from 1967 to 1975. *In* Cairns J, et al (eds): Banbury Report 4. Cancer Incidence in Defined Populations. Cold Spring Harbor, NY, Cold Spring Harbor Laboratory, pp. 3–30.

LYON JL, KLAUBER MR, GARDNER JW, et al. 1976. Cancer incidence in Mormons and non-Mormons in Utah, 1966–1970. N Engl J Med 294:129–133.

MAANI R, TOWNSEND CM, GOMEZ G, et al. 1988. A potent CCK receptor antagonist (L-364, 718) inhibits the growth of human pancreatic cancer in nude mice. (Abstract). Gastroenterology 94:274.

MACCORNACK FA. 1977. The effects of coffee drinking on the cardiovascular system: Experimental and epidemiological research. Prev Med 6:104–119.

MACDERMOTT RP, KRAMER P. 1973. Adenocarcinoma of the pancreas in four siblings. Gastroenterology 65:137–139.

MACK TM, PAGANINI-HILL A. 1981. Epidemiology of pancreas cancer in Los Angeles. Cancer 47:1474–1483.

MACK TM, PETERS JM, YU MC, et al. 1985. Pancreas cancer is unrelated to the workplace in Los Angeles. Am J Ind Med 7:253–266.

MACK TM, YU MC, HANISCH R, et al. 1986. Pancreas cancer and smoking, beverage consumption and past medical history. J Natl Cancer Inst 76:49–60.

MCGUINESS EE, HOPWOOD D, WORMSLEY KG. 1982. Further studies of the effects of raw soya flour on the rat pancreas. Scand J Gastroenterol 17:273–277.

MCLEAN-ROSS AH, SMITH MA, ANDERSON JR, et al. 1982. Late mortality after surgery for peptic ulcer. N Engl J Med 307:519–522.

MACMAHON B. 1960. The ethnic distribution of cancer mortality in New York City, 1955. Acta Un Int Cancer 16:1716–1724.

MACMAHON B, YEN S, TRICHOPOULOS C, et al. 1981. Coffee and cancer of the pancreas. N Engl J Med 304:630–633.

MCMICHAEL AJ. 1981. Coffee, soya and pancreatic cancer. Lancet 2:689–690.

MCMICHAEL AJ, MCCALL MG, HARTSHORNE JM, et al. 1980. Patterns of gastro-intestinal cancer in European migrants to Australia: The role of dietary change. Int J Cancer 25:431–437.

MCMICHAEL AJ, SPIRTAS R, KUPPER LL. 1974. An epidemiologic study of mortality within a cohort of rubber workers, 1964–72. Occup Med 16:458–464.

MAGNANI C, COGGON D, OSMOND C, et al. 1987. Occupation and five cancers: A case-control study using death certificates. Br J Ind Med 44:769–776.

MAINZ DL, BLACK O, WEBSTER PD. 1973. Hormonal control of pancreatic growth. J Clin Invest 52:2300–2304.

MALAGELADA JR. 1979. Pancreatic cancer. Mayo Clin Proc 54:459–467.

MALLIN K, RUBIN M, JOO E. 1989. Occupational cancer mortality in Illinois white and black males, 1979–1984 for seven cancer sites. Am J Ind Med 15:699–717.

MANCUSO TF, EL-ATTAR AA. 1967. Cohort study of workers exposed to betanaphthylamine and benzidine. J Occup Med 9:277–285.

MANCUSO TF, STEWART A, KNEALE G. 1977. Radiation exposures of Hanford workers dying from cancer and other causes. Health Physics 33:369–385.

MARBLE A. 1934. Diabetes and cancer. N Engl J Med 211:339–349.

MARINGHINI A, THIRUVENGADAM R, MELTON LJ, et al. 1987. Pancreatic cancer risk following gastric surgery. Cancer 60:245–247.

MARIYAMA M, KISHI K, NAKAMURA K, et al. 1989. Frequency and types of point mutation at the 12th codon of the c-Ki-*ras* gene found in pancreatic cancers from Japanese patients. Jpn J Cancer Res 80:622–626.

MARSHALL CJ, LLOYD AC, MORRIS JDH, et al. 1989. Signal transduction by p21*ras*. Int J Cancer 4 (Suppl):29–31.

MARUCHI N, BRIAN D, LUDWIG J, et al. 1979. Cancer of the pancreas in Olmsted County, Minnesota, 1935–1974. Mayo Clin Proc 54:245–249.

MATANOSKI GM, SELSTER R, SARTWELL PE, et al. 1975. The current mortality rates of radiologists and other physician specialists: Specific causes of death. Am J Epidemiol 101:199–210.

MEERS PD. 1973. Allergy and cancer. Lancet 1:884–885.

MENCK HR, HENDERSON BE, PIKE MC, et al. 1975. Cancer incidence in the Mexican-American. J Natl Cancer Inst 55:531–536.

MIKAL S, CAMPBELL AJA. 1950. Carcinoma of the pancreas. Surgery 28:963–969.

MILHAM S JR. 1976. Occupational Mortality in Washington State 1950–1971. Washington, DC, U.S. Government Printing Office, NIOSH Pub No. 76-175A.

MILITELLO C, SPERTI C, FORESTA C, et al. 1984. Plasma levels of testosterone and hypophyseal gonadotrophins in men affected by pancreatic cancer. (Abstract). Digestion 30:122.

MILLER BA, RIES LAG, HANKEY BF, et al (eds). 1992. Cancer Statistics Review: 1973–1989. National Cancer Institute. NIH Pub No. 92-2789.

MILLS PK, BEESON L, ABBEY DE, et al. 1988. Dietary habits and past medical history as related to fatal pancreas cancer risk among Adventists. Cancer 61:2578–2585.

MIRVISH SS. 1986. Effects of vitamins C and E on *N*-nitroso compound formation, carcinogenesis, and cancer. Cancer 58 (Suppl 8):1842–1850.

MIZUNO S, WATANABE S, NAKAMURA K, et al. 1992. A multi-institute case-control study on the risk factors of developing pancreatic cancer. Jpn J Clin Oncol 22:286–291.

MOLDOW RE, CONNELLY RR. 1968. Epidemiology of pancreatic cancer in Connecticut. Gastroenterology 55:667–686.

MØOLLER H, TOFTGAARD C. 1991. Cancer occurrence in a cohort of patients surgically treated for peptic ulcer. Gut 32:740–744.

MONSON RR, FINE LA. 1978. Cancer mortality and morbidity among rubber workers. J Natl Cancer Inst 61:1047–1053.

MONSON RR, LYON JL. 1975. Proportional mortality among alcoholics. Cancer 36:1077–1079.

MORSE MA, WANG C-X, STONER GD, et al. 1989. Inhibition of 4-

(methylnitrosamino)-1-(3-pyridyl)-1-butanone-induced DNA adduct formation and tumorigenicity in the lung of F344 rats by dietary phenethyl isothiocyanate. Cancer Res 49:549–553.

MOYNAN RW, NEERHOUT RC, JOHNSON TS. 1964. Pancreatic carcinoma in childhood: Case report and review. J Pediatri 65:711–719.

MUIR C, WATERHOUSE J, MACK T, et al (eds). 1987. Cancer Incidence in Five Continents, vol. V. IARC Sci Pub No. 88. Lyon, International Agency for Research on Cancer.

MULVIHILL JJ. 1985. Familial aspects of pancreatic cancer. *In* Müller HJ, Weber W (eds): Familial Cancer. 1st Int Res Conf. Basel, Karger, pp. 88–89.

NADER CJ, SPENCER LK, WELLER RA. 1981. Mutagen production during pan-broiling compared with microwave irradiation of beef. Cancer Lett 13:147–151.

NAGATA Y, ABE M, MOTOSHIMA K, et al. 1990. Frequent glycine-to-aspartic acid mutations at codon 12 of c-Ki-*ras* gene in human pancreatic cancer in Japanese. Jpn J Cancer Res 81:135–140.

NASCA PC, BURNETT WS, GREENWALD P, et al. 1980. Population density as an indicator of urban-rural differences in cancer incidence, upstate New York, 1968–72. Am J Epidemiol 112:362–375.

NATIONAL RESEARCH COUNCIL (U.S.), COMMITTEE ON DIET AND HEALTH. 1989. Diet and Health: Implications for Reducing Chronic Disease Risk. Washington, DC, National Academy Press.

NELSON NA, VAN PEENEN PFD, BLANCHARD AG. 1987. Mortality in a recent oil refinery cohort. J Occup Med 29:610–612.

NEUMAN WL, WASYLYSHYN ML, JACOBY R, et al. 1991. Evidence for a common molecular pathogenesis in colorectal, gastric and pancreatic cancer. Genes, Chromosomes Cancer 3:468–473.

NEWHOUSE ML, MATHEWS G, SHEIKH K, et al. 1988. Mortality of workers at acetylene production plants. Br J Ind Med 45:63–69.

NEWILL VA. 1961. Distribution of cancer mortality among ethnic subgroups of the white population of New York City. J Natl Cancer Inst 26:405–417.

NIEDERAU C, GRENDELL JH. 1992. Diagnosis of pancreatic carcinoma: Imaging techniques and tumor markers. Pancreas 7:66–86.

NORELL SE, AHLBOM A, ERWALD R, et al. 1986a. Diet and pancreatic cancer: A case-control study. Am J Epidemiol 124:894–902.

NORELL SE, AHLBOM A, ERWALD R, et al. 1986b. Diabetes, gall stone disease, and pancreatic cancer. Br J Cancer 54:377–378.

NORELL SE, AHLBOM A, OLIN R, et al. 1986c. Occupational factors and pancreatic cancer. Br J Ind Med 43:775–778.

O'CONNOR TP, ROEBUCK BD, PETERSON FJ, et al. 1989. Effect of dietary omega-3 and omega-6 fatty acids on development of azaserine-induced preneoplastic lesions in rat pancreas. J Natl Cancer Inst 81:858–863.

OFFERHAUS JGA, GIARDIELLO FM, MOORE GW, et al. 1987. Partial gastrectomy: A risk factor for carcinoma of the pancreas? Hum Pathol 18:285–288.

OLSEN GW, MANDEL JS, GIBSON RW, et al. 1989. A case-control study of pancreatic cancer and cigarettes, alcohol, coffee and diet. Am J Public Health 79:1016–1019.

OLSEN GW, MANDEL JS, GIBSON RW, et al. 1991. Nutrients and pancreatic cancer: A population-based case-control study. Cancer Causes Control 2:291–297.

OLSEN JH, JENSEN OM. 1987. Occupation and risk of cancer in Denmark: An analysis of 93,810 cancer cases, 1970–1979. Scand J Work Environ Health 13 (Suppl) 7–91.

ORNITZ DM, HAMMER RE, MESSING A, et al. 1987. Pancreatic neoplasia induced by SV40T-antigen expression in acinar cells of transgenic mice. Science 238:188–193.

OTTERLAND A. 1967. A sociomedical study of the mortality in merchant seafarers. Acta Med Scand 357:5–277, 293–300.

PARIZA MW. 1987. Dietary fat, calorie restriction, *ad libitum* feeding and cancer risk. Nutr Rev 45:1–7.

PARIZA MW. 1988. Dietary fat and cancer risk: Evidence and research needs. Annu Rev Nutr 8:167–183.

PARKIN DM, MUIR CS, WHELAN SL, et al (eds). 1992. Cancer Incidence in Five Continents, vol. VI. IARC Sci Pub No. 120. Lyon, International Agency for Research on Cancer.

PARSA I, POUR PM, CLEARY CM, et al. 1988. Amplification of *c*-Ki-*ras*-2 oncogene sequences in human carcinoma of the pancreas. Int J Pancreatol 3:45–51.

PATRIANAKOS C, HOFFMAN D. 1979. Chemical studies on tobacco smoke. LXIV. On the analysis of aromatic amines in cigarette smoke. J Anal Toxicol 3:150–159.

PAULINO-NETTO AP, DREILING DA, BARONOFSKY ID. 1960. The relationship between pancreatic calcification and cancer of the pancreas. Ann Surg 151:530–537.

PETERSEN GR, MILHAM S JR. 1980. Occupational Mortality in California 1959–61. Washington, U.S. Government Printing Office, NIOSH Pub No 80–104.

PETERSON H, SOLOMON T, GROSSMAN MI. 1978. Effect of chronic pentagastrin, cholecystokinin and secretin on pancreas of rats. Am J Physiol 234:E286–293.

PHILLIPS RL. 1975. Role of life-style and dietary habits in risk of cancer among Seventh-Day Adventists. Cancer Res 35:3513–3522.

PHILLIPS RL, et al. 1980. Mortality among California Seventh-Day Adventists for selected cancer sites. J Natl Cancer Inst 65:1097–1107.

PICKLE LW, GOTTLIEB MS. 1980. Pancreatic cancer mortality in Louisiana. Am J Public Health 70:256–259.

PICTET RL, CLARK WR, WILLIAMS RH, et al. 1972. An ultrastructural analysis of the developing embryonic pancreas. Develop Biol 29:436–467.

PIETRI F, CLAVEL F. 1991. Occupational exposure and cancer of the pancreas: A review. Br J Ind Med 48:583–587.

PIETRI F, CLAVEL F, AUQUIER A, et al. 1990. Occupational risk factors for cancer of the pancreas: A case-control study. Br J Ind Med 47:425–428.

POIRIER LA, WEISBURGER JH. 1974. Enzymatic reduction of carcinogenic aromatic nitro compounds by rat and mouse liver fractions. Biochem Pharmacol 23:661–669.

POLEDNAK AP, STEHNEY AF, LUCAS HF. 1983. Mortality among male workers at a thorium processing plant. Health Physics 44 (Suppl 1):239–251.

POLISSAR L, SEVERSON RK, BOATMAN ES. 1984. A case-control study of asbestos in drinking water and cancer risk. Am J Epidemiol 119:456–471.

POSTON GJ, GILLESPIE J, GUILLOU PJ. 1991. Biology of pancreatic cancer. Gut 32:800–812.

POTTER JD. 1990. The epidemiology and prevention of pancreas cancer. *In* Zatonski W, Boyle P, Tyczynski J (eds): Cancer Prevention, Vital Statistics to Intervention. Warsaw, PA Interpress.

POTTER JD. 1992. Epidemiology of diet and cancer: Evidence of human maladaptation. *In* Micozzi MS, Moon TE (eds): Macronutrients: Investigating Their Role in Cancer. New York, Marcel Dekker, pp. 55–84.

POTTER JD, ALBERTS DS, BYERS TE, et al. 1993. Report of group A of the American Cancer Society research workshop on cancer and nutrition: Panel on human studies. Cancer Res (Suppl.) 53:2449s–2451s.

POUR P. 1980. Experimental pancreatic ductal (ductular) tumors. *In* Fitzgerald PJ, Morrison AB (eds): The Pancreas. Baltimore, Williams & Wilkins, pp. 111–139.

POUR PM. 1989. Experimental pancreatic cancer. Am J Surg Pathol 13 (Suppl 1):96–103.

POUR PM, BIRT DF. 1983. Modifying factors in pancreatic carcinogenesis in the hamster model. IV. Effects of dietary protein. J Natl Cancer Inst 71:347–353.

POUR P, KRÜGER FW, ALTOFF J, et al. 1975a. A new approach for induction of pancreatic neoplasms. Cancer Res 35:2259–2268.

POUR P, MOHR, U, CARDESA A, et al. 1975b. Pancreatic neoplasms in an animal model: Morphological, biological and comparative studies. Cancer 36:379–389.

POUR PM, REBER HA, STEPAN K. 1983a. Modification of pancreatic carcinogeneis in the hamster model. XII. Dose-related effect of ethanol. J Natl Cancer Inst 71:1085–1087.

POUR PM, TAHAHASHI M, CONELLY T, et al. 1983b. Modification of pancreatic carcinogenesis in the hamster model. IX. Effect of pancreatitis. J Natl Cancer Inst 71:607–613.

PRIESTER WA. 1974. Data from eleven United States and Canadian Colleges of Veterinary Medicine on pancreatic carcinoma in domestic animals. Cancer Res 34:1372–1375.

PROBST MR, BLUM M, FASSHAUER I, et al. 1992. The role of the human acetylation polymorphism in the metabolic activation of the food carcinogen 2-amino-3- methylimidazo[4,5-*f*]quinoline (IQ). Carcinogenesis 13:1713–1717.

PUKKALA E, NOKSO-KOIVISTO P, ROPONEN P. 1992. Changing cancer risk pattern among Finnish hairdressers. Int Arch Occup Environ Health 64:39–42.

RAGOZZINO M, MELTON LJ, CHU C-P, et al. 1982. Subsequent cancer risk in the incidence cohort of Rochester, Minnesota, residents with diabetes mellitus. J Chronic Dis 35:13–19.

RAO MS. et al. 1974. The ultrastructural effects of aflatoxin B in the rat pancreas. Virchows Arch B Cell Path 17:149–157.

RASTOGI H, BROWN CH. 1967. Carcinoma of the pancreas. A review of one hundred cases. Cleveland Clin Q 34:243–263.

RAYMOND L, BOUCHARDY C. 1990. Les facteurs de risque du cancer du pancréas d'après les études épidémiologiques analytiques. Bull Cancer 77:47–68.

RAYMOND L, INFANTE F, TUYNS AJ, et al. 1987. Alimentation et cancer du pancréas. Gatroenterol Clin Biol 11:488–492.

REDDING TW, SCHALLY, AV. 1984. Inhibition of growth of pancreatic carcinomas in animal models by analogues of hypothalmic hormones. Proc Natl Acad Sci USA 81:248–252.

REDDY JK, RAO MS. 1975. Pancreatic adenocarcinoma in guinea pigs induced by V-methyl-N-nitrosourea. Cancer Res 35:2269–2277.

REDDY JK, RAO MS. 1977. Transplantable pancreatic carcinoma of the rat. Science 198:78–80.

REDMOND CK. 1983. Cancer mortality among coke oven workers. Environ Health Perspect 52:67–73.

REDMOND CK, STROBINO BR, CYPRESS RH. 1976. Cancer experience among coke by-product workers. Ann NY Acad Sci 271:102–115.

REGISTRAR GENERAL'S DECENNIAL SUPPLEMENT FOR ENGLAND AND WALES, 1931. 1938. Occupational Mortality. London, HM Stat Off.

REGISTRAR GENERAL'S DECENNIAL SUPPLEMENT FOR ENGLAND AND WALES, 1951. 1954. Occupational Mortality Tables, Part 1. London, HM Stat Off.

REGISTRAR GENERAL'S DECENNIAL SUPPLEMENT FOR ENGLAND AND WALES, 1961. 1971. Occupational Mortality Tables. London, HM Stat Off.

REGISTRAR GENERAL'S DECENNIAL SUPPLEMENT FOR ENGLAND AND WALES, 1970–72. 1978. Occupational Mortality. London, HM Stat Off.

RIBOLI E, STANTA G, DELENDI M, et al. 1991. Comparison between diagnoses of cancers of the stomach, colon, rectum, gall-bladder, liver and pancreas on death certificates and at autopsy in Trieste, 1970–1984. IARC Sci Pub No. 112. Lyon, International Agency for Research on Cancer, pp. 45–54.

RICHARD L, COHN J. 1969. Cancer of the pancreas. Am Surg 35:95–103.

RIELA A, ZINSMEISTER AR, MELTON LJ D, et al. 1992. Increasing incidence of pancreatic cancer among women in Olmsted County, Minnesota, 1940 through 1988. Mayo Clin Proc 67:839–845.

RIVENSON A, HOFFMANN D, PROKOPCZYK B, et al. 1988. Induction of lung and exocrine pancreas tumors in F344 rats by tobacco-specific and areca-derived *N*-nitrosamines. Cancer Res 48:6912–6917.

ROBBINS SL, COTRAN RS. 1979. Pathologic Basis of Disease, 2nd ed. Philadelphia, W. B. Saunders, pp. 1104–1114.

ROBINETTE CD, FRAUMENI JF JR. 1978. Asthma and subsequent mortality in World War II veterans. J Chronic Dis 31:619–624.

ROBINSON AB, et al. 1970. The occurrence of carcinoma of the pancreas in chronic pancreatitis. Radiology 94:289–290.

ROCKETTE HE, ARENA VC. 1983. Mortality studies of aluminium reduction plant workers: Portroom and carbon department. J Occup Med 25:549–557.

ROEBUCK BD. 1992. Dietary fat and the development of pancreatic cancer. Lipids 27:804–806.

ROEBUCK BD, BAUMGARTNER KJ, MACMILLAN DL. 1993. Caloric restriction and intervention in pancreatic carcinogenesis in the rat. Cancer Res 53:46–52.

ROEBUCK BD, BAUMGARTNER KJ, THRON CD, et al. 1984a. Inhibition by retinoids of the growth of azaserine-induced foci in the rat pancreas. J Natl Cancer Inst 73:233–236.

ROEBUCK BD, MACMILLAN DL, BUSH DM, et al. 1984b. Modulation of azaserine-induced pancreatic foci by phenolic antioxidants in rats. J Natl Cancer Inst 72:1405–1410.

ROEBUCK BD, KAPLITA PV, EDWARDS BR, et al. 1987. Effects of dietary fats and soybean protein on azaserine-induced pancreatic carcinogenesis and plasma cholecystokinin in the rat. Cancer Res 47:1333–1338.

ROEBUCK BD, LONGNECKER DS, BAUMGARTNER KJ, et al. 1985. Carcinogen-induced lesions in the rat pancreas: Effects of varying levels of essential fatty acid. Cancer Res 45:5252–5256.

ROEBUCK BD, LONGNECKER DS, BIRT DF. 1989. Role of dietary fat in experimental pancreatic carcinogenesis. *In* Abraham S (ed): Carcinogenesis and Dietary Fat. Boston, Kluwer Academic Publishers, pp. 135–150.

ROEBUCK BD, YAGER JD JR, LONGNECKER DS. 1981a. Dietary modulation of azaserine-induced pancreatic carcinogenesis in the rat. Cancer Res 41:888–893.

ROEBUCK BD, YAGER JD JR, LONGNECKER DS, et al. 1981b. Promotion by unsaturated fat of azaserine-induced pancreatic carcinogenesis in the rat. Cancer Res 41:3961–3966.

RÖSCH T, BRAIG C, GAIN T, et al. 1992. Staging of pancreatic and ampullary carcinoma by endoscopic ultrasonography: Comparison with conventional sonography, computed tomography, and angiography. Gastroenterology 102:188–199.

ROWLATT U. 1967. Spontaneous epithelial tumors of the pancreas of mammals. Br J Cancer 21:82–107.

RUBIO V, RODRIGUEZ JI. 1989. Near-simultaneous adenocarcinoma of the pancreas in husband and wife. Lancet 1:166–167.

RUSHTON L, ALDERSON MR. 1981. An epidemiological survey of eight oil refineries in Britain. Br J Ind Med 38:225–234.

RUTTER WJ. 1980. The development of the endocrine and exocrine pancreas. *In* Fitzgerald PJ, Morrison AB (eds): The Pancreas. Baltimore, Williams & Wilkins, pp. 30–38.

SAFTLAS AF, BLAIR A, CANTOR KP, et al. 1987. Cancer and other causes of death among Wisconsin Farmers. Am J Ind Med 11:119–129.

SAITO K, YAMAZOE Y, KAMATAKE T, et al. 1983. Activation and detoxication of *N*-hydroxy-Trp-2 by glutathione and glutathione transferases. Carcinogenesis 4:1551–1557.

SANDGREN EP, LUETTKE NC, PALMITER RD, et al. 1990. Overexpression of TGF-alpha in transgenic mice: Induction of epithelial hyperplasia, pancreatic metaplasia and carcinoma of the breast. Cell 61:1121–1135.

SARLES H. 1973. An international survey on nutrition and pancreatitis. Digestion 9:389–403.

SARLES H, FIGARELLA C, TISCORNIA O, et al. 1980. Chronic calcifying pancreatitis (CCP), mechanism of formation of the lesions. New data and critical study. *In* Fitzgerald PJ, Morrison AB (eds): The Pancreas. Baltimore, Williams & Wilkins, pp. 48–66.

SARLES H, TISCORNIA O. 1974. Ethanol and chronic calcifying pancreatitis. Med Clin North Am 58:1333–1346.

SCARPELLI DG. 1975. Preliminary observations on the mitogenic effect of cyclopropenoid fatty acids on rat pancreas. Cancer Res 35:2278–2283.

SCHAEFFER BK, ZURLO J, LONGNECKER DS. 1990. Activation of *c-*Ki-*ras* not detectable in adenomas or adenocarcinomas arising in rat pancreas. Mol Carcinog 3:165–170.

SCHIFFMAN MH, FELTON JS. 1990. RE: Fried foods and the risk of colon cancer. (Letter). Am J Epidemiol 131:376–378.

SCHLAG P, ULRICH H, NERKLE P, et al. 1980. Are nitrite and *N-*nitroso compounds in gastric juice risk factors for carcinoma in the operated stomach? Lancet 1:727–729.

SCHOTTENFELD D, WARSHAUER ME, ZAUBER AG, et al. 1981. A prospective study of morbidity and mortality in petroleum industry employees in the United States—A preliminary report. *In* Peto R, Schneiderman M (eds): Banbury Report 9. Quantification of Occupational Cancer. Cold Spring Harbor, NY, Cold Spring Harbor Laboratory, pp. 247–265.

SEARLE CE, WATERHOUSE JAH, HENMAN BA, et al. 1981. Epidemiological study of the mortality of British chemists. Br J Cancer 38:192–193.

SEGI M, KURIHARA M. 1972. Cancer Mortality for Selected Sites in 24 Countries. No. 6 (1966–1967). Nagoya, Japan, Japan Cancer Society.

SEIDMAN H. 1970. Cancer death rates by site and sex for religious and socioeconomic groups in New York City. Environ Res 3:234–250.

SELIKOFF IJ, SEIDMAN H. 1981. Cancer of the pancreas among asbestos insulation workers. Cancer 47:1469–1473.

SENER SF, FREMGEN A, IMPERATO JP, et al. 1991. Pancreatic cancer in Illinois: A report by 88 hospitals on 2,401 patients diagnosed 1978–84. Am Surg 57:490–495.

SHAPIRO S, HEINONEN OP, SISKIND V. 1971. Cancer and allergy. Cancer 28:396–400.

SHEFFET A, THIND I, MILLER AM, et al. 1982. Cancer mortality in a pigment plant utilizing lead and zinc chromates. Arch Environ Health 37:44–52.

SHIBATA D, ALMOGUERA C, FORRESTER K, et al. 1990a. Detection of c-K-*ras* mutations in fine needle aspirates from human pancreatic adenocarcinomas. Cancer Res 4:1279–1283.

SHIBATA D, CAPELLA G, PERUCHO M. 1990b. Mutational activation of the c-K-*ras* gene in human pancreatic carcinoma. Baillières Clin Gastroenterol 4:151–169.

SILVERSTEIN M, PARK R, MARMOR M, et al. 1988. Mortality among bearing plant workers exposed to metal-working fluids and abrasives. J Occup Med 30:706–714.

SINDELAR WF, KINSELLA TJ, MAYER RJ. 1985. Cancer of the pancreas. *In* DeVita VT Jr, Hellman S, Tosenberg SA (eds): Cancer: Principles and Practice of Oncology, 2nd ed. Philadelphia, J.B. Lippincott, pp. 691–739.

SLYE M, HOLMES HF, WELLS HG. 1935. The comparative pathology of carcinoma of the pancreas, with report of two cases in mice. Am J Cancer 23:81–86.

SMIT VTHBM, BOOT AJM, SMITS AMM, et al. 1988. KRAS codon 12 mutations occur very frequently in pancreatic adenocarcinomas. Nucleic Acids Res 16:7773–7782.

SMITH JP, BARRETT, B, SOLOMON TE. 1987. CCK stimulates growth of five human pancreatic cancer cell lines in serum-free medium. (Abstract). Gastroenterology 92:1646.

SMITH JP, KRAMER S, BAGHERI S. 1990. Effects of a high-fat diet and L364,718 on growth of human pancreas cancer. Dig Dis Sci 35:726–732.

SMITH PG, DOLL R. 1981. Mortality from cancer and all causes among British radiologists. Br J Radiol 54:187–194.

SMITH RL. 1956. Recorded and expected mortality among the Japanese of the United States and Hawaii, with special reference to cancer. J Natl Cancer Inst 17:459–473.

SPARKS PJ, WEGMAN DH. 1980. Cause of death among jewelry workers. J Occup Med 22:733–735.

SPINGARN NE, WEISBURGER JH. 1979. Formation of mutagens in cooked foods. I. Beef. Cancer Lett 7:259–264.

STEINECK G, GERHARDSSON DE VERDIER M, ÖVERVIK E. 1993. The epidemiological evidence concerning intake of mutagenic activity from the fried surface and the risk of cancer cannot justify preventive measures. Eur J Cancer Prev 2:293–300.

STEINMETZ KA, POTTER JD. 1991a. Vegetables, fruit, and cancer. I. Epidemiology. Cancer Causes Control 2:325–357.

STEINMETZ KA, POTTER JD. 1991b. Vegetables, fruit, and cancer. II. Mechanisms. Cancer Causes Control 2:427–442.

STERNBY NH. 1991. The role of autopsy in cancer registration in Sweden, with particular reference to findings in Malmö. IARC Sci Publ No. 112. Lyon, International Agency for Research on Cancer, pp. 217–222.

STOCKS P. 1970. Cancer mortality in relation to national consumption of cigarettes, solid fuel, tea and coffee. Br J Cancer 24:215–225.

SUGIMURA T. 1985. Carcinogenicity of mutagenic heterocyclic amines formed during the cooking process. Mutat Res 150:33–41.

SUGIMURA T, SATO S. 1983. Mutagens-carcinogens in foods. Cancer Res 43:2415s–2421s.

SUGUITAN EA, et al. 1973. Pancreatic carcinoma: A statistical dilemma. Gastroenterology 64:A-125-808.

TADA M, OMATA M, KAWAI S, et al. 1993. Detection of *ras* gene mutations in pancreatic juice and peripheral blood of patients with pancreatic adenocarcinoma. Cancer Res 53:2472–2474.

TADA M, OMATA M, OHOTO M. 1991. Clinical application of *ras* gene mutation for diagnosis of pancreatic adenocarcinoma. Gastroenterology 100:233–238.

TADA M, YOSOSUKA O, OMATA M, et al. 1990. Analysis of *ras* gene mutations in biliary and pancreatic tumors by polymerase chain reaction and direct sequencing. Cancer 66:930–935.

TANAKA T, BARNES WS, WILLIAMS GM, et al. 1985. Multipotential carcinogenicity of the fried food mutagen 2-amino-3-methylimidazo[4,5-*f*]quinoline in rats. Jpn J Cancer Res (Gann) 76:570–576.

TANNENBAUM A. 1959. Nutrition and Cancer. *In* Homburger F (ed): The Physiopathology of Cancer. New York, Hoeber-Harper, pp. 517–562.

TAXY JB. 1976. Adenocarcinoma of the pancreas in childhood. Cancer 37:1508–1518.

TERSMETTE A, OFFERHAUS JA, GIARDIELLO FM, et al. 1990. Occurrence of non-gastric cancer in the digestive tract after remote partial gastrectomy: Analysis of an Amsterdam cohort. Int J Cancer 46:792–795.

THERIAULT G, PROVENCHER S. 1987. Mortality study of oil refinery workers: Five year follow-up. J Occup Med 29:357–360.

THEVE NO, POUSETTE A, CARLSTROM K. 1983. Adenocarcinoma of the pancreas—a hormone sensitive tumor? A preliminary report of volvadex treatment. Clin Oncol 9:193–197.

THOMAS TL, DECOUFLÉ P, MOURE-ERASO R. 1980. Mortality among workers employed in petroleum refining and petrochemical plants. J Occup Med 22:97–103.

THOMAS TL, MAXWEILER RJ, MOURE-ERASON R, et al. 1982. Mortality patterns among workers in three Texas oil refineries. J Occup Med 24:135–141.

TOLLEY HD, MARKS S, BUCHANAN JA, et al. 1983. A further update of the analysis of the mortality of workers in a nuclear facility. Radiat Res 95:211–213.

TRICKER AR, PREUSSMANN R. 1991. Carcinogenic *N*-nitrosamines in the diet: Occurrence, formation, mechanisms and carcinogenic potential. Mutat Res 259:277–289.

TSUKIMOTO I, WATANABE K, LIN JB, et al. 1973. Pancreatic carcinoma in children in Japan. Cancer 31:1203–1207.

TULASSAY Z, SANDO Z, BODROGI L, et al. 1988. An endocrine model for pancreatic cancer. Br Med J 297:1447–1448.

TURESKY RJ, LANG NP, BUTLER MA, et al. 1991. Metabolic activation of carcinogenic heterocyclic aromatic amines by human liver and colon. Carcinogenesis 12:1839–1845.

TURNER HM, GRACE HG. 1938. An investigation into cancer mortality among males in certain Sheffield trades. J Hygiene 38:90–103.

U.S. DEPARTMENT OF HEALTH AND HUMAN SERVICES. 1989. Reducing the Health Consequences of Smoking: 25 Years of Progress, A Report of the Surgeon General. USDHHS, PHS, Centers for Disease Control, Center for Chronic Disease Prevention and Health Promotion, Office on Smoking and Health. DHHS Pub No. (CDC) 89-8411.

U.S. DEPARTMENT OF HEALTH AND HUMAN SERVICES. 1990. Cancer Statistics Review 1973–1987. USDHHS, PHS, NCI, NIH publication No. 90-2789.

UPP JR, OLSON D, POSTON GJ, et al. 1988. Inhibition of growth of two human pancreatic adenocarcinomas in vivo by somatostatin analog SMS 201-995. Am J Surg 155:29–35.

VAN KRANEN HJ, VERMEULEN E, SCHOREN L, et al. 1991. Activation of c-K-*ras* is frequent in pancreatic carcinomas of Syrian hamsters, but is absent in pancreatic tumors of rats. Carcinogenesis 12:1477–1482.

VELEMA JP, WALKER AM, GOLD EB. 1986. Alcohol and pancreatic cancer, insufficient epidemiologic evidence for a causal relationship. Epidemiol Rev 8:28–41.

VENA JE, SULTZ HA, FIEDLER RC, et al. 1985. Mortality of workers in an automobile engine and parts manufacturing complex. Br J Ind Med 42:85–93.

VIADANA E, BROSS IDJ, HOUTEN L. 1976. Cancer experience of men exposed to inhalation of chemicals or to combustion products. J Occup Med 18:787–792.

VOIROL M, INFANTE F, RAYMOND L, et al. 1987. Nutrional profile of patients with cancer of the pancreas. Schweiz Med Wochenshr 117:1101–1104.

WALKER AM. 1990. Diabetes and pancreatic cancer. *In* Zatonski W, Boyle P, Tyczynski J (eds): Cancer Prevention, Vital Statistics to Intervention. Warsaw, PA Interpress, pp. 152–154.

WALKER ARP, WALKER BF, SEGAL I. 1993. Cancer patterns in three African populations compared with the United States Black population. Eur J Cancer Prev 2:313–320.

WARSHAW AL, FERNÁNDEZ-DEL CASTILLO C. 1992. Pancreatic carcinoma. N Engl J Med 326:455–465.

WATANAPA P, WILLIAMSON RCN. 1993. Experimental pancreatic hyperplasia and neoplasia: Effects of dietary and surgical manipulation. Br J Cancer 67:877–884.

WATERHOUSE J, MUIR C, CORREA P, et al (eds). 1976. Cancer Incidence in Five Continents, vol III. IARC Sci Pub No. 15. Lyon, International Agency for Research on Cancer.

WATTENBERG LW. 1985. Chemoprevention of cancer. Cancer Res 45:1–8.

WEINBERG RA. 1991. Tumor suppressor genes. Science 254:1138–1146.

WEIR JM, DUNN JE JR. 1970. Smoking and mortality: A prospective study. Cancer 25:105–112.

WEISBURGER JH. 1991. Carcinogenesis in our food and cancer prevention. *In* Friedman M (ed): Nutritional and Toxicological Consequences of Food Processing. New York, Plenum Press, pp. 137–151.

WEISBURGER JH. 1993. Heterocyclic amines in cooked foods: Possible human carcinogens. (Meeting report). Cancer Res 53:2422–2424.

WEISS W, BERNARDE MA. 1983. The temporal relation between cigarette smoking and pancreatic cancer. Am J Public Health 73:1403–1404.

WELCH RM, HSU SY, DE ANGELIS RL. 1977. Effect of Aroclor 1254, phenobarbital, and polycyclic aromatic hydrocarbons on the plasma clearance of caffeine in the rat. Clin Pharmacol Ther 22:791–798.

WEN CP, TSAI SP, MCCLELLAN WA, et al. 1983. Long-term mortality study of oil refinery workers. I. Mortality of hourly and salaried workers. Am J Epidemiol 118:526–542.

WHITTEMORE AS, PAFFENBARGER RS, ANDERSON K, et al. 1983. Early precursors of pancreatic cancer in college men. J Chronic Dis 36:251–256.

WIKLUND K, DICH J, HOLM L-E, et al. 1989. Risk of cancer in pesticide applicators in Swedish agriculture. Br J Ind Med 46:809–814.

WIKLUND K, HOLM L-E. 1986. Trends in cancer risks among Swedish agricultural workers. J Natl Cancer Inst 77:657–664.

WILLETT W. 1990. Nutritional Epidemiology. New York, Oxford University Press.

WILLETT WC, MACMAHON B. 1984a. Diet and cancer—an overview. (First of two parts.) N Engl J Med 310:633–638.

WILLETT WC, MACMAHON B. 1984b. Diet and cancer—An overview. (Second of two parts.) N Engl J Med 310:697–703.

WILLETT WC, STAMPFER MJ. 1986. Total energy intake: Implications for epidemiologic analyses. Am J Epidemiol 124:17–27.

WILLIAMS AJ, CUBILLA A, MADEAN BJ, et al. 1979. Twenty-two years experience with periampullary carcinoma at Memorial Sloan-Kettering Cancer Center. Am J Surg 138:662–665.

WILLIAMS JA. 1987. Role of receptors in mediating trophic stimuli in the pancreas. Gut 28:(Suppl)45–49.

WILLIAMS JA, HOOTMAN SR. 1986. Stimulus-secretion coupling in pancreatic acinar cells. *In* Go VLW (ed): The Exocrine Pancreas: Biology, Pathophysiology and Disease. New York, Raven Press, pp. 123–139.

WILLIAMS RR, HORM JW. 1977. Association of cancer sites with tobacco and alcohol consumption and socioeconomic status of patients: Interview study from the Third National Cancer Survey. J Natl Cancer Inst 58:525–547.

WILLIAMS RR, STEGENS NL, GOLDSMITH JR. 1977. Associations of cancer site and type with occupation and industry from the Third National Cancer Survey Interview. J Natl Cancer Inst 59:1147–1185.

WONG O, BROCKER W, DAVIS HV, et al. 1984. Mortality of workers potentially exposed to organic and inorganic brominated chemicals, DBCP, TRIS, PBB, and DDT. Br J Ind Med 41:15–24.

WONG O, MORGAN RW, BAILEY WJ, et al. 1986. An epidemiological study of petroleum refinery employees. Br J Ind Med 43:6–17.

WOUTERSEN RA, VAN GARDEREN-HOETMER A. 1988a. Inhibition of dietary fat promoted development of (pre)neoplastic lesions in exocrine pancreas of rats and hamsters by supplemental selenium and β-carotene. Cancer Lett 42:79–85.

WOUTERSEN RA, VAN GARDEREN-HOETMER A. 1988b. Inhibition of dietary fat promoted development of (pre)neoplastic lesions in exocrine pancreas of rats and hamsters by supplemental vitamins A, C and E. Cancer Lett 41:179–189.

WYNDER EL, DIECK GS, HALL NEL. 1986. Case-control study of decaffeinated coffee consumption and pancreatic cancer. Cancer Res 46:5360–5363.

WYNDER EL, HALL NEL, POLANSKY M. 1983. Epidemiology of coffee and pancreatic cancer. Cancer Res 43:3900–3906.

WYNDER EL, MABUCHI K, MARUCHI N, et al. 1973a. A case control study of cancer of the pancreas. Cancer 31:641–648.

WYNDER EL, MABUCHI K, MARUCHI N, et al. 1973b. Epidemiology of cancer of the pancreas. J Natl Cancer Inst 50:645–667.

YAMADA H, SAKAMOTO H, TAIRA M, et al. 1986. Amplification of both *c*-Ki-*ras* with a point mutation and *c-myc* in a primary pancreatic cancer and its metastatic tumors in lymph nodes. Jpn J Cancer Res (Gann) 77:370–375.

YANAI H, et al. 1979. Multivariate analysis of cancer mortalities for selected sites in 24 countries. Environ Health Perspect 32:83–101.

YOUNG JL, DEVESA SS, CULTER SJ. 1975. Incidence of cancer in United States blacks. Cancer Res 35:3523–3526.

YOUNG JL, et al. 1978. SEER Program: Cancer Incidence and Mortality in the United States. 1973–1976. Washington, DC, U.S. Government Printing Office, DHEW Pub No. (NIH) 78–1834.

ZATONSKI W, BOYLE P, PREZEWOZNIAK K, et al. 1993. Cigarette smoking, alcohol, tea and coffee consumption and pancreas cancer risk: A case-control study from Opole, Poland. Int J Cancer 53:601–607.

ZATONSKI W, PRZEWOZNIAK K, HOWE GR, et al. 1991. Nutritional factors and pancreatic cancer: A case-control study from Opole, Poland. Int J Cancer 48:390–394.

ZOLOTH SR, MICHAELS DM, VILLALBI JR, et al. 1986. Patterns of mortality among commercial pressmen. J Natl Cancer Inst 76:1047–1051.

36 Liver cancer

W. THOMAS LONDON
KATHERINE A. McGLYNN

A number of tumor types occur in the liver, but except for primary hepatocellular carcinoma (HCC), all are rare. HCC, on the other hand, is one of the three most common causes of cancer mortality in the world, accounting for 250,000 to 1,000,000 deaths per year. Precise estimates have not been established because the tumor occurs most commonly in Asia and Africa, areas lacking good tumor registries. HCC is almost always lethal. The median survival from time of diagnosis is less than 6 months (Falkson et al, 1988). Hence, mortality and incidence can be equated.

About 80% of HCCs are etiologically associated with chronic infection with hepatitis B virus (HBV) (WHO, 1983). In those areas where HCC is endemic, most chronic HBV infections are acquired perinatally or in early childhood. With the advent of safe, effective hepatitis B vaccines and the introduction of routine vaccination of newborns in high-risk areas, it is likely that the incidence of HCC will decrease markedly over the next four decades (see Chapter 24).

HISTOPATHOLOGY

The liver is a common site of metastasis for tumors originating in other organs. Death certificates and hospital charts cannot be relied on to accurately distinguish primary from secondary tumors. Therefore, statistics that are not based on histopathologic diagnoses are suspect.

Both benign and malignant tumors occur in the liver, but benign tumors are quite rare. Table 36–1 provides a simplified classification of liver tumors, with a brief description of histopathology and, when known, etiology and epidemiology.

ANATOMIC DISTRIBUTION

Hepatocellular adenomas are usually 5 to 15 cm in diameter, subcapsular tumors. They may bleed into the peritoneal cavity and can present with acute abdominal pain. Bile duct adenomas are also found most commonly under the liver capsule. Typically, they are trivial lesions, 1 cm in diameter or less, found incidentally at autopsy. Hemangiomas are usually solitary tumors, less than 4 cm in diameter, which can occur anywhere in the liver. Infantile hemangioendotheliomas may also occur anywhere in the liver, but they may be solitary or multicentric and vary in size from less than 1 cm to 15 cm in diameter. Mesenchymal hamartomas are solitary tumors found in young children. They range in size from 15 cm to 30 cm in diameter and may occur in any part of the liver.

Hepatoblastomas are usually solitary tumors varying in size from 5 cm to 17 cm. The right lobe alone is the site of 58% of the tumors, whereas 15% involve only the left lobe; 27% affect both lobes (Stocker and Ishak, 1987). Angiosarcomas are most often multifocal, involving the entire liver (Ishak, 1987).

Cholangiocarcinomas, which may arise from any part of the intrahepatic bile duct epithelium, have been classified into massive (or infiltrative), nodular, diffuse types, and periductal types. The infiltrative and diffuse types invade the entire liver. The periductal type infiltrates throughout the liver but also infiltrates and proliferates along the extrahepatic bile duct. Solitary and multiple nodular tumors occur at any site in the liver (Edmondson, 1958; Sugihara and Kojiro, 1987).

In the past it was thought that HCCs were largely multicentric. Recent evidence, obtained from prospective studies of hepatitis B carriers in China, Japan, and Alaska and early intervention studies in China, indicate that all such tumors begin as solitary nodules (Tang, 1985). The old classification of nodular, diffuse, and massive types is descriptive of advanced cases and, therefore, not particularly informative. These tumors originate in all parts of the liver but are found more frequently in the right lobe, perhaps because it is larger than the left. Hepatocellular carcinoma commonly invades the portal and hepatic venous systems, producing

TABLE 36–1. *Classification of Primary Liver Tumors*

Liver Tumors	*Histologic Characteristics*	*Etiology/Epidemiology*
BENIGN		
Hepatocellular adenoma	Well-differentiated cells with abundant eosinophilic cytoplasm arranged in sheets, cords. Lobules, portal areas, bile ducts absent. Clearly demarcated from surrounding liver, but unencapsulated.	Almost all cases in females. Exposure to androgens, oral contraceptives, clomiphene. Associated with glycogen storage disease Type I, galactosemia.
Hemangioma	Differentiated endothelial cells.	Congenital. Most common benign liver tumor.
Infantile hemangioendothelioma	Abnormal endothelial cells.	
Epithelioid hemangioendothelioma	Dendritic and epithelioid cells. (Not totally benign, may invade hepatic veins.)	
Mixed hamartoma	Clusters of "embryonal" hepatocytes.	
Mesenchymal hamartoma	Well-differentiated bile ducts and extensive mesenchymal stroma.	
MALIGNANT		
Hepatoblastoma	Epithelial type—fetal and/or embryonal hepatocytes. Mixed type—fetal hepatocytes plus mesenchymal elements. Osteoid often present.	Most common hepatic tumor of childhood. Associated with biliary atresia, Beckwith-Weidemann syndrome. Age: < 3 years.
Bile duct (cholangio-) carcinoma	Infiltrative, nodular, and diffuse types. Glandular structures surrounded by abundant fibrous stroma.	M:F = 1–2:1. Infestation with liver flukes, *Clonorchis sinensis*, *Opistorchis viverini.* Exposure to thorotrast. In U.S. associated with ulcerative colitis, cystic dilation of bile duct.
Angiosarcoma	Multicentric, ill-defined hemorrhagic nodules. Anaplastic, spindle cells form a roof over the surface of liver cell trabeculae.	M:F = 3:1. In adults, exposure to thorotrast, arsenicals, vinyl chloride monomer.
Hepatocellular carcinoma	Well, moderately or poorly differentiated parenchymal cells. Trabeculae ranging in thickness from two to eight cells separated by sinusoids. Clear cell variant contains excess glycogen; fibrolamellar variant—large, polygonal, eosinophilic cells.	M:F = 4–5:1. Chronic infection with hepatitis B virus. Exposure to mycotoxins, alcohol, androgens, tobacco.
TUMORLIKE NON-NEOPLASMS		
Focal nodular hyperplasia	Well-circumscribed, unencapsulated solitary nodule. Cut surface contains a central "stellate" scar with radiating fibrous septae.	M:F = 1:2. Not associated with oral contraceptives, but they may stimulate growth of lesion.
Nodular regenerative hyperplasic	Scattered multiple hepatocellular nodules with intervening areas of hepatic atrophy. (Possibly preneoplastic.)	M:F = 1:1. Associated with myeloproliferative, lymphoproliferative, and collagen-vascular diseases.

(See Edmondson, 1958; Anthony, 1979; Goodman, 1987; Stocker and Ishak, 1987; Sugihara and Kojiro, 1987; Ishak, 1987.)

tumor thrombi in the portal vein and its tributaries; tumor thrombi in the hepatic veins undoubtedly occur but are more difficult to identify (Kojiro and Nakashima, 1987).

INCIDENCE AND MORTALITY IN THE UNITED STATES

Hepatocellular carcinoma is an uncommon tumor among persons born in the United States. Of 1,208,000 estimated incident cancers in 1994, only 1.3% will be of the liver and intrahepatic bile duct (ACS, 1994). Incidence rates are higher for males (4.0/100,000) than females (1.4/100,000) and higher for African Americans than for whites (1.9/100,000 vs. 4.2/100,000) (SEER, 1993).

The survival time of patients with clinically detectable HCC is exceedingly poor. The American Cancer Society estimates that the 5-year survival in the UnitedStates is approximately 6% of cases and this rate has only marginally improved in 25 years (ACS, 1994). Because the survival of HCC patients is so poor, mortality and incidence are virtually identical. However, the 30-year time trends (1960–1990) in liver cancer mortality in the United States are encouraging (ACS, 1994). Among men, the rate has shown an overall 8% decline, although the rate appears to have plateaued in recent years, or even increased slightly. Among women, the downward trend is more pronounced with a 45% decline and with no sign of a leveling off. The cause of the decline is still a matter of debate.

INCIDENCE AND MORTALITY THROUGHOUT THE WORLD

Hepatocellular carcinoma has one of the greatest geographical variations of any major cancer. While it is a very rare tumor in the United States and in western Europe, liver cancer is one of the most common malignancies in eastern Asia and sub-Saharan Africa. Due to the population size in these latter areas, HCC ranks as one of the most common cancers in the world (Parkin et al, 1993). Among the areas listed in *Cancer Incidence in Five Continents*, Qidong, China, and Khon Kaen, Thailand, have the world's highest rates at 89.9/100,000 and 90.0/100,000, respectively. Forty-four percent of the world's cases occur in China alone (Parkin et al, 1993). Ireland and the United Kingdom have rates which are among the lowest at 1.1/100,000 and 1.4–2.0/100,000, respectively (IARC, 1992).

Unlike Western nations, in high-incidence areas the incidence of liver cancer does not appear to be declining, although time trends are hard to estimate because of the lack of long-established tumor registries. Of two studies examining worldwide trends, one reported an increasing incidence (Stevens et al, 1984) and one, no change in incidence (Muñoz and Bosch, 1987). Reports from individual countries have noted an increasing incidence in Taiwan (Lin et al, 1986) and Japan (Okuda et al, 1987), a flat trend in Singapore (Lee et al, 1988), and possibly a declining trend in South Africa (Robertson et al, 1971; Harington et al, 1975; Bradshaw et al, 1982; Van Rensburg et al, 1985).

While there is large geographic variation in incidence, there is little worldwide difference in survival and mortality. Studies among Japanese and African nations indicate that the median survival is only 2 to 4 months (Okuda et al, 1985; Kew and Geddes, 1982). The reason that survival is so poor is that the majority of patients are asymptomatic until the tumor has grown too large to be resectable. If the tumor can be detected when it is small enough (<3 cm) to be resected, the prognosis is much more favorable (Tang and Yang, 1985; Okuda et al, 1985).

MIGRATION

The changes in HCC incidence with migration are not consistent. Among Chinese males recorded in the San Francisco Bay Area tumor registry, the annual rate of liver cancer is 22.1 cases per 100,000 persons. While this is lower than the incidence in Shanghai (37.1/100,000), it is seven times as great as the rate among white males in San Francisco (Muir et al, 1987). In contrast, Chinese migrants to Singapore have the same HCC rate as Chinese in China (Lee et al, 1988). One postulated explanation for the difference in rates between the Chinese migrants to the United States and to Singapore is that the U. S. immigrants may come from a low-incidence area of China and the Singapore immigrants from a high-incidence area (Muñoz and Bosch, 1987). This hypothesis is not substantiated by data from China that lists the home province of the majority of U. S. immigrants, Guangdong, as one of the highest incidence areas in China (Chinese Academy of Medical Sciences, 1981). Also counter to the hypothesis are data from Singapore that detail liver cancer risk among Chinese and show no significant difference by ethnic groups from diverse provinces (Lee et al, 1988).

AGE

The peak age incidence of HCC is geographically variable. In South Africa, patients have the greatest incidence between the ages of 35 and 45, while patients in Asia are roughly ten years older, and those in the United States and Europe, yet another ten years older (Kew and Geddes, 1982; Ferenci et al, 1984; Zaman et al, 1985). In all geographic areas, the incidence increases with age and then plateaus once the peak is reached. In low-incidence areas, it is exceedingly rare to see cases in persons younger than 40 years of age, while high-incidence areas report cases in persons younger than age 20 (Lanier et al, 1987). This difference in the age distribution of cases may reflect, in part, a difference in age of exposure to HBV.

SEX

Worldwide, the male:female ratio is heavily biased toward males, with a preponderance of between 4:1 and 9:1 (Szmuness, 1978). The discrepancy between males and females is especially marked in high-incidence areas (Muir et al, 1987). The reason that males have a higher HCC rate is not resolved, but may be explained by such factors as a greater likelihood among males to become HBV carriers, genetic susceptibility, androgenic steroids, and higher body iron stores (Israel et al, 1989).

ETHNICITY

In those regions of the world where liver cancer is endemic, not all ethnic groups are equally affected. In sub-

Saharan Africa, only the black population is at a high risk of HCC. Similarly, while there is a high rate of HCC in Alaska, the elevated risk is only among the Alaska Native population (Eskimos, North American Indians, and Aleuts) (Heyward et al, 1985). In Singapore, the Chinese population has rates that are twice those of the Malay or Indian populations, and in New Zealand, the Maori rates are three times those of the non-Maori (Pearce et al, 1985; Muir et al, 1987). This ethnic variation in rates may reflect genetic susceptibility to HCC or differences in exposure or susceptibility to HBV.

FAMILIAL CLUSTERING

An argument similar to that of ethnic clustering can be made for familial clustering of HCC. While numerous familial HCC clusters have been reported (Ohbayashi, 1982; Scobie et al, 1983; Lynch et al, 1984; Lok and Lai, 1988a; Alberts et al, 1991), such families also tend to show clustering of hepatitis B carriers. However, two analyses have found evidence of genetic susceptibility to HCC, while taking into account HBV infection. In 1990, Yang et al reported an analysis of HCC in the Alaskan Native population which demonstrated that risk of HCC could be explained by the interaction of HBV infection and a major gene. In 1991, Shen et al also demonstrated an HBV-major gene interaction in an analysis of data from Chinese families. The only discrepancy between the two reports was that the analysis of Yang and colleagues (1990) indicated that the major gene was likely to be dominant and Shen et al (1991) found the gene to be recessive.

URBANIZATION

Besides ethnic and familial differences in HCC rates, there are urban-rural differences within populations. Kew et al (1983) found the rate in rural blacks in South Africa to be higher than the rate in urban blacks and the peak age incidence to be younger. The investigators compared HCC patients who had been raised in a rural area before moving to an urban area with HCC patients who did not migrate. After adjusting for age, the authors found that there was no significant difference in the prevalence of hepatitis B infection between the urban and rural groups. They suggested that a carcinogenic cofactor was present in rural areas that was absent from urban areas. The same group of researchers has reported that urban black HCC cases are more likely to be alcohol related than the rural cases, which is similar to the situation in Western countries (Paterson et al, 1985).

HEPATITIS B VIRUS (HBV)

The biology and epidemiology of HBV are reviewed in Chapter 24. Here we will expand on the relationship of chronic HBV infection with HCC.

In the 1950s several pathologists emphasized the close association of HCC with cirrhosis of the liver (Edmondson and Steiner, 1954; Edmondson, 1958; Higginson et al, 1957). At least 80% of liver cancers occurred in cirrhotic livers. Edmondson (1958) noted that in the United States and western Europe, 3% to 10% of men with cirrhosis developed HCC; whereas in Africa and Asia, 15% to 50% of cirrhotic patients developed liver cancer. In addition, these pathologists observed that cirrhosis in Western countries was related mainly to abuse of alcohol, but in Africa and Asia cirrhosis was caused by some agent other than alcohol. Nutritional deficiencies, ingestion of toxins, and chronic viral infections were all mentioned.

These early investigators were on the right track. A different agent, the hepatitis B virus, is responsible for most of the cases of cirrhosis in the areas of the world where HCC is endemic. The evidence, which has been gathered over the past 20 years, that chronic infection with HBV is also the major factor in the etiology of HCC is reviewed elsewhere (London, 1981; Szmuness, 1978; Beasley, 1988) and summarized below.

1. Areas of the world with high mortality rates for HCC also have high HBV infection rates. The reverse is also true. Every country in the world with a prevalence of HBV carriers greater than 2% has an increased mortality from HCC. The only exception may be among the small population of Eskimos in Greenland where chronic infection with HBV is common but HCC has not been observed (Melbye et al, 1984).
2. As suspected by liver pathologists in the 1950s, cross-sectional studies in the areas of the world where HCC is endemic have shown that cirrhosis is closely associated with chronic HBV infection (Hann et al, 1982; Yang and Tang, 1985).
3. Case-control studies in all regions of the world have consistently shown that chronic HBV infection (seropositivity for hepatitis B surface antigen, HBsAg) is much more common among HCC cases than controls. Odds ratios have ranged from approximately 5:1 to 65:1 (London, 1981; IARC, 1994).
4. Prospective studies of chronic carriers have demonstrated very high relative risks for HCC (Beasley et al, 1981; Ijima et al, 1984; Heyward et al, 1985). Table 36–2 summarizes the results of almost 9 years of follow-up of a large cohort of government workers in Taiwan (Beasley, 1988). The annual incidence of HCC among chronic carriers in the reported prospective studies has ranged between 400 and 500 per 100,000 per year com-

TABLE 36–2. *Incidence and Relative Risk of HCC among Chinese Male Government Workers in Taiwan after 11 Years of Follow-up*[*]

Recruitment Status	*Population at Risk*	*Cases of HCC*	*Cases of HCC per 100,000 per yr*	*Relative Risk (95% confidence interval)*
HBsAg(+)	3454	184	474	103 (57.2–204.8)
HBsAg(−)				
anti-HBs(+)/anti-HBc(+)	15,570	8	5	
anti-HBs(−)/anti-HBc(+)	2411	2	8	
anti-HBs(−)/anti-HBc(−)	1272	0	0	
Total	22,707	194	76	

[*]Beasley and Hwang, 1991.

pared with less than five per 100,000 per year in HBsAg negative controls (see Chapter 24 for definitions of HBV antigens). A very important observation from the Taiwan study is that 1272 men with no serologic evidence of previous HBV infection have not experienced any cases of liver cancer in 9 years of observation.

5. Cirrhosis is a well-documented risk factor for HCC. The hypothesis has been frequently stated that cirrhosis of any etiology is a precursor to cancer and that HBV infection is carcinogenic only in so far as it gives rise to cirrhosis. This hypothesis has been tested in Japan (Obata et al, 1980), Taiwan (Beasley, 1988), and Austria (Ferenci et al, 1984) by following patients with cirrhosis who were or were not HBV carriers. In the HCC endemic nations of Japan and Taiwan (Table 36–3), carriers with cirrhosis were at four- to sixfold greater risk than noncarriers with cirrhosis; but an increased risk for carriers was not detected in Austria, a nonendemic area.

6. In the areas of the world with high incidences of HCC and high prevalences of HBV, about half of all chronic HBV infections are acquired perinatally or in early childhood (Stevens et al, 1975; Okada et al, 1976; Marinier et al, 1985; Feret et al, 1987). Since persons who were chronic carriers the longest were likely to be at the greatest risk of liver cancer, it was predicted that mothers of patients with HCC were likely to be chronic HBV carriers. This hypothesis was supported in Senegal (Larouze et al, 1976), Korea (Hann et al, 1982), and Taiwan (Beasley, 1988). Seventy-one percent to 86% of mothers of cases were HBsAg positive compared with 10% to 35% of mothers of asymptomatic chronic carriers (Senegal and Taiwan). In Korea, 40% of mothers of HCC cases were HBsAg positive compared with none among age-matched controls.

TABLE 36–3. *Incidence of HCC in Patients with Cirrhosis with Respect to HBV Status*

	HBV Status	*Population at Risk*	*Cases of HCC*	*Relative Risk HBsAg(+) vs. HBsAg(−)*
Taiwan[a]	HBsAg(+)	40	9	6.75
	HBsAg(−)	30	1	
Japan[b]	HBsAg(+)	30	7	5
	HBsAg(−)	85	5	

[a]11 yrs of follow-up (Beasley and Hwang, 1991).
[b]4.5 yrs of follow-up (Obata et al, 1980).

7. Immunohistopathologic studies of liver tissues from HCC cases and controls obtained at autopsy or surgery have revealed HBsAg in 50% to 90% of nonneoplastic tissues of cases compared with less than 10% for controls (Nayak et al, 1977; Tan et al, 1977; Thung et al, 1979).

8. At the molecular level, HBV DNA is found in the tumor tissue of virtually all HCC patients with HBsAg in their serum and 10% to 20% of those who do not have detectable HBsAg but are positive for anti-HBs and/or anti-HBc (Shafritz et al, 1981; Brechot et al, 1985; Yokosuka et al, 1986).

9. Chronic infection with viruses belonging to the same family as HBV, hepadnaviruses (see Chapter 24), causes hepatocellular carcinoma in their natural hosts—woodchucks, ground squirrels, and possibly ducks (Summers et al, 1978; Marion et al, 1986; Omata et al, 1987). Under experimental conditions, liver cancer has been induced in woodchucks by inoculating newborn animals with the woodchuck hepadnavirus, WHV (Popper et al, 1987).

From the above nine lines of evidence, it is abundantly clear that the chronic HBV infection/HCC relationship satisfies the usual criteria for causation of disease: consistency, strength, specificity, temporal relationship, and coherence (biological plausibility) of the association (Advisory Committee to the Surgeon General of the Public Health Service, 1964). Other factors such as aflatoxins, androgens, iron stores, and alcohol may also be independent carcinogens or they may accelerate the development and increase the risk of HCC in HBV carriers; but chronic HBV infection is the major etiologic factor for HCC in humans. A working group of the International Agency for Research on Cancer

(IARC) concluded that chronic infection with HBV is carcinogenic to humans (IARC, 1994).

HEPATITIS C VIRUS (HCV)

The virology and general epidemiology of HCV is discussed in Chapter 24. Here we present additional information on the strong link of HCV with HCC.

Before the development of serologic assays for HCV infection, descriptive epidemiologic studies in Japan supported the hypothesis that infection with a non-A, non-B virus was a significant cause of liver cancer in that country (Liver Cancer Study Group of Japan, 1984; Okuda et al, 1987). The annual incidence of HCC, as recorded in the Osaka Cancer Registry, had risen from 16.3 per 100,000 men in 1966–1968 to 35.6 in 1983. Increased deaths from HCC recorded in the annual vital statistics of Japan and the increasing frequency of HCC among all autopsies performed in Japan supported the tumor registry data. As the incidence of HCC had risen, the proportion of cases associated with HBV infection had declined from 50% to 30% (Liver Cancer Study Group of Japan, 1984). Okuda and his colleagues (1987) proposed that chronic non-A, non-B hepatitis acquired from blood transfusions during the post World War II years was responsible for the increasing incidence of HCC.

Kiyosawa et al (1990) provided strong support for Okuda's hypothesis. They found that 94% of 54 Japanese patients with HCC, without markers of HBV infection in their serum or liver, had antibodies to HCV compared with 35% of 29 patients with HBV-associated HCC. Furthermore, 42% of the patients with HCV-associated HCC had received blood transfusions in the past, whereas none of the patients with HBV-associated HCC had been transfused. The interval from transfusion to diagnosis of HCC ranged from 15 to 60 years with a median interval of 29 years. More than 85% of the patients with HCV-associated HCC had cirrhosis at the time of diagnosis of cancer. Most of these patients had liver biopsies in the years between transfusion and development of HCC. These tissue specimens revealed a slow evolution from chronic persistent hepatitis to chronic active hepatitis to cirrhosis to HCC.

More than 20 case series and case-control studies have confirmed the association of HCV with HCC, not only in Japan (Miyamura et al, 1991) but also in the United States (Yu et al, 1990), Europe (Bruix et al, 1989; Colombo et al, 1989; Ducreux et al, 1990; Tremolada et al, 1990; Kaklamani et al, 1991), and Africa (Kew et al, 1990a, see IARC, 1994 for a summary). The early studies used first generation assays for anti-HCV that depended on detecting antibodies to a single HCV antigen (c-100). Second generation enzyme immunoassays that used two or more antigens and immunoblot assays that also incorporated multiple HCV antigens were more specific than the first generation tests. Of six case-control studies that used second generation assays, three reported significant odds ratios ranging from 10 to 77 (Tanaka et al, 1991; Stroffolini et al, 1992; Zavitsanos et al, 1992). In the three locations (Mozambique, Senegal, and Vietnam, HBV endemic areas) where the odds ratios were not significant, the prevalences of anti-HCV antibodies were very low in both the case and control populations (Dazza et al, 1993; Coursaget et al, 1992; Cordier et al, 1993).

Three additional cohort studies have been reported. In a clinic-based study from Sweden, 566 patients (331 men, 235 women) with chronic liver disease, established by biopsy, were followed for varying time intervals up to 11 years. Anti-HCV antibodies were ascertained by second generation tests in sera collected at the time of biopsy. Among 153 patients who died during follow-up, HCC occurred more commonly in the HCV antibody positive group (5/23) compared with the seronegative patients (6/130) (Verbaan et al, 1992). In a study of 9691 adult men from Taiwan, followed from 4 to 6 years, 35 cases of HCC developed. Seven of the 35 cases compared with four of 160 matched controls were HCV seropositive at enrollment. The adjusted relative risk was 12 (95% C.I. = 2.4-58) (Yu and Chen, 1993). The third cohort (Seeff et al, 1992) was a long-term follow-up of transfused patients from five prospective studies. Five hundred and sixty-eight (568) patients who developed acute non-A, non-B (NANB) posttransfusion hepatitis between 1967 and 1980 were compared with 984 controls who were not diagnosed with NANB. The mortality and cause-specific mortality after 18 years of follow-up of the NANB cases and the controls were very similar. Mortality due to liver disease was slightly higher among the NANB patients. Three cases of HCC occurred; one among the NANB cases and two among the controls. The relation of anti-HCV antibodies to these outcomes was not reported. Even if all three cases of HCC were associated with HCV infection, this study would suggest that HCC rarely occurs during the first 15 years of infection with HCV. The studies from Japan would suggest that many cases of HCC will occur in the next 15 (or more) years.

The specificity of the association of HCV with HCC was further confirmed by the detection of HCV RNA in the tumor and nontumor cirrhotic liver tissue of patients with HCC (Yoneyama et al, 1990). More recent studies have demonstrated HCV RNA plus and minus strands (replicating forms) in tumor and adjacent nontumor tissue (Haruna et al, 1994; Kobayashi et al, 1994).

No naturally occurring hepatitis C-like virus has been discovered among free-living animals. One chimpanzee which was inoculated with serum from a patient with

NANB hepatitis and subsequently with several other blood products developed chronic hepatitis. HCC was diagnosed 7 years after the initial inoculation. The animal remained seronegative for markers of HBV infection. HCV assays were not available at the time of the report (Muchmore et al, 1988).

Based on the epidemiologic and molecular evidence, an IARC working group determined that "chronic infection with hepatitis C virus is carcinogenic to humans" and fulfills the criteria of a Group 1 carcinogen (IARC, 1994). Thus, HCV is probably the major viral cause of HCC in areas of the world with low prevalences of HBV carriers. In both HBV endemic and nonendemic areas, dual infections with HCV may occur and may increase the risk of HCC beyond that imparted by either virus alone (Yu et al, 1990; Kaklamani et al, 1991; Stroffolini et al, 1992).

ALCOHOL AND CIRRHOSIS

Alcohol consumption has received extensive scrutiny as a putative risk factor for liver cancer. Most studies support a positive association, particularly in low-incidence areas, but questions remain concerning the nature of the relationship. Two models of association have been proposed: (1) alcohol causes cirrhosis, which predisposes to cancer, and (2) alcohol is, itself, carcinogenic.

Evidence in favor of the former model is based on both epidemiologic and laboratory data. It is estimated that 60% to 90% of HCC occurs in cirrhotic livers, depending on whether the tumor occurs in a high- or low-incidence area (Shikata, 1976). In low-incidence areas, HCC seems to occur as a consequence of chronic, clinical cirrhosis of alcoholic etiology and is usually of micronodular morphology (Kew and Paterson, 1985; Hoofnagle et al, 1987; Tuyns and Obradovic, 1975). In contrast, in high-incidence areas, cirrhosis is often only discovered during the work-up for HCC and is more likely to be macronodular (Kew, 1981; Nonomura et al, 1986a). Micronodular cirrhosis can progress, however, to the macronodular type (Kojiro and Nakashima, 1987).

There are several possible reasons that HCC is more rarely seen in conjunction with alcohol-associated micronodular cirrhosis than with macronodular cirrhosis. It has been estimated that, on average, HCC does not appear until approximately 8 years after a diagnosis of cirrhosis (Purtilo and Gottlieb, 1973). In a prospective study of alcoholics, the mean survival from the diagnosis of cirrhosis was 5.5 years (Schmidt and Popham, 1981). Therefore, alcoholics with cirrhosis may simply not live long enough to develop HCC. Alcoholics also have many other nonhepatic competing risks for mortality, e.g., accidents (Rothman, 1980). Ethanol may also kill too many hepatocytes to permit tumor growth. This hypothesis is supported by studies which found that alcoholics who continued to drink had a lower risk of both macronodular cirrhosis and HCC than alcoholics who stopped drinking (Lee, 1966; Nonomura et al, 1986b).

Geographically, there is a poor correlation between countries with high rates of cirrhosis and those with high rates of HCC. While cirrhosis rates are high in Chile, Mexico, Portugal, France, Puerto Rico, Italy, Ireland, and Austria, none of these countries rank as high-incidence areas for HCC. Conversely, Thailand, Hong Kong, and Greece have high HCC rates, but low cirrhosis rates (WHO, 1982). The most likely explanation of these data is that areas with high cirrhosis rates tend to be the areas of micronodular cirrhosis associated with alcoholism. Similarly, the high HCC areas tend to be areas where macronodular cirrhosis is diagnosed in conjunction with a symptomatic tumor.

The weight of the evidence is clearly in favor of a positive association between alcohol and cirrhosis, and cirrhosis and HCC. The question remaining is whether there is also an association of alcohol and HCC, independent of cirrhosis. Experimental studies argue against alcohol being directly carcinogenic (Schottenfeld, 1979; McCoy et al, 1981), even though it may be related to chromosomal damage (Obe and Herha, 1975). Significantly, although there is an animal model for alcohol-induced cirrhosis in the baboon, there is no comparable animal model for alcohol-induced cancer (Rubin and Lieber, 1974). However, alcohol may promote oncogenesis through a number of mechanisms, including: the induction of enzymes which activate procarcinogens, interference with the repair of carcinogen-mediated DNA alkylation, exacerbation of malnutrition, exacerbation of hepatitis B- and hepatitis C-related liver damage, and alteration of the metabolism and distribution of carcinogens (Lieber et al, 1986).

Epidemiologic studies conducted in high-incidence (Chen et al, 1991), moderate-incidence (Onishi et al, 1982, 1987; Kono et al, 1987; Tanaka et al, 1988; Shibata et al, 1990; Vall Mayans et al, 1990; Hiyama et al, 1990; Tsukuma et al, 1990), and low-incidence areas (Yu et al, 1983; Stemhagen et al, 1983; Hardell et al, 1984; Austin et al, 1986; Mirkin et al, 1990) have found alcohol to be a significant risk factor for liver cancer. Studies which show no significant association between alcohol and HCC include three from high-incidence areas, Hong Kong (Lam et al, 1982), Thailand (Srivatanakul et al, 1991), and Nigeria (Olubuyide et al, 1990), and two from a moderate-incidence area, Greece (Trichopoulos et al, 1980, 1987). Thus alcoholic cirrhosis is probably the most important risk factor for HCC in low-incidence areas. In high-incidence areas, alcohol may exacerbate HBV- and HCV-related liver damage and thereby promote the development of a tumor.

AFLATOXINS

Aflatoxins are mycotoxins produced by the fungi *Aspergillis flavus* and *A. parasiticus*. With the exception of very cold climates, these fungi are virtually ubiquitous (IARC, 1976). Concern about the toxicity of aflatoxins began in 1960 following an epizootic of mycotoxicosis among turkey poults in Britain (Blount, 1961; Asplin and Carnaghan, 1961) and the discovery of liver cancer in aflatoxin-exposed rainbow trout in the United States (Halver, 1965). The principal human exposure to aflatoxins is from food (e.g., peanuts, corn, and cassava) and, to a much lesser extent, through inhalation in certain workplaces (Hayes et al, 1984; McLaughlin et al, 1987; Olsen et al, 1988).

Although there are four principal aflatoxins, B_1, B_2, G_1, and G_2, aflatoxin B_1 (AFB_1) has been shown to be the most potent in animal studies (IARC, 1987b). Liver tumors have been produced in rats (Butler and Hempsall, 1981), infant mice (Vesselinovitch et al, 1972), fish (Sinnhuber et al, 1968; Wales and Sinnhuber, 1972; Sato et al, 1973), ducks (Carnaghan, 1965), marmosets (Lin et al, 1974), tree shrews (Reddy et al, 1976), and monkeys (Adamson et al, 1976; Sieber et al, 1979). These data have led IARC to conclude that there is sufficient evidence to classify aflatoxin as a carcinogen (IARC, 1987a).

While the experimental data on carcinogenicity are strong, the human data, until recently, lagged behind. The epidemiology suffered from the lack of a biological marker to determine past aflatoxin ingestion (Bennet et al, 1981). Consequently, researchers relied either on correlation studies or on dietary questionnaires concerning foods that may have been contaminated with aflatoxins in the past. Although the problem of estimating past aflatoxin exposure has not been solved, there are now methods to measure aflatoxin metabolites (Garner et al, 1985; Groopman et al, 1986), aflatoxin-DNA adducts in tissues and AFB_1-albumin adducts in serum (Wild et al, 1986; Sabbioni et al, 1987). Metabolites and adducts reflect exposures over days to a few months, making both methods more appropriate for prospective than case-control studies. Demonstrations that serum AFB_1-albumin adducts correlate closely with AFB_1 intake (Gan et al, 1988) and with AFB_1 bound to DNA (Wild et al 1986) make serum measurements of AFB_1-albumin adducts particularly amenable to longitudinal research.

Prior to the development of AFB_1 biomarkers, most epidemiologic studies correlated the incidence of HCC in a defined area with the amount of AFB_1 contamination found in typical foodstuffs or the estimated current AFB_1 intake of the population. Studies reporting a positive correlation between AFB_1 levels and HCC were completed in Uganda (Alpert et al, 1971), Thailand (Shank et al, 1972), Kenya (Peers and Linsell, 1973), Swaziland (Keen and Martin, 1971; Peers and Linsell, 1973; Peers et al, 1987), Mozambique (Purchase and Goncalves, 1971; Van Rensburg et al, 1974, 1985), and China (Armstrong, 1980; Yaobin et al, 1983; Yeh et al, 1985, 1989). Two studies which contrasted AFB_1 adducts with HCC incidence found no association. One study, conducted in Kenya, correlated the incidence of HCC with the urinary excretion of AFB_1-guanine adducts among volunteers (Autrup et al, 1987) and one study in Thailand examined AFB_1-albumin adducts in cases of HCC and controls (Srivatanakul et al, 1991).

There are, however, methodological problems associated with the aforementioned studies. The assessment of contemporary AFB_1 exposure was correlated with the incidence of a cancer that was initiated some decades in the past. While the argument is often made that the lifestyle in many of these countries has not changed for many years, past exposure cannot be estimated reliably from current levels of contamination by assuming dietary stability. A second problem is one inherent in correlation studies: two variables having elevated levels in a population is not equivalent to two variables having elevated levels in the same individual. A third problem is the failure to account for confounding variables, principally HBV infection. With the exception of three studies done in China (Yaobin et al, 1983; Yeh et al, 1985, 1989) and three in Africa (Van Rensburg et al, 1985; Peers et al, 1987; Autrup et al, 1987), HBV has not been considered in the aflatoxin studies. Of the three studies in Africa, one mentions HBV solely in the Discussion section (Van Rensburg et al, 1985), one reports such a high level of chronic HBV infection that it is probably unrepresentative of the general population (Peers et al, 1987), and one reports no synergistic or additive effect of HBV and AFB_1 on liver cancer rates (Autrup et al, 1987). In China, Yaobin et al (1983) found that HCC was associated with both AFB_1 in foodstuffs and HBV infection; and Yeh et al (1985) reported that the HCC mortality rate was higher among HBV carriers in villages with heavy AFB_1 contamination.

Case-control studies of AFB_1 and HCC have yielded inconsistent results. In Hong Kong, the outcome of a dietary questionnaire revealed no differences between cases and controls (Lam et al, 1982), while a similarly designed study conducted in the Philippines reported a positive association between possible AFB_1 intake and HCC (Bulatao-Jayme et al, 1982). In a third case-control study in Japan, Indonesia, and the Philippines, the serum and urine levels of AFB_1 were actually lower in HCC cases than in several control groups (Tsuboi et al,

1985). Among three studies of occupational exposures to AFB_1, one reported an elevated HCC risk among grain-mill workers (McLaughlin et al, 1987) and a second, an increased risk among livestock feed processing workers (Olsen et al, 1988), but a third study found no increased risk among oilpress workers (Hayes et al, 1984).

Several studies have been carried out in geographic areas where the effects of AFB_1 and HBV can be distinguished. The Alaskan native population has a high rate of HBV infection and HCC, but lacks exposure to AFB_1 (Alward et al, 1985, 1986). Conversely, there have been reports of aflatoxin contamination in crops in Latin America (De Campos and Olszyma-Marzys, 1979), but no elevation of either HBV or HCC rates (Muir et al, 1987). Aflatoxin contamination is a concern in India, as evidenced by an outbreak of acute aflatoxicosis, but neither the HBV nor the HCC rate is high (Krishnamachari et al, 1975). In the United States, where HBV infection, AFB_1 exposure, and HCC are all uncommon, a weak correlation between AFB_1 and HCC has been reported, which was not of the magnitude anticipated by the correlation studies done in Africa and Asia (Stoloff, 1983).

The 1989 study of Yeh et al was a more rigorous examination of the HCC risk factors. A large cohort of men from five communities was prospectively followed for 3 years after ascertainment of HBV status. AFB_1 was determined in food staples of each community to estimate annual per capita intake. At the end of the study, all HCC cases were matched to men who had not developed HCC during the course of follow-up. The authors concluded that (1) the cases were significantly more likely to be HBsAg(+) than the noncases, and (2) there was a direct community association between HCC rate and AFB_1 in foodstuffs.

In support of these findings have been the preliminary results of one of the first prospective studies to examine AFB_1 biomarkers. In 1992, Ross et al first estimated the risk of developing HCC among 18,244 men in Shanghai who were examined for levels of urinary AFB_1 biomarkers at study inception. In both the initial report and in a subsequent follow-up (Qian et al, 1994), the investigators found a significantly increased risk of HCC with increased levels of urinary AFB_1 biomarkers. Significantly, the authors also found that the relative risk of HCC was synergistically elevated among men who were also hepatitis B virus carriers. Using the HBsAg(−)/AFB1(−) men as the referent group, the relative risks of HCC were 7.3 in the HBsAg(+)/AFB1(−) men, 3.4 in the HBsAg(−)/AFB1(+) men and 59.4 in the HBsAg(+)/AFB1(+) men. Importantly, the investigators found no correlation between urinary AFB_1 biomarkers and dietary AFB_1 intake determined by questionnaire. This finding may indicate the importance of AFB_1 metabolism in increasing risk.

If AFB_1 has a major role in the pathogenesis of HCC in humans, its mode of action is thought to be related to its effects on DNA. AFB_1 binds covalently to guanine (G) residues in DNA and has been shown to induce G to T (thymidine) transversions (Foster et al, 1983). In certain HCC high-risk areas, a high rate of G to T transversions has been reported in codon 249 of the p53 tumor suppressor gene, leading to speculation that AFB_1 causes the p53 mutations (Hsu et al, 1991; Bressac et al, 1991). In the initial reports, Hsu and colleagues reported 8 codon 249 mutations of the p53 gene among 16 tumors from Qidong, China, while Bressac et al found 4 G to T transversions among 10 tumors examined from South Africa. In general, the high rate of codon 249 mutations has been confirmed in tumors originating from the AFB_1 endemic areas of China and South Africa (Scorsone et al, 1992; Hsia et al, 1992; Li, 1993; Ozturk, 1991), while HCC tumors originating from other areas have a low rate of codon 249 mutations (Murakami et al, 1991; Hayward et al, 1991; Buetow et al, 1992; Kress, 1992; Oda et al, 1992; Patel et al, 1992; Shen et al, 1992; Hosono et al, 1993). Support for the AFB_1-p53 mutation link has recently been provided by the in vitro demonstration of codon 249 preferential mutability by rat liver microsome-activated AFB_1 in HepG2 cells (Aguilar et al, 1993).

In addition to evidence of a role of AFB_1 in HCC is evidence that all individuals, as determined by their inherent ability to metabolize AFB_1, may not be equally susceptible to its effects. A study reported by McGlynn et al (1994) examined the influence of constitutional genotype at two AFB_1 detoxification loci on both the presence of serum AFB_1-albumin adducts and on HCC. The authors found a significant association between the allelic distributions of epoxide hydrolase (EPHX) and glutathione-s-transferase M1 (GSTM1) and the presence of serum AFB_1-albumin adducts. The genotypes at the two loci that correlated with AFB_1 adducts also correlated with the presence of HCC in a case-control study.

Taken together, the epidemiologic evidence supports AFB_1 and differential ability to metabolize AFB_1 as risk factors in the causation of HCC. Several prospective studies currently underway that measure both AFB_1 biomarkers and genetic susceptibility should provide a definitive answer to the AFB_1-p53-HCC puzzle in the coming years.

THOROTRAST

Thorotrast (colloidal 232 thorium dioxide, ThO_2) was the trade name of an x-ray contrast medium which was used for cerebral angiography and liver-spleen scans in Japan and Europe from 1930 to 1955. After injection, ThO_2 accumulates in the reticuloendothelial system where it continues to emit radioactive alpha-particles at an annual dose rate of about 25 rad. The half-life of Th-232 is greater than 10^{10} years. Fifty-nine percent of an intravenous dose is sequestered in the liver (Kaul and Noffz, 1978). Thus thorotrast-exposed persons receive chronic, low-level, internal alpha-particle radiation throughout the liver. In comparison with gamma and x-rays, alpha radiation is weakly penetrating and mainly affects cells very close to the source of emission.

Exposure to Thorotrast is a major risk factor for the development of hemangiosarcoma and also increases the risk of cholangiocarcinoma and HCC. In 1980, the Committee on the Biological Effects of Ionizing Radiation of the National Academy of Sciences, using data compiled from many long-term cohort studies of thorotrast-exposed patients (Faber, 1979; Motta et al, 1979; Mori et al, 1983; Van Kaick et al, 1983), estimated that about 300 liver cancers would be caused per million persons exposed per rad of alpha radiation to the liver (National Academy of Sciences, 1980). The total number of patients exposed is estimated to be in the tens of thousands (Anthony, 1988). The latency period from exposure to tumor development is approximately 20–25 years. Follow-up data from the Japanese thorotrast cohort indicate that, compared to the general population, the exposed group has 47 times the risk of liver cancer, 20 times the risk of cirrhosis, 12 times the risk of leukemia, and 3 times the risk of death from all causes (Kato and Kido, 1987). The risk of liver cancer in the exposed cohort, by histological type, is 21 times greater for HCC, 303 times greater for cholangiocarcinoma, and 3129 times greater for hemangiosarcoma. Data from the German cohort show a linear dose-response of cumulative tumor incidence to exposure, a greater risk among male patients than among female patients, and a greater risk for younger persons (Van Kaick et al, 1986). In the Japanese cohort, an age at exposure effect has not been demonstrated (Kato and Kido, 1987). Both the Japanese and German cohorts failed to identify HBV as a cofactor (Van Kaick et al, 1986; Kato and Kido, 1987).

VINYL CHLORIDE

In the early 1970s, laboratory animal studies revealed that vinyl chloride monomer was carcinogenic to rats (Viola, 1970), mice, and hamsters (Maltoni, 1977). Shortly after the appearance of the first report of angiosarcoma of the liver (ASL) in occupationally exposed humans (Creech and Johnson, 1974), an ASL registry was established to document tumors in polyvinyl chloride (PVC) workers worldwide (Forman et al, 1985). As of 1985, the registry had documented a total of 120 cases. Based on these data, the incidence of ASL reaches a peak 20 to 30 years after first exposure to vinyl chloride monomer. The mean age at diagnosis is 52 years, and the occupational group, within the PVC industry, at greatest risk of ASL is autoclave cleaners.

Extremely high levels of exposure are probably necessary for tumor induction. First, the tumors have predominated in those occupations with the highest exposure levels, and second, the cases have clustered in specific factories. Third, ASL is a rare tumor even among exposed workers, though its background rate is so low that the risk ratio in PVC workers is on the order of 400:1 (Tamburro, 1984). Given the number of diagnosed tumors and number of exposed workers prior to the reduction in allowable levels, it can be estimated that approximately 200 to 250 new tumors have yet to be diagnosed in the next 30 years. Although ASL is the predominant tumor type in PVC workers, a few cases of cholangiosarcoma (Forman et al, 1985) and HCC (Evans et al, 1983) have been documented.

STEROID HORMONES

A relationship between oral contraceptive (OC) use and benign hepatic adenomas has been well established (Edmondson et al, 1976; Klatskin, 1977; Rooks et al, 1979; Christopherson et al, 1980; Mettlin and Natarajan, 1981; Mays and Christopherson, 1984). An OC-HCC association, however, is less clear. There have now been over 100 case reports, as well as several case-control studies, which suggest that there is a small risk of HCC in OC users compared with nonusers (Vana et al, 1977; Christopherson et al, 1978; Goodman and Ishak, 1982; Henderson et al, 1983; Neuberger et al, 1986; Forman et al, 1983, 1986; Petitti, 1986; Palmer et al, 1989; La Vecchia et al, 1989). Results of the case-control studies, all conducted in developed countries with low HBV rates, indicate that risk increases with long-term use ($\geq$ 8 years) and is on the order of 7 in non-HBV carriers (Neuberger et al, 1986). This contrasts with the risk of hepatic adenoma of 100 to 500 after 5 years of OC use (Edmondson et al, 1976; Rooks et al, 1979). Given the rarity of the tumor in low-incidence areas, Neuberger et al (1986) estimate that 12 cases of HCC per year may be attributable to long-term OC use in Britain and Wales. There is some indication that the increased risk may be confined to the subset of users who took OCs containing mestranol (Keifer and Scott, 1977). Because these pills were largely replaced by other types of OCs in the late 1970s (Iversen, 1986), the risk of HCC in OC users may have been eliminated. In countries where HBV is endemic, two reports (WHO Collaborative Study, 1989; Kew et al, 1990b) found no association between OC use and HCC.

No studies of exogenous hormone replacement therapy and HCC have yet been conducted.

Anabolic steroids are derivatives of testosterone that were developed to decrease the androgenic side effects of the parent compound. There are two accepted medical uses for anabolic steroids: treatment of certain types of anemia because of their stimulatory effect on erythropoiesis and replacement therapy for hypogonadal males (Goodman and Gilman, 1975). Nontherapeutic use of these steroids was first reported in World War II, when they were administered to German troops to foster aggressiveness (Wade, 1972). Use by athletes began in the mid-1950s among Russian competitors and has since become widespread (Wade, 1972).

Cases of hepatoma, peliosis hepatitis, HCC, and cholangiocarcinoma have been reported in conjunction with anabolic steroid, principally oxymetholone, use (IARC, 1977, 1987). In most instances, the steroids were prescribed for therapeutic reasons over a long duration, though cases of liver cancer have appeared in as little as 2 months (Mokrohisky et al, 1977). Reports of spontaneous remission have, at times, accompanied the cessation of treatment (Farrell et al, 1975; Johnson et al, 1972; Mulvihill et al, 1975). There has been at least one case of liver cancer (combined cholangiocarcinoma and HCC) reported in an athlete (Overly et al, 1984). As in the majority of cases, the tumor developed after prolonged use of an orally active anabolic steroid.

While these case reports imply an etiologic association of anabolic steroids with HCC, establishment of such an association will have to await carefully designed epidemiologic studies.

IRON

Levels of serum ferritin, the principal iron storage protein, are raised in many liver diseases, including some cases of HCC (Prieto et al, 1975). Likely explanations for these elevated levels are that the tumor secretes ferritin (Kew et al, 1978), or that iron overload in an individual predisposes to HCC (Cohen et al, 1984; Weinberg, 1984) or, alternatively, a combination of the two. Evidence supporting the iron overload hypothesis is that HCC has been observed in persons suffering from siderosis because of excessive ingested iron and/or inordinate absorption of the metal (Berman, 1958; Robertson et al, 1971; Weinberg, 1981). HCC has also been demonstrated in a noncirrhotic patient with excess hepatic iron as a result of hereditary spherocytosis (Barry et al, 1968). Furthermore, hemochromatosis, a genetic disease of iron overload, is associated with an increased incidence of primary liver cancer (Bomford and Williams, 1976). The increased incidence has become even more prominent in the last decade, as the survival of treated hemochromatotic patients has lengthened (Niederau et al, 1985). Prior to recent reports, it was felt that iron predisposed hemochromatotics to cirrhosis, which in turn predisposed them to HCC. More current reports (Fellows et al, 1988; Blumberg et al, 1988; Sheehan et al, 1989) demonstrate that HCC occurs in hemochromatotics even in the absence of cirrhosis. As demonstrated by Niederau and colleagues (1985), the hemochromatotic patients most likely to develop HCC are those with the highest mobilizable iron levels. Among hepatitis B virus carriers, Stevens et al (1986) and Hann et al (1989) have reported higher serum ferritin levels in persons destined to develop HCC than in other carriers.

While the assessment of iron as a risk factor for HCC has not been as extensively examined as other factors, it appears that higher body iron stores may predispose persons to the development of HCC. The role of iron may be particularly important in hepatitis B carriers, who have higher mean iron levels than the general population (Israel et al, 1989) and are likely to have ongoing liver damage.

Recent evidence suggests that increased iron may also be important in individuals infected with hepatitis C virus. In large part the evidence rests on therapeutic response studies demonstrating increased effectiveness of α-interferon when accompanied by iron depletion (Van Thiel et al, 1992; Piperno et al, 1993; Olynyk et al, 1993; Bacon et al, 1993; Guptas et al, 1994). Even iron depletion alone, without concomitant α-interferon, appears to benefit patients as measured by significantly reduced serum aminotransferase levels (Hayashi et al, 1994). Though the iron-viral infection association is not yet well understood, the data suggest that increased iron stores may have a role in the path from viral infection to malignancy.

SMOKING

Smoking has been studied widely as a risk factor for HCC in both high- and low-incidence areas. Representative studies are those from Hong Kong (Lam et al, 1982), the United States (Yu et al, 1983, 1988; Stemhagen et al, 1983; Austin et al, 1986; Hsing et al, 1990), Greece (Trichopoulos et al, 1980, 1987), Italy (Filippazzo et al, 1985; La Vecchia et al, 1988), Sweden (Hardell et al, 1984), Japan (Oshima et al, 1984; Shibata et al, 1986, 1990; Kono et al, 1987; Tanaka et al, 1988; Hirayama 1989), China (Tu et al, 1985), Taiwan (Lu et al, 1988; Chen et al, 1991), Nigeria (Olubuyide and

Bamgboye, 1990), and South Africa (Kew et al, 1985). Its role as a risk factor has often been evaluated while controlling for alcohol consumption, and somewhat less frequently, while controlling for HBV infection. The results of these studies are summarized in Table 36–4.

Of the 22 studies examined, 11 reported a positive association and 11, no association. Among the studies with positive results, three found a relative risk whose 95% confidence interval included 1.0; four found an association only among HBV(−) persons; one found an association only among elderly women who currently smoked; and one reported a decrease in the relative risk once adjustment for alcohol was made. Among the negative studies, five used hospitalized controls, and so, should be accepted somewhat cautiously (Doll and Hill, 1952). Only the studies of Trichopoulos et al (1980, 1987) and Hirayama (1989) reveal a strong association of cigarette smoking with HCC.

The accumulated body of evidence on an association between smoking and HCC remains equivocal. If there is a smoking effect, it is most likely limited to an undefined subpopulation, or is a minor effect which can only be discerned with large sample sizes and in the absence of major risk factors.

CONCEPTS OF PATHOGENESIS

Experiments involving chemical induction of liver tumors in animals indicate two types of events are required for hepatocarcinogenesis—initiation and promotion. Initiators affect, in some undefined way, the genetic makeup of a cell, whereas promoters affect cell division. Chemical hepatocarcinogens (initiators) are also hepatotoxins. Many liver cells are killed by exposure to these substances, whereas other hepatocytes are resistant and proliferate in response to the death of the susceptible cells. There is considerable evidence that the resistant, proliferating cells are also the initiated cells (Solt et al, 1977; Farber and Cameron, 1980). Such cells

TABLE 36–4. *Studies on PHC and Smoking*

Reference & Location	*Design*	*Number of Cases*	*Relative Risk*	*95% C.I.*	*Comment*
Lam et al, 1982 Hong Kong	Case control	107	3.3	(1.0–13.4)	Association confined to HBV(−) persons
Yu et al, 1983 United States	Case control	78	2.6	(1.0–6.7)	RR in heavy smokers/light drinkers = 1.8 (0.1–4.6)
Hardell et al, 1984 Sweden	Case control	102	No association		
Kew et al, 1985 South Africa	Case control	240	No association		
Trichopoulos et al, 1980 Greece	Case control	79	5.5	(2.0–15.6)	Association confined to HBV(−) persons
Trichopoulos et al, 1987 Greece	Case control	194	χ^2 for trend 17.4	$p < .05$	Association confined to HBV(−) persons
Filippazzo et al, 1985 Italy	Case control	120	0.8	(0.4–1.5)	
La Vecchia et al, 1988 Italy	Case control	151	0.9	(0.6–1.5)	
Lu et al, 1988 Taiwan	Case control	131	No association		
Austin et al, 1986 United States	Case control	86	1.0	(0.5–1.8)	
Yu et al, 1988 United States	Case control	165	3.3	$p < .05$	Association only in elderly women who currently smoked
Stemhagen et al, 1983 United States	Case control	265	0.7 M 1.0 F	(0.4–1.1) M (0.6–1.7) F	
Tu et al, 1985 China	Cohort	70	4.6	$p < .05$	Cohort all HBV(+) persons
Oshima et al, 1984 Japan	Cohort	20	5.8	(1.0–34.2)	
Shibata et al, 1986 Japan	Cohort	22	No association		
Kono et al, 1987 Japan	Cohort	51	No association		

express altered enzyme patterns, and some foci of these altered cells will progress to form frank cancers, but only if a second process, promotion, is introduced which increases cell division. Otherwise, the foci of initiated cells will regress. Partial hepatectomy, phenobarbital, and alcohol are examples of effective promoters.

Chronic HBV infection has both initiator and promoter properties. The host cell genome is altered by the process of integration of HBV DNA sequences. Not only is viral genetic information added, but host genes are frequently rearranged or deleted. The promoter effects are provided by the host response to HBV-infected hepatocytes, i.e., cell death and cell proliferation.

Because HBV has both initiator and promoter properties, its carcinogenic effects can be enhanced by exposure to agents which have either of these properties. Hence exposure of HBV carriers to aflatoxins, alcohol, nitrosamines, carbon tetrachloride, and other hepatotoxins may increase their risk of developing HCC.

HCV, on the other hand, is an RNA virus that does not replicate through a DNA intermediate (Choo et al, 1989). Therefore, if it has an effect on cellular DNA, it must be by some mechanism other than integration. Chronic infection with HCV does cause chronic hepatitis and cirrhosis, suggesting that the increased cell division and the accompanying increased risk of mutations associated with these diseases may be sufficient to induce HCC. To investigate whether the rate of cell division affects the risk of developing HCC, Tarao et al (1993) studied 28 patients with early cirrhosis (Child's stage A) who also had anti-HCV antibodies. The investigators measured the uptake of bromodeoxyuridine (BrdU, a thymidine analogue) in liver biopsy specimens from the patients at entry to the study. Fourteen patients had normal labeling indices ($\leq 1.1\%$ of the cells); the remaining 14 had elevated labeling indices ($\geq 1.6\%$). During a 3-year follow-up, nine of the 14 patients with high DNA synthesis developed HCC compared with two of the 14 patients with normal DNA synthesis. This study provides strong support for the cell proliferation hypothesis.

The major unsolved question in hepatocarcinogenesis is what is the specific change (or changes) in the hepatocyte genome that leads to cancer? Several models have been explored in recent years. Some evidence for each model has been reported, but no single model has received compelling support.

Direct transformation by the entire HBV genome or one of the four HBV genes has been tested in several experimental systems. Transfection of immortalized murine hepatocytes with either the complete HBV genome or hepatitis B X gene sequences resulted in malignant transformation, but transforming activity was much weaker in mouse fibroblasts (Seifer et al, 1991). Incorporation of either hepatitis B S or X DNA sequences in transgenic mice has resulted in the development of HCC (Chisari et al, 1987; Kim et al, 1991). The mechanisms by which this occurs in this experimental system may not be relevant, however, to what occurs in nature. Furthermore, in humans and woodchucks, integrated HBV DNA sequences are frequently extensively rearranged, rendering these viral genes nonfunctional (Ogston et al, 1982).

A second hypothesis proposes that integrated viral sequences activate a cellular proto-oncogene. Support for this model is also weak. Rearrangement with enhanced expression of the *c*-myc proto-oncogene has been demonstrated in liver cancers in woodchucks infected with woodchuck hepatitis virus (Moroy et al, 1986). *c*-myc is apparently not activated in humans, however (Lee et al, 1988). The hepatitis B X gene has transactivating properties (Seto et al, 1988; Colgrove et al, 1989) and has the potential of influencing the expression of many cellular genes. No specific target of such transactivation has been reported. HBV DNA integrates either at random sites in the cellular genome or possibly nonrandomly at many different sites. Transforming cellular DNA sequences have been isolated from some human tumors (Ochiya et al, 1986), but neither increased expression nor mutation of the same oncogene has been found in a majority of HCCs.

More recently, interest has turned to recessive oncogenesis. In this model, a class of genes is postulated which acts recessively at the cell level to induce neoplastic transformation (Knudson, 1973). A tumor arises when both alleles at a critical locus are inactivated or lost within a single cell. This model has been tested on human HCCs from several different ethnic groups and geographic sites. Studies, thus far, have reported complicated loss patterns, often involving multiple chromosomes (Wang and Rogler, 1988; Buetow et al, 1989; Zhang et al, 1990; Fujimori et al, 1991). Three chromosome arms, however, have demonstrated higher loss rates; 4q, 16q, and 17p. Other chromosome arms, such as 11p and 13q, have had less consistently elevated loss rates. The basis of these variable results is unknown.

One hypothesis that has received considerable attention is that a specific codon of the p53 gene is mutated in regions of high exposure to aflatoxins. Mutational inactivation of p53 is the most common identified genetic alteration in human cancer (Hollstein et al, 1991). Studies of p53 mutations in HCCs from various geographic locations showed low prevalences in most parts of the world; high rates in Qidong, China, Mozambique, and parts of South Africa; and intermediate rates in Japan and other parts of China (Hsu et al, 1991; Bressac et al, 1991; Ozturk et al, 1991). Overall, only a minority of HCC cases are associated with p53 mutations at codon 249 or elsewhere in the genome (Hosono et al, 1991; Buetow et al, 1992; Hollstein et al 1993). There is no association of HBsAg seropositivity with p53 mutations (Oda et al, 1992; Sheu et al, 1992; Hollstein et al, 1993). The association of point mutations at codon 249 with aflatoxin exposure has not, at this writing, been tested directly. That is, AFB_1-DNA or -albumin adduct levels have not been assessed in persons with p53 mutations at codon 249.

It may be that different tumor suppressor genes are important in different tumors depending on the state of differentiation of the transformed hepatocyte (London and Buetow, 1988). Alterations in the hepatocyte genome leading to loss of both functional alleles could occur as a direct result of the effects of HBV DNA integration and/or excision. Alternatively, chronic HBV or HCV infection could influence allele loss by generating a high cell turnover rate which would increase rare events such as point mutations and somatic recombinations. The same mechanisms could explain the effects of other hepatocarcinogens. Aflatoxins, chemical carcinogens, and perhaps iron could induce HCC either through direct effects on the hepatocyte genome or by increasing cell division, whereas alcohol and steroid hormones would probably operate solely by promoting cell division.

PREVENTIVE MEASURES

Primary and secondary prevention measures have been applied to liver cancer. At the primary level, the U.S. government acting through the Environmental Protection Agency, the Occupational Safety and Health Administration, the Department of Agriculture, and the Food and Drug Administration has tried to limit the exposure of the general population and workers in certain industries to hepatocarcinogens. Specifically, aflatoxin concentration in foodstuffs must be below 20 parts per billion (ppb) (Center for Food Safety and Applied Nutrition, 1985). In practice, aflatoxin concentrations in peanut butter sold in the United States have averaged less than 1 ppb (Bureau of Foods, 1978).

Since chronic HBV infection is the major cause of HCC, the most important primary prevention measure is the prevention of HBV infection. A safe, effective vaccine, derived from the plasma of human HBV carriers, was approved in the United States in 1982 and recombinant vaccines have since been licensed (Centers for Disease Control, 1987).

From the viewpoint of preventing HCC, the most important time to introduce hepatitis B immunization is in the perinatal period. Up to 90% of infections acquired in early infancy become chronic and ultimately carry the highest risk of HCC. Babies born to HBV carrier mothers should receive hepatitis B immune globulin at birth and vaccination subsequently. Universal hepatitis B vaccination of newborns in the United States has been recommended by the Immunization Practices Advisory Committee to the Centers for Disease Control and Prevention (ACIP, 1991). Hepatitis B vaccination is rapidly becoming one of the routine, universally applied immunizations of childhood in both endemic and nonendemic areas. National programs for the vaccination of newborns and infants have already been instituted in many countries in Asia and southern Europe and in some countries in Africa. A controlled study of the introduction of vaccination in Gambia should allow evaluation of the effectiveness of this primary preventive measure in 15 to 40 years (Gambia Hepatitis Study Group, 1987).

Secondary prevention of HCC depends on early detection and surgical resection of asymptomatic liver cancers. Alpha-fetoprotein (AFP) is a fetal antigen synthesized by 40% to 75% of HCCs, but not by the normal adult liver. Therefore, screening high-risk populations for elevated AFP levels has been used as an early detection device. Tang and his associates in Shanghai have reported a 73% 5-year survival among 60 resected, asymptomatic patients detected by AFP screening, compared with no 5-year survivals among 40 asymptomatic patients detected in the same way, who refused resection (Tang, 1985; Tang and Yang, 1985).

AFP screening of HBV carriers has been applied systematically to all HBV carriers older than 5 years of age among the Native American populations in Alaska (McMahon et al, 1991). Two-thirds of the tumors detected in this program have been asymptomatic, and two-thirds of these have been successfully resected. Both in China and in Alaska, either new primary tumors or recurrences of the original tumors have occurred, necessitating second and even third resections. Additional prospective intervention studies of other populations are needed to evaluate the risks and benefits of this approach (McMahon and London, 1991).

Medical therapies of chronic HBV carriers are also being tried. Alpha-interferon appears to be the most effective of the currently available agents (Thomas, 1988; Wong et al, 1993). Because it produces flulike symptoms and must be administered intramuscularly, it is not suitable for the treatment of large numbers of carriers. The major beneficial effect has been a decrease or loss of viral replication in 33% of treated patients, but most of the responding patients have not become HBsAg negative. HBsAg positive persons infected in early childhood or perinatally have shown the least benefit (Lok et al, 1988b; Lai et al, 1988). There is no information as to whether α-interferon treatment alters the risk of HCC, although when successful, it does appear to decrease inflammatory liver disease (Thomas, 1988; Wong et al, 1993). Alpha-interferon is also being used to treat chronic HCV infections. The results are similar to those with HBV infections (DiBisceglie, 1991).

FUTURE RESEARCH

The major unsolved problems in liver cancer research concern:

1. The pathogenesis of HCC at the molecular genetic level
2. The degree and nature of interactions between HBV, aflatoxins, alcohol, iron, and other possible cofactors
3. The factors which increase or decrease the risk of HCC in persons chronically infected with HBV or HCV

The molecular biology of HCC is being actively pursued in many laboratories around the world. It is likely that this research will yield within the next decade a much deeper understanding of the mechanism of induction of HCC.

The epidemiologic studies needed to examine interactions between HBV or HCV and cofactors require observations of individuals over time and laboratory measurements of their exposure to these agents. Until now, the bulk of research has focused on one factor at a time. In those instances where multiple factors were evaluated, HBV factors were usually assayed in the study subjects, but aflatoxin ingestion, iron nutrition, and alcohol consumption, were estimated in the general populations from which the subjects were drawn. There are several prospective studies of HCC that have been in progress for up to 10 years, and during this time new methods of measuring exposure have been developed (e.g., aflatoxin adducts with serum albumin or leukocyte DNA). It may be possible to go back to the initially collected serum samples and assay, for example, aflatoxin-albumin adducts. Such adducts are supposed to represent cumulative aflatoxin exposure over the 2 months preceding sample collection. Studies of this type could begin to estimate whether the various postulated factors act independently as carcinogens or only increase the carcinogenicity of chronic HBV or HCV infections.

There are more than 250 million chronic carriers of HBV in the world. According to Beasley's projections, 25% to 40% of these individuals will eventually die of cirrhosis or HCC (Beasley, 1982). A more optimistic view of the same observations is that at least half of all chronic carriers will never develop a life-threatening liver disease. The current dilemma is that the factors which increase or decrease the risk of liver disease and liver cancer in these individuals are not understood. Some factors are undoubtedly environmental, as described above. Others may be genetic. A goal of this research would be to develop methods of reducing the risk of serious liver disease in HBV carriers that could be applied to large populations. Given the progress in understanding the etiology, pathogenesis, and prevention of HCC over the past 20 years, it is likely that the remaining problems will be addressed and largely solved over the next 10 years.

REFERENCES

ACIP. 1991. Hepatitis B virus: A comprehensive strategy for eliminating transmission in the United States through universal childhood vaccination— Recommendations of the Immunization Practices Advisory Committee (ACIP). Morbidity and Mortality Weekly Report 40:RR 13:11–14.

Adamson R, Correa P, Sieber S, et al. 1976. Carcinogenicity of aflatoxin B_1 in rhesus monkeys: Two additional cases of primary liver cancer. J Natl Cancer Inst 57:67–78.

Advisory Committee to the Surgeon General of the Public Health Service. 1964. Criteria for judgment. *In* Smoking and Health. Washington DC, US Government Printing Office, pp. 19–21.

Aguilar F, Hussain SP, Cerutti P. 1993. Aflatoxin B_1 induces the transversion of G → T in codon 249 of the p53 tumor suppressor gene in human hepatocytes. Proc Natl Acad Sci USA 90:8586–8590.

Alberts SR, Lanier AP, McMahon BJ, et al. 1991. Clustering of hepatocellular carcinoma in Alaska Native families. Genet Epidemiol 8:127–139.

Alpert M, Hutt M, Wogan G, et al. 1971. The association between aflatoxin content of food and hepatoma frequency in Uganda. Cancer 28:253–260.

Alward W, McMahon B, Hall D, et al. 1985. The long-term serological course of asymptomatic hepatitis B virus carriers and the development of primary hepatocellular carcinoma. J Infect Dis 151:604–609.

Alward W, McMahon B, Hall D, et al. 1986. The hepatitis B carrier state and the development of primary hepatocellular carcinoma—Reply to a letter. J Infect Dis 153:171–172.

American Cancer Society. 1991. Cancer Facts and Figures—1991. Atlanta.

American Cancer Society. 1994. Cancer Facts and Figures—1994. Atlanta.

Anthony PP. 1979. Hepatic neoplasms. *In* MacSween RNM, Anthony PP, Scheuer PJ, (eds): Pathology of the Liver. Edinburgh, Churchill Livingstone, pp. 387–413.

Anthony P. 1988. Liver Tumors. Baillieres Clin Gastroenterol 2:501–522.

Armstrong B. 1980. The epidemiology of cancer in the People's Republic of China. Int J Epidemiol 9:305–315.

Asplin F, Carnaghan R. 1961. The toxicity of certain groundnut meals for poultry with special references to their effect on ducklings and chickens. Vet Rec 73:1215–1219.

Austin H, Delzell E, Grufferman S, et al. 1986. A case-control study of hepatocellular carcinoma and the hepatitis B virus, cigarette smoking and alcohol consumption. Cancer Res 46:962–966.

Autrup H, Seremet T, Wakhisi J, et al. 1987. Aflatoxin exposure measured by urinary excretion of aflatoxin B_1-guanine adduct and hepatitis B virus infection in areas with different liver cancer incidence in Kenya. Cancer Res 47:3430–3433.

Bacon RB, Rebholz AE, Fried M, et al. 1993. Beneficial effect of iron reduction therapy in patients with chronic hepatitis C who failed to respond to interferon alpha. Hepatology 18:150.

Barry M, Scheuer PJ, Sherlock S, et al. 1968. Hereditary spherocytosis with secondary haemochromatosis. Lancet 2:481–485.

Beasley RP. 1982. Hepatitis B virus as the etiologic agent in hepatocellular carcinoma. Epidemiologic considerations. Hepatology 2:21S–26S.

BEASLEY RP. 1988. Hepatitis B virus, the major etiology of hepatocellular carcinoma. Cancer 61:1942–1956.

BEASLEY RP, LIN CC, HWANG LY. 1981. Hepatocellular carcinoma and hepatitis B virus. A prospective study of 22,707 men in Taiwan. Lancet 2:1129–1133.

BEASLEY RP, HWANG L-Y. 1991. Overview on the epidemiology of hepatocellular carcinoma. *In* Hollinger FB, Lemon SM, Margolis HS (eds): Viral Hepatitis and Liver Disease. Baltimore, Williams & Wilkins, pp. 532–535.

BENNET R, ESSIGNMANN J, WOGAN GN. 1981. Excretion of an aflatoxin-guanine adduct in the urine of aflatoxin B_1-treated rats. Cancer Res 41:650–654.

BERMAN C. 1958. Primary carcinoma of the liver. Adv Cancer Res 5:55–96.

BLOUNT W. 1961. Turkey "X" disease. Turkeys (Journal of the British Turkey Federation) 9:55–58.

BLUMBERG RS, CHOPRA S, IBRAHIM R, et al. 1988. Primary hepatocellular carcinoma in idiopathic hemochromatosis after reversal of cirrhosis. Gastroenterology 95:1399–1402.

BOMFORD A, WILLIAMS R. 1976. Long term results of venesection therapy in idiopathic haemochromatosis. Q J Med 45:611–623.

BRADSHAW E, MCGLASHAND N, FITZGERALD D, et al. 1982. Analyses of cancer incidence in black gold miners from South Africa (1964–79). Br J Cancer 46:737–748.

BRECHOT C, DEGOS F, LUGASSY C, et al. 1985. Hepatitis B virus DNA in patients with chronic liver disease and negative tests for hepatitis B surface antigen. N Engl J Med 312:270–276.

BRESSAC B, KEW M, WANDS J, OZTURK M. 1991. Selective G to T mutations of p53 gene in hepatocellular carcinoma from southern Africa. Nature 350:429–431.

BRUIX J, BARRERA JM, CALVET X, et al. 1989. Prevalence of antibodies to hepatitis C virus in Spanish patients with hepatocellular carcinoma and hepatic cirrhosis. Lancet 2:1004–1006.

BUETOW KH, MURRAY JC, ISRAEL JL, et al. 1989. Loss of heterozygosity suggests tumor suppressor gene responsible for primary hepatocellular carcinoma. Proc Natl Acad Sci USA 86:8852–8856.

BUETOW KH, SHEFFIELD VC, ZHU M, et al. 1992. Low frequency of p53 mutations observed in a diverse collection of primary hepatocellular carcinomas. Proc Natl Acad Sci USA 89:9622–9626.

BULATAO-JAYME J, ALMERO E, CASTRO M, et al. 1982. A case-control dietary study of primary liver cancer risk from aflatoxin exposure. Int J Epidemiol 11:112–119.

BUREAU OF FOODS. 1978. Assessment of estimated risk resulting from aflatoxin in consumer peanut products and other commodities. Food and Drug Administration. Washington, DC, US Government Printing Office.

BUTLER H, HEMPSALL V. 1981. Histochemical studies of hepatocellular carcinomas in the rat induced by aflatoxin. J Pathol 134:157–170.

CARNAGHAN R. 1965. Hepatic tumors in ducks fed a low level of toxic ground-nut meal. Nature 208:308.

CENTER FOR FOOD SAFETY AND APPLIED NUTRITION. 1985. Action levels for poisonous or deleterious substances in human food and animal feed. Food and Drug Administration. Washington, DC, US Government Printing Office.

CENTERS FOR DISEASE CONTROL. 1987. Update on hepatitis B prevention. Morbidity and Mortality Weekly Report 36:353–360, 366.

CHEN C-J, LIANG K-Y, CHANG A-S, et al. 1991. Effects of hepatitis B virus, alcohol drinking, cigarette smoking and familial tendency on hepatocellular carcinoma. Hepatology 13:398–406.

CHINESE ACADEMY OF MEDICAL SCIENCES. 1981. Atlas of cancer mortality in the People's Republic of China. Beijing, China Map Press.

CHISARI FV, FILIPPI P, BURAS J, et al. 1987. Structural and pathological effects of synthesis of hepatitis B virus large envelope polypeptide in transgenic mice. Proc Natl Acad Sci USA 84:6909–6913.

CHOO QL, KUO G, WEINER J, et al. 1989. Isolation of a cDNA clone derived from a bloodborne non-A, non-B viral hepatitis genome. Science 244:359–362.

CHRISTOPHERSON W, MAYS E, BARROWS G. 1978. Hepatocellular carcinoma in young women on oral contraceptives. Lancet 2:38–40.

CHRISTOPHERSON W, MAYS E, BARROWS G. 1980. Liver tumours in young women. *In* Fenoglis CM, Wolff R (eds): Progress in Surgical Pathology, Vol. 2. New York, Masson Publishing UK, pp. 187–205.

COHEN C, BERSON S, SHULMAN G, et al. 1984. Immunohistochemical ferritin in hepatocellular carcinoma. Cancer 53:1931–1935.

COLGROVE R, SIMON G, GANEM D. 1989. Transcriptional activation of homologous and heterologous genes by the hepatitis B virus X gene product in cells permissive for viral replication. J Virol 63:4019–4026.

COLOMBO M, KUO G, CHOO QL, et al. 1989. Prevalence of antibodies to hepatitis C virus inItalian patients with hepatocellular carcinoma. Lancet 2:1006–1008.

CORDIER S, THUY LTB, VERGER P, et al. 1993. Risk factors for hepatocellular carcinoma in Vietnam. Int J Epidemiol 55:196–201.

COURSAGET P, LEBOULLEUX D, LE CANN P, et al. 1992. Hepatitis C virus infection in cirrhosis and primary hepatocellular carcinoma in Senegal. Trans R Soc Trop Med Hyg 86: 552–553.

CREECH J, JOHNSON M. 1974. Angiosarcoma of the liver in the manufacture of PVC. J Occup Med 16:150–151.

DAZZA MC, VALDEMAR MENESES L, GIRARD PM, et al. 1993. Absence of a relationship between antibodies to hepatitis C virus and hepatocellular carcinoma in Mozambique. J Trop Med Hyg 48:237–242.

DE CAMPOS M, OLSZYMA-MARZYS A. 1979. Aflatoxin contamination in grains and grain products during the dry season in Guatemala. Bull Environ Contam Toxicol 22:350–356.

DI BISCEGLIE A. 1991. Treatment of chronic non-A, non-B (type C) hepatitis. *In* Hollinger FB, Lemon SM, Margolis (eds): Viral Hepatitis and Liver Disease. Baltimore, Williams & Wilkins, pp. 623–626.

DOLL R, HILL A. 1952. A study of the etiology of carcinoma of the lung. Br Med J 2:1271–1286.

DUCREUX M, BUFFET C, DUSSAIX E, et al. 1990. Antibody to hepatitis C virus in hepatocellular carcinoma. Lancet 335:301.

EDMONDSON H, HENDERSON B, BENTON B. 1976. Liver cell adenomas associated with the use of the oral contraceptive. N Engl J Med 294:470–472.

EDMONDSON HA, STEINER PE. 1954. Primary carcinoma of the liver. A study of 100 cases among 48,000 autopsies. Cancer 7:462–503.

EDMONDSON HA. 1958. *In* Tumors of the Liver and Intrahepatic Bile Ducts. Washington, Armed Forces Institute of Pathology, pp. 32–33.

EVANS D, WILLIAMS W, KUNG I. 1983. Angiosarcoma and hepatocellular carcinoma in vinyl chloride workers. Histopathology 7:377–388.

FABER M. 1979. Twenty-eight years of continuous follow-up of patients injected with thorotrast for cerebral angiography. Environ Res 18:37–43.

FALKSON G, CNAAN A, SCHUTT AJ, et al. 1988. Prognostic factors for survival in hepatocellular carcinoma. Cancer Res 48:7314–7318.

FARBER E, CAMERON R. 1980. The sequential analysis of cancer development. Adv CancerRes 31:125–226.

FARRELL G, JOSHUA D, UREN R, et al. 1975. Androgen-induced hepatoma. Lancet 1:430–431.

FELLOWS IW, STEWART M, JEFFCOATE WJ, et al. 1988. Hepatocellular carcinoma in primary haemochromatosis in the absence of cirrhosis. Gut 29:1603–1606.

FERENCI P, DRAGOSICS B, MAROSI L, et al. 1984. Relative incidence of primary liver cancer in cirrhosis in Austria. Etiologic considerations. Liver 4:7–14.

FERET E, LAROUZE B, DIOP B, et al. 1987. Epidemiology of hepatitis B virus infection in the rural community of Tip, Senegal. Am J Epidemiol 125:140–149.

FILIPPAZZO M, ARAGONA E, COTTONE M, et al. 1985. Assessment of some risk factors for hepatocellular carcinoma: A case-control study. Stat Med 4:345–351.

FORMAN D, BENNETT B, STAFFORD J, et al. 1985. Exposure to vinyl chloride and angiosarcoma of the liver: A report of the register of cases. Br J Ind Med 42:750–753.

FORMAN D, DOLL R, PETO R. 1983. Trends in mortality from carcinoma of the liver and use of oral contraceptives. Br J Cancer 48:349–352.

FORMAN D, VINCENT TJ, DOLL R. 1986. Cancer of the liver and use of oral contraceptives. Br Med J Clinical Research Ed 292:1357–1361.

FOSTER PL, EISENSTADT E, MILLER JH. 1983. Base substitution mutations induced by metabolically activated aflatoxin B_1. Proc Natl Acad Sci USA 80:2695–2698.

FUJIMORI M, TOKINO T, HINO O, et al. 1991. Allelotype study of primary hepatocellular carcinoma. Cancer Res 51:89–93.

GAMBIA HEPATITIS STUDY GROUP. 1987. The Gambia hepatitis intervention study. Cancer Res 47:5782–5787.

GAN L-S, SKIPPER PL, PENG X, et al. 1988. Serum albumin adducts in the molecular epidemiology of aflatoxin carcinogenesis: Correlation with aflatoxin B_1 intake and urinary excretion of aflatoxin M_1. Carcinogenesis 9:1323–1325.

GARNER C, RYDER R, MONTESANO R. 1985. Monitoring of aflatoxins in human body fluids and application to field studies. Cancer Res 45:922–928.

GOODMAN L, GILMAN A. 1975. The Pharmacological Basis of Therapeutics. 5th ed New York, Macmillan Publishing, pp. 1451–1471.

GOODMAN ZD. 1987. Benign tumors of the liver. *In* Okuda K, Ishaka KG (eds): Neoplastic Diseases of the Liver. Berlin, Springer-Verlag, pp. 105–126.

GOODMAN Z, ISHAK G. 1982. Hepatocellular carcinoma in women—Probable lack of etiologic association with oral contraceptive steroids. Hepatology 2:440–444.

GROOPMAN J, BUSBY W, DONAHUE P, et al. 1986. Aflatoxins as risk factors for human cancer: An application of monoclonal antibodies to monitor human exposure. *In* Harris C (ed): Biochemical and Molecular Epidemiology of Cancer. New York, Alan R. Liss, pp. 233–256.

GUPTAS RC, MULHOTRA S, LEHANDEKAR P, et al. January 26–29, 1994. Influence of low iron diet on the efficacy of interferon therapy in patients with chronic liver disease. Proc. IX Bicentennial Meeting of the Asian Pacific Association for the study of the liver. Kuala Lumpur, Malaysia.

HALVER J. 1965. Hepatomas in fish. *In* Burdette, W (ed): Primary Hepatoma. Utah, Utah Press, pp. 103–112.

HANN HL, KIM CY, LONDON WT, et al. 1982. Hepatitis B virus and primary hepatocellular carcinoma: Family studies in Korea. Int J Cancer 30:47–51.

HANN HL, KIM C, LONDON WT, BLUMBERG B. 1989. Increased serum ferritin in chronic liver disease: A risk factor for primary hepatocellular carcinoma. Int J Cancer 43:376–379.

HARDELL L, BENGTSSON N, JONSSON U, et al. 1984. Aetiological aspects on primary liver cancer with special regard to alcohol, organic solvents and acute intermittent porphyria—An epidemiological investigation. Br J Cancer 50:389–397.

HARINGTON J, MCGLASHAN N, BRADSHAW E, et al. 1975. A spatial and temporal analysis of four cancers in African gold miners from Southern Africa. Br J Cancer 31:665–678.

HARUNA Y, HAYASHI N, KAMADA T, et al. 1994. Expression of hepatitis C virus in hepatocellular carcinoma. Cancer 73:2253–2258.

HAYASHI H, TAKIKAWA T, NISHIMURA N, et al. 1994. Improvement of serum aminotransferase levels following phlebotomy in patients with chronic active hepatitis C and excess hepatic iron. Am J Gastroenterol 89:986–988.

HAYES R, VAN NIEUWENHUIZE J, RAATGEVER J, et al. 1984. Aflatoxin exposures in the industrial setting: An epidemiological study of mortality. Food Chem Toxicol 22:39–43.

HAYWARD NK, WALKER GJ, GRAHAM W, et al. 1991. Hepatocellular carcinoma mutation. Nature 352:764.

HENDERSON B, PRESTON-MARTIN S, EDMONDSON H, et al. 1983. Hepatocellular carcinoma associated with use of oral contraceptives. Br J Cancer 48:437–440.

HEYWARD WL, LANIER AP, MCMAHON BJ, et al. 1985. Early detection of primary hepatocellular carcinoma. Screening for primary hepatocellular carcinoma among persons infected with hepatitis B virus. JAMA 254:3052–3054.

HIGGINSON J, GROBBELAAR BG, WALKER ARP. 1957. Hepatic fibrosis and cirrhosis in man in relation to malnutrition. Am J Pathol 33:29–54.

HIRAYAMA T. 1989. A large-scale cohort study on risk factors for primary liver cancer, with special reference to the role of cigarette smoking. Cancer Chemother Pharmacol 23S:114–117.

HIYAMA T, TSUKUMA H, OSHIMA A, et al. 1990. Liver cancer and life style—drinking habits and smoking habits. Jpn J Cancer Clin (Spec):249–256.

HOLLSTEIN MC, SIRANSKY D, VOGELSTEIN B, HARRIS C. 1991. p53 mutations in human cancers. Science 253:51–55.

HOLLSTEIN MC, WILD CP, BLEICHER F, et al. 1993. p53 mutations and aflatoxin B1 exposure in hepatocellular carcinoma patients from Thailand. Int J Cancer 53:51–55.

HOOFNAGLE J, SHAFRITZ D, POPPER H. 1987. Chronic type B hepatitis and the 'healthy' hepatitis B surface antigen carrier state. Hepatology 7:758–763.

HOSONO S, CHOU M-J, LEE C-S, et al. 1993. Infrequent mutation of p53 gene in hepatitis B virus positive primary hepatocellular carcinomas. Oncogene 8:491–496.

HOSONO S, LEE C-S, CHOU M-J, et al. 1991. Molecular analysis of the p53 alleles in primary hepatocellular carcinomas and cell lines. Oncogene 6:237–243.

HSIA CC, KLEINER DE, AXIOTIS CA, et al. 1992. Mutations of p53 gene in hepatocellular carcinoma: Roles of hepatatitis B virus and aflatoxin contamination in the diet. J Natl Cancer Inst 21:1638–1641.

HSING AW, MCLAUGHLIN JK, HRUBEC Z, et al. 1990. Cigarette smoking and liver cancer among US veterans. Cancer Causes & Control 1:217–221.

HSU IC, METCALF RA, SUN T, et al. 1991. Mutational hotspot in the p53 gene in human hepatocellular carcinomas. Nature 350:427–428.

IARC MONOGRAPHS. 1976. Vol. 10, 51–72.

IARC MONOGRAPHS. 1977. Vol. 13, 131–139.

IARC MONOGRAPHS. 1987a. Suppl. 7, 83–87.

IARC MONOGRAPHS. 1987b. Suppl. 7, 96–98.

IARC MONOGRAPHS. 1994. Vol. 59, 45–221.

IARC SCIENTIFIC PUBLICATION NO. 120. 1992. Cancer Incidence in Five Continents, Vol. VI.

IJIMA T, SAITOH N, NOBOTUMO K, et al. 1984. A prospective cohort study of hepatitis B surface antigen carriers in a working population. Gann 75:571–573.

ISHAK KG. 1987. Malignant mesenchymal tumors of the liver. *In* Okuda K, Ishak KG (eds): Neoplastic Diseases of the Liver. Berlin, Springer-Verlag, pp. 159–176.

ISRAEL J, MCGLYNN K, HANN H, et al. 1989. Iron related markers in liver cancer. *In* de Sousa M, Brock JH (eds): Iron in Immunity, Cancer and Inflammation. New York, John Wiley & Sons Ltd, pp. 301–316.

IVERSEN O. 1986. Oral contraceptives and hepatocellular carcinoma. (Letter). Br Med J 292:1668.

JOHNSON F, FEAGLER J, LERNER K, et al. 1972. Association of androgenic-anabolic steroid therapy with development of hepatocellular carcinoma. Lancet 2:1273–1276.

KAKLAMANI E, TRICHOPOULOS D, TZONOU A, et al. 1991. Hepatitis B and C viruses and their interaction in the origin of hepatocellular carcinoma. JAMA 265:1974–1976.

KATO I, KIDO C. 1987. Increased risk of death in thorotrast-exposed patients during the late follow-up period. Jpn J Cancer Res 78:1187–1192.

KAUL A, NOFFZ W. 1978. Tissue dose in thorotrast patients. Health Physics 35:113–121.

KEEN P, MARTIN P. 1971. Is aflatoxin carcinogenic in man? The evidence in Swaziland. Trop Geogr Med 23:44–53.

KEIFER W, SCOTT J. 1977. Liver neoplasms and the oral contraceptives. Am J Obstet Gynecol 128:448–454.

KEW M. 1981. Clinical, pathological and etiological heterogeneity in HCC: Evidence from southern Africa. Hepatology 1:366–369.

KEW M, DI BISCEGLIE A, PATERSON A. 1985. Smoking as a risk factor in hepatocellular carcinoma. A case-control study in southern African blacks. Cancer 56:2315–2317.

KEW M, GEDDES E. 1982. Hepatocellular carcinoma in rural southern African blacks. Medicine 61:98–108.

KEW M, PATERSON A. 1985. Unusual clinical presentations of hepatocellular carcinoma. Trop Gastroenterol 6:10–22.

KEW M, ROSSOUW E, HODKINSON J, et al. 1983. Hepatitis B virus status of southern African blacks with hepatocellular carcinoma: Comparison between rural and urban patients. Hepatology 3:65–68.

KEW MC, HOUGHTON M, CHOO QL et al. 1990a. Hepatitis C virus antibodies in southern African blacks with hepatocellular carcinoma. Lancet 335:873–874.

KEW M, SONG E, MOHAMMED A, et al. 1990b. Contraceptive steroids as a risk factor for hepatocellular carcinoma: A case/control study in south African black women. Hepatology 11:298–302.

KEW M, TORRANCE J, DERMNA D, et al. 1978. Serum and tumour ferritins in primary liver cancer. Gut 19:294–299.

KIM CM, KOIKE K, SAITO I, et al. 1991. HBx gene of hepatitis B virus induces liver cancer in transgenic mice. Nature 351:317–320.

KIYOSAWA K, SODEYAMA T, TANAKA E, et al. 1990. Interrelationship of blood transfusion, non-A, non-B hepatitis and hepatocellular carcinoma: Analysis by detection of antibody to hepatitis C virus. Hepatology 12:671–675.

KLATSKIN G. 1977. Hepatic tumors—possible relationship to use of oral contraceptives. Gastroenterology 73:386–394.

KNUDSON AG. 1973. Mutation and human cancer. Adv Cancer Res 17:317–352.

KOBAYASHI S, HAYASHI H, ITOH Y, et al. 1994. Detection of minus-strand hepatitis C virus RNA in tumor tissues of hepatocellular carcinoma. Cancer 73:48–52.

KOJIRO M, NAKASHIMA T. 1987. Pathology of hepatocellular carcinoma. *In* Okuda K, Ishak KG (eds): Neoplastic Diseases of the Liver. Berlin, Springer-Verlag, pp. 81–104.

KONO S, IKEDA M, TOKUDOME S, et al. 1987. Cigarette smoking, alcohol and cancer mortality: A cohort study of male Japanese physicians. Jpn J Cancer Res 78:1323–1328.

KRESS S, JAHN U-R, BUCHMANN A, et al. 1992. p53 mutations in human hepatocellular carcinomas from Germany. Cancer Res 52:3220–3223.

KRISHNAMACHARI K, BHAT R, NAGARAJAN V, et al. 1975. Hepatitis due to aflatoxicosis inWestern India. Lancet 1:1061–1063.

LAI CL, LOK ASF, HSIANG-JU L, et al. 1988. Effect of recombinant alpha-2-interferon in Chinese hepatitis B surface antigen carrier children: A prospective controlled trial. *In* Zuckerman AJ (ed): Viral Hepatitis and Liver Disease. New York, Alan R. Liss, p. 850.

LAM K, YU M, LEUNG J, et al. 1982. Hepatitis B virus and cigarette smoking: Risk factors for hepatocellular carcinoma in Hong Kong. Cancer Res 42:5246–5248.

LANIER A, MCMAHON B, ALBERTS S, et al. 1987. Primary liver cancer in Alaskan natives, 1980–1985. Cancer 60:1915–1920.

LAROUZE B, LONDON WT, SAIMOT G, et al. 1976. Host responses to hepatitis B infection in patients with primary hepatic carcinoma and their families. A case/control study in Senegal, West Africa. Lancet 2:534–538.

LA VECCHIA C, NEGRI E, DECARLI A, et al. 1988. Risk factors for hepatocellular carcinoma in northern Italy. Int J Cancer 42:872–876.

LA VECCHIA C, NEGRI E, PARAZZINE F. 1989. Oral contraceptives and primary liver cancer. Br J Cancer 59:460–461.

LEE F. 1966. Cirrhosis and hepatoma in alcoholics. Gut 7:77–85.

LEE H, DAY N, SHANMUGARATNAM K. 1988. Trends in Cancer Incidence in Singapore 1968–1982 (IARC Scientific Publications No. 91), Lyon, International Agency for Research on Cancer.

LI D, CAO Y, HE L, et al. 1993. Aberrations of p53 gene in human hepatocellular carcinoma from China. Carcinogenesis 14:169–173.

LIEBER C, GARRO A, LEO M, et al. 1986. Alcohol and cancer. Hepatology 6:1005–1019.

LIN J, LIU C, SVOBODA D. 1974. Long term effects of aflatoxin B_1 and viral hepatitis on marmoset liver: A preliminary report. Lab Invest 30:267–278.

LIN T, TSU W, CHEN C. 1986. Mortality of hepatoma and cirrhosis of liver in Taiwan. Br J Cancer 54:969–976.

LIVER CANCER STUDY GROUP OF JAPAN. 1984. Primary liver cancer in Japan. Cancer 54:1747–1755.

LOK A, LAI C-C. 1988a. Factors determining the development of hepatocellular carcinoma in hepatitis B surface antigen carriers: A comparison between families with clusters and solitary cases. Cancer 61:1287–1291.

LOK ASF, LAI CL, WU PC, et al. 1988b. A randomized controlled trial of recombinant α-2 interferon in Chinese patients with chronic hepatitis B virus infection: An interim report. *In* Zuckerman AJ (ed): Viral Hepatitis and Liver Disease. New York, Alan R. Liss, pp. 848–849.

LONDON WT. 1981. Primary hepatocellular carcinoma—Etiology, pathogenesis and prevention. Hum Pathol 12:1085–1097.

LONDON WT, BUETOW K. 1988. Hepatitis B virus and primary hepatocellular carcinoma. Cancer Invest 6:317–326.

LU S, LIN T, CHEN C, et al. 1988. A case-control study of primary hepatocellular carcinoma in Taiwan. Cancer 62:2051–2055.

LYNCH H, SRIVATANSKUL P, PHORNTHUTKUL K, et al. 1984. Familial hepatocellular carcinoma in an endemic area of Thailand. Cancer Genet Cytogenet 11:11–18.

MALTONI C. 1977. Occupational carcinogenesis. *In* Advances in tumour prevention, detection, and characterization. Second International Symposium on Cancer Detection and Prevention, Bologna, 1974. Amsterdam, Excerpta Medica, Vol. 2.

MARINIER E, BARROIS V, LAROUZE B, et al. 1985. Lack of perinatal transmission of hepatitis B virus infection in Senegal, West Africa. J Pediatr 106:843–849.

MARION PL, VAN DAVELAAR MJ, KNIGHTS SS, et al. 1986. Hepatocellular carcinoma in ground squirrels persistently infected with ground squirrel hepatitis virus. Proc Natl Acad Sci USA 83:4543–4546.

MAYS E, CHRISTOPHERSON W. 1984. Hepatic tumors induced by sex steroids. Semin Liver Dis 4:147–157.

MCCOY G, HECHT S, KATAYAMA S, et al. 1981. Differential effect of chronic ethanol consumption on the carcinogenicity of *N*-nitrosopyrrolidine and *N'*-nitrosonornicotine in male Syrian golden hamsters. Cancer Res 41:2849–2854.

MCGLYNN KA, HU Y, SHEN FM, et al. 1994. Genetic susceptibility to primary liver cancer. Abstract Proc Am Assoc Cancer Res 35:293.

MCLAUGHLIN J, MALKER H, MALKER B, et al. 1987. Registry-based analysis of occupational risks for primary liver cancer in Sweden. Cancer Res 47:287–291.

MCMAHON BJ, LONDON T. 1991. Workshop on screening for hepatocellular carcinoma. J Natl Cancer Inst 83:916–919.

MCMAHON BJ, WAINWRIGHT RW, LANIER, AP. 1991. The Alaska Native HCC Screening Program: A population-based screening program for hepatocellular carcinoma. *In* Tabor E, Di Bisceglie AM, Purcell RH (eds). Etiology, Pathology and Treatment of Hepatocellular Carcinoma in North America. Advances in Applied Biotechnology Series, Vol. 13, Houston, Gulf Publishing Co, pp. 231–242.

MELBYE M, SKINHOJ P, NIELSEN NH, et al. 1984. Virus-associated cancers in Greenland: Frequent hepatitis B virus infection but low primary hepatocellular carcinoma incidence. J Natl Cancer Inst 73:1267–1272.

METTLIN L, NATARAJAN N. 1981. Studies on the role of oral contraceptive use in the etiology of benign and malignant liver tumors. J Surg Oncol 18:73–85.

MIRKIN IR, REMINGTON PL, MOSS M, et al. 1990. Liver cancer in Wisconsin: The potential for prevention. Wisc Med J 89:49–53.

MIYAMURA T, SAITO I, YONEYAMA T, et al. 1991. Role of hepatitis C virus in hepatocellular carcinoma. *In* FB Hollinger, SM Lemon, HS Margolis (eds): Viral Hepatitis and Liver Disease. Baltimore, Williams & Wilkins, pp. 559–562.

MOKROHISKY S, AMBRUSO D, HATHAWAY W. 1977. Fulminant hepatic neoplasia after androgen therapy. N Engl J Med 296:1411–1412.

MORI T, KATO Y, KUMATORI T, et al. 1983. Epidemiological follow-up study of Japanese thorotrast cases—1980. Health Physics 44:261–272.

MOROY T, MARCHIO A, ETIEMBLE J, et al. 1986. Rearrangement and enhanced expression of c-myc in hepatocellular carcinoma of hepatitis infected woodchucks. Nature 324:276–279.

MOTTA L, HORTA J, TAVARES M. 1979. Prospective epidemiological study of thorotrast-exposed patients in Portugal. Environ Res 18:152–172.

MUCHMORE E, POPPER H, PETERSON DA, et al. 1988. Non-A, non-B hepatitis-related hepatocellular carcinoma in a chimpanzee. J Med Primatol 17:235–246.

MUIR C, WATERHOUSE J, MACK T, et al. (eds). 1987. Cancer Incidence in Five Continents, Vol. V. IARC Scientific Publications No. 88, Lyon, International Agency for Research on Cancer.

MULVIHILL J, RIDOLFI R, SCHULTZ F, et al. 1975. Hepatoma adenoma in Fanconi anemia treated with oxymetholone. J Pediatr 87:122–124.

MUÑOZ N, BOSCH X. 1987. Epidemiology of hepatocellular carcinoma. *In* Okuda K, Ishak K (eds): Neoplasms of the Liver. Tokyo, Springer-Verlag, pp. 3–19.

MURAKAMI Y, HAYASHI K, HIROHASHI S, et al. 1991. Aberrations of the tumor suppressor p53 and retinoblastoma genes in human hepatocellular carcinomas. Cancer Res 51:5520–5525.

NATIONAL ACADEMY OF SCIENCES, COMMITTEE ON THE BIOLOGICAL EFFECTS OF IONIZING RADIATION. 1980. The effects on populations of exposure to low levels of ionizing radiation. Washington, DC, National Academy of Sciences.

NAYAK NC, DHAR A, SACHDEVA R. 1977. Association of human hepatocellular carcinoma and cirrhosis with hepatitis B virus surface and core antigens in the liver. Int J Cancer 20:643–654.

NEUBERGER J, FORMAN D, DOLL R, et al. 1986. Oral contraceptives and hepatocellular carcinoma. Br Med J 292:1355–1357.

NIEDERAU C, FISCHER R, SONNENBERG A, et al. 1985. Survival and causes of death in cirrhotic and in noncirrhotic patients with primary hemochromatosis. N Engl J Med 313:1256–1262.

NONOMURA A, HAYASHI M, TAKAYANAGI N, et al. 1986a. Correlation of morphologic subtypes of liver cirrhosis with excess alcohol intake, HBV infections, age at death, and hepatocellular carcinoma. A study of 234 autopsy cases in Japan. Acta Pathol Jpn 36:631–640.

NONOMURA A, HAYASHI M, WATANABE K, et al. 1986b. Studies on the pathogenesis of hepatocellular carcinoma in HBV-negative alcoholic cirrhotics. Acta Pathol Jpn 36:1297–1305.

OBATA H, HAYASHI N, HISAMITSU T, et al. 1980. A prospective study on the development of hepatocellular carcinoma from liver cirrhosis with persistent hepatitis B virus infection. Int J Cancer 25:741–747.

OBE G, HERHA J. 1975. Chromosomal damage in chronic alcohol users. Humangenetik 29:191–200.

OCHIYA T, FUJIYAMA A, FUKUSHIGE S, et al. 1986. Molecular cloning of an oncogene from a human hepatocellular carcinoma. Proc Natl Acad Sci USA 83:4993–4997.

ODA T, TSUDA H, SCARPA A. et al. 1992. p53 gene mutation spectrum in hepatocellular carcinoma. Cancer Res 52:6358–6364.

OGSTON CW, JONAK CJ, ROGLER CE, et al. 1982. Cloning and structural analysis of integrated woodchuck hepatitis virus sequences from hepatocellular carcinomas of woodchucks. Cell 29:385–394.

OHBAYASHI A. 1982. Considerations on familial clustering of liver cirrhosis and hepatocellular carcinoma. Gan To Kagaku Ryoho 1982:799–807.

OKADA K, KAMIYAMA I, INOMATA M, et al. 1976. e Antigen and anti-e in the serum of asymptomatic carrier mothers as indicators of positive and negative transmission of hepatitis B virus to their infants. N Engl J Med 294:746–749.

OKUDA K, FUJIMOTO I, HANAI A, et al. 1987. Changing incidence of hepatocellular carcinoma in Japan. Cancer Res 47:4967–4972.

OKUDA K, OHTSUKI T, OBATA H, et al. 1985. Natural history of hepatocellular carcinoma and prognosis in relation to treatment. Study of 850 patients. Cancer 56:918–928.

OLSEN J, DRAGSTED L, AUTRUP H. 1988. Cancer risk and occupational exposure to aflatoxins in Denmark. Br J Cancer 58:392–396.

OLUBUYIDE IO, BAMGBOYE EA. 1990. A case-controlled study of the current role of cigarette smoking and alcohol consumption in primary liver cell carcinoma in Nigerians. Afr J Med and Med Sci 19:191–194.

OLYNYK J, REDDY R, DIBISCEGLIE AM, et al. 1993. Hepatic iron concentration as a predictor of response to alpha-interferon therapy in chronic hepatitis C. Hepatology 18:90(A).

OMATA M, ZHOU YZ, UCHIUMI K, et al. 1987. Hepatitis B virus DNA, antigens and liver pathology in ducks: An animal model of human liver disease. *In* Robinson W, Koike K, Will H (eds): Hepadna Viruses, UCLA Symposia on Molecular and Cellular Biology. New York, Alan R. Liss, pp. 349–356.

ONISHI K, HIDETAKA T, UNUMA T, et al. 1987. Effects of habitual alcohol intake and cigarette smoking on the development of hepatocellular carcinoma. Alcoholism, Clin Exp Res 11:45–48.

ONISHI K, IIDA S, IWAMA S, et al. 1982. The effect of chronic habitual alcohol intake on the development of liver cirrhosis and hepatocellular carcinoma: Relation to hepatitis B surface antigen carriage. Cancer 49:672–677.

OSHIMA A, TSUKUMA H, HIYAMA T, et al. 1984. Follow-up study of HBsAg-positive blood donors with special reference to the effect of drinking and smoking on the development of liver cancer. Int J Cancer 34:775–779.

OVERLY W, DANKOFF J, WANG B, et al. 1984. Androgens and hepatocellular carcinoma in an athlete. (Letter). Ann Intern Med 100:158–159.

OZTURK M, et al. 1991. p53 mutation in hepatocellular carcinoma after aflatoxin exposure. Lancet 338:1356–1359.

PALMER JR, ROSENBERG L, KAUFMAN DW, et al. 1989. Oral contraceptive use and liver cancer. Am J Epidemiol 130:878–882.

PARKIN D, PISANI P, FERLAY, J. 1993. Estimates of the worldwide incidence of 18 major cancers in 1985. Int J Cancer 54:594–606.

PATEL P, STEPHENSON J, SCHEURR PJ, et al. 1992. p53 codon 249ser mutations in hepatocellular carcinoma patients with low aflatoxin exposure. Lancet 330:881.

PATERSON A, KEW M, HERMAN A, et al. 1985. Liver morphology in southern African blacks with hepatocellular carcinoma: A study within the urban environment. Hepatology 5:72–78.

PEARCE N, NEWELL K, CARTER H. 1985. Incidence of hepatocellular carcinoma in New Zealand, 1974–78: Ethnic, sex and geographical differences. NZ Med J 98:1033–1036.

PEERS F, BOSCH X, KALDOR J, et al. 1987. Aflatoxin exposure, hepatitis B infection and liver cancer in Swaziland. Int J Cancer 39:545–553.

PEERS F, GILMAN G, LINSELL C. 1976. Dietary aflatoxins and human liver cancer. A study in Swaziland. Int J Cancer 17:167–176.

PEERS F, LINSELL C. 1973. Dietary aflatoxins and liver cancer—A population based study in Kenya. Br J Cancer 27:473–484.

PETITTI D. 1986. Oral contraceptives and liver cancer. (Letter). Br Med J 293:204.

PIPERNO A, D'ALBA R, ROFFI L, et al. 1993. Relation between alpha-interferon therapy response and liver iron stores in chronic hepatitis C. Hepatology 18:250(A).

POPPER H, ROTH L, PURCELL RH, et al. 1987. Hepatocarcinogenicity of the woodchuck hepatitis virus. Proc Natl Acad Sci USA 84:866–870.

PRIETO J, BARRY M, SHERLOCK S. 1975. Serum ferritin in patients with iron overload and with acute and chronic liver diseases. Gastroenterology 68:525–533.

PURCHASE I, GONCALVES T. 1971. Primary results from food analyses in the Inhambane area. *In* Purchase I (ed): Proceedings: Symposium on Viral Hepatitis. London, Macmillan Press, pp. 263–269.

PURTILO D, GOTTLIEB L. 1973. Cirrhosis and hepatoma occurring at Boston City Hospital, 1917 to 1968. Cancer 32:458–462.

QIAN G-S, ROSS RK, YU MC, et al. 1994. A follow-up study of urinary markers of aflatoxin exposure and liver cancer risk in Shanghai, People's Republic of China. Cancer Epidemiol Biomark Prev 3:3–10.

REDDY J, SVOBODA D, RAO M. 1976. Induction of liver tumors by aflatoxin B_1 in the tree shrew (*Tupaia glis*), a nonhuman primate. Cancer Res 36:151–160.

ROBERTSON M, HARINGTON J, BRADSHAW E. 1971. The cancer pattern in Africans at Baragwanath Hospital, Johannesburg. Br J Cancer 25:377–384.

ROOKS J, ORY A, ISHAK K, et al. 1979. Epidemiology of hepatocellular adenoma. JAMA 242:644–648.

ROSS RK, YUAN J-M, YU MC, et al. 1992. Urinary aflatoxin biomarkers and risk of hepatocellular carcinoma. Lancet 339:943–946.

ROTHMAN K. 1980. The proportion of cancer attributable to alcohol consumption. Prev Med 9:174–179.

RUBIN E, LIEBER C. 1974. Fatty liver, alcoholic hepatitis and cirrhosis produced by alcohol in primates. N Engl J Med 290:128–135.

SABBIONI G, SKIPPER R, BUCHI G, et al. 1987. Isolation and characterization of the major serum albumin adduct formed by aflatoxin B_1 *in vivo* in rats. Carcinogenesis 8:819–824.

SATO S, MATSUSHIMA T, TANAKA N, et al. 1973. Hepatic tumors in the guppy (*Lebistes reticulatus*) induced by aflatoxin B_1, dimethylnitrosamine, and 2-acetylaminofluorene. J Natl Cancer Inst 50:765–778.

SCHMIDT W, POPHAM R. 1981. The role of drinking and smoking in mortality from cancer and other causes in male alcoholics. Cancer 47:1031–1041.

SCHOTTENFELD D. 1979. Alcohol as a co-factor in the etiology of cancer. Cancer 43:1962–1966.

SCOBIE B, WOODFIELD D, FONG R. 1983. Familial hepatocellular carcinoma and hepatitis B antigenemia in a New Zealand Chinese family. Aust NZ J Med 13:236–239.

SCORSONE KA, ZHOU Y-Z, BUTEL JS, et al. 1992. p53 mutations cluster at codon 249 in hepatitis B virus-positive hepatocellular carcinomas from China. Cancer Res 52:1635–1638.

SEEFF LB, BUSKELL-BALES Z, WRIGHT EC, et al. 1992. Long term mortality after transfusion associated non-A, non-B hepatitis. N Engl J Med 327:1906–1911.

SEER CANCER STATISTICS REVIEW: 1973–1990. 1993. National Institutes of Health Publication No. 93–2789.

SEIFER M, HÖHNE M, SCHAEFER S, et al. 1991. Malignant transformation of immortalized cells by hepatitis B virus DNA. *In* Hollinger FB, Lemoon SM, Margolis HM (eds): Viral Hepatitis and Liver Disease. Baltimore, Williams & Wilkins, pp. 586–588.

SETO E, YEN TSB, PETERLIN BM, et al. 1988. Transactivation of the human immunodeficiency virus long terminal repeat by the hepatitis B virus X protein. Proc Natl Acad Sci USA 85:8286–8290.

SHAFRITZ DA, SHOUVAL D, SHERMAN HI, et al. 1981. Integration of hepatitis B virus DNA into the genome of liver cells in chronic liver disease and hepatocellular carcinoma. N Engl J Med 305:1067–1073.

SHANK R, GORDON J, WOGAN G, et al. 1972. Dietary aflatoxins and human liver cancer. III. Field survey of rural Thai families for ingested aflatoxins. Food Cosmet Toxicol 10:71–84.

SHEEHAN F, CONNOLLY CE, MCCARTHY CF. 1989. Hepatocellular carcinoma in idiopathic haemochromatosis. Gut 30:889.

SHEN F-M, LEE MK, GONG H-M, et al. 1991. Complex segregation analysis of primary hepatocellular carcinoma in Chinese families: Interaction of inherited susceptibility and hepatitis B viral infection. Am J Hum Genet 49:88–93.

SHEU JC, HUANG GT, LEE PH, et al. 1992. Mutation of p53 gene in hepatocellular carcinoma in Taiwan. Cancer Res 52:6098–6700.

SHIBATA A, FUKUDA K, TOSHIMA H, et al. 1990. The role of cigarette smoking and drinking in the development of liver cancer: 28 years of observations on male cohort members in a farming and fishing area. Cancer Detect Prev 14:617–623.

SHIBATA A, HIROHATA T, TOSHIMA H, et al. 1986. The role of drinking and cigarette smoking in the excess deaths from liver cancer. Jpn J Cancer Res 77:287–295.

SHIKATA T. 1976. Hepatocellular Carcinoma. New York, John Wiley & Sons, p. 53.

SIEBER S, CORREA P, DALGARD D, et al. 1979. Induction of osteogenic sarcomas and tumors of the hepatobiliary system in nonhuman primates with aflatoxin B_1. Cancer Res 39:4545–4554.

SINNHUBER R, LEE D, WALES J, et al. 1968. Dietary factors and hepatoma in rainbow trout *(Salmo gairdneri)*. II. Co-carcinogenesis by cyclopropenoid fatty acids and the effect of gossypol and altered lipids on aflatoxin-induced liver cancer. J Natl Cancer Inst 41:1293–1301.

SOLT DB, MEDLINE A, FARBER E. 1977. Rapid emergence of carcinogen-induced hyperplastic lesions in a new model for the sequential analysis of liver cancer. Am J Pathol 88:595–618.

SRIVATANAKUL P, PARKIN DM, KHLAT M, et al. 1991. Liver cancer in Thailand. II. A case-control study of hepatocellular carcinoma. Int J Cancer 48:329–332.

STEMHAGEN A, SLADE J, ALTMAN R, et al. 1983. Occupational risk factors and liver cancer: A retrospective case-control study of primary liver cancer in New Jersey. Am J Epidemiol 117:443–454.

STEVENS C, BEASLEY RP, TSUI J, et al. 1975. Vertical transmission of hepatitis B antigen in Taiwan. N Engl J Med 292:771–774.

STEVENS R, BEASLEY RP, BLUMBERG B. 1986. Iron-binding proteins and risk of cancer in Taiwan. J Natl Cancer Inst 76:605–610.

STEVENS R, MERKLE E, LUSTBADER E. 1984. Age and cohort effects in primary liver cancer. Int J Cancer 33:453–458.

STOCKER JT, ISHAK KG. 1987. Hepatoblastoma. *In* Okuda K, Ishak KG (eds): Neoplastic Diseases of the Liver. Berlin, Springer-Verlag, pp. 127–136.

STOLOFF L. 1983. Aflatoxin as a cause of primary liver-cell cancer in the United States: A probability study. Nutr Cancer 5:165–186.

STROFFOLINI T, CHIARAMONTE M, TIRIBELLI C, et al. 1992. Hepatitis C virus infection, HBsAg carrier state and hepatocellular carcinoma: Relative risk and population attributable risk from a case-control study in Italy. J Hepatol 16:360–363.

SUGIHARA S, KOJIRO M. 1987. Pathology of cholangiocarcinoma.

In Okuda K, Ishak KG (eds): Neoplastic Diseases of the Liver. Berlin, Springer-Verlag, pp. 143–158.

SUMMERS J, SMOLEC JM, SNYDER R. 1978. A virus similar to hepatitis B associated with hepatitis and hepatoma in woodchucks. Proc Natl Acad Sci USA 75:4533–4537.

SZMUNESS W. 1978. Hepatocellular carcinoma and hepatitis B virus: Evidence for a causal association. Prog Med Virol 24:40–69.

TAMBURRO C. 1984. Relationship of vinyl monomers and liver cancers: Angiosarcoma and hepatocellular carcinoma. Semin Liver Dis 4:158–169.

TAN AY, LAO CH, LEE YS. 1977. Hepatitis B antigen in the liver cells in cirrhosis and hepatocellular carcinoma. Pathology 9:57–64.

TANAKA K, HIROHATA T, TAKASHITA S. 1988. Blood transfusion, alcohol consumption, and cigarette smoking in causation of hepatocellular carcinoma: A case-control study in Fukuoka, Japan. Jpn J Cancer Res (Gann) 79:1075–1082.

TANAKA K, HIROHATA T, KOGA S, et al. 1991. Hepatitis C and hepatitis B in the etiology of hepatocellular carcinoma in the Japanese population. Cancer Res 51:2842–2847.

TANG Z-Y. 1985. Prognosis of hepatocellular carcinoma and factors influencing it. *In* Tang Z-Y (ed): Subclinical Hepatocellular Carcinoma. Berlin, Springer-Verlag, pp. 179–187.

TANG Z-Y, YANG B-H. 1985. Early detection of subclinical hepatocellular carcinoma. *In* Tang Z-Y (ed): Subclinical Hepatocellular Carcinoma. Berlin, Springer-Verlag, pp. 12–21.

TARAO K, OHKAWA S, SHIMIZU A, et al. 1994. Significance of hepatocellular proliferation in the development of hepatocellular carcinoma from anti-hepatitis C virus-positive cirrhotic patients. Cancer 73:1149–1154.

THOMAS HC. 1988. Treatment of hepatitis B viral infection. *In* Zuckerman AJ (ed): Viral Hepatitis and Liver Disease. New York, Alan R. Liss, pp. 817–822.

THUNG SN, GERBER MA, SARNO E, et al. 1979. Distribution of five antigens in hepatocellular carcinoma. Lab Invest 41:101–105.

TREMOLADA F, BENVEGNU L, CASARIN C, et al. 1990. Antibody to hepatitis C virus in hepatocellular carcinoma. Lancet 335:300–301.

TRICHOPOULOS D, DAY N, KAKLAMANI E, et al. 1987. Hepatitis B virus, tobacco smoking and ethanol consumption in the etiology of hepatocellular carcinoma. Int J Cancer 39:45–49.

TRICHOPOULOS D, MACMAHON B, SPARROS L, et al. 1980. Smoking and hepatitis B-negative primary hepatocellular carcinoma. J Natl Cancer Inst 65:111–114.

TSUBOI S, KAWAMURA K, CRUZ M, et al. 1985. Aflatoxin B_1 and primary hepatocellular carcinoma in Japan, Indonesia and the Philippines: Detection of aflatoxin B_1 in human serum and urine samples. *In* Hepatocellular Carcinoma in Asia. Kobe, Japan, International Center for Medical Research, pp. 135–146.

TSUKUMA H, HIYAMA T, OSHIMA A, et al. 1990. A case-control study of hepatocellular carcinoma in Osaka, Japan. Intl J Cancer 45:231–236.

TU J, GAO R, ZHANG D, et al. 1985. Hepatitis B virus and primary liver cancer on Chongming Island, People's Republic of China. Natl Cancer Inst Monogr 69:213–215.

TUYNS A, OBRADOVIC M. 1975. Unexpected high incidence of primary liver cancer in Geneva, Switzerland. J Natl Cancer Inst 54:61–64.

VALL MAYANS M, CALVET X, BRUIX J, et al. 1990. Risk factors for hepatocellular carcinoma in Catalonia, Spain. Int J Cancer 46:378–381.

VANA J, MURPHY G, ARONOFF B, et al. 1977. Primary liver tumors and oral contraceptives—Results of a survey. JAMA 238:2154–2158.

VAN KAICK G, MUTH H, KAUL A, et al. 1983. Recent results of the German thorotrast study—Epidemiological results and dose effect relationships in thorotrast patients. Health Physics 44:299–306.

VAN KAICK G, WESCH H, LUHRS H, et al. 1986. Radiation-induced primary liver tumors in "thorotrast patients." Recent Results Cancer Res 100:16–22.

VAN RENSBURG S, COOK-MOZAFFARI P, VAN SCHALKWYK D, et al. 1985. Hepatocellular carcinoma and dietary aflatoxin in Mozambique and Transkei. Br J Cancer 51:713–726.

VAN RENSBURG S, VAN DER WATT J, PURCHASE I, et al. 1974. Primary liver cancer rate and aflatoxin intake in a high cancer area. S Afr Med J 48:2508a–2508d.

VAN THIEL DH, GAVALER JS, WRIGHT HI, et al. 1992. Responses to alpha-interferon therapy are influenced by the iron content of the liver. Gastroenterology 102:904.

VERBAAN H, WIDELL A, LINDGREN S, et al. 1992. Hepatitis C in chronic liver disease: An epidemiological study based on 566 consecutive cases undergoing liver biopsy during a 10-year period. J Intern Med 232:33–42.

VESSELINOVITCH S, MIHAILOVICH N, WOGAN G, et al. 1972. Aflatoxin B_1, a hepatocarcinogen in the infant mouse. Cancer Res 32:2289–2291.

VIOLA PL. 1970. Pathology of vinyl chloride. Med Lav 61:147–180.

WADE N. 1972. Anabolic steroids (news). Science 176:1399–1403.

WALES J, SINNHUBER R. 1972. Hepatomas induced by aflatoxin in the sockeye salmon (*Oncorhgrachus nerka*). J Natl Cancer Inst 48:1529–1530.

WANG HP, ROGLER CE. 1988. Deletions in human chromosome arms 11p and 13q in primary hepatocellular carcinomas. Cytogenet Cell Genet 48:72–78.

WEINBERG E. 1981. Iron and neoplasia. Biol Trace Element Res 3:55–80.

WEINBERG E. 1984. Iron withholding: A defense against infection and neoplasia. Physiol Rev 64:65–102.

WILD C, GARNER R, MONTESANO R, et al. 1986. Aflatoxin B_1 binding to plasma albumin and liver DNA upon chronic administration to rats. Carcinogenesis 7:853–858.

WONG DK, CHEUNG AM, O'ROURKE K, et al. 1993. Effect of alpha-interferon treatment in patients with hepatitis B e antigen-positive chronic hepatitis B. A meta-analysis. Ann Intern Med 119(4):312–23.

WHO COLLABORATIVE STUDY OF NEOPLASIA AND STEROID CONTRACEPTIVES. 1989. Combined oral contraceptives and liver cancer. Int J Cancer 43:254–259.

WORLD HEALTH ORGANIZATION. 1982. World health statistics annual, 1978–1982. Vital statistics and causes of death. Geneva, WHO.

WORLD HEALTH ORGANIZATION. 1983. Report of WHO meeting. Prevention of Liver Cancer. WHO Technical Series, 691, Geneva.

YANG B-H, TANG Z-Y. 1985. Hepatitis B virus and hepatocellular carcinoma—Clinical and serological aspects. *In* Tang Z-Y (ed): Subclinical Hepatocellular Carcinoma. Berlin, Springer-Verlag, pp. 212–217.

YANG P, BUETOW KH, LUSTBADER ED, et al. 1990. Evidence for a major locus modifying risk for primary hepatocellular carcinoma. Am J Hum Genet 47:A25.

YAOBIN W, LIZUN L, BENFA Y, et al. 1983. Relation between geographical distribution of liver cancer and climate—Aflatoxin B_1 in China. Sci Sin (Ser B) 26:1166–1175.

YEH F, MO C, YEN R. 1985. Risk factors for hepatocellular carcinoma in Guangxi, People's Republic of China. Natl Cancer Inst Monogr 69:47–48.

YEH F, YU MC, MO C-C, et al. 1989. Hepatitis B virus, aflatoxins, and hepatocellular carcinoma in southern Guangxi, China. Cancer Res 49:2506–2509.

YOKOSUKA O, OMATA M, IMAZEKI F, et al. 1986. Hepatitis B virus RNA transcripts and DNA in chronic liver disease. N Engl J Med 315:1187–1192.

YONEYAMA T, TAKEUCHI K, HARADA H, et al. 1990. Detection of hepatitis C viral sequences in non-B hepatocellular carcinoma. Jpn J Med Sci Biol 43:89–94.

YU H, HARRIS R, KABAT G, et al. 1988. Cigarette smoking, alcohol consumption and primary liver cancer: A case-control study in the U.S.A. Int J Cancer 42:325–328.

YU M, MACK T, HANISH R, et al. 1983. Hepatitis, alcohol consumption, cigarette smoking, and hepatocellular carcinoma in Los Angeles. Cancer Res 43:6077–6079.

YU MC, TONG MJ, COURSAGET P, et al. 1990. Prevalence of hepatitis B and C viral markers in black and white populations with hepatocellular carcinoma in the United States. J Natl Cancer Inst 82:1038–1041.

YU MW, CHEN CJ. 1993. Elevated serum testosterone levels and risk of hepatocellular carcinoma. Cancer Res 53:790–794.

ZAMAN S, MELIA W, JOHNSON R, et al. 1985. Risk factors in development of hepatocellular carcinoma in cirrhosis: Prospective study of 613 patients. Lancet 2:1357–1359.

ZAVITSANOS X, HATZAKIS A, KAKLAMANI E, et al. 1992. Association between hepatitis C virus and hepatocellular carcinoma using assays based on structural and nonstructural hepatitis C virus peptides. Cancer Res 52:5364–5367.

ZHANG W, HIROHASKI S, TSUDA H, et al. 1990. Frequent loss of heterozygosity on Chromosomes 16 and 4 in human hepatocellular carcinoma. Jpn J Cancer Res 81:108–111.

37 Biliary tract cancer

JOSEPH F. FRAUMENI, JR.
SUSAN S. DEVESA
JOSEPH K. McLAUGHLIN
JANET L. STANFORD

Cancers of the biliary tract encompass tumors arising from the gallbladder, extrahepatic bile ducts, and ampulla of Vater, according to the International Classification of Diseases. Not included in this category are tumors of the intrahepatic bile ducts, which are classified with primary liver cancer. The prognosis of biliary tract cancers is generally poor. They account for about 4,300 deaths per year in the United States, or almost 1% of all deaths due to cancer, and nearly all are adenocarcinomas. Microscopic confirmation of the diagnosis occurs in more than 96% of gallbladder cancer cases and about 86% of other biliary tract sites, according to data from the Surveillance, Epidemiology, and End Results (SEER) program of the United States (Miller et al, 1993). While gallbladder cancer occurs more often in women, other biliary tract tumors are more common in men. In the SEER program, about two-thirds of other biliary tumors arise in the extrahepatic bile ducts and about one-third in the ampulla of Vater, while only a small proportion of cases have an unspecified subsite. Biliary tract tumors can be difficult to diagnose and may be wrongly classified. In particular, biliary tumors may be confused with pancreatic cancer on clinical grounds, while ampullary tumors may be mistakingly assigned to the duodenum rather than the biliary tract.

Many of the etiologic leads to biliary tract cancers have come from clinical observations, autopsy series, and descriptive epidemiologic studies. While a significant fraction of these tumors appears causally related to gallstones, only limited etiologic information is otherwise available, owing to the rarity of the tumors, the often rapidly fatal course, and the small number of analytical studies conducted to date.

DEMOGRAPHIC CHARACTERISTICS

Around the world the most common type of biliary tract cancer is gallbladder cancer, which is among the few forms of cancer that occur more frequently in women than men. International variation in age-adjusted incidence rates among women is presented in Figure 37-1a, based generally on 1983–87 data in the most recent volume of Cancer Incidence in Five Continents (Parkin et al, 1992). The selected registries are listed in rank order for gallbladder cancer in various regions of the world. The rates for gallbladder cancer are highest in countries such as Poland and Hungary in eastern Europe and Colombia and Costa Rica in Latin America. Notably high rates are also reported in Peru and Ecuador (not shown), but not in Puerto Rico, suggesting that the high rates observed in Latin America are primarily in populations with Indian admixture. In the United States, rates are elevated among Spanish-surnamed whites and are low among blacks. Except for some high-risk areas in the Middle and Far East, the rates in other regions of the world are generally low.

For other biliary tract cancers, the international variation in incidence among women is less pronounced than for gallbladder cancer. Since cancer of the biliary tract not otherwise specified (NOS) is categorized with other biliary tract tumors, the elevated rates in some populations may actually reflect a high risk of gallbladder cancer. This problem appears most evident in registries of Colombia and Spain, where more than 80% of other biliary tract cancers represent tumors of the biliary tract NOS. Cancer of extrahepatic bile ducts is less common than gallbladder cancer. Although the annual rates for cancer of the bile ducts in women are generally less than one per 100,000, rates in Japan are notably higher. Cancer of the ampulla of Vater is the least common in all populations. In studying the international variation of biliary tract cancer, Strom et al (1985) concluded that cancers of the gallbladder, extrahepatic bile duct, and ampulla of Vater have distinct demographic patterns and should be regarded as separate disease entities.

Geographic differences in gallbladder cancer rates among men (Fig. 37-1b) are less striking than among

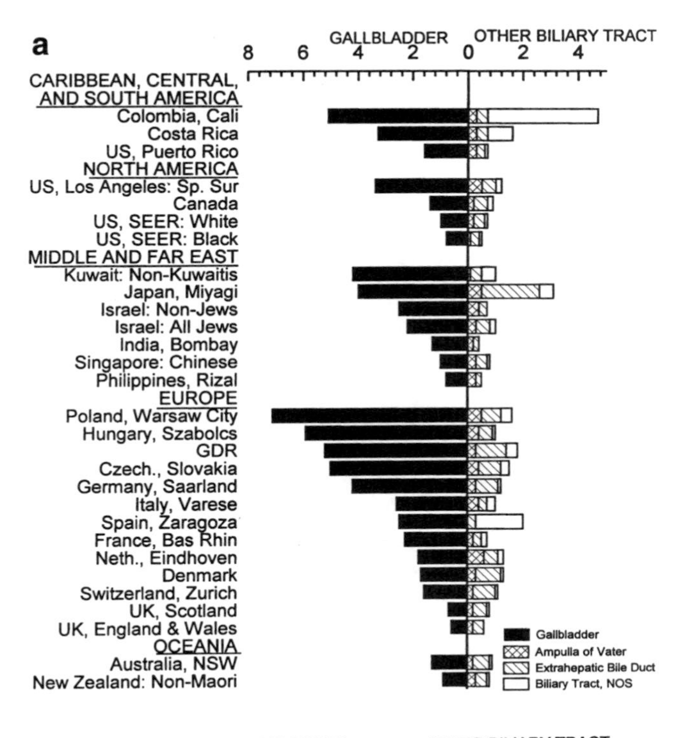

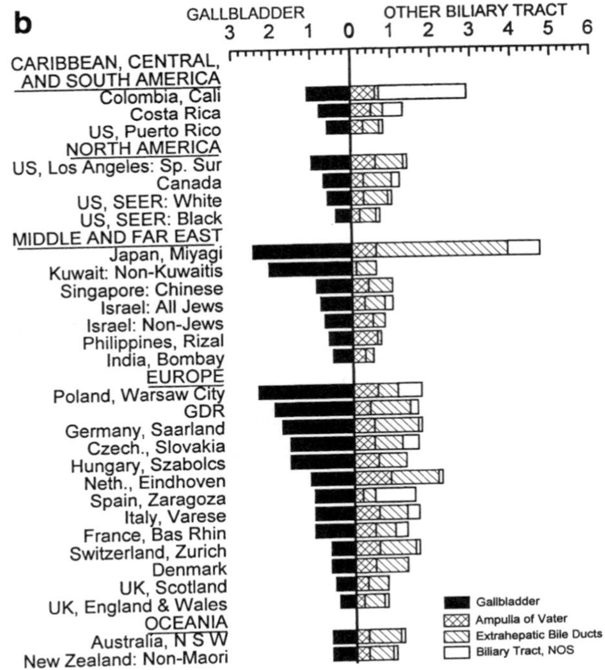

FIG. 37–1. International variation in biliary tract cancer incidence rates by subsite (per 100,000 person-years, age-standardized to the world population) among women (*a*) and men (*b*), circa 1985. Source: Parkin et al, 1992.

women. The highest rates for men are seen in eastern Europe, while the rates in Latin America are much less remarkable than the female pattern. Although subsite comparisons are limited by the high proportion of cases with cancer of the biliary tract NOS, the rates for bile duct cancer are especially high in Miyagi and other cities in Japan and among Japanese in Hawaii and Los Angeles (not shown). The high risk of this tumor in Japanese men does not appear to extend to other Asian populations. Around the world the annual rates per 100,000 for bile duct cancer in men range from 0.1 to 3.3, while rates for tumors of the ampulla of Vater are generally lower than 1.0. In contrast to gallbladder cancer, the rates for bile duct and ampullary cancers are generally higher in men than women.

In the United States, incidence data from the SEER program indicate substantial variations by racial/ethnic group, sex, and location within the biliary tract (Table 37-1). For gallbladder cancer, rates are especially high among American Indians of both sexes and among Hispanic women, with a female excess in all groups except the Chinese and Japanese. The rates are higher in married, widowed, and divorced women than in single women, with a clear increase in risk associated with a higher number of pregnancies (Moerman et al, 1994a). Some studies of gallbladder cancer in the United States and elsewhere have suggested an inverse association with socioeconomic status (Zatonski et al, 1992). For other biliary tract cancers, the rates are highest among Japanese and American Indians of both sexes, as well as among Hispanic men, with a male excess in all groups except American Indians.

TABLE 37–1. *Incidence Rates* for Biliary Tract Cancer by Subsite, Sex, and Ethnic Group (SEER program, 1977–83)*

	Males		*Females*	
	No.	*Rate*	*No.*	*Rate*
GALLBLADDER				
White[a]	274	0.9	751	1.6
Black[a]	34	0.8	68	1.2
American Indian[b]	27	5.9	72	13.6
Chinese American[c]	9	1.3	6	0.8
Japanese American[c]	16	1.5	21	1.5
Hispanic American[b]	12	1.2	87	7.6
OTHER BILIARY TRACT				
White[a]	520	1.7	490	1.1
Black[a]	41	1.0	43	0.8
American Indian[b]	11	2.6	16	3.0
Chinese American[c]	12	1.8	13	1.6
Japanese American[c]	34	3.4	33	2.5
Hispanic American[b]	27	2.8	15	1.3

*Per 100,000 person years, age-adjusted based on the 1970 U.S. standard.

[a]Atlanta, Detroit, San Francisco, Connecticut.

[b]New Mexico.

[c]Hawaii and San Francisco–Oakland.

Source: Adapted from Horm et al (this volume) and unpublished data.

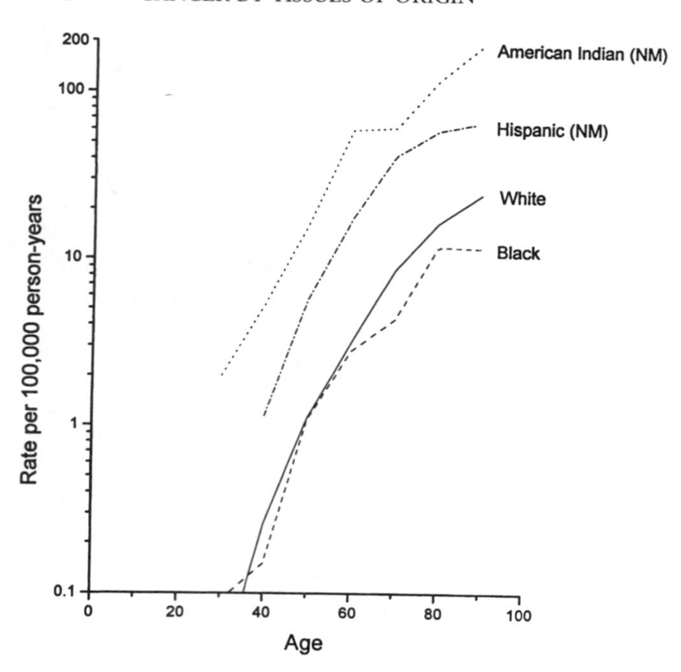

FIG. 37–2. Age-specific incidence rates for gallbladder cancer among U.S. women by racial/ethnic group, SEER program, 1975–85.

For U.S. women, the age curves for gallbladder cancer reveal sharply increasing incidence rates before age 50 among American Indians, ten years earlier than other racial/ethnic groups (Fig. 37-2). The age pattern for Hispanic women is similar. Rates among black and white women increase at a slower rate, with the excess among whites occurring primarily over the age of 60. Figure 37-3 shows the age curves for gallbladder and other biliary tract cancers among U.S. white men and women. The rates for gallbladder cancer are higher among women at all ages, although the sex ratio decreases slightly with increasing age. For other biliary tract tumors, the male excess is apparent by age 45 and persists through life. Around the world, the increase in rates with age is most pronounced for gallbladder cancer and least evident for ampullary cancer (Strom et al, 1985).

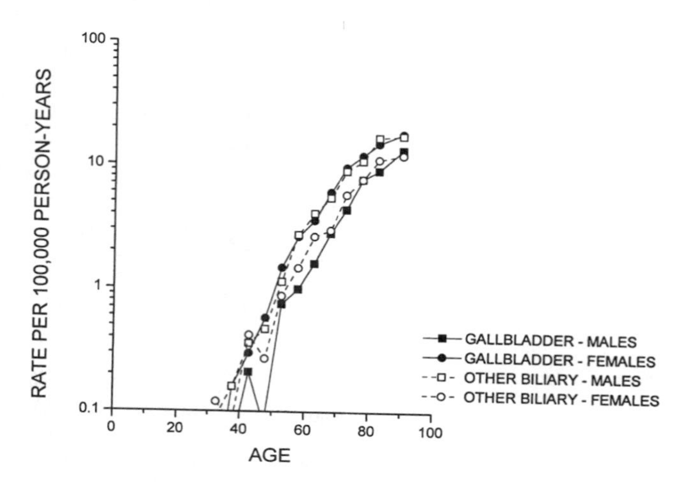

FIG. 37–3. Age-specific incidence rates for gallbladder and other biliary tract cancers by sex among U.S. whites, SEER program, 1986–90.

Evaluation of time trends has been impaired by the failure of the International Classification of Diseases to distinguish between cancers of the liver and the biliary system until the 7th revision in 1958, while cancers of the gallbladder and other biliary tract were not separately reported until the 8th revision in 1967. During the 1970s and 1980s, based on data from five geographic areas of the United States (Devesa et al, 1987), gallbladder cancer incidence and mortality rates decreased among white men and women, with mortality rates declining more steeply (42%–50%) than incidence rates (33%–34%) (Fig. 37-4a). Rates for gallbladder cancer among women were consistently about twice those reported among men. For other biliary tract cancers, the rates decreased less rapidly (16%–22% for incidence and 28%–29% for mortality) and remained 30%–60% higher among men than women (Fig. 37-4b). Of the deaths attributed to other biliary tract cancers, 60%–70% were due to extrahepatic bile duct cancer, about 15% to ampulla of Vater cancer, and the remainder to biliary tract cancer NOS.

The downward trends for biliary tract cancer appear related at least partly to the increasing number of cholecystectomies performed annually for gallbladder disease in the United States (Blanken, 1976), thus reducing the number of gallbladders at risk of developing cancer. A similar trend has been noted in other countries, including the United Kingdom (Diehl and Beral, 1981) and Czechoslovakia (Plesko et al, 1985a). The reduced risk after cholecystectomy extends to bile duct cancer, which is consistent with the role of gallstones in this tumor (Ekbom et al, 1993a). In Sweden, where the reported number of cholecystectomies performed was reported to decrease (Ahlberg et al, 1978), gallbladder and bile duct cancers were found to increase (Diehl and Beral, 1981), particularly among older women (Broden et al, 1978). A similar pattern has been reported in Chile (Serra et al, 1990). During the 1970s and 1980s, cholecystectomy rates in the United States increased mainly among persons aged 65 and older, whereas rates among younger persons did not change greatly (Diehl, 1987, 1991). The introduction of gallstone lithotripsy in 1986 may have temporarily reduced cholecystectomy rates, but during the late 1980s laparoscopic cholecystectomy became increasingly popular, due to its lowered morbidity when compared to open cholecystectomy (Johnston and Kaplan, 1993). The resulting increases in cholecystectomy rates have now been documented at all ages in the United States (Diehl, 1994; Legorreta et al, 1993), suggesting that the rates for biliary tract cancer should continue to decline. In Shanghai, a remarkable increase in the incidence of biliary tract cancer was reported recently and warrants further study (Jin et al, 1993).

The prognosis for patients with biliary tract cancer is unfavorable, with 5-year relative survival rates of only 16%–18% (Table 37-2). Among those few patients diagnosed with in situ tumors, survival rates are 80% or greater. Similar proportions of cases are diagnosed with localized, regional, or distant disease. Of those with localized disease, survival rates range from 40% to 55% for those with gallbladder cancer and from 27% to 33% for those with other biliary tract cancer. Once the disease has spread regionally, survival rates decline substantially, falling to 3% or below among those with distant disease. Survival is affected also by histologic grade and type, with papillary carcinomas having the most favorable prognosis (Henson et al, 1992).

TABLE 37–2. *Stage Distribution of Biliary Tract Cancers and Corresponding 5-year Relative Survival Rates among Whites by Subsite and Sex (SEER program, 1983–87)*

	Gallbladder		*Other Biliary Tract*	
	Males	*Females*	*Males*	*Females*
Number of cases	425	1136	717	722
DISTRIBUTION (%)				
In situ	3	4	1	1
Localized	27	24	26	21
Regional	28	30	35	34
Distant	36	38	20	24
Unknown	6	4	19	20
FIVE-YEAR RELATIVE SURVIVAL (%)				
Total	18	16	16	16
In situ	83	91	—	80
Localized	55	40	27	33
Regional	1	6	16	18
Distant	0	1	3	1
Unknown	0	—	4	8

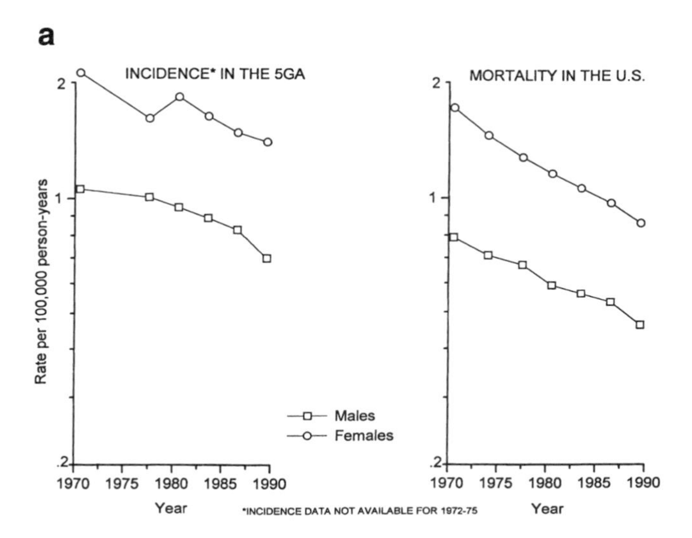

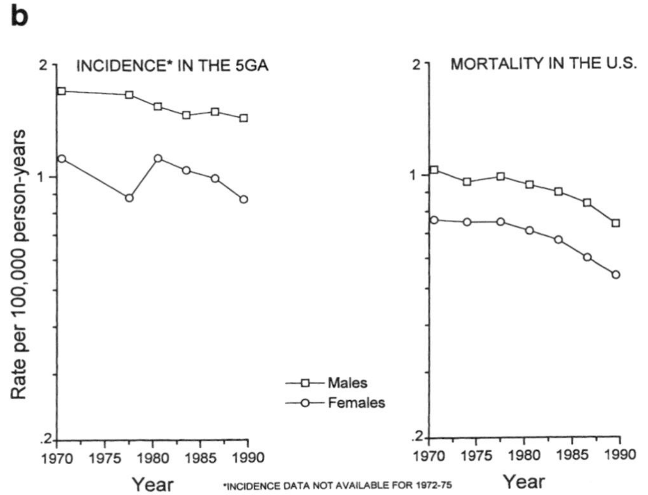

FIG. 37–4. Trends in incidence and mortality rates (per 100,000 person-years, age-standardized to the 1970 U.S. population) for cancers of the gallbladder (*a*) and other biliary tract (*b*) by sex among U.S. whites, 1969–71 to 1988–90. The five geographic areas (5GA) include Atlanta, Detroit, San Francisco–Oakland, Connecticut, and Iowa.

Analyses of U.S. mortality data by state economic area reveal a 5-fold variation in rates of gallbladder cancer among white women, with generally low rates across the Southeast and high rates in parts of the Southwest, the Appalachian region, the Midwest, and the upper north central states (Fig. 37-5). The reason for this pattern is not clear, although high rates in the Southwest are consistent with the susceptibility of Hispanic Americans. The patterns of gallbladder cancer for white men are similar but less striking. The distribution of other biliary tract tumors resembles that for gallbladder cancer, although the variation is less pronounced.

In various populations around the world there is remarkable concordance in the incidence of gallbladder cancer and gallstones. At one extreme, for example, the elevated risk of gallbladder cancer among American Indians appears part of a spectrum of gallstone-related disease endemic in this population (Morris et al, 1978). Also prone to both conditions are Alaskan natives, including Inuits (Nutting et al, 1993), and Hispanic populations with an admixture of American Indian genes, with stones being especially common in young women (Wiggins et al, 1993). In Israel the rates of gallbladder cancer and gallstones are higher among women born in Europe than those born in Asia or Africa (Hart et al, 1971). At the other extreme, in sub-Saharan Africa, both gallbladder cancer and gallstones are rarely reported (Heaton, 1973).

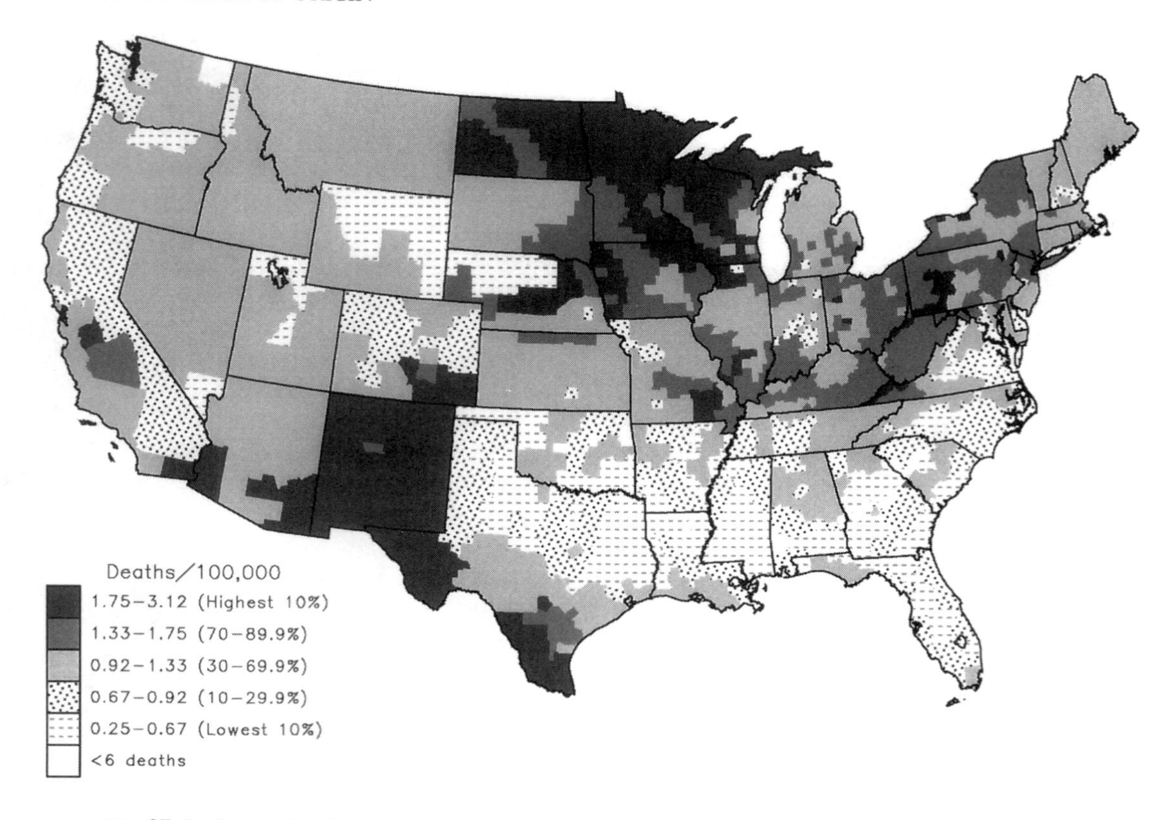

FIG. 37–5. Geographic variation in mortality rates (per 100,000 person-years, age-standardized to the 1970 U.S. population) for gallbladder cancer among U.S. white women by state economic area, 1970–89.

Tumors of the biliary tract are rarely found in domestic or exotic animals, but a high rate of extrahepatic bile duct cancer has been seen in captive bears (Gosselin and Kramer, 1984).

GALLSTONES

In the United States about 10%–15% of men and 25% of women over age 50 have gallstones, but the absolute risk of developing biliary tract cancer is very low (Diehl, 1991; Ransohoff and Gracie, 1993). However, in various series of gallbladder cancer, stones have been reported in about 60%–90% of cases, a rate several times higher than expected, while in bile duct cancer the percentage of cases with stones is usually less than 30%. Furthermore, gallbladder cancer is nearly always fatal and is reported to account for about one-third to one-half of gallstone-related deaths in the United States (American College of Physicians, 1993). To a remarkable degree, gallbladder cancer and gallstones share demographic characteristics, including female predominance, racial and ethnic susceptibility, and geographic variation, with especially high rates reported in selected populations in Latin America (Nervi et al, 1988; Weiss et al, 1984; Rios-Dalenz et al, 1985) and in central and eastern Europe (Zatonski et al, 1992; Plesko et al, 1985a). The similarity extends to geographic patterns even within the United States. Despite the rarity of deaths from gallstones, pronounced variation according to state economic area is evident among U.S. white women, with high mortality rates in parts of the Southwest, Midwest, and Appalachia (Fig. 37-6). It is noteworthy that a high incidence of gallstones has been reported in the Appalachian area (Richardson et al, 1973).

Based mainly on autopsy surveys and hospital-based case-control studies, a relation has been established between gallstones and the subsequent occurrence of gallbladder cancer (Nervi et al, 1988; WHO, 1989). In a cohort study of gallstone patients who did not have a cholecystectomy, Maringhini et al (1987) estimated the cumulative incidence of gallbladder cancer after 20 years to be about 1%, with a 3-fold elevation in the relative risk. The risk of gallbladder cancer is clearly related to gallstone size. Subjects with stones over 3 cm in diameter have shown a risk that is ten times that seen with stones under 1 cm (Diehl, 1983; Lowenfels et al, 1989). Further increases in the risk of gallbladder cancer have been associated also with long duration of stones,

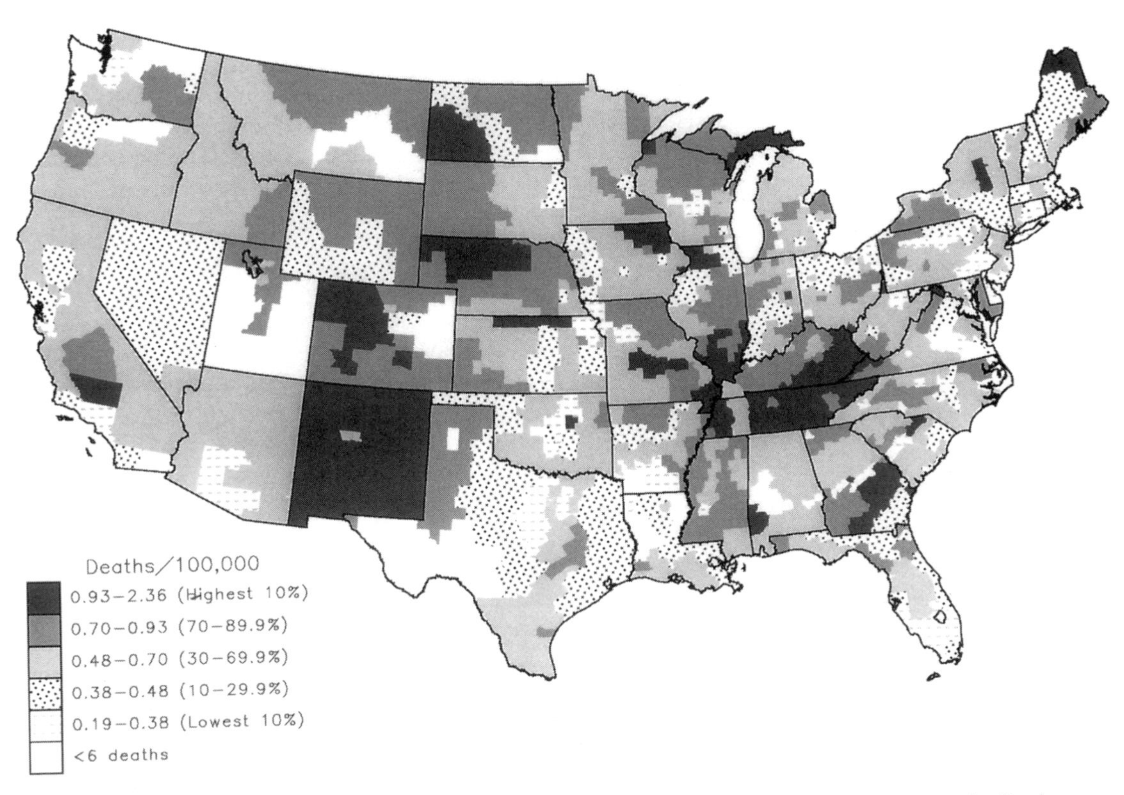

FIG. 37–6. Geographic variation in gallstone mortality rates (per 100,000 person-years, age-standardized to the 1970 U.S. population) among U.S. white women by state economic area, 1970–89.

symptomatic disease, occurrence in a New World Indian, calcification in the gallbladder wall (porcelain gallbladder), and anomalies of the pancreaticobiliary junction (So et al, 1990). For bile duct cancer, case-control studies have documented an elevated risk associated with prior gallbladder disease, including stones (Yen et al, 1987; Chow et al, 1994).

Several risk factors have been identified for cholesterol gallstones, the type that prevails in Western countries, as compared with the high frequency in Asia of pigment stones containing calcium salts of bilirubin (Guo et al, 1991). Individuals predisposed to cholesterol stones tend to have a "lithogenic" bile in which cholesterol is supersaturated, due either to increased hepatic secretion of cholesterol or diminished secretion of bile salts and phospholipids that maintain the solubility of cholesterol (Paumgartner and Sauerbruch, 1991). The formation of stones is enhanced also by destabilization and stasis of bile in the gallbladder. Since cholesterol gallstones and biliary tract cancer are so closely linked, it is clear that understanding the origins of gallstones is important in elucidating the causes of biliary tract cancer.

Most of the risk factors for cholesterol gallstones are associated with hypersecretion and saturation of cholesterol in the bile. These factors include the steady increase in risk with age, the differential susceptibility of females, and associations observed with obesity, multiple pregnancies, and use of exogenous estrogens (Diehl, 1991; Johnston and Kaplan, 1993). A genetic susceptibility may also help explain the very high rates of gallstones occurring among native Americans and Hispanic populations as well as the familial tendency to stones noted in some studies (Diehl, 1991). A candidate gene for gallstone disease has emerged with the recent localization and characterization of cholesterol 7α-hydroxylase, a microsomal cytochrome P450 mapped to chromosome 8q11–q12 that catalyzes the first stage of bile acid synthesis (Cohen et al, 1992). Cholesterol saturation of bile may also explain the elevated rates of gallstones associated with nonvegetarian and fiber-depleted diets, with use of clofibrate and other drugs to lower serum cholesterol, and with loss of ileal function following bowel resection or inflammatory disease (Paumgartner and Sauerbruch, 1991; Johnston and Kaplan, 1993). Data on the relation between serum cholesterol and gallstones are inconsistent, but there is some evidence that high serum triglycerides and low high-density-lipoprotein levels may be risk factors (Diehl, 1991). In addition, an effect of gallbladder hypomotility and stasis is suggested by the elevated risk of gallstones associated with pregnancy, fasting, total parenteral nutrition, thiazide use (Kakar et al, 1986), and gastric resection (Caygill et al, 1988).

The mechanisms linking gallstones to biliary tract cancer are not clear, and it is not possible to distinguish stones from a common underlying property of bile as the major cause. However, precancerous changes of the gallbladder mucosa, including dysplasia, have been described in areas adjacent to stones as well as tumors (Dowling and Kelly, 1986; Nakajo et al, 1990).

In contrast to cholesterol stones, the relation of pigment stones to biliary tract cancer is unclear and deserves further study (Trotman and Soloway, 1982). The risk factors for pigment stones include age, Asian residence, bacterial infections of the biliary system, low-protein diet, hemolytic anemia, and cirrhosis.

OTHER RISK FACTORS

Although cholesterol gallstones represent the most important risk factor in biliary tract cancers, especially of the gallbladder, it is important to consider other risk factors that may be responsible for tumors arising in the absence of stones or that may interact with stones or lithogenic bile to produce tumors. The information available is limited by the relatively small number of epidemiologic studies, and it is often difficult to gauge the extent to which the risk factors for biliary tract cancer simply overlap with the risk factors for gallstones.

Inflammation and Infection

It has been suggested that, with or without gallstones, inflammatory processes of the biliary tract may progress to dysplastic and neoplastic changes. This notion is supported by the reported prominence of cholecystitis among patients with gallstones who develop gallbladder cancer, by the greater risk associated with atrophic late stages of cholecystitis as compared with earlier stages (Levine, 1975), and by neoplasms reported with inflammatory conditions of the gallbladder in the absence of stones (Bengmark, 1968). Examination of cholecystectomy specimens removed for gallstones or cholecystitis suggest a sequence of precursor epithelial changes evolving through hyperplasia, atypical hyperplasia, metaplasia, dysplasia, and carcinoma in situ (Albores-Saavedra et al, 1980; Dowling and Kelly, 1986).

Biliary stasis and infection may also contribute to the risk of biliary tract cancer, particularly when it arises as a complication of biliary obstruction by cysts or other benign growths (Flanigan, 1977). Of special interest is the large excess risk of biliary tract tumors that has been observed among chronic typhoid and paratyphoid carriers (Caygill et al, 1994). The carrier state typically results from biliary tract colonization, and it is often accompanied by gallstones that may influence the susceptibility to biliary tumors. It is possible, however, that bacterial flora are involved in converting bile acids to carcinogenic metabolites (Shukla et al, 1993) or perhaps in directly inducing preneoplastic changes in the biliary mucosa.

Liver Flukes

In certain Asian countries, bile duct carcinomas occur excessively in populations infested with liver flukes, including *Clonorchis sinensis, Opisthorchis viverrini,* and *Opisthorchis felineus* (Schwartz, 1986; Srivatanakul et al, 1991). These infections cause a proliferative inflammatory reaction in the biliary system, which may progress to cancers that affect mainly the intrahepatic bile ducts (cholangiocarcinoma) but occasionally the extrahepatic ducts. Reports have occurred also among Asian immigrants in the United States. Similar tumors have been seen in infected cats and dogs and in hamsters exposed to metacercaria of *O. viverrini* plus dimethylnitrosamine (Thamavit et al, 1978). It is of interest that high levels of nitrosamines are present in fermented fish products and preserved protein foods that are widely used in the endemic areas.

Ulcerative Colitis

In patients with ulcerative colitis, the risk of biliary tract tumors is substantially higher than in the general population (Ritchie et al, 1974). Usually arising in the extrahepatic bile ducts, the tumors develop in about 1% of colitis patients and show a male excess (Christophi and Hughes, 1985). In a case-control study of bile duct cancer, the relative risk was 3.6 among individuals with a history of ulcerative colitis, after controlling for age and sex (Yen et al, 1987). In a series from the Mayo Clinic, the biliary tumors with colitis arose three decades earlier than usual but did not appear influenced by the extent, severity, or form of treatment of the colitis (Akwari et al, 1975). However, in a study from St. Mark's Hospital in London, the tumors occurred more often in patients with total colitis of long duration (Ritchie et al, 1974). The biliary tumors tend to arise without gallstones or the usual hepatobiliary manifestations of colitis (e.g., sclerosing cholangitis), so that the pathogenic mechanisms are obscure.

Partial Gastrectomy

An excess risk of biliary tract and pancreatic cancer has been reported after partial gastrectomy (Tersmette et al, 1990). The finding may be related to the high frequency of gallstones after gastrectomy or possibly to biliary excretion of N-nitroso compounds that are formed in the gastric remnant (Caygill et al, 1988).

Occupation

Environmental chemicals were implicated in 1970, when a study of workers in a rubber plant showed an excess of gallbladder and bile duct tumors (Mancuso and Brennan, 1970). Occupational mortality statistics for California suggested that automotive and rubber plant workers are prone to gallbladder and bile duct cancers (Krain, 1972). In the same survey, gallbladder cancers were increased in textile and metal workers, while bile duct cancers were prominent in workers from the aircraft, chemical, and wood-finishing industries. More recently, excess risks of biliary tract cancer have been observed in chemical workers (Bond et al, 1990), painters (Guberan et al, 1989), pesticide manufacturers (Brown, 1992), vinyl chloride workers (Wong et al, 1991), munitions workers exposed to dinitrotoluene (Stayner et al, 1993), and synthetic textile workers involved in cellulose triacetate fiber manufacturing (Lanes et al, 1990; Goldberg and Theriault, 1994). In Sweden, a linked-registry analysis of occupational tumors revealed excesses of gallbladder cancer associated with employment in petroleum refining, paper mills, chemical processing, shoemaking and repairing, and textile work, as well as excesses of bile duct cancer with asbestos-related occupations such as shipbuilding and insulation work (Malker et al, 1986). These epidemiologic observations, although based on small numbers and not definitive, are consistent with the capacity of several chemicals to produce hepatobiliary tumors and precursor lesions in laboratory animals (Diehl, 1980).

Reproductive and Hormonal Factors

A strong positive relation has been consistently observed between a higher number of pregnancies and risk of gallbladder cancer (Plesko et al, 1985b; WHO, 1989; Lambe et al, 1993). A recent case-control study of biliary tract cancer in the Netherlands also indicated an association with parity, as well as early age at menarche, early age at first pregnancy, and prolonged fertility (Moerman et al, 1994a). The authors attributed these associations to increased levels or duration of exposure to endogenous estrogens and progesterone. The hormonal changes may both alter the composition of bile and impair biliary motility to promote the development of gallstones (Kritz-Silverstein et al, 1990), although a direct effect of estrogens or secondary bile acids on the biliary epithelium is possible. In addition, hormonal factors may contribute to the slow colonic transit reported among women with gallstones and thus increase the absorption of secondary bile salts that may enhance the hepatobiliary secretion of cholesterol (Heaton et al, 1993).

Despite reports that oral contraceptive use and supplemental estrogens accelerate the development of gallstones (Petitti et al, 1988; Milne and Vessey, 1991; Thijs and Knipschild, 1993), analytical studies of biliary tract tumors have shown no clear association with exogenous hormones (WHO, 1989; Milne and Vessey, 1991; Moerman et al, 1994a; Chow et al, 1994). In addition, a possible role of gonadotropins has been suggested by an excess risk of pancreatic and biliary cancers observed in the mothers of dizygotic twins (Wyshak et al, 1983).

Obesity

A strong relation has been observed between risk of gallbladder cancer and high relative weight, particularly among women (Garfinkel, 1986; Zatonski et al, 1992). Obesity has been linked also to the risk of extrahepatic bile duct cancer in men and women, but not cancer of the ampulla of Vater (Chow et al, 1994). The risks associated with obesity may reflect well-established associations with antecedent gallstones (Petitti and Sidney, 1988) and the tendency for obese subjects to have high levels of endogenous estrogens (Kritz-Silverstein et al, 1990) as well as bile that is supersaturated with cholesterol (Bennion and Grundy, 1978). In addition, the pattern of body fat may be an independent risk factor, based on associations with the ratio of waist-to-hip girth (Hartz et al, 1984) and with the ratio of subscapular-to-triceps skinfold thickness (Haffner et al, 1989). In the management of obesity, a high rate of symptomatic gallstones has been reported during rapid weight loss (Everhart, 1993).

Dietary Habits

Dietary risk factors in biliary tract cancer are difficult to identify since the symptoms associated with biliary disease may induce changes in diet and nutritional status. However, the limited data available suggest a positive association with total caloric intake, along with protective effects from dietary fiber and micronutrients in vegetables and fruits (Zatonski et al, 1992; Moerman et al, 1993). Similar findings have been reported for gallstones, but the available evidence suggests that diet plays a comparatively small role compared to obesity (Diehl, 1991; Maclure et al, 1990). Recently a protective effect of calcium intake was suggested (Moerman et al, 1994c), while another study of gallstone patients showed a negative relation to serum concentrations of ionized calcium and a positive relation to total calcium, magnesium, bicarbonate and parathyroid hormone (Rudnicki et al, 1993).

Tobacco and Alcohol

The roles of tobacco smoking and alcohol consumption are unclear, but a recent case-control study of biliary tract cancer suggested a protective effect associated with long-term use of alcohol and an increased risk among smokers who did not drink alcohol (Moerman et al, 1994b). In a recent case-control investigation of extrahepatic bile duct cancer, Chow et al (1994) found that heavy smokers had a risk three times that of nonsmokers, while alcohol drinkers had a slightly reduced risk but no consistent trend with amount consumed. If confirmed, the association between smoking and bile duct cancer may contribute to the male predominance of this tumor. However, a cohort study suggested an excess risk of biliary tract cancer associated with heavy alcohol drinking after adjusting for smoking (Kato et al, 1992). Although the data on tobacco and alcohol in the formation of gallstones are inconsistent, a review of available data suggests that smoking, despite its antiestrogenic effect, slightly increases the risk of symptomatic stones (Baron and Logan, 1990), whereas alcohol lowers the risk, perhaps by reducing the cholesterol saturation of bile (Diehl, 1991).

Radiation

There is little evidence that ionizing radiation causes biliary tract tumors except for the elevated risks of intrahepatic and extrahepatic bile duct cancers reported among patients injected with the X-ray diagnostic contrast medium, Thorotrast (Andersson and Storm, 1992), and a possible excess of biliary tract cancer among underground miners exposed to radon (Tomasek et al, 1993).

Genetic Factors

There are several clues to genetic determinants of biliary tract tumors in addition to the striking susceptibility of American Indians and Hispanic populations. A familial tendency to biliary tract cancer has been suggested by several case reports (Garber and Shipley, 1989) and by recent epidemiologic studies (Fernandez et al, 1994; Cannon-Albright et al, 1994), although the available data on familial occurrence are insufficient to derive relative- or population-attributable risk estimates. Reports of ethnic and familial predisposition usually extend to gallstone formation and may involve a genetic defect of cholesterol and bile acid metabolism (Cohen et al, 1992).

In hereditary polyposis of the colon, including Gardner's syndrome, up to 12% of patients develop neoplasms of the ampulla of Vater (Harned et al, 1991). An excess of these tumors also appears with hereditary nonpolyposis colon cancer (Hatch et al, 1992). To a lesser degree, tumors of the extrahepatic bile ducts may occur with polyposis coli (Walsh et al, 1987). In addition, periampullary tumors, mainly of the carcinoid type, seem to be excessive among patients with neurofibromatosis (Klein et al, 1989).

A prospective study of families affected by ataxia-telangiectasia (A-T) has revealed an excess risk of breast and certain other cancers, including the gallbladder (Swift et al, 1991). Since heterozygous carriers of the A-T gene may constitute about 1% of the general population, it will be important to test this association as soon as DNA testing can be reliably used to detect A-T heterozygotes.

Congenital Defects

Various congenital biliary anomalies such as cystic dilatation of the bile duct (choledochal cysts) have been associated with biliary tract tumors in case reports. Such occurrences were once thought to be rare, but clinical surveys have suggested a close relation to anomalous union of the pancreaticobiliary duct (APBD), raising the possibility that reflux of pancreatic juice may be an etiologic factor (Kimura et al, 1985; Yamauchi et al, 1987). A disproportionate number of these tumors are papillary adenocarcinomas with multicentric involvement of the biliary and pancreatic tracts (Morohoshi et al, 1990). Although cases are usually sporadic, a genetic component is suggested by a report of familial aggregation of APBD associated with biliary neoplasia (Miyazaki et al, 1989).

PREVENTIVE MEASURES

Although biliary tract tumors are relatively uncommon in the United States, increased rates are seen in certain areas and ethnic groups, notably American Indians and Hispanic Americans. In Mexico and other Latin American countries, gallbladder cancer accounts for 5% or more of malignant neoplasms in women and is surpassed only by cancers of the cervix, breast, and stomach (Albores-Saavedra et al, 1980). High rates are also seen in some central and eastern European countries, but it is unclear whether elevated risks extend to corresponding ethnic groups in the United States. Unlike most other tumors, there is a female preponderance of gallbladder cancer around the world, and its demographic characteristics closely resemble the patterns for cholesterol gallstones, which represent the major risk factor for gallbladder and bile duct tumors. Further studies are needed to clarify the risk estimates of biliary tract neoplasms following gallstones and to identify the factors and mechanisms contributing to the risk. The information would help in evaluating prospects for controlling these tumors, such as cholecystectomy or use of stone-dissolving agents (e.g., chenodeoxycholic acid) in treatment or even in prophylaxis among susceptible populations (Black et al, 1977; Grundy and Kalser, 1987).

However, nonsurgical approaches to gallstones such as dissolution therapy or shock-wave lithotripsy have generally been replaced by the availability of laparoscopic cholecystectomy, except for certain high-risk patients who may not tolerate laparoscopy (Johnston and Kaplan, 1993). Treatment of stones has been recommended mainly for symptomatic patients (American College of Physicians, 1993), but cholecystectomy may be indicated also for asymptomatic stones when the cancer risk is substantial (e.g., with large stones, calcified gallbladder). Cholecystectomy is effective not only in preventing gallbladder cancer but also in lowering the risk of extrahepatic bile duct cancer (Ekbom et al, 1993a). There is little question that the risk of biliary tract cancer can be reduced also by controlling the risk factors for gallstones, especially through lifestyle changes similar to those recommended for prevention of coronary heart disease (Diehl, 1991).

Further leads to the prevention of biliary tract cancer are likely to come from epidemiologic research into the nutritional, metabolic, hormonal, and genetic determinants of cholesterol stones, utilizing biomarkers whenever possible. By linking risk factors to mechanisms of stone formation (e.g., increased biliary cholesterol, decreased bile acids, destabilization and stasis of bile), it should be possible to clarify the origins of biliary tumors and the means of prevention. Further studies of gallstones may also reveal insights into the causes of more common tumors, such as colon cancer, which appears to occur in excess after cholecystectomy (Ekbom et al, 1993b).

Future etiologic studies of biliary tract cancer should carefully distinguish between cancers of the gallbladder, bile duct, and ampulla of Vater, which have important epidemiologic dissimilarities. In addition, case-control studies should consider abdominal ultrasound examinations whenever possible to help corroborate the diagnoses of tumors and stones in cases (Shea et al, 1994) and to rule out asymptomatic stones in the reference group. Since a high proportion of individuals with gallstones are unaware of the condition, ultrasonography permits more precise classification of disease status, reducing potential misclassification that may obscure associations or result in spurious findings. A major challenge is to determine how cancer risk factors differ from those of gallstones, since many people have stones but few develop cancer. Use of an additional comparison group of patients with symptomatic gallstones may help shed light on this issue.

REFERENCES

Ahlberg J, Ewerth S, Hellers G, Holmstrom B. 1978. Decreasing frequency of cholecystectomies in the counties of Stockholm and Uppsala, Sweden. Acta Chir Scand Suppl 482:21–23.

Akwari OE, Van Heerden JA, Foulk WT, Baggenstoss AH. 1975. Cancer of the bile ducts associated with ulcerative colitis. Ann Surg 181:303–309.

Albores-Saavedra J, Alcantra-Vazquez A, Cruz-Ortiz H, Herrara-Goepfert R. 1980. The precursor lesions of invasive gallbladder carcinoma: Hyperplasia, atypical hyperplasia and carcinoma in situ. Cancer 45:919–927.

American College of Physicians. 1993. Guidelines for the treatment of gallstones. Ann Intern Med 119:620–622.

Andersson M, Storm HH. 1992. Cancer incidence among Danish Thorotrast-exposed patients. J Natl Cancer Inst 84:1318–1325.

Baron JA, Logan RFA. 1990. Smoking and gallstones. In Wald N, Baron J (eds): Smoking and Hormone-Related Disorders. Oxford: Oxford University Press, pp. 103–110.

Bengmark S. 1968. Carcinoma of the gallbladder. In Engel A, Larsson T (eds): Thule International Symposium on Cancer and Aging. Stockholm: Nordiska Bokhandlns Forlag, pp. 261–270.

Bennion LJ, Grundy SM. 1978. Risk factors for the development of cholelithiasis in man. N Engl J Med 299:1161–1167, 1221–1227.

Black WC, Key CR, Carmany TB, Herman D. 1977. Carcinoma of the gallbladder in a population of southwestern American Indians. Cancer 39:1267–1279.

Blanken A. 1976. Hospital discharges and length of stay: Short-stay hospitals, United States, 1972. Vital Health Stat (1); Series 10(107):1–66.

Bond GG, McLaren EA, Sabel FL, et al. 1990. Liver and biliary tract cancer among chemical workers. Am J Ind Med 18:19–24.

Broden G, Ahlberg J, Bengtsson L, Hellers G. 1978. The incidence of carcinoma of the gallbladder and bile ducts in Sweden, 1958 to 1972. Acta Chir Scand Suppl 482:24–25.

Brown DP. 1992. Mortality of workers employed at organochlorine pesticide manufacturing plants—An update. Scand J Work Environ Health 18:155–161.

Cannon-Albright LA, Thomas A, Goldgar DE, et al. 1994. Familiality of cancer in Utah. Cancer Res 54:2378–2385.

Caygill CPJ, Hill MJ, Braddick M, Sharp JCM. 1994. Cancer mortality in chronic typhoid and paratyphoid carriers. Lancet 343:83–84.

Caygill C, Hill M, Kirkham J, Northfield TC. 1988. Increased risk of biliary tract cancer following gastric surgery. Br J Cancer 57:434–436.

Chow WH, McLaughlin JK, Menck HR, Mack TM. 1994. Risk factors for extrahepatic bile duct cancers: Los Angeles County, California (USA). Cancer Causes Control 5:267–272.

Christophi C, Hughes ER. 1985. Hepatobiliary disorders in inflammatory bowel disease. Surg Gynecol Obstet 160:187–193.

Cohen JC, Cali JJ, Jelinek DF, et al. 1992. Cloning of the human cholesterol 7α-hydroxylase gene (CYP7) and localization to chromosome 8q11-q12. Genomics 14:153–161.

Devesa SS, Silverman DT, Young JL Jr, et al. 1987. Cancer incidence and mortality trends among whites in the United States, 1947-84. J Natl Cancer Inst 79:701–770.

DIEHL AK. 1980. Epidemiology of gallbladder cancer: A synthesis of recent data. J Natl Cancer Inst 65:1209–1214.

DIEHL AK. 1983. Gallstone size and the risk of gallbladder cancer. JAMA 250:2323–2326.

DIEHL AK. 1987. Trends in cholecystectomy rates in the United States. Lancet 2:683.

DIEHL AK. 1991. Epidemiology and natural history of gallstone disease. Gastroenterol Clin North Am 20:1–19.

DIEHL AK. 1994. Increased cholecystectomy rate after introduction of laparoscopic cholecystectomy. JAMA 271:501.

DIEHL AK, BERAL V. 1981. Cholecystectomy and changing mortality from gallbladder cancer. Lancet 2:187–189.

DOWLING GP, KELLY JK. 1986. The histogenesis of adenocarcinoma of the gallbladder. Cancer 58:1702–1708.

EKBOM A, HSIEH CC, YUEN J, et al. 1993a. Risk of extrahepatic bileduct cancer after cholecystectomy. Lancet 342:1262–1265.

EKBOM A, YUEN J, ADAMI HO, et al. 1993b. Cholecystectomy and colorectal cancer. Gastroenterology 105:142–147.

EVERHART JE. 1993. Contributions of obesity and weight loss to gallstone disease. Ann Intern Med 119:1029–1035.

FERNANDEZ E, LA VECCHIA C, D'AVANZO B, et al. 1994. Family history and the risk of liver, gallbladder, and pancreatic cancer. Cancer Epidemiol Biomarkers Prev 3:209–212.

FLANIGAN DP. 1977. Biliary carcinoma associated with biliary cysts. Cancer 40:880–883.

GARBER JE, SHIPLEY W. 1989. Carcinoma of the gall bladder in three members of a family. Cancer Genet Cytogenet 39:141–142.

GARFINKEL L. 1986. Overweight and mortality. Cancer 58:1826–1829.

GOLDBERG MS, THERIAULT G. 1994. Retrospective cohort study of workers of a synthetic textiles plant in Quebec: I. General mortality. Am J Ind Med 25:889–907.

GOSSELIN SJ, KRAMER LW. 1984. Extrahepatic biliary carcinoma in sloth bears. J Am Vet Med Assoc 185:1314–1316.

GRUNDY SM, KALSER SC. 1987. Highlights of the meeting on prevention of gallstones. Hepatology 7:946–951.

GUBERAN E, USEL M, RAYMOND L, et al. 1989. Disability, mortality, and incidence of cancer among Geneva painters and electricians: A historical prospective study. Br J Ind Med 46:16–23.

GUO RX, HE SG, SHEN K. 1991. The bacteriology of cholelithiasis—China versus Japan. Jpn J Surg 21:606–612.

HAFFNER SM, DIEHL AK, STERN MP, HAZUDA HP. 1989. Central adiposity and gallbladder disease in Mexican Americans. Am J Epidemiol 129:587–595.

HARNED RK, BUCK JL, OLMSTED WW, et al. 1991. Extracolonic manifestations of the familial adenomatous polyposis syndromes. Am J Roentgenol 156:481–485.

HART J, MODAN B, SHANI M. 1971. Cholelithiasis in the aetiology of gallbladder neoplasms. Lancet 1:1151–1153.

HARTZ AJ, RUPLEY DC, RIMM AA. 1984. The association of girth measurements with disease in 32,856 women. Am J Epidemiol 119:71–80.

HATCH EE, CURTIS RE, BOICE JD, FRAUMENI JF JR. 1992. Malignant neoplasms associated with cancer of the ampulla of Vater. Br J Cancer 66:1204.

HEATON KW. 1973. The epidemiology of gallstones and suggested etiology. Clin Gastroenterol 2:67–83.

HEATON KW, EMMETT PM, SYMES CL, BRADDON FEM. 1993. An explanation for gallstones in normal-weight women: Slow intestinal transit. Lancet 341:8–10.

HENSON DE, ALBORES-SAAVEDRA J, CORLE D. 1992. Carcinoma of the gallbladder: Histologic types, stage of disease, grade, and survival rates. Cancer 70:1493–1497.

JIN F, DEVESA SS, ZHENG W, et al. 1993. Cancer incidence trends in urban Shanghai, 1972–1989. Int J Cancer 53:764–770.

JOHNSTON DE, KAPLAN MM. 1993. Pathogenesis and treatment of gallstones. N Engl J Med 328:412–421.

KAKAR F, WEISS NS, STRITE SA. 1986. Thiazide use and the risk of cholecystectomy in women. Am J Epidemiol 124:428–433.

KATO I, NOMURA AMY, STEMMERMANN GN, CHYOU PH. 1992. Prospective study of the association of alcohol with cancer of the upper aerodigestive tract and other sites. Cancer Causes Control 3:145–151.

KIMURA K, OHTO M, SAISHO H, et al. 1985. Association of gallbladder carcinoma and anomalous pancreaticobiliary ductal union. Gastroenterology 89:1258–1265.

KLEIN A, CLEMENS J, CAMERON J. 1989. Periampullary neoplasms in von Recklinghausen's disease. Surgery 106:815–819.

KRAIN LS. 1972. Gallbladder and extrahepatic bile duct carcinoma: Analysis of 1,808 cases. Geriatrics 27:111–117.

KRITZ-SILVERSTEIN D, BARRETT-CONNOR E, WINGARD DL. 1990. The relation between reproductive history and cholecystectomy in older women. J Clin Epidemiol 43:687–692.

LAMBE M, TRICHOPOULOS D, HSIEH CC, et al. 1993. Parity and cancers of the gallbladder and the extrahepatic bile ducts. Int J Cancer 54:941–944.

LANES SF, COHEN A, ROTHMAN KJ, et al. 1990. Mortality of cellulose fiber production workers. Scand J Work Environ Health 16:247–251.

LEGORRETA AP, SILBER JH, COSTANTINO GN, et al. 1993. Increased cholecystectomy rate after the introduction of laparoscopic cholecystectomy. JAMA 270:1429–1432.

LEVINE T. 1975. Chronic Cholecystitis. New York: John Wiley and Sons, pp. 207–208.

LOWENFELS AB, WALKER AM, ALTHAUS DP, et al. 1989. Gallstone growth, size, and risk of gallbladder cancer: An interracial study. Int J Epidemiol 18:50–54.

MACLURE KM, HAYES KC, COLDITZ GA, et al. 1990. Dietary predictions of symptom-associated gallstones in middle-aged women. Am J Clin Nutr 52:916–922.

MALKER HSR, MCLAUGHLIN JK, MALKER BK, et al. 1986. Biliary tract cancer and occupation in Sweden. Br J Ind Med 43:257–262.

MANCUSO TF, BRENNAN MJ. 1970. Epidemiological considerations of cancer of the gallbladder, bile ducts and salivary glands in the rubber industry. J Occup Med 12:333–341.

MARINGHINI A, MOREAU JA, MELTON LJ, et al. 1987. Gallstones, gallbladder cancer, and other gastrointestinal malignancies: An epidemiologic study in Rochester, Minnesota. Ann Intern Med 107:30–35.

MILLER BA, RIES LAG, HANKEY BF, et al (eds). 1993. SEER Cancer Statistics Review: 1973–1990. NIH Publ. No. 93-2789. Bethesda, MD: National Cancer Institute.

MILNE R, VESSEY M. 1991. The association of oral contraception with kidney cancer, colon cancer, gallbladder cancer (including extrahepatic bile duct cancer) and pituitary tumours. Contraception 43:667–693.

MIYAZAKI K, DATE K, IMAMURA S, et al. 1989. Familial occurrence of anomalous pancreaticobiliary duct union associated with gallbladder neoplasms. Am J Gastroenterol 84:176–181.

MOERMAN CJ, BUENO DE MESQUITA HB, RUNIA S. 1993. Dietary sugar intake in the aetiology of biliary tract cancer. Int J Epidemiol 22:207–214.

MOERMAN CJ, BERNS MPH, BUENO DE MESQUITA HB, RUNIA S. 1994a. Reproductive history and cancer of the biliary tract in women. Int J Cancer 57:146–153.

MOERMAN CJ, BUENO DE MESQUITA HB, RUNIA S. 1994b. Smoking, alcohol consumption and the risk of cancer of the biliary tract; a population-based case-control study in the Netherlands. Eur J Cancer Prev 3:427–436.

MOERMAN CJ, SMEETS FW, KROMHOUT D. 1994c. Dietary risk

factors for clinically diagnosed gallstones in middle-aged men: A 25-year follow-up study (the Zutphen Study). Ann Epidemiol 4: 248–254.

Morohoshi T, Kunimura T, Kanda M, et al. 1990. Multiple carcinomata associated with anomalous arrangement of the biliary and pancreatic duct system. Acta Pathol Jpn 40:755–763.

Morris DL, Buechley RW, Key CR, Morgan MV. 1978. Gallbladder disease and gallbladder cancer among American Indians in tricultural New Mexico. Cancer 42:2472–2477.

Nakajo S, Yamamoto M, Tahara E. 1990. Morphometrical analysis of gall-bladder adenoma and adenocarcinoma with reference to histogenesis and adenoma-carcinoma sequence. Virchows Arch [A] Pathol Anat Histopathol 417:49–56.

Nervi F, Duarte I, Gomez G, et al. 1988. Frequency of gallbladder cancer in Chile, a high-risk area. Int J Cancer 41:657–660.

Nutting PA, Freeman WL, Risser DR, et al. 1993. Cancer incidence among American Indians and Alaska Natives, 1980 through 1987. Am J Public Health 83:1589–1598.

Parkin DM, Muir CS, Whalen SL, et al (eds). 1992. Cancer Incidence in Five Continents, Vol VI. IARC Sci Publ. No. 120. Lyon: International Agency for Research on Cancer.

Paumgartner G, Sauerbruch T. 1991. Gallstones: pathogenesis. Lancet 338:1117–1121.

Petitti DB, Sidney S. 1988. Obesity and cholecystectomy among women: Implications for prevention. Am J Prev Med 4:327–330.

Petitti DB, Sidney S, Perlman JA. 1988. Increased risk of cholecystectomy in users of supplemental estrogen. Gastroenterology 94:91–95.

Plesko I, Somogyi J, Dimitrova E, et al. 1985a. Epidemiological features of biliary tract cancer incidence in Slovakia. Neoplasma 32:125–134.

Plesko I, Preston-Martin S, Day NE, et al. 1985b. Parity and cancer risk in Slovakia. Int J Cancer 36:529–533.

Ransohoff DF, Gracie WA. 1993. Treatment of gallstones. Ann Intern Med 119:606–619.

Richardson JD, Scutchfield FD, Proudfoot WH, Benenson AS. 1973. Epidemiology of gallbladder disease in an Appalachian community. Health Serv Rep 88:241–246.

Rios-Dalenz J, Takabayashi A, Henson DE, et al. 1985. Cancer of the gallbladder in Bolivia: Suggestions concerning etiology. Am J Gastroenterol 80:371–375.

Ritchie JK, Allan RN, Macartney J, et al. 1974. Biliary tract carcinoma associated with ulcerative colitis. Q J Med 43:263–279.

Rudnicki M, Jorgensen T, Jensen KH, and Thode J. 1993. Calcium, magnesium, and free fatty acids in the formation of gallstones: A nested case-control study. Am J Epidemiol 137:404–408.

Schwartz DA. 1986. Cholangiocarcinoma associated with liver fluke infection: A preventable source of morbidity in Asian immigrants. Am J Gastroenterol 81:76–79.

Serra I, Calvo A, Maturana M, Sharp A. 1990. Biliary-tract cancer in Chile. Int J Cancer 46:965–971.

Shea JA, Berlin JA, Escarce JJ, et al. 1994. Revised estimates of diagnostic test sensitivity and specificity in suspected biliary tract disease. Arch Intern Med 154:2573–2581.

Shukla VK, Tiwari SC, Roy SK. 1993. Biliary bile acids in cholelithiasis and carcinoma of the gall bladder. Eur J Cancer Prev 2:155–160.

So CB, Gibney RG, Scudamore CH. 1990. Carcinoma of the gallbladder: A risk associated with gallbladder-preserving treatments for cholelithiasis. Radiology 174:127–130.

Srivatanakul P, Parkin DM, Jiang YZ, et al. 1991. The role of infection by Opisthorchis viverrini, hepatitis B virus, and aflatoxin exposure in the etiology of liver cancer in Thailand. Cancer 68:2411–2417.

Stayner LT, Dannenberg AL, Bloom T, Thun M. 1993. Excess hepatobiliary cancer mortality among munitions workers exposed to dinitrotoluene. J Occup Med 35:291–296.

Strom BL, Hibberd PL, Soper KA, et al. 1985. International variations in epidemiology of cancers of the extrahepatic biliary tract. Cancer Res 45:5165–5168.

Swift M, Morrell D, Massey RB, Chase CL. 1991. Incidence of cancer in 161 families affected by ataxia-telangiectasia. N Engl J Med 325:1831–1836.

Tersmette AC, Offerhaus GJA, Giardiello FM, et al. 1990. Occurrence of non-gastric cancer in the digestive tract after remote partial gastrectomy: Analysis of an Amsterdam cohort. Int J Cancer 46:792–795.

Thamavit W, Bhamarapravati N, Sahaphong S, et al. 1978. Effects of dimethylnitrosamine on induction of cholangiocarcinoma in Opisthorchis viverrini–infected Syrian golden hamsters. Cancer Res 38:4634–4639.

Thijs C, Knipschild P. 1993. Oral contraceptives and the risk of gallbladder disease: A meta-analysis. Am J Public Health 83:1113–1120.

Tomasek L, Darby SC, Swerdlow AJ, et al. 1993. Radon exposure and cancers other than lung cancer among uranium miners in West Bohemia. Lancet 341:919–923.

Trotman BW, Soloway RD. 1982. Pigment gallstone disease: Summary of the National Institutes of Health-International workshop. Hepatology 2:879–884.

Walsh N, Qizilbash A, Banerjee R, Waugh GA. 1987. Biliary neoplasia in Gardner's syndrome. Arch Pathol Lab Med 111:76–77.

Weiss KM, Ferrell RE, Hanis CL, Styne PN. 1984. Genetics and epidemiology of gallbladder disease in New World native peoples. Am J Hum Genet 36:1259–1278.

WHO Collaborative Study of Neoplasia and Steroid Contraceptives. 1989. Combined oral contraceptives and gallbladder cancer. Int J Epidemiol 18:309–314.

Wiggins CL, Becker TM, Key CR, Samet JM. 1993. Cancer mortality among New Mexico's Hispanics, American Indians, and non-Hispanic Whites, 1958–1987. J Natl Cancer Inst 85:1670–1678.

Wong O, Whorton MD, Foliart DE, Ragland D. 1991. An industry-wide epidemiologic study of vinyl chloride workers, 1942–1982. Am J Ind Med 20:317–334.

Wyshak G, Honeyman MS, Flannery JT, Beck AS. 1983. Cancer in mothers of dizygotic twins. J Natl Cancer Inst 70:593–599.

Yamauchi S, Koga A, Matsumoto S, et al. 1987. Anomalous junction of pancreaticobiliary duct without congenital choledochal cyst: A possible risk factor for gallbladder cancer. Am J Gastroenterol 82:20–24.

Yen S, Hsieh CC, MacMahon B. 1987. Extrahepatic bile duct cancer and smoking, beverage consumption, past medical history, and oral-contraceptive use. Cancer 59:2112–2116.

Zatonski WA, La Vecchia C, Przewozniak K, et al. 1992. Risk factors for gallbladder cancer: A Polish case-control study. Int J Cancer 51:707–711.

38 Cancers of the small intestine

DAVID SCHOTTENFELD
SYED S. ISLAM

Malignant neoplasms of the small intestine are relatively rare in the United States, with an estimated 1900 cases in males and 1500 cases in females in 1992; the average annual age-adjusted incidence, 1.2 per 100,000, is about 1/50th the incidence of colorectal cancer in the United States. There are fewer than 1000 deaths each year in the United States attributed to cancers of the small intestine; the age-adjusted mortality per 100,000 (1970 U. S. standard) during 1985–1989 was 0.4 in males and 0.3 in females (Miller et al, Cancer Statistics Review, 1992). The small intestine, consisting of the duodenum, jejunum, and ileum, represents 75% of the length and 90% of the absorptive surface area of the entire gastrointestinal tract, but is the location for only 1%–3% of all gastrointestinal cancers. International age-standardized incidence rates per 100,000 for all malignant neoplasms of the small intestine varied in males from 4.2 (New Zealand:Maori) to 0.1 (Jews born in Israel); the rates in females ranged more narrowly from 2.3 (United States:Hawaiian) to 0.1 (Iceland and eastern European countries) (Parkin et al, 1992).

ANATOMY AND PATHOLOGY

The adult small intestine is an elongated tube about 12 feet (360 cm) to 22 feet (660 cm) long, its length depending in part on the tone of the muscular wall. The duodenum constitutes the proximal 25 to 30 cm, adhering to the posterior abdominal wall and encircling the head of the pancreas in a horseshoe fashion. Bile and pancreatic secretions enter the duodenum in the region of the ampulla of Vater. Unlike the fixed retroperitoneal duodenum, the jejunum and ileum are suspended by an extensive mesentery and have considerable mobility within the abdominal cavity. The jejunum constitutes the next segment and is approximately 2.5 meters in length. No specific anatomic structure serves to delineate the end of the jejunum and the beginning of the ileum, which constitutes about the distal 3.5 meters of the small intestine. The diameter of the proximal jejunum is almost twice that of the distal ileum, and its wall considerably thicker due to the circumferential mucosal and submucosal folds, the plicae circulares. The distal half of the ileum contains prominent elliptical aggregates of lymphoid follicles (Peyer's patches).

The innermost tissue layer of the small intestine is the mucosa consisting of absorptive cells and intestinal glands that line the crypts and villi. The crypt epithelium functions in cell proliferation and renewal and is comprised of Paneth, goblet, undifferentiated, and endocrine cells; the villi normally do not participate in cell renewal and proliferation but function as absorptive cells (Madara and Trier, 1987). The intestinal glandular cells give rise to adenocarcinomas, and the enteroendocrine cells, also called enterochromaffin or argentaffin cells, are the cells of origin for benign and malignant carcinoid tumors (Ashley and Wells, 1988).

Beneath the mucosa is the submucosa, consisting of dense connective tissue, sparsely infiltrated by cells, including fibroblasts, lymphocytes, macrophages, mast cells, and plasma cells. The submucosa contains lymphatic and venous plexuses, and an extensive network of arterioles, ganglion cells, and nerve fibers. The submucosa of the proximal half of the duodenum contains small islands of Brunner's glands, which contain both mucous and serous secretory cells. Beneath and within the submucosa, lymphoid nodules throughout the small intestine can give rise to malignant lymphomas. The muscularis, located beneath the serosal outer layer, is the tissue of origin for leiomyosarcomas.

INCIDENCE AND MORTALITY

The age-specific incidence rates, after age 30, increased proportionately with increasing age for adenocarcinomas, carcinoids, and lymphomas; sarcomas, including leiomyosarcomas, appeared to level off after age 70 (Fig. 38–1). The age-adjusted incidence per 100,000 (1970 U.S. standard) during 1985–1989 was 1.5 in

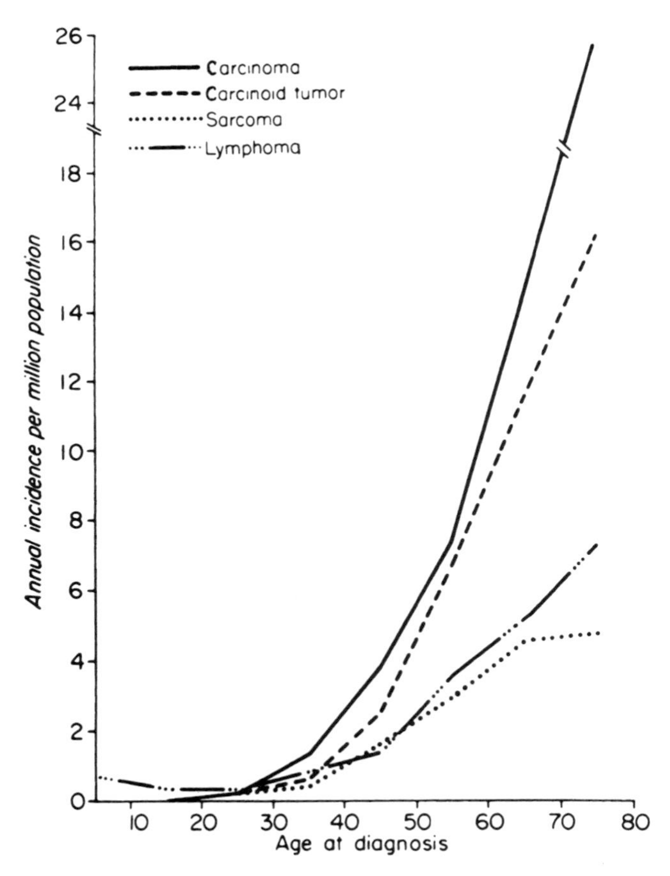

FIG. 38–1. Age-specific incidence per million population for adenocarcinoma, carcinoid, lymphoma, and sarcoma of the small intestine (Weiss and Yang, 1987).

males and 0.9 in females. The age-adjusted mortality (0.5×10^{-5}) and incidence (2.0×10^{-5}) in U.S. blacks reflected slightly higher risks compared to U.S. whites (Table 38–1). The 25-year trend of age-adjusted incidence in Connecticut since 1960 indicated for each 5-year period about a 50% excess in males compared to females, but without any indication of significant temporal variation.

TABLE 38–1. *Age-adjusted* Incidence and Mortality Rates per 100,000 Population for Cancer of the Small Intestine, Males and Females, Whites and Blacks, United States, 1985–1989*

	Whites		*Blacks*	
Small Intestine	*Males*	*Females*	*Males*	*Females*
Mortality	0.4	0.2	0.6	0.4
Incidence	1.4	0.9	2.7	1.5

*Age-adjusted to 1970 U. S. standard population.

The patterns of age-standardized international incidence rates (1983–1987) suggested that small intestinal cancer risks were generally higher in men than in women for each racial and ethnic group comparison, and somewhat higher in North American and western European countries (Fig. 38–2). Lowenfels (1973) has indicated that international incidence rates for cancer of the small intestine are positively correlated (r = +0.79) with cancer of the colon incidence rates; no correlation exists between stomach cancer and small intestinal cancer incidence rates. In Israel, the lowest rates were described for the Jews born in Israel (Table 38–2). Among the Japanese residing in the United States, the age-standardized incidence rates in males and females (Hawaii and Los Angeles) were closer to those registered in Japan (Miyagi) than in U.S. whites and blacks (Table 38–2).

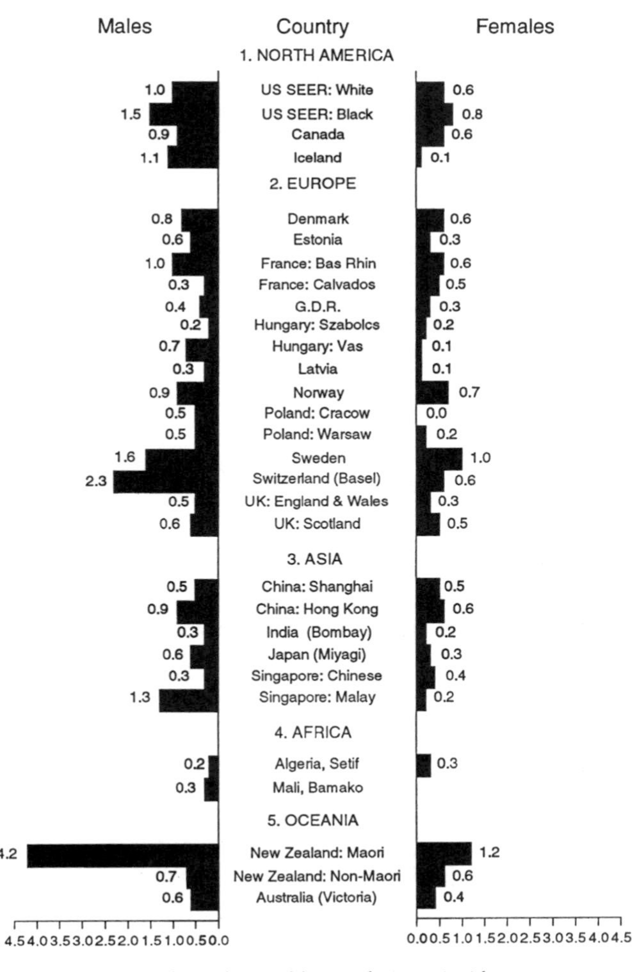

FIG. 38–2. Age-adjusted (world population) incidence rates per 100,000 population for cancer of the small intestine, males and females, selected countries, 1983–1987.

TABLE 38–2. *Age-Adjusted (World Population) Incidence Rates per 100,000 Population for Cancer of the Small Intestine, Males and Females, by Ethnicity in Selected Countries, 1983–1987*

Population	Males	Females
UNITED STATES		
Los Angeles:		
White	0.9	0.6
Spanish	0.5	0.5
Black	1.5	1.0
Japanese	0.4	0.3
Chinese	1.1	0.8
Filipino	0.2	1.0
Korean	0.7	0.8
Hawaii:		
White	0.7	0.7
Japanese	0.3	0.3
Hawaiian	0.7	2.3
Filipino	1.2	0.7
Chinese	—	0.3
ISRAEL		
All Jews:	0.4	0.4
Born in Israel	0.1	0.2
European/American	0.5	0.5
African/Asian	0.3	0.4
Non-Jews	0.4	0.4

Source: Cancer Incidence In Five Continents, Vol. VI, 1992.

RISK FACTORS AND HISTOPATHOLOGY

Adenocarcinoma

About 40%–50% of all small intestinal cancers are adenocarcinomas, with 75%–80% of the glandular neoplasms distributed in the duodenum and adjacent jejunum. The distal jejunum and proximal ileum, for unexplained reasons, are generally spared. The average annual incidence rate per 100,000 (adjusted to the 1980 U. S. population) was 0.46 in males and 0.33 in females (Weiss and Yang, 1987).

Adenoma. Adenomas of the small intestine are premalignant lesions (Sellner, 1990). Three types of adenomas are found in the small intestine: Brunner's gland in the submucosa of the duodenum, islet-cell, and polypoid. Most adenomatous polyps occur in the periampullary region of the duodenum, where bile and pancreatic secretions enter the small intestine, and proximal jejunum. As in the colon, the risk of adenocarcinoma increases in relation to increasing polyp size, the predominance of villous features, and the extent of epithelial dysplasia.

Gastrointestinal polyposis refers to the presence of multiple polypoid lesions throughout the gastrointestinal tract. Familial adenomatous polyposis (FAP) and Gardner's syndrome are attributed to a germ line mutation or deletion in the 5q21-q22 chromosomal region (Groden et al, 1991). The FAP locus is adjacent to the "mutated in colorectal cancer" (MCC) gene, which appears as a somatic cell mutation in sporadic colorectal cancer. Colorectal cancer is generally considered an inevitable consequence in the natural history of FAP, appearing 10 to 15 years after the clinical diagnosis of polyposis. Polyps are present in the upper gastrointestinal tract in nearly all FAP patients. The duodenum, and in particular the periampullary region, may contain multiple adenomas; in such patients, the prevalence of adenocarcinoma may be as high as 10% to 15% (MacDonald et al, 1967; Bussey, 1990; Melmed and Bouchier, 1972; Qizilbash, 1976).

Peutz-Jeghers syndrome is an example of a familial hamartomatous polyposis syndrome in which there is an increased risk of adenocarcinoma of the small intestine (Dozois et al, 1969). Peutz-Jeghers syndrome consists of mucocutaneous pigmentation and gastrointestinal polyposis. The syndrome appears to be inherited as a single pleiotropic autosomal dominant gene with variable penetrance. The gene for this syndrome has not been identified. The histological framework for the Peutz-Jeghers polyp consists of a central core of broad bands of smooth muscle that are contiguous with the muscularis mucosae. The melanin deposits in the syndrome are distributed around the mouth, nose, lips, buccal mucosa, hands, feet, and the anogenital region. While the Peutz-Jeghers polyps are not true adenomas, carcinomas in the small intestine may arise from foci of adenomatous epithelium. The cumulative lifetime incidence of small intestinal adenocarcinomas in Peutz-Jeghers patients has been estimated as 2.4%. In addition, the gene for Peutz-Jeghers syndrome confers an increased risk of breast cancer and ovarian germ cell tumors in young women; Sertoli cell testicular tumors with feminizing features in young boys; and polyps and carcinomas in the biliary tree, gallbladder, and pancreas (Giardello et al, 1987; Konishi et al, 1989; Spigelman et al, 1990).

The risk of a metachronous primary adenocarcinoma in the large intestine was found to be significantly increased in patients with an index primary adenocarcinoma in the small intestine. The Standardized Incidence Ratio (SIR) was 5.0 (95% C.I., 2.3–9.4) in men, and 3.7 (95% C.I., 1.3–8.0) in women. The relative risks were mutually increased; in men with colorectal cancer, the SIR for adenocarcinoma in the small intestine was 7.1 (95% C.I., 4.7–10.3), and in women with colorectal cancer, the SIR for adenocarcinoma in the small intestine was 9.0 (6.0–12.9). There were no apparent associations between adenocarcinoma in the small intestine and second primary cancers in the stomach, female breast, ovary, or endometrium (Neugut and Santos, 1993). Adenocarcinoma of the small intestine has been reported in members of families with Lynch syndrome II, or hereditary nonpolyposis colorectal cancer (Lynch et al, 1989).

Regional Enteritis (Crohn's Disease). Inflammatory bowel disease (IBD) includes two related but clinically and histologically separate entities: ulcerative colitis (UC) and Crohn's disease (CD), also classified as regional enteritis or enterocolitis. CD is a chronic, recurrent transmural inflammation of the alimentary tract that usually affects the ileum, colon, and/or perianal region. The transmural inflammatory process commonly begins with focal microscopic mucosal crypt abscesses. The focal lesions are accompanied by an inflammatory response and the aggregation of macrophages, lymphocytes, and plasma cells. Progression of the disease is accompanied by segmental ulcerations, fissures, and fistulae, and subsequently by fibrotic thickening of the intestinal wall and its mesentery with regional narrowing of the lumen.

While CD may affect any segment of the gastrointestinal tract, the most common anatomic distributions are small intestine alone (30% to 40%), both small and large intestine (40% to 55%), and large intestine alone (15% to 25%). In those patients with CD involving the small intestine, the terminal ileum will be affected in at least 90%. The determination of the true incidence of CD may be problematic because of the delay between onset of symptoms and the date of clinical diagnosis; the absence of population-based registration data; and the potential for misclassification or in distinguishing CD from other inflammatory or noninfectious diseases of the small bowel. Both CD and UC incidence rates are highest in the United States, Canada, northern and western European countries, American- or European-born Jews rather than Israeli-born Jews, and in the Caucasian populations of Australia, New Zealand, and South Africa. The estimated age-standardized annual incidence of CD ranges from 1 to 15 per 100,000; the primary, peak age-specific interval is 15–35 years, and is similar in males and females.

Many family studies have shown a significantly elevated risk of CD among the relatives of patients with IFB. Studies of familial aggregation, in monozygotic twin pairs, and of genetic immunologic markers underscore genetic influences in CD. Siblings of patients with CD are 20–30 times more likely to develop CD than siblings of the general population. Many of the extraintestinal manifestations of IBD, (i.e., sclerosing cholangitis, ankylosing spondylitis—especially in conjunction with the HLA-B27 haplotype, and erythema nodosum) suggest that immune mechanisms are important in disease pathogenesis. The early events in the mucosa and submucosa of CD appear to represent an impaired ability to regulate immune mechanisms that accompany the inflammatory response to the luminal stream of microbial, dietary, and other exogenous antigens (Kornbluth et al, 1993).

Adenocarcinomas in the small intestine and colon occur with increased frequency in patients with CD (Fielding et al, 1972; Greenstein et al, 1980; Hawker et al, 1982; Richards et al, 1989). In comparing de novo adenocarcinomas in the small intestine, carcinomas associated with Crohn's disease: occur at a younger mean age, or after an average interval of follow-up of 15–20 years; occur predominantly in the terminal ileum or generally in areas where CD has been active for many years; tend to be multifocal; and in approximately 30% to 40% of the total of reported cases the carcinomas developed in surgically excluded or by-passed segments of small intestine. Although the incidence of adenocarcinoma of the small intestine is rare, the relative risk in patients with CD is increased more than 10-fold (Lightdale et al, 1975; Nesbit et al, 1976; Korelitz, 1983).

Carcinoid

The second most commonly reported cancer in the small intestine is the carcinoid tumor, or the argentaffinoma. The average annual incidence rate per 100,000 (adjusted to the 1980 U. S. population) is 0.33 in males and 0.26 in females (Weiss and Yang, 1987). Malignant carcinoid tumors account for approximately 35% of all malignant neoplasms in the small intestine; 90% of the carcinoid tumors of the small intestine originate in the ileum, and in at least one-third of the patients are multicentric (Gabos et al, 1993). The production of serotonin by the neoplastic cells, and the urinary excretion of its metabolite, 5-hydroxyindoleacetic acid, represent an important biologic marker for recurrent tumor growth and metastatic disease. The carcinoid tumor is classified as a neuroendocrine tumor with the capability of producing biogenic amines and polypeptide hormones.

Lymphoma

Lymphomas of the small intestine, which are less common than gastric lymphomas, must be evaluated carefully to determine if the tumor has originated in the small intestine or whether the small intestine is involved secondarily in conjunction with disseminated disease. The average annual incidence rate per 100,000 (adjusted to the 1980 U. S. population) is 0.22 in males and 0.12 in females (Weiss and Yang, 1987). In Western industrialized nations, 15%–30% of all small bowel cancers are classified as non-Hodgkin's and Hodgkin's lymphomas, in contrast to less than 0.5% of colon cancers. The small intestine is the most common site of origin for extranodal immunoproliferative lymphoma, which has been described in the Arabs and Jews in the Middle East (Mediterranean lymphoma) and North Africa, and in South African blacks. Mediterranean lymphoma, an immunoblastic B-cell lymphoma, is commonly associated with clonal expression of Ig A heavy chain immunoglobulin, macroscopic presentation in the jejunum or duodenum, and the occurrence in patients who are 10–29 years of age (Al-Saleem and Al-Bahrani, 1973; Isaacson et al, 1979).

The pathologic classification of small intestinal non-Hodgkin's lymphomas (NHL) consists of diffuse histiocytic (B-cell diffuse large cell lymphoma more commonly than immunoblastic), lymphocytic, and mixed types. Primary Hodgkin's disease of the small intestine accounts for less than 3% of all small bowel lymphomas (Freeman et al, 1977).

An increased incidence of NHL has been observed among patients with acquired immunodeficiency syndrome (AIDS), which may be manifested as a systemic disease or as a primary extranodal lymphoma, as, for example, gastrointestinal lymphoma. NHL in AIDS patients is usually classified as poorly differentiated, diffuse B-cell lymphoma. The molecular basis for AIDS-associated lymphoma, in a number of instances, is distinguished by rearrangement of the *c-myc* proto-oncogene and DNA integration of the lymphotropic Epstein-Barr virus (Lister and Armitage, 1995).

Celiac sprue or gluten-sensitive enteropathy is characterized by blunting and clubbing of the villous mucosal folds of the small intestine, lymphoid and plasma cell infiltration of the lamina propria, and hyperplasia of the crypt epithelium. These architectural distortions decrease the mucosal surface area and functional activity of mucosal enzymes that are normally available for digestion and absorption. Celiac sprue usually affects the proximal small intestine to a greater degree than the ileum. The interaction of the water-insoluble, alcohol-soluble, gluten fractions of proteins of cereal grains, namely, of wheat, barley, and rye, with the mucosa of the small intestine is fundamental in the pathogenesis of celiac sprue. Possible mechanisms for the clinical and pathologic sequelae of the gluten interaction with the intestinal mucosa are enzyme deficiency with incomplete digestion of toxic products (prolamins) of grains such as the gliadins in wheat that are damaging to a susceptible mucosa; toxicity mediated by a lectinlike interaction between toxic products of gluten and intestinal cells due to abnormal glycosylation of epithelial cell apical membrane glycoproteins; and genetically determined, antibody and cell-mediated aberrant immune responses resulting in the overproduction of cytokines and activated T lymphocytes. The class I histocompatibility antigen, HLA-B8, and the class II histocompatibility antigens, HLA-DR3 and HLA-DQw2, are associated with 60% to 90% of celiac sprue patients, compared with 20% or less in normal controls, studied in the United States and northern Europe. There is little evidence that celiac sprue represents an inherited or constitutive metabolic disorder of peptidases important in the digestion of gluten products. However, with respect to the consideration of immunologic, genetic, and environmental (e.g., dietary) factors, it has been hypothesized that a specific "trigger" may be an infectious agent, with homology to the antigenic determinants in gluten. (Trier, 1993).

Patients with celiac sprue are at increased risk of T-cell lymphomas, and possibly adenocarcinomas, in the small intestine (Petreshock et al, 1975; Brandt et al, 1978; Swanson et al, 1983; Trier, 1993). Holmes et al (1976) evaluated a cohort of 202 patients with celiac sprue, and after more than 30 years of follow-up, observed that 12 patients (5.9%) developed small intestinal histiocytic lymphomas.

SMALL INTESTINAL CARCINOGENESIS: THE INFREQUENCY OF ADENOCARCINOMAS

Although adenocarcinoma is the most common histopathologic subgroup of the malignant neoplasms occurring in the small intestine, the incidence in Western industrialized nations is about 1/50th the incidence of colorectal cancer. International patterns of age-standardized incidence rates indicate that the risks of small intestinal and colorectal cancers are positively correlated (Lowenfels, 1973). Per capita consumption of animal protein and fat are positively correlated (+0.61) with international age-standardized small intestinal and colorectal cancer incidence rates (Chow et al, 1993). The risks of second primary adenocarcinomas of the small intestine and of the large intestine are mutually increased (Neugut and Santos, 1993). These observations would suggest that there are common causal determinants for adenocarcinomas, and for the precursor lesions (e.g., adenomas and dysplasias), throughout the intestinal tract. In advancing a unifying hypothesis that accounts for contrasting mucosal susceptibilities, the biochemistry and microbial flora of the fecal stream, enterohepatic bile acid metabolism, mucosal cell proliferation kinetics and intestinal motility will be reviewed.

The contents of the small intestine remain liquid throughout, and then beyond the ileum, the luminal contents become increasingly dehydrated and more concentrated. Transit time through the small intestine is generally much faster per unit length than through the large intestine, which may further limit the exposure of the lining epithelium of the small intestine to ingested mutagens and carcinogens. The peristaltic "ring" contractions in the small intestine occur with greater frequency per unit time in the duodenum, and then progressively diminish in the jejunum and ileum. Overall transit time in the large intestine is slow. It may require as long as one week for solid radiopaque markers to pass through the colon. The principal points of delay are in the cecum and ascending colon, and in the sigmoid colon and rectum (Christensen, 1993).

The epithelial cells lining the mucosal crypts of the small and large intestine are rapidly proliferating. Mitoses are not seen normally in the absorptive cells of small intestinal villi or colorectal surface epithelium. As new progenitor cells are formed within the crypts, they migrate to and terminally differentiate at the level of villous tips in the small intestine, or onto the flat absorptive surface in the colon, after a 4- to 7-day proliferation and maturation cycle throughout the intestinal tract. Because of this significant regenerative potential, the intestinal epithelium is potentially susceptible to damage by genotoxic agents. Given the similarities in the dynamics of cell renewal in the small and large intestine, the contrasting cancer incidence patterns requires consideration of other microecologic and metabolic differences (Lipkin and Higgins, 1988).

The small intestine normally contains relatively small numbers of bacteria. When bacteria are present, they are usually lactobacilli and enterococci, gram-positive aerobes, or facultative anaerobes that are present in concentrations not exceeding 10,000 viable organisms per gram of jejunal contents. Anaerobic bacteroides organisms do not reside in the proximal small intestine. The pH in the jejunum is around 6.0–7.0, but is maintained above 7.0 in the distal ileum. The pH of the cecum is generally around 6.8–7.3. In the ileum, the concentration of microorganisms increases up to levels of one billion organisms per gram of contents. Strict anaerobes, which normally cannot survive in the jejunum, frequently colonize the ileum at concentrations around one million organisms per gram of contents. Beyond the ileocecal valve, the bacerial flora of the large intestine increase up to one millionfold and are composed of anaerobic organisms such as bacteroides and clostridia, which outnumber aerobic and facultative organisms by 10,000:1 (Wilkins et al, 1983; Venitt, 1988).

The intestinal anaerobic microorganisms generate various metabolic enzymes, such as beta-glucuronidases, sulfatases, reductases, and decarboxylases, which act, for example, on cholesterol, bile acids, fatty acids, androgens, and estrogens substrates. Dietary fat increases the metabolic activity of gut bacteria and bile acid secretion (Reddy and Ohmori, 1981). The pathogenic mechanism of metabolic activation of ingested chemicals by the indigenous intestinal bacterial flora, and their conversion to mutagens or electrophilic molecules, has been derived mainly from animal studies. In such studies, the rate of chemically induced tumor development in germ-free and antibiotic-treated rodents is compared with that in untreated rodents. For example, cycasin, methylazoxymethanol (MAM) glucoside, found in Cycadeceae plants, is not tumorigenic when given parenterally or orally to germ-free rats (Laquer, 1964). However, when fed orally to rats with normal intestinal microflora, less than 50% of the conjugated compound was recovered in the feces and urine, and adenocarcinomas appeared in the large intestine, liver, biliary passages, and kidney (Bull et al, 1979). Microbial beta-glucosidase converts cycasin to MAM, an active mutagen that is tumorigenic. Tumor induction by dimethylhydrazine (DMH) and 2,3′-dimethyl 4-aminobiphenyl is enhanced by the beta-glucuronidase enzymatic activity of intestinal bacteria (Weisburger and Fiala, 1983). The increased risk of adenocarcinoma of the small intestine in patients with Crohn's disease occurring in segments of surgically bypassed loops of chronically inflamed ileum is attributed to stagnation of intestinal contents accompanied by bacterial multiplication (Kornbluth et al, 1993).

Bile acids are the water-soluble end products of cholesterol metabolism that are essential for lipid digestion and absorption in the proximal small intestine. More than 90% of the bile acids discharged into the duodenum are absorbed in the terminal segment of the ileum, transported in the portal venous blood back to the liver, extracted by the liver, and then resecreted into bile (Hofmann, 1977, 1993). The active transport mechanism in the terminal ileum is specific and efficient for unconjugated bile acids but is inefficient in the absorption of glucuronide, sulfate, and glycine conjugates of bile acids. The primary bile acids formed from cholesterol in the liver are the 3,7 dihydroxy derivative, chenodeoxycholic acid, and cholic acid (3,7,12 trihydroxy bile acid).

The bile acids that are not absorbed in the terminal ileum enter the cecum by passing through the ileocecal valve. In the cecum, the anaerobic bacterial enzymes dehydrogenate the hydroxy substituents at the 3, 7, and 12 positions on the primary bile acids. The 7-dehydroxylation of cholic acid results in the formation of deoxycholic acid, and 7-dehydroxylation of chenodeoxycholic acid results in the formation of lithocholic acid. These secondary bile acids formed by the action of colonic bacteria may be passively absorbed from the colon, to some degree, and recycled with the primary bile acids. However, bacterial deconjugation in the colon of residual bile acids results in the fecal passage of unconjugated secondary bile acids. In experimental animal models, the unconjugated secondary bile acids act as potent promoters of colonic carcinogenesis (Ross et al, 1991). These pathophysiologic interrelationships will be discussed in more detail in the chapter on the large intestine.

REFERENCES

AL-SALEEM T, AL-BAHRANI Z. 1973. Malignant lymphoma of the small intestine in Iraq (Middle East lymphoma). Cancer 31:291–294.

ASHLEY SW, WELLS SA JR. 1988. Tumors of the small intestine. Semin Oncol 15:115–128.

BRANDT L, HAGANDER B, NORDEN A, et al. 1978. Lymphoma of the small intestine in adult celiac disease. Acta Med Scand 204:467–470.

BULL AW, BURD AD, NIGRO ND. 1979. Promotion of azoxymethane-induced intestinal cancer by high fat diets in rats. Cancer Res 39:4956–4959.

BUSSEY HJR. 1990. Historical developments in familial adenomatous polyposis. *In* Herrera L (ed): Familial Adenomatous Polyposis, New York, Alan R Liss, pp. 1–7.

CHOW W-H, LINET MS, MCLAUGHLIN JK, et al. 1993. Risk factors for small intestine cancer. Cancer Causes Control 4:163–169.

CHRISTENSEN J. 1993. Motility of the intestine. *In* Sleisenger MH, Fordtran JS (eds): Gastrointestinal Disease Pathophysiology/Diagnosis/Management, 5th ed. Philadelphia, W. B. Saunders, pp. 822–837.

DOZOIS RR, JUDD ES, DAHLIN DC, et al. 1969. The Peutz-Jeghers syndrome. Is there a predisposition to the development of intestinal malignancy? Arch Surg 98:509–515.

FIELDING JR, PRIOR P, WATERHOUSE JA, et al. 1972. Malignancy in Crohn's disease. Scand J Gastroenterol 7:3–7.

FREEMAN HJ, WEINSTEIN WM, SHNITKA TK, et al. 1977. Primary abdominal lymphoma. Am J Med 63:585–594.

GABOS S, BERKEL J, BAND P, et al. 1993. Small bowel cancer in western Canada. Int J Epidemiol 22:198–206.

GIARDELLO FM, WELSH SB, HAMILTON SD, et al. 1987. Increased risk of cancer in the Peutz-Jeghers syndrome. N Engl J Med 316:1511–1514.

GREENSTEIN AJ, SACHAR DB, SMITH H, et al. 1980. Patterns of neoplasia in Crohn's disease and ulcerative colitis. Cancer 46:403–407.

GRODEN J, THLIVERIS A, SAMOWITZ W, et al. 1991. Identification and characterization of the familial adenomatous polyposis coli gene. Cell 66:589–600.

HAWKER PC, GYDE SN, THOMPSON H, et al. 1982. Adenocarcinoma of the small intestine complicating Crohn's disease. Gut 23:188–193.

HOFMANN AF. 1977. The enterohepatic circulation of bile acids in man. Clin Gastroenterol 6:3–24.

HOFMANN AF. 1993. The enterohepatic circulation of bile acids in health and disease. *In* Sleisenger MH, Fordtran JS (eds): Gastrointestinal Disease Pathophysiology/Diagnosis/Management, 5th ed. Philadelphia, W. B. Saunders, pp. 127–150.

HOLMES GKT, STOKES PL, SORAHAN TM, et al. 1976. Celiac disease, gluten-free diet, and malignancy. Gut 17:612–619.

ISAACSON P, WRIGHT DH, JUDD MA, et al. 1979. Primary gastrointestinal lymphomas. Cancer 43:1805–1819.

KONISHI F, WYSE NE, MUTO T, et al. 1989. Peutz-Jeghers polyposis associated with carcinoma of the digestive organs. Dis Colon Rectum 30:790–799.

KORELITZ BI. 1983. Carcinoma of the intestinal tract in Crohn's disease: Results of a survey conducted by the National Foundation for Ileitis and Colitis. Am J Gastroenterol 78:44–46.

KORNBLUTH A, SALOMON P, SACHAR DB. 1993. Crohn's disease. *In* Sleisenger MH, Fordtran JS (eds): Gastrointestinal Disease Pathophysiology/Diagnosis/Management, 5th ed. Philadelphia, W. B. Saunders, pp. 1270–1292.

LAQUER GL. 1964. Carcinogenic effects of cycad meal and cycasin, methylazoxymethanol glycoside, in rats and effects of cycasin in germfree rats. Fed Proc 23:1386–1387.

LIGHTDALE CJ, STERNBERG SS, POSNER G, et al. 1975. Carcinoma complicating Crohn's disease. Report of seven cases and a review of the literature. Am J Med 59:262–268.

LIPKIN M, HIGGINS P. 1988. Biological markers of cell proliferation and differentiation in human gastrointestinal diseases. Adv Cancer Res 50:1–24.

LISTER TA, ARMITAGE JO. 1995. Non-Hodgkin's lymphomas. *In* Abeloff MD, Armitage JO, Lichter AS, Niederhuber JE (eds): Clinical Oncology, New York, Churchill Livingstone, pp. 2109–2147.

LOWENFELS AB. 1973. Why are small bowel tumors so rare? Lancet 1:24–26.

LYNCH HT, SMYRK TC, LYNCH PM, et al. 1989. Adenocarcinoma of the small bowel in Lynch syndrome II. Cancer 64:2178–2183.

MACDONALD JM, DAVIS WC, CRAGO HR, et al. 1967. Gardner's syndrome and periampullary malignancy. Am J Surg 113:425–430.

MADARA JL, TRIER JS. 1987. Functional morphology of the mucosa of the small intestine. *In* Johnson LR (ed): Physiology of the Gastrointestinal Tract, 2nd ed. New York, Raven Press, pp. 1209–1249.

MELMED RN, BOUCHIER IAD. 1972. Duodenal involvement in Gardner's syndrome. Gut 13:524–527.

MILLER BA, RIES LAG, HANKEY BF, et al. 1992. Cancer Statistics Review: 1973–1989, National Cancer Institute. NIH Pub. No. 92-2789.

NESBIT RR, ELBADAW NA, MORTON JH, et al. 1976. Carcinoma of the small bowel. A complication of regional enteritis. Cancer 37:2948–2959.

NEUGUT AI, SANTOS J. 1993. The associations between cancers of the small and large bowel. Cancer Epidemiol Biomarkers Prev 2:551–553.

PARKIN DM, MUIR CS, WHELAN SL. 1992. Cancer Incidence in Five Continents, Vol. VI. IARC Scientific Publications No. 120, Lyon.

PETRESHOCK EP, PESSAH M, MENACHEMI E. 1975. Adenocarcinoma of the jejunum associated with nontropical sprue. Am J Dig Dis 20:796–802.

QIZILBASH AH. 1976. Familial polyposis coli and periampullary carcinoma. Can J Surg 19:166–168.

REDDY BS, OHMORI T. 1981. Effect of intestinal microflora and dietary fat on 3,2′-dimethyl-4-aminobiphenyl-induced colon carcinogenesis in F344 rats. Cancer Res 41:1363–1367.

RICHARDS ME, RICKERT RR, NANCE FC. 1989. Crohn's disease-associated carcinoma. Ann Surg 209:764–773.

ROSS RK, HARTNETT NM, BERNSTEIN L, et al. 1991. Epidemiology of adenocarcinomas of the small intestine: Is bile a small bowel carcinogen? Br J Cancer 63:143–145.

SELLNER F. 1990. Investigations on the significance of the adenoma-carcinoma sequence in the small bowel. Cancer 66:702–715.

SPIGELMAN AD, MURDAY V, PHILLIPS RKS. 1990. Cancer and the Peutz-Jeghers syndrome. Gut 30:1588–1590.

SWANSON CM, SLAVIN G, COLES EC, et al. 1983. Celiac disease and malignancy. Lancet 1:111–115.

TRIER JS. 1993. Celiac sprue. *In* Sleisenger MH, Fordtran JS (eds): Gastrointestinal Disease Pathophysiology/Diagnosis/Management, 5th ed. Philadelphia, W. B. Saunders, pp. 1078–1096.

VENITT S. 1988. Mutagens in human feces and cancer of the large bowel. *In* Venitt S (ed): Role of the Gut Flora in Toxicity and Cancer. New York, Academic Press, pp. 399–460.

WEISBURGER JH, FIALA ES. 1983. Experimental colon carcinogens and their mode of action. *In* Autrup H, Williams GM (eds): Experimental Colon Carcinogenesis. Boca Raton, CRC Press, pp. 27–50.

WEISS NS, YANG CT. 1987. Incidence of histologic types of cancer of the small intestine. J Natl Cancer Inst 78:653–656.

WILKINS TD, VAN TASSELL RL. 1983. Bacterial mutagens in the human colon. *In* Hentges DJ (ed): Human Intestinal Microflora in Health and Disease. New York, Academic Press, pp. 265–288.

39 Cancers of the large intestine

DAVID SCHOTTENFELD
SYDNEY J. WINAWER

Cancer of the large intestine accounted for 13%–15% of all incident cancers in the United States, or approximately 152,000 cases in 1993. Colorectal cancer is the second most common cancer in women (after breast cancer) and the third most frequently occurring cancer in men (after cancer of the prostate and lung). When the vital statistics for women and men are combined, cancer of the large intestine is second only to lung cancer as the leading cause of cancer mortality. The average annual age-adjusted colonic cancer incidence per 100,000 in the United States for 1985–1989 was 34% higher in males (41.9), when compared as a ratio of rates with that in females (31.3); the male predominance was more evident for rectal cancer incidence (73%) (Table 39–1). In the late 1980s, the lifetime probability of developing colorectal cancer was estimated to be 6.0% for women and 6.2% for men. The estimation of lifetime probability is based upon lifetable projections of current annual age-, sex-, site-specific incidence rates and consideration of competing causes of death that serve to remove individuals from subsequent risks of developing cancer. By way of comparison, the cumulative lifetime risk of developing invasive cancer in the total of anatomic sites and tissues was estimated to be 39.2% for women and 42.5% for men. Between 1973 and 1985, the age-adjusted incidence of colorectal cancer in the United States increased relatively by about 19% in males (Fig. 39–1); during the subsequent 5-year interval (1985–1989), the incidence declined by 6%. For females, the incidence of colorectal cancer increased by 9% during 1973–1985; then, during 1985–1989, it declined by almost 10% (National Cancer Institute, 1992).

ANATOMIC DISTRIBUTION

The average length of the adult large intestine is 4 feet to 5 feet. More than half of all colonic cancers occur either in the sigmoid (35%) or cecum (22%). The distribution throughout the remaining colon is as follows: ascending colon (12%), transverse colon (10%), and descending colon (7%). The incidence of colonic cancer (36.2 per 100,000) in the United States is about $2\frac{1}{2}$ times that reported for rectal cancer (14.6 per 100,000). Within the large intestine, 69% of cancers are in the colon and 31% are in the rectum and rectosigmoid junction.

Internationally, there is a positive correlation between the age-adjusted incidence of colonic and rectal cancer (correlation coefficient exceeds 0.85 for males and females). Countries in which colonic cancer incidence is high demonstrate a relatively higher proportion of sigmoid cancers, whereas in countries with a lower incidence, cancers of the cecum and ascending colon predominate. In countries with low incidence rates of colorectal cancer, the incidence of colonic cancer is lower than that of rectal cancer because of a deficit in the incidence of sigmoid cancer (Ziegler et al, 1986).

The distribution of neoplasms in the large intestine may also be viewed as either right-sided (i.e., including cecum, ascending colon, hepatic flexure, and transverse colon) or left-sided (i.e., including splenic flexure, descending colon, sigmoid, rectosigmoid, and rectum). DeJong et al (1972) in their examination of the subsite distribution of cancers of the large intestine in various populations, described the male preponderance at ages above 65 years for neoplasms in the left side, including the rectum, and the female preponderance at ages below 65 years for all subsites in the colon, but excluding the rectum. In a similar analysis based upon the population-based Danish Cancer Registry, Jensen (1984) reported that the male:female ratio of age-standardized incidence rates increased in relation to the more distal location of left-sided lesions.

In an analysis of the anatomic distribution of carcinomas diagnosed throughout the large intestine based upon information from the Connecticut Tumor Registry, Snyder et al (1977) reported that the proportion of colorectal cancers occurring in the right colon increased gradually over the period 1940–1973. During the period 1940–1944, 26% of tumors were located in the cecum, ascending colon, and transverse colon, and 74% in the descending colon, sigmoid colon, and rectum. During the period 1970–1973, left-sided lesions de-

TABLE 39–1. *Average Annual Age-Adjusted* Incidence per 100,000 Population, for Colorectal Cancer, All Races, United States, 1985–1989*

	Incidence†		
	Males	Females	Male/Female
Colon and rectum	60.8	42.3	1.44
Colon	41.9	31.3	1.34
Rectum	19.0	11.0	1.73

*Age-adjusted to 1970 United States standard population.
†SEER, National Cancer Institute, Cancer Stat Rev.

creased proportionally to 66%. The analysis of the Connecticut experience has been updated by Vukasin et al (1990), who have questioned the appropriateness in various studies of interpreting the true magnitude of a left-to-right shift based upon the proportional distribution of lesions without concomitant measurements of temporal trends in site-specific incidence rates.

During the period 1935–1985 in Connecticut, the age-adjusted annual incidence of cancers of the cecum and ascending colon increased from 3.6 to 16.7 per 100,000 in men, and from 4.9 to 14.2 per 100,000 in women; during the same time period, the annual incidence of cancer of the sigmoid colon increased from 8.8 to 18.7 per 100,000 in men, and from 7.7 to 12.8 per 100,000 in women. While the age-adjusted incidence of colonic cancer in Connecticut increased proportionally for right-sided and sigmoid lesions, the rates for cancers of the descending colon and rectum did not change significantly over a 50-year period.

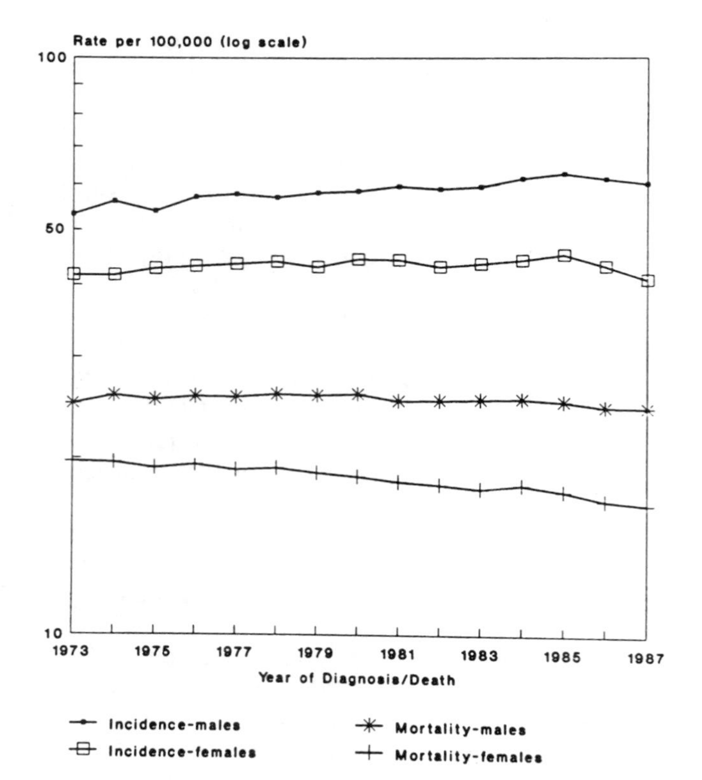

FIG. 39–1. Cancer of the colon and rectum. Age-adjusted (1970 Standard) SEER incidence and U. S. mortality rates per 100,000 by sex, 1973–1987.

INCIDENCE AND MORTALITY IN THE UNITED STATES

The age-adjusted colorectal cancer mortality (per 100,000) in the United States for 1985–1989 was highest in black males (27.6) and exceeded by 33% the mortality in black females (20.8); the corresponding rate in white males (24.2) exceeded by 48% the mortality in white females (16.4). The incidence rates for colorectal cancer were similar for white (61.0) and black males (60.5). The male:female age-adjusted colorectal cancer incidence ratios exceeded 1.0 by 30% in blacks and by 45% in whites (Table 39–2).

During the period 1973–1989, colorectal cancer mortality decreased by 20% in white females and by 8.5% in white males; in contrast, mortality increased in black males by 22.5%, and by 2.6% in black females. For whites, the decreases in mortality rates occurred in all age groups, except in the age group, 85 and above. For blacks, only females under 65 years of age showed a decrease in mortality, which was most evident over the period, 1985–1989. The mortality rate for cancer of the rectum, including the rectosigmoid junction, decreased among each of the four race-gender subgroups, and particularly in those 70 and above. One important caveat in reporting rectal cancer mortality trends in the United States is that there is substantial misclassification of sigmoid colon versus rectum (including rectosigmoid junction) on the death certificate. The rectosigmoid junction is located at or above the peritoneal reflection, or approximately 15 cm from the anal orifice. The surgeon generally locates the junction at the level of the lower margin of the sacral promontory; at this junction, the mucosa changes, becoming smoother in the rectum. An analysis by Percy et al (1981) indicated that as a result of inaccuracies in certification, the mortality rate for colonic cancer is generally overestimated, and that for can-

TABLE 39–2. *Average Annual Age-Adjusted* Mortality and Incidence per 100,000 Population for Colorectal Cancer, Whites and Blacks, Males and Females, United States, 1985–1989†*

	Whites		Blacks	
Colon and Rectum	Males	Females	Males	Females
Mortality	24.2	16.4	27.6	20.8
Incidence	61.0	42.1	60.5	46.4

*Age-adjusted to 1970 United States standard population.
†SEER, National Cancer Institute.

cer of the rectum and rectosigmoid is generally underestimated by approximately 30%. In evaluating the accuracy of death certificates in the United States, Chow and Devesa (1992) compared each death certificate with the codified information of the SEER registry. The authors estimated that during 1980–1986, deaths from colonic cancer were overreported by 26%, and those from rectal cancer were underreported by 53%. As a result, the reported decline in rectal cancer mortality between 1950 and 1988 (−65%) was, after correcting for underreporting, reduced by about one-half (−31%). In contrast to the mortality trends just described for cancer of the rectum, the age-standardized incidence rates for cancer of the rectum have been quite stable in the four race-gender subgroups since 1973, which does underscore the cogency of reporting mortality trends for colon and rectum combined. However, as emphasized by Funkhouser and Cole (1992), even after assuming significant misclassification bias, there has been a residual real decline in the mortality rate for cancer of the rectum, which may have resulted in part from improved survival. From the early 1960s through the 1980s, the relative 5-year survival rate, combining all stages, has increased from 38% to 55% for white patients and from 27% to 44% for black patients.

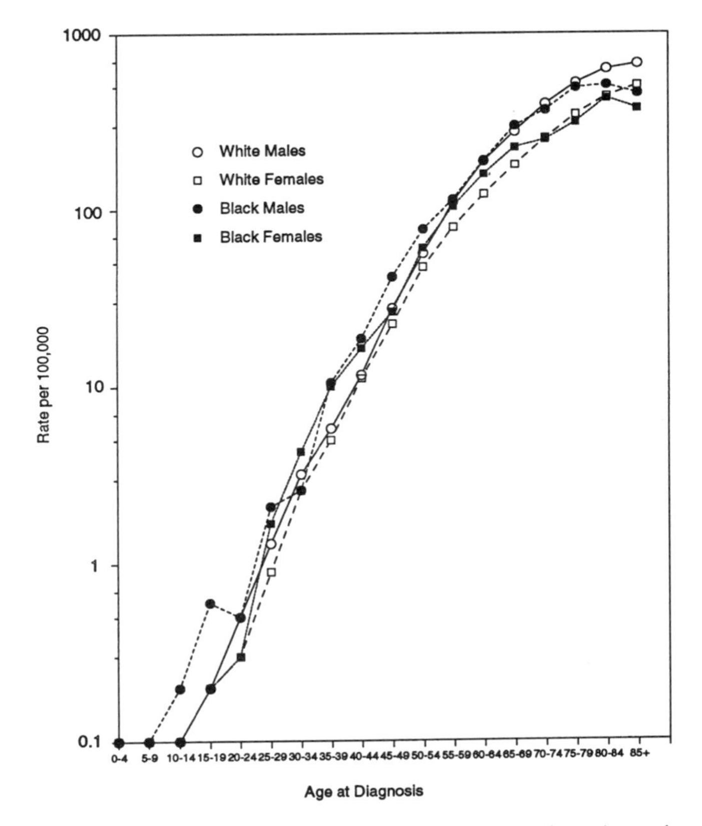

FIG. 39–2. Age-specific incidence rates (per 100,000) for colorectal cancer, by race and sex, United States, 1985–1989.

Age-specific incidence of colorectal cancer in the United States rises sharply after age 35 years, with 90% of cancers occurring in persons 50 years and older (Fig. 39–2). The incidence trends from 1973 to 1989 indicated a relative decline under age 65 years of 13.5% in white females, in contrast to an increase of 15.6% in black females; the decrease in white males was minimal, 1.0%, in contrast to the increase in black males of 32.4%. At 65 years and above, from 1973 to 1989, there were relative increases of 38.4% in black males, 16.5% in black females, 8.8% in white males, and 1.8% in white females. Blacks had higher rates than whites below age 70, and whites exhibited higher rates than blacks above age 70.

Race/Ethnicity

The comparison of incidence rates among racial and ethnic groups in the United States reveals the influence of cultural and socioeconomic differences such as lifestyle practices (e.g., dietary habits, use of tobacco and/or alcohol, reproductive history, physical activity, high-risk occupations), or possibly the interaction of genetic and environmental factors. Incidence, mortality, and survival patterns in racial and ethnic minorities may be influenced by access to, and availability and utilization of quality health care and preventive medical services. In Table 39–3, the distribution of average annual incidence rates during 1977–1983 by racial/ethnic groups suggested three levels of risk for colorectal cancer in males and females. The highest risk level was exhibited in Japanese Americans, and United States whites and blacks; the intermediate level in Chinese Americans and Filipino Americans; and the lowest level in Mexican Americans and Native Americans. During 1986–1988, age-adjusted mortality in Mexican Americans that was attributed to colorectal cancer was less than one half that in Puerto Rican Americans (Table 39–4) (Desenclos and Hahn, 1992).

TABLE 39–3. *Average Annual Age-Adjusted* Incidence per 100,000 Population, for Colorectal Cancer, by Race, United States, 1977–1983*[†]

Race	*Males*	*Females*
Japanese	62.3	37.5
White	59.6	41.9
Black	56.5	46.0
Chinese	48.8	33.0
Filipino	36.7	18.3
Mexican American	28.9	23.9
Native American (New Mexico)	10.4	9.1

*Age-adjusted to 1970 United States standard population.
[†]SEER, National Cancer Institute.

TABLE 39–4. *Age-Adjusted* Mortality Rates per 100,000 Population for Colorectal Cancer, by Race and Hispanic Origin, Males and Females, United States, 1986–1988*

Race	*Male*	*Female*
Total	27.7	19.8
Whites	27.9	19.4
Blacks	30.4	23.3
Hispanics	13.6	8.9
Puerto Ricans	18.9	13.8
Mexican Americans	8.3	6.7
Native Americans/Alaskan Americans	12.5	11.5

*Age-adjusted to 1970 U.S. standard population.
Source: Morbidity and Mortality Weekly Report, 1992.

INTERNATIONAL INCIDENCE

Colorectal cancer is the third ranking cancer in the world, accounting for about 9% (more than 570,000 new cases) of the estimated 6.35 million invasive cancers occurring each year throughout the world. The substantial international variation in incidence rates, and the observation that patterns change dramatically after migration, indicate the importance of environmental factors, particularly those related to lifestyle (Armstrong and Doll, 1975). For example, the age-standardized incidence of colonic cancer in Connecticut white males and females is almost 10 times greater than that reported in Bombay, India; the rate for rectal cancer is more than four times higher in Connecticut than in Bombay (Parkin et al, 1992).

The highest incidence rates for colonic cancer are reported in North America, Australia, and New Zealand. In countries at high risk, the incidence rates between the ages 35 and 60 years are generally higher in females, whereas the rates in males are higher above age 60 (Kune et al, 1986). The rates in western European countries are uniformly lower than those in North America, but are consistently higher than those in eastern European countries. The lowest rates are generally reported in Africa, Asia, and Latin America. Incidence rates in Asia vary considerably in that the rates in the Chinese of Singapore and Hong Kong are approximately twice the rate in the Shanghai Chinese, but are comparable to the rates in western Europeans, Hawaiian Chinese, and Jews of Israel. The age-standardized rates in India and among the non-Jews in Israel are among the lowest in the world (Fig. 39–3). In general, colonic cancer is relatively more common in economically advantaged populations exhibiting Westernized lifestyle practices.

The incidence of colonic cancer varies internationally to a greater extent than that of rectal cancer. In contrast to colonic cancer, rectal cancer is usually more common in males at all ages, with an age-standardized male:female incidence rate ratio of 1.5 to 2.0. In areas with low incidence rates for colorectal cancer—such as India, Senegal, and countries in eastern Europe—the rates for rectal cancer may exceed those for colonic cancer (Fig. 39–4).

International trends of age-standardized (world population) incidence rates for cancers of the colon and rectum in men are summarized in Tables 39–5 and 39–6 for a 20-year period, 1967 to 1987. Throughout this

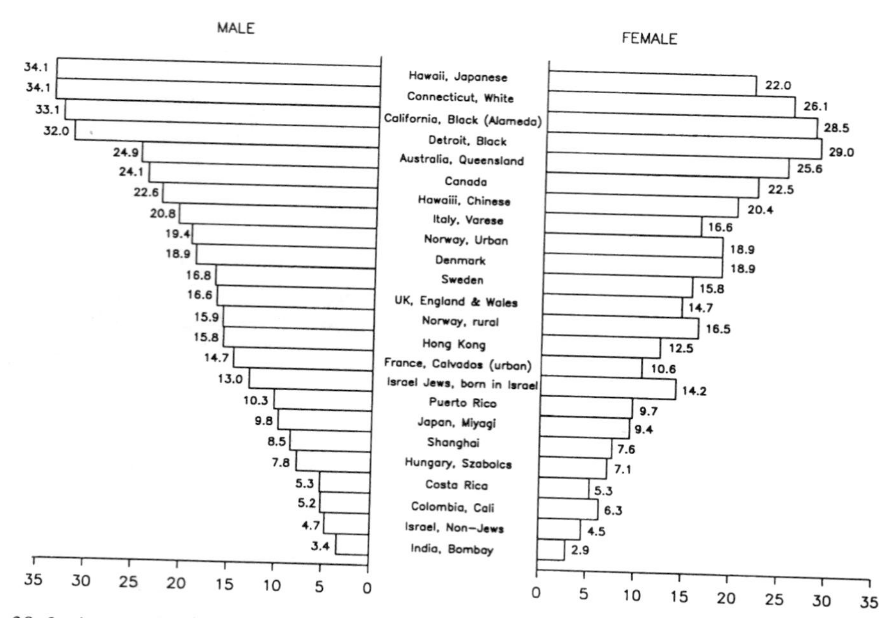

FIG. 39–3. Age-standardized incidence rates per 100,000 (world population) for colonic cancer in 24 selected countries, 1978–1982. Source: Cancer Incidence in Five Continents, Vol. VI, 1992.

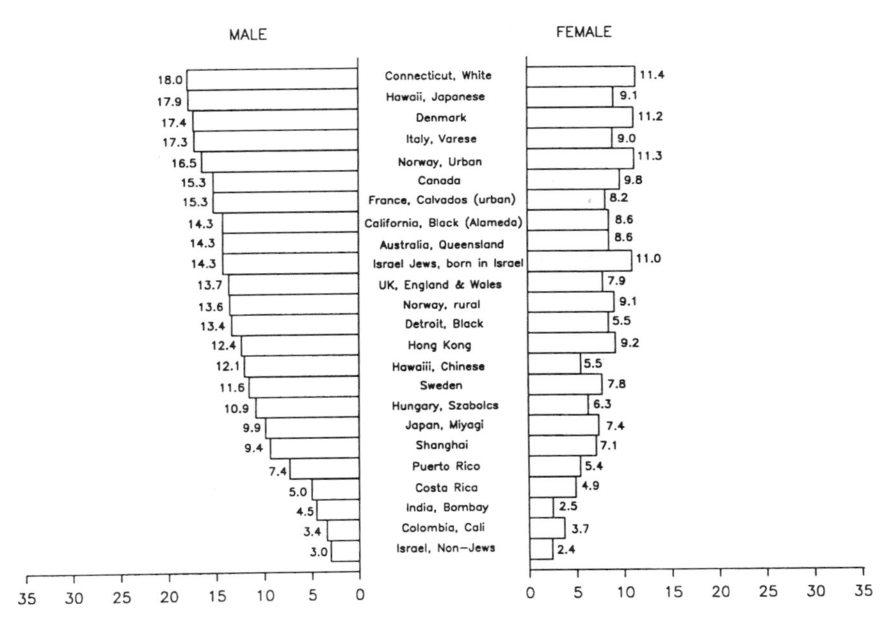

FIG. 39–4. Age-standardized incidence rates per 100,000 (world population) for cancer of rectum (including rectosigmoid junction) in 24 selected countries, 1978–1982. Source: Cancer Incidence in Five Continents, Vol. VI, 1992.

TABLE 39–5. *Age-Standardized (World Population) Incidence per 100,000 for Colonic Cancer in Men, Selected Countries, 1967–1987*

Country	*1967–1971*	*1978–1982*	*1983–1987*
USA, Connecticut (White)	30.1	34.1	35.9
Canada, Newfoundland	24.7	24.2	32.5
USA, California (Black)	23.0	33.1	35.8
New Zealand, non-Maori	23.0	26.5	30.9
Canada, Alberta	17.1	18.6	21.8
United Kingdom, Birmingham	16.5	16.9	19.6
Denmark	16.2	18.9	20.3
Sweden	15.8	16.8	17.5
Germany, Saarland	15.5	21.1	23.7
Norway	15.0	17.4	20.9
Iceland	12.3	14.5	19.8
Finland	7.9	10.0	11.9
New Zealand, Maori	7.4	10.5	11.4
Puerto Rico	6.0	10.3	12.3
Japan, Miyagi	5.6	9.8	17.1
India, Bombay	4.6	3.4	3.2
Colombia, Cali	3.2	5.2	4.4

Source: Cancer Incidence in Five Continents, Vols. III, V, and VI.

period, in the selected countries with population-based cancer registries, the ranges of geographic variations in incidence rates persisted as tenfold for cancer of the colon and fivefold for cancer of the rectum. When compared with the baseline, 1967–1971, for the countries at highest risk of colonic cancer, (i.e., United States, Canada, New Zealand [non-Maori] and United Kingdom), the rate ratios in 1983–1987 varied from 1.13 to 1.55; the relative pattern of increases was similar for the countries at intermediate risk, (i.e., Denmark, Sweden, Germany, Norway, and Iceland), and, as a result, the rank order and level of risk among the countries was unchanged. There appeared to be greater volatility for several of the geographic areas, such as Japan and

TABLE 39–6. *Age-Standardized (World Population) Incidence per 100,000 for Rectal Cancer in Men, Selected Countries, 1967–1987*

Country	*1967–1971*	*1978–1982*	*1983–1987*
USA, Connecticut (White)	18.2	18.0	17.2
Germany, Saarland	16.9	16.9	16.9
Denmark	16.7	17.4	17.3
United Kingdom, Birmingham	16.1	15.3	18.4
New Zealand, non-Maori	15.4	17.1	20.4
Canada, Newfoundland	13.1	16.4	14.9
Norway	11.2	14.8	14.6
USA, California (Black)	10.7	14.3	12.1
Canada, Alberta	10.6	14.3	16.2
Sweden	10.5	11.6	11.9
Iceland	7.9	7.7	7.9
Finland	7.7	10.1	10.2
Japan, Miyagi	6.8	9.9	12.8
New Zealand, Maori	4.6	11.6	12.2
India, Bombay	4.4	4.5	3.2
Puerto Rico	4.2	7.4	7.4
Colombia, Cali	3.1	3.4	3.6

Source: Cancer Incidence in Five Continents, Vols. III, V, and VI.

Puerto Rico, that were at the lowest level of risk in 1967–1971; whereas for other countries such as Colombia and India, the rates persisted among the lowest. In the Miyagi prefecture, the increased rate ratio was 3.05, and in Puerto Rico, 2.05. The incidence patterns for cancer of the rectum exhibited, in most instances, a narrow range of temporal variation—the rate ratios were close to the null value in the United States, Canada, Denmark, Iceland, Sweden, Germany, India, and Colombia. The more significant increases in relative risk for cancer of the rectum were registered in Japan (1.88), Puerto Rico (1.76), and New Zealand (Maori) (2.65). The increasing trend for cancer of the rectum that was described among the male Maoris in New Zealand, an indigenous population of low socioeconomic status, was not accompanied by a similar proportional increase for colonic cancer; the annual age-adjusted incidence rates in male and female Maoris for cancer of the large intestine were only 40% of the incidence in the total population in New Zealand (Sutton et al, 1993).

Migrants

In migrant studies, the age-standardized mortality (or incidence) in a specific racial or ethnic group attributed to a disease is compared in the country of origin or birth with that in the country of adoption or host country. Migrants may be described as *first-generation* (e.g., Issei Japanese), or with respect to their offspring who reside in the country of adoption as *second-generation* (e.g., Nisei Japanese), or as third and future generations; those who are of uncertain generation are referred to collectively as *descendants of migrants*. Migrant studies are of particular interest in estimating latency periods and in assessing the association with environmental factors. Migrants make up a subset of the country of origin population who seek residence in the country of adoption for reasons of economic opportunity, freedom from oppression, or for reasons associated with aging and familial dependency. These selective forces may bear on future health risks. With respect to the patterns of displacement of cancer rates, the migrant population is characterized by specific geographic location in the country of origin, age at migration, duration of residence in the country of adoption, and extent of cultural assimilation. Migrant studies are experiments of nature where the populations to be studied are characterized by marked differences in rates at baseline (or prior to migration) and where subsequently, in the current and future generations of migrants, the long-term health effects of transition from one culture to another may be assessed.

A mortality survey of generations of Japanese Americans during 1949–1952 revealed that colorectal cancer mortality among the Japanese Americans, although lower than that in United States whites, was significantly higher than that among the Japanese in Japan. The upward trend was more apparent in the males. These trends continued, so that by the early 1970s, colorectal cancer mortality in Japanese men and women in Hawaii was similar to that in the United States whites for the ages up to 70 years, but continued to be lower for the group over age 70. It should be noted that over a 25-year period, 1960–1985, colorectal cancer mortality increased 2.5-fold in Japan. The transitional pattern in the Japanese migrants was associated with a right-to-left shift in anatomic distribution, with a proportionally greater concentration of carcinomas and adenomatous polyps in the sigmoid colon (Wynder et al, 1991).

The majority of Chinese migrating to the United States have come from Guangzhou province and are identified by their Cantonese dialect. The age-adjusted rates of mortality for cancer in the large intestine in 1970 among first-generation Chinese-American men and women were, respectively, 5.6 and 2.7 times the rates in men and women in Guangzhou province (King et al, 1985).

In 1978–1982, among Israeli Jews who were born in Europe or North America, colonic cancer incidence in the men was more than twice that in Israeli Jews born in Africa or Asia, and more than four times that in Israeli non-Jews. The rates in Israeli-born Jews, men and women, were intermediate between those in the European/American and African/Asian Jews (Table 39–7). Similar patterns were evident for rectal cancer.

Cancer mortality rates in migrants to Australia from southern and eastern Europe and from the United Kingdom have been reviewed for the period 1962–1982. The migrant groups from Poland, Yugoslavia, Greece, and Italy had premigration risks of dying of colonic cancer that were from 0.3 to 0.7 times those in Australia. After living in Australia for 16 years or more, the relative risk of dying of colonic cancer in the Polish migrants reached the level of risk in the Australian-born, however, the migrating populations from Yugoslavia, Greece, and It-

TABLE 39–7. *Average Annual Age-Adjusted (World Population) Incidence per 100,000 for Colonic and Rectal Cancer in Israel, by Religion and Place of Birth, 1978–1982*

	Males		*Females*	
Israeli Population	*Colon*	*Rectum*	*Colon*	*Rectum*
All Jews	19.7	16.3	16.9	13.6
Jews born in Europe or America	22.5	19.0	19.7	16.1
Jews born in Africa or Asia	13.2	11.0	11.1	9.2
Jews born in Israel	18.1	12.8	20.5	11.0
Non-Jews	4.6	3.6	4.6	2.9

Source: Cancer Incidence in Five Continents, Vol. VI, 1992.

aly exhibited risks that were 0.7 times that of the Australian-born. In contrast to the demographic characteristics of the Polish migrants to the United States, Polish migrants to Australia were, in general, of a higher socioeconomic status and drawn predominantly from urban residential areas. This would have affected the baseline premigration level of colorectal cancer mortality (McMichael et al, 1980).

The vast majority of Puerto Rican migrants to the United States arrived after 1945. Unlike the Japanese, Chinese, and Europeans, the Puerto Rican migrants traveled back and forth between the mainland and Puerto Rico, so that environmental and lifestyle exposures accompanied by changing cultural practices were intermittent and of variable duration. Reverse migration was so common that in the 1970s there was a net migration from the United States to Puerto Rico. Warshauer et al (1986) examined age-adjusted incidence and mortality rates for colorectal cancer during 1975–1979 among Puerto Rican–born residents of New York City. Incidence and mortality for Puerto Rican men and women living in New York City were about twice the rates reported in Puerto Rico and one-half to two-thirds the rates of non-Hispanic white men and women in New York City.

The studies of migrant populations in the United States have demonstrated that, for many racial and ethnic groups throughout the world, the risks of colonic and rectal cancer approach those of the United States–born whites in the first generation, or after 20 or more years of residence in the country of adoption. The transition for some groups, however, such as those originating in Mexico or Puerto Rico, may not be complete in the first generation. However, the risks of rectal and colonic cancer appear to change more rapidly and extensively in the first migrating generation than has been evident for gastric, breast, or prostatic cancers. These differences may reflect the relative importance of earlier versus later exposures to putative carcinogens, genetic factors that influence metabolic processes, and/or the rapidity and degree of acculturation that is correlated with determinants of the carcinogenic process. The observations from ecologic and descriptive studies influence the focus of case-control and cohort analytic studies that are seeking to identify the major differences in dietary practices and their implications with respect to anatomic displacement of neoplasms in the colon, shifts in age-specific incidence and mortality rates of precursor lesions and carcinomas, or biomarker indicators of aberrant epithelial stem cell proliferation (Weisburger and Wynder, 1987).

Urbanization and Socioeconomic Status

In countries throughout the world, colorectal cancer incidence rates are consistently higher among urban residents. The urban excess is more apparent for men than for women, and for colonic more than for rectal cancer. Current residence in an urban area is a stronger determinant or predictor of colorectal cancer risk than is place of birth. That is, whereas the risk for persons born in rural areas and migrating to large cities resembles that for persons born and currently residing in large cities, the risk for persons born and currently residing in rural areas is about 30% less than that for urban residents (Ziegler et al, 1986).

Mortality from colorectal cancer by county in the United States during 1950–1969 was positively correlated with indices of socioeconomic status; namely, that the highest risk was demonstrated in the areas of highest income and highest median years of education. Socioeconomic factors, as they are related to access to and quality of medical care, are an important independent predictor of survival in patients with colorectal cancer. In an analysis of colorectal cancer incidence in the United States based upon the Third National Cancer Survey (1969–1971), the correlation of socioeconomic factors was demonstrable only in white males with colonic cancer; the age-adjusted relative risks were increased by 30% to 40% in the subgroups with the highest income and median number of years of education (Cutler and Young, 1975; Ziegler et al, 1986). In an analysis of the SEER cancer incidence in three United States metropolitan areas between 1978 and 1982, Baquet et al (1991) reported a positive association for cancer of the colon, and rectum and rectosigmoid, with population density, which is a measure of urbanization. The incidence of colonic cancer in either blacks or whites was not correlated with educational level or median family income based upon data from the 1980 census. The incidence rates for cancer of the rectum were significantly higher for whites than for blacks at every educational level. In summary, in contrast to the international incidence patterns of upper digestive tract squamous cell carcinomas and gastric adenocarcinomas which demonstrate significant inverse correlations with socioeconomic factors, the current relative risks of colorectal adenocarcinomas in the United States and in other industrialized countries are not uniformly associated with indices of social and economic advancement.

Occupation

Colorectal cancer is generally not viewed as an occupational disease. A statistically significant relationship with a particular occupational group may be confounded by social class and lifestyle risk factors, or may be due to a specific exposure in the work setting. A causal association has been suggested in the studies of pattern and model makers in the automobile manufacturing industry. Twofold to threefold increases in risk of colorectal cancer incidence and mortality have been described among these skilled workers who were exposed to woods, metals, plastics, fiberglass, and a variety of fumes and solvents (Schottenfeld et al, 1980; Swanson et al, 1985).

Epidemiologic studies have suggested that there is a weak association between asbestos exposure, in particular to chrysotile and amosite fibers, and colonic cancer (Morgan et al, 1985). Asbestos fibers and the formation of asbestos bodies have been demonstrated by light and electron microscopy in tumor tissue in the colons of patients with occupational asbestos exposure (Ehrlich et al, 1991). In a population-based case-control study in Los Angeles County, Garabrant et al (1992) reported that there was no association between colonic cancer and the intensity, duration, or latency of reported asbestos exposure. In a meta-analysis based on 20 published reports of asbestos-exposed cohorts, the summary standarized mortality ratio (SMR) for colorectal cancer in the cohorts exposed to amphibole asbestos was 1.47 (95% C.I., 1.09–2.00); in the cohorts exposed to serpentine asbestos, the summary SMR was 1.04 (95% C.I., 0.81–1.33) (Homa et al, 1994). In a cohort study of asbestos cement workers conducted in Sweden, Albin et al (1990) reported that there was a relationship between cumulative dose and the relative risk of colorectal cancer. For workers with a minimum latency period of 20 years, the relative risks were 1.3 (0.5–2.9) at a cumulative dose level <15 fiber-years per ml; 1.1 (0.3–3.9) at 15–39 fiber-years per ml; and 3.4 (1.2–9.5) at ≥ 40 fiber-years per ml. Spiegelman and Wegman (1985), after controlling for diet and physical activity, were not able to detect an elevated odds ratio for work-related asbestos exposure and colonic cancer.

Persky et al (1981) reported that baseline heart rate, which is inversely associated with level of physical activity, was a predictor of colonic cancer mortality. In a population-based case-control study of risk factors for colorectal cancer in males, ages 20–64 years, Garabrant et al (1984) observed that men with sedentary jobs (i.e., less than 20% of work time required physical activity) experienced a risk of colonic cancer (excluding rectum and rectosigmoid junction) at least 1.6 times that of men whose jobs required a high level (i.e., more than 80% of work time) of activity. The risk ratios particularly for cancers located in the transverse, descending, and sigmoid colon increased significantly in a stepwise manner as occupational physical activity level decreased. The protective effect of physical activity was not evident for cancers located in the proximal colon or rectum. The relationship of occupational physical activity as a risk factor was evident after controlling for race, ethnicity, and socioeconomic status; it did not appear to reflect common environmental chemical exposures. The observed negative association between the risk of colon cancer and physical activity has been corroborated by numerous epidemiologic studies that have been conducted in various countries (Vena et al, 1985; Gerhardsson et al, 1986; Wu et al, 1987; Fredriksson et al, 1989; Ballard-Barbasch et al, 1990; Chow et al, 1993; Arbman et al, 1993). Several of these studies have demonstrated a protective effect of avocational physical activity for distal colonic cancer in men and women. Dietary factors, in particular the average daily consumption of total calories and total fat (saturated and unsaturated), did not confound or obscure the independent association of physical activity as a risk factor for colorectal cancer. In the comparative study of colorectal cancer among Chinese in North America and China, Whittemore et al (1990) inferred that saturated fat intakes exceeding 10 g/day in combination with physical inactivity accounted for 60% of colorectal cancer incidence among Chinese-American men and 40% among Chinese-American women.

A plausible physiological explanation has been advanced to reconcile the differential effects of physical activity on the distribution of neoplasms in the proximal and distal colon. Increased physical activity, perhaps through the release of paracrine hormones, such as the prostaglandins, accompanied by neural reflex mechanisms, enhances propagative peristalsis in the colon (Holdstock et al, 1970; Demers et al, 1981). The accelerated transit time reduces the likeihood of contact at the interface of the fecal stream containing putative mutagens and bile acids and the colonic mucosa. The physiologic effect of physical activity would be experienced in the descending and sigmoid colon where the stool is semisolid and the transit time responsive to extrinsic and endogenous factors.

RISK FACTORS

Adenomatous Polyp

The precursor neoplastic lesion of colorectal carcinoma may be either an adenoma or nonpolypoid flat mucosa exhibiting epithelial dysplasia of various grades of severity. Neoplastic polyps, namely, tubular and villous adenomas, and the smaller "flat adenomas," are associated with perturbations in the mucosal epithelium of the regulation of stem cell renewal, proliferation, and differentiation. The non-neoplastic polyps include hyperplastic polyps; inflammatory polyps; and juvenile polyps, which have been classified as hamartomas.

Tubular adenomas are characterized by a complex network of branching adenomatous glands and account for about 80% of adenomas prevalent in the large intestine. The adenomatous glands in villous adenomas extend from the mucosal surface to the center of the polyp as relatively straight fingerlike projections. Tubulovillous adenomas are characterized by a combination of these two histologic types. Villous adenomas accounting for about 10% of adenomas tend to be larger than tubular adenomas and more often associated with high-grade dysplasia. Adenomas with high-grade dysplasia are more likely to contain foci of invasive cancer.

The flat absorptive mucosa lining the large intestine differs from that of the small intestine in that the fingerlike villi are absent. However, numerous straight tubular crypts are normally present and extend from the muscularis mucosa to the absorptive surface; both are lined by columnar epithelial cells. Thymidine-labeling studies have shown aberrant patterns of DNA synthesis along the crypts of the surface epithelium in patients with dysplastic lesions and adenomas (Lipkin and Higgins, 1988). The initial aberration in the morphogenesis of an adenomatous polyp appears to arise in the colonic crypt. The DNA-synthesizing cells expand throughout the entire crypt and continue to proliferate at the surface, ultimately exhibiting a pattern of downward infolding, branching, and connective tissue reaction. The malignant potential of an adenoma may be predicted by: (1) its size—namely, whether it is 1.0 cm or larger in surface diameter; (2) the presence of high-grade dysplasia; and (3) the predominance of villous features (O'Brien et al, 1992; Simons et al, 1992; Winawer et al, 1993). Morson (1984) reported that in patients with an adenoma 1.0 cm or larger, the cumulative incidence of colorectal cancer was 10% over 15 years of follow-up. The relative risk of developing colorectal cancer in patients with a single adenoma of 1.0 cm or larger may be increased from 1.5 to 3.6 times that expected in a control population. This level of estimated relative risk is multiplied by a factor of approximately two in the presence of multiple adenomas and/or a significant component of villous histology. Familial aggregation of colorectal cancer has been described in the families of probands with adenomatous polyps (Burt et al, 1992). In a prospective observational study of patients who had colonoscopy during which one or more adenomas of the colon or rectum were removed, subsequent colonoscopic surveillance and polypectomy resulted, during an average follow-up of almost 6 years, in a 90% reduction in the incidence of colorectal cancer (Winawer et al, 1993).

The frequency of adenomas in various populations parallels the level of colorectal cancer incidence. The positive correlation coefficient worldwide for men and women combined is about 0.7. In cross-sectional studies, the prevalence of colorectal adenomas is reported to be higher in males than in females, and increases with age; larger adenomas are observed more frequently distal to the transverse colon, although an increasing proportion of adenomas have been found on colonoscopy in the cecum and ascending colon concurrently with the shifting anatomic distribution of carcinomas (Neugut et al, 1993). Giovannucci et al (1992) in a prospective study of male health professionals provided evidence in support of the hypothesis that a diet high in saturated fat, or in the ratio of the intake of red meat to the combined intake of chicken and fish, after adjustment for total energy intake or amount of kilocalories, was positively associated with the risk of colorectal adenoma. Conversely, a high-fiber diet, provided by the regular intake of vegetables, fruits, and grains, was associated with a decreased risk of adenoma. The apparent protective relationship with fiber persisted after adjustment for saturated fat, total calories, and micronutrients commonly found in fruits and vegetables (i.e., vitamins C, E, and beta-carotene).

Five published clinical trials, with inconsistent conclusions, tested the efficacy of antioxidant vitamins to prevent the occurrence of new colorectal adenomas (Bussey et al, 1982; McKeown-Eyssen et al, 1988; DeCosse et al, 1989; Roncucci et al, 1993; Greenberg et al, 1994). In the study of Greenberg et al (1994), after 4 years of daily treatment with either beta-carotene (25 mg/day), or vitamins C (1 g/day) and E (400 mg d-alpha tocopherol/day), there was no apparent reduction in the incidence of colorectal adenomas in patients who had had an adenoma removed recently before entering the study. The authors speculated about the disappointing or inconsistent results of trials that have used supplementation with antioxidant vitamins, in light of the results of epidemiologic studies that have suggested a protective effect of the consumption of vegetables and fruits; apart from methodological limitations with respect to sample size, and adherence to and length of endoscopic surveillance and follow-up, a fundamental consideration is whether the chemopreventive effect of vegetables and fruits in patients at increased risk of colorectal adenomas may be attributed to ingestion of fiber or folate, rather than beta-carotene, or vitamins C and E.

Familial and Hereditary Factors

In addition to the rare autosomal dominant syndrome of familial adenomatous polyposis (FAP) and of Gardner, and the hereditary nonpolyposis colorectal cancer syndromes (Lynch I and II), it is well established that first-degree relatives of patients with large bowel cancer or with adenomatous polyps—in the absence of a well-defined monogenic syndrome—have a two- to threefold increased relative risk of colorectal cancer (St. John et al, 1993). In the latter more common instances of familial large bowel cancer, where specific inheritance patterns are not apparent, other mechanisms have been suggested such as polygenic inheritance, shared environmental factors, the interactions of genetic and environmental factors, and/or the partial penetrance of an autosomal dominant susceptibility gene (Lev, 1990).

Inherited conditions, as currently defined, account for

approximately 10%–15% of colorectal carcinomas in the general population (Lynch and Lynch, 1985; Peltomaki et al, 1993). An unknown dimension of genetic susceptibility in the general population is the prevalence of polymorphic germline mutations at the loci of tumor suppressor genes that have been identified in somatic tumor cells of colorectal adenomas and carcinomas. Familial adenomatous polyposis is prototypic of the polyposis-related colorectal cancer syndromes occurring with a frequency of about 1 per 5000 or 1 per 10,000 live births, and accounting for less than 1% of colorectal cancers in adult life. Penetrance has been variously estimated at 80%–100%. About one-third of cases do not present with a family history and are assumed to represent new germline mutants of the APC (adenomatous polyposis coli) gene locus mapped at 5q21. The localization of the APC gene was facilitated by recognition of an interstitial deletion of 5q in a patient with adenomatous polyposis of Gardner syndrome and mental retardation (Herrera et al, 1986; Groden et al, 1991). The cumulative incidence of colorectal carcinoma approaches 100% by age 55. Adenocarcinoma of the large intestine develops approximately 20 years earlier in FAP patients than in the general population and is commonly associated with synchronous multicentric carcinomas in the large intestine. In addition, both FAP and Gardner syndrome are characterized by an increased risk of adenomas and carcinomas in the stomach and proximal small intestine (Bulow, 1990). Numerous point or frameshift mutations of the APC gene have been identified, but it has been suggested that the site of mutation, for example, a deletion in codon 1309 in exon 15, may be an unfavorable prognostic biomarker of severity of neoplastic disease (Caspari et al, 1994; Mandl et al, 1994).

In the adenomatous polyposis of Gardner syndrome, various extraintestinal lesions and benign tumors have been identified—osteomas, epidermal inclusion cysts, cutaneous fibromas, abnormal dentition, and dentigerous cysts. Other lesions include pigmented ocular fundus lesions, characterized by hyperplasia and hypertrophy of the retinal pigment epithelium. Turcot syndrome is a rare autosomal recessive syndrome associated with adenomatous polyposis of the large intestine, astrocytomas of the central nervous system, and basal cell carcinomas of the skin (Murday and Slack, 1989).

A variety of mucosal hyperproliferation and differentiation biomarkers has been explored in FAP patients. These have included the use of tritiated thymidine incorporation, immunohistochemistry, and flow cytometry. Hyperproliferative activity may be evidenced by elevated mucosal activity of ornithine decarboxylase, a rate-limiting enzyme in polyamine biosynthesis (Luk and Baylin, 1984); and altered glycoprotein cell surface biochemistry detected by aberrant lectin binding and the expression of abnormal carbohydrate antigens. Molecular genetic alterations, in addition to that of the 5q21 locus, appear to be necessary in the pathogenesis of colorectal neoplasia in FAP patients. These include deletion of the DCC gene (deleted in colorectal carcinoma) on chromosome 18q, mutation of the *ras* proto-oncogene, overexpression of *myc* and *src* oncogenes, and mutation and deletion of the p53 gene on chromosome 17p (Bos et al, 1987; Fearon et al, 1990; Fearon and Vogelstein, 1990; Finley et al, 1990).

Puetz-Jeghers syndrome segregates in an autosomal dominant pattern and has the phenotypic characteristics of hamartomatous polyps of the gastrointestinal tract and mucocutaneous melanin pigmentation. The hamartomas are most frequent in the small intestine but also occur in the colon and stomach. The hamartomatous polyps are characterized by proliferation of histopathologically normal epithelial and smooth muscle elements. The incidence of Peutz-Jeghers syndrome has been estimated to be less than that of FAP syndrome. Adenomas and adenocarcinomas of the large intestine have been reported with increased frequency in the syndrome; in addition, adenocarcinomas in the small intestine, pancreas, breast, ovary, and uterus have contributed to the estimated 18-fold increased risk of cancer in affected patients (Watanabe et al, 1990).

The relatively rare juvenile polyposis syndrome segregates in an autosomal dominant pattern and is associated with multiple juvenile or retention polyps. The polyps occur most commonly in the large intestine but may be found in the small intestine and stomach. The morphology of the polyp consists of dilated, mucus-filled glands, lined with attenuated epithelium surrounded by inflamed granulation tissue. The presence of multiple polyps in the intestinal tract and familial history serve to distinguish persons with the syndrome from those with a sporadic solitary juvenile polyp. Adenomas, dysplastic polyps, and adenocarcinoma of the large intestine are phenotypic features of the syndrome (Hamilton, 1990).

The autosomal dominant hereditary nonpolyposis colorectal cancer syndrome (HNPCC) is manifested in the absence of familial polyposis and includes hereditary site-specific colonic cancer (Lynch syndrome I) and the cancer family syndrome (Lynch syndrome II). HNPCC is more common than FAP and may account for 5% to 10% of colorectal cancer in the United States (Lynch et al, 1992; Lynch et al, 1993). In families with Lynch syndrome I, the increased risk of colorectal cancer is expressed 15 years to 20 years earlier than in the general population. Two-thirds of the malignant neoplasms, often as synchronous and metachronous multiple primaries, occur in the proximal or right half of the colon. A mutated genetic locus (hMSH2) has been mapped on chromosome 2p15-16 with linkage to microsatellite DNA makers, and associated with perhaps 60% of familial colonic cancer (FCC) of the HNPCC syndrome

(Peltomaki et al, 1993; Aaltonen et al, 1993; Thibodeau et al, 1993). Preliminary studies have suggested that the mutated "FCC" locus of a mismatch repair gene gives rise to alterations in short repeated DNA sequences, and confers on germ and somatic cells a mutator phenotype which affects the inherent mutability of the human genome. A second mismatch repair gene was subsequently identified, hMLH1, residing on chromosome 3p 21, which when mutated may account for 30% of cases of HNPCC. The two genes, on chromosomes 2 and 3, respectively, encode enzymes that ensure the integrity of the DNA repair pathway and are homologous to the genetic sequences in bacteria and yeast (Papadopoulos et al, 1994). Family members of pedigrees with Lynch syndrome II are distinguished by the increased occurrences of extracolonic cancers, most commonly of the endometrium and ovary, but also of other sites in the gastrointestinal, urinary, and biliary tracts (Watson and Lynch, 1993). A subset of the families with type II syndrome manifest sebaceous adenomas and keratoacanthomas of the skin, and are classified under the Muir-Torre syndrome.

Examination of familial clustering of colorectal cancers in population-based studies indicated that they were not limited to cases characterized by either proximal colonic distribution or early age at onset. However, tumor location proximal to the splenic flexure in the probands identified by population-based tumor registries appeared to be correlated with a higher risk of extracolonic multiple primary cancers in the relatives, when compared with the pedigrees of probands with more distal or left-sided cancers (Cannon-Albright et al, 1989). Bulfill (1990) has suggested that the neoplasms occurring in the right colon, whether sporadically or in an inherited segregation pattern, appear to be genetically more stable than neoplasms occurring in the distal colon and rectum. Preliminary cytogenetic, flow cytometric, and molecular genetic studies have begun to explore mechanistic differences by distinguishing proximal and distal tumors with respect to polyploidy, aneuploidy, chromosomal abnormalities, c-myc oncogene expression, and allelic deletions (Delattre et al, 1989).

Inflammatory Bowel Disease

Inflammatory bowel disease (IBD) includes two related, but clinically and histologically separate entities: ulcerative colitis and Crohn's disease. Worldwide, the annual incidence of IBD varies from 0.5 to 30 per 100,000, with high-risk areas where the incidence of ulcerative colitis is about 26×10^{-5} and Crohn's disease about 5×10^{-5}, in northern Europe, the United States, United Kingdom, Canada, and Israel; intermediate risk exists in central Europe and Australia; and low risk in South America, Asia, and Africa. In Israel, eastern European Jews are at greater risk than Jews born in Asia or Africa. Both African-born and African-American blacks experience risks that are only one-fifth the incidence in United States whites.

Patients with IBD are at increased risk of colorectal carcinoma; the magnitude of relative and/or absolute risk increases in relation to early age at diagnosis, duration of symptoms, the extent of mucosal involvement, and the demonstration by biopsy of multicentric foci of dysplasia in flat mucosa, or less commonly, adenomatous polyps. In the colonoscopic surveillance of patients with IBD, the predictive value for colorectal cancer of a positive biopsy of dysplasia ranged from 15% to 20%; severe, or high-grade, dysplasia was associated with a higher predictive value than low-grade, or mild, dysplasia (Waye, 1986; Collins et al, 1987; Riddell, 1995). The overall increase in relative risk for cancer of the large intestine in patients with IBD has been estimated between 4- and 20-fold. In general, the mean age at diagnosis of colorectal cancer in patients with IBD is about 20–30 years younger than the mean age at diagnosis in the general population at risk of colorectal cancer. The cumulative incidence of colorectal cancer in patients with ulcerative colitis has been reported to vary in different population groups (Freeman, 1989). Most studies of cumulative incidence have shown an annual increase of 0.5% to 1.0%, after 10–15 years from onset of colitis (Ekbom et al, 1990; Lennard-Jones et al, 1990). The cumulative incidence, 25 to 35 years after diagnosis, has ranged from 7% (Katzka et al, 1983) to 49% (Podolsky, 1991). The extent to which genetic predisposition and environmental or lifestyle factors such as diet modify risk is as yet unknown. Crohn's disease involves the colon in 67%–70% of patients; the relative risk (5.6) of colorectal cancer is substantially increased in relation to the extent of inflammatory disease and severity of dysplasia (Hamilton, 1989; Ekbom et al, 1990).

Second Primary Cancers

In the analysis of incidence patterns of multiple primary cancers in a total of 26,804 persons with an index primary cancer of the colon reported by the Connecticut Tumor Registry, the relative risk of a metachronous primary cancer in the remaining large intestine was more than double the incidence expected in the general population. The risk of a second primary varied with age at the time of diagnosis of the index primary: 8.7 when the age was below 45; 3.7 at ages 45 to 54; and 1.8 at 55 and above. The cumulative incidence of a metachronous primary cancer in the colon and rectum after 10 years of follow-up from the diagnosis of the index primary cancer of the colon was 1.9%. Significant increases in relative risk of metachronous primary cancers of the ovary, corpus uteri, and breast have been observed in women with colorectal cancer; the observed increases in relative risk (i.e., at least 50%–100%) were mutual, in that women with cancer of the endometrium, ovary, or breast were at increased risk of developing colorectal cancer (Schottenfeld et al, 1969). The patterns of multiple primary cancers of the reproductive organs and large intestine in women have stimulated epidemiologic investigations of the potential significance of nulliparity, age at first birth, and use of exogenous estrogens as risk factors for colonic cancer (McMichael and Potter 1980; Marcus et al, 1995). McMichael and Potter (1985) speculated that if there is a protective mechanism associated with the level of endogenous or exogenous estrogens, it may be related to altered hepatic production of cholesterol and decreased concentration of secondary bile acids in the colon. Although recent studies have suggested that current and protracted exposure to estrogen replacement therapy in postmenopausal women is accompanied by a significant reduction in the risk of colonic cancer (Chute et al, 1991; Calle et al, 1995; Newcomb et al, 1995), other studies (Howe et al, 1985; Furner et al, 1989; Kune et al, 1989; Wu-Williams et al, 1991; Marcus et al, 1995) have not demonstrated consistent risk patterns of reproductive practices, menstrual activity, and/or exogenous estrogen consumption in women with colorectal cancer. Future studies should continue to explore common genetic determinants and the relationship of physical activity, and energy and micronutrient consumption, to endogenous estrogen synthesis and excretion, and bile acid metabolism.

MOLECULAR GENETICS OF COLORECTAL NEOPLASIA

The incidence of colorectal cancer increases exponentially in the general population with age raised to a power of four or five. There are undoubtedly multiple genetic events required for somatic stem cell initiation, transformation, and clonal progression in carcinogenesis. In their multistage theoretical model, Moolgavkar and Luebeck (1992) concluded that there were at least three essential rate-limiting or mutational steps in the genesis of colorectal cancer. Whether or not the proposed construct adequately explains the cascade of molecular genetic and epigenetic events in colorectal neoplasia, it is clear that tumorigenesis involves extensive alteration of the genome (Vogelstein et al, 1988). The total number of genetic alterations, whether inherited or acquired, and to a lesser extent the chronological sequence in which these events occur, influence the biological properties of the neoplasm.

Knudson (1971) postulated that the inherited and sporadic occurrences of each specific form of human cancer resulted from mutations or deletions in the same gene. Knudson further hypothesized that many of these mutations were recessive at the cellular level, which he characterized as antioncogenes (tumor suppressor genes), and that both copies of the gene must be lost. Powell et al (1992) observed, for example, that somatic mutations in the APC gene at chromosome 5q21, namely, mutations in tumor tissue DNA and not in the germline DNA, were detected in 60% of patients with colorectal cancer, and in a similar proportion of patients with colorectal adenomas, including adenomas as small as 0.5 cm in diameter. Mutation and ablation of the APC gene is an early determinant of the upward shift in the zone of proliferation in the colonic crypt, and the persistence of immature, proliferating cells that tend to lose the ability to accumulate intracellular mucin. It has not been established that all mutations of the APC gene are recessive, requiring a second genetic event, rather than, for example, functioning as dominant-negative or codominant mutations at the cellular level. In experimental studies in athymic nude mice, the replacement of mutated APC function by transfer of a normal wild type chromosome 5 into a colorectal tumor cell line markedly reduced tumorigenicity, which would support the theory that APC is a tumor suppressor gene (Goyette et al, 1992). It has also been suggested that loss of function or truncation of the APC gene translation product may also occur in noncolonic tumors in the gastrointestinal tract, such as in the stomach and pancreas (Horii et al, 1992). The mutated colorectal cancer (MCC) gene, located only 150 kilobases centromeric to the APC gene, was found to be mutated in a small percentage of sporadic colorectal carcinomas (Kinzler et al, 1991). Loss of heterozygosity (LOH) in the region of the MCC locus (5q21) has also been detected in patients with esophageal, and small cell and non–small cell lung cancers. It is currently unclear if LOH at the MCC locus contributes to the neoplastic phenotype or is a marker of proximity to APC or other tumor suppressor genes.

The accumulation of epithelial cells throughout the crypt capable of continued proliferation results in the formation of the adenomatous polyp. The adenoma may progress gradually as evidenced by a continuum of increasing size, number of dysplastic cells and villous architectural features. The growth and neoplastic conversion of an adenoma is accompanied by aberrations in DNA methylation, and mutations of the K-ras or N-ras proto-oncogene (Jones, 1986; Fearon, 1994). The ras genes are a family of proto-oncogenes that are commonly mutated in solid tumors. Mutations of K-ras have been identified in at least 40% of colorectal adenomas (greater than 1 cm in diameter) and carcinomas (Bos, 1989). The encoded ras proteins are located on the inner surface of the plasma membrane and participate in signal transduction from membrane receptors (Prendergast and Gibbs, 1993). Mutations of the Kirsten variant of the ras gene, in particular at codons 12 or 13, may, using the polymerase chain reaction technique, be detected in stool samples of patients with early stage colorectal cancer (Sidransky et al, 1992).

In addition to the APC gene, allelic losses have been reported in neoplastic somatic cells on chromosomes 17p and 18q. Loss of heterozygosity and decreased levels of mRNA involving chromosome 18q have been detected in approximately 70% of invasive colorectal carcinomas; but such abnormalities are relatively infrequent in adenomas or preinvasive colonic neoplasms (Kikuchi-Yanoshita et al, 1992). Allelic loss of chromosome 18q may have adverse prognostic significance in stage II colorectal cancer (Jen et al, 1994). Fearon et al (1990) identified a candidate tumor suppressor gene on chromosome 18q, the DCC gene ("deleted in colorectal carcinoma"). It is speculated that the DCC gene encodes a cell adhesion molecule. In neoplastic transformation, there is deregulated expression of cell adhesion molecules or of the receptors that mediate cellular adhesion.

Allelic losses of 17p, the locus of another tumor suppressor gene, have been detected in 70%–80% of early invasive colorectal cancers (Baker et al, 1991). Inactivation of the p53 tumor suppressor gene on chromosome 17p13.1, as a result of point mutation, and deletion ("loss of heterozygosity") of the second allele, is one of the most common genetic abnormalities demonstrable in human cancers. More than 350 independent point mutations of the p53 gene have been discovered in a wide variety of human cancers (deFromentel and Soussi, 1992). The temporal sequence, however, of inactivation of both alleles of p53 in oncogenesis is not the same for different organs and tissues, and thus may be coincident with the earlier event of dysplasia in esophageal and bronchial tissues (Rotter and Prokocimer, 1991). Mutations in the p53 gene are generally missense mutations that produce faulty proteins, which in some instances can be dominantly transforming but may also result in the encoding of nonsense truncated proteins. Cells expressing mutant p53 protein do not pause in G1 but continue into S phase before completing the repair of DNA abnormalities (Vile, 1993). Normally, p53 would keep in check the inherent mutability of somatic cells because of its controlling functions with respect to DNA replication and repair, and in cellular differentiation and apoptosis (Harris and Hollstein, 1993).

EXPERIMENTAL CARCINOGENESIS

Animal experiments are assumed to simulate or at least provide plausible explanations for pathophysiological mechanisms in human carcinogenesis. Various interpretive problems arise in long-term bioassays of putative carcinogens in rodents owing to species differences in susceptibility; confounding or interactive influences of dietary parameters; using the maximum tolerated dose which exceeds significantly the range of exposure levels relevant to humans; selection of a particular dose-response extrapolation model that impacts risk assessment, and may be at variance with the inference based on the use of a different extrapolation model; possible existence of a threshold dose below which no carcinogenic effect is observed; and failure of the controlled experimental conditions to assess adequately in humans the effects of genetic heterogeneity, varying exposure intensities, and concurrent exposures to other environmental agents (O'Connor and Campbell, 1987).

Experimental systems of colorectal carcinogenesis were introduced when compounds with selective action on the intestinal mucosa of rodents were identified. The earliest use of chemical carcinogens to produce intestinal neoplasia involved the oral administration of dibenzanthracene and methylcholanthrene. Laqueur et al (1963) observed that cycasin, found in the Cycadeceae plant, was a potent carcinogen in rat colon. The proximate carcinogen in cycasin is a hydrazine compound, the beta-glucoside of methylazoxymethanol (MAM). The related hydrazines, azoxymethane (AOM) and 1,2 dimethylhydrazine (DMH), require metabolic degradation to the active electrophilic compound. MAM undergoes metabolic degradation to formaldehyde and a highly reactive and unstable methyldiazonium ion which can alkylate or bind covalently with nucleic acids. Other generic compounds capable of tumorigenic activity include *N*-methylnitrosourea (NMU) and *N*-methyl-*N*-nitro-*N*-nitrosoguanidine (MNNG), examples of alkylnitrosoureas which act directly on intrarectal instillation. With respect to the hydrazines, while their concentration in the fecal stream is correlated with the risk of tumor induction, parenteral or vascular delivery of DMH or MAM can induce tumors in surgically isolated segments of the large intestine (Rubio and Nylander, 1981). For rodents, the effective parenteral dose range for DMH is 10–20 mg/kg body weight, given once a week for about 10–15 weeks. Colonic tumors appear about 6 months after the initial injection; in general, the higher the total dose administered, the higher the cumulative incidence of colonic tumors, the shorter the latency period, and the higher the incidence of extracolonic primary tumors. Male animals appear to be more susceptible than females to DMH-induced adenomas and carcinomas.

Preneoplastic changes have been demonstrated in the colonic crypt columns of the experimental animals; namely, there is an expansion of epithelial proliferative activity into the middle one-third segment of the column accompanied by cellular atypia (Lipkin and Deschner, 1976). Tumorigenesis originates in a single aberrant crypt and evolves by clonal proliferation of transformed cells (Bird et al, 1989). In the hydrazine rat model, there are changes in epithelial surface carbohydrate expression and the expression of oncofetal antigens, accompanied by an altered pattern of lectin binding (Boland et al, 1982). Aberrations in mucosal lectin histochemistry and the appearance of abnormal sialomucins suggest that alterations occur in the cell membrane and in the synthesis of mucin glycoconjugates in colonic tumor formation (Freeman, 1983).

The metabolic activity of intestinal bacteria may enhance (or inhibit) the action of generic types of carcinogens. Various bacterial enzymes have been implicated in generating mutagens, carcinogens, and tumor promoters—e.g., beta-glucuronidase, beta-glucosidase, beta-galactosidase, nitroreductase, and azoreductase. Conjugated metabolites of exogenous and endogenous compounds secreted in the bile may be activated, or their biologic activity altered, by the microflora in the colon. Cycasin, or MAM glucoside, is not tumorigenic when given parenterally or orally to germ-free adult rats. However, when cycasin is fed to infant rats with indigenous intestinal microflora, adenocarcinomas are induced in the large intestine, liver, and biliary ducts; and renal sarcomas and squamous cell carcinomas of the ear duct are observed. As reviewed by Weisburger and Fiala (1983), the enzymatic activity of intestinal bacteria (beta-glucosidase) is required to cleave the glucoside bond of cycasin and release the active aglycone and proximate carcinogen, MAM. Goldin and Gorbach (1981), in using a DMH model, discovered that the incidence of colonic tumors was reduced by more than two-thirds when rats were treated concurrently with oral broad spectrum antibiotics. Apparently, tumor induction by DMH is facilitated by the beta-glucuronidase activity of intestinal anaerobic bacteria.

Nutrient and caloric intake may be as rate-limiting in experimental tumorigenesis as the dose of the carcinogen. A diet high in animal fat when compared with a diet low in fat enhances the occurrence and metastatic potential of colonic tumors induced by DMH, MAM, or NMU. Under such experimental conditions it is necessary to formulate a high fat diet that is comparable to the low fat diet with respect to total calories, and the composition of protein, fiber, minerals, and vitamins.

The animal studies provide evidence that both the total amount of fat and fatty acid composition determine the cumulative risk of colonic tumors. Diets high in omega-6 fatty acids (e.g., linoleic acid) are tumor-enhancing when ingested after the administration of the carcinogen. High fat diets containing high levels of fish oil rich in omega-3 fatty acids (docosahexanoic acid and eicosapentanoic acid) exhibit no tumor-promoting effects when administered after the genotoxic carcinogen (Reddy, 1987; Reddy, 1992).

The dominant dietary hypothesis for colonic cancer derives from the relationship between dietary fat intake and bile acid metabolism (Reddy et al, 1989). Cholic acid, mainly derived from endogenous cholesterol, and chenodeoxycholic acid, from dietary cholesterol, are the major primary bile acids excreted from the liver. Through 7 alpha-dehydroxylation, colonic bacteria convert primary bile acids to fecal secondary bile acids, lithocholic (LA) and deoxycholic (DA) acids. The secondary bile acids have been shown in experimental models to stimulate colonic crypt epithelial cell proliferation and to promote tumorigenesis. It has been suggested that the LA to DA concentration ratio may be more predictive as a risk marker than the total concentration of bile acids (Owen et al, 1987). Surgical diversion of the biliary effluent from the duodenum into the middle segment of the small intestine potentiates the carcinogenicity of AOM in the large intestine (Williamson et al, 1979).

Dietary fiber includes a wide variety of plants that contain storage carbohydrates and cell walls resistant to digestive enzymes. Most dietary fibers are polysaccharides and can be classified as either pectin, hemicellulose, or cellulose. The other major component is lignin, which is a nonpolysaccharide, phenylpropane polymer. Cellulose, lignin, and some hemicelluloses are structural fibers and tend to be nonfermentable by colonic bacteria and insoluble in water; whereas pectins, gums, mucilages, and the other hemicelluloses are natural gel-forming fibers that are fermentable and water-soluble. The degradation products resulting from bacterial digestion include gases (i.e., hydrogen, methane, and carbon dioxide) and short-chain fatty acids (i.e., acetic, propionic, and butyric). Foods vary with respect to the density and types of fiber that may be derived from them. Cereals may contain soluble oats and barley but are especially concentrated in hemicelluloses; vegetables and fruits tend to be higher in cellulose than most cereals and contain a range of soluble and insoluble fibers. Lignin is highest in fruits with edible seeds or in root vegetables. Fiber has been postulated to reduce the adverse effects of dietary fat and fecal bile acids by: increasing fecal bulk and reducing transit time; physical dilution of fecal contents by water absorption; altering the metabolic activity and composition of colonic microflora; binding bile acids and bile salts; and lowering colonic pH, by increasing fermentation and short-chain fatty acid production. At an increased pH, the bile acids and free fatty acids are relatively more solubilized and more damaging to the bowel mucosa, whereas reduction in pH reduces the conversion of primary to secondary bile acids and facilitates binding of free fatty acids with calcium and other salts (Cummings, 1983; Lanza et al, 1992). Stool weight reflects residual fiber concentration and adherent bacteria. Fiber particle size affects transit time and fecal mass; coarse bran is more effective than fine bran in reducing transit time and increasing fecal mass.

Animal studies of dietary fiber and colonic cancer

have provided inconsistent results, presumably because of variations in the macro- and micronutrient composition of the diet, qualitative and quantitative differences in the fibers administered, the nature and dose of the carcinogen used, and the timing of onset and duration of the fiber feeding in relation to the administration of the genotoxic agent. In general, fibers that are water-insoluble and less fermentable in the colon (e.g., cellulose and wheat bran) have been more consistently effective in inhibiting tumorigenesis. The relative protective effect of fiber has been evident with a restricted fat diet: when administered during the promotional, as distinguished from the initiational, stage of carcinogenesis; and when given in conjunction with an indirect-acting carcinogenic agent that requires microsomal activation (Galloway, 1989).

DIETARY FACTORS

Dietary macronutrient and micronutrient factors may enhance or inhibit carcinogenesis in the colon and rectum. The in vivo and in vitro experimental studies, and the comparative international, case-control, and cohort epidemiologic studies, have proposed a multiplex causal pathway that appears to be compatible with the multistep molecular biology of colorectal cancer (Potter, 1992). The general mechanistic framework of diet and digestive processes was recently summarized without assigning hierarchical significance or assuming mutual exclusivity: (1) mutagens appear naturally in foods, or as a result of cooking meat proteins at a high temperature (heterocyclic amines); (2) conversion of bile acids to tumor-promoting chemicals by normal colonic bacteria, which is enhanced by a high fat and low fiber diet; (3) formation of oxygen radicals and lipid peroxidation products by diet-induced metabolic activation of procarcinogens; or (4) the inhibition of toxicity by the action of nutrient antioxidants, minerals, and trace elements that quench free radicals, enhance cell-mediated immunity or the ability of cells to repair damaged DNA, or modulate prostaglandin synthesis or cell proliferation (Surgeon General's Report on Nutrition and Health, 1988).

In reviewing the results of nutritional epidemiologic studies of cancer of the large intestine that have been conducted in various countries, there is a general impression of inconsistency and continuing controversy. Exposures to nutrients may be measured with instruments of uncertain reliability and validity; dose-response relationships frequently are not compatible with the assumption of linearity and/or the absence of a threshold; and the degree of confounding by other nutrients and total energy consumption is not adequately controlled for and may vary with race, ethnicity, and sociocultural factors. The basis for inconsistencies in the reported results may be intrinsic to the methodology of recording previous or baseline usual food consumption patterns, and the limited sensitivity of the study design to detect small differences in mean intake of nutrients or food groups between study and comparison subjects selected from a relatively homogenous population.

FAT AND ENERGY

In a number of experimental animal studies, increasing caloric intake, regardless of the nutrient source (i.e., fat, protein, or carbohydrate), potentiated the incidence of tumors induced by a carcinogen (Tannenbaum, 1945; Kritchevsky et al, 1986). In many epidemiologic studies reporting a positive association of meat or animal fat with colonic cancer, the authors have also described a positive association with total energy intake (Jain et al, 1980; Potter and McMichael, 1986; Lyon et al, 1987; Graham et al, 1988; Willett and Stampfer, 1986). Macronutrient associations that have been observed in epidemiologic studies of cancer patients are potentially confounded by energy intake, and thus it is essential to adjust for caloric intake by stratified analysis or regression models in attempting to establish whether there is a unique association with the highly correlated macronutrient. The regression models are ultimately needed when controlling simultaneously for multiple dietary and nondietary covariates, and in examining for interactions (Willett and Stampfer, 1986).

Jain et al (1980) observed a positive association of increased energy consumption and colorectal cancer in men and women in a population-based study that was conducted in Canada. For example, odds ratios of 1.5 and 1.8 were derived for men in the middle (2485–3255 kilocalories) and high (> 3255 kilocalories) tertiles, respectively, when compared with the low intake group (< 2485 kilocalories). Similarly, Lyon et al (1987) noted higher energy intake among colon cancer cases in a population-based case-control study in Utah; odds ratios ranged from 2.0 to 3.6 in women (high tertile > 1800 kilocalories), and up to 2.5 in men (high tertile > 2600 kilocalories). In a hospital-based study of colonic cancer cases conducted in western New York (Graham et al, 1988), a positive association in a logistic regression analysis was reported with a significant trend in men (but not in women) among the quartile boundaries of total calories; the odds ratios ranged from 1.45 to 1.99 among men, and from 1.09 to 1.52 among women. However, in other case-control studies conducted in Hawaii (Stemmermann et al, 1984) and in Australia (Kune et al, 1987), the differences in caloric intake were not significant or did not demonstrate a consistent pattern by gender or level of consumption. In their cohort study of nurses, Willett et al (1990) were not able to demonstrate an independent relationship of energy intake and colon cancer. In a summary review of nine epidemiologic studies of energy intake and the risk of cancer of the colon and rectum, Albanes (1992) concluded that six demonstrated a positive association and three no association.

The demonstration of an association with total energy intake raises additional questions about the biologic importance of energy balance between intake and expenditure or physical activity; body composition and distribution of adiposity; individual variation in metabolic efficiency; the independent relationship with fat as an energy-providing macronutrient; or other lifestyle factors associated with energy output. Methodologic questions persist about the validity of measurement of dietary intake and of analytical regression models that attempt to resolve the collinearity of total energy intake and its component macronutrients (Willett and Stampfer, 1986; Marshall and Zielezny, 1993).

The hypothesis that diets high in animal fat and meats (and low in plant fiber, fruits, and vegetables) were a cause of colorectal cancer was partly derived from the correlation coefficient as high as 0.89 between per capita consumption of animal fat and international age-adjusted colorectal cancer incidence rates. From the various ecologic studies it was estimated that "food disappearance" data for total fat and fiber consumption accounted for 67% of the variance in international colonic cancer mortality (Potter et al, 1993). Subsequently, there have been numerous case-control studies and at least five cohort studies that have attempted to test the "fat/fiber" hypothesis (Potter, 1992; Thun et al, 1992). A case-control study conducted in Canada and reviewed by Miller (1992) used a logistic regression model to analyze the effects of saturated fats, and calories from sources other than saturated fats. The odds ratio for the highest level relative to the referent low consumption level of saturated fats was 2.0 for males and 2.3 for females. In a case-control study of colonic and rectal cancer conducted in western New York State, the initial analysis by Graham et al (1988) suggested that both saturated fats and total calories were independent but highly correlated risk factors. On reanalysis using both the method of Willett and Stampfer (1986), namely, the calorie-adjusted nutrient residual approach, and the logistic regression method of Howe et al (1986), Marshall and Zielezny (1993) concluded that fat intake was a significant independent predictor of risk of colorectal cancer. In the Nurses' Health Study, Willett et al (1990) examined prospectively the relationship of fat and fiber on the incidence of colonic cancer during 6 years of follow-up. Neither total energy intake nor body mass index was a predictor of risk. The relative risk of colonic cancer for the highest quintile of animal fat compared with the lowest quintile, after adjustment for total energy intake, was 1.89 (95% C.I., 1.13–3.15). The relative risk in women who ate beef, pork, or lamb every day was 2.49 (95% C.I., 1.24–5.03), when compared with women who reported eating meat less than once a month. A positive association and linear trend was also noted for processed meats; similar results were reported by Bjelke (1980) in Norway, in the American Cancer Society Cancer Prevention Study II (Thun et al, 1992), and in the case-control study in the Netherlands (Goldbohm et al, 1994).

Cholecystectomy and Right-Sided Colonic Cancer

In humans and laboratory animals, maintaining isocaloric diets high in animal fat results in the: increased excretion of bile acids; predominance of anaerobic microbial enzymatic activity in the colon; and inversely lower levels of dietary fiber (Reddy, 1981). An association between cholecystectomy and colonic cancer was first reported by Capron et al (1978), and subsequently by Vernick et al (1980). Since then more than 60 studies have attempted to confirm whether cholecystectomy increases the risk for colonic cancer. A proposed biological mechanism is the continuous secretion of bile into the gut as a result of the absence of a gallbladder. Giovannucci et al (1993) combined the results of 38 cohort and case-control studies and determined that the pooled relative risk for colorectal cancer after cholecystectomy for men was 1.21 (95% C.I., 1.04–1.40), and for women was 1.24 (95% C.I., 1.10–1.40). The meta-analysis for the risk of right-sided colonic cancer, based on reviewing hospital-based case-control studies, concluded that the pooled relative risk was 1.88 (95% C.I., 1.54–2.30); the review of population-based case-control studies resulted in the estimated pooled relative risk of 1.33 (95%, C.I., 1.09–1.62). In a cohort study conducted in Sweden by Ekbom et al (1993), women had an increased risk for right-sided colonic cancer after cholecystectomy (Standardized Incidence Ratio, 1.24; 95% C.I., 1.03–1.48). During the follow-up interval, which exceeded 20 years, the excess risk observed in women appeared to increase with the increasing interval of latency. Friedman et al (1987) in reviewing the records of the Kaiser Permanente Medical Care Program in northern California concluded that in cases with colonic cancer, there was no apparent association with prior cholecystectomy. For women with right-sided colonic cancer, the odds ratio was not significantly elevated, and there was no consistent effect of latency interval. Friedman et al (1987) recommended that future studies should be restricted to fatal cases of colorectal cancer, because of their concern for the potential confounding factor of surveillance bias. The general conclusion, however, would be that cholecystectomy may be associated with a small increase in relative risk of proximal colonic cancer that is perhaps less than 50%.

Mutagens Formed in Cooking

Most epidemiologic studies have focused on nutrient excesses or deficiencies, and not on methods of cooking or preparation. Sugimura et al (1977) reported on the formation of mutagenic and carcinogenic compounds, generic heterocyclic aromatic amines (HAA), under ordinary cooking conditions. The HAA mutagens detected in cooked foods can be classified into two types: (1) imidazole subgroup, where the amino group is attached to the 2-position of an imidazole ring (e.g., 2-amino-3 methyl-3H-imidazo[4,5-f]quinoline); (2) nonimidazole subgroup, where an amino group is attached to the pyridine ring (e.g., 2-amino-5-phenylpyridine).

The formation of HAA in cooked food is influenced by the type of food, which serves as a source of protein, or of sugars and amino acids, and the cooking method, time, and temperature. Mutagenic activity of the imidazole subgroup of HAA has been detected in beef, pork, lamb, chicken, and fish after cooking at temperatures above 100°C. The imidazole HAA mutagens are generated in cooked meat from the reaction of creatinine with an amino acid. Cooking methods such as frying, broiling, and barbecuing that reach temperatures over 100°C produce the highest levels of HAA (imidazole subgroup) mutagenicity; negligible amounts are formed during microwaving, or by poaching, boiling, or stewing (Adamson, 1990). The primary route of metabolic activation of HAA is by cytochrome P-450IA2, which leads to hydroxyamino derivatives; and through *O*-acetylation and *O*-sulfation, the ultimate reactive mutagen and clastogen binds at the C-8 position of DNA guanine (Sugimura et al, 1994). In feeding experiments in rodents, the reactive metabolites of HAA produce cancers in the liver, small intestine and large intestine, forestomach, mammary gland, lymphoid tissue, urinary bladder, oral cavity, lung, skin, and Zymbal glands (ear duct). Weisburger et al (1994) in a bioassay for genotoxicity and carcinogenicity underscored the significance of the microsomal P-450 bioactivation pathway for heterocyclic aromatic amines, mediated in liver and extrahepatic tissues, rather than metabolic activation by intestinal microflora as previously hypothesized (Kadlubar, 1994). A potential genetic interaction has been suggested by Kadlubar et al (1992) in that individuals at increased risk may be characterized as "rapid" acetylators and *N*-oxidizers of heterocyclic amines.

Epidemiologic studies up until now have not measured directly the dietary intake of heterocyclic aromatic amines or the concentration of blood leukocyte and colonic tissue HAA-DNA adducts. The assessment of risks has distinguished the intake of barbecued, smoked, or cured meats (Willett et al, 1990; Verdier et al, 1991; Thun et al, 1992; Goldbohm et al, 1994), or of broiled fish (Kuratsune et al, 1986). Although exposure to sources of pyrolysis mutagens in cooked foods is universal, the design of epidemiologic studies to estimate potential heterogeneity of exposure levels in relation to colorectal cancer should focus on comparing cooking methods and the preparation and preservation of meat (i.e., how well done, curing or smoking, and inclusion of gravy), and the use of biomarkers of HAA genotoxic exposure.

FIBER, FRUITS, AND VEGETABLES

The concept of fiber deficiency as an etiologic factor in cancer of the large intestine evolved on the basis of broadly drawn comparisons of patterns of large intestinal diseases in Western and traditional African societies (Higginson and Oettle, 1960; McKeown-Eyssen, 1987). Observers of clinical disease in diverse parts of Africa affirmed the rarity of appendicitis, diverticular disease of the colon, colonic adenomas and carcinomas, and inflammatory bowel disease in rural African populations with high fiber intake (Painter and Burkitt, 1971). An inverse correlation ($r = -0.49$) between dietary fiber consumption in different countries and age-adjusted colonic cancer mortality rates was derived by McKeown-Eyssen and Bright-See (1985); fiber availability was measured for cereal fiber per 1000 kilocalories and adjusted for fats, meats, or energy. A systematic effort to test the hypothesis of dietary fiber as a risk factor for colorectal cancer was coordinated by the International Agency for Research on Cancer (IARC). Two areas were selected for detailed study of diet, transit time, and stool bacterial content: Kuopio, a rural farming area of Finland, and Copenhagen, Denmark, which has colorectal cancer incidence rates four times those of Kuopio. Diet histories, including 5-day diaries of food intake, were taken on a random sample of males, aged 55 to 64, drawn from population listings. The results of this investigation documented higher meat intake and beer consumption in Copenhagen, and higher fiber intake and milk consumption in Kuopio (Jensen et al, 1974). In a study of African Americans in the San Francisco Bay area, the highest risk of colorectal cancer was observed in those with a high consumption of saturated fat-containing foods and a low consumption of fiber-containing foods (Dales et al, 1979).

In their review of 24 case-control studies that assessed the role of fiber or fiber-containing foods in reducing the risk of colonic cancer in different populations, Lanza and Greenwald (1989) concluded that 17 showed an inverse association, 4 no association, and 3 a positive association. In a related review and meta-analysis of dietary fiber, vegetables, and colonic cancer, Trock et al (1990) concluded that the aggregated assessment gave support for a protective effect associated with fiber-rich diets; the estimated combined odds ratio was 0.57 (95% C.I. = 0.50–0.64), based on the comparison of the highest and lowest quantiles or extremes of intake. Howe et al (1992) reported on the combined analysis of 13 case-control studies conducted in various countries. Instead of pooling the summary results of published studies as in the usual meta-analysis, the investigators examined and combined the original data records for 5287 colorectal cancer cases and 10,470 control subjects. Two logistic regression models were used to examine the effect (relative risk) of dietary fiber, which was represented either in relation to the median value of each quintile distribution of intake among all study subjects, or as a continuous variable for each subject. The analysis concluded that in 12 of the 13 studies, the consumption of fiber-containing foods was protective in men and women, without a differential effect by age, and for proximal and distal colonic and rectal cancer. The decreasing monotonic dose-response trend was statistically significant; the relative risk, adjusted for total energy intake, case-control study, age group, and gender was 0.53 (95% C.I., 0.47–0.61) for the highest quintile of intake (median 31.2 g/day) compared to the lowest quintile (median 10.1 g/day). In the combined analysis, the protective effect demonstrated for fiber was unaltered by adjusting for the intake of vitamin C and beta-carotene.

It is important to distinguish the putative chemopreventive properties of dietary fiber in colorectal cancer from those that may be assigned to vegetables and fruits, which contribute to approximately 50% of the total fiber intake in the United States. High or moderate levels of consumption of fruits and vegetables, when compared with the lowest level, have been associated in case-control and cohort studies with diminished risks of carcinomas in the large intestine (Steinmetz and Potter, 1991). However, after adjustment for energy and fiber intake, a number of studies have recorded only weak inverse associations between the consumption of vegetables and fruits and colorectal cancer (Howe et al, 1992; Steinmetz et al, 1994). Fruits and vegetables are the major dietary sources of antioxidants (i.e., carotenoids, vitamins C and E, selenium), folic acid, dithiolthiones, protease inhibitors, phenols, flavonoids, thiocyanates and isothiocyanates, allium, and indoles (Block, 1993). Various chemopreventive mechanisms of action by micronutrients and non-nutritive phytochemicals in fruits and vegetables have been suggested by in vitro and animal feeding experimental studies. Wattenberg (1985) has assessed these chemopreventive actions with respect to blocking the biochemical pathway of interaction of the carcinogen and the target locus on DNA or a critical macromolecule, or suppressing the clonal expression of neoplasia in previously initiated cells. The complex interrelated mechanisms by which substances in vegetables and fruits may inhibit carcinogenesis include: regulation of cell differentiation; "quenching" or "trapping" of oxygen or hydroxyl free radicals; preventing the formation of electrophilic metabolites from precursor compounds by inhibiting the enzymatic activation pathway or by inducing the detoxification pathway (e.g., glutathione S-transferase, cytochrome P450 mixed-function oxidases); enhancing DNA methylation; inhibiting the expression of oncogenes; and stimulating immune function.

In 11 of the 14 case-control studies reviewed by Steinmetz and Potter (1991), the investigators reported that there was a significant inverse relationship between colonic cancer and at least one index measure of vegetable and fruit consumption; 2 studies did not report any significant associations, and 1 observed paradoxically positive associations with multiple food items. A methodologic concern in the study that reported positive associations with multiple vegetables and fruits consumed in Japan was the selection of control patients with polyps, ulcers, gastritis, and other gastrointestinal disorders (Tajima and Tominaga, 1985). In seven of nine case-control studies, a similar inverse or apparently protective association was reported between rectal cancer and at least one index measure of vegetable and fruit consumption (Steinmetz and Potter, 1991). The studies reporting an inverse relationship by type of vegetable or fruit emphasized, in general, a pattern of consumption of raw or fresh vegetables; leafy green vegetables; cruciferous vegetables or specifically broccoli; carrots; raw or fresh fruit, including citrus fruit; and/or allium vegetables. The cruciferous vegetables contain a variety of phytochemicals, including sulforaphane, dithiolthiones, isothiocyanates, and glucobrassicin, a complex alkaloid which yields a variety of indolemethylene compounds, including indole-3-carbinol. A metabolite of indole-3-carbinol, 3,3′-diindolylmethane, is an active inducer of cytochrome P450 phase II enzymes which detoxify carcinogens (Bjeldanes et al, 1991). The allium vegetables, including onion, garlic, and chives, contain chemical compounds which induce such enzymes as glutathione S-transferase that are involved in detoxification of electrophilic metabolites.

The antioxidant micronutrients include vitamins E and C, the carotenoids, selenium, and zinc, which trap or neutralize free radicals and reactive oxygen molecules. Superoxide radicals, hydroxyl radicals, and hydrogen peroxide are reactive oxygen species that can induce mutagenic alterations in DNA. A combined analysis of 13 case-control studies by Howe et al (1992), which pooled data on 4326 patients with colorectal cancer and 8946 control subjects, concluded that there was a weak inverse association between the estimated beta-carotene intake and the risk of colorectal cancer; after adjusting for fiber intake, the relative risk for the highest quintile compared to the lowest quintile of consumption level was 0.89 (95% C.I., 0.75–1.05). In the Iowa

Women's Health Study Cohort, the multivariate adjusted relative risk of colonic cancer for the highest compared to the lowest quintile of total (i.e., dietary and daily supplements) vitamin E intake was 0.32 (95% C.I., 0.19–0.54). The inverse association was evident only in the women under 65 years of age. The relative risks among women with higher total intakes of vitamins A and C, and beta-carotene were not significantly different from 1.0 (Bostick et al, 1993). In a pooled analysis of five cohort studies which compared the highest quartile of serum alpha-tocopherol concentration to the lowest, Longnecker et al (1992), estimated the odds ratio for colorectal cancer as 0.6 (95% C.I., 0.4–1.0). The antioxidant property of vitamin E resides in the phenolic hydroxyl group at C-6 on the aromatic ring. Vitamin E also interrupts the chain of membrane lipid peroxidation and radical formation in membrane systems at cell surfaces and in microsomes and mitochondria (Packer and Fuchs, 1992).

Folic acid is required for DNA synthesis and cell replication. Fresh fruits and vegetables are the major sources of folate, an essential cofactor in the production of S-adenosylmethionine, which is required for DNA methylation. In the Nurses Health Study and the Health Professionals Follow-up Study, high dietary and supplemental use of folate was inversely associated with the subsequent risk of colorectal adenoma in women and men. In a multiple logistic model, the relative risk of adenoma in the distal colon and rectum was reduced to 0.65 (95% C.I., 0.49–0.85), in the highest quintile of folate intake from diet and supplements, when compared with the lowest quintile (Giovannucci et al, 1993).

CALCIUM AND VITAMIN D

In the experimental studies following the administration of 1,2-dimethylhdrazine or intestinal bypass surgery in rats, supplemental dietary calcium suppresses aberrant colonic epithelial cell proliferation and mucosal ornithine decarboxylase activity, and decreases the bacterial production of diacylglycerol (Appleton et al, 1987; Lans et al, 1991, Steinbach et al, 1994). Various mechanisms for the antiproliferative effects of ionized calcium on colonic epithelial cells have been proposed. The solubilizing function of bile acids interacts with fecal lipids, which results in the enhancement of enzymatic degradation and mucosal absorption of fatty acids. The ionized forms of fatty acids and bile acids, which are not bound to calcium, apparently are toxic to the colonic epithelium; the administration of calcium has been shown to sequester and complex with fatty acids and bile acids. Administering supplemental dietary calcium or vitamin D3 (1,25-dihydroxy-vitamin D3 or calcitriol) inhibited ornithine decarboxylase activity and induced terminal differentiation in rat colonic epithelium (Newmark and Lipkin, 1992). In subjects from high-risk families (familial colonic cancer syndrome), the prevalence and distribution of proliferating cells lining the colonic crypts were studied both before and after oral calcium supplementation (1250 mg calcium carbonate each day for 2 to 3 months). Supplemental calcium was observed to down-regulate the hyperproliferative pattern, or tritiated thymidine labeling index, observed at baseline (Lipkin and Newmark, 1985).

The epidemiologic studies have not been consistent in establishing an inverse or protective association between dietary and supplemental levels of calcium or vitamin D and colorectal cancer. Ecological comparisons within and between countries of calcium intake, and the availability of milk and milk products, in relationship to age-standardized colonic or rectal mortality, have served to generate hypotheses (Sorenson et al, 1988). Garland et al (1991) asserted that the decreasing north to south gradient of colonic cancer mortality in the United States would be correlated with increasing opportunities for exposure to ultraviolet radiation and increasing serum concentration of 25-hydroxy vitamin D. However, support for an inverse association between calcium consumption and colorectal cancer was reported in four case-control studies (Macquart-Moulin et al, 1986; Kune et al, 1987; Slattery et al, 1988; Peters et al, 1991); and one cohort study (Garland and Garland, 1986); but not in three case-control studies (Tuyns et al, 1987; Graham et al, 1988; Freudenheim et al, 1990); and two cohort studies (Heilbrun et al, 1986; Stemmermann et al, 1990). In the Health Professionals Follow-up Study and the Nurses' Health Study, the dietary intake of calcium, vitamin D, and dairy products was not significantly associated with the incidence of colorectal adenomas; nor was there any interaction of calcium intake at different levels of consumption of saturated fat or dietary fiber (Kampman et al, 1994). In a randomized trial, Alder et al (1993) were not able to validate the hypothesis that calcium supplementation would decrease the concentration of fecal aqueous phase bile acids.

ALCOHOL AND TOBACCO

In the report of the International Agency For Research On Cancer Working Group (1988) on cumulative exposure to alcohol and cancer of the large intestine, the concluding statement was: "Overall, some of the epidemiologic studies provide suggestive but inconclusive data for a causal role of drinking of alcoholic beverages, most often beer consumption, in rectal cancer." In a meta-analysis of 27 published cohort and case-control studies of alcohol consumption in association with colonic and/or rectal cancer, Longnecker et al (1990) concluded that: a causal role of alcoholic beverage consumption, by amount or type, could not be established; the association did not vary significantly by gender or anatomic site in the large intestine; and a weak association at best may be inferred from a least-squares regression model with an overall summary relative risk of 1.10 (95% C.I., 1.05–1.14). In the published case-control studies of total alcohol and beer consumption and the risk of rectal cancer, the results have been inconsistent, or limited to men, heavy drinkers of beer, or in conjunction with dietary deficiencies, as in calcium, vitamin D, or folate and methionine (Potter et al, 1993). In their report of a positive association with rectal cancer of lifetime total intake of alcohol, but in particular with heavy beer consumption by men (odds ratio = 1.80; 95% C.I., 1.12–2.89), Freudenheim et al (1990) observed that inconsistencies in the published literature of case-control studies appeared to be due to the uncontrolled confounding or selection bias that may have arisen in the selection of hospital-based controls; and that modest increases in risk were generally reported when population-based controls served as the referent group. In a case-control study of Wisconsin women, Newcomb et al (1993) reported that an alcohol consumption level of 11 or more drinks per week was associated with an elevated adjusted odds ratio of 1.47 (95% C.I., 1.0–2.2) for cancer of the large intestine; however, only rectal cancer exhibited a significant linear trend with level of alcohol consumption, and particularly with the consumption of beer. In a review of seven prospective studies that examined the relationship of alcohol and colonic and rectal cancer, Hiatt (1992) concluded that the association was weak, but because of the substantial fraction of the population exposed, perhaps 25% of rectal cancers in the United States may be attributable to alcohol. Of additional interest is the prospective study of health professionals by Giovannucci et al (1993), in which, relative to nondrinkers, average daily exposure of more than 30 grams of alcohol was associated with an increased risk of colorectal adenoma in women (relative risk = 1.84; 95% C.I., 1.19–2.86) and in men (relative risk = 1.64; 95% C.I., 0.92–2.93). Other studies have reported a positive association between alcohol intake and colorectal adenoma (Diamond, 1952; Stemmermann et al, 1988; Kono et al, 1990; Cope et al, 1991; Kikendall et al, 1989; Kune et al, 1991; Honjo et al, 1992); while others (Lee et al, 1993; Riboli et al, 1991) have not.

Studies of cigarette smoking as a risk factor for colorectal cancer in men have either described a modest association (Doll and Peto, 1976; Carstensen et al, 1987; Wu et al, 1987; Rogot and Murray, 1980); or an association only with pipe tobacco smoking (Slattery et al, 1990); or no association (Schwartz et al, 1961; Haenszel et al, 1980; Choi and Kahyo, 1991). In the follow-up study of male health professionals, cumulative exposure to cigarette smoking (≥ 16 pack-years) was associated with an elevated risk of colorectal cancer (relative risk = 1.94; 95% C.I., 1.13–3.35), after allowing for an induction-latency period of at least 35 years (Giovannucci et al, 1994); similarly, among women in the Nurses' Health Study who were cigarette smokers of more than one-half pack per day, the risk of colorectal cancer increased significantly (47% to 100%) after a minimal interval of 35 years from the initiation of smoking (Giovannuci et al, 1994). The estimated relative risks of smoking were computed by use of multivariate logistic regression which controlled for age, family history of colorectal cancer, body mass, physical activity, and intake of saturated fat, dietary fiber, folate, and alcohol.

The studies of cigarette smoking and the risk of adenomatous polyps in the colon and rectum are generally supportive of a causal relationship (Lee et al, 1993; Giovannucci et al, 1994). The reported associations of cigarette smoking with colorectal adenomas have been consistent with respect to: men and women; both proximal and distal locations in the large intestine; small (< 1 cm) and large (≥ 1 cm) adenomas; dose-response gradients or monotonic trends in risk; and an induction-latency period of less than 20 years from the initiation of smoking for small adenomas, and of at least 20 years or longer for large adenomas.

We may only speculate why the association of cigarette smoking appears to be compelling and consistent in studies of colorectal adenoma, and conflicting in studies of colorectal carcinoma. A proposed biologic explanation is that exposure to tobacco smoke occurs in the large intestine, either systemically or through gastrointestinal transport. The reported temporal relationships would suggest that tobacco may trigger an early event in the multistep process, prior to neoplastic transformation, and in the adenoma-carcinoma pathogenic sequence (Lee et al, 1993; Giovannucci et al, 1994). The inconsistencies in prior studies of cigarette smoking and colorectal cancer may have been due in part to the failure to consider an optimal induction-latency period that appears to be at least 30–40 years; selection bias in using hospital-based controls as the sole referent group for estimating the prevalence of cigarette smoking exposure in the population; and/or detection bias due to differential cancer surveillance and detection practices exhibited by smokers compared to non-smokers.

NONSTEROIDAL ANTIINFLAMMATORY PHARMACEUTICALS

Experimental animal studies (Pollard and Luckert, 1983; Metzger et al, 1984; Reddy et al, 1987; Craven and DeRubertis, 1992), clinical trials (Waddell et al, 1989; Rigau et al, 1991; Giardiello et al, 1993) and epidemiologic analytic studies (Greenberg et al, 1993; Kune et al, 1988; Rosenberg et al, 1991; Paganini-Hill et al, 1991; Thun et al, 1992; Gridley et al, 1993; Logan et al, 1993; Peleg et al, 1994) have addressed the nature of the association and potential mechanisms of action of the nonsteroidal antiinflammatory drugs (NSAIDs) in reducing the risk of colorectal adenoma and cancer. The pharmaceuticals under investigation include aspirin, ibuprofen, sulindac, indomethacin, and piroxicam. NSAIDs inhibit cyclooxygenase activity, the synthesis of prostaglandins, and the cascade of arachidonic acid metabolites, which may play an activating role in cell transformation, tumor growth, and metastasis. Each prostaglandin which functions in intercellular and intracellular signal transduction has its own range of biological activities in a given tissue. In rat models of colonic carcinogenesis, indomethacin, piroxicam, and sulindac, which are inhibitors of cyclooxygenase, exhibit chemopreventive activity when administered concurrently with dimethylhydrazine or methylnitrosourea (Marnett, 1992). In the case-control studies of Kune et al (1988) and Rosenberg et al (1991), regular and recent use of aspirin was accompanied by about a 50% reduction in risk of colonic and rectal cancer. In the Cancer Prevention Study II of the American Cancer Society, the adjusted relative risks of dying of colonic cancer decreased with more frequent aspirin use; use of aspirin, 16 or more times per month, was associated with an adjusted relative risk of 0.56 (95% C.I., 0.35–0.91) in men; and of 0.48 (95% C.I., 0.29–0.78) in women (Thun et al, 1992). In the study by Paganini-Hill et al (1991), daily use of aspirin was not accompanied by any reduction in risk of colonic cancer. Future epidemiologic studies that explore the anticancer effects of NSAIDs should evaluate carefully the temporal aspects of starting and stopping use of the medication; average intensity and duration of exposure; indication for use and type of NSAID; interaction with other established risk factors; assessment of confounding by underlying medical condition for which regular use of NSAID was prescribed; and differential medical surveillance in those exposed when compared to those not exposed to NSAIDs.

CANCER OF THE ANAL REGION

In the United States, the average annual age-adjusted incidence of cancer of the anal region (i.e., anal canal and anal margin) is 0.6 per 100,000. Only 1%–2% of cancers of the large intestine are located in the anal region. The annual age-adjusted incidence (1970 U.S. standard) per 100,000 for cancer of the anal region in 1985–1989 was 40% higher in women; namely, the incidence in white females (0.7) exceeded that in white males (0.5), and, similarly, the rate in nonwhite females (0.9) was higher than that in nonwhite males (0.7). In women, the age-specific incidence of invasive anal cancer increases with age in a logarithmic pattern similar to that of the rectum, colon, or vulva, rather than that of the uterine cervix, which tends to peak in the fifth decade (Melbye and Sprogel, 1991). Since 1960, age-adjusted anal cancer incidence in Connecticut increased 1.9-fold among men and 2.3-fold among women (Melbye et al, 1994). During the past decade, an increasing incidence of squamous cell and transitional cell carcinomas of the anal region has been described in homosexual males younger than 45 years (Austin, 1982). Similar patterns of increasing incidence have been described in Sweden (Goldman et al, 1989) and in Denmark (Frisch et al, 1993).

Anatomy

Cancers in the anal region may occur either in the anal margin (perianal cancer) or in the anal canal. The anal margin is located within the 5 cm cutaneous area surrounding the anal orifice and consists of stratified squamous epithelium with keratinization, hair, and sweat glands. The anal canal, which is about 2.5–4.0 cm in length, extends proximally from the anus to the lower boundary of the rectum and above the dentate or pectinate line. The dentate line represents the embryonic junction between the ectodermal and endodermal layers of the hindgut. The lumen of the anal canal presents in its upper half a number of vertical mucosal folds known as the rectal columns of Morgagni. The histologic lining of the anal canal is composed of nonkeratinizing squamous epithelium. At about the level of the dentate line, the mucosa assumes a transitional-cell pattern, not unlike the pattern in the lower urinary tract, which then emerges as simple columnar epithelium in the rectum.

Pathology

More than 60% of the anal cancers are squamous cell or epidermoid carcinomas, and 20%–25% are transitional cell or cloacogenic carcinomas. (The cloaca or cloacogenic membrane in mammalian embryology develops from the terminal end of the hindgut and forms the urogenital sinus before dividing into the rectum, urinary bladder, and genital primordia.) Adenocarcinomas account for about 7% of all anal cancers, and melanomas for about 1%–2%. Mucinous adenocarcinomas are especially rare but have been reported in patients with a prior history of anal fistula (Getz et al, 1981; Frisch et al, 1994). Anal margin cancers are viewed biologically and morphologically as skin cancers (Mitchell, 1988). The cell types for anal margin cancers, in addition to keratinizing squamous cell carcinoma, include basal cell carcinoma; Bowen's intraepithelial squamous cell carcinoma; and Paget's disease, an adenocarcinoma arising from an apocrine sweat gland. Bowenoid papulosis or multicentric pigmented Bowen's disease combines features of multicentric intraepithelial neoplasia and condylomata acuminata, or wartlike papules (Bhawan, 1980).

Risk Factors

Anal canal tumors are more common in women, whereas anal margin tumors are more common in men. Never married young men, and separated or divorced men and women, are at increased risk of anal cancer and anal intraepithelial neoplasia (AIN) (Peters and Mack, 1983; Wexner et al, 1987). In the San Francisco Bay area, the relative risk of anal cancer among never married men increased from 6.7 (95% C.I., 4.7–9.5) in 1979–1984 to 10.3 (95% C.I., 7.5–14.1) in 1985–1989. Cooper et al (1979) hypothesized that the epidemiology of anal cancer may be viewed as that of a sexually transmitted disease, and Scholefield et al (1989) underscored the similarities with the natural history of cervical intraepithelial neoplasia (CIN). Peters et al (1984) reviewed the similarities in the descriptive epidemiology of squamous and transitional cell carcinomas of the uterine cervix, vagina, vulva, anus, and penis—increasing incidence with decreasing social class, low risk among Jews, and elevated risk among separated and divorced persons of both sexes. Women with a previous primary invasive carcinoma of the uterine cervix were at significantly increased relative risk of developing a metachronous primary carcinoma of the anus, vulva, and vagina (Rabkin et al, 1992). In a cohort study of patients with anal cancer, the relative risks of metachronous second primary cancers, when compared with the expected incidence in the general population of Denmark, were significantly increased for uterine cervix, vagina, vulva, respiratory system, urinary bladder, and breast in women; there were fewer than expected cancers of the uterine corpus and ovary (Frisch et al, 1994). The common embryologic origin and anatomic continuity of the anogenital epithelium appears to be associated with a shared susceptibility and potential for exposure to a putative carcinogenic agent (Scholefield et al, 1992) (Fig. 39–5).

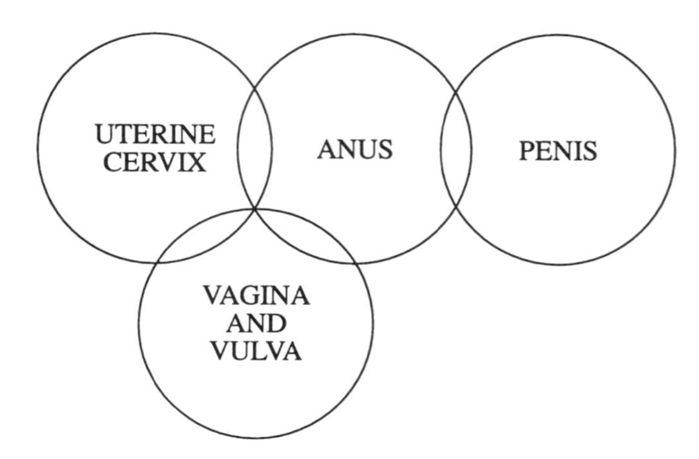

FIG. 39–5. Mutually increased risks of second primary epidermoid (squamous cell) carcinomas of the anus and lower genital tract in females and males, respectively.

Risk factors for anal cancer are correlated with sexual behavior and may include a history of sexually transmitted infectious diseases; homosexual preference; marital instability or multiple sexual partners; receptive anal intercourse; anogenital condylomata or genital warts; and chronic anal inflammatory conditions such as proctitis, fissures, or fistulas (Daling et al, 1987; Holly et al, 1989). Current cigarette smoking and cumulative exposure of 20 pack-years or more (Holly et al, 1989), and immunosuppression, as in transplant patients or in patients with human immunodeficiency virus infection (Palefsky et al, 1991), are associated independently with an increased risk of anal neoplasia. Prospective surveillance of AIDS patients by linkage with cancer registries in different regions of the United States has estimated that the cumulative incidence of epidermoid carcinoma of the anus is about one per 1000 cases; however, anal dysplasia, including carcinoma-in-situ, may occur in up to 15% of HIV-infected homosexual men. The relative risk of epidermoid anal cancer is increased significantly both before and after the diagnosis of AIDS (Critchlow et al, 1992; Melbye et al, 1994).

Most anogenital squamous cell carcinomas, including cervical intraepithelial neoplasia, have been causally linked with specific human papillomavirus (HPV) serotypes, and in particular types 16 and 18; types 6 and 11 have been associated with genital warts or condylomata. A history of genital warts in homosexuals or heterosexuals identifies individuals at increased risk of concomitant infection with other HPV types that may express transforming and integrating oncogenic characteristics. HPV DNA has been detected in the tissues of most cases with anal intraepithelial neoplasia, the precursor lesion of invasive anal cancer, and HPV RNA expression has been detected in anal cancer tissues (Zachow et al, 1982; Beckmann et al, 1989; Duggan et al, 1989; Gal et al, 1989). Palefsky et al (1991) reported that by using the polymerase chain reaction technique they were able to demonstrate the presence of HPV 16 DNA in over 75% (10/13) of subjects with invasive anal carcinoma. In contrast, types 6 and 11 were associated only with low grade anal intraepithelial neoplasia and/or condyloma. Herpes simplex (HSV) DNA was also detected in almost one-half of the subjects with invasive anal cancer and high-grade intraepithelial neoplasia.

The oncogenic role of type-specific HPV is suggested by persistence of HPV DNA in the host genome in primary and metastatic neoplastic tissues. Integration of the viral DNA in the host genome presumably disrupts the E2 open reading frame and leads to unregulated production of the E6 and E7 open reading frames. The continued expression of E6 and E7 results in unregulated cell growth and the potential for cell transformation. Cofactors, such as HSV infection, cigarette smoking, immunosuppression, and chronic infection, appear to be essential for the neoplastic conversion, promotion, and progression of HPV DNA-harboring cells (zur Hausen, 1989).

REFERENCES

AALTONEN LA, PELTOMAKI P, LEACH FS, et al. 1993. Clues to the pathogenesis of familial colorectal cancer. Science 260:812–816.

ADAMSON RH. 1990. Mutagens and carcinogens formed during cooking of foods and methods to minimize their formation. *In* DeVita VT Jr, Hellman S, Rosenberg SA (eds): Cancer Prevention. Philadelphia, J. B. Lippincott, pp. 1–7.

ALBANES D. 1992. Energy intake and cancer. *In* Micozzi MS, Moon TE (eds): Macronutrients: Investigating Their Role in Cancer. New York, Marcel Dekker, pp. 205–229.

ALBIN M, JAKOBSSON K, ATTEWELL R, et al. 1990. Mortality and cancer morbidity in cohort of asbestos cement workers and referents. Br J Ind Med 47:602–610.

ALDER RJ, MCKEOWN-EYSSEN G, BRIGHT-SEE E. 1993. Randomized trial of the effect of calcium supplementation on fecal risk factors for colorectal cancer. Am J Epidemiol 138:804–814.

APPLETON GV, DAVIES PW, BRISTOL JB, et al. 1987. Inhibition of intestinal carcinogenesis by dietary supplementation with calcium. Br J Surg 74:523–525.

ARBMAN G, AXELSON O, FREDRIKSSON M, et al. 1993. Do occupational factors influence the risk of colon and rectal cancer in different ways? Cancer 72:2543–2549.

ARMSTRONG B, DOLL R. 1975. Environmental factors and cancer incidence and mortality in different countries, with special reference to dietary practices. Int J Cancer 15:617–631.

AUSTIN DF. 1982. Etiological clues from descriptive epidemiology: squamous carcinoma of the rectum or anus. Natl Cancer Inst Monogr 62:89–90.

BAKER SJ, FEARON ER, NIGRO JM, et al. 1991. Chromosome 17 deletions and p53 gene mutations in colorectal cancer. Science 244:217–221.

BALLARD-BARBASCH R, SCHATZKIN A, ALBANES D, et al. 1990. Physical activity and risk of large bowel cancer in the Framingham study. Cancer Res 50:3610–3613.

BAQUET CR, HORM JW, GIBBS T, et al. 1991. Socioeconomic factors and cancer incidence among blacks and whites. J Natl Cancer Inst 83:551–557.

BECKMANN AM, DALING JR, SHERMAN KJ, et al. 1989. Human papillomavirus infection and anal cancer. Int J Cancer 43:1042–1049.

BHAWAN J. 1980. Multicentric pigmented Bowen's disease: A clinically benign squamous cell carcinoma in situ. Gynecol Oncol 10:201–205.

BIRD RP, MCLELLAN EA, BRUCE WR. 1989. Aberrant crypts, putative precancerous lesions, in the study of the role of diet in the etiology of colon cancer. Cancer Surv 8:189–200.

BJELDANES LF, KIM J-Y, GROSE KR, et al. 1991. Aromatic hydrocarbon responsiveness-receptor agonists generated from indole-3-carbinol in vitro and in vivo: Comparisons with 2,3,7,8-tetrachlordibenzo-p-dioxin. Proc Natl Acad Sci USA 88:9543–9547.

BJELKE E. 1980. Epidemiology of colorectal cancer, with emphasis on diet. *In* Maltoni C (ed): Advances in Tumor Prevention, Detection and Characterization. Amsterdam, Excerpta Medica, pp. 158–174.

BLOCK G. 1993. Micronutrients and cancer: Time for action? J Natl Cancer Inst 85:846–848.

BOLAND CR, MONTGOMERY CK, KIM YS. 1982. A cancer-associated mucin alteration in benign colonic polyps. Gastroenterology 82:664–672.

BOS JL, FEARON ER, HAMILTON SR, et al. 1987. Prevalence of ras gene mutations in human colorectal cancers. Nature 327:293–297.

BOS JL. 1989. Ras oncogenes in human cancer: A review. Cancer Res 49:4682–4689.

BOSTICK RM, POTTER JD, SELLERS TA, et al. 1993. Relation of calcium, vitamin D, and dairy food intake to incidence of colon cancer among older women. Am J Epidemiol 137:1302–1317.

BOSTICK RM, POTTER JD, MCKENZIE DR, et al. 1993. Reduced risk of colon cancer with high intake of vitamin E: The Iowa Women's Health Study. Cancer Res 53:4230–4237.

BULFILL JA. 1990. Colorectal cancer: Evidence for distinct genetic categories based on proximal or distal tumor location. Ann Intern Med 113:779–788.

BULOW S. 1990. Extracolonic manifestations of familial adenomatous polyposis. *In* Herrera L (ed): Familial Adenomatous Polyposis. New York, Alan R Liss, pp. 109–114.

BURT RW, BISHOP DT, CANNON-ALBRIGHT L, et al. 1992. Hereditary aspects of colorectal adenomas. Cancer 70:1296–1299.

BUSSEY HJ, DECOSSE JJ, DESCHNER EE, et al. 1982. A randomized trial of ascorbic acid in polyposis coli. Cancer 50:1434–1439.

CALLE EE, MIRACLE-MCMAHILL HL, THUN MJ, et al. 1995. Estrogen replacement therapy and risk of fatal colon cancer in a prospective cohort of postmenopausal women. J Natl Cancer Inst 87:517–523.

CANNON-ALBRIGHT LA, THOMAS TC, BISHOP T, et al. 1989. Characteristics of familial colon cancer in a large population data base. Cancer 64:1971–1975.

CAPRON JP, DELAMARRE J, CANARELLI JP, et al. 1978. Cholecystectomy and colon cancer. Gastroenterol Clin Biol 2:383–389.

CARSTENSEN JM, PERSHAGEN G, EKLUND G. 1987. Mortality in relation to cigarette and pipe smoking: 16 years' observation of 25,000 Swedish men. J Epidemiol Community Health 41:166–172.

CASPARI R, FRIEDL W, MANDL M, et al. 1994. Familial adenomatous polyposis: Mutation at codon 1309 and early onset of colon cancer. Lancet 343:629–632.

CHOI SY, KAHYO H. 1991. Effect of cigarette smoking and alcohol consumption in the etiology of cancers of the digestive tract. Int J Cancer 49:381–386.

CHOW WH, DEVESA SS. 1992. Death certificate reporting of colon and rectal cancers. JAMA 267:3028.

CHOW W-HO, DOSEMECI M, ZHENG W, et al. 1993. Physical activity and occupational risk of colon cancer in Shanghai, China. Int J Epidemiol 22:23–29.

CHUTE CG, WILLETT WC, COLDITZ GA, et al. 1991. A prospective study of reproductive history and exogenous estrogens on the risk of colorectal cancer in women. Epidemiology 2:201–207.

COLLINS RH, FELDMAN M, FORDTRAN JS. 1987. Colon cancer, dysplasia, and surveillance in patients with ulcerative colitis: A critical review. N Engl J Med 316:1654–1658.

COOPER HS, PATCHEVSKY AS, MARKS G. 1979. Cloacogenic carcinoma of the anorectum in homosexual men. Dis Colon Rectum 22:557–558.

COPE GF, WYATT JI, PINDER IF, et al. 1991. Alcohol consumption in patients with colorectal adenomatous polyps. Gut 32:70–72.

CRAVEN PA, DERUBERTIS FR. 1992. Effects of aspirin on 1,2-dimethylhydrazine-induced colonic carcinogenesis. Carcinogenesis 13:541–546.

CRITCHLOW CW, HOLMES KK, WOOD R, et al. 1992. Association of human immunodeficiency virus and anal human papillomavirus infection among homosexual men. Arch Intern Med 152:1673–1676.

CUMMINGS J. 1983. Fermentation in the human large intestine: Evidence and implications for health. Lancet 1:1206–1209.

CUTLER SJ, YOUNG JL. 1975. Third National Cancer Survey: Incidence Data. National Cancer Institute Monograph 41. Washington, D. C., U. S. Government Printing Office.

DALES LG, FRIEDMAN GD, URY HK, et al. 1979. A case-control study of relationships of diet and other traits to colorectal cancer in American Blacks. Am J Epidemiol 109:132–144.

DALING JR, SHERMAN KJ, HISLOP TG, et al. 1992. Cigarette smoking and the risk of anogenital cancer. Am J Epidemiol 135:180–189.

DECOSSE JJ, MILLER HH, LESSER ML. 1989. Effect of wheat fiber and vitamins C and E on rectal polyps in patients with familal adenomatous polyposis. J Natl Cancer Inst 81:1290–1297.

DEFROMENTEL CC, SOUSSI T. 1992. Tp53 tumor suppressor gene: A model for investigating human mutagenesis. Genes Chromosomes Cancer 4:1–15.

DEJONG UW, DAY NE, MUIR CS, et al. 1972. The distribution of cancer within the large bowel. Int J Cancer 10:463–477.

DELATTRE O, OLSCHWANG S, LAW DJ, et al. 1989. Multiple genetic alterations in distal and proximal colorectal cancer. Lancet 2:353–356.

DEMERS LM, HARRISON TS, HALBERT DR, et al. 1981. Effect of prolonged exercise on plasma prostaglandin levels. Prostaglandins Med 6:413–418.

DESENCLOS JA, HAHN RA. 1992. Years of potential life lost before age 65, by race, Hispanic origin, and sex—United States, 1986–1988. MMWR 41:13–23.

DIAMOND M. 1952. Adenomas of the rectum and sigmoid in alcoholics: A sigmoidoscopic study. Am J Dig Dis 19:47–50.

DOLL R, PETO R. 1976. Mortality in relation to smoking: 20 years observation on male British doctors. Br Med J 2:1525–1536.

DUGGAN MA, BORAS VF, INOUE M, et al. 1989. Human papillomavirus DNA determination of anal condylomata, dysplasias, and squamous carcinomas with in-situ hybridization. Am J Clin Pathol 92:16–21.

EHRLICH A, GORDON RE, DIKMAN SH. 1991. Carcinoma of the colon in asbestos-exposed workers: Analysis of asbestos content in colon tissue. Am J Ind Med 19:629–636.

EKBOM A, HELMICK C, ZACK M, et al. 1990. Increased risk of large bowel cancer in Crohn's disease with colonic involvement. Lancet 336:357–359.

EKBOM A, HELMICK C, ZACK M, et al. 1990. Ulcerative colitis and colorectal cancer: A population-based study. N Engl J Med 323:1228–1233.

EKBOM A, YUEN J, ADAMI H, et al. 1993. Cholecystectomy and colorectal cancer. Gastroenterology 105:142–147.

FEARON ER. 1994. Molecular genetic studies of the adenoma-carcinoma sequence. Adv Intern Med 39:123–147.

FEARON ER, CHO KR, NIGRO JM, et al. 1990. Identification of a chromosome 18q gene that is altered in colorectal cancers. Science 247:49–56.

FEARON ER, VOGELSTEIN B. 1990. A genetic model for colorectal tumorigenesis. Cell 61:759–767.

FINLEY GG, SCHULZ NT, HILL SA, et al. 1990. Expression of the myc gene family in different stages of human colorectal cancer. Oncogene 4:963–971.

FREDRIKSSON M, BENGTSSON NO, HARDELL L, et al. 1989. Colon cancer, physical activity and occupational exposures. A case-control study. Cancer 63:1838–1842.

FREEMAN HJ. 1983. Lectin histochemistry of 1,2-dimethylhydrazine induced rat colon neoplasia. J Histochem Cytochem 31:1241–1245.

FREEMAN HJ. 1989. Neoplastic complications of inflammatory bowel disease. *In* Freemen HJ (ed): Inflammatory Bowel Disease, Vol. II. Boca Raton, Florida, CRC Press, pp. 24–35.

FREUDENHEIM JL, GRAHAM S, MARSHALL JR, et al. 1990. A case-control study of diet and rectal cancer in Western New York. Am J Epidemiol 131:612–624.

FREUDENHEIM JL, GRAHAM S, MARSHALL JR, et al. 1990. Lifetime alcohol intake and risk of rectal cancer in Western New York. Nutr Cancer 13:101–109.

FRIEDMAN GD, GOLDHABER MK, QUESENBERRY CP JR. 1987. Cholecystectomy and large bowel cancer. Lancet 1:906–908.

FRISCH M, MELBYE M, MOLLER H. 1993. Trends in incidence of anal cancer in Denmark. Br Med J 306:419–422.

FRISCH M, OLSEN JH, MELBYE M. 1994. Malignancies that occur before and after anal cancer: Clues to their etiology. Am J Epidemiol 140:12–19.

FRISCH M, OLSEN JH, BAUTZ A, et al. 1994. Benign anal lesions and the risk of anal cancer. N Engl J Med 331:300–302.

FUNKHOUSER E, COLE P. 1992. Declining mortality rates for cancer of the rectum in the United States: 1940–1985. Cancer 70:2597–2601.

FURNER SE, DAVIS FG, NELSON RL, et al. 1989. A case-control study of large bowel cancer and hormone exposure in women. Cancer Res 49:4936–4940.

GAL AA, SAUL SH, STOLER MH. 1989. In situ hybridization analysis of human papillomavirus in anal squamous cell carcinoma. Mod Pathol 2:439–443.

GALLOWAY DJ. 1989. Animal models in the study of colorectal cancer. Cancer Surv 8:169–188.

GARABRANT DH, PETERS JM, MACK TM, et al. 1984. Job activity and colon cancer risk. Am J Epidemiol 119:1005–1014.

GARABRANT DH, PETERS RK, HOMA DM. 1992. Asbestos and colon cancer: Lack of association in a large case-control study. Am J Epidemiol 135:843–853.

GARLAND CF, GARLAND FC. 1986. Calcium and colon cancer Clin Nutr 5:161–166.

GARLAND CF, GARLAND FC, GORHAM ED. 1991. Can colon cancer incidence and death rates be reduced with calcium and vitamin D? Am J Clin Nutr 54:193S–201S.

GERHARDSSON M, NORELL SE, KIVIRANTA H, et al. 1986. Sedentary jobs and colon cancer. Am J Epidemiol 123:775–780.

GETZ SB, OUGH YD, PATTERSON RB, et al. 1981. Mucinous adenocarcinoma developing in chronic anal fistula: Report of two cases and review of literature. Dis Colon Rectum 24:562–566.

GIARDELLO FM, HAMILTON SR, KRUSH AJ, et al. 1993. Treatment of colonic and rectal adenomas with sulindac in familial adenomatous polyposis. N Engl J Med 328:1313–1316.

GIOVANNUCCI E, COLDITZ GA, STAMPFER MJ. 1993. A meta-analysis of cholecystectomy and risk of colorectal cancer. Gastroenterology 105:130–141.

GIOVANNUCCI E, COLDITZ GA, STAMPFER MJ, et al. 1994. A prospective study of cigarette smoking and risk of colorectal adenoma and colorectal cancer in U.S. women. J Natl Cancer Inst 86:192–199.

GIOVANNUCCI E, RIMM EB, STAMPFER MJ, et al. 1994. A prospective study of cigarette smoking and risk of colorectal adenoma and colorectal cancer in U.S. men. J Natl Cancer Inst 86:183–191.

GIOVANNUCCI E, STAMPFER MJ, COLDITZ GA, et al. 1993. Folate, methionine and alcohol intake and risk of colorectal adenoma. J Natl Cancer Inst 85:875–884.

GIOVANNUCCI E, STAMPFER MJ, COLDITZ G, et al. 1992. Relationship of diet to risk of colorectal adenoma in men. J Natl Cancer Inst 84:91–98.

GOLDBOHM RA, BRANDT VAN DEN PA, VEER P, et al. 1994. A prospective cohort study on the relation between meat consumption and the risk of colon cancer. Cancer Res 54:718–723.

GOLDIN BR, GORBACH SL. 1981. Effect of antibiotics on incidence of rat intestinal tumors induced by 1,2-dimethylhydrazine dihydrochloride. J Natl Cancer Inst 67:877–880.

GOLDMAN S, GLIMELIUS B, NILSSON B, et al. 1989. Incidence of anal epidermoid carcinoma in Sweden 1970–1984. Acta Chir Scand 155:191–197.

GOYETTE MC, CHO K, FASCHING CL, et al. 1992. Progression of colorectal cancer is associated with multiple tumor suppressor gene defects but inhibition of tumorigenicity is accomplished by correction of any single defect via chromosome transfer. Mol Cell Biol 12:1387–1395.

GRAHAM S, MARSHALL JR, HAUGHEY B, et al. 1988. Dietary epidemiology of cancer of the colon in Western New York. Am J Epidemiol 128:490–503.

GREENBERG ER, BARON JA, FREEMAN DH JR, et al. 1993. Reduced risk of large bowel adenomas among aspirin users. J Natl Cancer Inst 85:912–916.

GREENBERG ER, BARON JA, TOSTESON TD, et al. 1994. A clinical trial of antioxidant vitamins to prevent colorectal adenoma. N Engl J Med 331:141–147.

GRIDLEY GG, MCLAUGHLIN JK, EKBOM A, et al. 1993. Incidence of cancer among patients with rheumatoid arthritis. J Natl Cancer Inst 85:307–311.

GRODEN J, THLIVERIS A, SAMOWITZ W. 1991. Identification and characterization of the familial adenomatous polyposis coli gene. Cell 66:589–600.

HAENSZEL W, LOCKE FB, SEGI M. 1980. A case-control study of large bowel cancer in Japan. J Natl Cancer Inst 64:17–22.

HAMILTON SR. 1989. Colorectal carcinoma in patients with Crohn's disease. Gastroenterology 89:398–407.

HAMILTON SR. 1990. Genetic susceptibility to colorectal carcinoma. *In* DeVita VT Jr, Hellman S, Rosenberg SA (eds): Cancer Prevention. Philadelphia, J. B. Lippincott, pp. 1–11.

HARRIS CC, HOLLSTEIN M. 1993. Clinical implications of the p53 tumor-suppressor gene. N Engl J Med 329:1318–1327.

HEILBRUN LK, HANKIN JH, NOMURA AMY, et al. 1986. Colon cancer and dietary fat, phosphorus, and calcium in Hawaiian-Japanese men. Am J Clin Nutr 43:306–309.

HERRERA L, KAKATI S, GIBAS L, et al. 1986. Gardner's syndrome in a man with an interstitial deletion of 5q. Am J Med Genet 25:473–476.

HIATT RA. 1992. Alcohol. *In* Micozzi MS, Moon TE (eds): Macronutrients: Investigating Their Role in Cancer. New York, Marcel Dekker, pp. 245–282.

HIGGINSON J, OETTLE AG. 1960. Cancer incidence in the Bantu and "Cape Colored" races of South Africa: Report of a cancer survey in the Transvaal (1953–55). J Natl Cancer Inst 24:589–671.

HOLDSTOCK DJ, MISIEWICZ JJ, SMITH T, et al. 1970. Propulsion (mass movements) in the human colon and its relationship to meals and somatic activity. Gut 11:91–99.

HOLLY EA, WHITTEMORE AS, ASTON DA, et al. 1989. Anal cancer incidence: genital warts, anal fissure or fistula, hemorrhoids, and smoking. J Natl Cancer Inst 81:1726–1731.

HOMA DM, GARABRANT DH, GILLESPIE BW. 1994. A meta-analysis of colorectal cancer and asbestos exposure. Am J Epidemiol 139:1210–1222.

HONJO S, KONO S, SHINCHI K, et al. 1992. Cigarette smoking, alcohol use and adenomatous polyps of the sigmoid colon. Jpn J Cancer Res 83:806–811.

HORII A, NAKATSURU S, MIYOSHI Y, et al. 1992. The APC gene, responsible for familial adenomatous polyposis, is mutated in human gastric cancer. Cancer Res 52:3231–3233.

HOWE GR, BENITO E, CASTELLETO R, et al. 1992. Dietary intake of fiber and decreased risk of cancers of the colon and rectum: Evidence from the combined analysis of 13 case-control studies. J Natl Cancer Inst 84:1887–1896.

HOWE GR, CRAIB KJP, MILLER AB. 1985. Age at first pregnancy and risk of colorectal cancer: A case-control study. J Natl Cancer Inst 74:1155–1159.

HOWE GR, MILLER AB, JAIN M. 1986. Total energy intake: Implications for epidemiologic analysis. Am J Epidemiol 124:156–157.

INTERNATIONAL AGENCY FOR RESEARCH ON CANCER. 1988. Alcohol Drinking. IARC Monographs on the Evaluation of Carcinogenic Risks to Humans. Vol 44. Lyon, WHO, p. 255.

JAIN M, COOK GM, DAVIS FG, et al. 1980. A case-control study of diet and colorectal cancer. Int J Cancer 26:757–768.

JEN J, KIM H, PIANTADOSI S, et al. 1994. Allelic loss of chromosome 18q and prognosis in colorectal cancer. N Engl J Med 331:213–221.

JENSEN OM. 1984. Different age and sex relationship for cancer of subsites of the large bowel. Br J Cancer 50:825–829.

JENSEN OM, MOSBECH J, SALASPURO M, et al. 1974. A comparative study of the diagnostic basis for cancer of the colon and cancer of the rectum in Denmark and Finland. Int J Epidemiol 3:183–186.

JONES P. 1986. DNA methylation and cancer. Cancer Res 46:461–466.

KADLUBAR FF. 1994. Rethinking the role of intestinal microflora in bioactivation of food-borne heterocyclic amine carcinogens. J Natl Cancer Inst 1:5.

KADLUBAR FF, BUTLER MA, KADERLIK KR, et al. 1992. Polymorphisms for aromatic amine metabolism in humans: Relevance for human carcinogenesis. Environ Health Perspect 98:69–74.

KAMPMAN E, GIOVANNUCCI E, VAN'T VEER P, et al. 1994. Calcium, vitamin D, dairy foods, and the occurrence of colorectal adenomas among men and women in two prospective studies. Am J Epidemiol 139:16–29.

KATZKA I, BRODY RS, MORRIS E, et al. 1983. Assessment of colorectal cancer risk in patients with ulcerative colitis: Experience from a private practice. Gastroenterology 85:22–29.

KIKENDALL JW, BOWEN PE, BURGESS MB, et al. 1989. Cigarettes and alcohol as independent risk factors for colonic adenomas. Gastroenterology 97:660–664.

KIKUCHI-YANOSHITA R, KONISHI M, FUKUNARI H, et al. 1992. Loss of expression of the DCC gene during progression of colorectal carcinomas in familial adenomatous polyposis and non-familial adenomatous polyposis patients. Cancer Res 52:3801–3803.

KING H, LI JY, LOCKE FB, et al. 1985. Patterns of site-specific displacement in cancer mortality among migrants: The Chinese in the United States. Am J Public Health 75:237–242.

KINZLER KW, NILBERT MC, VOGELSTEIN B, et al. 1991. Identification of a gene located at chromosome 5q21 that is mutated in colorectal cancers. Science 251:1366–1370.

KNUDSON AG. 1971. Mutation and cancer: Statistical study of retinoblastoma. Proc Natl Acad Sci USA 68:820–823.

KONO S, IKEDA N, YANAI F, et al. 1990. Alcoholic beverages and adenomatous polyps of the sigmoid colon: A study of male self-defense officials in Japan. Int J Epidemiol 19:848–852.

KRITCHEVSKY D, WEBER MM, BUCK CL, et al. 1986. Calories, fat and cancer. Lipids 21:272–274.

KUNE GA, KUNE S, READ A, et al. 1991. Colorectal polyps, diet, alcohol, and family history of colorectal cancer: A case-control study. Nutr Cancer 16:25–30.

KUNE GA, KUNE S, WATSON LF. 1989. Children, age at first birth, and colorectal cancer risk: Data from the Melbourne colorectal cancer study. Am J Epidemiol 129:533–542.

KUNE GA, KUNE S, WATSON LF. 1988. Colorectal cancer risk, chronic illnesses, operations, and medications: Case-control results from the Melbourne colorectal cancer study. Cancer Res 48:4399–4404.

KUNE S, KUNE GA, WATSON LF. 1987. Case-control study of dietary etiological factors: The Melbourne colorectal cancer study. Nutr Cancer 9:21–42.

KUNE S, KUNE GA, WATSON LF. 1986. The Melbourne colorectal cancer study: Incidence findings by age, sex, site, migrants and religion. Int J Epidemiol 15:483–493.

KURATSUNE M, IKEDA M, HAYASHI T. 1986. Epidemiologic studies on possible health effects of intake of pyrolyzates of foods, with reference to mortality among Japanese Seventh-Day Adventists. Environ Health Perspect 67:143–146.

LANS JI, JASZEWSKI R, ARLOW FL, et al. 1991. Supplemental calcium suppresses colonic mucosal ornithine decarboxylase activity in elderly patients with adenomatous polyps. Cancer Res 51:3416–3419.

LANZA E, GREENWALD P. 1989. The role of dietary fiber in cancer prevention. *In* DeVita VT Jr, Hellman S, Rosenberg SA (eds): Cancer Prevention. Philadelphia, J. B. Lippincott, pp. 1–9.

LANZA E, SHANKAR S, TROCK B. 1992. Dietary fiber. *In* Micozzi MS, Moon TE (eds): Macronutrients: Investigating Their Role in Cancer. New York, Marcel Dekker, pp. 293–319.

LAQUEUR GL, MICKELSON O, WHITING MG. 1963. Carcinogenic properties of nuts from cycas circinalis indigenous to Guam. J Natl Cancer Inst 31:919–951.

LEE WC, NEUGUT AI, GARBOWSKI GC, et al. 1993. Cigarettes, alcohol, coffee, and caffeine as risk factors for colorectal adenomatous polyps. Ann Epidemiol 3:239–244.

LENNARD-JONES JE, MELVILLE DM, MORSON BC, et al. 1990. Precancer and cancer in extensive ulcerative colitis: Findings among 401 patients over 22 years. Gut 31:800–806.

LEV R. 1990. Adenomatous Polyps of the Colon. New York, Springer-Verlag, pp. 45–52.

LIPKIN M, DESCHNER E. 1976. Early proliferative changes in intestinal cells. Cancer Res 36:2665–2668.

LIPKIN M, HIGGINS P. 1988. Biological markers of cell proliferation and differentiation in human gastrointestinal diseases. Adv Cancer Res 50:1–24.

LIPKIN M, NEWMARK H. 1985. Effect of added dietary calcium on colonic epithelial cell proliferation in subjects at high risk for familial colonic cancer. N Engl J Med 313:1381–1384.

LOGAN RFA, LITTLE J, HAWTIN PG, et al. 1993. Effect of aspirin and non-steroidal anti-inflammatory drugs on colorectal adenomas: A case-control study of subjects participating in the Nottingham fecal occult blood screening program. Br Med J 307:285–289.

LONGNECKER MP, MARTIN-MORENO J, KNEKT P, et al. 1992. Serum alpha-tocopherol concentration in relation to subsequent colorectal cancer: Pooled data from five cohorts. J Natl Cancer Inst 84:430–435.

LONGNECKER MP, ORZA MJ, ADAMS ME, et al. 1990. A meta-analysis of alcoholic beverage consumption in relation to risk of colorectal cancer. Cancer Causes Control 1:59–68.

LUK GD, BAYLIN SB. 1984. Ornithine decarboxylase as a biologic marker in familial colonic polyposis. N Engl J Med 311:80–83.

LYNCH HT, SMYRK TC, WATSON P, et al. 1993. Genetics, natural history, tumor spectrum, and pathology of hereditary nonpolyposis colorectal cancer: An updated review. Gastroenterology 104:1535–1549.

LYNCH HT, WATSON P, SMYRK TC, et al. 1992. Colon cancer genetics. Cancer 70:1300–1312.

LYNCH PM, LYNCH HT. 1985. Colon Cancer Genetics. New York, Van Nostrand Reinhold.

LYON JL, MAHONEY AW, WEST DW, et al. 1987. Energy intake: Its relationship to colon cancer risk. J Natl Cancer Inst 78:853–861.

MACQUART-MOULIN G, RIBOLI E, CORNEE J, et al. 1986. Case-control study on colorectal cancer and diet in Marseilles. Int J Cancer 38:183–191.

MANDL M, FRIEDL W, PAFFENHOLZ R, et al. 1994. Frequency of common and novel inactivating APC mutations in 202 families with familial adenomatous polyposis. Hum Mol Genet 3:181–184.

MARCUS PM, NEWCOMB PA, YOUNG T, et al. 1995. The association of reproductive and menstrual characteristics and colon and rectal cancer risk in Wisconsin women. Ann Epidemiology 5:303–309.

MARNETT LJ. 1992. Aspirin and the potential role of prostaglandins in colon cancer. Cancer Res 52:5575–5589.

MARSHALL JR, ZIELEZNY MA. 1993. Fat and calories in the epidemiology of colon cancer in Western New York. Prev Med 22:775–782.

MCKEOWN-EYSSEN GE. 1987. Fiber intake in different populations and colon cancer risk. Prev Med 16:532–539.

MCKEOWN-EYSSEN GE, BRIGHT-SEE E. 1985. Dietary factors in colon cancer: International relationships. An update. Nutr Cancer 7:251–253.

MCKEOWN-EYSSEN GE, HOLLOWAY C, JAZMAJI V, et al. 1988. A randomized trial of vitamins C and E in the prevention of recurrence of colorectal polyps. Cancer Res 48:4701–4705.

MCMICHAEL AJ, MCCALL MG, HARTSHORNE JM, et al. 1980. Patterns of gastrointestinal change in European migrants to Australia: The role of dietary change. Int J Cancer (Suppl)25:431–437.

MCMICHAEL AJ, POTTER JD. 1980. Reproduction, endogenous and exogenous sex hormones, and colon cancer: A review and hypothesis. J Natl Cancer Inst 65:1201–1207.

MCMICHAEL AJ, POTTER JD. 1985. Host factors in carcinogenesis: Certain bile-acid metabolic profiles that selectively increase the risk of proximal colon cancer. J Natl Cancer Inst 75:185–191.

MELBYE M, SPROGEL P. 1991. Etiological parallel between anal cancer and cervical cancer. Lancet 338:657–659.

MELBYE M, COTÉ TR, KESSLER L, et al. 1994. High incidence of anal cancer among AIDS patients. Lancet 343:636–639.

MELBYE M, RABKIN C, FRISCH M, et al. 1994. Changing patterns of anal cancer incidence in the United States, 1940–1989. Am J Epidemiol 139:772–780.

METZGER U, MEIER J, UHLSCHMID G, WEIHE H. 1984. Influence of various prostaglandin synthesis inhibitors on DMH-induced rat colon cancer. Dis Colon Rectum 27:366–369.

MILLER AB. 1992. Dietary fat. *In* Micozzi MS, Moon TE (eds): Macronutrients: Investigating Their Role in Cancer. New York, Marcel Dekker, pp. 231–243.

MITCHELL EP. 1988. Carcinoma of the anal region. Semin Oncol 15:146–153.

MOOLGAVKAR SH, LUEBECK EG. 1992. Multistage carcinogenesis: Population-based model for colon cancer. J Natl Cancer Inst 84:610–618.

MORGAN RW, FOLIART DE, WONG O. 1985. Asbestos and gastrointestinal cancer.West J Med 143:60–65.

MORSON BC. 1984. The evolution of colorectal carcinoma. Clin Radiol 35:425–431.

MUIR C, WATERHOUSE J, MACK T, et al. 1987. Cancer Incidence in Five Continents, Vol. V, IARC Scientific Publication No. 88, Lyon, France, International Agency for Research on Cancer.

MURDAY V, SLACK J. 1989. Inherited disorders associated with colorectal cancer. Cancer Surv 8:139–157.

NATIONAL CANCER INSTITUTE. 1992. Cancer Statistics Review, 1973–1989. DHHS Publ No. (NIH) 92-2789, Bethesda, MD.

NEUGUT AI, JACOBSON JS, DEVIVO I. 1993. Epidemiology of colorectal adenomatous polyps. Cancer Epidemiol Biomarkers Prev 2:159–176.

NEWCOMB PA, STORER BE, MARCUS PM. 1993. Cancer of the large bowel in women in relation to alcohol consumption: A case-control study in Wisconsin (United States). Cancer Causes Control 4:405–411.

NEWCOMB PA, STORER BE. 1995. Postmenopausal hormone use and risk of large bowel cancer. J Natl Cancer Inst 87:1067–1071.

NEWMARK HL, LIPKIN M. 1992. Calcium, vitamin D, and colon cancer. Cancer Res 52:2067s–2070s.

O'BRIEN MJ, O'KEANE JC, ZAUBER AG, et al. 1992. Precursors of colorectal carcinoma: Biopsy and biologic markers. Cancer 70:1317–1327.

O'CONNOR TP, CAMPBELL TC. 1987. The contribution of animal experiments to knowledge of the relationship between diet and cancer risk in humans. Cancer Surv 6:573–583.

OWEN RW, THOMPSON MH, HILL MJ, et al. 1987. The importance of the ratio of lithocholic to deoxycholic acid in large bowel carcinogenesis. Nutr Cancer 9:67–71.

PACKER L, FUCHS J (EDS). 1992. Vitamin E in Health and Disease. New York, Marcel Dekker.

PAGANINI-HILL A, HSU G, ROSS RK, et al. 1991. Aspirin use and incidence of large bowel cancer in a California retirement community. J Natl Cancer Inst 83:1182–1183.

PAINTER NS, BURKITT DP. 1971. Diverticular disease of the colon:

A deficiency disease of Western civilization. Br Med J 2:450–454.

PALEFSKY JM, HOLLY EA, GONZALEZ J, et al. 1991. Detection of human papillomavirus DNA in anal intraepithelial neoplasia and anal cancer. Cancer Res 51:1014–1019.

PAPADOPOULOS N, NICOLAIDES NC, YING-FEI W, et al. 1994. Mutation of a mutL homolog in hereditary colon cancer. Science 263:1625–1629.

PARKIN DM, MUIR CS, WHELAN SL, GAO Y-T, FERLAY J, POWELL J. 1992. Cancer Incidence in Five Continents, Volume VI, Lyon, IARC Scientific Publications, Number 120, pp. 928–929.

PELEG II, MAIBACH HT, BROWN SH, et al. 1994. Aspirin and nonsteroidal anti-inflammatory drug use and the risk of subsequent colorectal cancer. Arch Intern Med 154:394–399.

PELTOMAKI P, AALTONEN LA, SISTONEN P, et al. 1993. Genetic mapping of a locus predisposing to human colorectal cancer. Science 260:810–812.

PERCY C, STANEK E III, GLOECKLER L. 1981. Accuracy of cancer death certificates and its effect on cancer mortality statistics. Am J Public Health 71:242–250.

PERSKY V, DYER AR, LEONAS J, et al. 1981. Heart rate: A risk factor for cancer? Am J Epidemiol 114:477–487.

PETERS RK, MACK TM. 1983. Patterns of anal carcinoma by gender and marital status in Los Angeles county. Br J Cancer 48:629–636.

PETERS RK, MACK TM, BERSTEIN L. 1984. Parallels in epidemiology of selected anogenital carcinomas. J Natl Cancer Inst 72:609–615.

PETERS RK, MACK TM, GARABRANT DH, et al. 1991. Calcium and colon cancer in Los Angeles County. *In* Lipkin M, Newmark HL, Kelloff G (eds): Calcium, Vitamin D and Prevention of Colon Cancer. Boca Raton, CRC Press, pp. 113–118.

PODOLSKY DK. 1991. Inflammatory bowel disease. N Engl J Med 325:1008–1016.

POLLARD M, LUCKERT PH. 1983. Prolonged antitumor effect of indomethacin on autochthonous intestinal tumors in rats. J Natl Cancer Inst 70:1103–1105.

POTTER JD. 1992. Reconciling the epidemiology, physiology, and molecular biology of colon cancer. JAMA 268:1573–1577.

POTTER JD, MCMICHAEL AJ. 1983. Large bowel cancer in women in relation to reproductive and hormonal factors: A case-control study. J Natl Cancer Inst 71:703–709.

POTTER JD, MCMICHAEL AJ. 1986. Diet and cancer of the colon and rectum: A case-control study. J Natl Cancer Inst 76:557–569.

POTTER JD, SLATTERY ML, BOSTICK RM, et al. 1993. Colon cancer: A review of the epidemiology. Epidemiol Rev 15:499–545.

POWELL SM, ZILZ N, BEAZER-BARCLAY Y, et al. 1992. APC mutations occur early during colorectal tumorigenesis. Nature 359:235–237.

PRENDERGAST GC, GIBBS JB. 1993. Pathways of ras function: Connections to the actin cytoskeleton. Adv Cancer Res 62:19–64.

RABKIN CS, BIGGAR RJ, MELBYE M, et al. 1992. Second primary cancers following anal and cervical carcinoma: Evidence of shared etiologic factors. Am J Epidemiol 136:54–58.

REDDY BS. 1992. Animal experimental evidence on macronutrients and cancer. *In* Micozzi MS, Moon TE (eds): Macronutrients: Investigating Their Role in Cancer. New York, Marcel Dekker, pp. 33–54.

REDDY BS. 1987. Dietary fat and colon cancer: Animal models. Prev Med 16:460–467.

REDDY BS. 1981. Diet and excretion of bile acids. Cancer Res 41:3766–3768.

REDDY BS, ENGLE A, KATSIFIS S, et al. 1989. Biochemical epidemiology of colon cancer: Effects of types of dietary fiber on fecal mutagens, acid and neutral sterols in healthy subjects. Cancer Res 49:4629–4635.

REDDY BS, MARUYAMA H, KELLOFF G. 1987. Dose-related inhibition of colon carcinogenesis by dietary piroxicam, a nonsteroidal antiinflammatory drug, during different stages of rat colon tumor development. CancerRes 47:5340–5346.

RIBOLI E, CORNEE J, MACQUART-MOULIN G, et al. 1991. Cancer and polyps of the colorectum and lifetime consumption of beer and other alcoholic beverages. Am J Epidemiol 134:157–166.

RIDDELL RH. 1995. Inflammatory bowel disease and colorectal cancer. *In* Cohen AM, Winawer SJ, Friedman MA, Gunderson LL (eds): Cancer of the Colon, Rectum, and Anus. New York, McGraw-Hill, pp. 105–119.

RIGAU J, PIQUE JM, RUBIO E, et al. 1991. Effects of long-term sulindac therapy on colonic polyposis. Ann Intern Med 115:952–954.

ROGOT E, MURRAY JL. 1980. Smoking and causes of death among U.S. veterans: 16 years of observation. Public Health Rep 95:213–222.

RONCUCCI L, DIDONATO P, CARATI L, et al. 1993. Antioxidant vitamins or lactulose for the prevention of the recurrence of colorectal adenomas. Dis Colon Rectum 36:227–234.

ROSENBERG L, PALMER JR, ZAUBER AG, et al. 1991. A hypothesis: Nonsteroidal anti-inflammatory drugs reduce the incidence of large bowel cancer. J Natl Cancer Inst 83:355–358.

ROTTER V, PROKOCIMER M. 1991. p53 and human malignancies. Adv CancerRes 57:257–272.

RUBIO CA, NYLANDER G. 1981. Further studies on the carcinogenesis of the colon of the rat with special reference to the absence of intestinal contents. Cancer 48:951–953.

SCHOLEFIELD JH, SONNEX C, TALBOT IC, et al. 1989. Anal and cervical intraepithelial neoplasia: possible parallel. Lancet 2:765–769.

SCHOLEFIELD JH, HICKSON WGE, SMITH JHF, et al. 1992. Anal intraepithelial neoplasia: part of a multifocal disease process. Lancet 340:1271–1273.

SCHOTTENFELD D, BERG JW, VITSKY B. 1969. Incidence of multiple primary cancers. II. Index cancers arising in the stomach and lower digestive system. J Natl Cancer Inst 43:77–86.

SCHOTTENFELD D, WARSHAUER ME, ZAUBER AG, et al. 1980. Study of cancer mortality and incidence in wood shop workers of the General Motors Corporation. Report prepared for the Occupational Health Advisory Board of United Auto Workers; April 18, 1980.

SCHWARTZ D, FLAMANT R, LELLOUCH J, et al. 1961. Results of a French survey on the role of tobacco, particularly inhalation, in different cancer sites. J Natl Cancer Inst 26:1085–1108.

SIDRANSKY D, TOKINO T, HAMILTON SR, et al. 1992. Identification of ras oncogene mutations in the stool of patients with curable colorectal tumors. Science 256:102–105.

SIMONS BD, MORRISON AS, LEV R, et al. 1992. Relationships of polyps to cancer of the large intestine. J Natl Cancer Inst 84:962–966.

SLATTERY ML, SORENSON AW, MAHONEY AW, et al. 1988. Diet and colon cancer: Assessment of risk by fiber type and food source. J Natl Cancer Inst 80:1474–1480.

SLATTERY ML, SORENSON AW, FORD MH. 1988. Dietary calcium intake as a mitigating factor in colon cancer. Am J Epidemiol 128:504–514.

SLATTERY ML, WEST DW, ROBISON LM, et al. 1990. Tobacco, alcohol, coffee and caffeine as risk factors for colon cancer in a low-risk population. Epidemiology 1:141–145.

SNYDER DN, HESTON JF, MEIGS JW, et al. 1977. Changes in site distribution of colorectal carcinoma in Connecticut, 1940–1973. Dig Dis 22:791–797.

SORENSON AW, SLATTERY ML, FORD MH. 1988. Calcium and colon cancer: A review. Nutr Cancer 11:135–145.

SPIEGELMAN D, WEGMAN DH. 1985. Occupation-related risks for colorectal cancer. J Natl Cancer Inst 75:813–821.

STEINBACH G, MOROTOMI M, NOMOTO K, et al. 1994. Calcium reduces the increased fecal 1,2-SN-diacylglycerol content in intestinal bypass patients: a possible mechanism for altering colonic hyperproliferation. Cancer Research 54:1216–1219.

STEINMETZ KA, POTTER JD. 1991. Vegetables, fruit and cancer. I. Epidemiology. Cancer Causes Control 2:325–357.

STEINMETZ KA, POTTER JD. 1991. Vegetables, fruit, and cancer. II. Mechanisms. Cancer Causes Control 2:427–442.

STEINMETZ KA, KUSHI LH, BOSTICK RM, et al. 1994. Vegetables, fruit and colon cancer in the Iowa Women's Health Study. Am J Epidemiol 139:1–15.

STEMMERMANN GN, NOMURA AMY, HEILBRUN LK. 1984. Dietary fat and risk of colorectal cancer. Cancer Res 44:4633–4637.

STEMMERMANN GN, NOMURA AMY, CHYOU PH. 1990. The influence of dairy and nondairy calcium on subsite large bowel cancer risk. Dis Colon Rectum 33:190–194.

STEMMERMANN GN, HEILBRUN LK, NOMURA AMY. 1988. Association of diet and other factors with adenomatous polyps of the large bowel: A prospective autopsy study. Am J Clin Nutr 47:312–317.

ST. JOHN DJB, MCDERMOTT FT, HOPPER JL, et al. 1993. Cancer risk in relatives of patients with common colorectal cancer. Ann Intern Med 118:785–790.

SUGIMURA T, NAGAO M, WAKABAYASHI K. 1994. Heterocyclic amines in cooked foods: Candidates for causation of common cancers. J Natl Cancer Inst 86:2–4.

SUGIMURA T, NAGO M, KAWACHI T, et al. 1977. Mutagens and carcinogens in foods with special reference to highly mutagenic pyrolytic production in broiled foods. *In* Hiatt HH, Watson JD, Winsten JA (eds): Origins of Human Cancer. Cold Spring Harbor, New York, pp. 1561–1577.

SURGEON GENERAL'S REPORT ON NUTRITION AND HEALTH. 1988. U.S. Department of Health and Human Services, Public Health Service, DHHS (PHS) Publication No. 88-50210, pp. 177–247.

SUTTON TD, EIDE TJ, JASS JR. 1993. Trends in colorectal cancer incidence and histologic findings in Maori and Polynesian residents in New Zealand. Cancer 71:3839–3845.

SWANSON GM, BELLE SH, BURROWS RW. 1985. Colon cancer incidence among model makers and pattern makers in the automobile manufacturing industry: A continuing dilemma. J Occup Med 27:567–569.

TAJIMA K, TOMINAGA S. 1985. Dietary habits and gastro-intestinal cancers: A comparative case-control study of stomach and large intestinal cancers in Nagoya, Japan. Jpn J Cancer Res 76:705–716.

TANNENBAUM A. 1945. The dependence of tumor formation on the degree of caloric restriction. Cancer Res 5:609–615.

THIBODEAU SN, BREN G, SCHAID D. 1993. Microsatellite instability in cancer of the proximal colon. Science 260:816–819.

THUN MJ, CALLE EE, NAMBOODIRI MM, et al. 1992. Risk factors for fatal colon cancer in a large prospective study. J Natl Cancer Inst 84:1491–1500.

TROCK B, LANZA E, GREENWALD P. 1990. Dietary fiber, vegetables, and colon cancer: Critical review and meta-analyses of the epidemiologic evidence. J Natl Cancer Inst 82:650–661.

TUYNS AJ, HAELTERMAN M, KAAKS R. 1987. Colorectal cancer and the intake of nutrients: Oligosaccharides are a risk factor, fats are not. Nutr Cancer 10:181–196.

VENA JE, GRAHAM S, ZIELEZNY M, et al. 1985. Lifetime occupational exercise and colon cancer. Am J Epidemiol 122:357–365.

VERDIER DEG, HAGMAN U, PETERS RK, et al. 1991. Meat, cooking methods and colorectal cancer: A case-referent study in Stockholm. Int J Cancer 49:520–525.

VERNICK LJ, KULLER LK, LOHSOONTHORN P, et al. 1980. Relationship between cholecystectomy and ascending colon cancer. Cancer 45:392–395.

VILE R. 1993. p53: a gene for all tumors? Br Med J 307:1226–1227.

VOGELSTEIN B, FEARON ER, HAMILTON SR, et al. 1988. Genetic alterations during colorectal tumor development. N Engl J Med 319:525–532.

VUKASIN AP, BALLANTYNE GH, FLANNERY JT, et al. 1990. Increasing incidence of cecal and sigmoid carcinoma. Data from the Connecticut tumor registry. Cancer 66:2442–2449.

WADDELL WR, GANSER GF, CERISE EJ, et al. 1989. Sulindac for polyposis of the colon. Am J Surg 157:175–179.

WARSHAUER ME, SILVERMAN DT, SCHOTTENFELD D, et al. 1986. Stomach and colorectal cancer incidence and mortality in Puerto Rican-born residents in New York City. J Natl Cancer Inst 76:591–595.

WATANABE H, AJIOKA Y, IWAFUCHI M, et al. 1990. Histogenesis of gastrointestinal carcinoma in Peutz-Jegher's polyp. *In* Utsunomiya J, Lynch HT (eds): Hereditary Colorectal Cancer. Tokyo, Springer-Verlag, pp. 337–342.

WATSON P, LYNCH HT. 1993. Extracolonic cancer in hereditary nonpolyposis colorectal cancer. Cancer 71:677–685.

WATTENBERG LW. 1985. Chemoprevention of cancer. Cancer Res 45:1–8.

WAYE JD. 1986. Screening for cancer in ulcerative colitis. Front GastrointestRes 10:243–256.

WEISBURGER JH, FIALA ES. 1983. Experimental colon carcinogens and their mode of action. *In* Autrup H, Williams GM (eds): Experimental Colon Carcinogenesis. Boca Raton, CRC Press, pp. 27–50.

WEISBURGER JH, RIVENSON A, REINHARDT J, et al. 1994. Genotoxicity and carcinogenicity in rats and mice of 2-amino-3,6-dihydro-3-methyl-7H-imidazole [4,5-f] quinolin-7-one: An intestinal bacterial metabolite of 2-amino-3-methyl-3H-imidazo [4,5-f] quinoline. J Natl Cancer Inst 86:25–30.

WEISBURGER JH, WYNDER EL. 1987. Etiology of colorectal cancer with emphasis on mechanism of action and prevention. *In* DeVita VT Jr, Hellman S, Rosenberg SA (eds): Important Advances in Oncology. Philadelphia, J. B. Lippincott, pp. 197–220.

WEXNER SD, MILSOM JW, DAILEY TH. 1987. The demographics of anal cancer are changing. Dis Colon Rectum 30:942–946.

WHITTEMORE AS, WU-WILLIAMS AH, LEE M. et al. 1990. Diet, physical activity and colorectal cancer among Chinese in North America and China. J Natl Cancer Inst 82:915–926.

WILLETT W, STAMPFER MJ. 1986. Total energy intake: Implications for epidemiologic analyses. Am J Epidemiol 124:17–27.

WILLETT W, STAMPFER MJ, COLDITZ GA, et al. 1990. Relation of meat, fat, and fiber intake to the risk of colon cancer in a prospective study among women. N Engl J Med 323:1664–1672.

WILLIAMSON RCN, BAUER FLR, ROSS JS, et al. 1979. Enhanced colonic carcinogenesis with azoxymethane in rats after pancreatico-biliary diversion to mid small bowel. Gastroenterology 76:1386–1392.

WINAWER SJ, ZAUBER AG, HO MN, et al. 1993. Prevention of colorectal cancer by colonoscopic polypectomy. N Engl J Med 329:1977–1981.

WINAWER SJ, ZAUBER AG, O'BRIEN MJ, et al. 1993. Randomized comparison of surveillance intervals after colonoscopic removal of newly diagnosed adenomatous polyps. N Engl J Med 328:901–906.

WU AH, PAGANINI-HILL A, ROSS RK, et al. 1987. Alcohol, physical activity and other risk factors for colorectal cancer: A prospective study. Br J Cancer 55:687–694.

WU-WILLIAMS AH, LEE M, WHITTEMORE AS. 1991. Reproductive factors and colorectal cancer risk among Chinese females. Cancer Res 51:2307–2311.

WYNDER EL, FUJITA Y, HARRIS RE, et al. 1991. Comparative epidemiology of cancer between the United States and Japan. Cancer 67:746–763.

ZACHOW KR, OSTROW RS, BENDER M, et al. 1982. Detection of human papillomavirus DNA in anogenital neoplasia. Nature 300:771–773.

ZIEGLER RC, DEVESA SS, FRAUMENI JF JR. 1986. Epidemiologic patterns of colorectal cancer. *In* DeVita VT Jr, Hellman S, Rosenberg SA (eds): Important Advances in Oncology. Philadelphia, J. B. Lippincott, pp. 209–232.

ZUR HAUSEN H. 1989. Papillomaviruses in anogenital cancer as a model to understand the role of viruses in human cancer. Cancer Res 49:4677–4681.

40 The leukemias

MARTHA S. LINET
RAYMOND A. CARTWRIGHT

The leukemias constitute less than 5% of malignancies in most countries, but include a wide diversity of biologically and clinically distinct subtypes. Understanding of the steps in leukemogenic transformation of hematopoietic system cells has rapidly expanded in recent years owing to advances in molecular biology and immunology, but elucidation of risk factors has been hampered by the rarity of individual leukemia subtypes and limitations of the classification criteria employed. Epidemiologic studies of the leukemias prior to the early 1980s and associated methodologic problems have been previously reviewed (Cartwright and Bernard, 1985; Linet, 1985; Linet and Blattner, 1988; Linet and Devesa, 1990; Cartwright and Staines, 1992; Finch and Linet, 1992). This chapter emphasizes recent research, highlighting leukemia subtype differences in patterns of occurrence and etiology, while recognizing similarities in risk profiles among subtypes and among related lymphoproliferative malignancies and myelodysplastic syndromes.

HISTOLOGY AND CLASSIFICATION SYSTEMS

Implementation of the Eighth Revision of the International Classification of Diseases (World Health Organization, 1967) resulted in increasing consideration of four leukemia cell type groupings: acute lymphoblastic leukemia (ALL), chronic lymphocytic leukemia (CLL), acute myeloid leukemia (AML, used interchangeably with acute nonlymphoblastic or ANLL), and chronic myeloid or granulocytic leukemia (CML or CGL). The Seventh Revision (World Health Organization, 1957) did not differentiate acute and chronic forms of lymphoid and myeloid leukemia, whereas the Sixth Revision assigned a single code to all leukemias (World Health Organization, 1947). Newer approaches for distinguishing additional leukemia subtypes within the four major cell type categories appear to have biologic and etiologic relevance based on preliminary data (Ramot and Magrath, 1982; Greaves et al, 1985; McKinney et al, 1987; Matsuo et al, 1988; Robison et al, 1989; Buckley et al, 1989; Nishi and Miyake, 1989). Since 1976 the French-American-British (FAB) collaborative hematology group has proposed classifications utilizing morphologic and cytochemical features to more fully characterize ALL (Bennett et al, 1976; Catovsky et al, 1991), AML (Bennett et al, 1985a, b, 1991; Cheson et al, 1990), and chronic B and T lymphoid leukemias, with the latter group incorporating membrane phenotype characteristics (Bennett et al, 1989). Immunophenotyping, based on the reactions of monoclonal antibodies directed against cell surface B and T cell antigens and cytoplasmic proteins, has been used to define subtypes of ALL, each comprised of leukemic cells designated by their relationship to normal cellular differentiation (Greaves, 1986). Subtypes of B-CLL have also been defined by expression of cell surface immunoglobulins and other receptors (Freedman and Nadler, 1988). High resolution chromosomal banding techniques, in conjunction with molecular probes, have identified consistent karyotypic abnormalities specific to ALL (Copelan and McGuire, 1995), CLL (Croce and Nowell, 1985; Brito-Babapulle et al, 1987), AML (Yunis et al, 1984; Le Beau et al, 1986), and CML (Burkhardt et al, 1984).

A classification incorporating morphologic, immunophenotypic, and cytogenetic features has been proposed for ALL (First MIC Cooperative Study Group, 1986; Heim and Mitelman, 1987), and similar efforts have been undertaken for the chronic B- and T-cell leukemias (Bennett et al, 1990). Epidemiologic studies may also contribute by testing risk factor associations with various morphologic, immunophenotypic, and cytogenetic categories and identifying links between specific agents and particular leukemia cell types. Detailed morphologic (and, if possible, immunophenotypic and cytogenetic) review of leukemia cases should be undertaken routinely in epidemiologic studies to ascertain

We are grateful to Drs. Susan Devesa and Frank Groves and to the publishers of the British Journal of Cancer (Macmillan Press, Ltd.) and the European Journal of Cancer (Pergamon) for allowing us to reprint the three figures. Dr. Joseph Fraumeni Jr. critically reviewed several drafts of this chapter and made many helpful comments.

whether unique forms with features characteristic of specific exposures can be identified (Toolis et al, 1981; Finch and Finch, 1990).

DEMOGRAPHIC PATTERNS

Incidence Statistics

Incidence data provide better estimates of risk than mortality rates, because of differing survival patterns and inadequate specification of leukemia deaths by cell type. Also, the level of specification varies considerably among and within countries. Therefore, mortality data are not presented, except for description of time trends. For additional information on mortality, the reader is referred to Segi et al, 1977; Gardner et al, 1983; Selvin et al, 1983; Linet, 1985; Linet and Devesa, 1990; Wingren and Karlsson, 1990; Aoki et al, 1992; Coleman et al, 1993; Kinlen, 1994.

Internationally, lymphoid leukemias and myeloid leukemias each account for approximately 44% of all cases, and other and unspecified leukemias comprise the remaining 12% (Parkin et al, 1992). Leukemia incidence rates derived from data routinely reported to population-based registries may be 18%–23% lower than rates determined from special case-finding approaches (Mattson and Wallgren, 1984; Bowie, 1987; Alexander et al, 1989). To determine leukemia and lymphoma incidence rates by histopathologic subtype more accurately, a special surveillance network was established in the early 1980s in parts of England and Wales and data for 1984–88 have been published (Cartwright et al, 1990). Incomplete characterization or misclassification may also affect registered cases. Rates for leukemia incompletely specified or not otherwise specified (NOS) vary considerably by registry, which may affect the precision of the observed histologic type-specific rates. Thus, comparisons of type-specific incidence rates should be interpreted cautiously.

Acute Lymphoblastic Leukemia. ALL comprises only 5% of leukemias in persons aged 40 and older but is the most common childhood cancer except in Africa and the Middle East (Muir et al, 1987; Parkin et al, 1988, 1992). There is little variation in age-adjusted rates among populations, and the differences between countries are similar for males and females. Highest rates for both sexes occur in Spain, among Hispanics or Latinos in Los Angeles, in Caucasians in New Zealand and in Quebec and Ontario in Canada; among females, high rates are also found in Puerto Rico and in Cali, Colombia. Lowest rates are observed among U. S. blacks and Israeli Jews (Groves et al, 1995) (Fig. 40–1). Incidence varies more than threefold within England and Wales (Cartwright et al, 1990), with high rates observed in relatively isolated communities of higher socioeconomic status, farthest from urban centers (Alexander et al, 1990b).

Childhood ALL rates vary more than fourfold, with highest incidence in Costa Rica and among Hispanics in Los Angeles, and lowest rates among American blacks, in the Middle East, and in India (Linet and Devesa, 1991) (Fig. 40–2). Histopathologic misclassification (Bessho, 1989) may explain most of the apparent deficit of childhood ALL previously described for Japan (Nishiyama, 1969; Fraumeni and Miller, 1967). Preliminary data suggest a higher frequency of the subtype of T-ALL in Japan, India, Nigeria, Kenya, and South Africa than in most Western countries (Greaves et al, 1985; Bhargava et al, 1988), and a marked selective deficit in occurrence of the common (B-cell precursor) subset of ALL among black childhood populations in parts of Africa (Greaves et al, 1993). It has been proposed that the higher occurrence of T-ALL in these populations (if confirmed in population-based incidence data by immunophenotypic subtype) may reflect lower socioeconomic status. More detailed information about childhood ALL descriptive epidemiology can be found in the chapter on childhood cancers in this volume.

Childhood and adult ALL rates, based on data from the Surveillance, Epidemiology, and End Results (SEER) Program in the United States, are consistently higher among males than females in each age group, except among young persons under age 20 (Groves et al, 1995) (Fig. 40–3). Age-specific patterns in the United States, the United Kingdom, and many other countries show a peak among children ages 2–4, with a subsequent decline in rates to a low at ages 25–59, followed by an increase to a second slightly lower peak at ages 85+ (Fig. 40–3) (McKinney et al, 1989a; Linet and Devesa, 1990, 1991; Miller et al, 1993; Groves et al, 1995). ALL is rare in Africa, particularly among persons aged 40 and older, and no peak is observed among children under age 5; case series suggest that ALL is more common among children 5–14 than among children 0–4 years old (Fleming, 1985; Williams et al, 1984a).

Chronic Lymphocytic Leukemia. It is difficult to interpret international or even within-country variation in CLL because it is often diagnosed incidentally in the course of evaluating older individuals for other conditions. Thus, differences in level of medical care among populations may substantially bias CLL incidence data. Reported CLL rates differ more than 30-fold among populations, the greatest variation among all leukemia types. Geographic patterns are similar for both sexes. Rates (see Fig. 40–1) are highest in the north central United States and the contiguous central provinces in Canada; lower in South America and the Caribbean;

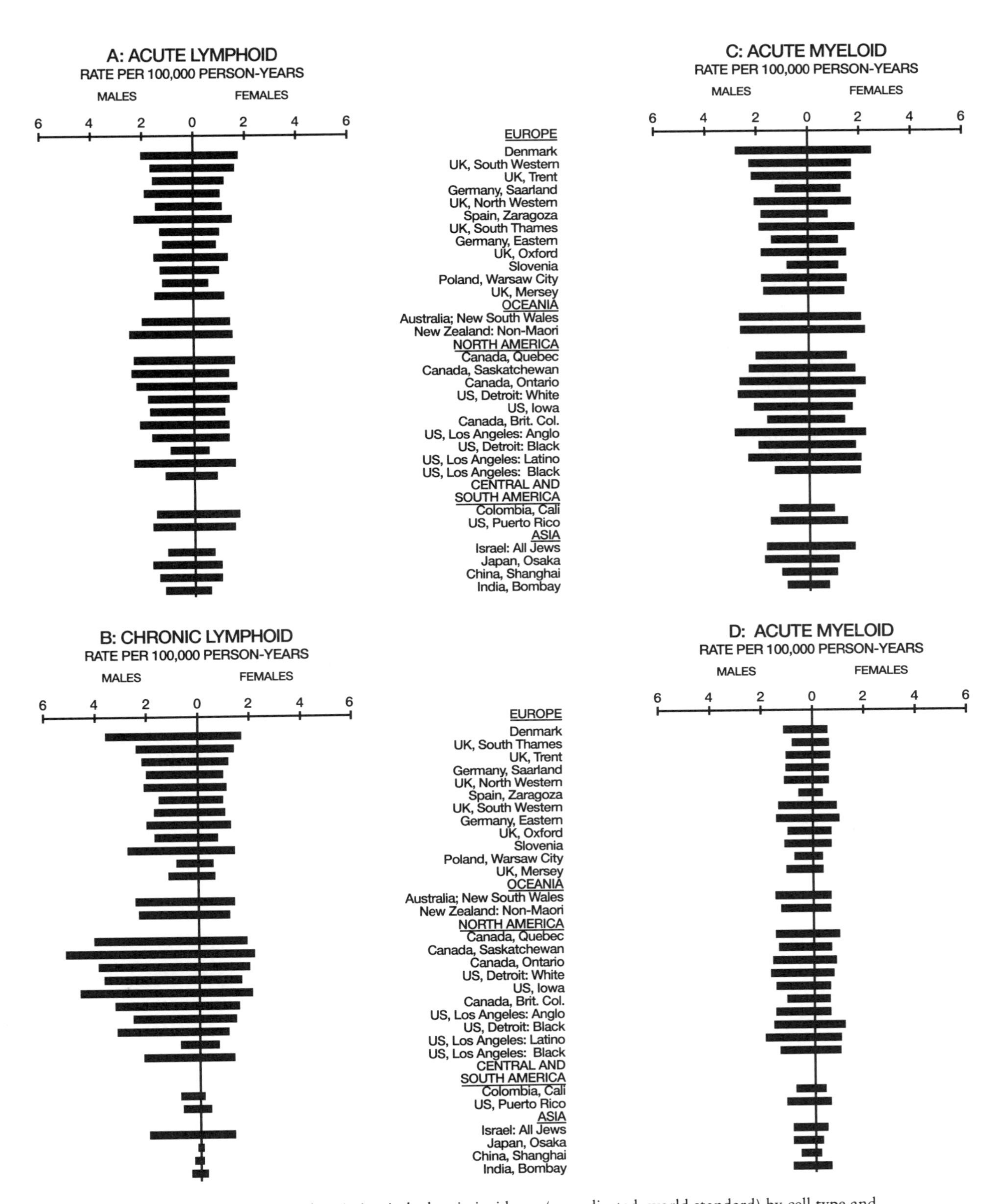

FIG. 40–1. International variation in leukemia incidence (age-adjusted, world standard) by cell type and sex, 1983–87. (Reprinted from European Journal of Cancer, Volume 31A, F.D. Groves et al, "Patterns of occurrence of the leukemias," pages 941–949, 1995, with kind permission from Elsevier Science Ltd, The Boulevard, Langford Lane, Kidlington OX5 1GB, UK. Source of data shown in figure is Parkin et al, 1992.)

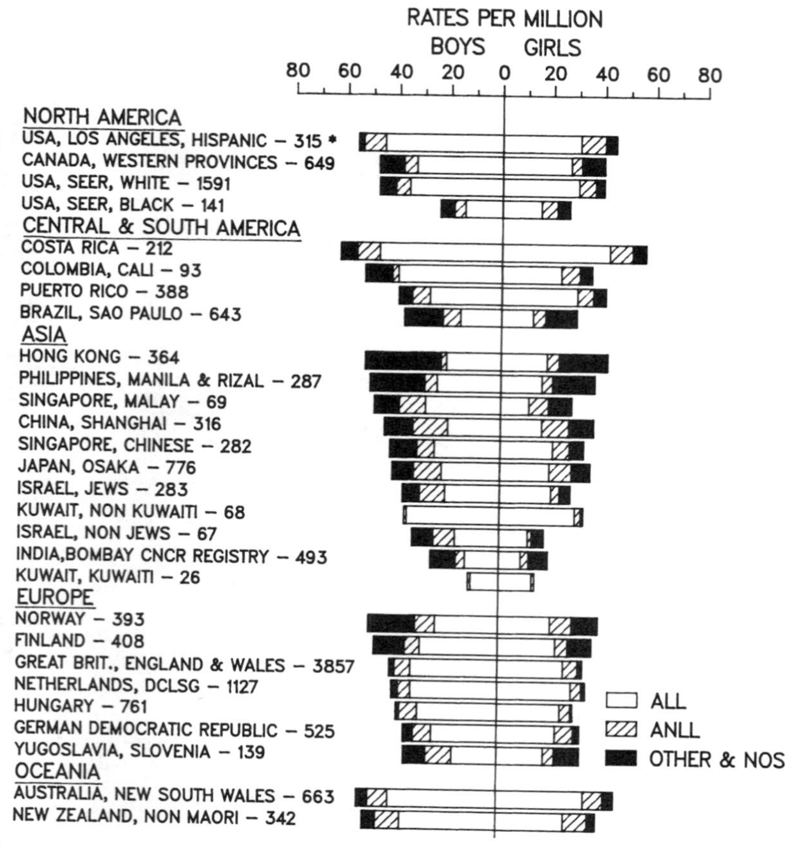

FIG. 40–2. International childhood leukemia incidence rates (age-adjusted, world standard) by cell type, circa 1970–79. Note: ANLL (acute nonlymphocytic leukemia) = AML (acute myeloid leukemia and related subtypes). (Reprinted from British Journal of Cancer, Volume 63, M.S. Linet and S.S. Devesa, "Descriptive epidemiology of childhood leukemia," pages 424–429, 1991, with kind permission from Stockton Press, Houndmills, Basingstoke, Hampshire RG21 6XS, UK. Source of data shown in figure is Parkin et al, 1988.) *Total number of boys and girls on which the rates are based.

and exceptionally low in Japan, India, and China (Muir et al, 1987; Yang and Zhang, 1991; Parkin et al, 1992), due to a marked deficit among persons aged 55 and older (T- and B-Cell Malignancy Study Group, 1988; Kushwaha et al, 1985; Muir et al, 1987). The rare occurrence of CLL in many African populations may reflect an overall shorter lifespan, although underdiagnosis and lower incidence at older ages may also contribute (Fleming, 1988).

Rates are consistently lower in females, although the sex ratio varies among geographic areas (see Fig. 40–1, 40–3) (Parkin et al, 1992). An unusual series of young (aged 35–50), mainly female cases of CLL (or possibly the related prolymphocytic leukemia) was reported from Nigeria, where older cases showed the usual male excess (Fleming, 1985, 1990; Okpala, 1990). In contrast, no young CLL cases of either sex were identified in a hospital series from Kenya (Oloo and Ogada, 1984). In most countries, CLL is extremely rare under age 30, though SEER Program incidence increases 350-fold between the ages of 25 to 29 and 80 to 84 (BA Miller et al, 1993) (see Fig. 40–3), similar to the age-specific pattern in most Western nations (Parkin et al, 1992). Differences between U. S. whites and blacks for the same sex are inconsistent (Groves et al, 1995).

Acute Myeloid Leukemia. AML is generally the most common of the specified leukemia types, and geographic patterns are similar for both sexes (see Fig. 40–1). Age-adjusted rates are consistently higher in more developed countries (Parkin et al, 1992) and in metropolitan areas of the United States than are AML rates in less developed nations and in rural areas of the United States (Linet and Devesa, 1990). This pattern was not observed

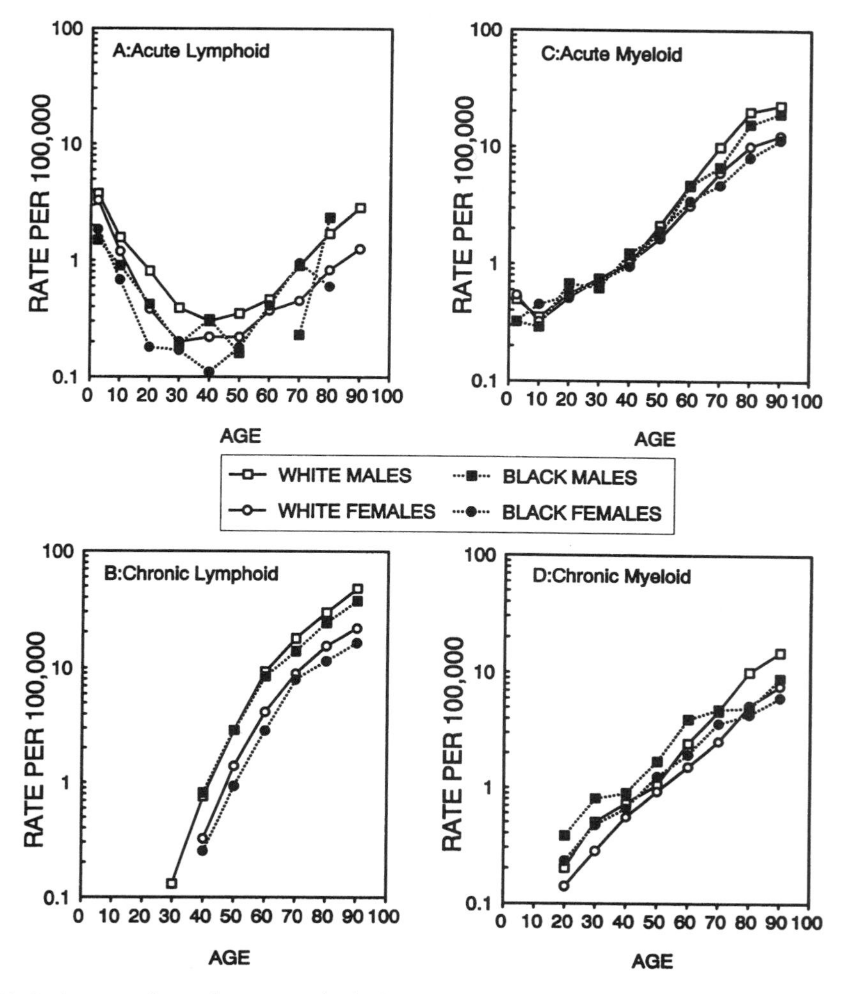

FIG. 40–3. Age-specific incidence rates for leukemia by cell type, race, and sex for nine SEER areas, 1973–87. (*A:* Acute Lymphoid Leukemia; *B:* Chronic Lymphoid Leukemia; *C:* Acute Myeloid Leukemia; *D:* Chronic Myeloid Leukemia.) (Reprinted from European Journal of Cancer, Volume 31A, F.D. Groves et al, "Patterns of occurrence of the leukemias," pages 941–949, 1995, with kind permission from Elsevier Science Ltd, The Boulevard, Langford Lane, Kidlington OX5 1GB UK.)

in the United Kingdom although there is considerable heterogeneity within different geographic areas of the country (McKinney et al, 1989b).

AML accounts for 15%–25% of childhood leukemia and 20%–40% in children aged 4 and younger in most white populations (see Fig. 40–2) (Parkin et al, 1988; Neglia and Robison, 1988). Internationally, rates range more than sixfold among boys and threefold among girls, with the male/female ratio varying from 0.8 to 2.6 (see Fig. 40–2) (Parkin et al, 1988). Despite lack of reliable incidence data for most African populations, occurrence of AML appears to be similar to or higher than that for ALL because the latter is quite uncommon (Waterhouse, 1982; Parkin et al, 1988). Estimated rates for Nigerian children aged 5–9 are higher than corresponding rates among U. S. black or white children (Williams et al, 1982; Fleming, 1988). AML rates are quite variable among Asian children, with rates in Shanghai the highest internationally (see Fig. 40–2).

Among adults in SEER Program data in the United States and elsewhere, rates for females are lower at age 55 and older than those for males (see Fig. 40–3). Age-specific rates show a small peak in children under 5 years of age followed by a slight decline until age 10, then a continuous rise, increasing in slope at age 50 and leveling off among the very elderly (see Fig. 40–3). This pattern is similar for both sexes and for U. S. whites and blacks (Cutler and Young, 1975; Young et al, 1981; BA Miller et al, 1993) and may indicate that risk factors for young children differ from those of older individuals.

For children under age 10 and adults over 55, rates are higher in U. S. whites than blacks, whereas incidence is similar in both races for the age range 10–54 (see Fig. 40–3) (BA Miller et al, 1993; Groves et al, 1995).

Chronic Myeloid Leukemia. Age-adjusted rates for CML vary little internationally or by geographic area in the United States or the United Kingdom (see Fig. 40–1) (Cutler and Young, 1975; Young et al, 1981; Cartwright et al, 1990). For example, CML rates among Nigerians are similar to those among U. S. whites and blacks (Williams and Bamgboye, 1983).

CML generally accounts for only 1%–3% of childhood leukemia in Western countries (Court Brown and Doll, 1959; Hansen et al, 1983), but an apparently higher proportion in African countries (Essien, 1976; Fleming, 1985). Internationally, white males under age 5 have a small peak in incidence rates, while juvenile CML is extremely rare among white females or U. S. blacks of either sex (Neglia and Robison, 1988).

Incidence is higher in males than females; unlike the other leukemia types, rates are higher in blacks than in whites in the United States (see Fig. 40–3) (Finch and Linet, 1992; Groves et al, 1995). In SEER Program data in the United States and other Western nations, CML first becomes apparent in the mid-teens, followed by a rapid rise in early adulthood; rates continue to rise throughout middle age and among the elderly, though CLL predominates among persons aged 65 and older (see Fig. 40–3) (BA Miller et al, 1993). In contrast, highest rates occur in black Africans in the third and fourth decades (Lowenthal, 1976; Okany and Akinyanju, 1989).

Time Trends

Total Leukemia. A dramatic decrease in U. S. childhood leukemia mortality since the mid-1960s (seen in whites and nonwhites, but most pronounced among the youngest children), attributed to therapeutic advances (Miller and McKay, 1984; Linet and Devesa, 1991; Groves et al, 1995), has similarly been observed in most countries (Kinlen, 1994). A smaller decline in mortality occurred among young adults in the United States (Groves et al, 1995) and internationally (Kinlen, 1994), while there was little change among middle-aged persons. Rates have increased among the elderly in the United States, particularly nonwhites (Groves et al, 1995), and in most other countries between the 1950s and the mid-1970s, when the increase began to taper off (Kinlen, 1994).

Acute Lymphoblastic Leukemia. Childhood leukemia (primarily ALL where designated by cell type) mortality increased during the first half of the century in England and Wales (Court Brown and Doll, 1959), Scotland (Hems, 1972), and Saskatchewan (Klassen, 1969). In the United Kingdom, United States, and Australia, a mortality increase among children age 4 and younger during 1935–51 was partially attributed to improvements in diagnosis and early (prediagnostic) treatment of infections. The increase was followed by a decline among children of the same age born in 1952 and later, believed to be associated with therapy-related improvements in survival (Adelstein and White, 1976).

Incidence of childhood ALL has increased primarily among boys age 5 and younger during the past few decades in Great Britain (Stiller and Draper, 1982), Connecticut (van Hoff et al, 1988), and for a few years during the late 1970s and early 1980s in the Netherlands (Coebergh et al, 1989). No increase occurred in Sweden (Ericsson et al, 1978), Denmark (Brown et al, 1989) or Scotland (Hems, 1972). Patterns in the United States during the 1970s are difficult to interpret because of incomplete ascertainment of cases during the initial years of the Surveillance Epidemiology and End Results (SEER) Program data collection, and the decrease in the proportion of not otherwise specified cases in the mid-1970s as treatments specifically effective against childhood ALL became available and the level of specification subsequently improved (Linet and Devesa, 1991; RW Miller, 1992); ALL rates have risen in children since 1980. In the 1960s Arab and Oriental Jewish children were more likely to develop Burkitt's lymphoma than ALL, but in the 1970s ALL incidence rose in these groups while Burkitt's lymphoma declined (Virag and Modan, 1969; Ramot et al, 1985).

Since the late 1970s, there has been an apparent decline in ALL among white male farmers in rural Iowa counties (Donham et al, 1980, 1987). In contrast, age-adjusted incidence rates increased 24%–43% among whites and blacks, males and females in the U. S. SEER population during 1973–90 (Groves et al, 1995). Environmental influences are believed to be responsible for each of these patterns, but specific factors have not been identified.

Chronic Lymphocytic Leukemia. Earlier in the century, the male predominance of CLL in Western countries was more pronounced (reported male:female ratios ranged from 2.5 to 3.0) than that reported in more recent studies (male:female ratio ranging from 1.6 to 1.9), although reasons are unknown (Von Gross et al, 1958; Hansen, 1983). CLL mortality increased among males age 45 and older and to a lesser extent among females 60 and older during the 1940s and 1950s in England and Wales (Court Brown and Doll, 1959), Australia (Keogh and McCall, 1958), and New Zealand (Gunz, 1964). Increases in incidence have been reported among the elderly of both sexes since the start of population-based registries in 1943 in Denmark (Hansen et al, 1983) and in 1935 in Connecticut (Heston et al, 1986), but rates have declined among both whites and blacks in the U. S. SEER populations between 1973 and 1990 (Groves et al, 1995).

Acute Myeloid Leukemia. AML mortality rates increased among both sexes in the 1940s in England and Wales (Court Brown and Doll, 1959), and incidence rose in the 1960s and 1970s in Somerset, England (Bowie, 1987), Scotland (Heasman et al, 1987), and the Netherlands (Huisman et al, 1981). These findings may have represented true increases or improvements in reporting. Incidence has increased among men aged 50 since population data collection began in 1935 in Olmstead County, Minnesota (Linos et al, 1978), and also in Connecticut (Heston et al, 1986). However, SEER population trends show generally little change between 1973 and 1990, except for an increase among black males (Groves et al, 1995). Similar trends arose in 1943 in Denmark (Hansen et al, 1983), and more recently in Sweden (Brandt et al, 1979). The consistent increase among older males in many geographic areas, together with the higher incidence of AML in developed countries and industrial metropolitan areas in the U. S., suggest the influence of occupational or environmental factors. Data from the Connecticut tumor registry show a fall in rates since 1970 (Stevens, 1986).

Chronic Myeloid Leukemia. A twofold increase occurred in Lancashire, England, between 1965–70 and 1971–76, although rates remained stable between these time periods throughout England and Wales (Geary et al, 1979) and in Denmark during 1943–77 (Hansen et al, 1983). CML incidence rose among elderly males and females in Connecticut during 1935–80 (Heston et al, 1986), possibly reflecting changes in diagnostic practice. A recent decline in CML rates in the U. S., greater for whites than blacks (Groves et al, 1995), and parts of England and Wales (Cartwright et al, 1990), may reflect an increasing tendency to classify chronic myelomonocytic leukemia with the myelodysplastic syndromes. While rates were higher among U. S. whites than blacks prior to the mid-1970s, an excess of CML has been observed among blacks since then due to a more rapid decline of age-adjusted CML incidence rates among whites compared to blacks (Groves et al, 1995).

Survival

Based on the SEER program data in the U. S., the 5-year relative survival rates during 1983–89 for persons of all ages with all leukemia types combined range from 38.9% among white males and 38.4% among white females to 29.6% among black males and 31.4% among black females (BA Miller et al, 1993). Most notable are improvements among white children ages 0–14 with acute lymphocytic leukemia, with 5-year relative survival increasing from 4% among children diagnosed in 1960–63 to 72.4% among those diagnosed during 1983–89. The corresponding increase among white children ages 0–14 with acute myeloid leukemia during the same time period has been less dramatic, rising from 3% to 31.1% alive at 5 years post diagnosis (Miller et al, 1993). In population-based data from the U. K., 5-year relative survival for childhood ALL cases increased from 2% to 47% between 1954–63 and 1974–83, and from 37% to 70% between 1971–73 and 1983–85, whereas a smaller improvement (from 2% to 21% between 1954–63 and 1974–83 and 4% to 26% between 1971–73 and 1983–85) was observed for childhood AML (Birch et al, 1988; Stiller and Bunch, 1990). CLL cases diagnosed during 1974–1989 show little change in 5-year relative survival, but neither stage nor other prognostic factors were considered (Miller et al, 1993). In hospital-based CLL series, 5-year survival ranged from 30% to 70%, with stage at diagnosis clearly the major prognostic factor, although age, sex, and response to treatment were also important (Catovsky et al, 1988). Five-year survival rates for AML have improved among children and adolescents but have otherwise remained essentially unchanged among adults in the U. S. general population. No apparent improvements occurred among CML cases in the U. S. (Miller et al, 1993).

ENVIRONMENTAL FACTORS

Occupation

Occupational exposure to benzene and radiation has been implicated in the etiology of leukemia for more than 50 years. Evaluation of occupation–leukemia associations may be difficult due to the limited size of many occupational cohorts and the large number of recognized leukemia subtypes, only one or a few of which may be associated with a specific exposure. Some occupational cohorts with elevated leukemia risk also have an excess of other types of hematolymphoproliferative neoplasms. Findings are often inconsistent within a specific industry, and specific leukemogenic exposures have not been identified for many occupations. The latency period for leukemia onset (other than CLL, perhaps) subsequent to occupational exposure appears shorter than that of solid tumors, if the model for occupational leukemogenesis is similar to those for high-level radiation exposures or antineoplastic agents.

Workers Exposed to Ionizing Radiation.

Radiologists and x-ray technicians. Physicians joining a British radiological society during 1897–1921 experienced a six-fold leukemia mortality excess, whereas leukemia deaths were not increased among radiologists obtaining membership after 1921 (Smith and Doll, 1981). United States radiologists entering a specialty society in 1920–29 had an 8.8-fold elevated leukemia mortality and those becoming members in 1930–39 a 3.4-fold increase (primarily acute and myeloid leukemias), whereas no excess deaths from leukemia occurred in later cohorts (Seltser and Sartwell, 1965; Matanoski et al, 1975, 1984), nor in other groups of American physicians recently joining radiologic societies (Logue et al, 1986). Leukemia (except CLL) incidence was significantly elevated among 27,011 diagnostic x-ray workers followed-up during 1950–80 in China (Wang et al, 1988, 1990), but leukemia deaths were not increased among U. S. Army x-ray technicians followed-up during 1946–74 (Jablon and Miller, 1978). The Chinese technicians appear to have had higher radiation exposures. Studies of medical workers exposed to radiation generally lack exposure estimates.

Nuclear industry workers. Many studies of nuclear industry and weapons production workers (Acquavella et al, 1985; Beral et al, 1985; Checkoway et al, 1985; Smith and Douglas, 1986; Wilkinson et al, 1987; Beral et al, 1988; Gilbert et al, 1989a, b; Gilbert et al, 1993a, b; Wing et al, 1993) and nuclear shipyard workers (Rinsky et al, 1981a; Greenberg et al, 1985; Stern et al, 1986) have reported no increases of leukemia or only small, nonsignificant excesses. The findings from some of the initial studies were difficult to interpret because of very low recorded radiation doses (Checkoway et al, 1985), elevated risk only when exposure was lagged 15 years (Smith and Douglas, 1986; Beral et al, 1988), or increases confined to one subgroup of employees (Cragle et al, 1988). Excess leukemia risks based on small numbers of leukemia cases in some studies are also problematic (Gribbin et al, 1993). Kendall et al (1992), however, found a positive dose-response relationship associated with leukemia risk in a follow-up of 95,217 radiation workers employed at major sites of the nuclear industry in the United Kingdom, and a significantly elevated relative risk of 1.8 for leukemia mortality was shown in a comparison of workers who received a cumulative dose of 10–50 mSv with those exposed to less than 10 mSv in a meta-analysis of seven U. K. and U. S. studies (Wilkinson and Dreyer, 1991). Also, a relative risk of 1.2 was observed for leukemia mortality excluding CLL for a cumulative protracted dose of 100 mSv compared to 0 mSv and an excess relative risk of 2.2 for leukemia excluding CLL in a combined analysis of 95,673 workers employed for 6 months or longer in the nuclear industry from seven U.S., U.K. and Canadian facilities (Cardis et al, 1995). In contrast, a follow-up of United Kingdom Atomic Energy Authority employees showed no association between measured radiation exposures and leukemia mortality (Fraser et al, 1993). Also, no excess was seen in a cohort of U. S. nuclear power plant workers (Jablon and Boice, 1993).

Radium dial workers and underground miners. No significant increase in leukemia has been noted among several cohorts of U. S. and U. K. radium dial workers (Spiers et al, 1983; Stebbings et al, 1984; Baverstock and Papworth, 1986), but a borderline significant increase of myeloid leukemia was observed among U. K. tin miners who had worked 10–20 years underground (Hodgson and Jones, 1990). Uranium miners, who are heavily exposed to radon and related decay products, have not been reported at elevated risk of leukemia occurrence (Waxweiler et al, 1981; Morrison et al, 1988; Sevc et al, 1988; National Research Council, 1988).

Participants in atmospheric nuclear tests. Although a 2.5-fold leukemia excess (primarily AML and CML) was reported among 3741 American servicemen exposed to one aboveground 1957 nuclear detonation ("SMOKY") (Caldwell et al, 1983), leukemia mortality was not elevated among 46,186 U. S. military participants in several other atmospheric nuclear tests between 1951 and 1958 (Robinette et al, 1985). The elevated leukemia risk confined to a single test may have been related to circumstances peculiar to that detonation, or influenced by inclusion of the index case instigating the investigation as well as a secondary leukemia case (arising in a serviceman irradiated for lymphoma), or possibly related to concomitant widespread publicity (Rothman, 1984). Leukemia mortality and incidence were elevated among 528 New Zealand military participants in British atomic weapons tests (Pearce et al, 1990). Leukemia and multiple myeloma mortality, but not death rates for other radiation-related malignancies, were also significantly increased among 22,347 British participants in nuclear tests in relation to mortality of an unexposed comparison group (Darby et al, 1988). Compared to national mortality rates for these hematologic malignancies, however, risk was not elevated among the exposed, but rather it was substantially lower among the unexposed comparison group, and no association was found with type or degree of radiation exposure.

Workers Exposed to Nonionizing Electromagnetic Fields.

Death certificate (Milham, 1982, 1988), PMR (Wright et al, 1982; McDowall, 1983; Coleman et al, 1983; Robinson et al, 1991), case-control (Stern et al, 1986; Flodin et al, 1986, 1990; Pearce, 1988; Preston-Martin et al, 1998a; Pearce et al, 1989; Matanoski et al, 1993; London et al, 1994), and linked registry (Linet et al, 1988a; Juutilainen et al, 1990; Tornqvist et al, 1991; Tynes et al, 1992; Guenel et al, 1993; Floderus et al, 1994) investigations have shown increased leukemia (primarily AML, although Swedish and New Zealand workers had excesses of CLL) among radio/television repairmen, electricians, electrical/electronic engineers, electric and gas utilities workers, electrical equipment assemblers, railway engine drivers and conductors, aluminum workers, photographic equipment manufacturing workers, electrical technicians, computer and telephone mechanics, communications equipment operators, power line workers, and miners. A nonsignificant leukemia increase was observed among telephone linemen, with higher risks among workers employed for long durations in jobs with intermittent peak exposures, particularly those in cable splicing or old telephone switching offices (Matanoski et al, 1993). A small increase in leukemia occurrence was found among electricians' mates in a follow-up of U. S. Navy personnel (Garland et al, 1990), but other investigations of electrical workers have shown no excess risk (McDowall, 1983; Olin et al, 1985; Wiklund et al, 1981; Tornqvist et al, 1986; Tynes et al, 1994), including a recent large cohort and nested case-control studies of U. S. electrical utility workers that included a measurement component (Sahl et al, 1993). Combining the results of 11 investigations, total leukemia was estimated to be 18% increased, primarily related to a 46% AML excess among electrical workers (Coleman and Beral, 1988), although another meta-analysis incorporating an adjustment for heterogeneity reported a lower 95% confidence limit closer to unity (Shore, 1988). Preliminary data suggest wide variability in field exposures among different types of electrical workers and over time (Bowman et al, 1988; Gamberale et al, 1989). A large cohort study of Canadian and French utility workers, which included an extensive measurement component, showed an excess of AML, but no dose-response relationship (Theriault et al, 1994), whereas a Swedish case-control study of leukemia and brain tumors showed a positive dose-response relationship between magnetic field measurements and CLL, but no increase of AML (Floderus et al, 1993). Among close to 139,000 men employed at five large electric power companies in the U.S., leukemia mortality was not significantly increased nor were significant excesses observed for specific leukemia cell types (Savitz and Loomis, 1995). Interpretation is uncertain, however, in the absence of magnetic field exposure data and information on chemical exposures for the implicated job titles in most studies (Savitz and Calle, 1987; Ahlbom, 1988; Cartwright, 1989).

Benzene-Exposed Workers

History and quantification of leukemia risk. Since 1928 there have been many reports of acute leukemia occurring in benzene-exposed shoe, leather, rubber, and rotoprinting workers in Italy, France, and Turkey (Delore and Borgomano, 1928; Vigliani and Forni, 1976; Goguel et al, 1967; Girard and Revol, 1970; Aksoy et al, 1974; Paci et al, 1989). Case-control investigations have noted approximately threefold leukemia excesses among persons with a past history of benzene exposure (Girard and Revol, 1970; Linos et al, 1980). Cohort studies of benzene-exposed pliofilm (Infante et al, 1977; Rinsky et al, 1981b) and chemical manufacturing workers (Ott et al, 1978) showed significantly increased risk ratios of 3.8–5.6 for all leukemias and up to 10.0 for AML. These data were concluded to be sufficient evidence that benzene causes AML in humans (IARC, 1981).

Subsequent cohort investigations among benzene-exposed chemical manufacturing, refinery, and other workers in the United States (Decoufle et al, 1983; McCraw et al, 1985; Wong, 1987; Olsen et al, 1989), the United Kingdom (Rushton and Alderson, 1981), and China (Yin et al, 1987) have confirmed the benzene-leukemia association, with total leukemia increased 1.9- to 7.0-fold and AML 3.9- to 10.0-fold (McCraw et al, 1985; Bond et al, 1986; Rinsky et al, 1987). Erythroleukemia and unusual variants of AML appeared to occur disproportionately in studies of benzene-related leukemia, although newer histopathologic methods should enable more accurate classification of AML subtypes as well as correct designation of myelodysplastic syndromes, aplastic anemia, and other hematopoietic disorders which may precede AML in some benzene-exposed workers (Aksoy and Erdem, 1978; Aksoy, 1988; Yin et al, 1989; Travis et al, 1994). Neither the incidence of preleukemias and related disorders nor the steps in leukemogenesis has been systematically evaluated.

Risk assessment and sources of benzene exposures. Workers with higher, continuous, or longer duration exposures appear to have a greater risk of developing leukemia (Wong, 1987; Rinsky et al, 1987; Austin et al, 1988). Approximately 45–50 excess leukemias (with a range of 5–250) would be expected per 1000 deaths among workers exposed to a time-weighted average of 10 ppm benzene during the usual 30-year working life (Crump and Allen, 1984; Rinsky et al, 1987; Austin et al, 1988; Swaen and Meijers, 1989). Risks of total leukemia and of myeloid leukemia among benzene-exposed workers have been found to be similar for females and males in a large cohort study in China (Li et al, 1994). Most epidemiologic studies assessing benzene-related leukemogenicity have focused on certain occupational cohorts, but a U. S. Environmental Protection Agency survey suggests that the workplace may account for only 1% of benzene exposures (Wallace, 1989). More important sources appear to be cigarette smoking (with mainstream and passive smoking exposures responsible for an estimated 55% of the total), residential exposures from various consumer products (accounting for 20%), and automobile-related exposures (comprising most of the remainder).

Rubber manufacturing workers. Benzene was used extensively in the rubber industry in earlier years, although other chemicals (some contaminated with a small amount of benzene) have been used as replacements in recent times. Studies of large cohorts of rubber manufacturing workers in the United Kingdom (Fox and Collier, 1976; Parkes et al, 1982) and the United States (Mancuso, 1975; Monson and Nakano, 1976; Delzell and Monson, 1981) have shown a 1.4- to 4.0-fold increase in leukemia, although no leukemia excess was observed in a more recent follow-up of one of the U. K. cohorts (Sorahan et al, 1989). Preliminary data implicate certain jobs (Delzell and Monson, 1982, 1984) and suggest a link between lymphocytic leukemia and solvent exposures (McMichael et al, 1976) including notably benzene, but also carbon disulfide, carbon tetrachloride, xylene, and others (Arp et al, 1983; Wilcosky et al, 1984; Checkoway et al, 1984).

Petroleum refinery workers. Efforts to identify high-risk job titles among petroleum refinery workers have generally not been successful (McCraw et al, 1985; Austin et al, 1986), although process changes increasing benzene exposure have resulted in a rise in AML occurrence (Wongsrichanalai et al, 1989). Increased rates of leukemia (Marsh et al, 1991), and, in particular, lymphocytic leukemia have also been reported among some long-term workers (Wong and Raabe, 1989; Wongsrichanalai et al, 1989; Bertazzi et al, 1989), whereas other large studies have shown no leukemia excess (Thorpe, 1974; Rushton and Alderson, 1981; Hanis et al, 1982; Waxweiler et al, 1983; Kaplan, 1986; Rushton, 1993a, b). Although leukemia mortality overall was not significantly elevated among approximately 23,000 workers employed for at least one year in oil distribution centers in the United Kingdom, mortality was elevated at one of the three companies evaluated and acute myeloid leukemia increased among drivers (Rushton 1993a, b). Two comprehensive assessments of the epidemiologic data have concluded that there is a small excess of total leukemia (meta-analysis SMR = 1.10, p = .10) (Wong and Raabe, 1989) and that occupational exposures in this industry are probably carcinogenic based on limited evidence for leukemia and skin cancer (IARC, 1989). Evaluation of cell-type-specific leukemia risk among 208,000 petroleum workers in the U.S. and U.K. has shown no evidence of increased risks for AML, CML or CLL, and only a small nonsignificant excess of ALL (Wong and Raabe, 1995).

Pressmen. Leukemia was increased among pressmen and printers (Registrar General, 1958; Viadana and Bross, 1972; Lloyd et al, 1977). Excess myelomonocytic leukemia (Paganini-Hill et al, 1980) and myelofibrosis (Zoloth et al, 1986) have been noted. Possible leukemogenic exposures include benzene, toluene, cutting oils, carbon tetrachloride, carbon disulfide, and methylene chloride (Kay, 1976).

Painters. High rates of leukemia among painters (Viadana and Bross, 1972; RR Williams et al, 1977a; Matanoski et al, 1986; Lindqvist et al, 1987) and lacquer workers (Morgan et al, 1981a; Morgan et al, 1985) may also be related to benzene, currently found in measurable amounts in latex paints (Wallace, 1989). The lack of a leukemia excess in other studies may reflect variation in the composition of paint used by different occupational groups (Bethwaite et al, 1990).

Farmers. Despite some negative studies in the United States and Sweden (Decoufle et al, 1977; Linos et al, 1980; Delzell and Grufferman, 1985; Wiklund and Holm, 1986), investigations in Washington State and Oregon (Milham, 1971), Iowa (Donham et al, 1980; Burmeister et al, 1982), Nebraska (Blair and White, 1985a), Wisconsin (Blair and White, 1981), British Columbia, Canada (Gallagher et al, 1984), and New Zealand (Pearce et al, 1986) have shown associations between farming and leukemia. One study revealed increased risk of leukemia only among Italian female farmers and Danish female farm owners; Italian and Danish male farmers or farm owners did not experience an elevated risk (Ronco et al, 1992).

Leukemia types linked with farming include ALL (Donham et al, 1980), CLL (Blair and White, 1985a; Brown et al, 1990), AML (Pearce et al, 1986), and CML (Blair and White, 1981). Farmers also have higher rates of non-Hodgkin's lymphoma, multiple myeloma, and aplastic anemia (Gallagher et al, 1984; Hoar et al, 1986; Wiklund and Holm, 1986; Cuzick et al, 1987), suggesting overlap of risk factors among these hematologic conditions. Agricultural extension agents (who disseminate information from agricultural researchers to individual farmers in the United States) have increased leukemia mortality that rises significantly with longer duration of employment, with risk of both myeloid and lymphatic leukemia increased four- to fivefold among workers employed 15 or more years (Alavanja et al, 1988). AML mortality is increased among U. S. veterinarians (Blair and Hayes, 1980, 1982), and AML incidence among New Zealand abattoir workers (Pearce et al, 1988), both of which may be consistent with a viral etiology (Pearce and Reif, 1990). Risk ratios are generally less than 1.5, with the greatest excess among younger farmers in later time periods, possibly implicating more recent agricultural practices in some areas (Burmeister et al, 1982; Blair et al, 1980; Blair and White, 1985a) but not others (Wiklund and Holm, 1986).

Agricultural exposures related to poultry and dairy farming, livestock production, certain crops (e.g., soybeans, corn, and other cereal grains), various agrichemicals (including crop and animal insecticides, herbicides, and fertilizers), and viruses have been associated with elevated leukemia risk (Blair et al, 1985b; Linet, 1985; Brown et al, 1990; Pearce and Reif, 1990; Viel and Richardson, 1991; Blair and Zahm, 1991; Richardson et al, 1992; Blair and Zahm, 1995). Workers exposed to pesticides in the U. S. flour industry also have increased leukemia occurrence (Alavanja et al, 1990).

Other Suspect Occupations

Styrene and butadiene manufacture. Elevated leukemia and lymphoma have been reported among generally small cohorts of workers in plants producing, polymerizing, and/or processing styrene monomers and butadiene (Leman and Young, 1976; McMichael et al, 1976; Monson and Nakano, 1976; Nicholson et al, 1978; Ott et al, 1980a; Hodgson and Jones, 1985; Downs et al, 1987), with monomeric styrene and butadiene implicated in some studies (Spirtas et al, 1976; Ott et al, 1980a), whereas benzene or other solvents were more clearly linked in other investigations (Monson and Fine, 1978). However, no leukemia excesses were observed in small (Cowles et al, 1994) or large cohorts of workers employed in styrene-butadiene polymer manufacturing and reinforced plastics and composites (styrene-exposed) manufacturing plants, respectively (Matanoski et al, 1990; Wong, 1990; Cole et al, 1993). Small leukemia excesses at one of two plants evaluated during 1943–76 among workers with shorter, but not longer duration exposure seem inconsistent with a causal association (Lemen et al, 1990). A notable excess of leukemia among workers exposed to butadiene, but not styrene, in a nested case-control study of 59 cases (26 leukemias) and 193 controls may indicate a causal association or possibly chance or confounding (Santos-Burgoa et al, 1992). A recent meta-analysis suggests little evidence of excess leukemia risk in the styrene and butadiene industries (Cole et al, 1993).

Ethylene oxide and related chemicals. Ethylene oxide has been designated as a probable human carcinogen (IARC, 1985) based on leukemia and lymphoma excesses in three small Swedish cohort studies (Hogstedt et al, 1979a, b, 1984, 1986), cytogenetic abnormalities of exposed workers (Stolley et al, 1984), and animal carcinogenicity data (Snellings et al, 1984). Since then, a significant dose-response relationship was seen for lymphoid leukemias and lymphomas among ethylene oxide sterilization workers in a U. S. plant (Stayner et al, 1993), and a nonsignificant leukemia excess found among Italian workers (Bisanti et al, 1993). Yet, deaths from leukemia were not increased among 18,000 exposed U. S. workers employed in 14 plants producing sterilized medical supplies, although non-Hodgkin's lymphoma was significantly elevated (Steenland et al, 1991). Elevated leukemia risks observed among workers in two U. S. facilities were specifically linked with production of ethylene or propylene chlorhydrin rather than ethylene oxide (Greenberg et al, 1990; Benson and Teta, 1993). Leukemia mortality was unremarkable in German (Theiss et al, 1981) and British (Gardner et al, 1989) cohorts, and no cases were found in two U. S. plants (Morgan et al, 1981b; Teta et al, 1993). A comprehensive assessment of the epidemiological evidence concludes that the available data do not provide consistent and convincing evidence of leukemogenicity (Shore et al, 1993). It is interesting to note that shipyard painters exposed to ethylene glycol, from which ethylene oxide is derived, were found to have anemia and granulocytopenia in a survey (Welch and Cullen, 1988).

Garage and transport maintenance. Maintenance workers in bus garages (Rushton et al, 1983), railway workers (Schenker et al, 1984), highway maintenance workers (Bender et al, 1989), and professional drivers exposed to petroleum products in fuels and exhaust (Lindqvist et al, 1991) appear to have an increased leukemia risk. If the findings are confirmed, benzene and/or diesel exhaust may be responsible (Holmberg and Lundberg, 1985; Boffetta et al, 1988; Flodin et al, 1988; Wallace, 1989). The latter contains polynuclear aromatic hydrocarbons and other carcinogenic heterocyclic compounds.

Others. Elevated leukemia risk has been reported among workers in other occupations including excess myeloid (primarily acute) leukemia among embalmers, anatomists, and pathologists (Walrath and Fraumeni, 1984; Harrington and Oakes, 1984; Stroup et al, 1986; Linos et al, 1989; Matanoski, 1989; Hayes et al, 1990); abattoir workers with excess AML (Johnson et al, 1986; Pearce et al, 1988); nurses handling antineoplastic drugs (Skov et al, 1992); welders with an increase of myeloid leukemia (Stern et al, 1987), particularly CML (Preston-Martin and Peters, 1988a); metal mill (Gallagher and Threlfall, 1983), aluminum (Rockette and Arena, 1983), and foundry workers (Decoufle and Wood, 1979); grain industry workers with increased AML (Thomas et al, 1985; Alavanja et al, 1987); male barbers and hairdressers with increased lymphocytic and myelocytic leukemia (Milham, 1976; Teta et al, 1984; Spinelli et al, 1984); dry cleaners with excess leukemia (Blair et al, 1979; Katz and Jowett, 1981; Brown and Kaplan, 1987); carpet manufacturing workers with a higher incidence of lymphocytic leukemia (Cartwright et al, 1987a; O'Brien and Decoufle, 1988); workers in the sawmill, lumber, and wood products industries (IARC, 1981; Burkhardt, 1982; Lynge, 1985; Flodin et al, 1988; BA Miller et al, 1989); underground coal miners with an excess of CLL and myeloid leukemia (Gilman et al, 1985); firefighters with an excess of leukemia and multiple myeloma (Heyer et al, 1990), and asbestos-exposed workers with an elevated occurrence of CLL (Schwartz et al, 1988).

Parental Occupation. Although findings conflict, childhood leukemia has been associated with paternal and maternal employment in hydrocarbon-related occupations and the chemical industry (Vianna et al, 1984; Lowengart et al, 1987; Shu et al, 1988). Excesses of ALL were observed among children of fathers working in rubber manufacturing (Olsen et al, 1991) and in farming (Magnani et al, 1990), and of mothers producing piecework by machine sewing at home Infante-Rivard et al, 1991). AML was significantly higher among offspring of mothers employed in metal refining and processing (Shu et al, 1988) and occupationally exposed to metal dusts (Buckley et al, 1989), of fathers working in construction and tire production (Magnani et al, 1990) or exposed to solvents and petroleum products (Buckley et al, 1989). Excess AML occurred among children of parents employed in the textile industry (Magnani et al, 1990). Also implicated are maternal exposures to benzene (linked with AML), petroleum products, paint, organic (cotton, wool, synthetic fibers) and wood dusts, food-related exposures and pesticides (associated with ALL and AML, particularly the monocytic and myelomonocytic subtypes) (Van Steensel-Moll et al, 1985; Shu et al, 1988; Laval and Tuyns, 1988; Savitz and Chen, 1990; Olsen et al, 1991; McKinney et al, 1991). Fathers' occupational exposures to benzene, radiation, and wood dust have also been associated with excess childhood leukemia risk (McKinney et al, 1991). Methodologic issues related to interpretation of this literature are discussed more fully in the chapter on cancers in children in this volume.

For young persons ages 0–24 residing in Seascale near the Sellafield nuclear fuels reprocessing plant in the United Kingdom, a statistical association has been described between fathers' employment in this plant (4 of 46 fathers of cases received 10 mSv or more during the 6 months prior to conception and 100 mSv or higher in the decade prior to conception based on film badge readings) and the development of several types of leukemia (Gardner et al, 1990). Paternal employment in farming and mining was also implicated, but these associations were based on small numbers and are difficult to interpret. Kinlen noted that children in Seascale with unexposed fathers had increased rates of leukemia (Kinlen, 1993). In another investigation among fathers employed at Sellafield whose children were born in the surrounding region, the mean individual radiation doses of fathers whose children were born in Seascale were lower than those of fathers whose children were born further away, suggesting that the preconception occupational ionizing radiation exposures were unlikely to explain the leukemia excess observed among children residing in Seascale (Parker et al, 1992). However, the excess leukemia and non-Hodgkin's lymphoma among children residing in proximity to the Dounreay nuclear installation in Scotland were not linked with either parental employment at this facility or father's dose of ionizing radiation preconception or prediagnosis (Urquhart et al, 1991). Also, case-control studies in other regions of the United Kingdom were unable to confirm the hypothesis that paternal preconception exposure to ionizing radiation was linked with elevated risks of childhood leukemia (McKinney et al, 1991; Alexander et al, 1992; Sorahan et al, 1993; Roman et al, 1993; Kinlen et al, 1993). In addition, childhood leukemia was not associated with preconception paternal occupational exposure to ionizing radiation among fathers residing near nuclear facilities in Ontario, Canada (McLaughlin et al, 1993).

Ionizing Radiation (Nonoccupational)

Japanese Atomic Bomb Survivors. Leukemia mortality has been systematically evaluated among approximately 120,000 atomic bomb survivors residing in Hiroshima or Nagasaki, 93,000 of whom were exposed when the bombs were detonated in 1945 (National Research Council, 1990). From approximately 2 million person-years of follow-up, 202 leukemia deaths had been registered by 1985, with mortality significantly elevated for AML, CML, ALL, and myelodysplastic syndromes (Shimizu et al, 1989; Matsuo et al, 1988). ALL was the type most likely to occur in subjects under age 30 at the time of the bomb, and AML in those aged 45 and older. Early CML peaked within 5 years of exposure, and the relative risk of developing CML was greater in younger (< age 15 years) than in older individuals. However, there were no time-related differences between older versus younger individuals in occurrence of the CML excess (Finch, 1984). Within 5–10 years after the bombs, overall leukemia incidence was notably higher among younger males (under age 45 at the time of the detonations) who were heavily exposed. Compared with younger persons, the leukemogenic effect occurred later among older persons and decreased more slowly. During 1950–84, only two leukemia cases (not a significant increase) occurred among the 1630 offspring in utero when the bombs were detonated, and neither of the mothers of the leukemia cases had received high radiation doses. Similarly, no excess of leukemia has been observed up to the age of 20 among the first generation of children born to the Japanese A-bomb survivors (Yoshimoto, 1990).

Leukemia mortality was significantly elevated among survivors exposed to radiation doses of 0.4 Gray (Gy) and above. Mortality rose with increasing radiation exposures, with highest rates among those exposed to 3–4 Gy, and a decline in rates at higher exposures, attributed to cell killing or reduced survival of potentially transformed myeloblasts (United Nations, 1986). The summary relative risk estimate for the excess leukemia mortality observed among atomic bomb survivors from both Hiroshima and Nagasaki was 6.2 per Gray (1 Gray = 100 rads) (Shimizu et al, 1990). Leukemia was the earliest radiation-related malignancy, with a 2-year minimum latent interval, and an average of about 10 years after exposure, followed by declining occurrence. By the late 1970s most of the excess leukemia risk had disappeared (Preston et al, 1987, 1994; National Research Council, 1990). Dose-response estimates based on the 1986 dosimetry show no significant difference between the two cities, although leukemia mortality per unit dose equivalent is still somewhat lower in Nagasaki than in Hiroshima (Shimuzu et al, 1989). Recent histologic reevaluation indicated that the original CML diagnoses were generally correct (e.g., the low frequency of radiation-induced CML in Nagasaki compared with Hiroshima remained unchanged), although approximately 25% of acute leukemias have been reclassified from the original designations (Ishimaru et al, 1979; Moloney, 1987; Matsuo et al, 1988). Histologically, A-bomb-induced leukemia cases were similar to those of de novo leukemia (Matsuo et al, 1988).

About 55% of the leukemia occurrence in the two cities during 1950–85 was attributable to radiation exposure from the bombs, a proportion far greater than that estimated for other malignancies (Shimuzu et al, 1989).

A lower proportion of healthy young adult males were residing in Hiroshima and Nagasaki at the time of the atomic bomb blasts than before World War II, since many young men were away in the military. There were also decreased proportions of children and the elderly among the survivors compared with the frequency among those exposed, since these groups were more likely to die immediately after the bombing (Jablon et al, 1965). Other unusual features of leukemia occurrence among Japanese, such as the virtual absence of CLL among persons over age 55, may also affect interpretation of the findings. Currently efforts are focusing on the analysis of leukemia, lymphoma, and multiple myeloma incidence data from the Life Span Study cohort of atomic bomb survivors during 1950–87 (Preston et al, 1994).

Fallout from Nuclear Weapons. A study in Utah ascribed elevated childhood leukemia mortality to exposure from radiation due to aboveground nuclear weapons tests in Nevada (Lyon et al, 1979). However, this finding was not supported in a subsequent investigation (Land et al, 1984). Other studies of leukemia in Utah among all age groups were also conflicting (Johnson et al, 1984; Machado et al, 1987), but there appeared to be a nearly threefold elevated rate of leukemia deaths among children born in southwestern Utah during the peak fallout period (Machado et al, 1987). Methodologic differences and limitations of these studies have been reviewed (Land, 1979; Enstrom, 1979; Beck and Krey, 1983; Lyon and Schuman, 1984). A case-control study of leukemia deaths during 1952–1981 among Utah residents, however, reported a weak dose-response relationship between estimated bone marrow radiation dose and all types of leukemia, with the greatest excess risk found among persons with ALL under age 20 at the time of death (Machado et al, 1987; Stevens et al, 1990).

In an ecologic trends comparison in the United States, mortality from acute myeloid leukemia was increased during 1960–69 among children ages 5–9, and leukemia mortality was reported to be elevated among persons of all ages residing in states with high strontium^{90} levels (Archer, 1987). No association was identified in a more rigorous study comparing childhood leukemia incidence patterns with trends in fallout exposures in England and Wales, Norway, and Denmark (Darby and Doll, 1987), but there was some evidence that the rates of childhood leukemia were increased in Nordic countries (Denmark, Sweden, Norway, Finland, and Iceland) during the late 1960s when effects of fallout doses to the red bone marrow would be at a maximum, with stronger effects observed among children ages 0–4, although these data revealed some inconsistencies (Darby et al, 1992). Overall, there appears to be a small excess of childhood leukemia in populations exposed to fallout from nuclear weapons testing. The level of the excess is consistent with risk estimates from the Japanese atomic bomb survivors study extrapolating to low exposure levels.

Proximity to Nuclear Plants. A leukemia excess observed among children born and residing in proximity to the Sellafield nuclear reprocessing plant was described above. Measured radiation levels in proximity to this and other nuclear facilities were believed to be too low to ascribe the leukemia excess to postnatal exposures (Darby and Doll, 1987; Black, 1984). There was also no evidence of more complete ascertainment of childhood leukemia cases near nuclear installations (Draper et al, 1989). Further surveys among children living near nuclear sites in the United Kingdom (Hole and Gillis,

1986; Roman et al, 1987) revealed consistently significant excesses only in proximity to Sellafield (Bithell et al, 1994), persistance of the increase during 1984–90 (Draper et al, 1993), a deficit of deaths from lymphoid leukemia among persons ages 25–64 (Cook-Mozaffari et al, 1989a), lower than expected mortality in control areas (Cook-Mozaffari et al, 1987; Forman et al, 1987), and absence of a decline in mortality with increasing distance from the nuclear installations (Beral, 1987).

In the largest study to date in the United States, there was no increase of childhood or adult leukemia deaths in 113 counties adjacent to 62 nuclear facilities, compared with the rate in control counties having similar population and socioeconomic characteristics (Jablon et al, 1990, 1991). In addition, no significant childhood leukemia excesses have been identified in proximity to plants in California (Enstrom, 1983), Pennsylvania (Berkheiser, 1986; Hatch et al, 1990), Colorado (Crump et al, 1987), or Massachusetts (Poole et al, 1988). An excess of adult leukemia among a population proximate to a nuclear power plant in Massachusetts was restricted to a period of a few years (Morris and Knorr, 1990).

No increase in leukemia mortality was observed among persons under age 25 living in proximity to nuclear plants in France (Hill and Laplanche, 1990; Viel and Richardson, 1990). An elevated risk of acute leukemia among children aged 0–5 residing within 5 kilometers of nuclear facilities in West Germany beginning operations before 1970 was, for the most part, attributed to an unexpectedly low incidence in control regions (Michaelis et al, 1992). A slight but nonsignificant increase in childhood leukemia was observed in five regions in Ontario in proximity to nuclear plants (McLaughlin et al, 1993).

In view of uncertainties about the role of prenatal and preconception radiation exposure, it is difficult to envision biologic mechanisms which might account for elevated leukemia risks among children residing near nuclear facilities in the United Kingdom. Paternal germ-cell injury from occupational radiation exposure has been postulated (Wheldon et al, 1989), but most studies subsequent to the investigation by Gardner and colleagues (1990) have been negative (see above), and analyses drawing on results of experimental mammalian studies and accepted notions of radiobiology suggest that the doses to the Sellafield workers were too low to result in childhood leukemia (Abrahamson, 1990). Kinlen has alternatively proposed that these childhood leukemia excesses may represent a rare response to a new infection being introduced to the previously isolated communities surrounding nuclear installations (Kinlen, 1988), and that population movement into rural areas changes the pattern of infection (Kinlen et al, 1991; Kinlen and Hudson, 1991; Kinlen, 1993). Some support for this theory is provided by the age-related patterns of leukemia found among children residing in British New Towns established in rural areas, but a responsible infectious agent has not been identified (Kinlen et al, 1990). It is also noteworthy that excess leukemia deaths have occurred among young people living near sites in the United Kingdom where nuclear facilities had been planned but not built or where plants were constructed *subsequent* to the occurrence of increased leukemia mortality (Cook-Mozaffari et al, 1989b). These data similarly suggest etiologies other than radiation exposures from nuclear plants.

Accidents Involving Nuclear Plants. The 1986 accident at the Chernobyl nuclear plant in the Ukraine has resulted in substantial public concern among workers who survived the accident, clean-up workers, and proximate populations in the former Soviet Union and Europe. No childhood leukemia excesses have been identified to date in studies in Europe utilizing cancer registries (Parkin et al, 1993; Auvinen et al, 1994; Hjalmars et al, 1994), but the estimated population exposure was less than that of background radiation, the length of follow-up has been quite short, and the ecologic nature of the studies limits interpretation (Linet and Boice, 1993; Boice and Linet, 1994). Efforts are underway to study clean-up workers, but the organization and conduct of such studies are complex.

High Levels of Naturally-Occurring Radiation. Regions with high natural gamma-radiation levels in the United Kingdom (Court Brown et al, 1960) and Sweden (Flodin et al, 1981, 1986, 1990) have been reported to have elevated leukemia rates, particularly AML, although no increase has been noted in other studies in the United Kingdom (Stewart, 1986), Sweden (Stjernfeldt et al, 1987), Japan (Sakka, 1979), China (Wei et al, 1990), and Connecticut (Walter et al, 1986).

Although areas in Florida with high levels of radium^{226} in drinking water have shown elevated incidence rates of AML and total leukemia (Lyman et al, 1985), AML was not associated with drinking-water radium content in Iowa (Fuortes et al, 1990). Recent international correlation studies linking radon with AML and ALL (Henshaw et al, 1990; Alexander et al, 1990a), a U. S. investigation of 1600 counties correlating leukemia increases with high average indoor radon levels (Cohen, 1993), and a study in North Carolina reporting an increase in childhood leukemia mortality in relation to elevated radon levels in drinking water (Collman et al, 1991), require further evaluation. Muirhead et al (1991) have shown conflicting results for between-county and within-county analyses for both radon and indoor gamma radiation in the United Kingdom, suggesting that between-county analysis may be affected by geographical confounding factors. These investigators suggest that ecologic investigations of natural background radiation and leukemia risk may be problematic; studies should instead focus on small areas, or preferably should employ case-control or cohort methodology.

It has been estimated that 3%–5% of all cancers may be attributable to all sources of radiation, including medical, occupational, and environmental exposures (National Research Council, 1990). While large doses of radiation have clearly been shown to cause leukemia, there is no consistent evidence that the low levels of natural background radiation affect risk.

Nonionizing Electromagnetic Radiation (Nonoccupational)

A case-control investigation in Denver first linked childhood cancer mortality with wiring configurations of residentially proximate electric power lines, noting correlations between the current flow along power lines, their wiring configurations, and magnetic field exposures within residences (Wertheimer and Leeper, 1979). Findings were conflicting among eight subsequent childhood cancer case-control studies (Fulton et al, 1980; Tomenius, 1986; Savitz et al, 1988; Myers et al, 1990; London et al, 1991; Feychting and Ahlbom, 1993; Olsen et al, 1993; Verkasalo et al, 1993), six of which described results specific to childhood leukemia (Fulton et al, 1980; Savitz et al, 1988; London et al, 1991; Feychting and Ahlbom, 1993; Olsen et al, 1993; Verkasalo et al, 1993). Magnetic field measurements, obtained in five studies of childhood leukemia, were weakly related to leukemia risk in three of these; the association in one of these (Savitz et al, 1988) was stronger for low power than for high power magnetic fields. In the two U. S. investigations, 2.9-fold (Savitz et al, 1988) and 2.2-fold (London et al, 1991) leukemia excesses were observed among children whose residences were proximate to the highest level of wire configuration patterns. The Swedish investigation reported a 2.7-fold increase of childhood leukemia, based on seven cases, among children residing in homes with an estimated annual level of exposure ≥ 0.2 μT, but there was an inverse association with spot measurements made in homes (Feychting and Ahlbom, 1993). Interpretation is difficult because of limitations in exposure assessment, case-control differences in participation and residential mobility characteristics, weaker associations of leukemia with measured magnetic fields than with wire code configurations, small numbers of leukemia cases, and other methodologic problems (Savitz et al, 1989; Cartwright, 1989; Poole and Trichopoulos, 1991; National Radiological Protection Board, 1992).

Adult acute nonlymphocytic leukemia was not linked with directly measured magnetic fields in Seattle residences (Severson et al, 1988), nor was a significant excess of leukemia associated with residential proximity to electrical transmission facilities (particularly low voltage substations) in East Anglia (McDowall, 1986), overhead power lines and electricity substations in London (Coleman et al, 1989), nor myeloid leukemia with maximum load currents carried by overhead power lines in the Northwest and Yorkshire regions of England (Youngson et al, 1991). However, acute and chronic myeloid leukemia, but not CLL, were nonsignificantly increased among Swedish adults who resided in homes (at diagnosis or reference date) with estimated magnetic field levels of 0.2 μT or who had the highest estimated cumulative exposure to magnetic fields (Feychting and Ahlbom, 1994).

Prenatal and postnatal electric blanket exposures were associated with small, nonsignificant increases in the incidence of childhood leukemia (Savitz et al, 1990). Neither AML nor CML in adults have been linked with electric blanket use (Preston-Martin et al, 1988b). Prenatal and postnatal exposures to other electrical appliances have not been studied to the same extent as electric blankets (Savitz et al, 1990; London et al, 1991).

Environmental Pesticide Exposure

Subsequent to a chemical manufacturing plant explosion near Seveso, Italy, with widespread contamination of the surrounding area by 2,3,7,8-tetrachlorodibenzo-p-dioxin (TCDD), a 10-year follow-up revealed elevated leukemia mortality among males but not females residing in close proximity (Bertazzi et al, 1989). However, neither occupation of the affected men nor other potentially confounding exposures were considered. A nonsignificant excess of myeloid leukemia was more recently reported based on three cases identified from hospital discharges during the 10-year follow-up (Pesatori et al, 1993). Increased leukemia has not been reported among manufacturing workers or those otherwise occupationally exposed to chlorinated phenoxyacetic acid or derivatives contaminated with TCDD (Cook et al, 1980; Ott et al, 1980b; Axelson et al, 1980; Riihimaki et al, 1983; Lynge, 1985; Coggon et al, 1986).

Clinical reports (Infante et al, 1978; Reeves et al, 1989) and case-control studies (Lowengart et al, 1987) have linked childhood leukemia with postnatal residential pesticide exposures. Pregnancy-related occupational exposure to pesticides and maternal employment in agriculture were significantly associated with increased risk of childhood ALL in Shanghai (Shu et al, 1988). Occupational pesticide exposures of mother and father (both pre- and postnatal) and application of pesticides within homes and gardens (postnatal) have been linked with elevated risk of AML (particularly the FAB subtypes M4 and M5) among American children (Buckley et al, 1989). Interview-derived pesticide exposure information may be affected by recall bias and absence of detail about specific products applied.

Cigarette Smoking

Cigarette smoking has been established as an important risk factor for lung cancer since 1950, and also linked with several other cancers, but an association with leukemia was not recognized until recently. Austin and Cole (1986) reexamined the relationship of cigarette smoking and leukemia, noting a 50% mortality excess for smokers compared with nonsmokers in two large cohort investigations, with one showing a possible dose-response relationship for current smokers (Hammond, 1966; Kahn, 1966). Smoking was also associated with myelocytic leukemia in a third cohort (Paffenbarger et al, 1978), and with acute and chronic myelocytic leukemia in a case-control study (Williams et al, 1977b).

In 16-year (Kinlen and Rogot, 1988) and 26-year (McLaughlin et al, 1989) follow-ups of more than 240,000 U. S. veterans, leukemia mortality was significantly increased among smokers, with a positive dose-response relationship. Risks were 60% higher for monocytic and myeloid subtypes among current smokers, with smoking estimated to account for about 24% of myeloid leukemia deaths (McLaughlin et al, 1989). Myeloid leukemia was also significantly elevated among college graduates (Paffenbarger et al, 1978), Seventh-Day Adventists (Mills et al, 1990), and among men but not women smokers in two U. S. populations of more than a million subjects each enrolled in prospective cancer prevention follow-up surveys (Garfinkel and Boffetta, 1990). Cigarette smokers in three cohorts (Kinlen and Rogot, 1988; Garfinkel and Boffetta, 1990; Linet et al, 1991) were found to have an elevated risk of lymphatic leukemia, and a significant excess of CLL was observed in a case-control study of white males in Iowa and Minnesota (Brown et al, 1992a). In contrast, leukemia was not increased among smokers in a 20-year follow-up of British physicians (Doll and Peto, 1976) nor among Japanese smokers (Hirayama, 1990).

AML was significantly associated with cigarette smoking in population-based case-control studies in Missouri (Brownson, 1989) and in western Washington State (Severson, 1987); the latter noted a dose-response relationship for duration of exposure and a population attributable risk of 31%. In a large case-control study of acute leukemia, risks of both AML and ALL were increased among cigarette smokers, particularly among older persons, and acute leukemia was associated with both duration and amount of smoking. Smoking was linked with higher risks of the French-American-British M2 subtype of AML and the L2 subtype of ALL in patients over age 60, and with specific chromosomal abnormalities in AML and ALL (Sandler et al, 1993). Adults exposed in childhood to smoking parents also had an elevated leukemia risk (Sandler et al, 1985). No relationship was found between AML and cigarette smoking in other case-control investigations (Flodin et al, 1986; Kabat et al, 1988; Cartwright et al, 1988). Cigarette smokers reporting the longest duration of smoking had a significantly increased risk of CML among men in the population-based Iowa and Minnesota study (Brown et al, 1992a). Although the elevated leukemia risks among smokers were virtually all observed in epidemiologic investigations of other hypotheses, most studies support an association, particularly with AML (Wald, 1988; Brownson et al, 1993; Siegel, 1993). Childhood AML was not increased overall among offspring of mothers who smoked during pregnancy, but a small excess occurred among children under age 2 of mothers who both smoked and consumed alcohol (Severson et al, 1992). Known and suspected leukemogenic constituents of cigarette smoke include benzene, polonium-210, agricultural chemicals, nitrosamines, and hydrocarbons.

Hair Dyes

Leukemia and myelodysplastic syndromes have been reported with personal and occupational exposure to hair dyes among men (Cantor et al, 1988), and AML with personal exposures in both sexes (Markowitz et al, 1985). Acute leukemia was associated with long-term use of dark hair dye (Mele et al, 1994). Risk of CLL was not elevated among men or women using hair dyes in a population-based study in Nebraska (Zahm et al, 1992), nor in a large study of fatal cancers among more than half a million U. S. women (Thun et al, 1994). Neither CLL nor other leukemias were linked with permanent hair dye use among close to 100,000 women enrolled in the Nurses Health Study (Grodstein et al, 1994). Elevated leukemia risks among hairdressers and cosmetologists (Teta et al, 1984; Spinelli et al, 1984), and laboratory evidence of carcinogenicity (IARC, 1977; Sontag, 1981) and mutagenicity (Ames et al, 1975) of hair dye components suggest the need for further studies.

Alcohol

Although alcohol consumption has not generally been linked with elevated leukemia risk, a population survey in Hawaii found a significant association between beer consumption and leukemia (Hinds et al, 1980) and a case-control interview study of a sample of subjects in the U. S. Third National Cancer Survey revealed nonsignificant elevations in risks of ALL among females, AML and CML among males with moderate alcohol consumption (but no significant dose-response effect) (Williams and Horm, 1977b). In addition, a relatively high mean alcohol intake was observed among men of Japanese origin dying of hematopoietic and lymphatic cancers in the Honolulu Heart Study (Blackwelder et al, 1980), and a significantly high risk of leukemia occurred among a cohort of Swedish brewery workers (Carstensen et al, 1990). However, leukemia was not increased among men belonging to the Danish Brewery Workers Union (Jensen, 1979), male alcoholics treated in Ontario, Canada (Schmidt and Popham, 1981), or among males in a large population-based case-control study in Iowa and Minnesota (Brown et al, 1992b). An elevated risk and dose-response relationship was observed for AML (particularly M2) among children under 18 months whose mothers drank alcohol during pregnancy (Shu et al, 1996), but this finding requires confirmation in other populations.

Diet

There have been few studies assessing the role of dietary factors, micronutrients, or vitamins in the etiology of leukemia. A case-control study of childhood leukemia in China found a protective effect associated with consumption of cod liver oil, which contains high levels of vitamins A and D (Shu et al, 1988). Two U. S. case-control studies reported associations of childhood leukemia with consumption of processed meats, but controls may have been of higher socioeconomic status than cases, perhaps explaining the finding (Peters et al, 1994; Sarasua and Savitz, 1994).

Leukemia Clusters

There has been considerable historical interest in leukemia aggregations since the last century, especially in regard to childhood leukemia. Until recently concern was centered on the possible role of infectious agents. Studies prior to the early 1980s have been previously reviewed (Cartwright and Bernard, 1985; Linet, 1985). The reader is also referred to early papers (Obrastzow, 1890; Pearson, 1913; Ward, 1917; Aubertin, 1923); initial population-based investigations (Pinkel and Nefzger, 1954; Heath and Hasterlik, 1963; Lingeman, 1963; Wood, 1960, 1963); studies evaluating space-time clustering (Knox, 1963; Ederer et al, 1964, 1965; Barton et al, 1965; Lundin, 1966; Stark and Mantel, 1967; Glass and Mantel, 1964); analyses using a regression model (Mantel, 1967; Pike and Smith, 1968); methodologies emphasizing latency (Smith et al, 1976); acquaintance linkage approaches (Greenwald et al, 1979); investigations utilizing case-control methods (Halperin et al, 1980); and analyses of spatial clustering without time considerations (Lewis, 1980). The findings prior to the early 1980s (reviewed in Linet, 1985) appeared to be inconclusive.

Some investigations showing evidence of clustering (Flynn, 1970; Evatt et al, 1973; Gorst et al, 1987) have been counterbalanced by a series of negative studies (Corbett and Schey, 1981; Van Steensel-Moll et al, 1983; Pinder, 1985; Gerrard and Eden, 1986; Gilbert et al, 1987; Muir et al, 1990; Selvin et al, 1992). Kinlen and colleagues have suggested that incidence of childhood leukemia can be increased by population mixing, particularly in rural areas (Kinlen et al, 1993, 1995; Kinlen, 1995).

Since the late 1970s, attention has increasingly focused on environmental hypotheses, including ionizing radiation from nuclear power facilities, chemical manufacturing facilities, hazardous waste sites, and contaminated drinking wells. The cause of a prolonged leukemia cluster of childhood leukemia in Woburn, Massachusetts, remains unknown, despite detailed investigation of a hypothesis regarding chemical contamination of well-water (Lagakos et al, 1986; MacMahon et al, 1986; Swan and Robins, 1986; Rogan, 1986). Family members of affected cases have been shown to have immunologic abnormalities (Byers et al, 1988).

Some of the newer approaches currently being evaluated for identifying and investigating possible clusters include a nearest neighbor method using a case-control approach (Cuzick and Edwards, 1989; Alexander et al, 1992); use of small-area population census data to compute expected case numbers (Clayton and Kaldor, 1987); improvement of small area estimates through use of more precise measures from other appropriate areas within the region being plotted (Kaldor and Clayton, 1989); and mapping by an isotronic regression model (Bithell and Stone, 1989). High quality leukemia incidence data, obtained by special case-surveillance approaches (Baijal et al, 1989), should be independently evaluated using several of the newer analytic methods to assess whether leukemia subtypes display generalized clustering (Chen et al, 1984).

Viruses

HTLV-I and Related Human Retroviruses. For more than 80 years, information has accumulated on the viral etiology of leukemia and other hematopoietic cancers in a variety of species, including mice, chicken, cats, cattle, sheep, and primates (Gross, 1978). Retroviruses, long suspected as a cause of human leukemias, were first associated with human leukemia/lymphoma in 1980 with the description of the human T-cell lymphotropic virus type I (HTLV-I) (Poiesz et al, 1980). Soon after, HTLV-I was more closely linked with the rare adult T-cell leukemia/lymphoma (ATL), a disease entity with geographic clustering first identified in southern Japan (Uchiyama et al, 1977; Yoshida et al, 1982). ATL is an aggressive form of leukemia characterized by skin manifestations, lymphadenopathy, hypercalcemia, bone marrow involvement, and a uniformly fatal outcome (Blattner, 1989).

Descriptive epidemiologic studies (reviewed in Murphy and Blattner, 1988; Blattner, 1989; Manns and Blattner, 1991; Wiktor and Blattner, 1991) have begun to clarify patterns of occurrence of ATL and its relationship with HTLV-I infection in endemic areas of southern Japan (Hinuma et al, 1981, 1982; Clark et al, 1985a; T- and B-Cell Malignancy Study Group, 1988; Tajima et al, 1990), Jamaica (Blattner et al, 1983; Clark et al, 1985b; Gibbs et al, 1987; Kamihira et al, 1992), Trinidad (Bartholomew et al, 1985), among Israeli patients of Iranian origin (Sidi et al, 1990), and parts of Africa including Ghana, Nigeria, the Ivory Coast, Zaire, and Rwanda (Williams et al, 1984b, c; Biggar et al, 1984; Fleming et al, 1986; Verdier et al, 1989; Rwandan HIV Seroprevalence Study Group, 1989; Wiktor et al, 1990; Williams et al, 1994).

Improvements in specificity of HTLV-I serologic assays have enabled more accurate description of HTLV-I seroprevalence in Africa where relatively little is known (Blattner, 1989). In Trinidad, seropositivity is limited almost exclusively to individuals of African descent, even though persons of African and Indian descent have shared a common environment for more than 100 years (GJ Miller et al, 1986). HTLV-I has also been identified among blacks in the southeastern United States (Blayney et al, 1983) and among intravenous drug abusers in the northeastern United States and in New Orleans (Weiss et al, 1987; Robert-Guroff et al, 1986).

A latent, persistent infection is established in peripheral blood T lymphocytes of individuals following primary infection with HTLV-I, and virus can be demonstrated by co-cultivation from the cells of carriers. There is some evidence of diminished cellular immunity (Mueller, 1991). HTLV-I is highly cell-associated, unlike other retroviral infections in which circulating viral products can be detected. The prevalence among apparently healthy individuals in endemic areas ranges between 2% and 12%. In addition to variation in seropositivity rates among broader geographic areas, microgeographic clustering has been observed, with highest infection rates often found in more isolated communities (Kamihira et al, 1992). In geographic areas where historical collections of blood specimens are available, there has been little change over time in patterns of infection (Kashiwagi et al, 1986; Blattner, 1989). Based on cross-sectional data from endemic areas and a few longitudinal seroprevalence studies, a low prevalence of HTLV-I infection is first noted among young children between ages 1 and 2 (approximately 1%) and is consistent with transmission via breast-feeding (Kajiyama et al, 1986; Kinoshita et al, 1987; Kusuhara et al, 1987). Subsequently, there is a consistent age-dependent rise in seropositivity, plateauing among males at around age 50 (Clark et al, 1985a), and declining after age 60. Among older females, rates continue to increase with age. At ages 30–40 a female excess is first apparent, probably reflecting greater efficiency of sexual transmission from men to women (Tajima et al, 1982; Kajiyama et al, 1986; Murphy et al, 1989a; Mueller, 1991). Additional sexually-related risk factors include male homosexual activity and female prostitution (Bartholomew et al, 1987; Khabbaz et al, 1990).

Transmission has also been shown to occur from transfusion of cellular blood components (Okochi et al, 1984; Sato et al, 1986; Kamihira et al, 1987; Manns et al, 1988, 1992), and by intravenous drug abuse (Robert-Guroff et al, 1986; Lee et al, 1989). Only 0.025% tested positive in a 1988 survey of 30,000 blood donors (AE Williams et al, 1988), and only 0.014% were positive among 6.4 million donations to the American Red Cross (MMWR, 1990). Positives were likely to be black, born in or having sexual contact with a person from the Caribbean or Japan, or a history of intravenous drug use or a blood transfusion (AE Williams et al, 1988). Approximately 16%–21% of intravenous drug abusers have been found to be positive for HTLV-I (Mayer and Ebbesen, 1991; Briggs et al, 1995). HTLV-I/II infection may also be endemic among American Indians; prevalence of this infection was 1.0%–1.6% among blood donors from this population compared with 0.16%–0.27% among Hispanic donors and 0.0009%–0.06% among non-Hispanic white donors in New Mexico (Hielle et al, 1991). In addition, almost 3% of 211 U. S. adult leukemia patients (Minamoto et al, 1988) and 49% of black intravenous drug abusers attending a methadone clinic in New Orleans were seropositive (Wiktor and Blattner, 1990). Insect vectors seem unlikely (Blattner, 1989; Wiktor and Blattner, 1990).

Eight percent (6) of 75 T-cell neoplasms from the New York City area evaluated by polymerase chain reaction for the presence of integrated HTLV-I proviral sequences were found to be HTLV-I positive, and 5 of the 6 were from HTLV-I endemic areas with 5 each being black, female, and less than 45 years old (Chadburn et al, 1991). Among 15 patients with ATL in Brooklyn, New York, all were black, 9 originated from the Caribbean islands, 6 from the southern United States, and 2 were father and daughter (Dosik et al,

1988). Further investigations have confirmed an endemic clustering of HTLV-I-associated ATL in a black community in Brooklyn (Welles et al, 1994). Data from a registry of cases diagnosed in the United States have shown that patients of Japanese ancestry were generally older than black patients and presented more often with leukemia. Close to half were born in the United States (Levine et al, 1994).

Virtually all seropositive Japanese migrants residing in Hawaii and Brazil were born in or had maternal ancestral links to viral endemic areas of Japan where infection was apparently acquired (Blattner et al, 1986; Blattner, 1989), and most, but not all, patients with ATL in metropolitan areas in Japan were born in endemic areas (Tajima et al, 1990). Among family members of 77 patients with ATL, 34% of children, 64% of siblings, 61% of spouses, and 81% of parents had anti-HTLV-I antibodies (Momita et al, 1990). Longitudinal data from Japan have been interpreted as showing a cohort effect, with older individuals more likely to have been exposed to the virus at earlier ages than are young people at the present time (Ueda et al, 1989). Based on a follow-up study of Jamaican food handlers, however, seroconversion was observed among young persons associated with multiple sexual partners and/or a history of blood transfusion (Coté et al, 1995).

The age-standardized incidence rate of ATL is estimated to range from 1.9 to 2.9 per 100,000 person-years based on data from Jamaica and Trinidad (Cleghorn et al, 1995), with highest risk observed among individuals who acquired HTLV-I in childhood. Lifetime risk of ATL is estimated as 1%–4% (Kondo et al, 1989; Murphy et al, 1989b). It is noteworthy that females have higher levels of HTLV-I seropositivity than males after age 30–40, whereas the annual incidence of ATL is 1.5- to 3-fold higher for males than females (Kondo et al, 1989; Tajima et al, 1990). In Kyushu, incidence increases steeply with age until the age of 70, then decreases markedly in both sexes (Tajima et al, 1990). Murphy et al (1989b) have postulated that infection during early childhood (when the prevalence of seropositivity is similar between the sexes) may be the most important determinant of ATL incidence and that infection acquired in young adulthood and later is probably associated with a lower risk ATL.

Other important genetic and environmental risk factors have not been identified. It has been suggested that perinatal infection may be an important modifier of risk or infections such as filariasis or strongyloidiasis (Tajima, 1988), although the association of disseminated filariasis and other serious infections with ATL may not be a primary event but rather a consequence of immunosuppression occurring in the premalignant as well as the malignant phase of this hematologic neoplasm (Nakada et al, 1987). Occupations such as farming and furniture manufacturing have been found to be associated with both ATL and non-Hodgkin's lymphoma in case-control studies of these two malignancies in Jamaica and Trinidad-Tobago (Manns et al, 1990, 1992). Childhood infective dermatitis has also been reported to be a potential predictor of later development of ATL during adulthood (LaGrenade et al, 1990). Functional impairment of the T-cell system in patients with ATL, and to a lesser extent healthy seropositive persons, may also result in an unusual immune response of antibodies to EBV-associated antigens (Imai and Hinuma, 1983). In the United States, there appears to be overlap in lifestyle risk factors for HTLV-I and HIV-I, with preliminary data showing elevated rates of HTLV-I in parental drug abusers and male homosexuals (Blattner, 1989). Approximately 16% of intravenous drug abusers have been found to be positive for HTLV-I (Mayer and Ebbesen, 1991).

HTLV-I has also been linked with an HTLV-associated myelopathy or tropical spastic paraparesis, with neurologic symptoms related to demyelination of long motor tracts in the spinal cord (Gessain et al, 1985; Osame and Igata, 1989). This condition has a similar age and geographic distribution as ATLL, but females are predominantly affected. HTLV-associated myelopathy resulting from transfusion-acquired infection appears to have a shorter latent period and a somewhat younger age distribution, based on case reports (Osame and Igata, 1989).

HTLV-II was first isolated from a patient with a T-cell variant of hairy cell leukemia (Kalyanaraman et al, 1982). Little is known of the epidemiology, although this may be the predominant retrovirus in some U. S. drug abuser populations (Wiktor and Blattner, 1991; Murphy, 1993). This virus has also been found to be endemic in Guaymi Indians in Panama (Lairmore et al, 1990). Although initially believed to be harmless, viral infection with HTLV-II has more recently been associated with occurrence of leukemias/lymphomas and neurologic or dermatologic conditions (Murphy, 1993).

Bovine Leukemia Virus. Ecologic studies have linked lymphoid leukemias with exposure to cattle, particularly those with bovine lymphosarcoma (Fasal et al, 1968; Kvarnfors et al, 1975; Donham et al, 1980, 1987; Burmeister et al, 1982). Bovine leukemia virus is a retrovirus related to HTLV-I and HTLV-II and is readily transmitted among cattle through milk, and possibly by insects (Dutcher et al, 1964; Piper et al, 1975; Buxton et al, 1982; Burny et al, 1987). A case-control study showed that leukemia patients had lower-than-expected contact with herds infected with bovine leukemia virus (Donham et al, 1987). A negative case-control serologic study of childhood leukemia also suggests lack of an association (Bender et al, 1988).

Feline Leukemia Virus. Evidence for a relationship of feline leukemia virus with leukemia is also not persuasive in view of a negative serologic study (Sordillo et al, 1982), despite an earlier report that leukemia patients, particularly those with CLL, were more likely to describe a history of a sick cat in the household prior to leukemia onset (Bross and Gibson, 1980; Bross et al, 1972).

Epstein-Barr Virus. Case reports have linked the Epstein-Barr virus (EBV, a herpes virus) to a lymphoproliferative disorder with associated defects in cell-mediated immunity and hemopoiesis. Subsequently, the lymphoproliferative state may evolve into ALL (Finlay et al, 1986) or CML (Mecucci et al, 1986). Some cases appear to complicate an infectious mononucleosis syndrome, which may actually represent an early manifestation of leukemia.

Hepatitis B Virus. An atypical hepatitis B virus (HBV) serologic profile has been observed in adults with AML who were not previously transfused (Markowitz, 1984) and among children with leukemia (Locasciulli et al, 1985). HBV-DNA sequences have also been identified in bone marrow at diagnosis in five of nine children with AML prior to treatment or blood transfusion (Pontisso et al, 1987). No correlation was observed between HTLV-I carrier status and infection with HBV among healthy inhabitants in an ATL-endemic area in Japan (Tachibana et al, 1991).

Nonspecific Infections and Immunizations. Some studies of ALL in children have suggested a relation to nonspecific postnatal viral (McKinney et al, 1987; Petridou et al, 1993) and/or bacterial infections (Shu et al, 1988), while others have described a decreased occurrence of infections within the first year of live (van Steensel-Moll et al, 1986). There are limited data to suggest that the common B-cell precursor form of childhood ALL is increased by higher socioeconomic status, isolation, and other evidence of abnormal infection patterns during infancy (Greaves and Alexander, 1993). A deficit of routine childhood vaccinations has also been reported among ALL patients in some studies (Kneale et al, 1986; McKinney et al, 1987; Nishi and Miyake, 1989).

MEDICAL AND IATROGENIC EVENTS

Medical Conditions

Case reports have described CLL cases with prior history of rheumatoid arthritis, thyroid disease, pernicious anemia, myasthenia gravis, autoimmune hemolytic anemia, and other autoimmune conditions (Conley et al, 1980). Large population-based cohorts of persons with rheumatoid arthritis in Finland had elevated risks of CLL and AML (Isomaki et al, 1982; Hakulinen et al, 1985). An increase in AML subsequent to rheumatoid arthritis had been related to the use of cytotoxic drugs (Hazleman, 1982; Hakulinen et al, 1985). In two surveys of rheumatoid arthritis in the United Kingdom, only non-Hodgkin's lymphomas occurred in excess (Kinlen et al, 1985; Symmons, 1985), but in a third cohort CLL was increased (Taylor et al, 1989) and this leukemia type was also associated with a prior history of rheumatism and arthritis among U. S. males (Gibson et al, 1976). A linked registry study of a large cohort of patients hospitalized with rheumatoid arthritis in Sweden showed nonsignificant increases of all leukemia, particularly CLL, and a significant excess of lymphoma (Gridley et al, 1993). Possible explanations for this association include genetic predisposition, proliferation of a forbidden clone or other common etiology for both diseases; chronic immune stimulation resulting in malignant transformation of B cells; lymphoproliferation resulting from treatment for rheumatoid arthritis; prolonged reduction in natural killer cell activity allowing a normally suppressed B-cell subpopulation to proliferate and/or spontaneously transform; or a bias as a result of intensive medical surveillance (Symmons, 1988; Taylor et al, 1989). No increase of leukemia has been seen in other rheumatoid arthritis cohorts (Hazleman, 1982).

Excess myeloid leukemia has been found in cohorts with other autoimmune diseases including pernicious anemia (Blackburn et al, 1968; Brinton et al, 1989; Hsing et al, 1993), inflammatory bowel disease (Cuttner, 1982; Mir-Madjlessi et al, 1986; Halme et al, 1990), and psoriasis (Zheng et al, 1993). The possible association of pernicious anemia with myeloid leukemia may, however, be spurious if a substantial proportion of the pernicious anemia diagnoses were a result of misclassification of one or more subtypes of myelodysplastic syndromes. CLL was also increased among persons with scleroderma (Doyle et al, 1985), idiopathic thrombocytopenic purpura (Carey et al, 1976; Wang et al, 1984), diabetes (Gibson et al, 1976), and allergy-related conditions (Gibson et al, 1976). Other studies have reported inverse relationships of allergy-related disorders with CLL (McCormick et al, 1971; Linet et al, 1986) and AML (Cartwright et al, 1988; Severson et al, 1989; Zheng et al, 1993), although one study found a positive association of hay fever with AML based on medical record data (Doody et al, 1992). Neither kidney transplant patients (Hoover and Fraumeni, 1973; Penn, 1984) nor patients treated with immunosuppressive drugs (Kinlen et al, 1979) had a notably elevated risk of leukemia; a slight increase was ascribed to the effect of therapeutic radiation.

CLL has been associated with history of prior skin

cancers, heart disease, migraine, and use of antihypertensive agents (Cartwright et al, 1987b), and with syphilis, tuberculosis, and urinary tract infections (Rosenblatt et al, 1991). In addition, AML has been reported in association with systemic mast cell disease (Cooper et al, 1982; Travis et al, 1989) and Sweet's syndrome (Cooper et al, 1983; Vestey et al, 1986), with either of these two diseases often occurring simultaneously with onset of AML. It is often not clear whether the reported association of leukemia with prior illnesses represents a causal relationship to the underlying condition or reflects heightened surveillance, treatment effects, or chance events.

Surgical excision of lymphoid tissue has been inversely correlated with CLL (Linet et al, 1986), but studies reporting leukemia risk subsequent to appendectomy have described conflicting findings (Cartwright et al, 1987b; Zheng et al, 1993).

Iatrogenic Exposures

Diagnostic X-Rays. Mortality from childhood ALL (OR = 1.6) and AML (OR = 1.6) has been associated with pregnancy-related diagnostic x-ray exposure in the U. K. nationwide Oxford Childhood Cancer Study (Stewart et al, 1958; Bithell and Stewart, 1975) and for all childhood leukemia, types not specified, in New England and the mid-Atlantic states (MacMahon, 1962; Monson and MacMahon, 1984). Other studies have confirmed these findings (Graham et al, 1966; Diamond et al, 1973; Harvey et al, 1985; Shu et al, 1994), with risk confined to first trimester exposure in some studies (McWhirter and Chant, 1990), but more often late in the third trimester (Monson and MacMahon, 1984), fetal exposures estimated to be in the range of 5–50 mGy (Monson and MacMahon, 1984) and the excess subsequent leukemia risk estimated to be approximately 40%. The lack of an elevated leukemia risk among black children who were prenatally exposed (Diamond et al, 1973), the occurrence of an unremarkable incidence of childhood cancers in atomic bomb survivors heavily exposed in utero (Yoshimoto, 1990), and the absence of leukemia occurrence in animals following fetal irradiation (United Nations, 1986) are puzzling. The discrepant findings suggest that host susceptibility characteristics or selection factors may be involved. Paternal preconception exposure has also been linked with both ALL and AML (Graham et al, 1966; Shu et al, 1988), although recall bias is a likely explanation (Shu et al, 1994). Childhood leukemia has also been associated with postnatal diagnostic x-ray exposures in some studies (Stewart et al, 1958; Graham et al, 1966; Shu et al, 1988).

Among adults, leukemia in males (Gibson et al, 1972) and myeloid leukemia and CML in both sexes (Gunz and Atkinson, 1964; Preston-Martin et al, 1989; Flodin et al, 1990) have been linked with diagnostic x-rays, particularly of the back and gastrointestinal tract. Other investigations have shown no relationship (Linos et al, 1980; Boice et al, 1981; Evans et al, 1986) or an excess of diagnostic radiography only within 2–5 years of leukemia diagnosis (Stewart et al, 1962; Stewart, 1973; Boice et al, 1991), suggesting that the diagnostic x-rays may have been obtained for early manifestations of leukemia.

In studies of patients repeatedly x-rayed or fluoroscoped for chronic conditions, leukemia was not elevated among patients with tuberculosis (Davis et al, 1989), women monitored for scoliosis (Hoffman et al, 1989), or children undergoing cardiac catheterization (Spengler et al, 1983). In addition, no excess was observed among patients receiving I^{131} for diagnostic purposes (Holm et al, 1989), despite an estimated mean absorbed dose to the bone marrow of 14 mGy (Hall et al, 1992). Patients injected with the contrast medium Thorotrast (containing the alpha-emitter, thorium dioxide) had elevated risks of AML and CML, with rates continuing to increase up to 40 years after exposure (Faber, 1978; van Kaick et al, 1986; Mori et al, 1983; Andersson and Storm, 1992; Andersson et al, 1993). Negative studies must be cautiously interpreted since large numbers of subjects are required to adequately evaluate leukemia risk from diagnostic x-ray exposure (Kumamoto, 1985). It has been estimated that 1% of all leukemia cases in the general population may be attributable to diagnostic radiography (Evans et al, 1986).

Radiation Therapy.

Ankylosing spondylitis. Increased mortality from AML, CML, aplastic anemia, and lymphoma was observed among 14,106 ankylosing spondylitis patients treated with a single course of x-ray therapy (Court Brown and Doll, 1965, Smith et al, 1982; Darby et al, 1987), but not among spondylitis patients who were not given radiation (Radford et al, 1977). The increase in risk (estimated overall to be 0.45 additional leukemia cases per 10^4 PYGy) first became apparent within 2 years after irradiation, attained a peak at 5 years, then declined, with rates somewhat above baseline levels approximately 20–25 years after treatment (Smith and Doll, 1982; Darby et al, 1987). The leukemia excess in this population was not as great as that among atomic bomb survivors (Smith and Doll, 1982; Lewis et al, 1988). In Germany, spondylitis patients treated with Ra^{224} also had excess leukemia (Speiss, 1989).

Cervical and uterine cancer and benign gynecologic disorders. In a follow-up of 182,040 women with cervical cancer, 82,616 of whom were treated with fractionated doses of radiation during 1935–70, a 1.3-fold excess of acute and nonlymphocytic leukemias was found (Boice et al, 1985). In a more detailed case-control study of nonlymphocytic leukemia cases identified within this cohort, risk was elevated 2-fold among exposed women and the absolute risk estimated as 0.48×10^{-6} PY-cGy (Boice et al, 1987). Risk was highest within 1–14 years after irradiation, greater in women under age 45 at exposure, and notable for all cell types except CLL (Boice et al, 1987), but these findings based on subgroup results need to be confirmed. Highest rates occurred among women receiving an average bone marrow dose of 2.5–5.0 Gy, whereas rates were lower among women receiving higher doses. This decrease was ascribed to cell killing in the irradiated bone marrow.

A nested case-control investigation was carried out in a cohort of 110,000 women with uterine corpus cancer in nine areas of the United States to assess the relationship of radiation theapy to leukemia. A 90% significant increase of leukemia was observed, but the dose-response relationship was inconsistent. Elevated risks were seen for patients irradiated at age 65 or older (Curtis et al, 1994).

A 70% excess leukemia mortality was seen among approximately 13,000 women treated with radiation for benign gynecologic disorders in New England and New York State (Inskip et al, 1993). No clear dose-response effect was observed. Risk of leukemia was highest within 5 years after irradiation, but remained elevated even after 30 years.

Elevated risks of AML (Curtis et al, 1984) and non-CLL leukemias (Boivin et al, 1986) were found among women treated with radiation for uterine corpus cancer. Pelvic irradiation given in the past to control menorrhagia not associated with malignancy was also associated with elevated risk of leukemia among Scottish (Smith and Doll, 1976) and U. S. women (Wagoner, 1984; Inskip et al, 1990).

Breast cancer. Excess AML has been reported among breast cancer patients treated with radiotherapy in clinical trials (Fisher et al, 1985; Andersson et al, 1991) and among patients reported to population-based cancer registries (Curtis et al, 1984, 1992; Boivin et al, 1986). However, there was no increase in risk and no dose-response effect in a case-control study in which radiation doses were carefully estimated (Curtis et al, 1989).

Hodgkin's disease. Most studies of Hodgkin's disease patients given high voltage radiotherapy alone have shown no excess of AML (Coltman and Dixon, 1982; Boivin et al, 1984; Valagussa et al, 1986; Pedersen-Bjergaard et al, 1987), although a few studies have reported elevated risks in a small number of patients (Tucker et al, 1988; Kaldor et al, 1990a). Patients treated with both radiotherapy and chemotherapy have a substantial risk of developing AML, with combined regimens yielding a rate that is 3- to 12-fold higher than that observed for chemotherapy alone (Papa et al, 1984; Tester et al, 1984; Valagussa et al, 1986; Blayney et al, 1987; Andrieu et al, 1990). The mechanisms of carcinogenesis in patients treated with both of these modalities are unknown, but one possibility is immunologic alteration. Therapeutic lymphoid irradiation has been shown to produce important long-term alterations in lymphocyte subpopulations and immunologic responsiveness, particularly in the notable long-term increase in natural killer cells (Macklis et al, 1992).

Other adult malignant and benign conditions. Among patients with non-Hodgkin's lymphoma (NHL), only one of 305 treated with radiation therapy alone developed secondary AML (Lavey et al, 1990). In contrast, a high AML risk and evidence of dose-response effects were associated with total body and hemibody irradiation of NHL cases in which large volumes of bone marrow were exposed to relatively low cumulative doses of radiation therapy (Greene et al, 1983). Small leukemia excesses occurred among patients receiving I^{131} for thyroid cancer (Brincker et al, 1973; Edmonds and Smith, 1986), but not those treated with this radionuclide for hyperthyroidism (Saenger et al, 1969; Hoffman et al, 1982; Holm, 1984; Holm et al, 1991). Risk of leukemia was increased more than three-fold among 1831 patients with peptic ulcer treated with radiotherapy compared with risk among 1778 patients receiving other treatments (Griem et al, 1994). Acute leukemia was significantly increased among patients with polycythemia vera receiving P^{32} compared with those treated with phlebotomy (Modan and Lilienfeld, 1965). In general, the risk of leukemia associated with partial body high-dose radiotherapy is less than that observed among groups receiving lower doses, and there is uncertainty about possible synergistic effects of radiotherapy and chemotherapy.

Childhood disorders. An increased risk of leukemia has been seen among American and Israeli children treated with radiation to the scalp for tinea capitis (Albert and Omram, 1968; Hurley et al, 1976; Shore et al, 1976; Ron et al, 1988). Leukemia was also elevated among children irradiated in infancy for enlarged thymuses (Hempelmann et al, 1975; Hildreth et al, 1985), but not among children treated with nasopharyngeal radium for adenoid hypertrophy (Sandler et al, 1982). In surveys of children treated with radiotherapy alone for malignancy, there has been no clear evidence of excess leukemia occurrence (Draper et al, 1986; Meadows et al, 1986; Tucker et al, 1987).

Alkylating Drugs and Other Chemotherapy Agents. An increased risk of AML as a second malignancy was first described among multiple myeloma patients (Kyle et al, 1970; Andersen and Videbaek, 1970), and linked with the use of alkylating agents, melphalan, and cyclophosphamide (Gonzales et al, 1977; Kyle, 1982; Cuzick et al, 1987). Some of the secondary AML may be part of the natural history of the initial hematologic malignancy, particularly if the secondary AML arises early in the course of the initial malignancy, if markers characteristic of AML cells are also found on cells of the initial hematologic malignancy, and if cells of the initial malignancy show lineage infidelity suggesting an early hematopoietic stem cell origin. Subsequent to the initial reports linking melphalan and cyclophosphamide with AML, other agents have been implicated in AML including mechlorethamine, chlorambucil, busulfan, dihydroxybusulphan, carmustine, lomustine and semustine, epipodophyllotoxins, and possibly others (Najean, 1987; Pedersen-Bjersgaard and Philip, 1989; Giles and Koeffer, 1994). Unfortunately, the median survival subsequent to secondary AML is 3–6 months, with a poor response to therapy.

Alkylating agents are linked with a 10- to 300-fold increased risk of secondary AML among patients treated for various lymphatic and hematopoietic malignancies including Hodgkin's disease among adults (Arsenau et al, 1972; Coltman and Dixon, 1982; Boivin et al, 1984; Tucker et al, 1988; Kaldor et al, 1990a; Devereaux et al, 1990; Cimino et al, 1991; Swerdlow et al, 1992; van Leeuwen et al, 1994), non-Hodgkin's lymphoma in adults (Greene et al, 1983; Pedersen-Bjergaard et al, 1985; Lavey et al, 1990; Travis et al, 1993) and children (Ingram et al, 1987; Pui et al, 1990; Rivera et al, 1993), Waldenstrom's macroglobulinemia (Rosner and Grunwald, 1980), polycythemia vera (Berk et al, 1981; Haanen et al, 1981; Ellis et al, 1986), and chronic lymphocytic leukemia (Zarrabi et al, 1977; Teichmann et al, 1986).

Alkylating agents have also been linked with secondary AML among patients with solid tumors including ovarian cancer (Reimer et al, 1977; Greene et al, 1982; Haas et al, 1987; Kaldor et al, 1990b), small cell carcinoma of the lung (Stott et al, 1977; Osterlind et al, 1986), gastrointestinal malignancies (Boice et al, 1983), male germ cell tumors (Redman et al, 1983), and female breast cancer (Portugal et al, 1979; Curtis et al, 1984, 1990, 1992; Fisher et al, 1985; Haas et al, 1987; Andersson et al, 1990).

Among the few large cohorts of childhood ALL cases with substantial follow-up, most investigators (Hawkins et al, 1987; Tucker et al, 1987; Neglia et al, 1991) have not reported a significant excess of secondary AML. A substantially elevated cumulative risk (3.8% at 6 years; 95% CI = 2.3%–6.1%) was found in one cohort and linked with schedule of drug administration, but not dose, of epipodophyllotoxin (Pui et al, 1991); further clarification is needed of the relationship of this agent with secondary AML, subsequent to treatment of childhood ALL. A recent detailed evaluation of the results of treatment of childhood ALL during four time periods at a major referral hospital in the United States has shown 5-year risk of secondary AML to be 0.5% among 825 children treating during 1967–79, 2.3% among 428 children treated during 1979–83, and 3.6% among 358 children treated during 1984–88 (Rivera et al, 1993).

In many surveys, risk was generally greater among patients treated with higher doses of alkylating agents (particularly cyclophosphamide), those receiving more than one alkylating agent, those given more than one course of treatment, and those treated after 1970. It is not clear whether older patients have a higher risk, or whether females are more likely to develop secondary AML than males (Swerdlow et al, 1992; Tarbell et al, 1993). The addition of radiotherapy to chemotherapy regimens did not generally increase leukemia risk (Levine and Bloomfield, 1986; Brusamolino et al, 1986; Pedersen-Bjersgaard et al, 1987; Kaldor et al, 1990a; Devereaux et al, 1990). Among Hodgkin's disease patients, splenectomy seemed to enhance risk of leukemia (Kaldor et al, 1990a). Secondary leukemia incidence has appeared to be notably higher following treatment with melphalan (Greene et al, 1986; Cuzick et al, 1987; Kaldor et al, 1990b; Curtis et al, 1990, 1992), and also somewhat higher for busulfan (Stott et al, 1977), lomustine, and chlorambucil (Najean, 1987; Kaldor et al, 1990a) than with cyclophosphamide. Hodgkin's disease patients treated with mechlorethamine, vincristine, prednisone, and procarbazine (MOPP) have a higher risk of secondary leukemia than those treated with adriamycin, bleomycin, vinblastine, and dacarbazine (ABVD) (Valagussa et al, 1986; Cimino et al, 1991), possibly related to the high risk associated with use of mechlorethamine (Henry-Amar et al, 1989).

A myelodysplastic phase is observed in 70% of patients who developed therapy-related leukemia (Giles and Koeffer, 1994). The majority of patients developing secondary leukemia subsequent to treatment of Hodgkin's or non-Hodgkin's disease have a chromosomally abnormal clone; most commonly there is loss of part or all of chromosomes 5 and 7 (Rowley et al, 1977; Levine and Bloomfield, 1986; Whang-Peng et al, 1988). Other karyotypic abnormalities may involve chromosomes 1, 3, 4, 8, 11, 12, 14, 17, 18, and 21. Abnormalities of chromosome 17 are most frequent in secondary leukemia among patients treated for solid tumors (Giles and Koeffer, 1994). Patients with therapy-related AML with t(8;21), inv(16), t(8;16), t(15;17) or balanced translocations involving 11q23 appear to belong to a subset of secondary AML cases not preceded by myelodysplastic syndrome (Quesnel et al, 1993). Leukemia as a secondary malignancy first becomes apparent within 1–2 years after treatment initiation, with incidence continuing to rise for at least 9–10 years (Tucker et al, 1988). Although data from two series of Hodgkin's disease patients with prolonged follow-up suggest that secondary AML continues to occur more than 10 years after initial treatment (Van Leeuwen et al, 1994; Cimino et al, 1991), there are few data available for patients followed more than 10 years. Cumulative risks for secondary AML generally ranged from 0.2% to 4.0% per year, reaching totals as high as 10%–15%, but even higher for multiple myeloma and polycythemia vera (Ellis et al, 1986; Najean, 1987). The actuarial risk of secondary leukemia may reach 25% among patients treated for small cell lung cancer, owing to the use of multiple alkylating agents in conjunction with high-dose cranial irradiation (Chak et al, 1984).

AML has also been noted among persons given alkylating agents for various nonmalignant conditions including psoriasis, rheumatoid arthritis, and multiple sclerosis, and Wegener's granulomatosis (Grunwald and Rosner, 1979; Aymard et al, 1983; Baltus et al, 1983; Rieche, 1984; Lee et al, 1991).

Although most secondary leukemias are nonlymphoblastic in phenotype, some cases of secondary ALL have been described (Grunwald and Rosner, 1979; Kyle, 1984; Tucker et al, 1987; Felix et al, 1994), a few linked with the t(4;11) chromosomal abnormality (Secker-Walker et al, 1985; Archimbaud et al, 1988). Most of these patients have been treated with topoisomerase II inhibitors (such as epipodophyllotoxins, anthracyclines, or derivatives (Giles and Koeffler, 1994). Some secondary leukemias are biphenotypic (Chen et al, 1989).

Other Drugs. A population-based case-control study of childhood leukemia in Shanghai revealed a relationship to the use of antibiotics, chloramphenicol, and syntomycin, which is pharmacologically related to chloramphenicol (Shu et al, 1987). Previous clinical surveys have suggested that patients with chloramphenicol-induced aplastic anemia may be at elevated risk of AML (Fraumeni, 1967; Adamson and Sieber, 1981).

Childhood leukemia, notably ALL, has been associated with pregnancy-related use of narcotic analgesics in one case-control study (McKinney et al, 1987), and sedatives and tranquilizers during the first trimester in another (McWhirter and Chant, 1990). A population-based nested case-control study in Sweden implicated nitrous oxide anesthesia during delivery, and use of supplemental oxygen for newborns (Zack et al, 1991). A U. S. investigation suggested a relation between childhood ANLL and maternal use of marijuana during pregnancy, with the risk highest for the myelomonocytic and monocytic subtypes (Robison et al, 1989). The same study also suggested that prolonged use of antinausea drugs during pregnancy may be a risk factor for ANLL.

Case reports have linked growth hormone therapy with subsequent development of leukemia, primarily ALL, among children and adolescents in Japan and other countries (Watanabe et al, 1988; Stahnke and Zeisel, 1989). Most of these patients were treated after 1975, and about half had additional leukemia risk factors. The rarity of the exposure and outcome makes it difficult to quantify risk, although scintigraphy for thyroid function using radioactive iodide and associated chromosomal breakage syndrome among cases may be responsible for the elevated risk (Watanabe et al, 1989). Although a cohort of growth hormone recipients in the United States had a nearly two-fold excess of leukemia, most had received radiation therapy for intracranial tumors (Fradkin et al, 1993). No new cases of leukemia occurred among 1908 patients treated with human pituitary growth hormone in the United Kingdom during 1959–95 (Buchanan et al, 1991).

Phenylbutazone has been suggested as a leukemogen in case reports, but no excess of leukemia was seen among 3660 health plan members receiving phenylbutazone prescriptions (Friedman and Ury, 1980). The relationship between AML and phenylbutazone use in some reports appears to be confounded by the musculoskeletal symptoms that occur as an early manifestation of leukemia (Friedman, 1982). In a population-based case-control study of CLL in the United Kingdom, an association was found with phenylbutazone use for arthritic conditions (Cartwright et al, 1987b).

There have been two reports from the United Kingdom linking childhood leukemia with neonatal injection with vitamin K (Golding et al, 1990, 1992). Yet, no association was observed in a large nested case-control study in the United States (Klebanoff et al, 1993).

Bacillus Calmette-Guérin (BCG) Vaccination. Initial reports of reduced leukemia mortality among children vaccinated with BCG in Quebec (Davignon et al, 1970) and Chicago (Rosenthal et al, 1972) were criticized because of methodologic problems (Stewart and Draper, 1970, 1971; Hoover, 1976). A second study comparing Quebec with the rest of Canada did not find a protective effect (Kinlen and Pike, 1971), nor was leukemia reduced among children receiving BCG in controlled trials (Comstock et al, 1975; Snider et al, 1978). Protective effects in reports from Finland (Haro, 1986) and Japan (Nishi and Miyake, 1989) are difficult to interpret in light of the negative clinical trial data.

Bone Marrow Transplants. Among more than 2000 patients with leukemia and aplastic anemia treated at a single center with bone marrow transplant over a 17-year period, 1.6% developed a secondary cancer after 1.5 to 13.9 years, including 0.3% with secondary leukemia (Witherspoon et al, 1989). The secondary leukemias post transplant were generally ALL, most arising in donor cells of patients whose initial primaries were ALL or CML. An apparent excess of AML occurred among patients treated with bone marrow transplant for advanced lymphomas (Marolleau et al, 1993). Although secondary NHL was linked with acute graft-versus-host disease and treatment of this with anti-T-cell monoclonal antibody, total body irradiation, and HLA mismatch, none of these factors were associated with secondary leukemia. It is possible that the original etiologic agents persist and cause a second primary leukemia in donor cells. As bone marrow transplantation is used more widely (Gratwohl et al, 1993), the elucidation of factors responsible for leukemia development in donor cells may be helpful in understanding basic mechanisms of leukemogenesis.

FAMILIAL AND GENETIC FACTORS

Familial Aggregation

Case reports of families in which two or more members developed leukemia (Anderson, 1951; Gunz et al, 1966, 1978; Fraumeni et al, 1969; Schweitzer et al, 1973; Gunz, 1977; Cuttner, 1992) have been confirmed in case-control studies showing excess leukemia among family members of cases (Vidabaek, 1947; Gunz, 1964; Gunz and Veale, 1969; Gunz et al, 1975; Cartwright et al, 1987b, 1988; Linet et al, 1989; Pottern et al, 1991). Most reports describe concordant leukemia cell types among affected members (Blattner et al, 1976; Gunz, 1977; Gunz et al, 1978; Lillicrap and Sterndale, 1984), but a small proportion have discordant leukemia types (Heath, 1975; Gunz et al, 1978). Relatives of leukemia cases also appear to be at higher risk of other hematolymphoproliferative malignancies (Rigby et al, 1968; Gunz and Veale, 1969; Blattner et al, 1979; Bourguet et al, 1985; Bjerrum et al, 1986; Gerncik et al, 1987; Linet al, 1988b, 1989; Cartwright et al, 1990; Cuttner, 1992). CLL is the type most consistently associated with other hematolymphoproliferative malignancies in families (Dameshek and Gunz, 1964; Rigby et al, 1968; Gunz et al, 1969, 1975; Zuelzer and Cox, 1969; Pottern et al, 1991). Risk appears to be highest for siblings, although parental excess has also been found (Linet et al, 1989; McKinney et al, 1990). A fourfold excess risk of childhood leukemia was estimated among siblings of ALL cases in one study (Miller, 1963), and a 2.3-fold risk in another (Draper et al, 1977). Childhood leukemia has also been identified as part of the Li-Fraumeni cancer family syndrome, which features sarcomas and breast cancer (Li and Fraumeni, 1982). There have been a few reports of immune abnormalities among unaffected members of leukemia-prone families (Potolsky et al, 1971; Blattner et al, 1979).

Although the mechanisms for familial leukemia are unclear, there may be some involvement of inherited chromosomal defects (Fitzgerald and Hamer, 1976; Cervenka et al, 1977) or specific genetic mutations that may be linked with related or unrelated conditions (Al-Jader et al, 1990), primary immunologic alterations (Hann et al, 1975; Blattner et al, 1976), sharing of a common haplotype (Fazekas et al, 1978; Conley et al, 1980), consanguinity (Heath, 1975; Blattner et al, 1979), similar environmental influences (Blattner et al, 1976; Linet et al, 1989), or combined effects.

Family members of CLL probands may also have an elevated risk of nonmalignant autoimmune conditions among close relatives, with or without increased occurrence of other hematolymphoproliferative malignancies (Reilly et al, 1952; Issitt, 1977; Conley et al, 1980). In addition, an excess of multiple sclerosis has been suggested among blood relatives and spouses of CLL cases (Bernard et al, 1987).

Twin Studies

Case reports (Jelke, 1939; Anderson and Herman, 1955; Pearson et al, 1963), death certificate studies (Court Brown and Doll, 1961; MacMahon and Levy, 1964; Miller, 1971), and analytic investigations of siblings (Draper et al, 1977) and twins (Jackson et al, 1969; Harvey et al, 1985; Cnattingius et al, 1995a) have described elevated leukemia risk for the twin of an affected child. Investigators have reported a 17%–25% concordance for leukemia (virtually all acute lymphoblastic leukemia) among identical twins, with onset under age one in the majority of cases, and a male-to-female ratio of 7:9 (Court Brown and Doll, 1961; MacMahon and Levy, 1964; Zuelzer and Cox, 1969; Miller, 1971; Inskip et al, 1991). In one study of 4679 childhood leukemia deaths, 72 involved one member of a twin pair; both members were affected in 5 of the 72 sets (MacMahon and Levy, 1964). Among 30,925 twins born in Connecticut between 1930 and 1969, 13 leukemia cases (4 in two female twin pairs) were identified in a linking of the twin roster with the Connecticut Tumor Registry, although the leukemia risk appeared to be somewhat decreased in this population (Inskip et al, 1991). Risk was also not increased among more than 35,000 Swedish twins (Rodvall et al, 1992). Leukemia in both members of an identical twin pair may originate from a single mutation affecting one of the twin fetuses and passed to the cotwin by cross-placental transfusion of cells (Chaganti et al, 1979; Hartley and Sainsbury,

1981; Pombo de Oliveira et al, 1986). Karyotypic and molecular data support this sequence of events. The absence of 100% concordance suggests that the intrauterine transfer does not always occur or that other promoting factors may be important (Greaves, 1989).

The age distribution in affected dizygous twin pairs is closer to that of nontwin children, while males predominate (Zuelzer and Cox, 1969). Concordance of leukemia has rarely been observed in adult twin populations (Harnden, 1985).

Chromosomal Syndromes

Children with certain hereditary or congenital conditions accompanied by a tendency to chromosomal abnormalities or breaks have an elevated risk of leukemia. Estimates of leukemia risk, derived from case reports in the absence of population-based data, are affected by the greater likelihood that individuals with both conditions will be reported in the literature (Miller, 1967).

The most common genetic condition linked with childhood leukemia is Down syndrome, diagnosed in more than 90% of children with both a genetic disorder and leukemia in a large population-based series (Narod et al, 1991). Persons with Down syndrome (trisomy 21) have an estimated 20- to 30-fold increased risk of developing acute leukemia of various cell types (Holland et al, 1962; Miller, 1968; Jackson et al, 1968; Fabia and Drollette, 1970; Scholl et al, 1982; Robison and Neglia, 1987; Fong and Brodeur, 1987; Zack et al, 1991; Cnattingius et al, 1995a, b). Among 1036 children with newly diagnosed non-T, non-B acute lymphoblastic leukemia and a demonstrated cytogenetic abnormality, there were 33 patients with trisomy 21 as the single abnormality; 14 of these 33 had Down syndrome (Watson et al, 1993). Among 131 Down syndrome–associated leukemias of 5564 diagnosed during 1971–83 and reported to the National Registry of Childhood Tumors in the United Kingdom, 73 were ALL (1.7% of the ALL cases) and 49 were AML (5.3% of the AML cases) (Narod et al, 1991). The age distribution at diagnosis for ALL cases with and without Down syndrome is similar, but AML cases with Down syndrome are significantly younger (Robison and Neglia, 1987; Narod et al, 1991). Since techniques for identifying megakaryoblasts have become available, a noteworthy excess of acute megakaryoblastic leukemia (AML M7) in children with Down syndrome has been recognized, and it is likely that earlier cases diagnosed as ALL were actually AML M7 (Zipursky et al, 1987). Both childhood acute leukemia and Down syndrome have similar risk factors, including associations with prenatal radiation exposure, older maternal age at birth, higher risk among first-born, and abnormal maternal reproductive history (Robison and Neglia, 1987). Some studies have also described familial clustering of Down syndrome and childhood leukemia (Verresen et al, 1964; Ebbin et al, 1968).

Among 24 cases with both Down syndrome and acute leukemia studied with chromosome banding, two-thirds had extra chromosomes in their malignant cells (often extra chromosome 8, 21, 19, and 22), while 9 cases had chromosome rearrangements (Hecht et al, 1986). The precise basis of the etiologic association is unclear (Hecht et al, 1986; Robison and Neglia, 1987), although acquired trisomy 21 is among the common cytogenetic abnormalities seen in ALL and AML (Heim and Mitelman, 1987). Transient leukemia (incidence unknown) occurs in neonates with Down syndrome or in normal children with a cell line trisomic for chromosome 21 (Iselius et al, 1990). Although this disorder usually disappears without treatment within 1–2 months, in about 25% of cases true leukemia occurs later in early childhood (Zipursky et al, 1987). It is noteworthy that patients with transient leukemia are born to significantly younger mothers than patients with true leukemia, suggesting differing etiologies (Iselius et al, 1990).

Other congenital disorders with extra chromosomes associated with leukemia are Klinefelter's syndrome (XXY) (linked with AML generally) (Fraumeni and Miller, 1967; Oguma et al, 1989) and D-trisomy (Schade et al, 1962; Zuelzer et al, 1968).

Also prone to acute leukemia are congenital disorders characterized by chromosome breakage such as Bloom's syndrome (linked with ALL in younger persons, AML in older individuals), ataxia-telangiectasia (associated with ALL), and Fanconi's anemia (10%–20% of persons with this disorder develop AML) (Bloom et al, 1966; Sawitsky et al, 1966; Miller, 1967, 1968; Toledano and Lange, 1980; Spector et al, 1982; Morrell et al, 1986; Gretzula et al, 1987; Hecht and Hecht, 1990). Ataxia-telangiectasia, a recessively inherited disorder characterized cytogenetically by a translocation involving chromosomes 7 and 14 (Taylor, 1992), also has a functional immunodeficiency which may contribute to the elevated risk (cumulative risk of a childhood malignancy among A-T homozygotes has been estimated as 10%) of lymphoid leukemias and non-Hodgkin's lymphoma (Spector et al, 1978). A substantial proportion of ALL cases have been found to have markers for T-cell leukemia (Taylor, 1992). Black patients with this disorder seem at particular risk in some studies (Sugimoto et al, 1982; Morrell et al, 1986), but not others (Pippard et al, 1988).

Other Congenital Disorders

Leukemia, particularly the rare juvenile CML, has been linked in clinical reports with neurofibromatosis (Hardisty et al, 1964; McWhirter et al, 1971; Bader and Miller, 1978; Clark and Hutter, 1982; Matsui et al, 1993), although follow-up studies of probands and their relatives have not consistently shown leukemia excesses (Voutsinas and Wynne-Davies, 1983; Sorensen et al, 1986). A study of children with neurofibromatosis-I who developed a myeloid malignancy suggests that the product of the gene that is mutated in patients with the autosomal dominant neurofibromatosis-I functions as a tumor suppressor, and that the normal product of this gene plays an important role in controlling growth of myeloid cells; mutations in this gene can subsequently result in the abnormal cellular proliferation seen in childhood malignant myeloid diseases (Shannon et al, 1994).

There have also been reports of acute leukemia (generally ALL, occasionally AML) (Gilman and Miller, 1982; Sackey et al, 1984) and CML (Costa et al, 1991) among children with Poland syndrome and those with Schwachman syndrome (both ALL and AML) (Caselitz et al, 1979; Woods et al, 1981). An excess of ALL and non-Hodgkin's lymphoma has been described in a syndrome consisting of familial microcephaly, normal intelligence, and immunodeficiency (Seemanova et al, 1985). Although non-Hodgkin's lymphoma predominates in primary immunodeficiency syndromes, there are reports indicating excesses of lymphoid leukemias (Spector et al, 1978; Kinlen et al, 1985) and myeloid leukemias (Spector et al, 1978). In addition, immunologic abnormalities have been described among mothers and siblings of leukemic children in small studies (Sutton et al, 1969; Chandra, 1972; Till et al, 1975, 1979; Hann et al, 1975). Relatives of patients with cystic fibrosis may also be at increased risk of leukemia (Al-Jader et al, 1989). The cystic fibrosis gene and the met-oncogene are closely linked on the long arm of chromosome 7, mapped to a region associated with nonrandom chromosomal deletions in some patients with AML (Dean et al, 1985).

Since 1985, the rare nonseminomatous germ cell tumors arising within the mediastinum have been linked with subsequent occurrence of AML (particularly acute megakaryocytic leukemia), and less commonly with malignant histiocytosis and ALL, in as many as 10%–20% of patients (Nichols, 1991, 1993; Bajorin et al, 1993). It has been suggested that the germ cell and hematologic malignancies are closely related biologically and that the hematologic malignancy may result from differentiation of the multipotent malignant germ cell, based on the short interval between the two disorders, the explosive onset of the hematologic malignancy, and cytogenetic findings (of the same abnormality in both germ cell tumor and hematologic tumor in one patient and chromosomal abnormalities in the hematologic tumors of others that are not typically chemotherapy-related (Nichols, 1991). However, the association of AML and myelodysplastic syndrome in a cohort of 212 patients with germ cell tumors was ascribed to etoposide-containing chemotherapy instead (Pedersen-Bjergaard et al, 1991). Etoposides used in treatment of children with ALL has also been linked with an excess of secondary AML in some (Winick et al, 1993), but not all (Pui et al, 1991) studies. Additional research is needed to clarify the mechanisms of the association of germ cell tumors, etoposide-containing therapy, and AML, and the relationship of etoposides with secondary AML among children with other types of malignancies.

Clonal Chromosomal Abnormalities

Refinements in laboratory techniques have confirmed that most patients with acute leukemias at diagnosis have nonrandom, primary karyotypic anomalies which are thought to be associated with the molecular events involved in leukemogenesis (Yunis et al, 1984; Sandberg, 1986). The subtypes defined by these primary karyotypic abnormalities may be useful for diagnostic classification (Linet, 1985; Sandler and Collman, 1987).

The Ph^1 chromosome was the first cytogenetic abnormality linked to the majority of cases with a disease entity, CML. Although the Ph^1 chromosome has been found in dividing marrow or peripheral-blood blasts of 85% of the approximately 1000 CML patients cytogenetically studied, factors responsible for the 9/22 translocation (found in 92% of CML cases with the Ph^1 chromosome) or other translocations are unknown (Chaganti, 1987). The key chromosome event in Ph^1-positive CML is the transposition of part of the oncogene *abl* from chromosome 9 to an abbreviated gene within the breakage cluster region (*bcr*) at band q11 on chromosome 22, leading to the creation of a new gene (*bcr/c-abl*) with abnormal messenger RNA and a resultant abnormal protein product. Although this chromosome translocation appears associated with an early step in leukemogenesis, clinical and cytogenetic data show that the presence of the Ph^1 chromosome alone is not sufficient for transformation of CML to the acute phase. It is noteworthy that chronic myeloid leukemia can be induced by *c-abl* variants in mice (Daley et al, 1990). Other oncogenes frequently implicated in the leukemias and other hematologic malignancies include *h-ras* and *c-myc*. Taylor et al (1992) found that ras mutation-positive AML was strongly associated with employment in any of 32 a priori occupations reported to be associated with increased risk of this leukemia type. Patients with ras-positive AML also had a significantly higher frequency of working 5 or more years in an a priori high-risk occupation than did population-based controls, and were more likely than control subjects to have had dermal exposure or to have breathed chemical vapors on the job.

Structural alterations of the p53 tumor suppressor gene are rare in patients in the chronic phase of CML, but when the disease starts to progress, acquisition of p53 abnormalities occurs concomitantly, with gross abnormalities or mutations of p53 observed in 40%–60% of cases in blast crisis (Cline and Ahuja, 1991). The genetic and environmental factors that mediate the acquisition of abnormalities of p53 and the transformation are unknown.

Follow-up studies of patients with certain preleukemic disorders have also shown increasing acquisition of genetic abnormalities that are hastened by treatment by myelosuppresive agents or onset of leukemia (Swolin et al, 1988). The specific mechanisms by which polycythemia vera, essential thrombocythemia, or myelodysplastic syndromes may transform to AML or CML have also not been determined (Swolin et al, 1988; Stoll et al, 1988).

Certain nonrandom chromosomal abnormalities have been linked with exposure to ionizing radiation (Tanaka et al, 1983; Stricker and Linder, 1983; Tanaka and Kamada, 1985; Rowley, 1985; Yokota et al, 1989; Ishihara et al, 1990); to benzene (Picciani, 1979; Tice et al, 1980; Infante and White, 1983); to solvents, insecticides, petroleum products, and related chemicals (Mitelman et al, 1981; Golomb et al, 1982; Fagioli et al, 1992; Cuneo et al, 1992; Ciccone et al, 1993); to employment in chemical laboratories and rotoprinting (Funes-Cravioto et al, 1977); and to treatment with alkylating agents (Rowley, 1985). Atomic bomb survivors with high exposure levels have shown a greater number of chromosome aberrations, and a diversity of complex changes (Tanaka and Kamada, 1985). Clinical series have described chromosomal abnormalities in AML patients occupationally exposed to mutagens (Mitelman et al, 1981; Golomb et al, 1982; Fourth International Workshop, 1984; Narod and Dube, 1989; Crane et al, 1989), and to cigarettes and alcohol (Crane et al, 1989) as well as the loss of all or part of chromosomes 5 and 7 following treatment with cytotoxic agents (Whang-Peng et al, 1988; Pedersen-Bjergaard and Philip, 1989; Narod and Dube, 1989). Geographic heterogeneity in frequency of nonrandom chromosome aberrations (Mitelman, 1986) may be influenced by selective reporting.

Elucidation of the relationships between primary nonrandom chromosomal abnormalities, basic molecular events, and risk factors is a major objective in understanding leukemia pathogenesis. Also to be determined is whether secondary karyotypic abnormalities are nonrandom and how these relate to molecular changes and leukemia risk factors. An important current issue is whether oncogenes near any of the breakpoints play a role in leukemogenesis (Bishop, 1988; Rowley, 1988; Cimino et al, 1993; Thirman et al, 1993; Chen et al, 1993; Ford et al, 1993).

HLA Associations

The HLA (human leukocyte antigen) system is the major histocompatibility complex in humans and consists of a large group of antigenic specificities. Studies in the mouse have shown a relationship between its transplantation antigen system and susceptibility to virus-induced leukemia. With the possible exception of some relationships with ALL, the generally weak and inconsistent associations between HLA and leukemia have not helped to clarify etiology.

ALL has been linked with A2 (Rogentine et al, 1973; Gluckman et al, 1976), 5a (Warren et al, 1977, 1981), Cw2 and Cw3 (D'Amaro et al, 1984), Cw7 (linked with adult ALL) (Muller et al, 1988), and inversely with A9 (Sanderson et al, 1973; Klouda et al, 1974). ALL cases with A9 have a longer first remission (Davey et al, 1974) and improved survival (Klouda et al, 1974; Cohen et al, 1977). A restricted heterogeneity has been found in parents of ALL cases (MacSween et al, 1980; van Fliedner et al, 1983), who are also more likely to share at least two common antigens than parents of controls (Werner-Favre and Jeannet, 1979). Four ALL cases in one family all shared the same haplotype (Kato et al, 1983). These data suggest a role for immunogenetic factors in etiology or progression of ALL.

Although some studies have linked A9 with CLL (Jeannet and Magnin, 1971; Pollak and DuBois, 1976), others have been unremarkable (Richter et al, 1973; Pollak and DuBois, 1976; Dyer et al, 1986; Linet et al, 1988c). In one report, HLA-B8 appeared to be a marker of mild disease, whereas A2 and the closely associated antigens B12(44) and DR7 were related to more severe disease (Dyer et al, 1986).

B17 has been weakly linked with AML (Heise et al, 1979; Jeannet and Magnin, 1971; Hester et al, 1977; Albert et al, 1977); remission is induced less often in patients with this antigen (Heise et al, 1979). AML cases are more likely to have B12 (Oliver et al, 1976), and patients with this antigen appear to experience improved survival (Oliver et al, 1976; Harris et al, 1978). No significant HLA associations have been observed for CML (Hester et al, 1977) or for ATLL (Tajima, 1988).

The lack of consistency of HLA associations may be partly due to the heterogeneity of leukemia subtypes and the presence of both short- and long-term survivors in most case groups studied; inadequate sample size; technical problems in defining HLA types particularly during relapse; and inappropriate methods used for statistical analysis.

PREVENTION

Despite extensive epidemiologic study, prospects for prevention of the leukemias are limited because etiologic factors are largely unknown. Clearly it would be prudent to limit the occupational, environmental, and medical exposures to radiation and chemicals that have been implicated in leukemia. In the use of cytotoxic agents as well as radiotherapy, physicians should clearly weight the leukemia risks against the benefits of particular treatment regimens. The number, dose, and duration of use of alkylating agents should be minimized to the extent feasible, particularly for older patients. Identification of efficacious drugs associated with lower toxicity should be high priorities. Although further research is required to confirm associations of leukemia with drugs other than cytotoxic agents, physicians should limit prescriptions of chloramphenicol in all forms (including ophthalmic preparations) unless no other options are available.

Most efforts to reduce benzene-related exposures have been directed at the workplace. However, if cigarette smoking, and residence- and automobile-related exposures are confirmed as important sources, public health measures should include vigorous pursuit of smoking cessation, installation of devices for minimizing exposure to gasoline at service stations, and reduction of the percent of benzene in gasoline, paints, solvents, and other sources. Clarification of possible leukemogenic factors in the rubber, styrene, butadiene, and petrochemical industries, and among farmers, pressmen, printers, painters, and those exposed to ethylene oxide is also necessary.

The detection of a retrovirus as a cause of adult T-cell leukemia has expanded opportunities for prevention. Transmission of HTLV-I from mother to child via breast-feeding can be avoided, and screening of blood products is now standard practice. It will be more difficult to halt spread through sexual activity and drug abuse, but such efforts are clearly needed.

FUTURE DIRECTIONS

Because of the rarity of the leukemias and the biologic and epidemiologic evidence that each of the major categories is composed of distinct subtypes, many of the etiologic leads described in this review should be pursued in large case-control studies in conjunction with detailed morphologic, immunophenotypic, cytogenetic, and oncogene characterization. Nested case-control studies within occupational cohorts may be particularly useful for evaluating the role of specific exposures to cytogenetic or oncogene-activated subtypes of leukemia. Examination of unifying hypotheses that apply to particular subtypes may be the best approach to minimize the problem of multiple comparisons.

To evaluate the leukemogenic risk of suspected occupational, environmental, or medical exposures, large populations with valid dosimetry or exposure information should be sought and the role of host factors and interactions carefully examined. Similar approaches should be used to clarify the mechanisms of action of known leukemogens.

Further studies of benzene-exposed groups are needed to evaluate the risks of leukemia types exclusive of AML and to determine whether other hematolymphoproliferative tumors occur excessively. Registries could be established for key industries (petrochemical, rubber manufacturing, farming) to enable complete ascertainment and evaluation of hematologic neoplasms and related disorders, as well as more detailed assessment of benzene exposures and other risk factors.

Familial aggregation of leukemias, other hematologic malignancies, autoimmune conditions, and immunologic abnormalities suggests the need for detailed genetic studies along with evaluation of environmental exposures. International registries of various congenital disorders, particularly those accompanied by chromosomal breaks or immunodeficiency, should be encouraged to generate sufficient numbers of cases to pursue detailed epidemiologic investigations in conjunction with state-of-the-art karyotypic and molecular genetic studies.

Finally, the discovery of a retrovirus as a cause of one form of leukemia suggests that other leukemogenic viruses remain to be identified. Recent interest has centered on the human herpesvirus-6 (HHV-6) as a possible risk factor for leukemia and lymphoma (Clark et al, 1990). Further research on the role of HTLV-I and HTLV-II in populations at high risk of ATLL, and the identification of cofactors, may prove useful as a model for more fully elucidating the causes of leukemia, and the means of prevention.

REFERENCES

ABRAHAMSON S. 1990. Childhood leukemia at Sellafield. Radiat Res 123:237–238.

ACQUAVELLA JF, WIGGS LD, WAXWEILER RJ, et al. 1985. Mortality among workers at the Pantex weapons facility. Health Physics 48:735–746.

ADAMSON RH, SIEBER SM. 1981. Chemically induced leukemia in humans. Environ Health Perspect 39:93–103.

ADELSTEIN A, WHITE G. 1976. Leukaemia 1911–1973: Cohort analysis. Population Trends 3:9–13.

AHLBOM A. 1988. A review of the epidemiologic literature on magnetic fields and cancer. Scand J Work Environ Health 14:337–343.

AKSOY M. 1988. Benzene hematotoxicity. *In* Aksoy M (ed): Benzene Carcinogenicity. Boca Raton: CRC Press, pp. 59–112.

AKSOY M, ERDEM S. 1978. A follow-up study on the mortality and the development of leukemia in pancytopenic patients associated with long-term exposure to benzene. Blood 44:285–292.

AKSOY M, ERDEM S, DINCOL G. 1974. Leukemia in shoe workers exposed chronically to benzene. Blood 44:837–841.

ALAVANJA MCR, BLAIR A, MASTERS MN. 1990. Cancer mortality in the flour industry. J Natl Cancer Inst 82:840–848.

ALAVANJA MCR, BLAIR A, MERKLE S, et al. 1988. Mortality among agricultural extension agents. Am J Ind Med 14:167–176.

ALAVANJA MCR, RUSH GA, STEWART P, et al. 1987. Proportionate mortality study of workers in the grain industry. J Natl Cancer Inst 78:247–252.

ALBERT ED, NISPEROS B, THOMAS ED. 1977. HLA antigens and haplotypes in acute leukemia. Leuk Res 1:261–269.

ALBERT RE, OMRAM AR. 1968. Follow-up study of patients treated by x-ray epilation for tinea capitis. Arch Environ Health 17:899–918.

ALEXANDER FE, CARTWRIGHT RA, MCKINNEY PA. 1992. Paternal occupation of children with leukaemia. Br Med J 305:715–716.

ALEXANDER FE, MCKINNEY PA, MONCRIEFF KC, et al. 1992. Residential proximity of children with leukaemia and non-Hodgkin's lymphoma in three areas in Northern England. Br J Cancer 65:583–588.

ALEXANDER F, RICKETTS TJ, MCKINNEY PA, et al. 1989. Cancer registration of leukaemias and lymphomas: Results of a comparison with a specialist registry. Community Med 11:81–89.

ALEXANDER FE, MCKINNEY PA, CARTWRIGHT RA. 1990a. Radon and leukaemia. Lancet 335:1336–1337.

ALEXANDER FE, RICKETTS TJ, MCKINNEY PA, et al. 1990b. Community lifestyle characteristics and risk of acute lymphoblastic leukaemia in children. Lancet 336:1461–1465.

AL-JADER LN, WEST RR, GOODCHILD MC, et al. 1989. Mortality from leukaemia among relatives of patients with cystic fibrosis. Br Med J 298:164.

AL-JADER LN, WEST RR, HOLMES JA, et al. 1990. Leukaemia mortality among relatives of cystic fibrosis patients. Arch Dis Child 65:317–319.

AMES BN, KAMMEN H, YAMASAKI E. 1975. Hair dyes are mutagenic: identification of a variety of mutagenic ingredients. Proc Natl Acad Sci USA 72:2423–2427.

ANDERSEN E, VIDEBACK AA. 1970. Stem cell leukemia in myelomatosis. Scand J Haematol 7:201–207.

ANDERSON RC. 1951. Familial leukemia. A report of leukemia in five siblings with a brief review of the genetic aspects of the disease. Am J Dis Child 81:313–322.

ANDERSON RC, HERMANN HW. 1955. Leukemia in twin children. JAMA 158:652–654.

ANDERSSON M, CARSTENSON B, VISFELDT J. 1993. Leukemia and other related hematological disorders among Danish patients exposed to Thorotrast. Radiat Res 134:224–233.

ANDERSSON M, PHILIP P, PEDERSEN-BJERGAARD J. 1990. High risk of therapy-related leukemia and preleukemia after therapy with prednimustine, methotrexate, 5-fluorouracil, mitoxantrone, and tamoxifen for advanced breast cancer. Cancer 65:2460–2464.

ANDERSSON M, STORM HH. 1992. Cancer incidence among Danish Thoratrast exposed patients. J Natl Cancer Inst 84:1318–1325.

ANDERSSON M, STORM HH, MOURIDSEN HT. 1991. Incidence of new primary cancers after adjuvant Tamoxifen therapy and radiotherapy for early breast cancer. J Natl Cancer Inst 83:1013–1017.

ANDRIEU J-M, IFRAH N, PAYEN C, et al. 1990. Increased risk of secondary acute nonlymphocytic leukemia after extended-field radiation therapy combined with MOPP chemotherapy for Hodgkin's disease. J Clin Oncol 8:1148–1154.

AOKI K, KURIHARA M, HAYAKAWA N, SUSUKI S. 1992. Death rates for malignant neoplasms for selected sites by sex and five-year age group in 33 countries 1953–57 to 1983–87. Nagoya, University of Nagoya Press, pp. 503–536.

ARCHER VE. 1987. Association of nuclear fallout with leukemia in the United States. Arch Environ Health 42:263–271.

ARCHER VE, GILLIAN JD, WAGNER JK. 1976. Respiratory disease mortality among uranium miners. Ann NY Acad Sci 271:280–293.

ARCHIMBAUD E, CHASSIN C, GYOTAT, et al. 1988. Acute leukaemia with t(4;11) in patients previously exposed to carcinogens. Br J Haematol 69:467–470.

ARP EW, WOLFE PH, CHECKOWAY H. 1983. Lymphocytic leukemia and exposures to benzene and other solvents in the rubber industry. J Occup Med 25:598–602.

ARSENAU JC, SPONZO RW, LEVIN DL, et al. 1972. Non-lymphomatous malignant tumors complicating Hodgkin's disease. N Engl J Med 287:1119–1122.

AUBERTIN CH, GRELLETY BOSVIEL P. 1923. Contribution a l'etude de la leucemie aigue. Arch Mal Coeur 16:696–713.

AUSTIN H, COLE P. 1986. Cigarette smoking and leukemia. J Chronic Dis 39:417–421.

AUSTIN H, COLE P, MCCRAW DS. 1986. A case-control study of leukemia at an oil refinery. J Occup Med 28:1169–1173.

AUSTIN H, DELZELL E, COLE P. 1988. Benzene and leukemia. A review of the literature and a risk assessment. Am J Epidemiol 127:419–439.

AUVINEN A, HAKAMA M, ARVELA H, et al. 1994. Fallout from Chernobyl and incidence of childhood leukemia in Finland, 1976–92. Br Med J 309:151–154.

AXELSON O, SUNDELL L, ANDERSSON K, et al. 1980. Herbicide exposure and tumor mortality: An updated epidemiologic investigation on Swedish railroad workers. Scand J Work Environ Health 6:73–79.

AYMARD JP, LEDERLIN P, WITZ F, et al. 1983. Acute leukemia following prolonged chlorambucil treatment for non-neoplastic disease: A study of two cases and literature review. Clin Belg 38:228–234.

BADER JL, MILLER RW. 1978. Neurofibromatosis and childhood leukemia. J Pediatr 92:925–929.

BAIJAL E, ROWORTH M, WALKER D, et al. 1989. An investigation of apparent leukaemia clusters in Fife by validation of cancer register data and a case-control study. Public Health 103:91–97.

BAJORIN DF, MOTZER RJ, RODRIGUEZ E, et al. 1993. Acute nonlymphocytic leukemia in germ cell tumor patients treated with Etoposide-containing chemotherapy. J Natl Cancer Inst 85:60–62.

BALTUS JAM, BOERSMO JW, HARTMAN AP, et al. 1983. The occurrence of malignancies in patients with rheumatoid arthritis treated with cyclophosphamide. Ann Rheum Dis 42:268–273.

BARTHOLOMEW C, SAXINGER WC, CLARK JW, et al. 1987. Transmission of HTLV-I and HIV among homosexual men in Trinidad. JAMA 257:2604–2608.

BARTON DE, DAVID FN, MERRINGTON M. 1965. A criterion for testing contagion in time and space. Ann Hum Genet (London) 29:97–102.

BAVERSTOCK KF. 1991. DNA instability, paternal irradiation, and leukaemia in children around Sellafield. Int J Radiat Biol 60:581–595.

BAVERSTOCK KF, PAPWORTH DG. 1986. The UK radium luminiser survey. *In* Gossner W, Gerber GB (eds): The Radiobiology of Radium Thorotrast. Munich, Urban, pp. 22–28.

BECK HL, KREY PW. 1983. Radiation exposures in Utah from Nevada nuclear tests. Science 20:18–24.

BENDER AP, ROBISON LL, KASHMIRI SVS, et al. 1988. No involvement of bovine leukemia virus in childhood acute lymphoblastic leukemia and non-Hodgkin's lymphoma. Cancer Res 48:2919–2922.

BENDER AP, PARKER DL, JOHNSON RA, et al. 1989. Minnesota highway maintenance worker study: Cancer mortality. Am J Ind Med 15:545–556.

BENNETT JM, CATOVSKY D, DANIEL M-T, et al. 1976. Proposals for the classification of the acute leukemias. Br J Hematol 33:451–458.

BENNETT JM, CATOVSKY D, DANIEL MT, et al. 1985a. Criteria for the diagnosis of acute leukemia of megakaryocytic lineage (M7): A report of the French-American-British Cooperative Group. Ann Intern Med 103:460–462.

BENNETT JM, CATOVSKY D, DANIEL MT, et al. 1985b. Proposed revised criteria for the classification of acute myeloid leukemia. Ann Intern Med 103:626–629.

BENNETT JM, CATOVSKY D, DANIEL M-T, et al. 1989. Proposals for the classification of chronic (mature) B and T lymphocytic leukaemias. J Clin Pathol 42:567–584.

BENNETT JM, CATOVSKY D, DANIEL M-T, et al. 1991. Proposal for the recognition of minimally differentiated acute myeloid leukemia (AML-M0). Br J Haemotol 78:325–329.

BENNETT JM, JULIUSSON G, MECUCCI C. 1990. Morphologic, immunologic, and cytogenetic classification of the chronic (mature) B and T lymphoid leukemias: Fourth Meeting of the MIC Cooperative Study Group. Cancer Res 50:2212.

BENSON LO, TETA MJ. 1993. Mortality due to pancreatic and lymphopoietic cancers in chlorhydrin production workers. Br J Ind Med 50:710–716.

BERAL V. 1987. Cancer near nuclear installations. Lancet 1:556.

BERAL V, FRASER P, CARPENTER L, et al. 1988. Mortality of employees at the Atomic Weapons Establishment 1951–1982. Br Med J 297:757–770.

BERAL V, INSKIP H, FRASER P, et al. 1985. Mortality of employees of the United Kingdom Atomic Energy Authority, 1946–1979. Br Med J 291:440–447.

BERK PD, GOLDBERG JD, SILVERSTEIN MN, et al. 1981. Increased incidence of acute leukemia in polycythemia vera associated with chlorambucil therapy. N Engl J Med 304:441–447.

BERKHEISER SW. 1986. Review of leukemia, lymphoma, and myeloma before and after the TMI accident. Pa Med 89:50–52.

BERNARD SM, CARWRIGHT RA, DARWIN CM, et al. 1987. A possible epidemiological association between multiple sclerosis and leukaemia/lymphoma. Br J Haematol 65:122–123.

BERTAZZI PA, ZOCCHETTI C, PESATORI AC, et al. 1989. Ten-year mortality study of the population involved in the Seveso incident in 1976. Am J Epidemiol 129:1187–1200.

BESSHO F. 1989. Acute non-lymphocytic leukemia is not a major type of childhood leukemia in Japan. Eur J Cancer Clin Oncol 25:729–732.

BETHWAITE PB, PEARCE N, FRASER J. 1990. Cancer risks in painters: Study based on the New Zealand Cancer Registry. Br J Ind Med 47:742–746.

BHARGAVA M, KUMAN R, KARAK A. 1988. Immunological subtypes of acute lymphoblastic leukemia in North India. Leuk Res 12:673–678.

BIGGAR RJ, SAXINGER C, GARINER C, et al. 1984. Type-I HTLV antibody in urban and rural Ghana, West Africa. Int J Cancer 34:215–219.

BIRCH JM, MARSDEN HB, MORRIS JONES PH, et al. 1988. Improvements in survival from childhood cancer: Results of a population-based survey over 30 years. Br Med J 296:1372–1376.

BISANTI L, MAGGINI M, RASCHETTI R, et al. 1993. Cancer mortality in ethylene oxide workers. Br J Ind Med 50:317–324.

BISHOP JM. 1988. The molecular genetics of cancer. Science 235:305–311.

BITHELL J, STEWART A. 1975. Prenatal irradiation and childhood malignancy: A review of British data from the Oxford survey. Br J Cancer 31:271–287.

BITHELL JF, DUTTON SJ, DRAPER GJ, et al. 1994. Distribution of childhood leukaemias and non-Hodgkin's lymphomas near nuclear installations in England and Wales. Br Med J 309:501–505.

BITHELL JF, STONE RA. 1989. On statistical methods for analyzing the geographical distribution of cancer cases near nuclear installations. J Epidemiol Community Health 43:79–85.

BJERRUM OW, HASSELBALCH HC, DRIVESHOLM A, et al. 1986. Non-Hodgkin malignant lymphomas and Hodgkin's disease in first-degree relatives. Scand J Haematol 36:398–401.

BLACK D. 1984. Investigation of the Possible Increased Incidence of Cancer in West Cumbria. London, HMSO.

BLACKBURN ER, CALLENDAR ST, DACIE JV, et al. 1968. Possible association between pernicious anemia and leukaemia: A prospective study of 1,625 patients with a note on the very high incidence of stomach cancer. Int J Cancer 3:163–170.

BLACKWELDER WC, YANO K, RHOADS GG, et al. 1980. Alcohol and mortality: The Honolulu Heart Study. Am J Med 68:164–169.

BLAIR A, DECOUFLE P, GRAUMAN DJ. 1979. Causes of death among laundry and dry cleaning workers. Am J Public Health 69:508–511.

BLAIR A, FRAUMENI JF JR, MASON TJ. 1980. Geographic patterns of leukemia in the United States. J Chronic Dis 33:251–260.

BLAIR A, HAYES HM JR. 1980. Cancer and other causes of death among U.S. veterinarians. Int J Cancer 25:181–185.

BLAIR A, HAYES HM JR. 1982. Mortality patterns among United States veterinarians 1947–1977: An expanded study. Int J Epidemiol 2:391–397.

BLAIR A, WHITE DW. 1981. Death certificate study of leukemia among farmers from Wisconsin. J Natl Cancer Inst 66:1027–1030.

BLAIR A, WHITE D. 1985a. Leukemia cell types and agricultural practices in Nebraska. Arch Environ Health 40:211–214.

BLAIR A, MALKER H, CANTOR KP, et al. 1985b. Cancer among farmers. A review. Scand J Work Environ Health 11:397–407.

BLAIR A, ZAHM SH. 1991. Cancer among farmers. Occup Med 6:335–354.

BLAIR A, ZAHM SH. 1995. Agricultural exposures and cancer. Environ Health Perspect 103(Suppl 8):205–208.

BLATTNER WA. 1989. Retroviruses. *In* Evans AS (ed): Viral Infections in Humans, 3rd ed. New York, Plenum Medical Book Co., pp. 545–592.

BLATTNER WA, DEAN JH, FRAUMENI JF JR. 1979. Familial lymphoproliferative malignancy: Clinical and laboratory follow-up. Ann Intern Med 90:943–947.

BLATTNER WA, GIBBS WN, SAXINGER WC, et al. 1983. Human T-cell leukemia/lymphoma virus-associated lymphoreticular neoplasia in Jamaica. Lancet 2:61–64.

BLATTNER WA, NOMURA A, CLARK JW, et al. 1986. Modes of transmission and evidence for viral latency from studies of HTLV-I in Japanese migrant populations in Hawaii. Proc Natl Acad Sci USA 83:4895–4898.

BLATTNER WA, STROBER W, MUCHMORE AV, et al. 1976. Familial chronic lymphocytic leukemia. Ann Intern Med 84:554–557.

BLAYNEY DW, BLATTNER WA, ROBERT-GUROFF M, et al. 1983. The human T cell leukemia-lymphoma virus (HTLV) in the Southeastern United States. JAMA 250:1048–1052.

BLAYNEY DW, LONGO DL, YOUNG RC, et al. 1987. Decreasing risk of leukemia with prolonged follow-up after chemotherapy and radiotherapy for Hodgkin's disease. N Engl J Med 316:710–714.

BLOOM GE, WARNER S, GERLAND PS, et al. 1966. Chromosome abnormalities in constitutional aplastic anemia. N Engl J Med 274:8–14.

BOFFETTA P, STELLMAN S, GARFINKEL L. 1988. Diesel exhaust exposure and mortality among males in the American Cancer Society prospective study. Am J Ind Med 14:403–415.

BOICE JD JR, BLETTNER M, KLEINERMAN RA, et al. 1987. Radiation dose and leukemia risk in patients treated for cancer of the cervix. J Natl Cancer Inst 79:1295–1311.

BOICE JD JR, DAY NE, ANDERSEN A, et al. 1985. Second cancers following radiation treatment for cervical cancer. An international collaboration among cancer registries. J Natl Cancer Inst 74:955–975.

BOICE JD JR, ENGHOLM G, KLEINERMAN RA, et al. 1988. Radiation dose and second cancer risk in patients treated for cancer of the cervix. Radiat Res 116:3–55.

BOICE JD JR, GREEN MH, KILLEN JY, et al. 1983. Leukemia and

preleukemia after adjuvant treatment of gastrointestinal cancer with semustine (methyl-CCNU). N Engl J Med 309:1079–1084.

BOICE JD JR, LINET MS. 1994. Chernobyl, childhood cancer, and chromosome 21. Br Med J 309:139–140.

BOICE JD JR, MONSON RR, ROSENSTEIN M, et al. 1981. Cancer mortality in women after repeated fluoroscopic examinations of the chest. J Natl Cancer Inst 66:863–867.

BOICE JD JR, MORIN MM, GLASS AG, et al. 1991. Diagnostic x-rays and risk of leukemia, lymphoma, and multiple myeloma. JAMA 265:1290–1294.

BOIVIN JA, HUTCHINSON GB, LYDEN M, et al. 1984. Second primary cancers following treatment of Hodgkins disease. J Natl Cancer Inst 72:233–241.

BOIVIN JF, HUTCHINSON GB, EVANS FB, et al. 1986. Leukemia after radiotherapy for first primary cancers of various anatomic sites. Am J Epidemiol 123:993–1003.

BOND GG, MCLAREN EA, BALDWIN CL, et al. 1986. An update of mortality among chemical workers exposed to benzene. Br J Ind Med 43:685–691.

BOURGUET CC, GRUFFERMAN S, DELZELL E, et al. 1985. Multiple myeloma and family history of cancer. Cancer 56:2133–2139.

BOWIE C. 1987. The validity of a cancer register in leukemia epidemiology. Community Med 9:152–159.

BOWMAN JD, GARABRANT DH, SOBEL E, et al. 1988. Exposures to extremely low frequency (ELF) electromagnetic fields in occupations with elevated leukemia rates. Appl Ind Hyg 3:189–194.

BRANDT L, NILSSON PG, MITELMAN F. 1979. Trends in incidence of acute leukemia. Lancet 2:1069–1071.

BRINCKER H, HANSEN HS, ANDERSEN AP. 1973. Induction of leukaemia by ^{131}I treatment of thyroid carcinoma. Br J Cancer 23:232–237.

BRIGGS NC, BATTJES RJ, CANTOR KP, ET AL. 1995. Sero-prevalance of human T cell lymphotropic virus type II infection with or without human immunodeficiency virus type I coinfection among U.S. intravenous drug users. J Infec Dis 172:51–58.

BRINTON LA, GRIDLEY G, HRUBEC Z, et al. 1989. Cancer risk following pernicious anemia. Br J Cancer 59:810–813.

BRITO-BABAPULLE V, PITTMAN S, MELO JV, et al. 1987. Cytogenetic studies on prolymphocytic leukemia. I. B-cell prolymphocytic leukemia. Hematol Pathol 1:27–33.

BROSS IDJ, GIBSON R. 1980. Cats and childhood leukemia. J Med 1:180–187.

BROSS IDJ, BEITELL R, GIBSON R. 1972. Pets and adult leukemia. Am J Public Health 62:1520–1531.

BROWN DP, KAPLAN SD. 1987. Retrospective cohort mortality study of dry cleaning workers using perchlorethylene. J Occup Med 29:535–541.

BROWN LM, BLAIR A, GIBSON R, et al. 1990. Pesticide exposures and other agricultural risk factors for leukemia among men in Iowa and Minnesota. Cancer Res 50:6585–6591.

BROWN LM, GIBSON R, BLAIR A, et al. 1992a. Smoking and risk of leukemia. Am J Epidemiol 135:763–768.

BROWN LM, GIBSON R, BURMEISTER LF, et al. 1992b. Alcohol consumption and risk of leukemia, non-Hodgkin's lymphoma, and multiple myeloma. Leuk Res 16:979–984.

BROWN PDN, HERTZ H, OLSEN JH, et al. 1989. Incidence of childhood cancer in Denmark 1943–1984. Int J Epidemiol 18:546–555.

BROWNSON RC. 1989. Cigarette smoking and risk of leukemia. J Clin Epidemiol 42:1025–1026.

BROWNSON RC, NOVOTNY TE, PERRY MC. 1993. Cigarette smoking and adult leukemia. A meta-analysis. Arch Intern Med 153:469–475.

BRUSAMOLINO E, PAGNUCCO G, BERNASCONI C. 1986. Acute leukemia occurring in a primary neoplasia (secondary leukemia). A review in biological, epidemiological and clinical aspects. Haematologica 71:60–83.

BUCHANAN CR, PREECE MA, MILNER RDG. 1991. Mortality, neoplasia, and Creutzfeldt-Jakob disease in patients treated with known pituitary growth hormone in the United Kingdom. Br Med J 302:824–828.

BUCKLEY JD, ROBISON LL, SWOTINSKY R, et al. 1989. Occupational exposures of parents of children with acute nonlymphocytic leukemia. A report from the Children's Cancer Study Group. Cancer Res 49:4030–4037.

BURBANK F. 1971. Patterns in Cancer Mortality in the United States: 1950–67. Natl Cancer Inst Monogr 33. Washington, D.C., U.S. Government Printing Office.

BURKHARDT JA. 1982. Leukemia in hospital patients with occupational exposure to the sawmill industry. West J Med 137:440–441.

BURKHARDT R, BARTL R, JAGER K, et al. 1984. Chronic myeloproliferative disorders (CMPD). Pathol Res Pract 179:131–186.

BURMEISTER LF, VAN LIER SF, ISACSON P. 1982. Leukemia and farm practices in Iowa. Am J Epidemiol 115:720–728.

BURNEY A, CLENTER Y, KETTMANN R, et al. 1987. Bovine leukaemia: Facts and hypothesis derived from the study of an infectious cancer. Cancer Surv 6:139–159.

BUTTURINI A, GALE RP. 1989. Age of onset and type of leukaemia Lancet 2:789–791.

BUXTON BA, SCHULTZ RD, COLLINS WE. 1982. Role of insects in the transmission of bovine leukosis virus. Am J Vet Res 43:1458–1459.

BYERS VS, LEVIN AS, OZONOFF DM, et al. 1988. Association between clinical symptoms and lymphocytic abnormalities in a population with chronic domestic exposure to industrial solvent-contaminated domestic water supply and a high incidence of leukaemia. Cancer Immunol Immunother 27:77–81.

CALDWELL GG, KELLEY D, HEATH CW JR, et al. 1983. Mortality and cancer frequency among military nuclear test (Smoky) participants 1957 through 1979. JAMA 250:620–624.

CANTOR KP, BLAIR A, EVERETT G, et al. 1988. Hair dye use and risk of leukemia and lymphoma. Am J Public Health 78:570–571.

CARDIS E, GILBERT ES, CARPENTER L, ET AL. 1995. Effects of low doses and low dose rates of external ionizing radiation: Cancer mortality among nuclear industry workers in three countries. Radiat Res 142:117–132.

CAREY R, MCGINNIS A, JACOBSON B, et al. 1976. Idiopathic thrombocytopenic purpura complicating chronic lymphocytic leukemia. Ann Intern Med 136:62–66.

CARSTENSEN JM, BYGREN LO, HATSCHEK T. 1990. Cancer incidence among Swedish brewery workers. Int J Cancer 45:393–396.

CARTWRIGHT RA. 1989. Low frequency alternating electromagnetic fields and leukemia: The saga so far. Br J Cancer 60:649–651.

CARTWRIGHT RA, ALEXANDER FE, MCKINNEY PA, et al. 1990. Leukaemia and Lymphoma. An Atlas of Distribution Within Areas of England and Wales 1984–88. London, Leukaemia Research Fund.

CARTWRIGHT RA, BERNARD SM. 1985. Epidemiology. *In* Whittaker JA, Delamore IW (eds): Leukaemia. Oxford, Blackwell Scientific Publications, pp. 3–23.

CARTWRIGHT RA, DARWIN C, MCKINNEY PA, et al. 1988. Acute myeloid leukemia in adults: Control study in Yorkshire. Leukemia 2:687–690.

CARTWRIGHT RA, MILLER JG, SCARISBRICK DA. 1987a. Leukaemia in a carpet factory: An epidemiological investigation. J Soc Occup Med 37:42–43.

CARTWRIGHT RA, BERNARD SM, BIRD CC, et al. 1987b. Chronic lymphocytic leukemia: Case-control epidemiological study in Yorkshire. Br J Cancer 56:79–82.

CARTWRIGHT RA, STAINES A. 1992. Acute leukemias. *In* Fleming AF (ed): Epidemiology of Haematological Disease. Part I. London, Bailliere Tindal, pp. 1–26.

CASELITZ J, KLOPPEL G, DELLING G, et al. 1979. Schwachman's syndrome and leukaemia. Virchows Arch [A] 385:109–116.

CATOVSKY D, FOOKS J, RICHARDS S. 1988. The UK Medical Research Council CLL trials 1 and 2. Nouv Rev Fr Hematol 30:423–427.

CATOVSKY D, MATUTES E, BUCCHERI V, et al. 1991. A classification of acute leukaemia for the 1990s. Ann Hematol 62:16–21.

CERVENKA J, ANDERSON RS, NESBIT ME, et al. 1977. Familial leukemia and inherited chromosomal aberration. Int J Cancer 19:783–788.

CHADBURN A, ATHAN E, WIECZOREK R, et al. 1991. Detection and characterization of human T-cell lymphotropic virus type I (HTLV-I) associated T-cell neoplasms in an HTLV-I nonendemic region by polymerase chain reaction. Blood 77:2419–2430.

CHAGANTI RSK. 1987. Cytogenetics of leukemia and lymphoma. Monogr Pathol 29:184–203.

CHAGANTI RSK, MILLER DR, MEYERS PA, et al. 1979. Cytogenetic evidence of the intrauterine origin of acute leukemia in monozygotic twins. N Engl J Med 300:1032–1034.

CHAK LY, SIKIC BI, TUCKER MA. 1984. Increased incidence of acute nonlymphocytic leukemia following therapy in patients with small cell carcinoma of the lung. J Clin Oncol 2:385–390.

CHANDRA RK. 1972. Serum immunoglobulin levels in children with acute lymphoblastic leukemia and their mothers and sibs. Arch Dis Child 47:618–620.

CHECKOWAY H, WILCOSKY T, WOLF P, TYROLER H. 1984. An evaluation of the associations of leukemia and rubber industry solvent exposures. Am J Ind Med 5:239–249.

CHECKOWAY H, MATTHEW RM, SHY CM, et al. 1985. Radiation, work experience, and cause-specific mortality among workers at an energy research laboratory. Br J Ind Med 42:525–533.

CHEN CS, SORENSEN PH, DOMER PH, et al. 1993. Molecular reaarangements on chromosome 11q23 predominate in infant acute lymphoblastic leukemia and are associated with specific biologic variables and poor outcome. Blood 81:2386–2393.

CHEN R, MANTEL N, et al. 1984. A study of 3 techniques for time-space clustering in Hodgkin's Disease. Stat Med 3:173–184.

CHEN S-J, CHEN Z, DERRE J, et al. 1989. Are most secondary acute lymphoblastic leukemias mixed acute leukemias? Nouv Rev Fr Hematol 31:17–22.

CHESON BD, CASSILETH PA, HEAD DR, et al. 1990. Report of the National Cancer Institute-Sponsored Workshop on definitions of diagnosis and response in acute myeloid leukemia. J Clin Oncol 8:813–819.

CHRISTIE D, ROBINSON K, GORDON I, et al. 1991. A prospective study in the Australian petroleum industry. II. Incidence of Cancer. Br J Ind Med 48:511–514.

CICCONE G, MIRABELLI D, LEVIS A, et al. 1993. Myeloid leukemias and myelodysplastic syndromes: Chemical exposure, histologic subtype and cytogenetics in a case-control study. Cancer Genet Cytogenet 68:135–139.

CIMINO G, LO COCCO F, BIONDI A, et al. 1993. ALL-1 gene at chromosome 11q23 is consistently altered in acute leukemia of early infancy. Blood 82:544–546.

CIMINO G, PAPA G, TURA S, et al. 1991. Second primary cancer following Hodgkin's disease: Updated results of an Italian multicentric study. J Clin Oncol 9:432–437.

CLARK DA, ALEXANDER FE, MCKINNEY PA, et al. 1990. The seroepidemiology of human herpesvirus-6 (HHV-6) from a case-control study of leukaemia and lymphoma. Int J Cancer 45:829–833.

CLARK JW, ROBERT-GUROFF M, IKEHARA M, et al. 1985a. The human T-cell leukemia/lymphoma virus type-I (HTLV-I) in Okinawa. Cancer Res 45:2849–2852.

CLARK J, SAXINGER C, GIBBS WN, et al. 1985b. Seroepidemiologic studies of human T-cell leukemia/lymphoma virus type-I in Jamaica. Int J Cancer 36:37–41.

CLARK RD, HUTTER JJ JR. 1982. Familial neurofibromatosis and juvenile chronic myelogenous leukemia. Hum Genet 60:230–232.

CLAYTON D, KALDOR J. 1987. Empirical Bayes estimates of age-standardized relative risks for use in disease mapping. Biometrics 43:671–681.

CLEGHORN FR, MANNS A, FALK R, et al. Effect of human T-lymphotropic virus type I infection in non-Hodgkin's lymphoma incidence. J Natl Cancer Inst 87:1009–1014.

CLINE MJ, AHUJA H. 1991. Oncogenes and anti-concogenes in the evaluation of human leukemia/lymphoma. Leuk Lymph 4:153–158.

CNATTINGIUS S, ZACK MM, EKBOM A, et al. 1995a. Prenatal and neonatal risk factors for childhood lymphatic leukemia. J Natl Cancer Inst 87:908–914.

CNATTINGIUS S, ZACK M, EKBOM A, et al. 1995b. Prenatal and neonatal risk factors for childhood myeloid leukemia. Cancer Epidemiol Biomark Prev 4:441–445.

COEBERGH JWW, VAN DER DOES-VANDEN BERG A, VAN WERING ER, et al. 1989. Childhood leukemia in The Netherlands, 1973–1986: Temporary variation in the incidence of acute lymphocytic leukaemia in young children. Br J Cancer 59:100–105.

COGGON D, PANNETT B, WINTER PD, et al. 1986. Mortality of workers exposed to 2-methyl-4-chlorophenoxyacetic acid. Scand J Work Environ Health 12:448–454.

COHEN BL. 1993. Relationship between exposure to radon and various types of cancer. Health Physics 65:529–531.

COHEN E, SINGAL DP, KHURANA U, et al. 1977. HLA-A9 and survival in acute lymphocytic leukemia and myelocytic leukemia. *In* Murphy GP, Cohen E, Fitzpatrick JE, Pressman D (eds): HLA and Malignancy. Progress in Clinical and Biological Research, Vol 16. New York, Alan Liss, pp. 65–70.

COLE P, DELZELL E, ACQUAVELLA J. 1993. Exposure to butadiene and lymphatic and hematopoietic cancer. Epidemiology 4:96–103.

COLEMAN MC, BELL J, SKEET R, et al. 1983. Leukaemia incidence in electrical workers in England and Wales. Lancet 1:246.

COLEMAN MP, BELL CMJ, TAYLOR H-L, et al. 1989. Leukaemia and residence near electricity transmission equipment: A case-control study. Br J Cancer 60:793–798.

COLEMAN M, BERAL V. 1988. A review of epidemiological studies of the health effects of living near or working with electricity generation and transmission equipment. Int J Epidemiol 17:1–13.

COLEMAN MP, ESTEVE J, DAMIECKI P, et al. 1993. Trends in Cancer Incidence and Mortality. Lyon, France: IARC Scientific Publications No. 121, pp. 737–768.

COLLMAN GW, LOOMIS DP, SANDLER DP. 1991. Childhood cancer mortality and radon concentration in drinking water in North Carolina. Br J Cancer 63:626–629.

COLTMAN CA, DIXON DO. 1982. Second malignancies complicating Hodgkin's disease: A Southwest Oncology Group 10-year follow-up. Cancer Treat Rep 66:1023–1033.

COMMITTEE ON MEDICAL ASPECTS OF RADIATION IN THE ENVIRONMENT. 1988. Second Report. Report on the incidence of childhood cancer in the West Berkshire and North Hampshire area. London, HMSO.

COMMITTEE ON MEDICAL ASPECTS OF RADIATION IN THE ENVIRONMENT. 1989. Third Report. Report on the incidence of childhood cancer in the West Berkshire and North Hampshire area. London, HMSO.

COMSTOCK GW, MARTINEZ I, LIVESAY VT. 1975. Efficacy of BCG vaccination in prevention of cancer. J Natl Cancer Inst 54:835–839.

CONLEY CL, MISITI J, LASTER AJ, et al. 1980. Genetic factors predisposing to CLL and to autoimmune disease. Medicine 59:323–331.

COOK RR, TOWNSEND JC, OTT MG, et al. 1980. Mortality experience of employees exposed to 2,3,7,8-tetrachlorodibenzo-p-dioxin (TCDD). J Occup Med 22:530–532.

COOK-MOZAFFARI PJ, ASHWOOD FL, VINCENT T, et al. 1987. Cancer Incidence and Mortality in the Vicinity of Nuclear Installations, England and Wales 1959–1980. Studies on Medical and Population Subjects, No. 51. London, HMSO.

COOK-MOZAFFARI PJ, DARBY SC, DOLL R, et al. 1989a. Geographical variation in mortality from leukaemia and other cancers in England and Wales in relation to proximity to nuclear installations, 1969–78. Br J Cancer 59:476–485.

COOK-MOZAFFARI P, DARBY S, DOLL R. 1989b. Cancer near potential sites of nuclear installations. Lancet 2:1145–1147.

COOPER AJ, WINKELMANN RK, WILTSIC JC. 1982. Hematologic malignancies occurring in patients with urticaria pigmentosa. J Am Acad Dermatol 7:215–220.

COOPER PH, INNES DJ, GREER KE. 1983. Acute febrile neutrophilic dermatosis (Sweet's syndrome) and myeloproliferative disorders. Cancer 51:1518–1526.

COPELAN EA, MCGUIRE EA. 1995. The biology and treatment of acute lymphoblastic leukemia in adults. Blood 85:1151–1168.

CORBETT WT, SCHEY HM. 1981. A study of leukaemia clustering in Albermarle, North Carolina, 1968–1978. Cancer 47:2952–2954.

COSTA R, AFONSO E, BENEDITO M, et al. 1991. Poland's syndrome associated with chronic granulocytic leukemia. Pol Hematol 36:417–418.

COTÉ T, MANNS A, HANCHARD B, et al. 1995. HTLV-I sero-incidence among Jamaican food handlers. *Proceedings of the American Society for Clinical Oncology Meeting,* 14:484.

COURT BROWN WM, DOLL R. 1958. Expectation of life and mortality from cancer among British radiologists. Br Med J 2:181–187.

COURT BROWN WM, DOLL R. 1959. Adult leukaemia. Br Med J 1:1063–1066.

COURT BROWN WM, DOLL R. 1961. Leukemia in childhood and young adult life. Trends in mortality in relation to aetiology. Br Med J 1:981–988.

COURT BROWN WM, DOLL R. 1965. Mortality from cancer and other causes after radiotherapy for ankylosing spondylitis. Br Med J 2:1327–1332.

COURT BROWN WM, SPIERS FW, DOLL R, et al. 1960. Geographical variation in leukaemia mortality in relation to background radiation and other factors. Br Med J 1:1753–1759.

COWLES SR, TSAI SP, SNYDER PJ, et al. 1994. Mortality, morbidity, and haematological results from a cohort of long term workers involved in 1, 3 butadiene monomer production. Occup Environ Med 51:323–329.

CRAGLE DL, MCLAIN RW, QUALTERS JR, et al. 1988. Mortality among workers at nuclear fuels production facility. Am J Ind Med 14:379–401.

CRANE MM, KEATING MJ, TRUJILLO JM, et al. 1989. Environmental exposures in cytogenetically defined subsets of acute nonlymphocytic leukemia. JAMA 262:634–639.

CROCE CM, NOWELL PC. 1985. Molecular basis of human B cell neoplasia. Blood 65:1–7.

CROSBY WH. 1969. Acute granulocytic leukemia, a complication of therapy in Hodgkin's disease. Clin Res 17:463.

CRUMP KS, ALLEN BC. 1984. Quantitative estimates of risk of leukemia from occupational exposure to benzene. Occupational Safety and Health Administration, Docket H-059 B, Exhibit 152.

CRUMP KS, NG TH, CUDDIHY RG. 1987. Cancer incidence patterns in the Denver metropolitan area in relation to the Rocky Flats plant. Am J Epidemiol 126:127–135.

CUNEO A, FAGIOLI F, PAZZI I, et al. 1992. Morphologic, immunologic and cytogenetic studies in acute myeloid leukemia following occupational exposure to pesticides and organic solvents. Leuk Res 16:789–796.

CURTIS RE, BOICE JD JR, MOLONEY WC, et al. 1990. Leukemia following chemotherapy for breast cancer. Cancer Res 50:2741–2746.

CURTIS RE, BOICE JD JR, STOVALL M, et al. 1989. Leukemia risk following radiotherapy for breast cancer. J Clin Oncol 17:21–29.

CURTIS RE, BOICE JD JR, STOVALL M, et al. 1992. Risk of leukemia after chemotherapy and radiation treatment for breast cancer. N Engl J Med 326:1745–1751.

CURTIS RE, BOICE JD JR, STOVALL M, et al. 1994. Relationship of leukemia risk to radiation dose following cancer of the uterine corpus. J Natl Cancer Inst 86:1315–1324.

CURTIS RE, HANKEY BF, MYERS MH, et al. 1984. Risk of leukemia associated with the first course of cancer treatment: An analysis of the Surveillance, Epidemiology, and End Results Program Experience. J Natl Cancer Inst 72:531–544.

CUTLER SJ, YOUNG JL JR. 1975. Third National Cancer Survey: Incidence data. Natl Cancer Inst Monogr 41. DHEW Publication No. (NIH) 75-787.

CUTTNER J. 1982. Increased incidence of acute promyelocytic leukemia in patients with ulcerative colitis. J Clin Gastroenterol 2:225–227.

CUTTNER J. 1992. Increased incidence of hematology malignancies in first-degree relatives of patients with chronic lymphocytic leukemia. Cancer Invest 10:103–109.

CUZICK J, EDWARDS R. 1989. Tests for spatial clustering in inhomogeneous populations. J R Stat Soc 86:70–79.

CUZICK J, ERSKINE S, EDELMAN D, et al. 1987. A comparison of the incidence of the myelodysplastic syndrome and acute myeloid leukemia following melphalan and cyclophosphamide treatment for myelomatosis. Br J Cancer 55:523–529.

DALEY GQ, VAN ETTEN RA, BALTIMORE D. 1990. Induction of chronic myelogenous leukemia in males by the p210 bcr/abl gene of the Philadelphia chromosome. Science 247:824–828.

D'AMARO, BACH F, VAN ROOD JJ, et al. 1984. HLA-C associations with acute leukemia. Lancet 2:1176–1178.

DAMESHEK W, GUNZ F. 1964. Leukemia, 2nd ed. New York, Grune & Stratton, pp. 63–72.

DARBY SC, DOLL R. 1987. Fallout, radiation doses near Dounreay, and childhood leukaemia. Br Med J 294:603–607.

DARBY SC, DOLL R, GILL SR, et al. 1987. Long-term mortality after a single treatment course with x-rays in patients treated for ankylosing spondylitis. Br J Cancer 55:179–190.

DARBY SC, KENDALL GM, FELL TP, et al. 1988. A summary of mortality and incidence of cancer in men from the United Kingdom who participated in the United Kingdom's atmospheric nuclear weapon tests and experimental programmes. Br Med J 296:332–338.

DARBY SC, OLSEN JH, DOLL R, et al. 1992. Trends in childhood leukaemia in the Nordic countries in relation to fallout from atmosphere nuclear weapons testing. Br Med J 304:1005–1009.

DAVEY FR, HENRY JB, GOTTLIEB AJ. 1974. HL-A antigens and acute lymphocytic leukemia. Am J Clin Pathol 61:662–665.

DAVIGNON L, LEMONDE P, ROBILLARD P, et al. 1970. BCG vaccination and leukaemia mortality. Lancet 2:638.

DAVIS FG, BOICE JD, KELSEY JL, et al. 1989. Cancer mortality in a radiation-exposed cohort of Massachusetts tuberculosis patients. Cancer Res 49:6130–6136.

DAY NE, BOICE JD JR. 1983. Second Cancer in Relation to Radiation Treatment for Cervical Cancer. IARC Publication No. 52. Lyon, IARC.

DEAN M, PARK M, LEBEAU M, et al. 1985. The human met-oncogene is related to tyrosine kinase oncogenes. Nature 318:385–388.

DECOUFLE P, BLATTNER WA, BLAIR A. 1983. Mortality among chemical workers exposed to benzene and other agents. Environ Res 30:16–25.

DECOUFLE P, STANISLAWIZYK K, HOUTEN L, et al. 1977. A Retrospective Survey of Cancer in Relation to Occupation. National Institute for Occupational Safety and Health. Cincinnati, OH. DHEW (NIOSH) Publication no. 77–178.

DECOUFLE P, WOOD DJ. 1979. Mortality patterns among workers in a grey iron foundry. Am J Epidemiol 109:667–675.

DELORE P, BORGOMANO C. 1928. Leukemia aigue un cour de l'intoxication benzenique, sur l'origine toxique de certains leukemies aigues et leurs relations avec les anemies graves. J Med Lyon 9:227–233.

DELZELL E, GRUFFERMAN S. 1985. Mortality among white and non-white farmers in North Carolina, 1976–1978. Am J Epidemiol 121:391–402.

DELZELL E, MONSON RR. 1981. Mortality among rubber workers. II. Cause-specific mortality, 1940–1978. J Occup Med 23:677–684.

DELZELL E, MONSON RR. 1982. Mortality patterns among rubber workers. V. Processing workers. J Occup Med 24:539–545.

DELZELL E, MONSON RR. 1984. Mortality among rubber workers. VII. Aerospace workers. Am J Ind Med 6:265–271.

DEVEREAUX S, SELASSIE TG, VAUGHN HUDSON G, et al. 1990. Leukaemia complicating treatment for Hodgkin's disease: The experience of the British National Lymphoma Investigation. Br Med J 301:1077–1080.

DEVESA SS, SILVERMAN DT, YOUNG JL JR, et al. 1987. Cancer incidence and mortality trends among whites in the United States, 1947–84. J Natl Cancer Inst 79:701–745.

DIAMOND EL, SCHMERLER H, LILIENFELD AM. 1973. The relationship of intra-uterine radiation to subsequent mortality and development of leukaemia in children. Am J Epidemiol 97:283–313.

DOLL R, PETO R. 1976. Mortality in relation to smoking. 20 years observations on male British doctors. Br Med J 2:1525–1536.

DONHAM KJ, BERG JW, SAWIN RS. 1980. Epidemiologic relationships of the bovine population and human leukemia in Iowa. Am J Epidemiol 112:80–92.

DONHAM KJ, BURMEISTER LF, VAN LIER SF, et al. 1987. Relationships of bovine leukemia virus prevalence in dairy herds and density of dairy cattle to human lymphocytic leukemia. J Vet Res 48:235–238.

DOODY MM, LINET MS, GLASS AG, et al. 1992. Leukemia, lymphoma and multiple myeloma following selected medical conditions. Cancer Causes Control 3:449–456.

DOSIK H, DENIC S, PATEL N, et al. 1988. Adult T-cell leukemia/lymphoma in Brooklyn. JAMA 259:2255–2257.

DOWNS TD, CRANE MM, KIM KW. 1987. Mortality among workers at a butadiene facility. Am J Ind Med 12:311–329.

DOYLE JA, CONNOLLY SM, HAAGLAND HC. 1985. Hematologic disease in scleroderma syndromes. Acta Derm Venereol 65:521–525.

DRAPER GJ, BOWER BD, DARBY SC, et al. 1989. Completeness of registration of childhood leukaemia near nuclear installations and elsewhere in the Oxford region. Br Med J 299:952.

DRAPER GJ, HEAF MM, KINNEAR-WILSON LM. 1977. Occurrence of childhood cancers among sibs and estimation of familial risks. J Med Genet 14:81–90.

DRAPER GJ, SANDERS BM, KINGSTON JE. 1986. Second primary neoplasm in patients with retinoblastoma. Br J Cancer 53:661.

DRAPER GJ, STILLER CA, CARTWRIGHT RA, et al. 1993. Cancer in Cumbria and in the vicinity of the Sellafield nuclear installation, 1963–90. Br Med J 306:89–94.

DUTCHER RM, LARKIN EP, MARSHAK RR. 1964. Virus-like particles in cow's milk from a herd with high incidence of lymphosarcoma. J Natl Cancer Inst 33:1055–1064.

DYER PA, RIDWAY JC, FLANAGAN NG. 1986. HLA-A, B and DR antigens in chronic lymphocytic leukaemia. Dis Mark 4:231–237.

EBBIN AJ, HEATH CW JR, MOLDOW RE, et al. 1968. Down's syndrome and leukemia in a family. J Pediatr 73:917–920.

EDERER F, MYERS MH, MANTEL N. 1964. A statistical problem in space time clustering: Do leukemia cases come in clusters? Biometrics 20:626–638.

EDERER F, MYERS MH, MANTEL N. 1965. Temporal spatial distribution of leukemia and lymphoma in Connecticut. J Natl Cancer Inst 35:625–629.

EDMONDS CJ, SMITH T. 1986. The long-term hazards of the treatment of thyroid cancer with radioiodine. Br J Radiol 59:45–51.

ELLIS JT, PETERSON P, GELLER SA, et al. 1986. Studies of the bone marrow in polycythemia vera and the evolution of myelofibrosis and second hematologic malignancies. Semin Hematol 23:144–155.

ENSTROM JE. 1979. Leukemia from atomic fallout. N Engl J Med 300:1491.

ENSTROM JE. 1983. Cancer mortality patterns around the San Onofre nuclear power plant, 1960–1978. Am J Public Health 73:83–92.

ERICSSON JL-E, KARNSTROM L, MATTSON B. 1978. Childhood cancer in Sweden, 1958–74. I. Incidence and mortality. Acta Pediatr Scand 67:425–436.

ESSIEN EM. 1976. Leukaemia in Nigerians. II. The chronic leukaemias. E Afr Med J 53:96–104.

EVANS JS, WENNBERG JE, MCNEIL BJ. 1986. The influence of diagnostic radiography on the incidence of breast cancer and leukemia. N Engl J Med 315:800–815.

EVATT BL, CHASE GA, HEATH CW JR. 1973. Time space clustering among cases of acute leukemia in two Georgia counties. Blood 41:265–272.

EWINGS PD, BOWIE C, PHILLIPS MJ, et al. 1989. Incidence of leukaemia in young people in the vicinity of Hinkley Point nuclear power station, 1959–86. Br Med J 299:289–293.

FABER M. 1978. Malignancies in Danish Thorotrast patients. Health Physics 35:153–162.

FABIA J, DROLLETTE M. 1970. Malformations and leukemia in children with Down's syndrome. Pediatrics 45:60–70.

FAGIOLI F, CUNEO A, PIVA N, et al. 1992. Distinct cytogenetic and clinicopathologic features in acute myeloid leukemia after occupational exposure to pesticides and organic solvents. Cancer 70:77–85.

FASAL E, JACKSON EW, KLAUBER MR. 1968. Leukemia and lymphoma mortality and farm residence. Am J Epidemiol 87:267–274.

FAZEKAS VT, BACH K, TOTH S, et al. 1978. Familiares Borkomen von chronisher lymphatischer Leukamie. HLA-Antigen-und zytogenetische Untersurhungen. Wien Med Wochenschr 9:262–273.

FELIX CA, WINICJ NJ, NEGRINI M, et al. 1994. Common region of ALL-1 gene disrupted in epipodophyllotoxin-related secondary acute myeloid leukemia. Cancer Res 53:2954–2956.

FEYCHTING M, AHLBOM A. 1993. Magnetic fields and cancer in children residing near Swedish high voltage power lines. Am J Epidemiol 138:467–481.

FEYCHTING M, AHLBOM A. 1994. Magnetic fields, leukemia, and central nervous system tumors in Swedish adults residing near high-voltage power lines. Epidemiology 5:501–509.

FINCH S. 1984. Leukemia and lymphoma in atomic bomb survivors. *In* Boice JD Jr, Fraumeni JF Jr (eds): Radiation Carcinogenesis: Epidemiology and Biological Significance. New York, Raven Press, pp. 37–44.

FINCH SC, FINCH CA. 1990. Summary of the studies at ABCC-RERF concerning the late hematologic effects of atomic bomb exposure in Hiroshima and Nagasaki. Technical Report RERF TR 23-88. Hiroshima, Japan, Radiation Effects Research Foundation.

FINCH SC, LINET MS. 1992. Chronic leukaemias. *In* Fleming AF (ed): Epidemiology of Haematological Disease. Part I. London, Bailliere Tindal, pp. 27–56.

FINLAY J, LUFT B, YOUSEM S, et al. 1986. Chronic infectious mononucleosis syndrome, pancytopenia, and polyclonal B-lymphoproliferation terminating in acute lymphoblastic leukemia. Am J Pediatr Hematol/Oncol 8:18–27.

FIRST MIC COOPERATIVE STUDY GROUP. 1986. Morphologic, immunologic, and cytogenetic (MIC) working classification of acute lymphoblastic leukemias. Cancer Genet Cytogenet 23:189–197.

FISHER B, ROCKETTE H, FISHER ER, et al. 1985. Leukemia in breast cancer patients following adjuvant chemotherapy or postoperative radiation: The NSABP experience. J Clin Oncol 3:1640–1658.

FITZGERALD PH, HAMER JW. 1976. Karyotype and survival in human acute leukemia. J Natl Cancer Inst 56:459–462.

FLEMING AF. 1985. The epidemiology of lymphomas and leukaemias in Africa—An overview. Leuk Res 9:735–740.

FLEMING AF. 1988. Possible aetiological factors in leukaemias in Africa. Leuk Res 12:33–43.

FLEMING AF. 1990. Chronic lymphocytic leukaemia in tropical Africa. A review. Leuk Lymph 1:169–173.

FLEMING AF, MAHARAJAN R, ABRAHAM M, et al. 1986. Antibodies to HTLV-I in Nigerian blood donors and their relatives and patients with leukemias, lymphomas and other diseases. Int J Cancer 38:809–813.

FLODERUS B, PERSSON T, STENLUND C, et al. 1993. Occupational exposure to electromagnetic fields in relation to leukemia and brain tumors. Cancer Causes Control 4:465–476.

FLODERUS B, TÖRNQVIST S, STENLUND C. 1994. Incidence of selected cancers in Swedish railway workers. Cancer Causes Control 5:189–194.

FLODIN U, ANDERSSON L, ANJOU D-G, et al. 1981. A case-referent study on acute myeloid leukemia, background radiation and exposure to solvents and other agents. Scand J Work Environ Health 7:169–178.

FLODIN U, FREDRIKSON M, AXELSON O, et al. 1986. Background radiation, electrical work, and some other exposures associated with acute myeloid leukemia in a case-referent study. Arch Environ Health 41:77–84.

FLODIN U, FREDRIKSON M, PERSSON B, et al. 1988. Chronic lymphocytic leukemia and engine exhausts, fresh wood, and DDT: A case-referent study. Br J Ind Med 45:33–38.

FLODIN U, FREDRIKSON M, PERSSON B, et al. 1990. Acute myeloid leukemia and background radiation in an expanded case-referent study. Arch Environ Health 45:364–366.

FLYNN JW. 1970. Epidemiological studies of childhood leukemia in Green Bay, Wisconsin. J Natl Cancer Inst 44:489–495.

FONG C-T, BRODEUR GM. 1987. Down's syndrome and leukemia: Epidemiology, genetics, cytogenetics, and mechanisms of leukemogenesis. Cancer Genet Cytogenet 28:55–76.

FORU AM, RIDGE SA, CABRERA ME, et al. 1993. In utero rearrangements in the trithorax-related oncogene in infant leukemia. Nature 363:358–360.

FORMAN D, COOK-MOZAFFARI P, DARBY S, et al. 1987. Cancer near nuclear installations. Nature 329:499–505.

FOURTH INTERNATIONAL WORKSHOP ON CHROMOSOMES IN LEUKEMIA. 1984. The correlation of karyotype and occupational exposure to potential mutagenic/carcinogenic agents in acute nonlymphocytic leukemia. Cancer Genet Cytogenet 11:326–331.

FOX AJ, COLLIER PF. 1976. A survey of occupational cancer in the rubber and cable-making industries: Analysis of deaths occurring in 1972–74. Br J Ind Med 33:249–264.

FRADKIN JF, MILLS JL, SCHONBERGER LB, et al. 1993. Risk of leukemia after treatment with pituitary growth hormone. JAMA 270:2829–2832.

FRASER P, CARPENTER L, MACONOCHIE, et al. 1993. Cancer mortality and morbidity in employees of the United Kingdom Atomic Energy Authority, 1946–1986. Br J Cancer 67:615–624.

FRAUMENI JF JR. 1967. Bone marrow depression induced by chloramphenicol or phenylbutazone. JAMA 201:828–834.

FRAUMENI JF JR, MILLER RW. 1967. Epidemiology of leukemia: Recent observations. J Natl Cancer Inst 38:593–605.

FRAUMENI JF JR, VOGEL CL, DEVITA VT. 1969. Familial chronic lymphocytic leukemia. Ann Intern Med 71:279–284.

FREEDMAN AS, NADLER LM. 1988. Chronic lymphocytic leukemia: Cell surface phenotype and normal cellular counterparts. *In* Polliack A, Catovsky D (eds): Chronic Lymphocytic Leukemia. Chur, Switzerland, Harwood Academic Publishers, pp. 47–66.

FRIEDMAN GD. 1982. Phenylbutazone, musculoskeletal disease, and leukemia. J Chronic Dis 35:233–243.

FRIEDMAN GD, URY H. 1980. Initial screening for carcinogenicity of commonly used drugs. J Natl Cancer Inst 65:723–733.

FULTON JF, COBB S, PREBLE L, et al. 1980. Electrical wiring configurations and childhood leukemia in Rhode Island. Am J Epidemiol 111:292–296.

FUNES-CRAVIOTO F, ZAPATA-GAYON C, KOLMODIN-HEDMAN B, et al. 1977. Chromosome aberrations and sister chromatid exchange in workers in chemical laboratories and a rotoprinting factory and in children of women laboratory workers. Lancet 2:322–325.

FUORTES L, MCNUTT L, LYNCH C. 1990. Leukemia incidence and radioactivity in drinking water in 59 Iowa towns. Am J Public Health 80:1261–1262.

GALLAGHER RP, THRELFALL WJ. 1983. Cancer mortality in metal workers. Can Med Assoc J 129:1191–1194.

GALLAGHER RP, THELFALL WJ, JEFFRIES E, et al. 1984. Cancer and aplastic anemia in British Columbia farmers. J Natl Cancer Inst 72:1311–1315.

GALLO RC, SLISKI A. 1986. Origins of human T-lymphotropic viruses. Nature 320:219.

GAMBERALE F, ANSHELM OLSEN B, ENEROTH P, et al. 1989. Acute effects of ELF electromagnetic fields: A field study of linesmen working with kV powerlines. Br J Ind Med 46:729–737.

GARDNER MJ, COGGON D, PANNETT B, et al. 1989. Workers exposed to ethylene oxide: A follow-up study. Br J Ind Med 46:860–865.

GARDNER MJ, HALL AJ, DOWNES S, et al. 1987a. Follow up study of children born to mothers resident in Seascale, West Cumbria (birth cohort). Br Med J 295:822–827.

GARDNER MJ, HALL AJ, DOWNES S, et al. 1987b. Follow up study of children born elsewhere but attending schools in Seascale, West Cumbria (schools cohort). Br Med J 295:819–822.

GARDNER MJ, SNEE MP, HALL AJ, et al. 1990. Results of case-control study of leukaemia and lymphoma among young people near Sellafield nuclear plant in West Cumbria. Br Med J 300:423–434.

GARDNER MJ, WINTER PD. 1984. Mortality in Cumbria during 1978 with reference to cancer in young people around Windscale. Lancet 1:216–217.

GARDNER MJ, WINTER PD, TAYLOR CD, et al. 1983. Atlas of Cancer Mortality. Chichester, John Wiley and Sons.

GARFINKEL L, BOFFETTA P. 1990. Association between smoking and leukemia in two American Cancer Society prospective studies. Cancer 65:2356–2360.

GARLAND FC, SHAW E, GORHAM ED, et al. 1990. Incidence of leukemia in occupations with potential electromagnetic field exposure in United States Navy personnel. Am J Epidemiol 132:293–303.

GEARY CG, BENN RT, LECK I. 1979. Incidence of myeloid leukemia in Lancashire. Lancet 2:549–551.

GERNCIK A, BUSER M, TEMMINCK B, et al. 1987. High incidence of stomach cancer in relatives of patients with malignant lymphoproliferative disorders. Cancer Detect Prevent (Suppl) 1:121–129.

GERRARD M, EDEN OB. 1986. Variations in incidence of childhood leukaemia in South East Scotland (1970–1984). Leuk Res 10:561–564.

GESSAIN A, BARIN F, VERNANT JC, et al. 1985. Antibodies to human T-lymphotropic virus type I in patients with tropical spastic paraparesis. Lancet 2:407–410.

GIBBS WN, LOFTERS WS, CAMPBELL M, et al. 1987. Non-Hodgkin's lymphoma in Jamaica and its relation to adult-T cell leukemia-lymphoma. Ann Intern Med 106:361–368.

GIBSON E, GRAHAM S, LILIENFELD A, et al. 1976. Epidemiology of diseases in adult males with leukemia. J Natl Cancer Inst 56:891–898.

GIBSON R, GRAHAM S, LILIENFELD A, et al. 1972. Irradiation in the epidemiology of leukemia among adults. J Natl Cancer Inst 48:301–311.

GILBERT ES, MARKS S. 1979. An analysis of the mortality of workers in a nuclear facility. Radiat Res 79:122–148.

GILBERT ES, FRY SA, WIGGS LD, et al. 1989a. Analyses of combined mortality data on workers at the Hanford site, Oak Ridge National Laboratory, and Rocky Flats Nuclear Weapons Plant. Radiat Res 120:19–35.

GILBERT ES, PETERSEN GR, BUCHANAN JA. 1989b. Mortality of workers at the Hanford site: 1945–1981. Health Physics 56:11–25.

GILBERT ES, OMOHUNDRO E, BUCHANAN JA, et al. 1993a. Mortality of workers at the Hanford site: 1945–1986. Health Phys 64:577–590.

GILBERT ES, CRAGLE DL, WIGGS LD. 1993b. Updated analyses of combined mortality data for workers at the Hanford site, Oak Ridge National Laboratory, and Rocky Flats Weapons Plant. Radiat Res 136:408–421.

GILBERT RD, KARABUS CD, MILLS AE. 1987. Acute promyelocytic leukemia. A childhood cluster. Cancer 59:933–935.

GILES FJ, KOEFFLER HP. 1994. Secondary myelodysplastic syndromes and leukemias. Curr Opin Hematol 1:256–260.

GILLIAM AG, WALTER WA. 1958. Trends of mortality from leukemia in the United States, 1921–55. Public Health Rep 73:773–784.

GILMAN PA, AMES RG, MCCAWLEY MA. 1985. Leukemia risk among U.S. white male coal miners. J Occup Med 27:669–671.

GILMAN PA, MILLER RW. 1982. No link between Poland syndrome and leukemia? Am J Dis Child 136:176.

GIRARD PR, REVOL L. 1970. La Frequence d'une exposition benzenique au cours des hemopathies graves. Nouv Rev Fr Hematol 10:477–484.

GLASS AG, MANTEL N. 1964. Lack of time space clustering of childhood leukemia in Los Angeles County 1960–1964. Cancer Res 29:1995–2001.

GLUCKMAN E, LEMARCHAND F, NUNEZ-ROLDAN A, et al. 1976. Possible excess of HLA-A2 homozygous among aplastic anemia and acute lymphoblastic leukaemia (ALL). *In* HLA and Disease. Paris, Inserm, pp. 226.

GOGUEL A, CAVIGNEAUX A, BERNARD J. 1967. Les leucemies benzeniques de la region Parisienne entre 1950 et 1965. (Etude de 50 observations). Nouv Rev Fr Hematol 7:465–480.

GOLDING J, GREENWOOD R, BIRMINGHAM K, MOTT M. 1992. Childhood cancer, intramuscular vitamin K, and pethidine given during labour. Br Med J 305:341–246.

GOLDING J, PATERSON M, KINLEN LJ. 1990. Factors associated with childhood cancer in a national cohort study. Br J Cancer 62:304–308.

GOLOMB HM, ALIMENA G, ROWLEY JD, et al. 1982. Correlation of occupation and karyotype in adults with acute nonlymphocytic leukemia. Blood 60:404–411.

GONZALES F, TRUJILLO JM, ALEXANIAN R. 1977. Acute leukemia in multiple myeloma. Ann Intern Med 86:440–443.

GORST DW, ATKINSON C, MORRIS JA. 1987. A temporal cluster of acute leukemia. Clin Lab Haematol 9:211–213.

GRACE M, LARSON M, HANSON J. 1980. Bronchogenic carcinoma among former uranium mine workers at Port Radium, Canada. A pilot study. Health Physics 38:657–661.

GRAHAM S, LEVIN M, LILIENFELD A, et al. 1966. Pre-conception, intrauterine, and postnatal irradiation as related to leukemia. Natl Cancer Inst Monogr 19:347–371.

GRATWOHL A, HERMANS J, GOLDMAN JM, et al. 1993. Bone marrow transplantation in Europe: Major geographical differences. J Int Med 233:333–341.

GREAVES MF. 1986. Differentiation-linked leukemogenesis in lymphocytes. Science 234:697–701.

GREAVES MF. 1989. Etiology of childhood acute lymphoblastic leukemia: A soluble problem? *In* Gale RP and Hoelzer D (eds): Acute Lymphoblastic Leukemia. UCLA Symposium on Molecular and Cellular Biology. New Series Vol. 108. New York, Alan Liss.

GREAVES MF, ALEXANDER FE. 1993. An infectious etiology for common acute lymphoblastic leukemia in childhood? Leukemia 7:349–360.

GREAVES MF, COLMAN SM, BEARD MEJ, et al. 1993. Geographical distribution of acute lymphoblastic leukaemia subtypes: Second report of the Collaborative Group Study. Leukemia 7:27–34.

GREAVES MF, PEGRAM SM, CHAN LC. 1985. Collaborative group study of the epidemiology of acute lymphoblastic leukemia subtypes: Background and first report. Leuk Res 9:715–733.

GREENBERG ER, ROSNER B, HENNEKENS C, et al. 1985. An investigation of bias in a study of nuclear shipyard workers. Am J Epidemiol 121:301–308.

GREENBERG HL, OTT MG, SHORE RE. 1990. Men assigned to ethylene oxide or other ethylene oxide related chemical manufacturing: A mortality study. Br J Ind Med 47:221–230.

GREENE MH, BOICE JD JR, GREER BE, et al. 1982. Acute nonlymphocytic leukemia after therapy with alkylating agents for ovarian cancer. A study of five randomized clinical trials. N Engl J Med 307:1416–1421.

GREENE MH, HARRIS EL, GERSHENSON DM, et al. 1986. Melphalan may be a more potent leukemogen than cyclophosphamide. Ann Intern Med 105:360–367.

GREENE MH, HOOVER RN, ELK RL, et al. 1979. Cancer mortality among printing plant workers. Environ Res 20:66–73.

GREENE MH, YOUNG RC, MERRILL JM, et al. 1983. Evidence of a treatment dose response in acute nonlymphocytic leukemias which occur after therapy of non-Hodgkin's lymphoma. Cancer Res 43:1891–1898.

GREENWALD P, ROSE JS, DAITCH PB. 1979. Acquaintance networks among leukemia and lymphoma patients. Am J Epidemiol 110:162–177.

GRETZULA JC, OSCAR HEVIA DO, WEBER BS, et al. 1987. Bloom's syndrome. J Am Acad Dermatol 17:479–488.

GRIBBIN MA, WEEKS JL, HOWE GR. 1993. Cancer mortality (1956–1985) among male employees of Atomic Energy of Canada Limited with respect to occupational exposure to external low-linear-energy-transfer ionizing radiation. Radiat Res 133:375–380.

GRIDLEY G, MCLAUGHLIN EKBOM A, et al. 1993. Incidence of cancer among patients with rheumatoid arthritis. J Natl Cancer Inst 85:307–311.

GRIEM ML, KLEINERMAN RA, BOICE JD JR, et al. 1994. Cancer following radiotherapy for peptic ulcer. J Natl Cancer Inst 86:842–849.

GRODSTEIN F, HENNEKENS CH, COLDITZ GA, et al. 1994. A prospective study of permanent hair dye use and hematopoietic cancer. J Natl Cancer Inst 86:1466–1470.

GROSS L. 1978. Viral etiology of cancer and leukemia: A look into the past, present, and future—GHA Clowes Memorial Lecture. Cancer Res 38:485–493.

GROVES FD, LINET MS, DEVESA SS. 1995. Patterns of occurrence of the leukemias. Eur J Cancer 31A:941–949.

GRUNWALD H, ROSNER R. 1979. Acute leukemia and immune suppressive drug use. Arch Intern Med 139:461–466.

GUENEL P, RASKMARK P, ANDERSON JB, et al. 1993. Incidence of cancer in persons with occupational exposure to electromagnetic fields in Denmark. Br J Ind Med 50:758–764.

GUNZ FW. 1964. Leukemia in New Zealand and Australia. Pathol Microbiol 27:697–704.

GUNZ FW. 1977. The epidemiology and genetics of the chronic leukaemias. Clin Haematol 6:3–20.

GUNZ F, ATKINSON H. 1964. Medical radiation and leukemia: A retrospective survey. Br Med J 5380:389–396.

GUNZ FW, FITZGERALD PH, CROSSEN PE, et al. 1966. Multiple cases of leukemia in a sibship. Blood 27:482–489.

GUNZ FW, GUNZ JP, VEALE AMO, et al. 1975. Familial leukaemia: A study of 909 families. Scand J Haematol 15:117–131.

GUNZ FW, GUNZ JP, VINCENT PC, et al. 1978. Thirteen cases of leukemia in a family. J Natl Cancer Inst 60:1243–1250.

GUNZ FW, VEALE AMO. 1969. Leukemia in close relatives—accident or predisposition? J Natl Cancer Inst 42:517–524.

HAANEN G, MATHE G, HAYAT M. 1981. Treatment of polycythemia vera by radio-phosphorus or busulphan: A randomized trial. Br J Cancer 44:75–80.

HAAS JF, KITTELMANN B, MEHNERT WH, et al. 1987. Risk of leukemia in ovarian tumor and breast cancer patients following treatment by cyclophosphamide. Br J Cancer 55:213–218.

HADJIMICHAEL OC, OSTFELD AM, D'ATRI DA, et al. 1983. Mortality and cancer incidence experience of employees in a nuclear fuels fabrication plant. J Occup Med 25:48–61.

HAENSZEL W, KURIHARA M. 1968. Studies of Japanese migrants. I. Mortality from cancer and other diseases among Japanese in the United States. J Natl Cancer Inst 40:43–68.

HAKULINEN T, ISOMAKI H, KNEKT P. 1985. Rheumatoid arthritis and cancer studies based on linking nationwide registries in Finland. Am J Med 78(Suppl 1A):29–32.

HALL P, BOICE JD JR, BERG G, et al. 1992. Leukaemia incidence after iodine[1]31 exposure. Lancet 340:1–4.

HALME L, VON KNORRIN J, ELONEN E. 1990. Development of acute myelocytic leukemia in patients with Crohn's disease. Dig Dis Sci 35:1553–1556.

HALPERIN W, ALTMAN R, STEMHAGEN A, et al. 1980. Epidemiologic investigation of clusters of leukemia and Hodgkin's disease in Rutherford, New Jersey. J Med Soc NJ 77:267–273.

HAMMOND EC. 1966. Smoking in relation to death rates of one million men and women. Natl Cancer Inst Monogr 19:127–204.

HANIS NM, HOLMES TM, SHALLENBERGER LG, et al. 1982. Epidemiologic study of refinery and chemical plant workers. J Occup Med 24:203–212.

HANN HWL, LONDON WT, SUTNICK AI, et al. 1975. Studies of parents of children with acute leukemia. J Natl Cancer Inst 54:1299–1305.

HANSEN NE, KARLE H, JENSEN OM. 1983. Trends in the incidence of leukemia in Denmark, 1943–77: An epidemiologic study of 14,000 patients. J Natl Cancer Inst 71:697–701.

HARDISTY RM, SPEED DE, TILL M. 1964. Granulocytic leukaemia in childhood. Br J Haematol 10:551–566.

HARNDEN DG. 1985. Inherited factors in leukemia and lymphoma. Leuk Res 9:705–707.

HARO AS. 1986. The effect of BCG-vaccination and tuberculosis on the risk of leukaemia. Dev Biol Stand 58(part A):433–449.

HARRINGTON JM, OAKES D. 1984. Mortality study of British pathologists 1974–80. Br J Ind Med 41:188–191.

HARRIS R, LAWLER SD, OLIVER RTD. 1978. The HLA system in acute leukaemia and Hodgkin's disease. Br Med Bull 34:301–304.

HARTLEY SE, SAINSBURY C. 1981. Acute leukemia and the same chromosome abnormality in monozygotic twins. Hum Genet 58:408–410.

HARVEY EB, BOICE JD, HAREGMAN M, et al. 1985. Prenatal X-ray exposure and childhood cancer in twins. N Engl J Med 312:541–545.

HATCH MC, BEYEA J, NIEVES JW, et al. 1990. Cancer near the Three Mile Island nuclear plant: Radiation emissions. Am J Epidemiol 132:397–412.

HAWKINS MM, DRAPER GJ, KINGSTON JE. 1987. Incidence of second primary tumours among childhood cancer survivors. Br J Cancer 56:339–347.

HAYES RB, BLAIR A, STEWART PA, et al. 1990. Mortality of U.S. embalmers and funeral directors. Am J Ind Med 18:641–652.

HAZLEMAN BL. 1982. Comparative incidence of malignant disease in rheumatoid arthritis patients exposed to different treatment regimens. Ann Rheum Dis 41(Suppl):12–17.

HEASMAN MA, URQUHART JD, BLACK RJ, et al. 1987. Leukaemia in young persons in Scotland: A study of its geographical distribution and relationship to nuclear installations. Health Bull 45:147–151.

HEATH CW JR. 1975. The epidemiology of leukemia. *In* Schottenfeld D (ed): Cancer Epidemiology and Prevention: Current Concepts. Springfield, Illinois, Charles C Thomas, pp. 318–350.

HEATH CW JR, HASTERLIK RJ. 1963. Leukemia among children in a suburban community. Am J Med 34:796–812.

HECHT F, HECHT B, MORGAN R, et al. 1986. Chromosome clues to acute leukemia in Down's syndrome. Cancer Genet Cytogenet 21:93–98.

HECHT F, HECHT BK. 1990. Cancer in ataxia telangiectasia patients. Cancer Genet Cytogenet 46:9–19.

HEIM S, MITELMAN F. 1987. Cancer Cytogenetics. New York, Alan Liss, pp. 65–110, 141–174.

HEISE E, PARRISH E, COOPER R. 1979. HLA-B17 and the HLA-A1, B17 haplotype in acute myelogenous leukemia. Tissue Antigens 14:98–104.

HEMPELMANN L, HALE W, PHILLIPS M, et al. 1975. Neoplasms in persons treated with x-ray in infancy: Fourth survey in 20 years. J Natl Cancer Inst 55:519–530.

HEMS G, STEWART A. 1972. Childhood leukemia in Scotland, 1939–68. Scott Med J 17:13–19.

HENRY-AMAR M, PELLAE-COSSET B, BAYLE-WEISGERBER C, et al. 1989. Risk of secondary acute leukemia and preleukemia after Hodgkin's disease: The Institute Gustave-Roussy experience. Recent Res Cancer Res 117:270–283.

HENSHAW DL, EATOUGH JP, RICHARDSON RB. 1990. Radon as a causative factor in induction of myeloid leukaemia and other cancers. Lancet 1:1008–1012.

HESTER JP, ROSSEN R, TRUIJILLO J. 1977. Frequency of HLA antigens in chronic myelocytic leukemia. South Med J 70:691–693.

HESTON JF, KELLY JB, MEIGS JW, et al. 1986. Forty-five Years of Cancer Incidence in Connecticut: 1935–79. Natl Cancer Inst Monogr 70. PHS (NIH). Bethesda, MD. U.S. DHHS 86-2652.

HEYER N, WEISS NS, DEMERS P, et al. 1990. Cohort mortality study of Seattle fire fighters: 1945–1983. Am J Ind Med 17:493–504.

HIELLE B, MILLS R, SWENSON S, et al. 1991. Incidence of hairy cell leukemia, mycosis fungoides, and chronic lymphocytic leukemia in the first known HTLV-II-endemic population. J Infect Dis 163:435–440.

HILDRETH NG, SHORE RE, HEMPELMANN LH, et al. 1985. Risk of extrathyroid tumors following radiation treatment in infancy for thymic enlargement. Radiat Res 102:378–391.

HILL C, LAPLANCHE A. 1990. Overall mortality and cancer mortality around French nuclear sites. Nature 347:755–757.

HINDS MW, KOLONEL LN, LEU T, et al. 1980. Associations between cancer incidence and alcohol and cigarette consumption among five ethnic groups in Hawaii. Br J Cancer 41:929–940.

HINUMA Y, KOMODA H, CHOSA T, et al. 1982. Antibodies to adult T-cell leukemia-virus-associated antigen (ATLA) in sera from patients with ATL and controls in Japan: A nation-wide seroepidemiologic study. Int J Cancer 29:631–635.

HINUMA Y, NAGATA K, HANAOKA M, et al. 1981. Adult T-cell leukemia: Antigen in an ATL cell line and detection of antibodies to the antigen in human sera. Proc Natl Acad Sci USA 78:6476–6480.

HIRAYAMA T. 1990. Smoking and mortality. *In* Harayama T (ed): Life Style and Mortality: A Large-Scale Census-Based Cohort Study in Japan. Basel, S. Karger, pp. 28–59.

HJALMARS U, KULLDORFF M, GUSTAFSSON G, AND THE SWEDISH CHILD LEUKAEMIA GROUP. 1994. Risk of acute childhood leukaemia in Sweden after the Chernobyl reactor accident. Br Med J 309:154–157.

HOAR SK, BLAIR A, HOLMES FF, et al. 1986. Agricultural herbicide use and risk of lymphoma and soft tissue sarcoma. JAMA 256:1141–1147.

HODGSON JT, JONES RD. 1985. Mortality of styrene production, polymerization and processing workers at a site in northwest England. Scand J Work Environ Health 11:347–352.

HODGSON JT, JONES RD. 1990. Mortality of a cohort of tin miners 1941–86. Br J Ind Med 47:665–676.

HOFFMAN DA, LONSTEIN JE, MORIN MM, et al. 1989. Breast cancer in women with scoliosis exposed to multiple diagnostic x-rays. J Natl Cancer Inst 81:1307–1312.

HOFFMAN DA, MCCONAHEY WM, FRAUMENI JF JR, et al. 1982. Cancer incidence following treatment of hyperthyroidism. Int J Epidemiol 11:218–224.

HOGSTEDT C, ARRINGER L, GUSTAVSSON A. 1984. Ethylene oxide and cancer—review of the literature and follow-up of two studies. Arbete Halsa 49:1–32.

HOGSTEDT C, ARRINGER L, GUSTAVSSON A. 1986. Epidemiologic support for ethylene oxide as a cancer-causing agent. JAMA 255:1575–1578.

HOGSTEDT C, MALINQVIST N, WADMAN B. 1979. Leukemia in workers exposed to ethylene oxide. JAMA 241:1132–1133.

HOGSTEDT C, ROHLEN O, BERNDTSSON BS, et al. 1979b. A cohort study of mortality and cancer incidence in ethylene oxide production workers. Br J Ind Med 36:276–280.

HOLE DJ, GILLIS CR. 1986. Childhood leukaemia in the west of Scotland. Lancet 2:524–525.

HOLLAND WW, DOLL R, CARTER CO. 1962. The mortality from leukaemia and other cancers among patients with Down's syndrome and among their parents. Br J Cancer 16:177–184.

HOLM L-E. 1984. Malignant disease following iodine-131 therapy in Sweden. *In* Boice JD Jr, Fraumeni JF Jr (eds): Radiation Carcinogenesis: Epidemiology and Biological Significance. New York, Raven Press, pp. 263–271.

HOLM L-E, HALL P, WIKLUND K, et al. 1991. Cancer risk after iodine-131 therapy for hyperthyroidism. J Natl Cancer Inst 83:1072–1077.

HOLM L-E, WIKLUND KE, LUNDELL GE, et al. 1989. Cancer risk in populations examined with diagnostic doses of ^{131}I. J Natl Cancer Inst 81:302–306.

HOLMBERG B, LUNDBERG P. 1985. Benzene: Standards, occurrence and exposure. Am J Ind Med 7:375–383.

HOOVER RN. 1976. Bacillus Calmette-Guerin vaccination and cancer prevention: A critical review of the human experience. Cancer Res 36:652–654.

HOOVER R, FRAUMENI JF JR. 1973. Risk of cancer in renal transplant recipients. Lancet 2:55–57.

HSING AW, HANSSON L-E, MCLAUGHLIN JK, et al. 1993. Pernicious anemia and subsequent cancer. Cancer 71:745–750.

HUISMAN CH, VAN DEN WIELEN AW, TEN THIJ AC. 1981. Incidence of leukaemia. Lancet 1:673–676.

HURLEY N, ALBERT R, SHONE R, et al. 1976. Follow-up study of patients treated by x-ray epilation for tinea capitis. Estimation of the dose to the thyroid and pituitary gland and other structures in the head and neck. Phys Med Biol 21:631–642.

HUTCHISON GB, MACMAHON B, JABLON S, et al. 1979. Review of report by Mancuso, Stewart, and Kneale of radiation exposure of Hanford workers. Health Physics 37:207–220.

IMAI J, HINUMA Y. 1983. Epstein-Barr virus-specific antibodies in patients with adult T-cell leukemia (ATL) and healthy ATL virus-carriers. Int J Cancer 31:197–200.

INFANTE PF, RINSKY RA, WAGONER JR, et al. 1977. Leukemia in benzene workers. Lancet 2:76–78.

INFANTE PF, EPSTEIN SS, NEWTON WA JR. 1978. Blood dyscrasias and childhood tumors and exposure to chlordane and heptachlor. Scand J Work Environ Health 4:137–150.

INFANTE PF, WHITE MC. 1983. Benzene: Epidemiologic observations of leukemia by cell type and adverse health effects associated with low-level exposure. Environ Health Perspect 52:75–82.

INFANTE-RIVARD C, MUR P, ARMSTRONG B, et al. 1991. Acute lymphoblastic leukaemia among Spanish children and mothers' occupation: A case-control study. J Epidemiol Community Health 45:11–15.

INGRAM L, MOTT MG, MANN JR, et al. 1987. Second malignancies in children treated for non-Hodgkin's lymphoma and T-cell leukemia in the UKCCSG regimens. Br J Cancer 55:463–466.

INSKIP PD, HARVEY EB, BOICE JD JR, et al. 1991. Incidence of childhood cancer in twins. Cancer Causes Control 2:315–324.

INSKIP PD, KLEINERMAN RA, STOVALL M, et al. 1993. Leukemia, lymphoma, and multiple myeloma after pelvic radiotherapy for benign disease. Radiat Res 135:108–124.

INSKIP PD, MONSON RR, WAGONER JK, et al. 1990. Leukemia following radiotherapy for uterine bleeding. Radiat Res 122:107–119.

INTERNATIONAL AGENCY FOR RESEARCH ON CANCER. 1977. Monographs on the Evaluation of the Carcinogenic Risk of Chemicals to Man. Some Aromatic Amines and Related Nitro Compounds-Hair Dyes, Colouring Agents, and Miscellaneous Chemicals. Volume 16. Lyon: IARC, pp. 25–47.

INTERNATIONAL AGENCY FOR RESEARCH ON CANCER. 1981. Monographs on the Evaluation of the Carcinogenic Risk of Chemicals to Man. Wood, Leather, and Some Associated Industries. Volume 25. Lyon: IARC, pp. 1–97.

INTERNATIONAL AGENCY FOR RESEARCH ON CANCER. 1982. Monographs on the Evaluation of the Carcinogenic Risk of Chemicals to Man. Some Industrial Chemicals and Dyestuffs. Volume 29. Lyon: IARC, pp. 93–148.

INTERNATIONAL AGENCY FOR RESEARCH ON CANCER. 1985. Monographs on the Evaluation of the Carcinogenic Risk of Chemicals to Man. Allyl Compounds, Aldehydes, Epoxides, and Peroxides. Volume 36. Lyon: IARC, pp. 189–226.

INTERNATIONAL AGENCY FOR RESEARCH ON CANCER. 1989. Monographs on the Evaluation of the Carcinogenic Risk of Chemicals to Man. Occupational Exposures in Petroleum Refining: Crude Oil and Major Petroleum Fuels. Volume 45. Lyon: IARC, pp. 39–117.

ISELIUS L, JACOBS P, MORTON N. 1990. Leukaemia and transient leukaemia in Down Syndrome. Hum Genet 85:477–485.

ISHIHARA T, KOHNO S, MINAMIHISAMATSU M. 1990. Radiation exposure and chromosome abnormalities. Human cytogenetic studies at the Institute of Radiological Sciences, Japan, 1963–1988. Cancer Genet Cytogenet 45:13–33.

ISHIMARU T, OTAKE M, ICHIMARU M. 1979. Dose-response relationship of neutrons and gamma rays to leukemia incidence among atomic bomb survivors in Hiroshima and Nagasaki by type of leukemia, 1950–1971. Radiat Res 77:377–394.

ISOMAKI HA, HAKULINEN T, JOUSENLAHTI U. 1982. Excess risk of lymphomas, leukemia and myeloma in patients with rheumatoid arthritis. Ann Rheum Dis 41 (Suppl):34–36.

ISSITT PD. 1977. Autoimmune hemolytic anemia and cold hemagglutinin disease. Clinical disease and laboratory findings. Prog Clin Pathol 7:137–141.

JABLON S, BOICE JD JR. 1993. Mortality among workers at a nuclear power plant in the United States. Cancer Causes Control 4:427–430.

JABLON S, HRUBEC Z, BOICE JD JR. 1991. Cancer in populations living near nuclear facilities. JAMA 265:1403–1408.

JABLON S, HRUBEC Z, STONE BJ, BOICE JD JR. 1990. Cancer in Populations Living Near Nuclear Facilities. NIH Publ 90-874. Washington, D.C., U.S. Government Printing Office.

JABLON S, ISHIDA M, YAMASAKI M. 1965. Studies of the mortality of A-bomb survivors. 3. Description of the sample and mortality, 1950–1960. Radiat Res 25:25–52.

JABLON S, KATO H. 1970. Childhood cancer in relation to pre-natal exposure to atomic-bomb radiation. Lancet 2:1000–1002.

JABLON S, MILLER RW. 1978. Army technologists: 29-year follow up for cause of death. Radiology 126:677–679.

JACKSON EW, NORRIS FD, KLAUBER MR. 1969. Childhood leukemia in California-born twins. Cancer 23:913–919.

JACKSON EW, TURNER JH, KLAUBER MR, et al. 1968. Down's syndrome: Variation of leukemia occurrence in institutionalized populations. J Chronic Dis 21:247–253.

JEANNET M, MAGNIN C. 1971. HLA antigens in malignant diseases. Transplant Proc 3:1301–1303.

JELKE H. 1939. Acute lymphatisch Leukamie bei eineiigen Zwillingen. Acta Paediatr 27:87–136.

JENSEN OM. 1979. Cancer morbidity and causes of death among Danish brewery workers. Int J Cancer 23:454–463.

JOHNSON CJ. 1987. A cohort study of cancer incidence in Mormon families exposed to nuclear fallout versus an area-based study of cancer deaths in whites in Southwestern Utah. Am J Epidemiol 125:166–168.

JOHNSON CJ. 1984. Cancer incidence in an area of radioactive fallout downwind from the Nevada test site. JAMA 251:230–236.

JOHNSON ES, FISCHMAN HK, MATANOSKI GM. 1986. Occurrence of cancer in women in the meat industry. Br J Ind Med 43:597–604.

JUUTILAINEN J, LAARA E, PUKKALA E. 1990. Incidence of leukemia and brain tumors in Finnish workers exposed to ELF magnetic fields. Int Arch Occup Environ Health 62:289–293.

KABAT GC, AUGUSTINE A, HEBERT JR. 1988. Smoking and adult leukemia: A case-control study. J Clin Epidemiol 41:907–914.

KAHN HA. 1966. The Dorn study of smoking and mortality among U.S. Veterans. Report on 8.5 years of observation. Natl Cancer Inst Monogr 19:1–125.

KAJIYAMA W, KASHIWAGI S, IKEMATSU H, et al. 1986. Intra familial transmission of adult T-cell leukemia virus. J Infect Dis 154:851–857.

KALDOR J, CLAYTON D. 1989. Role of advanced statistical techniques in cancer mapping. Recent Results Cancer Res 114:87–91.

KALDOR JM, DAY NE, CLARKE EA, et al. 1990a. Leukemia following Hodgkin's disease. N Engl J Med 322:7–13.

KALDOR JM, DAY NE, PETTERSON F, et al. 1990b. Leukemia following chemotherapy for ovarian cancer. N Engl J Med 322:1–6.

KALYANARAMAN US, SARNGADHARAN MG, ROBERT-GUROFF M, et al. 1982. A new subtype of human T-cell leukemia virus (HTLV-II) associated with a T-cell variant of hairy cell leukemia. Science 218:571–573.

KAMIHIRA S, NAKASOMA S, OYAKOWA Y, et al. 1987. Transmission of human T cell lymphotropic virus type I by blood transfusion before and after mass screening of sera from seropositive donors. Vox Sang 52:43–44.

KAMIHIRA S, YAMADA Y, IKEDA S, et al. 1992. Risk of adult T-cell leukemia developing in individuals with HTLV-I infection. Leuk Lymph 6:437–439.

KAPLAN SD. 1986. Update of a monthly study of workers in petrochemical refineries. J Occup Med 28:514–516.

KASHIWAGI S, KAJIYAMA W, HAYASHI J, et al. 1986. No significant changes in adult T-cell leukemia virus infection in Okinawa after intervals of 13 and 15 years. Jpn J Cancer Res 77:452–455.

KATO S, TSUJI K, TSUNEMATSU Y, et al. 1983. Familial leukemia HLA system and leukemia predisposition in a family. Am J Dis Child 137:641–644.

KATZ RM, JOWETT D. 1981. Female laundry and dry cleaning workers in Wisconsin: A mortality analysis. Am J Public Health 71:305–307.

KAY K. 1976. Toxicologic and carcinogenic evaluation of chemicals used in the graphic arts industries. Clin Toxicol 9:359–390.

KENDALL GM, MUIRHEAD CR, MACGIBBON BH, et al. 1992. Mortality and occupational exposure to radiation: First analysis of the National Registry for Radiation Workers. Br Med J 304:220–225.

KEOGH EV, MCCALL. 1958. Mortality from leukemia in Victoria, 1946–1955: A report from the Central Cancer Registry, Melbourne. Med J Aust 2:632–639.

KHABBAZ RF, DARROW WW, HARTLEY TM, et al. 1990. Seroprevalence and risk factors for HTLV-I/II infection among female prostitutes in the United States. JAMA 263:555–560.

KINLEN L. 1985. Incidence of cancer in rheumatoid arthritis patients and other disorders after immunosuppression therapy. Am J Med 78(Suppl):44–49.

KINLEN L. 1988. Evidence for an infective cause of childhood leukaemia: Comparison of a Scottish New Town with nuclear reprocessing sites in Britain. Lancet 2:1323–1326.

KINLEN LJ. 1993. Can paternal preconceptional radiation account for the increase of leukaemia and non-Hodgkin's lymphoma in Seascale? Br Med J 306:1718–1721.

KINLEN LJ. 1994. Leukaemia. *In* Doll R, Fraumeni JF Jr, Muir CS (eds): Trends in Cancer Incidence and Mortality. New York, Cold Spring Harbor Laboratory Press, pp. 475–491.

KINLEN LJ. 1995. Epidemiological evidence for an infective basis in childhood leukaemia. Br J Cancer 71:1–5.

KINLEN LJ, CLARKE K, BALKWILL A. 1993. Paternal preconceptional radiation exposure in the nuclear industry and leukaemia and non-Hodgkin's lymphoma in young people in Scotland. Br Med J 306:1153–1158.

KINLEN LJ, CLARKE K, HUDSON C. 1990. Evidence from population mixing in British New Towns 1946–85 of an infective basis for childhood leukaemia. Lancet 336:577–582.

KINLEN LJ, DICKSON M, STILLER CA. 1995. Childhood leukaemia and non-Hodgkin's lymphoma near large rural construction sites, with a comparison with Sellafield nuclear site. Br Med J 310:763–768.

KINLEN LJ, HUDSON C. 1991. Childhood leukaemia and poliomyelitis in relation to military encampments in England and Wales in the period of national military service 1950–63. Br Med J 303:1357–1362.

KINLEN LJ, HUDSON C, STILLER CA. 1991. Contrasts between adults as evidence for an infective origin of childhood leukaemia: An explanation for the excess near nuclear establishments in West Berkshire? Br J Cancer 64:549–554.

KINLEN LJ, O'BRIEN F, CLARKE K, et al. 1993. Rural population mixing and childhood leukaemia: Effects of the North Sea oil industry in Scotland, including the area near Dounreay nuclear site. Br Med J 306:743–748.

KINLEN LJ, PIKE MC. 1971. BCG vaccination and leukaemia. Evidence of vital statistics. Lancet 2:398–402.

KINLEN LJ, ROGOT E. 1988. Leukaemia and smoking habits among United States veterans. Br Med J 297:657–659.

KINLEN LJ, SHEIL AGR, PETO J, et al. 1979. Collaborative United Kingdom Australasian study of cancer in patients treated with immunosuppressive drugs. Br Med J 2:1461–1466.

KINLEN LJ, WEBSTER ADB, BIRD AG, et al. 1985. Prospective study of cancer in patients with hypogammaglobulinemia. Lancet 1:263–265.

KINOSHITA K, AMAGASAKI T, HIRO S, et al. 1987. Milk-borne transmission of HTLV-I from carrier mothers to their children. Jpn J Cancer Res 78:674–680.

KLASSEN DJ. 1969. Acute leukemia in children in the province of Saskatchewan, 1961–66. Can Med Assoc J 101:87–90.

KLEBANOFF MA, READ JS, MILLS JL, et al. 1993. The risk of childhood cancer after neonatal exposure to vitamin K. N Engl J Med 329:905–908.

KLOUDA PT, LAWLER SD, TILL MM, et al. 1974. Acute lymphoblastic leukaemia and HL-A: A prospective study. Tissue Antigens 4:262–265.

KNEALE GW, STEWART AM, KINNEAR WILSON LM. 1986. Immunizations against infectious diseases and childhood cancers. Cancer Immunol Immunother 21:129–132.

KNOX G. 1963. Detection of low intensity epidemicity: Application to cleft lip and palate. Br J Prev Soc Med 17:121–129.

KONDO T, KONO H, MIYAMOTO N, et al. 1989. Age- and sex-specific cumulative rate and risk of ATLL for HTLV-I carriers. Int J Cancer 43:1061–1064.

KUMAMOTO Y. 1985. Population doses, excess deaths and loss of life expectancy from mass chest x-ray examinations in Japan-1980. Health Physics 49:37–48.

KURIHARA M, AOKI K, TOMINAGA S. 1984. Cancer Mortality Statistics in the World. Nagoya, The University of Nagoya Press.

KUSHWAHA MRS, CHANDRA D, MISRA NC, et al. 1985. Leukemias and lymphomas at Lucknow. Leuk Res 9:799–802.

KUSUHARA K, SONODA S, TAKAHASHI K, et al. 1987. Mother-to-child transmission of human T cell leukemia virus type I (HTLV-I): A fifteen-year follow-up study in Okinawa, Japan. Int J Cancer 40:755–757.

KVARNFORS B, HENRICSON B, HUGOSON G. 1975. A statistical study on farm and village level in the possible relations between human leukemia and bovine leukosis. Acta Vet Scand 16:163–169.

KYLE RA. 1982. Second malignancies associated with chemotherapeutic agents. Semin Oncol 9:131–142.

KYLE RA. 1984. Second malignancies associated with chemotherapy. *In* Perry MC, Yarbro W (eds): Toxicity of Chemotherapy. Orlando, Grune & Stratton, pp. 479–506.

KYLE RA, PIERRE RV, BAYRD ED. 1970. Multiple myeloma and acute myelomonocytic leukemia: Report of four cases possibly related to melphalan. N Engl J Med 283:1121–1125.

LAGAKOS SW, WESSEN BJ, ZELEN M. 1986. An analysis of contaminated well water and health effects in Woburn, Massachusetts. J Am Stat Assoc 81:583–596.

LAGRENADE L, HANCHARD B, FLETCHER V, et al. 1990. Infective dermatitis of Jamaican children: A marker for HTLV-I infection. Lancet 336:1345–1347.

LAIRMORE MD, JACOBSON S, GRACIA F, et al. 1990. Isolation of human T-lymphotropic virus type 2 from Guaymi Indians in Panama. Proc Natl Acad Sci USA 87:8840–8844.

LAND CE. 1979. The hazards of fallout or of epidemiologic research. N Engl J Med 300:431–432.

LAND CE, MCKAY FW, MACHADO SG, et al. 1984. Childhood leukemia and fallout from the Nevada nuclear tests. Science 223:139–144.

LAVAL G, TUYNS AJ. 1988. Environmental factors in childhood leukemia. Br J Ind Med 45:843–844.

LAVEY RS, EBY NL, PROSNITZ LR. 1990. Impact on second malignancy risk of the combined use of radiation and chemotherapy for lymphomas. Cancer 66:80–88.

LE BEAU MM, ALBAIN KS, LARSON RA, et al. 1986. Clinical and cytogenetic correlations in 63 patients with therapy-related myelodysplastic syndromes and acute nonlymphocytic leukemia: Further evidence for characteristic abnormalities of chromosomes No. 5 and 7. J Clin Oncol 4:325–345.

LEE H, SWANSON P, SHORTY V, et al. 1989. High rate of HTLV-II infection in seropositive IV drug abusers in New Orleans. Science 244:471–475.

LEE K, BAGLIN TP, MARCUS RE. 1991. Therapy-related leukaemia in Wegener's granulomatosis. Clin Lab Haemotol 13:207–209.

LEMAN RA, YOUNG R. 1976. Investigations of health hazards in SBR facilities. *In* Proceedings of the NIOSH Styrene-Butadiene Briefing, Covington, Kentucky, April 30, 1976. DHEW Publ No. (NIOSH) 77-129, pp. 3–8.

LEMEN RA, MEINHARDT TJ, CRANDALE MS, et al. 1990. Environmental epidemiologic investigations in the styrene-butadiene rubber production industry. Environ Health Perspect 86:103–106.

LEVINE EG, BLOOMFIELD CD. 1986. Secondary myelodysplastic syndromes and leukemias. Clin Haematol 15:1037–1080.

LEVINE PH, MANNS A, JAFFE ES, et al. 1994. The effect of ethnic differences on the patterns of HTLV-I-associated T-cell leukemia/lymphoma in the United States. Int J Cancer 56:177–181.

LEWIS CA, SMITH PG, STRATTON IM, et al. 1988. Estimated radiation doses to different organs among patients treated for ankylosing spondylitis with a single course of x-rays. Br J Radiol 61:212–220.

LEWIS MS. 1980. Spatial clustering in childhood leukaemia. J Chronic Dis 33:703–712.

LI FP, FRAUMENI JF JR. 1982. Prospective study of a cancer family syndrome. JAMA 247:2692–2694.

LI GL, LINET MS, HAYES RB, et al. 1994. Gender differences in hematopoietic and lymphoproliferative and other cancer risk by major occupational group among workers exposed to benzene in China. I. Descriptive findings. J Occup Med 36:875–881.

LILLEYMAN JS. 1978. Schwachman's syndrome and acute lymphoblastic leukaemia. Br Med J 2:6129.

LILLICRAP DA, STERNDALE H. 1984. Familial chronic myeloid leukaemia. Lancet 2:699.

LINDQVIST R, NILSSON B, EKLUND G, et al. 1987. Increased risk of developing acute leukemia after employment as a painter. Cancer 60:1378–1384.

LINDQVIST R, NILSSON B, EKLUND G, et al. 1991. Acute leukemia in professional drivers exposed to gasoline and diesel. Eur J Haematol 47:98–103.

LINET MS. 1985. The Leukemias: Epidemiologic Aspects. New York, Oxford University Press.

LINET MS, BLATTNER WA. 1988. The epidemiology of chronic lymphocytic leukemia. *In* Polliack A, Catovsky D (eds): Chronic Lymphocytic Leukemia. Chur, Switzerland, Harwood Academic Press, pp. 11–32.

LINET MS, BOICE JD JR. 1993. Radiation from Chernobyl and risk of childhood leukemia. Eur J Cancer 29A:1–3.

LINET MS, DEVESA SS. 1990. Descriptive epidemiology of the leukemias. *In* Henderson ES, Lister TA (eds): Leukemia, 5th ed. Philadelphia, WB Saunders, pp. 207–224.

LINET MS, DEVESA SS. 1991. Descriptive epidemiology of childhood leukaemia. Br J Cancer 63:424–429.

LINET MS, MCCAFFREY LD, HYMPHREY RL, et al. 1986. Chronic lymphocytic leukemia and acquired disorders affecting the immune system: A case-control study. J Natl Cancer Inst 77:371–378.

LINET MS, MALKER HSR, MCLAUGHLIN JK, et al. 1988a. Leukemias and occupation in Sweden: A registry-based analysis. Am J Ind Med 14:319–330.

LINET MS, MCLAUGHLIN JK, HARLOW SD, et al. 1988b. Family history of autoimmune disorders and cancer in multiple myeloma. Int J Epidemiol 17:512–513.

LINET MS, BIAS WB, DORGAN JF, et al. 1988c. HLA antigens in chronic lymphocytic leukemia. Tissue Antigens 31:71–78.

LINET MS, MCLAUGHLIN JK, HSING AW, et al. 1991. Relationship of cigarette smoking and leukemia: Results from the Lutheran Brotherhood cohort study. Cancer Causes Control 2:413–417.

LINET MS, VAN NATTA ML, BROOKMEYER R, et al. 1989. Familial cancer history and chronic lymphocytic leukemia. A case-control study. Am J Epidemiol 130:655–664.

LINGEMAN CH. 1963. The epidemiologic approach to leukemia. II. Geographic distribution in Indiana 1951–1960. J Indiana State Med Assoc 56:405–411.

LINOS A, BLAIR A, CANTOR KP, et al. 1989. Leukemia and non-Hodgkin's lymphoma among embalmers and funeral directors. J Natl Cancer Inst 82:66.

LINOS A, KYLE RA, ELVEBACK LR, et al. 1978. Leukemia in Olmstead County, Minnesota, 1965–74. Mayo Clin Proc 53:714–720.

LINOS A, KYLE RA, O'FALLON WM, et al. 1980. A case-control study of occupational exposures and leukemia. Int J Epidemiol 9:131–135.

LINOS A, KYLE R, O'FALLON WM. 1981. Leukemia and prior malignant and hematologic diseases: A case-control study. Am J Epidemiol 113:285–289.

LLOYD JW, DECOUFLE P, SALVIN LG. 1977. Unusual mortality experience of printing pressmen. J Occup Med 19:543–550.

LOCASCIULLI A, SANTARRARIA M, MASERA G, et al. 1985. Hepatitis B virus markers in children with acute leukemia. The effect of chemotherapy. J Med Virol 15:29–33.

LOGUE JN, BARRICK MK, JESSUP GL. 1986. Mortality of radiologists and pathologists in the radiation registry of physicians. J Occup Med 28:91–99.

LONDON SJ, BOWMAN JD, SOBEL E, et al. 1994. Exposure to magnetic fields among electrical workers in relation to leukemia risk in Los Angeles County. Am J Ind Med 26:47–60.

LONDON SJ, THOMAS DC, BOWMAN JD, et al. 1991. Exposure to residential electric and magnetic fields and risk of childhood leukemia. Am J Epidemiol 134:923–937.

LOWENGART RA, PETERS JM, CICCIONI C, et al. 1987. Childhood leukemia and parents' occupational and home exposures. J Natl Cancer Inst 79:39–46.

LOWENTHAL MN. 1976. Chronic myeloid leukemia in Zambians. Trop Geogr Med 27:132–137.

LUNDIN F, FRAUMENI J, LLOYD WJ, et al. 1966. Temporal relationship of leukemia and lymphoma deaths in neighborhoods. J Natl Cancer Inst 37:123–133.

LYMAN GH, LYMAN CG, JOHNSON W. 1985. Association of leukemia with radium groundwater contamination. JAMA 254:621–626.

LYNGE E. 1985. A follow-up study of cancer incidence among workers in manufacture of phenoxy herbicides in Denmark. Br J Cancer 52:259–270.

LYON JL, KLAUBER MR, GARDNER J, et al. 1979. Childhood leukemias associated with fallout from nuclear testing. N Engl J Med 300:397–402.

LYON JL, SCHUMAN KL. 1984. Radioactive fallout and cancer. JAMA 252:1854–1855.

MACHADO SG, LAND CE, MCKAY FW. 1987. Cancer mortality and radioactive fallout in southwestern Utah. Am J Epidemiol 125:44–61.

MACKLIS RM, MAUCH PM, BURAKOFF SJ, et al. 1992. Lymphoid irradiation results in long-term increases in natural killer cells in patients treated for Hodgkin's disease. Cancer 69:778–783.

MACMAHON B. 1962. Prenatal x-ray exposure and childhood cancer. J Natl Cancer Inst 28:1173–1191.

MACMAHON B, LEVY M. 1964. Prenatal origin of childhood leukemia: Evidence from twins. N Engl J Med 270:1082–1085.

MACMAHON B, PRENTICE RL, ROGAN WJ, et al. 1986. Comment. J Am Stat Assoc 81:597–610.

MACSWEEN JM, FERNANDEZ LA, EASTWOOD SL, et al. 1980. Restricted genetic heterogeneity in families of patients with acute lymphocytic leukemia. Tissue Antigens 16:70–72.

MAGNANI C, PASTORE G, LUZZATTO L, et al. 1990. Parental occupation and other environmental factors in the etiology of leukaemias and non-Hodgkin's lymphomas in childhood: A case-control study. Tumori 76:413–419.

MANCUSO TF. 1975. Epidemiological investigation of occupational cancers in the rubber industry. *In* Levinson C (ed): The New Multinational Health Hazards. Geneva, ICF, pp. 80–136.

MANN DL, DESANTIS P, MARK G, et al. 1987. HTLV-I associated B-cell CLL: Indirect role for retrovirus in leukemogenesis. Science 236:1103–1106.

MANNS A. 1994. Natural history of HTLV-I infection: Relationship to leukemogenesis. Leukemia 7(Suppl 2):575–577.

MANNS A, BLATTNER WA. 1991. The epidemiology of HTLV-I and HTLV-II: Etiologic role in human disease. Transfusion 31:67–75.

MANNS A, FALK R, MURPHY EL, et al. 1990. Risk factors for development of non-Hodgkin's lymphoma in Jamaica. *Proceedings of the American Association for Cancer Research,* 31:229 (Abstract 1358).

MANNS A, MURPHY EL, WILKS R, et al. 1988. Transfusion transmission HTLV-I: Seroconversion in a prospective cohort of recipients. Blood 72(Suppl 1):72:356A.

MANNS A, WILKS RJ, MURPHY EL, et al. 1992. A prospective study of transmission by transfusion of HTLV-I and risk factors associated with seroconversion. Int J Cancer 51:886–891.

MANTEL N. 1967. The detection of disease clustering and a generalized regression approach. Cancer Res 27:209–222.

MARKOWITZ J. 1984. Acute nonlymphocytic leukemia: Population-based epidemiologic study. Doctoral thesis. The Johns Hopkins University, Baltimore.

MARKOWITZ JA, SZKLO M, SENSENBRENNER LL, et al. 1985. Hair dyes and acute nonlymphoctic leukemia (ANLL). Am J Epidemiol 122:523.

MAROLLEAU JP, BRICE P, MOREL P, et al. 1993. Secondary acute myeloid leukemia after autologous bone marrow transplantation for malignant lymphomas. J Clin Oncol 11:590–591.

MARSH GM, ENTERLINE PE, MCGRAW D. 1991. Mortality patterns among petroleum refinery and chemical plant workers. Am J Ind Med 19:29–42.

MASON TJ, MCKAY FW, HOOVER R, et al. 1975. Atlas of Cancer Mortality in US Counties, 1950–69. DHEW (NIH) Pub No. 76-1204. Washington, DC: U.S. Government Printing Office.

MATANOSKI GM. 1989. Risk of Pathologists Exposed to Formaldehyde. Final Report. DHHS Grant No. 5 RO1OH01511-03. Cincinnati, OH: National Institute for Occupational Safety and Health. Centers for Disease Control.

MATANOSKI GM, ELLIOTT EA, BREYSSE PN, et al. 1993. Leukemia in telephone linemen. Am J Epidemiol 137:609–619.

MATANOSKI GM, SANTOS-BURGOA C, SCHWARTZ L. 1990. Mortality of a cohort of workers in the styrene-butadiene polymer manufacturing industry (1943–1982). Environ Health Perspect 86:107–117.

MATANOSKI GM, SARTWELL P, ELLIOTT E, et al. 1984. Cancer risks in radiologists and radiation workers. *In* Boice JD Jr, Fraumeni JF Jr (eds): Radiation Carcinogenesis: Epidemiology and Biological Significance. New York, Raven Press, pp. 83–96.

MATANOSKI GM, SELTSER R, SARTWELL PE, et al. 1975. The current mortality rates of radiologists and other physician specialists. Am J Epidemiol 101:188–210.

MATANOSKI GM, STOCKWELL HG, DIAMOND EL, et al. 1986. A cohort mortality study of painters and allied tradesmen. Scand J Work Environ Health 12:16–21.

MATSUI I, TANIMURA M, KOBAYASHI N, et al. 1993. Neurofibromatosis type 1 and childhood cancer. Cancer 72:2746–2754.

MATSUO T, TOMONAGA M, BENNETT JM, et al. 1988. Reclassification of leukemia among A-bomb survivors in Nagasaki using French-American-British (FAB) classification for acute leukemia. Jpn J Clin Oncol 18:91–96.

MATTSON B, WALLGREN J. 1984. Completeness of registration in the Swedish Cancer Registry. Non-notified cancer recorded on death certificates in 1978. Acta Radiol (Oncol) 23:305–131.

MAYER V, EBBESSEN P. 1991. HTLV-I virus in Europeans: The continuous spread. A meta-analysis. Acta Virol 25:472–495.

MCCORMICK DP, AMMANN AJ, ISHIZAKA K, et al. 1971. A study of allergy in patients with malignant lymphoma and chronic lymphocytic leukemia. Cancer 27:93–99.

MCCRAW DS, JOYNER RE, COLE P, et al. 1985. Excess leukemia in a refinery population. J Occup Med 27:220–222.

MCDOWALL ME. 1983. Leukaemia mortality in electrical workers in England and Wales. Lancet 1:246.

MCDOWALL ME. 1986. Mortality of persons resident in the vicinity of electricity transmission facilities. Br J Cancer 53:271–279.

MCKINNEY PA, ALEXANDER FE, CARTWRIGHT RA, et al. 1989a. The Leukaemia Research Fund Data Collection Study: Descriptive epidemiology of acute lymphoblastic leukemia. Leukemia 3:880–885.

MCKINNEY PA, ALEXANDER FE, CARTWRIGHT RA, et al. 1989b. The Leukaemia Research Fund Data Collection Survey: The incidence and geographical distribution of acute myeloid leukemia. Leukemia 3:875–879.

McKinney PA, Alexander FE, Cartwright RA. 1991. Parental occupation of children with leukaemia in west Cumbria, North Humberside, and Gateshead. Br Med J 302:681–687.

McKinney PA, Alexander FE, Roberts BE, et al. 1990. Yorkshire case control study of leukemias and lymphomas: Parallel multivariate analysis of seven disease categories. Leuk Lymph 2:67–80.

McKinney PA, Cartwright RA, Saiu JMT, et al. 1987. The inter-regional epidemiological study of childhood cancer (IRESCC): A case control study of etiological factors in leukemia and lymphoma. Arch Dis Child 62:279–287.

McLaughlin JK, Hrubec Z, Linet MS, et al. 1989. Cigarette smoking and leukemia. J Natl Cancer Inst 81:1262–1263.

McLaughlin JR, Clarke EA, Nishri ED, et al. 1993. Childhood leukemia in the vicinity of Canadian nuclear facilities. Cancer Causes Control 4:51–58.

McLaughlin JR, King WD, Anderson TW, et al. 1992. Paternal radiation exposure among leukemia in offspring: The Ontario case-control study. Br Med J 307:959–966.

McMichael AJ, Spirtas R, Gamble JF, et al. 1976. Mortality among rubber workers: Relationship to specific jobs. J Occup Med 18:178–185.

McWhirter WR, Chant DC. 1990. A study of antenatal factors associated with the occurrence of childhood leukemia. Cancer Ther Control 1:133–139.

McWhirter WR, Savage DC, Williams BM. 1971. Neurofibromatosis with leukaemia. Br Med J 4:114–115.

Mecucci C, Ghione F, Louwagie A, et al. 1986. Variant translocation t(7;9;22) during lymphoid blastic crisis in a case of Ph^1 positive chronic myelogenous leukemia with previous EBV infection. Acta Haematol 75:46–48.

Mele A, Szklo M, Visani G, et al. 1994. Hair dye use and other risk factors for leukemia and pre-leukemia. Am J Epidemiol 139:609–619.

Michaelis J, Keller B, Haaf G, et al. 1992. Incidence of childhood malignancies in the vicinity of West German nuclear power plants. Cancer Causes Control 3:255–263.

Milham S Jr. 1971. Leukemia and multiple myeloma in farmers. Am J Epidemiol 92:307–310.

Milham S Jr. 1982. Mortality from leukemia in workers exposed to electrical and magnetic fields. N Engl J Med 307:249.

Milham S Jr. 1988. Increased mortality in amateur radio operators due to lymphatic and hematopoietic neoplasms. Am J Epidemiol 127:50–54.

Milham S Jr. 1976. Occupational Mortality in Washington State, 1950–71, Vols. 1-3. DHEW, PHS. Washington, D.C.: U.S. Government Printing Office.

Miller BA, Blair AE, Raynor HL, et al. 1989. Cancer and other mortality patterns among United States furniture workers. Br J Ind Med 46:508–515.

Miller BA, Linet MS, Cheson BD. 1993. Leukemias. *In* Miller BA, Ries LAG, Hankey BH, et al (eds): Cancer Statistics Review 1973–1990. Bethesda, National Cancer Institute NIH Pub. No. 93-2789, pp. XIII.1–23.

Miller GJ, Pegram SM, Kirkwood BR, et al. 1986. The composition, age, and sex, together with location and type of housing as determinants of HTLV-I infection in a Trinidadian Community. Int J Cancer 38:801–807.

Miller RW. 1963. Down's syndrome (mongolism), other congenital malformations and cancers among sibs of leukemic children. N Engl J Med 268:393–401.

Miller RW. 1967. Persons at exceptionally high risk of leukemia. Cancer Res 27:2420–2423.

Miller RW. 1968. Relation between cancer and congenital defects: An epidemiologic evaluation. J Natl Cancer Inst 40:1079–1085.

Miller RW. 1971. Deaths from childhood leukemia and solid tumors among twins and other sibs in the United States, 1960–67. J Natl Cancer Inst 46:203–209.

Miller RW. 1992. Childhood leukemia and neonatal exposure to lighting in nurseries. Cancer Causes Control (letter) 3:581–582.

Miller RW, McKay FW. 1984. Decline in U.S. childhood cancer mortality, 1950 through 1980. JAMA 251:1567–1570.

Mills PK, Newell GR, Beeson WL, et al. 1990. History of cigarette smoking and risk of leukemia and myeloma: Results from the Adventist health study. J Natl Cancer Inst 82:1832–1836.

Minamoto GY, Gold JWM, Scheinberg DA, et al. 1988. Infection with human T-cell leukemia virus type I in patients with leukemia. N Engl J Med 318:219–222.

Mir-Madjlessi SHM, Farmer RG, Weick JK. 1986. Inflammatory bowel disease and leukemia. Dig Dis Sci 31:1025–1031.

Mitelman F. 1986. Geographic heterogeneity of chromosome aberrations in hematologic disorders. Cancer Genet Cytogenet 20:203–208.

Mitelman F, Nilsson PG, Brandt L, et al. 1981. Chromosome pattern, occupation, and clinical features in patients with acute nonlymphocytic leukemia. Cancer Genet Cytogenet 4:197–214.

Modan B, Lilienfeld AM. 1965. Polycythemia vera and leukemia—the role of radiation treatment: A study of 1222 patients. Medicine 44:305–344.

Mole RH. 1974. Antenatal irradiation and childhood cancer: Causation or coincidence? Br J Cancer 30:199–208.

Moloney WC. 1987. Radiogenic leukemia revisited. Blood 70:905–908.

Momita S, Ikeda S, Amagasaki T, et al. 1990. Survey of anti-human T-cell leukemia virus type I antibody in family members of patients with adult T-cell leukemia. Jpn J Cancer Res 81:884–889.

Monson RR, Fine LJ. 1978. Cancer mortality and morbidity among rubber workers. J Natl Cancer Inst 61:1047–1053.

Monson RR, MacMahon B. 1984. Prenatal x-ray exposure and cancer in children. *In* Boice JD Jr, Fraumeni JF Jr (eds): Radiation Carcinogenesis: Epidemiology and Biological Significance. New York, Raven Press, pp. 107–118.

Monson RR, Nakano KK. 1976. Mortality among rubber workers. I. White male union employees in Akron, Ohio. Am J Epidemiol 103:284–296.

Morbidity and Mortality Weekly Report. 1990. Human T-Lymphotropic Virus Type I screening in volunteer blood donors—United States, 1989. MMWR 39:915–924.

Morgan RW, Kaplan SD, Gaffey WR. 1981a. A general mortality study of production workers in the paint and coatings manufacturing industry: A preliminary report. J Occup Med 23:13–21.

Morgan RW, Claxton KW, Divine BJ, et al. 1981b. Mortality among ethylene oxide workers. J Occup Med 25:767–770.

Morgan RW, Claxton KW, Kaplan SD, et al. 1985. Mortality of paint and coatings industry workers. J Occup Med 27:377–378.

Mori T, Kato Y, Aoki N, et al. 1983. Statistical analysis of Japanese Thorotrast-administered autopsy cases-1980. Health Physics 44:281–292.

Morrell D, Cromartic E, Swift M. 1986. Mortality and cancer incidence in 263 patients with ataxia-telangiectasia. J Natl Cancer Inst 77:89–92.

Morris M, Knorr RS. 1990. Southeastern Massachusetts Health Study 1975–1990. Boston, MA: Division of Environmental Health Assessment, Department of Public Health, Commonwealth of Massachusetts: October 1990.

Morrison HI, Semenciw RM, Mao Y, et al. 1988. Cancer mortality among a group of fluorspar miners exposed to radon progeny. Am J Epidemiol 128:1266–1275.

Mueller N. 1991. The epidemiology of HTLV-I infection. Cancer Causes Control 2:37–52.

Muir C, Waterhouse J, Mack T, et al. 1987. Cancer Incidence

in Five Continents. Volume 5. IARC Scientific Publications No. 88. Lyon: IARC.

MUIR KR, PARKES SE, MANN JR, et al. 1990. 'Clustering'—real or apparent? Probability maps of childhood cancer in the West Midlands Health Authority region. Int J Epidemiol 19:853–859.

MUIRHEAD CR, BUTLAND BK, GREEN BMR, et al. 1991. Childhood leukaemia and natural radiation. Lancet 337:503–504.

MULLER CA, HASMAN R, GROSSE-WILDE H, et al. 1988. Significant association of acute lymphoblastic leukemia with HLA-Cw7. Genet Epidemiol 5:453–461.

MURPHY EL. 1993. HTLV-II disease. Lancet 341:888.

MURPHY EL, BLATTNER WA. 1988. HTLV-I associated leukemia: A model for chronic retroviral disease. Ann Neuro 23(Suppl):S174–S180.

MURPHY EL, FIGUEROA JP, GIBBS WN, et al. 1989a. Sexual transmission of HTLV-I. Ann Intern Med 111:555–560.

MURPHY EL, HANCHARD B, FIGUEROA JP, et al. 1989b. Modelling the risk of adult T-cell leukemia/lymphoma in persons infected with human T-lymphotropic virus type I. Int J Cancer 43:250–252.

MYERS A, CLAYDEN AD, CARTWRIGHT RA, et al. 1990. Childhood cancer and overhead powerlines: A case-control study. Br J Cancer 62:1008–1014.

NAJEAN Y. 1987. The iatrogenic leukemias induced by radio- and/or chemotherapy. Med Oncol Tumor Pharmacother 4:245–257.

NAKADA K, YAMAGUCHI K, FURUNGEN S, et al. 1987. Monoclonal integration of HTLV-I proviral DNA in patients with strongyloidiasis. Int J Cancer 40:145–148.

NAROD SA, DUBE ID. 1989. Occupational history and involvement of chromosomes 5 and 7 in acute nonlymphocytic leukemia. Cancer Genet Cytogenet 38:261–269.

NAROD SA, STILLER C, LENOIR GM. 1991. An estimate of the heritable fraction of childhood cancer. Br J Cancer 63:993–999.

NATIONAL RADIOLOGICAL PROTECTION BOARD. 1992. Electromagnetic Fields and the Risk of Cancer. Report of an Advisory Group on Non-Ionizing Radiation. Vol. 3, No. 1. Chilton, Didcot, Oxon, National Radiological Protection Board.

NATIONAL RESEARCH COUNCIL COMMITTEE ON THE BIOLOGIC EFFECTS OF IONIZING RADIATION. 1980. The Effects on Populations of Exposure to Low Levels of Ionizing Radiation (BEIR III). Washington, DC, National Academy Press.

NATIONAL RESEARCH COUNCIL COMMITTEE ON THE BIOLOGIC EFFECTS OF IONIZING RADIATION. 1988. Health Risks of Radon and Other Internally Deposited Alpha-Emitters (BEIR IV). Washington, DC, National Academy Press.

NATIONAL RESEARCH COUNCIL COMMITTEE ON THE BIOLOGIC EFFECTS OF IONIZING RADIATION. 1990. The Effects on Populations of Exposure to Low Levels of Ionizing Radiation (BEIR V). Washington, DC, National Academy Press.

NEEL JV, SCHULL WJ, AWA A, et al. 1990. The children of parents exposed to atomic bombs: Estimates of the genetic doubling dose of radiation for humans. Am J Hum Genet 46:1053–1072.

NEGLIA JP, MEADOWS AT, ROBISON LL, et al. 1991. Second neoplasms after acute lymphoblastic leukemia in childhood. N Engl J Med 325:1330–1336.

NEGLIA JP, ROBISON LL. 1988. Epidemiology of childhood acute leukemias. Pediatr Clin N Am 35:675–692.

NEGLIA JP, SEVERSON RK, LINET MS. 1990. Toward a testable etiology of childhood acute lymphocytic leukemia. Leukemia 4:517–521.

NEULAND CY, BLATTNER WA, MANN DL, et al. 1983. Familial chronic lymphocytic leukemia. J Natl Cancer Inst 71:1143–1150.

NICHOLS CR. 1991. Malignant hematologic disorders arising from industrial germ cell tumors. A review of clinical and biologic features. Leuk Lymph 4:221–229.

NICHOLS CR, BREEDEN ES, LOEHRER PJ, et al. 1993. Secondary leukemia associated with a conventional dose of Etoposide: Review of serial germ cell tumor protocols. J Natl Cancer Inst 85:36–40.

NICHOLSON WJ, SELIKOFF IJ, SEIDMAN H. 1978. Mortality experience of styrene-polystyrene polymerization workers. Scand J Work Environ Health 4(Suppl 2):247–252.

NISHI M, MIYAKE H. 1989. A case-control study of non-T cell acute lymphoblastic leukaemia of children in Hokkaido, Japan. J Epidemiol Community Health 43:352–355.

NISHIYAMA H. 1969. Relative frequency and mortality rate of various types of leukemia in Japan. Gann 60:71–81.

OBRASTZOW V. 1890. Zwei Falle von actuer Leukamie. Deutsch Med Wochenschr 16:44.

O'BRIEN TR, DECOUFLE P. 1988. Cancer mortality among northern Georgia carpet and textile workers. Am J Ind Med 14:15–24.

OGUMA N, TAKEMOTO M, ODA K, et al. 1989. Chronic myelogenous leukemia and Klinefelter's syndrome. Eur J Haematol 42:207–208.

OKANY CC, AKINYANJU OO. 1989. Chronic leukemia: An African experience. Med Oncol Tumor Pharmacother 6:189–194.

OKOCHI K, SATO H, HINUMA Y. 1984. A retrospective study on transmission of adult T cell leukemia virus by blood transfusion: Seroconversion in recipients. Vox Sang 46:245–253.

OKPALA I. 1990. Contrasting sex distribution of chronic lymphocytic leukaemia and well-differentiated diffuse lymphocytic lymphoma in India, Nigeria. Eur J Cancer 26:1105.

OLIN R, VAGERO O, AHLBOM A. 1985. Mortality experience of electrical engineers. Br J Ind Med 42:211–216.

OLIVER RTD, KLOUDA P, LAUDER S. 1976. HLA associated resistance factors and myelogenous leukemia. *In* HLA and Disease. Paris, Inserm, p. 231.

OLOO AJ, OGADA TA. 1984. Chronic lymphocytic leukemia (CLL): Clinical study at Kenyatta National Hospital (KNH). East Afr Med J 61:797–801.

OLSEN GW, HEARN S, COOK RR, et al. 1989. Mortality experience of a cohort of Louisiana chemical workers. J Occup Med 31:32–34.

OLSEN JH, DE NULLY BROWN P, SCHULGEN G, et al. 1991. Parental employment at time of conception and risk of cancer in offspring. Eur J Cancer 27:958–965.

OLSEN JH, NIELSEN A, SCHULGEN G. 1993. Residence near high voltage facilities and risk of cancer in children. Br Med J 307:891–895.

OSAME M, IGATA A. 1989. The history of discovery and clinico-epidemiology of HTLV-I-associated myelopathy (HAM). Jpn J Med 28:412–414.

OSTERLIND K, HANSEN HH, HANSEN M, et al. 1986. Mortality and morbidity in long-term surviving patients treated with chemotherapy with or without irradiation for small-cell long cancer. J Clin Oncol 4:1044–1052.

OTT MG, KOLESAR RC, SCHARNWEBER HC, et al. 1980a. A mortality survey of employees engaged in the development or manufacture of styrene-based products. J Occup Med 22:445–460.

OTT MG, HOLDER BB, OLSON RD. 1980b. A mortality analysis of employees engaged in the manufacture of 2,4,5-trichlorophenoxyacetic acid. J Occup Med 22:47–50.

OTT MG, TOWNSEND JC, FISHBACK WA, et al. 1978. Mortality among individuals occupationally exposed to benzene. Arch Environ Health 33:3–10.

PACI E, BUIATTI E, COSTANTINI AS, et al. 1989. Aplastic anemia, leukemia and other cancer mortality in a cohort of shoe workers exposed to benzene. Scand J Work Environ Health 15:313–318.

PAFFENBARGER RS, WING AL, HYDE RT. 1978. Characteristics in youth predictive of adult-onset malignant lymphomas, melanomas, and leukemias: Brief communication. J Natl Cancer Inst 60: 89–92.

PAGANINI-HILL A, GLAZER E, HENDERSON BE, et al. 1980. Cause-specific mortality among newspaper web pressman. J Occup Med 22:542–544.

PAPA G, MAURO FR, ANSELMO AP, et al. 1984. Acute leukemia in patients treated for Hodgkin's disease. Br J Haematol 54:43–52.

PARKER L, CRAFT AW, SMITH J, et al. 1992. Geographical distribution of preconceptional radiation doses to fathers employed at the Sellafield nuclear installation, West Cumbria. Br Med J 307:966–971.

PARKES HG, VEYS CA, WATERHOUSE JAH, et al. 1982. Cancer mortality in the British rubber industry. Br J Ind Med 39:209–220.

PARKIN DM, CARDIS E, MASUYER E, et al. 1993. Childhood leukaemia following the Chernobyl accident: The European Childhood Leukaemia-Lymphoma Incidence Study (ECLIS). Eur J Cancer 29A:87–95.

PARKIN DM, MUIR CS, WHELAN SL, et al. 1992. Cancer Incidence in Five Continents, vol 6. Lyon, IARC Scientific Publications No. 120.

PARKIN DM, STILLER CA, DRAPER GJ, et al. 1988. International Incidence of Childhood Cancer. IARC Scientific Publications No. 87. Lyon, IARC.

PEARCE NE. 1988. Leukemia in electrical workers in New Zealand: A correction. Lancet 2:48.

PEARCE N, PRIOR I, METHVEN D, et al. 1990. Follow up of New Zealand participants in British atmospheric nuclear weapons tests in the Pacific. Br Med J 300:1161–1166.

PEARCE N, REIF J, FRASER J. 1989. Case-control studies of cancer in New Zealand electrical workers. Int J Epidemiol 18:55–59.

PEARCE N, REIF JS. 1990. Epidemiologic studies of cancer in agricultural workers. Am J Ind Med 18:133–142.

PEARCE NE, SHEPPARD RA, HOWARD JK, et al. 1986. Leukemia among New Zealand agricultural workers. A cancer registry-based study. Am J Epidemiol 124:402–409.

PEARCE NE, SMITH AH, REIF JS. 1988. Increased risks of soft tissue sarcoma, malignant lymphoma, and acute myeloid leukemia in abattoir workers. Am J Ind Med 14:63–72.

PEARSON HW, GRELLO FW, CONE TE JR. 1963. Leukemia in identical twins. N Engl J Med 268:1151–1156.

PEARSON K, WEBB T. 1913. Multiple cases of disease in the same house. Biometrika 8:430–435.

PEDERSEN-BJERGAARD J, DAUGAARD G, HANSEN SW, et al. 1991. Increased risk of myelodysplasia and leukaemia after etoposide, cisplatin, and bleomycin for germ-cell tumors. Lancet 338:359–363.

PEDERSEN-BJERGAARD J, ERSBOLL J, SORENSEN HM, et al. 1985. Risk of acute nonlymphocytic leukemia and preleukemia in patients treated with cyclophosphamide for non-Hodgkin's lymphoma. Ann Intern Med 103:195–200.

PEDERSEN-BJERGAARD J, PHILIP P. 1989. Therapy-related malignancies: A review. Eur J Haematol 42(Suppl 48):39–47.

PEDERSEN-BJERGAARD J, SPECHT L, LARSEN SO, et al. 1987. Risk of therapy-related leukemia and preleukemia after Hodgkin's disease. Lancet 2:83–88.

PENN I. 1984. Cancer in immunosuppressed patients. Transplant Proc 16:492–494.

PESATORI AC, CONSONNI D, TIRONI A, et al. 1993. Cancer in a young population in a dioxin-contaminated area. Int J Epidemiol 22:1010–1013.

PETERS JM, PRESTON-MARTIN S, LONDON SJ, et al. 1994. Processed meats and risk of childhood leukemia (California, USA). Cancer Causes Control 5:195–202.

PETRIDOU E, MASSIMOS D, KALMANTI M, et al. 1993. Age of exposure to infections and risk of childhood leukaemia. Br Med J 307:774.

PICCIANI D. 1979. Cytogenetic study of workers exposed to benzene. Environ Res 19:33–38.

PIFER JW, HEMPELMANN LH, DODGE HJ, et al. 1968. Neoplasms in the Ann Arbor series of thymus-irradiated children: A second survey. Am J Roentgenol 103:13–18.

PIKE MC, SMITH PG. 1968. Disease clustering: A generalization of Knox's approach to the detection of space-time interactions. Biometrics 24:541–556.

PINDER DC. 1985. Trends and clusters of leukaemia in the Mersey region. Community Med 1:272–277.

PINKEL D, NEFZGER D. 1954. Some epidemiological features of childhood leukemia in the Buffalo, NY area. Cancer 12:352–358.

PIPER CE, ABT DA, FERRER JF, et al. 1975. Sero-epidemiological evidence for horizontal transmission of bovine C-type virus. Cancer Res 35:2714–2716.

PIPPARD EC, HALL AJ, BARKER DJP, et al. 1988. Cancer in homozygotes and heterozygotes of ataxia telangiectasia and xeroderma pigmentosum in Britain. Cancer Res 48:2929–2932.

POCHIN EE. 1969. Long-term hazards of radioiodine treatment of thyroid carcinoma. *In* Hedinger J (ed): Thyroid Cancer. UICC Monograph Series 12. Berlin, Springer-Verlag, pp. 293–304.

POIESZ BJ, RUSCATTI FW, GAZDAR AF, et al. 1980. Detection and isolation of type-C retrovirus particles from fresh and cultured lymphocytes of a patients with cutaneous T-cell lymphoma. Proc Natl Acad Sci USA 77:7415–7419.

POLLAK MS, DUBOIS D. 1976. Non-HLA antibodies in common typing sera: Effects on HLA frequency data in leukemia. *In* HLA and Disease. Paris, Inserm, p. 232.

POMBO DE OLIVEIRA MS, AWAD EL SEED FER, FORONI L, et al. 1986. Lymphoblastic leukaemia in Siamese twins: Evidence for identity. Lancet 2:969–970.

PONTISSO P, LOCASCIULLI A, SCHIAVON E, et al. 1987. Detection of hepatitis B virus DNA sequences in bone marrow of children with leukemia. Cancer 59:292–296.

POOLE C, ROTHMAN KJ, DREYER NA. 1988. Leukaemia near Pilgrim nuclear power plant, Massachusetts. Lancet 2:1308.

POOLE C, TRICHOPOULOS D. 1991. Extremely low frequency electric and magnetic fields and cancer. Cancer Causes Control 2:267–276.

PORTUGAL MA, FALKSON HC, STEVENS K, et al. 1979. Acute leukemia as a complication of long term treatment of advanced breast cancer. Cancer Treat Rep 63:177–181.

POTOLSKY AI, HEATH CW JR, BUCKLEY CE, et al. 1971. Lymphoreticular malignancies and immunologic abnormalities in a sibship. Am J Med 50:42–51.

POTTERN LM, LINET M, BLAIR A, et al. 1991. Familial cancers associated with subtypes of leukemia and lymphoma. Leuk Res 15:305–314.

PRESTON DL, KATO H, KOPECKY KJ, et al. 1987. Studies of the mortality of A-bomb survivors. Cancer mortality 1950–1982. Radiat Res 111:151–178.

PRESTON DL, KUSUMI S. TOMONAGA M, et al. 1994. Cancer incidence in A-bomb survivors. III. Leukemia, lymphoma, and multiple myeloma, 1950–1987. Radiat Res 137(Suppl):68–97.

PRESTON-MARTIN S, PETERS JM. 1988a. Prior employment as a welder associated with the development of chronic myeloid leukemia. Br J Cancer 58:105–108.

PRESTON-MARTIN S, PETERS, JM, YU MC, et al. 1988b. Myelogenous leukemia and electric blanket use. Bioelectromagnetics 9:207–213.

PRESTON-MARTIN S, THOMAS DC, YU MC, et al. 1989. Diagnostic radiography as a risk factor for chronic myeloid and monocytic leukaemia. Br J Cancer 59:639–644.

PUI CH, HANCOCK ML, RAIMONDI SC, et al. 1990. Myeloid neoplasia in children treated for solid tumors. Lancet 336:417–421.

PUI C-H, RIBEIRO RC, HANCOCK ML, et al. 1991. Acute myeloid leukemia in children treated with Epipodophyllotoxin for acute lymphoblastic leukemia. N Engl J Med 325:1682–1687.

QUESNEL B, KANTARAJAN H, BJERGAARD-PETERSON J, et al. 1993. Therapy-related acute myeloid leukemia with t(8;21) inv(16) and t(8;

16). A report on 25 cases and review of the literature. J Clin Oncol 11:2370–2379.

RADFORD EP, DOLL R, SMITH PG. 1977. Mortality among patients with ankylosing spondylitis not given x-ray therapy. N Engl J Med 297:572–576.

RAMOT B, BEN-BASSET I, BINIAMINOV M. 1985. Observations on the epidemiology and subtypes of lymphatic malignancies in Israel. Leuk Res 9:769–774.

RAMOT B, MAGRATH I. 1982. Hypothesis: The environment is a major determinant of the immunologic subtype of lymphoma and acute lymphoblastic leukemia in children. Br J Hematol 52:183–189.

RANDALL CL, PALONCEK FP, GRAHAM JB, et al. 1964. Causes of death in cases of preclimacteric menorrhagia. Am J Obstet Gynecol 88:880–897.

REDMAN JR, VUGRIN D, ARLIN ZA, et al. 1983. Leukemia following treatment of germ cell tumors in men. J Clin Oncol 2:1080–1087.

REEVES JD, DRIGGERS DA, KILEY VA. 1989. Household insecticide associated aplastic anaemia and leukaemia in children. Lancet 2:300–301.

REEVES WC, SAXINGER C, BRENES MM, et al. 1988. Human T-cell Lymphotropic Virus Type I (HTLV-I) seroepidemiology and risk factors in metropolitan Panama. Am J Epidemiol 127:532–539.

REGISTRAR GENERAL. 1958. The Registrar General's Decennial Supplement, England and Wales, 1951. Part II, Vol 2. Occupational Mortality Tables. London, Her Majesty's Stationary Office.

REILLY EB, RAPAPORT SI, KARR NW. 1952. Familial chronic lymphocytic leukemia. Arch Intern Med 90:87–95.

REIMER RR, HOOVER R, FRAUMENI JF JR, et al. 1977. Acute leukemia after alkylating agent therapy of ovarian cancer. N Engl J Med 297:177–181.

RICHARDSON S, ZITTOUN R, BASTUJI-GARIN S, et al. 1992. Occupational risk factors for acute leukaemia: A case-control study. Int J Epidemiol 21:1063–1073.

RICHTER KV, FISCHER G, MENZEL GR, et al. 1973. HLA antigene und Disposition fur hamatologische Maligne Erkrankungen. Haematologia 7:203–209.

RIECHE K. 1984. Carcinogenicity of anti-neoplastic agents in man. Cancer Treat Rev 11:39–67.

RIGBY PG, PRATT PT, ROSENLOF RC, et al. 1968. Genetic relationships in familial leukemia and lymphoma. Arch Intern Med 121:67–70.

RIIHIMAKI V, ASP S, PUKKALA E, et al. 1983. Mortality and cancer morbidity among chlorinated phenoxyacid applicators in Finland. Chemosphere 12:779–784.

RINSKY RA, SMITH AB, HORNUNG R, et al. 1987. Benzene and leukemia. An epidemiologic risk assessment. N Engl J Med 316:1044–1050.

RINSKY RA, ZUMWALDE RD, WAXWEILER RJ, et al. 1981a. Cancer mortality at a naval nuclear shipyard. Lancet 1:231–235.

RINSKY RA, YOUNG RJ, SMITH AB. 1981b. Leukemia in benzene workers. Am J Ind Med 2:217–245.

RIVERA GK, PINKEL D, SIMONE JV, et al. 1993. Treatment of acute lymphoblastic leukemia, 30 year's experience at St. Jude's Children's Research Hospital. N Engl J Med 329:1289–1295.

ROBERT-GUROFF M, WEISS SH, GIRON JA, et al. 1986. Prevalence of antibodies to HTLV-I II and III in intravenous drug abusers from an AIDS epidemic region. JAMA 255:3133–3137.

ROBINETTE CD, JABLON S, PRESTON TL. 1985. Mortality of Nuclear Weapons Test Participants. Medical Follow Up Agency, National Research Council. Washington, DC, National Academy Press.

ROBINSON CF, LALICH NR, BURNETT CA, et al. 1991. Electromagnetic field exposure and leukemia mortality in the United States. J Occup Med 33:160–162.

ROBISON LL, BUCKLEY JD, DAIGLE A, et al. 1989. Maternal drug use and risk of childhood nonlymphoblastic leukemia among offspring. Cancer 63:1904–1911.

ROBISON LL, NEGLIA JP. 1987. Epidemiology of Down syndrome and childhood acute leukemia. *In* McCoy EE, Epstein CJ (eds): Oncology and Immunology of Down Syndrome. New York, Alan Liss, pp. 19–32.

ROCKETTE HE, ARENA VC. 1983. Mortality studies of aluminum reduction plant workers: Potroom and carbon department. J Occup Med 25:549–557.

RODVALL Y, HRUBEC Z, PERSHAGEN G, et al. 1992. Childhood cancer among Swedish twins. Cancer Causes Control 3:527–532.

ROGAN WJ. 1986. An analysis of contaminated well water and health effects in Woburn, Massachusetts. J Am Stat Assoc 81:602–603.

ROGENTINE GN, TRAPANI RJ, YANKEE RA, et al. 1973. HLA antigens and acute lymphocytic leukemia: The nature of the HL-A2 association. Tissue Antigens 3:470–476.

ROMAN E, BERAL V, CARPENTER L, et al. 1987. Childhood leukaemia in the West Berkshire and Basingstoke and North Hampshire District Health Authorities in relation to nuclear establishments in the vicinity. Br Med J 294:597–602.

ROMAN E, WATSON A, BERAL V, et al. 1993. Case-control study of leukaemia and non-Hodgkin's lymphoma among children aged 0–4 years living in West Berkshire and North Hampshire health districts. Br Med J 306:615–621.

RON E, MODAN B. 1984. Thyroid and other neoplasms following childhood scalp irradiation. *In* Boice JD Jr, Fraumeni JF Jr (eds): Radiation Carcinogenesis: Epidemiology and Biologic Significance. New York, Raven Press, pp. 139–151.

RON E, MODAN B, BOICE JD JR. 1988. Mortality after radiotherapy for ringworm of the scalp. Am J Epidemiol 127:713–725.

RONCO G, COSTA G, LYNGE E. 1992. Cancer risk among Danish and Italian farmers. Br J Ind Med 49:220–225.

ROSENBLATT KA, KOEPSELL TD, DALING JR, et al. 1991. Antigenic stimulation and the occurrence of chronic lymphocytic leukemia. Am J Epidemiol 134:22–28.

ROSENTHAL SR, CRISPEN RG, THORNE MG, et al. 1972. BCG vaccination and leukemia mortality. JAMA 222:1543–1544.

ROSNER F, GRUNWALD HW. 1980. Multiple myeloma and Waldenstrom's macroglobulinemia terminating in acute leukemia. A review with an emphasis on karyotypic and ultrastructural abnormalities. NY State J Med 80:558–568.

ROTHMAN KJ. 1984. Significance of studies of low-dose radiation fallout in the western United States. *In* Boice JD Jr, Fraumeni JF Jr (eds): Radiation Carcinogenesis: Epidemiology and Biological Significance. New York, Raven Press, pp. 73–82.

ROWLEY JD. 1988. Chromosome abnormalities in leukemia. J Clin Oncol 6:194–202.

ROWLEY JD. 1985. Chromosome abnormalities in human leukemia as indicators of mutagenic exposure. *In* Huberman E (ed): The Role of Chemicals and Radiation in the Etiology of Cancer. New York, Alan Liss, pp. 409–419.

ROWLEY JD. 1981. Down's syndrome and acute leukaemia: Increased risk may be due to Trisomy 21. Lancet 1:1020–1022.

ROWLEY JD, GOLOMB HM, VARDIMAN J. 1977. Nonrandom chromosomal abnormalities in acute nonlymphocytic leukemia in patients treated for Hodgkin's disease and non-Hodgkin's lymphomas. Blood 50:759–770.

RUSHTON L. 1993a. Further follow-up of mortality in a United Kingdom oil distribution centre cohort. Br J Ind Med 50:549–560.

RUSHTON L. 1993b. A 39 year follow-up of the UK oil refinery and distribution centre studies: Results for kidney cancer and leukaemia. Environ Health Perspect 101(Suppl 6):77–84.

RUSHTON L, ALDERSON MR. 1981. Case-control study to investigate the association between exposure to benzene and deaths from leukaemia in oil refinery workers. Br J Cancer 43:77–84.

RUSHTON L, ALDERSON MR, NAGARAJAH CR. 1983. Epidemiological survey of maintenance workers in London transport bus garages and Chiswick works. Br J Ind Med 40:340–345.

RWANDAN HIV SEROPREVALENCE STUDY GROUP. 1989. Nationwide community-based serological survey of HIV-1 and other human retrovirus infections in a central African country. Lancet 1:941–943.

SACKEY K, ODONE V, GEORGE SL, et al. 1984. Poland's syndrome associated with childhood non-Hodgkin's lymphoma. Am J Dis Child 138:600–601.

SAENGER EL, THOMAS GE, THOMPKINS EA. 1969. Incidence of leukemia following treatment of hyperthyroidism. Preliminary report of the Cooperative Thyrotoxicosis Therapy Follow-up Study. JAMA 205:855–862.

SAHL JD, KELSH MA, GREENLAND S. 1993. Cohort and nested case-control studies of hematopoietic cancers and brain cancer among electric utility workers. Epidemiology 4:104–114.

SAKKA M. 1979. Background radiation and childhood cancer mortality. Nippon Igaku Hoshasen Gakkai Zasshi 39:536–539.

SANDBERG A. 1986. The chromosomes in human leukemia. Semin Hematol 23:201–217.

SANDERSON AR, MAHOUR GH, JAFFE N, et al. 1973. Incidence of HLA in acute lymphocytic leukemia. Transplant 16:672–674.

SANDLER DP, COLLMAN GW. 1987. Cytogenetic and environmental factors in the etiology of the acute leukemias in adults. Am J Epidemiol 126:1017–1032.

SANDLER DP, COMSTOCK GN, MATANOSKI GM. 1982. Neoplasms following childhood irradiation of the nasopharynx. J Natl Cancer Inst 68:3–8.

SANDLER DP, EVERSON RB, WILCOX AJ, et al. 1985. Cancer risk in adulthood from early life exposure to parents' smoking. Am J Public Health 75:487–492.

SANDLER DP, SHORE DL, ANDERSON JR, et al. 1993. Cigarette-smoking and risk of acute leukemia: Associations with morphology and cytogenetic abnormalities in bone marrow. J Natl Cancer Inst 85:1994–2003.

SANTOS-BURGOA C, MATANOSKI GM, ZEGER S, et al. 1992. Lymphohematopoietic cancer in styrene-butadiene polymerization workers. Am J Epidemiol 136:843–854.

SARASUA S, SAVITZ DA. 1994. Cured and broiled meat consumption in relation to childhood cancer. Cancer Causes Control 5:141–148.

SATO H, OKOCHI K. 1986. Transmission of human T-cell leukemia virus (HTLV-I) by blood transfusion: Demonstration of proviral DNA in recipients's blood lymphocytes. Int J Cancer 7:395–400.

SAVITZ DA, CALLE EE. 1987. Leukemia and occupational exposure to electromagnetic fields: Review of epidemiologic surveys. J Occup Med 29:47–51.

SAVITZ DA, CHEN JH. 1990. Parental occupation and childhood cancer: Review of epidemiologic studies. Environ Health Perspect 88:325–337.

SAVITZ DA, JOHN EM, KLECKNER RC. 1990. Magnetic field exposure from electric appliances and childhood cancer. Am J Epidemiol 131:763–773.

SAVITZ DA, LOOMIS DP. 1995. Magnetic field exposure in relation to leukemia and brain cancer mortality. Am J Epidemiol 141:123–134.

SAVITZ DA, PEARCE NE, POOLE C. 1989. Methodological issues in the epidemiology of electromagnetic fields and cancer. Epidemiol Rev 11:59–78.

SAVITZ DA, WACHTEL H, BARNES FA, et al. 1988. Case-control study of childhood cancer and exposure to 60-Hz magnetic fields. Am J Epidemiol 128:21–38.

SAWITSKY A, BLOOM D, GERMAN J. 1966. Chromosomal breakage and acute leukemia in congenital telangiectatic: Erythema and stunted growth. Ann Intern Med 65:487–495.

SCHADE H, SCHOELLER L, SCHULTZE KW. 1962. D-Trisomis (Patau-Syndrome) mit kongenitler myeloischer Leukamie. Med Welt 50:2690–2692.

SCHENKER MB, SMITH T, MUNOZ A, et al. 1984. Diesel exposure and mortality among railway workers: Results of a pilot study. Br J Ind Med 41:320–327.

SCHMIDT W, POPHAM RE. 1981. The role of drinking and smoking in mortality from cancer and other causes in male alcoholics. Cancer 47:1031–1041.

SCHOLL T, STEIN Z, HANSEN H. 1982. Leukemia and other cancers, anomalies and infections as causes of death in Down's syndrome in the United States during 1976. Dev Med Child Neurol 24:817–829.

SCHOTTENFELD D, WARSHAUER ME, ZAUBER AG, et al. 1981. A prospective study of morbidity and mortality in petroleum industry employees in the United States—a preliminary report. *In* Peto R, Schneiderman M (eds): Banbury Report 9—Quantitation of Occupational Cancer. New York, Cold Spring Harbor Laboratory, pp. 247–265.

SCHWARTZ DA, VAUGHAN TL, HEYER NJ, et al. 1988. B cell neoplasms and occupational asbestos exposure. Am J Ind Med 14:661–671.

SCHWEITZER M, MELIEF CJM, PLOEM JE. 1973. Chronic lymphocytic leukemia in 5 siblings. Scand J Haematol 11:97–105.

SECKER-WALKER LM, STEWART EL, TODD A. 1985. Acute lymphoblastic leukemia with t(4;11) follows neuroblastoma: A late effect of treatment? Med Pediatr Oncol 13:48–50.

SEEMANOVA E, PASSARGE E, BENESKOVA D, et al. 1985. Familial microcephaly with normal intelligence, immunodeficiency, and risk for lymphoreticular malignancies: A new autosomal recessive disorder. Am J Hum Gen 20:639–648.

SEGI M, NOYE H, SEGI R. 1977. Age Adjusted Death Rates for Cancer for Selected Sites (A-Classification) in 43 Countries in 1972. Nagoya, Japan, Segi Institute of Cancer Epidemiology.

SELTSER R, SARTWELL PE. 1965. The influence of occupational exposure on the mortality of American radiologists and other medical specialists. Am J Epidemiol 101:188–198.

SELVIN S, LEVIN LI, MERRILL DW, et al. 1983. Selected epidemiologic observations of cell-specific leukemia mortality in the United States, 1969–77. Am J Epidemiol 117:140–152.

SELVIN S, SCHULMAN J, MERRILL DW. 1992. Distance and risk measures for the analysis of spatial data: A study of childhood cancers. Soc Sci Med 34:769–777.

SEVC J, KUNZ E, TOMASEK L, et al. 1988. Cancer in man and exposure to Rn daughters. Health Physics 54:27–46.

SEVERSON RK. 1987. Cigarette smoking and leukemia. Cancer 60:141–144.

SEVERSON RK, BUCKLEY JD, WOODS WG, et al. 1992. Cigarette smoking and alcohol consumption by parents of children with acute myeloid leukemia: An analysis within morphological subgroups—A report from the Children's Cancer Group. Cancer Epidemiol Biomarkers Prevent 2:433–439.

SEVERSON RK, DAVIS S, THOMAS DB, et al. 1989. Acute myelocytic leukemia and prior allergies. J Clin Epidemiol 42:995–1001.

SEVERSON RK, STEVENS RG, KAUNE WT, et al. 1988. Acute nonlymphocytic leukemia and residential exposure to power frequency magnetic fields. Am J Epidemiol 128:10–20.

SHANNON KM, O'CONNELL P, MARTIN GA, et al. 1994. Loss of the normal NF-1 allele from the bone marrow of children with type 1 neurofibromatosis and malignant myeloid disorders. N Engl J Med 330:597–601.

SHIMIZU Y, KATO H, SCHULL W, et al. 1989. Studies of the mortality of A-bomb survivors. Mortality, 1950–1985. Part 1. Comparison of the risk coefficients for site-specific cancer mortality based on DS86 and T65DR shielded kerma and organ doses. Radiat Res 118:502–524.

SHIMIZU Y, KATO H, SCHULL W, et al. 1990. Studies of the mortality of A-bomb survivors. Mortality, 1950–1985. Part 2. Cancer mortality based on recently revised doses (DS86). Radiat Res 122:120–141.

SHORE RE. 1988. Electromagnetic radiations and cancer. Cause and Prevention. Cancer 62:1747–1754.

SHORE RE, ALBERT RE, PASTERNACK BJ. 1976. Follow up study of patients treated by x-ray epilation for tinea capitis. Arch Environ Health 31:21–30.

SHORE RE, GARDNER MJ, PANNETT B. 1993. Ethylene oxide: An assessment of the epidemiological evidence on carcinogenicity. Br J Ind Med 50:971–997.

SHU X-O, GAO Y-T, BRINTON LA, et al. 1988. A population-based case-control study of childhood leukemia in Shanghai. Cancer 62:635–644.

SHU X-O, GAO Y-T, LINET MS, et al. 1987. Chloramphenicol use and childhood leukaemia in Shanghai. Lancet 2:934–937.

SHU X-O, JIN F, LINET MS, et al. 1994. Diagnostic x-ray and ultrasound exposure and risk of childhood cancers. Br J Cancer 70:531–536.

SHU X-O, ROSS JA, PENDERGRASS TW, et al. 1996. Parental alcohol consumption, cigarette smoking, and risk of infant leukemia: A Childrens Cancer Group Study. J Natl Cancer Inst 88:24–31.

SIDI Y, MEYTES D, SHOHAT B, et al. 1990. Adult T-cell lymphoma in Israeli patients of Iranian origin. Cancer 65:590–593.

SIEGEL M. 1993. Smoking and leukemia: Evaluation of a causal hypothesis. Am J Epidemiol 138:1–9.

SKOV T, MAARUP B, OLSEN J, et al. 1992. Leukaemia and reproductive outcome among nurses handling antineoplastic drugs. Br J Ind Med 49:855–861.

SMITH PG, DOLL R. 1976. Late effects of X irradiation in patients treated for metropathia hemorrhagica. Br J Radiol 49:224–232.

SMITH PG, DOLL R. 1981. Mortality from cancer and all causes among British radiologists. Br J Radiol 54:187–194.

SMITH PG, DOLL R. 1982. Mortality among patients with ankylosing spondylitis after a single treatment course with X-ray. Br Med J 284:449–460.

SMITH PG, DOUGLAS AJ. 1986. Mortality of workers at the Sellafield plant of British Nuclear Fuels. Br Med J 293:845–854.

SMITH PG, PIKE MC, TILL MM, et al. 1976. Epidemiology of childhood leukaemia in greater London: A search for evidence of transmission assuming a long latent period. Br J Cancer 33:1–8.

SNELLINGS WM, WEIL CS, MARONPOT RR. 1984. A two-year inhalation study of the carcinogenic potential of ethylene oxide in Fischer 344 rats. Toxicol Appl Pharmacol 75:105–117.

SNIDER DE, COMSTOCK GW, MARTINEZ I, et al. 1978. Efficiency of BCG vaccination in prevention of cancer: An update. J Natl Cancer Inst 60:785–88.

SONTAG JM. 1981. Carcinogenicity of substituted benzene diamines (phenylene diamines) in rats and mice. J Natl Cancer Inst 66:591–602.

SORAHAN T, PARKES HG, VEYS CA. 1989. Mortality in the British rubber industry 1946–85. Br J Ind Med 46:1–11.

SORAHAN T, ROBERTS PJ. 1993. Childhood cancer and paternal exposure to ionizing radiation: Preliminary findings from the Oxford survey of childhood cancers. Am J Ind Med 23:343–354.

SORDILLO PP, MARCOVICH RP, HARDY WD JR. 1982. Search for evidence of feline leukemia virus infection in humans with leukemias, lymphomas, or soft tissue sarcomas. J Natl Cancer Inst 69:333–337.

SORENSEN SA, MULVIHILL JJ, NIELSEN A. 1986. Long-term follow-up of von Recklinghausen neurofibromatosis. Survival and malignant neoplasms. N Engl J Med 314:1010–1015.

SPECTOR BD, FILIPOVICH AH, PERRY GS III, et al. 1982. Epidemiology of cancer in ataxia-telangiectasia. *In* Bridges BA, Harnden DC (eds): Ataxia-Telangiectasia: A Cellular and Molecular Link Between Cancer, Neuropathology, and Immune Deficiency. New York, Wiley.

SPECTOR BD, PERRY G III, KERSEY J, et al. 1978. Genetically determined immunodeficiency diseases (GDID) and malignancy: Report from the Immunodeficiency Cancer Registry. Clin Immunol Immunopathol 11:12–29.

SPEISS H, MAYS CW, CHMELEVSKY D. 1989. Malignancies in patients injected with radium 224. *In* Taylor DM, Mays CW, Gerber GB, Thomas RG (eds): Risks from Radium and Thorotrast. BIR Report 21. London, British Institute of Radiology, pp. 7–12.

SPENGLER RF, COOK DH, CLARKE EA, et al. 1983. Cancer mortality following cardiac catheterization: A preliminary follow up on 4891 irradiated children. Pediatrics 71:235–244.

SPIERS FW, LUCAS HF, RUNDO J, et al. 1983. Leukemia incidence in the U.S. dial workers. Health Physics 44:65–72.

SPINELLI JJ, GALLAGHER RP, BAND PR, et al. 1984. Multiple myeloma, leukemia, and cancer of the ovary in cosmetologists and hair dressers. Am J Ind Med 6:97–102.

SPIRTAS R, VAN ERT M, GAMBLE J, et al. 1976. Toxicologic, industrial hygiene and epidemiologic considerations in the possible association between SBR manufacturing and neoplasms of lymphatic and hematopoietic tissues. *In* Proceedings of NISH Syrene-Butadiene Briefing, Covington, Kentucky, April 30, 1976. DHEW publication no. (NIOSH) 77-129.

STAHNKE N, ZEISEL HJ. 1989. Growth hormone therapy and leukaemia. Eur J Pediatr 148:591–596.

STARK CR, MANTEL N. 1967. Temporal spatial distribution of birth dates for Michigan children with leukemia. Cancer Res 27:1749–1775.

STAYNER L, STEENLAND K, GREIFE A, et al. 1993. Exposure-response analysis of cancer mortality in a cohort of workers exposed to ethylene oxide. Am J Epidemiol 138:787–798.

STEBBINGS JH, LUCAS HF, STENNEY AF. 1984. Mortality from cancers of major sites in female radium dial workers. Am J Ind Med 5:435–459.

STEENLAND K, STAYNER L, GREIFE A, et al. 1991. Mortality among workers exposed to ethylene oxide. N Engl J Med 324:1402–1407.

STERN FB, WAXWEIFER RA, BEAUMONT JJ, et al. 1986. A case-control study of leukemia at a naval nuclear shipyard. Am J Epidemiol 123:980–992.

STERN RM. 1987. Cancer incidence among welders: Possible effects of exposure to extremely low frequency electromagnetic radiation (ELF) and to welding fumes. Environ Health Perspect 76:221–229.

STEVENS RG. 1986. Age and risk of leukemia. J Natl Cancer Inst 76:845–848.

STEVENS W, THOMAS DC, LYON JL, et al. 1990. Leukemia in Utah and radioactive fallout from the Nevada test site. JAMA 264:585–591.

STEWART A. 1973. The carcinogenic effects of low level radiation. A reappraisal of epidemiologists' methods and observations. Health Physics 24:223–240.

STEWART A. 1986. Background radiation and childhood cancer. Proceedings of the 20th Meeting of the European Society of Radiation Biology. Pisa, Italy.

STEWART AM, DRAPER G. 1970. BCG vaccination and leukaemia mortality. Lancet 1:983.

STEWART AM, DRAPER G. 1971. BCG vaccination and leukaemia mortality. Lancet 1:799.

STEWART A, PENNYPACKER W, BARBER R. 1962. Adult leukaemia and diagnostic X-rays. Br Med J 5309:882–890.

STEWART A, WEBB J, MERITT D. 1958. A survey of childhood malignancies. Br Med J 2:1495–1508.

STILLER CA, BUNCH KJ. 1990. Trends in survival for childhood cancer in Britain diagnosed 1971–85. Br J Cancer 62:806–815.

STILLER CA, DRAPER GJ. 1982. Trends in childhood leukemia in Britain 1968–78. Br J Cancer 45:543–551.

STJERNFELDT M, SAMUELSSON L, LUDVIGSSON J. 1987. Radiation in dwellings and cancer in children. Pediatr Hematol Oncol 4:55–61.

STOLL DB, PETERSON P, EXTEN R, et al. 1988. Clinical presentation and natural history of patients with essential thrombocythemia and the Philadelphia chromosome. Am J Hematol 27:77–83.

STOLLEY PD, SOPER KA, GALLOWAY SM, et al. 1984. Sister-chromatid exchanges in association with occupational exposure to ethylene oxide. Mutat Res 129:89–102.

STORM HH. 1988. Second primary cancer after treatment for cervical cancer. Cancer 61:679–688.

STOTT H, FOX W, GIRLING DJ, et al. 1977. Acute leukaemia after busulphan. Br Med J 2:1513–1517.

STRICKER RB, LINDER CA. 1983. Acute lymphoblastic leukemia with monosomy 7 in a Hiroshima survivor 37 years after the bomb. JAMA 250:640–641.

STROUP NE, BLAIR A, ERIKSON GE. 1986. Brain cancer and other causes of death in anatomists. J Natl Cancer Inst 77:1217–1224.

SUGIMOTO T, KIDOWAKI K, SAWADA T, et al. 1982. Ataxia-telangiectasia associated with non-T, non-B cell acute lymphocytic leukemia. Acta Pediatr Scand 71:509–510.

SUTHERLAND GR, MATTEI JF. 1987. Report of the Committee on Cytogenetic Markers. Human Gene Mapping 9. Ninth International Workshop on Human Gene Mapping. Cytogenet Cell Genet 46:316–324.

SUTTON RNP, BISHON NP, SOOTHILL JF. 1969. Immunological and chromosomal studies in first-degree relatives of children with acute lymphoblastic leukaemia. Br J Haematol 17:113–119.

SWAEN GMH, MEIJERS JMM. 1989. Risk assessment of leukaemia and occupational exposure to benzene. Br J Ind Med 46:826–830.

SWAN SH, ROBINS JM. 1986. An analysis of contaminated well water and health effects in Woburn, Massachusetts (comment). J Am Stat Assoc 81:604–609.

SWERDLOW AJ, DOUGLAS AJ, VAUGHAN HUDSON G, et al. 1992. Risk of second primary cancers after Hodgkin's disease by type of treatment: Analysis of 2846 patients in the British National Investigation. Br J Med 304:1137–1143.

SWOLIN B, WEINFELD A, WESTIN J. 1988. A prospective long-term cytogenetic study of polycythemia vera in relation to treatment and clinical course. Blood 72:386–395.

SYMMONS D. 1985. Neoplasms of the immune system in rheumatoid arthritis. Am J Med 78(Suppl 1A):22–27.

SYMMONS DPM. 1988. Neoplasia in rheumatoid arthritis. J Rheumatol 15:1319–1322.

TACHIBANA K, ITO S, SHIRAHAMA S, et al. 1991. Epidemic patterns of hepatitis type B virus (HBV) and human T lymphotropic virus type I (HTLV-I) in two ATL-endemic islands in Kyushu, Japan. Nagoya J Med Sci 53:23–32.

TAJIMA K. 1988. Malignant lymphomas in Japan: Epidemiological analysis of adult T-cell leukemia/lymphoma (ATL) Cancer Metastasis Rev 7:223–241.

TAJIMA K, T- AND B-CELL MALIGNANCY STUDY GROUP, AND CO-AUTHORS. 1990. The 4th nationwide study of adult T-cell leukemia/lymphoma (ATL) in Japan: Estimates of risk of ATL and its geographical and clinical features. Int J Cancer 45:237–243.

TAJIMA K, HINAWA Y. 1989. Epidemiological features of adult T-cell leukemia virus. *In* Mathe G, Ricenstein P (eds): Pathophysiological Aspects of Cancer Epidemiology. Oxford, Pergamon Press, pp. 75–87.

TAJIMA K, TOMINAGA S, SUCHI T, et al. 1982. Epidemiological analysis of the distribution of antibody to adult T-cell leukemia-lymphoma virus-associated antigen: Possible horizontal transmission of adult T-cell leukemia virus. Jpn J Cancer Res 73:893–901.

TANAKA K, KAMADA N. 1985. Leukemogenesis and chromosome aberrations: De novo leukemia in humans—with special reference to atomic bomb survivors. Acta Haematol Jpn 48:1830–1842.

TANAKA K, KAMADA N, OHKITA T, et al. 1983. Non-random distribution of chromosome breaks in lymphocytes of atomic bomb survivors. J Radiat Res 24:291–304.

TARBELL NJ, GELBER RD, WEINSTEIN HJ, et al. 1993. Sex differences in risk of second malignant tumors after Hodgkin's disease in childhood. Lancet 341:1428–1432.

T- AND B-CELL MALIGNANCY STUDY GROUP. 1988. The third nation-wide study on adult T-cell leukemia/lymphoma (ATL) in Japan: Characteristic patterns of HLA antigen and HTLV-I infection in ATL patients and their relatives. Int J Cancer 41:505–512.

TAYLOR AMR. 1992. Ataxia telangiectasia genes and predisposition to leukaemia, lymphoma, and breast cancer. Br J Cancer 66:5–9.

TAYLOR HG, NIXON N, SHEERAN TP, et al. 1989. Rheumatoid arthritis and chronic lymphatic leukaemia. Clin Exp Rheumatol 7:529–532.

TAYLOR JA, SANDLER DP, BLOOMFIELD CD, et al. 1992. *ras* oncogene activation and occupational exposures in acute myeloid leukemia. J Natl Cancer Inst 84:1626–1632.

TEICHMANN JV, SIEBER S, LUDWIG WD, et al. 1986. Chronic myelocytic leukemia as a second neoplasm in the course of chronic lymphocytic leukemia. Leuk Res 10:361–368.

TESTER WJ, KINSELLA TJ, WALLER B, et al. 1984. Second malignant neoplasms complicating Hodgkin's disease: The National Cancer Institute experience. J Clin Oncol 2:762–769.

TETA MJ, WALRATH J, MEIGS JW, et al. 1984. Cancer incidence among cosmetologists. J Natl Cancer Inst 72:1051–1057.

TETA MJ, BENSON LO, VITALE JN. 1993. Mortality study of ethylene oxide workers in chemical manufacturing: A 10-year update. Br J Ind Med 50:704–709.

THEISS AM, FRENTZEL-BEYME R, LINK R, et al. 1981. Mortality study on employees exposed to alkylene oxides (ethylene oxide/propylene oxide) and their derivatives. *In* Prevention of Occupational Cancer-International Symposium. Occupational and Health Series No. 46. Geneva, International Labour Office, pp. 249–259.

THERIAULT G, GOLDBERG M, MILLER AB, et al. 1994. Cancer risks associated with occupational exposure to magnetic fields among electric utility workers in Ontario and Quebec, Canada, and France: 1970–89. Am J Epidemiol 139:550–572.

THIRMAN MJ, GILL HJ, BURNETT RC, et al. 1993. Rearrangement of the MLL gene in acute lymphoblastic and acute myeloid leukemias with 11q23 chromosomal translocations. N Engl J Med 329:909–914.

THOMAS TL, KREKEL S, HEID M. 1985. Proportionate mortality among male corn wet-milling workers. Int J Epidemiol 14:432–437.

THORPE JJ. 1974. Epidemiologic survey of leukemia in persons potentially exposed to benzene. J Occup Med 16:375–382.

THUN MJ, ALTERKRUSE SF, NAMBOODIRI MM, et al. 1994. Hair dye use and risk of fatal cancers in U.S. women. J Natl Cancer Inst 86:210–215.

TICE R, COSTA D, DREW R. 1980. Cytogenetic effects of inhaled benzene in murine bone marrow: Induction of sister chromatid exchanges, chromosomal aberrations, and cellular proliferation. Inhibition in DBA/2 mice. Proc Natl Acad Sci USA 77:2148–2151.

TILL MM, JONES LH, PENTYCROSS CR. 1975. Leukaemia in children and their grandparents: Studies of immune function in six families. Br J Haematol 29:575–586.

TILL M, RAPSON N, SMITH PG. 1979. Family studies in acute leukaemia in childhood: A possible association with autoimmune disease. Br J Cancer 40:62–71.

TOLEDANO SR, LANGE BJ. 1980. Ataxia-telangiectasia and acute lymphoblastic leukemia. Cancer 45:1675–1678.

TOMENIUS L. 1986. 50-Hz electromagnetic environment and the incidence of childhood tumors in Stockholm County. Bioelectromagnetics 7:191–207.

TOOLIS F, POTTER B, ALLAN NC, et al. 1981. Radiation induced leukemias in ankylosing spondylitis. Cancer 48:1582–1585.

TORNQVIST S, KNAVE B, AHLBOM A, et al. 1991. Incidence of leukaemia and brain tumors in some electrical occupations. Br J Ind Med 48:597–603.

TORNQVIST S, NORELL S, AHLBOM A. 1986. Mortality experience of electrical engineers. Br J Ind Med 42:211–212.

TRAVIS LB, CURTIS RE, GLIMELIUS B, et al. 1993. Second cancers after non-Hodgkin's lymphoma. J Natl Cancer Inst 85:1932–1937.

TRAVIS LB, LI C-Y, ZHANG Z-N, et al. 1994. Hematopoietic malignancies and related disorders among benzene-exposed workers in China. Leuk Lymph 14:91–102.

TRAVIS WD, LI C-Y, BERGSTVALH EJ. 1989. Solid and hematologic malignancies in 60 patients with systemic mast cell disease. Arch Pathol Lab Med 113:365–368.

TUCKER MA, COLEMAN CN, COX RS, et al. 1988. Risk of second cancers after treatment for Hodgkin's disease. N Engl J Med 318:76–81.

TUCKER MA, MEADOWS AT, BOICE JD JR. 1987. Leukemia after therapy with alkylating agents for childhood cancer. J Natl Cancer Inst 78:459–464.

TYNES T, ANDERSSEN A, LANGMARK F. 1992. Incidence of cancer in Norwegian workers potentially exposed to electromagnetic fields. Am J Epidemiol 136:81–88.

TYNES T, JYNGE H, VISTNES AI. 1994. Leukemia and brain tumors in Norwegian railway workers, a nested case-control study. Am J Epidemiol 139:645–653.

UCHIYAMA T, YODOI J, SAGAWA K, et al. 1977. Adult T-cell leukemia: Clinical and hematologic features of 15 cases. Blood 50:481–492.

UEDA K, KUSUHARA K, TOKUGAWA K, et al. 1989. Cohort effect on HTLV-I seroprevalence in southern Japan. Lancet 2:979–982.

UNITED NATIONS SCIENTIFIC COMMITTEE ON THE EFFECTS OF IONIZING RADIATION. 1986. Genetic and Somatic Effects of Ionizing Radiation. New York, United Nations.

URQUHART JD, BLACK RJ, MUIRHEAD MJ, et al. 1991. Case-control study of leukaemia and non-Hodgkin's lymphoma in children in Caithness near the Dounreay nuclear installation. Br Med J 302:687–692.

VALAGUSSA P, SANTORO A, FOSSATI-BELLANI F, et al. 1986. Second acute leukemia and other malignancies following treatment for Hodgkin's disease. J Clin Oncol 4:830–837.

VAN FLIEDNER VE, MERICA H, JEANNET M, et al. 1983. Evidence for HLA-linked susceptibility factors in childhood leukemia. Hum Immunol 8:183–193.

VAN HOFF J, SCHYMURA MJ, CURRAN MGM. 1988. Trends in the incidence of childhood and adolescent cancer in Connecticut 1935–1979. Med Pediatr Oncol 16:78–87.

VAN KAICK G, MUTH R, KAUL A. 1986. Report on the German Thorotrast study. *In* Gossner W, Gerber GB, Hagen U, Luz A (eds): The Radiobiology of Radium and Thorotrast. Munich, Urban, pp. 114–126.

VAN LEEUWEN FE, CHORUS AMJ, VAN DEN BELT-DUSEBOUT, et al. 1994. Leukemia risk following Hodgkin's disease: Relation to relative dose of alkylating agents, treatment with teniposide combinations, number of episodes of chemotherapy, and bone marrow damage. J Clin Oncol 12:1063–1073.

VAN STEENSEL-MOLL HA, VALKENBURG HA, VANDERBROUCKE JP, et al. 1983. Time space distribution of childhood leukaemia in the Netherlands. J Epidemiol Community Health 37:145–148.

VAN STEENSEL-MOLL HA, VALKENBURG HA, VAN ZANEN GE. 1985. Childhood leukemia and parental occupation: A register-based case-control study. Am J Epidemiol 121:216–224.

VAN STEENSEL-MOLL HA, VALKENBURG HA, VAN ZANEN GE. 1986. Childhood leukemia and infectious diseases in the first year of life: A register-based case-control study. Am J Epidemiol 124:590–594.

VERDIER M, DENIS F, SANGARE A, et al. 1989. Prevalence of antibody to human T-cell leukemia virus type 1 (HTLV-I) in populations of Ivory Coast, West Africa. J Infect Dis 160:363–370.

VERKASALO PK, PUKKALA E, HONGISTO MY, et al. 1993. Cancer in Finnish children living close to power lines. Br Med J 307:895.

VERRESEN H, VAN DEN BERGHE H, CREEMERO J. 1964. Mosaic trisomy in phenotypically normal mothers of mongols. Lancet 1:526–527.

VESTEY JP, JUDGE M, SAVIN JA. 1986. Sweet's syndrome followed by acute myelomonocytic leukaemia: The need for follow-up. Scott Med J 31:184–186.

VIADANA E, BROSS IDJ. 1972. Leukemia and occupations. Prev Med 1:513–521.

VIANNA NJ, KOVASZNAY B, POLAN A, et al. 1984. Infant leukemia and parental exposure to motor vehicle exhaust fumes. J Occup Med 26:679–682.

VIDEBAEK A. 1947. Familial leukemia. A preliminary report. Acta Med Scand 127:26–52.

VIEL JF, RICHARDSON ST. 1990. Childhood leukaemia around the La Hague nuclear waste reprocessing plant. Br Med J 300:580–581.

VIEL JF, RICHARDSON ST. 1991. Adult leukemia and farm practices: An alternative approach for assessing geographical pesticide exposure. Soc Sci Med 32:1067–1073.

VIGLIANI EC, FORNI A. 1976. Benzene and leukemia. Environ Res 11:122–127.

VIRAG I, MODAN B. 1969. Epidemiologic aspects of neoplastic disease in an Israeli immigrant population. Cancer 23:137–144.

VON GROSS R, WILDHACK R, STEINER H. 1958. Klinisch statistische uber sich uber 900 Leukosen. Dtsch Med Wochenschr 83:1974–1981.

VOUTSINAS S, WYNNE-DAVIES R. 1983. The infrequency of malignant disease in diaphyseal aclasis and neurofibromatosis. J Med Genet 20:345–349.

WAGONER JK. 1984. Leukemia and other malignancies following radiation therapy for gynecological disorders. *In* Boice JD Jr, Fraumeni JF Jr (eds): Radiation Carcinogenesis: Epidemiology and Biological Significance. New York, Raven Press, pp. 153–159.

WALD N. 1988. Smoking and leukaemia. Br Med J 297:638.

WALLACE LA. 1989. Major sources of benzene exposure. Environ Health Perspect 82:165–169.

WALRATH J, FRAUMENI JF JR. 1984. Cancer and other causes of death among embalmers. Cancer Res 44:4638–4641.

WALTER SD, MEIGS JW, HESTON JF. 1986. The relationship of cancer incidence to terrestrial radiation and population density in Connecticut, 1935–1974. Am J Epidemiol 123:1–14.

WANG G, AHN YS, WHITCOMB CC, et al. 1984. Development of polycythemia vera and chronic lymphocytic leukemia during the course of refractory idiopathic thrombocytopenic purpura. Cancer 53:1770–1776.

WANG J-X, BOICE JD JR, LI B-X, et al. 1988. Cancer among medical diagnostic x-ray workers in China. J Natl Cancer Inst 80:344–350.

WANG J-X, INSKIP PD, BOICE JD JR, et al. 1990. Cancer incidence among medical diagnostic x-ray workers in China, 1950 to 1985. Int J Cancer 45:889–895.

WARD G. 1917. The infection theory of acute leukaemia. Br J Childh Dis 14:10–20.

WARREN RP, STORB R, NELSON NJ, et al. 1981. Increased frequency of the group 5a antigen in patients in the hematologic malignancies. Tissue Antigens 18:85–91.

WARREN RP, STORB R, NGUYEN DD, et al. 1977. Association between leucocyte group 5a antigen and acute lymphoblastic leukemia. Lancet 1:509–510.

WATANABE S, TSUNEMATSU Y, FUJIMOTO J, et al. 1988. Leukaemia in patients treated with growth hormone. Lancet 1:1159–1162.

WATANABE S, YAMAGUCHI N, TSUNEMATSU Y, et al. 1989. Risk factors for leukemia occurrence among growth hormone users. Jpn J Cancer Res 80:822–825.

WATERHOUSE J, MUIR C, SHANMUGARATNUM K, et al. 1982. Cancer Incidence in Five Continents. Vol. IV. Lyon, IARC.

WATSON MM, CARROLL AJ, SHUSTER CP, et al. 1993. Trisomy 21 in childhood acute lymphoblastic leukemia: A Pediatric Oncology Group Study (8602). Blood 82:3098–3102.

WAXWEILER RJ, ROSCOE RJ, ARCHER VA, et al. 1981. Mortality

follow-up through 1977 of the white underground uranium miners cohort examined by the United States Public Health Service. *In* Gomez M (ed): International Conference, Radiation Hazards in Mining-Control, Measurements, and Medical Aspects. Golden, Colorado, Colorado School of Mines.

WAXWEILER RJ, ALEXANDER V, LEFFINGWELL SS, et al. 1983. Mortality from brain tumor and other causes in a cohort of petrochemical workers. J Natl Cancer Inst 70:75–81.

WEI L, ZHA U, TAO Z, et al. 1990. Epidemiological investigation of radiological effects in high background radiation areas of Yangjiang, China. J Radiat Res 31:119–136.

WEISS SH, GINZBURG HM, SAXINGER WC, et al. 1987. Emerging high rates of human T-cell lymphotropic virus type I (HTLV-I) and HIV infection among U.S. drug abusers. Proceedings, Third International AIDS Conference, Paris, June, p. 211.

WELCH LS, CULLEN MR. 1988. Effect of exposure to ethylene glycol ethers on shipyard painters. III. Hematologic effects. Am J Ind Med 14:527–536.

WELLES SL, LEVINE PH, JOSEPH EM, et al. 1994. An enhanced surveillance program for adult T-cell leukemia in central Brooklyn. Leukemia 8(Suppl 1):S111–S115.

WERNER-FAVRE C, JEANNET M. 1979. HLA compatibility in couples with children suffering from acute leukemia or aplastic anemia. Tissue Antigens 13:307–309.

WERTHEIMER N, LEEPER E. 1979. Electrical wiring configurations and childhood cancer. Am J Epidemiol 109:273–284.

WHANG-PENG J, YOUNG RC, LEE EC, et al. 1988. Cytogenetic studies in patients with secondary leukemia/dysmyelopoietic syndrome after different treatment modalities. Blood 71:403–414.

WHELDON TE, MAIRS R, BARRETT A. 1989. Germ cell injury and childhood leukaemia clusters. Lancet 1:792–793.

WICH RR, CLINELEVSKY D, GOSSNER W. 1986. Ra^{224} risk to bone and hematopoietic tissue in ankylosing spondylitis patients. *In* Gossner W, Gerber GB, Hazen U, Luz A (eds): The Radiobiology of Radium and Thorotrast. Munich, Urban, pp. 38–49.

WIGGS LD, COX-DEVORE CA, WILKINSON GS, et al. 1991. Mortality among workers exposed to external ionizing radiation at a nuclear facility in Ohio. J Occup Med 33:632–637.

WIKLUND K, EINHORN J, EIKLUND G. 1981. An application of the Swedish Cancer-Environment registry. Leukemia among telephone operators at the Telecommunications Administration in Sweden. Int J Epidemiol 10:373–376.

WIKLUND K, HOLM L-H. 1986. Trends in cancer risks among Swedish agricultural workers. J Natl Cancer Inst 77:657–664.

WIKTOR SZ, BLATTNER WA. 1991. Epidemiology of HTLV-I. *In* Gallo RC, Jay G (eds): The Human Retrovirus. San Diego, Academic Press, pp. 175–192.

WIKTOR SZ, MANN JM, NZILABMI N, et al. 1990. Human T-cell lymphotropic virus type I (HTLV-I) among female prostitutes in Kinshasa, Zaire. J Infect Dis 161:1073–1077.

WILCOSKY TC, CHECKOWAY H, MARSHALL EG, et al. 1984. Cancer mortality and solvent exposures in the rubber industry. Am Ind Hyg Assoc J 45:809–811.

WILKINSON GS, DREYER NA. 1991. Leukemia among nuclear workers with protracted exposure to low-dose ionizing radiation. Epidemiology 2:305–309.

WILKINSON GS, TEITJEN GL, WIGGS LD. 1987. Mortality among plutonium and other radiation workers at a plutonium weapons facility. Am J Epidemiol 125:231–250.

WILLIAMS AE, FANG CT, SLAMON DJ, et al. 1988. Seroprevalence and epidemiologic correlates of HTLV-I infection in U.S. blood donors. Science 240:643–646.

WILLIAMS CKO, BAMGBOYE EA. 1983. Estimation of incidence of human leukemia subtypes in an urban African population. Oncology 40:381–386.

WILLIAMS CKO, DADA A, BLATTNER WA. 1994. Some epidemiological features of the Human T-cell Lymphotropic Virus Type I (HTLV-I) and ATL in Nigerians. Leukemia 8(Suppl 1):577–582.

WILLIAMS CKO, ESSIEN EM, BAMGBOYE E. 1984a. Trends in leukemia incidence in Ibadan, Nigeria. *In* Magrath I, O'Conor GT, Ramot B (eds): Pathogenesis of Leukemias and Lymphomas: Environmental Influence. New York, Raven Press, pp. 17–27.

WILLIAMS CKO, ALABI GO, JUNAID TA, et al. 1984b. Human T-cell leukaemia virus associated lymphoproliferative disease: Report of two cases in Nigeria. Br Med J 288:1495–1496.

WILLIAMS CKO, JOHNSON AOK, BLATTNER WA. 1984c. Human T-cell leukaemia virus in Africa: Possible roles in health and disease. IARC Scientific Publication No. 63. Lyon, IARC, pp. 713–726.

WILLIAMS CKO, FOLAMI AO, LADITAN AAO, et al. 1982. Childhood acute leukaemia in a tropical population. Br J Cancer 46:89–94.

WILLIAMS RR, STEGENS NL, GOLDSMITH JR. 1977a. Associations of cancer site and type with occupation and industry from the Third National Cancer Survey Interview. J Natl Cancer Inst 59:1147–1185.

WILLIAMS RR, HORM JW. 1977b. Association of cancer sites with tobacco and alcohol consumption and socioeconomic status of patients: Interview study from the Third National Cancer Survey. J Natl Cancer Inst 58:525–547.

WING S, SHY CM, WOOD JL, et al. 1993. Job factors, radiation and cancer mortality at Oak Ridge National Laboratory. Follow-up through 1984. Am J Ind Med 23:265–279.

WING S, SHY CM, WOOD JL, et al. 1991. Mortality among workers at Oak Ridge National Laboratory. Evidence of radiation effects in follow-up through 1984. JAMA 65:1397–1402.

WINGREN G, KARLSSON M. 1990. Mortality trends for leukemia in selected countries. *In* Davis DL, Hoel D (eds): Trends in Cancer Mortality in Industrial Countries. New York, New York Academy of Sciences, pp. 280–286.

WINICK NJ, MCKENNA RW, SHUSTER JJ, et al. 1993. Secondary acute myeloid leukemia in children with acute lymphoblastic leukemia treated with Etoposide. J Clin Oncol 11:209–217.

WITHERSPOON RP, FISHER LD, SCHOCH G, et al. 1989. Secondary cancers after bone marrow transplantation for leukemia or aplastic anemia. N Engl J Med 321:784–789.

WONG O. 1987. An industry wide mortality study of chemical workers occupationally exposed to benzene. II. Dose response analyses. Br J Ind Med 44:382–395.

WONG O. 1990. A cohort mortality study and a case-control study of workers potentially exposed to styrene in the reinforced plastics and composites industry. Br J Ind Med 47:753–762.

WONG O, RAABE GK. 1989. Critical review of cancer epidemiology in petroleum industry employees, with a quantitative meta-analysis by cancer site. Am J Ind Med 15:283–310.

WONG O, RAABE GK. 1995. Cell-type-specific leukemia analyses in a combined cohort of more than 208,000 petroleum workers in the United States and the United Kingdom, 1937–1989. Reg Toxicol Pharmacol 21:307–321.

WONGSRICHANALAI C, DELZELL E, COLE P. 1989. Mortality from leukemia and other diseases among workers at a petroleum refinery. J Occup Med 31:106–111.

WOOD EE. 1963. Leukemia clusters. Lancet 2:583.

WOOD EE. 1960. A survey of leukaemia in Cornwall 1948–1959. Br Med J 1:1760–1764.

WOODS WG, ROLOFF JS, LUKENS JN, et al. 1981. The occurrence of leukemia in patients with Schwachman's syndrome. J Pediatr 99:425–428.

WORLD HEALTH ORGANIZATION. 1947. International Classification of Diseases (Sixth Revision). Geneva, WHO.

WORLD HEALTH ORGANIZATION. 1957. International Classification of Diseases (Seventh Revision). Geneva, WHO.

WORLD HEALTH ORGANIZATION. 1967. International Classification of Diseases (Eighth Revision). Geneva, WHO.

WRIGHT WE, PETERS JM, MACK TM. 1982. Leukaemia in workers exposed to electrical and magnetic fields. Lancet 2:1160–1161.

YANG C, ZHANG X. 1991. Incidence survey of leukemia in China. Chin Med Sci J 6:65–70.

YIN S-N, LI G-L, TAIN F-D, et al. 1987. Leukaemia in benzene workers: A retrospective cohort study. Br J Ind Med 44:124–128.

YIN S-N, LI G-L, TAIN F-D, et al. 1989. A retrospective cohort study of leukemia and other cancers in benzene workers. Environ Health Perspect 82:207–213.

YOKOTA S, TANIWAKI M, OKUDA T, et al. 1989. Acute nonlymphocytic leukemia (M2) with chromosome abnormality trisomy 4 developing eight years after radiation therapy for breast cancer. Blut 58:27–31.

YOSHIDA M, MIYOSHI I, HINUMA Y. 1982. Isolation and characterization of retrovirus from cell lines of human adult T-cell leukemia and its implication in the disease. Proc Natl Acad Sci USA 79:2031.

YOSHIMOTO Y. 1990. Cancer risk among children of atomic bomb survivors. A review of RERF epidemiologic studies. JAMA 264:596–600.

YOUNG JL JR, PERCY CL, ASIRE AJ. 1981. Surveillance, Epidemiology and End Results: Incidence and Mortality Data, 1973–77. Natl Cancer Inst Monogr 57.

YOUNGSON JHAM, CLAYDEN AD, MYERS A, et al. 1991. A case/control study of haematological malignancies in relation to overhead powerlines. Br J Cancer 63:977–985.

YUNIS JJ, BRUNNING RD, HOWE RB, et al. 1984. High-resolution chromosomes as an independent prognostic indicator in adult acute nonlymphocytic leukemia. N Engl J Med 311:812–818.

ZACK M, ADAMI H-O, ERICSON A. 1991. Maternal and perinatal risk factors for childhood leukemia. Cancer Res 51:3696–3701.

ZAHM SH, WEISENBURGER DD, BABBITT PA, et al. 1992. Use of hair coloring products and the risk of lymphoma, multiple myeloma, and chronic lymphocytic leukemia. Am J Public Hlth 82:990–997.

ZARRABI MH, GRUNWALD HW, ROSNER F. 1977. Chronic lymphocytic leukemia terminating in acute leukemia. Arch Intern Med 137:1059–1064.

ZHENG W, LINET MS, SHU X-O, et al. 1993. Prior medical conditions and the risk of adult leukemia in Shangai, People's Republic of China. Cancer Causes Control 4:361–368.

ZIPURSKY A, PEETERS M, POON A. 1987. Megakaryoblastic leukemia and Down's syndrome—a review. *In* McCoy EE, Epstein CJ (eds): Oncology and Immunology of Down's Syndrome. New York, Alan Liss, pp. 33–56.

ZOLOTH SR, MICHAELS DM, VILLALBI JR, et al. 1986. Patterns of mortality among commercial pressmen. J Natl Cancer Inst 76:1047–1051.

ZUELZER WW, COX DE. 1969. Genetic aspects of leukemia. Semin Hematol 6:4–25.

ZUELZER WW, THOMPSON RI, MOSTANGELO R. 1968. Evidence for a genetic factor related to leukemogenesis and congenital anomalies: Chromosomal aberrations and pedigree of an infant with partial D-trisomy. J Pediatr 72:367–376.

41 Hodgkin's disease

NANCY E. MUELLER

Hodgkin's disease (HD), a malignancy of the immune system, is distinguished by its atypical clinical features and unusual epidemiology. Biologically, the co-existing features of a chronic granulomatous infection, a complex immunologic disorder, and a malignant lymphoid neoplasm suggest that the pathogenesis of the disease is exceptional from what is generally true of cancer and likely involves an infectious process (Kaplan, 1981). Epidemiologically, the bimodal age incidence curve suggests that it is a disease syndrome which results from two age-dependent etiologic pathways (MacMahon, 1957). The lineage of the Reed-Sternberg cell (RSC)—the presumed malignant cell—continues to be a matter of debate. With the advent of molecular biology, however, new tools are now available to address many persisting questions about the fundamental nature of this disease and, in particular, its relationship with the Epstein-Barr virus (EBV) (Ford, 1988; Mueller, 1991). We may now be entering a period when the relationship between the epidemiology and biology of HD will become clear.

DEMOGRAPHIC PATTERNS

Biologic Features

The clinical and histologic features of HD suggest a chronic infectious process. Patients characteristically present with cervical lymphadenopathy often accompanied by splenic enlargement; mediastinal, axillary, and inguinal nodes may also be involved. Fever, night sweats, and unexplained weight loss are common and indicate a less favorable prognosis. Leukocytoses, including eosinophilia and monocytosis, often occur. The disease spreads contiguously in the lymphatic system.

The pathologic appearance of involved lymph nodes is that of a highly mixed and reactive process. The diagnosis of HD is based on the presence of the giant polynuclear RSC. However, very few of these cells and their apparent precursor mononuclear variant, "Hodgkin's cells," are evident. The diagnosis is also based on the characteristic reactive cellular environment of the RSC predominated by rosetting, activated T-helper cells as well as eosinophils, macrophages, histiocytes, interdigitating reticulum cells, plasma cells, and fibroblasts (Morris and Stuart, 1984; Romagnani et al, 1985; Ree and Kadin, 1985; Carbone et al, 1987). The highly reactive cellular microenvironment in involved nodes has been reported to be accompanied by a reciprocal reduction of circulating T-helper cells, apparently due to displacement from the peripheral blood to lymphoid organs, suggesting a sustained immune response to chronic tissue-based antigen (Romagnani et al, 1983).

Based on histological features, the disease is classified into four major categories: *lymphocyte predominance* (LP), *nodular sclerosis* (NS), *mixed cellularity* (MC), and *lymphocyte depletion* (LD). Of these, LP—the most infrequent subtype (~5%)—differs in many aspects from the others and likely represents an independent entity (Poppema et al, 1979). The other three can be viewed as on a continuum of increasing clinical aggressiveness with NS being the most favorable and LD, the least. In a study of 719 patients, Mauch et al (1993) found that NS- and MC-HD most frequently arise in the triad formed by the mediastinum and low cervical/supraclavicular nodes, which is consistent with an infectious etiology. In contrast, LD is the most likely to have abdominal involvement, to be accompanied by "B" symptoms, and to occur at an older age.

The disease is accompanied by a complex deficiency in cellular immunity. This impairment is evident prior to treatment and persists to some degree following remission. As extensively reviewed by Romagnani et al (1985) and Slivnick et al (1990), the spectrum of immune alterations includes impairment of delayed cutaneous hypersensitivity, enhanced immunoglobulin production, high levels of circulating immune complexes, production of anti-lymphocyte and anti-Ia (class II antigen) antibodies, decreased natural killer cell cytotoxicity, enhanced sensitivity to suppressor monocytes and

Dr. Mueller was a recipient of an American Cancer Faculty Research Award. The editorial assistance of Ms. Sara Vargas and Ms. Sandra Chinn is greatly appreciated. This chapter is dedicated to the memory of Bill Soiffer, author of *Life in the Shadow*, a guide for living with Hodgkin's disease.

T-suppressor cells, and a variety of serum factor abnormalities. In vitro, peripheral blood lymphocytes evidence spontaneous DNA and IgG synthesis. However, these cells exhibit a depressed proliferative response to T-cell mitogen stimulation with concomitant impairment of lymphokine production.

To help explain these findings, Ford et al (1984, 1988) had proposed that the primary immune defect is the deficiency of interleukin-2 (IL-2) production by T cells upon activation by macrophage-processed antigen. IL-2 plays a central role in immune response by stimulating the clonal expansion of activated T cells bearing IL-2 receptors, activating cytotoxic lymphocytes, and inducing the synthesis of other lymphokines (Dinarello and Mier, 1987). Pizzolo et al (1987) have observed that the majority of HD patients with active disease have significantly higher than normal serum levels of soluble IL-2 receptors. This suggests that there is, in fact, a chronic stimulation by IL-2 in these patients. Thus the inability of HD patients' T cells to produce IL-2 may be due to feedback down-regulation by continuous endogenous exposure in vivo (Fuchs et al, 1987).

This view of a chronic production of immune mediators as central to the pathogenesis of HD is supported by the detection of a range of cytokines in biopsy material as reviewed by Drexler (1992) and Gruss et al (1994), and in Hodgkin cell cultures as reviewed by Diehl et al, 1990.

The malignant characteristics of HD include aneuploidy, clonality, metastatic spread, and heterotransplantability (Kaplan, 1980). Cabanillas (1988) and Thangavelu and LeBeau (1989) have reviewed the results of studies of cytogenetic abnormalities identified in involved tissue. Not all specimens have evidence of chromosomal abnormality, and none of those found are universal (Mueller, 1991). The most common abnormalities seen are at chromosome sites 14q, 11q, 6p, and 8, with frequent involvement of 14q32—the site of the immunoglobulin heavy-chain genes. The other structural abnormalities generally correspond to those seen in other immunologic disorders. There is no consistent expression of oncogene expression; altered *p53* is found in about one-third of HD cases (Drexler, 1992; Doussis et al, 1993).

Griesser and Mak (1988) reviewed the results of immunogenotyping findings in 112 HD cases. Four types of gene rearrangement patterns were found: T-cell receptor γ and β chain genes, and immunoglobulin heavy and light chain genes in a minority of cases. Subsequent studies found similar results (Mueller, 1991; Drexler, 1992). No one pattern is uniformly present, nor are gene rearrangements detected frequently—generally less than 15%. Because of the mixed cellular environment of lesions, these rearrangements may not necessarily occur in the RSC or Hodgkin's cell populations themselves but may reflect clonal expansion of reactive lymphoid cell populations.

Attempts to establish continuing cultures of the Reed-Sternberg and Hodgkin's cells have been fraught with failures, with few apparent successes (Diehl et al, 1982). The few cell lines which have been established are from atypical cases and are themselves heterogenous in character (Drexler, 1993). The difficulty in establishing cell lines has been attributed to the exceedingly low mitotic activity of these cells (Rowley, 1982). Anastasi et al (1987) have pointed out that the aneuploidy seen in HD appears to represent replication of DNA without accompanying nuclear division. This "dead-end-cell"–like behavior is dramatically different from the monoclonal proliferation which characterizes the other lymphomas.

The lineage of the RSC is uncertain and has been a matter of continuing debate for several decades (Drexler, 1992). (It should be noted that in LP (nodular) HD, the Hodgkin's cells stain for pan B-cell markers (Pinkus and Said, 1988).) As reviewed by Romagnani et al in 1985, this question has not been resolved by phenotyping of the apparent HD cell lines because of the difficulty in proving that the cells are in fact the progeny of the RSC. Monoclonal antibody phenotyping of fixed RSCs suggests two candidates as possible cells of origin: an activated T cell, because of the presence of the activation markers Ki-1 antigen and IL-2 receptor (CD25) (Kadin et al, 1988; Stein, et al, 1985; Pizzolo et al, 1984); and an interdigitating reticulum cell or histiocyte, due to the presence of prostaglandin H synthase (Hsu et al, 1988). Following a symposium on this question, Drexler and Leber (1987) concluded that phenotypically, the RSC are lymphoid cells "frozen in a state of activation." The observations of clonal genetic rearrangements in both B and T lymphocytes suggest that the ultimate lesion is in neither one. Rather, these clonal rearrangements and the bizarre nature of the RSC may be secondary effects of chronic antigen stimulation.

DESCRIPTIVE EPIDEMIOLOGY: USA

HD accounts for less than 1% of all new cancers diagnosed in the United States. Based on the Surveillance, Epidemiology and End Results (SEER) Program of the National Cancer Institute, the age-adjusted incidence rate for the period 1986–90 was 2.8 per 100,000 person-years (Miller et al, 1993). Incidence was more common among males than females, and was more common among whites than blacks (Table 41–1). Between 1973 and 1990 there was an overall decrease of 8.3% (Miller et al, 1993). This decrease was not uniform across age-groups; rather, there was an increase of HD incidence among young adults and a greater decrease among persons older than age 40 (Glaser, 1986; Hartge et al,

TABLE 41–1. *Incidence and Mortality Rates of Hodgkin's Disease from 1989 to 1990 and Percent Changes between 1973–74 and 1990**

	Total Population		*Blacks*		*Whites*	
	Males	*Females*	*Males*	*Females*	*Males*	*Females*
Incidence rate (1989–90)	3.3[a]	2.5	2.9	2.1	3.6	2.7
Percent change (1973–85)	−14.7	−6.2	−25.1	−40.1	−11.8	+0.6
Percent change (1986–90)	1.9	6.5	19.5	34.7	3.7	3.7
Mortality rate (1989–90)	0.8	0.5	0.8	0.4	0.8	0.5
Percent change (1973–85)	−44.9	−47.4	−30.3	−24.1	−45.6	−48.8
Percent change (1986–90)	−10.0	−11.0	−2.7	−11.5	−10.8	−10.3

*From Miller et al (1993) with permission.
[a]Cases per 100,000 person-years.

1994). The decrease in incidence among the older ages appears to reflect a reduction in the number of misdiagnosed cases (Glaser and Swartz, 1990; Dige et al, 1991).

During the period 1986–90, the age-adjusted mortality rate was 0.6 per 100,000 person-years. Between 1973 and 1990 there was a decrease of 54.6% in mortality rates, reflecting the substantial improvement in treatment over the past two decades. The 5-year relative survival rate for the patients diagnosed between 1983 and 1989 was 74.1% for blacks and 78.6% for whites (Miller et al, 1993).

The distinguishing epidemiological feature of HD—its bimodal age-incidence curve—is characteristically seen among "developed" or, more precisely, economically advantaged populations (Fig. 41–1). In such populations there are very few cases occurring among children, a rapid increase of incidence among teenagers which peaks about age 25, and then a decrease to a plateau through middle-age, after which rates increase

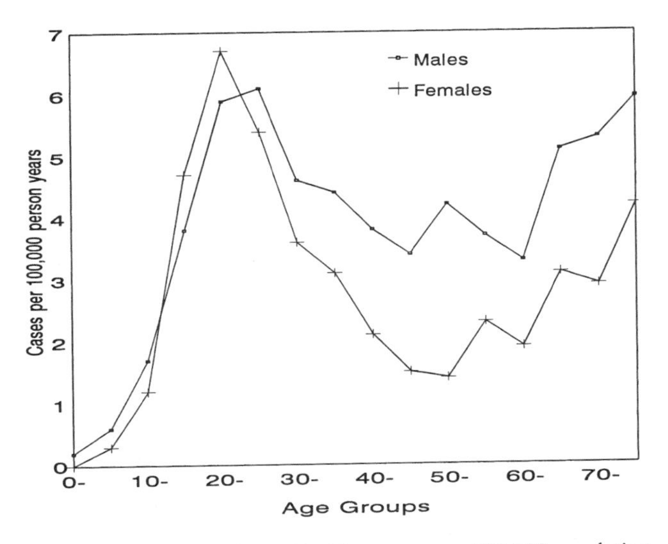

FIG. 41–1. Age-specific annual incidence rates per 100,000 population of Hodgkin's disease for whites by sex, 1981–1985, in the SEER Program (Miller et al, 1993).

with advancing age to the second peak. There is generally an excess among males in both age peaks. MacMahon (1957) proposed that the bimodality results from the overlap of two disease distributions with differing age peaks. Specifically, he proposed that among young adults, HD is caused by a biological agent of low infectivity, and that among the elderly, the cause is probably similar to those of the other lymphomas (MacMahon, 1966).

In 1971 Correa and O'Conor noted that among economically disadvantaged populations, a different age pattern is evident. In this case there is an initial peak during childhood only for boys (Parkin et al, 1988), and relatively low rates among young adults, followed by the late peak among those of advanced age. An example of this pattern is apparent in incidence data for Cali, Colombia in the early 1960s (Fig. 41–2). By 1970 the pattern for Cali had evolved from the developing pattern to what Correa and O'Connor termed an "intermediate" pattern. A similar shift is evident in data from Puerto Rico and Bombay for males between 1970 and 1985 (Hartge et al, 1994). A notable exception to these observations has been in Japan, where HD has been extremely rare before age 50. Recent data from Osaka, however, indicate that the disease has become more frequent among young adults (Aozasa et al, 1986).

Currently, essentially all majority populations in Europe and North America have a well-defined developed pattern of HD incidence. The height of peak occurrence during young adulthood varies within this set of countries with rates being high in Canada, the United States, Switzerland, and France, and lower in southern Europe. The pattern within the former Eastern Bloc countries is variable. In contrast, the pattern in Asia and Africa is generally intermediate or developing (Parkin et al, 1992).

Within the same population, the age pattern will differ between population subgroups with major differences in socioeconomic level. An example of this was observed in Norway during the early 1960s in relation to urbanization, where the pattern in rural areas was

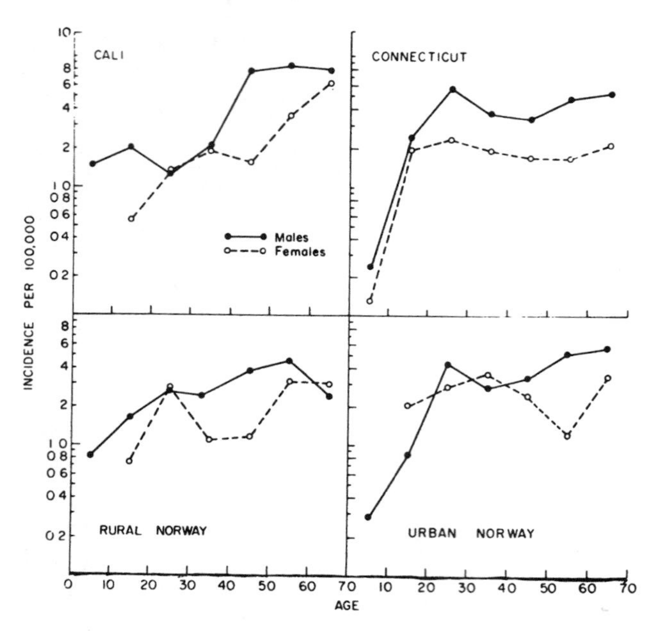

FIG. 41–2. Age-specific average annual incidence rates per 100,000 population of Hodgkin's disease by sex in *(a)* Cali, Colombia (1962–1966); *(b)* Connecticut, USA (1960–1962); *(c)* rural Norway (1964–1966); and *(d)* urban Norway (1964–1966). From Correa and O'Conor, 1971, with permission.

intermediate and that in urban areas was developed (Fig. 41–2). An example of this variation between races was reported by Cohen and Hamilton (1980) for patients diagnosed in Johannesburg, South Africa. The age–incidence pattern among blacks was characterized as "developing-intermediate" and that among whites, "intermediate-developed." The predominant pattern among blacks in America at present is best characterized as intermediate-developed, based on national statistics from 1973 to 1981 (Horm et al, 1985). As recently reviewed by Glaser (1990a), the secular changes in HD mortality in blacks and whites in America is consistent with their respective general socioeconomic conditions. Spitz et al (1986) evaluated the age–incidence data for white, black, and Hispanic American children and adolescents. Again, the data are generally in keeping with the pattern of general socioeconomic level. Examination of longitudinal data from the Connecticut Cancer Registry reveals the evolution from an intermediate to a typical developed pattern between 1935 and 1980 (Fig. 41–3). The data suggest a childhood peak among boys in the late 1930s. Clemmesen (1981) has noted the existence of a secondary peak among middle-aged males in some economically advantaged populations. That secondary peak is apparent in Figure 41–3.

From social class–specific incidence data there has been evidence that rates of HD are higher among adults from a higher social class. However, the data have not always been consistent (Mueller, 1987). When the data

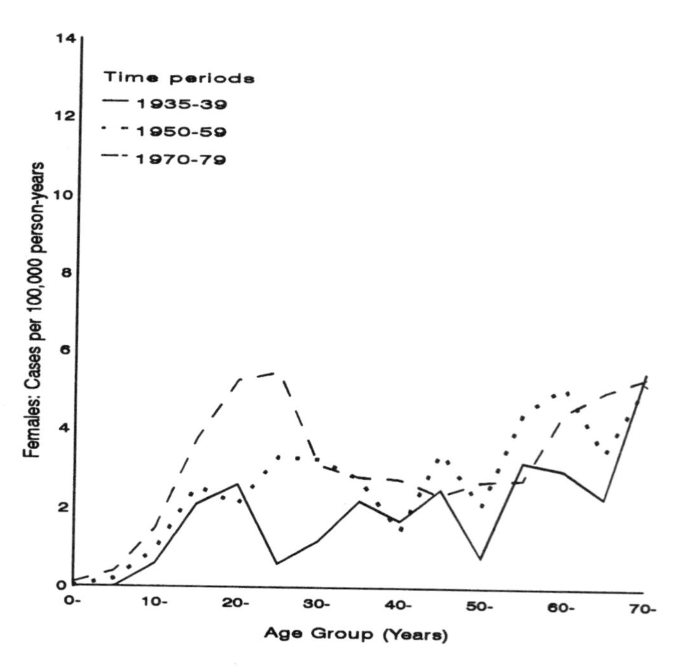

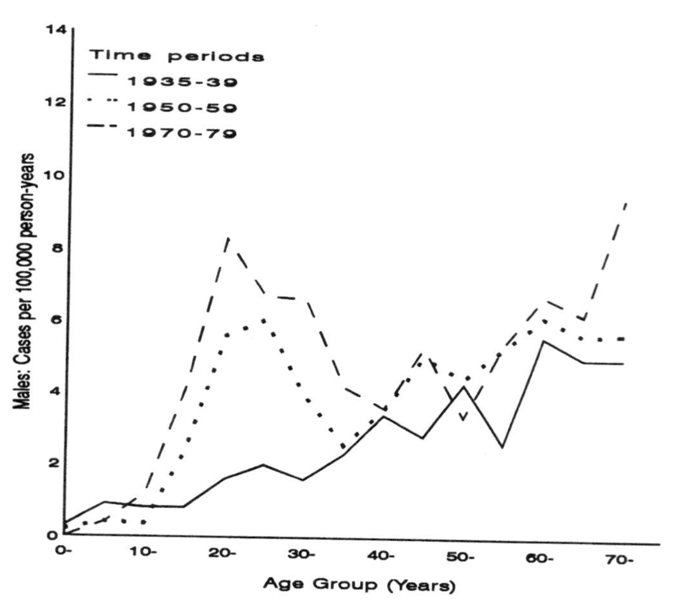

FIG. 41–3. Age-specific incidence rates for Hodgkin's disease in the state of Connecticut (USA) for three time periods, 1935 through 1979, according to sex (Cusano and Young, 1986).

are examined separately by respective age-group corresponding to the two major age peaks, a clearer picture emerges. Glaser (1987) evaluated U.S. incidence data from 1969 to 1980. She found that rates for young adults were correlated with community-level social class indicators. She also reported that the incidence of NS type HD, the most common histologic type diagnosed in young adults, increased with regional social class indices. Henderson et al (1979) computed histologic-specific incidence rates for HD in Los Angeles County from 1972 to 1975 by social class. They reported that the incidence of NS was directly related to social class, but there was no consistent association for the other histological types. These data were extended through 1985 by Cozen et al (1992) who confirmed the initial observation. In addition, they found that the risk pattern for MC was quite distinct and was negatively associated with social class, suggesting that the two histologic subtypes had separate etiologies.

As part of a large, population-based leukemia/lymphoma registry covering about half of the United Kingdom over a 5-year period, Alexander and colleagues have evaluated the characteristics of over 1,800 HD cases by area-based socioeconomic and population density indices. They reported that, of the 486 cases diagnosed under age 25, the rates were significantly greater in the high socioeconomic areas (relative risk [RR] = 1.22), and there was a significant trend toward increased rates in areas closer to built-up areas, with mutual adjustment for type of area (Alexander et al, 1991b). They also reported that for ages < 35 yr at diagnosis, there was a significantly positive association for social class; while a negative association was found for cases grouped by ages 35–49 and 50–79, with the trend for the latter being significant (Alexander, 1991a).

Using SEER data from 1969 to 1980, Glaser and Swartz (1990) analyzed the secular trends in HD incidence among U.S. whites by age-group with adjustment for diagnostic error. The adjustments were based on the database from the Repository Center for Lymphoma Clinical Studies which include original and expert review diagnoses on about 16,000 patients with presumed lymphoma seen between 1967 and 1986. Of these, 2,670 cases had an original and/or an expert diagnosis of HD and had complete demographic data. Analysis of diagnostic accuracy found that the percentage of original HD diagnoses confirmed on expert review decreased with age and increased over the time period. With correction, there was a slight increase in HD incidence among young adults over the time period. For older adults, rates were lower than those reported and showed no secular changes. It is noteworthy that in SEER data from Los Angeles County, there was a secular increase in NS-HD but not in other subtypes between 1971 and 1985 (Cozen et al, 1992).

A general observation is that HD cases occurring in economically developing populations (Mueller, 1987) and among lower social class groups in developed populations (Hu et al, 1988) are predominantly of the MC and LD subtypes. These subtypes are associated with an advanced stage of disease. The social class differences seen in the histologic presentation of HD may reflect a mix of age-dependent host responses related to environmental exposures.

Taken together, these observations are consistent with the hypothesis that HD may develop as a rare consequence of a common infection, with risk increasing if infection is delayed until adolescence or young adulthood (Gutensohn and Cole, 1977). With more clinically severe infection, which often occurs when the infections normally encountered in childhood are experienced instead during adulthood, the immunological control of a latent virus may be altered. This may result in more chronic viral expression and continuing antigenic stimulation. This hypothesis is based on the observations of Newell in 1970 and Abramson in 1974 of the similarity between the geographical distribution of HD with that of a highly prevalent infection for which early infection was protective and generally mild, as in paralytic poliomyelitis.

The epidemiology of HD and that of paralytic polio in the prevaccine era are clearly analogous. For both diseases, age–incidence patterns vary with level of economic development, internationally and regionally. Among young children, the risk of both diseases is greater in the least favorable environment, and among adolescents and young adults, the risk is greater in the most favorable environment. For both diseases, there has been a shift in the age–incidence pattern over time that is coincident with socioeconomic development. Finally, risk of both diseases increases directly with social class. If this analogy is correct, then factors in the childhood social environment such as family size and general hygiene, which influence the age of exposure to infectious agents, should be associated with risk of HD. As will be shown subsequently, there is substantial epidemiological evidence to support the hypothesis.

An interesting feature of the descriptive epidemiology of HD is the variation in sex ratio by age. As Glaser (1994) has pointed out, there appears to be a deficit of cases among women in their late thirties and forties in recent data from the United States and elsewhere. Glaser proposes that this may represent a protective effect from childbearing, perhaps mediated by estrogens.

ANALYTICAL EPIDEMIOLOGY

Because of the variation in incidence of HD with age, the following review of the analytical epidemiological features of the disease will be divided where appropriate into four age-groups: *children* (0–14 yr), *young adults* (15–39 yr), *middle-aged* (40–54 yr), and *older* (≥ 55 yr).

Social Class and Childhood Environment

Children. Relatively little analytical work has dealt with social class characteristics of children with HD. Because the disease in children occurs primarily in developing countries, it is likely, in general, that the children at risk are those of lower social class. In a small study done in the north of Portugal of 28 children under age 10 compared to 22 similarly aged children whose presumptive diagnosis of HD was not confirmed, it was found that the cases were more likely to have been diagnosed in a free general hospital than in a private clinic. The RR was 5.8. These cases also came from larger families than was expected (Sobrinho-Simoes and Areias, 1978). Bogger-Goren et al (1983) reported on 21 Israeli-born children diagnosed in one pediatric oncology-hematology center between 1971 and 1981. They noted that a disproportionate number of patients came from large families (average of 5.5 children) and from either a Jewish African-Asian or Arab ethnic origin, which may reflect a lower socioeconomic status in that population. Vianna and Polan (1978) reported the sibship size distribution of 90 cases of ages < 12 yr in upstate New York. Analysis of their data suggests that there was no consistent association of disease with family size (Gutensohn and Cole, 1979).

We addressed this question of whether lower social class children have a higher risk of HD by evaluating the social class characteristics of 66 families with children diagnosed with HD from 1959 through 1977 in a population-based study in eastern Massachusetts (Gutensohn and Shapiro, 1982). This study was based on data for 14 children who were diagnosed under the age of 10, and 52 children who were diagnosed between 10 and 14 years. Unlike the three previous studies cited, there was no strong male predominance. Characteristics of these cases were compared to those of 182 control families identified by a random process from the population base. Comparison information was based on occupational class of head of household as listed in population registries and U.S. census tract data for median income, percentage of single-unit housing, and percentage of residents below the poverty level of income. The 14 youngest children were of somewhat lower social class backgrounds than their 37 controls; the RR for children from tracts in the lowest third of median income was 3.6. In contrast, the social class of the 52 cases who were aged 10–14 yr was very similar to that of their 145 population controls.

If an infection does play a role in the etiology of HD, this apparent shift from lower to average social class between the younger and older children with the disease may reflect a shift in their age of exposure to common infections, since such infections generally occur earlier in life under more crowded and less hygienic conditions.

Young Adults. Cohen et al (1964) studied nearly 400 U.S. Army soldiers who developed HD during World War II. Before induction, these men had held occupations of higher social class than had another comparable group of soldiers. In addition, there was a twofold gradient of risk of the disease which increased with their level of education.

Among a prevalent series of young adult HD cases followed by a major treatment facility in Boston in 1974, the level of education, when compared with that of the general population, showed a risk gradient of 2.6 which increased with education level (Gutensohn and Cole 1977). More interestingly, an inverse association of risk was found in the family size distribution of these cases when compared to population data, as shown in Table 41–2. There was nearly a twofold gradient of risk, with risk among the largest families being half that of persons from the smallest families. In addition, those

TABLE 41–2. *Distribution of Hodgkin's Disease Cases and Population Data or Controls and the Relative Risk According to Sibship Size**

Study Population	*Sibship Size*	*Cases (%)*	*Population (%)*	*Relative Risk*	
				Crude	*Adjusted*
PREVALENT CASES[a]	1–2	39.7	28.7	1.00[b]	
	3	27.9	25.0	0.81	
	4	11.8	18.2	0.47	
	5+	20.6	28.1	0.53	
Total		100.0	100.0		
INCIDENCE CASES[c]	1–2	33.8	23.1	1.00[b]	1.00[b,d]
	3	25.8	27.4	0.64	0.64
	4–5	27.1	30.7	0.60	0.64
	6	13.3	18.8	0.48	0.56
Total		100.0	100.0		

*Adjusted for housing, religion, number of playmates, and infectious mononucleosis. From Gutensohn and Cole (1977, 1981) with permission.
[a]136 cases, Boston area, compared to population data, 1974.
[b]Referent category.
[c]225 cases, 447 population controls, Boston-Worcester, Massachusetts, 1973–1977.
[d]P-value for trend = 0.02 (one-tail).

persons in the fifth or later birth-order positions of large families were at lower risk than those born earlier.

To determine whether family size itself was a primary risk factor or simply another marker for social class, we conducted a population-based case–control study in the combined Boston and Worcester metropolitan areas of Massachusetts in which we attempted to identify and interview all newly diagnosed cases among the 3,098,000 residents over a 4 1/2-year period. For comparison, a control group randomly selected from the population base was also interviewed. (See Gutensohn and Cole [1981] for a detailed description of study procedures.) Among young adults in this population, a similar inverse gradient of risk with sibship size was found (Table 41–2). When the effects of other related factors—including education, parental social class, housing, religion, number of playmates, and infectious mononucleosis (IM) history—were adjusted for, effects that may be mixed with (or confound) the relationship, there was little change in the association (Table 41–2). In addition, risk was reduced among persons with late birth positions in large families. Other studies have shown a similar gradient of risk for young adult cases (T. Mack, P. Smith, personal communications).

Bernard et al (1987) have reported the results of a population-based case–control study of 248 HD patients and 489 hospital controls in the Yorkshire Health Region, UK, in which they found a similar gradient of risk. The majority of these cases were likely to be young adults. This English study also found a significant negative association with smoking (RR = 0.7). Since smoking behavior is inversely related to social class in the UK (Pocock et al, 1987), this finding suggests that the HD patients are of a higher social class.

Further, the type of childhood housing for cases in the Boston-Worcester study differed significantly from that of the controls. Persons who had lived in dwellings of three or more units had half the risk of those living in single-family homes. Cases also reported having fewer neighborhood playmates as a child, and their parents had more education than the parents of the population controls (Gutensohn and Cole, 1981).

A similar population-based study was conducted in Israel by Abramson et al (1978), based on 473 Jewish residents diagnosed between 1960 and 1970 and controls matched for sex, year and country of birth, and year of immigration. In this study, young adult cases were more likely to be high school graduates (RR = 1.4). Cases also reported somewhat more frequently than controls that their childhood homes contained a flush toilet (RR = 1.2). No data were available on family size, and the authors reported that there were no noteworthy differences in either childhood household crowding or in social class.

Two recent case–control studies from Italy looked at social class risk factors. Both studies used hospital controls. The study by Bonelli et al (1990) in Genoa found a significant inverse relation with sibship size for all ages; among young adults (97 cases, 87 controls), the association became non-significant when education level was controlled. In a case–control study conducted in Pordenone in northeastern Italy involving 152 HD cases of all ages and 613 hospital controls, there was no association with sibship size or birth order. Among the NS cases alone, which should include primarily young adults, there was a strong association with increasing education (Serraino et al, 1991).

In summary, there is evidence that risk of HD in young adults is associated with higher education, higher social class, smaller sibship, less crowded housing, and early birth position. All of these factors foster susceptibility to late infections with the common childhood infections.

In agreement with Glaser's hypothesis that parity is protective for woman in the first age peak, Kravdal and Hansen (1993) evaluated the effect of parity and HD within the Norwegian population for cohorts born between 1935 and 1974 using population registries for all data. Most of these cases were diagnosed among young adults. In their analysis there was no association of risk for parity for men but an increasingly protective effect for women; for women with ≥ 3 births, the RR was 0.46. Adjustment for social class as indexed by either the cases' or their fathers' educational level did not modify this finding, although each of these social class measures as positively associated with risk, as would be predicted. The relationship between HD risk in women and parity was also examined by Franceschi et al (1994), who used data from an earlier hospital-based case–control study in northern Italy (Franceschi et al 1991). They found a small protective association with ≥ 3 pregnancies (RR = 0.77) and a nearly significant effect of ≥ 1 abortions (RR = 0.46), with control for education.

Middle-aged Adults. Among middle-aged persons, increased risk of HD was also found to be associated with factors that reflect susceptibility to late infections in the Boston-Worcester study (Table 41–3). However, the mix of these factors differed somewhat from that seen among the young adults. In the middle-aged group there was a threefold inverse gradient of risk associated with family size, which is a somewhat greater range than that among young adults. However, the gradient of risk was lost when the confounding effects of other factors were controlled. In contrast to the young adults, neither birth order nor number of playmates was a risk factor for the middle-aged subjects (Gutensohn, 1982).

Although cases were more likely to have lived in a single-family or two-family home than were controls, this association was much weaker among the middle-

TABLE 41–3. *Percent Distribution of Middle-aged Subjects and the Relative Risk of Hodgkin's Disease According to Childhood Social Class Risk Factors**

	Percent of Subjects		*Relative Risk*	
Risk Factor	*Patients (n = 53)*	*Controls (n = 106)*	*Crude*	*Adjusted*
SIBSHIP SIZE				
1–2	40	29	1.00[a]	1.00[a,b]
3–5	49	45	0.80	1.21
6+	11	25	0.33	0.70
HOUSING				
1-family	38	33	1.00[a]	1.00[a,c]
2-family	30	24	0.62 (2-family and ≥ 3 units)	0.69 (2-family and ≥ 3 units)
≥ 3 units	32	43		
MOTHER'S EDUCATION (YR)				
≥ 13	16	7	1.00[a]	1.00[a,d]
12	44	25	0.80	0.99
9–11	16	15	0.47	0.47
≤ 8	24	53	0.21	0.15

*From Gutensohn (1982) with permission.
[a]Referent category.
[b]Adjusted for maternal education and number of children sharing bedroom.
[c]Adjusted for mother's education.
[d]Adjusted for sibship size and housing; *P*-value for trend = 0.004 (two-tail).

aged than among young adults. However, whether subjects had shared their bedroom with other children was of some importance; 57% of the HD patients had their own bedrooms when they were 11 years old, as compared to 33% of controls; the crude RR = 2.7. When controlled for sibship size, the association of risk with having one's own bedroom was evident only among subjects in families with 3–5 children (RR = 5.2).

The most important risk factor in this age-group was maternal education. Risk among persons whose mothers had more than a high school education was five times that of people whose mothers had not attended high school. Although maternal education was clearly associated with the other social class factors, its association with disease risk was quite primary. Higher paternal social class was also associated with HD risk; however, it had no independent effect once maternal education was taken into account.

In the Israeli study (Abramson et al, 1978), middle-aged cases were more likely to have a high school education and to have had a flush toilet in their childhood home; the RR for each factor was 2.0. In both of these populations, middle-aged cases appeared to be individuals whose childhood provided some protection from early infection, an observation which suggests that these may be susceptible individuals who were infected as adults, perhaps by their children. (The two recent Italian studies did not provide data for middle-aged vs. older subjects.)

Older Adult Patients. Among the oldest persons in the Boston-Worcester population, risk was not directly associated with social class (Gutensohn 1982). If anything, patients came from a somewhat lower social class than their controls. Among older men there was increased risk among those who had lived in multiple-family housing as children relative to those who had lived in single- or two-family homes. However, no difference was evident among women. For both sexes, risk was neither associated with maternal education nor with paternal social class (Table 41–4). Within the Israeli population, however, (Abramson et al, 1978), older cases again appeared to come from a somewhat higher social class as evidenced by level of education (RR = 2.1) and by the presence of a flush toilet in their childhood home (RR = 1.6).

In summary, children with relatively poor living conditions are at risk of HD. For both young adult and middle-aged persons, there is evidence that HD may be the result of an age-related host response to a common infection. Among older Americans risk appears to be independent of factors associated with age at infection, although among older Israelis, risk is associated with higher social class. Whether this latter observation is in some way confounded by the apparent general increased risk of HD among adult Jews is unknown.

TABLE 41–4. *Percent Distribution of Older Subjects and the Relative Risk of Hodgkin's Disease According to Childhood Social Risk Factors**

	Percent of Subjects		*Relative Risk*			
Risk Factor	*Patients (n = 47)*	*Controls (n = 93)*	*Crude*		*Adjusted*	
SIBSHIP SIZE						
1–2	11	17	1.0[a]		1.0[a,b]	
3–5	47	51	1.5		1.4	
6+	43	32	2.1		1.8	
HOUSING			M	F	M	F
1-family	36	48	1.0[a] (1-family and 2-family)	1.0[a] (1-family and 2-family)	1.0[a,c] (1-family and 2-family)	— (1-family and 2-family)
2-family	21	24				
≥3-unit	43	28	3.1	1.2	6.2	—
MATERNAL EDUCATION (YR)						
≥9	39	37	1.0[a]			—
8	33	29	1.1			—
≤7	28	33	0.80			—

*From Gutensohn (1982) with permission.
[a]Referent category.
[b]Adjusted for education and sex; *P*-value = 25 (two-tail).
[c]Adjusted for sibship size and education for 23 male patients, 46 controls; *P*-value = 0.008 (two-tail).

VIRAL INFECTIONS

Epstein-Barr Virus

The major candidate as an etiological infectious agent for HD is the ubiquitous herpesvirus, the EBV (Evans, 1971). This was first suggested by the ability of the virus to transform B lymphocytes, by finding Reed-Sternberg cells in lymphoid tissue of patients with IM (Lukes et al, 1969), and by recognition of the epidemiological similarities between HD and IM. Subsequent epidemiologic, serologic, and molecular biologic data have supported the association.

There have been several case reports of HD developing in close association with serologically documented EBV primary infection (Henle and Henle, 1973; Greene et al, 1979; Veltri et al, 1983). Further, in 6 cohort studies involving nearly 42,000 young adults with serologically confirmed IM who were followed, a consistent threefold excess of HD incidence was found (Miller and Beebe, 1973; Rosdahl et al, 1974; Connelly and Christine, 1974; Carter et al, 1977; Muñoz et al, 1978; Kvale et al, 1979). In the case–control study conducted in the Boston-Worcester population, significantly more young adult cases reported a history of IM than did population controls (RR = 1.8; adjusted for family size, birth order and housing) and in comparison to their own siblings (RR = 1.5) (Gutensohn and Cole, 1981; Evans and Gutensohn, 1984). In the Yorkshire study, no association was found overall. However, the authors note a significantly greater number of young adult men with HD than expected, who had IM within five years prior to diagnosis, (RR = 4.9) (Bernard et al, 1987). In the case–control study conducted in northeastern Italy (Serraino et al, 1991), 4 of 152 cases reported a history of IM compared to 1 of 613 controls; all 4 cases were young adults.

In studies of more than 1,900 HD cases of all ages, the proportion who have IgG antibody to the EBV viral capsid antigen (VCA), which is indicative of prior infection, has been quite similar to that of controls. However, the cases have consistently higher mean antibody titers than controls. Further, more of the cases have antibodies (as well as higher titers) against the early antigen (EA) of EBV, which is indicative of viral replication (Mueller, 1987).

In the Boston-Worcester case–control study, Evans and Gutensohn (1984) compared the antibody profiles of 304 cases to those of 276 of their siblings. Of particular interest was the observation that those young adult cases with a history of IM had a significantly higher geometric mean titer (GMT) of antibodies against VCA (239) than cases who did not report a history (159). Similarly, sibling controls in this age group with a history of IM had a GMT of 71, as compared to 57 for the other siblings. Since the subjects with IM were likely to have had their primary EBV infection somewhat later in life, the elevated titers seen among cases may reflect their generally late EBV infection.

Since all these results were based on blood specimens collected after the diagnosis of the disease, the findings may simply reflect the reactivation of latent EBV as a result of the immune dysfunction characteristically seen in HD. To clarify the temporal relationship between altered antibody patterns against the EBV and HD, we undertook a collaborative serologic case–control study in which we consolidated the resources of five serum banks with specimens from over 240,000 persons (Mueller et al, 1989). In these populations, we identified 43 patients from whom blood had been drawn and stored for an average of 50.5 mo before diagnosis. For comparison, we selected 96 matched controls who had blood drawn at the same time. All blood specimens were assayed for antibodies against the VCA (IgG, IgA, IgM), the EA (both the diffuse and restricted form), and the EB nuclear antigen complex (EBNA).

As shown in Table 41–5, the previous findings of elevated IgG titers against the VCA (RR = 2.6) and EA-diffuse (RR = 2.6), EA-restricted (RR = 1.9) among the cases were confirmed. In addition, a greater proportion of cases had elevated titers of IgA against the VCA than did the controls (RR = 3.7), and substantially fewer had IgM antibody (RR = 0.22). When all antibodies were simultaneously controlled for, the most significant findings were for the prevalence of higher titers for anti-EBNA (RR = 6.7) and an inverse association for IgM (RR = 0.07); this pattern is the reverse of what was seen for similar serologic specimens from non-Hodgkin's lymphoma patients prior to diagnosis (see Chapter 42). These findings for altered EBV antibody patterns before

TABLE 41–5. *Relative Risk of Hodgkin's Disease Associated with Elevated Titers of Antibodies against EBV in Blood Samples Drawn Prior to Diagnosis**

	Relative Risk (90% Confidence Interval)			
EBV Antibody	*Adjusted for IgM*		*Full Model*[a]	
VCA				
IgG (≥1:320)[b]	2.6	(1.1–6.1)	1.7	(0.52–5.4)
IgA (≥1:20)	3.7	(1.4–9.3)	4.1	(1.3–12.9)
IgM (≥1:5)	0.22	(0.04–1.3)	0.07	(0.01–0.53)
EBNA				
(≥1:80)	4.0	(1.4–11.4)	6.7	(1.8–24.5)
EA				
Diffuse (≥1:5)	2.6	(1.1–6.1)	1.5	(0.55–4.2)
Restricted (≥1:40)	1.9	(0.90–4.0)	1.2	(0.41–3.4)

*From Mueller et al (1989) with permission.
[a]Adjusted for all other antibodies against EBV.
[b]Referent category for all antibodies less than elevated.

the diagnosis of HD were generally stronger in blood specimens drawn at least three years before diagnosis than in those tested closer to the time of diagnosis.

Lehtinen et al (1993) conducted a similar study in a cohort of 39,000 healthy Finnish adults followed for 12 years. Of these, 6 adults were subsequently diagnosed with HD. Although the data are not shown, the authors report that risk for HD was associated with increased antibody response to the EBNA complex and to the EA, which is consistent with our findings (Mueller et al, 1989). The combination of both elevated anti-EA and elevated anti-EBNA is aberrant, based on present knowledge of normative host control of EBV. The presence of anti-EA is thought to reflect virus replication and is negatively associated with the frequency of EBV-specific, cytotoxic T cells. Elevated anti-EBNA is thought to reflect the level of *in vivo* destruction of virus-infected cells by T cells, and is positively associated with the frequency of EBV-specific cytotoxic T cells (Kusunoki et al, 1994). The observations from these two pre-diagnosis serologic studies imply that for a subset of cases, the development of HD is preceded over an extended period of time by endogenous EBV activation coupled with an unusual host response.

More recently, with the advent of highly sensitive molecular probes, assays for the direct detection of viral genome or of viral-encoded proteins or transcripts have been used to evaluate the relationship of EBV with HD. These include the slot blot and Southern blot (Weiss et al, 1987), in situ hybridization (Anagnostopoulos et al, 1989), and polymerase chain reaction (PCR) (Uhara et al, 1990) assays to detect the presence of viral genome fragments; PCR and in situ hybridization to detect the abundant small EB-encoded nuclear RNA transcripts termed *EBERs* (Wu et al, 1990), which are actively transcribed in latently infected cells; and in situ hybridization with monoclonal antibodies to test for the presence of the latent viral gene products, latent membrane protein 1 (LMP1) and EBNA2 (Pallesen et al, 1991a). In addition, the clonality of the episomal EBV genome has been assayed using probes for the EBV terminal repeats (Weiss et al, 1987). The EBER-1 probes are viewed as the most sensitive in detecting EBV genome in paraffin-embedded tissues, and the most specific when combined with in situ hybridization to the RSC. The presence of LMP1, which has become a fingerprint of EBV-associated HD, is not universally detected in EBV-positive RSC and is therefore somewhat less sensitive as a sole assay (Herbst et al, 1992).

Table 41–6 summarizes the plethora of studies looking for EBV fingerprints in HD tissue through 1993. The reports by Weiss et al (1987, 1991) provided the first concrete evidence that monoclonal episomal EBV was detectable in HD tissue and localized to the RSC in 4 of 21 specimens tested. This discovery has been confirmed in a large number of subsequent reports. The detection rate increased with the use of more sensitive methods. Overall, the findings suggest that about 30%–50% of HD cases are EBV-genome positive.

Pallesen et al (1991a) further demonstrated that the EBV-genome positive RSC express an altered latent infection phenotype of LMP1+/EBNA2−, both viral gene products being normally co-expressed in latently infected lymphocytes (Kieff and Liebowitz, 1990). This important finding has been confirmed by subsequent investigators. This latent phenotype of EBV is also found in EBV-genome positive nasopharyngeal carcinoma; these two malignancies share similar transcriptional programs (Deacon et al, 1993) and similar serologic patterns of elevated anti-EA-diffuse and IgA antibodies against the VCA (Evans and Mueller, 1990). A similar latent phenotype of EBV has also been reported in a small proportion of T-cell non-Hodgkin's lymphoma (Hamilton-Dutoit and Pallesen, 1992).

EBV-genome status appears to be stable over time. Delsol et al (1992) reported that EBV-genome status was quite consistent in subsequent biopsies at relapse (range 14–126 mo) in 12 cases of which 7 were initially positive. Two EBV-genome positive cases showed substantial reduction or loss of LMP1 staining in their later biopsy and all 5 initially EBV-genome negative cases were negative at relapse. Coates et al (1991) evaluated sequential biopsies in three EBV-genome positive patients (range 2–10 yr) and found all remained positive at about the same level of the initial biopsy. In terms of EBV strains in HD, almost all those typed were type 1 (Jarrett et al, 1991; Ambinder et al, 1993; Boyle et al, 1993), although 3 type B and 4 hybrid strains have been reported (Boyle et al, 1993; Lin et al, 1993). In general, the number of virus episomes per cell is low (Staal et al, 1989).

The question of the specificity of the EBV-genome positivity was raised by reports of EBV-genome positive (but LMP1−) small lymphocytes in both EBV-genome positive and negative HD (Masih et al, 1991; Weiss et al, 1991; Herbst et al, 1992; Khan et al, 1992; Ambinder et al, 1993; Chang et al, 1993; Jiwa et al, 1993; Bhagat et al, 1993), which are also found at a low frequency in normal lymph nodes (Niedobitek al, 1992). Further, clonal EBV has been detected in reactive hyperplasia biopsies (Libetta et al, 1990: Masih et al, 1991). However, the consistent finding of clonal EBV of a restricted phenotype expressing LMP1 with its oncogene-like properties (Knecht et al, 1993b) in a substantial proportion of HD cases studied throughout the world argues strongly for a causal role in these cases (Herbst and Niedobitek, 1993). The presence of the viral products LMP1 and EBER indicate that the episomal viral genome is not silent but that the latent state of the virus is actively maintained. EBNA1, the virus genome

TABLE 41–6. *Summary of Studies on Detection of Epstein-Barr Viral Genome or Gene Products in Tissue from HIV-I–Negative Hodgkin's Disease Cases**

Reference	*Number of Cases*	*Number Positive (%)*	*Method Used*	*Specific for RSC?*	*Clonal EBV?*	*Notes*
Weiss et al (1987)	21	4 (19)	SB; slot blot	—	3 of 4	Positivity increased with histologic grade; CMV−; overlaps with next study.
Weiss et al (1989)	16	3 (19)	SB; slot blot; in situ	Yes		Includes 7 cases selected for numerous RSC.
Staal et al (1989)	28	8 (29)	SB	—	1 of 8	Positivity increased with histologic grade.
Uccini et al (1989)	32	6 (19)	SB; in situ	Yes	—	
Boiocchi et al (1989)	17	7 (41)	SB	—	6 of 7	
Herbst et al (1989)	39	5 (13)	SB	—	—	Overlaps with next study.
Anagnostopoulos et al (1989)	42	7 (17)	SB; in situ	Yes	Yes.	
Uhara et al (1990)	31	8 (26)	PCR; in situ	Yes	—	Positivity increased with histologic grade.
Bignon et al (1990)	16	8 (50)	PCR	—	—	Mostly young adult cases.
Wu et al (1990)	8	6 (75)	in situ EBER	Yes	—	Cases were positives from Staal, 1989.
Herbst et al (1990)	198	114 (58)	PCR; in situ	19/28	—	No variation by age and sex.
Libetta et al (1990)	34	15 (44)	SB	—	—	No variation with age.
Uccini et al (1990)	20	3 (15)	SB; in situ	Yes	—	None positive for VCA or EA; all positives were MC.
Ohshima et al (1990)	17	2 (29)	SB; PCR	Yes	Yes	Serology available on 1 case: high titer anti-VCA and EA IgG, positive for anti-VCA IgM and IgA.
Pallesen et al (1991a)	84	40 (48)	in situ LMP-1 and EBNA2	Yes	—	Positive only for LMP-1; positivity increased with histologic grade.
Gledhill et al (1991)	35	12 (34)	PCR	—	Yes	8 of 8 type 1; based on data presented, no association with histology and little with age.
Brousset et al (1991)	54	16 (30)	in situ "mRNA"	Yes	—	Positivity increased with histologic grade; no correlation with serology with one case seronegative; results later interpreted as detecting EBV-DNA (Delsol, 1992).
Herbst et al (1991)	47	32 (68) DNA 18 (38) LMP	PCR in situ LMP-1, EBNA2, and gp350/250	Yes	—	Positive only for LMP-1; all LMP-1+ were PCR+; no variation with histology for PCR.
Knecht et al (1991)	48	32 (67)	PCR (semiquantitative)	—	Yes	Approximately 2/3 of cases selected for numerous RSC; no association with histology or proportion of RSC.
Masih et al (1991)	52	30 (58)	PCR; slot blot; SB	—	7 of 13	Positivity increased with histologic grade; 43% of hyperplastic lymph node controls were EBV+ with 2 clonal of 6 tested.
Pallesen et al (1991b)	96	47 (49)	in situ LMP-1, ZEBRA, EA, VCA, MA	Yes	—	Includes cases from Pallesen, 1991a; all cases negative for CMV; 3 LMP-1+ are ZEBRA+; none positive for EA, VCA, MA.
Vestler et al (1992)	66	27 (41)	Follow-up of cases from above			LMP-1+ cases more likely to be MC, male, and less likely to have mediastinal involvement; LMP-1 status not associated with prognosis.

(continued)

TABLE 41–6. *Summary of Studies on Detection of Epstein-Barr Viral Genome or Gene Products in Tissue from HIV-I–Negative Hodgkin's Disease Cases** (*Continued*)

Reference	*Number of Cases*	*Number Positive (%)*	*Method Used*	*Specific for RSC?*	*Clonal EBV?*	*Notes*
Jarrett et al (1991)	95	43 (45)	SB	—	25 of 26	48 cases selected for age and histology; includes cases from Gledhill, 1991; positivity highest among children and older adults; 30 of 30 type 1.
Weiss et al (1991)	40	14 (39)	PCR; in situ EBER	Yes	—	Positivity varied with histologic grade; some background B and T cells positive.
Coates et al (1991)	55	9 (16)	in situ	Yes	—	Positivity higher among NS cases (7/24) than MC (2/16); no difference in mean age of EBV+ and EBV− cases; variation in amount of virus between cases; no association with age; 3 patients with sequential biopsies (≤10 yr) were positive at same level in all specimens; in 8 other cases, EBV found only in non-RSC.
Brocksmith et al (1991)	57	33 (58)	SB; PCR	—	—	Positivity increased with histologic grade; no variation with age.
Delsol et al (1992)	107	37 (35)	in situ; in situ LMP-1, EBNA2	Yes	—	Overlaps with Brousset, 1991a; positivity highest in MC; of 12 cases tested at diagnosis and relapse, all remained concordant for EBV except 1 LMP-1+ became LMP− and 1 LMP-1+ became +/−; no correlation with serology or short-term prognosis; of 13 positive cases, all EBNA2 were negative.
Khan et al (1992)	33	12 (36)	in situ EBER	6 of 12	—	6 positives localized only to small lymphocytes.
Herbst et al (1992)	46	26 (57)	in situ EBER, LMP-1	23 of 26		18 (39%) positive for LMP-1 (all EBER-positive); EBER+ small lymphocytes found in 39 cases at low levels, 3 at high levels.
Fellbaum et al (1992)	187	66 (35)	PCR	—	—	Positivity highest in MC; no association with survival.
Murray et al (1992)	46	22 (48)	in situ LMP-1	Yes	—	Positivity and the proportion of RSC which were LMP-1+ increased with histologic grade.
Ambinder et al (1993)	36	20 (56)	in situ EBER, LMP	Yes	—	All cases <15 years; 11 of 11 cases from Honduras and 9 of 25 from U.S. were positive, all type A; all CMV−; positive small lymphocytes also seen in 9 positive cases; positivity increased with histologic grade in U.S. cases.
Boyle et al (1993)	27	8 (30)	PCR; in situ	Yes	—	1 type 1, 1 type 2; positivity associated with younger age.

(*continued*)

TABLE 41–6. (*Continued*)

Reference	Number of Cases	Number Positive (%)	Method Used	Specific for RSC?	Clonal EBV?	Notes
Chang et al (1993)	32	30 (94)	in situ EBER, LMP-1, MA			Patients from Peru; positivity by age: 19 of 19 <15, 1 of 9 were 15–39 years, 4 of 4 were older; some small lymphocytes positive.
Carbone et al (1993)	39	15 (38)	in situ; in situ LMP-1, vimentin	Yes	—	Positivity increased with histologic grade; vimentin localized to RSC found in 24 cases including all 11 LMP-1+ cases.
Deacon et al (1993)	23	16 (70)	in situ EBER, LMP-1	Yes	—	Transcription analysis demonstrated the EBV latency pattern found in NPC.
Jiwa et al (1993)	33	19 (58)	PCR; in situ EBER, LMP, *bcl*-2, c-*myc*	Yes	—	Almost all cases NS; some small lymphocytes also positive; 20 of 29 cases expressed *bcl*-2 and 30 of 32 expressed c-*myc* in RSC independent of EBV status.
Niedobitek et al (1993)	116	33 (28)	in situ EBER, *p53*	Yes	—	Positivity increased with histologic grade; 37 positive for *p53* in RSC independent of histology, less frequent in EBV+ (21%) then EBV− (36%) (P = 0.12).
Lin et al (1993)	23	16 (70)	PCR for EBER (multiple gene loci)	—	Yes	Of 6 MC cases, 4 were type 1, 1 was 1/2 hybrid; of 14 NS cases 4 were type 1, 4 were 1/2 hybrid, 2 were type 2; of 3 LP cases, 1 was type 1; 2 of 10 reactive hyperplasia control nodes were EBV+.
Bhagat et al (1993)	13	4 of 11 (36)	in situ EBER, *bcl*-2	Yes	—	Cases selected for equal numbers of t(14;18) and high RSC content, most were NS; 3 of 7 with t(14;12) were *bcl*-2+ and 5 of 6 without t(14;18); *bcl*-2 found in RSC but also in majority of small lymphocytes; EBV positivity did not correlate with presence of t(14;18) or *bcl*-2.
Khan et al (1993)	77	25 (32)	in situ EBER, LMP-1			Cases selected on basis of histology and age; positivity highest in MC (68%); some increase with age; some small lymphocytes positive; no case positive for CMV or HHV-6.

* CMV = cytomegalovirus; EA = early antigen; EBER = small EBV-encoded nuclear RNA; EBNA2 = EBV nuclear antigen 2; gp350/250 = envelope glycoprotein; LMP-1 = latent membrane protein-1; LP = lymphocyte predominance; MA = membrane antigen; MC = mixed cellularity; NS = nodular sclerosis; PCR = polymerase chain reaction; RSC = Reed-Sternberg cells; SB = Southern blot; VCA = viral capsid antigen; ZEBRA = replication-inducing protein; in situ hybridization is for EBV genome probe unless specified.

maintenance protein, is also apparently expressed (Deacon et al, 1993; Young, 1994), although this point has been challenged (Kahn and Naase, 1995).

Pallesen et al (1991b) evaluated whether the BZLF1 gene product ZEBRA was expressed in 47 HD-genome positive biopsies. This product induces the switch from latency to the lytic cycle and virus replication. They found that it was rarely expressed—only 3 biopsies were positive—and no structural viral proteins were detected. This finding was replicated by Bibeau et al (1994). This observation suggested to these investigators that the latent state of the EBV genome in HD is not severely impaired; rather, the infrequent activation of replication is impaired, resulting in an abortive viral productive cycle.

Thus the apparent mechanism of EBV in HD is not related to viral replication *per se*, but may be due to the transforming properties of LMP1 in combination with a mutation which allows it to escape immune regulation (Klein, 1994). Given the highly reactive cellular environment of the RSC, the pervasive immune dysfunction, and the array of cytokine production and receptors detected in RSC (Drexler, 1992), the EBV phenotype could be related to protracted cytokine production. The lack of expression of EBNA2, a target for cytotoxic T cells, places HD in the family of EBV-associated malignancies with restricted patterns of latent gene expression.

The data concerning histology and EBV-genome status from studies with at least 30 specimens are summarized in Table 41–7. Since the sensitivity of assays varies between studies, the most valid comparison is within studies. When the histologic subtypes are viewed as representing a continuum of increasing clinical aggressiveness from LP, NS, MC, to LD, the EBV-genome positivity rate increases with the histologic grade, although the data for LD cases are sparse and somewhat inconsistent. Of the two most common subtypes, NS and MC, MC cases generally had higher rates than NS cases with a range 10–100% in studies with at least 10 MC cases tested; however, the rates among NS cases were sometimes high and covered the same range. In the two studies involving cases from economically developing countries, Honduras (Ambinder et al, 1993) and Peru (Chang et al, 1993), where patients generally present with more advanced disease, the positivity rate was notably high. Guilley et al (1994) compared 125 cases from the United States, Mexico, and Costa Rica and found in multivariate analysis that Hispanic ethnicity *per se* was an independent predictor (RR = 4.3) of EBV genome positivity. Murray et al, (1992) noted that among EBV-genome positive specimens, the proportion of RSC that are positive for LMP1 increased in parallel to the histologic grade. Thus based on both histology and economic background, EBV-genome positivity appears to be higher among cases with a poorer host response to their disease.

TABLE 41–7. *Summary of Larger Studies on Prevalence of Epstein-Barr Virus Genome or Gene Products Detected in Tissue HIV-Negative Hodgkin's Disease Cases by Histologic Classification*

Reference	*Lymphocyte Predominance % + (No.)*	*Nodular Sclerosis % + (No.)*	*Mixed Cellularity % + (No.)*	*Lymphocyte Depletion % + (No.)*
Herbst et al (1989)	33 (3)	15 (26)	0 (10)	—
Uhara et al (1990)	25 (4)	24 (17)	33 (9)	0 (1)
Herbst et al (1990)	50 (12)	61 (109)	58 (64)	25 (4)
Libetta et al (1990)	60 (5)	41 (22)	50 (6)	0 (1)
Pallasen et al (1991a)	10 (10)	32 (50)	96 (24)	—
Brousset et al (1991)	0 (5)	18 (22)	46 (26)	—
Herbst et al (1991)	0 (1)	70 (27)	72 (18)	0 (1)
Masih et al (1991)	42 (12)	52 (21)	69 (13)	83 (6)
Jarrett et al (1991)	NS[a]	40 (45)	52 (25)	NS
Gledhill et al (1991)[b]	100 (2)	27 (26)	17 (6)	100 (1)
Weiss et al (1991)	0 (14)	33 (12)	75 (8)	50 (2)
Coates et al (1991)	0 (7)	29 (24)	13 (16)	0 (8)
Brocksmith et al (1991)	60 (5)	54 (41)	73 (11)	—
Delsol et al (1992)	0 (10)	10 (40)	60 (55)	—
Khan et al (1992)	0 (2)	15 (26)	67 (3)	0 (2)
Herbst et al (1992)	100 (2)	42 (24)	56 (18)	50 (2)
Fellbaum et al (1992)	31 (13)	28 (98)	50 (68)	12 (8)
Murray et al (1992)	8 (12)	50 (24)	86 (7)	100 (3)
Ambinder et al (1993)[c]				
Honduras	100 (1)	100 (3)	100 (6)	—
U.S.	0 (2)	13 (15)	86 (7)	—
Chang et al (1993)[d]	—	100 (7)	100 (20)	60 (5)
Carbone et al (1993)	(5) (0)	10 (20)	64 (11)	100 (3)
Niedobitek et al (1993)	11 (9)	27 (75)	39 (31)	0 (1)
Khan et al (1993)	0 (10)	24 (38)	68 (22)	14 (7)

[a]NS = not stated.
[b]Subset of above.
[c]Pediatric cases.
[d]Cases from Peru.

Table 41–8 summarizes data on EBV-genome positivity and age. In general, positivity does not appear to vary substantially with age. In a study of 198 patients, Herbst et al (1990) reported that there was no significant association between EBV-genome status and age, as did Brocksmith et al (1991) in a study of 57 patients. Further, in a study of 55 patients, Coates et al (1991) reported that the mean age of EBV-genome positive cases was 36 yr (range 18–56), which did not differ from that of negative cases, or 34 yr (12–63). The very high rate of positivity in children from economically developing populations is noteworthy.

These observations suggest that the factors affecting or reflecting immune competency are associated with EBV-genome status. These include having a more ad-

TABLE 41–8. *Summary of Studies on Prevalence of Epstein-Barr Virus Genomes or Gene Products Detected in Tissue from HIV-Negative Hodgkin's Disease Cases by Broad Age Groups*

		Children/ Adolescents (< 15 years)	*Young Adults (15–39 years)*	*Middle-aged (40–49 years)*	*Older Adults (≥ 50 years)*
Reference	*Population*	*% (No.)*	*% (No.)*	*% (No.)*	*% (No.)*
Bignon et al (1990)	France		55 (11)	50 (2)	33 (3)
Libetta et al (1990)	UK	38 (16)		50 (10)	
Jarrett et al (1991)	UK	54 (13)	20 (44)		71 (38)
Gledhill et al (1991)[a]		100 (2)	26 (23)	0 (3)	43 (7)
Ambinder et al (1993)	Peru USA	100 (11) 56 (16)			
Boyle et al (1993)	Australia		37 (19)	0 (1)	14 (7)
Chang et al (1993)	Peru	100 (19)	83 (6)	80 (5)	100 (2)
Khan et al (1993)	UK	24 (25)	33 (36)		41 (17)

[a]Subset of above.

vanced stage as indicated by histology, living in economically disadvantaged settings, and developing HD in early childhood. It is conceivable that EBV plays a pathogenic role in all of HD, but the LMP1 is excised from lesions in persons with a more vigorous immune response, leaving no viral "footprint" behind. Alternatively, in progressive disease, mutations occur in the LMP1 protein which render it non-immunogenic. Knecht et al (1993a) have reported that of 52 HD cases evaluated that were LMP1, 5 have detectable deletions in LMP1 which clustered in the 3′ end of the LMP1 gene and showed homology with deletions seen in nasopharyngeal carcinoma.

Alternatively, these findings imply that there are two types of HD: EBV-genome positive and EBV-genome negative. In this case the variation in histology and ethnicity reflects two causal pathways in the development of the disease. Consistent with this hypothesis is O'Grady et al's (1994) report that in stage I disease, EBV positivity is associated with neck node presentation. However, a number of characteristics of the disease appear to be independent of EBV-genome status. EBV-genome status has not been found to be an independent predictor of prognosis (Vestlev et al, 1992; Delsol et al, 1992; Fellbaum et al, 1992). In addition, EBV-genome status does not appear to be associated with the presence of HLA-A2, *bcl-2*, c-*myc*, or *p-53* overexpression, nor with the presence of the t (14;18) translocation (Jiwa et al, 1993; Niedobitek, 1993; Bhagat et al, 1993; Poppema and Visser, 1994).

Few data are available on EBV serology and the presence of EBV genome or gene products. Ohshima et al (1990) reported a single case of an 8-year-old boy with EBV-genome positive HD. His detailed serologic pattern (anti-VCA-IgG 1:1280,-IgA 1:10, -IgM 1:10; anti-EA 160; anti-EBNA 1:40) was consistent with that reported in our prediagnosis study (Mueller et al, 1989). In an overlapping series of 107 cases, Brousset et al (1991) and Delsol et al (1992) concluded that there was no association with EBV-genome positivity and a serologic pattern of reactivation which they defined as anti-VCA > 1:640, anti-EA > 1:40, anti-EBNA > 1:160. Of data shown however, only 1 of 35 EBV-negative and none of 16 EBV-positive cases had this rather extreme pattern. Thus there have been insufficient data to evaluate the correlation between EBV serology and viral genome status in HD specimens. In addition, no individual risk factor data related to age at infection have been published in relation to EBV-genome status in HD.

Other Viruses

A second lymphotropic herpesvirus which has been considered as a factor in the development of HD is the cytomegalovirus (CMV). However, results of antibody studies involving over 900 diagnosed cases have been inconsistent (Mueller, 1987). In addition, in our study involving serum specimens collected prior to diagnosis, no consistent association between antibodies against the CMV and HD was found (Mueller et al, 1989). Weiss et al (1987) screened for CMV genome in 21 HD biopsies by molecular hybridization; none were positive. The recently identified lymphotropic human herpesvirus type 6 also does not appear to be related to risk of HD (Salahuddin et al, 1986; Levine et al, 1992).

THE CONTAGION HYPOTHESIS

The hypothesis that HD is a contagious disease transmitted by case-to-case contact was first put forth by Vianna et al's reports (1971, 1972) of an "extended epidemic" of 31 HD cases who were either members of or could be linked by social contact to one high school graduating class in upstate New York. A second investigation by the same group conducted in Nassau and Suffolk Counties of New York State found that more HD cases than expected developed among students and teachers from a high school in which a first case had already been present (Vianna and Polan, 1973). However, these findings have not been confirmed in other school-based populations nor has excess risk been confirmed among medical personnel occupationally exposed to HD cases (Grufferman and Delzell, 1984; Mueller, 1987).

Reports of patient clusters, such as that by Klinger and Minton (1973), also sparked interest in the spatial clustering of cases. However, these early studies of clusters based on population data have yielded either negative, inconsistent, or only weakly positive results (Mueller, 1987). More recently, newer statistical methodology has been applied in evaluating case-clustering in three population-based studies. Using data from the specialist leukemia/lymphoma registry in the United Kingdom, Alexander et al (1989) tested for global evidence for localized clustering of cases' residence at diagnosis. They reported some evidence of spatial clustering among younger patients with NS-HD but that it was not consistent. Ross and Davis (1990) used point pattern analysis of spatial clustering of residences over a range of time preceding diagnosis of cases from northwestern Washington State. No evidence was found for significant clustering; cases ≥ 40 yr of age at diagnosis were significantly less clustered than expected in the 15 years prior to diagnosis but were closer than expected during childhood. In contrast, Glaser (1990b) evaluated spatial clustering of cases' residence at diagnosis in San Francisco-Oakland, California. She reported evidence of small, widely dispersed clusters.

On balance, there is little to support the hypothesis that HD is a contagious disease that is primarily transmitted by person-to-person contact. This is not inconsistent, however, with an infectious etiology. That is, a disease may be initiated by an infection but may not itself be transmissible. For example, subacute sclerosing panencephalitis has an infectious etiology; it is an age-dependent consequence of measles infection. However, it is not a contagious disease; it is not transmitted within a population by case-to-case contact.

OCCUPATIONAL EXPOSURES

Few analytical epidemiologic studies on HD have addressed issues other than those related to a viral exposure. Two occupational exposures have been investigated to some degree: wood and chemical exposure. Grufferman and Delzell (1984) have reviewed these reports in detail.

Occupational exposure in wood-related industries has been most extensively studied. As shown in Table 41–9, the results of case–control studies have been generally positive, with RR estimates up to 7.2 (Milham and Hesser, 1967; Petersen and Milham, 1974; Grufferman et al, 1976; Abramson et al, 1978; Greene et al, 1978; Kirchoff et al, 1980; Fonte et al, 1982). In a study in Yorkshire, England, however, (Bernard et al, 1987), no association with wood-related occupation or with self-reported contact with wood dust was found. In Matté and Mueller's study (unpublished) in the Boston-Worcester area, no association with occupation was found overall. There was an association with self-reported exposure to dust or sawdust which increased with age; for subjects aged 15–39 yr, RR = 1.1; ages 40–54 yr, RR = 2.1; ages ≥ 55 yr, RR = 2.7. However, no dose–response was evident.

The results of three studies of mortality among men employed in the carpentry or furniture-making occupations have been mixed. Olsen and Sabroe (1979) found a deficit of deaths from HD among 40,000 carpenters. Milham (1974) found no association overall among over 16,000 union carpenters, but found an excess of HD deaths among men over age 60. Acheson et al (1984) evaluated mortality among 5,000 furniture makers and found one HD death with 4.0 expected. However, there was a significant excess of deaths attributed to "other and unspecified lymphoma" (8 observed and 2.3 expected), which suggests the presence of diagnostic misclassification. In summary, although it is not consistent, there is some evidence of a moderate association between occupational exposure to wood and dust.

Turning to occupational exposure to chemicals, the findings are more varied (Table 41–10). There have been three case–control studies in Sweden. Olsson and Brandt (1979) first reported a RR of 9.0 associated with employment in any of seven chemical-related occupations. In a second study published in 1980, they reported a RR of 6.6 associated with occupational exposure to organic solvents. In 1983, Hardell and Bengtsson evaluated exposure to phenoxy acids (RR = 4.0), to chlorophenols (RR = 6.5), and to organic solvents (RR = 3.0). Early case–control studies conducted in Great Britain (Benn et al, 1979) and in Italy (Fonte et al, 1982) found no association with employment in chemical industries. But a more recent study in Yorkshire (Bernard et al, 1987) did report a significant association between HD and occupation as a worker in rubber or plastic (RR = 3.2), and a more recent study conducted in the greater Milan area also found a positive association (RR = 4.3) between HD and an occupation in chemical industries (LaVecchia et al (1989). Franceschi et al (1991) conducted a case–control study of occupation and HD risk in northern Italy; they reported a significant excess of cases who were employed in agriculture with more than a threefold risk associated with herbicide and pesticide exposure. In the United States Matté and Mueller (unpublished report) found an association with employment in the rubber, plastics, or synthetics industry, especially among older men (RR = 11.7) in eastern Massachusetts.

The finding that links HD with chlorophenoxy her-

TABLE 41–9. *Studies of Hodgkin's Disease and Wood-Related Exposure**

Study Area and Reference	*Study Design (Time Period)*	*Subjects*	*(a) Exposure Definition (b) Source of Data*	*Relative Risk*	*P Value or 95% Confidence Interval(I)*
Upstate New York Milham and Hesser (1967)	Case–control (1940–1964)	1,549 white male HD deaths; 1,549 controls with other causes of death	(a) Employment in wood-working or wood-related industries (b) Death certificates	2.3	<0.001
Washington State Petersen and Milham (1974)	Case–control (1950–1971)	707 male HD deaths; 707 controls with other causes of death	(a) Employment in wood-related industries (b) Death certificates, next-of-kin interviews for deaths in 1965–1970	1.8	<0.05
United States Milham (1974)	Mortality survey (1969–1970)	Members of the Brotherhood of Carpenters and Joiners of America Union (16,443 deaths); referent rate: US age- and sex-specific mortality rates in 1968	(a) Union membership (b) Union records	All Ages	
				0.9	(0.16–1.2)
				≥ 60+ yr	
				1.8	(1.2–2.6)
Boston Grufferman et al (1976)	Incidence survey (1959–1973)	1,577 incident HD cases; referent rate: census data on population	(a) Employment in wood-related industries (b) Medical records	1.6	(0.9–2.6)
Israel Abramson et al (1978)	Case–control (1960–1972)	397 HD cases; 397 general population controls	(a) Work with wood or trees (b) Interviews	1.1	Not stated
				Mixed Cell	
				5.2	0.0005
				1.4	(0.8–2.5)
North Carolina Greene et al (1978)	Case–control (1956–1974)	167 white male HD deaths; 334 controls with other causes of death	(a) Occupations with wood or paper exposure (b) Death certificates	Carpentry/Lumber	
				4.2	(1.4–15.0)
Denmark Olsen and Sabroe (1979)	Retrospective cohort (1971–1976)	40,428 members of the Carpenters/Cabinet Makers' Trade Union; referent rate: mortality of all Danish men	(a) Union membership (b) Union records	0.6	Not stated
Brazil Kirchoff et al (1980)	Case–control (1976)	38 ever-employed HD cases; 42 ever-employed hospital controls with neoplastic diseases	(a) Occupational exposure to wood or wood products (b) Interviews	2.9	(0.7–12.0)
Italy Fonte et al (1982)	Case–control (1972–1979)	387 HD cases; 771 hospital controls	(a) Occupation in the wood industry (b) Medical records	7.2	(2.3–22.2)
Buckinghamshire, UK Acheson et al (1984)	Retrospective cohort (?–1982)	5,108 male furniture workers, mortality; Referent rates: area-corrected England and Wales, age- and sex-specific mortality rates, 1968–1978	(a) Occupation within industry (b) Industry records	0.3	Not stated
				Other/unspecified lymphoma	
				3.5	(1.5–6.9)
Yorkshire, UK Bernard et al (1987)	Case–control (1979–1984)	248 incident cases; 489 hospital controls	(a) Occupation as woodworker Industry employment as woodworker Self-reported contact with wood dust (b) Interviews	1.1 0.8 1.0	Not stated Not stated Not stated
Boston-Worcester metropolin areas Matté and Mueller (unpublished)	Case–control (1973–1977)	181 incident male cases; 345 population controls	(a) Occupation in paper and wood industry Self-reported wood-related occupation Self-reported exposure to dust or sawdust (b) Interviews	1.0 0.9 1.8	(0.5–1.9) (0.6–1.6) (1.2–2.7)
Milan area, Italy LaVecchia et al (1989)	Case–control (1983–1988)	69 cases; 396 hospital controls	(a) Self-reported exposure to wood dust for >10 years (b) Interviews	0.46	Not stated

*Adapted from Grufferman and Delzell, 1984.

TABLE 41–10. *Studies of Hodgkin's Disease and Occupational Exposure to Chemicals**

Study Area and Reference	*Study Design (Time Period)*	*Subjects*	*(a) Exposure Definition (b) Source of Data*	*Relative Risk*	*P value or 95% Confidence Interval(/)*
Upstate New York Vianna and Polan (1979)	Mortality survey (1950–1969)	216 HD deaths ≥ age 20; referent rate: male population of Upstate New York, 1960	(a) employed in one of 14 occupations with potential exposure to benzene (b) Death certificates	1.6	Not stated
Sweden Olsson and Brandt (1979)	Case–control (1973–1978)	88 male HD cases aged 20–65; 323 hospital controls	(a) Employed in one of 7 occupations involving chemicals (b) Medical records	9.0	<0.01
Great Britain Benn et al (1979)	Case–control (1962–1976)	588 male HD cases aged 16+ years; controls: 33,097 men with other neoplasms reported in 1972–1975 to Northwestern Regional Cancer Registry	(a) Employed in occupations that entail chemicals (b) Cancer Registry records	1.0	Not stated
Sweden Olin and Ahlbom (1980)	Retrospective cohort (1930–1977)	822 male graduates of chemical engineering school (three HD deaths); referent group: general male population of Sweden	(a) Graduation from a school of chemical engineering (b) University records	4.3	0.3
Sweden Olsson and Brandt (1980)	Case–control (1978–1979)	25 male HD cases, aged 20–65 years; 50 general population controls	(a) Occupational exposure to organic solvents daily for at least one year (b) Interviews	6.6	(1.8–24.0)
Italy Fonte et al (1982)	Case–control (1972–1979)	387 HD cases; 771 hospital controls	(a) Occupation in the chemical or pharmaceutical industry Occupation in the rubber or plastics industry (b) Medical records	0.2 0.1	Not stated Not stated
Sweden Hardell and Bengtsson (1983)	Case–control (1974–1978)	60 male HD cases, aged 25–85 years (median 65.4); 335 general population controls	(a) Occupational exposure to phenoxy acids Chlorophenols (high exposure) Organic solvents (high exposure) (b) Self-administered questionnaire plus supplemental telephone interviews	5.0 6.5 3.0	(2.4–10.2) (2.2–19.0) (1.4–6.1)
Kansas Hoar et al (1986)	Case–control (1976–1982)	173 male incident HD cases; 488 (est.) population controls	(a) Farm herbicide use on 4 specific crops (b) Interviews	0.9 No trend with duration or frequency	(0.5–1.5)
Yorkshire, UK Bernard et al (1987)	Case–control (1979–1984)	248 incident cases; 489 hospital controls	(a) Occupation as dye or chemical worker Occupation rubber or plastic industry Chemical industry (b) Interviews	1.2 3.2 1.2	Not stated 0.03 Not stated
Boston-Worcester metropolitan areas Matté and Mueller (unpublished)	Case–control (1973–1977)	181 incident male cases; 345 population controls	(a) Occupation in rubber, plastics, or synthetics industry (b) Interviews	2.7 Age >55 Years 11.7	(1.1–6.7) <0.02
Milan area, Italy LaVecchia et al (1989)	Case–control (1983–1988)	69 cases: 396 hospital controls	(a) Occupation in chemical industry Occupation in agriculture (b) Interviews	4.3 2.1	(1.4–10.2) (1.0–3.8)
Pordenonc Province, Italy Franceschi et al (1991)	Case–control (1985–1990)	152 cases, 613 hospital controls	(a) Occupational exposure to herbicides/pesticides for >10 years (b) Interviews	3.2	(1.6–6.5)
United States Selected Cancers Cooperative Study Group (1990)	Case–control (1984–1988)	310 cases; 1,776 controls (all male Vietnam veterans)	(a) Military exposure to Agent Orange (b) Military records	1.1	(0.71–1.8)
United States Fingerhut et al (1991)	Retrospective cohort (1942–1987)	5,172 male employees (3 HD deaths); referent group: general U.S. male population	(a) Worked in chemical manufacture involving dioxin (b) Company records	SMR[a] = 119	(25–349)
Multinational Saracci et al (1991)	Retrospective cohort (1955–1987)	18,390 employees; internal comparison	(a) Worked in production or spraying of herbicides (b) Company records	SMR = 39	(5–141)

*Adapted from Grufferman and Delzell (1984) with permission. [a] SMR = Standardized Mortality Ratio.

bicides and chlorophenols was not been confirmed (Zahm, 1995). Hoar et al (1986) found no association between herbicide exposure (primarily chlorophenols) and HD in a population-based case–control study in Kansas. In a large case–control study of HD among Vietnam veterans exposed to Agent Orange no association was found (RR = 1.1; not significant) (The Selected Cancers Cooperative Study Group, 1990). Nor was a positive association found in two occupational cohort studies of chlorophenoxy herbicide manufacturing (Fingerhut et al, 1991; Saracci et al, 1991). In summary, there is some evidence implicating exposure to chemicals as a risk factor for HD, but no specific compounds have been identified and the data are not consistent.

HOST FACTORS

Genetic Factors

Many investigators have dealt with the question of whether genetic factors play a role in the etiology of HD. These include case reports of HD occurring among family members in association with immune deficiency (Creagan and Fraumeni, 1972; Buehler et al, 1975; McBride and Fennelly, 1977; Greene et al, 1978). Several cases have been reported in association with a high degree of inbreeding among the Amish population in the United States (Halazun et al, 1972; Maldonado et al, 1972). Robertson et al (1987) have reported a family in which all four siblings developed HD. Recently, Mack et al (1995) identified and followed 366 sets of twins in which at least one had HD and evaluated the subsequent risk of the second to develop HD before age 50 by zygosity. Among the 179 monozygotic twin sets, 10 became concordant for the disease compared to none of the 187 dizygotic twin sets—a highly significant difference.

Kerzin-Storrar et al (1983) evaluated the incidence of HD among 2,517 first and second degree relatives of 131 Scottish cases. Six familial cases were identified with 1.4 expected. Bernard et al (1987) found that nine of 248 cases in their population-based incidence series reported having a relative with HD, compared to only one of 489 controls. In a population-based incidence survey which identified 1577 cases, Grufferman et al (1977) found 13 sibling cases. They reported that siblings of a young adult with HD have, overall, a roughly sevenfold higher risk than do members of the general population. In addition, their findings suggest that the excess risk among siblings is concentrated among those of the same sex as the first affected. That is, if a male is affected, his brothers have about a ninefold increased risk, while his sisters have a fivefold increased risk. If a female is affected, the reverse applies. More recently, Grufferman et al (1987) have reviewed all published data on HD occurring among young adult siblings. The data include 85 reported sibling pairs. These data confirm their observation of a significant excess of same-sex sibling pairs. They note that this phenomenon is also true for three other diseases involving immune dysfunction which are suspected to have a viral etiology: Bechet's disease, multiple sclerosis, and sarcoidosis. (It is tempting to speculate that this phenomenon may be an earmark for virally induced diseases where age-related immune response plays a major role.) This observation argues against the theory that genetic factors play a major role in the etiology of HD since it may be explained by childhood environmental exposures that are more likely to be shared by siblings of the same sex.

Several investigations have addressed the question of whether relatives of HD patients show evidence of immune dysfunction. Bjorkholm et al (1977) found that of 6 healthy twins of HD cases, 3 had reduced in vitro lymphocyte response to mitogens. They reported similar findings in both first degree relatives and spouses of patients (Bjorkholm et al, 1978). This impairment among relatives was confirmed in one study (del Giacco et al, 1985) but not in another (Ricci and Romagnani, 1980).

Hors and Dausset (1983) have extensively reviewed the evidence concerning the role of human leukocyte antigen (HLA) haplotypes, or genetic markers of immune responsiveness, in relation to susceptibility to HD. They conclude that among multicase families involving both siblings and cousins, there is a higher concordance of haplotypes than expected. Chakravarti et al (1986) reanalyzed HLA data from 41 multicase families and concluded that the data support a recessive mode of inheritance for susceptibility, but that other factors are necessary. Hors and Dausett (1983) also concluded that susceptibility to HD is clearly associated with the haplotypes A1 and probably with B5 and B18, and that the haplotypes A1 and B8 predominate in long-term survivors. Thus there is some evidence that genetic factors associated with immune competence play a role in the etiology of HD as well as in influencing survival.

In addition, as is generally recognized for most hematopoietic malignancies, Jews are at somewhat higher risk for HD than non-Jews (MacMahon, 1960). In the Boston-Worcester population-based case–control study conducted in the 1970's, we found that Jewish people in the population were at particularly high risk at all ages (Gutensohn and Cole, 1981). In a 1957 study of cases occurring in Brooklyn, New York, MacMahon reported that older Jews were at increased risk, but younger Jews were not. Bernard et al (1984, 1987) have also noted an excess of Jewish cases in their more recent population-based studies in Yorkshire, England. Similarly, an increased incidence among Jews was documented in Los Angeles County (Cozen et al, 1992). These observations may reflect the effects of both genetic and life style factors.

Tonsillectomy

A considerable number of epidemiologic studies have addressed the question of whether tonsillectomy is a risk factor for HD. This relates to the broader question of the role of a virus in the etiology of the disease. Tonsillectomy is a risk factor for two diseases that share epidemiological characteristics with HD: paralytic poliomyelitis (Paffenbarger and Wilson, 1955) and multiple sclerosis (Poskanzer, 1965). The RR of HD among persons with prior tonsillectomy relative to those without one has ranged from 0.7 to 3.6 in 14 published studies. (Bonelli et al [1990] in their recent case–control study in Italy found no association overall, but they did find a significant deficit of cases having a tonsillectomy prior to age 10 [RR = 0.46]). There is also great variation in the prevalence of tonsillectomy among the populations studied, from 9% in Denmark to 74% among Boston area cases (Mueller, 1987).

The explanation of this variability of association is uncertain. Part of the difficulty in evaluating the relationship involves the comparability of the case and control groups, since risk of tonsillectomy varies appreciably with local medical practice (Gittelsohn and Wennberg, 1977). Siblings are suitable controls as they do not differ from cases on extraneous factors that may influence their risk of tonsillectomy. In all four of the published studies using sibling controls, a positive association was found. However, in two of the three of these that involved adult cases, the association was not uniformly present within all family-size groups (Gutensohn et al, 1975). This lack of uniform association suggests either that tonsillectomy is not a causal factor or, if it is, its effect is complex and modified by factors related to family size. The former explanation is favored by our findings from two companion population-based case–control studies on this issue (Mueller et al, 1987). These studies involved 556 cases and 1499 siblings from the metropolitan areas of Boston and Worcester, Massachusetts, and Detroit, Michigan. There was no evidence among young adults that prior tonsillectomy was a risk factor (RR = 1.0). Among middle-aged persons, the RR was 1.5 and not significant. Among older persons, the RR (3.0), was significantly elevated, but the data are sparse. Based on these data, it appears unlikely that prior tonsillectomy is a causal factor in the development of HD in young and middle-aged adulthood. Whether it is associated with risk among older persons is unclear (Mueller, 1987).

IMMUNODEFICIENCY

There is some evidence that the risk of HD is increased among patients with certain primary immunodeficiencies. Although there is a substantial risk of lymphoma strongly associated with loss of control of EBV among such patients (List et al, 1987), the number diagnosed with HD is relatively small, or about 10% of all malignancies (Filipovich et al, 1980). These cases are seen in children with ataxia telangiectasia (10 of 59 lymphomas), a complex deficiency involving a DNA repair defect (Rosen et al, 1984). These patients have defects in EBV-specific T-cell suppression which predisposes them to viral reactivation marked by elevated antibodies to VCA and EA with low or absent anti-EBNA. Of 40 lymphomas diagnosed in children with Wiskott-Aldrich syndrome, four were HD. This syndrome is an X-linked trait marked by a progressive decline in T-cell number and function; susceptibility to opportunistic infections is a major complication. Five HD cases among 41 malignancies diagnosed in patients with common variable immunodeficiency have been reported. These patients have a mixed immunodeficiency which characteristically develops in the sixth decade of life.

HD is even less common among the malignancies occurring in renal transplant patients, in whom it comprises about 2% of all lymphomas. (Sheil, 1984; Doyle et al, 1983). Whether this is greater than expected is not clear, as generally the number of patients and length of follow-up are not stated. In one report which did calculate the expected value, no HD case occurred, with 0.2 cases expected (Kinlen et al, 1979).

Finally, it is of interest that HD appears to be part of the spectrum of opportunistic malignancies occurring in the natural history of human immunodeficiency virus-I (HIV-I) infection. This occurrence has been discussed in a series of case reports (Robert and Schneiderman, 1984; Ioachim et al, 1984; Schoeppel et al, 1985; Scheib and Siegel, 1985; Temple and Andes, 1986; Unger and Strauchen, 1986; Cid et al, 1986; Prior et al, 1986; Tirelli et al, 1988; Knowles et al, 1988). Hessol et al (1992) has reported a significant increase of HD in a cohort of HIV-1–infected homosexual men. Uccini et al (1989) reported that the EBV genome was detected by in situ hybridization in 10 of 12 HD patients who were infected with HIV-I. This detection rate was substantially higher than that of 6 of 32 HIV-I–negative HD patients matched for age, sex, histology, and time of diagnosis. This finding of a very high EBV-positivity rate in HIV-1–positive HD cases has been verified in additional studies (Audouin et al, 1992, Boiocchi et al, 1993, Hamilton-Dutoit et al, 1993). In general, these HIV-I–infected patients present with advanced HD and exhibit a poor prognosis. In many of these patients HD appears to spread noncontiguously—without mediastinal or splenic involvement (Knowles et al, 1988). This alteration in the natural history of HD has been attributed to the loss of T-helper cells.

PATHOGENESIS

In 1972 Order and Hellman likened HD to a civil war and suggested that the underlying pathogenesis involved a graft versus host interaction. The evolving picture of HD revealed through use of newly available tools of molecular biology is also that of a protracted civil engagement with both sides firmly entrenched, in which much of the immune dysfunction is explicable by lymphocyte hyperactivity induced by chronic antigenic stimulation (Romagnani et al, 1985). The question then becomes, what is the nature of the tenacious intruder that generates such a sustained immunologic response?

Much of the epidemiologic and molecular biologic evidence points to dysfunctional immunologic control of a latent lymphotropic viral infection. The epidemiologic evidence points to age at infection as an important modifier of risk. Among young adults and middle-aged persons in economically advantaged populations, risk of HD is indexed by factors associated with susceptibility for late infections with common viruses. In economically disadvantaged populations, risk is instead seen in children. As Abramson (1973) and T. Mack (personal communication) have pointed out, the parallel between the bimodality of HD and mortality from tuberculosis suggests that endogenous reactivation of a latent infection among older persons may be of relevance in the etiology of HD. Such endogenous reactivation may be enhanced by chronic occupational exposures. Genetic factors may also, to some degree, modify disease risk, apparently in relation to immunocompetency.

The EBV has become clearly an involved agent in the pathogenesis of at least half of HD cases, as evidenced by both altered antibody status of cases prior to and following diagnosis suggestive of chronic viral expression, by the increased risk seen among persons with a history of IM, and by the evidence of integrated EBV genome in lesions with a specific phenotype of LMP1 expression. Smithers (1983) has postulated a mechanism by which chronic antigenic stimulation could act in the pathogenesis of HD. He commented that "... we are bound to look at the evidence for the effect of prolonged pressures on the cell-mediated arm of the immune system and for feedback failure of restraint in influencing the development of this disease." It may be that in HD, an alteration in normal gene expression occurs as a consequence of continuing antigenic stimulation of such cells. In this case, however, the gene involved is not one controlling proliferation, but rather one controlling the expression of the normal, functionally active mediators released by antigen-stimulated cells. Gene expression may be quantitatively altered, resulting in a greatly amplified message. Alternatively, it may be that the gene which normally shuts down the messages by feedback inhibition is translocated and underexpressed. Either case could result in an immune system which is continually "turned on," that is, an immune system that is perpetually mobilized in response to a chronic antigen, and thus unable to respond appropriately to others. The mechanism underlying such an alteration in gene expression could be triggered by the continuing antigenic stimulation of the cells, in which case there would have to be a selective advantage for the altered cells to remain viable. In any case, the result is the immortalization not of the target cells but rather of their message. This could explain the many failures to establish cell cultures (Gutensohn, 1984).

This hypothesis can be used to explain the biological paradox of HD: the malignant properties reflect the underlying genetic changes; the histological features reflect the response of normal immune cells to the perpetual stimulation; and the immune defects reflect the resulting imbalance in the immune response system (Mueller, 1987).

PREVENTION AND FUTURE RESEARCH

Although much has been learned about the epidemiology and biology of HD, no clear strategies for prevention have emerged. This is unfortunate in view of the substantial decrease in family size which has occurred in the United States since the mid-1960s (Fig. 41–4). This will result in a cohort of adolescents and young adults who are relatively more susceptible to late infections. If the inverse association between HD risk and sibship size is in fact primary (and the effects not modified by social changes such as increased use of day care), then we would predict an increased incidence of young adult HD in the next decade. Further evaluation of the family size relationship with HD with current data and more importantly, of the effect of age on host response to infection with the EBV, should prove valuable. The intriguing finding relating parity and risk in young women needs to be addressed in relation to potential confounding by social class correlates in childhood.

Continued studies using molecular biologic techniques in combination with serology and risk factor information are a priority. Such studies should clarify the role of EBV in the pathogenesis of the disease. This ap-

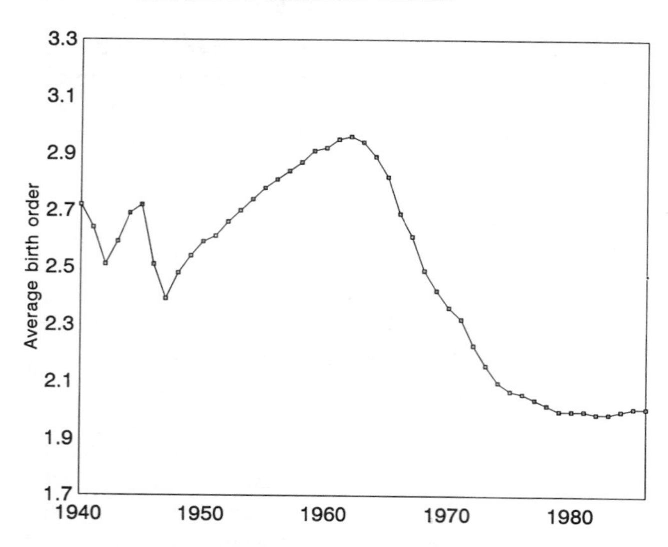

FIG. 41–4. Average birth order for live-born children, United States, 1940–1986. (Vital Statistics of the United States, 1986).

proach will also highlight the EBV-negative cases and may provide evidence of other possible causal pathways. Finally, the AIDS epidemic offers at least two opportunities to increase our understanding of the pathogenesis of HD. The first is the opportunity to verify our findings of altered antibody patterns to EBV prior to HD diagnosis. Since serum banks have been established on many HIV-1–infected cohorts, nested case–control studies could be done comparing antibody status for those who later develop HD to comparable individuals who do not. This could be linked with molecular probes for EBV in diagnostic biopsies. Secondly, the substantial insight into human immune function which has come from AIDS research may provide new strategies for directly measuring the expression of genes involved in the immune dysfunction in HD, as is being done for oncogenes. This in turn may provide a means of identifying whether altered genetic expression could explain the pathogenesis of this disease. If this is the case, then following the proposal of Davies et al (1990) for paracrine cytokine-mediated diseases, a strategy for treatment may be to suppress the cytokines that are responsible for the symptoms.

REFERENCES

ABRAMSON JH. 1973. Infective agents in the causation of Hodgkin's disease: A review of the empidemiologic evidence. Isr J Med Sci 9:932–953.

ABRAMSON JH. 1974. Childhood experience and Hodgkin's disease in adults. An interpretation of incidence data. Isr J Med Sci 10:1365–1370.

ABRAMSON JH, PRIDAN H, SACKS MI, et al. 1978. A case–control study of Hodgkin's disease in Israel. J Natl Cancer Inst 61:307–314.

ACHESON ED, PIPPARD EC, WINTER PD. 1984. Mortality of English furniture makers. Scand J Work Environ Health 10:211–217.

ALEXANDER FE, MCKINNEY PA, WILLIAMS J, et al. 1991a. Epidemiological evidence for the 'two-disease hypothesis' in Hodgkin's disease. Int J Epidemiol 20:354–361.

ALEXANDER FE, RICKETTS TJ, MCKINNEY PA, et al. 1991b. Community lifestyle characteristics and incidence of Hodgkin's disease in young people. Int J Cancer 48:10–14.

ALEXANDER FE, WILLIAMS J, MCKINNEY PA, et al. 1989. A specialist leukaemia/lymphoma registry in the UK. Part 2: clustering of Hodgkin's disease. Br J Cancer 60:948–952.

AMBINDER RA, BROWNING PJ, LORENZANA I, et al. 1993. Epstein-Barr virus and childhood Hodgkin's disease in Honduras and the United States. Blood 81:462–467.

ANAGNOSTOPOULOS I, HERBST H, NIEDOBITEK G, et al. 1989. Demonstration of monoclonal EBV genomes in Hodgkin's disease and Ki-1-positive anaplastic large cell lymphoma by combined southern blot and in situ hybridization. Blood 74:810–816.

ANASTASI J, BAUER KD, VARIAKOJIS D. 1987. DNA aneuploidy in Hodgkin's disease: A multiparameter flow-cytometric analysis with cytologic correlation. Am J Pathol 128:573–582.

AOZASA K, UEDA T, TAMAI M, et al. 1986. Hodgkin's disease in Osaka, Japan (1964–1985). Eur J Cancer Clin Oncol 22:1117–1119.

AUDOUIN J, DIEBOLD J, PALLESEN G. 1992. Frequent expression of Epstein-Barr virus latent membrane protein-1 in tumour cells of Hodgkin's disease in HIV-positive patients. J Pathol 167:381–384.

BENN RT, MANGOOD A, SMITH A. 1979. Hodgkin's disease and occupational exposure to chemicals. Br Med J 2:1143.

BERNARD SM, CARTWRIGHT RA, BIRD CC, et al. 1984. Aetiologic factors in lymphoid malignancies: A case–control epidemiological study. Leuk Res 8:681–689.

BERNARD SM, CARTWRIGHT RA, DARWIN CM, et al. 1987. Hodgkin's Disease: Case control epidemiological study in Yorkshire. Br J Cancer 55:85–90.

BHAGAT SKM, MEDEIROS LJ, WEISS LM, et al. 1993. *Bcl-2* expression in Hodgkin's disease: Correlation with the t(14,18) translocation and Epstein-Barr virus. Am J Clin Pathol 99:604–608.

BIBEAU F, BROUSSET P, KNECHT H, et al. 1994. Epstein-Barr virus replication in Hodgkin's disease. Bull Cancer 81:114–118.

BIGNON Y-J, BERNARD D, CURÉ H, et al. 1990. Detection of Epstein-Barr viral genomes in lymphnodes of Hodgkin's disease patients. Mol Carcinog 3:9–11.

BJORKHOLM M, HOLM G, DE FAIRE U, et al. 1977. Immunological defects in healthy twin siblings to patients with Hodgkin's disease. Scand J Haematol 19:396–404.

BJORKHOLM M, HOLM G, MELLSTEDT H. 1978. Immunological family studies in Hodgkin's disease. Scand J Haematol 20:297–305.

BOGGER-GOREN S, ZAIZOV R, VOGEL R, et al. 1983. Clinical and virological observations in childhood Hodgkin's disease in Israel. Isr J Med Sci 19:989–991.

BOIOCCHI M, CARBONE A, DERE V, et al. 1989. Is the Epstein-Barr virus involved in Hodgkin's disease? Tumori 75:345–350.

BOIOCCHI M, DERE V, GLOGHINI A, et al. 1993. High incidence of monoclonal EBV episomes in Hodgkin's disease and anaplastic large-cell KI-1-positive lymphomas in HIV-1-positive patients. Int J Cancer 54:53–59.

BONELLI L, VITALE V, BISTOLFI F, et al. 1990. Hodgkin's disease in adults: Association with social factors and age at tonsillectomy. A case–control study. Int J Cancer 45:423–427.

BOYLE MJ, VASAK E, TSCHUCHNIGG M, et al. 1993. Subtypes of Epstein-Barr virus (EBV) in Hodgkin's disease: Association between B-type EBV and immunocompromise. Blood 81:468–474.

BROCKSMITH D, ANGEL CA, PRINGLE JH, et al. 1991. Epstein-Barr viral DNA in Hodgkin's disease: Amplification and detection using the polymerase chain reaction. J Pathol 165:11–15.

BROUSSET P, CHITTAL S, SCHLEIFER D, et al. 1991. Detection of Epstein-Barr virus messenger RNA in Reed-Sternberg cells of Hodgkin's disease by in situ hybridization with biotinylated probes on specially modified acetone methyl benzoate xylene (ModAmex) sections. Blood 77:1781–1786.

BUEHLER SK, FODOR G, MARSHALL WH, et al. 1975. Common variable immunodeficiency, Hodgkin's disease, and other malignancies in a Newfoundland family. Lancet 1:195–197.

CABANILLAS F. 1988. A review and interpretation of cytogenetic abnormalities identified in Hodgkin's disease. Hematol Oncol 6:271–274.

CARBONE A, GLOGHINI A, ZANETTE I, et al. 1993. Co-expression of Epstein-Barr virus latent membrane protein and vimentin in "aggressive" histological subtypes of Hodgkin's disease. Virchows Arch A Pathol Anat Histopathol 422:39–45.

CARBONE A, MANCONI R, POLETTI A, et al. 1987. Reed-Sternberg cells and their cell microenvironment in Hodgkin's disease with reference to macrophage and histiocytes and interdigitating reticulum cells. Cancer 60:2662–2668.

CARTER CD, BROWN TM JR, HERBERT JT, et al. 1977. Cancer incidence following infectious mononucleosis. Am J Epidemiol 105:30–36.

CHAKRAVARTI A, HALLORAN SL, BALE SJ, et al. 1986. Etiological heterogeneity in Hodgkin's disease: HLA linked and unlinked determinants of susceptibility independent of histological concordance. Genet Epidemiol 3:407–415.

CHANG KL, ALBÚJAR PF, CHEN Y-Y, et al. 1993. High prevalence of Epstein-Barr virus in the Reed-Sternberg cells of Hodgkin's disease occurring in Peru. Blood 81:496–501.

CID JAL-H, CID JL-H, SANUDO EF, et al. 1986. AIDS and Hodgkin's disease. Lancet ii:1104–1105.

CLEMMESEN J. 1981. To the epidemiology of Hodgkin's lymphogranulomatosis. J Belge Radiol 3:263–271.

COATES PJ, SLAVIN G, D'ARDENNE AJ. 1991. Persistence of Epstein-Barr virus in Reed-Sternberg cells throughout the course of Hodgkin's disease. J Pathol 164:291–297.

COHEN C, HAMILTON DG. 1980. Epidemiologic and histiologic patterns of Hodgkin's disease: Comparison of the Black and White populations of Johannesburg, South Africa. Cancer 46:186–189.

COHEN BM, SMETANA HE, MILLER RW. 1964. Hodgkin's disease: Long survival in a study of 388 World War II army cases. Cancer 17:856–866.

CONNELLY RR, CHRISTINE BW. 1974. A cohort study of cancer following infectious mononucleosis. Cancer Res 34:1172–1178.

CORREA P, O'CONOR GT. 1971. Epidemiologic patterns of Hodgkin's disease. Int J Cancer 8:192–201.

COZEN W, KATZ J, MACK T. 1992. Risk patterns of Hodgkin's disease in Los Angeles vary by cell type. Cancer Epidemiol Biomarkers Prev 1:261–268.

CREAGAN ET, FRAUMENI JT JR. 1972. Familial Hodgkin's disease. Lancet 2:547.

CUSANO MM, YOUNG JL JR. 1986. Forty-five Years of Cancer Incidence in Connecticut: 1935–79. NIH publ. no. 86-2652. Bethesda MD, National Cancer Institute, U.S. Department of Health and Human Service.

DAVIES AJS, WALLIS VJ, MORRISON WI. 1990. The trouble with T cells. Lancet 335:1574–1576.

DEACON EM, PALLESEN G, NIEDOBITEK G, et al. 1993. Epstein-Barr virus and Hodgkin's disease: Transcriptional analysis of virus latency in the malignant cells. J Exp Med 177:339–349.

DEL GIACCO GS, CENGIAROTTI L, MANTOVANI G, et al. 1985. Quantitative and functional abnormalities of total T lymphocytes in relatives of patients with Hodgkin's disease. Eur J Cancer Clin Oncol 21:793–801.

DELSOL G, BROUSSET P, CHITTAL S, et al. 1992. Correlation of the expression of Epstein-Barr virus latent membrane protein and *in situ* hybridization with biotinylated *Bam* HI-W probes in Hodgkin's disease. Am J Pathol 140:247–253.

DIEHL V, KIRCHNER HH, BURRICHTER H, et al. 1982. Characteristics of Hodgkin's disease-derived cell lines. Cancer Treat Rep 66:615–632.

DIEHL V, VON KALLE C, FONATSCH C, et al. 1990. The cell of origin in Hodgkin's disease. Semin Oncol 17:660–672.

DIGE U, JOHANSSON H, LENNER P, et al. 1991. Hodgkin's disease in northern Sweden 1971–1981. Acta Oncol 30:593–596.

DINARELLO CA, MIER JW. 1987. Current concepts: Lymphokines. N Engl J Med 317:940–945.

DOUSSIS IA, PEZZELLA F, LANE DP, et al. 1993. An immunocytochemical study of p53 and *bcl*-2 protein expression in Hodgkin's disease. Am J Clin Pathol 99:663–667.

DOYLE TJ, KUMARAPURAM KV, MAEDA K, et al. 1983. Hodgkin's disease in renal transplant recipients. Cancer 51:245–247.

DREXLER HG. 1992. Recent results on the biology of Hodgkin and Reed-Sternberg cells I. Biopsy material. Leuk Lymphoma 8:283–313.

DREXLER HG. 1993. Recent results on the biology of Hodgkin and Reed-Sternberg cells II. Continuous cell lines. Leuk Lymphoma 9:1–25.

DREXLER HG, LEBER BF. 1987. The nature of the Hodgkin cell. Report of the First International Symposium on Hodgkin's Lymphoma, Kohl, FRG, October 2–3, 1987. Blut 56:135–137.

EVANS AS. 1971. The spectrum of infections with Epstein-Barr virus: A hypothesis. J Infect Dis 124:330–337.

EVANS AS, GUTENSOHN (MUELLER) N. 1984. A population-based case–control study of EBV and other viral antibodies among persons with Hodgkin's disease and their siblings. Int J Cancer 34:149–157.

EVANS AS, MUELLER N. 1990. Viruses and cancer: Causal associations. Ann Epidemiol 1:71–92.

FELLBAUM C, HANSMANN M-L, NIEDERMEYER H, et al. 1992. Influence of Epstein-Barr virus genomes on patient survival in Hodgkin's disease. Am J Clin Pathol 98:319–323.

FILIPOVICH AH, SPECTOR BC, KERSEY J. 1980. Immunodeficiency in humans as a risk factor in the development of malignancy. Prev Med 9:252–259.

FINGERHUT MA, HALPERIN WE, MARLOW DA, et al. 1991. Cancer mortality in workers exposed to 2,3,7,8-tetrachlorodibenzo-*p*-dioxin. N Engl J Med 324:212–218.

FONTE R, GRIGIS L, GRIGIS P, et al. 1982. Chemicals and Hodgkin's disease. Lancet 2:50.

FORD RJ. 1988. Hodgkin's disease in 1987—Is history repeating itself? Hematol Oncol 6:201–204.

FORD RJ, RAJARAMAN C, LU M, et al. 1988. *In vitro* analysis of cell populations involved in Hodgkin's disease lesions and in the characteristic T cell immunodeficiency. Hematol Oncol 6:247–255.

FORD RJ, TSAO J, KOUTTAB NM, et al. 1984. Association of an interleukin abnormality with the T cell defect in Hodgkin's disease. Blood 64:386–392.

FRANCESCHI S, BIDOLI E, LA VECCHIA C. 1994. Pregnancy and Hodgkin's disease. Int J Cancer 58:465–466.

FRANCESCHI S, SERRAINO D, LA VECCHIA C, et al. 1991. Occupation and risk of Hodgkin's disease in north-east Italy. Int J Cancer 48:831–835.

FUCHS D, HAUSEN A, HENGSTER P, et al. 1987. *In vivo* activation of CD4+ cells in AIDS. Science 235:356.

GITTELSOHN AM, WENNBERG JE. 1977. On the incidence of tonsillectomy and other surgical procedures. *In* Bunker JP, Barnes BA, Mosteller F (eds): Costs, Risks and Benefits of Surgery. New York, Oxford University Press, pp. 91–106.

GLASER SL. 1986. Recent incidence and secular trends in Hodgkin's disease and its histologic subtypes. J Chron Dis 39:789–798.

GLASER SL. 1987. Regional variation in Hodgkin's disease incidence by histologic subtype in the US. Cancer 60:2841–2847.

GLASER SL. 1990a. Hodgkin's disease in black populations: A review of the epidemiologic literature. Semin Oncol 17:643–659.

GLASER SL. 1990b. Spatial clustering of Hodgkin's disease in the San Francisco Bay Area. Am J Epidemiol 132 (Suppl.):S167–S177.

GLASER SL. 1994. Reproductive factors in Hodgkin's disease in women: a review. Am J Epidemiol 139:237–246.

GLASER SL, SWARTZ WG. 1990. Time trends in Hodgkin's disease incidence: The role of diagnostic accuracy. Cancer 66:2196–2204.

GLEDHILL S, GALLAGHER A, JONES DB, et al. 1991. Viral involvement in Hodgkin's disease: Detection of clonal type A Epstein-Barr virus genomes in tumour samples. Br J Cancer 64:227–232.

GREEN JA, DAWSON AA, VALERIO D. 1979. Hodgkin's disease and infectious mononucleosis. Scand J Haematol 23:313–314.

GREENE MH, BRINTON LA, FRAUMENI JH JR, et al. 1978. Familial and sporadic Hodgkin's disease associated with occupational wood exposure. Lancet 2:626–627.

GRIESSER H, MAK TW. 1988. Immunogenotyping in Hodgkin's disease. Hematol Oncol 6:239–245.

GRUFFERMAN S, BARTON JW III, EBY NL. 1987. Increased sex concordance of sibling pairs with Behcet's disease, Hodgkin's disease, multiple sclerosis and sarcoidosis. Am J Epidemiol 126:365–369.

GRUFFERMAN S, COLE P, SMITH PG, et al. 1977. Hodgkin's disease in siblings. N Engl J Med 296:248–250.

GRUFFERMAN S, DELZELL E. 1984. Epidemiology of Hodgkin's disease. Epidemiol Rev 6:76–106.

GRUFFERMAN S, DUONG T, COLE P. 1976. Occupation and Hodgkin's disease. J Natl Cancer Inst 57:1193–1195.

GRUSS H-J, HERRMAN F, DREXLER HG. 1994. Hodgkin's disease: A cytokine-producing tumor—A review. Crit Rev Oncogenesis 5:473–538.

GUILLEY ML, EAGAN PA, QUINTANILLA-MARTINEZ L, et al. 1994. Epstein-Barr virus DNA is abundant and monoclonal in the Reed-Sternberg cells of Hodgkin's disease: association mixed cellularity subtype and hispanic American ethnicity. Blood 83:1595–1602.

GUTENSOHN (MUELLER) N. 1982. Social class and age at diagnosis of Hodgkin's disease: New epidemiologic evidence on the "two-disease" hypothesis. Cancer Treat Rep 66:689–695.

GUTENSOHN (MUELLER) N. 1984. The epidemiology of Hodgkin's disease: Clues to etiology. *In* Ford RJ, Fuller LM, Hagemeister FB (eds): New Perspectives in Human Lymphomas. New York, Raven Press, pp. 3–10.

GUTENSOHN (MUELLER) N, COLE P. 1977. Epidemiology of Hodgkin's disease in the young. Int J Cancer 19:595–604.

GUTENSOHN (MUELLER) N, COLE P. 1981. Childhood social environment and Hodgkin's disease. N Engl J Med 304:135–140.

GUTENSOHN (MUELLER) N, COLE P. 1979. Immunity in Hodgkin's disease: Importance of age at exposure. Ann Intern Med 91:316–317.

GUTENSOHN (MUELLER) N, LI FP, JOHNSON RE, et al. 1975. Hodgkin's disease, tonsillectomy and family size. N Engl J Med 292:22–25.

GUTENSOHN (MUELLER) N, SHAPIRO D. 1982. Social class risk factors among children with Hodgkin's disease. Int J Cancer 30:433–435.

HALAZUN JF, KERR SE, LUKENS JN. 1972. Hodgkin's disease in three children from an Amish kindred. J Pediatr 80:289–291.

HAMILTON-DUTOIT SJ, RAPHAEL M, AUDOUIN J, et al. 1993. In situ demonstration of Epstein-Barr virus small RNAs (EBER 1) in acquired immunodeficiency syndrome-related lymphomas: correlation with tumor morphology and primary site. Blood 82:619–624.

HAMILTON-DUTOIT SJ, PALLESEN G. 1992. A survey of Epstein-Barr virus gene expression in sporadic non-Hodgkin's lymphoma. Am J Pathol 140:1315–1325.

HARDELL L, BENGTSSON NO. 1983. Epidemiologic study of socioeconomic factors and clinical findings in Hodgkin's disease, and reanalysis of previous data regarding chemical exposure. Br J Cancer 48:217–225.

HARTGE P, DEVESA SS, FRAUMENI JF JR. 1994. Hodgkin's disease and non-Hodgkin's lymphomas. Cancer Surv 19/20:423–453.

HENDERSON BE, DWORSKY R, PIKE MC, et al. 1979. Risk factors for nodular sclerosis and other types of Hodgkin's disease. Cancer Res 39:4507–4511.

HENLE W, HENLE G. 1973. Epstein-Barr virus-related serology in Hodgkin's disease. Natl Cancer Inst Monog 36:79–84.

HERBST H, DALLENBACH F, HUMMEL M, et al. 1991. Epstein-Barr virus latent membrane protein expression in Hodgkin and Reed-Sternberg cells. Proc Natl Acad Sci USA 88:4766–4770.

HERBST H, NIEDOBITEK G. 1993. Epstein-Barr virus and Hodgkin's disease. Int J Clin Lab Res 23:13–16.

HERBST H, NIEDOBITEK G, KNEBA M, et al. 1990. High incidence of Epstein-Barr virus genomes in Hodgkin's disease. Am J Pathol 137:13–18.

HERBST H, STEINBRECHER E, NIEDOBITEK G, et al. 1992. Distribution and phenotype of Epstein-Barr virus-harboring cells in Hodgkin's disease. Blood 80:484–491.

HERBST H, TIPPELMANN G, ARAGNOSTOPOULOS I, et al. 1989. Immunoglobin and T-cell receptor gene rearrangements in Hodgkin's disease and ki-1-positive anaplastic large cell lymphoma: Dissociation between phenotype and genotype. Leuk Res 13:103–116.

HESSOL NA, KATZ MH, LIU JY, et al. 1992. Increased incidence of Hodgkin disease in homosexual men with HIV infection. Ann Intern Med 117:309–311.

HOAR SK, BLAIR A, HOLMES EF, et al. 1986. Agricultural herbicide use and risk of lymphoma and soft-tissue sarcoma. JAMA 256:1141–1147.

HORM JW, ASIRE AJ, YOUNG JL JR, et al. 1985. SEER Program: Cancer Incidence and Mortality in the United States, 1973–81. NIH publ. no. 85-1837, National Cancer Institute, Bethesda, MD, U.S. Department of Health and Human Services.

HORS J, DAUSSET J. 1983. HLA and susceptibility to Hodgkin's disease. Immunol Rev 70:167–191.

HSU S-M, HSU P-L, LO S-S, et al. 1988. Expression of prostaglandin H synthase (cyclooxygenase) in Hodgkin's mononuclear and Reed-Sternberg cells: Functional resemblance between H-RS cells and histocytes or interdigitating reticulum cells. Am J Pathol 133:5–12.

HU E, HUFFORD S, LUKES R, et al. 1988. Third-world Hodgkin's disease at Los Angeles County–University of Southern California Medical Center. J Clin Oncol 6:1285–1292.

IOACHIM HL, COOPER MC, HELLMAN GC. 1984. Hodgkin's disease and the Acquired Immunodeficiency Syndrome. Ann Intern Med 101:876–877.

JARRETT RF, GALLAGHER A, JONES DB, et al. 1991. Detection of Epstein-Barr virus genomes in Hodgkin's disease: Relation to age. J Clin Pathol 44:844–848.

JIWA NM, KANAVAROS P, VAN DER VALK P, et al. 1993. Expression of c-myc and bcl-2 oncogene products in Reed-Sternberg cells independent of presence of Epstein-Barr virus. J Clin Pathol 46:211–217.

KADIN ME, MURAMOTO L, SAID J. 1988. Expression of T-cell antigens on Reed-Sternberg cells in a subset of patients with nodular sclerosing and mixed cellularity Hodgkin's disease. Am J Pathol 130:345–353.

KAHN G, NAASE MA. 1995. Down-regulation of Epstein-Barr virus nuclear antigen 1 in Reed-Sternberg cells of Hodgkin's disease. J Clin Pathol 48:845–848.

KAPLAN HS. 1980. Hodgkin's disease: Unfolding concepts concerning its nature, management and prognosis. Cancer 45:2439–2474.

KAPLAN HS. 1981. Hodgkin's disease. Biology, treatment, prognosis. Blood 57:813–822.

KERZIN-STORRAR L, FAED MJW, MACGILLIVRAY JB, SMITH PG. 1983. Incidence of familial Hodgkin's disease. Br J Cancer 47:707–712.

KHAN G, COATES PJ, GUPTA RK, et al. 1992. Presence of Epstein-Barr virus in Hodgkin's disease is not exclusive to Reed-Sternberg cells. Am J Pathol 140:757–762.

KHAN G, NORTON AJ, SLAVIN G. 1993. Epstein-Barr virus in Hodgkin disease: Relation to age and subtype. Cancer 71:3124–3129.

KIEFF E, LIEBOWITZ D. 1990. Epstein-Barr virus and its replication. *In* Fields B, Knipe DM (eds): Virology, 2nd ed. New York, Raven Press, pp. 1889–1920.

KINLEN LJ, SHEIL AGR, PETO J, et al. 1979. Collaborative United Kingdom-Australasian study of cancer in patients treated with immunosuppressive drugs. BMJ ii:1461–1466.

KIRCHOFF LV, EVANS AS, MCCLELLAND KE, et al. 1980. A case–control study of Hodgkin's disease in Brazil. I. Epidemiologic aspects. Am J Epidemiol 112:595–608.

KLEIN G. 1994. The paradoxical coexistence of the EBV and the human species. Epstein-Barr Virus Reports 1:5–9.

KLINGER RJ, MINTON JP. 1973. Case clustering of Hodgkin's disease in a small rural community, with associations among cases. Lancet 1:168–171.

KNECHT H, BACHMANN E, BROUSSET P, et al. 1993a. Deletions within the LMP1 oncogene of Epstein-Barr virus are clustered in Hodgkin's disease and identical to those observed in nasopharyngeal carcinoma. Blood 82:2937–2943.

KNECHT H, BROUSSET P, BACHMANN E, et al. 1993b. Latent membrane protein 1: a key oncogene in EBV-related carcinogenesis? Acta Hematol 90:167–171.

KNECHT H, ODERMATT BF, BACHMANN E, et al. 1991. Frequent detection of Epstein-Barr virus DNA by the polymerase chain reaction in lymph node biopsies from patients with Hodgkin's disease without genomic evidence of B- or T-cell clonality. Blood 78:760–767.

KNOWLES DE, CHAMULAK GA, SUBAR M, et al. 1988. Lymphoid neoplasia associated with the Acquired Immunodeficiency Syndrome (AIDS): The New York University Medical Center experience with 105 patients (1981–1986). Ann Intern Med 108:744–753.

KRAVDAL Ø, HANSEN S. 1993. Hodgkin's disease: the protective effect of childbearing. Int J Cancer 55:909–914.

KUSUNOKI Y, KYOIZUMI S, FUKUDA Y, et al. 1994. Immune responses to Epstein-Barr virus in atomic bomb survivors: study of precursor frequency of cytotoxic lymphocytes and titer levels of anti-Epstein-Barr virus-related antibodies. Radiat Res 138:127–132.

KVALE G, HOIBY EA, PEDERSEN E. 1979. Hodgkin's disease in patients with previous infectious mononucleosis. Int J Cancer 23:593–597.

LAVECCHIA C, NEGRI E, D'ARANZO B, et al. 1989. Occupation and lymphoid neoplasms. Br J Cancer 60:385–388.

LEHTINEN T, LUMIO J, DILLNER J, et al. 1993. Increased risk of malignant lymphoma indicated by elevated Epstein-Barr virus antibodies—a prospective study. Cancer Causes Control 4:187–193.

LEVINE P, EBBESEN P, ABLASHI DV, et al. 1992. Antibodies to human herpes virus-6 and clinical course in patients with Hodgkin's disease. Int J Cancer 51:53–57.

LIBETTA CM, PRINGLE JH, ANGEL CA, et al. 1990. Demonstration of Epstein-Barr viral DNA in formalin-fixed paraffin-embedded samples Hodgkin's disease. J Pathol 161:255–260.

LIN J-C, LIN S-C, DE BK, et al. 1993. Precision of genotyping of Epstein-Barr virus by polymerase chain reaction using three gene loci (EBNA-2, EBNA-3C, and EBER): Predominance of Type A virus associated with Hodgkin's disease. Blood 81:3372–3381.

LIST AF, GRECO FA, VOGLER LB. 1987. Lymphoproliferative diseases in immunocompromised hosts: The role of Epstein-Barr virus. J Clin Oncol 5:1673–1689.

LUKES RJ, TINDLE BH, PARKER JW. 1969. Reed-Sternberg-like cells in infectious mononucleosis. Lancet 2:1003–1004.

MACK TM, COZEN W, SHIBATA DK, et al. 1995. Concordance for Hodgkin's disease in identical twins suggesting genetic susceptibility to the young-adult form of the disease. N Engl J Med 332:413–418.

MACMAHON B. 1957. Epidemiological evidence on the nature of Hodgkin's disease. Cancer 10:1045–1054.

MACMAHON B. 1960. The ethnic distribution of cancer mortality in New York City, 1955. Acto Unio Internat Contra Cancrum 16:1716–1724.

MACMAHON B. 1966. Epidemiology of Hodgkin's disease. Cancer Res 26:1189–1200.

MALDONADO JE, TASWELL HF, KIELY JM. 1972. Familial Hodgkin's disease. Lancet 2:1259.

MASIH A, WEISENBURGER D, DUGGAN M, et al. 1991. Epstein-Barr viral genome in lymph nodes from patients with Hodgkin's disease may not be specific to Reed-Sternberg cells. Am J Pathol 139:37–43.

MAUCH PM, KALISH LA, KADIN M, et al. 1993. Patterns of presentation of Hodgkin disease. Cancer 71:2062–2071.

MCBRIDE A, FENNELLY JJ. 1977. Immunological depletion contributing to familial Hodgkin's disease. Eur J Cancer 13:549–554.

MILHAM S JR. 1974. Mortality experience of the AFL-CIO United Brotherhood of Carpenters and Joiners of America, 1969–1970. DHEW publ. no. (NIOSH) 174-129. Cincinnati, OH, Office of Technical Publications.

MILHAM S JR, HESSER JE. 1967. Hodgkin's disease in woodworkers. Lancet 2:136–137.

MILLER BA, RIES LAG, HANKEY BF, et al (eds). 1993. SEER Cancer Statistics Review: 1973–1990. NIH publ. no. 93-2789. Bethesda, National Cancer Institute.

MILLER RW, BEEBE GW. 1973. Infectious mononucleosis and the empirical risk of cancer. J Natl Cancer Inst 50:315–321.

MORRIS CS, STUART AE. 1984. Reed-Sternberg/lymphocyte rosette: Lymphocyte sub-populations as defined by monoclonal antibodies. J Clin Pathol 37:761–771.

MUELLER N. 1991. An epidemiologist's view of the new molecular biology findings in Hodgkin's disease. Ann Oncol 2 (Suppl. 2):23–28.

MUELLER N, EVANS A, HARRIS NL, et al. 1989. Hodgkin's disease and Epstein-Barr virus: Altered antibody pattern before diagnosis. N Engl J Med 320:689–695.

MUELLER N, SWANSON GM, HSIEH C-C, et al. 1987. Tonsillectomy and Hodgkin's disease: Results from companion population-based studies. J Natl Cancer Inst 78:1–5.

MUELLER NE. 1987. The epidemiology of Hodgkin's disease. *In* Selby D, McElwain TJ (eds): Hodgkin's Disease. Oxford, Blackwell Scientific Publications, pp. 68–93.

MUÑOZ N, DAVIDSON RJL, WITTHOFF B, et al. 1978. Infectious mononucleosis and Hodgkin's disease. Int J Cancer 22:10–13.

MURRAY PG, YOUNG LS, ROWE M, et al. 1992. Immunohistochemical demonstration of the Epstein-Barr virus-encoded latent membrane protein in paraffin sections of Hodgkin's disease. J Pathol 166:1–5.

NEWELL G. 1970. Etiology of multiple sclerosis and Hodgkin's disease. Am J Epidemiol 91:119–122.

NIEDOBITEK G, ROWLANDS DC, YOUNG LS, et al. 1993. Overexpression of p53 in Hodgkin's disease: Lack of correlation with Epstein-Barr virus infection. J Pathol 169:207–212.

NIEDOBITEK G, HERBST H, YOUNG LS, et al. 1992. Patterns of Epstein-Barr virus infection in non-neoplastic lymphoid tissue. Blood 79:2520–252.

O'GRADY J, STEWART S, ELTON RA, et al. 1994. Epstein-Barr virus in Hodgkin's disease and site of origin of tumour. Lancet 343:265–266.

OHSHIMA K, KIKUCHI M, EGUCHI F, et al. 1990. Analysis of Epstein-Barr viral genomes in lymphoid malignancy using southern blotting, polymerase chain reaction and in situ hybridization. Virchows Archiv B 59:383–390.

OLIN GR, AHLBOM A. 1980. The cancer mortality among Swedish chemists graduated during three decades: A comparison with the general population and with a cohort of architects. Environ Res 22:154–161.

OLSEN J, SABROE S. 1979. A follow-up study of non-retired and retired members of the Danish Carpenters/Cabinet Markers' Trade Union. Int J Epidemiol 8:375–382.

OLSSON H, BRANDT L. 1979. Occupational handling of chemicals preceding Hodgkin's disease in men. BMJ 2:580–581.

OLSSON H, BRANDT L. 1980. Occupational exposure to organic

solvents and Hodgkin's disease in men: A case–referent study. Scand J Work Environ Health 7:302–305.

ORDER SE, HELLMAN S. 1972. Pathogenesis of Hodgkin's disease. Lancet i:57:1–3.

PAFFENBARGER RS JR, WILSON VO. 1955. Previous tonsillectomy and current pregnancy as they affect risk of poliomyelitis attack. Ann N Y Acad Sci 61:856–868.

PALLESEN G, HAMILTON-DUTOIT SJ, ROWE M, et al. 1991a. Expression of Epstein-Barr virus latent gene products in tumour cells of Hodgkin's disease. Lancet 337:320–322.

PALLESEN G, SANDVEJ K, HAMILTON-DUTOIT SJ, et al. 1991b. Activation of Epstein-Barr virus replication in Hodgkin and Reed-Sternberg cells. Blood 78:1162–1165.

PARKIN DM, MUIR CS, WHELAN SL, et al (eds). 1992. Cancer Incidence in Five Continents, Vol VI. IARC publ. no. 120. Lyon, International Agency for Research on Cancer.

PARKIN DM, STILLER CA, DRAPER GJ, et al. 1988. The international incidence of childhood cancer. Int J Cancer 41:511–520.

PETERSEN GR, MILHAM S JR. 1974. Hodgkin's disease mortality and occupational exposure to wood. J Natl Cancer Inst 53:957–958.

PINKUS GS, SAID JW. 1988. Hodgkin's disease, lymphocyte predominance type, nodular—Further evidence for a B cell derivation: L and H variants of Reed-Sternberg cells express L26, a pan B cell marker. Am J Pathol 133:211–217.

PIZZOLO G, CHILOSI M, SEMENZATO G, et al. 1984. Immunohistological analysis of Tac antigen expression in tissues involved by Hodgkin's disease. Br J Cancer 50:415–417.

PIZZOLO G, CHILOSI M, VINANTE F, et al. 1987. Soluble interleukin-2 receptors in the serum of patients with Hodgkin's disease. Br J Cancer 55:427–428.

POCOCK SJ, COOK DG, SHAPER AG, et al. 1987. Social class differences in ischaemic heart disease in British men. Lancet ii:197–201.

POPPEMA S, KAISERLING E, LENNERT K. 1979. Hodgkin's disease with lymphocytic predominance, nodular type (nodular paragranuloma) and progressively transformed germinal centres: A cytohistological study. Histopathology 3:295–308.

POPPEMA S, VISSER L. 1994. Epstein-Barr virus positivity in Hodgkin's disease does not correlate with an HLA A2-negative phenotype. Cancer 73:3059–3063.

POSKANZER DC. 1965. Tonsillectomy and multiple sclerosis. Lancet 2:1264–1266.

PRIOR E, GOLDBERG AF, CONJALKA MS, et al. 1986. Hodgkin's disease in homosexual men: An AIDS-related phenomenon? Am J Med 81:1085–1088.

REE HJ, KADIN E. 1985. Macrophage-histocytes in Hodgkin's disease: The relation of peanut-agglutin-binding macrophage-histiocytes to clinicopathologic presentation and course of disease. Cancer 56:333–338.

RICCI M, ROMAGNANI S. 1980. Immune status in Hodgkin's disease. *In* Doria G, Eskol A (eds): The Immune System: Function and Therapy of Dysfunctions. New York, Academic Press, p. 105.

ROBERT NJ, SCHNEIDERMAN H. 1984. Hodgkin's disease and the Acquired Immunodeficiency Syndrome. Ann Intern Med 101:142–143.

ROBERTSON SJ, LOWMAN JT, GRUFFERMAN S, et al. 1987. Familial Hodgkin's disease: A clinical and laboratory investigation. Cancer 59:1314–1319.

ROMAGNANI S, DELPRETE GF, MAGGI E, et al. 1983. Displacement of T lymphocytes with the "Helper/Inducer" phenotype from peripheral blood to lymphoid organs in untreated patients with Hodgkin's disease. Scand J Haematol 31:305–314.

ROMAGNANI S, FERRINI PLS, RICCI M. 1985. The immune derangement in Hodgkin's disease. Semin Hematol 22:41–55.

ROSDAHL N, LARSEN SO, CLEMMESEN J. 1974. Hodgkin's disease in patients with previous infectious mononucleosis: 30 years' experience. BMJ 2:253–256.

ROSEN FS, COOPER MD, WEDGWOOD RJP. 1984. The primary immuno-deficiencies. N Engl J Med 311:235–242, 300–309.

ROSS A, DAVIS S. 1990. Point pattern analysis of the spatial proximity of residences prior to diagnosis of persons with Hodgkin's disease. Am J Epidemiol 132 (Suppl.):S53–S62.

ROWLEY JD. 1982. Chromosomes in Hodgkin's disease. Cancer Treat Rep 66:639–643.

SALAHUDDIN SZ, ABLASHI DV, MARKHAM PD, et al. 1986. Isolation of a new virus, HBLV, in patients with lymphoproliferative disorders. Science 243:596–601.

SARACCI R, KOGEVINAS M, BERTAZZI P-A, et al. 1991. Cancer mortality in workers exposed to chlorophenoxy herbicides and chlorophenols. Lancet 338:1027–1032.

SCHEIB RC, SIEGEL RS. 1985. Atypical Hodgkin's disease and the Acquired Immunodeficiency Syndrome. Ann Intern Med 102:554.

SCHOEPPEL SL, HOPPE RT, DORFMAN RF, et al. 1985. Hodgkin's disease in homosexual men with generalized lymphadenopathy. Ann Intern Med 102:68–70.

SERRAINO D, FRANCESCHI S, TALAMINI, et al. 1991. Socioeconomic indicators, infectious diseases and Hodgkin's disease. Int J Cancer 47:352–357.

SHEIL AGR. 1984. Cancer in organ transplant recipients: Part of an induced immune deficiency syndrome. BMJ 288:659–661.

SLIVNICK DJ, ELLIS TM, NAWROCKI JF, et al. 1990. The impact of Hodgkin's disease on the immune system. Semin Oncol 17:673–682.

SMITHERS D. 1983. On some general concepts in oncology with special references to Hodgkin's disease. Int J Radiat Oncol Biol Phys 9:731–738.

SOBRINHO-SIMOES MA, AREIAS MA. 1978. Relative high frequency of childhood Hodgkin's disease in the north of Portugal. Cancer 42:1952–1956.

SPITZ MR, SIDER JG, JOHNSON CC, et al. 1986. Ethnic patterns of Hodgkin's disease incidence among children and adolescents in the United States, 1973–82. J Natl Cancer Inst 76:235–239.

STAAL SD, AMBINDER R, BESCHORNER WE, et al. 1989. A survey of Epstein-Barr virus DNA in lymphoid tissue: Frequent detection in Hodgkin's disease. Am J Clin Pathol 91:1–5.

STEIN H, MASON DY, GERDES J, et al. 1985. The expression of the Hodgkin's disease associated antigen Ki-1 in reactive and neoplastic lymphoid tissue: Evidence that Reed-Sternberg cells and histiocytic malignancies are derived from activated lymphoid cells. Blood 66:848–858.

TAKAHASHI K, TAKEZAKI T, OKI T, KAWAKAMI K, YASHIKI S, FUJIYOSHI T, USUKU K, MUELLER N, et al. 1991. Inhibitory effect of maternal antibody on mother-to-child transmission of human T-lymphotropic virus type I. Int J Cancer 49:673–677.

TEMPLE JJ, ANDES WA. 1986. AIDS and Hodgkin's disease. Lancet ii:454–455.

THANGAVELU M, LEBEAU MM. 1989. Chromosomal abnormalities in Hodgkin's disease. Hematol Oncol Clin North Am 3:221–236.

SELECTED CANCERS COOPERATIVE STUDY GROUP, THE. 1990. The association of selected cancers with service in the US military in Vietnam III. Hodgkin's disease, nasal cancer, nasopharyngeal cancer, and primary liver cancer. Arch Intern Med 150:2495–2505.

TIRELLI U, VACCHER E, AMBROSINI A, et al. 1988. HIV-related malignant lymphoma: A report of 46 cases observed in Italy. Acta Haematol 80:49–51.

UCCINI S, MONARDO F, RUCO LP, et al. 1989. High frequency of Epstein-Barr virus genome in HIV-positive patients with Hodgkin's disease. Lancet 333:1458.

UCCINI S, MONARDO F, STOPPACCIARO A, et al. 1990. High frequency of Epstein-Barr virus genome detection in Hodgkin's disease of HIV-positive patients. Int J Cancer 46:581–585.

UHARA H, SATO Y, MUKAI K, et al. 1990. Detection of Epstein-Barr virus DNA in Reed-Sternberg cells of Hodgkin's disease using the polymerase chain reaction and in situ hybridization. Jpn J Cancer Res 81:272–278.

UNGER PD, STRAUCHEN JA. 1986. Hodgkin's disease in AIDS complex patients: Report of four cases and tissue immunologic marker studies. Cancer 58:821–825.

U.S. DEPARTMENT OF HEALTH AND HUMAN SERVICES. 1988. Hyattsville, MD, Vital Statistics of the United States, 1986, Vol. 1. Natality. Public Health Service, Centers for Disease Control, National Center for Health Statistics.

VELTRI RW, SHAH SH, MCCLUNG JE, et al. 1983. Epstein-Barr virus, fatal infectious mononucleosis, and Hodgkin's disease in siblings. Cancer 51:509–520.

VESTLEV PM, PALLESEN G, SANDVEJ K, et al. 1992. Prognosis of Hodgkin's disease is not influenced by Epstein-Barr virus latent membrane protein. Int J Cancer 50:670–671.

VIANNA NJ, GREENWALD P, BRADY J, et al. 1972. Hodgkin's disease: Cases with feature of a community outbreak. Ann Intern Med 77:169–180.

VIANNA NJ, GREENWALD P, DAVIES JNP. 1971. Extended epidemic of Hodgkin's disease in high school students. Lancet 1:1209–1211.

VIANNA NJ, POLAN AK. 1978. Immunity in Hodgkin's disease: Importance of age at exposure. Ann Intern Med 89:550–556.

VIANNA NJ, POLAN A. 1979. Lymphomas and occupational benzene exposure. Lancet i:1394–1395.

VIANNA NJ, POLAN AK. 1973. Epidemiologic evidence for transmission of Hodgkin's disease. N Engl Med 289:499–502.

WEISS LM, CHEN Y-Y, LIU X-F, et al. 1991. Epstein-Barr virus and Hodgkin's disease: A correlative *in situ* hybridization and polymerase chain reaction study. Am J Pathol 139:1259–1265.

WEISS LM, MOVAHED LA, WARNKE RA, et al. 1989. Detection of Epstein-Barr viral genomes in Reed-Sternberg cells of Hodgkin's disease. N Engl J Med 320:502–506.

WEISS LM, STRICKLER JG, WARNKE RA, et al. 1987. Epstein-Barr viral DNA in tissue of Hodgkin's disease. Am J Pathol 129:86–91.

WU T-C, MANN RB, CHARACHE P, et al. 1990. Detection of EBV gene expression in Reed-Sternberg cells of Hodgkin's disease. Int J Cancer 46:801–804.

YANAGIHARA R. 1992. Human T-cell lymphotropic virus type I infection and disease in the Pacific basin. Hum Biol 64:843–854.

YOSHIDA M, FUJISAWA T-I. 1992. Positive and negative regulation of HTLV-I gene expression and their roles in leukemogenesis in ATL. *In* Takatsuki K, Hinuma Y, Yoshida M (eds): Advances in Adult T-cell Leukemia and HTLV-I Research. Gann Monograph on Cancer Research no. 39. Tokyo, Japan Scientific Societies Press, and Boca Raton, CRC Press, pp. 217–235.

YOUNG LS. 1994. Ludwig/CRC EBV Meeting. Epstein-Barr Virus Report 1:10–12.

ZANINOVIC V, SANZON F, LOPEZ F, VELANDIA G, BLANK A, BLANK M, FUJIYAMA C, YASHIKI S, MATSUMOTO D, KATAHIRA Y, MIYASHITA H, FUJIYOSHI T, CHAN L, SAWADA T, MIURA T, HATAMI M, TAJIMA K, SONODA S. 1994. Geographic independence of HTLV-I and HTLV-II foci in the Andes Highland, the Atlantic coast, and the Orinoco of Colombia. AIDS Res Hum Retroviruses 10:97–101.

ZAHM SH. 1995. Epidemiologic research on Vietnam veterans: Difficulties and lessons learned. Ann Epidemiol 5:414–416.

42 Non-Hodgkin's lymphomas

PAUL A. SCHERR
NANCY E. MUELLER

Since the term *malignant lymphoma* was first introduced by Billroth in 1871, there has been continuing confusion as to the classification of this group of diseases. The identification of Reed-Sternberg cells distinguished Hodgkin's disease from the other lymphomas, leaving a collection of diseases regarded as non-Hodgkin's lymphomas (NHL). In the ninth revision of the International Classification of Diseases (World Health Organization, 1977), non-Hodgkin's disease includes lymphosarcoma and reticulosarcoma (code 200), nodular lymphoma (202.0), mycosis fungoides (202.1), other lymphomas (202.8), and other and unspecified (202.9).

PATHOLOGY

Before 1966, NHL were divided into two main cytologic groups of reticulum cell sarcoma and lymphosarcoma. The Rappaport classification system (Rappaport, 1966) became the standard system for the classification of NHL (Table 42–1) and remains as one of the classification systems frequently used today. Subsequently, advances in morphologic classification and in immunology led to the development of no less than six additional classification schemes. These classification schemes can be arranged according to the major criterion selected for classification (Nathwani, 1987). The Dorfman (1974, 1975), British or Bennett (1974; Henry et al, 1978), and World Health Organization (Mathé et al, 1976) classifications are based on the morphologic pattern; the Lukes and Collins (1974), according to immunologic origin; the Kiel (Gerard-Marchant et al, 1974; Lennert et al, 1975), according to histologic grade; and the Working Formulation (National Cancer Institute [NCI], 1982), according to prognosis.

The Working Formulation was developed as a means of translating from one classification scheme to another. The hope was that studies that used the Working Formulation to classify pathology could be easily compared to studies that used another classification scheme. Pathologists who played major roles in developing the other classification schemes were members of the committee that developed the Working Formulation. The major factor used to discriminate pathologic groups was detectable differences in survival. The major classification groups are low grade (median survival of subgroups 5.1 to 7.2 yr), intermediate grade (1.5 to 3.0 yr), high grade (0.7 to 2.0 yr), and miscellaneous (Table 42–2). Provision was made for the inclusion of subtypes under each major type, such as plasmacytoid differentiation and sclerosis. These features may have clinical relevance, but did not relate to differences in survival. Insufficiencies of the system were noted among the major participants. These include the fact that entities which are biologically closely related are separated, and entities biologically unrelated are grouped together. In addition, the formulation does not distinguish the cell of origin of the lymphoma as B cell, T cell, non-B or T cell, and histiocyte; although most NHL appear to be B cell in origin.

The various histologies of NHL can be related to stages in the development of normal lymphocytes. Normal lymphocytes originate from a multipotential stem cell and pass through a series of developmental stages as they differentiate into mature lymphocytes or plasma cells. Through the use of immunologic cell marker studies, the cell surface markers for each stage in the development of normal cells were found to correspond with those for the histologies of NHL and some leukemias. For example, the cell markers for acute lymphoblastic leukemia were found to be similar to those on normal cells that had differentiated just past the multipotential stem cell state (Magrath 1981). In the Rappaport scheme, the observed diseases that correspond to successive stages in the normal maturation process are undifferentiated lymphomas of the Burkitt's and non-Burkitt's type, poorly differentiated lymphocytic lymphoma, mixed lymphocytic-histiocytic lymphoma, histiocytic lymphoma, and both well-differentiated lymphocytic lymphoma and myeloma. It has been suggested that the lymphomas and leukemias represent neoplastic lymphocytes that are blocked at different stages of differentiation (Warnke and Weiss, 1987).

At a symposium sponsored by the U.S. National Can-

TABLE 42–1. *Modified Rappaport Classification and Relative Frequency of Histologic Subtypes of NHL**

NODULAR	FREQUENCY (%)
Lymphocytic, well differentiated	0 to 1.6[a]
Lymphocytic, poorly differentiated	18.4
Mixed, lymphocytic and histiocytic	7.9
Histiocytic	1.7
DIFFUSE	
Lymphocytic, well differentiated without plasmacytoid features with plasmacytoid features	4.0
Lymphocytic, poorly differentiated without plasmacytoid features with plasmacytoid features	9.1
Lymphoblastic convoluted non-convoluted	8.3
Mixed, lymphocytic and histiocytic	4.4
Histiocytic without sclerosis	24.9
Histiocytic with sclerosis	2.9
Burkitt's tumor Undifferentiated	2.0
MALIGNANT LYMPHOMA, UNCLASSIFIED COMPOSITE LYMPHOMA	14.7 to 16.4

*From National Cancer Institute (1982) with permission.
[a]Data on categories with few cases not reported in detail. Distribution based on 1175 consecutive patients at four hospitals.

TABLE 42–2. *Working Formulation and Relative Frequency of Histologic Subtypes of NHL (NCI, 1982) and United States SEER Incidence Rates, 1977–1985**

Histology	*Frequency (%)*	*Incidence Rates (100,000 PY)*
LOW GRADE		
Small lymphocytic NOS consistent with chronic lymphocytic leukemia plasmacytoid	3.5	1.03
Follicular predominantly small cleaved cell NOS with diffuse areas with sclerosis	22.0	1.31
Follicular mixed, small cleaved and large cell NOS with diffuse areas with sclerosis	7.6	0.50
INTERMEDIATE GRADE		
Follicular predominantly large cell NOS with diffuse areas with sclerosis	3.7	0.23
Diffuse small cleaved cell NOS with sclerosis	6.7	1.48
Diffuse mixed, small and large cell NOS with sclerosis with epitheloioid cell component	6.6	0.76
Diffuse large cell NOS with cleaved cell with noncleaved cell with sclerosis	19.3	2.89
HIGH GRADE		
Large cell, immunoblastic NOS with plasmacytoid with clear cell with polymorphous with epithelioid cell component	7.7	0.36
Lymphoblastic NOS with convoluted cell with non-convoluted cell	4.2	0.13
Small noncleaved cell NOS Burkitt's with follicular areas	4.9	0.30
MISCELLANEOUS Composite Mycosis fungoides Histiocytic Extramedullary plasmacytoma Unclassifiable Other	13.7	1.60

*NOS = not otherwise specified; PY = person-years.

cer Institute on "The Emerging Epidemic of NHL," Jaffe et al (1992) proposed that NHL could be classified by integrating morphological, immunophenotypical, and molecular information to delineate individual diseases which are likely to have different etiologies. The broad categories which they proposed include the low-grade B-cell lymphomas, the aggressive B-cell lymphomas (which can occur *de novo* or evolve from the latter), the post-thymic T-cell malignancies, and the lymphoblastic malignancies. As an example of the specificity of this scheme from among the low-grade B-cell lymphomas, the follicular lymphomas appear to form a distinct epidemiologic entity. These represent nearly half of all NHL, occur in adults, and have an equal sex ratio. Characteristically, the malignant cells form follicular aggregates held together by dendritic reticulum cells. Further, 90% of these cells share a characteristic cytogenetic translocation of the immunoglobulin heavy chain locus on chromosome 14 and the *bcl*-2 gene on chromosome 18. These characteristics suggest common etiologic factors related to antigen selection (Bahler et al, 1992).

Unfortunately, most epidemiologic studies do not use the current classification systems to differentiate the various histologies of NHL. At the extreme, some of the epidemiologic literature refers to lymphomas, which includes both Hodgkin's disease and NHL. Other reports refer to NHL, which include all types of lymphoma with the exclusion of Hodgkin's disease. A few studies will distinguish between lymphosarcoma or reticulum cell sarcoma and other lymphomas. Only the most recent literature has begun to use classification schemes such as that of Rappaport. One reason for not using a detailed classification scheme may be the size of the study that would be required to have a sufficient number of cases of even a few of the various histologies that would achieve statistical significance for a twofold relative risk (RR) or less. To the extent that various histologic entities represent different diseases with different etiologies, progress in our understanding of the cause of NHL has been greatly limited.

DEMOGRAPHY

U.S. Mortality

The mortality rate for NHL in the United States in 1990 was 6.3 deaths per 100,000 population. The annual age-specific mortality rates by race and sex for the period 1982–1986 (NCI, 1993) are shown in Figure 42–1. Below age 40, the rates for males and females do not differ substantially with race. Above that age, however, differences in mortality rates by race can be noted.

Between 1950 and 1985, the United States mortality rate had doubled from 2.9 deaths per 100,000 population in 1950 (Fig. 42–2) (NCI, 1988). Over these 35 years, the highest rate of increase occurred among the elderly, while a decline in mortality rates in the youngest age-groups occurred (Devesa et al, 1987). These secular trends in mortality rates can reflect trends in incidence rates, inaccuracy of diagnosis, or improved treatments for specific histologies. Cantor and Fraumeni (1980) noted that the mortality rates for reticulum cell sarcoma more than doubled from 1950 to 1965, while the rates for lymphosarcoma remained nearly constant.

U.S. Incidence

The annual incidence rate of NHL in the period 1986–1990 estimated from the Surveillance, Epidemiology and End Results (SEER) sites is 13.9 cases per 100,000

FIG. 42–1. Averaged annual age-specific mortality rates for NHL per 100,000 population among white males (*WM*), white females (*WF*), black males (*BM*), and black females (*BF*) in the United States, 1986–1990. (National Cancer Institute, 1993.)

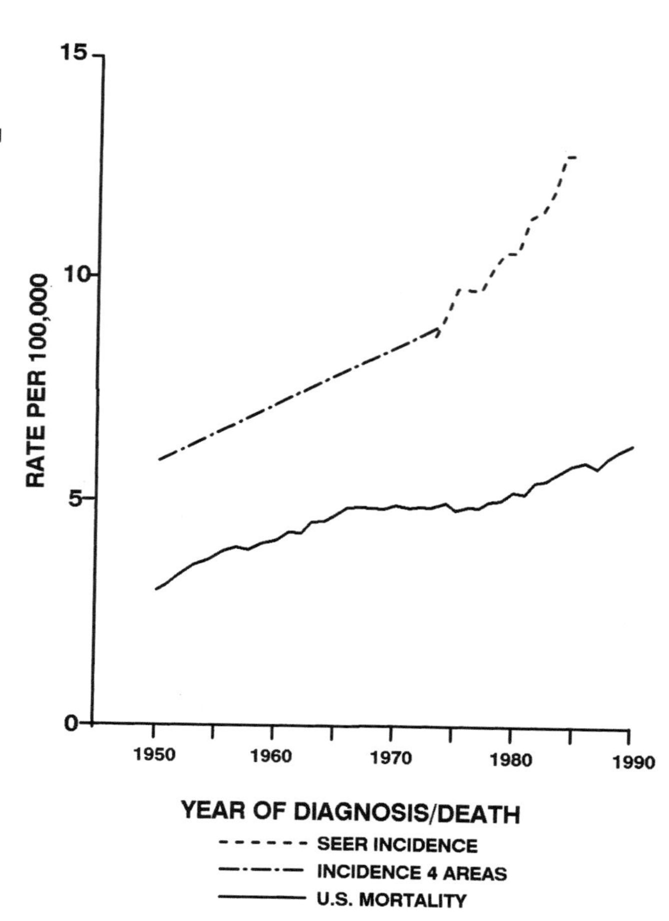

FIG. 42–2. Age-adjusted annual incidence rates of NHL estimated from rates in four survey areas (Atlanta, Connecticut, Detroit, San Francisco–Oakland) and the SEER cancer registry areas. Cancer mortality rates for the U.S. population, 1950–1980. (National Cancer Institute, 1988; National Cancer Institute, 1993.)

persons (NCI, 1993). Age-specific incidence rates (Fig. 42–3) show an exponentially increasing rate for both sexes. Based on the 1979–91 incidence rates, approximately 50,900 cases occurred in the United States in 1995 (Wingo et al, 1995).

The incidence of NHL has been markedly increasing over time. After ranking all cancers by the rate of increase in the U.S. population between 1973 and 1990, NHL rank third among males and third among females (NCI, 1993). For the four locations in the United States (Atlanta, Connecticut, Detroit, and San Francisco-Oakland) that have had cancer incidence rates determined at several points in time from 1950 to the present, the overall annual incidence rate per 100,000 people has risen from 5.9 in 1950, to 9.9 in 1975, and to 13.1 in 1985 (Fig. 42–2) (NCI, 1988). This represents more than a doubling of the incidence rate of disease over the 35-year period. These increases have been largest among those aged 65 and older and intermediate among those aged 35 to 64, while the rates among young adults have not changed substantially (Devesa et al, 1987). Some of the increase in rates among the elderly is thought to be due to better diagnosis in the elderly, particularly during the 1950s and 1960s (Devesa et al, 1987). In a recent review of the descriptive epidemiology of NHL, Devesa and Fears (1992) concluded that this increase has occurred for both sexes and among both whites and blacks in the United States, as well as internationally.

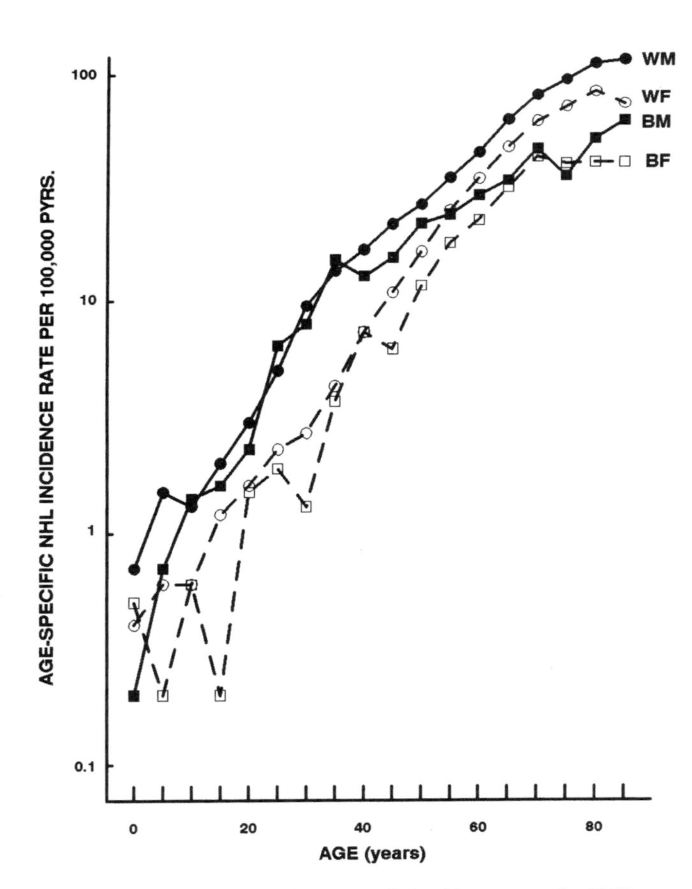

FIG. 42–3. Average, annual age-specific incidence rates for NHL per 100,000 population among white males (*WM*), white females (*WF*), black males (*BM*), and black females (*BF*) in the United States, 1986–1990, as estimated from the SEER Cancer Registries. (National Cancer Institute, 1993.)

As part of the SEER program, NHL cases have been classified according to the Working Formulation since 1977. The average incidence rates for 1977 to 1985 by these histologic subtypes are given in Table 42–2. Since 1977, the incidence rate of all subtypes of lymphoma have increased, with the largest rate of increase occurring among high-grade lymphomas (NCI, 1988).

U.S. Survival

The one-year survival rate for all NHL diagnosed in 1984 was 73.1%, and the 5-year survival rate for those diagnosed from 1983 through 1989 was 51.7%. Historically, the 5-year survival rate for NHL remained at 28% for cases diagnosed from 1950 through 1964, increased to 47% for cases diagnosed from 1974 through 1976, and rose slowly to 51.7% for the period 1983 through 1989 (NCI, 1993). Survival by subtype according to the Working Formulation is presented in Table 42–3 (NCI, 1988). One of the defining characteristics of this classification system is survival, with low grade (A–C) having the highest survival rates, intermediate grade (D–G) having intermediate survival rates, and high grade (H–J) having the poorest survival rates. Since 1977, statistically significant increases in survival rates have only been noted for follicular, large cell, immunoblastic, and small noncleaved, Burkitt's lymphoma (NCI, 1988).

TABLE 42–3. *Relative Survival Rates (%) for Non-Hodgkin's Lymphomas Classified by the Working Formulation by Year of Diagnosis*

Histology	*1-year (1979–80)*	*5-year (1983–84)*
Small lymphocytic	89.6	54.0
Follicular, small cleaved	94.6	68.6
Follicular, mixed small cleaved and large cell	87.1	68.5
Follicular, large cell	78.1	67.4
Diffuse, small cleaved	77.6	42.1
Diffuse, mixed small and large cell	71.8	44.7
Diffuse, large cell	64.1	39.1
Large cell, immunoblastic	52.7	35.2
Lymphoblastic[a]	63.3	33.6
Small noncleaved; Burkitt's	51.7	36.0

[a]Data aggregated for the years 1977–84 due to small numbers.

International Patterns

The geographic variation of incidence rates is often useful in providing clues to the etiology of disease. For NHL, the United States, Switzerland, and Canada have the highest reported rates while Mali, Gambia, and Poland ("rural" Warsaw) report the lowest rates (Parkin et al, 1992), with an approximately tenfold difference between the two sets of rates (Table 42–4). Comparison of the rates of histologic subtypes of lymphoma between countries or over time is complicated by the secular changes in terminology and classification (Muir et al, 1987). In general, the incidence of NHL appears to be associated with level of economic development, although exceptions do occur.

Age and Sex

In essentially all countries, the incidence rate among males is higher than that among females (Table 42–4). In averaging the data from 1986 to 1990 for all races in the United States, the annual incidence rate of NHL is 17.1 cases per 100,000 males and 11.2 cases per 100,000 females. The corresponding mortality rates are 7.5 deaths per 100,000 males and 4.9 deaths per 100,000 females (NCI, 1993).

Race and Ethnicity

Variation of disease rates within a country by racial and ethnic groups has been reported for NHL. Seidman (1970) and Newill (1961) noted higher mortality rates of lymphosarcoma and reticulosarcoma among Jews in New York City relative to other religious groups. In Israel, a higher incidence of NHL has been reported among Jews (9.5/100,000 person-years for males, 6.9/100,000 person-years for females) relative to non-Jews (6.3/100,000 person-years for males, 4.0/100,000 person-years for females) (Muir et al, 1987). Two geo-

TABLE 42–4. *High and Low Age-Standardized Annual Incidence Rates and Standard Errors for Non-Hodgkin's Lymphomas (ICD-9, 200+202) per 100,000 Person-Years**

Area	Males		Females	
	Rate	Standard Error	Rate	Standard Error
San Francisco Bay Area, USA (white)	17.4	0.5	9.1	0.3
New York City, USA	14.3	0.3	8.2	0.2
Seattle, WA, USA	14.1	0.4	9.1	0.3
Detroit, MI, USA (white)	13.9	0.4	9.6	0.3
SEER, USA (white)	13.6	0.2	8.9	0.1
New Orleans, LA, USA (white)	13.6	0.9	9.0	0.6
Iowa, USA	13.0	0.4	8.7	0.3
Los Angeles, CA, USA (white and other)	13.0	0.3	8.1	0.2
St. Gall, Switzerland	12.7	1.0	8.7	0.7
Connecticut, USA (white)	12.6	0.4	9.4	0.3
Manitoba, Canada	12.5	0.6	10.6	0.6
Quebec, Canada	12.5	0.3	9.6	0.2
Ontario, Canada	12.5	0.2	8.8	0.2
St. Petersburg, Russia	3.2	0.2	2.1	0.1
Qidong, China	3.2	0.4	1.5	0.2
Bermuda (white and other)	3.1	1.6	3.4	1.4
Kyrgyzstan	3.1	0.3	1.6	0.2
Ahmedabad, India	3.0	0.2	1.6	0.2
Bangalore, India	2.9	0.2	1.8	0.2
Belarus	2.9	0.1	1.6	0.1
Setif, Algeria	2.7	0.5	1.4	0.3
Country Cluj, Rumania	2.7	0.4	1.1	0.2
Madras, India	2.6	0.2	1.2	0.1
Khon Kaen, Thailand	2.5	0.5	3.6	0.6
Warsaw ("Rural"), Poland	2.4	0.4	1.9	0.3
Gambia	2.4	0.6	1.3	0.4
Bamako, Mali	1.4	0.5	0.4	0.3

*From Parkin et al, 1992, with permission.

graphic areas containing subgroups with highly divergent rates (Table 42–4) are the Kuwaitis and non-Kuwaitis in Kuwait and the American Indians and non-Hispanic whites in New Mexico. In the United States, the incidence and mortality rates for the period 1986–1990 are lower for blacks (9.5 and 4.2 per 100,000 person-years, respectively) than for whites (14.6 and 6.3 per 100,000 person-years, respectively) (NCI, 1993).

Socioeconomic Status and Urbanization

In general, mortality rates for NHL increase directly with the level of socioeconomic status and urbanization (Registrar General, 1958; Guralnick, 1963; Hoover et al, 1975; Cantor and Fraumeni, 1980). Hoover et al (1975), using the U.S. cancer mortality data by county from 1950 to 1969 (Mason and McKay, 1974), contrasted the age-adjusted mortality rates of NHL in 957 counties listed as totally rural with 13 counties listed as totally urban and found an urban–rural ratio of 1.4 for both males and females. Excluding those used in the urban–rural comparison, the counties were ranked by median educational attainment, an indicator of socioeconomic status. By contrasting the upper 10% of the distribution with the lowest 10%, a social class ratio of 1.4 was observed for males and that of 1.5 for females. However, in a study of mortality rates in New York City, Seidman (1970) found no significant trend with socioeconomic status. In a case–control study in northern Italy, La Vecchia et al (1992) found that those with 12 or more years of education had lower rates of NHL relative to those with fewer than 7 years (RR 0.6, 95% confidence interval [CI] 0.4, 1.0).

The relationship of socioeconomic status and incidence rates was investigated as part of the Third National Cancer Survey (Williams et al, 1977). No consistent pattern was observed between socioeconomic status and either lymphosarcoma or reticulum cell sarcoma, but there was a suggestion of increased rates for other lymphoma with increasing socioeconomic status, although the relationship was not statistically significant.

Familial Aggregation

The hypothesis that NHL would tend to aggregate in families seems plausible since an inherited defect of immune function might place all members of a family at increased risk of the disease. In a review of the literature, Greene (1982) identified 38 families with multiple cases of NHL. Many of these families could be classified into two general categories according to the characteristics of the lymphoma. One type includes preadolescent male sibships with extra-nodal NHL occurring primarily in the gastrointestinal tract. This type involves an inherited immune deficiency resulting in an inability to control infection with the Epstein-Barr virus (EBV) (Purtilo et al, 1978), as discussed below. The second type consists of adult siblings, mainly females, with nodal NHL (Greene, 1982). Linet and Pottern (1992) have noted that in some reported families with multiple NHL cases, other hematopoietic malignancies are also present. Even though family members may have a genetic predisposition to NHL, exposure to latent tumor viruses or other environmental factors may be required for the expression of the disease (Potolsky et al, 1971).

Although these case reports of familial aggregation can further our understanding of the disease process, a genetic predisposition may only account for a small proportion of NHL. As part of a larger study at Memorial Sloan-Kettering Cancer Center in New York (Razis et al, 1959), 1,269 cases with lymphosarcoma were interviewed regarding first degree blood relatives with a number of diseases including lymphosarcoma. The study did not find a statistically significant excess of families with multiple cases of lymphosarcoma. In a study by Ross et al (1983), all newly diagnosed lymphoreticular and hematological malignancies that occurred among the 7 million residents of Los Angeles County from 1972 to 1979 were reviewed to identify multiple malignancies that occurred in the same household. From 5,106 cases of NHL identified by the Cancer Surveillance Program, three pairs were observed. The expected number was 2.8 or 2.9, depending on the requirements of the model. A study of incident cases diagnosed between 1972 and 1980 in Tasmania (Giles et al, 1984) identified 241 cases of NHL of whom 8 had a first degree relative with the same diagnosis. For 532 cases of NHL treated from 1960 to 1980 at the Rambam Medical Center, Haifa, Israel from 1960 to 1980, three pairs of NHL cases were observed in close relatives while 3.86 were expected. In conclusion, there seems to be little evidence that a major proportion of cases of NHL have a strong genetic basis.

PRIMARY AND ACQUIRED IMMUNOSUPPRESSION

Persons with congenital immunodeficiency are at greatly increased risk of developing cancer, especially NHL, before they reach adulthood. (See Chapter 24 for an extensive review.) In data collected by the Immunodeficiency Cancer Registry, almost half of the reported malignancies are NHL (Table 42–5) (Filipovich et al, 1984, 1992). Since the underlying population base of persons with primary immunodeficiency is unenumerated, the actual risk of NHL in the population is not calculable, but its proportion of all reported malignancies is substantially higher than expected. An unusual

TABLE 42–5. *Cancer Cases by Disease Category from the Immunodeficiency-Cancer Registry**

Immunodeficiency Disease	*Total Cancer Cases*	*Non-Hodgkin's Lymphoma*	*Hodgkin's Disease*	*Leukemia*	*Other*
Ataxia telangiectasia	150	69	16	32	33
Common variable immunodeficiency	120	55	8	8	49
Wiskott-Aldrich syndrome	78	59	3	7	9
Severe combined immunodeficiency	42	31	4	5	2
Other	100	34	11	11	44
Totals	490	248	42	63	137

*Modified from Filipovich et al (1992).

pathologic feature of these lymphomas is the large proportion which are B-immunoblastic sarcomas, similar to what is seen in post-transplant lymphomas (Frizzera et al, 1980). Four of 13 tissue specimens tested for the presence of the EBV genome were positive. Serum cytokine assays from primary immunodeficiency patients with EBV-associated B-cell lymphoproliferative disorders suggest that cytokine immunoregulation of B-cell proliferation is abnormal in these patients, as indexed by high levels of interleukin-4 (IL-4) and low levels of interferon-alpha (IFN-α), (Filipovich et al, 1992).

A low, but clearly excessive risk of NHL is seen among patients who are therapeutically immunosuppressed in conjunction with organ or bone marrow transplantation. Among 6,297 patients who received renal transplants between 1951 and 1971 in the United States, 25 lymphomas were diagnosed, or a 35-fold excess risk (Hoover and Fraumeni, 1973). In the final follow-up of this cohort (total number unstated), 54 NHL were observed (Hoover, 1992). The RR was substantially higher, or 25, among those whose first transplant was before 1968 when tissue typing was less advanced, than for those transplanted in the early 1970s, or 10.5. The RR also increased with the number of transplants, from 13.5 for those with one kidney transplant to 100 for those with three or more transplants. On follow-up of 3,823 renal transplant recipients in the United Kingdom and Australia through 1978, 34 NHL cases were diagnosed, or a nearly 60-fold excess (Kinlen et al, 1979). Among 2,915 organ transplant patients seen at the University of Cincinnati through early 1987, 396 were subsequently diagnosed with NHL; these occurred more frequently in non-renal transplant patients (Penn, 1988). Similarly, in a large series reported by the Collaborative Transplant Study of 45,141 kidney and 7,634 heart recipients, the risk of developing NHL in the first transplant year was 0.2% and 1.2%, respectively. This risk diminished substantially and stabilized in subsequent years (Opeiz et al, 1993).

Among 506 bone marrow transplant recipients treated at the University of Minnesota between 1968 and 1986, 8 developed B-cell lymphoproliferative disorders. Six of these cases developed among the 25 patients who received T cell–depleted marrow from a human lymphocyte antigen (HLA) mismatched donor (Shapiro et al, 1988). Similarly, among 2,246 patients who received bone marrow transplants at the University of Washington between 1970 and early 1987, 16 NHL cases were diagnosed, with 0.045 cases expected (Witherspoon et al, 1989). Risk was also found to be associated with T-cell depletion of donor marrow and HLA mismatching, as well as with use of anti-T-cell monoclonal antibody or anti-thymocyte globulin to treat acute graft-vs.-host disease. More recently, Swinnen et al (1990) reported a substantial increase in the incidence of NHL among cardiac transplant recipients who were treated with the monoclonal antibody OKT3, which profoundly depletes circulating CD3+ T lymphocytes, in comparison to that expected based on other immunosuppressive regimens. This finding of increased risk of NHL in patients who received more aggressive immunosuppression was echoed in the study by Opeiz et al (1993).

In all of these groups of immunosuppressed patients, the great majority of NHL cases were diagnosed within a few years following transplant. Extranodal involvement—especially of the central nervous system—is common (Penn, 1986). Histologically, the tumors tend to be diffuse large cell, often immunoblastic lymphomas (Weintraub and Warnke, 1982).

Other Conditions

The occurrence of NHL has been reported for a variety of conditions which are either autoimmune in nature or require immunosuppressive treatment (Penn, 1986). Again, most reports are only of cases and the number of persons at risk is unknown; in such instances, the magnitude of the association cannot be estimated. For a few populations, however, estimates are available. Kinlen et al (1979) followed 1,349 non-transplant patients who were treated with immunosuppressive drugs for a variety of conditions. They reported that 4 cases of NHL developed, with 0.34 cases expected. Among 1,651 dialysis patients who had not received immunosuppressive treatment, Kinlen et al (1980) evaluated the occurrence of malignancy over a 10-year period. They reported an excess of NHL, or 4 cases vs. the 0.15 cases expected.

Kassan et al (1978) followed 136 women with Sjögren's syndrome treated at the National Institutes of Health for an average of 8.1 years. Of these patients, 7 developed NHL with only 0.16 cases expected. A series of 182 female and 23 male patients with systemic lupus erythematosus were followed for subsequent cancer using the Finnish Cancer Registry (Pettersson, 1992). Four cases of NHL occurred among the females while 0.09 cases were expected.

Gridley et al (1994) used the discharge records from a Veteran's Affairs hospital to identify 906 men with Felty syndrome. The risk of subsequent NHL among these patients was 12.8 (95% CI 7.7, 20.0), which is much higher than the risk usually observed for rheumatoid arthritis. Silman et al (1988) followed 202 patients with rheumatoid arthritis who had been treated with azathioprine for up to 20 years. A matched number of patients who were not treated with the drug were also followed. Four cases of NHL occurred in the treated group and 2 occurred in the untreated group. The expected number based on population data was 0.40 and 0.42, respectively. The overall finding was consistent with that of Symmons et al (1984) who reported 6 cases of NHL occurring among 489 rheumatoid arthritis patients. After reviewing the data on NHL incidence among patients with this condition, Kinlen (1992) estimated that the overall risk among those patients treated with azathioprine or cyclophosphamide was tenfold and those without, 2.5-fold.

The association between celiac disease and related conditions with the occurrence of NHL of the intestinal tract has long been noted (Swinson et al, 1983). Holmes et al (1976) followed 210 patients with biopsy-diagnosed celiac disease for subsequent malignancy. Thirteen cases were observed, with 0.11 cases expected. Among 109 patients with dermatitis herpetiformis, 3 developed NHL, with 0.03 cases expected (Leonard et al, 1983). These researchers also reported that those who adopted a gluten-free diet had a lower risk of developing NHL than those who did not. Sigurgeirsson et al (1994) followed 976 patients with dermatitis herpetiformis without clinical signs of coeliac disease. An increased risk of NHL (RR = 5.4, 95% CI = 2.2–11.1) was found, but only among male patients.

This observation is reinforced by the opportunistic occurrence of lymphoma among acquired immunodeficiency syndrome (AIDS) patients (see Chapter 24). NHL are the most frequent opportunistic malignancies seen in HIV-I–infected persons. These lymphomas are typically of B-cell origin with high-grade histology, primarily immunoblastic and Burkitt's lymphoma (BL), with primary lymphoma of the brain not uncommon. These lymphomas appear to occur independent of risk factors for HIV infection, in proportion with the risk of non-HIV–infected populations in terms of sex and race, and risk of occurrence increases along with decreasing immune function (Obrams and Grufferman, 1991; Beral et al, 1991; Biggar and Rabkin, 1992; Levine, 1993). Occult NHL are not unusual at autopsy (Obrams and Grufferman, 1991; Mohar et al, 1992). It is estimated that with antiviral therapy, the probability of developing NHL is 29% after 36 mo of treatment (Pluda et al, 1993). About half of the NHL in AIDS patients are EBV-genome positive. These includes virtually all primary CNS lymphomas, 35%–40% of BL, and 50%–60% of other lymphomas (Borisch-Chappuis et al, 1990; MacMahon et al, 1991; Hamilton-Dutoit et al, 1991, 1993).

In sum, for patients with a variety of conditions involving substantial immune dysfunction, there is a consistent finding of an excess risk of developing NHL. This risk is generally greater in conditions where chronic antigenic stimulation is present; for example, post- vs. pretransplant, the presence of an incompatible organ graft, normal diet vs. gluten-free diet in celiac disease; or when these is a severe depletion of T cells.

In 1975 Matas et al speculated that among organ transplant recipients, the chronic antigenic stimulation induced by both the graft and by the reactivation of latent herpesvirus infections led to the development of NHL. This hypothesis is consistent with the relatively rapid onset of these malignancies (Hoover and Fraumeni, 1973). More recent evidence points to loss of cell-mediated immune control of reactivated EBV as part of this process (Anonymous, 1984).

Recent studies have provided a picture of the natural history of what occurs in some patients. Polyclonal B-cell proliferation is often seen among transplant recipients (Hanto et al, 1981; Starzl et al, 1984; Cleary et al, 1984; Touraine et al, 1989). In some cases this process is reversible by the cessation of immunosuppressive treatment, but in other cases it persists and can evolve into a monoclonal proliferation. As reviewed by List et al (1987), the EBV appears to be intimately involved in this process. In brief, the immunosuppression necessary for the tolerance of the transplant results in a loss of control of persistent EBV infection. Serologically, this is reflected in the enhanced production of antibodies against the viral capsid antigen (VCA) (and the early antigen), but low or absent antibodies against the EB nuclear antigen (EBNA).

This process was evaluated prospectively by the analysis of serial blood specimens for 14 transplant patients who developed B-cell lymphomas or lymphoproliferative disease (Ho et al, 1985). Six of these patients had primary EBV infection in conjunction with transplantation and 8 patients had reactivated EBV infection. The general serologic pattern for these patients following transplant and prior to malignancy was that of elevated IgG, IgM, and IgA antibodies against the VCA, and low or absent anti-EBNA. All but one of these tumors were found to contain either EBNA or EBV-DNA genome. Similar findings have been reported for 3 Japanese patients with primary immunodeficiencies who developed NHL (Okano et al, 1986). In addition, Purtilo et al (1988) have documented the development of NHL in males with the X-linked lymphoproliferative syndrome following primary EBV infection. Such patients fail to develop anti-EBNA antibodies. Among 13 NHL cases which occurred following bone marrow transplantation, 11 tumors were positive for EBV-specific antigens (Witherspoon et al, 1989). The causal role of EBV in this process is reflected in the finding of clonal EBV in post-transplant NHL (Patton et al, 1990), and in the demonstration that EBV-associated lymphoproliferation in bone marrow recipients can be reversed with the infusion of lymphocytes from the seropositive donor (Papadopoulos et al, 1994).

VIRUSES

Since oncogenic viruses are known to cause lymphoma in a variety of animal models, it is reasonable to propose that they also play a role in the development of NHL outside of immunodeficiency. Evidence for this assertion is provided by the human retrovirus HTLV-I, which has been demonstrated to cause adult T-cell lymphoma (Mueller, 1991). However, this is a relatively rare infection and contributes little to overall NHL incidence. In contrast, the EBV is an ubiquitous infection and it is present in essentially all cases of "endemic" BL occurring in children in areas with holoendemic malaria, as well as in about half of non-endemic BL (Evans and Mueller, 1995). In endemic BL, it appears that early EBV infection combined with the chronic antigenic stimulation of malaria, can lead to the c-*myc*/immunoglobulin translocation which is the hallmark of BL (Magrath, 1992). Since EBV plays an intimate role in the evolution of most transplant-related NHL and many of those seen in AIDS, the question arises whether it also is involved in de novo NHL other than for the rare cases of BL. We evaluated this question in a collaborative case–control study involving four large serum banks established from normal populations, in which subsequent diagnoses of malignancy could be identified (Mueller et al, 1991). One hundred and four patients were identified who developed NHL, on average 63 mo following the collection and storage of blood specimens. Compared to controls from the same populations, the case specimens were more likely to have elevated IgG antibodies (RR = 2.4), and IgM antibodies (RR = 3.1) against the VCA, but less likely to have either elevated antibody titers (RR = 0.5) or low titers (RR = 0.5) against EBNA. This finding suggests that for some cases of "spontaneous" NHL, a causal pathway is shared with or is quite similar to that seen in immunosuppressed patients. The antibody response to the EBV is intimately involved in this process, but whether it is a direct causal factor is not clear from these data.

Based on molecular biologic studies to detect the presence of EBV genome, only a subset of "spontaneous" NHL cases are positive for EBV. For example, Staal et al (1989) found 4 of 100 samples EBV-genome positive, Herbst et al (1990) found 27 of 151 positive, and Levine et al (1992) found 3 of 20 samples positive. Surprisingly, it has recently been recognized that among NHL, EBV-positivity appears to be concentrated in the T-cell rather than the B-cell derived entities. Pallesen et al (1993) recently reviewed the data for EBV in peripheral T-cell NHL. In these cases, there is heterogeneity of EBV-positivity by histologic type, by geographic area, as well as by the proportion of cells which are positive. CD30-positive lymphomas, which appear to represent the interface of Hodgkin's disease and NHL, have also been recognized as an entity in which a proportion of cases (~ 20%) are EBV-associated (Herbst et al, 1993). In summary, although it is clear that viruses are causal factors for some specific NHL subtypes, their role in NHL as a whole appears to be minor.

VACCINATIONS AND MEDICATIONS

Several medical exposures have been associated with risk of lymphoma and lymphadenopathy. Within several large clinical trials of the effect of Bacillus Calmette-Guerin (BCG) vaccinations involving thousands of children, an increased occurrence of NHL was found among the treatment group. The observed-to-expected ratios were 2.9 for the study in Muscogee Country, Georgia, and Russell County, Alabama (Kendrick and Comstock, 1981); 4.0 for Puerto Rico (Comstock et al, 1975); and 2.1 (mortality) for the North Island of New Zealand (Skegg, 1978). In the second phase of the New Zealand study, an increased rate of the disease was found in the North Island where vaccination continued, while only the expected number of cases were observed in the South Island following cessation of vaccinations. This increased risk of NHL has been attributed to chronic antigenic stimulation from the vaccinations.

Dilantin is a medication used to treat epilepsy and known to produce lymphadenopathy in patients. The condition usually resolves upon the cessation of the drug. There is evidence that the condition may progress to lymphoma in some instances (Harrington et al, 1962). An increased risk of lymphoma has been supported in studies by Anthony (1970) and Li et al (1975) with the later study reported a threefold relative risk. However, a follow-up study of a large series of epileptic patients found no increased risk of the disease (Clemmesen, 1974). Immunologically, the drug inhibits delayed hypersensitivity responses by an effect either on the mast cells or the sensitized T cells (Mekori et al, 1985).

NHL has been observed to occur after cancer chemotherapy. Krikorian et al (1979) and Henry-Amar (1983) reported a higher than expected number of cases of NHL subsequent to treatment for Hodgkin's disease. Later, a cooperative study of 11 population-based registries (Kaldor et al, 1987) identified a cohort of 133,411 cases of testicular cancer, ovarian cancer, and Hodgkin's disease who were followed for the occurrence of subsequent cancers. Increased risk of NHL was observed for patients with testicular cancer (RR = 2.7) and Hodgkin's disease (RR = 3.0) but not those with ovarian cancer (RR = 1.3). The excess cases of NHL tended to occur within 5 years of the diagnosis of the initial cancer. The British National Lymphoma Investigation (Swerdlow, 1993) followed 2,846 Hodgkin's disease patients for subsequent cancer. The observed NHL risk was 16.8 (95% CI = 9.8, 26.9) relative to the general population. The risk was highest among those with lymphocyte predominant Hodgkin's disease. An even higher rate of NHL (106 cases, 3.34 expected) was observed among the 12,411 Hodgkin's disease patients enrolled in the International Database on Hodgkin's Disease (Henry-Amar, 1992). In another study which followed 1,507 patients with Hodgkin's disease, Tucker et al (1988) also found an increased risk of NHL (observed-to-expected ratio = 18.0) and also noted that approximately half of the patients had radiation therapy without adjuvant chemotherapy. This is consistent with the hypothesis that it may be the immune suppression seen in patients with Hodgkin's disease rather than its treatment which is a risk factor for subsequent NHL (Rosenberg et al, 1982).

Several studies have evaluated the risk of NHL among people receiving blood transfusions. In a study by Blomberg et al (1993), a cohort of 3,177 blood recipients was identified by the hospital blood center, in-patient, and discharge registers. Thirteen cases of NHL were observed with 4.8 cases expected (Standardized Mortality Ratio [SMR] = 2.7, 95% CI = 144, 4.62). In the second part of the study, 28,338 patients not receiving a transfusion and 1,572 patients who received a transfusion were followed from 3 to 9 years. An incidence rate ratio for NHL of 3.1 (95% CI 1.56, 6.20) was observed between these two groups. In another study, Cerhan et al (1993) identified a cohort of 37,337 cancer-free women in Iowa and assessed their transfusion history by a mail questionnaire. After five years of follow-up, those reporting a transfusion had a relative risk of NHL that was 2.2 times (95% CI 1.35, 3.58) the risk of those that did not report a transfusion. The risk seemed to diminish with time since first transfusion.

RADIATION

When studying the effects of ionizing radiation, the dosage level, type of radiation, and duration of exposure could modify the relationship of the occurrence of NHL with exposure. However, even with the consideration of the characteristics of the exposure, few studies suggest an increased risk of NHL from radiation. One of the few studies that support a relationship showed an excess of NHL among patients receiving radiotherapy for ankylosing spondylitis (Court-Brown and Doll, 1965). Among studies that did not quantify the dosage of radiation, studies among uranium mill workers (Archer et al, 1973), thorium processing plant workers (Polednak et al, 1983), radiologists (Matanoski et al, 1975), and people residing near nuclear installations (Forman et al, 1987), no significant excess of NHL was observed. At exposure levels of less than 100 rems, studies of 39,548 employees of an atomic energy authority (Beral et al, 1985) and of 8,375 employees at an energy research laboratory (Checkoway et al, 1985) found no increased risk of disease. At radiation levels in excess of 100 rads with a long duration of exposure, the study of over 5,000 Thorotrast patients and controls (Van Kaick et al, 1983) found an odds ratio for NHL of 1.4, which was not significant. No excess of NHL was found among the Japanese survivors of the atomic bomb explosions (Shimizu et al, 1990). In a study in Utah of diseases associated with radioactive fallout, an increased risk of lymphoma was noted, but it was limited only to women (Johnson, 1984). A study of exposure to diagnostic X rays (Boice, 1991) concluded that there was little evidence that these X rays can cause NHL. Reviews by Miller (1974) and Boice (Chapter 16) conclude that there is no reliable estimate of the effect of radiation and that the effect, if any, is small. Perhaps the ionizing radiation dose required to cause cell mutation is larger than the dose that results in cell death.

For lower energy electromagnetic radiation, a study by Milham (1988) noted no increased risk of mortality due to lymphosarcoma or reticulosarcoma among amateur radio operators licensees. For 60-Hz magnetic fields from power lines, there is a suggestion of an increase risk of childhood lymphomas (Wertheimer and Leeper, 1979; Savitz et al, 1988), but the findings were not statistically significant. However, the study of cancers among workers in a Swedish electronic industry, among electrical engineers, and among power linesman and power station operators showed no increase risk of lymphoma (Coleman and Beral, 1988). In conclusion, there is little convincing evidence for an increased risk of lymphoma due to any form of radiation.

OCCUPATION

Tables 42–6 and 42–7 summarize a large number of reports concerning occupational exposures and the risk of NHL. Except for some early reports, studies that aggregate NHL with other diseases are omitted from the tables. Table 42–6 includes studies that have looked at the distribution of occupations among NHL patients. Several of these are based only on a review of death certificates. In general, occupations of somewhat higher social class are associated with a higher risk of the disease, similar to the descriptive epidemiology. Although the data are not entirely consistent, occupations dealing with chemicals and agriculture appear to be associated with NHL in studies of incident cases.

Table 42–7 summarizes research based on the occurrence of NHL in specific occupational groups. A major group of interest includes farmers, herbicide and pesticide appliers, and grain workers. The earlier studies among farmers were based on mortality reports in which no specific exposure was examined or exposures were inferred by specific farming practices within the county of death. Subsequent studies have attempted to identify particular exposures that place farmers at increased risk of NHL. Studies of incident cases did find a higher risk among those using herbicide for more than 20 days per year (odds ratio [OR] = 6.0); mixing and applying herbicide themselves (OR = 8.0) (Hoar, 1986); 2,4-dichlorophenoxyacetic acid use for more than 20 days per year (OR = 2.4); using organophosphate insecticides (OR = 2.4) (Zahm, 1990). Higher risk was also found among those doing fence work, orchard workers, and meat works employees (Pearce et al, 1987).

A Swedish case–control study of malignant lymphoma showed an increased risk of lymphoma with exposure to phenoxy acids (RR = 4.8) and chlorophenols (RR = 4.3). Similar results were obtained when the data for Hodgkin's disease and NHL were analyzed separately. This report had major implications since these chemicals are widely used as pesticides and herbicides (Hardell et al, 1981). Subsequent case–control studies of NHL in western Washington State (Woods et al, 1987) and in New Zealand (Pearce et al, 1986), and studies of lymphoma among Swedish workers in agriculture or forestry and among pesticide appliers (Wiklund et al, 1987, 1988) did not report an increased risk of disease. Several more recent studies have supported an association (Bond et al, 1988; Perrson et al, 1989; Wigle et al, 1990; Coggon et al, 1991; Scherr et al, 1992), although others have not (Fingerhut et al, 1991; Saracci et al, 1991). In studies of phenoxy acids or chlorophenols exposure, the increased risk of lymphoma has been attributed to the contaminant 2,3,7,8-tetrachlorodibenzo-p-dioxin (2,3,7,8-TCDD). The concentration of this impurity may differ depending on production methods. The difference in NHL risks among studies may, in part, be explained by the differing exposures to TCDD. Reports of accidental industrial exposures to TCDD have not demonstrated an increased risk of NHL, but the number of individuals exposed was small. Alternately, the differences in risk may depend on differences in the particular phenoxy acid or chlorophenols used between studies with risk most consistently found with exposure to 2,4-dichlorophenoxyacetic acid. Additional evidence supporting this association is the finding of Hayes et al (1991) in a case–control study of canine malignant lymphoma and the owners' application of 2,4-dichlorophenoxyacetic acid herbicides to their lawns. Overall, there was a RR of 1.3 (1.04–1.67) and a significant trend with increasing yearly applications. A possible mechanism is suggested by the findings of a pilot study by Lipkowitz et al (1992) of an increased level of T cell–specific chromosomal aberrations in a sample of 12 agricultural workers which varied with seasonal exposure.

Several studies have reported on the risk of NHL among Vietnam veterans, particularly those exposed to Agent Orange. Most studies (Project Ranch Hand, 1983; Clapp et al, 1991; Dalager et al, 1991; Watanabe et al, 1991) did not find an increased risk. Several studies (O'Brien et al, 1991; Anonymous, 1990) did find an increased risk for Vietnam veterans, but it was not associated with Agent Orange exposure. A mortality study by Breslin et al (1988) did observe an increased risk of NHL with exposure of Agent Orange for Marines, but not for the Army.

A number of solvents have been studied as possible risk factors for NHL. Benzene received early attention due to its association with an increased risk of leukemia and some case reports. A study of NHL mortality and occupational benzene exposures (Vianna and Polan, 1979) found increased relative risks for reticulum cell sarcoma and lymphosarcoma. The methods used in this study have been criticized and three other mortality studies (Enterline, 1979; Smith and Lickiss, 1980; Wong, 1987) showed no increased risk of lymphoma. A number of other studies (Table 42–7) have found an increased risk of NHL with exposure to other solvents,

TABLE 42–6. *Studies of Multiple Occupations**

Reference	Study Type	Histology	(95% Confidence Intervals) Relative Risk	Occupation
Milham (1976c)	Mortality	LS, RC	1.7 (1.04–2.62)	Accountant
		LS, RC	3.9 (1.56–8.01)	Professor/instructor
		LS, RC	2.2 (0.88–4.51)	Aluminum worker
		LS, RC	2.0 (1.03–3.49)	Guard
		LS	1.4 (0.96–2.09)	All engineers
		LS	1.5 (0.95–2.26)	Misc. engineers
		LS	1.61 (1.07–2.33)	Electrical exposure
		LS	1.82 (0.87–3.35)	Pulp/paper
		LS	2.55 (0.94–5.56)	Bookkeeper
		LS	2.96 (1.09–6.47)	Mail carrier
		LS	2.79 (1.02–6.07)	Postal clerk
		LS	1.94 (0.97–3.47)	Real estate agent
		LS	1.82 (0.94–3.18)	Building contractor
		LS	1.31 (0.48–2.85)	Orchardist
		LS	1.28 (0.55–2.52)	Wheat farmer
		LS	0.85 (0.34–1.75)	Farm labor
Goldsmith and Guidotti (1975)	Mortality 1959–61	LS	2.62 (1.05–5.40)	Civil engineer
		LS	3.65 (1.34–7.96)	Food delivery
		LS	0.82 (0.51–1.25)	Farmer
		LS	0.42 (0.17–0.86)	Farm laborer
		LS	1.77 (0.85–3.25)	Electrician
		LS	3.51 (0.96–8.98)	Plasterer
	Mortality 1971–72	LS	1.50 (0.99–2.16)	Engineer
		LS	0.38 (0.10–0.98)	Technician
		LS	1.36 (1.14–1.62)	Craftsman
		LS	0.56 (0.40–0.75)	Operative
		LS	0.57 (0.33–0.91)	Laborers except farmers
		LS	0.81 (0.57–1.13)	Farmer
Blair et al, (1985)	Mortality	NHL, HD	1.94 (1.06–3.26)	Foreman (NEC)
			1.32 (0.53–2.72)	Chemist
			1.31 (0.57–2.58)	Typesetter
			1.29 (0.74–2.10)	Electrical engineer
			1.17 (0.60–2.04)	Physician
			1.10 (0.85–1.40)	Farmer
			0.72 (0.34–1.32)	Carpenter
			0.17 (0.04–9.61)	Plumber
Schumacher and Delzell (1988)	Mortality Case–control	NHL	0.86 (0.62–1.18) 90% CI	Agriculture (W)
			0.65 (0.33–1.27)	Agriculture (B)
			0.66 (0.36–1.21)	Farmer, high herbicide (W)
			1.11 (0.37–3.28)	Farmer, high herbicide (B)
			1.22 (0.82–1.82)	Construction (W)
			0.95 (0.33–2.70)	Construction (B)
			0.79 (0.54–1.17)	Paper, wood Furniture (W)
			1.17 (0.79–1.73)	Trucking (W)
			0.60 (0.25–1.46)	Trucking (B)
			0.64 (0.30–1.35)	Medicine (W)
			0.81 (0.59–1.12)	Textile (W)
			2.67 (0.98–7.29)	Textile (B)
			2.70 (1.95–3.72)	Professional (W)
			1.40 (0.99–1.99)	Clerical, sales (W)
			0.52 (0.32–0.85)	Machine trades (W)
			3.63 (1.32–9.97)	Machine trades (B)
			0.78 (0.59–1.03)	Asbestos (W)
			1.16 (0.58–2.30)	Asbestos (B)
			0.77 (0.56–1.07)	Benzene (W)
			0.94 (0.47–1.87)	Benzene (B)
Ng (1988)	Mortality	NHL	1.50 (1.08–7.78)	Artists
			5.08 (0.43–2.57)	Production foreman
			14.7 (1.21–2.68)	Construction worker
Williams et al (1977)	Incidence Case–control	LS, RC	1.14 (0.03–6.33)	Coal mine
		LS, RC	4.00 (0.10–22.29)	Metal
		LS, RC	6.54 (2.63–13.48)	Transportation
		LS, RC	3.00 (0.08–16.88)	Trucking (M)
		LS, RC	3.50 (0.09–19.21)	Communications (M)
		LS, RC	0.22 (0.05–0.64)	Retail stores (M)
		Other	5.25 (0.13–29.32)	Education (M)
		LS, RC	4.39 (0.91–12.89)	Food products (F)
		LS, RC	1.94 (0.05–10.82)	Textile (F)
		LS, RC	0.0	Education (F)
		LS, RC	14.4 (2.97–42.03)	Agriculture (M)

(continued)

TABLE 42–6. *Studies of Multiple Occupations* (Continued)*

Reference	Study Type	Histology	(95% Confidence Intervals) Relative Risk	Occupation
Brownson and Reif (1988)	Incidence Case–control	NHL	2.72 (0.96–7.69)	Printing
		NHL	1.11 (0.70–1.77)	Farming
		RS	1.99 (0.93–4.25)	Farming
		LS	0.95 (0.48–1.89)	Farming
		Other	0.73 (0.28–1.86)	Farming
Bernard et al (1984)	Incidence Case–control	NHL	1.30 (0.49–3.50)	Electricity
			0.58 (0.23–1.48)	Metal dust and paint
			7.71 (1.24–47.9)	Solvents (F)
			0.49 (0.21–2.00)	Benzene (M)
			4.67 (1.50–13.6)	Hairsprays (F)
			1.49 (0.75–2.95)	Hairsprays (F, age > 65)
Giles et al (1984)	Incidence Case–control	NHL	1.9 (1.06–3.47)	Professions
			8.0 (1.07–356.)	Metal, foundry worker
			1.9 (1.0–3.29)	Farmer
			5 cases, no controls	Hairdressers
Perrson et al (1989)	Case–control	NHL	1.9 (1.1–3.2) 90% CI	Solvents
			2.8 (1.1–7.1)	Carpentry
			2.2 (0.9–5.2)	Plastic/rubber chemicals
			2.2 (0.2–19)	Hairdressers
			0.3 (0.1–0.7)	Farmers
			0.4 (0.04–3.0)	Other pesticides
			9.4 (1.2–69)	Creosote
LaVecchia et al (1989)	Case–control	NHL	1.9 (1.2–3.0)	Agriculture
Hall and Rosenman (1991)	Incidence	NHL	1.61 (1.0–2.4)	Apparel manufacture (WF)
			2.17 (0.9–4.5)	Bakery products (WM)
			1.33 (1.0–1.8)	Electrical equipment mfg. (WM)
			1.66 (0.9–2.7)	Instrument mfg. (WM)
			1.98 (1.1–3.2)	Printing industry (WF)
Blair et al (1993a,b)	Case–control	NHL	2.3 (0.9–5.8)	Agriculture
			1.9 (0.9–3.8)	Painting/papering
			2.6 (0.9–3.8)	Masonry/tiler
			1.4 (0.96–2.0)	Metal fabrication
			2.0 (0.97–4.3)	Laundry/garments
			2.7 (0.9–8.7)	Barber shops
Scherr et al (1992)	Case–control	NHL	3.4 (1.1–10.8)	Agriculture
			2.1 (1.0–4.6)	Construction
			0.3 (0.1–0.9)	Chemical-related
			2.1 (0.9–4.8)	Leather
Blair (1993b)	Case–control	NHL	9.6 (1.1–80.6)	Special industrial machinery
			3.9 (1.01–14.8)	Real estate
			1.9 (1.1–3.2)	Personal services
Linet et al (1993)	Incidence	NHL	1.6 (1.1–2.4)	Dairy
			1.8 (1.2–2.7)	Shoe repair
			1.9 (1.1–3.3)	Porcelain and earthenware
			2.0 (1.2–3.3)	Wholesale paper
			1.8 (1.2–2.6)	Banking
			3.5 (1.9–6.0)	Research and scientific institute
			2.7 (1.3–5.0)	Other public jobs
			1.9 (1.2–3.0)	Engineers, technicians in mining
			2.1 (1.1–3.5)	School teachers
			1.6 (1.0–2.4)	Special teachers
			3.3 (1.2–7.4)	Bank cashier
			2.1 (1.0–3.7)	Secretaries, typists
			3.2 (1.3–6.6)	Health insurance clerks
			1.7 (1.1–2.6)	Shoemakers
			1.4 (1.0–1.9)	Lorry drivers
Persson et al (1993)	Case–control	NHL	2.3 (1.0–5.1)	Welding
			6.0 (1.1–31)	Lumberjacks
			5.6 (1.2–3.8)	Nursing

*Abbreviations: B = black; F = female; HD = Hodgkin's disease; LS = lymphosarcoma; M = male; MM = multiple myeloma; NEC = not elsewhere classified; NHL = non-Hodgkin's lymphomas; other = other lymphomas, usually ICD 202; RC = reticulum cell sarcoma; W = white. 95% confidence intervals calculated from observed and expected cases (Rothman and Boice, 1979).

TABLE 42–7. *Selected Studies**

Reference	Occupation Group	Study Type	Histology	Relative Risk	Possible Exposure and Comments
FARMERS, HERBICIDE AND PESTICIDE APPLIERS, GRAIN WORKERS					
Fasal et al (1968)	Farmers	Mortality	LS, RC	0.79 (not significant)	None
Burmeister (1981)	Farmers	Mortality	NHL	1.14 $P < 0.05$	None
Cantor et al (1982)	Farmers	Mortality Case–control	NHL RC LS Other	1.22 (0.98, 1.51) 1.41 (1.00, 1.98) 1.19 (0.86, 1.65) 1.10 (0.78, 1.55)	Cattle, insecticides, wheat acreage
Burmeister et al (1983)	Farmers	Mortality Case–control	NHL	$P < 0.05$	Chicken, milk, hogs, herbicide, insecticide
Schumacher (1985)	Farmers	Mortality Case–control	NHL LS Histio	1.3 (0.9–2.3) 1.9 (1.1–3.3) 0.9 (0.4–2.3)	None
Pearce et al (1985)	Farmers	Case–control	LS, RC LS, RC Other Other	1.13 (0.67–1.90) 0.87 (0.49–1.54) 1.76 (1.03–3.02) 1.15 (0.63–2.11)	age <65 age 65+ age <65 age 65+
Gallagher et al (1985)	Farmers	Mortality	NHL	0.93 (0.59–1.37)	
Hoar et al (1986)	Farmers	Interview	NHL	1.4 (0.9–2.1) 6.0 (1.9–19.5) 8.0 (2.3–27.9)	 Herbicide 20 days/yr Herbicide mixed, apply phenoxyacetic acid
Pearce et al (1987)	Farmers	Interview Case–control	NHL	1.0 (0.8–1.4) 1.0 (0.7–1.5) 3.7 (1.1–12.1) 1.4 (1.0–2.0)	 Phenoxy herbicides Orchard lead arsenate Fencing (arsenic, pentachlorophenol)
Woods et al (1987)	Farmers	Case–control	NHL	1.33 (1.03–1.7)	
Dubrow et al (1988)	Farmers	Mortality Case–control	NHL	1.6 (0.8–3.4)	
Wiklund et al (1988)	Farmers	Follow-up	NHL	0.97 (0.89–1.06)	
Ritter et al (1990)	Farmers	Mortality	NHL	0.9 (0.8–1.1) 2.2 (1.0–4.6)	 Herbicides, 250+ acres sprayed
Weisenburger (1990)	Farmers	Case–control	NHL	1.5 (0.9–2.4) 1.9 (1.1–3.1) 1.8 (1.0–3.2) 1.4 (0.8–2.3)	2,4-dichlorophenoxyacetic acid Organophosphates Carbamates Chlorinated hydrocarbons
Wigle et al (1990)	Farmers	Mortality	NHL	0.9 (0.8–1.1) 2.2 (1.0–4.6)	 Herbicides, 250+ acres sprayed
Zahm et al (1990)	Farmers	Interview Case–control	NHL	2.4 2.1	Organophosphate insecticide 2,4-dichlorophenoxyacetic acid
Zahm et al (1990)	Farmers	Case–control	NHL	0.9 (0.6–1.4) 1.1 (0.7–1.6) 1.3 (0.8–2.0) 1.5 (0.9–2.5)	Lived or worked on farm Insecticides Herbicides 2,4-dichlorophenoxyacetic acid
Cantor et al (1992)	Farmers	Case–control	NHL	1.2 (1.0–1.5) 1.2 (0.9–1.4) 1.1 (0.9–1.4) 1.2 (0.9–1.5) 1.3 (1.0–1.6) 1.3 (0.8–2.0)	 Pesticide ever Livestock insecticides Crop insecticide Herbicide Fungicide
			Diffuse NHL	2.3 (1.4–3.8) 2.2 (1.3–3.8) 2.2 (1.1–4.5) 1.6 (1.0–2.6)	Organophosphates Non-halogenated aliphatic organophosphates Cyclodiene chlorinated hydrocarbons Triazine herbicides
			Sm. Lympho	2.4 (1.1–5.2) 5.2 (1.9–14.3)	Natural product insecticides Halogenated aromatic organophosphates
Hansen (1992)	Gardeners	Incidence	NHL	2.0 (0.9–3.9)	

(continued)

TABLE 42–7. *Selected Studies* (Continued)*

Reference	Occupation Group	Study Type	Histology	Relative Risk	Possible Exposure and Comments
Ronco et al, (1992)	Farmers	Incidence	NHL	1.0 (0.8–1.2) 1.0 (0.7–1.5) 1.3 (0.6–2.4) 1.3 (0.5–3.0) 0.8 (0.5–1.2) 1.2 (0.3–3.4)	Denmark, self-employed, M Denmark, employees, M Italy, self-employed, M Italy, employees, M Denmark, F Italy, F
Blair et al (1993)	Farmers	Mortality	NHL	1.2 (1.1–1.3) 1.1 (0.6–1.7) 0.7 (0.5–1.1) 1.1 (0.4–2.3)	WM WF Non-white M Non-white F
Franceschi et al (1993)	Farmers	Case–control	NHL	0.8 (0.6–1.1)	
Zahm et al, (1993b)	Farmers	Case–control	NHL	1.1 (0.7–1.4)	F
Zahm et al, (1993a)	Farmers	Case–control	NHL	1.4 (1.1–1.8)	Atrazine (herbicide)
Riihimaki et al, (1982)	Herbicide appliers	Follow-up	NHL	0.0	2,4-dichlorophenoxyacetic acid 2,4,5-trichlorophenoxyactic acid
Woods et al, (1987)	Herbicide appliers	Case–control	NHL	4.80 (1.2–19.4)	
Wiklund et al, (1987)	Pesticide appliers	Follow-up	NHL	1.01 (0.63–1.54)	Phenoxy herbicides
Woods et al, (1987)	Various	Case–control	NHL	1.82 (1.04–3.2)	Organochlorine insecticides
Alavanja et al, (1987)	Grain industry	Mortality	LS, RC Other	1.88 (0.91–3.88) 1.77 (1.02–3.09)	Pesticides
Breslin et al, (1988)	Vietnam veterans	Mortality Follow-up	NHL	0.81 (0.63–1.04) 2.10 (1.17–3.79)	Army, Agent Orange Marines, Agent Orange
Project Ranch Hand (1983)	Vietnam veterans	Mortality Follow-up	NHL	0.0	Herbicide
CHEMICALS—TCDD, PHENOXY ACIDS, CHLOROPHENOLS					
Cook et al, (1980)	Chemical	Follow-up	NHL	0.0 (small number)	TCDD
Zack and Suskind, (1980)	Chemical	Follow-up	NHL	0.0 (small number)	TGDD
Hardell et al, (1981)	Various	Case–control	NHL, HD	4.8 (2.9–8.1) 8.4 (4.2–16.9)	Phenoxy acids Chlorophenols (high level)
Thiess et al, (1982)	Chemical	Follow-up	NHL	0.0 (small number)	TCDD
Lynge (1985)	Chemical	Follow-up	NHL, HD	1.3 (0.52–2.69)	Phenoxy herbicides
Pearce et al, (1986)	Various	Case–control	Other	1.4 (0.7–2.5) 1.3 (0.6–2.7)	Phenoxyherbicides Chlorophenols
Woods et al, (1987)	Various	Case–control	NHL	1.07 (0.8–1.4) 0.99 (0.8–1.2)	Phenoxyherbicides Chlorophenol
Hardell (1979)	Various	Case–control	Histio	6.0	Phenoxyacetic acid Chlorophenols
Bond et al, (1988)	Manufacture	Follow-up	NHL	2.0 (0.84–4.8)	2,4-dichlorophenoxyacetic acid
Perrson et al (1989)	Population	Case–control	NHL	4.9 (1.3–18)	Phenoxyacids
Wigle et al (1990)	Farmers	Mortality Follow-up	NHL	2.2 (1.0–4.6)	Herbicide use, high level: mainly 2,4 dichlorophenoxyacetic acid
Coggan et al (1991)	Manufacture	Mortality Follow-up	NHL	2.7 (0.33–9.8)	Phenoxy herbicides
Fingerhut et al (1991)	Manufacture	Mortality Follow-up	NHL	1.4 (0.66–2.5)	TCDD
Saracci et al (1991)	Manufacture Sprayers	Mortality Follow-up	NHL	1.5 (0.64–2.9) 0.5 (0.10–1.4)	Phenoxy herbicides
Eriksson et al (1992)	Carpenters Forestry	Incidence Incidence	NHL NHL	1.2 (1.0–1.5) 0.8 (0.6–1.0)	Phenoxyacetic acids or dioxins Phenoxyacetic acids or dioxins
Lampi et al (1992)	Community	Incidence	NHL	2.8 (1.4–5.6)	Chlorophenol
Scherr et al (1992)	Various	Case–control	NHL	1.8 (0.9–3.7)	Pesticides/insecticides
Bertazzi et al (1993)	Community	Incidence	LS, RC	5.7 (1.7–19.0)	2,3,7,8-tetrachlorodibenzo-para-dioxin
Bloemem et al (1993)	Manufacture	Mortality	NHL	1.96 (0.2–7.1)	2,4 dichlorophenoxyacetic acid
Hardell et al (1994)	Various	Case–control	NHL	4.8 (2.7–8.8) 5.5 (2.7–11.)	Chlorophenols Phenoxy acids

(continued)

TABLE 42–7. *(Continued)*

Reference	Occupation Group	Study Type	Histology	Relative Risk	Possible Exposure and Comments
CHEMICALS—BENZENE, STYRENE, VINYL CHLORIDE, ETHYLENE OXIDE					
Nicholson et al (1978)	Chemical	Follow-up	NHL, HD	0.8 (0.02–4.46)	Styrene, benzene
Tabershaw and Gaffey (1974)	Chemical	Follow-up	NHL, HD	0.99 (0.36–2.15)	Vinyl chloride
Ott and Kolesar (1980)	Styrene	Mortality Follow-up	NHL, HD	1.32 (0.53–2.72)	Vinyl chloride, asbestos, arsenic
Hardel et al (1981)	Various	Case–control	NHL, HD	4.6 (1.9–11.4)	Styrene, benzene trichloroethylene, perchlor
				2.8 (1.6–4.8)	Other organic solvents
Hodgson and Jones (1985)	Styrene	Mortality Follow-up	NHL	5.4 (1.10–15.7)	Styrene
Vianna and Polan (1979)	Various	Mortality Mortality	RC LS	1.6 (1.29–1.85) 2.0 (1.77–2.23)	Benzene Benzene
Scherr et al (1992)	Various	Case–control	NHL	1.2 (0.5–2.6)	Benzene
Blair et al (1993b)	Various	Case–control	NHL	1.5 (0.7–3.1)	Benzene, high level
Steenland et al (1991)	Workers	Mortality	NHL	1.2 (0.6–2.3)	Ethylene oxide
Bisanti et al (1993)	Workers	Mortality	LS, RC	6.8 (1.8–17.5)	Ethylene oxide
Wong and Trent (1993)	Workers	Mortality	LS, RC	1.1 (0.5–2.1)	Ethylene oxide
Teta et al (1993)	Chemical	Mortality	LS, RC	1.0 (0.1–3.6)	Ethylene oxide
CHEMICALS—CHEMICAL SOLVENTS					
Capurro and Eldridge (1978)	Population nearby	Mortality	RC	73.0 (15.1–214)	Solvents
		Incidence	NHL, HD	11.0 (5.3–20.3)	Solvents
Wilcosky et al (1984)	Rubber	Case–control	LS	4.2 ($P < 0.05$) 3.7 ($P < 0.05$) 5.6 ($P < 0.01$) 4.0 ($P < 0.05$)	Carbon tetrachloride Xylenes Carbon disulfide Hexane
Woods et al (1987)	Various	Case–control	NHL	1.35 (1.06–1.7)	Organic solvents
Scherr et al (1992)	Various	Case–control	NHL	1.2 (0.8–1.8)	Chlorinated
Blair et al (1993b)	Various	Case–control	NHL	1.4 (0.8–2.5)	Non-benzene, high level
Hardell et al (1994)	Various	Case–control	NHL	2.4 (1.4–3.9)	Organic solvents
RUBBER MANUFACTURE AND PROCESSING					
Monson and Fine (1978)	Chemical	Follow-up	NHL	2.5 (1.08–4.93)	Tire-building
Delzell and Monson (1984)	Rubber	Mortality Mortality	RC, LS NHL	1.0 (0.5–1.9) 2.4 (1.12–4.28)	 (1970–78 deaths)
Meinhardt et al (1982)	Rubber	Mortality Follow-up	RC, LS	1.81 (0.37–5.28) (small number)	Styrene, butadiene
McMichael et al (1976)	Rubber	Mortality Follow-up	NHL, HD	1.29	
Hagmar et al (1993)	Polyurethane	Incidence	NHL	1.5 (0.4–3.9)	
OIL					
Divine et al (1985)	Oil	Mortality Follow-up	LS	0.9 (0.55–1.39)	
Wong et al (1986)	Oil	Mortality	LS, RC	1.27 (0.74–2.03)	
Kaplan (1986)	Oil	Mortality Follow-up	LS, RC	0.90 (0.51–1.46)	
			Other	1.12 (0.43–1.64)	
Marsh et al (1991)	Oil	Mortality	LS, RC	1.9 (0.8–3.7)	
Dagg et al (1992)	Oil	Mortality	LS, RC	1.1 (0.6–1.7)	
LOGGING, PULP, AND PAPER					
Gallagher et al (1985)	Woodworkers	Mortality	NHL	1.39 (1.02–1.88)	Chlorophenols
Gallagher et al (1985)	Loggers	Mortality	NHL	0.89 (0.53–1.40)	

(continued)

TABLE 42–7. *Selected Studies* (Continued)*

Reference	*Occupation Group*	*Study Type*	*Histology*	*Relative Risk*	*Possible Exposure and Comments*
Wiklund (1988)	Loggers	Follow-up	NHL	0.87 (0.72–1.05)	
Milham (1976b)	Wood and Pulp	Mortality	LS	1.82 (0.89–3.41)	Paper and pulp
Milham and Demers (1984)	Pulp and paper	Mortality	RC, LS	1.64 (0.82–2.94)	
Partanen et al (1993)	Wood industry	Case–control	NHL	4.2 (0.7–26.6) 2.1 (0.2–19.7)	Formaldehyde Wood dust
MEAT INDUSTRY					
Pearce et al (1987)	Meat work	Interview	NHL	1.8 (1.2–2.6)	Chlorophenol, zoonotic virus
Pearce et al (1986)	Meat work	Case–control	Other	1.8 (1.3–3.1)	2,4,6-trichlorophenol
Pearce et al (1988)	Meat industry	Case–control	LS, RC Other	1.8 (1.1–2.9 [90%]) 1.7 (1.0–2.8 [90%])	Viruses, trichlorophenol
Johnson et al (1986)	Meat industry	Mortality Follow-up	LS	0.61 (0.20–1.42)	Viruses, nitrosamines butylated hydroxyanisole (BHA), butylated hydroxy toluene (BHT), heated plastic films
METAL INDUSTRY					
Milham (1976a)	Aluminum	Mortality	NHL	2.5 (1.20–4.60)	Coal tar pitch
Milham (1976c)	Plumbers	Mortality	NHL	1.46 (0.92–2.22)	
Milham (1979)	Aluminum	Mortality Follow-up	RC, LS	3.16 (1.28–6.56)	
Gallagher and Threlfall (1983)	Metal workers	Mortality	NHL	0.82 (0.59–1.12)	
Dolan et al (1983)	Plumbers	Incidence	SCFCC (Lukes Collins)	4.62 (1.69–10.05)	
LABORATORY WORKERS					
Li et al (1969)	Chemists	Mortality Follow-up	NHL, HD, MM, MF	1.79 (1.37–2.30)	
Harrington and Shannon (1975)	Pathologists	Mortality Follow-up	NHL, MM, PV	3.53 (1.30–7.68)	
	Lab. technicians			1.18 (0.14–4.25)	
Hoar and Pell (1981)	Chemists	Incidence Follow-up	LS, RC	1.42 (0.36–3.85)	
			Other	0.67 (0.03–3.32)	
		Mortality Follow-up	LS, RC	0.85 (0.04–4.11)	
Stroup et al (1986)	Anatomists	Mortality Follow-up	LS, RC	0.7 (0.1–2.5)	Formaldehyde, solvents
OTHER OCCUPATIONS					
Blair et al (1986)	Various	Mortality Follow-up	LS, RC	0.52 (0.21–1.06)	Formaldehyde
Rinsky et al (1988)	Chemicals	Mortality Follow-up	LS, RC	1.40 (1.04–1.87)	
Okun et al (1985)	Boat-building	Mortality	NHL	0.0	
Rinsky et al (1981)	Shipyard	Mortality Follow-up	RC, LS	0.44 (0.09–1.29)	Radiation
Graham et al (1977)	Asbestos mining country	Incidence	RC, LS Other	1.15 (0.46–2.37) 0.65 (0.08–2.35)	Males only Males only
Robinson (1982)	Asbestos products	Mortality Follow-up	NHL	2.13 (0.82–4.05)	Chrysotile asbestos
Delzell and Grufferman (1983)	Textile	Mortality	NHL	1.7 (1.2–2.3)	
Dubrow et al (1988)	Textile	Mortality	NHL	0.92 (0.65–1.29)	

(continued)

TABLE 42–7. (*Continued*)

Reference	*Occupation Group*	*Study Type*	*Histology*	*Relative Risk*	*Possible Exposure and Comments*
Siemiatycki et al (1986)	Various	Incidence Case–Control	NHL	0.5 (0.2–0.9)	Wood dust
				0.7 (0.2–1.8)	Paper dust
				0.5 (0.1–1.7)	Grain dust
				0.3 (0.0–1.3)	Flour dust
				0.9 (0.4–1.9)	Fabric dust
				1.6 (0.9–2.8)	Cotton dust
				1.0 (0.4–2.6)	Wool dust
				0.7 (0.2–2.2)	Synthetic fiber dust
				1.3 (0.4–4.8)	Fur dust
Zoloth et al (1986)	Pressman	Mortality	NHL	2.09 (1.31–4.69)	Solvents, dyes
Wong (1987)	Various	Mortality Follow-up	LS, RS	0.91 (0.29–2.11)	
Pearce et al (1986)	Fencing work	Case–control	Other	2.0 (1.3–3.0)	Arsenic, sodium pentachlorophenate
Wegman and Eisen (1981)	Synthetic abrasive	Mortality	RC, LS	0.77 (0.16–2.25)	
Teta et al (1984)	Cosmetologists	Incidence Follow-up	NHL, HD	1.29 (0.81–1.95)	
Cantor et al (1988)	Population	Incidence Case–control	NHL	2.0 (1.3–3.0)	Hair dye
Ross et al (1982)	Various	Incidence Case–control	Large-cell (GI or oral)	12.0 (1.37–3 × 10⁶)	
Alavanja et al (1990)	Flour	Mortality	NHL	4.2 (1.2–14.2)	
Hayes et al (1990)	Embalmers Funeral directors	Mortality	NHL	1.3 (0.9–1.8)	
Linos et al (1990)	Embalmers Funeral directors	Case–control	NHL	3.2 (0.8–13.4)	
Sama et al (1990)	Firefighters	Case–control	NHL	3.2 (1.2–9.0)	Policemen referent
				1.6 (0.9–2.8)	Population referent
Linos et al (1991)	Community	Case–control	NHL	1.5 (1.1–1.9)	Living within one-half mile of an industrial plant
Benson and Teta (1993)	Manufacture	Mortality	NHL	3.0 (0.9–7.2)	Chlorohydrin
Walker et al (1993)	Shoe	Mortality	NHL	0.7 (0.2–1.8)	

*Abbreviations: F = female; GI = gastrointestinal; HD = Hodgkin's disease; Histio = histiocytic lymphoma; LS = lymphosarcoma; M = male; MF = mycosis fungoides; MM = multiple myeloma; NHL = non-Hodgkin's lymphomas; Other = other lymphomas, usually ICD 202; PV = Polycythemia Vera; RC = Reticulum cell sarcoma; SCFF = Small cleaved follicular centered cell; TCDD = 2,3,7,8-tetrachlorodibenzo-p-dioxin; W = white. 95% confidence intervals calculated from observed and expected cases (Rothman and Boice, 1979).

which suggests that this may be a fruitful area for further investigation.

A fairly large number of studies have been conducted in three industries. For the manufacture of plastics from styrene and from vinyl chloride, most studies did not find an increased risk of NHL. In the styrene-butadiene rubber industry, elevated risks of NHL are observed more consistently, however, the risks did not appear to be elevated significantly among petroleum refiners. Other industries with reported increased risks of NHL are woodworkers, meat workers, and metal workers.

ANIMAL EXPOSURES

One mechanism by which animal exposures could increase the risk of lymphoma in humans is by exposure to viruses that cause lymphoma in animals such as feline leukemia virus (FeLV) and bovine leukemia virus (Donham et al, 1977). In the United States, 400,000 to 800,000 cat owners and 100,000 veterinarians are exposed to cats that continuously shed FeLV (Gutensohn et al, 1980). However, a small study of members of 221 households containing cats with malignant lymphoma presumably caused by FeLV did not demonstrate an increased risk of NHL relative to members in control households containing cats without malignant lymphoma (Schneider, 1972).

Studies of the mortality experience of veterinarians have been used to evaluate the effect of animal exposures. A study of the causes of death among white male veterinarians who died in the United States between 1966 and 1977 found a proportional mortality ratio for NHL of 162 for all veterinarians and 195 for practicing veterinarians (Blair and Hayes, 1980). These findings, however, did not reach statistical significance. Mortality studies of veterinarians in California (Fasal et al, 1966) and Missouri (Botts et al, 1966) also were consistent with no excess mortality from NHL. Other groups that have been studied include approximately 50,000 children who were bitten by dogs and followed for 5 or more years to assess their mortality experience (Norris et al, 1971). There was no evidence that mortality due to NHL was elevated among these children. Also, the causes of death of 580 beekeepers were investigated (McDonald et al, 1979). These workers receive antigenic challenges from 10 to 100 bee stings per week for years and develop high levels of antibodies to the venom. The findings of 4 deaths from NHL relative to 2 deaths expected were not statistically significant. In conclusion, there is no evidence of an increased risk of NHL due to animal exposures at this time.

OTHER EXPOSURES

Little is known concerning the role of diet in the etiology of NHL (Davis, 1992). In 1976 Cunningham reported a ecologic correlation between per capita consumption of bovine protein and the occurrence of lymphoma. In a hospital-based case–control study of NHL conducted in northeastern Italy, Franceschi et al (1989a) reported on dietary habits of 208 cases and 401 controls. They reported a RR of 2.2 associated with a high level of consumption of milk, and a protective effect of a high level of consumption of whole-grain bread or pasta, or RR = 0.44. In a prospective cohort study of 15,914 Norwegians followed for more than 11 years, a RR of 3.4 associated with drinking more than one daily glass of milk was reported for the incidence of lymphoma based on 36 observed cases. However, this risk varied considerably with a variety of demographic features (Ursin et al, 1990). A study of vegetable and fruit consumption (Negri et al, 1991) found an increased risk of NHL (RR 1.5, 95% CI 1.0, 2.2) in the highest tertile of green vegetable consumption and a non-significant decreased risk with fruit consumption.

Recently there have been several reports of an association between the use of hair dyes and risk of NHL. Cantor et al (1988) conducted a population-based case–control study of men in Iowa and non-metropolitan Minnesota involving 622 cases and 1,245 controls. They found a RR of 2.0 for ever-use. In a similar study conducted in Nebraska, Zahm et al (1992) found an association of 1.5 among women (184 cases, 707 controls) which was higher for use of permanent hair coloring and for darker colors. However, there was no association among the men (201 cases, 725 controls). A study of hairdressers in Denmark, Sweden, Norway, and Finland (Boffetta et al, 1994) found an overall standardized incidence ratio of 1.2 (95% CI 0.84, 1.16) for NHL with an excess risk (1.92) in Denmark and a decreased risk (0.63) in Sweden. The American Cancer Society study (Thun et al, 1994) and the Nurses Health Study (Grodstein et al, 1994) did not find an increased risk with the use of permanent hair dyes.

Several studies have investigated the relationship between smoking and NHL. A hospital-based study of 208 cases of NHL and 401 controls (Franceschi et al, 1989b) found a non-significant increased risk for those with a history of smoking versus those who never smoked (RR = 1.5, 95% CI = 1.0, 2.3). A population-based case–control study by Brown et al (1992) in Iowa and Minnesota found an increased risk for all lymphoma (OR = 1.4, 95% CI = 1.1–1.8), high-grade lymphoma (OR = 2.3, CI = 1.0–5.1) and unclassified lymphoma (OR = 2.7, CI = 1.3, 5.6). A significant dose–response relationship was not observed. In another study (Linet et al, 1992), the history of tobacco use was obtained for 17,633 U.S. white males in 1966. In the following 20 years, there were 49 deaths due to NHL. People who had ever smoked had an increased risk of 2.1 (CI = 0.9–4.9) of dying from NHL relative to never-smokers. The relative risk was 3.8 (CI = 1.4–10.1) for the heaviest smokers.

CONCLUSIONS

One recurring theme for factors that increase the risk of NHL is the chronic antigenic stimulation of the immune system which may then compromise the control of latent oncogenic infections. Individuals at increased risk of the NHL include those with primary immunodeficiency diseases, acquired immunodeficiency diseases, and patients who are immunosuppressed subsequent to transplantation. An increased risk of NHL has been noted among AIDS patients where incidence rates of NHL approaching 50% have been reported among patients with who survived 3 months of anti-retroviral treatment with azidothymidine (Pluda et al, 1990).

Another group who appears to be at increased risk are individuals with occupational exposures to chemicals. There is mounting evidence implicating phenoxy herbicide exposures, although the evidence is still not conclusive.

Thus the etiology of most of the cases of NHL remains unknown. The proportion of cases attributable to established or suspected causes is very small (Hartge and Devesa, 1992). Although cases occurring in AIDS patients will contribute to increasing rates of NHL in the future, the secular increase in NHL rates was noted well before the AIDS epidemic. The factors leading to the earlier increase in disease rates have yet to be identified.

REFERENCES

ANONYMOUS. 1984. Lymphoma in organ transplant recipients. Lancet i:601–603.

ANONYMOUS. 1990. The association of selected cancers with service in the US military in Vietnam. I. Non-Hodgkin's lymphoma. The Selected Cancers Cooperative Study Group: Arch Intern Med 150:2473–2483.

ALAVANJA MC, BLAIR A, MASTERS MN. 1990. Cancer mortality in the U.S. flour industry. J Natl Cancer Inst 82:840–848.

ALAVANJA MC, RUSH GA, STEWART P, et al. 1987. Proportionate mortality study of workers in the grain industry. J Natl Cancer Inst 78:247–252.

ANTHONY JJ. 1970. Malignant lymphoma associated with hydantoin drugs. Arch Neurol 22:450–454.

ARCHER VE, WAGONER JK, LUNDIN FE. 1973. Cancer mortality among uranium mill workers. J Occup Med 15:11–14.

BAHLER DW, ZELENETZ AD, CHEN TT, LEVY R. 1992. Antigen selection in human lymphomagenesis. Cancer Res (Suppl.) 52:5547s–5551s.

BENNETT MH, FARRER-BROWN G, HENRY K, et al. 1974. Classification of non-Hodgkin's lymphomas. Lancet 2:405–406.

BENSON LO, TETA MJ. 1993. Mortality due to pancreatic and lymphopoietic cancers in chlorohydrin production workers. Br J Ind Med 50:710–716.

BERAL V, INSKIP H, FRASER P, et al. 1985. Mortality of employees of the United Kingdom Atomic Energy Authority, 1946–1979. BMJ 291:440–447.

BERAL V, PETERMAN T, BERKELMAN R, et al. 1991. AIDS-associated non-Hodgkin lymphoma. Lancet 337:805–809.

BERNARD SM, CARTWRIGHT RA, BIRD CC. 1984. Aetiologic factors in lymphoid malignancies: a case-control epidemiological study. Leuk Res 8:681–689.

BERTAZZI PA, PESATORI AC, CONSONNI D, et al. 1993. Cancer incidence in a population accidentally exposed to 2,3,7,8-tetrachlorodibenzo-para-dioxin. Epidemiology 4:398–406.

BIGGAR RJ, RABKIN CS. 1992. The epidemiology of acquired immunodeficiency syndrome-related lymphomas. Curr Opin Oncol 4:883–892.

BILROTH T. 1871. Multiple Lymphome. Erfolgreiche Behandlung mit Arsenik. Wien Med Wochenschr 21:1066–1067.

BISANTI L, MAGGINI M, RASCHETTI R, et al. 1993. Cancer mortality in ethylene oxide workers. Br J Ind Med 50:317–324.

BLAIR A, DOSEMECI M, HEINEMAN EF. 1993a. Cancer and other causes of death among male and female farmers from twenty-three states. Am J Ind Med 23:729–742.

BLAIR A, HAYES HM. 1980. Cancer and other causes of death among U.S. veterans, 1966–1977. Int J Cancer 25:181–185.

BLAIR A, LINOS A, STEWART P. 1993b. Evaluation of risks for non-Hodgkin's lymphoma by occupation and industry exposures from a case-control study. Am J Ind Med 23:301–312.

BLAIR A, STEWART P, OBERG M, et al. 1986. Mortality among industrial workers exposed to formaldehyde. J Natl Cancer Inst 76:1071–1084.

BLAIR A, WALRATH J, ROGOT E. 1985. Mortality patterns among U.S. veterans by occupation. 1. Cancer. J Natl Cancer Inst 75:1039–1047.

BLOEMEN LJ, MANDEL JS, BOND GG, et al. 1993. An update of mortality among chemical workers potentially exposed to the herbicide 2,4-dichlorophenoxyacetic acid and its derivatives. J Occup Med 35:1208–1212.

BLOMBERG J, MOLLER T, OLSSON H, et al. 1993. Cancer morbidity in blood recipients—results of a cohort study. Eur J Cancer 29A:2101–2105.

BOFFETTA P, ANDERSEN A, LYNGE E, et al. 1994. Employment as hairdresser and risk of ovarian cancer and non-Hodgkin's lymphoma among women. J Occup Med 36:61–65.

BOICE JD JR, MORIN MM, GLASS AG, et al. 1991. Diagnostic x-ray procedures and risk of leukemia, lymphoma, and multiple myeloma. JAMA 265:1290–1294.

BOND GG, WETTERSTROEM NH, ROUSH GJ, MCLAREN EA, LIPPS TE, COOK RR. 1988. Cause specific mortality among employees engaged in the manufacture, formulation, or packaging of 2,4-dichlorophenoxyacetic acid and related salts. Br J Ind Med 45:98–105.

BORISCH-CHAPPUIS B, MÜLLER H, STUTTE J, et al. 1990. Identification of EBV-DNA in lymph nodes from patients with lymphadenopathy and lymphomas associated with AIDS. Virchows Arch B Cell Pathol Incl Mol Pathol 58:199–205.

BOTTS RP, EDLAVITCH S, PAYNE G. 1966. Mortality of Missouri veterinarians. J Am Vet Med Assoc 149:499–504.

BRESLIN P, KANG HK, LEE Y, et al. 1988. Proportionate mortality study of US Army and US Marine Corps veterans of the Vietnam War. J Occup Med 30:412–419.

BROWN LM, EVERETT GD, GIBSON R, et al. 1992. Smoking and risk of non-Hodgkin's lymphoma and multiple myeloma. Cancer Causes Control 3:49–55.

BROWNSON RC, REIF JS. 1988. A cancer registry-based study of occupational risk for lymphoma, multiple myeloma and leukaemia. Int J Epidemiol 17:27–32.

BURMEISTER LF. 1981. Cancer mortality in Iowa Farmers. J Natl Cancer Inst 66:461–464.

BURMEISTER LF, EVERETT GD, VAN LIER SF, et al. 1983. Selected cancer mortality and farm practices in Iowa. Am J Epidemiol 118:72–77.

CANTOR KP. 1982. Farming and mortality from non-Hodgkin's lymphoma: a case-control study. Int J Cancer 29:239–247.

CANTOR KP, BLAIR A, EVERETT G, et al. 1988. Hair dye use and risk of leukemia and lymphoma. Am J Public Health 78:570–571.

CANTOR KP, BLAIR A, EVERETT G, et al. 1992. Pesticides and other agricultural risk factors for non-Hodgkin's lymphoma among men in Iowa and Minnesota. Cancer Res 52:2447–2455.

CANTOR KP, FRAUMENI JF. 1980. Distribution of non-Hodgkin's lymphoma in the United States between 1950 and 1975. Cancer Res 40:2645–2652.

CAPURRO PU, ELDRIDGE JE. 1978. Solvent exposure and cancer. Lancet 1:942.

CERHAN JR, WALLACE RB, FOLSOM AR, et al. 1993. Transfusion history and cancer risk in older women. Ann Intern Med 119:8–15.

CHECKOWAY H, MATHEW RM, SHY CM, et al. 1985. Radiation, work experience, and cause specific mortality among workers at an energy research laboratory. Br J Ind Med 42:525–533.

CLAPP RW, COUPLES LA, COLTON T, et al. 1991. Cancer surveillance of Veterans in Massachusetts, USA, 1982–1988. Int J Epidemiol 20:7–12.

CLEARY ML, WARNKE R, SKLAR J. 1984. Monoclonality of lymphoproliferative lesions in cardiac-transplant recipients: Clonal analysis based on immunoglobulin-gene rearrangements. N Engl J Med 310:477–482.

CLEMMESEN J. 1974. Are anticonvulsants oncogenic? Lancet 1:705–707.

COGGON D, OSMOND C, PANNETT B, et al. 1987. Mortality of workers exposed to styrene in the manufacture of glass-reinforced plastics. Scand J Work Environ Health 13:94–99.

COGGON D, PANNETT B, WINTER P. 1991. Mortality and incidence of cancer at four factories making phenoxy herbicides. Br J Ind Med 48:173–178.

COLEMAN M, BERAL V. 1988. A review of epidemiological studies of the health effects of living near or working with electricity generation and transmission equipment. Int J Epidemiol 17:1–13.

COMSTOCK GW, MARTINEZ I, LIVESAY VT. 1975. Efficacy of BCG vaccination in prevention of cancer. J Natl Cancer Inst 54:835–839.

COOK RR, TOWNSEND JC, OTT MG, et al. 1980. Mortality experience of employees exposed to 2,3,7,8-tetrachlorodibenzo-p-dioxin (TCDD). J Occup Med 22:530–532.

COURT-BROWN WM, DOLL R. 1965. Mortality from cancer and other causes after radiotherapy for ankylosing spondylitis. BMJ 2:1327–1332.

CUNNINGHAM AS. 1976. Lymphomas and animal-protein consumption. Lancet 2(7996):1184–1186.

DAGG TG, SATIN KP, BAILEY WJ, et al. 1992. An updated cause specific mortality study of petroleum refinery workers. Br J Ind Med 49:203–212.

DALAGER NA, KANG HK, BURT VL, et al. 1991. Non-Hodgkin's lymphoma among Vietnam veterans. J Occup Med 33:774–779.

DAVIS S. 1992. Nutritional factors and the development of non-Hodgkin's lymphoma: A review of the evidence. Cancer Res (Suppl.) 52:5492s–5495s.

DELZELL E, GRUFFERMAN S. 1983. Cancer and other causes of death among female textile workers, 1976–78. J Natl Cancer Inst 71:735–740.

DELZELL E, MONSON RR. 1984. Mortality among rubber workers: VII. Industrial products workers. Am J Ind Med 6:273–279.

DEVESA SS, FEARS T. 1992. Non-Hodgkin's lymphoma time trends: United States and international data. Cancer Res (Suppl.) 52:5432s–5440s.

DEVESA SS, SILVERMAN DT, YOUNG JL, et al. 1987. Cancer incidence and mortality trends among whites in the United States, 1947–84. J Natl Cancer Inst 79:701–770.

DIVINE BJ, BARRON V, KAPLAN SD. 1985. Texaco mortality study. I. Mortality among refinery, petrochemical, and research workers. J Occup Med 27:445–447.

DOLAN BP, LEVINE AM, DOLAN DC. 1983. Small cleaved follicular center cell lymphoma: seven cases in California plumbers. J Occup Med 25:613–615.

DONHAM KJ, VAN DER MAATEN MJ, MILLER JM, et al. 1977. Seroepidemiologic studies on the possible relationships of human and bovine leukemia: brief communication. J Natl Cancer Inst 59:851–853.

DORFMAN RF. 1974. Classification of non-Hodgkin's lymphomas. Lancet 1:1295–1296.

DORFMAN RF. 1975. The non-Hodgkin's lymphomas. *In* The Reticuloendothelial System. International Academy of Pathology Monograph No 16. Baltimore, Williams and Wilkins.

DUBROW R, PAULSON JO, INDIAN RW. 1988. Farming and malignant lymphoma in Hancock County, Ohio. Br J Ind Med 45:25–28.

ENTERLINE PE. 1979. Lymphoma and benzene. Lancet ii:1021.

ERIKSSON M, HARDELL L, MALKER H, et al. 1992. Malignant lymphoproliferative diseases in occupations with potential exposure to phenoxyacetic acids or dioxins: a register-based study. Am J Ind Med 22:305–312.

EVANS AS, MUELLER N. 1995. Malignant lymphomas. *In* Evans AS, Kaslow R (eds): Viral Infections of Humans: Epidemiology and Control, fourth ed. New York, Plenum Medical Book, (in press).

FASAL E, JACKSON EW, KLAUBER MR. 1966. Mortality in California veterinarians. J Chron Dis 19:293–306.

FASAL E, JACKSON EW, KLAUBER MR. 1968. Leukemia and lymphoma mortality and farm residence. Am J Epidemiol 87:267–274.

FILIPOVICH AH, MATHUR A, KAMAT D, et al. 1992. Primary immunodeficiencies: Genetic risk for lymphoma. Cancer Res (Suppl.) 52:5465s–5467s.

FILIPOVICH AH, ZERBE D, SPECTOR BD, et al. 1984. Lymphomas in persons with naturally occurring immunodeficiency disorders. *In* Magrath IT, O'Connor GT, Ramot B (eds): Pathogenesis of Leukemias and Lymphomas: Environmental Influences. New York, Raven Press, pp. 225–234.

FINGERHUT MA, HALPERIN WE, MARLOW DA, PIACITELLI LA, HONCHAR PA, SWEENEY MH, GREIFE AL, DILL PA, STEENLAND K, SURUDA AJ. 1991. Cancer mortality in workers exposed to 2,3,7,8-tetrachlorodibenzo-p-dioxin. N Engl J Med 324:121–128.

FORMAN D, COOK-MOZAFFARI P, DARBY S, et al. 1987. Cancer near nuclear installations. Nature 329:499–505.

FRANCESCHI S, BARBONE F, BIDOLI E, et al. 1993. Cancer risk in farmers: results from a multi-site case–control study in north-eastern Italy. Int J Cancer 53:740–745.

FRANCESCHI S, SERRAINO D, ANTONINO C, TALAMINI R, LA VECCHIA C. 1989a. Dietary factors and non-Hodgkin's lymphoma: A case–control study in the northeastern part of Italy. Nutr Cancer 12:333–341.

FRANCESCHI A, SERRAINO D, BIDOLI E, et al. 1989b. The epidemiology of non-Hodgkin's lymphoma in the north-east of Italy: a hospital-based case-control study. Leuk Res 13:465–472.

FRIZZERA G, ROSAI J, DEHNER LP, et al. 1980. Lymphoreticular disorders in primary immunodeficiencies: New findings based on an up-to-date histologic classification of 35 cases. Cancer 46:692–699.

GALLAGHER RP, THRELFALL WJ. 1983. Cancer mortality in metal workers. Can Med Assoc J 129:1191–1194.

GALLAGHER RP, THRELFALL WJ, BAND PR, et al. 1985. Cancer mortality experience of woodworkers, loggers, fishermen, farmers, and miners in British Columbia. Natl Cancer Inst Monogr 69:163–167.

GERARD-MARCHANT, HAMLIN R, LENNERT K, et al. 1974. Classification of non-Hodgkin's lymphomas. Lancet 2:406–408.

GILES GG, LICKLISS, BAIKIE JN. 1984. Myeloproliferative and lymphoproliferative disorders in Tasmania, 1972–1980: occupational and familial aspects. J Natl Cancer Inst 72:1233–1240.

GOLDSMITH JR, GUIDOTTI TL. 1975. Environmental factors in the epidemiology of lymphosarcoma. Pathol Annu 12:411–425.

GRAHAM S, BLANCHET M, ROHRER T. 1977. Cancer in asbestos-mining and other areas of Quebec. J Natl Cancer Inst 59:1139–1145.

GREENE MH. 1982. Non-Hodgkin's lymphoma and mycosis fungoides. *In* Scottenfeld D, Fraumeni JF Jr, (eds): Cancer Epidemiology and Prevention. Philadelphia, WB Saunders Co., pp. 754–778.

GRIDLEY G, KLIPPEL JH, HOOVER RN, et al. 1994. Incidence of cancer among men with Felty Syndrome. Ann Intern Med 120:35–39.

GRODSTEIN F, HENNEKENS CH, COLDITZ GA, et al. 1994. A prospective study of permanent hair dye use and hematopoietic cancer. J Natl Cancer Inst 86:1466–1470.

GURALNICK L. 1963. Mortality by occupation (or industry) and cause of death among men 20–64 years of age: United States, 1950. Vital Statistics Special Report 53:95–433.

GUTENSOHN (MUELLER) N, ESSEX M, TODARO GJ, ZUR HAUSEN H. 1980. Risk to humans from exposure to feline leukemia virus: epidemiological considerations. *In* Viruses in Naturally Occurring Cancers, Cold Spring Harbor Conferences on Cell Proliferation, Vol 7. Cold Spring Harbor Laboratory, pp. 699–706.

HAGMAR L, WELINDER H, MIKOCZY Z. 1993. Cancer incidence and mortality in the Swedish polyurethane foam manufacturing industry. Br J Ind Med 50:437–443.

HAIM N, COHEN Y, ROBINSON E. 1982. Malignant lymphoma in first-degree blood relatives. Cancer 49:2197–2200.

HALL NEL, ROSENMAN KD. 1991. Cancer by industry: analysis of a population-based cancer registry with an emphasis on blue-collar workers. Am J Ind Med 19:145–159.

HAMILTON-DUTOIT SJ, PALLESEN G, FRANZMANN MB, et al. 1991. AIDS-related lymphoma: Histopathology, immunophenotype, and association with Epstein-Barr virus as demonstrated by in situ nucleic acid hybridization. Am J Pathol 138:149–163.

HAMILTON-DUTOIT SJ, RAPHAEL M, AUDOUIN J, et al. 1993. In situ demonstration of Epstein-Barr virus small RNAs (EBER1) in acquired immunodeficiency syndrome-related lymphomas: Correlation with tumor morphology and primary site. Blood 82:619–624.

HANSEN ES, HASLE H, FLEMMING L. 1992. A cohort study on cancer incidence among Danish gardeners. Am J Ind Med 21:651–660.

HANTO DW, SAKAMOTO K, PURTILO DT, et al. 1981. The Epstein-Barr virus in the pathogenesis of post-transplant lymphoproliferative disorders: Clinical, pathologic, and virologic correlation. Surgery 90:204–213.

HARDELL L. 1979. Malignant lymphoma of histiocytic type and exposure to phenoxyacetic acids or chlorophenols. Lancet 1:55–56.

HARDELL L, ERIKSSON M, DEGERMAN A. 1994. Exposure to phenoxyacetic acids, chlorophenols, or organic solvents in relation to histopathology, stage, and anatomical localization of non-Hodgkin's lymphoma. Cancer Res 54:2386–2389.

HARDELL L, ERIKSSON, LENNER P, et al. 1981. Malignant lymphoma and exposure to chemicals especially organic solvents, chlorophenols and phenoxy acids: a case–control study. Br J Cancer 43:169–176.

HARRINGTON WJ, MCALISTER WH, SALTZSTEIN SL, et al. 1962. A clinicopathologic conference on lymphoma or drug reaction occurring during hydantoin therapy for epilepsy. Am J Med 32:286–297.

HARRINGTON JM, SHANNON HS. 1975. Mortality study of pathologists and medical laboratory technicians. Br Med J 4:329–332.

HARTGE P, DEVESA SS. 1992. Quantification of the impact of known risk factors on time trends in non-Hodgkin's lymphoma incidence. Cancer Res (Suppl.) 52:5566s–5569s.

HAYES HM, TARONE RE, CANTOR KP, JESSEN CR, MCCURNIN DM, RICHARDSON RC. 1991. Case-control study of canine malignant lymphoma: Positive association with dog owner's use of 2,4-dichlorophenoxyacetic acid herbicides. J Natl Cancer Inst 83:1226–1231.

HAYES RB, BLAIR A, STEWART PA, et al. 1990. Mortality of U.S. embalmers and funeral directors. Am J Ind Med 18:641–652.

HENRY K, BENNETT MH, FARRER-BROWN G. 1978. Morphologic classification of non-Hodgkin's lymphomas. *In* Seligmann M, Tubiana M (eds): Recent Results in Cancer Research. New York, Springer-Verlag.

HENRY-AMAR M. 1983. Second cancers after radiotherapy and chemotherapy for early stages of Hodgkin's disease. J Natl Cancer Inst 71:911–916.

HENRY-AMAR M. 1992. Second cancer after the treatment for Hodgkin's disease: a report from the International Database on Hodgkin's Disease. Ann Oncol 3 (Suppl) 4:117–128.

HERBST H, NIEDOBITEK G, KNEBA M, et al. 1990. High incidence of Epstein-Barr virus genomes in Hodgkin's disease. Am J Pathol 137:13–18.

HERBST H, STEIN H, NIEDOBITEK G. 1993. Epstein-Barr virus and CD30+ malignant lymphomas. Crit Rev Oncog 4:191–239.

HO M, MILLER G, ATCHISON RW, et al. 1985. Epstein-Barr virus infection and DNA hybridization studies in post-transplantation lymphoma and lymphoproliferative lesions: The role of primary infection. J Infect Dis 152:876–886.

HOAR SK, BLAIR A, HOLMES FF, et al. 1986. Agricultural herbicide use and risk of lymphoma and soft-tissue sarcoma. JAMA 256:1141–1147.

HOAR SK, PELL S. 1981. A retrospective cohort study of mortality and cancer incidence among chemists. J Occup Med 23:485–494.

HODGSON JT, JONES RD. 1985. Mortality of styrene production, polymerization and processing workers at a site in northwest England. Scand J Work Environ Health 11:347–352.

HOLMES GKT, STOKES PL, SORAHAN TM, et al. 1976. Coeliac disease, gluten-free diet, and malignancy. Gut 17:612–619.

HOOVER R, FRAUMENI JF JR. 1973. Risk of cancer in renal-transplant recipients. Lancet 2:55–57.

HOOVER R, MASON TJ, MCKAY FW, et al. 1975. Geographic patterns of cancer mortality in the U.S. *In* Fraumeni JF Jr (ed): Persons at High Risk of Cancer. New York, Academic Press, pp. 343–360.

HOOVER RN. 1992. Lymphoma risks in populations with altered immunity: A search for mechanism. Cancer Res (Suppl.) 52:5477s–5478s.

JAFFE ES, RAFFELD M, MADEIROS LJ, STETLER-STEVENSON M. 1992. An overview of the classification of non-Hodgkin's lymphomas: An integration of morphological and phenotypical concepts. Cancer Res (Suppl.) 52:5447s–5452s.

JOHNSON CJ. 1984. Cancer incidence in an area of radioactive fallout downwind from the Nevada test site. JAMA 251:230–236.

JOHNSON ES, FISCHMAN HR, MATANOSKI GM, et al. 1986. Cancer mortality among white males in the meat industry. J Occup Med 28:23–32.

KALDOR JM, DAY NE, BAND P, et al. 1987. Second malignancies following testicular cancer, ovarian cancer and Hodgkin's disease: an international collaborative study among cancer registries. Int J Cancer 39:571–585.

KAPLAN SD. 1986. Update of a mortality study of workers in petroleum refineries. J Occup Med 28:514–516.

KASSAN SS, THOMAS TL, MOUTSOPOULOS HM, et al. 1978. Increased risk of lymphoma in Sicca Syndrome. Ann Intern Med 89:888–892.

KENDRICK MA, COMSTOCK GW. 1981. BCG vaccination and the subsequent development of cancer in humans. J Natl Cancer Inst 66:431–437.

KINLEN L. 1992. Immunosuppressive therapy and acquired immunological disorders. Cancer Res (Suppl.) 52:5474s–5476s.

KINLEN LJ, EASTWOOD JB, KERR DNS, et al. 1980. Cancer in patients receiving dialysis. BMJ 1:1401–1403.

KINLEN LJ, SHEIL AGR, PETO J, et al. 1979. Collaborative United Kingdom-Australasian study of cancer in patients treated with immunosuppressive drugs. BMJ 2:1461–1466.

KRIKORIAN JG, BURKE JS, ROSENBERG SA, et al. 1979. Occurrence of non-Hodgkin's lymphoma after therapy for Hodgkin's disease. N Engl J Med 300:452–458.

LA VECCHIA C, NEGRI E, D'AVANZO B, FRANCESCHI S. 1989. Occupation and lymphoid neoplasms. Br J Cancer 60:385–388.

LA VECCHIA C, NEGRI E, FRANCESCHI S. 1992. Education and cancer risk. Cancer 70:2935–2941.

LAMPI P, HAKULINEN T, LUOSTARINEN T, et al. 1992. Cancer incidence following chlorophenol exposure in a community in southern Finland. Arch Environ Health 47:167–75.

LENNERT K, STEIN H, KAISERLING E. 1975. Cytological and functional criteria for the classification of malignant lymphomata. Br J Cancer 31(Suppl. II):29–43.

LEONARD JN, TUCKER WFG, FRY JS, et al. 1983. Increased incidence of malignancy in dermatitis herpetiformis. BMJ 1:16–18.

LEVINE AM. 1993. AIDS-related malignancies: The emerging epidemic, J Natl Cancer Inst 85:1382–1397.

LEVINE PH, PETERSON D, MCNAMEE FL, O'BRIEN K, GRIDLEY G, HAGERTY M, BRADY J, FEARS T, ATHERTON M, HOOVER R. 1992. Does chronic fatigue syndrome predispose to non-Hodgkin's lymphoma? Cancer Res (Suppl.) 52:5516s–5518s.

LI FP, FRAUMENI JF, MANTEL N, et al. 1969. Cancer mortality among chemists. J Natl Cancer Inst 43:1159–1164.

LI FP, WILLARD DR, GOODMAN R, et al. 1975. Malignant lymphoma after diphenylhydantoin (dilantin) therapy. Cancer 36:1359–1362.

LINET MS, MALKER HSR, MCLAUGHLIN JK, et al. 1993. Non-Hodgkin's lymphoma and occupation in Sweden: a registry based analysis. Br J Ind Med 50:79–84.

LINET MS, MCLAUGHLIN JK, HSING AW, et al. 1992. Is cigarette smoking a risk factor for non-Hodgkin's lymphoma or multiple myeloma? Results from the Lutheran Brotherhood Cohort Study. Leuk Res 16:621–624.

LINET MS, POTTERN LM. 1992. Familial aggregation of hematopoietic malignancies and risk of non-Hodgkin's lymphoma. Cancer Res (Suppl.) 52:5468s–5473s.

LINOS A, BLAIR A, CANTOR KP, et al. 1990. Leukemia and non-Hodgkin's lymphoma among embalmers and funeral directors. J Natl Cancer Inst 82:66.

LINOS A, BLAIR A, GIBSON R, et al. 1991. Leukemia and non-Hodgkin's lymphoma and residential proximity to industrial plants. Arch Environ Health 46:70–74.

LIPKOWITZ S, GARRY VF, KIRSCH IR. 1992. Interlocus V-J recombination measures genomic instability in agriculture workers at risk for lymphoid malignancies. Proc Natl Acad Sci USA 89:5301–5305.

LIST AF, GRECO A, VOGLER LB. 1987. Lymphoproliferative diseases in immunocompromised hosts: The role of Epstein-Barr virus. J Clin Oncol 5:1673–1689.

LUKES RJ, COLLINS RD. 1974. Immunologic characterization of human malignant lymphomas. Cancer 34:1488–1503.

LUKES RJ, COLLINS RD. 1975. New approaches to the classification of the lymphomata. Br J Cancer 31(Suppl. II):1–28.

LYNGE E. 1985. A follow-up study of cancer incidence among workers in manufacture of phenoxy herbicides in Denmark. Br J Cancer 52:259–270.

MACMAHON EME, GLASS JD, HAYWARD SD, et al. 1991. Epstein-Barr virus in AIDS-related primary central nervous system lymphoma. Lancet 338:969–973.

MAGRATH I. 1981. Lymphocyte precursors and neoplastic counterparts in vivo and in vitro. *In* Berard CW (moderator): A multidisciplinary approach to non-Hodgkin's lymphomas. Ann Intern Med 94:218–235.

MAGRATH I. 1992. Molecular basis of lymphomagenesis. Cancer Res (Suppl.) 52:5529s–5540s.

MARSH GM, ENTERLINE PE, MCCRAW D. 1991. Mortality patterns among petroleum refinery and chemical plant workers. Am J Ind Med 19:29–42.

MASON TJ, MCKAY FW. 1974. U. S. Cancer Mortality by County, 1950–69. DHDW Publication No. (NIH) 74-615. Washington, D.C., U.S. Government Printing Office.

MATANOSKI GM, SELTSER R, SARTWELL PE, et al. 1975. The current mortality rates of radiologists and other physician specialists: specific causes of death. Am J Epidemiol 101:199–210.

MATAS AJ, SIMMONS RL, NAJARIAN JS. 1975. Chronic antigenic stimulation, herpes virus infection, and cancer in transplant recipients. Lancet i:1277–1279.

MATHÉ G, RAPPAPORT H, O'CONOR GT, et al. 1976. Histological and cytological typing of neoplastic diseases of hematopoietic and lymphoid tissues. *In* WHO International Histological Classification of Tumours, No 13. Geneva, World Health Organization.

MCDONALD JA, LI FP, MEHTA CR. 1979. Cancer mortality among beekeepers. J Occup Med 21:811–813.

MCMICHAEL AJ, ANDJELKOVIC DA, TYROLER HA. 1976. Cancer mortality among rubber workers: an epidemiologic study. Ann N Y Acad Sci 271:125–137.

MEINHARDT TJ, LEMEN RA, CRANDALL MS, et al. 1982. Environmental epidemiologic investigation of the styrene-butadiene rubber industry. Mortality patterns with discussion of the hematopoietic and lymphatic malignancies. Scand J Environ Health 8:250–259.

MEKORI YA, WEITZMAN GL, GALLI SJ. 1985. Reevaluation of reserpine-induced suppression of contact sensitivity. J Exp Med 162:1935–1953.

MILHAM S. 1988. Increased mortality in amateur radio operators due to lymphatic and hematopoietic malignancies. Am J Epidemiol 127:50–54.

MILHAM S JR. 1976a. Cancer mortality patterns associated with exposure to metals. Ann N Y Acal Sci 271:243–249.

MILHAM S JR. 1976b. Neoplasia in the wood and pulp industry. Ann N Y Acad Sci 271:294–300.

MILHAM S JR. 1976c. Occupational Mortality in Washington State, 1950–1971. DHEW Publication No. (NIOSH) 76-175. Washington, D.C., U.S. Government Printing Office.

MILHAM S JR. 1979. Mortality in aluminum reduction plant workers. J Occup Med 21:475–480.

MILHAM S JR, DEMERS RY. 1984. Mortality among pulp and paper workers. J Occup Med 26:844–846.

MILLER RW. 1974. Late radiation effects: status and needs of epidemiologic research. Environ Res 8:221–233.

MOHAR A, ROMO J, SALIDO F, et al. 1992. The spectrum of clinical and pathological manifestations of AIDS in a consecutive series of autopsied patients in Mexico, AIDS 6:467–473.

MONSON RR, FINE LJ. 1978. Cancer mortality and morbidity among rubber workers. J Natl Cancer Inst 61:1047–1053.

MUELLER N. 1991. The epidemiology of HTLV-I infection. Cancer Causes Control 2:37–52.

MUELLER N, MOHAR A, EVANS A, et al. 1991. Epstein-Barr virus antibody patterns preceeding diagnosis of non-Hodgkin's lymphoma. Int J Cancer 49:387–393.

MUIR C, WATERHOUSE J, MACK T, et al. (eds). 1987. Cancer Incidence in Five Continents Vol. V. IARC Scientific Publication No. 88. Lyon, International Agency for Research on Cancer.

NATHWANI B. 1987. Classifying non-Hodgkin's lymphomas. *In* Berard CW, Dorfman RF, Kaufman N (eds): Malignant Lymphoma. Baltimore MD, Williams and Wilkins.

NATIONAL CANCER INSTITUTE (NCI). 1982. Non-Hodgkin's lymphoma pathologic classification project writing group: National Cancer Institute sponsored study of classifications of non-Hodgkin's lymphomas. Summary and description of a working formulation for clinical usage. Cancer 49:2112–2135.

NATIONAL CANCER INSTITUTE (NCI). 1988. 1987 Annual Cancer Statistics Review. NIH Publication No. 88-2789. Bethesda, MD, National Cancer Institute.

NATIONAL CANCER INSTITUTE (NCI). 1993. SEER Cancer Statistics Review 1973–1990. NIH Publication No. 93-2789. Bethesda, MD, National Cancer Institute.

NEGRI E, LA VECCHIA C, FRANCESCHI S, et al. 1991. Vegetable and fruit consumption and cancer risk. Int J Cancer 48:350–354.

NEWILL VA. 1961. Distribution of cancer mortality among ethnic subgroups of the white population of New York City, 1953–58. J Natl Cancer Inst 26:405–417.

NG TP. 1988. Occupational mortality in Hong Kong, 1979–1983. Int J Epidemiol 17:105–110.

NICHOLSON WJ, SELIKOFF IJ, SEIDMAN H. 1978. Mortality experience of styrene-polystyrene polymerization workers. Initial findings. Scand J Work Environ Health 4 (Suppl. 2):247–252.

NORRIS FD, JACKSON EW, AARON E. 1971. Prospective study of dog bite and childhood cancer. Cancer Res 31:383–386.

OBRAMS GI, GRUFFERMAN S. 1991. Epidemiology of HIV associated non-Hodgkin lymphoma. Cancer Surv 10:91–102.

O'BRIEN TR, DECOUFLE P, BOYLE CA. 1991. Non-Hodgkin's lymphoma in a cohort of Vietnam veterans. Am J Public Health 81:758–760.

OKANO M, OSATO T, KOIZUMI S, et al. 1986. Epstein-Barr virus infection and oncogenesis in primary immunodeficiency. AIDS Res 2(S1):S115–119.

OKUN AH, BEAUMONT JJ, MEINHARDT TJ, et al. 1985. Mortality patterns among styrene-exposed boatbuilders. Am J Ind Med 8:193–205.

OPEIZ G, HENDERSON R, FOR THE COLLABORATIVE TRANSPLANT STUDY. 1993. Incidence of non-Hodgkin lymphoma in kidney and heart transplant recipients. Lancet 342:1514–1516.

OTT MG, HOLDER BB, GORDON HL. 1974. Respiratory cancer and occupational exposure to arsenicals. Arch Environ Health 29:250–255.

OTT MG, KOLESAR RC, SCHARNWEBER HC, et al. 1980. A mortality survey of employees engaged in the development or manufacture of styrene-based products. J Occup Med 22:445–460.

PALLESEN G, HAMILTON-DUTOIT SJ, ZHOU X. 1993. The association of Epstein-Barr virus (EBV) with T cell lymphoproliferations and Hodgkin's disease: Two new developments in the EBV field. Adv Cancer Res 62:179–239.

PAPADOPOULOS EB, LADANYI M, EMANUEL D, et al. 1994. Infusions of donor leukocytes to treat Epstein-Barr virus-associated lymphoproliferative disorders after allogenic bone marrow transplantation. N Engl J Med 330:1185–1191.

PARKIN DM, MUIR CS, WHELAN SL, et al. 1992. Cancer Incidence in Five Continents Vol. VI. IARC Scientific Publication No. 120. Lyon, International Agency for Research on Cancer.

PARTANEN T, KAUPPINEN T, LUUKKONEN R. 1993. Malignant lymphomas and leukemias, and exposures in the wood industry: an industry-based case-referent study. Int Arch Occup Environ Health 64:593–596.

PATTON, DF, WILKOWSKI CW, HANSON CA, et al. 1990. Epstein-Barr virus-determined clonality in posttransplant lymphoproliferation disease. Transplantation 49:1080–1084.

PEARCE NE, SHEPPARD RA, SMITH AH, et al. 1987. Non-Hodgkin's lymphoma and farming: an expanded case–control study. Int J Cancer 39:155–161.

PEARCE NE, SMITH AH, FISHER DO. 1985. Malignant lymphoma and multiple myeloma linked with agricultural occupations in a New Zealand Cancer Registry–based study. Am J Epidemiol 121:225–237.

PEARCE NE, SMITH AH, HOWARD K, et al. 1986. Non-Hodgkin's lymphoma and exposure to phenoxyherbicides, chlorophenols, fencing work, and meat works employment: a case–control study. Br J Ind Med 43:75–83.

PEARCE N, SMITH AH, REIF JS. 1988. Increased risks of soft tissue sarcoma, malignant lymphoma, and acute myeloid leukemia in abattoir workers. Am J Ind Med 14:63–72.

PENN I. 1986. The occurrence of malignant tumors in immunosuppressed states. *In* Klein E (ed): Acquired Immunodeficiency Syndrome. Progress in Allergy vol. 37. Basel, Karger, pp. 259–300.

PENN I. 1988. Secondary neoplasms as a consequence of transplantation and cancer therapy. Cancer Detect Prev 12:39–57.

PERSSON B, DAHLANDER AM, FREDRIKSSON M, BRAGE HN, OHLSON CG, AXELSON O. 1989. Malignant lymphomas and occupational exposures. Br J Ind Med 46:516–520.

PERSSON B, FREDRIKSSON M, OLSEN K. 1993. Some occupational exposures as risk factors for malignant lymphomas. Cancer 72:1773–1778.

PETTERSSON T, PUKKALA E, TEPPO L, et al. 1992. Increased risk of cancer in patients with systemic lupus erythematosus. Ann Rheum Dis 51:437–439.

PLUDA JM, VENSON DJ, TOSATO G, et al. 1993. Parameters affecting the development of non-Hodgkin's lymphoma in patients with severe human immunodeficiency virus infection receiving antiretroviral therapy, J Clin Oncol 11:1099–1107.

PLUDA JM, YARCHOAN R, JAFFEE ES, et al. 1990. Development of non-Hodgkin lymphoma in a cohort of patients with severe human immunodeficiency virus (HIV) infection on long-term antiretroviral therapy. Ann Intern Med 133:276–282.

POLEDNAK AP, STEHNEY AF, LUCAS HF. 1983. Mortality among male workers at a thorium-processing plant. Health Phys 44 (Suppl. 1):239–251.

POTOLSKY AI, HEATH CW, BUCKLEY CE, et al. 1971. Lymphoreticular malignancies and immunologic abnormalities in a sibship. Am J Med 50:42–48.

PROJECT RANCH HAND II: An Epidemiologic Investigation of Health Effects in Air Force Personnel Following Exposure to Herbicides, Baseline Mortality Study Results. 1983. Brooks Air Force Base, TX, Epidemiology Division, Data Sciences Division, U.S. Air Force School of Aerospace Medicine.

PURTILO DT, BHAWAN J, HUTT LM, et al. 1978. Epstein-Barr virus infections in the X-linked recessive lymphoproliferative syndrome. Lancet 1:798–801.

PURTILO DT, YASUDA N, GRIERSON HL, et al. 1988. X-linked lymphoproliferative syndrome provides clues to the pathogenesis of Epstein-Barr virus-induced lymphomagenesis. *In* Miller RW et al (eds): Unusual Occurrences as Clues to Cancer Etiology. Tokyo, Japan, Sci Soc Press, pp. 149–158.

RAPPAPORT H. 1966. Tumors of the hematopoietic system. Atlas of Tumor Pathology. Section 3, Fascicle 8. Washington, D.C., Armed Forces Institute of Pathology.

RAZIS DV, DIAMOND HD, CRAVER LF. 1959. Familial Hodgkin's disease: its significance and implications. Ann Intern Med 51:933–971.

REGISTRAR GENERAL FOR ENGLAND AND WALES. 1958. The Registrar General's Decennial Supplement. England and Wales: 1951. Occupational Mortality, Part II, Vol. 2. London, His Majesty's Stationery Office.

RIIHIMAKI V, ASP S, HERNBERG S. 1982. Mortality of 2,4-dichlorophenoxyacetic acid and 2,4,5-trichlorophenoxyacetic acid herbicide applicators in Finland. Scand J Work Environ Health 8:37–42.

RINSKY RA, OTT G, WARD E, et al. 1988. Study of mortality among chemical workers in the Kanawha Valley of West Virginia. Am J Ind Med 13:429–438.

RINSKY RA, ZUMWALDE RD, WAXWEILER RJ, et al. 1981. Cancer mortality at a naval nuclear shipyard. Lancet 1(8214):231–235.

RITTER L, WIGLE DT, SEMENCIW RM, et al. 1990. Mortality study of Canadian male farm operators: cancer mortality and agricultural practices in Saskatchewan. Med Lav 81:499–505.

ROBINSON JE. 1982. The biology of circulating B lymphocytes infected with Epstein-Barr virus during infectious mononucleosis. Yale J Biol Med 55:311–316.

RONCO G, COSTA G, LYNGE E. 1992. Cancer risk among Danish and Italian farmers. Br J Ind Med 49:220–225.

ROSENBERG W, OKEN MM, RYDELL RE, et al. 1982. Non-Hodgkin's lymphoma after treatment for Hodgkin's disease. Oncology 39:216–217.

ROSS R, DWORSKY R, NICHOLS P, et al. 1982. Asbestos exposure and lymphomas of the gastrointestinal tract and oral cavity. Lancet 2(8308):1118–1120.

ROSS R, DWORSKY R, PAGANINI-HILL A, et al. 1983. The occurrence of multiple lymphoreticular and hematological malignancies in the same households. Br J Cancer 47:853–856.

ROTHMAN KJ, BOICE JD. 1979. Epidemiologic analysis with a programmable calculator. NIH No. 79-1649. Washington, D.C., U.S. Government Printing Office.

SAMA SR, MARTIN TR, DAVIS LK, et al. 1990. Cancer incidence among Massachusetts firefighters, 1982–1986. Am J Ind Med 18:47–54.

SARACCI R, KOGEVINAS M, BERTAZZI P-A, BUENO DE MESQUITA BH, COGGON D, GREEN LM, KAUPPINEN T, L'ABBÉ KA, LITTORIN M, LYNGE E, MATHEWS JD, NEUBERGER M, OSMAN J, PEARCE N, WINKELMANN R. 1991. Cancer mortality in workers exposed to chlorophenoxy herbicides and chlorophenols. Lancet 338:1027–1032.

SAVITZ DA, WACHTEL H, BARNES FA, et al. 1988. Case–control study of childhood cancer and exposure to 60-hz magnetic fields. Am J Epidemiol 128:21–38.

SCHERR PA, HUTCHISON GB, NEIMAN RS. 1992. Non-Hodgkin's lymphoma and occupational exposure. Cancer Res (Suppl.) 52:5503s–5509s.

SCHNEIDER R. 1972. Human cancer in households containing cats with malignant lymphoma. Int J Cancer 10:338–344.

SCHUMACHER MC. 1985. Farming occupations and mortality from non-Hodgkin's lymphoma in Utah. J Occup Med 27:580–584.

SCHUMACHER MC, DELZELL E. 1988. A death-certificate case–control study of non-Hodgkin's lymphoma and occupation in men in North Carolina. Am J Ind Med 13:317–330.

SEIDMAN H. 1970. Cancer death rates by site and sex for religious and socioeconomic groups in New York City. Environ Res 3:234–250.

SHAPIRO RS, MCCLAIN K, FRIZZERA G, et al. 1988. Epstein-Barr virus associated B cell lymphoproliferative disorders following bone marrow transplantation. Blood 71:1234–1243.

SHIMIZU Y, KATO H, SCHULL WJ. 1990. Studies of the mortality of A-bomb survivors. 9. Mortality, 1950–1985: part 2. Cancer mortality based on the recently revised doses (DS86). Radiat Res 121:120–141.

SIEMIATYCKI J, RICHARDSON L, GERIN M, et al. 1986. Associations between several sites of cancer and nine organic dusts: results from an hypothesis-generating case–control study in Montreal, 1979–1983. Am J Epidemiol 123:235–249.

SIGURGEIRSSON B, AGNARSSON BA, LINDELOF B. 1994. Risk of lymphoma in patients with dermatitis herpetiformis. BMJ 308:13–15.

SILMAN AJ, PETRIE J, HAZLEMAN B, et al. 1988. Lymphoproliferative cancer and other malignancy in patients with rheumatoid arthritis treated with azathioprine: a 20 year follow-up study. Ann Rheum Dis 47:988–992.

SKEGG DCG. 1978. BCG vaccination and the incidence of lymphomas and leukaemia. Int J Cancer 21:18–21.

SMITH PR, LICKISS JN. 1980. Benzene and lymphoma. Lancet 1080 (i):719.

STAAL SD, AMBINDER R, BESCHORNER WE, et al. 1989. A survey of Epstein-Barr virus DNA in lymphoid tissue: Frequent detection in Hodgkin's disease. Am J Clin Path 91:1–5.

STARZL TE, PORTER KA, IWATSUKI S, et al. 1984. Reversibility of lymphomas and lymphoproliferative lesions developing under cyclosporin-steroid therapy. Lancet i:583–587.

STEENLAND K, STAYNER L, GREIFE A, et al. 1991. Mortality among workers exposed to ethylene oxide. N Engl J Med 324:1402–1407.

STROUP NE, BLAIR A, ERIKSON GE. 1986. Brain cancer and other causes of death in anatomists. J Natl Cancer Inst 77:1217–1224.

SWERDLOW AJ, DOUGLAS AJ, VAUGHAN HG, et al. 1993. Risk of second primary cancers after Hodgkin's disease in patients in the British National Lymphoma Investigation: relationships to host factors, histology and stage of Hodgkin's disease, and splenectomy. Br J Cancer 68:1006–1011.

SWINNEN LJ, COSTANZO-NORDIN MR, FISHER SG, et al. 1990. Increased incidence of lymphoproliferative disorder after immunosuppression with the monoclonal antibody OKT3 in cardiac-transplant recipients. N Engl J Med 323:1723–1728.

SWINSON CM, COLES EC, SLAVIN G, et al. 1983. Coeliac disease and malignancy. Lancet i:111–115.

SYMMONS DPM, AHERN M, BACON PA, et al. 1984. Lymphoproliferative malignancy in rheumatoid arthritis: A study of 20 cases. Ann Rheum Dis 43:132–135.

TABERSHAW IR, GAFFEY WR. 1974. Mortality study of workers in the manufacture of vinyl chloride and its polymers. J Occup Med 16:509–518.

TETA MJ, BENSON LO, VITALE JN. 1993. Mortality study of ethylene oxide workers in chemical manufacturing: a 10 year update. Br J Ind Med 50:704–709.

TETA MJ, WALRATH J, MEIGS JW, et al. 1984. Cancer incidence among cosmetologists. J Natl Cancer Inst 72:1051–1057.

THIESS AS, FRENTZEL-BEYME R, LINK R. 1982. Mortality study of persons exposed to dioxin in a trichlorophenol-process accident that occurred in the BASF AG on November 17, 1953. Am J Ind Med 3:179–189.

THUN MJ, ALTEKRUSE SF, NAMBOODIRI MM, et al. 1994. Hair dye use and risk of fatal cancers in U.S. women. J Natl Cancer Inst 86:210–215.

TOURAINE JL, GARNIER JL, LEFRANCOIS N, et al. 1989. Severe lymphoproliferative disease and Kaposi's sarcoma in transplant patients. Transplant Proc 21:3197–3198.

TUCKER MA, COLEMAN CN, COX RS, et al. 1988. Risk of second cancers after treatment for Hodgkin's disease. N Engl J Med 318:76–81.

URSIN G, BJELKE E, HEUCH I, VOLLSET SE. 1990. Milk consumption and cancer incidence: A Norwegian prospective study. Br J Cancer 61:454–459.

VAN KAICK G, LIEVERMAN D, LORENZ D, et al. 1983. Recent results of the German thorotrast study—epidemiological results and dose effect relationships in thorotrast patients. Health Phys 44 (Suppl. 1):299–306.

VIANNA NJ, POLAN A. 1979. Lymphomas and occupational benzene exposure. Lancet 1(8131):1394–1395.

WALKER JT, BLOOM TF, STERN FB, et al. 1993. Mortality of workers employed in shoe manufacturing. Scand J Work Environ Health 19:89–95.

WARNKE RA, WEISS LM. 1987. B-cell malignant lymphomas: an immunologic perspective. *In* Berard CW, Dorfman RF, Kaufman N (eds): Malignant Lymphoma. Baltimore, Williams and Wilkins.

WATANABE KK, KANG HK, THOMAS TL. 1991. Mortality among Vietnam veterans: with methodological considerations. J Occup Med 33:780–785.

WEGMAN DH, EISEN EA. 1981. Causes of death among employees of a synthetic abrasive product manufacturing company. J Occup Med 23:748–754.

WEINTRAUB J, WARNKE RA. 1982. Lymphoma in cardiac allotransplant recipients. Transplantation 33:347–351.

WEISENBURGER DD. 1990. Environmental epidemiology of non-Hodgkin's lymphoma in eastern Nebraska. Am J Ind Med 18:303–305.

WERTHEIMER N, LEEPER E. 1979. Electrical wiring configurations and childhood cancer. Am J Epidemiol 109:273–284.

WIGLE DT, SEMENCIW RM, WILKINS K, RIEDEL D, RITTER L, MORRISON HI, YANG M. 1990. Mortality study of Canadian male farm operators: Non-Hodgkin's lymphoma mortality and agricultural practices in Saskatchewan. J Natl Cancer Inst 82:575–582.

WIKLUND K, DICH J, HOLM LE. 1987. Risk of malignant lymphoma in Swedish pesticide appliers. Br J Cancer 56:505–508.

WIKLUND K, LINDEFORS BM, HOLM LE. 1988. Risk of malignant lymphoma in Swedish agricultural and forestry workers. Br J Ind Med 45:19–24.

WILCOSKY TC, CHECKOWAY H, MARSHALL EG, et al. 1984. Cancer mortality and solvent exposures in the rubber industry. Am Ind Hyg Assoc J 45:809–811.

WILLIAMS RR, STEGENS NL, GOLDSMITH JR. 1977. Associations of cancer site and type with occupation and industry from the Third National Cancer Survey Interview. J Natl Cancer Inst 59:1147–1185.

WINGO PA, TONG T, BOLDEN S. 1995. Cancer statistics, 1995. Ca Cancer J Clin 45:8–30.

WITHERSPOON RP, FISHER LD, SCHOCH G, et al. 1989. Secondary cancers after bone marrow transplantation for leukemia or aplastic anemia. N Engl J Med 321:784–789.

WONG O. 1987. An industry wide mortality study of chemical workers occupationally exposed to benzene. I. general results. Br J Ind Med 44:365–381.

WONG O, MORGAN RW, BAILEY WJ, et al. 1986. An epidemiological study of petroleum refinery employees. Br J Ind Med 43:6–17.

WONG O, TRENT LS. 1993. An epidemiological study of workers potentially exposed to ethylene oxide. Br J Ind Med 50:308–316.

WOODS JS, POLISSAR L, SEVERSON RK, et al. 1987. Soft tissue sarcoma and non-Hodgkin's lymphoma in relation to phenoxyherbicide and chlorinated phenol exposure in western Washington. J Natl Cancer Inst 78:899–910.

World Health Organization. 1977. International Classification of Diseases. Manual of the International Statistical Classification of Diseases, Injuries, and Causes of Death, Ninth Revision. Geneva, World Health Organization.

Zack JA, Suskind RR. 1980. The mortality experience of workers exposed to tetrachlorodibenzodioxin in a trichlorophenol process accident. J Occup Med 22:11–14.

Zahm SH, Weisenburger DD, Babbitt PA, et al. 1990. A case–control study of non-Hodgkin's lymphoma and the herbicide 2,4-dichlorophenoxyacetic acid (2,4-D) in eastern Nebraska. Epidemiology 1:349–356.

Zahm SH, Weisenburger DD, Babbitt PA, Saal RC, Vaught JB, Blair A. 1992. Use of hair coloring products and the risk of lymphoma, multiple myeloma, and chronic lymphocytic leukemia. Am J Public Health 82:990–997.

Zahm SH, Weisenburger DD, Cantor KP, et al. 1993a. Role of the herbicide atrazine in the development of non-Hodgkin's lymphoma. Scand J Work Environ Health 19:108–14.

Zahm SH, Weisenburger DD, Saal RC, et al. 1993b. The role of agricultural pesticide use in the development of non-Hodgkin's lymphoma in women. Arch Environ Health 48:353–358.

Zoloth SR, Michaels DM, Villalbi JR, et al. 1986. Patterns of mortality among commercial pressmen. J Natl Cancer Inst 76:1047–1051.

43 Multiple myeloma

LISA J. HERRINTON
NOEL S. WEISS
ANDREW F. OLSHAN

Plasma cells, the final products of B-cell differentiation, synthesize and release immunoglobulins (Ig) and Ig subunits (light and heavy chains). Plasma cell malignancies, which are characterized by the presence of elevated numbers of plasma cells in bone marrow and, very often, elevated levels of monoclonal protein in serum and urine, include the following: Waldenström's macroglobulinemia, in which there is production of IgM; multiple myeloma, in which there is production of IgA, IgD, IgE, IgG, or light chains; and the heavy-chain diseases, in which there is production of the heavy chains (gamma, mu, and delta) (Osserman et al, 1987). Because they occur relatively infrequently, neither descriptive nor analytical studies of the heavy-chain diseases have been reported. Consequently, this chapter is restricted to multiple myeloma and Waldenström's macroglobulinemia.

Recent studies provide strong evidence that the malignant transformation causing multiple myeloma occurs not at the terminally differentiated B cell, but rather at the early B-cell or lymphoid stem cell (Barlogie et al, 1989). B-cell precursors express specific antigens during discrete stages of maturation, and early B-cell and T-cell antigens have been identified from tumor cells (Barlogie et al, 1989). Furthermore, cytogenetic abnormalities of transformed plasma cells from one multiple myeloma patient were also evident in the patient's early B cells (MacKenzie and Lewis, 1985).

The manifestation of multiple myeloma is variable and the disease can be difficult to diagnose (Kyle and Greipp, 1988). Excluding nonsecretory myeloma, the diagnosis is based on the presence of monoclonal protein in serum or urine and more than 10% atypical plasma cells in bone marrow (Kyle and Greipp, 1988) with additional symptoms, which may include osteolytic lesions, renal insufficiency, hypercalcemia, anemia, and increased susceptibility to infections. When a heavy chain other than delta is present, monoclonal protein can be detected using serum protein electrophoresis; however, in approximately 15% of patients, the only manifestation of disease is light chains (Bence Jones protein). Detection of light chains requires immunoelectrophoresis or immunofixation, methods that are more expensive and less available than serum protein electrophoresis. The availability and use of serum protein electrophoresis, immunoelectrophoresis, and immunofixation have increased over time and vary by location, and this variation probably accounts for part of the temporal and geographic variability in the reported incidence of the disease.

DEMOGRAPHIC CORRELATES OF INCIDENCE

Internationally, the reported incidence of multiple myeloma varies substantially, as shown in Table 43–1 for the years 1982–1986. The availability and use of serum protein electrophoresis, immunoelectrophoresis, and immunofixation—all relatively sensitive diagnostic methods—vary by location. This variation probably accounts for part of the geographic variability in the reported incidence of and mortality from the disease, particularly in older persons. Therefore, the table provides incidence rates only for individuals aged 35–64 years. The highest incidence rates have been reported for African Americans and native Pacific Islanders; Europeans and North American Caucasians have intermediate rates; while generally low rates have been reported for Asians living in Asia and the United States. It should be noted that some of the estimates reported in Table 43–1 are based on small numbers of occurrences.

Age-, sex-, and race-specific incidence rates from the U.S. Surveillance, Epidemiology, and End Results (SEER) program are shown in Figure 43–1 for 1986–1990. The incidence of multiple myeloma increased rapidly with age and men had higher rates than women; this sex difference has been observed consistently in international comparisons (Levi et al, 1992). African Americans had higher rates than Caucasians; the cumulative incidence (ages 0–74 years) in African Ameri-

TABLE 43–1. *Annual Age-standardized* Incidence Rate of Multiple Myeloma by Geographic Location, 1983–1987*

Location	*Ethnicity*	*Men*	*Women*
AMERICA			
Bermuda	Black	0.0	3.6
	Other	2.8	2.0
Brazil		1.6–2.4	0.6–2.5
Canada		4.9	3.6
Colombia		2.0	1.9
Costa Rica		3.3	2.6
Cuba		3.0	2.8
Equador		3.6	1.9
Martinique		8.3	8.0
Peru		2.9	0.0
Puerto Rico		4.8	2.8
USA	White	4.7	3.2
	Spanish-surname White	5.4	3.2
	Black	10.3	7.1
	Chinese	2.1	2.1
	Japanese	2.0	0.8
	Filipino	3.1	0.5
ASIA			
China		1.1–2.9	0.5–1.5
Hong Kong		2.7	1.6
India		1.3–1.8	1.0–1.5
Israel	Jews born in Israel	6.5	3.7
	Jews, African or Asian	3.2	2.5
	Jews, European or American	4.7	2.8
	Non-Jews	4.2	1.7
Japan		1.6–2.6	1.1–2.2
Kuwait	Kuwaitis	1.9	2.6
	Non-Kuwaitis	4.8	3.8
Philippines		1.1–1.4	1.1
Singapore	Chinese	2.7	1.5
	Malay	4.5	1.8
	Indian	2.0	1.8
EUROPE			
Czechoslovakia		4.0	2.8
Denmark		3.5	2.9
Estonia		2.4	2.7
Finland		4.4	2.8
France		2.3–9.4	1.3–7.4
German Democratic Republic		2.9–3.0	1.8–2.4
Hungary		1.0–1.4	1.5–2.9
Iceland		5.7	5.9
Ireland, Southern		5.3	3.3
Italy		2.8–5.5	1.0–3.4
Latvia		3.1	2.2
Netherlands		2.5–4.0	1.3–3.5
Norway		5.2	3.6
Poland		1.4–3.3	1.2–2.5
Portugal		2.7	2.0
Romania		1.7	1.1
Slovenia		2.8	2.2
Spain		1.9–4.2	2.2–3.4
Sweden		5.2	3.3
Switzerland		1.9–6.3	2.5–4.3
Britain		3.4–4.5	2.2–3.7
Scotland		3.2–4.2	1.9–4.1
OCEANIA			
Australia		3.7–4.8	2.2–4.9
Hawaii	White	4.4	1.5
	Japanese	2.6	0.9
	Hawaiian	7.4	5.6
	Filipino	4.0	2.9
	Chinese	3.0	1.9
New Zealand	Maori	8.4	7.8
	Non-Maori	5.3	3.4

*Standardized to the age distribution of the world population, per 100,000, aged 35–64 years.
Adapted from Parker et al, 1993.

can men was reported to be 10 per thousand; in African American women, Caucasian men, and Caucasian women, the corresponding rates were seven, four, and three per thousand, respectively (Miller et al, 1993). Although comparable data for Asians living in the USA were not available for the period 1986–1990, the data shown in Table 43–1 suggest that, as with international rates, myeloma incidence in the United States is relatively low among Asians. Using data from the São Paulo, Brazil, cancer registry, Bouchardy et al (1991) observed that a larger proportion of myeloma patients than other cancer patients were black (black compared with white race, OR = 2.8, 95% CI, 1.4–5.5). In addition, British migrants from West Africa, East Africa, and the Caribbean were at higher risk of myeloma than native-born British residents (Grulich et al, 1992). The respective relative risks (RR) and 95% confidence intervals (CI) comparing migrants to native-born Britons were as follows: men, 4.1 (2.2–7.6), 1.9 (1.0–3.7), and 2.2 (1.7–2.7); women, 1.6 (0.2–12), 1.7 (0.7–4.1), and 2.0 (1.5–2.7).

The incidence of Waldenström's macroglobulinemia has been estimated using SEER data collected for only a limited population base (western Washington, 1978–89, and the eight other SEER areas, 1988–89). In Caucasian men and women, the age-standardized incidence rates were 6.1 and 2.5 per million person-years, respectively (1980 U.S. standard). No cases were diagnosed in African American men, but in African American women, the incidence rate was 3.6 per million person-years (Herrinton and Weiss, 1993).

In nine studies the secular changes in myeloma inci-

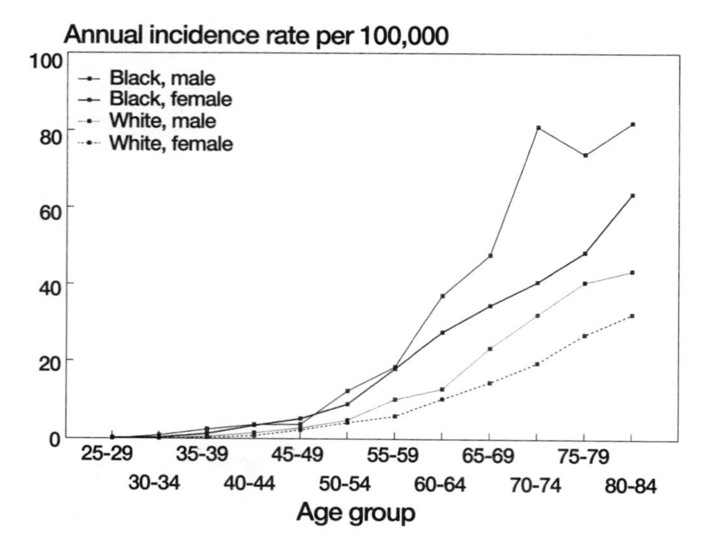

FIG. 43–1. Age-, sex-, and race-specific incidence rates of multiple myeloma, SEER program, USA, 1986–90. (From data reported by Miller et al 1993.)

dence have been examined. Three of these were conducted in areas in which a particularly high level of case ascertainment might have been expected: one in Olmsted County, Minnesota, where the Mayo Clinic is located; another in Malmö, Sweden, where the medical community has had an interest in multiple myeloma dating to the 1960s; and the other in the Canton of Vaud, Switzerland. In Olmsted County, the annual age-standardized incidence of multiple myeloma remained constant from 1945 to 1977 at approximately 35 per million among men and 22 per million among women (1950 U.S. standard) (Linos et al, 1981). In Malmö, the incidence rate in men increased by 60% between 1950 and 1979 to an annual rate of 46 per million (1950 U.S. standard) and all age groups were affected. In contrast, no increase was observed in the rate among women (average annual incidence was 27 per million) (Turesson et al, 1984). In the Canton of Vaud, no changes in incidence were noted between 1978 and 1987 (average annual incidence rates were 48 per million in men and 27 per million in women, European standard) (Levi and LaVecchia, 1990).

Secular changes in incidence among Caucasian residents of four geographic areas of the United States that had participated in national cancer surveys or had established tumor registries (Atlanta, Connecticut, Detroit, San Francisco/Oakland) were examined by Devesa et al (1987) for the period 1947–1984. The reported annual incidence rates increased between 1947 and 1975 by about 150% to 38 per million in men and 26 per million in women (1950 U.S. standard). No increases were observed between 1975 and 1985. The age-adjusted incidence of myeloma among African Americans did not change appreciably from 1973 to 1990 (Miller et al, 1993).

Other studies of changes in incidence rates over time have been conducted using data from Denmark, Connecticut, New Zealand, Western Australia, and Israel. In Denmark, the reported annual incidence increased between 1943 and 1962 from 13 to 33 per million in men and from 12 to 25 per million in women (European standard); no increase was observed between 1963 and 1982 (Hansen et al, 1989). In Connecticut, the reported annual incidence rates in men and women rose nearly 10-fold between 1935 and 1975 to approximately 47 and 38 per million, respectively (Zheng et al, 1992). In the three other studies, the annual incidence increased throughout the 1970s (Nandakumar et al, 1988; Pearce et al, 1985; Shapira and Carter, 1986). Five studies have also reported secular increases in mortality (Blattner et al, 1981; Cuzick, 1990; Cuzick et al, 1983; Kato et al, 1985; Ludwig et al, 1982; Velez et al, 1982).

Several lines of evidence suggest that the reported secular increase in the incidence of multiple myeloma was predominantly the result of changes in ascertainment of the disease, including the following:

1. There was no increase in the incidence of multiple myeloma in Olmsted County or the Canton of Vaud, areas with good surveillance for myeloma.
2. In countries with relatively high incidence, rates stabilized since the 1970s.
3. When reported, increases in incidence were greatest among older individuals, a group in whom a laboratory diagnosis might less commonly have been sought in the past than in the present.

Thus, changes in the availability and use of serum protein electrophoresis were likely to account for the reported increases in incidence in some locations. Conversely, the finding of an increase in the incidence of myeloma in men, but not women, of all ages who resided in Malmö is consistent with the possible introduction of an occupational agent causing multiple myeloma (Turesson et al, 1984).

Seven studies have examined multiple myeloma incidence in relation to socioeconomic status. In a hospital-based case-control study conducted at Duke University during the period 1976–1982, the odds ratio (OR) for the association of home ownership with myeloma incidence was 1.6 (95% CI, 1.0–2.6), and there was a weak trend of increasing risk with occupational level. However, family income and education were unrelated to risk of the disease (Johnston et al, 1985). Five studies that were conducted in Europe, the United States and Australia, with various study periods set between 1961 and 1984, observed no relationship between various indices of socioeconomic status (including occupational and educational level, income, and social class) and myeloma incidence (Boffetta et al, 1989; Cuzick and De Stavola, 1988; McWhorter et al, 1989; Nandakumar et al, 1986; Vågerö and Persson, 1986). A sixth study (Williams and Horm, 1977) reported a "suggestive" positive relationship. The association of socioeconomic status with multiple myeloma that was reported in earlier studies of mortality (Blattner et al, 1981; Hoover et al, 1975; MacMahon, 1966; Velez et al, 1982) was possibly the result of better access to sensitive diagnostic methods by individuals of higher socioeconomic status.

EPIDEMIOLOGIC RISK FACTORS

Individuals with monoclonal gammopathy of unknown significance (MGUS) are predisposed to developing multiple myeloma. MGUS is an asymptomatic, non-malignant disorder involving proliferation of plasma cells and production of M-components. In addition, autoimmune disorders, chronic immune stimulation, exposure to ionizing radiation, occupational exposures, exposure to hair-coloring products, consumption of alcohol and tobacco, and a family history of myeloma and other diseases also have been examined as risk factors for multiple myeloma in humans. The possibility of etiologic heterogeneity of myeloma of various M-component types has been investigated. The occurrence of Waldenström's macroglobulinemia has been examined only in relation to autoimmune disorders, chronic immune stimulation, and the family history of disease.

Monoclonal Gammopathy of Unknown Significance

In a large, population-based prevalence survey in the Värmland district of Sweden, 61 individuals with MGUS who were initially free of myeloma were identified and followed for up to 20 years; two went on to develop multiple myeloma (Axelsson, 1986) (annual incidence rate of 2.2 per thousand), although only 0.2 cases were expected (Turesson et al, 1984). At the Mayo Clinic, 47 patients developed multiple myeloma or Waldenström's macroglobulinemia from a series of 241 initially diagnosed with MGUS who were followed for a median of 7 years (Kyle, 1993) (annual incidence rate of 1.9 percent compared with 0.02 percent expected in similarly aged persons in the general population), while at the University of Barcelona, 10 patients developed multiple myeloma during 20 years of follow-up of 128 persons initially diagnosed with MGUS (Blade et al, 1992) (annual incidence rate of 1.9 percent compared with approximately 0.01 percent expected). The difference in the incidence of multiple myeloma in the first and latter two cohorts is probably attributable to the manner in which cohort members were identified. In the Värmland study, a population-based survey was used, while the Mayo Clinic and University of Barcelona patients had been referred as a consequence of having elevated monoclonal proteins determined in the course of their clinical care.

The prevalence of MGUS has been characterized in three large, population-based studies: the original Värmland study (Axelsson et al, 1966), and in studies conducted in the town of Thief River Falls, Minnesota (Kyle et al, 1972) and in the Finistère region of France (Saleun et al, 1982). The studies were consistent in revealing an age-related increase in the prevalence of MGUS, which reached 4%–5% among persons aged 80 years and over. There was also a marked sex differential, with men being 1.5 to 2.0 times more likely (after adjustment for age) to have the condition. The study of Saleun et al (1982) also revealed a 40% excess prevalence of the condition among farmers relative to people in other occupations (after adjustment for age and sex). All three studies used paper electrophoresis, a relatively insensitive method (Kyle and Greipp, 1988), to detect monoclonal proteins; the true prevalence may be higher (Axelsson, 1986).

Saleun et al (1982) reported the distribution of M-components in MGUS to be as follows: IgG, 68%; IgM, 23%; IgA, 6%; other M-components, less than 1%; two components, 2%; light chains only, 1%. Nevertheless, the investigators reported that the proportion of persons with only light chains probably was artifically low because of the laboratory method used. It has also been reported that the age-specific prevalence of MGUS in 1,864 African American veterans was higher than that in 857 Caucasian veterans (age 50 years and younger, 2.4% in African Americans compared with 0% in Caucasians; age 51–60 years, 2.1% compared with 1.8%; age 61–70 years, 4.6% compared with 1.6%; age 70 years and older, 6.5% compared with 4.8%) (Schechter et al, 1991). In addition, the prevalence in Japanese residents aged 70-80 years (3%) was lower than that in similarly aged American residents (10%) (Bowden et al, 1993).

The production of monoclonal protein as a response to chronic disease and infection has been studied epidemiologically only to a very limited extent. In a cohort of patients with infections, increased levels of monoclonal proteins were found to be present in persons with leishmaniasis (16/20) and cytomegalovirus (8/18), but not in those with echinococcosis (1/18), nor infectious mononucleosis (0/30), nor among healthy control subjects (1/39) (Haas et al, 1990). In this study, most monoclonal protein produced in leishmaniasis patients did not bind to *Leishmania* antigens. The duration of the increase in monoclonal protein was studied in seven patients; its maximum was 18 months.

Autoimmune Disorders

The relationship between rheumatoid arthritis and multiple myeloma has been investigated in four cohort and five case-control studies. In a Finnish rheumatoid arthritis cohort followed from 1967 through 1973, the relative risk of myeloma was 3.3 in men (n = 7) and 9.5 in women (n = 21) compared with the incidence in the general population (Isomäki et al, 1978). A Mayo clinic cohort followed from 1950 through 1974 revealed a relative risk of 5.0 (95% CI, 1.4–13) (Katusic et al, 1985). While none of the members of a Birmingham, UK, cohort with rheumatoid arthritis, followed from 1964 through 1978, died of myeloma, the expected number of deaths was only 0.2 (Prior et al, 1984). Compared with the general population, rheumatoid arthritis patients enrolled in a Toronto treatment registry were at 8.1-fold (95% CI, 3.3–21) increased risk of "lymphoproliferative disorders and myeloma"; two of the four incident tumors in this category were myeloma (Matteson et al, 1991). A New Zealand case-control study in which cancer patients were selected from a tumor registry to serve as controls yielded a 2.3-fold (95% CI, 0.6–8.0) excess risk of myeloma among rheumatoid arthritis patients (Pearce et al, 1986). A medical-record-based study set at Kaiser Permanente (Doody et al, 1992) and a population-based study in northern Sweden (Eriksson, 1993) found small (OR = 1.2, 95% CI, 0.4–4.3) and large (OR = 4.0, no. of exposed cases = 9) excesses in risk, respectively. Two hospital-based case-control studies reported no association of rheumatoid arthritis or autoimmune disease with myeloma (Gramenzi et al, 1991, Linet et al, 1987); however, selecting controls from among hospitalized patients may have introduced a bias that obscured an actual association. An additional hospital-based case-control study (Cuzick and De Stavola, 1989) and a population-based case-control study (Lewis et al, 1994) also observed no relationship, but the prevalences of rheumatoid arthritis in the two studies were notably elevated (9% and 14%, respectively, compared with 2% or less in the other studies), suggesting some degree of misclassification with osteoarthritis.

Pernicious anemia has been examined in relation to subsequent myeloma risk in three studies. U.S. male veterans hospitalized for pernicious anemia during 1969–1985 were at 2-fold (95% CI, 1.0–4.0) increased risk of myeloma (Brinton et al, 1989). Follow-up through 1984 of patients in the Uppsala health care region in Sweden who had been diagnosed with pernicious anemia during 1965 through 1983 resulted in a relative risk of 1.0 in men (95% CI, 0.2–2.8) and 2.5 in women (95% CI, 1.1–4.9) (Hsing et al, 1993). A modest association of prior pernicious anemia with myeloma was observed in black (OR = 1.5, 95% CI, 0.5–4.5) but not white (OR = 0.8, 95% CI, 0.3–2.2) persons in a population-based case-control study set in three metropolitan areas of the United States (Lewis et al, 1994). The same study also examined a history of psoriasis, which was not associated with myeloma, and a history of any autoimmune disorder, which was modestly related to myeloma risk in blacks (OR = 1.7, 95% CI, 0.7–3.7) but not whites (OR = 1.0, 95% CI, 0.5–1.8) (Lewis et al, 1994).

Linet et al (1993) observed no relationship between a history of autoimmune and connective tissue disorders and Waldenström's macroglobulinemia, but only one case reported a history.

A possible basis for the relationship of autoimmune disease with myeloma risk concerns the cytokine interleukin-6 (IL-6). IL-6 is a potent stimulator of B-cell differentiation and a promoter of myeloma cell growth (Hirano, 1991; Wolvekamp and Marquet, 1990). IL-6 is produced by a wide variety of cell types in response to bacterial products, trauma, viruses, and other stimuli (Wolvekamp and Marquet, 1990). Hirano (1991) notes that IL-6 gene deregulation may occur from insertion of viral DNA in the promoter region of the IL-6 gene, by a cytokine cascade induced by an inflammatory reaction, or by other mechanisms. Apart from multiple myeloma, IL-6 production has been noted to increase substantially in association with rheumatoid arthritis and systemic lupus erythematosus, acute infectious neural diseases, trauma, cardiac myxoma, and transplantation (Wolvekamp and Marquet, 1990). As more information becomes known about the causes of abnormally high IL-6 levels, it may lead to identification of specific new exposures that could be examined in future epidemiologic studies of possible myeloma risk factors.

Chronic Immune Stimulation

When first put forth, the hypothesis that chronic immune stimulation could cause multiple myeloma was based on the assumption that antigenic stimulation could increase the likelihood of a malignant transformation in a mature B cell. Since then, evidence has accumulated that the malignant transformation in myeloma occurs at the level of a pre-B or stem cell (Barlogie and Epstein, 1990); these cells are not stimulated by antigen. Nonetheless, chronic immune stimulation could have a promotional effect on myeloma, although there is no experimental evidence to support this hypothesis.

The hypothesis that chronic immune stimulation increases myeloma risk has been examined in 11 epidemiologic studies. (The study by Cohen et al (1987) used hospital outpatients for controls and is not presented here.) Characteristics of the design of these studies are summarized in Table 43–2, and the study results are summarized in Table 43–3. The interpretation of the results shown in Table 43–3 is somewhat difficult for several reasons:

1. Interviews of unknown and differing sensitivity and specificity were used in the various studies to measure chronic immune stimulation.
2. Because of the large numbers of conditions examined, many comparisons were made, and some spurious associations may have been identified.
3. Various studies categorized immunologic challenges differently, and it is not possible to make direct comparisons between studies.
4. Multiple myeloma may have a prolonged prodromal period during which there may be increased susceptibility to infections.

Nonetheless, some limited inferences are possible.

In five case-control studies and a cohort study, a history of asthma was not found to be related to the risk of multiple myeloma (Boffetta et al, 1989; Cuzick and De Stavola, 1988; Doody et al, 1992; Lewis et al, 1994; Pearce et al, 1986; Vesterinen et al, 1993). The study of Doody et al (1992) was based on medical-record reviews for information on prior illnesses, while the other case-control studies were based on interview.

A possible association between myeloma and a history of allergies has been examined in ten case-control studies. A modest association between a history of hay fever and myeloma was found in the New Zealand study (OR = 1.9, 95% CI, 1.0–3.5) (Pearce et al, 1986), the Kaiser Permanente study (OR = 1.3, 95% CI, 0.6–2.7) (Doody et al, 1992), and the American Cancer Society study (OR = 1.6, 95% CI, 0.8–2.9) (Boffetta et al, 1989), but not in the others. Gallagher et al (1983) found a 3.1-fold increase (95% CI, 1.6–6.3) in risk associated with a history of allergies (all types combined), in contrast to four other studies (Cuzick and De Stavola, 1988; Gramenzi et al, 1991; Linet et al, 1987; Lewis et al, 1994) and in contrast to two studies that observed no relationship with a history of allergy desensitization shots (Koepsell et al, 1987; Lewis et al, 1994). A positive association with a history of eczema was observed by Doody et al (1992) (OR = 2.0, 95% CI, 1.1–4.0), but not three other groups of investigators (Cuzick and De Stavola, 1988; Lewis et al, 1994; Pearce et al, 1986).

Other chronic conditions have been examined in relation to multiple myeloma in eight studies; in at least one, relative risks above 1.4 have been reported for a history of allergies to drugs and household products, as well as a history of hyperthyroidism, hepatitis, osteomyelitis, chronic bronchitis, malaria, sinus infection, tuberculosis, disc disease and other musculoskeletal conditions, diabetes, gastric ulcer, myxedema, pyelonephritis, embedded shrapnel, and syphilis (Boffetta et al, 1989; Cuzick and De Stavola, 1988; Doody et al, 1992; Eriksson, 1993; Gallagher et al, 1983; Gramenzi et al, 1991; Koepsell et al, 1987; Lewis et al, 1994).

TABLE 43–2. *Design Characteristics of Studies That Have Assessed the Risk of Myeloma in Relation to Chronic Immune Stimulation*

Study	*Reference to Table 43–3*	*Study Design*	*Study Population*	*Study Period*
Vesterinen et al, 1993	1	Cohort incidence	Finland, asthma patients	1970–85
Lewis et al, 1994	2 (white) 3 (black)	Population-based case-control	Three metropolitan areas, USA	1986–89
Boffetta et al, 1989	4	Case-control, mortality	American Cancer Society members	1982–86
Cuzick and De Stavola, 1988	5, 6	Hospital-based case-control	Six areas in England and Wales	1978–84
Doody et al, 1992	7	Population-based case-control	Kaiser Permanente, Oregon, California	1956–82
Eriksson, 1993	8	Population-based case-control	Northern Sweden	1982–86
Gallagher et al, 1983	9	Tumor-registry-based case-control[a]	Vancouver, BC	1972–81
Gramenzi et al, 1991	10	Hospital-based case-control	Greater Milan area, northern Italy	1983–89
Koepsell et al, 1987	11	Population-based case-control	Four SEER areas, USA	1977–81
Linet et al, 1987, 1988	12	Hospital-based case-control	Baltimore, MD	1975–82
Pearce et al, 1986	13	Tumor-registry-based case-control[a]	New Zealand	1977–81

[a]Controls were registered with cancers other than multiple myeloma.

TABLE 43–3. *Summary of Studies That Have Assessed the Risk of Multiple Myeloma in Relation to Chronic Immune Stimulation*

Category	Reference from Table 43–2	Prevalence of Exposure in Controls (%)	No. of Exposed Cases	Relative Risk[a]	95% CI
ASTHMA					
Asthma	4	0.4	5	1.0	0.3–2.7
	5	7	19	0.7[b]	—
	13	9	9	1.3	0.6–2.9
	7	4	9	1.4	0.5–3.8
	1	—	38	0.5–1.1	—
	2	5	22	1.2	0.7–2.1
	3	6	16	1.3	0.7–2.3
ALLERGIES AND ALLERGY TREATMENTS					
Hay fever	4	7	14	1.6	0.8–2.9
	5	4	15	1.0[b]	—
	7	8	18	1.3	0.6–2.7
	13	15	19	1.9	1.0–3.5
	2	21	54	0.9	0.7–2.0
	3	18	40	1.1	0.7–1.6
"Allergies"	5	31	139	1.2[b]	—
	8	7	20	1.1	0.5–2.3
	9	11	24	3.1	1.6–6.3
	10	21	17	0.6	0.3–1.0
	12	22[c]	21[d]	1.0	0.5–2.3
Severe allergic reaction	2	11	35	0.9	0.6–1.4
	3	6	18	1.1	0.8–1.5
Allergy shots	2	8	18	0.7	0.4–1.3
	3	4	8	0.9	0.4–20
No. of allergy desensitization shots:					
1–99 vs. 0	11	2	4	0.5	0.1–1.6
≥100 vs. 0		2	9	1.2	0.6–2.6
Drug allergies	2	14	53	1.1	0.8–1.5
	3	5	18	1.6	0.9–2.9
Dust allergy	2	5	13	0.8	0.4–1.5
	3	4	9	1.2	0.5–2.5
Eczema	5	3	11	0.7[b]	—
	7	25	2	1.1–4.0	
	13	6	4	0.9	0.3–2.8
	2	5	19	1.2	0.7–2.0
	3	3	6	1.1	0.4–2.7
Household-products allergies	2	2	21	0.9	0.3–2.4
	3	18	40	1.1	0.7–1.6
Psoriasis	7	1	2	1.4	0.2–10
OTHER CHRONIC CONDITIONS					
Arthritis	4	32	39	0.9	0.6–1.5
	7	44	85	1.4	0.9–2.2
	8	3	9	1.4[b]	—
Bursitis	7	9	10	0.6	0.2–1.3
Chronic bronchitis	7	10	27	2.0	1.0–3.9
	10	11	15	1.3	0.7–2.4
	11	10	46	0.9	0.6–1.3
Chronic lung disease	2	6	21	0.8	0.5–1.4
	3	4	8	1.0	0.5–2.4
Colitis	2	5	18	0.9	0.5–1.5
	3	2	1	0.3	0.1–2.1
Diabetes	4	7	17	1.9	1.1–3.4
	8	14	22	0.7	0.3–1.4
	2	9	38	1.1	0.7–1.7
	3	16	36	1.0	0.6–1.4
Disc and other musculoskeletal disease	7	12	36	2.3	1.2–4.1
Gallbladder disease	8	5	10	1.0	0.4–2.7
Gastric ulcer	8	5	14	1.5	0.6–3.7
Gout	7	2	5	1.3	0.3–4.7
Hyperlipidemia	8	2	10	1.1	0.4–3.1
Hypertension	8	30	62	0.9	0.6–1.4

(continued)

TABLE 43–3. (*Continued*)

Category	Reference from Table 43–2	Prevalence of Exposure in Controls (%)	No. of Exposed Cases	Relative Risk[a]	95% CI
Hyperthyroidism	2	2	5	0.4	0.2–1.1
	3	2	7	1.5	0.6–3.7
Hypothyroidism	2	4	18	1.1	0.6–1.9
	3	2	2	0.5	0.1–2.3
Inflammatory bowel disease	8	6	9	0.6	0.2–1.5
Kidney disease	4	3	5	1.4	0.5–4.0
Malaria	10	4	7	1.8	0.7–4.5
	11	1	5	1.0	0.3–3.2
Use of a medical implant	11	7	32	1.0	0.6–1.6
Myxedema	9	1	6	5.0	1.0–25.7
Pyelonephritis	10	1	3	2.0	0.5–8.4
Embedded shrapnel	11	2	15	1.8	0.9–3.7
	2	6	16	0.8	0.4–1.4
	3	4	3	0.4	0.1–1.3
Sinus infection	7	4	5	0.8	0.3–2.5
	11	3	15	1.7	0.9–3.3
	2	12	32	0.8	0.5–1.2
	3	7	12	0.6	0.3–1.2
Syphilis	11	1	10	2.4	0.8–6.7
	2	0	2	11.6	0.8–173
	3	2	6	1.5	0.6–4.0
Thrombosis	8	9	19	0.8	0.4–1.6
Tuberculosis	7	5	11	2.0	0.8–5.5
	8	5	12	1.1	0.4–2.8
	10	3	8	2.3	0.9–5.7
	11	2	17	1.7	0.9–3.2
	2	2	5	0.8	0.3–2.2
	3	3	2	0.3	0.1–1.3
ACUTE CONDITIONS					
Blood transfusion	11	25	129	1.1	0.8–1.4
	2	19	83	1.1	0.8–1.5
	3	19	45	1.0	0.7–1.5
Chicken pox	5	68	198	1.0[b]	—
	10	47	42	0.7	0.5–1.1
	11	70	334	0.9	0.7–1.2
	2	70	235	0.8	0.6–1.1
	3	66	131	0.9	0.6–1.2
Ear infection	2	9	22	0.7	0.4–1.2
	3	2	2	0.4	0.1–1.6
Gonorrhea	11	4	18	0.7	0.4–1.3
	2	2	7	1.6	0.6–3.9
	3	12	2	0.4	0.1–1.6
Hepatitis	11	2	4	0.3	0.1–1.0
	2	4	8	0.7	0.3–1.6
	3	1	3	1.5	0.4–5.4
Horse serum injections	11	4	22	1.3	0.7–2.5
Infectious mononucleosis	5	4	9	0.5[b]	—
	10	1	2	0.4	0.1–2.6
	11	1	4	0.8	0.1–3.5
	2	2	6	1.2	0.5–3.0
Insect sting	11	79	397	1.1	0.8–1.5
Lymphoid tissue surgery	12	20	25	1.2[b]	0.6–2.6
Measles	5	83	259	0.8[b]	—
	10	60	69	1.0	0.6–1.5
	11	89	424	1.1	0.7–1.6
Mumps	5	58	184	1.1[b]	—
	10	41	45	1.0	0.7–1.6
	11	73	364	1.2	0.9–1.6
	2	64	221	1.0	0.8–1.3
	3	69	134	0.8	0.6–1.2

(continued)

TABLE 43–3. *Summary of Studies That Have Assessed the Risk of Multiple Myeloma in Relation to Chronic Immune Stimulation* (*Continued*)

Category	Reference from Table 43–2	Prevalence of Exposure in Controls (%)	No. of Exposed Cases	Relative Risk[a]	95% CI
Osteomyelitis	11	1	11	1.4	0.6–3.1
	2	0.4	3	1.7	0.4–7.9
	3	0.6	3	2.3	0.6–9.4
Pelvic infection	7	3	7	2.1	0.5–8.5
Pneumonia	11	0.3	3	1.2	0.3–5.3
	2	2	9	1.1	0.5–2.4
	3	1	4	2.6	0.7–9.2
Polio	11	1	3	0.7	0.2–2.3
	2	2	5	0.9	0.3–2.5
Rheumatic fever	5	5	9	1.4	0.6–3.2
	7	1	3	1.5	0.3–9.0
	8	1	2	0.9[b]	—
	11	3	21	1.6	0.9–2.7
	2	3	15	1.4	0.7–2.7
	3	4	7	0.7	0.3–1.6
Rubella	5	26	71	1.0[b]	—
	10	14	15	0.8	0.5–1.4
Scarlet fever	5	16	61	1.0[b]	—
	10	8	17	2.0	1.1–3.9
	11	14	54	0.9	0.6–1.3
	2	10	36	0.9	0.6–1.4
	3	3	6	1.0	0.4–2.4
Shingles	5	15	101	1.9[b]	—
	7	1	7	2.7	0.7–11
	8	3	5	0.7	0.2–2.3
	10	6	13	1.6	0.8–3.3
	11	8	50	1.3	0.9–1.9
	2	10	39	1.0	0.7–1.5
	3	3	11	1.7	0.8–3.6
Snakebite	11	3	6	0.4	0.2–1.0
Strep throat	2	7	19	0.9	0.5–1.5
	3	3	1	0.2	0.0–1.3
Throat, tonsil, or ear infection	11	2	14	1.8	0.8–3.9
Tonsillitis	2	10	25	0.8	0.5–1.2
	3	5	7	0.6	0.3–1.3
Tonsillectomy	5	29	90	0.9[b]	—
	2	54	166	0.8	0.6–1.0
	3	22	38	0.8	0.5–1.1
Tooth abscess	11	49	255	1.2	1.0–1.5
Typhus	10	6	9	1.2	0.6–2.6
Whooping cough	5	30	92	1.0[b]	—
	10	28	35	1.1	0.7–1.7
Urinary tract infection	7	4	7	1.3	0.5–3.5
	11	24	138	1.3	1.0–1.7
	2 (men)	10	37	1.0	0.7–1.5
	2 (women)	19	24	0.9	0.5–1.5
	3 (men)	9	15	2.0	1.1–3.8
	3 (women)	8	8	1.0	0.4–2.3
IMMUNIZATIONS					
BCG	5	7	27	1.0[b]	—
	10	5	11	3.0	1.4–6.4
Cholera	5	10	45	1.2[b]	—
Diphtheria	5	4	28	1.8[b]	—
	10	14	10	0.9	0.4–1.8
Influenza	11	60	259	0.8	0.7–1.0
	2	59	220	1.1	0.8–1.4
	3	51	100	0.9	0.7–1.2
Polio	5	13	48	0.9[b]	—
	10	24	28	0.9	0.6–1.4
	11	54	215	0.9	0.7–1.2
	2	63	213	1.0	0.8–1.4
	3	46	82	0.8	0.6–1.1

(continued)

TABLE 43–3. (*Continued*)

Category	Reference from Table 43–2	Prevalence of Exposure in Controls (%)	No. of Exposed Cases	Relative Risk[a]	95% CI
Scarlet fever	5	1	7	2.2[b]	—
Smallpox	5	62	255	1.1[b]	—
	10	83	91	0.7	0.4–1.3
	11	91	419	0.8	0.5–1.1
	2	76	277	1.0	0.7–1.4
	3	66	138	1.1	0.7–1.5
Tetanus	5	47	177	1.0[b]	—
	10	78	70	0.6	0.4–1.0
	11	59	262	0.8	0.6–1.0
	2	76	262	1.0	0.8–1.4
	3	57	119	1.2	0.8–1.7
Typhoid	5	15	61	1.0[b]	—
Typhus	5	6	28	1.1[b]	—
Whooping cough	5	2	12	1.7[b]	—
Yellow fever	5	7	35	1.3[b]	—

[a]Comparison is ever vs. never unless otherwise specified.
[b]Unadjusted odds ratio.
[c]Included hay fever, asthma, eczema, recurrent hives, insect sting allergy, and treatment with desensitization procedures.
[d]No. of discordant pairs in which only the case was exposed.

Most of these associations were unconfirmed in a second report; however, one merits closer attention. For a history of tuberculosis, relative risks of 1.7 to 2.3 were reported in three studies (Doody et al, 1992; Gramenzi et al, 1991; Koepsell et al, 1987), although two others reported odds ratios closer to 1.0 (Eriksson, 1993; Lewis et al, 1994).

Other chronic conditions that have been examined and observed not to be associated with myeloma include a history of bursitis, degenerative joint disease, gallbladder disease, chronic lung disease, hypothyroidism, gout, hyperlipidemia, hypertension, inflammatory bowel disease, kidney disease, use of a medical implant, and thrombosis (Boffetta et al, 1989; Doody et al, 1992; Eriksson, 1992; Gramenzi et al, 1991; Koepsell et al, 1987; Lewis et al, 1994).

Prior histories of specific acute conditions have been examined in six studies, and associations greater than 1.4 have been reported in one or more studies for pneumonia; urinary tract infection; pelvic infections; scarlet fever; throat, tonsil, or ear infection; acute or chronic rheumatic fever; and shingles (Cuzick and De Stavola, 1988; Doody et al, 1992; Gramenzi et al, 1991; Koepsell et al, 1987; Lewis et al, 1994; Linet et al, 1987), of which the former three have not been confirmed. With respect to a history of rheumatic fever, four studies found odds ratios of 1.4–1.6 (Lewis et al, 1994; Gramenzi et al, 1991; Doody et al, 1991; Koepsell et al, 1987), although a fifth study reported an odds ratio of 0.9 (Eriksson, 1993). In three of five studies that ascertained a history of shingles, it was noted to be more prevalent among myeloma cases than controls; however, most investigators suggested that because of the temporal proximity of the infection to the recognition of myeloma it most likely was a manifestation of the as-yet-undiagnosed malignancy.

Other acute conditions that have been examined and observed not to be associated with myeloma include a history of blood transfusion, chicken pox, gonorrhea, hepatitis, horse serum injections, infectious mononucleosis, insect sting, lymphoid tissue surgery, measles, mumps, osteomyelitis, pneumonia, polio, Rubella, snakebite, tonsillectomy, tooth abscess, typhus, urinary tract infection, and whooping cough (Cuzick and De Stavola, 1988; Doody et al, 1992; Gramenzi et al, 1991; Koepsell et al, 1987; Linet et al, 1987; Lewis et al, 1994).

Immunization histories have been examined in four studies, and odds ratios exceeding 1.4 have been reported for a history of BCG, diphtheria, scarlet fever, and whooping cough vaccines (Cuzick and De Stavola, 1988; Gramenzi et al, 1991; Koepsell et al, 1987; Lewis et al, 1994), but none of the positive associations has been confirmed in a second study. Vaccines that have been observed not to be related to myeloma risk include cholera, influenza, polio, smallpox, tetanus, typhoid, typhus, and yellow fever (Cuzick and De Stavola, 1988; Gramenzi et al, 1991; Koepsell et al, 1987; Lewis et al, 1994).

With respect to Waldenström's macroglobulinemia, Linet and coworkers (1993) observed no relationship of the disease with a history of the following: chronic bacterial infections (OR = 1.0, 95% CI, 0.5–2.1), subacute viral disease (OR = 0.5, 95% CI, 0.1–3.8), allergy-related conditions (OR = 1.1, 95% CI, 0.5–2.1), or surgical excision of lymphoid tissue (OR = 1.1, 95% CI, 0.5–2.4).

In summary, there is little evidence that chronic immune stimulation increases myeloma risk, although specific diseases may play a role.

Ionizing Radiation

Studies of persons exposed to the atomic bombs, of nuclear workers, of radiology workers, and of recipients of therapeutic and diagnostic radiation have been reported and are summarized in Table 43–4.

Two studies have been published of myeloma risk in Japanese survivors of the atomic bombs detonated in Hiroshima and Nagasaki in 1945. The study of Shimizu et al (1990) was of myeloma mortality during the period 1950 through 1985, while that of Preston et al (1994) was of incidence from 1950 through 1987. The design and methods differed appreciably between the two studies, as did the findings. Shimizu et al (1990) ascertained 36 persons whose primary cause of death was myeloma and for whom DS86 revised doses had been estimated among the approximately 75,000 persons who were in the cities at the time of the bomb, and they observed a slope in the relationship of radiation dose and myeloma risk such that the RR was 3.29 (90% CI, 1.67–6.31) following exposure to 1 Gray (Gy) bone marrow dose (see notes to Table 43–4 regarding units of dose). The mean bone marrow dose in the cohort was 0.14 Gy (corresponding RR of 1.18). Preston et al (1994) ascertained 59 persons whose first cancer diagnosis was myeloma and whose DS86 kerma doses were estimated to be less than 4 Gy. After adjusting for age at diagnosis and age at the time of the bomb, they observed a relative risk of 1.25 ($p > 0.05$) per Sievert (Sv). Including persons whose myeloma was a second primary or whose doses exceeded 4 Gy increased the RR to 1.9 ($p = 0.02$). More than 99% of the radiation from the atomic bomb was reported as gamma radiation, so the dose in Sv would be approximately equal to the dose in Gy in this study.

Radiation-exposed workers at three U.S. nuclear weapons plants were found to be at increased risk of death relative to their unexposed peers (Gilbert et al, 1989). A direct relationship between dose and mortality was observed, with workers who received 0.050–0.099, 0.010–0.199, and 0.200 Sv or more of external radiation being at 3.3-fold (n = 1), 5.0-fold (n = 1), and 33-fold (n = 1) increased risk, respectively, relative to the general population. British radiation workers at major sites of the nuclear industry were at lower risk of death from myeloma than the general population, with a standard mortality ratio (SMR) of 71 (no. of exposed cases = 17), but there was a trend ($p = 0.06$) of increasing risk with increasing level of exposure such that workers exposed to 0.400 or more Sv (n = 2) were at 3.4-fold higher risk than those exposed to less than 0.010 Sv (n = 5) (Kendall et al, 1992). A study conducted at the Sellafield nuclear fuels plant, in which there were seven deaths from myeloma, also showed a direct relationship between dose and mortality, with workers receiving an external dose of 0.200 Sv or more being at 5.0-fold (n = 2) increased risk relative to the general population (Smith and Douglas, 1986). A study of persons exposed occupationally to considerably lower levels of radiation (< 0.01 Sv) observed no excess risk (Beral et al, 1985). British workers who participated in atmospheric nuclear weapons testing were at 50% increased risk of death from multiple myeloma (90% CI, 0.55–4.26); their radiation doses were not estimated (Darby et al, 1993). New Zealand participants in the same testing were not at increased risk (SIR = 0 vs. 5.56 in unexposed workers, 90% CI, 0.0–3.1) (Pearce et al, 1990). Czech uranium miners with cumulative radon exposures of 210–329 and 330 or more "working level months" were at 1.9-fold (n = 1) and 4.4-fold (n = 2) excess risk of myeloma (Tomášek et al, 1993). In addition, the American Cancer Society case-control study noted a 1.9-fold excess in mortality (95% CI, 0.8–4.8) following occupational exposure to X rays and radioactive materials (Boffetta et al, 1989).

Two cohort studies of medical radiology workers have been conducted. In China, no myeloma cases were diagnosed, though only 0.5 were expected, among 27,000 radiology workers (Wang et al, 1988). In the United States, physicians listed by the American Board of Radiologists in 1950 or 1960 were at a 5-fold increased risk of dying from multiple myeloma (95% CI, 1.6–12) (Lewis, 1963).

Doses received during therapeutic irradiation can be high. However, both therapeutic and diagnostic irradiation are directed to a focal area, whereas the doses received by the atomic bomb survivors and by occupational cohorts were relatively uniform over the body. Three cohort studies and five case-control studies of the relationship between multiple myeloma and therapeutic irradiation have been reported. Risk of multiple myeloma was increased among women who were estimated to have received a mean bone marrow dose of 10 Gy during therapy for cervical cancer; after 15 years, there was a 2.0-fold excess (95% CI, 1.1–3.2) (Boice et al, 1985). Boice et al (1988) also conducted a nested case-control study using the cervical cancer cohort described above, along with additional subjects, to obtain more-precise information on radiation exposures. In the case-control study, no excess risk was noted among women who received an average marrow dose of 7.1 Gy compared to those who received less than 2.0 Gy (OR = 0.3, 90% CI, 0.1–1.4); no relationship was ob-

TABLE 43–4. *Summary of Studies That Have Assessed the Risk of Multiple Myeloma in Relation to Ionizing Radiation*

Study	*Study Location and Design*	*Study Period*	*Comparison*[a]	*No. of Exposed Cases*	*Relative Risk*	*95% CI*
A-BOMB SURVIVORS						
Shimizu et al, 1990	Japan, cohort mortality	1950–85	Increased risk per 1 Gy bone marrow dose	23	3.3	1.7–6.3
Preston et al, 1994	Japan, cohort incidence	1950–87	Increased risk per Sv bone marrow dose	59	1.25	—
NUCLEAR WORKERS						
Gilbert et al, 1989	Three U.S. nuclear weapons plants, cohort mortality	1943–81	External dose ≥10 years earlier, Sv 0.001–0.009 vs. general population 0.010–0.049 0.050–0.099 0.100–0.199 ≥0.200	8 1 1 1 1	0.9 0.4 3.3 5.0 33	— — — — —
Kendall et al, 1992	National Registry for Radiation Workers, UK, cohort mortality	1976–83	Registered persons vs. general population	17	0.71	—
Smith and Douglas, 1986	Sellafield plant, UK, cohort mortality	1947–83	External dose ≥15 years earlier, Sv <0.050 vs. general population 0.050–0.199 ≥0.200 Sv	3 2 2	0.7 1.3 5.0	— — —
Beral et al, 1985	UK Atomic Energy Authority, cohort mortality	1946–79	Employed by AEA vs. general population, median external dose <0.010 Sv	8	0.8	0.4–1.6
Pearce et al, 1990	New Zealand, cohort mortality	1957–87	Nuclear weapons test workers vs. unexposed workers; doses not estimated	0	0.0	0.0–3.1(b)
Darby et al, 1993	UK, case-control	1952–90	Nuclear weapons test workers vs. unexposed workers; doses not estimated	6	1.51	0.55–4.26 (b)
Boffetta et al, 1989	American Cancer Society, U.S., nested case-control	1982–86	Ever vs. never occupationally exposed to X rays or radioactive materials	7	1.9	0.8–4.8
RADIOLOGY WORKERS						
Wang et al, 1988	China, cohort incidence	1950–80	Diagnostic X-ray workers vs. general population	0	0.0	0–6.0
Lewis, 1963	U.S. radiologists, cohort mortality	1948–61	Employed as radiologist vs. general population	5	5.0	1.6–12
THERAPEUTIC IRRADIATION						
Boice et al, 1985	International, cohort incidence	—	Exposed to cervical radiation ≥15 years vs. unexposed; average bone marrow dose approximately 10 Gy	33	2.0	1.1–3.2
Darby et al, 1987	England and N. Ireland ankylosing spondylitis patients, cohort mortality	1935–83	Single course of X-ray treatment ≥5 years earlier vs. none; skeletal dose approx. 3 Gy	8	1.7	—
Boice et al, 1988	International, case-control of cervical cancer patients	—	Bone marrow dose: 2–4 vs. <2 Gy 5–9 vs. <2 Gy ≥10 vs. <2 Gy	12 23 11	0.3 0.2 0.6	0.0–2.6[b] 0.0–1.4[b] 0.1–5.2[b]
Boffetta et al, 1989	See above	See above	X-ray treatment vs. none	14	1.6	0.8–3.0
Darby et al, 1994	Scotland, metropathia hemorrhagica patients, cohort mortality	1940–86	Radiographic treatment ≤5 years earlier vs. general population, mean bone marrow dose = 1.3 Gy	9	2.6	1.2–4.9
Eriksson et al, 1993	Northern Sweden, population-based case-control	1982–86	Ever vs. never received radiotherapy	10	0.7	0.3–1.8

(continued)

TABLE 43–4. *Summary of Studies That Have Assessed the Risk of Multiple Myeloma in Relation to Ionizing Radiation (Continued)*

Study	*Study Location and Design*	*Study Period*	*Comparison*[a]	*No. of Exposed Cases*	*Relative Risk*	*95% CI*
Flodin et al, 1987	Southeast Sweden, population-based case-control	1973–83	X-ray treatment vs. none	4	0.9	0.3–2.7
Friedman, 1986	Kaiser Permanente, northern California, population-based case-control	1969–82	Ever vs. never exposed to X-ray therapy	9(c)	1.9	0.9–4.2
DIAGNOSTIC IRRADIATION						
Andersson and Storm, 1992	Danish neurology patients, cohort mortality	1946–88	Thorotrast injection vs. general population	4	4.6	1.2–12
Davis et al, 1989	Massachusetts tuberculosis patients, cohort mortality	1925–86	Ever vs. never received X-ray fluoroscopy exam; mean dose = 0.09 Gy	2	0.4	0.1–1.8
Boffetta et al, 1989	See above	See above	Diagnostic X-rays, above vs. below median number, median not reported	62	0.9	0.6–1.4
Boice et al, 1991	Kaiser Permanente, population-based case-control	1956–82	Bone marrow dose > 2 years earlier:	198 exposed to ≥ 0.01 Gy		
			0.01 vs. 0 Gy		1.3	—
			0.02 vs. 0 Gy		1.5	—
			0.03 vs. 0 Gy		1.3	—
			0.04 vs. 0 Gy		3.9	—
Cuzick and De Stavola, 1988	England and Wales, hospital-based case-control	1978–84	Number of diagnostic X rays:			
			1–4 vs. 0	86	0.8[d]	—
			5–8 vs. 0	79	0.7[d]	—
			≥ 9 vs. 0	181	0.7[d]	—
Eriksson, 1993	See above	See above	≥ 5 vs. ≤ 4	65	0.6	0.3–1.1
			6–10 vs. ≤ 4	29	0.5	0.3–0.9
			11–20 vs. ≤ 4	20	0.8	0.4–1.5
			≥ 21 vs. ≤ 4	16	0.9	0.4–2.1
Flodin et al, 1987	See above	See above	Heavy vs. light X-ray exam 10–30 years earlier	2	2.9	0.4–19

[a]Studies of ionizing radiation use various units of dose, including Sievert (Sv) and Gray (Gy), which are Standard International units, and rem (1 Sv = 100 rem) and rad (1 Gy = 100 rad). Sv is related to Gy as follows: Sv = Gy × Q, where Q is the "quality factor," i.e., the biological potency of the specific type of radiation relative to orthovoltage X rays; although not standardized, gamma rays are often assigned a Q of 1, and fast neutrons a Q of 10. Dose can be expressed as external radiation dose (whole body dose, shielded kerma) or organ dose.
[b]90% confidence interval.
[c]No. of discordant pairs in which only the case was exposed.
[d]Unadjusted odds ratio.

served even after excluding women who had been followed for less than 15 years. Furthermore, the investigators found no evidence that risk increased with increasing radiation dose above 2 Gy. The authors stated that the only differences between the case-control and cohort studies were:

1. The number of women with multiple myeloma—34 in the cohort and 46 in the case-control study.
2. The comparison group—population rates were used for the cohort study, while cervical cancer patients who did not undergo radiotherapy were used for the case-control study.

Compared with individuals who had never undergone X-ray therapy, myeloma mortality was modestly elevated in a cohort of patients receiving a single course of X-ray treatment for ankylosing spondylitis (RR = 1.7, n = 8) (Darby et al, 1987) or metropathia hemorrhagica (RR = 2.6, 95% CI, 1.2–4.9) (Darby et al, 1994), among American Cancer Society subjects who had received X-ray treatment for any condition (OR = 1.6, 95% CI, 0.8–3.0) (Boffetta et al, 1989), and among Kaiser Permanente members who had received X-ray treatment for any condition (OR = 1.9, 95% CI, 0.9–4.2) (Friedman, 1986), but not among subjects who reported a history of radiotherapy for any condition in two Swedish population-based case-control studies, however (OR = 0.9, 95% CI, 0.3–2.7; OR = 0.7, 95% CI, 0.3–2.7) (Flodin et al, 1987; Eriksson, 1993, respectively).

Compared with the general population, myeloma incidence was elevated 4.6-fold (95% CI, 1.2–12) among

1,095 Danish patients exposed to alpha-emitting Thorotrast used with cerebral arteriography (Andersson and Storm, 1992). A single, diagnostic X-ray received by Massachusetts tuberculosis patients did not increase their risk of multiple myeloma (RR = 0.4, 95% CI, 0.1–1.8) (Davis et al, 1989). Having a relatively large number of diagnostic X rays (more than the median) did not increase myeloma risk among American Cancer Society members (OR = 0.9, 95% CI, 0.6–1.4) (Boffetta et al, 1989); nor did having nine or more diagnostic X rays in a UK case-control study (unadjusted OR = 0.7 relative to having no exams, no. of exposed individuals = 81) (Cuzick and De Stavola, 1988). In a Swedish case-control study conducted between 1973 and 1983, individuals who received "heavy" levels of X-ray examinations were at 2.9-fold excess risk of myeloma (95% CI, 0.4–19) relative to individuals who received "light" levels (Flodin et al, 1987). In a later study set in northern Sweden, risk was reduced among persons who reported a history of five or more X rays compared to those who reported a history of four or fewer; however, risk increased with increasing numbers of examinations such that exposure to 21 or more resulted in an odds ratio of 0.9 (95% CI, 0.4–2.1), compared to the odds ratio of 0.5 (95% CI, 0.3–0.9) for exposure to 6 to 10 examinations (Eriksson, 1993). At Kaiser Permanente, bone marrow doses of 0.04 Gy or more were related to a 3.9-fold increased risk of myeloma, and there was some evidence that increasing doses were related to increasing risk (see Table 43–4) (Boice et al, 1991). The authors remarked that categorizing the data on the basis of number of procedures resulted in substantial misclassification; for example, five or fewer X-ray procedures led to a range in the bone marrow dose of 0.00001–0.03 Gy, while the range for 15 or more procedures was 0.001–0.23 Gy. The discordance between the number of prior X-ray examinations and bone marrow dose was caused by differences in procedures; for example, an upper gastrointestinal procedure contributed 60 times more radiation to the bone marrow than a chest roentgenogram (Boice et al, 1991). Failure to take into account this source of misclassification may account for the negative findings in the studies of Boffetta et al (1989), Cuzick and De Stavola (1988), and Eriksson (1993).

There is evidence from studies of atomic bomb survivors, occupational groups with exposure to approximately 0.05 Sv or more, persons exposed to therapeutic radiation, and from a carefully conducted study of diagnostic procedures (Boice et al, 1991) that ionizing radiation causes multiple myeloma. It has also been reported that ionizing radiation caused MGUS and multiple myeloma in rhesus monkeys (Radl et al, 1991). However, there are inconsistencies in the body of evidence—for example, from the two studies of the atomic bomb survivors and from the two studies of women who received radiotherapy for cervical cancer. There are also differences in the reported dose-response relationships, but this could be related to differences in the quality and timing of exposure.

Occupational Exposures

Since myeloma is a relatively rare cancer, cohort studies of the relation between occupational exposures and multiple myeloma have generally provided only limited information. The only cohort studies in which there were large numbers of myeloma cases have been those using census data; in such studies job title as recorded in the census was the only occupational exposure variable that could be evaluated. Although respondents in most interview-based case-control studies were asked whether they had ever been exposed to specific chemical and physical agents, it is possible that they knew the agents by different names. Also, it is possible that cases, particularly those exposed to agents known to be hazardous, better recalled their exposures than controls. An additional difficulty in summarizing over many studies concerns the varied occupational standards and practices in use over time and place. The case-control studies generally were of limited power as well, in that only a small number of subjects had worked in the occupations and industries of interest and only abbreviated occupational histories could be obtained. An exception is the case-control study reported by Heineman et al (1992a) and Pottern et al (1992b); it was based on work histories recorded in a national pension plan and included approximately 800 men and 600 women with myeloma.

Occupational cohort studies in which workers were exposed to only a limited number of chemical and physical agents and case-control studies that elicited information concerning both occupational and leisure-time exposures to such agents have provided information concerning the relationship between exposure to specific agents and multiple myeloma occurrence. Characteristics of case-control studies that have evaluated the relation between occupational exposures and multiple myeloma are summarized in Table 43–5. Results concerning specific agents are discussed first. Results from occupational cohort studies in which specific agents could not be isolated, and from case-control studies of job title and industry group, are discussed in the subsequent section.

Specific Chemical and Physical Agents. Numerous reports of the relationship between multiple myeloma and exposure to asbestos, benzene, pesticides, paints and solvents, engine exhaust, and metals have been published.

Asbestos. Asbestos was postulated as a lymphoid-sys-

TABLE 43–5. *Design Characteristics of Case-control Studies That Have Assessed the Risk of Multiple Myeloma in Relation to Chemical and Physical Agents, Job Title, or Industry Group**

Study	*Study Population and Period*	*Ascertainment of Exposure*
Alavanja et al, 1988	Death certificates of persons who were employed at the U.S. Department of Agriculture	History of employment as an agricultural extension agent ascertained from work records, 1970–79
Bethwaite et al, 1990	Persons registered with the New Zealand tumor registry, 1981–84	Most recent occupation at time of registration
Boffetta et al, 1989	American Cancer Society members, 1982–86	Most recent occupation, occupation held for the longest period, and occupational and leisure-time exposure to 12 groups of agents recorded on a mailed questionnaire completed in 1982
Brownson et al, 1989	Persons registered with the Missouri tumor registry, 1984–88	Most recent occupation at time of registration
Burmeister et al, 1983	Death certificates, Iowa, 1964–78	Most recent occupation as recorded on the death certificate
Burmeister, 1990	Persons registered with myeloma in the Iowa tumor registry and persons from the general population, 1982–84	Exposure to various pesticides ascertained during interview (not further described)
Cantor and Blair, 1984	Death certificates, Wisconsin, 1968–76	Most recent occupation as recorded on the death certificate
Cuzick and De Stavola, 1988	Hospital patients, six areas in England and Wales, 1978–84	Occupational history and occupational exposure to various agents ascertained during interview
Demers et al, 1992	Persons registered with myeloma and persons from the general population, four SEER areas, U.S., 1977–81	Work history categorized by job title and industry as ascertained during interview
Eriksson and Karlsson, 1992	Persons registered with myeloma and persons from the general population, northern Sweden, 1982–86	Occupational history and occupational exposure to various agents ascertained during interview
Flodin et al, 1987	Persons with myeloma admitted to three hospitals and persons from the general population, southeast Sweden, 1973–83	Occupational history and occupational exposure to various agents ascertained from a mailed questionnaire
Friedman, 1986	Kaiser Permanante members, northern California, 1969–82	Occupation recorded on the medical chart ≥ 6 months prior to reference date
Gallagher et al, 1983	Patients admitted to a Vancouver, BC, cancer center, 1972–81	Occupational history ascertained from interview
Heineman et al, 1992a	Men identified with myeloma and persons from the general population, Denmark, 1970–84	Industrial history recorded since 1964 in the nationwide pension fund program; occupation recorded on the most recent tax records; industrial-hygienist-developed job-exposure matrix
Kawachi et al, 1989	Persons registered with the New Zealand tumor registry, 1980–84	Most recent occupation at time of registration
LaVecchia et al, 1989	Hospital patients, Milan, 1983–88	Occupational history and occupational exposures to various agents ascertained during interview
Linet et al, 1987	Hospital patients, Baltimore, Maryland, 1975–82	Occupational history and occupational exposure to various agents ascertained during interview
Milham, 1971	Death certificates, Washington and Oregon, 1950–67	Most recent occupation as recorded on the death certificate
Morris et al, 1986	Persons identified with myeloma and persons from the general population, four SEER areas, U.S., 1977–81	Formation of ever/never categories of exposure to various agents from responses to specific questions about a history of "high" exposure to various substances, open-ended questions about a history of exposure to "other" agents and occupational history ascertained during interview
Nandakumar et al, 1986	Death certificates, Western Australia, 1975–84	Most recent occupation as recorded on the death certificate
Pasqualetti et al, 1990	Hospital patients resident in the referral basin of Aquila and Avezzano, Italy, 1970–88	Occupational history and ever exposure to classes of chemicals ascertained during interview

(continued)

TABLE 43–5. (*Continued*)

Study	Study Population and Period	Ascertainment of Exposure
Pottern et al, 1992b	Women identified with myeloma and persons from the general population, Denmark, 1970–84	Industrial history recorded since 1964 in the nationwide pension fund program; occupation recorded on the most recent tax records; industrial-hygienist-developed job-exposure matrix
Reif et al, 1989a	Persons registered with the New Zealand tumor registry, 1980–84	Most recent occupation at time of registration
Reif et al, 1989b	Persons registered with the New Zealand tumor registry, 1980–84	Most recent occupation at time of registration
Schwartz et al, 1988	Persons identified with myeloma and persons from the general population, four SEER areas, U.S., 1977–81	Probability and intensity of exposure to low, medium, and high levels of asbestos based on a job-exposure matrix from an occupational history ascertained during interview
Tollerud et al, 1985	Death certificates, North Carolina, 1956–80	Most recent occupation as recorded on the death certificate

*Excluding occupations and occupational exposures related to ionizing radiation.

tem carcinogen following the publication of case reports of men with both asbestosis and B-cell neoplasms, as well as animal and human studies that demonstrated increased production of M-components in relation to asbestosis and asbestos exposure (Kagan, 1985). Nine epidemiological studies have examined the relationship between a history of asbestos exposure and multiple myeloma. A Danish cohort of all employees in an asbestos-cement plant, followed from their employment as early as 1928 through 1984, noted a 1.7-fold increased risk of myeloma (95% CI, 0.7–3.3) (Raffin et al, 1989). In interview-based case-control studies conducted in the UK (OR = 3.6, no. of exposed cases = 1) (Cuzick and De Stavola, 1988), Italy (OR = 6.1, no. of exposed cases = 2) (LaVecchia et al, 1989) (OR = 4.0, 95% CI, 2.0–8.1) (Pasqualetti et al, 1990), and Baltimore (OR = 3.5, 95% CI, 1.0–12) (Linet et al, 1987), individuals with a history of occupational exposure to asbestos had a 3- to 6-fold increased risk of myeloma, but in four other case-control studies, no evidence for a relationship was found (Boffetta et al, 1989; Eriksson and Karlsson, 1992; Heineman et al, 1992a; Schwartz et al, 1988).

Benzene. Rinsky et al (1987) developed a job-exposure matrix using industrial hygiene data from an Ohio rubber plant and found a 4.1-fold increased risk (95% CI, 1.1–11) of multiple myeloma among benzene-exposed workers followed from 1950 to 1981. All of the myeloma cases were diagnosed 20 years or later after first exposure, but no patterns of risk with cumulative level of benzene exposure were apparent. Decouflé et al (1983) identified two cases of multiple myeloma in a cohort of chemical workers principally exposed to benzene (total number of lymphatic and hematopoietic tissue cancers expected was 1.1). In case-control studies, however, neither Linet et al (1987) nor Heineman et al (1992a) found a relationship between a history of occupational exposure to benzene and myeloma occurrence (OR = 1.2, 95% CI, 0.4–3.6; OR = 1.0, 95% CI, 0.6–1.7, respectively).

Pesticides. Following the observation that agricultural workers were at increased risk of multiple myeloma (discussed later), it was hypothesized that exposure to pesticides was the basis for the association. A history of pesticide exposure in relation to multiple myeloma has been examined in 14 reports.

In Seveso, Italy, where an industrial accident in 1976 exposed the local population to 2,3,7,8-tetrachlorodibenzo-*p*-dioxin, the risk of myeloma in the subsequent 10 years was elevated in both men (RR = 3.2, 95% CI, 0.8–13.3) and women (RR = 5.2, 95% CI, 1.2–22.6) (Bertazzi et al, 1993). Concentrations of the chemical in serum taken from 13 persons soon after the accident ranged from 74 to 526 parts per trillion. In a cohort study of Dutch licensed herbicide applicators, myeloma mortality was elevated by a factor of 8.2 (95% CI, 1.6–23) compared with the general population (Swaen et al, 1992). The most heavily used herbicides to which the applicators were exposed during the time period of interest were simazine, chlorothiamide, dalapon, dichlorbenil, and diuron. In a cohort study set from 1965 to 1982 in which Swedish agricultural pesticide applicators licensed during 1965–1976 were compared with agricultural workers who had not been exposed to pesticides, Wiklund et al (1989) did not find an increased risk of multiple myeloma (OR = 1.0, 95% CI, 0.5–1.9). Two case-control studies that also took into account a history of agricultural work when examining the relation between pesticide use and myeloma occurrence observed that myeloma risk was greater among individuals exposed to both factors than among individuals exposed to either factor alone. Boffetta et al (1989) reported the following results: compared with neither exposure—pesticides alone, OR = 1.0; farming alone, OR = 1.7, both pesticides and farming, OR = 4.3. The results of Demers et al (1992) were as follows: pesticides alone, OR = 2.1; farming alone, OR = 1.4; both pesticides and farming, OR = 7.9. Four other case-control studies, which did not take into account possible bias caused by the relationship between other aspects of agricultural work and pesticide use, also provided evidence for a positive association of pesticide use with multiple myeloma (Burmeister, 1990; Eriksson and Karlsson, 1992; Flodin et al, 1987; Pasqualetti et al, 1990). In Denmark, a relationship was found in women (OR = 1.9, 95% CI, 0.4–8.4) (Pottern et al, 1992b) but not men (OR = 0.9, 95% CI, 0.5–1.5) (Heineman et al, 1992a). Besides the cohort study of Wiklund et al (1989), the only other studies that observed no relationship between a history of exposure to pesticides and myeloma occurrence were those of LaVecchia et al (1989) (unadjusted OR = 0.9; no. of exposed cases = 4) and Pearce et al (1986) (phenoxyherbicides, OR = 1.3, 95% CI, 0.8–2.5; chlorophenols, OR = 1.1, 95% CI, 0.4–2.7).

Paints and solvents. Painters are exposed to dyes and pigments, dusts, aromatic and aliphatic hydrocarbons, and low-molecular-weight solvents such as trichloroethylene and methylethyl ketone (Bethwaite et al, 1990). Six of the eight epidemiologic studies that have assessed it provide evidence for a relationship between a history of exposure to paint and solvents and multiple myeloma risk. A cohort study of Swedish production workers in nine paint-manufacturing companies who were employed for five years or longer during 1955–1975 observed a 5.5-fold elevated risk (95% CI, 1.1–16) of myeloma among paint-industry workers; all of the workers who developed myeloma had received "high" exposures (RR = 10, n = 3) (Lundberg, 1986). A second Swedish cohort study using census information on occupation observed a 1.7-fold excess risk (n = 7) (McLaughlin et al, 1988). In four case-control studies, odds ratios of 1.9–3.0 were reported (Bethwaite et al, 1990; Cuzick and De Stavola, 1988; Demers et al, 1992; Friedman, 1986) but no association was observed in studies conducted in Italy (unadjusted OR = 0.9, no. of exposed cases = 5) (LaVecchia et al, 1989) or Denmark (women, OR = 0.7, 95% CI, 0.3–1.7; men, OR = 1.0, 95% CI, 0.5–2.1) (Pottern et al, 1992b; Heineman et al, 1992a). One study reported that risk increased with duration of employment (less than 10 years, OR = 1.4, 95% CI, 0.6–2.8; 10 years or longer, OR = 4.1, 95% CI, 1.8–10) and was stronger for individuals who reported relatively high exposure (compared with low leisure-time exposure: high leisure-time exposure, OR = 1.6, 95% CI, 1.0–3.2); low occupational exposure, OR = 1.9, 95% CI, 0.6–5.5); high occupational exposure, OR = 3.1, 95% CI, 1.5–7.5) (Demers et al, 1992), while another noted that the relationship was stronger among younger men (less than 60 years old, OR = 4.2, 95% CI, 1.8–9.9; 60 years older or older, OR = 1.3, 95% CI, 0.5–3.1) (Bethwaite et al, 1990).

In addition, a history of exposure to dyes and inks has been noted to be related to multiple myeloma in the U.S. in studies by Boffetta et al (1989) (OR = 2.7, 95% CI, 0.9–8.6) and Morris et al (1986) (OR = 1.9, 95% CI, 0.7–5.3), but not in studies conducted in the U.K., Italy, or Denmark (Cuzick and De Stavola, 1988; LaVecchia et al, 1989; and Heineman et al, 1992a and Pottern et al, 1992b, respectively).

Engine exhaust. Myeloma risk was related to a history of occupational exposure to diesel or engine exhaust in one cohort and six case-control studies. Self-reported occupation as a truck driver in the 1970 Swedish census was related to myeloma mortality in the subsequent 10 years (SMR = 439, 95% CI, 142–1020) (Hansen, 1993), while in the case-control studies odds ratios ranged from 1.4 to 2.1 (Boffetta et al, 1989; Flodin et al, 1987; Eriksson and Karlsson, 1992; Pottern et al, 1992b; Heineman et al, 1992a; Van Den Eeden and Friedman, 1993). Risk was also related to prior carbon monoxide exposure in two studies, with odds ratios of 1.9 (95% CI, 1.1–3.2) (Morris et al, 1986) and 1.5 (95% CI, 1.2–2.2) (Pasqualetti et al, 1990).

Metals. In a cohort study, Teta and Ott (1988) noted that male hourly workers employed at a New York metal-fabrication facility and followed during 1946–1981 were at slightly increased risk of myeloma (RR = 1.4, no. of exposed cases = 3). In two case-control studies, a history of exposure to metals (not otherwise specified) was related to myeloma risk, with odds ratios of 1.8 (95% CI, 1.1–2.9) (Morris et al, 1986) and 1.5 (no. of exposed cases = 81) (Cuzick and De Stavola, 1988). In four other reports, there was no relationship (Heineman et al, 1992a; LaVecchia et al, 1989; Pasqualetti et al, 1990; Pottern et al, 1992b). There is only limited information about exposure to specific metals in relation to the disease (Egedahl et al, 1993; Eriksson and Karlsson, 1992; Linet et al, 1987).

Other specific chemical and physical substances. Other substances that have been found to be associated with multiple myeloma in at least one study include textile fibers (Boffetta et al, 1989; Delzell and Grufferman, 1983; Dubrow and Gute, 1988); formaldehyde (Boffetta et al, 1989; Hayes et al, 1990; Pottern et al, 1992b); phthalates and vinyl chloride (Heineman et al, 1992a); styrene (Bond et al, 1992); solvents (Cuzick and De Stavola, 1988; Flodin et al, 1987; LaVecchia et al, 1989; Pasqualetti et al, 1990; Spirtas et al, 1991); sulfonylurea, creosote, and fresh wood (Flodin et al, 1987); wood dust (Boffetta et al, 1989; Pottern et al, 1992b); coal-tar (Boffetta et al, 1989); acids (Morris et al, 1986);

alkalis (Pasqualetti et al, 1990); and fertilizer (Morris et al, 1986; Pasqualetti et al, 1990).

Job Title and Industry Group. Agricultural workers and workers in the petroleum refining, rubber and plastics manufacturing, and wood products industries have been reported to be at increased risk of myeloma. Several studies have reported on cosmetologists and hairdressers as well; they are discussed in a later section concerning personal and occupational exposure to hair-coloring products.

Agricultural workers. Two cohort (Stark et al, 1990; Steineck and Wiklund, 1986) and 19 case-control studies of agricultural work in relation to multiple myeloma occurrence have been conducted and all but one observed the relative risk to exceed 1.0 (Table 43–6), although some to only a very limited extent. The only study that did not observe a positive relationship was that of Tollerud et al (1985), which was one of several that ascertained occupational information from death certificates.

Four studies considered duration of employment as a farmer. A trend of increasing relative risk with duration was noted by Demers et al (1992) (less than 10 years, OR = 1.1; 10 years or longer, OR = 1.3), Alavanja et al (1988) (less than 15 years, OR = 0.2; 15 years or longer, OR = 2.6), and Boffetta et al (1989) (20 years or less, OR = 0.0; 21-40 years, OR = 1.7; longer than 40 years, OR = 4.3), but not by Heineman et al (1992a) (5 years or less, OR = 1.1; more than 5 years, OR = 0.8).

As discussed in the previous section, a history of pesticide exposure has been examined as a risk factor for myeloma and may play a role in the disease. However, only two studies have sought to exclude the effects of pesticide use when considering the relation between agricultural work and myeloma risk. In neither did pesticide use appear to explain completely the relationship between agricultural work and the disease (Boffetta et al, 1989; Demers et al, 1992).

Other specific exposures that may increase myeloma risk among farmers include paints and solvents, wood-treatment chemicals used for fencing, engine exhaust, welding fumes, dusts, animals, zoonotic infections, and pollen (Blair et al, 1985; Pearce and Reif, 1990). Among farmers, these exposures are difficult to measure reliably, and efforts to identify which exposures increase myeloma risk have been made in only two studies. Both ascertained exposure by asking specific questions during interview. In the study of Pearce et al (1986), in which 36% of the controls reported having a history of employment as a farmer, the magnitude of the relationship between farming and multiple myeloma occurrence varied somewhat by type of farming (categories not mutually exclusive), as follows: orchard farmers, OR = 2.8 (95% CI, 0.5–16.9); produce farmers, OR = 2.0 (95% CI, 0.6–6.0); sheep farmers, OR = 1.9 (95% CI, 1.0–3.6); dairy farmers, OR = 1.4 (95% CI, 0.8–2.5); mixed sheep and beef farmers, OR = 1.3 (95% CI, 0.6–2.6); and poultry farmers, OR = 0.9 (95% CI, 0.1–8.4). The relationship between a history of occupational exposure to specific animals and multiple myeloma was as follows: sheep, OR = 1.4 (95% CI, 0.9–2.4); cows, OR = 1.3 (95% CI, 0.9–2.1); beef cattle, OR = 1.7 (95% CI, 1.0–2.9); poultry, OR = 1.3 (95% CI, 0.8–2.1), and pigs, OR = 1.3 (95% CI, 0.8–2.3). Many of the respondents who did not report a history of agricultural

TABLE 43–6. *Summary of Studies That Have Assessed the Risk of Multiple Myeloma in Relation to Agricultural Work*

Study	*Prevalence of Exposure in Controls (%)*	*No. of Exposed Cases*	*Relative Risk*	*95% CI*
COHORT STUDIES[a]				
Stark et al, 1990	—	11	1.1	—
Steineck and Wiklund, 1986	—	568	1.2	1.1–1.3
CASE-CONTROL STUDIES[b]				
Alavanja et al, 1988	—	7	1.1	0.4–2.9
Boffetta et al, 1989	1	16	3.4	1.5–7.5
Brownson et al, 1989	11	24	1.4	0.9–2.2
Burmeister et al, 1983	—	550	1.5	—
Cantor and Blair, 1984	22	110	1.4	1.0–1.8
Cuzick and De Stavola, 1988	10	28	1.8[c,d]	—
Demers et al, 1992	2	19	1.4	0.9–3.3
Eriksson and Karlsson, 1992	44	151	1.7	1.2–2.3
Flodin et al, 1987	12	29	1.4	0.8–2.5
Franceschi et al, 1993	2	20	1.3	0.7–2.3
Gallagher et al, 1983	23	30	2.2	1.2–4.0
Heineman et al, 1992a	5	45	1.1	0.8–1.5
LaVecchia et al, 1989	14	25	2.0[c,d]	1.1–3.5
Milham, 1971	7	60	1.8	—
Nandakumar et al, 1986	11	21	1.4	0.8–2.5
Pasqualetti et al, 1990	19	44	2.7	1.9–4.4
Pearce et al, 1986	36	43	1.7	1.0–2.9
Pottern et al, 1992b	3	14	1.5	0.8–2.8
Reif et al, 1989a	15	54	1.2	0.9–1.6
Tollerud et al, 1985	19	39	0.6	—

[a]Expected numbers were based on rates in the general population.
[b]Comparison was a history of agricultural work vs. no history unless otherwise specified.
[c]Comparison was a history of food processing/agriculture vs. no history.
[d]Unadjusted odds ratio.

employment nonetheless reported prior exposure to farm animals (for example, 23% of controls reported a history of employment on a dairy farm, while 40% reported a history of contact with dairy cows).

In the study of Eriksson and Karlsson (1992), in which 47% of respondents reported having a history of agricultural employment, the relationship between exposure to specific farm animals and myeloma occurrence was evaluated after taking into consideration exposure to other farm animals, with the following results: horses, OR = 1.6 (no. of exposed cases = 137); cattle, OR = 1.5 (no. of exposed cases = 152); goats, OR = 1.5 (no. of exposed cases = 24); hogs, OR = 0.9 (no. of exposed cases = 124); and poultry, OR = 0.9 (no. of exposed cases = 86).

Petroleum refining. Known carcinogens to which petroleum workers are exposed include polycyclic aromatic hydrocarbons and various solvents, which in the past may have included benzene. Five cohort and four case-control studies of the relationship between previous work in the petroleum industry and multiple myeloma risk have been published. Four of the cohort studies found that petroleum workers were at little or no increased risk of death from myeloma (Kaplan, 1986; McLaughlin et al, 1988; Rushton and Alderson, 1983; Schnatter et al, 1992), while the fifth observed a 2.2-fold (95% CI, 0.6–5.6) increased risk for all men employed 5 years or longer in any department (Christie et al, 1991). The case-control study of Cuzick and De Stavola (1988) noted that four cases but no controls had worked in the petroleum industry; however, three other case-control studies found no evidence for a relationship (Demers et al, 1992; Eriksson and Karlsson, 1992; LaVecchia et al, 1989).

Rubber and plastics manufacturing. Rubber workers can be exposed to organic solvents, plastic monomers, rubber additives, and asbestos, among other agents, and in the past, exposure to benzene was relatively high. Six studies of myeloma risk among workers in the rubber and plastics industry have been reported. Female workers from a cohort of rubber workers in the United States exposed during 1967–1973 were observed to be at increased risk of myeloma (RR = 2.3, n = 2) (Andjelkovic et al, 1978), but male members of the cohort were not (RR = 0.8, n = 5) (Andjelkovic et al, 1976). In addition, two Swedish cohort studies with overlapping sampling frames set during 1952–1981 (Gustavsson et al, 1986; McLaughlin et al, 1988), a British cohort study set during 1946–1985 (Sorahan and Cooke, 1989), and six case-control studies (Cuzick and De Stavola, 1988; Demers et al, 1992; Flodin et al, 1987; Heineman et al, 1992a; LaVecchia et al, 1989; Pottern et al, 1992b) have observed no association between a history of work in rubber or plastics manufacturing and multiple myeloma occurrence.

Wood products industries. This category includes manufacturing of lumber, wood products, furniture and fixtures, as well as the forestry industries, and may involve exposure to wood dust and chemicals used to treat wood, adhesives, and paint and stains. The ten studies of myeloma among workers in these industries suggest little or no altered risk, with the possible exception of forestry workers (Cuzick and De Stavola, 1988; Heineman et al, 1992a; Kawachi et al, 1989; LaVecchia et al, 1989; McLaughlin et al, 1988; Miller et al, 1989; Nandakumar et al, 1986; Pottern et al, 1992b; Reif et al, 1989b; Tollerud et al, 1985). Demers et al (1992) reported a 2.3-fold (95% CI, 0.9–15) excess risk for forestry workers, while Eriksson and Karlsson (1992) reported a 1.5-fold excess (95% CI, 1.0–2.3) for lumberjacks and a 1.4-fold excess (95% CI, 0.9–2.3) for afforestation workers.

Other job title and industry groups. Occupational cohort studies have also noted associations of myeloma incidence with fishing (Hagmar et al, 1992), and of mortality with the job title "stoker" (Hansen, 1992). In case-control studies, odds ratios exceeding 2.0 have been observed for the following job-title and industry groups (only categories with at least five exposed cases are presented): photography (unadjusted OR = 6.1, no. of exposed cases = 7) (Cuzick and De Stavola, 1988); longshoremen (unadjusted OR = 2.2, no. of exposed cases = 15) (Friedman, 1986); bricklayer/concrete workers (OR = 2.2, 95% CI, 0.7–7.5) (Flodin et al, 1987); industrial mechanics and maintenance workers (OR = 2.2, 95% CI, 0.6–8.5) (Demers et al, 1992); workers in the chemical industry (unadjusted OR = 2.1, no. of exposed cases = 28) (Cuzick and De Stavola, 1988), (OR = 2.2, 95% CI, 0.6–7.2) (Heineman et al, 1992a); and wool spinners and weavers (OR = 2.9, 95% CI, 0.9–9.3) (Heineman et al, 1992a).

Summary. There is some evidence from cohort studies that benzene causes multiple myeloma; however, other chemical exposures that occurred with exposure to benzene may have been responsible for the elevated risk noted in those studies. It should be noted that benzene was used as a solvent by painters and in various industries in which myeloma excesses have been noted. Other solvents used in paints also appear to increase myeloma risk, however, as evidenced by the elevated risk among painters in Sweden, where benzene has been banned for many years. Multiple studies have provided evidence that pesticide use is associated with myeloma risk. Unfortunately, there is little data concerning the specific classes of pesticides that should be targeted for further investigation. Pesticide use may account for part of the association of agricultural work with myeloma, but there is also some evidence that other agricultural exposures increase risk.

Hair-coloring Products

Personal use of hair-coloring products has been examined as an etiologic factor for myeloma occurrence in the American Cancer Society cohort study and in three population-based case-control studies, while a history of employment as a hairdresser or cosmetologist has been examined in one cohort study and two population-based case-control studies. In the American Cancer Society cohort, there was no relation between duration of use of permanent hair dyes for less than 20 years and death from myeloma, although there was a slight association with use for 20 years or longer (RR = 1.40, 95% CI, 0.85–2.29) (Thun et al, 1994) that was most apparent in women who had used black dyes (RR = 4.39, 95% CI, 1.1–18.3). Personal use of hair dyes was related to myeloma risk in both women (OR = 1.8, 95% CI, 0.9–3.7; OR = 1.5, 95% CI, 0.8–2.9) (Zahm et al, 1992; Herrinton et al, 1994) and men (OR = 1.8, 95% CI, 0.5–5.7; OR = 1.9, 95% CI, 1.0–3.6; OR = 1.5, 95% CI, 0.8–2.9) (Zahm et al, 1992; Brown et al, 1992a; Herrinton et al, 1994, respectively). In contrast, a Connecticut cohort of women holding hairdresser licenses for 5 years or longer was not at increased risk of myeloma compared with the general population (RR = 0.7, 95% CI, 0.1–2.0) (Teta et al, 1984). Neither was a relationship with occupation as a hairdresser observed in a Swedish case-control study of men and women (OR = 0.7, 95% CI, 0.2–2.7) (Eriksson and Karlsson, 1992), nor in a case-control study of four SEER areas (women, OR = 1.1, 95% CI, 0.4–2.7; men OR = 2.2, 95% CI, 0.2–27) (Herrinton et al, 1994). A possible explanation for the different results obtained by comparing personal versus occupational exposure is that the former was reported more completely by cases than by controls in the retrospective case-control studies. Nevertheless, the relatively high prevalence of personal use of hair dyes argues for further study of this question.

Alcohol Intake and Use of Tobacco

Four studies observed no relationship between alcohol intake and risk of myeloma (Boffetta et al, 1989; Brown et al, 1992c; Linet et al, 1992; Williams and Horm, 1977).

In ten recent studies that have investigated the role of tobacco use in relation to myeloma occurrence, only one found evidence for an increased risk among smokers. In a prospective cohort study of Seventh Day Adventists, the risk of myeloma was increased among current smokers (OR = 6.8, 95% CI, 1.4–33.6) and past smokers (OR = 3.0, 95% CI, 1.1–8.1) relative to individuals who had never smoked, and there was a trend of increasing risk with maximum number of cigarettes regularly smoked per day (1–14 cigarettes/day, OR = 1.4, 95% CI, 0.3–6.8; 15–24 cigarettes/day, OR = 5.6, 95% CI, 1.7–18.1; 25 cigarettes/day or more, OR = 4.7, 95% CI, 1.3–17.3) (Mills et al, 1990). However, no trend with years of cigarette smoking was observed. None of the other nine studies found any indication of an association between multiple myeloma and cigarette smoking (Boffetta et al, 1989; Brown et al, 1992b; Brownson, 1991; Flodin et al, 1987; Friedman, 1993; Heineman et al, 1992b; Herrinton et al, 1992; Linet et al, 1987; Williams and Horm, 1977). It is possible that Seventh Day Adventists who smoke differ from those who do not in one or more ways that bear on the incidence of myeloma.

Familial and Genetic Influences

There have been numerous case reports of multiple myeloma occurring in two or more members of a family and of multiple myeloma occurring with MGUS in families (for a review, see Olshan, 1991), and two case-control studies observed a relationship between a first-degree family history of multiple myeloma with multiple myeloma occurrence (OR = 5.6, 90% CI, 1.2–28; OR = 2.3, 95% CI, 0.5–10.1) (Eriksson and Hållberg 1992; Bourguet et al, 1985, respectively).

Olshan (1991) compared the distributions of age, heavy chain components, and light chain components of familial myeloma cases reported in the literature with data from the SEER program and the Mayo Clinic, but found no evidence that familial cases had different characteristics than other cases.

An epidemiologic study of healthy African and Caucasian Americans observed that the ratio of B to T cells was higher among African Americans, and that African Americans had a higher proportion of HLA-DR positive cells and activated T cells (Tollerud et al, 1991). The investigators hypothesized that these differences may be related to the observed difference in myeloma incidence in these two groups. A case-control study of 46 African American men and 85 Caucasian men found a strong association between the HLA-Cw2 allele and the incidence of myeloma in both racial groups (African American, OR = 5.7, 95% CI, 1.0–7.2; Caucasian, OR = 2.6, 95% CI, 1.0–7.2) (Pottern et al, 1992a). This association does not explain the racial difference in incidence, however, and larger studies with additional markers are required to evaluate the role of immunogenetic factors. A study of African Americans noted that HLA-Cw5 and Cw6 antigens were associated with myeloma risk (Leech et al, 1983).

Average serum immunoglobulin levels were elevated in 200 first-degree relatives, but not spouses, of multiple myeloma patients compared with numerous controls selected from blood donors and clinic patients (Festen et al, 1977).

Linet et al (1988) investigated the relationship between a history of autoimmune disorders in first-degree relatives and the occurrence of multiple myeloma; they observed an odds ratio of 3.0 (95% CI, 1.3–7.1). In a later study, Linet et al (1993) observed that a family history of pneumonia (OR = 2.5, 95% CI, 1.3–4.7) and rheumatic fever (OR = 4.9, 95% CI, 1.1–22) were associated with an increased risk of Waldenström's macroglobulinemia. The significance of these findings is not clear.

ETIOLOGIC HETEROGENEITY OF M-COMPONENT SUBTYPES

Owing to known differences in the normal physiological function of immunoglobulins of different classes, it has been hypothesized that environmental factors that trigger malignant growth of the various classes of M-components might also differ. It has been observed that IgD myeloma may differ epidemiologically from other types of myeloma, with an earlier age at onset and a higher male-to-female incidence ratio (Jancelewicz et al, 1975). However, only IgG, IgA, and light-chain myeloma have been examined in epidemiologic studies, because the occurrence of the other M-component-type myelomas is relatively uncommon (percent of cases: IgG, 55.8; IgA, 22.0; light chains, 16.7; IgM, 2.8; IgD, 0.2; IgE, 0.3; two components, 2.2) (Herrinton et al, 1993). The distribution of M-component types in Taiwanese myeloma patients (Wang et al, 1992) was similar to that for U.S. patients (Herrinton et al, 1992), although 4.8% of the 227 cases were of IgD M-component type. In analytical studies in which the M-component type was determined, the incidence of light chain myeloma was observed to have a lower male-to-female ratio than the IgG or IgA subtypes, and IgA myeloma was somewhat more strongly related to a history of diagnostic X rays (Williams et al, 1989; Herrinton et al, 1993), but no other differences with respect to chronic immune stimulation or occupational history have been observed (Herrinton et al, 1993; Lewis et al, 1994).

RECOMMENDATIONS FOR FUTURE RESEARCH

From the research completed to date, it appears that the question "What causes multiple myeloma?" will not be easy to answer. In areas where there are indicators—for example, associations with exposure to radiation and pesticides or a history of farming—the difficulty of more precisely measuring potential etiologic factors has limited our understanding of the nature of the associations. One promising avenue for future research is based on the acceptance of MGUS as a strong predictor of myeloma risk, and would involve studying the causes of MGUS. In addition, among other persons at increased risk of myeloma, such as farmers or African Americans, it might prove useful to investigate immune system characteristics that might be relevant to the development of multiple myeloma.

REFERENCES

ALAVANJA MCR, BLAIR A, MERKLE S, TESKE J, EATON B. 1988. Mortality among agricultural extension agents. Am J Ind Med 14:167–176.

ANDERSSON M, STORM HH. 1992. Cancer incidence among Danish Thorotrast-exposed patients. J Natl Cancer Inst 84:1318–1325.

ANDJELKOVIC D, TAULBEE J, SYMONS M. 1976. Mortality experience of a cohort of rubber workers, 1964–1973. J Occup Med 18:387–394.

ANDJELKOVICH D, TAULBEE J, BLUM S. 1978. Mortality of female workers in a rubber manufacturing plant. J Occup Med 20:409–413.

AXELSSON U. 1986. A 20-year follow-up study of 64 subjects with M-components. Acta Med Scand 219:519–522.

AXELSSON U, BACHMANN R, HÄLLÉN J. 1966. Frequency of pathological proteins (M-components) in 6,995 sera from an adult population. Acta Med Scand 179:235–247.

BARLOGIE B, EPSTEIN J, SELVANAYAGAM P, ALEXANIAN R. 1989. Plasma cell myeloma—new biological insights and advances in therapy. Blood 73:865–879.

BARLOGIE B, EPSTEIN J. 1990. Multiple myeloma: biology and therapy. Cancer Res Clin Oncol 116:109–111.

BERAL V, INSKIP H, FRASER P, BOOTH M, COLEMAN D, ROSE G. 1985. Mortality of employees of the United Kingdom Atomic Energy Authority, 1946–1979. BMJ 291:440–447.

BERTAZZI PA, PESATORI AC, CONSONNI D, TIRONI A, LANDI MT, ZOCCHETTI C. 1993. Cancer incidence in a population accidentally exposed to 2,3,7,8-tetrachlorodibenzo-para-dioxin. Epidemiology 4:398–406.

BETHWAITE PB, PEARCE N, FRASER J. 1990. Cancer risks in painters: study based on the New Zealand cancer registry. Br J Ind Med 47:742–746.

BLADE J, LOPEZ-GUILLERMO A, ROZMAN C, CERVANTES F, SALGADO C, AGUILAR JL, et al. 1992. Malignant transformation and life expectancy in monoclonal gammopathy of undetermined significance. Br J Haematol 81:391–394.

BLAIR A, MALKER H, CANTOR KP, BURMEISTER L, WIKLUND K. 1985. Cancer among farmers. Scand J Work Environ Health 11:397–407.

BLATTNER WA, BLAIR A, MASON TJ. 1981. Multiple myeloma in the United States, 1950–1975. Cancer 48:2547–2554.

BOFFETTA P, STELLMAN SD, GARFINKEL L. 1989. A case-control study of multiple myeloma nested in the American Cancer Society prospective study. Int J Cancer 43:554–559.

BOICE JD, DAY NE, ANDERSON A, BRINTON LA, BROWN R, CHOI NW, et al. 1985. Second cancers following radiation treatment for cervical cancer. An international collaboration among cancer registries. J Natl Cancer Inst 74:955–975.

BOICE JD, ENGHOLM G, KLEINERMAN RA, BLETTNER M, STOVALL M, LISCO H, et al. 1988. Radiation dose and second cancer risk in patients treated for cancer of the cervix. Radiat Res 116:3–55.

BOICE JD, MORIN MM, GLASS AG, FRIEDMAN GD, STOVALL M, HOOVER RN, et al. 1991. Diagnostic X-ray procedures and risk of leukemia, lymphoma, and multiple myeloma. JAMA 265:1290–1294.

BOND GG, BODNER KM, OLSEN GW, COOK RR. 1992. Mortality among workers engaged in the development or manufacture of styrene-based products—an update. Scand J Work Environ Health 18:145–154.

BOUCHARDY C, MIRRA AP, KHLAT M, PARKIN DM, PACHECO DE SOUZA JM, GOTLIEB SLD. 1991. Ethnicity and cancer risk in São Paulo, Brazil. Cancer Epidemiol Biomarkers Prev 1:21–27.

BOURGUET CC, GRUFFERMAN S, DELZELL E, DELONG ER, COHEN HJ. 1985. Multiple myeloma and family history of cancer: a case-control study. Cancer 56:2133–2139.

BOWDEN M, CRAWFORD J, COHEN HJ, NOYAMA O. 1993. A comparative study of monoclonal gammopathies and immunoglobulin levels in Japanese and United States elderly. J Am Geriatr Soc 41:11–14.

BRINTON LA, GRIDLEY G, HRUBEC Z, HOOVER R, FRAUMENI JF JR. 1989. Cancer risk following pernicious anemia. Br J Cancer 59:810–813.

BROWN LM, EVERETT GD, BURMEISTER LF, BLAIR A. 1992a. Hair dye use and multiple myeloma in White men. Am J Public Health 82:1673–1674.

BROWN LM, EVERETT GD, GIBSON R, BURMEISTER LF, SCHUMAN LM, BLAIR A. 1992b. Smoking and risk of non-Hodgkin's lymphoma and multiple myeloma. Cancer Causes Control 3:49–55.

BROWN LM, GIBSON R, BURMEISTER LF, SCHUMAN LM, EVERETT GD, BLAIR A. 1992c. Alcohol consumption and risk of leukemia, non-Hodgkin's lymphoma, and multiple myeloma. Leuk Res 16:979–984.

BROWNSON R. 1991. Cigarette smoking and risk of myeloma. J Natl Cancer Inst 83:1036–1037.

BROWNSON RC, REIF JS, CHANG JC, DAVIS JR. 1989. Cancer risks among Missouri farmers. Cancer 64:2381–2386.

BURMEISTER LF. 1990. Cancer in Iowa farmers: recent results. Am J Ind Med 18:295–301.

BURMEISTER LF, EVERETT GD, VAN LIER SF, ISACSON P. 1983. Selected cancer mortality and farm practices in Iowa. Am J Epidemiol 118:72–77.

CANTOR KP, BLAIR A. 1984. Farming and mortality from multiple myeloma: a case-control study with the use of death certificates. J Natl Cancer Inst 72:251–255.

CHRISTIE D, ROBINSON K, GORDON I, BISBY J. 1991. A prospective study in the Australian petroleum industry. II Incidence of cancer. Br J Ind Med 48:511–514.

COHEN HJ, BERNSTEIN RJ, GRUFFERMAN S. 1987. Role of immune stimulation in the etiology of multiple myeloma: a case-control study. Am J Hematol 24:119–126.

CUZICK J. 1990. International time trends for multiple myeloma. Ann NY Acad Sci 609:205–214.

CUZICK J, DE STAVOLA B. 1988. Multiple myeloma—a case-control study. Br J Cancer 57:516–520.

CUZICK J, DE STAVOLA BL. 1989. Autoimmune disorders and multiple myeloma (letter). Int J Epidemiol 18:283.

CUZICK J, VELEZ R, DOLL R. 1983. International variations and temporal trends in mortality from multiple myeloma. Int J Cancer 32:13–19.

DARBY SC, DOLL R, GILL SK, SMITH PG. 1987. Long term mortality after a single treatment course with X-rays in patients treated for ankylosing spondylitis. Br J Cancer 55:179–190.

DARBY SC, KENDALL GM, FELL TP, DOLL R, GOODILL AA, CONQUEST AJ, et al. 1993. Further follow up of mortality and incidence of cancer in men from the United Kingdom who participated in the United Kingdom's atmospheric nuclear weapon tests and experimental programmes. BMJ 307:1530–1535.

DARBY SC, REEVES G, KEY T, DOLL R, STOVALL M. 1994. Mortality in a cohort of women given X-ray therapy for metropathia haemorrhagica. Int J Cancer 56:793–801.

DAVIS FG, BOICE JD, HRUBEC Z, MONSON RR. 1989. Cancer mortality in a radiation-exposed cohort of Massachusetts tuberculosis patients. Cancer Res 49:6130–6136.

DECOUFLÉ P, BLATTNER WA, BLAIR A. 1983. Mortality among chemical workers exposed to benzene and other agents. Environ Res 30:16–25.

DELZELL E, GRUFFERMAN S. 1983. Cancer and other causes of death among female textile workers, 1976–78. J Natl Cancer Inst 71:735–740.

DEMERS PA, VAUGHAN TL, KOEPSELL TD, LYON JL, SWANSON GM, GREENBERG RS, et al. 1992. A case-control study of multiple myeloma and occupation. Am J Ind Med 23:629–639.

DEVESA SS, SILVERMAN DT, YOUNG JL, POLLACK ES, BROWN CC, HORM JW, et al. 1987. Cancer incidence and mortality trends among Whites in the United States, 1947–84. J Natl Cancer Inst 79:701–770.

DOODY MM, LINET MS, GLASS AG, FRIEDMAN GD, POTTERN LM, BOICE JD, et al. 1992. Leukemia, lymphoma, and multiple myeloma following selected medical conditions. Cancer Causes Control 3:449–456.

DUBROW R, GUTE DM. 1988. Cause-specific mortality among male textile workers in Rhode Island. Am J Ind Med 13:439–454.

EGEDAHL RD, CARPENTER M, HORNIK R. 1993. An update of an epidemiology study at a hydrometallurgical nickel refinery in Fort Saskatchewan, Alberta. Statistics Canada, Health Reports 5:291–302.

ERIKSSON E, HÅLLBERG B. 1992. Familial occurrence of hematologic malignancies and other diseases in multiple myeloma: a case-control study. Cancer Causes Control 3:63–67.

ERIKSSON M, KARLSSON M. 1992. Occupation and other environmental factors and multiple myeloma: a population-based case-control study. Br J Ind Med 49:95–103.

ERIKSSON M. 1993. Rheumatoid arthritis as a risk factors for multiple myeloma: a case-control study. Eur J Cancer 29A:259–263.

FESTEN JJM, MARRINK J, DE WAARD-KUIPER EH, MANDEMA E. 1977. Immunoglobulins in families of myeloma patients. Scand J Immunol 6:887–896.

FLODIN U, FREDRIKSSON M, PERSSON B. 1987. Multiple myeloma and engine exhausts, fresh wood, and creosote: a case-referent study. Am J Ind Med 12:519–529.

FRIEDMAN GD. 1986. Multiple myeloma: relation to propoxyphene and other drugs, radiation and occupation. Int J Epidemiol 15:423–425.

FRIEDMAN GD. 1993. Cigarette smoking, leukemia, and multiple myeloma. Ann Epidemiol 3:425–428.

GALLAGHER RP, SPINELLI JJ, ELWOOD JM, SKIPPEN DH. 1983. Allergies and agricultural exposure as risk factors for multiple myeloma. Br J Cancer 48:853–857.

GILBERT ES, FRY SA, WIGGS LD, VOELZ GL, CRAGLE DL, PETERSEN GR. 1989. Analyses of combined mortality data on workers at the Hanford site, Oak Ridge National Laboratory, and Rocky Flats Nuclear Weapons Plant. Radiat Res 120:19–35.

GRAMENZI A, BUTTINO I, D'AVANZO B, NEGRI E, FRANCESCHI S, LAVECCHIA C. 1991. Medical history and the risk of multiple myeloma. Br J Cancer 63:769–772.

GRULICH AE, SWERDLOW AJ, HEAD J, MARMOT MG. 1992. Cancer mortality in African and Caribbean migrants to England and Wales. Br J Cancer 66:905–911.

GUSTAVSSON P, HOGSTEDT C, HOLMBERG B. 1986. Mortality and incidence of cancer among Swedish rubber workers, 1952–81. Scand J Work Environ Health 12:538–544.

HAAS H, ANDERS S, BORNKAMM GW, MANNWEILER E, SCHMITZ H, RADL J, et al. 1990. Do infections induce monoclonal immunoglobulin components? Clin Exper Immunol 81:435–440.

HAGMAR L, LINDÉN K, NILSSON A, NORRVING B, ÅKESSON B, SCHÜTZ A, et al. 1992. Cancer incidence and mortality among Swedish Baltic Sea fisherman. Scand J Work Environ Health 18:217–224.

HANSEN NE, KARLE H, OLSEN JH. 1989. Trends in the incidence of multiple myeloma in Denmark 1943–1982: a study of 5500 patients. Eur J Haematol 42:72–76.

HANSEN ES. 1992. A mortality study of Danish stokers. Br J Ind Med 49:48–52.

HANSEN ES. 1993. A follow-up study on the mortality of truck drivers. Am J Ind Med 23:811–821.

HAYES RB, BLAIR A, STEWART PA, HERRICK RF, MAHAR H. 1990. Mortality of U.S. embalmers and funeral directors. Am J Ind Med 18:641–652.

HEINEMAN EF, OLSEN JH, POTTERN LM, GOMEZ M, RAFFN E, BLAIR A. 1992a. Occupational risk factors for multiple myeloma among Danish men. Cancer Causes Control 3:555–568.

HEINEMAN EF, ZAHM SH, MCLAUGHLIN JK, VAUGHT JB, HRUBEC Z. 1992b. A prospective study of tobacco use and multiple myeloma: evidence against an association. Cancer Causes Control 3:555–568.

HERRINTON LJ, KOEPSELL TD, WEISS NS. 1992. Smoking and multiple myeloma. Cancer Causes Control 3:391–392.

HERRINTON LJ, WEISS NS. 1993. Incidence of Waldenström's macroglobulinemia. Blood 82:3148–3150.

HERRINTON LJ, DEMERS PA, KOEPSELL TD, WEISS NS, DALING JR, TAYLOR JW, et al. 1993. Epidemiology of the M-components immunoglobulin type of multiple myeloma. Cancer Causes Control 4:83–92.

HERRINTON LJ, WEISS NS, KOEPSELL TD, DALING JR, TAYLOR JW, LYON JL, et al. 1994. Exposure to hair-coloring products in relation to the risk of multiple myeloma. Am J Public Health 84:1142–1144.

HIRANO T. 1991. Interleukin 6 (IL-6) and its receptor: their role in plasma cell neoplasias. Int J Cell Cloning 9:166–184.

HOOVER RN, MASON TJ, MCKAY FW, FRAUMENI JF. 1975. Geographic patterns of cancer mortality in the United States. In Fraumeni J (ed): Persons at High Risk of Cancer, An Approach to Cancer Etiology and Control. New York: Academic Press, pp. 343–360.

HSING AW, HANSSON LE, MCLAUGHLIN JK, NYREN O, BLOT WJ, EKBOM A, FRAUMENI JF JR. 1993. Pernicious anemia and subsequent cancer: a population-based cohort study. Cancer 71:745–750.

ISOMÄKI HA, HAKULINEN T, JOUTSENLAHTI U. 1978. Excess risk of lymphomas, leukemia and myeloma in patients with rheumatoid arthritis. J Chron Dis 31:691–696.

JANCELEWICZ Z, TAKATSUKI K, SUGAI S, PRUZANSKI W. 1975. IgD multiple myeloma: review of 133 cases. Arch Intern Med 135:87–93.

JOHNSTON JM, GRUFFERMAN S, BOURGUET CC, DELZELL E, DELONG ER, COHEN HJ. 1985. Socioeconomic status and risk of multiple myeloma. J Epidemiol Community Health 39:175–178.

KAGAN E. 1985. Current perspectives in asbestosis. Ann Allergy 54:464–474.

KAPLAN SD. 1986. Update of a mortality study of workers in petroleum refineries. J Occup Med 28:514–516.

KATO I, TAJIMA K, HIROSE K, NAKAGAWA N, KUROISHI T, TOMINAGA S. 1985. A descriptive epidemiological study of hematopoietic neoplasms in Japan. Jpn J Clin Oncol 15:347–364.

KATUSIC S, BEARD CM, KURLAND L, WEIS JW, BERGSTRALH E. 1985. Occurrence of malignant neoplasms in the Rochester, Minnesota, rheumatoid arthritis cohort. Am J Med 78 (Suppl 1A):50–55.

KAWACHI I, PEARCE N, FRASER J. 1989. A New Zealand cancer registry-based study of cancer in wood workers. Cancer 64:2609–2613.

KENDALL GM, MUIRHEAD CR, MACGIBBON BH, O'HAGAN JA, CONQUEST AJ, GOODILL AA, et al. 1992. Mortality and occupational exposure to radiation: first analysis of National Registry for Radiation Workers. BMJ 304:220–225.

KOEPSELL TD, DALING JR, WEISS NS, TAYLOR JW, OLSHAN AF, LYON JL, et al. 1987. Antigenic stimulation and the occurrence of multiple myeloma. Am J Epidemiol 126:1051–1062.

KYLE RA. 1993. "Benign" monoclonal gammopathy—after 20 to 35 years of follow-up. Mayo Clin Proc 68:26–36.

KYLE RA, FINKELSTEIN S, ELVEBACK LR, KURLAND LT. 1972. Incidence of monoclonal proteins in a Minnesota community with a cluster of multiple myeloma. Blood 40:719–724.

KYLE RA, GREIPP PR. 1988. Plasma cell dyscrasias: current status. Crit Rev Oncol Hematol 8:93–153.

LAVECCHIA C, NEGRI E, D'AVANZO B, FRANCESCHI S. 1989. Occupation and lymphoid neoplasms. Br J Cancer 60:385–388.

LEECH SH, BRYAN CF, ELSTON RC, RAINEY J, BICKERS JN, PELIAS MZ. 1983. Genetic studies in multiple myeloma: 1. Association with HLA-Cw5. Cancer 51:1408–1411.

LEVI F, LAVECCHIA C. 1990. Trends in multiple myeloma (letter). Int J Cancer 46:755–756.

LEVI F, LAVECCHIA C, LUCCHINI F, NEGRI E. 1992. Trends in cancer mortality sex ratios in Europe, 1950–89. World Health Stat Q 45:117–164.

LEWIS EB. 1963. Leukemia, multiple myeloma, and aplastic anemia in American radiologists. Science 142:1492–1494.

LEWIS DR, POTTERN LM, BROWN LM, SILVERMAN DT, HAYES RB, SHOENBERG JB, et al. 1994. Multiple myeloma among US blacks and whites: the role of chronic antigenic stimulation. Cancer Causes Control, In press.

LINET MS, HARLOW SD, MCLAUGHLIN JK. 1987. A case-control study of multiple myeloma in Whites: chronic antigenic stimulation, occupation, and drug use. Cancer Res 47:2978–2981.

LINET MS, MCLAUGHLIN JK, HARLOW SD, FRAUMENI JF. 1988. Family history of autoimmune disorders and cancer in multiple myeloma. Int J Epidemiol 17:512–513.

LINET MS, MCLAUGHLIN JK, HSING AW, WACHOLDER S, CO CHIEN HT, SCHUMAN LM, et al. 1992. Is cigarette smoking a risk factor for non-Hodgkin's lymphoma or multiple myeloma? Results from the Lutheran Brotherhood Cohort Study. Leuk Res 16:621–624.

LINET MS, HUMPHREY RL, MEHL ES, BROWN LM, POTTERN LM, BIAS WB, et al. 1993. A case-control and family study of Waldenström's macroglobulinemia. Leukemia 7:1363–1369.

LINOS A, KYLE RA, O'FALLON WM, KURLAND LT. 1981. Incidence and secular trend of multiple myeloma in Olmsted County, Minnesota: 1965–77. J Natl Cancer Inst 66:17–20.

LUDWIG H, FRITZ E, FRIEDL HP. 1982. Epidemiologic and age-dependent data on multiple myeloma in Austria. J Natl Cancer Inst 68:729–733.

LUNDBERG I. 1986. Mortality and cancer incidence among Swedish paint industry workers with long-term exposure to organic solvents. Scand J Work Environ Health 12:108–113.

MACKENZIE MR, LEWIS JP. 1985. Cytogenetic evidence that the malignant event in multiple myeloma occurs in a precursor lymphocyte. Cancer Genet Cytogenet 17:13–20.

MACMAHON B. 1966. Epidemiology of Hodgkin's disease. Cancer Res 26:1189–1200.

MATTESON EL, HICKEY AR, MAGUIRE L, TILSON HH, UROWITZ MB. 1991. Occurrence of neoplasia in patients with rheumatoid arthritis enrolled in a DMARD registry. Rheumatoid Arthritis Azathioprine Registry Steering Committee. J Rheumatol 18:809–814.

MCLAUGHLIN JK, LINET MS, STONE BJ, BLOT WJ, FRAUMENI JF, MALKER HSR, et al. 1988. Multiple myeloma and occupation in Sweden. Arch Environ Health 43:7–10.

MCWHORTER WP, SCHATZKIN AG, HORM JW, BROWN CC. 1989. Contribution of socioeconomic status to Black/White differences in cancer incidence. Cancer 63:982–987.

MILHAM S. 1971. Leukemia and multiple myeloma in farmers. Am J Epidemiol 94:307–310.

MILLER BA, BLAIR AE, RAYNOR HL, STEWART PA, ZAHM S, FRAUMENI JF JR. 1989. Cancer and other mortality patterns among United States furniture workers. Br J Ind Med 46:508–515.

MILLER BA, RIES LAG, HANKEY BF, KOSARY CL, HARRAS A, DEVESA SS, et al. 1993. SEER Cancer Statistics: Review 1973–1990. National Cancer Institute. NIH Publ. No. 93-2789.

MILLS PK, NEWELL GR, BEESON WL, FRASER GE, PHILLIPS RLP. 1990. History of cigarette smoking and risk of leukemia and myeloma: results from the Adventist Health Study. J Natl Cancer Inst 82:1832–1836.

MORRIS PD, KOEPSELL TD, DALING JR, TAYLOR JW, LYON JL,

SWANSON GM, et al. 1986. Toxic substance exposure and multiple myeloma: a case-control study. J Natl Cancer Inst 76:987–994.

NANDAKUMAR A, ARMSTRONG BK, DEKLERK NH. 1986. Multiple myeloma in Western Australia: a case-control study in relation to occupation, father's occupation, socioeconomic status and country of birth. Int J Cancer 37:223–226.

NANDAKUMAR A, ENGLISH DR, DOUGAN LE, ARMSTRONG BK. 1988. Incidence and outcome of multiple myeloma in Western Australia, 1960 to 1984. Aust N Z J Med 18:774–779.

OLSHAN AF. 1991. Familial and genetic associations. In Obrams GI, Potter M (eds): Epidemiology and Biology of Multiple Myeloma New York: Springer, pp. 31–39.

OSSERMAN EF, MERLINI G, BUTLER VP. 1987. Multiple myeloma and related plasma cell dyscrasias. JAMA 258:2930–2937.

PARKER DM, MUIR CS, WHELAN SL, GAO YT, FERLAY J, POWELL J. 1993. Cancer Incidence in Five Continents, Volume VI. IARC Scientific Publications 120. Lyon, France: International Agency for Research on Cancer.

PASQUALETTI P, CASALE R, COLLACCIANI A, COLANTONIO D. 1990. Occupation and multiple myeloma risk: a case-control study. Med Lav 81:309–319.

PEARCE NE, SMITH AH, FISHER DO. 1985. Malignant lymphoma and multiple myeloma linked with agricultural occupations in a New Zealand cancer registry-based study. Am J Epidemiol 121:225–237.

PEARCE NE, SMITH AH, HOWARD JK, SHEPPARD RA, GILES HJ, TEAGUE CA. 1986. Case-control study of multiple myeloma and farming. Br J Cancer 54:493–500.

PEARCE N, REIF JS. 1990. Epidemiologic studies of cancer in agricultural workers. Am J Ind Med 18:133–148.

PEARCE N, PRIOR I, METHVEN D, CULLING C, MARSHALL S, AULD J, et al. 1990. Follow up of New Zealand participants in British atmospheric nuclear weapons tests in the Pacific. BMJ 300:1161–1166.

POTTERN LM, GART JJ, NAM JM, DUNSTON G, WILSON J, GREENBERG R, et al. 1992a. HLA and multiple myeloma among Black and White men: evidence of a genetic association. Cancer Epidemiol Biomarkers Prev 1:177–182.

POTTERN LM, HEINEMAN EF, OLSEN JH, RAFFN E, BLAIR A. 1992b. Multiple myeloma among Danish women: employment history and workplace exposures. Cancer Causes Control 3:427–432.

PRESTON DL, KUSUMI S, TOMONAGA M, IZUMI S, RON E, KURAMOTO A, et al. 1994. Cancer incidence in atomic bomb survivors, Part III: leukemia, lymphoma and multiple myeloma, 1950–1987. Radiat Res 137:S68–S97.

PRIOR P, SYMMONS DPM, HAWKINS CF, SCOTT DL, BROWN R. 1984. Cancer morbidity in rheumatoid arthritis. Ann Rheum Dis 43:128–131.

RADL J, LIU M, HOOGEVEEN CM, VAN DEN BERG P, MINKMAN-BRONDIJK RJ, BROERSE JJ, et al. 1991. Monoclonal gammapathies (sic) in long-term surviving Rhesus monkeys after lethal irradiation and bone marrow transplantation. Clin Immunol Immunopathol 60:305–309.

RAFFN E, LYNGE E, JUEL K, KORSGAARD B. 1989. Incidence of cancer and mortality among employees in the asbestos cement industry in Denmark. Br J Ind Med 46:90–96.

REIF J, PEARCE N, FRASER J. 1989a. Cancer risks in New Zealand farmers. Int J Epidemiol 18:768–774.

REIF JS, PEARCE N, KAWACHI I, FRASER JO. 1989b. Soft-tissue sarcoma, non-Hodgkin's lymphoma, and multiple myeloma in New Zealand forestry workers. Int J Cancer 43:49–54.

RINSKY RA, SMITH AB, HORNUNG R, FILLOON TG, YOUNG RJ, OKUN AH, et al. 1987. Benzene and leukemia: an epidemiologic risk assessment. N Engl J Med 316:1044–1050.

RUSHTON L, ALDERSON M. 1983. Epidemiological survey of oil distribution centres in Britain. Br J Ind Med 40:330–339.

SALEUN JP, VICARIOT M, DEROFF P, MORIN JF. 1982. Monoclonal gammopathies in the adult population of Finistère, France. J Clin Pathol 35:63–68.

SCHECHTER GP, SHOFF N, CHAN C, MCMANUS CD, HAWLEY HP. 1991. The frequency of monoclonal gammopathy of unknown significance in Black and Caucasian veterans in a hospital population. In Obrams GI, Potter M (eds): Epidemiology and Biology of Multiple Myeloma. New York: Springer-Verlag, pp. 83–85.

SCHNATTER AR, THÉRIAULT G, KATZ AM, THOMPSON FS, DONALESKI D, MURRAY N. 1992. A retrospective mortality study within operating segments of a petroleum company. Am J Ind Med 22:209–229.

SCHWARTZ DA, VAUGHAN TL, HEYER NJ, KOEPSELL TD, LYON JL, SWANSON GM, et al. 1988. B cell neoplasms and occupational asbestos exposure. Am J Ind Med 14:661–671.

SHAPIRA R, CARTER A. 1986. Multiple myeloma in northern Israel, 1970–1979. Cancer 58:206–209.

SHIMIZU Y, KATO H, SCHULL WJ. 1990. Studies of the mortality of A-bomb survivors. 9. Mortality, 1950–1985: Part 2. Cancer mortality based on the recently revised doses (DS86). Radiat Res 121:120–141.

SMITH PG, DOUGLAS AJ. 1986. Mortality of workers at the Sellafield plant of British Nuclear Fuels. BMJ 293:845–854.

SORAHAN T, COOKE MA. 1989. Cancer mortality in a cohort of United Kingdom steel foundry workers, 1946–85. Br J Ind Med 46:74–81.

SORAHAN T, PARKES HG, VEYS CA, WATERHOUSE JAH, STRAUGHAN JK, NUTT A. 1989. Mortality in the British rubber industry 1946–85. Br J Ind Med 46:1–11.

SPIRTAS R, STEWART PA, LEE JS, MARANO DE, FORBES CD, GRAUMAN DJ, et al. 1991. Retrospective cohort mortality study of workers at an aircraft maintenance facility. I. Epidemiological results. Br J Ind Med 48:515–530.

STARK AD, CHANG HG, FITZGERALD EF, RICCARDI K, STONE RR. 1990. A retrospective cohort study of cancer incidence among New York State Farm Bureau members. Arch Environ Health 45:155–162.

STEINECK G, WIKLUND K. 1986. Multiple myeloma in Swedish agricultural workers. Int J Epidemiol 15:321–325.

SWAEN GMH, VAN VLIET C, SLANGEN JJM, STURMAS F. 1992. Cancer mortality among licensed herbicide applicators. Scand J Work Environ Health 18:201–204.

TETA MJ, OTT MG. 1988. A mortality study of a research, engineering, and metal fabrication facility in western New York state. Am J Epidemiol 127:540–551.

TETA MJ, WALRATH J, MEIGS JW, FLANNERY JT. 1984. Cancer incidence among cosmetologists. J Natl Cancer Inst 72:1051–1057.

THUN MJ, ALTEKRUSE SF, NAMBOODIRI MM, CALLE EE, MYERS DG, HEATH CW JR. 1994. Hair dye use and risk of fatal cancers in US women. J Natl Cancer Inst 86:210–215.

TOLLERUD DJ, BRINTON LA, STONE BJ, TOBACMAN JK, BLATTNER WA. 1985. Mortality from multiple myeloma among North Carolina furniture workers. J Natl Cancer Inst 74:799–801.

TOLLERUD DJ, BROWN LM, BLATTNER WA, HOOVER RN. 1991. The influence of race on T-cell subset distributions. In Obrams GI, Potter M (eds): Epidemiology and Biology of Multiple Myeloma, New York: Springer-Verlag, pp. 45–49.

TOMÁŠEK L, DARBY SC, SWERDLOW AJ, PLACEK V, KUNZ E. 1993. Radon exposure and cancers other than lung cancer among uranium miners in West Bohemia. Lancet 341:919–923.

TURESSON I, ZETTERVALL O, CUZICK J, WALDENSTROM JG, VELEZ R. 1984. Comparison of trends in the incidence of multiple myeloma in Malmö, Sweden, and other countries, 1950–1979. N Engl J Med 310:421–424.

VÅGERÖ D, PERSSON G. 1986. Occurrence of cancer in socioeconomic groups in Sweden. Scand J Soc Med 14:151–160.

VAN DEN EEDEN SK, FRIEDMAN GD. 1993. Exposure to engine exhaust and risk of subsequent cancer. J Occup Med 35:307–311.

VELEZ R, BERAL V, CUZICK J. 1982. Increasing trends of multiple myeloma mortality in England and Wales; 1950–79: are the changes real? J Natl Cancer Inst 69:387–392.

VESTERINEN E, PUKKALA E, TIMONEN T, AROMAA A. 1993. Cancer incidence among 78,000 asthmatic patients. Int J Epidemiol 22:976–982.

WANG JX, BOICE JD, LI BX, ZHANG JY, FRAUMENI JF JR. 1988. Cancer among medical diagnostic X-ray workers in China. J Natl Cancer Inst 80:344–350.

WANG CR, CHUANG CY, LIN KT, CHEN MY, LEE GL, HSIEH RP, et al. 1992. Monoclonal gammopathies and the related autoimmune manifestations in Taiwan. Asian Pac J Allergy Immunol 10:123–128.

WIKLUND K, DICH J, HOLM LE, EKLUND G. 1989. Risk of cancer in pesticide applicators in Swedish agriculture. Br J Ind Med 46:809–814.

WILLIAMS RR, HORM JW. 1977. Association of cancer sites with tobacco and alcohol consumption and socioeconomic status of patients: interview study from the Third National Cancer Survey. J Natl Cancer Inst 58:525–547.

WILLIAMS AR, WEISS NS, KOEPSELL TD, LYON JL, SWANSON GM. 1989. Infectious and noninfectious exposures in the etiology of light chain myeloma: a case-control study. Cancer Res 49:4038–4041.

WOLVEKAMP MCJ, MARQUET RL. 1990. Interleukin-6: historical background, genetics and biological significance. Immunol Lett 24:1–10.

ZAHM SH, WEISENBURGER DD, BABBITT PA, SAAL RC, VAUGHT JB, BLAIR A. 1992. Use of hair coloring products and the risk of lymphoma, multiple myeloma, and chronic lymphocytic leukemia. Am J Public Health 82:990–997.

ZHENG T, MAYNE ST, FLANNERY J. 1992. The time trends of multiple myeloma in Connecticut, 1935–1987 (letter). Int J Cancer 50:163–164.

44 Bone cancer

ROBERT W. MILLER
JOHN D. BOICE, JR.
ROCHELLE E. CURTIS

Cancers that arise from bone or cartilage account for about 0.5% of all malignant neoplasms in the human. As with other neoplasms, much more research has been devoted to diagnosis and therapy than to causation. This chapter reviews the epidemiologic observations on bone cancer that have provided clues to its origins.

DEMOGRAPHIC CHARACTERISTICS

Descriptive studies in the past have been handicapped by the use of a single code number in the International Classification of Diseases, which groups all cell types of bone cancer. The three main subtypes are osteosarcoma, which arises most often from the growing ends of long bones; chondrosarcoma, which develops in cartilage; and Ewing's sarcoma, which according to recent evidence may arise from primitive nervous tissue (Cavazzana et al, 1987; Ewing's Tumour Workshop, 1990; Horowitz et al, 1993), most commonly in the shafts of the axial skeleton.

The cell types should be studied separately, because they have marked demographic differences that are of etiologic significance. Histologic diagnoses are thus required, as from population-based cancer registries. Of particular value in this regard are data from the Surveillance, Epidemiology and End-Results (SEER) Program of the National Cancer Institute (Percy et al, 1995), which has covered about 10% of the U.S. population since 1973. Ninety-five percent of bone cancers were histologically confirmed. The geographic areas covered and distribution by cell type are shown in Table 44–1.

Of the 1961 cases among whites and 163 among blacks registered in the SEER Program from 1973 through 1985, osteosarcoma was reported in 36%, chondrosarcoma in 26%, and Ewing's sarcoma in 16%. Age-adjusted rates by histologic type are presented in Figure 44–1.

Age, Sex, and Race-Specific Incidence

Osteosarcoma has a bimodal age distribution, with peaks in adolescence and late in life (Fig. 44–2). It is rare early in life, but the rate increases rapidly in late childhood. In 1950–1959, before improved therapy increased survival, mortality and incidence rates were similar. There were enough deaths in the United States during this ten-year interval to allow study of the distribution by single year of age (Fig. 44–3). At age 13 the rate for males rose higher than that for females, and remained elevated for a longer time, suggesting that bone cancer is related to the adolescent growth spurt. (Price, 1958; Fraumeni, 1967; Glass and Fraumeni, 1970).

Chondrosarcoma is rare in childhood and rises with advancing age, for unknown reasons (Young et al, 1990). The age distribution of Ewing's sarcoma resembles that of osteosarcoma early in life, but rarely develops over 35 years of age (Fig. 44–2). Apparently, malignant change of the primitive tissue from which it arises does not occur later in life.

There is a male predominance of each major form of bone cancer among whites and blacks (Fig. 44–1). The two races have similar incidence rates for childhood osteosarcoma, but blacks have almost no cases of Ewing's sarcoma, either in the United States (Figs. 44–1 and 44–4) or Africa (Parkin et al, 1988). Rates of Ewing's sarcoma are also low among Asians, but less so than in blacks. A possible explanation for these racial differences is that a gene for osteosarcoma is equally mutable among the various races, but that for Ewing's sarcoma resists mutation in blacks and Asians.

Table 44–1 shows an absence of chordoma, when about 10 cases were expected if blacks had 12% of the total, as they did for osteosarcoma. Among blacks there is also a rarity of giant cell and blood-vessel tumors. These racial differences have not previously been recognized, and need further investigation.

TABLE 44–1. *Number of Patients with Primary Bone Cancer Among Whites and Blacks According to Histologic Type, SEER Cancer Registries[a], 1973–85*

	Number of Cases						
	Whites			*Blacks*			
Histology	*M*	*F*	*Total*	*M*	*F*	*Total*	*%[c]*
Osteosarcoma	379	287	666	51	42	93	12.3
Chondrosarcoma	295	248	543	18	14	32	5.6
Ewing's sarcoma	218	121	339	2	3	5	1.5
Chordoma	55	31	86	0	0	0	—
Fibrous histiocytoma[b]	35	21	56	1	4	5	8.2
Fibrosarcoma	27	26	53	2	5	7	11.7
Sarcoma, NOS	26	19	45	3	1	4	8.2
Giant cell tumor	22	22	44	0	1	1	2.2
Blood vessel tumors	15	19	34	0	1	1	2.9
Odontogenic tumors[b]	12	14	26	4	1	5	16.1
Other types	11	16	27	2	2	4	12.9
Malignant neoplasm, NOS	24	18	42	1	5	6	12.5
Total	1119	842	1961	84	79	163	100
Percent histologically confirmed			95%		94%		

[a]SEER areas include the states of Connecticut, Hawaii, Iowa, New Mexico, Utah and the metropolitan areas of Detroit, Atlanta (1975–1985), Seattle (1974–1985), and San Francisco-Oakland.
[b]Includes morphology categories in use since only 1977.
[c]For a given subtype, % that were Black; e.g., osteosarcoma = 93/(666 + 93) × 100 = 12.3%.

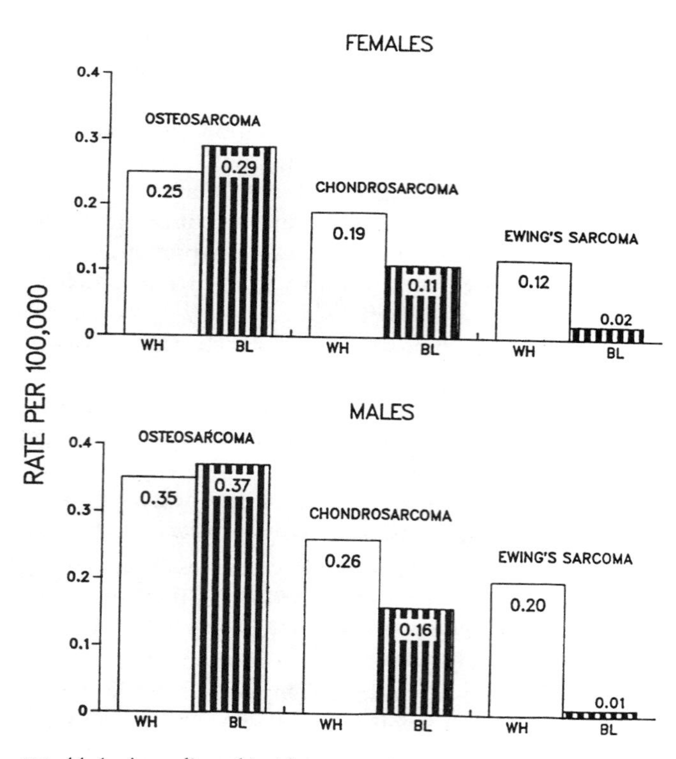

FIG. 44–1. Age-adjusted incidence rates (per 100,000, 1970 standard) for bone cancer, by sex, race, and histologic type (SEER 1973–85, WH=whites, BL=blacks).

Table 44–2 summarizes SEER data concerning the distribution of the seven main bone cancers among whites with respect to age, sex, and anatomic site. It shows that osteosarcoma most often arises from long bones of the lower limbs, whereas chondrosarcoma and Ewing's sarcoma most often arise from flat bones. Chordoma, presumably arising from remnants of the embryologic notochord, is a tumor of the flat bones of the trunk and head, and of the lower limbs. The lower limbs are the principal sites for fibrosarcoma, giant cell tumors, and malignant fibrous histiocytoma, which has recently gained attention as a clinical entity, especially as a complication of Paget's disease.

Geographic Variation

Little geographic variation is seen worldwide in the incidence of bone cancer, all forms combined (Muir et al., 1987). Incidence rates that differ by more than 2-fold are rare in the few populations of sufficient size to ensure stable estimates. No clues to etiology are apparent from international comparisons of age-adjusted rates. With few exceptions, rates are higher among males than females, with ranges of 0.8 to 1.6 and 0.6 to 1.2 per 100,000, respectively.

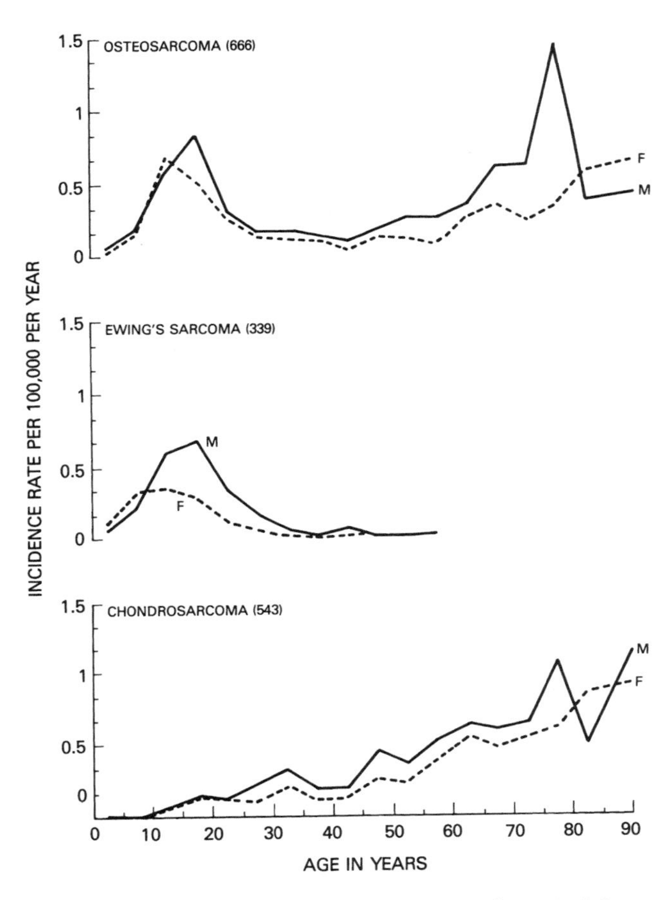

FIG. 44–2. Age- and sex-specific incidence rates for United States whites for three major types of bone cancer (SEER 1973–85).

FIG. 44–3. Comparison of stature with bone cancer mortality by single year of age and sex among United States whites, 1950–59. From Miller, 1981.

Time Trends in Mortality and Incidence

Mortality rates for bone cancer, all forms combined, in the United States (Fig. 44–5) and other countries have declined steadily from the 1950s to the mid-1980s, largely attributable to improved diagnosis and treatment (Pickle et al, 1987; Miller and McKay, 1984; Decarli et al, 1987; La Vecchia and Decarli, 1988; Ericsson et al, 1978). Using SEER incidence data, Hoover et al (1991) found that between 1973–1980 and 1981–1987 there was an unexplained increase in the annual incidence rates of osteosarcoma in males under 20 years of age, from 3.6 to 5.5 cases per million people. Among females the corresponding annual rates were 3.8 and 3.7 cases per million.

Figures 44–6 and 44–7 show survival rates for the three main cell types for males and females, respectively (SEER data, 1980–1989, all races combined). Survival was by far the best for chondrosarcoma, and, for all 3 cell types, was substantially better in females than in males.

ENVIRONMENTAL FACTORS

Radiation

Ionizing radiation is one of the few environmental agents known to induce certain bone cancers, particularly osteosarcoma, chondrosarcoma, and fibrosarcoma. In 1925, Martland linked bone cancer to occupational exposure to radium. In subsequent studies (see Table 44–3) an excess risk of bone cancer was found following brief exposure to high-dose radiation therapy (Robinson et al, 1988) and following continuous exposure to internally deposited radionuclides injected to treat bone disease or to provide a contrast medium in diagnostic radiography (Mays, 1988). Investigations of radiogenic bone cancer have enabled researchers to develop an elegant theory of the induction of osteosarcoma (Marshall and Groer, 1977); models in which genetic-environmental interactions can be evaluated (Knudson, 1985); and guidelines for protecting against the effects of internally deposited radionuclides, especially plutonium (Healy, 1975).

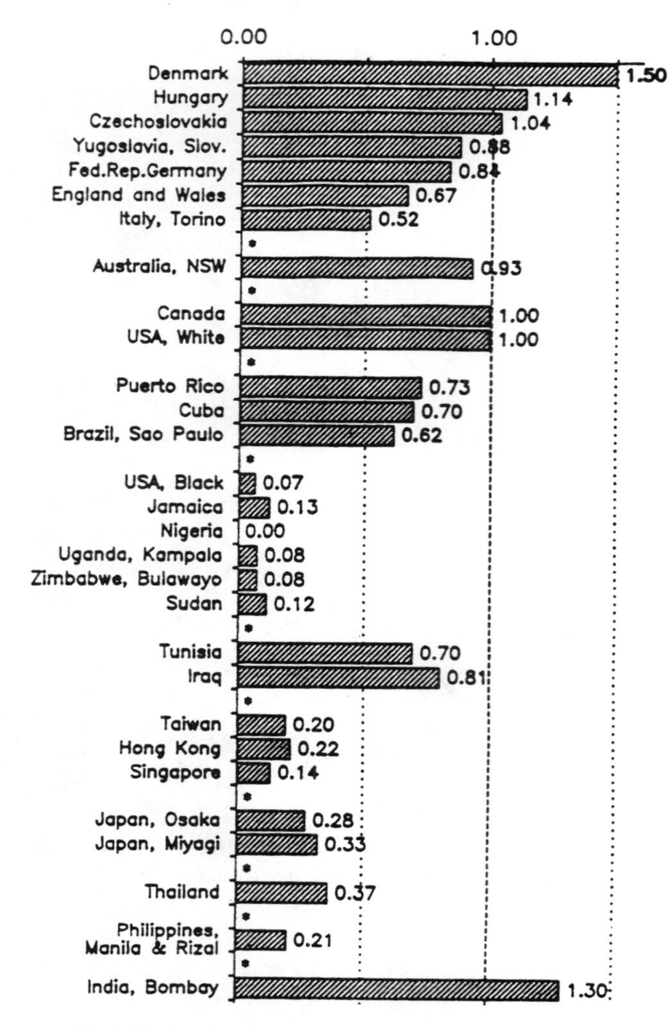

FIG. 44–4. Ratio of Ewing's sarcoma to osteosarcoma (number of cases registered). From Parkin et al, 1988.

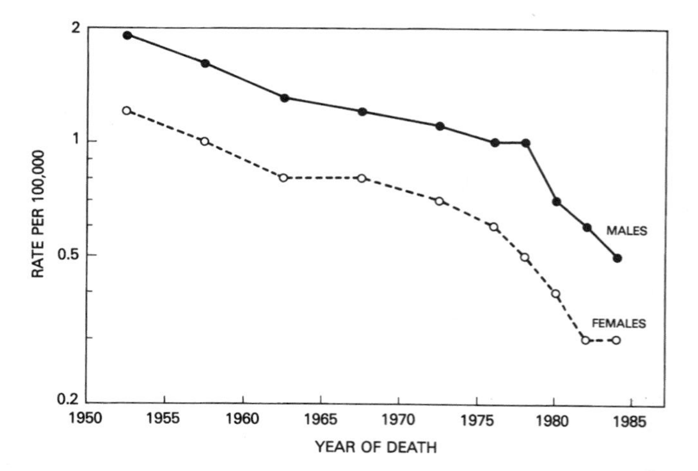

FIG. 44–5. Age-adjusted mortality rates (per 100,000, 1970 standard) for cancer of the bone and joints among the white population in the United States, by sex (1950–84). (Data from Devesa et al, 1987).

Although primary cancers of bone have been associated with external high-dose radiation, used especially in the therapy of various cancers, the fraction of bone cancers that result from this exposure appears to be small, i.e., less than 0.05% to 0.2% of patients treated (Boice et al, 1985a, 1985b; Robinson et al, 1988). Between 1935 and 1982 in Connecticut 30 bone cancers developed vs. 17 expected in 253,536 patients treated for cancer (30.8% of whom received radiotherapy) (Boice et al, 1985b). Among 379,941 cancer patients in Denmark treated between 1946 and 1980, 43 bone cancers occurred vs. 23 expected. Among 82,616 patients with cervical cancer treated with high-dose pelvic radiation, only 11 bone cancers were reported vs. 5.7 expected (Boice et al, 1985a); the dose to exposed bone was estimated to be 2,200 cGy (rad) on average (Boice et al, 1988). In each of these three studies, 0.01% of the patients given radiotherapy developed bone sarcoma,

TABLE 44–2. *Age, Sex, and Site Distribution of Primary Bone Cancer Among Whites According to Histologic Type, SEER Cancer Registries, 1973–85*

		Age Distribution			
Histology	*No. Patients*	*Median Age*	*Peak Incidence*	*Percent Male*	*Major Sites (%)*[a]
Osteosarcoma	759	23	10–19, M 65–79, F 80+	57	170.7 (59%), 170.6 (12%), 170.4 (11%)
Chondrosarcoma	575	55	M 60–85+	54	170.7 (30%), 170.6 (21%), 170.3 (16%)
Ewing's sarcoma	344	15	M 10–19, F 5–14	64	170.7 (32%), 170.6 (23%), 170.3 (19%)
Chordoma	86	62	M 50–79 F 70–84	64	170.6 (45%), 170.2 (35%), 170.0 (20%)
Fibrous histiocytoma	61	61	60–79	63	170.7 (54%), 170.6 (14%)
Fibrosarcoma	60	59	60–79	51	170.7 (47%), 170.4 (13%)
Giant cell tumor	45	28	20–29, 70–79	50	170.7 (52%), 170.4 (20%)

[a]International Classification of Diseases for Oncology (1976) site code definitions: 170.0 skull, face; 170.2 vertebra; 170.3 rib, sternum, clavicle; 170.4 upper limb, long bones, scapula; 170.6 pelvic bones, sacrum, coccyx; 170.7 lower limb, long bones.

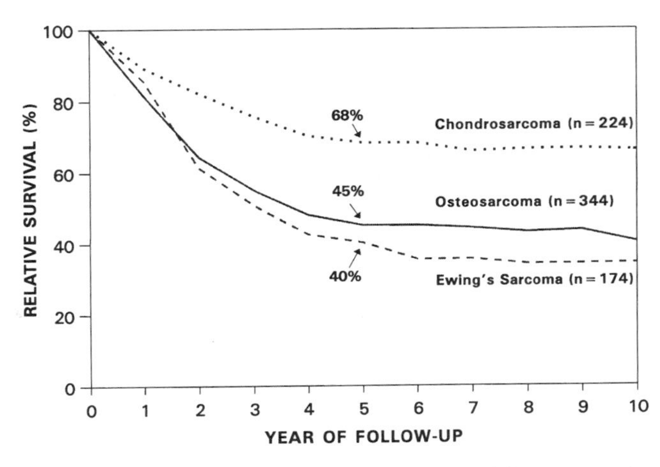

FIG. 44–6. Relative survival rates (%) for males with bone cancer, by histological type (all races, SEER 1980–89).

about twice the expected frequency. Excess bone cancers have also been reported following radiotherapy for breast cancer (Doherty et al, 1986) and Hodgkin's disease (Woodard et al, 1988).

Children with certain cancers, however, seem to be particularly susceptible to radiogenic bone cancer (Hawkins et al, 1987). High risks have been reported following treatment, primarily with radiation, for retinoblastoma (12 vs. 0.01 expected), Wilms' tumor (6 vs. 0.05), Hodgkin's disease (5 vs. 0.05), neuroblastoma (4 vs. 0.03) and Ewing's sarcoma (7 vs. 0.01) (Tucker et al, 1984). Among 1,603 children with retinoblastoma, 36 developed and died from bone cancer, whereas less than 1 death was expected (Eng et al, 1993). The excess bone cancers occurred only among patients with inherited germline retinoblastoma, and radiotherapy appeared to interact with genetic susceptibility to cancer

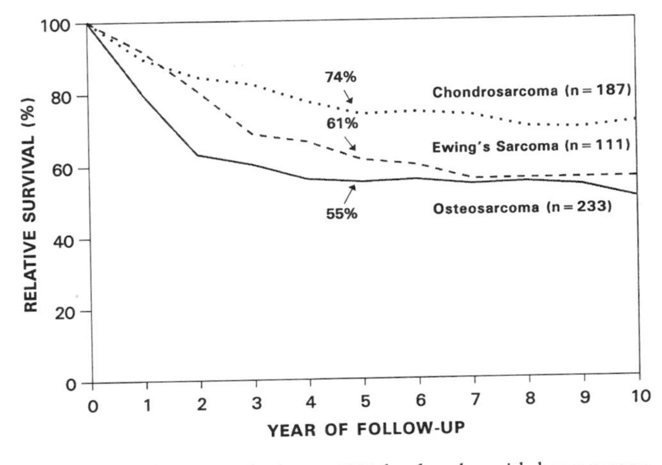

FIG. 44–7. Relative survival rates (%) for females with bone cancer, by histological type (all races, SEER 1980–89).

development. A cumulative risk of second primary tumor development of 7.9% (6% for osteosarcoma) was seen in a cancer registry investigation of 303 children with retinoblastoma (Draper et al, 1986).

Radiotherapy in childhood was linked to a 2.7-fold overall risk of bone cancer in a matched case-control study that took into account the underlying risk associated with the disease being treated (Tucker et al, 1987). Risk increased with estimated dose to bone (mean, 2,690 cGy) and reached 40-fold at 6,000 cGy. This is one of the few studies with individual dosimetry. The relative dose-response effect among patients treated for retinoblastoma resembled that among children with all other types of initial tumors, but the cumulative risk of bone cancer in the retinoblastoma group at 20 years was much higher than that for the entire cohort of children with cancer (14.1% vs. 2.8%). This implies that radiation must interact with underlying susceptibilities in a multiplicative, rather than additive fashion, the higher cumulative risk among retinoblastoma patients being due to the much higher background rate. The risk of bone cancer also rose significantly with time, up through 20 years after initial treatment. This pattern is similar to that seen for other radiogenic solid tumors, but different from the wavelike pattern seen for radiogenic leukemia (Boice et al, 1985a) and for ^{224}Ra-induced bone cancer (Mays and Spiess, 1984).

Although few studies have been able to quantify the risk of radiogenic bone cancer in man, children are apparently at much higher risk than adults, possibly due to their bone growth. For cervical cancer patients the relative risk for bone doses above 1,000 cGy was estimated to be 3.1 (Boice et al, 1988), whereas following childhood cancer the relative risk ranged from 6.0 to 38 (Sagerman et al, 1969; Tucker et al, 1987).

Relatively small increases of benign and malignant bone tumors have also been reported following X-ray therapy for non-neoplastic diseases such as ankylosing spondylitis (Darby et al, 1987; Weiss et al, 1994), ringworm of the scalp (Shore et al, 1976; Ron et al, 1988), and enlarged thymus glands (Pifer et al, 1963; Hildreth et al, 1985). No excess has been reported following whole-body exposure received by the atomic-bomb survivors in Japan (Shimizu, 1990), or among tuberculosis patients given massive numbers of chest fluoroscopies (Davis et al, 1989). Bone is considered relatively insensitive to the carcinogenic action of radiation, with excesses apparently occurring only after very high therapeutic doses on the order of 1,000 or more cGy (Boice et al, 1996—this volume).

Bone-seeking radium isotopes have been conclusively linked to bone cancer other than Ewing's sarcoma. Among 1,474 women employed as radium dial painters before 1930 in the United States, 61 (4%) developed bone sarcoma (Rowland et al, 1978). Large quantities

TABLE 44–3. *Epidemiologic Studies of Radiation-Induced Bone Cancer*

Study	*Type of Exposure*	*Number Exposed*	*Duration of Follow-up (years)*	*Person–Years at Risk*	*Average Bone Dose (cGy)*	*Relative Risk (O/E)*
Adult—external radiation						
1. Cervical cancer (Boice et al, 1985a, 1988)	External radiotherapy, Brachytherapy	82,616	1–35	547,222	2,200	11/5.7
2. Ankylosing spondylitis (Darby et al, 1987)	External radiotherapy	14,106	1–39	183,749	372	4/1.4
3. Atomic bomb survivors (Shimizu et al, 1990)	Gamma rays, neutrons	41,719	5–40	1,200,000	~25	13/17
Childhood/fetal—external radiation						
4. Childhood cancer—LESG (Tucker et al, 1984)	External radiotherapy	9,170[a]	2–29	50,609	0–7,000	48/0.36
5. Childhood cancer—UK (Hawkins et al, 1987)	External radiotherapy	10,100[a]	3–35	78,483	0–7,000	28/0.65
6. Retinoblastoma—NY (Abramson et al, 1984)	External radiotherapy, Radium placque	688[b]	1–32	~5,000	3,000–15,000	45/small
7. Retinoblastoma—UK (Hawkins et al, 1987; Draper et al, 1986)	External radiotherapy, Radium plaque	303[b]	3–35	~2,300	~2,000	13/0.03
8. Childhood cancer—LESG (Tucker et al, 1987)	External radiotherapy	84% of 64 cases 73% of 209 controls	NA	NA	2,690	2.7
9. Oxford survey (Bithell and Stewart, 1975)	Prenatal X-ray	10.7% of 244 cases 9% of 244 controls	NA	NA	<10	1.11
Radionuclides—internal radiation						
10. Radium-dial painters[c] (Rowland et al, 1978; Polednak et al, 1978)	^{226}Radium, ^{228}Radium	757	1–56	33,597	1,700	38/0.4
11. Bone disease—Germany (Spiess et al, 1989)	^{224}Radium	900	1–43	21,600	416	56/0.25
12. Ankylosing spondylitis—Germany (Wick and Gössner, 1989)	^{224}Radium	1,473	1–38	~25,000	56–67	1/small
13. Thorotrast patients—Portugal (da Motta et al, 1979)	^{232}Thorium (translocating ^{224}Ra, ^{228}Th, ^{228}Ra)	1,244	1–45	~19,000	~400	5/small
14. Thorotrast patients—Germany (van Kaick et al, 1989)	as above	2,326	1–45	>20,000	~400	4/1.2
15. Thorotrast patients—Denmark (Faber, 1979)	as above	1,012	1–36	18,000	~400	0/0.2

[a]Radiotherapy status not reported. Approximately 73–84% exposed. Includes children with genetic predisposition to develop osteosarcoma.
[b]Genetic retinoblastoma; these children are genetically predisposed to develop osteosarcoma.
[c]Only data for women with known doses are presented. Overall 61 bone sarcomas have occurred in 1,474 women employed prior to 1930.
NA = Not applicable.
~ = Estimated.

of ^{226}Ra and ^{228}Ra (mesothorium) were ingested due to the habit of licking paintbrushes to make fine tips. Radium decays by emitting high-LET alpha particles, and the resulting bone dose can be very high. Among 759 women whose bone doses have been determined (1,700 cGy average) an S-shaped dose-effect curve was observed. A linear relationship could be rejected. The downturn at very high doses may be due to an inability of cells to divide. Interestingly, no osteosarcomas occurred below a dose of about 1,000 cGy. It has been suggested that a threshold could exist for cancer induced by radium isotopes (NAS, 1972), which was consistent with recent evaluations of the U.S. radium dial study (Rowland, 1995). A threshold would explain why only 1 osteosarcoma was reported among 1,203 radium luminizers studied in the U.K. who ingested much lower amounts of ^{226,228}Ra than U.S. dial painters (Baverstock and Papworth, 1989).

Another bone-seeking radium isotope, ^{224}Ra, was used in Germany after World War II to treat bone tuberculosis and ankylosing spondylitis. Among 900 patients injected with ^{224}Ra, 56 (6%) developed bone cancer, particularly osteosarcoma, with latent periods from 4 to 22 years (Spiess et al, 1989). The average dose to bone was approximately 420 cGy. The pattern of incidence over time for ^{224}Ra-induced bone sarcomas was generally similar to that observed for leukemia in A-bomb survivors, spondylitis patients given radiotherapy, and cervical cancer patients treated with radiation. This wave of induced cancers is contrary to observations on all other forms of cancer, which have a sustained rise. Excess bone sarcomas appeared within 5 years after injection, peaked between 6 to 8 years, and decreased to normal levels after about 33 years. The lowest skeletal dose was 90 cGy. No excess bone sarcomas were found in a series of 1,501 patients treated with lower doses of ^{224}Ra (Wick and Gössman, 1989).

Also, contrary to the experience following exposure to sparsely ionizing radiation such as X or gamma rays, protracted exposures to radium alpha particles appeared to increase the carcinogenic effect; that is, for the same total dose, injections spread over long time periods were more carcinogenic. This protraction-enhancement effect may be due to (a) killing fewer premalignant cells, (b) exposing more cells, (c) increasing the stimulus for cell division, or (d) preventing repair of local damage (Mays and Spiess, 1984). The dose-response effect was best described by a linear-quadratic-exponential equation (Chmelevsky et al, 1988). It is noteworthy that bone sarcomas appeared at doses about 10 times lower, on average, than in the ^{226}Ra dial painters.

This difference in carcinogenic effectiveness, as well as in latency period and shape of the dose-effect curve, appears to be related to the different radium isotopes involved. The dial painters ingested predominantly ^{226}Ra, a bone-volume seeker, whereas the German patients were injected with ^{224}Ra, a bone-surface seeker. The isotope ^{226}Ra has a long half-life (1,600 years) and deposits its energy throughout the entire bone. The long latent periods observed are probably related to the ^{226}Ra continually irradiating tissue throughout life. The shape of the dose-effect curve and the carcinogenic efficiency would be expected to differ from ^{224}Ra if the cells at risk for osteosarcoma are assumed to be the surface endosteal cells. Much of the dose from ^{226}Ra would be "wasted" in the nonactive mineral component of bone. For the German patients, however, the short-lived ^{224}Ra (3.8 days) would give up its energy quickly and mainly on the bone surface, and the endosteal cells would thus receive more exposure per average bone dose. When endosteal doses are in fact computed, the minimum doses for development of osteosarcoma are comparable for ^{224}Ra and ^{226}Ra; i.e., 810 cGy and 760 cGy respectively (UNSCEAR, 1977).

Thorotrast, used in radiographic studies in the past, causes hepatic angiosarcomas and leukemia. Evidence is now mounting to support an excess of bone sarcoma apparently due to ^{224}Ra, which is deposited in bone after being given off as a decay product from deposits of Thorotrast in the reticuloendothelial system (NAS, 1988). Studies of workers exposed to plutonium have yet to reveal a significant increase in bone cancer (Boice et al, 1996—see pp 334–335).

Chemicals

Treatment of childhood cancer with alkylating agents has been linked to a 4.7-fold risk of bone cancer, with risk increasing as cumulative drug exposure rose (Tucker et al, 1987; Kingston et al, 1987; Newton et al, 1991). Half of the 64 children who developed bone cancer as a second malignancy received chemotherapeutic agents, most commonly cyclophosphamide, triethylenemelamine, and chlorambucil. Radiotherapy and hereditary retinoblastoma were ruled out as potential confounders. Associations between chemical agents and bone cancers, independent of radiation exposure, have not been previously reported. Studies of retinoblastoma (Draper et al, 1986) and Ewing's sarcoma (Strong et al, 1979) have suggested that cyclophosphamide may potentiate the effect of radiotherapy in the development of osteosarcomas. Neither fluoridated drinking water (Hoover et al, 1991) nor occupational exposures to chemicals have been implicated in the genesis of osteosarcomas.

Viruses

Osteosarcomas and other cancers of connective tissue have been induced in experimental animals since Rous's work in 1912. Recent human studies have shown viruslike particles in osteosarcoma cells, and immunological peculiarities related to the presence of this neoplasm (reviewed by Silcocks and Murrells, 1987). Studies of time-space clustering of osteosarcoma or Ewing's sarcoma, however, have shown no evidence of horizontal spread in the United States (Fraumeni and Glass, 1970) or England (Silcocks and Murrells, 1987). Occasionally clusters of bone cancer have been reported, but virtually all forms of cancer, no matter how rare, may cluster geographically by chance, given that in the United States alone, for example, there are 29,000 towns (Neutra et al, 1990)—plus a large number of neighborhoods in cities.

Trauma and Metal Implants

Trauma, of interest in the past, is rarely suggested as a cause of bone cancer today, despite a few persuasive cases (Berry et al, 1980). By contrast, metal nails and implants, as in hip replacement, are more often associated with cancers in bone and other adjacent tissues. Recently, case reports have accumulated sufficiently to suggest an etiologic relationship. Seventeen cases through 1988 (excluding two lymphomas) were cited in a case presentation at the Massachusetts General Hospital (1991), to which must be added the case presented, and four others published since 1988 (Haag and Adler, 1989; Harris, 1989; Brien et al, 1990, Khurana et al, 1991)), which brings the total to 22. Seventeen of these cases were reported since 1980. The tumor types were mixed, and included two with Ewing's sarcoma, six with osteosarcoma, and, since 1984, five with malignant fibrous histiocytoma. The patients were over 40 years of age at implant except for an 8-year-old with Morquio syndrome, and an 11-year-old. The interval from implant to diagnosis of the cancer was 15 months to 30 years; seven had intervals of less than four years. These intervals were shorter than usual for occupationally or drug-induced solid cancers except for lymphoma. The implants were of metals in various combinations. Among them were chromium, a known human carcinogen, and nickel, a suspected carcinogen (Tomatis et al, 1989; IARC Monographs, 1990). Malignant fibrous histiocytoma has also been described in association with bone infarcts, caisson workers, and sickle-cell anemia (Heater et al, 1987). Metal implants have induced cancer experimentally in dogs (Harrison et al, 1976; Sinibaldi et al, 1976). The etiologic role of bone cement must also be considered, but it was not used in all cases. Throughout the literature the association of metal implants and adjacent sarcoma is attributed to chance, but there is now suggestive evidence of an association. The establishment of a registry of cases should provide information on details of the relationship.

HOST FACTORS

Preexisting Bone Defects

Certain syndromes of skeletal maldevelopment are prone to bone cancer (Fraumeni, 1973). Multiple exostoses (diaphyseal aclasia) are osteochondromas on the surfaces of growing bone. This dominantly inherited condition may produce severe deformities, and transformation to chondrosarcoma has been reported in 5% to 11% of patients. Chondrosarcoma also occurs excessively with enchondromatosis (Ollier's syndrome) or with the combination of enchondromatosis and skin hemangiomas (Maffucci's syndrome), but neither syndrome is inherited in a simple Mendelian fashion (Schwartz et al, 1987). Case reports also indicate an excess of osteosarcoma and fibrosarcoma with polyostotic fibrous dysplasia (Yabut et al, 1988), and osteogenesis imperfecta (Lasson et al, 1978). Osteosarcoma has been described with Hutchinson-Gilford progeria (King et al, 1978) and with incompletely defined syndromes involving growth disturbances (Parry et al, 1978; Schuman and Burton, 1979).

Of special importance is Paget's disease (osteitis deformans), which predisposes mainly to osteosarcoma, but also to fibrosarcoma, chondrosarcoma, and giant cell tumor (Haibach et al, 1985). The legs are much more often affected than the arms (McKusick, 1972). Localized bone destruction occurs for an unknown reason, which makes the bone susceptible to the effects of stress. Repair occurs almost simultaneously with resorption, and the bone enlarges (Fallon and Schwamm, 1989). The skull is commonly involved, and one sign of the disease is the need for a larger hat size than before. Of 101 osteosarcomas in a series of patients older than 60 years of age, 55 percent were associated with Paget's disease (Huvos, 1986).

When the disease is familial, which is not uncommon, it is transmitted as an autosomal dominant trait (McKusick, 1994). In one family, three siblings with polyostotic Paget's disease developed osteosarcoma at 67–77 years of age (Brenton et al, 1980), and in another family three siblings developed Paget's disease, two of whom died of osteosarcoma at 55 and 57 years of age (Wu et al, 1991). In a case-control study, a history of Paget's disease in parents or siblings was given by 12.3% of 788 cases as compared with 2.1% of 387 spouse controls (Siris et al, 1991). Among relatives of cases, the cumulative risk was highest when the case was diagnosed under 55 years of age and had bone deformity, an indication of severity of the disease.

Sarcoma occurs in about 0.7% of patients with Paget's disease (Hadjipavlou et al, 1992), and is thought to account for the rise in bone sarcoma late in life (Boyd et al, 1969). In the United Kingdom, a radiologic survey showed that 5.4% of people over 55 years had Paget's disease (Barker et al, 1977). The disorder is usually silent. In one study, only 3 of 85 patients with the disease had complaints referable to bone (Monroe, 1951). Men are affected 1.5–2 times more often than women. Cancer may arise from Paget's disease limited to one bone, such as a vertebra (Groh, 1988).

Osteosarcoma in Paget's disease develops most frequently in the femur, followed by the humerus, pelvis, and calvarium (Haibach et al, 1985). The neoplasm may occur at several sites in polyostotic Paget's disease, perhaps due to metastases related to the highly vascular nature of the underlying disorder (Schajowicz et al, 1983). Viral-like inclusions in osteoclasts are found in some, but by no means all cases, suggesting that Paget's disease may have an infectious etiology (Mirra, 1987), but the evidence to date is conflicting (reviewed by Posen, 1992). Occasional geographic clustering of cases has occurred as in Lancashire, England (Barker et al, 1980), and in a few small towns in New South Wales (Posen, 1992).

Some cases have angioid streaks in the fundus of the eye as seen in pseudoxanthoma elasticum, an inherited disease of connective tissue. Biochemical studies suggest that Paget's disease may also belong to this group of hereditary disorders (Francis and Smith, 1974).

Environmental influences may also be involved, as suggested by the declining trend and substantial international variation, including the higher incidence reported in the United Kingdom than in the United States and Scandinavian countries (Gardner and Barker, 1978). Regional variation has been reported within the United Kingdom (Barker et al, 1977). Among migrants from the United Kingdom to Australia, the radiologic prevalence of subclinical Paget's disease was intermediate between the rates prevailing in the countries of origin and destination (Gardner et al, 1978). Although Paget's disease is reported to be rare in Africa, radiographic surveys in the United States suggest no difference in prevalence between blacks and whites (Rosenkrantz et al, 1952).

Factors responsible for the malignant transformation of Paget's disease are obscure, but in Australia a latitudinal gradient was reported in the proportion of males affected with Paget's sarcoma of the skull (Brackenridge, 1979). This pattern appeared to correspond to the intensity of sunlight exposure. Genetic factors may also contribute to the severity of Paget's disease, including familial occurrences complicated by giant cell tumors (Jacobs et al, 1979). It remains to be seen whether the risk of malignant degeneration will diminish with the wider treatment of Paget's disease by suppressive amounts of calcitonins and diphosphonates.

Apart from Paget's disease, solitary skeletal defects have been reported with increased frequency in patients with bone cancer, but the risk is difficult to evaluate, since the anomaly may be obliterated during tumor growth. Cancers of various types have been observed on the walls of bone cysts, and have arisen from benign giant cell tumors, osteomas and osteoblastomas, bone infarcts, fibrous dysplasia, and chronic osteomyelitic sinuses (Unni and Dahlin, 1978). Such observations prompted the hypothesis by Johnson (1953) that bone disorders with prolonged periods of excessive cell activity are prone to neoplastic change. In certain benign lesions, notably giant cell tumors, radiation therapy may promote malignant transformation or may induce sarcomas independent of the original condition (Nascimento et al, 1979).

Familial Aggregation and Multiple Neoplasms

In addition to its appearance in several genetic syndromes that affect bone, as noted above, osteosarcoma occasionally aggregates in families. Children who survive bilateral (hereditary) retinoblastoma have an increased frequency of osteosarcoma (36 cases all with bilateral retinoblastoma, as compared with 0.1 expected), unrelated to radiotherapy or chemotherapy (Eng et al, 1993). Earlier recognition of this concurrence led to the realization that the retinoblastoma susceptibility gene (Rb-1), located at chromosome 13q14, is also important in the development of osteosarcomas that are secondary to retinoblastoma (Benedict et al, 1990). Alterations of the Rb-1 gene have also been found in only the tumor tissue of sporadic cases of osteosarcoma and soft-tissue sarcomas (Wunder et al, 1991); inactivation of this gene may be involved in the genesis and progression of mesenchymal tumors in general. Osteosarcoma and retinoblastoma also tend to aggregate individually among close relatives. Such observations have prompted the generalization that cancers occurring excessively as double primaries may also aggregate excessively in families. These clinical observations provide clues for laboratory scientists in their search for genes of diverse cancers that are familial or occur as multiple primaries.

A spectacular example of familial aggregation of cancer has been delineated as the Li-Fraumeni syndrome (Li et al, 1988). About 100 affected families have been identified to date. The cancers that occur singly or in combination include osteosarcoma, soft-tissue sarcomas, carcinoma of the breast, brain cancer, adrenocortical carcinoma, and leukemia. In five of these families that have been evaluated in molecular studies, germ-line mutation of the tumor-suppressor gene, p53, located at chromosome 17p13, has been found (Malkin et al, 1990). The normal function of the Rb-1 gene and the p53 gene is to regulate normal growth of specific organs; when the function is inactivated, as by chromosomal deletion or degradation, growth becomes abnormal and cancerous. This class of genes, first recognized in rare cancers of childhood, now has counterparts in certain adult cancers that are far more common. Discovery of these genes should lead to new means for cancer prevention, early detection, and treatment. When the aggregation of cancer is limited by small family size, or occurs in a single member with multiple primary cancers of types found in the Li-Fraumeni syndrome, the mutated gene can be sought as a means for diagnosing the syndrome.

Recent evidence points to a neural origin for Ewing's sarcoma (reviewed by Horowitz et al, 1993), which rarely aggregates in families (Zamora et al, 1989). In about 85% of cases the tumor cells show a translocation

TABLE 44–4. *Epidemiologic Comparisons of Osteogenic Sarcoma (OS) and Ewing's Sarcoma (ES)*[a]

Feature	*OS*	*ES*
Radiation-related	Yes	No
Age peaks	Early and late	Early
Rarity in blacks	No	Yes
Relation to precursor bone syndromes	Yes	No
Correlation with growth patterns	Yes	Possibly
Familial tendency	Yes	Rare
Multiple primary cancer syndromes	Yes	No
Relation to retinoblastoma	Yes	No
Occurrence in other species	Common	Rare
Susceptibility of large dogs	High	None

[a]Adapted from Miller (1981).

involving chromosomes 11q24 and 22q12 (Ewing's Tumour Workshop, 1990). A principal gene locus for Ewing's sarcoma is near 22q12; some cases have a deletion here with no translocation. The same translocation is consistently seen in peripheral primitive neuroectodermal tumors. An origin in common would signify that the tumor can present in an undifferentiated form (Ewing's sarcoma), or with varying degrees of neural differentiation, culminating in peripheral primitive neuroectodermal tumors.

The contrast between osteosarcoma and Ewing's sarcoma goes well beyond morphologic and genetic differences, as summarized in Table 44–4. Ewing's sarcoma is among the cancers that have not been induced by exposure to ionizing radiation. No new leads to etiology were found in a case-control study of 208 patients with Ewing's sarcoma, with data on demography, maternal reproduction, child health, parental occupation, and family history (Winn et al, 1992). The main epidemiologic clue to its origin remains its rarity among nonwhites.

CONCLUSIONS

Studies of bone cancer have provided many epidemiologic leads to etiology. The dissimilarities by cell type, particularly between osteosarcoma and Ewing's sarcoma, indicate that the origins of these tumors are different. Laboratory studies have shown that both cell types have genetic origins but involve different loci. Other types of bone cancer, such as chondrosarcoma and fibrosarcoma, are epidemiologically dissimilar to osteosarcoma.

The adolescent peak for osteosarcoma appears to be related to the pubertal growth spurt, and the rising incidence after middle age has been linked to Paget's disease. Animal experimentation has shown that certain viruses can cause osteosarcoma, but there is no evidence that they can do so in the human. Recent observations of cancer in bone and soft tissue adjacent to metal implants containing chromium has been reproduced experimentally in dogs. Thus, chromium, a known human carcinogen, and perhaps other metals in the implant may be responsible.

The role of genetic susceptibility is clear from (a) molecular and cytogenetic studies of the gene loci for osteosarcoma and Ewing's sarcoma; (b) the linkages of osteosarcoma with hereditary retinoblastoma and the Li-Fraumeni syndrome; (c) the association of osteosarcomas with several genetic disorders of bone; and (d) the near-absence of Ewing's sarcoma in blacks and Asians, presumably due to diminished mutability of a gene for this neoplasm.

The identification of high-risk groups has important implications for the detection and prevention of bone cancer. Persons with predisposing conditions should be followed regularly for early diagnosis and treatment of bone cancer; e.g., patients with Paget's disease, enchondromas, other benign growths, heavy radiation exposures, or familial aggregation involving osteosarcoma, retinoblastoma, or the diverse neoplasms of the Li-Fraumeni syndrome. Appropriate steps should be taken, of course, to reduce exposures to ionizing radiation, and, in families with Li-Fraumeni syndrome, to known human carcinogens. Further study of the molecular genetics of type-specific bone cancers should lead to improved methods of cancer prevention and control.

REFERENCES

ABRAMSON DH, ELLSWORTH RM, KITCHIN FD, TUNG G. 1984. Second monocular tumors in retinoblastoma survivors: Are they radiation-induced? Ophthalmology 91:1351–1355.

BARKER DJP, CHAMBERLAIN AT, GUYER PB, et al. 1980. Paget's disease of bone: the Lancashire focus. Brit Med J 280:1105–1107.

BARKER DJP, CLOUGH PWL, GUYER PB, et al. 1977. Paget's disease of bone in 14 British towns. Br Med J 1:1181–1183.

BAVERSTOCK KF, PAPWORTH DG. 1989. The UK radium luminiser survey. *In*: Taylor DM, Mays CW, Gerber GB, Thomas RG (eds). Risks from Radium and Thorotrast. BIR Report 21. London, Br Inst Radiol, pp. 72–76.

BENEDICT WF, XU H-J, TAKAHASHI R. 1990. The retinoblastoma gene: its role in human malignancies. Cancer Investigation 8:535–540.

BERRY MP, JENKIN DT, FORNASIER VL, et al. 1980. Osteosarcoma at the site of previous fracture. J Bone Joint Surg 62-A:1216–1218.

BITHELL JF, STEWART AM. 1975. Pre-natal irradiation and childhood malignancy: a review of the British data from the Oxford Survey. Br J Cancer 31:271–287.

BOICE JD JR, DAY NE, ANDERSEN A, et al. 1985a. Second cancers following radiation treatment for cervical cancer. An international collaboration among cancer registries. JNCI 74:955–975.

BOICE JD JR, ENGHOLM G, KLEINERMAN RA, et al. 1988. Radiation dose and second cancer risk in patients treated for cancer of the cervix. Radiat Res 116:3–55.

BOICE JD JR, LAND CE, PRESTON DL. 1996. Ionizing radiation. *In*: Schottenfeld D, Fraumeni JF Jr (eds): Cancer Epidemiology and Prevention. New York, Oxford University Press.

BOICE JD JR, STORM HH, CURTIS RE, et al (eds). 1985b. Multiple Primary Cancers in Connecticut and Denmark. Natl Cancer Inst Monogr 68. Washington D.C., U.S. Govt Print Off, pp. 1–437.

BOYD JT, DOLL R, HILL GB, et al. 1969. Mortality from primary tumours of bone in England and Wales, 1961–63. Br J Prev Soc Med 23:12–22.

BRACKENRIDGE CJ. 1979. A statistical study of sarcoma complicating Paget's disease of bone in three countries. Br J Cancer 40:194–200.

BRENTON DP, ISENBERG DA, BERTRAM J. 1980. Osteosarcoma complicating familial Paget's disease. Postgrad Med J 56:238–243.

BRIEN WW, SALVATI EA, HEALEY JH. 1990. Osteogenic sarcoma arising in the area of a total hip replacement. J Bone Joint Surg 72-A:1097.

CAVAZZANA A, TRICHE TJ, TSOKOS M, et al. 1987. Experimental evidence for the neural origin of Ewing's sarcoma. Am J Pathol 127:507–518.

CHMELEVSKY D, KELLERER AM, LAND CE, et al. 1988. Time and dose dependency of bone sarcomas in patients injected with radium-224. Radiat Environ Biophys 27:103–114.

DA MOTTA LC, DA SILVA HORTA J, TAVARES MH. 1979. Prospective epidemiologic study of Thorotrast-exposed patients in Portugal. Environ Res 18:152–172.

DAHLIN DC. 1978. Osteosarcoma of bone and a consideration of prognostic variables. Cancer Treat Rep 62:189–192.

DARBY SC, DOLL R, GILL SK, et al. 1987. Long term mortality after a single treatment course with X-rays in patients treated for ankylosing spondylitis. Br J Cancer 55:179–190.

DAVIS FG, BOICE JD JR, HRUBEC Z, MONSON RR. 1989. Lung cancer mortality in a radiation-exposed cohort of Massachusetts tuberculosis patients. Cancer Res 49:6130–6136.

DAVISON EV, PEARSON ADJ, EMSLIE J, et al. 1989. Chromosome 22 abnormalities in Ewing's sarcoma. J Clin Pathol 42:797–799.

DECARLI A, LA VECCHIA C, MEZZANOTTE G. 1987. Birth cohort, time, and age effects in Italian mortality. Cancer 59:1221–1232.

DEVESA SS, SILVERMAN DT, YOUNG JL JR, et al. 1987. Cancer incidence and mortality trends among whites in the United States, 1947–84. JNCI 79:701–770.

DOHERTY MA, RODGER A, LANGLANDS AO. 1986. Sarcoma of bone following therapeutic irradiation for breast carcinoma. Int J Radiat Oncol Biol Phys 12:103–106.

DRAPER GJ, SANDERS BM, KINGSTON JE. 1986. Second primary neoplasms in patients with retinoblastoma. Br J Cancer 53:661–671.

ENG C, LI FP, ABRAMSON DH, ELLSWORTH RM, WONG FL, GOLDMAN MB, SEDDON J, TARBELL N, BOICE JD JR. 1993. Mortality from second tumors among long-term survivors of retinoblastoma. J Natl Cancer Inst 85:1121–1128.

ERICSSON JL-E, KARNSTRÖM L, MATTSSON B. 1978. Childhood cancer in Sweden, 1958–1974. I. Incidence and mortality. Acta Paediat Scand 67:425–432.

EWING'S TUMOUR WORKSHOP. 1990. First children's solid tumour group workshop in Ewing's sarcoma 30 June to 1 July 1989. Br J Cancer 62:326–330.

FABER M. 1979. Twenty-eight years of continuous follow-up of patients injected with Thorotrast for cerebral angiography. Environ Res 18:37–43.

FALLON MD, SCHWAMM HA. 1989. Paget's disease of bone. An update on the pathogenesis, pathophysiology, and treatment of osteitis deformans. Pathol Annu 1:115–159.

FRANCIS MJO, SMITH R. 1974. Evidence of a generalised connective-tissue defect in Paget's disease of bone. Lancet 1:841–842.

FRAUMENI JF JR. 1967. Stature and malignant tumors of bone in childhood and adolescence. Cancer 20:967–973.

FRAUMENI JF JR. 1973. Genetic factors. *In* Holland JF, Frei E (eds): Cancer Medicine. Philadelphia, Lea and Febiger, pp. 7–15.

FRAUMENI JF JR, GLASS AG. 1970. Rarity of Ewing's sarcoma among US Negro Children. Lancet 1:366–367.

GARDNER MJ, BARKER DJP. 1978. Mortality from malignant tumours of bone and Paget's disease in the United States and in England and Wales. Int J Epidemiol 7:121–130.

GARDNER MJ, GUYER PB, BARKER DJP. 1978. Radiological prevalence of Paget's disease of bone in British migrants to Australia. Br Med J 1:1655–1657.

GLASS AG, FRAUMENI JF JR. 1970. Epidemiology of bone cancer in children. J Natl Cancer Inst 44:187–199.

GROH JA. 1988. Mono-osteotic Paget's disease as a clinical entity. Roentgenologic observations in nine cases. Am J Roentgenol 150:235–248.

HAAG M, ADLER CP. 1989. Malignant fibrous histiocytoma in association with hip replacement. J Bone Joint Surg 71B:701.

HADJIPAVLOU A, LANDER P, SROLOVITZ H, ENKER IP. 1992. Malignant transformation of Paget disease of bone. Cancer 70:2802–2808.

HAIBACH H, FARRELL C, DITTRICH FJ. 1985. Neoplasms arising in Paget's disease of bone: A study of 82 cases. Am J Clin Pathol 83:594–600.

HARRIS WR. 1990. Chondrosarcoma complicating total hip arthroplasty in Maffucci's syndrome. Clin Orthopaed Rel Res Number 260:212–214.

HARRISON JW, MCLAIN DL, HOHN RB, et al. 1976. Osteosarcoma associated with metal implants: report of two cases in dogs. Clin Orthop 116:253–257.

HAWKINS MM, DRAPER GJ, KINGSTON JE. 1987. Incidence of second primary tumours among childhood cancer survivors. Br J Cancer 56:339–347.

HEALY JW. 1975. The origin of current standards. Health Phys 29:489–494.

HEATER K, COLLINS PA. 1987. Osteosarcoma in association with infarction of bone. J Bone Joint Surg 69A:300–302.

HILDRETH NG, SHORE RE, HEMPELMANN LH, ROSENSTEIN M. 1985. Risk of extrathyroid tumors following radiation treatment in infancy for thymic enlargement. Radiat Res 102:378–391.

HOOVER RN, DEVESA SS, CANTOR KP, et al. 1991. Fluoridation of drinking water and subsequent cancer incidence and mortality. *In*: Report of the ad hoc Subcommittee on Fluoride of the Committee to Coordinate Environmental Health and Related Programs: Review on Fluoride, Benefits and Risks. DHHS PHS February, Apps. E and F.

HOROWITZ ME, DELANEY TF, MALAWER MM, TSOKOS MG. 1993. Ewing's sarcoma family of tumors: Ewing's sarcoma of bone and soft tissue and the peripheral primitive neuroectodermal tumors. In Pizzo PA, Poplack DG: Principles and Practice of Pediatric Oncology. Second edition. Philadelphia, JB Lippincott, pp. 795–821.

HUVOS AG. 1986. Osteogenic sarcoma of bones and soft tissues in older persons. A clinicopathologic analysis of 117 patients older than 60 years. Cancer 57:1442–1449.

IARC. 1990. IARC Monographs on the Evaluation of Carcinogenic Risks to Humans. Chromium, Nickel and Welding. v. 49.

JACOBS TP, MICHELSEN J, POLAY JS, et al. 1979. Giant cell tumor in Paget's disease of bone. Cancer 44:742–747.

JOHNSON LC. 1953. A general theory of bone tumors. Bull NY Acad Med 164–171.

KHURANA JS, ROSENBERG AE, KATTAPURAM SV, et al. 1991. Malignancy supervening on an intramedullary nail. Clin Orthop 267:251–254.

KING CR, LEMMER J, CAMPBELL JR, et al. 1978. Osteosarcoma in a patient with Hutchinson-Gilford progeria. J Med Genet 15:481–484.

KINGSTON JE, HAWKINS MM, DRAPER GJ, et al. 1987. Patterns of multiple primary tumours in patients treated for cancer during childhood. Br J Cancer 56:331–338.

KLEINERMAN RA, LITTLEFIELD LG, TARONE RE, et al. 1990. Chromosome aberrations in relation to radiation dose following partial-body exposures in three populations. Radiat Res. 123:93–101.

KNUDSON AG. 1985. Hereditary cancer, oncogenes, antioncogenes. Cancer Res 45:1437–1443.

LASSON U, HARMS D, WIEDERMANN HR. 1978. Osteogenic sarcoma complicating osteogenesis imperfecta tarda. Eur J Pediatr 129:215–218.

LA VECCHIA C, DECARLI A. 1988. Decline of childhood cancer mortality in Italy, 1955–80. Oncology 45:93–97.

LEVI F, LA VECCHIA C. 1988. Childhood cancer in Switzerland: Mortality from 1951 to 1984. Oncol 45:313–317.

LI FP, FRAUMENI JF JR, MULVIHILL JJ, et al. 1988. A cancer family syndrome in twenty-four kindreds. Cancer Res 48:5358–5362.

MALKIN D, LI FP, STRONG LC, et al. 1990. Germ line p53 mutations in a family syndrome of breast cancer, sarcomas and other neoplasms. Science 250:1233–1238.

MARSHALL JH, GROER PG. 1977. A theory of the induction of bone cancer by alpha radiation. Radiat Res 71:149–192.

MARTLAND HS, CONLON P, KNEF JP. 1925. Some unrecognized dangers in the use and handling of radioactive substances. JAMA 85:1769–1776.

MASSACHUSETTS GENERAL HOSPITAL. 1991. Case record 4-1991. New Engl J Med 324:251–259.

MAYS CW. 1988. Alpha-particle-induced cancer in humans. Health Phys 55:637–652.

MAYS CW, SPIESS H. 1984. Bone sarcomas in patients given radium-224. *In:* Boice JD Jr, Fraumeni JF Jr (eds): Radiation Carcinogenesis: Epidemiology and Biological Significance. New York, Raven Press, pp. 241–252.

MCKUSICK VA. 1972. Paget's disease of the bone. *In:* McKusick VA: Heritable Disorders of Connective Tissue. St Louis, CV Mosby Co, (4th ed). pp 718–723.

MCKUSICK VA. 1994. Mendelian Inheritance in Man. Eleventh edition, Johns Hopkins Baltimore, University Press.

MILLER RW. 1981. Contrasting epidemiology of childhood osteosarcoma, Ewing's tumor, and rhabdomyosarcoma. Natl Cancer Inst Monogr 56:9–14.

MILLER RW, MCKAY FW. 1984. Decline in US childhood cancer mortality 1950 through 1980. JAMA 251:1567–1570.

MIRRA JM. 1987. Pathogenesis of Paget's disease based on viral etiology. Clin Orthop Related Res 217:162–170.

MONROE RT. 1951. Diseases of Old Age. Cambridge, Harvard Univ Press.

MUIR C, WATERHOUSE J, MACK T, et al. 1987. Cancer Incidence in Five Continents. Vol. V. International Agency for Research on Cancer, Lyon.

NAS (NATIONAL ACADEMY OF SCIENCES). 1972. Advisory Committee on the Biological Effects of Ionizing Radiations (The BEIR Report): The Effects on Populations of Exposure to Low Levels of Ionizing Radiation. Washington D.C., U.S. Government Printing Office.

NASCIMENTO AG, HUVOS AG, MARCOVE RC. 1979. Primary malignant giant cell tumor of bone. Cancer 44:1393–1402.

NEUTRA RR, SWAN S, FREEDMAN D, et al. 1990. Clusters galore. Arch Environ Health 45:314.

NEWTON WA, MEADOWS AT, SHIMADA H, et al. 1991. Bone sarcomas as second malignant neoplasms following childhood cancer. Cancer 67:193–201.

PARKIN DM, STILLER CA, DRAPER GJ, et al. 1988. International Incidence of Childhood Cancer. IARC Sci Publ 87:1–401.

PARRY DM, SAFYER AW, MULVIHILL JJ. 1978. Waardenburg-like features with cataracts, small head size, joint abnormalities, hypogonadism, and osteosarcoma. J Med Genet 15:66–69.

PERCY C, YOUNG JL JR, MUIR C, et al. 1995. Histology of Cancer: SEER Population-Based Data, 1973–87. Cancer (Suppl) 75:139–422.

PICKLE LW, MASON TJ, HOWARD N, et al. 1987. Atlas of U.S. cancer mortality among whites: 1950–1980. DHHS Publ No (NIH) 87-2900, Washington, D.C., U.S. Government Printing Office.

PIFER JW, TOYOOKA ET, MURRAY RW, et al. 1963. Neoplasms in children treated with x-rays for thymic enlargement. 1. Neoplasms and mortality. JNCI 31:1333–1356.

POLEDNAK AP. 1978. Bone cancer among female radium workers. Latency periods and incidence rates by time after exposure. J Natl Cancer Inst 60:77–82.

POSEN S. 1992. Paget's disease: current concepts. Aust N Z J Surg 62:17–23.

PRICE CHG. 1958. Primary bone-forming tumours and their relationship to skeletal growth. J Bone Jt Surg 40B:574–593.

ROBINSON E, NEUGUT A, WYLIE P. 1988. Clinical aspects of post-irradiation sarcomas. J Natl Cancer Inst 80:233–240.

RON E, MODAN B, BOICE JD JR. 1988. Mortality after radiotherapy for ringworm of the scalp. Am J Epidemiol 127:713–725.

ROSENKRANTZ JA, WOLK J, KAICHER JJ. 1952. Paget's disease (osteitis deformans). Arch Intern Med 90:610–633.

ROWLAND RE. 1995. Dose-response relationships for female radium dial workers: a new look. *In:* Health Effects of Internally Deposited Radionuclides: Emphasis on Radium and Thorium, van Kaick G, Karaoglou A, Kellerer AM (eds). Singapore: World Scientific, pp 135–143.

ROWLAND RE, STEHNEY AF, LUCAS HF JR. 1978. Dose-response relationships for female radium dial workers. Radiat Res 76:368–383.

SAGERMAN RH, CASSIDY JR, TRETTER P, et al. 1969. Radiation-induced neoplasia following external beam therapy for children with retinoblastoma. Am J Roentgenol 105:529–535.

SCHAJOWICZ F, ARAUJO ES, BERENSTEIN M. 1983. Sarcoma complicating Paget's disease of bone. J Bone Joint Surg 65-B:299–306.

SCHUMAN SH, BURTON WE. 1979. A new osteosarcoma/malformation syndrome. Clin Genet 15:462–463.

SCHWARTZ HS, ZIMMERMAN NB, SIMON MA, et al. 1987. The malignant potential of enchondromatosis. J Bone Joint Surg 69-A:269–274.

SHIMIZU Y, KATO H, SCHULL WJ. 1990. Studies of the mortality of A-bomb survivors. 9. Mortality, 1950–1985: Part 2. Cancer mortality based on the recently revised doses (DS86). Rad Res 121:120–141.

SHORE RE, ALBERT RE, PASTERNACK BS. 1976. Follow-up study of patients treated by x-ray epilation for tinea capitis: resurvey of post-treatment illness and mortality experience. Arch Environ Health 31:17–24.

SILCOCKS PBS, MURRELLS T. 1987. Space-time clustering and bone tumours: Application of Knox's method to data from a population-based cancer registry. Int J Cancer 40:769–771.

SINIBALDI K, ROSEN H, LIU SK, et al. 1976. Tumors associated with metallic implants in animals. Clin Orthop 118:257–276.

SIRIS ES, OTTMAN R, FLASTER E, KELSEY JL. 1991. Familial aggregation of Paget's disease. J Bone Miner Res 6:495–500.

SPIESS H, MAYS CW, CHMELEVSKY D. 1989. Malignancies in patients injected with radium 224. *In:* Taylor DM, Mays CW, Gerber GB (eds): Risks from Radium and Thorotrast. BIR Report 21. London, Br Inst Radiol, pp. 7–12.

STRONG LC, HERSON J, OSBORNE BM, et al. 1979. Risk of radiation-related subsequent malignant neoplasms in survivors of Ewing's sarcoma. JNCI 62:1401–1406.

TOMATIS L, AITIO A, WILBOURN J, et al. 1989. Human carcinogens so far identified. Jpn J Cancer Res 80:795–807.

TUCKER MA, MEADOWS AT, BOICE JD JR, et al. 1984. Cancer risk following treatment of childhood cancer. *In:* Boice JD Jr, Fraumeni JF Jr (eds): Radiation Carcinogenesis: Epidemiology and Biological Significance. New York, Raven Press, pp. 211–224.

TUCKER MA, D'ANGIO GJ, BOICE JD JR, et al. 1987. Bone sarcoma linked to radiotherapy and chemotherapy in children. N Engl J Med 317:588–593.

UNNI KK, DAHLIN DC. 1979. Premalignant tumors and conditions of bone. Am J Surg Pathol 3:47–60.

UNSCEAR (UNITED NATIONS SCIENTIFIC COMMITTEE ON THE EFFECTS OF ATOMIC RADIATION). 1977. Sources and Effects of Ionizing Radiation. Publ E.77.XI.1. New York, United Nations, pp. 399–401.

VAN KAICK G, WESCH H, LÜHRS H, et al. 1989. The German Thorotrast Study-report on 20 years follow-up. *In*: Taylor DM, Mays CW, Gerber GB, Thomas RG (eds): Risks from Radium and Thorotrast. BIR Report 21. London, Br Inst Radiol, pp. 98–104.

WEISS HA, DARBY SC, DOLL R. 1994. Cancer mortality following x-ray treatment for ankylosing spondylitis. Int J Cancer 59:327–338.

WICK RR, GÖSSNER W. 1989. Recent results of the follow-up of radium-224-treated ankylosing spondylitis patients. *In*: Taylor DM, Mays CW, Gerber GB (eds): Risks from Radium and Thorotrast. BIR Report 21. London. Br Inst Radiol, pp. 25–28.

WINN DM, LI FP, ROBISON LL, et al. 1992. A case-control study of the etiology of Ewing's tumor. Cancer Epidemiol Biomarkers Prev 1:525–532.

WOODARD HQ, HUVOS AG, SMITH J. 1988. Radiation-induced malignant tumors of bone in patients with Hodgkin's disease. Health Phys, 55:615–620.

WU RK, TRUMBLE TE, RUWE PA. 1991. Familial incidence of Paget's disease and secondary osteosarcoma. A report of three cases from a single family. Clin Orthop 265:306–309.

WUNDER JS, CZITROM AA, KANDEL R, et al. 1991. Analysis of alterations in the retinoblastoma gene and tumor grade in bone and soft-tissue sarcomas. J Natl Cancer Inst 83:194–200.

YABUT SM JR, KENAN S, SISSONS HA, et al. 1988. Malignant transformation of fibrous dysplasia. A case report and review of the literature. Clin Orthop 228:281–289.

YOUNG CL, SIM FH, UNNI KK, MCLEOD RA. 1990. Chondrosarcoma of bone in children. Cancer 66:1641–1648.

ZAMORA P, GARCÍA DE PAREDES ML, GONZÁLEZ BARÓN M, et al. 1986. Ewing's tumour in brothers: An unusual observation. Am J Clin Oncol 9:358–360.

45 Soft tissue sarcomas

SHELIA HOAR ZAHM
MARGARET A. TUCKER
JOSEPH F. FRAUMENI, JR.

Cancers of soft tissue account for about 1% of all malignant neoplasms and for about 1% of all cancer deaths (Silverberg and Lubera, 1988). The tumors are derived from mesenchymal tissues other than bone and cartilage, and are by definition sarcomas. A diversity of cell types are seen, with tumors originating from muscle, fat, blood vessels, fibrous tissue, or other supporting tissue (Enzinger and Weiss, 1988a). Most soft tissue sarcomas (STS) are located in the space between the skin and visceral organs, where the tissue mass accounts for over 50% of the body weight, but they may also arise from the mesenchyme in any part of the body exclusive of bony structures.

DEMOGRAPHIC PATTERNS

Histopathology and Anatomic Distribution

The cell of origin and the site distribution of STS, by histologic type, are presented in Table 45–1.

Blood vessel sarcomas are currently the most commonly reported STS. This group includes Kaposi's sarcoma, hemangioendothelioma, and hemangiopericytoma. Kaposi's sarcoma, which has increased dramatically in recent years as a result of the acquired immunodeficiency syndrome (AIDS) epidemic, is characterized by spindle cells and vascular channels and slits (Safai, 1987). Although the precise cell of origin is uncertain, it is most likely the endothelial cell (Werner et al, 1989). Historically, the tumor was rare in Western countries, occurred mainly in men of Italian or Jewish background, and had an indolent clinical course. The incidence rose progressively with advancing age, with 70% to 90% of cases occurring in men, usually arising on the legs (Templeton, 1973). The classical form of Kaposi's sarcoma is uncommon in African Americans, but accounts for about 5% to 12% of all cancer in some African countries. In the 1980s, however, Kaposi's sarcoma was found increasingly in young and middle-aged men in association with AIDS (Biggar et al, 1984). These epidemic cases typically have a more aggressive clinical course than the classical or endemic form of Kaposi's sarcoma (Safai, 1987).

Hemangioendotheliomas are characterized by atypical endothelial cells lining vascular channels with anastomosing lumens (Stout, 1943). In children, the male-to-female ratio is 0.8. Hepatic hemangioendotheliomas often develop in the first year of life and are associated with cutaneous hemangiomas (Chabalko and Fraumeni, 1975). Hemangiopericytomas are characterized by malignant round cells outside the basement membrane of endothelial lined vascular channels. The most common site is the lower extremity, followed by the pelvic fossa (Enzinger and Smith, 1976).

Fibrosarcomas, the next most commonly reported STS, are confounded by uncertainties and variations in pathologic classification. Two types are generally recognized. The adult form consists of cells ranging from fibroblasts to anaplastic spindle cells. The tumors occur mainly at 40 to 70 years of age, and may follow an aggressive course depending on the histologic grade (Pritchard et al, 1974). In the infantile form the cells are similar but less mature, with an onset usually under 2 years of age and with a better prognosis (Chung and Enzinger, 1976). Adult sarcomas occur mainly on the trunk, followed by the extremities; the infantile tumors occur most often on the extremities (Iwasaki and Enjoji, 1979). There is a male predominance at all ages.

Leiomyosarcomas are composed of a continuum of cells, from smooth muscle cells to anaplastic spindle cells (Yannopoulos and Stout, 1962). The incidence of leiomyosarcoma of the uterus, the most common site of origin, is highest in the third and fourth decades of life and declines thereafter (Fig. 45–1). The rates for uterine leiomyosarcomas are much higher among African Americans than whites (Harlow et al, 1986). The next most common site is the gastrointestinal tract, with a male predominance in both races. Only about 1% of tumors arising from the prostate, bladder, and gastrointestinal tract occur in children. Most leiomyosarco-

TABLE 45–1. *Cell of Origin and Site Distribution of Soft Tissue Sarcomas by Histologic Type*

Histology	*Malignant Cell*	*Major Sites*
Blood Vessel Sarcomas		
Kaposi's sarcoma	Endothelial cells, spindle cells, vascular channels, and vascular slits	Extremities
Hemangioendothelioma	Atypical endothelial cells lining vascular channels with anastomosing lumens	Head and neck, trunk, extremities, liver
Hemangiopericytoma	Ovoid or round cells outside the basement membrane with endothelial lined vascular channels	Lower extremity, pelvic fossa and retroperitoneum, head and neck
Fibrosarcoma		
Infantile	Neoplastic spindle cells to primitive mesenchymal cells	Extremities
Adult	Fibroblasts to anaplastic spindle cells	Trunk, extremities
Leiomyosarcoma	Smooth muscle cells to anaplastic spindle cells	Uterus, gastrointestinal tract
Liposarcoma	Lipoblasts, adult fat cells, embryonal fat cells	Lower extremity, upper extremity, trunk
Rhabdomyosarcoma		
Embryonal	Small embryonal rhabdomyoblasts	Head and neck, genitourinary tract
Pleiomorphic	Rhabdomyoblasts	Extremities, trunk, head and neck, genitourinary tract
Synovial sarcoma	Spindle cells and epithelioid cells without basement membrane	Extremities
Mesenchymoma	More than 2 neoplastic mesenchymal cell types, excluding fibroblasts	Extremities
Lymphangiosarcoma	Endothelium of proliferated lymphatics	Extremities

mas occur in visceral organs and are missed entirely by classifications that rely on site-oriented codes.

Liposarcomas are composed of adult or embryonal fat cells or lipoblasts (Pack and Pierson, 1954). There is a male predominance at all ages and about 1% to 3% of tumors occur in children. The most common sites are the legs, arms, and trunk, in that order.

Rhabdomyosarcomas consist of primitive striated muscle cells and are the most common childhood STS. As shown in Figure 45–1, there is a peak incidence under age 5 and a smaller peak at 15 to 19 years. Embryonal tumors prevail in childhood and adolescence (Mahour et al, 1967). In early childhood the tumors arise in the head and neck, and genitourinary tract, especially the testis and paratesticular tissue. The male-to-female ratio is 1.2 for head and neck tumors and 2.0 for genitourinary tumors (Miller and Dalager, 1974). In adults the risk increases with age and is greater in men than women; the major cell type is pleiomorphic rhabdomyosarcoma. Tumors tend to develop in the legs, followed by the arms, trunk, head and neck, and genitourinary tract (Keyhani and Booher, 1968).

Mortality

A special handicap to the study of STS has been the failure of the International Classification of Diseases to categorize these tumors in a meaningful way. The site-oriented code for "connective tissue cancers" excludes mesenchymal tumors arising in parenchymatous organs and does not distinguish between the heterogeneous cell types. Tabulations based on topography and histology lead to considerably different results (Lynge et al, 1987). Since most sources of mortality data rarely contain or code histologic type, the reported death rates underestimate the true mortality of STS, perhaps by as much as one-half. In the United States, mortality rates are higher among nonwhites than whites and among men than women (Table 45–2).

Incidence

Like mortality, incidence data are affected by the assignment of STS to sites other than connective tissue. Examination of data from the National Cancer Institute Surveillance, Epidemiology, and End Results (SEER) Program reveals that approximately one-half of the cases deemed to be STS, based on histologic data, are attributed to sites other than "connective tissue." For some cell types, the percent assigned to sites other than connective tissue is even greater. For example, approximately two-thirds of Kaposi's sarcoma cases are designated as malignancies of the skin. Age-adjusted incidence rates for STS, based on all cases in the SEER

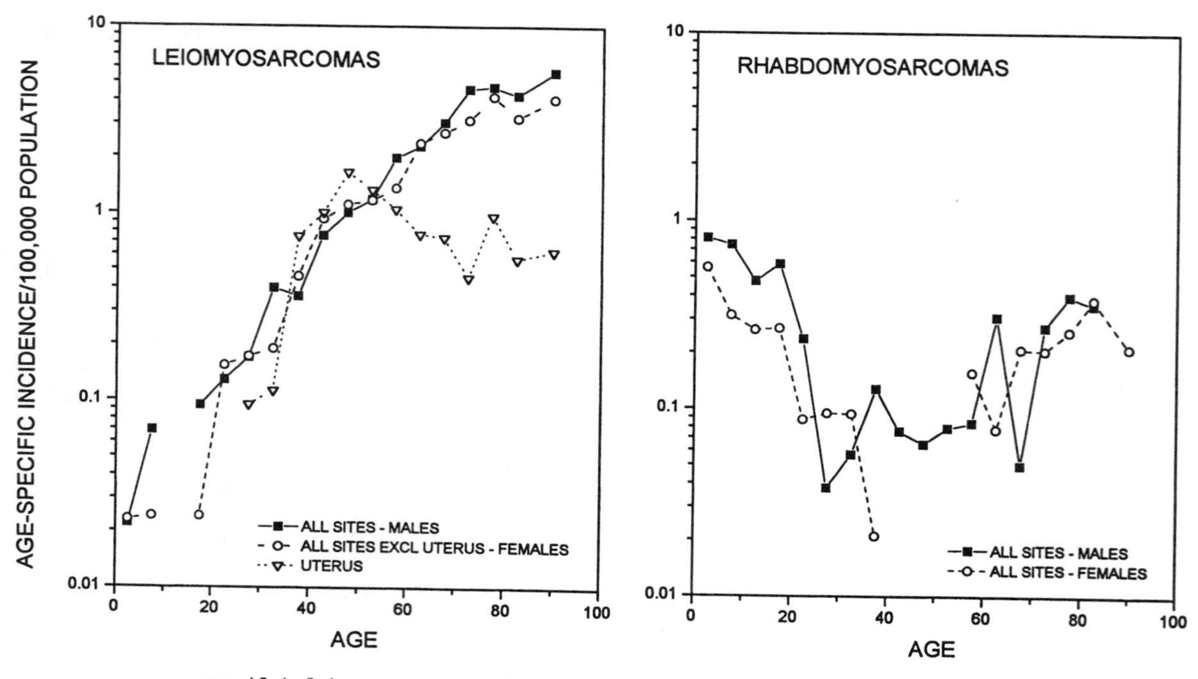

FIG. 45–1. Leiomyosarcomas and rhabdomyosarcomas in the 9 SEER areas, 1986–90.

program during 1986–1990, are presented in Table 45–3. The most common cell types are blood vessel sarcomas, fibrosarcoma, leiomyosarcoma, and liposarcoma, in that order. For all cell types combined and most individual cell types, there is a male excess. In particular, blood vessel sarcomas (primarily Kaposi's sarcoma) are over 20 times more common among white men than women. Leiomyosarcoma, on the other hand, is more common among women. The rates are generally higher among African Americans than whites, except for blood vessel sarcomas in men and liposarcoma in women. The largest racial difference is for leiomyosarcoma, particularly among women, which is consistent with incidence surveys from New York State (Polednak, 1986).

Since the SEER program covers about 10% of the U.S. population, it is usually possible to easily estimate the number of cancer cases expected to be diagnosed each year in the country. For STS, however, recent SEER data may overestimate the true national experience because SEER includes San Francisco, a geographic area with extremely high rates of AIDS and Kaposi's sarcoma.

Survival

The National Cancer Institute has evaluated the survival experience of cancer patients in the United States since 1950 (Axtell et al, 1976). As shown in Table 45–4, the 5-year relative survival rate was 36% for white patients with STS diagnosed during 1984–1989 (67% for localized and 34% for regional disease). The corresponding survival rate for African American patients was 38% (64% for localized and 46% for regional disease). The 5-year survival rates were highest for liposarcoma (whites: 73%; African Americans: 76%), and lowest for blood vessel sarcomas (whites: 13%; African Americans: 17%).

The survival rate for all STS combined has decreased

TABLE 45–2. *Average Annual Age-Adjusted Mortality Rates (per 100,000) for Connective Tissue Cancer in the United States by Pentad, Gender, and Race, 1950–1989**

	1950–54	*1955–59*	*1960–64*	*1965–69*	*1970–74*	*1975–79*	*1980–84*	*1985–89*
White men	0.49	0.60	0.71	0.81	0.85	0.85	1.19	1.23
White women	0.36	0.44	0.52	0.59	0.62	0.68	0.96	1.00
Nonwhite men	0.40	0.52	0.61	0.79	0.80	0.81	1.21	1.27
Nonwhite women	0.27	0.45	0.58	0.64	0.74	0.86	1.17	1.27

*Mortality rates are adjusted to the 1970 United States standard population.

over time due to the increased number of Kaposi's sarcoma cases, which have very low 5-year relative survival rates. There has been little to no change over time in the survival rates for the other histology types.

It has been suggested that the presence of estrogen receptors in leiomyosarcomas and liposarcomas might result in better survival among women than men (Chaudhuri et al, 1981). Among whites, there is little difference in 5-year relative survival by gender for leiomyosarcoma (women: 51%, men: 47%) or liposarcoma (women: 74%, men: 72%). Larger gender differences are observed among African Americans, however. African American women with leiomyosarcoma experience a 5-year relative survival rate of 43% while men have 17% survival. Similarly, the survival rate of African American women with liposarcoma (87%) is higher than for African American men (62%). Survival for women with fibrosarcoma is also better than for men (white women: 75%, white men: 69%, African American women: 78%, African American men: 62%).

The 5-year relative survival rates for all STS combined are significantly different for white men (27%) and women (56%), which is almost entirely attributable to the difference in survival rates for blood vessel sarcomas (e.g., Kaposi's sarcoma) (white men: 11%, white women: 53%). White men with rhabdomyosarcoma had better survival (56%) than women (48%). For most other types of STS, the survival is similar for both genders. Among African Americans, women also have higher survival than men for all types of STS combined (51% and 28%, respectively), primarily due to the large number and poor survival of male Kaposi's sarcoma cases (men: 14%, women: 55%).

Other factors thought to influence survival include histologic grade of malignancy, mitotic activity, presence of necrosis, tumor size, depth of tumors, bone and neurovascular structure infiltration, regional lymph node and distant metastases, anatomic location, adequacy of original surgery, local recurrence, altered expression of the retinoblastoma-susceptibility gene product, and socioeconomic status (Emrich et al, 1989; Tsujimoto et al, 1988; Mandard et al, 1989; Cance et al, 1990; El-Jabbour et al, 1990; Ciccone et al, 1991; Casson et al, 1992; El-Naggar and Garcia, 1992; Hashimoto et al, 1992; Pezzi et al, 1992).

Time Trends

Evaluation of time trends in the occurrence of STS is hindered by lack of long-existing databases with histology information (Lynge et al, 1987). Trends seen in site-oriented data may not accurately reflect changes in all

TABLE 45–3. *Average Annual Age-Adjusted Incidence Rates (per 100,000) for Soft Tissue Sarcomas by Histologic Type, Race, and Gender**

Histology and Number of Cases	White		African American	
	Men	Women	Men	Women
Blood vessel sarcoma (4,843)	6.81	0.28	5.04	0.32
Fibrosarcoma (1,688)	1.54	1.09	1.88	1.48
Leiomyosarcoma (1,265)	0.80	1.10	1.22	2.01
Sarcoma, NOS (595)	0.53	0.44	0.72	0.50
Liposarcoma (573)	0.60	0.35	0.79	0.31
Rhabdomyosarcoma (259)	0.32	0.17	0.43	0.22
Stromal sarcoma (172)	0.02	0.23	0.03	0.34
Synovial sarcoma (120)	0.10	0.09	0.17	0.07
Meningiosarcoma (113)	0.07	0.09	0.20	0.08
Mesenchymoma (11)	0.01	<0.01	0.03	0.04
Lymphangiosarcoma (7)	<0.01	0.01	—	—
Others (661)	0.35	0.67	0.23	1.06
Total (10,307)	11.15	4.53	10.73	6.43

*From the Survival, Epidemiology, and End Results Program, 1986–1990, adjusted to the 1970 United States standard population. Case selection was based on histology codes.

TABLE 45–4. *Five-Year Relative Survival Rates (%) for Patients with Soft Tissue Sarcoma Diagnosed in 1984–1989, by Histology, Race, and Stage[a]*

	All	Localized	Regional
White Patients (Number of Cases)			
All types (10,952)	36	67	34
Blood vessel sarcoma (5,025)	13	29	9
Fibrosarcoma (1,810)	71	82	74
Leiomyosarcoma (1,340)	50	70	38
Sarcoma, NOS (643)	35	65	37[b]
Liposarcoma (658)	73	82	72[b]
Rhabdomyosarcoma (274)	52	67[b]	61[b]
Stromal sarcoma (183)	69	83[b]	—[c]
Synovial sarcoma (138)	64[b]	77[b]	—[c]
Meningiosarcoma (117)	54[b]	—[c]	—[c]
African American Patients (Number of Cases)			
All types (1,263)	38	64	46[b]
Blood vessel sarcoma (408)	17	29[b]	20[b]
Fibrosarcoma (255)	70	77[b]	77[b]
Leiomyosarcoma (218)	36	54[b]	—[c]
Sarcoma, NOS (93)	21[b]	—[c]	—[c]
Liposarcoma (61)	76[b]	—[c]	—[c]
Rhabdomyosarcoma (46)	44[b]	—[c]	—[c]

[a]From the Survival, Epidemiology, and End Results Program. Case selection was based on histology codes, not site.

[b]Standard error between 5% and 10%.

[c]Number of cases too small to yield reliable rates; standard error greater than 10%.

TABLE 45–5. *Number of Cases and Average Annual Age-Adjusted Incidence Rates (per 100,000) for Kaposi's Sarcomas among Men by Calendar Period, Geographic Area, and Race*[a]

Race and Geographic Area	1975–1979		1980–1984		1985–1989	
	Count	Rate	Count	Rate	Count	Rate
White men						
9 SEER areas[b]	115	0.30	699	1.36	3,607	6.10
San Francisco	25	0.44	491	5.86	2,490	26.96
African American men						
9 SEER areas[b]	6	0.21	45	0.85	291	4.27
San Francisco	4	0.61	28	2.55	192	15.05

[a]From the Survival, Epidemiology, and End Results Program, 1975–1989, adjusted to the 1970 United States standard population.
[b]The nine Survival, Epidemiology, and End Results Program areas are the state of Connecticut; the Detroit, Michigan metropolitan area; the state of Iowa; the Atlanta, Georgia metropolitan area; the state of New Mexico; the state of Utah; the Seattle–Puget Sound, Washington area; the San Francisco–Oakland, California area; and the state of Hawaii.

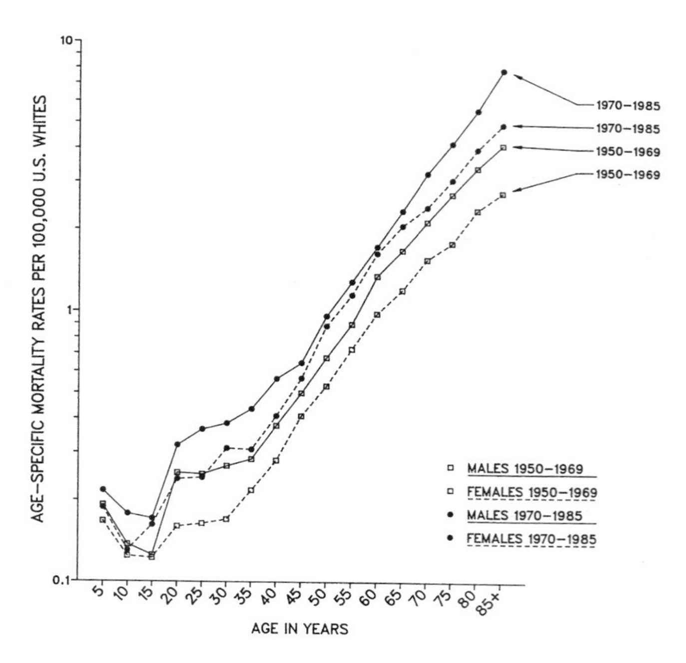

FIG. 45–2. Age-specific mortality rates per 100,000 for connective tissue cancers in the white population of the United States, by gender and calendar period, 1950–1969 and 1970–1985.

STS, because of the variable assignment of certain morphologic types to sites other than connective tissue. For example, in the SEER data, approximately two-thirds of cases of Kaposi's sarcoma, which rapidly increased as a result of the AIDS epidemic (Table 45–5), are assigned to the skin, whereas about one-half of all STS combined are assigned to sites other than connective tissue. Therefore, it is likely that reliance upon site-oriented data dampens observed trends for STS. In addition, large increases of Kaposi's sarcoma in high-risk areas, such as San Francisco, may be diluted in national statistics (Biggar et al, 1985).

Despite these limitations, upward trends in STS can be observed in both incidence and mortality statistics. Using data from the Connecticut Tumor Registry covering the years 1935–1989, an upward trend in incidence is seen for both genders, with a greater increase among men (Table 45–6). The increase in Kaposi's sarcoma peaked in the later 1980s, with declines in 1989 and 1990 (Ries et al, 1993). Based on HIV infection patterns, the Kaposi's sarcoma rates are expected to decline throughout the 1990s.

An upward trend for STS is seen in U.S. mortality statistics during 1950–1989, with the rate of increase being greater in nonwhites than whites (Table 45–2). Among men, the death rates were consistently higher in whites than nonwhites until the two most recent time periods, 1980–1984 and 1985–1989. Among women, the rates were higher in nonwhites starting in 1955–1959. As shown in Figure 45–2, the mortality rates among whites for 1970–1985 exceeded those for 1950–1969 in both genders. The increase affected all age groups. Similar increases in incidence and mortality in both genders have been reported in Canada (Ayiomamitis, 1988). Although the reported incidence and mortality rates have risen in a manner suggesting environmental influences, it is not possible to exclude the role of diagnostic and reporting practices. Because of the inherent problems in classifying STS, one cannot evaluate international variation or other geographic patterns in a meaningful way.

TABLE 45–6. *Average Annual Age-Adjusted Incidence Rates (per 100,000) for Connective Tissue Cancer in Connecticut by Calendar Period and Gender, 1935–1989**

	1935–39	1940–44	1945–49	1950–54	1955–59	1960–64	1965–69	1970–74	1975–79	1980–84	1985–89
Men	1.6	1.8	1.9	2.0	2.4	3.1	2.8	2.5	2.7	2.8	2.6
Women	1.5	1.7	1.4	1.7	1.8	2.0	1.7	1.7	1.5	2.1	1.6

*Incidence rates are adjusted to the 1970 United States standard population. Case selection was based on ICDO site code 171 only, not histology. STS of the heart are excluded.

ENVIRONMENTAL FACTORS

Radiation

A small fraction of STS is induced by external radiation therapy for various benign disorders and malignant tumors. In a study of multiple primary cancers in Connecticut, elevated risks of STS were observed in women who received radiation therapy for cancers of the breast and ovary. After at least ten years of follow-up, the risks for STS were elevated almost 8- and 25-fold, respectively, in the irradiated women (Harvey and Brinton, 1985; Curtis et al, 1985). In other tumor registry and cohort studies, significant increases in connective tissue tumors were reported following cancers of the breast, ovary, and testes and non-Hodgkin's lymphoma, while nonsignificantly elevated risks were noted following Hodgkin's disease (Taghian et al, 1991; Kaldor et al, 1987; Greene and Wilson, 1985). However, in hospital-based cohort studies of both children and adults treated for Hodgkin's disease, 40- and 15-fold increased risks of STS, respectively, were found (Tucker et al, 1984, 1988). In these two studies, all patients developing STS had received radiation to the anatomic site of the sarcoma.

The risk of uterine sarcoma is increased among women irradiated for cancer of the cervix (Czesnin and Wronkowski, 1978). A very high risk of radiogenic sarcoma with short latent periods (4 to 6 years) has been described in the orbital field of children treated for bilateral or familial retinoblastoma (Strong, 1977) and also in family members prone to sarcomas as part of Li-Fraumeni syndrome (Li et al, 1988).

In a series of 53 patients submitted to the Armed Forces Institute of Pathology, the latent period for post-irradiation STS varied from 2 to 40 years, with a mean of 10 years and a median of 8 years (Laskin et al, 1988). Other case series have similar range and mean latent periods (Kim et al, 1978; Davidson et al, 1986; Taghian et al, 1991; Mark et al, 1993). Nearly all cell types of STS have been described following radiation, the most common being malignant fibrous histiocytoma (Davidson et al, 1986; Laskin et al, 1988). Sarcomas secondary to radiation are usually diagnosed at a more advanced stage with higher grade and poorer prognosis than other sarcomas (Davidson et al, 1986; Robinson et al, 1988).

Few studies have assessed the risk of sarcoma according to the actual radiation dose delivered to the site of the sarcoma. In a study of STS following treatment for childhood cancer, 60% of the sarcomas arose within the field of radiation. Individual dosimetry to the site of the second sarcomas was determined. The risk of sarcoma was related to the total radiation dose to the site, with a greater than 50-fold excess in patients receiving over 50 Gy (Tucker MA, personal communication). It has been suggested that the level of risk of second tumors may be lower in patients treated with megavoltage than in those treated with orthovoltage (Potish et al, 1985). Total radiation dose, however, may be more important than the modality by which the radiation is delivered.

Thorotrast (colloidal thorium dioxide) is an alpha-emitting radioisotope once used for radiographic delineation of blood vessels. Its use was abandoned around 1955 when it produced several forms of cancer, most notably hepatic angiosarcomas (Locker et al, 1979; Van Kaick et al, 1983; Kato and Kido, 1987; Mays, 1988). The cumulative risk of liver cancers (angiosarcomas and carcinomas) is related to the dose rate to the liver tissue, reaching 30% at 40 years in the group receiving over 20 ml (approximately 30 rad/year) (Van Kaick et al, 1983). In the United States, the number of Thorotrast-induced angiosarcomas increased in the 1970s, resulting from the cumulative effects of low-dose procedures and prolonged latent periods (Falk et al, 1979a). Sarcomas of various types have also developed on the edge of Thorotrast deposits and granulomas, usually at injection sites (da Motta et al, 1979; Van Kaick et al, 1983). Other radioactive materials may induce sarcomas at or near sites of deposition, as suggested by a report of laryngeal sarcoma arising eight years after treatment of thyrotoxicosis by ^{125}iodine, which gives a higher extrathyroidal dose than ^{131}iodine (McKillop et al, 1978).

In one study of low-frequency electromagnetic fields and childhood cancer, a nonsignificant association was observed between STS and measured magnetic fields in houses under low power use (Savitz et al, 1988). However, risk was lower for magnetic fields under high power use conditions. Excess incidence of STS was also observed in a cohort study of male Norwegian electrical workers potentially exposed to electromagnetic fields (Tynes et al, 1992). The authors noted that immunosuppression is a known etiologic factor for STS and that exposure to electromagnetic fields can alter the circadian cycle of pineal melatonin and affect immune function in animals.

Occupational Exposures

In Sweden, clinical observations (Hardell, 1977) prompted a case-control study that related STS to herbicide exposures (Hardell and Sandstrom, 1979). Among 52 patients with STS, a 6-fold increased risk was associated with occupational exposure to phenoxyacetic acids or chlorophenols. Because of the magnitude of the reported risk and the widespread potential for exposure, numerous studies were then conducted around the world. Results from these investigations, which have employed both case-control and cohort design and have focused on several exposure scenarios, have been inconsistent. Associations between STS and phenoxyacetic acid herbicides and chlorophenols used primarily in agriculture and forestry were observed among men in four additional case-control studies in Sweden (Eriksson et al, 1981; Hardell and Eriksson, 1988; Eriksson et al, 1990; Wingren et al, 1990) and among women employed as rice weeders in Italy (Vineis et al, 1987). In addition, farmers were reported at excess risk for STS in England and Wales (Balarajan and Acheson, 1984). However, several studies, some with detailed exposure histories, have not shown any excess risk (Milham, 1982; Smith et al, 1982, 1983, 1984; Gallagher and Threlfall, 1984; Hoar et al, 1986; Wiklund and Holm, 1986; Woods et al, 1987; Wiklund et al, 1988; Serraino et al, 1992).

There have been several clinical surveys and cohort studies of manufacturing workers exposed to phenoxyacetic acid herbicides, chlorophenols, and their contaminants, such as 2,3,7,8-tetrachlorodibenzo-para-dioxin (2,3,7,8-TCDD) (Honchar and Halperin, 1981; Johnson et al, 1981). There has also been a case report of STS in a hospital worker exposed to hexachlorophene, a polychlorinated biphenyl detergent, produced from 2,4,5-trichlorophenol and contaminated by 2,3,7,8-TCDD (Hardell, 1992). Excesses of STS were found among manufacturing workers presumably exposed to 2,3,7,8-TCDD in the manufacture of trichlorophenols (Zack and Suskind, 1980; Cook et al, 1980; Cook, 1981; Johnson et al, 1981; Fingerhut et al, 1991) and among workers whose exposure to 2,4-dichlorophenoxyacetic acid (2,4-D), 2 methyl-4-chlorophenoxy acid (MCPA), and other phenoxyacetic acids were unlikely to be contaminated by 2,3,7,8-TCDD (Lynge, 1985, 1987). Chlorophenols may be responsible for an excess of STS observed in a small cohort of Italian leather tannery workers (Seniori Costantino et al, 1989). A review of the cases in some of the American cohorts, however, failed to confirm the diagnosis of STS or the exposure status of many of the cases (Fingerhut et al, 1984). In addition, other studies of chemical workers producing higher chlorinated phenols (Sobel et al, 1986; Ott et al, 1987), 2,4,5-trichlorophenoxyacetic acid (2,4,5-T) (Ott et al, 1980), MCPA (Coggon et al, 1986) and 2,4-D (Bond et al, 1988) did not detect excess STS.

Persons living in the vicinity of an Italian factory that accidentally released 2,3,7,8-TCDD into the environment were found to have a higher incidence rate of STS than residents in adjacent areas unaffected by the accident and in other parts of Italy (Puntoni et al, 1986; Bertazzi et al, 1989).

Excesses of STS have also been observed in several proportional mortality studies and clinical surveys of Vietnam veterans (Sarma and Jacobs, 1982; Anderson et al, 1986; Holmes et al, 1986; Kogan and Clapp, 1988), some of whom were exposed to Agent Orange, an herbicide mixture of 50% 2,4,5-T and 50% 2,4-D. However, other proportional mortality studies and several case-control studies have not observed any significant increases in STS risk for Vietnam veterans (Greenwald et al, 1984; Lawrence et al, 1985; Kang et al, 1986, 1987; Breslin et al, 1988; Goun and Kuller, 1988; Selected Cancers Cooperative Study Group, 1990b), including the Project Ranch Hand members who were directly involved with spraying Agent Orange (Lathrop et al, 1984). Verification of exposure has been extremely difficult in the veteran studies (Booth, 1987) and complex indices of exposure based on proximity to herbicide spraying in Vietnam have shown no meaningful correlation with 2,3,7,8-TCDD serum levels (Stellman and Stellman, 1986; Centers for Disease Control, 1989; Selected Cancers Cooperative Study Group, 1990a).

The reasons for the inconsistent results from studies of populations exposed to phenoxy herbicides or their contaminants are not known. Possible explanations include lack of comparable type and extent of exposure, differences in relevant contaminants, varying definitions of sarcomas under study, underascertainment of cases, recall bias, lack of sufficient latency, inherent susceptibility of study populations (e.g., Scandinavians), and chance (Blair and Zahm, 1990; Coggon and Acheson, 1982; Hardell and Axelson, 1982; Constable et al, 1987; Woods et al, 1987; Bond et al, 1989). To resolve these issues, improvements in exposure assessment and other study design features are needed.

The mechanism for an association between STS and phenoxy herbicides has been the subject of debate, especially for the herbicides not known to be contaminated by 2,3,7,8-TCDD. Immunosuppression, peroxisome proliferation, genotoxicity as evidenced by increased rates of sister chromatid exchanges, or inhibition of gap-junctional intercellular communication may play a role (Blair et al, 1990; Vineis and Zahm, 1988; Jennings et al, 1988; Tucker et al, 1986; Turkula and Jalal, 1985; Vainio et al, 1982; Korte and Jalal, 1982).

STS has also been associated with exposure to insecticides used on animals prior to the mid-1950s, in particular chlorinated hydrocarbon insecticides (Zahm et al, 1988). The excess risk appeared to be primarily for fibrous and myomatous sarcomas. Inorganic arsenical insecticides are a well-established cause of angiosarcomas of the liver (Popper et al, 1978).

Angiosarcomas of the liver are also caused by vinyl chloride exposures during the manufacturing of polyvinyl chloride plastics (Popper et al, 1978). A fibrotic precursor stage in the liver has been identified among individuals exposed to vinyl chloride, inorganic arsenic compounds, and Thorotrast. A survey of deaths from hepatic angiosarcoma in the United States during 1964–1974 recorded 168 cases, of which 37 (22%) were associated with vinyl chloride, Thorotrast, or inorganic arsenic (Falk et al, 1979b).

Two New Zealand case-control studies of cancer and

occupation found an association between STS and employment in an abattoir (Pearce et al, 1988). Abattoir workers may be exposed to plastics used to wrap meat (e.g., polyvinyl chloride), zoonotic oncogenic viruses, and various chemicals, including 2,4,6-trichlorophenol, which is used in the treatment of pelts.

An increased risk of STS observed among New Zealand forestry workers seemed related not to phenoxy herbicides, but possibly to the use of chain saws or other equipment (Reif et al, 1989). In addition, workers exposed to formaldehyde had excess mortality from cancers of the connective tissue in one study (Stayner et al, 1988), but not in others (Acheson et al, 1984; Blair et al, 1986).

Medicinal Agents

Angiosarcomas of the liver have been associated with inorganic arsenical medications (Fowler's solution) (Falk et al, 1981; Kasper et al, 1984) and with androgenic-anabolic steroids (Falk et al, 1979b), and possibly with estrogenic compounds (Ham et al, 1980).

Although an increased risk of STS following cancer chemotherapy is not well established, there is suggestive evidence for a relation to bone sarcomas and STS (Halperin et al, 1984; Tucker et al, 1987). Most treatment-related sarcomas are considered radiogenic whether or not chemotherapy is used (Laskin et al, 1988; Halperin et al, 1984; Tucker et al, 1988); but an excess risk of STS was reported after chemotherapy when used alone for Hodgkin's disease (Halperin et al, 1984). In a recent case-control study of second childhood cancers, the risk of STS was approximately 2-fold higher among patients receiving both radiation and alkylating agent chemotherapy than in subjects receiving only radiation (Tucker MA, personal communication). Doxorubicin has induced rhabdomyosarcoma following isolated limb perfusions in rats and the effect appeared to be dose dependent (Van't Hoff et al, 1986), but no data exist for humans. Further studies are needed to clarify whether alkylating agents or anthracyclines contribute to treatment-related sarcomas.

Various forms of STS, including Kaposi's sarcoma, have developed excessively after the use of immunosuppressive drugs, especially for renal transplantation, but also for other conditions (Kinlen et al, 1979). In addition, a survey of Kaposi's sarcoma in Norway over a 5-year period revealed that 6 of the 41 patients (15%) had taken immunosuppressive drugs for conditions other than cancer or transplants, while none of 242 control patients with basal-cell skin carcinomas used these drugs (Klepp et al, 1978).

In several case reports, sarcomas have arisen at the sites of previous iron-dextran injections (McIllmurray and Langman, 1978; Weinbren et al, 1978). Although these preparations have induced sarcomas in laboratory animals, the risk in man appears to be extremely small. Also, certain aluminum compounds, used as adjuvants in vaccines and allergenic extracts, have induced injection-site sarcomas in mice. An analysis of incidence trends in Connecticut, however, has revealed no increase in STS of the upper arms since 1963, when alum-adsorbed allergenic extracts were introduced (Jekel et al, 1978).

A number of chemicals have induced sarcomas in laboratory animals after subcutaneous or intramuscular injections. Although the significance of injection-site sarcomas has been debated, it is noteworthy that many of these compounds are also carcinogenic when tested experimentally by other routes (Boyland, 1980).

Parental use of the illegal drugs marijuana and cocaine has been linked to rhabdomyosarcoma in children (Grufferman et al, 1993). Use during the year preceding the child's birth was associated with a 2-fold to 5-fold increase in risk.

Viruses

More than a decade ago, a viral etiology of endemic Kaposi's sarcoma was hypothesized for several reasons. The geographic distribution in Africa resembled that of Burkitt's lymphoma; virus particles were identified in cell lines from African cases, which were later identified as cytomegalovirus (CMV); and serologic studies linked CMV to Kaposi's sarcoma in African, European, and North American cases (Giraldo et al, 1980; Giraldo et al, 1989; Safai, 1987). Studies of endemic African Kaposi's sarcoma have revealed no underlying immunodeficiency state (Kestens et al, 1985).

With the recognition of Kaposi's sarcoma in association with acquired immunodeficiency syndrome (AIDS), interest in the potential viral etiology of this tumor has intensified. Epidemic Kaposi's sarcoma is a more aggressive disease and tends to arise in younger individuals than the endemic variety (Safai, 1987). Relatively early in the AIDS outbreak, it was recognized that Kaposi's sarcoma was much more frequent in homosexuals with AIDS than in other risk groups, such as intravenous drug users, hemophiliacs, or transfusion recipients (Safai, 1987). The epidemiologic features of epidemic Kaposi's sarcoma suggest a sexually transmissable agent (Giraldo et al, 1989; Beral et al, 1992), particularly through anal intercourse with homosexual or bisexual men with AIDS. There is also some evidence that the incidence of Kaposi's sarcoma among homosexuals with AIDS has decreased somewhat in recent years (Des Jarlais et al, 1987), perhaps due to changing sexual practices. Although extensive laboratory investigations have attempted to isolate viruses from epidemic and endemic Kaposi's sarcoma, none have been successful to date. Efforts to identify viral sequences have yielded inconsistent results (Roth et al, 1988; Werner et al, 1989; Van Den Berg et al, 1989; Huang et al, 1992; Nickoloff et al, 1992; Biggar et al, 1992; Chang et al, 1994; Collandre et al, 1995; Boshoff et al, 1995), but epidemiologic and molecular studies are continuing to search for a viral agent that may be transmitted by fecal-oral contact or blood products.

Although a viral etiology of other sarcomas has been hypothesized because of animal models, the epidemiologic data are very limited. One case-control study from Italy found slightly elevated risks of STS associated with a history of childhood chicken pox or mumps (Serraino et al, 1991). There was also an increased risk of sarcoma associated with a history of herpes zoster, particularly in the three years prior to diagnosis. This association may be due to an underlying immune deficiency, which predisposes both to infection and to the development of sarcoma.

Other Environmental Factors

It has been suggested that trauma may increase the risk of STS, but the available evidence suggests that local injury only calls attention to a preexisting tumor and perhaps accelerates its growth. Sarcomas have been reported at the sites of surgical scars (Ott, 1970), burn scars (Enzinger and Weiss, 1988b), and in the soft tissue near metals used for bone fracture fixation (Dube and Fisher, 1972; Lee et al, 1984), and more recently at the site of total hip arthroplasty (Swann, 1984; Ryu et al, 1987). Although such occurrences appear to be rare, clinical reports of sarcomas at the site of bone implants have raised concern (Rock and Unni, 1990). To date, epidemiologic studies have revealed no excess risk of STS or bone cancer after hip replacement with metal implants (Nyren et al, 1995).

The risk of breast sarcomas among women with silicone breast implants is under investigation (Brinton, 1993), although examination of SEER incidence rates of breast sarcomas shows little or no change over time (May and Stroup, 1991; Engel and Lamm, 1992). Given the low incidence of the disease and the low prevalence of the exposure, however, examination of incidence rates in the general population is limited in its ability to assess an association.

There has been one case-control study relating STS to the use of smokeless tobacco (Zahm et al, 1989). The risk associated with chewing tobacco or snuff was more pronounced for sarcomas of the upper gastrointestinal tract, the lung and pleura, and the head, neck, and face region than for lower regions of the body. Lip sarcomas and other tumors have been reported in rats exposed to snuff, possibly a consequence of N-nitrosamines (Johansson et al, 1989). A cohort study of U.S. veterans, however, showed only a nonsignificant 40% excess of mortality from STS among smokeless tobacco users with no striking risk patterns by characteristics of use, although frequent users had a slightly higher risk than infrequent users (Zahm et al, 1992).

Cigarette smoking has not been linked with STS (Hardell and Sandstrom, 1979; Gebauer, 1982; Kang et al, 1987; Vineis et al, 1987; Woods et al, 1987; Hardell and Eriksson, 1988; Zahm et al, 1989; Serraino et al, 1991). However, a study of rhabdomyosarcoma among children revealed an excess risk associated with paternal (but not maternal) smoking (Grufferman et al, 1982). An interaction between cigarette smoking and occupational exposure to 2,3,7,8-TCDD in the development of STS has been suggested among heavily exposed workers (Cook, 1981).

Information on the role of dietary factors in STS is very scarce. One case-control study suggested an increased risk associated with a high intake of dairy products and oil (i.e., mostly seed oil) and a decreased risk associated with whole-grain bread and pasta (Serraino et al, 1991). In another study, rhabdomyosarcoma in childhood was related to diets that included organ meats (e.g., liver, brain, and tongue) (Grufferman et al, 1982).

HOST FACTORS

Precursor Lesions

Sarcomas generally have benign counterparts (e.g., lipomas), which are at least five times as common, but nearly all sarcomas appear to be malignant from the start and do not evolve from precursor tumors (Morton, 1973). Although malignant change of benign tumors is a rare event, transformation can be promoted by ionizing radiation as used in therapy of angiomas (King et al, 1979).

Genetic Factors

Li-Fraumeni syndrome was initially recognized in four families with an autosomal dominant pattern of STS, breast cancer, and other tumors in children and young adults (Li and Fraumeni, 1969). Subsequent experience with nearly 100 families with Li-Fraumeni syndrome have expanded the tumor phenotype to encompass osteosarcoma, brain tumor, leukemia, adrenocortical carcinoma, and germ cell tumors (Blattner et al, 1979; Strong et al, 1987; Li et al, 1988; Hartley et al, 1989). Another feature is the tendency for multiple primary tumors to occur in individual family members, including a susceptibility to second cancers, notably STS, arising in the radiotherapy field. Epidemiologic studies have excluded the role of chance and selection or referral bias as an explanation for the familial aggregations. Prospective studies of Li-Fraumeni kindreds have revealed continued expression of the component tumors, with the greatest risk among those under age 20 (Li and Fraumeni, 1982; Garber et al, 1991). Other surveys have shown excesses of breast cancer in the mothers of patients with STS, osteosarcoma, or chondrosarcoma (Birch et al, 1990; Hartley et al, 1986). Furthermore, segregation analysis of several families of children with STS have confirmed an autosomal dominant pattern of the various tumors characteristic of Li-Fraumeni syndrome (Williams and Strong, 1985). In affected families, the recent discovery of germ line mutations of the tumor-suppressor gene, p53, which is located on chromosome 17p13, has important implications to the origins and prevention of STS as well as other component tumors of the syndrome (Malkin et al, 1990). Recommendations for predictive p53 testing of at-risk individuals in Li-Fraumeni families should be useful in strategies for testing other cancer susceptibility genes that are discovered (Li et al, 1992).

Along with osteosarcoma, STS occurs more often than expected in survivors of the hereditary form of retinoblastoma (Sanders et al, 1989). The mesenchymal tumors often arise in the lower extremities, but also develop excessively in the irradiated field around the orbit. Mutations of the retinoblastoma gene (Rb-1), which has been mapped to chromosome 13q14, appear to account for the heritable retinoblastomas as well as subsequent sarcomas (Hansen et al, 1985). Rb-1, a tumor-suppressor gene, is altered also in the tumor tissue of some sporadic sarcomas (Cance et al, 1990), while specific morphologic subtypes show a number of genetic defects, including chromosomal translocations, point mutations, and allele loss (Knight, 1990; Li, 1988). Although Rb-1 appears to be implicated in adult sarcomas, one study of childhood rhabdomyosarcoma did not observe any structural or functional abnormalities in Rb-1 (De Chiara et al, 1993).

Another dominantly inherited trait predisposing to STS is neurofibromatosis type 1. Neurogenic sarcomas (e.g., neurofibrosarcoma) occur with excess frequency, especially in adults (Hope and Mulvihill, 1981; Bader, 1987). In children, rhabdomyosarcomas arise excessively (McKeen et al, 1978), along with fibrosarcomas and liposarcomas. In Gardner's syndrome, familial polyposis occurs with a spectrum of mesenchymal lesions, including desmoid tumors, aggressive fibromatosis, and rarely fibrosarcoma.

In addition, clinical reports have linked the nevoid basal cell carcinoma syndrome to fibrosarcoma and rhabdomyosarcoma, tuberous sclerosis to rhabdomyosarcoma, and familial hydronephrosis to congenital renal sarcomas (Mulvihill, 1975). A familial syndrome of cutaneous and uterine leiomyomas, sometimes complicated by uterine leiomyosarcomas, has been described (Walker and Reed, 1973). Carney's triad is a syndrome of gastric leiomyosarcoma, pulmonary chondroma, and extra-adrenal paraganglioma, which has been reported in a series of young women (Margulies and Sheps, 1988). The tumors tend to be multicentric, but familial occurrences are yet to be seen. A few patients with genetic hemochromatosis have developed hepatic angiosarcomas (Sussman et al, 1974), although hepatocellular carcinoma occurs more often as a complication. An association between melanoma and STS has been reported recently, but the mechanism involved is unclear (Garber et al, 1990). The association may be due to the same mechanism as the newly described familial constellation of Ewing's sarcoma family of tumors, melanoma, brain cancer, and possibly stomach cancer (Novakovic et al, 1994).

Werner's syndrome (adult progeria) is a recessively inherited disorder featuring a shortened life span due to early atherosclerosis and cancer. Most common are sarcomas, perhaps related to the retarded growth of skin fibroblasts in vitro (Lutzner, 1977). Congenital multiple fibromatosis, which appears inherited in some cases, resembles low-grade fibrosarcoma, although the tumors regress and eventually disappear a few months after birth (Baird and Worth, 1976).

Immunologic Defects

An STS excess has been reported in patients receiving therapeutic immunosuppression for renal transplantation and other conditions, although the risks are not nearly as high as for non-Hodgkin's lymphoma (Hoover and Fraumeni, 1973; Kinlen et al, 1979). In the genetic immunodeficiency syndromes, there is also a predominance of lymphoid tumors and a suggestion that STS is overrepresented among the other tumors reported (Spector et al, 1978). Patients with chronic lymphocytic leukemia are also prone to STS, apparently as a result of the immunodeficiency state associated with this form of leukemia (Greene et al, 1978). Similarly, the immunodeficiency associated with non-Hodgkin's lymphoma and Hodgkin's disease may contribute to the excess risk of STS (Tucker et al, 1988; Halperin et al 1984; Greene and Wilson, 1985; Kaldor et al, 1987).

Kaposi's sarcoma is especially prominent among the posttransplant cases of STS (Harwood et al, 1979), and this tumor also develops excessively among patients with lymphoproliferative neoplasms (Safai et al, 1980) or autoimmune hemolytic anemia (Hammond et al, 1977). It is noteworthy that various immunodeficiency states, including AIDS and the use of immunosuppressive drugs, predispose to STS as well as lymphoma, so that intact immunosurveillance mechanisms may be important in controlling both kinds of tumors.

Other Host Factors

Lymphangiosarcomas may arise in the chronically edematous arms of women who have undergone radical mastectomy for breast cancer (Stewart-Treves syndrome). Several cases of lymphangiosarcoma have also been reported following long-standing lymphedema of a congenital or heritable nature (Dubin et al, 1974). Sarcomas have appeared as well in families with the lymphedema-distichiasis syndrome (Falls and Kerlesz, 1964). In addition, sarcomas have arisen at the site of chronic skin ulcers (Routh et al, 1985; Fletcher, 1987).

Childhood rhabdomyosarcoma has been linked in one study to maternal history of stillbirth with risk increasing with the number of prior stillbirths (Ghali et al, 1992). The data suggest that rhabdomyosarcoma and stillbirths may share a common risk factor that is either genetic or may involve in utero exposure to an exogenous or endogenous agent. Rhabdomyosarcoma also shows a rise in risk at puberty, with the peak for girls occurring about two years earlier than that for boys, coincident with differences in muscle growth patterns, suggesting that hormones may play a role (dos Santos Silva and Swerdlow, 1993).

PREVENTIVE MEASURES

The present state of knowledge of STS risk factors, although incomplete, has important implications for the detection and prevention of these tumors. Persons at high risk (e.g., as a result of radiation exposure, immunosuppression, or genetic susceptibility) need appropriate medical surveillance, including the judicious use of computed tomography or magnetic resonance imaging aimed at the early diagnosis and characterization of soft tissue tumors. Appropriate steps should be taken, of course, to reduce potentially hazardous exposures to ionizing radiation and certain chemicals, such as vinyl chloride, arsenic, and phenoxyacetic acid herbicides. Adherence to the recommendations to inhibit the transmission of the human immunodeficiency virus (Goedert, 1987) would decrease the risk of Kaposi's sarcoma associated with AIDS.

FUTURE RESEARCH

Epidemiologic progress in understanding STS has been hindered by uncertainties in the morphologic classification of this diverse group of neoplasms, and it is hoped that refinements in diagnostic criteria will strengthen the basis for further studies. The epidemiologic variation by cell type have suggested some degree of etiologic heterogeneity, although there is evidence that some risk factors are shared by different forms of STS.

Ionizing radiation at high doses is known to produce a variety of sarcomas, but accounts for only a small fraction of cases. Thorotrast, vinyl chloride, inorganic arsenic, and androgenic steroids can induce hepatic angiosarcomas, and recent studies have linked STS with occupational exposure to herbicides, mainly phenoxyacetic acids and chlorophenols. Further case-control studies of STS are obviously indicated, particularly in view of the climbing incidence and mortality rates for these tumors. More research is needed on the etiologic role of chemotherapy, immunosuppressive drugs, and orthopedic implants in sarcomas, while future studies on the effects of pesticides and other environmental exposures will require improved methods for assessing historical exposures. Research is also needed to pursue the suggested associations between STS and use of smokeless tobacco, exposure to electromagnetic radiation, and the possible role of nutritional factors.

The bimodal age curve for STS includes an initial peak in early childhood that has long suggested the role of prenatal factors. In Li-Fraumeni syndrome, the tendency for childhood sarcomas and other tumors to cluster in families has provided direction for molecular research to probe into genetic mechanisms of carcinogenesis, including the role of the tumor-suppressor gene, p53, in various forms of STS. Further work is needed on genetic-environment interactions, as illustrated by the excess of radiogenic sarcomas in Li-Fraumeni syndrome and in heritable retinoblastoma. The higher incidence of STS in African Americans than in whites may also reflect genetic determinants underlying the risk and biologic behavior of certain STS subtypes, although other risk factors need to be evaluated as well.

Recent evidence suggests that various states of immunosuppression, particularly T-cell abnormalities, predispose to STS, although the risks are not nearly as high as for lymphoproliferative neoplasms. Kaposi's sarcoma is conspicuous among the tumors complicating immunosuppression, most notably AIDS, and occurs excessively in patients with lymphoid neoplasms. These observations suggest common or related etiologies for lymphoma and STS, especially the Kaposi type. Further research into AIDS-associated tumors should clarify the role of oncogenic viruses, immune defects, growth factors, and other mechanisms of carcinogenesis. Based on recent progress, it seems likely that interdisciplinary approaches aimed at clarifying host and environmental determinants of STS will contribute more broadly to a better understanding of cancer biology, etiology, and prevention.

REFERENCES

ACHESON ED, BARNES HR, GARDNER MJ, et al. 1984. Formaldehyde in the British chemical industry: An occupational cohort study. Lancet 1:611–616.

ANDERSON HA, HANRAHAN LP, JENSEN M, et al. 1986. Wisconsin Vietnam veteran mortality study. Madison, Wisconsin Department of Health and Social Services.

AXTELL LM, ASIRE AJ, MYERS MH (eds). 1976. Cancer Patient Survival, Report No. 5 DHEW Publ. No. (NIH) 77-992. Washington, D.C.: U.S. Government Printing Office. pp. 253–258.

AYIOMAMITIS A. 1988. Epidemiology of cancer of the connective tissue in Canada during the period 1950–1985. Cancer Detect Prev 13:149–156.

BADER JL. 1987. Neurofibromatosis and cancer: An overview. Dysmorph Clin Gen 1:43–48.

BALARAJAN R, ACHESON ED. 1984. Soft tissue sarcomas in agriculture and forestry workers. J Epidemiol Community Health 38:113–116.

BAIRD PA, WORTH AJ. 1976. Congenital generalized fibromatosis: An autosomal recessive condition? Clin Genet 9:488–494.

BERAL V, BULL D, DARBY S, et al. 1992. Risk of Kaposi's sarcoma and sexual practices associated with faecal contact in homosexual or bisexualmen with AIDS. Lancet 339:632–635.

BERTAZZI PA, ZOCCHETTI C, PESATORI AC, et al. 1989. Ten-year mortality study of the population involved in the Seveso incident in 1976. Am J Epidemiol 129:1187–1200.

BIGGAR RJ, DUNSMORE N, KURMAN RJ, et al. 1992. Failure to detect human papillomavirus in Kaposi's sarcoma. Lancet 339:1605–1605.

BIGGAR RJ, HORM J, FRAUMENI JF JR, et al. 1984. Incidence of Kaposi's sarcoma and mycosis fungoides in the United States including Puerto Rico, 1973–1981. J Natl Cancer Inst 73:89–94.

BIGGAR RJ, HORM J, LUBIN JH, et al. 1985. Cancer trends in a population at risk of acquired immunodeficiency syndrome. J Natl Cancer Inst 74:793–797.

BIRCH JM, HARTLEY AL, BLAIR V, et al. 1990. Identification of factors associated with high breast cancer risk in the mothers of children with soft tissue sarcoma. J Clin Oncol 8:583–590.

BLAIR A, STEWART P, O'BERG M, et al. 1986. Mortality among industrial workers exposed to formaldehyde. J Natl Cancer Inst 57:487–492.

BLAIR A, AXELSON O, FRANKLIN C, et al. 1990. Carcinogenic effects of pesticides. In Baker SR, Wilkinson CF (eds): Advances in Modern Environmental Toxicology: The Effects of Pesticides on Human Health. Princeton, NJ: Princeton Scientific Publ. Co., 18:201–260.

BLAIR A, ZAHM SH. 1990. Herbicides and cancer: A review and discussion of methodologic issues. In Band P (ed): Recent Results in Cancer Research: Occupational Cancer Epidemiology. New York: Springer-Verlag, 120:132–145.

BLATTNER WA, MCGUIRE DB, MULVIHILL JJ, et al. 1979. Genealogy of cancer in a family. JAMA 241:259–261.

BOND GG, BODNER KM, COOK RR. 1989. Phenoxyherbicides and cancer: Insufficient epidemiologic evidence for a causal relationship. Fundam Appl Toxicol 12:172–188.

BOND GG, WETTERSTROEM NH, ROUSH GJ, et al. 1988. Cause specific mortality among employees engaged in the manufacture, formulation, or packaging of 2,4-dichlorophenoxyacetic acid and related salts. Br J Ind Med 45:98–105.

BOOTH W. 1987. Agent Orange study hits brick wall. Science 237:1285–1286.

BOSHOFF C, WHITBY D, HATZIIOANNOU T, et al. 1995. Kaposi's-sarcoma-associated herpesvirus in HIV-negative Kaposi's sarcoma. Lancet 345:1043–1044.

BOYLAND E. 1980. The history and future of chemical carcinogenesis. Br Med Bull 36:5–10.

BRESLIN P, KANG HK, LEE Y, et al. 1988. Proportionate mortality study of US Army and US Marine Corps veterans of the Vietnam war. J Occup Med 30:412–419.

BRINTON LA. 1993. Protocol for a follow-up study of women with augmentation mammoplasty. National Cancer Institute, Protocol.

CANCE WG, BRENNAN MF, DUDAS ME, et al. 1990. Altered expression of the retinoblastoma gene product in human sarcomas. N Engl J Med 323:1457–1462.

CASSON AG, PUTNAM JB, NATARAJAN G, et al. 1992. Five-year survival after pulmonary metastasectomy for adult soft tissue sarcoma. Cancer 69:662–668.

CENTERS FOR DISEASE CONTROL. 1989. Comparison of serum levels of 2,3,7,8-tetrachlorodibenzo-*p*-dioxin with indirect estimates of Agent Orange exposure among Vietnam veterans: Final report. Atlanta: U.S. Dept. of Health and Human Service.

CHABALKO JJ, FRAUMENI JF JR. 1975. Blood vessel neoplasms in children: Epidemiologic aspects. Med Pediatr Oncol 1:135–141.

CHANG Y, CESARMAN E, PESSIN MS, et al. 1994. Identification of herpes-like DNA sequences in AIDS-associated Kaposi's sarcoma. Science 266:1865–1869.

CHAUDHURI PK, WALKER MJ, BEATTIE CW, et al. 1981. Distribution of steroid hormone receptors in human soft tissue sarcomas. Surgery 90:149–153.

CHUNG FB, ENZINGER FM. 1976. Infantile fibrosarcoma. Cancer 38:729–739.

CICCONE G, MAGNANI C, DELSEDIME L, VINEIS P. 1991. Socioeconomic status and survival from soft-tissue sarcomas: A population-based study in Northern Italy. Am J Public Health 81:747–749.

COGGON D, ACHESON ED. 1982. Do phenoxy herbicides cause cancer in man? Lancet 1:1057–1059.

COGGON D, PANNETT B, WINTER PD, et al. 1986. Mortality of workers exposed to 2 methyl-4 chlorophenoxyacetic acid. Scand J Work Environ Health 12:448–454.

COLLANDRE H, FERRIS S, GRAV O, et al. 1995. Kaposi's sarcoma and new herpesvirus. Lancet 345:1043, 1995.

CONSTABLE JD, TIMPERI R, CLAPP R, et al. 1987. Vietnam veterans and soft tissue sarcoma. J Occup Med 29:726.

COOK RR. 1981. Dioxin, chloracne, and soft tissue sarcoma. Lancet 1:618–619.

COOK RR, TOWNSEND JC, OTT MG, et al. 1980. Mortality experience of employees exposed to 2,3,7,8-tetrachlorodibenzo-p-dioxin (TCDD). J Occup Med 22:530–532.

CURTIS RE, HOOVER RN, KLEINERMAN RA, et al. 1985. Second cancer following cancer of the female genital system. Natl Cancer Inst Monogr 68:113–137.

CZESNIN K, WRONKOWSKI Z. 1978. Second malignancies of the irradiated area in patients treated for uterine cervix cancer. Gynecol Oncol 6:309–315.

DA MOTTA LC, DA SILVA HORTA J, TAVARES MH. 1979. Prospective epidemiologic study of thorotrast-exposed patients in Portugal. Environ Res 18:152–172.

DAVIDSON T, WESTBURY G, HARMER CL. 1986. Radiation-induced soft-tissue sarcoma. Br J Surg 73:308–309.

DE CHIARA A, T'ANG A, TRICHE TJ. 1993. Expression of the retinoblastoma susceptibility gene in childhood rhabdomyosarcomas. J Natl Cancer Inst 85:152–157.

DES JARLAIS DC, STONEBURNER R, THOMAS P, FRIEDMAN SR. 1987. Declines in proportion of Kaposi's sarcoma among cases of AIDS in multiple risk groups in New York City. Lancet ii:1024–1025.

DOS SANTOS SILVA I, SWERDLOW AJ. 1993. Sex differences in the risks of hormone-dependent cancers. Am J Epidemiol 138:10–28.

DUBE VE, FISHER DE. 1972. Hemangioendothelioma of the leg following metallic fixation of the tibia. Cancer 30:1260–1266.

DUBIN HV, CREEHAN EP, HEADINGTON JT. 1974. Lymphangiosarcoma and congenital lymphedema of the extremity. Arch Dermatol 110:608–614.

EL-JABBOUR JN, AKHTAR SS, KERR GR, et al. 1990. Prognostic factors for survival in soft tissue sarcoma. Br J Cancer 62:857–861.

EL-NAGGAR AK, GARCIA GM. 1992. Epithelioid sarcoma: flow cytometric study of DNA content and regional DNA heterogeneity. Cancer 69:1721–1728.

EMRICH LJ, RUKA W, DRISCOLL DL, et al. 1989. The effect of local recurrence on survival time in adult high-grade soft tissue sarcomas. J Clin Epidemiol 42:105–110.

ENGEL A, LAMM SH. 1992. Risks of sarcomas of the breast among women with breast augmentation. Plast Reconstr Surg 89:571–572.

ENZINGER FM, SMITH BH. 1976. Hemangiopericytoma: An analysis of 106 cases. Hum Pathol 7:61–82.

ENZINGER FM, WEISS SW. 1988a. General considerations. In Enzinger FM, Weiss SW (eds): Soft Tissue Tumors. St. Louis, C.V. Mosby, pp. 1–18.

ENZINGER FM, WEISS SW. 1988b. Fibrosarcoma. In Enzinger FM, Weiss SW (eds): Soft Tissue Tumors. St. Louis, C.V. Mosby, p. 213.

ERIKSSON M, HARDELL L, BERG NO, et al. 1981. Soft-tissue sarcomas and exposure to chemical substances: A case-referent study. Br J Ind Med 38:27–33.

ERIKSSON M, HARDELL L, ADAMI H-O. 1990. Exposure to dioxins as a risk factor for soft tissue sarcoma: A population-based case-control study. J Natl Cancer Inst 82:486–490.

FALK H, TELLES NC, ISHAK KG, et al. 1979a. Epidemiology of thorotrast-induced hepatic angiosarcoma in the United States. Environ Res 18:65–73.

FALK H, THOMAS LB, POPPER H, et al. 1979b. Hepatic angiosarcoma associated with androgenic-anabolic steroids. Lancet 2:1120–1123.

FALK H, CALDWELL GG, ISHAK KG, et al. 1981. Arsenic-related hepatic angiosarcoma. Am J Ind Med 2:43–50.

FALLS HF, KERLESZ ED. 1964. A new syndrome combining pterygium colli with developmental anomalies of the eyelids and lymphatic of the lower extremities. Trans Am Ophthalmol Soc 62:248–275.

FINGERHUT MA, HALPERIN WE, HONCHAR PA, et al. 1984. An evaluation of reports of dioxin exposure and soft tissue sarcoma pathology among chemical workers in the United States. Scand J Work Environ Health 10:299–303.

FINGERHUT MA, HALPERIN WE, MARLOW DA, et al. 1991. Cancer mortality in workers exposed to 2,3,7,8-tetrachlorodibenzo-*p*-dioxin. N Engl J Med 324:212–218.

FLETCHER CDM. 1987. Soft tissue sarcomas apparently arising in chronic tropical ulcers. Histopathology 11:501–510.

GALLAGHER RP, THRELFALL WJ. 1984. Cancer and occupational exposure to chlorophenols. Lancet 2:48.

GARBER JE, GOLDSTEIN AM, KANTOR AF, et al. 1991. Follow-up study of twenty-four families with Li-Fraumeni syndrome. Cancer Res 51:6094–6097.

GARBER JE, LIEPMAN MK, GELLES EJ, CORSON JM, ANTMAN KH. 1990. Melanoma and soft tissue sarcoma in seven patients. Cancer 66:2432–2434.

GEBAUER C. 1982. Primary pulmonary sarcomas. 1982. Etiology, clinical assessment and prognosis with a comparison to pulmonary carcinomas—A review of 41 cases and 394 other cases of the literature. Jpn J Surg 12:148–159.

GHALI MH, YOO K-Y, FLANNERY JT, et al. 1992. Association between childhood rhabdomyosarcoma and maternal history of stillbirths. Int J Cancer 50:365–368.

GIRALDO G, BETH E, HUANG E-S. 1980. Kaposi's sarcoma and its relationship to cytomegalovirus (CMV): III. CMV DNA and CMV early antigens in Kaposi's sarcoma. Int J Cancer 26:23–29.

GIRALDO G, BUONAGURO FM, BETH-GIRALDO E. 1989. The role of opportunistic viruses in Kaposi's sarcoma (KS) evolution. APMIS (Suppl.) 8:62–70.

GOEDERT JJ. 1987. What is safe sex? Suggested standards linked to testing for human immunodeficiency virus. N Engl J Med 316:1339–1342.

GOUN B, KULLER L. 1988. Vietnam military service and risk of selected cancers. Am J Epidemiol 128:901.

GREENE MH, HOOVER RN, FRAUMENI JF JR. 1978. Subsequent cancer in patients with chronic lymphocytic leukemia—a possible immunologic mechanism. J Natl Cancer Inst 61:337–340.

GREENE MH, WILSON J. 1985. Second cancer following lymphatic and hematopoietic cancers in Connecticut, 1935–1982. Natl Cancer Inst Monogr 68:191–197.

GREENWALD P, KOVASZNAY B, COLLIN DN, THERRIAULT G. 1984. Sarcomas of soft tissues after Vietnam service. J Natl Cancer Inst 73:1107–1109.

GRUFFERMAN S, SCHWARTZ AG, RUYMANN FB, et al. 1993. Parents' use of cocaine and marijuana and increased risk of rhabdomyosarcoma in their children. Cancer Causes Control 4:217–224.

GRUFFERMAN S, WANG HH, DELONG ER, et al. 1982. Environmental factors in the etiology of rhabdomyosarcoma in childhood. J Natl Cancer Inst 68:107–113.

HALPERIN EC, GREENBERG MS, SUIT HD. 1984. Sarcoma of bone and soft tissue following treatment of Hodgkin's disease. Cancer 53:232–236.

HAM JM, PIROLA RC, CROUCH RL. 1980. Hemangioendothelial sarcoma of the liver associated with long-term estrogen therapy in a man. Dig Dis Sci 25:879–883.

HAMMOND DB, ELLMAN L, SIROTA RL. 1977. Kaposi's sarcoma presenting as autoimmune hemolytic anemia. Am J Hematol 2:393–396.

HANSEN MR, KOUFOS A, GALLIE BL, et al. 1985. Osteosarcoma and retinoblastoma: A shared chromosomal mechanism revealing recessive predisposition. Proc Natl Acad Sci USA 82:6216–6220.

HARDELL L. 1977. Soft tissue sarcomas and exposure to phenoxy acids—a clinical observation. Lakartidningen 74:2753–2754.

HARDELL L. 1992. Hexachlorophene exposure in a young patient with soft tissue sarcoma. Br J Ind Med 49:743–744.

HARDELL L, AXELSON O. 1982. Soft-tissue sarcoma, malignant lymphoma, and exposure to phenoxyacids or chlorophenols. Lancet 1:1408–1409.

HARDELL L, ERIKSSON M. 1988. The association between soft tissue sarcomas and exposure to phenoxyacetic acids: A new case-referent study. Cancer 62:652–656.

HARDELL L, SANDSTROM A. 1979. Case-control study: Soft-tissue sarcomas and exposure to phenoxyacetic acids or chlorophenols. Br J Cancer 39:711–717.

HARLOW BL, WEISS NS, LOFTON S. 1986. The epidemiology of sarcomas of the uterus. J Natl Cancer Inst 76:399–402.

HARTLEY AL, BIRCH JM, MARSDEN HB, HARRIS M. 1986. Breast cancer risk in mothers of children with osteosarcoma and chondrosarcoma. Br J Cancer 54:819–823.

HARTLEY AL, BIRCH JM, KELSEY AM, et al. 1989. Are germ cell tumors part of the Li-Fraumeni cancer family syndrome? Cancer Genet Cytogenet 42:221–226.

HARVEY EB, BRINTON LA. 1985. Second cancer following cancer of the breast in Connecticut, 1935–82. Natl Cancer Inst Monogr 68:99–112.

HARWOOD AR, OSOBA D, HOFSTADER SL, et al. 1979. Kaposi's sarcoma in recipients of renal transplants. Am J Med 67:759–765.

HASHIMOTO H, DAIMARU Y, TAKESHITA S, et al. 1992. Prognostic significance of histologic parameters of soft tissue sarcomas. Cancer 70:2816–2822.

HOAR SK, BLAIR A, HOLMES FF, et al. 1986. Agricultural herbicide use and risk of lymphoma and soft-tissue sarcoma. JAMA 256:1141–1147.

HOLMES AP, BARLEY C, BARON RC, et al. 1986. Vietnam-era veterans mortality study-West Virginia residents 1968–1983. Charleston, West Virginia Department of Health.

HONCHAR PA, HALPERIN WE. 1981. 2,4,5-T, trichlorophenol and soft tissue sarcoma. Lancet 1:268–269.

HOOVER R, FRAUMENI JF JR. 1973. Risk of cancer in renal transplant recipients. Lancet 2:55–57.

HOPE DG, MULVIHILL JJ. 1981. Malignancy in neurofibromatosis. Adv Neurol 29:33–56.

HUANG YQ, LI JJ, RUSH MG, et al. 1992. HPV-16-related DNA sequences in Kaposi's sarcoma. Lancet 339:515–518.

IWASAKI H, ENJOJI M. 1979. Infantile and adult fibrosarcomas of the soft tissues. Acta Pathol Jpn 29:377–388.

JEKEL JF, FREEMAN DH, MEIGS JW. 1978. A study of trends in upper arm soft tissue sarcomas in the state of Connecticut following the introduction of alum-absorbed allergenic extract. Ann Allergy 40:28–31.

JENNINGS AM, WILD G, WARD JD, WARD AM. 1988. Immunological abnormalities 17 years after accidental exposure to 2,3,7,8-tetrachlorodibenzo-p-dioxin. Br J Ind Med 45:710–704.

JOHANSSON SL, HIRSCH JM, LARSSON P-A, et al. 1989. Snuff-induced carcinogenesis: Effect of snuff in rats initiated with 4-nitroquinoline-N-oxide. Cancer Res 49:3063–3069.

JOHNSON FE, KUGLER AM, BROWN SM. 1981. Soft tissue sarcomas and chlorinated phenols. Lancet 2:40.

KALDOR JM, DAY NE, BAND P, et al. 1987. Second malignancies following testicular cancer, ovarian cancer, and Hodgkin's disease: An international collaborative study among cancer registries. Int J Cancer 39:571–585.

KANG H, ENZINGER F, BRESLIN P, et al. 1987. Soft tissue sarcoma and military service in Vietnam: A case-control study. J Natl Cancer Inst 79:693–699.

KANG HK, WEATHERBEE L, BRESLIN PP, et al. 1986. Soft tissue sarcomas and military service in Vietnam: A case comparison group analysis of hospital patients. J Occup Med 28:1215–1218.

KASPER ML, SCHOENFIELD L, STROM RL, et al. 1984. Hepatic angiosarcoma and bronchioloalveolar carcinoma induced by Fowler's solution. JAMA 252:3407–3408.

KATO I, KIDO C. 1987. Increased risk of death in thorotrast-exposed patients during the late followup period. Jpn J Cancer Res 78:1187–1192.

KESTENS L, MELBYE M, BIGGAR RJ, STEVENS WJ, PIOT P, MUYNCK AD, TAELMAN H, DE FEYTER M, PALUKU L, GIGASE PL. 1985. Endemic African Kaposi's sarcoma is not associated with immunodeficiency. Int J Cancer 36:49–54.

KEYHANI A, BOOHER RJ. 1968. Pleiomorphic rhabdomyosarcoma. Cancer 22:956–967.

KIM JH, CHU FC, WOODWARD HO, et al. 1978. Radiation-induced soft-tissue and bone sarcoma. Radiology 129:501–508.

KING DT, DUFFY DM, HIROSE FM, et al. 1979. Lymphangiosarcoma arising from lymphangioma circumscriptum. Arch Dermatol 115:969–972.

KINLEN LJ, SHEIL AGR, PETO J, et al. 1979. Collaborative United Kingdom—Australian study of cancer in patients treated with immunosuppressive drugs. BMJ 2:1461–1466.

KLEPP O, DAHL O, STENWIG JT. 1978. Association of Kaposi's sarcoma and prior immunosuppressive therapy. Cancer 42:2626–2630.

KNIGHT JC. 1990. The molecular genetics of soft tissue sarcoma. Eur J Cancer 26:511–513.

KOGAN MD, CLAPP RW. 1988. Soft tissue sarcoma mortality among Vietnam veterans in Massachusetts, 1972 to 1983. Int J Epidemiol 17:39–43.

KORTE C, JALAL SM. 1982. 2,4-D induced clastogenicity and elevated rates of sister chromatid exchanges in cultured human lymphocytes. J Hered 73:224–226.

LASKIN WB, SILVERMAN TA, ENZINGER FM. 1988. Postradiation soft tissue sarcomas: An analysis of 53 cases. Cancer 62:2330–2340.

LATHROP GD, WOLFE WH, ALBANESE RA, MOYNAHAN PM. Project Ranch Hand II. 1984. An epidemiologic investigation of health effects in Air Force personnel following exposure to herbicides—Baseline mortality study results. Brooks Air Force Base, Texas: U.S. Air Force School of Aerospace Medicine.

LAWRENCE CE, REILLY AA, QUICKENTON P, et al. 1985. Mortality patterns of New York State Vietnam veterans. Am J Public Health 75:277–279.

LEE YS, PHO RWH, NATHER A. 1984. Malignant fibrous histiocytoma at site of metal implant. Cancer 54:2286–2289.

LI FP. 1988. Cancer families: Human models of susceptibility to neoplasia. Cancer Res 48:5381–5386.

LI FP, FRAUMENI JF. 1969. Rhabdomyosarcoma in children: Epidemiologic study and identification of a familial cancer syndrome. J Natl Cancer Inst 43:1365–1373.

LI FP, FRAUMENI JF JR. 1982. Prospective study of a family cancer syndrome. JAMA 247:2692–2694.

LI FP, FRAUMENI JF JR, MULVIHILL JJ, et al. 1988. A cancer family syndrome in twenty-four kindreds. Cancer Res 48:5358–5362.

LI FP, GARBER JE, FRIEND SH, et al. 1992. Recommendations on predictive testing for germ line p53 mutations among cancer-prone individuals. J Natl Cancer Inst 84:1156–1160.

LOCKER GY, DOROSHOW JH, ZWELLING LA, et al. 1979. The clinical features of hepatic angiosarcoma: A report of four cases and a review of the English literature. Medicine 58:48–64.

LUTZNER MA. 1977. Nosology among the neoplastic genodermatoses. In Mulvihill JJ, Miller RW, Fraumeni JF Jr (eds): Genetics of Human Cancer. New York: Raven Press, pp. 145–168.

LYNGE E. 1985. A follow-up study of cancer incidence among workers in manufacture of phenoxy herbicides in Denmark. Br J Cancer 52:259–270.

LYNGE E. 1987. Background and design of a Danish cohort study of workers in phenoxy herbicide manufacture. Am J Ind Med 11:427–437.

LYNGE E, STORM HH, JENSEN OM. 1987. The evaluation of trends in soft tissue sarcoma according to diagnostic criteria and consumption of phenoxy herbicides. Cancer 60:1896–1901.

MAHOUR GH, SOULE EH, MILLS SD, et al. 1967. Rhabdomyosarcoma in infants and children: A clinicopathologic study of 75 cases. J Pediatr Surg 2:402–409.

MALKIN D, LI FP, STRONG LC, et al. 1990. Germ line p53 mutations in a familial syndrome of breast cancer, sarcomas, and other neoplasms. Science 250:1233–1238.

MANDARD AM, PETIOT JF, MARNAY J, et al. 1989. Prognostic factors in soft tissue sarcomas: A multivariate analysis of 109 cases. Cancer 63:1437–1451.

MARGULIES KB, SHEPS SG. 1988. Carney's triad: Guidelines for management. Mayo Clin Proc 63:496–502.

MARK RJ, BAILET JW, POEN J, et al. 1993. Postirradiation sarcoma of the head and neck. Cancer 72:887–893.

MAY DS, STROUP NE. 1991. The incidence of sarcomas of the breast among women in the United States, 1973–1986. Plast Reconstr Surg 87:193.

MAYS CW. 1988. Alpha-particle-induced cancer in humans. Health Phys 55:637–652.

MCKEEN EA, BODURTHA J, MEADOWS AT, DOUGLASS EC, MULVIHILL JJ. 1978. Rhabdomyosarcoma complicating multiple neurofibromatosis. J Pediatr 93:992–993.

MCKILLOP JH, DOIG JA, KENNEDY JS, et al. 1978. Laryngeal malignancy following iodine-125 therapy for thyrotoxicosis. Lancet 2:1177–1179.

MCILLMURRAY MB, LANGMAN MJS. 1978. Soft tissue sarcomas and intramuscular injections: An epidemiological survey. BMJ 2:864–865.

MILHAM S JR. 1982. Herbicides, occupation, and cancer. Lancet 1:1464–1465.

MILLER RW, DALAGER NA. 1974. Fatal rhabdomyosarcoma among children in the United States, 1960–1969. Cancer 34:1897–1900.

MORTON DL. 1973. Soft tissue sarcomas. In Holland JF, Frei E (eds): Cancer Medicine. Philadelphia: Lea and Febiger, pp. 1845–1861.

MULVIHILL JJ. 1975. Congenital and genetic diseases. In Fraumeni JF Jr (ed): Persons at High Risk of Cancer: An Approach to Cancer Etiology and Control. New York: Academic Press, pp. 3–39.

NICKOLOFF BJ, HUANG YQ, LI JJ, et al. 1992. Immunohistochemical detection of papillomavirus antigens in Kaposi's sarcoma. Lancet 339:548–549.

NOVAKOVIC B, GOLDSTEIN AM, WEXLER LH, et al. 1994. Increased risk of neuroectodermal tumors and stomach cancer in relatives of patients with Ewing's sarcoma family of tumors. J Natl Cancer Inst, 86:1702–1706.

NYREN O, MCLAUGHLIN JK, GRIDLEY G, et al. 1995. Cancer risk after hip replacement with metal implants: a population-based cohort study in Sweden. J Natl Cancer Inst, 87:28–33.

OTT G. 1970. Fremdkorpersarkome. In Leuthardt HvF, Schoen R, Schwiegk H, et al (eds): Experimentelle Medezin, Pathologie, und Klinik. Berlin: Springer-Verlag, Vol. 32.

OTT MG, HOLDER BB, OLSON RD. 1980. A mortality analysis of employees engaged in the manufacture of 2,4,5-trichlorophenoxyacetic acid. J Occup Med 22:47–50.

OTT MG, OLSON RA, COOK RR, et al. 1987. Cohort mortality study of chemical workers with potential exposure to the higher chlorinated dioxins. J Occup Med 29:422–429.

PACK GT, PIERSON JC. 1954. Liposarcoma: A study of 105 cases. Surgery 36:687–712.

PEARCE N, SMITH AH, REIF JS. 1988. Increased risks of soft tissue sarcoma, malignant lymphoma, and acute myeloid leukemia in abattoir workers. Am J Ind Med 14:63–72.

PEZZI CM, RAWLINGS MS JR, ESGRO JJ, et al. 1992. Prognostic factors in 227 patients with malignant fibrous histiocytoma. Cancer 69:2098–2103.

POLEDNAK AP. 1986. Incidence of soft-tissue cancers in blacks and whites in New York State. Int J Cancer 38:21–26.

POPPER H, THOMAS LB, TELLES NC, et al. 1978. Development of hepatic angiosarcoma in man induced by vinyl chloride, thorotrast, and arsenic. Am J Pathol 92:349–376.

POTISH RA, DEHNER LP, HASELOW RE, et al. 1985. The incidence of second neoplasms following megavoltage radiation for pediatric tumors. Cancer 56:1534–1537.

PRITCHARD DJ, SOULE EH, TAYLOR WF, et al. 1974. Fibrosarcoma—a clinicopathologic and statistical study of 199 tumors of the soft tissues of the extremities and trunk. Cancer 33:888–897.

PUNTONI R, MERLO F, FINI A, et al. 1986. Soft tissue sarcomas in Seveso. Lancet 2:525.

REIF J, PEARCE N, KAWACHI I, FRASER J. 1989. Soft-tissue sarcoma, non-Hodgkin's lymphoma and other cancers in New Zealand forestry workers. Int J Cancer 43:49–54.

RIES LAG, BIGGAR RJ, FEIGAL E. 1993. Kaposi's sarcoma. In Miller BA, Ries LAG, Hankey BF, et al (eds): SEER Cancer Statistics Review: 1973–1990, National Cancer Institute. NIH Publ. No. 93-2789.

ROBINSON E, NEUGUT AJ, WYLIE P. 1988. Clinical aspects of post-irradiation sarcomas. J Natl Cancer Inst 80:233–240.

ROCK MG, UNNI KK. 1990. Iatrogenic bone malignancy and pseudomalignancy. Curr Opin Rheumatol 2:138–144.

ROTH WK, WERNER S, RISAU W, PEMBERGER K, HOFSCHNEIDER PH. 1988. Cultured, AIDS-related Kaposi's sarcoma cells express endothelial cell markers and are weakly malignant in vitro. Int J Cancer 42:767–773.

ROUTH A, HICKMAN BT, JOHNSON WW. 1985. Malignant fibrous histiocytoma arising from chronic ulcer. Arch Dermatol 121:529–531.

RYU RKN, BOVILL EG, SKINNER HB, MURRAY WR. 1987. Soft tissue sarcoma associated with aluminum oxide ceramic total hip arthroplasty: A case report. Clin Orthop 216:207–212.

SAFAI B. 1987. Pathophysiology and epidemiology of epidemic Kaposi's sarcoma. Semin Oncol 14:7–12.

SAFAI B, MIKE V, GIRALDO G, et al. 1980. Association of Kaposi's sarcoma with second primary malignancies: Possible etiopathogenic implications. Cancer 45:1472–1479.

SANDERS BM, JAY M, DRAPER GJ, et al. 1989. Non-ocular cancer in relatives of retinoblastoma patients. Br J Cancer 60:358–365.

SARMA PR, JACOBS J. 1982. Thoracic soft-tissue sarcoma in Vietnam veterans exposed to Agent Orange. N Engl J Med 306:1109.

SAVITZ DA, WACHTEL H, BARNES FA, et al. 1988. Case-control study of childhood cancer and exposure to 60-Hz magnetic fields. Am J Epidemiol 128:21–38.

SELECTED CANCERS COOPERATIVE STUDY GROUP. 1990a. The association of selected cancers with service in the US military in Vietnam. I. Non-Hodgkin's lymphoma. Arch Intern Med 150:2473–2483.

SELECTED CANCERS COOPERATIVE STUDY GROUP. 1990b. The association of selected cancers with service in the US military in Vietnam. II. Soft tissue and other sarcomas. Arch Intern Med 150:2485–2492.

SENIORI COSTANTINO A, PACI E, MILIGI L, et al. 1989. Cancer mortality among workers in the Tuscan tanning industry. Br J Ind Med 36:384–388.

SERRAINO D, FRANCESCHI S, LAVECCHIA C, et al. 1992. Occupation and soft-tissue sarcoma in northeastern Italy. Cancer Causes Control 3:25–30.

SERRAINO D, FRANCESCHI S, TALAMINI R, et al. 1991. Non-occupational risk factors for adult soft-tissue sarcoma in northern Italy. Cancer Causes Control 2:157–164.

SILVERBERG E, LUBERA JA. 1988. Cancer statistics, 1988. CA Cancer J Clin 38:5–22.

SMITH AH, FISHER DO, GILES HJ, PEARCE NE. 1983. The New Zealand soft tissue sarcoma case-control study: Interview findings concerning phenoxyacetic acid exposure. Chemosphere 12:565–571.

SMITH AH, FISHER DO, PEARCE N, TEAGUE CA. 1982. Do agricultural chemicals cause soft tissue sarcoma? Initial findings of a case-control study in New Zealand. Community Health Stud 6:114–119.

SMITH AH, PEARCE NE, FISHER DO, et al. 1984. Soft tissue sarcoma and exposure to phenoxyherbicides and chlorophenols in New Zealand. J Natl Cancer Inst 73:1111–1117.

SOBEL W, BOND GG, SKOWRONSKI BJ, et al. 1986. Soft-tissue sarcoma: Case-control study. J Occup Med 28:804–807.

SPECTOR BD, PERRY GS, KERSEY JH. 1978. Genetically determined immunodeficiency diseases (GDID) and malignancy: Report from the immunodeficiency-cancer registry. Clin Immunol Immunopathol 11:12–29.

STAYNER LT, ELLIOTT L, BLADE L, et al. 1988. A retrospective cohort mortality study of workers exposed to formaldehyde in the garment industry. Am J Ind Med 13:667–681.

STELLMAN SD, STELLMAN JM. 1986. Estimation of exposure to Agent Orange and other defoliants among American troops in Vietnam: A methodological approach. Am J Ind Med 9:305–321.

STOUT AP. 1943. Hemangioendothelioma: A tumor of blood vessels featuring vascular endothelial cells. Ann Surg 118:445–464.

STRONG LC. 1977. Theories of pathogenesis: Mutation and cancer. In Mulvihill JJ, Miller RW, Fraumeni JF Jr (eds): Genetics of Human Cancer. New York: Raven Press, pp. 401–415.

STRONG LC, STINE M, NORSTED TL. 1987. Cancer in survivors of childhood soft tissue sarcoma and their relatives. J Natl Cancer Inst 79:1213–1220.

SUSSMAN EB, NYDICK I, GRAY GF. 1974. Hemangioendothelial sarcoma of the liver and hemochromatosis. Arch Pathol 97:39–42.

SWANN M. 1984. Malignant soft-tissue tumour at the site of a total hip replacement. J Bone Joint Surg [Br] 66:629–631.

TAGHIAN A, DE VATHAIRE F, TERRIER P, et al. 1991. Long-term risk of sarcoma following radiation treatment for breast cancer. Int J Radiat Oncol Biol Phys 21:361–367.

TEMPLETON AC. 1973. Soft tissue sarcoma. In Templeton AC (ed): Recent Results in Cancer Research. New York: Springer-Verlag, Vol. 41, pp. 234–296.

TSUJIMOTO M, AOZASA K, VEDA T, et al. 1988. Multivariate analysis for histologic prognostic factors in soft tissue sarcomas. Cancer 62:994–998.

TUCKER AH, VORE SJ, LUSTER MI. 1986. Suppression of B cell differentiation by 2,3,7,8-tetrachlorodibenzo-p-dioxin. Mol Pharmacol 29:372–377.

TUCKER MA, COLEMAN CN, COS RS, et al. 1988. Risk of second cancers after treatment for Hodgkin's disease. N Engl J Med 318:76–81.

TUCKER MA, D'ANGIO GJ, BOICE JC JR, et al. 1987. Bone sarcomas linked to radiotherapy and chemotherapy in children. N Engl J Med 317:588–593.

TUCKER MA, MEADOWS AT, BOICE JD JR, et al. 1984. Cancer risk following treatment of childhood cancer. In Boice JD Jr, Fraumeni JF Jr, (eds): Radiation Carcinogenesis: Epidemiology and Biological Significance. New York: Raven Press, pp. 211–224.

TURKULA TE, JALAL SM. 1985. Increased rates of sister chromatid exchanges induced by the herbicide 2,4-D. J Hered 76:213–214.

TYNES T, ANDERSEN A, LANGMARK F. 1992. Incidence of cancer in Norwegian workers potentially exposed to electromagnetic fields. Am J Epidemiol 136:81–88.

VAINIO H, NICKELS J, LINNAINMAA K. 1982. Phenoxy acid herbicides cause peroxisome proliferation in Chinese hamsters. Scand J Work Environ Health 8:70–73.

VAN DEN BERG F, SCHIPPER M, JIWA M, ROOK R, VAN DE RIJKE F, TIGGES B. 1989. Implausibility of an aetiological association between cytomegalovirus and Kaposi's sarcoma shown by four techniques. J Clin Pathol 42:128–131.

VAN KAICK G, LIEBERMAN D, LORENZ D, et al. 1983. Recent results of the German thorotrast study—Epidemiologic results and dose effect relationships in thorotrast patients. Health Phys 44:299–306.

VAN'T HOFF SC, VAN DIJK WJ, BUYS W-J, et al. 1986. Conditional oncogenicity of perfused adriamycin in the tourniquet-isolated rat limb. Carcinogenesis 7:178–189.

VINEIS P, TERRACINI B, CICCONE G, et al. 1987. Phenoxy herbicides and soft-tissue sarcomas in female rice weeders: A population-based case-referent study. Scand J Work Environ Health 13:9–17.

VINEIS P, ZAHM SH. 1988. Immunosuppressive effects of dioxin in the development of Kaposi's sarcoma and non-Hodgkin's lymphoma. Lancet 1:55.

WALKER RH, REED WB. 1973. Genetic cutaneous disorders with gynecologic tumors. Am J Obstet Gynecol 4:485–492.

WEINBREN K, SALM R, GREENBERG G. 1978. Intramuscular injections of iron compounds and oncogenesis in man. BMJ 1:683–685.

WERNER S, HOFSCHNEIDER PH, ROTH WK. 1989. Cells derived from sporadic and AIDS-related Kaposi's sarcoma reveal identical cytochemical and molecular properties in vitro. Int J Cancer 43:1137–1144.

WIKLUND K, DICH J, HOLM L-E. 1988. Soft tissue sarcoma risk in Swedish licensed pesticide applicators. J Occup Med 30:801–804.

WIKLUND K, HOLM L-E. 1986. Soft tissue sarcoma risk in Swedish agricultural and forestry workers. J Natl Cancer Inst 76:229–234.

WILLIAMS WR, STRONG LC. 1985. Genetic epidemiology of soft tissue sarcomas in children. In Muller HR, Weber W (eds): Familial Cancer, First International Conference. Basel: S. Karger AG, pp. 151–153.

WINGREN G, FREDRIKSON M, BRAGE HN, et al. 1990. Soft tissue sarcoma and occupational exposures. Cancer 66:806–811.

WOODS JS, POLISSAR L, SEVERSON RK, et al. 1987. Soft tissue sarcoma and non-Hodgkin's lymphoma in relation to phenoxyherbicide and chlorinated phenol exposure in Western Washington. J Natl Cancer Inst 78:899–910.

YANNOPOULOS K, STOUT AP. 1962. Smooth muscle tumors in children. Cancer 15:958–971.

ZACK JA, SUSKIND RR. 1980. The mortality experience of workers exposed to tetrachlorodibenzodioxin in a trichlorophenol process accident. J Occup Med 22:11–14.

ZAHM SH, BLAIR A, HOLMES FF, et al. 1988. A case-referent study of soft-tissue sarcoma and Hodgkin's disease: Farming and insecticide use. Scand J Work Environ Health 14:224–230.

ZAHM SH, BLAIR A, HOLMES FF, et al. 1989. A case-control study of soft-tissue sarcoma. Am J Epidemiol 130:665–674.

ZAHM SH, HEINEMAN EF, VAUGHT JB. 1992. Soft tissue sarcoma and tobacco use: data from a prospective cohort study of United States veterans. Cancer Causes Control 3:371–376.

46 Thyroid cancer

ELAINE RON

Cancer of the thyroid is relatively uncommon. The prognosis is extremely good for papillary and follicular carcinoma and extremely poor for anaplastic carcinoma. Other than ionizing radiation, the causes of thyroid cancer remain relatively obscure, but results from several recently published epidemiologic studies have implicated benign thyroid nodules and goiter, hormonal and reproductive variables, dietary intake, and genetic factors. The study of thyroid cancer is complicated by the different demographic, etiologic, and survival patterns of each histologic type. This chapter reviews the epidemiology of thyroid cancer, taking histology into account whenever possible. Because thyroid cancer is a rare disease, however, the number of cases included in individual studies generally is too small to allow systematic analysis by histology.

DEMOGRAPHIC PATTERNS

Histopathology

The large majority (95%) of thyroid cancers originates in cells derived from the epithelium. The revised World Health Organization (WHO) classification includes papillary (including mixed papillary-follicular), follicular, medullary, and undifferentiated (anaplastic) carcinomas as epithelial tumors (Hedinger et al, 1988). Papillary, follicular, and anaplastic cancers all arise from follicular cells, but medullary carcinoma arises from parafollicular or C cells. Epithelial tumors are also divided into well-differentiated (papillary and follicular) and poorly differentiated tumors (anaplastic). Medullary carcinoma appears to be intermediate between well differentiated and poorly differentiated. Non-epithelial thyroid tumors are infrequent and are now grouped together, except for malignant lymphomas which have been added as a major separate class. The majority of small-cell carcinomas are thought to be malignant lymphomas (Hedinger et al, 1988).

The most common histologic type of thyroid cancer is by far, papillary carcinoma (between 50% and 80% of the cases) (Table 46–1). Variants of papillary carcinoma include papillary microcarcinoma (formerly called focal sclerosing or occult papillary carcinoma), follicular variant, and diffuse sclerosing type (Hedinger et al, 1988). Most often there are no clinical manifestations of papillary microcarcinoma, so that generally it is diagnosed in early detection screening programs, incidentally during surgery, or at autopsy. Typically, follicular carcinoma represents about 20% of thyroid malignancies (range, 10–40%), and anaplastic and medullary carcinomas account for between 5% and 15% of thyroid cancer incidence. The relative frequency of papillary and follicular thyroid cancer is complicated by qualitative differences in diagnosis. Because it can be difficult to distinguish between benign and highly differentiated malignant follicular neoplasms, there may be some underreporting of follicular thyroid cancer. On the other hand, it is relatively easy to diagnose papillary carcinoma and ascertainment is more complete (Hedinger, 1985; Rojeski and Gharib, 1985; Ron et al, 1986).

The female-to-male ratio is approximately 3:1 among patients with papillary and follicular cell types, whereas medullary carcinoma occurs almost equally among males and females. Consistent with the epidemiology data is the finding of a high frequency of estrogen receptors in differentiated carcinomas but not in medullary carcinoma (Chaudhuri and Prinz, 1989). The mean age at diagnosis is mid-forties to early fifties for papillary carcinoma, fifties for follicular and medullary, and sixties for anaplastic carcinoma. Children and adolescents most frequently have papillary cancer. Over 80% of thyroid cancers diagnosed under age 40 are of the papillary type (LiVolsi, 1978; Robbins et al, 1984). Medullary carcinoma occurs both sporadically and as a familial disease.

Incidence and Mortality in the United States

The thyroid is one of the least cancer-prone organs in the body, representing only 0.54% of cancers occurring among U.S. males and 1.7% among U.S. females as compared to, for example, 16% for male and 13% for female occurrence of lung cancer, or 12% and 13%, respectively, for male and female colorectal cancer in-

TABLE 46–1. *Distribution of Thyroid Cancer by Histologic Type in Selected Population Surveys*

Study Location and Reference	*Years of Study*	*No. of Cases*	*Source of Data*	*Histology (%)*				
				Papillary	*Follicular*	*Medullary*	*Anaplastic*	*Other*
Minnesota, USA Verby et al (1969)	1935–65	46	hospital and death certificate	60.0[a]	20.0	7.0	13.0	7.0
Connecticut, USA Pottern et al (1980)	1935–75	1,915	cancer registry	52.1	13.3	10.3	9.4	14.9
Iceland Hrafnkelsson et al (1988)	1955–84	392	cancer registry	76.8[a]	13.8	1.5	7.4	0.5
Israel Modan et al (1969)	1960–65	323	hospital and cancer registry	54.8	18.3	0	11.5	15.4
Malmo, Sweden Borup Christensen et al (1984)	1960–77	104	hospital records	63.5	21.2	3.8	11.5	0
Singapore Lee (1982)	1968–77	346	cancer registry	70.0	22.5	1.2	4.6	1.7
Hawaii, USA Goodman et al (1988)	1969–84	1,110	cancer registry	74.3	17.5	1.9	1.5	4.8
Los Angeles, CA, USA Preston-Martin and Menck (1979)	1972–76	1,574	county cancer registry	69.6	17.2	2.4	10.8	
SEER, USA Correa and Chen (1995)	1973–87	13,791	cancer registries	73.0	17.3	3.2	2.3	4.2

[a]Excluding papillary microcarcinomas (occult).

cidence (Boring et al, 1994). The 1987–1991 age-standardized incidence rates for thyroid cancer in the U.S. Surveillance, Epidemiology and End Results (SEER) cancer registries were 2.5 and 6.4 per 100,000 males and females, respectively (Ries et al, 1994).

Because long-term survival is exceptionally good, only 0.14% of male and 0.25% of female cancer mortality is due to thyroid cancer. The number of incident cases is more than ten times higher than the number of deaths: 13,000 new cases and 1,025 thyroid cancer deaths were projected for 1994 (Boring et al, 1994). The ratio of incidence to mortality decreases, however, with age. This is partially because anaplastic thyroid cancer, which has a high fatality rate, occurs among older patients. Overall, the 1987–1991 age-adjusted U.S. mortality rates were 0.3 and 0.4 per 100,000 males and females, respectively. Mortality rates were high in Hawaii, New Jersey, New Hampshire, Colorado, and New York (Ries et al, 1994).

Thyroid cancer incidence and mortality rates measure different types of disease. Incidence rates are heavily weighted with young women with papillary or follicular carcinoma, whereas mortality statistics reflect elderly males and females with a relatively high proportion of undifferentiated carcinomas.

International Patterns

With the exception of Hawaii and Iceland, where thyroid cancer incidence is particularly high, incidence rates (world adjusted) from much of the world range between 1 and 2 cases per 100,000 males and between 2 and 6 cases per 100,000 females. The variation that is seen does not conform to usual patterns. Low rates occur both in developed and developing countries, although high rates are generally confined to developed nations with good medical systems (Table 46–2). While data are sparse, no significant difference in incidence has been observed between urban and rural areas in Europe.

Proposed explanations for geographic variation include a possible association with endemic goiter, volcanic lava, dietary patterns, or differences in reporting or case ascertainment. In regard to thyroid cancer, international comparisons are particularly subject to a wide diversity in diagnostic, treatment, and reporting practices. Furthermore, because thyroid cancer is a rare malignancy, many of the reported low-incidence rates are based on few cases, often less than 10, making them unstable. In addition, the data from several of the Asian and South American registries may not be complete, and only three African registries reported to the latest volume of Cancer Incidence in Five Continents (Parkin et al, 1992).

In a study of thyroid cancer incidence in the Nordic countries, the rate for Iceland was five times higher than that for Finland, whereas rates for Sweden and Norway fell between those of Iceland and Finland. Differences were apparent for both sexes, all age-groups, and all histological types, although the variation was widest for papillary thyroid cancer. These results are notable because pathologic material was reclassified by study pathologists, and because similar standards of medical

TABLE 46–2. *Age-Standardized Incidence of Thyroid Cancer in Selected Populations, 1983–87*

Continent	Country	Area	Population	Incidence[a] Male	Female
Asia	China[b]	Shanghai	6,594,100	0.9	2.2
	Hong Kong[b]	All	5,469,000	1.5	5.7
	India[b]	Bombay	8,813,700	0.8	1.5
	Israel	All (Jews only)	3,439,400	2.5	5.9
	Japan	Osaka Prefecture	8,668,100	1.1	3.3
	Kuwait[b]	All (Kuwaitis)	686,400	1.4	5.0
	Philippines[b]	Rizal Province	3,303,000	2.1	7.7
	Singapore	All (Chinese)	1,915,500	2.0	5.9
Europe	Denmark	All	5,117,400	1.0	2.0
	Estonia	All	1,529,600	0.6	2.8
	Finland	All	4,889,400	1.8	5.8
	France	Bas-Rhin region	931,300	1.5	2.9
	GDR	All	16,655,900	1.3	2.9
	Iceland	All	241,400	6.2	8.3
	Italy	Lombardy region	791,400	2.0	4.9
	Norway	All	4,162,300	1.6	5.1
	Poland	Cracow City	739,900	0.9	2.3
	Slovenia	All	1,957,400	1.0	1.9
	Spain	Murcia Province	1,001,400	1.1	3.6
	Sweden	All	8,365,400	1.6	3.8
	Switzerland	Vaud	533,500	1.8	4.3
	UK	England/Wales	49,925,000	0.7	1.5
North America	Canada	All	25,037,800	1.7	4.3
	United States	SEER (white)	18,318,700	2.2	5.8
		SEER (black)	2,856,100	1.0	2.7
South America	Colombia[b]	Cali	1,324,500	1.8	6.6
	Costa Rica	All	2,678,700	1.1	3.9
	Cuba[b]	All	10,245,900	1.1	3.6
	Ecuador[b]	Quito	1,038,000	2.9	6.3
Oceania	Australia	NSW	5,472,800	1.3	3.6
	New Zealand	All (Non-Maori)	2,976,500	1.1	3.0
		All (Maori)	293,400	1.6	4.0
	Hawaii	Filipino	116,200	6.6	24.2
		Hawaiian	199,500	5.4	9.6

[a]Annual rate per 100,000 population standardized to the World Standard Population. Data from Parkin et al, 1992.
[b]Quality indicators suggest that data from these registries may be incomplete.

care and reporting in the Nordic countries reduce the limitations associated with other intercountry comparisons (Franssila et al, 1981). The reasons for the variation in incidence among the Nordic countries are presently unknown, although differences in iodine intake may play some role.

In contrast to the low incidence and mortality rates of thyroid cancer, prevalence of occult thyroid cancer at autopsy occasionally can be quite high, and the epidemiologic patterns differ. Among autopsied cases, the sex ratio is equal and geographic variation can be extreme. The prevalence of occult papillary thyroid cancer at autopsy was 36% in Finland (Harach et al, 1985), 35% for Japanese living in Japan or Hawaii (Fukunaga and Lockett, 1971; Fukunaga and Yatani, 1975), 3–13% in Canada, the United States, Poland, Israel, and Argentina (Fukunaga and Yatani, 1975; Ottino et al, 1989; Sampson et al, 1974; Siegal and Modan, 1981; Silverberg and Vidone, 1966), and less than 1% in Switzerland (Heitz et al, 1976). While some variation can be attributed to the extent of thyroid examination, geographic differences also were found when comparisons were made by the same pathologists (Fukunaga and Yatani, 1975). Franssila and Harach (1986) observed a high prevalence of occult thyroid cancer during adolescence. They postulated that hormonal factors may act as promoters. With the exception of Switzerland (Heitz et al, 1976), papillary carcinoma is the predominant histologic type in most autopsy series, probably reflecting its slow-growing behavior.

Survival

With the exception of non-melanoma skin cancer, survival for thyroid cancer is better than for all other cancer sites. In the U.S., the 1983–90 all-stage relative 5-year survival rate was 94.6%. Survival was slightly better for women (95.4%) than for men (92.2%) and for whites (94.7%) than for blacks (90.2%). During the same time period, the survival rate was 99.6% for localized thyroid cancer. Although thyroid cancer with distant metastases has a poor survival rate (49.3%), only 5% of thyroid cancers are diagnosed at this stage, compared to 34% at the regional stage and 56% at the local stage (Ries et al, 1994).

Survival rates are highly correlated with histologic type and the degree of thyroid differentiation. Differentiated thyroid cancers have good survival rates whereas undifferentiated cancers are almost uniformly fatal. Papillary carcinoma has the best prognosis of all histopathologic types. Follicular carcinoma also has a good prognosis, except when distant metastases are present. Papillary carcinoma spreads locally through the lymphatics, whereas follicular carcinoma metastasizes widely via the blood stream. Survival is extremely poor for anaplastic cancer. In Malmo, Sweden, the 5-year relative survival rate for patients with papillary and follicular carcinoma was 95% and 70%, respectively; but the 1-year rate for anaplastic cancer was less than 1% (Borup Christensen et al, 1984). Taking histology into account, survival is inversely correlated with age at diagnosis, size of tumor, degree of local invasion, and extent of distant metastases (Akslen et al, 1991; Borup Christensen et al, 1984; Hrafnkelsson et al, 1988; Levi et al, 1990; Mazzaferri and Young, 1981; Schindler et al, 1991).

Time Trends

Papillary and follicular thyroid cancer incidence increased until about 1980 (Franeschi and La Vecchia, 1994; Glattre et al, 1990; Hrafnkelsson et al, 1988; Pettersson et al, 1991; Pottern et al, 1980; Sprøgel and Storm, 1989). Based on five geographic areas in the U.S., incidence increased between 1947 and 1978, particularly among 25–54-year-olds, but the rates appeared to plateau or slightly decline between 1979 and 1984 (Devesa et al, 1987) (Figure 46–1). These time trends

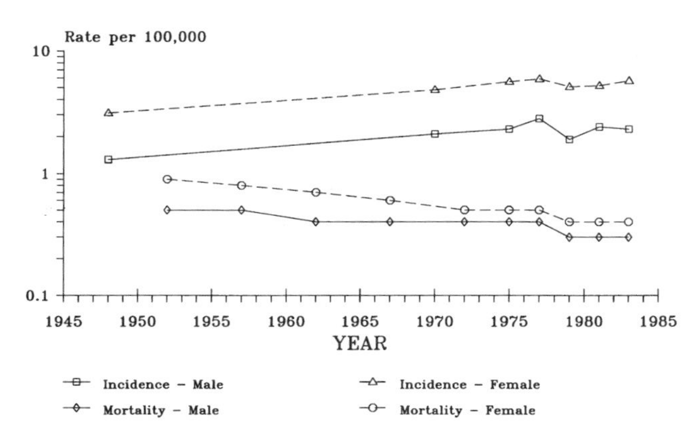

FIG. 46–1. Thyroid cancer incidence and mortality trends by sex, 1945–1985. United States white, age-standardized (1970 standard) rates. Data from Devesa et al, 1987.

are consistent with the wide use of radiation treatment for benign head and neck conditions between 1930 and 1960. Radiation-associated thyroid cancers would be expected to begin to occur around 1940 and to decline starting around 1980. Indeed, in a birth cohort analysis, Pottern et al (1980) demonstrated that the slopes of the curves for birth cohorts from 1870 to 1910 were similar, increased substantially for cohorts from 1920 to 1950, and began to decline for the 1960 cohort. However, the increase in incidence was also seen in the Nordic countries, where radiation therapy for benign conditions was used infrequently. In Finland, incidence rates have been increasing about 20% every 5 years (Coleman et al, 1993). Glattre et al (1990) hypothesized that the increase in incidence seen until 1980 and the subsequent decrease may be associated with changes in fish consumption in Norway. More recent data from the U.S. SEER program indicate that thyroid cancer is again increasing. From 1987 to 1991, incidence increased 7.6% (Ries et al, 1994). Incidence also continued to rise in Switzerland after 1980 (Levi et al, 1990).

Mortality, on the other hand, has decreased in most countries (Coleman et al, 1993; Franceschi and La Vecchia, 1994; La Vecchia et al, 1992; Ries et al, 1994). U.S. mortality rates for white females decreased more than 50% in the last 40 years, from 0.8/100,000 in the period 1950–54, to 0.4/100,000 in 1976–80, to 0.3/100,000 in 1988–1991. Among males there was also a marked decline, but it was less dramatic—from 0.5/100,000 to 0.3/100,000 during the same time period (Pickle et al, 1987; Ries et al, 1994). As a result, the sex differential in mortality rates has diminished since 1970 (Fig. 46–1). Since incidence has increased, it follows that mortality declined due to better survival. Possible reasons for the improved survival include increased incidence of histologic types (papillary and follicular) with good prognosis, earlier diagnosis, and more effective treatment.

Age and Sex

Thyroid cancer has an unusual age distribution (Fig. 46–2). About 10% of all thyroid cancer occurs in patients less than 21 years of age and incidence rises comparatively slowly with age. However, the incidence of thyroid cancer is relatively high between the ages of 15 and 39 years, when thyroid cancer accounts for 8.7% of all newly diagnosed cancers, as compared to 0.7% between the ages of 55 and 64, and 0.3% at age 80 and above. In fact, thyroid cancer was ranked as one of the five most frequent cancers among persons aged 15–39 (Myers and Ries, 1989).

Females consistently have a higher frequency of thyroid cancer than males (Muir et al, 1987; Devesa et al, 1987; Parkin et al, 1992). The female-to-male ratio is high (>3) after puberty and during the reproductive years, and then declines at the time of menopause (Fig. 46–2). Although the incidence of thyroid cancer is roughly two to three times more common among females, mortality rates are nearly equal until about age 60. At that time, female mortality increases and the difference between males and females becomes more evident (Fig. 46–3).

Socioeconomic Status, Race, Ethnicity, and Religion

Patterns relating to socioeconomic status, race, ethnicity, and religion are inconsistent, except that the incidence of thyroid cancer is about two times greater among whites than among blacks (Table 46–3), and persons of Asian origin have elevated rates compared to persons of other ethnic backgrounds living in the same areas (Goodman et al, 1988; Preston-Martin and Menck, 1979; Spitz et al, 1988). Further analysis indicates that the higher incidence of thyroid cancer among whites is confined to papillary carcinoma (Correa and Chen, 1995).

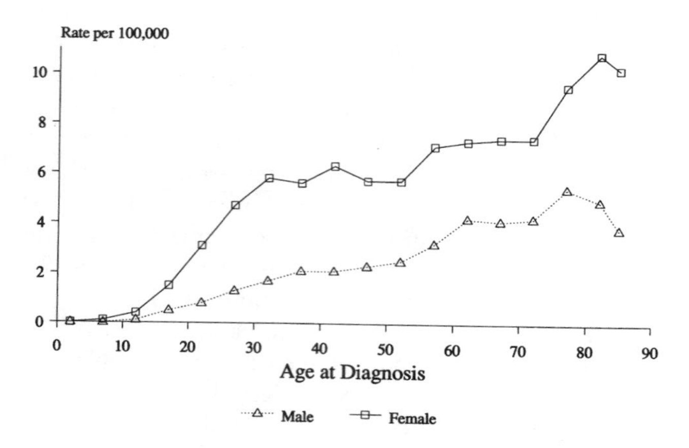

FIG. 46–2. Age-specific thyroid cancer incidence in Canada by sex, 1978–1982. Data from Muir et al, 1987.

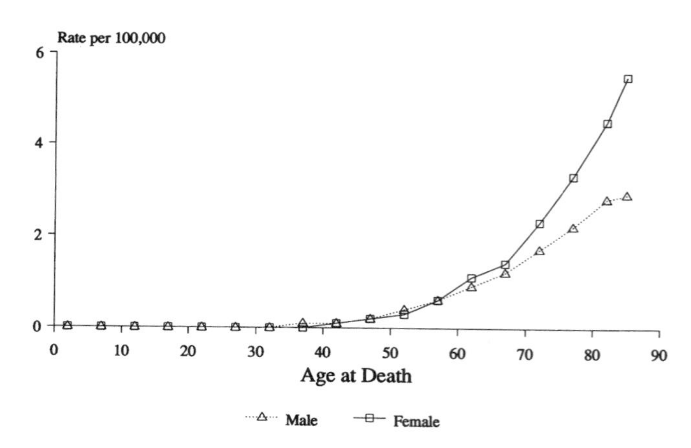

FIG. 46–3. Age-specific United States thyroid cancer mortality, 1982–1986. Data from National Cancer Institute, 1989.

Neither social class nor education appear to be important risk factors for thyroid cancer (Franceschi et al, 1989; Kolonel et al, 1990; McTiernan et al, 1984b; Ron et al, 1987a; Vågerö and Persson, 1986), although the incidence of thyroid cancer was elevated among persons with high socioeconomic occupations in Los Angeles (Preston-Martin and Menck, 1979) and was lower among male blue collar workers than other men in Sweden (Carstensen et al, 1990). In Switzerland, thyroid cancer cases occurred among better educated persons and more often among those who belonged to a higher socioeconomic class than controls (Levi et al, 1991). Persons of higher socioeconomic status may consult doctors more frequently than other individuals, which may lead to a detection bias. In contrast, elderly Hispanics in Florida have significantly higher thyroid cancer incidence rates than non-Hispanics (Trapido et al, 1990); in Hawaii, Filipinos and Hawaiians, who have the lowest socioeconomic levels, have particularly high rates of thyroid cancer (Goodman et al, 1988); and a strong negative correlation between social class and thyroid cancer mortality was noted in Switzerland (Levi et al, 1988).

Thyroid cancer incidence rates are extremely high in Hawaii, and Hawaiian residents often have rates greater than members of the same ethnic group living elsewhere. For example, Chinese women resident in Hawaii have an incidence rate of 12.1/100,000 as compared to 9.6, 5.3, and 3.7/100,000 for those living in San Francisco, Los Angeles, and Singapore, respectively (Goodman et al, 1988). The substantially elevated rates of thyroid cancer among Filipinos living outside of their country are striking. Filipino women living in Hawaii, San Francisco, and Los Angeles have incidence rates between two and four times that of women in Rizal, Philippines (Muir et al, 1987). Thyroid cancer incidence is also elevated in several other Pacific Island populations. Samoa is one of the few South Pacific Islands that does

TABLE 46–3. *Age-Standardized Incidence of Thyroid Cancer in Selected U.S. Areas by Race and Sex, 1983–1987**

Area	White		Black		White:Black Ratio	
	Female	Male	Female	Male	Female	Male
Atlanta, Georgia	5.4	2.0	2.4	0.7[a]	2.2	2.9
Alameda, California	5.1	2.5	2.7	1.2[a]	1.9	2.1
Bay Area, California	5.6	2.6	3.3	0.9	1.7	2.9
Detroit, Michigan	6.7	2.9	3.5	1.4	1.9	2.1
Los Angeles, California	5.9	2.3	3.2	1.2	1.8	1.9
New Orleans, Louisiana	5.4	2.2	3.9	1.6	1.4	1.4

*Annual rate per 100,000 population standardized to the World Standard Population. Data from Parkin et al, 1992.
[a]Based on <10 cases.

not have a high frequency of thyroid cancer (Henderson et al, 1985; Paksoy et al, 1990; Paksoy et al, 1991).

The hypothesis that Jews are more susceptible to both naturally occurring (Bross et al, 1971) and radiation-associated (Hempelmann et al, 1975; Shore et al, 1985; 1993) thyroid cancer has prompted other investigators to examine religion as a risk factor. The majority of studies did not indicate a significantly increased risk among Jews as compared to that among Catholic or Protestant subjects (Greenwald et al, 1975; McTiernan et al, 1984b; Pottern et al, 1990; Ron et al, 1987a). But an elevated incidence of thyroid cancer among Jews was observed in Los Angeles (Preston-Martin and Menck, 1979) and Jews in Israel have a high incidence of thyroid cancer (Table 46–2). Non-Jewish Israelis have only one-half the incidence of Israeli Jews, but this difference may be due to poor case ascertainment in the non-Jewish population.

ENVIRONMENTAL FACTORS

Radiation

Between 1920 and 1960, radiotherapy was widely used to treat benign conditions, such as tinea capitis, thymic enlargement, cervical lymphadenopathy, tonsillar hypertrophy, and skin disorders. Studies of these populations (Albert et al, 1968; DeGroot and Paloyan, 1973; Favus et al, 1976; Fürst et al, 1988; Hempelmann et al, 1975; Janower and Miettinen, 1971; Lundell et al, 1994; Maxon et al, 1980; Modan et al, 1974; Pottern et al, 1990; Ron et al, 1989; Schneider et al, 1985, 1986, 1993; Shore et al, 1976, 1985, 1986), as well as of patients treated for a first primary cancer (Boice et al, 1988; de Vathaire et al, 1988; Hancock et al, 1991; Hawkins and Kingston, 1988; Tucker et al, 1988, 1991), and of survivors of the atomic bombings in Hiroshima and Nagasaki (Ezaki et al, 1986; Nagataki et al, 1994; Prentice et al, 1982; Thompson et al, 1994; Wakabayashi et al, 1983) have contributed much to what is known about radiation-induced thyroid cancer. Although the studies employed different methodologies and included populations from many countries who were exposed to a large range of doses, all have demonstrated significantly increased risks of thyroid carcinomas following radiation exposure during childhood. In contrast, external exposure during adulthood (Thompson et al, 1994) and internal exposure to therapeutic or diagnostic doses of ^{131}I (Dobyns et al, 1974; Hall et al, 1992; Holm et al, 1988; Glöbel et al, 1984) have not been linked convincingly to thyroid cancer.

Acute External Exposures. Based on a small case series, an association between radiation and thyroid cancer was first suggested by Duffy and Fitzgerald in 1950. Soon after, Clark (1955) found that all of a series of 15 children with thyroid cancer had previous irradiation to their head or chest. In 1970 Winship and Rosvoll (1970) summarized the literature on childhood thyroid cancer and found that over 70% of the patients had a history of radiation exposure. The first comprehensive study of this subject was started in the 1950s by Hempelmann and colleagues (Hempelmann et al, 1975; Shore et al, 1985). Since then, numerous epidemiologic studies have been conducted and the thyroid gland has been shown to be as highly sensitive to the carcinogenic effects of acute, external low-LET (linear energy transfer) ionizing radiation as the female breast (Committee on the Biological Effects of Ionizing Radiation [BEIR], 1990; Shore, 1992; United Nations Scientific Committee on the Effects of Atomic Radiation [UNSCEAR], 1994). It has been suggested that the extreme radiosensitivity of the thyroid is related to its superficial site, its high degree of oxygenation, and the high rate of cell division (Barnes, 1988).

More recently, a pooled analysis of seven studies of external radiation was undertaken to better quantify the risk and to evaluate modifying influences on risk (Ron et al, 1995). Only the following published studies with estimated individual thyroid doses were included in the analysis: atomic bomb survivors (Thompson et al, 1994); infants irradiated for an enlarged thymus gland (Shore et al, 1985); children irradiated for tinea capitis in Israel (Ron et al, 1989); children treated with radiation for benign head and neck conditions, mostly enlarged tonsils, in Chicago (Schneider et al, 1993) and in Boston (Pottern et al, 1990); women irradiated for cervical cancer (Boice et al, 1988); and childhood cancer patients (Tucker et al, 1991) (Table 46–4). Approximately 700 thyroid cancers occurred among almost 120,000 persons. A significant dose–response was observed in each study of childhood exposure, and even at doses as low as 0.10 gray (Gy), the dose–response relationship was consistent with linearity. At doses as high as > 10 Gy, risk appeared to level off. Individual excess relative risks (ERR) per Gy ranged from 1.1 (95% confidence interval [CI] = 0.4, 29.4) following high-dose radiotherapy for childhood cancer, to 32 (95% CI = 14.0, 57.1) following relatively low-dose treatment for tinea capitis.

When data for childhood exposure from the five cohort studies were combined, the pooled ERR/Gy was 7.7 (95% CI = 2.1, 28.7). Although the ERR estimates for the individual cohorts differed ($P < 0.001$), none of the studies had a statistically significant influence on the pooled risk estimate. Persons exposed as young children (<5 years) had an ERR of more than twice as high as that of children exposed between 5 and 15 years of age. The pooled ERR/Gy was twice as high for women as for men (P = 0.07), but the results from the individual studies were not consistent. The ERR was highest at 15–29 years after exposure, but continued to be elevated at 40 or more years. Based on limited data, there was some suggestion that risk may be reduced somewhat when exposure is fractionated. For childhood exposure the pooled excess absolute risk was 4.4 per 10^4 person-year (PY) Gy (95% CI = 1.9, 10.1) and the attributable risk per Gy was 88%. In contrast, based on data from two studies, the ERR/Gy was not significantly elevated following adult exposure (Fig. 46–4). These findings are

TABLE 46–4. *Summary of Studies Used in Pooled Analysis of External Radiation Exposure and Thyroid Cancer*

Study and Location	*Reference*	*Study Population Number (Person-Years)*[a]		*No. of Thyroid Cancers*		*Mean Dose (Gy)*	*ERR/Gy (95% CI)*	*EAR/10^4PY-Gy (95% CI)*
COHORT STUDIES		EXPOSED	NON-EXPOSED	EXPOSED	NON-EXPOSED			
Atomic bomb survivors Hiroshima and Nagasaki, Japan	Thompson et al (1994)	41,234[b] (859,475)[b]	38,738[b] (817,556)[b]	132	93	0.27	4.7 (1.7, 10.9)[c] 0.4 (−0.1, 1.2)[c]	2.7 (1.2, 4.6)[c] 0.4 (−0.1, 1.4)[c]
Enlarged thymus gland Rochester, New York	Shore et al (1985)	2,475 (87,556)	4,991 (176,133)	38	5	1.36	9.1 (3.6, 28.8)	2.6 (1.7, 3.6)
Tinea capitis Israel	Ron et al (1989)	10,834 (328,092)	16,226 (493,080)	44	16	0.09	32 (14.0, 57.1)	7.6 (2.7, 13.0)
Enlarged tonsils (MRH)[d] Chicago, Illinois	Schneider et al (1993)	2,634 (88,100)	0 0	309	0	0.59	2.5 (0.6, 26.0)	3.0 (0.5, 17.1)[e]
Enlarged tonsils (CHMC)[d] Boston, Massachusetts	Pottern et al (1990)	1,192 (34,527)	1,063 (31,474)	10	0	0.24	—[f]	—[f]
CASE-CONTROL STUDIES		CASES	CONTROLS	% EXPOSED[g]	% NON-EXPOSED[g]			
Cervical cancer International	Boice et al (1988)	43	81	88.4	84.0	0.11	35 (−2.2, infinity)	
Childhood cancer International	Tucker et al (1991)	22	82	86.4	51.2	12.5	1.1 (0.4, 29.4)	

[a]Persons included in the present analysis (excludes people without follow-up or thyroid dose estimates).
[b]Exposed defined as ≥ 0.01 Sv to the thyroid, non-exposed defined as < 0.01 Sv; person-years take migration adjustment into account.
[c]ERR/Gy for persons exposed < 15 yrs (top line), and exposed ≥ 15 years (bottom line).
[d]MRH = Michael Reese Hospital; CHMC = Children's Hospital Medical Center.
[e]This is the average EAR, however, the EAR/10^4PY-Gy was 2.4 (95% CI = undetermined, 10.4) for follow-up until 1974 and 45 (95% CI = −3.2, 89.0) for follow-up after 1974. The EAR/10^4PY-Gy estimates in this study are subject to large variability because of the influence of extreme dose points. These points, however, appeared to have little influence on the ERR/Gy.
[f]Can't be estimated because there were no comparison subjects with thyroid cancer.
[g]Exposed defined as ≥ 0.05 Gy for cervical cancer study and ≥ 2.0 Gy for childhood cancer study.

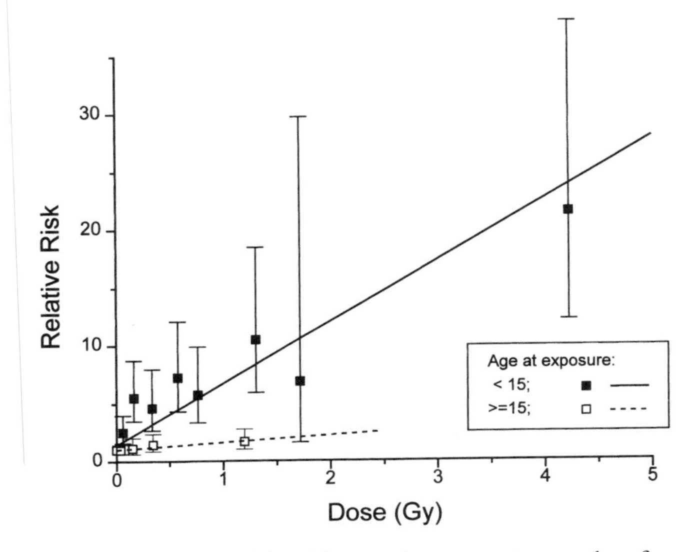

FIG. 46–4. Pooled fitted thyroid cancer dose–response curves from five cohort studies of childhood exposure (<15 years) and two studies of adult exposure (≥15 years). Adapted from Ron et al, 1995.

consistent with recently published summaries of the literature (Shore, 1992; UNSCEAR, 1994).

The clinical course of radiation-associated cancers is similar to spontaneous cancers, even though radiation-induced tumors are more often bilateral (Samaan et al, 1987; Schneider et al, 1985, 1986; Turrin et al, 1985), and an excess of multiple tumors was noted (Schneider et al, 1985, 1986). Well-differentiated papillary adenocarcinoma is the principal cell type induced by radiation, but there may be an increase in follicular and anaplastic carcinoma as exposed persons reach the natural ages to develop these histologic types (DeGroot et al, 1983; Ron et al, 1989, 1995; Samaan et al, 1987; Schneider et al, 1985, 1993).

Protracted Exposures

Medical. The widespread medical use of ^{131}I, the 1986 Chernobyl nuclear reactor accident, and the reported Hanford nuclear facility releases of large quantities of ^{131}I have focused attention on radioactive iodides. In animals, high-dose experiments have indicated that ^{131}I is much less effective than X rays in the induction of thyroid tumors (National Council on Radiation Protection and Measurement [NCRP], 1985). However, a large study of 3,000 female rats has suggested that at doses of about 300–400 centigray (cGy), the risks from external X rays and ^{131}I may be roughly equal (Lee et al, 1982). This study has highlighted the need to explore this topic further. Human studies comparing ^{131}I to external gamma or X-ray exposure have been limited and the results equivocal. In the older literature, ^{131}I was estimated to be from one-fifteenth to one-half as effective at inducing thyroid cancer as external X radiation (NCRP, 1985). It was thought that the difference in the carcinogenic effects of the two types of radiation was due to the lower dose rate of ^{131}I. The 7-day half-life of ^{131}I allows time for repair of radiation damage.

There have been numerous case reports of thyroid cancer occurring subsequent to ^{131}I treatment for hyperthyroidism (Adamson and Gardham, 1991; Araki and Oshiro, 1970; Gossage et al, 1984; Kogut et al, 1965; McDougall et al, 1971; Ozaki, 1994; Pilch et al, 1973; Sheline et al, 1962). Epidemiologic studies, however, have largely been negative (Dobyns et al, 1974; Glöbel et al, 1984; Hall et al, 1992; Hoffman et al, 1982; Holm et al, 1991; Safa et al, 1975). Dobyns et al (1974) studied about 35,000 hyperthyroid patients treated between 1946 and 1964. When follow-up ended in 1968, they reported no significant excess of thyroid cancer among the ^{131}I treated patients. These data, however, have also been interpreted as showing an increased incidence of anaplastic cancer, possibly as a result of progression from undetected differentiated thyroid cancer (Williams, 1986). Case reports of adults treated with ^{131}I and who have developed anaplastic carcinoma have been published (Gossage et al, 1984; Shimaoka et al, 1979). Approximately 10,000 hyperthyroid patients treated with a mean dose of >10,000 cGy were followed in Sweden for an average of 15 years. When compared to age, sex, region, and calendar-year–specific incidence rates for Sweden, the risk of thyroid cancer was not significantly elevated 10 or more years after treatment (Holm et al, 1991; Hall et al, 1992). Because these studies were composed of persons with underlying thyroid disease, did not include childhood exposure, and had fairly short follow-up periods, their results can not be considered definitive. However, they provide little evidence that radio-iodine therapy is an important cause of thyroid carcinoma.

Thus far, the risks of thyroid cancer following diagnostic doses of ^{131}I have not been studied extensively, although it is this low-dose range which is most important from a public health standpoint. Holm et al (1988) studied over 35,000 Swedish patients (approximately 2,000 patients were under age 20) examined with ^{131}I for suspected thyroid disorders between 1951 and 1969, and followed them through 1984. The mean radiation dose to the thyroid was approximately 50 cGy, yet no significant excess risk of thyroid cancer was demonstrated. Glöbel et al (1984) also found no excess risk of thyroid cancer among approximately 14,000 Germans receiving ^{131}I uptake examinations. In a preliminary study of 3,500 children receiving diagnostic ^{131}I exams (median dose 35 cGy; range, 10–2000 cGy) and 2,600 controls, the risk of thyroid cancer was not significantly elevated based on 5 observed thyroid cancers (Hamilton et al, 1989).

The data on both therapeutic and diagnostic ^{131}I exposure suggest that in humans ^{131}I has less of a carcinogenic effect than external X rays. However, the fact that most persons exposed to ^{131}I were adults with thyroid disease, whereas the majority of persons exposed to X rays were children with normal thyroids, complicates the comparison. In a statistical evaluation of one epidemiologic study of persons exposed to diagnostic ^{131}I, one experimental study of rats exposed to ^{131}I, and six epidemiologic studies of humans exposed to external radiation, the risk associated with ^{131}I was approximately 66% of the risk from external radiation, but the confidence interval was large (Laird, 1987). Clearly, more data from populations, particularly children, exposed to a range of doses of ^{131}I, are needed.

Accidental nuclear releases. During the 1950s and 60s, the U.S. conducted a large number of above-ground nuclear weapons tests. In a clinical study of 1,378 children in Utah exposed to a mean dose of about 120 cGy of ^{131}I from fallout during weapons testing and 3,801 non-exposed children from neighboring counties, no evidence of ^{131}I-induced thyroid carcinomas was found (BEIR, 1980; Rallison et al, 1975). A more recent follow-up of approximately 75% of this cohort has been completed (Kerber et al, 1993). Comprehensive dose reconstruction was performed and thyroid doses were estimated to range from 0 to 4.6 Gy. Based on 19 cases, a significant excess for all thyroid neoplasms combined was observed, but the dose–response for only the 8 malignant tumors did not reach significance. Zieghami and Morris (1986) compared the incidence of thyroid cancer in Utah to the incidence in other western states and in the entire United States. They reported an excess of thyroid cancer in Utah compared to the entire United States, but not compared to the other western states.

In 1954 one of the nuclear tests in the Pacific Ocean accidentally exposed people living in the Marshall Islands to large doses of both short- and long-lived radioisotopes and gamma radiation (Conard, 1984; Hamilton et al, 1987; Robbins and Adams, 1989). The Marshall Islanders have exhibited an excess of thyroid carcinoma and other thyroid abnormalities following radiation doses to the thyroid of 700 to 1400 cGy for young children and approximately 2000 cGy for infants. The cancer risk was calculated to be 1.5 per 10^6 PY-cGy (Robbins and Adams, 1989). This estimate is similar to the A-bomb absolute risk estimate, but because 80–90% of the dose absorbed by the thyroid was from the short-lived radioisotopes, this study does not provide much information on the risks from ^{131}I.

Following the Chernobyl reactor accident, radioactive nuclides were released into the atmosphere, resulting in millions of people being exposed to substantial internal and external radiation to the thyroid in the most contaminated areas of the former Soviet Union (Likhtarev et al, 1994; UNSCEAR, 1988). When the thyroid glands of 1,060 children living in Belarus, the Ukraine, or Russia were examined in 1990 by palpation and ultrasonography, there was no difference in the prevalence of thyroid nodules between the group residing in contaminated areas and non-contaminated areas (Mettler et al, 1992). Over the last few years, however, the incidence of childhood thyroid cancer, particularly papillary carcinoma, has increased dramatically in Belarus and the Ukraine (Abelin et al, 1994; Commission of the European Communities [CEC], 1993; Kazakov et al, 1992; Prisyazhiuk et al, 1991). While better reporting and screening might be partly responsible for the large number of thyroid cancers ascertained (Ron et al, 1992), more than 50% of the cases diagnosed in one group of patients were not detected as a result of screening (CEC, 1993). Although the increased incidence appears to be related to the Chernobyl accident, a causal association between the ^{131}I exposure and thyroid cancer has not been established. It may never be possible to conclusively establish whether ^{131}I, other radiation, or other consequences of the Chernobyl accident are related to the excess childhood thyroid cancer, but it is clearly important to carefully monitor the long-term risks of thyroid cancer associated with Chernobyl. Molecular studies may be helpful in identifying the causative agent.

The carcinogenic potential of continuous low-dose radionuclide exposure has been studied among persons living near nuclear plants and waste sites. One thyroid cancer was observed among 200 screened women living close to a uranium waste site in Pennsylvania which had gamma radiation levels two times higher than background levels. No thyroid cancers were detected among 150 similarly screened women living 5 miles away (Radford et al, 1983). In another study, levels of ^{129}I activity increased with proximity to the Sellafield fuel reprocessing plant in England ($P < 0.001$), yet thyroid cancer incidence increased with greater distance from Sellafield ($P = 0.0007$) (Bowlt and Tiplady, 1989). Additional information about low-dose, highly fractionated exposures of ^{131}I is expected from an investigation currently underway of people living in the vicinity of the Hanford nuclear facility in Washington State (Cate et al, 1990).

Background Radiation. Studies of residents in areas of high natural background radiation have generally been negative, partly because of their low statistical power. Close to 13,000 people living in the high background area of Kerala, India and about 6,000 people living in a comparable village with normal radiation levels were examined (Pillaj et al, 1976). No thyroid cancers were detected in either group.

In China 1,000 women, aged 45–64 and living in a region of elevated background radiation were compared to an equal number of women living in an area of normal radiation levels (Wang et al, 1990b). The mean cumulative thyroid dose for the high and normal background groups was 14 cGy and 5 cGy, respectively. No excess of malignant thyroid neoplasia was found, even though all women were intensively examined.

Occupational exposures. Low-dose fractionated occupational exposures are most relevant for setting radiation exposure standards. Unfortunately, data from studies of workers have yielded little information in regard to thyroid cancer for a number of reasons: the rarity of the disease; the predominance of male workers studied; and the reliance on mortality data which are of limited value in terms of thyroid cancer. Given these limitations, the majority of studies did not find a statistically significant relation between occupational exposure and thyroid cancer (Matanoski et al, 1984), but recent studies have reported some positive associations.

Among 686 female radium dial workers employed before 1930, 2 thyroid cancers developed, yielding a significant excess absolute risk (excess cases per 10^6 person-rem = 46; 95% Cl = 19, 101) (Polednak, 1986). Kendall et al (1992) examined cancer mortality in over 95,000 United Kingdom radiation workers. This study combined and updated previous British radiation worker studies. Thyroid cancer mortality (n = 9) was significantly elevated, but no dose–response was observed based on recorded external radiation doses. The small number of thyroid cancer cases makes it difficult to draw inferences from these studies.

In a study of 27,000 X-ray workers and 26,000 other medical specialists in China, 8 thyroid cancers were observed compared to 4.5 expected (RR = 1.7; 95% Cl = 0.6–4.7). Risk was most pronounced among employees who worked before 1960 when exposures were highest, and decreased with increasing age at first exposure (Wang et al, 1990a). Consistent with these data is the preliminary finding of 220 thyroid cancers observed among over 100,000 American radiologic technicians compared to 100 expected, based on Connecticut incidence rates (Boice et al, 1992). Similarly, in a hypothesis generating record-linkage study, a significant twofold risk of thyroid cancer was seen among Swedish X-ray operators and laboratory assistants as compared to the general population of Sweden (Carstensen et al, 1990). Since individual doses were not available in any of these studies, the level of cancer ascertainment was uncertain in some cases, risk estimates were not always significant, and multiple comparisons were made, these results should be interpreted with caution.

Iodine and Endemic Goiter

Iodine is essential in the regulation of thyroid hormones. In animals iodine deficiency has been shown to act as both a carcinogen and as a tumor promoter by inhibiting excess thyroid-stimulating hormone (TSH) secretion (Isler, 1959; Ohshima and Ward, 1986; Ward and Ohshima, 1986). In humans the role of iodine is not so clear. In 1928 Wegelin reported that the prevalence of thyroid cancer at autopsy was ten times higher in Bern, an endemic goiter area, than in Berlin, a non-endemic goiter area. Since then, endemic goiter and/or iodine deficiency have been considered possible risk factors for thyroid cancer. This hypothesis is supported by the finding of a decline in thyroid cancer mortality in Switzerland after iodine supplementation (Wynder, 1952). Furthermore, thyroid cancer mortality rates in the endemic goiter belt of northern Italy are two times higher than the national average (Franceschi et al, 1989). On the other hand, in the United States, no decrease in thyroid cancer mortality or incidence was observed after the introduction of iodized salt (Pendergrast et al, 1961). Moreover, in the Nordic countries, thyroid cancer rates are not correlated with the occurrence of endemic goiters (Franssila et al, 1981; Saxen and Saxen, 1954).

These contradictory findings may stem from differences in histology. Endemic goiter areas seem to be associated with an elevated risk of follicular and, perhaps, anaplastic thyroid cancer (Belfiore et al, 1987; Correa et al, 1969; Doniach, 1969; McGill, 1978; Wahner et al, 1966; Williams et al, 1977), whereas iodine-rich areas have been associated with an enhanced risk of papillary carcinoma (Doniach, 1971; Williams et al, 1977). Thus a change in iodine intake may increase the frequency of one cell type while decreasing the frequency of the other, resulting in no net change in incidence.

Diet

Until recently, diet has seldom been studied in relation to thyroid cancer, although dietary iodine (Williams et al, 1977), goitrogens (Hempelmann and Furth, 1978), calcium and vitamin D (Williams, 1979), and alcohol (Breslow and Enstrom, 1974; Williams, 1976) have been proposed as possible risk factors. During the last decade several epidemiologic studies collected data regarding diet. Since these studies will be referred to frequently in this and subsequent sections of this chapter, they are briefly summarized in Table 46–5.

In the Connecticut and Southeastern Sweden studies (Ron et al, 1987a; Wingren et al, 1993), approximately ten food items were included in the questionnaire. A non-significant inverse association between thyroid cancer and the consumption of cruciferous vegetables was noted. In the Connecticut study, there was also a slight indication of a positive association with fish and vitamin D intake. The Italian study (Franceschi et al, 1989, 1990b) included 31 food items and revealed a significantly decreased risk associated with high consumption

TABLE 46–5. *Brief Description of Thyroid Cancer Case–Control Studies*

Study Location and References	Years of Diagnosis	Cases		Controls		Summarized Results
		Females	Males	Females	Males	
Northern Italy Franceschi et al (1989, 1990a, 1990b, 1991)	1985–89	219	80	343	138	Protective effect of vegetables and fish, possibly fruit; positive association with first and last birth, menstrual irregularity, and history of benign thyroid disease.
Vaud, Switzerland Levi et al (1991, 1993)	1987–94	100	23	318	91	Weak association with parity and miscarriage; strong association with artificial menopause and history of benign thyroid disease.
Norway Glattre et al (1989, 1993)	1955–89	71	21	355	105	Protective effect of serum selenium.
Southeastern Sweden Wingren et al (1993)	1977–87	93	11	187	200	Weak protective effect of cruciferous vegetables; weak association with parity; significant association with family history of goiter.
Northern Sweden Hallquist et al (1994)	1980–89	123	48	240	85	Weak association with parity; protective effect of smoking.
Shanghai, China Preston-Martin et al (1993)	1981–84	207	0	207	0	Positive association with seafood; weak association with parity; strong association with miscarriage, benign thyroid disease, and family history of thyroid disease.
Hawaii, USA Kolonel et al (1990)	1980–87	140	51	328	113	Detailed dietary history showed protective effect of goitrogenic vegetables and increased risk with seafood intake; no association with parity, but association with miscarriage and fertility drugs.
Los Angeles, CA, USA Preston-Martin et al (1987)	1980–83	293	0	293	0	Association with parity, miscarriage, and history of benign thyroid disease.
Connecticut, USA Ron et al (1987a)	1978–80	109	50	209	76	Weak inverse association with cruciferous vegetables; positive association with fish and vitamin D, parity, miscarriage, and history of benign thyroid disease.
Washington, USA McTiernan et al (1984a, 1984b, 1987)	1974–79	183	0	394	0	Association with estrogen-containing drugs, history of benign thyroid disease, and breast cancer.

of carrots and green vegetables, fruit, ham and fish, and an increased risk with bread, polenta, potatoes, poultry, salami, cheese and butter. The results of the Italian study were pooled with those from a study conducted in Switzerland (Franceschi et al, 1991), but since the Italian study contributed 80% of the cases, the findings tended to mirror those noted in the Italian study. An additional analysis of a subset of the Italian data was also conducted and a strong protective effect of vegetable consumption was observed, but no association with fruit was reported (Negri et al, 1991). The questionnaire used in Hawaii contained a detailed quantitative dietary history (Kolonel et al, 1990). Consistent with the Connecticut study, a higher intake of seafood and lower intake of goitrogenic vegetables was associated with thyroid cancer among females. Cases also consumed more harm ha (a pigmented fish paste commonly eaten by Asians) which may contain nitrosamines.

The finding of a reduced risk associated with vegetable intake was common to all studies, while the results regarding fish intake were inconsistent. Data from a small prospective study in Norway (Glattre et al, 1993) and a case–control study in Shanghai (Preston-Martin et al, 1993) support a positive association between seafood and thyroid cancer. Since northern Italy is an endemic goiter area, whereas Hawaii and Connecticut are not, it is possible that the increased iodine associated with seafood intake would reduce the risk of thyroid cancer in Italy but would be unimportant in the United States.

Vegetable consumption has been reported to have a protective effect on a wide range of tumors (Negri et al, 1991). Several of the vegetables studied, however, were from the cruciferous family which contains thioglucosides that may be degraded to form goitrogens. In laboratory animals, goitrogens can promote thyroid cancer by causing the pituitary gland to increase TSH secretion. On the other hand, cruciferous vegetables also contain indole components, isothiocyanates, and phenols that may inhibit the development of certain cancers by blocking the activation of hydrocarbons and perhaps other agents (National Academy of Sciences [NAS], 1983). Furthermore, diets rich in vitamin A have been associated with reduced risks of cancers of the oral cavity, larynx, esophagus, large intestine, and lung (Metlin, 1986; Peto et al, 1981). This antitumor effect may also extend to the thyroid gland. In China a lower risk of thyroid nodules was associated with high intake of allium vegetables such as garlic and onions (Wang et al, 1990b).

In the Connecticut study (Ron et al, 1987a), the use

of vitamin D but not calcium supplements was significantly linked with medullary carcinoma, a tumor of the calcitonin-secreting C cells. Although C-cell production of calcitonin is influenced by serum calcium levels, studies of laboratory animals have shown that dietary calcium does not increase the incidence of medullary-like tumors, whereas vitamin D increases both calcitonin production and a precursor lesion called C-cell hyperplasia (Williams et al, 1977; Williams, 1979).

Glattre et al (1989) studied 43 thyroid cancer cases and 129 controls selected from a large Norwegian prospective study. Serum selenium was significantly higher among the controls, but this effect was limited to 7 years before diagnosis. Dietary information was available for 29 cases and 87 controls, but intake of the major dietary sources of selenium did not differ in the two groups.

A correlation between U.S. thyroid cancer mortality and alcohol consumption was reported by Breslow and Enstrom (1974). In addition, an analysis of interview data from the Third National Cancer Survey revealed a positive association between thyroid cancer and wine, beer, and hard liquor (Cutler and Young, 1975). Williams (1976) suggested that alcohol could promote thyroid cancer by inducing TSH secretion. While Ron et al (1987a) could not confirm this hypothesis, Franceschi et al (1989) reported a significant association with regular use of hard liquor (RR = 1.8; 95% Cl 1.0–3.2) and an association of borderline significance with wine consumption (RR = 1.4; 95% Cl 0.9–2.2).

In a Greek study of 61 thyroid cancer cases and an equal number of controls, controls drank significantly more coffee than cases (Linos et al, 1989). There also was some evidence of a protective effect of coffee from the pooled Italian and Swiss analysis (Franceschi et al, 1991).

Volcanic Activity

In a correlation study of thyroid cancer incidence and ecologic factors, Kung et al (1981) noted that Hawaii and Iceland, the two regions with strikingly high thyroid cancer incidence, both have frequently erupting volcanoes that produce hugh quantities of basaltic lava. However, Arnbjörnsson et al (1986) were unable to relate the incidence of thyroid cancer to 13 major volcanic eruptions occurring in Iceland during the past 80 years.

Prescription Drugs

Epidemiologic surveys of prescription drug use have reported statistically significant associations between thyroid cancer and pentobarbital (barbiturate), meclizine (antihistamine used for motion sickness), diphenoxylate (antidiarrheal), dicyclomine (antispasmodic used for gastrointestinal disorders), griseofulvin (antifungal antibiotic), bisacodyl (cathartic), and senna (cathartic) (Friedman and Ury, 1980, 1983; Selby et al, 1989). These associations have not been confirmed in analytic studies (Kolonel et al, 1990; Olsen et al, 1989; Ron et al, 1987a), but use of spironolactone conveyed a fourfold risk of borderline significance in one study (Ron et al, 1987a).

HOST FACTORS

Hormonal and Reproductive Factors

In humans elevated levels of TSH are associated with thyroid growth and are thought to increase the risk of thyroid carcinoma (Henderson et al, 1982; Williams, 1990). In rodents increased TSH secretion induces thyroid tumors (Hempelmann and Furth, 1978; Williams, 1979). Several possible mechanisms in which TSH interacts with other risk factors have been considered. Elevated TSH secretion occurs during puberty, pregnancy, and delivery, as well as while using oral contraceptives (Chan et al, 1975; Malkesian and Mayberry, 1970; Pacchiarotti et al, 1986; Rastogi et al, 1974; Weeke and Hanson, 1975); and partial thyroidectomy for benign thyroid disease (Němec et al, 1980), goitrogen intake (Paynter et al, 1988), and radiation to the neck (Williams, 1990) may raise TSH levels.

The role of hormonal factors in female thyroid cancer has been suspected on the basis of the high female-to-male incidence ratio, the better survival of women, the possible association of thyroid and breast cancers (Ron et al, 1984), and the presence of estrogen receptors in differentiated thyroid cancers (Chaudhuri and Prinz, 1989). In women the peak occurrence of thyroid cancer is during the reproductive years. Thus it is of note that the thyroid gland becomes enlarged during puberty and pregnancy and may change in size and activity during the menstrual cycle (Robbins et al, 1984). Estrogen receptor immunoreactivity has also been positively correlated with the degree of differentiation in thyroid cancer (Takeichi et al, 1991). In male rats castration reduces the incidence of thyroid cancer (Paloyan et al, 1982), while testosterone promotes radiation-induced thyroid tumors by increasing TSH levels (Hofmann et al, 1986).

Most of the data currently available (Franceschi et al, 1990a; Galanti et al, 1995; Hallquist et al, 1994; Kravdal et al, 1991; Levi et al, 1993; Miller et al, 1980; McTiernan et al, 1984b; Ron et al, 1987a; Preston-Martin et al, 1987; Preston-Martin et al, 1993; Wingren et al, 1993) but not all available data (Akslen et al, 1992; Kolonel et al, 1990), provide some evidence that women with thyroid cancer have had more pregnancies and/or live births than controls (Table 46–5). In a prospective study of 1.1 million Norwegian women of reproductive age, the risk of thyroid cancer increased from 1.0 for nulliparous women to 1.13, 1.30, 1.39, and 1.46 for women with 1, 2, 3, and 4+ children, respectively. In several studies (Kolonel et al, 1990; Levi et al, 1993; Ron et al, 1987a; Preston-Martin et al, 1987; Preston-Martin et al, 1993), women who had a history of a miscarriage were at increased risk of thyroid cancer, which might suggest that changes which occur early in pregnancy are important. A suggestion of an elevated risk of thyroid cancer among two cohorts of infertile women has been reported (Brinton et al, 1989; Ron et al, 1987b), and in one case–control study, cases used fertility drugs significantly more often than controls (Kolonel et al, 1990). If the infertility was due to habitual abortion, then these data would be consistent with studies implicating miscarriage in thyroid cancer. During pregnancy the ratio of malignant to benign thyroid tumors is higher than at other times in a woman's life (Rosen and Walfish, 1986).

Artificial menopause (Levi et al, 1993) and use of oral contraceptives (McTiernan et al, 1984b; Preston-Martin et al, 1987; Preston-Martin et al, 1993) have been associated with thyroid cancer in some studies. The association with oral contraceptives was strongest for recent use, which suggests promotion rather than initiation.

The current data suggest an influence of hormonal and reproductive events in the etiology of thyroid cancer. The studies conducted to date, however, were fairly small, and results were generally weak and not always consistent.

Predisposing Thyroid Disease

There is no simple way to describe the relationship between thyroid cancer and nonmalignant thyroid diseases. While there have been reports of positive associations between thyroid cancer and adenoma, simple or endemic goiter, multiple nodular goiter, thyrotoxicosis and Hashimoto's thyroiditis, there have also been a number of negative studies. The role of endemic goiter was discussed previously and will not be considered here.

The relationship between thyroid nodules and subsequent cancer is still not clear. A strong link between benign thyroid nodules or goiter and thyroid cancer has been demonstrated in numerous epidemiologic studies (Franceschi et al, 1989; Goldman et al, 1990; Kolonel et al, 1990; Levi et al, 1991; McTiernan et al, 1984a; Preston-Martin et al, 1987; Preston-Martin et al, 1993; Ron et al, 1987a; Wingren et al, 1993). In most case–control studies, the odds ratios associated with a history of benign thyroid nodules and goiter were about 10 and 5, respectively, and the association was found for both papillary and follicular carcinomas. In the population-based Connecticut study, 17% of the thyroid cancer cases could be attributed to previous thyroid nodules and 4% to goiter (Ron et al, 1987a). Although case–control studies are always subject to recall bias, the strength of the association, the consistency of the results over all studies, and the lack of an association with other thyroid diseases support the view that a history of thyroid adenoma, nodule, or goiter confers an enhanced risk of thyroid cancer. This association may reflect a true causal relation, a precursor lesion, an effect of treatment, similar risk factors exerting independent effects, close medical surveillance, or misdiagnosis of the earlier disease. Experimentally, a transition from adenoma to carcinoma has been shown (Meissner and Warren, 1969), and more recently, it has been suggested that genetic mutations are associated with thyroid tumor progression (Fagin 1994, Farid et al, 1994). Further genetic research is needed to better understand this process.

The role of thyrotoxicosis in the etiology of thyroid cancer is also uncertain. Over the last forty years, several studies have addressed this issue, but most have determined the frequency of thyroid carcinoma at the time of thyroidectomy. Furthermore, since most did not have a comparison group or calculate expected values, it is difficult to judge whether the occurrence of thyroid cancer exceeded expectation.

Autoimmune thyroiditis (Hashimoto's thyroiditis) is frequently accompanied by years of subclinical hypothyroidism with elevated TSH levels. Studies assessing the relationship between thyroid cancer and autoimmune thyroiditis have most often examined coexistent disease, thus complicating interpretation of the findings; however, a significant excess risk of thyroid lymphomas was reported in two prospective studies of thyroiditis patients (Aozosa, 1990; Holm et al, 1985). Although fewer in number, there have also been studies reporting no association between Hashimoto's thyroiditis and thyroid cancer (Crile and Hazard, 1962; Maceri et al, 1986).

Associated Neoplasms and Other Diseases

Several studies of multiple primaries have shown an excess of thyroid cancer among patients with breast cancer (Harvey and Brinton, 1985; Iwasa et al, 1986; Ron et al, 1984; Schenker et al, 1984; Schottenfeld and Berg, 1971; Teppo et al, 1985), as well as the inverse relationship, i.e., an excess of breast cancer among women with thyroid cancer (Chalstrey and Benjamin, 1966; Ron et al, 1984; Schoenberg, 1977; Shands and Gatling, 1970; Shimaoka et al, 1967; Tucker et al, 1985). These results, however, were not replicated in similar studies conducted in Denmark (Ewertz and Mouridsen, 1985; Østerlind et al, 1985) or in Sweden (Hall et al, 1990). A history of breast cancer was evaluated in several case–control studies, but a higher frequency among cases was found only in one study (McTiernan et al, 1987). Although thyroid and breast cancer do not share many of the same risk factors, extreme radiosensitivity is common to both cancer sites.

In addition, there are reports of thyroid cancer patients developing leukemia (Teppo et al, 1985), cancers of the kidney (Hall et al, 1990; Tucker et al, 1985), connective tissue (Tucker et al, 1985), brain and nervous system (Hall et al, 1990; Østerlind et al, 1985), and endocrine glands (Hall et al, 1990), as well as non-Hodgkin's lymphoma (Østerlind et al, 1985), more often than the general population. An increased frequency of thyroid cancer among patients with renal cancer (Teppo et al, 1985) and Hodgkin's disease (Greene and Wilson, 1985) has also been observed. But since the thyroid of the majority of the Hodgkin's patients received large doses of radiation, the association may be treatment related.

Hyperparathyroidism has been related to thyroid cancer (Al-Jurf et al, 1979; Kaplan et al, 1971; LiVolsi and Feind, 1976). The long-term exposure to hypercalcemia, acting as a goitrogen, has been proposed as the mechanism for this association. Alternatively, radiation exposure may induce both the hyperparathyroidism and thyroid cancer.

Associations between carcinoma of the thyroid and aplastic anemia (Neglia et al, 1986), acromegaly (Barzilay et al, 1991), and ataxia telangiectasia (Narita and Takagi, 1984; Ohta et al, 1986) have been reported. Previous tonsillectomy and allergy and skin disorders have also been suggested as possible thyroid cancer risk factors (Bross et al, 1971), but they have not been substantiated in other studies (Kolonel et al, 1990; Levi et al, 1991; Ron et al, 1987a).

Familial Aggregation and Heritable Conditions

Approximately 20% of all medullary thyroid carcinomas appear to be of the familial form (Block 1969; Block et al, 1967). Familial medullary thyroid carcinoma is inherited in an autosomal dominant pattern with penetrance of nearly 100%. It can occur alone or as part of a multiple endocrine neoplasia (MEN) syndrome, including medullary thyroid cancer and pheochromocytoma, in association with parathyroid adenoma or hyperplasia (MEN 2A), or mucosal neuromas (MEN 2B) (Schimke et al, 1968). Hereditary medullary thyroid cancer generally occurs at an earlier age than sporadic medullary cancer and the incidence of bilateral and multiple tumors is increased (Jackson et al, 1979). Papillary thyroid cancer is most often sporadic, but Nakamura et al (1987) suggested that a MEN syndrome might also predispose to papillary thyroid cancer.

Numerous case reports (Fischer et al, 1989; Flannigan et al, 1983; Lote et al, 1980; Němec et al, 1975; Ozaki et al, 1988; Szántó et al, 1990) and two larger studies (Stoffer et al, 1986; Ron et al, 1991) implicate genetic factors in the pathogenesis of papillary cancer. The extremely high incidence of papillary thyroid cancer in Iceland, which has a small isolated population, is consistent with a genetic influence.

Familial polyposis coli has been associated with papillary thyroid cancer. Although based on a small number of cases, excess risks of over 100 have been noted among female polyposis coli patients (Bülow et al, 1988; Plail et al, 1987). Thyroid cancers that developed in conjunction with polyposis coli tended to occur before age 35, were often multicentric, and occurred more frequently among women. Recently, mutations in the adenomatous polyposis coli (APC) gene were found also in sporadic papillary thyroid tumors (Fagin, 1994).

Growth Factors and Oncogenes

New developments in molecular biology indicate a role for growth factors, growth factor receptors, oncogenes, and tumor suppressor genes in the development of human thyroid carcinoma. Growth factors can stimulate or inhibit cell growth and can influence cell differentiation. Insulin growth factors (IGF), transforming growth factor beta (TGF-β), epidermal growth factor (EGF), interleukin-1 (IL-1), platelet-derived growth factor (PDGF) and fibroblast growth factor (FGF), alone or in conjunction with oncogenes, all may be involved in the regulation of thyroid cell growth. Studies of TSH in cultured thyroid cells have been contradictory and species specific. In human thyroid cells in culture, TSH has sometimes been identified as a growth factor. At this time, however, the function of growth factors in human thyroid carcinogenesis is still not well understood (Aaronson, 1991; Farid, 1994; Frauman and Moses, 1990; Melmed, 1988).

Mutations, abnormal expression, and amplification of oncogenes are associated with abnormal cell growth and the partial blockage of terminal differentiation, whereas inactivation of tumor suppressor genes can prevent necessary repair to genetically damaged cells. Several oncogenes have been studied in relation to thyroid cancer and specific patterns of oncogene expression appear to be associated with different histologic types of thyroid cancer.

Papillary carcinoma was first associated with a thyroid-specific transforming gene, the PTC/*ret* oncogene, but prevalence of this gene is only about 25% and varies geographically (Bongarzone et al, 1989; Donghi et al, 1989; Fagin, 1994; Fusco et al, 1987; Grieco et al, 1990). The PTC/*ret* oncogene appears to be an intrachromosomal rearranged form of the *ret* proto-oncogene (Grieco et al, 1990). PTC/*ret* is a member of the family of genes with tyrosine kinase-associated activity and has been localized to a region on chromosome 10, proximal to the region linked with MEN 2A (Donghi et al, 1989). Bongarzone et al (1989) reported a high frequency of mutational activation of *trk*, another tyrosine kinase oncogene, in papillary carcinoma. Recently, germline mutations of the *ret* proto-oncogene on chromosome 10 were found in individuals with MEN 2A, MEN 2B, and familial medullary thyroid cancer (Donis-Keller et al, 1993; Hofstra et al, 1994; Mulligan et al, 1993). In families with these syndromes, detection of specific germline mutations in the *ret* proto-oncogene allows early identification of gene carriers and is now being used to screen children (Lips et al, 1994). Performing thyroidectomy on gene carriers at a very early age has been recommended as a method to prevent medullary thyroid cancer (Utiger, 1994).

Activation of *ras* (H-*ras*, K-*ras*, and N-*ras*) oncogenes has been found in all stages of thyroid tumorigenesis (Lemoine et al 1988, 1989; Namba et al, 1990) which suggests that the *ras* oncogene plays a part during the early stage of tumor development. *Ras* mutations are found in up to 50% of thyroid tumors and appear to be most common in follicular carcinomas, although they also occur in papillary carcinomas (Karga et al, 1991; Lemoine et al, 1988, 1989; Suárez et al, 1990; Wright et al, 1989). In one study, the mutation rate of the *ras* oncogene in follicular tumors was substantially higher in an iodine-deficient area than an iodine-rich area, suggesting that iodine may influence oncogene activation (Shi et al, 1991). Another study indicated that radiation may interact with *ras* oncogene activation (Wright et al, 1991). Although the prevalence of *ras* activation was the same in human follicular carcinomas that occurred spontaneously and those which were radiation induced, the type of *ras* oncogene activated differed. As in rodents, K-*ras* was activated significantly more often in the radiation-induced tumors than in the spontaneous ones.

Del Senna and colleagues (1987) reported the c-*myc* oncogene to be modified in structure, dosage, and methylation in thyroid carcinomas and Terrier et al (1988) described an increased amount of c-*myc* and c-*fos*. They also found that c-*myc* occurred more frequently in thyroid cancers with poor prognosis. On the other hand, failure to find amplification or rearrangement of c-*myc* was reported by Wyllie et al (1989) and Aasland et al (1988). Boultwood et al (1988) found increased N-*myc* expression in thyroid tumors derived from C cells which is consistent with reports of N-*myc* expression in other neuroendocrine tumors.

Inactivation of the *p53* tumor suppressor gene appears to be involved in thyroid carcinogenesis. Zou et al (1993) described *p53* mutations in differentiated thyroid cancer, while others have reported these mutations only in poorly or undifferentiated thyroid carcinomas (Ito et al, 1992; Fagin et al, 1993).

The field of oncogenes and growth factors in relation to thyroid cancer is progressing rapidly and further advances are expected in the future. While the presence of molecular defects has been seen in a variety of thyroid neoplasia, they are not very prevalent, and their role in thyroid carcinogenesis has not yet been clarified. At present, the theoretical possibilities are exciting, but other than screening for specific germline mutations in *ret* in members of families with MEN 2A and B and familial medullary thyroid carcinoma, few concrete clinical applications have been developed. A better understanding of the role of *p53* might result in the development of a prognostic marker and possibly in a method to reduce dedifferentiation. Further understanding is also needed of how oncogenes interact with other oncogenes, tumor suppressor genes, growth factors, or exogenous factors during the complex carcinogenic process. Of particular interest in thyroid cancer is how genes respond to radiation damage. This is an area where clinical, experimental, and epidemiologic collaboration should be encouraged.

PROSPECTS

Despite the recent improved understanding of the etiology of thyroid cancer (Table 46–6), several areas remain where further research would be valuable. While radiation has been studied extensively, the risk associated with adult exposure to external radiation and childhood exposure to ^{131}I is still not well described. Moreover, little is known about dose–rate effects in humans and additional data on the effects of radiation on gene regulation are needed.

Recent epidemiologic studies have suggested an influence of diet on thyroid carcinoma. A protective effect of cruciferous vegetables has been observed and consumption of certain seafoods has been linked with thyroid cancer in some studies. But at present, the data on dietary factors are relatively crude. Reproductive factors have been examined in women and a role for endogenous and possibly exogenous hormones has been postulated. Findings from several studies underscore the influence of TSH in the development of thyroid cancer. Further investigation of hormonal influences in the pathogenesis of thyroid cancer is warranted. A number

TABLE 46–6. *Summary of Risk Factors for Thyroid Cancer*

Risk Factor	*Comment*
Radiation	External, acute, childhood X-radiation is carcinogenic for long periods of time. The dose–response relationship is consistent with linearity. Papillary carcinoma is the type most often caused by radiation.
Diet	Both iodine deficiency and iodine excess can cause thyroid cancer, depending on histology. Cruciferous vegetables appear to be protective. Seafood may be a risk factor.
TSH	Elevated TSH is associated with thyroid growth and possibly thyroid cancer.
Parity and miscarriage	A weak association between both parity and miscarriage and thyroid cancer has been reported in several studies.
Benign thyroid nodules	Benign thyroid nodules appear to be associated with thyroid cancer and some types may be precursor lesions.
Familial syndromes	Thyroid cancer occurs as part of Gardner's syndrome, Crowden's disease, and MEN I and II.
Oncogene and tumor suppressor genes	Mutations, abnormal expression or amplification of *ras*, PTC-*ret*, c-*myc*, and c-*fos*, as well as inactivation of *p53* have been reported.

of investigations have shown thyroid adenomas, nodules, and goiters, as well as Hashimoto's thyroiditis to be associated with later development of thyroid cancer, so that prospective studies might be directed at examining the issue of precursor lesions. Genetics may be a more important determinant of papillary cancer than once thought, and family studies may be helpful in this area. Recent research on thyroid oncogenes may be helpful in elucidating mechanisms of thyroid carcinogenesis, developing genetic markers, and intervening to prevent tumor progression. Research on specific histologic types has been limited because the number of cases is usually insufficient to provide stable risk estimates. In the future, special emphasis should be given to the various histologic types of thyroid cancer, which may reflect etiologic differences.

REFERENCES

AARONSON SA. 1991. Growth factors and cancer. Science 254:1146–1153.

AASLAND R, LILLEHAUG JR, MALE R, et al. 1988. Expression of oncogenes in thyroid tumours: Coexpression of c-*erbB2/neu* and c-*erbB*. Br J Cancer 57:358–363.

ABELIN T, EGGER M, RUCHTI C. 1994. Belarus increase was probably caused by Chernobyl. BMJ 309:1298.

ADAMSON AS, GARDHAM JRC. 1991. Post ^{131}I carcinoma of the thyroid. Postgrad Med J 67:289–290.

AKSLEN LA, HALDORSEN T, THORESEN SØ, et al. 1991. Survival and causes of death in thyroid cancer: a population-based study of 2479 cases from Norway. Cancer Res 51:1234–1241.

AKSLEN LA, NILSSEN S, KVÅLE G. 1992. Reproductive factors and risk of thyroid cancer. A prospective study of 63,090 women from Norway. Br J Cancer 65:772–774.

ALBERT RE, OMRAN AR. 1968. Follow-up of patients treated by x-ray epilation for tinea capitis. I. Population characteristics, post-treatment illness, and mortality experience. Arch Environ Health 17:899–918.

AL-JURF A, ESSELSTYN CB, CRILE G JR. 1979. Thyroid lesions in patients with hyperparathyroidism. Int Surg 64:33–36.

AOZASA K. 1990. Hashimoto's thyroiditis as a risk factor of thyroid lymphoma. Acta Pathol Jpn 40:459–468.

ARAKI M, OSHIRO K. 1970. Papillary adenocarcinoma of the thyroid developing after treatment of hyperthyroidism with ^{131}I. Gann 61:267–269.

ARNBJÖRNSSON E, ARNBJÖRNSSON A, ÓLAFSSON A. 1986. Thyroid cancer incidence in relation to volcanic activity. Arch Environ Health 41:36–40.

BARNES ND. 1988. Effects of external irradiation on the thyroid gland in childhood. Horm Res 30:84–89.

BARZILAY J, HEATLEY GJ, CUSHING GW. 1991. Benign and malignant tumors in patients with acromegaly. Arch Intern Med 151:1629–1632.

BELFIORE A, LA ROSA GL, PADOVA G, et al. 1987. The frequency of cold thyroid nodules and thyroid malignancies in patients from an iodine-deficient area. Cancer 60:3096–3102.

BLOCK MA. 1969. Familial medullary carcinoma of the thyroid. Gen Prac 39:105–107.

BLOCK MA, HORN RC, MILLER JM, et al. 1967. Familial medullary carcinoma of the thyroid. Ann Surg 166:403–411.

BOICE JD JR, ENGHOLM G, KLEINERMAN RA, et al. 1988. Radiation dose and second cancer risk in patients treated for cancer of the cervix. Radiat Res 116:3–55.

BOICE JD JR, MANDEL JS, DOODY MM, et al. 1992. A health survey of radiologic technologists. Cancer 69:686–698.

BONGARZONE I, PIEROTTI MA, MONZINI N, et al. 1989. High frequency of activation of tyrosine kinase oncogenes in human papillary thyroid carcinoma. Oncogene 4:1457–1462.

BORING CC, SQUIRES TS, TONG T, et al. 1994. Cancer statistics, 1994. CA Cancer J Clin 44:7–26.

BORUP CHRISTENSEN S, LJUNGBERG O, TIBBLIN S. 1984. A clinical epidemiologic study of thyroid carcinoma in Malmö, Sweden. Curr Probl Cancer 8:1–49.

BOULTWOOD J, WYLLIE FS, WILLIAMS ED, et al. 1988. N-*myc* expression in neoplasia of human thyroid c-cells. Cancer Res 48:4073–4077.

BOWLT C, TIPLADY P. 1989. Radioiodine in human thyroid glands and incidence of thyroid cancer in Cumbria. BMJ 299:301–302.

BRESLOW NE, ENSTROM JE. 1974. Geographic correlations between cancer mortality rates and alcohol-tobacco consumption in the United States. J Natl Cancer Inst 53:631–639.

BRINTON LA, MELTON J, MALKASIAN GD JR, et al. 1989. Cancer risk after evaluation for infertility. Am J Epidemiol 129:712–722.

BROSS ID, SHIMAOKA K, TIDINGS J. 1971. Some epidemiological clues in thyroid cancer. Arch Intern Med 128:755–760.

BÜLOW S, HOLM NV, MELLAMGAARD A. 1988. Papillary thyroid carcinoma in Danish patients with familial adenomatous polyposis. Int J Colorect Dis 3:29–31.

CARSTENSEN JM, WINGREN G, HATSCHEK T, et al. 1990. Occupational risks of thyroid cancer: data from the Swedish Cancer Environment Register, 1961–1979. Am J Indust Med 18:535–540.

CATE S, RUTTENBER AJ, CONKLIN AW. 1990. Feasibility of an epidemiologic study of thyroid neoplasia in persons exposed to radionuclides from the Hanford nuclear facility between 1944 and 1956. Health Physics 59:169–178.

CHALSTREY LJ, BENJAMIN B. 1966. High incidence of breast cancer in thyroid cancer patients. Br J Cancer 20:670.

CHAN V, PARASKEVAIDES CA, HALE JF. 1975. Assessment of thyroid function during pregnancy. Br J Obstet Gynaecol 82:137–141.

CHAUDHURI PK, PRINZ R. 1989. Estrogen receptor in normal and neoplastic human thyroid tissue. Am J Otolaryngol 10:322–326.

CLARK DE. 1955. Association of irradiation with cancer of the thyroid in children and adolescents. JAMA 159:1007–1009.

COLEMAN MP, ESTÈVE J, DAMIECKI P, et al. 1993. Trends in cancer incidence and mortality. IARC Publication No. 121. Lyon, International Agency for Research on Cancer. pp. 609–640.

COMMISSION OF THE EUROPEAN COMMUNITIES (CEC). 1993. Thyroid cancer in children living near Chernobyl. Expert panel report on the consequences of the Chernobyl accident. EUR 15248EN. Brussels, CEC.

COMMITTEE ON THE BIOLOGICAL EFFECTS OF IONIZING RADIATION (BEIR). 1980. The effects on populations of exposure to low levels of ionizing radiation (BEIR III). Washington, D.C., National Academy Press.

COMMITTEE ON THE BIOLOGICAL EFFECTS OF IONIZING RADIATIONS (BEIR). 1990. Health effects of exposure to low levels of ionizing radiation (BEIR V). Washington, D.C., National Academy Press.

CONRAD RA. 1984. Late radiation effects in Marshall Islanders exposed to fallout 28 years ago. *In* Boice JD Jr, Fraumeni JF Jr (eds): Radiation Carcinogenesis: Epidemiology and Biological Significance. New York, Raven Press, pp. 57–71.

CORREA P, CHEN VW. 1995. Endocrine gland cancer. Cancer 75:338–352.

CORREA P, CUELLO C, EISENBERG H. 1969. Epidemiology of different types of thyroid cancer. *In* Hedinger C (ed): Thyroid Cancer. UICC Monograph Series, Vol. 12. New York, Springer-Verlag, pp. 81–93.

CRILE G JR, HAZARD JB. 1962. Incidence of cancer in struma lymphomatosa. Surg Gynecol Obst 115:101–103.

CUTLER SJ, YOUNG JL (EDS). 1975. Third National Cancer Survey: Incidence Data. Natl Cancer Inst Monogr 41.

DEGROOT L, PALOYAN E. 1973. Thyroid carcinoma and radiation: a Chicago endemic. JAMA 225:487–491.

DEGROOT LJ, REILLY M, PINNAMENENI K, et al. 1983. Retrospective and prospective study of radiation-induced thyroid disease. Am J Med 74:852–862.

DEL SENNA L, GAMBARI R, DEGLI UBERTI E, et al. 1987. C-myc oncogene alterations in human thyroid carcinomas. Cancer Detect Prev 10:159–166.

DE VATHAIRE F, FRANÇOIS P, SCHWEISGUTH O, et al. 1988. Irradiated neuroblastoma in childhood as potential risk factor for subsequent thyroid tumour. Lancet 2:455.

DEVESA SS, SILVERMAN DT, YOUNG JL JR, et al. 1987. Cancer incidence and mortality trends among whites in the United States, 1947-84. J Natl Cancer Inst 79:701–770.

DOBYNS BM, SHELINE GE, WORKMAN JB, et al. 1974. Malignant and benign neoplasms of the thyroid in patients treated for hyperthyroidism: A report of the Cooperative Thyrotoxicosis Therapy Follow-up Study. J Clin Endocrinol Metab 38:976–998.

DONGHI R, SOZZI G, PIEROTTI MA, et al. 1989. The oncogene associated with human papillary thyroid carcinoma (PTC) is assigned to chromosome 10 q11-q12 in the same region as multiple endocrine neoplasia type 2A (MEN2A). Oncogene 4:521–523.

DONIACH I. 1971. Aetiological considerations of thyroid cancer. Br J Radiol 44:819.

DONIACH I. 1969. The thyroid: Epidemiology of thyroid cancer. J R Coll Surg Edinb 14:261–262.

DONIS-KELLER H, DOU S, CHI D, et al. 1993. Mutations in the RET proto-oncogene are associated with MEN 2A and FMTC. Hum Mol Genet 2:851–6.

DUFFY BJ JR, FITZGERALD PJ. 1950. Cancer of the thyroid in children: A report of 28 cases. J Clin Endocrinol Metab 10:1296–1308.

EWERTZ M, MOURIDSEN HT. 1985. Second cancer following cancer of the female breast in Denmark, 1943–80. Natl Cancer Inst Monogr 68:325–329.

EZAKI H, ISHIMARU T, HAYASHI Y, et al. 1986. Cancer of the thyroid and salivary glands. Gann Monogr 32:129–139.

FAGIN JA. 1994. Molecular pathogenesis of human thyroid neoplasms. Thyroid Today 17:1–7.

FAGIN JA, MATSUO K, KARMARKER A, et al. 1993. High prevalence of mutations of the p53 gene in poorly differentiated human thyroid carcinomas. J Clin Invest 91:179–184.

FARID NR, SHI Y, ZOU M. 1994. Molecular basis of thyroid cancer. Endocrine Rev 15:202–232.

FAVUS MJ, SCHNEIDER AB, STACHURAS ME, et al. 1976. Thyroid cancer occurring as a late consequence of head and neck irradiation. Evaluation of 1056 patients. N Engl J Med 294:1019–1025.

FISCHER DK, GROVES MD, THOMAS SJ, et al. 1989. Papillary carcinoma of the thyroid: Additional evidence in support of a familial component. Cancer Invest 7:323–325.

FLANNIGAN GM, CLIFFORD RP, WINSLET M, et al. 1983. Simultaneous presentation of papillary carcinoma of thyroid in a father and son. Br J Surg 70:181–182.

FRANCESCHI S, FASSINA A, TALAMINI R, et al. 1989. Risk factors for thyroid cancer in North Italy. Int J Epidemiol 18:578–584.

FRANCESCHI S, FASSINA A, TALAMINI R, et al. 1990a. The influence of reproductive and hormonal factors on thyroid cancer in women. Rev Epidemiol Sante Publique 38:27–34.

FRANCESCHI S, LA VECCHIA C. 1994. Cancer of the thyroid. *In* Doll R, Fraumeni JF Jr, Muir CS (eds): Trends in Cancer Incidence and Mortality, Vol. 19/20. Cold Spring Harbor, Cold Spring Harbor Press, pp. 393–424.

FRANCESCHI S, LEVI F, NEGRI E, et al. 1991. Diet and thyroid cancer: a pooled analysis of four European case–control studies. Int J Cancer 48:395–398.

FRANCESCHI S, TALAMINI R, FASSINA A, et al. 1990b. Diet and epithelial cancer of the thyroid gland. Tumori 76:331–338.

FRANSSILA K, SAXÉN E, TEPPO L, et al. 1981. Incidence of different morphological types of thyroid cancer in the Nordic countries. APMS 89:49–55.

FRANSSILA KO, HARACH HR. 1986. Occult papillary carcinoma of the thyroid in children and young adults: a systemic autopsy study in Finland. Cancer 58:715–719.

FRAUMAN AG, MOSES AC. 1990. Oncogenes and growth factors in thyroid carcinogenesis. Endocrinol Metab Clin North Am 19:479–493.

FRIEDMAN G, URY HK. 1980. Initial screening for carcinogenicity of commonly used drugs. J Natl Cancer Inst 65:723–733.

FRIEDMAN GD, URY HK. 1983. Screening for possible drug carcinogenicity: Second report of findings. J Natl Cancer Inst 71:1165–1175.

FUKUNAGA FH, LOCKETT LJ. 1971. Thyroid carcinoma in the Japanese in Hawaii. Arch Pathol 92:6–13.

FUKUNAGA FH, YATANI R. 1975. Geographic pathology of occult thyroid carcinomas. Cancer 36:1095–1099.

FÜRST CJ, LUNDELL M, HOLM L-E, et al. 1988. Cancer incidence after radiotherapy for skin hemangioma: A retrospective cohort study in Sweden. J Natl Cancer Inst 80:1387–1392.

FUSCO A, GRIECO M, SANTORO M, et al. 1987. A new oncogene in human thyroid papillary carcinomas and their lymph-nodal metastases. Nature 328:170–172.

GALANTI MR, LAMBE M, EKBOM A, et al. 1995. Parity and risk of thyroid cancers: a nested case–control study of a nationwide Swedish cohort. Cancer Causes Control 6:37–44.

GLATTRE E, AKSLEN LA, THORESEN SØ, et al. 1990. Geographic patterns and trends in the incidence of thyroid cancer in Norway 1970–1986. Cancer Detect Prev 14:625–631.

GLATTRE E, HALDORSEN T, BERG JP, et al. 1993. Norwegian case–control study testing the hypothesis that seafood increases the risk of thyroid cancer. Cancer Causes Control 4:11–16.

GLATTRE E, THOMASSEN Y, THORESEN SØ, et al. 1989. Prediagnostic serum selenium in a case–control study of thyroid cancer. Int J Epidemiol 18:45–49.

GLÖBEL B, GLÖBEL H, OBERHAUSEN E. 1984. Epidemiologic studies on patients with iodine-131 diagnostic and therapy. *In* Kaul A, Neider R, Pensko J, et al, (eds.): Radiation-Risk-Protection, Vol II. International Radiation Protection Association. Köln: Fachverband für Strahlenschutz e.V., pp. 565–568.

GOLDMAN MB, MONSON RR, MALOOF F. 1990. Cancer mortality in women with thyroid disease. Cancer Res 50:2283–2289.

GOODMAN MT, YOSHIZAWA CN, KOLONEL LN. 1988. Descriptive epidemiology of thyroid cancer in Hawaii. Cancer 61:1272–1281.

GOSSAGE AAR, NEAL FE, ROSS CMD, et al. 1984. Cases of carcinoma of thyroid following Iodine-131 therapy for hyperthyroidism. Oncology 41:8–12.

GREENE MH, WILSON J. 1985. Second cancer following lymphatic and hematopoietic cancers in Connecticut, 1935–82. Natl Cancer Inst Monogr 68:191–218.

GREENWALD P, KORNS RF, NASCA PC, et al. 1975. Cancer in United States Jews. Cancer Res 35:3507–3512.

GRIECO M, SANTORO M, BERLINGIERI MT, et al. 1990. PTC is a novel rearranged form of the *ret* proto-oncoene and is frequently detected *in vivo* in human thyroid papillary carcinoma. Cell 60:557–563.

HALL P, BERG G, BJELKENGREN G, et al. 1992. Cancer mortality after iodine-131 therapy for hyperthyroidism. Int J Cancer 50:886–890.

HALL P, HOLM L-E, LUNDELL G. 1990. Second primary tumors following thyroid cancer. A Swedish record-linkage study. Acta Oncol 29:869–873.

HALLQUIST A, HARDELL L, DEGERMAN A, et al. 1994. Thyroid cancer: reproductive factors, previous thyroid diseases, drug intake, family history and diet. A case–control study. Eur J Cancer Prev 3:481–488.

HAMILTON PM, CHIACCHIERINI RP, KACZMAREK RG. 1989. A follow-up study of persons who had iodine-131 and other diagnostic procedures during childhood and adolescence. FDA Publication 89-8276. Washington, DC, U.S. Dept of Health and Human Services.

HAMILTON TE, VAN BELLE G, LOGERFO JP. 1987. Thyroid neoplasia in Marshall Islanders exposed to nuclear fallout. JAMA 258:629–636.

HANCOCK SL, COX RS, MCDOUGALL IE. 1991. Thyroid diseases after treatment of Hodgkin's disease. N Engl J Med 325:599–605.

HARACH HR, FRANSSILA KO, WASENIUS V-M. 1985. Occult papillary carcinoma of the thyroid. Cancer 56:531–538.

HARVEY EB, BRINTON LA. 1985. Second cancer following cancer of the breast in Connecticut, 1935–82. Natl Cancer Inst Monogr 68:99–112.

HAWKINS MM, KINGSTON JE. 1988. Malignant thyroid tumours following childhood cancer. Lancet 2:804.

HEDINGER C, WILLIAMS ED, SOBIN LH. 1988. Histological Typing of Thyroid Tumours, Second ed. International Histological Classification of Tumours. World Health Organization. No. 11. Berlin, Springer-Verlag.

HEDINGER CE. 1985. Epidemiology of thyroid cancer. *In* Jaffiol C, Milhaud G (eds): Thyroid Cancer. New York, Elsevier Science Publishers, pp. 3–9.

HEITZ P, MOSER H, STAUB JJ. 1976. Thyroid cancer: A study of 573 thyroid tumors and 161 autopsy cases observed over a thirty-year period. Cancer 37:2329–2337.

HEMPELMANN LH, FURTH J. 1978. Etiology of thyroid cancer. *In* Greenfield LD (ed): Thyroid Cancer. West Palm Beach, FL, CRC Press, pp. 37–49.

HEMPELMANN LH, HALL WJ, PHILLIPS M, et al. 1975. Neoplasms in persons treated with x-rays in infancy: Fourth survey in 20 years. J Natl Cancer Inst 55:519–530.

HENDERSON BE, KOLONEL LN, DWORSKY R, et al. 1985. Cancer incidence in the islands of the Pacific. Natl Cancer Inst Monogr 69:73–81.

HENDERSON BE, ROSS RK, PIKE MC, et al. 1982. Endogenous hormones as a major factor in human cancer. Cancer Res 42:3232–3239.

HOFFMAN DA, MCCONAHEY WM, FRAUMENI JF, et al. 1982. Cancer incidence following treatment of hyperthyroidism. Int J Epidemiol 11:218–224.

HOFMANN C, OSLAPAS R, NAYYAR R, et al. 1986. Testosterone enhancement of thyroid carcinoma in rats: The role of TSH. Surgery 100:1078–1085.

HOFSTRA RMW, LANDSVATER RM, CECCHERINI I, et al. 1994. A mutation in the *RET* proto-oncogene associated with multiple endocrine neoplasia type 2B and sporadic medullary thyroid carcinoma. Nature 367:375–376.

HOLM L-E, BLOMGREN H, LÖWHAGEN T. 1985. Cancer risks in patients with chronic lymphocytic thyroiditis. N Engl J Med 312:601–604.

HOLM L-E, HALL P, WIKLUND KE, et al. 1991. Cancer risk after iodine-131 therapy for hyperthyroidism. J Natl Cancer Inst 83:1072–1077.

HOLM L-E, WIKLUND KE, LUNDELL GE, et al. 1988. Thyroid cancer after diagnostic doses of Iodine-131: A retrospective cohort study. J Natl Cancer Inst 80:1132–1138.

HRAFNKELSSON J, JONASSON JG, SIGURDSSON G, et al. 1988. Thyroid cancer in Iceland 1955–1984. Acta Endocrinol (Copenh) 118:566–572.

ISLER H. 1959. Effect of iodine on thyroid tumors induced in the rat by a low-iodine diet. J Natl Cancer Inst 23:675–693.

ITO T, SEYAMA T, MIZUNO T, et al. 1992. Unique association of *p53* mutations with undifferentiated but not with differentiated carcinomas of the thyroid gland. Cancer Res 52:1369–1371.

IWASA Z, JINNAI D, KOYAMA H, et al. 1986. Second primary cancer following adjuvant chemotherapy, radiotherapy and endocrine therapy for breast cancer: A nationwide survey on 47,005 Japanese patients who underwent mastectomy from 1963–1982. Jpn J Surg 16:262–271.

JACKSON CE, BLOCK MA, GREENWALD KA, et al. 1979. The two mutational-event theory in modelling thyroid cancer. Am J Hum Genet 31:704–710.

JANOWER ML, MIETTINEN OS. 1971. Neoplasms after childhood irradiation of the thymus gland. JAMA 212:753–756.

KAPLAN L, KATZ AD, BEN-ISAAC C, et al. 1971. Malignant neoplasms and parathyroid adenoma. Cancer 28:401–407.

KARGA H, LEE J-K, VICKERY AL, et al. 1991. Ras oncogene mutations in benign and malignant thyroid tumors. J Clin Endocrinol Metab 73:832–836.

KAZAKOV VS, DEMIDCHIK EP, ASTAKHOVA LN. 1992. Thyroid cancer after Chernobyl. Nature 359:21.

KENDALL GM, MUIRHEAD CR, MACGIBBON BH, et al. 1992. Mortality and occupational exposure to radiation: first analysis of the National Registry for Radiation Workers. Br Med J 304:220–225.

KERBER RA, TILL JE, SIMON SL, et al. 1993. A cohort study of thyroid disease in relation to fallout from nuclear weapons testing. JAMA 270:2076–2082.

KOGUT MD, KAPLAN SA, COLLIPP PJ, et al. 1965. Treatment of hyperthyroidism in children: analysis of 45 patients. N Engl J Med 272:217–221.

KOLONEL LN, HANKIN JH, WILKENS LR, et al. 1990. An epidemiologic study of thyroid cancer in Hawaii. Cancer Causes Control 1:223–234.

KRAVDAL Ø, GLATTRE E, HALDORSEN T. 1991. Positive correlation between parity and incidence of thyroid cancer: new evidence based on complete Norwegian birth cohorts. Int J Cancer 49:831–836.

KUNG T-M, NG W-L, GIBSON JB. 1981. Volcanoes and carcinoma of the thyroid: a possible association. Arch Environ Health 36:265–267.

LAIRD NM. 1987. Thyroid cancer risk from exposure to ionizing radiation: A case study in the comparative potency model. Risk Anal 7:299–309.

LA VECCHIA C, LUCCHINI F, NEGRI E, et al. 1992. Trends of cancer mortality in Europe, 1955–1989: IV, urinary tract, eye, brain and nerves, and thyroid. Eur J Cancer 28A:1210–1281.

LEE W, CHIACCHIERINI RP, SHLEIEN B, et al. 1982. Thyroid tumors following ^{131}I or localized X irradiation to the thyroid and pituitary glands in rats. Radiat Res 92:307–319.

LEMOINE NR, MAYALL ES, WYLLIE FS, et al. 1988. Activated *ras* oncogenes in human cancers. Cancer Res 48:4459–4463.

LEMOINE NR, MAYALL ES, WYLLIE FS, et al. 1989. High frequency of *ras* oncogene activation in all stages of human thyroid tumorigenesis. Oncogene 4:159–164.

LEVI F, FRANCESCHI S, GULIE C, et al. 1993. Female thyroid cancer: the role of reproductive and hormonal factors in Switzerland. Oncology 50:309–315.

LEVI F, FRANCESCHI S, LA VECCHIA C, et al. 1991. Previous thyroid disease and risk of thyroid cancer in Switzerland. Eur J Cancer 27:85–88.

LEVI F, FRANCESCHI S, TE VC, et al. 1990. Descriptive epidemiology of thyroid cancer in the Swiss canton of Vaud. J Cancer Res Clin Oncol 116:639–647.

LEVI F, NEGRI E, LA VECCHIA C, et al. 1988. Socioeconomic groups and cancer risk at death in the Swiss Canton of Vaud. Int J Epidemiol 17:711–717.

LIKHTAREV IA, CHUMACK VV, REPIN VS. 1994. Retrospective reconstruction of individual and collective external gamma doses of population evacuated after the Chernobyl accident. Health Phys 66:643–652.

LINOS A, LINOS DA, VGOTZA N, et al. 1989. Does coffee consumption protect against thyroid disease? Acta Chir Scand 155:317–320.

LIPS CJM, LANDSVAATER RM, HÖPPENER JWM, et al. 1994. Clinical screening as compared with DNA analysis in families with multiple endocrine neoplasia type 2A. N Engl J Med 331:828–835.

LIVOLSI VA. 1978. Pathology of thyroid cancer. *In* Greenfield LD (ed): Thyroid Cancer. West Palm Beach, FL, CRC Press, pp. 85–141.

LIVOLSI VA, FEIND CR. 1976. Parathyroid adenoma and non-medullary thyroid carcinoma. Cancer 38:1391–1393.

LOTE K, ANDERSON K, NORDAL E, et al. 1980. Familial occurrence of papillary thyroid carcinoma. Cancer 46:1291–1297.

LUNDELL M, HAKULINEN T, HOLM L-E. 1994. Thyroid cancer after radiotherapy for skin hemangioma in infancy. Radiat Res 140:334–339.

MACERI DR, SULLIVAN MJ, MCCLATCHNEY KD. 1986. Autoimmune thyroiditis: Pathophysiology and relationship to thyroid cancer. Laryngoscope 96:82–86.

MALKASIAN GD, MAYBERRY WE. 1970. Serum total and free thyroxine and thyrotropin in normal and pregnant women, neonates, and women receiving progestogens. Am J Obstet Gynecol 108:1234–1238.

MATANOSKI GM, SARTWELL P, ELLIOTT E, et al. 1984. Cancer risks in radiologists and radiation workers. *In* Boice JD Jr, Fraumeni JF Jr (eds): Radiation Carcinogenesis. Epidemiology and Biological Significance. New York, Raven Press, pp. 83–96.

MAXON HR, SAENGER EL, THOMAS SR, et al. 1980. Clinically important radiation-associated thyroid disease. JAMA 244:1802–1805.

MAZZAFERRI EL, YOUNG RL. 1981. Papillary thyroid carcinoma: A ten year follow-up report of the impact of therapy in 576 patients. Am J Med 70:511–518.

MCDOUGALL IR, KENNEDY JS, THOMSON JA. 1971. Thyroid carcinoma following iodine-131 therapy: Report of a case and review of the literature. J Clin Endocrinol Metab 33:287–292.

MCGILL PE. 1978. Thyroid carcinoma in Kenya. Trop Geogr Med 30:81–86.

MCTIERNAN AM, WEISS NS, DALING JR. 1984a. Incidence of thyroid cancer in women in relation to previous exposure to radiation therapy and history of thyroid disease. J Natl Cancer Inst 73:575–581.

MCTIERNAN AM, WEISS NS, DALING JR. 1984b. Incidence of thyroid cancer in women in relation to reproductive and hormonal factors. Am J Epidemiol 120:423–435.

MCTIERNAN AM, WEISS NS, DALING JR. 1987. Incidence of thyroid cancer in women in relation to known or suspected risk factors for breast cancer. Cancer Res 47:292–295.

MEISSNER WA, WARREN S. 1969. Tumors of the Thyroid Gland. Fascicle No. 4, Second Series. Washington, D.C., Armed Forces Institute of Pathology.

MELMED S. 1988. Oncogenes and the thyroid. Thyroid Today 11:1–7.

METTLER FA, WILLIAMSON MR, ROYAL HD, et al. 1992. Thyroid nodules in the population living around Chernobyl. JAMA 268:616–619.

METTLIN C. 1986. Dietary factors for cancer of specific sites. Surg Clin North Am 66:917–929.

MILLER AB, BARCLAY TH, CHOI NW, et al. 1980. A study of cancer, parity and age at first pregnancy. J Chron Dis 33:595–605.

MODAN B, BAIDATZ D, MART H, et al. 1974. Radiation-induced head and neck tumours. Lancet 1:277–279.

MUIR C, WATERHOUSE J, MACK T, et al. 1987. Cancer Incidence in Five Continents, Vol V. IARC Scientific Publication No. 88. Lyon, International Agency for Research on Cancer.

MULLIGAN LM, KWOK JBJ, HEALTY CS, et al. 1993. Germ-line mutations of the *RET* proto-oncogene in multiple endocrine neoplasia type 2A. Nature 363:458–460.

MYERS M, RIES LAG. 1989. Cancer patient survival rates: SEER program results for 10 years of follow-up. Ca 39:21–32.

NAGATAKI S, SHIBATA Y, INOUE S, et al. 1994. Thyroid disease among atomic bomb survivors in Nagasaki. JAMA 272:364–370.

NAKAMURA H, KOGA M, HIGA S, et al. 1987. A case of von Recklinghausen's disease associated with pheochromocytoma and papillary carcinoma of the thyroid gland. Endocrinol Japan 34:545–551.

NAMBA H, RUBIN SA, FAGIN JA. 1990. Point mutations of ras oncogenes are an early event in thyroid tumorigenesis. Mol Endocrinol 4:1474–1479.

NARITA T, TAKAGI K. 1984. Ataxia-telangiectasia with dysgerminoma of right ovary, papillary carcinoma of thyroid, and adenocarcinoma of pancreas. Cancer 54:1113–1116.

NATIONAL ACADEMY OF SCIENCES (NAS). 1983. Committee on Diet, Nutrition, and Cancer. Diet, nutrition, and cancer: Interim dietary guidelines. J Natl Cancer Inst 70:1151–1170.

NATIONAL CANCER INSTITUTE (NCI). 1989. Statistics Review, 1973–1986. NIH Publication No. 89-2789. Bethesda, MD, U.S. Department of Health and Human Services.

NATIONAL COUNCIL ON RADIATION PROTECTION AND MEASUREMENT (NCRP). 1985. Induction of thyroid cancer by ionizing radiation. Report No. 80. Bethesda, MD, NCRP.

NEGLIA JP, RAMSAY NK, MCGLAVE PB, et al. 1986. Increased occurrence of thyroid cancer among patients with severe aplastic anemia (meeting abstract). Proc Ann Meet Am Assoc Cancer Res 27:231.

NEGRI E, LA VECCHIA C, FRANCESCHI S, et al. 1991. Vegetable and fruit consumption and cancer risk. Int J Cancer 48:350–354.

NĚMEC J, SOUMAR J, ZAMRAZIL V, et al. 1975. Familial occurrence of differentiated (non-medullary) thyroid cancer. Oncology 32:151–157.

NĚMEC J, ZAMRAZIL V, POHUNKOVÁ D, et al. 1980. Thyroidectomy as a pathogenic factor in the evolution of thyroid cancer. Neoplasma 27:595–599.

OHSHIMA M, WARD JM. 1986. Dietary iodine deficiency as a tumor promoter and carcinogen in male F344/NCR rats. Cancer Res 46:877–883.

OHTA S, KATSURA T, SHIMADA M, et al. 1986. Ataxia-telangiectasia with papillary carcinoma of the thyroid. Am J Pediat Hemat/Oncol 8:255–268.

OLSEN JH, BOICE JD JR, JENSEN JPA, et al. 1989. Cancer among epileptics exposed to anti-convulsant drugs. J Natl Cancer Inst 81:803–808.

ØSTERLIND A, OLSEN JH, LYNGE E, et al. 1985. Second cancer following cutaneous melanoma and cancers of the brain, thyroid, connective tissue, bone, and eye in Denmark, 1943–80. Natl Cancer Inst Monogr 68:361–388.

OTTINO A, PIANZOLA HM, CASTELLETTO RH. 1989. Occult papillary thyroid carcinoma at autopsy in La Plata, Argentina. Cancer 64:547–551.

OZAKI O. 1994. Thyroid carcinoma following radio-active iodine therapy for Grave's disease. Cancer J 7:98.

OZAKI O, ITO K, KOBAYASHI K, et al. 1988. Familial occurrence of differentiated, nonmedullary thyroid carcinoma. World J Surg 12:565–571.

PACCHIAROTTI A, MARTINO E, BARTALENA L, et al. 1986. Serum thyrotropin by ultrasensitive immunoradiometric assay and serum free thyroid hormones in pregnancy. J Endocrinol Invest 9:185–189.

PAKSOY N, BOUCHARDY C, PARKIN DM. 1991. Cancer incidence in Western Samoa. Int J Epidemiol 20:634–641.

PAKSOY N, MONTAVILLE B, MCCARTHY SW. 1990. Cancer occurrence in Vanuatu in the South Pacific, 1980–86. Trop Geogr Med 42:157–161.

PALOYAN E, HOFMANN C, PRINZ R, et al. 1982. Castration induces a marked reduction in the incidence of thyroid cancers. Surgery 92:839–848.

PARKIN DM, MUIR CS, WHELAN SL, et al. 1992. Cancer Incidence in Five Continents, Vol VI. IARC Scientific Publication No. 120. Lyon, International Agency for Research on Cancer.

PAYNTER OE, BURIN GJ, JAEGER RB, et al. 1988. Goitrogens and thyroid follicular cell neoplasia: evidence for a threshold process. Regul Toxicol Pharmocol 8:102–119.

PENDERGRAST WJ, MILMORE BK, MARCUS SC. 1961. Thyroid cancer and thyrotoxicosis in the United States: their relation to endemic goiter. J Chron Dis 13:22–38.

PETO R, DOLL R, BUCKLEY JD, et al. 1981. Can dietary beta-carotene materially reduce human cancer rates? Nature 290:201–208.

PETTERSSON B, ADAMI H-O, WILANDER E, et al. 1991. Trends in thyroid cancer incidence in Sweden, 1958–1981, by histopathologic type. Int J Cancer 48:28–33.

PICKLE LW, MASON TJ, HOWARD N, et al. 1987. Atlas of U.S. mortality among whites: 1930–1980. NIH Publication No. 87-2900. Washington, D.C., U.S. Govt. Printing Office.

PILCH BZ, KAHN CR, KETCHAM AS, et al. 1973. Thyroid cancer after radioactive iodine diagnostic procedures in childhood. Pediatrics 51:898–902.

PILLAJ NK, THANGAVELU M, RAMALINGASWAMI V. 1976. Nodular lesions of the thyroid in an area of high background radiation in coastal Kerala, India. Indian J Med Res 64:537–544.

PLAIL RO, BUSSEY HJR, GLAZER G, et al. 1987. Adenomatous polyposis: an association with carcinoma of the thyroid. Br J Surg 74:377–380.

POLEDNAK AP. 1986. Thyroid tumors and thyroid function in women exposed to internal and external radiation. J Environ Pathol Toxicol Oncol 7:53–64.

POTTERN LM, KAPLAN MM, LARSEN PR, et al. 1990. Thyroid nodularity after irradiation for lymphoid hyperplasia: a comparison of questionnaire and clinical findings. J Clin Epidemiol 43:449–460.

POTTERN LM, STONE BJ, DAY NE, et al. 1980. Thyroid cancer in Connecticut, 1935–1975: An analysis by cell type. Am J Epidemiol, 112:764–774.

PRENTICE RL, KATO H, YOSHIMOTO K, et al. 1982. Radiation exposure and thyroid cancer incidence among Hiroshima and Nagasaki residents. Natl Cancer Inst Monogr 62:207–212.

PRESTON-MARTIN S, BERNSTEIN L, PIKE MC, et al. 1987. Thyroid cancer among young women related to prior thyroid disease. Br J Cancer 55:191–195.

PRESTON-MARTIN S, JIN F, DUDA MJ, et al. 1993. A case–control study of thyroid cancer in women under age 55 in Shanghai (People's Republic of China). Cancer Causes Control 4:431–440.

PRESTON-MARTIN S, MENCK HR. 1979. The epidemiology of thyroid cancer in Los Angeles county. West J Med 131:369–372.

PRISYAZHIUK A, PJATAK OA, BUZANOV VA, et al. 1991. Cancer in the Ukraine, post-Chernobyl. Lancet 338:1334–1335.

RADFORD E, TALBOTT E, SCHMELTZ R, et al. 1983. Effects of elevated gamma-ray exposures on the prevalence of thyroid abnormalities in a community. *In* Broerse J, Barendsen G, Kal H, et al (eds): Radiation Research: Somatic and Genetic Effects. Proc. 7th Intl Congr Radiat Res. The Hague, Martinus Nijhoff, C8–12.

RALLISON ML, DOBYNS BM, KEATING RF, et al. 1975. Thyroid nodularity in children. JAMA 233:1069–1072.

RASTOGI GK, SAWHNEY RC, SINHA MK, et al. 1974. Serum and urinary levels of thyroid hormones in normal pregnancy. Obstet Gynecol 44:176–180.

RIES LAG, MILLER BA, HANKEY BF, et al (eds.). 1994. SEER Cancer Statistics Review, 1973–1991: tables and graphs. NIH publ. no. 94-2789. Bethesda, National Cancer Institute.

ROBBINS J, ADAMS WH. 1989. Radiation effects in the Marshall Islands. *In* Nagataki S (ed): Radiation and the Thyroid. Amsterdam, Excerpta Medica, pp. 11–24.

ROBBINS SL, COTRAM RS, KUMAR V. 1984. Pathologic Basis of Disease. Thyroid Gland. Philadelphia, WB Saunders, pp. 1201–1225.

ROJESKI MT, GHARIB H. 1985. Nodular thyroid disease. Evaluation and management. N Engl J Med 313:428–436.

RON E, CURTIS R, HOFFMAN DA, et al. 1984. Multiple primary breast and thyroid cancer. Br J Cancer 49:87–92.

RON E, GRIFFEL B, LIBAN E, et al. 1986. Histopathologic reproducibility of thyroid disease in an epidemiologic study. Cancer 57:1056–1059.

RON E, KLEINERMAN RA, BOICE JD JR, et al. 1987a. A population-based case–control study of thyroid cancer. J Natl Cancer Inst 79:1–12.

RON E, KLEINERMAN RA, LIVOLSI VA, et al. 1991. Familial non-medullary thyroid cancer. Oncology 48:309–311.

RON E, LUBIN J, SCHNEIDER AB. 1992. Thyroid cancer incidence. Nature 360:113.

RON E, LUBIN JH, SHORE RE, et al. 1995. Thyroid cancer following exposure to external radiation: a pooled analysis of seven studies. Radiat Res 141:255–273.

RON E, LUNENFELD B, MENCZER J, et al. 1987b. Cancer incidence in a cohort of infertile women. Am J Epidemiol 125:780–790.

RON E, MODAN B, PRESTON D, et al. 1989. Thyroid neoplasia following low-dose radiation in childhood. Radiat Res 120:516–531.

ROSEN IB, WALFISH PG. 1986. Pregnancy as a predisposing factor in thyroid neoplasia. Arch Surg 121:1287–1290.

SAFA AM, SCHUMACHER OP, RODRIGUEZ-ANTUNEZ A. 1975. Long-term follow-up results in children and adolescents treated with radioactive iodine (^{131}I) for hyperthyroidism. N Engl J Med 292:167–171.

SAMAAN NA, SCHULTZ PN, ORDONEZ NG, et al. 1987. A comparison of thyroid carcinoma in those who have and have not had head and neck irradiation in childhood. J Clin Endocrinol Metab 64:219–223.

SAMPSON RJ, WOOLNER LB, BAHN RC, et al. 1974. Occult thyroid carcinoma in Olmstead County, Minnesota. Prevalence at autopsy compared with that in Hiroshima and Nagasaki, Japan. Cancer 34:2072–2076.

SAXEN EA, SAXEN LO. 1954. Mortality from thyroid disease in an endemic goitre area. Studies in Finland. Doc Med Geogr Trop (Amst) 6:335–341.

SCHENKER JC, LEVINSKY R, OHEL G. 1984. Multiple primary malignant neoplasms in breast cancer patients in Israel. Cancer 54:145–150.

SCHIMKE RN, HARTMANN WH, PROUT TE, et al. 1968. Syndrome of bilateral pheochromocytoma, medullary carcinoma and multiple neuromas. N Engl J Med 279:1–7.

SCHINDLER A-M, VAN MELLE G, EVEQUOZ B, et al. 1991. Prognostic factors in papillary carcinoma of the thyroid. Cancer 68:324–330.

SCHNEIDER AB, RON E, LUBIN J, et al. 1993. Dose–response relationships for radiation-induced thyroid cancer and thyroid nodules: evidence for the prolonged effects of radiation on the thyroid. J Clin Endocrinol Metab 77:362–369.

SCHNEIDER AB, SHORE-FREEDMAN E, RYO UY, et al. 1985. Radiation-induced tumors of the head and neck following childhood irradiation: Medicine 64:1–15.

SCHNEIDER AB, SHORE-FREEDMAN E, WEINSTEIN RA. 1986. Radiation-induced thyroid and other head and neck tumors: Occurrence of multiple tumors and analysis of risk factors. J Clin Endocrinol Metab 63:107–112.

SCHOENBERG B. 1977. Multiple Primary Malignant Neoplasms. The Connecticut Experience, 1935–1964. New York, Springer-Verlag.

SCHOTTENFELD D, BERG JW. 1971. Incidence of multiple primary cancers. IV. Cancers of the female breast and genital organs. J Natl Cancer Inst 46:161–170.

SELBY JV, FRIEDMAN GD, FIREMAN BH. 1989. Screening prescription drugs for possible carcinogenicity: eleven to fifteen years of follow-up. Cancer Res 49:5736–5747.

SHANDS WC, GATLING RR. 1970. Cancer of the thyroid: Review of 109 cases. Ann Surg 171:735–745.

SHELINE GE, LINDSAY S, MCCORMACK KR, et al. 1962. Thyroid nodules occurring late after treatment of thyrotoxicosis with radioiodine. J Clin Endocrinol Metab 22:8–18.

SHI Y, ZOU M, SCHMIDT H, et al. 1991. High rates of *ras* codon 61 mutation in thyroid tumors in an iodide-deficient area. Cancer Res 51:2690–2693.

SHIMAOKA K, GETAZ EP, RAO U. 1979. Anaplastic carcinoma of thyroid. NY State J Med 79:874–877.

SHIMAOKA K, TAKEICHI S, PICKREN JW. 1967. Carcinoma of thyroid associated with other primary malignant tumors. Cancer 30:1000–1005.

SHORE RE. 1992. Issues and epidemiological evidence regarding radiation-induced thyroid cancer. Radiat Res 131:98–111.

SHORE RE, ALBERT RE, PASTERNACK BD. 1976. Follow-up study of patients treated by X-ray epilation for tinea capitis. IV. Resurvey of post-treatment illness and mortality. Arch Environ Health 31:21–28.

SHORE RE, HEMPELMANN LH, WOODWARD ED. 1986. Carcinogenic effects of radiation on the human thyroid gland. *In* Upton AC, Albert RE, Burns FJ, et al (eds): Radiation Carcinogenesis. New York, Elsevier, pp. 293–310.

SHORE RE, HILDRETH N, DVORETSKY E, et al. 1993. Thyroid cancer among persons given X-ray treatment in infancy for an enlarged thymus gland. Am J Epidemiol 137:1068–1080.

SHORE RE, WOODARD E, HILDRETH N, et al. 1985. Thyroid tumors following thymus irradiation. J Natl Cancer Inst 74:1177–1184.

SIEGAL A, MODAN M. 1981. Latent carcinoma of thyroid in Israel: a study of 260 autopsies. Isr J Med Sci 17:249–253.

SILVERBERG SG, VIDONE RA. 1966. Carcinoma of the thyroid in surgical and postmortem material. Analysis of 300 cases at autopsy and literature review. Ann Surg 164:291–299.

SPITZ MR, SIDER JG, KATZ RL, et al. 1988. Ethnic patterns of thyroid cancer incidence in the United States, 1973–1981. Int J Cancer 42:549–553.

SPRØGEL P, STORM HH. 1989. Thyroid cancer: incidence, mortality and histological pattern in Denmark. Int J Epidemiol 18:990–992.

STOFFER SS, VAN DYKE DL, BACH JV, et al. 1986. Familial papillary carcinoma of the thyroid. Am J Med Genet 25:775–782.

SUÁREZ HG, DU VILLARD JA, SEVERINO M, et al. 1990. Presence of mutations in all three *ras* genes in human thyroid tumors. Oncogene 5:565–570.

SZÁNTÓ J, GUNDY C, TÓTH K, et al. 1990. Coincidental papillary carcinoma of the thyroid in two sisters. Oncology 47:992–994.

TAKEICHI N, ITO H, HARUTA R, et al. 1991. Relation between estrogen receptor and malignancy of thyroid cancer. Jpn J Cancer Res 82:19–22.

TEPPO L, PUKKALA E, SAXÉN E. 1985. Multiple cancer—an epidemiologic exercise in Finland. J Natl Cancer Inst 75:207–217.

TERRIER P, SHENG Z-M, SCHLUMBERGER M, et al. 1988. Structure and expression of c-*myc* and c-*fos* proto-oncogenes in thyroid carcinomas. Br J Cancer 57:43–47.

THOMPSON D, MABUCHI K, RON E, et al. 1994. Cancer incidence in a-bomb survivors, 1958–87. Part II: Solid tumors. Rad Res 137:S17–S67.

TRAPIDO EJ, MCCOY CB, STEIN NS, et al. 1990. The epidemiology of cancer among Hispanic women. Cancer 66:2435–2441.

TUCKER MA, BOICE JD JR, HOFFMAN DA. 1985. Second cancer following cutaneous melanoma and cancers of the brain, thyroid, connective tissue, bone and eye in Connecticut, 1935–82. Natl Cancer Inst Monogr 68:161–189.

TUCKER MA, COLEMAN CN, COX RS, et al. 1988. Risk of second malignancies after treatment for Hodgkin's disease. N Engl J Med 318:76–81.

TUCKER MA, MORRIS JONES PH, BOICE JD JR, et al. 1991. Therapeutic radiation at a young age is linked to secondary thyroid cancer. Cancer Res 51:2885–2888.

TURRIN A, PILOTTI S, RICCI SB. 1985. Characteristics of thyroid cancer following irradiation. Int J Radiat Oncol Biol Phys 11:2149–2154.

UNITED NATIONS SCIENTIFIC COMMITTEE ON THE EFFECTS OF ATOMIC RADIATION (UNSCEAR). 1988. Sources, Effects and Risks of Ionizing Radiation. Publ. E88.IX.7. New York, United Nations.

UNITED NATIONS SCIENTIFIC COMMITTEE ON THE EFFECTS OF ATOMIC RADIATION (UNSCEAR). 1994. Sources and Effects of Ionizing Radiation. Publ. E94.IX.11. New York, United Nations.

UTIGER RD. 1994. Medullary thyroid carcinoma, genes, and the prevention of cancer. N Engl J Med 331:870–871.

VÅGERÖ D, PERSSON G. 1986. Occurrence of cancer in socioeconomic groups in Sweden. An analysis based on the Swedish Cancer Environment Registry. Scand J Soc Med 14:151–160.

VERBY JE, WOOLNER LB, NOBREGA FT, et al. 1969. Thyroid cancer in Olmsted County 1935-1965. JNCI 43:813–820.

WAHNER HW, CUELLO C, CORREA P, et al. 1966. Thyroid carcinoma in an endemic goiter area, Cali, Colombia. Am J Med 40:58–66.

WAKABAYASHI T, KATO H, IKEDA T, et al. 1983. Studies of the mortality of A-bomb survivors, Report 7. Part III. Incidence of cancer in 1959–1978, based on the tumor registry, Nagasaki. Radiat Res 93:112–146.

WANG J-X, INSKIP PD, BOICE JD JR, et al. 1990a. Cancer incidence among medical diagnostic x-ray workers in China, 1950 to 1985. Int J Cancer 45:889–895.

WANG Z, BOICE JD JR, LUXIN W, et al. 1990b. Thyroid nodularity and chromosome aberrations among women in areas of high background radiation in China. J Natl Cancer Inst 82:478–485.

WARD JM, OHSHIMA M. 1986. The role of iodine in carcinogenesis. Adv Exp Med Biol 206:529–542.

WEEKE J, HANSEN AP. 1975. Serum TSH and serum T_3 levels during normal menstrual cycles and during cycles on oral contraceptives. Acta Endocrinol 79:431–438.

WEGELIN C. 1928. Malignant disease of the thyroid gland and its relation to goitre in man and animal. Cancer Rev 3:297–313.

WILLIAMS ED. 1979. The aetiology of thyroid tumors. Clin Endocrinol Metab 8:193–207.

WILLIAMS ED. 1986. Relation between 131-I therapy for thyrotoxicosis and development of thyroid carcinoma. Lancet 2:456.

WILLIAMS ED. 1990. TSH and thyroid cancer. Horm Metab Res Suppl 23:72–75.

WILLIAMS ED, DONIACH I, BJARNASON O, et al. 1977. Thyroid cancer in an iodine-rich area. A histopathological study. Cancer 39:215–222.

WILLIAMS RR. 1976. Breast and thyroid cancer and malignant melanoma promoted by alcohol-induced pituitary secretion of prolactin, TSH and MSH. Lancet 1:996–999.

WINGREN G, HATSCHEK T, AXELSON O. 1993. Determinants of papillary cancer of the thyroid. Am J Epidemiol 138:482–491.

WINSHIP T, ROSVOLL RV. 1970. Thyroid carcinoma in childhood: Final report on a 20 year study. Clin Proc Children's Hosp 26:327–348.

WRIGHT PA, LEMOINE NR, MAYALL ES, et al. 1989. Papillary and follicular thyroid carcinomas show a different pattern of *ras* oncogene mutation. Br J Cancer 60:576–577.

WRIGHT PA, WILLIAMS ED, LEMOINE NR, et al. 1991. Radiation-associated and "spontaneous" human thyroid carcinomas show a difference pattern of *ras* oncogene mutation. Oncogene 6:471–473.

WYLLIE FS, LEMOINE NR, WILLIAMS ED, et al. 1989. Structure and expression of nuclear oncogenes in multi-stage thyroid tumorigenesis. Br J Cancer 60:561–565.

WYNDER EL. 1952. Some practical aspects of cancer prevention (concluded). N Engl J Med 246:573–582.

ZEIGHAMI EA, MORRIS MD. 1986. Thyroid cancer risk in the population around the Nevada Test Site. Health Phys 50:19–32.

ZOU M, SHI Y, FARID NR. 1993. p53 mutations in all stages of thyroid carcinomas. J Clin Endocrinol Metab 77:1054–1058.

47 Breast cancer

BRIAN E. HENDERSON
MALCOLM C. PIKE
LESLIE BERNSTEIN
RONALD K. ROSS

Breast cancer is the most common cancer among women in the United States, accounting for almost 30% of all newly diagnosed cancers. It is also the most common cancer in women worldwide (Parkin et al, 1984). There have been sustained increases in the incidence of this cancer in developing countries in recent years. It has been estimated that if these increasing rates persist, the annual worldwide incidence of breast cancer will be over one million by the year 2000 (Miller and Bulbrook, 1986). Male breast cancer is rare compared to female breast cancer. Female-to-male incidence ratios vary from 70 to 130 around the world (Shelan et al, 1990).

A substantial body of experimental, clinical, and epidemiologic evidence indicates that hormones play a major role in the etiology of breast cancer (Henderson et al, 1988; Henderson et al, 1982). The known risk factors for breast cancer (Table 47–1) can be understood as measures of the cumulative exposure of the breast to estrogen and, perhaps, progesterone. The actions of these ovarian hormones (and the hormones used in combination oral contraceptives [COCs] and hormone replacement therapy [HRT]) on the breast do not appear to be genotoxic, but they do affect the rate of cell division. Their effects on breast cancer rates are thus manifest in their effects on proliferation of the breast epithelial cell. Recent advances in the molecular genetics of cancer have provided a molecular basis for the concept that cell division is essential in the genesis of human cancer.

The activation of oncogenes and inactivation of tumor-suppressor genes (e.g., *BRCA1*, *TP53*) produce a sequence of genetic changes that lead to a malignant phenotype (Fig. 47–1). The activation of oncogenes, whether by mutation, translocation, or amplification, requires cell division. Genetic errors that precede the development of a fully malignant tumor also include the loss or inactivation during mitosis of several tumor-suppressor genes that function to control normal cellular behavior (Fearon et al, 1990; Sager, 1989; Stanbridge, 1990). Most of the models currently favored suggest that the first hit is the inactivation by a mutational event of one of the two alleles of a tumor-suppressor gene present in diploid cells, followed by a reduction to homozygosity of the faulty chromosome (Knudson, 1971). The initial mutagenic event and the loss of the wild-type allele of the tumor-suppressor gene both require cell division. Thus, for expression of the full malignant phenotype, cells are absolutely required to divide.

Since endogenous hormones directly affect the risk of breast cancer, there is reason for concern about the effects on breast cancer risk if the same or closely related hormones are administered for therapeutic purposes (e.g., as contraceptives or as hormone replacement therapy). It also follows that approaches to the prevention of breast cancer should focus on reducing the lifetime exposure of the breast to estrogen and progesterone, e.g., reducing the number of ovulations through exercise or perhaps lowering of steroid hormone levels by increasing the fiber content of the diet or by pharmacological means.

HISTOPATHOLOGY

Carcinoma of the breast develops as a neoplasm of the ductal epithelium in over 90% of cases, with the remainder developing as lower grade neoplasms from lobular epithelium. A variable degree of adjacent connective tissue proliferation produces the cirrhotic nature of breast cancer. Inflammatory carcinoma represents an unusually malignant variety of ductal carcinoma, in which anaplastic tumor cells invade and obstruct the dermal lymphocytes (Canellos, 1985).

Approximately 60% of breast cancers have measur-

TABLE 47–1. *Breast Cancer Risk Factors*

Risk Factors—Increased Exposure to Estrogen and/or Progesterone
Early menarche
Late menopause
Obesity (postmenopausal women)
Hormone replacement therapy
Protective Factors—Decreased Exposure to Estrogen and/or Progesterone
Early first-term pregnancy
Lactation
Physical activity

able estrogen receptor protein (ERP), a cytoplasmic protein which binds and transfers estrogen to the nucleus. The presence of ERP varies markedly with ovulation, with less than 30% of cancers diagnosed in ovulating women demonstrating ERP compared to more than 60% in postmenopausal women (McCarty et al, 1983).

Survival rates across all stages of breast cancer have been slowly but steadily increasing during the past two decades (Myers and Gloeckler Ries, 1989). The 5-year relative survival rate for whites has increased from 63% in 1960 to 80% by 1983–1989. Some, if not most of this increased survival is a consequence of secular changes in screening (Hankey et al, 1993). Young women have poorer survival rates and there remains a significant gap in breast cancer survival for blacks compared to whites. The 5-year survival rate for blacks in 1983–1989 was only 63%.

Descriptive Factors

As for other epithelial cancers, the most important demographic risk factor is increasing age. By the late teenage years the first cases of breast cancer occur, and thereafter, there is a rapid rise in the age-specific rates. Up to age 50 the rate of increase is very high; after this, the rate of increase slows dramatically (Pike, 1987).

There is substantial variation in breast cancer rates among different countries. Rates are some six times higher in the U.S., Canada, or Northern Europe than in Asia (Fig. 47–2) or in black populations in Africa. These international differences in breast cancer rates do not appear to be determined primarily by variation in genetic susceptibility (Haenszel and Kurihara, 1968). Breast cancer rates for U.S. blacks are quite similar to rates for U.S. whites, not to rates for African blacks (Shelan et al, 1990). Furthermore, Japanese migrants to Hawaii and California have increased rates of breast cancer compared to their counterparts in Japan (Buell, 1973). Those Japanese women who are born in Japan and migrate to the U.S. as young adults experience only a modest increase in their breast cancer rates, whereas Japanese women born in the U.S. have rates approaching their white counterparts (Shimizu et al, 1991). Thus the risk of breast cancer seems at least partly related to early life experiences. Nonetheless, Polish and Italian migrants to the U.S. and Australia appear to have substantial increases in breast cancer mortality within 20–25 years of migration (Prentice et al, 1988).

Age-adjusted breast cancer mortality rates have remained fairly stable among white women in the U.S. during the past several decades, whereas incidence rates have risen slowly but steadily during the same time period (Glass, 1988). Between 1973 and 1987 there was a 20% overall increase in incidence, but breast cancer mortality increased only 2% during the same period (Ries et al, 1990). Increased detection by mammogra-

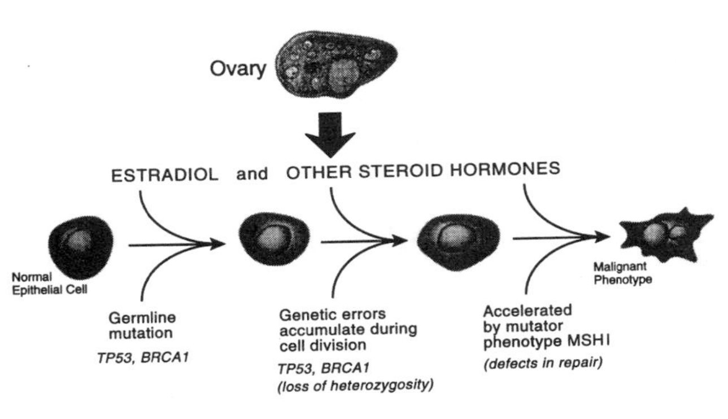

FIG. 47–1. Estradiol, and to a lesser degree, other steroid hormones (e.g. progesterone) drive cell proliferation, which facilitates fixation of genetic errors by loss of heterozygosity or leads to genetic changes that facilitate mutation by defects in DNA repair enzymes. Germline mutations in relevant tumor suppressor genes accelerate the transformation into the malignant phenotype.

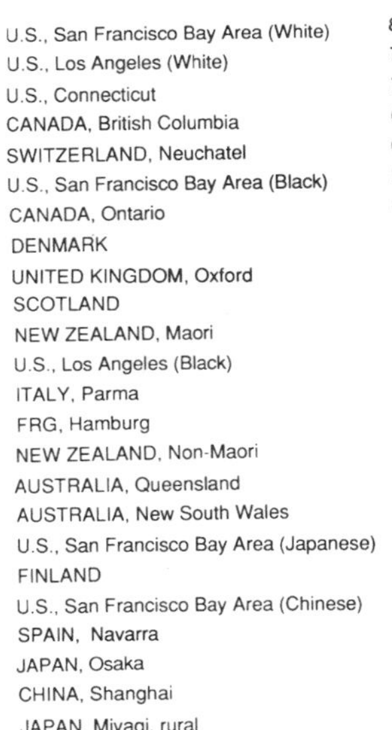

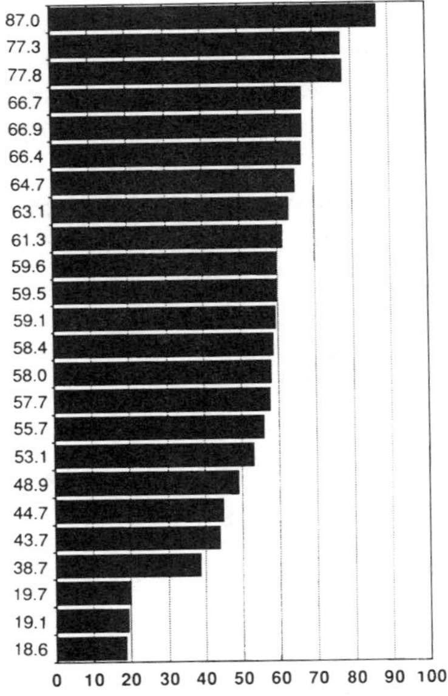

FIG. 47–2. Breast cancer incidence in different countries.

phy may be responsible for this increase in incidence as it is largely confined to early stage disease (White et al, 1990). In fact, it appears that incidence rates have plateaued through 1990 (Boring et al, 1993; Hankey et al, 1993).

Breast cancer incidence rates are strongly associated with social class; rates in the highest quintile of social class are almost 50% higher than those in the lowest quintile (Henderson et al, 1984). This relationship appears to be explicable largely on the basis of reproductive risk factors, described below.

ANALYTIC FACTORS

Age at Menarche

Early age at menarche has been demonstrated as a risk factor for breast cancer in most case–control studies. In general, an approximately 20% decrease in breast cancer risk results from each year that menarche is delayed. In a study of young women, we recorded not only age at onset of menstruation, but also age when "regular" (i.e., predictable) menstruation was first established (Henderson et al, 1981). For a fixed age at menarche, women who established regular menstrual cycles within 1 year of the first menstrual period had more than double the risk of breast cancer of women with a 5-year or longer delay in onset of regular cycles. Women with early menarche (age 12 or younger) and rapid establishment of regular cycles had an almost fourfold increased risk of breast cancer when compared with women with late menarche (age 13 or older) and long duration of irregular cycles.

These observations suggested that regular ovulatory cycles increase a woman's risk of breast cancer (Henderson et al, 1985) and supported results from an earlier study of circulating hormone levels in daughters of breast cancer patients and in age-matched daughters of controls. The daughters of the breast cancer patients, who as a group have at least twice the breast cancer risk of the general population, had higher levels of circulating estrogen and progesterone on day 22 of the menstrual cycle than did the controls (Henderson et al, 1975). This result was later confirmed (Trichopoulos et al, 1981). Since cumulative estrogen levels are greater during the normal luteal phase than during a comparable period of nonovulatory cycle, cumulative frequency of ovulatory cycles is an index of cumulative estrogen exposure (and of progesterone exposure as well).

Other supportive evidence for the concept that the cumulative number of ovulatory cycles (i.e., cumulative estrogen exposure) is a major determinant of breast cancer risk comes from international studies of the frequency of ovulation in relation to age at menarche and the number of years since menarche in girls ages 15 to 19 years, selected from several populations at varying risk of breast cancer (MacMahon et al, 1982). In all of these populations, women with later menarche were more likely to have anovular cycles than women with early menarche, given the same number of elapsed years since menarche. Adjusting for years since menarche, the highest frequency of ovulatory cycles was observed in those populations with the highest breast cancer rates. Apter and Vihko (1983), in a longitudinal study of 200 schoolgirls, also found that those with early menarche establish ovulatory cycles more quickly than girls with later onset of menstruation.

Over the past 100 years, age at menarche has progressively decreased in both the U.S. and in most other areas of the world. In a series of extensive cross-sectional studies, it has been demonstrated that age at menarche is directly related to childhood growth patterns (Tanner, 1962). Attainment of a critical body weight: height ratio appears necessary for menarche to occur (Frisch and McArthur, 1974). Chronic malnutrition during childhood delays the age at menarche, whereas the improved nutrition and control of infectious diseases of childhood of the past decades have combined to lower it.

Physical Activity

Strenuous physical activity may delay menarche. Girls who engage in regular ballet dancing, swimming, or running have a considerable delay in the onset of menses. In one study, ballet dancers had a mean age at menarche of 15.4 years, compared with 12.5 years for controls (Frisch et al, 1981). Breast development was also delayed in the dancers, and they experienced intermittent amenorrhea through their teenage years, as long as they remained active dancers. Even moderate physical activity during adolescence can lead to anovular cycles. Girls who engaged in regular, moderate physical activity (averaging at least 600 Kcal of energy expended per week) were 2.9 times more likely to be anovular than were girls who engaged in lesser amounts of physical activity (Bernstein et al, 1987) (Fig. 47–3). More recently, we reported that adolescent and adult physical activity significantly reduces the risk of breast cancer in young women (≤ or 40 years of age) (Bernstein et al, 1994). The risk of breast cancer among women who averaged four or more hours of exercise activity during their reproductive years was nearly 60% lower than that of inactive women (Fig. 47–4).

Age at Menopause

The relationship between menopause and breast cancer risk has been known for some time. The rate of increase

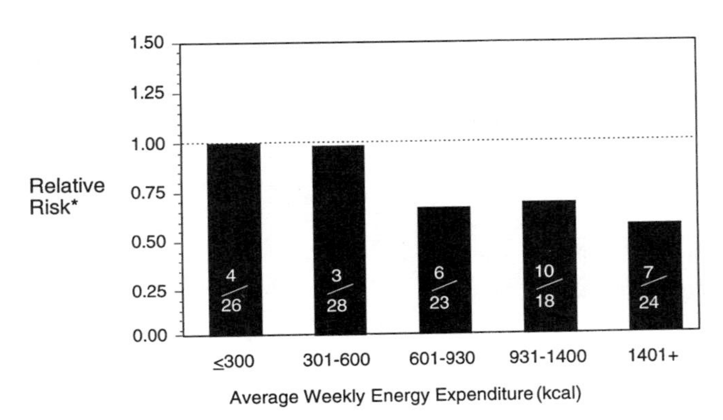

FIG. 47–3. Relative risk of ovulatory menstrual cycles in teenage girls by physical activity.[33] *Adjusted for gynecological age and age at menarche. Test for trend: one-sided $P = 0.03$. (From Bernstein et al, 1987.)

in the age-specific incidence rate of breast cancer slows markedly at the time of menopause, and the rate of increase in the postmenopausal period is only about one-sixth the rate of increase in the premenopausal period.

It has been estimated that women who experience natural menopause (defined as cessation of periods) before age 45 have only one-half the breast cancer risk of those whose menopause occurs after age 55 (Trichopoulos et al, 1972) (Table 47–2). Another way of expressing this result is that women with 40 or more years of active menstruation have twice the breast cancer risk of those with fewer than 30 years of menstrual activity. Artificial menopause, by either bilateral oophorectomy or pelvic irradiation, also markedly reduces breast cancer risk. The effect appears to be just slightly greater than that of natural menopause, probably because surgical removal of the ovaries causes an abrupt cessation of hormone production whereas some hormone production continues for a few months or years after the

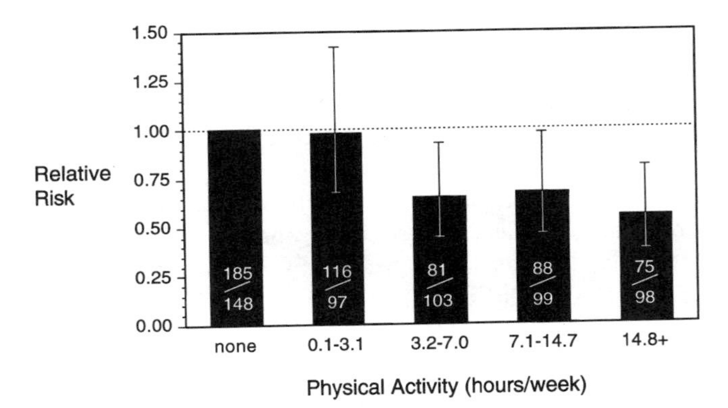

FIG. 47–4. Average hours of intense physical activity per week, breast cancer cases aged 40 and under and controls.[34] $P = 0.0004$ (trend).

TABLE 47–2. *Relative Risk of Breast Cancer by Age at Menopause**

	Age at Menopause			
	<44	45–49	50–54	≥55
Artificial menopause[a]	0.77	1.00	1.34	—
Natural menopause	1.00	1.27	1.47	2.03

*From Trichopoulos et al, 1972.
[a]Bilateral oophorectomy.

natural cessation of menses at the menopause. Feinleib (1968) showed that unilateral oophorectomy or a simple hysterectomy produced little change in risk.

Pregnancy

Two of the earliest known and most reproducible features of breast cancer epidemiology are the decreased risk associated with increased parity and the increased risk of single women.

MacMahon et al (1970) made a major advance in our understanding of the role of pregnancy in altering breast cancer risk through their analysis of an international collaborative case–control study. Single and nulliparous married women were found to have the same increased risk of breast cancer, approximately 1.4 times the risk of parous married women. Among married women in each country, parous cases had fewer children than parous controls. These authors clearly demonstrated, however, that this protective effect of parity was totally due to a protective effect of early age at first birth. Those women with a first birth under age 20 had about one-half the risk of nulliparous women. Controlling for age at first birth, subsequent births had no influence on the risk of developing breast cancer. More recent studies in other populations have observed a small residual protective effect of an increasing number of births, suggesting that, under certain circumstances, multiparity does offer some further protection. In a study in Shanghai, we observed a protective effect of multiple pregnancies, which was most notable after the fifth pregnancy (Yuan et al, 1988) (Table 47–3). The main protective effect is, however, undoubtedly associated with the first full-term pregnancy.

Married women who have a late first full-term pregnancy are actually at an elevated risk of breast cancer, compared with nulliparous women (MacMahon et al, 1970). This paradoxical effect of a late first full-term pregnancy has been confirmed repeatedly. A possible explanation for this effect is suggested by several related observations. In a hospital-based case–control study, the risk of breast cancer was substantially higher among women who had given birth during the 3 years before

TABLE 47–3. *Relative Risk of Breast Cancer by Number of Full-Term Pregnancies Among Parous Cases and Controls**

Number of FTP	*Cases*	*Controls*	*Relative Risk (RR) (95% CI)*	*Adjusted RR (95% CI)*
1	116	77	1.00	1.00[a]
2	113	100	0.61 (0.39, 0.96)	0.72 (0.45, 1.16)
3	78	74	0.47 (0.28, 0.79)	0.67 (0.38, 1.21)
4	55	61	0.33 (0.11, 0.34)	0.59 (0.30, 1.16)
5+	67	117	0.19 (0.11, 0.34)	0.39 (0.19, 0.80)

*From Yuan et al, 1988.
[a]One-sided significance levels after adjustment by analysis of covariance for cycle length (days) and age (yr), and for weight for SHBG.

TABLE 47–4. *Geometric Mean Levels of Plasma and Urinary Hormones and Relevant Characteristics of Nulliparous and Parous Women with 24- to 32-day Menstrual Cycles at Time of Sampling**

Variable	*Nulliparous Women, n = 59*	*Parous Women, n = 47*	*P-value*[a]
PLASMA HORMONE			
Prolactin, ng/ml	23.2	17.1	.001
E_1, ng/100 ml	8.7	8.0	.079
E_2, ng/100 ml	14.8	12.0	.001
SHBG, 10^{-8} *M*	3.8	4.2	.099
Urinary hormone, *pg*/12 hr			
E_1	4.9	4.0	.018
E_2	2.6	2.1	.008
E_3	5.7	4.6	.029
$E_1 + E_2 + E_3$	13.7	11.1	.010
CHARACTERISTIC			
Age, yr	33.3	33.3	.499
Weight, lbs	137.9	134.1	.200
Cycle length, days	28.2	28.0	.307

*From Bernstein et al, 1985.
[a]One-sided significance levels after adjustment by analysis of covariance for cycle length (days) and age (yr), and in addition for weight for SHBG.

the interview than among comparable women whose last birth occurred 10 years earlier (relative risk [RR] = 2.66) (Bruzzi et al, 1988). We found that a first-trimester abortion, whether spontaneous or induced, before the first full-term pregnancy, was associated with an increased risk of breast cancer (Pike et al, 1981). This observation has been confirmed in cohorts of Connecticut and New York women (Hadjimichael et al, 1986; Howe et al, 1989). Furthermore, concurrent or recent previous pregnancy appears to contribute to poor breast cancer survival (Guinee et al, 1994).

We concluded that pregnancy has two contradictory effects on breast cancer risk which are particularly notable in the first pregnancy. This apparent paradox actually has a physiologic explanation that is based on estrogen and prolactin secretion and metabolism during pregnancy. During the first trimester of pregnancy there is a rapid rise in the level of "free" estradiol, an effect that is more apparent in the first, compared with subsequent pregnancies (Bernstein et al, 1986). The net effect of this early part of pregnancy, in terms of estrogen exposure to the breast, is equivalent to several ovulatory cycles over a relatively short time.

However, in the long run, this negative effect of early pregnancy on breast cancer risk can be overridden by two beneficial consequences of a completed pregnancy. Several years ago we reported (Yu et al, 1981) that prolactin levels were substantially lower in parous compared with nulliparous women, an observation that has been replicated recently (Musey et al, 1987). In addition, we found that parous women had higher levels of sex hormone–binding globulin (SHBG) and lower levels of free (non–protein-bound) estradiol than their nulliparous counterparts (Bernstein et al, 1985) (Table 47–4).

Lactation

Lactation has been increasingly reported to protect against breast cancer development. If the cumulative number of ovulatory cycles is directly related to breast cancer risk, a beneficial effect of long duration of nursing would be expected, because nursing results in a substantial delay in re-establishing ovulation following a completed pregnancy. With only a small proportion of mothers having a large cumulative number of nursing months, most previous epidemiologic studies have been unable to provide precise estimates of the effects of lactation on breast cancer risk. We recently completed a population-based case–control study in China, a population in which long-duration nursing is the norm. In that study a progressive reduction in breast cancer risk was observed with an increasing number of years of nursing experience (Ross and Yu, 1994; Yuan et al, 1988) (Fig. 47–5).

Weight

In addition to the menstrual and reproductive risk factors described in the foregoing, there is a strong relationship between weight and breast cancer risk. The relationship is critically dependent on age. For women under age 50 there is little or no increased risk associated with increased weight, but by age 60, a 10-kg increment in weight results in approximately an 80% increase in breast cancer risk (de Waard et al, 1977) (Table 47–5).

Whether this weight effect is one of excess weight (body fat) or weight per se is unclear. Contradictory results have been reported, for example, on whether

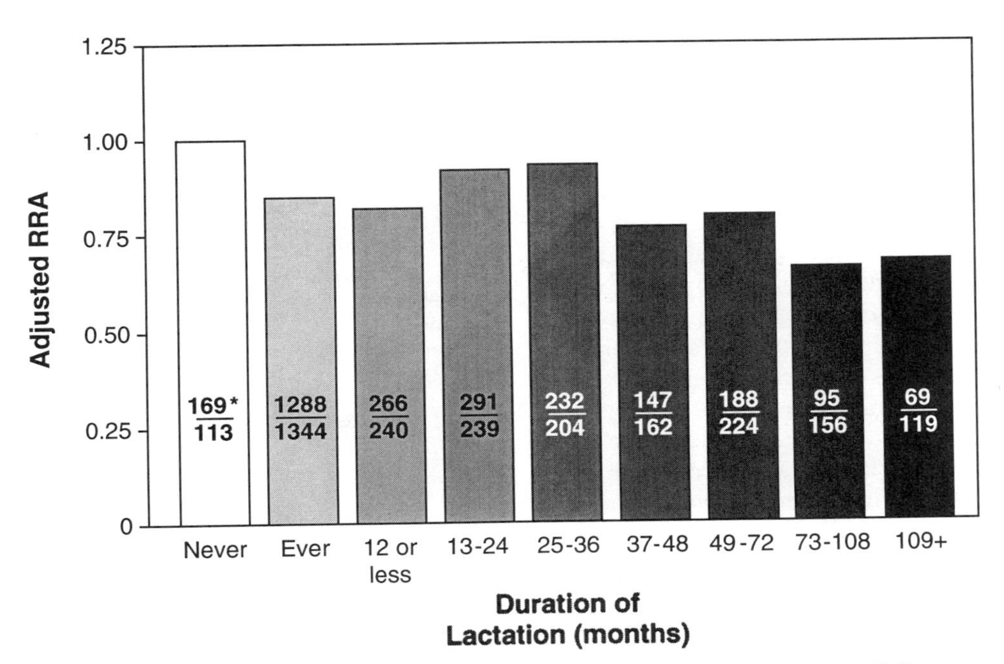

FIG. 47–5. Duration of lactation among parous breast cancer cases and controls in China.[38, 48] *Case/controls; test for trend: two-sided $P < 0.01$.

Quetelet's index (a measure of body mass) is correlated with breast cancer risk. Unadjusted weight appears to be as good an indicator of risk as any function of weight and height. In the postmenopausal period the major source of estrogen is from extraglandular (largely adipose tissue) conversion of the adrenal androgen, androstenedione, to estrone (Siiteri et al, 1981).

Menstrual Cycle Length

Long menstrual cycles generally have the same luteal phase as short cycles (Aksel, 1981), i.e., the length of the luteal phase is approximately 14 days irrespective of the length of the follicular (preovulatory) phase. If the cumulative frequency of ovulatory cycles is a primary determinant of breast cancer risk, then women with short (ovulatory) cycles should be at increased risk of breast cancer. Furthermore, women in countries with high breast cancer rates might be expected to have shorter average cycles than women in countries with low breast cancer rates.

Olsson et al (1983) made a retrospective assessment of menstrual cycle length in breast cancer cases and controls. There was a highly significant difference between the two groups; the average cycle length of the breast cancer patients was 26.4 days compared to 28.6 days for the controls. These findings were later confirmed by LaVecchia and colleagues (1985). Studies of menstrual cycle length in Japanese and U.S. women suggest that Japanese women also have longer cycles than U.S. women—28.8 days versus 27.1 days at age 30 (Matsumoto et al, 1962; Treloar et al, 1967).

TABLE 47–5. *Relative Risk of Breast Cancer by Body Weight**

	Weight (kg)		
Age at Diagnosis	*<60*	*60–69*	*≥70*
35–49	1.00	0.94	1.16
50–59	1.00	1.22	1.43
60–69	1.00	1.61	1.81

*From de Waard et al, 1977.

Exogenous Estrogens

There is evidence that long-term use of exogenous estrogens, given as hormone replacement therapy to postmenopausal women, increases the risk of breast cancer (Henderson et al, 1993). The magnitude of this increased risk is considerably less than for endometrial cancer among women exposed to exogenous estrogens. This issue is carefully reviewed in Chapter 49 and will not be discussed further here.

A MODEL OF BREAST CANCER PATHOGENESIS

Pike and co-workers (1983) developed a model of breast cancer incidence that incorporates all of the reproductive and endocrine risk factors and provides an excellent fit to the actual age-specific incidence curves for breast cancer in different populations (Figs. 47–6 and 47–7). This model is based on the concept that breast cancer incidence does not increase proportionally with calendar age, but rather with breast tissue age raised to the power 4.5. The concept of breast tissue age is closely associated with the cell kinetics of breast tissue stem cells, which, in turn, are closely associated with exposure of breast tissue to ovarian hormones. The model predicts relative risks that are remarkably consistent with the observed values for each of these risk factors, including the two contradictory effects of pregnancy. This model allows us to explore the degree to which variations in these risk factors among different populations may explain the large international variation in breast cancer rates, e.g., such as those between Japan and the United States.

As of 1970, age-adjusted incidence rates of breast cancer were some five to six times higher in the United States than in Japan. Data on average age at menarche, first birth, and menopause among Japanese are available

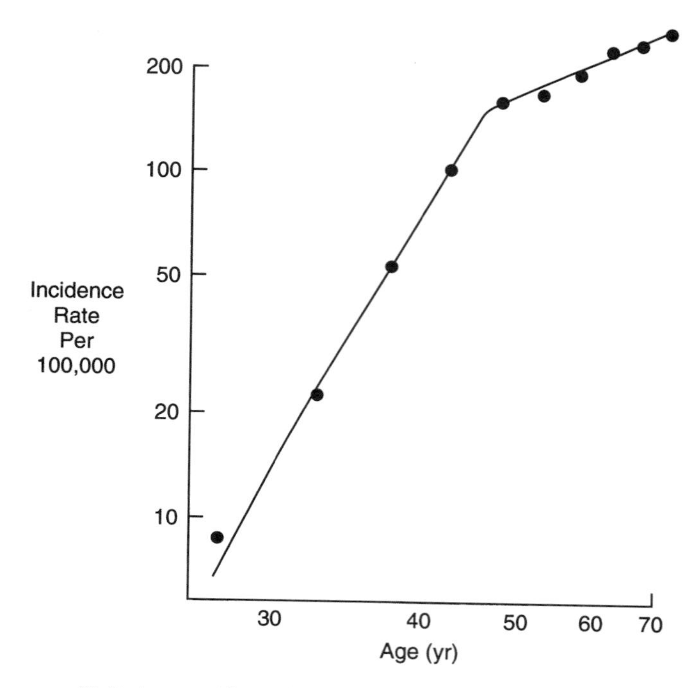

FIG. 47–7. Age-specific incidence rates for breast cancer in U.S. white women from Third National Cancer Survey, National Cancer Institute, 1969–1971. The dots are the actual incidence data and the solid line marks the expected incidence rates calculated from the model in Figure 47–6.

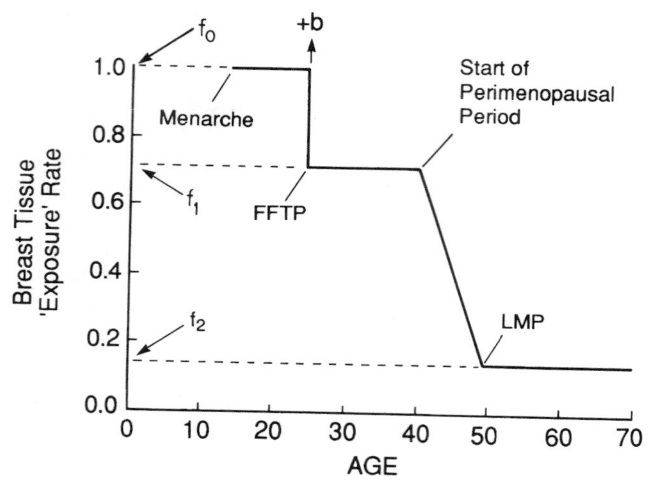

FIG. 47–6. Model of rate of breast tissue aging. For most hormone-dependent cancers the relationship between incidence, I, and age, t, can be represented by the equation $I(t) = at^k$ which produces a straight line with slope k when the logarithm of incidence is plotted against the logarithm of age (t). Breast cancer incidence can be reconciled with a linear log = log plot of incidence against age if t in the formula is considered to be the cumulative "effective mitotic rate" of the breast epithelium. The fundamental idea is that "aging" of the breast relates directly to its cell kinetics. When the tissue is not undergoing cell division, the rate of aging is zero, whereas aging is maximum when the mitotic rate is maximal. To adapt the above equation to breast cancer incidence, a simple model assumes aging begins at menarche with rate $f_0 = 1$, is modified by first full-term pregnancy (FFTP) to $f_1 = 0.7$, is reduced further by the onset of the premenopause at age 40, and eventually slows at the last menstrual period (LMP) to $f_2 = 0.1$. A small increase in risk of the initial part of pregnancy is represented by the value b. The value of k is set at 4.5. For further details see Pike et al (1983).

from a 1970 survey (Hoel et al, 1983). The average age at natural menopause of Japanese women is similar to that of American women for these age-groups, but fewer Japanese women have had a surgical menopause. The data on menarche favor a lower breast cancer incidence rate for Japanese women: older Japanese women had a much later menarche than American women, but the data on age at first birth and nulliparity show that none of the decreased breast cancer rates in Japan can be attributed to these factors.

Japanese breast cancer rates remain almost constant after age 50 (Hoel et al, 1983). In model terms, this implies that no further breast tissue aging occurs in Japanese women in the postmenopausal period. This is, in all probability, a reflection of body weight. In 1970 the average weight of postmenopausal women was less than 50 kg and these women were unlikely to have been producing significant amounts of estrogen.

The model-predicted breast cancer incidence rates of Japanese women, which allow for their actual distribution of the established breast cancer risk factors, are still considerably lower than the observed rates for U.S. whites, whereas they are between 2.4- and 3.8-fold greater than observed Japanese rates. The very late menarche in Japanese women would be expected to result in a substantial delay in the establishment of regular menstrual cycles compared with U.S. women. After allowing for this delay and incorporating the differences in average cycle length and the lower estrogen levels (see below) actually achieved during a typical ovulatory cycle in Asian women compared with U.S. white women (Bernstein et al, 1990; MacMahon et al, 1974), the predicted Japanese rates are essentially identical to those observed in United States whites.

HORMONAL DATA

Estrogens

The association of breast cancer with cyclic ovarian activity implies that estrogen is important in the pathogenesis of this disease. We have discussed the rationale that hormones, and in particular, estradiol, can directly increase the incidence of breast cancer (Henderson et al, 1988). A substantial amount of experimental work demonstrates the critical role of estrogens in breast cancer in experimental animals. Exogenous estrone, estradiol, and under some conditions, estriol, increase the incidence of mammary tumors in mice and rats. They also increase the tumor yield and decrease the time to induction following administration of dimethylbenzanthracine. Removing the ovaries or administering an antiestrogenic drug has the opposite effect (Dao, 1981).

Attempts to understand and quantify the role of estrogen in breast cancer development have been limited to some extent by our technical capability for measuring steroid hormones in human blood. A few studies of estrogen levels in premenopausal patients and controls have been reported. England and co-workers (1974) found a 15% average elevation of plasma total estrogens in patients with breast cancer, and a similar increase was reported by others for total urinary estrogens (England et al, 1974; MacMahon et al, 1982). Problems with such studies have been discussed. In particular, it has been pointed out that, in a number of studies, urine collection was neither done on a fixed day of the cycle nor in a similar manner for cases and controls (Bernstein and Ross, 1993). It was also noted that very close age matching is probably required in the premenopausal period.

The first substantial study of plasma estrogen levels in postmenopausal breast cancer cases and controls was reported by England et al (England et al, 1974). They studied the estradiol levels of 25 cases and 25 controls and found that, on average, the levels were 30% higher in cases. There have been at least 12 additional studies on plasma estrogens and 7 on urinary estrogens in postmenopausal breast cancer cases and controls (Bernstein and Ross, 1993). Taken together, these studies support the finding of increased levels of estrogen and in particular, estradiol, found by England and associates (1974).

Recent findings emphasize the possible importance of bioavailable estradiol fractions in the etiology of breast cancer. Siiteri and colleagues (1981) studied a small group of breast cancer patients and controls matched on age, weight, height, and menopausal status; they found the known relationship between obesity, SHBG, and increased free estradiol in both patients and controls. They also found that some "normal-weight" breast cancer patients with normal SHBG levels had an elevated percentage of free estradiol. These results suggest that in breast cancer patients, free estradiol in serum may be elevated by factors unrelated to SHBG concentration.

Moore and co-authors (1982) compared total and non–protein-bound estradiol levels of 38 postmenopausal women with breast cancer with those of 38 controls of similar age and weight. Breast cancer patients had significantly higher levels of total estradiol and free estradiol than controls, and significantly less SHBG. In fact, the level of free estradiol in patients was nearly four times that of controls. Jones et al (1987) reported similar results in comparing 32 women with breast cancer and 188 controls. The mean percentage free estradiol and percentage albumin-bound estradiol were significantly higher in the patients.

The most carefully done international studies comparing estrogen levels in populations at differing risks of breast cancer also support a role of estrogens, particularly estradiol, in the pathogenesis of breast cancer. In the early 1970s, MacMahon et al 1974) conducted a series of studies on teenagers and young women to investigate whether some aspect of estrogen metabolism was responsible for the large differences in breast cancer rates between Asia and North America. They found that, in overnight urine samples collected on the morning of day 21 of the menstrual cycle, total urinary estrogen levels were 36% higher in the North American teenagers. In nulliparous women aged 20 to 24, total urinary estrogen levels were 49% higher on day 21 and 38% higher on day 10; similar differences were found among parous women aged 30 to 39. In two more recent studies, we have characterized the relationship between serum estradiol levels and the international differences in breast cancer risk (Bernstein et al, 1990; Shimizu et al, 1990). Geometric mean estradiol levels were higher in breast cancer cases than in controls in Shanghai and Los Angeles and estradiol levels were 20% higher in Los Angeles compared to Shanghai controls (Bernstein et al, 1990) (Table 47–6). In a comparison of postmenopausal women, the differences were even more striking with estradiol levels 36% higher in Los Angeles women than their age-matched Japanese counterparts (Shimizu et al, 1990). There are at least two possible explanations for these differences in estradiol levels: (1) physical activity, e.g. greater physical activity among Asians, which might alter the frequency or

TABLE 47–6. *Geometric Mean Values (with 95% Confidence Intervals) for Serum Estradiol and SHBG on Premenopausal Women with Breast Cancer and Individually Matched Control Women in Shanghai, China (39 pairs) and Los Angeles, California (42 pairs)*†

Variable	*Study Group*	*Cases*	*Controls*	*P-value** *Case vs. Control*
Estradiol (pmol/L)	Shanghai Chinese	584 (509–671)	501 (444–565)	0.089
	Los Angeles whites	669 (586–761)	604 (530–687)	0.23
	P-value* (control comparison)		0.036	
SHBG (nmol/L)	Shanghai Chinese	59.4 (50.3–70.2)	61.6 (55.4–68.6)	0.71
	Los Angeles whites	54.1 (46.4–63.0)	59.1 (51.5–68.0)	0.28
	P-value* (control comparison)		0.63	

†From Bernstein et al, 1990.
*Two-sided *P*-value; paired *t*-test for matched case–control comparisons and Student's *t*-test for comparison of controls.

length of ovulatory cycles; and (2) higher dietary fiber intake among Asians, which might alter fecal excretion of enterohepatic steroids and thereby lower plasma estradiol levels (Aldercreutz et al, 1987).

More recently, much interest has focused on the issue of the relationship of increased breast cancer risk and exposure to certain organochlorine compounds (particularly those commonly used in pesticides) and possibly to other halogenated compounds (Davis et al, 1993). The assumed mechanism by which these compounds influence breast cancer risk is their estrogenic effects. However, the observed estrogenicity of these compounds is relatively low. Hence it has been suggested that they would provide only a small increase in exposure to estrogen among women. It has been proposed that differences in two alternative pathways of estradiol metabolism are associated with risk of breast cancer, with 16-alpha-hydroxylation (vs. 2-hydroxylation) associated with elevated risk (Fishman et al, 1983; Schneider et al, 1982). Metabolites resulting from these two metabolic pathways differ in biologic properties. 16-alpha-hydroxyestrone (16-OHE1) is a potent estrogen whereas 2-hydroxyestrone (2-OHE1) is not. Several small studies have suggested that the extent of 16-alpha-hydroxylation is greater among breast cancer cases than among controls (Fishman et al, 1983; Osborne et al, 1993; Schneider et al, 1982). Highly trained athletes who are amenorrheic also appear to metabolize more readily along the 2-hydroxylation pathway (Snow et al, 1989). Although not all researchers agree that 16-alpha-hydroxylation is the critical pathway (Aldercreutz et al, 1989; Lemon et al, 1993) for breast cancer risk, variations in estrogen metabolism could substantially influence the estrogenic effects of phytoestrogens and organochlorine compounds.

Progesterone

Evidence that elevated levels of the other major ovarian hormone, progesterone, may also be an important factor in increasing breast cancer risk has only recently been summarized (Key and Pike, 1988). The mitotic activity of breast epithelium varies markedly during the normal menstrual cycle, with peak activity occurring late in the luteal phase (Ferguson and Anderson, 1981; Potten et al, 1988). This suggests that progesterone, at least in the presence of estrogen, induces mitotic activity in breast epithelium. This effect of progesterone would be in sharp contrast to its effect on endometrial tissue, in which the peak mitotic activity occurs in the estrogen-dominated follicular phase of the cycle. It strongly agrees, however, with the experimental findings that progesterone induces ductal growth in rodent breast tissue (Dulbecco et al, 1982). If progesterone does increase breast cancer risk, then regular ovulatory cycles should be more common in breast cancer patients than in controls. Breast cancer patients would be expected to have shorter cycles on average than controls, because differences in cycle length are almost completely due to differences in the length of the follicular phase. In ovulatory menstrual cycles, the shorter the cycle length, the greater the proportion of time a women spends in the luteal phase with its associated high progesterone level (Aksel, 1981). Although few studies have addressed these issues, they all provide support for this role for progesterone (Henderson et al, 1975; Olsson et al, 1983).

Several studies have measured progesterone, or its major urinary metabolite pregnanediol, in premenopausal women. All four studies of pregnanediol, and five of six studies of progesterone, found lower levels in breast cancer cases than in controls (Key and Pike, 1988). There is reason to suspect, however, that early in the clinical course of breast cancer, the regularity of ovulation is disrupted, so that such case–control comparisons may be misleading (Bernstein et al, 1990). Furthermore, luteal-phase progesterone levels are difficult to quantitate with spot samples because the amount of progesterone detected in plasma or the amount of progesterone metabolites in urine depends specifically on the day of sampling in relation to the luteal phase peak. Three prospective studies have examined breast cancer incidence in women with clinical evidence of progesterone deficiency and all report elevated risks (Key and Pike, 1988). Overall, there is little objective evidence supporting the role of progesterone in the pathogenesis of breast cancer. More direct evidence to support or refute the role of progesterone should come from surveillance of women receiving medroxyprogesterone as a form of contraception or hormone replacement therapy.

Prolactin

One of the hormone changes that accompanies puberty is an increase in prolactin levels. Prolactin is a critically important hormone in mammary carcinogenesis in the rat. In humans, prolactin, in association with estrogen, directly affects the growth of breast epithelium. A decrease in prolactin levels appears to be part of the mechanism by which pregnancy reduces breast cancer risk (Musey et al, 1987; Yu et al, 1981). Case–control studies of breast cancer patients provide some support for a role of prolactin in the etiology of breast cancer (Henderson et al, 1984; Levin and Malarkey, 1981). Such studies have consistently found higher prolactin levels in premenopausal cases but not among postmenopausal women (Henderson et al, 1984). The finding of higher prolactin levels in post- compared to premastectomy breast cancer patients (Rose and Pruitt, 1981) emphasizes the caution required in evaluating these case–control comparisons.

Studies comparing prolactin levels among women in countries with different breast cancer rates have not found any substantial differences in daytime prolactin levels (Gray et al, 1982). Prolactin levels have marked diurnal variation, and further work is needed before one can be certain that there are not major differences in peak prolactin levels which occur a few hours before waking.

For a time it appeared that prolactin might provide the link between dietary fat and breast cancer. Rats fed a high-fat diet have elevated prolactin levels, and drugs which block prolactin secretion abolish the difference in tumor yield which normally occurs between rats on low and high-fat diets when they are given a carcinogen (Carroll, 1975). Hill and Wynder (1976) found that peak nocturnal prolaction levels fell by half in seven female nurses who reduced their fat intake from 40% to 33% of calories for two weeks, but another small study failed to confirm this finding (Gray et al, 1981). An international study found no difference in circulating prolactin levels between Japanese and American girls with a twofold difference in fat consumption (Gray et al, 1982).

Various drugs, including reserpine, phenothiazines, methyldopa, and tricyclic antidepressants, are known to increase prolactin secretion. Several case–control studies of reserpine and breast cancer have reported small to moderate increases (1.5- to 2.0-fold) in risk (Anonymous, 1974; Armstrong et al, 1974; Heinen et al, 1974), and it has been suggested that even this modest increased risk may be due to confounding by socioeconomic status or other breast cancer risk factors (Armstrong et al, 1976). Ross et al (1984) have demonstrated that long-term reserpine users have approximately 50% higher levels of prolactin. They have argued that the observed small increases in risk associated with long-term reserpine use are consistent with predicted relative risks based on these prolactin changes.

OTHER POSSIBLE RISK FACTORS

Dietary Factors

Much attention has been focused on dietary differences, particularly fat consumption, to explain both the international pattern of breast cancer occurrence and the changes in rates of breast cancer with migration (Armstrong and Doll, 1975; Carroll, 1975; Gray et al, 1979; Prentice et al, 1988). International breast cancer mortality rates are highly correlated with per capita consumption of fat ($r = 0.93$) (Gray et al, 1979). There is a wealth of evidence that nutrition profoundly influences breast cancer occurrence by modifying age at menarche and weight, but the correlation of fat with international breast cancer mortality remains highly significant after statistical adjustment for those factors. Hirayama (1978) reported that breast cancer mortality rates in various regions of Japan are highly correlated with fat consumption. When international breast cancer incidence rates rather than mortality rates are considered, the magnitude of the correlation coefficient is still very high ($r = 0.84$) (Gray et al, 1979).

Many case–control studies of fat consumption and breast cancer have found only small differences between cases and controls—generally no larger than the differences in total calorie consumption (Miller and Bulbrook, 1986; Nomura et al, 1978). However, Howe and colleagues (1990) recently conducted a combined analysis of dietary risk factors for breast cancer from 12 large case–control studies representing populations with a wide range of dietary habits and underlying breast cancer rates. They found a positive association between both total fat and saturated fat intake and breast cancer risk among postmenopausal women (approximately 50% difference in risk among individuals in the highest versus lowest quintile of intake). Nonetheless, the three cohort studies that have used food-frequency questionnaires to study the relationship of diet and breast cancer have found no clear or consistent relationship with either total fat, saturated fat, or vegetable fat (Howe et al, 1991b; Hunter and Willett, 1994; Mills et al, 1989; Willett et al, 1987).

Albanes (1987) has summarized an extensive number of animal experiments on the interrelationships of caloric and fat intake, weight, and mammary tumor incidence. He showed that in the face of the limited physical activity of a laboratory animal, caloric intake was highly correlated with both weight and increased mammary cancer risk (Table 47–7). Fat per se was clearly unimportant in these studies, outside of its contribution to total caloric intake.

Prentice et al (1988) have attempted to reconcile these inconsistent observations on the possible role of dietary fat by arguing that the narrow range of fat intake within any population and the measurement error associated with retrospective or prospective dietary assessment instruments bias relative risk estimates towards 1.0. The effect of dietary change on hormonal profiles in healthy women is not well studied. There is some evidence that a reduction in fat intake may reduce circulating estradiol levels in postmenopausal women (Prentice et al, 1990).

Diets high in fiber may protect against breast cancer, perhaps because fiber may reduce the intestinal reabsorption of estrogens excreted via the biliary system (Aldercreutz et al, 1987; Goldin et al, 1982). In one animal study (Cohen et al, 1991), a high-fiber diet was associated with reduced incidence of mammary cancer. Assessment of fiber intake in epidemiologic studies has been problematic because of a paucity of data on the fiber content of individual foods and disagreement about the most appropriate methods of biochemical analysis to determine different types of fiber. In their meta-analysis of ten case–control studies that included data on dietary fiber intake, Howe et al (1990) reported a statistically significant 15% reduction in risk for a 20 g/day increase in dietary fiber. In a case–control study of 519 cases nested in a prospective cohort, Rohan et al (1993) observed a marginally significant inverse association between dietary fiber and breast cancer risk, but this finding was no longer significant after controlling for vitamin A intake. Graham et al (1992) observed no suggestion of a protective association in another prospective cohort with 344 cases. The relationship between total dietary fiber intake and subsequent breast cancer incidence in a large prospective investigation was very close to null (Willett et al, 1992), which suggests that any protective effect of dietary fiber is likely to be small.

TABLE 47–7. *Effect of Dietary Fat and Total Calories on Breast Tumor Incidence in Mice**

Diet			
Calories	*Fat*	*Body wt (g)*	*Tumor Incidence (%)*
Low	Low	20.2 ± 1.0[a]	34.4 ± 4.3
Low	High	20.9 ± 1.1	23.1 ± 4.7
High	Low	29.0 ± 1.1	52.4 ± 4.7
High	High	32.6 ± 0.8	54.4 ± 3.4

*Modified from Albanes (1987), summarizing 82 experiments in the literature

[a]Mean ± SE.

Micronutrient intake and breast cancer risk has been the subject of several studies (Hunter and Willett, 1994), but no consistent relationship has emerged. Perhaps the most interesting results suggest a protective effect of vitamin A (Hunter et al, 1993). Randomized clinical trials utilizing various micronutrients are underway and should provide more definitive information on this issue.

Finally, foods rich in phytoestrogens, in particular soy protein, have been found in a study in Singapore to be protective (Lee et al, 1991). However, two case–control studies in the Peoples Republic of China show no evidence of such protection (Yuan, 1995). The presumed mechanism by which phytoestrogens influence breast cancer risk is their estrogenic effects, i.e., competition for metabolites or binding sites with estradiol as discussed above for the organochlorine compounds.

Family History

A family history of breast cancer is associated with an increased risk of the disease. This is particularly so if the family history includes a woman who was affected at an early age or had bilateral disease. Whereas overall, two- to threefold increased risk of the disease has been observed in first degree relatives of breast cancer cases, a ninefold increased risk has been found in first degree relatives of premenopausal women with bilateral breast cancer (Anderson, 1974). High risks (fivefold increases) have also been found for women with multiple first degree relatives with breast cancer.

The patterns of risks observed among the relatives of breast cancer cases in epidemiologic studies are consistent with a genetic model. More formal genetic analyses corroborate the genetic hypothesis. The majority of segregation analyses of breast cancer pedigrees has provided evidence for the existence of one or more rare autosomal dominant genes leading to increased susceptibility to breast cancer (Bishop et al, 1988; Claus et al, 1991; Iselius et al, 1991; Newman et al, 1988; Williams and Anderson, 1984), including a recent segregation analysis of the 4,730 breast cancer cases from the Cancer and Steroid Hormone (CASH) study (Claus et al, 1991).

The results of segregation analyses have been confirmed by recent linkage analyses. These analyses provide strong evidence for the existence of a breast cancer susceptibility gene (or genes) located on the long arm of chromosome 17 (Easton et al, 1993; Hall et al, 1990, 1992; Narod et al, 1991). In the families for whom linkage has been found, the transmission of breast cancer is consistent with an autosomal dominant inheritance pattern. Hall et al (1990), the first group to report linkage of breast cancer to chromosome 17q21, found particularly strong evidence of linkage in families with an early age at onset. In 1991 Narod et al (1991) showed that both breast and ovarian cancer were linked to chromosome 17q12-23 by examining five families characterized by multiple cases of early-onset breast and ovarian cancer. The authors did find evidence of genetic heterogeneity, however, as only three of the five families appeared to be linked to chromosome 17.

In an effort to confirm the aforementioned linkage results as well as to attempt to localize a breast cancer gene, called *BRCA1*, members of the Breast Cancer Consortium (Easton et al, 1993) recently analyzed 214 extensive breast cancer pedigrees, including 57 families characterized by both breast and ovarian cancer. Current estimates of the gene frequency from the Consortium and additional analyses indicate, however, that the *BRCA1* gene is likely to account for approximately 5–7% of all breast cancers. This gene has been recently characterized and various mutations described in some of the breast and ovarian cancer kindred, but not in sporadic cases (Futreal et al, 1994; Miki et al, 1994). A second breast cancer susceptibility locus, BRCA2, has been localized on chromosome 13q12-13 (Wooster et al, 1994) and a third locus proposed (Cornelis et al, 1994).

The recent finding of germline *TP53* mutations in the Li-Fraumini syndrome suggests another potential mechanism of genetic susceptibility (Malkin et al, 1992). Breast cancer is a common feature of this syndrome. The other genes critical to breast cancer risk are those that control the metabolism of estradiol (e.g., 17 hydroxysteroid dehydrogenase [17HSD] and the activity of the estrogen receptor in the breast epithelial cell (Fig. 47–8). In breast tissue there are at least two forms of 17HSD (Types I and II), one of which seems to favor the reductive conversion of estrone to estradiol (Poutanen et al, 1993). The *EDH17B2* (which codes for 17HSD I) gene is encoded by two autosomal codominant alleles and there is some suggestion of an association between differences in exon 6 polymorphisms and the risk of breast cancer in a Finnish population (Mannermaa et al, 1994). The estrogen receptor gene is a large gene (> 140 kb in length) (Piva et al, 1992; Ponglikitmongkol et al, 1988) and several polymorphisms and mutations have been described (Yaich et al, 1992; Zuppan et al, 1991). Substantial polymorphism has been reported for a TA

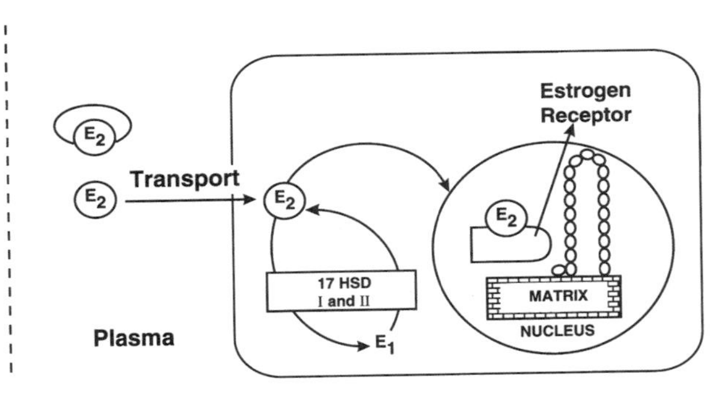

FIG. 47–8. Metabolism and transport of estradiol (E_2) in breast epithelial cells (17 HSD = 17 hydroxysteroid dehydrogenase, E_1 = estrone).

repeat in the upstream promoter region of the gene as well (del Senno et al, 1992). The functional significance of these and presumably other yet-to-be-described polymorphisms needs to be clarified.

Benign Breast Disease

The most common type of benign breast disease is chronic cystic or fibrocystic disease. This lesion is clinically recognized when a cystic dilatation of a duct becomes large enough to be palpable and is most commonly diagnosed in middle-aged women (Cole et al, 1978). Women with cystic breast disease have a two- to threefold elevated risk of developing breast cancer (Kodlin et al, 1977).

Fibroadenoma is the second most common histologic type of benign breast lesion. These tumors are usually solitary and are diagnosed most often in young women (Cole et al, 1978). The breast cancer risk associated with fibroadenoma is not well established, but Kodlin et al (1977) found a sevenfold increased risk in a follow-up study of women with this condition. Subsequent studies have indicated that the overall risk is actually closer to twofold, although some groups of fibroadenomas carry a somewhat higher risk (Dupont et al, 1994; Levi et al, 1994).

For both fibrocystic disease and fibroadenoma it is probably not the lesion per se that is the precursor of the breast cancer but the epithelial proliferative lesions that are associated with these benign changes. Black et al (1972) found that they could distinguish a subgroup of women with benign breast disease with "atypical" epithelial changes; these women had a fivefold increased risk of breast cancer compared to other women with benign breast disease. This relationship has been further clarified and quantified by Dupont and Page (1985) and London and colleagues (1992). These investigators have demonstrated that there is little or no increase in risk for women with non-proliferative benign breast disease, a modest increase in risk among women with proliferative disease with no atypia, and, verifying the results of Black et al (1972), a four- to fivefold increase in risk for women with atypical hyperplasia.

Benign breast disease has been defined in a useful way radiologically as well as histologically. Wolfe et al (1982) showed that women whose mammograms show "dysplasia" (DY pattern) or a greater than normal amount of "prominent ducts" (P_2 pattern) are at an increased risk of breast cancer (Wolfe et al, 1982). These findings have been reproduced by others (Saftlas et al, 1989; Wilkinson et al, 1977). These mammographic patterns are related to established breast cancer risk factors such as age at first birth, age at menopause, and family history of breast cancer (Wilkinson et al, 1977), but these associations are not large enough to explain totally the association of breast mammographic patterns with risk of breast cancer.

Fuller definition of the varieties of benign breast disease and clarification of their relationship with breast cancer should permit the reliable identification of subgroups of the population of women with benign breast disease at very different risks of breast cancer.

Cigarette Smoking

Baron (1984) and MacMahon (1990) have recently reviewed the epidemiologic evidence on the association of cigarette smoking and breast cancer. Smoking produces an anti-estrogenic effect, altering the risk of several estrogen-related diseases including osteoporotic fractures (increased risk in smokers) and endometrial cancer (decreased risk in smokers) (Baron, 1984). The exact mechanism for the anti-estrogenic effect of smoking is unclear. Published data do not suggest large differences in circulating estrogen levels in postmenopausal smokers compared to non-smokers (Barrett-Conner, 1990). There are some data to suggest that smokers have increased hydroxylation of estradiol to inactive metabolites (Michnovicz et al, 1986).

Alcohol Consumption

A positive association between alcohol consumption and breast cancer has been reported in a large series of recent studies. These have been extensively reviewed and summarized in meta-analyses conducted by Longnecker and colleagues (1988) and more recently by Howe et al (1991a). The summary data suggest that women who consume three or more alcoholic drinks per day have about 50–70% increase in breast cancer risk compared to non-drinkers. This association is not due to confounding by other dietary factors, including total caloric or fat consumption. For lower levels of consumption the risks are correspondingly lower and confidence intervals generally include 1.0. It is presumed that self-reporting of alcohol consumption is not entirely reliable and that the actual risks of breast cancer could be higher than have been observed. Several possible explanations for the association between alcohol and breast cancer have been suggested. These include altered hepatic function which could increase estrogen levels (Swann et al, 1984) or a direct mitogenic effect of alcohol on breast epithelium (Wickramasinghe et al, 1986). There appear to be few data on the effect of ethanol on female pituitary–gonadal function, although elevated basal prolactin levels have been described in alcoholics (Ylikahari et al, 1980). More recently, Reichman et al (1993) provided evidence that twice daily alcohol intake increases estrogen levels.

Male Breast Cancer

In one of the largest case–control studies conducted to date on male breast cancer, the only statistically significant risk factor identified was higher reported weight by cases in young adulthood (Casagrande et al, 1988). Cases with weight greater than 90 kg at age 30 had 5.5 times the risk of those weighing less than 60 kg. Serum hormone levels were measured in cases and controls in this study. As in women, serum estrone levels were positively and sex hormone–globulin levels negatively correlated with body weight. This suggests that the underlying risk factor to explain an association with body weight may be increased exposure to bioavailable estrogens. Although there were no statistically significant difference in serum or urinary estrogen levels between cases and controls, at the time of sampling there was little difference in weight between the two groups. Other small studies of urinary or serum estrogen levels in male breast cancer patients and controls have provided inconsistent results; some have found evidence of higher levels in cases (Calabresi et al, 1976; Dao et al, 1973), whereas others have detected no differences (Scheike et al, 1973).

Gynecomastia (Casagrande et al, 1988; Scheike and Visfeldt, 1973) and sex chromatin positivity (Casagrande et al, 1988; Nadel and Koss, 1967) appear to be risk factors for male breast cancer, and there is evidence that both of these conditions are associated with estrogen excess. In a recent multicenter study by Thomas et al (Thomas et al, 1992), an increased risk of breast cancer was associated with undescended testes which further suggests an underlying neuroendocrine basis for this cancer in men.

Bernstein et al (1989) have utilized the breast tissue

aging model described above to show that differences in urinary estrogen levels in men compared to women are large enough to explain entirely the large differences in breast cancer incidence between the sexes.

Implications for Cancer Prevention

For women, breast cancer risk appears to be determined in large part by the cumulative exposure of breast epithelium to estrogen and progesterone. Most of this exposure is accumulated during the years of active ovarian function. Possible approaches to primary prevention require a detailed understanding of the factors that influence the onset, regularity, and quality of ovarian activity.

Differences in childhood nutrition patterns and energy balance seem to be reasonable explanations for much of the international differences in breast cancer risk but require further exploration. Regular participation in moderate physical activity, thus reducing the frequency of ovulatory cycles, may provide an opportunity for the primary prevention of breast cancer (Bernstein et al, 1987, 1994). Using the breast cancer incidence model discussed above, it is possible to demonstrate the considerable impact of modest changes in the ovulatory frequency at a young age. Reducing by one-half the number of ovulatory cycles between menarche at age 12 and first full-term pregnancy at age 22 could lower a women's lifetime risk of breast cancer by more than 50%.

Chemoprevention of breast cancer via hormonal manipulation has received much recent attention (Henderson et al, 1993). One such formulation using luteinizing hormone-releasing hormone agonist to totally suppress endogenous estrogen and progesterone production, coupled with a low-dose conjugated equine estrogen, has been proposed by Pike et al (1989). The potential benefits of such a regimen, particularly in women at increased risk of breast cancer, should spur efficacy studies.

Tamoxifen, a synthetic non-steroidal "anti-estrogen" that is a widely used chemotheraputic agent for postmenopausal breast cancer, has been advocated for chemoprevention (Cuzick et al, 1986). When used for chemotherapy of postmenopausal breast cancer, there is strong evidence of a lower incidence of breast cancer in the contralateral breast (Fornander et al, 1989). Tamoxifen-treated versus control patients show a 38% reduction in risk of contralateral breast cancer (Henderson et al, 1993). Tamoxifen treatment, despite being anti-estrogenic for the breast, results in substantial increases in circulating estrogen levels. This effect has spurred concerns about possible adverse consequences of tamoxifen therapy on other organs, especially the endometrium (Henderson et al, 1993; VanLeeuwen et al, 1994). Nonetheless, recruitment has begun for a large national trial for the hormonal chemoprevention of breast cancer in healthy women using tamoxifen.

There has been considerable discussion about the usefulness and feasibility of dietary fat reduction intervention in middle-aged women as a method of reducing the incidence of breast cancer. Prentice et al (1988) have argued that the international variation in breast cancer rates are likely due mainly to variations in dietary fat consumption. They have proposed a large, 10-year intervention trial with a goal of reducing dietary fat from 40% to 20% of calories. They believe that such a reduction would achieve a 17% reduction in breast cancer incidence. The accuracy of this figure has been questioned as it assumes that the postmenopausal rate of breast cancer would actually decline to a level below that of a women passing through menopause. The time interval required to achieve such reduction has also been seriously questioned. To the extent that a fat reduction diet results in weight loss or maintenance of an ideal body weight, such a diet would be expected to reduce breast cancer incidence.

Until suitable avenues for primary prevention of breast cancer are established, the most viable approach to reducing breast cancer mortality for the postmenopausal patient is through regular mammography and physician breast examination (Habbema et al, 1986; Tabar et al, 1985). The benefit of mammography in reducing breast cancer mortality in premenopausal women remains controversial.

The characterization of mutations in *BRCA1* and other candidate breast cancer susceptibility genes opens the door to the real possibility that individual susceptibility can be more precisely determined. Potential polymorphisms in genes that control estradiol metabolism and cellular transport can further define the polygenic nature of breast cancer and lead to genetic counseling, earlier diagnosis and potentially, genetic therapeutic manipulation.

REFERENCES

ASKEL S. 1981. Hormonal characteristics of long cycles in fertile women. Fertil Steril 36:521–523.

ALBANES D. 1987. Total calories, body weight, and tumor incidence in mice. Cancer Res 47:1987–1992.

ALDERCREUTZ H, FOTSIS T, et al. 1989. Diet and urinary estrogen profile in premenopausal omnivorous and vegetarian women and in premenopausal women with breast cancer. J Steroid Biochem 34:527–530.

ALDERCREUTZ H, HOCKERSTEDT K, et al. 1987. Effect of dietary components, including ligands and phytoestrogens, on enterohepatic circulation and liver metabolism of estrogens and on sex hormone binding globulin (SHBG). J Steroid Biochem 27:1135–1144.

ANDERSON DE. 1974. Genetic study of breast cancer: identification of a high risk group. Cancer 34:1090–1097.

ANONYMOUS. 1974. Boston Collaborative Drug Surveillance Program: Reserpine and breast cancer. Lancet 2:669–671.

APTER D, VIHKO R. 1983. Early menarche, a risk factor for breast cancer, indicates early onset of ovulatory cycles. J Clin Endocrinol Metab 57:82.

ARMSTRONG B, DOLL R. 1975. Environmental factors and cancer incidence and mortality in different countries, with special reference to dietary practices. Int J Cancer 15:617–631.

ARMSTRONG B, SKEGG D, et al. 1976. Rauwolfia derivatives and breast cancer in hypertensive women. Lancet 2:8–12.

ARMSTRONG B, STEVENS W, et al. 1974. Retrospective study of the association between use of Rauwolfia derivatives and breast cancer in English women. Lancet 2:672–755.

BARON JA. 1984. Smoking and estrogen-related disease. Am J Epidemiol 119:9–22.

BARRETT-CONNER E. 1990. Smoking and endogenous sex hormones in men and women. *In* Wald N, Baron J. (eds): Smoking and Hormone-related Disorders. Oxford, Oxford University Press, pp. 183–196.

BERNSTEIN L, DEPUE RH, et al. 1986. Higher maternal levels of free estradiol in first compared to second pregnancy: a study of early gestational differences. J Natl Cancer Inst 76:1035–1039.

BERNSTEIN L, HENDERSON BE, et al. 1994. Physical exercise activity reduces the risk of breast cancer in young women. J Natl Cancer Inst 86:1403–1408.

BERNSTEIN L, PIKE MC, et al. 1985. Estrogen and sex hormone-binding globulin levels in nulliparous and parous women. J Natl Cancer Inst 74:741–745.

BERNSTEIN L, ROSS R. 1993. Hormones and breast cancer. Epidemiol Rev 15:48–65.

BERNSTEIN L, ROSS RK, et al. 1987. Effects of moderate physical activity on menstrual cycle patterns in adolescence: implications for breast cancer prevention. Br J Cancer 55:681–685.

BERNSTEIN L, ROSS RK, et al. 1989. Urinary estrogens and male-to-female breast cancer ratios [letter]. Int J Cancer 44:954–956.

BERNSTEIN L, YUAN JM, et al. 1990. Serum hormone levels in premenopausal Chinese women in Shanghai and white women in Los Angeles: results from two breast cancer case-control studies. Cancer Causes Control 1:51–58.

BISHOP DT, CANNON-ALBRIGHT L, et al. 1988. Segregation and linkage analysis of nine Utah breast cancer pedigrees. Genet Epidemiol 5:151–159.

BLACK MM, BARCLAY THC, et al. 1972. Association of atypical characteristics of benign breast lesions with subsequent risk of breast cancer. Cancer 29:338–343.

BORING CC, SQUIRES TS, et al. 1993. Cancer Statistics, 1993. CA Cancer J Clin 43:7–26.

BRUZZI P, NEGRI E, et al. 1988. Short term increase in risk of breast cancer after full term pregnancy. BMJ 197:1096.

BUELL P. 1973. Changing incidence of breast cancer in Japanese-American women. J Natl Cancer Inst 51:1479–1483.

CALABRESI E, DEGIULI G, et al. 1976. Plasma estrogens and androgens in male breast cancer. J Steroid Biochem 7:605–609.

CANELLOS G. 1985. Carcinoma of the Breast. *In* Wyngaarden JB, Smith LJ (eds): Cecil Textbook of Medicine. Philadelphia, W.B. Saunders Co., pp. 1402–1405.

CARROLL KK. 1975. Experimental evidence of dietary factors and hormone-dependent cancers. Cancer Res 35:3374–3383.

CASAGRANDE JT, HANISCH R, et al. 1988. A case–control study of male breast cancer. Cancer Res 48:1326–1330.

CLAUS EB, RISCH N, et al. 1991. Genetic analysis of breast cancer in the Cancer and Steroid Hormone study. Am J Hum Genet 48:232–242.

COHEN LA, KENDALL ME, et al. 1991. Modulation of N-nitrosomethylurea-induced mammary tumor promotion by dietary fiber and fat. J Natl Cancer Inst 83:496–501.

COLE P, ELWOOD JM, et al. 1978. Incidence rates and risk factors of benign breast neoplasms. Am J Epidemiol 108:112–120.

CORNELIS RS, CORNELISSE CJ, et al. 1994. Selection of families for predictive testing for breast cancer [letter]. Lancet 344:1151.

CUZICK J, WANG DY, et al. 1986. The prevention of breast cancer. Lancet i:83–86.

DAO T. 1981. The role of ovarian steroid hormones in mammary carcinogenesis. *In* Pike M, Siiteri P, Welsh C (eds): Hormones and Breast Cancer. Cold Spring Harbor, NY, Cold Spring Harbor Laboratories, pp. 281–298.

DAO TL, MOREAL C, et al. 1973. Urinary estrogen excretion in men with breast cancer. N Engl J Med 289:138–140.

DAVIS DL, BRADLOW HL, et al. 1993. Medical hypothesis: xenoestrogens as preventable causes of breast cancer. Environ Health Perspect 101:372–377.

DE WAARD FJ, CORNELIS J, et al. 1977. Breast cancer incidence according to weight and height in two cities of the Netherlands and in Aichi Prefecture, Japan. Cancer 40:1269.

DEL SENNO L, AGUIARI G, et al. 1992. Dinucleotide repeat polymorphism in the human estrogen receptor (ESR) gene. Hum Molec Genet 1:354.

DULBECCO R, HWENAHAN M, et al. 1982. Cell types of morphogenesis in the mammary gland. Proc Natl Acad Sci USA 79:7346.

DUPONT WD, PAGE DL. 1985. Risk factors for breast cancer in women with proliferative breast disease. N Engl J Med 312:146–155.

DUPONT W, PAGE DL, et al. 1994. Long-term risk of breast cancer in women with fibroadenoma. N Engl J Med 331:10–15.

EASTON DF, BISHOP DT, et al. 1993. Genetic linkage analysis in familial breast and ovarian cancer: results from 214. Am J Hum Genet 52:678–701.

ENGLAND P, SKINNER L, et al. 1974. Serum oestradiol-17β in women with benign and malignant breast disease. Br J Cancer 30:571.

FEARON E, CHO K, et al. 1990. Identification of a chromosome 18q gene that is altered on colorectal cancers. Science 247:49–56.

FEINLEIB M. 1968. Breast cancer and artificial menopause: a cohort study. J Natl Cancer Inst 41:315.

FERGUSON D, ANDERSON T. 1981. Morphological evaluation of cell turnover in relation to the menstrual cycle in the "resting" human breast. Br J Cancer 44:177.

FISHMAN J, SCHNEIDER J, et al. 1983. Increased estrogen 16-alpha-hydroxylase activity in women with breast and endometrial cancer. J Steroid Biochem 20:1077–1081.

FORNANDER T, RUTQVIST LE, et al. 1989. Adjuvant tamoxifen in early breast cancer: occurrence of new primary cancers. Lancet i:117–120.

FRISCH R, GOTZ-WELBERGEN A, et al. 1981. Delayed menarche and amenorrhea of college athletes in relation to age at onset of training. JAMA 246:1559.

FRISCH R, MCARTHUR J. 1974. Menstrual cycles: fatness as a determinant of minimum weight for height necessary for their maintenance or onset. Science 185:949.

FUTREAL PA, LIU Q, et al. 1994. BRCA1 mutations in primary breast and ovarian carcinomas. Science 266:120–122.

GLASS A. 1988. Changing incidence of breast cancer [letter]. J Natl Cancer Inst 80:1076.

GOLDIN BR, ALDERCREUTZ H, et al. 1982. Estrogen excretion patterns and plasma levels in vegetarian and omnivorous women. N Engl J Med 307:1542–1547.

GRAHAM S, ZIELEZNY M, et al. 1992. Diet in the epidemiology of postmenopausal breast cancer in the New York State cohort. Am J Epidemiol 136:1327–1337.

GRAY GE, PIKE MC, et al. 1979. Breast cancer incidence and mortality rates in different countries in relation to known risk factors and dietary practices. Br J Cancer 39:1–7.

GRAY GE, PIKE MC, et al. 1981. Dietary fat and plasma prolactin. Am J Clin Nutr 34:1160–1162.

GRAY G, PIKE MC, et al. 1982. Diet and hormone profiles in teenage girls in four countries at different risk to breast cancer. Prev Med 11:108–113.

GUINEE VF, OLSSON H, et al. 1994. Effect of pregnancy on prognosis for young women with breast cancer. Lancet 343:1587–1589.

HABBEMA JDF, VAN OORTMARSSEN GJ, et al. 1986. Age-specific reduction in breast cancer mortality by screening. An analysis of the results of the Health Insurance Plan of Greater New York. J Natl Cancer Inst 77:317–320.

HADJIMICHAEL O, BOYLE C, et al. 1986. Abortion before first live birth and risk of breast cancer. Br J Cancer 53:281.

HAENSZEL W, KURIHARA M. 1968. Studies of Japanese migrants. 1. Mortality from cancer and other diseases among Japanese in the United States. J Natl Cancer Inst 40:43–68.

HALL J, LEE M, et al. 1990. Linkage of early-onset familial breast cancer to chromosome 17q21. Science 250:1684–1689.

HALL JM, FRIEDMAN L, et al. 1992. Closing in on a breast cancer gene on chromosome 17q. Am J Hum Genet 50:1235–1242.

HANKEY BF, BRINTON LA, et al. 1993. Breast. *In* Miller BA, Ries LAG, Hankey BF, et al (eds): SEER Cancer Statistics Review: 1973–1990, National Cancer Institute. NIH Pub. No. 93-2789. Bethesda, National Cancer Institute, pp. IV1–IV24.

HEINEN OP, SHAPIRO S, et al. 1974. Reserpine use in relation to breast cancer. Lancet 2:675–677.

HENDERSON BE, GERKINS VR, et al. 1975. Elevated serum levels of estrogen and prolactin in daughters of patients with breast cancer. N Engl J Med 293:790–795.

HENDERSON BE, PIKE MC, et al. 1981. Breast cancer and the oestrogen window hypothesis [letter]. Lancet ii:363–364.

HENDERSON BE, PIKE MC, et al. 1984. Epidemiology and Risk Factors. *In* Bonadonna G, et al (eds): Breast Disease: Recent Advances in Diagnosis and Management. New York, John Wiley and Sons, Inc., pp. 15–33.

HENDERSON BE, ROSS RK, et al. 1982. Endogenous hormones as a major factor in human cancer. Cancer Res 42:3232–3239.

HENDERSON BE, ROSS RK, et al. 1985. Do regular ovulatory cycles increase breast cancer risk? Cancer 56:1206–1208.

HENDERSON BE, ROSS RK, et al. 1988. Estrogens as a cause of human cancer: The Richard and Hinda Rosenthal Foundation Award Lecture. Cancer Res 48:246–253.

HENDERSON BE, ROSS RK, et al. 1993. Hormonal chemoprevention of cancer in women. Science 259:633–638.

HILL P, WYNDER EL. 1976. Diet and prolactin release. Lancet 2:806–807.

HIRAYAMA T. 1978. Epidemiology of breast cancer with special reference to the role of diet. Prev Med 7:173–195.

HOEL D, WAKABAYASHI T, et al. 1983. Secular trends in the distributions of the breast cancer risk factors—menarche, first birth, menopause, and weight—in Hiroshima and Nagasaki, Japan. Am J Epidemiol 118:79–89.

HOWE G, ROHAN T, et al. 1991a. The association between alcohol and breast cancer risk: evidence from the combined analysis of six dietary case-control studies. Int J Cancer 47:707–710.

HOWE GR, FRIEDERREICH CM, et al. 1991b. A cohort study of fat intake and risk of breast cancer. J Natl Cancer Inst 83:336–340.

HOWE GR, HIROHATA T, et al. 1990. Dietary factors and risk of breast cancer: combined analysis of 12 case–control studies. J Natl Cancer Inst 82:561–569.

HOWE H, SENIE R, et al. 1989. Early abortion and breast cancer risk among women under age 40. Int J Epidemiol 18:300.

HUNTER D, MANSON J, et al. 1993. A prospective study of the intake of vitamins C, E, and A and the risk of breast cancer. N Engl J Med 329:234–240.

HUNTER DJ, WILLETT WC. 1994. Diet, body build, and breast cancer. Annu Rev Nutr 14:393–418.

ISELIUS L, SLACK J, et al. 1991. Genetic epidemiology of breast cancer in Britain. Ann Hum Genet 55:151–159.

JONES L, OTA D, et al. 1987. Bioavailability of estradiol as a marker for breast cancer risk assessment. Cancer Res 47:5224.

KEY T, PIKE M. 1988. The role of oestrogens and progestogens in the epidemiology and prevention of breast disease. Eur J Cancer Clin Oncol 24:29.

KNUDSON A. 1971. Mutation and cancer: statistical study of retinoblastoma. Proc Natl Acad Sci USA 68:820–823.

KODLIN D, WINGER EE, et al. 1977. Chronic mastopathy and breast cancer. Cancer 39:2603–2607.

LAVECCHIA C, DECARLI A, et al. 1985. Menstrual cycle patterns and the risk of breast cancer. Eur J Cancer Onc 21:417–422.

LEE HP, GOURLEY L, et al. 1991. Dietary effects on breast cancer risk in Singapore. Lancet 337:1197–1200.

LEMON HM, HEIDEL JW, et al. 1993. Increased catechol estrogen metabolism as a risk factor for nonfamilial breast cancer. Cancer 85:648–652.

LEVI F, RANDIMBISON L, et al. 1994. Incidence of breast cancer in women with fibroadenoma. Int J Cancer 57:681–683.

LEVIN PA, MALARKEY WB. 1981. Daughters of women with breast cancer have elevated mean 24-hour prolactin (PRL) levels and a partial resistance of PRL to dopamine suppression. J Clin Endocrinol 53:179–184.

LONDON SL, CONNOLLY JL, et al. 1992. A prospective study of benign breast disease and the risk of breast cancer. JAMA 267:941–944.

LONGNECKER MP, BERLIN JA, et al. 1988. A meta-analysis of alcohol consumption in relation to risk of breast cancer. JAMA 260:652–656.

MACMAHON B. 1990. Cigarette smoking and cancer of the breast. In Wald N, Baron J (eds). Smoking and Hormone-Related Disorders. Oxford, Oxford University Press, pp 154–166.

MACMAHON B, COLE P, et al. 1970. Age at first birth and cancer of the breast. A summary of an international study. Bull World Health Organ 43:209.

MACMAHON B, COLE P, et al. 1974. Urine oestrogen profiles of Asian and North American women. Int J Cancer 14:161–167.

MACMAHON B, TRICHOPOULOS D, et al. 1982. Age at menarche, probability of ovulation and breast cancer risk. Int J Cancer 29:13.

MALKIN D, LI FP, et al. 1992. Germline p53 mutations in a familial syndrome of breast cancer, sarcomas and other neoplasms. Science 250:1233–1238.

MANNERMAA A, PELTOKETO H, et al. 1994. Human familial and sporadic breast cancer: analysis of the coding regions of the 17β-hydroxysteroid dyhydrogenase 2 gene (EDH17B2) using a single-strand conformation polymorphism assay. Hum Genet 93:319–324.

MATSUMOTO S, NOGAMI Y, et al. 1962. Statistical studies of menstruation: criticism of the definition of normal menstruation. Gunma J Med Sci 11:294–318.

MCCARTY KSJ, SILVA JS, et al. 1983. Relationship of age and menopausal status to estrogen receptor content in primary carcinoma of the breast. Ann Surg 197:123–127.

MICHNOVICZ JJ, HERSHCOPF RJ, et al. 1986. Increased 2-hydroxylation of estradiol as a possible mechanism for the anti-estrogenic effect of cigarette smoking. N Engl J Med 315:1305–1309.

MIKI Y, SWENSEN J, et al. 1994. A strong candidate for the breast and ovarian cancer susceptibility gene BRCA1. Science 266:66–71.

MILLER AB, BULBROOK RD. 1986. UICC multidisciplinary project on breast cancer: the epidemiology, aetiology and prevention of breast cancer. Int J Cancer 37:173–177.

MILLS PK, BEESON WL, et al. 1989. Dietary habits and breast cancer incidence among Seventh-Day Adventists. Cancer 64:582–590.

MOORE J, CLARK G, et al. 1982. Serum concentrations of total and non-protein bound oestradiol in patients with breast cancer and in normal controls. Int J Cancer 29:17.

MUSEY V, COLLINS D, et al. 1987. Long-term effect of a first pregnancy on the secretion of prolactin. N Engl J Med 316:229.

MYERS MH, GLOECKLER RIESE LA. 1989. Cancer patient survival rates: SEER program results for 10 years of follow-up. CA Cancer J Clin 39:21–32.

NADEL M, KOSS LG. 1967. Klinefelter's syndrome and male breast cancer. Lancet ii:366.

NAROD SA, FEUTEUN J, et al. 1991. Familial breast-ovarian cancer locus on chromosome 17q12-q23. Lancet 338:82–83.

NEWMAN B, AUSTIN MA, et al. 1988. Inheritance of human breast cancer: evidence for autosomal dominant transmission in high risk families. Proc Natl Acad Sci USA 85:1–5.

NOMURA A, HENDERSON BE, et al. 1978. Breast cancer and diet among the Japanese in Hawaii. Am J Clin Nutr 31:2020–2025.

OLSSON H, LANDIN-OLSSON M, et al. 1983. Retrospective assessment of menstrual cycle length in patients with breast cancer, in patients with benign breast disease, and in women without breast disease. J Natl Cancer Inst 70:17.

OSBORNE MP, BRADLOW HL, et al. 1993. Upregulation of estradiol C16α-hydroxylation in human breast tissue: a potential biomarker of breast cancer risk. J Natl Cancer Inst 85:1917–1920.

PARKIN DM, STJERNSWARD J, et al. 1984. Estimates of worldwide frequency of twelve major cancers. Bull World Health Organ 62:163–182.

PIKE MC. 1987. Age-related factors in cancer of the breast, ovary, and endometrium. J Chron Dis 40(Suppl 2):595–695.

PIKE MC, HENDERSON BE, et al. 1981. Oral contraceptive use and early abortion as risk factors for breast cancer in young women. Br J Cancer 43:72–76.

PIKE MC, KRAILO MD, et al. 1983. Hormonal risk factors, breast tissue age and the age-incidence of breast cancer. Nature 303:767–770.

PIKE MC, ROSS RK, et al. 1989. LHRH agonists and the prevention of breast and ovarian cancer. Br J Cancer 60:142–148.

PIVA R, GAMBARI R, et al. 1992. Analysis of upstream sequences of the human estrogen receptor gene. Biochem Biophys Res Commun 183:996–1002.

PONGLIKITMONGKOL M, GREEN S, et al. 1988. Genomic organization of the human oestrogen receptor gene. EMBO 7:3385–3388.

POTTEN C, WATSON R, et al. 1988. The effect of age and menstrual cycle upon proliferative activity of the normal human breast. Br J Cancer 58:163.

POUTANEN M, MIETTINEN M, et al. 1993. Differential estrogen substrate specificities for transiently expressed human placental 17β-hydroxysteroid dehydrogenase and an endogenous enzyme expressed in cultured COS-m6 cells. Endocrinology 133:2639–2644.

PRENTICE RL, KAKAR F, et al. 1988. Aspects of the rationale for the women's health trial. J Natl Cancer Inst 80:802–814.

PRENTICE RL, THOMPSON D, et al. 1990. Dietary fat reduction and plasma estradiol concentration in healthy postmenopausal women. J Natl Cancer Inst 82:129.

REICHMAN M, JUDD J, et al. 1993. Effects of alcohol consumption on plasma and urinary hormone concentrations in premenopausal women. J Natl Cancer Inst 85:722–727.

RIES LAG, HUNKEY BF, et al. (eds). 1990. Cancer Statistic Review 1973–1987. NIH Publ 90:2789. Bethesda, MD, National Institutes.

ROHAN TE, HOWE GR, et al. 1993. Dietary fiber, vitamins A, C and E, and risk of breast cancer: a cohort study. Cancer Causes Control 4:29–37.

ROSE DP, PRUITT BT. 1981. Plasma prolactin levels in patients with breast cancer. Cancer 48:2687–2691.

ROSS R, YU M. 1994. Breast Feeding and Breast Cancer [Letter to the editor]. N Engl J Med 330:1683.

ROSS RK, PAGANINI-HILL A, et al. 1984. Effects of reserpine on prolactin levels and incidence of breast cancer in postmenopausal women. Cancer Res 44:3106–3108.

SAFTLAS AF, WOLFE JN, et al. 1989. Mammographic parenchymal patterns as indicators of breast cancer risk. Am J Epidemiol 129:518–526.

SAGER R. 1989. Tumor-suppressor genes: the puzzle and the promise. Science 246:1406–1412.

SCHEIKE O, SVENSTRUP B, et al. 1973. A male breast cancer. 2. Metabolism of oestradiol-17beta in men with breast cancer. J Steroid Biochem 4:489–501.

SCHEIKE O, VISFELDT J. 1973. Male breast cancer. 4. Gynecomastia in patients with breast cancer. APMIS 81:359–365.

SCHNEIDER J, KINNE D, et al. 1982. Abnormal oxidative metabolism in women with breast cancer. PNAS 79:3047–3051.

SHELAN SL, PARKIN DM, et al. (eds). 1990. Patterns of Cancer in Five Continents. IARC Scientific Publications No. 102. Lyon, International Agency for Research on Cancer.

SHIMIZU H, ROSS RK, et al. 1990. Serum oestrogen levels in postmenopausal women: comparison of American whites and Japanese in Japan. Br J Cancer 62:451–453.

SHIMIZU H, ROSS RK, et al. 1991. Cancers of the prostate and breast among Japanese and white immigrants in Los Angeles County. Br J Cancer 63:963–966.

SIITERI P, HAMMOND G, et al. 1981. Increased availability of serum estrogens in breast cancer: A new hypothesis. Pike M, Siiteri P, Welsh C (eds): Hormones and Breast Cancer. Cold Spring Harbor, NY, Cold Spring Harbor Laboratories, pp. 87–106.

SNOW RC, BARBIERI RL, et al. 1989. Estrogen II—hydroxylase oxidation and menstral function among elite oarswomen. J Clin Endocrinol Metab 315:369–376.

STANBRIDGE E. 1990. Identifying tumor-suppressor genes in human colorectal cancer. Science 247:12–13.

SWANN PF, COE AM, et al. 1984. Ethanol and dimethylnitrosamine and diethylnitrosamine metabolism and disposition in the rat: possible relevance to the influence of ethanol on human cancer incidence. Carcinogenesis (Lond) 5:1337–1343.

TABAR L, FAGERBERG CJ, et al. 1985. Reduction in mortality from breast cancer after mass screening with mammography. Lancet i:829–832.

TANNER J. 1962. Growth at Adolescence. Oxford, Blackwell Scientific Publishers.

THOMAS DB, JIMENEZ LM, et al. 1992. Breast cancer in men: risk factors with hormonal implications. Am J Epidemiol 135:734–748.

TRELOAR AE, BOYNTON RE, et al. 1967. Variation of the human menstrual cycle through reproductive life. Int J Fertil 12:77–126.

TRICHOPOULOS D, BROWN J, et al. 1981. Elevated urine estrogen and pregnanediol levels in daughters of breast cancer patients. J Natl Cancer Inst 67:603.

TRICHOPOULOS D, MACMAHON B, et al. 1972. The menopause and breast cancer risk. J Natl Cancer Inst 48:605.

VANLEEUWEN FE, BENRAADT J, et al. 1994. Risk of endometrial cancer after tamoxifen treatment of breast cancer. Lancet 343:448–452.

WHITE EW, LEE CY, et al. 1990. Evolution of the increase in breast cancer incidence in relation to mammography use. J Natl Cancer Inst 82:1546–1552.

WICKRAMASINGHE SN, GARDNER B, et al. 1986. Cytotoxic protein molecules generated as a consequence of ethanol metabolism *in vitro* and *in vivo*. Lancet 2:823–826.

WILKINSON E, CLOPTON C, et al. 1977. Mammographic parenchymal pattern and the risk of breast cancer. J Natl Cancer Inst 59:1397–1400.

WILLETT WC, HUNTER DJ, et al. 1992. Dietary fat and fiber in relation to risk of breast cancer. JAMA 268:2037–2044.

WILLETT WC, STAMPFER MJ, et al. 1987. Dietary fat and risk of breast cancer. N Engl J Med 316:22–28.

WILLIAMS WR, ANDERSON DE. 1984. Genetic epidemiology of

breast cancer: segregation analysis of 200 Danish pedigrees. Genet Epidemiol 1:7–20.

WOLFE JN, ALBERT S, et al. 1982. Breast parenchymal patterns: analysis of 332 incident breast carcinomas. Am J Roentgenol 138:113–118.

WOOSTER R, NEUHAUSEN SL, et al. 1994. Localization of a breast cancer susceptibility gene, BRCA2, to chromosome 13q12-13. Science 265:2088–2090.

YAICH L, DUPONT W, et al. 1992. Analysis of the *Pvu*II restriction fragment-length polymorphism and exon structure of the estrogen receptor gene in breast cancer and peripheral blood. Cancer Res 52:77–83.

YLIKAHARI RH, HUTTUNEN MO, et al. 1980. Hormonal changes during alcohol intoxication and withdrawal. Pharmacol Biochem Behav 13(Suppl.):131–137.

YU MC, GERKINS VR, et al. 1981. Elevated levels of prolactin in nulliparous women. Br J Cancer 43:826–831.

YUAN JC. 1995. Diet and breast cancer in Shanghai and Tianjin, China. Br J Cancer: 71:1353–1358.

YUAN JM, YU MC, et al. 1988. Risk factors for breast cancer in Chinese women in Shanghai. Cancer Res 48:1949–1953.

ZUPPAN P, HALL J, et al. 1991. Possible linkage of the estrogen receptor gene to breast cancer in a family with late-onset disease. Am J Hum Genet 48:1065–1068.

48 Ovarian cancer

NOEL S. WEISS
LINDA S. COOK
DIANA C. FARROW
KARIN A. ROSENBLATT

Cancer of the ovary will strike 1%–2% of women in developed countries in their lifetime, and will be responsible for the death of most women it strikes. Almost all the neoplasms that arise in the ovary have their origin in and resemble one of three cell types: germ cells, follicular cells, and coelomic epithelial cells. The current state of knowledge of the epidemiology of ovarian tumors suggests that each tumor type has some etiologic factors separate from the others.

DEMOGRAPHIC CORRELATES OF OVARIAN CANCER OCCURRENCE

Germ Cell Tumors

This category comprises a number of types of rare tumors—dysgerminomas, teratomas (embryonal, adult)—and others still more rare (Scully, 1963). Based on cross-sectional data, the incidence of these tumors peaks in young adulthood, falls, rises again, and levels off after middle age (Fig. 48–1). The annual incidence does not exceed one per 100,000 at any age.

Mortality from germ cell tumors in the United States during the 1950s and 1960s was relatively constant (Li et al, 1973). Additionally, there has been little or no change in incidence rates of ovarian germ cell tumors since the early 1970s (Table 48–1). One report found that the incidence of germ cell tumors among 15–34-year-old women in Los Angeles rose severalfold between 1972–76 and 1977–81, with no appreciable change in other age groups (Walker et al, 1984). National figures (unpublished data, SEER program), however, were far less dramatic for women aged 15–34 years; the rate rose from 5.9 to 7.3 per million between 1973–76 and 1977–80, to 7.8 per million in 1981–84, then declined to 7.0 per million in 1985–87.

Some 13%–15% of all ovarian tumors that arise in African and Asian populations are of germ cell origin (Bhoola and Bhamjee, 1976), in contrast to a figure of less than 5% for European and North American populations (Weiss et al, 1977). However, this difference in proportional incidence may be a poor indicator of a difference in absolute incidence between the countries, since:

1. the incidence of ovarian tumors other than those of germ cell origin is lower in Africa and Asia than in Europe and North America;
2. the differing age distributions of the populations have not been accounted for in these comparisons; and
3. it is possible that the ascertainment of ovarian tumors in older women (in whom the proportional incidence of germ cell tumors is lowest) was relatively less complete in the African and Asian populations.

Sex Cord–Stromal Tumors

Tumors rarely arise in follicular cells and other tissues derived from the sex cords or mesenchyme of the embryonic gonad. More than 90% of the malignant tumors are granulosa cell tumors (Cutler and Young, 1975). In the United States, the incidence of malignant sex cord–stromal tumors rises with age to reach a maximum in middle age of 0.5–1.0 per 100,000 per year, after which the rates plateau (Fig. 48–1). The reported incidence of these tumors in the U.S. has declined substantially during the past 10–20 years (Table 48–1).

The incidence of sex cord–stromal and germ cell tumors was found to be similar among women of the major racial/ethnic groups of the United States (Weiss and Peterson, 1978). However, because of the small number of cases that were identified in that study, moderate differences in incidence could well exist. Among Israeli Jews, for example, the incidence of malignant sex cord–stromal tumors in women born in Europe or America was about twice that of women born in Asia or Africa (Ohel et al, 1983).

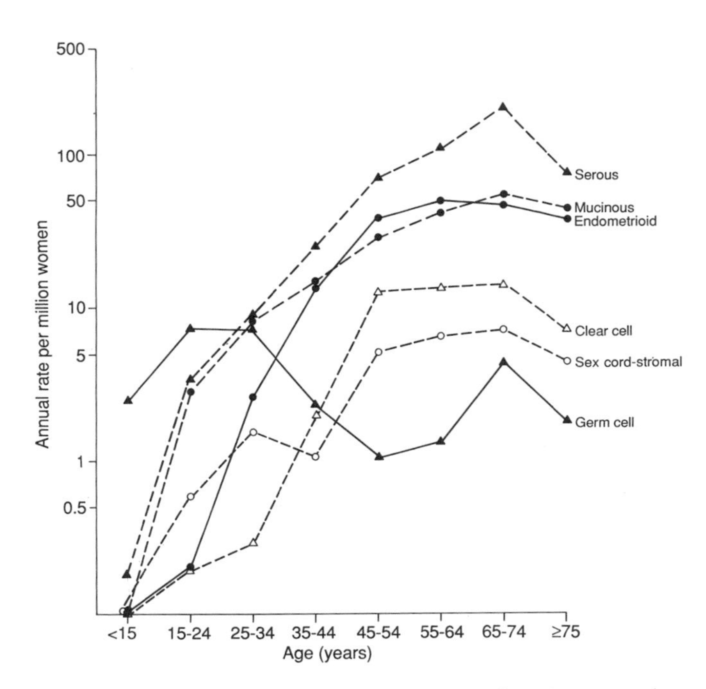

FIG. 48–1. Incidence of selected histologic types of ovarian cancer, by age: United States, 1980–84. (Source: The Surveillance Epidemiology and End Results Program, National Cancer Institute.

Epithelial Tumors

The majority of malignant ovarian tumors originate in cells derived from coelomic epithelium. Thus, the incidence of these epithelial neoplasms is closely approximated by the incidence of ovarian cancer as a whole. Since far more data are available for the latter than for individual histologic types, the descriptive epidemiology of epithelial ovarian tumors is better known than that of germ cell or sex cord–stromal tumors.

Important reservations exist regarding the quality of the data on the incidence of ovarian epithelial tumors. These tumors can be difficult to diagnose, particularly when the malignant process is widespread; the diagnosis of ovarian cancer is only an educated guess in many women with advanced abdominal malignancy. There may also be uncertainty in the diagnosis of lesions that exhibit various microscopic features of malignancy (such as substantial nuclear atypia and mitotic activity) but do not appear to have invaded the stroma. These tumors of low malignant potential (or "borderline" tumors) are often not included in the published statistics of most cancer-reporting systems. However, the degree of invasion of a given tumor can be difficult to determine, and the criteria for this may vary among pathologists. Since borderline tumors may be widely implanted on the peritoneum, they could be termed "carcinoma" in the absence of a careful histologic assessment. The determination of the specific histologic type among epithelial tumors is also highly variable. An internationally accepted classification, that of the International Federation of Gynecology and Obstetrics, was devised several decades ago, but not all pathologists employ it. Furthermore, the tumors themselves can be hard to classify, as some may include several different types of malignant cells.

Despite these problems in ascertainment and classification, variation in the reported incidence of epithelial tumors is sufficiently large so as to provide us with some etiologic clues. Table 48–2 documents the incidence of ovarian cancer in a number of areas of the world. Rates are given for women ages 35–64 years only, as: (a) almost all ovarian tumors that are diagnosed in them are epithelial in nature; and (b) the diagnosis and ascertainment of ovarian cancer is better in women of these ages than in older women. The highest rates are found in white women in Europe and North America, with particularly high rates in Scandinavia. Women in Central and South America tend to have relatively low rates. The incidence of ovarian cancer in Hispanic women in the U.S. is nearly as high as that of white women of other ethnicity.

In general, Asian women have a relatively low incidence of epithelial ovarian tumors. Though women of Chinese and Japanese descent who reside in the United States tend to have higher rates than their Asian counterparts, the disease is still less common in them than in the native white population overall (Herrinton et al, 1994). However, subgroups of these Asian-Americans appear to have rates comparable to those among U.S. white women. In women aged 20 to 49, the incidence of ovarian tumors is similar in U.S. white women, U.S.-born Chinese women, and Japanese women born either in the U.S. or Japan (Herrinton et al, 1994).

The only published data available on racial variation in incidence rates of specific histologic types of ovarian cancer come from the United States. The rate in members of racial minorities was found to be lower than that of white women for each class of epithelial tumor (Weiss and Peterson, 1978). The difference in the incidence be-

TABLE 48–1. *Time Trends in the Incidence of Ovarian Malignant Nonepithelial Tumors: United States, 1973–87.*

	Incidence Rates[a]			
Histologic Category	*1973–76*	*1977–80*	*1981–84*	*1985–87*
Germ cell	4.2 (160)[b]	4.4 (189)	3.9 (190)	3.9 (147)
Sex cord–stromal	3.6 (135)	2.8 (117)	2.5 (114)	1.1 (49)

[a]Rate per million females under age 85 years, adjusted to the age distribution of the 1980 U.S. population.
[b]Number of cases in parentheses.
Source: The Surveillance, Epidemiology, and End Results Program, National Cancer Institute.

TABLE 48–2. *Incidence of Cancer of the Ovary in Selected Populations in Recent Years**

Continent	Country	Area	Race	"Truncated" Incidence[a]
South and Central America	Brazil	Goiania	All	7.7
	Costa Rica	All	All	10.6
North America	Canada	All	All	22.6
	United States	All	White	24.7
		Los Angeles	White, Spanish surname	20.4
			White, other	24.4
Asia	China	Tianjin	All	9.2
	Japan	Hiroshima	All	12.4
	Singapore	All	Chinese	18.0
			Malay	23.6
			Indian	22.1
	Thailand	Chiang Mai	All	12.1
Europe	Denmark	All	All	30.5
	Finland	All	All	19.9
	France	Bas Rhin	All	24.7
		Calvados	All	19.7
	Italy	Varese	All	23.3
	Netherlands	Eindhoven	All	20.9
	Norway	All	All	30.6
	Spain	Tarragona	All	14.2
	Sweden	All	All	30.4
	Switzerland	Zurich	All	20.3
	UK	All	All	23.7
Oceania	United States	Hawaii	White	24.9
			Japanese	14.6
			Hawaiian	17.9
			Filipino	19.4
			Chinese	22.4
	Australia	Western Australia	All	19.1
	New Zealand	All	Maori	20.3
			Non-Maori	20.2

*From Parkin et al (1992).
[a]Annual rate per 100,000 population ages 35 to 64 years, standardized to the age distribution of the world standard population.

TABLE 48–3. *Incidence of Ovarian Cancer by Histologic Type, Age, and Race (Third National Cancer Survey, 1968–71)**

Histologic Type	Age (years)	Race: White	Black	White/Black
All[a]	≤39	1.7	2.0	0.9
	40–59	27.9	20.4	1.4
	≥60	46.3	32.2	1.4
Epithelial	≤39	1.4	1.4	1.0
	40–59	26.0	17.7	1.5
	≥60	38.4	24.3	1.6
Nonepithelial[b]	≤39	0.3	0.5	0.7
	40–59	0.9	1.1	0.9
	≥60	1.2	1.2	1.0

*From Weiss et al (1977). Annual rate per 100,000 women. Data from Colorado, Iowa, and Minneapolis–St. Paul are not included in this table owing to the small size of their nonwhite population.
[a]Includes clinical, autopsy, and nonspecific histologic diagnoses.
[b]Germ cell and sex cord–stromal tumors only.

tween blacks and whites depended on age (or birth cohort). Rates were identical prior to age 40, after which the white excess incidence emerged (Table 48–3).

Epithelial tumors are rare in girls and young women. Their incidence rises rapidly with increasing age until the 50s and 60s, after which it plateaus (Fig. 48–1). This pattern applies to each of the major categories of epithelial tumors (serous, mucinous, endometrioid, clear cell), as well as to the incidence of borderline ovarian tumors (Harlow et al, 1987).

In most parts of Europe and North America, the incidence of ovarian cancer has remained nearly constant for several decades (Coleman et al, 1993; Ewertz and Kjaer, 1988; Adami et al, 1990). In several parts of Asia, the reported rates increased 50% to 100% during the 1970s and 1980s (Coleman et al, 1993).

Epithelial tumors develop in the two ovaries with equal frequency. The right-left percentages were equal in women with one involved ovary who were diagnosed in Western Washington in the past decade. Both ovaries were observed to be involved in about 34% of cases. Data from cytogenetic studies suggest that, of this group, few if any tumors arise from independent foci of cancer (Pejovic et al, 1991).

THE DEVELOPMENT OF OVARIAN TUMORS IN OTHER MAMMALS

Several mechanisms that appear to operate in ovarian tumor occurrence in other species may play a role in women as well; these mechanisms are discussed in detail here.

Oocyte Depletion

X-irradiation of the ovaries of mice and rats can induce tumors, as can the administration of certain chemicals to mice, notably 7,12-dimethylbenz(a)anthracene (DMBA). The action of these agents results in the loss of oocytes and follicles, after which the tumors appear (Bonser and Jull, 1977). The observation that the ovaries of mice with the W-W genotype, which are congenitally deficient in oocytes, are also prone to develop tumors suggests that oocyte loss is a requisite for tumor production. In addition, DMBA administration has little if any impact on the oocytes of rats, and does not induce ovarian tumors in that species (Bonser and Jull, 1977).

Gonadotropin Stimulation

Pituitary secretions have been shown to play a role in both DMBA and X-ray models of ovarian tumor induction. For example, ovaries exposed to DMBA will produce tumors when transplanted into hosts that have undergone oophorectomy, but not in those that have undergone hypophysectomy (Marchant, 1961). Irradiated ovaries often develop tumors when transplanted into oophorectomized hosts, but remain tumor-free when the host retains her ovaries (Kaplan, 1950). Presumably the secretions of the normal ovarian tissue are adequate to prevent the excess gonadotropin secretion needed for tumor growth.

Anatomic alterations in rats and mice that bring about an increase in gonadotropin secretion can lead to increased ovarian tumor incidence in the absence of any external carcinogen. This has been observed by implanting a rodent's ovaries into her spleen, causing the ovarian secretions to enter the portal circulation and be deactivated in the liver. A high frequency of tumors often follows. There is reason to believe that the high gonadotropin levels (in response to low peripheral estrogen levels) are responsible, since:

1. the development of such tumors is prevented by the administration of estrogens;
2. implants of intrasplenic ovaries in a rodent with one ovary remaining in its normal position will not develop tumors; and
3. exogenous gonadotropins can speed the development of tumors in intrasplenic transplants (Shimkin, 1960).

A clue to the stages in tumor development in which gonadotropins play a role comes from studies of mice that are deficient in gonadotropin secretion because of a deficiency in the production of hypothalamic gonadotropin-releasing hormone. Irradiation of these mice causes oocyte destruction, but the subsequent changes that lead to tumor occurrence that have been seen in other rodent models (i.e., follicular atresia and stromal hypertrophy) take place only if exogenous gonadotropin is administered (Tennent and Beamer, 1986). (Actual tumors do not develop in this particular strain. Presumably, these mice are lacking at least one other necessary characteristic that prompts the next event in tumor development—invagination and penetration of the ovary by surface epithelium.)

Nature of the Ovarian Tumors Induced in Rodents

Most tumors that can be experimentally induced in rodents are types that are either uncommon in women (e.g., granulosa cell tumors) or have no apparent human analog at all (tubular adenomas). Thus, it is possible that the observations in rodents have little relevance to our understanding of the etiology of ovarian epithelial tumors, which are the predominant type in humans. Nonetheless, some parallels may exist since the same carcinogenic stimulus given to different strains of rodents can produce tumors of considerably different histologic appearance (Bosner and Jull, 1977), and some of the requirements for the development of tumors in rodents, such as oocyte depletion and gonadotropin stimulation, appear to be present in women.

RISK FACTORS FOR HUMANS OVARIAN TUMORS

Aging

The human female possesses some 7 million oocytes midway through fetal life, virtually all of which have disappeared by the time of menopause. About 95% are lost before menstrual activity even begins, and the remainder are eliminated either during ovulation or through atresia (Baker, 1972). The variation in incidence of epithelial ovarian tumors with age (see Fig. 48–1) is inversely related to the number of oocytes: rates are low early in life, rising rapidly into midlife when, at about the time there are no further oocytes left to lose, the rates plateau.

Ionizing Radiation

Among female residents of Hiroshima and Nagasaki who survived the atomic bomb detonations of 1945, those who received an estimated dose of 100 or more rads had about twice the incidence of ovarian cancer as unexposed Japanese women (Tokuoka et al, 1987). No increased risk was evident among women who received an estimated dose less than 100 rads. The elevated incidence in heavily exposed women did not begin to be evident until 20 years following exposure. The size of the relative risk in these women also was inversely related to their age in 1945; women 50 years and older at that time had no increase in risk.

No excess incidence of ovarian cancer (2 observed, 1.9 expected) was present in Chinese diagnostic X-ray workers with five or more years employment, whereas these women had severalfold increases in risk of leukemia and thyroid cancer (Wang et al, 1988). Also, British women whose ovaries were "heavily irradiated" as a result of X-ray treatment for ankylosing spondylitis were observed (Darby et al, 1987) to have no increase in mortality from ovarian cancer (five cases observed, 5.4 cases expected, beginning five years from the time of treatment). On the other hand, two studies of women who underwent X-ray therapy for ostensibly benign pelvic conditions found a 70%–90% increase in the risk of ovarian cancer (Doll and Smith, 1968; Wagoner, 1984). While a large cohort of women with cervical cancer who had received X-ray therapy has been assembled and followed for the occurrence of subsequent cancer (Boice et al, 1985), the lack of data on oophorectomy status of these women precludes a meaningful calculation of an expected number of ovarian cancers. Nonetheless, the presence of long-term increased risk is supported by the experience of the subcohort of women under 30 years of age, a group most likely to have intact ovaries, in whom five developed ovarian cancer whereas 1.6 cases would have been expected. Additional support is provided by the observation that the average dose received by cohort members who developed ovarian cancer 10 or more years after treatment was greater than that received by a sample of subjects with intact ovaries who remained free of a second cancer (Boice et al, 1988).

It appears that high doses of radiation may induce ovarian cancer in women, but that the absolute magnitude of the effect is not great. If a linear dose-response curve exists, or one not too different than linear, the relatively small amounts of X-irradiation to which women are ordinarily exposed should have little bearing on their chances of developing ovarian cancer.

Chemical Carcinogens

Asbestos. Three occupational cohorts of women who were exposed to sufficient asbestos to produce large excesses of lung cancer and mesothelioma have also been monitored for their mortality from ovarian cancer. Two of these cohorts were involved in the assembly of gas masks in England prior to and during the Second World War (Wignall and Fox, 1982; Acheson et al, 1982); in them, a total of 23 ovarian cancer deaths occurred compared to 10.6 expected. The third group of women had been employed at an asbestos factory beginning in 1936–42 (Newhouse et al, 1985); nine deaths from ovarian cancer occurred, compared to the 3.6 expected. The observed/expected ratio increased both with increasing intensity and increasing duration of exposure in two of these cohorts in which it could be evaluated (Wignall and Fox, 1982; Newhouse et al, 1985).

Several pathologists have argued that some lesions diagnosed as ovarian cancer are peritoneal mesotheliomas that only incidentally involve the ovary (Parmley and Woodruff, 1974). The association of ovarian cancer with asbestos exposure tends to support such an assertion, as do the following observations:

1. Among the gas mask assemblers, those who worked with products containing crocidolite had a relative risk of ovarian cancer of 3.0, a value which exceeded that of assemblers who were exposed only to other forms of asbestos (relative risk = 1.7) (Acheson et al, 1982). The risk of mesothelioma has been found to be substantially greater for persons exposed to crocidolite than to other forms of asbestos (Doll and Peto, 1985).
2. Tumors morphologically indistinguishable from epithelial ovarian cancer have developed in the peritoneum of a number of women while being absent in their ovaries (Foyle et al, 1981).
3. Three of 28 women who had undergone bilateral oophorectomy as a prophylactic measure, because of a strong positive family history of ovarian cancer, nonetheless developed disseminated intraabdominal malignancy that strongly resembled ovarian cancer (Tobacman et al, 1982).

It would appear that the much smaller levels of asbestos to which women are exposed outside the industrial setting are of little consequence in determining the occurrence of ovarian cancer. The excess risk of lung cancer and mesothelioma in industrially exposed women is far higher than that for ovarian cancer, and rates of these diseases in women without occupational exposure to asbestos (or exposure to other known carcinogens) are very low. If the relation of ovarian cancer incidence to asbestos dose parallels that of lung cancer or mesothelioma, only a small fraction of the variation in ovarian cancer occurrence is attributable to variation in exposure to environmental asbestos.

Talc. Talc has certain mineralogical similarities to asbestos, and it is frequently contaminated with asbestos (Paoletti et al, 1984). Talc is commonly applied to the perineal area, and other substances have been demonstrated to migrate from the vagina to the peritoneal cavity and ovaries (Venter, 1981). As a result there has been concern that talc exposure may increase a woman's risk of developing ovarian cancer. Studies in experimental animals have been largely negative regarding the carcinogenicity of talc (Hildick-Smith, 1976). For example, none of 48 rats developed a mesothelioma following intrapleural administration of cosmetic talc, versus 18 of 48 rats similarly exposed to chrysotile asbestos. Nonetheless, the results of studies in women, while far from definitive, have suggested a positive association. Henderson et al (1971) found that particles with the appearance of talc were more prevalent in ovarian and other gynecologic tumors than in normal human ovarian tissue. In six of seven interview studies, a greater percentage of women with ovarian cancer than controls reported a history of perineal application of talc (Table 48–4). A similar association with perineal use of talc was found in a study of borderline ovarian tumors (relative risk of 1.5 based on 34 exposed cases) (Harlow and Weiss, 1989). Other genital exposures to talc have also been investigated. For example, the results of two studies suggest an excess risk of ovarian cancer associated with the use of diaphragms dusted with talc (Whittemore et al, 1988; Rosenblatt et al, 1992), whereas four other studies did not observe such an association (Cramer et al, 1982; Hartge et al, 1983; Booth et al, 1989; Harlow et al, 1992). There is little consistency between studies for other genital exposures to talc, such as talc dusting of sanitary napkins or undergarments (Cramer et al, 1982; Whittemore et al, 1988; Harlow et al, 1992; Rosenblatt et al, 1992).

Other Chemicals. Evidence in support of a modest increased risk of ovarian cancer among hairdressers has been summarized by Boffetta et al (1994). It is unknown at present whether these associations are due to the carcinogenic effects of one or more chemicals encountered in this particular profession, or instead to the confounding influence of other risk factors for ovarian cancer. There is one study that suggests that the use of hair dyes may influence risk; Tzonou et al (1993b) found that there was a higher proportion of women who dyed their hair five or more times per year among ovarian cancer cases than controls (relative risk = 2.2).

TABLE 48–4. *Relative Risk of Ovarian Cancer in Relation to Perineal Talc Exposure*

Reference	Talc Exposure to the Perineum[a]	Number of Subjects: Cases	Number of Subjects: Controls	Relative Risk
Cramer et al (1982)	None	123	154	1.0
	Yes	75	47	2.3[c]
Whittemore et al (1988)	None	91	292	1.0
	Yes	97	247	1.4[d]
Booth et al (1989)	None	76	178	1.0
	Yes	141	256	1.5[e]
Chen et al (1992)	None	105	219	1.0
	Yes	7	5	3.9[f]
Harlow et al (1992)	None	121	145	1.0
	Yes	85	61	1.7[g]
Rosenblatt et al (1992)	None[b]	54	35	1.0
	Yes	22	8	1.7[h]
Tzonou et al (1993a)	None	183	193	1.0
	Yes	6	7	1.1[i]

[a]Exposure defined as application of dusting powder or talc to the perineal area.
[b]May include individuals with other genital exposures to talc (e.g., dusting of undergarments).
[c]Adjusted for parity and menopausal status.
[d]Adjusted for parity.
[e]Adjusted for age and social class.
[f]Adjusted for education and parity.
[g]Adjusted for parity, marital status, religion, use of sanitary napkins, douching, age, weight, and education.
[h]Adjusted for age and race.
[i]Adjusted for age, education, weight, age at menarche, menopausal status, parity, smoking, coffee and alcohol consumption, hair dyeing, and use of tranquilizers/hypnotics.

A possible etiologic role for exposure to herbicides has been suggested by a study in Milan (Donna et al, 1984), in which cases and controls were queried about residential and occupational use. "Definite" or "probable" exposure to herbicides was claimed by 18 of 60 cases but only 14 of 127 control women (relative risk = 4.4). This issue needs to be addressed in other studies.

Pituitary Gonadotropin Stimulation

Pregnancy. Pregnancy causes a sharp reduction in secretion of pituitary gonadotropins. By the time of delivery, serum levels are nearly zero (Parlow et al, 1970), and require several weeks to months to return to normal (Said and Wide, 1973; Jeppsson et al, 1977). The effect of having been pregnant on ovarian cancer risk can be gauged indirectly from examination of incidence rates in never-married women, which are about 50% greater than in ever-married women (Dorn and Cutler, 1955). Parous women were found to be at decreased risk of ovarian cancer relative to nulliparous women in all but one of the 20 published studies in which the effect of

TABLE 48–5. *Relative Risk of Ovarian Cancer in Relation to Number of Full-term Pregnancies*

Reference	*Number of Full-term Pregnancies*		
	None	*1–2*	*≥3*
Wynder et al (1969)[a]	1	1.4	1.5
Joly et al (1974)[a]	1	0.8	0.4
Newhouse et al (1977)	1	0.5	0.3
Casagrande et al (1979)	1	0.8	0.6
McGowan et al (1979)	1	0.4	0.5
Hildreth et al (1981)[a]	1	0.6	0.6
Franceschi et al (1982a)	1	0.8	0.5
Cramer et al (1983a)	1	0.5	0.3
Risch et al (1983)	1	1.0	0.7
Tzonou et al (1984)	1	0.8[b]	0.6[b]
Nasca et al (1984)	1	0.6	0.5
Centers for Disease Control Cancer and Steroid Hormone Study (1987)	1	0.7	0.4
Kvale et al (1988)	1	0.7	0.5
Wu et al (1988)	1	0.7	0.6
Hartge et al (1989)	1	0.9	0.7
Shu et al (1989a)	1	0.8	0.3
Booth et al (1989)	1	0.7	0.4
Chen et al (1992)	1	0.4	0.1
Rosenberg et al (1994)	1	1.0	0.7

[a]All pregnancies included.
[b]Categories represent 1–3 and ≥4 births, respectively.

the number of full-term pregnancies could be examined (Table 48–5). While this effect is observed across all age groups, in relative terms it appears to be most pronounced in younger women (Whittemore et al, 1992b). A pooled analysis of seven case-control studies (John et al, 1993) suggests that nulliparity is associated with an increased risk of ovarian cancer in black as well as white women.

The apparent effect of increasing parity in lowering ovarian cancer risk probably cannot be attributed to a confounding effect of age at first birth, since nine of the ten studies that adjusted for any differences in the distribution of age at first birth between cases and controls continued to find an association with parity or gravidity (Lesher et al, 1985; Cramer et al, 1983a; Joly et al, 1974; LaVecchia et al, 1984a; Voigt et al, 1986; Kvale et al, 1988; Mori et al, 1988; Wu et al, 1988; Shu et al, 1989a; Booth et al, 1989). On the other hand, these nine studies observed little or no influence of age at first birth on the risk of ovarian cancer, once the confounding effect of parity was controlled. These same relationships to parity and age at first birth also appear to be present for borderline tumors (Harlow et al, 1988; Parazzini et al, 1991b; Harris et al, 1992). While increasing parity may lower ovarian cancer risk for some nonepithelial tumors (Kvale et al, 1988; Horn-Ross et al, 1992), it may increase the risk for sex cord–stromal tumors (Horn-Ross et al, 1992). However, the rarity of nonepithelial tumors has prevented anything more than a superficial inquiry into the relationship of their incidence to reproductive events.

It is unlikely that the reduced risk of ovarian cancer among parous women is due only to the association of low parity with one or more forms of infertility that independently predispose to ovarian cancer (Weiss, 1988). First, the risk progressively declines with each additional birth, even among women who have already borne several children (Table 48–5). It is improbable that there is an appreciable frequency of some condition (e.g., endometriosis or a hormonal abnormality) that can cause both infertility and ovarian cancer in these women, or that the frequency of that condition would differ between women who had given birth to two or to more than two children. Second, two studies (Nasca et al, 1984; Booth et al, 1989) found that there remained a steadily declining risk of ovarian cancer with increasing number of pregnancies even after adjusting for the number of contraceptive-free years of sexual activity.

Lactation. Because breast-feeding retards the return of gonadotropin secretion (Yen, 1991) and ovulation (Perez et al, 1972) to their prepregnancy status, women who have nursed might be expected to be at reduced risk of developing ovarian cancer. The results of some studies tend to support this expectation (Risch et al, 1983; Centers for Disease Control Cancer and Steroid Hormone Study, 1987; Hartge et al, 1989), with relative risks of 0.6–0.7 (adjusted for parity) associated with a history of any or more-than-minimal breast-feeding. However, six studies of invasive tumors (Wynder et al, 1969; Hildreth et al, 1981; Cramer et al, 1983a; Kvale and Heuch, 1988; Booth et al, 1989; Chen et al, 1992), as well as a pooled analysis of studies evaluating borderline tumors (Harris et al, 1992), found no such association. The relationship of long periods of nursing to subsequent ovarian cancer risk is no better resolved. A history of nursing for relatively long periods was more common in cases than controls in both a Japanese and a British study (Mori et al, 1984; Mori et al, 1988; Booth et al, 1989). In contrast, in the U.S. Cancer and Steroid Hormone Study (Gwinn et al, 1990), women who had nursed a total of two or more years were estimated to be at but 30% the risk of parous women who had not nursed. Yet other studies indicate a modest reduction in ovarian cancer risk associated with 6 to 12 months of breast-feeding, but no further reduction in risk with longer durations of breast-feeding (Whittemore et al, 1992a; Rosenblatt et al, 1993). Clearly, more work will be needed before the influence of lactation on the risk of ovarian cancer is understood.

Interruption of Gonadotropin Stimulation by Exogenous Ovarian Hormones. Since estrogen-containing oral contraceptives (OCs) reduce gonadotropin secretion by the pituitary (Lauritzen, 1967), these agents might be expected to exert an effect similar to that of pregnancy on the development of ovarian cancer. Nearly every study that has investigated this question has found prior use of OCs to have been less common among women with ovarian cancer than among controls. This case-control difference has been greatest, in general, for durations of use of several years or more (Table 48–6). A meta-analysis of 14 of the studies in Table 48–6, which also included a study of borderline tumors (Harlow et al, 1988), estimated that each additional year of OC use was associated with an 11% reduction in ovarian cancer risk (Hankinson et al, 1992). While not all studies are in accord, the relatively low risk among OC users appears to be present at all intervals from first or last use, and across all age groups or levels of parity (Prentice and Thomas, 1987), although the effect appears to be most pronounced in women age 55 and older (Whittemore et al, 1992b). A similar negative association has been found among black women (John et al, 1993), for malignant epithelial tumors (Centers for Disease Control Cancer and Steroid Hormone Study, 1987), for borderline tumors (Harlow et al, 1988; The WHO Collaborative Study of Neoplasia and Steroid Contraceptives, 1989; Parazzini et al, 1991b; Harris et al, 1992), and for sex cord–stromal tumors (but not for germ cell tumors) (Horn-Ross et al, 1992).

While it is likely that this consistently observed negative association represents a protective effect of oral contraceptive use on the incidence of ovarian cancer, the interruption of pituitary gonadotropin stimulation may not be the sole means by which the protection is produced. It is possible that ovulation is a factor in tumor initiation. Interruption of ovulation (during OC use, or during pregnancy) could lessen the amount of potential "irritation" to the surface epithelium; or it could lessen the chances of developing an ovarian inclusion cyst, the epithelial lining of which may be susceptible to malignant transformation (Cramer and Welch, 1983).

The impact on risk from using postmenopausal estrogens would be difficult to predict even if pituitary gonadotropin stimulation is a component of one or more causal pathways leading to ovarian cancer. These exogenous hormones lower the elevated gonadotropin levels characteristic of postmenopausal women, but the resulting levels are still higher than those of premenopausal women (Mathur et al, 1985). This decrease in gonadotropins could possibly interfere with the development of some ovarian tumors. However, postmenopausal gonadotropin levels may be beyond some sort of "threshold" necessary for cancer promotion regardless of the presence or absence of exogenous estrogens.

Results of epidemiologic studies suggest that the use of postmenopausal estrogens has little or no effect on the incidence of ovarian cancer. While some studies have reported approximately a 50% increase in risk among estrogen users (Weiss et al, 1982; Cramer et al, 1983a; Tzonou et al, 1984; Booth et al, 1989), several others have found no association (Annegers et al, 1979; Hildreth et al, 1981; Franceschi et al, 1982a; Wu et al, 1988; Polychronopoulou et al, 1993) and two studies have reported a reduced risk among users (Smith et al, 1984; Hartge et al, 1988). Early suggestions that a particular histologic type (endometrioid tumors) might be influenced more than others (Weiss et al, 1982; LaVecchia et al, 1982), or that a particular type of estrogen (stilbestrol) might carry an unusually high risk when taken by postmenopausal women (Hoover et al, 1977), do not appear to have been confirmed. However, it should be noted that two studies of women who had taken stilbestrol while pregnant (Bibbo et al, 1978; Hadjimichael et al, 1984) collectively observed 10 subsequent cases of ovarian cancer, whereas only 3.9 would have been expected.

Infertility. Until recently, only surrogate measures of infertility have been used to investigate the relationship with ovarian cancer. For example, ovarian cancer occurrence has been noted to be higher among childless women who tried to conceive (presumably infertile) than among childless women who did not (most of whom were probably fertile) (Hartge et al, 1989; Booth et al, 1989; Chen et al, 1992). This relationship was further investigated in a pooled analysis of 12 U.S. case-control studies (Whittemore et al, 1992a). A slightly higher risk of ovarian cancer was found in nulligravid women who tried to conceive for more than two years compared to nulligravid women who had never tried for more than one year. Additionally, women who had been infertile and reported having received "fertility drugs" had a increased risk of both invasive and borderline ovarian tumors relative to women either with no clinical history of infertility or with infertility who were not treated with fertility drugs (Whittemore et al, 1992a; Harris et al, 1992).

In a cohort of infertile women, Rossing et al (1994) found that infertile women who had taken clomiphene, an ovulation-induction agent, had 2.3 times the incidence of malignant or borderline ovarian tumors than did infertile women who had not taken this drug. The association was present in women with and without ovulatory abnormalities as the basis for their infertility. The increased risk was restricted to women who took clomiphene for 12 or more menstrual cycles (relative risk = 11.1). These findings need to be confirmed in other studies that are able to characterize the types of infertility in study subjects and to identify specific treatments received for infertility.

TABLE 48–6. *Relative Risk of Ovarian Cancer in Relation to Duration of Oral Contraceptive Use*

Reference	*Duration of Use (years)*	*Number of Subjects*		*Relative Risk*
		Cases	*Controls*	
Casagrande et al (1979)	<0.5	109	100	1
	0.5–6	31	36	0.7
	≥7	10	14	0.6
Willett et al (1981)	0	34	311	1
	<3	7	87	0.7
	≥3	6	65	0.8
Weiss et al (1981)	<1	91	345	1
	1–3	14	79	1.0
	4–8	3	83	0.2
	≥9	4	45	0.4
Cramer et al (1982b)	0	110	91	1
	<1	11	13	0.9
	1–3	13	11	1.1
	4–5	3	11	0.3
	≥6	7	11	0.6
LaVecchia et al (1986)	0	367	1104	1
	≤2	29	109	0.8
	>2	10	69	0.5
Centers for Disease Control Cancer and Steroid Hormone Study (1987)	0	242	1532	1
	<0.5	26	280	0.6
	0.5–0.9	14	134	0.7
	1–2	65	602	0.7
	3–4	40	397	0.6
	5–9	39	594	0.4
	≥10	13	328	0.2
Wu et al (1988)	0	188	619	1
	<1	51	136	1.0
	1–3	24	69	0.8
	≥4	28	169	0.4
Beral et al (1988)	0	(cohort study)		1
	<5			0.8
	≥5			0.3
Shu et al (1989a)	0	149	160	1
	<1	6	2	4.4
	1–5	8	6	0.8
	>5	7	4	1.9
The WHO Collaborative Study of Neoplasia and Steroid Contraceptives (1989)	0	286	1635	1
	<1	38	312	0.9
	1–4	26	258	0.7
	≥5	10	146	0.5
Hartge et al (1989)	0	115	131	1
	<1	23	16	1.6
	1–2	16	19	1.0
	3–4	10	12	0.8
	≥5	25	31	0.8
Booth et al (1989)	0	178	306	1
	≤5	24	70	0.6
	6–10	10	29	0.6
	>10	1	15	0.1
Parazzini et al (1991a)	0	464	1183	1
	<2	22	78	0.9
	≥2	19	111	0.5
Chen et al (1992)	0	<1	1–2	≥3
	<1	9	30	0.7
	1–2	12	20	1.4
	≥3	10	21	1.1
Rosenberg et al (1994)	0	304	1271	1
	<0.5	30	143	1.1
	0.5–0.9	16	85	0.9
	1	28	104	1.3
	2	19	81	1.2
	3–4	11	88	0.5
	5–9	22	150	0.7
	>10	11	99	0.5

Other Factors

Hormone Levels and Events of Reproductive Life

Germ cell tumors. A greater percentage of mothers of girls and young women with malignant ovarian germ cell tumors, as opposed to mothers of controls (14% vs. 6%), were exposed to exogenous hormones while the subject was in utero (Walker et al, 1988). Likewise, it was observed that a very high prepregnancy relative weight (> 25 kg/m^2) among mothers (which is predictive of high estrogen and low progesterone levels) was also associated with an increased risk of germ cell tumors in their daughters (2.7 times the risk of daughters of less heavy women). The investigators also found a disproportionately large fraction of cases born to young mothers (relative risk of 2.8 comparing maternal ages < 20 versus ≥ 20 years).

Epithelial tumors. There has been little interest in attaching any etiologic significance to relative levels of pituitary, ovarian, or adrenal hormones in cases and controls because of the substantial systemic changes that have occurred by the time ovarian cancer is commonly diagnosed. There has been one report of prediagnostic hormone levels in 12 women who developed ovarian cancer 1.5 to 19 years later (Cuzick et al, 1983). The cases tended to have a lower output of three androgen metabolites (dehydroepiandrosterone, androsterone, and etiocholanolone) compared to a sample of women who did not go on to develop ovarian cancer. While the interpretation of this observation is unclear, it should be noted that a roughly similar difference in this pattern of excretion has been found between women who later develop breast cancer and those who do not (Bulbrook et al, 1971). However, in a mouse model, the spontaneous high incidence of malignant granulosa cell tumors is not decreased, but actually increased, when exogenous dehydroepiandrosterone or testosterone is administered (Beamer et al, 1988).

Shu et al (1989a) found that the risk of ovarian cancer in the small proportion of Shanghai residents whose menarche did not occur until 18 or more years of age was one-third to one-quarter that of other women. However, within the range of ages at menarche more commonly encountered, three studies (Casagrande et al, 1979; LaVecchia et al, 1986; Wynder et al, 1969) have observed a negative association and three studies observed a positive association (Szamborski, 1981; Tzonou et al, 1984; Wu et al, 1988), while still others found little or no association with invasive tumors (Newhouse et al, 1977; McGowan et al, 1979; Hildreth et al, 1981; Willett et al, 1981; Cramer et al, 1983b; Mori et al, 1984; Booth et al, 1989; Chen et al, 1992; Polychronopoulou et al, 1993) or borderline tumors (Harris et al, 1992). This pattern of results suggests that no important relation exists between age at menarche (at least through age 18) and the risk of ovarian cancer.

Hartge et al (1988) found no difference between cases and controls with regard to their median age at menopause using a life-table approach. Other studies that have examined this issue have not used the life-table approach, and have instead contrasted the distribution of age at menopause, or the percent of subjects still menstruating, between cases and controls. No consistent findings have emerged.

It is possible to evaluate the influence of hysterectomy on the subsequent risk of ovarian cancer, since many physicians do not routinely remove both ovaries at the time of hysterectomy for a nonmalignant uterine condition. Most studies have found that prior hysterectomy is reported less often by women with ovarian cancer than by controls (Wynder et al, 1969; Annegers et al, 1979; Cramer et al, 1983a; McGowan et al, 1979; Hartge et al, 1988; Booth et al, 1989; Hankinson et al, 1993; Parazzini et al, 1993; Rosenberg et al, 1994), though some found no difference (Newhouse et al, 1977; Casagrande et al, 1979; Hildreth et al, 1981).

It has been proposed (Weiss and Harlow, 1986) that the relatively low incidence of ovarian cancer following hysterectomy may not be related to the removal of the uterus per se. Rather, the reduced risk could result because women with subclinical ovarian tumors generally have them removed at the time of hysterectomy. For some period of time afterward, the remaining women with normal-appearing ovaries would be expected to have a deficit in diagnosed ovarian cancer, relative to women who had not been "screened" in this way, even if the absence of the uterus has no effect. In support of this proposal is the finding in one study (Weiss and Harlow, 1986) of a sizable reduction in risk of ovarian cancer in the first three years following hysterectomy, but not thereafter. However, some studies have noted a reduced risk more than 5–10 years after hysterectomy (Hartge et al, 1988; Whittemore et al, 1988; Irwin et al, 1991; Hankinson et al, 1993; Parazzini et al, 1993). It remains uncertain whether the reduced long-term incidence of ovarian cancer seen in these studies results from the hysterectomy itself, or is in some way related to the reasons for the hysterectomy.

Similarly, there is mounting evidence that women who have undergone a tubal ligation are at relatively low risk of ovarian cancer (Mori et al, 1988; Whittemore et al, 1988; Booth et al, 1989; Irwin et al, 1991; Hankinson et al, 1993; Rosenberg et al, 1994). While the screening bias described above could be partially responsible, it is unlikely that this could account for the long-term reduction in ovarian cancer risk found in a few studies. Irwin et al (1991) and Hankinson et al (1993) found a persistent decrease in ovarian cancer incidence 5 or more years following tubal sterilization (although this effect appeared to diminish after 15 years in the former study). Moreover, in the study by Whittemore et al (1988), a reduction in ovarian cancer risk was noted only 10 or more years after tubal ligation. These results argue that tubal sterilization reduces ovarian cancer incidence, although the means by which it does so have not yet been identified.

Physical Characteristics

Weight/Quetelet's Index. A number of investigators have evaluated body weight (relative or absolute) as a possible risk factor for ovarian cancer because of the differences between lean and obese women with regard to levels of endogenous sex hormones. The results of these studies have not been uniform. Byers et al (1983), Mori et al (1984; 1988), and Engle et al (1991) found that women with ovarian cancer were generally leaner than controls, and Hildreth et al (1981), Hartge et al (1989), Chen et al (1992), and Polychronopoulou et al (1993) found no case-control difference. However, four studies have noted a positive association with usual adult weight/Quetelet's index (Casagrande et al, 1979; Trichopoulos et al, 1981; Annegers et al, 1979; Centers for Disease Control Cancer and Steroid Hormone Study, 1987), and three others found elevations of risk of 40%–70% largely confined to the heaviest group (upper quartile or upper quintile) of women (Cramer et al, 1984; Garfinkel, 1985; Farrow et al, 1989). In the study of Farrow et al (1989), the elevated risk among heavy women was further confined to those who were premenopausal and who had a serous or an endometrioid tumor, a finding that is yet to be confirmed in other studies. Borderline ovarian tumors have also been associated with higher relative weights (Harris et al, 1992).

Height. Three studies (Hildreth et al, 1981; Cramer et al, 1984; Mori et al, 1984) noted the mean height of women with ovarian cancer to be slightly greater than that of controls. Tzonou et al (1984) found a modest excess of tall women (≥ 165 cm) among cases in Greece (risk = 1.8 times that of shorter women), whereas a subsequent study of Greek women found no excess risk (Polychronopoulou et al, 1993). Further assessment of height as a possible risk factor for ovarian cancer could probably be readily accomplished through additional analyses of existing data sets.

Genetic Factors. The presence of dysgenetic gonads in phenotypic females with an XY karyotype predisposes to the development of germ cell tumors (Teter and Boczkowski, 1967). Nevertheless, fewer than 5% of germ cell tumors can be accounted for by this abnormality (Li et al, 1973).

A hereditary condition known to predispose to the development of sex cord–stromal tumors is the Peutz-Jeghers syndrome (characterized by mucocutaneous pigmentation and intestinal polyps). Of 115 girls and women with the syndrome, five were observed to have tumors of this type (Dozois et al, 1970). Epithelial ovarian tumors occurred with increased frequency as well. The reasons for the increase are unknown. Unlike breast tumors, epithelial ovarian tumors do not appear to occur with increased frequency in female relatives of persons with ataxia telangiectasia, an autosomal recessive condition (Swift et al, 1991).

Apart from the abnormalities underlying the Peutz-Jeghers syndrome, there are likely to be other genetic influences on the development of epithelial ovarian tumors. Numerous reports of families with two or more women affected by ovarian cancer have been published. It seems likely that more than chance played a role in producing such clusters, since in such families virtually none of the tumors of known histology were of the mucinous type (Lurain and Piver, 1979; Franceschi et al, 1982b). In a group of 30 women with ovarian cancer who were members of twin pairs, none had a twin sister with the disease (Harvald and Hauge, 1963). However, even a strong genetic effect may not have been detected in such a small sample, particularly since not all the twins were monozygous. Case-control studies should be able to determine whether ovarian cancer is more common than expected in the families of cases, but difficulties in diagnosis, particularly in the era of mothers and grandmothers of contemporary cases, limit the sensitivity of such investigations. Of the eight studies that did examine the question, two found no difference in the family histories of cases and controls (Lau et al, 1977; Wynder et al, 1969). However, the six other studies noted a strong association. Cramer et al (1983a) found that four of 213 cases, but none of a similar number of controls, reported ovarian cancer occurrence in a "primary" female relative. These four cases had either serous or endometrioid tumors. Tzonou et al (1984) found a positive history of ovarian cancer in a mother or sister from nine of 146 cases, in contrast to zero of 243 controls. In the study of Hartge et al (1989), the corresponding numbers were 13 of 296 cases and five of 343 controls (relative risk = 3.3). Based on 62 total cases and over 1,000 controls, Hildreth et al (1981) estimated a relative risk of 18.2 associated with a history of ovarian cancer in a mother or sister (numbers with a positive family history were not provided). Casagrande et al (1979) found that neither cases nor controls had any relatives on the paternal side of their families with a history of ovarian cancer. On the maternal side, however, seven of 150 cases had a positive history, in contrast to zero of 150 controls. Finally, in the Cancer and Steroid Hormone Study (Schildkraut and Thompson, 1988) 16 of 493 women (3.2%) with an epithelial tumor reported ovarian cancer in a mother or sister, in contrast to 0.9% of controls (relative risk = 3.6). In this study there was also a 3-fold increase in risk associated with a history of ovarian cancer in a grandmother or aunt, whether on the maternal or paternal side.

The genetic basis for this familial clustering is not clear at present, although there is evidence that at least one germline mutation may play a role. Among women with breast cancer who have several female relatives with breast or ovarian cancer, some have evidence of a germline mutation in a gene (BRCA 1) on chromosome 17. The subsequent incidence of ovarian cancer in these women is extremely high, about 44% by age 70 years (Ford et al, 1994).

A clue to another possible genetic basis for the multiple occurrence of ovarian cancer in some families comes from the observation of abnormally low serum levels of the enzyme α-L-fucosidase in women with ovarian cancer (Barlow et al, 1981). Levels of this enzyme, which are believed to be largely under genetic control, are also lower than average in members of families in which there had been multiple cases of ovarian cancer (Lynch et al, 1985), though they do not appear to be low in nonfamilial cases with borderline tumors (Harlow et al, 1990). However, it has been argued that a low level of α-L-fucosidase is unlikely to be in the causal pathway leading to cancer occurrence, but merely represents a correlate of a cause (Wells et al, 1987).

Blood type has also been linked with ovarian cancer in several studies. Bjorkholm (1984) and Henderson et al (1993) noted that ovarian cancer cases were slightly more likely to have blood type A relative to type O than control women (relative risk = 1.19 and 1.17, respectively). However, Chen et al (1992) found no case-control difference.

Infectious Agents. At present there is no clear evidence to indicate that ovarian infection by any microorganism plays a role in carcinogenesis. Mumps virus infection, which can affect the ovaries, is reported less commonly by women with ovarian cancer than controls in most studies (Menczer et al, 1979; Newhouse et al, 1977; Wynder et al, 1969; West, 1966; Cramer et al, 1983b; Schiffman et al, 1985; McGowan et al, 1979; Hartge et al, 1989). In one study (Golan et al, 1979), women with ovarian cancer had similar levels of neutralizing antibody titers against mumps virus to controls.

Human papillomavirus, which almost certainly plays a role in the etiology of several other gynecologic cancers, has been sought and not detected in epithelial ovarian tumors (Beckmann et al, 1991).

Food, Beverage, and Tobacco Consumption A reduced risk of ovarian cancer has been reported among Mormons (Lyon et al, 1976) and Seventh Day Adventists (Phillips et al, 1980), persons who tend to consume very low quantities of alcohol, tobacco, and coffee. A number of studies have attempted to identify which of those factors may be associated with an altered risk of ovarian cancer.

Alcohol. Findings with respect to alcohol consumption are inconsistent, but taken in aggregate do not suggest an association. Three studies reported increased risk with increasing alcohol consumption (Tzonou et al, 1984; Hartge et al, 1989; LaVecchia et al, 1992), one study reported a decreased risk only in drinkers of more than 20 drinks per week (Gwinn et al, 1986), and five studies found no association (Trichopoulos et al, 1981; Byers et al, 1983; Cramer et al, 1984; Whittemore et al, 1988; Polychronopoulou et al, 1993).

Tobacco. With one exception (Doll et al, 1980), studies have failed to find an association between smoking and ovarian cancer risk (Baron et al, 1986; Byers et al, 1983; Cramer et al, 1984; Trichopoulos et al, 1981; Tzonou et al, 1984; Franks et al, 1987; Whittemore et al, 1988; Hartge et al, 1989; Booth et al, 1989; Polychronopoulou et al, 1993).

Coffee. Case-control studies in Greece and Italy (Trichopoulos et al, 1981; LaVecchia et al, 1984b) found an increase in risk with increasing per-day coffee consumption (Table 48–7). A second study in Greece (Tzonou et al, 1984) and one in the U.S. (Whittemore et al, 1988) also noted an association, though the excess risk did not rise with increasing amount consumed.

However, other American case-control studies (Hartge et al, 1982; Byers et al, 1983; Miller et al, 1987), two American cohort studies (Jacobsen et al, 1986; Snowdon et al, 1984), and one Greek study (Polychronopoulou et al, 1993) failed to observe any consistent association. Differences between European and American coffee-drinking habits, including types of beans, brewing methods, and usual coffee strength, may account for some of the differences in these studies' results. Consumption of decaffeinated coffee was found not to be associated with the incidence of ovarian cancer (Miller et al, 1987).

Diet. Stimulated by the correlation between international ovarian cancer occurrence and dietary fat intake (Armstrong and Doll, 1975), several studies have sought to identify dietary components associated with an altered risk of ovarian cancer. In case-control studies, Cramer et al (1984), LaVecchia et al (1987), and Shu et al (1989b) found a trend of increasing risk with increasing animal fat intake, and Risch et al (1994) noted a similar trend with increasing saturated-fat intake. In a cohort study among Seventh Day Adventists (Snowdon et al, 1985), frequent consumption of eggs and fried foods was associated with an increased risk. A Canadian case-control study specifically noted higher intakes of cholesterol from eggs among ovarian cancer cases

TABLE 48–7. *Case-control Studies of Ovarian Cancer in Relation to Coffee Consumption*

Reference	*Location*	*Coffee Consumption (cups per day)*	*Relative Risk*[a]
Trichopoulos et al (1981)	Greece	≤1	1.1
		≥2	2.2
Hartge et al (1982)	U.S.	<2	1.0
		2–3	1.8
		≥4	1.4
Byers et al (1983)	U.S.	<2	1.3
		≥3	1.0
Cramer et al (1984)	U.S.	1–2	1.1
		3–4	1.1
		≥5	1.5
LaVecchia et al (1984b)	Italy	<2	1.3
		2–3	1.7
		≥4	1.8
Tzonou et al (1984)	Greece	.5–1	0.9
		1.5–2	1.6
		2.5–3	0.9
		≥3.5	1.5
Miller et al (1987)	U.S.	1	1.0, 1.6[b]
		2	0.9, 1.5
		3	0.9, 1.6
		4	1.6, 1.7
		≥5	1.0, 1.1
Whittemore et al (1988)	U.S.	1	1.9, 2.4[b]
		2–3	1.6, 2.3
		≥4	1.6, 2.1
Polychronopoulou et al (1993)	Greece	≤1	1.3 or 1.0
		1–2	1.6 or 1.3
		>2	1.2 or 1.1

[a]Relative to nondrinkers of coffee.
[b]Relative risks estimated from each of two control groups.

compared to controls (Risch et al, 1994). On the other hand, no association with total fat or protein intake was found in case-control studies by Byers et al (1983), Slattery et al (1989), and Tzonou et al (1993a), although in the latter study women with ovarian cancer had diets lower in monounsaturated fats than the diets of control women.

The high levels of gonadotropins in women with galactosemia (Kaufman et al, 1981), along with the suspected role of gonadotropin levels in the genesis of ovarian cancer, has prompted interest in galactose consumption and metabolism as a possible influence on the occurrence of ovarian cancer. Galactose, a component of lactose, is obtained when the latter is hydrolyzed. This can occur in the intestines of some, but not all, adults, or in certain dairy products (e.g., yogurt) prior to their being eaten. Conceivably, gonadotropin levels are higher and tumor development more likely among women who consume higher than average amounts of lactose and/or have a decreased capacity to metabolize galactose.

Cramer et al (1989) addressed this question and found that both yogurt consumption and higher levels of total lactose consumption were reported more commonly by women with ovarian cancer than by controls, whereas other dairy products were consumed to a similar degree. However, Engle et al (1991) and Herrinton et al (1994) did not find higher lactose consumption among women with ovarian cancer compared to controls. Cramer et al (1989) also found that women who consumed greater than average amounts of lactose from all sources combined, especially those with below average red-cell levels of galactose-1-phosphate uridyl transferase (a key enzyme in galactose metabolism), appeared to be at increased risk of ovarian cancer. This was not confirmed in the study by Herrinton et al (1994), which also evaluated lactose consumption in relation to galactose-1-phosphate uridyl transferase activity. Additionally, the latter study determined galactose-1-phosphate uridyl transferase genotypes, and found that the presence of the low-activity variant was, if anything, slightly less common among the women with ovarian cancer than among controls.

Other evidence suggests that the potential relationship between consumption of dairy products and ovarian cancer could be due to consumption of dairy fat. In a population of Caucasian women, most of whom would be expected not to be lactose-deficient, Mettlin and Piver (1990) observed no difference in consumption of low- or nonfat milk between cases and controls; in contrast, there was a severalfold increase in risk associated with regular drinking of whole milk. Cramer and Harlow (1991) did not find such a difference in risk associated with milk fat content. Nonetheless, it is possible that a 6-fold increase in risk (Ursin et al, 1990) among Norwegian women who reported in the 1960s that they drank two or more glasses of milk each day (relative to those who drank less than one glass per day), was due less to an effect of lactose than to an effect of fat intake, as it seems likely that most milk consumed by Norwegians during the 1960s was whole milk. From the foregoing, it is evident that some aspect of fat or galactose intake/metabolism could well influence ovarian cancer risk. Unfortunately, it is equally evident that at present we do not have a clear idea as to what that aspect might be or how it might operate.

The studies of Engle et al (1991), Slattery et al (1989), LaVecchia et al (1987), and Byers et al (1983) have noted that women with ovarian cancer had, on average, diets lower in beta-carotene than controls, though in the latter study this association was restricted to women 30–49 years of age. Shu et al (1989b) observed no such relationship. Risch et al (1994) also noted an inverse relationship; however, when beta-carotene consumption was considered simultaneously with vegetable fiber intake, beta-carotene consumption had little influence on the risk of ovarian cancer, whereas a strong inverse relationship was noted between vegetable fiber intake and ovarian cancer risk. In a Finnish study (Knekt et al, 1990) in which serum samples drawn and frozen up to eight years earlier on a group of 12 cases with ovarian cancer and 23 controls were thawed and analyzed, the distribution of beta-carotene levels were nearly the same in the two groups. In contrast, the authors estimated the risk among women in the lowest quintile of serum retinol levels to be 4–7 times that of women in the highest quintile. This issue should be pursued in other studies of cancer in women whose serum has been stored.

OUTLOOK

Among the approaches recommended for enhancing the ability of epidemiologic studies to identify etiologic relationships (Weiss and Liff, 1983), several are appropriate to consider in future studies of ovarian cancer.

1. A division should be made of individuals who are diagnosed as having a particular "disease" into subgroups within which there is a greater degree of etiologic homogeneity. One of the problems hindering epidemiologic studies of ovarian cancer arises from the ambiguity that often surrounds the diagnosis of this tumor, particularly when the disease is in its very earliest or very latest stages. The development of additional methods for determining whether a given ovarian tumor is benign, malignant, or of low malignant potential, or whether the tissue of origin is indeed ovarian or not in women with widely metastatic disease, will enable future epidemiologic studies to avoid the misclassification that results from the inclusion of women who have other conditions.

In a similar way, the separation of women with bona fide ovarian tumors into smaller subcategories (based on morphology or some other characteristic) might allow the identification of a factor that influences the occurrence of tumors in only one of the subcategories. Several epidemiologic studies have already explored the separate histologic types for variation in their relation to some risk factors (e.g., oral contraceptive use and parity). While some variation did emerge, the pattern has not been consistent across studies. Part of the lack of consistency could relate to the ambiguity that can arise in trying to make a single histologic diagnosis and the nonuniformity among pathologists in doing so. Possibly, some different criteria for the classification of ovarian tumors other than those available now would produce a greater yield in terms of a differential relationship to known risk factors.

2. The separation of cases into those with and without a strong risk factor for disease occurrence should be made for purposes of analysis. This approach, useful in the study of many other diseases, is at present not practical in ovarian cancer, since we have not yet been successful in identifying a potent risk factor for the disease. Possibly, studies of women with ovarian cancer with a strongly positive family history of that disease will enable discovery of a genetic marker that predicts its occurrence. Subsequently, it might be possible to investigate whether the risk of ovarian cancer among women possessing this marker is particularly influenced by selected features of reproductive history (e.g., low parity) or by exposure to various environmental factors (e.g., talc).

3. The improved ability to measure environmental exposures themselves is important. It is clear that historical assessment of many environmental exposures is limited in sensitivity. The development of assays for the presence of these environmental factors, or of any persistent biological effect they may reliably produce in the body, will greatly enhance studies of their relationship with ovarian cancer.

The past few years have seen, in relative terms, an "explosion" of epidemiologic research devoted to ovarian cancer. We have a better understanding of which factors increase a woman's risk of developing this disease as a result of this research. Nonetheless, the gaps in our knowledge concerning the reasons for ovarian cancer development are enormous. In terms of prevention, we can offer no practical strategies, save those whose benefits to most women might be exceeded by their deleterious effects, such as prolonged oral contraceptive use or prophylactic oophorectomy. The research approaches outlined in the preceding text offer some ideas for moving beyond where we are at present, but all require initiatives by investigators outside the field of epidemiology. Those epidemiologists interested in learning more about the reasons for the occurrence of cancer of the ovary would be well advised to keep abreast of these fields for means by which we can strengthen our own research.

REFERENCES

ACHESON ED, GARDNER MJ, PIPPARD EC, et al. 1982. Mortality of two groups of women who manufactured gas masks from chrysotile and crocidolite asbestos: A 40-year follow-up. Br J Ind Med 39:344–348.

ADAMI H-O, BERGSTROM R, PERSSON I, SPAREN P. 1990. The incidence of ovarian cancer in Sweden, 1960–1984. Am J Epidemiol 132:446–452.

ANNEGERS JF, STROM H, DECKER DG, et al. 1979. Ovarian cancer: Incidence and case-control study. Cancer 43:723–729.

ARMSTRONG B, DOLL R. 1975. Environmental factors and cancer incidence in different countries, with special reference to dietary factors. Int J Cancer 15:617–631.

BAKER TG. 1972. Oogenesis and ovarian development. In: Bolin H, Glasser S (eds): Reproductive Biology. Amsterdam; Excerpta Medica.

BARLOW JJ, DICIOCCIO RA, DILLARD PH, et al. 1981. Frequency of an allele for low activity of a-L-fucosidase in sera: Possible increase in epithelial ovarian cancer patients. J Natl Cancer Inst 67:1005–1009.

BARON JA, BYERS T, GREENBERG ER, et al. 1986. Cigarette smoking in women with cancers of the breast and reproductive organs. J Natl Cancer Inst 77:677–680.

BEAMER WG, SHULTZ KL, TENNENT BJ. 1988. Induction of ovarian granulosa cell tumors in SWXJ-9 mice with dehydroepiandrosterone. Cancer Res 48:2788–2792.

BECKMANN AM, SHERMAN KJ, SARAN L, et al. 1991. Genital type human papillomavirus infection is not associated with surface epithelial ovarian carcinoma. Gynecol Oncol 43:247–251.

BERAL V, HANNAFORD P, KAY C. 1988. Oral contraceptive use and malignancies of the genital tract. Lancet 2:1331–1336.

BHOOLA KD, BHAMJEE A. 1976. A comparative study of ovarian tumors in black and Indian patients. S Afr Med J 50:1935–1936.

BIBBO M, HAENSZEL WM, WIED GL, et al. 1978. A twenty-five-year follow-up study of women exposed to diethylstilbestrol during pregnancy. N Engl J Med 298:763–767.

BJORKHOLM E. 1984. Blood group distribution in women with ovarian cancer. Int J Epidemiol 13:15–17.

BOFFETTA P, ANDERSEN A, LYNGE E, et al. 1994. Employment as hairdresser and risk of ovarian cancer and non-hodgkin's lymphomas among women. J Occup Med 36:61–65.

BOICE JD JR, DAY NE, ANDERSEN A, et al. 1985. Second cancers following radiation treatment for cervical cancer. An international collaboration among cancer registries. J Natl Cancer Inst 74:955–975.

BOICE JD JR, ENGHOLM G, KLEINERMAN RA, et al. 1988. Radiation dose and second cancer risk in patients treated for cancer of the cervix. Radiat Res 116:3–55.

BONSER GM, JULL JW. 1977. Tumors of the ovary. In Zuckerman S, Weir BJ (eds): The Ovary, Vol. II. New York: Academic Press.

BOOTH M, BERAL V, SMITH P. 1989. Risk factors for ovarian cancer: A case-control study. Br J Cancer 60:592–598.

BULBROOK RD, HAYWARD JL, SPICER CC. 1971. Relation between urinary androgen and corticoid excretion and subsequent breast cancer. Lancet 2:395–398.

BYERS T, MARSHALL J, GRAHAM S, et al. 1983. A case-control study of dietary and nondietary factors in ovarian cancer. J Natl Cancer Inst 71:681–686.

CASAGRANDE JT, PIKE MC, ROSS RK, et al. 1979. "Incessant ovulation" and ovarian cancer. Lancet 2:170–173.

CENTERS FOR DISEASE CONTROL CANCER AND STEROID HORMONE STUDY. 1987. The reduction in risk of ovarian cancer associated with oral-contraceptive use. N Engl J Med 316:650–655.

CHEN Y, WU PC, LANG JH, et al. 1992. Risk factors for epithelial ovarian cancer in Beijing, China. Int J Epidemiol 21:23–29.

COLEMAN MP, ESTEVE J, DAMIECKI P, ARSLAN A, RENARD H. 1993. Trends in Cancer Incidence and Mortality. IARC Scientific Publications No. 121, Lyon.

CRAMER DW, HUTCHISON GB, WELCH WR, et al. 1982a. Factors affecting the association of oral contraceptives and ovarian cancer. N Engl J Med 307:1047–1051.

CRAMER DW, WELCH WR, SCULLY RE, et al. 1982b. Ovarian cancer and talc: A case-control study. Cancer 50:372–376.

CRAMER DW, WELCH WR. 1983. Determinants of ovarian cancer risk. II. Inferences regarding pathogenesis. J Natl Cancer Inst 71:717–721.

CRAMER DW, HUTCHISON GB, WELCH WR, et al. 1983a. Determinants of ovarian cancer risk. I. Reproductive experiences and family history. J Natl Cancer Inst 71:711–716.

CRAMER DW, WELCH WR, CASSELLS S, et al. 1983b. Mumps, menarche, menopause, and ovarian cancer. Am J Obstet Gynecol 147:1–6.

CRAMER DW, WELCH WR, HUTCHISON GB, et al. 1984. Dietary animal fat in relation to ovarian cancer risk. Obstet Gynecol 63:833–838.

CRAMER DW, HARLOW BL, WILLETT WC, et al. 1989. Galactose consumption and metabolism in relation to the risk of ovarian cancer. Lancet 2:66–71.

CRAMER DW, HARLOW BL. 1991. Commentary: A case-control study of milk drinking and ovarian cancer risk. Am J Epidemiol 134:454–456.

CUTLER SJ, YOUNG JL JR (EDS). 1975. Third National Cancer Survey: Incidence data. Natl Cancer Inst Monogr 41:1–454.

CUZICK J, BULSTRODE JC, STRATTON I, et al. 1983. A prospective study of urinary androgen levels and ovarian cancer. Int J Cancer 32:723–726.

DARBY SC, DOLL R, GILL SK, et al. 1987. Long term mortality after a single treatment course with X-rays in patients treated for ankylosing spondylitis. Br J Cancer 55:179–190.

DOLL R, GRAY R, HAFNER B, et al. 1980. Mortality in relation to smoking: 22 years' observations on female British doctors. BMJ 1:967–971.

DOLL R, PETO J. 1985. Effects on health of exposure to asbestos. Health and Safety Commission. London: Her Majesty's Stationery Office.

DOLL R, SMITH PG. 1968. The long-term effects of X irradiation in patients treated for metropathia haemorrhagica. Br J Radiol 41:362–368.

DONNA A, BETA P-G, ROBUTTI F, et al. 1984. Ovarian mesothelial tumors and herbicides: A case-control study. Carcinogenesis 5:941–942.

DORN HF, CUTLER SJ. 1955. Morbidity from cancer in the United States. U.S. Department of Health, Education, and Welfare, Public Health Monogr 29. Washington D.C. U.S. Government Printing Office.

DOZOIS RR, KEMPERS RD, DAHLIN DC, et al. 1970. Ovarian tumors associated with the Peutz-Jeghers syndrome. Ann Surg 172:233–238.

ENGLE A, MUSCAT JE, HARRIS RE. 1991. Nutritional risk factors and ovarian cancer. Nutr Cancer 15:239–247.

EWERTZ M, KJAER SK. 1988. Ovarian cancer incidence and mortality in Denmark, 1943–1982. Int J Cancer 42:690–696.

FARROW DC, WEISS NS, LYON JL, et al. 1989. Association of obesity and ovarian cancer in a case-control study. Am J Epidemiol 129:1300–1304.

FORD D, EASTON DF, BISHOP DT, et al. 1994. Risks of cancer in BRCA1-mutations carriers. Lancet 343:692–695.

FOYLE A, AL-JABI M, MCCAUGHEY WTE. 1981. Papillary peritoneal tumors in women. Am J Surg Pathol 5:241–249.

FRANCESCHI S, LAVECCHIA C, HELMRICH SP, et al. 1982a. Risk factors for epithelial ovarian cancer in Italy. Am J Epidemiol 115:714–719.

FRANCESCHI S, LAVECCHIA C, MANGIONI C. 1982b. Familial ovarian cancer: Eight more families. Gynecol Oncol 13:31–36.

FRANKS AL, LEE NC, KENDRICK JS, et al. 1987. Cigarette smoking and the risk of epithelial ovarian cancer. Am J Epidemiol 126:112–117.

GARFINKEL L. 1985. Overweight and cancer. Ann Intern Med 103:1034–1036.

GOLAN A, JOOSTING ACC, ORCHARD ME. 1979. Mumps virus and ovarian cancer. S Afr Med J 56:18–20.

GWINN ML, LEE NC, RHODES PH, et al. 1990. Pregnancy, breast feeding, and oral contraceptives and the risk of epithelial ovarian cancer. J Clin Epidemiol 43:559–568.

GWINN ML, WEBSTER LA, LEE NC, et al. 1986. Alcohol consumption and ovarian cancer risk. Am J Epidemiol 123:759–766.

HADJIMICHAEL OC, MEIGS JW, FALCIER FW, et al. 1984. Cancer risk among women exposed to exogenous estrogens during pregnancy. J Natl Cancer Inst 73:831–834.

HANKINSON SE, COLDITZ GA, HUNTER DJ, et al. 1992. A quantitative assessment of oral contraceptive use and risk of ovarian cancer. Obstet Gynecol 80:708–714.

HANKINSON SE, HUNTER DJ, COLDITZ GA, et al. 1993. Tubal ligation, hysterectomy, and risk of ovarian cancer. JAMA 270:2813–2818.

HARLOW BL, CRAMER DW, BELL DA, WELCH WR. 1992. Perineal exposure to talc and ovarian cancer risk. Obstet Gynecol 80:19–26.

HARLOW BL, WEISS NS, LOFTON S. 1987. Epidemiology of borderline ovarian tumors. J Natl Cancer Inst 78:71–74.

HARLOW BL, WEISS NS, ROTH GJ, et al. 1988. Case-control study of borderline ovarian tumors: Reproductive history and exposure to exogenous female hormones. Cancer Res 48:5849–5852.

HARLOW BL, WEISS NS. 1989. A case-control study of borderline ovarian tumors: The influence of perineal exposure to talc. Am J Epidemiol 130:390–394.

HARLOW BL, WEISS NS, HOLMES EH. 1990. Plasma alpha-L-Fucosidase activity and the risk of borderline epithelial ovarian tumors. Cancer Res 50:4702–4703.

HARRIS R, WHITTEMORE AS, ITNYRE J, AND THE COLLABORATIVE OVARIAN CANCER GROUP. 1992. Characteristics relating to ovarian cancer risk: collaborative analysis of 12 case-control studies. III. Epithelial tumors of low malignant potential in white women. Am J Epidemiol 136:1204–1211.

HARTGE P, SCHIFFMAN MH, HOOVER R, et al. 1989. A case-control study of epithelial ovarian cancer. Am J Obstet Gynecol 161:10–16.

HARTGE P, HOOVER R, LESHER LP, et al. 1983. Talc and ovarian cancer. JAMA 250:1844.

HARTGE P, HOOVER R, MCGOWAN L, et al. 1988. Menopause and ovarian cancer. Am J Epidemiol 127:990–998.

HARTGE P, LESHER LP, MCGOWAN L, et al. 1982. Coffee and ovarian cancer. Int J Cancer 30:531–532.

HARVALD B, HAUGE M. 1963. Heredity of cancer elucidated by a study of unselected twins. JAMA 186:89–93.

HENDERSON J, SRAGROATT V, GOLDACRE M. 1993. Ovarian cancer and ABO blood groups. J Epidemiol Community Health 47:287–289.

HENDERSON WJ, JOSLIN CAF, TURNVULL AC, et al. 1971. Talc and carcinoma of the ovary and cervix. J Obstet Gynecol Br Commw 78:266–272.

HERRINTON LJ, STANFORD JL, SCHWARTZ SM, WEISS NS. 1994. Ovarian cancer incidence among Asian migrants to the United States and their descendents. J Natl Cancer Inst 86:1336–1339.

HERRINTON LJ, WEISS NS, BERESFORD SAA, et al. Lactose and galactose intake and metabolism in relation to the risk of epithelial ovarian cancer. Am J Epidemiol 1995; 141:407–16.

HILDICK-SMITH GY. 1976. The biology of talc. Br J Ind Med 33:217–229.

HILDRETH NG, KELSEY JL, LIVOLSI VA, et al. 1981. An epidemiologic study of epithelial carcinoma of the ovary. Am J Epidemiol 114:398–405.

HOOVER R, GRAY LA, FRAUMENI JF. 1977. Stilboestrol (diethylstilbestrol) and the risk of ovarian cancer. Lancet 2:533–534.

HORN-ROSS PL, WHITTEMORE AS, HARRIS R, et al. 1992. Characteristics relating to ovarian cancer risk: collaborative analysis of 12 case-control studies. VI. Nonepithelial cancers among adults. Epidemiology 3:490–495.

IRWIN KL, WEISS NS, LEE NC, et al. 1991. Tubal sterilization, hysterectomy, and the subsequent occurrence of epithelial ovarian cancer. Am J Epidemiol 134:362–369.

JACOBSEN BK, BJELKE E, KVALE G, et al. 1986. Coffee drinking, mortality, and cancer incidence: Results from a Norwegian Prospective study. J Natl Cancer Inst 76:823–831.

JEPPSSON S, RANNEVIK G, THORELL JI, et al. 1977. Influence of LH/FSH releasing hormone (LRH) on the basal secretion of gonadotropins in relation to plasma levels of oestradiol, progesterone and prolactin during the post-partum period in lactating and non-lactating women. Acta Endocrinol (Copenh), 84:713–728.

JOHN EM, WHITTEMORE AS, HARRIS R, et al. 1993. Characteristics relating to ovarian cancer: collaborative analysis of seven U.S. case-control studies. Epithelial ovarian cancer in black women. J Natl Cancer Inst 85:142–147.

JOLY DJ, LILIENFELD AM, DIAMOND EL, et al. 1974. An epidemiologic study of the relationship of reproductive experience to cancer of the ovary. Am J Epidemiol 99:190–209.

KAPLAN HS. 1950. Influence of ovarian function on incidence of radiation-induced ovarian tumors in mice. J Natl Cancer Inst 11:125–132.

KAUFMAN FR, KOGUT MD, DONNELL GN, et al. 1981. Hypergonadotropic hypogonadism in female patients with galactosemia. N Engl J Med 304:994–998.

KNEKT P, AROMAA A, MAATELA J, et al. 1990. Serum vitamin A an subsequent risk of cancer: Cancer incidence follow-up of the Finnish Mobile Clinic Health Examination Survey. Am J Epidemiol 132:857–870.

KVALE G, HEUCH I, NILSSEN S, et al. 1988. Reproductive factors and risk of ovarian cancer: A prospective study. Int J Cancer 42:246–251.

KVALE G, HEUCH I. 1988. Lactation and cancer risk: Is there a relation specific to breast cancer? J Epidemiol Community Health 42:30–37.

LAU HU, PETSCHELT E, POEHLS H, et al. 1977. Zur epidemiologie des ovarialkarzinoms. Arch Geschwulstforsch 47:57–66.

LAURITZEN C. 1967. On endocrine effects of oral contraceptives. Acta Endocrinol 124 (Suppl):87–100.

LAVECCHIA C, LIBERATI A, FRANCESCHI S. 1982. Noncontraceptive estrogen use and the occurrence of ovarian cancer. J Natl Cancer Inst 69:1207.

LAVECCHIA C, DECARLI A, FRANCESCHI S, et al. 1984a. Age at first birth and the risk of ovarian cancer. J Natl Cancer Inst 73:663–666.

LAVECCHIA C, FRANCESCHI S, DECARLI A, et al. 1984b. Coffee drinking and the risk of epithelial ovarian cancer. Int J Cancer 33:559–562.

LAVECCHIA C, DECARLI A, FASOLI M, et al. 1986. Oral contraceptives and cancers of the breast and of the female genital tract. Interim results from a case-control study. Br J Cancer 54:311–317.

LAVECCHIA C, DECARLI A, NEGRI E, et al. 1987. Dietary factors and risk of epithelial ovarian cancer. J Natl Cancer Inst 79:663–669.

LAVECCHIA C, NEGRI E, FRANCESCHI S, et al. 1992. Alcohol and epithelial ovarian cancer. J Clin Epidemiol 45:1035–1030.

LESHER L, MCGOWAN L, HARTGE P, et al. 1985. Age at first birth and risk of epithelial ovarian cancer. J Natl Cancer Inst 74:1361.

LI FP, FRAUMENI JF, DALAGER N. 1973. Ovarian cancers in the young: Epidemologic observations. Cancer 32:969–972.

LURAIN JR, PIVER MS. 1979. Familial ovarian cancer. Gynecol Oncol 8:185–192.

LYNCH HT, SCHUELKE GS, WELLS IC, et al. 1985. Hereditary ovarian carcinoma: Biomarker studies. Cancer 55:410–415.

LYON JL, KLAUBER MR, GARDNER JW, et al. 1976. Cancer incidence in Mormons and non-Mormons in Utah, 1966–1970. N Engl J Med 294:129–133.

MARCHANT J. 1961. The effect of hypophysectomy on the development of ovarian tumors in mice treated with dimethylbenzanthrocene. Br J Cancer 15:821–827.

MATHUR RS, LANDGREBE SC, MOODY LO, et al. 1985. The effect of estrogen treatment on plasma concentrations of steroid hormones, gonadotropins, prolactin and sex hormone-binding globulin in postmenopausal women. Maturitas 7:129–133.

MCGOWAN L, PARENT L, LEDNAR W, et al. 1979. The woman at risk for developing ovarian cancer. Gynecol Oncol 7:325–344.

MENCZER J, MODAN M, RANON L, et al. 1979. Possible role of

mumps virus in the etiology of ovarian cancer. Cancer 43:1375–1379.

METTLIN CJ, PIVER MS. 1990. A case-control study of milk-drinking and ovarian cancer risk. Am J Epidemiol 132:871–876.

MILLER DR, ROSENBERG L, KAUFMAN DW, et al. 1987. Epithelial ovarian cancer and coffee drinking. Int J Epidemiol 16:13–17.

MORI M, HARABUCHI I, MIYAKE H, et al. 1988. Reproductive, genetic, and dietary risk factors for ovarian cancer. Am J Epidemiol 128:771–777.

MORI M, KIYOSAWA H, MIYAKE H. 1984. Case-control study of ovarian cancer in Japan. Cancer 53:2746–2752.

NASCA PC, GREENWALD P, CHOROST S, et al. 1984. An epidemiologic case-control study of ovarian cancer and reproductive factors. Am J Epidemiol 119:705–713.

NEWHOUSE ML, BERRY G, WAGNER JC. 1985. Mortality of factory workers in east London 1933–80. Br J Ind Med 42:4–11.

NEWHOUSE ML, PEARSON RM, FULLERTON JM, et al. 1977. A case-control study of carcinoma of the ovary. Br J Prev Soc Med 31:148–153.

OHEL G, KANETI H, SCHENKER JG. 1983. Granulosa cell tumors in Israel: A study of 172 cases. Gynecol Oncol 15:278–286.

PAOLETTI L, CHIAZZA S, DONELLI G, et al. 1984. Evaluation by electron microscopy techniques of asbestos contamination in industrial, cosmetic, and pharmaceutical talcs. Regul Toxicol Pharmacol 4:222–235.

PARAZZINI F, LAVECCHIA C, NEGRI E, et al. 1991a. Oral contraceptive use and the risk of ovarian cancer: An Italian case-control study. Eur J Cancer 27:594–598.

PARAZZINI F, RESTELLI C, LAVECCHIA C, et al. 1991b. Risk factors for epithelial ovarian tumors of borderline malignancy. Int J Epidemiol 20:871–877.

PARAZZINI F, NEGRI E, LAVECCHIA C, et al. 1993. Hysterectomy, oophorectomy, and subsequent ovarian cancer risk. Obstet Gynecol 81:363–366.

PARKIN ET AL (EDS). 1992. Cancer Incidence in Five Continents. Volume VI. IARC Scientific Publications No. 120, Lyon.

PARLOW AF, DAANE TA, DIGNAM WJ. 1970. On the concentration of radioimmunoassayable FSH circulating in blood throughout human pregnancy. J Clin Endocrinol 31:213–214.

PARMLEY TH, WOODRUFF JD. 1974. The ovarian mesothelioma. Am J Obstet Gynecol 120:234–241.

PEJOVIC T, HEIM S, MANDAHL N, et al. 1991. Bilateral ovarian carcinoma: Cytogenetic evidence of unicentric origin. Int J Cancer 47:358–361.

PEREZ A, VELA P, MASNICK GS, et al. 1972. First ovulation after childbirth: The effect of breastfeeding. Am J Obstet Gynecol 114:1041–1047.

PHILLIPS RL, GARFINKEL L, KUZMA JW, et al. 1980. Mortality among Seventh-Day Adventists for selected cancer sites. J Natl Cancer Inst 65:1097–1107.

POLYCHRONOPOULOU A, TZONOU A, HSIEH C, et al. 1993. Reproductive variables, tobacco, ethanol, coffee and somatometry as risk factors for ovarian cancer. Int J Cancer 55:402–407.

PRENTICE RL, THOMAS DB. 1987. On the epidemiology of oral contraceptives and disease. Adv Cancer Res 49:285–401.

RISCH HA, WEISS NS, LYON JL, et al. 1983. Events of reproductive life and the incidence of epithelial ovarian cancer. Am J Epidemiol 117:128–139.

RISCH HA, JAIN M, MARRETT LD, HOWE GR. 1994. Dietary fat intake and risk of epithelial ovarian cancer. J Natl Cancer Inst 86:1409–1415.

ROSENBERG L, PALMER JR, ZAUBER AG, et al. 1994. A case-control study of oral contraceptive use and invasive epithelial ovarian cancer. Am J Epidemiol 139:654–661.

ROSENBLATT KA, SZKLO M, ROSENSHEIN NB. 1992. Mineral fiber exposure and the development of ovarian cancer. Gynecol Oncol 45:20–25.

ROSENBLATT KA, THOMAS DB, AND THE WHO COLLABORATIVE STUDY OF NEOPLASIA AND STEROID CONTRACEPTIVES. 1993. Lactation and the risk of epithelial ovarian cancer. Int J Cancer 22:192–197.

ROSSING MA, DALING JR, WIESS NS, et al. 1994. Ovarian tumors in a cohort of infertile women. N Engl J Med 331:771–776.

SAID SAH, WIDE L. 1973. Serum levels of FSH and LH following normal parturition. Acta Obstet Gynecol Scand 52:361–365.

SCHIFFMAN MH, HARTGE P, LESHER LP, et al. 1985. Mumps and postmenopausal ovarian cancer. Am J Obstet Gynecol 152:116–117.

SCHILDKRAUT JM, THOMPSON WD. 1988. Familial ovarian cancer: A population-based case-control study. Am J Epidemiol 128:456–466.

SCULLY RE. 1963. Germ cell tumors of the ovary and fallopian tube. Prog Gynecol 4:335–347.

SHIMKIN MB. 1960. Hormones and neoplasia. In Raven RW (ed): Cancer, Vol. 1. London: Butterworth and Co.

SHU XO, BRINTON LA, GAO YT, et al. 1989a. Population-based case-control study of ovarian cancer in Shanghai. Cancer Res 49:3670–3674.

SHU XO, GAO YT, YUAN JM, et al. 1989b. Dietary factors and epithelial ovarian cancer. Br J Cancer 59:92–96.

SLATTERY ML, SCHUMAN KL, WEST DW, et al. 1989. Nutrient intake and ovarian cancer. Am J Epidemiol 130:497–502.

SMITH EM, SOWERS MF, BURNS TL. 1984. Effects of smoking on the development of female reproductive cancers. J Natl Cancer Inst 73:371–376.

SNOWDON DA. 1985. Diet and ovarian cancer. JAMA 254:356–357.

SNOWDON DA, PHILLIPS RL. 1984. Coffee consumption and risk of fatal cancers. Am J Public Health 74:820–823.

SWIFT M, MORRELL D, MASSEY RB, et al. 1991. Incidence of cancer in 161 families affected by ataxia-telangiectasia. N Engl J Med 325:1831–1836.

SZAMBORSKI J, CZERWINSKI W, GADOMSKA H, et al. 1981. Case control study of high-risk factors in ovarian carcinomas. Gynecol Oncol 11:8–16.

TENNENT BJ, BEAMER WG. 1986. Ovarian tumors not induced by irradiation and gonadotropins in hypogonadal (hpg) mice. Biol Reprod 34:751–760.

TETER J, BOCZKOWSKI K. 1967. Occurrence of tumors in dysgenetic gonads. Cancer 20:1301–1310.

TOBACMAN JK, GREENE MH, TUCKER MA, et al. 1982. Intra-abdominal carcinomatosis after prophylactic oophorectomy in ovarian-cancer-prone families. Lancet 795–797.

TOKUOKA S, KAWAI K, SHIMIZU Y, et al. 1987. Malignant and benign ovarian neoplasms among atomic bomb survivors, Hiroshima and Nagasaki, 1950–80. J Natl Cancer Inst 79:47–57.

TRICHOPOULOS D, PAPAPOSTOLOU M, POLYCHRONOPOULOU A. 1981. Coffee and ovarian cancer. Int J Cancer 28:691–693.

TZONOU A, DAY NE, TRICHOPOULOS D, et al. 1984. The epidemiology of ovarian cancer in Greece: A case-control study. Eur J Cancer Clin Oncol 20:1045–1052.

TZONOU A, HSIEH C, POLYCHRONOPOULOU A, et al. 1993a. Diet and ovarian cancer: a case-control study in Greece. Int J Cancer 55:411–414.

TZONOU A, POLYCHRONOPOULOU A, HSIEH C, et al. 1993b. Hair dyes, analgesics, tranquilizers and perineal talc application as risk factors for ovarian cancer. Int J Cancer 55:408–410.

URSIN G, BJELKE E, VOLLSET SE. 1990. Milk consumption and cancer incidence: A Norwegian prospective study. Br J Cancer 61:454–459.

VENTER PF. 1981. Ovarian epithelial cancer and chemical carcinogenesis. Gynecol Oncol 12:281–285.

VOIGT LF, HARLOW BL, WEISS NS. 1986. The influence of age at first birth and parity on ovarian cancer risk. Am J Epidemiol 124:490–491.

WAGONER JK. 1984. Leukemia and other malignancies following radiation therapy for gynecological disorders. In Boice JD Jr, Fraumeni JF Jr (eds): Radiation Carcinogenesis: Epidemiology and Biological Significance. New York: Raven Press.

WALKER AH, ROSS RK, HAILE RWC, et al. 1988. Hormonal factors and risk of ovarian germ cell cancer in young women. Br J Cancer 57:418–422.

WALKER AH, ROSS RK, PIKE MC, et al. 1984. A possible rising incidence of malignant germ cell tumours in young women. Br J Cancer 49:669–672.

WANG J-X, BOICE JD JR, LI B-X, et al. 1988. Cancer among medifjcal diagnostic X-ray workers in China. J Natl Cancer Inst 80:344–350.

WEISS NS. 1988. Measuring the separate effects of low parity and its antecedents on the incidence of ovarian cancer. Am J Epidemiol 128:451–455.

WEISS NS, HARLOW BL. 1986. Why does hysterectomy without bilateral oophorectomy influence the subsequent incidence of ovarian cancer? Am J Epidemiol 124:856–858.

WEISS NS, HOMONCHUCK T, YOUNG JL. 1977. Incidence of histologic types of ovarian cancer: The U.S. Third National Cancer Survey, 1969–71. Gynecol Oncol 5:161–167.

WEISS NS, LIFF JM. 1983. Accounting for the multicausal nature of disease in the design and analysis of epidemiologic studies. Am J Epidemiol 117:14–18.

WEISS NS, LYON JL, KRISHNAMURTHY S, et al. 1982. Noncontraceptive estrogen use and the occurrence of ovarian cancer. J Natl Cancer Inst 68:95–98.

WEISS NS, LYON JL, LIFF JM, et al. 1981. Incidence of ovarian cancer in relation to the use of oral contraceptives. Int J Cancer 28:669–671.

WEISS NS, PETERSON AS. 1978. Racial variation in the incidence of ovarian cancer in the United States. Am J Epidemiol 107:91–95.

WELLS IC, LYNCH HT, LYNCH JF. 1987. a-L-fucosidase variant and lipid-associated sialic acid in hereditary ovarian cancer. Cancer Genet Cytogenet 25:247–251.

WEST RO. 1966. Epidemiologic study of malignancies of the ovaries. Cancer 19:1001–1007.

WHITTEMORE AS, WU ML, PAFFENBARGER RS JR, et al. 1988. Personal and environmental characteristics related to epithelial ovarian cancer. II. Exposures to talcum powder, tobacco, alcohol, and coffee. Am J Epidemiol 128:1228–1240.

WHITTEMORE AS, HARRIS R, ITNYRE J, AND THE COLLABORATIVE OVARIAN CANCER GROUP. 1992a. Characteristics relating to ovarian cancer risk: collaborative analysis of 12 case-control studies. II. Invasive epithelial ovarian cancers in white women. Am J Epidemiol 136:1204–1211.

WHITTEMORE AS, HARRIS R, ITNYRE J, AND THE COLLABORATIVE OVARIAN CANCER GROUP. 1992b. Characteristics relating to ovarian cancer risk: collaborative analysis of 12 case-control studies. IV. The pathogenesis of epithelial ovarian cancer. Am J Epidemiol 136:1212–1220.

WIGNALL BK, FOX AJ. 1982. Mortality of female gas mask assemblers. Br J Ind Med 39:34–38.

WILLETT WC, BAIN C, HENNEKENS CH, et al. 1981. Oral contraceptives and risk of ovarian cancer. Cancer 48:1684–1687.

WHO COLLABORATIVE STUDY OF NEOPLASIA AND STEROID CONTRACEPTIVES. 1989. Epithelial ovarian cancer and combined oral contraceptives. Int J Epidemiol 18:538–545.

WU ML, WHITTEMORE AS, PAFFENBARGER RS JR, et al. 1988. Personal and environmental characteristics related to epithelial ovarian cancer. I. Reproductive and menstrual events and oral contraceptive use. Am J Epidemiol 128:1216–1227.

WYNDER EL, DODO H, BAYER HR. 1969. Epidemiology of cancer of the ovary. Cancer 23:352–370.

YEN SSC. 1991. Prolactin in human reproduction. In Yen SSC, Jaffe RB (eds): Reproductive Endocrinology. London; Philadelphia: W.B. Saunders Co., pp. 357–388.

49 Endometrial cancer

DEBORAH GRADY
VIRGINIA L. ERNSTER

Endometrial cancer ranks fourth in age-adjusted cancer incidence among women in the United States and is the most common gynecologic cancer. Because it is usually not fatal, it ranks only about fourteenth in age-adjusted cancer mortality rates. In 1994, uterine corpus cancer accounted for about 5.4% of female cancer incidence (an estimated 31,000 cases) and 2.3% of female cancer mortality (an estimated 5,900 deaths) in the United States (Boring et al, 1994; Ries et al, 1994). Death rates for the disease have declined by over 60% since the 1950s. Incidence, however, showed a marked increase during the 1970s, followed by a reduction to earlier levels. The increase appears to have been related to an increase in the use by menopausal women of relatively high dose unopposed estrogens during that period. Factors shown to affect risk of endometrial cancer include menstrual and reproductive characteristics, obesity and other measures of body size, use of hormones, certain medical conditions, smoking, and possibly dietary factors.

HISTOPATHOLOGY AND STAGING

The uterine corpus includes the endometrium (lining of the uterine corpus) and the myometrium (the muscular tissue of the uterine corpus). In white women, the vast majority of cancers of the uterine corpus affect the endometrium. Adenocarcinoma is the predominant histologic type of endometrial cancer. Cancers of the myometrium, almost entirely sarcomas, are rare. In blacks, the majority of uterine corpus cancers are also of the endometrium, but cancers of the myometrium are relatively more common than in whites (Kelsey and Hildreth, 1983; Cramer et al, 1974). The histologic distribution of uterine corpus cancer cases diagnosed in areas participating in the National Cancer Institute's (NCI) Surveillance, Epidemiology, and End Results (SEER) population-based cancer incidence program during 1983–1987 is shown in Table 49–1. Because most analytic epidemiological studies have been confined to endometrial cancer, the discussion of risk factors in this chapter does not apply to the sarcomas. Only recently have attempts been made to examine demographic and reproductive characteristics specific to women with uterine sarcomas. Black and never-married women appear to be at higher risk for the sarcomas than white or ever-married women (Harlow et al, 1986; Schwartz and Weiss, 1990), but the relation of various reproductive characteristics to the sarcomas is less certain (Krale et al, 1988; Schwartz and Thomas, 1989).

The severity of endometrial cancers is defined by stage and histologic grade; higher scores on each are associated with poorer prognosis. The stages are I—tumor limited to endometrium or myometrium; II—endocervical or cervical stromal invasion; III—invasion of the serosa or adnexae, positive peritoneal cytology, or metastases to the vagina or to pelvic or para-aortic lymph nodes; and IV—invasion of bladder or bowel mucosa or distant metastases. The three histologic grades are based on percent of the tumor with undifferentiated or solid growth pattern: 1—5% or less; 2—6%–50%; and 3—greater than 50% (Photopulos, 1994).

DEMOGRAPHIC PATTERNS

Incidence and Mortality

Incidence and mortality data for cancers of the uterus are conventionally reported in three categories: cervix, corpus, and uterus "not otherwise specified" (NOS). Reflecting better classification of disease over time, mortality rates for the NOS category have been dropping dramatically, while death rates based on the corpus component alone have increased slightly (Fig. 49–1). Studies that have examined medical records for patients whose deaths are recorded as "uterus, NOS" show that the proportion of deaths within the NOS category that are actually due to corpus cancer rose from 20% to

Supported in part by USPHS grant PO1 CA 13556-18 from the National Cancer Institute, Bethesda, Maryland.
The authors thank Maureen Morris for assistance.

TABLE 49–1. *Percent Distribution of Uterine Corpus Cancer Cases by Histologic Type, White and Black Women, 1983–1987*

Histologic Type	*White (n = 12,516)*	*Black (n = 701)*
Carcinoma	94.1	79.7
Sarcoma and other soft tissue tumors	1.7	6.4
Other specified	4.2	13.8
	100.0	99.9

Source: From Ries et al, 1991.

75% between 1950 and the late 1970s (Percy et al, 1983). An analysis of 377 death certificates coded "uterus, NOS" for individuals who died in SEER program areas in 1985–1986 and who had a microscopically confirmed diagnosis of cancer reported to the SEER registry between 1973 and 1986 found that 78% were corpus cancers, 11% cervical cancers, and, for lack of better information, 4% remained uterus, NOS; an additional 7% were other cancers (Percy et al, 1990). Because in recent years the majority of cancers in the NOS category have been corpus cancers (Cramer et al, 1974; Weiss, 1978; Percy et al, 1983), the two categories are often combined for reporting of corpus cancer rates and time trends (Devesa and Silverman, 1978; Pollack and Horm, 1980; 1987 Annual Cancer Statistics Review, 1988). However, to the extent that cervical cancer cases are included in the NOS category, rates are overestimated, and, given the changing proportion over time (Table 49–2), caution is warranted in interpreting time trends in death rates. In sum, mortality trends based on the combination of corpus and NOS deaths have been heavily weighted by the changing NOS component and do not accurately reflect trends specific to corpus cancer. In contrast, corpus cancer incidence based on current SEER program data is affected only slightly, because the proportion of NOS cases in the SEER data is low (1.9% of all uterine corpus cancer cases in whites and 2.0% in blacks in 1986) (National Cancer Institute).

The prevalence of hysterectomy in the population should also be considered in interpreting rates and time trends for cancer of the uterine corpus. Because women in whom the uterus has been removed are not at risk for the disease, their inclusion in the calculation of population-based cancer rates artificially lowers estimates of disease occurrence. The prevalence of hysterectomy increased in recent decades; by the mid-1970s, approximately one-third of U.S. women aged 50 and over had undergone hysterectomy, although the exact proportion varied by age and geographic area (Walker and Jick, 1979; Walker and Jick, 1980; Howe, 1984; Koepsell et al, 1980). Several authors have estimated the impact of the changing frequency of hysterectomy on trends in corpus cancer rates. Thus, corrected mortality rates (based on removing hysterectomized women from the population at risk) for U.S. whites during 1960–1973 showed a decline that was 30% less than that seen with

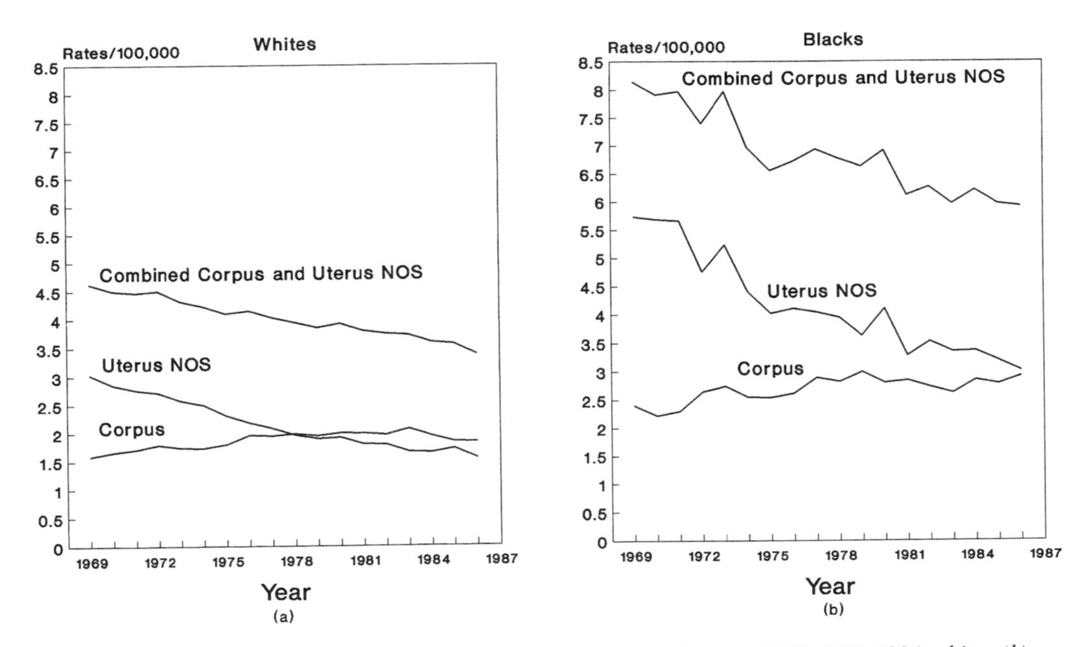

FIG. 49–1 (*a*) Mortality rates for cancers of the uterine corpus and uterus, NOS, 1969–1986, whites; (*b*) Mortality rates for cancers of the uterine corpus and uterus, NOS, 1969–1986, blacks. (Source: National Cancer Institute.)

TABLE 49–2. *Percent of Total Uterine Corpus Cancer Deaths and Incident Cases Actually Classified as "Uterus, Not Otherwise Specified," 1969–1986*

	Deaths (% Uterus, NOS)		*Incident Cases (% Uterus, NOS)*	
Year	*Whites*	*Blacks*	*Whites*	*Blacks*
1969	65.6%	70.5%	—	—
1970	63.3	71.9	—	—
1975	56.3	61.3	1.3%	4.1%
1980	49.0	59.5	1.9	5.5
1985	48.3	53.4	1.0	2.0
1986	45.9	50.8	1.1	2.0

Source: National Cancer Institute, unpublished data.

uncorrected rates. Similarly, the increase in incidence of uterine corpus cancer for whites in Alameda County, California, during 1960–1973, based on corrected rates was estimated to be 25%–45% higher than that based on uncorrected rates (Lyon and Gardner, 1977). Later work, incorporating more accurate estimates of the prevalence of hysterectomy, suggests that the effects may be of even greater magnitude (Marrett, 1980). Apparent declines in hysterectomy rates in the United States since the mid-1970s should be taken into account in future analyses of corpus cancer time trends (Pokras, 1984).

The issues discussed above make it difficult to draw precise conclusions about trends in corpus cancer rates over time or to correlate changes in risk factor exposure to the disease experience. They suggest caution in interpreting published rates, which, in the case of death rates, are often based on combined corpus and uterus, NOS, statistics and are unadjusted for the prevalence of hysterectomy in the population.

Age. Age-specific incidence and mortality rates for cancers of the corpus and uterus, NOS, separately were published by the NCI for the period 1984–1988 and are shown in Figure 49–2. In both whites and blacks, incidence for corpus cancer rises steadily until around age 65 or 70 and then declines. Incidence for uterus, NOS, is low at all ages in both racial groups but shows an upward trend with age. Mortality rates for corpus cancer and for uterus, NOS, are close to zero until ages 45–49 in both racial groups and then increase, but at much lower levels than incidence. In late life, mortality rates for uterus, NOS, are actually higher than for corpus cancer in both whites and blacks.

Race. Age-adjusted incidence for cancer of the uterine corpus is higher in white than in black or Asian women in the United States (Fig. 49–3). This difference is unexplained but may relate in part to differences in exogenous estrogen use or utilization of diagnostic services. In contrast, mortality rates are highest in blacks, followed by whites and Asians. The higher mortality rate among blacks compared with whites probably reflects a combination of less favorable histologic types of corpus cancer and more advanced disease at diagnosis, as well as possible treatment differences.

Geographic Area. It is noteworthy that international cancer registry data generally show much higher incidence for cancer of the uterine corpus for white, black,

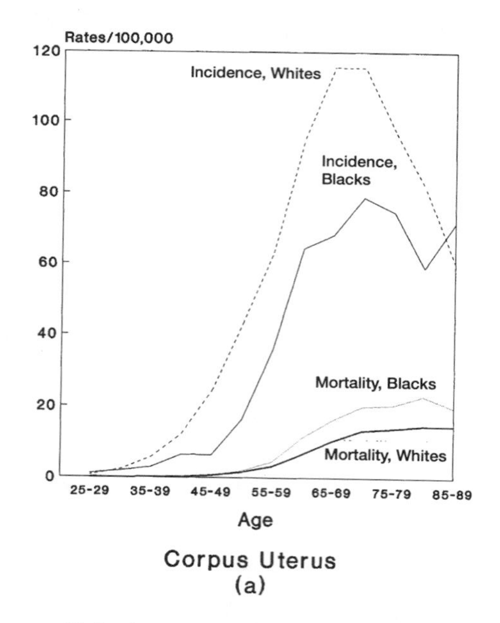

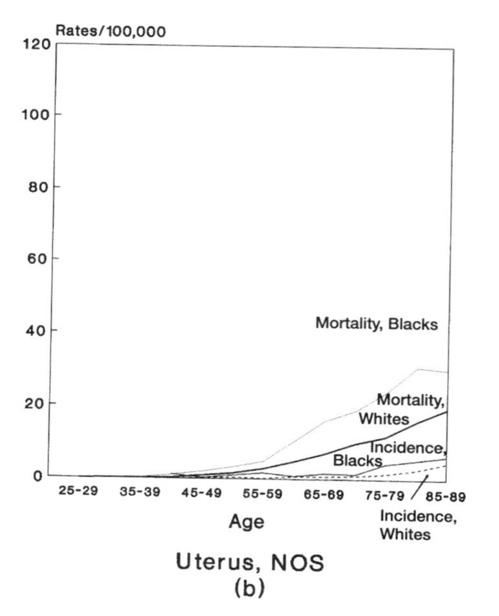

FIG. 49–2. Average annual age-specific incidence and mortality rates for cancers of the (*a*) uterine corpus and (*b*) uterus, NOS, whites and blacks, 1984–1988. (Source: Ries et al, 1991.)

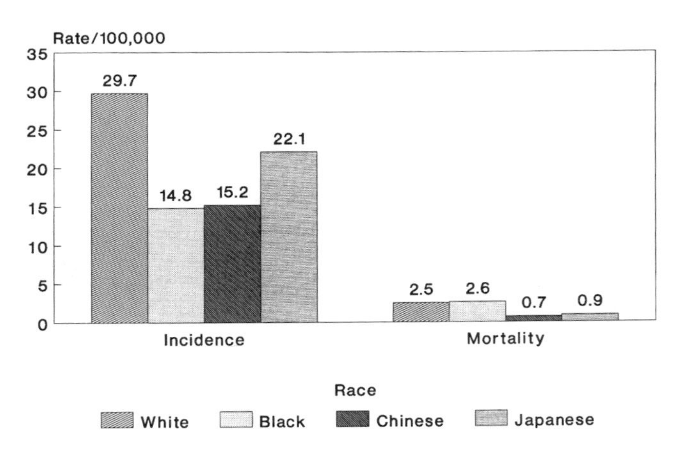

FIG. 49–3. Average annual age-adjusted incidence and mortality rates for cancer of the uterine corpus (corpus and uterus, NOS, combined) by race, San Francisco–Oakland SMSA, 1978–1981. (Source: Horm et al, 1984.)

and Asian women in the United States than for their racial counterparts in other countries. For example, incidence in whites in the United States is generally two- to threefold higher than in Europeans, and rates in Japanese in the United States are several-fold higher than in Japan (Parkin et al, 1992).

Time Trends. Overall age-adjusted mortality rates for uterine corpus cancer (which includes cancers of the uterus, NOS) declined steadily until the early to mid 1980s in blacks and until the late 1980s in whites (Devesa and Silverman, 1978; Pollack and Horm, 1980; SEER Cancer Statistics Review, 1973–1991). In whites, for example, rates declined by 66.8% between 1950 and 1991, from 8.9 to 3.1 deaths per 100,000 population (1987 Annual Cancer Statistics Review, 1988; SEER Cancer Statistics Review, 1973–1991). The decline in mortality suggests earlier detection or improved treatment for uterine cancer over time. However, as discussed above, it is possible that the decreasing mortality rates are due in part to the increasingly correct classification of cervical cancers that were previously included in the NOS group.

In contrast to the downward trend in mortality rates, incidence among whites was stable between 1947 and 1970 (the dates of the first two national cancer surveys in the United States), then increased during the early 1970s, and subsequently declined and plateaued in recent years at lower levels (Devesa and Silverman, 1978; Pollack and Horm, 1980; 1987 Annual Cancer Statistics Review, 1988; SEER Cancer Statistics Review, 1973–1991). The epidemic of endometrial cancer incidence in the early to mid-1970s was most marked in menopausal age groups, and the increase and subsequent decline in rates paralleled increases and then reductions in the use of relatively high dose unopposed estrogen replacement therapy (Weiss et al, 1976; Walker and Jick, 1980; Marrett et al, 1982; Austin and Roe, 1982). An analysis of time trends in uterine corpus cancer incidence based on SEER data for 1979–1986 suggests an acceleration in the decline in rates during the latter years of that period, mostly confined to women aged 45–64; the declines might be explained by coincident increases in the use of exogenous progestins among those women (Persky et al, 1990). Because trends for incidence and mortality have been somewhat divergent, it appears that some factors that influence incidence of uterine cancer (eg, estrogen replacement therapy) may have little effect on mortality from the disease.

In recent years, trends in rates for women over the age of 50 have differed for white and black women. As noted above, rates have declined in whites; however, they have increased in black women (by 16% between 1973 and 1990), with most of the increase seen in black women 50–64 years of age (Miller et al, 1993).

Survival

Among women diagnosed with uterine corpus cancer (including uterus, NOS) between 1983 and 1990, the 5-year overall survival rate for all stages combined was 85% for whites and 55% for blacks (SEER Cancer Statistics Review, 1973–1991). There are marked differences between whites and blacks in the distribution of cases by stage at diagnosis (Table 49–3). Fully 75% of whites diagnosed with uterine corpus cancer during 1983–1990 had localized disease, compared with only 52% of blacks. Stage at diagnosis is strongly related to probability of 5-year survival. Among whites, those diagnosed with localized disease between 1983 and 1990 had 5-year survival rates of 95%, compared to only 29% for those diagnosed with distant-stage disease; among blacks, 5-year survival for women with localized disease was 79.7%, compared with 12.4% for those with distant disease (Table 49–3). That whites experience more favorable survival rates within staging categories than blacks suggests less advanced disease within stage, more favorable histologic types of corpus cancer, or better access to quality medical treatment following diagnosis.

An analysis of uterine corpus cancer cases diagnosed during 1973–1977 in three geographic areas in the SEER program found that, among women with adenocarcinomas, racial differences in survival were reduced but persisted even after adjustment for stage and age at diagnosis, family income, and education. Interestingly, race was not independently associated with survival among women with sarcomas (Steinhorn et al, 1986).

TABLE 49–3. *Distribution and 5-Year Relative Survival Rates by Stage and Race, Uterine Corpus Cancer Cases (Including Uterus, NOS), 1983–1990*

	Percent Distribution						*Percent 5-Year Survival*					
	Whites			*Blacks*			*Whites*			*Blacks*		
Stage	*All*	*<50*	*≥50*	*All*	*<50*	*≥50*	*All*	*<50*	*≥50*	*All*	*<50*	*≥50*
Localized	75	81	74	52	68	50	95.1	96.9	94.9	79.7	92.3	77.3
Regional	12	10	12	20	15	21	70.4	82.4	69.2	40.7[a]	—	37.2
Distant	9	5	10	19	8	21	29.1	55.8	27.1	12.4	—	11.1
Unknown	4	4	4	8	8	8	59.0	79.0	56.1	27.2	—	19.7

Source: From National Cancer Institute (NCI), SEER Cancer Statistics Review, 1973–1991, 1994.
[a]Standard error between 5 and 10 percentage points

Overall 5-year survival rates for uterine corpus cancer increased steadily between the early 1960s and the mid-1970s and then declined slightly (Fig. 49–4). Among whites, 5-year survival was 73% for women diagnosed between 1960 and 1963 and 85% for those diagnosed between 1983 and 1990. Among blacks, 5-year survival improved more dramatically, from 31% to 55% over the same period. The more favorable prognosis for women diagnosed in the mid-1970s is attributed to the higher proportion of estrogen-associated cases in that time period; such cases tend to be early-stage, well-differentiated tumors that are rarely fatal (Chu et al, 1982).

Socioeconomic Status

A small increase in risk for endometrial cancer in women of higher compared to lower socioeconomic status (SES) has been reported by some (Armstrong and Doll, 1975; Elwood et al, 1977; Kelsey et al, 1982) but not all (Shapiro et al, 1980; La Vecchia et al, 1984; Ewertz et al, 1988) investigators. An analysis of trends in uterine corpus cancer incidence between 1969 and 1975 among women 50–74 years of age in the San Francisco–Oakland area showed an association between affluence (measured by median income of census tract of residence) and incidence of corpus cancer in 1969. There was also a much greater increase in incidence over the study period for women residing in the two upper SES census quartiles compared with those in the two lower quartiles (Austin and Roe, 1979). The association of socioeconomic status with endometrial cancer may be explained by greater use of estrogen replacement among better educated women (Weiss et al, 1979; Kelsey et al, 1982) or the association may be due to better access to medical care and more complete diagnosis and reporting of endometrial cancer among women of higher SES.

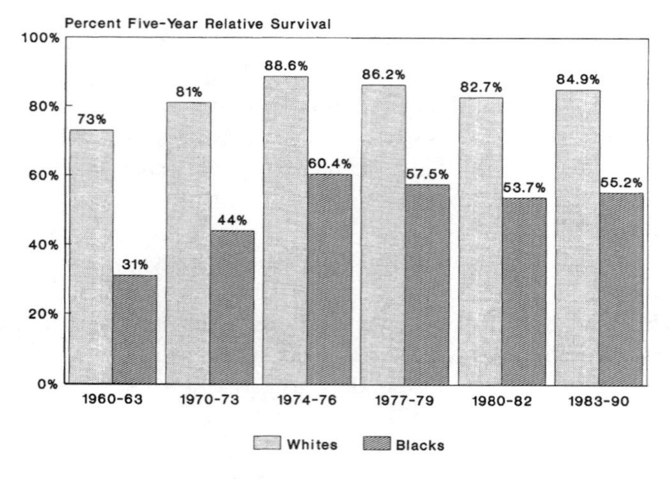

FIG. 49–4. Five-year relative survival rates for uterine corpus cancer, U.S. whites and blacks, 1960–1963 to 1983–1990. (Source: Ries et al, 1994.)

HOST AND ENVIRONMENTAL FACTORS

Menstrual and Reproductive Factors

Many aspects of menstrual and reproductive history have been examined in relation to endometrial cancer risk, including age at menarche, parity, age at first birth, age at last birth, menstrual irregularities, infertility, duration of menses, menopausal symptoms, and age at menopause. Several decades ago it was observed that single women and married women without children in England and Wales had higher deaths rates from uterine corpus cancer than married parous women (Logan, 1953). More recent U.S. cancer survey data also show higher incidence of the disease in single than in married women (Ernster et al, 1979). Case-control studies consistently have shown that nulliparity is associated with a two- to threefold increased risk of endometrial cancer and most but not all show that risk decreases with increasing number of children (MacMahon et al, 1974; Kelsey et al, 1982; Henderson et al, 1983; La Vecchia et al, 1984; Pettersson et al, 1986; Brinton et al, 1992; Kvale et al, 1991; Parazzini et al, 1991).

Most studies have not found a reduction in endometrial cancer risk associated with early age at first birth such as has been found for breast cancer (MacMahon et al, 1974; Elwood et al, 1977; Henderson et al, 1983; Pettersson et al, 1986; Lesko et al, 1991; Brinton et al, 1992). However, late age at first birth may reduce risk (Kvale et al, 1991); in two studies, risk for women whose last delivery occurred after age 35 or 40 was about half that of women whose last delivery occurred before age 20 or 25 (Parazzini et al, 1991; Lesko et al, 1991). In some studies, the protective effect of parity (La Vecchia et al, 1984) or age at last birth (Parazzini et al, 1991) appears limited to premenopausal women. Infertility, defined as a recognized inability to become pregnant for three or more years, was associated with a 3.5-fold increased risk in one case-control study (Henderson et al, 1983), and in another study nulliparous women who had sought medical advice for infertility had a significantly elevated risk compared with nulliparous women who had no difficulty conceiving (Brinton et al, 1992).

Later age at menopause has been found to be a risk factor for endometrial cancer in most (Wynder et al, 1966; MacMahon et al, 1974; Elwood et al, 1977; Kelsey et al, 1982; Pettersson et al, 1986; Kvale et al, 1991) but not all (Brinton et al, 1992) studies. The relation of age at menarche to endometrial cancer is less clear. Earlier age at menarche has been associated with increased risk for the disease (Elwood et al, 1977; Brinton et al, 1992; Kvale, 1991), although this association may be limited to premenopausal women (La Vecchia et al, 1984) or obese women (Henderson et al, 1983). One study found no differences between cases and controls in age at menarche but noted a significantly longer "menstruation span" (years between menarche and menopause, excluding pregnancy-related time) in women with endometrial cancer compared to controls (Pettersson et al, 1986). Finally, an association of irregular menses with endometrial cancer in young women has been reported (Henderson et al, 1983).

Hormones

Estrogens

Endogenous estrogens. Women with elevated endogenous estrogen levels have been reported to have an increased risk of endometrial cancer. Estrogen-secreting tumors and polycystic ovarian syndrome (Stein-Leventhal syndrome) are associated with high endogenous estrogen levels (Jackson et al, 1957; Wood et al, 1976).

Young women with estrogen-secreting (feminizing) ovarian tumors have a high frequency of endometrial hyperplasia and carcinoma (Mansell and Hertig, 1955). The prevalence of endometrial carcinoma in these women ranges from 4% to 17% (Diddle, 1952; Larson, 1954; Salerno, 1962; Kjellgren, 1977).

Women with polycystic ovarian syndrome have chronically elevated levels of luteinizing hormone (LH) without the cyclic peaks usually associated with ovulation. Chronic hyperstimulation of the ovary by LH results in abnormally increased secretion of androstenedione (Wood and Boronow, 1976), which is aromatized peripherally to estrone (MacDonald et al, 1967). There have been several case reports (Sommers et al, 1949; Speert, 1949; DeVere and Dempster, 1953; Castleman and McNeely, 1966; Wood and Boronow, 1976) and one series of 16 patients (Jackson and Dockerty, 1957) with polycystic ovarian syndrome who developed endometrial cancer. Although such case series provide no comparison group, most of these reported endometrial cancers occurred in women under 40 years of age, when endometrial cancer is uncommon. The diagnosis of polycystic ovarian syndrome may be made in up to 30% of cases of endometrial cancer in selected groups of premenopausal women (Gallup and Stock, 1984).

The evidence concerning the association of blood steroid hormone levels and endometrial cancer is conflicting. Some investigators have found higher levels of serum estrogens in women with endometrial cancer compared to controls (Carlstrom et al, 1979; Benjamin and Deutsch, 1976; Nisker et al, 1980; Pettersson et al, 1986). Other investigators have found no differences in levels of estradiol-17B and estrone in postmenopausal women with endometrial cancer compared with controls (Schenker et al, 1979; von Holst et al, 1981).

Exogenous estrogens. Several lines of evidence indicate that exogenous estrogen treatment increases the risk of endometrial cancer.

Oral contraceptives. Prior to the mid-1970s, oral contraceptive pills (OCPs) were available as either sequential (estrogen followed by a progestin) or combination pills (estrogen plus progestin). In the 1970s, an increased risk of endometrial cancer was reported in women using sequential oral contraceptives, particularly Oracon (a sequential pill with relatively high dose, long-duration estrogen and low-dose, short-duration progestin) (Lyon, 1975; Silverberg and Makowski, 1975; Cohen and Deppe, 1977; Silverberg et al, 1977; Weiss and Sayvetz, 1980; Henderson et al, 1983). For this reason, sequential OCPs were removed from the market in the mid-1970s.

In contrast, the risk of endometrial cancer in women who have used combination OCPs is decreased by about 50% compared with that of nonusers (Gray et al, 1977; Weiss and Sayvetz, 1980; Kaufman et al, 1980a; Hulka et al, 1982; Kelsey et al, 1982; Centers for Disease Control, 1987; La Vecchia et al, 1984; La Vecchia et al, 1986a; World Health Organization, 1988; Voigt, 1994; Jick et al, 1993b). The protective effect of OCPs is evident after a relatively short interval of use (ie, 1 to 3 years), is dose-related (Kaufman et al, 1980a; Hulka et al, 1982; Henderson et al, 1983), and persists for at least 5 years even after discontinuing the pills (Weiss et al,

1980; Schlesselman, 1991). Some investigators have reported greater protection against endometrial cancer with pills in which progesterone effects predominate (Hulka et al, 1982) while others have found no difference (Voigt, 1994). The apparent protective effect of OCPs may be due to the fact that women who take OCPs have fewer children (Henderson et al, 1983; Centers for Disease Control, 1987) or other confounding factors (Weiss et al, 1980), but most studies have shown an independent protective effect after controlling for multiple potential confounders (Weiss et al, 1980; Kaufman et al, 1980a; Hulka et al, 1982; Centers for Disease Control, 1987; World Health Organization, 1988).

Estrogen replacement therapy. Cutler and coworkers (1972) reported two patients with endometrial cancer among 24 women with gonadal dysgenesis who were treated with stilbestrol (a synthetic, nonsteroidal estrogen) for 5 years or more. Although there was no comparison group, the early ages at which these tumors were detected suggested that estrogens might play a causal role in the disease. An increased incidence of endometrial cancer in women with breast cancer was reported in the 1960s and early 1970s (Bailar, 1963; Schoenberg et al, 1969; MacMahon, 1974). Because many women with breast cancer were treated with estrogens at that time, hormone therapy was thought responsible for the increased risk. In a large retrospective study, patients with breast cancer who were treated with stilbestrol had about twice the expected incidence of endometrial cancer compared to the general population, whereas those not treated with hormones had no increased incidence (Hoover et al, 1976).

During the past few decades, women have been treated with estrogen replacement therapy (ERT) for menopausal symptoms such as hot flushes and to prevent osteoporosis and coronary heart disease. Some women treated with estrogens were found to have adenomatous hyperplasia of the endometrium (Gusberg, 1947) that regressed or disappeared after estrogen treatment was discontinued (Kistner, 1973). Adenomatous hyperplasia frequently coexists with endometrial cancer and has been noted to precede the appearance of carcinoma (Gusberg and Hall, 1961; Gusberg and Kaplan, 1963; Wentz, 1974; Sherman and Brown, 1979). These findings strengthened the suspicion that exogenous estrogen treatment might cause endometrial cancer.

A fourfold increase in sales of estrogens in the United States occurring from 1962 to 1975 was paralleled by a marked increase in the incidence of endometrial cancer in the 1970s (Kennedy et al, 1985). However, this increase in incidence of endometrial cancer was not accompanied by an increase in mortality from the disease. Rates of prescription of estrogens began to decline in the late 1970s (Jick et al, 1979; Kennedy, 1985), presumably due to concern over the association with endometrial cancer. This decline in rates of estrogen prescription was followed by a decrease in endometrial cancer incidence. Although rates of estrogen prescription have risen again since 1980, the incidence of endometrial cancer has remained stable, possibly because estrogen doses are lower than previously and because progestins are now commonly added to the hormone replacement regimen in women with a uterus (Hemminki, 1988).

The first cases of endometrial cancer in women using chronic estrogen replacement were reported in the early 1960s (Gusberg and Hall, 1961). Since 1970, at least 29 case-control studies have examined the association of exogenous estrogen treatment and cancer of the endometrium (Smith et al, 1975; Ziel and Finkle, 1975; Mack et al, 1976; Gray et al, 1977; McDonald et al, 1977; Horwitz and Feinstein, 1978; Hoogerland et al, 1978; Wigle et al, 1978; Antunes et al, 1979; Jick et al, 1979; Weiss et al, 1979; Shapiro et al, 1980; Hulka et al, 1980a, b; Jelovsek et al, 1980; Salmi, 1980; Spengler et al, 1981; Stavraky et al, 1981; Kelsey et al, 1982; Henderson et al, 1983; La Vecchia et al, 1984; Shapiro et al, 1985; Buring et al, 1986; Ewertz et al, 1988; Rubin et al, 1990; Voigt et al, 1991; Jick et al, 1993a; Levi et al, 1993; Brinton and Hoover, 1993). Most of these studies have shown increased odds ratios for endometrial cancer in women who have taken estrogen replacement therapy (Table 49–4). Two of the studies that did not find an elevated odds ratio (OR) for overall estrogen use noted an increased risk for prolonged duration of use (McDonald et al, 1977; Hulka et al, 1980a). One study from Finland showed a significant decrease in risk for endometrial cancer in estrogen users (OR=0.4) (Salmi, 1980). In contrast to the United States, where conjugated estrogens are primarily used, women in the Finnish study used primarily nonconjugated estrogens (see below), and the average duration of use was short (10.2 months).

Each of 11 cohort studies (Hoover, 1976; Hammond, 1979; Gambrell, 1980; Vakil, 1983; Lafferty, 1985; Stampfer, 1986; Hunt et al, 1987; Petitti, 1987; Ettinger, 1988; Paganini-Hill, 1989; Persson, 1989) shows an increased relative risk for endometrial cancer among estrogen users, ranging from 1.4 (Gambrell, 1980; Persson, 1989) to 10.0 (Paganini-Hill, 1989) (Table 49–5). A meta-analysis that included risk ratios from case-control and cohort studies found a summary relative risk of 2.3 (95% confidence interval 2.1–2.5) for endometrial cancer comparing ever-users of estrogen to non-users (Table 49–6) (Grady et al, 1995).

The increased incidence of endometrial cancer in the United States in the 1970s clearly paralleled increasing estrogen use, but mortality from endometrial cancer did not (Kennedy, 1985). The reason for this is not entirely clear but may be because endometrial cancers associated

TABLE 49–4. *Case-Control Studies of Estrogen Replacement Therapy and Cancer of the Corpus Uterus since 1970 and Risk (Odds Ratio or Relative Risk) of Endometrial Cancer Due to ERT: Effect of Duration, Type, Dosing Regimen, Time Since Last Use, and Stage/Grade*

Reference	*Cases/Controls Source of Controls*	*Case Pathology Reviewed*	*Data Source*	*Definition of Estrogen Replacement Therapy (ERT)*	*Odds Ratio*	
					Ever Use	*Conjugated Estrogen (mg)*
Smith (1975)	317/317 other gynecologic cancers	no	medical records	any estrogen ≥6 months of use	4.5[a]	
Ziel (1975)	94/188 other Kaiser-Permanente members	no	medical records	any conjugated estrogens except within 1 year of diagnosis	7.6[a]	
Mack (1976)	63/396 community controls	no	medical records, pharmacy records, some telephone interviews	any estrogen except within 6 months of diagnosis	8.0[a]	≤.625 5.0[a] >.625 9.4[a]
Grey (1977)	205/205 hysterectomy for benign conditions	no	medical records	any estrogen ≥3 months duration	2.1[a]	
McDonald (1977)	145/580 community controls	yes	medical records	conjugated estrogen ≥6 months' duration	4.9[a]	.625 1.4 ≥1.25 7.2[a]
Horwitz (1978)	119/119 other gynecologic cancers	no		at least .3 mg conjugated estrogens for at least 3 months	12.0[a]	
	149/149 D&C or hysterectomy for benign condition	no		at least .3 mg conjugated estrogens for at least 3 months	2.3[a]	
Hoogerland (1978)	587/587 other gynecologic cancers	no	medical records	any estrogen	2.2[a]	
Wigle (1978)	202/1243 cancer other than breast or gynecologic	no	interview	any estrogen	2.5[a]	
Antunes (1979)	451/888 hospitalized 444 gynecologic problems, 444 nongynecologic problems	10%	medical records, some interviews	any estrogen except combination OCP's	5.5[a] nongyn. 2.4[a] gyn.	
Weiss (1979)	322/289 population-based	yes	interview	any estrogen	4.5	≤.5 2.5[a] .6–1.2 8.8[a] ≥1.25 7.6[a]
Jick (1979)	67/122 members of Group Health Cooperative of Puget Sound	no	interview, medical records	any estrogen	11.2[a]	.3 12.0 .625 15.0[a] 1.25 37.5[a]
Shapiro (1980)	149/453 hospitalized	no	interview	any estrogen ≥3 months' duration except within 2 years of diagnosis	3.9[a]	
Hulka (1980a,b)	256 invasive cancers/321 community controls, 224 hospitalized with gynecologic problems except D&C or uterine biopsy	yes	medical records and interview	any estrogen	*white*: comm. 1.4 gyn. 1.8 *black*: comm. 1.5 gyn. 0.7	*comm. gyn.* ≤.625 2.3, 1.6 >.625 1.4, 1.8

(continued)

TABLE 49–4. *Case-Control Studies of Estrogen Replacement Therapy and Cancer of the Corpus Uterus since 1970 and Risk (Odds Ratio or Relative Risk) of Endometrial Cancer Due to ERT: Effect of Duration, Type, Dosing Regimen, Time Since Last Use, and Stage/Grade (Continued)*

Reference	*Cases/Controls Source of Controls*	*Case Pathology Reviewed*	*Data Source*	*Definition of Estrogen Replacement Therapy (ERT)*	*Odds Ratio*		
					Ever Use	*Conjugated Estrogen (mg)*	
Jelovsek (1980)	431 invasive cancers/431 hospitalized and clinic	yes	medical records	any estrogen	2.4[a]		
Salmi (1980)	282/282 volunteers in a screening program	no	interview	any estrogen but mostly unconjugated	0.4		
Spengler (1981)	88/177 neighborhood	yes	interview	any estrogen ≥1 month duration postmenopause	2.9[a]	≤1 >1	2.0 4.0[a]
Stavraky (1981)	206/191 nonmalignant gynecologic disease, 199 nongynecologic disease	76%	interview	any estrogen ≥6 months' duration	2.4[a] gynecologic disease 4.3[a] nongynecologic disease	 ≤.625 >.625	*Gyn* *Non-Gyn* 1.9 2.9[a] 3.1 6.4[a] *P*<.05 trend *P*<.05 trend
Kelsey (1982)	167/903 hospitalized surgical patients without gynecologic problems	yes	interview	any estrogen	1.6[a] for ≥ 5 years of use		
Henderson (1983)	127 ≤ 45 years of age/132 neighborhood	yes		any estrogen	1.8		
La Vecchia (1984)	283/566 hospitalized	no	interview	any estrogen	2.3[a]		
Shapiro (1985)	425/792 hospitalized	no	interview	any estrogen beginning at least 2 years before interview	3.5[a]		
Buring (1986)	188/428 hospitalized	yes	medical records	any estrogen	2.4[a]	.3–.625 1.25–2.5	2.7 3.8[a]
Ewertz (1988)	149/157 cervical cancer	yes	medical records	any noncontraceptive estrogen	4.7[a]		
Rubin (1990)	196/986	yes	interview	any noncontraceptive estrogen except vaginal cream ≥3 months	1.9[a]	<.625 >1.25	1.2 3.8[a]
Voigt (1991)	158/182 population-based	no	interview	any noncontraceptive estrogen	3.1[a]		
Jick (1993)	172/1720 members of Group Health Cooperative of Puget Sound	no	computer records, questionnaire	any estrogen	6.5[a]	.3 .625 1.25	4.3[a] 7.1[a] 8.4[a]
Levi (1993)	158/468 hospitalized for acute, nonneoplastic, non-hormone-related conditions in Switzerland	yes	interview	replacement estrogen	2.7[a]		
Brinton (1993)	300/207 population-based	no	interview	any menopausal estrogen	3.0[a]	.3 .625 ≥1.25	2.8 4.0[a] 2.8

Reference	Duration (Years)	Type of Estrogen	Dosing Regimen	Time Since Last Used (Years)	Stage/Grade
Ziel (1975)	<1 3.0 1.0–4.9 5.6[a] 5.0–6.9 7.2[a] >7 13.9[a]				
Mack (1976)	conjugated estrogen <1 2.8 1–5 4.5[a] 5–8 9.3[a] >8 8.8[a]	conjugated estrogen 5.6[a] any estrogen 8.0[a]	free interval 0–1 days/mo. 4.4 2–3 days/mo. 6.5 ≥4 days/mo. 3.3	0–2 7.2 ≥2 3.4	invasive 3.2 noninvasive 5.0 Grades I,II 12.9 Grade III 4.0
Gray (1977)	conjugated estrogen 0–4 1.2 5–9 4.1 ≥10 11.6[a]	conjugated estrogen 3.1[a] other oral 2.9 intramuscular 2.3 vaginal 0.7			
McDonald (1977)	conjugated estrogen ≥.5 4.9[a] ≥1 5.3[a] ≥2 8.3[a] ≥3 7.9[a]	conjugated estrogen 4.9[a] all estrogen 0.9	conjugated estrogen ≥6 mo. intermittent 1.6 cyclic 3.3[a] continuous 7.9		depth of invasion ≤5 mm 7.9[a] >5 mm 1.3 Stage I 6.0[a] Stages II–IV 2.2 Grade I 6.0[a] Grades II–IV3.8[a]
Hoogerland (1978)	any estrogen ≤.5 1.2 .5–1 1.8 1–3 3.6[a] 3–5 3.9[a] 5–10 3.3[a] ≥10 6.7[a]				
Wigle (1978)	any estrogen 1–4 1.8 ≥5 5.2				
Antunes (1974)	<1 2.2 1–5 2.9[a] >5 15.0[a]	conjugated estrogen 4.9[a] DES 9.0[a]	intermittent 3.5[a] cyclic 5.4[a] continuous 4.4[a]		Stage 0 10.0[a] Stage I 7.2[a] Stages II–IV 4.0 noninvasive 5.3[a] invasive 7.2[a]
Weiss (1979)	1–2 1.2 3–4 5.4[a] 5–7 4.7[a] 8–10 11.7[a] 11–14 24.2[a] 15–19 10.2[a] ≥20 8.3[a]	no difference between all estrogen vs. conjugated estrogen	weeks estrogen/mo. 3 8.1[a] 4 4.8[a] other 4.7[a]	current 8.7[a] 1–2 5.3[a] 3–7 3.8[a] ≥8 3.0	CIS 6.1[a] invasive 5.3
Jick (1979)	0–4 3.0 5–8 36.0[a] 9–12 63.0[a] ≥13 21.0[a]	conjugated 21.0[a] other 24.0[a]	cyclic 29.0[a] continuous 6.0		

(continued)

TABLE 49–4. *Case-Control Studies of Estrogen Replacement Therapy and Cancer of the Corpus Uterus since 1970 and Risk (Odds Ratio or Relative Risk) of Endometrial Cancer Due to ERT: Effect of Duration, Type, Dosing Regimen, Time Since Last Use, and Stage/Grade* (Continued)

Reference	*Duration (Years)*	*Type of Estrogen*	*Dosing Regimen*	*Time Since Last Used (Years)*	*Stage/Grade*
Shapiro (1980)	<1 0.9	conjugated estrogen 3.9[a]		<1 8.8	
	1–4 2.6	nonconjugated estrogen 0.9		≥1 3.6	
	≥5 6.0			≥2 3.3	
	P<.05 trend			≥3 2.7	
				≥4 2.7	
				≥5 2.6	
Hulka (1980a,b)	*comm.* *gyn.*	*comm* *gyn.*	*comm.* *gyn.*	risk decreased to	Stage IA 7.6[a]
	<3.5 0.7 0.8	conjugated 1.8 1.9	cyclic 1.8 1.5	baseline after	Stage II 3.3[a]
	≥3.5 3.6[a] 4.1	other 0.8 0.9	continuous 1.6 2.0	2 years	Stages III–IV 1.5
				estrogen free	Grade 1 5.5
					Grade 2 1.9
					Grade 3 2.9
					invasive 2.5
					noninvasive 5.2
Jelovsek (1980)	.5–3 1.4				Stage IA 5.5
	3–5 1.4				Stage IB 3.2
	5–10 4.8[a]				noninvasive 4.7
	>10 2.6[a]				invasive 10.8
Salmi (1980)		estradiol ± androgen 0.3[a]			
		estriol 0.4[a]			
		conjugated estrogen 5.0			
		others 0.6			
Spengler (1981)	≤.5 1.4				
	.5–2.0 2.6				
	2–5 2.2				
	>5 8.6[a]				
Stavraky (1981)	*Gynecol Dis* *Non-Gyn Dis*	*Gyn* *Non-Gyn*		*Gyn*[b] *Non-Gyn*[b]	
	<2 0.7 1.6	cont. 3.7 5.6			
	2–4 1.0 4.0[a]	cyclic 2.9 4.3		≤11.3 11.3	
	5–9 1.7 5.3[a]	other 1.2 3.4		>10.5 2.3	
	≥10 6.4[b] 14.4[a]				
Kelsey (1982)	<1 1.1				Stage I 3.7
	1–2.5 1.0				Stages II, III 1.5
	2.6–5 2.9[a]				
	5.1–7.5 4.3[a]				
	7.6–10 8.2[a]				
	>10 2.7[a]				
	P<.05 trend				

(continued)

Henderson (1983)	<2	1.3						
	≥2	3.2						
La Vecchia (1984)	significant increased risk for increasing duration $P<.05$ trend							
Shapiro (1985)	<1	0.9			no clear decrease in risk after 10 years' estrogen free		localized	5.2
	1–4	2.9[a]					extrauterine	3.1
	5–9	5.6[a]						
	≥10	10.0[2a]						
Buring (1986)	<1	1.4	continuous	2.4[b]	<1	2.4	Grade I	4.8[b]
	1–4	2.4	cyclic	3.6[b]	1–2	4.2	Grades II, III	1.3
	5–9	6.4[a]	P = .13 for continuous vs. cyclic; difference remains after adjustment for dose and regimen		3–4	5.9	Stage I	3.1[b]
	≥10	7.6[a]			≥	4.5	Grade 1	5.5[b]
							Grades 2,3	1.5
							Stages II–IV	0.7
							noninvasive	4.6
							invasive:	
							proximal ½	2.2
							distal ½	0.7
Rubin (1990)	<2	1.3						
	2–5	2.1[a]						
	≥6	3.5[a]						
Jick (1993)	<3	3.6						
	3–4	1.9						
	≥5	22.0[a]						
Levi (1993)	>5	5.1[a]			≤2	2.5[a]		
					2–9	3.4[a]		
					≥10	2.3[a]		
Brinton (1993)	<5	1.4			<5	4.0[a]		
	≥5	1.9			≥5	1.9		
	≥10	16.1[a]						

[a] $P < 0.05$.
[b] Odds ratios for users of ≥5 years.

TABLE 49–5. *Cohort Studies of Estrogen Replacement Therapy and Cancer of the Corpus Uterus Since 1970*

Reference	Cohort	Case Pathology Reviewed	Definition of Estrogen Replacement Therapy (ERT)	Odds Ratio				
				Ever Use	Dose Conjugated Estrogen (mg)		Duration (years)	
Hoover (1976)	19 cases/4212 users with breast cancer compared to population rates; follow-up 1–37 years	no	received "hormones" for breast cancer	2.3				
Vakil (1983)	8 cases/1483 users; postmenopausal patients of 20 Toronto gynecologists compared to population rates; 44% used a progestin or androgen with estrogen; mean follow-up ≥17 yrs	no	conjugated or synthetic estrogens for ≥3 months	1.3				
Hunt (1987)	12 cases/4544 users; women in British menopause clinics treated with hormones compared to population rates; 43% used a progestin with estrogen; mean follow-up 5.6 years	yes	"hormone replacement therapy" for at least one year	2.8[a]				
Hammond (1979)	14 cases/516 hypoestrogenic women; mean follow-up ≥5 years	yes	any estrogen therapy ≥5 years	5.8[a]				
Gambrell (1980)	13 cases/4242 person-years at risk among women in a gynecologic clinic; mean follow-up 4 years	no	"postmenopausal estrogen"	1.4				
Lafferty (1985)	4 cases/124 women patients of one physician; mean follow-up 8.6 years	NA	Premarin .625 mg daily; 3 out of 4 weeks	3.1				
Stampfer (1986)	70 cases/114,896 person-years at risk; U.S. Nurses' Health Study; mean follow-up 4 years	yes	"postmenopausal hormone use"	4.4[a]			<1 ≥5	3.5[a] 6.9[a]
Petitti (1987)	6 cases/6093 HMO members; Walnut Creek Contraceptive Drug Study; mean follow-up 10–13 years	no	"estrogen user"	2.6				
Ettinger (1988)	21 cases/401 HMO members; mean follow-up 15–19 yrs	yes	oral estrogen preparation	7.7[a]				
Paganini-Hill (1989)	50 cases/5153 women; Leisure World Study; mean follow-up 2–6 yrs	no	any estrogen	10.0[a]	≤0.625 ≥1.25	15.0[a] 11.0[a]	≤2 3–7 8–14 ≥15	5.2[a] 7.0[a] 4.0[a] 20.0[a]
Persson (1986/ 1989)	48 cases/121,190 person-years at risk among users in Uppsala health care region compared to the remaining female population of Uppsala; 31% used a progestin with estrogen	yes	noncontraceptive estrogens	1.4[a]			≤.5 .5–3 3–6 ≥6	1.1 1.4 1.2 1.8[a]

[a]$P < 0.05$.

with estrogen use are not as aggressive as spontaneously occurring cancers or because women who take estrogen are likely to have their tumors discovered at a more curable stage. Estrogen may cause early bleeding from endometrial tumors and women taking estrogen often undergo regular examination and endometrial tissue sampling. At diagnosis, endometrial cancers in women who have used estrogen are generally of earlier stage and lower grade and show less myometrial invasion than tumors in women who have not used estrogen (Mack, 1976; McDonald, 1977; Antunes, 1979; Hulka et al, 1980; Collins, 1980; Jelovsek, 1980; Kelsey, 1982; Buring, 1986). As would be expected from the lower grade and earlier stage of cancers in estrogen users, survival is better than in nonusers with the disease (Robboy, 1979; Collins, 1980; Chu, 1982). However, several studies have also shown estrogen use to be associated with late-stage, high-grade invasive tumors (Shapiro et al, 1985; Ewertz, 1988; Rubin, 1990) and a nonsignificant increased risk for endometrial cancer death in estrogen users has been reported (Mack, 1976; Lafferty, 1985; Petitti, 1987; Ettinger, 1988; Paganini-Hill,

TABLE 49–6. *Summary Relative Risk for Developing Endometrial Cancer among Estrogen Users (Compared with Nonusers)*

Estrogen Use	RR[a] for Developing Endometrial Cancer	95% CI[a]	Number of Studies[b]
EVER USE OF ESTROGENS			
All eligible studies	2.3	2.1– 2.5	29
Cohort studies	1.7	1.3– 2.1	4
Case-control studies	2.4	2.2– 2.6	25
Hospital controls	2.2	2.0– 2.5	10
Gynecologic controls	3.3	2.7– 4.0	6
Community controls[c]	2.4	2.0– 2.9	10
DOSE OF CONJUGATED ESTROGEN			
0.3 mg	3.9	1.6–9.5	3
0.625 mg	3.4	2.0–5.6	4
≥1.25 mg	5.8	4.5–7.5	9
DURATION OF USE			
≤1 year	1.4	1.0– 1.8	9
1–5 years	2.8	2.3– 3.5	12
5–10 years	5.9	4.7– 7.5	10
≥10 years	9.5	7.4–12.3	10
TIME SINCE LAST USE			
≤1 year	4.1	2.9– 5.7	3
1–4 years	3.7	2.5– 5.5	3
≥5 years	2.3	1.8– 3.1	5
REGIMEN			
Intermittent or cyclic	3.0	2.4– 3.8	8
Daily	2.9	2.2– 3.8	8
TYPE OF ESTROGEN			
Conjugated	2.5	2.1– 2.9	9
Synthetic	1.3	1.1– 1.6	7
STAGE/INVASIVENESS OF CANCER			
Stage 0–1	4.2	3.1– 5.7	3
Stage 2–4	1.4	0.8– 2.4	3
Noninvasive	6.2	4.5– 8.4	4
Invasive	3.8	2.9– 5.1	6
	RR[a] for Dying of Endometrial Cancer		
Ever use of estrogens: All eligible studies	2.7	0.9– 8.0	3

[a]Summary relative risk (RR) and 95% confidence interval (CI) from meta-analysis
[b]Number of study findings that were included in the meta-analysis
[c]Community controls include residential, neighborhood, and population-based controls
Source: Adapted from a meta-analysis by Grady et al, 1995.

1989). Summary relative risks by stage and invasiveness and for endometrial cancer death are given in Table 49–6.

Dose-response relation. In the dosage range commonly prescribed (0.3–2.50 mg/day of conjugated estrogens), the risk of endometrial cancer is elevated for all doses and increases somewhat with increasing dose (Mack et al, 1976; Gray et al, 1977; McDonald et al, 1977; Weiss et al, 1979; Hulka et al, 1980a; Stavraky, 1981; Buring et al, 1986) (Table 49–6).

Duration of use. Risk of endometrial cancer increases with increasing duration of estrogen use (Ziel and Finkle, 1975; Mack et al, 1976; McDonald et al, 1977; Hoogerland et al, 1978; Wigle et al, 1978; Shapiro et al, 1980; Hulka et al, 1980a; Jelovsek et al, 1980; Spengler et al, 1981; Stavraky, 1981; Shapiro et al, 1985; Buring et al, 1986; Stampfer, 1986; Paganini-Hill, 1989; Persson, 1989). Several studies show increased risk only after 2 to 6 years of estrogen therapy (Ziel and Finkle, 1975; Gray et al, 1977; Hulka et al, 1980a; Jelovsek et al, 1980; Spengler et al, 1981; Kelsey et al, 1982; Shapiro et al, 1985; Persson, 1989); other studies suggest an increased risk even for short-term use of less than 1 year (Mack et al, 1976; McDonald et al, 1977; Hoogerland et al, 1978). Summary relative risk estimates suggest about a 40% increase in endometrial cancer risk even with a year or less of estrogen therapy and a 10-fold increase with 10 or more years of use (Grady et al, 1995) (Table 49–6).

Persistence of risk after discontinuation of ERT. Some studies noted a decrease in the elevated risk of endometrial cancer soon after estrogen use was stopped (Weiss et al, 1979; Shapiro et al, 1980; Hulka et al, 1980b; Stavraky, 1981); other studies found that the increased risk persists for several years (Mack et al, 1976; Shapiro et al, 1985; Buring et al, 1986). Summary data suggest that risk of endometrial cancer remains increased about twofold, even 5 years after cessation of therapy (Grady et al, 1995) (Table 49–6).

Type of estrogen used. Subjects in most epidemiological studies have taken oral conjugated natural estrogen, which is the predominant type of estrogen prescribed in the United States for ERT. Most studies that have examined these preparations have shown an increased risk of endometrial cancer (Ziel and Finkle, 1975; Mack et al, 1976; Gray et al, 1977; McDonald et al, 1977; Horwitz and Feinstein, 1978; Antunes et al, 1979; Shapiro et al, 1980; Hulka et al, 1980a, b; Buring et al, 1986; Persson, 1989). Increased incidence of endometrial cancer has also been shown among women who used diethylstilbestrol, a synthetic estrogen (Antunes et al, 1979) and ethinyl estradiol (Persson, 1989). Some investigators have reported no difference in risk between users and nonusers of nonconjugated estrogens (Shapiro et al, 1980), and one Finnish study reported a significant decrease in risk among users (Salmi, 1980). Use of vaginal estrogens results in systemic absorption of estrogen. One study in which vaginal estrogen use was examined separately showed no increase in risk, but the number of women using vaginal estrogens was small and there was no adjustment for dose and duration of use (Gray et al, 1977).

Dosing regimen. Exogenous estrogens are usually taken orally once a day. Many clinicians prescribe cyclic therapy (no treatment for 5 to 7 days each month) in the belief that endometrial stimulation is lessened. However, this regimen is often associated with estrogen-deficiency symptoms during the "off period" and is difficult for patients to follow. Daily (continuous) therapy is an easier regimen to follow. Several studies have compared women on both dosing regimens to controls with no clear difference between the regimens in risk of endometrial cancer (Mack et al, 1976; McDonald et al, 1977; Hulka et al, 1980a; Stavraky, 1981; Antunes et al, 1979; Weiss et al, 1979) (Table 49–6). Only one study directly compared women on the two regimens (Buring et al, 1986) and showed that women using cyclic therapy had slightly higher risk of endometrial cancer than those using continuous therapy (OR=3.6 vs 2.4; P=0.13).

Methodological issues. Questions have been raised concerning the validity of studies that report an increased risk for endometrial cancer in women using ERT. Misclassification due to inclusion of women with endometrial hyperplasia among endometrial cancer cases could spuriously increase risk (Shanklin, 1976). Studies based on careful review of pathological slides, however, still show an increased risk of endometrial cancer in women who have taken estrogens (Gordon et al, 1977; Horwitz and Feinstein, 1978; Bhagavan et al, 1984). The finding of increased risk of endometrial cancer in women who have taken estrogens might be due to biased selection of controls, recall bias among the women with cancer, and surveillance bias among women using ERT (Horwitz et al, 1978, 1986). However, the consistently increased risk reported despite differing control groups, the increased risk with increasing duration of use, the clear dose-response relation, and increased risk despite adjustment for multiple confounding variables make it unlikely that the reported association is due to bias.

Summary. Randomized controlled trials are lacking, but the fact that exogenous estrogens can produce endometrial hyperplasia, the increased incidence of endometrial cancer in relation to trends in estrogen use in the United States and Canada, and the consistent results of case-control and cohort studies of ERT strongly argue that exogenous estrogens are a cause of endometrial cancer. Risk of mortality from endometrial cancer among estrogen users is probably also increased slightly. Increased risk of endometrial cancer in women who use exogenous estrogens is related to dose and duration of therapy. Current doses (usually 0.625 mg conjugated estrogen daily) are lower than doses used in the past and should be associated with lower risks. However, ERT as now prescribed for prevention of coronary heart disease and osteoporosis will typically continue for 15–20 years, significantly longer than ERT was given in the past for perimenopausal symptoms.

Progestins. Unopposed estrogens may increase risk of endometrial cancer by causing continuous mitotic stimulation and incomplete shedding of the endometrium. Progesterone antagonizes the effects of estrogen by decreasing estrogen receptors (Hsueh et al, 1975) and increasing the activity of enzymes that metabolize estradiol to less potent metabolites (Tseng et al, 1975). Progesterone secretion during the luteal phase of the menstrual cycle ends estrogenic mitotic stimulation and cellular replication, and causes endometrial cells to differentiate to a secretory state (Novak et al, 1979). Progesterone withdrawal at the end of the menstrual cycle leads to cyclic sloughing of the endometrium. These effects of progesterone probably prevent the continuous proliferation that results in endometrial hyperplasia or neoplasia.

Endometrial hyperplasia. Endometrial hyperplasia, especially adenomatous or atypical hyperplasia, may be a precursor of endometrial cancer (McBride et al, 1959; Gusberg, 1976). Endometrial hyperplasia can be successfully treated with progestins (Gambrell et al, 1978; Ferenczy, 1978; Thom et al, 1979), and about 30% of women with metastatic adenocarcinoma of the endometrium respond to treatment with progestins (Reifenstein et al, 1974). Endometrial hyperplasia is less common in women taking estrogen and progestins compared with women taking estrogen alone (Whitehead and Fraser, 1987; Whitehead et al, 1979; Paterson et al, 1980; Varma, 1985; Persson et al, 1986; Gelfand, 1989). Whitehead and Fraser (1987) reported that after 18 months of therapy with unopposed estrogen, approximately 30% of women had endometrial hyperplasia on aspiration biopsy. In women taking estrogen and progestins, the incidence of endometrial hyperplasia was lower (7 days per month of progestin was associated with a 4% incidence of hyperplasia, 10 days per month with a 2% incidence, and 12 days per month with no endometrial hyperplasia).

Endometrial cancer. That endometrial hyperplasia and cancer can be treated with progestins and the decreased risk of endometrial cancer in users of combination oral contraceptive suggest that progestin added to estrogen therapy may protect against endometrial cancer. Three small cohort studies and one randomized trial (total number of endometrial cancers in all four studies = 19) have reported decreased risk of endometrial cancer in users of estrogen and progestins compared with nonusers (Table 49–7) (Hammond, 1979; Nachtigall, 1979; Gambrell, 1980; Persson, 1989).

Three more recent case-control studies each showed a small, nonsignificantly increased risk for endometrial cancer among estrogen plus progestin users compared with nonusers (Table 49–7). In one study that evaluated the number of days per month that a progestin was used, estrogen users who added progestin for 10 or more days per month had no increased risk of endometrial cancer (Voigt et al, 1991). Because prevention of endometrial hyperplasia appears to depend on adequate dose and duration of progestin use, the increased risk noted in the case-control studies might be due to the lower doses of progestins now in common use or to lack of compliance with the prescribed progestin.

Summary. Although large randomized controlled trials are lacking, biochemical, histologic, and clinical data suggest that adding progestins to estrogen replacement therapy reduces the increased risk of endometrial cancer caused by treatment with unopposed estrogen. Based on these data, a progestin is typically added to estrogen therapy for 10–14 days per month in women with a uterus. Epidemiological evidence regarding the effect of added progestins on endometrial cancer risk are conflicting and the long-term effects of progestin therapy are unknown. Estrogen therapy may reduce the incidence of coronary artery disease in postmenopausal women (Stampfer and Colditz, 1991; Grady et al, 1992). Progestins may reverse some of this beneficial effect of estrogens on the lipid profile, or antagonize other beneficial cardiovascular effects of estrogen, reducing the favorable effects of estrogens on coronary artery disease risk (Hirvonen et al, 1981; Ottosson et al, 1985; Jensen, 1986). Given the high incidence and mortality of coronary artery disease in postmenopausal women, a small increase in the risk of this disease could outweigh the benefits of progestins in preventing endometrial cancer. The effect of progestin treatment on risk of breast cancer is currently unknown (Ernster and Cummings, 1986; Grady and Ernster, 1991; Grady, 1992).

Tamoxifen. Tamoxifen is a nonsteroidal hormone that has both antiestrogenic and estrogenic properties. It is effective for treatment of advanced breast cancer and has been used for that purpose since its introduction in the early 1970s. In the 1980s, it was proven to be effective adjuvant therapy for women with early-stage breast cancer (Early Breast Cancer Trialists' Collaborative Group, 1988). Women with breast cancer who are treated with tamoxifen have a lower risk of developing cancer in the contralateral breast (Fisher et al, 1989), suggesting that tamoxifen might also be effective in primary prevention of breast cancer. Based on this theory, tamoxifen is currently being studied in large randomized trials for the prevention of breast cancer in healthy women who are at increased risk for the disease.

Uterine cancer. Tamoxifen has partial estrogen agonist effects in the uterus. It has been shown to enhance growth of human endometrial carcinoma cells trans-

TABLE 49–7. *Postmenopausal Estrogen Plus Progestin Use and Endometrial Cancer*

Reference	*Study Design*	*Population*	*Relative Risk*
Nachtigall (1979)	randomized control trial; mean follow-up 10 years	1 case; 168 women; 84 pairs of institutionalized women matched for age and diagnosis, randomized to estrogen plus progestin or placebo	[a]
Hammond (1979)	cohort; mean follow-up ≥5 years	3 cases; 381 hypoestrogenic women	[a]
Gambrell (1980)	cohort; mean follow-up 4 years	8 cases; 7,337 person-years at risk; women in gynecologic clinic	0.2[b]
Persson (1989)	cohort; mean follow-up 5.7 years	7 cases; 35,318 person-years at risk; women >35 years in Uppsala health care region prescribed estrogen plus progestin compared with the remaining female population of Uppsala	0.9
Voigt (1991)	case-control	158 cases; 182 population-based controls	1.6
Jick (1993)	case-control	172 cases; 1720 from Group Health Cooperative of Puget Sound	1.9
Brinton (1993)	case-control	300 cases; 207 population-based controls	1.8

[a]No cancers observed in the estrogen plus progestin group.
[b]$P < 0.05$.

planted into athymic mice (Satayaswaroop et al, 1984; Gourtadis et al, 1988) and to cause proliferation of the endometrium and estrogenization of the vagina in women (Boccardo et al, 1984). Endometrial hyperplasia has been reported in postmenopausal breast cancer patients taking tamoxifen (Gal et al, 1991). In the mid-1980s, cases of uterine cancer among women with breast cancer being treated with tamoxifen were reported (Killackey et al, 1985; Neven et al, 1985; Magriples et al, 1993; Seoud et al, 1993), including high-grade, aggressive tumors (Magriples et al, 1993).

Information on uterine cancer risk is now available from five major randomized trials of tamoxifen as adjuvant therapy for breast cancer (Table 49–8). Swedish and Danish trials reported a substantial increased risk of endometrial cancer among treated women (relative risk 6.4 and 3.3, respectively). In contrast, Scottish and British trials found no increased risk of endometrial cancer, although three cases of uterine sarcoma occurred in the tamoxifen-treated group in the Scottish trial (Malfetano, 1990). Some investigators felt that the difference in these findings was explained by the fact that higher doses of tamoxifen were used in the Swedish and Danish trials (40 and 30 mg/day, respectively) compared with the Scottish and British trials, in which the currently recommended dose of 20 mg/day was used. However, the U.S. National Surgical Adjuvant Breast and Bowel Project (NSABP) B-14 trial, which randomly assigned 2843 women with estrogen receptor–positive, node-negative breast cancer to tamoxifen at 20 mg/day or placebo for 5 years, also reported a substantial increase in risk for endometrial cancer among treated women (relative risk 7.4; 95% C.I.: 1.7-32.7) (Fisher et al, 1994). Fifteen endometrial cancers occurred in the tamoxifen-treated group, compared to two in the placebo group, and both endometrial cancers that occurred in the placebo group were in women who required tamoxifen treatment after randomization. At least four women in the tamoxifen group died of their endometrial cancer, compared to none in the placebo group (Fisher et al, 1994).

Summary. Two randomized trials showed no increased risk of uterine cancer among women treated with tamoxifen, but three other larger trials each showed a substantially increased risk. There is some suggestion that risk is increased only with higher doses of tamoxifen, but the largest trial to date showed a statistically significant sevenfold increased risk of endometrial cancer in women taking 20 mg of tamoxifen daily (Fisher et al, 1994), the dose currently used for adjuvant therapy and the dose under study in primary prevention trials. In the NSABP B-14 trial, the cumulative hazard rate for endometrial cancer at 1 year was 1.2 and at 5 years 6.3, suggesting that risk increases with increasing duration of tamoxifen therapy (Fisher et al, 1994). One case-control study also suggested that risk for endometrial cancer increases with increasing dose and duration of use of tamoxifen (van Leeuwen et al, 1994), but the data are limited. Some investigators have assumed that tamoxifen-associated endometrial cancers are less aggressive than endometrial cancers in untreated women, but data do not support this claim (Magriples et al, 1993). In the NSABP B-14 trial, four of the 15 women assigned to tamoxifen treatment who developed endometrial cancer died of their disease (Fisher et al, 1994).

In women with breast cancer, the benefits of tamoxifen therapy clearly outweigh the risks. In women at high risk for developing breast cancer (such as those with one or more first-degree relatives with breast can-

TABLE 49–8. *Randomized Controlled Trials of Tamoxifen as Adjuvant Therapy for Breast Cancer: Endometrial Cancer Risk*

Trial (reference)	*Number of Subjects*	*Tamoxifen Dose (mg/day)*	*Duration of Therapy (years)*	*Follow-up (years)*	*Relative Risk (95% CI)*
Swedish (Fornander, 1989)	1846 postmenopausal women; operable breast cancer	40	5	4.5	6.4 (1.4–28)
Danish (Andersson, 1991)	1710 postmenopausal women; operable breast cancer	30	1	7.9	3.3 (0.6–32.4)
Scottish (Stewart, 1992)	747 pre- and postmenopausal women; lymph node negative breast cancer	20	5	5.0	NA[a]
British (Ribeiro, 1992)	961 pre- and postmenopausal women; operable breast cancer	20	1	13.0	NA[a]
NSABP-14 (Fisher, 1994)	2843 pre- and postmenopausal women; lymph node negative breast cancer	20	5	6.8	7.5 (1.7–32.7)

[a]One endometrial cancer occurred in the tamoxifen-treated group and one in the placebo-treated group.

cer), the benefits of therapy may also outweigh the risks of developing uterine cancer. If tamoxifen therapy increases uterine cancer risk as much as sevenfold, women whose underlying risk of breast cancer is only moderately high may not benefit (Bush and Helzlsouer, 1993).

Obesity and Related Measures

Obesity, measured in various ways, is associated with increased risk of endometrial cancer. Risk has been shown to increase with body weight (Mack, 1976; McDonald et al, 1977; Horwitz and Feinstein, 1978; Weiss and Sayvetz, 1980; Hulka et al, 1980a; Jelovsek et al, 1980; Kelsey et al, 1982; Henderson et al, 1983), body mass index (Ziel and Finkle, 1975; Elwood et al, 1977; Hoogerland et al, 1978; Ewertz et al, 1988; Shapiro et al, 1980; Spengler et al, 1981; La Vecchia et al, 1984, 1986b; Törnberg and Carstensen, 1994), and waist-to-thigh circumference ratio (Swanson et al, 1993; Elliott et al, 1990) or waist-to-hip circumference ratio (Schapira et al, 1991). Two cohort studies suggest that these effects may be largely confined to older women. One found positive associations of endometrial cancer with adult weight and gain in body mass only in women 60 years and older at the time of diagnosis (Le Marchand et al, 1991), and the other reported a strong positive gradient for Quetelet Index among women 55 years of age or older at diagnosis, but among women under the age of 55 risk was increased only for the most obese (Törnberg and Carstensen, 1994). The range for increased risk of endometrial cancer attributed to these various measures is shown in Table 49–9.

The increase in risk of endometrial cancer associated with body weight may not be linear. Risk is generally small for moderate increases in weight but may be significantly elevated when the most obese women are compared with those of normal weight (Kelsey et al, 1982; Henderson et al, 1983; La Vecchia et al, 1984; Swanson et al, 1993).

In many populations, obesity may account for a large etiologic fraction of endometrial cancer. McDonald and coworkers (1977) estimated that obesity (weight more than 30% above ideal) accounted for 25% of endometrial cancer in their study population from the Mayo Clinic. La Vecchia and coworkers (1984) concluded that obesity is the major cause of endometrial cancer in northern Italy.

Obesity may increase the risk of endometrial cancer by altering estrogen metabolism. Peripheral conversion of androstenedione to estrone is increased in obese women (MacDonald and Siiteri, 1974; MacDonald et al, 1978) and concentrations of sex hormone–binding globulin are decreased (Anderson et al, 1974), thereby increasing levels of bioavailable estrogens. Whether lack of physical activity plays a role in the association of obesity with endometrial cancer has received little attention. One case-control study in China found that women with sedentary lifestyles were at somewhat increased risk for the disease; however, this result was unaffected when body mass index and caloric intake were controlled, suggesting that lack of physical activity may be an independent risk factor (Shu et al, 1993).

Among women who have endometrial cancer, the risk of dying of the disease is markedly increased in obese women. In a large prospective study of body weight and mortality, the most obese women were five times more likely to die of endometrial cancer compared with women of average weight (Lew and Garfinkel, 1979).

Diet and Alcohol Consumption

Armstrong and Doll (1975) studied the incidence of various cancers in relation to dietary intake in 23 countries. The incidence of endometrial cancer was higher in areas with high total dietary fat consumption. Analysis of dietary profiles among women in Hawaii showed a positive association of endometrial cancer with high average daily intake of fat and protein, and a protective effect of high daily intake of complex carbohydrates (Kolonel et al, 1981), and an Italian case-control study also reported that risk was increased among women reporting greater intake of dietary fat (OR=5.65). The latter study also reported that lower intake of green vegetables, fruit, milk, liver, and fish was associated with increased risk of the disease (La Vecchia et al, 1986b). A population-based case-control study conducted in five areas of the United States also reported increased risk associated with higher fat intakes, a reduced risk with intake of complex carbohydrates, and no association with carotenoids—findings that were independent of one another and were adjusted for body mass and other risk factors (Potischman et al, 1993). However, a smaller case-control study conducted in Alabama did not find an association with total fat intake, nor a protective effect for complex carbohydrates; it did find reduced risks associated with consumption of certain vegetables and dairy products (Barbone et al, 1993). Thus, although few studies of diet and endometrial cancer have been conducted and the results are not entirely consistent, the evidence to date suggests that high dietary fat intake may increase the risk of endometrial cancer and that complex carbohydrates may reduce risk.

Several studies have examined the association between alcohol consumption and endometrial cancer risk, with inconsistent results. Based on the evidence to date, alcohol appears to have little, if any, relation to

TABLE 49–9. *Risk of Endometrial Cancer in Women with Obesity, Diabetes, Hypertension, and Gallbladder Disease (Relative Risks or Odds Ratios and 95% Confidence Intervals or P-Values unless otherwise indicated)*

Reference	*Body Weight or Obesity*[a]	*Diabetes Mellitus*	*Hypertension*	*Gallbladder Disease*
Ziel and Finkle (1975)	~2 (CI not given) for upper third Quetelet index vs lower third			
Mack et al (1976)	1.5 (NS)[b] for weight in excess of standard for frame	0.9 (NS)	1.5 (NS)	3.7 (95% CI excludes 1.0)
Gray et al (1977)	Cases = 148.3 lb; Controls = 141 lb ($P<0.01$)	9.8 (1.1–369.4)	Diastolic blood pressure: no case-control differences; Systolic blood pressure: cases 146.6 mm Hg; controls 141.5 mm Hg ($P<0.05$)	
McDonald et al (1977)	3.5 (2.3–11.5) for 30% > ideal body weight vs normal body weight	0.7 (0.3–1.4)		1.2 (0.7–1.8)
Elwood et al (1977)	Quetelet index: <22 1.0 22–24 1.0 25–27 1.2 ≥28 1.9 (*P* for trend = 0.004)	2.3 (0.9–5.8)	1.7 (1.0–2.7)	
Horwitz and Feinstein (1978)	Percent obese significantly higher in cases than controls (*P* not given)	NS	NS	
Hoogerland et al (1978)	2.7 ($P<0.001$) for Quetelet index ≥40	2.1 ($P<0.001$)	2.1 ($P<0.001$)	
Weiss et al (1980)	Weight (lb) / No Estrogen Use or >1 Year / 1–7 Years' Estrogen Use <120 / 1.0 / 3.2 (1.5–6.8) 120–159 / 0.8 (0.3–2.3) / 6.0 (1.8–20.3) ≥160 / 2.2 (1.1–4.5) / 3.5 (1.3–9.4)		If no estrogen use or <1 year of use: 2.0 (1.0–3.9); If 1–7 years use: 4.0 (1.9–8.4)	
Shapiro et al (1980)	Ponderal index ≥40 in 34% of cases; 24% of controls[c]	5% of cases; 2% of controls[c]		
Hulka et al (1980a)	Weight >170 lb in 51.6% of cases; 39.9% of gynecologic controls; 31.4% of community controls[c]	19.4% of cases; 17% of gynecologic controls; 6.8% of community controls[c]	51.1% of cases; 47.7% of gynecologic controls; 33.5% of community controls[c]	17.7% of cases 25.5% of gynecologic controls 12.3% of community controls[c]
Jelovsek et al (1980)	Weight ≥200 lb in 23.2% of cases; 9.3% of controls ($P<0.001$)	22.5% of cases; 13% of controls ($P<0.001$)	61.5% of cases; 43.8% of controls ($P<0.001$)	
Spengler et al (1981)	Ponderal index ≥40 in 24% of cases; 26% of controls (NS)	9% of cases; 4% of controls (NS)	32% of cases; 33% of controls (NS)	29% of cases; 17% of controls ($P<0.05$)
Kelsey[d] et al (1982)	Weight (lb): <125 1.0 126–145 1.3 146–165 1.3 ≥166 2.3 (*P* for trend = 0.001)	1.3 (0.7–2.3)	1.0 (NS)	

Henderson et al (1983)	Weight (lb): <129 1.0 129–150 1.4 150–170 1.9 170–190 9.6 >190 17.7 $P<0.001$ for trend		
La Vecchia et al (1986b)	Body mass index: <20 0.43 (0.21–0.91) 20–24 1.00 (referent) 25–29 1.82 (1.11–2.99) ≥30 3.10 (1.80–5.33)	2.77 (1.61–4.75)	2.08 (1.35–3.20)
Ewertz et al (1988)	Quetelet index: <22 1.0 22– 1.5 (0.8–2.7) 25– 2.3 (1.2–4.4) ≥28 2.6 (1.3–4.7)		1.2 (0.6–2.2)
Elliott[e] et al (1990)	Waist-to-hip circumference: <0.78 1.0 0.78–0.83 2.6 (0.88–7.9) ≥0.84 3.0 (1.02–9.0)		
Le Marchand[f] et al (1991)	Weight in 1992 of women ages ≥60 when diagnosed from 1972–1986: 1st tertile 1.0 2nd tertile 1.2 3rd tertile 2.3 (P = 0.04 for trend)		
Schapira[g] et al (1991)	15.0 (1.98–58.0) for waist-to-hip circumference ratio of >1.14 vs ≤1.14		
Swanson[h] et al (1993)	Weight (kg): <58.6 1.0 58.6–68.8 1.0 (0.6–1.6) 68.9–78.3 0.7 (0.4–1.1) >78.3 2.3 (1.4–3.7) Waist-to-thigh circumference: <1.62 1.0 1.62–1.78 1.5 (0.8–2.5) 1.79–1.99 1.8 (1.1–3.2) >1.99 2.6 (1.5–4.5)		
Törnberg and Carstensen (1994)	Quetelet index <55 Years / ≥55 Years <22 1.0 / 1.0 22–23.9 1.06 / 1.52 24–25.9 1.06 / 2.05 26–27.9 0.72 / 2.17 ≥28 1.64 / 3.16 (P for trend=0.33) / (P for trend <0.0001)		

(continued)

TABLE 49–9. *Risk of Endometrial Cancer in Women with Obesity, Diabetes, Hypertension, and Gallbladder Disease (Relative Risks or Odds Ratios and 95% Confidence Intervals or P-Values unless otherwise indicated) (Continued)*

Reference	*Body Weight or Obesity*[a]	*Diabetes Mellitus*	*Hypertension*	*Gallbladder Disease*
Brinton[i] et al (1992)	Weight (lb): <125 1.00 125–149 1.12 (1.7–1.8) 150–174 0.91 (0.5–1.6) 175–199 1.94 (1.1–3.5) ≥200 7.18 (3.9–13.3) Body Mass Index <23 1.0 23–25 0.82 (0.5–1.3) 26–28 0.88 (0.5–1.5) 29–31 2.70 (1.5–4.9) >32 4.15 (2.5–6.8)	1.95 (1.1–3.6)	0.94 (0.6–1.4)	1.41 (0.8–2.3)

[a]Variously measured as weight, body mass index (ie, Quetelet index or Ponderal index), waist-to-hip circumference, or waist-to-thigh circumference, as indicated.
[b]NS = not significant (if so stated by authors and *P* value not given).
[c]Statistical significance not given.
[d]Odds ratios adjusted for multiple risk factors.
[e]Odds ratios adjusted for age, parity, and smoking status. Risk increased more dramatically with increasing waist-to-hip circumference in obese than nonobese women.
[f]No association of adult body weight seen in women less than 60 years of age at diagnosis, nor was there a significant effect for Quetelet index in any age group. Adult weight gain was also significant for women age 60 or older.
[g]Controls matched to cases on age and Quetelet index.
[h]Adjusted for age, education, number of births, menopausal estrogen use, and smoking status. Weight was further adjusted for weight-to-thigh circumference and vice versa.
[i]All analyses adjusted for age at interview, years of education, number of births, oral contraceptive use, and menopausal estrogen use. The relative risks for diabetes, hypertension, and gallbladder disease were further adjusted for recent weight gain.

risk of the disease (Gapstur et al, 1993; Austin et al, 1993).

Diabetes

An increased frequency of diabetes mellitus or abnormal glucose tolerance among women with endometrial cancer has been reported. As summarized in Table 49–9, most of the case-control studies performed since 1970 that have examined this relationship show an increased risk of endometrial cancer in women with diabetes (Gray et al, 1977; Elwood et al, 1977; Hoogerland et al, 1978; Shapiro et al, 1980; Hulka et al, 1980a; Jelovsek et al, 1980; Spengler et al, 1981; Kelsey et al, 1982; La Vecchia et al, 1986b; Brinton et al, 1992). Interpretation of these studies is complicated by the difficulty of diagnosing diabetes from retrospective data, and the absence in most studies of adjustment for confounding factors, especially body weight. When evidence is limited to those studies that appropriately adjusted for body weight, findings are conflicting (Elwood et al, 1977; Hoogerland et al, 1978; Hulka et al, 1980a; Kelsey et al, 1982; Brinton et al, 1992). In sum, there may be an increase in risk of endometrial cancer among women with diabetes, but it is not clear whether this increased risk is at least partly explained by obesity (Kelsey et al, 1982).

Hypertension

Hypertension, like diabetes, has been reported to be common among women with endometrial cancer. As reviewed in Table 49–9, several studies have shown an increased risk of endometrial cancer among women with hypertension (Mack et al, 1976; Gray et al, 1977; Elwood et al, 1977; Hoogerland et al, 1978; Weiss et al, 1980; Jelovsek et al, 1980; La Vecchia et al, 1986b). However, inaccuracies in the retrospective assessment of blood pressure and lack of adjustment for confounding variables such as body weight and estrogen use make the association difficult to interpret. Studies have shown that the increased risk for endometrial cancer among hypertensive women may be due to estrogen use (Mack et al, 1976; Hoogerland et al, 1978) or to obesity (Kelsey et al, 1982). No increased risk was found to be associated with hypertension in a study that controlled for multiple potential confounding variables, including parity, estrogen use, and recent weight gain (Brinton et al, 1992).

Gallbladder Disease

The finding of an increased risk of endometrial cancer among women with gallbladder disease (Table 49–9) could potentially be due to an association of gallbladder disease with obesity or estrogen replacement therapy. The increased risk persisted in an analysis confined to estrogen users (Mack et al, 1976), but in a study that controlled for both estrogen use and body weight, as well as other risk factors, the excess risk of endometrial cancer associated with gallbladder disease was no longer statistically significant (Brinton et al, 1992).

Smoking

The results of a case-control study reported by Weiss and coworkers (1980) suggested that cigarette smoking might be associated with a reduced risk of endometrial cancer. In that study, women who had ever smoked were found to have lower risks of the disease than nonsmokers, and this was true for both users and nonusers of estrogen replacement therapy. Since that time, additional case-control studies of smoking and endometrial cancer have been reported. All large studies but one confirm the protective effect of smoking (Table 49–10). One study that did not find an association included only women aged 20–54 years (Tyler et al, 1985); a later report from the same study confined to postmenopausal women aged 40–55 years found a significant protective effect associated with smoking after menopause (Franks et al, 1987). That the effect might be confined to postmenopausal women was also suggested by studies that stratified by menopausal status (Smith et al, 1984; Lesko et al, 1986; Kouimantaki et al, 1989) or age (Stockwell and Lyman, 1987). The early study by Weiss and coworkers (1980) that reported significantly reduced risks included only postmenopausal women. However, reduced risks for both pre- and postmenopausal women were found in two studies (Lawrence et al, 1987; Levi et al, 1987).

Evidence with respect to a dose-response relation between smoking and endometrial cancer to date is inconsistent. Three studies found decreases in risk with amount smoked (Baron et al, 1986; Lawrence et al, 1987; Stockwell and Lyman, 1987), one found the protective effect to be limited to women who smoked more than 25 cigarettes per day (Lesko et al, 1985), and several found little or no evidence of a dose-response relation (Weiss et al, 1980; Levi et al, 1987; Brinton et al, 1993).

It is not clear whether the protective effect of smoking applies to former smokers. One study found a significantly reduced risk for former smokers (Stockwell and Lyman, 1987), and another reported a reduced risk for former smokers of more than one pack per day (Lawrence et al, 1987). Other studies reported no significant reduction in risk for former smokers (Tyler et al, 1985; Lesko et al, 1985; Levi et al, 1987; Austin et al, 1993;

TABLE 49–10. *Studies of Smoking and Endometrial Cancer*

Reference	*Study Design and Subjects*	*Relative Risk and 95% Confidence Interval (by menopausal status or age when given)*	*Effect in Ex-Smokers*	*Dose-Response Effect*	*Comments/Other Variables Controlled/ Modifying Effects*
Weiss et al (1980a)	Population-based case-control (N=322 and 289); women aged 50–74 years	0.4 (0.2–0.7) for ever vs never smokers among nonusers of menopausal estrogens	Not available separately	No relation to daily maximum number of cigarettes smoked	The increased risk of endometrial cancer associated with estrogens was much greater in nonsmokers than smokers
Smith et al (1984)	Population-based case-control (N=70 and 612); women aged 20–54 years	1.27 (0.65–2.5) for premenopausal smokers vs nonsmokers; 0.41 (0.16–1.04) for menopausal women	Not available separately	Increase in risk with pack-years of smoking, premenopausal women; decrease in postmenopausal women; neither statistically significant	
Tyler et al (1985)	Population-based case-control (N=437 and 3200); women aged 24–54 years	0.8 (0.7–1.1) for current smokers vs never smokers; 0.7 (0.5–1.0) in women aged 50–54 years	No effect (1.0 for former vs never smokers)	No effect by pack-years of smoking	Study confined to women <55 years of age. Logistic regression to control for numerous variables. In estrogen users, RR of 0.4 (0.2–0.9) for smokers vs nonsmokers
Lesko et al (1985)	Hospital-based case-control (N=510 and 727); women aged 18–69 years	0.5 (0.3–0.8) for all current smokers of ≥ 25 cigarettes per day vs never smokers; 0.9 (0.4–2.2) in premenopausal women; 0.5 (0.2–0.9) in postmenopausal women	No effect (0.9 for former vs never smokers)	No effect for smokers of <25 cigarettes per day	Multiple logistic regression to control for numerous variables
Baron et al (1986)	Cancer hospital–based case-control (N=476 and 2128); women aged 40–89 years	0.57 (0.37–0.86) for smokers of ≥ 15 cumulative pack-years vs never smokers; 0.78 (0.54–1.14) for smokers of 1–14 pack-years vs never smokers	Not available separately	Yes (measured by pack-years of smoking)	Multiple logistic regression to control for age, marital status, number of pregnancies, and Quetelet index
Franks et al (1987)	Population-based case-control (N=79 and 416); women aged 40–55 years who had undergone natural menopause after age 40	0.5 (0.3–0.8) for women who smoked after menopause vs nonsmokers	Not available separately	Not given	Subset of the Tyler et al (1985) study. Logistic regression to adjust for numerous variables. Increased risk of endometrial cancer associated with estrogens was greater in nonsmokers than smokers. Decreased risk associated with smoking was greater in estrogen users than nonusers.

Lawrence et al (1987)	Population-based case-control (N=200 and 200); women aged 40–69 years	0.47 for current smokers of >1 pack per day (linear trend test P<0.025, one-sided); no difference by menopausal status	0.58 for former smokers of >1 pack per day	Yes (measured by packs per day)	Confined to early stage disease. Matched logistic regression. Increased risk of endometrial cancer with body weight was confined to nonsmoking postmenopausal women who did not use exogenous estrogens.
Stockwell and Lyman (1987)	Population-based case-control (N=1374 and 3921); controls = women with cancers of the colon or rectum, cutaneous melanoma, or endocrine neoplasms	No association for women <50 years. In women ≥50 years, 0.9 (0.7–1.2) for current smokers of <20 cigarettes per day; 0.6 (0.4–0.9) for 20–40 cigarettes/day; 0.4 (0.2–0.8) for >40 cigarettes/day	0.6 (0.4–0.8) in former vs never smokers	Yes (measured by number of cigarettes per day)	Smoking status unknown for 28% of cases and 25% of controls. Multiple logistic regression to control for age, race, tobacco use, and marital status.
Levi et al (1987)	Hospital-based case-control (N=357 and 1122); women aged 25–74 years (Milan, Italy)	0.45 (0.3–0.7) in current smokers vs never smokers; 0.46 (0.23–0.93) in premenopausal women; 0.44 (0.28–0.70) in postmenopausal women	0.82 (0.49–1.35) for ex-smokers vs never smokers	No differences between smokers of <15 and ≥15 cigarettes per day	Multiple logistic regression to control for numerous variables
Koumantaki et al (1989)	Hospital-based case-control (N=83 and 164) (Athens, Greece)	0.49 (90% CI: .26–.93) in smokers of 15-20 cigarettes daily per 20 years of smoking	Not available	Not available	Effect seen only in postmenopausal women
Elliott et al (1990)	Hospital-based cases (N=46) and community-based controls (N=140)	0.17 (0.05–0.62) for current vs never smokers	1.4 (0.56–3.5) in former vs never smokers	Not available	Adjusted for age, parity, and wasit-to-hip circumference/body mass index
Brinton et al (1993)	Hospital-based cases (N=405) and population-based controls (N=297); women 20–74	0.5 (0.1–1.7) for premenopausal current vs never smokers; 0.4 (0.2–0.7) for postmenopausal women	Increased risk for former smokers among premenopausal women; little effect in postmenopausal women	No	Adjusted for age, education, number of births, recent weight, use of oral contraceptives, and use of menopausal estrogens
Austin et al (1993)	Hospital-based case-control (N=168 and 334)	0.69 (0.4–1.19) in current vs nonsmokers	No	No	Adjusted for race, years of schooling, body mass, index of central obesity, replacement estrogen use, and number of pregnancies

Elliott et al, 1990), and one reported an increased risk for former smokers among premenopausal women (Brinton et al, 1993).

Cigarette smoking may modify the relation between other risk factors and endometrial cancer. The increased risk associated with estrogen use may be greater in nonsmokers than in smokers (Weiss et al, 1980), and the increased risk associated with obesity may be greater in postmenopausal women who do not smoke or use exogenous estrogens (Lawrence et al, 1987; Elliott et al, 1990).

The reduced risk of endometrial cancer in smokers has been interpreted as evidence of an anti-estrogenic effect of smoking. This hypothesis is supported by other epidemiological studies that show smoking to be related to earlier age at menopause (Kaufman et al, 1980b; Willett et al, 1983) and increased risk of osteoporosis (Daniell, 1976; Williams et al, 1982), both of which are associated with decreased estrogen levels. Although one study reported lower levels of urinary estrogens in premenopausal smokers compared with nonsmokers (MacMahon et al, 1982), most studies of postmenopausal women have found no differences in circulating estrogens between smokers and nonsmokers (Jensen et al, 1985; Friedman et al, 1987; Austin et al, 1993). One study of postmenopausal women that found no difference in mean plasma levels of estrogens between smokers and nonsmokers (Khaw et al, 1988) did report significantly elevated levels of adrenal androgens in smokers. The authors suggested that increased androgenic activity, rather than decreased estrogenic activity, might be responsible for the protective effect of smoking on endometrial cancer risk.

It should be noted that two prospective studies, one in the United States (Garfinkel, 1980) and the other in Sweden (Cederlof et al, 1975), found no significant difference between smokers and nonsmokers in death rates for cancer of the uterine corpus, suggesting that smoking may reduce risk of developing nonfatal disease but have little effect on corpus cancer mortality. In any event, the dramatic increases in risk of other cancers, cardiovascular diseases, and other fatal conditions far outweigh any benefits of smoking for endometrial cancer.

Family History and History of Other Cancers

Few studies have addressed the question of whether women with a family history of endometrial cancer are at increased risk for the disease. Evidence supporting an association includes one study of a large cancer-prone family (Lynch et al, 1966) and a hospital-based case-control study that found an increased risk for women whose mothers or sisters had a history of endometrial or ovarian cancer (Kelsey et al, 1982); an earlier case-control study found no evidence of an association (Wynder et al, 1966). If an association exists, it is likely to be weak and does not account for a large fraction of cases of the disease.

Rates for cancers of the breast, ovary, and endometrium are strongly correlated across populations (Wynder et al, 1967; Dunn, 1974; Winkelstein et al, 1977; Howe et al, 1984). In addition, women with any one of these cancers appear to be at increased risk for developing a second cancer of the other sites (Bailer, 1963; Lynch et al, 1966; Schoenberg, 1969; Schottenfeld, 1971; Nelson et al, 1993; Tulinius et al, 1992), although the association for endometrial cancer is probably not strong and may be explained by other shared risk factors, such as nulliparity and late age at menopause.

RELATION OF RISK FACTORS TO EXCESS ESTROGEN

Most of the major risk factors for endometrial cancer can be characterized as states of excess unopposed estrogenic stimulation of the endometrium. Menopausal estrogen replacement therapy is associated with a significantly increased risk of endometrial cancer. Women who are nulliparous and those who undergo menopause late in life are also exposed to a long period of estrogen exposure uninterrupted by pregnancy. The association of hypertension and gallbladder disease with endometrial cancer might be explained by the fact that these diseases are more common in women with excess estrogen states. Polycystic ovarian syndrome and feminizing ovarian tumors are diseases associated with excess endogenous estrogen production and endometrial cancer. Obesity is also a condition of excess estrogen exposure produced by peripheral conversion of androstenedione to estrone.

The role of progesterone in modulating the stimulatory effect of estrogens on the endometrium and reducing the risk of endometrial cancer is demonstrated by the efficacy of progestins in the treatment of endometrial hyperplasia and endometrial cancer, by the reduced risk of endometrial cancer among women taking combination oral contraceptive pills, and by the attenuation of risk of endometrial cancer among women treated with estrogens and concomitant progestin therapy.

SCREENING AND PREVENTION

Multiple screening procedures for endometrial cancer have been suggested, but none has been proven to be sufficiently accurate, cost-effective, and acceptable (Pritchard, 1989). Endometrial biopsy techniques have been evaluated in symptomatic women, with accuracy ranging from 85%–93% (Vuopala, 1977), but these techniques are relatively uncomfortable and are not acceptable for mass screening. The routine cervical Papanicolaou smear is inaccurate for detection of corpus cancers (Burk et al, 1974). Endometrial cytologic sampling is relatively painless and safe, but efficacy has not been studied in a randomized trial. One large cohort study using this technique to screen asymptomatic women has been performed but did not include comparison to a "gold standard" tissue-sampling technique or sufficient follow-up time to determine the accuracy of the test (Kass et al, 1984). Although the American Cancer Society (1980) has recommended endometrial sampling at menopause in high-risk women (those with a history of infertility, obesity, failure to ovulate, abnormal uterine bleeding, or estrogen therapy), at the present time no screening method for endometrial cancer has proven to be effective in any group (Eddy et al, 1980; Canadian Task Force on the Periodic Health Examination, 1987; Pritchard et al, 1989). The U.S. Preventive Services Task Force makes no recommendation regarding screening for endometrial cancer (U.S. Preventive Services Task Force, 1989).

With regard to primary prevention, observational data suggest that decreasing body weight, minimizing estrogen dose, and adding a progestin to estrogen regimens may decrease risk of endometrial cancer, but no randomized controlled trials of such interventions have been published.

FUTURE RESEARCH

Our current knowledge of risk factors for cancer of the uterine corpus suggests a variety of research opportunities to better understand the etiology, prevention, and control of the disease. The strong association of exogenous menopausal estrogen use with increased risk of endometrial cancer is tempered by evidence of the benefits of such estrogens in reducing risk of other common and serious diseases, including osteoporosis and coronary heart disease. The addition of progestins to the estrogen regimen appears to reduce the risk of endometrial cancer associated with estrogens, although this practice may reduce the beneficial effects of estrogen on coronary heart disease (Barrett-Connor and Bush, 1991). Thus, it is very important to determine the types of estrogens and progestins, the minimal doses, the dosing regimens, and the modes of administration that will optimize cancer prevention while providing protection for osteoporosis and cardiovascular disease.

Racial differences in occurrence of and survival from uterine corpus cancer require further investigation. Although incidence of the disease is much higher in whites than blacks, mortality rates are considerably higher in blacks. The difference in 5-year relative survival between whites (85%) and blacks (55%) in 1983–1990 (SEER Cancer Statistics Review, 1973–1991) is greater than for any other major cancer. This might be explained in part by racial differences in histopathologic types of uterine corpus cancer, as well as by differences in stage at diagnosis and medical treatment. That the gap in survival rates between whites and blacks has narrowed somewhat over time suggests the potential for secondary prevention.

Although some screening modalities such as cytologic sampling have strong proponents, evidence is lacking for a beneficial effect of such methods as the basis for large-scale screening programs. Given that endometrial cancer is relatively uncommon and that survival rates for the disease are already high, it may be difficult to demonstrate major survival benefits associated with screening. That the fluctuation in rates with changes in estrogen use during the 1970s was seen only for incidence, not mortality, suggests that some factors that affect development of the disease may have little impact on risk of death. A potential limitation of improved screening and early detection efforts is that many endometrial cancers detected through such programs may be clinically unimportant cases. It would be of great benefit to detect early cancers that have the poorest potential for survival. These issues should receive careful attention.

Finally, the accuracy of mortality statistics for uterine corpus cancer should be improved. Currently, as many as one half of deaths counted as corpus cancer may actually have been certified at the time of death as "uterine, not otherwise specified." Although the great majority of these are corpus cancers, some are cervical cancers. Because the proportion that the NOS group represents of all corpus cancer deaths has declined over time, it is difficult to draw any meaningful conclusions regarding secular trends in uterine cancer mortality and to assess accurately the extent of progress in reducing mortality from the disease. Efforts to determine precisely the distribution of deaths in the NOS category (corpus vs cervix) in the past and present, as well as educational efforts to improve the certification of such deaths in the future, are needed.

REFERENCES

AMERICAN CANCER SOCIETY. 1980. Guidelines for the cancer-related checkup: recommendations and rationale. CA 30:193–240.

ANDERSON DC. 1974. Sex-hormone-binding globulin. Clin Endocrinol 3:69–72.

ANDERSSON M, STORM H, MOURIDSEN H. 1991. Incidence of new

primary cancers after adjuvant tamoxifen therapy and radiotherapy for early breast cancer. J Natl Cancer Inst 83:1013–1017.

1987 Annual Cancer Statistics Review, Including Cancer Trends: 1950–1985. 1988. Bethesda, MD: NIH Publication No. 88-2789.

Antunes CMF, Stolley PD, Rosenshein NB, Davies JL, Tonascia JA, Brown C, Burnett L, Rutledge A, Pokempner M, Garcia R. 1979. Endometrial cancer and estrogen use. N Engl J Med 300:9–13.

Armstrong B, Doll R. 1975. Environmental factors and cancer incidence and mortality in different countries, with special reference to dietary practices. Int J Cancer 15:617–631.

Austin H, Drews C, Partridge EE. 1993. A case-control study of endometrial cancer in relation to cigarette smoking, serum estrogen levels and alcohol use. Am J Obstet Gynecol 169:1086–1081.

Austin DF, Roe KM. 1979. Increase in cancer of the corpus uteri in the San Francisco–Oakland Standard Metropolitan Statistics Area, 1960–75. J Natl Cancer Inst 62:13–16.

Austin DF, Roe KM. 1982. The decreasing incidence of endometrial cancer: public health implications. Am J Public Health 72:65–68.

Bailar JC III. 1963. The incidence of independent tumors among uterine cancer patients. Cancer 16:842–853.

Barbone F, Austin H, Partridge EE. 1993. Diet and endometrial cancer: a case-control study. Am J Epidemiol 137:393–403.

Baron JA, Byers T, Greenberg ER, Cummings KM, Swanson M. 1986. Cigarette smoking in women with cancers of the breast and reproductive organs. J Natl Cancer Inst 77:677–680.

Barrett-Connor E, Bush TL. 1991. Estrogen and coronary heart disease in women. JAMA 265:1861–1867.

Benjamin F, Deutsch S. 1976. Plasma levels of fractionated estrogens and pituitary hormones in endometrial carcinoma. Am J Obstet Gynecol 126:638–647.

Bhagavan BS, Parmly TH, Rosenshein NB, Jefferys JL, Grisso JA, Stolley PD. 1984. Comparison of estrogen induced hyperplasia to endometrial cancer. Obstet Gynecol 64:12–15.

Boccardo F, Guarneri D, Rubagotti A, et al. 1984. Endocrine effects of tamoxifen in post-menopausal breast cancer patients. Tumori 70:61–68.

Boring CC, Squires TS, Tong T. 1994. Cancer statistics, 1994. CA 44:7–26.

Brinton LA, Barrett RJ, Berman ML, Mortel R, Twiggs LB, Wilbanks GD. 1993. Cigarette smoking and the risk of endometrial cancer. Am J Epidemiol 137:281–291.

Brinton LA, Hoover RN. 1993. Estrogen replacement therapy and endometrial cancer risk: unresolved issues. Obstet Gynecol 81:265–271.

Brinton LA, Berman ML, Mortel R, Twiggs LB, Barrett RJ, Wilbanks GD, Lannom L, Hoover RN. 1992. Reproductive, menstrual, and medical risk factors for endometrial cancer: results from a case-control study. Am J Obstet Gynecol 167:1317–1325.

Buring JE, Bain CJ, Ehrmann RL. 1986. Conjugated estrogen use and risk of endometrial cancer. Am J Epidemiol 124:434–441.

Burk JR, Lehman HF, Wolf FS. 1974. Inadequacy of Papanicolaou smears in the detection of endometrial cancer. N Engl J Med 291:191–192.

Bush T, Helzlsouer K. 1993. Tamoxifen for the primary prevention of breast cancer: a review and critique of the concept and trial. Epidemiol Rev 15:233–243.

Canadian Task Force on the Periodic Health Examination. 1987. The periodic health examination. 1. Introduction. 2. 1987 update. Can Med Assoc J 138:617–618; 618–626.

Carlstrom K, Damber M-G, Furuhjelm M, Joelsson I, Lunell N-O, von Schoultz B. 1979. Serum levels of total dehydroepiandrosterone and total estrone in postmenopausal women with special regard to carcinoma of the uterine corpus. Acta Obstet Gynecol Scand 58:179–181.

Castleman B, McNeely BU, eds. 1966. Case records of the Massachusetts General Hospital. N Engl J Med 274:1139–1145.

Cederlof R, et al. 1975. The relationship of smoking and social covariables to mortality and cancer morbidity: a ten-year follow-up in a probability sample of 55,000 Swedish subjects aged 18 to 69. Stockholm: Karolinska Institute.

Centers for Disease Control. 1987. Combination oral contraceptive use and the risk of endometrial cancer. JAMA 257:796–800.

Chu J, Schweid AI, Weiss WS. 1982. Survival among women with endometrial cancer: a comparison of estrogen users and nonusers. Am J Obstet Gynecol 143:569–573.

Cohen CJ, Deppe G. 1977. Endometrial carcinoma and oral contraceptive agents. Obstet Gynecol 49:390–392.

Collins J, Allen LH, Donner A, Adams O. 1980. Oestrogen use and survival in endometrial cancer. Lancet 1:901–963.

Cramer DW, Cutler SJ, Christine B. 1974. Trends in the incidence of endometrial cancer in the United States. Gynecol Oncol 2:130–143.

Cutler BS, Forbes AB, Ingersoll FM. 1972. Endometrial cancer after stilbesterol therapy in gonadal dysgenesis. N Engl J Med 287:628–631.

Daniell HW. 1976. Osteoporosis of the slender smoker: vertebral compression factors and loss of metacarpal cortex in relation to postmenopausal cigarette smoking and lack of obesity. Arch Intern Med 136:298–304.

DeVere RD, Dempster DR. 1953. A case of the Stein-Leventhal syndrome associated with carcinoma of the endometrium. J Obstet Gynaecol Br Emp 60:865–867.

Devesa SS, Silverman DT. 1978. Cancer incidence and mortality trends in the United States: 1935–74. J Natl Cancer Inst 60:545–571.

Diddle AW. 1952. Granulosa and theca cell ovarian tumors: Prognosis. Cancer 5:215–228.

Dunn JE. 1974. Geographic considerations of endometrial cancer. Gynecol Oncol 2:114–121.

Early Breast Cancer Trialists' Collaborative Group. 1988. Effects of adjuvant tamoxifen and of cytotoxic therapy on mortality in early breast cancer. N Engl J Med 319:1681–1692.

Eddy D. 1980. ACS report on the cancer-related health checkup. CA 30:193–240.

Elliott EA, Matanoski GM, Rosenshein NB, Grumbine FC, Diamond EL. 1990. Body fat patterning in women with endometrial cancer. Gyencol Oncol 39:253–258.

Elwood JM, Cole P, Rothman KJ, Kaplan SD. 1977. Epidemiology of endometrial cancer. J Natl Cancer Inst 59:1055–1060.

Ernster VL, Sacks ST, Selvin S, Petrakis NL. 1979. Cancer incidence by marital status: U.S. Third National Cancer Survey. J Natl Cancer Inst 63:567–585.

Ernster VL, Bush TL, Huggins GR, Hulka BS, Kelsey JL, Schottenfeld D. 1988. Benefits and risks of postmenopausal estrogen and/or progestin hormone use. Prev Med 17:201–223.

Ernster VL, Cummings S. 1986. Progesterone and breast cancer. Obstet Gynecol 68:715–717.

Ettinger B, Golditch IM, Friedman G. 1988. Gynecologic consequences of long-term, unopposed estrogen replacement therapy. Maturitas 10:271–282.

Ewertz M, Schou G, Boice JD Jr. 1988. The joint effect of risk factors on endometrial cancer. Eur J Cancer 24:189–194.

Ferenczy A. 1978. How progestogens affect endometrial hyperplasia and neoplasia. Contemp Obstet Gynecol 11:137–143.

Fisher B, Costantino J, Redmond C, et al. 1989. A randomized clinical trial evaluating tamoxifen in the treatment of patients with node-negative breast cancer who have estrogen-receptor-positive tumors. N Engl J Med 320:479–484.

Fisher B, Costantino J, Redmond C, Fisher E, Wickerham L, Cronin W. 1994. Endometrial cancer in tamoxifen-treated breast cancer patients: findings from the National Surgical Adjuvant

Breast and Bowel Project (NSABP) B-14. J Natl Cancer Inst 86:527–537.

FORNANDER T, RUTQVIST L, CEDERMARK B, et al. 1989. Adjuvant tamoxifen in early breast cancer: occurrence of new primary cancers. Lancet 1:117–120.

FRANKS AL, KENDRICK JS, TYLER CW JR, THE CANCER AND STEROID HORMONE STUDY GROUP. 1987. Postmenopausal smoking, estrogen replacement therapy, and the risk of endometrial cancer. Am J Obstet Gynecol 156:20–23.

FRIEDMAN AJ, RAVNIKAR VA, BARBIERI RL. 1987. Serum steroid hormone profiles in postmenopausal smokers and nonsmokers. Fertil Steril 47:398–401.

GAL D, KOPEL S, BASHEVKIN M, LEBOWITZ J, LEV R, TANCER L. 1991. Oncogenic potential of tamoxifen on endometria of postmenopausal women with breast cancer: preliminary report. Gynecol Oncol 42:120–123.

GALLUP DG, STOCK RJ. 1984. Adenocarcinoma of the endometrium in women 40 years of age or younger. Obstet Gynecol 64:417–420.

GAMBRELL RD JR. 1986. Prevention of endometrial cancer with progestogens. Maturitas 8:159–168.

GAMBRELL RD JR, MASSEY FM, CASTANEDA TN, UGENAS AJ, RICCA CA, WRIGHT JM. 1980. Use of the progesterone challenge test to reduce the risk of endometrial cancer. Obstet Gynecol 55:732–738.

GAMBRELL RD JR, CASTANEDA TA, RICCI CA. 1978. Management of postmenopausal bleeding to prevent endometrial cancer. Maturitas 1:99–106.

GAPSTUR SM, POTTER JD, SELLERS TA, KUSHI LH, FOLSOM AR. 1993. Alcohol consumption and postmenopausal endometrial cancer: results from the Iowa Women's Health Study. Cancer Causes Control 4:323–329.

GARFINKEL L. 1980. Cancer mortality in nonsmokers: prospective study by the American Cancer Society. J Natl Cancer Inst 65:1169–1173.

GELFAND MM, FERENCZY A. 1989. A prospective 1-year study of estrogen and progestin in postmenopausal women: effects on the endometrium. Obstet Gynecol 398–402.

GORDON J, REAGAN JW, FINKLE WD, ZIEL HK. 1977. Estrogen and endometrial carcinoma: an independent pathology review supporting original risk estimate. N Engl J Med 297:570–571.

GOURTADIS M, ROBINSON S, SATYASWAROOP P, JORDAN V. 1988. Contrasting actions of tamoxifen on endometrial and breast tumor growth in the athymic mouse. Cancer Res 48:812–815.

GRADY D, RUBIN SM, PETITTI DB, FOX CS, BLOCK D, ETTINGER B, ERNSTER VL, CUMMINGS SR. 1992. Hormone therapy to prevent disease and prolong life in postmenopausal women. Ann Intern Med 117:1016–1037.

GRADY D, GEBRETSADIK T, KERLIKOWSKE K, ERNSTER V, PETITTI D. 1995. Hormone replacement therapy and endometrial cancer risk: a meta-analysis. Obstet Gynecol 85:304–313.

GRADY D, ERNSTER VL. 1991. Does postmenopausal hormone therapy cause breast cancer? Am J Epidemiol 134:1396–1400.

GRAY LA SR, CHRISTOPHERSON WM, HOOVER RN. 1977. Estrogens and endometrial carcinoma. Obstet Gynecol 49:385–389.

GUSBERG SB. 1947. Precursors of corpus carcinoma and adenomatous hyperplasia. Am J Obstet Gynecol 54:905–927.

GUSBERG SB, HALL RE. 1961. Precursors of corpus cancer. III. The appearance of cancer of the endometrium in estrogenically conditioned patients. Obstet Gynecol 17:397–412.

GUSBERG SB, KAPLAN AI. 1963. Precursors of corpus cancer. IV. Adenomatous hyperplasia as stage D of carcinoma of the endometrium. Am J Obstet Gynecol 87:662–676.

GUSBERG S. 1976. The individual at high risk for endometrial carcinoma. Am J Obstet Gynecol 126:535–539.

HAMMOND CB, JELOVSEK FR, LEE KL, CREASMAN WT, PARKER RT. 1979. Effects of long-term estrogen replacement therapy. II. Neoplasia. Am J Obstet Gynecol 133:537–547.

HARLOW BL, WEISS NS, LOFTON S. 1986. The epidemiology of sarcomas of the uterus. J Natl Cancer Inst 76:399–402.

HEMMINKI E, KENNEDY DL, BAUM C, MCKINLAY SM. 1988. Prescribing of noncontraceptive estrogens and progestins in the United States, 1974–86. Am J Public Health 78:1479–1481.

HENDERSON BE, CASAGRANDE JT, PIKE MC, MACK T, ROSARIO I, DUKE A. 1983. The epidemiology of endometrial cancer in young women. Br J Cancer 47:749–756.

HIRVONEN E, MALKONEN M, MANNINEN V. 1981. Effects of different progestogens on lipoproteins during postmenopausal replacement therapy. N Engl J Med 304:560–563.

HOOGERLAND DL, BUCHLER DA, CROWLEY JJ, CARR WF. 1978. Estrogen use—risk of endometrial carcinoma. Gynecol Oncol 6:451–458.

HOOVER R, FRAUMENI JF, EVERSON R. 1976. Cancer of the uterine corpus after hormonal treatment for breast cancer. Lancet 1:885.

HORM JW, ASIRE AJ, YOUNG JL JR, POLLACK ES. 1984. SEER Program: Cancer Incidence and Mortality in the United States 1973–81. Bethesda, MD: US DHHS (PHS).

HORWITZ RI, FEINSTEIN AR. 1978. Alternative analytic methods for case-control studies of estrogens and endometrial cancer. N Engl J Med 299:1089–1094.

HORWITZ RI, FEINSTEIN AR. 1986. Estrogens and endometrial cancer. Response to arguments and current status of an epidemiologic controversy. Am J Med 81:503–507.

HOWE GR, SHERMAN GJ, MALHOTRA A. 1984. Correlations between cancer incidence rates from the Canadian National Cancer Incidence Reporting System, 1969–78. J Natl Cancer Inst 72:585–591.

HOWE HL. 1984. Age-specific hysterectomy and oophorectomy prevalence rates and the risks for cancer of the reproductive system. Am J Public Health 74:560–563.

HSUEH AJW, PECK EJ, CLARK JH. 1975. Progesterone antagonism of the estrogen receptor and estrogen-induced uterine growth. Nature 254:337–340.

HULKA BS, FOWLER WC JR, KAUFMAN DG, GRIMSON RC, GREENBERG BG, HOGUE CJR, BERGER GS, PULLIAM CC. 1980a. Estrogen and endometrial cancer: cases and two control groups from North Carolina. Am J Obstet Gynecol 137:92–101.

HULKA BS, KAUFMAN DG, FOWLER WC JR, GRIMSON RC, GREENBERG BG. 1980b. Predominance of early endometrial cancers after long-term estrogen use. JAMA 244:2419–2422.

HULKA BS, CHAMBLESS LE, KAUFMAN DG, FOWLER WC JR, GREENBERG BG. 1982. Protection against endometrial carcinoma by combination-product oral contraceptives. JAMA 247:475–477.

HUNT K, VESSEY M, MCPHERSON K, COLEMAN M. 1987. Long-term surveillance of mortality and cancer incidence in women receiving hormone replacement therapy. Br J Obstet Gynaecol 94:620–635.

JACKSON RL, DOCKERTY MB. 1957. The Stein-Leventhal syndrome: analysis of 43 cases with special reference to association with endometrial carcinoma. Am J Obstet Gynecol 73:161–173.

JELOVSEK FR, HAMMOND CB, WOODARD BH, DRAFFIN R, LEE KL, CREASMAN WT, PARKER RT. 1980. Risk of exogenous estrogen therapy and endometrial cancer. Am J Obstet Gynecol 137:85–91.

JENSEN J, CHRISTIANSEN C, RODBRO P. 1985. Cigarette smoking, serum estrogens, and bone loss during hormone replacement therapy early after menopause. N Engl J Med 313:973–975.

JENSEN J, NILAS L, CHRISTIANSEN C. 1986. Cyclic changes in serum cholesterol and lipoprotein following different doses of combined postmenopausal hormone replacement therapy. Br J Obstet Gynecol 93:613–618.

JICK H, WALKER AM, ROTHMAN KJ. 1980. The epidemic of endometrial cancer: a commentary. Am J Public Health 70:264–267.

JICK H, WATKINS RN, HUNTER JR, et al. 1979. Replacement estrogens and endometrial cancer. N Engl J Med 300:218–222.

JICK S, WALKER A, JICK H. 1993a. Estrogens, progesterone, and endometrial cancer. Epidemiology 4:20–24.

JICK SS, WALKER AM, JICK H. 1993b. Oral contraceptives and endometrial cancer. Obstet Gynecol 82:931–935.

KASS LG, SCHREIBER K, OBERLANDER SG, MOUSSOURIS HF, LESSER M. 1984. Detection of endometrial carcinoma and hyperplasia in asymptomatic women. Obstet Gynecol 64:1–11.

KAUFMAN DW, SHAPIRO S, SLONE D, ROSENBERG L, MIETTINEN O, STOLLEY PD, KNAPP RC, LEAVITT T JR, WATRING WG, ROSENSHEIN NB, LEWIS JC JR, SCHOTTENFELD D, ENGLE RL JR. 1980a. Decreased risk of endometrial cancer among oral contraceptive users. N Engl J Med 303:1045–1048.

KAUFMAN DW, SLONE D, ROSENBERG L, MIETTINEN OS, SHAPIRO S. 1980b. Cigarette smoking and age at natural menopause. Am J Public Health 70:420–422.

KELSEY JL, HILDRETH NG. 1983. Cancer of the corpus uteri. In: *Breast and Gynecologic Cancer Epidemiology,* Chapter 3. Boca Raton, FL: CRC Press.

KELSEY JL, LIVOLSI VA, HOLFORD TR, FISCHER DB, MOSTOW ED, SCHWARTZ PE, O'CONNOR T, WHITE C. 1982. A case-control study of cancer of the endometrium. Am J Epidemiol 116:333–342.

KENNEDY DL, BAUM C, FORBES MB. 1985. Noncontraceptive estrogens and progestins: use patterns over time. Obstet Gynecol 65:441–446.

KHAW K-T, TAZUKE S, BARRETT-CONNOR E. 1988. Cigarette smoking and levels of adrenal androgens in postmenopausal women. N Engl J Med 318:1705–1709.

KILLACKEY M, HAKES T, et al. 1985. Endometrial adenocarcinoma in breast cancer patients receiving antiestrogens. Cancer Treat Rep 69:237–238.

KING RJB, WHITEHEAD MI, CAMPBELL S. 1979. Effect of estrogen and progestin treatments on endometria from postmenopausal women. Cancer Res 39:1094–1098.

KISTNER RW. 1973. Endometrial alterations associated with estrogens and estrogen-progestin combinations. In: *The Uterus.* Morris HJ, Hertig AT, Abell MR (eds). Baltimore: Williams and Wilkins.

KJELLGREN O. 1977. Epidemiology and pathophysiology of corpus carcinoma. Acta Obstet Gynecol Scand 65 (Suppl):77–82.

KOEPSELL TD, WEISS NS, THOMPSON DJ, MARTIN DP. 1980. Prevalence of prior hysterectomy in the Seattle-Tacoma area. Am J Public Health 70:40–47.

KOLONEL LN, HANKIN JH, LEE J, CHU SY, NOMURA AM, HINDS MW. 1981. Nutrient intakes in relation to cancer incidence in Hawaii. Br J Cancer 44:332–339.

KOUMANTAKI Y, TZONOU A, LOUMANTAKIS E, KAKLAMANI E, ARAVANTINOS D, TRICHOPOULOS D. 1989. A case-control study of cancer of endometrium in Athens. Int J Cancer 43:795–799.

KRALE G, HEUCH I, URSIN G. 1988. Reproductive factors and risk of cancer of the uterine corpus: a prospective study. Cancer Res 48:6217–6221.

KVALE S, HEUCH I, NILSSEN S. 1991. Reproductive factors and cancers of the breast and genital organs—are the different cancer sites similarly affected? Cancer Detect Prev 15:369–377.

LAFFERTY F, HELMUTH D. 1985. Postmenopausal estrogen replacement: the prevention of osteoporosis and systemic effects. Maturitas 7:147–159.

LARSON JA. 1954. Estrogens and endometrial cancer. Obstet Gynecol 3:551–572.

LA VECCHIA C, FRANCESCHI S, DECARLI A, GALLUS G, TOGNONI G. 1984. Risk factors for endometrial cancer at different ages. J Natl Cancer Inst 73:667–671.

LA VECCHIA C, DECARLI A, FASOLI M, FRANCESCHI S, GENTILE A, NEGRI E, PARAZZINI F, TOGNONI G. 1986a. Oral contraceptives and cancers of the breast and of the female genital tract: interim results from a case-control study. Br J Cancer 54:311–317.

LA VECCHIA C, DECARLI A, FASOLI M, GENTILE A. 1986b. Nutrition and diet in the etiology of endometrial cancer. Cancer 57:1248–1253.

LAWRENCE C, TESSARO I, DURGERIAN S, CAPUTO T, RICHART R, JACOBSON H, GREENWALD P. 1987. Smoking, body weight, and early-stage endometrial cancer. Cancer 59:1665–1669.

LE MARCHAND L, WILKENS LR, MI M-P. 1991. Early-age body size, adult weight gain and endometrial cancer risk. Int J Cancer 48:807–811.

LESKO SM, ROSENBERG L, KAUFMAN DW, STOLLEY P, WARSHAUER ME, LEWIS JL JR, SHAPIRO S. 1991. Endometrial cancer and age at last delivery: evidence for an association. Am J Epidemiol 133:554–559.

LESKO SM, ROSENBERG L, KAUFMAN DW, HELMRICH SP, MILLER DR, STROM B, SCHOTTENFELD D, ROSENSHEIN NB, KNAPP RC, LEWIS J, SHAPIRO S. 1985. Cigarette smoking and the risk of endometrial cancer. N Engl J Med 313:593–596.

LESKO SM, ROSENBERG L, KAUFMAN DW, SHAPIRO S. 1986. Cigarette smoking and endometrial cancer (Letter). N Engl J Med 315:646.

LEVI F, LA VECCHIA C, DECARLI A. 1987. Cigarette smoking and the risk of endometrial cancer. Eur J Cancer Clin Oncol 23:1025–1029.

LEVI F, LA VECCHIA C, GULIE C, FRANCHESCHI S, NEGRI E. 1993. Oestrogen replacement treatment and the risk of endometrial cancer: an assessment of the role of covariates. Eur J Cancer 29:1445–1449.

LEW EA, GARFINKEL L. 1979. Variations in mortality by weight among 750,000 men and women. J Chron Dis 32:563–576.

LOGAN WPD. 1953. Marriage and childbearing in relation to cancer of the breast and uterus. Lancet 2:1199–1202.

LYNCH HT, KRUSH AJ, LARSEN AL, MAGNUSON CW. 1966. Endometrial carcinoma: multiple primary malignancies, constitutional factors, and heredity. Am J Med Sci 252:381–390.

LYON FA. 1975. The development of adenocarcinoma of the endometrium in young women receiving long-term sequential contraception. Am J Obstet Gynecol 123:299–301.

LYON JL, GARDNER JW. 1977. The rising frequency of hysterectomy: its effect on uterine cancer rates. Am J Epidemiol 105:439–443.

MACDONALD PC, EDMAN CD, HANSELL DL, PORTER SC, SIITERI PK. 1978. Effect of obesity on conversion of plasma androstenedione to estrone in postmenopausal women with and without endometrial cancer. Am J Obstet Gynecol 130:448–455.

MACDONALD PC, ROMBAUT BP, SIITERI PK. 1967. Plasma precursors of estrogen. I. Extent of conversion of plasma androstenedione to estrone in normal males and nonpregnant, normal castrate and adrenalectomized females. J Clin Endocrinol Metab 27:1103–1110.

MACDONALD PC, SIITERI PK. 1974. Relationship between extraglandular production of estrone and the occurrence of endometrial neoplasia. Gynecol Oncol 2:2159–2163.

MACK TM, PIKE MC, HENDERSON BE, PFEFFER RI, GERKINS VR, ARTHUR M, BROWN SE. 1976. Estrogens and endometrial cancer in a retirement community. N Engl J Med 294:1262–1267.

MACMAHON B. 1974. Risk factors for endometrial cancer. Gynecol Oncol 2:122–129.

MACMAHON B, TRICHOPOULOUS D, COLE P, BROWN J. 1982. Cigarette smoking and urinary estrogens. N Engl J Med 307:1062–1065.

MAGRIPLES U, NAFTOLIN F, SCHWARTZ P, et al. 1993. High-grade endometrial carcinoma in tamoxifen-treated breast cancer patients. J Clin Oncol 11:485–490.

MALFETANO J. 1990. Tamoxifen-associated endometrial carcinoma in postmenopausal breast cancer patients. Gynecol Oncol 39:82–84.

MANSELL H, HERTIG AT. 1955. Granulosa–theca cell tumors and

endometrial carcinoma: a study of their relationship and a survey of 80 cases. Obstet Gynecol 6:385–394.

MARRETT LD. 1980. Estimates of the true population at risk of uterine disease and an application to incidence data for cancer of the uterine corpus in Connecticut. Am J Epidemiol 111:373–378.

MARRETT LD, MEIGS JW, FLANNERY JT. 1982. Trends in the incidence of cancer of the corpus uteri in Connecticut, 1964–1979, in relation to consumption of exogenous estrogens. Am J Epidemiol 116:57–67.

MCBRIDE JM. 1959. Premenopausal cystic hyperplasia and endometrial carcinoma. J Obstet Gynecol Br Commonw 54:521–525.

MCDONALD TW, ANNEGERS JF, O'FALLON WM, DOCKERTY MB, MALKASIAN GD JR, KURLAND LT. 1977. Exogenous estrogen and endometrial carcinoma: case-control and incidence study. Am J Obstet Gynecol 127:572–579.

MILLER BA, GLOECKLER LA, HANKEY BF, KOSARY CL, HARRAS A, DEVESA SS, EDWARDS BK. 1993. SEER Cancer Statistics Review 1973–1990. National Cancer Institute. NIH Publication No. 93-2789.

NACHTIGALL LE, NACHTIGALL RH, NACHTIGALL RB, BECKMAN EM. 1976. Estrogens and endometrial carcinoma (Letter). N Engl J Med 294:848.

NACHTIGALL LE, NACHTIGALL RH, NACHTIGALL RD, BECKMAN EM. 1979. Estrogen replacement therapy. II. A prospective study in the relationship to carcinoma and cardiovascular and metabolic problems. Obstet Gynecol 54:74–79.

NATIONAL CANCER INSTITUTE. Unpublished data from the Surveillance, Epidemiology, and End Results (SEER) program, provided by E. Sondik and B. Hankey of NCI's Division of Cancer Prevention and Control.

NELSON CL, SELLERS TA, RICH SS, POTTER JD, MCGOVERN PG, KUSHI LH. 1993. Familial clustering of colon, breast, uterine, and ovarian cancers as assessed by family history. Genet Epidemiol 10:235–244.

NEVEN P, DE MUYLDER X, VAN BELLE Y, BANDERICK G, DE MUYLDER E. 1985. Tamoxifen and the uterus and endometrium (Letter). Lancet 1:375.

NISKER JA, HAMMOND GL, DAVIDSON BJ, FRUMAR AM, TAKAKI NK, JUDD HL, SIITERI PK. 1980. Serum sex hormone-binding globulin capacity and the percentage of free estradiol in postmenopausal women with and without endometrial cancer. Am J Obstet Gynecol 138:637–642.

NOVAK ER, WOODRUFF JD. 1979. Novak's Gynecologic and Obstetric Pathology, 8th ed. Philadelphia: WB Saunders, p 260.

OTTOSSON UB, JOHANSSON BG, VON SCHOULTZ B. 1985. Subfractions of high-density lipoprotein cholesterol during estrogen replacement therapy: a comparison between progestogins and natural progesterone. Am J Obstet Gynecol 151:746–750.

PAGANINI-HILL A, ROSS RK, HENDERSON BE. 1989. Endometrial cancer and patterns of use of oestrogen replacement therapy: a cohort study. Br J Cancer 59:445–447.

PARAZZINI F, LA VECCHIA C, BOCCIOLONE L, FRANCESCHI S. 1991. The epidemiology of endometrial cancer. Gynecol Oncol 41:1–16.

PARAZZINI F, LA VECCHIA C, NEGRI E, FEDELE L, BALOTTA F. 1991. Reproductive factors and risk of endometrial cancer. Am J Obstet Gynecol 164:522–527.

PARKIN DM, MUIR CS, WHELAN SL, GAO YT, FERLAY J, POWELL J. 1992. Cancer Incidence in Five Continents, Vol. VI. Lyon: International Agency for Research on Cancer.

PATERSON ME, WADE-EVANS T, STURDEE WD, THOM MH, STUDD JW. 1980. Endometrial disease after treatment with oestrogens and progestogens in the climacteric. Br Med J 280:822–824.

PERCY CL, HORM JW, YOUNG JL JR, ASIRE AJ. 1983. Uterine cancers of unspecified origin—a reassessment. Public Health Rep 98:176–180.

PERCY CL, MILLER BA, GLOECKLER RIES LA. 1990. Effect of changes in cancer classification and the accuracy of cancer death certificates on trends in cancer mortality. Ann NY Acad Sci 609:87–97.

PERSKY V, DAVIS F, BARRETT R, RUBY E, SAILER C, LEVY P. 1990. Recent time trends in uterine cancer. Am J Public Health 80:935–939.

PERSSON I, ADAMI H-O, BERGKVIST L, LINDGREN A, PETTERSSON B, HOOVER R, SCHAIRER C. 1989. Risk of endometrial cancer after treatment with oestrogens alone or in conjunction with progestogens: results of a prospective study. Br Med J 298:147–151.

PERSSON IR, ADAMI H-O, EKLUND G, JOHANSSON EDB, LINDBERG BS, LINDGREN A. 1986. The risk of endometrial neoplasia and treatment with estrogens and estrogen-progestogen combinations. Acta Obstet Gynecol Scand 65:211–217.

PETITTI DB, PERLMAN JA, SIDNEY S. 1987. Noncontraceptive Estrogens and Mortality: Long-term follow-up of Women in the Walnut Creek Study. Obstet Gynecol 70:289–93.

PETTERSSON B, BERGSTROM R, JOHANSSON EDB. 1986. Serum estrogens and androgens in women with endometrial carcinoma. Gynecol Oncol 25:223–233.

PHOTOPULOS GJ. 1994. Surgicopathologic staging of endometrial adenocarcinoma. Curr Opin Obstet Gynecol 6:92–97.

POKRAS R. 1984. Hysterectomies in the United States, 1965–1984. Vital Health Stat [13] No. 92.

POLLACK ES, HORM JW. 1980. Trends in cancer incidence and mortality in the United States, 1969–76. J Natl Cancer Inst 64:1091–1103.

POTISCHMAN N, SWANSON CA, BRINTON LA, MCADAMS M, BARRETT RJ, BERMAN ML, MORTEL R, TWIGGS LB, WILBANKS GD, HOOVER RN. 1993. Dietary associations in a case-control study of endometrial cancer. Cancer Causes Control 4:239–250.

PRITCHARD KI. 1989. Screening for endometrial cancer: is it effective? Ann Intern Med 110:177–179.

REIFENSTEIN EC. 1974. The treatment of advanced endometrial cancer with hydroxyprogesterone caproate. Gynecol Oncol 2:377–414.

RIBEIRO G, SWINDELL R. 1992. The Christie Hospital adjuvant tamoxifen trial. NCI Monogr 11:121–125.

RIES LAG, HANKEY BF, MILLER BA, HARTMAN AM, EDWARDS BK. 1991. Cancer Statistics Review 1973–1988. National Cancer Institute. NIH Pub. No. 91-2789.

RIES LA, MILLER BA, HANKEY BF, KOSARY CL, HARRAS A, EDWARDS BK. 1994. SEER Cancer Statistics Review, 1973–1991. National Cancer Institute. NIH Pub. No. 94-2789.

ROBBOY SJ, BRADLEY R. 1979. Changing trends and prognostic features in endometrial cancer associated with exogenous estrogen therapy. Obstet Gynecol 54:269–277.

RUBIN G, PETERSON H, LEE N, MAES E, WINGO P, BECKER S. 1990. Estrogen replacement therapy and the risk of endometrial cancer: remaining controversies. Am J Obstet Gynecol 162:148–154.

SALERNO IJ. 1962. Feminizing mesenchymomas of the ovary: an analysis of 28 granulosa–theca cell tumors and their relationship to coexistent carcinoma. Am J Obstet Gynecol 84:731–738.

SALMI T. 1980. Endometrial carcinoma risk factors, with special reference to the use of oestrogens. Acta Endocrinol Suppl (Copenh) 233:37–43.

SATYASWAROOP P, ZAINO R, MORTEL R. 1984. Estrogen-like effects of tamoxifen on human endometrial carcinoma transplanted into nude mice. Cancer Res 44:4006–4010.

SCHAPIRA DV, KUMAR NB, LYMAN GH, CAVANAGH D, ROBERTS WS, LA POLLA J. 1991. Upper-body fat distribution and endometrial cancer risk. JAMA 266:1808–1811.

SCHENKER JG, WEINSTEIN D, OKON E. 1979. Estradiol and testosterone levels in the peripheral and ovarian circulations in patients with endometrial cancer. Cancer 44:1809–1812.

SCHLESSELMAN JJ. 1991. Oral contraceptives and neoplasia of the uterine corpus. Contraception 43:557–559.

SCHOENBERG BS, GREENBERG RA, EISENBERG H. 1969. Occurrence of certain multiple primary cancers in females. J Natl Cancer Inst 43:15–32.

SCHOTTENFELD D, BERG J. 1971. Incidence of multiple primary cancers. IV. Cancers of the female breast and genital organs. J Natl Cancer Inst 46:161–170.

SCHWARTZ SM, THOMAS DB. 1989. A case-control study of risk factors for sarcomas of the uterus: The World Health Organization Collaborative Study of Neoplasia and Steroid Contraceptives. Cancer 64:2487–2492.

SCHWARTZ SM, WEISS NS. 1990. Marital status and the incidence of sarcomas of the uterus. Cancer Res 50:1886–1889.

SEOUD M-F, JOHNSON J, WEED J JR. 1993. Gynecologic tumors in tamoxifen-treated women with breast cancer. Obstet Gynecol 82:165–169.

SHANKLIN DR. 1976. Estrogens and endometrial carcinoma (Letter). N Engl J Med 294:847.

SHAPIRO S, KAUFMAN DW, SLONE D, ROSENBERG L, MIETTINEN OS, STOLLEY PD, ROSENSHEIN NB, WATRING WG, LEAVITT T JR, KNAPP RC. 1980. Recent and past use of conjugated estrogens in relation to adenocarcinoma of the endometrium. N Engl J Med 303:485–489.

SHAPIRO S, KELLY JP, ROSENBERG L, KAUFMAN DW, HELMRICH SP, ROSENSHEIN NB, LEWIS JL JR, KNAPP RC, STOLLEY PD, SCHOTTENFELD D. 1985. Risk of localized and widespread endometrial cancer in relation to recent and discontinued use of conjugated estrogens. N Engl J Med 313:969–972.

SHERMAN AI, BROWN S. 1979. The precursors of endometrial carcinoma. Am J Obstet Gynecol 135:947–954.

SHU XO, HATCH MC, ZHENG W, GAO YT, BRINTON LA. 1993. Physical activity and risk of endometrial cancer. Epidemiology 4:342–349.

SILVERBERG E, LUBERA JA. 1989. Cancer statistics, 1989. CA 39:3–20.

SILVERBERG SG, MAKOWSKI EL. 1975. Endometrial carcinoma in young women taking oral contraceptive agents. Obstet Gynecol 46:503–506.

SILVERBERG SG, MAKOWSKI EL, ROCHE WD. 1977. Endometrial cancer in women under 40 years of age: comparison of cases in oral contraceptive users and nonusers. Cancer 39:592–598.

SMITH DC, PRENTICE R, THOMPSON DJ, HERRMANN WL. 1975. Association of exogenous estrogen and endometrial carcinoma. N Engl J Med 293:1164–1167.

SMITH EM, SOWERS MF, BURNS TL. 1984. Effects of smoking on the development of female reproductive cancers. J Natl Cancer Inst 73:371–376.

SOMMERS SC, HERTIG AT, BENGLOFF H. 1949. Genesis of endometrial carcinoma. II. Cases 19 to 35 years old. Cancer 2:957–963.

SPEERT H. 1949. Carcinoma of the endometrium in young women. Surg Gynecol Obstet 88:332–336.

SPENGLER RF, CLARKE EA, WOOLEVER CA, NEWMAN AM, OSBORN RW. 1981. Exogenous estrogens and endometrial cancer: a case-control study and assessment of potential biases. Am J Epidemiol 114:497–506.

STAMPFER M, COLDITZ G, WILLETT W, ROSNER B, HENNEKENS C, SPEIZER F. 1986. A prospective study of exogenous hormones and risk of endometrial cancer (Abstract). Am J Epidemiol 124:520.

STAMPFER MJ, COLDITZ GA. 1991. Estrogen replacement therapy and coronary heart disease: a quantitative assessment of the epidemiologic evidence. Prev Med 20:47–63.

STAVRAKY KM, COLLINS JA, DONNER A, WELLS GA. 1981. A comparison of estrogen use by women with endometrial cancer, gynecologic disorders, and other illnesses. Am J Obstet Gynecol 141:547–555.

STEIN IF, LEVENTHAL ML. 1935. Amenorrhea associated with bilateral polycystic ovaries. Am J Obstet Gynecol 29:181–191.

STEINHORN SC, MYERS MH, HANKEY BF, PELHAM VF. 1986. Factors associated with survival differences between black women and white women with cancer of the uterine corpus. Am J Epidemiol 124:85–93.

STEWART H. 1992. The Scottish trial of adjuvant tamoxifen in node-negative breast cancer: Scottish Cancer Trials Breast Group. NCI Monogr 11:117–120.

STOCKWELL HG, LYMAN GH. 1987. Cigarette smoking and the risk of female reproductive cancer. Am J Obstet Gynecol 157:35–40.

SWANSON CA, POTISCHMAN N, WILBANKS GD, TWIGGS LB, MORTEL R, BERMAN ML, BARRETT RJ, BAUMGARTNER RN, BRINTON LA. 1993. Relation of endometrial cancer risk to past and contemporary body size and body fat distribution. Cancer Epidemiol Biomark Prev 2:321–327.

THOM MH, WHITE RJ, WILLIAMS RM, PATERSON MEL, WADE-EVANS T, STUDD JWW. 1979. Prevention and treatment of endometrial disease in climacteric women receiving estrogen therapy. Lancet 2:455–457.

TÖRNBERG SA, CARSTENSEN JM. 1994. Relationship between Quetelet's index and cancer of breast and female genital tract in 47,000 women followed for 25 years. Br J Cancer 69:358–361.

TSENG L, GURPIDE E. 1975. Induction of human endometrial estradiol dehydrogenase by progestins. Endocrinology 97:825–833.

TULINIUS H, EGILSSON V, OLAFSDOTTIR GH, SIGVALDASON H. 1992. Risk of prostate, ovarian, and endometrial cancer among relatives of women with breast cancer. Br Med J 305:855–857.

TYLER CW JR, WEBSTER LA, ORY HW, RUBIN GL. 1985. Endometrial cancer: how does cigarette smoking influence the risk of women under age 55 years having this tumor? Am J Obstet Gynecol 151:899–905.

U.S. PREVENTIVE SERVICES TASK FORCE. 1989. Guide to Clinical Preventive Services: An Assessment of the Effectiveness of 169 Interventions. Baltimore: Williams & Wilkins.

VAKIL D, MORGAN R, HALIDAY M. 1983. Exogenous estrogens and development of breast and endometrial cancer. Cancer Detect Prev 6:415–424.

VAN LEEUWEN F, BENRAADT J, COEBERGH J, et al. 1994. Risk of endometrial cancer after tamoxifen treatment of breast cancer. Lancet 343:448–452.

VARMA TR. 1985. Effect of long-term therapy with estrogen and progesterone on the endometrium of postmenopausal women. Acta Obstet Gynecol Scand 64:41–46.

VOIGT L, WEISS N, CHU J, DALING J, MCKNIGHT B, VAN BELLE G. 1991. Progestagen supplementation of exogenous oestrogens and risk of endometrial cancer. Lancet 338:274–277.

VOIGT LF, DENG Q, WEISS NS. 1994. Recency, duration, and progestin content of oral contraceptives in relation to the incidence of endometrial cancer. Cancer Causes Control 5:227–233.

VON HOLST T, KLINGA K, RUNNEBAUM B. 1981. Hormone levels in healthy post-menopausal women and in women with post-menopausal bleeding with or without endometrial carcinoma. Maturitas 138:637–642.

VUOPALA S. 1977. Diagnostic accuracy and clinical application of cytological and histological methods for investigating endometrial carcinoma. Acta Scand Obstet Gynecol 79 (Suppl):1–72.

WALKER AM, JICK H. 1979. Temporal and regional variation in hysterectomy rates in the United States, 1970–1975. Am J Epidemiol 110:41–46.

WALKER AM, JICK H. 1980. Declining rates of endometrial cancer. Obstet Gynecol 56:733–736.

WEISS NS. 1978. Assessing the risks from menopausal estrogen use: what can we learn from trends in mortality from uterine cancer? J Chron Dis 31:705–708.

WEISS NS, SZEKELY DR, AUSTIN DF. 1976. Increasing incidence of endometrial cancer in the United States. N Engl J Med 294:1259–1262.

WEISS NS, SZEKELY DR, ENGLISH DR, SCHWEID AI. 1979. Endometrial cancer in relation to patterns of menopausal estrogen use. JAMA 242:261–264.

WEISS NS, FAREWELL VT, SZEKELY DR, ENGLISH DR, KIVIAT N. 1980a. Oestrogens and endometrial cancer: effects of other risk factors in the association. Maturitas 2:185–190.

WEISS NS, SAYVETZ TA. 1980b. Incidence of endometrial cancer in relation to the use of oral contraceptives. N Engl J Med 302:551–554.

WENTZ WB. 1974. Progestin therapy in endometrial hyperplasia. Gynecol Oncol 2:362–367.

WHITEHEAD MI, KING RJB, MCQUEEN J. 1979. Endometrial histology and biochemistry in climacteric women during estrogen and estrogen/progestin therapy. J R Soc Med 73:222–226.

WHITEHEAD MI, FRASER D. 1987. The effects of estrogens and progestogens on the endometrium. Obstet Gynecol Clin North Am 14:299–320.

WIGLE DT, GRACE M, SMITH SO. 1978. Estrogen use and cancer of the uterine corpus in Alberta. Can Med Assoc J 118:1276–1278.

WILLETT W, STAMPFER MJ, BAIN C, LIPNICK R, SPEIZER FE, ROSNER B, CRAMER D, HENNEKENS CH. 1983. Cigarette smoking, relative weight and menopause. Am J Epidemiol 117:651–658.

WILLIAMS AR, WEISS NS, URE CL, BALLARD J, DALING JA. 1982. Effect of weight, smoking, and estrogen use on the risk of hip and forearm fractures in postmenopausal women. Obstet Gynecol 60:695–699.

WINKELSTEIN W, SACKS ST, ERNSTER VL, SELVIN S. 1977. Correlations of incidence rates for selected cancers in the nine areas of the Third National Cancer Survey. Am J Epidemiol 105:407–419.

WOOD GP, BORONOW RC. 1976. Endometrial adenocarcinoma and the polycystic ovarian syndrome. Am J Obstet Gynecol 124:140–142.

WORLD HEALTH ORGANIZATION. 1988. Endometrial cancer and combined oral contraceptives. Int J Epidemiol 17:263–269.

WYNDER EL, ESCHER GC, MANTEL N. 1966. An epidemiological investigation of cancer of the endometrium. Cancer 19:489–520.

WYNDER EL, HYAMS L, SHIGEMATSU T. 1967. Correlations of international cancer death rates. Cancer 20:113–126.

ZIEL HK, FINKLE WD. 1975. Increased risk of endometrial carcinoma among users of conjugated estrogens. N Engl J Med 293:1167–1170.

50 Cervical cancer

MARK H. SCHIFFMAN
LOUISE A. BRINTON
SUSAN S. DEVESA
JOSEPH F. FRAUMENI, JR.

Cervical cancer is an important public health problem worldwide. It is the second most common cancer among women, ranking first in many developing countries (Parkin et al, 1993). In the United States and other countries with broad-coverage, cervical cytologic screening ("Pap smear") programs, there has been a marked decline in cervical cancer incidence and mortality over recent decades (Coleman et al, 1993; Beral et al, 1994). The reduction has apparently been due to detection and treatment of intraepithelial, preinvasive lesions. Nonetheless, rates of invasive cancer have recently started to increase again among young women in several countries, including white women in the United States, despite costly and laborious screening programs. At present in the United States, there are approximately 15,000 cases of invasive cervical cancer per year, and about 4600 deaths (Boring et al, 1994). Carcinoma in situ, the most severe intraepithelial precursor detected through cytologic screening, accounts for another 55,000 cases yearly.

The success of cervical cytologic screening in the past led to decreased epidemiological study of cervical cancer. Recently, however, there has been renewed research interest in cervical cancer, particularly after the discovery of an etiologic role for the human papillomaviruses (HPV). It now appears that the large majority of cases of cervical cancer worldwide can be attributed to HPV infection. However, cervical infection with HPV is extremely common compared to the relatively rare development of cervical cancer. Thus, additional critical etiologic factors must be involved, such as HPV type and intensity of infection, variability in the host immunologic response, co-infection with other viral or bacterial agents, parity, cigarette smoking, oral contraceptive use, and diet. Behavioral characteristics of male sexual partners also may play an etiologic role, adding a further level of complexity to epidemiological investigations.

We thank Ms. Joan Hertel for computer programming and graphics preparation, and Mr. Dan Grauman for the map.

Although there are still major challenges in clarifying the multistage pathogenesis of cervical cancer, epidemiological understanding of this tumor now rivals our understanding of any other malignancy. As a result, it may soon be possible, using a variety of molecular epidemiological approaches, to define new prevention strategies that will be even more effective than cervical cytologic screening alone. For example, HPV DNA testing may prove to be a useful adjunct to Pap smears. In the long term, the most exciting possibility is the primary prevention of cervical neoplasia via HPV immunization of the general population.

BACKGROUND

The Cervical Transformation Zone

The cervix is the cylindrically shaped lower third of the uterus extending into the vagina from the anterior vaginal wall (Fig. 50–1). The cervical epithelium is derived from two embryologically distinct sources. The part of the cervix that projects into the vagina, called the *portio*, is covered by nonkeratinized stratified squamous epithelium similar to the neighboring lining of the vagina. The endocervical canal is covered by tall, mucus-secreting columnar cells of the same embryologic derivation as the uterine endometrium. At birth, the columnar epithelium extends out onto the portio, but with age the squamocolumnar junction recedes into the endocervical canal, as columnar epithelium is replaced by squamous epithelium in a process called *squamous metaplasia*. The metaplastic area adjacent to the receding squamocolumnar junction is called the transformation zone, and it is this area that appears to have a unique sensitivity for neoplastic events (Fenoglio and Ferenczy, 1982). Accordingly, women with an increased area of squamous metaplasia, such as diethylstilbestrol (DES)-exposed daughters, may have an increased incidence of

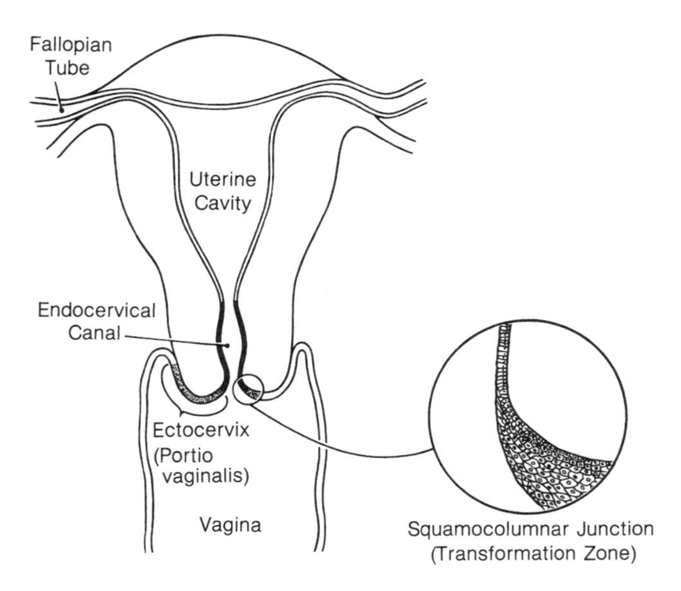

FIG. 50–1. Diagrammatic representation of cervical anatomy.

cervical neoplasia (Robboy et al, 1984). As the great majority of cervical cancers arise in the transformation zone, treatment of this ring of epithelium by cryotherapy, laser surgery or, most recently, loop electrical excision (LEEP) is the mainstay of clinical intervention when preinvasive lesions are found (Ferenczy and Wright, 1993).

Classifying the Intraepithelial Precursors of Cervical Cancer

Squamous carcinomas of the cervix result from the progression of preinvasive precursor lesions called cervical intraepithelial neoplasia (CIN), dysplasia, dyskaryosis (British), or a variety of other names (see Table 50–1 for a comparison of common classification schemes in the United States).

To bring order to the diagnostic confusion, a new cytology classification called the Bethesda System was recently introduced in the United States (Kurman and Solomon, 1994; National Cancer Institute Workshop, 1989). The Bethesda System combines clinically similar intraepithelial diagnoses into broad categories, specifically, low-grade squamous intraepithelial lesions (SIL) and high-grade SIL. The new classification was designed for use in cytologic screening. It remains technically more correct to use the more detailed CIN scale when discussing histopathology (ie, biopsies). Nonetheless, the Bethesda System will be employed primarily for this discussion, because it has proven very useful for epidemiological studies of multistage cervical carcinogenesis.

Low-grade SIL combines CIN 1 (mild dysplasia) with the cytologic diagnosis of HPV infection (Meisels and Fortin, 1976), called koilocytotic (or condylomatous) atypia. The two older categories shared virtually the same epidemiological and HPV DNA profiles and were so overlapping morphologically as to be indivisible. Typically, koilocytotic atypia was about two to three times as common a diagnosis as CIN 1. Of the two diagnoses, CIN 1 was thought to be slightly more severe and more closely linked to "pre-cancer." Accordingly, the new category of low-grade SIL is much larger and, on average, slightly less severe than CIN 1.

The distinction between low-grade SIL and high-grade SIL (Table 50–1) is quite important for epidemiologists studying cervical carcinogenesis. Low-grade SIL is common and represents the usually benign cytopathologic signs of HPV infection. In contrast, high-grade SIL is rare and represents a truly premalignant lesion in the most severe cases (carcinoma in situ). Whereas low-grade SIL can be viewed as an epidemiological "exposure" or risk factor for cervical cancer, high-grade SIL

TABLE 50–1. *Common Classifications of Cervical Squamous Neoplasia*

Dysplasia Scale	*Pap Smear Class*[a]	*CIN*[b] *Scale*	*Bethesda*[c] *System*
Normal	1	Normal	Normal
Inflammatory or reactive atypia	2a	Inflammatory or reactive atypia	Normal or ASCUS[d]
Koilocytotic or condylomatous atypia	2b	Koilocytotic or condylomatous atypia	Low-grade SIL[e]
Mild dysplasia	3	CIN 1	Low-grade SIL
Moderate dysplasia	3	CIN 2	High-grade SIL
Severe dysplasia	3	CIN 3	High-grade SIL
Carcinoma in situ (CIS)	4	CIN 3	High-grade SIL
Invasive squamous carcinoma	5	Invasive squamous carcinoma	Invasive squamous carcinoma

[a]Numeric scale still in widespread use, but not recommended.
[b]CIN = cervical intraepithelial neoplasia.
[c]Recommendations of the 1988 Bethesda System (National Cancer Institute Workshop, 1989).
[d]ASCUS = atypical squamous cells of undetermined significance.
[e]SIL = squamous intraepithelial lesion.

can be viewed as more tightly linked to the cancer "outcome."

This useful conceptual distinction is not perfect, however, because there exists a continuum of changes encompassing low-grade and high-grade SIL, without a clear cut point. At the microscopic level, for example, the characteristic cells of low-grade SIL are abnormal but terminally differentiated (Fig. 50–2). The atypical cells progress to the surface, produce keratins, die, and slough, as would normal cells. The gradient from low-grade SIL to high-grade SIL (CIN 2–3) is characterized by increasing nuclear atypia and failure of cellular differentiation in progressively more superficial levels of epithelium, with carcinoma in situ representing full thickness replacement with undifferentiated, immortalized, atypical cells. Despite inevitable misclassification from such a continuum of changes, the Bethesda System remains the best available simplifying schema for epidemiological research.

HPV Infection

HPV infection is the primary risk factor for cervical cancer and for certain other anogenital cancers (Barrasso et al, 1987; Kurman et al, 1993; Reid et al, 1987; Stanbridge and Butler, 1983). Interested readers are referred elsewhere for a thorough review of papillomavirus biology (Shah and Howley, 1995) or the epidemiology of HPV infection itself apart from cervical neoplasia outcomes (Schiffman and Burk, in press).

Human papillomaviruses are non-enveloped, double-stranded DNA viruses of approximately 8000 base pairs, part of a large group of papillomaviruses that includes wart viruses of cattle, cotton-tailed rabbits, deer, and horses. There are over 70 types of human papillomaviruses characterized according to DNA sequence homology, with a few more identified every year. The types are numbered sequentially as they are characterized. Each type has its own tissue predilection and disease spectrum. For example, HPV 1 is the major cause of deep plantar warts; HPV 2 and 4 cause mainly common skin warts; and types 6 and 11 are the most common agents of venereal warts (condyloma acuminatum) as well as laryngeal polyps. Based on current data, types 6, 11, 16, 18, 26, 31, 33, 35, 39, 42, 43, 44, 45, 51, 52, 53, 54, 55, 56, 58, 59, 64, 66, and 68 are the types most commonly found to infect cervical epithelia.

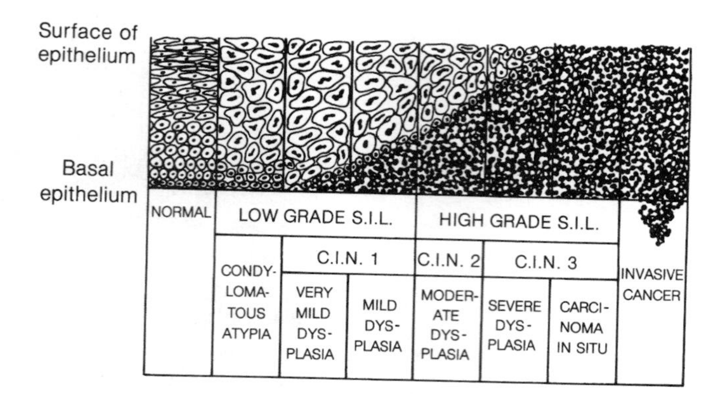

FIG. 50–2. Cervical cancer precursor lesions (adapted from Fenoglio and Ferenczy, 1982). Early cervical cancer precursors are characterized by superficial cellular abnormalities that represent the koilocytotic changes of human papillomavirus infection. More severe precursors demonstrate a progressive increase in undifferentiated, malignant-appearing cells.

The epidemiological study of HPV has been limited by HPV measurement techniques. Reliable serologic assays are not available to define cumulative lifetime incidence of HPV infection (Galloway, 1992), although serologic tests that detect the majority of recent infections have just been developed (Kirnbauer et al, 1994). At present, cervical HPV infection is still most accurately measured by current detection of HPV DNA sequences in infected tissues.

Epidemiologists studying cervical HPV infection have relied on DNA testing of cervical specimens obtained noninvasively using swabs, scrapes, brushings, and lavages. HPV prevalence estimates have varied accordingly, due to differences in cell sampling (Vermund et al, 1989), the poorly understood intermittency of viral DNA detectability (de Villiers et al, 1987) and, most importantly, the choice of DNA detection method (Schiffman, 1992a). Misclassification resulting from the first, poorly validated DNA tests severely limited early epidemiological studies of HPV infection (Franco, 1991).

Essentially there are two categories of HPV DNA detection methods used in population studies: those that identify the nucleic acids directly and those that amplify nucleic acids first and then detect the amplified product (Gravitt and Manos, 1992; Lorincz, 1992; Schiffman, 1992a). In the first category are Southern blot hybridization, dot blot hybridization (eg, ViraPap and Profile kits), and Hybrid Capture liquid hybridization kit. The only amplification methods currently used for HPV epidemiology are polymerase chain reaction (PCR)-based techniques. In general, PCR-based tests yield HPV population prevalence estimates about two to three times higher than those of nonamplified tests. However, if ample specimen is tested, the detection of HPV DNA in prevalent cases of SIL or cancer is similar regardless of whether nonamplified or amplified tests are used, because viral load is typically much higher in cases than in infected but cytologically normal controls.

DEMOGRAPHIC PATTERNS

Histopathology

Consistent with their origin in the transformation zone, most cervical cancers (80% or more) are squamous cell carcinomas, with adenocarcinomas and mixed adenosquamous tumors accounting for most of the remainder. Other histologic types, such as melanomas, sarcomas, and metastatic tumors, are very rare. The relative and absolute frequencies of adenocarcinomas are rising, particularly among younger women, for reasons that are only partly understood (Kjaer and Brinton, 1993). Almost all epidemiological studies of cervical cancer have focused on squamous carcinomas or have ignored histologic distinctions altogether.

Incidence and Mortality of Invasive Cervical Cancer in the United States

Figure 50–3 illustrates the historically downward trend for invasive cervical cancer in the United States through the early 1990s (updated from Devesa et al, 1987). In whites, incidence per 100,000 declined 76%, from 32.6 in the late 1940s to 7.9 in 1989–1991. Mortality rates in whites also declined, especially during the 1960s and 1970s. Average decreases in both incidence and mortality were about 4% per year until the 1980s, when rates started to level or, most recently, perhaps increase slightly. Although mortality and incidence declined also

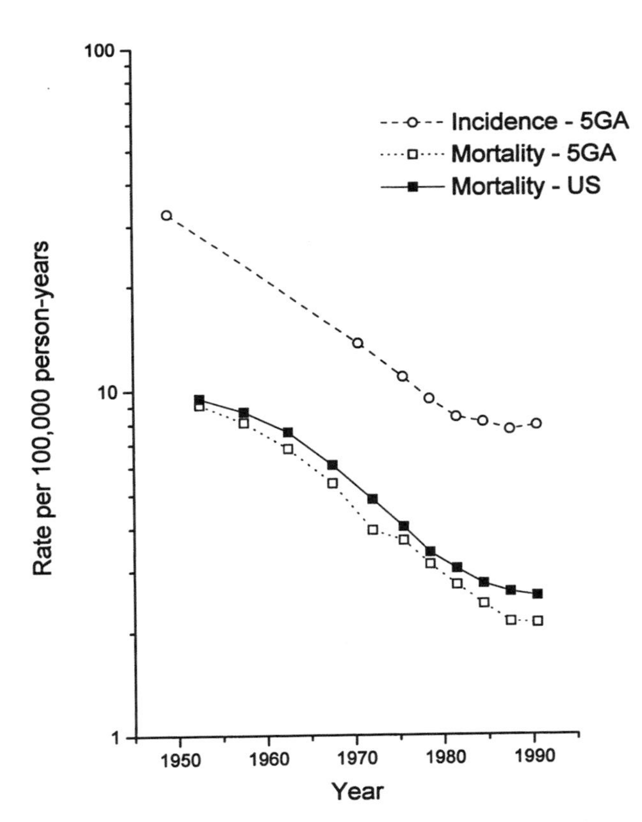

FIG. 50–3. Incidence and mortality trends for invasive cervical cancer in the United States (rates age-adjusted using the 1970 U.S. population; data from five geographic areas [5GA] of the National Cancer Surveys, the SEER program of National Cancer Institute, and the National Center for Health Statistics; updated from Devesa et al, 1987).

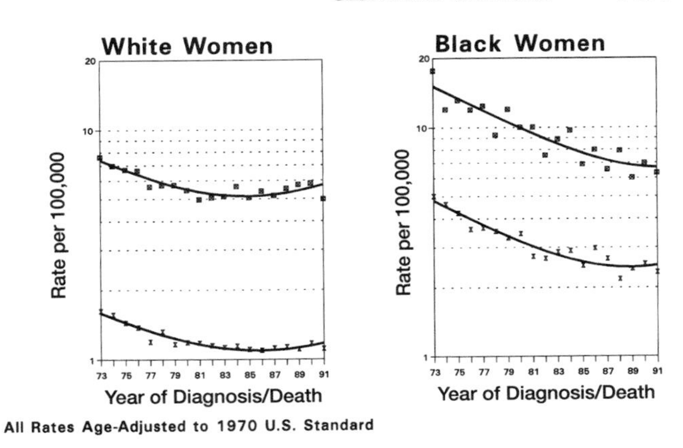

FIG. 50–4. Recent annual incidence and mortality rates for invasive cervical cancer, U.S. whites and African Americans under age 50 (from Ries et al, 1994).

among African Americans in the past decades, the decrease in mortality started later than among whites.

As shown in Figure 50–4, since the mid-1980s, among white women under age 50 years, the long decline in cervical cancer incidence has stopped and even reversed (Ries et al, 1994). Similar but weaker trends are evident in older white women. In contrast, cervical cancer incidence has continued to fall among African American women. Although data for 1987–1991 from the Surveillance, Epidemiology, and End Results (SEER) Program indicate an 80% excess in age-adjusted incidence of invasive cervical cancer in African Americans compared to whites (Ries et al, 1994), this differential appears restricted now to older women. Specifically, the incidence of cervical cancer continues to rise with age among African Americans (Fig. 50–5). Among whites, there is a plateauing of rates after age 40, an unusual pattern of risk compared to that of other epithelial tumors.

Examined by race and histology (Table 50–2), invasive cervical carcinoma incidence declined from 9.8 to 7.6 among whites and from 23.4 to 14.3 among blacks from 1975–1979 to 1985–1989, respectively. The majority of cervical carcinomas were squamous cell carcinomas, for which the rates continued to decrease among both races. Adenocarcinomas of the cervix are relatively rare, and adenosquamous carcinomas are even less frequent. Some increases in adenocarcinoma were suggested, at least among whites. These were seen primarily among young and middle-aged women (Devesa et al, 1989; Beral et al, 1994).

In addition to black-white differences, the incidence of cervical cancer is also about twice as high among Hispanics and even higher among Native Americans, while most Asian-American groups experience rates similar to those of whites (National Cancer Institute, 1984). The racial-ethnic differences in cervical cancer incidence are paralleled by differences in the incidence

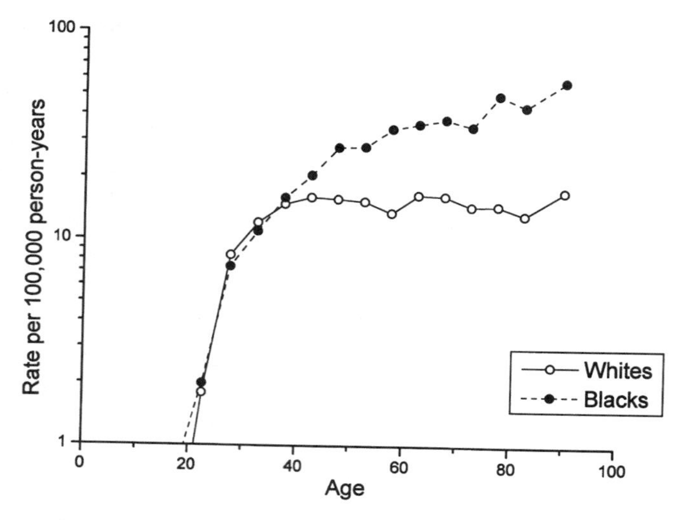

FIG. 50–5. Age-specific incidence of invasive cervical cancer, U.S. whites and African Americans, 1987–1991 (data from Ries et al, 1994).

and prevalence of SIL (Schiffman et al, unpublished data).

Moreover, racial differences also exist in survival experience (Ries et al, 1994). Women diagnosed with invasive cervical cancer in the United States experienced 5-year relative rates of 70% among whites and 56% among blacks, based on about 8000 cases diagnosed during 1983–1990 (Table 50–3). More than half of all cases among whites were diagnosed at a localized stage and about one third at a regional stage, in contrast to about 40% at each of these stages among blacks. The differences in stage distribution partly explained the difference in overall survival, but survival rates were more favorable for whites than blacks at each stage of diagnosis. Among both whites and blacks, stage at diagnosis strongly influenced subsequent survival experience, ranging from 86% to 91% among those diagnosed at a localized stage to 11% to 12% with distant disease. Age at diagnosis also strongly influenced survival, with rates declining from 70% to 80% among women under age 45 years to 30% to 40% among those age 75 and older.

At least some of the racial/ethnic differences in demographic patterns can be explained by the strong inverse associations observed between socioeconomic indicators and the risk of invasive cervical cancer. These inverse relationships with income and education prevail among both whites and African Americans. In one analysis, when adjustment was made for socioeconomic

TABLE 50–2. *Trends in Microscopically Confirmed Invasive Cervical Carcinoma Incidence by Histologic Type, SEER Program*

	1975–1979		1980–1984		1985–1989	
	No.	Rate[a]	No.	Rate[a]	No.	Rate[a]
WHITES						
squamous	3747	7.63	3307	6.24	3236	5.71
adenosquamous	107	0.23	122	0.24	145	0.25
adenocarcinoma	508	1.02	535	1.01	694	1.23
Total[b]	4827	9.80	4251	8.02	4331	7.64
BLACKS						
squamous	868	19.44	731	14.07	681	11.61
adenosquamous	22	0.49	24	0.48	38	0.63
adenocarcinoma	51	1.20	63	1.28	72	1.23
Total[b]	1046	23.35	877	16.91	842	14.34

[a]Per 100,000 woman-years, age-adjusted using the 1970 U.S. population.
[b]Includes carcinoma, not otherwise specified.

TABLE 50–3. *Stage Distribution and Relative Survival Rates for White and Black Patients Diagnosed with Invasive Cervical Cancer, SEER Program, 1983–1990*

Number of Cases	*Whites* (n=6599)	*Blacks* (n=1319)
STAGE DISTRIBUTION (%)		
localized	53	39
regional	32	40
distant	9	13
unstaged	7	9
FIVE-YEAR RELATIVE SURVIVAL RATES (%) BY STAGE		
all stages	69.9	56.4
localized	91.1	86.1
regional	52.7	42.7
distant	11.8	11.2
unstaged	59.4	58.9
FIVE-YEAR RELATIVE SURVIVAL RATES (%) BY AGE		
<45	81.1	68.6
45–54	68.7	55.6
55–64	64.0	52.4
65–74	55.1	47.8
75+	42.5	29.7

Source: Based on data from Ries et al, 1994; n = number of cases.

variables, the excess risk of cervical cancer among African Americans was substantially reduced, from more than 70% to less than 30% (Devesa and Diamond, 1980).

In addition to racial and socioeconomic differences, there are distinct geographic patterns in the United States (Fig. 50–6), with mortality rates ranging from 1.5 to 6.8 per 100,000 woman-years. High mortality rates are scattered throughout the South, and particularly in Appalachia and the Midwest (NCI, unpublished data). This reflects the tendency of the disease to affect rural women in lower socioeconomic classes and possible differences in screening practices and subsequent survival experience.

The upturn in cervical cancer incidence among younger white women in the United States occurred more recently than the trend in other countries, and this delay may reflect the effectiveness of aggressive U.S. screening and treatment programs that have counteracted anticipated increases from changes in the prevalence of risk factors (Devesa et al, 1989). In particular, it is possible that spread of genital HPV infections into the general population during the "sexual revolution" of the 1960s–1970s might account for the recent increases in cervical cancer reported among younger women, with the lag time reflecting the long latency period in the development of cervical cancer. As would be expected with this hypothesis, intermediate increases in the rates of low-grade SIL and HPV-induced venereal warts were reported in the 1970s and 1980s (Koutsky et al, 1988; Evans and Dowling, 1990).

International Patterns

Cervical cancer is the second most common cancer of women worldwide, and the fifth most common cancer in humans (Parkin et al, 1993). The worldwide incidence of cervical cancer is about 440,000 cases per year. The incidence rate per 100,000 woman-years for invasive cervical cancer in various geographic areas is shown

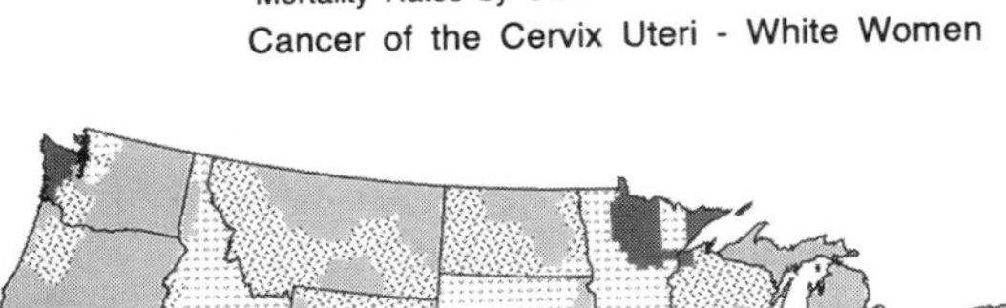

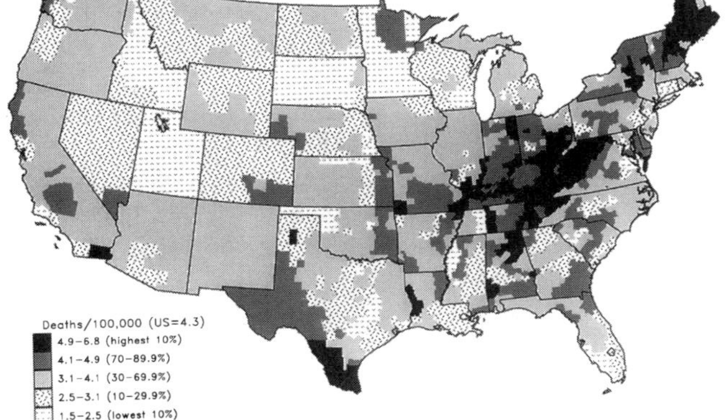

FIG. 50–6. Geographic patterns of cervical cancer mortality among white females according to state economic areas of the United States, 1970–1989 (rates age-adjusted using the 1970 U.S. population; based on data from the National Center for Health Statistics).

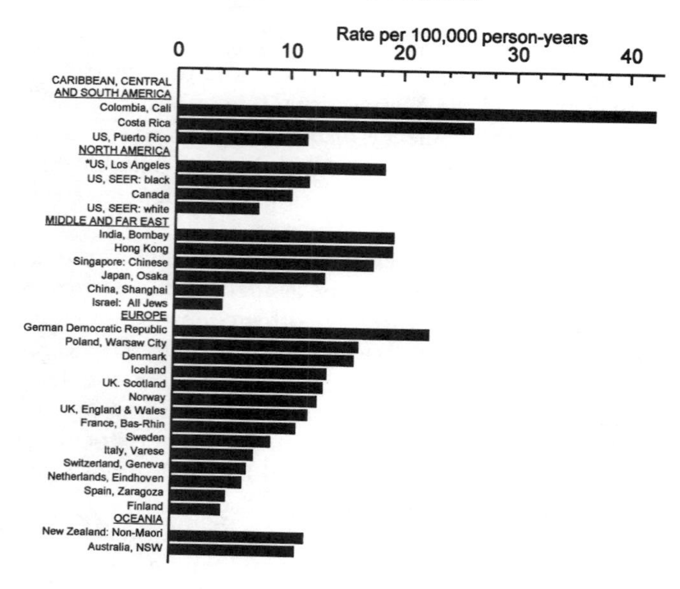

FIG. 50–7. Age-adjusted (world standard) incidence per 100,000 women for invasive cervical cancer by selected geographic areas (from Parkin et al, 1992).

in Figure 50–7 (Parkin et al, 1992). The highest rate was reported from Cali, Colombia, where the risk was almost six times that of U.S. whites, whose rate is among the lowest in the world. High rates were also reported in Costa Rica, among Spanish-surnamed whites in Los Angeles, in parts of Asia, and in eastern Europe. Notably low rates were reported for Jewish women in Israel, Chinese women in Shanghai, and women in Finland. However, the incidence and mortality rates of cervical cancer are profoundly influenced by the efficacy of available screening and treatment programs. Thus, the geographic variation in rates may not necessarily be useful in generating etiologic hypotheses.

Recent upturns in incidence and mortality rates among young women, preceding similar trends in the United States mentioned above, have been observed in a number of countries (Coleman et al, 1993; Beral et al, 1994), including Canada (Carmichael et al, 1986), Great Britain (Parkin et al, 1985), New Zealand (Green, 1979), and Australia (Holman and Armstrong, 1987).

The geographic distribution of HPV infection has been studied mainly in correlation with cervical cancer incidence rates, to determine whether variation in prevalences of HPV measured by DNA would be reflected in cancer rates. Recent geographic studies using sensitive PCR DNA testing methods to detect a wide spectrum of HPV types have generally observed HPV prevalences to correlate with the population risks of cervical cancer, although it has not been possible to take into account the relative efficacy of regional screening programs (Munoz et al, 1992).

HPV INFECTION AS THE MAJOR CAUSE OF CERVICAL CANCER

The epidemiological association between HPV infection and cervical cancer fulfills all of the established epidemiological criteria for causality (Hill, 1965). These criteria include strength and consistency of the epidemiological association, time sequence, specificity of the association, and coherence with existing biological and epidemiological evidence.

The association between HPV infection and cervical cancer is remarkably strong and consistent, with virtually no negative studies. Selected case-control studies of invasive cervical cancer are summarized in Table 50–4, with relative risks ranging from about 4 to more than 40. Although not shown here, similar risks have been observed in studies of SIL that included expert cytopathology review to minimize misclassification of low-grade cases (Schiffman et al, 1993). Thus, the great majority of women with cervical cancer and/or SIL have detectable HPV DNA, compared to a consistently lower percentage of control women.

In case series worldwide, most squamous cervical cancers and adenocarcinomas, and their metastases, have been found to contain HPV of the same types (Lancaster et al, 1986). The most definitive study of invasive cervical cancer included 1050 cervical cancers from over 20 countries, tested for all known HPV types by PCR (Bosch et al, 1995). Over 85% of cervical cancers from each country contained HPV DNA, with the inclusion of "possible" infections raising the proportions even higher.

Accordingly, the cancer-associated group of genital HPV types is defined as those found with appreciable prevalence in invasive cervical cancers (Fuchs et al, 1988; Lorincz et al, 1992; Bosch et al, 1995). Based on this definition, the current list of cancer-associated HPV types includes at least types 16, 18, 26, 31, 33, 35, 39, 45, 51, 52, 54, 55, 56, 58, 59, 64, and 68. Other, more restrictive definitions of "high-risk" types, based on relative risk or attributable proportion calculations, may be more useful for some purposes. By most definitions, HPV 16 is the most important cancer-associated type in almost all regions, along with HPVs 18, 31, and 45 (Bosch et al, 1995).

With regard to a logical time sequence, HPV infection (as measured by DNA) tends to precede and predict incident cervical neoplasia. Early results from large prospective studies of cytologically normal women show substantially elevated relative (>10) and absolute (>30%) risks of incident SIL, including high-grade SIL, within a few years of viral DNA detection (Koutsky et al, 1992; Schiffman et al, unpublished data). Cancer-associated HPV types are associated with a higher risk of developing cytologically evident lesions than are

TABLE 50–4. *Selected Case-Control Studies Assessing the Relation between HPV DNA Detection and Invasive Cervical Cancer*

			Testing Methods		*Invasive Cancer*		*Controls*		
Reference Year	*Area*	*Adjustment Factors*[1]	*Cell Sampling*	*DNA Hybridization*[2]	*No.*	*Percent HPV Pos.*	*No.*	*Percent HPV Pos.*	*Relative Risk*[3]
de Villiers, 1987	Germany	a	Swab	FISH	62	40	8755	9	10.3
Eluf-Neto, 1994	Brazil	a,b	Swab	PCR	199	84	225	17	37.1
Fuchs, 1988	Germany	None	Biopsy	Southern	44	72	31	10	23.1
Lorincz, 1987	North/South America	None	Biopsy	Southern	39	82	31	19	19.2
McCance, 1985	England	None	Biopsy	Southern	13	92	17	18	52.4
Meanwell, 1987	England	a	Biopsy	Southern	47	66	26	35	3.6[4]
Munoz, 1992	Spain	a,b,c,d,e	Swab	PCR	142	69	130	5	46.2
	Colombia	a,b,c,d,e	Swab	PCR	87	72	98	13	15.6
Peng, 1991	China	a,b,f,i	Swab	PCR	101	35	146	1	32.9
Reeves, 1989	Latin America	a,b,c,e,g,h	Swab	FISH	759	62	1467	32	9.1[5]

[1]a = age, b = socioeconomic status, c = number of sexual partners, d = age at first birth, e = Pap smear screening history, f = smoking, g = age at first intercourse, h = parity, i = age at first marriage.
[2]FISH = filter in situ hybridization, PCR = polymerase chain reaction, Southern = Southern blot hybridization.
[3]Relative risk calculated by DNA prevalence odds ratio P_{ca} $(1-P_{co})/P_{co}$ $(1-P_{ca})$ where P_{ca} is proportion of cases with DNA detected and P_{co} is proportion of controls. When adjustment factors were taken into account, adjusted RR is shown, although most varied little from the crude estimates.
[4]An interaction with age was observed, with RR = 10.5 under 40 years of age and RR = 1.2 for 40 or older.
[5]Relative risk associated with high levels of HPV types 16 or 18.

other HPV types (Stellato et al, 1994; Schiffman et al, unpublished data). Additionally, follow-up studies of women with low-grade SIL have observed that the finding of cancer-associated HPV types predicts an elevated risk of progression to high-grade SIL (Campion et al, 1986; Kataja et al, 1990). Finally, several small follow-up studies of women with invasive cancer have suggested that the presence or type of HPV might predict prognosis (Barnes et al, 1988; Walker et al, 1989; Riou et al, 1990; Higgins et al, 1991; Franco, 1992).

HPV infection causes a specific set of carcinomas of mucocutaneous epithelia (Daling et al, 1992), particularly anogenital tumors (cervical carcinoma, and some types of vulvar, vaginal, penile, and anal carcinomas). To a lesser extent, some subsets of head and neck carcinomas may also be associated with HPV. Numerous anecdotal reports of associations with a wide variety of tumor types, such as adenocarcinoma of the colon and Kaposi's sarcoma, have not been confirmed.

The animal data and experimental evidence for HPV carcinogenicity are strong, satisfying the causal criterion of "coherence." In fact, the potential for malignant transformation of papillomavirus-induced lesions has long been recognized. Cotton-tailed rabbit papillomavirus causes skin cancers in conjunction with exposure to coal tar (Rous and Kidd, 1938), and bovine papillomavirus causes alimentary tract cancers in cows ingesting the co-carcinogen bracken fern (Jarrett et al, 1978). In the rare genetic disorder epidermodysplasia verruciformis, patients develop multiple HPV-induced cutaneous warts that are prone to squamous cell carcinomas, especially in sun-exposed areas (Orth et al, 1980).

Cellular and molecular biological evidence for the oncogenic potential of human papillomaviruses is especially compelling (zur Hausen, 1994). Certain types of HPV have been shown to transform human cell lines in culture (Yasumoto et al, 1986) and to cause growth abnormalities that stimulate low-grade SIL (Kreider et al, 1985; McCance et al, 1988). The types with the strongest known transforming abilities in vitro (16 and 18) are also the most important cancer-associated types defined epidemiologically. In addition, the cancer-associated types are observed to be genetically related when "phylogenetic trees" are constructed that categorize HPV types by DNA sequence homology (Van Ranst et al, 1992). In mechanistic studies, HPV DNA, though found in an episomal (nonintegrated) form in early cervical lesions, is often integrated into the cellular genome in cervical cancers and derived cancer cell lines; integration may therefore play a role in progression and maintenance of neoplasia (Cullen et al, 1991). Protein products of HPV early genes (E6, E7) have been identified that interact with growth-regulatory proteins of the human cell (p53, pRb), providing a possible mechanism for an HPV oncogenic effect (Dyson et al, 1989; Werness et al, 1990). Finally, as shown below, HPV infection explains much of the established epidemiology of cervical cancer, meeting the criterion of "coherence with existing epidemiologic knowledge," and it is now generally accepted to be the major causal factor for most cases of cervical cancer in the world (IARC Working Group, 1995; Munoz et al, 1992; zur Hausen, 1994).

OTHER RISK FACTORS FOR CERVICAL CANCER

The recognition of the key etiologic role of HPV infection has profoundly altered the epidemiological study of cervical cancer. Yet this shift in theoretical paradigms to include HPV infection is still new and incomplete. Specifically, it is not yet clear which "established" risk factors for cervical cancer are mere correlates of HPV infection, which are HPV cofactors operating only in the presence of infection, and which are independent risk factors. As a result of the uncertainty, it is important to start by summarizing the established epidemiological risk factors for cervical cancer without consideration of HPV infection, analogous to a "crude" statistical analysis that precedes consideration of confounding and causal intermediacy. In each section, there will be an attempt to reconsider each of the established risk factors in light of the central role for HPV.

Sociodemographic Factors

Both descriptive and analytic studies have demonstrated that cervical cancer predominantly affects women in lower social classes, as defined by levels of income and education (Brinton et al, 1987a; Fasal et al, 1981; Jones et al, 1958; West et al, 1984). As a partial explanation, cervical HPV infections appear to be more prevalent in women of lower educational and income levels (Hildesheim et al, 1993). Other correlates of low socioeconomic level, including deficient nutrition, multiparity, and concurrent genital infections, could also be involved.

Religion

Low cervical cancer risks have been recorded among Catholic nuns (Fraumeni et al, 1969), the Amish (Cross et al, 1968), Mormons (Lyon et al, 1994), and Jews (Boyd and Doll, 1964; Graham and Schotz, 1979). It is probable that a reduced number of sexual partners and subsequently lowered risk of HPV infection among these groups accounts for their historically lower cancer risk. However, no study of religion and cervical cancer incorporating accurate HPV testing has been reported.

Marital and Sexual Factors

Early studies (Boyd and Doll, 1964; Jones et al, 1958) revealed that the risk of cervical cancer is especially high among women marrying at young ages. Subsequent investigations indicated the importance of sexual activity (Kessler et al, 1977; Martin, 1967; Pridan and Lilienfeld, 1971; Rotkin, 1967; Terris et al, 1967), with women who have sexual relationships at early ages being at higher risk than either virgins or women whose sexual experiences began later in life. Thus, it has been shown in a variety of case-control studies that women who become sexually active before age 16 have about a twofold or greater risk compared with women who start after the age of 20 years (Table 50–5).

The risk of cervical cancer is also influenced by the number of sexual partners, often indexed by multiple marriages, separations, and divorces. A number of stud-

TABLE 50–5. *Selected Case-Control Studies Assessing the Relation between Age at First Sexual Intercourse and Invasive Cervical Cancer*

Reference Year	*No. of Cases*	*No. of Controls*	*Type of Controls*	*Adjustment Factors*[1]	*Relative Risk*	*Comparison Categories*
Bosch, 1992	436	387	Population	a,c,d,g,h,p	4.3	<16 vs ≥24
Brinton, 1987a	418	704	Community	a,c,g,h,i,j,k,l	2.3	<16 vs ≥22
Clarke, 1982	178	855	Neighborhood	c,g[2],k	1.8	≤19 vs ≥20
Ebeling, 1987	129	275	Hospital	a,g,h,j,k	2.0	≤16 vs ≥20
Eluf-Neto, 1994	199	225	Hospital	a,c,g,h,j,l,p	1.3	≤14 vs ≥20
Herrero, 1990b	759	1430	Hosp/Comm	a,c,g,h,j,p	1.8	14–15 vs ≥20
Kjaer, 1992	59	614	Population	a,c,g,i,l	3.7	≤13 vs ≥20
La Vecchia, 1986b	327	327	Hospital	a,g	5.4	≤17 vs ≥23
Peters, 1986b	200	200	Neighborhood	a,b	16.1	<16 vs ≥23

[1]a = age, b = race, c = socioeconomic status or religion, d = country of origin or residence, e = marital status or age at marriage, f = age at first intercourse, g = number of sexual partners, h = Pap smear screening history, i = genital infection, j = menstrual and reproductive factors, k = smoking, l = contraceptive use, m = noncontraceptive hormone use, n = anthropometric or dietary factors, o = male partner characteristics, p = HPV.

[2]"Sexual stability" rather than number of sexual partners.

TABLE 50–6. *Selected Case-Control Studies Assessing the Relation between Number of Sexual Partners and Invasive Cervical Cancer*

Reference Year	*No. of Cases*	*No. of Controls*	*Type of Controls*	*Adjustment Factors*[1]	*Relative Risk*	*Comparison Categories*
Bosch, 1992	436	387	Population	a,c,d,g,h,j,p	5.6	≥6 vs 1
Brinton, 1987a	418	704	Community	a,c,f,h,i,j,k,l	2.8	≥10 vs 1
Ebeling, 1987	129	275	Hospital	f,h,i,j,k	3.9	≥5 vs 1
Eluf-Neto, 1994	199	225	Hospital	a,c,f,h,j,l,p	3.4	≥4 vs 1
Herrero, 1990b	759	1430	Hosp./Comm.	a,c,f,h,j,p	1.7	≥6 vs 1
Kjaer, 1992	59	614	Population	a,c,f,i,l	3.0	≥5 vs 0–1
La Vecchia, 1986b	327	327	Hospital	a,f	2.7	≥3 vs 0–1
Peters, 1986b	200	200	Neighborhood	a,b	2.6	≥10 vs 0–1

[1]a = age, b = race, c = socioeconomic status or religion, d = country of origin or residence, e = marital status or age at marriage, f = age at first intercourse, g = number of sexual partners, h = Pap smear screening history, i = genital infection, j = menstrual and reproductive factors, k = smoking, l = contraceptive use, m = non-contraceptive hormone use, n = anthropometric or dietary factors, o = male partner characteristics, p = HPV.

ies (Martin, 1967; Pridan and Lilienfeld, 1971; Rotkin, 1967; Terris et al, 1967) have shown that women with cervical cancer more frequently report multiple sexual partners than control subjects. Furthermore, within many data sets, risk appears to increase directly with the number of sexual partners reported. Selected recent studies are shown in Table 50–6.

When HPV infection is taken into account, the effect of lifetime number of partners is weakened but still apparent, especially in the HPV-negative group (Bosch et al, 1992; Eluf-Neto et al, 1994). This residual effect could reflect false-negative HPV testing of some cases or might indicate an independent role for other sexually transmitted agents. Age at first intercourse (or the correlated variable, age at first birth) also remains a weak risk factor even after HPV positivity is taken into account (Bosch et al, 1992; Eluf-Neto et al, 1994). Age at first intercourse might be viewed logically as a proxy for time of HPV infection; that is, the start of "latency." However, it might also suggest a "vulnerable period" of the cervix when the transforming effect of HPV is greatest.

In view of suggestions that the cervix may be more vulnerable at early ages, when the transformation zone is more exposed, the number of different sexual partners at specific ages has been of interest. Brinton and colleagues (1987a) and Herrero and colleagues (1990b) failed to find that number of partners before age 20 was more of a risk discriminator than lifetime number of partners, but Peters and colleagues (1986b) observed that the effect of lifetime number of partners was totally attributable to effects associated with number of sexual relationships before the age of 20. Peters and colleagues (1986b) also found some evidence that subjects with short intervals between menarche and initiation of sexual intercourse were at elevated risk (with associations stronger than those observed with age at first intercourse alone), but this effect was not subsequently confirmed (Brinton et al, 1989a).

Most investigations have failed to note any effect of frequency of intercourse on risk after accounting for the effects of number of partners (Boyd and Doll, 1964; Brinton et al, 1987a; Herrero et al, 1990b; Jones et al, 1958; Martin, 1967; Rotkin, 1967; Terris et al, 1967). This would be concordant with the assumption that HPV is relatively easily transmitted during vaginal intercourse. In one of the few age-specific studies of frequency of intercourse and cervical cancer (Herrero et al, 1990b), high frequency was a significant risk factor only before age 20, supporting the notion of a vulnerable period.

The number of steady sexual partners (relationships lasting more than 3 months) was more related to risk of cervical cancer than the number of non-steady partners in the studies of Brinton and colleagues (1987a) and Herrero and colleagues (1990b). However, there are HPV data suggesting that the total lifetime number of sexual partners might be a better predictor of HPV infection than number of steady partners (Schiffman et al, 1993).

Gynecologic and Obstetrical Events

There is little evidence that the risk of cervical cancer is affected by age at menarche, age at menopause, or character of menses (Boyd and Doll, 1964; Brinton et al, 1987a; Fasal et al, 1981; Jones et al, 1958; Rotkin, 1967; Wynder et al, 1954), or by hygiene factors (Brinton et al, 1987a; Herrero et al, 1990b).

Early reports suggested that poorly managed parturition may increase risk (Smith, 1931), but subsequent studies dismissed a true effect because of the presumed correlation of pregnancy with sexual activity. However, several recent studies controlling for the separate effects of reproductive and sexual factors, including HPV infection, have found a persistent influence of multiparity (Brinton et al, 1987a; Brinton et al, 1989b; Kjaer et al, 1992; Parazzini et al, 1989).

In a Latin American study in which multiparity was commonly observed, the adjusted relative risk rose steadily to over 5 for those with 14 or more pregnancies, with effects relating primarily to live births rather than to short-term pregnancies (Brinton et al, 1989a). Two other recent studies in Latin America showed a relation of risk with multiparity independent of HPV infection (Bosch et al, 1992; Eluf-Neto et al, 1994).

It has been suggested that pregnancy could influence cell growth either directly or indirectly through immunologic or hormone-dependent influences on HPV (Pater et al, 1990). Although HPV detection rates may increase slightly during current pregnancies (Schneider et al, 1987; Hildesheim et al, 1993), the prevalence of HPV infection is not increased in multiparous women. Thus, whether there is any interaction between HPV and multiparity is unclear. Alternatively, the effect of pregnancy could reflect cervical trauma during parturition; this is supported by findings from two studies of reduced cervical cancer risk associated with a caesarean section (Brinton et al, 1989b; Bosch et al, 1992). Finally, nutritional effects of reproduction deserve attention.

Characteristics of the Male Sexual Partner

Despite extensive evidence implicating sexual factors in the etiology of cervical cancer, until recently there has been little attention given to a role of the male partner. Geographic clusters of cervical and penile cancers (Cartwright and Sinson, 1980; Li et al, 1982; MacGregor and Innes, 1980), as well as elevated rates of cervical cancer among the wives of men with penile cancer (Graham et al, 1979; Martinez, 1969; Smith et al, 1980), provided the first suspicion that a "male factor" might be important. This notion was supported by a follow-up study in which the wives of men previously married to cervical cancer patients were found to have elevated rates of cervical neoplasia compared to control wives (Kessler, 1977). Further interest in the role of a male factor derives from findings that some female populations exhibit high incidence rates of cervical cancer, despite traditions of having few sexual contacts—for example, many Latin American populations (Skegg et al, 1982).

Most recently, the role of the male in the etiology of cervical cancer has been examined by comparing the sexual and other behavioral characteristics of husbands of cervical cancer patients with husbands of control patients (Brinton et al, 1989c; Buckley et al, 1981; Kjaer et al, 1991; Niruthisard and Trisukosol, 1991; Pridan and Lilienfeld, 1971; Zunzunegui et al, 1986). In all of these studies, the husbands of case patients were found to report significantly more sexual partners than husbands of control patients. In several of the studies, husbands of patients with cervical cancer were also more likely to report histories of various genital conditions, including venereal warts (caused by HPV types 6 and 11), gonorrhea, and herpes. Consistent with these associations was a low relative risk of cervical cancer when husbands reported frequent usage of condoms (Kjaer et al, 1991).

Of specific interest in these studies has been the relation of cervical cancer risk to the type of sexual activity engaged in by the husbands. Some studies (Buckley et al, 1981; Kjaer et al, 1991; Niruthisard and Trisukosol, 1991) have found visits by the male partners to prostitutes to relate to cervical cancer risk, but other studies have failed to confirm this association (Brinton et al, 1989c; Agarwal et al, 1993). This may relate to differences in types of prostitutes visited (eg, streetwalkers, house prostitutes, "cabaret entertainers"), since these groups have been found to differ in the prevalence of sexually transmitted diseases (Reeves and Quiroz, 1987).

Reliable prevalence estimates for genital HPV infections in males are more difficult to obtain than those for females. It appears from the available data that genital HPV infections are about equally common in both sexes, although the HPV-containing penile lesions are usually very subtle and difficult to detect (Barrasso et al, 1987; Barrasso, 1992; Bergman and Nalick, 1992).

Apart from HPV infection, poor hygiene of the male partner has been postulated to play a role in the etiology of cervical cancer, with special attention given to the effects of circumcision. Lilienfeld and Graham (1958) discussed the difficulties of defining circumcision status by interview, a problem confirmed in a recent study where there was limited agreement between interview and clinical reports (Brinton et al, 1989c). Despite several reports of a protective effect associated with circumcision of the partner (Agarwal et al, 1993; Kjaer et al, 1991; Terris and Oalmann, 1960; Wynder et al, 1954), many other studies have shown no substantial differences between case and control husbands (Boyd and Doll, 1964; Brinton et al, 1989c; Jones et al, 1958; Rotkin, 1967). Studies with good clinical documentation of circumcision status and penile HPV infections are needed to address this issue further.

Infectious Agents Other Than HPV

Despite the evidence linking HPV to cervical cancer, it would be premature to conclude that HPV is the only agent involved. Of the other agents examined, most attention has been focused on herpes simplex virus 2 (HSV-2) and chlamydia.

Laboratory studies have demonstrated that HSV-2 infection can transform cells in culture and that HSV-2 proteins and integrated DNA can be found in some cervical cancers (McDougall et al, 1986). Multiple serologic studies have observed higher prevalence of antibody to HSV-2, unadjusted for HPV, among cases of cervical neoplasia than controls (Adam et al, 1973; Jha et al, 1993). This association has been documented in many geographic areas, using various assay methods.

Research interest in the oncogenic potential of HSV-2 declined when HSV-2 DNA and protein were not detected consistently in tumors and when a large follow-up study of Czechoslovakian women failed to demonstrate a significantly increased risk of cervical neoplasia related to HSV-2 serology at enrollment (Vonka et al, 1984). It is possible that the serologic evidence of elevated exposure to HSV-2 among cases could represent an immunosuppressive effect of cancer or a noncausal association resulting from the correlation of HSV-2 with sexual activity and HPV infection. The association of HSV-2 with risk of cervical cancer has been weak and inconsistent when HPV infection has been taken into account (Hildesheim et al, 1991; de Sanjose et al, 1994).

Chlamydial cervicitis has been suspected to be a risk factor for cervical cancer, based on case-control comparisons of serology (Schachter et al, 1982) and of chlamydia-associated changes seen on stored cervical smears (Allerding et al, 1985). Again, however, the risk of cervical cancer associated with chlamydia seropositivity has been inconsistent after adjusting for HPV infection (de Sanjose et al, 1994).

Additional infections that have been studied include syphilis, gonorrhea, cytomegalovirus, Epstein-Barr virus, and bacterial vaginosis. No consistent association with cervical cancer risk has been observed for any one of these agents. One investigation (Schmauz et al, 1989) but not another (de Sanjose et al, 1994) noted a rise in risk of cervical cancer with multiple, concurrent infections, consistent with the hypothesis that chronic cervicovaginal inflammation might increase the oncogenicity of HPV infection.

Smoking

A correlation between the distribution of cervical cancer and other smoking-related cancers prompted Winkelstein (1977) to suggest that cigarette smoking may affect the risk of cervical cancer. A number of case-control studies (Table 50–7) and one cohort investigation (Greenberg et al, 1985) subsequently demonstrated excess risks of cervical cancer (and SIL) among smokers. A number of the investigations that were able to control for age at first intercourse, number of sexual partners, and/or social class found the associations with smoking to persist (Brinton et al, 1986b; Clarke et al, 1982; Harris et al, 1980; Hellberg et al, 1983; La Vecchia et al, 1986a; Lyon et al, 1983; Peters et al, 1986b; Slattery et al, 1989b; Trevathan et al, 1983).

In most studies not adjusted for HPV, the relative risks for smokers have been around twofold, with the

TABLE 50–7. *Selected Case-Control Studies Assessing the Relation between Smoking and Invasive Cervical Cancer*

Reference Year	*No. of Cases*	*No. of Controls*	*Type of Controls*	*Adjustment Factors*[1]	*Relative Risk*	*Measure of Exposure*
Baron, 1986	1174	2128	Hospital	a,e,j,n	1.8	≥15 pack-years
Bosch, 1992	436	387	Population	a,c,d,g,h,j,p	1.5	Ever smoked
Brinton, 1986b	480	797	Community	a,b,c,f,g,	2.4	≥40 cigs/day
Clarke, 1982	178	855	Neighborhood	a,c,f,g[2]	2.2	Current smokers
Daling, 1992	207	426	Random-digit dialing	a,d,g	3.1	Current ≥40 cigs/day
Eluf-Neto, 1994	157[3]	32[3]	Hospital	a,c,f,g,h,j,l,p	<1.0	Ever smoked
Herrero, 1989	667	1430	Hosp/Comm	a,g,n	1.5	≥40 years
LaVecchia, 1986a	230	230	Hospital	j,l	1.8	Current ≥15 cigs/day
Marshall, 1983	513	490	Hospital		1.6	Current smokers
Peng, 1991	101	146	Hospital	a,c,e,p	1.2	Ever smoked
Peters, 1986b	200	200	Neighborhood	a,b	3.7	≥20 cigs/day

[1]a = age, b = race, c = socioeconomic status or religion, d = country of origin or residence, e = marital status or age at marriage, f = age—at first intercourse, g = number of sexual partners, h = Pap smear screening history, i = genital infection, j = menstrual and reproductive factors, k = smoking, l = contraceptive use, m = noncontraceptive hormone use, n = anthropometric or dietary factors, o = male partner characteristics, p = HPV.

[2]"Sexual stability" rather than number of sexual partners.

[3]HPV-positive subjects only; exact RR cannot be calculated from data presented.

highest risks generally observed for long-term or high-intensity smokers. In several studies, the smoking relation was restricted to current smokers; in one investigation, the effect was further limited to continuous smokers and those who started smoking later in life (Herrero et al, 1989). It is noteworthy that the smoking effect is restricted to squamous cell carcinoma, with no relation observed for the rarer occurrences of adenocarcinoma or adenosquamous carcinoma (Brinton et al, 1986b).

In the most definitive case-control studies of cervical cancer to date, taking HPV infection into account, the role of smoking has been practically null (Bosch et al, 1992; Eluf-Neto et al, 1994). These studies were conducted mainly in Latin America, where even crude smoking effects on cervical cancer are often weak. Perhaps the full influence of smoking on risk of cervical cancer could only be observed in regions where prolonged, heavy smoking among women is prevalent, such as in the United States.

Recently, several investigations have attempted to define possible mechanisms by which smoking might alter cervical epithelium. Smoking is not strongly associated with risk of cervical HPV infection once correlations with sexual behavior are taken into account (Hildesheim et al, 1993). However, several studies have demonstrated high rates of smoke-derived nicotine and cotinine in the cervical mucus of smokers (McCann et al, 1992; Sasson et al, 1985; Schiffman et al, 1987). The immunosuppressive effects of smoking (Barton et al, 1988; Phillips et al, 1985) could theoretically enhance the persistence of HPV infection (Burger et al, 1993; zur Hausen, 1982).

Oral Contraceptives

Studies examining the relation between oral contraceptive use and cervical cancer risk are especially complex, with questions arising about the potential for confounding, particularly by sexual and screening behavior (Brinton et al, 1986a; Brinton et al, 1990; Brinton, 1991; Piper, 1985).

Because of limited information on potential confounding factors, prospective studies (Andolsek et al, 1983; Beral et al, 1988; Peritz et al, 1977; Vessey et al, 1983a) are difficult to interpret. In the study of Vessey and colleagues (1983a), the incidence of cervical neoplasia (preinvasive and invasive) rose from 0.9 per 1000 woman-years among those with up to 2 years of oral contraceptive use to 2.2 among those with more than 8 years' use. Of note in this prospective study, as well as another (Andolsek et al, 1983), was that all cases of invasive cancer occurred among oral contraceptive users. In the study of Beral and colleagues (1988), the incidence of cervical cancer after 10 years of use was more than four times that of nonusers. It did not appear from a sub-study conducted by Vessey and colleagues (1983b) that oral contraceptive users were different in their sexual histories from the comparison group (IUD users). Swan and Brown (1981), however, concluded that the excess risk associated with long-term oral contraceptive use in their prospective study (Peritz et al, 1977) was likely to be highly confounded by sexual activity.

Results from recent case-control studies, mainly without consideration of HPV, are summarized in Table 50–8. Although several studies have noted no relation between oral contraceptives and cervical cancer risk, the majority of studies indicate that long-term users are at excess risk, even after adjustment for sexual and social factors. Studies showing no relation of risk to oral contraceptive use are generally those that have used neighborhood controls (Celentano et al, 1987; Peters et al, 1986b), which may reflect overmatching, or those that have included noninvasive abnormalities, presenting difficulties for interpretation because of possible detection biases (Coker et al, 1992; Irwin et al, 1988; Molina et al, 1988). In addition, the absence of an effect in several studies may merely reflect the limited number of long-term oral contraceptive users. In a recent, large study by the World Health Organization (1993), a risk of 2.2 was associated with contraceptive use of 8 or more years.

The effects of oral contraceptive use may be somewhat stronger for adenocarcinomas than for squamous cell neoplasms (Brinton et al, 1986a; Ursin et al, 1994), in line with descriptive surveys showing increasing rates of cervical adenocarcinoma among young women (Chilvers et al, 1987; Peters et al, 1986a; Schwartz and Weiss, 1986; Beral et al, 1994). In view of clinical studies suggesting that cervical adenocarcinoma may result from exogenous hormones (Chumas et al, 1985; Dallenbach-Hellweg, 1984), further investigation appears warranted.

Recent interest has focused on possible interactive effects of oral contraceptives and HPV, especially in view of studies showing that the transcriptional regulatory regions of HPV DNA contain hormone-recognition elements and that transformation of cells in vitro with viral DNA is enhanced by hormones (Auborn et al, 1991; Monsonego et al, 1991, Pater et al, 1990). Oral contraceptive use has been only inconsistently associated with increased rates of HPV infection (Hildesheim et al, 1993; Lorincz et al, 1990; Ley et al, 1991; Moscicki et al, 1993). However, two recent studies found an especially elevated risk of invasive cervical cancer among HPV-positive women who used oral contraceptives (Bosch et al, 1992; Eluf-Neto et al, 1994). Perhaps oral contraceptive use promotes the activity of HPV once infection has occurred.

TABLE 50–8. *Selected Case-Control Studies Assessing the Relation between Oral Contraceptives and Invasive Cervical Cancer*

Reference Year	*No. of Cases*	*No. of Controls*	*Type of Controls*	*Adjustment Factors*[1]	*Relative Risk*	*Measure of Exposure*
Bosch, 1992	436	387	Population	a,c,d,g,h,j,p	1.3	Ever use
Brinton, 1986a	479	789	Community	a,b,c,f,g,h,i	1.8	≥10 years' use
Brinton, 1990	759	1430	Hosp/Comm	a,b,d,f,g,h,i,j	1.2	≥10 years' use
Celentano, 1987	153	153	Assorted	a,b,f,h,j,k	0.7	Ever use
Ebeling, 1987	129	275	Hospital	f,g,h,i,j,k	1.8	≥7 years' use
Eluf-Neto, 1994	199	225	Hospital	a,c,f,g,h,j,p	2.5	≥5 years' use
Irwin, 1988	149	764	Community	a,f,g,h,i,j	0.9	≥5 years' use
Kjaer, 1993	59	614	Population	a,g,h,i,j,l	1.3	≥6 years' use
Parazzini, 1990	367	323	Hospital	a,c,e,f,g,h,j,k,l	2.5	≥2 years' use
Peters, 1986b	200	200	Neighborhood	a,b	1.1	≥10 years' use
WHO, 1993	2361	13644	Hospital	a,d,h,j	2.2	>8 years' use

[1]a = age, b = race, c = socioeconomic status or religion, d = country of origin or residence, e = marital status or age at marriage, f = age at first intercourse, g = number of sexual partners, h = Pap smear screening history, i = genital infection, j = menstrual and reproductive factors, k = smoking, l = contraceptive use, m = noncontraceptive hormone use, n = anthropometric or dietary factors, o = male partner characteristics, p = HPV.

Other Hormonal Contraceptives

Evidence linking oral contraceptives to cervical abnormalities has raised concern about long-acting steroid preparations, notably depot-medroxyprogesterone acetate (DMPA). Although these agents are widely used in many countries, studies evaluating their effects are limited. Two studies conducted in the United States (Powell and Seymour, 1971; Litt, 1975) have reported the prevalence of SIL to be elevated in DMPA users, but information on other risk factors was not available. A study in Chile (Dabancens et al, 1974), which was able to account for other factors, failed to find any effect on cervical neoplasia of either DMPA or chlormadinone acetate. Data from the WHO Collaborative Study of Neoplasia and Steroid Contraceptives also failed to confirm any significant relation (Thomas et al, 1989). However, a study from Latin America showed an approximate doubling of risk of invasive cervical cancer associated with use of injectable contraceptives for 5 or more years, with the risk particularly enhanced among women with limited screening histories (Herrero et al, 1990a). These findings support the need for further monitoring of cervical cancer risks among users of injectable contraceptives, taking HPV infection into account. Additional studies of HPV infection in the context of hormone replacement therapy and menopause are also indicated.

Other Contraceptive Methods

In a number of studies, users of barrier methods of contraception (diaphragm and condom) were found to have a low risk of cervical cancer (Boyce et al, 1977; Boyd and Doll, 1964; Fasal et al, 1981; Martin, 1967; Melamed et al, 1969; Terris and Oalmann, 1960; Worth and Boyes, 1972). The apparent protective effect, however, has usually been small with limited information on other risk factors. The most convincing evidence derives from the Oxford–Family Planning Association Contraceptive Study (Wright et al, 1978) in which the incidence of cervical neoplasia (per 1000 woman-years of observation) was 0.17 among diaphragm users compared to 0.95 and 0.87 among oral contraceptive and IUD users, respectively. Because this difference could not be explained by other risk factors, it is plausible that the diaphragm (like the condom) may protect the cervix from venereally transmitted agents like HPV. It has also been suggested that part of the protection associated with diaphragm use may reflect concurrent use of spermicides, which have anti-viral properties (Hildesheim et al, 1990). However, the most common spermicide has no appreciable anti-HPV activity in vitro (Hermonat et al, 1992).

Several studies (Brinton et al, 1987a; Graham and Schotz, 1979; Peters et al, 1986b) have found frequent vaginal douching, especially with other than vinegar or water, associated with increased cervical cancer risk. If real, the douching association could possibly relate to local irritation or to the destruction of normal vaginal flora.

Occupational Factors

Findings regarding the role of occupational factors in the etiology of cervical cancer have been limited to high rates among prostitutes (Moghissi et al, 1968; Rojel, 1952), cleaners and food preparation workers (Savitz et al, 1995), and waitresses (Kjaerheim and Andersen, 1994), most likely reflecting the effects of correlated sexual behavior linked to HPV infection. Of note, the point prevalences of HPV DNA found in surveys of immunocompetent (HIV-uninfected) prostitutes have not necessarily been elevated (Kreiss et al, 1992), possibly suggesting immunity in some women following intense exposure.

Other occupational studies have centered on the male partner. Beral (1974) found a high rate of cervical cancer among spouses of men whose work necessitated prolonged absences from home, and postulated that male extramarital affairs might be responsible. Robinson (1982) proposed a more direct effect of the male occupation, with certain dusts, metals, chemicals, tar, or machine oils as possible risk factors for cervical cancer in the wives. Zakelj and colleagues (1984), however, found no support for this hypothesis when British cervical cancer mortality data were examined in relation to occupational classification.

Dietary Factors

The influence of nutrient status on risk of cervical neoplasia has received substantial research attention (reviewed in Potischman, 1993). Most studies have utilized case-control approaches, assessing dietary intake or blood levels at the time of diagnosis, but some prospective studies have been completed. No study to date has taken HPV infection properly into account, and firm associations between nutritional status and HPV infection have yet to be found.

The majority of case-control studies have shown no relation between preformed vitamin A intake and either SIL or invasive disease (Brock et al, 1988; de Vet et al, 1991; Harris et al, 1986; La Vecchia et al, 1988). However, direct (topical) application of a vitamin A analogue to high-grade SIL in a randomized trial was shown to influence favorably the natural history (Meyskens et al, 1994), analogous to the dermatologic use of similar compounds to suppress flat facial warts.

In some studies, but not others, low dietary intake of carotenoids (provitamin A) has been found to increase the risk of SIL (Brock et al, 1988; Liu et al, 1993; Van Eenwynk et al, 1991; de Vet et al, 1991; La Vecchia et al, 1988; Ziegler et al, 1991) and cervical cancer (Herrero et al, 1991; La Vecchia et al, 1988; Marshall et al, 1983; Verreault et al, 1989; Slattery et al, 1990; Ziegler et al, 1990). Studies that have focused on blood carotenoids provide additional support for a protective effect of carotenoids on both SIL (Batieha et al, 1993; Brock et al, 1988; Harris et al, 1986; Palan et al, 1991; Van Eenwyk et al, 1991) and invasive cancer (Potischman et al, 1991), although the studies are not entirely consistent (Cuzick et al, 1990). In a study of SIL that measured a variety of serum carotenoids, the component most strongly related to reduced risk was serum lycopene, with ambiguous findings for alpha-carotene, beta-carotene and cryptoxanthin (Van Eenwyk et al, 1991).

Vitamin C has been of interest because of its role in the healing process and its antioxidant function. Several studies of SIL have shown reduced risks associated with high plasma levels of ascorbic acid (Basu et al, 1991; Romney et al, 1985), a relation for which there is support from dietary intake data for both SIL (Liu et al, 1993; Van Eenwyk et al, 1991; Wassertheil-Smoller et al, 1981) and invasive cancer (Herrero et al, 1991). Two studies that showed no overall effect did observe a reduced risk associated with vitamin C intake among smokers (Slattery et al, 1990; Ziegler et al, 1990), suggesting that an antioxidant function might underlie the association.

Because vitamin E is poorly measured through dietary intake data, most studies have focused on blood measures. Prospective studies have shown either a weak protective effect of serum alpha-tocopherol levels (Knekt, 1988) or no effect (Batieha et al, 1993). Case-control studies support an effect for SIL (Cuzick et al, 1990; Palan et al, 1991) but not for invasive cancer (Potischman et al, 1991).

Folate deficiency has also been suggested as a cervical cancer risk factor on the basis of megaloblastic features in cervical cells of oral contraceptive users (Whitehead et al, 1973) and findings that folate supplementation among oral contraceptive users with SIL leads to marked cellular improvement (Butterworth et al, 1982). One case-control study supported an etiologic role for folates as a cofactor of HPV 16 (Butterworth et al, 1992a). However, a subsequent intervention trial by these same investigators failed to show that folate supplementation altered the clinical course of SIL (Butterworth et al, 1992b). Further, most epidemiological studies employing dietary questionnaires have shown no relation between estimated folate intake or folate-rich foods and either high-grade SIL (Brock et al, 1988; Ziegler et al, 1991) or invasive cervical cancer (Herrero et al, 1991; Ziegler et al, 1990). One recent study, however, did find higher rates of SIL linked with low dietary and serologic folate (Van Eenwyk et al, 1992). The folate hypothesis deserves further attention, especially since folate depletion, which occurs during pregnancy, has been hypothesized as a possible explanation for high cervical cancer risks associated with multiparity.

Genetics

Little attention has been given to familial occurrences of cervical cancer, although some reports suggest that a familial tendency exists (Bender et al, 1976; Brinton et al, 1987b; Furgyik et al, 1986). Whether this tendency reflects environmental or genetic factors is yet to be resolved.

Several investigators have observed associations of human leukocyte antigen (HLA) alleles or haplotypes with invasive cervical cancer. Most current interest is focused on genotypes of the HLA-D loci (Apple et al, 1994). However, none of the reported associations have been consistently observed, raising concern of a multiple comparison problem.

Immunosuppression

Much of what is known about HPV immunology derives from small investigations of HPV infections in immunodeficient individuals (Evans and Mueller, 1990). Cervical SIL rates are elevated among immunosuppressed women with renal transplants (Hoover, 1977; Matas et al, 1975; Porreco et al, 1975), who are prone to a variety of genital infections, including HPV and HSV-2 (Matas et al, 1975; Schneider et al, 1983; Sillman et al, 1984). However, the excess risks observed among patients with renal transplants are complicated by close medical surveillance and difficulties in obtaining reliable expected values (Hoover, 1977).

HIV infection provides perhaps the most important example of the effect of immunosuppression on HPV infection. Individuals infected with HIV through sexual contacts are likely also to be exposed to genital HPV. However, the increased diagnosis of HPV in HIV-infected individuals is so striking that the increase is apparently real and related to immunosuppression. Specifically, HIV infection is associated with a very high prevalence of HPV DNA detection, especially in immunosuppressed women with low CD4 counts (Ho et al, 1994; Maiman et al, 1991; Vermund et al, 1991). In such women, SIL is very commonly diagnosed. It is not known whether HIV immunosuppression permits reactivation of previously suppressed HPV infection, as opposed to allowing rapid infection or reinfection.

Although the association between HIV infection, HPV infection, and SIL is established, a causal role for immunosuppression in the risk of progression of SIL to invasive carcinoma is less clear. Anal carcinoma rates are increasing in the homosexual male population, probably related to HIV infection (Palefsky et al, 1991). In contrast, cervical cancer rates are not greatly elevated in HIV-infected female cohorts, possibly reflecting more limited follow-up time (Cote et al, unpublished data). It is unclear whether HIV immunosuppression could speed the normally long progression from SIL to invasive carcinoma, or whether it mainly increases the prevalence and persistence of SIL precursors. Of note, a mildly immunosuppressive retrovirus, HTLV-1, has recently been linked to an increased risk of high-grade SIL and cancer among HPV-infected women (Strickler et al, 1995).

Based on animal experiments and the immunosuppression data, it is assumed that the key immune response involved in the clearance of HPV infections is cell-mediated (Lancaster and Olson, 1982; Sundberg, 1987). The two classes of cells thought to be involved in the cellular immune response to HPV are antigen-presenting cells (Langerhans cells) and cytotoxic T lymphocytes (Crawford, 1993; McArdle and Muller, 1986).

Risk Factors by Cell Type

The vast majority of cervical cancers are HPV-containing, squamous cell tumors, but some important exceptions should be mentioned. Adenocarcinomas are increasing in absolute and relative frequency in the United States, especially among younger women (Kjaer and Brinton, 1993). As a result, adenocarcinomas are approaching 15%–20% of cervical cancer cases in the United States.

Although the comparison of risk factors by cell type has received little attention, there is some evidence that cervical adenocarcinoma may resemble endometrial adenocarcinoma, particularly with respect to associations with nulliparity and obesity (Brinton et al, 1987b; Parazzini et al, 1988; Kjaer and Brinton, 1993). Since adenocarcinomas are more likely to contain HPV 18 than squamous carcinomas, HPV type may be a determinant of histologic type (Shroyer, 1993).

CONCEPTS OF PATHOGENESIS

The multistep pathogenesis of cervical cancer is understood more fully than for most cancers. Greater knowledge of pathogenesis implies increased complexity for the epidemiologist, in that the epidemiology of invasive cancer now includes the natural history of its precursor lesions, starting with the transmission of cervical HPV infection.

The Transmission of Cervical HPV Infection

The epidemiology of cervical HPV infections can be studied either on the molecular level (DNA detection) or the microscopic level (low-grade SIL). Cytologic diagnoses of low-grade SIL represent only about 10%–30% of molecularly detectable HPV infections, depending on the DNA test method. (Schiffman, 1992b) However, 30% of the women in whom molecular evidence of HPV infection is found, using a non-amplified test method, develop incident low-grade SIL within 4 years of viral detection (Schiffman et al, unpublished data). Thus, there is great overlap between microscopic and molecular diagnoses. This is logical because, from the point of view of the HPV life cycle, the atypical cells recognized microscopically as low-grade SIL are the production and assembly sites of new virions.

HPV infections are usually transmitted by person-to-person contact. Specifically, it is clear that cervical HPV infection is usually sexually transmitted (Fisher et al, 1991; Ley et al, 1991; Hildesheim et al, 1993). HPV infection of the cervix is rare in virgins (Fairley et al, 1992). The prevalence of cervical HPV DNA increases with reported numbers of different sexual partners, particularly recent partners because infection is often transient (Hildesheim et al, 1994).

Although proper transmission studies have not been done, it appears that genital HPV infections are transmitted rather easily between sexual partners. For example, the scant HPV DNA acquisition data suggest that among HPV-negative women, having new male sexual partners is associated with a high prevalence of cervical HPV (DNA) within months. Also, the age curve of cervical HPV prevalence, with a peak at ages 16–25, suggests that the transmission of HPV infection to the cervix occurs soon after the initiation of sexual intercourse (Schiffman, 1992b).

Although sexual transmission is the most important route, fomite transmission of HPV to the cervix appears theoretically possible based on findings of HPV DNA on underclothes and gynecologic equipment (Ferenczy et al, 1989; Ferenczy et al, 1990). Vertical transmission of genital types of HPV is certainly possible, although the frequency is unknown (Roman and Fife, 1986; Shah et al, 1986).

The Descriptive Epidemiology of Cervical HPV Infection

The cumulative lifetime probability of cervical infection with at least one type of HPV is extremely high for sexually active individuals (Schiffman, 1992b; Schneider et al, 1992). Because the typical detectable duration of HPV infection is short (less than 2–3 years), estimates of HPV incidence are similar to prevalence, but both grossly underestimate the cumulative incidence.

The HPV prevalence of a given population depends most strongly on the age and sexual practices of the population. Young sexually active women have the highest HPV prevalences (Fisher et al, 1991; Ley et al, 1991; Melkert et al, 1993; Moscicki et al, 1990; Rosenfeld et al, 1989). Although cervical HPV prevalence is highly influenced by age and sexual behavior (as well as diagnostic definition), estimates generally range from 1% to 3% based on screening diagnoses of low-grade SIL, 5% to 10% using non-amplified DNA tests, and 15% to 30% using PCR-based surveys. Published HPV DNA prevalences can range from 1% to nearly 100%, however, depending on the analytic sensitivity of the assay and the risk profile of the study group (Guerrero et al, 1992).

Most HPV prevalence studies, apart from case series of SIL and cancer, have not distinguished between the different genital HPV types. The many types of cervical HPV can only be distinguished at the molecular level. Based on scant data, HPV 16 is probably the most common type among normal women (2.4% of cytologically normal women in one large series) (Schiffman, 1994). Most of the still uncharacterized types of HPV are found among normal women and probably have virtually no oncogenic potential. Among infected women, the proportion with multiple infections typically approaches 20%–30% using PCR (Bauer et al, 1993).

As mentioned, the prevalence of cervical HPV infection declines sharply with age, from a peak prevalence at 16–25 years of age (Schiffman, 1992b). This age trend is seen for both HPV DNA detection and low-grade SIL in parallel. The very high prevalence of HPV in young, sexually active women is consistent with an "epidemic curve," a rapid rise in prevalence following first (sexual) exposure. The subsequent profound drop in cervical HPV prevalence in women over 30 might be due to immunologic clearance or suppression of existing infections, combined with less exposure to new HPV types because of fewer new sexual partners. The decrease in HPV prevalence with age might also be due partly to a "cohort effect," with an increase over time in the amount of cervical HPV infection among young female populations. Both the immunologic and cohort explanations for the decrease in cervical infection rates with age have scientific support (Schiffman and Burk, in press).

Progression to High-Grade SIL

Most HPV infections disappear within months to a few years after diagnosis. This is true for infections detected only by HPV DNA tests (Hildesheim et al, 1994) and for low-grade SIL, which tends to regress to cytologic normalcy. Uncommonly, however, HPV infections progress to high-grade SIL. The absolute risk of progression from low-grade to high-grade SIL is about 15%–25% over 2–4 years.

The prospective data generating the estimates of progression rates from low-grade to high-grade SIL are somewhat conflicting because of different diagnostic terminology and study methods (eg, cytologic versus histologic definitions of low-grade disease at enrollment). For example, in a 1–3 year study, Richart and Baron (1969) found a progression rate of 20.3% from what they termed "mild" to severe dysplasia. Using different pathologic criteria more akin to current terminology, Nasiell and colleagues (1986) observed that only 16% of 555 women with CIN 1 progressed to CIN 3 or invasive cancer (n = 2), despite a longer median observation period of 4 years. A recent British study documented a 35% rate of progression to CIN 3 over 1–2 years among 538 women with mild "dyskaryosis," a slightly more severe start point than low-grade SIL (Flannelly et al, 1994). Whichever estimates of absolute risk are accepted, women with low-grade SIL are at a substantially (over 16-fold) increased risk of developing high-grade SIL and invasive cervical cancer, compared with women with normal cytologic diagnoses (Soutter and Fletcher, 1994).

Nonetheless, the overall incidence of high-grade SIL is much less than 1% in most cervical cytologic screening series, at least in the United States. When divided, CIN 2 and CIN 3 are typically about equally diagnosed. The low prevalence of high-grade SIL compared with low-grade SIL is not as pronounced in regions with deficient cervical cancer screening and treatment, where high-grade lesions can develop and accumulate.

The three kinds of risk factors postulated to influence the risk of progression to high-grade SIL are the same as the established risk factors for cervical cancer: viral factors, host factors, and environmental cofactors.

With regard to viral factors, the most obvious is HPV type. Among women with low-grade SIL, the cancer-associated types of HPV (about two thirds of infections) predict a higher risk of progression than either the non-cancer-associated types or HPV negativity (Kataja et al, 1990; Campion et al, 1986). Apart from viral type, it appears from cross-sectional analyses that high levels of HPV DNA are closely linked to high-grade SIL (Morrison et al, 1991; Cuzick et al, 1992). Time since first infection may also be important (Munoz et al, 1993), because the degree of nuclear atypia may increase with the duration of infection (zur Hausen, 1994).

The most important host factors related to progression from low-grade to high-grade SIL are probably immunologic. Another host factor could be parity, which might act by influencing immunity or by hormonal, nutritional, or traumatic mechanisms (Munoz et al, 1993). Age has not been shown to be a strong predictor of risk of progression to high-grade SIL, once the severity of the initial diagnosis is taken into account (Nasiell et al, 1986).

The most likely environmental cofactors for the development of high-grade SIL are the established risk factors for cervical cancer that do not appear to be mere proxies for HPV infection. A role for smoking has some epidemiological support (Schiffman et al, 1993), but smoking has not been found to be associated with the development of high-grade SIL in a few recent, well-designed studies (Koutsky et al, 1992; Munoz et al, 1993). Other possible cofactors for the development of high-grade SIL include multiparity (Munoz et al, 1993), oral contraceptive use (Schiffman et al, 1993), deficiencies of folate, carotenoids, retinoids, or vitamin C (Butterworth et al, 1992a), and concurrent infection with other sexually transmitted agents such as chlamydia (Koutsky et al, 1992; de Sanjose et al, 1994).

It is unclear whether all cases of cervical cancer pass through each stage of the preinvasive continuum. For example, some cases of high-grade SIL arise in HPV-infected women within 1–2 years, without an appreciable intervening diagnosis of low-grade SIL (Koutsky et al, 1992), or adjacent to rather than arising directly from low-grade lesions (Kiviat et al, 1992). However, along with cohort studies, some "ecologic" support for a continuum of disease is provided by the observation that HPV infection and low-grade SIL are usually diagnosed among women in their late teens and early 20s, high-grade SIL in 25–35-year-olds, and invasive cancer after the age of 35–40 years.

High-Grade SIL to Invasive Cancer

The invasive potential of high-grade SIL (particularly carcinoma in situ) is very high, and women with high-grade SIL are less likely to regress than those with low-grade SIL. Peterson (1956) noted a 33% progression rate after 9 years among 127 women with untreated carcinoma in situ. Longer follow-up would presumably have led to even higher progression rates, given that regression of carcinoma in situ is not typical (Kinlen and Spriggs, 1978).

No risk factors have been found in case-control studies to distinguish invasive cancer from high-grade SIL, with the sole exception of age. Women with invasive cancer are 10 or more years older on average than women with high-grade SIL (Devesa et al, 1984). It may be that invasion is related to molecular events (eg, integration of HPV DNA into the host genome) that occur with low, nearly random frequency in the setting of persistent high-grade SIL.

PREVENTIVE MEASURES

The Papanicolaou (Pap) Smear

Because of the continuum of cervical neoplasia, there is little doubt that exfoliative cytology (the Pap smear), used to detect treatable cervical cancer precursors, can have profound effects on incidence and mortality. The eradication of precursor lesions has resulted in significant declines in cervical cancer rates in areas where screening has been widespread and prolonged, such as

Kentucky (Christopherson et al, 1970) and British Columbia (Boyes, 1981). In contrast, the rates for cervical cancer have not declined in regions or countries with limited screening programs (Hill, 1975).

A number of case-control studies have evaluated the role of Pap smear screening in preventing invasive cervical cancer. Clarke and Anderson (1979) found a relative risk of 0.37 associated with screening within the past 5 years; La Vecchia and colleagues (1984) found a risk of 0.18 if the patient had been screened within 3–5 years. In a Finnish study, even patients who had been screened more than 5 years previously had a relative risk of 0.67 compared to those who had never been screened (Olesen, 1988).

Although there is little doubt that cytology is an effective means of preventing cervical cancer, there is still extensive debate regarding the optimal interval of population-screening efforts. The American Cancer Society currently recommends that all women who are, or who have been, sexually active, or have reached 18 years of age, have an annual Pap test and pelvic examination. After a woman has had three or more consecutive satisfactory normal annual examinations, the Pap test may be performed less frequently at the discretion of her physician (Fink, 1988).

Ancillary Screening Methods

Because Pap smear screening is imperfect and not feasible in many resource-poor countries, refinements of the Pap smear or ancillary screening methods are continually being proposed. Screening methods can be categorized as clinical (visual), microscopic, or molecular.

Clinical screening denotes the detection of cervical lesions by inspection, sometimes aided by a magnifying eyepiece and tissue stains. In some very poor regions, clinical inspection may be the only currently affordable strategy, although it is not accurate. A currently promising clinical screening test is cervicography, which relies on photography of the cervix after staining with acetic acid to highlight visible abnormalities. The resultant images are magnified by projection onto a screen and read by experts, a procedure analogous to radiology. Cervicography is especially useful in detecting high-grade SIL and cancer, but its detection of low-grade SIL tends to have low specificity.

The Pap smear continues to be the major microscopic technique. Promising refinements now under evaluation are (1) new cell collection instruments designed to improve sampling of the cervical transformation zone, (2) transport of cell specimens in liquid media permitting automation of slide preparation, and (3) computer-assisted screening or rescreening of smears.

On the molecular level, HPV testing can be used to clarify and triage inconclusive Pap smear diagnoses (Cox et al, 1992; Schiffman and Sherman, 1994; Sherman et al, 1994). The borderline between normal and abnormal (SIL) cervical cytologic diagnoses has never been clear, as indicated by the plethora of uninformative terms such as "Class 2 Pap" or "atypia," which can account for up to 10% or more of diagnoses in some centers. HPV testing can be used as an independent reference standard for improving the diagnosis of equivocal smears in cytopathology laboratories.

More data are needed to establish whether HPV testing can be useful in two other important and theoretically appealing applications: general screening of older women and triage of low-grade SIL. HPV screening at older ages could be used to supplement Pap smears as a means of defining women at high risk (Melkert et al, 1993; Morrison et al, 1991). Because HPV DNA prevalence in cytologically normal women declines sharply with age, while HPV prevalence in women with cervical neoplasia remains very high regardless of age, the positive predictive value of finding HPV DNA rises with age (Morrison et al, 1991). Moreover, the use and accuracy of the Pap smear decline with age, due to inadequate sampling of receding transformation zones (false negatives) and overdiagnosis of atrophy-related changes (false positives). Thus, HPV detection and typing in older women might define a small subset of patients who remain at appreciable risk and could benefit from closer surveillance. Older women who are cytologically normal and have a negative HPV DNA test might be at very low risk for the development of cervical cancer and could be screened infrequently.

The diagnosis of low-grade SIL, by cytology or histology, is a poor marker of risk for the development of cervical cancer, because progression to invasive carcinoma is rare, even in untreated women. Many lesions regress spontaneously within months of detection. Colposcopically directed biopsy and ablation of all low-grade SIL represents possible overtreatment, with high costs and some associated morbidity. Natural history studies indicate that lesions associated with cancer-associated types of HPV are the most likely to progress (Campion et al, 1986; Kataja et al, 1990). A prospective clinical trial is needed to determine whether testing patients with low-grade SIL for both HPV type and a measure of viral load could result in safe and cost-effective clinical management, reducing the morbidity that can result from treatment. Cervicography might also be useful for this purpose.

Prevention of HPV Transmission

Prevention of transmission of HPV infections appears to be nearly unachievable, given current patterns of sexual activity. The exception may be that genital HPV transmission might be reduced by condom use, although this has not been proven. Condom use cannot entirely prevent the spread of genital HPV infections, because genital HPV infections in the male are not limited to the penile skin. Viral spread from scrotal and perineal lesions cannot be prevented by condom use, although it appears that these sites of infection are uncommon compared to lesions on the glans, foreskin, urethral meatus, or shaft (Rosemberg, 1991).

FUTURE RESEARCH

Multidisciplinary teams of investigators are attempting to piece together a coherent picture of HPV natural history and cervical carcinogenesis. Through large investigations that focus on increasing grades of neoplasia and time-related exposures, the multistage processes involved in tumor development and progression can be examined and factors that promote or inhibit transition to higher grades can be clarified.

Active areas of research include (1) validating reliable and inexpensive HPV test methods, to permit larger studies than are possible using intensive research techniques; (2) defining the epidemiology of HPV infection as a sexually transmitted disease, particularly the distribution of the different cancer-associated HPV types and the risk factors for transmission; (3) clarifying prospectively the natural history of HPV infections, focusing on viral persistence, disappearance, and latency; and (4) defining cofactors that may interact with HPV in the development of high-grade SIL and cancer.

The search for important HPV cofactors for high-grade SIL and cancer is likely to dominate future epidemiological research on cervical cancer. Although HPV infection explains much of what is known about classic risk factors for cervical neoplasia, particularly its venereal transmission, we still know little about potential cofactors. Therefore, even if HPV infection is the unifying, central risk factor for cervical neoplasia throughout the world, it is worth considering that necessary cofactors could vary considerably across different geographic regions. Smoking, for example, might be a cofactor in the United States, but as studies in Latin America have already demonstrated, it is unlikely to explain the occurrence of cervical cancer where heavy smoking among women is rare.

The importance of HPV persistence in the pathogenesis of high-grade SIL and cancer must be verified, and the determinants of persistence identified. If carcinomas arise only from persistent infections, not from molecularly inapparent ("latent") infections that suddenly reactivate, then prevention of carcinomas should be achievable by screening for virus at ages preceding the usual onset of carcinoma. The study of HPV persistence requires repeated measurements and extremely reliable HPV testing. It will be necessary to distinguish variants of HPV types (Chan et al, 1992) to permit, for example, the distinction of new HPV 16 infections from recurrent ones.

Through continued descriptive analyses and cohort studies, the decrease in cervical HPV infection rates with increasing age should be better understood. The separate contributions to the age trend of cohort effects and immunologic suppression must be distinguished because any cohort effect of increasing HPV infection in currently younger women might predict further increases in invasive cervical cancer in the future.

Although the study of cervical neoplasia is now inextricably linked to HPV infection, it will be important to define separately the epidemiology of the minority (15% or less) of cervical cancers that do not contain HPV-related DNA. It is possible that unknown HPV types may account for some of these tumors, but recent molecular studies have suggested that HPV-negative cancers may be an etiologically distinct group, perhaps associated with somatic mutations in tumor suppressor genes (Scheffner et al, 1991). Moreover, HPV-negative cervical cancer might have a worse prognosis (Riou et al, 1990; Higgins et al, 1991; de Britton et al, 1993). If cervical cancer can arise, albeit rarely, from precursor lesions not associated with HPV infection, the morphologic appearance and natural history of those precursor lesions must be defined. Also needed are studies to define hormonal and other risk factors for the rarely occurring adenocarcinomas and adenosquamous carcinomas of the cervix, whose epidemiology is poorly understood.

It will be important to verify or exclude the role of HPV in carcinomas of other sites. The natural history of HPV infection in the cervix should be compared to its natural history in the vagina, vulva, and anus. In particular, why the transformation zone of the cervix is so prone to HPV carcinogenesis should be addressed.

As the highest priority, HPV immunology is likely to occupy epidemiologists studying cervical cancer etiology and prevention over the next decade. In the immediate future, the interactions of multiple HPV types in mixed cervical infections should be clarified, as one pathway to understanding HPV immunity. Assays of cell-mediated immunity must be developed and applied. The ultimate goal will be to define the successful immune response to HPV infection, in the hope that cancer-preventive immunity can be stimulated by vaccination (Crawford, 1993).

Because HPV is a central cause of most cervical neoplasia, it is reasonable to consider HPV immunization as the ultimate primary preventive strategy for eliminating most cervical cancer. The protection of cattle herds from bovine papillomavirus infection by vaccination serves as a successful animal model (Campo et al, 1993). Use of the hepatitis B vaccine in Asia to reduce the incidence of hepatocellular carcinoma may serve as a public health model.

REFERENCES

ADAM E, KAUFMAN RH, MELNICK JL, et al. 1973. Seroepidemiologic studies of herpesvirus type 2 and carcinoma of the cervix. III. Houston, Texas. Am J Epidemiol 96:427–442.

AGARWAL SS, SEHGAL A, SARDANA S, et al. 1993. Role of male behavior in cervical carcinogenesis among women with one lifetime sexual partner. Cancer 72:1666–1669.

ALLERDING TJ, JORDAN, SW, BOARDMAN RE. 1985. Association of human papillomavirus and chlamydia infections with incidence cervical neoplasia. Acta Cytol 29:653–660.

AMBURGEY CF, VANEENWYK J, DAVIS FG, et al. 1993. Undernutrition as a risk factor for cervical intraepithelial neoplasia: a case-control analysis. Nutr Cancer 20:51–60.

ANDOLSEK L, KOVACIC J, KOZUH M, et al. 1983. Influence of oral contraceptives on the incidence of premalignant and malignant lesions of the cervix. Contraception 28:505–519.

APPLE RJ, ERLICH HA, KLITZ W, et al. 1994. HLA DR-DQ associations with cervical carcinoma show papillomavirus-type specificity. Nature Genet 6:157–162.

AUBORN KJ, WOODWORTH C, DIPAOLO JA, et al. 1991. The interaction between HPV infection and estrogen metabolism in cervical carcinogenesis. Int J Cancer 49:867–869.

BARNES W, DELGADO G, KURMAN RJ, et al. 1988. Possible prognostic significance of human papillomavirus type in cervical cancer. Gynecol Oncol 29:267–273.

BARON JA, BYERS T, GREENBERG ER. 1986. Cigarette smoking in women with cancers of the breast and reproductive organs. J Natl Cancer Inst 77:677–680.

BARRASSO R. 1992. HPV-related genital lesions in men. In: Munoz N, Bosch FX, Shah KV, et al (eds). The Epidemiology of Human Papillomavirus and Cervical Cancer. Lyon, IARC Monograph, pp 85–92.

BARRASSO R, DE BRUX J, CROISSANT O, et al. 1987. High prevalence of papillomavirus-associated penile intraepithelial neoplasia in sexual partners of women with cervical intraepithelial neoplasia. N Engl J Med 317:916–923.

BARTON SE, JENKINS D, CUZICK J, et al. 1988. Effect of cigarette smoking on cervical epithelial immunity: mechanism for neoplastic change? Lancet 2:652–654.

BASU J, PALAN PR, VERMUND SH, et al. 1991. Plasma ascorbic acid and beta-carotene levels in women evaluated for HPV infection, smoking, and cervix dysplasia. Cancer Detect Prev 15:165–170.

BATIEHA AM, ARMENIAN HK, NORKUS EP, et al. 1993. Serum micronutrients and the subsequent risk of cervical cancer in a population-based nested case-control study. Cancer Epidemiol Biomark Prev 2:335–339.

BAUER HM, TING Y, GREER CE, et al. 1991. Genital HPV infection in female university students as determined by a PCR-based method. JAMA 265:472–477.

BENDER S. 1976. Carcinoma in situ of cervix and sisters. Br Med J 502.

BERAL V. 1974. Cancer of the cervix: a sexually-transmitted infection? Lancet 1:1037–1040.

BERAL V, HANNAFORD P, KAY C. 1988. Oral contraceptive use and malignancies of the genital tract: results from The Royal College of General Practitioners' Oral Contraceptive Study. Lancet 2:1331–1335.

BERAL V, HERMON C, MUNOZ N, et al. 1994. Cervical cancer. Cancer Surveys Volume 19/20: Trends in Cancer Incidence and Mortality, pp 265–285.

BERGMAN A, NALICK R. 1992. Prevalence of human papillomavirus infection in men: comparison of the partners of infected and uninfected women. J Reprod Med 37:710–712.

BORING CC, SQUIRES TS, TONG T, et al. 1994. Cancer statistics, 1994. CA 44:7–26.

BOSCH FX, MANOS MM, MUNOZ N, et al. 1995. Prevalence of human papillomavirus in cervical cancer: a worldwide perspective. J Natl Cancer Inst 87:796–802.

BOSCH FX, MUNOZ N, DE SANJOSE S, et al. 1992. Risk factors for cervical cancer in Colombia and Spain. Int J Cancer 52:750–758.

BOYCE JG, LU T, NELSON JH, et al. 1977. Oral contraceptives and cervical carcinoma. Am J Obstet Gynecol 128:761–766.

BOYD JT, DOLL R. 1964. A study of the aetiology of carcinoma of the cervix uteri. Br J Cancer 18:419–434.

BOYES DA. 1981. The value of a pap smear program and suggestions for its implementation. Cancer 48:613–621.

BRINTON LA, HAMMAN RF, HUGGINS GR, et al. 1987a. Sexual and reproductive risk factors for invasive squamous cell cervical cancer. J Natl Cancer Inst 79:23–30.

BRINTON LA, HERRERO R, FRAUMENI JF JR. 1989a. Response. J Clin Epidemiol 42:927–928.

BRINTON LA, HUGGINS GR, LEHMAN HF, et al. 1986a. Long-term use of oral contraceptives and risk of invasive cervical cancer. Int J Cancer 38:339–344.

BRINTON LA, REEVES WC, BRENES MM, et al. 1989c. The male factor in the etiology of cervical cancer among sexually monogamous women. Int J Cancer 44:199–203.

BRINTON LA, REEVES WC, BRENES MM, et al. 1989b. Parity as a risk factor for cervical cancer. Am J Epidemiol 130:486–496.

BRINTON LA, REEVES WC, BRENES MM, et al. 1990. Oral contraceptive use and risk of invasive cervical cancer. Int J Epidemiol 19:4–11.

BRINTON LA, SCHAIRER C, HAENSZEL W, et al. 1986b. Cigarette smoking and invasive cervical cancer. JAMA 255:3265–3269.

BRINTON LA, TASHIMA KT, LEHMAN HF, et al. 1987b. Epidemiology of cervical cancer by cell type. Cancer Res 47:1706–1711.

BRINTON LA. 1991. Oral contraceptives and cervical neoplasia. Contraception 43:581–595.

BROCK KE, BERRY G, BRINTON LA, et al. 1989a. Sexual, reproductive and contraceptive risk factors for carcinoma-in-situ of the uterine cervix in Sydney. Med J Aust 150:125–130.

BROCK KE, BERRY G, MOCK PA, et al. 1988. Nutrients in diet and plasma and risk of in situ cervical cancer. J Natl Cancer Inst 80:580–585.

BROCK KE, MACLENNAN R, BRINTON LA, et al. 1989b. Smoking and infectious agents and risk of in situ cervical cancer in Sydney, Australia. Cancer Res 49:4925–4928.

BUCKLEY JD, HARRIS RWC, DOLL R, et al. 1981. Case-control study of the husbands of women with dysplasia or carcinoma of the cervix uteri. Lancet 2:1010–1015.

BURGER MPM, HOLLEMA H, GOUW ASH, et al. 1993. Cigarette smoking and human papillomavirus in patients with reported cervical cytological abnormality. Br Med J 306:749–752.

BUTTERWORTH CE JR, HATCH KD, MACALUSO M, et al. 1992a. Folate deficiency and cervical dysplasia. JAMA 267:528–533.

BUTTERWORTH CE JR, HATCH KD, SOONG S-J, et al. 1992b. Oral folic acid supplementation for cervical dysplasia: a clinical intervention trial. Am J Obstet Gynecol 166:803–809.

BUTTERWORTH CE JR, HATCH KD, GORE H, et al. 1982. Improvement in cervical dysplasia associated with folic acid therapy in users of oral contraceptives. Am J Clin Nutr 35:73–82.

CAMPION MJ, MCCANCE DJ, CUZICK J, et al. 1986. Progressive potential of mild cervical atypia: prospective cytological, colposcopic, and virological study. Lancet 2:237–240.

CAMPION MJ, SINGER A, CLARKSON PK, et al. 1985. Increased risk of cervical neoplasia in consorts of men with penile condylomata acuminata. Lancet 1:943–946.

CAMPO MS, GRINDLAY GJ, O'NEIL BW, et al. 1993. Prophylactic and therapeutic vaccination against a mucosal papillomavirus. J Gen Viro 74:945–953.

CARMICHAEL JA, CLARKE DH, MOHER D, et al. 1986. Cervical carcinoma in women aged 34 and younger. Am J Obstet Gynecol 154:264–269.

CARTWRIGHT RA, SINSON JD. 1980. Carcinoma of penis and cervix. Lancet 1(8159):97.

CELENTANO DD, KLASSEN AC, WEISMAN CS, et al. 1987. The role of contraceptive use in cervical cancer: the Maryland cervical cancer case-control study. Am J Epidemiol 126:592–604.

CHAN SY, HO L, ONG CK, et al. 1992. Molecular variants of human papillomavirus type 16 from four continents suggest ancient pandemic spread of the virus and its coevolution with humankind. J Viro 66:2057–2066.

CHILVERS C, MANT D, PIKE MC. 1987. Cervical adenocarcinoma and oral contraceptives. Br Med J 295:1446–1447.

CHRISTOPHERSON WM, PARKER JE, MENDEZ WM, et al. 1970. Cervix cancer death rates and mass cytologic screening. Cancer 26:808–811.

CHUMAS JC, NELSON B, MANN WJ, et al. 1985. Microglandular hyperplasia of the uterine cervix. Obstet Gynecol 66:406–409.

CLARKE EA, ANDERSON TW. 1979. Does screening by "pap" smears help prevent cervical cancer? A case-control study. Lancet 2:1–4.

CLARKE EA, MORGAN RW, NEWMAN AM. 1982. Smoking as a risk factor in cancer of the cervix: additional evidence from a case-control study. Am J Epidemiol 115:59–66.

COKER AL, MCCANN MF, HULKA BS, et al. 1992. Oral contraceptive use and cervical intraepithelial neoplasia. J Clin Epidemiol 45:1111–1118.

COLEMAN MP, ESTEVE J, DAMIECKI P, et al. 1993. Trends in cancer incidence and mortality. IARC Scientific Publications No 121. Lyon: IARC.

COX JT, SCHIFFMAN MH, WINZELBERG AJ, et al. 1992. An evaluation of HPV testing as a part of referral to colposcopy clinic. Obstet Gynecol 80:389–395.

CRAWFORD L. 1993. Prospects for cervical cancer vaccines. Cancer Surv 16:215–229.

CROSS HE, KENNEL EE, LILIENFELD AM. 1968. Cancer of the cervix in an Amish population. Cancer 21:102–108.

CULLEN AP, REID R, CAMPION M, et al. 1991. Analysis of the physical state of different human papillomavirus DNAs in intraepithelial and invasive cervical neoplasms. J Virol 65:605–612.

CUZICK J, SINGER A, DE STAVOLA BL, et al. 1990. Case-control study of risk factors for cervical intraepithelial neoplasia in young women. Eur J Cancer 26:684–890.

CUZICK J, TERRY G, HO L, et al. 1992. Human papillomavirus type 16 DNA in cervical smears as a predictor of high-grade cervical intraepithelial neoplasia. Lancet 339:959–960.

DABANCENS A, PRADO R, LARRAGUIBEL R, et al. 1974. Intraepithelial cervical neoplasia in women using intrauterine devices and long-acting injectable progestogens as contraceptives. Am J Obstet Gynecol 119:1052–1056.

DALING JR, SHERMAN KJ, HISLOP TG, et al. 1992. Cigarette smoking and the risk of anogenital cancer. Am J Epidemiol 135:180–189.

DALLENBACH-HELLWEG G. 1984. On the origin and histological structure of adenocarcinoma in women under 50 years of age. Pathol Res Pract 179:38–50.

DE BRITTON RC, HILDESHEIM A, DELAO SL, et al. 1993. Human papillomavirus and other influences on survival from cervical cancer in Panama. Obstet Gynecol 81:19–24.

DE SANJOSE S, MUNOZ N, BOSCH FX, et al. 1994. Sexually transmitted agents and cervical neoplasia in Colombia and Spain. Int J Cancer 56:358–363.

DE VET HCW, KNIPSCHILD PG, GROL MEC, et al. 1991. The role of beta-carotene and other dietary factors in the aetiology of cervical dysplasia: results of a case-control study. Int J Epidemiol 20:603–610.

DE VILLIERS EM, SCHNEIDER A, MIKLAW H, et al. 1987. Human papillomavirus infections in women with and without abnormal cervical cytology. Lancet 2:703–706.

DEVESA SS, DIAMOND EL. 1980. Association of breast cancer and cervical cancer incidences with income and education among whites and blacks. J Natl Cancer Inst 65:515–528.

DEVESA SS. 1984. Descriptive epidemiology of cancer of the uterine cervix. Obstet Gynecol 63:605.

DEVESA SS, SILVERMAN DT, YOUNG JL JR, et al. 1987. Cancer incidence and mortality trends among whites in the United States, 1947–84. J Natl Cancer Inst 79:701–770.

DEVESA SS, YOUNG JL JR, BRINTON LA, et al. 1989. Recent trends in cervix uteri cancer. Cancer 64:2184–2190.

DYSON N, HOWLEY PM, MUNGER K, et al. 1989. The human papilloma virus-16 E7 oncoprotein is able to bind to the retinoblastoma gene product. Science 243:934–937.

EBELING K, NISCHAN P, SCHINDLER CH. 1987. Use of oral contraceptives and risk of invasive cervical cancer in previously screened women. Int J Cancer 39:427–430.

ELUF-NETO J, BOOTH M, MUNOZ N, et al. 1994. Human papillomavirus and invasive cancer in Brazil. Br J Cancer 69:114–119.

EVANS AS, MUELLER NE. 1990. Viruses and cancer: causal associations. Ann Epidemiol 1:71–92.

EVANS S, DOWLING K. 1990. The changing prevalence of cervical human papilloma virus infection. Aust N Z J Obstet Gynaecol 30:375–377.

FAIRLEY CK, CHEN S, TABRIZI SN, et al. 1992. The absence of genital human papillomavirus DNA in virginal women. Int J STD AIDS 3:414–417.

FASAL E, SIMMONS ME, KAMPERT JB. 1981. Factors associated with high and low risk of cervical neoplasia. J Natl Cancer Inst 66:631–636.

FERENCZY A, BERGERON C, RICHART RM. 1989. Human papillomavirus DNA in fomites on objects used for the management of patients with genital human papillomavirus infections. Obstet Gynecol 74:950–954.

FERENCZY A, BERGERON C, RICHART RM. 1990. Human papillomavirus DNA in CO2 laser-generated plume of smoke and its consequences to the surgeon. Obstet Gynecol 75:114–118.

FERENCZY A, WRIGHT TC. 1993. Managing abnormal Papanicolaou results — large-loop excision of the transformation zone. Female Patient 18:37–44.

FENOGLIO CM, FERENCZY A. 1982. Etiologic factors in cervical neoplasia. Semin Oncol 9:349–372.

FINK DJ. 1988. Change in American Cancer Society guidelines for detection of cervical cancer. CA 38:127–128.

FISHER M, ROSENFELD WD, BURK RD. 1991. Cervicovaginal human papillomavirus infection in suburban adolescents and young adults. J Pediatr 119:821–825.

FLANNELLY G, ANDERSON D, KITCHENER HC, et al. 1994. Management of woman with mild and moderate cervical dyskaryosis. Br Med J 308:1399–1403.

FRANCO EL. 1991. The sexually transmitted disease model for cervical cancer: incoherent epidemiologic findings and the role of misclassification of human papillomavirus infection. Epidemiology 2:98–106.

FRANCO EL. 1992. Prognostic value of human papillomavirus in the survival of cervical cancer patients: an overview of the evidence. Cancer Epidemiol Biomark Prev 1:499–504.

FRAUMENI JF JR, LLOYD JW, SMITH EM, et al. 1969. Cancer mortality among nuns: Role of marital status in etiology of neoplastic disease in women. J Natl Cancer Inst 42:455–468.

FUCHS PG, GIRARDI F, PFISTER H. 1988. Human papillomavirus DNA in normal, metaplastic, preneoplastic and neoplastic epithelia of the cervix uteri. Int J Cancer 41:41–45.

FURGYIK S, GRUBB R, KULLANDER S, et al. 1986. Familial occurrence of cervical cancer, stages 0–IV. Acta Obstet Gynecol Scand 65:223–227.

GALLOWAY D. 1992. Serological assays for the detection of HPV antibodies. In: The Epidemiology of Human Papillomavirus and Cervical Cancer, Vol 119, Munoz N, Bosch FX, Shah KV, et al (eds). Lyon, IARC Scientific Publications, pp 147–161.

GRAHAM S, PRIORE R, GRAHAM M, et al. 1979. Genital cancer in wives of penile cancer patients. Cancer 44:1870–1874.

GRAHAM S, SCHOTZ W. 1979. Epidemiology of cancer of the cervix in Buffalo, New York. J Natl Cancer Inst 63:23–27.

GRAVITT PE, MANOS MM. 1992. Polymerase chain reaction-based methods for the detection of human papillomavirus DNA. In: The Epidemiology of Human Papillomavirus and Cervical Cancer, Vol 119, Munoz N, Bosch FX, Shah KV, et al (eds). Lyon, IARC Scientific Publications, pp 121–133.

GREEN GH. 1979. Rising cervical cancer mortality in young New Zealand women. N Z Med J 89:89–91.

GREENBERG ER, VESSEY M, MCPHERSON K, et al. 1985. Cigarette smoking and cancer of the uterine cervix. Br J Cancer 51:139–141.

GUERRERO E, DANIEL RW, BOSCH X, et al. 1992. Comparison of virapap, Southern hybridization, and polymerase chain reaction methods for human papillomavirus identification in an epidemiological investigation of cervical cancer. J Clin Microbiol 30:2951–2959.

HAKAMA M, LEHTINEN M, KNEKT P, et al. 1993. Serum antibodies and subsequent cervical neoplasms: a prospective study with 12 years of follow-up. Am J Epidemiol 137:166–170.

HARRIS RWC, FORMAN D, DOLL R, et al. 1986. Cancer of the cervix uteri and vitamin A. Br J Cancer 53:653–659.

HARRIS RWC, BRINTON LA, COWDELL RH, et al. 1980. Characteristics of women with dysplasia or carcinoma in situ of the cervix uteri. Br J Cancer 42:359–369.

HARRIS RW, SCOTT WA. 1979. Vasectomy and cancer of the cervix. N Engl J Med 301:1064–1065.

HELLBERG D, VALENTIN J, NILSSON S. 1983. Smoking as risk factor in cervical neoplasia. Lancet 2:1497.

HERMONAT PL, DANIEL RW, SHAH KV. 1992. The spermicide nonoxynol-9 does not inactivate papillomavirus. Sex Transm Dis 19:203–205.

HERRERO R, BRINTON LA, REEVES WC, et al. 1989. Invasive cervical cancer and smoking in Latin America. J Natl Cancer Inst 81:205–211.

HERRERO R, BRINTON LA, REEVES WC, et al. 1990a. Injectable contraceptives and risk of invasive cervical cancer: evidence of an association. Int J Cancer 46:5–7.

HERRERO R, BRINTON LA, REEVES WC, et al. 1990b. Sexual behavior, venereal diseases, hygiene practices, and invasive cervical cancer in a high-risk population. Cancer 65:380–386.

HERRERO R, POTISCHMAN N, BRINTON LA, et al. 1991. A case-control study of nutrient status and invasive cervical cancer. I. Dietary indicators. Am J Epidemiol 134:1335–1346.

HIGGINS GD, DAVY M, RODER D, et al. 1991. Increased age and mortality associated with cervical carcinomas negative for human papillomavirus RNA. Lancet 338:910–913.

HILDESHEIM A, BRINTON LA, MALLIN K, et al. 1990. Barrier and spermicidal contraceptive methods and risk of invasive cervical cancer. Epidemiology 1:266–272.

HILDESHEIM A, GRAVITT P, SCHIFFMAN MH, et al. 1993. Determinants of genital human papillomavirus infection in low-income women in Washington, D.C. Sex Transm Dis 20:279–285.

HILDESHEIM A, MANN V, BRINTON LA, et al. 1991. Herpes simplex virus type 2: a possible interaction with human papillomavirus types 16/18 in the development of cervical cancer. Int J Cancer 38:335–341.

HILDESHEIM A, SCHIFFMAN MH, GRAVITT P, et al. 1994. Persistence of type-specific human papillomavirus infection among cytologically normal women in Portland, Oregon. J Infect Dis 169:235–240.

HILL AB. 1965. Environment and disease: association or causation? Proc R Soc Med 58:295–300.

HILL GB. 1975. Mortality from malignant neoplasm of the uterus since 1950. World Health Stat Rep 28:323–327.

HO GYF, BURK RD, FLEMING I, et al. 1994. Risk for human papillomavirus infection in women with human immunodeficiency virus-induced immunosuppression. Int J Cancer 56:788–792.

HOLMAN CDJ, ARMSTRONG BK. 1987. Cervical cancer mortality trends in Australia—an update. Med J Aust 146:410–412.

HOOVER R. 1977. Effects of drugs—immunosuppression. In: Origins of Human Cancer, Hiatt HH, Watson JD, Winsten JA (eds). Cold Spring Harbor Conferences on Cell Proliferation 4. Cold Spring Harbor Laboratory, pp 369–379.

IARC WORKING GROUP. 1995. IARC Monographs on the Evaluation of Carcinogenic Risks to Humans Vol. 64: Human papillomaviruses. International Agency for Research on Cancer, Lyon, France.

IRWIN KL, ROSERO-BIXBY L, OBERLE MW, et al. 1988. Oral contraceptives and cervical cancer risk in Costa Rica: detection bias or causal association? JAMA 259:59–64.

JARRETT WFH, MCNEIL PE, GRIMSHAW WTR, et al. 1978. High incidence area of cattle cancer with a possible interaction between an environmental carcinogen and a papilloma virus. Nature 274:215–217.

JHA PKS, BERAL V, PETO J, et al. 1993. Antibodies to human papillomavirus and to other genital infectious agents and invasive cervical cancer risk. Lancet 341:1116–1118.

JONES EG, MACDONALD I, BRESLOW L. 1958. A study of epidemiologic factors in carcinoma of the uterine cervix. Am J Obstet Gynecol 76:1–10.

KAEBLING M, BURK RD, ATKIN NB, et al. 1992. Loss of heterozygosity in the region of the TP53 gene on chromosome 17p in HPV-negative human cervical carcinomas. Lancet 340:140–142.

KATAJA V, SYRJANEN K, SYRJANEN S, et al. 1990. Prospective follow-up of genital HPV infections: survival analysis of the HPV typing data. Eur J Epidemiol 6:9–14.

KESSLER II. 1977. Venereal factors in human cervical cancer: evidence from marital clusters. Cancer 39:1912–1919.

KINLEN LJ, SPRIGGS AI. 1978. Women with positive cervical smears but without surgical intervention: a follow-up study. Lancet 2:463–465.

KIRNBAUER R, HUBBERT NL, WHEELER CM, et al. 1994. A virus-like particle ELISA detects serum antibodies in a majority of women infected with human papillomavirus type 16. J Natl Cancer Inst 86:494–499.

KIVIAT NB, KOUTSKY LA, PAAVONEN JA, et al. 1989. Prevalence of genital papillomavirus infection among women attending a college student health clinic or a sexually transmitted disease clinic. J Infect Dis 159:293–302.

KIVIAT NB, CRITCHLOW CW, KURMAN RJ. 1992. Reassessment of the morphological continuum of cervical intraepithelial lesions: does it relfect different stages in the progression to cervical carcinoma? In: The Epidemiology of Human Papillomavirus and Cervical Cancer, Munoz N, Bosch FX, Shah KV, et al (eds). Lyon: IARC Scientific Publications, pp 59–66.

KJAER SK, BRINTON LA. 1993. Adenocarcinomas of the uterine cervix: the epidemiology of an increasing problem. Epidemiol Rev 15:486–498.

KJAER SK, DAHL C, ENGHOLM G, et al. 1992. Case-control study of risk factors for cervical neoplasia in Denmark. II. Role of sexual activity, reproductive factors, and venereal infections. Cancer Causes Control 3:339–348.

Kjaer SK, de Villiers EM, Dahl C, et al. 1991. Case-control study of risk factors for cervical neoplasia in Denmark. I. Role of the "male factor" in women with one lifetime sexual partner. Int J Cancer 48:29–44.

Kjaer SK, Engholm G, Dahl C, et al. 1993. Case-control study of risk factors for cervical squamous-cell neoplasia in Denmark. III. Role of oral contraceptive use. Cancer Causes Control 4:513–519.

Kjaerheim K, Andersen A. 1994. Cancer incidence among waitresses in Norway. Cancer Causes Control 5:31–37.

Knekt P. 1988. Serum vitamin E level and risk of female cancers. Int J Epidemiol 17:281–286.

Koutsky LA, Galloway DA, Holmes KK. 1988. Epidemiology of genital human papillomavirus infection. Epidemiol Rev 10:122–163.

Koutsky LA, Holmes KK, Critchlow CW, et al. 1992. A cohort study of the risk of cervical intraepithelial neoplasia grade 2 or 3 in relation to papillomavirus infection. N Engl J Med 327:1272–1278.

Kreider JW, Howett MK, Wolfe SA, et al. 1985. Morphological transformation in vivo of human uterine cervix with papillomavirus from condylomata acuminata. Nature 317:639–641.

Kreiss JK, Kiviat NB, Plummer FA, et al. 1992. Human immunodeficiency virus, human papillomavirus, and cervical intraepithelial neoplasia in Nairobi prostitutes. Sex Trans Dis 19:54–59.

Kurman RJ, Solomon D. 1994. The Bethesda System for Reporting Cervical/Vaginal Cytologic Diagnoses. New York: Springer-Verlag.

Kurman RJ, Toki T, Schiffman MH. 1993. Basaloid and warty carcinomas of the vulva: Distinctive types of squamous cell carcinoma frequently associated with human papillomavirus. Am J Surg Pathol 17:133–145.

La Vecchia C, Decarli A, Fasoli M, et al. 1988. Dietary vitamin A and the risk of intraepithelial and invasive neoplasia. Gynecol Oncol 30:187–195.

La Vecchia C, Decarli A, Gentile A, et al. 1984. "Pap" smear and the risk of cervical neoplasia: quantitative estimates from a case-control study. Lancet 2:779–782.

La Vecchia C, Franceschi S, Decarli A, et al. 1986a. Cigarette smoking and the risk of cervical neoplasia. Am J Epidemiol 123:22–29.

La Vecchia C, Franceschi S, Decarli A, et al. 1986b. Sexual factors, venereal diseases, and the risk of intraepithelial and invasive cervical neoplasia. Cancer 58:935–941.

Lancaster WD, Castellano C, Santos C, et al. 1986. Human papillomavirus deoxyribonucleic acid in cervical carcinoma from primary and metastatic sites. Am J Obstet Gynecol 154:115–119.

Lancaster WD, Olson C. 1982. Animal papillomaviruses. Microbiol Rev 46:191–207.

Ley C, Bauer HM, Reingold A, et al. 1991. Determinants of genital papillomavirus infection in young women. J Natl Cancer Inst 83:997–1003.

Lorincz AT, Reid R, Jenson B, et al. 1992. Human papillomavirus infection of the cervix: relative risk associations of 15 common anogenital types. Obstet Gynecol 79:328–337.

Lorincz AT, Schiffman MH, Jaffurs WJ, et al. 1990. Temporal associations of human papillomavirus infection with cervical cytologic abnormalities. Am J Obstet Gynecol 162:645–651.

Ley C, Bauer HM, Reingold A, et al. 1991. Determinants of genital human papillomavirus infection in young women. J Natl Cancer Inst 83:997–1003.

Li JY, Li FP, Blot WJ, et al. 1982. Correlation between cancers of the uterine cervix and penis in China. J Natl Cancer Inst 69:1063–1065.

Lilienfeld AM, Graham S. 1958. Validity of determining circumcision status by questionnaire as related to epidemiological studies of cancer of the cervix. J Natl Cancer Inst 21:713–720.

Litt BP. 1975. Statistical review of carcinoma in situ reported among contraceptive users of Depoprovera. Memorandum of 17 June 1974 to United States Food and Drug Administration hearing on Depoprovera.

Liu T, Soong S-J, Wilson NP, et al. 1993. A case control study of nutritional factors and cervical dysplasia. Cancer Epidemiol Biomark Prev 2:525–530.

Lorincz AT. 1992. Detection of human papillomavirus DNA without amplification: prospects for clinical utility. In: *The Epidemiology of Human Papillomavirus and Cervical Cancer*, Vol 119, Munoz N, Bosch FX, Shah KV, et al (eds). Lyon: IARC Scientific Publications, pp 135–145.

Lorincz AT, Reid R, Jenson AB, et al. 1992. Human papillomavirus infection of the cervix: relative risk associations of 15 common anogenital types. Obstet Gynecol 79:328–337.

Lorincz AT, Schiffman MH, Jaffurs WJ, et al. 1990. Temporal associations of human papillomavirus infection with cervical cytologic abnormalities. Am J Obstet Gynecol 162:645–651.

Lyon JL, Gardner K, Gress RE. 1994. Cancer incidence among Mormons and non-Mormons in Utah (United States) 1971–85. Cancer Causes Control 5:149–156.

Lyon JL, Gardner JW, West DW, et al. 1983. Smoking and carcinoma in situ of the uterine cervix. Am J Public Health 73:558–562.

MacGregor JE, Innes G. 1980. Carcinoma of penis and cervix (Letter). Lancet 1:1246–1247.

Maiman M, Tarricone N, Vieira J, et al. 1991. Colposcopic evaluation of human immunodeficiency virus-seropositive women. Obstet Gynecol 78:84–88.

Marshall JR, Graham S, Byers T, et al. 1983. Diet and smoking in the epidemiology of cancer of the cervix. J Natl Cancer Inst 70:847–851.

Martin CE. 1967. Marital and coital factors in cervical cancer. Am J Public Health 57:803–814.

Martinez I. 1969. Relationship of squamous cell carcinoma of the cervix uteri to squamous cell carcinoma of the penis among Puerto Rican women married to men with penile carcinoma. Cancer 24:777–780.

Matas AJ, Simmons RL, Kjellstrand CM, et al. 1975. Increased incidence of malignancy during chronic renal failure. Lancet 1:883–885.

McArdle JP, Muller HK. 1986. Quantitative assessment of Langerhans' cells in human cervical intraepithelial neoplasia and wart virus infection. Am J Obstet Gynecol 154:509–515.

McCance DJ, Clarkson PK, Chesters PM, et al. 1985. Prevalence of human papillomavirus type 16 DNA sequences in cervical intraepithelial neoplasia and invasive carcinoma of the cervix. Br J Obstet Gynaecol 92:1101–1105.

McCance DJ, Kopan R, Fuchs E, et al. 1988. Human papillomavirus type 16 alters human epithelial cell differentiation in vitro. Proc Natl Acad Sci U S A 85:7169–7173.

McCann MF, Irwin DE, Walton LA, et al. 1992. Nicotine and cotinine in the cervical mucus of smokers, passive smokers, and nonsmokers. Cancer Epidemiol Biomark Prev 1:125–129.

McDougall JK, Beckmann AM, Galloway DA. 1986. The enigma of viral nucleic acids in genital neoplasia. In: *Viral Etiology of Cervical Cancer*, Banbury Report 21, Peto R, zur Hausen H (eds). Cold Spring Harbor Laboratory, pp 199–210.

Meanwell CA, Blackledge G, Cox MF, et al. 1987. HPV 16 DNA in normal and malignant cervical epithelium: implications for the aetiology and behaviour of cervical neoplasia. Lancet 1:703–707.

Meisels A, Fortin R. 1976. Condylomatous lesions of the cervix and vagina. I. Cytologic patterns. Acta Cytol 20:505–509.

Melamed MR, Koss LG, Flehinger BJ, et al. 1969. Prevalence

rates of uterine cervical carcinoma in situ for women using the diaphragm or contraceptive oral steroids. Br Med J 3:195–200.

MELKERT PWJ, HOPMAN E, VAN DEN BRULE AJC, et al. 1993. Prevalence of HPV in cytomorphologically normal cervical smears, as determined by the polymerase chain reaction, is age-dependent. Int J Cancer 53:919–923.

MEYSKENS FL JR, SURWIT E, MOON TE, et al. 1994. Enhancement of regression of cervical intraepithelial neoplasia II (moderate dysplasia) with topically applied all-trans-retinoic acid: a randomized trial. J Natl Cancer Inst 86:539–543.

MOGHISSI KS, MACK HC, PORZAK JP. 1968. Epidemiology of cervical cancer: study of a prison population. Am J Obstet Gynecol 100:607–612.

MOLINA R, THOMAS DB, DABANCENS A, et al. 1988. Oral contraceptives and cervical carcinoma in situ in Chile. Cancer Res 48:1011–1015.

MONSONEGO J, MAGDALENAT H, CATALAN F, et al. 1991. Estrogen and progesterone receptors in cervical human papillomavirus related lesions. Int J Cancer 48:533–539.

MORRISON EAB, BURK RD. 1993. Classification of human papillomavirus infection. JAMA 270:453.

MORRISON EAB, HO GYF, VERMUND SH, et al. 1991. Human papillomavirus infection and other risk factors for cervical neoplasia: a case-control study. Int J Cancer 49:6–13.

MOSCICKI A-B, PALEFSKY J, GONZALES J, et al. 1990. Human papillomavirus infection in sexually active adolescent females: prevalence and risk factors. Pediatr Res 28:507–513.

MOSCICKI AB, PALEFSKY J, SMITH G, et al. 1993. Variability of human papillomavirus DNA testing in a longitudinal cohort of young women. Obstet Gynecol 82:578–585.

MUNOZ N. 1992. HPV and cervical cancer: review of case-control and cohort studies. In: *The Epidemiology of Human Papillomavirus and Cervical Cancer*, Vol 119, Munoz N, Bosch FX, Shah KV, et al (eds). Lyon: IARC Scientific Publications, pp 251–261.

MUNOZ N, BOSCH FX, DE SANJOSE S, et al. 1992. The causal link between human papillomavirus and invasive cervical cancer: a population-based case-control study in Colombia and Spain. Int J Cancer 52:743–749.

MUNOZ N, BOSCH FX, DE SANJOSE S, et al. 1993. Risk factors for cervical intraepithelial neoplasia grade III/ carcinoma in situ in Spain and Colombia. Cancer Epidemiol Biomark Prev 2:423–431.

NASIELL K, ROGER V, NASIELL M. 1986. Behavior of mild cervical dysplasia during long-term follow-up. Obstet Gynecol 67:665–669.

NATIONAL CANCER INSTITUTE WORKSHOP. 1989. The 1988 Bethesda system for reporting cervical/vaginal cytologic diagnoses. JAMA 262:931–934.

NATIONAL CANCER INSTITUTE. 1984. Cancer Among Blacks and Other Minorities: Statistical Profiles. U.S. Dept. of Health and Human Services, Public Health Service, National Institutes of Health.

NIRUTHISARD S, TRISUKOSOL D. 1991. Male sexual behavior as risk factor in cervical cancer. J Med Assoc Thai 10:507–512.

OLESEN F. 1988. A case-control study of cervical cytology before diagnosis of cervical cancer in Denmark. Int J Epidemiol 17:501–508.

ORTH G, FAVRE M, BREITBURD F, et al. 1980. Epidermodysplasia verruciformis: a model for the role of papilloma viruses in human cancer. In: Viruses in Naturally Occurring Cancers, Essex M, Todaro G, zur Hausen H (eds). Cold Spring Harbor Conferences on Cell Proliferation 7, Cold Spring Harbor Laboratory, pp 259–282.

PALAN PR, MIKHAIL MS, BASU J, et al. 1991. Plasma levels of antioxidant beta-carotene and alpha-tocopherol in uterine cervix dysplasias and cancer. Nutr Cancer 15:13–20.

PALEFSKY JM, HOLLY EA, GONZALES J, et al. 1991. Detection of human papillomavirus DNA in anal intraepithelial neoplasia and anal cancer. Cancer Res 51:1014–1019.

PARAZZINI F, LA VECCHIA C, NEGRI E, et al. 1989. Reproductive factors and the risk of invasive and intraepithelial cervical neoplasia. Br J Cancer 59:805–809.

PARAZZINI F, LA VECCHIA C, NEGRI E, et al. 1988. Risk factors for adenocarcinoma of the cervix: a case-control study. Br J Cancer 57:201–204.

PARAZZINI F, LA VECCHIA C, NEGRI E, et al. 1990. Oral contraceptive use and invasive cervical cancer. Int J Epidemiol 19:259–263.

PARKIN DM, MUIR CS, WHELAN SL, et al. 1992. Cancer Incidence in Five Continents, Vol VI. IARC Publ No. 120. Lyon: International Agency for Research on Cancer.

PARKIN DM, NGUYEN-DINH X, DAY NE. 1985. The impact of screening on the incidence of cervical cancer in England and Wales. Br J Obstet Gynecol 92:150–157.

PARKIN DM, PISANI P, FERLAY J. 1993. Estimates of the worldwide frequency of eighteen major cancers in 1985. Int J Cancer 54:594–606.

PATER A, BAYATPOUR M, PATER MM. 1990. Oncogenic transformation by human papillomavirus type 16 deoxyribonucleic acid in the presence of progesterone or progestins from oral contraceptives. Am J Obstet Gynecol 162:1099–1103.

PENG H, LIU S, MANN V et al. 1991. Human papillomavirus types 16 and 33, Herpes simplex virus type 2 and other risk factors for cervical cancer in Sichuan Province, China. Int J Cancer 47:711–716.

PERITZ E, RAMCHARAN S, FRANK J, et al. 1977. The incidence of cervical cancer and duration of oral contraceptive use. Am J Epidemiol 106:462–469.

PETERS RK, CHAO A, MACK TM, et al. 1986a. Increased frequency of adenocarcinoma of the uterine cervix in young women in Los Angeles County. J Natl Cancer Inst 76:423–428.

PETERS RK, THOMAS D, HAGAN DG, et al. 1986b. Risk factors for invasive cervical cancer among Latinas and non-Latinas in Los Angeles County. J Natl Cancer Inst 77:1063–1077.

PETERSON O. 1956. Spontaneous course of cervical precancerous conditions. Am J Obstet Gynecol 72:1063–1071.

PHILLIPS B, MARSHALL ME, BROWN S, et al. 1985. Effect of smoking on human natural killer cell activity. Cancer 56:2789–2792.

PICKLE LW, MASON TJ, HOWARD N, HOOVER R, FRAUMENI JF, JR EDS. 1987. Atlas of U.S. Cancer Mortality Among Whites: 1950–1980. U.S. Dept of Health and Human Services, Public Health Service, National Institutes of Health, DHHS Publication No. (NIH) 87-2900.

PIPER JM. 1985. Oral contraceptives and cervical cancer. Gynecol Oncol 22:1–14.

PORRECO R, PENN I, DROEGEMUELLER W, et al. 1975. Gynecologic malignancies in immunosuppressed organ homograft recipients. Obstet Gynecol 45:359–364.

POTISCHMAN N. 1993. Nutritional epidemiology of cervical neoplasia. J Nutr 123:424–429.

POTISCHMAN N, HERRERO R, BRINTON LA, et al. 1991. A case-control study of nutrient status and invasive cervical cancer. II. Serologic indicators. Am J Epidemiol 134:1347–1355.

POWELL LC, SEYMOUR RJ. 1971. Effects of depo-medroxyprogesterone acetate as a contraceptive agent. Am J Obstet Gynecol 110:36–41.

PRIDAN H, LILIENFELD AM. 1971. Carcinoma of the cervix in Jewish women in Israel, 1960–1967: An epidemiological study. Isr J Med Sci 7:1465–1470.

REEVES WC, BRINTON LA, GARCIA M, et al. 1989. Human papillomavirus (HPV) infection and cervical cancer in Latin America. N Engl J Med 320:1436–1441.

REEVES WC, CAUSSY D, BRINTON LA, et al. 1987. Case-control study of human papillomaviruses and cervical cancer in Latin America. Int J Cancer 40:450–454.

REEVES WC, QUIROZ E. 1987. Prevalence of sexually transmitted diseases in high-risk women in the Republic of Panama. Sex Trans Dis 14:69–74.

REID R, GREENBERG MD, JENSON AB, et al. 1987. Sexually transmitted papillomaviral infections. I. The anatomic distribution and pathologic grade of neoplastic lesions associated with different viral types. Am J Obstet Gynecol 156:212–222.

RICHART RM, BARRON BA. 1969. A follow-up study of patients with cervical dysplasia. Am J Obstet Gynecol 105:386–393.

RIES LAG, MILLER BA, HANKEY BF, et al eds. 1994. SEER Cancer Statistics Review: 1973–1991—Tables and Graphs. NIH Pub. No. 94-2789, Bethesda, MD: National Cancer Institute.

RIOU G, FAVRE M, JEANNEL D, et al. 1990. Association between poor prognosis in early-stage invasive cervical carcinomas and non-detection of HPV DNA. Lancet 335:1171–1174.

ROBBOY SJ, NOLLER KL, O'BRIEN P, et al. 1984. Increased incidence of cervical and vaginal dysplasia in 3980 diethylstilbestrol-exposed young women. JAMA 252:2979–2983.

ROBINSON J. 1982. Cancer of the cervix: occupational risk of husbands and wives and possible preventive strategies. In: *Preclinical Neoplasia of the Cervix*, Jordan JA, Sharp F, Singer A (eds). Proc Ninth Study Group of the Royal College of Obstetricians and Gynaecologists, London, pp 11–27.

ROJEL J. 1952. The interrelation between uterine cancer and syphilis: a patho-demographic study. Acta Pathol Microbiol Scand (Suppl) 97:11–82.

ROMAN A, FIFE K. 1986. Human papillomavirus DNA associated with foreskins of normal newborns. J Infect Dis 153:855–861.

ROMNEY SL, DUTTAGUPTA C, BASU J, et al. 1985. Plasma vitamin C and uterine cervical dysplasia. Am J Obstet Gynecol 151:976–980.

ROSEMBERG SK. 1991. Sexually transmitted papillomaviral infection in men. Dermatol Clin 9(2):317–331.

ROSENFELD WD, VERMUND SH, WENTZ SJ, et al. 1989. High prevalence rate of human papillomavirus infection and association with abnormal Papanicolaou smears in sexually active adolescents. Am J Dis Child 143:1443–1447.

ROTKIN ID. 1967. Adolescent coitus and cervical cancer: associations of related events with increased risk. Cancer Res 27:603–617.

ROTKIN ID, CAMERON JR. 1968. Clusters of variables influencing risk of cervical cancer. Cancer 21:663–671.

ROUS P, KIDD JG. 1938. The carcinogenic effect of papilloma virus on the tarred skin of rabbits. I. Description of the phenomenon. J Exp Med 67:399–428.

ROYSTON I, AURELIAN L. 1970. The association of genital herpesvirus with cervical atypia and carcinoma in situ. Am J Epidemiol 91:531–538.

SASSON IM, HALEY NJ, HOFFMANN D, et al. 1985. Cigarette smoking and neoplasia of the uterine cervix: smoke constituents in cervical mucus. N Engl J Med 312:315–316.

SAVITZ DA, ANDREWS KA, BRINTON LA. 1995. Occupation and cervical cancer. J Occup Environ Med 37:357–361.

SCHACHTER J, HILL EC, KING EB, et al. 1982. Chlamydia trachomatis and cervical neoplasia. JAMA 248:2134–2138.

SCHEFFNER M, MUNGER K, BYRNE JC, et al. 1991. The state of the p53 and retinoblastoma genes in human cervical carcinoma cell lines. Proc Natl Acad Sci USA 88:5523–5527.

SCHIFFMAN MH. 1992a. Validation of HPV hybridization assays: Correlation of FISH, dot blot, and PCR with Southern blot. In: The Epidemiology of Human Papillomavirus and Cervical Cancer, Munoz N, Bosch FX, Shah KV, et al (eds). Lyon, IARC Monograph, pp 169–179.

SCHIFFMAN MH. 1992b. Recent progress in defining the epidemiology of human papillomavirus infection and cervical neoplasia. J Natl Cancer Inst 84:394–398.

SCHIFFMAN MH. 1994. Epidemiology of cervical human papillomaviruses. In: Human Pathogenic Papillomaviruses, zur Hausen H (ed). Heidelberg: Springer Verlag, pp 55–81.

SCHIFFMAN MH, BAUER HM, HOOVER RN, et al. 1993. Epidemiologic evidence showing that human papillomavirus infection causes most cervical intraepithelial neoplasia. J Natl Cancer Inst 85:958–964.

SCHIFFMAN MH, BURK RD. In press. Human papillomaviruses and cervical neoplasia. In: *Viral Infections of Humans, Epidemiology and Control*, 4th Edition, Evans A, Kaslow R (eds). New York: Plenum.

SCHIFFMAN MH, HALEY NJ, FELTON JS, et al. 1987. Biochemical epidemiology of cervical neoplasia: measuring cigarette smoke constituents in the cervix. Cancer Res 47:3886–3888.

SCHIFFMAN MH, SHERMAN ME. 1994. HPV testing can be used to improve cervical cancer screening. In: *Molecular Markers of Early Detection of Cancer*, Srivastava S (ed). Armonk, NY: Futura Publishing Co, pp 265–277.

SCHMAUZ R, OKONG P, DE VILLIERS EM, et al. 1989. Multiple infections in cases of cervical cancer from a high-incidence area in tropical Africa. Int J Cancer 43:805–809.

SCHNEIDER A, HOTZ M, GISSMANN L. 1987. Increased prevalence of human papillomaviruses in the lower genital tract of pregnant women. Int J Cancer 40:198–201.

SCHNEIDER A, KIRCHHOFF T, MEINHARDT G, et al. 1992. Repeated evaluation of human papillomavirus 16 status in cervical swabs of young women with a history of normal Papanicolaou smears. Obstet Gynecol 79:683–688.

SCHNEIDER V, KAY S, LEE HM. 1983. Immunosuppression as a high-risk factor in the development of condyloma acuminatum and squamous neoplasia of the cervix. Acta Cytol 27:220–224.

SCHWARTZ SM, WEISS NS. 1986. Increased incidence of adenocarcinoma of the cervix in young women in the United States. Am J Epidemiol 124:1045–1047.

SETH P, PRAKASH SS, GHOSH D. 1978. Antibodies to herpes simplex virus types 1 and 2 in patients with squamous-cell carcinoma of uterine cervix in India. Int J Cancer 22:708–714.

SHAH K, KASHIMA H, POLK F, et al. 1986. Rarity of cesarean delivery in cases of juvenile-onset respiratory papillomatosis. Obstet Gynecol 68:795–799.

SHAH KV, HOWLEY P. 1995. Papillomaviruses. In: *Virology*, Fields BN, Knipe DM (eds). New York: Raven Press.

SHERMAN ME, SCHIFFMAN MH, LORINCZ AT, et al. 1994. Towards objective quality assurance in cervical cytopathology: correlation of cytopathologic diagnoses with detection of high risk HPV types. Am J Clin Pathol 101:182–187.

SHROYER KR. 1993. Human papillomavirus and endocervical adenocarcinoma. Human Pathol 24:119–120.

SILLMAN F, STANEK A, SEDLIS A, et al. 1984. The relationship between human papillomavirus and lower genital intraepithelial neoplasia in immunosuppressed women. Am J Obstet Gynecol 150:300–308.

SINGER A. 1975. The uterine cervix from adolescence to the menopause. Br J Obstet Gynaecol 82:81–99.

SKEGG DCG, CORWIN PA, PAUL C, et al. 1982. Importance of the male factor in cancer of the cervix. Lancet 2:581–583.

SLATTERY ML, ABBOTT TM, OVERALL JC, et al. 1990. Dietary vitamins A, C, and E and selenium as risk factors for cervical cancer. Epidemiology 1:8–15.

SLATTERY ML, OVERALL JC, ABBOTT TM, et al. 1989a. Sexual activity, contraception, genital infections, and cervical cancer: support for a sexually transmitted disease hypothesis. Am J Epidemiol 130:248–258.

SLATTERY ML, ROBISON LM, SCHUMAN KL, et al. 1989b. Cigarette smoking and exposure to passive smoke are risk factors for cervical cancer. JAMA 261:1593–1598.

SMITH FR. 1931. Etiologic factors in carcinoma of the cervix. Am J Obstet Gynecol 21:18–25.

SMITH PG, KINLEN LJ, WHITE GC, et al. 1980. Mortality of wives of men dying with cancer of the penis. Br J Cancer 41:422–428.

SOUTTER WP, FLETCHER A. 1994. Invasive cancer of the cervix in women with mild dyskaryosis followed up cytologically. Br Med J 308:1421–1423.

STANBRIDGE CM, BUTLER EB. 1983. Human papillomavirus infection of the lower female genital tract: association with multicentric neoplasia. Int J Gynecol Pathol 2:264–274.

STELLATO G, NIEMINEN P, AHO H, et al. 1994. Human papillomavirus infection of the female genital tract: correlation of HPV DNA with cytologic, colposcopic, and natural history findings. Eur J Gynaecol Oncol 13:262–267.

STRICKLER HD, RATTRAY C, ESCOFFREY C, et al. 1995. Human T-cell lymphotropic virus type I and severe neoplasia of the cervix in Jamaica. Int J Cancer 60:1–4.

SUNDBERG JP. 1987. Papillomavirus infections in animals. In: Papillomaviruses and Human Disease, Syrjanen K, Gissmann L, Koss L (eds). Heidelberg: Springer-Verlag, pp 40–103.

SWAN SH, BROWN WL. 1981. Oral contraceptive use, sexual activity, and cervical carcinoma. Am J Obstet Gynecol 139:52–57.

TERRIS M, OALMANN MC. 1960. Carcinoma of the cervix: an epidemiologic study. JAMA 174:1847–1851.

TERRIS M, WILSON F, SMITH H, et al. 1967. The relationship of coitus to carcinoma of the cervix. Am J Public Health 57:840–847.

THOMAS DB, MOLINA R, CUEVAS HR, et al. 1989. Monthly injectable steroid contraceptives and cervical cancer. Am J Epidemiol 130:237–247.

TREVATHAN E, LAYDE P, WEBSTER LA, et al. 1983. Cigarette smoking and dysplasia and carcinoma in situ of the uterine cervix. JAMA 250:499–502.

URSIN G, PETERS RK, HENDERSON BE, et al. 1994. Oral contraceptive use and adenocarcinoma of cervix. Lancet 344:1390–1379.

VAN EENWYK J, DAVIS FG, BOWEN PE. 1991. Dietary and serum carotenoids and cervical intraepithelial neoplasia. Int J Cancer 48:34–38.

VAN EENWYK J, DAVIS FG, COLMAN N. 1992. Folate, vitamin C, and cervical intraepithelial neoplasia. Cancer Epidemiol Biomark Prev 1:119–124.

VAN RANST M, KAPLAN JB, BURK RD. 1992. Phylogenetic classification of human papillomaviruses: correlation with clinical manifestations. J Gen Virol 73:2653–2660.

VERMUND SH, KELLY KF, KLEIN RS, et al. 1991. High risk of human papillomavirus infection and cervical squamous intraepithelial lesions among women with symptomatic human immunodeficiency virus infection. Am J Obstet Gynecol 165:392–400.

VERMUND SH, SCHIFFMAN MH, GOLDBERG GL, et al. 1989. Molecular diagnosis of genital human papillomavirus infection: comparison of two methods used to collect exfoliated cervical cells. Am J Obstet Gynecol 160:304–308.

VERREAULT R, CHU J, MANDELSON M, et al. 1989. A case-control study of diet and invasive cervical cancer. Int J Cancer 43:1050–1054.

VESSEY MP, LAWLESS M, MCPHERSON K, et al. 1983a. Neoplasia of the cervix uteri and contraception: a possible adverse effect of the pill. Lancet 2:930–934.

VESSEY MP, LAWLESS M, MCPHERSON K, et al. 1983b. Oral contraceptives and cervical cancer (Letter). Lancet 2:1358–1359.

VONKA V, KANKA J, HIRSCH I, et al. 1984. Prospective study on the relationship between cervical neoplasia and herpes simplex type-2 virus. II. Herpes simplex type-2 antibody presence in sera taken at enrollment. Int J Cancer 33:61–66.

WALKER J, BLOSS JD, LIAO SY, et al. 1989. Human papillomavirus genotype as a prognostic indicator in carcinoma of the uterine cervix. Obstet Gynecol 74:781–785.

WASSERTHEIL-SMOLLER S, ROMNEY SL, WYLIE-ROSETT J, et al. 1981. Dietary vitamin C and uterine cervical dysplasia. Am J Epidemiol 114:714–24.

WERNESS BA, LEVINE AJ, HOWLEY PM. 1990. Association of human papillomavirus types 16 and 18 E6 proteins with p53. Science 248:76–79.

WEST DW, SCHUMAN KL, LYON JL, et al. 1984. Differences in risk estimations from a hospital and a population-based case-control study. Int J Epidemiol 13:235–239.

WHITEHEAD N, REYNER F, LINDENBAUM J. 1973. Megaloblastic changes in the cervical epithelium: association with oral contraceptive therapy and reversal with folic acid. JAMA 226:1421–1424.

WHO COLLABORATIVE STUDY OF NEOPLASIA AND STEROID CONTRACEPTIVES. 1993. Invasive squamous-cell cervical carcinoma and combined oral contraceptives: results from a multi-national study. Int J Cancer 55:228–236.

WINKELSTEIN W JR. 1977. Smoking and cancer of the uterine cervix: hypothesis. Am J Epidemiol 106:257–259.

WORTH AJ, BOYES DA. 1972. A case control study into the possible effects of birth control pills on pre-clinical carcinoma of the cervix. J Obstet Gynaecol Br Commonw 79:673–679.

WRIGHT NH, VESSEY MP, KENWARD B, et al. 1978. Neoplasia and dysplasia of the cervix uteri and contraception: a possible protective effect of the diaphragm. Br J Cancer 38:273–279.

WYNDER EL, CORNFIELD J, SCHROFF PD, et al. 1954. A study of environmental factors in carcinoma of the cervix. Am J Obstet Gynecol 68:1016–1052.

YASUMOTO S, BURKHARDT AL, DONIGER J, et al. 1986. Human papillomavirus type 16 DNA-induced malignant transformation of NIH 3T3 cells. J Virol 57:572–577.

ZAKELJ MP, FRASER P, INSKIP H. 1984. Cervical cancer and husband's occupation. Lancet 1:510.

ZIEGLER RG, BRINTON LA, HAMMAN RF, et al. 1990. Diet and the risk of invasive cervical cancer among white women in the United States. Am J Epidemiol 132:432–445.

ZIEGLER RG, JONES CJ, BRINTON LA, et al. 1991. Diet and the risk of in situ cervical cancer among white women in the United States. Cancer Causes Control 2:17–29.

ZUNZUNEGUI MV, KING MC, CORIA CF, et al. 1986. Male influences on cervical cancer risk. Am J Epidemiol 123:302–307.

ZUR HAUSEN H. 1982. Human genital cancer: synergism between two virus infections or synergism between a virus infection and initiating events? Lancet 2:1370–1372.

ZUR HAUSEN H, ED. 1994. Current Topics in Microbiology and Immunology, Vol. 186, Human Pathogenic Papillomaviruses. Heidelberg: Springer-Verlag.

51 Cancers of the vulva and vagina

JANET R. DALING
KAREN J. SHERMAN

Vulvar and vaginal cancers are both uncommon malignancies that primarily afflict elderly women. Little is known about the causes of these diseases, although the role of human papillomavirus in the etiology of vulvar cancer and the role of in utero exposure to diethylstilbestrol in the genesis of clear cell adenocarcinoma of the vagina have received attention.

Both vaginal and vulvar cancers may share some etiologic features with cervical cancer, which often precedes, coincides with, or follows the development of vulvar or vaginal neoplasia. When appropriate, findings from the cervical cancer literature that may supplement our current understanding of these diseases will be included.

Carcinoma in situ of the vulva is a lesion often detected more commonly than its invasive counterpart in situations where all occurrences of these neoplasms are recorded. Information on both of these lesions of the vulva and vagina will be presented in this chapter. Unless otherwise specified, information will pertain to the invasive form of these diseases, and the term *neoplasm* will be used when referring to both the invasive and in situ lesions.

DEMOGRAPHIC PATTERNS

Histopathology

Most vulvar cancers are squamous cell in origin; these account for some 80%–90% of all histologic types (Berg and Lampe, 1981; Peters et al, 1984). Melanomas are the next most common vulvar malignancy (5%–10%), sarcomas occur less frequently (3%–5%), and adenocarcinomas, primarily of Bartholin's gland, are quite rare.

Among the squamous cell cancers, several pathologically and clinically distinct entities exist. Verrucous carcinomas are wartlike proliferative lesions that frequently recur, are locally aggressive, but rarely metastasize (Crowther et al, 1988). Condylomatous carcinomas are invasive squamous cell cancers that arise in either condylomata or giant condylomata (Downey et al, 1988).

Most preinvasive tumors of the vulva are of the squamous cell type; Bowen's disease and vulvar intraepithelial neoplasia III are other terms used to describe this disease (Campion and Singer, 1987). Lesions may be unifocal or multifocal; the latter are also known as bowenoid papulosis and occur usually in women under 40 years of age.

Most vaginal cancers are squamous cell (Peters et al, 1984). Among teens and young women, however, clear cell adenocarcinoma is the most common. Infants primarily have embryonal cell rhabdomyosarcomas.

Anatomic Distribution

Vulvar tumors are most likely to arise in the labia majora. The second most common sites are the labia minora and the clitoris (Woodcock, 1976). In most series, the majority of squamous cell vaginal tumors arise in the upper third of the vagina and the posterior wall (Wade-Evans, 1976).

Geographic Distribution

Vulvar and vaginal cancers are uncommon tumors in all areas of the world where incidence has been reported from tumor registries (Muir et al., 1987). Incidence is highest in Recife, Brazil, with an age-standardized rate of 2.1 vaginal and 3.4 vulvar cancers per 100,000 women per year. The lowest rates of vaginal cancer (0.1–0.3 cases annually/100,000 women) have been reported from Israel and Japan. The province of Rizal in the Philippines has reported the lowest rates of vulvar cancer (0.3 cases yearly/100,000 women). Incidence tends to be highest in South and Central America and lowest in East Asia. No information on incidence is available from Africa.

This work was supported in part by Grants 5 R01 CA 35881 and 1 P01 CA 42792 and Contract NO. NO1-CN-05230 from the National Cancer Institute.

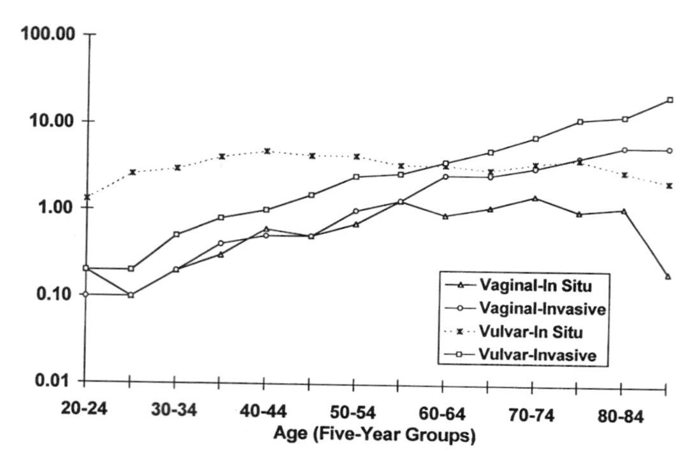

FIG. 51–1. Incidence of vulvar and vaginal neoplasia by age, from populations served by the Surveillance, Epidemiology, and End Results Program (SEER), 1983–87.

Incidence, Mortality, and Survival

In the United States, the incidence of invasive vulvar and vaginal cancers, as reported by cancer registries participating in the Surveillance, Epidemiology, and End Results Program (SEER) of the National Cancer Institute, is 1.7 and 0.6 per 100,000 females, respectively (NCI, 1994).

The average annual age-adjusted mortality rate per 100,000 women is 0.3 for cancer of the vulva and 0.2 for cancer of the vagina (NCI, 1994). The relative 5-year survival rate for vulvar cancer is 73%, whereas the rate for cancer of the vagina is 46%. The lower survival rate for cancer of the vagina probably reflects a larger proportion of women diagnosed with distant metastases.

Time Trends

The incidence of vaginal cancer decreased 17% from 1973 through 1991, whereas vulvar cancer increased 20% (NCI, 1994) in the same time period. Reported rates of in situ vulvar cancer increased from 0.02 to 0.81 per 100,000 women between 1945–49 and 1975–79 (Schwartz and Naftolin, 1981). Though the rising incidence could reflect increased surveillance of individuals, the observation that more women under age 40 were diagnosed recently and that a higher proportion of women were asymptomatic at diagnosis argues that artifact is not explaining the entire increase (Schwartz and Naftolin, 1981).

More recent data, available from all participants in the SEER program, show incidence of in situ vulvar cancer nearly doubled between 1973–1976 and 1986–1987 (Sturgeon et al, 1992).

Age

In the United States, all vaginal neoplasms are rare before age 45. In situ lesions reach their highest incidence between age 55 and 70, whereas invasive lesions continue to increase in incidence exponentially throughout life. The incidence of vulvar neoplasms follows a similar pattern, although the rates rise more rapidly and begin to increase at younger ages (Fig. 51–1). The median age of vulvar cancer patients was 71 during the time period 1987–1991, whereas the median age of patients with vaginal cancer was 69 (NCI, 1994).

Race and Ethnicity

Black women tend to develop vaginal neoplasms, especially of an invasive nature, more often than white women (Young et al, 1981; Peters et al, 1984). Their incidence of in situ and invasive vulvar cancer is rather similar to that of white women. Women of Asian ancestry have uniformly lower occurrence rates of both of these malignancies and their preinvasive stages than do white women (Muir et al, 1987; Young et al, 1981). Women with Spanish surnames have lower rates of in situ and invasive vulvar cancers than do white women (Young et al, 1981; Peters et al, 1984; Muir et al, 1987). In a study of vulvar cancer in Israel, Menczer et al (1982) found that Jewish women born in North Africa or Israel had higher rates of this disease than Jewish women born in Europe or Asia.

Socioeconomic Status

Vulvar cancer is more common among women of low socioeconomic status. When census tracts were divided into quintiles based on average family income, years of schooling, and median rental costs, women residing in areas in the lowest quintile had a 23% higher incidence rate of vulvar cancer compared to women residing in areas found in the highest quintile (Berg and Lampe, 1981). This same association was also noted by Peters et al (1984), who found that the incidence of vulvar cancer in the census tracts with the lowest socioeconomic status was three times that of women in the highest census tracts; they found a more modest difference in rates of vaginal cancer between high and low census tracts. Newcomb et al (1984) found that, after adjusting for age, a greater proportion of women with in situ vulvar cancer resided in low-income areas than did controls. They found no association with income for invasive disease. Brinton et al (1990a) and Sherman et al (1991) found that women with vulvar cancer had somewhat lower educational levels and income than did controls. Women with vaginal cancer in the case-control study by Brinton et al (1990b) were more poorly educated and had lower incomes than did the controls.

RISK FACTORS

Only a handful of case-control studies of these neoplasms has been conducted, and most of them are plagued by small sample sizes, which limits the robustness of the findings. What little else is known of the causes of these malignancies has come essentially from case series. Since comparison groups are lacking from virtually all such studies, conclusions can be regarded as tentative at best for most purported risk factors.

ENVIRONMENTAL FACTORS

Infection with Human Papillomavirus

Multiple lines of evidence suggest that the human papillomavirus (HPV), a group of viruses that cause condylomata as well as subclinical lesions, is associated with vulvar cancer. In a study using cases from a population-based cancer registry, Daling et al (1984) reported that 19.5% of 221 women diagnosed with squamous cell vulvar carcinoma in situ in western Washington had coexisting condyloma described on their cancer registry report. The comparable figure for women with squamous cell invasive vulvar tumors was 12.1%. By contrast, none of the 49 women with other histologic types of vulvar cancer had a coexistent condyloma denoted on their abstract. As mention of the condyloma was optional, the proportion of individuals who had vulvar neoplasms and condyloma could well have been higher. Reports of case series typically indicate that 20%–35% of patients with vulvar carcinoma in situ have coexistent condyloma, as do 5%–10% of patients with invasive vulvar carcinoma (Rutledge et al, 1970; Friedrich et al, 1980a; Buscema et al, 1980a). This figure is considerably higher when microscopic features of condyloma are also included (Rueda-Leverone et al, 1987; Crum et al, 1982). In addition, reports exist of condyloma preceding carcinoma (Rhatigan and Saffos, 1977; Downey et al, 1988), as do reports of carcinoma arising in a condylomata (Charleswood and Shippel, 1953; Boxer and Skinner, 1977; Schmauz and Owor, 1980; Downey et al, 1988). In two case-control studies of vulvar cancer, women with either in situ or invasive vulvar cancer were 15 times more likely to report a prior history of condyloma than were controls (Brinton et al, 1990a; Sherman et al, 1991).

With the use of electron microscopy, virus particles have been found in both carcinoma in situ and "warty" carcinoma of the vulva (Pilotti et al, 1984; Rastkar et al, 1982). In a small proportion (16%) of intraepithelial neoplasia of the vulva selected for study because they had histologic evidence of HPV infection, HPV antigens were detected by immunoperoxidase staining (Crum et al, 1982; Pilotti et al, 1984; Rueda-Leverone et al, 1987). None of the six cases of invasive vulvar cancer tested was positive for HPV capsid antigens. Since these antigens can be detected only if virus was replicating (a process that requires mature, well-differentiated epithelial cells), the low rate of detection in carcinoma in situ and the absence of detection in invasive vulvar cancer are not surprising.

More recently, four techniques of DNA hybridization (in situ hybridization, dot hybridization, Southern hybridization, and amplification by polymerase chain reaction) have been used to detect specific genotypes of HPV in vulvar neoplasms. HPV has been found in vulvar intraepithelial neoplasia, invasive vulvar cancers, condylomatous cancers, bowenoid papulosis progressing to invasive cancer, and verrucous carcinomas. The proportion of lesions that were positive for HPV has varied among studies, from less than 25% (Carson et al, 1988) to more than 75% (Buscema et al, 1988, Daling et al, 1992), no doubt depending upon the sensitivity of the detection method used, the number of specific types of HPV used as probes, and variation in other aspects of the biochemical assays, such as temperature. In two studies reporting HPV results from the same laboratory on both in situ and invasive lesions, the in situ lesions were more likely to contain HPV DNA (Buscema et al, 1988; Pilotti et al, 1990). Park et al (1991) and Toki et al (1991) have suggested that HPV DNA is commonly found in only a portion of squamous cell carcinoma in situ and invasive cancer of the vulva that have distinct histologic features. Among those lesions that have been analyzed for specific types of HPV, HPV 16 is most often found in both vulvar intraepithelial neoplasia and invasive cancer in the majority of case series (e.g., Di Luca et al, 1987; Buscema et al, 1988; Jones et al, 1990; Pilotti et al, 1990; Park et al, 1991; Toki et al, 1991; Daling et al, 1992). By contrast, those few verrucous carcinomas that have been analyzed to date contained types 6 or 11, types that are most often associated with condylomata (Crowther et al, 1988). In one study of condylomatous carcinoma, types 2, 6, and 16 were each found in one of five tumors with HPV (Downey et al, 1988). Because all lesions have not been tested for all HPV types known to date and because new HPV types are continually being characterized, the possibility exists that other or additional types of HPV may play an important role in the development of vulvar tumors.

Fewer studies have examined the role of HPV in the development of vaginal cancer. Nonetheless, results from these studies are consistent with the evidence that links HPV to other anogenital cancers. Condylomata, and especially subclinical HPV infections, do occur in the vagina and also have been observed to coexist with carcinoma in situ of the vagina (Campion, 1987). Brinton et al (1990b) reported that 26% of women with vaginal carcinoma in situ, compared with 4% of controls, gave a history of condyloma. Daling et al (1992) found that women with vaginal cancer were more likely to report a history of genital warts than were controls (20.2% cases, 4.7% controls). Malignant transformation of vaginal condylomata to invasive vaginal cancer has been reported as well (Beck, 1984). Okagaki et al (1984) found HPV DNA in two verrucous carcinomas of the vagina, and Okagaki (1984) reported HPV DNA in several vaginal intraepithelial neoplasia. Ostrow et al (1988), Kiyabu et al (1989), and Ikenberg et al (1990) have reported detecting HPV DNA in invasive squamous cell vaginal cancers, with the most prevalent HPV type being HPV 16.

Multiple Primary Tumors of the Genital Tract

Using data on cancer incidence rates from the Connecticut Tumor Registry, Schoenberg (1977) showed that women who had had cervical cancer were at greater risk for other anogenital malignancies. In a hospital-based case-control study of invasive vulvar cancer, Mabuchi et al (1985) found that six of 149 women with vulvar cancer but none of 149 controls had a history of prior urogenital cancer. In a population-based case-control study, women with vulvar neoplasms were more likely to report a history of other anogenital cancers than were controls, with relative risks of 30 and 19 for women with in situ and invasive disease, respectively (Sherman et al, 1988).

In addition, there have been numerous reports of women with squamous cell cancer of the vulva who have had one or more second primary malignancies of the anogenital tract (Taussig, 1940; Cromer, 1963; Day, 1958; Rose et al, 1987), especially the cervix (Franklin and Rutledge, 1972; Friedrich et al, 1980a) that were detected before (McPherson et al, 1963), simultaneous with (Eichner, 1956), or after a vulvar tumor (Diehl et al, 1951). In situ and invasive vaginal cancers are also more common in women with prior, concurrent, or subsequent malignancies of the anogenital tract (Benedet and Sanders, 1984; Rose et al, 1987).

Few studies have looked for evidence of HPV in those individuals with multiple primary tumors of the anogenital tract. In a study of six women with vulvar carcinoma in situ and a second intraepithelial neoplasia, four had evidence of HPV infection in both tumors (Beckmann et al, 1988). McCance et al (1985) found HPV DNA in the cervix, vagina, and vulva of five women who had intraepithelial neoplasia in at least two of those sites.

Ionizing Radiation

In a large multinational study of second cancers following radiation treatment for cervical cancer, Boice et al (1985) found that women who were treated with radiation for cervical cancer were nearly three times as likely to develop a second tumor of the vulva or vagina as expected based on age- and calendar year-specific incidence rates of these diseases from the population served by the registries. By contrast, they found no excess risk among women treated for cervical cancer without radiation. Pride and Buchler (1977) found that 1.3% of patients who were treated with pelvic irradiation for cervical cancer developed a vaginal neoplasm 10 or more years after treatment.

Other Sexually Transmitted Diseases and Vulvar Cancer

In their case-control study of invasive vulvar cancer, Mabuchi et al (1985) found that 3% of cases but none of the controls reported a history of syphilis. A history of syphilis (or positive serology) has also been recalled in a substantial proportion of cases in some series (Japaze et al, 1977; Friedrich et al, 1980a; Rutledge et al, 1970). In fact, in a study of women with vulvar cancer in Jamaica, 52% of the cases had evidence of prior exposure to treponemes, a figure that was much higher than the 15% of women attending the antenatal clinic (Sengupta, 1980). Nonetheless, other case series have reported that fewer than 5% of cases had such a history (Green, 1978; Buscema et al, 1981; Figge and Gaudenz, 1974). The lack of appropriate comparison data and failure to adjust for confounding variables makes any conclusions difficult. Only a few women with vulvar cancer and controls reported a history of syphilis in two recently conducted case-control studies (Brinton et al, 1990a; Sherman et al, 1991).

Recent series from the United States found fewer than 5% of women with vulvar cancer who had a history of granulomatous vulvar diseases, such as chancroid, lymphogranuloma venereum, and granuloma inguinale (Buscema et al, 1981; Figge and Gaudenz, 1974; Parker et al, 1975; Rutledge et al, 1970); these sexually transmitted diseases are quite rare in the U.S. No cases or controls gave a history of granulomatous vulvar disease in the case-control study reported by Sherman et al (1991). In a study of women with vulvar cancer in Jamaica, Sengupta (1980) found that 70% of the patients had prior granuloma inguinale and/or lymphogranuloma venereum. Consequently, these diseases may be important in the etiology of vulvar cancer in countries where they are common.

Evidence implicating herpes simplex type II (HSV-2) as a risk factor for vulvar cancer is inconsistent. Kaufman et al (1981) found HSV-2–induced antigens in seven of nine vulvar in situ carcinomas but none in four normal tissues from a subset of these individuals. Cabral et al (1982) found nonstructural HSV-2 proteins in biopsy specimens from carcinoma in situ of the vulva, but were unable to culture the virus. In an editorial, Schwartz and Naftolin (1981) reported that HSV-specific DNA polymerase was present in invasive vulvar cancer and metastases, but gave no details.

More recently, HSV-2 antigens have been found in both in situ and invasive vulvar cancers (Costa et al, 1990). Homology to HSV-2 DNA from a transforming region was detected in three of 10 specimens of carcinoma in situ and none of 10 specimens of invasive cancer in one study (Pilotti et al, 1990), whereas in a second study none of four specimens of carcinoma in situ and one of nine specimens of invasive vulvar cancer had evidence of HSV-2 DNA from a transforming region (Costa et al, 1990). Brinton et al (1990a) reported that fewer than 1% of women in their case-control study gave a history of genital herpes. Cases, however, were over eight times more likely to give such a history than controls. Sherman et al (1991) found a positive association between seropositivity to HSV-2 and a diagnosis of vulvar carcinoma in situ.

Cigarette Smoking

Although few studies have examined cigarette smoking as a potential risk factor for vulvar cancer, an increased risk was seen in all five of the studies where it has been considered. In the study by Newcomb et al (1984), women who were smokers at diagnosis, as well as those who were former smokers, were at increased risk of both in situ and invasive vulvar cancers. Mabuchi et al (1985) found that current smokers were at increased risk for invasive vulvar cancer; they found a dose-response relationship as well. Cook et al (1986) reported that a greater proportion of cases with vulvar intraepithelial neoplasia smoked than would be expected in the general population. In the studies by Brinton et al (1990a) and Daling et al (1992), women who were smokers at diagnosis were more likely to develop in situ or invasive vulvar cancer, particularly if they began smoking when they were young adolescents (less than 17 years of age). Neither study found that the number of years a woman smoked influenced her risk of vulvar cancer, and only one study found that the average daily number of cigarettes smoked influenced risk (Daling et al, 1992). In contrast to these reports, Parazzini et al (1993) reported no association of vulvar cancer to smoking in a case-control study in Italy. The use of hospital controls may be one reason these investigators failed to show an association. That these data support a causal relationship is made more plausible by the association between smoking and cervical cancer (Brinton et al, 1986; Winkelstein, 1990), as well as other cancers (Daling et al, 1992).

Two small case-control studies have examined smoking as a possible risk factor for vaginal cancer (Brinton et al, 1990b; Daling et al, 1992). In both studies, the relative risk associated with smoking at diagnosis was quite modest (1.3–1.4) and the confidence intervals included one.

Oral Contraceptive Use

Newcomb et al (1984) found that women who had ever used oral contraceptives were at increased risk for in situ vulvar cancer. They were, however, unable to evaluate oral contraceptives as a risk factor for invasive disease because those cases, for the most part, spent their reproductive years in an era before oral contraceptives were used. Brinton et al (1990a,b) found no relationship between years of oral contraceptive use and either vulvar or vaginal cancer. Sherman et al (1994) did not find an association with ever use or duration of use of oral contraceptives, in either in situ or invasive vulvar cancer. These investigators also failed to show any relationship of hormone replacement therapy to vulvar cancer. Nonetheless, the observation that prolonged use of oral contraceptives may result in a slightly increased risk of cervical cancer suggests that this exposure is worthy of further study (Vessey, 1986).

Sexual Activity

Age at first intercourse was not associated with the risk of vulvar cancer in the three studies that examined this variable (Mabuchi et al, 1985; Brinton et al, 1990a; Sherman et al, 1991). In addition, a small but definite proportion of women without a history of sexual intercourse develop vulvar tumors (Cario, 1984; Valente et al, 1991). In both studies where the number of sexual partners was investigated as a possible risk factor for vulvar cancer, relative risk increased with an increasing number of reported partners (Brinton et al, 1990a; Sherman et al, 1991). By contrast, women with vaginal cancer did not differ from controls in either their age at first intercourse (Brinton et al, 1990b; Daling et al, 1992) or the number of sexual partners (Brinton et al, 1990b) they had prior to diagnosis. Parazzini et al (1993) did not find any relationship of indicators of sexual habits with vulvar cancer in their hospital-based case-control study.

Occupation and Vulvar Cancer

Occupational exposures have rarely been examined. Mabuchi et al (1985) found that women with vulvar cancer worked as private household maids or servants and as laundry workers more often than did controls. Friedrich et al (1980a) published a report of twins who, as children on a farm, were exposed to Paris Green, an arsenical insecticide, and later developed vulvar carcinoma in situ.

Diet and Vulvar Cancer

Only one study has explored the possibility that dietary factors, notably those that are implicated as risk factors for cervical neoplasms, may play a role in the etiology of vulvar cancer. Sturgeon et al (1991) did not find that women with high levels of vitamin A, beta-carotene, vitamin C, folate, or high intake of foods that are high in these micronutrients were less likely to develop vulvar cancer. An unexpected finding was that increasing intake of dark yellow-orange vegetables and beta-carotene was related to lower risks of vulvar cancer.

Diethylstilbestrol and Vaginal Cancer

Both clear cell adenocarcinoma and, more recently, squamous cell carcinoma of the vagina have been linked with in utero exposure to diethylstilbestrol (DES), a synthetic estrogen used between 1940 and 1970 to prevent spontaneous abortion and premature delivery (Gunning, 1976; Bornstein et al, 1988). Many of these studies have included both vaginal and cervical carcinomas of the appropriate cell type because, in many women who have been exposed to DES, there are structural abnormalities of the vagina and cervix that make the origin of these tumors difficult, if not impossible, to establish precisely.

Observations supporting the involvement of DES with clear cell adenocarcinoma include:

1. This cancer virtually never occurred in adolescents born before 1945 (Gunning, 1976).
2. This malignancy has not been reported in adolescents or young women from countries where DES was not prescribed for pregnant women (Ulfelder et al, 1971).
3. The incidence of this tumor by birth year cohort paralleled sales of DES from one manufacturer in the prior year (Melnick et al, 1987).
4. Two case-control studies found that seven of eight and five of five patients with this tumor were exposed, compared with none of 32 or eight controls, respectively (Herbst et al, 1971; Greenwald et al, 1971).
5. Among women exposed in utero, those who developed a cancer were more likely to be exposed before the twelfth week of pregnancy (Herbst et al, 1986).

Clear cell adenocarcinoma of the vagina is rare, even among women exposed to DES. The most recent report from the Registry for Research on Hormonal Transplacental Carcinogenesis, a registry that collects information on all cases of these cancers, estimated that an exposed woman had about one chance in 1,000 of developing this disease by her mid-30s (Melnick et al, 1987). The observation that none of these tumors developed in a cohort of 1580 women who were prenatally exposed to DES and who were assembled by record review at selected hospitals is compatible with this risk (McFarlane et al, 1986).

DES is believed to act as a teratogen on the developing embryonic reproductive tract, in that benign vaginal adenosis and structural alterations are found in some adolescents exposed in utero (Robboy et al, 1981). Most clear cell adenocarcinomas arise in areas of adenosis (Prins et al, 1976). Other factors, possibly including hormonal events triggered by puberty, are hypothesized to actually induce tumor development.

Stafl and Mattingly (1974) predicted a 20-fold increase in cervical and vaginal intraepithelial neoplasia among DES-exposed women as they reached the age when these diseases occurred most frequently. Subsequent reports from screening clinics had inconsistent findings, with the proportion of intraepithelial neoplasia ranging from none to 16%. A large collaborative cohort study of DES-exposed women found that dysplasia and carcinoma in situ were twice as frequent in those women as in the matched controls (Robboy et al, 1984). No cases of invasive carcinoma were found (Bornstein et al, 1988). The reason for this excess of tumors is not yet clear; the most plausible explanation is that the cervical transformation zone in a DES-exposed woman, which frequently extends into the vagina, offers a larger area of high susceptibility to carcinogens. As women exposed to DES reach the ages where squamous cell carcinoma in situ and invasive cancers are common, further follow-up will be necessary to determine if their risk of developing these neoplasms is elevated (Bornstein et al, 1988).

Chronic Irritation and Vaginal Cancer

Chronic irritation may play a role in the genesis of vaginal cancer. Kaiser (1952) found that nine of 55 patients with this malignancy either had worn a pessary or had severe procidentia. Pessary use occurred in over 10% of the patients reviewed by Rutledge (1967). While several other series found similar results (Way, 1948; Herbst et al, 1970; Johnston et al, 1983), more recent studies report little or no pessary use by their patients (Gallup et al, 1987; Manetta et al, 1988), suggesting that this source of vaginal irritation is of largely historical interest. Women who were diagnosed with vaginal cancer were more likely to recall a history of vaginal discharge or irritation in the study reported by Brinton et al (1990b).

Hysterectomy for Benign Conditions and Vaginal Cancer

In many series, a substantial proportion of cases with vaginal cancer have had a prior hysterectomy (Lee and Symmonds, 1976; Stuart et al, 1981; Bell et al, 1984; Ruiz-Moreno et al, 1987). While some of these hysterectomies were treatments for cervical neoplasia, a high prevalence of prior hysterectomy for benign conditions has been reported from some series (Stuart et al, 1981; Bell et al, 1984). In the case-control study reported by Brinton et al (1990b), a history of hysterectomy was more common in women with vaginal cancer than in controls, even after excluding women with a history of cervical cancer. However, in a clinic-based case-control study, Herman et al (1986) found that women with vaginal cancer and controls were equally likely to have had a prior hysterectomy, even when they examined only the subset of women without prior cervical neoplasia.

HOST FACTORS

Immunosuppression

Immunodeficient patients develop intraepithelial neoplasia of the anogenital tract much more frequently than do healthy people in the general population (Sillman and Sedlis, 1987). These neoplasias often recur, tend to be found at several anatomic sites, and frequently progress to malignancy.

A study of 934 patients with renal transplants in Sweden between 1965 and 1981 found three patients with vulvar or anal cancer, but expected only 0.3 (Blohme and Brynger, 1985). These patients received azathioprine and prednisone as their immunosuppressive therapy.

The Cincinnati Transplant Tumor Registry, which collects information on cancer in all types of organ-transplant recipients, found that 4% of the malignancies reported (excluding cervical carcinoma in situ and non-melanoma skin cancer) were of the vulva and perineum; this is a much larger figure than that for the general population (Penn, 1988).

Sillman and Sedlis (1987) suggested that HPV infections, which are common among transplant recipients, may contribute to the high incidence of anogenital cancers seen in these patients. Caterson et al (1984) found that two of 200 renal transplant recipients from an Australian hospital developed vulvar cancer associated with HPV after immunosuppressive therapy. Among 105 renal transplant patients from a New York hospital, one each developed vulvar and vaginal carcinoma in situ, both of which were associated with HPV infection (Halpert et al, 1986).

Numerous case reports exist of women who are immunodeficient for a variety of reasons and who have developed vulvar or vaginal neoplasms (Shokri-Tabibzadeh et al, 1981; Kennedy and Hart, 1982; Katz et al, 1987; Lindeque et al, 1987).

Women with HIV infection have been shown to have a high prevalence of anogenital HPV infections (Schrager et al, 1989; Palefsky, 1991). With the onset of immune deficiencies due to the HIV infection, they may be at particularly high risk for developing HPV-associated neoplasms. To date, rates of cervical and other anogenital cancers apparently have not increased among HIV-infected women, but this could be because HIV-infected women usually die of other causes before anogenital cancers have a chance to develop. As women with HIV-associated immunodeficiency receive treatment that prolongs their lives, the incidence of HPV-associated cancers may increase substantially in this group.

Reproductive Factors

Brinton et al (1990a) found a slightly reduced risk of vulvar cancer among women who had ever been pregnant. Newcomb et al (1984) found fewer nulliparous women than expected among women with either in situ or invasive vulvar cancer. By contrast, Mabuchi et al (1985) and Sherman et al (1994) found that women with invasive vulvar cancer were nulliparous more often than were controls, findings that could have been due to chance.

Case series have reported a highly variable proportion of nulliparous women (ranging from 11% to 38%), though the few that have compared their patients with a similar group of healthy women have not found a substantial excess of nulliparous women.

Newcomb et al (1984) reported that women with in situ vulvar cancer were more likely to have an early age at first birth. By contrast, they, Mabuchi et al (1985), and Sherman et al (1994) found that women who had a first birth (pregnancy) at an older age were at increased risk for invasive vulvar cancer. Parazzini et al (1993) found the opposite to be true.

Women who had more live births were at increased risk of in situ vulvar cancer, but not of invasive vulvar malignancy (Newcomb et al, 1984). Women with invasive vulvar disease were less likely to have multiple pregnancies in the study reported by Mabuchi et al (1985). The number of pregnancies or live births was not clearly related to vulvar cancer in the studies reported by Brinton et al (1990a), Sherman et al (1994), and Parazzini et al (1993).

Although trauma from childbirth has been suggested as a risk factor for vaginal cancer, Brinton et al (1990b) did not find a relationship between the number of live births and a diagnosis of vaginal cancer.

Obesity

Although some case series have contained a considerable proportion (30% or more) of obese women (Japaze et al, 1977; Rutledge et al, 1970; Kelsey and Hildreth, 1983), Newcomb et al (1984) and Brinton et al (1990a) failed to find a relation between body mass index or weight and in situ or invasive vulvar cancer in their case-control studies. In contrast to these reports, Sherman et al (1994), in the largest population-based case-control study to date, found a significant 2-fold risk with weight for invasive vulvar cancer, but there was no association for in situ disease. An even stronger association was found for women in the highest versus lowest Quetelet's index. In the study by Parazzini et al (1993), the risk of vulvar cancer increased with body mass index, but the trend in risk was not significant after taking into account potential confounders in a multivariate analysis. Brinton et al (1990b) found no relation between body mass index and vaginal cancer. However, Sharp and Cole (1991), in describing risks factors for clear cell adenocarcinoma of the vagina in women with in utero exposure to diethylstilbestrol, found women in the highest compared to lowest tertile of body mass index had a 2.8-fold risk of disease.

Early Menopause

Some 40%–55% of women with vulvar cancer experienced menopause at an early age in several series where such information was reported (Franklin and Rutledge, 1972; Green, 1978). Voliovitch et al (1984) noted that more women with vulvar cancer reported menopause before age 45 than in the general population. In a case-control study, Newcomb et al (1984) reported no relationship between age at menopause and either in situ or invasive vulvar cancer. Brinton et al (1990a) found that women with earlier menopause, regardless of whether it was surgically determined, were at higher risk of vulvar cancer.

Late menopause has been suggested as a risk factor for vaginal cancer. The study reported by Brinton et al (1990b), however, found that women with either surgical or natural menopause at a young age were at highest risk for this neoplasm.

Medical Conditions

In a case-control study of cancers at all sites from western New York State, women with diabetes were found to have an increased risk for vulvar and vaginal cancer. The risk was greatest for women who were diagnosed with diabetes before age 29 (O'Mara et al, 1985). Newcomb et al (1984) found that women with invasive vulvar cancer gave a history of diabetes more frequently than controls. Mabuchi et al (1985) found fewer diabetics among cases, and Brinton et al (1990a) found no relation between diabetes and vulvar cancer. In a study of Jewish women with vulvar cancer in Israel, Voliovitch et al (1984) found a greater proportion of patients who had diabetes diagnosed prior to their vulvar cancer than expected. In many but not all case series, at least 10% of the cases had diabetes as well as vulvar cancer. Diabetes is often associated with both vulvar dystrophies and chronic dermatitis, conditions that are both risk factors for invasive vulvar cancer, indicating that this relationship may be of etiologic importance. Diabetes was less common among cases than among controls in the study of vaginal cancer reported by Brinton et al (1990b).

A history of hypertension and cardiovascular disease has been common in some series of vulvar cancer patients (Rutledge et al, 1970; Voliovitch et al, 1984). This might be expected, because such patients are typically elderly. Indeed, case-control studies have not found a substantial association between these conditions and either in situ or invasive vulvar malignancy (Newcomb et al, 1984; Mabuchi et al, 1985; Brinton et al, 1990a).

Vulvar Dystrophies

The classification of nonmalignant vulvar lesions that appear as ill-defined and variable changes in the vulvar skin has been confusing because it has been based on clinical appearances (Lavery, 1984). In addition, the same term has had various definitions, depending on the author, and different terms have been used by separate authors to describe the same lesion. Consequently, studies of whether these lesions are actually premalignant are difficult to interpret accurately.

In the early part of this century, the vulvar dystrophies, then termed "leukoplakia," and most recently called "non-neoplastic epithelial disorders of the skin and mucosa" (Ridley et al, 1989), were thought by many authors to be premalignant. Nonetheless, Jeffcoate (1966) found only four cancers (2.9%) of the vulva developing among 138 women followed up for three to 25 years who had "chronic vulvar dystrophy." Hart et al (1975) summarized the results of 10 case series of lichen sclerosis, a form of vulvar dystrophy; out of 465 patients, 16 (3.4%) developed vulvar cancer. No invasive cancers developed among the 28 patients with vulvar dystrophy followed by Lavery (1984). These studies are in contrast to that of Rodke et al (1988), who found that three of 18 (16.7%) selected women who had histologic evidence of both hyperplastic dystrophy (now called squamous cell hyperplasias) and lichen sclerosis later developed squamous cell vulvar cancer.

On the other hand, dystrophies are often found adjacent to invasive cancer in case series. Borgno et al (1988), for example, found that some 60% of women in their series with invasive vulvar cancer had histologic changes consistent with dystrophies adjacent to their vulvar tumor. In a series from the Johns Hopkins Hospital, the comparable figure was 52% (Buscema et al, 1980b). Lichen sclerosis has been found adjacent to 4% of 98 vulvar cancers in one recent series, 53% in another, and 60% in a third (Buscema et al, 1980b; Punnonen et al, 1985; Neill et al, 1990).

In a case-control study of invasive vulvar cancer, Mabuchi et al (1985) found that 13 of 148 women with cancer and none of the matched controls reported a prior history of "leukoplakia."

CONCEPTS OF PATHOGENESIS

Carcinoma In Situ as a Precursor to Invasive Cancer

The question of whether vulvar carcinoma in situ is truly a precursor to invasive cancer remains unresolved. Observations suggesting a low malignant potential for carcinoma in situ of the vulva include:

1. Spontaneous regression of bowenoid atypia and Bowen's disease (carcinoma in situ) (Friedrich et al, 1980b; Buscema et al, 1980a; Kimura, 1982).

2. Only 15% to 30% of patients with invasive vulvar cancer have adjacent carcinoma in situ present upon histologic examination (Buscema et al, 1980b; Becagli et al, 1983), whereas the comparable figure for cervical carcinoma in situ adjacent to invasive disease is 80% to 100% (Park et al, 1991).

3. Fewer than 5% of cases with carcinoma in situ progress to malignancy in most series (Buscema et al, 1980a; Friedrich et al, 1980a; Jones and McLean, 1986). But because patients in these studies are treated for their carcinoma in situ, these studies do not necessarily reflect the true risk of progression.

Nonetheless, at least some patients with Bowen's disease who are treated for it do develop invasive cancer; this is particularly true among patients who are immunosuppressed and among women who are older. Of the four patients with vulvar carcinoma in situ who developed invasive vulvar cancer after treatment for their initial lesion reported by Buscema et al (1980a), two of these patients were immunosuppressed and two were over 70 years old. Jones and McLean (1986) found one of 31 treated patients with carcinoma in situ of the vulva developed an invasive malignancy but that all of the four patients managed by limited biopsy eventually developed invasive disease. These four patients had a history of other neoplasms in the genital tract as well and may not characterize the situation for all women with vulvar in situ cancer. Karyotypic analyses of biopsies from vulvar carcinoma in situ typically show aneuploid DNA content, which suggests a malignant potential for these lesions (Campion and Singer, 1987). More recently, Toki et al (1991) suggested that there are three pathologically distinct types of invasive squamous cell carcinomas, two of which are highly associated with vulvar intraepithelial neoplasia.

The invasive potential for vaginal intraepithelial neoplasia is also uncertain, although progression to malignancy does occur (Campion, 1987). Aho et al (1991) demonstrated this by following 23 untreated patients with vaginal intraepithelial neoplasia for three years. Two patients (9%) progressed to invasive vaginal carcinoma. Benedet and Sanders (1984) found that one of four patients with untreated carcinoma of the vagina progressed to invasive disease, but none of 44 patients with completely excised carcinoma in situ developed invasive vaginal cancer.

Papillomavirus in the Pathogenesis of Neoplasia

Recently, several studies (reviewed in Toki et al, 1991) have suggested that only a subset of in situ and invasive squamous cell vulvar cancers, which can be distinguished by specific pathologic and clinical characteristics, are related to HPV infection. In these studies, women who had tumors lacking HPV were older than those with HPV-associated lesions.

Even in HPV-associated cancers, both epidemiologic and laboratory observations support the idea that additional agents are needed for an anogenital cancer to develop. Zur Hausen (1986) has noted that anogenital HPV infections in women are relatively common compared to the incidence of cancers at those sites. In experimental systems, HPV 16 and 18 are able to immortalize cell lines, but those cell lines do not cause tumor formation in nude mice without the addition of an activated oncogene, such as Ha-ras or c-myc, suggesting that additional changes are necessary for that to occur (Matlashewski et al, 1988; Zur Hausen, 1989; Wright and Richart, 1990). Zur Hausen (1986) has postulated that cellular factors usually control the expression of the early genes of HPV in an infected cell. When a cell fails to regulate HPV transcription, due to modifications of the host genome by cofactors, a tumor develops. Potential cofactors include carcinogens found in cigarette smoke (Daling et al, 1992), infection with other viruses (including herpes virus type 2), chronic infections, use of oral contraceptives and hormones, and immunosuppression (reviewed in Zur Hausen, 1989). Dyson et al (1989) reported that the protein product of the E7-transforming region of HPV can bind to the protein product of the retinoblastoma gene, a tumor suppressor. They suggested that the formation of a complex between these two proteins might lead to the inactivation of the retinoblastoma gene, and with that, a loss of cellular growth control leading to the development of a tumor. More recently, it has been shown that cells infected with HPV produce a viral protein (E6), which binds to and causes rapid degeneration of p53, possibly contributing to cellular transformation (DiPaolo et al, 1993).

In invasive cancers, HPV types 16 and 18 typically are found integrated into the human genome, although not at specific places on certain chromosomes. However, integration does normally interrupt the HPV genome in the E1/E2 region, and leaves the regulatory and transforming regions intact. One consequence of this is that two HPV genes thought to encode a transforming function are expressed in a deregulated manner (Howley and Schlegel, 1988; Venuti et al, 1989).

In cell lines established from cervical cancer, Cannizzaro et al (1988) reported that HPV DNA integrated near regions of the chromosome that are known to break. In one cervical cancer specimen, HPV DNA had integrated near the location of a known oncogene and also a fragile site.

PREVENTIVE MEASURES

Although the causes of these neoplasms are not well understood, the association of HPV with both vulvar and vaginal cancers indicates that women who have had genital warts, a subclinical HPV infection, other anogenital cancers, or multiple sexual partners should be screened on a frequent basis. In addition, the development of a vaccine against types of HPV that commonly infect the anogenital area might reduce the incidence of vulvar and vaginal cancer. The consistency of the finding that women with vulvar cancer are current smokers argues that smoking-cessation programs may lead to some decrease in the incidence of this disease.

Future Research

The number of etiologic case-control studies of both vulvar and vaginal cancer has been limited as a consequence of the low incidence of these tumors. However, recent interest in the role of HPV in the genesis of genital cancers has stimulated research on vulvar cancer, and data from at least two population-based case-control studies are currently being analyzed. Important questions that remain unanswered include the role of specific types of HPV in the development of these cancers as well as the identification of specific cofactors that participate in the neoplastic process. In this context, examination of the role of cigarette smoking and its potential interaction with HPV would be particularly fruitful. Additional agents that need to be explored in more detail as possible risk factors include exogenous hormones, diet, diabetes, and other sexually transmitted diseases.

REFERENCES

Aho M, Vesterinen E, Meyer B, Purola E, Paavonen J. 1991. Natural history of vaginal intraepithelial neoplasia. Cancer 68(1):195–197.

Becagli L, Scrimin F, De Bastiani B, De Salvia D, Nardelli GB, Ambrosini A. 1983. Vulvar carcinoma: natural history. Eur J Gynaecol Oncol 4:229–233.

Beck I. 1984. Vaginal carcinoma arising in vaginal condylomata. Case report. Br J Obstet Gynaecol 91:503–505.

Beckmann AM, Kiviat NB, Daling JR, Sherman KJ, McDougall JM. 1988. Human papillomavirus type 16 in multifocal neoplasis of the female genital tract. Int J Gynecol Pathol 7:39–47.

Bell J, Sevin B, Averette H, Nadji M. 1984. Vaginal cancer after hysterectomy for benign disease: value of cytologic screening. Obstet Gynecol 64:699–701.

Benedet JL, Sanders BH. 1984. Carcinoma in situ of the vagina. Am J Obstet Gynecol 148:695–700.

Berg JW, Lampe JG. 1981. High-risk factors in gynecologic cancer. Cancer 48 (Suppl):429–441.

Blohme I, Brynger H. 1985. Malignant disease in renal transplant patients. Transplantation 39:23–25.

Boice JD, Day NE, Andersen A, et al. 1985. Second cancers following radiation treatment for cervical cancer. An international collaboration among cancer registries. J Natl Cancer Inst 74:955–975.

Borgno G, Micheletti L, Barbero M, Preti M, Cavanna L, Ghiringhello B. 1988. Epithelial alterations adjacent to 111 vulvar carcinomas. J Reprod Med 33:500–502.

Bornstein J, Adam E, Adler-Storthz K, Kaufman RH. 1988. Development of cervical and vaginal squamous cell neoplasia as a late consequence of in utero exposure to diethylstilbestrol. Obstet Gynecol Surv 43:15–21.

Boxer RJ, Skinner DG. 1977. Condylomata acuminata and squamous cell carcinoma. Urology 9:72–78.

Brinton LA, Schairer C, Haenszel W, Stolley P, Lehman HF, Levine R, Savitz DA. 1986. Smoking and invasive cervical cancer. JAMA 255:3265–3269.

Brinton LA, Nasca PC, Mallin K, Baptiste MS, Wilbanks GD, Richard RM. 1990a. Case-control study of cancer of the vulva. Obstet Gynecol 75:859–865.

Brinton LA, Nasca PC, Mallin K, Schairer C, Rosenthal J, Rothenberg R, Yordan E, Richart RM. 1990b. Case-control study of in-situ and invasive carcinoma of the vagina. Gynecol Oncol 38:49–56.

Buscema J, Woodruff J, Parmley TH, Genadry R. 1980a. Carcinoma in situ of the vulva. Obstet Gynecol 55:225–230.

Buscema J, Stern J, Woodruff JD. 1990b. The significance of the histologic alterations adjacent to invasive vulvar carcinoma. Am J Obstet Gynecol 137:902–909.

Buscema J, Stern JL, Woodruff JD. 1981. Early invasive carcinoma of the vulva. Am J Obstet Gynecol 140:563–569.

Buscema J, Naghashfar Z, Sawada E, Daniel R, Woodruff JD, Shah K. 1988. The predominance of human papillomavirus type 16 in vulvar neoplasia. Obstet Gynecol 71:601–606.

Cabral CA, Marciario-Cabral F, Fry D, Lumpkin CK, Mercer L, Gopelrud S. 1982. Expression of herpes simplex virus type 2 antigens in premalignant human vulvar cells. Am J Obstet Gynecol 143:814–820.

Campion MJ. 1987. Clinical manifestations and natural history of genital human papillomavirus infection. Obstet Gynecol Clin North Am 14:363–387.

Campion MJ, Singer A. 1987. Vulval intraepithelial neoplasia: clinical review. Genitourin Med 63:147–152.

Cannizzaro LA, Durst M, Mendez MJ, Hecht BK, Hecht F. 1988. Regional chromosome localization of human papillomavirus integration sites near fragile site, oncogenes, and cancer chromosome breakpoints. Cancer Genet Cytogenet 33:93–98.

Cario GM. 1984. Squamous cell carcinoma of the vulva in association with mixed vulvar dystrophy in an 18-year-old girl. Case report. Br J Obstet Gynaecol 91:87–90.

Carson LF, Twiggs LB, Okagaki T, Clark BA, Ostrow RS, Faras AJ. 1988. Human papillomavirus DNA in adenosquamous carcinoma and squamous cell carcinoma of the vulva. Obstet Gynecol 72:63–67.

Caterson RJ, Furber J, Murray J, McCarthy W, Mahony JF, Sheil GR. 1984. Carcinoma of the vulva in two young renal allograft recipients. Transplant Proc 16:559–561.

Charleswood GP, Shippel S. 1953. Vulval condyloma acuminata as a pre-malignant lesion in the Bantu. S Afr Med J 27:149–151.

Cook JC, Wilkinson EJ, Friedrich EG, Massay JR. 1986. Vulvar intraepithelial neoplasia and smoking. Presented at Human Papillomavirus and Squamous Cancer, Second International Conference, Chicago.

Costa S, Rotola A, Terzano P, Poggi MG, Di Luca D, Aurelian L, Cassa E, Orlandi C. 1990. Search for herpes simplex virus and human papillomavirus genetic expression in vulvar neoplasia. J Reprod Med 35:1108–1112.

Cromer JK. 1963. Further observations on the multicentric origin of carcinomas of the female anogenital tract. Am Surg 29:793–798.

Crowther ME, Lowe DG, Shepherd JH. 1988. Verrucous carcinoma of the female genital tract: a review. Obstet Gynecol Survey 43:263–280.

Crum CP, Braun LA, Shah KV, Fu Y, Levine RU, Fenoglio CM, Richart RM, Townsend DE. 1982. Vulvar intraepithelial neoplasia: correlation of nuclear DNA content and the presence of a human papilloma virus (HPV) structural antigen. Cancer 49:468–471.

Daling JR, Chu J, Weiss NS, Emel L, Tamimi HK. 1984. The association of condylomata acuminata and squamous carcinoma of the vulva. Br J Cancer 50:533–535.

Daling JR, Sherman KJ, Hislop TG, Maden C, Mandelson MT, Beckmann AM, Weiss NS. 1992. Cigarette smoking and the risk of anogenital cancer. Am J Epidemiol 135(2):180–189.

Day JC. 1958. Second primary malignant tumor in gynecology. Am J Obstet Gynecol 75:976–982.

Diehl WK, Baggett JW, Shell JH. 1951. Vulvar cancer. Am J Obstet Gynecol 62:1209–1224.

DiPaolo JA, Popescu NC, Alvarez L, Woodworth CD. 1993. Cellular and molecular alterations in human epithelial cells transformed by recombinant human papillomavirus DNA. Crit Rev Oncogen 4(4):337–360.

Di Luca D, Rotola A, Pilotti S, Monini P, Caselli E, Rilke F, Cassai E. 1987. Simultaneous presence of herpes simplex and human papillomavirus sequences in human genital tumors. Int J Cancer 40:763–768.

Downey GO, Okagaki T, Ostrow RS, Clark BA, Twiggs LB, Faras AJ. 1988. Condylomatous carcinoma of the vulva with special reference to human papillomavirus DNA. Obstet Gynecol 72:68–73.

Dyson N, Howley PM, Munger K, Harlow E. 1989. The human papillomavirus 16 E7 oncoprotein is able to bind to the retinoblastoma gene product. Science 243:934–937.

Eichner E. 1956. Multiple carcinoma in situ. Obstet Gynecol 8:508–511.

Figge DC, Gaudenz R. 1974. Invasive carcinoma of the vulva. Am J Obstet Gynecol 119:382–395.

Franklin EW, Rutledge FD. 1972. Epidemiology of epidermoid carcinoma of the vulva. Obstet Gynecol 39:165–172.

Friedrich EG, Wilkinson EJ, Fu YS. 1980a. Carcinoma in situ of the vulva: a continuing challenge. Am J Obstet Gynecol 136:830–843.

Friedrich EG, Wilkinson EJ, Fu YS. 1980b. Carcinoma in situ of the vulva: a continuing challenge. Am J Obstet Gynecol 136:523–525.

Gallup DG, Talledo OE, Shah KJ, Hayes C. 1987. Invasive squamous cell carcinoma of the vagina: a 14-year study. Obstet Gynecol 69:782–785.

Green TH. 1978. Carcinoma of the vulva. A reassessment. Obstet Gynecol 52:462–469.

Greenwald P, Barlow JJ, Nasca PC, Burnett WS. 1971. Vaginal cancer after maternal treatment with synthetic estrogens. N Engl J Med 285:390–392.

Gunning JE. 1976. Supplement: The DES story. Obstet Gynecol Surv 31:827–833.

Halpert R, Fruchter RG, Sedlis A, Butt K, Boyce JG, Sillman FH. 1986. Human papillomavirus and lower genital neoplasia in renal transplant patients. Obstet Gynecol 68:251–258.

Hart WR, Norris HJ, Helwig EB. 1975. Relation of lichen sclerosus etatrophicus of the vulva to development of carcinoma. Obstet Gynecol 45:369–377.

Herbst AL, Green TH, Ulfelder H. 1970. Primary carcinoma of the vagina. Am J Obstet Gynecol 106:210–218.

Herbst AL, Ulfelder H, Poskanzer DC. 1971. Adenocarcinoma of the vagina: association of maternal stilbestrol therapy with tumor appearance in young women. N Engl J Med 284:878–881.

Herbst AL, Anderson S, Hubby MM, Haenszel WM, Kaufman RH, Noller KL. 1986. Risk factors for the development of diethylstilbestrol-associated clear cell adenocarcinoma: a case-control study. Am J Obstet Gynecol 154:814–822.

Herman JM, Homesley HD, Dignan MB. 1986. Is hysterectomy a risk factor for vaginal cancer? JAMA 256:601–603.

Heston JF, Kelly JB, Meig JW, Flannery JT. 1986. Forty-five years of incidence in Connecticut: 1935–79. National Cancer Institute Monograph No. 70, DHHS Public Health Service Publ. No. 86-2652.

Howley PM, Schlegel R. 1988. The human papillomaviruses. An overview. Am J Med 85 (Suppl 2A):155–158.

Ikenberg H, Runge M, Goppinger A, Pfleiderer A. 1990. Human papillomavirus DNA in invasive carcinoma of the vagina. Obstet Gynecol 76:432–438.

Japaze H, Garcia-Bunuel R, Woodruff JD. 1977. Primary vulvar neoplasia. A review of in situ and invasive carcinoma, 1935–1972. Obstet Gynecol 49:404–411.

Jeffcoate TNA. 1966. Chronic vulval dystrophies. Am J Obstet Gynecol 95:61–74.

Johnston GA, Klotz J, Boutselis JG. 1983. Primary invasive carcinoma of the vagina. Am J Obstet Gynecol 154:34–39.

Jones RW, McLean MR. 1986. Carcinoma in situ of the vulva: a review of 31 treated and five untreated cases. Obstet Gynecol 68:499–503.

Jones RW, Park JS, McLean MR, Shah KV. 1990. Human papillomavirus in women with vulvar intraepithelial neoplasia. J Reprod Med 35:1124–1126.

Kaiser IH. 1952. Primary carcinoma of the vagina. Cancer 5:1146–1150.

Kasher MS, Roman A. 1988. Characterization of human papillomavirus type 6b DNA isolated from an invasive squamous carcinoma of the vulva. Virology 165:225–233.

Katz RL, Veanattukalathil S, Weiss KM. 1987. Human papillomavirus infection and neoplasia of the cervix and anogenital region in women with Hodgkin's disease. Acta Cytol 31:845–854.

Kaufman RH, Dreesman GR, Burek J, Korhonen MO, Matson DO, Melnick JL, Powell KL, Purifoy DJM, Courtney RJ, Adam E. 1981. Herpesvirus-induced antigens in squamous-cell carcinoma in situ of the vulva. N Engl J Med 305:483–488.

Kelsey JL, Hildreth NG. 1983. Breast and gynecologic cancer epidemiology. Boca Raton, FL: CRC Press, pp. 143–151.

Kennedy AW, Hart WR. 1982. Multiple squamous-cell carcinomas in Fanconi's anemia. Cancer 50:811–814.

Kimura S. 1982. Bowenoid papulosis of the genitalia. Int J Dermatol 21:432–436.

Kiyabu MT, Shibata M, Arnheim N, Martin WJ, Fitzgibbons P. 1989. Detection of human papillomavirus in formalin-fixed, invasive squamous carcinomas using the polymerase chain reaction. Am J Surg Pathol 13:221–224.

Lavery HA. 1984. Vulval dystrophies: new approaches. Clin Obstet Gynecol 11:155–169.

Lee RA, Symmonds RE. 1976. Recurrent carcinoma in situ of the vagina in patients previously treated for in situ carcinoma of the cervix. Obstet Gynecol 48:61–64.

Lindeque BG, Nel AE, du Toit JP. 1987. Immune deficiency and invasive carcinoma of the vulva in a young woman: a case report. Gynecol Oncol 26:112–118.

Mabuchi K, Bross DS, Kessler II. 1985. Epidemiology of cancer of the vulva. A case-control study. Cancer 55:1843–1848.

Manetta A, Pinto JL, Larson JE, Stevens CW, Pinto JS, Podczaski ES. 1988. Primary invasive carcinoma of the vagina. Obstet Gynecol 72:77–81.

Matlashewski G, Osborn K, Banks L, Stanley M, Crawford L. 1988. Transformation of primary human fibroblast cells with human papillomavirus type 16 DNA and EJ-ras. Int J Cancer 42:232–238.

McCance DJ, Clarkson PK, Dyson JL, Walker PG, Singer A. 1985. Human papillomavirus types 6 and 16 in multifocal intraepithelial neoplasias of the female lower genital tract. Br J Obstet Gynaecol 92:1093–1100.

McFarlane MJ, Feinstein AR, Horwitz RI. 1986. Diethylstilbestrol and clear cell vaginal carcinoma: reappraisal of the epidemiologic evidence. Am J Med 81:855–863.

McPherson HA, Diddle AW, Gardner WH, Williamson PJ. 1963. Epidermoid carcinoma of the cervix, vagina, and vulva: a regional disease. Obstet Gynecol 21:145–149.

Melnick S, Cole P, Anderson D, Herbst A. 1987. Rates and risks of diethylstilbestrol-related clear-cell adenocarcinoma of the vagina and cervix: an update. N Engl J Med 316:514–516.

Menczer J, Voliovitch Y, Modan B, Modan M, Steinitz R. 1982. Some epidemiologic aspects of carcinoma of the vulva in Israel. Am J Obstet Gynecol 143:893–896.

Muir C, Waterhouse J, Mack T, et al. 1987. Cancer Incidence in Five Continents, Volume V. IARC Scientific Publications No. 88, Lyon.

National Cancer Institute (Division of Cancer Prevention and Control, Division of Cancer Treatment). 1994. SEER Cancer Statistics Review, 1973–1991. DHHS NCI Publ. No. 94-2789.

Neill SM, Lessana-Leibowitch M, Plesse M, Moyal-Barracco M. 1990. Lichen sclerosis, invasive squamous cell carcinoma, and human papillomavirus. Am J Obstet Gynecol 162:1633–1634.

Newcomb PA, Weiss NS, Daling JR. 1984. Incidence of vulvar carcinoma in relation to menstrual, reproductive, and medical factors. J Natl Cancer Inst 73:391–396.

Okagaki T. 1984. Female genital tumors associated with human papillomavirus infection, and the concept of genital neoplasia-papilloma syndrome (GENPS). Pathol Annu 19:31–62.

Okagaki T, Clark BA, Zachow KR, Twiggs LB, Ostrow RS, Pass F, Faras AJ. 1984. Presence of human papillomavirus in verrucous carcinoma (Akerman) of the vagina. Arch Pathol Lab Med 108:567–570.

O'Mara BA, Byers T, Schoenfeld E. 1985. Diabetes mellitus and cancer risk: A multisite case-control study. J Chron Dis 38:435–441.

Ostrow RS, Manias DA, Clark BA, Fukushima M, Okagaki T, Twiggs LB, Faras AJ. 1988. The analysis of carcinoma of the vagina for human papillomavirus DNA. Int J Gynecol Pathol 7:308–314.

Palefsky J. 1991. HPV infection among HIV-infected individuals. Hematol Oncol Clin North Am 5:357–370.

Parazzini F, LaVecchia C, Garsia S, Negri E, Sideri M, Rognoni MT, Origoni M. 1993. Determinants of invasive vulvar cancer risk: an Italian case-control study. Gynecol Oncol 48(1):50–55.

Park JS, Jones RW, McClean MR, et al. 1991. Possible etiologic heterogeneity of vulvar intraepithelial neoplasia. Cancer 67:1599–1607.

Parker RT, Duncan I, Rampone JR, Creasman W. 1975. Operative management of early invasive epidermoid carcinoma of the vulva. Am J Obstet Gynecol 123:349–355.

Penn I. 1988. Tumors of the immunocompromised patient. Annu Rev Med 39:63–73.

Peters RK, Mack TM, Bernstein L. 1984. Parallels in the epidemiology of selected anogenital carcinomas. J Natl Cancer Inst 72:609–615.

Pilotti S, Rilke F, Shah KV, Delle Torre G, De Palo G. 1984. Immunohistochemical and ultrastructural evidence of papilloma virus infection associated with in situ and microinvasive squamous cell carcinoma of the vulva. Am J Surg Pathol 8:751–761.

Pilotti S, Rotola A, D'Amato L, Di Luca D, Shah KV, Cassai E, Rilke F. 1990. Vulvar carcinomas: search for sequences homologous to human papillomavirus and herpes simplex virus DNA. Mod Pathol 3:442–448.

Pride GL, Buchler DA. 1977. Carcinoma of vagina 10 or more years following pelvic irradiation therapy. Am J Obstet Gynecol 127:513–517.

Prins RP, Morrow CP, Townsend DE, Disaia PJ. 1976. Vaginal embryogenesis, estrogens, and adenosis. Obstet Gynecol 48:246–250.

Punnonen R, Soidinmaki H, Kauppila O, Pystynen P. 1985. Relationship of vulvar lichen sclerosus et atrophicus to carcinoma. Annales Chirurgiae et Gynaecologiae 74 (Suppl. 197):23–26.

Rastkar G, Okagaki T, Twiggs LB, Clark BA. 1982. Early invasive and in situ warty carcinoma of the vulva: clinical, histologic, and electron microscopic study with particular reference to viral association. Am J Obstet Gynecol 143:814–820.

Rhatigan RM, Saffos RO. 1977. Condyloma acuminatum and squamous carcinoma of the vulva. South Med J 70:591–594.

Ridley CR, Frankman O, Joens ISC, Pincus SH, Wilkinson EJ. 1989. New nomenclature for the study of vulvar disease: International society for the study of vulvar disease. Hum Pathol 20:495–496.

Robboy SJ, Truslow GY, Anton J, Richart RM. 1981. Role of hormones including diethylstilbestrol (DES) in the pathogenesis of cervical and vaginal intraepithelial neoplasia. Gynecol Oncol 12:S98–S110.

Robboy SJ, Noller KL, O'Brien P, Kaufman RH, Townsend D, Barnes AB, Gundersen J, Lawrence D, Bergstrahl E, McGorray S, Tilley BC, Anton J, Chazen G. 1984. Increased incidence of cervical and vaginal dysplasia in 3,980 diethylstilbestrol-exposed young women. JAMA 252:2979–2983.

Rodke G, Friedrich EG, Wilkinson EJ. 1988. Malignant potential of mixed vulvar dystrophy (lichen sclerosus associated with squamous cell hyperplasia). J Reprod Med 33:545–550.

Rose PG, Herterick EE, Boutselis JG, Moeshberger M, Sachs L. 1987. Multiple primary gynecologic neoplasms. Am J Obstet Gynecol 157:261–267.

Rueda-Leverone NG, Di Paola GR, Meiss RP, Vighi SG, Llamosas F. 1987. Association of human papillomavirus and vulvar intraepithelial neoplasia: a morphological and immunohistochemical study of 30 cases. Gynecol Oncology 26:331–339.

Ruiz-Moreno JA, Garcia-Gomez R, Vargas-Solano A, Alonso P. 1987. Vaginal intraepithelial neoplasia. Report of 14 cases. Int J Gynaecol Obstet 25:359–362.

Rutledge F. 1967. Cancer of the vagina. Am J Obstet Gynecol 97:635–655.

Rutledge F, Smith JP, Franklin EW. 1970. Carcinoma of the vulva. Am J Obstet Gynecol 106:1117–1130.

Schmauz R, Owor R. 1980. Epidemiology of malignant degeneration of condylomata acuminata in Uganda. Pathol Res Pract 91:103.

Schoenberg BS. 1977. Multiple primary malignant neoplasms: the Connecticut experience 1935–1964. Recent results. Cancer Res 58:1–173.

Schrager LK, Friedland GH, Maude D, Schreiber K, Adachi A, Pizzuti DJ, Koss LG, Klein RS. 1989. Cervical and vaginal squamous cell abnormalities in women infected with human immunodeficiency virus. J Acquired Immune Deficiency Syndrome 2:570–575.

Schwartz PE, Naftolin F. 1981. Type 2 herpes simplex virus and vulvar carcinoma in situ. Editorial. N Engl J Med 305:517–518.

Sengupta BS. 1980. Vulvar carcinoma in premenopausal Jamaican women. Int J Gynaecol Obstet 17:526–530.

Sharp GB, Cole P. 1991. Identification of risk factors for diethylstilbestrol-associated clear cell adenocarcinoma of the vagina: similarities to endometrial cancer. Am J Epidemiol 134(11):1316–1324.

Sherman KJ, Daling JR, Chu J, McKnight B, Weiss NS. 1988. Multiple primary tumors in women with vulvar neoplasms: A case-control study. Br J Cancer 57:423–427.

Sherman KJ, Daling JR, Chu J, Weiss NS, Ashley RL, Corey L. 1991. Genital warts, other sexually transmitted diseases, and vulvar cancer. Epidemiology 2:257–262.

Sherman KJ, Daling JR, McKnight B, et al. 1994. Hormonal factors in vulvar cancer: A case-control study. J Reprod Med 39:857–861.

Shokri-Tabibzadeh S, Koss LG, Molnar J, Romney S. 1981. Association of human papillomavirus with neoplastic processes in the genital tract of four women with impaired immunity. Gynecol Oncol 12:S129–S140.

Sillman FH, Sedlis A. 1987. Anogenital papillomavirus infection and neoplasia in immunodeficient women. Obstet Gynecol Clin North Am 14:537–559.

Stafl A, Mattingly RF. 1974. Vaginal adenosis: a precancerous lesion? Am J Obstet Gynecol 120:666–677.

Stuart GC, Allen HH, Anderson RJ. 1981. Squamous cell carcinoma of the vagina following hysterectomy. Am J Obstet Gynecol 139:311–315.

Sturgeon SR, Ziegler RG, Brinton LA, Nasca PC, Mallin K, Gridley G. 1991. Diet and the risk of vulvar cancer. Ann Epidemiol 1:427–437.

Sturgeon SR, Brinton LA, Devesa SS, Kurman RJ. 1992. In situ and invasive vulvar cancer incidence trends (1973 to 1987). Am J Obstet Gynecol 166:1482–1485.

Taussig FL. 1940. Cancer of the vulva: analysis of 155 cases (1911–1940). Am J Obstet Gynecol 40:764–779.

Toki T, Kurman RJ, Park JS, Kessis T, Daniel RW, Shah KV. 1991. Probable nonpapillomavirus etiology of squamous cell carcinoma of the vulva in older women: A clinicopathologic study using in situ hybridization and polymerase chain reaction. Int J Gynecol Pathol 10:107–125.

Ulfelder H, Poskanzer D, Herbst AL. 1971. Stilbestrol-adenosis-carcinoma syndrome: geographic distribution. Letter. N Engl J Med 285:619.

Valente PT, Hurt MA, Jelan I. 1991. Human papillomavirus-associated vulvar verrucous carcinoma in a 20-year-old with an intact hymen. J Reprod Med 36:213–216.

Venuti A, Marcante ML. 1989. Presence of human papillomavirus type 18 DNA in vulvar carcinomas and its integration into the cell genome. J Gen Virol 70:1587–1592.

Vessey MP. 1986. Epidemiology of cervical cancer: role of hormonal factors, cigarette smoking and occupation. In Peto R, zur Hausen H (eds): Viral etiology of cervical cancer. New York: Cold Springs Harbor Laboratory, pp. 29–44.

Voliovitch Y, Menczer J, Modan M, Modan B. 1984. Clinical features of Jewish Israeli patients with squamous cell carcinoma of the vulva. Israel J Med Sci 20:421–425.

Wade-Evans T. 1976. The aetiology and pathology of cancer of the vagina. Clin Obstet Gynecol 3:229–241.

Way S. 1948. Primary carcinoma of the vagina. J Obstet Gynecol Br Commonw 55:739–755.

Winkelstein W. 1990. Smoking and cervical cancer—current status: a review. Am J Epidemiol 131:945–957.

Woodcock AS. 1976. The aetiology and pathology of cancer of the vulva. Clin Obstet Gynecol 3:201–216.

Wright TC, Richart RM. 1990. Role of human papillomavirus in the pathogenesis of genital tract warts and cancer. Gynecol Oncol 37:151–164.

Young JL, Percy CL, Asire AJ. 1981. Surveillance, Epidemiology and End Results: Incidence and Mortality Data, 1973–1977. Natl Cancer Inst Monogr No. 57. NIH Publ. No. 81-2330.

zur Hausen H. 1982. Human genital cancer: synergism between two virus infections or synergism between a virus infection and initiating events? Lancet 2:1370–1371.

zur Hausen H. 1986. Intracellular surveillance of persisting viral infections. Lancet 2:489–491.

zur Hausen H. 1989. Papillomaviruses as carcinomaviruses. In Klein G (ed): Adv Virol Oncol. Vol. 8. New York: Raven Press, pp. 1–26.

52 Choriocarcinoma

JONATHAN BUCKLEY

Gestational choriocarcinoma is an unusual tumor in many respects. Perhaps the most remarkable feature is that it is a malignant allograft, being genetically distinct from its host. Gestational choriocarcinoma derives from trophoblastic epithelium of the placenta and thus arises from a conceptus, and it is usually diagnosed within a few months of a normal delivery, an abortion, an ectopic pregnancy, or the expulsion of a hydatidiform mole. Of these precursors, the most important is the hydatidiform mole, a developmental abnormality of the trophoblast, since the risk of choriocarcinoma is at least 1,000 times higher following a hydatidiform mole than following other types of pregnancy (Park and Lees, 1950). A consequence of this exceedingly high relative risk is that the descriptive epidemiology of choriocarcinoma and hydatidiform mole are similar.

Choriocarcinoma is a very rare malignancy, with an incidence of 1.4 per million population in the United States (Brinton et al, 1986), making epidemiological investigation difficult. Attention has tended to focus more on the precursor conditions, such as the hydatidiform mole, in the hope that these will shed light on the pathogenesis of choriocarcinoma, and this review presents the epidemiological features of hydatidiform mole alongside those of choriocarcinoma for the same reason. This is not to imply that choriocarcinoma and hydatidiform mole form part of a continuous spectrum of trophoblastic disease, nor that they necessarily share risk factors. However, whether the diseases are developmentally related or not, the epidemiology of hydatidiform mole is highly relevant if only because choriocarcinoma so often follows a molar pregnancy, and risk factors for hydatidiform mole will have (at a minimum) a strong secondary effect on choriocarcinoma risk (Palmer, 1994).

A small proportion of choriocarcinomas are nongestational, usually arising from the ovary or testis. However, this chapter will follow common practice in using the term choriocarcinoma to refer to the gestational form of the disease, unless otherwise stated.

DEMOGRAPHIC PATTERNS

Histopathology and Diagnosis

The histopathology of choriocarcinoma is characterized by a layered arrangement of the same cell types found in the developing trophoblast (cytotrophoblastic, syncytiotrophoblastic, and intermediate cells), absence of chorionic villi, and, commonly, extensive areas of hemorrhage and necrosis. The cells may be pleomorphic, with enlarged nuclei, and abnormal mitotic figures (Ober, 1971). While the microscopic appearance of the tumor is quite characteristic and usually permits a definitive diagnosis, the most important feature of the malignant cells from a diagnostic viewpoint is probably not their morphology but their ability to secrete human chorionic gonadotrophin (hCG). Thus, a firm diagnosis of choriocarcinoma may not depend on histological confirmation, but instead be based on the obstetric history, presenting features, and presence of an elevated hCG level.

The greatest diagnostic difficulties are to distinguish choriocarcinoma from the benign forms of trophoblastic disease, most notably invasive hydatidiform mole, in which molar tissue persists after the pregnancy terminates. These conditions, although ultimately self-limiting, can mimic choriocarcinoma in producing local invasion, metastases, and elevated hCG levels, and in having shared histological features (Lurain and Brewer, 1982). Important features of the nonmalignant trophoblastic conditions that help to differentiate them from choriocarcinoma are that they always follow a molar pregnancy, rarely spread beyond the uterus, its adnexae, or the lungs, and spontaneously resolve within 4 to 6 months (Park and Lees, 1950). The presence of hydatidiform villi is an important differentiating feature, since it almost guarantees benignity (Novak and Seah, 1954); the converse is not true, however, since absence of villi may result from collection of an inadequate or unrepresentative sample (Elston and Bagshawe, 1972).

Since invasive moles are more common than choriocarcinoma and thus more easily studied, an important question is whether the invasive mole represents a self-limiting variant of choriocarcinoma, or is better characterized as a form of hydatidiform mole. Its behavior would certainly suggest a close relationship with choriocarcinoma. On the other hand, the frequency of choriocarcinoma after an invasive mole appears to be similar to that following a hydatidiform mole (Park and Lees, 1950; Hunt et al, 1953), and tissue from invasive moles when transplanted to a nude mouse does not show the aggressively malignant behavior characteristic of choriocarcinoma (Kato et al, 1982). Until more is known about the relationship of choriocarcinoma and invasive mole, these conditions should be considered as quite distinct entities.

Whether or not invasive moles and choriocarcinoma are biologically related, they have come to be grouped together clinically, for entirely practical reasons. The importance of instituting early treatment for choriocarcinoma (and the small but definite risk of serious complications of invasive moles) is viewed by many as outweighing any immediate or long-term risks of chemotherapy. As a result, many patients receive a nonspecific diagnosis of "residual trophoblastic disease." Blurring of the distinction between choriocarcinoma and nonmalignant residual trophoblastic disease makes epidemiological study of these diseases particularly difficult, and inevitably complicates efforts to determine their individual risk factors.

In recent years the importance of distinguishing between different types of hydatidiform moles has been recognized. The traditional division of moles into "complete," in which no fetal tissue is present, and "partial," in which both trophoblastic and fetal or embryonal tissues are present, has been shown to be based on a fundamental genetic difference between the two forms (Szulman and Surti, 1978). Most attention is now focused on complete moles, which are the group most likely to progress to choriocarcinoma (Wake et al, 1984). The genetics of hydatidiform mole and choriocarcinoma are described in more detail below.

Incidence—United States

Incidence of choriocarcinoma is commonly expressed as a rate per 100,000 pregnancies, since a preceding conception is an absolute requirement and any factors that are related solely to differences in pregnancy rates are usually not of interest. Determination of pregnancy rates in a population is problematic, however, as official statistics may not include counts of induced and spontaneous abortions or molar pregnancies. The number of live births in the population under study has been used by many investigators as a useful surrogate for the number of pregnancies, when reliable information on other forms of pregnancy has not been available. Obviously an adjustment is needed if these rates are to be compared to pregnancy-based estimates, and when rates based on live births are to be compared some consideration must be given to possible differences in the numbers of other types of pregnancy, particularly induced abortions.

The most comprehensive study of choriocarcinoma incidence in the United States was based on SEER Program data for 1973–1982 (Brinton et al, 1986). In this period, there were 80 cases reported from Connecticut, Iowa, New Mexico, Utah and Hawaii, and the rate per 100,000 pregnancies was 4.15 (95% CI, 3.3–5.2), or one case per 24,100 pregnancies. The denominator used in the calculation was an underestimate of the total pregnancies, since only births and induced abortions were counted. The investigators also considered the numerator to be an underestimate of the true figure, due to incomplete reporting of cases. Earlier population-based studies of choriocarcinoma incidence in the United States produced estimates of 1.9 per 100,000 live births in Connecticut (1935–1964) and 2.2 per 100,000 pregnancies for Rhode Island (1956–1965), although these were based on only 23 and 4 cases, respectively (Shanmugaratnam et al, 1971; Yen and MacMahon, 1968).

By comparison, the incidence of hydatidiform mole is approximately 1 per 1,000 pregnancies in the United States (Hayashi et al, 1982).

Survival—United States

Before the development of effective chemotherapy, the mortality rate was over 90%, with death generally occurring within the first year, due to early metastasis and rapid progression. The introduction of methotrexate for treatment of choriocarcinoma in 1956 (Hertz et al, 1959), and the subsequent use of combination chemotherapy for high-risk patients, has completely reversed this picture such that the current cure rate now exceeds 80%. The success of chemotherapy reflects an unusual sensitivity of choriocarcinoma cells to antineoplastic agents, greatly aided by the availability of hCG as a sensitive and specific marker for the presence of residual trophoblastic tissue. Measurement of hCG levels, particularly following evacuation of a hydatidiform mole, provides for early detection of the disease and is used during chemotherapy to monitor the response.

Time Trends—United States

The small number of cases reported in most studies of choriocarcinoma incidence do not permit an analysis of seasonal or secular trends. An exception is the report based on SEER data for 1973 to 1982, which included

203 choriocarcinoma cases, and which found no evidence for a trend in incidence over this period (Brinton et al, 1986).

An alternative approach is to examine trends for hydatidiform mole and assume a relatively constant ratio of choriocarcinoma to hydatidiform mole incidence over the study period. Two studies have shown apparent seasonal variations in the incidence of hydatidiform mole, although in neither case was the statistical significance of the variation reported. In Guangxi province, China, molar pregnancies occurred most frequently following conceptions between March and July (Shang et al, 1982), and in Singapore molar pregnancies were more common in the first six months of the year (Teoh et al, 1971).

A secular trend has been observed in a number of countries. The incidence of hydatidiform mole in Jewish women in Israel increased significantly, from 1:2400 births for 1950–1954 to 1:900 births for 1960–1965 (Matalon and Modan, 1972). This study also provided data on choriocarcinoma incidence, which appeared to decrease by a factor of three over the same period, from 1:11,700 to 1:40,000 live births (Matalon et al, 1972). The inverse relationship of choriocarcinoma and hydatidiform mole incidence either suggests that the trends were due to changes in diagnosis and disease classification, or that these diseases have quite different determinants. The incidence of hydatidiform mole in Greenland more than doubled from 1950 to 1974, due in large part to an increase in the rate for teenage women (Nielsen and Hansen, 1979).

Studies in the United States raise the possibility that the incidence of hydatidiform mole may be increasing, although the data are rather limited. Yen and MacMahon (1968) reported that the incidence of moles increased from 64 per 100,000 pregnancies in 1930–1934 to 88 per 100,000 in 1960–1964; there was, however, a substantial drop in incidence in the 1940s, with rates of 29 and 39 per 100,000 in 1940–1944 and 1945–1949, respectively. An 8-fold increase in incidence of molar pregnancies over the period 1957–1959 to 1966–1968 for young women treated at a New York hospital led to the suggestion that a sexually transmissible agent might be responsible (Slocumb and Lund, 1969). Finally, a study of Hayashi et al (1982), based on diagnoses from a random sample of hospital admissions for 1970 to 1977, showed an increase in incidence from 80 per 100,000 pregnancies in 1970–1971 to 131 per 100,000 in 1974–1975. However, the incidence for 1976–1977 decreased to 121 per 100,000 pregnancies.

International Patterns

Based on figures derived from both hospital-based and population-based studies, the incidence of hydatidiform mole and choriocarcinoma varies by a factor of fifty or more from country to country. However, the highest rates, mostly from Asia (Wei and Ouyang, 1963; Poen and Djojoprantoto, 1965, Anh et al, 1993; Cheah et al, 1993), Latin America (Marquez-Monter et al, 1968), and the Middle East (Saleh et al, 1966) have been based generally on hospital series that use as a denominator the number of deliveries at the hospital over the period of case accrual. There is obviously a potential for substantial overestimation of trophoblastic disease incidence in such studies, particularly in countries in which home delivery is common and there is differential referral of complicated pregnancies to the major hospitals. The disparity of results from hospital and population-based studies in the same country provides evidence for this bias: for example, the incidence of hydatidiform mole based on data from 47 major hospitals throughout China was 6.7 per 1,000 pregnancies (Song et al, 1981), compared to a figure of 0.78 per 1,000 found by a national population-based study (National Coordination Research Group, 1980).

Selected estimates of choriocarcinoma incidence are presented in Table 52–1, with values from 2.2 per 100,000 pregnancies in Rhode Island to 35 per 100,000 in Greenland. Similar, although less extreme, variation is seen for hydatidiform mole incidence (Table 52–2). The estimates presented are limited to those based on reasonably well-defined populations. Although the Asian rates are less than those previously reported from hospital-based studies, they remain higher than those reported for the U.S. or Europe. Possible explanations that have been advanced for international variations in incidence include socioeconomic or nutritional factors (Poen and Djojoprantoto, 1965), and genetic predisposition (Martin, 1978; Miller and Barnhardt, 1975; Iliya et al, 1967).

In studies that provide reasonably reliable estimates for both hydatidiform mole and choriocarcinoma incidence the ratio of choriocarcinoma to hydatidiform mole generally lies between 0.05 and 0.10. Exceptions are ratios of 0.03 in the U.S. (Yen and MacMahon, 1968) and 0.30 in Greenland (Nielson and Hansen, 1979), suggesting the possibility of case ascertainment biases in these two studies.

Migration

The only migrant groups studied in any detail are the Asian populations of Hawaii (McCorriston, 1968), and here the relatively small population restricts the comparison to hydatidiform mole incidence. The rate for Japanese Hawaiians is substantially lower than that reported for Japanese in Japan (Nakano et al, 1980), while the incidence in Chinese women is higher in Hawaii than in China (National Coordination Research

TABLE 52–1. *Estimates of Choriocarcinoma Incidence from Selected Population-Based Studies*

Region	Period	Ethnic Subgroup	Incidence[a] (per 100,000)	Reference
United States				
SEER Program[b]	1973–82	White	4.4 (60)	Brinton et al (1986)
		Black	9.3 (NS)	
		Other	8.1 (NS)	
Rhode Island[b]	1956–65	—	2.2 (4)	Yen and MacMahon (1968)
Connecticut[c]	1935–64	—	1.9 (23)	Shanmugaratnam et al (1971)
Greenland[c]	1950–74	Eskimo-Caucasian	35.0 (11)	Nielsen and Hansen (1979)
Paraguay[b]	1960–69	—	2.3 (21)	Rolon and de Lopez (1979)
Jamaica[c]	1958–73	—	13.5 (52)	Sengupta et al
Israel[c]	1950–65	Jewish	5.1 (36)	Matalon et al (1972)
Sweden[b]	1958–65	—	3.9 (40)	Ringertz (1970)
Norway[c]	1957–66	—	4.6 (29)	Shanmugaratnam et al (1971)
Singapore[c]	1960–70	—	20.4 (122)	Teoh et al (1971)
	1959–64	Chinese	12.1 (30)	Shanmugaratnam et al (1971)
		Malay	8.9 (6)	
Malaysia[b]	1958–63	—	12.5 (18)	Llewellyn-Jones (1965)
Philippines[b]	1970–74	—	15.6 (91)	Baltazar (1976)
Japan[b]	1972–77	—	12.1 (18)	Nakano et al (1980)

[a]Number of cases in parentheses for each study.
[b]Incidence per 100,000 pregnancies.
[c]Incidence per 100,000 deliveries.
NS, Not stated.

Group, 1980). Caucasian rates are low compared to figures reported elsewhere in the United States. These rather discrepant results, showing no clear pattern, tend to reinforce the view that methodological differences may limit the value of comparisons between studies and populations.

In another study from Hawaii, restricted to complete moles, it was reported that Hawaiian-born women of Asian descent had an incidence rate similar to that seen in the countries of origin, although only limited data were presented to support this conclusion (Matsuura et al, 1984).

Age

One of the most striking features of both hydatidiform mole and choriocarcinoma is the rapidly increasing risk for women who become pregnant late in their reproductive life. Since most reported choriocarcinoma series include relatively few cases, estimates of the effect of maternal age vary considerably from study to study. In particular, data relating to the risk for women under 20 have been inconsistent, with only some studies showing an increased risk. Some of the variation can be attributed to small-sample fluctuations, and the remainder to methodological differences and shortcomings, such as the difficulty of accurately enumerating the denominator. Pooled estimates of age-specific incidence across many studies have the advantage of averaging out the effects of methodological differences and providing more-precise estimates. Table 52–3 shows estimates of age-specific incidence of choriocarcinoma and hydatidiform mole, relative to the incidence for the 20–24-year-old group, based on a loglinear Poisson regression model using data from 18 studies (Nielson and Hansen, 1979; Song et al, 1981; Rolon and Lopez 1977, 1979; Llewellyn-Jones, 1965; Teoh et al, 1971; Shanmugaratnam et al, 1971; Ringertz, 1970; Matalon et al, 1972; Baltazar, 1976; Wei and Ouyang, 1963; Leighton, 1973; Yen and MacMahon, 1968; Nakano et al, 1980; Matalon and Modan, 1972; Marquez-Monter et al, 1968; Bagshawe and Lawler, 1982; Brinton et al, 1986). A separate stratum coefficient was included in the model for each study to allow for interregional differences. An underlying assumption in the analysis is that the relationship of maternal age to risk is consistent across the studies.

From this analysis it can be seen that the relative risk for hydatidiform mole remains near unity until after age 39, and then rises rapidly. For choriocarcinoma the pat-

TABLE 52–2. *Estimates of Hydatidiform Mole Incidence from Selected Population-Based Studies*

Region	Period	Ethnic Subgroup	Incidence[a] (per 100,000)		Reference
United States					
All states[b]	1970–77	White	118.0	(139)	Hayashi et al (1982)
		Black	58.2	(16)	
Rhode Island[b]	1956–65	—	66.1	(122)	Yen and MacMahon (1968)
Honolulu[b]	1951–65	Japanese	130.8	(51)	McCorriston (1968)
		Chinese	136.6	(10)	
		Filipino	52.2	(7)	
		Caucasian	35.5	(13)	
		Hawaiian	36.9	(9)	
Greenland[c]	1950–74	Eskimo-Caucasians	117.6	(37)	Nielsen and Hansen (1979)
Paraguay[b]	1960–69	—	22.9	(209)	Rolon and de Lopez (1979)
Israel[c]	1950–65	Jewish	75.0	(534)	Matalon and Modan (1972)
Norway[c]	1953–61	—	75.0	(405)	Holstad and Hognestad
Sweden[b]	1958–65	—	64.8	(654)	Ringertz (1970)
China[b]	NS	—	77.5	(5863)	Song et al (1971)
Singapore[c]	1963–65	Chinese	123.3	(151)	Teoh et al (1971)
		Malay	113.8	(39)	
		Indian	147.2	(20)	
Malaysia[b]	1958–63	—	136.5	(196)	Llewellyn-Jones (1965)
Japan[b]	1972–77	—	214.6	(318)	Nakano et al (1980)

[a]Number of cases in parenthesis for each study.
[b]Incidence per 100,000 pregnancies.
[c]Incidence per 100,000 deliveries.
NS, Not stated.

tern is similar, although risk appears to increase progressively after age 25, and is also significantly higher for women under age 20 than for the reference group. Some of the increase in risk with age could reflect biases, such as the possibility of underascertainment of spontaneous or induced abortions in some age groups. While this is not likely to be an adequate explanation for the dramatic increase at older age, it is certainly a possibility for the much smaller increase seen at young maternal age. There were few women over age 50 in any of the studies (31 hydatidiform mole and 5 choriocarcinoma in total), and very few pregnancies to women at this advanced age, making estimates for the oldest age category particularly susceptible to bias. Two factors could have artifically inflated the risk estimates. First, most investigators classified cases by age at diagnosis. Since diagnosis can follow pregnancy by a year or more, some cases whose pregnancy occurred between the ages of 45 and 49 may have been diagnosed after age 50, and consequently counted in the 50+ age division. Second, while inclusion of small numbers of women with nongestational choriocarcinoma would have little impact on choriocarcinoma risk estimates for the younger age groups, even a single such case in the 50+ age group would substantially increase the calculated age-specific risk.

TABLE 52–3. *Estimated Age-Specific Risk of Hydatidiform Mole and Choriocarcinoma, Based on Data from 18 Studies (Calculated Relative to Risk of Women Aged 20–24)*

	Hydatidiform Mole		Choriocarcinoma	
Age Group	Risk	95% Confidence Interval	Risk	95% Confidence Interval
Under 20	1.06	0.94–1.21	1.46	1.06–2.00
20–24	1.00	—	1.00	—
25–29	1.00	0.92–1.08	1.41	1.16–1.72
30–34	0.90	0.81–1.00	1.75	1.42–2.15
35–39	1.07	1.42–2.15	2.51	2.02–3.16
40–44	3.05	2.68–3.47	10.77	8.67–13.4
45–59	15.00	12.5–18.0	63.67	46.5–87.2
50 and older	280.98	195.7–403.3	840.79	331.7–2131.3

Paternal age is highly correlated with maternal age, and it is particularly difficult to determine their independent effects. Yen and MacMahon (1968) concluded that maternal age was the more important factor and that paternal age was probably not an independent risk factor. In contrast, LaVecchia et al (1984) found relatively small risks for women in the oldest age categories when the analysis was adjusted for paternal age, but found large and significant relative risks for older men even when adjusted for maternal age.

Race and Ethnicity

The question of the effect of ethnicity on risk is related to issues of international variation and migration (see discussions earlier in this chapter), since regional differences could be attributed to racial differences in susceptibility. Data on migrant populations, which could help distinguish a genetic susceptibility from a cultural effect, are unfortunately too confused to be very helpful. The only other relevant information comes from internal comparisons of the few multiracial communities that have been adequately studied. Tables 52–1 and 52–2 give incidence figures for racial subgroups in Singapore (Chinese and Malay, and Indians), Hawaii (Japanese, Chinese, Filipinos, Caucasians, and Hawaiians) and the United States (whites and blacks). The statistical uncertainties that result from subdivision of small case series into even smaller racial subgroups make interpretation of the differences difficult. Nevertheless, rates appear to differ substantially by race within some communities; for example, rates of hydatidiform mole in the Japanese and Chinese of Honolulu are more than twice that seen in Filipinos and three to four times greater than those for Caucasians and Hawaiians (McCorriston, 1968).

Socioeconomic Status

Although many of the high-risk populations around the world are those with relatively low median incomes and, frequently, a protein-deficient diet, the earlier reports of association with socioeconomic status have not been more generally substantiated (Marques-Monter, 1968; Acosta-Sison, 1959; Hsu et al, 1963). In Hawaii, the Japanese have both a higher standard of living and a higher incidence of molar pregnancy than do the Caucasian population of the island (McCorriston, 1968). In Mexico, estimates of mean caloric intake in 145 patients with a molar pregnancy showed no difference from means for a normal control group (McGregor et al, 1969). Berkowitz et al (1985) reported that cases in their study consumed less carotene and animal fat than did control women, but found no difference in intake of protein.

ENVIRONMENTAL FACTORS

Exogenous Hormones

Of the seven case-control studies published to date, four found a significant risk associated with oral contraceptive use: Baltazar (1976) reported a relative risk of 6.4 for a small sample of choriocarcinoma patients, Berkowitz et al (1985) reported a relative risk of 2.1 for oral contraceptive use in women with complete molar pregnancies, Brinton et al (1989) found a relative risk of 5.5 for complete moles but no increase in risk for invasive moles, and Palmer (1991) reported a relative risk of 6.0 for choriocarcinoma for five or more years of use, with smaller risks of 2.8 and 1.6 for invasive mole and hydatidiform mole, respectively. The findings of Berkowitz were not found to be significant in a multivariate analysis that included the more significant (and independent) risk factors relating to diet, birthplace, age, and IUD use.

Since it is desirable for women to avoid pregnancy for several months after a molar pregnancy, in order that any abnormal persistence of elevated hCG may be detected and unambiguously interpreted, the effect of the oral contraceptive on the risk of sequelae is an important issue. Until very recently, this was very much an open question, with some studies showing an apparent effect of oral contraceptive use on postmolar sequelae (Stone and Bagshawe, 1979; Stone et al, 1976; Yuen and Birch, 1983) and others failing to do so (Berkowitz et al, 1981; Morrow et al, 1985). The issue has now been largely resolved by the results of a randomized intervention study in which no effect of oral contraceptive use on the risk of sequelae was seen (Curry et al, 1989).

An observation of two molar pregnancies in 129 women who had been exposed in utero to diethylstilbestrol (Schmidt et al, 1980) is significantly greater than expected, assuming a population incidence of one per thousand. A case report of two hydatidiform moles following treatment with bromocriptine for infertility could be interpreted as an association with either the drug or the underlying reproductive problem, or indeed as a chance observation (Ogborn, 1977).

Infection

The high incidence in regions of the world with poor nutrition and relatively poor sanitary conditions has suggested to some researchers that infections may play a role in the pathogenesis. Increasing incidence rates for women under 20 years of age in New York (Slocomb and Lund, 1969) and Greenland (Nielsen and Hansen, 1979) raises the possibility that a sexually transmissible agent is involved. In a recent case-control study of choriocarcinoma the strongest single risk factor was multiple marriage, a finding that would also be consistent with an infectious etiology. However, no significant differences were found in the number of women with histories of venereal disease in that study, and no information was collected on nonmarital sexual partners, so this remains an open question.

HOST FACTORS

Personal and Familial Tendency

Multiple occurrence of molar pregnancies in one woman is rare, but does appear to occur with greater frequency than expected. Approximately 0.5%–2% of women with hydatidiform mole have had a previous molar pregnancy, and some women have had five or more hydatidiform moles (Federschneider et al, 1980). Spontaneous abortion is common in women who have had moles, particularly those women who have had recurrent moles (Goldstein et al, 1984). There may also be an association between the mechanisms responsible for twinning and molar pregnancies (see "Pregnancy History, Infertility, and Twinning," later in this chapter).

The available data suggest that maternal rather than paternal factors are important for women with a familial predisposition. For example, one woman delivered 10 hydatidiform moles by two husbands. For families that appear to be at particular risk of trophoblastic disease, the clustering generally occurs on the maternal side. Ambani et al (1980) described three families with hydatidiform mole and/or choriocarcinoma occurring in sisters. In one, a woman with two moles had a sister with one mole and three abortions, and a cousin with a mole. The second family consisted of a woman who had had three molar pregnancies and a sister with a hydatidiform mole and subsequent amenorrhea and sterility, and the third familial cluster included a woman with three moles, a sister with two moles and choriocarcinoma, and a second sister who had had a hydatidiform mole. A hydatidiform mole and hydatidiform mole followed by choriocarcinoma have been reported for a pair of female homozygous twins (LaVecchia et al, 1982). The simple explanation of such observations is that some women have a genetic susceptibility to trophoblastic disease, but a role for shared environmental influences cannot be entirely ruled out.

Preceding Pregnancy

By far the most important risk factor for choriocarcinoma is the nature of the preceding pregnancy. This is best illustrated by Figure 52–1, which attempts to relate the frequency of live births, abortions, and molar pregnancies to the likelihood of proliferative sequelae. In compiling these data it was assumed that approximately 15% of pregnancies will be spontaneously aborted and that another 15% of pregnancies will be electively terminated. Other numerical estimates are based on data pooled from a variety of sources, with the emphasis on data reported from studies conducted in the United States. Figure 52–1 illustrates several important points. First, while complete moles appear to be the more common subtype, representing approximately 65% of all moles, careful study of abortuses reveals that a significant number of these pregnancies are partial moles, and in fact partial moles outnumber complete moles by

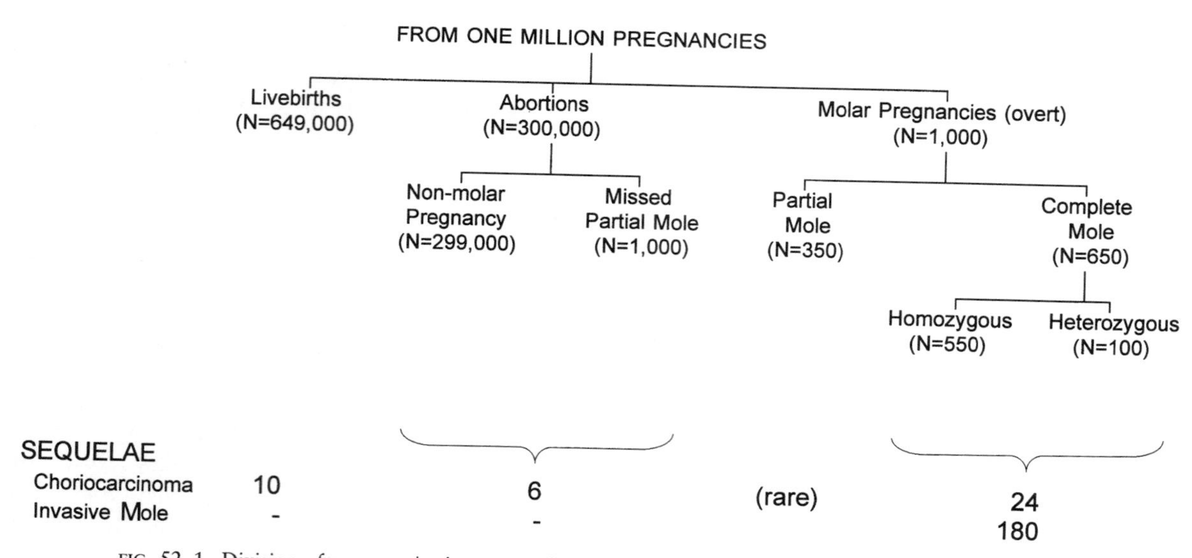

FIG. 52–1. Division of pregnancies into normal delivery, abortion, and hydatidiform mole, with further subdivision into mole type and relation to invasive sequelae.

about 2:1. Proliferative sequelae have been reported following a partial mole (Berkowitz et al, 1979), but it is clear that the risk is very much less than following complete moles. Trophoblastic disease has been noted to be more common after a spontaneous abortion than after a normal delivery (Teoh et al, 1971). It has yet to be determined whether the abnormal termination of pregnancy affects risk per se, or whether in these instances choriocarcinoma arises from a molar pregnancy that is unrecognized owing to early abortion. Figure 52–1 also highlights one of the most important unresolved questions at this time, which is the relative propensity of homozygous and heterozygous moles to invade or progress to choriocarcinoma. Based on the few, very small, published series of cases in which the genetic composition of the moles have been determined, it appears that heterozygous moles are more likely to persist and require treatment (Davis et al, 1984; Kajii et al, 1984; Wake et al, 1984). This is consistent with the observation that seven of seven choriocarcinoma cell lines examined to date are heterozygous.

Estimates for the proportion of choriocarcinoma cases that follow live births, abortions, and molar pregnancies vary from study to study; 25%, 15%, and 60% are the values used in Figure 52–1. Using these figures, the risk of choriocarcinoma following a molar pregnancy is 1,680 times than that following a livebirth. The risk following a complete mole is even higher—over 2,500—and may be greater still for heterozygous complete moles.

Immunology

The ABO blood groups of the parents appear to be a factor for choriocarcinoma development. While women of blood group A have been shown to have a greater risk than group O women, the most striking difference is seen for the particular mating combination of group A women married to group O men, which is associated with a 10-fold greater risk of choriocarcinoma, compared to A × A matings (Bagshawe et al, 1971). The reasons for these specific associations have remained obscure. Of interest is the fact that ABO associations have not been found for hydatidiform mole (Dawood et al, 1971).

Studies of HLA-A and -B locus antigens in women with choriocarcinoma, their husbands, and their children have failed to detect any specific antigens associated with the disease. Neither are there data to suggest that mating combinations which would be expected to produce conceptuses that were more (or less) closely HLA-matched to the mother than average are at any increased risk (Yamashita et al, 1981; Lawler, 1978; Lawler et al, 1971). The product of a consanguineous mating would tend to be more antigenically similar to the mother than average, and would be more likely to be homozygous for an uncommon recessive gene. Consanguinity has been suggested as a factor in the pathogenesis of the trophoblastic diseases (Iliya et al, 1967), but there is little evidence in support of this hypothesis. When choriocarcinoma follows a live birth, it is possible to type the cancer indirectly by typing the child (assuming a common origin), and no statistically significant relationship of mother to child HLA has been demonstrated (Bagshawe and Lawler, 1982).

Body Build/Menstrual Patterns

Several studies have compared menstrual characteristics of women with trophoblastic disease to those of control women. A related factor is body build, which can play a role in determining patterns of menstruation and ovulation (Frisch, 1984). Only two small case-control studies of choriocarcinoma have been conducted. The first, including only 28 Filipino women, found no significant differences in body weight or age at menarche (Baltazar, 1976). The second included 75 cases and obtained quite detailed information on menstrual history and related factors (Buckley et al, 1988). In this study, women with choriocarcinoma had a later age at menarche, were lighter in build, and reported lighter menses. There was no significant difference in the frequency or regularity of menstruation. Since the cases reported low-calorie dieting and regular exercise significantly less often than controls, the suggestion was that they were inherently lighter in build.

Body build and menstrual factors were not reported for the three more general case-control studies of women with trophoblastic disease, although it is not clear whether these factors were examined in detail (Messerli et al, 1985; Berkowitz et al, 1985; LaVecchia et al, 1985). The three studies included 90, 190, and 100 cases respectively, but only 0, 8, and 20 cases of choriocarcinoma, and one explanation for lack of agreement with the findings above is that these associations are specific to choriocarcinoma.

Pregnancy History, Infertility, and Twinning

Maternal parity is confounded with maternal age, and it is difficult to establish a relationship of parity to disease risk in the presence of the strong maternal age effect. In studies of trophoblastic disease that have controlled for maternal age, parity has not been a significant risk factor (Matalon and Modan, 1972; Yen and MacMahon, 1968). On the other hand, some studies have shown that a previous live birth is associated with a reduced risk, and a previous miscarriage is associated with an increased risk, of hydatidiform mole (Messerli et al, 1985; Parazzini et al, 1985; Brinton et al, 1989). In the study of Brinton et al, an increase in risk was seen for women with invasive mole who had had either an induced or spontaneous abortion, and no increase was seen for women with noninvasive (complete) mole.

A relationship of infertility to trophoblastic disease has been reported from two studies, but in one case the relative risk was 3.7 (LaVecchia et al, 1985), while in the other it was protective with a relative risk of 0.5 (Brinton et al, 1989). Buckley et al (1988) and Messerli et al (1985) did not find any significant association with a prior history of infertility.

Buckley et al (1988) found that there were more twins born to cases of choriocarcinoma and their first-degree relatives, than to controls: 12 case families with 13 sets of twins compared to 3 control sets (OR = 6.4, p = 0.0009). De George (1970) had previously described an unusually high number of hydatidiform moles (4) in 898 pregnancies of mothers of twins, and it has been noted that in a third of cases in which a hydatidiform mole coexists with a fetus, the fetus is a dizygous twin.

CONCEPTS OF PATHOGENESIS

Cytogenetics

The first clue to the curious genetics of hydatidiform moles was the observation that molar tissues generally contained sex chromatin, or Barr bodies, indicating an XX or female genetic composition (Baggish et al, 1968). When large series of moles was karyotyped, it appeared that complete moles usually had a normal 46,XX chromosome complement, while partial moles were very commonly trisomic 69,XXY. Use of cytogenetic heteromorphisms and polymorphic biochemical markers revealed that the complete mole was not genetically normal, however, in that only paternal chromosomes were present in most complete moles. In fact, there are at least two distinct mechanisms through which complete moles arise. The most common is duplication of a haploid (23,X) genome of a single sperm in an ovum that has lost its maternal complement of DNA. Since 46,YY moles have not been seen, it is presumed that duplication of a 23,Y sperm either cannot occur or, more probably, leads to a nonviable zygote.

Less frequently, complete moles are heterozygous with a 46,XY chromosomal complement, that arises from double fertilization and the loss of the maternal DNA. Again, the absence of 46,YY moles indicates that this is not a viable genetic complement.

In addition to the above, a number of unusual karyotypes have proved helpful in our understanding of the genetic basis of the molar phenotype. A trisomic complete mole in which all three haploid sets were derived from the father (Vejerslev et al, 1984) provides evidence that it is the presence of a maternal haploid set in the trisomic partial moles that distinguishes them from complete moles (and not trisomy per se). Consistent with this is the observation of a tetraploid partial mole in which there were three paternal haploid sets and one maternal set (Surti et al, 1986). Since a tetraploid conceptus arising from duplication of a diploid zygote has a nonmolar placenta, the evidence suggests that partial moles arise when paternal haploid sets outnumber maternal sets, and complete moles arise when no maternal chromosomes are retained. This model is supported by nuclear transplantation experiments on mice that indicate the paternal chromosomes play a key role in trophoblastic development: introduction of two female pronuclei into an enucleated egg produced a conceptus with a poorly developed trophoblast, while introduction of two male pronuclei produced a conceptus with much better development of the placenta than of the embryo (Barton et al, 1984). This model for the development of hydatidiform moles is both simple and intellectually satisfying, but it should be noted that there have been two reported cases of complete moles with apparently normal maternal and paternal haploid sets (Jacobs et al, 1980; Szulman and Surti, 1978).

Less is known about the genetics of choriocarcinoma and about the malignant potential of the various types of hydatidiform mole. Choriocarcinoma cell lines tend to develop multiple chromosomal abnormalities including rearrangements, duplications, translocations, and deletions and commonly have modal chromosome numbers from 50 to 80 (Surti, 1987). Three cell lines from choriocarcinomas that followed a term delivery were heterozygous, as would be expected if the tumor arose from the identified pregnancy. In addition, four choriocarcinoma cell lines from tumors that appeared after molar pregnancies (three cases) or spontaneous abortion (one case) have been shown to be heterozygous (Wake et al, 1981; Sasaki et al, 1982; Sheppard et al, 1985). The implications of these observations are not clear, since the sample is small and biases may result from the selection of established cell lines to study, but there is certainly a suggestion that choriocarcinomas may derive preferentially from heterozygous moles. One question that has been little addressed is whether choriocarcinoma is a single entity, or whether postmolar choriocarcinoma and choriocarcinoma arising from other types of pregnancy are genetically (and presumably etiologically) different. The only study to examine risk factors separately for the two groups was unable to detect any difference (Buckley et al, 1988), although the power of this study to demonstrate heterogeneity was very limited.

Azuma et al (1990) used an RLFP analysis to determine parental origin of the DNA in three complete moles and three choriocarcinomas. As expected the complete moles contained only paternal DNA, but the results for the choriocarcinomas were surprising: in two choriocarcinomas, which followed a complete mole and a normal pregnancy respectively, the DNA content of the tumor was of maternal origin. Although these data could be explained by contamination of the sample by normal maternal tissues, the investigators expressed confidence that this was not the case.

Immunology

The normal fetus and trophoblast carry both maternal and paternal genes and represent a natural allograft. The mechanisms that prevent immunological rejection of this antigenically foreign tissue presumably play a role in the growth and spread of invasive mole and choriocarcinoma. It might be anticipated that the risk of trophoblastic disease, and particularly of persistent or invasive disease, be related in part to the degree of mismatch between mother and conceptus, and there have been a number of studies that have looked at histocompatibility antigen (HLA) and ABO blood group similarities of the parents: unfortunately, tissue typing of trophoblastic tissue itself is generally not possible, since surface antigens are either not expressed or are poorly expressed and difficult to detect (Lawler et al, 1974; Loke et al, 1971; Jones and Bodmer, 1980). Based on the data presented earlier in this chapter, under "Immunology," the most that can be said is that while immunogenetic factors appear to be relevant, the mechanism of action is not understood.

Ovulatory Disorder

The cytogenetic data suggest that complete hydatidiform mole development starts with an abnormal ovum that lacks (or loses) functional maternal DNA and/or permits double fertilization. Observations on familial clusters of trophoblastic disease, and the relationship of choriocarcinoma to increased twinning, further suggest that genetic factors are important (although possibly only in a subset of patients). This is consistent with the data on body build, delayed menarche, and light menses (Buckley et al, 1988). The data relating to prior infertility are conflicting, but it would be reasonable to expect that women at particular risk for trophoblastic disease might have disturbances of fertility. Similarly, significant associations with a history of a prior live birth or spontaneous abortion might reflect fertility (and ovulatory) disturbances, although data relating a history of a prior induced abortion to increased risk (Brinton et al, 1989) would suggest a different mechanism of action.

It is not known whether the factors that determine progression of a hydatidiform mole to choriocarcinoma are present in the abnormal ovum prior to fertilization, are a consequence of genetic factors, or result from later environmental influences. The observation that heterozygous complete moles have greater malignant potential tends to implicate genetic determinants.

Environmental Factors

While many environmental factors, including diet (Berkowitz et al, 1985), occupation (Messerli et al, 1985), smoking habit (LaVecchia et al, 1985), contraceptive practice (LaVecchia et al, 1985; Baltazar 1976; Berkowitz et al, 1985; Brinton et al, 1989), and infection (Baltazar, 1976), have been associated with hydatidiform mole or choriocarcinoma, the findings have been inconsistent and often contradictory. While it is reasonable to suppose that some of the ethnic and geographic variations are attributable to environmental differences, the factors that influence trophoblastic disease risk have yet to be clearly identified.

PREVENTIVE MEASURES

Until more is known about the pathogenesis of both hydatidiform mole and choriocarcinoma there is little that can be recommended by way of preventive measures. Women in high-risk categories, such as those becoming pregnant after age 45 or, for choriocarcinoma, women who have a molar pregnancy, should be monitored to ensure that the hCG level returns to normal. If the suggested difference in risk of choriocarcinoma following homozygous and heterozygous moles is substantiated, it will be possible to tailor treatment more accurately, adopting a far more conservative policy for follow-up of women with homozygous moles, and a very aggressive treatment policy for women with dizygous moles.

FUTURE RESEARCH

The most important questions to be addressed at this time are the following: (1) What determines whether or not a hydatidiform mole will become invasive and/or malignant? (2) Since most complete moles include only paternal DNA, is the same true for most postmolar choriocarcinomas; if so, does this imply that choriocarcinoma appearing after other types of pregnancies has a completely different pathogenesis? (3) What is the abnormality in the ovum that permits double fertilization and causes loss of maternal DNA? (4) What (if anything) do women from high-incidence areas, women becoming pregnant late in life, and women with a family history of hydatidiform mole or dizygotic twinning have in common that predisposes them to trophoblastic disease? (5) Can factors related to menstruation, body build, and oral contraceptive use be confirmed as risk factors for hydatidiform mole and/or choriocarcinoma, and if so how do these factors act?

Much of the progress in recent years in the understanding of the pathogenesis of the trophoblastic diseases has come from the laboratory, particularly from studies of the genetics of hydatidiform mole and choriocarcinoma. The comparative rarity of choriocarcinoma, and methodological difficulties related to case identification and the selection of appropriate controls, makes epidemiological study more difficult for this tumor than for many other human cancers. On the positive side, however, the epidemiologist interested in the causes of the trophoblastic diseases now has a much better understanding of the cellular and genetic mechanisms that are involved. As the techniques used to examine the genetic origin of hydatidiform moles become more routinely available, it will become feasible to focus on the environmental and familial risk factors for specific subgroups of patients and to address many of the questions outlined above.

REFERENCES

Acosta-Sison H. 1959. The chance of malignancy in a repeated hydatidiform mole. Am J Obstet Gynecol 78:876–877.

Ambani LM, Vaidya RA, Rao CS, et al. 1980. Familial occurrence of trophoblastic disease-report of recurrent molar pregnancies in sisters in three families. Clin Genet 18:27–29.

Anh PT, Parkin DM, Hanh NT, et al. 1993. Cancer in the population of Hanoi, Vietnam, 1988–1990. Br J Cancer 68:1236–1242.

Azuma C, Saji F, Nobunaga T, et al. 1990. Studies of the pathogenesis of choriocarcinoma by analysis of restriction fragment length polymorphisms. Cancer Res 50:488–491.

Baggish MS, Woodruff JD, Tow SH, et al. 1968. Sex chromatin pattern in hydatidiform mole. Am J Obstet Gynecol 102:362–370.

Bagshawe KD, Lawler SD. 1982. Choriocarcinoma. In Schottenfeld D, Fraumeni JF (eds): Cancer Epidemiology and Prevention. Philadelphia, W. B. Saunders, pp. 909–924.

Bagshawe KD, Rawlins G, Pike MC, et al. 1971. ABO blood-groups in trophoblastic neoplasia. Lancet 1:553–557.

Baltazar JC. 1976. Epidemiological features of choriocarcinoma. Bull World Health Organ 54:523–532.

Barton SC, Surani AH, Norris ML. 1984. Role of paternal and maternal genomes in mouse development. Nature 311:374–376.

Berkowitz RS, Goldstein DP, Marean AR, et al. 1979. Proliferative sequelae after evacuation of partial hydatidiform mole. Lancet 2:804.

Berkowitz RS, Goldstein DP, Marean AR, et al. 1981. Oral contraceptives and postmolar trophoblastic disease. Obstet Gynecol 58:474–477.

Berkowitz RS, Cramer DW, Bernstein MR, et al. 1985. Risk factors for complete molar pregnancy from a case-control study. Am J Obstet Gynecol 152:1016–1020.

Brinton LA, Bracken MB, Connelly RR. 1986. Choriocarcinoma incidence in the United States. Am J Epidemiol 123:1094–1100.

Brinton LA, Wu BC, Wang W, et al. 1989. Gestational trophoblastic disease: a case-control study from the People's Republic of China. Am J Obstet Gynecol 161:121–127.

Buckley JD, Henderson BE, Morrow CP, et al. 1988. Case-control study of gestational choriocarcinoma. Cancer Res 48:1004–1010.

Cheah PL, Looi LM, Sivan Esaratnam V. 1993. Hydatidiform molar pregnancy in Malaysian women: a histopathological study from the University Hospital, Kuala Lumpur. Malays J Pathol 15:59–63.

Curry SL, Schlaerth JB, Boyce JB, et al. 1989. Hormonal contraception and trophoblastic sequelae after hydatidiform mole. Am J Obstet Gynecol 160:805–811.

Davis JR, Surwit EA, Perada GJ, et al. 1984. Sex assignment in gestational trophoblastic disease. Am J Obstet Gynecol 148:722–725.

Dawood MY, Teoh ES, Ratnam SS. 1971. ABO blood group in trophoblastic disease. J Obstet Gynecol Br Commonw 78:918–923.

De George FV. 1970. Hydatidiform moles in other pregnancies of mothers of twins. Am J Obstet Gynecol 108:369–371.

Elston CW, Bagshawe KD. 1972. The diagnosis of trophoblastic tumours from uterine curettings. J Clin Pathol 25:111–118.

Federschneider JM, Goldstein DP, Berkowitz RS, et al. 1980. Natural history of recurrent molar pregnancy. Obstet Gynecol 55:457–459.

Frisch RE. 1984. Body fat, puberty and fertility. Biol Rev 59:161–188.

Goldstein DP, Berkowitz RS, Bernstein MR. 1984. Reproductive performance after molar pregnancy and gestational trophoblastic tumors. Clin Obstet Gynecol 27:221–227.

Hayashi K, Bracken MB, Freeman DH, et al. 1982. Hydatidiform mole in the United States (1970–1977): a statistical and theoretical analysis. Am J Epidemiol 115:67–77.

Hertz R, Bergenstal DM, Lipsett MB, et al. 1959. Chemotherapy of choriocarcinoma and related trophoblastic tumours in women. Ann NY Acad Sci 80:262–277.

Hsu CT, Lai CH, Changchien CL, et al. 1963. Repeat hydatidiform moles—report of seven cases. Am J Obstet Gynecol 87:543–547.

Hunt W, Dockerty MB, Randall LM. 1953. Hydatidiform mole: a clinicopathologic study involving "grading" as a measure of possible malignant change. Obstet Oncol 1:593–609.

Iliya FA, Williamson S, Azar HA. 1967. Choriocarcinoma in the Near East: consanguinity as a possible etiologic factor. Cancer 20:144–149.

Jacobs PA, Wilson CM, Sprenkle JA, et al. 1980. Mechanism of origin of complete hydatidiform moles. Nature 286:714–715.

Jones EA, Bodmer WF. 1980. Lack of expression of HLA antigens on choriocarcinoma cell lines. Tissue Antigens 16:195–202.

Kajii T, Kurashige H, Ohama K, et al. 1984. XY and XX complete moles: clinical and morphologic correlations. Am J Obstet Gynecol 150:57–64.

Kato M, Tanaka D, Takeuchi S. 1982. The nature of trophoblastic disease initiated by transplantation into immunosuppressed animals. Am J Obstet Gynecol 142:497–505.

LaVecchia C, Franceschi S, Fasoli M, et al. 1982. Gestational trophoblastic neoplasms in homozygous twins. Obstet Gynecol 60:250–252.

LaVecchia C, Parazzini F, Decarli A, et al. 1984. Age of parents and risk of gestational trophoblastic disease. J Natl Cancer Inst 73:639–642.

LaVecchia C, Franceschi S, Parazzini F, et al. 1985. Risk factors for gestational trophoblastic disease in Italy. Am J Epidemiol 121:457–464.

Lawler SD, Klouda PT, Bagshawe KD. 1971. The HLA system in trophoblastic neoplasia. Lancet 2:834–837.

Lawler SD, Lkouda PT, Bagshawe KD. 1974. Immunogenicity of molar pregnancies in the HLA system. Am J Obstet Gynecol 120:857–861.

Lawler SD. 1978. HLA and trophoblastic tumours. Br Med Bull 34:305–308.

LEIGHTON PC. 1973. Trophoblastic disease in Uganda. Am J Obstet Gynecol 117:341–344.

LLEWELLYN-JONES D. 1965. Trophoblastic tumours: geographical variations in incidence and possible aetiological factors. J Obstet Gynecol Br Commonw 72:242–248.

LOKE YW, JOYSEY VC, BORLAND R. 1971. HLA antigens on human trophoblast cells. Nature 232:403–405.

LURAIN JR, BREWER JI. 1982. Invasive mole. Semin Oncol 9:174–180.

MARQUEZ-MONTER H, DE LA VEGA GA, RIDAURA C, et al. 1968. Gestational choriocarcinoma in the general hospital of Mexico. Cancer 22:91–98.

MARTIN PM. 1978. High frequency of hydatidiform mole in native Alaskans. Int J Gynaecol Obstet 15:395–396.

MATALON M, MODAN B. 1972. Epidemiologic aspects of hydatidform mole in Israel. Am J Obstet Gynecol 112:107–112.

MATALON M, PAZ B, MODAN M, et al. 1972. Malignant trophoblastic disorders. Am J Obstet Gynecol 112:101–106.

MATSUURA J, CHIU D, JACOBS A, et al. 1984. Complete hydatidiform mole in Hawaii: an epidemiological study. Genet Epidemiol 1:271–284.

MCCORRISTON CC. 1968. Racial incidence of hydatidiform mole. Am J Obstet Gynecol 101:377–382.

MCGREGOR C, ONTIVEROS EC, VARGAS EL, et al. 1969. Hydatidiform mole: analysis of 145 patients. Obstet Gynecol 33:343–351.

MESSERLI ML, LILLIENFELD AM, PARMLEY T, et al. 1985. Risk factors for gestational trophoblastic disease. Am J Obstet Gynecol 153:294–300.

MILLER FL, BARNHARDT RJ. 1975. Mixed marriage may offer Asian women protection against hydatidiform mole. Ob Gyn News 10:16.

MORROW P, NAKAMURA R, SCHLAERTH J, et al. 1985. The influence of oral contraceptives on the postmolar human chorionic gonadotropin regression curve. Am J Obstet Gynecol 151:906–914.

NAKANO R, SASAKI K, YAMOTO M, et al. 1980. Trophoblastic Disease: analysis of 342 patients. Gynecol Obstet Invest 11:237–242.

NATIONAL COORDINATION RESEARCH GROUP OF CHORIOCARCINOMA. 1980. Incidence of hydatidiform mole (a retrograde study of 2,023,621 women in 23 providences). Zhonghua Yixue Zazhi 60:641–644.

NIELSEN NH, HANSEN JPH. 1979. Trophoblastic tumours in Greenland. J Cancer Res Clin Oncol 95:177–186.

NOVAK E, SEAH CS. 1954. Benign trophoblastic lesions in Mathieu chorionephithelioma registry (hyaditidiform mole, syncytial endometritis). Am J Obstet Gynecol 68:376–390.

OBER WB. 1971. The pathology of choriocarcinoma. Ann NY Acad Sci 179:299–321.

OGBORN ADR. 1977. Hydatidiform mole arising twice during bromocriptine therapy. Br J Obstet Gynaecol 84:717–718.

PALMER JR. 1991. Oral contraceptive use and gestational choriocarcinoma. Cancer Detect Prev 15:45–48.

PALMER JR. 1994. Advances in the epidemiology of gestational trophoblastic disease. J Reprod Med 39:155–162.

PARAZZINI F, LAVECCHIA C, PAMPALLONA S, et al. 1985. Reproductive patterns and the risk of gestational trophoblastic disease. Am J Obstet Gynecol 152:866–870.

PARK WW, LEES JC. 1950. Choriocarcinoma. A general review, with analysis of 516 cases. Arch Pathol 49:73–104.

POEN HT, DJOJOPRANOTO M. 1965. The possible etiologic factors of hydatidiform mole and choriocarcinoma. Am J Obstet Gynecol 92:510–512.

RINGERTZ N. 1970. Hydadidiform mole, invasive mole and choriocarcinoma in Sweden 1958–1965. Acta Obstet Gynecol Scand 49:195–203.

ROLON PA, LOPEZ BH. 1977. Epidemiological aspects of hydatidiform mole in the republic of Paraguay (South America). Br J Obstet Gynecol 84:862–864.

ROLON PA, LOPEZ BH. 1979. Malignant trophoblastic disease in Paraguay. J Reprod Med 23:94–96.

SALEH JS, POURMAND K, MOJARADI N. 1966. A study of the trophoblastic disease among the Iranian population. Br J Clin Pract 20:119–127.

SASAKI S, KATAYAMA PK, ROESLER M, et al. 1982. Cytogenetic analysis of choriocarcinoma cell lines. Acta Obstet Gynaecol Jpn 1982:2253–2256.

SCHMIDT G, FOWLER WC, TALBERT LM. 1980. Reproductive history of women exposed to diethylstilbestrol in utero. Fertil Steril 33:21–24.

SHANG E, XU L, WEI M. 1982. A retrospective study on incidence of hydatidiform mole in 20,548 fertile women. Zhonghua Yixue Zazhi 62:282–285.

SHANMUGARATNAM D, MUIR CS, TOW SH, et al. 1971. Rates per 100,000 births and incidence of choriocarcinoma and malignant mole in Singapore Chinese and Malays. Comparison with Connecticut, Norway and Sweden. Int J Cancer 8:165–175.

SHEPPARD DM, FISHER RA, LAWLER SD. 1985. Karyotypic analysis and chromosome polymorphisms in four choriocarcinoma cell lines. Cancer Genet Cytogenet 16:251–258.

SLOCUMB JC, LUND CJ. 1969. Incidence of trophoblastic disease: increased rate in youngest age group. Am J Obstet Gynecol 104:421–423.

SONG H, WU B, TANG M, et al. 1971. Trophoblastic tumors: diagnosis and treatment. Technical report, Department of Obstetrics and Gynecology, Capital Hospital, Beijing, China.

STONE M, BAGSHAWE KD. 1979. An analysis of the influence of maternal age, gestational age, contraceptive method, and the mode of primary treatment of patients with hydatidiform moles on the incidence of subsequent chemotherapy. Br J Obstet Gynaecol 86:782–792.

STONE M, DENT J, KARDANA A, et al. 1976. Relationship of oral contraception to development of trophoblastic tumour after evacuation of a hydatidiform mole. Br J Obstet Gynaecol 83:913–916.

SURTI U. 1987. Genetic concepts and techniques. In Szulman AE, Buchsbaum HJ (eds): Gestational Trophoblastic Disease. New York Springer-Verlag, pp. 111–121.

SURTI U, SZULMAN AE, WAGENER K, et al. 1986. Tetraploid partial hydatidiform moles: two cases with a triple paternal contribution and a 92,XXXY karyotype. Hum Genet 72:15–21.

SZULMAN AE, SURTI U. 1978. The syndromes of hydatidiform mole. I Cytogenetic and morphologic correlations. Am J Obstet Gynecol 131:665–671.

TEOH ES, DAWOOD MY, RATNAM SS. 1971. Epidemiology of hydatidiform mole in Singapore. Am J Obstet Gynecol 110:415–420.

VEJERSLEV LO, FISHER RA, SURTI U, et al. 1987. Hydatidiform mole: cytogenetically unusual cases and their implications for present classification. Am J Obstet Gynecol 157:180–184.

WAKE N, SEKI T, FUJITA H, et al. 1984. Malignant potential of homozygous and heterzygous complete moles. Cancer Res 44:1226–1230.

WAKE N, TANAKA K, CHAPMAN V, et al. 1981. Chromosomes and cellular origin of choriocarcinoma. Cancer Res 41:3137–3140.

WEI PY, OUYANG PC. 1963. Trophoblastic diseases in Taiwan. Am J Obstet Gynecol 85:844–849.

YAMASHITA K, ISHIKAWA M, SHIMIZU T, et al. 1981. HLA antigens in husband-wife pairs with trophoblastic tumor. Gynecol Oncol 12:68–74.

YEN S, MACMAHON B. 1968. Epidemiologic features of trophoblastic disease. Am J Obstet Gynecol 101:126–132.

YUEN BH, BIRCH P. 1983. Relationship of oral contraceptive devices to the regression of concentrations of human chorionic gonadotrophin and invasive complications after molar pregnancy. Am J Obstet Gynecol 145:214–217.

53 Renal cancer

JOSEPH K. McLAUGHLIN
WILLIAM J. BLOT
SUSAN S. DEVESA
JOSEPH F. FRAUMENI, JR.

Malignant tumors of the kidney account for about 2% of all new cancer cases and deaths each year in the United States, making this site the twelfth most common cancer (Boring et al, 1994). Data from the Surveillance, Epidemiology and End Results (SEER) program for ICD-189 (renal and urinary tract cancers other than bladder) for the years 1975–1985 show that renal parenchyma (renal cell) cancer accounts for 70% of the total, renal pelvis cancer 15%, ureter cancer 8%, urethra cancer 4%, and other sites about 3% (Devesa et al, 1990). Nearly all renal cell cancers are adenocarcinomas, whereas the vast majority of cancers of the renal pelvis, ureter, and urethra are transitional cell carcinomas. Wilms' tumor (nephroblastoma), an embryonal neoplasm, is reviewed in the chapter on childhood cancer.

The etiology of kidney cancer remains enigmatic for the most part, except for renal pelvis and ureter cancers, the majority of which are related to cigarette smoking. In this review, information on renal cell cancer will be presented separately, whenever possible, from data on renal pelvis and ureter cancers. In many descriptive and some analytical studies, however, the available data pertain to all kidney cancers combined and do not permit further analyses by site.

DEMOGRAPHIC PATTERNS

Incidence in the United States

Incidence rates for renal cell cancer have risen about 2% per year among the four major race/sex groups since 1970 (Fig. 53–1), based on data from five U.S. registries (Devesa et al, 1987; Devesa et al, 1990). Increases have been more rapid among blacks than whites, resulting in a recent shift in excess from among whites to among blacks (Kosary and McLaughlin, 1993). Age-adjusted rates among whites, blacks, and Hispanics during 1975–1985 were similar, although elevated rates were found among American Indian women, based on small numbers (Table 53–1). Alaskan natives have also been reported to have increased rates of renal cell cancer (Lanier et al, 1980). Rates among Asians of both sexes were about half those of other racial groups. With the exception of American Indians, rates among men are more than twice those among women. Incidence rates of renal cell cancer rise with increasing age before plateauing around age 70 (Fig. 53–2). The recent excess among blacks is less apparent at older ages compared to younger ages, whereas the excess among males is most notable at ages 50 years and older (Fig. 53–2).

For cancers of the renal pelvis, rates rose almost 3% per year during the 1970s and less rapidly thereafter (Fig. 53–1). There is a suggestive decrease in rates among blacks starting in the late 1970s, but the numbers involved are small. Rates among white men for these cancers are 2.5 times those among white women, black men, and Hispanic men, whereas the rates for Asians are intermediate (Table 53–1).

International Patterns

Figure 53–3 presents kidney cancer rates from selected cancer registries around the world, as reported in Volume 6 of *Cancer Incidence in Five Continents* (Parkin et al, 1992). The rates, shown here in descending order within continent among men, vary more than 10-fold. Incidence is highest in Bas-Rhin, France, with relatively high rates in several Scandinavian countries, and other parts of northern Europe, but not England and Wales. The lowest rates are reported in India, among Chinese and Japanese populations, and in areas of Central and South America.

Many registries provide data separately for renal cell and renal pelvis cancers (using the fourth digit level of the International Classification of Diseases). The incidence of renal cell cancer is elevated in several areas of

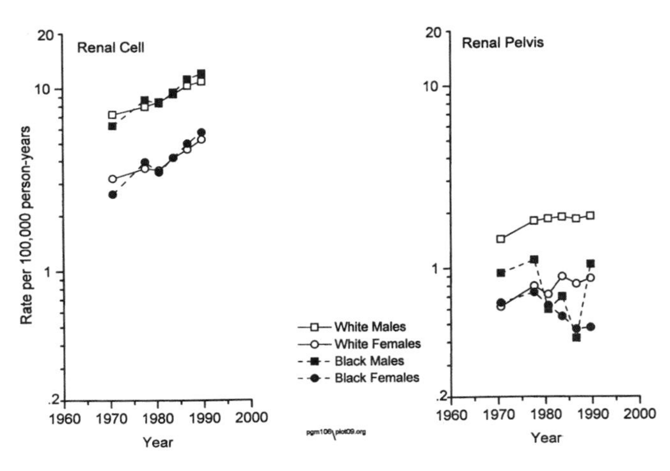

FIG. 53–1. Trends in age-adjusted (1970 standard) incidence of renal cell cancer and renal pelvis cancer in five geographic areas of the United States (Atlanta, Detroit, San Francisco, Connecticut, Iowa) by race and sex, 1969–1990. (Based on data from the Third National Cancer Survey, the Connecticut Tumor Registry, and the SEER Program.)

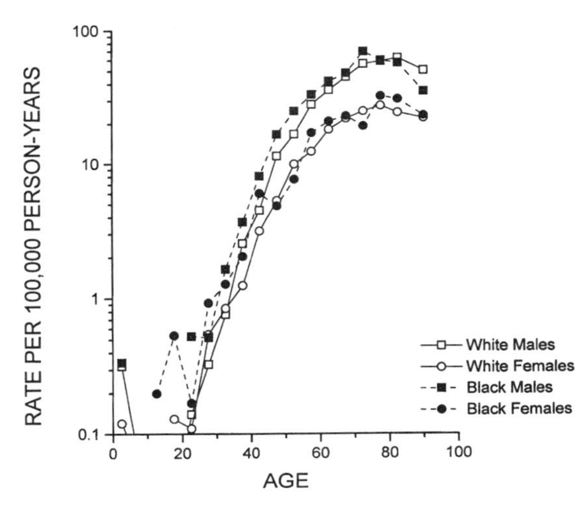

FIG. 53–2. Age-specific incidence of renal cell cancer in the United States by race and sex, 1986–1990. (Based on Kosary and McLaughlin, 1993.)

northern Europe; the rates for renal pelvis cancer appear high in Switzerland, Denmark, and among U.S. whites (Fig. 53–3). The proportion specified as renal pelvis cancer varies considerably by registry. This may partly reflect variations in reporting and classification, as well as actual differences in cancer rates. In certain rural parts of Bulgaria, Yugoslavia, and Romania, rates for renal pelvis and ureter cancers are exceptionally high because of a predisposing condition called Balkan nephropathy, which is endemic in these areas (Stoyanov et al, 1978). In general, the descriptive patterns for cancer of the renal pelvis (and ureter) resemble those of bladder cancer more than renal cell cancer (Devesa et al, 1990).

TABLE 53–1. *Incidence Rates* for Cancers of the Renal Parenchyma, Renal Pelvis, and Ureter, by Racial/Ethnic Group and Sex, SEER Program, 1975–1985*

	Males		*Females*	
	No.	*Rate*	*No.*	*Rate*
Renal parenchyma[a]				
Whites (9 SEER areas)	7717	8.42	4307	3.69
Blacks (9 SEER areas)	677	8.62	379	3.78
Hispanics (New Mexico)	130	7.91	67	3.70
American Indians (New Mexico)	24	8.43	19	5.85
Asians (San Francisco and Hawaii)[b]	163	4.26	64	1.70
Native Hawaiians	29	5.73	14	2.42
Renal pelvis and ureter				
Whites (9 SEER areas)	2564	2.85	1421	1.14
Blacks (9 SEER areas)	77	1.04	69	0.71
Hispanics (New Mexico)	17	1.14	15	0.85
Asians (San Francisco and Hawaii)[b]	58	1.67	34	0.84

*Rates per 100,000 person-years, age-adjusted using 1970 U.S. standard.
[a]Transitional, papillary, and squamous cell cancers of the kidney (ICD 189.0) are grouped with renal pelvis tumors.
[b]Includes Japanese, Chinese, Filipino.
Source: Unpublished SEER data; Devesa et al, 1990.

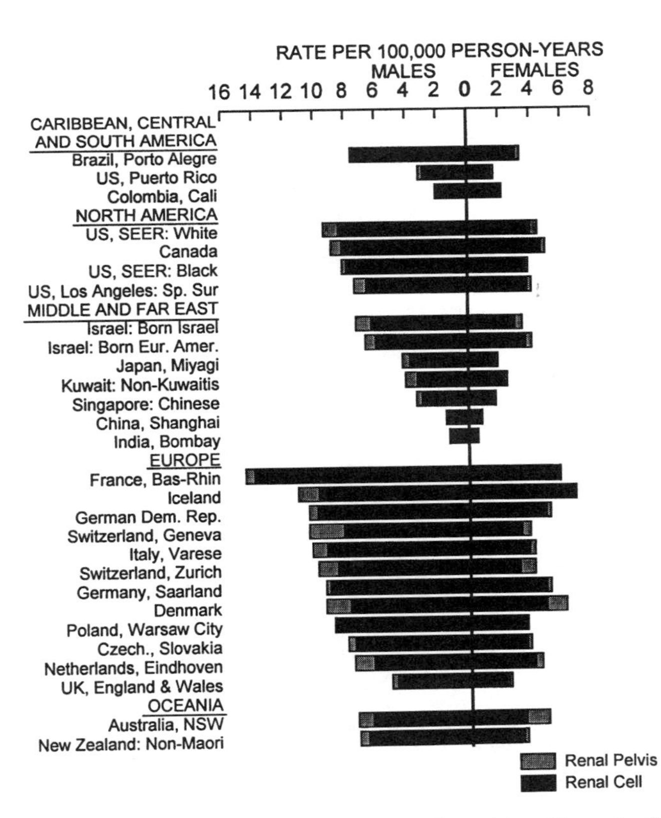

FIG. 53–3. International variation in age-adjusted (world standard) incidence of total kidney cancer, renal cell cancer, and cancers of the renal pelvis and ureter by sex, 1983–1987. (Based on Parkin et al, 1992.)

Survival

The prognosis of patients diagnosed with kidney cancer has improved in recent times, with 5-year relative survival rates increasing from 36% to 39% in the early 1960s to over 50% in the 1980s (Axtell et al, 1976; National Cancer Institute, 1989; Kosary and McLaughlin, 1993). Table 53–2 presents 5-year relative survival rates by site, race, and sex. Survival rates are generally better for cancers of the renal pelvis than renal cell cancer for men; for women, the rates are similar. Blacks tend to have poorer survival rates for renal cell cancer, although they have better rates for renal pelvis cancer.

Urbanization and Socioeconomic Factors

Mortality and incidence rates for kidney cancer are generally higher in urban than rural areas in the United States, England and Wales, and Norway and Denmark (McLaughlin and Schuman, 1983; Muir et al, 1987). The urban-rural differential is mainly among men, and probably reflects past levels of cigarette smoking. The pattern is influenced also by the greater availability of medical care and diagnostic services in urban than rural areas.

Kidney cancer mortality statistics from the United States and other countries have shown no clear relation with educational achievement (McLaughlin and Schuman, 1983). Case-control studies of renal cell cancer have not indicated an effect of social class variables such as education (Wynder et al, 1974; Armstrong et al, 1976; McLaughlin et al, 1984; Goodman et al, 1986; McCredie et al, 1988; Talamini et al, 1991; Maclure and Willett, 1990; McCredie and Stewart, 1993; Kreiger et al, 1993), although studies in Oklahoma (Asal et al, 1988a) and Denmark (Mellemgaard et al, 1994a) have reported an inverse trend with education. In a recent case-control study from France, patients were significantly better educated than the control subjects (Benhamou et al, 1993). Except for the new study from Australia (McCredie and Stewart, 1993), investigations of renal pelvis and ureter cancers have also reported no major differences in education between patients and control subjects (Armstrong et al, 1976; McCredie et al, 1982, 1983a,b; McLaughlin et al, 1983; Jensen et al, 1988; Ross et al, 1989; McLaughlin et al, 1992c). When available, kidney cancer data have shown little relation to income level (McLaughlin and Schuman, 1983), although one correlation study reported a weakly positive association (Blot and Fraumeni, 1979).

TABLE 53–2. *Five-Year Relative Survival Rates (percent) for Cancer of the Renal Parenchyma and Renal Pelvis, by Race and Sex, SEER Program, 1983–1989*

	Males Rate	*Females Rate*
Renal parenchyma		
Whites	58	59
Blacks	50	55
Renal pelvis		
Whites	62	55
Blacks	71	57

Source: Kosary and McLaughlin, 1993.

RENAL CELL CANCER

Virtually all information on risk factors for renal cell cancer has come from case-control studies (Table 53–3). These studies have been conducted in a number of countries, including the United States, Canada, England, Australia, Italy, Finland, France, Denmark, and China; the studies ranged in size from 64 cases and 197 controls to 690 cases and 707 controls.

Cigarette Use

Although results from case-control studies are not entirely consistent, a convincing relation between cigarette smoking and renal cell cancer has emerged (Wynder et al, 1974; McLaughlin et al, 1984; Yu et al, 1986; Brownson, 1988; McCredie et al, 1988; La Vecchia et al, 1990; Maclure and Willett, 1990; McLaughlin et al, 1992a; McCredie and Stewart, 1992a; Kreiger et al, 1993; Mellemgaard et al, 1994a). Cohort studies also support this association (McLaughlin and Schuman, 1983), with the most recent and largest study, a 26-year follow-up of U.S. veterans (719 kidney cancer deaths), showing a strong dose-response relation (McLaughlin et al, 1990). The relative risks among smokers from case-control and cohort studies range from 1.2 to 2.3, although a small chart-review study in the 1960s reported a five-fold increase in risk (Bennington and Laubscher, 1968). A number of the case-control studies have demonstrated a dose-response relation in men (Wynder et al, 1974; McLaughlin et al, 1984; Yu et al, 1986; Brownson, 1988; McCredie et al, 1988; La Vecchia et al, 1990; Maclure and Willett, 1990; McLaughlin et al, 1992a; McCredie and Stewart; 1992a; Kreiger et al, 1993; Mellemgaard et al, 1994a) as well as in women (Wynder et al, 1974; McLaughlin et al, 1984; Yu et al, 1986; La Vecchia et al, 1990; Maclure and Willett, 1990; McLaughlin et al, 1992a; McCredie and Stewart, 1992a; Kreiger et al, 1993), with risks for heavy smokers ranging from 2.0 to 3.0. Use of hospital controls or small sample size is the likely explanation for the absence of a statistically significant cigarette as-

TABLE 53–3. *Published Case-Control Studies of Renal Cell Cancer*

Authors	*Year*	*Source of Controls*	*Number of Cases/Controls*	*Location*
Bennington and Laubacher	1968	hospital	100/190	Washington
Wynder et al	1974	hospital	202/394	3 U.S. cities
Armstrong et al	1976	hospital	106/106	England
Kolonel	1976	hospital	64/197	New York
McLaughlin et al	1984	population	495/697	Minneapolis
Yu et al	1986	neighborhood	160/160	Los Angeles
Goodman et al	1986	hospital	267/267	6 U.S. cities
Brownson	1988	cancer registry	326/978	Missouri
Asal et al	1988a	hospital/population	315/313/336	Oklahoma
McCredie et al	1988	population	360/985	New South Wales
Sharpe et al	1989	urologic patients	164/161	Montreal
La Vecchia et al	1990	hospital	131/394	Northern Italy
Maclure and Willett	1990	population	410/605	Boston
Talamini et al	1991	hospital	240/665	Northern Italy
Partanen et al	1991	population	338/484	Finland
McCredie and Stewart	1992a,b	population	489/523	New South Wales
McLaughlin et al	1992a	population	154/157	Shanghai
Kreiger et al	1993	population	518/1381	Ontario
Finkle et al	1993	medical plan	191/191	Los Angeles
Benhamou et al	1993	hospital	196/347	France
Mellemgaard et al	1994a,b,c,d	population	368/396	Denmark
Hiatt et al	1994	medical plan	257/257	San Francisco
Chow et al	1994a,b	population	690/707	Minnesota

sociation in some case-control studies (Schwartz et al, 1961; Armstrong et al, 1976; Kolonel, 1976; Goodman et al, 1986; Asal et al, 1988a; Talamini et al, 1991; Benhamou et al, 1993). The moderate risk of renal cell cancer associated with cigarette smoking would be difficult to detect in a small study and could easily be obscured with the use of control subjects who have an elevated prevalence of smoking.

The risk associated with cigarette smoking has been shown to decline significantly with years of cessation (McLaughlin et al, 1984). More recent studies in Italy and Australia have confirmed the effect of cessation (LaVecchia et al, 1990; McCredie and Stewart, 1992a). Population-based attributable risks indicate that between approximately 30% and 37% of the renal cell cancers among men and 14% to 24% among women could be due to cigarette smoking (McLaughlin et al, 1984; McCredie and Stewart, 1992a). A recent study has reported a suggestive association of passive smoking with renal cell cancer (Kreiger et al, 1993).

Drugs

Although heavy use of phenacetin-containing drugs has been clearly linked to renal pelvis tumors (International Agency for Research on Cancer [IARC], 1987), an association has been reported also for renal cell cancer (McLaughlin et al, 1984, 1985; Maclure and MacMahon, 1985; McCredie et al, 1988; McLaughlin et al, 1992a; Kreiger et al, 1993). Confounding does not explain the association, because the studies adjusted for cigarette smoking and the use of other types of analgesics. These studies revealed no increased risk associated with aspirin or acetaminophen, but a cohort study of retirees reported a significant six-fold increased risk for daily aspirin use (Paganini-Hill et al, 1989). This finding is preliminary, because it was based on nine cases, apparent only among men, and not adjusted for prior use of phenacetin-containing analgesics, relative weight, or smoking habits. A new large-scale population-based case-control study in an area of the world known for heavy analgesic consumption confirmed the relation of phenacetin to renal cell cancer, but found no evidence that aspirin increases the risk of renal cell cancer (McCredie et al, 1993). In the same study, a link with acetaminophen analgesics was suggested. In the large Canadian study an association was also observed for phenacetin use but none with acetaminophen (Kreiger et al, 1993). The recent large-scale study in Minnesota observed no relation with regular use or duration of use for aspirin, acetaminophen, or phenacetin (Chow et al, 1994a), however, in Denmark, women who were heavy users of phenacetin had a significant five-fold risk of renal cell cancer (Mellemgaard et al, 1994b). This study observed no significantly increased risk for aspirin or acetominophen users. Linked-registry studies of patients with diseases that require treatment with analgesics have reported increased risks of renal cell cancer, although the type of analgesic was unknown and control of confounding factors was not possible (Mellemgaard et al, 1992b; Gridley et al, 1993; Lindblad et al, 1993).

Diuretic use has been associated with a five-fold increase in the risk of renal cell cancer among women (Yu et al, 1986). Adjustment for blood pressure status made little difference, because both hypertensives and nonhypertensives were at elevated risk. This finding was confirmed by a larger case-control study, although the excess risk was confined to nonhypertensive women (McLaughlin et al, 1988). Recent cohort studies have also linked renal cell cancer with diuretic use (Fraser et al, 1990; Grove et al, 1991; Mellemgaard et al, 1992a; Lindblad et al, 1993). The recent Australian study did not confirm the association with diuretics, but rather found an increased risk with nondiuretic antihypertensive medications (McCredie and Stewart, 1992b). One screening study of prescription drug–cancer associations did not observe a significantly elevated risk (Selby et al, 1989). But recent medical records–based case-control studies using prescription data from patients' charts have found three- to four-fold increased risks among women after adjustment for known confounders, including hypertension (Finkle et al, 1993; Hiatt et al, 1994). It is noteworthy that animal studies have linked hydrochlorothiazide and furosemide, the most commonly used diuretics, with tubular cell adenomas and adenocarcinomas of the kidney in rats and hepatocellular tumors in mice (Lijinsky and Reuber, 1987; National Toxicology Program, 1989a,b). Moreover, these compounds act on the renal tubules (Laski, 1986), the site of origin for renal cell cancers. In the United States, the use of diuretics increased by 40% between 1975 and 1984 and is especially common among the elderly (Baum et al, 1988). Future analytical studies of renal cell cancer should strive to clarify the role of diuretics, because an association, if causal, would have major public health implications as a result of the widespread use of these drugs (National Center for Health Statistics, 1987, 1993).

Although estrogens have induced renal cell carcinomas in laboratory animals, particularly Syrian golden hamsters, there is little epidemiological evidence supporting an association in humans (McLaughlin and Schuman, 1983; Newsom and Vurgin, 1987). Weakly positive findings have been reported for menopausal estrogen use (Asal et al, 1988b; McLaughlin et al, 1992a; McCredie and Stewart, 1992b) and oral contraceptives (McLaughlin et al, 1992a; Kreiger et al, 1993). The relation in humans between hormone-related variables and renal cell cancer remains unclear.

Coffee, Alcohol, and Other Beverages

Although correlation studies have suggested a relation between the distribution of kidney cancer and per capita consumption of coffee (Shennan, 1973; Armstrong and Doll, 1975), the finding has not been confirmed by case-control studies of renal cell cancer, when adjustment is made for the confounding effect of cigarette use (Wynder et al, 1974; Armstrong et al, 1976; McLaughlin et al, 1984; Asal et al, 1988a; McCredie et al, 1988; Maclure and Willett, 1990; Talamini et al, 1991; Partanen et al, 1991; Kreiger et al, 1993; Benhamou et al, 1993; Mellemgaard et al, 1994a; Chow et al, 1994b). However, two studies have suggested a positive association. A two-fold risk in both sexes combined was associated with use of decaffeinated coffee without dose-response relation (Goodman et al, 1986), while an increased risk for regular coffee use was seen among women only, again with no dose-response relation (Yu et al, 1986). On the other hand, results from a cohort study in Norway, an area of heavy coffee intake, showed a significant inverse trend, with consumers of seven or more cups having one fourth the risk of those drinking two or fewer cups daily (Jacobsen et al, 1986). Overall, the results from analytical studies indicate that coffee consumption does not increase the risk of renal cell cancer.

Correlation studies have also reported a relation between per capita intake of alcohol and kidney cancer mortality (Breslow and Enstrom, 1974; Hinds et al, 1980). Analytical studies of renal cell cancer do not support these findings, with cases and controls consuming similar amounts of alcohol (Wynder et al, 1974; Armstrong et al, 1976; McLaughlin et al, 1984; Goodman et al, 1986; Yu et al, 1986; Brownson, 1988; Asal et al, 1988a; Maclure and Willett, 1990; Talamini et al, 1991; Kreiger et al, 1993; Benhamou et al, 1993; Chow et al, 1994b). The recent Danish case-control study observed a statistically significant inverse association of alcohol consumption with renal cell cancer risk (Mellemgaard et al, 1994a). Moreover, cohort studies of alcoholics and brewery workers have reported no excess mortality from kidney cancer (Schmidt and De Lint, 1972; Pell and Alonzo, 1973; Monson and Lyon, 1975; Jensen, 1979; Schmidt and Popham, 1981; Adami et al, 1992).

An increased risk among tea drinkers has been reported in a few studies of renal cell cancer, particularly among women (McLaughlin et al, 1984; Goodman et al, 1986; Asal et al, 1988a). Also, a mortality follow-up of 20,000 London men revealed a dose-response relation between tea consumption and kidney cancer mortality (Kinlen et al, 1988). Although some teas have been found to be mutagenic (Uyeta et al, 1981) and contain tannins that appear carcinogenic in laboratory animals (IARC, 1976), the etiologic significance of these findings is not clear.

Diet

Correlation studies in the 1970s pointed to an association of kidney cancer mortality with per capita consumption of fat and protein (Wynder et al, 1974; Armstrong and Doll, 1975). Case-control studies of renal cell cancer, however, have found relatively few significant differences in dietary factors (Armstrong et al, 1976; Yu et al, 1986; McLaughlin et al, 1984; McCredie et al, 1988; Maclure and Willett, 1990; Talamini et al, 1991; Kreiger et al, 1993). However, elevated risks have been reported with consumption of meat (McLaughlin et al, 1984; Maclure and Willett, 1990; Kreiger et al, 1993), milk (McCredie et al, 1988), and margarine and oils (Talamini et al, 1991). Reduced risks have been observed with increased intake of vegetables (Maclure and Willett, 1990; McLaughlin et al, 1992a), carrots (Talamini et al, 1991), and fruits (McLaughlin et al, 1992a). Recently, an association with high dietary protein consumption independent of fat and caloric intake has been shown (Chow et al, 1994b). There may be some biologic plausibility to a high protein diet affecting risk of renal cell cancer, because animal studies have shown protein intake can induce renal tubular hypertrophy (Smith et al, 1993).

Occupation

Unlike bladder cancer, the most common tumor of the urinary tract, renal cell cancer is not generally considered an occupationally associated tumor. However, asbestos has been linked to kidney cancer in several studies. Two cohort studies, one of insulators (Selikoff et al, 1979) and one of asbestos products workers (Enterline et al, 1987), reported significantly elevated mortality rates for kidney cancer. An association between asbestos exposure, mostly from work in shipyards, and renal cell cancer was suggested in a Boston-area case-control study (Maclure, 1987). There is some evidence from autopsy surveys and animal studies that asbestos fibers can be deposited in the kidney (Smith et al, 1989). Most case-control studies of renal cell cancer have found no association with asbestos exposure (McLaughlin et al, 1984; Yu et al, 1986; Goodman et al, 1986; Asal et al, 1988b; Brownson, 1988; Partanen et al, 1991), although their power to detect risks for asbestos exposure is generally low because of the small number of exposed workers. However, case-control studies from Australia (McCredie and Stewart, 1993) and Denmark (Mellemgaard et al, 1994d) observed elevated risks for self-reported exposure to asbestos.

Coke-oven workers exposed to high levels of polycyclic aromatic hydrocarbons have been reported to be at increased risk for kidney cancer (Redmond et al, 1972), although this finding is based on small numbers (eight deaths), with no clear evidence of a dose-response or duration-of-employment effect (Redmond, 1983). Two recent case-control studies observed little excess risk for coke-oven workers (McCredie and Stewart, 1993; Mellemgaard et al, 1994c). More general exposure to hydrocarbons was linked to renal cell cancer in two small case-control studies (Sharpe et al, 1989; Kadamani et al, 1989), but was not associated with risk in a large case-control study in Finland (Partanen et al, 1991).

Cadmium exposure was estimated from employment, food, and cigarettes, and linked to renal cell cancer in a case-control study from Roswell Park Memorial Institute in New York (Kolonel et al, 1976). Subsequent case-control studies and occupational cohort investigations have shown no relation between cadmium exposure and renal cancer (McLaughlin et al, 1984; Elinder et al, 1985; Thun et al, 1985; Yu et al, 1986; Brownson, 1988; Asal et al, 1988b; McCredie and Stewart, 1993). Although inorganic lead has induced renal tumors in laboratory animals, there is little epidemiological evidence of an association in humans (IARC, 1987). However, a recent update of lead smelter workers did detect an excess mortality from kidney cancer (including renal pelvis and ureter cancers) (Steenland et al, 1992). It is not clear, however, how many of the nine deaths were caused by transitional cell tumors, and the kidney cancer excess was not clearly related to duration of exposure.

Proportional mortality studies have suggested that laundry and dry cleaning workers may be at increased risk for kidney cancer (Blair et al, 1979; Katz and Jowett, 1981; Duh and Asal, 1984; Brown and Kaplan, 1987), and case-control studies of renal cell cancer in Oklahoma (Asal et al, 1988b) and Australia (McCredie and Stewart, 1993) indicated an excess risk among dry cleaners. However, a recent large-scale cohort study of these workers showed no increased mortality from kidney cancer (Blair et al, 1990). Dry cleaners have been exposed to a large number of chemicals, notably tetrachloroethylene, which has produced hepatocellular carcinomas in laboratory animals (IARC, 1987).

It has been suggested that kidney cancers occur excessively among oil refinery workers (Savitz and Moure, 1984). A case-control study of renal cell cancer in Oklahoma reported an excess risk associated with employment in petroleum refining work (Asal et al, 1988b). Recent reviews of cohort studies of petroleum refinery workers find little or no evidence of an excess risk of kidney cancer (Wong and Raabe, 1989; IARC, 1989).

Gasoline came under suspicion as a risk factor for renal cell cancer when male rats exposed long-term to vapors of unleaded gasoline developed a significant excess of renal cancers (MacFarland et al, 1984). As a result of this finding, a number of epidemiological studies examined the effect of gasoline exposure. In a case-control study of renal cell cancer in Minnesota, service station attendants experienced a slight upward trend in risk with duration of employment (McLaughlin et al, 1985b). No association with gasoline was observed in case-control studies in New York (Domiano et al, 1985), Los Angeles (Yu et al, 1986), or Australia (McCredie and Stewart, 1993). Exposure to aviation and jet fuels was related to kidney cancer risk in a case-control screening study of occupational exposures and cancers (Siemiatycki et al, 1987), but a later cohort study of aviation maintenance workers showed no association with risk (Spirtas et al, 1991). Case-control studies in Finland (Partanen et al, 1991) and Denmark (Mellemgaard et al, 1994c) have reported a significant association with gasoline exposure. However, studies of gasoline-exposed workers in the petroleum industry have not found an association (McLaughlin, 1993). In addition, recent nested case-control and cohort studies of gasoline exposure among industry workers have not observed a significantly increased risk of kidney cancer (Poole et al, 1993; Wong et al, 1993; Rushton, 1993; Schnatter et al, 1993).

Several other occupational associations have been reported. One cohort study found newspaper pressmen at elevated risk for kidney cancer (Paganini-Hill et al, 1980), although the association has not been confirmed (Alderson, 1986; McCredie and Stewart, 1993; Mellemgaard et al, 1994d). Swedish lumberjacks were reported at increased risk for kidney cancer in a pilot study of forestry workers (Edling and Granstam, 1980), but a nationwide survey of renal cell cancer incidence and occupation in Sweden showed no increased risk in this particular industry (McLaughlin et al, 1987). The same survey found an excess risk among health care workers, including physicians. An elevated risk of renal cell cancer among truck drivers was reported in a Missouri case-control study (Brownson, 1988), and more recently in Denmark (Mellemgaard et al, 1994d). A link between renal cell cancer and exposure to polychlorinated biphenyls was suggested when a cluster of three cases occurred among electric power utility workers (Shalat et al, 1989). Inorganic arsenic has been linked to kidney cancer, although mainly through drinking water in one area of Taiwan (Bates et al, 1992). Architects were reported to be at excess risk for renal cell cancer (Lowry et al, 1991), although no other reports support this observation (McLaughlin et al, 1992b). Another study has reported that paperboard printing workers have an elevated risk (Sinks et al, 1992).

Obesity

Virtually every study that has examined body weight and renal cell cancer has observed a positive association. Earlier studies noted the association primarily in women (Whisenand et al, 1962; Wynder et al, 1974; Lew and Garfinkel, 1979; McLaughlin et al, 1984), but more recent studies have found an effect in both sexes, although it is usually more pronounced in women (Whittemore et al, 1985; Yu et al, 1986; Goodman et al, 1986; Asal et al, 1988a; Maclure and Willett, 1990; McCredie and Stewart, 1992b; McLaughlin et al, 1992a; Kreiger et al, 1993; Benhamou et al, 1993; Mellemgaard et al, 1994c). One study reported that the association was primarily for weight gained in later adulthood (McLaughlin et al, 1984), but other studies have not supported this finding (Yu et al, 1986; Asal et al, 1988a). A linked-registry study of Danish patients discharged with a diagnosis of obesity reported significantly elevated risks for renal cell cancer in both sexes (Mellemgaard et al, 1991).

The mechanism responsible for the obesity effect is unclear. Because the association with renal cell cancer is most pronounced in women, it is believed that obesity may act by promoting hormonal changes, such as increased levels of endogenous estrogens. Although estrogens induce renal cancer in certain laboratory animals (Newsom and Vurgin, 1987), there is scant epidemiological evidence linking hormone-associated variables to renal cell cancer. Obesity may also predispose to arterionephrosclerosis, which may, in turn, render the renal tubules more susceptible to carcinogenesis. Moreover, obestity is sometimes treated with diuretics, which are under evaluation as a potential risk factor.

Radiation

Ionizing radiation appears to increase the risk of renal cell cancer, especially among patients treated for ankylosing spondylitis and cervical cancer, but the effects are weak (Land, 1986; Boice et al, 1988). An increased risk has also been described among patients receiving radium 224 for bone tuberculosis and ankylosing spondylitis (Spiess et al, 1989). In one case-control study, significantly more female patients than control subjects reported receiving diagnostic or therapeutic radiation (Asal et al, 1988b).

Hemodialysis

Among patients undergoing renal dialysis, there is an increased incidence of acquired cystic disease of the kidney, which predisposes to renal cell cancer, especially in men (Ishikawa, 1987). Although the carcinogenic mechanism is uncertain, some aspect of the uremic process appears involved.

Genetic Susceptibility

There have been several reports of familial clustering of renal cell cancer. Cohen and colleagues (1979) described a family with an inborn chromosomal defect and renal cell cancer affecting seven members of three generations. The pattern of tumors suggested an autosomal dominant mode of inheritance. Surveillance of remaining family members uncovered bilateral renal cancers in three young women, who were treated with surgical resection. The cytogenetic defect in lymphocytes was a balanced reciprocal translocation between chromosomes 3 and 8, with breakpoints determined at bands 3p14.2 and 8q24.1 (Wang and Perkins, 1984). This constitutional rearrangement prompted cytogenetic and molecular studies of tumor cells in unselected patients with renal cell cancer, which have consistently revealed deletions of distal chromosome 3p (Kovacs et al, 1988; Zbar et al, 1987). These findings have been extended by molecular studies of von Hippel-Lindau disease (featuring angiomatosis of the retina and cerebellum), an autosomal dominant condition that predisposes to renal cell cancer. The gene for this disorder has been linked to c-*raf*-1 on chromosome 3p25 (Seizinger et al, 1988). Recent work has cloned and characterized the tumor suppressor gene for von Hippel-Lindau disease (Latif et al, 1993).

These observations, taken together, suggest that the origins of renal cell cancer may involve several tumor suppressor genes on the short arm of chromosome 3. This concept has been further extended by studies of the nonheritable form of renal cell cancer (Gnarra et al, 1994). However, hereditary papillary renal cell cancer, a rare histologic subtype, may not be linked to chromosome 3 (Zbar et al, 1994). The role of developmental defects in renal cell cancer is suggested also by reports of associated renal anomalies, including polycystic kidneys (McFarland et al, 1972) and horseshoe kidneys (Blackard and Mellinger, 1968). In addition, an excess frequency of polymastia or supernumerary nipples has been noted with renal cell cancer (Goedert et al, 1981; Asal et al, 1988b), as well as with various renal anomalies (Pellegrini and Wagner, 1983).

CANCERS OF THE RENAL PELVIS AND URETER

As with renal cell cancer, the identification of risk factors for renal pelvis and ureter cancers has come mainly from case-control studies, summarized in Table 53–4. As a result of the relative infrequency of renal pelvis and ureter tumors, these studies are typically smaller than those for renal cell cancer, ranging in size from 27 to 502 cases.

Cigarette Use

Case-control studies have generally reported smoking-related risks that are higher than those for renal cell cancer or bladder cancer (Schmauz and Cole, 1974; Armstrong et al, 1976; McCredie et al, 1982, 1983a,b; McLaughlin et al, 1983; Jensen et al, 1988; Ross et al, 1989; McLaughlin et al, 1992c; McCredie and Stewart, 1992a). The risks for smokers are 2.5 to 7 times those for nonsmokers, with heavy smokers having risks of five- to 11-fold. This variation in reported risks proba-

TABLE 53–4. *Published Case-Control Studies of Renal Pelvis and Ureter Cancers*

Authors	*Year*	*Source of Controls*	*Number of Cases/Controls*	*Location*
Schmauz and Cole	1974	population	17 renal pelvis 10 ureter/451	Massachusetts
Armstrong et al	1976	hospital	33 renal pelvis/33	England
McCredie et al	1982	friend/clinic	67 renal pelvis/84/96	New South Wales
McCredie et al	1983a	population	29 renal pelvis 36 ureter/307	New South Wales
McCredie et al	1983b	population	31 renal pelvis/400	New South Wales
McLaughlin et al	1983	population	74 renal pelvis/697	Minnesota
Jensen et al	1988	hospital	76 renal pelvis 20 ureter/294	Denmark
Ross et al	1989	neighborhood	121 renal pelvis 66 ureter/187	Los Angeles
McLaughlin et al	1992c	population	308 renal pelvis 194 ureter/496	3 areas in United States
McCredie and Stewart	1992a,b	population	147 renal pelvis/523	New South Wales

bly reflects the relatively small number of cases in most of the studies. In the largest study of these cancers, cigarette smokers had a 3.2-fold risk, with current smokers at a 4.4-fold risk (McLaughlin et al, 1992c). Cessation of smoking for 10 years or longer reduced the risks for these tumors 60% to 70% relative to current smokers (McLaughlin et al, 1992c). Similar reductions in risk were seen among quitters in Australia (McCredie and Stewart, 1992a). This steep decline in risk suggests that smoking affects a relatively late stage in carcinogenesis, thus making it possible for smoking cessation to lower the risk for these tumors. Population-based attributable risk estimates for cigarette smoking and renal pelvis and ureter cancers in the United States have suggested that 70% to 82% of the cases among men and 37% to 61% among women are due to smoking (McLaughlin et al, 1983; McLaughlin et al, 1992c). Results from Denmark indicate that smoking accounts for 56% of the cases of renal pelvis and ureter cancers among men and 40% among women (Jensen et al, 1988). In Australia, 46% of the cases among men and 35% among women are attributable to cigarette smoking (McCredie and Stewart, 1992a). Thus, cigarette smoking appears to be the strongest risk factor for these tumors and accounts for the majority of cases in most areas of the world.

Drugs

The relation between heavy use of phenacetin-containing analgesics and cancers of the renal pelvis, ureter, and bladder is well established (IARC, 1980, 1987). Case reports and clinical surveys starting in the mid-1960s and continuing through the 1970s linked phenacetin use to analgesic nephropathy, and an accompanying excess of renal pelvis cancer (Hultengren et al, 1965). In a series of case-control studies in New South Wales, Australia, where analgesic abuse is relatively common, McCredie and colleagues (1982, 1983a,b, 1993) reported three- to 12-fold increased risks for renal pelvis and ureter cancers among men and women using phenacetin analgesics. In the United States, where analgesic abuse is relatively uncommon (Murray and Goldberg, 1978), two case-control studies were limited by the small number of exposed subjects. In the Minnesota study of renal pelvis cancer, long-term use (over 3 years) of phenacetin was related to an eight-fold risk for men and a four-fold risk for women (McLaughlin et al, 1985a). In the Los Angeles study, the risk for renal pelvis and ureter cancers was only slightly elevated after use of phenacetin analgesics over 30 consecutive days (Ross et al, 1989). In Denmark, use of phenacetin-containing analgesics was associated with risks of 2.4 among men and 4.2 among women after adjustment for use of other analgesics, cigarettes, and occupation (Jensen et al, 1989). Phenacetin has also been shown to induce urinary tract tumors in laboratory animals (Nakanishi et al, 1982; IARC, 1987). In future studies, detection of risk for phenacetin use may be difficult, because phenacetin was removed from analgesics in most industrial countries starting in the late 1960s.

There are some limited data suggesting that acetaminophen, a relatively recent addition to over-the-counter analgesics, may increase risk of renal pelvis cancer. Acetaminophen is the major metabolite of phenacetin (Hinsen, 1981). Although a few clinical and experimental findings have linked heavy acetaminophen intake with renal papillary necrosis (Nanra, 1983), the primary lesion of analgesic nephropathy, a population-based case-control evaluation of this condition in Australia showed no association (McCredie and Stewart, 1988). Results of animal studies have been mixed, with two studies suggesting carcinogenic effects (Flaks and Flaks, 1983; Flaks et al, 1985) and two being negative (Hiraga and Fujii, 1985; Amo and Matsuyama, 1985). The Minnesota case-control study of renal pelvis cancer reported a positive association with acetaminophen, although only a few patients took acetaminophen-containing analgesics exclusively (McLaughlin et al, 1983, 1985a). In Australia, no increase in risk was observed for cancer of the renal pelvis among acetaminophen users, but a significant 2.5-fold increase in risk was found for ureter cancer (McCredie and Stewart, 1988). In a larger and more recent Australian study, acetaminophen use was not related to risk (McCredie et al, 1993). The Los Angeles case-control study reported a two-fold risk for acetaminophen use, but again, the number of users was small. Use of acetaminophen-containing analgesics in the United States did not become widespread until the mid-1970s—hence it may be too early to detect tumors with long latency periods and the number of exclusive users of these products may be too small to evaluate risks presently. Moreover, heavy users of acetaminophen products were often past users of phenacetin-containing analgesics, further confounding the association (McLaughlin et al, 1985a).

Experimental, clinical, and most epidemiological studies have shown no relation between aspirin intake and cancers of the renal pelvis or ureter (Emkey, 1983; Patierno et al, 1989; Armstrong et al, 1976; McCredie et al, 1982, 1983a,b; McLaughlin et al, 1985a). One study, however, has reported a significant two-fold risk for aspirin use, with the excess mainly among women with renal pelvis tumors (Ross et al, 1989). The Danish study also reported a significant association among women who took aspirin, which the authors attributed to prior or concomitant phenacetin use (Jensen et al, 1989). By contrast, the recent Australian study found aspirin use associated with a decreased risk of renal pelvis cancer (McCredie et al, 1993).

Overall, the available evidence on analgesics indicates a causal relation between phenacetin intake and cancers of the renal pelvis and ureter. Evidence for acetaminophen is weak, but suggestive because of its biochemical resemblance to phenacetin. The relatively recent introduction of this widely used analgesic warrants close monitoring for possible carcinogenic effects. The limited positive findings for aspirin probably reflect confounding by earlier phenacetin use or a chance event, but further study appears indicated.

Coffee, Alcohol, and Other Beverages

There are few data to indicate that coffee or alcohol is related to renal pelvis and ureter cancers (Armstrong et al, 1976; McLaughlin et al, 1983; Ross et al, 1989). One study found a 15-fold increased risk for drinkers of over seven cups of coffee per day, but this observation was based on two cases (Schmauz and Cole, 1974). Another study reported a significant inverse relation between coffee intake and risk of renal pelvis cancer (Armstrong et al, 1976). No case-control differences have been observed for alcohol consumption (Armstrong et al, 1976; McLaughlin et al, 1983; Ross et al, 1989). An excess risk has been reported among heavy consumers of tea, particularly women, which may deserve further study (McLaughlin et al, 1983).

Occupation

There are few occupational associations for renal pelvis and ureter cancers because of their relative rarity and frequent inclusion with renal cell cancers in occupational cohort studies. Early case reports linked renal pelvis and ureter tumors with exposure to dyes (Macalpine, 1947; Poole-Wilson, 1969). A significant excess of employment in the leather industry was reported in Massachusetts (Schmauz and Cole, 1974), but was not confirmed in the British case-control study, which included an area with a concentration of boot and shoe manufacturing (Armstrong et al, 1976). Case-control studies in Australia (McCredie et al, 1982) and the United States (McLaughlin et al, 1983) have revealed no significant occupational associations. However, in the U.S. study, significant increases in risk were associated with exposure to high-risk materials such as coal, natural gas, and mineral oils (McLaughlin et al, 1983). In the recent Australian case-control study, employment in the dry cleaning, iron and steel, and petroleum refining industries was related to an increased risk (McCredie and Stewart, 1993). The Danish case-control study found significantly increased risks for employment in the chemical, petrochemical, and plastics industries, and for exposures to coal and coke, and to asphalt and tar (Jensen et al, 1988). A record-linkage survey of occupation and cancer incidence in Denmark found significantly elevated risks for renal pelvis and ureter cancers in a number of industries, including forestry and logging; slaughtering, preparing and preserving meat; and printing and publishing (Olsen and Jensen, 1987). A Swedish record-linkage study reported a significant excess risk among machinists and plumbers (McLaughlin et al, 1987), but adjustment for smoking was not possible in either Scandinavian survey. Although the available data are limited, the work-related risks observed for cancers of the renal pelvis and ureter resemble the occupational associations that are more clearly established for bladder cancer.

Radiation

The carcinogenic influence of ionizing radiation appears stronger for the renal pelvis and ureter than the renal parenchyma. The effect is seen especially in cervical cancer patients treated with radiation (Boice et al, 1988). Renal pelvis cancer has also been a consequence of Thorotrast administration during retrograde pyelography (Verhaak et al, 1965).

Multicentric Tumors

Transitional epithelial tumors of the lower urinary tract have a tendency to arise at multicentric sites, due partly to shared risk factors such as smoking (Kantor and McLaughlin, 1985). This pattern suggests the need for screening patients with renal pelvis and ureter cancers (eg, urinary cytology) for new tumors arising along the urinary tract, including the bladder.

PREVENTIVE MEASURES

It may be possible to prevent—through elimination of cigarette smoking—the majority of renal pelvis and ureter cancers and a smaller fraction of renal cell cancers. Hence, measures aimed at persuading current smokers to quit and encouraging nonsmokers, particularly young people, not to start should have a substantial impact on subsequent renal cancer incidence and mortality. The exclusion of phenacetin from analgesic products, an action already taken by most Western countries, should contribute to a reduction of renal tumors. Further research into the environmental and genetic determinants of renal cancer will augment the means of primary prevention and target high-risk groups for screening aimed at early detection and treatment.

REFERENCES

ADAMI H-O, MCLAUGHLIN JK, HSING AW, et al. 1992. Alcoholism and cancer risk: a population-based study. Cancer Causes Control 3:419–425.

ALDERSON M. 1986. *Occupational Cancer*. London: Butterworth, pp 108–110.

AMO H, MATSUYAMA M. 1985. Subchronic and chronic effects of feeding large amounts of acetaminophen in B6C3F1 mice. Jpn J Hyg 40:567–574.

ARMSTRONG B, DOLL R. 1975. Environmental factors and cancer incidence and mortality in different countries, with special reference to dietary practices. Br J Cancer 15:617–631.

ARMSTRONG B, GARROD A, DOLL R. 1976. A retrospective study of renal cancer with special reference to coffee and animal protein consumption. Br J Cancer 33:127–136.

ASAL NR, RISSER DR, KADAMANI S, et al. 1988a. Risk factors in renal cell carcinoma. I. Methodology, demographics, tobacco, beverage use, and obesity. Cancer Detect Prev 11:359–377.

ASAL NR, GEYER JR, RISSER DR, et al. 1988b. Risk factors in renal cell carcinoma. II. Medical history, occupation, multivariate analysis, and conclusion. Cancer Detect Prev 13:263–279.

AXTELL LM, ASIRE AJ, MYERS MH. 1976. Cancer Patient Survival. Report No. 5. Bethesda, MD: National Institutes of Health, DHEW publication no. (NIH) 77–992.

BATES MN, SMITH AH, HOPENHAYEN-RICH C. 1992. Arsenic ingestion and internal cancers: a review. Am J Epidemiol 135:462–476.

BAUM C, KENNEDY KC, KNOPP DE, et al. 1988. Prescription drug use in 1984 and changes over time. Med Care 26:105–114.

BENHAMOU S, LENFANT M-H, ORY-PAOLETTI C, et al. 1993. Risk factors for renal cell carcinoma in a French case-control study. Int J Cancer 55:32–36.

BENNINGTON JL, LAUBSCHER FA. 1968. Epidemiologic studies of carcinoma of the kidney. I. Association of renal adenocarcinoma with smoking. Cancer 21:1069–1071.

BLACKARD CE, MELLINGER GT. 1968. Cancer in a horseshoe kidney: a report of two cases. Arch Surg 97:616–627.

BLAIR A, DECOUFLE P, GRAUMAN D. 1979. Causes of death among laundry and dry cleaning workers. Am J Public Health 69:508–511.

BLAIR A, STEWART PA, TOLBERT PE, et al. 1990. Cancer and other causes of death among a cohort of dry cleaners. Br J Ind Med 47:162–168.

BLOT WJ, LANIER A, FRAUMENI JF JR, et al. 1975. Cancer mortality among Alaskan natives, 1960–1969. J Natl Cancer Inst 55:547–554.

BLOT WJ, FRAUMENI JF JR. 1979. Geographic patterns of renal cancer in the United States. J Natl Cancer Inst 63:363–366.

BOICE JD, ENGHOLM G, KLEINERMAN RA, et al. 1988. Radiation dose and second-cancer risk in patients treated for cancer of the cervix. Radiat Res 116:3–55.

BORING CC, SQUIRES TS, TONG T. 1994. Cancer statistics, 1994. CA Cancer J Clin 44:7–26.

BRESLOW NE, ENSTROM JE. 1974. Geographic correlations between cancer mortality rates and alcohol-tobacco consumption in the United States. J Natl Cancer Inst 53:631–639.

BRESLOW NE, DAY NE. 1980. Statistical methods in cancer research. Vol I. The Analysis of Case-control Studies. Lyon: France, IARC Pub No 32.

BROWN DP, KAPLAN SD. 1987. Retrospective cohort mortality study of dry cleaning workers using perchloroethylene. J Occup Med 29:535–541.

BROWNSON RC. 1988. A case-control study of renal cell carcinoma in relation to occupation, smoking, and alcohol consumption. Arch Environ Health 43:238–241.

BRUZZI P, GREEN SB, BEZAR DP, BRINTON LA AND SCHAIRER C. 1985. Estimating the population attributable risk for multiple risk factors using case-control data. Am J Epidemiol, 122:904–914.

CHOW W-H, MCLAUGHLIN JK, LINET MS, et al. 1994a. Use of analgesics and risk of renal cell cancer. Int J Cancer 59:467–470.

CHOW W-H, GRIDLEY G, MCLAUGHLIN JK, et al. 1994b. Protein intake and risk of renal cell cancer. J Natl Cancer Inst 86:1131–1139.

COHEN AJ, LI FP, BERG S, et al. 1979. Hereditary renal-cell carcinoma associated with a chromosomal translocation. N Engl J Med 301:592–595.

DECOUFLE P, STANISLAWCZYK K. 1977. A Retrospective Survey of Cancer in Relation to Occupation. U.S. Department of Health, Education, and Welfare: Washington, DC.

DEVESA SS, SILVERMAN DT, YOUNG JL JR, et al. 1987. Cancer incidence and mortality trends among whites in the United States, 1974–84. J Natl Cancer Inst 79:701–770.

DEVESA SS, SILVERMAN DT, MCLAUGHLIN JK, et al. 1990. Comparison of the descriptive epidemiology of urinary tract cancer. Cancer Causes Control 1:133–141.

DOLL R, PETO R. 1976. Mortality in relation to smoking: 20 years' observations on male British doctors. Br Med J 2:1525–1536.

DOMIANO SF, VENA JE, SWANSON MK. 1985. Gasoline exposure, smoking, and kidney cancer. J Occup Med 27:398–399.

DUH RW, ASAL NR. 1984. Mortality among laundry and dry cleaning workers in Oklahoma. Am J Public Health 74:1278–1280.

EDLING C, GRANSTAM S. 1980. Causes of death among lumberjacks—a pilot study. J Occup Med 22:403–406.

ELINDER CG, KJELLSTROM T, HOGSTEDT C, et al. 1985. Cancer mortality of cadmium workers. Br J Ind Med 42:651–655.

EMKEY RD. 1983. Aspirin and renal disease. Am J Med 74(suppl 6A):97–101.

ENTERLINE PE, VIREN J. 1985. Epidemiologic evidence of an association between gasoline and kidney cancer. Environ Health Perspect 62:303–312.

ENTERLINE PE, HARTLEY J, HENDERSON V. 1987. Asbestos and cancer: a cohort followup to death. Am J Ind Med 44:396–401.

FINKLE WD, MCLAUGHLIN JK, RASGON SA, YEOH HH, LOW JE. 1993. Increased risk of renal cell cancer among women using diuretics in the United States. Cancer Causes Control 4:555–558.

FLAKS A, FLAKS B. 1983. Induction of liver cell tumor in 1F mice by paracetamol. Carcinogenesis 4:363–368.

FLAKS B, FLAKS A, SHAW APW. 1985. Induction by paracetamol of bladder and liver tumors in the rat. Acta Pathol Microbiol Immunol Scand (Section A) 93:367–377.

FRASER GE, PHILLIPS RL, BEESON WL. 1990. Hypertension, antihypertensive medication and risk of renal carcinoma in California Seventh-Day Adventists. Int J Epidemiol 19:832–838.

FRAUMENI JF JR. 1968. Cigarette smoking and cancers of the urinary tract: geographic variation in the United States. J Natl Cancer Inst 41:1205–1211.

GART JJ. 1970. Point and interval estimation of the common odds ratio in the combination of 2×2 tables with fixed marginals. Biometrika 57:471–475.

GNARRA JR, TORY K, WENG Y, et al. 1994. Mutation of the VHL tumor suppressor gene in renal carcinoma. Nat Genet 7:85–90.

GOEDERT JJ, MCKEEN EA, FRAUMENI JF JR. 1981. Polymastia and renal adenocarcinoma. Ann Intern Med 95:182–184.

GOODMAN MT, MORGENSTERN H, WYNDER EL. 1986. A case-control study of factors affecting the development of renal cell cancer. Am J Epidemiol 124:926–941.

GRAHAM S, BLANCHET M, ROHRER T. 1977. Cancer in asbestos-mining and other areas of Quebec. J Natl Cancer Inst 59:1139–1145.

GREENE MH, HOOVER RN, ECK RL, et al. 1979. Cancer mortality among printing plant workers. Environ Res 20:66–73.

GRIDLEY G, MCLAUGHLIN JK, EKBOM A, et al. 1993. Incidence of cancer among patients with rheumatoid arthritis. J Natl Cancer Inst 85:307–311.

GROVE JS, NOMURA A, SEVERSON RK, et al. 1991. The association of blood pressure with cancer incidence in a prospective study. Am J Epidemiol 134:942–947.

HAMILTON JM. 1975. Renal carcinogenesis. Adv Cancer Rev 22:1–56.

HAMMOND EC. 1966. Smoking in relation to the death rates of 1 million men and women. NCI Monogr 19:127–204.

HIATT RA, TOLAN K, QUESENBERG CP. 1994. Renal cell carcinoma and thiazide use: a historical case-control study. Cancer Causes Control 5:319–325.

HINDS MW, KOLONEL LM, LEE J, et al. 1980. Association between cancer incidence and alcohol/cigarette consumption among five ethnic groups in Hawaii. Br J Cancer 41:929–940.

HINSEN JA. 1981. Biochemical toxicology of acetaminophen. In: Hodgson E, Bend JR, Philpot RM (eds). Reviews in Biochemical Toxicology. Vol 2. New York: Elsevier/North Holland, pp 103–129.

HIRAGA K, FUJII T. 1985. Carcinogenicity testing of acetaminophen in F344 rats Jpn J Cancer Res 76:79–85.

HIRAYAMA T. 1977. Changing patterns in Japan with special reference to the decrease in stomach cancer mortality. In: Hiatt HH, Watson JD, Winsten JA (eds). Origins of Human Cancer, Book A. New York: Cold Spring Harbor Laboratory, pp 55–75.

HULTENGREN N, LAGERGREN C, LJUNGQVIST A. 1965. Carcinoma of the renal pelvis in renal papillary necrosis. Acta Chir Scand 130:314–320.

INTERNATIONAL AGENCY FOR RESEARCH ON CANCER. 1976. Tannic acid and tannins. IARC Monogr Eval Carcinog Risks Hum 10:253–262.

INTERNATIONAL AGENCY FOR RESEARCH ON CANCER. 1980. Some pharmaceutical drugs. IARC Monogr Eval Carcinog Risks Hum 24:135–161.

INTERNATIONAL AGENCY FOR RESEARCH ON CANCER. 1987. Overall Evaluations of Carcinogenicity: An Updating of IARC Monographs, Volumes 1 to 42. IARC Monogr Eval Carcinog Risks Hum Suppl 7.

INTERNATIONAL AGENCY FOR RESEARCH ON CANCER. 1989. Occupational exposures in petroleum refining; crude oil and major petroleum fuels. IARC Monogr Eval Carcinog Risks Hum 45:39–117.

ISHIKAWA I. 1987. Development of adenocarcinoma and acquired cystic disease of the kidney in hemodialysis patients. In: Miller RW, Watanabe S, Fraumeni JF Jr, et al (eds). Unusual Occurrences as Clues to Cancer Etiology. Tokyo: Japan Scientific Societies Press, pp 77–86.

JACOBSEN BK, BJELKE E, KVALE G, et al. 1986. Coffee drinking, mortality, and cancer incidence: results from a Norwegian prospective study. J Natl Cancer Inst 76:823–841.

JENSEN OM. 1979. Cancer morbidity and causes of death among Danish brewery workers. Int J Cancer 23:454–463.

JENSEN OM, KNUDSEN JB, MCLAUGHLIN JK, et al. 1988. The Copenhagen case-control study of renal pelvis and ureter cancer: role of smoking and occupational exposures. Int J Cancer 41:557–561.

JENSEN OM, KNUDSEN JB, TOMASSON H, et al. 1989. The Copenhagen case-control study of renal pelvis and ureter cancer: role of analgesics. Int J Cancer 44:965–968.

KADAMANI S, ASAL NR, NELSON RY. 1989. Occupational hydrocarbon exposure and risk of renal cell carcinoma. Am J Ind Med 15:131–141.

KAHN HA. 1966. The Dorn study of smoking and mortality among U.S. veterans: report on 8 1/2 years of observation. NCI Monogr 19:1–125.

KANTOR AF, MCLAUGHLIN JK. 1985. Second cancer following cancer of the urinary system in Connecticut, 1935–82. NCI Monogr 68:149–159.

KATZ RM, JOWETT D. 1981. Female laundry and dry cleaning workers in Wisconsin: a mortality analysis. Am J Public Health 71:305–307.

KINLEN LJ, WILLOWS AN, GOLDBLATT P, et al. 1988. Tea consumption and cancer. Br J Cancer 58:397–401.

KJELLSTROM T, FRIBERG L, RAHNSTER B. 1979. Mortality and cancer morbidity among cadmium-exposed workers. Environ Health Perspect 28:199–204.

KOLONEL LN. 1976. Association of cadmium with renal cancer. Cancer 37:1782–1787.

KOSARY CL, MCLAUGHLIN JK. 1993. Kidney and renal pelvis. In: Miller BA, Ries LAG, Hankey BF, et al (eds). Cancer Statistics Review: 1973–1990. National Cancer Institute. NIH Pub. No. 93–2789, X1–X22.

KOVACS G, ERLANDSSON R, BOLDOY F, et al. 1988. Consistent chromosome 3p deletion and loss of heterozygosity in renal cell carcinoma. Proc Natl Acad Sci U S A 85:1571–1575.

KREIGER N, MARETT LD, DODDS L, et al. 1993. Risk factors for renal cell carcinoma: results of a population-based case-control study. Cancer Causes Control 4:101–110.

LAND CE. 1986. Carcinogenic effects of radiation on the human digestive tract and other organs. In: Cyston AC, Albert RE, Burns FJ, et al (eds). Radiation Carcinogenesis. New York: Elsevier, pp 347–378.

LANIER AP, BLOT WJ, BENDER TR, et al. 1980. Cancer in Alaskan Indians, Eskimos, and Aleuts. J Natl Cancer Inst 65:1157–1159.

LASKI ME. 1986. Diuretics: mechanism of action and therapy. Semin Nephrol 6:210–223.

LATIF F, TORY K, GNARRA JR, et al. 1993. Identification of the von Hippel-Lindau disease tumor suppressor gene. Science 260:1317–1320.

LA VECCHIA C, NEGRI E, D'AVANZO B, et al. 1990. Smoking and renal cell carcinoma. Cancer Res 50:5231–5233.

LEW EA, GARFINKEL L. 1979. Variations in mortality by weight among 750,000 men and women. J Chron Dis 32:563–576.

LIJINSKY W, REUBER MD. 1987. Pathologic effects of chronic administration of hydrochlorothiazide, with and without sodium nitrate, to 344 rats. Toxicol Ind Health 3:413–422.

LINDBLAD P, MCLAUGHLIN JK, MELLEMGAARD A, et al. 1993. Risk of kidney cancer among patients using analgesics and diuretics: a population-based cohort study. Int J Cancer 55:5–9.

LOWRY JT, PETERS JM, DEAPEN D, et al. 1991. Renal cell carcinoma among architects. Am J Ind Med 20:123–125.

MACLURE M, MACMAHON B. 1985. Phenacetin and cancer of the urinary tract. N Engl J Med 313:1479.

MACLURE M. 1987. Asbestos and renal adenocarcinoma: a case-control study. Environ Res 42:353–361.

MACLURE M, WILLETT W. 1990. A case-control study of diet and risk of renal adenocarcinoma. Epidemiology 1:430–440.

MACFARLAND HN, ULRICH CF, HOLDSWORTH CE, et al. 1984. A chronic inhalation study with unleaded gasoline vapor. J Am Coll Toxicol 3:231–248.

MACALPINE JB. 1947. Papilloma of the renal pelvis in dye workers: two cases, one of which shows bilateral growth. Br J Surg 35:137–140.

MCCREDIE M, FORD JM, TAYLOR JS, et al. 1982. Analgesics and cancer of the renal pelvis in New South Wales. Cancer 49:2617–2625.

MCCREDIE M, STEWART JH, FORD JM. 1983a. Analgesics and tobacco as risk factors for cancer of the ureter and renal pelvis. J Urol 130:28–30.

MCCREDIE M, STEWART JH, FORD JM, et al. 1983b. Phenacetin-containing analgesics and cancers of the bladder and renal pelvis in women. Br J Urol 55:220–224.

MCCREDIE M, FORD JM, STEWART JH. 1988. Risk factors for cancer of the renal parenchyma. Int J Cancer 42:13–16.

MCCREDIE M, STEWART JH. 1988. Does paracetamol cause urothelial cancer or renal papillary necrosis? Nephron 49:296–300.

MCCREDIE M, STEWART JH. 1992a. Risk factors for kidney cancer in New South Wales: I. Cigarette smoking. Eur J Cancer 28A:2050–2054.

MCCREDIE M, STEWART JH. 1992b. Risk factors for kidney cancer in New South Wales. II. Urological disease, hypertension, obesity and hormonal factors. Cancer Causes Control 3:323–331.

McCredie M, Stewart JH. 1993. Risk factors for kidney cancer in New South Wales: IV. Occupation. Br J Ind Med 50:349–354.

McCredie M, Stewart JH, Day NE. 1993. Different roles for phenacetin and paracetamol in cancer of the kidney and renal pelvis. Int J Cancer 53:245–249.

McFarland WL, Wallace S, Johnson DE. 1972. Renal carcinoma and polycystic disease. J Urol 107:530–532.

McLaughlin JK, Schuman LM. 1983. Epidemiology of renal cell carcinoma. In: Lilienfeld AM (ed). Reviews in Cancer Epidemiology. Vol 2. New York: Elsevier/North Holland, pp 170–210.

McLaughlin JK, Blot WJ, Mandel JS, et al. 1983. Etiology of cancer of the renal pelvis. J Natl Cancer Inst 71:287–291.

McLaughlin JK, Mandel JS, Blot WJ, et al. 1984. Population-based case-control study of renal cell carcinoma. J Natl Cancer Inst 72:275–284.

McLaughlin JK, Blot WJ, Mehl ES, et al. 1985a. Relation of analgesic use to renal cancer: population-based findings. NCI Monogr 69:213–215.

McLaughlin JK, Blot WJ, Mehl ES, et al. 1985b. Petroleum-related employment and renal cell cancer. J Occup Med 27:672–674.

McLaughlin JK, Malker HSR, Stone BJ, et al. 1987. Occupational risks for renal cancer in Sweden. Br J Ind Med 44:119–123.

McLaughlin JK, Blot WJ, Fraumeni JF Jr. 1988. Diuretics and renal cell cancer. J Natl Cancer Inst 80:378.

McLaughlin JK, Hrubec Z, Heineman EF, et al. 1990. Renal cancer and cigarette smoking: 26-year followup of U.S. veterans. Public Health Rep 105:535–537.

McLaughlin JK, Gao Y-T, Gao R-N, et al. 1992a. Risk factors for renal cell cancer in Shanghai, China. Int J Cancer 52:562–565.

McLaughlin JK, Malker HSR, Blot WJ, et al. 1992b. Renal cell cancer among architects and allied professionals in Sweden. Am J Ind Med 21:873–876.

McLaughlin JK, Silverman DT, Hsing AW, et al. 1992c. Cigarette smoking and cancers of the renal pelvis and ureter. Cancer Res 52:254–257.

McLaughlin JK. 1993. Renal cell cancer and exposure to gasoline: a review. Environ Health Perspect Suppl 101(suppl 6):111–114.

Mellemgaard A, Moller H, Olsen JH, et al. 1991. Increased risk of renal cell carcinoma among obese women. J Natl Cancer Inst 21:1581–1582.

Mellemgaard A, Moller H, Olsen JH. 1992a. Diuretics may increase risk of renal cell carcinoma. Cancer Causes Control 3:309–312.

Mellemgaard A, Moller H, Jensen OM, et al. 1992b. Risk of kidney cancer in analgesics users. J Clin Epidemiol 45:1021–1024.

Mellemgaard A, Engholm G, McLaughlin JK, et al. 1994a. Risk of renal cell carcinoma in Denmark. I. Role of socioeconomic status, tobacco use, beverages, and family history. Cancer Causes Control 5:105–113.

Mellemgaard A, Niwa S, Mehl ES, et al. 1994b. Risk factors for renal cell carcinoma in Denmark. II. Role of medication and medical history. Int J Epidemiol 23:923–930.

Mellemgaard A, Engholm G, McLaughlin JK, et al. 1994c. Risk of renal cell carcinoma in Denmark. III. Role of weight, physical activity, and reproductive factors. Int J Cancer 56:66–71.

Mellemgaard A, Engholm G, McLaughlin JK, et al. 1994d. Risk of renal cell carcinoma in Denmark. IV. Role of occupation. Scand J Work Environ Health 20:160–165.

Monson RR, Lyon JL. 1975. Proportional mortality among alcoholics. Cancer 36:1077–1079.

Muir C, Waterhouse J, Mack T, et al. 1987. Cancer Incidence in Five Continents. Volume V. IARC Sci. Pub. No. 88 Lyon, France: International Agency for Research on Cancer.

Murray TG, Goldberg M. 1978. Analgesic-associated nephropathy in the U.S.A.: epidemiologic, clinical, and pathogenetic features. Kidney Int 13:64–71.

Nakanishi K, Kurata Y, Oshima M, et al. 1982. Carcinogenicity of phenacetin: long-term feeding study in B6C3F1 mice. Int J Cancer 29:439–444.

Nanra RS. 1983. Renal effects of antipyretic analgesics. Am J Med 75:70–81.

National Cancer Institute. 1989. Cancer Statistics Review, 1973–1986. Bethesda, MD, NIH publication no. 89–2789.

National Center for Health Statistics. 1987. Highlights of drug utilization in office practice: National Ambulatory Care Survey, 1985. Adv Data Vital Health Stat, No. 134.

National Center for Health Statistics. 1993. Drug utilization in office practice: National Ambulatory Medical Care Survey, 1990. Adv Data Vital Health Stat, No 232.

National Toxicology Program. 1989a. Toxicology and carcinogenesis studies of furosemide in F344/N rats and B6C3F mice. NTP Technical Report No. 356, Research Triangle Park, North Carolina.

National Toxicology Program. 1989b. Toxicology and carcinogenesis studies of hydrochlorothiazide in F344/N rats and B6C3F mice. NTP Technical Report No. 357, Research Triangle Park, North Carolina.

Newsom GD, Vurgin D. 1987. Etiologic factors in renal cell adenocarcinoma. Semin Nephrol 7:109–116.

Olsen JH, Jensen OM. 1987. Occupation and risk of cancer in Denmark: an analysis of 93,810 cancer cases, 1970–1979. Scand J Work Environ Health 13 (suppl 1):1–91.

Paganini-Hill A, Glazer E, Henderson BE, et al. 1980. Cause-specific mortality among newspaper web pressmen. J Occup Med 22:542–544.

Paganini-Hill A, Chao A, Ross RK, et al. 1989. Aspirin use and chronic disease: a cohort study of the elderly. Br Med J 299:1247–1250.

Parkin DM, Muir CS, Whelan SL, et al. 1992. Cancer Incidence in Five Continents, Volume VI. IARC Sci. Pub. No. 120 Lyon, France: International Agency for Research on Cancer.

Partanen T, Heikkila P, Hernberg S, et al. 1991. Renal cell cancer and occupational exposure to chemical agents. Scand J Work Environ Health 17:231–239.

Patierno SR, Lehman NL, Henderson BE, et al. 1989. Study of the ability of phenacetin, acetaminophen, and aspirin to induce cytotoxicity, mutation, and morphological transformation in C3H/10T1/2 clone 8 mouse embryo cells. Cancer Res 49:1038–1044.

Pell S, Alonzo CA. 1973. A five-year mortality study of alcoholics. J Occup Med 15:120–125.

Pellegrini JR, Wagner RF. 1983. Polythelia and associated conditions. Am Fam Physician 28:129–132.

Poole C, Dreyer NA, Satterfield MH, et al. 1993. Kidney cancer and hydrocarbon exposures among petroleum refinery workers. Environ Health Perspect 101 (suppl 6):53–62.

Poole-Wilson DB. 1969. Occupational tumours of the renal pelvis and ureter arising in the dye-making industry. Proc R Soc Med 62:93–94.

Redmond CK, Ciocco A, Lloyd W, et al. 1972. Long-term mortality study of steelworkers. VI. Mortality from malignant neoplasms among coke oven workers. J Occup Med 14:621–629.

Redmond CK. 1983. Cancer mortality among coke oven workers. Environ Health Perspect 52:67–73.

Ross RK, Paganini-Hill A, Landolph J, et al. 1989. Analgesics, cigarette smoking, and other risk factors in cancer of the renal pelvis and ureter. Cancer Res 49:1045–1048.

Rushton L. 1993. The U.K. oil refinery and distribution centre studies: a 39-year follow-up. Environ Health Perspect 101 (suppl 6):77–84.

Savitz D, Moure R. 1984. Cancer risk among oil refinery workers: a review of epidemiologic studies. J Occup Med 26:662–670.

SCHMAUZ R, COLE P. 1974. Epidemiology of cancer of the renal pelvis and ureter. J Natl Cancer Inst 52:1431–1434.

SCHMIDT W, DE LINT. 1972. Causes of death of alcoholics. Q J Stud Alcohol 33:171–185.

SCHMIDT W, POPHAM RE. 1981. The role of drinking and smoking in mortality from cancer and other causes in male alcoholics. Cancer 47:1031–1041.

SCHNATTER AR, KATZ AM, NICOLICH MJ, et al. 1993. A retrospective mortality study among Canadian petroleum marketing and distribution workers. Environ Health Perspect 101 (suppl 6):85–99.

SCHWARTZ V, FLAMANT R, LELLOUCH J, et al. 1961. Results of a French survey on the role of tobacco, particularly inhalation in different cancer sites. J Natl Cancer Inst 26:1085–1108.

SEIZINGER BR, ROULEAU GA, OZELIUS LJ, et al. 1988. Von Hippel-Landau disease maps to the region of chromosome 3 associated with renal cell carcinoma. Nature 332:268–269.

SELBY JV, FRIEDMAN GD, FIREMAN BH. 1989. Screening prescription drugs for possible carcinogenicity: Eleven to fifteen years of follow-up. Cancer Res 49:5736–5747.

SELIKOFF IJ, HAMMOND EC, SEIDMAN H. 1979. Mortality experience of insulation workers in the United States and Canada, 1943–1976. Ann NY Acad Sci 330:91–116.

SHALAT SC, TRUE LD, FLEMING LE, et al. 1989. Kidney cancer in utility workers exposed to polychlorinated biphenyls (PCBs). Br J Ind Med 46:823–824.

SHARPE CR, ROCHON JE, ADAM JM, et al. 1989. Case-control study of hydrocarbon exposures in patients with renal cell carcinoma. Can Med Assoc J 140:1309–1318.

SHENNAN DH. 1973. Renal carcinoma and coffee consumption in 16 countries. Br J Cancer 28:473–474.

SIEMIATYCKI J, DEWAR R, NADON L, et al. 1987. Associations between several sites of cancer and twelve petroleum-derived liquids. Scand J Work Environ Health 13:493–504.

SINKS T, LUSHNIAK B, HAUSSLER BJ, et al. 1992. Renal cell cancer among paperboard printing workers. Epidemiology 3:483–489.

SMITH AH, SHEARN VI, WOOD R. 1989. Asbestos and kidney cancer: the evidence supports a causal association. Am J Ind Med 16:159–166.

SMITH LJ, ROSENBERG ME, HOSTETTER TH. 1993. Effect of angiotensin II blockade on dietary protein-induced renal growth. Am J Kidney Dis 22:120–127.

SPIESS H, MAYS CW, CHMELVESKY B. 1989. Radium 224 in humans. In: Taylor DM, Mays CW, Gerber GB, et al (eds). Risks from Radium and Thorotrast. BIR Report 21:7–12.

SPIRTAS R, STEWART PA, LEE JS, et al. 1991. Retrospective cohort mortality study of workers at an aircraft maintenance facility. I. Epidemiologic results. Br J Ind Med 48:515–530.

STEENLAND K, SELVAN S, LANDRIGAN P. 1992. The mortality of lead smelter workers: an update. Am J Public Health 82:1641–1644.

STOYANOV IS, CHERNOZEMSKY IN, NICOLOV IG, et al. 1978. Epidemiologic association between endemic nephropathy and urinary system tumors in an endemic region. J Chron Dis 31:721–724.

TALAMINI R, BARON AE, BARRA S, et al. 1991. A case-control study of risk factors for renal cell cancer in northern Italy. Cancer Causes Control 1:125–131.

THOMAS TL, DECOUFLE P, MOURE-ERASO R. 1980. Mortality among workers employed in petroleum refining and petrochemical plants. J Occup Med 22:97–103.

THUN MJ, SCHNORR TM, SMITH AB, et al. 1985. Mortality among a cohort of U.S. cadmium production workers—an update. J Natl Cancer Inst 74:325–333.

UYETA M, TAUE S, MEZAKI M. 1981. Mutagenicity of hydrolysates of tea infusions. Mutat Res 88:233–240.

VERHAAK R. 1965. Tumor induction in a thorotrast kidney. Oncologica 19:20–32.

WANG N, PERKINS KL. 1984. Involvement of band 3p14 in *i*(3;8) hereditary renal carcinoma. Cancer Genet Cytogenet 11:479–481.

WEIR JM, DUNN JE. 1970. Smoking and mortality: a prospective study. Cancer 25:105–112.

WEN CP, TSAI SP, GIBSON RL, et al. 1984. Epidemiologic studies of the role of gasoline (hydrocarbon) exposure in kidney cancer risk. In: Mehlman MA (ed). *Advances in Modern Environmental Toxicology.* Vol VIII. Princeton, NJ: Princeton Scientific Pub, pp 245–257.

WHISENAND JM, KOSTOS D, SOMMERS SC. 1962. Some host factors in the development of renal cell carcinoma. West J Surg Gynecol 70:284–285.

WHITTEMORE AS, PAFFENBARGER RS JR, ANDERSON K, et al. 1985. Early precursors of site-specific cancers in college men and women. J Natl Cancer Inst 74:43–51.

WONG O, RAABE GK. 1989. Critical review of cancer epidemiology in petroleum industry employees, with a quantitative meta-analysis by cancer site. Am J Ind Med 15:283–310.

WONG O, HARRIS F, SMITH TJ. 1993. Health effects of gasoline exposure. II. Mortality patterns among petroleum refinery workers. Environ Health Perspect 101 (suppl 6):63–76.

WYNDER EL, MABUCHI K, WHITMORE WF. 1974. Epidemiology of adenocarcinoma of the kidney. J Natl Cancer Inst 53:1619–1634.

YAMASAKI E, AMES BN. 1977. Concentration of mutagens from urine by absorption with the nonpolar resin XAD-2: cigarette smokers have mutagenic urine. Proc Natl Acad Sci U S A 74:3555–3559.

YU MC, MACK TM, HANESCH R, et al. 1986. Cigarette smoking, obesity, diuretic use, and coffee consumption as risk factors for renal cell carcinoma. J Natl Cancer Inst 77:351–356.

ZBAR B, BRAUCH H, TALMADGE C, et al. 1987. Loss of alleles of loci in the short arm of chromosome 3 in renal cell carcinoma. Nature 327:721–724.

ZBAR B, TORY K, MERINO M, et al. 1994. Hereditary papillary renal cell carcinoma. J Urol 151:561–566.

54 Bladder cancer

DEBRA T. SILVERMAN
ALAN S. MORRISON
SUSAN S. DEVESA

In the United States, an estimated 51,200 cases of cancer of the urinary bladder are diagnosed and 10,600 deaths from the disease occur each year (Boring et al, 1994). These account for 6% of all new cases of cancer among men and 2% of cases among women, as well as 2% of cancer deaths among men and 1% among women.

DESCRIPTIVE FACTORS

Histopathology and Anatomic Distribution

More than 98% of bladder cancers diagnosed in the United States are histologically confirmed (Devesa, unpublished data from the Surveillance, Epidemiology, and End Results [SEER] program; Young et al, 1981). Most of these are transitional cell carcinomas (93%); 2% are squamous cell carcinomas and 1% are adenocarcinomas. About 43% do not have a subsite within the bladder specified, and 13% arise in more than one subsite. Of bladder cancers for which a single subsite is specified, most occur on one of the bladder walls, with three times as many on the lateral walls (40%) as on the anterior (3%) or posterior (11%) walls combined. Less common subsites include the ureteric orifice (17%), followed by the trigone, dome, and neck (13%, 9%, and 7%, respectively).

Geographic Variation

Internationally, incidence rates of bladder cancer vary almost 10-fold (Parkin et al, 1992). High rates occur in western Europe and North America; relatively low rates are found in eastern Europe and several areas of Asia (Fig. 54–1). Some of the geographic variation may be the result of differing practices regarding the registration of "benign" tumors or "papillomas" as cancer, although rates reported by registries that include these categories are not consistently high compared to rates reported by other registries. Within the United States, bladder cancer mortality is relatively high in parts of the Northeast and upper Midwest, and generally lower in the South (Mason et al, 1975; Pickle et al, 1987). During 1970–1989, mortality rates varied geographically by as much as three- to four-fold (Fig. 54–2). These patterns are consistent with incidence data, with rates in Con-

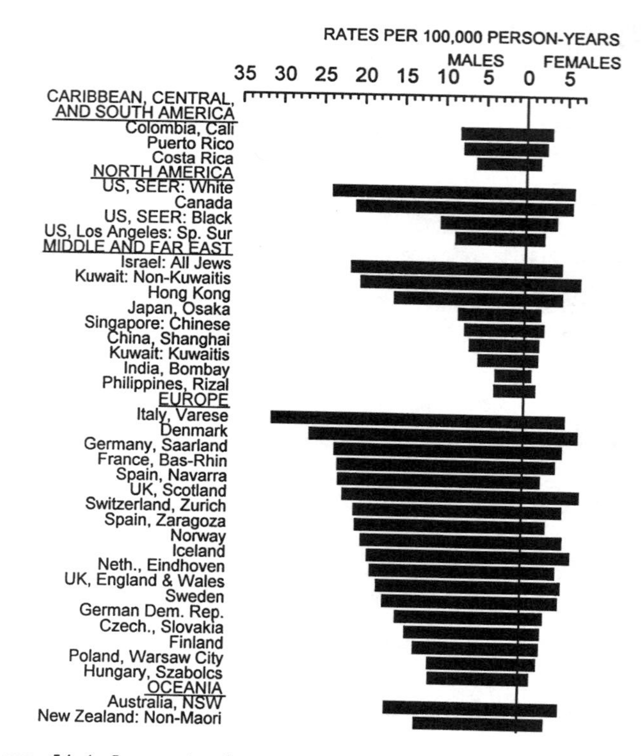

FIG. 54–1. International variation in age-adjusted (world standard) bladder cancer incidence rates per 100,000 person-years by sex, circa 1985. (Based on data from Parkin et al, 1992.)

This chapter is dedicated to the late Dr. Alan Morrison in recognition of his many contributions to cancer epidemiology.

The authors thank Drs. Neil Caporaso, Richard Hayes, and Nathaniel Rothman for their comments on the section on biomarkers, and Dr. Kenneth Cantor for his advice on the section on drinking water.

TABLE 54–1. *Bladder Cancer Incidence among Whites by Area and Sex, U.S. SEER Program, 1986–1990**,†

	Males		*Females*	
Geographic Area	*Cases*	*Rate*	*Cases*	*Rate*
Connecticut	2937	37.0	1021	9.2
Detroit	2621	36.4	932	9.0
Seattle	2325	33.7	721	7.9
San Francisco	2107	31.7	788	8.3
Iowa	2393	30.7	793	6.9
Atlanta	776	30.0	268	6.8
Hawaii	208	26.9	59	6.9
New Mexico	800	26.1	259	6.6
Utah	684	23.0	185	4.8
All areas	14851	32.4	5026	7.8

*Unpublished data from the SEER program.
†Rates per 100,000 person-years, age-adjusted by the direct method using the 1970 U.S. population standard.

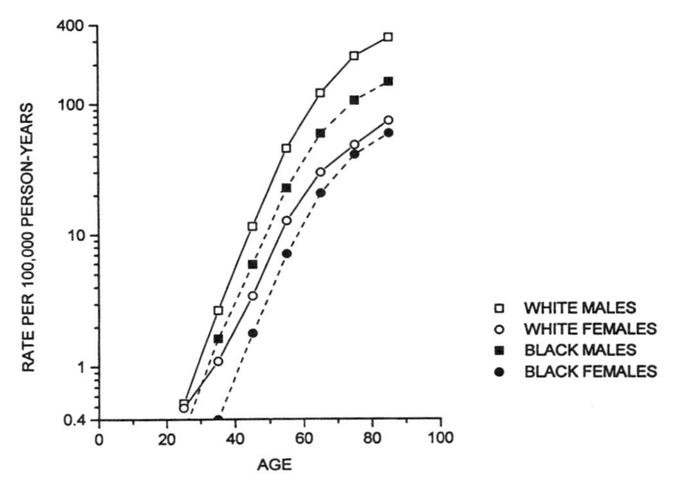

FIG. 54–3. Age-specific incidence rates for bladder cancer in the U.S. SEER Program by race and sex, 1986–1990. (Based on data from Hankey et al, 1993.)

necticut and Detroit about 50% higher than those in New Mexico and Utah (Table 54–1).

Bladder cancer mortality in the United States had been considerably higher in urban than rural areas, but these differences have diminished (Blot and Fraumeni, 1978; Greenberg, 1983). More recent international incidence data indicate, however, that urban-rural differences persist in many other countries (Muir et al, 1987).

Sex, Race, and Age

Cancer of the bladder occurs primarily among white men (Table 54–2). In most racial groups, the male to female rate ratio is at least three to one, approaching four to one among whites. The incidence rate among black men is about 50% of that among whites. Rates are somewhat lower among Asian and Hispanic groups than among blacks, and very low among American Indians. There is little or no association between socioeconomic status (SES) and bladder cancer (Devesa, 1979; Logan, 1982; McWhorter et al, 1989). Adjustment for SES has little effect on the black-white difference in bladder cancer incidence (Devesa, 1979; McWhorter et al, 1989).

Incidence and mortality rates rise sharply with age (Figs. 54–3 and 54–4); about two-thirds of cases occur among persons aged 65 years and older. Incidence is higher among whites than blacks over the entire age range (Fig. 54–3). Higher mortality in whites than

TABLE 54–2. *Bladder Cancer Incidence by Racial/Ethnic Group and Sex, U.S. SEER Program, 1977–1983**,†

	Males		*Females*	
Racial/Ethnic Group	*Cases*	*Rate*	*Cases*	*Rate*
White[a]	10005	31.9	3722	8.3
Black[a]	635	15.3	313	5.5
Chinese[b]	108	14.7	30	3.7
Hispanic[c]	128	12.8	43	3.7
Hawaiian[d]	33	12.4	18	5.7
Japanese[b]	133	12.0	64	4.6
Filipino[b]	40	5.4	14	2.9
American Indian[c]	11	2.8	2	0.2

*Adapted from Horm et al, 1996.
†Rates per 100,000 person-years, age-adjusted by the direct method using the 1970 U.S. population standard.
[a]Atlanta, Detroit, San Francisco, Connecticut.
[b]San Francisco and Hawaii.
[c]New Mexico.
[d]Hawaii only.

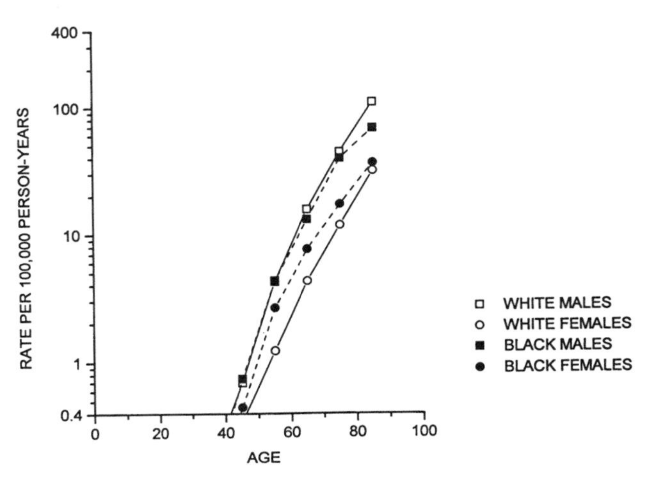

FIG. 54–4. Age-specific mortality rates for bladder cancer in the total United States by race and sex, 1986–1990. (Based on data from Hankey et al, 1993.)

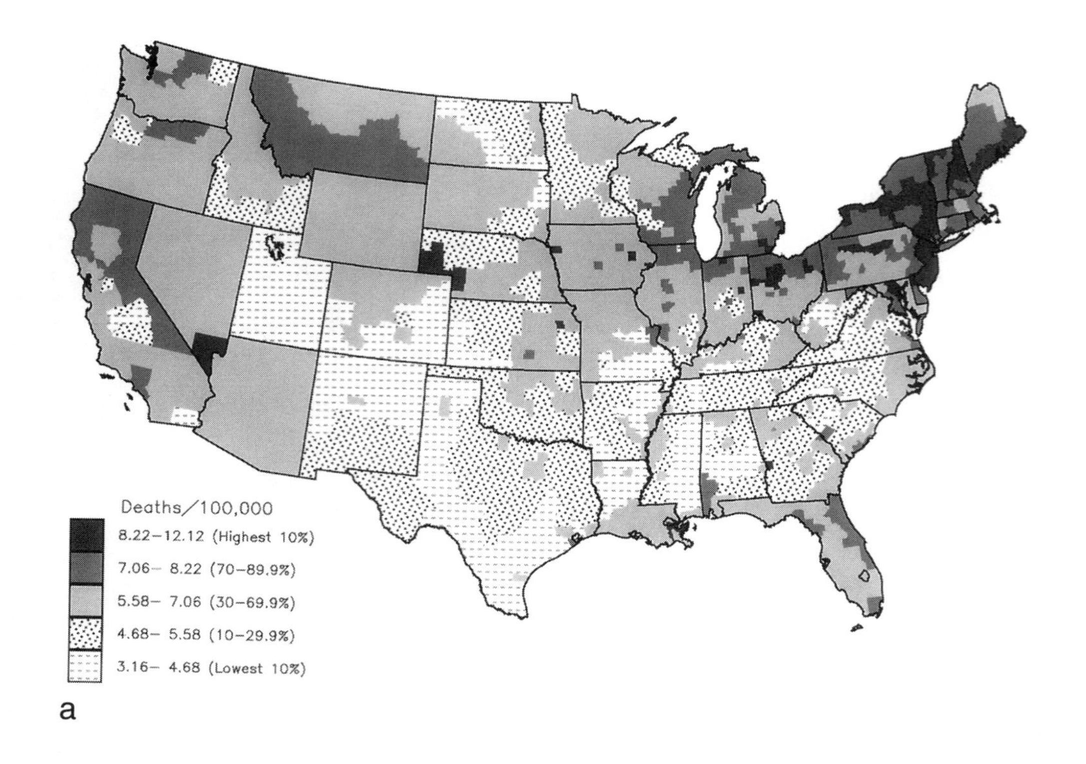

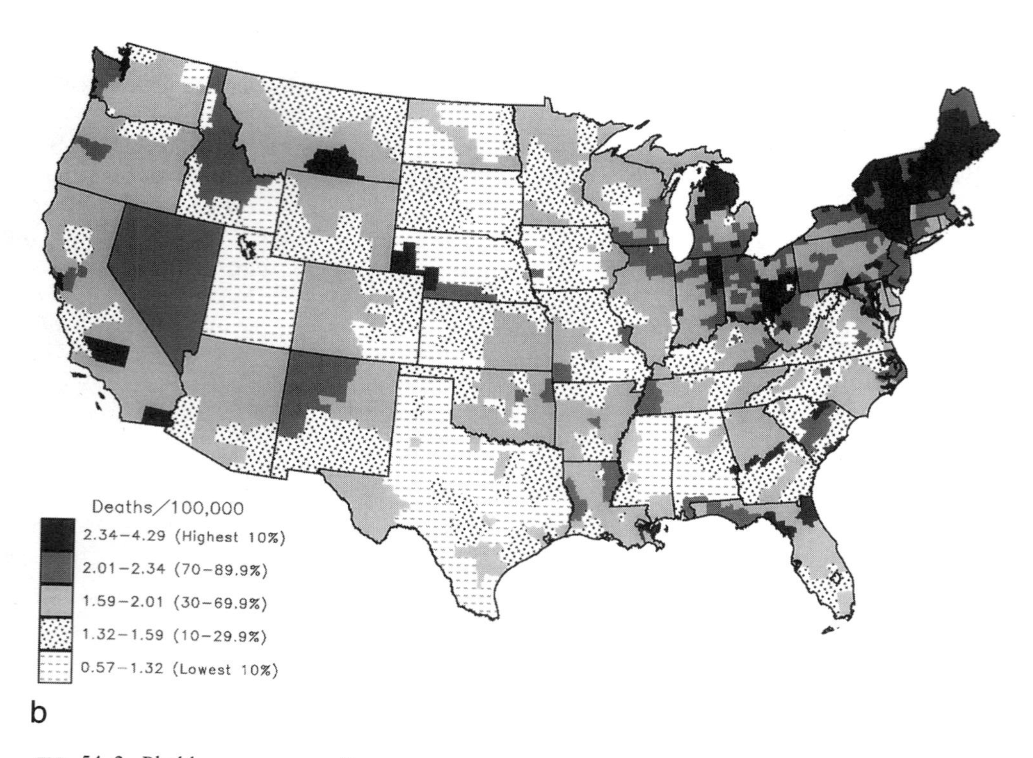

FIG. 54–2. Bladder cancer mortality rates among whites by state economic area, United States, 1970–1989: (*a*) males; (*b*) females. (Based on data from the National Center for Health Statistics and the Census Bureau.)

blacks is seen only among men aged 60 years and older (Fig. 54–4). Among women, mortality rates are higher in blacks than whites at all ages.

Stage of Disease

The stage of bladder cancer at diagnosis varies by age, sex, and race. The proportion of cases diagnosed as localized declines with age from 82% among patients aged 40–44 years to 70% among those 70–74 and 61% among those over 84 years (Devesa, unpublished data from the SEER program). The proportion localized is 76% among white men, 71% among white women, 64% among black men, and 46% among black women (Hankey et al, 1993). The higher incidence among whites compared to blacks is limited to localized cases, with blacks and whites having similar risk of more advanced tumors (Schairer et al, 1988).

Time Trends

From 1969–1971 to 1988–1990, incidence rates increased 31%–37% among whites and 15%–21% among blacks (Fig. 54–5). Increases were greater during the 1970s than during the 1980s. During this period of increasing incidence, mortality rates declined 18%–24%.

The observed increases in incidence may be partly explained by changes in diagnostic practice. The distinction between in situ and invasive disease may be difficult to make. The proportion of bladder tumors classified as "carcinoma in situ" increased from less than 1% in 1969–1971 to more than 7% around 1980, and considerably more in recent years (Cutler and Young, 1975; Devesa, unpublished data from the SEER program; Lynch et al, 1991). Much of the observed rise in incidence appears to be a result of an increase in the incidence of bladder cancer diagnosed at a localized stage (including in situ), with the rate of localized disease rising from 10.3 in 1975–1978 to 11.8 in 1982–1985 (Devesa, unpublished SEER data). This increase was accompanied, however, by a decrease in the incidence of unstaged bladder cancer (1.7 to 0.7), suggesting that some of the apparent increase in localized disease was the result of a reduction in the frequency of unstaged cases. Incidence rates of regional- and distant-stage bladder cancer remained virtually constant.

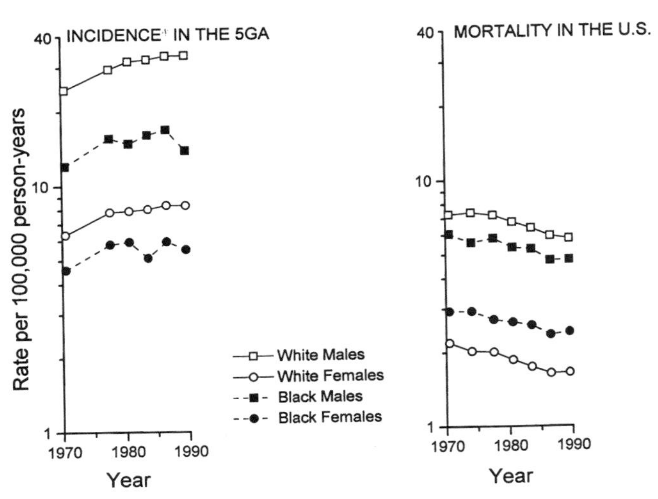

FIG. 54–5. Trends in age-adjusted (1970 standard) bladder cancer incidence and mortality rates in the United States by race and sex, 1969–1990. (Based on data from the Third National Cancer Survey, the SEER Program, the Connecticut Tumor Registry, and the National Center for Health Statistics as in Devesa et al, 1987.) The five geographic areas (5GA) are Atlanta, Connecticut, Detroit, Iowa, and San Francisco. Incidence data are not available for 1972–1974.

Survival

Five-year relative survival rates among bladder cancer patients range from 91% for those diagnosed with localized disease to 9% for those with distant disease (Table 54–3). For cases diagnosed at the localized or regional stages, whites have a better prognosis than blacks, whereas survival varies little among patients with distant disease. The relative survival is higher for white men than white women among regional-stage cases, and higher for black men than black women among localized-stage cases. Overall black-white survival differences are only partly explained by differences in stage at diagnosis; racial disparities in survival rates persist after adjustment for stage, histologic type, grade, and socioeconomic status (Hankey and Myers, 1987; Page and Kuntz, 1980).

Survival among patients with bladder cancer has increased more than 50% since the early 1960s (Hankey et al, 1993). In the period from 1974–1976 to 1983–1989, 5-year survival increased more among blacks (47.8% to 60.9%) than among whites (73.7% to 79.9%).

TABLE 54–3. *Five-Year Relative Survival Rates (Percent) among Bladder Cancer Patients by Stage at Diagnosis, Race, and Sex, U.S. SEER Program, 1983–1987**

		Five-Year Relative Survival Rate (%)				
Race and Sex	*Cases*	*Total*	*Local*	*Regional*	*Distant*	*Unknown*
Total	17309	79	91	46	9	60
White males	12141	81	92	48	11	66
White females	4020	75	89	43	4	50
Black males	497	65	82	35	0	64
Black females	246	48	70	31	—[a]	—[a]

*Data from Hankey et al, 1993.
[a]Statistic could not be calculated.

RISK FACTORS

Occupation

Following a number of clinical observations and mortality surveys, the study of occupational causes of bladder cancer gained momentum in the 1950s with the identification of bladder cancer hazards in the British dyestuffs and rubber industries (Case et al, 1954; Case and Hosker, 1954). During the subsequent three decades, scores of studies have suggested approximately 40 potentially high-risk occupations. Despite this effort, the relations of many of these occupations to bladder cancer risk are unclear. Observed relative risks typically have been less than two, based on a small number of exposed subjects. Further, many reported associations have not been consistently found (Silverman et al, 1989b). Strong evidence of increased risk is apparent for very few occupational groups.

Dyestuffs Workers and Dye Users. In 1895, Rehn suggested that men employed in the dyestuffs industry had increased risk of bladder cancer. It was not until 1954, however, that Case and colleagues (1954) showed that dyestuffs workers in England and Wales had a 10- to 50-fold increased risk of death from bladder cancer due to exposure to two aromatic amines, 2-naphthylamine and benzidine. Exposure to a third aromatic amine, 1-naphthylamine, also appeared related to risk, but this elevation may have been caused by contamination with 2-naphthylamine. No excess risk was associated with exposure to aniline.

Two reports based on a cohort of dyestuffs workers in northern Italy (Decarli et al, 1985; Rubino et al, 1982) confirmed the increased risk from exposure to 2-naphthylamine and benzidine. A positive trend in bladder cancer mortality with increasing duration of employment was apparent; observed/expected ratios of 13, 34, and 71 were associated with employment as a dyestuffs worker for 10 years or less, 11 to 20 years, and more than 20 years, respectively. Dyestuffs workers involved in fuchsin and safranine T manufacturing also experienced high mortality (observed/expected = 62.5), which may have been the result of exposure to two precursors, *o*-toluidine and 4,4′-methylene bis(2-methylaniline).

The increased risk among dyestuffs workers also has been observed in case-control studies (Boyko et al, 1985; La Vecchia et al, 1990; Morrison et al, 1985; Najem et al, 1982; Puntoni et al, 1988; Risch et al, 1988a; Vineis and Magnani, 1985), with relative risks ranging from 1.7 to 8.8. Data from the United Kingdom indicate that bladder cancer risk among dyestuffs workers has been reduced since the introduction of protective measures and the subsequent banning of the industrial use of 2-naphthylamine and benzidine in 1950 and 1962, respectively (Boyko et al, 1985; Morrison et al, 1985).

Studies of the Italian cohort of dyestuffs workers have provided additional information on temporal patterns of risk (Decarli et al, 1985; Piolatto et al, 1991; Rubino et al, 1982). First, the mean time from start of exposure to death was 25 years, with a range of 12 to 41 years. Second, an inverse relationship between age at first exposure and risk was observed; risk was greatest for workers who started before age 25 years (observed/expected = 200.0). Third, a negative trend in relative risk with increasing time since last exposure was observed.

Users of finished dyes also may have an increased risk of bladder cancer, but the evidence is not as persuasive as that for dyestuffs manufacturing workers. Kimono painters, many of whom ingest benzidine-based dyes by licking the brush, have been found to have seven times the expected rate of bladder cancer (Yoshida et al, 1971). Coarse fishermen who use chrysoidine azo dyes to stain maggot bait have been reported to have an increased risk of bladder cancer (relative risk = 3.0 for fishermen who used bronze dyes for 5 or more years) (Sole and Sorahan, 1985), although a more recent case-control study did not confirm this observation (Sorahan and Sole, 1990). Canadian dyers of cloth were reported to have a relative risk of 4.6 (Risch et al, 1988a), and British textile dyers with more than 20 years of employment had a relative risk of 3.4 (Antony, 1974). Two other studies, however, found no excess risk for dye users (Cartwright et al, 1979b; Silverman et al, 1989b).

Aromatic Amine Manufacturing Workers. Evidence that 2-naphthylamine and benzidine are human bladder carcinogens extends beyond the dyestuffs industry into the chemical industry where these aromatic amines, as well as a third bladder carcinogen, 4-aminobiphenyl, were manufactured (International Agency for Research on Cancer [IARC], 1987). A fourfold risk was observed among 2-naphthylamine-exposed chemical workers in the United States (Schulte et al, 1986). The observation of an increased risk of bladder cancer among workers involved in the commercial preparation of 4-aminobiphenyl resulted in the discontinuation of production of this aromatic amine, thus averting its widespread use (IARC, 1987). In a cohort of workers at a benzidine manufacturing facility, an overall excess of bladder cancer cases was apparent (standardized incidence ratio [SIR] = 343) (Meigs et al, 1986). Risk was greatest among those in the highest exposure category (SIR = 1303); little or no excess was observed for those in the low or medium exposure categories. Corresponding to the introduction of preventive measures in the plant, a reduction in risk was observed for those first employed in 1950 or later compared to those first employed in 1945–1949. In a cohort of benzidine-exposed workers in China, an overall SIR of 25 was reported, with risk ranging from 4.8 for those with low exposure to 158.4 for those with high exposure (Bi et al, 1992). Risks were elevated for producers of benzidine (SIR = 45.7) as well as for users of benzidine-based dyes (SIR = 20.9).

Two structural analogues of benzidine, MDA (4,4′-methylene-dianiline) and MBOCA (4,4′-methylene-bis(2-chloroaniline)), are carcinogenic in animals (Schulte et al, 1987), and possibly in humans, as well. MDA, a curing agent for certain resins, was associated with a threefold elevation of proportional mortality from bladder cancer (Schulte et al, 1987). MBOCA, a curing agent used in the manufacture of rigid plastics, has been suggested as the exposure responsible for two noninvasive papillary tumors of the bladder in workers in a MBOCA production plant, although no invasive bladder tumors have been identified in the cohort (Ward et al, 1988). Manufacturing of another aromatic amine, 4-chloro-*o*-toluidine (4-COT), has been associated with excess bladder cancer mortality in a cohort of chemical workers in Germany (relative risk = 72.7) (Stasik, 1988). This large excess in bladder cancer mortality has been confirmed recently in another cohort of German chemical workers exposed to 4-COT (Popp et al, 1992). In New York State, a cohort of chemical workers exposed to both *o*-toluidine and aniline also experienced elevated risk of bladder cancer (SIR = 360), which was probably attributable to exposure to *o*-toludine (Ward et al, 1991).

Rubber Workers. Antioxidants containing 2-naphthylamine were used in the rubber and electric-cable manufacturing industries in Great Britain (Baus Subcommittee on Industrial Bladder Cancer, 1988). Case and Hosker (1954) observed that the bladder cancer mortality among British rubber workers was twice the expected level. This excess was observed only among rubber workers employed before 1950; 2-naphthylamine was withdrawn from use in the British rubber industry in 1949 (Parkes et al, 1982).

Excess risk of bladder cancer also has been reported among rubber workers in the United States (Alderson, 1986; IARC, 1982) and Italy (Negri et al, 1989), although a few studies of rubber workers found no excess (Jensen et al, 1987b; La Vecchia et al, 1990; McMichael et al, 1976; Morrison et al, 1985). The elevation of risk reported in most American studies (Checkoway et al, 1981; Delzell and Monson, 1981; Monson and Nakano, 1976) is less than that reported in the British and Italian studies. There was little exposure to 2-naphthylamine in the U.S. rubber industry (Checkoway et al, 1981), but many workers were exposed to another antioxidant, phenyl-β-naphthylamine (PBNA), which can be metabolized to 2-naphthylamine (IARC, 1987).

Leather Workers. An increased risk of bladder cancer among leather workers has been observed in at least 10 studies (Baxter and McDowall, 1986; Cole et al, 1972; Decoufle, 1979; Dolin and Cook-Mozaffari, 1992; Garabrant and Wegman, 1984; Henry et al, 1931; Marrett et al, 1986; Morrison et al, 1985; Seniori Costantini et al, 1989; Vineis and Magnani, 1985; Wynder et al, 1963), although no increased risk was observed in two studies of leather tanners (Edling et al, 1986; Stern et al, 1987). Most of the positive results are from case-control studies; the relative risk varied from 1.4 to 6.3. The definition of "leather worker" was not consistent among studies. Some reported increased risks for shoe makers and shoe repairers (Dolin and Cook-Mozaffari, 1992; Garabrant and Wegman, 1984; Wynder et al, 1963), whereas others reported elevations for workers in leather products manufacturing (Decoufle, 1979) or, more broadly, for workers exposed to leather or leather products (Cole et al, 1972; Marrett et al, 1986; Morrison et al, 1985).

The exposure responsible for the increased risk among leather workers is not known. Cole and colleagues (1972) reported that the excess was associated with jobs that involved finishing and related processes, including cutting and assembling leather pieces. In a large case-control study in 10 areas of the United States (Marrett et al, 1986), risk was found to be slightly higher for workers with possible exposure to leather dust compared to other types of leather exposure. In addition to leather dust, leather workers also are exposed to dyes, their solvents, and unreacted intermediates (Risch et al, 1988a). Identification of carcinogens in the leather industry may require chemical analysis of substances encountered in the industry in combination with biologic monitoring of workers (Marrett et al, 1986).

Painters. Bladder cancer risk has been elevated among painters in many studies (Bethwaite et al, 1990; Claude et al, 1988; Cole et al, 1972; Decoufle et al, 1977; Dolin and Cook-Mozaffari, 1992; Guberan et al, 1989; Henry et al, 1931; Jensen et al, 1987b; La Vecchia et al, 1990; Malker et al, 1987; Matanoski et al, 1986; Miller et al, 1986; Morrison et al, 1985 (Boston); Myslak et al, 1991; Siemiatychi et al, 1994; Silverman et al, 1989b; Wynder et al, 1963), although a few studies have suggested no excess risk (Englund, 1980; Morrison et al, 1985 (Manchester, UK, and Nagoya, Japan)). Most of the observed relative risks have been 1.2 to 1.5. Jensen and coworkers (1987b) reported a positive trend in risk with increasing duration of employment; painters employed 20 years or more had a relative risk of 4.1. In a large case-control study in the United States (Silverman et al, 1989b), painters experienced a 50% increased risk. Among those who started working before 1930, a trend in risk with increasing duration of employment was apparent; the relative risk for such painters employed 10 years or more was 3.0. Painters may be exposed to many known or suspected carcinogens in paints (eg, benzidine, polychlorinated biphenyls, formaldehyde, and asbestos) and solvents (eg, benzene, dioxane, and methylene chloride) (Miller et al, 1986).

Drivers of Trucks and Other Motor Vehicles. Excess risk of bladder cancer has been observed frequently among drivers of trucks, buses, or taxi cabs (Baxter and McDowall, 1986; Claude et al, 1988; Decoufle et al, 1977; Dubrow and Wegman, 1984; Hoar and Hoover, 1985; Iscovich et al, 1987; Jensen et al, 1987b; Logan, 1982; Milham, 1976; Schifflers et al, 1987; Siemiatychi et al, 1994; Silverman et al, 1983; 1986; Steenland et al, 1987), although one Swedish study found no elevation in risk for truck drivers (Malker et al, 1987). Overall relative risks varied from 1.3 to 2.2. A positive trend in risk with increasing duration of employment was observed for drivers in most studies, with relative risks for long-term drivers ranging from 2.2 to 12.0 (Claude et al, 1988; Hoar and Hoover, 1985; Jensen et al, 1987b; Silverman et al, 1983, 1986; Steenland et al, 1987). In the largest study of bladder cancer among truck drivers, the trend in risk by duration of employment was most consistent for those first employed at least 50 years before observation (Silverman et al, 1986) (Table 54–4). Although the specific exposure responsible for the elevation of risk among drivers has not been identified, one likely candidate is motor exhaust. Exhaust emissions contain polycyclic aromatic hydrocarbons (PAHs) and nitro-PAHs, which are highly mutagenic, as well as carcinogenic in laboratory animals (Silverman et al, 1986).

TABLE 54–4. *Numbers of Cases and Controls and Relative Risk According to Duration of Employment as a Truck Driver or Deliveryman among Those First Employed at Least 50 Years Before Observation**,†

Duration of Employment (years)	*Cases*	*Controls*	*Relative Risk*[a]
Never any motor exhaust-related occupation	1353	2724	1.0
<5	74	129	1.2
5–9	32	45	1.4
10–24	33	31	2.1
25+	22	19	2.2
		(χ = 3.93; $P < 0.0001$)	

*Data from Silverman et al, 1986. The time of observation was the date of diagnosis for cases and the date of interview for controls.
†Males with unknown smoking history, duration of employment, or date started employment were excluded.
[a]Relative to a risk of 1.0 for males never employed in a motor exhaust-related occupation; adjusted for age and smoking.

Aluminum Workers. Wigle (1977) suggested that an elevated incidence of bladder cancer among men in the Chicoutimi census division of the Province of Quebec was the result of exposures incurred in the aluminum refining industry. Subsequently, increased bladder cancer mortality was observed in three cohort studies of aluminum smelter workers (Gibbs, 1985; Rockette and Arena, 1983; Spinelli et al, 1991). The elevated risk in the aluminum industry has been associated with employment in the Soderberg potrooms (relative risk = 2.4) (Theriault et al, 1981, 1984). Risk increased with increasing duration of employment in this department. Relative risks were 1.0 for less than 1 year, 1.9 for 1–9 years, 3.0 for 10–19 years, 3.2 for 20–29 years, and 4.5 for 30 years or more (Theriault et al, 1984). Armstrong and coworkers (1986) used historical data on workplace exposures to better quantify exposure-response relationships (Table 54–5).

Coal-tar pitch volatiles emitted from anodes in the Soderberg electrolytic reduction process may be responsible for the observed bladder cancer excess (Theriault et al, 1984). The bladder carcinogens within tar volatiles are unknown, but aromatic amines (particularly 2-naphthylamine) are suspected (Armstrong et al, 1986).

Other Occupations. Employment as a machinist has been associated with bladder cancer risk in many studies (Silverman et al, 1989b), although the increase in risk has not been consistently linked to a specific type of work. Machinists are exposed to mists from oils used as coolants and lubricants in metal machining processes (Silverman et al, 1983; Vineis and DiPrima, 1983). Some cutting and lubricating oils contain potentially

TABLE 54–5. *Relative Risks Predicted Following 40 Years of Exposure to Tar Volatiles**,†

BSM			*BaP*		
Concentration (mg/m³)	*Relative Risk*[a]	*95% CI*	*Concentration (ug/m³)*	*Relative Risk*[a]	*95% CI*
1.0	8.1	3.8 –17.4	10	10.2	4.6 –21.8
0.5	4.5	2.40–9.2	5	5.6	2.8 –11.4
0.2	2.42	1.56–4.3	2	2.84	1.72–5.2
0.1	1.71	1.28–2.64	1	1.92	1.36–2.15
0.05	1.35	1.14–1.82	0.5	1.46	1.18–2.04
0.02	1.14	1.06–1.33	0.2	1.18	1.07–1.42
0.01	1.07	1.03–1.16	0.1	1.09	1.04–1.21

*Data from Armstrong et al, 1986.
†Assumes that a minimum of 10 years elapses before an effect of exposure occurs.
[a]Estimates of risk are relative to a risk of 1.0 for unexposed persons.
BSM = benzene-soluble matter; BaP = benzo-a-pyrene; CI = confidence interval.

carcinogenic PAHs (Silverman et al, 1983) and nitrosamines (Fan et al, 1977).

Increased risk of bladder cancer has also been reported for many other occupational groups: metal workers, printers, chemical workers (other than those involved in manufacturing aromatic amines), hairdressers, dry cleaners, carpenters, construction workers, miners, gas workers, coke plant workers, auto mechanics, petroleum workers, railroad workers, textile workers, tailors, engineers, butchers, clerical workers, cooks and kitchen workers, food processing workers, electricians, gas station attendants, medical workers, pharmacists, glass processors, nurserymen, photographic workers, security guards and watchmen, welders, sailors, stationary firemen or furnace operators, stationary engineers, paper and pulp workers, roofers, gardeners, bootblacks, and asbestos workers (Alderson, 1986; Matanoski and Elliot, 1981; Silverman et al, 1989a,b). Findings for most of these occupations are not as persuasive as those discussed earlier, and require corroboration.

The relation between occupation and bladder cancer risk is dynamic (Silverman et al, 1989b). With the elimination of bladder carcinogens from the workplace and the advent of new chemicals, changing worker exposures are generating shifts in "high-risk occupations." For example, risks among rubber and leather workers have diminished over time (Marrett et al, 1986; Parkes et al, 1982), whereas new high-risk occupations, such as truck driver and aluminum smelter worker (Silverman et al, 1986; Wigle, 1977), have emerged. Thus, occupational bladder cancer continues to be a public health problem, with risks changing over time and from population to population.

Tobacco

Cigarettes. Cigarette smoking is well established as a cause of bladder cancer, although the association is not as strong as that observed for smoking and several other cancers. An association between cigarette smoking and bladder cancer has been observed in more than 30 case-control studies and in 10 cohort studies (Augustine et al, 1988; Brownson et al, 1987; Burch et al, 1989; Claude et al, 1986; Clavel et al, 1989; D'Avanzo et al, 1990; Gonzalez et al, 1985; Hartge et al, 1987; IARC, 1986; Iscovich et al, 1987; Jensen et al, 1987a; Mills et al, 1991; Nomura et al, 1989; Rebelakos et al, 1985; Schifflers et al, 1987). Overall, smokers appear to have two to three times the risk of nonsmokers. Data from correlational studies also are consistent with a smoking–bladder cancer association. In the United States, bladder cancer mortality rates at the state level are highly correlated with per capita cigarette sales (Fraumeni, 1968). Birth cohort–specific patterns of bladder cancer incidence and mortality parallel the smoking patterns of those cohorts (Armstrong and Doll, 1974; Hoover and Cole, 1971).

Risk increases with increasing intensity of smoking (packs per day), with relative risk estimates for moderate to heavy smokers typically ranging from about 2.0 to 5.0, compared to nonsmokers (Augustine et al, 1988; Burch et al, 1989; Claude et al, 1986; Clavel et al, 1989; D'Avanzo et al, 1990; Hartge et al, 1987; IARC, 1986; Rebelakos et al, 1985; Schifflers et al, 1987; Vineis et al, 1988). The shape of the dose-response curve has varied among the studies, however. Some have reported a regular gradient in risk with amount smoked, whereas others have reported little change in risk from moderate to heavy smoking levels (Augustine et al, 1988; D'Avanzo et al, 1990; Hartge et al, 1987; IARC, 1986; Schifflers et al, 1987). Duration of smoking has been evaluated less often than intensity, but a regular duration-response relationship has been observed in most studies that investigated the issue (Augustine et al, 1988; Burch et al, 1989; Claude et al, 1986; Clavel et al, 1989; D'Avanzo et al, 1990; Hartge et al, 1987; IARC, 1986; Vineis et al, 1988).

Cessation. Cessation of cigarette smoking has been associated with a 30% to 60% reduction in bladder cancer risk in many studies (IARC, 1986). The pattern of change in risk in relation to time since quitting is less clear, however (Table 54–6). Three studies suggested that the risk of former smokers who stopped smoking for many years approximates that of nonsmokers (Cartwright et al, 1983; D'Avanzo et al, 1990; Wynder and Stellman, 1977). Other studies indicate that a reduction in risk occurs within the first 2–4 years after stopping, but that risk does not continue to decline with increasing time since quitting (Augustine et al, 1988; Burch et al, 1989; Hartge et al, 1987; Vineis et al, 1988). In most of these studies, the effect of time since quitting was not adjusted for the effects of age at starting and duration of smoking. Hartge and coworkers (1987), however, estimated relative risk by length of time since quitting among intermittent former smokers (ie, smokers who quit for at least 6 months, started again, and subsequently quit) with adjustment for age at starting and duration of smoking, as well as age at observation. Among all former smokers, the pattern of risk by time since quitting was weak and inconsistent (Table 54–6). When this analysis was restricted to intermittent former smokers, risk declined 50% within the first 4 years of stopping, but did not continue to decrease with increasing time since quitting. The almost immediate reduction in risk within the first few years after quitting suggests that cigarette smoke contains agents that act at a late stage of bladder carcinogenesis (Hartge et al, 1987).

TABLE 54–6. *Relative Risks of Bladder Cancer According to Time Since Quitting Smoking, Males*

Reference	*Years Since Quitting*	*Relative Risk*		*Comments*
Wynder and Stellman (1977)	0 1–3 4–6 7–10 11–15 16+	2.7 2.9 1.9 1.4 1.6 1.1		Risks relative to a risk of 1.0 for nonsmokers, adjusted for age at observation and race
Howe et al (1980)	0 2–15 15+	1.0 0.6 0.5		Risks relative to a risk of 1.0 for current smokers, adjusted for age at observation and lifetime cigarette consumption
Cartwright et al (1983)	0–5 6–15 16–25 26–35	1.7 1.0 1.1 0.9		Risks relative to a risk of 1.0 for nonsmokers, adjusted for age at observation
Claude et al (1986)	0 2–15 15+	1.0 0.6 0.4		Risks relative to a risk of 1.0 for current smokers, adjusted for age at observation and lifetime consumption
Hartge et al (1987)		All Smokers	Intermittent Smokers	Includes women; risks relative to a risk of 1.0 for current smokers, adjusted for age at observation, sex, race, duration (all smokers); and age at observation, sex, race, duration, age started (intermittent smokers)
	0 1 2–4 5–9 10–19 20+	1.0 0.9 0.6 0.8 0.7 0.9	1.0 0.7 0.5 0.4 0.4 0.5	
Iscovich et al (1987)	0 2–4 5–9 10–19 20+	1.0 0.6 0.3 0.2 0.2		Risks relative to a risk of 1.0 for current smokers or those who stopped less than 2 years before diagnosis/interview, adjusted for age at observation, intensity, duration
Vineis et al (1988)	0 <3 3–9 10+	1.0 0.4 0.4 0.6		Risks relative to a risk of 1.0 for current smokers, adjusted for age at observation, duration, intensity
Augustine et al (1988)	0 ≤6 7–12 13+	1.0 0.7 0.7 0.7		Risks relative to a risk of 1.0 for current smokers, adjusted for age at observation, intensity, duration, education, race, and marital status
Burch et al (1989)	0 >1–≤5 >5–≤10 10+	1.6 1.1 0.8 1.4		Risks relative to a risk of 1.0 for nonsmokers, adjusted for age at observation and lifetime cigarette consumption
D'Avanzo et al (1990)	2–4 5–14 15+	2.8 1.9 1.0		Risks relative to a risk of 1.0 for nonsmokers, adjusted for age at observation and sex

Filtration. People who smoke unfiltered cigarettes exclusively have been reported to experience about a 35% to 50% higher risk of bladder cancer than those who smoke filtered cigarettes exclusively (Hartge et al, 1987; Wynder et al, 1988). Switching to filtered cigarettes does not appear to reduce the excess risk, however (Burch et al, 1989; Hartge et al, 1987; Wynder et al, 1988) (Table 54–7). There are several possible explanations for these inconsistent findings. First, people who smoke filtered cigarettes exclusively may have different smoking histories or habits than do people who first smoked unfiltered cigarettes. For example, the latter group may start smoking earlier, or take more puffs of smoke per cigarette. Second, the effect of changing from unfiltered to filtered cigarettes may be quite small, given the small difference between the risk for smokers of only filtered cigarettes and that for smokers of only unfiltered cigarettes. Third, interview data on changing from unfiltered to filtered cigarettes may contain inaccuracies that mask a real, but small, reduction in excess risk. Fourth, smokers of only filtered cigarettes may not, in fact, have a lower risk than smokers of only unfiltered cigarettes; any observed reduction in risk may have been a chance effect.

TABLE 54–7. *Estimated Relative Risks of Bladder Cancer, According to Use of Filtered and Unfiltered Cigarettes, among Current Smokers*

Filtered Cigarettes/ Day	Unfiltered Cigarettes/Day			
	None[a]	1–19	20–39	>40
None		2.4 (1.3–4.5)	3.1 (1.7–5.6)	3.6 (1.8–6.9)
1–19	1.0	2.4 (1.4–4.1)	2.7 (1.3–5.5)	2.7 (0.8–8.5)
20–39	1.9 (1.1–3.3)	2.1 (1.2–3.7)	3.2 (1.9–5.5)	3.2 (1.5–6.7)
≥40	3.0 (1.4–6.5)	2.9 (1.2–7.0)	3.6 (2.0–6.6)	3.9 (2.1–7.1)
	No. of Controls/Cases			
None		87/56	172/40	61/57
1–19	102/29	165/122	35/28	8/6
20–39	90/48	100/68	328/321	26/26
≥40	24/21	16/15	71/79	73/85

Source: Data from Hartge et al, 1987.
[a]Reference category is <20 filtered cigarettes per day, never smoked unfiltered. Estimates are adjusted for age, sex, race, and duration of smoking. 95% confidence intervals are shown in parentheses.

Inhalation. Cigarette smokers who inhale deeply may have a greater risk than those who do not (Burch et al, 1989; Clavel et al, 1989; Cole et al, 1971; Lopez-Abente et al, 1991). Morrison and colleagues (1984b) observed 30% to 40% elevation of risk for male cigarette smokers who inhaled deeply compared to those who inhaled somewhat or not at all. An association between inhalation and risk has not been observed, however, in some other studies (Hartge et al, 1987; Howe et al, 1980; Lockwood, 1961).

Black versus Blond Tobacco. Smokers of black tobacco have a risk of bladder cancer two to three times higher than the risk in smokers of blond tobacco (Clavel et al, 1989; De Stefani et al, 1991; Iscovich et al, 1987; Vineis et al, 1984, 1988). Three laboratory observations support this epidemiological observation. First, black tobacco has higher concentrations of aromatic amines, some of which are human bladder carcinogens, than does blond tobacco (Vineis et al, 1988). Second, blood levels of 4-aminobiphenyl hemoglobin adducts, as well as adducts of several other aromatic amines, are higher for smokers of black than of blond tobacco (Bryant et al, 1988). Third, the urine of smokers of black tobacco is more mutagenic than is the urine of smokers of blond tobacco (Malaveille et al, 1989; Mohtashamipur et al, 1987).

Pipes, Cigars, and Smokeless Tobacco. The roles of pipes, cigars, snuff, and chewing tobacco in the etiology of bladder cancer are unclear. Evidence of increased risk is strongest for pipe smokers, particularly those who never smoked any other type of tobacco. At least 10 studies have suggested that pipe smokers experience elevated risk compared to nonsmokers (relative risks typically ranged from 1.3 to 3.9) (Claude et al, 1986; Hartge et al, 1985; Howe et al, 1980; Jensen et al, 1987a; Lockwood, 1961; Mommsen and Aagaard, 1983; Morrison et al, 1984b; Slattery et al, 1988a; Williams and Horm, 1977; Wynder et al, 1963), whereas three studies have suggested no association (Burch et al, 1989; Cole et al, 1971; Wynder and Goldsmith, 1977). A dose-response relation has been found only rarely, although pipe smokers who inhale deeply do appear to be at greatest risk (Hartge et al, 1985; Howe et al, 1980).

Weak and inconsistent relations have been observed between bladder cancer risk and the other forms of tobacco use. For cigars, some studies have been positive (Hartge et al, 1985; Lockwood, 1961; Mommsen and Aagard, 1983; Slattery et al, 1988a), whereas others have shown little or no association (Burch et al, 1989; Cole et al, 1971; Howe et al, 1980; Jensen et al, 1987a; Kahn, 1966; Kunze et al, 1992; Williams and Horm, 1977; Wynder et al, 1963; Wynder and Goldsmith, 1977). In the positive studies, relative risks for cigar smokers compared to nonsmokers varied from about 1.3 to 2.5. Risks associated with the use of snuff or chewing tobacco have been assessed in a small number of studies (Burch et al, 1989; Cole et al, 1971; Hartge et al, 1985; Howe et al, 1980; Mommsen and Aagard, 1983; Wynder et al, 1963). Of these studies, an increased risk of bladder cancer for snuff users who never smoked cigarettes has been observed in only one (Slattery et al, 1988a), and for users of chewing tobacco in only two (Mommsen and Aagaard, 1983; Slattery et al, 1988a).

Dietary Factors

Coffee Drinking. An association between coffee drinking and bladder cancer was suggested by a population-based, case-control study conducted in Massachusetts (relative risk 1.3 for men and 2.5 for women) (Cole, 1971). Since that report, many studies have evaluated this association. Ten studies indicated little or no overall association in either sex (Cartwright et al, 1981; Ciccone and Vineis, 1988; Gonzalez et al, 1985; Jensen et al, 1986; Kabat, 1986; Morrison et al, 1982a; Piper et al, 1986 [women only]; Pujolar et al, 1993; Rebelakos et al, 1985; Slattery et al, 1988a [men only]); seven studies showed positive results for men, but not for women (Bross and Tidings, 1973; Clavel and Cordier, 1991; Fraumeni et al, 1971; Hartge et al, 1983; Howe et al, 1980; Mettlin and Graham, 1979; Wynder and Goldsmith, 1977); four studies gave positive results for women, but not for men (Miller et al, 1978; Morgan and Jain, 1974; Simon et al, 1975 [women only]; Risch et al, 1988b); one study reported positive results for both men and women (Kunze et al, 1992); and five studies suggested an overall positive association, but sex-specific risks were not examined (D'Avanzo et al, 1992; Iscovich et al, 1987; La Vecchia et al, 1989; Mills et al, 1991; Najem et al, 1982). In most of the studies reported as positive, however, the relative risk of bladder cancer in coffee drinkers compared to nondrinkers has been less than two. A regular dose-response relation has been observed only infrequently (Bross and Tidings, 1973; Clavel and Cordier, 1991; Iscovich et al, 1987; Kunze et al, 1992; Piper et al, 1986; Wynder and Goldsmith, 1977), although risk was elevated among drinkers of large amounts of coffee in several studies (Hartge et al, 1983; Jensen et al, 1986; Morrison et al, 1982a; Rebelakos et al, 1985). The weakness and inconsistency of the observed associations indicate that if coffee is a bladder carcinogen, it is a weak one. Alternatively, associations between coffee drinking and bladder cancer could be the result of residual confounding by smoking (Hartge et al, 1983; Morrison, 1982a, 1984a). Because cigarette smoking is both an important risk factor for bladder cancer and a strong correlate of coffee drinking, tight control for smoking is required to estimate the bladder cancer risk associated with coffee drinking alone. Although relative risk estimates in nearly all cited studies were adjusted for smoking, adjustment may have been inadequate if smoking categories were too broad. Confounding by smoking also could be introduced by inaccurate recall of smoking habits. In this instance, it might not be possible to completely control the effect of smoking in estimating the risk of bladder cancer associated with coffee drinking.

To avoid residual confounding by smoking, the effect of coffee drinking on bladder cancer risk can be evaluated in lifelong nonsmokers. Few studies, however, have had adequate numbers of nonsmokers to estimate this risk with reasonable precision. Of these, some indicated no increased risk associated with coffee drinking (Bross and Tidings, 1973; Howe et al, 1980; Kabat et al, 1986; Morrison et al, 1982a), whereas others suggested an increased risk (Ciccone and Vineis, 1988; Clavel and Cordier, 1991; D'Avanzo et al, 1992; Hartge et al, 1983; Mills et al, 1991; Pujolar et al, 1993; Rebelakos et al, 1985; Risch et al, 1988b; Slattery et al, 1988a). Of the positive studies that distinguished between men and women in examining the coffee drinking effect, one is positive in both men and women (Rebelakos et al, 1985), three are positive in men but not in women (Ciccone and Vineis, 1988; Clavel and Cordier, 1991; Hartge et al, 1983), and one is positive in women but not in men (Risch et al, 1988b).

Artificial Sweeteners. Artificial sweeteners were suggested as potential human bladder carcinogens by the results of animal experiments. The most important evidence was an excess of bladder cancer in rats exposed to high doses of saccharin in utero and weaned to a saccharin-containing diet (U.S. Congress, Office of Technology Assessment, 1977). Saccharin did not induce bladder cancer in rats or other animals fed saccharin only after birth (Council on Scientific Affairs, 1985).

Epidemiological studies have not substantiated a relation between artificial sweeteners and bladder cancer. Bladder cancer mortality rates were found not to be elevated among diabetics in the United States (Kessler, 1970) or Great Britain (Armstrong and Doll, 1975). The time trend in bladder cancer mortality in England and Wales has not appeared related to saccharin consumption (Armstrong and Doll, 1974). Bladder cancer incidence among the Danish population born during World War II, a group with higher in utero saccharin exposure than previous birth cohorts, was not increased in either men or women during the first 30–35 years of life (Jensen and Kamby, 1982).

Several case-control studies have provided data on the relation between artificial sweeteners and bladder cancer. Results of most studies have been negative (Cartwright et al, 1981; Iscovich et al, 1987; Jensen et al, 1983; Kabat, 1986; Kessler and Clark, 1978; Morgan and Jain, 1974; Morrison and Buring, 1980; Najem et al, 1982; Piper et al, 1986; Risch et al, 1988b; Simon et al, 1975; Wynder and Goldsmith, 1977; Wynder and Stellman, 1980). One study suggested a positive association in men (relative risk = 1.6) (Howe et al, 1977; Miller and Howe, 1977), but there was an inverse association in women (relative risk = 0.6). Moreover, a weak inverse association between use of artificially sweetened beverages and bladder cancer was apparent in both men and women. In a large U.S. population-based, case-control study, the relative risk for subjects who had ever used artificial sweeteners was 1.0 (Hoover et al, 1980). Those who reported very frequent use of artificial sweeteners appeared to have a small elevation in risk, but the dose-response pattern was irregular. A positive association was observed in two study subgroups, white male heavy smokers and nonsmoking white females with no known exposure to bladder carcinogens. The reason for these associations is uncertain, however (Hoover and Hartge, 1982; Walker et al, 1982).

It is difficult to separate the effects of saccharin and cyclamates in the United States and Canada because both substances were used extensively in both countries. Studies conducted in England and Japan, however, pertain primarily to the use of saccharin (Morrison et al, 1982b). Results of the latter studies suggested that use of saccharin is not associated with increased bladder cancer risk.

The findings of nearly all studies indicate that the use of artificial sweeteners confers little or no excess risk of human bladder cancer. If, in fact, saccharin is a very weak carcinogen, such a low-level effect may not be detectable in epidemiological studies (Hoover and Hartge, 1982).

Alcohol Drinking. Most studies that have evaluated alcohol drinking as a risk factor for bladder cancer have not supported a positive association (Brownson et al, 1987; Cartwright et al, 1981; Howe et al, 1980; Kabat et al, 1986; Mills et al, 1991; Najem et al, 1982; Thomas et al, 1983; Wynder et al, 1963; Wynder and Goldsmith, 1977). Elevated risks related to consumption of specific types of alcoholic beverages have been reported in a few studies (Iscovich et al, 1987; Kunze et al, 1992; Mommsen et al, 1982a; Morgan and Jain, 1974; Risch et al, 1988b; Slattery et al, 1988a), but these findings have not been consistent with respect to type of beverage or sex, and regular dose-response relations have not been apparent. Thus, the positive findings are likely to be the result of chance or residual confounding by smoking.

Other Dietary Factors. The role of dietary factors in human bladder carcinogenesis is unclear. Dietary supplements of natural and synthetic retinoids inhibit bladder carcinogenesis in laboratory animals (Hicks, 1983). However, results of epidemiological studies are inconsistent. Increasing intake of foods that contain vitamin A, particularly milk, has been associated with decreasing risk of bladder cancer in three case-control studies (La Vecchia et al, 1989; Mettlin and Graham, 1979; Slattery et al, 1988a) and one cohort study (Chyou et al, 1993), but two other case-control studies have not supported this relation (Risch et al, 1988b; Tyler et al, 1986). The use of vitamin A supplements also has been associated with decreased risk (Steineck et al, 1990). Serum levels of retinol, retinol-binding protein, and carotenoids do not appear related to risk (Helzlsouer et al, 1989; Nomura et al, 1985; Tyler et al, 1986), although a recent study reported a decreased risk associated with increased carotenoid consumption in subjects under 65 years of age (Vena et al, 1992). Relatively high fruit and vegetable consumption has been associated with relatively low risk in some studies (Chyou et al, 1993 [fruits only]; Claude et al, 1986; La Vecchia et al, 1989; Mettlin and Graham, 1979; Mills et al, 1991), but not in others (Steinbeck et al, 1988).

In addition, increased bladder cancer risk has been associated with a relatively high intake of cholesterol (Risch et al, 1988b), with total fat (Vena et al, 1992) and saturated fat (Riboli et al, 1991), with fatty meals (Claude et al, 1986), with fried foods (Steineck et al, 1990), and with relatively high pork and beef consumption (Steineck et al, 1988). A nearly linear increasing trend in risk with decreasing serum levels of selenium was observed in a nested case-control study in Washington County, Maryland (Helzlsouer et al, 1989).

Drugs

Analgesics. Heavy consumption of phenacetin-containing analgesics was first linked to cancers of the renal pelvis, ureter, and bladder by a series of case reports (IARC, 1980). There have been only a few case-control studies in which the relation between use of phenacetin and risk of bladder cancer has been evaluated (Fokkens, 1979; McCredie et al, 1983; McCredie and Stewart, 1988; Piper et al, 1985). Fokkens (1979) reported that Dutch subjects who had a lifetime consumption of at least 2 kg had a relative risk of 4.1 compared to incidental users or nonusers. McCredie and coworkers (1983, 1988) found a relative risk of 2.0 in Australian women aged 45–85 years who had a lifetime consumption of at least 1 kg. Piper and coworkers (1985) reported a relative risk of 6.5 in U.S. women aged 20–44 years who had used phenacetin-containing compounds for at least 30 days in a year. Despite these fairly strong associations, a regular gradient in risk with increasing dose was demonstrated only in the Australian study (McCredie et al, 1983). Further study of the relation between phenacetin and bladder cancer will be difficult because most western countries no longer allow phenacetin-containing analgesics to be sold.

Acetaminophen was assessed as a risk factor in the Australian and U.S. studies (McCredie and Stewart, 1988; Piper et al, 1985). Results of both studies suggested that heavy use of acetaminophen-containing analgesics does not increase risk. However, acetaminophen did not become popular until the 1970s. Thus, subjects in both these studies may not have had sufficient time since initial exposure for bladder cancer to develop.

Cyclophosphamide and Chlornaphazine. Cyclophosphamide, an alkylating agent that has been used to treat both malignant and nonmalignant diseases since the early 1950s, has been linked to risk of bladder cancer in many case reports and case series (IARC, 1981; Levine and Richie, 1989). Cyclophosphamide has been shown to produce bladder tumors in both rats and mice (IARC, 1981). Patients with non-Hodgkin's lymphoma who were treated with cyclophosphamide experienced a sevenfold risk of bladder cancer in a Danish study (Pedersen-Bjergaard et al, 1988). A report of bladder cancer risk among patients with non-Hodgkin's lymphoma who received chemotherapy, based on data from the SEER program and the Connecticut Tumor Registry, also was positive (observed/expected = 1.7) (Travis et al, 1989). Findings from an international case-control study of urinary tract cancer in a cohort of two-year survivors of non-Hodgkin's lymphoma indicated a 4.5-fold risk of bladder cancer associated with cyclophosphamide therapy (Travis et al, 1995). A dose-response relation was observed, with the relative risk peaking at 14.5 for heavily exposed subjects. Additional groups of patients, such as long-term survivors of breast cancer who were treated with cyclophosphamide as adjuvant chemotherapy, should be studied in order to clarify the extent of the carcinogenic risk associated with use of this important antineoplastic drug.

In the 1960s, the antineoplastic drug chlornaphazine was linked to the development of bladder cancer (Thiede and Christensen, 1969). Chlornaphazine is related chemically to 2-naphthylamine. This drug was never used in the United States and probably is not widely used elsewhere (IARC, 1974).

Urologic Conditions

Urinary Tract Infection. A positive association between urinary bladder infection and risk of bladder cancer has been reported in a number of case-control studies (Dunham et al, 1968; Howe et al, 1980; Kantor et al, 1984; La Vecchia et al, 1991; Piper et al, 1986; Wynder et al, 1963), although two studies found no support for a causal association (Gonzalez et al, 1991; Kjaer et al, 1989). In the United States, Kantor and colleagues (1984) found an increased risk associated with urinary tract infections in both men and women; subjects with a history of at least three infections had a relative risk of 2.0, compared to those with no infections. In addition, bladder infection was more strongly associated with squamous cell than with transitional cell cancer, a striking parallel to the relation between schistosomiasis and squamous cell bladder cancer. However, information on dates of the bladder infections was not obtained in most of the reported studies. Thus, the occurrence or diagnosis of infections may have been the consequence of early bladder cancer, rather than a cause of the disease.

Urinary Stasis. If carcinogens are present in urine, urinary retention or stasis might increase the risk of developing bladder cancer by increasing the duration of contact of the carcinogens with the bladder mucosa (Parkash and Kiesswetter, 1976). Although urinary stasis has not been investigated directly as a risk factor, several findings are consistent with the hypothesis that stasis is related to risk. First, conditions that cause stasis, such as benign prostatic hypertrophy, have been associated with increased risk (Dunham et al, 1968; Fellows, 1978; Mommsen and Sell, 1983). It is uncertain, however, whether these conditions preceded the bladder cancer or were related to its diagnosis. Second, infrequent micturition and high urine concentration, both of which increase urine contact with bladder epithelium, were more prevalent in high-risk areas of Israel than in low-risk areas (Braver et al, 1987). Third, the upper hemisphere of the bladder (dome), which has less contact with urine than the rest of the bladder, is a relatively infrequent site of bladder tumors (Parkash and Kiesswetter, 1976). Fourth, dogs exposed to 2-naphthylamine do not develop tumors in bladders that have not been in contact with urine (McDonald and Lund, 1954). Finally, urine itself appears to be a promoter of bladder carcinogenesis in the rat (Oyasu et al, 1981; Rowland et al, 1980).

Schistosoma Haematobium. For 80 years it has been thought that *S. haematobium* infection is related to increased risk of bladder cancer (Ferguson, 1911). Although there is little evidence that contradicts the suspected association, few convincing epidemiological findings are available. The proportional incidence of bladder cancer is high in developing countries where schistosomiasis is endemic (Tawfik, 1988). The percentage of bladder cancers that are squamous cell tumors is also much higher in endemic areas than it is in nonendemic areas. In Egypt, 70% or more of bladder cancers are squamous cell (Tawfik, 1988), compared to about 2% in the United States. However, bladder cancer incidence rates appear similar in areas of Africa where schistosomiasis is endemic, infrequent, or absent (Payet, 1962).

In two hospital-based studies, the prevalence of schistosome infection was higher among bladder cancer patients than among control patients (Gelfand et al, 1967; Mustacchi and Shimkin, 1958). Results of a registry-based, case-control study conducted in Zimbabwe from 1963 to 1977 indicated that the presence of schistosomiasis, evaluated from past history of bilharzia or hematuria, was associated with increased risk of bladder cancer in both men (odds ratio [OR] = 3.9) and women (OR = 5.7) (Vizcaino et al, 1994). In series of cases from South Africa and Zambia, *S. haematobium* ova were found in higher proportions of patients with squamous cell than with transitional cell tumors (Bhagwandeen, 1976; Hinder and Schmaman, 1969). Bladder tumors have been produced in monkeys infected with *S. haematobium* (Kuntz et al, 1972), but these were transitional cell rather than squamous cell tumors. Squamous metaplasia has been observed in the bladders of hamsters infected experimentally with *S. haematobium* (El-Morsi et al, 1974).

Several mechanisms by which schistosomiasis infection predisposes to bladder cancer have been suggested. First, chronic inflammation by calcific ova and urinary retention caused by infection might affect the absorption of carcinogens from the urine (Cheever, 1978). Second, the urine of patients infected with *S. haematobium* or bacteria might have greater amounts of potentially carcinogenic nitroso compounds than that of noninfected patients (Tawfik, 1988). Third, the schistosoma antigen might depress the immunocompetence of infected patients (Mee, 1982).

Radiation

Ionizing radiation causes bladder cancer, although this exposure contributes very little to bladder cancer incidence in the general population. Women who received therapeutic pelvic radiation for dysfunctional uterine bleeding appear to have a two- to fourfold risk of bladder cancer (Inskip et al, 1990; Wagoner, 1970). In a large international study of cervical cancer patients treated with radiation, high-dose radiotherapy was associated with a fourfold risk of bladder cancer (Boice et al, 1988). Higher risks were experienced by women under age 55 years when first treated, compared to those age 55 or older. Risk increased with increasing dose to the bladder. Risk also increased with time since exposure, with the relative risk reaching 8.7 for patients treated at least 20 years earlier.

Radioactive iodine (iodine 131) exposure has also been associated with elevated bladder cancer risk. A threefold risk was found among women who had a thyroid uptake procedure with iodine 131 (Piper et al, 1986). A cohort of patients treated with high-dose iodine 131 for thyroid cancer also experienced excess risk (Edmonds and Smith, 1986).

Follow-up of atomic bomb survivors in Hiroshima and Nagasaki revealed a dose-response relation between radiation exposure and bladder cancer mortality (National Academy of Sciences [NAS], 1990). Bladder cancer mortality also appeared to be elevated in two groups of workers at nuclear installations in the United Kingdom (Inskip et al, 1987; Smith and Douglas, 1986), but an excess was not apparent in U.S. nuclear workers (Gilbert et al, 1989).

Drinking Water and Fluid Intake

An association between by-products of chlorination in drinking water and bladder cancer risk was first suggested by ecological studies (National Research Council, 1980), and later by two case-control studies based on death certificates (Crump and Guess, 1982).

In four investigations, detailed information was available on water quality and temporal aspects of exposure. These studies support the association between chlorination by-product levels in drinking water sources and bladder cancer risk. In Washington County, Maryland, residents supplied with chlorinated surface water had higher bladder cancer incidence rates than did those who consumed unchlorinated deep well water (relative risks were 1.8 and 1.6 for men and women, respectively) (Wilkins and Comstock, 1981). In the National Cancer Institute (NCI) study conducted in 10 areas of the United States, risk increased with level of intake of beverages made with tap water (Cantor et al, 1987). The gradient was restricted to subjects with at least 40 years of exposure to chlorinated surface water and was not observed among long-term consumers of nonchlorinated groundwater. Among subjects whose residences were served by a chlorinated surface water source for at least 60 years, a relative risk of 2.0 was estimated for heavy consumers compared with low consumers of tap water. In a study in Massachusetts, residents of communities supplied with chlorinated drinking water experienced higher bladder cancer mortality than did those of communities exposed to water containing lower concentrations of chlorination by-products (mortality odds ratio = 1.6) (Zierler et al, 1988). In a Colorado study, years of exposure to chlorinated surface water was significantly associated with increased bladder cancer risk (McGeehin et al, 1993). The relative risk for those exposed for more than 30 years to chlorinated surface water was 1.8 compared to subjects with no exposure.

A relation between exposure to high levels of arsenic in well water and bladder cancer mortality has been suggested in Argentina (Hopenhayn-Rich et al, in press) and by surveys conducted in an endemic area of chronic arsenic toxicity, manifested by skin cancer and blackfoot disease in Taiwan (Chen et al, 1985, 1986; Chiang et al, 1993; Wu et al, 1989). Ingestion of arsenic also has been associated with an increase in micronuclei in exfoliated bladder cells (Warner et al, 1994) and increased bladder cancer mortality among a cohort of patients treated with Fowler's solution (potassium arsenite) (Cuzick et al, 1992).

Total fluid intake may be related to bladder cancer risk, but the results have been equivocal. Increased total fluid consumption has been associated with decreased risk (Dunham et al, 1968); with a positive trend in risk (Cantor et al, 1987; Claude et al, 1986; Jensen et al, 1986; Vena et al, 1993); and with no excess risk (Slattery et al, 1988b; Wynder et al, 1963).

Hair Dyes

Three lines of evidence suggest that the use of hair dyes may be associated with increased bladder cancer risk. First, hairdressers and barbers have been reported to be at elevated risk (Clemmesen, 1981). Second, findings from mutagenicity tests and animal experiments indicate that some compounds in hair dyes are mutagens and possible bladder carcinogens (Hartge et al, 1982). Third, people who dye their hair appear to excrete dye compounds in their urine (Hartge et al, 1982). Results of several epidemiological studies, however, are negative (Hartge et al, 1982).

Familial Occurrence

Evidence for familial predisposition to bladder cancer comes mainly from clinical reports, but elevated risks among persons with bladder cancers in close relatives have been identified in a few case-control studies (Cartwright, 1979a; Kantor et al, 1985; Kramer et al, 1991; Kunze et al, 1992; Piper et al, 1986). In the largest case-control study to date (Kantor et al, 1985), familial risks were especially high among those with environmental exposures, such as heavy cigarette smoking, suggesting genetic and environmental interactions. Familial occurrences provide an opportunity to identify genetic markers of susceptibility, including metabolic polymorphisms, pharmacogenetic traits, or oncogene expression.

BIOMARKERS

Markers of Exposure

Urinary Mutagens. Investigations of urinary mutagenicity in relation to bladder cancer have focused on correlating exposure to bladder cancer risk factors with the presence of mutagens in the urine. Cigarette smoking has been found to be associated with mutagenic activity in the urine (Menon and Bhide, 1984; Yamasaki and Ames, 1977). The level of mutagenic activity has been observed to be higher for smokers of black tobacco than for smokers of blond tobacco (Malaveille et al, 1989). The relation of urinary mutagenic activity to the tar level of cigarettes is uncertain (Kriebel et al, 1985; Mohtashamipur et al, 1987). Other risk factors that have been studied in relation to urinary mutagenicity include employment as a rubber worker (Falck et al, 1980) and cyclophosphamide exposure (Falck et al, 1979). Only one study, however, has attempted to directly link urinary mutagenicity with risk of bladder cancer. Garner and coworkers (1982) reported an association of mutagenic urine with bladder cancer in a comparison of cases and controls. The design of the study precluded the possibility of determining whether the appearance of mutagenicity in urine preceded the onset of disease.

Hemoglobin and DNA Adducts. Hemoglobin adducts of aromatic amines have been related to cigarette smoking, but the levels of adducts have not yet been related to the occurrence of bladder cancer. Bryant and coworkers (1988) found that smokers have higher levels of hemoglobin adducts of several aromatic amines, including the carcinogens 4-aminobiphenyl and 2-naphthylamine. The levels of adducts of 4-aminobiphenyl and 3-aminobiphenyl were correlated with the number of cigarettes smoked per day. Smokers of black tobacco had a higher mean level of adducts of 4-aminobiphenyl, as well as several other aromatic amines, than smokers of blond tobacco (Bryant et al, 1988). Maclure and coworkers (1990) reported that the levels of the adduct of 4-aminobiphenyl declined after the cessation of smoking. Recently, carcinogen–DNA adducts have been identified in human bladder biopsy samples (Talaska et al, 1991a) and in exfoliated urothelial cells (Talaska et al, 1991b), providing new techniques for the identification of human bladder carcinogens.

Susceptibility Factors

Acetylation Genotype/Phenotype. Some of the aromatic amines that are carcinogenic for the bladder are detoxified in acetylation reactions involving the liver enzyme *N*-acetyltransferase. Persons can be classified as "slow acetylators" or "rapid acetylators" by measurement of the extent of acetylation of a drug such as sulfamethazine (Lower et al, 1979), or caffeine (Grant et al, 1984). The *NAT2* genotype associated with *N*-acetylation of these drugs has been described and polymerase chain reaction-based tests have been developed for its characterization (Deguchi et al, 1990; Agundez et al, 1994). The distribution of acetylator status has been compared between bladder cancer cases and controls (Bicho et al, 1988; Cartwright et al, 1982, 1984; Evans et al, 1983; Hanssen et al, 1985; Karakaya et al, 1986; Ladero et al, 1985; Lower et al, 1979; Miller and Cosgriff, 1983; Mommsen et al, 1982b; Woodhouse, 1982). In most of the reported studies, a modest positive association has been found between the slow acetylator status and bladder cancer (relative risks typically ranged from 1.1 and 1.9, compared to rapid acetylators). The individual studies have been small, but the association is statistically significant in combined data from most of the studies (Evans, 1986). Despite uncertainties related to the suitability of control series, and the use of "prevalent" (surviving) rather than "incident" (newly diagnosed) case series (Evans, 1984, 1986), the observed association is intriguing. Yu and coworkers (1994) have suggested that acetylator phenotype may play a role in the racial/ethnic differences in bladder cancer risk. They found that the proportion of slow acetylators was highest among whites, intermediate among blacks, and lowest among Asians, closely paralleling the racial/ethnic variation in risk. Acetylator status also has been analyzed in relation to the histologic grade or the stage at diagnosis of bladder tumors (Cartwright et al, 1982; Hanssen et al, 1985; Mommsen and Aagaard, 1986), but the results are inconsistent.

Among smokers, slow acetylators have been reported to have a higher mean level of the hemoglobin adduct of 4-aminobiphenyl than do rapid acetylators (Vineis et al, 1990; Yu et al, 1994). This difference was most pronounced at low exposure levels (Vineis et al, 1994).

Among persons occupationally exposed to aromatic amines, several studies have shown an excess of the slow acetylator phenotype among cases compared to controls (Cartwright et al, 1982; Hanke et al, 1990; Ladero et al, 1985; Weber et al, 1983), but workers in these studies may have been exposed to a mixture of aromatic amines. In contrast, a more recent study in Chinese workers with an increased risk of bladder cancer (Bi et al, 1992) who were exposed exclusively to benzidine did not demonstrate an excess of slow acetylators among bladder cancer cases, based on both phenotype and *NAT2* genotype analysis (Hayes et al, 1993). This finding suggests that the association between *N*-acetylation and bladder cancer risk may be specific to certain aromatic amines.

In a cross-sectional study of workers currently exposed to benzidine and benzidine-based dyes, the predominant DNA adduct in exfoliated urothelial cells was acetylated, providing evidence that acetylation represents an activation rather than a detoxification step in benzidine-induced bladder carcinogenesis (Rothman et al, in press).

Glutathione *S*-Transferase μ Genotype. Findings from six case-control studies also have suggested that glutathione *S*-transferase μ (GSTμ) gene deficiency may predispose individuals to bladder cancer (Bell et al, 1993; Brockmöller et al, 1994; Daly et al, 1993; Katoh et al, 1995; Lin et al, 1994; Lafuente et al, 1993), although no association between the GSTμ gene and bladder cancer risk was observed in one study (Zhong et al, 1993). Bell and coworkers (1993) found that the absence of the GSTμ gene significantly increased risk to smokers but posed little increased risk to nonsmokers, whereas Brockmöller et al (1994) reported that the risk associated with the GSTμ null genotype was highest in nonsmokers. Among smokers, the GSTμ null genotype has been associated with increased urine mutagenicity (Hirvonen et al, 1994) and increased levels of 3- and 4-aminobiphenyl adducts (Yu et al, 1995).

Cytochrome P-450 Enzymes. Initially, it was suggested (Cartwright et al, 1984) that the rate of oxidation of the antihypertensive drug, debrisoquine, by a cytochrome P-450 enzyme (P-450IID6) might reflect the rate at which carcinogenic aromatic amines are oxidized to their active forms. Benitez and coworkers (1990) found a tendency toward lower values of metabolic ratio of debrisoquine in bladder cancer patients than in control patients. Results of two other studies do not support this hypothesis, however. Cartwright and coworkers (1984) found only small differences between bladder cancer cases and controls in the distribution of the oxidation rate of debrisoquine. Kaisary and coworkers (1987) found a tendency toward more rapid oxidation among advanced cases of bladder cancer compared to controls, but not among less advanced cases. It is uncertain whether the extent of the tumor might have an effect on the measured rate of metabolism of the drug. Kaisary and coworkers also found that the mephenytoin oxidation phenotype was similar in case and controls.

More recently, Butler and coworkers (1989) have identified a cytochrome P-450 enzyme, P-450IA2, that is responsible for the metabolic activation of 4-aminobiphenyl and 2-naphthylamine. Susceptibility to aromatic amine-induced bladder cancer may thus vary with an individual's level of P-450IA2. It is unclear, however, whether the activity of this enzyme is determined by genotype and/or by enzyme induction from environmental exposures (eg, cigarette smoking, dietary factors, and drugs).

Tryptophan Metabolism. Laboratory and clinical studies suggested that metabolites of tryptophan are involved in the causation of bladder cancer (Allen et al, 1957; Benassi et al, 1963; Bonser et al, 1952; Boyland and Watson, 1956; Boyland and Williams, 1956; Brown et al, 1960, 1969; Bryan et al, 1964; Dunning et al, 1950; Dunning and Curtis, 1954; Gailani et al, 1973). The suspect metabolites have some chemical similarities to carcinogenic metabolites of aromatic amines. However, the data available do not support a specific relation between tryptophan metabolites and bladder cancer (Fraumeni and Thomas, 1967; Friedlander and Morrison, 1981; Price and Brown, 1962; Quagliariello et al, 1961).

Oncogenes

A variety of activated oncogenes and deletion of candidate tumor suppressor genes have been found in human bladder cancer, but the etiologic significance of these findings is unclear (Schulte, 1988).

PREVENTIVE MEASURES

In public health terms, avoidance of cigarette smoking is the most effective means available for the prevention of bladder cancer, because the proportion of cases attributable to smoking is greater than that for other risk factors (IARC, 1986; Silverman et al, 1989b). A further measure would be curtailment of hazardous occupational exposures.

Screening is appealing as a potential method of cancer control. Certain conditions must be met, however, for a cancer screening program to be successful. First, an adequate screening test must be available. Second, the prevalence of the detectable preclinical phase of the disease must be high. Third, a treatment must be available that is more effective for the screen-detected disease than for otherwise similar, routinely diagnosed disease (Morrison, 1985). It is uncertain whether all these conditions are met for bladder cancer.

Cytologic examination of the urine may be a satisfactory screening test. The sensitivity appears to be about 75% (Hutchison, 1977; Kern, 1985). The specificity is likely to be above 95% (Kern, 1985), and possibly as high as 99.9% (Hutchison, 1977). Furthermore, this test is relatively inexpensive and convenient, and is free of risk. Testing for asymptomatic hematuria also has been investigated as a method of screening for bladder cancer. Because a single test is not sensitive enough, repeated testing at short intervals such as a week has been advocated (Messing et al, 1987, 1989). The result of repeated testing, however, is excessive false positives.

The prevalence of preclinical bladder cancer is probably too low in the general population for large-scale screening programs to be rewarding (Morrison, 1979). On the other hand, certain occupational groups may have a sufficiently high prevalence of the disease to justify screening as a bladder cancer control measure for those groups (Kern, 1985), provided that early treatment is beneficial. Intervention trials are probably necessary to determine whether urine cytology, alone or in combination with other screening methods, leads to a reduction in mortality from bladder cancer among high-risk occupational groups (UICC, 1984).

The natural history of preclinical bladder cancer is poorly understood. In general, the survival of screen-detected cases of cancer is expected to be better than the survival of routinely diagnosed cases, even if screening confers no benefit in terms of reduced mortality from the disease (Morrison, 1985). For bladder cancer, however, the survival of screen-detected cases may be no better, and possibly is worse, than the survival of cases coming to medical attention as a result of symptoms (Shaw, 1977). In addition, screening for bladder cancer seems to detect preferentially cases with prognostically unfavorable histologic appearance (Farrow et al, 1979; Kern, 1985). Neither of these findings, by themselves, would negate the possible value of screening. However, they suggest that the gains may be small, and that particular care is needed in designing and evaluating bladder cancer screening programs (Hutchison, 1977).

Lastly, the effectiveness of the treatment of bladder cancer is uncertain. No data are available on the relative value of treating bladder cancer "early," as detected by screening, or "late," as it comes to medical attention as a result of symptoms.

FUTURE RESEARCH

Bladder cancer is known to be caused by cigarette smoking, occupational exposure to certain aromatic amines, and ionizing radiation. It is likely that phenacetin-containing analgesics, cyclophosphamide, and *S. haematobium* infection also cause the disease. The roles of a number of occupational exposures (eg, motor exhausts), urinary tract infections and stasis, dietary factors, chlorination by-products in drinking water, tobacco products other than cigarettes, and genetic susceptibility deserve further study.

Cigarette smoking accounts for an estimated 48% of bladder cancer diagnosed among men and 32% among women in the United States (Hartge et al, 1987). Occupational exposures have been estimated to be responsible for 21% to 25% of bladder cancer among U.S. white men (Silverman et al, 1989b) and 11% among white women (Silverman et al, 1990). Cigarette smoking and occupational exposures, however, explain only a small part of the large excess risk of bladder cancer among men (Hartge et al, 1990). Exploration of possible reasons for this male excess, such as gender differences in unidentified environmental risk factors, urination habits, or hormonal (Cantor et al, 1992) and metabolic determinants of risk, should enhance our understanding of the etiology of bladder cancer.

Finally, the identification of human bladder carcinogens provides an opportunity to conduct interdisciplinary studies that may help to explain the general mechanisms of carcinogenesis. Potentially useful approaches include acetylation and oxidation phenotyping, determination of hemoglobin- and DNA-adduct levels, and oncogene activation and suppression, and correlation of these measures with exposure to bladder carcinogens.

REFERENCES

AGUNDEZ JAG, MARTINEZ C, OLIVERA M, et al. 1994. Molecular analysis of the arylamine *N*-acetyltransferase polymorphism in a Spanish population. Clin Pharmacol Ther 56:202–209.

ALDERSON M. 1986. Occupational Cancer. London: Butterworth and Co. Ltd.

ALLEN MJ, BOYLAND E, DUKES CE, et al. 1957. Cancer of the urinary bladder induced in mice with metabolites of aromatic amines and tryptophan. Br J Cancer 11:212–228.

ANTONY HM. 1974. Industrial exposure in patients with carcinoma of the bladder. J Soc Occup Med 24:110.

ARMSTRONG B, DOLL R. 1974. Bladder cancer mortality in England and Wales in relation to cigarette smoking and saccharin consumption. Br J Prev Soc Med 28:233–240.

ARMSTRONG B, DOLL R. 1975. Bladder cancer mortality in diabetics in relation to saccharin consumption and smoking habits. Br J Prev Soc Med 29:73–81.

ARMSTRONG BG, TREMBLAY CG, CYR D, et al. 1986. Estimating the relationship between exposure to tar volatiles and the incidence of bladder cancer in aluminum smelter workers. Scand J Work Environ Health 12:486–493.

AUGUSTINE A, HEBERT JR, KABAT GC, et al. 1988. Bladder cancer in relation to cigarette smoking. Cancer Res 48:4405–4408.

BAUS SUBCOMMITTEE ON INDUSTRIAL BLADDER CANCER. 1988. Occupational bladder cancer: a guide for clinicians. Br J Urol 61:183–191.

BAXTER PJ, MCDOWALL ME. 1986. Occupation and cancer in London: an investigation into nasal and bladder cancer using the Cancer Atlas. Br J Ind Med 43:44–49.

BELL DA, TAYLOR JA, PAULSON DF, et al. 1993. Genetic risk and carcinogen exposure: a common inherited defect of the carcinogen-metabolism gene glutathione S-transferase M1 (GSTM1) that increases susceptibility to bladder cancer. J Natl Cancer Inst 85:1159–1164.

BENASSI C, PERISSINOTTO B, ALLEGRI G. 1963. The metabolism of tryptophan in patients with bladder cancer and other urological diseases. Clin Chim Acta 8:822–831.

BENITEZ J, LADERO JM, FERNANDEZ-GUNDIN MJ, et al. 1990. Polymorphic oxidation of debrisoquine in bladder cancer. Ann Med 22:157–160.

BETHWAITE PB, PEARCE N, FRASER J. 1990. Cancer risks in painters: study based on the New Zealand Cancer Registry. Br J Ind Med 47:742–746.

BHAGWANDEEN SB. 1976. Schistosomiasis and carcinoma of the bladder in Zambia. S Afr Med J 50:1616–1620.

BI W, HAYES RB, FENG P, et al. 1992. Mortality and incidence of bladder cancer in benzidine-exposed workers in China. Am J Ind Med 21:481–489.

BICHO MP, BREITENFELD L, CARVALLO AA, et al. 1988. Acetylation phenotypes in patients with bladder carcinoma. Ann Genet 31:167–171.

BLOT WJ, FRAUMENI JF, JR. 1978. Geographic patterns of bladder cancer in the United States. J Natl Cancer Inst 61:1017–1023.

BOICE JD, ENGHOLM G, KLEINERMAN RA, et al. 1988. Radiation dose and second cancer risk in patients treated for cancer of the cervix. Radiat Res 116:3–55.

BONSER GM, CLAYSON DB, JULL JW, et al. 1952. The carcinogenic properties of 2-amino-1-naphthol hydrochloride and its parent amine 2-naphthylamine. Br J Cancer 6:412–424.

BORING CC, SQUIRES TS, TONG T, et al. 1994. Cancer Statistics, 1994. CA 4:7–26.

BOYKO RW, CARTWRIGHT RA, GLASHAN RW. 1985. Bladder cancer in dye manufacturing workers. J Occup Med 27:799–803.

BOYLAND E, WATSON G. 1956. 3-Hydroxyanthranilic acid, a carcinogen produced by endogenous metabolism. Nature 177:837–838.

BOYLAND E, WILLIAMS D. 1956. The metabolism of tryptophan. II. The metabolism of tryptophan in patients suffering from cancer of the bladder. Biochem J 64:578–582.

BRAVER DJ, MODAN M, CHETRIT A, et al. 1987. Drinking, micturition habits, and urine concentration as potential risk factors in urinary bladder cancer. J Natl Cancer Inst 78:437–440.

BROCKMÖLLER J, KERB R, DRAKOULIS N, et al. 1994. Glutathione S-transferase M1 and its variants A and B as host factors of bladder cancer susceptibility: a case-control study. Cancer Res 54:4103–4111.

BROSS ID, TIDINGS J. 1973. Another look at coffee drinking and cancer of the urinary bladder. Prev Med 2:445–451.

BROWN RR, PRICE JM, FRIEDELL GH, et al. 1969. Tryptophan metabolism in patients with bladder cancer: geographical differences. J Natl Cancer Inst 43:295–301.

BROWN RR, PRICE JM, SATTER EJ, et al. 1960. The metabolism of tryptophan in patients with bladder cancer. Acta Unio Int Contra Cancrum 16:299–303.

BROWNSON RC, CHANG JC, DAVIS JR. 1987. Occupation, smoking, and alcohol in the epidemiology of bladder cancer. Am J Prev Med 77:1298–1300.

BRYAN GT, BROWN RR, PRICE JM. 1964. Mouse bladder carcinogenicity of certain tryptophan metabolites and other aromatic nitrogen compounds suspended in cholesterol. Cancer Res 24:596–602.

BRYANT MS, VINEIS P, SKIPPER PL, et al. 1988. Hemoglobin adducts of aromatic amines: associations with smoking status and type of tobacco. Proc Natl Acad Sci USA 85:9788–9791.

BURCH JD, ROHAN TE, HOWE GR, et al. 1989. Risk of bladder cancer by source and type of tobacco exposure: a case-control study. Int J Cancer 44:622–628.

BUTLER MA, IWASAKI M, GUENGERICH FP, et al. 1989. Human cytochrome P-450pa (P-450IA2), the phenacetin O-deethylase, is primarily responsible for the hepatic 3-demethylation of caffeine and N-oxidation of carcinogenic arylamines. Proc Natl Acad Sci USA 86:7696–7700.

CANTOR KP, HOOVER R, HARTGE P, et al. 1992. Bladder cancer, drinking water source, and tap water consumption: a case-control study. J Natl Cancer Inst 79:1269–1279.

CANTOR KP, LYNCH CF, JOHNSON D. 1992. Bladder cancer, parity, and age at first birth. Cancer Causes Control 3:57–62.

CARTWRIGHT RA. 1979a. Genetic association with bladder cancer. Br Med J 2:798.

CARTWRIGHT RA, ADIB R, APPLEYARD I, et al. 1983. Cigarette smoking and bladder cancer: an epidemiological inquiry in West Yorkshire. J Epidemiol Community Health 37:256–263.

CARTWRIGHT RA, ADIB R, GLASHAN R, et al. 1981. The epidemiology of bladder cancer in West Yorkshire: a preliminary report on non-occupational aetiologies. Carcinogenesis 2:343–347.

CARTWRIGHT RA, BERNARD SM, GLASHAN RW, et al. 1979b. Bladder cancer amongst dye users. Lancet 2:1073–1074.

CARTWRIGHT RA, GLASHAN RW, ROGERS HJ, et al. 1982. Role of N-acetyltransferase phenotypes in bladder carcinogenesis: a pharmacogenetic epidemiological approach to bladder cancer. Lancet 2:842–845.

CARTWRIGHT RA, PHILIP PA, ROGERS HJ, et al. 1984. Genetically determined debrisoquine oxidation capacity in bladder cancer. Carcinogenesis 5:1191–1192.

CASE RAM, HOSKER ME. 1954. Tumour of the urinary bladder as an occupational disease in the rubber industry in England and Wales. Br J Prev Soc Med 8:39–50.

CASE RAM, HOSKER ME, MCDONALD DB, et al. 1954. Tumours of the urinary bladder in workmen engaged in the manufacture and use of certain dyestuff intermediates in the British chemical industry. Br J Ind Med 11:75–104.

CHECKOWAY H, SMITH AH, MCMICHAEL AJ, et al. 1981. A case-control study of bladder cancer in the United States rubber and tire industry. Br J Ind Med 38:240–246.

CHEEVER AW. 1978. Schistosomiasis and neoplasia. J Natl Cancer Inst 61:13–18.

CHEN C-J, CHUANG Y-C, LIN T-M, et al. 1985. Malignant neoplasms among residents of a blackfoot disease-endemic area in Taiwan: high-arsenic artesian well water and cancers. Cancer Res 45:5895–5899.

CHEN C-J, CHUANG Y-C, YOU S-L, et al. 1986. A retrospective study on malignant neoplasms of bladder, lung and liver in blackfoot disease endemic area in Taiwan. Br J Cancer 53:399–405.

CHIANG HS, GUO HR, HONG CL, et al. 1993. The incidence of bladder cancer in the blackfoot disease endemic area in Taiwan. Br J Urol 71:274–278.

CHYOU PH, NOMURA AMY, STEMMERMANN GN. 1993. A prospective study of diet, smoking, and lower urinary tract cancer. Ann Epidemiol 3:211–216.

CICCONE G, VINEIS P. 1988. Coffee drinking and bladder cancer. Cancer Lett 41:45–52.

CLAUDE JC, FRENTZEL-BEYME RR, KUNZE E. 1988. Occupation and risk of cancer of the lower urinary tract among men: a case-control study. Int J Cancer 41:371–379.

CLAUDE J, KUNZE E, FRENTZEL-BEYME R, et al. 1986. Life-style and occupational risk factors in cancer of the lower urinary tract. Am J Epidemiol 124:578–589.

CLAVEL J, CORDIER S. 1991. Coffee consumption and bladder cancer risk. Int J Cancer 47:207–212.

CLAVEL J, CORDIER S, BOCCON-GIBOD L, et al. 1989. Tobacco and bladder cancer in males: increased risk for inhalers and smokers of black tobacco. Int J Cancer 44:605–610.

CLEMMESEN J. 1981. Epidemiological studies into the possible carcinogenicity of hair dyes. Mutat Res 87:65–79.

COLE P. 1971. Coffee drinking and cancer of the lower urinary tract. Lancet 1:1335–1337.

COLE P, HOOVER R, FRIEDELL G. 1972. Occupation and cancer of the lower urinary tract. Cancer 29:1250–1260.

COLE P, MONSON RR, HANING H, et al. 1971. Smoking and cancer of the lower urinary tract. N Engl J Med 284:129–134.

COUNCIL ON SCIENTIFIC AFFAIRS. 1985. Saccharin review of safety issues. JAMA 254:2622–2624.

CRUMP KS, GUESS HA. 1982. Drinking water and cancer: review of recent epidemiological findings and assessment of risks. Ann Rev Public Health 3:339–357.

CUTLER SJ, YOUNG JL JR, EDS. 1975. Third National Cancer Survey: incidence data. NCI Monogr 41:1–454.

CUZICK J, SASIENI P, EVANS S. 1992. Ingested arsenic, keratoses, and bladder cancer. Am J Epidemiol 136:417–421.

DALY AK, THOMAS DJ, COOPER J, et al. 1993. Homozygous deletion of gene for glutathione *S*-transferase M1 in bladder cancer. Br Med J 307:481–482.

D'AVANZO B, NEGRI E, LA VECCHIA C, et al. 1990. Cigarette smoking and bladder cancer. Eur J Cancer 26:714–718.

D'AVANZO B, LA VECCHIA C, FRANCESCHI S, et al. 1992. Coffee consumption and bladder cancer risk. Eur J Cancer 28:1480–1484.

DE STEFANI E, CORREA P, FIERRO L, et al. 1991. Black tobacco, mate, and bladder cancer. Cancer 67:536–540.

DECARLI A, PETO J, PIOLATTO G, et al. 1985. Bladder cancer mortality of workers exposed to aromatic amines: analysis of models of carcinogenesis. Br J Cancer 51:707–712.

DECOUFLE P. 1979. Cancer risks associated with employment in the leather and leather products industry. Arch Environ Health 34:33–37.

DECOUFLE P, STANISLAWCZYK K, HOUTEN L, et al. 1977. A Retrospective Survey of Cancer in Relation to Occupation. DHEW Publ No. (NIOSH) 77–178. Washington, DC, US Govt Print Office.

DEGUCHI T, MASHIMO M, SUZUKI T. 1990. Correlation between acetylator phenotypes and genotypes of polymorphic arylamine *N*-acetyltransferase in human liver. J Biol Chem 265:12757–12760.

DELZELL E, MONSON RR. 1981. Mortality among rubber workers, III: Cause-specific mortality, 1940–1978. J Occup Med 23:677–684.

DEVESA SS. 1979. The association of cancer incidence with income and education. Unpublished doctoral thesis, Johns Hopkins University, Baltimore.

DEVESA SS, SILVERMAN DT, YOUNG JL JR, et al. 1987. Cancer incidence and mortality trends among whites in the United States, 1947–84. J Natl Cancer Inst 79:701–770.

DOLIN PJ, COOK-MOZAFFARI P. 1992. Occupation and bladder cancer: a death-certificate study. Br J Cancer 66:568–578.

DUBROW R, WEGMAN DH. 1984. Cancer and occupation in Massachusetts: a death certificate study. Am J Ind Med 6:207–230.

DUNHAM LJ, RABSON AS, STEWART HL, et al. 1968. Rates, interview, and pathology study of cancer of the urinary bladder in New Orleans, Louisiana. J Natl Cancer Inst 41:683–709.

DUNNING WF, CURTIS MR. 1954. Further studies on the relation of dietary tryptophan to the induction of neoplasms in rats. Cancer Res 14:299–302.

DUNNING WF, CURTIS MR, MAUN ME. 1950. The effect of added dietary tryptophan on the occurrence of 2-acetylaminofluorene-induced liver and bladder cancer in rats. Cancer Res 10:454–459.

EDLING C, KLING H, FLODIN U, et al. 1986. Cancer mortality among leather tanners. Br J Ind Med 43:494–496.

EDMONDS CJ, SMITH T. 1986. The long-term hazards of the treatment of thyroid cancer with radioiodine. Br J Radiol 59:45–51.

EL-MORSI B, SHERIF M, EL-RAZIKI ES. 1974. Experimental bilharzia squamous metaplasia of the urinary bladder in hamsters. Eur J Cancer 11:199–201.

ENGLUND A. 1980. Cancer incidence among painters and some allied trades. J Toxicol Environ Health 6:1267–1273.

EVANS DAP. 1984. Survey of the human acetylator polymorphism in spontaneous disorders. J Med Genet 21:243–253.

EVANS DAP. 1986. Acetylation. In: Ethnic Differences in Reactions to Drugs and Menobiotics. New York, Alan R Liss Inc, pp 209–242.

EVANS DAP, EZE LC, WHIBLEY EJ. 1983. The association of the slow acetylator phenotype with bladder cancer. J Med Genet 20:330–333.

FALCK K, GROHN P, SORSA M, et al. 1979. Mutagenicity of urine of nurses handling cytostatic drugs. Lancet 1:1250–1251.

FALCK K, SORSA M, VAINIO H. 1980. Mutagenicity in urine of workers in rubber industry. Mutat Res 79:45–52.

FAN TY, MORRISON J, ROUNBEHLER DP, et al. 1977. N-Nitrosodiethanolamine in synthetic cutting fluids: a part-per-hundred impurity. Science 196:70–71.

FARROW GM. 1979. Pathologist's role in bladder cancer. Semin Oncol 6:198–206.

FELLOWS GJ. 1978. The association between vesical carcinoma and urinary obstruction. Eur Urol 4:187–188.

FERGUSON AR. 1911. Associated bilharziosis and primary malignant disease of the urinary bladder with observations in a series of forty cases. J Pathol Bacteriol 16:76–94.

FOKKENS W. 1979. Phenacetin abuse related to bladder cancer. Environ Res 20:192–198.

FRAUMENI JF, JR. 1968. Cigarette smoking and cancers of the urinary tract: geographic variation in the United States. J Natl Cancer Inst 41:1205–1211.

FRAUMENI JF JR, SCOTTO J, DUNHAM LF. 1971. Coffee drinking and bladder cancer. Lancet 2:1204.

FRAUMENI JF JR, THOMAS LB. 1967. Malignant bladder tumors in a man and his three sons. JAMA 201:507–509.

FRIEDLANDER E, MORRISON AS. 1981. Urinary tryptophan metabolites and cancer of the bladder in humans. J Natl Cancer Inst 67:347–351.

GAILANI S, MURPHY G, KENNY G, et al. 1973. Studies on tryptophan metabolism in patients with bladder cancer. Cancer Res 33:1071–1077.

GARABRANT DH, WEGMAN DH. 1984. Cancer mortality among shoe and leather workers in Massachusetts. Am J Ind Med 5:303–314.

GARNER RC, MOULD AJ, LINDSAU-SMITH V. 1982. Mutagenic urine from bladder cancer patients. Lancet 2:389.

GELFAND M, WEINBERG RW, CASTLE WM. 1967. Relation between carcinoma of the bladder and infestation with Schistosoma haematobium. Lancet 1:1249–1251.

GIBBS GW. 1985. Mortality of aluminum reduction plant workers, 1950 through 1957. J Occup Med 27:761–770.

GILBERT ES, FRY SA, WIGGS LD, et al. 1989. Analyses of combined mortality data on workers at the Hanford Site, Oak Ridge National Laboratory, and Rocky Flats Nuclear Weapons Plant. Radiat Res 120:19–35.

GONZALEZ CA, ERREZOLA M, IZARZUGAZA I, et al. 1991. Urinary infection, renal lithiasis and bladder cancer in Spain. Eur J Cancer 27:498–500.

GONZALEZ CA, LOPEZ-ABENTE G, ERREZOLA M, et al. 1985. Occupation, tobacco use, coffee, and bladder cancer in the county of Mataro (Spain). Cancer 55:2031–2034.

GRANT DM, TANG BK, KALOW W. 1984. A simple test for acetylation phenotype using caffeine. Br J Clin Pharmacol 17:459–464.

GREENBERG MR. 1983. Urbanization and cancer mortality: the United States experience, 1950–1975. Monographs in Epidemiology and Biostatistics, Vol 4. New York: Oxford University Press.

GUBERAN E, USEL M, RAYMOND L, et al. 1989. Disability, mortality, and incidence of cancer among Geneva painters and electricians: a historical prospective study. Br J Ind Med 46:16–23.

HANKE J, KRAJEWSKA B. 1990. Acetylation phenotypes and bladder cancer. J Occup Med 32:917–918.

HANKEY BF, MYERS MH. 1987. Black/white differences in bladder cancer survival. J Chron Dis 40:65–73.

HANKEY BF, SILVERMAN DT, KAPLAN R. 1993. Urinary bladder. In: SEER Cancer Statistics Review: 1973–1990, Miller BA, Ries LAG, Hankey BF, et al (eds). NIH Pub. No. 93 789, Bethesda, MD: National Cancer Institute, pp XXXVI.1–17.

HANSSEN H-P, AGARWAL DP, GOEDDE HW, et al. 1985. Association of n-acetyltransferase polymorphism and environmental factors with bladder carcinogenesis. Eur Urol 11:263–266.

HARTGE P, HARVEY EB, LINEHAN WM, et al. 1990. Explaining the male excess in bladder cancer risk. J Natl Cancer Inst 82:1636–1640.

HARTGE P, HOOVER R, ALTMAN R, et al. 1982. Use of hair dyes and risk of bladder cancer. Cancer Res 42:4784–4787.

HARTGE P, HOOVER R, KANTOR A. 1985. Bladder cancer risk and pipes, cigars and smokeless tobacco. Cancer 55:901–906.

HARTGE P, HOOVER R, WEST DW, LYON JL. 1983. Coffee drinking and risk of bladder cancer. J Natl Cancer Inst 70:1021–1026.

HARTGE P, SILVERMAN D, HOOVER R, et al. 1987. Changing cigarette habits and bladder cancer risk: a case-control study. J Natl Cancer Inst 78:1119–1125.

HAYES RB, BI W, ROTHMAN N, et al. 1993. N-acetylation phenotype and genotype and risk of bladder cancer, in benzidine-exposed workers. Carcinogenesis 14:675–678.

HELZLSOUER KJ, COMSTOCK GW, MORRIS JS. 1989. Selenium, lycopene, α-tocopherol, β-carotene, retinol, and subsequent bladder cancer. Cancer Res 49:6144–6148.

HENRY SA, KENNAWAY NM, KENNAWAY EL. 1931. The incidence of cancer of the bladder and prostate in certain occupations. J Hyg 31:125–137.

HICKS RM. 1983. The scientific basis for regarding vitamin A and its analogues as anti-carcinogenic agents. Proc Nutr Soc 42:83–93.

HINDER RA, SCHMAMAN A. 1969. Bilharziasis and squamous carcinoma of the bladder. S Afr Med J 43:617–618.

HIRVONEN A, NYLUND L, KOCIBA P, et al. 1994. Modulation of urinary mutagenicity by genetically determined carcinogen metabolism in smokers. Carcinogenesis 15:813–815.

HOAR SK, HOOVER R. 1985. Truck driving and bladder cancer mortality in rural New England. J Natl Cancer Inst 74:771–774.

HOOVER R, COLE P. 1971. Population trends in cigarette smoking and bladder cancer. Am J Epidemiol 94:409–418.

HOOVER R, HARTGE P. 1982. Non-nutritive sweeteners and bladder cancer. Am J Public Health 72:382–383.

HOOVER RN, STRASSER PH, CHILD M, et al. 1980. Artificial sweeteners and human bladder cancer. Lancet 1:837–840.

HOPENHAYN-RICH C, BIGGS ML, FUCHS A, et al. Bladder cancer mortality associated with arsenic in drinking water in Argentina. Epidemiology (in press).

HORM JW, DEVESA SS, BURHANSSTIPANOV L. 1996. Cancer incidence, survival and mortality among social and ethnic minority groups in the United States. In: Cancer Epidemiology and Prevention, 2nd Ed, Schottenfeld D, Fraumeni JF, Jr (eds). New York: Oxford University Press.

HOWE GR, BURCH JD, MILLER AB, et al. 1977. Artificial sweeteners and human bladder cancer. Lancet 2:578–581.

HOWE GR, BURCH JD, MILLER AB, et al. 1980. Tobacco use, occupation, coffee, various nutrients, and bladder cancer. J Natl Cancer Inst 64:701–713.

HUTCHINSON GB. 1977. Summary: State-of-the-Art Conference on Bladder Cancer Screening. Washington, DC.

IARC. 1974. Evaluation of Carcinogenic Risk of Chemicals to Man: Some Aromatic Amines, Hydrazine and Related Substances, N-nitroso Compounds and Miscellaneous Alkylating Agents, Vol 4. Lyon: International Agency for Research on Cancer.

IARC. 1980. Evaluation of the Carcinogenic Risk of Chemicals to Humans: Some Pharmaceutical Drugs, Vol 24. Lyon: International Agency for Research on Cancer.

IARC. 1981. Evaluation of the Carcinogenic Risk of Chemicals to Humans: Some Antineoplastic and Immunosuppressive Agents, Vol 26. Lyon, International Agency for Research on Cancer.

IARC. 1982. Evaluation of the Carcinogenic Risk of Chemicals to Humans: Chemicals, Industrial Processes and Industries Associated with Cancer in Humans, Suppl 4. Lyon: International Agency for Research on Cancer.

IARC. 1986. Evaluation of the Carcinogenic Risk of Chemicals to Humans: Tobacco Smoking, Vol 38. Lyon: International Agency for Research on Cancer.

IARC. 1987. Overall Evaluations of Carcinogenicity: An Updating of IARC Monographs Volumes 1 to 42, Suppl 7, International Agency for Research on Cancer.

INSKIP H, BERAL V, FRASER P, et al. 1987. Further assessment of the effects of occupational radiation exposure in the United Kingdom Atomic Energy Authority mortality study. Br J Ind Med 44:149–160.

INSKIP PD, MONSON RR, WAGONER JK, et al. 1990. Cancer mortality following radiotherapy for uterine bleeding. Radiat Res 123:331–344.

ISCOVICH J, CASTELLETTO R, ESTEVE J, et al. 1987. Tobacco smoking, occupational exposure and bladder cancer in Argentina. Int J Cancer 40:734–740.

JENSEN OM, KAMBY C. 1982. Intra-uterine exposure to saccharine and risk of bladder cancer in man. Int J Cancer 29:507–509.

JENSEN OM, KNUDSEN JB, SORENSEN BL, et al. 1983. Artificial sweeteners and absence of bladder cancer risk in Copenhagen. Int J Cancer 32:577–582.

JENSEN OM, WAHRENDORF J, BLETTNER M, et al. 1987a. The Copenhagen case-control study of bladder cancer: role of smoking in invasive and non-invasive bladder tumours. J Epidemiol Community Health 41:30–36.

JENSEN OM, WAHRENDORF J, KNUDSEN JB, et al. 1986. The Copenhagen case-control study of bladder cancer, II: Effect of coffee and other beverages. Int J Cancer 37:651–657.

JENSEN OM, WAHRENDORF J, KNUDSEN JB, et al. 1987b. The Copenhagen case-referent study on bladder cancer: risks among drivers, painters and certain other occupations. Scand J Work Environ Health 13:129–134.

KABAT GC, DIECK GS, WYNDER EL. 1986. Bladder cancer in nonsmokers. Cancer 57:362–367.

KAHN HA. 1986. The Dorn study of smoking and mortality among U.S. veterans: report on eight and one-half years of observation. In: Epidemiological Approaches to the Study of Cancer and Other

Chronic Diseases, Haenszel W (ed). Natl Cancer Inst Monogr 19. Washington, DC: US Govt Print Office, pp 1–125.

KAISARY A, SMITH P, JACZQ, et al. 1987. Genetic predisposition to bladder cancer: ability to hydroxylate debrisoquine and mephenytoin as risk factors. Cancer Res 47:5488–5493.

KANTOR AF, HARTGE P, HOOVER RN, et al. 1984. Urinary tract infection and risk of bladder cancer. Am J Epidemiol 119:510–515.

KANTOR AF, HARTGE P, HOOVER RN, et al. 1985. Familial and environmental interactions in bladder cancer risk. Int J Cancer 35:703–706.

KARAKAYA AE, COK I, SARDAS S, et al. 1986. N-acetyltransferase of patients with bladder cancer. Hum Toxicol 5:333–335.

KATOH T, INATOMI H, NAGAOKA A, et al. 1995. Cytochrome P4501A1 gene polymorphism and homozygous deletion of the glutathione *S*-transferase M1 gene in urothelial cancer patients. Carcinogenesis 16:655–657.

KERN WH. 1985. Screening tests for bladder cancer. In: Screening for Cancer, Miller AB (ed). Academic Press, p 121.

KESSLER II. 1970. Cancer mortality among diabetics. J Natl Cancer Inst 44:673–686.

KESSLER II, CLARK JP. 1978. Saccharin, cyclamate, and human bladder cancer. JAMA 240:349–355.

KJAER SK, KNUDSEN JB, SORENSEN BL, et al. 1989. The Copenhagen case-control study of bladder cancer. Acta Oncol 28:631–636.

KRAMER AA, GRAHAM S, BURNETT WS, et al. 1991. Familial aggregation of bladder cancer stratified by smoking status. Epidemiology 2:145–148.

KRIEBEL D, HENRY J, GOLD JC, et al. 1985. The mutagenicity of cigarette smokers' urine. J Environ Pathol Toxicol Oncol 6:157–169.

KUNTZ RE, CHEEVER AW, MYERS BJ. 1972. Proliferative epithelial lesions of the urinary bladder of nonhuman primates infected with Schistosoma haematobium. J Natl Cancer Inst 48:223–235.

KUNZE E, CHANG-CLAUDE J, FRENTZEL-BEYME R. 1992. Life style and occupational risk factors for bladder cancer in Germany: a case-control study. Cancer 69:1776–1790.

LADERO JM, KWOK CK, JARA C, et al. 1985. Hepatic acetylator phenotype in bladder cancer patients. Ann Clin Res 17:96–99.

LAFUENTE A, PUJOL F, CARRETERO P, et al. 1993. Human glutathione *S*-transferase μ (GSTμ) deficiency as a marker for the susceptibility to bladder and larynx cancer among smokers. Cancer Lett 68:49–54.

LA VECCHIA C, NEGRI E, D'AVANZO B, et al. 1990. Occupation and the risk of bladder cancer. Int J Epidemiol 19:264–268.

LA VECCHIA C, NEGRI E, D'AVANZO B, et al. 1991. Genital and urinary tract diseases and bladder cancer. Cancer Res 51:629–631.

LA VECCHIA C, NEGRI E, DECARLI A, et al. 1989. Dietary factors in the risk of bladder cancer. Nutr Cancer 12:93–101.

LEVINE LA, RICHIE JP. 1989. Urological complications of cyclophosphamide. J Urol 141:1063–1069.

LIN HJ, HAN CY, BERNSTEIN DA, et al. 1994. Ethnic distribution of the glutathione transferase Mμ1-1 (GSTM1) null genotype in 1473 individuals and application to bladder cancer susceptibility. Carcinogenesis 15:1077–1081.

LOCKWOOD K. 1961. On the etiology of bladder tumors in København-Frederiksberg: an inquiry of 369 patients and 369 controls. Acta Pathol Microbiol Scand 51 (Suppl 145):1–166.

LOGAN WPD. 1982. Cancer Mortality by Occupation and Social Class, 1851–1971. IARC Publ No. 36. Lyon: International Agency for Research on Cancer.

LOPEZ-ABENTE G, GONZALEZ CA, ERREZOLA M, et al. 1991. Tobacco smoking inhalation pattern, tobacco type, and bladder cancer in Spain. Am J Epidemiol 134:830–839.

LOWER GM JR, NILSSON T, NELSON CE, et al. 1979. N-acetyltransferase phenotype and risk of urinary bladder cancer: approaches in molecular epidemiology. Preliminary results in Sweden and Denmark. Environ Health Perspect 29:71–79.

LYNCH CF, PLATZ CE, JONES MP, et al. 1991. Cancer Registry problems in classifying invasive bladder cancer. J Natl Cancer Inst 83:429–433.

MACLURE M, BRYANT MS, SKIPPER PL, et al. 1990. Decline of the hemoglobin adduct of 4-aminobiphenyl during withdrawal from smoking. Cancer Res 50:181–184.

MALAVEILLE C, VINEIS P, ESTEVE J, et al. 1989. Levels of mutagens in the urine of smokers of black and blond tobacco correlate with their risk of bladder cancer. Carcinogenesis 10:577–586.

MALKER HSR, MCLAUGHLIN JK, SILVERMAN DT, et al. 1987. Occupational risks for bladder cancer among men in Sweden. Cancer Res 47:6763–6766.

MARRETT LD, HARTGE P, MEIGS JW. 1986. Bladder cancer and occupational exposure to leather. Br J Ind Med 43:96–100.

MASON TJ, MCKAY F, HOOVER R, et al. 1975. Atlas of Cancer Mortality for US Counties: 1950–1969. DHEW Publ No. (NIH) 75-780. Washington, DC: US Govt Printing Office.

MATANOSKI GM, ELLIOT EA. 1981. Bladder cancer epidemiology. Epidemiol Rev 3:203–229.

MATANOSKI GM, STOCKWELL HG, DIAMOND EL, et al. 1986. A cohort mortality study of painters and allied tradesmen. Scand J Work Environ Health 12:16–21.

MCCREDIE M, STEWART JH. 1988. Does paracetamol cause urothelial cancer or renal papillary necrosis? Nephron 49:296–300.

MCCREDIE M, STEWART JH, FORD JM, et al. 1983. Phenacetin-containing analgesics and cancer of the bladder or renal pelvis in women. Br J Urol 55:220–224.

MCDONALD DF, LUND RR. 1954. The role of the urine in vesical neoplasm. 1. Experimental confirmation of the urogenous theory of pathogenesis. J Urol 71:560–570.

MCGEEHIN MA, REIF JS, BECHER JC, et al. 1993. Case-control study of bladder cancer and water disinfection methods in Colorado. Am J Epidemiol 138:492–501.

MCMICHAEL AJ, ANDJELKOVICH DA, TYROLER HA. 1976. Cancer mortality among rubber workers. Ann NY Acad Sci 271:125–137.

MCWHORTER WP, SCHATZKIN AG, HORM JW, et al. 1989. Contribution of socioeconomic status to black/white differences in cancer incidence. Cancer 63:982–987.

MEE AD. 1982. Aetiological aspects of bladder cancer in urinary bilharzia. Saudi Med J 3:123–128.

MEIGS JW, MARRETT LD, ULRICH FU, et al. 1986. Bladder tumor incidence among workers exposed to benzidine: a thirty-year follow-up. J Natl Cancer Inst 76:1–8.

MENON MM, BHIDE SY. 1984. Mutagenicity of urine of bidi and cigarette smokers and tobacco chewers. Carcinogenesis 5:1523–1524.

MESSING EM, YOUNG TB, HUNT VB, et al. 1987. The significance of asymptomatic microhematuria in men 50 or more years old: findings of a home screening study using urinary dipsticks. J Urol 137:919–922.

MESSING EM, YOUNG TB, HUNT VB, et al. 1989. Urinary tract cancers found by home screening with hematuria dipsticks in healthy men over 50 years of age. Cancer 64:2361–2367.

METTLIN C, GRAHAM S. 1979. Dietary risk factors in human bladder cancer. Am J Epidemiol 110:255–263.

MILHAM S, JR. 1976. Occupational mortality in Washington State, 1950–1971. DHEW Publ No. (NIOSH) 76-175-C. Washington, DC: US Govt Print Office.

MILLER AB, HOWE G. 1977. Artificial sweeteners and bladder cancer. Lancet 2:1221–1222.

MILLER BA, SILVERMAN DT, HOOVER RN, et al. 1986. Cancer risk among artistic painters. Am J Ind Med 9:281–287.

MILLER CT, NEUTEL CI, NAIR RC, et al. 1978. Relative importance of risk factors in bladder carcinogenesis. J Chronic Dis 31:51–56.

MILLER ME, COSGRIFF JM. 1983. Acetylator phenotype in human bladder cancer. J Urol 130:65–66.

MILLS PK, BEESON L, PHILLIPS RL, et al. 1991. Bladder cancer in a low risk population: results from the Adventist Health Study. Am J Epidemiol 133:230–239.

MOHTASHAMIPUR E, NORPOTH K, LIEDER F. 1987. Urinary excretion of mutagens in smokers of cigarettes with various tar and nicotine yields, black tobacco, and cigars. Cancer Lett 34:103–112.

MOMMSEN S, AAGAARD J. 1983. Tobacco as a risk factor in bladder cancer. Carcinogenesis 4:335–338.

MOMMSEN S AND AAGAARD J. 1986. Susceptibility in urinary bladder cancer; acetyltransferase phenotypes and related risk factors. Cancer Lett 32:199–205.

MOMMSEN S, AAGAARD J, SELL A. 1982a. An epidemiological case-control study of bladder cancer in males from a predominantly rural district. Eur J Cancer Clin Oncol 18:1205–1210.

MOMMSEN S, SELL A. 1983. Prostatic hypertrophy and venereal disease as possible risk factors in the development of bladder cancer. Urol Res 11:49–52.

MOMMSEN S, SELL A, BARFOD N. 1982b. N-acetyltransferase phenotypes of bladder cancer patients in a low-risk population. Lancet 2:1228.

MONSON RR, NAKANO KK. 1976. Mortality among rubber workers. I. White male union employees in Akron, Ohio. Am J Epidemiol 103:284–296.

MORGAN RW, JAIN MG. 1974. Bladder cancer: smoking, beverages and artificial sweeteners. Can Med Assoc J 111:1067–1070.

MORRISON AS. 1979. The public health value of using epidemiologic information to identify high risk groups for bladder cancer screening. Semin Oncol 6:184–188.

MORRISON AS. 1984a. Control of cigarette smoking in evaluating the association of coffee drinking and bladder cancer. In: Coffee and Health, Banbury Report 17, MacMahon B, Sugimura T (eds). Cold Spring Harbor, NY: Cold Spring Harbor Laboratory, pp 127–136.

MORRISON AS. 1985. Screening in Chronic Disease. New York: Oxford University Press.

MORRISON AS, AHLBOM A, VERHOEK WG, et al. 1985. Occupation and bladder cancer in Boston, USA, Manchester, UK, and Nagoya, Japan. J Epidemiol Community Health 39:294–300.

MORRISON AS, BURING JE. 1980. Artificial sweeteners and cancer of the lower urinary tract. N Engl J Med 302:537–541.

MORRISON AS, BURING JE, VERHOEK WG, et al. 1982a. Coffee drinking and cancer of the lower urinary tract. J Natl Cancer Inst 68:91–94.

MORRISON AS, BURING JE, VERHOEK WG, et al. 1984b. An international study of smoking and bladder cancer. J Urol 131:650–654.

MORRISON AS, VERHOEK WG, LECK I, et al. 1982b. Artificial sweeteners and bladder cancer in Manchester, UK, and Nagoya, Japan. Br J Cancer 45:332–336.

MUIR C, WATERHOUSE J, MACK T, et al, eds. 1987. Cancer Incidence in Five Continents, Vol V. IARC Publ No. 88. Lyon: International Agency for Research on Cancer.

MUSTACCHI P, SHIMKIN MB. 1958. Cancer of the bladder and infestation with Schistosoma hematobium. J Natl Cancer Inst 20:825–842.

MYSLAK ZW, BOLT HM, BROCKMANN W. 1991. Tumors of the urinary bladder in painters: a case-control study. Am J Ind Med 19:705–713.

NAJEM GR, LOURIA DB, SEEBODE JJ, et al. 1982. Life time occupation, smoking, caffeine, saccharine, hair dyes and bladder carcinogenesis. Int J Epidemiol 11:212–217.

NAS (National Academy of Sciences). 1990. Health Risks of Exposure to Low Levels of Ionizing Radiation (BEIR V). Washington, DC: Natl Acad Press.

NATIONAL CANCER INSTITUTE. 1989. Cancer Statistics Review, 1973–1986, Including a Report on the Status of Cancer Control. NIH Publ No. 89–2789. Bethesda, Md: NCI.

NATIONAL RESEARCH COUNCIL. 1980. Drinking Water and Health, Vol 3. Washington, DC: Natl Acad Press, pp 5–21.

NEGRI E, PIOLATTO G, PIRA E, et al. 1989. Cancer mortality in a northern Italian cohort of rubber workers. Br J Ind Med 46:624–628.

NOMURA A, KOLONEL LN, YOSHIZAWA CN. 1989. Smoking, alcohol, occupation and hair dye use in cancer of the lower urinary tract. Am J Epidemiol 130:1159–1163.

NOMURA AMY, STEMMERMANN GN, HEILBRUN LK, et al. 1985. Serum vitamin levels and the risk of cancer of specific sites in men of Japanese ancestry in Hawaii. Cancer Res 45:2369–2372.

OYASU R, HIRAO Y, IZUMI K. 1981. Enhancement by urine of urinary bladder carcinogenesis. Cancer Res 41:478–481.

PAGE WF, KUNTZ AJ. 1980. Racial and socioeconomic factors in cancer survival: a comparison of Veterans Administration results with selected studies. Cancer 45:1029–1040.

PARKASH O, KIESSWETTER H. 1976. The role of urine in the etiology of cancer of the urinary bladder. Urol Int 31:343–348.

PARKES HG, VEYS CA, WATERHOUSE JAH, et al. 1982. Cancer mortality in the British rubber industry. Br J Ind Med 39:209–220.

PARKIN DM, MUIR CS, WHELAN SL, et al. 1992. Cancer Incidence in Five Continents, Vol VI. IARC Publ. No. 120. Lyon: International Agency for Research on Cancer.

PAYET M. 1962. Mortality and morbidity from bladder cancer in West Africa. Acta Unio Int Contra Cancrum 18:641–642.

PEDERSON-BJERGAARD J, ERSBOLL J, HANSEN VL, et al. 1988. Carcinoma of the urinary bladder after treatment with cyclophosphamide for non-Hodgkin's lymphoma. N Engl J Med 318:1028–1032.

PICKLE LW, MASON TJ, HOWARD N, et al. 1987. Atlas of US Cancer Mortality among Whites: 1950–80. DHHS Publ No. (NIH) 87-2900. Washington, DC: US Govt Print Office.

PIOLATTO G, NEGRI E, LA VECCHIA C, et al. 1991. Bladder cancer mortality of workers exposed to aromatic amines: an updated analysis. Br J Cancer 63:457–459.

PIPER JM, MATANOSKI GM, TONASCIA J. 1986. Bladder cancer in young women. Am J Epidemiol 123:1033–1042.

PIPER JM, TONASCIA J, MATANOSKI GM. 1985. Heavy phenacetin use and bladder cancer in women aged 20 to 49 years. N Engl J Med 313:292–295.

POPP W, SCHMIEDING W, SPECK M, et al. 1992. Incidence of bladder cancer in a cohort of workers exposed to 4-chloro-o-toluidine while synthesizing chlordimeform. Br J Ind Med 49:529–531.

PRICE JM, BROWN RR. 1962. Studies on the etiology of carcinoma of the urinary bladder. Acta Unio Int Contra Cancrum 18:684–688.

PUJOLAR AE, GONZALEZ CA, LOPEZ-ABENTE G, et al. 1993. Bladder cancer and coffee consumption in smokers and nonsmokers in Spain. Int J Epidemiol 22:38–44.

PUNTONI R, BOLOGNESI C, BONASSI S, et al. 1988. Cancer risk evaluation in an area with a high density of chemical plants: an interdisciplinary approach. Ann NY Acad Sci 534:808–816.

QUAGLIARIELLO E, TANCREDI F, FEDELE L, et al. 1961. Tryptophan–nicotinic acid metabolism in patients with tumors of the bladder: changes in the excretory products after treatment with nicotinamide and vitamin B6. Br J Cancer 15:367–372.

REBELAKOS A, TRICHOPOULOS D, TZONOU A, et al. 1985. Tobacco smoking, coffee drinking, and occupation as risk factors for bladder cancer in Greece. J Natl Cancer Inst 75:455–461.

RIBOLI E, GONZALEZ CA, LOPEZ-ABENTE G, et al. 1991. Diet and bladder cancer in Spain: a multi-centre case-control study. Int J Cancer 49:214–219.

RISCH HA, BURCH JD, MILLER AB, et al. 1988a. Occupational factors and the incidence of cancer of the bladder in Canada. Br J Ind Med 45:361–367.

RISCH HA, BURCH JD, MILLER AB, et al. 1988b. Dietary factors and the incidence of cancer of the urinary bladder. Am J Epidemiol 127:1179–1191.

ROCKETTE HE, ARENA VC. 1983. Mortality studies of aluminum reduction plant workers: potroom and carbon department. J Occup Med 25:549–557.

ROTHMAN N, BHATNAGAR YK, HAYES RB, et al. The impact of *NAT2* activity on benzidine urinary metabolites and urothelial DNA adducts in exposed workers. Proc Natl Acad Sci (in press).

ROWLAND RG, HENNEBERRY MO, OYASU R, et al. 1980. Effects of urine and continued exposure to carcinogen on progression of early neoplastic urinary bladder lesions. Cancer Res 40:4524–4527.

RUBINO GF, SCANSETTI G, PIOLATTO G, et al. 1982. The carcinogenic effect of aromatic amines: an epidemiological study on the role of O-toluidine and 4,4'-methylene bis(2-methylaniline) in inducing bladder cancer in man. Environ Res 27:241–254.

SCHAIRER C, HARTGE P, HOOVER RN, et al. 1988. Racial differences in bladder cancer risk: a case-control study. Am J Epidemiol 128:1027–1037.

SCHIFFLERS E, JAMART J, RENARD V. 1987. Tobacco and occupation as risk factors in bladder cancer: a case-control study in southern Belgium. Int J Cancer 39:287–292.

SCHULTE PA. 1988. The role of genetic factors in bladder cancer. Cancer Detect Prev 11:379–388.

SCHULTE PA, RINGEN K, HEMSTREET GP, et al. 1986. Risk factors for bladder cancer in a cohort exposed to aromatic amines. Cancer 58:2156–2162.

SCHULTE PA, RINGEN K, HEMSTREET GP, et al. 1987. Occupational cancer of the urinary tract. Occup Med 2:85–107.

SENIORI COSTANTINI A, PACI E, MILIGI L, et al. 1989. Cancer mortality among workers in the Tuscan tanning industry. Br J Ind Med 46:384–388.

SHAW GH. 1977. Use of Papanicolaou staining to predict urinary tract cancer. Paper presented at the State-of-the-Art Conference; Bladder Cancer Screening, Washington, DC.

SIEMIATYCHI J, DEWAR R, NADON L, et al. 1994. Occupational risk factors for bladder cancer: Results from a case-control study in Montreal, Quebec, Canada. Am J Epidemiol 140:1061–1080.

SILVERMAN DT, HOOVER RN, ALBERT S, et al. 1983. Occupation and cancer of the lower urinary tract in Detroit. J Natl Cancer Inst 70:237–245.

SILVERMAN DT, HOOVER RN, MASON TJ, et al. 1986. Motor exhaust-related occupations and bladder cancer. Cancer Res 46:2113–2116.

SILVERMAN DT, LEVIN LI, HOOVER RN. 1989a. Occupational risks of bladder cancer in the United States: II. Nonwhite men. J Natl Cancer Inst 81:1480–1483.

SILVERMAN DT, LEVIN LI, HOOVER RN. 1990. Occupational risks of bladder cancer among white women in the United States. Am J Epidemiol 132:453–461.

SILVERMAN DT, LEVIN LI, HOOVER RN, et al. 1989b. Occupational risks of bladder cancer in the United States: I. White men. J Natl Cancer Inst 81:1472–1480.

SIMON D, YEN S, COLE P. 1975. Coffee drinking and cancer of the lower urinary tract. J Natl Cancer Inst 54:587–591.

SLATTERY ML, SCHUMACHER MC, WEST DW, et al. 1988a. Smoking and bladder cancer: the modifying effect of cigarettes on other factors. Cancer 61:402–408.

SLATTERY ML, WEST DW, ROBISON LM. 1988b. Fluid intake and bladder cancer in Utah. Int J Cancer 42:17–22.

SMITH PG, DOUGLAS AJ. 1986. Mortality of workers at the Sellafield plant of British Nuclear Fuels. Br Med J 293:845–854.

SOLE G, SORAHAN T. 1985. Coarse fishing and risk of urothelial cancer. Lancet 1:1477–1479.

SORAHAN T, SOLE G. 1990. Coarse fishing and urothelial cancer: a regional case-control study. Br J Cancer 62:138–141.

SPINELLI JJ, BAND PR, SVIRCHEV LM, et al. 1991. Mortality and cancer incidence in aluminum reduction plant workers. J Occup Med 33:1150–1155.

STASIK MJ. 1988. Carcinomas of the urinary bladder in a 4-chloro-O-toluidine cohort. Int Arch Occup Environ Health 60:21–24.

STEENLAND K, BURNETT C, OSORIO AM. 1987. A case-control study of bladder cancer using city directories as a source of occupational data. Am J Epidemiol 126:247–257.

STEINECK G, HAGMAN V, GERHARDSSON M, et al. 1990. Vitamin A supplements, fried foods, fat and urothelial cancer: a case-referent study in Stockholm in 1985–87. Int J Cancer 45:1006–1011.

STEINECK G, NORELL SE, FEYCHTING M. 1988. Diet, tobacco and urothelial cancer: A 14-year follow-up of 16477 subjects. Acta Oncol 27:323–327.

STERN FB, BEAUMONT JJ, HALPERIN WE, et al. 1987. Mortality of chrome leather tannery workers and chemical exposures in tanneries. Scand J Work Environ Health 13:108–117.

TALASKA G, AL-JUBURI AZSS, KADLUBAR FF. 1991a. Smoking related carcinogen-DNA adducts in biopsy samples of human urinary bladder: identification of *N*-(deoxyquanosin-8-yl)-4-aminobiphenyl as a major adduct. Proc Natl Acad Sci U S A 88:5340–5354.

TALASKA G, SCHAMER M, SKIPPER P, et al. 1991b. Detection of carcinogen-DNA adducts in exfoliated urothelial cells of cigarette smokers: association with smoking, hemoglobin adducts, and urinary mutagenicity. Cancer Epidemiol Biomarkers Prev 1:61–66.

TAWFIK HN. 1988. Carcinoma of the urinary bladder associated with schistosomiasis in Egypt: The possible causal relationship. In: Unusual Occurrences as Clues to Cancer Etiology, Miller RW, et al (eds). Tokyo: Japan Sci Soc Press, pp 197–209.

THERIAULT G, DEGUIRE L, CORDIER S. 1981. Reducing aluminum: an occupation possibly associated with bladder cancer. Can Med Assoc J 124:419–425.

THERIAULT G, TREMBLAY C, CORDIER S, et al. 1984. Bladder cancer in the aluminum industry. Lancet 1:947–950.

THIEDE T, CHRISTENSEN BC. 1969. Bladder tumours induced by chlornaphazine. A five-year follow-up study of chlornaphazine-treated patients with polycythaemia. Acta Med Scand 185:133–137.

THOMAS DB, UHL CN, HARTGE P. 1983. Bladder cancer and alcoholic beverage consumption. Am J Epidemiol 118:720–727.

TRAVIS LB, CURTIS RE, BOICE JD JR, et al. 1989. Bladder cancer after chemotherapy for non-Hodgkin's lymphoma. N Engl J Med 321:544–545.

TRAVIS LB, CURTIS RE, GLIMELIUS B, et al. 1995. Bladder and kidney cancer following cyclophosphamide therapy for non-Hodgkin's lymphoma. J Natl Cancer Inst 87:524–530.

TYLER HA, NOTLEY RG, SCHWEITZER FAW, et al. 1986. Vitamin A status and bladder cancer. Eur J Surg Oncol 12:35–41.

UICC. 1984. Screening for Cancer. I. General Principles on Evaluation of Screening for Cancer and Screening for Lung, Bladder and Oral Cancer. UICC Technical Report Series, Vol 78. Geneva, International Union Against Cancer.

US CONGRESS, OFFICE OF TECHNOLOGY ASSESSMENT. 1977. Cancer Testing Technology and Saccharin. Washington, DC: US Govt Print Office.

VENA JE, GRAHAM S, FREUDENHEIM J, et al. 1992. Diet in the epidemiology of bladder cancer in western New York. Nutr Cancer 18:255–264.

VENA JE, GRAHAM S, FREUDENHEIM J, et al. 1993. Drinking water, fluid intake, and bladder cancer in western New York. Arch Environ Health 48:191–198.

VINEIS P, BARTSCH H, CAPORASO N, et al. 1994. Genetically based *N*-acetyltransferase metabolic polymorphism and low-level environmental exposure to carcinogens. Nature 369:154–156.

VINEIS P, CAPORASO N, TANNENBAUM S, et al. 1990. The acetylation phenotype, carcinogen-hemophobin adducts, and cigarette smoking. Cancer Res 50:3002–3004.

VINEIS P, DIPRIMA S. 1983. Cutting oils and bladder cancer. Scand J Work Environ Health 9:449–450.

VINEIS P, ESTEVE J, HARTGE P, et al. 1988. Effects of timing and type of tobacco in cigarette-induced bladder cancer. Cancer Res 48:3849–3852.

VINEIS P, ESTEVE J, TERRACINI B. 1984. Bladder cancer and smoking in males: types of cigarettes, age at start, effect of stopping and interaction with occupation. Int J Cancer 34:165–170.

VINEIS P, MAGNANI C. 1985. Occupation and bladder cancer in males: a case-control study. Int J Cancer 35:599–606.

VIZCAINO AP, PARKIN DM, BOFFETTA P, et al. 1994. Bladder cancer: epidemiology and risk factors in Bulawayo, Zimbabwe. Cancer Causes Control 5:517–522.

WAGONER JK. 1970. Leukemia and Other Malignancies Following Radiation Therapy for Gynecological Disorders. Unpublished doctoral thesis, Harvard School of Public Health, Boston.

WALKER AM, DREYER NA, FRIEDLANDER E, et al. 1982. An independent analysis of the National Cancer Institute Study on non-nutritive sweeteners and bladder cancer. Am J Public Health 72:376–381.

WARD E, CARPENTER A, MARKOWITZ S, et al. 1991. Excess number of bladder cancers in workers exposed to ortho-toluidine and aniline. J Natl Cancer Inst 83:501–506.

WARD E, HALPERIN W, THUN M, et al. 1988. Bladder tumors in two young males occupationally exposed to MBOCA. Am J Ind Med 14:267–272.

WARNER ML, MOORE LE, SMITH MT, et al. 1994. Increased micronuclei in exfoliated bladder cells of individuals who chronically ingest arsenic-contaminated water in Nevada. Cancer Epidemiol Biomarkers Prev 3:583–590.

WEBER WW, HEIN DW, LITWIN A, et al. 1983. Relationship of acetylator status to isoniazid toxicity, lupus erythematosus, and bladder cancer. Fed Proc 42:3086–3097.

WIGLE DT. 1977. Bladder cancer: possible new high-risk occupation. Lancet 2:83–84.

WILKINS JR III, COMSTOCK GW. 1981. Source of drinking water at home and site-specific cancer incidence in Washington County, Maryland. Am J Epidemiol 114:178–190.

WILLIAMS RR, HORM JW. 1977. Association of cancer sites with tobacco and alcohol consumption and socioeconomic status of patients: interview study from the Third National Cancer Survey. J Natl Cancer Inst 58:525–547.

WOODHOUSE KW, ADAMS PC, CLOTHIER A, et al. 1982. N-acetylation phenotype in bladder cancer. Hum Toxicol 1:443–445.

WU M-M, KUO T-L, HWANG Y-H, et al. 1989. Dose-response relation between arsenic concentration in well water and mortality from cancers and vascular diseases. Am J Epidemiol 130:1123–1132.

WYNDER EL, AUGUSTINE A, KABAT G, et al. 1988. Effect of the type of cigarette smoked on bladder cancer risk. Cancer 61:622–627.

WYNDER EL, GOLDSMITH R. 1977. The epidemiology of bladder cancer: a second look. Cancer 40:1246–1268.

WYNDER EL, ONDERDONK J, MANTEL N. 1963. An epidemiological investigation of cancer of the bladder. Cancer 16:1388–1407.

WYNDER EL, STELLMAN SD. 1977. Comparative epidemiology of tobacco-related cancers. Cancer Res 37:4608–4622.

WYNDER EL, STELLMAN SD. 1980. Artificial sweetener use and bladder cancer: a case-control study. Science 207:1214–1216.

YAMASAKI E, AMES BN. 1977. Concentration of mutagens from urine by absorption with the nonpolar resin XAD-2: cigarette smokers have mutagenic urine. Proc Natl Acad Sci U S A 74:3555–3559.

YOSHIDA O, HARADA T, MIYAGAWA M, et al. 1971. Bladder cancer in workers in the dyeing industry. Igaku No Ayumi (Jpn) 79:421.

YOUNG JL JR, PERCY CL, ASIRE AJ, EDS. 1981. Surveillance, Epidemiology, End Results: Incidence and Mortality Data, 1973–77. NCI Monogr 57:1–1082.

YU MC, ROSS RK, CHANK K, et al. 1995. Glutathione *S*-transferase M1 genotype affects aminobiphenyl-hemoglobin adduct levels in white, black, and Asian smokers and nonsmokers. Cancer Epidemiol Biomarkers Prev 4:861–864.

YU MC, SKIPPER PL, TAGHIZADEHK, et al. 1994. Acetylator phenotype, aminobiphenyl-hemoglobin adduct levels, and bladder cancer risk in white, black, and Asian men in Los Angeles, California. J Natl Cancer Inst 86:712–716.

ZHONG S, WYLLIE AH, BARNES, et al. 1993. Relationship between the GTSM1 genetic polymorphism and susceptibility to bladder, breast and colon cancer. Carcinogenesis 14:1821–1824.

ZIERLER S, FEINGOLD L, DANLEY RA, et al. 1988. Bladder cancer in Massachusetts related to chlorinated and chloraminated drinking water: a case-control study. Arch Environ Health 43:195–200.

55 Prostate cancer

RONALD K. ROSS
DAVID SCHOTTENFELD

Prostate cancer is now the most common cancer diagnosed among men in the United States, accounting for 27.5% of all cancer cases in men. Approximately 244,000 cases will be diagnosed in 1995, and 40,600 deaths are anticipated for that year. Prostate cancer ranks second after lung cancer as the underlying cause of cancer deaths in men, accounting for almost 13% of all cancer deaths and 2.5% of all deaths in U.S. men (Miller et al, 1993). Because 90% of deaths due to prostate cancer occur after age 65, or at a median age of 77 years, the major impact of the disease is on the subgroup in the population with relatively limited life expectancy (Whitmore, 1994). Although the etiology is unknown, the major credible hypotheses that have been proposed involve hormonal patterns, family history, and dietary practices.

ANATOMIC DISTRIBUTION AND HISTOPATHOLOGY

The prostate is a small accessory sex gland located at the base of the bladder (Clemente and Gray, 1985). The main function of prostatic fluid appears to be to aid sperm in traversing the female genital tract by adjusting the pH of semen and liquefying cervical mucus (Isaacs, 1983). The development and maintenance of the prostate is largely controlled by the male sex hormone testosterone, which diffuses from plasma into the prostate where it is converted to dihydrotestosterone (DHT) by the enzyme 5-alpha reductase. Dihydrotestosterone is bound to cytoplasmic receptors and translocated to cell nuclei where it controls cell replication (Coffey, 1979).

Prostate cancers are almost uniformly adenocarcinomas arising in glandular acini (Waisman, 1988). Benign histologic precursors of prostate cancer have not been well studied. However, atypical hyperplasia (adenosis) and especially prostatic intraepithelial neoplasia (PIN) frequently occur in conjunction with adenocarcinoma (Kastendieck and Helpap, 1989). High-grade PIN is frequently associated with DNA aneuploidy which is indicative of genetic instability (Prendergast and Walther, 1995). Transitional cell carcinomas, squamous cell carcinomas, and sarcomas combined comprise less than 1% of all prostatic cancers. Adenocarcinoma of the prostate spreads through lymphatics and blood. Metastases to bone occur in two-thirds of patients with advanced disease. Surveillance, Epidemiology and End Results (SEER) data for patients diagnosed in 1983–89 indicated a 79% 5-year relative survival rate for prostate cancer among whites across all stages of disease, compared to 64% for blacks (Miller et al, 1993). Five-year relative survival is strongly related to stage—92% for patients with disease confined to the prostate, 82% for patients with regional metastases, and 28% for patients presenting with distant metastases. There has been a gradual improvement in 5-year relative survival rates for prostate cancer overall among both whites and blacks in the United States in recent years, but the difference in survival rates between blacks and whites across all stages of disease has actually increased during the past two decades (i.e., 8% in 1970–73, and 15% in 1983–89) (Silverberg and Lubera, 1989; Myers and Ries, 1989; Boring et al, 1992).

Radical prostatectomy is generally recommended for localized disease and hormonal therapy for more advanced disease, although other potentially curative treatment strategies such as external beam radiation therapy are also widely used and some have questioned whether any treatment is required for early stage disease, particularly among elderly men (Trump and Robertson, 1993; Catalona, 1994).

DEMOGRAPHIC PATTERNS

Age

Prostate cancer is rare before age 40, and then incidence rates double for each subsequent decade of life (Ross et al, 1979). The age-specific incidence curve for prostate cancer has a steeper slope than for any other cancer, increasing at approximately the eighth or ninth power of age in men older than 50 years.

Race/International Variation

Although the prostate is the most common site of cancer in U.S. men, prostate cancer is the fifth most frequent cancer worldwide (Parkin et al, 1984). There is approximately a 30-fold difference internationally between the highest incidence rate among African-American men and the lowest rates in China and Japan (Muir et al, 1987). In 1990, age-adjusted incidence (per 100,000) among U.S. blacks (163.6) was about 27% higher than for U.S. whites (128.5). Although an excess among U.S. blacks, compared to U.S. whites, persists throughout the age range in which prostate cancer occurs, it appears to be of a lower magnitude at more advanced ages (Satariano and Swanson, 1988). The cumulative incidence rate for U.S. blacks approaches 30% by age 85 (Ross et al, 1988). The high incidence rate among blacks does not appear to have a strong genetic basis. Although exactly comparable incidence data for blacks in Africa are nonexistent, prostate cancer appears to be less common (Higginson and Oettle, 1960; Kovi and Heshmat, 1972).

Among countries with reasonably reliable cancer statistics, China and Japan have the lowest prostate cancer incidence rates. Asian-Americans have rates which are approximately one-third to one-half those of U.S. whites, but there is still a three- to five-fold excess risk among Japanese- and Chinese-Americans over native Japanese and Chinese, respectively. Although some of the difference in incidence between native Japanese, on the one hand, and Japanese-Americans and other Americans on the other, is due to differences in detection strategies for prostate cancer between countries (Shimizu et al, 1991a), the results of migrant studies appear to show some real shift in incidence toward rates in the new host country, providing evidence that these international and racial differences in prostate cancer incidence are not based entirely on genetic predisposition.

Rates for U.S. and other North American whites are substantially less than those for blacks, but they are higher than rates elsewhere in the world. Non-Hispanic whites in the U.S. have prostate cancer incidence rates somewhat higher than Hispanics (SEER, 1984; Bernstein and Ross, 1995). Incidence rates in the United Kingdom are, inexplicably, only roughly one-half those in U.S. whites. Incidence rates in Israel are among the lowest observed outside of the Orient.

The geographic pathology of latent or subclinical prostate cancer compared to clinical disease has been the subject of considerable epidemiologic study. The overall and age-specific prevalences of latent prostate cancer appear to have considerably less geographic and racial variation than clinical prostate cancer, but the observed trends are compatible with those of clinical disease. Yatani et al (1982) have observed, for example, using serially step-sectioned and microscopically examined prostate specimens from autopsy series, that the prevalence of latent carcinomas of the prostate is slightly higher for U.S. blacks (37%) than for U.S. whites (35%) which, in turn, is higher than that for Japanese migrants in Hawaii (26%) or for native Japanese (21%). These data also indicate the very high international prevalence of latent prostate cancer. The prevalence rate of latent carcinomas tends to increase with age in all populations. The frequency of latent carcinoma of the prostate in Japan, as with clinical prostate cancer, appears to be increasing and approaching the prevalence rate for U.S. whites (Yatani et al, 1988). These observations have been interpreted to be consistent with a two-step model of prostate carcinogenesis, with the prevalence of exposure to initiating factors showing less international diversity than exposure to the necessary promotional factors (Yatani et al, 1988). Although it is widely assumed that latent prostate cancer is a precursor of clinical disease, this assumption remains untested. Whittemore et al (1991) have provided evidence that the volume of low-grade, latent prostate cancer tissue at any age is a useful predictor of subsequent risk of aggressive symptomatic prostate cancer.

There is considerably less international variation in prostate cancer mortality than in prostate cancer incidence among those countries with both types of data available, although U.S. blacks, on the one hand, and Japanese, on the other, still represent the opposite ends of the spectrum for prostate cancer mortality. In the United States, age-adjusted prostate cancer mortality rates in 1977–83 demonstrated the following pattern by ethnic group: African-American (43.9); non-Hispanic white (21.1); Mexican-American (19.4); native Hawaiian (15.8); American Indian (11.7); Filipino (8.7); Japanese (8.4); and Chinese (7.4) (Reynolds, 1992). Mortality rates are also very high in Sweden, where incidence rates are comparable to those for U.S. whites, and in Switzerland, where incidence rates are somewhat lower. Mortality rates for U.S. whites are about 25% less than rates in these two high-risk countries (Segi, 1978). The highest mortality rates worldwide have been reported from Caribbean countries and the lowest from Central America and Southeast Asia, but none of these countries have population-based incidence data available for comparison. Zaridze et al (1984) have described the wide variation internationally in the ratio of prostatic cancer mortality to incidence rates. Mortality rates are about two-thirds or more of the incidence rates in Japan, England, and Eastern Europe, compared to one-third or less of the incidence rates in most U.S. populations. As calculated by Scardino et al (1992), for a 50-year-old U.S. man with a life expectancy of 25 years, the cumulative lifetime incidence of microscopic, clinical, or fatal prostatic cancer is approximately 42%, 9.5%, and 2.9%, respectively.

Migration

Migrant studies have evaluated prostate cancer risk among immigrants to the United States, where the prevailing rates of prostate cancer are high, who arrive in the United States from countries where the prevailing rates are substantially less, such as Poland or Japan (Table 55–1). All such analyses show a shift in risk toward the U.S. rate. For example, Haenszel and Kurihara (1968) found that Japanese migrants to the U.S. had almost four times the prostate cancer mortality rate of Japanese men, but still only 40% that of U.S. whites. In fact, there is no evidence that prostate cancer rates among Japanese-Americans ever approach those of U.S. whites, much less those of U.S. blacks. Lilienfeld et al (1972) reported that Polish migrants to the U.S. were three times as likely to die of prostate cancer as Polish residents in Poland, but 20% less than those of U.S. whites.

TABLE 55–1. *Age-Adjusted Death Rates for Prostate Cancer Per 100,000 Population of Selected Countries, 1982–1983**

Country	*Rate*	*Country*	*Rate*
Martinique[a]	52.1	Northern Ireland[b]	20.0
Switzerland	32.0	England and Wales	19.2
Luxembourg	31.3	Portugal	18.8
Barbados	30.0	Scotland	18.0
Norway	30.0	Venezuela[b]	18.0
Iceland	28.2	Czechoslovakia	17.9
Sweden	27.3	Chile	17.4
Denmark	26.4	Costa Rica	17.2
Belgium	26.3	Panama	16.5
Netherlands	26.0	Dominican Republic[a]	16.3
Germany, F.R.	24.7	Yugoslavia[a]	16.0
France	24.4	Germany, D.R.	15.5
Uruguay	24.1	Israel	13.5
New Zealand	24.1	Poland	13.0
Cuba	24.0	Paraguay	11.7
Finland	23.7	Greece	11.6
Surinam[a]	23.7	Mexico[a]	11.2
Hungary	23.4	Rumania	10.3
Australia	23.2	Bulgaria	10.3
Austria	23.2	Peru[a]	9.4
United States	23.1	Kuwait	9.1
Ireland	22.4	Mauritius	5.9
Canada	22.2	Singapore[b]	5.4
Malta and Gozo	21.5	Japan	4.6
Puerto Rico	20.6	El Salvador	3.3

*From CA—A Cancer Journal for Clinicians 39:16–17, 1989, as abstracted from the World Health Statistics Annual, 1983–1986.
[a]1982 only.
[b]1983 only.

Shimizu et al (1991b), in an analysis of prostate cancer incidence among Japanese in Los Angeles (LA) County, California, used social security numbers to distinguish those migrating to LA County earlier from those migrating later in adult life. Prostate cancer rates among Japanese in LA County were intermediate between those of LA County whites and those among Japanese in Japan. Furthermore, rates among "late" immigrants were almost as high as those among "early" immigrants.

Time Trends

It is generally accepted that both prostate cancer incidence and mortality rates have been increasing worldwide over the past several decades. Zaridze et al (1984) compared prostate cancer mortality in 42 countries between the 1950s and late 1970s. Only three countries (Egypt, Barbados, and Bulgaria) failed to show an increase over this period. The largest increases in mortality tended to occur among those countries with the lowest baseline prostate cancer mortality rates. For example, age-adjusted mortality rates increased almost eight-fold in Japan during a 3-decade period ending in 1978, whereas rates in Hong Kong tripled over a 2-decade period ending in the same year. By comparison, U.S. mortality rates increased only 6% overall during a comparable time period (Silverberg and Lubera, 1989). In the United States, the modest overall increase in mortality rates has been due almost entirely to a much larger increase among nonwhites; the mortality rates for whites were very stable from the 1950s through the early 1970s and then increased 18% from 1973–90 (Aoki et al, 1992; Miller et al, 1993).

When time trends in prostate cancer mortality worldwide are evaluated by age, it is clear that almost uniformly around the world much larger increases have occurred among men over age 65 than at younger ages (Zaridze et al, 1984). During the period 1973–1990, for men under age 65, mortality increased by 13% among U.S. whites and 6% among U.S. blacks; for men 65 and over, mortality increased by 19% among whites and 39% among blacks. Ernster et al (1977) conducted a birth cohort analysis of prostate cancer mortality among U.S. nonwhites and found that rates for all age-groups peaked in the birth cohort 1896–1900 and have since declined. In a more recent cohort mortality analysis based on 20 additional years of data, Hsing and Devesa (1994) observed that the peak reported previously in the 1896–1900 nonwhite birth cohort has not persisted. The age-specific rates for blacks 65 and over have continued to increase in cohorts born between 1900 and 1920.

Cancer Incidence in Five Continents has been published every 5 years over the past 25 years (Doll et al, 1966, 1970; Waterhouse et al, 1976, 1982; Muir et al, 1987; Parkin et al, 1992) and provides an excellent resource for monitoring secular trends in cancer incidence among selected populations, using data from population-based cancer registries worldwide. Zaridze et al (1984) have previously summarized trends in incidence through 1975 based on the first four volumes and have shown that, like mortality rates, incidence rates have increased almost uniformly (i.e., around 3% per year) around the world. Unlike mortality statistics, the largest increases have not necessarily been limited to those populations with the lowest rates initially (Boyle et al, 1995).

In Table 55–2, we have extended these comparisons to include data published from *Cancer Incidence in Five Continents*, Volumes V and VI (Muir et al, 1987; Parkin et al, 1992). Note that incidence rates for the most part have continued to increase around the world since 1975. Unlike mortality data, the observed increases in incidence rates have not been predictably greater among men over age 65, compared to younger age-groups. Using combined registry data from the SEER program, prostate cancer incidence in the U.S. increased 85% from 1973 to 1990 (Ries et al, 1990; Miller et al, 1993), or some four times greater than the percentage change in mortality (20%) during this period.

Doll and Peto (1981) have argued that much if not all of the increase in prostate cancer incidence over the last several decades is artifactual. They have noted the relatively stable mortality rates for men under age 65 in many populations, which have occurred in the face of substantial increases in incidence and with minimal changes in survival rates. They suggest that these increases in incidence might be due to more aggressive diagnosis and screening, using digital rectal examination (DRE), and more recently, prostate-specific antigen (PSA) and transrectal ultrasound, which would increase the discovery rate of latent carcinomas (Catalona et al, 1993). Potosky et al (1990) have argued that the nationwide increase in prostate cancer incidence during the 1970s and 1980s was due almost entirely to increasing rates of transurethral resection (TURP) for clinically benign prostatic hyperplastic disease (BPH) but with concurrent detection of prostate cancer. Transurethral resections for BPH have been associated with the incidental diagnosis of prostate cancer in 8% to 22% of procedures (Murphy et al, 1986).

Other Demographic Risk Factors

Other possible demographic risk factors, such as socioeconomic status, urban versus rural residence, religion, and marital status have been explored in relationship to prostate cancer risk. For the most part, any observed differences are small.

The possible relationship between socioeconomic characteristics and prostate cancer incidence and mortality has been explored in a variety of ways: e.g., using occupational data from death certificates or using median family income or educational level in the geographic area of residence to define socioeconomic class. These studies find that there are no large differences in prostate cancer risk between men in the highest versus those in the lowest socioeconomic strata, no matter how socioeconomic status is defined (Seidman, 1970; Ernster et al, 1977; Hoover et al, 1975; Richardson, 1965; Baquet et al, 1991). Ross et al (1979) have shown that the marked excess of prostate cancer in blacks persists across all socioeconomic strata, when socioeconomic status is defined by the median income and educational level of the census tract of residence at diagnosis.

Mandel and Schuman (1980) have summarized data on urban–rural comparisons of prostate cancer incidence and mortality. Most studies find a slight excess in urban areas; in the U.S., these differences appear to be at most 15%, and not all studies consistently report such an excess (Lilienfeld et al, 1972).

Despite substantially lower than expected incidence and mortality rates for cancer overall and for most cancer sites, Mormons in Utah have an approximately 10%–15% higher incidence and mortality rate from prostate cancer than do men in the U.S. as a whole (Lyon et al, 1976, 1977). Seventh Day Adventists (SDAs), who, like Mormons, proscribe use of alcohol, tobacco, and caffeine beverages, but who also advocate a lacto-ovo-vegetarian diet, appear to have a somewhat reduced incidence and mortality rate from prostate cancer compared to national data (Phillips, 1975; Phillips and Snowdon, 1983). Jewish men in the U.S. have been reported to have a reduced risk of prostate cancer (MacMahon, 1969). This observation is consistent with the quite low incidence of prostate cancer reported for Jews in Israel (Waterhouse et al, 1982).

Population-based cancer incidence and mortality analyses of whites consistently find a higher rate of prostate cancer among married compared to never-married men (Lilienfeld et al, 1972; Newell et al, 1987; Clemmesen, 1969; Ernster et al, 1979a), but data for nonwhites by marital status are inconsistent (Lilienfeld et al, 1972; Newell et al, 1987). Mortality data for whites suggest an even higher risk among divorcees and widowers than for those currently married (Lilienfeld et al, 1972; Wigle, 1978), but incidence data do not consistently support this observation (Newell et al, 1987).

TABLE 55–2. *Time Trends in Age-Adjusted Prostatic Cancer Incidence Among Selected Cancer Registries*†

Registry	Location[a]	Circa 1985	Circa 1980	Circa 1975	Circa 1970	Circa 1965	Circa 1960	Percentage Change 1960–1980	Percentage Change 1970–1980
USA, Alameda black	NA	93.5	87.8	100.2	75.0	65.3	*	—	17
USA, Bay Area black	NA	95.6	82.5	92.2	77.0	*	*	—	7
Hawaii, Caucasian	NA	62.8	58.3	59.8	42.3	43.4	40.9	43	38
Canada, Saskatchewan	NA	53.0	57.6	46.1	39.0	39.0	33.4	72	48
USA, Bay Area white	NA	57.8	50.0	47.4	44.6	*	*	—	12
USA, Alameda white	NA	55.2	49.6	44.5	40.4	38.0	*	—	23
USA, Connecticut white	NA	47.2	46.8	42.7	37.7	33.0	33.8	38	24
Sweden	WE	50.2	45.9	44.4	38.8	33.5	26.5	73	18
Canada, Alberta	NA	54.9	45.3	37.8	32.4	23.5	21.3	113	40
Canada, Manitoba	NA	54.7	44.4	43.2	37.6	31.1	30.6	45	18
USA, New York State (less New York City)	NA	48.9	42.6	39.9	29.4	*	23.5	81	45
Norway	WE	43.8	42.0	38.9	33.1	29.8	25.0	68	27
Canada, Quebec	NA	50.7	41.5	31.9	28.2	21.1	*	—	47
Hawaii, Hawaiian	NA	43.4	40.9	42.5	19.8	30.0	20.2	102	107
New Zealand, Maoris	O	37.3	35.4	39.8	34.6	40.3	*	—	2
Finland	WE	36.1	34.2	27.2	22.7	17.4	17.6	94	51
New Zealand, Non-Maoris	O	35.4	33.3	30.7	26.0	40.0	*	—	28
Hawaii, Japanese	NA	34.4	31.2	36.0	24.6	13.9	12.6	148	27
Puerto Rico	NA	33.1	30.7	25.0	21.4	17.2	16.5	86	43
Colombia, Cali	SA	26.1	30.6	21.9	19.9	23.2	22.4	37	54
Hawaii, Filipino	NA	36.5	30.6	30.6	14.0	17.6	*	—	119
Denmark	WE	29.9	27.7	23.6	21.8	19.5	17.7	57	27
Canada, Newfoundland	NA	34.4	27.4	27.4	21.6	17.0	12.6	117	27
FRG, Hamburg	WE	28.9	26.5	28.5	22.9	18.3	16.5	61	16
Hawaii, Chinese	NA	28.0	25.2	25.8	17.8	9.8	*	—	42
Israel, Jews born in Israel	A	18.6	24.3	12.9	9.7	10.8	*	—	151
UK, Oxford	WE	27.7	23.7	20.8	19.2	19.2	*	—	23
Israel, Jews born in NA/WE	A	17.5	22.5	12.4	12.6	13.2	*	—	79
UK, S. Thames	WE	24.8	21.4	20.1	16.4	19.3	14.8	45	30
Germany Dem. Rep.	EE	21.9	19.9	18.1	14.6	12.6	*	—	36
UK, Mersey	WE	23.1	19.2	18.1	17.5	18.2	17.1	12	11
UK, Birmingham	WE	25.0	18.9	18.6	17.7	18.4	17.3	9	7
Israel, all Jews	A	17.5	18.8	15.1	14.3	12.5	*	—	31
Yugoslavia, Slovenia	EE	18.6	18.7	15.8	16.8	13.1	10.9	72	11
Hungary, Vas	EE	20.1	16.9	13.3	16.1	19.5	*	—	5
Israel, Jews born in Africa, Asia	A	17.4	16.8	13.6	13.2	11.4	*	—	27
USA, Bay Area Chinese	NA	—	14.9	18.6	18.2	*	*	—	−18
Poland, Cracow	EE	10.5	13.8	11.0	8.0	4.9	*	—	73
Hungary, Szabolcs	EE	14.3	12.6	10.1	9.1	5.0	*	—	38
India, Bombay	A	6.9	8.2	6.9	8.0	6.5	*	—	3
Singapore, Chinese	A	7.6	6.6	4.8	3.6	*	0.9	633	83
Israel, non-Jews	A	7.7	6.5	4.9	4.3	3.1	*	—	50
Japan, Miyagi	A	7.8	6.3	4.9	2.7	3.2	3.8	66	133

†Ordered from high to low according to 1980 incidence rates; adapted from Zaridze (1984).
[a]NA = North America; SA = South America; A = Asia; WE = Western Europe; EE = Eastern Europe; O = Oceania.
[b]* = Data not available.

ENVIRONMENTAL FACTORS

Endocrine Factors

There has been a long-standing interest in the possible role of steroid hormones in the etiology of prostatic cancer (Henderson et al, 1982). Normal growth and function of prostatic tissue is under the control of testosterone through conversion to DHT by the enzyme 5-alpha reductase (Coffey, 1979; Griffiths et al, 1979). More than 95% of testosterone production occurs in the Leydig cells of the testis (Coffey, 1979). Testosterone is bound within the circulation to sex hormone–binding globulin (nearly 60%) or more weakly to albumin (nearly 40%), with a small fraction (about 2%) totally unbound to plasma proteins. About 90% of the testosterone which diffuses into the prostate is converted to DHT (Coffey, 1979). Ablation or antagonism of testosterone production, either through estrogen administration, orchiectomy, or treatment with luteinizing hormone–releasing hormone (LHRH) agonists or antiandrogens, is used to control disseminated prostate cancer (Murphy et al, 1982; Catalona, 1994).

A number of studies have compared circulating testosterone levels measured by radioimmunoassay in cases of prostate cancer with those in controls of similar age who had no known prostatic diseases (Table 55–3). Ghanadian and colleagues (1979) showed that patients with cancer of the prostate had higher levels of serum testosterone than did healthy controls. Seven of 33 cases but only one of 42 controls had serum testosterone levels greater than 30 nMol/dl. Ahluwalia and co-workers (1981) found levels of serum testosterone significantly higher in patients with prostatic cancer than in age-matched controls in the U.S., but not in African blacks. Drafta and colleagues (1982) also found significantly higher circulating testosterone levels in 23 patients with prostatic cancer, compared with 63 "normal ambulatory controls."

Other investigators have found no evidence or inconsistent evidence of alteration in circulating testosterone levels among prostate cancer cases. Wright and co-workers (1985) found no difference in circulating testosterone levels between 23 elderly French urology patients devoid of prostatic disease and 26 elderly men with well-differentiated cancer of the prostate. However, the cancer patients in this study were somewhat older than the controls. Zumoff and colleagues (1982) in a small study of 24-hour serum testosterone levels actually found prostatic cancer patients under age 65 to have a mean level significantly lower than that of controls without prostatic disease, whereas those over age 65 had a mean level which was 10% higher. It should be noted that the average age of the controls under age 65 was about 18 years less than that of the patients with prostatic cancer. Harper et al (1976) compared testosterone levels in 33 patients with prostate cancer with those in 35 hospitalized control men of roughly comparable age. Patients had a statistically non-significant 15% lower level of testosterone than controls. Bartsch et al (1977) in a study of comparable size but using "normal males" of similar age found a slight and also statistically non-significant deficit of circulating testosterone among the cases. The source and other characteristics of the control group are not provided in this study. Hulka et al (1987) found a statistically non-significant reduction in testosterone in 34 prostate cancer cases treated at the University of North Carolina Med-

TABLE 55–3. *Mean Levels of Serum Testosterone in Case–Control Studies of Prostate Cancer*

	Cases		Controls			
Reference	N	Value (pg/ml)	N	Value (pg/ml)	P	Difference (%)
STUDIES USING HEALTHY/POPULATION CONTROLS						
Bartsch et al (1977)	34	4730	29	5210	NS[a]	−9
Ghanadian et al (1979)	33	6030	42	4820	<0.01	+25
Ahluwalia et al (1981)						
U.S. Blacks	170	4200[b]	170	3500[b]	<0.05	+20
African Blacks	55	2000[b]	55	2200[b]	<0.05	−9
Drafta et al (1982)	23	6344	63	4011	<0.001	+58
STUDIES USING HOSPITAL/CLINIC CONTROLS						
Harper et al (1976)	33	5450	35	6400	NS	−15
Zumoff et al (1982)[c]	7	2820	36	4340	<0.001	−35
Wright et al (1985)	26	4440	23	4380	NS	+1
Hulka et al (1987)	34	3308	161	4052	NS	−18

[a]NS = not significant.
[b]Values not cited in text but interpolated from graphs.
[c]Subjects under 65 years of age.

ical Center over a 15-month period compared to 161 general medical clinic controls. Controls were about 5 years younger on average and had a somewhat higher proportion of smokers than the cases. Substantially lower testosterone levels were observed for that portion of the case group with the most advanced disease, and the authors thus interpreted the overall difference in testosterone levels as a consequence rather than as a cause of the disease. Hammond and co-workers (1978) also found no difference in circulating testosterone levels in their case–control study of only 11 patients with prostatic cancer. Meikle and Stanish (1982) found significantly lower testosterone levels in brothers and sons of prostatic cancer patients than in healthy, unrelated controls of comparable age.

Many of these same case–control studies which have evaluated possible alterations in circulating testosterone in relationship to prostate cancer have also considered possible abnormalities in plasma estrogens. Since estrogen therapy remains a major component of the therapeutic armamentarium for prostatic cancer and circulating estrogens can compete with androgens for binding to sex hormone–binding globulin, one might predict an inverse relationship between circulating estrogen levels and prostate cancer risk. In dogs, however, the only animal other than man with a relatively high incidence of spontaneous prostate cancer, estrogens enhance the effect of androgens on prostate growth by increasing androgen receptor content. Drafta et al (1982) have suggested that men at high risk of prostate cancer have a decreased ability to aromatize testosterone to estrogen, resulting in higher levels of the former and lower levels of the latter steroid. Case–control data are highly inconsistent with studies finding either evidence of reduced estrogen levels in cases (Drafta et al, 1982; Rannikko et al, 1989), increased levels in cases (Ahluwalia et al, 1981), or no differences between cases and controls (Harper et al, 1976; Bartsch et al, 1977; Nomura et al, 1988).

The possible role of other hormones, such as prolactin, in the development of prostate cancer has also been considered. Prolactin receptors have been identified in human prostate tissue (Keenan et al, 1979), and prolactin enhances testosterone activity in the prostatic tissue of animals (Grayhack, 1963). Nonetheless, there are few relevant human data on the possible role of prolactin in prostate cancer etiology and those that exist do not suggest an important relationship (Ahluwalia et al, 1981; Hammond et al, 1978).

Rose (1986) has recently reviewed some of the difficulties in interpreting case–control studies which evaluate plasma steroid hormones. These difficulties include appropriate control selection, especially the handling of variables known to be related to circulating testosterone levels such as weight, age, smoking, alcohol use, and use of certain medications (Dai et al, 1981; Deslypere and Vermeulen, 1984), and possible confounding by the presence of concurrent chronic diseases. Additional problems include the effects of the malignant process on the steroids of interest and of the timing of the relevant hormonal milieu relative to the timing of clinical detectability of prostate cancer. Prospective serological studies can overcome some of these methodological problems but few such studies related to prostate cancer have been published to date. Barrett-Conner et al (1990) found an increased risk of prostate cancer with increased circulating levels of the adrenal androgen, androstenedione, in a 14-year prospective study of 1,008 men, aged 40–79, living in a Southern California retirement community. Risk also tended to increase with increasing levels of estradiol but not testosterone; however, even the former result was not statistically significant. In a case–control study nested within a large prospective study in Hawaii, Nomura observed no differences in testosterone or DHT levels between 98 prostate cancer cases and age- and hour-of-sampling-matched controls (Nomura et al, 1988).

The hypothesis of a hormonal etiology for prostatic cancer would predict that healthy U.S. black males should have higher testosterone levels than U.S. white males. Ross et al (1986) studied circulating steroid hormone levels in white and black college students in Los Angeles. After adjustment by analysis of covariance for time of sampling, age, weight, alcohol use, cigarette smoking, and use of prescription drugs, the mean testosterone level in blacks was 15% higher than that in whites, and the "free" (i.e., nonprotein-bound) testosterone level was 13% higher. Ellis and Nyborg (1992) have also reported that U.S. black men have a higher mean testosterone level than U.S. white men, although the absolute difference in this study was small. Prostate cancer rates tend to increase at approximately the eighth or ninth power of "tissue age" (Pike et al, 1983). If this "tissue aging" for prostatic cancer begins at puberty, and if a 15% increase in testosterone translates into a 15% increase in "prostatic tissue aging," Ross and colleagues (1986) have argued that such an increase could readily explain the excess risk of prostatic cancer among U.S. blacks. Young black men also have higher estrogen levels than their white counterparts.

Black women have markedly higher serum levels of testosterone and estradiol during early pregnancy than do white women, averaging 50% and 40% higher, respectively (Henderson et al, 1988). It seems plausible that these higher steroid hormone levels *in utero* may contribute to the higher prostate cancer rate for black men by determining subsequent androgen production, or target tissue sensitivity (Ross and Henderson, 1994).

Ahluwalia et al (1981) have reported that both U.S. black prostate cancer patients and healthy U.S. blacks have substantially higher levels of testosterone than African black prostate cancer patients and healthy African blacks, respectively, of comparable age.

Serum testosterone levels in young adult native Japanese men do not differ from those in U.S. men (Ross et al, 1992). However, both native Japanese and Chinese men appear to have reduced 5-alpha reductase expression, the enzyme which converts testosterone to DHT. Circulating DHT levels unreliably reflect 5-alpha reductase activity in the prostate, since this hormone is mainly converted locally to androstanediol which circulates as its glucuronide conjugate. Native Japanese and Chinese men have markedly reduced levels of this hormonal metabolite compared to U.S. blacks and whites (Ross et al, 1992; Lookingbill et al, 1991). Levels of androsterone glucuronide, another index of this enzymatic activity, are also markedly reduced in these two groups of Asian men. These findings not only suggest an important role for 5-alpha reductase in prostatic carcinogenesis but also suggest a potential means for primary chemoprevention of prostate cancer. Five-alpha reductase inhibitors represent a newly developed class of drugs which selectively block this enzymatic activity without affecting other testosterone dependent processes. Recruitment in a 7-year national placebo-controlled prostate cancer chemoprevention trial of 18,000 healthy men is now under way utilizing finasteride, a 5-alpha reductase inhibitor, as the chemopreventive agent (Brawley et al, 1994).

The human androgen receptor (AR) gene is a nuclear hormone receptor (Parker and Schimmer, 1994). The AR binds DHT, and to a lesser degree testosterone, in the cytosol of prostate epithelial cells. The hormone receptor complex translocates to the nucleus for DNA binding and transactivation of androgen responsive genes. The physiologic control of prostatic growth by androgens is summarized in Figure 55–1. With the cloning of the AR gene, studies are emerging that are characterizing the heterogeneity of expression of the AR in human prostatic normal and neoplastic tissues (Wilding, 1992). AR content in epithelial, but not stromal cells, is positively correlated with the grade of tumor differentiation. Androgen sensitivity of prostate cancer cells can be diminished or lost as a result of point mutations or deletions in the AR gene. The AR gene is highly polymorphic in human populations as evidenced by variable trinucleotide microsatellite repeats in exon 1 (Edwards et al, 1992). Genetic variations at the AR locus, such as the number of repeats, may be correlated with transactivational androgenic function and serve as a biomarker of ethnic variations in risk of prostate cancer (Coetzee and Ross, 1994).

If androgens such as testosterone affect prostate cancer risk, then the recent explosion in use of anabolic steroids in young athletes could conceivably affect future prostate cancer incidence. A recent case report of prostatic cancer in a young body builder is of interest in this regard (Roberts and Essenhigh, 1986), although a recent review of prostate cancer incidence in young men (less than age 40) in one major urban area of the U.S. did not reveal an increasing trend through the late 1980s (Ross, unpublished results).

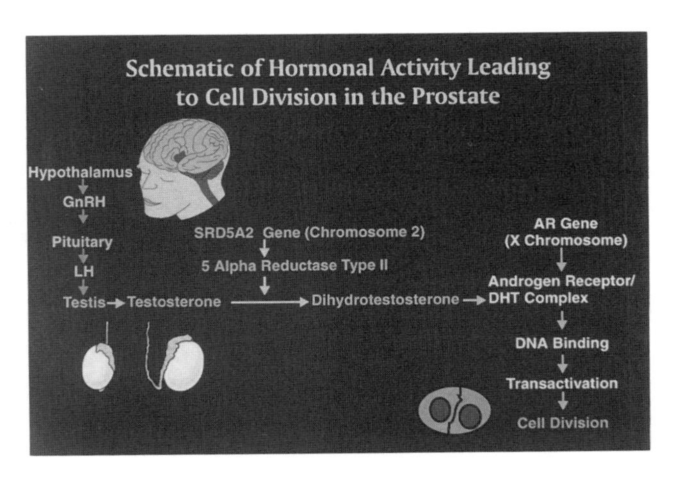

FIG. 55–1. Testosterone in the male is derived primarily from the testis which is stimulated by luteinizing hormone produced by the pituitary. Testosterone is metabolically activated intracellularly by the activity of the 5-alpha reductase type II enzyme whose expression is regulated by the SRD5A2 gene on the short arm of chromosome 2. Dihydrotestosterone is bound to the androgen receptor and this complex translocates to the nucleus for DNA binding and transactivation of androgen responsive genes. The androgen receptor gene is located on the long arm of the X chromosome.

There are few other epidemiologic data relevant to a hormonal etiologic hypothesis. It has long been known that castration produces a palliative effect on advanced prostate cancer (Huggins and Hodges, 1941) and that the disease is apparently rare in castrated subjects (Hovenian and Deming, 1948). In addition to an inverse correlation with age (Deslypere and Vermeulen, 1984), alcohol (inversely), cigarette smoking, and low weight are weak correlates of circulating testosterone levels (Dai et al, 1981). The epidemiologic evidence for an association between each of these factors and prostate cancer risk is reviewed below, and none appear to be a strong risk factor.

Laboratory animals have a very low spontaneous incidence of clinically detectable adenocarcinoma of the prostate (Rivenson and Silverman, 1979). Adenocarcinoma of the prostate has proven to be very difficult to produce experimentally. Although such tumors have been produced in low frequency by chemical carcinogens such as methylcholanthrene (Mirand and Staubitz, 1956), the most successful experimental model was produced by Noble (1977). The administration of testosterone and/or estrone pellets subcutaneously to Nb strain of rats increased markedly the incidence of adenocarcinoma of the prostate over the spontaneous rate of 0.5%. Testosterone alone induced tumors, with increasing incidence proportionate to the dose; however, it appeared that the greatest tumor yield occurred with administration of testosterone followed by estrone (Noble, 1980).

Brown and co-workers (1979) have induced adenocarcinomas of the prostate in male rats by joining such rats through parabiosis either to castrated male rats or to oophorectomized female rats, following unilateral nephrectomy in both partners. Very high circulating levels of testosterone were demonstrated in the target male prior to tumor development. In recently developed rodent models of chemical- or irradiation-induced prostatic carcinomas in rats, testosterone priming or adjuvant testosterone administration has proven critical (Takizawa and Hirose, 1978; Bosland et al, 1984; Pollard et al, 1989b), suggesting that active cell proliferation is an essential prerequisite for inducing prostate cancer by other carcinogens (Rivenson and Silverman, 1979).

NUTRITION

Although a number of dietary factors have been investigated in relationship to prostate cancer development, the two most extensively studied are vitamin A and its precursors, and fat consumption. There has also been increased attention to the possible role of vitamin D in modifying the growth and differentiation of prostate cancer cells.

Vitamin A

Vitamin A compounds (retinoids) have been extensively evaluated by epidemiologists in association with development of a number of epithelial tumors. Interest in these compounds has evolved because of their potential as chemopreventive agents (Peto et al, 1981). Retinoids are important in the normal differentiation of cells and in cell membrane permeability (Bates, 1995). Provitamin A compounds, such as beta-carotene, are able to deactivate free radicals, which are potentially genotoxic (Peto, 1983). Vitamin A and synthetic retinoids can inhibit carcinogen-induced anaplastic lesions in mouse prostate organ cultures (Chopra and Wilkoff, 1988). On the other hand, vitamin A may promote tumor progression of chemically induced tumors in some animal model systems (Quander et al, 1985). Some vitamin A analogues inhibit human prostate cell proliferation in low concentrations, but promote proliferation in higher doses (Chaproniere and Weber, 1985).

In 1979 Hirayama (1979a) reported results from a large prospective study involving 10 years of follow-up of 265,000 Japanese men and women. At the time of this report, there had been 63 prostate cancer deaths among a total of 4,373 male cancer deaths. Men who consumed green and yellow vegetables (cruciferous vegetables, asparagus, carrots, chicory, chives, green pepper, leeks, lettuce, parsley, pumpkin, and spinach) on a daily basis had a 60% reduction in risk of dying of prostate cancer, compared to men who rarely or never consumed such foods. Risk reduction was dose related, although a subsequent report of this cohort found that the effect dissipated in older age-groups (Hirayama, 1986). Green and yellow vegetable consumption accounted for nearly half the total intake of vitamin A compounds in this population (Hirayama, 1979b).

Subsequently, there have been a number of studies, mainly case–control in design, which have evaluated the association between vitamin A compounds and risk of prostate cancer (Table 55–4).The literature remains confused as to the precise effect of these compounds on prostate cancer risk. Other prospective studies were conducted by Paganini-Hill et al (1987) in a retirement community near Los Angeles, California; by Mills and colleagues (1989) of a cohort of Seventh Day Adventist men; and by Hsing et al (1990b) using the Lutheran Brotherhood cohort. In the study by Paganini-Hill et al (1987), a self-administered mailed questionnaire was completed by 4,280 men in 1981. The questionnaire contained a detailed dietary history including food frequency and vitamin supplementation. As of late 1986, 93 incident prostate cancers had occurred. Although there was no significant increase or decrease in risk associated with intake of beta-carotene, dietary vitamin A or total vitamin A, the data are most consistent with an increasing risk associated with increasing consumption of vitamin A from all sources. The food frequency questionnaire used in the prospective study of Seventh Day Adventists did not allow determination of total dietary beta-carotene or vitamin A consumption. Several foods with high vitamin A content were, however, protective against prostate cancer development in this analysis. As with the study by Paganini-Hill and colleagues, Hsing et al (1990b) found no relationship overall between vitamin A and beta-carotene intake and fatal prostate cancer based on 149 cases identified during follow-up of the 18,000 participants in the Lutheran Brotherhood cohort. This study was also limited by incomplete dietary histories.

The first case–control study of a positive association with consumption of vitamin A was reported by Graham and collagues (1983). In a hospital-based study of 260 white prostate cancer patients and 294 controls of similar age, risk increased with increasing consumption of vitamin A. Men consuming more than 150,500 In-

TABLE 55–4. *Summary of Studies Evaluating the Association of Dietary Intake of Vitamin A Compounds and Risk of Prostate Cancer**

Reference	*Site*	*Study Design*	*Size*	*Vitamin A Categories*	*Relative Risk*	*Remarks*
Hirayama (1979a,b)	Japan	Cohort (P)	63 Ca Deaths	Rare	1.0	Results for green and yellow vegetable intake only
				Occasional	0.7	
				Daily	0.4	
Graham et al (1983)	Buffalo, NY	Ca-Co (H)	260 Ca/294 Co	<50,500 IU/mo	1.0	Statistically significant ≥70 years of age only
				−100,500	1.4	
				−150,500	2.4	
				≥150,500	1.8	
Mishina et al (1985)	Japan	Ca-Co (SC)	100 Ca/100 Co	Never/occasional	1.0	Results for green and yellow vegetable intake only
				More often	0.5	
Heshmat et al (1985)	Washington, DC	Ca-Co (H)	181 Ca/181 Co	<50 Yrs $\bar{x}$ Ca = 5300 IU/Kcal	—	$P = 0.007$ (<50)
				$\bar{x}$ Co = 4352 IU/Kcal	—	
				≥50 Yrs $\bar{x}$ Ca = 6035 IU/Kcal	—	$P = 0.07$ (≥50)
				$\bar{x}$ Co = 5332 IU/Kcal	—	
Kaul et al (1987)	Washington, DC	Ca-Co (H)	55 Ca/55 Co	<50 Yrs $\bar{x}$ Ca = 5000 IU/Kcal	—	
				$\bar{x}$ Co = 4200 IU/Kcal	—	
				≥50 Yrs $\bar{x}$ Ca = 6200 IU/Kcal	—	
				$\bar{x}$ Co = 6800 IU/Kcal	—	
Kolonel et al (1987)	Hawaii	Ca-Co (P)	452 Ca/899 Co	<70 Yrs 1 (Low)	1.0	Similar results for Caucasians and Japanese; beta-carotene results less striking
				2	1.3	
				3	1.0	
				4 (High)	0.8	
				≥70 Yrs 1 (Low)	1.0	
				2	1.4	
				3	1.3	
				4 (High)	2.0	
Paganini-Hill et al (1987)	Laguna Hills, CA	Cohort (P)	93 Ca	Low	1.0	No association with beta-carotene
				Medium	1.4	
				High	1.4	
Honda et al (1988)	Los Angeles, CA	Ca-Co (P)	216 Ca/216 Co	1 (Low)	1.0	Results for total vitamin A including supplements; $P =$ 0.06 test for trend; inverse association for beta-carotene
				2	1.2	
				3	2.0	
				4 (High)	1.5	
Oishi et al (1988)	Japan	Ca-Co (H)	100 Ca/100 Co	>Median of Co (%) 37	0.6	Results stronger for beta-carotene
			100 Ca/100 BPH	>Median of Co (%) 34	0.5	
Ross et al (1988)	Los Angeles, CA	Ca-Co (P)	142 Ca/142 Co (B)	(B)Low	1.0	Incomplete dietary history; suggestion of inverse association for beta-carotene, in blacks only
				Medium	1.2	
				High	0.8	
			142 Ca/142 Co (W)	(W)Low	1.0	
				Medium	0.6	
				High	1.0	
Mettlin et al (1989)	Buffalo, NY	Ca-Co (H)	371 Ca/370 Co	1 (Low)	1.0	Results for beta-carotene only; highest quartile significantly different from 1.0
				2	0.9	
				3	0.7	
				4	0.9	
				5 (High)	0.6	
Fincham (1990)	Alberta, Canada	Ca-Co (P)	382 Ca/625 Co	1 (Low)	1.0	Notation that cases over age 70 consumed more vitamin A than controls (not significant)
				2	0.9	
				3	0.7	
				4 (High)	0.8	
Hsing et al (1990a)	U.S.	Cohort	149 Ca Deaths	1 (Low)	1.0	Retinol
				2	0.8	
				3	0.9	
				4 (High)	1.2	
				1 (Low)	1.0	Beta-carotene
				2	1.2	
				3	1.3	
				4 (High)	0.9	

(continued)

TABLE 55–4. *Summary of Studies Evaluating the Association of Dietary Intake of Vitamin A Compounds and Risk of Prostate Cancer* (Continued)*

Reference	*Site*	*Study Design*	*Size*	*Vitamin A Categories*	*Relative Risk*	*Remarks*
West et al (1991)	Utah	Ca-Co (P)	358 Ca/679 Co	<68 Yrs 1 (Low)	1.0	Results weaker for beta-carotene; suggestion of protective effect of vitamin A in younger men
				2	1.2	
				3	1.1	
				4 (High)	1.0	
				≥68 Yrs 1 (Low)	1.0	
				2	2.1	
				3	1.6	
				4 (High)	1.6	

*Abbreviations: B = blacks; BPH = benign prostatic hyperplasia; Ca = case(s); Co = control(s); H = hospital-based; IU = international unit(s); P = population-based; SC = screening clinic-based; W = whites; Yrs = years of age.

ternational Units (IU) monthly had 1.8 times the risk of those consuming less than 50,500 IU per month. When dichotomized by age, results were statistically significant for those over age 70 only, although the actual risk estimates did not differ greatly between the two age groups. Several other case–control studies conducted in the U.S. on this association also found results consistent with increasing risk with increasing consumption of vitamin A, but not beta-carotene. In a population-based case–control study in Hawaii, Kolonel et al (1987) found a significant association between total vitamin A and prostate cancer risk which was limited to men over 70 years of age. Honda et al (1986) found elevated risk estimates with higher intake of vitamin A in a population-based case–control study of men under 60 years of age in Los Angeles, but the results did not quite achieve statistical significance. However, when beta-carotene consumption was considered alone, the relative risk (RR) estimates were in the direction of a reduced risk with increased intake (RR = 0.7 for highest versus lowest quartile of intake). In case–control studies of older blacks and whites in Los Angeles, no association was found with vitamin A intake using a restricted food frequency dietary history (Ross et al, 1987). There was a suggestion of reduced risk with increasing beta-carotene intake among blacks but not whites. Mettlin et al (1989) found a substantial reduction in risk among men in the highest versus the lowest quintile of beta-carotene consumption in a large hospital-based case–control study in New York (RR = 0.60). Heshmat et al (1985) reported a significant positive association between vitamin A intake and prostate cancer in a case–control study among blacks in Washington, DC. The same group of investigators was later unable to confirm these findings in a somewhat smaller case–control study in the same population (Kaul et al, 1987).

Similar to the observations in cohort studies, case–control studies conducted in populations at low risk of prostate cancer have described a reduction in risk associated with high intake of beta-carotene from green and yellow vegetables. Oishi et al (1988) compared beta-carotene intake levels in 100 patients with prostate cancer with 100 patients each with either benign prostatic hyperplasia (BPH) or hospitalized for reasons unrelated to prostatic disease. Compared to either control group, men whose beta-carotene intake fell below the median intake of the controls had over twice the risk of prostate cancer as that of men with intake above the median. Compared to the hospital controls, there was a monotonic dose–response association from the highest to lowest quartile of beta-carotene intake, with a three-fold difference in risk between the extreme categories. For total retinol intake, the risk estimates were attenuated somewhat compared to those for beta-carotene and were statistically significant only in comparison to the BPH control group. Mishina et al (1985) found that, compared to more frequent consumption, persons consuming green and yellow vegetables occasionally or not at all had twice the risk of prostate cancer.

In addition to dietary studies of intake of vitamin A compounds and prostate cancer risk, four prospective studies—two of them of limited sample size, and one larger case–control study—have evaluated the relationship between serum retinol levels and the development of prostate cancer. Kark et al (1981) conducted a prospective study of cancer risk and serum retinol levels using frozen sera from a prospective study of heart disease in Evans County, Georgia. Although cancer cases overall had significantly lower retinol levels than controls, the mean level for the eight observed prostate cancers was only slightly reduced. In a similar study involving 111 participants in the Hypertension Detection and Follow-up Study who eventually developed cancer, and 210 controls who did not, there were only small, non-significant differences in serum retinol and carotenoids among the 11 prostate cancer cases as compared to controls (Willett et al, 1984). In a cohort of 26,000 persons followed for 13 years in Washington County, Maryland, serum levels of vitamin A and beta-carotene were compared in the 103 men who developed prostate cancer and 103 controls of the same age and race (Hsing et al, 1990a). There was no apparent relationship with beta-carotene, but for retinol, risk appeared to decrease with increasing serum levels. Compared to men in the lowest quartile, risk levels were 0.67, 0.39, and 0.40 for men in the second, third and fourth quartiles, respectively ($P = 0.01$). The other large prospective study that has evaluated this relationship was the National Health and Nutrition Examination Survey Epidemiologic Follow-up Study. During a 10-year follow-up of 2,440 men, 84 cases of prostate cancer were identified. The prediagnostic serum vitamin A level was significantly lower in cases than in men of similar age who did not develop prostate cancer (Reichman et al, 1990). Men in the lowest quartile had 2.2 times the risk of prostate cancer of men in the highest quartile. Hayes et al (1988) compared retinol levels in 94 clinical prostatic cancer cases with those in 40 men with focal prostatic cancer and with those in 130 hospital controls. Results were comparable for the two case groups and across all stages of disease. The two case groups combined had a 9% lower level of retinol than the controls ($P < 0.05$); there was some evidence of a dose–response effect with risk decreasing as circulating levels of retinol increased.

The serum studies to date seem to indicate, if anything, that a higher serum retinol level is associated with a lower risk of prostate cancer. The studies of serum retinol levels, however, are not consistent with the pattern of results from the dietary case–control and cohort studies.

Fat

There is a strong correlation between per capita fat consumption and international prostate cancer age-standardized mortality rates (Armstrong and Doll, 1975; Carroll and Khor, 1975) and prostate cancer incidence on a regional basis (Kolonel et al, 1983). Epidemiologic data generally support a positive association between dietary fat intake and prostate cancer risk (Table 55–5). Six of the seven largest case-control studies to date find that cases tend to consume more fat than controls. These six studies have involved U.S. blacks (Ross et al, 1987; Heshmat et al, 1985), U.S. whites (Graham et al, 1983; Ross et al, 1987; Heshmat et al, 1985; West et al, 1991), African blacks (Walker et al, 1992), and Asian-Americans (Kolonel et al, 1988), and they have utilized both population controls (Ross et al, 1987; Heshmat et al, 1985; West et al, 1991; Walker et al, 1992) and hospital controls (Graham et al, 1983; Heshmat et al, 1985). Four of these studies (Graham et al, 1983; Heshmat et al, 1985; Kolonel et al, 1988; West et al, 1991) evaluated risk by the source of dietary fat (animal versus other) or considered saturated versus unsaturated fat intake separately. These studies do not suggest systematic differences in risk of prostate cancer between animal or saturated fat versus total fat intake, although in the large case–control study of Kolonel et al (1988), the relative risks were slightly larger with saturated fat intake than with fat intake overall, and only the former produced statistically significant results. However, all associations with dietary fat intake in this study were limited to men age 70 or older. A large population-based case–control study in Canada found no association with fat intake overall or with animal fat evaluated separately. Vegetable fat consumption actually showed a statistically significant inverse association (Fincham et al, 1990). Similarly, in two smaller, hospital-based case–control studies conducted in the U.S. (Kaul et al, 1987) and Japan (Ohno et al, 1988), respectively, no clear association was observed between fat intake and prostate cancer risk.

Studies which have evaluated prostate cancer risk in association with intake of specific high-fat content foods (e.g., beef and pork, eggs, milk, butter and cheeses) rather than as a specific nutrient, generally find higher risks with increasing frequency of consumption (Mishina et al, 1985; Rotkin 1977; Talamani et al, 1986; Snowdon et al, 1984; Mettlin et al, 1989), although there have been exceptions (Hirayama, 1979b; Mills et al, 1989; Hsing et al, 1990a).

In addition to the case–control studies described above, there have been at least three prospective studies which have reported on the association between dietary fat intake and prostate cancer risk. Giovannucci et al (1993c) reported results from the Health Professionals Follow-up Study which examined the relationship between prostate cancer and dietary fat, including specific fatty acids and specific foods. Of the 47,855 participants (men aged 40–75 who completed a 131-item, food-frequency questionnaire in 1986), 300 prostate cancer cases had been diagnosed as of January 31, 1990. Total fat consumption was found to be associated with risk of advanced prostate cancer (defined as stages C and D and fatal cases), but not early stage disease. For advanced stage prostate cancer cases, the age- and energy-adjusted RR was 1.79 (95% CI = 1.04–3.07) for the highest compared with the lowest quintile of intake. This association was mainly due to animal fat, especially from red meat, and not vegetable fat.

Between 1975 and 1980, a cohort of 20,316 men of diverse ethnic origins in Hawaii completed questionnaires that recorded weekly frequency of intake of 13 food items (high-fat animal products and fresh fruits and vegetables) and were then followed until December 1989 (LeMarchand et al, 1994). There were 198 incident cases of invasive prostate cancer, as ascertained by the Hawaii SEER Cancer Registry. Risk (adjusted for

TABLE 55–5. *Summary of Results from Case-Control Studies of the Association of Fat Intake and Prostate Cancer Risk**

Reference	*No. of Cases/Controls*	*Dietary Fat Categories*	*Relative Risk*	*Remarks*
Graham et al (1983)	260/294	Total fat: ≤1200 g/mo	1.0	
		1201–1800 g/mo	1.0	
		1800+ g/mo	1.7	
		Animal fat: ≤1200 g/mo	1.0	
		1201–1800 g/mo	1.0	
		1800+ g/mo	1.7	
Kolonel et al (1988)	452/899	Total fat: Age <70 1 (Low)	1.0	Stronger, statistically significant association for saturated fat (men ≥70 only)
		2	0.9	
		3	0.8	
		4 (High)	1.0	
		Age ≥70 1 (Low)	1.0	
		2	1.0	
		3	1.1	
		4 (High)	1.5	
Heshmat et al (1985)	181/181	Age 30–49 $\bar{x}$ Cases 39.4 g/Kcal/day	—	Results similar for saturated fat
		$\bar{x}$ Controls 37.7 g/Kcal/day	—	
		Age 50+ $\bar{x}$ Cases 35.0 g/Kcal/day	—	Results similar for saturated fat
		$\bar{x}$ Controls 35.0 g/Kcal/day	—	
Ross et al (1987)	142/142 (blacks)	1 (Low)	1.0	Incomplete dietary histories
		2	1.4	
		3 (High)	1.9	
	142/142 (whites)	1 (Low)	1.0	
		2	1.8	
		3 (High)	1.6	
Kaul et al (1987)	55/55	Age 30–49 $\bar{x}$ Cases 40 g/Kcal/day	—	
		$\bar{x}$ Controls 38 g/Kcal/day	—	
		Age 50+ $\bar{x}$ Cases 36 g/Kcal/day	—	
		$\bar{x}$ Controls 34 g/Kcal/day	—	
Ohno et al (1988)	100/100 (H)	>Median intake of H (%) 52	1.3	
	100/100 (BPH)	>Median intake of BPH (%) 44	0.8	
Fincham et al (1990)	382/625	1 (Low)	1.0	Negative association with vegetable fat
		2	1.0	
		3	0.9	
		4 (High)	0.8	
West et al (1991)	358/679	Total fat: Age <68 1 (Low)	1.0	Results similar for saturated fat, monounsaturated fat, and polyunsaturated fat; confidence intervals exclude 1.0 for 3 highest quartiles in men ≥68 yrs old
		2	1.1	
		3	1.2	
		4 (High)	0.8	
		Age ≥68 1 (Low)	1.0	
		2	1.6	
		3	2.0	
		4 (High)	1.7	
Walker et al (1992)	166/166	<25% calories from fat	1.0	
		≥25% calories from fat	2.6	

*Abbreviations: BPH = benign prostatic hyperplasia controls; H = hospital controls.

age, ethnicity, and income) of prostate cancer was elevated with increasing consumption of beef (RR = 1.6; 95% CI = 1.1–2.4, for the highest compared with the lowest tertile of intake; P = .02 for trend); milk (RR = 1.4; 95% CI = 1.0–2.1, for the highest compared with the lowest tertile of intake; P = .04 for trend), and for a summary index of foods high in animal fat (RR = 1.6; 95% CI = 1.0–2.4, for the highest compared with the lowest quartile of intake; P = .05 for trend). These associations were stronger in the men who had been diagnosed with prostate cancer before the age of 73 years, the median age of the case group. There was no significant association between prostate cancer and the intake of fruits or vegetables.

A prospective study evaluating the relationship between total fat intake and prostate cancer in 8,000 Hawaiians of Japanese ancestry found no association. This study, which identified 174 cases of prostate cancer during follow-up, also found no relationship between saturated or unsaturated fat intake and prostate cancer risk (Severson et al, 1989).

In a nested case–control study, the relationship between fatty acid concentrations in plasma (including the essential fatty acids, linoleic and α-linolenic acids) and prostate cancer risk was examined (Gann et al, 1994). As part of the Physicians' Health Study initiated in 1982, 14,196 U.S. male physicians provided plasma samples and filled out questionnaires, including a limited food-frequency record. The plasma fatty acid compositions of 120 men who later developed prostate cancer were compared to those of 120 controls matched for age and smoking status. There was a significant association between plasma α-linolenic acid level and prostate cancer risk. The relative risks of prostate cancer for men in increasingly higher quartiles of plasma α-linolenic acid level, as compared to the men in the lowest quartile were as follows: 3.0 (95% CI = 1.2–7.3); 3.4 (95% CI = 1.6–7.5); and 2.1 (95% CI = 0.9–4.9) ($P = 0.03$ for trend). The risks were similar and still significant when adjusted for frequency of exercise, Quetelet's index, plasma linoleic acid level, and meat intake. The association between plasma linoleic acid and prostate cancer appeared to be protective, but was not statistically significant. There was no significant association between prostate cancer risk and plasma levels of marine oil fatty acids. There was, however, an association between red meat consumption and prostate cancer risk—the relative risk for eating red meat (a major source of α-linolenic acid) as a main dish five or more times per week, as compared to less than once a week, was 2.5 (95% CI = 0.9–6.7). No association between consumption of dairy products and prostate cancer risk was found.

The authors postulated four possible mechanisms by which essential fatty acid intake could have an impact on prostate cancer development: eicosanoid synthesis via the cyclooxygenase pathway; membrane phospholipid composition (which affects receptor activity); sex steroid hormone metabolism (for example, via an effect on 5-α-reductase activity in prostatic tissue); and free radical formation from oxidation of fatty acids.

It had been hypothesized previously that dietary fat might affect prostate cancer occurrence via alteration in the hormonal environment (Berg, 1975). In support of this hypothesis, Hill and Wynder (1979) found that 4 volunteers who switched from a Western diet (40% calories from fat) to an isocaloric vegetarian low-fat diet (25% calories from fat) had substantially reduced plasma testosterone levels during each of 6 daily sampling periods. An additional 11 men who switched from their usual diets to a vegetarian diet for 2 weeks had a 33% reduction in both mid-morning and late-afternoon testosterone levels ($P < 0.01$). In a study comparing circulating hormone levels in 12 Seventh Day Adventist men following a lacto-ovo-vegetarian diet and 10 nonvegetarian SDAs, the latter group was found to have significantly higher testosterone levels (10% difference overall).

Consistent with a fat hypothesis is Kolonel's (1980) observation that all four of the major non-Caucasian ethnic groups that compose the population of Hawaii (Japanese, Chinese, Filipinos, and Hawaiians) have a reduced incidence of prostate cancer compared to Caucasians in Hawaii (Standardized Incidence Ratios reduced between 40% and 58% with Caucasians as the referent group). All of these four groups have a lower dietary intake of both total and animal fat than Caucasians. Hawaiian-Japanese, for example, consume 23% less total fat and 26% less animal fat than Hawaiian-Caucasians and have a 43% lower incidence rate of prostate cancer. However, nutritional surveys have found little difference in dietary fat intake between black and white adults in the U.S. within a social class grouping (Mettlin, 1980), which argues against a major role of adult fat intake in explaining the high risk of prostate cancer among U.S. blacks.

In an experimental model in which dietary fat has been studied as a possible modifier of prostate cancer incidence, no difference in the rate of tumor development was observed in animals on a 10% versus 40% calories-as-fat diet or in animals fed lard versus those fed sunflower seed oil as the principal source of dietary fat (Kroes et al, 1986). However, Pollard et al (1989a) have reduced the incidence of metastatic adenocarcinoma of the prostate in rats through reduced total dietary intake. Reduced caloric intake in such rats may have resulted in reduced testosterone levels (Pollard et al, 1989b). Wang et al (1995) studied the influence of dietary fat content on the growth rate in athymic nude mice of androgen-sensitive human prostatic adenocarcinoma cells (LNCaP cells). Tumor growth rates, final tumor weights and serum prostate-specific antigen (PSA) levels were substantially greater in the subgroup of 15 mice fed the highest fat (40.5-kcal %) compared with 30.8 to 2.3-kcal % isocaloric fat diets. Among the five subgroups of experimental mice there were no significant differences in serum testosterone levels.

Vitamin D

Schwartz and Hulka (1990) have hypothesized that vitamin D deficiency increases the risk of invasive prostate cancer. In a prospective study of Kaiser Permanente Medical Care Plan members in Oakland and San Francisco, Corder et al (1993) reported that low serum levels of the active vitamin D metabolite, 1,25-dihydroxyvitamin D (1,25-D), were significantly associated with an increased risk of clinically detected prostate cancer. In this study, however, healthy African-American controls had somewhat higher 1,25-D levels than whites, which argues against this factor playing a role in determining black–white differences in risk. Peehl et al (1994) detected the presence of vitamin D receptors in cells cultured from human prostate tissue. Vitamin D3, or 1,25 dihydroxycholecalciferol, inhibits the proliferation of cultured normal, hyperplastic, and malignant prostatic epithelial cells (Nomura and Kolonel, 1993). Miller et al (1992) observed that the production of PSA, a protein produced by prostatic epithelial cells, was stimulated by 1α,25-dihydroxyvitamin D3, suggesting that vitamin D might be associated with the differentiation and function of prostate cells.

Other Dietary Factors

In a cohort study of 6,763 white male SDAs, Snowdon et al (1984) reported that overweight men (> 30% above ideal body weight) had a 2.5-fold increased risk of fatal prostate cancer compared to men near their desirable weight ($P < 0.01$), although this relationship did not hold when prostate cancer incidence as opposed to mortality was evaluated (Mills et al, 1989). Talamini et al (1986) in a hospital-based case–control study of 161 patients and 202 controls in Italy found a similarly strong association. Men in the highest quartile of body mass index had 4.4 times the risk of men in the lowest quartile ($P < 0.001$, test for trend). In a population-based case–control study in Canada, Fincham and colleagues (1990) also found a strong association between obesity measured by a ponderal index and prostate cancer risk. In the large American Cancer Society cohort study, overweight men had about a 30% higher mortality rate of prostate cancer (Lew and Garfinkel, 1979). In the cohort of 8,006 Japanese men living in Hawaii, Severson and colleagues (1989) found a weakly positive association between body mass index and prostate cancer risk based on the 174 cases identified during follow-up. This relationship was substantially stronger for muscle area in the arm (lean body mass) than for fat area in the arm. The investigators suggested that this relationship could be an index of androgen production. However, a series of other case–control studies have found no relationship with weight or indices of obesity (Graham et al, 1983; Ross et al, 1987; Wynder et al, 1971; Greenwald et al, 1974; Yu et al, 1988, Oishi et al, 1989), nor did a prospective study of prostate cancer occurrence in former college men (Whittemore et al, 1984).

Decreased regular physical activity is associated with positive energy balance, increased endogenous circulating testosterone levels, and increased fat distribution and body mass index (Thune and Lund, 1994). Previous studies, however, have reported conflicting conclusions about whether decreased self-reported recreational and occupational physical activity is an independent risk factor for prostate cancer (Albanes et al, 1989; Paffenbarger et al, 1987; Severson et al, 1989; LeMarchand et al, 1991; Hsing et al, 1994a).

Dietary intake of other specific nutrients has been investigated in relationship to prostate cancer development (Graham et al, 1983; Kaul et al, 1987; Oishi et al, 1988). Most such investigations have suffered from the lack of specific hypotheses and from small sample sizes. Graham et al (1983) found a positive association with increasing intake of vitamin C in men over 70 years of age but not in younger men, but Kolonel et al (1985) found no such association in their large case–control study in Hawaii.

SEXUAL AND REPRODUCTIVE FACTORS

Sexual Activity

A number of investigators have found evidence that factors associated with increased sexual activity are associated with increased prostate cancer risk. The first such evidence came from a small case–control study in Canada. Steele et al (1971) reported that prostate cancer cases had a greater number of sexual partners and more frequent sexual intercourse than did controls, a finding later confirmed in a larger case–control study conducted in Los Angeles (Krain, 1973). Ross et al (1987) reported a higher frequency of intercourse among black but not white prostate cancer cases than among race- and age-matched neighborhood controls in Los Angeles. Jackson and others (1980) reported similar results, comparing frequency of intercourse among black prostate cancer cases to that of hospital controls. Mandel and Schuman (1987) reported that prostate cancer cases had more sexual experiences with prostitutes than did controls, but also found a lower frequency of intercourse among the cases. Several studies have found an increased risk of prostate cancer associated with early first intercourse (Mishina et al, 1985; Honda et al, 1988), although this has not been a uniform finding (Ross et al, 1987). Fincham et al (1990) found that early age at marriage, but not age at first intercourse, was associated with an increased risk of prostate cancer in a population-based case–control study in Canada.

A fairly consistent finding among a large series of epidemiologic studies has been a higher prevalence of past venereal disease among prostate cancer cases than among controls (Steele et al, 1971; Krain, 1973; Heshmat et al, 1975; Lew and Garfinkel, 1979; Lees et al, 1985; Mishina et al, 1985; Mandel and Schuman, 1987; Ross et al, 1987; Honda et al, 1988). The results of studies of this association are shown in Table 55–6. Although relative risks as high as 5.6 have been observed for a history of all venereal diseases combined compared to no such history (Krain, 1973), risks tend to cluster between 2.0 and 3.0.

Since these types of sexual activity risk factors are similar to those observed for cervix cancer, it has been

TABLE 55–6. *Case–Control Studies of the Association of Venereal Disease and Cancer of the Prostate**

Author(s)	*Year*	*No. of Exposed Cases/ No. of Exposed Controls*	*Relative Risk*
Steele et al	1971	5/1	5.0
Wynder et al	1971	25/28 (W)	1.2
		12/19 (B)	0.7
Krain	1974	28/5	5.6**
Heshmat et al	1975	42/29 (B,G)	2.1**
Lees et al	1985	12/9 (S)	2.9**
		13/30 (G)	0.8
		29/41 (Any)	1.5
Mishina et al	1985	16/11 (G)	1.5
		18/11 (S)	1.5
Mandel and Schuman	1987	19/7 (H)	2.7**
		23/11 (N)	2.1**
Ross et al	1987	16/7 (W)	2.3
		70/53 (B)	1.7**
Honda et al	1988	33/25 (G)	1.4
		6/1 (S)	6.0
		35/25 (Any)	1.5

*Abbreviations: B = blacks; G = gonorrhea; H = hospital control series; N = neighborhood control series; S = syphilis; W = whites.
**$P \leq 0.05$.

hypothesized that prostate cancer might be caused by an infectious agent, possibly spread through sexual activity (Ross et al, 1983). Findings of viral-like particles in human prostatic cancer (Tannenbaum and Lattimer, 1970), the purported increased incidence of cervix cancer in spouses of prostatic cancer patients (Feminella and Lattimer, 1974), and the high rate of cervical cancer among black females in the U.S. (Muir et al, 1987) have suggested a possible common etiologic agent. However, unlike prostate cancer, cervix cancer rates are very high for Hispanics in the U.S. and are strongly associated with low social class. On an international basis, incidence rates for the two diseases are not highly correlated (Muir et al, 1987). Furthermore, the absence of a marked deficit of prostate cancer in Catholic priests is evidence against sexual transmission of the disease (Ross et al, 1981). Finally, studies of antibody titers to selected viruses, including herpes, cytomegalovirus, and Epstein-Barr, have, if anything, suggested lower titers in cases (Mandel and Schuman, 1987). An alternative explanation for the association between these indices of high levels of sexual activity and risk of prostate cancer is that they are indicators of circulating androgens (Honda et al, 1988).

Vasectomy

There has been much recent interest in the relationship of vasectomy to prostate cancer risk. In the early 1980s, it was estimated that over 50 million vasectomies had been performed worldwide and that 455,000 were being performed each year in the United States (Huber et al, 1986). Over 15% of U.S. men over the age of 40 have had a vasectomy. It was hypothesized originally that a vasectomy may lower the risk of prostate cancer (Sheth and Panse, 1982). This hypothesis was based in part on the observation that vasectomized rats have decreased prostate function and size (Kinson and Layberry, 1975; Pierrepoint and Davies, 1973). There is also evidence of increased levels of sperm-agglutinating antibodies and decreased prostatic secretory activity following vasectomy (Naik et al, 1980). On the other hand, there are studies which indicate that vasectomy may result in increased serum testosterone levels (Johnsonbaugh et al, 1975; Purvis et al, 1976; Smith et al, 1979), which might be expected to increase prostate cancer risk. Not all studies have reported such differences in testosterone levels between vasectomized and nonvasectomized men (DelaTorre et al, 1983; Skegg et al, 1976).

At least five case–control and four cohort studies have now reported on the relationship between vasectomy and prostate cancer risk. The first study to suggest this relationship was a population-based case–control study of prostate cancer in Los Angeles among men under age 60 conducted by Honda and colleagues (1985). In that study a past history of vasectomy was weakly and nonsignificantly associated with risk (RR = 1.4). Risk increased, however, with increasing interval from vasectomy (RR for 30+ years = 4.4 compared to no vasectomy; $P = 0.01$, test for trend). This finding was not confirmed in a cohort study of vasectomized and non-vasectomized men undergoing a multiphasic screening examination (Sidney, 1987; Sidney et al, 1991). In that study, the risk of prostate cancer was unrelated to vasectomy or to number of years elapsed since the procedure. Two hospital-based case–control studies have reported a strong positive association. Rosenberg and colleagues (1990) found a substantial elevation in prostate cancer risk associated with vasectomy. In this comparison of 220 men with prostate cancer and 571 non-cancer and 960 cancer controls, risk was increased 5.3-fold based on the non-cancer comparison group, and 3.5-fold when compared with other cancer patients. There was little evidence to suggest, however, that risk was modified by time since vasectomy. Mettlin et al (1990) compared the vasectomy histories of 614 prostate cancer patients seen at Roswell Park Memorial Institute with those of 2,588 patients seen with other cancers. Vasectomy was associated with increased risk (RR = 1.7) and, as in the study of Honda et al, the risk increased significantly in association with years since vasectomy.

A retrospective cohort study using linked medical record abstracts conducted in the Oxford region of England did not find an association between vasectomy and prostate cancer risk (Nienhuis et al, 1992). The cohort consisted of 13,246 men, 25–49 years of age who underwent vasectomy between 1970 and 1986, and a comparison group of 22,196 men who had been admitted to one of the same hospitals during the same time period for appendicitis, injuries, or one of three elective operations. Only six cases of prostate cancer were diagnosed during the follow-up period, which on average was 6.6 years for the men with vasectomy and 7.5 years for the comparison group. Hayes et al (1993) investigated the relationship between vasectomy and prostate cancer in black and white American men in a population-based case–control study. Vasectomy was associated with age, race, and education, and was less prevalent among blacks than whites. The risk for prostate cancer associated with vasectomy was increased among blacks, but the adjusted odds ratio (OR) was not statistically significant (OR = 1.6; 95% CI = 0.5, 4.8); however the risk was not increased among whites overall. Young age at vasectomy, namely before age 35, appeared to be a risk factor (OR = 2.0; 95% CI = 1.0, 4.0).

In China, about two million vasectomies have been performed each year since 1982. A hospital-based case–control study was conducted in 12 cities in China by Hsing et al (1994) to evaluate the relationship between vasectomy and the risk of prostate cancer. Vasectomy was performed at least 10 years prior to interview in 10% of 138 histologically confirmed cases, compared with 3% of 638 hospital and neighborhood controls. The odds ratios for prostate cancer associated with vasectomy varied between 2.0 and 6.7, depending on the comparison group: hospital cancer controls: OR = 2.0 (95% CI = 0.7, 6.1); hospital non-cancer controls: OR = 3.3 (95% CI = 1.0, 11.3); and neighborhood controls: OR = 6.7 (95% CI = 2.1, 21.6).

In a retrospective cohort study by Giovannucci et al (1993a,b), the age-adjusted relative risk for prostate cancer among husbands of nurses in the Nurses' Health Study was 1.56 (95% CI = 1.03,2.37), and in a companion report of a prospective study of male health professionals, the age-adjusted relative risk of prostate cancer associated with vasectomy was 1.66 (95% CI = 1.25, 2.21). The elevated risks persisted after eliminating the subgroup of cases with early stage lesions confined to the prostate. The relative risks were somewhat higher for the subcohorts who had had their vasectomy at least 20 years ago, and higher risk persisted after controlling for potential confounding by diet, level of physical activity, smoking, alcohol, body mass index, and educational level. Giovannucci and colleagues (1993a) summarized in these reports data from five case–control studies and one retrospective cohort study. In this meta-analysis, the overall risk of prostate cancer among vasectomized men was 1.5 ($P < 0.05$) and the risk was more pronounced among men who had their vasectomy for more than 20 years.

In the original case–control report by Honda et al (1988), vasectomized men had slightly higher testosterone levels ($P = 0.06$) and significantly higher testosterone/testosterone-binding globulin capacity ratios (a measure of bioavailable testosterone). Honda et al (1988) speculated that while these differences could be a result of the surgical procedure, alternatively it was also possible that the decision to have a vasectomy (especially in the distant past) might have been related to sexual practices, which might, in turn, have been related to bioavailable androgens.

In a position statement, the American Urological Association (AUA) (1993) recommended that men who had a vasectomy more than 20 years ago, or who were more than 40 years of age at the time of their vasectomy, should have an annual digital rectal examination and a determination of serum PSA level. Noting that the relationship between vasectomy and prostate cancer was unproven, the AUA does not recommend reversal of vasectomy.

Circumcision

Circumcision has been hypothesized to reduce risk of prostate cancer by reducing exposure to smegma and/or infectious agents collected by the foreskin. The consistent finding of a lower risk of prostate cancer for Jewish men (Waterhouse et al, 1982; Lilienfeld et al, 1972) has been interpreted to support this hypothesis. Most previous studies have found either no association (Wynder et al, 1971; Jackson et al, 1980) or a small reduction in risk (Rotkin, 1977). However, population-based case–control studies of prostate cancer among blacks and whites in Los Angeles found self-reported circumcision to be associated with a significant reduction in risk for both populations (RR = 0.6 in blacks; RR = 0.5 in whites) (Ross et al, 1987). A small hospital-based case–control study of prostate cancer found that circumcision was associated with a significant increase in risk (RR = 1.9) (Newell et al, 1989); however, failure to control for socioeconomic factors may have led to a spurious association.

OTHER POSSIBLE RISK FACTORS

Benign Prostatic Diseases

The probability that a 40-year-old man in the United States will undergo surgery for benign or malignant prostatic diseases by age 80 is 30% to 40% (Barry, 1990). In 10% of patients with benign prostatic hyperplasia who have undergone transurethral resection of the prostate (TURP), incidental prostate carcinoma was discovered on microscopic examination (Sheldon et al,

1980). Greenwald et al (1974) compared prostate cancer incidence among 838 men treated for BPH at a Boston clinic in the 1940s and 1950s, with 802 surgical controls of the same age treated during the same period. As of 1970, rates of prostate cancer development were similar between the two groups. The study has been criticized because the BPH cases had had partial removal of their prostates and therefore may have been at lower risk on this basis (Hodges and Wan, 1983). In addition, men with latent carcinomas were excluded from the BPH group, possibly leading to an underestimate of risk. In another prospective study, Armenian et al (1974) identified 338 men with BPH treated at Roswell Park Memorial Institute over a 20-year period and age-matched them to non-cancer hospital controls. Only about one-half of the BPH cases were histologically confirmed. As of 1972, the prostate cancer mortality rate among men with BPH was 3.5 times that of the controls. In a hospital-based case–control study conducted at the same center, men reporting past hospitalizations for BPH had 5.1 times the risk of developing prostatic cancer (Armenian et al, 1974). These findings were supported by case–control studies of prostate cancer in middle-aged men in Los Angeles (Honda et al, 1988); of older men in Japan (Mishina et al, 1985); and of men of all ages in Hawaii (Kolonel et al, 1988). In the study by Honda et al (1988), a population-based study involving 216 matched neighborhood control pairs, the prevalence of reported previous prostate problems in cases and the associated relative risks were as follows: prostatitis (17%, RR = 2.2); enlarged prostate (25%, RR = 3.6); and prostate surgery (9%, RR = 2.0). Mishina et al (1985) found an even higher risk for a past history of BPH in a case–control study in Japan (RR = 13.5, $P < 0.01$), but a statistically insignificant excess of prostatitis (RR = 1.6). Kolonel et al (1988) in a case–control study in Hawaii found a strong association with prior BPH in men under age 70 (RR = 10.5, $P < 0.01$), but minimal association in older men. In a prospective study of 35,000 Seventh Day Adventists, men who reported that a doctor had told them they had "prostate trouble" had a 1.6-fold increase in risk compared to men with no such history ($P = 0.04$) (Mills et al, 1989). Based on a 10-year follow-up study in Sweden, it was concluded that neither BPH nor TURP increased the risk of developing clinical prostate cancer; the control cohort consisted of age-matched men who underwent an operation for inguinal hernia (Hammarsten et al, 1994).

The total evidence suggests that previous prostatic diseases are associated with an increased risk of prostate cancer. BPH does not appear to be a major precancerous condition per se since it tends to arise more commonly in the periurethral area and transition zone of the prostate rather than in the peripheral zone where cancer occurs predominantly (McNeal, 1993). Conceivably, BPH could represent an entity in a neoplastic continuum or multistage process in relation to a subset of prostate cancer which arises in the transition zone (Bostwick et al, 1992), or BPH could occur together with prostate cancer in the same individual more often than expected due to a common hormonal etiology.

Family History

Available epidemiologic data strongly support a familial tendency toward prostate cancer occurrence. Woolf (1960) used the virtually complete genealogical records of the Mormon church to identify familial history of prostate cancer deaths among 228 men who died of prostate cancer and among a comparable number of men who died of other causes. Fifteen cases versus five controls had a family history of prostate cancer deaths ($P < 0.05$). Case–control studies which have collected family histories of prostate cancer in first-degree relatives have generally found comparable levels of risk (Kolonel et al, 1988; Honda et al, 1988; Krain, 1973; Jackson et al, 1980; Fincham et al, 1990; Ghadirian et al, 1991; Spitz et al, 1991). Steinberg and colleagues (1990) collected extensive cancer pedigrees on 691 men undergoing surgery for prostate cancer at the Johns Hopkins University Hospital, using the families of the patients' spouses for controls. Men with one first-degree relative with prostate cancer had a twofold increase in risk, whereas a positive family history for a second-degree relative was associated with a 70% increase in risk. A family history involving two first-degree relatives was associated with a fivefold increase, whereas a history in more than two first-degree relatives was associated with an 11-fold increase in risk. In their analysis, 15% of the first-degree relatives of patients with prostate cancer had a history of prostate cancer, compared with 8% of the control group's relatives.

Familial history of prostate cancer appears to be associated with earlier onset of disease in first-degree relatives. By means of segregation analysis, Carter et al (1992a) attributed familial aggregation to a rare, highly penetrant autosomal dominant allele. The theoretical model predicted that the inherited form of prostate cancer accounted for approximately 40% of cases diagnosed under 55 years of age, but for less than 10% of all cases. Mutation through deletion or unbalanced translocation with loss of heterozygosity of a putative tumor suppressor gene on chromosome 8p is currently under investigation in familial prostate cancer (MacGrogan et al, 1994). In a study of primary prostate tumors, the highest frequency (46%–65%) of allelic deletion was found on 8p (Bergerheim et al, 1991; Huncharek and Muscat, 1995).

Molecular Genetics

It has been hypothesized that progression from normal prostatic epithelium to prostatic intraepithelial neoplasia to invasive cancer occurs as a result of a "genetic cascade" of impaired control mechanisms for cell differentiation and proliferation. Sandberg (1992) has suggested a molecular model of prostate oncogenesis involving allelic losses of tumor suppressor genes on chromosomes 7q, 8p, 10q, 13q and 16q, and the overexpression of ras or myc oncogenes.

Little is known regarding the molecular basis of prostate cancer. Mutations in certain oncogenes such as *ras* (e.g., H-ras, K-ras and N-ras) have not commonly been described in prostate cancers in the United States, although *ras* mutations (e.g., codons 12, 13, and 61) appear to be more common in prostate cancer specimens from Japan (Isaacs and Carter, 1991; Isaacs et al, 1994; Konishi et al, 1992; Anwar et al, 1992). Mutations in the *p53* tumor suppressor gene, which normally encodes a nuclear phosphoprotein that regulates the cell cycle and induces apoptosis in DNA damaged cells, are common in many epithelial cancers; however, *p53* alterations have been described either as relatively infrequent (10%–20%) in some molecular studies of prostate cancer (Effert et al, 1993), or of a higher frequency (40%–50%) in others (Chi et al, 1994). Conceivably, radiation-resistant, androgen-independent, more aggressive lesions may be associated with an increased prevalence of p53 mutations (Prendergast and Walther, 1995).

Mutations in the androgen receptor gene are rare in prostate cancer and seem to occur only as somatic mutations during tumor progression which is refractory to hormone treatment, although it has been hypothesized that polymorphisms in the transcription modulatory domain of the AR gene might be related to variations in androgen activity and prostate cancer risk (Coetzee and Ross, 1994). Similar hypotheses are under exploration relating to expression of the 5-alpha reductase type II gene, which regulates metabolic activation of testosterone in prostate epithelium (Reichardt et al, 1995).

Allelic losses on chromosome 16q in approximately one-third of primary prostate tumor specimens and in a higher proportion of metastatic tumors have been correlated with poorly differentiated tumors of higher Gleason grade and with tumor progression. The locus of the E-cadherin gene on the long arm of chromosome 16 is of interest as it mediates the pathway of cell–cell adhesion (Isaacs et al, 1994). In studies using the Dunning rat prostate cancer model, reduction in E-cadherin protein levels was associated with enhanced invasive or metastatic potential, and transfection of invasive adenocarcinoma cells with E-cadherin cDNA limited or inhibited the invasive characteristics of tumor cells (Vleminckx et al, 1991; Bussemakers et al, 1992; Kallioniemi and Visakorpi, 1996).

Alcohol Use

Alcohol consumption is of interest as a possible risk factor for prostate cancer, primarily because of its acute depressant effect on circulating testosterone levels, and because of possible longer term reduction in sex steroid-binding globulin levels and relative hyperestrogenism associated with alcohol-induced chronic liver disease (Aldercreutz, 1974; Siiteri and MacDonald, 1973). Interest in this association was stimulated by an early report by Glantz (1964) that prostate cancer in an autopsy series of men with cirrhosis was one-third as common as in men without cirrhosis. However, prospective studies of men treated for alcoholism have found no significant excess or deficit of prostate cancer mortality compared with rates in the general population (Sundby, 1967; Schmidt and Delint, 1972; Pell and D'Alonza, 1973; Monson and Lyon, 1975). The results of case–control and other prospective studies are also compatible with little or no effect of alcohol consumption on risk, either overall or by amount consumed (Ross et al, 1987; Wynder et al, 1971; Rotkin, 1980; Yu et al, 1988; Mills et al, 1989; Tavani et al, 1994). In a study of U.S. blacks, Jackson et al (1980) found that significantly more controls than cases used alcohol ($P < 0.05$). Hirayama in a population-based prospective study in Japan found a significant association with alcohol intake that was present at all ages and unexplained by cigarette smoking (Ross et al, 1987). In a population-based case-control study, Hayes et al (1996) reported an increased risk of prostate cancer in U.S. white and black men with alcohol use in excess of 22 drinks per week, and unconfounded by tobacco use.

Cigarette Smoking

Studies of correlates of circulating testosterone levels find higher levels in cigarette smokers than in nonsmokers (Dai et al, 1981; Deslypere and Vermeulen, 1984), although these differences are not large and apparently are not dose related (Barrett-Conner and Khaw, 1990).

A number of previous studies including six large well-designed cohort studies have reported on the relationship between prostate cancer and cigarette smoking. Doll and Peto (1976) followed 34,000 male British physicians for approximately 20 years and observed 186 deaths from prostate cancer; smokers had a 23% reduction in risk, which was not statistically significant. In a report of the results of the American Cancer Society cohort study, Hammond (1966) found no alteration in risk among smokers in the 319 men who died of prostate cancer. In the Dorn study of 250,000 military veterans followed for 16 years, there were 1,020 prostate cancer deaths; smokers had a 31% increase and ex-smokers an 18% increase in risk of dying of prostate cancer, compared to non-smokers (Rogot and Murray, 1980). Ross et al (1990) studied the association of smoking and prostate cancer risk in 4,373 male residents of a retirement community near Los Angeles, California. Based on 138 prostate cancers identified during follow-up, current cigarette smokers had a slightly reduced risk of prostate cancer compared to lifetime non-smokers (RR = 0.9), but this reduction was not statistically significant. Men who smoked for more than 30 years had a significantly reduced risk of prostate cancer, compared to lifetime non-smokers (RR = 0.6, 95% CI = 0.4, 0.97), but risk in short-duration smokers was actually significantly increased (RR = 2.2, 95% CI = 1.2, 3.9). Hsing et al (1990b) reported a significant association between cigarette smoking (RR = 1.8, relative to non-smokers) and prostate cancer in a prospective study of 18,000 white male policy holders in the Lutheran Brotherhood Insurance Society. However, no dose–response relationship was apparent. This group also reported a small excess risk of prostate cancer in a 26-year follow-up study of 250,000 U.S. veterans (RR = 1.2) (Hsing et al, 1991). The relative risk increased to 1.5 for two-pack-a-day smokers.

Most of the case–control studies of the association between prostate cancer and smoking have been hospital based (Wynder et al, 1971; Armenian et al, 1974) and therefore difficult to interpret. Mandel (1981) examined the smoking habits of prostate cancer cases and of both hospital and neighborhood controls. The relative risks were 0.7 and 1.1, respectively, in smokers compared to non-smokers, which underscores the concern that use of hospital controls might bias studies of this association. In a population-based case–control study conducted in Los Angeles of males aged 60 or less, Honda et al (1988) found prostate cancer risk to be significantly related to smoking (RR = 1.9 for ever versus never smoked regularly; 95% CI = 1.2, 3.0). There was a positive relationship between prostate cancer risk and smoking duration ($P = 0.001$, test for trend); men who had smoked at least 40 years had 2.6 times the risk of men who had never smoked. It was hypothesized that sociocultural determinants of smoking in the U.S. might be age-related and that this might explain both an association between smoking and prostate cancer that is limited to young men and an association between smoking and testosterone levels that is non-causal (Honda et al, 1988).

Occupation

Occupational studies of prostate cancer have focused on cadmium. Cadmium, a non-essential trace element, is a zinc antagonist in biological systems (Gunn et al, 1961). Zinc, an essential trace element apparently involved in the regulation of cell growth, is concentrated more heavily in prostatic tissue than in any other organ (Kara and Chowdbury, 1968). It has been hypothesized that accumulation of cadmium in the prostate might interrupt normal cell growth and metabolism and result in neoplasia (Kolonel and Winkelstein, 1977).

Early epidemiological studies provided some limited support for this hypothesis. A small cohort study of smelter workers exposed to cadmium conducted by Lemen and colleagues (1976) found 4 deaths from prostate cancer among 92 decedents, compared to an expected 1.2 deaths. Kipling and Waterhouse (1967) found 4 prostate cancer cases compared to only 0.6 expected in a cohort of 248 workers exposed to cadmium oxide for a minimum of 1 year. In a subsequent case–control study, Kolonel and Winkelstein (1977) reported a relative risk of 1.6 for occupational histories entailing possible cadmium exposure, e.g., alkaline battery manufacturing, welding, and electroplating. However, in a report using data on occupation from a population-based cancer registry in Los Angeles, none of these occupations showed significantly higher than expected prostate cancer rates (Ross et al, 1979). Other studies have been unable to confirm any association between cadmium exposure and prostate cancer risk (Armstrong and Kazantzis, 1985).

Several studies have suggested that farmers are at high risk of prostate cancer (DeCoufle et al, 1977; Ernster et al, 1979b; Checkoway et al, 1987; Blair et al, 1985), although no specific explanation for this apparent high risk has been forthcoming and some large studies have been unable to confirm this observation (Pearce et al, 1987). Elevated rates of prostate cancer mortality since 1970, particularly among African-Americans, were described in the southeastern states, where approximately 38% of the excess mortality was attributed to farm-related occupations (Dosemeci et al, 1994). It has also been suggested that textile workers may be at high risk of prostate cancer (Checkoway et al, 1987; Blair and Fraumeni, 1978), but a case–control study in South Carolina based on review of death certificates could not confirm this (Hoar and Blair, 1984).

Increased risk of prostate cancer has been consistently reported for employees of rubber companies (Monson and Nakano, 1976a,b; Andjelkovic et al, 1976), but no specific etiologic exposure has been identified. A number of other occupations have been suggested to be associated with high risk in individual studies, but these results have been based on small numbers and should be considered preliminary (Ernster et al, 1979b; Williams et al, 1977; Logan, 1982).

If any of the occupational associations are real, it is likely that only a very small proportion of all prostate cancer cases can be attributed to a specific industrial chemical exposure.

PREVENTIVE MEASURES AND FUTURE RESEARCH

Our current knowledge of prostate cancer risk factors is insufficient to recommend confidently any strategies for primary prevention through lifestyle changes. Available data are highly suggestive that high fat intake leads to increased risk. Should the apparent association with fat become more firmly established, determining whether the association is mediated through hormonal alteration will prove important. Establishing such a mechanism may open other avenues of prevention as alternatives to dietary modification.

Further research will be required to clarify the possible association between intake of vitamin A compounds and prostate cancer risk, especially the discrepant findings between dietary survey and serum studies. Feeding of a synthetic retinoid, N-4-hydroxyphenyl retinamide, has been reported to inhibit the progression of prostate cancer in Lobund-Wistar or Dunning rats (Pollard et al, 1991; Pienta et al, 1993).

A better understanding of determinants of circulating testosterone levels will allow epidemiologists to evaluate an endocrine etiology of prostate cancer. Recent evidence that variability in 5-alpha reductase activity among populations may explain some of the international variations in prostatic cancer incidence has stimulated the experimental introduction of pharmaceuticals such as finasteride (proscar), a 5 alpha-reductase inhibitor, as potential chemopreventive agents in prostatic neoplasia (Gormley et al, 1992). As molecular technology has advanced, it has become possible to evaluate on a population basis whether prostate cancer risk might be related to sequence variations in genes associated with androgen secretion or metabolism, or in other genes that might affect biochemical functions (e.g., differentiation apoptosis, adhesion, DNA repair, genetic stability, angiogenesis) possibly related to prostate cancer.

There is no available testing method for prostate cancer that would ensure detection of a significant proportion of preclinical lesions at a potentially curable stage (Adami et al, 1994). Digital rectal examination, which examines the posterior and lateral surfaces of the prostate gland, has serious limitations; on a single, independent examination, the sensitivity is less than 50%, although specificity may be as high as 99%. The positive predictive value may vary between 10% and 35% (U.S. Preventive Services Task Force, 1994). Friedman et al (1991) inferred, based on a case–control study, that DRE was not effective in preventing metastatic prostatic cancer. The odds ratio for metastatic prostate cancer after one or more screening DRE, compared with men who had none during a 10-year period, was 0.9 (95% CI = 0.5,1.7).

Prostate-specific antigen (PSA) is a serine protease that is produced by the epithelial cells lining the acini and ducts of the prostate gland (Hara et al, 1971). PSA, although specific for prostatic tissue, lacks specificity for detecting prostate cancer (Stamey et al, 1987; Dorr et al, 1993; Stamey et al, 1993). In the American Cancer Society Prostate Cancer Detection Project in which the criterion for an abnormal PSA was > 4 ng/mL in men 50 to 70 years of age, the sensitivity for detecting prostate cancer was determined to be 67%, the specificity was 97%, and the positive predictive value was 43% (Babaian et al, 1992). Other studies that have evaluated the validity of PSA screening reported higher probability estimates of sensitivity from 83% to 96%, but much lower specificity, ranging from 38% to 56% (Canadian Task Force on the Periodic Health Examination, 1991; Catalona et al, 1991; Oesterling et al, 1993; Walther, 1995). Stenman et al (1991) demonstrated that the concentration of PSA complexed to alpha-1-antichymotrypsin (ACT) was higher in men with prostate cancer, compared with age-matched normal men, or men with only BPH. PSA complexed to ACT normally comprises about 85% of PSA in the serum; the ratio of free PSA to total PSA in prostate cancer patients is equal to or less than 0.18 (Lilja et al, 1991; Christensson et al, 1993).

To enhance the specificity of PSA, Benson et al (1992) suggested adjusting the measurement of serum PSA concentration by the prostatic volume. This concept of PSA density was advanced to help discriminate between prostatic hyperplasia and cancer for serum PSA concentrations in the elevated range of 4.0 to 10.0 ng/mL. However, the epithelium that produces PSA, in glands of similar volume, but with varying amounts of stromal compared to epithelial tissue, may produce substantially different amounts of PSA. In a longitudinal study, Carter et al (1992b) recorded patterns of variations in serum PSA on repeated measurements. The median increase in men without prostatic disease was 0.03 ng/mL per year; for men with symptomatic BPH, the PSA increased with age at a rate of 0.12 ng/mL per year; and for men with prostatic cancer, the yearly rate of increase was 0.75 ng/mL or higher. PSA in combination with DRE and transrectal ultrasound may result in enhanced sensitivity, but at the cost of increased false positivity. Because of the uncertainty surrounding the efficacy of screening for prostate cancer (Krahn et al, 1994; Waterbor and Bueschen, 1995), the National Cancer Institute has initiated a multicenter randomized trial (Kramer et al, 1993).

REFERENCES

ADAMI H-O, BARON JA, ROTHMAN KJ. 1994. Ethics of a prostate cancer screening trial. Lancet 343:958–960.

AHLUWALIA B, JACKSON MA, JONES GW, et al. 1981. Blood hormone profiles in prostate cancer patients in high risk and low risk populations. Cancer 48:2267–2273.

ALBANES D, BLAIR A, TAYLOR PR. 1989. Physical activity and risk of cancer in the NHANES I population. Am J Public Health 79:744–750.

ALDERCREUTZ N. 1974. Hepatic metabolism of estrogen in health and disease. N Engl J Med 290:1081–1083.

AMERICAN UROLOGICAL ASSOCIATION. 1993. Position statement. Cancer Epidemiol Biomarkers Prev 2:295.

ANDJELKOVIC D, TAULBEE J, SYMONS M. 1976. Mortality experience of a cohort of rubber workers, 1964–73. J Occup Med 18:387–394.

ANWAR K, NAKAKUKI K, SHIRAISHI T, et al. 1992. Presence of ras oncogene mutations and human papilloma virus DNA in human prostate carcinoma. Cancer Res 52:5991–5996.

AOKI K, KURIHARA M, HAYAKAWA N, SUZUKI S (eds). 1992. Death Rates for Malignant Neoplasms for Selected Sites by Sex and Five-Year Age Group in 33 Countries 1953–57 to 1983–87. International Union Against Cancer. Nagoya, Japan, University of Nagoya Coop. Press.

ARMENIAN HK, LILIENFELD AM, DIAMOND EL, et al. 1974. Relation between benign prostatic hyperplasia and cancer of the prostate. Lancet ii:115–117.

ARMSTRONG B, DOLL R. 1975. Environmental factors and cancer incidence and mortality in different countries, with special reference to dietary practices. Int J Cancer 15:617–631.

ARMSTRONG BG, KAZANTZIS G. 1985. Prostatic cancer and chronic respiratory and renal disease in British cadmium workers: a case-control study. Br J Ind Med 42:540–545.

BABAIAN RJ, METTLIN C, KANE R, et al. 1992. The relationship of prostate-specific antigen to digital examination and transrectal ultrasonography. Findings of the American Cancer Society National Prostate Cancer Detection Project. Cancer 69:1195–1200.

BAQUET CR, HORM JW, GIBBS T, et al. 1991. Socioeconomic factors and cancer incidence among blacks and whites. J Natl Cancer Inst 83:551–557.

BARRETT-CONNER E, KHAW KT. 1990. Smoking and endogenous sex hormones in men and women. Wald N, Baron J (eds). *In* Smoking and Hormone-Related Disorders. New York, Oxford University Press, pp. 183–196.

BARRY MJ. 1990. Epidemiology and natural history of benign prostatic hyperplasia. Urol Clin North Am 17:495–507.

BARTSCH W, HORST HJ, BECKER H, et al. 1977. Sex hormone binding globulin-binding capacity, testosterone, 5-α dihydrotestosterone, oestradiol and prolactin in plasma of patients with prostatic carcinoma under various types of hormonal treatment. Acta Endocrinol 85:650–654.

BATES CJ. 1995. Vitamin A. Lancet 345:31–35.

BENSON MC, WHANG JS, PONTUCK A, et al. 1992. Prostate-specific antigen density: a means of distinguishing benign prostatic hypertrophy and prostate cancer. J Urol 147:815–816.

BERG JW. 1975. Can nutrition explain the pattern of international epidemiology of hormone-dependent cancers? Cancer Res 35:3345–3350.

BERGERHEIM USR, KUNIMI K, COLLINS VP, et al. 1991. Deletion mapping of chromosomes 8, 10 and 6 in human prostatic carcinoma. Genes chromosomes and Cancer 3:215–220.

BERNSTEIN L, ROSS R. 1995. Cancer in Los Angeles County. A Portrait of Incidence and Mortality 1972–1987. Los Angeles, University of Southern California Press.

BLAIR A, FRAUMENI JF. 1978. Geographic patterns of prostate cancer in the United States. J Natl Cancer Inst 61:1379–1384.

BLAIR A, MALKER H, CANTOR KP, et al. 1985. Cancer among farmers: A review. Scand J Work Environ Health 11:397–407.

BORING CC, SQUIRES TS, TONG T. 1992. Cancer Statistics, 1992. Cancer J Clin 42:19–38.

BOSLAND MC, PRINSEN MK, KROES R. 1984. Chemical induction of prostatic adenocarcinomas in rats. AACR Abstracts, No. 103.

BOSTWICK DG, COONER WH, DENIS L, et al. 1992. The association of benign prostatic hyperplasia and cancer of the prostate. Cancer 70:291–301.

BOYLE P, MAISONNEUVE P, NAPALKOV P. 1995. Geographical and temporal patterns of incidence and mortality from prostate cancer. Urology 46:47–55.

BRAWLEY OW, FORD LG, THOMPSON I, et al. 1994. 5-α-reductase inhibition and prostate cancer prevention. Cancer Epidemiol, Biomarkers, Prev 3:177–182.

BROWN CE, WARREN S, CHUTE RN, et al. 1979. Hormonally induced tumors of the reproductive system of parabiosed male rats. Cancer Res 39:3971–3975.

BUSSEMAKERS MJG, VAN MOORSELAAR RJA, GIROLDI LA, et al. 1992. Decreased expression of E-cadherin in the progression of rat prostatic cancer. Cancer Res 52:2916–2922.

CANADIAN TASK FORCE ON THE PERIODIC HEALTH EXAMINATION. 1991. Periodic health examination, 1991 update: 3. Secondary prevention of prostate cancer. Can Med Assoc J 145:413–428.

CARROLL KK, KHOR HT. 1975. Dietary fat in relation to tumorigenesis. Prog Biochem Pharmacol 10:308–353.

CARTER BS, BEATY TH, STEINBERG GD, et al. 1992a. Mendelian inheritance of familial prostate cancer. Proc Natl Acad Sci USA 89:3367–3371.

CARTER HB, PEARSON JD, METTER EJ, et al. 1992b. Longitudinal evaluation of prostate-specific antigen levels in men with and without prostate disease. JAMA 267:2215–2220.

CATALONA WJ. 1994. Management of cancer of the prostate. N Engl J Med 331:996–1004.

CATALONA WJ, SMITH DS, RATLIFF T, et al. 1993. Detection of organ-confined prostate cancer is increased through prostate-specific antigen-based screening. JAMA 270:948–954.

CATALONA WJ, SMITH DS, RATLIFF TL, et al. 1991. Measurement of prostate-specific antigen in serum as a screening test for prostate cancer. New Engl J Med 324:1156–1161.

CHAPRONIERE DM, WEBER MM. 1985. Dexamethasone and retinol acetate similarly inhibit and stimulate EGF- or insulin-induced proliferation of prostatic epithelium. J Cell Physiol 122:249–253.

CHECKOWAY H, DIFERDINANDO G, HULKA BS, et al. 1987. Medical, lifestyle, and occupational risk factors for prostate cancer. Prostate 10:79–88.

CHI S-G, WHITE RWV, MEYERS FJ, et al. 1994. p53 in prostate cancer: frequent expressed transition mutations. J Natl Cancer Inst 86:926–933.

CHRISTENSSON A, BJÖRK T, NILSSON O, et al. 1993. Serum prostate-specific antigen complexed to alpha-1-antichymotrypsin as an indicator of prostate cancer. J Urol 150:100–105.

CLEMENTE CD, GRAY H. 1985. Anatomy of the Human Body. 30th American Ed. Philadelphia, Lea and Febiger. pp 1564–1566.

CLEMMESEN J. 1969. Statistical studies in the aetiology of malignant neoplasms. APMS Suppl 209:1–171.

COETZEE GA, ROSS RK. 1994. Re: Prostate cancer and the androgen receptor. J Natl Cancer Inst 86:872–873.

COFFEY DS. 1979. Physiological control of prostatic growth. An overview. In: Prostate Cancer. UICC Technical Report Series, Vol. 48. Geneva, International Union Against Cancer.

CORDER EH, GUESS HA, HULKA BS, et al. 1993. Vitamin D and prostate cancer: a prediagnostic study with stored sera. Cancer Epidemiol Biomarkers Prev 2:467–472.

DAI WS, KULLER LH, LAPORTE RE, et al. 1981. The epidemiology of plasma testosterone levels in middle-aged men. Am J Epidemiol 114:804–816.

DECOUFLE P, STANISLAWCZYK K, HOUTEN L, et al. 1977. A retrospective survey of cancer in relation to occupation. NIOSH Washington, D.C., Department of Health, Education and Welfare. Publ. No. 77-1788.

DELATORRE B, HEDMAN M, JENSEN F, et al. 1983. Lack of effect of vasectomy on peripheral gonadotrophin and steroid levels. Int J Androl 6:125–134.

DESLYPERE JP, VERMEULEN A. 1984. Leydig cell function in normal men: Effect of age, lifestyle, residence, diet, and activity. J Clin Endocrinol Metab 59:955–962.

DOLL R, MUIR C, WATERHOUSE J (eds). 1970. Cancer Incidence in Five Continents, Vol. II. New York, Springer-Verlag.

DOLL R, PAYNE P, WATERHOUSE J (eds). 1966. Cancer Incidence in Five Continents, Vol. I. New York, Springer-Verlag.

DOLL R, PETO R. 1976. Mortality in relation to smoking: 20 years' observations on male British doctors. BMJ 2:1525–1536.

DOLL R, PETO R. 1981. The causes of cancer: Quantitative estimates of avoidable risks of cancer in the United States today. New York, Oxford University Press.

DORR VJ, WILLIAMSON SK, STEPHENS RL. 1993. An evaluation of prostate-specific antigen as a screening test for prostate cancer. Arch Intern Med 153:2529–2537.

DOSEMECI M, HOOVER RN, BLAIR A, et al. 1994. Farming and prostate cancer among African-Americans in the southeastern United States. J Natl Cancer Inst 86:1718–1719.

DRAFTA D, PROCA E, ZAMFIR V, et al. 1982. Plasma steroids in benign prostatic hypertrophy and carcinoma of the prostate. J Steroid Biochem 17:689–693.

EDWARDS A, HAMMOND HA, JIN L, et al. 1992. Genetic variation at five trimeric and tetrameric tandem repeat loci in four human population groups. Genomics 12:241–253.

EFFERT PJ, MCCOY RH, WALTHER PJ, et al. 1992. p53 gene alterations in human prostate carcinoma. J Urol 150:257–261.

ELLIS L, NYBORG H. 1992. Racial/ethnic variations in male testosterone levels: a probable contributor to group differences in health. Steroids 57:72–75.

ERNSTER VL, SACKS ST, SELVIN S, et al. 1979a. Cancer incidence by marital status: U.S. Third National Cancer Survey. J Natl Cancer Inst 63:567–585.

ERNSTER VL, SELVIN S, BROWN SM, et al. 1979b. Occupation and prostatic cancer: A review and retrospective analysis based on death certificates in two California counties. J Occup Med 21:175–183.

ERNSTER VL, WINKELSTEIN W, SELVIN S, et al. 1977. Race, socioeconomic status and prostatic cancer. Cancer Treat Rep 61:187–191.

FEMINELLA JJ, LATTIMER JR. 1974. An apparent increase in genital carcinomas among wives of men with prostatic cancer: An epidemiologic survey. Pirquet Bull Clin Med 20:3–9.

FINCHAM SM, HILL GB, HANSON J, et al. 1990. Epidemiology of prostate cancer: A case–control study. Prostate 17:189–206.

FRIEDMAN GD, HIATT RA, QUESENBERRY CP, et al. 1991. Case–control study of screening for prostatic cancer by digital rectal examinations. Lancet 337:1526–1529.

GANN PH, HENNEKENS CH, SACKS FM, et al. 1994. Prospective study of plasma fatty acids and risk of prostate cancer. J Natl Cancer Inst 86:281–286.

GHADIRIAN P, CADOTTE M, LACROIX A, et al. 1991. Familial aggregation of cancer of the prostate in Quebec: The tip of the iceberg. Prostate 19:43–52.

GHANADIAN R, PUAH CM, O'DONOGHUE EPN. 1979. Serum testosterone and dihydrotestosterone in carcinoma of the prostate. Br J Cancer 39:696–699.

GIOVANNUCCI E, ASCHERIO A, RIMM E, et al. 1993a. A prospective cohort study of vasectomy and prostate cancer in U.S. men. JAMA 269:873–877.

GIOVANNUCCI E, ASCHERIO A, RIMM E, et al. 1993b. A retrospective cohort study of vasectomy and prostate cancer in U.S. men. JAMA 269:878–882.

GIOVANNUCCI E, RIMM EB, COLDITZ GA, et al. 1993c. A prospective study of dietary fat and risk of prostate cancer. J Natl Cancer Inst 85:1571–1579.

GLANTZ GM. 1964. Cirrhosis and carcinoma of the prostate gland. J Urol 91:291–293.

GORMLEY GJ, STONER E, BRUSKEWITZ RC, et al. 1992. The effect of finasteride in men with benign prostatic hyperplasia. N Engl J Med 327:1185–1191.

GRAHAM S, HAUGHEY B, MARSHALL J, et al. 1983. Diet in the epidemiology of carcinoma of the prostate gland. J Natl Cancer Inst 70:687–692.

GRAYHACK JT. 1963. Pituitary factors influencing growth of the prostate. Natl Cancer Inst Monogr 12:189–199.

GREENWALD P, DAMON A, KIRMSS V, et al. 1974. Physical and demographic features of men before developing cancer of the prostate. J Natl Cancer Inst 53:341–346.

GRIFFITHS R, DAVIES P, HARPER ME, et al. 1979. The etiology and endocrinology of prostatic cancer. *In* Rose DP (ed): Endocrinology of Cancer. Boca Raton, FL, CRC Press Inc.

GUNN SA, GOULD TC, ANDERSON WAD. 1961. Competition of cadmium for zinc in rat testis and dorsolateral prostate. Acta Endocrinol 37:24–30.

HAENSZEL W, KURIHARA M. 1968. Studies of Japanese migrants. I. Mortality from cancer and other diseases among Japanese in the United States. J Natl Cancer Inst 40:43–68.

HAMMARSTEN J, ANDERSON S, HOLMEN A, et al. 1994. Does transurethral resection of a clinically benign prostate gland increase the risk of developing clinical prostate cancer? Cancer 74:2347–2351.

HAMMOND EC. 1966. Smoking in relation to the death rates in one million men and women. Natl Cancer Inst Monogr 19:127–204.

HAMMOND GL, KONTTURI M, VIHKO R. 1978. Serum steroids in normal males and patients with prostatic diseases. Clin Endocrinol 9:113–121.

HARA M, INNORE T, FUKUYAMA T. 1971. Some physicochemical characteristics of gamma-seminoprotein, an antigenic component specific for human seminal plasma. Jpn J Leg Med 25:322–324.

HARPER ME, PEELING WB, COWLEY T, et al. 1976. Plasma steroid and protein hormone concentrations in patients with prostatic carcinoma, before and during estrogen therapy. Acta Endocrinol 81:409–426.

HAYES RB, BOGDANOVICZ FAT, SCHROEDER FH, et al. 1988. Serum retinol and prostate cancer. Cancer 62:2021–2026.

HAYES RB, POTTERN LM, GREENBERG R, et al. 1993. Vasectomy and prostate cancer in U.S. blacks and whites. Am J Epidemiol 137:263–269.

HAYES RB, BROWN LM, SCHOENBERG JB, et al. 1996. Alcohol use and prostate cancer risk in US blacks and whites. Am J Epidemiol 143:692–697.

HENDERSON BE, BERNSTEIN L, ROSS RK, et al. 1988. The early *in utero* oestrogen and testosterone environment of blacks and whites: Potential effects on male offspring. Br J Cancer 57:216–218.

HENDERSON BE, ROSS RK, CASAGRANDE JT. 1982. Endogenous hormones as a major factor in human cancer. Cancer Res 42:3232–3239.

HESHMAT NY, KAUL L, KOVI J, et al. 1985. Nutrition and prostate cancer. A case–control study. Prostate 6:7–17.

HESHMAT MY, KOVI J, HERSON J, et al. 1975. Epidemiologic association between gonorrhea and prostatic carcinoma. Urology 6:457–460.

HIGGINSON J, OETTLE AG. 1960. Cancer incidence in the Bantu and 'Cape-Colored' races of South Africa: Report of a cancer survey in the Transvaal 1953–1955. J Natl Cancer Inst 24:589–671.

HILL PB, WYNDER EL. 1979. Effect of vegetarian diet and dexamethasone on plasma prolactin, testosterone and dehydroepiandrosterone in men and women. Cancer Lett 7:273–282.

HIRAYAMA T. 1979a. Diet and cancer. Nutr Cancer 1:67–81.

HIRAYAMA T. 1979b. Epidemiology of prostate cancer with special reference to the role of diet. Natl Cancer Inst Mongr 53:149–155.

HIRAYAMA T. 1986. A large scale cohort study on cancer risk by diet with special reference to the risk reducing effect of green-yellow vegetable consumption. *In* Hayashi Y, Nagao M, Sugimura T, Takayama S, Tomatis L, Wattenberg LW, Wogan G (eds): Diet, Nutrition and Cancer. Tokyo, Japan Scientific Press.

HOAR SK, BLAIR A. 1984. Death certificate case–control study of cancers of the prostate and colon and employment in the textile industry. Arch Environ Health 39:280–283.

HODGES CV, WAN SP. 1983. The relationship between benign prostatic hyperplasia and prostatic carcinoma. *In* Hinman F Jr (ed): Benign Prostatic Hypertrophy. New York, Springer-Verlag.

HONDA GD. 1986. Vasectomy, cigarette smoking and other risk factors for prostate cancer in young men: a case–control study. Ph.D. Dissertation, UCLA.

HONDA GD, BERNSTEIN L, ROSS RK, et al. 1988. Vasectomy, cigarette smoking, and age at first sexual intercourse as risk factors for prostate cancer in middle-aged men. Br J Cancer 57:326–331.

HOOVER R, MASON TJ, MCKAY FW, et al. 1975. Geographic patterns of cancer mortality in the United States. *In* Fraumeni JF (ed): Persons at High Risk of Cancer. New York, Academic Press, pp. 343–360.

HSING WA, COMSTOCK GW, ABBEY H, et al. 1990a. Serologic precursors of cancer, retinol, carotenoids, and tocopherol and risk of prostate cancer. J Natl Cancer Inst 82:941–946.

HSING AW, DEVESA SS. 1994. Prostate cancer mortality in the United States by cohort year of birth, 1865–1940. Cancer Epidemiol Biomarkers Prev 3:527–530.

HSING AW, MCLAUGHLIN JR, HRUBEC Z, et al. 1991. Tobacco use and prostate cancer: 26-year follow-up of U.S. veterans. Am J Epidemiol 133:437–441.

HSING WA, MCLAUGHLIN JK, SCHUMAN LM, et al. 1990b. Diet, tobacco use, and fatal prostate cancer: Results from the Lutheran Brotherhood cohort study. Cancer Res 50:6836–6840.

HSING AW, MCLAUGHLIN JK, ZHENG W, et al. 1994a. Occupation, physical activity, and risk of prostate cancer in Shanghai, People's Republic of China. Cancer Causes Control 5:136–140.

HSING AW, WANG R-T, GU F-L, et al. 1994b. Vasectomy and prostate cancer risk in China. Cancer Epidemiol Biomarkers Prev 3:285–288.

HUBER DR, HONG S, ROSS JA. 1986. The international experience with vasectomy. *In* Zatuchni GI, Goldsmith A, Spieler JM, (eds): Male Contraception: Advances and Future Prospects. Philadelphia, Harper and Row, pp. 7–18.

HUGGINS C, HODGES CV. 1941. Studies on prostatic cancer: Effect of castration, of estrogen, and of androgen injection on serum phosphatases in metastatic carcinoma of the prostate. Cancer Res 1:293–297.

HULKA BS, HAMMOND JE, DIFERDINANADO G, et al. 1987. Serum hormone levels among patients with prostatic carcinoma or benign prostatic hyperplasia and clinic controls. Prostate 11:171–182.

HUNCHAREK M, MUSCAT J. 1995. Genetic characteristics of prostate cancer. Cancer Epidemiol Biomarkers Prev 4:681–687.

ISAACS JT. 1983. Prostatic structure and function in relation to the etiology of prostatic cancer. Prostate 4:351–366.

ISAACS WB, BOVA GS, MORTON RA, et al. 1994. Molecular biology of prostate cancer. Semin Oncol 21:514–521.

ISAACS WB, CARTER BS. 1991. Genetic changes associated with prostate cancer in humans. Cancer Surv 11:15–24.

JACKSON MA, KOVI J, HESHMAT MY, et al. 1980. Characterization of prostatic carcinoma among Blacks: A comparison between a low incidence area, Ibadan, Nigeria and a high incidence area, Washington DC. Prostate 1:185–205.

JOHNSONBAUGH RE, O'CONNELL K, ENGEL SB, et al. 1975. Plasma testosterone, luteinizing hormone, and follicle stimulating hormone after vasectomy. Fertil Steril 26:329–330.

KALLIONIEMI O-P, VISAKORPI T. 1966. Genetic basis and clonal evolution of human prostate cancer. Adv Cancer Res 68:225–255.

KARK JD, SMITH AH, SWITZER BR, et al. 1981. Serum vitamin A (retinol) and cancer incidence in Evans County, Georgia. J Natl Cancer Inst 66:7–16.

KASTENDIECK H, HELPAP B. 1989. Prostatic "dysplasia/atypical hyperplasia": terminology, histopathology, pathobiology, and significance. Urology (Suppl.) 34:28–42.

KAUL L, HESHMAT MY, KOVI J, et al. 1987. The role of diet in prostate cancer. Nutr Cancer 9:123–128.

KEENAN EJ, KEMP ED, RAMSEY EE, et al. 1979. Specific binding of prolactin by the prostate gland of the rat and man. J Urol 122:43–46.

KINSON GA, LAYBERRY RA. 1975. Long-term endocrine responses to vasectomy in the adult rat. Contraception 11:143–149.

KIPLING MD, WATERHOUSE JAH. 1967. Cadmium and prostatic carcinoma. Lancet i:730–731.

KOLONEL L, WINKELSTEIN W. 1977. Cadmium and prostatic carcinoma. Lancet ii:566–567.

KOLONEL LN. 1980. Cancer patterns of four ethnic groups in Hawaii. J Natl Cancer Inst 65:1127–1139.

KOLONEL LN, HANKIN JH, YOSHIZAWA CN. 1987. Vitamin A and prostate cancer in elderly men: Enhancement of risk. Cancer Res 47:2982–2985.

KOLONEL LN, HINDS MW, NOMURA AMY, et al. 1985. Relationship of dietary vitamin A and ascorbic acid intake to the risk for cancers of the lung, bladder, and prostate in Hawaii. Natl Cancer Inst Monogr 69:137–142.

KOLONEL LN, NOMURA A, HINDS MW, et al. 1983. Role of diet in cancer incidence in Hawaii. Cancer Res 43:2397s–2402s.

KOLONEL LN, YOSHIZAWA CN, HANKIN JH. 1988. Diet and prostatic cancer: A case–control study in Hawaii. Am J Epidemiol 127:999–1012.

KONISHI N, ENOMOTO T, BUZARD G, et al. 1992. K-ras activation and ras p21 expression in latent prostatic carcinoma in Japanese men. Cancer 69:2293–2299.

KOVI H, HESHMAT MY. 1972. Incidence of cancer in Negroes in Washington D.C. and selected African cities. Am J Epidemiol 96:401–403.

KRAHN MD, MAHONEY JE, ECKMAN MH, et al. 1994. Screening for prostate cancer: a decision analytic view. JAMA 272:773–780.

KRAIN LS. 1973. Epidemiologic variables in prostatic cancer. Geriatrics 28:93–98.

KRAIN LS. 1974. Some epidemiologic variables in prostatic carcinoma in California. Prev Med 3:154–159.

KRAMER BS, BROWN ML, PROROK PC, et al. 1993. Prostate cancer screening: what we know and what we need to know. Ann Intern Med 119:914–923.

KROES R, BEEMS RB, BOSLAND MC, et al. 1986. Nutritional factors in lung, colon, and prostate carcinogenesis in animal models. Federation Proc 45:136–141.

LEES REM, STEELE R, WARDLE D. 1985. Arsenic, syphilis, and cancer of the prostate. J Epidemiol Commun Med 39:227–230.

LEMARCHAND L, KOLONEL LN, WILKENS LR, et al. 1994. Animal fat consumption and prostate cancer: a prospective study in Hawaii. Epidemiology 5:276–282.

LEMARCHAND LL, KOLONEL LN, YOSHIZAWA CN. 1991. Lifetime occupational physical activity and prostate cancer risk. Am J Epidemiol 133:103–111.

LEMEN RA, LEE JS, WAGONER JR, et al. 1976. Cancer mortality among cadmium production workers. Ann NY Acad Sci 271:273–279.

LEW EA, GARFINKEL L. 1979. Variations in mortality by weight among 750,000 men and women. J Chron Dis 32:563–576.

LILIENFELD AM, LEVIN ML, KESSLER II. 1972. Cancer in the United States. APHA Monograph. Cambridge, Harvard University Press.

LILJA H, CHRISTENSSON A, DAHLÉN U, et al. 1991. Prostate-specific antigen in human serum occurs predominantly in complex with alpha-1-antichymotrypsin Clin Chem 37:1618–1625.

LOGAN WPP. 1982. Cancer mortality by occupation and social class, 1851–1971, (HMSO), Her Majesty's Stationery Office (HMSO), London.

LOOKINGBILL DP, DEMERS LM, WANG C, et al. 1991. Clinical and biological parameters of androgen action in normal healthy Caucasian versus Chinese subjects. J Clin Endocrinol Metab 72:1242–1248.

LYON JL, GARDNER JW, KLAUBER MR. 1977. Low cancer incidence and mortality in Utah. Cancer 39:2608–2618.

LYON JL, KLAUBER MR, GARDNER JW, et al. 1976. Cancer incidence in Mormons and non-Mormons in Utah, 1966-1970. N Engl J Med 294:129–133.

MACGROGAN D, LEVY A, BOSTWICK D, et al. 1994. Loss of chromosome arm 8p loci in prostate cancer: mapping by quantitative allelic imbalance. Genes Chromosome Cancer 10:151–159.

MANDEL JS. 1981. Epidemiologic study of etiologic factors in prostatic cancer. Ph.D. dissertation. University of Minnesota.

MANDEL JS, SCHUMAN LM. 1980. Epidemiology of cancer of the prostate. *In* Lilienfeld AM (ed): Reviews in Cancer Epidemiology, Vol. 1. New York, Elsevier/North-Holland, pp. 2–83.

MANDEL JS, SCHUMAN LN. 1987. Sexual factors and prostatic cancer: Results from a case–control study. J Gerontol 42:259–264.

MCNEAL JE. 1993. Prostatic microcarcinomas in relation to cancer origin and the evolution to clinical cancer. Cancer 71:984–991.

MEIKLE AW, STANISH WM. 1982. Familial prostatic cancer risk and low testosterone. J Clin Endocrinol Metab 54:1104–1108.

METTLIN C. 1980. Nutritional habits of blacks and whites. Prev Med 9:601–606.

METTLIN C, NATARAJAN N, RUBEN R. 1990. Vasectomy and prostate cancer risk. Am J Epidemiol 132:1056–1061.

METTLIN C, SELENSKAS S, NATARAJAN N, et al. 1989. Beta-carotene and animal fats and their relationship to prostate cancer risk. A case–control study. Cancer 64:605–612.

MILLER BA, RIES LAG, HANKEY BF, et al. 1993. SEER Cancer Statistics Review: 1973–1990. NIH Pub. No. 93-2789. Bethesda, National Cancer Institute.

MILLER GJ, STAPLETON GE, FERRARA JA, et al. 1992. The human prostatic carcinoma cell line LNCaP expresses biologically active, specific receptors for 1a, 25-dihydroxyvitamin D3. Cancer Res 52:515–520.

MILLS PK, BEESON L, PHILLIPS RL, et al. 1989. Cohort study of diet, lifestyle, and prostate cancer in Adventist men. Cancer 64:598–604.

MIRAND E, STAUBITZ W. 1956. Prostatic neoplasms of the Wistar rat induced with 20-methylcholanthrene. Proc Soc Exp Biol Med 93:457–462.

MISHINA T, WANTANABE T, ARAKI H, et al. 1985. Epidemiological study of prostatic cancer by matched pair analysis. Prostate 6:423–436.

MONSON RJ, LYON JL. 1975. Proportional mortality among alcoholics. Cancer 36:1077–1079.

MONSON RJ, NAKANO KK. 1976a. Mortality among rubber workers I. White male union employees in Akron, Ohio. Am J Epidemiol 103:288–296.

MONSON RJ, NAKANO KK. 1976b. Mortality among rubber workers II. Other employees. Am J Epidemiol 103:297–303.

MUIR C, WATERHOUSE J, MACK T, et al. (eds). 1987. Cancer Incidence in Five Continents, Vol. V. Lyon, International Agency for Research on Cancer.

MURPHY GP, NATARAJAN N, PONTES JE, et al. 1982. The national survey of prostate cancer in the United States by the American College of Surgeons. J Urol 127:928–934.

MURPHY WM, DEAN PJ, BRASFIELD JA, et al. 1986. Incidental carcinoma of the prostate. How much sampling is adequate? Am J Surg Pathol 10:170–174.

MYERS MH, RIES LA. 1989. Cancer patient survival rates: SEER program results for 10 years of follow-up. CA Cancer J Clin 39:21–32.

NAIK VK, JOSHI UM, SHETH AR. 1980. Long-term effects of vasectomy on prostatic function in men. J Reprod Fertil 58:289–293.

NEWELL GR, FUEGER JJ, SPITZ MR, et al. 1989. A case–control study of prostate cancer. Am J Epidemiol 130:395–398.

NEWELL GR, POLLACK ES, SPITZ MR, et al. 1987. Incidence of prostate cancer and marital status. J Natl Cancer Inst 79:259–262.

NIENHUIS H, GOLDACRE M, SEAGROATT V, et al. 1992. Incidence of disease after vasectomy: a record linkage retrospective cohort study. BMJ 304:743–746.

NOBLE RL. 1977. The development of prostatic adenocarcinoma in Nb rats following prolonged sex hormone administration. Cancer Res 37:1929–1933.

NOBLE RL. 1980. Production of Nb rat carcinoma of the dorsal prostate and response of estrogen dependent transplants to sex hormones and tamoxifen. Cancer Res 40:3547–3550.

NOMURA A, HEILBRUN LK, STEMMERMANN GN, et al. 1988. Prediagnostic serum hormones and the risk of prostate cancer. Cancer Res 48:3515–3517.

NOMURA A, KOLONEL LN. 1993. Shedding new light on the etiology of prostate cancer? Cancer Epidemiol Biomarkers Prev 2:409–410.

OESTERLING JE, JACOBSEN SJ, CHUTE CG, et al. 1993. Serum prostate-specific antigen in a community-based population of healthy men: establishment of age-specific reference ranges. JAMA 270:860–864.

OHNO Y, YOSHIDA O, OISHI K, et al. 1988. Dietary B-carotene and cancer of the prostate: A case–control study in Kyoto, Japan. Cancer Res 48:1331–1336.

OISHI R, OKADA K, YOSHIDA O, et al. 1988. A case–control study of prostatic cancer with reference to dietary habits. Prostate 12:179–190.

OISHI K, OKADA K, YOSHIDA S, et al. 1989. Case–control study of prostatic cancer in Kyoto, Japan: Demographic and some lifestyle risk factors. Prostate 14:117–122.

PAFFENBARGER RS, HYDE RT, WING AL. 1987. Physical activity and incidence of cancer in diverse populations: a preliminary report. Am J Clin Nutr 45:12–17.

PAGANINI-HILL A, CHAO A, ROSS RK, et al. 1987. Vitamin A, B-carotene and the risk of cancer. A prospective study. J Natl Cancer Inst 79:443–448.

PARKER KL, SCHIMMER BP. 1994. The role of nuclear receptors in steroid hormone production. Semin Cancer Biol 5:317–325.

NOMURA A, KOLONEL LN. 1993. Shedding new light on the etiology of prostate cancer? Cancer Epidemiol Biomarkers Prev 2:409–410.

PARKIN DM, MUIR CS, WHELAN SL, et al (eds). (1992). Cancer Incidence in Five Continents, Vol. VI. IARC Sci Publ 120. Lyon, International Agency for Research on Cancer.

PARKIN DM, STJERNSWARD J, MUIR CS. 1984. Estimates of the worldwide frequency of twelve major cancers. Bull World Health Organ 62:163–182.

PEARCE NE, SHEPPARD RA, FRASER J. 1987. Case–control study of occupation and cancer of the prostate in New Zealand. J Epidemiol Commun Health 41:130–132.

PEEHL DM, SKOWRONSKI RJ, LEUNG GK, et al. 1994. Antiproliferative effects of 1,25-dihydroxyvitamin D3 on primary cultures of human prostatic cells. Cancer Res 54:805–810.

PELL S, D'ALONZO CA. 1973. A five year mortality study of alcoholics. J Occup Med 15:120–125.

PETO R. 1983. The marked differences between carotenoids and retinoids: Methodological implications for biochemical epidemiology. Cancer Surv 2:327–340.

PETO R, DOLL R, BUCKLEY JD, et al. 1981. Can dietary beta-carotene materially reduce human cancer rates? Nature 290:201–208.

PHILLIPS RL. 1975. Role of life-style and dietary habits in risk of cancer among Seventh-Day Adventists. Cancer Res 35:3513–3522.

PHILLIPS RL, SNOWDON DA. 1983. Association of meat and coffee use with cancer of the large bowel, breast, and prostate among Seventh-Day Adventists: Preliminary results. Cancer Res 43:2403s–2408s.

PIENTA KJ, NGUYEN NM, LEHR JE. 1993. Treatment of prostate cancer in the rat with the synthetic retinoid fenretinide. Cancer Res 53:224–226.

PIERREPOINT CG, DAVIES P. 1973. The effect of vasectomy on the activty of prostatic RNA polymerase in rats. J Reprod Fertil 35:149–152.

PIKE MC, KRAILO MD, HENDERSON BE, et al. 1983. Hormonal risk factors, "breast tissue age," and the age-incidence of breast cancer. Nature 3030:767–770.

POLLARD M, LUCKERT PH, SYNDER DL. 1989a. Prevention of prostate cancer and liver tumors in L-W rats by moderate dietary restriction. Cancer 64:686–690.

POLLARD M, LUCKERT PH, SYNDER DL. 1989b. The promotional effect of testosterone on induction of prostate-cancer in MNU-sensitized L-W rats. Cancer Lett 45:209–212.

POLLARD M, LUCKERT PH, SPORN MB. 1991. Prevention of primary prostate cancer in Lobund-Wistar rats by N-(4-hydroxyphenyl)retinamide. Cancer Res 51:3610–3611.

POTOSKY AL, KESSLER L, GRIDLEY G, et al. 1990. Rise in prostatic cancer incidence associated with increased use of transurethral resection. J Natl Cancer Inst 82:1624–1628.

PRENDERGAST NJ, WALTHER PJ. 1995. Genetic alterations in prostate adenocarcinoma. Surg Oncol Clin North America 4:241–255.

PURVIS K, SAKSENA SK, CEKAN Z, et al. 1976. Endocrine effects of vasectomy. Clin Endocrinol 5:263–272.

QUANDER RV, LEARY SL, STANDBERG JD, et al. 1985. Long term effect of 2-hydroxyethyl retinamide on urinary bladder carcinogenesis and tumor transplantation in Fischer 344 rats. Cancer Res 45:5235–5239.

RANNIKKO KS, ADLERCREUTZ H, HAAPIANINEN R. 1989. Urinary oestrogen excretion in benign prostatic hyperplasia and prostate cancer. Br J Urol 64:172–175.

REICHARDT JKV, MAKRIDAKIS N, HENDERSON BE, et al. 1995. Genetic variability of the human SRD5A2 gene: Implications for prostate cancer risk. Cancer Res 55:3973–3975.

REICHMAN ME, HAYES RB, ZIEGLER RG, et al. 1990. Serum vitamin A and subsequent development of prostate cancer in the First National Health and Nutrition Examination Survey Epidemiologic Follow-up Study. Cancer Res 50:2311–2315.

REYNOLDS T. 1992. Stat bite: prostate cancer mortality by race/ethnic group, 1977–1983. J Natl Cancer Inst 84:997.

RICHARDSON IM. 1965. Prostatic cancer and social class. Br J Prev Med 19:140–142.

RIES LAG, HANKEY BD, EDWARDS BK (eds). 1990. Cancer Statistics Review, 1973–87. NIH Publ. 90:2789. Bethesda, MD, National Institutes of Health.

RIVENSON A, SILVERMAN J. 1979. Prostatic cancer in laboratory animals. *In* Rose DP (ed): Endocrinology of Cancer. Boca Raton, Florida, CRC Press, pp. 2–15.

ROBERTS JT, ESSENHIGH DM. 1986. Adenocarcinoma of prostate in 40-year old body builder. Lancet i:742.

ROGOT EM, MURRAY JL. 1980. Smoking and causes of death among U.S. veterans: 16 years of observation. Public Health Rep 95:213–222.

ROSE DP. 1986. The biochemical epidemiology of prostatic carcinoma. *In* Ip C, Birt DF, Rogers AE, Mettlin C (eds): Dietary Fat and Cancer. New York, Alan R. Liss, pp. 43–68.

ROSENBERG L, PALMER JR, ZAUBER AG, et al. 1990. Vasectomy and the risk of prostate cancer. Am J Epidemiol 132:1051–1055.

ROSS RK, BERNSTEIN L, JUDD H, et al. 1986. Serum testosterone levels in young black and white men. J Natl Cancer Inst. 76:45–48.

ROSS RK, BERNSTEIN L, LOBO RA, et al. 1992. 5-alpha-reductase activity and risk of prostate cancer among Japanese and U.S. white and black males. Lancet 339:887–890.

ROSS RK, BERNSTEIN L, PAGANINI-HILL, et al. 1990. Effects of cigarette smoking on "hormone-related" disease in a Southern California retirement community. *In* Wald N and Baron J (eds): Smoking and Hormone-Related Disorders. New York, Oxford University Press, pp. 32–54.

ROSS RK, DEAPEN DM, CASAGRANDE JT, et al. 1981. A cohort study of mortality from cancer of the prostate in Catholic priests. Br J Cancer 43:233–235.

ROSS RK, HENDERSON BE. 1994. Do diet and androgens alter prostate cancer risk via a common etiologic pathway? J Natl Cancer Inst 86:252–254.

ROSS RK, MCCURTIS JW, HENDERSON BE, et al. 1979. Descriptive epidemiology of testicular and prostatic cancer in Los Angeles. Br J Cancer 39:284–292.

ROSS RK, PAGANINI-HILL A, HENDERSON BE. 1988. Epidemiology of prostatic cancer. *In* Skinner DG, Lieskovsky G (eds): Diagnosis and Management of Genitourinary Cancer. Philadelphia, WB Saunders Co, pp. 40–45.

ROSS RK, PAGANINI-HILL A, HENDERSON BE. 1983. The etiology of prostate cancer: What does the epidemiology suggest? Prostate 4:333–344.

ROSS RK, SHIMIZU H, PAGANINI-HILL A, et al. 1987. Case–control studies of prostate cancer in blacks and whites in Southern California. J Natl Cancer Inst 78:869–874.

ROTKIN ID. 1977. Studies in the epidemiology of prostate cancer: Expanded sampling. Cancer Treat Rep 61:173–180.

ROTKIN ID. 1980. Epidemiologic clues to increased risk of prostatic cancer. *In* Spring-Mills E, Hafez ESE (eds): Male Accessory Sex Glands. New York, Elsevier/North-Holland Biomedical Press, pp. 289–309.

SANDBERG AA. 1992. Chromosomal abnormalities and related events in prostate cancer. Hum Pathol 23:368–380.

SATARIANO WA, SWANSON GM. 1988. Racial differences in cancer incidence: The significance of age-specific patterns. Cancer 62:2640–2653.

SCARDINO PT, WEAVER R, HUDSON MA. 1992. Early detection of prostate cancer. Hum Pathol 23:211–222.

SCHWARTZ GG, HULKA BS. 1990. Is vitamin D deficiency a risk factor for prostate cancer? (Hypothesis). Anticancer Res 10:1307–1312.

SEGI M. 1978. Age-adjusted Death Rates for Cancer for Selected Sites in 52 Countries in 1973. Segi, Japan, Segi Institute of Cancer Epidemiology.

SEIDMAN H. 1970. Cancer death rates by site and sex for religious and socioeconomic groups in New York City. Environ Res 3:235–250.

SEVERSON RK, NOMURA AMY, GROVE JS, et al. 1989. A prospective study of demographics, diet, and prostate cancer among men of Japanese ancestry in Hawaii. Cancer Res 49:1857–1860.

SEVERSON RK, NOMURA AMY, GROVE JS, et al. 1989. A prospective analysis of physical activity and cancer. Am J Epidemiol 130:522–529.

SHELDON CA, WILLIAMS RD, FRALEY EE. 1980. Incidental carcinoma of the prostate: a review of the literature and critical reappraisal of classification. J Urol 124:626–631.

SHETH AR, PANSE GT. 1982. Can vasectomy reduce the incidence of prostatic tumor? Med Hypotheses 89:237–241.

SHIMIZU H, ROSS RK, BERNSTEIN L, 1991a. Possible underestimation of incidence rate of prostate cancer in Japan. Jpn J Cancer Res 82:483–485.

SHIMIZU H, ROSS RK, BERNSTEIN L, et al. 1991b. Cancers of the prostate and breast among Japanese and white immigrants in Los Angeles County. Br J Cancer 63:963–966.

SIDNEY S. 1987. Vasectomy and the risk of prostatic cancer and benign prostatic hypertrophy. J Urol 138:795–797.

SIDNEY S, QUESENBERRY CP, SADLER MC, et al. 1991. Vasectomy and the risk of prostate cancer in a cohort of multiphasic health-checkup examinees: second report. Cancer Causes Control 2:113–116.

SIITERI PR, MACDONALD P. 1973. Role of extraglandular estrogen in human endocrinology. *In* Greep RD (ed): Handbook of Physiology. Washington DC, American Physiological Society, Sect. 7, Vol. 12, Part 1, pp. 615–629.

SILVERBERG BS, LUBERA JA. 1989. Cancer statistics, 1989. Cancer 39:3–20.

SKEGG DCG, MATTHEWS JD, GUILLEBAUD J, et al. 1976. Hormonal assessment before and after vasectomy. BMJ 1:621–622.

SMITH KD, TCHOLAKIAN RK, CHOWDHURY M, et al. 1979. Endocrine studies in vasectomized men. *In* Lepow IH, Crozier R (eds): Vasectomy: Immunologic and Pathophysiologic Effects in Animals and Man. New York, Academic Press, pp. 183–197.

SNOWDON DA, PHILLIPS RL, CHOI W. 1984. Diet, obesity, and risk of fatal prostate cancer. Am J Epidemiol 120:244–250.

SPITZ MR, CURRIET RD, FUEGER JJ, et al. 1991. Familial patterns of prostate cancer: A case–control analysis. J Urol 146:1305–1307.

STAMEY TA, FREIHA FS, MCNEAL JE, et al. 1993. Localized prostate cancer: relationship of the tumor volume to clinical significance for treatment of prostate cancer. Cancer 71:933–938.

STAMEY TA, YANG N, HAY AR, et al. 1987. Prostate-specific antigen as a serum marker for adenocarcinoma of the prostate. N Engl J Med 317:909–916.

STEELE R, LEES REM, KRAUS AS, et al. 1971. Sexual factors in the epidemiology of cancer of the prostate. J Chron Dis 24:29–37.

STEINBERG GD, CARTER BS, BEATY TH, et al. 1990. Family history and the risk of prostate cancer. Prostate 17:337–347.

SUNDBY P. ALCOHOLISM AND MORTALITY. 1967. National Institute for Alcohol Research, Publ. No. 6. Oslo, Universitetsforlaget.

SURVEILLANCE, EPIDEMIOLOGY AND END RESULTS (SEER) 1971–1981. Cancer Incidence and Mortality in the United States. U.S. Bethesda, MD, Department of Health and Human Services, Public Health Services, National Institutes of Health, 1984.

TAKIZAWA S, HIROSE F. 1978. Role of testosterone in the development of radiation-induced prostatic carcinomas in rats. Gann 69:72.

TALAMINI R, LAVECCHIA C, DECARLI A, et al. 1986. Nutrition, social factors and prostatic cancer in a Northern Italian population. Br J Cancer 53:817–821.

TANNENBAUM M, LATTIMER JK. 1970. Similar virus-like particles found in cancers of the prostate and breast. J Urol 103:471–475.

TAVANI A, NEGRI E, FRANCESCHI S, et al. 1994. Alcohol consumption and risk of prostate cancer. Nutr Cancer 21:25–31.

THUNE I, LUND E. 1994. Physical activity and the risk of prostate and testicular cancer: a cohort study of 53,000 Norwegian men. Cancer Causes and Control 5:549–556.

TRUMP DL, ROBERTSON CN. 1993. Neoplasms of the prostate. *In* Holland JF, Frei E III, Bast RC Jr, Kufe DW, Morton DL, Weichselbaum RR (eds): Cancer Medicine. Philadelphia, Lea & Febiger, pp. 1562–1586.

U.S. PREVENTIVE SERVICES TASK FORCE. 1994. Screening for prostate cancer: commentary on the recommendations of the Canadian Task Force on the Periodic Health Examination. Am J Prev Med 10:187–193.

VLEMINCKX K, VAKAET L, MAREEL M, et al. 1991. Genetic manipulation of E-cadherin expression by epithelial tumor cells reveals an invasion suppressor role. Cell 66:107–119.

WAISMAN J. 1988. Pathology of neoplasms of the prostatic gland. *In* Skinner DG, Lieskovsky G (eds): Diagnosis and Management of Genitourinary Cancer. Philadelphia, WB Saunders Co, pp. 150–194.

WALKER ARP, WALKER BF, TSOTETSI NG, et al. 1992. Case–control study of prostate cancer in black patients in Soweto, South Africa. Br J Cancer 65:438–441.

WALTHER PJ. 1995. Prostate cancer screening. Why the controversy? Surg Oncology Clin North America 4:315–334.

WANG Y, CORR JG, THALER HT, et al. 1995. Decreased growth of established human prostate LNCaP tumors in nude mice fed a low-fat diet. J Natl Cancer Inst 87:1456–1462.

WATERBOR JW, BUESCHEN AJ. 1995. Prostate cancer screening (United States). Cancer Causes and Control 6:267–274.

WATERHOUSE JAH, MUIR CS, CORREA P, POWELL J (eds). 1976. Cancer Incidence in Five Continents, Vol. III. IARC Sci. Publ. 26. Lyon, International Agency for Research on Cancer.

WATERHOUSE JAH, MUIR CS, SHANMUGARATNAM K, POWELL J (eds). 1982. Cancer Incidence in Five Continents, Vol. IV. IARC Sci. Publ. 42. Lyon, International Agency for Research on Cancer.

WEST DW, SLATTERY ML, ROBINSON LM, et al. 1991. Adult dietary intake and prostate cancer risk in Utah: a case–control study with special emphasis on aggressive tumors. Cancer Causes Control 2:85–94.

WHITMORE WF. 1994. Localized prostatic cancer: management and detection issues. Lancet 343:1263–1267.

WHITTEMORE AS, KELLER JB, BETENSKY R. 1991. Low-grade, latent prostate cancer volume: predictor of clinical cancer incidence. J Natl Cancer Inst 83:1231–1235.

WHITTEMORE AS, PAFFENBARGER RS, ANDERSON K, et al. 1984. Early precursors of urogenital cancers in former college men. J Urol 132:1256–1261.

WIGLE DT. 1978. Cancer patterns in Canada. Can J Public Health 69:113–120.

WILDING G. 1992. The importance of steroid hormones in prostate cancer. Cancer Surv 14:113–130.

WILLETT WC, POLK BF, UNDERWOOD BA, et al. 1984. Relation of serum vitamins A and E, and carotenoids to the risk of cancer. N Engl J Med 310:430–434.

WILLIAMS RR, STEGENS NL, GOLDSMITH JR. 1977. Associations of cancer site and type with occupation and industry from the Third National Cancer Survey. J Natl Cancer Inst 59:1147–1185.

WOOLF CM. 1960. An investigation of the familial aspects of cancer of the prostate. Cancer 13:739–743.

WRIGHT F, POIZAT R, BONGINI M, et al. 1985. Decreased urinary (5α-androstane-3α, 17-diol) glucuronide excretion in patients with benign prostatic hypertrophy. J Clin Endocrinol Metab 60:294–298.

WYNDER EL, MABUCHI K, WHITMORE WF. 1971. Epidemiology of cancer of the prostate. Cancer 28:344–360.

YATANI R, CHIGUSA I, AKAZAKI K, et al. 1982. Geographic pathology of latent prostatic carcinoma. Int J Cancer 29:611–616.

YATANI R, SHIRAISHI T, NAKAKUKI K, et al. 1988. Trends in frequency of latent prostate carcinoma in Japan from 1965–1979 to 1982–1986. J Natl Cancer Inst 80:683–687.

YU H, HARRIS RE, WYNDER EL. 1988. Case–control study of prostate cancer and socioeconomic factors. Prostate 13:317–325.

ZARIDZE DG, BOYLE P, SMANS M. 1984. International trends in prostatic cancer. Int J Cancer 33:223–230.

ZUMOFF B, LEVIN J, STRAIN GW, et al. 1982. Abnormal levels of plasma hormones in men with prostate cancer: Evidence towards a "two-disease" theory. Prostate 3:579–588.

56 Testicular cancer

DAVID SCHOTTENFELD

Cancer of the testis is relatively uncommon in the United States, with an annual age-adjusted incidence rate of 4.5 per 100,000 men, or about 6,500 cases per year. The lifetime probability of white men in the United States to develop testicular cancer is about 0.2%. Testicular cancer is most commonly diagnosed between the ages of 20 and 44 years (Table 56–1), and it is among this subgroup that the age-adjusted incidence has increased at least 50% over the period 1973–1990 (Fig. 56–1). The age-adjusted incidence in whites in 1986–1990 (5.1 per 100,000) was about seven times that in blacks (0.7 per 100,000) in the United States. During the period 1973–1990, the age-adjusted testicular cancer incidence in the United States increased 60% in whites but decreased 16% in blacks; concurrently, age-adjusted mortality declined 65% in whites and 37% in blacks (Fig. 56–2). Dramatic advances in the treatment of testicular cancer have been accompanied by declining age-adjusted mortality rates (per 100,000) in white males—from 0.8 in 1973 to 0.3 in 1990 (Miller et al, SEER Cancer Statistics Review, 1993). The 5-year relative survival rate in whites, all stages, was 72.0% for patients diagnosed in 1970–1973, and 93.0% for patients diagnosed in 1983–1989.

PATHOLOGY AND HISTOGENESIS

Most primary neoplasms of the testis arise from germinal elements, which account for 95% of all testicular tumors. Germinal neoplasms may be composed of embryonal and/or extraembryonal tissues and are divided clinically into the seminoma and a variety of pure and mixed types of nonseminomatous tumors (Table 56–2). Five basic cell types predominate either alone or in combination: seminoma (classic [90%–95%] and spermatocytic [5%–10%]); teratoma (mature, immature, with malignant transformation); choriocarcinoma; and yolk sac tumor (endodermal sinus tumor of Teilum), the cells of which stain immunohistochemically for alpha-fetoprotein (AFP). In patients under 15 years of age, yolk sac and teratoma neoplastic cell types predominate; during the peak incidence interval in young adults, between ages 20 and 40, the most common cell type is the seminoma. Dysgerminoma of the ovary is morphologically equivalent to seminoma of the testis, and both have been classified under germinoma. The relatively rare and clinically indolent spermatocytic seminoma, which represents only 2% to 3% of all testicular tumors, occurs usually over the age of 50 (Brodsky, 1991). Spermatocytic seminoma occurs only in man, is not associated with gonadal dysgenesis, and does not occur in association with intratubular seminoma or any other type of germ cell tumor.

Embryonal carcinoma appears to recapitulate the earliest phases of embryogenesis, and is interpreted as representing the primitive cell type from which further differentiation gives rise to choriocarcinoma, yolk sac carcinoma, and teratoma (Fig. 56–3). Embryonal carcinoma occurs rarely in pure form (< 5%) but is relatively common in mixed germ cell tumors.

The teratoma results from the differentiation of pluripotent embryonal carcinoma cells and is potentially derived from the three embryonic cell layers (Fig. 56–3). Teratomas of the testis, as pure lesions, represent the second most common germ cell tumor, after yolk sac tumors, in infancy and early childhood. Teratomas are benign unless they are immature and/or are composed of stem cells that have undergone malignant transformation. Stem cells are defined as renewing and replicating cell populations that are capable of differentiating into cells that are distinctive morphologically, functionally, and/or developmentally from the progenitor cells. In contrast to the mature teratoma, the immature teratoma may consist of epithelial tubular structures that are more primitive, stroma with loose spindle cells in a mucopolysaccharide matrix, and primitive myoblastic and neural elements. In the mature teratoma, the most common pattern includes cystic epithelial areas lined by respiratory, gastrointestinal, or squamous epithelium, with adjacent fibroblastic or smooth muscle stroma and an admixture of cartilaginous and nervous tissues.

Choriocarcinoma of the testis consists of both cytotrophoblastic cells and syncitiotrophoblastic giant cells. The syncytiotrophoblastic giant cells stain positively by immunohistochemical methods for the beta subunit of human chorionic gonadotropin (HCG). Both cytotro-

TABLE 56–1. *Rank Order of Most Common Cancers in Males 20–44 Years of Age, SEER Average Annual Incidence Rates (per 100,000), United States, 1986–1990**

Rank	Age (y) 20–24	Rate	Age (y) 25–29	Rate	Age (y) 30–34	Rate	Age (y) 35–39	Rate	Age (y) 40–44	Rate
1	Testis	8.7	Testis	12.3	Testis	13.5	Melanoma	13.5	Lung	16.7
2	Hodgkin's	5.2	Hodgkin's	5.5	Non-Hodgkin's lymphoma	8.9	Non-Hodgkin's lymphoma	13.3	Melanoma	16.4
3	Non-Hodgkin's lymphoma	2.7	Non-Hodgkin's lymphoma	5.0	Melanoma	8.7	Testis	11.3	Non-Hodgkin's lymphoma	16.0
4	Melanoma	2.7	Melanoma	5.0	Hodgkin's	4.3	Lung	6.7	Testis	8.1
5	Brain and nervous system	2.5	Thyroid	1.7	Thyroid	2.3	Brain and nervous system	4.8	Brain and nervous system	5.8

*Based on SEER Cancer Statistics Review: 1973–1990, all areas and races.

phoblastic and syncitiotrophoblastic cells stain for placental alkaline phosphatase. These serum tumor markers have been used in morphologic classification, monitoring treatment, and determining prognosis in patients with pure or mixed patterns of testicular neoplasms (Bates, 1991).

Sex cord–stromal tumors are frequently benign and constitute about 5% of testicular neoplasms, and include Leydig cell (derived from the stroma), Sertoli cell (derived from the sex cord), and granulosa cell tumors, which resemble the ovarian granulosa cell tumor, and presumably develop from fetal precursors of specialized stromal cells; gonadoblastoma; or a mixed pattern of germ cell, sex cord, and stromal tumors. The Sertoli cells line the basement membrane of the seminiferous tubules and are in close proximity to the germinal cells as they pass through various stages of spermatogenesis. The stroma that supports the seminiferous tubules is connected to tissue in which the interstitial, androgen-producing Leydig cells are arranged in clusters. The gonadoblastoma consists of seminoma-like germ cells, and cells derived from the gonadal stroma, including Sertoli cells, granulosa cells, Leydig cells and/or luteinized stromal cells. Gonadoblastomas occur almost exclusively in dysgenetic gonads.

Carcinoma in situ (CIS) of the testis is a preinvasive lesion of the seminiferous tubules that precedes all types of invasive germ cell tumors, with the possible exception of spermatocytic seminoma (Jorgensen et al, 1990). Intratubular neoplasia has been reported in the exami-

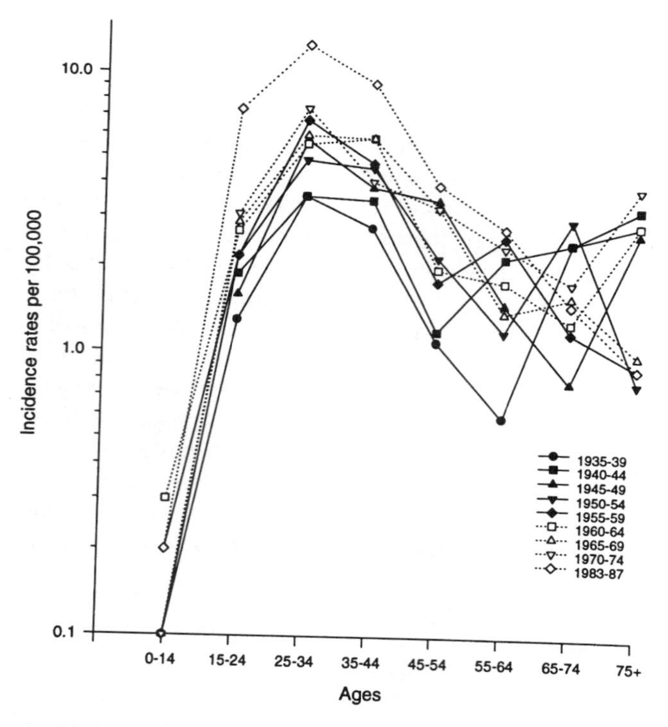

FIG. 56–1. Average annual age-specific incidence rates (per 100,000), testicular cancer, 5-year calendar intervals, Connecticut, 1935–1987.

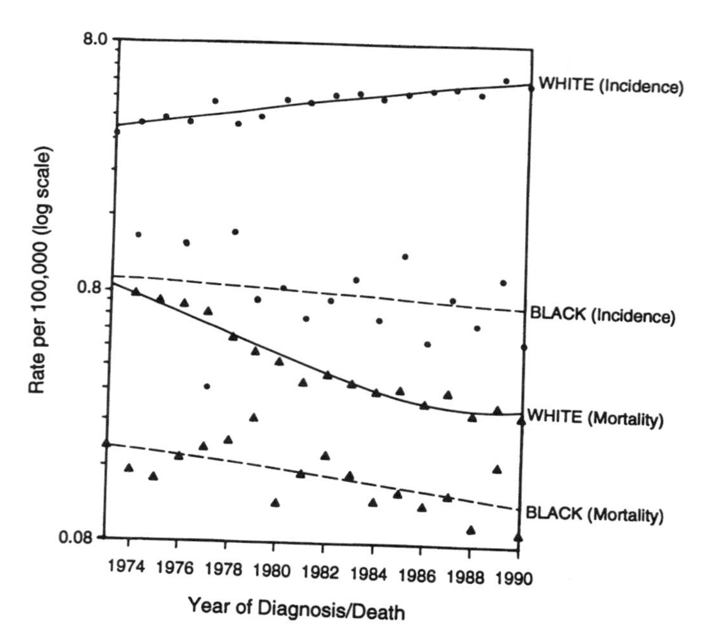

FIG. 56–2. Age-adjusted (under 65 years) annual incidence and mortality rates (per 100,000), testicular cancer, United States (SEER), white and black men, 1973–1990.

TABLE 56–2. *Pathologic Classification and Frequency Distribution (%) of Tumors of the Testis in the United States*

Nomenclature	*Frequency (%)*
GERM CELL NEOPLASMS	95
Seminoma	40–45
Spermatocytic seminoma	2–3
Teratoma	5–10
Mature	
Immature	
With malignant transformation	
Embryonal carcinoma[a]	<5 (pure cell type neoplasm)–25
Choriocarcinoma	≤1
Yolk sac (endodermal sinus tumor)[b]	<1
NON-GERMINAL NEOPLASMS	5
Gonadal stroma	
Leydig cell	1–3
Sertoli cell	
Androblastoma	
Gonadoblastoma	

[a]Combined histologic patterns may account for 40% to 50% of all germ cell tumors; for example, "teratocarcinoma" (embryonal carcinoma with teratoma) may account for 25% of cases in a clinical series.
[b]Pure yolk sac tumor is extremely rare in the adult testis, but it has been classified as a common component (about 30%) of mixed nonseminomatous germ cell tumors.

nation of tissues obtained from patients with infertility and oligospermia, gonadal dysplasia, hypogonadism with cryptorchidism, or in the contralateral testis of patients with invasive germ cell tumors (Scully, 1993). The cumulative risk of a metachronous contralateral *invasive* germ cell neoplasm, of the same or different cell

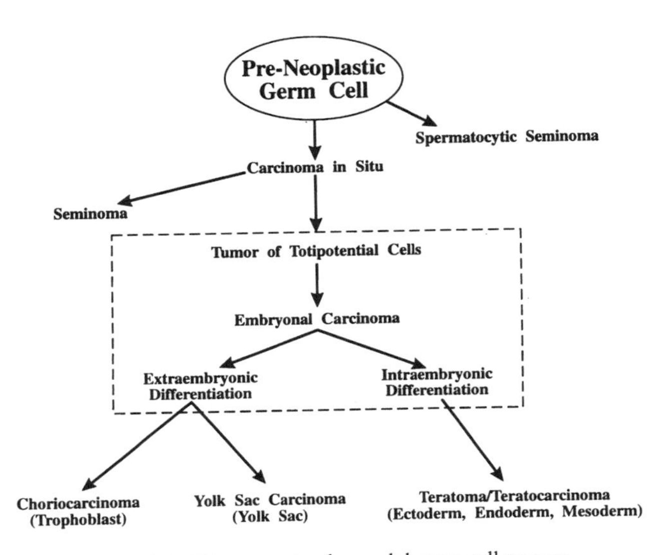

FIG. 56–3. Histogenesis of gonadal germ cell tumors.

type, has been estimated variously as 0.5% to 3.0%, or 500 times the risk in the general population of healthy males. The cumulative incidence of carcinoma in situ in the contralateral testis of patients with a previous history of invasive germ cell tumor of the testis has been reported to be 5% to 10% (Berthelsen et al, 1982; von der Maase, 1986, Reinberg et al, 1991).

DEMOGRAPHIC PATTERNS

United States

The average annual age-adjusted mortality rate per 100,000 for testicular cancer in whites declined from 0.6 in 1975–1979 to 0.3 in 1985–1990; concurrently, average annual mortality remained the same (0.2 per 100,000) in African American men. The age-specific mortality rates for whites are bimodal, with a prominent peak at 25 to 34 years and a lesser peak beginning after 70. The age-specific mortality rates for blacks do not demonstrate a similar peak in the early decades, but begin to increase after 65 years. In general, germ cell tumors constitute more than 90% of testicular cancer deaths in men under age 65, while poorly differentiated, non-Hodgkin's lymphomas account for at least 50% of testicular cancer deaths above age 65. During 1973–1990, testicular cancer mortality in white males declined 65% in all age groups; the rate of decline, however, has decreased in recent years (Miller et al, 1993).

During the period between 1975 and 1990, the age-adjusted annual incidence rate (per 100,000) increased from 3.7 to 5.2, or by 51%, in whites; which, when calculated from the slope of the regression line fitted to the yearly rates, represented an average annual percentage increase of 2.8%. The annual incidence rates in blacks during the same period fluctuated between 0.5 and 1.3 per 100,000. The age-specific incidence pattern demonstrates, for 1986–1990, a single peak in whites aged between 24 and 35 years; during this age interval, the risk of testicular cancer in United States whites is 15 times that in African Americans (Fig. 56–4).

The 5-year age-specific incidence rates in Connecticut for testicular cancer occurring between ages 15 and 44 may also be viewed in relation to birth cohort and the calendar period, 1935–1987 (Fig. 56–5, Table 56–3). For each of the birth cohorts, the peak age-specific interval was 30–34 years, which increased from 5.7 per 100,000 in the 1918–1922 cohort to 12.8 in the 1953–1957 cohort. When comparing the averages of the age-specific rates in the two earliest birth cohorts (1918–1922 and 1923–1927) with those in two later birth cohorts (1938–1942 and 1943–1947), the highest percentage increases were reflected at ages 20–24 (71%) and 15–19 (44%) years; the rates for the age-cohorts at 25–29 and 30–34 years were unchanged or failed to

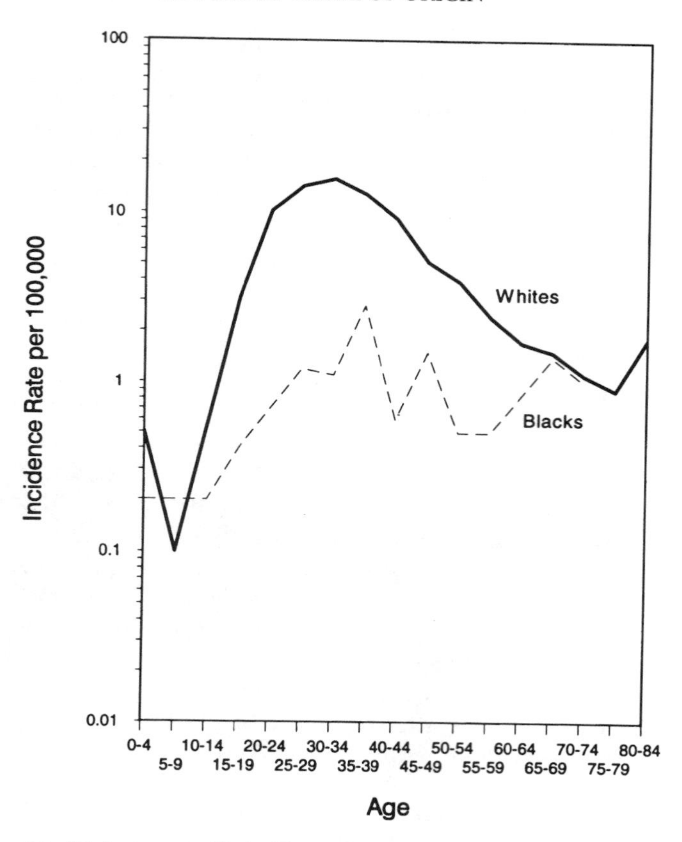

FIG. 56–4. Age-specific incidence rates (per 100,000) for testicular cancer by race, United States, 1986–1990.

exhibit any consistent trend, while increases were noted at ages 35–39 (30%) and 40–44 (29%) years. For the combined age group 15–24, the proportionate increase in incidence was composed mainly of non-seminomatous germ cell tumors (Pottern and Goedert, 1986). In a similar analysis of testicular cancer incidence in Denmark by Moller (1989), it was concluded that men born just before or during the Second World War appeared to be at lower risk than expected, based on the generally increasing age-cohort trends. The cumulative risk of testicular cancer for the age interval 20 to 34 years increased 25%–30% in successive 5-year cohorts born between 1920 and 1935.

International Patterns

Even though the age-adjusted incidence of testicular cancer is relatively low in all populations of the world, there is considerable geographic variation. Rates are four to nine times higher in Denmark, Norway, New Zealand, and North American whites, compared with the lower rates registered in Asian populations, African Americans, black populations in general, and non-Jews in Israel (Fig. 56–6). The incidence rates of testicular cancer in white males in the age group 25–44 have increased during the 1970s and 1980s in most countries in Europe and North America. The Japanese Americans residing in Hawaii or California tend to have incidence rates that are 40% to 100% higher than the rates determined for the Japanese residing in Japan; in contrast, the Chinese Americans residing in California have lower rates than those registered for the Chinese in Singapore or Hong Kong.

Socioeconomic Status

Most studies have shown that the incidence of testicular cancer is highest in the highest socioeconomic classes (eg, professional and skilled nonmanual occupations), and that the rates are approximately double the incidence in blue collar occupational groups, such as laborers, and other unskilled and partly skilled occupations (Graham and Gibson, 1972; Graham et al, 1977). The risk in relation to social class does not vary significantly by age at diagnosis, nor is the social class gradient limited to a particular histological type of testicular cancer (Swerdlow and Skeet, 1988). Thus, while Ross and coworkers (1979) described a steeper social class gradient for patients with embryonal carcinoma when compared

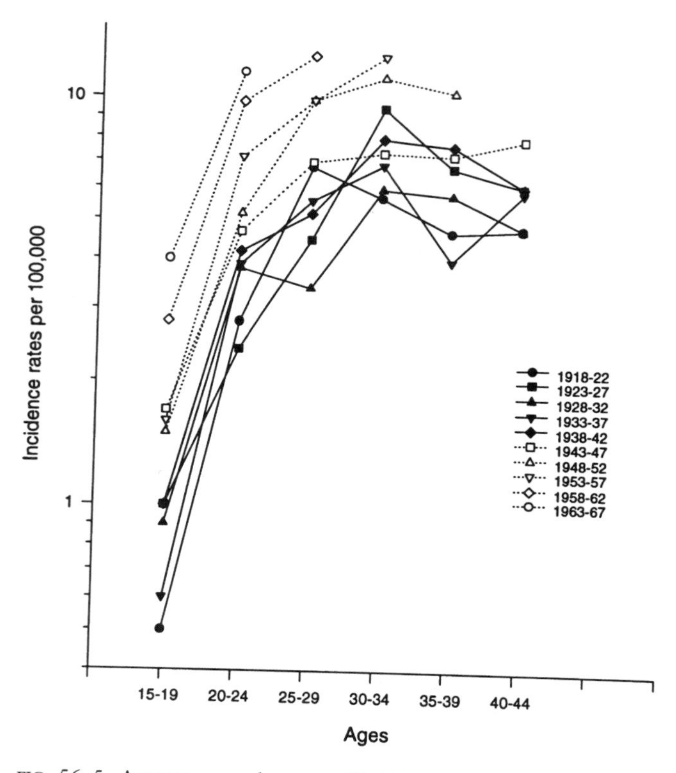

FIG. 56–5. Average annual age-specific (15–44 years) incidence rates (per 100,000), testicular cancer, 5-year birth cohorts, Connecticut, 1918–1967.

TABLE 56–3. *Age-Cohort–Specific Incidence Rates Per 100,000 for Testicular Cancer in Connecticut Based on Rates in 1935–1987*

	Age Group at Diagnosis					
Birth Cohort	*15–19*	*20–24*	*25–29*	*30–34*	*35–39*	*40–44*
1918–1922	0.5	2.8	6.8	5.7	4.7	4.8
1923–1927	1.0	2.4	4.5	9.5	6.8	6.1
1928–1932	0.9	3.8	3.4	6.0	5.8	4.8
1933–1937	0.6	3.9	5.6	6.9	4.0	5.9
1938–1942	1.0	4.2	5.2	8.0	7.7	6.1
1943–1947	1.7	4.7	7.0	7.4	7.3	8.0
1948–1952	1.5	5.2	9.9	11.3	10.4	
1953–1957	1.6	7.2	9.9	12.8		
1958–1962	2.8	9.8	12.8			
1963–1967	4.0	11.6				

with seminoma patients, other investigators (Morrison, 1976; Coldman et al, 1982) observed that the social class gradient was more evident in patients with seminoma than with other non-seminomatous histological types.

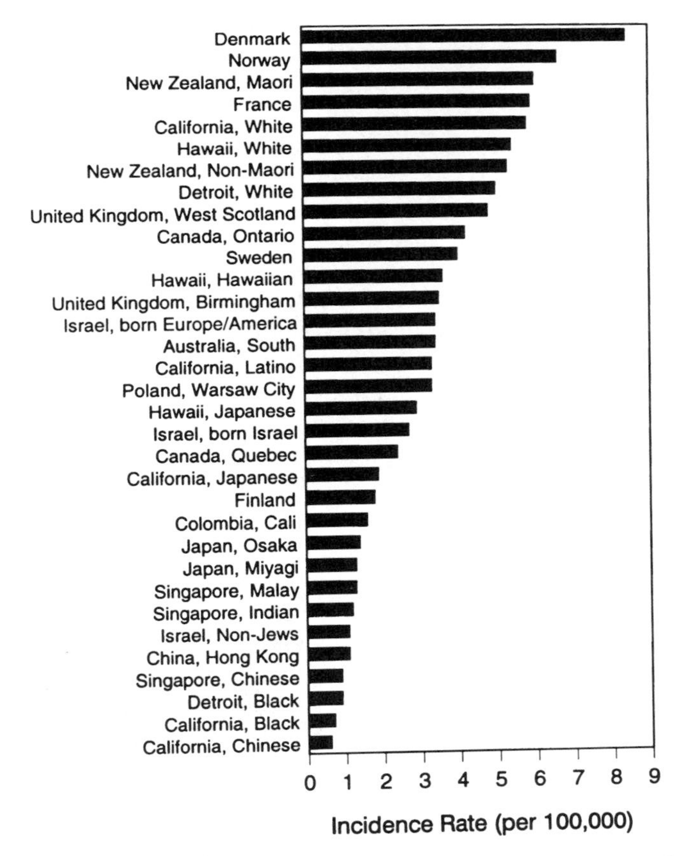

FIG. 56–6. Age-adjusted incidence rates per 100,000 (world standard population) for testicular cancer in selected countries (*Cancer Incidence in Five Continents*, Volume VI).

Occupation

The most consistent observation about occupation and testicular cancer incidence is that white collar or professional occupations have been associated with moderately elevated relative risks, in the range of 1.5 to 2.5. Such observations, however, do not suggest a specific environmental exposure, but may serve to indicate that other risk factors correlated with socioeconomic status and lifestyle are intrinsically linked in the causal pathway (Van den Eeden et al, 1991; Pearce et al, 1987). Excesses of testicular cancer have been reported in association with employment in the armed forces (Dubrow and Wegman, 1983); among aviation support equipment technicians and engineers (Garland et al, 1988); civilians engaged in repair of F4 Phantom jets (Ducatman et al, 1986); workers in the crude petroleum and natural gas extraction industry (Mills et al, 1984); occupations with exposure to polycyclic aromatic hydrocarbons (Milham, 1983); printing industry (McDowall and Balajaran, 1986); and the leather industry, particularly leather finishing (Marshall et al, 1990). In using a case-control approach to investigate a reported cluster of testicular cancer cases among leather workers in New York State, Marshall and coworkers (1990) determined that the odds ratio for exposure to leather processing or manufacturing was 7.16 (95% confidence interval: 1.89–27.72). The putative exposures in this investigation included dimethylformamide-containing dyes used in leather finishing or unspecified solvents and/or dyes. In a hospital-based case-control study conducted in Germany, Rhomberg et al (1995) observed that there was an elevated risk of seminomas of the testis in skilled workers exposed to metals, metal dusts, and possibly cutting oils.

A study of military working dogs used in Vietnam reported a statistically significant increased risk of testicular neoplasms and of testicular dysfunction (Hayes et al, 1990). The toxicologic risks in military dogs may have provided a surveillance marker of potential human risks in the military personnel who have served in Vietnam. Of particular concern was the intensity and duration of exposure to chemical agents such as to Agent Orange, which is a mixture of 2,4-dichlorophenoxyacetic acid (2,4-D) and 2,4,5-trichlorophenoxyacetic acid (2,4,5-T). The compound 2,4,5-T was contaminated with small amounts of dioxin, which has been shown to be teratogenic and carcinogenic in experimental animals (Poland and Knutson, 1981). Epidemiological investigation of the suspected increased risk of testicular cancer observed in Vietnam veterans, however, has not implicated a specific environmental factor related to military service (Tarone et al, 1991; Bullman et al, 1994).

ETIOLOGY AND PATHOGENESIS

Gonadal Embryogenesis

The human testis is composed of a system of tubules for the production and transport of sperm and clusters of interstitial or Leydig cells between the tubules that produce both androgenic and estrogenic steroids. The basic histological components of the tubules are the germ cells and Sertoli cells. Both the Leydig and the Sertoli cells are derived from the mesenchymal tissue of the urogenital ridge, whereas the primordial germ cells are derived from primitive ectodermal cells, originate from the yolk sac, and migrate into the urogenital ridge by the sixth week of gestation. At this stage of development, the gubernaculum first appears as a ridge of mesenchymal tissue extending from the genital ridge through an opening in the musculature of the anterior abdominal wall to the site of genital swellings, or the anlage of the fetal scrotum.

At fertilization, the genome of the zygote contains both paternally and maternally imprinted chromosomes. Sexual organization of the human gonad first becomes apparent with the appearance of seminiferous cords in the fetal testis by the seventh week of gestation. During gametogenesis the imprinting pattern of genes in differentiating testicular germ cells is changed to a completely paternal pattern (van Gurp et al, 1994). The genetic control of testicular differentiation resides on the short arm of the Y chromosome, and at a locus distinct from the gene that encodes the H-Y antigen. Morphological development of the testis is generally completed by the end of the 12th week, while descent of the testis from the abdominal cavity to the scrotum occurs during the remaining months of gestation (Jost and Magre, 1988).

In the human embryo the actual movement of the testis from the abdominal cavity through the inguinal canal and into the scrotum usually occurs during the seventh month. Hormonal, neurogenic, and mechanical factors are believed to control the process of testicular descent. During the eighth week of gestation in the male embryo, the fetal testis begins to secrete the Müllerian-inhibiting factor (MIF) and testosterone. MIF, which is secreted by the fetal Sertoli cells, causes regression of the Müllerian ducts and initiates descent to the inguinal region. By causing regression of Müllerian ducts in the male fetus, MIF permits differentiation of the male phenotype by preventing development of the female genitalia. MIF has been demonstrated to inhibit epidermal growth factor activity, and as a polypeptide growth modulator has structural and functional homology to the transforming growth factor β (Liu and Oliff, 1991). Testosterone, which is synthesized and secreted by the fetal Leydig cells, is converted to dihydrotestosterone (DHT) by the 5α-reductase enzyme, and both androgenic hormones control the transinguinal phase of testicular descent into the scrotum. DHT is the active androgenic hormone that induces differentiation of the male external genitalia. Movement of the gastrointestinal organs into the abdominal cavity causes an increase in intra-abdominal pressure, which causes physiological herniation of the processus vaginalis through the ventral abdominal wall along the course of each gubernaculum. Shortening of the gubernaculum, which may be induced by androgens, anchors the fetal testis to the inguinal region. Neurogenic factors may contribute to descent of the human testes; in the neonatal rat, transection of the genitofemoral nerve prevents growth and enlargement of the gubernaculum, and interferes with transinguinal movement of the testes. After 40 gestational weeks, descent is generally completed, and the gubernaculum is resorbed and shrinks to a fibrous remnant (Hutson, 1985; Moul and Belman, 1988).

Gonadal Dysgenesis and Cryptorchism

Not all mammals have scrotal testes, but presumably the migration of the testes into an external scrotum conferred some evolutionary advantage on the species with respect to fertility and the rate of spontaneous mutation. Cryptorchidism (cryptorchism), or failure of normal testicular descent, may result in the male gonad being intra-abdominal, typically located just above the internal inguinal ring (10%); intracanalicular, or beyond the internal inguinal ring (15%–20%); high scrotal, with limited range of motion so that it can retract into the groin but not past the internal inguinal ring (40%); and obstructed, or where there is a fascial barrier between the inguinal pouch, just distal to the external inguinal ring, and the inlet of the scrotum (30%). It is important to distinguish the cryptorchid testis from the absent testis (anorchia), and the temporarily retracted normal testis.

The incidence of cryptorchism in men in the United States is about 0.7% to 0.8% (Rajfer et al, 1986). Studies of the incidence of cryptorchism in England and Wales, comparing the rates in the late 1950s with those in the mid-1980s, have concluded that there has been an increase of 65%–100% (Chilvers et al, 1984; Jackson et al, 1986). In the Collaborative Perinatal Study sponsored by the NIH (United States), the incidence of cryptorchism up to one year of age during the period 1959–1965 was estimated to be 1.1% (Myrianthopoulos and Chung, 1974). During the period 1968–1977, the survey of all hospitals in the five counties of Atlanta, Georgia, described a significant linear trend for the increase in the reported incidence of cryptorchism, and hypospadias, in white males up to one year of age. Cryptorchism is diagnosed among 10% to 18% of males with hypospadias (Harris, 1990). Cryptorchism is about twice as common in premature as in full-term infants, and is commonly associated with an inguinal hernia. Heinonen and coworkers (1977) reported that there was a threefold excess risk of cryptorchism in U.S. whites compared with blacks. The incidence of cryptorchism is increased in disorders of pituitary gonadotropin deficiency (eg, Laurence-Moon-Biedl (polydactyly, obesity, hypogonadism), Kallmann's (hypogonadotropic hypogonadism and anosmia), and Prader-Labhart-Willi (cryptorchism, obesity, deletion of chromosome 15) syndromes; neural tube disorders such as myelomeningocele; syndromes involving abnormalities of testosterone biosynthesis, such as the syndrome of androgen resistance (testicular feminization) and deficiency of 5-α-reductase activity; and gonadal dysgenesis (Palmer, 1991).

The cryptorchid gonad is generally accompanied by significant structural and functional abnormalities. The gonad is smaller than normal, with microscopic areas of hypoplastic tubules and decreased spermatogenesis. Eventually the tubules appear as dense cords of hyaline connective tissue outlined by prominent basement membranes. There is evidence of delayed maturation of Sertoli cells, which synthesize estrogen under stimulation by the follicle-stimulating hormone. The interstitial stroma may appear quite cellular, and is characterized by hyperplasia of Leydig cells. Cryptorchism is associated with defective spermatogenesis, and in unilateral cryptorchism, spermatogenesis may be decreased in the normally descended testis. Commonly, infants and prepubertal children with cryptorchism manifest functional abnormalities in the hypothalamic-pituitary-gonadal axis. Endocrine dysfunction may consist of decreased blood levels of testosterone and luteinizing hormone (LH), and/or a blunted response to stimulation-testing with gonadotropin-releasing hormone (Job et al, 1979).

Clinical studies had estimated that the risk of testicular cancer in men with unilateral or bilateral cryptorchism was 20 to 40 times higher than normally expected. During the past 20 years, case-control and cohort epidemiological studies have established that the relative risk of testicular cancer in men with undescended testes was in the range of 2.5 to 11.4 (Table 56–4), and that cryptorchism accounted for approximately 10% of the incident cases of testicular cancer (Schottenfeld, et al 1980; United Kingdom Testicular Cancer Study Group, 1994). Approximately 10% to 25% of patients with a history of cryptorchism have been reported to develop cancer in the contralateral, normally descended gonad (Gehring et al, 1974; Batata et al, 1982). Is it the malposition of the testis and its greater exposure to heat and trauma, and/or a primary malformation with hypoplastic germinal epithelium and endocrine dysfunction, that provide the pathophysiologic mechanism for tumorigenesis? It has been noted that the risk of testicular cancer in patients with cryptorchism increased with increasing age of orchiopexy (Pottern et al, 1985). A summary estimate of the odds ratio for testicular cancer in the ipsilateral cryptorchid testis compared to the contralateral descended testis, was 2.7-fold higher for those undergoing orchiopexy after age 10 years, when compared to patients who were treated before age 10. Studies in men without testicular cancer, 15–30 years after unilateral orchiopexy, have shown persistent histological abnormalities in spermatogenesis in both testicles (Lipshultz et al, 1976). In a population-based case-control study conducted in the United Kingdom, it was inferred that surgical correction of unilateral cryptorchism before the age of 10 years was an effective preventive intervention for testicular cancer in young men (United Kingdom Testicular Cancer Study Group, 1994). The potential reversibility in risk with early surgical correction, and limited risk to the contralateral testis in unilateral cryptorchism, would argue in support of the hypothesis that the microenvironment of the undescended testis is a determining pathogenic factor.

Prenatal Exposure to Estrogens

Exposure to exogenous estrogens during fetal development will profoundly alter sexual differentiation. Experiments in pregnant rodents have shown that prenatal estrogen administration has resulted in an increased incidence of cryptorchism and dysgenetic gonads in the male offspring (McLachlan et al, 1975). Subsequent administration of androgens during gestational development has reversed or ameliorated the risk of testicular maldescent (Rajfer and Walsh, 1977). Mice exposed in utero to diethylstilbestrol (DES), a synthetic nonsteroidal, stilbene-derived estrogen, are at increased risk of malignant interstitial cell tumor of the testis and adenocarcinoma of the rete testis (Newbold and McLachlan, 1988; Bullock et al, 1988).

DES exposure in utero has been linked to a variety of structural and functional alterations in the human male genital tract. The lesions have ranged from relatively minor structural alterations, such as epididymal or spermatocele cysts, to more major anatomical abnormalities of testicular hypoplasia, cryptorchism, hypospadias, and microphallus. The historical use of estrogens, in particular DES, during the period 1945–1960, for threatened abortion and other complications of pregnancy, was a common practice in the United States (Giusti et al, 1995). It is estimated that there may have been up to two to four million mothers exposed to DES, or other nonsteroidal synthetic estrogens, like dienestrol, before the use of such drugs in pregnant women was proscribed in 1971 by the Food and Drug Administration. Exogenous estrogen (and progestin) exposure in utero may also occur as a result of pregnancy testing, or from the inadvertent use of oral contraceptives after conception. Studies of the potential teratogenic effects of estrogen and/or progestin preparations administered during pregnancy may be confounded by a preexisting condition for which the hormone(s) was given; such studies are required to evaluate the gestational interval, intensity, and duration of exposure. In the fetus, uncon-

TABLE 56–4. *Summary of Case-Control and Cohort Studies of Cryptorchism and Testicular Cancer*

CASE-CONTROL STUDIES

	History of Cryptorchism					
	Cases		*Controls*			
Authors (year of publication)	*No. Studied*	*%*	*No. Studied*	*%*	*Odds Ratio (95% confidence interval)*	*Comments*
Morrison (1976)	596	2.9	602	0.3	8.8 (2.3–56.3)	History of inguinal hernia operation was independent risk factor: odds ratio was 2.9 (1.3–7.0)
Henderson et al (1979)	79	12.7	79	2.5	5.0	$P = 0.02$ In cases with unilateral cryptorchism, the risk of testicular cancer in the undescended testis was more than four times greater than in the contralateral testis
Schottenfeld et al (1980)	190	11.6	166 142	3.6 (hospital) 4.9 (neighborhood)	3.5 (1.34, 8.10) 2.5 (1.02, 5.68)	In 21% of cases with unilateral cryptorchism, the testicular cancer was diagnosed in the contralateral testis. Inguinal hernia was not a significant risk factor
Pottern et al (1985)	271	9.2	259	2.7	3.7 (1.6–8.6)	Men without cryptorchism who underwent an inguinal herniorrhaphy experienced a non-significantly elevated risk [1.3 (0.6–2.5)]. Among those with unilateral cryptorchism, the risk was increased sixfold for the homolateral testis,; no increase in risk was observed for the contralateral testis
Moss et al (1986)	217	11.1	223	2.7	4.5 (1.7–13.7)	The odds ratio associated with cryptorchism was 8.3 (2.8–32.9) when based on sons' responses, compared with 4.5, when measured from mothers' responses. There was no independent association with inguinal hernia [odds ratio for hernia was 1.3 (0.8–2.1)]
Gershman and Stolley (1988)	79	9.1	79	1.4	7.3 (0.8–62.3)	Significant risk noted for premature birth in the cases. In the matched analysis based on discordant pairs the odds ratio was 6.0 (0.5–69.3)
	(unmatched analysis)					
Strader et al (1988)	333	12.0	675	2.2	5.9 (3.4–10.2)	The odds ratios were similar for seminomatous and nonseminomatous germ cell tumors. The risk of cancer in the cryptorchid testis was 8.0 (4.2–15.3); in the descended contralateral testis of men with cryptorchism, the risk was 1.6 (0.6–4.1), relative to the risk in men without cryptorchism
Haughey et al (1989)	247	12.6	247	2.4	5.2 (2.4–32.5)	Independent associations of "testis-related" abnormalities were also noted: low sperm count, fertility problems, and atrophic testis. In logistic regression analysis, cryptorchism and atrophy were significant. History of inguinal hernia was a significant risk factor after controlling for age and education [odds ratio was 2.26 (1.3–4.0)]
United Kingdom Testicular Cancer Study Group (1994)	794	8.2	794	2.1	3.8 (2.2–6.5)	With bilateral undescended testes, the odds ratio was 5.9, whereas, with unilateral undescended testis, the odds ratio was 2.7. Twelve of the 46 cases (26%) with unilateral undescended testis had cancer diagnosed in the contralateral testis (odds ratio, 1.4, compared with 4.0 for the risk to the cryptorchid testis). History of inguinal hernia diagnosed before the age of 15 years was significantly associated with risk of testicular cancer [odds ratio 2.6 (1.3–5.3)]

(continued)

TABLE 56–4. *(Continued)*

COHORT STUDIES

Authors (year of publication)	*Cryptorchid Study Group*	*Control Group*	*Relative Risk (95% confidence interval)*	*Comments*
Giwercman et al (1987)	6/506 = 11.9 per 1,000	1.3 cancers expected The lifetime risk in the Danish male population was estimated at 0.5 percent	4.7 (1.7–10.2)	Expected number of testicular cancers based on Danish Cancer Registry. In men with unilateral cryptorchism, the relative risk was 2.4 (0.3–8.7); with bilateral cryptorchism, the relative risk was 9.3 (2.6–23.7). The maximal standardized incidence ratio was in the age group, 30 to 39 years [8.3 (2.7–19.5)]
Benson et al (1991)	2/224 = 8.9 per 1,000	0.2 cancers expected	11.4 (1.4–41.1)	Expected number of testicular cancers based on Olmstead County/Rochester, MN age-specific cancer incidence rates. Prevalence of cryptorchism was estimated to be 8.6 per 1,000 male births. Three percent of cryptorchid males had hypospadias. When compared with all other male infants, the relative risk for inguinal hernia in cryptorchid males was significantly increased (4.4)
Pinczowski et al (1991)	4/2918 = 1.4 per 1,000	0.54 cancers expected	7.4 (2.0–19.0)	Follow-up (25,360 person-years) was achieved by record linkage to the Swedish Cancer Registry. A comparison cohort of 30,199 males operated on for an inguinal hernia did not evidence an increased risk of testicular cancer [1.1 (0.4–2.2)]. Three of the four testicular cancers occurred in males with bilateral intraabdominal testes

jugated estrogen can bind to target organ receptor sites in the male genital tract with resultant antagonistic or inhibitory effects on the pituitary-gonadal axis, and the normal production and distribution of testosterone from the fetal testis.

It has been postulated that exogenous estrogen hormone use during the first trimester of pregnancy may be associated with an increased risk of testicular cancer (Henderson et al, 1979; Schottenfeld et al, 1980; Depue et al, 1983). In those three case-control studies suggesting an association, the odds ratios ranged from 2.8 to 5.3, but in two of the studies (Henderson et al, 1979; Schottenfeld et al, 1980), the confidence intervals overlapped 1.0. In the study of Depue and coworkers (1983), hormone exposure began in the initial two months of pregnancy; nine of the 107 patients were exposed in utero, and in five of the patients' mothers, exposure resulted from a single pregnancy test. In none of the above studies was there an interaction between exogenous hormones and cryptorchism in the cases with testicular cancer. Brown and coworkers (1986) did not observe any association with exogenous estrogen or progestin hormone use in pregnancy, but noted a statistically significant twofold [RR=2.4 (1.2–5.1)] increase in risk associated with unusual bleeding or spotting during the index pregnancy, and a significantly lower mean birth weight in the case patients than in the control patients. The association with unusual bleeding or spotting was independent of use of any medication and was specific for the index pregnancy. Moss and coworkers (1986) found a significant association with cryptorchism (Table 56–4), but no association with DES or other hormonal exposures in pregnancy.

Henderson and coworkers (1988) have proposed that elevated levels of maternal bioavailable estrogens, from either exogenous or endogenous sources, exert a teratogenic or "arrested developmental" effect on the maturation of fetal primordial germ cells, which may serve as precursors of neoplastic cells. One or more clones of aberrant germ cells are subsequently stimulated by prepubertal rising levels of luteinizing hormone and follicle-stimulating hormone. The epidemiology of ovarian germ cell neoplasms appears to parallel that of testicular neoplasms (Santos Silva and Swerdlow, 1991). In a population-based case-control study in young women with ovarian germ cell neoplasms conducted in Los Angeles and Seattle, Walker and coworkers (1988) reported that the mother's use of exogenous hormones was associated with an increased odds ratio (OR = 3.60, 95 percent confidence interval: 1.2–13.1).

Familial and Hereditary Factors

The various risk factors of gonadal dysgenesis, hypogonadism, cryptorchism, and familial aggregation suggest that genetic influences may be important in the pathogenesis of testicular cancer. Gonadal dysgenesis is a rare genetic disorder of embryogenesis, often with

TABLE 56–5. *Testicular Tumors in Disorders of Gonadal Differentiation*

Congenital Disorder	*Chromosomal Anomaly*	*Associated Testicular Tumor*
1. Klinefelter syndrome: eunuchoidism, gynecomastia, azoospermia, elevated FSH, decreased testosterone, increased estradiol, increased estrodiol/testosterone ratio, small dysgenetic testes	47, XXY 46XY/ 47XXY mosaicism	breast cancer: 8 times risk in normal males gonadoblastoma, invasive germ cell cancer
2. Male pseudohermaphroditism cryptorchidism, hypospadias, variable internal genital organs	XY or mosaicism with Y chromosome	gonadoblastoma, invasive germ cell cancer
3. Testicular feminization: female habitus, but without uterus or fallopian tubes; cryptorchidism	46, XY	Sertoli cell tumor in dysgenetic gonad
4. Mixed gonadal dysgenesis: female habitus, but some degree of virilization; streak gonad	XO/XY	gonadoblastoma, invasive germ cell tumor

maldescent of the testis and incomplete masculinization of the external genitalia (Table 56–5). Among index cases with testicular cancer, the prevalence of a family history of testicular cancer among first-degree relatives has varied from 0.2% to 2.2% (Tollerud et al, 1985). Among such relatives there may be associated urogenital anomalies (Kratzik et al, 1991), polythelia or supernumerary nipples (Goedert et al, 1984), or rare genetic syndromes, such as the recessive X-linked ichthyosis (Lykkesfeldt et al, 1991). Testicular cancer has been reported in non-twin brothers, identical twin brothers, and in fathers and sons (Dieckmann et al, 1987). Concordance by cell type, average age at diagnosis, associated cryptorchism, or bilaterality, was highest for identical twin pairs (Pottern and Goedert, 1986; Patel et al, 1990; Goss and Bulbul, 1990). Kratzik and coworkers (1991) studied patients with bilateral testicular germ cell tumors, comparing histocompatibility antigen types (HLA) in cases and matched controls. There was an overrepresentation in the cases of HLA-B14, DR5, and DR7; and a decreased frequency in the bilateral testicular germ cell cases of HLA-DR1, DR3, and DR4. Although familial occurrences of testicular cancer are uncommon, it may be prudent to recommend testicular self-examination in young adults with affected first-degree relatives (Wardle et al, 1994). Using actuarial analysis and taking into account the number of brothers at risk to age 50 years, Forman et al (1992) estimated that the risk of testicular cancer in the brothers of cases was 2.2% (95% confidence interval 0.6 to 3.8%).

A specific cytogenetic abnormality, an isochromosome of 12p, i(12p), has been described in male germ cell cancers. The i(12p) occurs in gonadal and extragonadal tumors histopathologically diagnosed as seminoma, nonseminoma, or teratoma (Dmitrovsky et al, 1990). The chromosome anomaly has been identified in 80% to 90% of all testicular germ cell tumors, and, therefore, has value as a diagnostic biomarker in the analysis of tumors of uncertain histogenesis. Multiple copies of the i(12p) marker, which may result in the amplification of c-ki-*ras*2 oncogene, usually characterize tumors with an aggressive growth pattern (Ilson et al, 1991). The appearance of the cytogenetic abnormality may signal the neoplastic transformation process. In general, the formation of an isochromosome in diploid cells leads to the loss of the chromosomal arm not included in the anomaly. In the case of i(12p), this would result in the loss of heterozygosity of the genes on the q arm of chromosome 12. However, VanKessel and coworkers (1991) reported that loss of heterozygosity on the q arm of chromosome 12 was not an invariable characteristic of i(12p)-positive testicular germ cell tumors.

In addition to the presence of i(12p), nonrandom gains in chromosomes 1, 7, 12, 21, 22, and X have been reported in more than 70% of male germ cell tumors. A deletion in the long arm of chromosome 12, occurring between bands q13 and q22, has been identified in nonseminomatous germ cell tumors. Chromosomal breaks during tumor progression at 1p11, 7q22 and 12p have given rise to characteristic patterns of chromosomal rearrangements (Bosl et al, 1989; Samaniego et al, 1990; Rodriguez et al, 1992; Sinke et al, 1993). In contrast to normal gametogenesis, testicular germ cell tumors, in general, express both parental alleles, which is consistent with the potential of the cell of origin to differentiate into somatic (embryonic) and/or trophoblastic (extraembryonic) imprinted lineages (van Gurp et al, 1994).

Other Risk Factors

Patients with testicular cancer may recall a history of trauma to the affected testicle (Coldman et al, 1982; Pattern et al, 1985). However, the assessment of risk in case-control studies may be biased by selective recall of instances of trauma of ill-defined severity, or where the trauma called attention to the existing tumor. Severe trauma may require orchiectomy, or may lead to necrosis or infarction and subsequent degeneration and atrophy of gonadal tissue (Stone et al, 1991). Similarly, atrophy of the testicle may occur after orchitis, but no causal association with a specific infectious agent, such as the mumps paramyxovirus, has been established (Heinzer et al, 1993). Initial observations of the occurrence of testicular cancer in men with human immunodeficiency virus (HIV) infection resulted in hypothesizing that the infectious agent was a possible causal factor. Recent epidemiologic studies have failed to establish an association (Rabkin et al, 1991; Reynolds et al, 1993). The prominent peak in the incidence of testicular cancer between 25 and 34 years in U.S. whites of higher social class is suggestive of the pattern of Hodgkin's disease in young adults from economically advantaged populations (Mueller et al, 1988; Algood et al, 1988).

Vasectomy is a common and increasing form of male contraception used in the United States (about 500,000 vasectomies each year) and throughout the world. Following vasectomy, morphologic changes in the human testis have been observed, including focal interstitial fibrosis and thickening of the tunica propria of seminiferous tubules, dilatation of seminiferous tubules, and reduction in the numbers of germ and Sertoli's cells. Immunologic studies have shown that 50 to 70% of men have elevated antibodies to spermatocytes in the seminal fluid and serum following vasectomy (Jarow et al, 1985). Cohort studies in general have not described a significant association between vasectomy and testicular cancer, although the follow-up interval and statistical power have been limited in the individual studies (Goldacre et al, 1979; Walker et al, 1981; Petitti et al, 1983; Massey et al, 1984; Nienhuis et al, 1992). Cale et al (1990) reported an increased incidence of testicular cancer soon after vasectomy which suggested either that the neoplasm was present at the time of vasectomy and detected through more careful postoperative surveillance, or that the procedure accelerated the progression of neoplastic disease. Among 3 case-control studies, the reported odds ratios (95% confidence intervals) were 1.1 (0.6 to 2.0) (Swerdlow et al, 1987); 0.6 (0.3 to 1.2) (Moss et al, 1986); and 1.5 (1.0 to 2.2) (Strader et al, 1988). The available information would allow for a preliminary assessment that there is either no or a weak association between vasectomy and testicular cancer (West, 1992).

REFERENCES

Algood CB, Newell GR, Johnson DE. 1988. Viral etiology of testicular tumors. J Urol 139:308–310.

Batata MA, Chu FC, Hilaris BC, et al. 1982. Testicular cancer in cryptorchids. Cancer 49:1023–1030.

Bates SE. 1991. Clinical applications of serum tumor markers. Ann Intern Med 115:623–638.

Beard CM, Melton JL, O'Fallon WM, et al. 1984. Cryptorchism and maternal estrogen exposure. Am J Epidemiol 120:707–716.

Benson RC, Beard MC, Kelalis PP, et al. 1991. Malignant potential of the cryptorchid testis. Mayo Clin Proc 66:372–378.

Berthelsen JG, Skakkebaek NE, von der Maase H, et al. 1982. Screening for carcinoma in situ of the contralateral testis in patients with germinal testicular cancer. Br Med J 285:1683–1686.

Bosl GJ, Dmitrovsky E, Reuter VE, et al. 1989. Isochromosome of chromosome 12: clinically useful marker for male germ cell tumors. J Natl Cancer Inst 81:1874–1878.

Brodsky GL. 1991. Pathology of testicular germ cell tumors. Hematol Oncol Clin North Am 5:1095–1126.

Brown LM, Pottern LM, Hoover RN. 1986. Prenatal and perinatal risk factors for testicular cancer. Cancer Res 46:4812–4816.

Bullman TA, Watanabe KK, Kang HK. 1994. Risk of testicular cancer associated with surrogate measures of Agent Orange exposure among Vietnam veterans on the Agent Orange registry. Ann Epidemiol 4:11–16.

Bullock BC, Newbold RR, McLachlan JA. 1988. Lesions of testis and epididymis associated with prenatal diethylstilbestrol exposure. Environ Health Perspect 77:29–31.

Cale ARJ, Farouk M, Prescott RJ, et al. 1990. Does vasectomy accelerate testicular tumor? Importance of testicular examinations before and after vasectomy. Br M J 300:370.

Chilvers C, Pike MC, Forman D, et al. 1984. Apparent doubling of frequency of undescended testis in England and Wales in 1962–81. Lancet 1:330–332.

Coldman AJ, Elwood JM, Gallagher RP. 1982. Sports activities and risk of testicular cancer. Br J Cancer 46:749–756.

Decoufle P, Stanislawczyk K. 1977. A retrospective survey of cancer in relation to occupation. DHEW (NIOSH) Publication No. 77–178.

Depue RH, Pike M, Henderson BE. 1983. Estrogen exposure during gestation and risk of testicular cancer. J Natl Cancer Inst 71:1151–1155.

Depue RH. 1984. Maternal and gestational factors affecting the risk of cryptorchidism and inguinal hernia. Int J Epidemiol 13:311–318.

Depue RH, Bernstein L, Ross RK, et al. 1987. Hyperemesis gravidarum in relation to estradiol levels, pregnancy outcome, and other maternal factors: a seroepidemiologic study. Am J Obstet Gynecol 156:1137–1141.

Dieckmann K-P, Becker T, Jonas D, et al. 1987. Inheritance and testicular cancer: arguments based on a report of three cases and a review of the literature. Oncology 44:367–377.

Dmitrovsky E, Bosl GJ, Chaganti RSK. 1990. Clinical and genetic features of human germ cell cancer. Cancer Surv 9:369–386.

Dubrow R, Wegman DH. 1983. Setting priorities for occupational cancer research and control: synthesis of the results of occupational disease surveillance studies. J Natl Cancer Inst 71:1123–1142.

Ducatman AM, Conwill DE, Crawl J. 1986. Germ cell tumors of the testicle among aircraft repairmen. J Urol 136:834–836.

Forman D, Oliver RTD, Brett AR, et al. 1992. Familial testicular cancer: a report of the UK family register, estimation of risk and an HLA class I sib-pair analysis. Br J Cancer 65:255–262.

Garland FC, Gorham ED, Garland CF, et al. 1988. Testicular cancer in US Navy personnel. Am J Epidemiol 127:411–414.

Gehring GG, Rodriguez FR, Woodhead DM. 1974. Malignant degeneration of cryptorchid testes following orchiopexy. J Urol 112:354–356.

Gershman ST, Stolley PD. 1988. A case-control study of testicular cancer using Connecticut tumor registry data. Int J Epidemiol 17:738–742.

Ghosh SN, Shah PM, Gharpure HM. 1978. Absence of H-Y antigen in XY females with dysgenetic gonads. Nature 276:180–181.

Gill WB, Schumacher GFB, Bibbo M, et al. 1979. Association of diethylstilbestrol exposure in utero with cryptorchidism, testicular hypoplasia and semen abnormalities. J Urol 122:36–39.

GIUSTI RM, IWAMOTO K, HATCH EE. 1995. Diethylstilbestrol revisited: a review of the long-term health effects. Ann Intern Med 122:778–788.

GIWERCMAN A, GRINDSTED J, HANSEN B, et al. 1987. Testicular cancer risk in boys with maldescended testis: a cohort study. J Urol 138:1214–1216.

GOEDERT JJ, MCKEEN EA, JAVADPOUR N, et al. 1984. Polythelia and testicular cancer. Ann Intern Med 101:646–647.

GOLDACRE M, VESSEY M, CLARKE J, et al. 1979. Record linkage study of morbidity following vasectomy. In: Lepow IH, Grozler R, eds. Vasectomy: Immunologic and Pathophysiologic Effects in Animals and Man. New York, Academic Press pp 567–569.

GOSS PE, BULBUL MA. 1990. Familial testicular cancer in five members of a cancer-prone kindred. Cancer 66:2044–2046.

GRAHAM S, GIBSON RW. 1972. Social epidemiology of cancer of the testis. Cancer 29:1242–1249.

GRAHAM S, GIBSON R, WEST D, et al. 1977. Epidemiology of cancer of the testis in upstate New York. J Natl Cancer Inst 58:1255–1261.

GURP VAN RJHLM, OOSTERHUIS JW, KALSCHEUER V, et al. 1994. Biallelic expression of the H19 and IGF2 genes in human testicular germ cell tumors. J Natl Cancer Inst 86:1070–1075.

HADZISELIMORIC F. 1983. Cryptorchidism: Management and Implications. Berlin, Heidelberg, New York: Springer-Verlag.

HARRIS EL. 1990. Genetic epidemiology of hypospadias. Epidemiol Rev 12:29–40.

HAUGHEY BP, GRAHAM S, BRASURE J, et al. 1989. The epidemiology of testicular cancer in upstate New York. Am J Epidemiol 130:25–36.

HAYES HM, TARONE RE, CASEY HW, et al. 1990. Excess of seminomas observed in Vietnam service U.S. military working dogs. J Natl Cancer Inst 82:1042–1046.

HERBST AL, COLE P, NORASIS MJ, et al. 1979. Epidemiologic aspects and factors related to survival in 384 registry cases of clear cell adenocarcinoma of the vagina and cervix. Am J Obstet Gynecol 135:876–886.

HEINONEN OP, SLONE D, SHAPIRO S. 1977. Malformations of the genitourinary system. In: *Birth Defects and Drugs in Pregnancy*, Kaufmann DW (ed). Littleton, MA: Publishing Sciences Group, Inc., pp 176–199.

HEINZER H, DIECKMANN K, HULAND E. 1993. Virus-related serology and in situ hybridization for the detection of virus DNA among patients with testicular cancer. Eur Urol 24:271–276.

HENDERSON BE, BENTON B, JING J, et al. 1979. Risk factors for cancer of the testis in young men. Int J Cancer 23:598–602.

HENDERSON BE, ROSS RK, PIKE MC, et al. 1982. Endogenous hormones as a major factor in human cancer. Cancer Res 42:3232–3239.

HENDERSON BE, ROSS RK, BERNSTEIN L. 1988. Estrogens as a cause of human cancer: The Richard and Hinda Rosenthal Foundation Award Lecture. Cancer Res 48:246–253.

HUTSON JM. 1985. A biphasic model for the hormonal control of testicular descent. Lancet 2:419–421.

ILSON DH, BOSL GJ, MOTZER R, et al. 1991. Genetic analysis of germ cell tumors: current progress and future prospects. Hematol Oncol Clin North Am 5:1271–1283.

JACKSON MB, CHILVERS C, PIKE MC, et al. 1986. Cryptorchidism: an apparent substantial increase since 1960. John Radcliffe Hospital Cryptorchidism Study Group. Br Med J 293:1401–1404.

JAROW JP, BUDIN RE, DYM M, et al. 1985. Quantitative pathologic changes in the human testis after vasectomy: A controlled study. N Engl J Med 313:1252–1256.

JORGENSEN N, MÜLLER J, GIWERCMAN A, SKAKKEBAEK NE. 1990. Clinical and biological significance of carcinoma in situ of the testis. Cancer Surv 9:287–302.

JOST A, MAGRE S. 1988. Control mechanisms of testicular differentiation. Philos Trans R Soc Lond (Biol) 322:55–61.

KRATZIK C, AIGINGER P, KUBER W, et al. 1991. Risk factors for bilateral testicular germ cell tumors: does heredity play a role? Cancer 68:916–921.

LIPSHULTZ LI, CAMINOS-TORRES R, GREENSPAN CS, et al. 1976. Testicular function after orchiopexy for unilaterally undescended testis. N Engl J Med 295:15–18.

LIU MA, OLIFF A. 1991. Transforming growth factor-β-Müllerian inhibiting substance family of growth regulators. Cancer Invest 9:325–336.

LYKKESFELDT G, BENNETT P, LYKKESFELDT AE, et al. 1991. Testis cancer: ichthyosis constitutes a significant risk factor. Cancer 67:730–734.

LYNCH HT, KATZ D, BOGARD P, et al. 1985. Familial embryonal carcinoma in a cancer-prone kindred. Am J Med 78:891–896.

MARSHALL EG, MELIUS JM, LONDON MA, et al. 1990. Investigation of a testicular cancer cluster using a case-control approach. Int J Epidemiol 19:269–273.

MASSEY FJ, BERNSTEIN GS, O'FALLON WM, et al. 1984. Vasectomy and health: results from a large cohort study. JAMA 252:1023–1029.

MCDOWALL ME, BALARAJAN R. 1986. Testicular cancer mortality in England and Wales 1971–80: variations by occupation. J Epidemiol Community Health 40:26–29.

MCLACHLAN JA, NEWBOLD RR, BULLOCK B. 1975. Reproductive tract lesions in male mice exposed prenatally to diethylstilbestrol. Science 190:991–992.

MILHAM S. 1983. Occupational mortality in Washington State, 1950–1971. Cincinnati, Ohio: US Department of Health, Education and Welfare, NIOSH Research Report, vol 1.

MILLER BA, RIES LAG, HANKEY BF, KOSARY CL, HARRAS A, DEVESA SS, EDWARDS BK, EDS. 1993. SEER Cancer Statistics Review: 1973–1990, National Cancer Institute. NIH Pub. No. 90-2789.

MILLS PK, NEWELL GR, JOHNSON DE. 1984. Testicular cancer associated with employment in agriculture and oil and natural gas extraction. Lancet 1:207–210.

MOLLER H. 1989. Decreased testicular cancer risk in men born in wartime. J Natl Cancer Inst 81:1668–1669.

MORRISON AS. 1976. Some social and medical characteristics of army men with testicular cancer. Am J Epidemiol 104:511–516.

MORRISON AS. 1976. Cryptorchidism, hernia, and cancer of the testis. J Natl Cancer Inst 56:731–733.

MOSS AR, OSMOND D, BACCHETTI P, et al. 1986. Hormonal risk factors in testicular cancer. A case-control study. Am J Epidemiol 124:39–52.

MOUL JW, BELMAN AB. 1988. A review of surgical treatment of undescended testes with emphasis on anatomical position. J Urol 140:125–128.

MUELLER N, HINKULA J, WAHREN B. 1988. Elevated antibody titers against cytomegalovirus among patients with testicular cancer. Int J Cancer 41:399–403.

MYRIANTHOPOULOS NC, CHUNG CS. 1974. Congenital malformations in singletons: Epidemiologic survey. Birth Defects 10: Number 11.

NEWBOLD RR, MCLACHLAN JA. 1988. Neoplastic and non-neoplastic lesions in male reproductive organs following perinatal exposure to hormones and related substances. In: *Toxicity of Hormones in Perinatal Life*, Mori T, Nagasawa H (eds). Boca Raton, Florida: CRC Press, Inc, pp 89–109.

NIENHUIS H, GOLDACRE M, SEAGROATT V, et al. 1992. Incidence of disease after vasectomy: a record linkage retrospective cohort study. Br M J 304:743–746.

PALMER JM. 1991. The undescended testicle. Endocrinol Metab Clin North Am 20:231–240.

PATEL SR, KVOLS LK, RICHARDSON RL. 1990. Familial testicular cancer: report of six cases and review of literature. Mayo Clin Proc 65:804–808.

PEARCE N, SHEPPARD RA, HOWARD JK, et al. 1987. Time trends and occupational differences in cancer of the testis in New Zealand. Cancer 59:1677–1682.

PETITTI DB, KLEIN R, KIPP H, et al. 1983. Vasectomy and the incidence of hospitalized illness. J Urol 129:760–762.

PINCZOWSKI D, MCLAUGHLIN JK, LACKGREN G, et al. 1991. I: Occurrence of testicular cancer in patients operated on for cryptorchism and inguinal hernia. J Urol 146:1291–1294.

POLAND A, KNUTSON J. 1981. 2, 3, 7, 8-Tetrachlorodibenzo-p-dioxin and related halogenated hydrocarbons: examination of the mechanism of toxicity. Annu Rev Pharmacol Toxicol 22:517–554.

POTTERN LM, BROWN LM, HOOVER RN, et al. 1985. Testicular cancer risk among young men: role of cryptorchidism and inguinal hernia. J Natl Cancer Inst 74:377–381.

POTTERN LM, GOEDERT JJ. 1986. Epidemiology of testicular cancer. In: Principles and Management of Testicular Cancer, Javadpour N (ed). New York: Thieme, Inc, pp 108–119.

RABKIN CS, BIGGAR RJ, HORM JW. 1991. Increasing incidence of cancer associated with the human immunodeficiency virus epidemic. Int J Cancer 47:692–696.

RAJFER J, WALSH PC. 1977. Hormonal regulation of testicular descent: experimental and clinical observations. J Urol 118:985–990.

RAJFER J, HANDELSMAN DJ, SWERDLOFF RS, et al. 1986. Hormonal therapy of cryptorchidism: a randomized, double-blind study comparing human chorionic gonadotropin and gonadotropin-releasing hormone. N Engl J Med 314:466–470.

REINBERG Y, MANIVEL JC, ZHANG G, et al. 1991. Synchronous bilateral testicular germ cell tumors of different histologic type. Cancer 68:1082–1085.

REYNOLDS P, SAUNDERS LD, LAYEFSKY ME, et al. 1993. The spectrum of acquired immunodeficiency syndrome-associated malignancies in San Francisco, 1980–1987. Am J Epidemiol 137:19–30.

RHOMBERG W, SCHMOLL HJ, SCHNEIDER B. 1995. High frequency of metalworkers among patients with seminomatous tumors of the testis: A case-control study. Am J Indust Med 28:79–87.

RODRIGUEZ E, MATHEW S, REUTER V, et al. 1992. Cytogenetic analysis of 124 prospectively ascertained male germ cell tumors. Cancer Res 52:2285–2291.

ROSS RK, MCCURTIS JW, HENDERSON BE, et al. 1979. Descriptive epidemiology of testicular and prostatic cancer in Los Angeles. Br J Cancer 39:284–292.

SAMANIEGO F, RODRIGUEZ E, HOULDSWORTH J, et al. 1990. Cytogenetic and molecular analysis of human male germ cell tumors: chromosome 12 abnormalities and gene amplification. Genes, Chromosomes, Cancer 1:289–300.

SANTOS SILVA DOS I, SWERDLOW AJ. 1991. Ovarian germ cell malignancies in England: epidemiologic parallels with testicular cancer. Br J Cancer 63:814–818.

SCHOTTENFELD D, WARSHAUER ME, SHERLOCK S, et al. 1980. The epidemiology of testicular cancer in young adults. Am J Epidemiol 12:232–246.

SCULLY RE. 1993. Testis. In: Pathology of Incipient Neoplasia, 2nd ed, Henson DE, Albores-Saavedra J (eds). Philadelphia: W.B. Saunders Co., pp 384–400.

SINKE RJ, SUIJKERBUIJK RF, DEJONG B, et al. 1993. Uniparental origin of i (12p) in human germ cell tumors. Genes, Chromosomes, Cancer 6:161–165.

SPELEMAN F, DEPOTTER C, DAL CIN P, et al. 1990. i (12p) in a malignant ovarian tumor. Cancer Genet Cytogenet 45:49–53.

STONE JM, CRUICKSHANK DG, SANDEMAN TF, et al. 1991. Laterality, maldescent, trauma and other clinical factors in epidemiology of cancer of testis. Br J Cancer 64:132–138.

STRADER CH, WEISS NS, DALING JR, et al. 1988. Cryptorchidism, orchiopexy and the risk of testicular cancer. Am J Epidemiol 127:1013–1018.

STRADER CH, WEISS NS, DALING JR. 1988. Vasectomy and the incidence of testicular cancer. Am J Epidemiol 128:56–63.

SWERDLOW AJ, SKEET RG. 1988. Occupational associations of testicular cancer in southeast England. Br J Ind Med 45:225–230.

SWERDLOW AJ, HUTTLEY SRA, SMITH PG. 1987. Testicular cancer and antecedent disease. Br J Cancer 55:97–103.

TARONE RE, HAYES H, HOOVER R, et al. 1991. Service in Vietnam and risk of testicular cancer. J Natl Cancer Inst 83:1497–1499.

TOLLERUD DJ, BLATTNER WA, FRASER MC, et al. 1985. Familial testicular cancer and urogenital development anomalies. Cancer 55:1849–1854.

TORFS CP, MILKOVICH L, VAN DEN BERG BJ. 1981. The relationship between hormonal pregnancy tests and congenital anomalies: a prospective study. Am J Epidemiol 113:563–574.

UNITED KINGDOM TESTICULAR CANCER STUDY GROUP. 1994. Etiology of testicular cancer: association with congenital abnormalities, age at puberty, infertility, and exercise. Br Med J 308:1393–1399.

VAN DEN EEDEN SK, WEISS NS, STRADER CH, et al. 1991. Occupation and the occurrence of testicular cancer. Am J Ind Med 19:327–337.

VAN KESSEL AG, SUIJKERBUIJK R, DEJONG B, et al. 1991. Molecular analysis of isochromosome 12p in testicular germ cell tumors. In: Pathobiology of Human Germ Cell Neoplasia, Oosterhuis JW, Walt H, Damjanov I (eds). Berlin: Springer–Verlag, pp 113–118.

VON DER MAASE H, RORTH M, WALBOM-JORGENSEN S, et al. 1986. Carcinoma in situ of contralateral testis in patients with testicular germ cell cancer: study of 27 cases in 500 patients. Br Med J 293:1398–1401.

WALKER AM, JICK H, HUNTER JR, et al. 1981. Hospitalization rates in vasectomized men. JAMA 245:2315–2317.

WALKER AH, ROSS RK, HAILE RWC, et al. 1988. Hormonal factors and risk of ovarian germ cell cancer in young women. Br J Cancer 57:418–422.

WARDLE J, STEPTOE A, BURCKHARDT R, et al. 1994. Testicular self-examination: attitudes and practices among young men in Europe. Prev Med 23:206–210.

WEST RR. 1992. Vasectomy and testicular cancer: No association on current evidence. Br Med J 304:729–730.

ZEVALLOS M, SNYDER RN, SADOFF L, COOPER JF. 1983. Testicular neoplasm in identical twins: a case report. JAMA 250:645–646.

57 Penile cancer

LOUISE WIDEROFF
DAVID SCHOTTENFELD

Cancer of the penis is an uncommon disease in North America and Europe, and generally in populations and cultures that practice neonatal circumcision. Population-based incidence rates in South America, Africa, and Asia, however, indicate that penile cancer remains a significant public health problem there. One hypothesis advanced about etiology was that in the uncircumcised adult male, and particularly in association with phimosis (unretractable foreskin) and poor personal hygiene, the collection of secretions, detritus, and microorganisms within the preputial sac enhanced the risk of penile cancer (Brinton et al, 1991). A contemporary perspective on the multifaceted pathogenic pathway would encompass behavioral risk factors and conditions associated with chronic irritation, the absence or delay in circumcision, the number of sexual partners and the sexual transmission of an infectious agent such as the human papillomavirus (HPV), cigarette smoking, exposure to ultraviolet radiation, and host factors (Holly and Palefsky, 1993; Maden et al, 1993).

PATHOLOGY

Epidermoid or squamous cell carcinoma constitutes over 90% of the malignant lesions of the penis. A form of exophytic epidermoid carcinoma, verrucous carcinoma, accounts for approximately 5% of all penile cancers. The giant condyloma acuminata of Buschke-Lowenstein, associated with HPV of specific types, is classified as a verrucous carcinoma.

Intraepithelial epidermoid carcinoma may occur on various locations on the penis. Bowen's disease and erythroplasia of Queyrat are forms of epidermoid carcinoma in situ. Bowen's disease appears as a sharply demarcated, scaly, erythematous plaque on the penile shaft, whereas erythroplasia of Queyrat arises usually on the penile glans and foreskin. Erythroplasia of Queyrat may subsequently advance to invasive squamous cell carcinoma or may be associated with a concurrent lesion of invasive carcinoma, in 10%–20% of patients (Rosai, 1989) (Figs. 57–1 and 57–2).

Other uncommon malignant tumors of the penis, accounting for less than 10% of lesions, include adenocarcinoma arising from the periurethral or bulbo-urethral glands; transitional cell carcinoma arising from the prostatic urethra; malignant melanoma; Kaposi's sarcoma; Paget's disease, arising from the accessory skin glands and frequently associated with an underlying adenocarcinoma; and fibrosarcoma and leiomyosarcoma (Lucia and Miller, 1992).

MORTALITY AND INCIDENCE IN THE UNITED STATES

In the United States, the average annual age-adjusted mortality rate per 100,000 for penile cancer was 0.2 in 1986–1990; during the same period, the average annual age-adjusted incidence was 0.7 per 100,000, or approximately 750–1000 cases each year. The age-adjusted incidence in African Americans was 0.9, and in white males, 0.7; for the same calendar period, age-adjusted mortality per 100,000 was 0.3 in African Americans and 0.1 in white males. When all stages of penile cancer were combined, the 5-year relative survival rate during 1983–1989 was around 71%, and similar in African American and white males. Age-standardized incidence over the period 1973–1990 exhibited a 31% decline (Miller et al, 1993).

INTERNATIONAL PATTERNS

Penile cancer is rare in the industrialized countries of North America and Europe, with incidence rates generally less than 1.0 per 100,000, and representing 0.3%–0.6% of all cancers in men. The age-adjusted incidence in Jews and non-Jews in Israel is 0.3 per 100,000. Higher rates are reported in Africa, Asia, and South America. The highest average annual age-standardized incidence rates per 100,000 population are

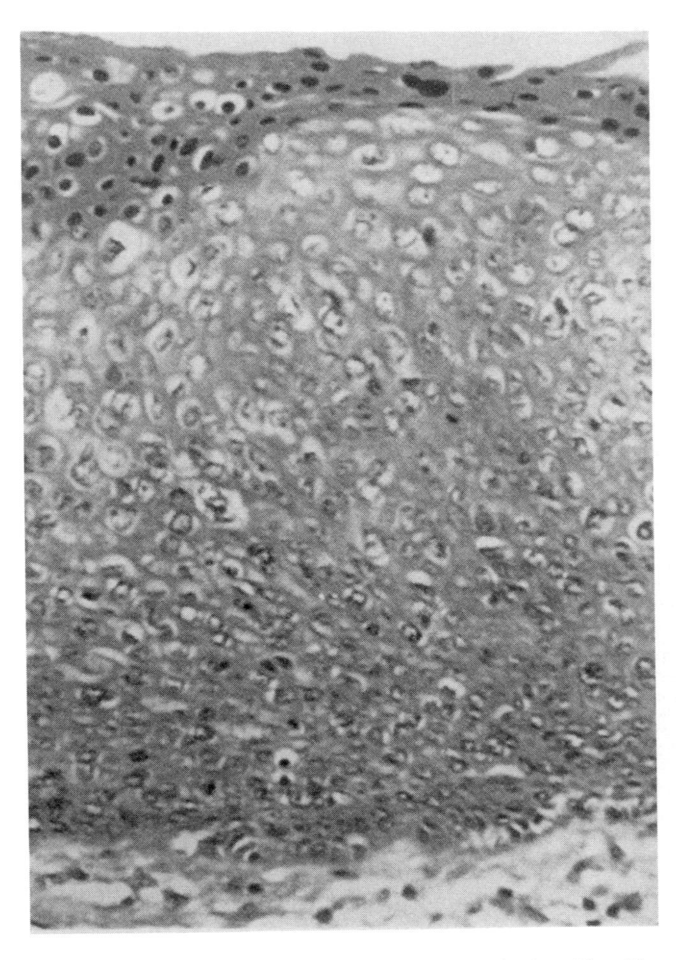

FIG. 57–1. Erythroplasia of Queyrat. Note acanthosis with widespread replacement of normal epithelium by anaplastic cells that have large nuclei surrounded by scanty cytoplasm.

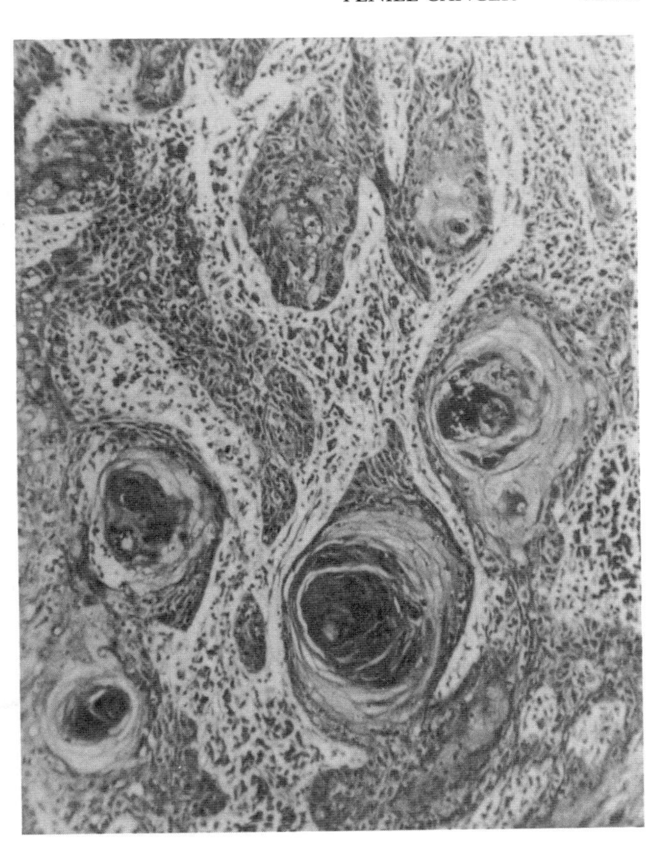

FIG. 57–2. Well-differentiated squamous cell carcinoma. Note formation of keratin and keratin pearls in infiltrative areas.

found in the population-based registries of Porto Alegre, Brazil (3.9); Martinique, France (3.3); Asuncion, Paraguay (4.2); Puerto Rico (3.3); Madras, India (2.7); and Chiang Mai, Thailand (3.1) (Parkin et al, 1993). The incidence in non-Muslims (ie, Hindus, Buddhists) in India is significantly higher than that reported in Muslims and Parsis (Muir and Nectoux, 1979). In general, the incidence rates do not vary in relation to urban or rural residence (Muir et al, 1987).

AGE

In white and African American males in the United States, the age-specific incidence per 100,000 ranges from 2.0 at 60–64 years to levels between 4.0 and 13.0 at 70 and over; the age-specific rates were uniformly higher in high-risk countries in South America, such as Asuncion, Paraguay, where the rate at 60–64 years was 32.4, and at age 70–74 years, 49.6 (Fig. 57–3). In Pan-

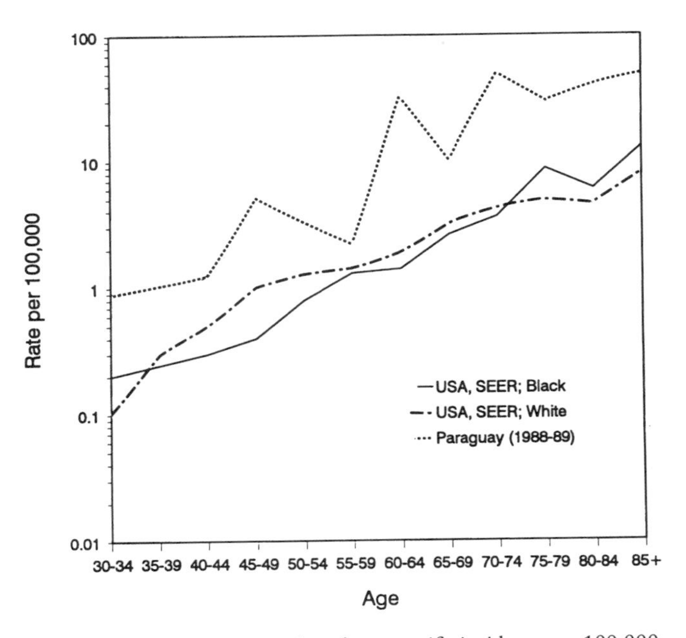

FIG. 57–3. Semilogarithmic plot of age-specific incidence per 100,000 of penile cancer. The rates in the United States are for 1983–1987.

ama, a high-prevalence area, the rise in incidence rates begins earlier, namely at 40–45 years (Reeves et al, 1982). In general, the age-specific incidence of penile cancer in high-risk countries is characterized by an earlier age peak than in countries at low risk. For example, in Denmark, the average age at diagnosis was 63.7 years and only 4% of patients were under age 40 (Jensen, 1977). In Puerto Rico, although penile cancer was diagnosed more frequently in men over 60, 11% of patients were under 40 (Martínez, 1969). In the state of Bahia, Brazil, the average age at diagnosis was 53 years, and 21% of patients were 40 or under (de Almeida Barbosa et al, 1984). In southern India, 30% of patients in one study were 40 or under, and 90% were 60 or under (Thomas and Small, 1968).

SOCIAL CLASS AND OCCUPATION

Most studies indicate that penile cancer occurs more frequently in countries with a relatively low standard of living (Persky, 1977). In England and Wales, a weak or inconsistent social class gradient has been reported for penile cancer mortality (Registrar General from England and Wales, 1978; Smith et al, 1980). Incidence data from the Los Angeles population-based registry suggest a weak inverse social class trend, based on census tract socioeconomic indicators (Peters et al, 1984).

In high-risk areas of China, an increased risk was observed with decreasing levels of education, although the trend was not statistically significant (Brinton et al, 1991). In Bahia, Brazil, the majority of cases were agricultural and industrial workers (de Almeida Barbosa et al, 1984). In a study of 23 Brazilian states, inverse correlations of −.64 to −.75 ($P<.001$) were demonstrated between the incidence of penile cancer and various socioeconomic indicators (Franco et al, 1988).

In a Danish study, the observed number of cases was significantly higher than that expected only in the middle social class stratum, although overestimation of social class for some occupational groups may have biased these results (Jensen, 1977). In a case-control study in Sweden, significant socioeconomic differences between cases and controls disappeared after controlling for smoking history (Hellberg et al, 1987).

The causal significance of the social class risk gradient may be in relation to poor personal hygiene, high-risk sexual practices, higher prevalence of cigarette smoking, or occupational factors (Brinton et al, 1991).

RISK FACTORS

Sexual Transmission of an Infectious Agent

The wives of men with penile cancer have a significantly increased risk of uterine cervical cancer. Mortality rates for cancers of the penis and cervix tend to be positively correlated (Li et al, 1982; Franco et al, 1988). In a case-control study conducted in Puerto Rico, Martínez (1969) was able to document eight cases of cervical cancer among wives of men with penile cancer, whereas there were no cases among the wives of controls. Graham and coworkers (1979) reported an elevated relative risk of 3.24 ($P<.01$) for the incidence of cervical cancer among the wives of a cohort of men with penile cancer, who were diagnosed in New York State. In a follow-up study conducted in England and Wales, Smith and coworkers (1980) estimated that the relative risk of dying of cancer of the uterine cervix was significantly increased in the wives of men who had died of cancer of the penis (relative risk = 2.8; $P<.01$). Thus, Smith and coworkers (1980) concluded that if the lifetime risk of developing cervical cancer in England and Wales was 1.5%, the wives of men with penile cancer would have a lifetime risk of 4.5%.

Various studies have reported on the association between penile cancer and a history of sexually transmitted diseases (Persky, 1977). Jensen (1977) noted that 9% of penile cancer cases in Denmark were also listed in a population-based registry of cases with syphilis, which was almost three times the frequency with which matched controls were cross-listed. A case-control study of penile cancer was undertaken in a high-risk area in China; an elevated risk was associated with reporting a history of more frequent premarital or extramarital affairs and of sexually transmitted genital diseases, including condyloma acuminata or genital warts (Brinton et al, 1991). In a population-based case-control study conducted in Washington state (USA) and in the province of British Columbia (Canada), Maden and coworkers (1993) reported that the risk of penile cancer was increased significantly in men who recalled having genital warts at least 5 years prior to diagnosis (odds ratio 4.5; 95 percent confidence interval [CI], 1.2–16.4). Although genital warts are most commonly associated with HPV types 6 and 11, which are not considered to be oncogenic in humans, the association in penile cancer cases may be interpreted as a marker of sexual activity and the probability of exposure to other sexually transmitted infectious agents.

Herpes simplex virus (HSV) Type II was investigated as a causal agent; however, HSV antigens were not detected in lesions of penile cancers (Raju and Lee, 1987; McCance et al, 1986), nor in bowenoid papulosis lesions (Patterson et al, 1986). Of current interest is human papillomavirus (HPV), a double-stranded DNA virus that infects epithelial cells of various organs. Specific types of HPV are associated with anogenital warts and carcinomas in both sexes, as well as with common warts, laryngeal papillomas, and skin, oral, and laryngeal carcinomas (McCance, 1986; zur Hausen, 1987).

Currently, at least 70 types of HPV have been identified, nearly 20 of which are found in preinvasive and invasive anogenital lesions. Evolutionary divergence has given rise to these genetically distinct HPV types, which have less than 90% nucleotide sequence homology in the L1, E6, and upstream regulatory regions of the viral genome (Van Ranst et al, 1993).

The viral genome consists of an early region that codes for proteins involved in viral replication, transcription, and transformation; a late region that codes for proteins involved in capsid formation; and a regulatory region. The early region has seven identified open reading frames, including E6 and E7. Viral DNA sequences of both regions have been demonstrated to be integrated into human chromosomes in uterine cervical cancers, and in transfection studies to result in the immortalization of cell lines. In vitro studies of HPV-immortalized cell lines have demonstrated that after transfection with the *ras* oncogene, the cells exhibit neoplastic characteristics. The E6 region of HPV types 16 and 18 encodes a protein that complexes with and inactivates the p53 tumor suppressor protein. The E7 oncogene protein is capable of binding with and inactivating the retinoblastoma (RB) protein, which functions to regulate intracellular signaling pathways (Werness et al, 1990; Howley, 1991; Pfister, 1992).

In the uterine cervix, the "low risk" types, 6, 11, 42, 43, and 44, are associated mainly with low-grade squamous intraepithelial neoplastic lesions; and the "intermediate risk" types, 31, 33, 35, 51, and 58, are associated with high-grade squamous intraepithelial neoplastic lesions. HPV 16, 18, 45, and 56 have been designated "high risk" types because of their strong association with high-grade lesions and invasive carcinomas (Lörincz et al, 1992). Viral DNA is regarded as the most sensitive and specific marker of HPV infection. It is identified through nucleic acid hybridization techniques, in which labeled nucleic acid probes of known genotypes anneal with complementary HPV DNA of unknown types present in biopsy samples or exfoliated cells (Lörincz, 1987). In recent years, the polymerase chain reaction (PCR) has also been used for detecting HPV DNA sequences in tissues (Resnick et al, 1990). PCR can be applied to archival or fresh tissue, or exfoliated tumor cells obtained by smear or lavage.

Several case series have examined the prevalence of selected HPV DNA types in benign and malignant lesions of the penis. Most studies probed simultaneously for more than one viral type, and thus reported a varying number of cases with multiple infections. The reported prevalence of HPV type 16 in penile cancers ranged from 0%–49%, and of type 18 from 9%–39%. HPV types 6 and 11 were detected infrequently. There is some suggestion of geographical variation by type, with HPV 18 DNA detected more frequently in genital tumors from Africa and Brazil than from Germany (Dürst et al, 1983; Lina Villa et al, 1986).

HPV 16 DNA has also been consistently identified in the preinvasive anogenital lesions, Bowen's disease and bowenoid papulosis. However, DNA prevalence estimates in male patients were highly variable, ranging from 6%–89% (Ikenberg et al, 1983; Gross et al, 1985; Obalek et al, 1986; Barrasso et al, 1987; Syrjänen et al, 1987; O'Brien et al, 1989; Nuovo et al, 1990). Other HPV types whose DNA was detected with varying frequency in preinvasive lesions included 6, 11, 18, 31, 33, and 35. In addition, type 39 has been cloned from a penile bowenoid lesion (Beaudenon et al, 1987). In contrast, penile condylomas, which generally show benign behavior, frequently contain types 6 and 11, but rarely harbor types 16 and 18 DNA.

Several studies have looked for HPV structural antigens in penile carcinomas, using a broadly cross-reactive antisera derived from bovine or rabbit papillomaviruses. HPV structural antigens are considered a less sensitive marker of HPV infection than viral DNA because structural antigen expression is negligible during latent infection, and also decreases with advancing stages of neoplasia (Koutsky et al, 1988). No HPV structural antigens were detected using immunoperoxidase methods in penile carcinomas (Raju and Lee, 1987), while antigens were detected in 5%–17% of anogenital bowenoid papulosis lesions (Gross et al, 1985; Patterson et al, 1986; Syrjänen et al, 1987).

The hypothesized sexual transmission of HPV through direct contact with infected epithelium, or possibly through infected semen (Green et al, 1989), has prompted studies that compare the prevalence of type-specific viral DNA in index cases and their long-term sexual partners. In several such studies, two thirds or more of HPV-positive couples harbored the same viral type (Schneider et al, 1987; Campion et al, 1985; Konno et al, 1990).

In most instances, some degree of intra-couple discordance in HPV status has been also observed, indicating that viral DNA is not always present in both partners, at least in readily detectable quantities. There are data to suggest that a protracted relationship, and the demonstration of a higher viral DNA copy concentration in genital tract tissues, enhance the risk of transmission of HPV to the sexual partner (Wickenden et al, 1988). Other studies of sexual partners have compared the prevalence of condylomas, or the extent of multicentric cervical and penile intraepithelial neoplasia, or CIN and PIN, respectively. The intraepithelial lesions are viewed as precursors of invasive genital cancer. Barrasso and coworkers (1987) reported PIN in 33% (61/186) of male partners of women with CIN. A histopathologic study of penile lesions, in which biopsies were obtained from 83 male partners of women with abnormal cervical smears (CIN I–III), found that only three lesions exhibited the severe cellular atypia characteristic of bowenoid papulosis; the other 80 lesions were diagnosed as condyloma acuminata (Krebs and Schneider, 1987).

The occurrence of PIN in a minority of the male partners of females with CIN (Barrasso et al, 1987) is consistent with the uniformly lower incidence rates of invasive penile cancer compared with that of invasive cervical cancer in high-risk populations. Although oncogenic HPVs have been associated with cancers of the cervix and other anogenital sites (Rabkin et al, 1992), differences in tissue susceptibilities may be attributed to the concurrence of exogenous and endogenous cofactors that are participating in transformation, promotion, and progression (Levine et al, 1984; Boon et al, 1988).

HPV type 16 has been found to induce histologic abnormalities resembling intraepithelial neoplasia when transfected into human foreskin keratinocytes (McCance et al, 1988). In malignant genital tumors and laboratory cell lines, HPV 16 DNA is covalently integrated into the host genome, whereas it is present in extrachromosomal form in benign and preinvasive lesions (Dürst et al, 1985; Gissman and Schwartz, 1986). Because integration causes a disruption in the host genome that may be critical to malignant transformation, the presence of integrated viral DNA implies an active role for HPV in carcinogenesis, rather than a mere opportunistic affinity for neoplastic cells (zur Hausen, 1994).

Methodological features, such as selection criteria and response rates for subjects, small sample sizes, and sampling error in tissue biopsies may account for the inconsistencies in published studies of HPV DNA. Differences in the sensitivity and specificity of the various molecular probes and PCR primers for viral DNA detection and typing have also contributed to variability in HPV prevalence estimates (Brandsma et al, 1989; Guerrero et al, 1992).

Photochemotherapy

An increased risk of penile and scrotal squamous cell carcinoma has been observed in a cohort of patients with psoriasis who were therapeutically exposed to oral 8-methoxypsoralen and ultraviolet A (UVA) radiation (Stern et al, 1980, 1990). This cohort participated in a multicenter clinical trial to evaluate the effects of photochemotherapy using UVA radiation (320–400 nanometers), which was administered in combination with the photosensitizing 8-methoxypsoralen, the combined therapy referred to as PUVA. In addition to PUVA treatment, many had at some point received ultraviolet B (UVB) radiation (290–320 nanometers), ionizing radiation, or topically applied coal tar.

In 892 PUVA-treated men, followed prospectively for an average of 12.3 years, unusually high, dose-dependent risks of penile and scrotal cancer were observed (Stern et al, 1990). The standardized morbidity ratio (SMR) for in situ and invasive penile cancer, which compared the observed incidence in the cohort to that expected in the general population, was 58.8 (95% CI, 26.9, 111.7). SMRs for low, medium, and high doses were 23.0 (2.80, 83.0), 34.5 (0.9, 192.1) and 162.2 (59.5, 353.0), respectively. After 12 years of follow-up, the cumulative incidence of penile and scrotal cancers was 1.6%; in the highest PUVA dose stratum, the subcohort experienced a cumulative risk of 6%. In a nested case-control analysis in this cohort, which included 14 genital cancer cases and 56 age-matched controls, Stern and coworkers (1990) reported, after controlling for the level of exposure to PUVA, a relative risk of 4.6 (1.4, 15.1) due to high versus low doses of UVB. Tar exposures were similar for cases and controls. The risk of squamous cell carcinoma of the penis and scrotum was 5–15 times greater than on other PUVA-exposed sites—a pattern observed consistently at each dose level. Patients who received more than 260 PUVA treatments had 11 times the risk of squamous cell carcinoma in all body sites, when compared with those patients who received 160 or fewer treatments.

It has been determined that patients with a history of psoriasis, a chronic inflammatory dermatosis that affects about 2% of the United States population, are not susceptible to cutaneous or genital squamous cell cancer in the absence of photochemotherapy (Stern et al, 1985). It is apparent that PUVA and ultraviolet B radiation are mutagenic and carcinogenic. In the study of Stern and coworkers (1990), the increased risk of cancer of the skin of the genitalia in the male patients with psoriasis was not noted in 488 female patients. This observation suggested that the male genitalia were particularly susceptible to these carcinogenic stimuli. In studies of UV radiation–induced skin cancers in mice (Kripke et al, 1983; Kripke and Morison, 1985; Kripke, 1989), there appear to be at least three important effects of exposure: antigenic changes on germinative cells in the skin; transformation of normal skin cells into cancer cells; and inhibition or blockage of the immune response to the cancer cells by inducing tumor-specific suppressor cells. Induction of immune suppressor pathways and depression of natural killer cell activity have been observed in humans exposed to UV radiation (Hersey et al, 1983). The methoxsalen molecule requires activation by UVA, and forms monofunctional and bifunctional photoproducts that insert onto pyrimidine bases in the DNA. An additional cofactor may be infection with human papillomavirus in those who develop neoplastic lesions.

Smoking

Chemical components of cigarette smoke have been detected in cervical mucus (Hellberg et al, 1988; Sasson et al, 1985; Schiffman, 1987), and cigarette smoking has been associated with cervical cancer in women (Winkelstein, 1990). Nitrosamine derivatives of cigarette smoke have been shown to concentrate in the preputial glands of the rat penis (Castonguay et al, 1983). An analogous mechanism in human smokers could result in exposure of the penile epithelium to cigarette carcinogens.

In a Swedish study of 232 penile cancer cases and age-matched controls, the odds ratio for smokers of more than 10 cigarettes per day, relative to nonsmokers, was 1.53 (95% confidence interval, 1.00–2.35). This analysis controlled for the presence of phimosis and balanitis, but only one fifth of the case patients were alive and available for interviewing (Hellberg et al, 1987). In a population-based case-control study conducted in western Washington State and in the province of British Columbia, the adjusted odds ratio for current cigarette smoking in penile cancer cases was 2.8 (95% confidence interval, 1.4–5.5) (Maden et al, 1993). Brinton and coworkers (1991) found no association of penile cancer with ever having smoked, current smoking, number of cigarettes per day, number of years of smoking, starting age of smoking, or inhalation. In a study of male partners of women with HPV-associated lesions, Schneider and coworkers (1988) found that 62% of HPV-positive men smoked regularly compared with 51% of HPV-negative men. Thus, future studies that examine the independent effect of smoking in penile cancer should explore potential confounding by HPV infection.

Immune System Impairment

Immune system impairment is a well-recognized risk factor for skin carcinogenesis. Renal transplant patients, in whom the immune system is suppressed by pharmaceuticals that prevent organ transplant rejection, show a much higher incidence of cutaneous malignancies than the general population (Editorial, 1987). A number of studies have examined cell-mediated immunity in relation to genital neoplasia, using lymphocyte counts, T-cell subset ratios, leukocyte migration inhibition assays, and delayed hypersensitivity skin tests. Impairment of the immune system of iatrogenic origin is associated with an elevated risk of anogenital warts and squamous cell carcinomas in males and females (Schneider et al, 1983; Halpert et al, 1985; Krebs et al, 1986; Penn, 1986). In women, alterations in cell-mediated immunity have been linked to the "genital neoplasia-papilloma" syndrome, which is characterized by multiple, recurring, HPV-associated lesions of high malignant potential (Carson et al, 1986). In one case series, males with therapy-resistant anogenital bowenoid papulosis were observed to have depleted T-helper lymphocytes and diminished reactivity to skin testing (Feldman et al, 1989). Conceivably, impairment of cell-mediated immunity predisposes to persistent HPV infection and enhanced risk of multicentric neoplasia.

Circumcision

For 5000 years or more, circumcision has been practiced across the world for religious and cultural reasons (Warner and Strashin, 1981). Although controversial, it has been widely recommended within sectors of the medical community as a means of promoting penile hygiene and reducing the risks of phimosis, posthitis (inflammation of the foreskin), sexually transmitted infections, and penile cancer (Schoen, 1990).

The preventive value of circumcision in the United States is suggested by the clinical observation that penile cancer occurs predominantly in noncircumcised males. In six major United States clinical studies of penile cancer that had been conducted since the early 1930s, none of the more than 1600 patients had undergone neonatal circumcision (Schoen, 1990). Erythroplasia of Queyrat also appears to predominate in uncircumcised males (Graham and Helwig, 1973), whereas bowenoid papulosis may occur independently of circumcision status (Wade et al, 1978). The benefit of circumcision appears to be correlated with age, with tumors occurring most frequently when circumcision is delayed until adulthood; the incidence is uncommon in those circumcised at puberty, and rare in those circumcised at birth (Schellhammer and Grabstald, 1986). Cases of penile cancer patients who were circumcised at birth have been reported only sporadically in the medical literature (Boczko and Freed, 1979).

Variability in circumcision practices in various countries and cultural groups has prompted population-based comparisons of penile cancer incidence rates. The disease is extremely rare among Jews, who traditionally circumcise infants at the end of the first week of life; it is also rare in Muslims, who are circumcised before puberty. In Africa and India, low incidence has been reported in populations where ritual circumcision is practiced, and high incidence reported where it is generally not practiced (Persky, 1977; Muir and Nectoux, 1979). The highest reported incidence rates in the world occur in Brazil, where circumcision is uncommon.

In Canada and the United States, where neonatal circumcision rates vary between 40% and 80%, incidence rates are relatively low (Warner and Strashin, 1981). However, incidence rates are also very low in Scandinavia and Japan, where circumcision is uncommon, raising questions about the cost-effectiveness or preventive value of this practice (Poland, 1990).

Circumcision is not a random practice, but instead predominates in certain religious, ethnic, and socioeconomic groups. Conceivably, low-risk sexual behaviors, social conditions that permit good penile hygiene, greater access to medical treatment for local infection, or other factors, could contribute to the low penile cancer incidence in these groups.

Originally, a reduced exposure to chemical carcinogens in smegma was considered responsible for the rare occurrence of penile cancer in circumcised men (Plaut and Kohn-Speyer, 1947). Smegma, which is formed from the bacterial breakdown of desquamated epithelium, begins to accumulate in the preputial sac in infancy (Shabad, 1964). No specific carcinogenic component has been identified in smegma, although sterol degradation products (Sobel and Plaut, 1949) and components of cigarette smoke (Hellberg et al, 1987) have been proposed. The outcomes of experimental models of cutaneous tumor induction by smegma in mice have been inconsistent or contradictory (Reddy and Baruah, 1963).

A more recent hypothesis invokes a predisposing role of the prepuce to sexually transmitted viral infection, by permitting accumulation of infectious vaginal secretions and increasing the surface area of exposed penile epithelium (Cameron et al, 1989). In several studies in Kenya, for example, lack of circumcision emerged as an independent risk factor for the prevalence of human immunodeficiency viral infection and seroconversion (Simonsen et al, 1988; Cameron et al, 1989). The prepuce, or foreskin, is the most common site of HPV-associated penile lesions in adult males (Krebs and Schneider, 1987; Syrjänen et al, 1987). Early preputial exposure to HPV infection is demonstrated by the identification of DNA from HPV types 6 and 16 in 4% of neonatal foreskins removed by routine circumcision (Roman and Fife, 1986).

Conceivably, circumcision may protect against penile cancer by reducing the risk of oncogenic HPV infection. However, it is also possible that populations whose sexual behaviors put them at low risk of HPV infection are more likely to be circumcised. Circumcision reduces the risk of phimosis, which has been consistently associated with the increased incidence of penile cancer.

Phimosis and Inflammation

Phimosis occurs when the orifice of the fully differentiated foreskin is too narrow or constricting to permit its retraction over the glans penis (Schoen et al, 1989). Although the separation of the glans from the prepuce is usually incomplete at birth, it is retractable in up to 90% of uncircumcised males in early childhood (Gairdner, 1949). Phimosis, which can be congenital or a sequela of inflammatory scarring involving the prepuce, interferes with adequate cleansing of the glans and prepuce.

Phimosis is often associated with balanoposthitis, the inflammation of the glans and prepuce, which usually results from bacterial infection (Cotran et al, 1989). Phimosis is consistently associated with an increased risk of penile carcinoma (Persky, 1977), with most studies reporting phimosis in more than half of all penile cancer cases (Shabad, 1964; Jensen, 1977). In a high-risk Hindu population, Reddy and coworkers (1977) found phimosis in 89% of penile cancer cases, compared to 18% of controls. In China, 73% of uncircumcised case patients had phimosis, compared to 7% of control patients (RR=37.2; 95 percent confidence interval, 11.9–116.1) (Brinton et al, 1991).

Although phimosis and balanoposthitis are often associated, the latter is also an independent risk factor for penile cancer (Jensen, 1977; Hellberg, 1987). Paraphimosis (retracted and inflamed prepuce with constriction of the glans penis) is an additional condition associated with increased risk (Brinton et al, 1991).

Phimosis is treated by circumcision, although therapeutic circumcision in adults with phimosis does not preclude the subsequent development of penile cancer (Tan, 1963; Thomas and Small, 1968; Jensen, 1977; Brinton et al, 1991). Neonatal circumcision eliminates the risk of phimosis and balanoposthitis. Thus, the strong inverse association of neonatal circumcision and penile cancer may be due to the elimination of these two risk factors.

PATHOGENESIS

Epidemiological evidence indicates that penile cancer is a disease of multifactorial etiology, which includes viral, chemical, and physical agents, as well as sociocultural practices and biological host factors. The viral model of pathogenesis hypothesizes that specific HPV types, which are able to integrate DNA into the infected host cell's genome, induce genetic alterations that lead to the abnormal and uncontrolled growth patterns characteristic of cancer cells. HPV DNA mainly persists within the infected cell as circular episomes physically separate from the host DNA, or in linear form covalently integrated into host DNA. Integration occurs at random sites in the host genome, but in a specific region of the viral genome that contains the E1 and E2 open reading frames (ORF) that code for viral proteins (Gissman and Schwartz, 1986).

HPV studies have consistently noted a correlation between the viral type, the physical state of the viral genome (integrated vs episomal), and the histologic nature of the lesion where viral DNA was detected. The genomes of types that are associated with benign anogenital lesions, such as HPV 6 and 11, persist in episomal form, in contrast to types 16 and 18, which are predominantly integrated in malignant anogenital tumors (Gissman and Schwartz, 1986). However, exceptions to the integrated state have been noted in HPV 18–associated penile carcinomas (McCance et al, 1986).

Molecular studies of the HPV 16 and 18 genomes indicate that the E6 and E7 ORF encode viral proteins associated with the regulation of cell growth and differentiation. In vitro, these proteins induce immortalization and resistance to differentiation in human foreskin keratinocytes (Munger et al, 1989). E6 and E7 proteins are expressed in most cervical carcinomas and derived cell lines that contain integrated HPV 16 or 18 DNA (Howley, 1990).

E6 and E7 gene expression is regulated by a promoter that, in turn, is repressed by protein products of the E2 ORF. During the process of viral DNA integration, the E2 ORF is disrupted, thus altering the expression of E2 regulatory proteins (Baker et al, 1987). The loss of this regulatory mechanism could lead to uncontrolled production of E6 and E7 transforming proteins.

Other cellular events that may foster malignant growth in HPV-infected cells include (1) the binding of E6 and E7 viral proteins to growth-regulating proteins in the host cell, such as the retinoblastoma and p53 gene products, causing loss of normal cellular protein functions (zur Hausen, 1991); (2) the activation of cellular proto-oncogenes, such as c-*myc,* following the integration of viral DNA (Dürst et al, 1987; Riou et al, 1987); and (3) the occurrence of human chromosomal aberrations that result in the deletion of genes coding for tumor-suppressing factors (Koi et al, 1989).

Sexually transmitted bacterial infections that cause genital ulceration and inflammation may increase susceptibility to HPV infection (Koutsky et al, 1988) because disruption in the integrity of the penile epithelium is likely to facilitate entry of virus into cells. The inflammatory response is accompanied by the generation of potentially carcinogenic cellular mutagens and mitogens. Inflammation may be an important intervening event in penile cancers associated with phimosis.

In addition to HPV infection, therapeutic UV radiation is a risk factor for penile cancer, although the proportion of total cases with this exposure would be influenced by cultural practices or limited to subgroups of patients, such as those with psoriasis. Ultraviolet A and B radiation cause direct damage to DNA, thus inhibiting the hyperproliferation of skin cells characteristic of psoriasis (Epstein, 1990). Methoxsalen, the active ingredient of the photosensitizing psoralens, potentiates this effect by covalently binding to DNA, forming adducts and cross-links when activated by UVA radiation. Unfortunately, the DNA damage induced by UVB and PUVA, which is beneficial in the treatment of hyperproliferative skin disease, is also potentially carcinogenic. The carcinogenic role of smegma has never been established. The intact prepuce is thought to facilitate accumulation of chemical carcinogens in smegma, at least where penile hygiene is deficient (Reddy et al, 1977). The detection of cigarette smoke carcinogens in rat preputial gland secretions is of potential significance in human chemical carcinogenesis.

The sharp increase of penile cancer in older age groups is consistent with the multi-hit model of carcinogenesis, in which multiple genetic and epigenetic events are required in cell transformation, promotion, and progression. Conceivably, these events could arise from exposure to a single etiologic agent, or to multiple agents or cofactors. Based on experimental evidence, zur Hausen (1991) has proposed that "high-risk" HPV types such as 16 and 18 can act as sole agents in the neoplastic process, whereas in the presence of other HPV types, cofactors assume a role of greater importance. Interactions of HPV infection and immunosuppression are causal factors for anogenital cancers in transplant patients.

PREVENTION

Given the predominance of penile cancer in uncircumcised males, neonatal circumcision has been recommended as an effective preventive measure, especially in populations where optimal genital hygiene is difficult to achieve (Schoen, 1990). Circumcision of boys with congenital phimosis may be particularly indicated, based on the strong association of phimosis and penile cancer.

However, the overall benefits of circumcision remain controversial in the medical community, and its general acceptance outside of specific ethnic or religious groups may be limited. Some argue that prevention of HPV infection, through condom use and limitation of sexual contacts, is a more effective means of preventing penile cancer (Poland, 1990).

The development of an HPV vaccine is considered an important long-term goal for the primary prevention of genital neoplasia (Schrier et al, 1988). Currently, much remains to be learned about the cell-mediated and humoral immune responses to HPV infection, before an effective candidate vaccine can be produced (Tindle and Frazier, 1990). In the absence of a vaccine, preventive measures for HPV-associated penile neoplasia must focus on the avoidance of high-risk sexual practices, and on efforts to detect and treat early viral lesions with malignant potential.

Screening the sexual partners of HPV-infected index

case patients for such lesions has been recommended, given that partners represent a group at high risk of infection and genital neoplasia (Bistoletti and Lidbrink, 1988; Barrasso et al, 1987). HPV-infected males are frequently asymptomatic, and over 40% of penile HPV lesions are subclinical (Barrasso et al, 1987). Subclinical lesions may be visualized by magnification with a colposcope after application of a 5% acetic acid solution, which confers a whitish appearance on the affected area (Sedlacek et al, 1986).

Biopsy is required to definitively diagnose HPV-associated precancerous penile lesions such as bowenoid populosis. The use of cytology to screen for such lesions is limited by difficulties in obtaining sufficient cellular material for cytologic evaluation on smears of external penile lesions (Krebs and Schneider, 1987). Where treatment of lesions is indicated, treatment modalities include excision, cryotherapy, CO_2 laser vaporization and topical chemotherapy (Krebs, 1989).

Penile skin, which is thin and tans poorly, is highly sensitive to the carcinogenic effects of therapeutic PUVA and UVB radiation. This sensitivity underscores the need for genital shielding of UV-treated patients whose skin conditions do not involve the genitals (Stern et al, 1990), or for new treatment modalities with reduced radiation dosages, if the genitals are involved (Epstein, 1990). The association of penile cancer and therapeutic UV radiation also has implications for individuals whose genitals are exposed to UV radiation in natural sunlight and commercial solariums.

REFERENCES

BAKER CC, PHELPS WC, LINDGREN V, et al. 1987. Structural and transitional analysis of human papillomavirus type 16 sequences in cervical carcinoma cell lines. J Virol 61:962–971.

BARRASSO R, DE BRUX J, CROISSANT O, et al. 1987. High prevalence of papillomavirus-associated penile intraepithelial neoplasia in sexual partners of women with cervical intraepithelial neoplasia. N Engl J Med 317:916–923.

BEAUDENON S, KREMSDORF D, OBALEK S, et al. 1987. Plurality of genital human papillomaviruses: characterization of two new types with distinct biological properties. Virology 161:374–384.

BISTOLETTI P, LIDBRINK P. 1988. Sexually transmitted diseases including genital papillomavirus infection in male sexual partners of women treated for cervical intraepithelial neoplasia III by conization. Br J Obstet Gynaecol 95:611–613.

BOCZKO S, FREED S. 1979. Penile carcinoma in circumcised males. N Y State J Med 79:1903–1904.

BOON ME, SCHNEIDER A, CORNELIS JA, et al. 1988. Penile studies and heterosexual partners peniscopy, cytology, histology, and immunocytochemistry. Cancer 61:1652–1659.

BRANDSMA J, BURK RD, LANCASTER WD, et al. 1989. Interlaboratory variation as an explanation for varying prevalence estimates of human papillomavirus infection. Int J Cancer 43:260–262.

BRINTON LA, JUN-YAO L, SHOU-DE R, et al. 1991. Risk factors for penile cancer: results from a case-control study in China. Int J Cancer 47:504–509.

CAMERON DW, D'COSTA LJ, MAITHA GM, et al. 1989. Female to male transmission of human immunodeficiency virus type I: risk factors for seroconversion in men. Lancet 2:403–407.

CAMPION MJ, SINGER A, CLARKSON PK, et al. 1985. Increased risk of cervical neoplasia in consorts of men with penile condylomata acuminata. Lancet 1:943–946.

CARSON LF, TWIGGS LB, FUKUSHIMA M, et al. 1986. Human genital papilloma infections: an evaluation of immunologic competence in the genital neoplasia-papilloma syndrome. Am J Obstet Gynecol 155:784–789.

CASTONGUAY A, TJALVE H, HECHT SS. 1983. Tissue distribution of the tobacco-specific carcinogen 4-(methylnitrosamino)-1-(3-pyridyl-)1-butanone and its metabolites in F344 rats. Cancer Res 43:630–638.

COTRAN RS, KUMAR V, ROBBINS SL. 1989. Male genital system. In: *Robbins Pathologic Basis of Disease,* 4th ed, Cotran RS, Kumar V, Robbins SL (eds). Philadelphia: WB Saunders Co., pp 1099–1103.

DE ALMEIDA BARBOSA JR A, FONTES ATHANAZIO PR, OLIVEIRA B. 1984. Câncer do pênis, estudo da sua patologia geográfica no Estado da Bahia, Brasil. Rev Saude Publica 18:429–435.

DÜRST M, GISSMAN L, IKENBERG H, et al. 1983. A papillomavirus DNA from a cervical carcinoma and its prevalence in cancer biopsy samples from different geographical regions. Proc Natl Acad Sci USA 80:3812–3815.

DÜRST M, KLEINHEINZ A, HOTZ M, et al. 1985. The physical state of human papillomavirus type 16 DNA in benign and malignant genital tumors. J Gen Virol 66:1515–1522.

DÜRST M, CROCE CM, GISSMAN L, et al. 1987. Papillomavirus sequences integrate near cellular oncogenes in some cervical carcinomas. Proc Natl Acad Sci USA 84:1070–1074.

EDITORIAL. 1987. Renal transplantation and the skin. Lancet 2:1312.

EPSTEIN JH. 1990. Phototherapy and photochemotherapy. N Engl J Med 322:1149–1151.

FELDMAN SB, SEXTON M, GLENN JD, et al. 1989. Immunosuppression in men with bowenoid papulosis. Arch Dermatol 125:651–654.

FRANCO EL, CAMPOS FILHO NC, VILLA LL, et al. 1988. Correlation patterns of cancer relative frequencies with some socioeconomic and demographic indicators in Brazil: an ecologic study. Int J Cancer 41:24–29.

GAIRDNER D. 1949. The fate of the foreskin: a study of circumcision. Br Med J 2:1433–1437.

GISSMAN L, SCHWARZ E. 1986. Persistance and expression of human papillomavirus and DNA in genital cancer. In: *Papillomaviruses* (Ciba Foundation Symposium 120), Evered D, Clark S (eds). Chichester: John Wiley and Sons, pp 190–207.

GRAHAM JH, HELWIG EB. 1973. Erythroplasia of Queyrat, a clinicopathologic and histochemical study. Cancer 32:1396–1414.

GRAHAM S, PRIORE R, GRAHAM M, et al. 1979. Genital cancer in wives of penile cancer patients. Cancer 44:1870–1874.

GREEN J, MONTEIRO E, GIBSON P. 1989. Detection of human papillomavirus DNA in semen from patients with intrameatal penile warts. Genitourin Med 65:357–360.

GROSS G, HAGEDORN M, IKENBERG H, et al. 1985. Bowenoid papulosis, presence of human papillomavirus (HPV) structural antigens and of HPV 16-related DNA sequences. Arch Dermatol 121:858–863.

GUERRERO E, DANIEL RW, BISCH FX, et al. 1992. Comparison of Virapap, southern hybridization, and polymerase chain reaction methods for human papillomavirus identification in an epidemiologic investigation of cervical cancer. J Clin Microbiol 30:2951–2959.

HALPERT R, BUTT AS, SEDLIS RG, et al. 1985. Human papillomavirus infection and lower genital neoplasia in female renal allograft recipients. Transplant Proc 17:93–95.

HELLBERG D, VALENTIN J, EKLUND T, et al. 1987. Penile cancer: is there an epidemiologic role for smoking and sexual behaviour? Br Med J 295:1306–1308.

HELLBERG D, NILSSON S, HALEY NJ, et al. 1988. Smoking and cervical intraepithelial neoplasia: nicotine and cotinine in serum and cervical mucus in smokers and non-smokers. Am J Obstet Gynecol 158:910–913.

HERSEY P, HARAN G, HASIC E, et al. 1983. Alteration of T cell subsets and induction of suppressor T cell activity in normal subjects after exposure to sunlight. J Immunol 31:171–174.

HOLLY EA, PALEFSKY JM. 1993. Factors related to risk of penile cancer: new evidence from a study in the Pacific northwest. J Natl Cancer Inst 85:2–4.

HOWLEY PM. 1990. Papillomavirinae and their replication. In: Fundamental Virology, 2nd ed., Fields BN, Knipe DM, Chanock RM, et al (eds). New York: Raven Press, pp 743–768.

HOWLEY PM. 1991. Role of the human papillomaviruses in human cancer. Cancer Res 51:5019s–5022s.

IKENBERG H, GISSMAN L, GROSS G, et al. 1983. Human papillomavirus type-16-related DNA in genital Bowen's disease and in bowenoid papulosis. Int J Cancer 32:563–565.

JENSEN MS. 1977. Cancer of the penis in Denmark 1942 to 1962. Danish Med Bull 24:66–72.

KOI M, MORITA H, YAMADA H, et al. 1989. Normal human chromosome 11 suppresses tumorigenicity of human cervical tumor cell line SiHa. Mol Carcinog 2:12–21.

KONNO R, SHIKANO K, HORIGUCHI M, et al. 1990. Detection of human papillomavirus DNA in genital condylomata in women and their male partners by using in situ hybridization with digoxygenin labeled probes. Tohoku J Exp Med 160:383–390.

KOUTSKY LA, GALLOWAY DA, HOLMES KK. 1988. Epidemiology of genital human papillomavirus infection. Epidemiol Rev 10:122–163.

KREBS HB, SCHNEIDER V, HURT WG, et al. 1986. Genital condylomas in immunosuppressed women: a therapeutic challenge. South Med J 79:183–187.

KREBS HB, SCHNEIDER V. 1987. Human papillomavirus-associated lesions of the penis: colposcopy, cytology and histology. Obstet Gynecol 70:299–304.

KREBS H. 1989. Genital HPV infections in men. Clin Obstet Gynecol 32:180–190.

KRIPKE ML, MORISON WL, PARRISH JA. 1983. Systemic suppression of contact hypersensitivity in mice by psoralen plus UVA radiation (PUVA). J Invest Dermatol 81:87–92.

KRIPKE ML, MORISON WL. 1985. Modulation of immune function by UV radiation. J Invest Dermatol 85:62s–66s.

KRIPKE ML. 1989. Sun and ultraviolet ray exposure. In: *Cancer Prevention*, DeVita VT, Hellman S, Rosenberg SA (eds). Philadelphia: JB Lippincott, pp 1–7.

LEVINE RU, CRUM C, HERMAN E, et al. 1984. Cervical papillomavirus infection and intraepithelial neoplasia: a study of male sexual partners. Obstet Gynecol 64:16–20.

LI JY, LI FP, BLOT WJ, et al. 1982. Correlation between cancers of the uterine cervix and penis in China. J Natl Cancer Inst 69:1063–1065.

LINA VILLA L, LOPES A. 1986. Human papillomavirus DNA sequences in penile carcinomas in Brazil. Int J Cancer 37:853–855.

LÖRINCZ AT. 1987. Detection of human papillomavirus infection by nucleic acid hybridization. Obstet Gynecol Clin North Am 14:451–469.

LÖRINCZ AT, REID R, JENSON B, et al. 1992. Human papillomavirus infection of the cervix: relative risk associations of 15 common anogenital types. Obstet Gynecol 79:328–337.

LUCIA MS, MILLER GJ. 1992. Histopathology of malignant lesions of the penis. Urol Clin North Am 19:227–246.

MADEN C, SHERMAN KJ, BECKMANN AM, et al. 1993. History of circumcision, medical conditions, and sexual activity and risk of penile cancer. J Natl Cancer Inst 85:19–24.

MARTÍNEZ I. 1969. Relationship of squamous cell carcinoma of the cervix uteri to squamous cell carcinoma of the penis among Puerto Rican women married to men with penile carcinoma. Cancer 24:777–780.

MCCANCE DJ. 1986. Human papillomaviruses and cancer. Biochim Biophys Acta 823:195–205.

MCCANCE DJ, KALACHE A, ASHDOWN K, et al. 1986. Human papillomavirus types 16 and 18 in carcinomas of the penis from Brazil. Int J Cancer 37:55–59.

MCCANCE DJ, KOPAN R, FUCHS E, et al. 1988. Human papillomavirus type 16 alters human epithelial cell differentiation in vitro. Proc Natl Acad Sci U S A 85:7169–7173.

MILLER BA, RIES LAG, HANKEY BF, et al. 1993. SEER Cancer Statistics Review: 1973–1990, National Cancer Institute. NIH Pub. No. 93-2789.

MUIR CS, NECTOUX J. 1979. Epidemiology of cancer of the testis and penis. NCI Monogr 53:157–164.

MUIR C, WATERHOUSE J, MACK T, et al. 1987. Cancer Incidence in Five Continents, Vol 5. IARC Scientific Publications No. 88. Lyon: International Agency for Research on Cancer.

MUNGER K, PHELPS WC, BUBB V, et al. 1989. The E6 and E7 genes of the human papillomavirus type 16 together are necessary and sufficient for transformation of primary human keratinocytes. J Virol 63:4417–4421.

NUOVO GJ, HOCHMAN HA, ELIEZRI YD, et al. 1990. Detection of human papillomavirus DNA in penile lesions histologically negative for condylomata: analysis by in situ hybridization and the polymerase chain reaction. Am J Surg Pathol 14:829–836.

OBALEK S, JABLONSKA S, BEAUDENON S, et al. 1986. Bowenoid papulosis of the male and female genitalia: risk of cervical neoplasia. J Am Acad Dermatol 14:433–444.

O'BRIEN WM, JENSON B, LANCASTER WD, et al. 1989. Human papillomavirus typing of penile condyloma. J Urol 141:863–865.

PARKIN DM, MUIR CS, WHELAN SL, et al. 1993. Cancer Incidence in Five Continents, Vol. 6. IARC Scientific Publications No. 120. Lyon: International Agency for Research on Cancer.

PATTERSON JW, KAO GF, GRAHAM JH, et al. 1986. Bowenoid papulosis, a clinicopathologic study with ultrastructural observations. Cancer 57:823–836.

PENN I. 1986. Cancers of the anogenital region in renal transplant recipients, analysis of 65 cases. Cancer 58:611–616.

PERSKY L. 1977. Epidemiology of cancer of the penis. Recent Results Cancer Res 60:97–100.

PETERS RK, MACK TM, BERNSTEIN L. 1984. Parallels in the epidemiology of selected anogenital carcinomas. J Natl Cancer Inst 72:609–615.

PFISTER H. 1992. Human papillomaviruses and skin cancer. Semin Cancer Biology 3:263–271.

PLAUT A, KOHN-SPEYER AC. 1947. The carcinogenic action of smegma. Science 105:391–392.

POLAND RL. 1990. The question of routine neonatal circumcision. N Engl J Med 322:1312–1315.

RABKIN CS, BIGGAR RJ, MELBYE M, et al. 1992. Second primary cancers following anal and cervical carcinoma: evidence of shared etiologic factors. Am J Epidemiol 136:54–58.

RAJU GC, LEE YS. 1987. Role of herpes simplex virus type-2 and human papillomavirus in penile cancers in Singapore. Ann Acad Med Singapore 16:550–551.

REDDY DG, BARUAH I. 1963. Carcinogenic action of human smegma. Arch Pathol 75:414–420.

REDDY CRRM, GOPAL RAO T, VENKATARATHNAM G, et al. 1977. A study of 80 patients with penile carcinoma combined with cervical biopsy study of their wives. Int Surg 62:549–553.

REEVES WC, VALDES PF, BRENES MM, et al. 1982. Cancer incidence in the republic of Panama, 1974–78. J Natl Cancer Inst 68:219–225.

REGISTRAR GENERAL FROM ENGLAND AND WALES. 1978. Occupational Mortality, The Registrar General's Decennial Supplement for England and Wales, 1970–72. Series DS no. 1. London: Her Majesty's Stationery Office.

Resnick RM, Cornelissen MTE, Wright DK, et al. 1990. Detection and typing of human papillomavirus in archival cervical cancer specimens by DNA amplification with consensus primers. J Natl Cancer Inst 82:1477–1484.

Riou G, Le MG, LeDoussal V, et al. 1987. C-myc proto-oncogene expression and prognosis in early carcinoma of the uterine cervix. Lancet 1:761–763.

Roman A, Fife K. 1986. Human papillomavirus DNA associated with foreskins of normal newborns. J Infect Dis 153:855–861.

Rosai J. 1989. Ackerman's Surgical Pathology, Seventh Ed. St. Louis: CV Mosby Co., pp 988–995.

Sasson IM, Hellberg D, Haley NJ, et al. 1985. Cigarette smoking and neoplasia of the uterine cervix: smoke constituents in cervical mucus. N Engl J Med 312:315–316.

Schellhammer PF, Grabstald H. 1986. Tumors of the penis. In: *Campbell's Urology,* Vol. 2, 5th Ed., Walsh PC, Gittes RF, Perlmutter AD, Stamey TA (eds). Philadelphia: WB Saunders Co., pp 1583–1606.

Schiffman MH, Haley NJ, Felton JS, et al. 1987. Biochemical epidemiology of cervical neoplasia: measuring cigarette constituents in the cervix. Cancer Res 47:3886–3888.

Schneider A, Sawada E, Gissman L, et al. 1987. Human papillomavirus in women with a history of abnormal papanicolaou smears and in their male partners. Obstet Gynecol 69:554–562.

Schneider A, Kirchmayr R, de Villiers EM, et al. 1988. Subclinical human papillomavirus infections in male sexual partners of female carriers. J Urol 140:1431–1434.

Schneider V, Kay S, Lee HM. 1983. Immunosuppression as a high-risk factor in the development of condyloma acuminatum and squamous neoplasia of the cervix. Acta Cytol 27:220–224.

Schoen EJ, Anderson G, Bohon C, et al. 1989. Report of the task force on circumcision. Pediatrics 84:388–391.

Schoen EJ. 1990. The status of circumcision of newborns. N Engl J Med 322:1308–1311.

Schreier AA, Allen WP, Laughlin C, et al. 1988. Prospects for human papillomavirus vaccines and immunotherapies. J Natl Cancer Inst 80:896–899.

Sedlacek TV, Cunnane M, Carpiniello V. 1986. Colposcopy in the diagnosis of penile condyloma. Am J Obstet Gynecol 154:494–496.

Shabad AL. 1964. Some aspects of etiology and prevention of penile cancer. J Urol 92:696–702.

Simonsen JN, Cameron DW, Gakinya MN, et al. 1988. Human immunodeficiency virus infection among men with sexually transmitted diseases: experience from a center in Africa. N Engl J Med 319:274–278.

Smith PG, Kinlen LJ, White GC, et al. 1980. Mortality of wives of men dying with cancer of the penis. Br J Cancer 41:422–428.

Sobel H, Plaut A. 1949. The assimilation of cholesterol by mycobacterium smegmatis. J Bacteriol 57:377–382.

Stern RS, Zierler S, Parrish JA. 1980. Skin carcinoma in patients with psoriasis treated with topical tar and artificial ultraviolet radiation. Lancet 1:732–735.

Stern RS, Scotto J, Fears TR. 1985. Psoriasis and susceptibility to nonmelanoma skin cancer. J Am Acad Dermatol 12:67–73.

Stern RS (and Members Photochemotherapy Follow-up Study). 1990. Genital tumors among men with psoriasis exposed to psoralens and ultraviolet A radiation (PUVA) and ultraviolet B radiation. N Engl J Med 322:1093–1097.

Syrjänen SM, von Krogh G, Syrjänen KJ. 1987. Detection of human papillomavirus DNA in anogenital condylomata in men using in situ DNA hybridization applied to paraffin sections. Genitourin Med 63:32–39.

Tan RE. 1963. Observations on the frequency of carcinoma of the penis at Macassar and its environs (South Celebs). J Urol 89:704–705.

Thomas JA, Small CS. 1968. Carcinoma of the penis in southern India. J Urol 100:520–526.

Tindle RW, Frazier IH. 1990. Immunology of anogenital human papillomavirus (HPV) infection. Aust NZ J Obstet Gynaecol 30:370–374.

Van Ranst MA, Tachezy R, Delius H, et al. 1993. Taxonomy of the Human Papillomaviruses. Papillomavirus Report 4:61–65.

Wade TR, Kopf AW, Ackerman AB. 1978. Bowenoid papulosis of the penis. Cancer 42:1890–1903.

Warner E, Strashin E. 1981. Benefits and risks of circumcision. Can Med Assoc J 125:967–976.

Werness BA, Levine AJ, Howley PM. 1990. Association of human papillomavirus types 16 and 18 E6 proteins with p53. Science 248:76–79.

Wickenden C, Hanna N, Taylor-Robinson D, et al. 1988. Sexual transmission of human papallomavirus in heterosexual couples, studied by DNA hybridization. Genitourin Med 64:34–38.

Winkelstein W. 1990. Smoking and cervical cancer—current status: a review. Am J Epidemiol 131:945–957.

zur Hausen H. 1987. Papillomaviruses in human cancer. Cancer 59:1692–1696.

zur Hausen H. 1991. Human papillomaviruses in the pathogenesis of anogenital cancer. Virology 184:9–13.

zur Hausen H. 1994. Molecular pathogenesis of cancer of the cervix and its causation by specific human papillomavirus types. In: Human Pathogenic Papillomaviruses. zur Hausen H (ed). Berlin/Heidelberg/New York: Springer-Verlag, pp 131–156.

58 Neoplasms of the nervous system

SUSAN PRESTON-MARTIN
WENDY J. MACK

About 17,000 new primary cancers of the central nervous system are diagnosed each year among residents of the United States (Boring et al, 1991). These are among the most rapidly fatal of all cancers, and only about half (52%) of patients are still alive one year after diagnosis (Ries et al, 1994). Controversy surrounds the issue of whether or not the incidence of brain tumors, particularly the more lethal subtypes, has increased in recent decades (Greig et al, 1990; Modan et al, 1992; Desmeules et al, 1992). This issue and the explosion of epidemiological and molecular genetic studies of brain tumors have focused attention on this important human cancer that until only a few decades ago was relatively little studied. Despite this surge of interest, the etiology of the majority of nervous system tumors remains unknown. Inherited syndromes that predispose individuals to brain tumor development appear to be present in fewer than 5% of brain tumor patients. Some environmental agents, in particular ionizing radiation, are clearly implicated in the etiology of brain tumors, but numerous other physical, chemical, and infectious agents long suspected of being risk factors have not yet been established as etiologically relevant. This chapter first addresses the classification of brain tumors and provides a brief discussion of their molecular genetic characteristics, which have been the subject of literally hundreds of papers in the past few years. Next we review the descriptive epidemiology of brain tumors and experimental findings from animal studies in some detail, with an eye to what clues these studies might give us about etiology. We then discuss findings from epidemiological studies relating to various established or suggested risk factors. In the final section we review where we stand and speculate on prospects for future research.

Our chapter will focus on tumors of the brain, cranial nerves, and cranial meninges, which account for 95% of tumors at this site. These tumors are unique because of their location within the bony structure of the cranium. Symptoms depend mainly on location, and histologically benign tumors can result in similar symptomatology and outcome as malignant tumors. For this reason many cancer registries have routinely included both benign and malignant intracranial tumors. For simplicity, this group of tumors will be called "brain tumors" or, when benign tumors are excluded, "brain cancer." The term "central nervous system tumors" (or "cancer") indicates that tumors of the spinal cord and spinal meninges are included along with brain tumors, and "nervous system tumors" indicates that tumors of the peripheral nerves are included as well.

The presenting symptom can be localized, as with a specific motor, speech, or sensory deficit resulting from compression of the corresponding region of the brain. More commonly, symptoms are generalized, as with headaches and seizures that result from an increase in intracranial pressure. A third of patients present with headaches and a fifth with seizures (Walker, 1975).

The presence of these symptoms often leads to a detailed neurological examination including brain imaging such as radioisotope scanning, computed tomography (CT), and magnetic resonance imaging (MRI). Although tumors of the brain and cranial meninges rarely metastasize outside the central nervous system, the brain is a common metastatic site for tumors arising at other anatomic locations, including the lung, breast, kidney, gastrointestinal tract, prostate, and skin (malignant melanoma) (Rubinstein, 1972). Diagnoses based solely on brain imaging and other noninvasive techniques are unreliable both in differentiating primary from metastatic tumors and in determining the histologic type of primary tumors (Todd et al, 1987). Therefore, histologic diagnosis is encouraged to allow for more appropriate patient management. New methods such as stereotactic brain biopsy reduce the risk to patients from such procedures (Bullard et al, 1984).

Brain tumors are the second leading cause of death from neurological disease—second only to stroke—and the tenth most common cause of death from cancer. It is estimated that in 1991, 11,500 U.S. residents died of primary nervous system tumors (Boring et al, 1991). This is similar to the number who died of cancers of the liver and biliary passages, and it exceeds the number who died of granulocytic leukemia, renal cancer, esophageal cancer, larynx cancer, malignant melanoma, all cancers of the buccal cavity and pharynx combined, or cancers of the cervix and endometrium combined (Boring et al, 1991).

CLASSIFICATION

Variation in Inclusion Criteria

The descriptive epidemiology of these tumors has been difficult to study because of the wide variation in specific tumors included in published rates. Quantitatively, the most important variation relates to the inclusion or exclusion of benign tumors. This critical difference has often been ignored in comparisons across geographic areas.

In Los Angeles County, 27% of brain tumors in men and 44% in women are meningiomas or nerve sheath tumors, two tumor types that are predominantly benign. Yet rates for Los Angeles and for other areas, such as Israel, that include benign tumors are often compared directly to rates from registries that include malignant tumors only (Velema and Walker, 1987). Further confusion has been caused by the fact that some registries that usually publish rates in one form sometimes include a different set of tumors without explicitly stating that they are doing so. Connecticut, for example, is one of the registries in the U.S. Surveillance, Epidemiology, and End Results (SEER) Program. As such it need only report malignant tumors. However, for many of the more than 50 years this registry has been in operation, reports on benign meningiomas have been collected, and in some published reports, unlike others, these benign tumors have been included. Since its beginning in 1972, the registry for Los Angeles County has included benign as well as malignant tumors of the central nervous system, and published rates for tumors at this site have usually combined benign and malignant tumors as in the fifth volume of *Cancer Incidence in Five Continents* (Muir et al, 1987). Los Angeles rates reported to the previous volume of *Cancer Incidence in Five Continents*, however, excluded benign tumors at this site, but these rates were erroneously cited as including them and this error was not noted in the subsequent volume (Waterhouse et al, 1982). The most recent volume of *Cancer Incidence in Five Continents* attempts to rectify this problem by publishing rates for malignant brain tumors only (Parkin et al, 1992), although some of the registries continue to include noninvasive tumors. Thus, geographical comparisons are more easily made using these data, but comparisons of rates over time must still be made with caution.

For international comparisons, this chapter uses data from registries that report rates for malignant tumors only. Although reporting of malignant tumors alone eases geographical comparisons, it is unfortunate that incidence of benign nervous system tumors is not also reported. For this reason, benign tumors will not be excluded from descriptive data shown for Los Angeles County. In fact, as will become clear from discussions of analytic studies below, more is known about the etiology of benign histologic types such as meningiomas than about the etiology of gliomas, which are more common than meningiomas and are usually malignant.

Anatomic Classification

Another difficulty in comparing various descriptive surveys and other studies of this group of tumors relates to the inconsistency with respect to what subsites are included. Tumors of the central nervous system include tumors of the brain, cranial nerves, cerebral meninges, spinal cord, and spinal meninges. These subsites are represented by the International Classification of Diseases for Oncology (ICD-O; World Health Organization [WHO], 1976; Percy et al, 1990) codes shown in Table 58–1. Unlike some surveys, we will not include tumors of sites such as the eye and the pituitary gland that appear to be etiologically distinct.

Our review will focus on benign and malignant tu-

TABLE 58–1. *Anatomic and Pathologic Classification of Tumors of the Central Nervous System*

Subsite	*ICD-O Codes, 1976*	*ICD-O Codes, 1991*
Brain	191.0–191.9	C-71.1–C-71.9
Cranial nerve	192.0	C-72.2–C-72.5
Cerebral meninges	192.1	C-70.0
Spinal cord	192.2	C-72.0
Spinal meninges	192.3	C-70.1
Histologic Type	*ICD-O Codes*	
Gliomas	9380–9481	
Astrocytoma	9384, 9400–21	
Glioblastoma multiforme	9440–42	
Ependymoma	9391–94	
Primitive Neuroectodermal Tumor (PNET)	9470–73	
Oligodendroglioma	9450–60	
Other gliomas	9380–83, 9390, 9422–30, 9443, 9472–81	
Meningioma	9530–39	
Nerve sheath tumors	9540–60	
Other	9120–61	
Unspecified	8000–02	
No microscopic confirmation	9990	

mors of the brain and cranial meninges, which account for most of the tumors at this site (95% of all central nervous system tumors; 93% of all nervous system tumors). Some data sets used in descriptive comparisons include tumors of the spine, which account for 5% of all nervous system tumors. Others, such as those compiled in volumes I through VI of *Cancer Incidence in Five Continents*, also include tumors of the peripheral nerves, which make up an even smaller proportion of the total (2% in our data for Los Angeles County). Few epidemiological studies (either descriptive or analytic) have investigated tumors of the spine or peripheral nerves per se.

Pathological Classification

Early classification systems for neoplasms of the central nervous system were based on the hypothesized "cell of origin" of each tumor type (Bailey and Cushing, 1926). In several fundamental ways, however, this "cytogenetic" approach does not jibe with pathologists' observations (Rorke, 1987, 1994). For this reason an alternative "phenotypic" approach is preferable, whereby tumors are classified based on their present appearance and characteristics rather than on uncertain assumptions about their origins (Rorke, 1987, 1994). A scheme used in some epidemiological studies uses clusters of equivalent diagnostic terms used by pathologists to determine histologic classification (Armstrong et al, 1990).

Currently, the classification scheme favored for cancers is the ICD-O. The histologic groups of tumors that occur within the central nervous system and their corresponding ICD-O codes are shown in Table 58–1. A modification of this scheme is proposed for classification of pediatric brain tumors (Rorke et al, 1985). In both children and adults, gliomas are the most common major histologic type; these are predominantly malignant tumors that arise in the glial cells, which constitute the supporting structure for the neurons or nerve cells in the brain. No tumors arise in the neurons themselves. In Los Angeles, gliomas account for 59% of primary tumors of the brain and cranial meninges among men and 42% among women. Over 80% of gliomas are astrocytic gliomas (ie, astrocytomas and glioblastoma multiforme). It has been generally accepted that astrocytic gliomas that are grades 1 and 2 are classified as astrocytomas, and those that are grades 3 and 4 are classified as glioblastomas. The possibility that this practice may not be followed consistently is suggested, however, by the considerable geographic variation in the relative proportions of astrocytic gliomas that are classified as glioblastomas. This variation is seen, for example, among the various U.S. registries in the SEER Program. In comparison with the other SEER registries, Connecticut has a considerably higher proportion of tumors classified as glioblastomas, and a correspondingly lower proportion of astrocytomas (Velema and Percy, 1987).

The other two most common major histologic types are both predominantly benign. Meningiomas arise in the cranial meninges and account for 20% of all primary brain tumors in men and 36% in women. Nerve sheath tumors, called neuromas, neurilemmomas, or schwannomas, arise in the Schwann cells of the nerve sheath. About 8% of brain tumors in both men and women are nerve sheath tumors. It is curious that about 90% arise in the eighth cranial nerve; these are known as acoustic neuromas.

Clinical Classification

Now that CT scanning is available in many general hospitals in the United States and other industrialized countries, the differential diagnosis of intracranial masses is often made by physicians who are not specialists in neurological disease. In a recent survey in the United Kingdom, fewer than half of patients with CT diagnoses were referred to neurosurgeons for histologic confirmation by surgery or biopsy, and the positive predictive value of the CT diagnosis was around 90% for gliomas and meningiomas but only 50% for metastatic tumors (Todd et al, 1987). MRI is superior to CT in CNS imaging but is not yet widely available (Brant-Zawadski and Norman, 1987). In geographic areas where CT scanning and MRI are not available, the accuracy of clinical diagnoses of primary brain tumors that are not histologically confirmed is likely to be much worse.

The rate of microscopic confirmation of brain and nervous system tumors included in the latest edition of *Cancer Incidence in Five Continents* varies widely across geographic areas from a high of 99% (eg, among Los Angeles County residents of Japanese or Korean ancestry) to a low of 0% (in Setifi, Algeria; Parkin et al, 1992). Rates vary considerably among registries as well as among specific population groups within a country. For example, the rates of histologic verification range from 76% to 95% in Switzerland, 27% to 91% in Canada, 45% to 87% in Brazil, 52% to 98% in Japan, and 63% to 99% in the United States (Parkin et al, 1992). Such wide variation suggests that caution in the interpretation of these rates is warranted. In general, for a relatively inaccessible cancer site such as the brain a higher rate of microscopic confirmation makes us more confident that the neoplasm actually existed and that it was correctly classified. In some registries, however, a high rate may indicate that only those tumors that received histologic verification were reported and that clinically diagnosed tumors may have been missed.

Molecular Genetic Characteristics

Studies of the molecular biology and cytogenetics of CNS tumors suggest that specific types of tumors have characteristic genetic abnormalities, which are summarized in recent review papers (Black, 1991a, b; Leon et al, 1994). Such characterization contributes importantly to our understanding of the pathogenesis of CNS tumors. Glioblastomas, for example, commonly show losses of chromosome 9p, 10, or 17p; gains of chromosome 7; and p53 mutations. Loss of alleles at 17p appear to be the earliest abnormalities that occur in the genesis of these tumors. Most of these tumors express the c-*sis* oncogene, and some express other oncogenes as well. Related characteristics include the synthesis and secretion of growth factors that influence mitotic activity (Jennings et al, 1991).

Various CNS tumors—in particular those of astrocytic origin—have been associated with loss or mutation of the p53 gene located on the short arm of chromosome 17 (Kleihues et al, 1994). P53 is a tumor suppressor gene, and mutations in this gene appear to play a role in the development of a number of human cancers (Nigro et al, 1989). P53 mutations have been observed in glioblastoma multiforme as noted above (Nigro et al, 1989), in neurofibrosarcoma occurring in association with neurofibromatosis 1 (Nigro et al, 1989; Menon et al, 1990), and in patients with Li-Fraumeni syndrome (Malkin et al, 1990). Li-Fraumeni syndrome is a rare autosomal dominant genetic syndrome that predisposes those affected to cancers of the brain and other sites (Garber et al, 1990). This predisposition may relate to germ cell mutations in the tumor suppressor gene p53 (Malkin et al, 1990). Because benign tumors from patients with neurofibromatosis 1 appear not to have p53 mutations, it is thought that inactivation of this gene may be associated with the malignant transformation of these tumors (Menon et al, 1990).

Other tumor types show distinct pathophysiological features; for example, loss of regions on chromosome 22 is the characteristic feature of meningiomas. Also, pediatric CNS tumors show different genetic patterns than adult tumors (Griffin et al, 1988; Crist and Kun, 1991). The characterization of the various types is still in progress and the etiologic, prognostic, and other implications of specific characteristics remain to be defined.

DESCRIPTIVE EPIDEMIOLOGY

Descriptive data are difficult to compare across time periods or across geographical areas because of major inconsistencies both in inclusion criteria and in diagnostic efficiency. Los Angeles County, however, has an unusual resource, the Cancer Surveillance Program (CSP), that enables us to study the distribution of these tumors by demographic characteristics and histologic type. The CSP has collected reports on all new central nervous system neoplasms diagnosed in the county population (now about 9 million) since the beginning of 1972 (Hisserich et al, 1975). Inclusion criteria have been consistent, and reporting of both benign and malignant tumors has been at least 95% complete since the beginning (Mack, 1977). In the following sections, data will be presented on the more than 14,000 cases diagnosed from 1972 through 1992. Specially trained CSP personnel abstract information from hospital charts that includes age, sex, race, address, religion, birthplace, occupation, and industry as well as details of the pathological diagnosis. More than 95% of these diagnoses were confirmed histologically.

Methods used in the calculation of rates are described in an earlier report (Preston-Martin et al, 1982a). In all sections we will also compare findings from our Los Angeles data to those reported in the literature. Comparisons are limited, however, because few registries have published incidence data for specific types of brain tumors even though the descriptive epidemiology of these tumors varies considerably by histologic type.

Age

The average annual age-specific incidence of brain tumors is shown in Figure 58–1. In both males and females, rates decline after a peak in childhood (under age 10 years), increase after age 25, and level off after age 75. An analysis of racial patterns in the incidence of childhood brain cancer in the United States shows a difference in the age-incidence curves for astrocytic glio-

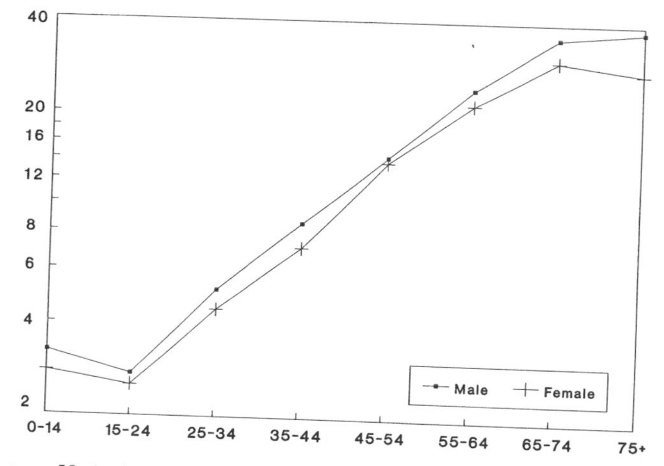

FIG. 58–1. Average annual age-specific incidence of tumors of the brain, cranial nerves, and cranial meninges (benign and malignant combined) in males and females, Los Angeles County, 1972–1992, whites (excluding Spanish-surnamed). Total cases: 5044 in males and 5212 in females.

mas in blacks and whites that seems unlikely to be explained by diagnostic delay in blacks (Bunin, 1987).

Comparisons of data from different areas of the United States have shown that the shape of the age-incidence curve after age 60 is highly dependent on the autopsy rate (Percy et al, 1972). Prior to 1955, rates among those over age 55 increased steeply with age in data from Rochester, Minnesota (location of the Mayo Clinic), but decreased in data from other areas (eg, the Second National Cancer Survey, Connecticut and Iowa). Subsequent analyses showed that the proportion of cases first diagnosed at death was considerably higher in Rochester than in Connecticut and that when these cases were excluded from the Rochester data, rates declined after age 65 rather than continuing to rise sharply (Schoenberg et al, 1978; Annegers et al, 1981). These comparisons suggest that brain tumor incidence continues to increase with age throughout life, but that there is often a significant under-ascertainment of cases in the oldest age groups. Comparisons of brain tumor rates from different registries might be more meaningful, therefore, if restricted to age groups under age 65.

Analyses of international data for ages 35–64 indicate that the shape of the age-incidence curve is similar across geographic areas although the level varies (Velema and Walker, 1987). This shape is a straight line on a log-log scale, and the slope (2.6) is the same for males and females, suggesting that incidence increases as a function of age to the 2.6 power. Slopes varied considerably by histologic type as follows: 0.4 for ependymoma; 1.0 for oligodendroglioma; 1.7 for astrocytoma; 2.8 for meningioma; and 3.9 for glioblastoma (Velema and Percy, 1987). The authors suggest that the significantly higher rate of increase with age seen for glioblastomas compared to other glial tumors is indicative of a different mechanism of carcinogenesis for these highly aggressive tumors.

Gender

In Figure 58–1 we see that for all types of brain tumors combined, rates are higher in males than in females at all ages. Figure 58–2 shows that males, regardless of ethnic group, have higher rates of gliomas but females consistently have higher meningioma rates. Table 58–2 shows the age-adjusted annual incidence for the major histologic groups of primary brain tumors by sex and ethnic group in Los Angeles County, 1972–1992. For all histologic types and races combined, the rate is higher in men than in women. For most ethnic groups, male rates for all histologic types combined are higher than female rates. The male to female sex ratio (SR) varies considerably, however, by histologic type. In each ethnic group, glioma rates are higher in males than in

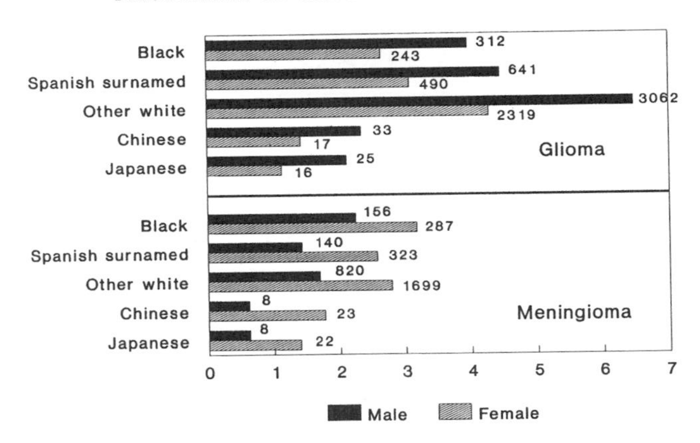

FIG. 58–2. Average annual age-adjusted incidence of gliomas and meningiomas by ethnic group and sex, Los Angeles County, 1972–1992.

females (SR for all races combined=1.5), and meningioma rates are higher in women (SR=0.6).

A comparison using international data on incidence of nervous system tumors of all histologic types combined found an average SR of 1.4 but noted significant variation in the SR with a range of 0.9 to 2.6 across geographic areas (Velema and Walker, 1987). The SR also varies considerably by age group and histologic type. The SR in children under age 15 is 1.2 for all tumor types combined. In contrast, primitive neuroectodermal tumors (PNET, formerly called medulloblastoma), which occur almost exclusively in children, have an SR of around 2 (Preston-Martin, 1985; Cruz, 1958), but no male excess is seen among U.S. black children (Bunin, 1987).

Sex ratios for specific histologic types also vary by anatomic subsite and by age group. One of the most interesting examples of this relates to meningiomas. Among non–Spanish-surnamed whites in Los Angeles County, spinal meningiomas are 3.5 (SR=0.3) times more common in women than in men, whereas cerebral meningiomas are only 1.5 (SR=0.7) times more common in women. Similar patterns are seen for meningiomas in Norway (Helseth et al, 1989b). Also, the female to male ratio for spinal meningiomas increases with age, whereas for cerebral meningiomas the female excess is greatest during the female reproductive years and declines after age 55. The sex differential for spinal meningiomas suggests the etiologic relevance of some factor related to aging in women; we hypothesize that this factor may be vertebral osteoporosis.

In data from the nine SEER registries on the incidence of nervous system tumors, differences in the SRs by histologic type range from 1.0 for malignant meningiomas to 1.6 for glioblastomas (Velema and Walker, 1987). The SR for all meningiomas (benign and malignant combined) is consistently less than 1. The SR for all tumor types combined is higher, therefore, for registries

TABLE 58–2. *Average Annual Age-Adjusted Incidence (Per 100,000) by Major Histologic Type of Primary Brain Tumor by Sex and Ethnic Group, Los Angeles County, 1972–1992*

	Gliomas	*Meningiomas*	*Nerve Sheath Tumors*	*All Histologic Types*	
					(Number)
MALES					
Black	4.0	2.2	0.2	7.4	(570)
Spanish surnamed	4.4	1.4	0.3	7.5	(1003)
Other whites	6.5	1.7	0.8	10.5	(5044)
Chinese	2.3	0.6	0.3	4.0	(54)
Japanese	2.1	0.6	0.6	4.0	(49)
Filipino	2.4	2.0	0.7	6.1	(69)
Korean	2.4	0.4	0.0	3.1	(26)
Other races	1.5	0.9	0.3	3.3	(62)
All races	5.5	1.6	0.6	9.2	(6877)
FEMALES					
Black	2.6	3.2	0.2	7.0	(635)
Spanish surnamed	3.1	2.6	0.4	6.9	(1000)
Other whites	4.3	2.8	0.8	9.1	(5212)
Chinese	1.4	1.8	0.4	4.2	(52)
Japanese	1.1	1.4	0.7	3.8	(58)
Filipino	1.7	2.3	0.4	4.9	(68)
Korean	1.9	1.4	0.4	5.0	(39)
Other races	1.5	1.6	0.7	4.1	(88)
All races	3.7	2.7	0.7	8.1	(7152)

that include only malignant tumors (SR=1.5) than for registries that include benign tumors as well (SR=1.3).

Race and Geography

Table 58–3 compares international data on the incidence of malignant brain and nervous system tumors included in the latest volume of *Cancer Incidence in Five Continents* (Parkin et al, 1992). These comparisons are limited to patients aged 35 to 64 years at diagnosis because it was thought that throughout the world, reporting of brain and nervous system tumors was likely to be most complete for this age group. All registries that had a rate of histologic verification of 55% or greater and had 10 or more cases each among males and among females are included. Certain registries meeting these two criteria were not included in Table 58–3 because their published rates included noninvasive tumors; thus, these rates are not directly comparable to registries including malignant tumors only. The methods used to calculate the standardized incidence ratios (SIRs) are described in detail elsewhere (Velema and Walker, 1987). In brief, the observed number of cases and person-years of observation in each of the six 5-year age groups were used to compute SIRs separately for males and females. Incidence among whites in the U.S. SEER registries is used as the baseline (SIR=100); for reference the age-adjusted annual incidence for U.S. SEER Registries for 1983–1987, ages 35–64, is 10.4 and 6.7 per 100,000 for males and females, respectively (Parkin et al, 1992).

In general, rates among whites in Canada, the United States, Europe, the United Kingdom, and Australia are relatively similar although rates are lower in certain eastern European countries and former Soviet republics (Russia, Belarus, Krygystan). An analysis of Canadian provincial rates found that the ratio of highest to lowest rates was 1.3 among females and 1.4 among males (Howe et al, 1984) suggesting that rates are relatively similar among provinces. Rates are lowest in Asian populations in Japan and India and among Chinese in Singapore. Rates are also lower in Puerto Rico, Costa Rica, and Brazil.

Table 58–3 shows lower rates for blacks than for whites in the same geographic area in the United States. Asian Americans and Latinos also have lower rates than whites in the same geographic area, although the number of cases among those aged 35–64 in these ethnic groups in several U.S. registries was too few for them to be included in Table 58–3. Some of these racial differences vary, however, from one histologic type of brain tumor to another. In Figure 58–2, we see that in Los Angeles County, the rate of gliomas is lower among black males and females than among whites but that the

TABLE 58–3. *Standardized Incidence Ratios (SIRs) and Number of Cases for Malignant Nervous System Tumors in Males and Females Aged 35–64, 1983–1987: U.S. SEER Whites Used as Referent**

Registry	Males		Females	
	SIR	*(Number)*	*SIR*	*(Number)*
Brazil, Goiania	54	(10)	93	(12)
Costa Rica	62	(68)	42	(30)
Puerto Rico	61	(140)	49	(87)
Canada	102	(2162)	107	(1528)
Canada, Alberta	86	(153)	81	(91)
Canada, British Columbia	96	(243)	85	(141)
Canada, Maritime Provinces	91	(112)	84	(70)
Canada, New Brunswick	87	(38)	71	(21)
Canada, Nova Scotia	95	(66)	98	(46)
Canada, Newfoundland	85	(35)	115	(30)
Canada, Ontario	108	(862)	125	(669)
Canada, Saskatchewan	88	(70)	103	(53)
Alameda County, White	97	(67)	120	(56)
Alameda County, Black	64	(10)	95	(11)
Los Angeles County, White	85	(360)	84	(246)
Los Angeles County, Latino	57	(66)	81	(64)
Los Angeles County, Black	81	(57)	75	(39)
San Francisco Bay, White	115	(261)	111	(166)
San Francisco Bay, Black	66	(21)	70	(16)
Connecticut, White	99	(256)	102	(185)
Atlanta, White	98	(108)	96	(74)
Atlanta, Black	61	(18)	46	(11)
Iowa	102	(235)	89	(142)
New Orleans, White	103	(59)	128	(52)
New Orleans, Black	76	(17)	54	(10)
Detroit, White	100	(258)	111	(200)
Detroit, Black	55	(35)	48	(24)
New Mexico	78	(86)	81	(62)
New York City	81	(476)	78	(362)
New York State (less NYC)	90	(822)	96	(620)
Seattle	91	(215)	96	(152)
Utah	93	(96)	89	(62)
U.S., Hawaii, White	118	(29)	82	(11)
U.S. SEER, White	100	(1528)	100	(1040)
U.S. SEER, Black	53	(94)	45	(60)
India, Ahmedabad	22	(40)	21	(20)
India, Bangalore	36	(72)	36	(37)
India, Bombay	31	(192)	36	(98)
India, Madras	39	(90)	29	(37)
Japan, Hiroshima	27	(23)	43	(25)
Japan, Miyagi	29	(62)	31	(46)
Kuwait, non-Kuwaitis	55	(47)	98	(20)
Kyrgystan	18	(17)	30	(21)
Singapore, Chinese	26	(35)	27	(24)
Belarus	57	(469)	54	(373)
Estonia	89	(118)	84	(93)
Finland	84	(377)	107	(339)
France, Bas-Rhin	103	(82)	97	(54)
France, Calvados	68	(35)	69	(25)
France, Isere	75	(65)	95	(54)
France, Somme	125	(23)	120	(15)
France, Tarn	69	(24)	42	(10)
Germany, Saarland	77	(83)	92	(72)
Hungary, Szabolcs	64	(35)	68	(27)
Ireland, Southern	92	(30)	114	(24)
Italy, Ragusa	106	(28)	75	(14)
Netherlands, Eindhoven	60	(47)	71	(36)
Poland, Cracow City	96	(50)	87	(34)
Spain, Basque Country	89	(74)	98	(53)
Spain, Granada	104	(41)	87	(24)
Spain, Murcia	82	(56)	83	(39)
Switzerland, Basel	88	(38)	82	(25)
Switzerland, Geneva	83	(31)	99	(26)
Switzerland, St. Gall	93	(38)	89	(25)
Switzerland, Vaud	97	(51)	79	(29)
Switzerland, Zurich	83	(93)	101	(78)
Russia, St. Petersburg	65	(259)	67	(252)
Slovenia	64	(130)	70	(107)
UK, Birmingham	88	(358)	82	(214)
UK, Mersey	94	(217)	105	(163)
UK, Northwestern	82	(310)	83	(208)
UK, Southwestern	91	(272)	92	(189)
UK, Trent	96	(434)	100	(293)
UK, Scotland	97	(457)	102	(334)
UK, Scotland, East	95	(35)	104	(27)
UK, Scotland, North	98	(21)	76	(10)
UK, Scotland, Northeast	106	(51)	110	(36)
UK, Scotland, Southeast	120	(130)	97	(73)
UK, Scotland, West	86	(221)	105	(188)
Australia, Capital Territory	84	(16)	115	(14)
Australia, New South Wales	98	(476)	105	(318)
Australia, South	97	(120)	109	(87)
Australia, Tasmania	130	(48)	80	(19)
Australia, Victoria	98	(349)	96	(221)
Australia, West	78	(92)	104	(76)
New Zealand, non-Maori	113	(284)	109	(176)
Czechoslovakia, Bohemia and Moravia	96	(921)	100	(683)
Czechoslovakia, Slovakia	83	(350)	99	(302)

*SIRs were derived from data reported to *Cancer Incidence in Five Continents*, Volume VI (Parkin et al, 1992), using a procedure described briefly in the text and in detail in a previous report (Velema and Walker, 1987). Any population was included if the registry had a microscopic confirmation rate of 55% or greater and if there were at least 10 cases in patients aged 35–64 of each sex.

reverse is true for meningiomas. This excess of meningiomas among blacks has been noted previously in other U.S. populations (Heshmat et al, 1976). In some African populations, meningioma is the most common type of brain tumor (Levy and Auchterlonie, 1975).

Latino males and females have lower rates of both gliomas and meningiomas than other white males and females (Fig. 58–2). Asians in Los Angeles have the lowest rates of both tumor types, but the differential in rates between Asians and whites is less for meningiomas (Fig. 58–2, Table 58–2). Although Filipinos have glioma rates equivalent to those of other Asian groups in Los Angeles County, meningioma rates are strikingly higher (Table 58–2). In fact, meningioma rates in Filipino males are higher than in white males.

Figure 58–3 shows rates for several racial groups and, for each race, includes rates for both native and migrant populations (except for blacks, because there were no registries on the African continent meeting the 55% histologic verification criterion). Registries reporting rates for malignant tumors alone are included. In general, rates of brain and nervous system tumors are highest among whites. Among each other racial group, rates are usually higher in migrant populations than in native populations that remain in the continent of origin. These differences between migrant and native populations suggest that some change in lifestyle may be occurring in migrant populations that places them at higher risk for brain tumors, although an increase in diagnostic efficiency may partially explain some of these differences.

Birthplace

Two studies in New York City found no major differences in brain cancer mortality rates by birthplace (MacMahon, 1960; Newill, 1961). Higher brain tumor mortality rates among foreign-born male and female residents of Minnesota were seen, however, especially in age groups under age 50 (Choi et al, 1970a). Another study found brain tumor mortality was significantly lower among U.S.-born males than among males born in countries in Scandinavia and eastern Europe, but U.S.-born females had higher mortality rates than those born in these areas (Lilienfeld et al, 1972). Male and female residents of Los Angeles County born in eastern Europe have a significantly elevated brain tumor incidence. This finding is likely related to the excess rates observed among Jewish residents of Los Angeles (see below). Among Los Angeles women, the excess in those born in southern Europe and the Middle East (observed in both sexes) is also statistically significant.

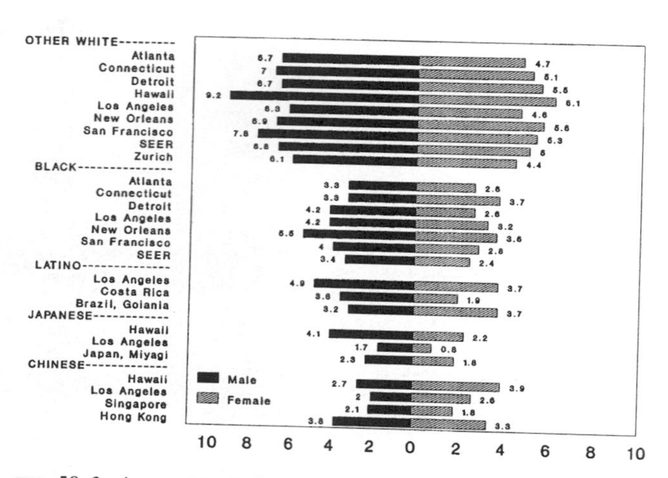

FIG. 58–3. Average annual age-adjusted incidence of nervous system tumors (benign and malignant) in males and females from native and migrant populations of five different ethnic groups, 1983–1987. Data from *Cancer Incidence in Five Continents*, Volume VI.

Religion

An excess of brain tumors was reported a few decades ago among adult Jewish residents of New York City (Newill, 1961). Another study in New York City around the same time found an excess of deaths from gliomas, but not other types of brain cancer among Jews (MacMahon, 1960). In Los Angeles, the association is weakest for gliomas and far stronger for meningiomas and nerve sheath tumors, two tumor types that are usually benign. The MacMahon study, because it was limited to cancer, lacked information on these benign histologic types.

An analysis of cancer incidence data for the state of Utah shows a statistically significant excess of brain cancer in Mormon compared to non-Mormon men and women (Lyon et al, 1976). This excess is of particular interest because, overall, Mormons have significantly less cancer (all sites combined) than do non-Mormons.

Marital Status

Analysis of data from the Third National Cancer Survey (TNCS, 1969–1971) showed brain cancer incidence was higher among single males and females aged 35–64 than among married people of the same age (Ernster et al, 1979). Data for Los Angeles County for 1972–1985 also show significantly higher incidence of tumors of the brain and cranial meninges among single men and women in the 35–64-year-old age group. In contrast, Los Angeles rates for all age groups combined are higher among married than among single men and women. Although different sources were used for information on marital status (the TNCS study used U.S. census data on marital status, whereas the study in Los Angeles used data from hospital charts), the above comparison suggests that apparent discrepancies between data sets looking at cancer incidence by marital status may be attributable to the different ages of the populations studied, rather than differences in data sources.

Urban versus Rural

A significantly higher proportion of male residents of Minnesota who died of brain tumors lived on farms compared to the general population of Minnesota (Choi et al, 1970a). A Norwegian study revealed that age-specific incidence of glial tumors was higher in rural compared to urban areas for age groups under 30 (Cancer Registry of Norway, 1961). However, a recent study showed that average annual incidence of all primary intracranial neoplasms in Oslo compared to that in other parts of Norway is similar under age 25, but is considerably higher among those over age 50 in Oslo, where the rate of histologic verification and the autopsy rate are much higher than in other areas (Helseth et al, 1988). A study in Italy found an excess risk among farmers, and a recent review discusses farming exposures that might contribute to these excesses (Musicco et al, 1982; Blair et al, 1985). Data from most registries that report rates separately for urban and rural areas, however, suggest higher incidence for all age groups combined in urban than in rural residents, but in some countries, these differences may be at least partially attributable to differences in diagnostic efficiency and completeness of case ascertainment (Waterhouse et al, 1982; Muir et al, 1987; Parkin et al, 1992).

A study of childhood central nervous system neoplasms in Manitoba reported that incidence of most gliomas—astrocytoma, glioblastoma, and ependymoma—was significantly higher in rural than in urban populations (Choi et al, 1977). One case-control study reported an association between brain tumors in children and a history of having lived on a farm or a history of exposure to farm animals (Gold et al, 1979). A study of a large cohort of Seventh-Day Adventists found that those living in rural areas were almost three times more likely to develop a glioma (Mills et al, 1989).

Social Class

Table 58–4 shows the proportional incidence ratios (PIRs) for primary tumors of the brain and cranial meninges by social class (as determined by census tract of residence) for Los Angeles County non–Spanish-surnamed whites. These age-adjusted PIRs represent the ratio of the number of cases observed to that expected in a subgroup. The expected number was calculated for each 5-year age group by assuming that the distribution of brain tumors by social class was the same as that for all other cancer sites combined. A summary chi-squared test was used to measure statistical significance (Mantel and Haentzel, 1959). There is a clear trend of increasing incidence with increasing social class. For males, this trend is evident for gliomas, meningiomas, and nerve sheath tumors. For females, this trend is clearly evident only for nerve sheath tumors. A similar trend of increasing brain cancer rates with increasing social class (as determined by occupation) was reported for men in England and Wales a few decades ago (Buell et al, 1960), in Washington State (Demers et al, 1991), and recently in New Zealand (Preston-Martin et al, 1993a). Because this trend occurs more strikingly among males than among females, it seems unlikely that it might relate to factors such as diagnostic efficiency or exposure to diagnostic radiography of the head (eg, dental x-rays), both of which might be expected to be greater among those in higher social classes.

TABLE 58–4. *Proportional Incidence Ratios for Primary Brain Tumors by Social Class and Total Number of Cases, Los Angeles County, 1972–1992, Non-Latino Whites*

	Proportional Incidence Ratios		
Socioeconomic Status	*Gliomas*	*Meningiomas*	*Nerve Sheath Tumors*
MALES			
1 (high)	132.8[a]	106.0	154.1[a]
2	99.6	101.5	107.0
3	96.8	100.7	90.0
4	87.5[a]	98.4	77.0[a]
5 (low)	95.3	53.5	44.7
FEMALES			
1	105.5	105.2	113.1
2	101.8	99.0	111.9
3	106.8	92.2	91.2
4	88.4[a]	108.0	85.8
5	60.3	106.5	88.5

[a] $P \leq 0.01$

Occupation and Industry

Although a myriad of epidemiological studies have investigated the relation between work in a variety of occupational/industrial settings and brain tumor incidence/mortality, repeated studies in various geographic areas have been reported for only a few occupations. Table 58–5 summarizes epidemiological studies of brain tumor risk in selected occupations and industries. For each occupation or industry considered, this table lists studies in descending order of publication date; negative studies are included in these listings. The relative risk estimates for descriptive studies and cohort studies are standardized mortality/incidence ratios (SMR or SIR), or proportionate mortality/incidence ratios (PMR or PIR). Case-control studies all used the odds ratio (OR) as the estimate of relative risk. Although many other studies have investigated brain tumor risk for specific occupations and occupational exposures, it is beyond

TABLE 58–5. *Summary of Epidemiologic Studies of Brain Tumor Risk in Selected Occupations and Industries*

Occupation/Industry	Risk Estimate	Number of Cases[a] Observed/Expected; Exposed/Total Cases	Study Period	Place	Reported by	Year
PETROCHEMICAL WORKERS						
Petroleum refinery workers	OR=8.8[b]		1969–78	Washington State	Demers et al	1991
Male employees of petrochemical plant	SMR=147	5/3.4	1941–83	United States	Teta et al	1991
Petroleum refining and chemical plant	SMR=76	8/10.5	1948–83	Texas	Marsh et al	1991
Chemical plant only	SMR=65	2/3.1				
Refinery only:						
Less than 20 years	SMR=59	2/3.4				
20–29 years	SMR=89	2/2.25				
30 or more years	SMR=211	2/0.95				
Petrochemical: hourly employees			1950–83	Texas	Teta et al	1991
Brain cancer	SMR=181[b]	17/9.4				
Benign/unspecified brain tumors	SMR=280[b]	7/2.5				
Ever worked with petroleum products such as gasoline or kerosene	OR=3.6[b]	18/70 meningiomas	1980–84	Los Angeles	Preston-Martin et al	1989a
Petroleum and coal products industry	PIR=113	12/10.6 gliomas	1972–85	Los Angeles	Preston-Martin	1989c
	PIR=252[b]	6/2.4 meningiomas				
Coal and petroleum refining industry	SIR=180	13/7.2	1961–79	Sweden	McLaughlin et al	1987a
Petroleum refining	SIR=120	5/4.2				
Other petroleum and coal industry	SIR=260[b]	8/3.1				
Coal and petroleum products	OR=3.5[b]	?/432	1959–63 and 1965–79	England	Magnani et al	1987
Petroleum refining: production & maintenance	OR=1.7	15/300 with astrocytomas	1978–80 or 1979–81	Northern New Jersey, Philadelphia, Louisiana Gulf Coast	Thomas et al	1987a
Oil refinery	SMR=126	22/17.5	1950–80	California	Wong et al	1986
Petrochemical: hourly employees	SMR=200[b]	10/5.0	1941–77	Texas	Austin and Schnatter	1983
	SMR=198[b]	19/9.6	1941–77	Texas	Waxweiler et al	1983
Oil refinery:			1937–78	Texas	Wen et al	1983
all workers	SMR=99	30/30.43				
white hourly	SMR=96	23/23.96				
nonwhite hourly	SMR=140	5/3.6				
salaried workers	SMR=67	2/2.99				
Oil refinery	PMR=221[b]	28/12.7	1943–79	Texas	Thomas et al	1982
Oil refinery and chemical plant	SMR=102	5/4.9	1970–77	Louisiana	Hanis et al	1982
Oil refinery	SMR=80	36/44.77	1950–75	England	Rushton and Alderson	1981
Oil refinery and petrochemical workers	PMR=176[b]	25/14.2	1947–77	Texas	Thomas et al	1980
Oil refinery	SMR=652[b]	3/0.46	1928–76	Montreal	Thériault and Goulet	1979
RUBBER INDUSTRY						
Rubber manufacturing: employed at least 10 years	SIR=500[b]		1979–88	Moscow	Solionova and Smulevich	1993
Male operatives in rubber industry	SMR=88	67/76.3	1946–85	United Kingdom	Sorahan et al	1989
Rubber and miscellaneous plastics industry	PIR=145	9/6.2 gliomas	1972–85	Los Angeles	Preston-Martin	1989c
	PIR=368[b]	5/1.4 meningiomas				

(continued)

TABLE 58–5. *(Continued)*

Occupation/Industry	Risk Estimate	Number of Cases[a] Observed/Expected — Exposed/Total Cases	Study Period	Place	Reported by	Year
Ever worked in rubber processing	OR=6.0	6/202 gliomas	1980–84	Los Angeles	Preston-Martin et al	1989a
Ever worked in rubber industry	OR=9.0[b]	9/251	1979–82	Toronto	Burch et al	1987
Rubber industry	SIR=110	18/16.4	1961–79	Sweden	McLaughlin et al	1987a
Tire assembly	SMR=400[b]	8/2.0	1940–76	Akron, Ohio	Monson and Fine	1978
Tire building	SMR=190	7/3.7	1940–73	Akron, Ohio	Monson and Nakano	1976
Rubber manufacturing	SMR=92	8/8.7	1964–73	Akron, Ohio	Andjelkovic et al	1976
Retired workers aged 40–64	SMR=323[b]					
Rubber industry (PMR elevated in some of 6 plants)	SMR=68	4/5.9	1964–72	United States	McMichael et al	1974
Rubber and cablemaking	SMR=108	14/13.0	1967–71	England	Fox et al	1974
Curing and tire building	RR=5.6	8 observed	1938–64	Ohio	Mancuso et al	1968
Tire manufacture plant	SMR=800[b]	2/0.25	1920–55	Summit, Ohio	Mancuso	1963
HEALTH PROFESSIONS						
Pathologists	SMR=240	6/2.5	1974–87	United Kingdom	Hall et al	1991
Physicians, dentists, and related professionals	PIR=152[b]	38/25.1, all histologic types	1972–85	Los Angeles	Preston-Martin	1989c
Registered nurses	PIR=278[b]	5/1.8, all histologic types	1972–85	Los Angeles	Preston-Martin	1989c
Female physicians	SIR=370[b]	4/1.08	1961–79	Sweden	McLaughlin et al	1987a
Male dentists	SIR=210[b]	12/5.7	1961–79	Sweden	McLaughlin et al	1987a
Female employees in health care industry	SIR=120[b]	121/100.83	1961–79	Sweden	McLaughlin et al	1987a
Health care industry, meningioma in males	SIR=170	?/?	1961–79	Sweden	McLaughlin et al	1987b
Dentists and dental nurses			1961–79	Sweden	Ahlbom et al	1986
Glioblastoma	SIR=213[b]	18/8.47				
Glioma	SIR=182	4/2.2				
Meningioma	SIR=131	6/4.59				
Health-diagnosing occupations	OR=6.8[b]	13/718	1978–81	Northern New Jersey, Philadelphia, Southern Louisiana	Thomas et al	1986
Pathologists	SMR=300[b]	6/2.0	1974–80	United Kingdom	Harrington and Oakes	1984
Veterinarians	PMR=261[b]	18/6.9	1966–77	United States	Blair and Hayes	1980
ELECTRICAL WORKERS/ELECTROMAGNETIC FIELD EXPOSURE						
Electric utility workers exposed to magnetic fields			1950–88	United States	Savitz and Loomis	1995
Employed at least 20 years	RR=1.4	27/NA				
Total estimated magnetic field exposure ≥4.3 microtesla	RR=2.3[b]	16/NA				
Electric utility workers: estimated cumulative exposure to magnetic fields			1970–89	Canada, France	Thériault et al	1994
≥90th percentile	OR=1.9	12/108				
≥50th percentile	OR=1.5	48/108				
Railway workers			1961–79	Sweden	Floderus et al	1994
1961–69	RR=1.2	31/256257 person-years				
1970–79	RR=0.9	39/284730 person-years				

(continued)

TABLE 58–5. *Summary of Epidemiologic Studies of Brain Tumor Risk in Selected Occupations and Industries (Continued)*

Occupation/Industry	*Risk Estimate*	*Number of Cases[a] Observed/Expected* *Exposed/Total Cases*	*Study Period*	*Place*	*Reported by*	*Year*
Electric utility workers						
Electric workers	RR=1.1	9/172062 person-years	1960–88	California	Sahl et al	1993
At least 10 years of exposure as an electrical worker	OR=1.0	12/32				
Electrical workers			1948–88	New Zealand	Preston-Martin et al	1993a
Electrical engineers	OR=8.2[b]	4/1113				
Electricians	OR=4.6[b]	7/1113				
Electrical workers with 10 or more years of employment	SIR=114	77/67.62	1971–85	Norway	Tynes et al	1992
Radio/TV assemblers and repair			1961–79	Sweden	Törnqvist et al	1991
All brain tumors	SIR=290[b]	7/2.41				
Glioblastoma	SIR=340[b]	5/1.47				
Welders:			1961–79	Sweden	Törnqvist et al	1991
All brain tumors	SIR=130	46/35.38				
Glioblastoma	SIR=150[b]	34/22.67				
Occupations with possible EM field exposure, more than 10 years:			1980–84	Los Angeles	Mack et al	1991
All brain tumors	OR=1.3	15/272				
Meningioma	OR=0.3	1/70				
Glioma	OR=1.7	14/202				
Astrocytoma	OR=10.3[b]	11/114				
Electrician, more than 5 years	OR=1.9	13/226	1987–88	Germany	Schlehofer et al	1990
Women	OR=5.2[b]	8/127				
Men	OR=0.9	5/99				
Any electrical occupation	OR=1.4[b]	75/2173	1985–86	United States	Loomis and Savitz	1990
Electrical engineers and technicians	OR=2.7[b]	29/2173				
Electrical workers in manufacturing industries	OR=2.1[b]	23/2173				
Electrical power workers	OR=1.7[b]	5/2173				
Telephone workers	OR=1.6[b]	9/2173				
Electricians	PIR=176[b]	20/11.4 gliomas	1972–85	Los Angeles	Preston-Martin	1989c
Electrical worker	OR=0.78	8/452	1980–84	New Zealand	Reif et al	1989
Electrical engineers	OR=4.74[b]	?/452				
Electricians	OR=1.91	?/452				
Electromagnetic field exposed occupations and utility workers	OR=3.9[b]	?/202	1969–78	East Texas	Speers et al	1988
Utility workers alone	OR=13.1[b]	?/202				
Transportation, communication, and utilities industries	OR=2.26[b]	?/202				
Electricians and electronic workers	SIR=90	75/83.3	1961–79	Sweden	McLaughlin et al	1987a
Electrical/electronic workers:			1979–81	Northern New Jersey, Philadelphia, Southern Louisiana	Thomas et al	1987b
Engineers, teachers, technicians	OR=3.9[b]	28/435				
Any microwave/radiofrequency radiation exposed job: 20+ years	OR=3.1[b]	22/435				
Design, manufacture, repair, or installation of electrical or electronic eqpt.	OR=2.3[b]	44/435				
Power linesmen	SMR=149	13/8.7	1961–79	Sweden	Törnqvist et al	1986
Power station operators	SMR=97	17/17.5				

TABLE 58–5. *(Continued)*

Occupation/Industry	Risk Estimate	Number of Cases[a] Observed/Expected; Exposed/Total Cases	Study Period	Place	Reported by	Year
Electromagnetic field exposure	PMR=123[b]	101/82	1950–82	Washington State	Milham	1985
EM field exposure only	PMR=89	19/21.3				
EM and other occupational exposure	PMR=136	82/60.5				
Electricity-related: electric/electronic engineer, utility company service worker (rated definite exposure)	OR=2.15[b]	27/951	1969–82	Maryland	Lin et al	1985
Electricians	PIR=142[b]	11/7.75	1972–77	Los Angeles County	Preston-Martin et al	1982a
AGRICULTURE						
Agricultural research institute; plant and soil science research	SMR=469[b]	4/0.85	1960–80	Ireland	Daly et al	1994
Agricultural workers			1948–88	New Zealand	Preston-Martin et al	1993a
Dairy farmers	OR=3.4[b]	17/1113				
Sheep handlers	OR=2.7[b]	13/1113				
Livestock workers	OR=3.8[b]	10/1113				
Farm managers	OR=3.2[b]	8/1113				
Male farmers: glioblastoma mortality in top quartile of fuel/oil expenditure	RR=1.9	25/595,879 person-years	1971–87	Canada	Morrison et al	1992
Male farmers licensed to use pesticides	SMR=169	11/6.5	1974–87	Northern Italy	Alberghini et al	1991
Forestry industry			1969–78	Washington State	Demers et al	1991
All brain tumors	OR=4.6	6/863				
Astrocytic tumors	OR=8.5[b]	3/282				
Agricultural industry	OR=1.1	72/863	1969–78	Washington State	Demers et al	1991
Farm Bureau members	SIR=87	12/13.8	1973–83	New York State	Stark et al	1990
Agricultural crop production	OR=1.5	22/312	1984–88	Missouri	Brownson et al	1990
Farming	OR=1.1	21/312				
Farmers	OR=1.33	74/452	1980–84	New Zealand	Reif et al	1989
Livestock farmer	OR=2.59[b]	11/452				
Dairy farmer	OR=1.61	9/452				
Orchard, vineyard	OR=1.29	6/452				
General farmer/farmworker	OR=1.11	41/452				
Field crop farmer	OR=1.08	4/452				
Farmers	OR=1.6[b]	61/240	1983–84	Milan, Italy	Musicco et al	1988
By use of agricultural chemicals:						
Nonusers	OR=1.2	19/240				
Chemical user	OR=1.6[b]	42/240				
Used insecticides/fungicides	OR=2.0[b]	37/240				
Used herbicides	OR=1.6	10/240				
Used fertilizers	OR=1.4	26/240				
Farmers, fishermen, and hunters	SIR=110	621/564.5	1961–79	Sweden	McLaughlin et al	1987a
Farming	OR=0.8	13/718	1978–81	Northern New Jersey, Philadelphia, Louisiana Gulf Coast	Thomas et al	1986
Farmers	OR=5.0[b]	15/42	1979–80	Milan, Italy	Musicco et al	1982

[a]Number of cases indicated is observed/expected for descriptive studies and cohort studies and exposed cases/total cases for case-control studies. Person-years are indicated for several studies.

[b]$P \leq .05$.

Abbreviations:
? = data not available
OR = odds ratio
PIR = proportionate incidence ratio
PMR = proportionate mortality ratio
RR = relative risk
SIR = standardized incidence ratio
SMR = standardized mortality ratio

the scope of this chapter to exhaustively summarize the literature in this area.

One specific occupational exposure of interest not reported in Table 58–5 is vinyl chloride. Motivated by experimental research on the induction of brain tumors in animals after exposure to vinyl chloride, several epidemiological studies of workers occupationally exposed to this chemical reported significantly elevated brain tumor mortality for vinyl chloride workers as a whole (Monson et al, 1974; Cooper, 1981), or for subgroups based on time since first exposure (Waxweiler et al, 1976). In addition, Infante (1976) reported elevated brain tumor mortality in communities surrounding vinyl chloride production facilities in the United States. More recent occupational studies have been conflicting. Many have found no significantly increased risk for brain tumors in these workers (Jones et al, 1988; Wu et al, 1989; Hagmar et al, 1990; Simonato et al, 1991), while a large industrywide cohort study found significantly elevated brain cancer mortality (Wong et al, 1991).

Epidemiological studies of possible brain tumor risk in the petrochemical industry, many initiated as a result of a cluster of cases identified at a Texas petrochemical plant in 1978, have repeatedly reported elevated risk in workers or subgroups of workers in this industry (Table 58–5). Elevated brain tumor risk is not, however, a consistent finding (Rushton and Alderson, 1981; Wen et al, 1983). A subsequent case-control study in one Texas petrochemical plant sought to identify any associations between exposure to suspected chemical carcinogens (including benzene, diethyl sulfate, ethylene dichloride, ethylene oxide, and vinyl chloride) and brain tumor deaths; no association was found with exposure to any of these chemicals (Austin and Schnatter, 1983). This study was hampered, however, by the inability to determine exposure status for over 50% of the cases and controls as well as the general limitation of occupational studies in accurately quantifying specific exposures based on a subject's history of work in particular departments of the plant. To date, no specific carcinogen has been implicated in the observed elevated risk in this industry; indeed, the conclusion of a true elevation in risk remains controversial.

Epidemiological studies of brain tumor deaths have reported elevated brain tumor risk for a variety of electricity-related occupations involving exposure to electromagnetic fields (EMF) (Table 58–5). These include electrical or electronic engineers, electronics teachers, electrical technicians and assemblers (Thomas et al, 1987b; Loomis and Savitz, 1990), utility company service workers (Lin et al, 1985; Speers et al, 1988; Loomis and Savitz, 1990), workers in the communications industry (Speers et al, 1988) and electrical workers in manufacturing industries (Loomis and Savitz, 1990). All but one of these studies (Thomas et al, 1987b) utilized information on the death certificate as to cause of death and occupation, and are thus limited by potential misclassification of a person's lifetime occupation. More recently, epidemiological studies of incident brain tumors and electricity-related occupations have been conducted. A New Zealand case-control study of brain cancer found no excess risk for electrical workers in total, but did find an elevated risk for electricians alone (Reif et al, 1989). This study was limited by the use of the most recent occupational title as an indicator of a subject's usual occupation. Two studies have obtained complete occupational histories on incident brain tumor cases and controls (Schlehofer et al, 1990; Mack et al, 1991). One of these found a significantly elevated risk for women employed more than 5 years in electrical occupations; however, this association was not apparent in men (Schlehofer et al, 1990). The second study of incident brain tumors in Los Angeles County males found a significantly elevated risk for men employed more than 10 years in occupations involving potential exposure to EM fields (Mack et al, 1991). The elevated risk was confined to astrocytomas, and the majority of exposed case patients had worked as electricians or electrical engineers. Los Angeles incidence data for 1972–1985 show a significantly elevated PIR for gliomas among male electricians aged 25–64 (PIR=176; 20 cases) but not for other types of brain tumors. A cohort study of Swedish railway workers, who are highly exposed to low-frequency EMF, reported elevated brain tumor incidence in subjects who were less than age 30 at the initiation of follow-up (Floderus et al, 1994). In contrast, other cohort studies of electrical workers have shown no increased risk of brain cancer (Törnqvist et al, 1986; Tynes et al, 1992). Recent cohort and nested case-control studies of electrical utility workers have estimated actual magnetic field exposures by linking subjects' occupational histories to samples of magnetic field levels by job category. While one study found no association between brain cancer mortality and estimated magnetic field exposure (Sahl et al, 1993), another study found non-significantly elevated risks for incident brain cancer in subjects above the median and above the 90th percentile of cumulative magnetic field exposure (Theriault et al, 1994). In a cohort study of over 138,000 male employees of electric power companies, a significant trend of increasing brain cancer risk by estimated cumulative magnetic field exposure was found (Savitz and Loomis, 1995). This trend was even more pronounced for more recent exposures (accrued in the past 2–10 years), and was independent of the subjects' potential exposure to polychlorinated biphenyls and solvents. Although the implication of electromagnetic field exposure as a risk factor for the occurrence of brain tumors is tempting based on these observations, the possible association between brain tumor risk and other exposures common to this industry (such as organic solvents) must be considered (Modan, 1988).

Other epidemiological studies have reported elevated risks for workers in certain health professions, agricultural workers, workers in the nuclear industry, and workers in the rubber industry, particularly those involved in the manufacture of tires (Table 58–5). Specific exposures underlying these associations have been suggested but not established.

Parental Occupation and Childhood Brain Tumors. Several studies have investigated possible associations between occupational exposures of parents and the development of brain tumors in their children. These studies have yielded inconsistent results. One study found that fathers of children with brain tumors who died before age 15 were more often paper- or pulp-mill workers than were control fathers (Kwa and Fine, 1980). Another study of Los Angeles children with brain tumors diagnosed at age 10 or younger found that case fathers more often had job exposure to chemical solvents, in particular to paint, and that more case fathers worked in the aircraft industry (Peters et al, 1981). The Los Angeles study also found case mothers more often had jobs where they inhaled chemical fumes or got chemicals on their skin (Peters et al, 1981). No clear associations with parental occupation were seen in another study that included children with brain tumors compared to normal control subjects (Gold et al, 1982). A study in Washington State confirmed the association with father's employment in the aircraft industry only for young children (less than age 10) with brain tumors (Olshan et al, 1986). A case-control study in Texas found an association between central nervous system tumors in children and fathers' employment in the Air Force; all childhood cancer, but not central nervous system tumors in particular, was associated with employment in the aircraft industry (Hicks et al, 1984). A case-control study in New York State failed to find any association with fathers' employment in the aerospace industry or pulp or paper manufacturing or with paternal job exposure to hydrocarbons or electric and magnetic fields (Nasca et al, 1988). A weakness of this study relates to its design; as in several of the earlier investigations, fathers' occupational exposures were determined only through interviews with their wives.

Two reports of a case-control sample of 499 childhood CNS tumor deaths used birth certificate data on parental occupation. No significant association with tumor risk was found for father's employment in any of a series of hydrocarbon-related occupations. However, an elevated risk was found for children whose father had been employed in the printing or graphic arts industry and also for fathers working in the chemical or petroleum industries (Johnson et al, 1987). A significantly elevated risk was also found for father's employment as an electrician and in the electronics manufacturing industry (Johnson and Spitz, 1989). A similar mortality-based case-control study utilizing birth certificate data for parental occupation found an elevated brain cancer risk for children whose fathers had been employed in agricultural jobs (primarily as farmers), metal-related jobs, electrical assembly, installation or repair in the machine industry, and in structural jobs in the construction industry (Wilkins and Koutras, 1988). Another study found no relationship between parents' usual occupation in hydrocarbon-related occupations and risk of childhood brain tumors (Howe et al, 1989).

A case-control study of incident childhood brain tumors identified elevated risk with fathers' employment in agricultural, construction, metal, and food and tobacco industries (Wilkins and Sinks, 1990). When reported occupations were clustered together by inferred common exposures, there was an elevated tumor risk for children whose fathers had worked in occupations associated with aromatic amino and aromatic nitro compounds, aromatic hydrocarbons, nonionizing radiation, and paints and metals. In general, elevated risks were more apparent when these occupational exposures occurred in the preconception period. Using a job exposure matrix, another study found parental occupational exposure to creosote was associated with an elevated risk of childhood brain cancer (Feingold et al, 1992).

In summary, although two or more of the studies reviewed did find associations with parents' employment in paint-related, aircraft, electricity-related, agricultural, metal, and construction industries, these studies have failed to implicate any particular exposure. The marked inconsistency of these studies may be partially attributed to the often small sample sizes (leading to imprecise risk estimates); the different geographic areas (with different major industries) studied; the fact that a variety of tumor sites, age cutoffs, and years of diagnosis are used in different studies; the different sources of occupational data; and the varying criteria used for classifying occupations. The relevant period of exposure is also uncertain; it may be preconception (presumably affecting the parents' genetic material), during gestation, or during early childhood. All studies are limited by the fact that occupation is acting as a surrogate for specific environmental agents, the true exposures of interest.

Median Survival

Recent relative 5-year survival rates for brain and nervous system cancer are around 25% (24% for whites and 32% for blacks among U.S. cases diagnosed from

1981–1986) compared to just under 20% 20 years earlier (18% for whites and 19% for blacks diagnosed in 1960–1963) (Boring et al, 1991). Survival rates vary considerably by histologic type and by age. The relative 5-year survival rate in children aged 0–14 is now 59% compared to 35% 20 years ago (Boring et al, 1991; Crist and Kun, 1991).

In a recent study in Victoria, Australia, 52% of female brain tumor patients, compared to 37% of male ones, are alive 5 years after diagnosis (Preston-Martin, 1993b). As might be expected, nerve sheath tumors, tumors in the "other" category (mostly hemangiomas and gangliogliomas not classified as malignant), and meningiomas, all of which are predominantly benign, have the best prognosis; 100%, 96%, and 92% of patients with tumors of these three types survive 5 years. Patients with glioblastoma multiforme have the poorest prognosis (5% survive 5 years), and the proportion who survive 5 years is also low for patients with unspecified tumors (20%) and those whose tumors were not confirmed microscopically (28%). Survival for the other subtypes of glial tumors varies considerably. The proportion who are alive 5 years after diagnosis is considerably greater for patients with ependymoma (65%) and oligodendroglioma (61%) than for those with medulloblastoma (43%) or astrocytoma (44%). For most individual histologic types, survival curves for the two sexes are similar. However, females who develop meningioma are more likely to have benign tumors and survive significantly longer than males with meningiomas (94% versus 87% 5-year survival in women and men).

Secular Trend

The significance of reported changes in brain tumor incidence over time is difficult to assess for several reasons. Improvements in case finding and reporting as well as changes in coding practices specific to a cancer registry will yield apparent changes in incidence in areas covered by this registry (Flannery et al, 1985). An illustration of this problem is provided by Devesa and Silverman (1978), who reported decreases in brain tumor incidence based on data from the Second and Third National Cancer Surveys (conducted in 1947–1948 and 1969–1971, respectively). However, direct comparison of the two surveys was not possible for two reasons. First, the Second National Cancer Survey (SNCS) included benign as well as malignant brain tumors, whereas the Third included malignant tumors only. Second, 36% of the brain tumors identified by the SNCS had a histology of "cancer, including brain tumor" (suggesting a possible metastatic tumor) and 18% were identified solely by death certificate report, leading the investigators to conclude that the SNCS had overstated brain tumor incidence.

A second problem in interpreting secular trends in incidence is that of assessing changes in medical and diagnostic practices over time. With substantial improvements in diagnostic technology and concomitant increases in microscopic verification of brain tumors, it is likely that some portion of any observed increase in brain tumor incidence is due to these factors. For example, changes in brain tumor incidence reported from the Connecticut Tumor Registry (from 1.5 per 100,000 in males in 1935–1939 to 6.5 per 100,000 in 1975–1979, with analogous increases observed in the female population) were influenced by improvements in medical diagnostics, illustrated by the rise in the percentage of microscopically verified tumors, from 40% of all tumors in 1935–1939 to 94% of all tumors in 1980–1982 (Flannery et al, 1985).

Other factors, such as temporal changes in autopsy rates and in death certificate reporting of brain tumors (which are subject to inaccuracy when not histologically verified) will also affect reported incidence. Incidence data from three population-based registries (Connecticut, Birmingham, and Sweden) for males from four calendar periods (reported in volumes I to IV of *Cancer Incidence in Five Continents*) show increasing rates specific to older age groups (males aged 60–84). Improvements in diagnostic procedures as well as higher autopsy rates specific to this age group (resulting in an increase in identified cases) were suggested as possible explanations of this trend. Simultaneous analysis of histology-specific and age-specific secular changes would be most informative but remain to be done.

The magnitude of the problem in the interpretation of secular trends in brain tumor incidence is illustrated by Devesa and coworkers (1987), who, in reporting trends in cancer incidence for a multitude of primary sites, excluded brain and other nervous system tumors because of the inability to identify comparable categories over time. In this context, although it is difficult to assess any real changes in brain tumor incidence that may relate to changes in exposure to risk factors over time, there are suggestions of increases in brain tumor incidence over time. For example, as mentioned above, incidence for Connecticut males increased from 1.5 to 6.5 per 100,000 during a 40-year period. It is not known how much of this increase is attributable to increases in diagnostic efficiency and how much, if any, is a true increase in disease occurrence.

During the period from 1973 to 1987 the incidence of cancer of the brain and nervous system in the United States rose 23% and mortality increased 9.4% (Stephens, 1991). International increases in CNS tumor mortality and incidence ranged from 40% to over 100% in the 15 years between 1951–1958 and 1967–1973; increases were more modest in countries that already had high standards of medical care in the 1950s (Bahemuka et al, 1988).

Increased Incidence of Primary Brain Tumors in the Elderly. The increases in brain tumor rates have been greatest among the elderly. The incidence of primary brain tumors among U.S. residents over age 75 more than doubled from 1968 to 1985 (Davis and Schwartz, 1988; Greig et al, 1990). Similar increases in brain cancer mortality among those over age 65 occurred in Europe, Japan, and the United States (Davis, 1990). In Los Angeles County, incidence of malignant brain tumors among persons over age 70 has shown a significantly increasing trend since the beginning of the countywide registry in 1972. Rates in the 1984 to 1988 period are almost double the rates in the 1972 to 1975 period (for males, this increase in rates represents an excess risk of 10.4 per 100,000; for females, the increase in rates represents an excess risk of 7.6 per 100,000). This trend of increasing tumor rates is not apparent in the 40- to 69-year-old age group. Less substantial increases are noted in males aged 20 to 39 (excess risk of 1.3 per 100,000 between rates in 1972–1975 and rates in 1984–1988) and females aged 0 to 19 (excess risk of 0.7 per 100,000).

Some of this apparent increase undoubtedly results from more complete diagnosis, but how much might be attributable to improved diagnosis has been the topic of considerable debate (Levi and La Vecchia, 1989; Ahlbom and Rodvall, 1989; Ben-Shlomo and Smith, 1989; Boyle et al, 1990; Modan et al, 1992; Desmeules et al, 1992). Advanced imaging techniques such as CT scans and MRI enable doctors to diagnose brain tumors that previously might have been incorrectly diagnosed as strokes, senile dementia, or other neurological disorders, and recent analyses attribute both the increase in glioma and the decline in stroke rates among the elderly to improved diagnostic accuracy (Riggs, 1991a, b). For decades, brain tumor age-specific incidence appeared to peak around age 60 in Los Angeles County and most other geographic areas; however, it seemed likely that this peak was an artifact of underdiagnosis among the elderly because rates continued to rise in older age groups in regions where autopsy rates are unusually high, such as Rochester County, Minnesota (Percy et al, 1972). An analysis of brain tumor data for Norway shows that the completeness of diagnosis, particularly among the elderly, depends heavily both on the autopsy rate and on the use of advanced imaging techniques (Helseth et al, 1988).

Increased Incidence of Brain Lymphomas. Primary CNS lymphoma is a rare tumor (<1% of all CNS tumors) that has been of interest because of its increasing incidence (Hochberg and Miller, 1988). It is known to occur in immunologically compromised patients such as organ transplant recipients (Schneck and Penn, 1971) and those with acquired immune deficiency syndrome (AIDS) (Gill et al, 1985). Analyses of SEER data show that U.S. rates of brain lymphoma almost tripled from 1973 to 1984 and that this increase occurred in age-sex groups (eg, elderly women) not at high risk of AIDS (Eby et al, 1988). Furthermore, the increase was not explained by a change in nosology (this tumor was formerly called microglioma). The increase was greater in those aged 60 or over (3.6-fold; from 7.9 to 28.7 per ten million) than in those under 60 (2.1-fold; from 1.9 to 3.9 per ten million, Eby et al, 1988). The extent to which increased diagnostic efficiency explains the rise in brain tumor rates, particularly among the elderly, needs to be evaluated, therefore, for lymphoma as well as for other specific histologic types.

Time and Space Clustering

Reports of community clusters of brain tumors have appeared in the literature (Brooks, 1972; Morantz et al, 1985), but several other studies have found no evidence for significant clustering (Kurtzke, 1969; Kurtzke and Stazio, 1967; Maroun and Jacob, 1973). Although the identification of such geographic concentrations of brain tumor cases allows the generation of hypotheses regarding potential environmental risk factors, most studies fail to implicate any suspected factors (Neuberger et al, 1991; Wilkins et al, 1991). One reported cluster identified six contiguous counties in eastern Kentucky with a brain tumor incidence 3.4 times that of the remainder of the state (with glioma incidence 4.4 times the remainder of the state). As this cluster area was relatively isolated from the rest of the state by rivers and mountains, and many of the cases had lived by tributaries of rivers, the area's rivers and streams were suspected to be a possible source of carcinogenic exposure. A subsequent investigation of incidence between 1969 and 1976 showed no difference in brain tumor rates between this area and the remainder of the state (Sims et al, 1979). It was concluded that the originally observed cluster was either a statistical fluctuation or that the exposures responsible for the cluster were no longer evident in this area.

A cluster reported in western Missouri in a town with a population of about 3000 (SMR=333.3 for a 10-year study period) was investigated through detailed interviews and site visits of possible places of exposure. The investigators hypothesized that direct or indirect exposures to pond water from an abandoned coal mining pit, chemicals in a local shoe factory, or pesticides in a local chicken hatchery were possible carcinogenic sources (Morantz et al, 1985). However, a later case-control study of this cluster failed to implicate any of these local environmental factors.

A number of apparent clusters of brain tumors or childhood cancer (including brain tumors) suspected to be related to higher than normal exposure to electric and magnetic fields are described in a recent review (Microwave News, 1990). Magnetic fields of greater than 10 mGauss (>2 mGauss is considered a high level of exposure for most residential studies) were found in and around the home of one of the four residents on a block in Milltown, NJ, who developed brain tumors. Four brain tumors occurred among residents on one block in Guilford, CT, where substation and high-voltage power lines are located. On the other hand, none of the homes of 11 brain tumor patients in a cluster in Monroe County, NY, were near high-voltage lines or substations. Two clusters of childhood cancer in California (one in San Francisco and one in MacFarland, a small agricultural town) are located near high-power radio transmitters, and radiofrequency radiation has been suggested as of possible etiologic relevance (Microwave News, 1990).

Another tumor cluster was reported in a Texas petrochemical plant in which 18 brain tumor deaths were identified in former employees of the plant (Morbidity Mortality Weekly Report, 1980). This initial identification led to a series of epidemiological studies of brain tumor risk at this and neighboring petrochemical plants in other geographic locations. Results of these studies are described in greater detail above in the Occupation and Industry section of this chapter and are summarized in Table 58–5. Findings of an elevated risk in this industry have failed to identify any specific exposures that might explain this observation.

In Ohio, a cluster of six children diagnosed with primary brain tumors was recently reported (Wilkins et al, 1991). Each child had one parent employed in the same electronics firm where more than 100 chemicals are used; all six parents were employed at the firm prior to, during, and after the index pregnancy. Attempts to identify common occupational exposures in these parents were not successful.

A recent report of a cluster of brain tumors in a New South Wales coal mine found that, in comparison to two control mines, a larger volume of solvents was used (Brown et al, 1993). The mine did not differ from the control mines on other environmental exposures (including ionizing and nonionizing radiation and other chemicals). In an agricultural research institute, a significant excess of brain tumor deaths in males was found, with all four cases occurring in research workers in the plant and soil science area (Daly et al, 1994). Specific causal exposures could not be identified.

Familiality

The numerous reports of families with two or more members who have nervous system tumors have been summarized in a review (Gold, 1980). There are few population-based studies of familial aggregation of central nervous system tumors. No difference was found in the incidence of intracranial tumors among relatives of 535 tumor patients compared to that of relatives of a control group (Hauge and Harvald, 1957). A study in Holland found the mortality rate from gliomas was four times higher among relatives of glioma patients than in the general population (van der Weil, 1959). In a death certificate study of children who died of cancer in the United States between 1960 and 1975, eight pairs of siblings (versus 0.9 pairs expected) died of brain tumors (Miller, 1968, 1971). One study found that Connecticut children with central nervous system tumors more often had relatives with nervous system tumors than did control children, but this familial occurrence, although statistically significant, was observed for fewer than 2% of the children with central nervous system tumors (Farwell and Flannery, 1984). Medulloblastoma and glioblastoma were overrepresented among children whose relatives had nervous system tumors (Farwell and Flannery, 1984). A large nationwide study found that children who had brain tumors and who also had relatives with CNS tumors had their tumors diagnosed at a younger age than average (Sussman et al, 1990). Another study found an excess of brain tumors among relatives of children with astrocytoma diagnosed before 5 years of age (Kuijten et al, 1990). What needs to be kept in mind is that population-based studies that have investigated associations of brain tumors with recognized predisposing genetic syndromes and/or with familial aggregations suggest that the proportion of brain tumors attributable to inheritance is no more than 4% (Bondy et al, 1991; Wrensch et al, 1990).

Clinical Associations

Brain tumors have been associated with various chronic diseases, but none of these suggested concordances have been investigated in more than one or two studies; they are, therefore, neither well established nor well understood. One study of glioma patients found that more case patients than control patients had a past history of tuberculosis (Ward et al, 1973), but a larger study that used more appropriate controls found no evidence to support this association (MacPherson, 1976). A Danish cohort of patients who had surgery for peptic ulcer was shown to have an excess of brain cancer (Toftgaard, 1988); this excess was observed in both men and women.

Gliomas, but not meningiomas, occur much less frequently in diabetic than in nondiabetic autopsied hospital patients (RR=0.2; Aronson and Aronson, 1965). This deficit of brain cancer deaths was confirmed in another cohort of diabetics (Kessler, 1970), and a case-control study of incident brain tumors has also reported reduced risk associated with diabetes (Schlehofer et al, 1992). Diabetics, in fact, have a lower frequency of all cancers at autopsy (Bell, 1957; Herdan, 1960).

In children with immunodeficiency diseases, there is an apparent excess of central nervous system neoplasms (Kersey et al, 1973; Kersey and Spector, 1975). Reticulum cell sarcoma, a normally rare cancer that occurs with much greater frequency in immunosuppressed transplant patients (Hoover and Fraumeni, 1973), occurs often as a brain tumor in this group of patients (Schneck and Penn, 1971).

Glioblastomas were diagnosed in two patients several months after the onset of stroke symptoms (Dobkin, 1985). Radiographic studies suggest that one tumor caused compressive occlusion mimicking embolism and the other surrounded a cerebral artery mimicking arteriosclerosis. A study of brain tumors in a cohort of Seventh-Day Adventists found an excess of meningioma patients had a history of stroke (Mills et al, 1989).

The clinical literature has described several patients with both multiple sclerosis (MS) and gliomas (Reagan and Freiman, 1973). A study of a cohort of MS patients in Sweden found no brain tumors among this group, but, because of the small size of the cohort, none would have been expected (Lindegård, 1985). It has been suggested that gliomas may develop in MS plaques, and a number of observations have been cited in support of this hypothesis. One such observation is that the proportion of gliomas that are multicentric is higher (28%) in MS patients with gliomas than in glioma patients without MS (2%–6%). It has not been clearly established, however, that MS patients have an excess glioma risk.

An excess of brain tumors has been reported in various cohorts of epileptics. A follow-up study of epileptics in Denmark found a marked excess of brain tumors among those who had been treated for seizures (with barbiturates) during the preceding 10 years and concluded that the tumor probably caused the seizures (Olsen et al, 1989). A U.S. study found no increase in risk related to in utero or childhood exposure to barbiturates after a history of epilepsy was considered (Goldhaber et al, 1990). The interpretation of these figures favored by the authors is that epilepsy was a sign of a slowly growing tumor and that there is no excess risk associated with treatment with anti-epileptic drugs. A 22-fold increase in brain tumor incidence was seen among residents of Rochester, Minnesota, who had seizure disorders (Shirts et al, 1986). Because most of the tumors occurred within 5 years after the onset of epilepsy, the seizures were likely to have been caused by the tumor. A study in Sweden found an almost 100-fold excess of brain tumors among younger epileptics, but no information was given on the number of years between the two diagnoses (Lindegård, 1985). Case-control studies have found elevated risks associated with prior epilepsy in adults (Schlehofer et al, 1992) and children (McCredie et al, 1994b), as would be expected because epilepsy is often an early brain tumor symptom. Studies have found no excess of CNS cancer in children born to epileptic mothers (Olsen et al, 1990) or children with a family history of epilepsy (Gold et al, 1994; McCredie et al, 1994a). One study however, has reported a significantly elevated risk of childhood astrocytoma related to family history of seizures (particularly childhood seizures) and epilepsy (Kuijten et al, 1993).

The best-established association of brain tumors with other primary neoplasms is the association of meningiomas with breast cancer. This association has been observed in a number of case reports, and an analysis of data from Connecticut and Norway showed that these two tumors occurred together in the same woman more frequently than would be expected by chance (Schoenberg et al, 1975; Helseth et al, 1989a). The Norwegian study also found that men with meningiomas were more likely to develop renal cancer (Helseth et al, 1989a). Clinicians should be aware of the meningioma/breast cancer association so that they will not assume that central nervous system lesions that are discovered after breast cancer diagnosis and treatment are metastatic (Mehta et al, 1983); this seems especially important because the breast cancer is usually diagnosed first (Knuckey et al, 1989). One large case series found that women with both breast cancer and meningioma were likely to have their meningioma located in the sphenoid ridge; they also sometimes had a third primary, which was often a genital cancer (Jacobs et al, 1987). The authors suggested that these three primary sites might be a combination of neoplasms that warrants further investigations. Tissues from meningiomas have been shown to contain hormone receptors but it is unclear whether or not this finding has etiologic implications (Halper et al, 1989).

The occurrence of multiple primary brain tumors of either similar or different histologic types is associated with the phakomatoses, but these tumors also occur in the absence of such syndromes (Deen and Laws, 1981). Several case reports have noted a brain tumor (often a meningioma) arising at the site of a prior brain tumor that was treated with radiation therapy, but only a small proportion of such double primary brain tumors in a clinical series were related to radiation treatment (Deen and Laws, 1981).

A deficit of allergic conditions has been found in two recent case-control studies for all brain tumors (Schlehofer et al, 1992) and glioma alone (Ryan et al, 1992a). Reduced brain tumor risk has also been noted for prior infections and colds, and elevated risk with meningitis (Schlehofer et al, 1992).

Summary of Descriptive Epidemiology

Perhaps the most important finding from our review of the descriptive epidemiology of brain tumors is that the pattern of occurrence varies considerably by histologic type. For gliomas: The sex ratio is greater than one; incidence declines after an early peak in individuals under age 10 and continues to rise again after age 25; rates are higher in whites than nonwhites and are lowest in Asians; and incidence increases with increasing social class, particularly in males. For meningiomas, the sex ratio is less than one, and the female excess is greatest from ages 25–54. These tumors first occur in the teenage years, and incidence increases with age. Rates in the oldest age groups would probably be considerably higher if a larger proportion of the population received cranial autopsies at death. Meningioma rates are higher in blacks than in whites and are higher in Jews than in non-Jews.

ETIOLOGIC HYPOTHESES

This section reviews findings from epidemiological studies that have investigated the possible association of human brain tumors with various suggested risk factors. Table 58–6 summarizes epidemiological studies of selected brain tumor risk factors. The numerous case reports and clinical series suggesting possible risk factors are not included in this table. Epidemiological studies investigating selected occupational exposures are reviewed in Table 58–5. Studies relating brain tumor risk to various chronic diseases are summarized in the Clinical Associations section of this chapter and are not included in Table 58–6. For each risk factor considered in Table 58–6, studies of childhood brain tumors, which have recently been reviewed (Kuijten and Bunin, 1993), are summarized first in order by publication date (most recent first), followed by studies of adult brain tumors and specific histologic types, which are also listed in reverse chronological order. Before beginning this review of risk factors summarized in Table 58–6, we will present in some detail a compelling etiologic hypothesis suggested by the experimental literature and discuss attempts to investigate this hypothesis epidemiologically.

Animal Models

A variety of chemical, physical, and biological agents can cause nervous system tumors in experimental animals. *N*-nitroso compounds (NOCs), in particular the nitrosoureas, are by far the most studied. These carcinogens show a striking nervous system selectivity in some species, including various primates, and tumors can be produced by relatively low levels of NOC precursors in the animals' food and drinking water. Because there is no reason to think that humans are less susceptible to these compounds, it is likely that NOCs cause cancer in them as well. Although NOC exposures in some occupational settings (eg, machine shops; tire and rubber factories) can be substantial most people have low-level, but virtually continuous, exposure to NOCs throughout life. But, because NOCs are the most potent of carcinogens in animals (and likely in humans as well), only small doses are needed to cause cancer.

N-Nitroso Compounds (NOCs)

Experimental Data. NOCs and their precursors are ubiquitous in our modern industrialized environment; they are also among the most potent experimental carcinogens (National Research Council [NRC], 1981; Lijinsky, 1992). This category of compounds contains two major subcategories—nitrosamines, which require metabolic activation, and nitrosamides, which do not. The nitrosamides, in particular the nitrosoureas, are effective nervous system carcinogens in a variety of species (Magee et al, 1976; Bogovski and Bogovski, 1981).

Neurogenic tumors can be caused by transplacental exposure to ethylnitrosourea (ENU) in various species, including the rat, mouse, rabbit, opossum, and monkey, through various routes of administration with either single-dose or chronic low-dose exposure (Rice and Ward, 1982). In rodents, these tumors occur in the brain, spinal cord, and peripheral nerves and are of various histologic types including gliomas, meningiomas, schwannomas, and sarcomas (Rice and Ward, 1982). In nonhuman primates, the nervous system tumors that are induced by transplacental exposure arise exclusively in the brain, have a histologic spectrum similar to that of pediatric brain tumors, and occur in young adult and immature monkeys (Rice, 1986).

If exposure is transplacental, only one fiftieth (1/50) of the dose of ENU required in adult animals is sufficient to cause 100% tumor induction (Ivankovic, 1979). This effect can be achieved if ENU precursors, ethyl urea, and

TABLE 58–6. *Summary of Selected Epidemiological Studies of Brain Tumor Risk Factors*

Risk Factor	*Study Design*	*Group Studied*	*Place*	*Risk Estimate*	*Reported by*	*Year*	*Comments*
TRAUMA	Case-control	Childhood brain tumors	New South Wales	OR=1.1	McCredie et al	1994b	Head injury seen by doctor/nurse
	Case-control	Astrocytomas, children	Delaware Valley	OR=0.7	Kuijten et al	1990	Head injury with loss of consciousness
	Case-control	Childhood brain tumors	Toronto	OR=2.2	Howe et al	1989	Birth injury or trauma
				OR=3.2[a]			Head and neck injury requiring medical attention
	Case-control	Childhood brain tumors	Los Angeles	OR=Infinite	Preston-Martin et al	1982b	Head, face severely bruised during delivery
	Case-control	Childhood brain tumors	Los Angeles	OR=3.0	Preston-Martin et al	1982b	Hospitalized for head injury
	Case-control	Childhood CNS tumors	Minneapolis	—[b]	Choi et al	1970b	Higher proportion of cases than controls had difficult delivery
	Case-control	Child and adult CNS tumors	Minneapolis		Choi et al	1970b	No association with head injury leading to hospitalization
	Case-control	Adult meningioma	Germany	OR=0.5	Schlehofer et al	1992	Any head injury with visit to a doctor, at least 5 years before diagnosis
		Adult glioma		OR=0.7			
	Case-control	Adult gliomas	Australia	OR=1.1	Ryan et al	1992a	Head injury with hospitalization
		Adult meningiomas		OR=1.7			
	Case-control	Meningiomas, men	Los Angeles	OR=2.3[a]	Preston-Martin et al	1989a	Serious head injury (ie, resulted in medical visit, loss of consciousness or dizziness). Significant dose-response by number of such injuries
	Case-control	Gliomas, men	Los Angeles	OR=0.8	Preston-Martin et al	1989a	Serious head injury
	Case-control	Acoustic neuromas, men	Los Angeles	OR=2.0	Preston-Martin et al	1989b	Had serious head injury ≥ 30 years before diagnosis
				OR=2.2[a]			Any job with loud noise ≥ 10 years prior to diagnosis; dose-response significant for years of exposure
	Case-control	Adult brain tumors	Toronto	OR=2.5[a]	Burch et al	1987	Significant association for any head injury/accident; not significant when restricted to accidents requiring medical attention
	Case-control	Meningiomas, men	Los Angeles	OR=1.9[a]	Preston-Martin et al	1983	Serious head injury
				OR=2.0[a]			Ever boxed as a sport
	Case-control	Meningiomas, women	Los Angeles	OR=2.0[a]	Preston-Martin et al	1980	Head injury treated medically

(continued)

TABLE 58–6. *Summary of Selected Epidemiological Studies of Brain Tumor Risk Factors (Continued)*

Risk Factor	*Study Design*	*Group Studied*	*Place*	*Risk Estimate*	*Reported by*	*Year*	*Comments*
	Cohort	Persons with head injuries followed for subsequent brain tumors	Minnesota	SIR=100	Annegers et al	1979	All brain tumors
				SIR=162			Meningiomas
							Average follow-up=10 years
DIAGNOSTIC X-RAY							
Dental	Case-control	Childhood brain tumors	New South Wales	OR=0.4	McCredie et al	1994b	Childhood dental x-rays
	Case-control	Astrocytomas, childhood	Delaware Valley	OR=0.9	Kuijten et al	1990	Childhood exposure
	Case-control	Brain tumors diagnosed at ages 15–24	Los Angeles	OR=2.5[a]	Preston-Martin et al	1982b	5 or more full-mouth x-rays 10 or more years before diagnosis
	Case-control	Adult glioma	Australia	OR=0.5[a]	Ryan et al	1992b	Exposure to amalgam fillings
				OR=0.4[a]			Exposure to diagnostic dental x-rays
	Case-control	Gliomas, men	Los Angeles	OR=3.0	Preston-Martin et al	1989a	Annual full-mouth x-rays after age 25 Significant frequency trend
	Case-control	Meningiomas, men	Los Angeles	OR=2.5	Preston-Martin et al	1989a	Annual full-mouth x-rays after age 25
	Case-control	Acoustic neuromas, men	Los Angeles	OR=2.4	Preston-Martin et al	1989b	Annual full-mouth x-rays after age 25
	Case-control	Adult brain tumors	Toronto	OR=1.2	Burch et al	1987	Ever versus never dental x-ray exposure
	Case-control	Meningiomas, men	Los Angeles	OR=2.7	Preston-Martin et al	1983	5 or more full-mouth dental x-rays before 1945
	Case-control	Meningiomas, women	Los Angeles	OR=4.0[a]	Preston-Martin et al	1980	Full-mouth x-ray before age 20; elevated but nonsignificant risks for other dental x-ray variables
Prenatal irradiation	Case-control	Childhood brain tumors	Sweden	OR=1.5	Rodvall et al	1990	No apparent confounding by obstetrical complications, mother's age or other factors
	Case-control	Astrocytomas, childhood	Delaware Valley	OR=0.9	Kuijten et al	1990	Mother had abdominal or pelvic x-ray during pregnancy
				OR=1.0			Child had head or neck x-ray not related to astrocytoma diagnosis or treatment
	Case-control	Childhood brain tumors	Los Angeles	OR=1.3	Preston-Martin et al	1982b	Prenatal exposure, maternal pelvic x-ray
	Case-control	Childhood cancer deaths	England, Wales	—[a,b]	Stewart et al	1958	Increased risk for prenatal x-ray exposure

(continued)

TABLE 58–6. *(Continued)*

Risk Factor	*Study Design*	*Group Studied*	*Place*	*Risk Estimate*	*Reported by*	*Year*	*Comments*
Medical	Case-control	Childhood brain tumors	New South Wales	OR=2.3	McCredie et al	1994b	Diagnostic x-rays to head
	Case-control	Childhood brain tumors	Toronto	OR=8.4[a]	Howe et al	1989	Skull x-rays 5 or more years before diagnosis
	Case-control	Adult meningioma	Germany	OR=0.6	Schlehofer et al	1992	Any diagnostic x-rays to head/neck, including dental x-rays
		Adult glioma		OR=1.2			
Radiation treatment to head	Cohort	Adults receiving radiation therapy for pituitary adenoma	Toronto	RR=16	Tsang et al	1993	
	Cohort	Persons with pituitary adenomas treated with surgery and radiation	U.K.	RR=9.4[a]	Brada et al	1992	Second brain tumors
	Case-control	Acoustic neuromas, men	Los Angeles	Infinite	Preston-Martin et al	1989b	Had ≥20 years before diagnosis
	Case-control	Adult brain tumors	Toronto	OR=2.7	Burch et al	1987	Ever x-rays to the head
	Cohort	Treated with radiation therapy for benign head, neck, and upper thoracic conditions	Chicago		Schneider et al	1985	66 neural tumors including peripheral neurilemmoma (25), acoustic neuroma (11), non-specified brain (7), meningioma (5), astrocytoma (4), glioma (3), others (11); relative risk not estimated
	Case-control	Meningiomas, men	Los Angeles	OR=7.0[a]	Preston-Martin et al	1983	X-ray treatment to head before age 20
	Cohort	Treated with nasopharyngeal radium irradiation to prevent deafness	Maryland	RR=Infinite	Sandler et al	1982	Brain cancer elevated in irradiated group, not statistically significant; 3 cases observed in irradiated group, none in nonirradiated group
	Cohort	Treated with scalp irradiation for tinea capitis as children	Israel	RR=8.4[a]	Ron et al	1988	All neural tumors of head and neck
							Strong dose response
				RR=33.1[a]			Nerve sheath tumors, all sites
				RR=18.8[a]			Nerve sheath tumors, head and neck
				RR=9.5[a]	Meningiomas		
				RR=2.6	Gliomas		
							Strong dose response

(continued)

TABLE 58–6. *Summary of Selected Epidemiological Studies of Brain Tumor Risk Factors (Continued)*

Risk Factor	Study Design	Group Studied	Place	Risk Estimate	Reported by	Year	Comments
	Cohort	Treated for tinea capitis as children: irradiated and nonirradiated groups	New York	RR=Infinite	Shore et al	1976	6 brain tumor cases in the irradiated group; no cases observed in the nonirradiated group
	Cohort	Treated with scalp irradiation for tinea capitis as children and two matched control groups	Israel	RR=7.0	Modan et al	1974	Referent nonirradiated population controls
				RR=3.5			Referent nonirradiated siblings
OTHER RADIATION	Cohort	A-bomb survivors	Japan	RR=4.8	Seyama et al	1979	Males in high-dose group (≥100 rads) No association in females
PARENTAL SMOKING	Case-control	Childhood brain tumors	Northern Italy	OR=1.7	Filippini et al	1994	Smoking during pregnancy
				OR=1.7			Nonsmoker exposed to light passive smoking during pregnancy
				OR=2.2[a]			Nonsmoker exposed to heavy passive smoking during pregnancy
	Case-control	Childhood brain tumors	New South Wales	OR=0.9	McCredie et al	1994a	Mother smoked during pregnancy
				OR=2.2[a]			Exposed to father's smoking during pregnancy
	Case-control	Childhood brain tumors	U.S.	OR=1.1	Gold et al	1993	Mother smoked during pregnancy
				OR=1.1			Father smoked >1 pack/day during year of child's birth
	Case-control	Astrocytomas, children	Delaware Valley	OR=1.0	Kuijten et al	1990	Mother smoked during pregnancy
				OR=0.8			Mother exposed to sidestream smoke during pregnancy
	Case-control	Childhood brain tumors	Toronto	OR=1.4	Howe et al	1989	Mother smoked during pregnancy
				OR=1.1			Father smoked during the pregnancy
	Case-control	Childhood brain tumors	Los Angeles	OR=1.5[a]	Preston-Martin et al	1982b	Prenatal exposure, maternal contact to sidestream smoke
				OR=1.1			Maternal smoking during pregnancy
	Case-control	Childhood brain tumors	Maryland	OR=5.0	Gold et al	1979	Continued maternal smoking during pregnancy
SMOKING	Case-control	Adult meningiomas	Australia	OR=1.9[a]	Ryan et al	1992a	Exposed to spouse's tobacco smoke
		Adult gliomas		OR=1.2			
	Case-control	Adult meningiomas	Australia	OR=1.8	Ryan et al	1992a	Any tobacco product
		Adult gliomas		OR=1.2			

(continued)

TABLE 58–6. *(Continued)*

Risk Factor	*Study Design*	*Group Studied*	*Place*	*Risk Estimate*	*Reported by*	*Year*	*Comments*
	Case-control	Gliomas, men	Los Angeles	OR=0.7	Preston-Martin et al	1989a	Ever smoked
		Meningiomas, men		OR=1.2			
	Case-control	Adult brain tumors	Toronto	OR=1.4	Burch et al	1987	Smoking plain (nonfilter) cigarettes, dose response significant
	Cohort	Adult brain tumor deaths	Japan	RR=3.0	Hirayama	1984	Nonsmoking wives, husband smoked 1–14 cigarettes/day
				RR=6.2			Husband smoked 15–19 cigarettes/day
				RR=4.3			Husband smoked 20+ cigarettes/day Significant dose response trend
	Case-control	Meningiomas, men	Los Angeles		Preston-Martin et al	1983	No association with tobacco use
	Case-control	Meningiomas, women	Los Angeles	OR=1.4	Preston-Martin et al	1980	Ever smoked more than 100 cigarettes; dose-response significant for amount smoked per day, not significant for total amount smoked (pack-years)
INCENSE BURNING	Case-control	Childhood brain tumors	New South Wales	OR=1.3	McCredie et al	1994a	Regular use during pregnancy
	Case-control	Astrocytomas, children	Delaware Valley	OR=1.4	Kuijten et al	1990	Prenatal exposure
	Case-control	Childhood brain tumors	Los Angeles	OR=3.3[a]	Preston-Martin et al	1982b	Prenatal exposure
DIETARY Nonpublic water	Case-control	Childhood brain tumors	Toronto	—[b]	Howe et al	1989	May contain higher levels of nitrates or nitrites
Spring water	Case-control	Adult brain tumors	Toronto	OR=4.3[a]	Burch et al	1987	Ever used spring water, dose-response significant for duration of use; other water sources not significantly associated
Alcohol	Case-control	Astrocytomas, childhood	Delaware Valley	OR=1.4	Kuijten et al	1990	Mother's use during pregnancy
	Case-control	Childhood brain tumors	Los Angeles		Preston-Martin et al	1982b	No association with alcohol use during mother's pregnancy
	Case-control	Adult brain tumors	Toronto	OR=2.1[a]	Burch et al	1987	Ever drank wine, significant dose-response trend; no association with other alcohol products
	Case-control	Adult CNS tumors	Minneapolis	—[a,c]	Choi et al	1970b	Significantly higher proportion of controls reported ever drinking alcoholic beverages
	Case-control	Meningiomas, men	Los Angeles		Preston-Martin et al	1983	No association with alcohol use

(continued)

TABLE 58–6. *Summary of Selected Epidemiological Studies of Brain Tumor Risk Factors (Continued)*

Risk Factor	Study Design	Group Studied	Place	Risk Estimate	Reported by	Year	Comments
Beer	Case-control	Gliomas, adults Meningiomas, adults	Australia	OR=0.8 OR=0.5	Ryan et al	1992a	Any use
	Case-control	Childhood brain tumors	Toronto	OR=3.5[a]	Howe et al	1989	Mother drank during pregnancy
	Case-control	Childhood brain tumors	Los Angeles	OR=1.0	Preston-Martin et al	1982b	Mother drank during pregnancy
	Case-control	Gliomas, men	Los Angeles	OR=0.7	Preston-Martin et al	1989a	Drank at least once a month
	Case-control	Gliomas, adults	Toronto	OR=1.2	Burch et al	1987	Ever drank
Wine	Case-control	Gliomas, adults Meningiomas, adults	Australia	OR=0.6[a] OR=0.5[a]	Ryan et al	1992a	Any use
	Case-control	Gliomas, men	Los Angeles	OR=0.7	Preston-Martin et al	1989a	Drank at least once a month
	Case-control	Gliomas, adults	Toronto	OR=2.1[a]	Burch et al	1987	Ever drank
Spirits	Case-control	Gliomas, adults	Australia	OR=0.8	Ryan et al	1992a	Any use
		Meningiomas, adults		OR=0.7			
	Case-control	Gliomas, men	Los Angeles	OR=1.3	Preston-Martin et al	1989a	Drank at least once a month
	Case-control	Gliomas, adults	Toronto	OR=1.0	Burch et al	1987	Ever drank
Cured meats/fish	Case-control	Astrocytoma, children	U.S. and Canada	OR=1.7	Bunin et al	1994	Highest quartile of mother's pregnancy diet
	Case-control	Childhood brain tumors	New South Wales	OR=2.5[a]	McCredie et al	1994a	Highest quartile of mother's pregnancy diet; trend significant
	Case-control	Childhood brain tumors	New South Wales	OR=2.0	McCredie et al	1994b	High vs no intake; child's diet in first year
	Case-control	Childhood brain tumors	Denver	OR=2.3	Sarasua and Savitz	1994	Mother ate hot dogs at least weekly during pregnancy
				OR=2.1			Child ate hot dogs at least weekly
	Case-control	Astrocytomas, childhood	Delaware Valley	OR=1.9	Kuijten et al	1990	Mother ate during pregnancy Significant trend for frequency
	Case-control	Childhood brain tumors	Toronto	OR=1.1	Howe et al	1989	Child ate >1 serving per week
	Case-control	Childhood brain tumors	Los Angeles	OR=1.2 (moderate consumption) OR=2.3 (high consumption)	Preston-Martin et al	1982b	Prenatal exposure (maternal consumption); significant dose-response relationship; also significant dose-response for childhood consumption, but not independent of maternal consumption
	Case-control	Gliomas, men	Australia	OR=3.1[a] OR=2.5[a]	Giles et al	1994	High intake of bacon High intake of corned meat
		Gliomas, women		OR=0.5			High intake of bacon

(continued)

TABLE 58–6. *(Continued)*

Risk Factor	Study Design	Group Studied	Place	Risk Estimate	Reported by	Year	Comments
				OR=0.8			High intake of corned meat
	Case-control	Adult glioma	Germany	OR=2.1[a]	Boeing et al	1993	Highest tertile of processed meat; significant trend
	Case-control	Meningiomas, men	Los Angeles	OR=1.6	Preston-Martin and Mack	1991	Daily consumption of cured meats
		Gliomas, men		OR=1.0			Daily consumption of cured meats
	Case-control	Adult brain tumors	Toronto	OR=7.0	Burch et al	1987	Regular consumption (at least once a month) of pickled fish, little excess for other processed meat and fish products
	Case-control	Meningiomas, men	Los Angeles		Preston-Martin et al	1983	No association with consumption of all types of cured meats
	Case-control	Meningiomas, women	Los Angeles	OR=2.8[a]	Preston-Martin et al	1980	Moderate or high consumption of high-nitrite meats, dose- response significant; OR=1.2 for childhood consumption
Fruits	Case-control	Childhood brain tumors	New South Wales	OR=1.5	McCredie et al	1994a	Highest quartile of mother's pregnancy diet; trend NS
	Case-control	Childhood brain tumors	New South Wales	OR=0.4	McCredie et al	1994b	Highest quartile of child's diet in 1st year, trend NS
	Case-control	PNET, children	U.S. and Canada	OR=0.3[a]	Bunin et al	1993	Highest quartile of mother's pregnancy diet; significant trend
	Case-control	Childhood brain tumors	Toronto	OR=0.2[a]	Howe et al	1989	Child drank >1 glass of fruit juice per week
	Case-control	Gliomas, men	Australia	OR=1.5	Giles et al	1994	Highest tertile of consumption
		Gliomas, women		OR=0.7			
	Case-control	Adult glioma	Germany	OR=1.1	Boeing et al	1993	Highest tertile of consumption
	Case-control	Meningiomas, men	Los Angeles	OR=0.4	Preston-Martin and Mack	1991	Ate citrus ≥5 times per week
		Gliomas, men		OR=0.8			Ate citrus ≥5 times per week
	Case-control	Gliomas, adult	Toronto	—[c]	Burch et al	1987	Protective effect (although significant only for oranges, peaches, bananas) for regular consumption of a variety of fruits
Vegetables	Case-control	Childhood brain tumors	New South Wales	OR=0.4	McCredie et al	1994a	Highest quartile of mother's pregnancy diet; P trend = 0.06
	Case-control	PNET, children	U.S. and Canada	OR=0.4[a]	Bunin et al	1993	Highest quartile of mother's pregnancy diet; significant trend

(continued)

TABLE 58–6. *Summary of Selected Epidemiological Studies of Brain Tumor Risk Factors (Continued)*

Risk Factor	Study Design	Group Studied	Place	Risk Estimate	Reported by	Year	Comments
	Case-control	Gliomas, men	Australia	OR=1.0	Giles et al	1994	Highest tertile of consumption
		Gliomas, women		OR=0.5[a]			
	Case-control	Adult glioma	Germany	OR=0.9	Boeing et al	1993	Highest tertile of consumption
NOC-RELATED NUTRIENTS							
Nitrate	Case-control	Astrocytoma, children	U.S. and Canada	OR=0.7	Bunin et al	1994	Highest quartile of mother's pregnancy diet; trend NS
	Case-control	PNET, children	U.S. and Canada	OR=0.4[a]	Bunin et al	1993	Highest quartile of mother's pregnancy diet; significant trend
	Case-control	Adult glioma	Germany	OR=0.9	Boeing et al	1993	Highest tertile of consumption
	Case-control	Gliomas, men	Australia	OR=1.1	Giles et al	1994	Highest tertile of consumption
		Gliomas, women		OR=0.5[a]			
Nitrite	Case-control	Astrocytoma, children	U.S. and Canada	OR=1.3	Bunin et al	1994	Highest quartile of mother's pregnancy diet; trend NS
	Case-control	PNET, children	U.S. and Canada	OR=1.1	Bunin et al	1993	Highest quartile of mother's pregnancy diet; trend NS
	Case-control	Gliomas, men	Australia	OR=1.6	Giles et al	1994	Highest tertile of consumption
		Gliomas, women		OR=1.0			
	Case-control	Adult glioma	Germany	OR=1.1	Boeing et al	1993	Highest tertile of consumption
Nitrosamines	Case-control	Astrocytoma, children	U.S. and Canada	OR =0.8	Bunin et al	1994	Highest quartile of mother's pregnancy diet; trend NS
	Case-control	PNET, children	U.S. and Canada	OR=1.6	Bunin et al	1993	Highest quartile of mother's pregnancy diet; trend NS
	Case-control	Gliomas, men	Australia	OR=1.8[a]	Giles et al	1994	Highest tertile of consumption of NDMA
		Gliomas, women		OR=1.4			
	Case-control	Adult glioma	Germany		Boeing et al	1993	Highest tertile of consumption:
				OR=2.8[a]			NDMA, significant trend
				OR=3.4[a]			NPYR, significant trend
				OR=2.7[a]			NPIP, significant trend
OTHER MICRO-NUTRIENTS	Case-control	PNET, children	U.S. and Canada		Bunin et al	1993	Highest quartile of mother's pregnancy diet; all trends significant:
				OR=0.6			Vitamin A
				OR=0.4[a]			Vitamin C
				OR=0.5			Beta-carotene
				OR=0.3[a]			Folate
	Case-control	Astrocytoma, children	U.S. and Canada		Bunin et al	1994	Highest quartile of mother's pregnancy diet; all trends NS
				OR=0.7			Vitamin A
				OR=0.7			Vitamin C
				OR=1.0			Beta-carotene
				OR=1.0			Folate

(continued)

TABLE 58–6. *(Continued)*

Risk Factor	Study Design	Group Studied	Place	Risk Estimate	Reported by	Year	Comments
	Case-control	Gliomas, men	Australia		Giles et al	1994	Highest tertile of consumption:
				OR=1.7[a]			Vitamin E
				OR=1.4			Vitamin C
				OR=1.0			Beta-carotene
		Gliomas, women		OR=1.1			Vitamin E
				OR=0.6			Vitamin C
				OR=0.7			Beta-carotene
	Case-control	Adult glioma	Germany	OR=0.9	Boeing et al	1993	Highest tertile of vitamin C consumption
VITAMIN SUPPLEMENTS	Case-control	Astrocytoma, children	U.S. and Canada		Bunin et al	1994	Any use during pregnancy:
				OR=0.5[a]			Iron
				OR=0.4			Calcium
				OR=0.6			Multivitamins
	Case-control	Childhood brain tumors	New South Wales		McCredie et al	1994b	Highest quartile of child's diet in 1st year:
				OR=0.9			Vitamin supplements
				OR=0.5			Vitamin syrup
	Case-control	PNET, children	U.S. and Canada		Bunin et al	1993	Any use during pregnancy:
				OR=0.4[a]			Iron
				OR=0.4[a]			Calcium
				OR=0.3[a]			Vitamin C
				OR=0.6[a]			Multivitamins, first 6 weeks of pregnancy
	Case-control	Childhood brain tumors	Toronto	OR=0.9	Howe et al	1989	Child used at least once a week
	Case-control	Childhood brain tumors	Los Angeles	OR=0.6	Preston-Martin et al	1982b	Maternal use during pregnancy; exposure information obtained by asking about "Other drug" use
	Case-control	Adult glioma	Germany	OR=1.2	Boeing et al	1993	High vitamin supplement use
	Case-control	Gliomas, men	Los Angeles	OR=0.6[a]	Preston-Martin and Mack	1991	Took vitamins ≥ twice a day
		Meningiomas, men					No association
	Case-control	Adult brain tumors	Toronto	OR=0.8	Burch et al	1987	Regular use of vitamin C
				OR=0.5			Regular use of vitamin A
				OR=0.4[a]			Regular use of vitamin E
LEAD	Case-control	Childhood brain tumors	Toronto	OR=0.9	Howe et al	1989	Child had contact with
	Case-control	Childhood brain tumors	Los Angeles	OR=1.4	Preston-Martin et al	1982b	Ate paint flakes
INSECTICIDES/ PESTICIDES	Case-control	Childhood brain tumors	New South Wales	OR=2.0	McCredie et al	1994a	House treated for pests during pregnancy
	Case-control	Childhood brain tumors	New South Wales	No association	McCredie et al	1994b	Child exposed to house treated for pests

(continued)

TABLE 58–6. *Summary of Selected Epidemiological Studies of Brain Tumor Risk Factors (Continued)*

Risk Factor	*Study Design*	*Group Studied*	*Place*	*Risk Estimate*	*Reported by*	*Year*	*Comments*
	Case-control	Childhood brain tumors	Missouri		Davis et al	1993	Range of ORs given for three exposure periods: pregnancy, 0-6 months, 7 months to diagnosis
				OR=1.8–3.4[a]			Pesticides for nuisance pests
				OR=1.1–2.1			Bombs used for nuisance pests
				OR=3.7[a]–5.2[a]			No-Pest Strips
				OR=2.9[a]			Any termite treatment
				OR=4.6[a]			Kwell shampoo for head lice
				OR=0.6–4.8			Exposed to pesticides for pets
				OR=0.9–5.5[a]			Exposed to flea collars on pets
				OR=0.5–4.2			Exposed to pet shampoo
				OR=1.5–2.3			Insecticides in garden/orchard
				OR=1.5			Carbaryl used in garden/orchard
				OR=4.6[a]			Diazinon used in garden/orchard
				OR=1.1–2.4			Herbicides used on yard
	Case-control	Childhood brain tumors	Los Angeles	OR=1.5	Preston-Martin et al	1982b	Prenatal exposure to pesticides
				OR=1.1			Childhood exposure to pesticides
	Case-control	Childhood brain tumors	Maryland	OR=2.3	Gold et al	1979	Exterminations in home prior to diagnosis
FARM RESIDENCE/ EXPOSURE TO ANIMALS	Case-control	Childhood brain tumors	New South Wales	OR=0.9	McCredie et al	1994a	Mother on farm during pregnancy
				OR=0.9			Cat in home during pregnancy
	Case-control	Childhood brain tumors	New South Wales	OR=0.6	McCredie et al	1994b	Child on farm>1 month
				OR=0.7			Regular contact with horses
	Case-control	Childhood brain tumors	Maryland	OR=4.0[a]	Gold et al	1979	Ever lived on farm and exposed to farm animals
				OR=4.5			Exposure to sick pets
	Case-control	Meningiomas, men	Los Angeles		Preston-Martin et al	1983	No association with farm residence after controlling for history of head injury
	Case-control	Meningiomas, women	Los Angeles	OR=0.8	Preston-Martin et al	1980	Ever lived on farm
MEDICATIONS	Case-control	Childhood brain tumors	New South Wales		McCredie et al	1994a	Mother used in month before or during pregnancy:
				OR=0.4			Fertility drugs
				OR=0.8			Oral contraceptives
				OR=0.5			Diuretics
				OR=0.7			Sleeping pills/ tranquilizers

(continued)

TABLE 58–6. *(Continued)*

Risk Factor	Study Design	Group Studied	Place	Risk Estimate	Reported by	Year	Comments
				OR=2.2			Nonprescription pain medication
				OR=0.8			Oral antihistamines
				OR=3.1			Cold/cough medications
	Case-control	Astrocytomas, childhood	Delaware Valley		Kuijten et al	1990	Prenatal exposure:
				OR=2.0[a]			Antinausea drugs
				OR=1.1			Neurally active drugs
				OR=0.9			Antihistamines
				OR=0.5			Diuretics
				OR=2.8			Marijuana
	Case-control	Childhood brain tumors	Toronto	OR=0.2	Howe et al	1989	Mother took barbiturates or Dilantin during pregnancy
	Case-control	Childhood brain tumors	Los Angeles		Preston-Martin et al	1982b	Prenatal exposure:
				OR=3.4[a]			Antihistamines
				OR=2.0[a]			Diuretics
				OR=Infinite[a]			General anesthesia
	Case-control	Childhood brain tumors	Maryland	OR=3.0	Gold et al	1978	Mother used barbiturates during pregnancy or child used barbiturates prior to diagnosis; normal control group
				OR=5.5[a]			Mother used barbiturates during pregnancy or child used barbiturates prior to diagnosis; other cancer control group
	Case-control	Adult brain tumors	Toronto	OR=0.7	Burch et al	1987	Regularly took medication for headaches, inability to sleep, aches and pains, etc.
				OR=0.5[a]			Ever treatment for hypertension
				OR=5.0[a]			Ever took Dilantin
HAIR DYES/HAIR SPRAYS	Case-control	Childhood brain tumors	New South Wales	OR=0.8	McCredie et al	1994a	Mother used hair dye during pregnancy
	Case-control	Astrocytomas, children	Delaware Valley	OR=0.9	Kuijten et al	1990	Mother used hair dye during pregnancy
	Case-control	Adult brain tumors	Toronto	OR=2.0[a]	Burch et al	1987	Ever used hair dye or hair spray
	Case-control	Meningiomas, women	Los Angeles	OR=1.0	Preston-Martin et al	1980	Ever used hair dyes or tints
FACE MAKEUP	Case-control	Childhood brain tumors	New South Wales	OR=0.4	McCredie et al	1994a	Mother used facial foundation during pregnancy
	Case-control	Astrocytomas, children	Delaware Valley	OR=0.7	Kuijten et al	1990	Mother used facial makeup during pregnancy
	Case-control	Childhood brain tumors	Los Angeles	OR=1.6[a]	Preston-Martin et al	1982b	Prenatal exposure; frequent maternal use

(continued)

TABLE 58–6. *Summary of Selected Epidemiological Studies of Brain Tumor Risk Factors (Continued)*

Risk Factor	*Study Design*	*Group Studied*	*Place*	*Risk Estimate*	*Reported by*	*Year*	*Comments*
ELECTRO-MAGNETIC FIELDS	Cohort	Incidence of nervous system tumors, children living close to overhead power lines	Finland		Verkasalo et al	1993	Exposed to calculated magnetic fields ≥0.20 microteslas:
				SIR=230			All children
				SIR=420[a]			Boys
				SIR=0			Girls
	Case-control	Childhood CNS tumors	Denmark	OR=1.0	Olsen et al	1993	Resided near high voltage installations of ≥0.1 calculated microteslas
	Case-control	Childhood CNS tumors	Sweden	OR=0.7	Feychting and Ahlbom	1993	Resided near power lines of ≥0.20 calculated microteslas
	Cohort	Persons residing near power lines and transformer substation	Netherlands		Schreiber et al	1993	
		Males		SMR=65			
		Females		SMR=175			
	Case-control	Astrocytomas, childhood	Delaware Valley	OR=1.6	Kuijten et al	1990	Mother used electric blanket during pregnancy
	Case-control	Childhood brain tumors	Colorado	OR=2.5[a]	Savitz et al	1990	Mother used electric blanket during pregnancy
	Case-control	Childhood brain tumors	Colorado	OR=2.0[a]	Savitz et al	1988	Wire configuration suggestive of high versus low magnetic field levels
				OR=1.0			Measured magnetic fields in home at 2.0 milligaus under low-power conditions
	Case-control	Childhood nervous system tumors	Sweden	OR=3.7[a]	Tomenius	1986	Measured magnetic field at least 3.0 milligaus at entrance to home
				OR=3.9			Visible 200-kV wires within 150 meters of home
	Case-control	Childhood nervous system tumor deaths	Colorado	—[b]	Wertheimer and Leeper	1979	Higher proportion of cases than controls lived near electrical wire configurations suggestive of high current flow
	Case-control	Gliomas, adults	Australia	OR=1.5	Ryan et al	1992a	Used electric blanket
				OR=0.7			Used electrically heated waterbed
		Meningiomas, adults		OR=0.9			Used electric blanket
				OR=1.3			Used electrically heated waterbed
	Case-control	Adult nervous system tumor deaths	Colorado	—[a,b]	Wertheimer and Leeper	1982	Significantly more case-control pairs with case having higher current configuration outside of home

(continued)

TABLE 58–6. *(Continued)*

Risk Factor	Study Design	Group Studied	Place	Risk Estimate	Reported by	Year	Comments
FAMILY HISTORY OF DISEASE	Case-control	Childhood brain tumors	U.S.	OR=0.8	Gold et al	1994	Parental history of epilepsy
				OR=1.6[a]			Mother had birth defect
				OR=2.1[a]			Maternal relatives with birth defects
				OR=1.4			Tumors in paternal relatives
				OR=1.0			Family history of brain tumors
	Case-control	Childhood brain tumors	New South Wales	OR=1.4	McCredie et al	1994a	Family history of NS tumors
				OR=1.0			Family history of epilepsy
				OR=1.2			Family history of any cancer
	Case-control	PNET, children	U.S. and Canada	OR=3.0	Kuijten et al	1993	Childhood cancers in relatives
		Astrocytoma, children		OR=2.5[a]			Relative with seizures
				OR=3.4[a]			Relative with childhood seizures
				OR=3.0			Relative with epilepsy
	Cohort	Relatives of children brain tumor subjects	Texas	SIR=88	Bondy et al	1991	No excess of all cancer
				SIR=310[a]			Colon cancer
	Case-control	Astrocytomas, children	Delaware Valley	OR=1.7[a]	Kuijten et al	1990	Had relative with cancer. Association strongest for cases ages 0–4 years and with second-degree relatives
				OR=4.5			Had relative with brain tumor Significant for cases ages 0–4
	Case-control	Childhood brain tumors	Maryland		Gold et al	1979	No association with family history of cancer or congenital disorders
	Case-control	Childhood and adult CNS tumors	Minneapolis	—[a,b]	Choi et al	1970b	Significantly higher rate of CNS tumors in families of cases (all CNS tumors and gliomas alone) than in families of controls
	Case-control	Adult meningioma	Australia	OR=1.3	Ryan et al	1992a	Family history of brain tumor
				OR=0.8			Family history of epilepsy
	Case-control	Gliomas, men	San Francisco	OR=1.6[a]	Wrensch and Barger	1990	Relative had cancer
	Case-control	Gliomas, men	Los Angeles	OR=1.0	Preston-Martin et al	1989a	Had first-degree blood relative with cancer.
		Meningiomas, men		OR=1.0			Had first-degree blood relative with cancer

(continued)

TABLE 58–6. *Summary of Selected Epidemiological Studies of Brain Tumor Risk Factors (Continued)*

Risk Factor	Study Design	Group Studied	Place	Risk Estimate	Reported by	Year	Comments
				OR=3.3[a]			Two or more of these relatives had cancer. Also, two cases had relatives with a meningioma
	Case-control	Adult brain tumors	Toronto	OR=1.5	Burch et al	1987	Any blood relatives with cancer
	Case-control	Meningiomas, women	Los Angeles	OR=1.0	Preston-Martin et al	1980	Any relatives with CNS tumors
				OR=0.9			Any relatives with cancer
TONSILLECTOMY	Case-control	Childhood brain tumors	Los Angeles	OR=1.0	Preston-Martin et al	1982b	
	Case-control	Childhood brain tumors	Maryland	OR=0.6	Gold et al	1979	
INFECTION	Case-control	Adult gliomas	Australia	OR=1.0	Ryan et al	1993	Test positive for *Toxoplasma gondii* infection
		Adult meningiomas		OR=2.1			
	Case-control	Adult and child brain tumors	Minnesota	—[a,b]	Schuman et al	1967	Higher proportion of cases than controls tested positive for *Toxoplasma gondii* infection; particularly evident for astrocytomas
BIRTH ORDER	Case-control	Childhood brain tumors	Australia	OR=1.1	McCredie et al	1994b	Firstborn
	Case-control	Astrocytomas, children	Delaware Valley	OR=1.0	Kuijten et al	1990	Firstborn
	Case-control	Childhood brain tumors	Toronto	OR=0.5[a]	Howe et al	1989	Firstborn
	Case-control	Childhood brain tumors	Los Angeles		Preston-Martin et al	1982b	No association
	Case-control	Childhood brain tumors	Maryland	OR=1.7	Gold et al	1979	Firstborn
	Case-control	Childhood CNS tumors (less than age 20)	Minneapolis	—[b]	Choi et al	1970b	Higher proportion of cases were firstborn; analysis included only 20 case-control pairs
	Case-control	Gliomas, men	San Francisco		Wrensch and Barger	1990	No association
	Case-control	Adult brain tumors	Toronto		Burch et al	1987	No association
BIRTH WEIGHT	Case-control	Childhood brain tumors	Australia	OR=0.9	McCredie et al	1994b	8 pounds or more
	Case-control	Childhood brain tumors	Washington State	OR=1.4	Emerson et al	1991	High birth weight
		Astrocytoma		OR=1.9[a]			High birth weight
	Case-control	Childhood brain tumors	Toronto	OR=1.1	Howe et al	1989	≥8.0 pounds versus <8.0 pounds
	Case-control	Childhood brain tumors	Washington State	OR=1.4	Emerson et al	1991	Birth weight ≥4000 g
				OR=1.9			Increased risk seen only in females
	Case-control	Childhood brain tumors	Los Angeles		Preston-Martin et al	1982b	No difference in mean birth weight
	Case-control	Childhood brain tumors	Maryland	OR=2.6[a]	Gold et al	1979	Birth weight 3629 grams or greater

(continued)

TABLE 58–6. (*Continued*)

Risk Factor	Study Design	Group Studied	Place	Risk Estimate	Reported by	Year	Comments
REPRODUCTIVE FACTORS	Case-control	Astrocytoma, children	Washington State	OR=1.9	Emerson et al	1991	History of prior fetal deaths
				OR=2.2[a]			Older maternal age
	Case-control	Brain cancers, women	Iowa	OR=0.4[a]	Cantor et al	1993	Ever parous
	Case-control	Brain tumors, women	Germany	OR=1.3	Schlehofer et al	1992	Ever parous
		Meningiomas		OR=0.6			Menopausal
				OR=0.1			Bilateral oophorectomy
		Gliomas, acoustic neuromas		OR=1.8			Menopausal
				OR=0.3			Bilateral oophorectomy

[a]$P \leq 0.05$.
[b]Positive association found, risk estimate not provided, or summarizes results for a number of related variables.
[c]Negative association found, risk estimate not provided, or summarizes results for a number of related variables.
Abbreviations: OR = odds ratio; RR = relative risk; SIR = standardized incidence ratios; SMR = standardized mortality ratios; NS = not significant

sodium nitrite, are added to the food and drinking water of a pregnant animal; however, no tumors develop if ascorbate (vitamin C) is also added to her diet (Mirvish, 1981). ENU exposure leads to the formation of O_6-ethylguanine, a mutagen removed more slowly from brain DNA than from DNA of other tissues (Rajewsky et al, 1976). The inability of the brain to remove this mutagen quickly coupled with the high rate of DNA replication in the fetal brain may explain why fetal animals are more sensitive than adults and why the brain is more sensitive than other tissues to the carcinogenic effects of ENU (Rajewsky et al, 1976); however, other investigators argue that this DNA alkylation may not be the key event in tumor development, although it may be a necessary one (Lijinsky, 1992). Other nitrosamides have also been shown to damage the DNA by production of an O_6-alkylguanine–DNA adduct (Craddock, 1983). It has also been suggested that these alkylated bases cause base mispairing and point mutations that lead to uncontrollable expression of oncogenes and growth factor receptors followed by permanently heightened cell proliferation (Bilzer et al, 1989).

Population Exposure to NOCs. Human exposure to NOCs is estimated to derive half from exogenously formed and half from endogenously formed compounds (National Research Council, 1981). Only levels of nitrosamines (not nitrosamides) have been widely measured in human environments and consumer products, even though many of these exposures probably involve both nitrosamines and nitrosamides. The major sources of population exposure to nitrosamines in the United States are tobacco smoke, cosmetics, automobile interiors, and cured meats (National Research Council, 1981). Only for a few individuals is the primary source of NOC exposure likely to be job related. Because the nitrosamines in cigarette smoke occur predominantly in the sidestream smoke (from the burning tip of the cigarette), a nonsmoker in close proximity to smokers could be almost as heavily exposed as the smoker to the nitrosamines in tobacco smoke. Many cosmetics, soaps, shampoos, and hand lotions are contaminated with *N*-nitrodiethanolamine (NDELA), but only face makeup—foundation cream or liquid—was consistently found to contain NDELA, and at levels that were 30–40 times higher than those found in other personal hygiene products (Fan et al, 1977). Low levels of NDELA cause cancer in rats (Lijinsky and Kovatch, 1985). Cosmetics are also known to contain high levels of amides and are likely to contain nitrosamides. *N*-nitroso compounds are also present in pacifiers and in rubber baby bottle nipples and in the liquids passed through them (Sen et al, 1984).

Endogenous formation of NOCs in humans occurs in the stomach or bladder when both an amino compound and a nitrosating agent are present simultaneously. Food is a primary source of both highly concentrated nitrite solutions (eg, from cured meats) and amino compounds (eg, in fish and other foods, but also in many drugs). Another source of nitrite is reduction (eg, in the saliva) from nitrate that comes predominantly from vegetables in the diet; this source is likely to be a far less important contributor to the NOC formed endogenously because it is highly diluted (and, therefore, less readily reactive) and because vegetables also contain vitamins that inhibit the nitrosation reaction. Drinking water also contains nitrate (in the absence of vitamins), but this is a minor source unless levels are extraordinarily high (Chilvers et al, 1984). When inhibitors such as ascorbate (vitamin C) or alpha tocopherol (vitamin

E), which are nitrite scavengers, are also present at high concentrations, NOCs are not formed (Tannenbaum and Mergens, 1980). Other compounds, such as caffeine, potentiate the NOC effect (Aida and Bodell, 1987). The level of NOCs in the human body is also influenced by other factors, such as which amino compounds are present, presence of bacteria or other nitrosation catalysts, gastric pH, and other physiologic factors. Uncertainty as to the simultaneous presence of NOC precursors and of inhibitors and/or catalysts of nitrosation make this hypothesis difficult to study epidemiologically. This difficulty is compounded by further uncertainty about what exposure period (during a person's life) is most likely to be etiologically relevant.

In summary, tobacco smoke and rubber products are major sources of population exposure to NOC in most parts of the world, but the particular foods, drugs, personal hygiene products, and so on that are important sources of NOC vary considerably from country to country. Increasingly complete information on dietary and other sources of NOC is available for the United States as well as most Western countries. Because NOCs are likely to be carcinogenic to humans, steps have been taken in recent years to reduce the levels of NOCs in consumer products such as cosmetics (Eisenbrand et al, 1991), and beer (Scanlan and Barbour, 1991) and in industrial environments such as rubber and tire plants (Wacker et al, 1991). Such steps have been taken before these exposures have been established epidemiologically to relate to risk.

Epidemiological Evidence. Findings from a preliminary study conducted in Los Angeles indicated that the hypothesis that NOCs cause brain tumors in humans deserves further investigation (Preston-Martin et al, 1982b). Other epidemiological studies of pediatric (Howe et al, 1989; Bunin et al, 1993; McCredie et al, 1994a) and adult (Burch et al, 1987; Preston-Martin and Mack, 1991; Boeing et al, 1993) patients have provided limited support for this hypothesis. Findings that use of vitamin supplements and/or high intake of fresh fruits or vegetables protect against brain tumor development might also be interpreted as supportive of the N-nitroso hypothesis, although this effect may be due to another mechanism (Preston-Martin et al, 1982b; Howe et al, 1989; Bunin et al, 1993; McCredie et al, 1994b; Preston-Martin and Mack, 1991; Bunin et al, 1994). The experimental model and its potential relevance to humans are sufficiently compelling to encourage further investigation of this hypothesis despite the fact that it is a difficult one to test epidemiologically. In the future, researchers must include more complete dietary histories if they hope to differentiate between findings supportive of the NOC/brain tumor hypothesis and those suggestive of other mechanisms for dietary effects.

Other Agents

Experimental work has demonstrated that other families of chemicals in addition to NOCs produce brain tumors. Early work with polycyclic aromatic hydrocarbons produced brain tumors at the site of implantation. It has recently been suggested, however, that many of these earlier experimental findings should be reevaluated to see if they meet various criteria of causality (Koestner, 1986; Swenberg, 1986). Other work has demonstrated that systemic administration of N-2-fluorenylacetamide, various triazenes, and symmetrical hydrazines produce brain tumors in mammalian species (Maltoni et al, 1982). Chemicals that produce brain tumors after inhalation include bis-chloromethyl ether, vinyl chloride and acrylonitrile, and ethylene oxide (Maltoni et al, 1992; Garman and Snellings, 1986).

Brain tumors occur after intracranial inoculation with various viruses and the histologic type of the tumor produced appears to depend on the site of inoculation and the age and species of the host animal (Bigner, 1978; Ohsumi et al, 1985). In addition, viruses and viruslike particles have been isolated from human nervous system tumors, but it is uncertain whether this finding has etiologic relevance (Bigner, 1978; Ohsumi et al, 1985; Corallini et al, 1987).

Experimental studies of the effects of high-dose whole-body irradiation in monkeys found the brain to be the most common site of the cancers that were produced (Traynor and Casey, 1971; Haymaker et al, 1972). Humans with high dose exposure are also at excess risk, and the epidemiological evidence that an environmental agent causes brain tumors appears strongest for ionizing radiation (see below).

INHERITANCE

Some central nervous system tumors have a relatively clear genetic character, particularly those that occur in association with neurofibromatosis and other phakomatoses, which often display an autosomal dominant pattern of inheritance with varying degrees of penetrance. Neurofibromatosis, the most common of these syndromes, is now recognized to be two genetically and clinically distinct disorders. Neurofibromatosis 1, also called classical or von Recklinghausen's neurofibromatosis, occurs in about 1 in 3000 people and has been linked to a gene near the centromere of chromosome 17 (Barker et al, 1987). About 5%–10% of those with the trait develop CNS tumors, including optic gliomas, other astrocytomas, acoustic neuromas, neurilemmomas, meningiomas, and neurofibromas (Riccardi, 1981). Among patients with severe cases who had been hospitalized for the disorder, 45% developed malignant or benign CNS tumors, and 20% developed multiple primary tumors (Sorensen et al, 1986). CNS tumors often occur during childhood among those affected (Sorensen et al, 1986; Blatt et al, 1986).

Neurofibromatosis 2 is called bilateral acoustic neurofibromatosis because of the tendency of those affected to develop bilateral acoustic neuromas around the time of puberty or later (Martuza and Eldridge, 1988). The long arm of chromosome 22 has been established as the locus for this disorder, and patients have also been found to develop multiple CNS tumors of various histologic types (Wertelecki et al, 1988).

Astrocytomas occur in association with tuberous sclerosis and hemangioblastomas with von Hippel-Lindau disease (Schoenberg, 1991). In addition, there are specific genetic multiple primary tumor syndromes that may involve the central nervous system, such as Turcot's syndrome and Turner's syndrome (Lewis et al, 1983; Wertelecki et al, 1970; Strong, 1977). Cancers of the brain and certain other sites occur in family members with Li-Fraumeni syndrome, which is thought to have an autosomal dominant basis (Garber et al, 1990). The proportion of brain tumor patients whose tumors occur in association with recognized genetic syndromes appears, however, to be small—fewer than 1% of children and adults with brain tumors in Los Angeles County (Preston-Martin et al, 1980, 1982b, 1983, 1989a). Even when the broadest definition of predisposing familial syndromes is applied, 4% or fewer of brain tumor patients have such predisposition (Bondy et al, 1991; Wrensch et al, 1990).

RADIATION

The occurrence of excess brain tumors after high-dose exposure to ionizing radiation is well established. Numerous cases have been reported of brain tumors arising at the site of radiation treatment either for an earlier head tumor or for a benign condition such as a facial birthmark. Meningiomas appear to be the most common tumor that results, but tumors of other histologic types have occurred, including gliomas in adults and in children who received radiation treatment for an earlier cancer (Rimm et al, 1987; Soffer et al, 1989; Shapiro et al, 1989; Brada et al, 1992; Tsang et al, 1993). Epidemiological studies of brain tumor risk associated with high-dose radiation exposure are summarized in Table 58–6. Mortality from brain tumors was elevated in survivors who were under age 10 when they were exposed to radiation from the atomic bombs in Hiroshima and Nagasaki (Jablon and Kato, 1971). A subsequent follow-up showed a fivefold increase in brain tumor incidence among males who had received 100 rads or more; in this high-dose group, glioma risk increased with younger age at exposure (Seyama et al, 1979). No increase was seen among females. Two large follow-up studies of children in Israel and New York given x-ray therapy for ringworm of the scalp show them to be at increased risk of both benign and malignant brain tumors (Modan et al, 1974; Shore et al, 1976). An updated follow-up of the Israeli cohort showed the relative risk is greatest for nerve sheath tumors of the head and neck (RR=33.1), intermediate for meningiomas (RR=9.5), and lowest for gliomas (RR=2.6; Ron et al, 1988). Persons given x-ray therapy to the tonsils and nasopharynx as children have also been shown to have an excess brain tumor risk, and each major histologic type, including several different types of gliomas, are represented among the tumors that occur (Schneider et al, 1985). An excess of benign CNS tumors has been observed among a cohort who received radiation treatment for thymic enlargement in infancy (Hildreth et al, 1985). Case-control studies of meningiomas and nerve sheath tumors in adults have found elevated risks associated with exposure to full-mouth dental x-rays decades ago, when doses were relatively high, as well as with prior radiation treatment to the head (Preston-Martin et al, 1980, 1983, 1989a; Ryan et al, 1992b).

The association with low-dose exposure is more controversial. Prenatal exposure from diagnostic radiography has been related to an excess of pediatric brain tumors in several studies. Stewart and colleagues (1958) and subsequently MacMahon (1962) found relative risks for brain tumors of about 1.5 among children exposed in utero to diagnostic x-rays when their mothers had x-ray pelvimetry late in pregnancy (Table 58–6). Studies of prenatal x-rays among twins have the advantage that x-ray pelvimetry late in pregnancy is less likely to relate to an unknown and possibly confounding reason for irradiation, because the indication for pelvimetry is usually just the fact that twins are expected. Such studies in twins have found an excess of brain tumors and other childhood cancers among twins who were irradiated compared with twins who were not (Mole, 1974; Harvey et al, 1985). Nonetheless, it was suggested that the studies in twins were not unequivocal because there might still be some unidentified confounding reason why pelvimetry was ordered for some twin pregnancies but not others (MacMahon, 1985). A case-control study of all childhood cancer deaths in England, Wales, and Scotland between 1953 and 1979 found further support for the association and no evidence for any systematic reduction in the rate of x-ray pelvimetry during pregnancy (Knox et al, 1987). This study has been criticized, however, because it failed to investigate other factors associated with an increased cancer rate and also failed to find a dose-response relation (Lancet, 1988). A study in Swedish twins found that abdominal x-rays of the mother during pregnancy were associated with an increase in CNS tumors, which appeared not to be confounded by mother's age, obstetrical complications, or other factors (Rodvall et al, 1990). Studies exploring the effects of low-dose radiation exposure are summarized in Table 58–6 only if brain tumors are specifically enumerated.

TRAUMA

The epidemiological evidence associating head trauma and brain tumors is strongest for meningiomas. A number of case reports present convincing circumstantial evidence (Reinhardt, 1928; Walsh et al, 1969). In a clinical series, presence of a scar or depressed fracture at the tumor site was noted for 8% of meningioma patients (Cushing and Eisenhardt, 1938). Three case-control studies found an excess risk of meningiomas: in women with histories of head trauma treated medically; in men who boxed as a sport; and in men with histories of serious head injuries (Preston-Martin et al, 1980, 1983, 1989a; Table 58–6). A study of patients treated for head injury who were followed an average of 10 years found no excess of brain tumors (Annegers et al, 1979; Table 58–6). However, the number of expected cases was small, and a 10-year follow-up period is inadequate to study the occurrence of slow-growing tumors such as meningiomas.

The relation of x-rays and trauma to the descriptive epidemiology of meningiomas is distinct. Dental x-rays account for more than 80% of all radiation exposure to the head in the U.S. population (Preston-Martin et al, 1988); women and those in the more affluent social classes have their teeth x-rayed more frequently than others in the U.S. population (USDHEW, 1973). Head trauma, in contrast, is more common among men and among nonwhites (Morbidity Mortality Weekly Report, 1986; Centers for Disease Control, 1986). It has been shown that the female excess of meningiomas, greatest in women aged 25 to 54, may be partially explained by the more frequent exposure of females to dental x-rays, particularly at ages 15 to 29 (USDHEW, 1973; Preston-Martin et al, 1984). Relatively high meningioma rates in blacks may be related to their higher rates of head trauma, although this has not been established. It is possible that no clear socioeconomic trend is seen for meningiomas because the demographic relationships of these two factors—x-rays and trauma—work at opposite ends of the demographic spectrum and, therefore, cancel each other out. The excess of meningiomas and nerve sheath tumors in Jews has not yet been explained; one possibility is that the rate of head x-rays is higher in Jews than non-Jews.

Limited experimental evidence suggests that trauma may act as a cocarcinogen in the induction of gliomas as well as meningiomas (Morantz and Shain, 1978). Childhood brain tumors, which are predominantly gliomas, have been associated with birth trauma (prolonged labor, forceps delivery, Caesarean section) in a study of 20 case-control pairs (Choi et al, 1970b). This and other studies have noted small excesses of risk for cerebral tumors among firstborn children, which investigators suggest may be attributable to perinatal trauma (MacMahon, 1962; Gold et al, 1979; Table 58–6). Other studies found either no association with birth order or a reduced risk among firstborns (Preston-Martin et al, 1982b; Kuijten et al, 1990; Howe et al, 1989; McCredie et al, 1994b). Some studies support an association with birth trauma or with head injury requiring medical attention (Table 58–6).

In studying this variable in retrospective case-control studies, investigators must remember that trauma is often regarded by lay persons as related to tumor development and is, therefore, susceptible to bias from differential recall. For this reason, an attempt must be made to limit reporting of trauma to injuries of a certain minimum severity (such as those requiring medical attention or hospitalization) and thereby limit recall bias.

Acoustic Trauma and Acoustic Neuromas

The observation that over 90% of all nerve sheath tumors arise in the eighth cranial nerve (the acoustic nerve) suggests an exposure unique to this nerve. A case–control study of acoustic neuromas in Los Angeles County residents supports the hypothesis that acoustic trauma may relate to the development of these tumors (Preston-Martin et al, 1989b, 1990). During the period 10 or more years prior to the year of diagnosis of the case, more case patients than control patients had a job involving exposure to extremely loud noise; noise exposure was determined by a blinded review of job histories and linkage to the National Occupational Hazards Survey database (odds ratio [OR]=2.2, 95% confidence interval [Cl]=1.12, 4.67). A dose-response analysis showed an increase in risk related to number of years of job exposure to extremely loud noise (*P* for trend=0.02) with an OR of 13.2 (Cl=2.01, 86.98) for exposure of 20 or more years accumulated up to 10 years before diagnosis. These findings may support the more general hypothesis that mechanical trauma may contribute to tumorigenesis (Preston-Martin et al, 1990). This contention is supported by experimental findings of tissue destruction and subsequent repair following acoustic trauma (Hamernik et al, 1984a, b; Corwin and Cotanche, 1988; Ryals and Rubel, 1988).

DIET

Investigations of possible associations between dietary exposures and brain tumor development have been conducted only relatively recently. Because the majority of these studies have focused on the possible role of dietary NOC exposures, food items have been primarily limited to include only those relevant to dietary NOCs. It should be noted that it is easier to study dietary NOCs in pediatric than in adult patients, because the most relevant exposure period (gestation) is clearly defined. Animal models also suggest that the relatively low levels of NOC exposure in humans may be more likely to relate to brain tumors in children (after transplacental exposure) than in adults. More recent epidemiological studies have begun to focus on the association between certain dietary micronutrients and brain tumor risk.

Case-control studies of brain tumors and dietary NOC exposures have provided some support for the NOC hypothesis (Table 58–6). Elevated risk has been linked to more frequent consumption of nitrite-cured or processed meats (including cooked ham, processed pork, corned beef, and fried bacon) in adults (Preston-Martin et al, 1980; Boeing et al, 1993; Giles et al, 1994), in children in relation to their own diets (Sarasua and Savitz, 1994), and in children in relation to the mother's diet during pregnancy (Preston-Martin et al, 1982b; Kuijten et al, 1990; Bunin et al, 1993; McCredie et al, 1994a; Bunin et al, 1994; Sarasua and Savitz, 1994). Other studies (mostly in adults) have found no clear association with consumption of cured meats (Preston-Martin, 1983; Burch et al, 1987; Howe et al, 1989; Preston-Martin et al, 1989a; Ryan et al, 1992a). Other food items involving dietary NOC found to be related to the risk of adult brain tumors include pickled or processed fish (Burch et al, 1987; Boeing et al, 1993), cheese (Boeing et al, 1993), and use of vegetable fat for deep frying (Boeing et al, 1993).

When calculated over all food items, intakes of nitrate and nitrite have not been found to relate to adult gliomas (Boeing et al, 1993; Giles et al, 1994) or childhood brain tumors (Bunin et al, 1993, 1994). In fact, two of these studies found a reduced risk of childhood PNET (Bunin et al, 1993), and risk of glioma in adult females (Giles et al, 1994) associated with total dietary nitrate. The lack of association with total dietary nitrate is likely due to the fact that vegetables are the primary source of nitrate for most people, but the nitrate in vegetables may not contribute substantially to endogenous NOC formation because vegetables also contain vitamins C and E, polyphenols, and other inhibitors of nitrosation (Pignatelli et al, 1984). Also, before endogenous NOC formation can occur the nitrate must be reduced to nitrite; this occurs in the saliva and results in a nitrite solution that is highly dilute and, therefore, less reactive. The intake of nitrosamines from processed meats (*N*-nitrosodimethylamine [NDMA], *N*-nitrosopyrrolidine [NPYR], and *N*-nitrosopiperidine [NPIP]) have been found to be strongly related to glioma risk, and to a lesser extent, meningioma risk in adults (Boeing et al, 1993; Giles et al, 1994).

Use of vitamin supplements, particularly vitamins C, E, and multivitamins, has been found to reduce brain tumor risk in adults (Preston-Martin and Mack, 1991; Burch et al, 1987); in children, risk is reduced by their personal vitamin use (McCredie et al, 1994b) and mother's use during pregnancy (Preston-Martin et al, 1982b; Bunin et al, 1993). This has not been supported in other case-control studies of adult brain tumors (Ryan et al, 1992a; Boeing et al, 1993). Increased consumption of fruit and fruit juice has been linked to reduced risk of meningiomas in males (Preston-Martin and Mack, 1991) and of childhood brain tumors (Howe et al, 1989; McCredie et al, 1994b). Higher vegetable consumption was found to reduce glioma risk in adult females, but not males (Giles et al, 1994). In addition, mothers' consumption during pregnancy of vegetables, fruits and fruit juices, and dietary vitamins C and E has been linked to reduced risk of brain tumors in their children (Preston-Martin et al, 1982b; Bunin et al, 1993, 1994; McCredie et al, 1994a).

Although the findings of reduced risk of brain tumors in children and adults associated with increased intake of vitamin supplements, fruits, and vegetables may be related to the *N*-nitroso hypothesis—namely, that these nutrients play a protective role by inhibiting endogenous formation of nitrosamines—it is important to consider other potential mechanisms of effect. In this respect, it is interesting that a study of childhood brain tumors reported higher relative risks associated with the consumption of cured meats when the children did not take multivitamins than when they did take multivitamins (Sarasua and Savitz, 1994).

Recent studies have investigated the possible associations of brain tumors with other dietary micronutrients (Bunin et al, 1993, 1994). In particular, a case-control study of childhood PNET found significant protective trends with increasing levels of dietary vitamins A and C, beta-carotene, and folate by the mother during pregnancy (Bunin et al, 1993). In a related study of childhood astrocytoma, reduced risks were evident for dietary vitamins A and C; however, these trends were not significant (Bunin et al, 1994). There was no relation between childhood astrocytoma and dietary beta-carotene or folate. Although these preliminary results suggest exciting prospects for the possible prevention of childhood brain tumors, interpretation is difficult because both studies were primarily focused on the evaluation of dietary NOCs. Thus, evaluation of other micronutrients was limited to the micronutrient composition of NOC-related food items. These results highlight the need to incorporate complete dietary evaluations in future epidemiological studies.

OTHER SUGGESTED RISK FACTORS

A number of other factors have been suggested in relation to brain tumor risk, including ABO blood type and exposure to infectious agents, barbiturates, electric and magnetic fields, alcohol, tobacco smoke, and pesticides. For the most part, these possible associations have not been studied often or very thoroughly. The few brain tumor studies that have investigated some factors (eg, alcohol, tobacco) have had conflicting findings. The best one can do in attempting to evaluate their etiologic relevance is to keep them in mind and hope that future brain tumor studies will also investigate possible associations with these factors.

Infectious Agents

Astrocytomas, but not other histologic types of brain tumors, appeared to be associated with positive antibody titers to *Toxoplasma gondii* (Schuman et al, 1967; Table 58–6), but a recent study failed to confirm this (Ryan et al, 1993). There are numerous reports in the literature of the isolation of viruses or viruslike particles from human cerebral tumors or tumor cell lines, but whether these findings may have etiologic implications is uncertain (Bigner, 1978; Corallini et al, 1987). People who received polio vaccine contaminated with SV40 did not develop more brain tumors in the 20 years after vaccination, although some histologic types (eg, spongioblastoma, medulloblastoma) did appear to occur more frequently (Geissler and Staneczek, 1988).

Neither prospective nor retrospective studies of maternal influenza infection during pregnancy have found a brain tumor excess in offspring (Fredrick and Alberman, 1972; Bithell et al, 1973). One study reported three medulloblastoma cases and no affected control subjects out of 9000 pairs studied whose mothers had chicken-pox during pregnancy (Bithell et al, 1973). Another study found no association between childhood brain tumors and maternal chicken pox, rubella, or mumps (Adelstein and Donovan, 1972).

ABO Blood Group

There are nine studies in the literature of the relation between blood group and brain tumors, but some have been poorly designed or have reported findings in such a way that they are difficult to interpret. For this reason, these studies have not been included in Table 58–6. What appears to emerge as a common finding is an excess of blood group A among astrocytoma patients (Yates and Pearce, 1960; Selverstone and Cooper, 1961) or with brain tumors of all types in men (Buckwalter et al, 1959; Strang et al, 1966). No explanation has been offered for this association, and recent studies relying on self reports of blood group failed to confirm these associations (Schlehofer et al, 1992; Ryan et al, 1992a). A smaller proportion of U.S. blacks compared to U.S. whites have blood group A (Garcia et al, 1963). Whether this relative deficit of type A among blacks may relate to their lower glioma incidence has not been investigated.

Barbiturates

Studies of childhood brain tumors have investigated their possible association with prenatal or childhood exposure to barbiturates. In the first study, the only barbiturate association that was statistically significant was that six mothers of case patients compared to no mothers of cancer control subjects used this drug during pregnancy (Gold et al, 1978; Table 58–6). A second larger study found no association with childhood exposure to barbiturates, other than to anti-epileptics (Preston-Martin et al, 1982b; Table 58–6). The only association with intrauterine exposure was with barbiturates administered to the mother for general anesthesia (Preston-Martin et al, 1982b). No association with barbiturate use was seen in recent studies (Howe et al, 1989; Kuijten et al, 1990; McCredie et al, 1994a). As mentioned above, epileptics who use barbiturates to control their seizure disorders have an excess of brain tumors. It seems likely, however, that the epilepsy is an early brain tumor symptom.

Phenobarbital and phenobarbital sodium, two common barbiturates, cause liver tumors but not nervous system tumors in experimental animals (IARC, 1977). The mode of action appears to be a powerful tumor-promoting effect (Goldsworthy et al, 1984; Schivapurkar et al, 1986).

Electric and Magnetic Fields

Recent research has explored the association between electromagnetic field (EMF) exposure and brain tumor risk and is summarized in Table 58–6. The first such study (Wertheimer and Leeper, 1979) compared electrical wiring configurations outside homes of 344 children in Denver who had died of cancer between 1950 and 1973 to that outside homes of matched control subjects. Although no risk estimates or confidence intervals were presented, a significantly higher proportion of case patients with nervous system tumors than control subjects lived near wiring configurations suggestive of high current flow. This association was observed for residences at both the birth and death of the case patient. A second case-control study conducted in Sweden (Tomenius, 1986) recorded the presence of visible electric structures within 150 meters of the home and measured EMF outside the entrance door of homes of children diagnosed with cancer (and matched control subjects). A significantly elevated risk of nervous system tumors was found for children with higher measured fields immediately outside the home. Savitz and coworkers (1988) measured both wire configuration codes and residential EMF in children diagnosed with cancer and matched control subjects. Brain tumor risk was found only to relate to residential wire codes, although the 95% confidence interval for the estimated odds ratio of 1.9 included 1.0. A case-control study of CNS tumors in Danish children found no elevated risk with estimated magnetic field levels in homes lived in from 9 months before the child's birth up to diagnosis (Olsen et al, 1993). Another case-control study of CNS tumors in Swedish children also found no association with estimated magnetic fields or spot measurements (Feychting and Ahlbom, 1993). A Finnish cohort study found a significantly elevated risk for nervous system tumors in boys (5 observed versus 1.18 expected cases), but not girls (0 observed versus 0.98 expected cases) exposed to higher estimated residential magnetic fields (Verkasalo et al, 1993). However, three of the five tumors observed in the boys occurred in one subject with neurofibromatosis. In a small cohort study of 1552 persons residing for at least 5 years within 100 meters of power lines or a transformer substation in an area of the Netherlands, no elevated brain cancer mortality was observed in men, and a non-significantly elevated brain cancer mortality rate was observed in women (Schreiber et al, 1993). Exposure assessment in all of these studies is hampered by the inability to measure the true exposure of interest, EMF prior to diagnosis. The extent to which measured EMF after diagnosis or death is accurately reflective of EMF prior to diagnosis cannot be completely determined. Both studies that asked about electric blanket use found elevated odds ratios for mother's use during the index pregnancy (Savitz et al, 1990; Kuijten et al, 1990).

An ecological study in Canada noted significant increases over time of both residential electric consumption and childhood brain cancer rates (Kraut et al, 1994). When provinces were ranked by their average residential electric consumption, a positive correlation was found between provincial electric consumption and brain cancer rates (Kraut et al, 1994).

Several epidemiological studies of brain tumor risk in electricity-related occupations have recently been reported, and there is some suggestion that this association may be strongest for astrocytomas (Thomas et al, 1987b; Mack et al, 1991). These are discussed above in the Occupation and Industry section of this chapter and are summarized in Table 58–5.

Alcohol

Table 58–6 summarizes studies that have investigated alcohol use as a possible brain tumor risk factor. No consistent association with risk is seen across studies for any type of alcoholic beverage or for all types combined. In an early case-control study of central nervous system tumors, significantly fewer case patients than control patients reported any past use of alcoholic beverages (Choi et al, 1970b); this finding was observed for a meningioma subgroup as well as for the group of all histologically verified brain tumors. Later studies found no association between alcohol consumption and meningioma risk or risk of all types of brain tumors in adult males (Preston-Martin et al, 1983, 1989a). A case-control study of gliomas in adults observed a significantly elevated risk for consumption of wine (with a significant dose-response trend such that those reporting greater amounts of wine consumption had greater brain tumor risk); however, no elevation in risk was observed for consumption of beer or liquor (Burch et al, 1987). The authors hypothesized that the nitrosamines contained in alcoholic beverages may have explained the observed association between wine consumption and brain tumor risk, although the fact that both beer and liquor are reported to have higher nitrosamine concentrations than wine mitigates against this interpretation.

Studies of childhood brain tumors have also been inconsistent as to whether or not an association was seen with mothers' consumption of alcohol during the index pregnancy. Two found no association with alcohol use (Preston-Martin et al, 1982b; Kuijten et al, 1990), but one found an elevated risk among the offspring of mothers who drank beer (Howe et al, 1989).

Tobacco Use

A significantly decreased risk for brain tumors among smokers was observed in an early case-control study of brain tumors (Choi et al, 1970b). However, the categorization of subjects as smokers based on their smoking status at the time of interview rather than at the time of diagnosis makes it difficult to interpret this observation. It is likely that this association was due to cessation of smoking in the case group after diagnosis of the tumor. Case-control studies in Los Angeles found no association between personal tobacco use and the occurrence of meningiomas or gliomas (Preston-Martin, 1980, 1983, 1989a). A case-control study of gliomas in adults in Toronto found elevated (although not significant) brain tumor risks for a variety of tobacco products (including plain cigarettes, cigars, pipes, and chewing tobacco), with a significant dose-response relation found for use of plain (nonfiltered) cigarettes (Burch et al, 1987).

Environmental Tobacco Smoke

Several studies in children have shown slightly elevated risks relating to smoking by either or both parents (Gold et al, 1979; Preston-Martin et al, 1982b; Howe et al, 1989; John et al, 1991; Filippini et al, 1994) but others found no increase in risk (Kuijten et al, 1990; Gold et al, 1993). A case-control study of childhood brain tumors found no association with mother's smoking during pregnancy, but reported a doubling of risk with mother's exposure during pregnancy to the father's tobacco smoke (McCredie et al, 1994a). A cohort study of over 91,000 non-smoking Japanese wives found significantly increased brain tumor mortality for women whose husbands smoked (Hirayama, 1984). A significant dose-response relation was observed, in that women whose husbands smoked more experienced greater excesses in brain tumor mortality. A case-control study found an increased risk of meningioma, particularly for females, in persons exposed to a smoking spouse (Ryan et al, 1992a).

Pesticides

Several epidemiological studies have investigated home and occupational use of pesticides, insecticides, or herbicides as possible etiologic factors for brain tumors. Case-control studies have linked household pest exterminations to the development of childhood brain tumors (Gold et al, 1979; McCredie et al, 1994a), while others have found no association with pesticide use (Preston-Martin et al, 1982b; Howe et al, 1989; McCredie et al, 1994b). In a cohort study of licensed pesticide applicators, an excess risk of brain cancer was found (SMR=200; Blair et al, 1983).

A recent case-control study of childhood brain tumors conducted in Missouri asked a series of detailed questions about household use of pesticides, insecticides, and herbicides (Davis et al, 1993) in a small sample of cases (N=45), friend controls, and cancer controls. Elevated risks were found for home use of pesticides, No-Pest strips, pesticides for termite control, personal use of Kwell shampoo, use of flea collars on pets to which the child was exposed, exposure to pet shampoo for the control of pests, and outside use of Diazinon, carbaryl, and herbicides to control weeds (Davis et al, 1993; Table 58–6). Although these findings are intriguing, they await confirmation in future epidemiological studies.

PROSPECTS

We simply have no idea what causes most nervous system tumors. Certain inherited syndromes can predispose individuals to the development of brain and other nervous system tumors. But, only a few percent, at most, of patients with nervous system tumors have one of these rare phakomatoses or a family member with a nervous system tumor. Studies of such patients and their families have described genetic events that are correlates of nervous system tumor pathogenesis, but the etiologic implications of these findings are unclear.

Ionizing radiation, the only well-established environmental risk factor for nervous system tumors, can cause all three major histologic types of brain tumors—gliomas, meningiomas, and nerve sheath tumors—but the association appears weakest for gliomas. Nonetheless, minimizing population exposure to x-rays of the head is, at this point, the best prospect for prevention of all three types of tumors. Beyond this, the etiology of gliomas remains largely unknown. New etiologic hypotheses are needed that might explain unusual features of the descriptive epidemiology such as the increasing incidence with increasing social class, a feature that is particularly striking in males. To date, no one has offered a hypothesis as to why glioma is commonly a disease of upper-class white males.

More is known about the etiology of meningiomas and nerve sheath tumors. Ionizing radiation and trauma appear to be important risk factors for both. Both tumors are related to prior radiation treatment to the head and to heavy exposure to dental x-rays several decades before diagnosis of these benign, slow-growing neoplasms. Head trauma appears to relate to both, although this factor appears to be more important in males than in females, as would be expected from the relatively higher prevalence of all types of accidental and violent injuries in men (Morbidity Mortality Weekly Report, 1986; Centers for Disease Control, 1986). Nerve sheath tumors, which are predominantly acoustic neuromas, appear to also relate to acoustic trauma, as from years of occupational exposure to extremely loud noise.

Nitrosamides, especially the nitrosoureas, are the most potent nervous system carcinogens used experimentally. It seems likely that these compounds may also cause nervous system tumors in humans. To date most epidemiologic studies of a possible association of brain tumors with *N*-nitroso exposures have focused on the other major group of these compounds, nitrosamines. Nitrosamines are easier to study because reliable assays exist for nitrosamines, unlike nitrosamides, and monitoring of human environments and consumer products for levels of nitrosamines has been done. But nitrosamines have not caused nervous system tumors in any of the many experimental species tested. Therefore, they seem far less likely than nitrosamides to be of etiologic relevance in humans. Because it seems likely that much of human exposure to nitrosoureas and other nitrosamides comes from compounds that are formed endogenously, it may still be possible to investigate associations with intake of precursors of these compounds such as nitrite (likely to be most important when in high concentration, as in cured meats) or with modulators of the nitrosation reaction such as vitamins C and E, which are effective nitrosation inhibitors.

For a number of other reasons, epidemiological studies of the hypothesis that nitrosamide exposures relate to brain tumors are very difficult. Human exposure to *N*-nitroso compounds and their precursors has been described as "ubiquitous" although the foods and other consumer products that are important sources varies considerably from country to country (NRC, 1981). Nonetheless, there are many unknowns about the sources of exposure both to exogenously formed nitrosamides and to sources of precursors, especially the alkylamides. Many questions also remain about the relevance of the various endogenous and exogenous sources of nitrogen compounds—nitrate, nitrite, and the oxides of nitrogen—and it may be difficult to classify individuals on levels of activity of macrophages that have been shown to play an important role in endogenous nitrosation. Another difficulty relates to defining the relevant time window of exposure. The relevant exposure period is more clearly defined for children (gestation and infancy, when the brain is developing rapidly and the rate of brain cell proliferation is high) than adults, and experimental findings suggest that the effect is stronger (even with exposure doses up to a hundred times lower) when exposure occurs during a period of rapid development of brain tissue. But, even with a relatively recent and well-defined exposure period such as gestation, the problem of poor recall and resulting misclassification remains. For this reason it is appealing to be able to rely on some biomarker of exposure. Unfortunately, finding a biomarker of *N*-nitroso exposure for use in brain tumor patients or their mothers when the relevant exposures occurred years earlier has not proved easy. Adduct formation by *N*-nitrosoureas in vivo is beginning to be studied, but the extent of damage induced in various tissues seems not to correlate well with tumorigenicity (Eisenbrand et al, 1994). What seems more promising is to identify a genetic polymorphism (one that could easily be assayed in epidemiological studies) for an enzyme or other system that regulates *N*-nitroso metabolism or detoxification or the repair of the molecular damage caused by nitroso compounds. One interesting candidate might be alkyltransferase, an enzyme involved in the repair of O_6-alkylguanine, which is formed and persists in brain DNA after exposure to alkylating agents such as the nitrosoureas (Pegg, 1990). Nitrosoureas produce different types of nervous system tumors in different species; identifying those histologic types in humans will also make future studies of nitrosamide exposures more efficient.

Many of the problems confronted by epidemiological studies of brain tumors and nitrosamides also apply to studies of other suspected brain carcinogens such as several investigated in occupational studies. Although a number of industries have long been noted to have an apparent excess of brain tumors among workers, it has proved difficult to implicate specific exposures. Simultaneous evaluation both of exposures to specific chemicals and of individual susceptibility to those chemicals may be the direction of the future.

Given that we are not yet at the point of incorporating assays of relevant genetic polymorphism into epidemiological studies of nervous system tumors, what further work seems indicated? Diet will be an important focus of the next generation of epidemiological studies of gliomas. Studies to date have included some questions about a limited number of dietary variables, such as the several studies that looked at foods thought likely to be relevant to the *N*-nitroso hypothesis. A number of intriguing associations are emerging from these and other studies, including the suggestion that intake of cured meats, fruits, and vitamin supplements all relate to glioma risk, with fruits and vitamins being protective. Future studies must include relatively complete dietary surveys in order to adequately evaluate associations with various micronutrients, cholesterol, nitrite from cured meats, and other suggested associations.

Are there additional etiologic clues to be gleaned from the descriptive epidemiology of brain tumors? The increase in incidence and mortality rates in recent decades was initially thought by some to suggest the effect of an environmental exposure, but on further consideration appears to be largely an artifact of improved diagnosis. Compared to other cancer sites, brain tumor rates show relatively little international variation. This suggests that either the relevant environmental exposures are ubiquitous or that endogenous factors are important. The gender differences in distribution by histologic type of brain tumor, namely the male predominance of glioma and the female predominance of meningioma, have long been noted and although evidence suggesting the importance of hormonal factors is weak, any compelling hypothesis related to this difference would be worth investigating. Most brain tumors in children are gliomas, and some types such as PNET occur predominantly in children under age 5 years. The observation that PNET rates, unlike rates of other pediatric brain tumors that are similar in the two genders, are up to two times higher in boys than in girls also remains unexplained. For gliomas as a major group as well as for specific glioma subtypes, it seems possible that some of the crucial etiologic questions have not yet been posed.

The etiology of the majority of nervous system tumors remains unexplained. Genetic predisposition, ionizing radiation, and the other suggested risk factors each seem to account for only a small proportion of total cases. It may be that there are numerous nervous system carcinogens, each with low attributable risk. Our continued investigation of suspected brain carcinogens needs to identify and focus on histology-specific associations and use improved methods of exposure assessment. In addition, we need to simultaneously consider host factors, in particular genetic polymorphisms, that may influence susceptibility.

REFERENCES

ADELSTEIN AM, DONOVAN JW. 1972. Malignant disease in children whose mothers had chickenpox, mumps or rubella in pregnancy. Br Med J 4:629–631.

AHLBOM A, NORELL S, RODVALL Y. 1986. Dentists, dental nurses, and brain tumors. Br Med J 292:662.

AHLBOM A, RODVALL Y. 1989. Brain tumour trends (Letter). Lancet 2:1272.

AIDA T, BODELL WJ. 1987. Effect of caffeine on cytotoxicity and sister chromatid exchange induction in sensitive and resistant rat brain tumor cells treated with 1,3-Bis(2-chloroethyl)-1-nitrosurea. Cancer Res 47:5052–5058.

ALBERGHINI V, LUBERTO F, GOBBA F, et al. 1991. Mortality among male farmers licensed to use pesticides. Med Lav 82:18–24.

ANDJELKOVIC D, TAULBEE J, SYMONS M. 1976. Mortality experience of a cohort of rubber workers, 1964–1973. J Occup Med 18:387–394.

ANNEGERS JF, LAWS ER, KURLAND LT, et al. 1979. Head trauma and subsequent brain tumors. Neurosurgery 4:203–206.

ANNEGERS JF, SCHOENBERG BS, OKAZAKI H, et al. 1981. Epidemiologic study of primary intracranial neoplasms. Arch Neurol 38:217–219.

ARMSTRONG DD, ALMES MJ, BUFFER P, et al. 1990. A cluster classification for histologic diagnosis of CNS tumors in epidemiologic study. Neuroepidemiology 9:2–16.

ARONSON SM, ARONSON BE. 1965. Central nervous system in diabetes mellitus. Lowered frequency of certain intracranial neoplasms. Arch Neurol 12:390–398.

AUSTIN SG, SCHNATTER AR. 1983. A case-control study of chemical exposures and brain tumors in petrochemical workers. J Occup Med 25:321.

BAHEMUKA M, MASSEY EW, SCHOENBERG BS. 1988. International mortality from primary nervous system neoplasms: distribution and trends. Int J Epidemiol 17:33–38.

BAILEY P, CUSHING H. 1926. A classification of tumors of the glioma group. Philadelphia: Lippincott.

BARKER D, WRIGHT T, NGUYEN K, et al. 1987. Gene for von Recklinghausen neurofibromatosis is in the pericentromeric region of chromosome 17. Science 236:1100–1102.

BELL ET. 1957. Carcinoma of pancreas: I. Clinical and pathological study of 609 necropsied cases. II. Relation to carcinoma of pancreas to diabetes mellitus. Am J Pathol 33:499–524.

BEN-SHLOMO Y, SMITH GD. 1989. Brain tumor trends (Letter). Lancet 2:1272–1273.

BIGNER DD. 1978. Role of viruses in the causation of neural neoplasia. In: *Biology of Brain Tumors*. Laerum OD, et al. (eds). Geneva, International Union Against Cancer.

BILZER T, REIFENBERGER G, WECHSLER W. 1989. Chemical induction of brain tumors in rats by nitrosoureas: molecular biology and neuropathology. Neurotoxicol Teratol 11:551.

BITHELL JF, DRAPER GJ, GORBACH PD. 1973. Association between malignant disease in children and maternal virus infections. Br Med J 1:706–708.

BLACK PM. 1991a. Brain tumors (Part 1). N Engl J Med 324:1471–1476.

BLACK PM. 1991b. Brain tumors (Part 2). N Engl J Med 324:1555–1564.

BLAIR A, GRAUMAN DJ, LUBIN JH, et al. 1983. Lung cancer and other causes of death among licensed pesticide applicators. J Natl Cancer Inst 71:31–37.

BLAIR A, HAYES HM JR. 1980. Cancer and other causes of death among U.S. veterinarians, 1966–1977. Int J Cancer 25:181–185.

BLAIR A, MALKER H, CANTOR KP, et al. 1985. Cancer among farmers: a review. Scand J Work Environ Health 11:397–407.

BLATT J, JAFFE R, DEUTSCH M, et al. 1986. Neurofibromatosis and childhood tumors. Cancer 57:1225–1229.

BOEING H, SCHLEHOFER B, BLETTNER M, et al. 1993. Dietary carcinogens and the risk for glioma and meningioma in Germany. Int J Cancer 53:561–565.

BOGOVSKI P, BOGOVSKI S. 1981. Animal species in which N-nitroso compounds induce cancer. Int J Cancer 27:471–474.

BONDY ML, LUSTBADER ED, BUFFLER PA, et al. 1991. Genetic epidemiology of childhood brain tumors. Genet Epidemiol 8:253–267.

BORING CC, SQUIRES TS, TONG T. 1991. Cancer statistics, 1991. CA 41:19–36.

BOYLE P, MAISSONNEUVE P, SARRACI R, et al. 1990. Is the increased incidence of primary malignant brain tumors in the elderly real? J Natl Cancer Inst 82:1594–1596.

BRADA M, FORD D, ASHLEY S, et al. 1992. Risk of second brain tumour after conservative surgery and radiotherapy for pituitary adenoma. Br Med J 304:1343–1346.

BRANT-ZAWADZKI M, NORMAN D. 1987. Magnetic resonance imaging of the central nervous system. New York: Raven Press.

BROOKS WH. 1972. Geographic clustering of brain tumors in Kentucky. Cancer 30:923–926.

BROWN AM, CHRISTIE D, DEVEY P, et al. 1993. A cluster of brain tumours in a New South Wales colliery: a problem in interpretation. Aust J Public Health 17:302–305.

BROWNSON RC, REIF JS, CHANG JC, et al. 1990. An analysis of occupational risks for brain cancer. Am J Public Health 80:169–172.

BUCKWALTER JA, TURNER JH, GAMBER HH. 1959. Psychoses, intracranial neoplasms and genetics. Arch Neurol Psychiatry 81:480–485.

BUELL P, DUNN JE, BRESLOW L. 1960. The occupational-social class risks of cancer mortality in men. Cancer 12:600–621.

BULLARD DE, NASHOLD BS, OSBORNE D, et al. 1984. CT-guided stereotactic biopsies using a modified frame and Gildenburg technique. J Neurol Neurosurg Psychiatry 47:590–595.

BUNIN G. 1987. Racial patterns of childhood brain cancer by histologic type. J Natl Cancer Inst 78:875–880.

BUNIN GR, KUITJEN RR, BOESEL CP, et al. 1994. Maternal diet and risk of astrocytic glioma in children: a report from the Childrens Cancer Group (United States and Canada). Cancer Causes Control 5:177–187.

BUNIN GR, KUITJEN RR, RORKE LB, et al. 1993. Evidence for a role of maternal diet in the etiology of primitive neuroectodermal tumor of brain in young children. N Engl J Med 329:536–541.

BURCH JD, CRAIB KJP, CHOI BCK, et al. 1987. An exploratory case-control study of brain tumors in adults. J Natl Cancer Inst 78:601–609.

CANCER REGISTRY OF NORWAY. 1961. Cancer Registration in Norway: the incidence of cancer in Norway, 1953–1958. Oslo, The Norwegian Cancer Society.

CANTOR KP, LYNCH CF, JOHNSON D. 1993. Reproductive factors and risk of brain, colon, and other malignancies in Iowa (United States). Cancer Causes Control 4:505–511.

CENTERS FOR DISEASE CONTROL, HOMICIDE SURVEILLANCE. 1986. High-risk racial and ethnic groups—Blacks and Hispanics, 1970–1983. Atlanta, Centers for Disease Control.

CHILVERS C, INSKIP H, CAYGILL C, et al. 1984. A survey of dietary nitrate in well-water users. Int J Epidemiol 13:324–331.

CHOI NW, HSU PH, NELSON NA, et al. 1977. Some descriptive epidemiologic features of central nervous system (CNS) neoplasms in childhood, in Manitoba Canada. Neurologia Neurocirugia Psiquiatria (Mexico) 18:199–210.

CHOI NW, SCHUMAN LM, GULLEN WH. 1970a. Epidemiology of primary central nervous system neoplasms. I. Mortality from primary central nervous system neoplasms in Minnesota. Am J Epidemiol 91:238–259.

CHOI NW, SCHUMAN LM, GULLEN WH. 1970b. Epidemiology of primary central nervous system neoplasms. II. Case-control study. Am J Epidemiol 91:467–485.

COOPER WC. 1981. Epidemiologic study of vinyl chloride workers: mortality through December 31, 1972. Environ Health Perspect 41:101–106.

CORALLINI A, PAGNANI M, VIADANA P, et al. 1987. Association of BK virus with human brain tumors and tumors of pancreatic islets. Int J Cancer 39:60–67.

CORWIN JT, COTANCHE DA. 1988. Regeneration of sensory hair cells after acoustic trauma. Science 240:1772–1774.

CRADDOCK VM. 1983. Nitrosamines and human cancer: proof of an association? Nature 306:638.

CRIST WM, KUN LE. 1991. Common solid tumors of childhood. N Engl J Med 324:461–471.

CRUZ BL. 1958. Medulloblastoma. Springfield: Charles C. Thomas.

CUSHING H, EISENHARDT L. 1938. Meningiomas, their classification, regional behavior, life history and surgical end results. Springfield: Thomas.

DALY L, HERITY B, BOURKE GJ. 1994. An investigation of brain tumours and other malignancies in an agricultural research institute. Occup Environ Med 51:295–298.

DAVIS DL, SCHWARTZ J. 1988. Trends in cancer mortality: US white males and females, 1968–83. Lancet 1:633–636.

DAVIS DL. 1990. International trends in cancer mortality in France, West Germany, Italy, Japan, England and Wales, and the USA. Lancet 336:474–481.

DAVIS JR, BROWNSON RC, GARCIA R, et al. 1993. Family pesticide use and childhood brain cancer. Arch Environ Contam Toxicol 24:87–92.

DEEN HG, LAWS ER. 1981. Multiple primary brain tumors of different cell types. Neurosurgery 8:20–25.

DEMERS PA, VAUGHAN TL, SCHOMMER RR. 1991. Occupation, socioeconomic status, and brain tumor mortality: a death certificate-based case-control study. J Occup Med 33:1001–1006.

DESMEULES M, MIKKELSEN T, MAO Y. 1992. Increasing incidence of primary brain tumors: influence of diagnostic methods. J Natl Cancer Inst 84:442–445.

DEVESA SS, SILVERMAN DT. 1978. Cancer incidence and mortality trends in the United States: 1935–1974. J Natl Cancer Inst 60:545–571.

DEVESA SS, SILVERMAN DT, YOUNG J, et al. 1987. Cancer incidence and mortality trends among whites in the United States, 1947–1984. J Natl Cancer Inst 79:701–745.

DOBKIN BH. 1985. Stroke associated with glioblastoma. Bull Clin Neurosci 50:111–118.

EBY NL, GRUFFERMAN S, FLANNELLY CM, et al. 1988. Increasing incidence of primary brain lymphoma in the US. Cancer 62:2461–2465.

EISENBRAND G, BLANKART M, SOMMER H, et al. 1991. N-nitrosoalkanolamines in cosmetics. In: Relevance to Human Cancer of N-nitroso Compounds, Tobacco and Mycotoxins, O'Neill IK, Chen J, Bartsch H (eds). IARC Scientific Publications, No. 105. Lyon: IARC, pp 238–241.

EISENBRAND G, PFEIFFER C, TANG W. 1994. DNA adducts of N-nitrosoureas. In: *DNA Adducts: Identification and Biological Significance*, Hemminkik, Dipple A, Shuker DEG, et al (eds). IARC Scientific Publications, No. 125. Lyon: IARC, pp 277–293.

EMERSON JC, MALONE KE, DALING JR, et al. 1991. Childhood brain tumor risk in relation to birth characteristics. J Clin Epidemiol 44:1159–1166.

ERNSTER WL, SACKS ST, SELVIN S, et al. 1979. Cancer incidence by marital status: U.S. Third National Cancer Survey. J Natl Cancer Inst 63:567–585.

FAN TY, GOFF U, SONG L, et al. 1977. N-nitrosodiethenolamine in cosmetics, lotions and shampoos. Food Cosmet Toxicol 15:423–430.

FARWELL J, FLANNERY JT. 1984. Cancer in relatives of children with central-nervous-system neoplasms. N Engl J Med 311:749–753.

FEINGOLD L, SAVITZ DA, JOHN EM. 1992. Use of a job-exposure matrix to evaluate parental occupation and childhood cancer. Cancer Causes Control 3:161–169.

FEYCHTING M, AHLBOM A. 1993. Magnetic fields and cancer in children residing near Swedish high-voltage power lines. Am J Epidemiol 138:467–481.

FILIPPINI G, FARINOTTI M, LOVICO G, et al. 1994. Mothers' active and passive smoking during pregnancy and risk of brain tumours in children. Int J Cancer 57:769–774.

FLANNERY JT, BOICE J JR, DEVESA SS, et al. 1985. Cancer registration in Connecticut and the study of multiple primary cancers, 1935–1982. NCI Monogr 68:13–24.

FLODERUS B, TORNQUIST S, STENLUND C. 1994. Incidence of selected cancers in Swedish railway workers, 1961–79. Cancer Causes Control 5:189–194.

FOX AJ, LINDARS DC, OWEN R. 1974. A survey of occupational cancer in the rubber and cablemaking industries: results of five year analysis, 1967–71. Br J Ind Med 31:140–151.

FREDRICK J, ALBERMAN ED. 1972. Reported influenza in pregnancy and subsequent cancer in the child. Br Med J 2:485–488.

GARBER JE, DREYFUS MG, KANTOR AF, et al. 1990. Abstract: Cancer occurrence on follow-up of 24 kindreds with the Li-Fraumeni syndrome. Proc Am Assoc Cancer Res 31:210.

GARCIA JH, OKAZAKI H, ARONSON SM. 1963. Blood group frequencies and astrocytoma. J Neurosurg 20:397–399.

GARMAN RH, SNELLINGS WM. 1986. Frequency, size and location of brain tumours in F-344 rats chronically exposed to ethylene oxide. Food Chem Toxicol 24:145–153.

GEISSLER E, STANECZEK W. 1988. SV40 and human brain tumors. Arch Geschwulstforsch 58:129–134.

GILES GG, MCNEIL JJ, DONNAN G, et al. 1994. Dietary factors and the risk of glioma in adults: results of a case-control study in Melbourne, Australia. Int J Cancer 59:357–362.

GILL PS, LEVINE AM, MEYER PR. 1985. Primary central nervous system lymphoma in homosexual men. Am J Med 78:742–748.

GOLD E, GORDIS L, TONASCIA J, et al. 1978. Increased risk of brain tumors in children exposed to barbiturates. J Natl Cancer Inst 61:1031–1034.

GOLD E, GORDIS L, TONASCIA L, et al. 1979. Risk factors for brain tumors in children. Am J Epidemiol 109:309–319.

GOLD EB. 1980. Epidemiology of brain tumors. In: *Reviews in Cancer Epidemiology*, Lilienfeld AM (ed). New York: Elsevier/North Holland.

GOLD EB, DIENER MD, SZKLO M. 1982. Parental occupations and cancer in children—a case-control study and review of the methodologic issues. J Occup Med 24:578–584.

GOLD EB, LEVITON A, LOPEZ R, et al. 1993. Parental smoking and risk of childhood brain tumors. Am J Epidemiol 137:620–628.

GOLD EB, LEVITON A, LOPEZ R, et al. 1994. The role of family history in risk of childhood brain tumors. Cancer 73:1302–1311.

GOLDHABER MK, SELBY JV, HIATT RA, et al. 1990. Exposure to barbiturates *in utero* and during childhood and risk of intracranial and spinal cord tumors. Cancer Res 50:4600–4603.

GOLDSWORTHY T, CAMPBELL HA, PITOT HC. 1984. The natural history and dose-response characteristics of enzyme-altered foci in rat liver following phenobarbital and diethylnitrosamine administration. Carcinogenesis 5:67–71.

GREIG NH, RIES LG, YANCIK R, et al. 1990. Increasing annual incidence of primary malignant brain tumors in the elderly. J Natl Cancer Inst 82:1621–1624.

GRIFFIN CA, HAWKINS AL, PACKER RJ, et al. 1988. Chromosome abnormalities in pediatric brain tumors. Cancer Res 48:175–180.

HAGMAR L, AKESSON B, NIELSEN J, et al. 1990. Mortality and cancer morbidity in workers exposed to low levels of vinyl chloride monomer at a polyvinyl chloride processing plant. Am J Indust Med 17:553–565.

HALL A, HARRINGTON JM, AW TC. 1991. Mortality study of British pathologists. Am J Ind Med 20:83–89.

HALPER J, COLVARD DS, SCHEITHAUER BW, et al. 1989. Estrogen and progesterone receptors in meningiomas: comparison of nuclear binding, dextran-coated charcoal, and immunoperoxidase staining assays. Neurosurgery 25:546–553.

HAMERNIK RP, TURRENTINE G, ROBERTO M, et al. 1984a. Anatomical correlates of impulse noise-induced mechanical damage in the cochlea. Hearing Res 13:229–247.

HAMERNIK RP, TURRENTINE G, WRIGHT GG. 1984b. Surface morphology of the inner sulcus and related epithelial cells of the cochlea following acoustic trauma. Hearing Res 16:143–160.

HANIS NM, HOLMES TM, SHALLENBERGER LG, et al. 1982. Epidemiologic study of refinery and chemical plant workers. J Occup Med 24:203–212.

HARRINGTON JM, OAKES D. 1984. Mortality study of British pathologists 1974–80. Br J Ind Med 41:188–191.

HARVEY EB, BOICE JD, HONEYMAN M, et al. 1985. Prenatal x-ray exposure and childhood cancer in twins. N Engl J Med 312:541–545.

HAUGE M, HARVALD B. 1957. Genetics in intracranial tumors. Acta Genet 7:573–591.

HAYMAKER W, RUBINSTEIN L, MIQUEL J. 1972. Brain tumors in irradiated monkeys. Acta Neuropathol 20:267–277.

HELSETH A, LANGMARK F, MORK SJ. 1988. Neoplasms of the central nervous system in Norway. II. Descriptive epidemiology of intracranial neoplasms 1955–1984. APMIS 96:1066–1074.

HELSETH A, MORK SJ, GLATTRE E. 1989a. Neoplasms of the central nervous system in Norway. V. Meningioma and cancer of other sites: an analysis of the occurrence of multiple primary neoplasms in meningioma patients in Norway from 1955 through 1986. APMIS 97:738–744.

HELSETH A, MORK SJ, JOHANSEN A, TRETLI S. 1989b. Neoplasms of the central nervous system in Norway: a population-based epidemiological study of meningiomas. APMIS 97:646–654.

HERDAN G. 1960. Frequency of cancer in diabetes mellitus. Br J Cancer 14:449–456.

HESHMAT MY, KOVI J, SIMPSON C, et al. 1976. Neoplasms of the central nervous system: incidence and population selectivity in the Washington, D.C. metropolitan area. Cancer 5:2135–2142.

HICKS N, ZACK M, CALDWELL GG, et al. 1984. Childhood cancer and occupational radiation exposure in parents. Cancer 53:1637–1643.

HILDRETH NG, SHORE RE, HEMPELMANN LH, et al. 1985. Risk of extrathyroid tumors following radiation treatment in infancy for thymic enlargement. Radiat Res 102:378–391.

HIRAYAMA T. 1984. Cancer mortality in nonsmoking women with smoking husbands based on a large scale cohort study in Japan. Prev Med 13:680–690.

HISSERICH JC, PRESTON-MARTIN S, HENDERSON BE. 1975. An areawide reporting network. Public Health Rep 90:15–17.

HOCHBERG FH, MILLER DC. 1988. Primary central nervous system lymphoma. J Neurosurg 68:835–853.

HOOVER R, FRAUMENI JF. 1973. Risk of cancer in renal-transplant recipients. Lancet 2:55–57.

HOWE GR, BURCH JD, CHIARELLI AM, et al. 1989. An exploratory case-control study of brain tumors in children. Cancer Res 49:4349–4352.

HOWE JR, SHERMAN GJ, MALHOTRA A. 1984. Correlations between cancer incidence rates from the Canadian National Cancer Incidence Reporting System, 1969–78. J Natl Cancer Inst 72:585–591.

IARC SCIENTIFIC PUBLICATIONS. 1977. Phenobarbital and phenobarbital sodium. IARC monographs on the evaluation of the carcinogenic effect of chemicals in humans. Lyon, IARC 13:157–182.

INFANTE PF. 1976. Oncogenic and mutagenic risks in communities with polyvinyl chloride production facilities. Ann NY Acad Sci 271:49–57.

IVANKOVIC S. 1979. Teratogenic and carcinogenic effects of some chemicals during prenatal life in rats, Syrian golden hamsters and minipigs. NCI Monogr 51:103–115.

JABLON S, KATO H. 1971. Mortality among atomic bomb survivors, 1950–1970. Atomic Bomb Casualty Commission Report (ABCC-TR):10–71.

JACOBS DH, MCFARLANE MJ, HOLMES FF. 1987. Female patients with meningioma of the sphenoid ridge and additional primary neoplasms of the breast and genital tract. Cancer 60:3080–3082.

JENNINGS MT, MACIUNAS RJ, CARVER R, et al. 1991. TGFb1 and TGFb2 are potential growth regulators for low-grade and malignant gliomas *in vitro*: evidence of an autocrine hypothesis. Int J Cancer 49:129–139.

JOHN EM, SAVITZ DA, SANDLER DP. 1991. Prenatal exposure to parents' smoking and childhood cancer. Am J Epidemiol 133:123–132.

JOHNSON CC, ANNEGERS JF, FRANKOWSKI RF, et al. 1987. Childhood nervous system tumors—an evaluation of the association with paternal occupational exposure to hydrocarbons. Am J Epidemiol 126:605–613.

JOHNSON CC, SPITZ MR. 1989. Childhood nervous system tumours: an assessment of risk associated with paternal occupations involving use, repair or manufacture of electrical and electronic equipment. Int J Epidemiol 18:756–762.

JONES RD, SMITH DM, THOMAS PG. 1988. A mortality study of vinyl chloride monomer workers employed in the United Kingdom in 1940–1974. Scand J Work Environ Health 14:153–160.

Kersey J, Spector BD, Good R. 1973. Primary immunodeficiency and cancer. Cancer Res 18:211–230.

Kersey JH, Spector BD. 1975. Persons at high risk of cancer. In: *Immune Deficiency Diseases*, Fraumeni JF (ed). New York: Academic Press.

Kessler IJ. 1970. Cancer mortality among diabetics. J Natl Cancer Inst 44:673–686.

Kleihues P, Ohgaki H, Eibl RH, et al. 1994. Type and frequency of p53 mutations in tumors of the nervous system and its coverings. Recent Results Cancer Res 135:25–31.

Knox EG, Stewart AM, Kneale GW, et al. 1987. Prenatal irradiation and childhood cancer. J Soc Radiol Prot 7:177–189.

Knuckey NW, Stoll J Jr, Epstein MH. 1989. Intracranial and spinal meningiomas in patients with breast carcinoma: case reports. Neurosurgery 25:112–117.

Koestner A. 1986. The brain-tumour issue in long-term toxicity studies in rats. Food Chem Toxicol 24:139–143.

Kraut A, Tate R, Tran N. 1994. Residential electric consumption and childhood cancer in Canada (1971–1986). Arch Environ Health 49:156–159.

Kuijten RR, Bunin GR. 1993. Risk factors for childhood brain tumors. Cancer Epidemiol Biomark Prev 2:277–288.

Kuijten RR, Bunin GR, Nass CC, et al. 1990. Gestational and familial risk factors for childhood astrocytoma: results of a case-control study. Cancer Res 50:2608–2612.

Kuijten RR, Strom SS, Rorke LB, et al. 1993. Family history of cancer and seizures in young children with brain tumors: a report from the Childrens Cancer Group (United States and Canada). Cancer Causes Control 4:455–464.

Kurtzke JF. 1969. Geographic pathology of brain tumors. Acta Neurol Scand 45:450–555.

Kurtzke JF, Stazio A. 1967. Geographic distribution of brain tumors. Trans Am Neurol Assoc 92:253–254.

Kwa SL, Fine LJ. 1980. The association between parental occupation and childhood malignancy. J Occup Med 22:792–794.

Lancet. 1988. Antenatal ionizing radiation and cancer. Vol. 1, pp 448–449.

Leon SP, Zhu J, Black PM. 1994. Genetic aberrations in human brain tumors. Neurosurgery 34:708–722.

Levi F, La Vecchia C. 1989. Trends in brain cancer (Letter). Lancet 1:917.

Levy LF, Auchterlonie WC. 1975. Primary cerebral neoplasia in Rhodesia. Intern Surg 60:286–292.

Lewis JH, Ginsberg AL, Toomey KE. 1983. Turcot's Syndrome. Cancer 51:524–528.

Lijinsky W. 1992. Chemistry and Biology of N-Nitroso Compounds. Cambridge University Press.

Lijinsky W, Kovatch RM. 1985. Induction of liver tumors in rats by nitrosodiethanolamine at low doses. Carcinogenesis 6:1679–1681.

Lilienfeld AM, Levin ML, Kessler II. 1972. Cancer in the United States. Cambridge, Harvard University Press.

Lin RS, Dischinger PC, Conde J, et al. 1985. Occupational exposure to electromagnetic fields and the occurrence of brain tumors: an analysis of possible associations. J Occup Med 27:413–419.

Lindegård B. 1985. Disease associated with multiple sclerosis and epilepsy. Acad Neurol Scand 71:267–277.

Loomis DP, Savitz DA. 1990. Mortality from brain cancer and leukaemia among electrical workers. Br J Ind Med 47:633–638.

Lyon JL, Klauber MR, Gardner JW, et al. 1976. Cancer incidence in Mormons and non-Mormons in Utah, 1966–70. N Engl J Med 294:129–133.

Mack T. 1977. Cancer surveillance program in Los Angeles County. NCI Monogr 47:99–101.

Mack W, Preston-Martin S, Peters JM. 1991. Astrocytoma risk related to job exposure to electric and magnetic fields. Bioelectromagnetics 12:57–66.

MacMahon B. 1960. The ethnic distribution of cancer mortality in New York City, 1955. Acta Unio Internat Contra Cancrum 16:1716–1724.

MacMahon B. 1962. Prenatal x-ray exposure and childhood cancer. J Natl Cancer Inst 28:1173–1191.

MacMahon B. 1985. Prenatal x-ray exposure and twins. N Engl J Med 312:576–577.

MacPherson P. 1976. Association between previous tuberculosis infection and glioma. Br Med J 2:1112.

Magee PN, Montesano R, Preusmann R. 1976. N-nitroso compounds and related carcinogens. In: *Chemical Carcinogens*, Searle ED (ed). Washington, DC, American Chemical Society.

Magnani C, Coggon D, Osmond C, et al. 1987. Occupation and five cancers: a case-control study using death certificates. Br J Ind Med 44:769–776.

Malkin D, Li FP, Strong LC, et al. 1990. Germ line p53 mutations in a familial syndrome of breast cancer, sarcomas and other neoplasms. Science 250:1233–1238.

Maltoni C, Ciliberti A, Carretti D. 1982. Experimental contributions in identifying brain potential carcinogens in the petrochemical industry. Ann NY Acad Sci 381:216–249.

Mancuso TF. 1963. Tumors of the central nervous system: industrial considerations. Acta U.N. Int Cancer 19:488–489.

Mancuso TF, Ciocco A, El-Attar AA. 1968. An epidemiological approach to the rubber industry: a study based on departmental experience. J Occup Med 10:213–232.

Mantel N, Haentzel W. 1959. Statistical aspects of the analysis of data from retrospective studies of disease. J Natl Cancer Inst 22:719–748.

Maroun FB, Jacob JC. 1973. The frequency of intracranial neoplasms in Newfoundland. Can J Public Health 64:53–67.

Marsh GM, Enterline PE, McCraw D. 1991. Mortality patterns among petroleum refinery and chemical plant workers. Am J Indus Med 19:29–42.

Martuza RL, Eldridge R. 1988. Neurofibromatosis 2. N Engl J Med 318:684–688.

McCredie M, Maisonneuve P, Boyle P. 1994a. Antenatal risk factors for malignant brain tumours in New South Wales children. Int J Cancer 56:6–10.

McCredie M, Maisonneuve P, Boyle P. 1994b. Perinatal and early postnatal risk factors for malignant brain tumours in New South Wales children. Int J Cancer 56:11–15.

McLaughlin JK, Malker HSR, Blot W, et al. 1987a. Occupational risks for intracranial gliomas in Sweden. J Natl Cancer Inst 78:253–257.

McLaughlin JK, Thomas TL, Stone BJ, et al. 1987b. Occupational risks for meningiomas of the CNS in Sweden. J Occup Med 29:66–68.

McMichael AJ, Spirtas R, Kupper LL. 1974. An epidemiologic study of mortality within a cohort of rubber workers, 1964–72. J Occup Med 16:458–464.

Mehta D, Khatib R, Patel S. 1983. Carcinoma of the breast and meningioma. Cancer 51:1937–1940.

Menon AG, Anderson KM, Riccardi VM, et al. 1990. Chromosome 17p deletions and p53 gene mutations associated with the formation of malignant neurofibrosarcomas in von Recklinghausen neurofibromatosis. Proc Natl Acad Sci U S A 87:5435–5439.

Microwave News. 1990. EMFs and cancer clusters: a true link or an epidemiologist's nightmare? X:8–11.

Milham S Jr. 1985. Mortality in workers exposed to electromagnetic fields. Environ Health Perspect 62:297–300.

Miller RW. 1968. Deaths from childhood cancers in sibs. N Engl J Med 279:122–126.

MILLER RW. 1971. Deaths from childhood leukaemia and solid tumours among twins and other sibs in the United States. J Natl Cancer Inst 46:203–209.

MILLS PK, PRESTON-MARTIN S, ANNEGERS JF, et al. 1989. Risk factors for tumors of the brain and cranial meninges in Seventh Day Adventists. Neuroepidemiology 8:266–275.

MIRVISH SS. 1981. Inhibition of the formation of carcinogenic N-nitroso compounds by ascorbic acid and other compounds. In: *Cancer: Achievements, Challenges and Prospects for the 1980's*, Burchenal JH et al (eds). New York: Grune & Stratton.

MODAN B. 1988. Exposure to electromagnetic fields and brain malignancy: a newly discovered menace? Am J Indus Med 13:625–627.

MODAN B, BAIDATZ D, MART H, et al. 1974. Radiation induced head and neck tumors. Lancet 1:277–279.

MODAN B, WAGENER DK, FELDMAN JJ, et al. 1992. Increased mortality from brain tumors: a combined outcome of diagnostic technology and change of attitude toward the elderly. Am J Epidemiol 135:1349–1357.

MOLE RH. 1974. Antenatal irradiation and childhood cancer: causation or coincidence? Br J Cancer 30:199–208.

MONSON RR, FINE LJ. 1978. Cancer mortality and morbidity among rubber workers. J Natl Cancer Inst 61:1047–1053.

MONSON RR, NAKANO KK. 1976. Mortality among rubber workers. I. White male union employees in Akron, Ohio. Am J Epidemiol 103:284–296.

MONSON RR, PETERS JM, JOHNSON MN. 1974. Proportional mortality among vinyl-chloride workers. Lancet 2:397–398.

MORANTZ RA, NEUBERGER JS, BAKER LH, et al. 1985. Epidemiological findings in a brain-tumor cluster in Western Missouri. J Neurosurg 62:856–860.

MORANTZ RA, SHAIN W. 1978. Trauma and brain tumors: an experimental study. Neurosurgery 3:181–186.

MORBIDITY MORTALITY WEEKLY REPORT. 1980. Glioblastoma cluster in a chemical plant—Texas. Vol. 29:359–362.

MORBIDITY MORTALITY WEEKLY REPORT. 1986. Premature mortality due to unintentional injuries—United States, 1983. Vol. 35:353–372.

MORRISON HI, SEMENCIW RM, MORISON D, et al. 1992. Brain cancer and farming in Western Canada. Neuroepidemiology 11:267–276.

MUIR C, MACK T, WATERHOUSE J, et al. 1987. Cancer Incidence in Five Continents. IARC Scientific Publications, No. 88. Lyon: IARC.

MUSICCO M, FILIPINI G, BORDO BM, et al. 1982. Gliomas and occupational exposure to carcinogens: case-control study. Am J Epidemiol 116:782–790.

MUSICCO M, SANT M, MOLINARI S, et al. 1988. A case-control study of brain gliomas and occupational exposure to chemical carcinogens: the risk to farmers. Am J Epidemiol 128:778–785.

NASCA PC, BAPTISTE MS, MACCUBBIN PA, et al. 1988. An epidemiologic case-control study of central nervous system tumors in children and parental occupational exposures. Am J Epidemiol 128:1256–1265.

NATIONAL RESEARCH COUNCIL (NRC). 1981. The health effects of nitrate, nitrite, and N-nitroso compounds. Part 1. Washington DC: National Academy Press.

NEUBERGER JS, BROWNSON RC, MORANTZ RA, et al. 1991. Association of brain cancer with dental x-rays and occupation in Missouri. Cancer Detect Prev 15:31–34.

NEWILL V. 1961. A distribution of cancer mortality among ethnic subgroups of the white population of New York City. J Natl Cancer Inst 26:405–417.

NIGRO JM, BAKER SJ, PREISINGER AC, et al. 1989. Mutations in the p53 gene occur in diverse tumor types. Nature 342:705–708.

OHSUMI S, IKEHARA I, MOTOI M, et al. 1985. Induction of undifferentiated brain tumors in rats by human polyomavirus (JC virus). Jpn J Cancer Res 76:429–431.

OLSEN JH, BOICE JD JR, JENSEN JPA, et al. 1989. Cancer among epileptic patients exposed to anticonvulsant drugs. J Natl Cancer Inst 81:803–808.

OLSEN JH, BOICE JD JR, FRAUMENI JF JR. 1990. Cancer in children of epileptic mothers and the possible relation to maternal anticonvulsant therapy. Br J Cancer 62:996–999.

OLSEN JH, NIELSEN A, SCHULGEN G. 1993. Residence near high voltage facilities and risk of cancer in children. Br Med J 307:891–895.

OLSHAN AF, BRESLOW NE, DALING JR, et al. 1986. Childhood brain tumors and paternal occupation in the aerospace industry. J Natl Cancer Inst 77:17–19.

PARKIN DM, MUIR CS, WHELAN SL, et al. 1992. Cancer Incidence in Five Continents, Volume VI. IARC Scientific Publications, No. 120. Lyon: IARC.

PEGG AE. 1990. Mammalian O^6-alkylguanine-DNA alkyltransferase: regulation and importance in response to alkylating carcinogenic and therapeutic agents. Cancer Res 50:6119–6129.

PERCY AK, ELVEBACK LR, OKAZAKI H, et al. 1972. Neoplasms of the central nervous system. Neurology 22:40–48.

PERCY C, VAN HOLTEN V, MUIR C, EDS. 1990. World Health Organization, International Classification of Diseases for Oncology, 2nd Edition. Geneva, Switzerland.

PETERS JM, PRESTON-MARTIN S, YU MC. 1981. Brain tumors in children and occupational exposure of parents. Science 213:235–237.

PIGNATELLI B, SCRIBAN R, DESCOTES G, et al. 1984. Modifying effects of polyphenols and other constituents of beer on the formation of N-nitroso compounds. Am Soc Brew Chem J 42:18–23.

PRESTON-MARTIN S. 1985. Epidemiology of childhood brain tumors. Ital J Neurol Sci 6:403–409.

PRESTON-MARTIN S. 1989c. Descriptive epidemiology of primary tumors of the brain, cranial nerves and cranial meninges in Los Angeles County. Neuroepidemiology 8:283–295.

PRESTON-MARTIN S, HENDERSON BE, PETERS JM. 1982a. Descriptive epidemiology of central nervous system neoplasms in Los Angeles County. Ann NY Acad Sci 381:202–208.

PRESTON-MARTIN S, HENDERSON BE, YU MC. 1984. The epidemiology of intracranial meningiomas in Los Angeles. Neuroepidemiology 2:164–178.

PRESTON-MARTIN S, LEWIS S, WINKELMANN R, et al. 1993a. Descriptive epidemiology of primary cancer of the brain, cranial nerves, and cranial meninges in New Zealand, 1948–1988. Cancer Causes Control 4:529–538.

PRESTON-MARTIN S, MACK W. 1991. Gliomas and meningiomas in men in Los Angeles County: investigation of exposures to n-nitroso compounds. In: *Relevance to Human Cancer of N-Nitroso Compounds, Tobacco Smoke and Mycotoxins*, O'Neill IK, et al (eds). IARC Scientific Publications, No. 105. Lyon: IARC, pp 197–203.

PRESTON-MARTIN S, MACK W, HENDERSON BE. 1989a. Risk factors for gliomas and meningiomas in males in Los Angeles County. Cancer Res 49:6137–6143.

PRESTON-MARTIN S, PAGANINI-HILL A, HENDERSON BE, et al. 1980. Case-control study of intracranial meningiomas in women in Los Angeles County. J Natl Cancer Inst 75:67–73.

PRESTON-MARTIN S, PIKE MC, ROSS RK, et al. 1990. Increased cell division as a cause of human cancer. Cancer Res 50:7413–7419.

PRESTON-MARTIN S, STAPLES M, FARRUGIA H, et al. 1993b. Primary tumors of the brain, cranial nerves and cranial meninges in Victoria Australia, 1982–1990: patterns of incidence and survival. Neuroepidemiology 12:270–279.

PRESTON-MARTIN S, THOMAS DC, WHITE SC, et al. 1988. Prior exposure to medical and dental x-rays related to tumors of the parotid gland. J Natl Cancer Inst 80:943–949.

PRESTON-MARTIN S, THOMAS DC, WRIGHT WE, et al. 1989b. Noise trauma in the aetiology of acoustic neuromas in men in Los Angeles County, 1978–1985. Br J Cancer 59:783–786.

PRESTON-MARTIN S, YU MC, BENTON B, et al. 1982b. N-nitroso compounds and childhood brain tumors: a case-control study. Cancer Res 42:5240–5245.

PRESTON-MARTIN S, YU MC, HENDERSON BE, et al. 1983. Risk factors for meningiomas in men in Los Angeles County. J Natl Cancer Inst 70:863–866.

RAJEWSKY MF, GOTH R, LAERUM OD, et al. 1976. Molecular and cellular mechanisms in nervous system-specific carcinogenesis by N-ethyl-N-nitrosourea. In: *Fundamentals in Cancer Prevention*, Magee PN, et al (eds). Baltimore: University Park Press.

REAGAN TJ, FREIMAN IS. 1973. Multiple cerebral gliomas in multiple sclerosis. J Neurol Neurosurg Psychiatry 36:523–528.

REIF JS, PEARCE N, FRASER J. 1989. Occupational risks for brain cancer: a New Zealand Cancer Registry-based study. J Occup Med 31:863–867.

REINHARDT G. 1928. Trauma-Fremdkorper-Hirngeschwulst. Munich Med Wochenschr 75:399–401.

RICCARDI VM. 1981. Von Recklinghausen neurofibromatosis. N Engl J Med 305:1617–1626.

RICE JM. 1986. Transplacental carcinogenesis in nonhuman primates: inferences for human risk assessment. Presented at workshop of transplacental carcinogenic risk to humans, Santa Margherita Ligure, Italy.

RICE JM, WARD JM. 1982. Age dependence of susceptibility to carcinogenesis in the nervous system. In: Brain Tumors in the Chemical Industry, Selikoff IJ, et al (eds). New York: Ann NY Acad Sci.

RIES LAG, MILLER BA, HANKEY BF, et al, eds. 1994. SEER Cancer Statistics Review 1973–1991: Tables and Graphs. NIH Pub. No. 94-2789. Bethesda: National Cancer Institute.

RIGGS JE. 1991a. The decline of mortality due to stroke: a competitive and deterministic perspective. Neurology 41:1135.

RIGGS JE. 1991b. Longitudinal Gompertzian analysis of primary malignant brain tumor mortality in the U.S., 1962–1987; rising mortality in the elderly is the natural consequence of competitive deterministic dynamics. Mech Ageing Dev 60:225.

RIMM IJ, LI FC, TARBELL NJ, et al. 1987. Brain tumors after cranial irradiation for childhood acute lymphoblastic leukemia. Cancer 59:1506–1508.

RODVALL Y, PERSHAGEN G, HRUBEC Z, et al. 1990. Prenatal x-ray exposure and childhood cancer in Swedish twins. Int J Cancer 46:362–365.

RON E, MODAN B, BOICE J, et al. 1988. Tumors of the brain and nervous system following radiotherapy in childhood. N Engl J Med 319:1033–1039.

RORKE LB, GILLES FH, DAVIS RL, et al. 1985. Revision of the World Health Organization classification of brain tumors for childhood brain tumors. Cancer 56:1869–1886.

RORKE LB. 1987. Editorial. NeuroOncol 5:95–97.

RORKE LB. 1994. Experimental production of primitive neuroectodermal tumors and its relevance to human neuro-oncology. Am J Patholol 144:444–448.

RUBINSTEIN LJ. 1972. Tumors of the central nervous system. In: *Atlas of Tumor Pathology*, Second Series, Fascicle 6, Washington, D.C., Armed Forces Institute of Pathology.

RUSHTON L, ALDERSON MR. 1981. An epidemiological survey of eight oil refineries in Britain. Br J Ind Med 38:225–234.

RYALS BM, RUBEL EW. 1988. Hair cell regeneration after acoustic trauma in adult coturnix quail. Science 240:1774–1776.

RYAN P, HURLEY SF, JOHNSON AM, et al. 1993. Tumors of the brain and presence of antibodies to *Toxoplasma gondii. Int J Epidemiol 22:412–419.*

RYAN P, LEE MW, NORTH B, et al. 1992a. Risk factors for tumors of the brain and meninges: results from the Adelaide Adult Brain Tumor Study. Int J Cancer 51:20–27.

RYAN P, LEE MW, NORTH B, et al. 1992b. Amalgam fillings, diagnostic dental x-rays and tumors of the brain and meninges. Eur J Cancer 28B:91–95.

SAHL JD, KELSH MA, GREENLAND S. 1993. Cohort and nested case-control studies of hematopoietic cancers and brain cancer among electric utility workers. Epidemiology 4:104–114.

SANDLER DP, COMSTOCK GW, MATANOSKI GM. 1982. Neoplasms following childhood irradiation of the nasopharynx. J Natl Cancer Inst 68:3–8.

SARASUA S, SAVITZ DA. 1994. Cured and broiled meat consumption in relation to childhood cancer: Denver, Colorado (United States). Cancer Causes Control 5:141–148.

SAVITZ DA, JOHN EM, KLECKNER RC. 1990. Magnetic field exposure from electric appliances and childhood cancer. Am J Epidemiol 131:763–773.

SAVITZ DA, LOOMIS DP. 1995. Magnetic field exposure in relation to leukemia and brain cancer mortality among electric utility workers. Am J Epidemiol 141:123–134.

SAVITZ DA, WACHTEL H, BARNES FA, et al. 1988. Case-control study of childhood cancer and exposure to 60-Hz magnetic fields. Am J Epidemiol 128:21–38.

SCANLAN RA, BARBOUR JF. 1991. N-nitrosodimethylamine content of US and Canadian beers. In: *Relevance to Human Cancer of N-Nitroso Compounds, Tobacco Smoke and Mycotoxins*, O'Neill IK et al (eds). IARC Scientific Publications, No. 105. Lyon: IARC, pp 242–243.

SCHIVAPURKAR M, HOOVER KL, POIRIER LA. 1986. Effect of methionine and choline on liver tumor promotion by phenobarbital and DDT in diethylnitrosamine-initiated rats. Carcinogenesis 7:547–550.

SCHLEHOFER B, KUNZE S, SACHSENHEIMER W, et al. 1990. Occupational risk factors for brain tumors: results from a population-based case-control study in Germany. Cancer Causes Control 1:209–215.

SCHLEHOFER B, BLETTNER M, BECKER N, et al. 1992. Medical risk factors and the development of brain tumors. Cancer 69:2541–2547.

SCHNECK SA, PENN I. 1971. *De novo* brain tumours in renal-transplant recipients. Lancet 1:983–986.

SCHNEIDER AB, SHORE-FREEDMAN E, RYO UY, et al. 1985. Radiation-induced tumors of the head and neck following childhood irradiation. Medicine 64:1–15.

SCHOENBERG BS, CHRISTINE BW, WHISNANT JP. 1975. Nervous system neoplasms and primary malignancies of other sites. Neurology 25:705–712.

SCHOENBERG BS, CHRISTINE BW, WHISNANT JP. 1978. The resolution of discrepancies in the reported incidence of primary brain tumors. Neurology 28:817–823.

SCHOENBERG BS. 1991. Epidemiology of primary intracranial neoplasms: disease distribution and risk factors. In: *Neurobiology of Brain Tumors*, Vol. 4 of Concepts in Neurosurgery, Salcman M (ed). Baltimore: Williams & Wilkins, pp 3–18.

SCHREIBER GH, SWAEN GM, MEIJERS JMM, et al. 1993. Cancer mortality and residence near electricity transmission equipment: a retrospective cohort study. Int J Epidemiol 22:9–15.

SCHUMAN LM, CHOI NW, GULLEN WH. 1967. Relationship of central nervous system neoplasms to *Toxoplasma gondii* infection. Am J Public Health 57:848–856.

SELVERSTONE B, COOPER DR. 1961. Astrocytoma and ABO blood groups. J Neurosurg 18:602–604.

SEN NP, SEAMAN S, CLARKSON S, et al. 1984. Volatile N-nitrosamines in baby bottle rubber nipples and pacifiers: analysis, occurrence and migration. In: N-Nitroso Compounds: Occurrence, Biological Effects and Relevance to Human Cancer, O'Neill IK, et al (eds). IARC Scientific Publications, No. 57 Lyon: IARC.

SEYAMA S, ISHIMARU T, IIJIMA S, et al. 1979. Primary intracranial tumors among atomic bomb survivors and controls, Hiroshima and Nagasaki, 1961–1975. Radiation Effects Research Foundation TR 15:1–19.

SHAPIRO S, MEALEY J, SARTORIUS C. 1989. Radiation-induced intracranial malignant gliomas. J Neurosurg 71:77–82.

SHIRTS SB, ANNEGERS JF, HAUSER WA, et al. 1986. Cancer incidence in a cohort of patients with seizure disorders. J Natl Cancer Inst 77:83–87.

SHORE RE, ALBERT RE, PASTERNACK BS. 1976. Follow-up study of patients treated by x-ray epilation for tinea capitis. Arch Environ Health 31:17–24.

SIMONATO L, L-ABBE KA, ANDERSON A, et al. 1991. A collaborative study of cancer incidence and mortality among vinyl chloride workers. Scand J Work Environ Health 17:156–169.

SIMS WL, MARX MB, BROOKS WH. 1979. A follow-up study of the geographic distribution of selected malignancies among Kentucky residents, 1969–1976. J Natl Med Assoc 71:685.

SOFFER D, GOMORI JM, SIEGAL T, et al. 1989. Intracranial meningiomas after high-dose irradiation. Cancer 63:1514–1519.

SOLIONOVA LG, SMULEVICH VB. 1993. Mortality and cancer incidence in a cohort of rubber workers in Moscow. Scand J Work Environ Health 19:96–101.

SORAHAN T, PARKES HG, VEYS CA, 1989. Mortality in the British rubber industry, 1946–85. Br J Ind Med 46:1–11.

SORENSEN SA, MULVIHILL JJ, NIELSEN A. 1986. Long-term follow-up of von Recklinghausen neurofibromatosis. N Engl J Med 314:1010–1015.

SPEERS MA, DOBBINS JG, MILLER VS. 1988. Occupational exposures and brain cancer mortality: a preliminary study of East Texas residents. Am J Ind Med 13:629–638.

STARK AD, CHANG HG, FITZGERALD EF, et al. 1990. A retrospective cohort study of cancer incidence among New York State Farm Bureau members. Arch Environ Health 45:155–162.

STEPHENS T. 1991. Special section: Cancer. A mixed bag of cancer trends. J NIH Res 3:71–72.

STEWART A, WEBB J, HEWITT D. 1958. A survey of childhood malignancies. Br Med J 1:1495–1508.

STRANG RR, TOVI D, LOPEZ J. 1966. Astrocytomas and the ABO blood groups. J Med Genet 3:274–275.

STRONG LC. 1977. Genetic and environmental interactions. Cancer 40:1861–1866.

SUSSMAN A, LEVITON A, ALLRED EN, et al. 1990. Childhood brain tumor: presentation at younger age is associated with a family tumor history. Cancer Causes Control 1:75–79.

SWENBERG JA. 1986. Brain tumours—problems and perspectives. Food Chem Toxicol 24:155–158.

TANNENBAUM SR, MERGENS W. 1980. Reaction of nitrite with vitamins C and E. Ann NY Acad Sci 355:267–277.

TETA MJ, OTT MG, SCHNATTER AR. 1991. An update of mortality due to brain neoplasms and other causes among employees of a petrochemical facility. J Occup Med 33:45–51.

THÉRIAULT G, GOLDBERG M, MILLER AB, et al. 1994. Cancer risks associated with occupational exposure to magnetic fields among electric utility workers in Ontario and Quebec, Canada, and France: 1970–1989. Am J Epidemiol 139:550–572.

THÉRIAULT G, GOULET L. 1979. A mortality study of oil refinery workers. J Occup Med 21:367–370.

THOMAS TL, DECOUFLE P, MOURE-ERASO R. 1980. Mortality among workers employed in petroleum refining and petrochemical plants. J Occup Med 22:97–103.

THOMAS TL, FONTHAM ETH, NORMAN SA, et al. 1986. Occupational risk factors for brain tumors: a case-referent death-certificate analysis. Scand J Work Environ Health 12:121–127.

THOMAS TL, STEWART PA, STEMHAGEN A, et al. 1987a. Risk of astrocytic tumors associated with occupational chemical exposures: a case-referent study. Scand J Work Environ Health 13:417–423.

THOMAS TL, STOLLEY PD, STEMHAGEN A, et al. 1987b. Brain tumor mortality risk among men with electrical and electronics jobs: a case-control study. J Natl Cancer Inst 79:233–238.

THOMAS TL, WAXWEILER RJ, MOURE-ERASO R, et al. 1982. Mortality patterns among workers in three Texas oil refineries. J Occup Med 24:135–141.

TODD NV, MCDONAGH T, MILLER JD. 1987. What follows diagnosis by computed tomography of solitary brain tumour? Lancet 1:611–612.

TOFTGAARD C. 1988. The overall cancer incidence after peptic ulcer surgery: a prospective cohort study. Cancer J 2:17–20.

TOMENIUS L. 1986. 50-Hz electromagnetic environment and the incidence of childhood tumors in Stockholm County. Bioelectromagnetics 7:191–207.

TÖRNQVIST S, KNAVE B, AHLBOM A, et al. 1991. Incidence of leukaemia and brain tumours in some "electrical occupations." Br J Ind Med 48:597–603.

TÖRNQVIST S, NORELL S, AHLBOM A, et al. 1986. Cancer in the electric power industry. Br J Ind Med 43:212–213.

TRAYNOR J, CASEY H. 1971. Five-year follow-up of primates exposed to 5 MeV protons. Radiat Res 47:143–148.

TSANG RW, LAPERRIERE NJ, SIMPSON WJ, et al. 1993. Glioma arising after radiation therapy for pituitary adenoma: a report of four patients and estimation of risk. Cancer 72:2227–2233.

TYNES T, ANDERSON A, LANGMARK F. 1992. Incidence of cancer in Norwegian workers potentially exposed to electromagnetic fields. Am J Epidemiol 136:81–88.

USDHEW. 1973. Public Health Service and Food and Drug Administration: Population exposure to x-rays: U.S.: 1970. DHEW Pub. No. (FDA) 73-8047.

VAN DER WEIL HJ. 1959. Inheritance of glioma: the genetic aspects of cerebral glioma and its relation to status dysgraphicus. Amsterdam: Elsevier.

VELEMA JP, PERCY CL. 1987. Age curves of central nervous system tumor incidence in adults: variation of shape by histologic type. J Natl Cancer Inst 79:623–629.

VELEMA JP, WALKER AM. 1987. The age curve of nervous system tumour incidence in adults: common shape but changing levels by sex, race and geographical location. Int J Epidemiol 16:177–183.

VERKASALO PK, PUKKALA E, HONGISTO MY, et al. 1993. Risk of cancer in Finnish children living close to power lines. Br Med J 307:895–899.

WACKER CD, SPIEGELHALDER B, PREUSSMANN R. 1991. New sulfenamide accelerators derived from 'safe' amines for the rubber and tyre industry. In: Relevance to Human Cancer of N-Nitroso Compounds, Tobacco Smoke and Mycotoxins, O'Neill IK, et al (eds). IARC Scientific Publications, No. 105. Lyon: IARC, pp 592–594.

WALKER MD. 1975. Malignant brain tumors—a synopsis. CA 25:114–120.

WALSH J, GYE B, CONNELLY TJ. 1969. Meningioma: a late complication of head injury. Med J Aust 1:906–908.

WARD RW, MATTISON ML, FINN R. 1973. Association between previous tuberculosis infection and cerebral glioma. Br Med J 1:83–84.

WATERHOUSE J, SHANMUGARATNAM K, MUIR C, et al, eds. 1982. Cancer Incidence in Five Continents. IARC Scientific Publications, No. 42. Lyon: IARC.

WAXWEILER RJ, ALEXANDER V, LEFFINGWELL SS, et al. 1983. Mortality from brain tumor and other causes in a cohort of petrochemical workers. J Natl Cancer Inst 70:75–81.

WAXWEILER RJ, STRINGER W, WAGONER JK, et al. 1976. Neoplastic risk among workers exposed to vinyl chloride. Ann NY Acad Sci 271:40–48.

WEN CP, TSAI SP, MCCLELLAN WA, et al. 1983. Long-term mortality study of oil refinery workers: 1. Mortality of hourly and salaried workers. Am J Epidemiol 118:526–541.

WERTELECKI W, FRAUMENI JF JR, MULVIHILL JJ. 1970. Nongonadal neoplasia in Turner's syndrome. Cancer 26:485–488.

WERTELECKI W, ROULEAU GA, SUPERNEAU DW, et al. 1988. Neurofibromatosis 2: clinical and DNA linkage studies of a large kindred. N Engl J Med 319:278–283.

WERTHEIMER N, LEEPER E. 1979. Electrical wiring configurations and childhood cancer. Am J Epidemiol 109:273–284.

WERTHEIMER N, LEEPER E. 1982. Adult cancer related to electrical wires near the home. Int J Epidemiol 11:345–355.

WORLD HEALTH ORGANIZATION. 1976. ICD-O International Classification of Diseases for Oncology, 1st Edition. Geneva, Switzerland.

WILKINS JR III, KOUTRAS RA. 1988. Paternal occupation and brain cancer in offspring: a mortality-based case-control study. Am J Ind Med 14:299–318.

WILKINS JR III, SINKS TH. 1990. Parental occupation and intracranial neoplasms of childhood: results of a case-control interview study. Am J Epidemiol 132:275–292.

WILKINS JR III, MCLAUGHLIN JA, SINKS TH. 1991. Parental occupation and intracranial neoplasms of childhood: anecdotal evidence from a unique occupational cancer cluster. Am J Ind Med 19:643–653.

WONG O, MORGAN RW, BAILEY WJ, et al. 1986. An epidemiologic study of petroleum refinery employees. Br J Ind Med 43:6–17.

WONG O, WHORTON MD, FOLIART DE, et al. 1991. An industry-wide epidemiologic study of vinyl chloride workers. Am J Ind Med 20:317–334.

WRENSCH M, BARGER GR. 1990. Familial factors associated with malignant gliomas. Genet Epidemiol 7:291–301.

WU W, STEENLAND K, BROWN D, et al. 1989. Cohort and case-control analyses of workers exposed to vinyl chloride: an update. J Occup Med 31:518–523.

YATES PO, PEARCE KM. 1960. Recent changes in blood-group distribution of astrocytomas. Lancet 1:194–195.

59 Cutaneous malignant melanoma

BRUCE K. ARMSTRONG
DALLAS R. ENGLISH

It was estimated that 92,000 new cases of cutaneous melanoma (referred to hereafter as melanoma) were diagnosed worldwide in 1985 (Parkin et al, 1993). This figure was 1.2% of the estimated total of all cancers diagnosed in that year. Although melanoma is a comparatively rare tumor in many populations, incidence rates are increasing around the world (Armstrong and Kricker, 1994a). Possible depletion of the stratospheric ozone layer may exacerbate these trends (Armstrong, 1994a). In the United States, melanoma is, after non-melanocytic skin cancer, now the commonest recorded cancer in men 35–44 years of age and is second only to breast cancer in women in this age group (Parkin et al, 1992). Identification of precise etiological mechanisms is therefore important for preventing a major public health hazard.

The descriptive epidemiology of melanoma suggests that exposure to sunlight is the major cause of the disease in susceptible populations (Armstrong and Kricker, 1994b). A number of recent case-control studies of sun exposure and melanoma have provided corroborating evidence for this view but have indicated that the exposure-response relationship is complex (Armstrong, 1988).

HISTOPATHOLOGY

Melanoma can usually be classified, according to the presence and pattern of intraepidermal growth, into one of three histopathological types—superficial spreading melanoma (SSM), lentigo maligna melanoma (LMM), which is also known as Hutchinson's melanotic freckle melanoma, and nodular melanoma (NM) (McGovern et al, 1986). A fourth and less frequent category, acral lentiginous melanoma (ALM) (McGovern et al, 1986), occurs on soles and palms and has a similar intraepidermal growth pattern to LMM. Melanomas that cannot be classified into any of these types are referred to as melanomas of unclassifiable type (UCM).

This histopathological classification is not universally accepted. Ackerman (1980) has proposed that the apparent histological differences are artefacts related to anatomic site and that all melanomas arise in the same way from epidermal melanocytes. Some epidemiological and histopathological data support this view (Heenan et al, 1987).

Superficial spreading melanoma is the most common type of melanoma, usually accounting for 50% or more of all tumors recorded in population-based series (MacKie and Hunter, 1982; Elwood et al, 1987; English et al, 1987a; Østerlind et al, 1988a). Nodular melanoma is usually the next most common and is defined as an invasive melanoma in which the intraepidermal spread does not extend more than three rete ridges beyond the perimeter of the invasive portion. As such, it may represent the end stages of one of the other types in which the intraepidermal portion has been obliterated (Heenan and Holman, 1982) and should, therefore, share many of the epidemiological features of the other types of melanoma, and of SSM in particular. There is limited evidence from its depth of invasion at diagnosis, pattern of age-specific incidence and body site distribution that this proposition is true (English et al, 1987a; Elwood et al, 1987). Lentigo maligna melanoma is relatively uncommon and is thought by some to be a distinct disease entity (McGovern et al, 1980).

When comparing results from different series of melanoma patients, whether in descriptive or analytical studies, it is important to be aware that differences in epidemiological features may be confounded by the differences in the mixture of lesions of different histological type. In particular, inclusion or exclusion of LMM may affect the results substantially, regardless of whether the present histological classification is meaningful, because most LMM occur on the head and neck, and to exclude them would mean that melanomas on these sites were underrepresented.

ANATOMIC DISTRIBUTION

In whites, melanomas occur most frequently on the trunk in males and the lower limbs in females. These patterns are present in populations at high risk, such as in Australia (Holman et al, 1980; Green et al, 1993a), and at lower risk, such as in Denmark and the United States (Østerlind et al, 1988a; Dennis et al, 1993). Lentigo maligna melanoma differs from the other types in occurring almost exclusively on the head and neck and other habitually exposed surfaces (McGovern et al, 1980; English et al, 1987a; Newell et al, 1988). It is strongly associated with sun damage in adjacent skin, partly, at least, because the diagnosis is influenced by the presence of sun damage (English et al, 1987a).

Superficial spreading melanoma and NM do not differ appreciably in their site distributions (Elwood and Gallagher, 1983; English et al, 1987a) and, in contrast to LMM, have incidence rates that are highest on body sites that are not habitually exposed to the sun—the trunk in men and the lower limbs in women (English et al, 1987a; Østerlind et al, 1988a). The legs in women and the back in men had the highest rates of these melanomas per unit area of body surface in Denmark (Østerlind et al, 1988a), although Elwood and Gallagher (1983) observed that the face in women had higher rates per unit area than the legs.

The anatomic site distribution of melanoma in blacks is quite different from that in whites. Most melanomas in blacks occur on the soles of the feet (Higginson and Oettlé, 1960; Fleming et al, 1975). This observation, first made among rural blacks in Africa, led to speculation that trauma was a cause of melanoma. However, Stevens and coworkers (1990) used SEER data to show that the excess on the soles in blacks, at least in the United States, was a *relative* excess but not an *absolute* excess, because the incidence rate on the soles in blacks was no higher than in whites.

DEMOGRAPHIC PATTERNS

Melanoma is primarily a disease of white populations. In the United States, the incidence in whites is approximately 10 times higher than in blacks living in the same areas (Parkin et al, 1992). The disease is least frequent in Asian populations.

Unless otherwise specified, patterns described below will relate to white populations in which the disease has been most extensively studied.

Mortality

Mortality from melanoma has been steadily increasing in most white populations for many years (Armstrong and Kricker, 1994a). For example, during the period 1950 to 1977, mortality from melanoma among whites in the United States increased from 1.04 per 100,000 person-years in men and 0.83 in women, to 2.64 in men and 1.59 in women (McKay et al, 1982). There is evidence from the United States and Sweden that this trend is now moderating or has come to an end (Roush et al, 1992; Thörn et al, 1992).

International Patterns of Incidence

The incidence of melanoma of the skin varies over 100-fold around the world. Among countries included in *Cancer Incidence in Five Continents*, Volume VI, the lowest rates reported around 1983–1987 were 0.5 per 100,000 person-years, or less, in parts of Asia (eg, China, Japan, Singapore, India, Philippines, Thailand) and in Asians and blacks in the United States; the highest were about 27 per 100,000 person years in the Australian Capital Territory (Parkin et al, 1992). In the continental United States, the incidence in the white population varied from 14.6 per 100,000 among males in Los Angeles to 5.3 in females in New Orleans (Parkin et al, 1992).

Although melanoma incidence increases with increasing proximity to the equator in many populations (Armstrong, 1984), this pattern is by no means consistent. In the first comprehensive analysis of the geography of melanoma in white races, Lancaster (1956) noted that mortality from the disease was higher in Australia and South Africa than in the parts of Europe from which their populations originated; that mortality in Australia, New Zealand, and the United States increased with proximity to the equator; but that within Europe it was higher in Norway and Sweden in the north than in France and Italy in the south. These patterns are also evident in more recent data (Armstrong, 1984). While Lancaster hypothesized from these data that sunlight is a cause of melanoma, he did not offer an explanation for the apparently anomalous relationship between latitude and melanoma in Europe.

These anomalies may be due, at least in part, to lack of a perfect correlation between latitude and exposure of human skin to ultraviolet B. Other factors may include the tendency for racial skin color to increase in darkness with increasing proximity to the equator and the influence of intermittent sun exposure from, for example, summer vacations in southern Europe in populations resident in northern Europe (Armstrong, 1984).

Survival

Five-year relative survival in the United States is about 85% in whites and 70% in blacks (Ries et al, 1994); and in Scotland it is 72% (MacKie et al, 1992). Differences in survival among populations and over time are probably due to differences in the distributions of thickness of melanomas at diagnosis (Heenan and Holman, 1983; Berwick et al, 1994). After adjustment for the substantial difference in thickness distributions between Oxford (an area of low incidence) and Western Australia (an area of high incidence), there was little difference between the two regions in survival rates (Heenan and Holman, 1983).

Time Trends in Incidence

In a comprehensive analysis of trends in the incidence of melanoma in populations represented in the first three volumes of *Cancer Incidence in Five Continents*, Muir and Nectoux (1982) reported that incidence had increased by about 5% a year from the early 1960s to about 1972 in most white populations. In contrast, increases in non-white populations were small and inconsistent.

Recent reports on the increasing incidence of melanoma in white populations have come from British Columbia, different parts of the United States, Denmark, Norway, Sweden, England and Wales, Scotland, Australia, and New Zealand (Armstrong and Kricker, 1994a). In some of these populations, notably in Scotland (MacKie et al, 1992), Australia (MacLennan et al, 1992; Burton et al, 1993), and New Zealand (Cooke et al, 1992), quite sharp increases were observed in recorded incidence rates in the 1980s, doubling in as short a period as 2 years in some cases. In other populations, such as Norway (Magnus, 1991), the increases have been reported to have become less steep recently and in the population covered by the U.S. SEER registries incidence rates actually fell in women and were relatively stable in men in the early 1980s (Scotto et al, 1991).

Table 59–1 summarizes the net trends in melanoma incidence between the early 1960s and about 1987 in white populations (ie, populations of mainly European origin) that were reported on in either Volume 1 or Volume 2 and Volume 6 of *Cancer Incidence in Five Continents* (Armstrong and Kricker, 1994a). The percentage trend per year in each population was calculated from the exponential of the difference in the logarithms of the first and last rates divided by the number of years between the midpoints of the periods on which they were based. This approach appeared reasonable because most of these populations showed linear trends when the logarithms of the rates were plotted against arithmetic values of calendar year.

The average increases in incidence in these populations almost all lay between 3% and 7% a year. There is little evident geographical pattern in these trends except that, when ranked by rate of increase, the Eastern European populations were concentrated among those with the lowest rates of change. This may suggest that the rate of increase in incidence of melanoma has been related to socioeconomic status.

TABLE 59–1. *Average Annual Percentage Increases in Incidence of Melanoma between the Early to Mid-1960s and the Mid-1980s in Populations of Mainly European Origin*

	Average Annual Percent Increase in Incidence		*Age-Standardized Incidence in Mid-1980s*	
Population	*Male*	*Female*	*Male*	*Female*
Canada, Alberta	4.5	3.8	6.3	6.7
Canada, Manitoba	5.2	4.1	5.1	6.1
Canada, Quebec	4.6	4.1	3.0	3.2
Canada, Saskatchewan	4.2	6.1	6.2	7.8
USA, Alameda County, white	5.3	4.7	12.3	10.8
USA, Connecticut	5.4	3.6	10.5	8.4
USA, Hawaii, white	8.9	8.9	22.2	14.9
USA, New York State	5.0	3.9	7.8	6.0
Israel, Jews	7.8	7.6	6.8	8.0
Denmark	5.4	5.1	7.7	9.8
Finland	5.3	4.5	6.6	6.0
Germany, East	3.8	3.5	3.8	4.4
Hungary, Szabolcs	2.7	0.9	2.8	2.3
Hungary, Vas	4.2	3.1	4.7	4.6
Iceland	6.3	4.5	3.4	5.7
Poland, Cracow City	8.2	6.0	4.0	4.2
Poland, Warsaw City	4.5	3.8	3.3	2.7
Norway	5.6	6.8	10.5	13.5
Slovenia	3.9	4.0	3.6	4.0
Sweden	5.6	5.0	9.5	9.6
UK, Birmingham	4.9	5.3	2.8	5.4
UK, Oxford	5.4	4.5	3.5	6.4
UK, South West	6.4	6.0	5.3	9.3
New Zealand, Non-Maori	5.4	4.5	18.6	23.0

Source: Reproduced with permission from Armstrong and Kricker, 1994a.

In contrast to populations of mainly European origin, there has been no consistent upward or downward trend over the full period from the early 1960s to the late 1980s in populations of mainly non-European origin (Armstrong and Kricker, 1994a). Only in Puerto Rico has there been a recent, steady increase in incidence rates based on sizeable numbers of cases. This lack of any consistent evidence of increasing melanoma rates in non-white populations, especially the black population of the United States that lives in the same environment as white populations experiencing the increase, would suggest that changes in sun exposure among susceptible populations may be responsible for the increases.

A review of age-standardized incidence rates of melanoma in four body-site groups (head and neck, trunk, upper limbs, and lower limbs) in 13 populations in North America, Scandinavia, the United Kingdom, and

Australia showed upwards trends in incidence of 2% to 7% a year (Armstrong and Kricker, 1994a). Increases in incidence were most pronounced on the trunk, particularly in men, while the incidence of melanoma of the face remained reasonably stable over time. An interesting trend has been reported from Norway. The incidence of melanoma on the breast has increased in young women since a specific code was allocated to this site in response to the advent of topless sunbathing around the end of the 1960s (Magnus, 1991).

Few data are available on tumor thickness in whole populations. The highest relative increases in seven populations (western Washington State, northern California, Scotland and, in Australia, the Hunter Area of New South Wales, Queensland, South Australia and Tasmania) were in the thinnest melanomas, except for males in Scotland and females in Queensland, where the highest increase was in the group of intermediate thickness (Armstrong and Kricker, 1994a).

Incidence and mortality rates in younger people have diverged recently from those in older people, with a flattening or downturn in rates in younger people in a number of populations (Kricker et al, 1993; Armstrong and Kricker, 1994a). This divergence is seen more clearly in mortality than incidence rates. In some populations, it is not seen at all in incidence rates, which continue to increase in all age groups (Armstrong and Kricker, 1994a).

These divergent trends are clearly seen in the comparison of age-specific trends in melanoma incidence and mortality by year of birth in Denmark shown in Figure 59–1. Incidence increased fairly consistently in all age groups except, perhaps, for a recent downturn in women under 35 years of age. Mortality, on the other hand, stopped rising or fell in men born after about 1935 and women born after about 1925 (ie, in those younger than about 55 years of age).

There are several possible reasons for these divergent patterns. First, the flattening or downturn in rates in younger people may indicate that the long-term increasing trend in incidence is coming to an end in recent birth cohorts. The absence of this pattern in incidence rates in some populations and, therefore, divergence of incidence and mortality rates may be explained by artifactual continuing increases in incidence due, for example, to advancement of the time of diagnosis of melanoma as a result of increased formal and informal screening. Second, it may be that a trend towards earlier diagnosis, more marked in younger people, has led to improvements in survival and a fall in mortality in the face of a continuing rise in incidence. These explanations cannot be readily distinguished and both may be contributing to the mixed trends observed (Armstrong and Kricker, 1994a).

That the former explanation is plausible is suggested by a detailed analysis of the recent sharp and substantial rises in observed incidence of melanoma observed in Australia, New Zealand, and Scotland (Burton et al, 1993; Burton and Armstrong, 1994). These increases lie outside the long-term trend, have been mainly in thin melanoma and, in Australia at least, have occurred in association with increased public and professional attention to melanoma and parallel sharp increases in the rates of excision of all kinds of skin lesions. This suggests that they are due, in part at least, to advancement of the time of diagnosis. The absence of a following fall in incidence in one population (Burton et al, 1993), even after a number of years of observation, may indicate that there has also been increasing ascertainment of a form of melanoma which appears innocuous clinically and is unlikely to cause death if not treated (Burton and Armstrong, 1994).

Notwithstanding possible recent trends toward advancement of the time of diagnosis of melanoma and diagnosis of previously unascertained melanoma, there is little doubt that much of the increase in incidence observed since the 1960s is real. First, the trend is evident in both incidence and mortality data and the trend in mortality cannot be explained by improved certification of cause of death on death certificates (Lee and Carter, 1970). Second, improved histopathological diagnosis cannot be responsible for much, if any, of the increases observed. A review of melanocytic nevi and malignant melanomas diagnosed in nine countries over a 50-year period showed only a very small change in the criteria for diagnosis of malignancy (van der Esch et al, 1991). In addition, where treatment of melanoma occurs largely on an outpatient basis, as is increasingly the case in many populations, underenumeration by cancer registries may be substantial and increasing, leading to underestimation rather than overestimation of increases in incidence (Karagas et al, 1991).

The reasons for this long-term trend toward increasing incidence of melanoma in populations of mainly European origin is not known with any certainty. While increasing recreational sun exposure, or a change from a predominantly occupational to a predominantly recreational pattern of sun exposure, may be the most likely cause (Armstrong and Kricker, 1994a), there are few data on population trends in sun exposure that would allow this hypothesis to be examined directly. Indirectly, it gains some support from the lack of increase in melanoma incidence in most populations of mainly non-European origin, the apparent lack of an increase in melanoma of nonexposed sites (eg, melanoma of the vulva, vagina, anus, and rectum; Ragnarsson-Olding et al, 1993; Weinstock, 1993), the comparatively high rates of increase on the trunk and low rates of increase on the face, and the lack of any plausible alternative explanation.

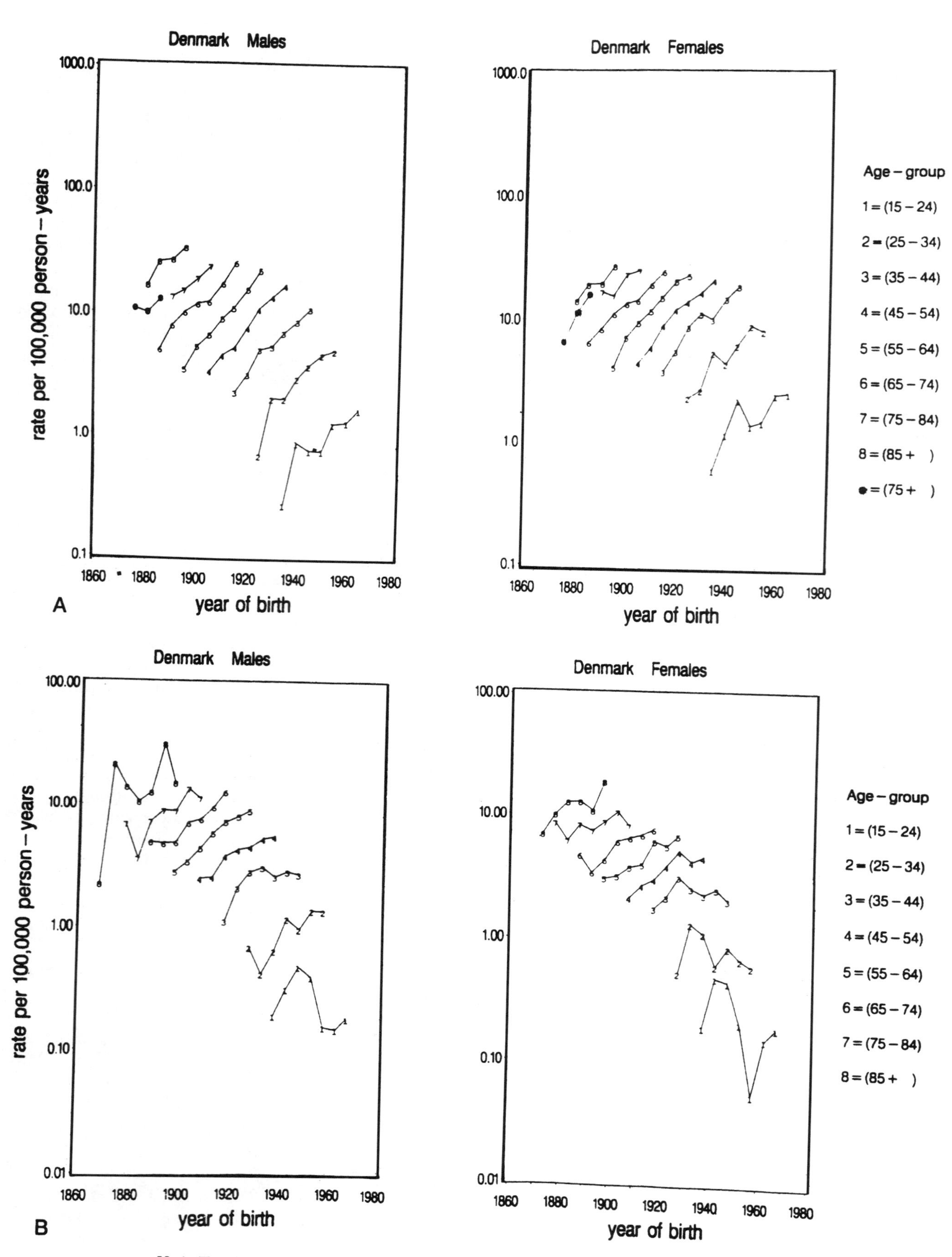

FIG. 59–1. Trends in incidence (A) of and mortality (B) from melanoma by sex, age, and year of birth in Denmark, 1953–1957 to 1983–1987. (Reproduced with permission from Kricker et al, 1993.)

Migration

Migrants who move from areas of low incidence to areas of high incidence with sunny climates, such as Australia, Israel, and New Zealand, generally have lower rates of melanoma than the native-born residents of the host countries (Katz et al, 1982; Cooke and Fraser, 1985; Khlat et al, 1992). Risk increased with increasing duration of residence and earlier age at migration in all these countries. A contradictory pattern was reported from Hawaii—incidence rates in white immigrants were substantially higher than in Hawaiian-born whites (Hinds and Kolonel, 1980). This apparent contradiction has been attributed to southern European or mixed-race ancestry in the Hawaiian-born.

British immigrants to Australia and New Zealand, where the populations are of predominantly British origin, had mortality rates about half those of the native-born residents (Cooke and Fraser, 1985; Khlat et al, 1992); similar differences were observed in incidence rates in Western Australia (Holman et al, 1980). Age at arrival in Australia appears to be a more powerful predictor of risk than duration of residence (Holman and Armstrong, 1984a; Khlat et al, 1992). Arrival before 10 years of age was associated with no decrease in risk of melanoma relative to that among the Australian-born, but arrival after that age had a relative risk of approximately 0.5. A similar conclusion was reached in a study of internal migration within the United States (Mack and Floderus, 1991).

Age

Unlike many tumors of adults, melanoma occurs frequently among the young and middle-aged. Incidence rates generally rise steeply until about 50 years of age, after which the rate of increase slows, particularly in women (Magnus, 1981). Data from the SEER program for 1983–1987 are shown in Figure 59–2. These overall patterns of age-specific incidence reflect a complex mixture of age-specific rates varying by anatomic site and histological type, which in turn may be affected by differing cohort-based incidence trends.

Melanomas occurring on the face show a near exponential increase in incidence with increasing age (Holman et al, 1980; Magnus, 1981; Newell et al, 1988), much as would be expected for a tumor caused by long-term exposure to an environmental agent. On other body sites, the incidence is highest among the middle-aged and declines thereafter (Holman et al, 1980; Magnus, 1981; Newell et al, 1988). Most, if not all, of the decline in old age may be due to rapid, cohort-based increases in incidence occurring for most of these sites (Magnus, 1981). With the evidence of falling incidence rates on the trunk and limbs in recent birth cohorts in the United States, particularly in women (Dennis et al, 1993), it will be of interest to see whether these site-specific patterns of incidence by age become concave up rather than concave down over time. This change would effectively exclude the possibility of age-limited exposure to the sun of body sites that are usually covered as an explanation for the middle-age peak in incidence (Holman et al, 1980).

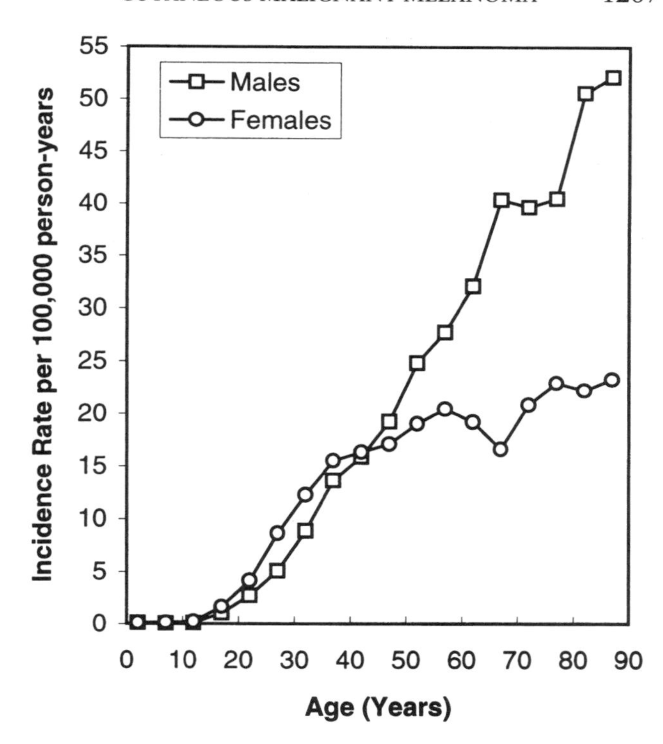

FIG. 59–2. Age-specific incidence of melanoma in whites in the United States. (Prepared from US SEER Registries' data in Parkin et al, 1992.)

Sex

The incidence of melanoma tends to be slightly higher in women than in men. Among 70 registries of white populations in Europe, North America, Australia, and New Zealand that were included in Volume V of *Cancer Incidence in Five Continents* (Muir et al, 1987), the average age-standardized incidence rate was 1.0 per 100,000 person-years higher in women (95% confidence interval, assuming normality of rates, 0.60 to 1.37 per 100,000) than in men. In addition, while the age-specific rate in men appears to increase throughout life, in women there appears to be little increase in incidence after middle age (see Figure 59–2).

Lee and Storer (1980) found that women of reproductive age had higher rates of melanoma than men in the British Isles but not in Scandinavia, where melanoma is more common. They suggested that there is a hormone-dependent factor in melanoma that is apparent when underlying disease rates are low (ie, when environmental factors are largely absent). To study this issue further, we examined the correlation between the average of and the difference between the two sex-specific incidence rates reported in *Cancer Incidence in Five Continents*, Volume V (Muir et al, 1987). Overall, the correlation coefficient was −0.18 (95% confidence interval −0.40 to 0.06), but between the ages of 20 and 49, the correlation was −0.72 (95% confidence interval −0.82 to −0.58), thus confirming the association between the magnitude of the incidence rates and the excess in females of reproductive age.

Survival after diagnosis is better in women than in men (Lemish et al, 1983; Ries et al, 1994; Thörn et al, 1987), thus men have a higher mortality than women. The death rate in men in the United States (3.5 per 100,000) in 1991 is more than double that in women (1.6) (Ries et al, 1994), whereas the incidence in men is about 35% more than that in women (Ries et al, 1994). These difference are at least partially, although perhaps not completely, explained by sex differences in thickness and site-distribution of melanoma (Vossaert et al, 1992; Thörn et al, 1994). Men generally have thicker melanomas at diagnosis than women (Jelfs et al, 1994).

Ethnicity

Among white populations, ethnic background is a determinant of melanoma incidence. The incidence is substantially lower among Hispanics than among other whites in the United States. For example, the incidence among those with Spanish surnames in Los Angeles was between 2 and 3 per 100,000 person-years, but in other whites it was over 11 per 100,000 (Parkin et al, 1992). In several case-control studies, subjects with a southern or eastern European background had lower risks than those of northern European or United Kingdom origins (Elwood et al, 1984; Holman and Armstrong, 1984b; Graham et al, 1985).

In a case-control study from western Canada (Elwood et al, 1984), the effect was not changed appreciably by adjustment for hair, eye, and skin color and the skin's reaction to sun exposure. In contrast, the effect of ethnic origin observed in a case-control study from western Australia was substantially reduced, although not removed completely, by adjustment for pigmentary characteristics (Holman and Armstrong, 1984b).

Socioeconomic Status

Incidence and mortality rates of melanoma are highest among high social classes (Holman et al, 1980; Lee and Strickland, 1980; Cooke et al 1984). Differences in rates among the social classes, imputed from occupation, vary up to twofold. Similar social class gradients have been observed in case-control and cohort studies in which measures of social class have been derived from occupation or education (MacKie and Aitchison, 1982; Gallagher et al, 1987; Østerlind et al, 1988b; Lee et al, 1992). An analysis from western Washington State, USA, showed the expected pattern of increasing melanoma incidence with increasing socioeconomic status (as assessed by mean household income of census tract of residence) at all ages, but the opposite in men greater than 70 years of age (Kirkpatrick et al, 1990). The latter effect was largely confined to melanomas occurring at sun-exposed sites.

Occupation, income, and education are confounded with sunlight exposure. High socioeconomic status is generally associated with indoor occupations, whereas a greater proportion of persons of low socioeconomic status is engaged in outdoor work. In two case-control studies, one from Canada and one from Denmark, in which socioeconomic status and known risk factors for melanoma were examined together, strong associations between high socioeconomic status and an increased risk of melanoma were partly explained by confounding with host factors such as skin, eye, and hair color and with occupational and recreational sun exposure (Gallagher et al, 1987; Østerlind et al, 1988b). Professionals and scientists had an odds ratio of 3.8 (95% confidence interval 2.0–7.4) relative to unskilled workers in the Canadian study, and 2.8 (95% confidence interval 1.5–5.3) in the Danish study. After adjustment, the odds ratios were reduced to 2.3 (95% confidence interval 1.0–5.1) and 1.9 (95% confidence interval 0.9–4.0) respectively.

It seems likely, then, that effects of social class are partly (if not wholly) due to differences in behavioral patterns and constitutional risk factors among the various social class groups, as has been suggested by several authors (Lee and Strickland, 1980; MacKie and Aitchison, 1982). This view is supported by the interaction between socioeconomic status, age, and site and histological type of melanoma observed by Kirkpatrick et al (1990).

ENVIRONMENTAL FACTORS

Sunlight

Attention has been drawn already to a number of observations that suggest a positive association between incidence of melanoma and exposure to the sun. They include the association of melanoma with latitude and measured ultraviolet B radiation, the apparent protective effect of racial pigmentation, the increasing incidence in white populations, and the effect on incidence of migration from an area of low to an area of high incidence.

A number of observations, however, are apparently inconsistent with a simple relationship between sun exposure and melanoma. In many populations, melanoma occurs as commonly in women as in men, although men are more likely to work outdoors. It shows a relative peak in incidence in middle life, which is not the pattern to be expected from lifelong exposure to an environmental agent, and it occurs frequently on the back in men and lower limbs in women, sites which are not maximally exposed. There are also, as noted above, a number of geographical areas in which the incidence of melanoma does not increase with increasing proximity to the equator. Of more significance, perhaps, is the relationship between incidence of melanoma and occupation and socioeconomic status—melanomas are more common in indoor than outdoor workers and are positively associated with socioeconomic status.

These observations led to postulation of the "intermittent exposure hypothesis" for the relationship of sunlight to melanoma (Fears et al, 1977; Holman et al, 1980). Briefly, this hypothesis states:

1. Incidence of melanoma is determined as much (or more) by the pattern of sun exposure as by the total accumulated "dose" of sun exposure.
2. Infrequent (intermittent) exposure of untanned skin to intense sunlight is particularly effective in increasing incidence of melanoma. Thus incidence rises initially as frequency of exposure increases but may fall as exposure becomes more continuous.

A simple rationalization for this complex hypothesis is that development and maintenance of a suntan is protective against the carcinogenic effects of continuing sun exposure. At low frequencies of sun exposure, a tan is not maintained (except in those with high natural skin pigmentation or who tan very easily), and the melanocytes are substantially unprotected from solar ultraviolet on each occasion of exposure.

Since the intermittent exposure hypothesis was put forward in the mid-1970s, a number of case-control studies of melanoma have been undertaken to see whether the disease can be related to sun exposure in individuals and whether this relationship takes the form suggested by the hypothesis. Characteristics of these studies are summarized in Table 59–2.

In interpreting these studies, a number of technical issues need to be kept in mind (Armstrong, 1988).

First, there is the issue of measurement error. The measurements used may be summarized as: measurement of potential for exposure to the sun (eg, age at arrival in a country with high ambient ultraviolet flux and average hours of bright sunlight at all places of residence); measurement of actual exposure to the sun (eg, by way of self-administered questionnaires of varying degrees of sophistication); and measurement of biological response to sun exposure (eg, by recall of sunburn and measurements of chronic skin damage presumed to be due to ultraviolet light).

A number of sources of error may affect these measurements. For example, unless actual outdoor exposure (in the case of measures of potential exposure) and protective behavior in the sun are documented, measures of both potential and actual exposure to the sun may substantially misclassify the true exposure of individual subjects. Measures of actual exposure to the sun are, however, generally dependent on subjective recall and may be substantially erroneous. Most of this error is likely to be non-differential (ie, similar in subjects with and without disease), leading to substantial attenuation of any real associations.

Second, there is the issue of confounding. The most important known confounder of sun exposure is "skin type" or the skin's reaction to sunlight (Holman et al, 1984a). People with sun-sensitive skin are at increased risk of melanoma (see below) but tend to avoid sun exposure or protect themselves when in the sun. The result will be negative confounding between sun sensitivity and sun exposure; that is, a positive association between sun exposure and melanoma unadjusted for sun sensitivity may appear weaker than it really is because of the association of sun sensitivity with low exposure and sun insensitivity with high exposure. Confounding with sun sensitivity should probably not be considered to be present, however, where the measure of sun exposure is a biological response to sunlight (Green and O'Rourke, 1985).

Some authors have adjusted for the number of benign melanocytic nevi on the skin (which correlates strongly with risk of melanoma; see below) when considering the association between melanoma and sun exposure (see, for example, Green et al, 1986). If nevi lie in the chain of effects between sun exposure and melanoma (Holman et al, 1983), control of their number as a confounding variable will bias the relative risk towards unity.

Third, it is important to appreciate that measurement error may have an effect on the control of confounding (Tzonou et al, 1986). This effect will be most important when controlling for sun sensitivity in examining relationships between sun exposure and melanoma. If there is error in the measurement of sun sensitivity, it will not be possible to control confounding between it and sun exposure. The residual confounding could partly mask associations between sun exposure and melanoma.

In describing the results of the studies summarized in Table 59–2, attention will be drawn to aspects of the control of confounding that are relevant to the points raised above. Unless stated otherwise, it may be as-

TABLE 59–2. *Case-Control Studies of Malignant Melanoma in Relationship to Sun Exposure Conducted or Reported after the "Intermittent Exposure" Hypothesis Was Advanced*

Reference	*Place*	*Period of Diagnosis*	*Cases*			*Controls*	
			No.	*Source*	*Type*[a]	*No.*	*Type and Source*
Klepp (1979)	Norway	1974–75	78	radium, hospital	not stated	131	hospital, other cancers
Adam (1981)	Parts of England	1971–76	111	population	not stated	342	general practice lists
MacKie and Aitchison (1982)	Western Scotland	1978–80	113	hospital	SSM or NM	113	hospital
Lew (1983)	Boston, USA	1978–79	111	clinic	not stated	107	friends of cases
Rigel (1983)	New York, USA	1978–81	114	clinic	not stated	228	clinic, staff
Brown (1984)	New York	1972–80	89	skin clinic	not stated	65	skin clinic
Elwood (1984, 1985, 1987)	Western Canada	1979–81	595	population	SSM, NM, or UCM	595	population
Green (1984, 1985b, 1986)	Queensland, Australia	1979–80	183	population	SSM, NM, or UCM	183	population
Holman (1984a, 1986b)	Western Australia	1980–81	511	population	all	511	population
Graham (1985)	Buffalo, USA	1974–80	404	hospital	not stated	521	hospital, cancer patients
Sorahan (1985)	Birmingham, UK	1980–82	58	hospital	not stated	333	hospital and population
Dubin (1986)	New York, USA	1972–82	1,103	hospital	not stated	585	skin clinic
Elwood (1986)	Nottingham, UK	1981–84	83	population	all	83	hospital
Cristofolini (1987)	Trento, Italy	1983–85	103	hospital	not stated	205	hospital
Holly (1987)	San Francisco	1984–85	121	melanoma clinic	SSM, NM, or UCM	139	clinic
Østerlind (1988b)	East Denmark	1982–85	474	population	SSM, NM, or UCM	926	population
Garbe (1989)	Berlin	1987	200	hospital	all	200	skin clinic
MacKie (1989)	Scotland	1987	280	population	all	280	hospital
Weinstock (1989a, 1991b)	USA	1976–84	130	cohort of nurses	all except ALM	300	cohort (nested)
Beitner (1990)	Stockholm	1978–83	525	hospital	all	525	population
Elwood (1990)	England	1984–86	195	population	SSM or NM	195	hospital
Grob (1990)	France	1986–88	207	hospital	not stated	295	clinic and hospital
Zanetti (1992)	Turin, Italy	1984–86	208	population	all	416	population
Zaridze (1992)	Moscow	not stated	96	hospital	all	96	hospital visitors
Dunn-Lane (1993)	Dublin	1985–86	100	hospital	SSM or NM	100	population
Nelemans (1993)	Netherlands	1988–90	141	population	SSM or NM	183	population, cancer patients
Garbe (1994a)	Germany and Switzerland	1990–91	513	hospital	all	498	skin clinic
White (1994)	Seattle, USA	1984–87	256	population	SSM	273	population

[a]SSM = superficial spreading melanoma, NM = nodular melanoma, UCM = unclassifiable melanoma, ALM = acral lentiginous melanoma.

sumed that age and sex were controlled in all studies. In this respect, another possible error in some studies is the performance of an "unmatched" analysis without control of the matching variables, after matching has been carried out in the design of the study. The effect of this error is usually to bias the measure of effect toward the null value.

Lifetime Total Exposure to the Sun. The commonly although not consistently observed gradient toward increasing incidence of melanoma with increasing proximity to the equator would suggest that, for the population as a whole, incidence of the disease increases with increasing lifetime exposure to the sun. A number of the case-control studies listed in Table 59–2 have included variables which could be taken as indicating lifetime accumulated exposure to the sun. The results obtained with these variables are summarized in Table 59–3.

The studies of potential lifetime exposure and biological responses thought to indicate lifetime exposure are consistent in showing an increased risk of melanoma with increased exposure or potential exposure to the sun. The evidence from the biological responses—his-

TABLE 59–3. *Associations between Individual Risk of Malignant Melanoma and Indicators of Lifetime Accumulated Exposure to the Sun*

Reference	*Measurement of Sun Exposure*	*Direction of Association*	*Relative Risk in Highest Category*	P *Value*
	POTENTIAL EXPOSURE			
Brown (1984)	World War II service in tropics	Up	8.0 (2.0–34.7)[a]	<0.001
Holman and Armstrong (1984a)	Age at arrival in Australia	Down	0.3 (0.1–1.1)	<0.001
	Mean annual hours of bright sunlight at places of residence	Up	2.8 (1.8–4.8)	<0.001
Graham (1985)	Ever resided below 40° N latitude	Up	1.4 (0.9–2.0)	NA[b]
Green (1986)	Migration to Australia	Down	0.3[c,f] (0.1–1.4)	NA
Østerlind (1988b)	Residence near coast	Up	1.7 (1.1–2.7)	0.006
MacKie (1989)	Tropical residence (males)	Up	2.6 (1.8–4.0)	NA
	Tropical residence (females)	Up	1.8 (0.8–4.0)	NA
Beitner (1990)	Residence near Mediterranean or in tropics	Up	1.9[c,d] (1.0–3.6)	NA
Weinstock (1989a)	Southerly latitude of residence age 15–20	Up	2.2[c] (1.1–4.2)	0.02
	Southerly latitude of residence age 30+	Up	1.6[c] (0.9–2.8)	0.12
	ACTUAL EXPOSURE			
Green (1984)	Total sun exposure throughout life	Up	5.3[c,d,e] (0.9–30.8)	NA
Graham (1985)	Total sun exposure throughout life	Down	0.6[c] (0.4–0.9)	<0.05
Dubin (1986)	Lifetime sun exposure	Up	1.1 (0.8–1.6)	>0.05
Grob (1990)	Cumulative sun exposure index	Up	3.4[c,d,e,] (1.6–7.1)	NA
Lê (1992)	Lifetime sun exposure	Up	5.4 (1.6–18.5)	0.01
	BIOLOGICAL RESPONSES			
Holman and Armstrong (1984a)	Cutaneous microtopography	Up	2.7 (1.4–5.0)	0.003
	History of non-melanocytic skin cancer	Up	3.7 (2.1–6.6)	<0.001
Green (1985)	Actinic tumors on face	Up	3.6 (1.8–7.3)	<0.001
Dubin (1986)	History of solar keratosis	Up	5.0 (2.3–10.5)	<0.01
Holly (1987)	History of non-melanocytic skin cancer	Up	3.8[d,e,f] (1.2–12.4)	0.03
Østerlind (1988b)	Cutaneous microtopography	Flat	1.1 (0.7–1.8)	NA
Garbe (1989)	Actinic lentigines	Up	6.2[c,e,f] (2.8–13.8)	NA
Garbe (1994a)	Actinic lentigines	Up	3.5[c,d,e] (2.3–5.4)	NA

[a]95% confidence interval in parentheses
[b]NA = not available
[c]Adjusted for cutaneous sensitivity to the sun
[d]Adjusted for pigmentary characteristics
[e]Adjusted for number or type of nevi
[f]Adjusted for some other measure(s) of sun exposure

tory of solar keratosis or non-melanocytic skin cancer, presence of solar keratoses or non-melanocytic skin cancer on the face at the time of interview, and cutaneous microtopography (a measure of loss of fine markings on the skin; Holman and Armstrong, 1984a)—is particularly strong in all studies except that of Østerlind and coworkers (1988b), with relative risks ranging from 2.7 to 6.2 and *P* values consistently very low.

On the other hand, the results from attempted measurement of actual lifetime exposure to the sun by interview are inconsistent, with relative risks for the highest exposure category ranging from 0.6 to 5.4. Recognizing the difficulty of measuring actual total lifetime exposure by means of a questionnaire or interview schedule and the fact that none of these analyses allowed for protective behaviors, it would seem reasonable to conclude that the evidence from measurement of potential exposure and biological responses is more reliable.

Total Exposure to the Sun in Specific Periods. It has been common in questionnaires on sun exposure to enquire about usual (presumably present) exposure to the sun, or exposure in some specific, limited period of life. Measurements based on such enquiries aim at actual exposure to the sun. "Total" is used here to distinguish these measurements from measures of occupational or recreational exposure. Results with such measurements in the case-control studies reviewed are summarized in Table 59–4.

There is little evidence, from these studies, of any effect of usual total exposure to the sun, or total exposure

TABLE 59–4. *Associations between Individual Risk of Melanoma and Measures of Recent or Usual Total Exposure to the Sun Based on Questionnaires*

Reference	*Measurement of Sun Exposure*	*Direction of Association*	*Relative Risk in Highest Category*	P *Value*
Rigel (1983)	Average daily sun exposure 1–5 years ago	Up	1.4 (NA)[a,b]	>.05
	Average daily sun exposure 11–20 years ago	Up	2.5 (NA)	<.001
Elwood (1985a)	Hours of sun exposure a year	Flat	1.2 (0.7–2.0)	>.1
Dubin (1986)	Hours of sun exposure a day 0–5 years ago	Flat	1.1 (0.6–2.1)	>.05
	Hours of sun exposure a day 11–20 years ago	Down	0.8 (0.5–1.4)	>.05
Holman (1986a)	Mean total outdoor hours a week in summer	Down	0.7[c,d] (0.4–1.1)	0.13
Cristofolini (1987)	Heavy or frequent exposure in past 20 years	Down	0.7[d,e,f] (0.4–1.1)	>.05
White (1994)	Average yearly hours of sun exposure in past 10 years	Flat	0.9[d,e,f]	0.5
	Sun exposure index[g] 2–10 years of age	Down	0.4[d,e,f]	0.001
	11–20 years of age	Down	0.5[d,e,f]	0.003

[a]95% confidence interval in parentheses
[b]NA = not available
[c]Adjusted for cutaneous sensitivity to the sun
[d]Adjusted for pigmentary characteristics
[e]Adjusted for number or type of nevi
[f]Adjusted for some other measure(s) of sun exposure
[g]Number of days a year in the sun divided by a measure of extent of usual clothing when exposed

in any specific period of life, to increase risk of melanoma. Paradoxically, White and coworkers (1994) found quite strong, apparent protection against melanoma of increasing sun exposure in childhood and adolescence. These results were apparently not due to negative confounding of measures of sun exposure with cutaneous sensitivity to the sun. However, an analysis of the interaction between sun exposure and cutaneous sensitivity to the sun showed that the apparent protective effect was confined to those who tanned well. Poor tanners, though, still did not show any consistent increase in risk of melanoma with increasing total exposure in the age ranges studied.

Occupational Exposure to the Sun. Most previous studies of occupation and melanoma have inferred occupational sun exposure from the occupational title. Several of the case-control studies sought information directly about occupational exposure to the sun; their results are summarized in Table 59–5. While there was some evidence of a fall in risk of melanoma with increasing occupational exposure in some studies, the evidence for it was not strong in any study and there were some quite strong associations in the opposite direction. The irregular patterns seen in the two studies conducted by Elwood and his colleagues (1985a, 1986) were contradictory. In the first (Elwood et al, 1985a), the relative risk was 1.8 (95% confidence interval [CI] 1.2–2.5) for 1–8 hours of exposure a week and approximately unity among those with no exposure or more than 8 hours a week of occupational exposure. In the second (Elwood et al, 1986), relative risk fell with increasing occupational exposure to 0.2 (95% CI 0.1–0.9) at 25,001 to 50,000 hours but rose to 1.7 (95% CI 0.3–8.6) with 50,000+ hours of exposure. One cohort study, of Harvard graduates, showed that men who had worked outdoors prior to commencing college had an increased mortality from melanoma (Paffenbarger et al, 1978).

There is, then, no consistent pattern of change in incidence of melanoma with increasing occupational exposure to the sun. Site of exposure, however, may be important. In a study based on cancer registry data and occupational titles, Vågerö et al (1986) observed the highest incidence of melanoma in office workers and the lowest in outdoor workers. This effect was restricted to melanomas on those body sites that were usually covered; melanomas on parts of the body that were usually exposed were more common in outdoor workers. Similarly, in New Zealand, incidence rates of melanoma on the upper limbs were higher among outdoor workers than indoor workers, but melanoma of the trunk was more common among indoor workers (Cooke et al, 1984). These observations are consistent with those of Cristofolini and coworkers (1987) with respect to "heavy or frequent" exposure to the sun. In addition, Holman and coworkers (1986a) found that among outdoor workers who, overall, had a lower incidence of melanoma than those who had not worked outdoors, incidence of melanoma was higher on sites that were sometimes or usually exposed than it was on sites that

TABLE 59–5. *Associations between Individual Risk of Melanoma and Measures of Occupational Exposure to the Sun Based on Questionnaires*

Reference	*Measurement of Sun Exposure*	*Direction of Association*	*Relative Risk in Highest Category*	P *Value*
Klepp (1979)	Hours of outdoor work a day	Up	1.4 (0.6–3.5)[a]	0.4
MacKie and Aitchison (1982)	Hours of outdoor occupation a week	Down	0.5[c,f] (0.2–1.2)	>0.05
Rigel (1983)	Outdoor occupation	Up	1.2 (NA[b])	>0.05
Elwood (1985a)	Hours of outdoor occupation a week in summer	Irreg	0.9[d] (0.6–1.5)	<0.01
Holman (1986a)	Mean hours of outdoor occupation a week in summer	Down	0.5[c,d] (NA)	0.04
Graham (1985)	Lifetime hours of outdoor occupation	Down	0.7[c] (0.3–1.3)	>0.05
Dubin (1986)	Occupation type	Up	2.4[c,d,f] (1.4–4.4)	<0.01
Elwood (1986)	Lifetime hours of outdoor occupation	Irreg	1.7 (0.3–8.6)	0.5
Østerlind (1988b)	Outdoor occupation	Down	0.7 (0.5–0.9)	NA
Garbe (1989)	Occupational sun exposure	Up	11.6[c,e,f] (2.1–63.3)	0.007
Beitner (1990)	Outdoor occupation	Down	0.6[d] (0.4–1.0)	NA
Grob (1990)	Outdoor occupation	Up	6.0[c,d,e] (2.1–17.4)	NA
Dunn-Lane (1993)	Hours of outdoor work a week	Up	1.3 (0.5–3.5)	0.7
Nelemans (1993)	Ever worked outdoors	Down	0.6[c,d] (0.3–1.0)	NA
White (1994)	Lifetime proportion of outdoor occupation	Down	0.6 (0.3–1.2)	0.13

[a]95% confidence interval in parentheses
[b]NA = not available
[c]Adjusted for cutaneous sensitivity to the sun
[d]Adjusted for pigmentary characteristics
[e]Adjusted for number or type of nevi
[f]Adjusted for some other measure(s) of sun exposure

were usually covered. This observation suggests the possibility that beyond some critical point, incidence of melanoma begins to increase with further increases in "dose" of sunlight. Thus the lack of any clear pattern of melanoma incidence with occupational sun exposure in Table 59–5 may be contributed to by failure to take site into consideration.

Intermittent or Recreational Exposure to the Sun. In most studies, intermittent exposure to the sun has been equated with recreational exposure. Thus results have been reported for various measures of recreational exposure to test the intermittent exposure hypothesis; they show a fairly consistent pattern (Table 59–6). Most showed convincing trends toward increasing risk of melanoma with increasing recreational exposure to the sun, including three of the largest and best of the studies reviewed (Elwood et al, 1985a; Holman et al, 1986a; Østerlind et al, 1988b). Two further studies (Klepp and Magnus, 1979; Sorahan and Grimley, 1985) showed an increasing risk with increasing recreational exposure to the sun although the P values were greater than 0.05. However, when deriving their P value Sorahan and Grimley (1985) included five covariates in a multivariate model based on only 53 cases and at least one of these covariates, number of moles, may be inappropriate. When only age and sex were controlled, the relative risk with 21+ days of holiday abroad in a hot climate was 6.5 ($P < 0.05$). The relative risk obtained by Klepp and Magnus (1979) may also be biased downward because they did not control for sun sensitivity.

Only one of the studies was frankly contradictory of the intermittent exposure hypothesis: MacKie and Aitchison (1982) found a relative risk of melanoma of less than unity (0.4) with 16+ hours of outdoor recreation a week. This relative risk, however, was derived from a model that also contained socioeconomic status and history of sunburn, both of which may be giving similar information to actual recreational exposure to the sun, so its meaning is uncertain. MacKie and Aitchison (1982) also stated that the total number of days spent in Mediterranean or warmer climates in the previous 5 years were "similar between cases and controls and not significant." Similarly, Graham and coworkers (1985) found "no relationship with number of weeks of vacation in southern regions." Adam and coworkers (1981) stated that there were "no differences between cases and controls in the amount of leisure time that they spent out of doors." Weinstock and coworkers (1991a), found increased risk of melanoma with increasing recreational exposure among sun-sensitive women (ie, those unable to tan), but decreasing risk with increasing recreational exposure among women able to tan readily, a pattern similar to that for total exposure in childhood and adolescence observed by White and coworkers (1994).

TABLE 59–6. *Associations between Individual Risk of Melanoma and Measures of Recreational Exposure to the Sun Based on Questionnaires*

Reference	Measurement of Sun Exposure	Direction of Association	Relative Risk in Highest Category	P Value
Klepp (1979)	Sunbathing holidays in southern Europe last 5 years	Up	2.4 (1.0–5.8)[a]	0.06
Adam (1981)	Spent some time deliberately tanning their legs	Up	1.5 (0.9–2.5)	0.16
	Spent some time deliberately tanning their trunk	Up	1.6 (1.0–2.5)	0.05
MacKie and Aitchison (1982)	Hours a week in outdoor recreation	Down	0.4[c,f] (0.2–0.9)	<0.05
Lew (1983)	Days of vacation in a sunny warm place in childhood	Up	2.5 (1.1–5.8)	<0.05
Rigel (1983)	Outdoor vs indoor recreation	Up	2.4 (NA[b])	0.01
Elwood (1985a)	Hours of high exposure recreational activities per week in summer	Up	1.7[d] (1.1–2.7)	<0.01
	Hours of high and moderate exposure recreational activities per day in summer vacations	Up	1.5[d] (1.0–2.3)	<0.01
	Number of sunny vacations per decade	Up	1.7[d] (1.2–2.3)	<0.001
Green (1986)	Recreational hours spent in sun on beach over whole of life	Irregular	1.9 (0.5–7.4)	0.62
Holman (1986a)	Recreational outdoor exposure proportion in summer at 10–24 years of age	Up	1.3[c,d] (0.8–1.9)	0.25
	Boating in summer	Up	2.4[c,d] (1.1–5.4)	0.04
	Fishing in summer	Up	2.7[c,d] (1.1–6.4)	0.07
	Swimming in summer	Irregular	1.1[c,d] (0.7–1.8)	0.66
	Sunbathing in summer at 15–24 years of age	Up	1.3[c,d] (0.8–2.2)	0.26
Sorahan (1985)	Number of holidays abroad in hot climate	Up	5.0[c,e,f] (NA)	>0.05
Dubin (1986)	Recreation type	Irregular	1.0[c,d,f] (NA)	NA
Østerlind (1988b)	Sunbathing	Up	1.9 (1.3–2.9)	0.004
	Boating	Up	1.7 (1.1–2.8)	0.012
	Skiing	Up	1.5 (0.9–2.4)	0.006
	Swimming	Up	1.5 (1.2–2.0)	0.004
	Vacations in sunny resorts	Up	1.7 (1.2–2.4)	0.01
Beitner (1990)	Frequency of sunbathing	Up	1.8[d] (1.2–2.6)	NA
	Sunbathing vacations abroad	Up	2.4[d] (1.5–3.8)	NA
Grob (1990)	Outdoor leisure exposure in last two years	Up	8.4[c,d,e] (3.6–19.7)	NA
Weinstock (1991a)	Type of swimsuit (bikini)	Up	1.8[c,f] (0.9–3.5)	0.065
	Annual frequency of swimsuit use by "sun resistant" women	Down	0.3[c,f] (0.1–0.8)	0.02
	Annual frequency of swimsuit use by "sun sensitive" women	Up	3.5[c,f] (0.1–0.8)	0.01
Zanetti (1992)	Number of weeks of beach holiday in childhood	Irregular	2.8 (1.6–4.6)	0.003
	Number of weeks of beach holiday in adulthood	Up	1.5 (0.9–2.4)	0.10
Zaridze (1992)	Frequency of sunbathing at 18–20 years of age	Up	3.4 (0.6–17.4)	0.03
Dunn-Lane (1993)	Any holiday in the sun	Up	1.3 (0.7–2.3)	0.5
	Any sunbathing	Up	1.2 (0.6–2.5)	0.7
Nelemans (1993)	Sunbathing, 15–25 years of age	Up	2.2[c,d] (1.2–3.8)	NA
	Water sports, 15–25 years of age	Up	1.6[c,d] (0.7–3.9)	NA
	Sunny vacations, 15–25 years of age	Up	1.4[c,d] (0.8–2.7)	NA

[a]95% confidence interval in parentheses
[b]NA = not available
[c]Adjusted for cutaneous sensitivity to the sun
[d]Adjusted for pigmentary characteristics
[e]Adjusted for number or type of nevi
[f]Adjusted for some other measure(s) of sun exposure

None of the results shown in Table 59–6 took specific account of the intermittency or otherwise of exposure of the site at which the melanoma arose. This failure could lead to substantial misclassification of exposure. An indication of the possible importance of this misclassification is given by some additional data from Holman and coworkers (1986a). While sunbathing at 15–24 years of age (the period of peak prevalence of this behavior) was only weakly associated with melanoma as a whole, a stronger association was observed for SSM of the back (relative risk for sunbathing once or more a week in summer, 2.6 with 95% CI 1.0–6.2, $P < 0.05$). Similarly, relative risk of melanoma of the trunk in women was strongly related to the type of bathing suit worn in summer at 15–24 years of age; with reference to a one-piece suit with a high back line, relative risk for a one-piece suit with a low back line was 4.0 (95% CI 0.6–25) and relative risk for wearing a two-piece bathing suit, or none at all, was 13.0 (95% CI 2.0–84). This finding was not confirmed, however, by Weinstock and coworkers (1991a), who found an odds ratio of 1.8 (95% CI 0.9–3.5) for predominant wearing of a bikini.

Sunburn is perhaps one of the most easily recalled and, therefore, least misclassified measures of intermittent sun exposure. It may also have the advantage of indicating dose received at the level of the basal layer of the skin, taking account of both intensity of exposure to the sun and degree of natural protection.

Sunburn has been more consistently associated with melanoma than has any other sun exposure variable (Table 59–7). In all except four of 20 relevant studies, a moderate to strongly positive relationship between

TABLE 59–7. *Associations between Individual Risk of Melanoma and History of Sunburn*

Reference	*Measurement of Sun Exposure*	*Direction of Association*	*Relative Risk in Highest Category*	P *Value*
MacKie and Aitchison (1982)	Blistering sunburn or erythema persisting more than one week	Up	2.8[c,f] (1.1–7.4)[a]	<0.05
Lew (1983)	Blistering sunburn during adolescence	Up	2.0 (1.2–3.6)	<0.05
Elwood (1985b)	Vacation sunburn score	Up	1.8 (1.1–3.0)	<0.01
Green (1985b)	Number of severe sunburns throughout life	Up	2.4[e] (1.0–6.1)	<0.05
Sorahan (1985)	Bouts of painful sunburn	Up	7.0 (NA[b])	<0.001
Holman (1986a)	Sunburn causing pain for 2+ days last 10 years	Irregular	0.9[g] (0.5–1.5)	0.43
	Sunburn causing pain for 2+ days <10 years of age	Up	1.2[g] (0.6–2.3)	0.10
	Blistering sunburn	Up	1.7[g] (1.0–2.9)	0.003
Elwood (1986)	Sunburn causing pain for 2+ days	Up	3.2 (1.7–5.9)	<0.001
Cristofolini (1987)	Severe sunburn in adolescence or early adult life	Down	0.7 (0.4–1.2)	>0.05
	Sunburn as an adult	Up	1.2 (0.7–2.1)	>0.05
Holly (1987)	Blistering sunburns up to adult age	Up	3.8[d,e,f] (1.4–10.4)	NA
Østerlind (1988b)	Sunburn causing pain for 2+ days <15 years of age	Up	3.7 (2.3–6.1)	<0.001
	Sunburn causing pain for 2+ days last 10 years	Up	3.0 (1.5–5.4)	<0.001
Zanetti (1988)	Sunburn in childhood (males)	Up	4.1 (1.8–9.2)	NA
	Sunburn in childhood (females)	Up	2.7 (1.3–4.3)	NA
Garbe (1989)	Number of sunburns	Flat	NA	NA
MacKie (1989)	Severe sunburn (males)	Up	9.2[c,e,f] (3.4–25)	NA
	Severe sunburn (females)	Up	3.6[c,e,f] (1.7–7.7)	NA
Weinstock (1989a)	Blistering sunburns ages 15–20 years	Up	1.9 (1.1–3.4)	0.03
	Blistering sunburns 30+ years of age	Irregular	1.1 (0.6–2.3)	0.3
Beitner (1990)	Erythema after sunbathing	Up	1.7[d] (1.0–2.9)	NA
Elwood (1990)	Severe sunburn age 8–12	Up	3.6	<0.01
Grob (1990)	Frequency of sunburns in recent years	Irregular	1.7[c,d,e] (0.6–4.6)	NA
	Severity of sunburn in recent years	Irregular	0.3[c,d,e] (0.1–2.0)	NA
Zanetti (1992)	Frequency of sunburn in childhood	Up	12.0 (4.6–31.0)	<0.001
	Frequency of severe sunburns lifelong	Irregular	1.7 (1.1–2.6)	0.04
Dunn-Lane (1993)	Bad sunburn at least once	Up	1.9	0.04
Nelemans (1993)	History of sunburn 15–25 years of age	Up	2.1[c,d] (1.2–3.6)	NA

[a]95% confidence interval in parentheses
[b]NA = not available
[c]Adjusted for cutaneous sensitivity to the sun
[d]Adjusted for pigmentary characteristics
[e]Adjusted for number or type of nevi
[f]Adjusted for some other measure(s) of sun exposure
[g]These results not previously published

sunburn and melanoma was observed. In one of the studies that did not follow this pattern consistently (Holman et al, 1986a), there was quite strong evidence for a relationship between number of blistering sunburns and incidence of melanoma. In another study not showing an effect, questions were asked about sunburns in recent years (Grob et al, 1990), whereas most of the other studies included sunburn in childhood and adolescence.

Intermittent or Total Accumulated Exposure to the Sun?

The studies summarized above show associations between both intermittent (as indicated by recreational exposure and sunburn) and total accumulated exposure to the sun (as indicated mainly by measures of potential for exposure to the sun and biological indicators of chronic sun-induced skin damage). There are a number of ways in which these relationships might be rationalized.

First, it may be that our assumptions about the meaning of some of these variables in terms of intermittent or accumulated exposure to the sun are incorrect. Thus, for example, while average annual hours of bright sunlight at places of residence might reasonably be expected to correlate with total accumulated exposure to the sun, it may be that it is more strongly correlated with recreational exposure because of the increased opportunities presented by long sunlight hours for outdoor recreation. Similarly, while it is generally believed that non-melanocytic skin cancers and solar keratoses correlate best with total accumulated exposure to the sun, there is now evidence that intermittent sun exposure may be important for basal cell carcinoma of the skin, at least (Kricker et al, 1995).

Among the large population-based studies, actinic skin damage generally had a stronger association with risk in areas of high incidence than in areas of low incidence. It may be that recreational exposure to the sun over long periods of time gives rise to severe damage to the skin in places where ultraviolet radiation is intense, such as in Australia. If this is true, biological effects of intermittent and total accumulated exposure to the sun may be more readily distinguished in regions of low ultraviolet radiation.

Second, it may be that only one of these groups of variables reflects the truth of the relationship of sunlight with melanoma and the other is confounded with it. Thus, since recreational exposure is a component of total exposure to the sun, a strong relationship between recreational exposure and melanoma would be expected to be reflected in a (probably) weaker relationship between total exposure and melanoma. Similarly, a person who had always lived in an area with many hours of bright sunshine annually would be more likely to have been sunburnt than a person who had lived in a place where bright sunshine was uncommon. We examined the effect of the latter relationship by including age at arrival in Australia (more or less than 10 years of age) in a logistic regression model with number of blistering sunburns. The negative association of melanoma with arrival after 10 years of age was hardly weakened at all (relative risk rose from 0.34 with 95% CI 0.24–0.48 to 0.36 with 95% CI 0.25–0.52) while its association with number of blistering sunburns was weakened (relative risk with 5+ blistering sunburns fell from 1.7 with 95% CI 1.0–2.9 to 1.3 with 95% CI 0.8–2.3). But does this mean that sunburn is not relevant to the association between sun exposure and melanoma? Not necessarily. The effect of residence in Australia in early life must be mediated in some way. It could simply be by way of total sun exposure without regard to peaks producing sunburn or it could be that it produces its effect through sunburn. If the latter were true, the effect of age at arrival in Australia should have been weakened in the above model to the same or to a greater extent than that of sunburn. However, the "measurement" of age at arrival in Australia is likely to be very much less in error than the measurement of number of blistering sunburns, either in total or in early life. This difference in measurement error could lead to the apparent dominance of the effect of age at arrival in Australia.

Third, the pattern of the relationship between melanoma and sun exposure may be even more complex than we have previously suggested (Holman et al, 1986a; Armstrong, 1988). Thus, while continuing exposure to the sun of a sufficient degree to produce persistent tanning may lead to a reduction in risk of melanoma below that observed with a more intermittent pattern of exposure, once more or less maximal tanning has been achieved risk of melanoma may begin to increase again in proportion to the total "dose" of sunlight received. As noted above, there is some evidence for this dose-response pattern in site-specific analyses of occupational sun exposure.

Our present concept of the relationship between risk of melanoma and total amount and intermittency (pattern) of sun exposure is illustrated in Figure 59–3. This figure suggests that risk of melanoma increases in those who tan poorly with increasing total exposure to the sun at all levels and in all patterns of exposure, whereas in those who tan well it falls with increasing exposure when the pattern of exposure is more or less continuous but increases when the pattern is very intermittent. In addition, risk of melanoma may increase in good tanners who are more or less continuously exposed when their total exposure goes beyond some critical level. This concept suggests that the overall relationship between total exposure and melanoma observed in any population will depend on the amount and pattern of exposure and the mix of good and poor tanners in the population

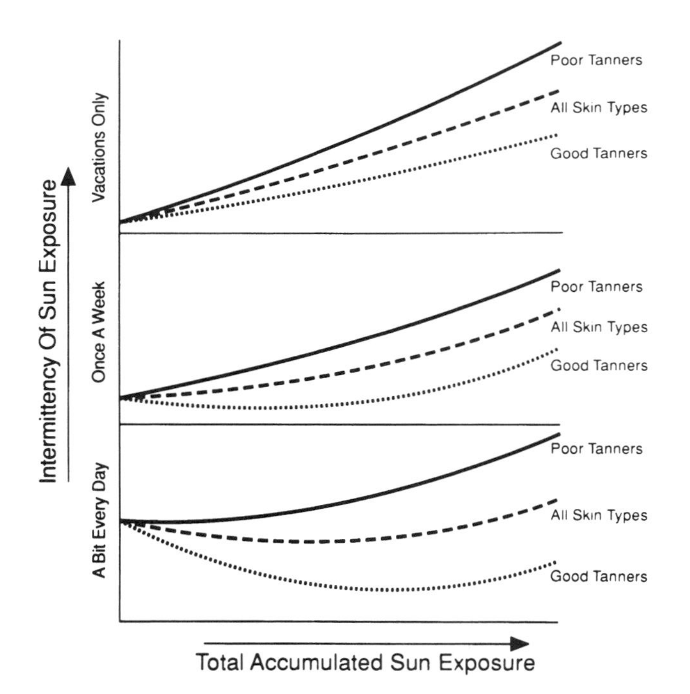

FIG. 59–3. Speculative representation of effects of amount and pattern of sun exposure on incidence of malignant melanoma in relation to cutaneous sensitivity to the sun. (Reproduced with permission from Armstrong, 1994b.)

and may, therefore, be quite variable from one population to another. The level of ambient solar UV radiation is likely to be another modifying factor.

Few studies have attempted to disentangle these variables and the capacity of epidemiological studies to do so is limited both by the numbers of subjects that would be required and the difficulty of making the measurements accurately. Among those who have tried to address the issue, Elwood and coworkers (1985a) did not find consistent evidence of modification of the effect of sun exposure by ability to tan. The observation of Weinstock and coworkers (1991a), however, that risk of melanoma was negatively associated with frequency of exposure in women who tan readily but positively associated in women who tan poorly is consistent with the effect modification postulated in Figure 59–3. Similarly, Nelemans and coworkers (1993) found much higher relative risks associated with sunbathing, water sports, vacations to sunny countries and history of sunburns in those who tanned poorly than those who tanned well. White and coworkers (1994) also found modification of the effect of estimated total sun exposure in adolescence and childhood by cutaneous sensitivity to the sun, although the finding that risk of melanoma did not increase with increasing estimated exposure to the sun even in those who tanned poorly is hard to explain. None of these studies attempted to analyze pattern and total amount of sun exposure together with cutaneous sensitivity in a single analysis. Such analyses will be necessary in studies carried out in comparable ways in populations at different levels of ambient UV radiation if these issues are to be clarified.

Fluorescent Lights and Other Sources of Artificial Ultraviolet Radiation

An association between exposure to fluorescent lights and melanoma risk has been regarded as plausible on the grounds that at short wave lengths (ie, < 295 nm), the absorbed dose of ultraviolet light from fluorescent lighting may be greater than that from a similar period in the sun (Maxwell and Elwood, 1983).

Beral and coworkers (1982) were the first to report an association between exposure to fluorescent lights and melanoma; women exposed at work had a twofold increase in risk of melanoma. They argued that fluorescent light exposure could account for the higher rate of melanoma among indoor workers than among outdoor workers. However, their argument was weakened because the increase in risk was restricted to the trunk, a site usually covered at work.

The results of case-control studies of exposure to fluorescent lights are summarized in Table 59–8. Adjustment for sun exposure was attempted only by Beral and coworkers (1982), English and coworkers (1985), Elwood and coworkers (1986), and Walter and coworkers (1992). The exposure data ranged from simple questions about whether fluorescent lights were "mainly on" at work (Sorahan and Grimley, 1985) to quantitative estimates of the actual number of hours of exposure (English et al, 1985; Elwood et al, 1986; Walter et al, 1992). Information on exposure was usually obtained from interview, but in one study a postal questionnaire was used (Sorahan and Grimley, 1985), and the source of information was unknown for one study (Rigel et al, 1983). Elwood and coworkers (1986) and Dubin and coworkers (1986) obtained primary information from interviews but also sent postal questionnaires to measure reproducibility.

Although plastic diffusers effectively prevent transmission of ultraviolet radiation (Maxwell and Elwood, 1983), only English and coworkers (1985) and Elwood and coworkers (1986) enquired about exposure to lights without diffusers. If exposure to fluorescent tubes is a cause of melanoma, the risk should only be present for tubes without diffusers. However, recall of exposure to fluorescent lights is probably poor (Dubin et al, 1986), and recall of whether there were diffusers fitted is likely to be even worse; thus, measurement error would be likely to lead to substantial weakening of any real positive effect.

Only the study of Beral and coworkers (1982) provides strong evidence for an effect of exposure to fluo-

TABLE 59–8. *Associations between Risk of Melanoma and Exposure to Fluorescent Lights*

Reference	Cases/ Controls	Odds Ratio[a]	Definition of Exposure
Beral (1982)	274/459	2.6[b] (1.2–5.9)	Indoor workers, 20+ years occupational exposure
		4.3[b] NA	Office workers, 20+ years occupational exposure
Rigel (1983)	114/228	0.7 NA	Any exposure
		0.6 NA	Any exposure, office workers
English (1985)	337/349	1.2[b] (0.8–1.9)	35,000+ hours exposure
		1.2[b] (0.7–1.9)	1600+ hours/year
		1.3[b] (0.8–1.9)	22,500+ hours undiffused lights
		1.2[b] (0.8–1.9)	1300+ hours/year undiffused lights
		1.2[b] (0.6–2.6)	22,500+ hours head, neck, upper limbs undiffused lights
Sorahan (1985)	58/333	0.6 NA	20+ years, occupational exposure
		0.5 NA	20+ years, indoor workers only
Dubin (1986)	1103/585	2.3[c] (1.0–5.8)	9+ hours/day 0–5 years ago
	508/222	0.6[d] (0.3–1.3)	9+ hours/day 0–5 years ago
Elwood (1986)	83/83	1.4[b,c] (0.4–5.1)	50,000+ hours occupational exposure
		4.0[b,c] (0.8–19)	50,000+ hours occupational exposure, undiffused lights
	67/66	1.2[b,d] (0.3–5.7)	50,000+ hours occupational exposure
		1.9[b,d] (0.4–8.4)	50,000+ hours occupational exposure, undiffused lights
Østerlind (1988b)	474/926	No association	Duration of exposure, age at first exposure, type of workplace
Swerdlow (1988)	180/197	1.2[b] (0.7–1.9)	Any occupational exposure ≤5 years ago
		0.8[b] (0.4–1.4)	Any exposure ≤5 years ago
		1.6[b] (0.9–2.6)	5+ hours/day ≤5 years ago
		1.4[b] (0.9–2.3)	Any occupational exposure > 5 years ago
		0.8[b] (0.4–1.4)	Any residential exposure > 5 years ago
Walter (1992)	583/608	1.9 (1.1–3.2)	Males—31+ years occupational exposure
		0.8 (0.5–1.2)	Females—21+ years occupational exposure

[a]Odds ratio for category with highest level of exposure; 95% confidence intervals in parentheses
[b]Adjusted for sun exposure
[c]Results obtained from interview
[d]Results obtained from postal questionnaire

rescent light on risk of melanoma although, implausibly, mainly in melanomas at unexposed sites. Evidence of an effect was also found by Walter and coworkers (1992) but only in men. This effect was mainly evident in melanoma of the head, neck, and upper limbs. The study of English and coworkers (1985) showed little effect of exposure to undiffused lights and no effect on rates of melanoma of the head, neck, or upper limbs, the sites most likely to be affected by fluorescent lights. Swerdlow and coworkers (1988) also reported no effect for any specific anatomic site, though they did find an association for SSM (odds ratio of 2.8 [95% CI 1.5–5.4]) for ≥5 hours' exposure per day within 5 years of interview). Although Elwood and coworkers (1986) found a relative risk of 4 for 50,000 hours or more exposure to undiffused lights, the number of subjects with this amount of exposure was small, the relative risk for the second highest exposure category was only 1.5, and the test for trend gave $P = 0.2$. In addition, the effect calculated from information obtained from postal questionnaires was much weaker. Dubin and coworkers (1986) also found a moderate positive association in interview data but a negative association in data obtained from postal questionnaire.

There are other sources of ultraviolet radiation to which people are exposed. These include sunlamps and sunbeds, ultraviolet lamps used for treating various skin conditions, and occupational sources (e.g., welding arcs).

Earlier case-control studies found no association between incidence of melanoma and use of sunbeds or sunlamps (Elwood et al, 1986 Gallagher et al, 1986b; Østerlind et al, 1988b; MacKie et al, 1989). However, several recent case-control studies that included extensive data on use of sunbeds and sunlamps found increasing risk of melanoma with increasing duration of use. In one, the odds ratio for any use was 2.9 (95% CI 1.3–6.4) (Swerdlow et al, 1988) and, in another, it was 1.9 (1.2–3.0) in men and 1.5 (1.0–2.1) in women (Swerdlow et al, 1988; Walter et al, 1990). In a third study, while risk was only moderately increased for more than 10 hours' exposure before 1980 (odds ratio 2.12, 95% CI 0.84–5.37), it was 7.35 (95% CI 1.67–32.3) in those who had also experienced skin burns (Autier et al, 1994). These results were adjusted for age, sex, hair color, and the average number of holiday weeks spent each year in sunny resorts. Elwood and coworkers (1986) reported a relative risk of 2.2 (95% CI 1.0–4.9) for occupational exposure to ultraviolet light from sources such as vacuum or discharge lamps, insecticidal or germicidal lamps, and printing or dyeline copying equipment. English and coworkers (1985), however, found no increased risk for exposure to a range of occupational sources of ultraviolet light.

Recently, the use of psoralens and ultraviolet A (UVA)—PUVA—for the treatment of psoriasis has become widespread. Several reports have been published of cases of melanoma in patients treated with PUVA, but the rates of melanoma in two cohorts of people treated with PUVA in the United States and Europe were little higher than would have been expected on the basis of population incidence rates. In the U.S. cohort the rate ratio was 1.46 (95% CI 0.3–7.3; Gupta et al, 1988), while in the European cohort the rate ratios were 1.1 (0.2–3.2) in men and 0.8 (0.1–3.0) in women (Lindelöf et al, 1991).

Occupation

Increased risks of melanoma have been observed in workers in the chemical, petrochemical, printing, aircraft, rubber, textiles, electronics, and telecommunications industries and in firemen and workers exposed to vinyl chloride, PCBs, and radiation (Austin and Reynolds, 1986; Gallagher et al, 1986a; Nelemans et al, 1992; Sinks et al, 1992; Lundberg et al, 1993, de Guire 1994). In most of these studies, the risk increases were small and based on small numbers of cases of melanoma; in addition, most associations have not been found consistently and possible confounding with sun exposure could not be controlled in most studies.

With respect to ionizing radiation, Holman and coworkers (1986b) found, by use of a job-exposure linkage scheme, a relative risk of 2.7 for LMM among those possibly exposed. In addition a significant excess of melanoma, based on only two cases, was observed in children irradiated in infancy for enlargement of the thymus gland (Krain, 1991). However, no appreciable increase in mortality from melanoma was observed in a large cohort of British radiation workers (Kendall et al, 1992).

Both chemicals and radiation have been implicated in the excess rates of melanoma among employees at the Lawrence Livermore National Laboratory in California. Employees at the facility had a fourfold increase in melanoma incidence rate over that prevailing in the surrounding area (Austin et al, 1981), and in a subsequent case-control study, elevated risks were noted for chemists and those exposed to volatile photographic chemicals or to radioactive materials, independently of consititutional risk factors and sun exposure habits (Austin and Reynolds, 1986). In contrast, the incidence among employees at a similar facility in New Mexico, the Los Alamos National Laboratory, was no higher than that observed in the surrounding region and not elevated among chemists or among those exposed to radiation (Acquavella et al, 1983). The usual excess of melanoma among professionals was seen in the Los Alamos study.

Oral Contraceptives and Reproductive Factors

There is a physiological basis for the hypothesis that melanoma risk is influenced by hormonal or reproductive factors. Estrogens alone, and in combination with progesterone, stimulate division of melanocytes and melanogenic activity in animals (Snell and Bischitz, 1960). These effects are presumably the cause of hyperpigmentation in women taking oral contraceptives (Jelinek, 1970). Sadoff and coworkers (1973) and Lee and Storer (1980) have proposed that a hormonal factor, possibly related to childbearing, may increase the risk of melanoma in premenopausal women. Their view is supported by the relative excess of melanoma among women in the later years of reproductive life.

The results of 15 reports of oral contraceptive use and melanoma are summarized in Table 59–9. The cohort study reported by Beral and coworkers in 1977 was later extended by Ramcharan and coworkers (1981). This study, which was part of the Walnut Creek Contraceptive Drug Study, was the only one in which there was strong evidence for an effect of ever use of oral contraceptives. The rate ratio reported by Ramcharan and coworkers (1981) was 3.5 (95% CI 1.4–9.0). All other studies yielded essentially negative results and a meta-analysis of those studies in Table 59–9 that reported estimates of the precision of relative risks gave a pooled estimate of relative risk for ever use of oral contraceptives of 1.04 (95% CI 0.92–1.18). The increase seen in the Walnut Creek study may have resulted from confounding, because women who used oral contraceptives had higher levels of recreational sun exposure than non-users. Furthermore, there was no increase in risk with increasing duration of use.

Long-term use of oral contraceptives was associated with about a twofold increased risk in the studies of Holly and coworkers (1983) and Lê and coworkers (1992), but with smaller or minimal increases in the other studies with data on long-term use (Table 59–9). A meta-analysis of the studies with long-term use data in Table 59–9 and estimates of the precision of relative risks gave a pooled estimate of relative risk for long-term use of 1.33 (95% CI 1.00–1.75). Confounding with sun exposure is a possible explanation for this small increase in risk.

Holly and coworkers (1983) found a stronger effect of long-term use for SSM than for all melanomas. For use of 10 years or more, the odds ratio was 3.6. In addition, the effect of long-term use on SSM was greater with increasing time since first or last use of oral contraceptives. No adjustment was made for sun exposure

TABLE 59–9. *Associations between Risk of Melanoma and Use of Oral Contraceptive Pills*

Reference	Type of Study	Ever Use[a]	Long-Term Use[b]	
			All Melanomas	Superficial Spreading Melanoma
Beral (1977)	Cohort	1.5	4+ years: 1.7 [0.5–5.5]	—
Beral (1977)	Case-control	1.8 [0.8–4.1]	—	—
Adam (1981)	Case-control	1.1 (0.7–1.8)	5+ years: 1.6 (0.6–3.0)	—
Kay (1981)	Cohort	1.5 (0.7–2.9)	—	—
Ramcharan (1981)	Cohort	3.5 (1.4–9.0)	—	—
Bain (1982)	Case-control	0.8 (0.5–1.3)	2+ years: 0.8 (0.5–1.5)	—
Holly (1983)	Case-control	1.2 (0.6–1.8)	10+ years: 2.1 [1.0–4.6]	10+: 3.6 [1.6–7.9]
Helmrich (1984)	Case-control	0.8 (0.5–1.3)	10+ years: 1.0 (0.4–2.9)	—
Beral (1984)	Case-control	1.0 [0.5–1.9]	5+ years: 1.6 [0.9–2.7]	—
Holman et al (1984b)	Case-control	1.0 (0.6–1.6)	5+ years: 1.1 (0.6–2.0)	5+ years: 1.5 (0.7–3.2)
Gallagher (1985)	Case-control	1.0	5+ years: 0.8	5+ years: 0.9
Østerlind (1988c)	Case-control	0.8 (0.6–1.1)	10+ years: 1.0 (0.6–1.7)	10+ years: 1.3 (0.7–2.2)
Zanetti (1990)	Case-control	1.0 (0.5–1.9)	3+ years: 1.0 (0.5–2.7)	—
Hannaford (1991)	Cohort	0.9 (0.6–1.5)	10+ years: 1.8 (0.8–3.9)	
	Cohort	0.9 (0.4–1.7)	10+ years: 1.0 (0.2–3.1)	
Lê (1992)	Case-control	NA[c]	10+ years: 2.1 (0.7–5.9)	
Palmer (1992)	Case-control	1.1[d] (0.8–1.5)	10+ years: 1.1 (0.6–2.1)	

[a]Rate-ratio for a cohort study, odds ratio for a case-control study. Figures in parentheses are 95% confidence intervals. Figures in square brackets are approximate intervals calculated by Prentice and Thomas (1987)
[b]Relative risk for category of longest duration of use
[c]Result not available
[d]Results are for patients with melanoma > 0.75 mm thick

or constitutional risk factors for melanoma. Lê and coworkers (1992) found a particularly strong effect of duration of use in women 30–40 years of age (RR 4.4, 95% CI 1.1–17.1, for 10-plus years of use; $P = 0.03$). No prior hypothesis was given for a specific effect in this age group.

Palmer and coworkers (1992) postulated in advance of their analysis that an increased risk of melanoma in oral contraceptive users would be confined to those with early disease on the grounds that the increase was due to surveillance bias rather than any causal effect of contraceptives. Consistent with their hypothesis, the odds ratio for early melanoma in oral contraceptive users was 1.5 (95% CI 1.1–2.4) whereas that for more advanced melanoma was 1.1 (95% CI 0.8–1.5). Surveillance bias could produce the observed weak association between melanoma and long-term use of oral contraceptives.

Use of replacement estrogens for 13 or more months appeared to increase risk of SSM (relative risk 2.3; 95% CI 0.8–6.2) in one study (Holman et al, 1984b), although the effect could have been due to chance. Beral and coworkers (1977, 1984) also reported higher rates of melanoma among users of estrogens, although again the increases could have occurred by chance alone. Gallagher and coworkers (1985) and Østerlind and coworkers (1988c) also examined estrogen use but found no association with melanoma.

Reproductive factors have been addressed in six case-control studies conducted in Seattle (Holly et al, 1983), Western Australia (Holman et al, 1984b) western Canada (Gallagher et al, 1985), Denmark (Østerlind et al, 1988c), northwestern Italy (Zanetti et al, 1990), and France (Lê et al, 1992) and in a Norwegian cohort study (Kvåle et al, 1994). High parity was protective in the Canadian and Italian studies, but not in the other five studies. Compared with nulliparous women, those having five or more births had relative risks of 0.3 (0.4 for SSM) in the Canadian study, 0.7 in the Norwegian study, 1.0 (0.6 for SSM) in the Seattle study, and 0.7 (0.9 for SSM) in the Australian study. In the Italian study the relative risk for three or more births was 0.3, in the French study it was 0.9, and in the Danish study, the relative risk for four or more births was 0.7. The relative risk for three-plus births increased to 0.6 in the Italian study and was no longer statistically significant (P for trend $= 0.22$) when potential confounding with education, sun sensitivity, and sun exposure variables was controlled in the analysis. Women whose first birth occurred after age 30 were at increased risk in the Seattle study (relative risk = 2.4 for all melanomas and 3.0 for SSM), but not in the Canadian, Danish, or Italian studies.

Age at menarche (Holman et al, 1984b; Gallagher et al, 1985; Østerlind et al, 1988c; Lê et al, 1992) and age at menopause (Holly et al, 1983; Gallagher et al, 1985; Østerlind et al, 1988c) have not been consistently related to melanoma, although early age at menarche showed a moderately strong relationship with melanoma in one study (RR 3.6, 95% CI 1.0–12.5, $P = 0.04$, for menarche at 10–13 years of age; Lê et al, 1992). Gallagher and coworkers (1985) reported a reduced risk for women with a bilateral oophorectomy (relative risk = 0.5), but Holly and coworkers (1983) found no association with type of menopause.

In summary, the direct evidence that sex hormones play a role in inducing melanoma is generally weak and inconsistent. Thus, the explanation for the comparatively high rates of melanoma in young women and the moderation in rise in incidence with age that is observed around the age of menopause in some populations must lie elsewhere. On present evidence, changes in patterns of sun-exposure with age provide the most likely explanation.

Other Factors

The role of several other, nonsolar factors, has been investigated.

Dietary intake of polyunsaturated fat was suggested as a risk factor (Mackie et al, 1980), but no positive associations were observed in six case-control studies (Gallagher et al, 1986b; Holman et al, 1986b; Østerlind et al, 1988d; Stryker et al, 1990; Bain et al, 1993; Kirkpatrick et al, 1994). Protective effects for anti-oxidant vitamins have also been postulated and Knekt and coworkers (1991) found significant and substantial falling risks of melanoma in association with increasing serum levels of vitamin E and beta-carotene (RRs of 0.20 and 0.03, respectively, per 1 standard deviation increase in serum levels; $P < 0.01$ in each case). These protective effects have been observed in several other studies, more consistently for vitamin E than for beta-carotene (Stryker et al, 1990; Bain et al, 1993; Kirkpatrick et al, 1994). Dietary or supplemental zinc also showed evidence of a protective effect in two studies (Bain et al, 1993; Kirkpatrick et al, 1994). Alcohol intake has shown a statistically significant positive association with melanoma in two studies (Knekt et al, 1991; Bain et al, 1993) but not in several others (Gallagher et al, 1986b; Holman et al, 1986b; Østerlind et al, 1988d; Kirkpatrick et al, 1994). Tobacco, coffee and tea consumption showed no consistent relationships with risk of melanoma (Gallagher et al, 1986b; Holman et al, 1986b; Østerlind et al, 1988d).

Somewhat inconsistent results have been obtained for the association between melanoma and anthropometric variables. Risk of melanoma has not been associated with obesity in women (Holman et al, 1984b; Gallagher et al, 1985; Østerlind et al, 1988c; Lê et al, 1992; Thune et al, 1993). However, in a very large Norwegian cohort study, the relative risk for the highest quintile of body mass index in men was 1.3 (95% CI 1.1–1.4) (Thune et al, 1993). Similarly, Kirkpatrick and coworkers (1994) found a significant positive association with body mass index in men and women together (odds ratio 1.9, 95% CI 1.1–3.3, for the highest quartile). Height was associated positively with melanoma in the Norwegian study (relative risk 1.6, 95% CI 1.4–1.8, in both men and women). These positive associations could be explained, perhaps, by the larger skin surface area in tall and obese people, although risk of melanoma of the face was also positively associated with height in the Norwegian study.

Immune suppression may increase risk of melanoma. Renal transplant patients have an increased incidence of melanoma (Hoover, 1977; Greene et al, 1981) and melanoma is increased in patients with lymphohematopoietic neoplasms that are associated with immune suppression (Greene and Wilson, 1985; Tucker et al, 1985; Travis et al, 1991, 1992). In addition, in patients infected with the human immunodeficiency virus, there have been reports of cases of melanoma (Tindall et al, 1989; McGregor et al, 1992), observation of an increased relative risk of melanoma in one cohort of infected individuals (Reynolds et al, 1993) and reports of the sudden appearance of typical and atypical melanocytic nevi (Duvic et al, 1989). Further, benign melanocytic nevi have apparently been induced in children receiving immunosuppressive therapy after renal transplantation and chemotherapy for cancer (Hughes et al, 1989; Smith et al, 1993). In a case-control study of survivors of childhood cancer, cases had no more nevi in total than matched controls, but more atypical and acral nevi (Green et al, 1993b).

Other factors that have been examined in case-control studies include use of hair dyes, which increased risk of LMM in one study (Holman and Armstrong, 1983) but not of all melanomas except LMM in a subsequent study (Østerlind et al, 1988d), surgery, prior skin problems, and some virus infections. On present evidence, no nonsolar factor appears to be an important risk factor.

HOST FACTORS

Family History

Melanoma has long been known to run in families (Cawley, 1952). Holman and Armstrong (1984b) reported a relative risk of 2.3 in patients who had one affected relative and 5.0 in those with two affected relatives; the effect appeared to be independent of other host factors and sun exposure.

In 1989, Bale and coworkers reported evidence of linkage between the combined trait of dysplastic nevi and melanoma and markers on the distal portion of the short arm of chromosome 1. Studies in other sets of families, however, including one from the Netherlands (van Haeringen et al, 1989), one from Utah (Cannon-Albright et al, 1990), and two from Australia (Kefford et al, 1991; Nancarrow et al, 1992), failed to find any evidence for linkage between markers on chromosome 1p and either melanoma alone, or melanoma and dysplastic nevi together.

Reports of rearrangements and deletions of parts of chromosome 9p in melanomas (Cowan et al, 1988, Petty et al, 1993) and analyses indicating loss of heterozygosity (Fountain et al, 1992) prompted speculation about the existence of a melanoma susceptibility gene, possibly a tumor suppressor gene, in the region 9p22 to 9p13. Two groups have reported linkage in familial melanoma to markers in the region (Cannon-Albright et al, 1992; Nancarrow et al, 1993). Most recently, there have been two analyses of mutations in a specific gene (CDKN2, also known as MTS1) in individuals from kindreds with melanoma (Hussussian et al, 1994; Kamb et al, 1994). The gene product of CDKN2, p16, inhibits a regulatory enzyme that is involved in cell division (Serrano et al, 1993). The first of these reports (Hussussian et al, 1994) found that a high proportion of subjects had germline mutations, whereas the second report (Kamb et al, 1994) did not. Although these studies present conflicting evidence, it appears likely that at least one susceptibility gene for melanoma will be identified shortly if it has not been identified already.

Genetic factors in the occurrence of acquired melanocytic nevi (which are strong predictors of risk of melanoma—see below) have been examined in one twin study from England and one family study from Utah. In the study of twins, the correlation between numbers of nevi in co-twins was considerably higher for monozygotic twins than for dizygotic twins, suggesting that genetic factors might be important (Easton et al, 1991; Risch and Sherman, 1992). Analyses of the family data by various investigators were inconsistent in showing evidence of genetic effects, although the analyses were consistent in showing that autosomal dominance was not a plausible model (Risch and Sherman, 1992).

Any conclusions regarding inheritance of nevi on the basis of these studies are limited by problems of study design. The twin study was small and data in it on sun exposure, which is related to prevalence of nevi, were crude. Data on sun exposure were not available in the Utah study and the method of ascertainment of the families complicated the analysis.

Pigmentary Traits and Reaction to Sunlight

Blue eyes, fair or red hair, and pale complexion are well known risk factors for melanoma. These pigmentary characteristics were documented in most of the case-control studies listed in Table 59–2. Eye color was generally a weak risk factor with relative risks usually less than 2, and its effect generally disappeared after adjustment for the other traits. Hair color was a stronger predictor of risk. Compared with those with dark brown to black hair, those with fair hair generally had a less than twofold increase in risk, but those with red hair usually had a two- to fourfold increase in risk. Relative risk for "light" skin color ranged from little more than unity to about 3.

The skin's reaction to sunlight is also an important risk factor for melanoma. Individuals who burn easily and tan poorly are at increased risk. Increased risks for these traits were observed in all the case-control studies of Table 59–2 in which sun sensitivity was examined (see for example, Holman and Armstrong, 1984b; Elwood et al, 1984; and Green et al, 1985a).

Sun exposure was rarely controlled in any of the studies. When considering sun sensitivity it is necessary to control sun exposure for the same reasons that it is necessary to control sensitivity when examining exposure—the two are negatively confounded. It is likely, therefore, that the real risks of sun sensitivity are higher than those observed in most studies.

The pigmentary traits of eye, hair, and skin color and propensity to burn and ability to tan are highly correlated. Therefore, separating their effects is difficult, if not impossible. Inclusion of one characteristic in a multivariate model almost invariably results in the other variables losing most if not all of their effect. With respect to skin reaction, the questions asked in many of the studies were not sufficiently detailed to identify the separate aspects of tanning and burning.

Because pigmentary traits and reaction to sunlight are important confounders of the relationship between sun exposure and melanoma risk, accurate measurements of these characteristics are necessary to obtain unbiased estimates of the effect of sun exposure. Questions on skin response to sunlight may be better than measurements of skin color (within the range observed in those of European origin), hair or eye color because, when sufficient detail is obtained, skin response generally shows a more consistent and strong relationship with melanoma (Holman and Armstrong, 1984b; Elwood et al, 1986; Østerlind et al, 1988e), although this is not always the case (Elwood et al, 1984). Part of the apparently stronger effect of reaction to sunlight might be due to recall bias. Weinstock and coworkers (1991b) asked questions about ability to tan on two questionnaires, and found that subjects who had had a melanoma during the intervening period were more likely to report decreased ability to tan on the later questionnaire. Control patients and case patients who had melanoma prior to the first questionnaire, were less likely to change their response. Hair color was reported similarly on both questionnaires by all groups. Because the questions on ability to tan in the two questionnaires were not identical, however, the results should be viewed with caution.

Freckles

Freckles, either in childhood, or as an adult, are associated with increased risk of melanoma. A tendency to freckle has usually been ascertained by self-report. The highest relative risks have been found in studies in which freckles, or a tendency to freckle, have been recorded in the greatest detail. Dubin and coworkers (1986) used a diagram of freckling density to obtain semi-quantitative measurements and found an odds ratio of 20 for a history of heavy freckling. In one study, in which propensity to freckle was classified simply as a dichotomous variable (ie, absent/present), its effect was weakened after adjustment for number of nevi (Green et al, 1985a). In other recent case-control studies, density of freckles has had a strong association with melanoma independently of the number of nevi (Elwood et al, 1986; Østerlind et al, 1988e; MacKie et al, 1989; Elwood et al, 1990). Thus, freckling is probably an independent risk factor for melanoma.

Acquired Melanocytic Nevi

Nevus remnants have been found in histological contiguity with up to 72% of melanomas (Elder et al, 1981), suggesting that some melanomas may arise in preexisting nevi. The prevalence of remnants falls, however, with increasing thickness of melanoma probably because of obliteration of nevi as the cancers grow (Sagebiel, 1993). In the case of the dysplastic nevus syndrome, the progression from normal skin to dysplastic nevus and, ultimately, histopathologically confirmed melanoma has been observed clinically (Greene et al, 1985a).

Apart from race and age, number of nevi is the strongest known risk factor for melanoma. Nevi have been considered in many case-control studies and the gradient in risk with increasing number of nevi has generally been steep with odds ratios typically of the order of 10 or more in the category with the highest number of nevi (Holman and Armstrong, 1984b; Reynolds and Austin, 1984; Green et al, 1985a; Elwood et al, 1986; Holly et al, 1987; Garbe et al, 1989; Grob et al, 1990; Garbe et al, 1994a). No increased risk was found in an Italian population (most of the others studied have been of northern or western European origin): the relative risk was only 1.2 for the presence of at least five nevi, relative to no nevi (Cristofolini et al, 1987).

Measurement of number of nevi in the various studies has varied in sophistication from subjective self-reports by participants to whole body counts by dermatologists. Given the difficulty in counting nevi (English and Armstrong, 1994a), and the obvious measurement error in many of these studies, the results indicate that the number of nevi a person has is a very powerful predictor of risk.

The high risks associated with number of nevi and the occurrence of melanoma in association with nevi suggest that the hypothesis that nevi are precursors for melanoma is plausible. Further epidemiological evidence to support this view would be the finding that nevi on a particular body site are more closely associated with melanoma on that site than on other sites. Neither of two case-control studies that reported on site-specificity of the association (Weinstock et al, 1989b; Swerdlow et al, 1986) found any evidence for site-specificity, but both were too small to be conclusive and one did not record nevi on the trunk (Weinstock et al, 1989b).

With respect to etiology, there is evidence that nevi have several risk factors in common with melanoma. Their numbers increase during childhood and adolescence and decrease during adult life (Nicholls, 1973; Cooke et al, 1985; Gallagher et al, 1990a; English and Armstrong, 1994b). Light skin and propensity to burn have been associated with increased numbers of nevi in children (Green et al, 1989; Gallagher et al, 1990b; Sorahan et al, 1990; English and Armstrong, 1994b). The association of nevi with skin color and reaction to sunlight is less consistent in adults than in children (MacKie et al, 1985b; Armstrong et al, 1986; Green et al, 1986; English et al, 1987b; Elwood et al, 1990).

Sun exposure may increase the prevalence of nevi in children. In Australia, the mean number of nevi on children aged 6 to 15 years increased with falling latitude (Kelly et al, 1994). More directly, number of nevi has been shown to be related to measures of sun exposure in individual children in several studies (Gallagher et al, 1990b; Pope et al, 1992; Coombs et al, 1992). Markers of intense, intermittent exposure, such as sunburn and holidays in sunny places, have shown the strongest relationships.

Sun exposure is also related to the prevalence of nevi in adults, but in an apparently more complex manner. Migrants to Australia and New Zealand had fewer nevi than the native born (Cooke et al, 1985; Armstrong et al, 1986). Positive associations between numbers of nevi and measures of sun exposure were found in Western Australia (Armstrong et al, 1986), and presence of more than 50 nevi was associated with the number of sunburns before 20 years of age in a European study (Garbe et al, 1994b). However, while nevi were more common on the lateral than the medial surfaces of the arms in a New York study (Kopf et al, 1978), estimated total sun exposure was negatively related to number of nevi. This finding caused the authors to speculate that "the sun not only elicits nevocytic nevi, but . . . excessive or cumulative exposure leads to their disappearance." This suggestion has been supported by studies that showed that the density of nevi was highest on intermittently exposed skin and least on chronically exposed skin (Augustsson et al, 1992) and that adults with solar keratoses had less nevi than those without keratoses (Harth et al, 1992).

Dysplastic Nevi

In 1978, Reimer and coworkers and Lynch and coworkers described a syndrome of numerous large and atypical nevi occurring in patients with familial melanoma. These nevi are now most commonly referred to as dysplastic nevi (Elder et al, 1981). Although they were first described clinically, the name implies the diagnosis is based on histology. The diagnosis, however, is controversial: not all pathologists agree with the concept (Ackerman, 1988) and the prevalence of the diagnosis can vary widely according to the histopathological criteria used. In 149 nevi, each examined by six pathologists, intra-observer agreement on the diagnosis of dysplasia was high, while inter-observer agreement was only fair; the estimated prevalence of dysplasia varied from 7% to 32% (Piepkorn et al, 1994).

In prospective follow-up of 77 patients with dysplastic nevi and familial melanoma, the incidence rate of new melanomas was 1430 per 100,000 person years (Greene et al, 1985b). These very high rates of melanoma have been confirmed in subsequent studies of the same and other cohorts (Rigel et al, 1988; Halpern et al, 1993; Tucker et al, 1993). No melanomas were identified in 125 members of melanoma-prone families without dysplastic nevi (Greene et al, 1985b; Tucker et al, 1993).

Not all familial melanoma is due to dysplastic nevi. We identified familial dysplastic nevus syndrome in only 25% of melanoma patients with a family history of the disease (English et al, 1986) and a family history of melanoma predicted risk of melanoma independently of mole proneness and pigmentary traits in a case-control study (Holman and Armstrong, 1984b).

Dysplastic nevi also occur in the absence of a family history of melanoma. Tiersten and coworkers (1991) followed 357 patients with the "classic" syndrome of atypical nevi (ie, numerous nevi, large nevi, and at least one atypical nevus), 70% of whom did not have a family history of melanoma. After an average of 49 months of follow-up, the rate of melanoma was 60 times higher than that expected on the basis of population rates. This figure was unaffected by the presence of a family or personal history of melanoma. A similarly high rate was observed by Halpern and coworkers (1993).

Whether risk of melanoma is also increased in those with one, or at most a few, clinically atypical nevi is not known. Another unresolved issue is whether the increased risk in persons with dysplastic nevi is explained simply by the increased numbers of nevi they usually have.

Several case-control studies have attempted to separate the effects of total number of nevi and number of (or presence of any) atypical nevi, but have produced inconsistent results. In four studies the number of atypical nevi (or presence of any atypical nevi) and the number of "normal" nevi appeared to have independent, strong effects (Holly et al, 1987; MacKie et al, 1989; Garbe et al, 1989, 1994a). Roush and coworkers (1988) and Halpern and coworkers (1991) also observed that the number of atypical nevi was a strong predictor of risk after adjustment for the total number of nevi; in the study of Roush and coworkers (1988), however, the odds ratio for the total number was reduced to 1.2 after adjustment for number of atypical nevi. In contrast, Swerdlow and coworkers (1986) found that number of nevi was strongly associated with risk of melanoma after excluding subjects having any large (>7mm) or atypical nevi. From a different perspective, Grob and coworkers (1990) found that the effect of atypical nevi was largely explained by the number of large nevi (5–10 mm in diameter).

Several factors could explain these discrepancies. The most important is probably measurement error, particularly with respect to the classification of atypical nevi. Large variations in the prevalence of any atypical nevi among controls in the various studies (from 5% to 21%; Garbe et al, 1989; Grob et al, 1990) suggests that the investigators were using different criteria for their identification. In most of the studies, cases and controls were examined by the same observer who was not blind to their status, and, in some of the studies, the examination of cases was for clinical purposes, so it is likely that bias with respect to classification of cases and controls occurred. The controls in at least two studies (Roush et al, 1988; Halpern et al, 1991) were unlikely to be representative of the population from which the cases arose. Finally, there were major differences in the various studies in the degree of accuracy in recording of, and adjusting for, total nevus counts. These difficulties and the inconsistent results prevent any conclusion as to the relative importance of number of nevi and atypical nevi in increasing risk of melanoma.

The observation of Grob and coworkers (1990) that the number of large nevi was a better predictor of risk than the presence of atypical nevi complements that of a clinicopathological study in which size of nevi was the clinical feature most highly correlated with histological dysplasia (Barnhill and Roush, 1991). Thus number of nevi according to size could be the best predictor of dysplasia and risk of melanoma. Whether or not it is, it is likely to be the least misclassified characteristic, and may prove to be the most simple, sensitive, and specific method of identifying persons at high risk.

CONCEPTS OF PATHOGENESIS

In 1967, Mishima reported that melanoma cells in LMM had ultrastructural features similar to those of normal melanocytes, whereas the subcellular features of other types of melanomas were more like those of cells found in nevi. On the basis of these observations he proposed that two distinct pathways existed for the pathogenesis of melanoma, one through transformation of solitary melanocytes, and the other through transformation of nevus cells. He considered that the precursors of nevus cells and melanocytes separated early during ontogeny. Not all dermatopathologists are in agreement with this theory: Ackerman (1980) and Crucioli and Stilwell (1982) have argued that melanomas rarely arise in association with preexisting nevi, and that the preexisting lesions reported by patients are, in fact, developing melanomas.

Descriptive studies of the epidemiology of LMM, and to a lesser extent analytical studies (Holman and Armstrong, 1984a,b; Holman et al, 1986a; Elwood et al, 1987), support the view that total accumulated exposure to the sun is the predominant cause of this type of melanoma. These lesions probably do arise from solitary melanocytes, since they are rarely found in association with nevi (English et al, 1987a; Gruber, et al, 1989). The most likely mechanism of pathogenesis is direct damage by ultraviolet radiation to DNA. It is possible, however, that ultraviolet-induced immune suppression may play a role because of the strong association of the LMM growth pattern with sun-damaged skin.

Although the proportion of melanomas that arise in conjunction with nevi is a matter of dispute, the hypothesis that nevi are precursors to SSM and NM is well substantiated. Clark and coworkers (1984) presented a model of tumor progression for SSM and NM in which they argued that these lesions arise from melanocytic dysplasia (nuclear atypia) occurring within melanocytic nevi, which in turn develop from normal epidermal melanocytes. In their model, development of dysplasia in nevi is an obligate step in the oncogenesis of melanoma. Present evidence suggests that ultraviolet radiation from sunlight may be important for this sequence of events to proceed. The prevalence of nevi is related to sun exposure, although not consistently. In addition, risk of a dysplastic nevus has been related to sun exposure variables (Titus-Ernstoff et al, 1991; Weinstock et al, 1991c).

We have previously argued that sun exposure may have a late-stage promotional effect on nevi on the basis of seasonality of diagnosis of nevi and melanoma (Holman et al, 1983). The results of several large case-control studies published since that time, especially our own study (Holman and Armstrong, 1984a; Holman et al, 1986a) suggest that the latent period may be longer. We found the strongest effect of sun exposure on melanoma risk to be during adolescence and early adulthood. We therefore conceive of at least three stages in the pathogenesis of melanoma: First, the stage of induction of nevi, which occurs mainly between the ages of 5 and 15 years; second, the stage of promotion of nevi when, under further exposure to the sun, mainly during adolescence and young adulthood, nevi undergo further mutational change and mature as intradermal nevi, or are destroyed by immunological attack (Wayte and Helwig, 1968), or persist with a junctional component; and third, the stage of progression to cancer by way of increasing dysplasia under influences that are not yet understood but which may include a further role for sun exposure.

The relation with sun exposure, therefore, is probably complex. It may well be involved in the etiology of nevi themselves, it may lead to changes in a nevus that either provoke maturation or destruction of the nevus or lead to persistence and dysplasia, and it may play a role in the further progression of the dysplastic nevus. Given the very small number of nevi that become melanomas, if indeed this is the truth of the pathogenesis of the disease, then factors that cause the maturation and disappearance of nevi may be as important in determining risk of melanoma as factors that cause their appearance and progression. The maturation and disappearance of nevi are phenomena that justify further study.

PREVENTIVE MEASURES

Primary Prevention

Total avoidance of sun exposure is likely to be the most effective way to prevent melanoma, regardless of what pattern of sun exposure is the most relevant etiologically. Avoiding sun exposure during the first decade of life may be particularly important (Holman and Armstrong, 1984a). How readily such behavior can be achieved in high-risk countries, where avoidance is most desirable, is uncertain. However, a reduction in the incidence of sunburn has been demonstrated in adults following a public education program aimed at reducing outdoor exposure in the middle of the day in summer and promoting the wearing of hats and protective clothing and the use of shade and, where necessary, chemical sunscreens (Hill et al, 1993). Whether or not chemical sunscreens are effective in preventing melanoma has not been established. Indeed, sunscreens have been associated with an increased risk in case-control studies (Holman et al, 1986b; Beitner et al, 1990) but this may have been due to incomplete control of confounding with sun sensitivity, sun exposure, or both.

If intermittent exposure to the sun is the major determinant of melanoma risk, the risk might actually be increased in certain groups if they reduce their total sun exposure without avoiding exposure completely. We have argued above (see Figure 59–3) that the development of a suntan may be protective in those who tan readily. If such people reduce their sun exposure to the extent that they do not develop a suntan, but do not avoid all exposure, their risk might be increased. Thus, we must be careful that public education programs do not, inadvertently, have the opposite effect to that intended. We need better information on the particular sun exposure patterns that determine melanoma risk before we can implement more specific health promotion programs.

Secondary Prevention

Early diagnosis of melanoma almost certainly has a beneficial effect on outcome. Mortality from melanoma, as from most cancers, increases with lateness at diagnosis—which, for melanoma, is indicated best by the thickness of the lesion (Lemish et al, 1983). Several approaches can be followed to achieve early diagnosis of melanoma.

Public education programs that highlight early signs and symptoms of melanoma, sometimes combined with education of doctors regarding early detection, appear to have proved successful. The thinness of lesions and favorable outcome of melanoma in Australia have generally been attributed to public education programs that have led to heightened awareness of the disease in the general public (Smith, 1979). An increase in the proportion of thin melanomas and a corresponding decrease in thick melanomas was seen following the introduction of an educational program in Scotland, together with a suggestion of a fall in melanoma mortality attributable to the program among women (MacKie and Hole, 1992). Evidence of moderation of melanoma mortality trends was also found following an educational program in Italy (Cristofolini et al, 1993).

Increased surveillance among people known to be at high risk of developing melanoma has been linked directly to earlier diagnosis of melanoma (Greene et al, 1985b; Schneider et al, 1987; Masri et al, 1990). Surveillance of people known to be at high risk could be a cost-effective preventive measure. English and Armstrong (1988) showed that a group constituting 16% of the population, identifiable by the number of raised nevi on the arms, age at arrival in Australia, history of nonmelanocytic skin cancer, mean time spent outdoors in summer at 10–24 years of age, and family history of melanoma, would give rise to 54% of all cases of melanoma. Similar methods of identifying high-risk groups have been reported by others (Rhodes et al, 1987; MacKie et al, 1989; Marrett et al, 1992; Garbe et al, 1994a) and there is evidence that subjects at high risk may be identifiable by self-examination (Gruber et al, 1993). While identification and surveillance of groups at high risk could be a useful public health measure, careful studies of effectiveness and cost should be performed before is implemented on any widespread basis.

Screening the whole population may not be cost effective because few people, about 1% in the United States (Ries et al, 1994), develop melanoma (Elwood, 1991). Moreover, the sensitivity and specificity of self-examination or examination by an appropriately trained observer have not been established. Further, evidence that there is a form of melanoma that is increasingly diagnosed when screening occurs but unlikely to ever metastasize or kill (Burton and Armstrong, 1994) casts doubt on the achievability of any acceptable level of specificity for potentially fatal melanoma.

FUTURE RESEARCH

Ultimately, the issue of whether intermittent bursts of intense sun exposure or chronic long-term exposure to the sun is more etiologically relevant will come only when and if we can produce measures of *site-specific* amounts and patterns of sun exposure that are less prone to error than those that have hitherto been used. It is doubtful whether this will be possible in case-control studies that depend on recall of behavior from the distant past. The way forward may be by way of a large cohort study with frequent resurvey of exposure patterns. Given that part of the origin of melanoma probably lies in the behaviors of childhood, this is a formidable prospect.

There is scope, though, for further case-control studies. Future case-control studies will need to pay careful attention to recording accurately exposure to the sun over the whole of life, paying particular attention to the nature of the exposure, whether it be intermittent or otherwise, and must include detailed information on site-specific exposures. The studies should be designed to minimize bias by appropriate choice of control groups, by unbiased ascertainment of accurate exposure information, and by control of confounding variables in their analysis.

Because the biological effects of intermittent exposure and chronic long-term exposure to the sun may be more readily separated in regions where ultraviolet radiation is low, case-control studies in areas with low to moderate incidence may be most useful in determining which type of exposure is the more etiologically important. However, full examination of the dose-response relationship for solar UV radiation and melanoma will require studies across a wide range of ambient solar UV irradiance as well as adequate documentation of amount and pattern of exposure. A large, international, collaborative study with each center using the same protocol could overcome many of the present deficiencies and provide sufficient statistical power to examine the details of the complex dose-response relationship.

Cohort studies of nevi could serve as proxies for cohort studies of melanoma itself, because nevi are strong determinants of risk of melanoma and probably precursors to melanoma. Studies of nevi have the advantage that nevi, unlike melanomas, are common, so the studies require smaller sample sizes. These studies of nevi should be conducted in children, particularly to examine the determinants of appearance of nevi, and in young adults, to examine the determinants of persistence and disappearance of nevi.

Another class of proxies for melanoma that might be exploited are biomarkers of the relevant effects of sun exposure in the skin, for example, dipyrimidine dimers in DNA and ultraviolet-induced mutations in the p53 gene (Freeman et al 1987; Nakazawa et al, 1994). Such markers might be used as short-term end points in experimental studies of administered ultraviolet radiation or sun exposure in humans, with the aim of documenting the relative roles of amount and pattern of exposure in causing biological changes relevant to melanoma.

Other potentially useful approaches would include conduct of a cohort study of melanoma in people over 35 years of age at high individual risk of melanoma in a high-incidence population, to examine the late-stage determinants of melanoma appearance (and, in particular, whether sun exposure has a late-stage role); and conduct of a multicenter, collaborative case-control study of melanoma developing in people under 30 years of age to examine the role of sun exposure in early life (which may still be recalled accurately at that age) and genetic and environmental interactions, particularly if one relevant genotype can now be measured (Hussussian et al, 1994; Kamb et al, 1994).

REFERENCES

Ackerman AB. 1980. Malignant melanoma: a unifying concept. Hum Pathol 11:591–595.

Ackerman AB. 1988. What naevus is dysplastic, a syndrome and the commonest precursor of malignant melanoma? A riddle and an answer. Histopathology 13:241–256.

Acquavella JF, Wilkinson GS, Tietjen GL. 1983. A melanoma case-control study at the Los Alamos National Laboratory. Health Phys 45:587–592.

Adam SA, Sheaves JK, Wright NH, et al. 1981. A case-control study of the possible association between oral contraceptives and malignant melanoma. Br J Cancer 44:45–50.

Armstrong BK. 1984. Melanoma of the skin. Br Med Bull 40:346–350.

Armstrong BK. 1988. Epidemiology of malignant melanoma: intermittent or total accumulated exposure to the sun? J Dermatol Surg Oncol 14:835–849.

Armstrong BK. 1994a. Stratospheric ozone and health. Int J Epidemiol 23:873–885.

Armstrong BK. 1994b. The epidemiology of melanoma: where do we go from here? In: Gallagher RP, Elwood JM (eds). Epidemiological Aspects of Cutaneous Malignant Melanoma, Boston: Kluwer Academic Publishers, pp 307–323.

Armstrong BK, Kricker A. 1994a. Cutaneous melanoma. Cancer Surv 19:219–240.

Armstrong BK, Kricker A. 1994b. How much melanoma is caused by sun exposure? Melanoma Research 3:395–401.

Armstrong BK, de Klerk NH, Holman CDJ. 1986. Etiology of common acquired melanocytic nevi: constitutional variables, sun exposure and diet. J Natl Cancer Inst 77:329–335.

Augustsson A, Stierner U, Rosdahl I, Suurküla M. 1992. Regional distribution of melanocytic naevi in relation to sun exposure, and site-specific counts predicting total number of naevi. Acta Derm Venereol 72:123–127.

Austin DF, Reynolds P. 1986. Occupation and malignant melanoma of the skin. Recent Results Cancer Res 102:98–107.

Austin DF, Reynolds PJ, Biggs MW, et al. 1981. Malignant melanoma among employees of Lawrence Livermore National Laboratory. Lancet 2:712–716.

Autier P, Doré J-F, Lejeune F, et al. 1994. Cutaneous malignant melanoma and exposure to sunlamps or sunbeds: An EORTC multicenter case-control study in Belgium, France and Germany. Int J Cancer, 58:809–813.

Bain C, Hennekins CH, Speizer FE, et al. 1982. Oral contraceptive use and malignant melanoma. J Natl Cancer Inst 68:537–539.

Bain C, Green A, Siskind Y, et al. 1993. Diet and melanoma. An exploratory case-control study. Ann Epidemiol 3:235–238.

Bale SJ, Dracopoli NC, Tucker MA, et al. 1989. Mapping the gene for hereditary cutaneous malignant melanoma-dysplastic nevus to chromosome 1p. N Engl J Med 320:1367–1372.

Barnhill RL, Roush GC. 1991. Correlation of clinical and histopathologic features in clinically atypical nevi. Cancer 67:3157–3164.

Beitner H, Norell SE, Ringborg U, Wennersten G, Mattson B. 1990. Malignant melanoma: aetiological importance of individual pigmentation and sun exposure. Br J Dermatol 122:43–51.

Beral V, Ramcharan S, Faris R. 1977. Malignant melanoma and oral contraceptive use among women in California. Br J Cancer 36:804–809.

Beral V, Shaw H, Evans S, et al. 1982. Malignant melanoma and exposure to fluorescent lighting at work. Lancet 2:290–293.

Beral V, Evans S, Shaw H. 1984. Oral contraceptive use and malignant melanoma in Australia. Br J Cancer 50:681–685.

Berwick M, Dubin N, Luo S-T, Flannery J. 1994. No improvement in survival from melanoma diagnosed from 1973 to 1984. Int J Epidemiol 23:673–681.

Brown J, Kopf AW, Rigel DS, Friedman RJ. 1984. Malignant melanoma in World War II veterans. Int J Dermatol 23:661–663.

Burton RC, Armstrong BK. 1994. Recent incidence trends imply a non-metastasizing form of invasive melanoma. Melanoma Research 4:107–113.

Burton RC, Coates MS, Hersey P, et al. 1993. An analysis of a melanoma epidemic. Int J Cancer 55:765–770.

Cannon-Albright LA, Goldgar DE, Wright EC, et al. 1990. Evidence against the reported linkage of the cutaneous melanoma-dysplastic nevus syndrome locus to chromosome 1p36. Am J Hum Genet 46:912–918.

Cannon-Albright LA, Godgar DE, Meyer LJ, et al. 1992. Assignment of a locus for familial melanoma, MLM, to chromsome 9p13-p22. Science 258:1148–1152.

Cawley EP. 1952. Genetic aspects of malignant melanoma. Arch Dermatol 65:440–450.

Clark WH, Elder DE, Guerry D. 1984. A study of tumor progression: the precursor lesions of superficial spreading and nodular melanoma. Hum Pathol 15:1147–1165.

Cooke KR, Fraser J. 1985. Migration and death from malignant melanoma. Int J Cancer 36:175–178.

Cooke KR, Skegg DCG, Fraser J. 1984. Socio-economic status, indoor and outdoor work, and malignant melanoma. Int J Cancer 34:57–62.

Cooke KR, Spears GFS, Skegg DCG. 1985. Frequency of moles in a defined population. J Epidemiol Community Health 39:48–52.

Cooke KR, McNoe B, Hursthouse M, Taylor R. 1992. Primary malignant melanoma of skin in four regions of New Zealand. N Z Med J 105:303–306.

Coombs BD, Sharples KJ, Cooke KR, Skegg DCG, Elwood JM. 1992. Variation and covariates of the number of benign nevi in adolescents. Am J Epidemiol 136:344–355.

Cowan JM, Halaban R, Franke U. 1988. Cytogenetic analysis of melanocytes from premalignant nevi and melanomas. J Natl Cancer Inst 80:1159–1164.

Cristofolini M, Franceschi S, Tasin L, et al. 1987. Risk factors for cutaneous malignant melanoma in a northern Italian population. Int J Cancer 39:150–154.

Cristofolini M, Bianchi R, Boi S, et al. 1993. Effectiveness of the health campaign for the early diagnosis of cutaneous melanoma in Trentino, Italy. J Dermatol Surg Oncol 19:117–120.

Crucioli V, Stilwell J. 1982. The histogenesis of malignant melanoma in relation to pre-existing pigmented lesions. J Cutan Pathol 9:396–404.

De Guire L. 1994. Malignant melanoma of the skin in the telecommunications industry. In: Epidemiological Aspects of Cutaneous Malignant Melanoma, Gallagher RP, Elwood JM (eds). Boston: Kluwer pp 175–185.

Dennis LK, White E, Lee JAH. 1993. Recent cohort trends in malignant melanoma by anatomic site in the United States. Cancer Causes Control 4:93–100.

Dubin N, Moseson M, Pasternack BS. 1986. Epidemiology of malignant melanoma: pigmentary traits, ultraviolet radiation, and the identification of high-risk populations. Recent Results Cancer Res 102:56–75.

Dunn-Lane J, Herity B, Moriarty MJ, Conroy R. 1993. A case-control study of malignant melanoma. Irish Med J 86:57–59.

Duvic M, Lowe L, Rapini RP, Rodriguez S, Levy ML. 1989. Eruptive dysplastic nevi associated with human immunodeficiency virus infection. Arch Dermatol 125:397–401.

Easton DF, Cox GM, Macdonald AM, Ponder BAJ. 1991. Genetic susceptibility to naevi—a twin study. Br J Cancer 64:1164–1167.

Elder D, Greene MH, Bondi EE, et al. 1981. Acquired melanocytic nevi and melanoma: the dysplastic nevus syndrome. In: Pathology of Malignant Melanoma, Ackerman AB (ed). New York: Masson, pp 185–215.

Elwood JM. 1991. Screening in the control of melanoma (Editorial). Med J Aust 155:654–656.

Elwood JM, Gallagher RP. 1983. Site distribution of malignant melanoma. Can Med Assoc J 128:1400–1404.

Elwood JM, Gallagher RP, Hill GB, et al. 1984. Pigmentation and skin reaction to sun as risk factors for cutaneous melanoma—Western Canada melanoma study. Br Med J 288:99–102.

Elwood JM, Gallagher RP, Hill GB. 1985a. Cutaneous melanoma in relation to intermittent and constant sun exposure—the Western Canada melanoma study. Int J Cancer 35:427–433.

Elwood JM, Gallagher RP, Hill GB. 1985b. Sunburn, suntan and the risk of cutaneous malignant melanoma—the Western Canada melanoma study. Br J Cancer 51:543–549.

Elwood JM, Williamson C, Stapleton PJ. 1986. Malignant melanoma in relation to moles, pigmentation, and exposure to fluorescent and other lighting sources. Br J Cancer 53:65–74.

Elwood JM, Gallagher RP, Worth AJ, et al. 1987. Etiological differences between subtypes of cutaneous malignant melanoma: Western Canada melanoma study. J Natl Cancer Inst 78:37–44.

Elwood JM, Whitehead SM, Davison J, Stewart M, Galt M. 1990. Malignant melanoma in England: risks associated with naevi, freckles, social class, hair colour, and sunburn. Int J Epidemiol 19:801–810.

English DR, Armstrong BK. 1988. Identifying people at high risk of cutaneous malignant melanoma: results from a case-control study in Western Australia. Br Med J 296:1285–1288.

English DR, Armstrong BK. 1994a. Melanocytic nevi in children II. Observer variation in counting nevi. Am J Epidemiol 139:402–407.

English DR, Armstrong BK. 1994b. Melanocytic nevi in children I. Anatomic sites and demographic and host factors. Am J Epidemiol 139:390–401.

English DR, Rouse IL, Xu Z, et al. 1985. Cutaneous malignant melanoma and fluorescent lighting. J Natl Cancer Inst 74:1191–1197.

English DR, Menz J, Heenan PJ, et al. 1986. The dysplastic naevus syndrome in patients with cutaneous malignant melanoma in Western Australia. Med J Aust 145:194–198.

English DR, Heenan PJ, Holman CDJ, et al. 1987a. Melanoma in Western Australia in 1981: incidence and characteristics of histological types. Pathology 19:383–392.

English JSC, Swerdlow AJ, MacKie RM, et al. 1987b. Relation between phenotype and banal melanocytic naevi. Br Med J 294:152–154.

Fears TR, Scotto J, Schneiderman MA. 1977. Mathematical models of age and ultraviolet effects on the incidence of skin cancer in the United States. Am J Epidemiol 105:420–427.

Fleming ID, Barnawell JR, Burlison PE, et al. 1975. Skin cancer in black patients. Cancer 35:600–605.

Fountain JW, Karayiorgou M, Ernstoff MS, et al. 1992. Homozygous deletions within human chromosome band 9p21 in melanoma. Proc Natl Acad Sci U S A 89:10557–10561.

Freeman SE, Gange RW, Sutherland JC, Sutherland BM. 1987. Pyrimidine dimer formation in human skin. Photochem Photobiol 46:207–212.

Gallagher RP, Elwood JM, Hill GB. 1985. Reproductive factors, oral contraceptives and risk of malignant melanoma—Western Canada melanoma study. Br J Cancer 52:901–907.

Gallagher RP, Elwood JM, Threlfall WJ. 1986a. Occupation and risk of cutaneous melanoma. Am J Ind Med 9:289–294.

Gallagher RP, Elwood JM, Hill GP. 1986b. Risk factors for cutaneous malignant melanoma—the Western Canada melanoma study. Recent Results Cancer Res 102:38–55.

Gallagher RP, Elwood JM, Threlfall WJ, et al. 1987. Socioeconomic status, sunlight exposure, and risk of malignant melanoma: the Western Canada melanoma study. J Natl Cancer Inst 79:647–652.

Gallagher RP, McLean DI, Yang CP, et al. 1990a. Anatomic distribution of acquired melanocytic nevi in white children: a comparison with melanoma: the Vancouver mole study. Arch Dermatol 126:466–471.

Gallagher RP, McLean DI, Yang CP, et al. 1990b. Suntan, sunburn, and pigmentation factors and the frequency of acquired melanocytic nevi in children. Arch Dermatol 126:770–776.

Garbe C, Krüger S, Stadler R, Guggenmoss-Holzmann I, Orfanos CE. 1989. Markers and relative risk in a German population for developing malignant melanoma. Int J Dermatol 28:517–523.

GARBE C, BÜTTNER P, WEISS J, et al. 1994a. Risk factors for developing cutaneos melanoma and criteria for identifying persons at risk: multicenter case-control study of the Central Malignant Melanoma Registry of the German Dermatological Society. J Invest Dermatol 102:695–699.

GARBE C, BÜTTNER P, WEISS J, et al. 1994b. Associated factors in the prevalence of more than 50 common melanocytic nevi, atypical melanocytic nevi, and actinic lentigines: multicenter case-control study of the Central Melanoma Registry of the German Dermatological Society. J Invest Dermatol 102:700–705.

GRAHAM S, MARSHALL J, HAUGHEY B, et al. 1985. An inquiry into the epidemiology of melanoma. Am J Epidemiol 122:606–619.

GREEN A. 1984. Sun exposure and the risk of melanoma. Aust J Dermatol 25:99–102.

GREEN A, MACLENNAN R, SISKIND V. 1985a. Common acquired naevi and the risk of malignant melanoma. Int J Cancer 35:297–300.

GREEN A, SISKIND V, BAIN C. 1985b. Sunburn and malignant melanoma. Br J Cancer 51:393–397.

GREEN A, BAIN C, MCLENNAN R. 1986. Risk factors for cutaneous melanoma in Queensland. Recent Results Cancer Res 102:76–97.

GREEN A, SISKIND V, HANSEN ME, HANSON L, LEECH P. 1989. Melanocytic nevi in schoolchildren in Queensland. J Am Acad Dermatol 20:1054–1060.

GREEN A, MACLENNAN R, YOUL P, MARTIN N. 1993a. Site distribution of cutaneous melanoma in Queensland. Int J Cancer 53:232–236.

GREEN A, SMITH P, MCWHIRTER W, et al. 1993b. Melanocytic naevi and melanoma in survivors of childhood cancer. Br J Cancer 67:1053–1057.

GREEN AC, O'ROURKE MGE. 1985. Cutaneous malignant melanoma in association with other skin cancers. J Natl Cancer Inst 74:977–980.

GREENE MH, WILSON J. 1985. Second cancer following lymphatic and hematopoietic cancers in Connecticut, 1935–82. NCI Monogr 68:191–217.

GREENE MH, YOUNG TI, CLARK WH. 1981. Malignant melanoma in renal-transplant recipients. Lancet 1:1196–1199.

GREENE MH, CLARK WH, TUCKER MA. 1985a. Acquired precursors of cutaneous malignant melanoma the familial dysplastic nevus syndrome. N Engl J Med 312:91–97.

GREENE MH, CLARK WH, TUCKER MA, et al. 1985b. High risk of malignant melanoma in melanoma-prone families with dysplastic nevi. Ann Intern Med 102:458–465.

GROB JJ, GOUVERNET J, AYMAR D, et al. 1990. Count of benign melanocytic nevi as a major indicator of risk for nonfamilial nodular and superficial spreading melanoma. Cancer 66:387–395.

GRUBER SB, BARNHILL RL, STENN K, ROUSH GC. 1989. Nevomelanocytic proliferations in association with cutaneous malignant melanoma: a multivariate analysis. J Am Acad Dermatol 21:773–780.

GRUBER SB, ROUSH GC, BARNHILL RL. 1993. Sensitivity and specificity of self-examination for cutaneous malignant melanoma risk factors. Am J Prev Med 9:50–54.

GUPTA AK, STERN RS, SWANSON NA, et al. 1988. Cutaneous melanomas in patients treated with psoralens plus ultraviolet A: a case report and the experience of the PUVA follow-up study. J Am Acad Dermatol 19:67–76.

HALPERN AC, GUERRY D, ELDER DE, et al. 1991. Dysplastic nevi as risk markers of sporadic (nonfamilial) melanoma. Arch Dermatol 127:995–999.

HALPERN AC, GUERRY D, ELDER DE, TROCK B, SYNNESTVEDT M. 1993. A cohort study of melanoma in patients with dysplastic nevi. J Invest Dermatol 100:346S–349S.

HANNAFORD PC, VILLARD-MACKINTOSH L, VESSEY MP, KAY CR. 1991. Oral contraceptives and malignant melanoma. Br J Cancer 63:430–433.

HARTH Y, FRIEDMAN-BIRNBAUM R, LINN S. 1992. Influence of cumulative sun exposure on the prevalence of common acquired nevi. J Am Acad Dermatol 27:21–24.

HEENAN PJ, HOLMAN CDJ. 1982. Nodular malignant melanoma: a distinct entity or a common end stage? Am J Dermatol 4:477–478.

HEENAN PJ, HOLMAN CDJ. 1983. Survival from invasive cutaneous malignant melanoma in Western Australia and the Oxford region: a comparative histological study of high and low incidence populations. Pathology 15:147–152.

HEENAN PJ, ARMSTRONG BK, ENGLISH DR, HOLMAN CDJ. 1987. Pathological and epidemiological variants of cutaneous malignant melanoma. Pigment Cell Res 8:107–146.

HELMRICH SP, ROSENBERG L, KAUFMAN DW, et al. 1984. Lack of an elevated risk of malignant melanoma in relation to oral contraceptives use. J Natl Cancer Inst 72:617–620.

HIGGINSON J, OETTLÉ AG. 1960. Cancer incidence in the Bantu and "Cape Colored" races of South Africa: report of a cancer survey in the Transvaal (1953–55). J Natl Cancer Inst 24:589–671.

HILL D, WHITE V, MARKS R, BORLAND R. 1993. Changes in sun-related attitudes and behaviours, and reduced sunburn prevalence in a population at high risk of melanoma. Eur J Cancer Prev 2:447–456.

HINDS MW, KOLONEL LN. 1980. Malignant melanoma of the skin in Hawaii 1960–1977. Cancer 45:81–817.

HOLLY EA, WEISS NS, LIFF JM. 1983. Cutaneous melanoma in relation to exogenous hormones and reproductive factors. J Natl Cancer Inst 70:827–831.

HOLLY EA, KELLY JW, SHPALL SN, et al. 1987. Number of melanocytic nevi as a major risk factor for malignant melanoma. J Am Acad Dermatol 17:459–468.

HOLMAN CDJ, ARMSTRONG BK. 1983. Hutchinson's melanotic freckle melanoma associated with non-permanent hair dyes. Br J Cancer 48:599–601.

HOLMAN CDJ, ARMSTRONG BK. 1984a. Cutaneous malignant melanoma and indicators of total accumulated exposure to the sun: an analysis separating histogenetic types. J Natl Cancer Inst 73:75–82.

HOLMAN CDJ, ARMSTRONG BK. 1984b. Pigmentary traits, ethnic origin, benign nevi, and family history as risk factors for cutaneous malignant melanoma. J Natl Cancer Inst 72:257–266.

HOLMAN CDJ, MULRONEY CD, ARMSTRONG BK. 1980. Epidemiology of pre-invasive and invasive malignant melanoma in Western Australia. Int J Cancer 25:317–323.

HOLMAN CDJ, ARMSTRONG BK, HEENAN PJ. 1983. A theory of the etiology and pathogenesis of human cutaneous malignant melanoma. J Natl Cancer Inst 71:651–656.

HOLMAN CDJ, EVANS PR, LUMSDEN GJ, et al. 1984a. The determinants of actinic skin damage: problems of confounding among environmental and constitutional variables. Am J Epidemiol 120:414–422.

HOLMAN CDJ, ARMSTRONG BK, HEENAN PJ. 1984b. Cutaneous malignant melanoma in women: exogenous sex hormones and reproductive factors. Br J Cancer 50:673–680.

HOLMAN CDJ, ARMSTRONG BK, HEENAN PJ. 1986a. Relationship of cutaneous malignant melanoma to individual sunlight-exposure habits. J Natl Cancer Inst 76:403–414.

HOLMAN CDJ, ARMSTRONG BK, HEENAN PJ, et al. 1986b. The causes of malignant melanoma: results from the West Australian Lions Melanoma Research Project. Recent Results Cancer Res 102:18–37.

HOOVER R. 1977. Effects of drugs—Immunosuppression. In: Origins of Human Cancer, Book A, Incidence of Cancer in Humans, Hiatt HH, Watson JD, Winsten JA (eds). New York: Cold Spring Harbor Laboratory, pp 369–380.

HUGHES BR, CUNLIFFE WJ, BAILEY CC. 1989. Excess benign melanocytic naevi after chemotherapy for malignancy in childhood. Br Med J 299:88–91.

HUSSUSSIAN CJ, STRUEWING JP, GOLDSTEIN AM, et al. 1994. Germline p16 mutations in familial melanoma. Nature Genetics 8:15–21.

JELFS PL, GILES G, SHUGG D, et al. 1994. Cutaneous malignant melanoma in Australia, 1989. Med J Aust 161:182–187.

JELINEK JE. 1970. Cutaneous side effects of oral contraceptives. Arch Dermatol 101:181–186.

KAMB A, SHATTUCK-EIDENS D, EELES R, et al. 1994. Analysis of CDKN2 (MTS1) as a candidate for the chromosome 9p melanoma susceptibility locus (MLM). Nature Genetics 8:22–26.

KARAGAS MR, THOMAS DB, ROTH GJ, JOHNSON LK, WEISS NS. 1991. The effects of changes in health care delivery on the reported incidence of cutaneous melanoma in Western Washington State. Am J Epidemiol 133:58–62.

KATZ L, BEN-TUVIA S, STEINITZ R. 1982. Malignant melanoma of the skin in Israel: effect of migration. In: Trends in Cancer Incidence: Causes and Practical Implications, Magnus K (ed). Washington: Hemisphere, pp 419–426.

KAY CR. 1981. Malignant melanoma and oral contraceptives. Br J Cancer 44:479.

KEFFORD RF, SALMON J, SHAW HM, DONALD JA, MCCARTHY WH. 1991. Hereditary melanoma in Australia: variable association with dysplastic nevi and absence of genetic linkage to chromosome 1p. Cancer Genet Cytogenet 51:45–55.

KELLY JW, RIVERS JK, MACLENNAN R. 1994. Sunlight: a major factor associated with the development of melanocytic nevi in Australian school children. J Am Acad Dermatol 30:40–48.

KENDALL GM, MUIRHEAD CR, MACGIBBON BH, et al. 1992. Mortality and occupational exposure to radiation: first analysis of the National Registry for Radiation Workers. Br Med J 304:220–225.

KHLAT M, VAIL A, PARKIN M, GREEN A. 1992. Mortality from melanoma among migrants to Australia: variation by age at arrival and duration of stay. Am J Epidemiol 135:1103–1113.

KIRKPATRICK CS, LEE JAH, WHITE E. 1990. Melanoma risk by age and socio-economic status. Int J Cancer 46:1–4.

KIRKPATRICK CS, WHITE E, LEE JAH. 1994. Case-control study of malignant melanoma in Washington State II. Diet, alcohol and obesity. Am J Epidemiol 139:869–880.

KLEPP O, MAGNUS K. 1979. Some environmental and bodily characteristics of melanoma patients: a case-control study. Int J Cancer 23:482–486.

KNEKT P, AROMAA A, MAATELA J, et al. 1991. Serum micronutrients and risk of cancers of low incidence in Finland. Am J Epidemiol 134:356–361.

KOPF AW, LAZAR M, BART RS, et al. 1978. Prevalence of nevocytic nevi on lateral and medial aspects of arms. J Dermatol Surg Oncol 4:153–158.

KRAIN LS. 1991. A commentary on an association of malignant melanoma with nonultraviolet radiation exposure. Health Phys 60:457–458.

KRICKER A, ARMSTRONG BK, ENGLISH DR, et al. 1995. Does intermittent sun exposure cause basal cell carcinoma? A case-control study in Western Australia. Int J Cancer 60:489–494.

KRICKER A, ARMSTRONG BK, JONES ME, BURTON RC. 1993. Health, Solar UV Radiation and Environmental Change, IARC Technical Report 13. Lyon: International Agency for Research on Cancer, pp 20–44.

KVÅLE G, HEUCH I, NILSSEN S. 1994. Parity in relation to mortality and cancer incidence: a prospective study of Norwegian women. Int J Epidemiol 23:691–699.

LANCASTER HO. 1956. Some geographical aspects of the mortality from melanoma in Europeans. Med J Aust 1:1082–1087.

LÊ MG, CABANES PA, DESVIGNES V, et al. 1992. Oral contraceptive use and risk of cutaneous malignant melanoma in a case-control study of French women. Cancer Causes Control 3:199–205.

LEE JAH, CARTER AP. 1970. Secular trends in mortality from malignant melanoma. J Natl Cancer Inst 45:91–97.

LEE JAH, STORER BE. 1980. Excess of malignant melanomas in women in the British Isles. Lancet 2:1337–1339.

LEE JAH, STRICKLAND D. 1980. Malignant melanoma: social status and outdoor work. Br J Cancer 41:757–763.

LEE PY, SILVERMAN MK, RIGEL DS, et al. 1992. Level of education and risk of malignant melanoma. J Am Acad Dermatol 26:59–63.

LEMISH WM, HEENAN PJ, HOLMAN CDJ, et al. 1983. Survival from preinvasive and invasive malignant melanoma in Western Australia. Cancer 52:580–585.

LEW RA, SOBER AJ, COOK N. 1983. Sun exposure habits in patients with cutaneous melanoma: a case control study. J Dermatol Surg Oncol 9:981–985.

LINDELÖF B, SIGURGEIRSSON B, TEGNER E, et al. 1991. PUVA and cancer: a large-scale epidemiological study. Lancet 338:91–93.

LUNDBERG I, GUSTAVSSON A, HOLMBERG B, MOLINA G, WESTERHOLM PAF. 1993. Mortality and cancer incidence among PVC-processing workers in Sweden. Am J Ind Med 23:313–319.

LYNCH HT, FRICHOT BC, LYNCH JF. 1978. Familial atypical multiple mole–melanoma syndrome. J Med Genet 15:352–356.

MACK TM, FLODERUS B. 1991. Malignant melanoma risk by nativity, place of residence at diagnosis, and age at migration. Cancer Causes Control 2:401–411.

MACKIE BS, JOHNSON AR, MACKIE LE, et al. 1980. Dietary polyunsaturated fats and malignant melanoma. Med J Aust 1:159–163.

MACKIE RM, AITCHISON T. 1982. Severe sunburn and subsequent risk of primary cutaneous malignant melanoma in Scotland. Br J Cancer 46:955–960.

MACKIE RM, HOLE D. 1992. Audit of public education campaign to encourage earlier detection of malignant melanoma. Br Med J 304:1012–1015.

MACKIE RM, HUNTER JAA. 1982. Cutaneous malignant melanoma in Scotland. Br J Cancer 46:75–80.

MACKIE RM, ENGLISH J, AITCHISON TC. 1985. The number and distribution of benign pigmented moles (melanocytic naevi) in a healthy British population. Br J Dermatol 113:167–174.

MACKIE RM, FREUDENBERGER T, AITCHISON TC. 1989. Personal risk-factor chart for cutaneous melanoma. Lancet 2:487–490.

MACKIE R, HUNTER JAA, AITCHISON TC, et al. 1992. Cutaneous malignant melanoma, Scotland, 1979–89. Lancet 339:971–975.

MACLENNAN R, GREEN AC, MCLEOD GRC, MARTIN NG. 1992. Increasing incidence of cutaneous melanoma in Queensland, Australia. J Natl Cancer Inst 84:1427–1432.

MAGNUS K. 1981. Habits of sun exposure and risk of malignant melanoma: an analysis of incidence rates in Norway 1955–1977 by cohort, sex, age and primary tumor site. Cancer 48:2329–2335.

MAGNUS K. 1991. The Nordic profile of skin cancer incidence: a comparative epidemiologial study of the three main types of skin cancer. Int J Cancer 47:12–19.

MARRETT LD, KING WD, WALTER SD, FROM L. 1992. Use of host factors to identify people at high risk for cutaneous melanoma. Can Med Assoc J 147:445–453.

MASRI GD, CLARK WH JR, GUERRY D, et al. 1990. Screening and surveillance of patients at high risk for malignant melanoma result in detection of earlier disease. J Am Acad Dermatol 22:1042–1048.

MAXWELL KJ, ELWOOD JM. 1983. UV radiation from fluorescent lights. Lancet 2:579.

MCGOVERN VJ, SHAW HM, MILTON GW, et al. 1980. Is malignant melanoma arising in a Hutchinson's melanotic freckle a separate disease entity? Histopathology 4:235–242.

MCGOVERN VJ, COCHRAN AJ, VAN DER ESCH EP, et al. 1986. The classification of malignant melanoma, its histological reporting and registration: a revision of the 1972 Sydney classification. Pathology 18:12–21.

MCGREGOR JM, NEWELL M, ROSS J, et al. 1992. Cutaneous malignant melanoma and human immunodeficiency virus (HIV) infection: a report of three cases. Br J Dermatol 126:516–519.

MCKAY FW, HANSON MR, MILLER RW. 1982. Cancer Mortality in the United States: 1950–1977. NCI Monograph No 59, NIH Publication No 82-2435, US Dept Health and Human Services, Bethesda, MD.

MISHIMA Y. 1967. Melanocytic and nevocytic malignant melanomas. Cancer 20:632–649.

MUIR CS, NECTOUX J. 1982. Time trends in malignant melanoma of the skin. In: Trends in Cancer Incidence: Causes and Practical Implications, Magnus K (ed). Washington: Hemisphere, pp 365–386.

MUIR CS, WATERHOUSE J, MACK T, et al. 1987. Cancer Incidence in Five Continents. Volume V. Lyon: International Agency for Research on Cancer.

NAKAZAWA H, ENGLISH D, RANDELL PL. 1994. UV and skin cancer: specific p53 gene mutation in normal skin as a biologically relevant exposure measurement. Proc Natl Acad Sci USA 91:360–364.

NANCARROW DJ, PALMER JM, WALTERS MK, et al. 1992. Exclusion of the familial melanoma locus (MLM) from the PND/D1S47 and MYCL1 regions of chromosome arm 1p in 7 Australian pedigrees. Genomics 12:18–25.

NANCARROW DJ, MANN GJ, HOLLAND EA, et al. 1993. Confirmation of chromosome 9p linkage in familial melanoma. Am J Hum Genet 53:936–942.

NELEMANS PJ, VERBEEK ALM, RAMPEN FHJ. 1992. Nonsolar factors in melanoma risk. Clin Dermatol 10:51–63.

NELEMANS PJ, GROENENDAL H, LAMBERTUS ALM, et al. 1993. Effect of intermittent exposure to sunlight on melanoma risk among indoor workers and sun-sensitive individuals. Environ Health Perspect 101:252–255.

NEWELL GR, SIDER JG, BERGFELT L, et al. 1988. Incidence of cutaneous melanoma in the United States by histology with special reference to the face. Cancer Res 48:5036–5041.

NICHOLLS EM. 1973. Development and elimination of pigmented moles, and the anatomical distribution of primary malignant melanoma. Cancer 32:191–195.

ØSTERLIND A, HOU-JENSEN K, MOLLER JENSEN O. 1988a. Incidence of cutaneous malignant melanoma in Denmark 1978–1982: anatomic site distribution, histologic types, and comparison with non-melanoma skin cancer. Br J Cancer 58:385–391.

ØSTERLIND A, TUCKER MA, STONE BJ, et al. 1988b. The Danish case-control study of cutaneous malignant melanoma. II. Importance of UV-light exposure. Int J Cancer 42:319–324.

ØSTERLIND A, TUCKER MA, STONE BJ, et al. 1988c. The Danish case-control study of cutaneous malignant melanoma. III. Hormonal and reproductive factors in women. Int J Cancer 42:821–824.

ØSTERLIND A, TUCKER MA, STONE BJ, et al. 1988d. The Danish case-control study of cutaneous malignant melanoma. IV. No association with nutritional factors, alcohol, smoking or hair dyes. Int J Cancer 42:825–828.

ØSTERLIND A, TUCKER MA, HOU-JENSEN K, et al. 1988e. The Danish case-control study of cutaneous malignant melanoma. I. Importance of host factors. Int J Cancer 42:200–206.

PAFFENBARGER RS, WING AL, HYDE RT. 1978. Characteristics in youth predictive of adult-onset malignant lymphomas, melanomas, and leukaemias: brief communication. J Natl Cancer Inst 60:89–92.

PALMER JR, ROSENBERG L, STROM BL, et al. 1992. Oral contraceptive use and risk of cutaneous malignant melanoma. Cancer Causes Control 3:547–554.

PARKIN DM, MUIR CS, WHELAN SL, et al. 1992. Cancer Incidence in Five Continents. Volume VI, Lyon: International Agency for Research on Cancer.

PARKIN DM, PISANI P, FERLAY J. 1993. Estimates of the worldwide incidence of eighteen major cancers in 1985. Int J Cancer 54:594–606.

PETTY EM, BOLOGNIA JL, BALE AE, YANG-FENG T. 1993. Cutaneous malignant melanoma and atypical moles associated with a constitutional rearrangement of chromosomes 5 and 9. Am J Med Genet 45:77–80.

PIEPKORN MW, BARNHILL RL, CANNON-ALBRIGHT LA. 1994. A multiobserver, population-based analysis of histologic dysplasia in melanocytic nevi. J Am Acad Dermatol 30:707–714.

POPE DJ, SORAHAN T, MARSDEN JR, et al. 1992. Benign pigmented nevi in children. Arch Dermatol 128:1201–1206.

RAGNARSSON-OLDING B, JOHANSSON H, RUTQVIST LE, RINGBORG U. 1993. Malignant melanoma of the vulva and vagina: trends in incidence, age distribution and long-term survival among 245 consecutive cases in Sweden 1960–1984. Cancer 71:1893–1897.

RAMCHARAN S, PELLEGRIN FA, RAY R, et al. 1981. The Walnut Creek Contraceptive Drug Study, Volume III An interim report. NIH Publication No 81-564. US Gov Printing Office, Washington.

REIMER RR, CLARK WH, GREENE MH, et al. 1978. Precursor lesions in familial melanoma—a new genetic preneoplastic syndrome. JAMA 139:744–746.

REYNOLDS P, AUSTIN DF. 1984. Epidemiologic-based screening strategies for malignant melanoma of the skin. In: Advances in Cancer Control: Epidemiology and Research, Engstrom PF, Anderson PN, Mortenson LE (eds). New York: Alan R Liss, pp 245–254.

REYNOLDS P, SAUNDERS LD, LAYEFSKY ME, LEMP GF. 1993. The spectrum of acquired immunodeficiency syndrome (AIDS)-associated malignancies in San Francisco, 1980–1987. Am J Epidemiol 137:19–30.

RHODES AR, WEINSTOCK MA, FITZPATRICK TB, et al. 1987. Risk factors for cutaneous melanoma: a practical method of recognizing predisposed individuals. JAMA 258:3146–3154.

RIES LAG, MILLER BA, HANKEY BF, et al. (eds). 1994. SEER Cancer Statistics Review, 1973–1991: Tables and Graphs, National Cancer Institute. NIH Pub No 94-2789, Bethesda, MD.

RIGEL DS, FRIEDMAN RJ, LEVENSTEIN MJ, et al. 1983. Relationship of fluorescent lights to malignant melanoma: another view. J Dermatol Surg Oncol 9:836–838.

RIGEL D, RIVERS JK, FRIEDMAN RJ, et al. 1988. Risk gradient for malignant melanoma in individuals with dysplastic naevi. Lancet 1:352–353.

RISCH N, SHERMAN S. 1992. Genetic Analysis Workshop 7: Summary of the melanoma workshop. Cytogenet Cell Genet 59:148–158.

ROUSH GC, NORDLUND JJ, FORGET B, et al. 1988. Independence of dysplastic nevi from total nevi in determining risk of nonfamilial melanoma. Prev Med 17:273–279.

ROUSH GC, MCKAY L, HOLFORD TR. 1992. A reversal in the long-term increase in deaths attributable to malignant melanoma. Cancer 69:1714–1720.

SADOFF L, WINKLEY J, TYSON S. 1973. Is malignant melanoma an endocrine-dependent tumor? The possible adverse effect of estrogen. Oncology 27:244–257.

SAGEBIEL RW. 1993. Melanocytic nevi in histologic association with primary cutaneous melanoma of superficial spreading and nodular types: effect of tumor thickness. J Invest Dermatol 100:322S–325S.

SCHNEIDER JS, SAGEBIEL RW, MOORE DH, et al. 1987. Melanoma surveillance and earlier diagnosis. Lancet 1:1435.

SCOTTO J, PITCHER H, LEE JAH. 1991. Indications of future decreasing trends in skin melanoma mortality among whites in the United States. Int J Cancer 49:490–497.

SERRANO M, HANNON GJ, BEACH D. 1993. A new regulatory motif in cell-cycle control causing specific inhibition of cyclin D/CDK4. Nature 366:704–707.

SINKS T, STEELE G, SMITH AB, WATKINS K, SHULTS RA. 1992. Mortality among workers exposed to polychlorinated biphenyls. Am J Epidemiol 136:389–398.

SMITH CH, MCGREGOR JM, BARKER JN, et al. 1993. Excess melanocytic nevi in children with renal allografts. J Am Acad Dermatol 28:51–55.

SMITH T. 1979. The Queensland melanoma project—an exercise in health education. Br Med J 1:253–254.

SNELL RS, BISCHITZ PG. 1960. The effect of large doses of estrogen and progesterone on melanin pigmentation. J Invest Dermatol 35:73–82.

SORAHAN T, GRIMLEY RP. 1985. The aetiological significance of sunlight and fluorescent lighting in malignant melanoma: a case-control study. Br J Cancer 52:765–769.

SORAHAN T, BALL PM, GRIMLEY RP, POPE D. 1990. Benign pigmented nevi in children from Kidderminster, England: prevalence and associated factors. J Am Acad Dermatol 22:747–750.

STEVENS NG, LIFF JM, WEISS NS. 1990. Plantar melanoma: is the incidence of melanoma of the sole of the foot really higher in blacks than whites? Int J Cancer 45:691–693.

STRYKER WS, STAMPFER MJ, STEIN EA, et al. 1990. Diet, plasma levels of beta-carotene and alpha-tocopherol, and risk of malignant melanoma. Am J Epidemiol 131:597–611.

SWERDLOW A, ENGLISH J, MACKIE M. 1986. Benign melanocytic naevi as a risk factor for malignant melanoma. Br Med J 292:1555–1559.

SWERDLOW AJ, ENGLISH JSC, MACKIE RM, et al. 1988. Fluorescent lights, ultraviolet lamps, and risk of cutaneous melanoma. Br Med J 297:647–649.

THÖRN M, ADAMI H, RINGBORG U, et al. 1987. Long-term survival in malignant melanoma with special reference to age and sex as prognostic factors. J Natl Cancer Inst 79:969–974.

THÖRN M, SPARÉN P, BERGSTRÖM R, ADAMI H-O. 1992. Trends in mortality rates from malignant melanoma in Sweden 1953–1987 and forecasts up to 2007. Br J Cancer 66:563–567.

THÖRN M, PONTÉN F, BERGSTRÖM R, SPARÉN P, ADAMI H-O. 1994. Clinical and histopathologic predictors of survival in patients with malignant melanoma: a population-based study in Sweden. J Natl Cancer Inst 86:761–769.

THUNE I, OLSEN A, ALBREKTSEN G, TRETLI S. 1993. Cutaneous malignant melanoma: association with height, weight and body-surface area; a prospective study in Norway. Int J Cancer 55:555–561.

TIERSTEN AD, GRIN CM, KOPF AW, et al. 1991. Prospective follow-up for malignant melanoma in patients with atypical-mole (dysplastic-nevus) syndrome. J Dermatol Surg Oncol 17:44–48.

TINDALL B, FINLAYSON R, MUTIMER K, et al. 1989. Malignant melanoma associated with human immunodeficiency virus infection in three homosexual men. J Am Acad Dermatol 20:587–591.

TITUS-ERNSTOFF L, ERNSTOFF MS, DURAY PH, et al. 1991. A relation between childhood sun exposure and dysplastic nevus syndrome among patients with nonfamilial melanoma. Epidemiology 2:210–214.

TRAVIS LB, CURTIS RE, BOICE JD, HANKEY BF, FRAUMENI JF. 1991. Second cancers following non Hodgkin's lymphoma: Cancer 67:2002–2009.

TRAVIS LB, CURTIS RE, HANKEY BF, FRAUMENI JF. 1992. Second cancers in patients with chronic lymphocytic leukaemia. J Natl Cancer Inst 84:1422–1427.

TUCKER MA, MISFELDT D, COLEMAN N. 1985. Cutaneous malignant melanoma after Hodgkin's disease. Ann Intern Med 102:37–41.

TUCKER MA, FRASER MC, GOLDSTEIN AM, et al. 1993. Risk of melanoma and other cancers in melanoma-prone families. J Invest Dermatol 100:350S–355S.

TZONOU A, KALDOR J, SMITH PG, DAY NE, TRICHOPOULOS D. 1986. Misclassification in case-control studies with two dichotomous risk factors. Rev Epidemiol Sante Publique 34:10–17.

VÅGERÖ D, RINGBÄCK G, KIVIRANTA H. 1986. Melanoma and other tumours of the skin among office, other indoor and outdoor workers in Sweden 1961–1979. Br J Cancer 53:507–512.

VAN DER ESCH EP, MUIR CS, NECTOUX J, et al. 1991. Temporal change in diagnostic criteria as a cause of the increase of malignant melanoma over time is unlikely. Int J Cancer 47:483–490.

VAN HAERINGEN A, BERGMAN W, NELEN MR, et al. 1989. Exclusion of the dysplastic nevus syndrome (DNS) locus from the short arm of chromosome 1 by linkage studies in Dutch families. Genomics 5:61–64.

VOSSAERT KA, SILVERMAN MK, KOPF AW, et al. 1992. Influence of gender on survival in patients with stage I malignant melanoma. J Am Acad Dermatol 26:429–440.

WALTER SD, MARRETT LD, FROM L, et al. 1990. The association of cutaneous malignant melanoma with the use of sunbeds and sunlamps. Am J Epidemiol 131:232–242.

WALTER SD, MARRETT LD, SHANNON HS, FROM L, HERTZMAN C. 1992. The association of cutaneous malignant melanoma and fluorescent light exposure. Am J Epidemiol 135:749–762.

WAYTE D, HELWIG E. 1968. Halo nevi. Cancer 22:69–90.

WEINSTOCK MA. 1993. Epidemiology and prognosis of anorectal melanoma. Gastroenterol 104:174–178.

WEINSTOCK MA, COLDITZ GA, WILLETT WC, et al. 1989a. Nonfamilial cutaneous melanoma incidence in women associated with sun exposure before 20 years of age. Pediatrics 84:199–204.

WEINSTOCK MA, COLDITZ GA, WILLETT WC, et al. 1989b. Moles and site-specific risk of nonfamilial cutaneous malignant melanoma in women. J Natl Cancer Inst 81:948–952.

WEINSTOCK MA, COLDITZ GA, WILLETT WC, et al. 1991a. Melanoma and the sun: the effect of swimsuits and a "healthy" tan on the risk of nonfamilial malignant melanoma in women. Am J Epidemiol 134:462–470.

WEINSTOCK MA, COLDITZ GA, WILLETT WC, et al. 1991b. Recall (report) bias and reliability in the retrospective assessment of melanoma risk. Am J Epidemiol 133:240–245.

WEINSTOCK MA, STAMPFER MJ, WILLETT WC. 1991c. Sunlight and dysplastic nevus risk: results of a clinic-based case-control study. Cancer 67:1701–1706.

WHITE E, KIRKPATRICK CS, LEE JAH. 1994. Case-control study of malignant melanoma in Washington State 1: Constitutional factors and sun exposure. Am J Epidemiol 139:857–868.

ZANETTI R, ROSSO S, FAGGIANO F, et al. 1988. A case-control study on malignant melanoma in the province of Torino Italy. Rev Epidem Sante Publ 36:309–319.

ZANETTI R, FRANCESCHI S, ROSSO S, BIDOLI E, COLONNA S. 1990. Cutaneous malignant melanoma in females: the role of hormonal and reproductive factors. Int J Epidemiol 19:522–526.

ZANETTI R, FRANCESCHI S, ROSSO S, COLONNA S, BIDOLI E. 1992. Cutaneous melanoma and sunburns in childhood in a southern European population. Eur J Cancer 28A:1172–1176.

ZARIDZE D, MUKERIA A, DUFFY SW. 1992. Risk factors for skin melanoma in Moscow. Int J Cancer 52:159–161.

60 Nonmelanoma skin cancer

JOSEPH SCOTTO
THOMAS R. FEARS
KENNETH H. KRAEMER
JOSEPH F. FRAUMENI, JR.

Nonmelanoma skin cancer (NMSC) is the most common malignant neoplasm in Caucasian populations around the world, and usually refers to either basal cell carcinoma (BCC) or squamous cell carcinoma (SCC) (Weinstock, 1994a). Although it is established that ultraviolet (UV) radiation from the sun is the dominant risk factor, epidemiologic study of these tumors has been limited by the fact that most patients are customarily seen and treated in the offices of physicians and not hospitalized (Scotto et al, 1983). Since the primary source of data for cancer registries is the inpatient hospital file, routinely collected statistics on NMSC are usually very incomplete and not comparable with other forms of cancer. Thus, population-based estimates of NMSC incidence require special surveys involving the collection of data from office records and outpatient files. These are formidable undertakings, especially in view of the large number of cases that are diagnosed in the general population.

Another obstacle to investigation is the perception that NMSC is a relatively trivial condition. The cure rates are close to 99%, with only a small percentage of cancers being metastatic or resulting in death (Preston and Stern, 1992), yet the tumors can result in substantial morbidity. The incidence rates for BCC and SCC have steadily increased with time, and these tumors represent a major health and economic problem in the United States and other parts of the world (National Institutes of Health [NIH], 1991; Miller and Weinstock, 1994; Marks, 1995). In addition, there is mounting concern about the future risks of all forms of skin cancer, including melanoma, in view of evidence that release of chlorofluorocarbons and other pollutants may deplete the stratospheric ozone layer that limits the amount of UV radiation reaching the earth's surface (Armstrong, 1994).

Both SCC and BCC of the skin are derived from keratinocytes (Preston and Stern, 1992; Sober and Borstein, 1995). While SCC develops from epidermal squamous cells that differentiate toward keratin formation, BCC is believed to arise from basal cells that differentiate toward glandular structures. BCC is generally more common, whereas SCC tends to be more invasive and accounts for most of the deaths attributed to these tumors (Weinstock, 1994b). It is estimated that less than one in 500 patients with SCC die of this cancer, thus causing about 1,500 deaths in the United States each year (Preston and Stern, 1992). This number is roughly one-fourth of the mortality attributed to melanoma, a less common but far more lethal tumor. Although the available statistics on NMSC often combine the cell types, epidemiologic distinctions are evident from the specially collected incidence data available in certain countries, including the United States. However, the potential for misclassification should be kept in mind, particularly when using routinely collected statistics that have recorded dramatic increases in incidence and mortality from NMSC resulting from the inclusion of AIDS-related Kaposi sarcoma (Weinstock, 1993; Devesa et al, 1995). When appropriate data collection and adjustments are made to ensure that the NMSC category includes only BCC and SCC, there is a consistent upward incidence trend (Miller and Weinstock, 1994) in the face of declining mortality (Weinstock, 1993).

DEMOGRAPHIC PATTERNS

Despite the inherent difficulties in assembling and comparing incidence data, the risks of BCC and SCC have consistently shown positive relationships with exposure to solar UV radiation and inverse relationships with the degree of skin pigmentation characteristic of the population (International Agency for Research on Cancer

[IARC], 1992). Thus in the United States, these tumors are much more common among whites than blacks, Asians, Hispanics, and Native Americans. Around the world, the highest rates have been reported in the white populations of Australia and South Africa, followed by Ireland, where there is comparatively low insolation but a susceptible skin phenotype related to Celtic ancestry (Giles et al, 1988; Green and Battistutta, 1990; Marks et al, 1993).

In the United States, the National Cancer Institute (NCI) has conducted two special surveys of NMSC utilizing the same protocol for identifying and recording cases (see further details in Chapter 17). The first survey covered four areas of the country over a 6-month period in 1971–72, while the second survey involved eight locations over a 1-year period in 1977–78, plus two more locations during 1979–80. An enormous racial differential was noted, with the annual average incidence rate for NMSC being 250 per 100,000 among whites compared with 3 to 4 per 100,000 among blacks. Using data from these surveys, incidence appeared to increase about 15–20% between 1971–72 and 1977–80. When rates from these surveys and others in the United States are projected to 1994 and 1995, the annual incidence of NMSC is estimated to be about 800,000 to 1.2 million cases, which nearly rivals the magnitude of all noncutaneous malignancies (Miller and Weinstock, 1994; American Cancer Society, 1995).

When the cell-type patterns for the white population are analyzed from the second skin cancer survey, 1977–80, the age-adjusted rates for BCC were about four times higher than the rates for SCC in males, and six times higher in females (Table 60–1). The male-to-female ratio was 1.6 for BCC and 2.8 for SCC. Similar ratios were noted in a skin cancer survey in Texas (Yiannias et al, 1988). As shown in Figure 60–1 (white males) and Figure 60–2 (white females), the rates in all parts of the country rose continuously with advancing age, with a tendency to level off in the oldest groups. The increase with age was more pronounced for SCC than BCC. Both cell types showed a latitudinal gradient, with higher rates and earlier onset in areas located in the South.

Figures 60–3 and 60–4 show the age-specific incidence rates for each cell type according to sex. The male and female rates for BCC were similar at younger ages, with a male predominance at older ages. The disparity between males and females tended to arise at an earlier age among those in southern areas. In contrast, the male excess of SCC was evident throughout life.

TABLE 60–1. *Annual Age-Adjusted Incidence Rates (per 100,000) for Nonmelanoma Skin Cancer by Cell Type and Sex, U.S. White Population, 1977–80*

	Basal Cell Carcinoma	*Squamous Cell Carcinoma*
Male	257.7	68.3
Female	154.8	23.9
Both sexes	198.5	42.7
Male/female ratio	1.6	2.8

Tumors arose on the face, head, and neck in about 80% of patients with NMSC (Table 60–2). This pattern contrasts with the more even anatomic distribution of melanoma, its frequency being highest on the trunk in males and the lower extremities in females (Scotto and Nam, 1980; Scotto et al, 1991). The anatomic distribution by sex is shown for BCC in Figure 60–5 and for SCC in Figure 60–6. The tendency to affect the face, head, and neck was greater for BCC than SCC. Both types showed a predilection for the ears in males and the nose in females. A male predominance for SCC of the lip was also seen, consistent with the risk factors of tobacco smoking and outdoor work (Lindqvist, 1979). Also noteworthy was the tendency for SCC to affect the upper extremities, especially in females, with the hands being most susceptible. However, the proportion of tumors arising on the trunk was somewhat greater for BCC than SCC.

Figures 60–7a and 60–7b show the age-adjusted incidence rates by sex and anatomic site for BCC and SCC, respectively. The male excess of both tumors affected all sites except the lower extremities. At this location, women have higher rates for all forms of skin cancer, including melanoma, which is consistent with the greater sunlight exposure of the lower legs among females (Lee and Yongchaiyudha, 1971; IARC, 1992). While the rates were generally lower for SCC than BCC, the rates for SCC of the upper extremities were higher. In the upper extremities, the risk of SCC on the hands was about twice that on the arms, whereas the risk of BCC on the hands was about six times lower than on the arms.

The age-adjusted incidence rates for BCC and SCC (Scotto, 1986), along with skin melanoma (Ries et al, 1990), are displayed by geographic area and estimated UVB exposure (Scotto et al, 1976a, 1988) in Figure 60–8 (white males) and Figure 60–9 (white females). The slopes are steeper for SCC than for BCC, which is consistent with international patterns showing that the ratio of BCC to SCC declines with decreasing latitude and increasing sunlight exposure (Urbach, 1971). The latitudinal gradient appears least pronounced for melanoma (Scotto and Fears, 1987), which is consistent with evidence that intermittent sunlight exposures and susceptibility factors such as dysplastic nevi are especially important in the development of this tumor (Greene and Fraumeni, 1979; IARC, 1992).

The UVB gradients in the incidence of NMSC are depicted according to anatomic site in Figures 60–10 and

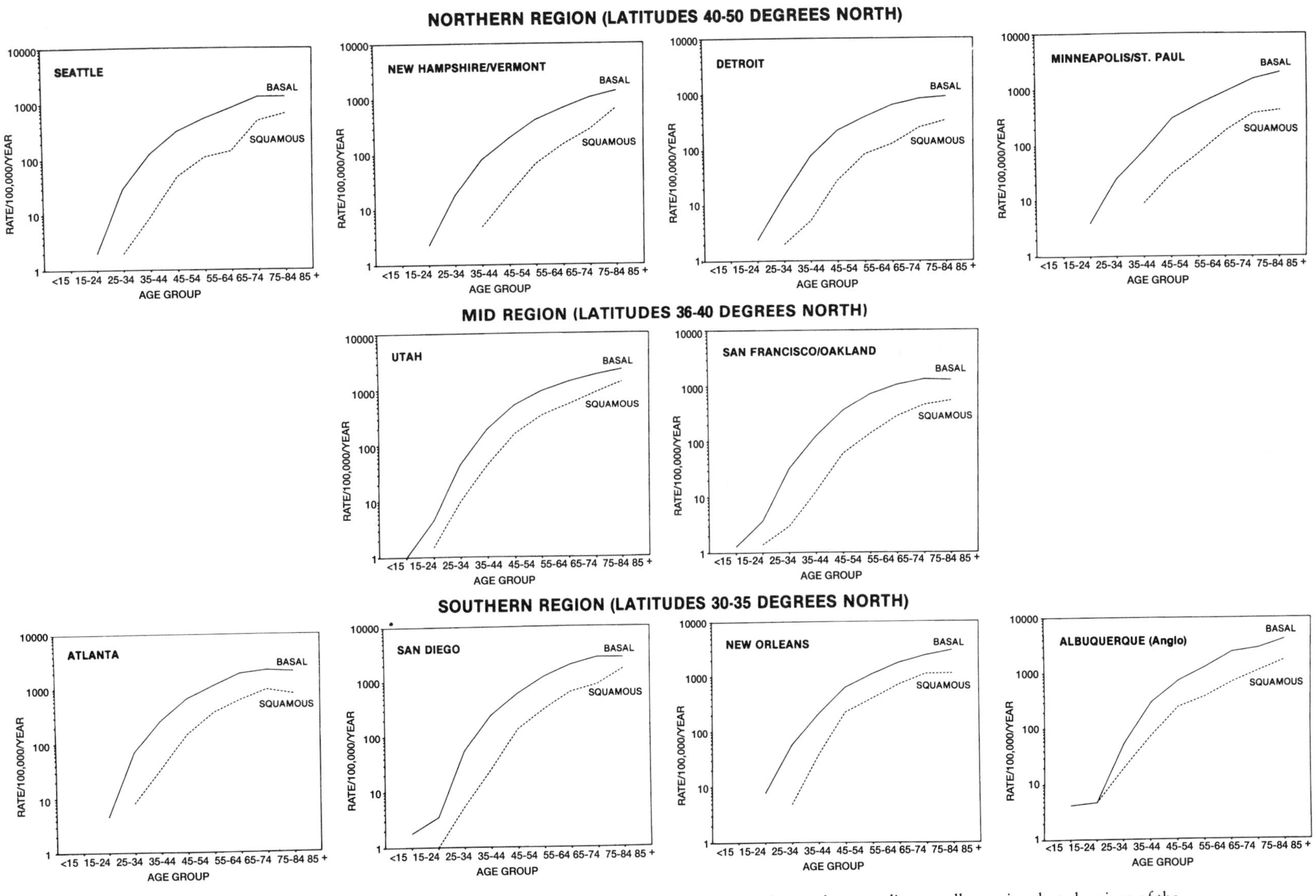

FIG. 60–1. Annual age-specific incidence rates for nonmelanoma skin cancer among white males according to cell type, in selected regions of the United States (1977–80).

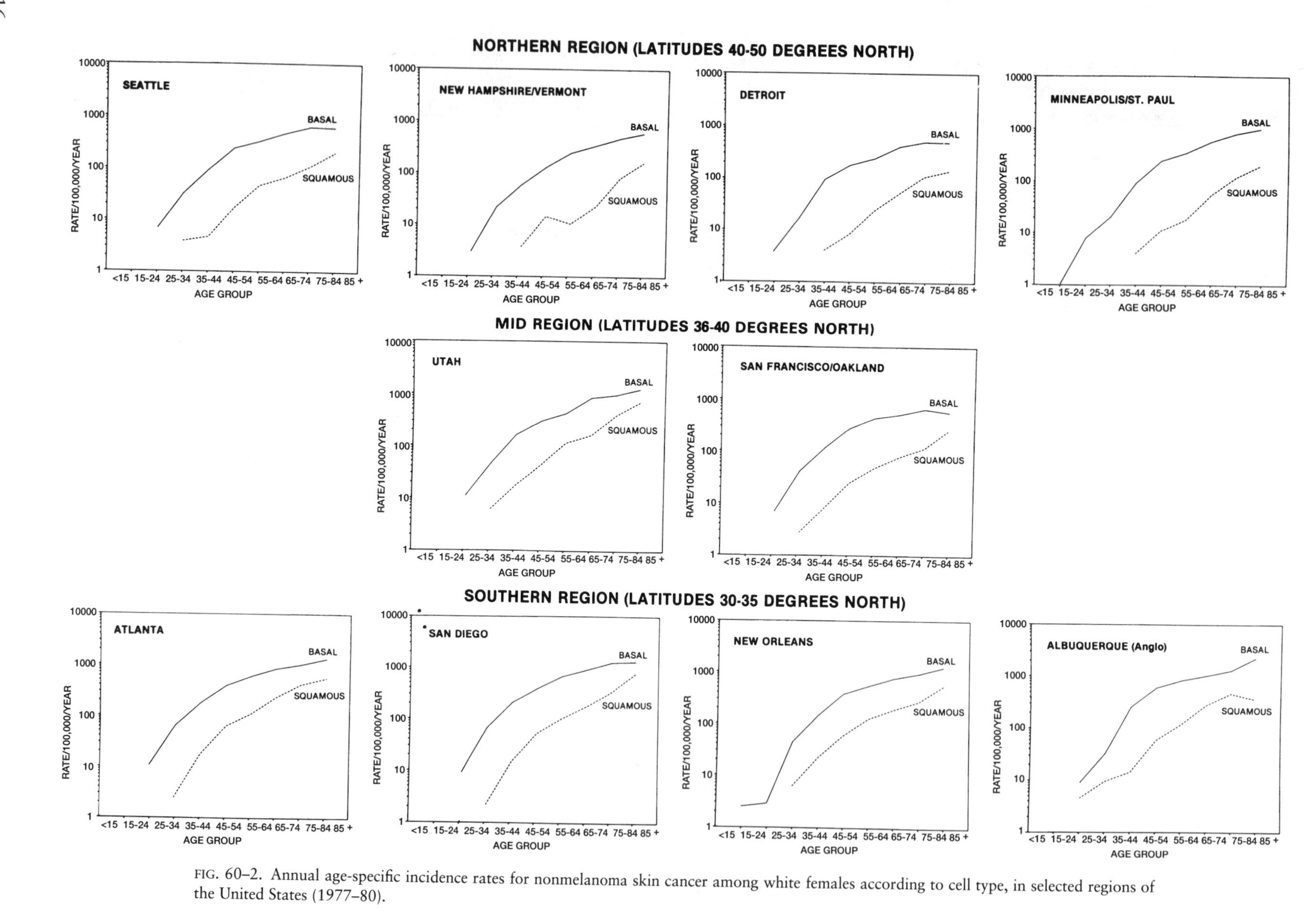

FIG. 60–2. Annual age-specific incidence rates for nonmelanoma skin cancer among white females according to cell type, in selected regions of the United States (1977–80).

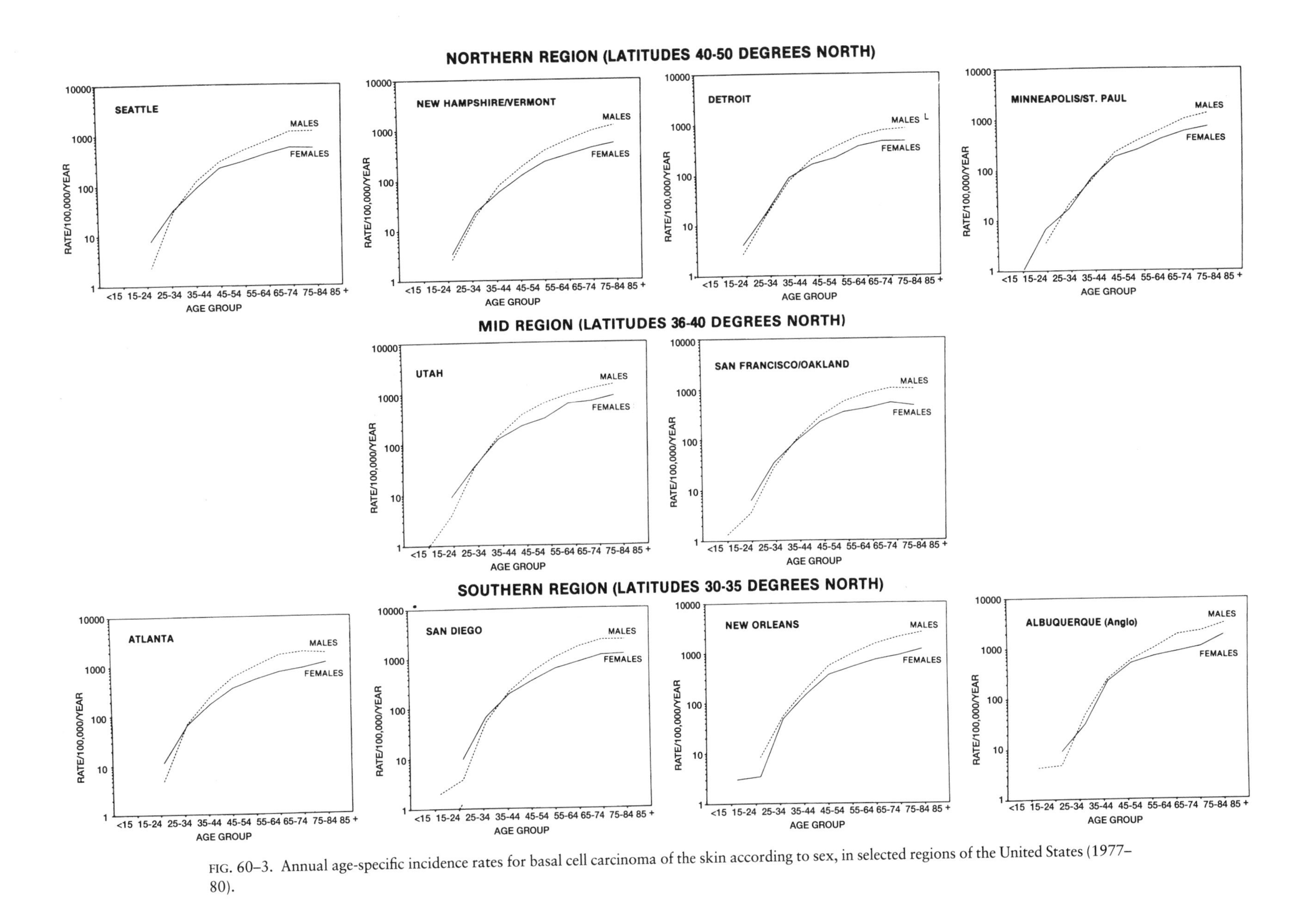

FIG. 60–3. Annual age-specific incidence rates for basal cell carcinoma of the skin according to sex, in selected regions of the United States (1977–80).

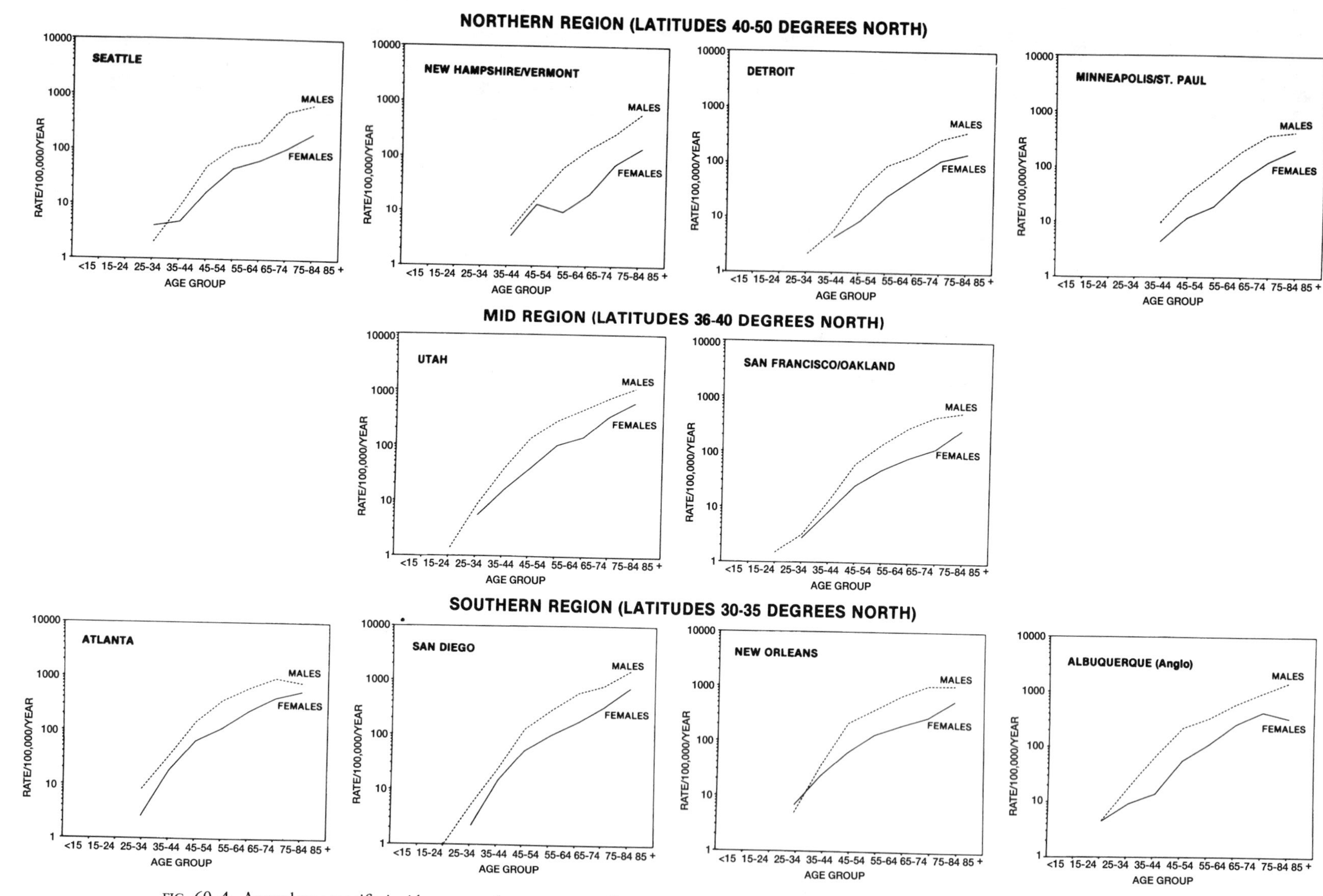

FIG. 60–4. Annual age-specific incidence rates for squamous cell carcinoma of the skin according to sex, in selected regions of the United States (1977–80).

TABLE 60–2. *Percentage of Tumors by Anatomic Site for Nonmelanoma Skin Cancer and Melanoma among White Males and Females in the United States*

	Nonmelanoma Skin Cancer (Percent)		*Melanoma*[a] *(Percent)*	
	Male	*Female*	*Male*	*Female*
Face, head, and neck	80	81	27	17
Upper extremities	11	9	22	26
Trunk	7	6	38	22
Lower extremities	2	4	13	35

[a]From Scotto and Nam (1980)

60–11 for white males and females, respectively. For each site, incidence rates rose as UVB increased, with dose–response slopes being steepest for tumors of the upper extremities among men and women. For tumors of the upper extremities, the biological amplification factor (BAF, i.e., the relative change in rate due to a relative change in dose) using a power model (Fears and Scotto, 1983) was estimated to be about 2.8 and 2.5 for males and females, respectively. In contrast, the slopes were most shallow for tumors of the trunk, with BAFs estimated around 1.2 for males and 1.0 for females. These findings suggest that NMSC of the trunk, like skin melanoma (Fears et al, 1977; Scotto et al, 1991), may be less influenced by changes in surface measurements of UVB radiation than by lifestyle variations in sun exposure habits.

As shown in Table 60–3, the rising incidence of NMSC in the United States during the 1970s was seen in both sexes and affected mainly BCC. An upward trend was apparent also when confining analysis to the two areas common to both NCI surveys (San Francisco-Oakland and Minneapolis-St. Paul), although it is difficult to exclude the possibility of more complete case findings. After adjusting for the month of diagnosis, the rise in incidence of BCC was about 15–20% over the 6-year period, with a slight increase in SCC among women only. When analyzed by anatomic site, the increase in BCC was greatest on the trunk of males, while an increase in SCC was apparent on the upper extremities of females. Incidence rates have also risen disproportionately for melanomas of the male trunk (Scotto et al, 1991). More recent surveys in the United States, Australia, and other countries have continued to show an upward trend for all types of skin cancer including

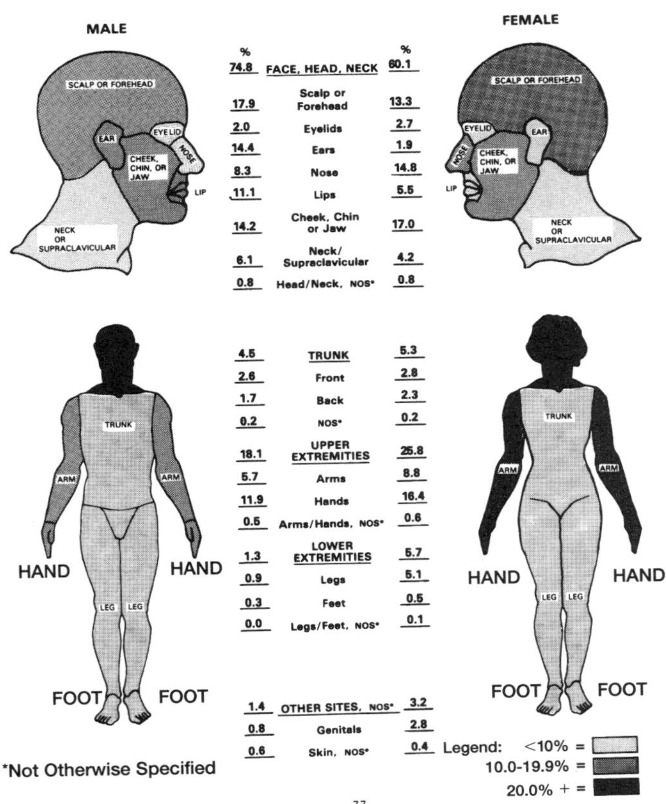

FIG. 60–6. Percentage of cases with squamous cell carcinoma of the skin by anatomic site among white males and females in the United States (1977–78).

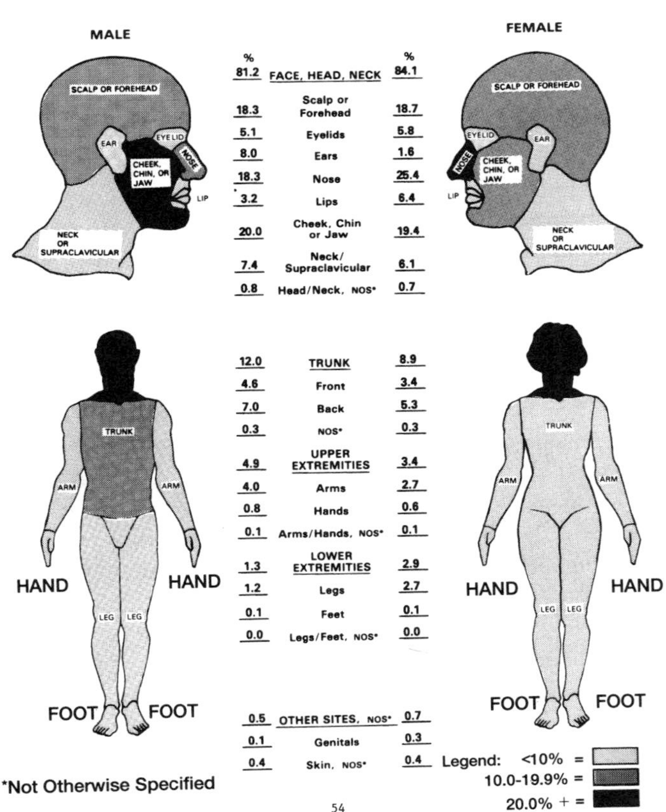

FIG. 60–5. Percentage of cases with basal cell carcinoma of the skin by anatomic site among white males and females in the United States (1977–78).

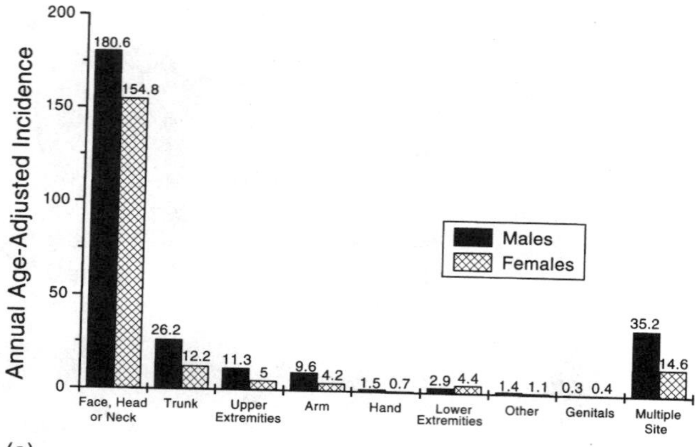

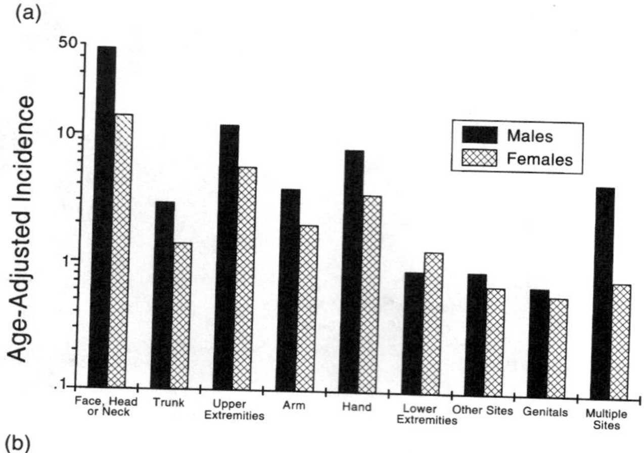

FIG. 60–7. *A:* Annual age-adjusted incidence rates for basal cell carcinoma of the skin by anatomic site among white males and females in the United States (1977–80). *B:* Annual age-adjusted incidence rates for squamous cell carcinoma of the skin by anatomic site among white males and females in the United States (1977–80).

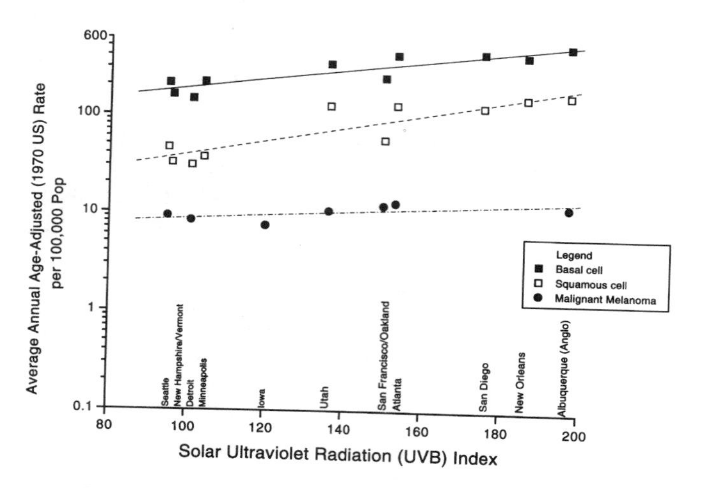

FIG. 60–8. Annual age-adjusted incidence rates for basal and squamous cell carcinomas (1977–80) and melanoma of the skin (SEER data, 1973–87) among white males according to UVB index at selected areas of the United States, with regression lines based on exponential models.

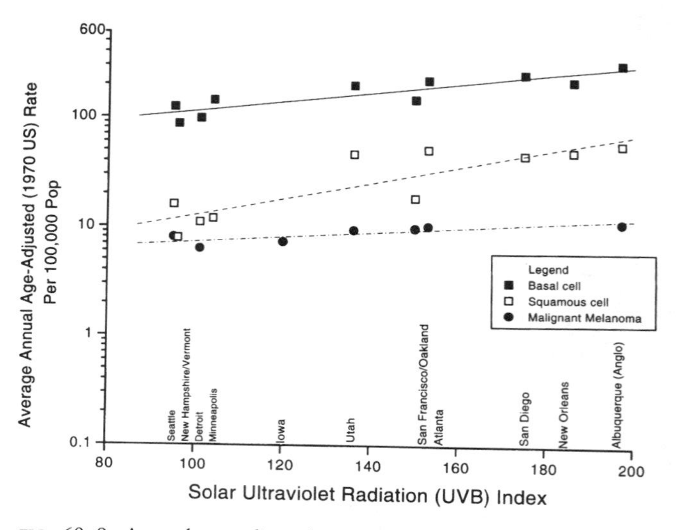

FIG. 60–9. Annual age-adjusted incidence rates for basal and squamous cell carcinomas (1977–80) and melanoma of the skin (SEER data, 1973–87) among white females according to UVB index at selected areas of the United States, with regression lines based on exponential models.

melanoma (Glass and Hoover, 1989; Gallagher et al, 1990; Chuang et al, 1990; Coebergh et al, 1991; Wallberg and Skog, 1991; Kaldor et al, 1993; Marks et al, 1993).

In the second NCI survey, only 68 black patients with NMSC were reported, with 67 being recorded as BCC or SCC (Table 60–4). The annual age-adjusted incidence rates for blacks varied from 6.1 per 100,000 population in Atlanta to 2.2 in Detroit. Although the number of cases is small, a latitudinal gradient was suggested for both cell types. A predominance of SCC was seen among blacks, with about 80% of the cases arising on the lower extremities. In addition, SCC rates were slightly higher among black females than males, resulting from a relative excess of tumors on the trunk, extremities, and genital area, while a deficit of SCC appeared on sun-exposed sites. A relative excess of SCC compared to BCC has previously been reported among blacks, particularly on covered areas of the skin and lower extremities (Halder and Bang, 1989). The tumors in blacks tend to be invasive and are often associated with predisposing conditions such as burn scars and chronic ulcers. The reason for the sex difference in the site distribution of SCC is unclear, although a high incidence of SCC involving the anal region has been reported among black women (Halder and Bang, 1988).

Also shown in Table 60–4 are the intermediate rates for BCC and SCC among Hispanics, as compared with non-Hispanic whites and blacks. The ethnic gradient was similar among men and women, but less pronounced for SCC than BCC. The anatomic distribution among Hispanics more closely resembled the pattern for whites than for blacks, with a particularly high proportion of tumors arising on the head, face, and neck.

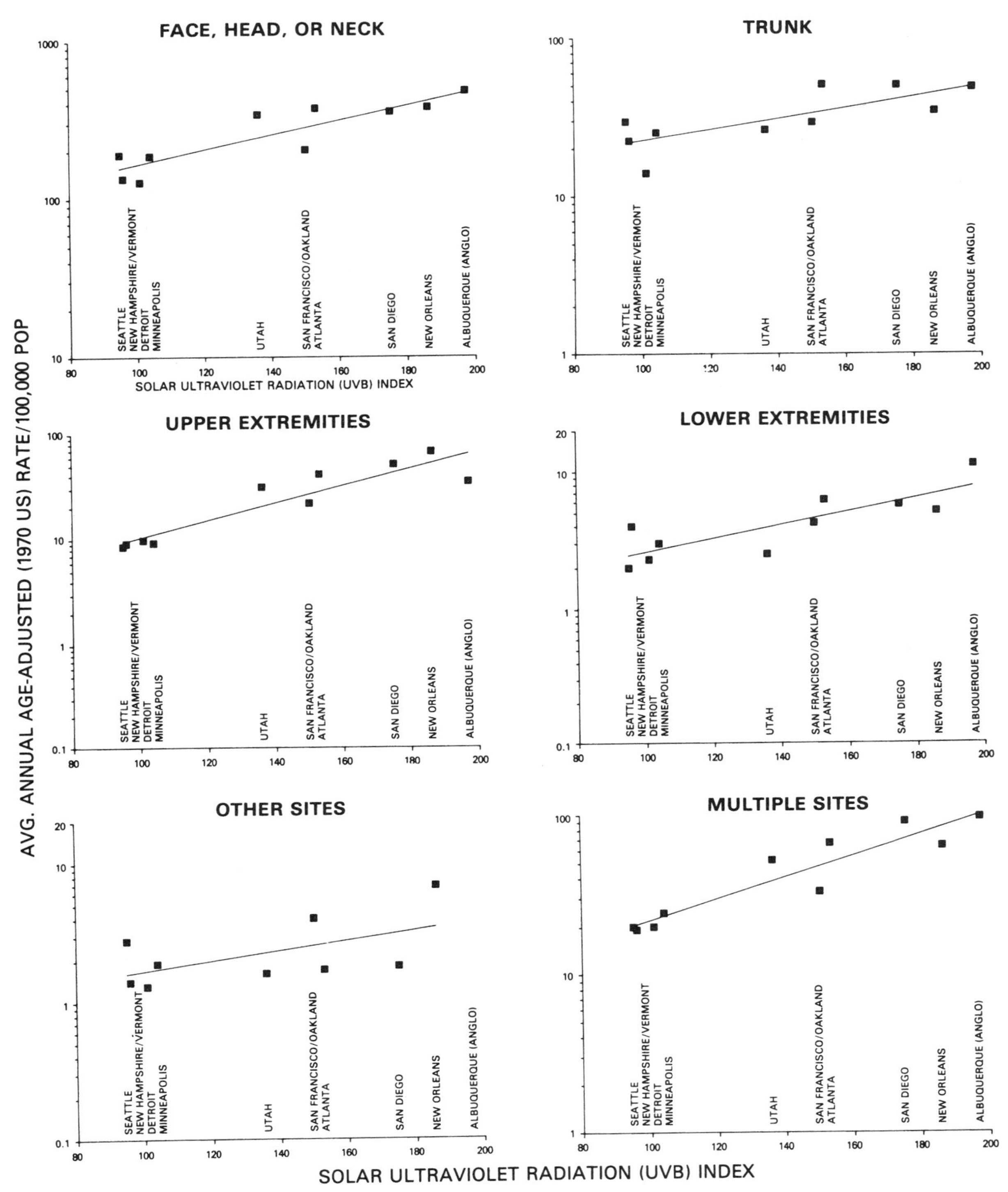

FIG. 60–10. Annual age-adjusted incidence rates for nonmelanoma skin cancer according to UVB index and anatomic site among white males in the United States (1977–80).

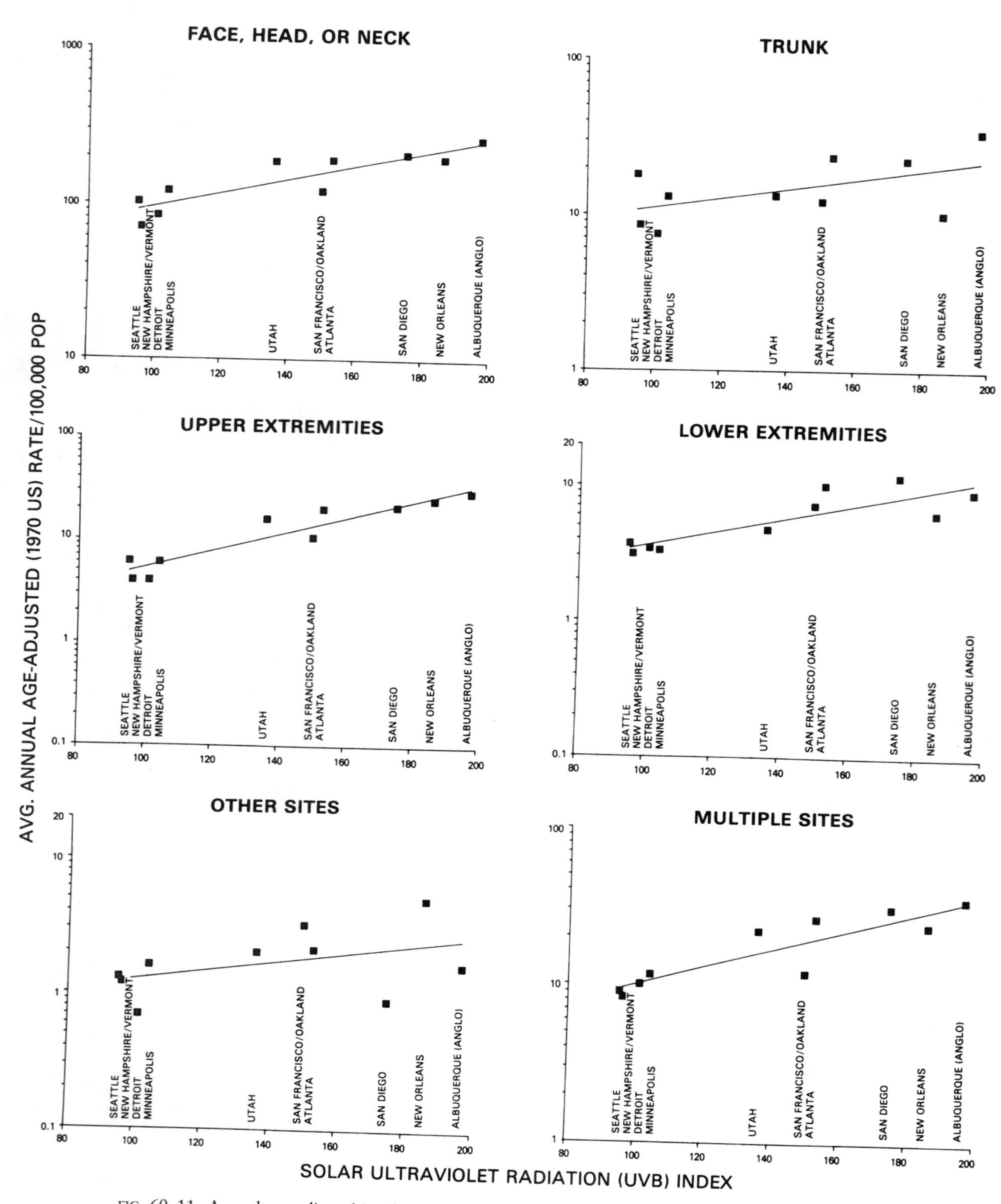

FIG. 60–11. Annual age-adjusted incidence rates for nonmelanoma skin cancer according to UVB index and anatomic site among white females in the United States (1977–80).

TABLE 60–3. *Annual Age-Adjusted Incidence Rates (per 100,000) for Nonmelanoma Skin Cancer among White Males and Females in the United States, 1971–1972 and 1977–1978*

	1971–1972 Survey[a]	*1977–1978 Survey*[b]
ALL SURVEY AREAS		
Basal Cell Carcinoma		
Male	202.1	246.6
Female	115.8	150.1
Squamous Cell Carcinoma		
Male	65.5	65.4
Female	21.8	23.6
SAN FRANCISCO-OAKLAND		
Basal Cell Carcinoma		
Male	197.9	239.0
Female	117.2	145.1
Squamous Cell Carcinoma		
Male	51.7	56.3
Female	15.8	18.4
MINNEAPOLIS-ST. PAUL		
Basal Cell Carcinoma		
Male	165.0	213.1
Female	102.8	144.0
Squamous Cell Carcinoma		
Male	36.5	36.6
Female	12.3	11.8

[a]Includes 4 areas
[b]Includes 8 areas

ENVIRONMENTAL FACTORS

Ultraviolet Radiation

The dominant risk factor for NMSC is UV radiation from the sun (IARC, 1992; Kricker et al, 1994). The evidence is based on (1) the tendency for tumors to arise on sun-exposed surfaces; (2) the high rates among occupational groups with outdoor exposures; (3) the generally inverse correlation between incidence rates and distance from the equator; (4) the predisposition of light-skinned populations, notably fair-complexioned people who sunburn easily, and the resistance of dark-skinned populations with protective melanin pigment; (5) the high rates among individuals with evidence of UV skin damage, actinic keratoses, and prior skin cancer; (6) the capacity of UV radiation in repeated doses to induce skin cancer in experimental animals, particularly in the UVB spectral range (290–320 nm) that causes delayed erythema in human skin; (7) the exceptionally high risk of skin cancer among persons with genetic diseases characterized by intolerance to sunlight (i.e., xeroderma pigmentosum and albinism); and (8) the highly specific mutations of the *p53* tumor-suppressor gene in SCC that are characteristic of UV-induced changes in model systems (Brash et al, 1991; Ziegler et al, 1994).

The available epidemiologic evidence suggests that the risk of NMSC is related to cumulative lifetime UV exposure (Fears et al, 1977; Hoffman, 1987; IARC, 1992), while studies in laboratory animals suggest that the risk is proportional to the square root of the annual dose (Blum, 1976; Kelfkens et al, 1990; United Nations Environmental Programme [UNEP], 1990). The effects of chronic, repeated exposures to UV radiation are most apparent for SCC, whereas intermittent sun-intensive exposures with sunburning tend to be associated with melanoma. However, a role for intermittent exposures in BCC is suggested by the temporal, geographic, and anatomic patterns of this tumor (Gallagher et al, 1990) and the reported absence of dose dependence at high exposure levels (Strickland et al, 1989). Recent studies also suggest that, like melanoma, the risk of BCC is related especially to sun exposures and sunburning during childhood, while the risk of SCC is not (Gallagher et al, 1995a, 1995b).

Whether the UVB exposure is cumulative or intermittent, its intensity is limited by the ozone layer in the stratosphere; however, this protective barrier may be impaired by various human activities, including the release of chlorofluorocarbons used in aerosol propellants, refrigerators, and air conditioners. Depletion of this layer is likely to enhance the penetration of UVB radiation that reaches the earth's surface and thus further increase the incidence of NMSC and melanoma (Armstrong, 1994). For each 1% relative decrease in stratospheric ozone, about a 4% or greater increase in NMSC may be expected, depending on cell type and anatomic site (see further details in Chapter 17).

Ionizing Radiation

Skin cancers were the first neoplasms related to ionizing radiation, with case reports in 1902 among early radiation workers, particularly in areas with chronic radiodermatitis. It has been difficult to evaluate skin cancer in studies of populations heavily exposed to ionizing radiation, because of the low case–fatality rate, the substantial underreporting of skin cancer to tumor registries, and the high background rate in the general population. Nevertheless, excess risks of NMSC have been described among radiologists, uranium miners, and atomic bomb survivors, and following X-ray therapy for tinea capitis of the scalp, enlargement of the thymus gland in infancy, lymphoid hyperplasia, and various benign skin diseases (Shore, 1990; United Nations, 1994). Taken together, the studies provide no indication of a dose threshold and suggest a dose–response relation that is linear in nature. The risks appear to be potenti-

TABLE 60–4. *Number of Cases and Annual Age-Adjusted Incidence Rates (per 100,000) for Nonmelanoma Skin Cancer by Cell Type and Sex among Non-Hispanic White, Hispanic, and Black Males and Females in the United States, 1977–1980, with Percentage Distribution of Cases by Anatomic Site*

	Basal Cell Carcinoma			*Squamous Cell Carcinoma*		
	Whites[a]	*Hispanics*[a]	*Blacks*[b]	*Whites*[a]	*Hispanics*[a]	*Blacks*[b]
MALES						
Face, head, or neck	68.1%	75.2%	69.2%	66.9%	77.4%	42.9%
Trunk	9.8	6.0	7.7	4.3	0.0	0.0
Upper extremities	5.7	4.0	0.0	18.9	9.7	7.1
Lower extremities	1.1	0.7	23.1	1.2	3.2	28.6
Other sites/NOS	0.6	2.0	0.0	1.1	9.7	7.1
Multiple sites	14.7	12.1	0.0	7.6	0.0	14.3
No. cases	8788	149	13	2425	31	14
Age-adjusted rate	360.1	51.6	1.9	101.1	10.0	2.2
(SE × 1.96)[c]	(7.6)	(8.5)	(1.1)	(4.0)	(3.9)	(1.2)
FEMALES						
Face, head, or neck	75.4%	83.8%	64.6%	57.1%	75.9%	17.4%
Trunk	6.9	2.8	5.9	5.8	3.4	21.7
Upper extremities	4.0	2.8	5.9	24.6	13.8	8.7
Lower extremities	3.3	1.4	11.8	5.5	0.0	30.5
Other sites/NOS	0.9	1.4	5.9	2.3	6.9	17.4
Multiple sites	9.5	7.8	5.9	4.7	0.0	4.3
No. cases	6446	142	17	1167	29	23
Age-adjusted rate	210.7	37.2	2.0	35.4	7.9	2.5
(SE × 1.96)[c]	(5.2)	(6.2)	(1.0)	(2.1)	(2.9)	(1.1)

[a]Includes San Francisco-Oakland, New Mexico, New Orleans, and San Diego
[b]Includes San Francisco-Oakland, Detroit, New Orleans, and Atlanta
[c]Standard error provides factor for 95% confidence limits on the mean of the age-adjusted rate

ated by exposure to UV radiation and by susceptible skin phenotype. The epidemiologic findings are consistent with the capacity of ionizing radiation to induce skin cancers in laboratory animals (National Research Council, 1990).

Chemicals

Studies of chemical skin carcinogenesis in rodents have provided important evidence for a multistage process of cancer development, and are yielding new insights into the genetic, biological, and biochemical alterations involved at various stages of carcinogenesis (Yuspa, 1994). The first stage, initiation, may result from limited exposure to a low dose of an agent given once or for a short time, and it rapidly produces an irreversible cellular change involving a mutation in the DNA. The next stage, promotion, follows repeated exposure to a tumor promoter that causes an expanded clone of initiated cells. Further genetic and epigenetic changes are needed for the subsequent stages of premalignant proliferation and malignant conversion. If a large dose or repeated exposure to an initiator results in tumor formation, the agent may be considered a complete carcinogen with both initiating and promoting activity. Table 60–5 lists some chemical and physical agents to which humans may be exposed and that have been identified as initiators or promoters of skin cancer in laboratory animals.

Several chemical carcinogens have been linked to an increased risk of skin cancer. Polycyclic aromatic hydrocarbons (PAHs), which are skin carcinogens in laboratory animals, occur as chemical mixtures in coal tars, pitch, asphalt, soot, creosotes, anthracenes, paraffin waxes, and lubricating and cutting oils. In 1775, Percivall Pott reported an excess of scrotal cancer among British chimney sweeps exposed to soot, the first recognition of an environmental cancer. In a series of studies from Great Britain over the past century, exposures to mineral oils have been linked to SSC of the skin and scrotum among shale oil workers, jute processors, tool setters operating automatic lathes, and mule spinners (Bingham et al, 1979). In the United States, an excess risk of skin and scrotal cancers has been reported among wax pressmen (Hendricks et al, 1959), while increases in risk have been documented among metal workers exposed to poorly refined cutting oils in France and among machine operators exposed to lubricating oils in Great Britain (Kipling and Waldron, 1976). Skin and lung

TABLE 60–5. *Chemical and Physical Agents that Initiate or Promote Nonmelanoma Skin Cancer in Laboratory Animals**

Initiators	*Promoters*
POLYCYCLIC AROMATIC HYDROCARBONS	*PHORBOL ESTERS*
Benz[a]pyrene	Croton oil
Tobacco tar	*AROMATICS*
Dibenz[a,h]anthracene	Phenol
NITROSAMINES	Anthralin
N,N′-Dimethylnitrosourea	*PHYSICAL AGENTS*
Methyl-nitro-nitrosoguanidine	Ultraviolet radiation
ALKYLATING AGENTS	Abrasion
β-Propriolactone	Wounding
Bis(chloromethyl) ether	*OTHERS*
Nitrogen mustard	Benzoyl peroxide
Cisplatin	Cigarette smoke condensate
PHYSICAL AGENTS	Retinoic acid
Ultraviolet radiation	Tetrachlorodibenzodioxin
Ionizing radiation	Dihydroteliocidin (fungal product)
OTHERS	
Urethane	
Dinitropyrene	

*Modified from Yuspa and Dlugosz (1991)

cancers also occur excessively among workers exposed to coal gas and tar (Doll et al, 1972), among roofers (Partanen and Boffetta, 1994), and among foundry workers (Partanen et al, 1994). The carcinogenicity of medicinal crude tar ointments has been argued for some time, and the epidemiologic evidence to date appears inconclusive based on studies of psoriasis patients treated with topical tar (Stern and Laird, 1994).

Inorganic arsenic, when taken internally for a prolonged time, is well-documented as a skin carcinogen (Brown et al, 1989; IARC, 1980). Exposure may result from medicinal agents used in the past (e.g., Fowler's solution), contaminated drinking water, or occupational exposures including agricultural pesticides. Arsenical skin cancers may be squamous or basal cell tumors and tend to arise at multiple sites, unexposed surfaces, and unusual locations, such as the palms and soles. It is also characteristic for the tumors to occur in association with hyperpigmentation and multiple keratoses of the skin. A dose–response relationship between chronic arsenic exposure and skin cancer prevalence has been reported in Taiwanese villages where artesian wells contain high levels of arsenic (Hsueh et al, 1995). It is noteworthy that arsenic has shown only limited evidence for carcinogenicity in laboratory studies, so that the carcinogenic mechanisms are probably different from those of other chemical carcinogens.

Psoralens, used in combination with UVA (long wavelength UV, 320–400 nm) for the treatment of psoriasis, have been linked to skin cancers, especially at sites not ordinarily exposed to the sun. In a recent follow-up averaging 13 years, Stern and Laird (1994) reported that one-fourth of the patients exposed to high doses of psoralens and UVA radiation (PUVA) developed SCC, with a relative risk six times higher than those exposed to lower doses of PUVA. This association has heightened concern about the potential hazards of photosensitizers in various preparations, including tanning aids, cosmetics, and medicines (Wei et al, 1994a). The use of methotrexate in treating psoriasis may also increase the risk of SCC (Stern and Laird, 1994).

An increased risk of NMSC has been reported in several occupational groups including pesticide applicators (Wang and MacMahon, 1979), chemical and printing workers (Whitaker et al, 1979), and hairdressers (Pukkala et al, 1992), but the specific exposures responsible for these associations are not clear.

Dietary Factors

Recent studies have suggested that the risk of NMSC may be decreased by low-fat diets or by micronutrients (Kune et al, 1992; Black et al, 1994; Wei et al, 1994b), but the findings have not been consistent (Hunter et al, 1992). The positive results, however, are in line with studies in laboratory animals and warrant further investigation.

Cigarette Smoking

An excess risk of squamous cancers of the lip has been documented among smokers, and there is some evidence that smoking may increase the risk of SCC at other cutaneous sites (Aubry and MacGibbon, 1985; Karagas et al, 1992). Further studies are needed to clarify this association and the mechanisms that may be involved.

Trauma, Burns and Scars

SCC may arise as a complication of tropical ulcers, burns and scars, sinuses and fistulas, or sites of chronic infection and inflammation (Kaplan, 1987). The formation of skin cancers in nonhealing scar tissue has been referred to as Marjolin's ulcer (Fleming et al, 1990). Although these predisposing conditions are seen especially in Africa and Asia, they play a role in some cases of SCC observed in African-Americans (Halder and Bridgeman-Shah, 1995). The spectrum of lesions includes tropical phagedenic ulcers in Africa which arise on the lower legs and feet from repeated trauma, become chronically infected, and often progress to SCC (Camain et al, 1972). The kangri cancer of Kashmir, India, complicates burn scars on the lower abdomen and thighs of people who warm themselves by baskets (kangri) containing clay pots with burning charcoal (Svindland, 1980). A related condition occurs in Japan, where kairo cancer results from woodburning heating devices (kairo) full of warm ashes (Everall and Dowd, 1978). Similarly, kang cancer has been reported among people who sleep on heated brick beds (kang) in northern China (Laycock, 1948). In these instances, the cancers associated with burn scars may be promoted by polycyclic hydrocarbons released from the heat-generating devices. In India, dhoti cancer develops on the groin, flank and buttocks of people who traditionally wrap loincloths (dhotis) tightly around their bodies (Mulay, 1963). In addition, case reports suggest that SCC may occur excessively in the scars of various inflammatory skin diseases such as tuberculosis, leprosy, syphilis, pemphigus vulgaris, and discoid lupus erythematosus (Halder and Bridgeman-Shah, 1995), although treatment with X rays, UV light, or certain drugs may contribute to the development of tumors.

HOST FACTORS

Pigmentation

Skin color is determined by the genetically regulated amount of melanin pigment produced by melanocytes. Depending on the quantity of pigment in these cells, the skin is protected from the cumulative damage produced by UV radiation (Marks, 1995). Thus dark-skinned individuals tend to be resistant to all forms of UV-induced skin cancer and precursor lesions, while light-skinned individuals are prone. Most susceptible are those with fair complexions that tend to freckle and burn rather than tan easily (Kricker et al, 1991). This phenotype is seen especially among persons of Celtic heritage, with some but not all studies suggesting an exceptional risk of skin cancer in relation to Celtic ancestry (Kricker et al, 1994).

Precursor Lesions

Actinic (solar) keratosis and Bowen's disease (SCC in situ) are precursor lesions for invasive SCC (Sober and Burstein, 1995). The progression rate of actinic keratosis is low, with about one keratosis per 1,000 per year converting to SCC. Actinic keratosis is associated with cumulative sunlight exposure and a susceptible skin phenotype, and occurs only on sun-exposed surfaces. Similar forms of keratosis can be produced by ionizing radiation, inorganic arsenic, and polycyclic hydrocarbons. Bowen's disease is an indolent lesion that mainly affects older people, with about three-fourths of the lesions occurring on sun-exposed surfaces. Progression to invasive SCC eventually occurs in about 5% of lesions. When Bowen's disease affects non–sun-exposed surfaces, inorganic arsenic may be the culprit. Some surveys have indicated that patients with Bowen's disease are prone to internal cancers, but recent population-based studies have revealed no excess risk of subsequent malignancies (Chute et al, 1991). In contrast to SCC, there is no known precursor lesion for BCC.

Genetic Predisposition

Several rare hereditary diseases predispose to NMSC, primarily by increasing susceptibility to the effects of UV radiation, and they provide important clues to mechanisms of skin carcinogenesis in the general population. The nevoid basal cell carcinoma syndrome is a dominantly inherited disorder consisting of multiple BCC and various developmental defects, including jaw cysts, skeletal anomalies, skin pits on the palms and soles, soft-tissue calcifications, and hypertelorism (Gorlin, 1987). A gene for this disorder has been located on chromosome 9q (Farndon et al, 1992). The basal cell tumors usually arise around puberty, but may appear as late as 40 years of age. It has been estimated that about one in 200 patients with BCC may have the syndrome, with the proportion rising to one in five when tumors develop before age 19 (Springate, 1986). There is a high risk of ovarian fibromas and medulloblastoma, which may be the presenting manifestation of the syndrome in children. The production of basal cell tumors in the syndrome is enhanced by exposure to sunlight and, most remarkably, to ionizing radiation that may be used to treat medulloblastoma (Strong, 1977). Another dominantly inherited condition is multiple self-healing squamous epitheliomata, which progress intermittently to invasive SCC but then spontaneously remit (Goudie et al, 1993). The mechanisms of tumor resolution are unclear, but the gene has been localized to a region of chromosome 9q that also contains the gene for nevoid basal cell carcinoma syndrome.

Xeroderma pigmentosum (XP) is a progressive sun-sensitive, autosomal recessive disease that develops during early childhood (Cleaver and Kraemer, 1995). In XP patients under age 20, there is a 1000-fold increased frequency of BCC, SCC, and melanoma on sun-exposed portions of the body, including the anterior eye and tongue (Kraemer et al, 1994). About 20% of patients have neurological abnormalities such as mental retardation, microcephaly, ataxia, choreoathetosis, and deafness (Kraemer et al, 1987). Despite extensive clinical and genetic heterogeneity in XP, all cases exhibit defects in the ability of cells to repair DNA damage induced by UV light (Bootsma, 1993). Using XP as a model, a recent population-based study in Maryland observed that non-XP patients with BCC have a reduced DNA repair capacity (Wei et al, 1993, 1994c). However, a subsequent study from Australia did not find these defects in patients with BCC or SCC (Hall et al, 1994).

Other recessively inherited states are prone to skin cancer. Since melanin pigment is absent, albinism greatly predisposes to skin cancer, especially SCC on sun-exposed areas (Witkop et al, 1989). Epidermodysplasia verruciformis consists of multiple benign verrucous tumors (warts) that develop in early childhood as a result of susceptibility to various types of human papillomaviruses (HPV) (Tyring, 1993). A high frequency of SCC has been reported, particularly in sun-exposed areas, with malignant conversion related mainly to HPV types 5 and 8. In the general population, HPVs are closely linked to squamous cancers involving anogenital skin, particularly HPV-16, but there has been no consistent association with other skin cancers except possibly in the setting of immunosuppression (Euvrard et al, 1993).

In addition, squamous cancers of the skin, mouth, and esophagus occur excessively in the scars of patients with the recessive and dominant types of dystrophic epidermolysis bullosa (Goldberg et al, 1988). Dyskeratosis congenita is a sex-linked recessive trait featuring skin pigmentation and atrophy, nail dysplasia, and leukoplakia of the mucous membranes (Sirinavin and Trowbridge, 1975). The condition often shows stigmata of Fanconi's aplastic anemia and carries a high risk of SCC involving the skin and mucous membranes.

In the general population, genetic determinants of skin color and complexion are responsible for the ethnic variations in NMSC, while other heritable factors may contribute to the familial tendency (Czarnecki et al, 1992; Wei et al, 1994a), the association reported with certain HLA antigens (Czarnecki et al, 1991), and possibly the increased risk with age (Wei et al, 1993).

Immunologic Factors

There is clear evidence that immunosuppressive states may predispose to various kinds of skin cancer, including melanoma. Most striking are the elevated risks of SCC among kidney transplant recipients receiving immunosuppressive drugs, including azathioprine and cyclosporine (Hoover and Fraumeni, 1973; Hartevelt et al, 1990). The excess risk is primarily on exposed areas of the skin and is further increased in sunny climates. To a lesser extent, an excess risk of SCC extends to other conditions that are treated with immunosuppressive drugs or are complicated by immunodeficiency (Kinlen, 1982). However, it is not clear whether the risk of NMSC is increased among patients infected with human immunodeficiency virus (HIV) (Lobo et al, 1992). The epidemiologic findings are intriguing in view of experimental evidence that UV radiation has an immunosuppressive effect that may promote its carcinogenic properties (Kripke, 1994).

PREVENTIVE MEASURES

The leading cause of nonmelanoma skin cancer is UV radiation from the sun, which accounts for the vast majority of SCC and BCC. Therefore, the risk of skin cancer can be substantially lowered by minimizing exposure to UV radiation. In particular, sunlight should be avoided during the middle of the day, especially between 11 a.m. to 1 p.m., when UVB exposures can be reduced by nearly 50% (Scotto et al, 1976b). The "shadow rule" may be used as a simple guide: Protect yourself from sunlight when your shadow is shorter than your height (Holloway et al, 1992). This rule avoids the need for watches, can be taught to children, holds true in all time zones, and is independent of daylight savings time. Also recommended are protective clothing and sunscreens with a sun protection factor (SPF) of at least 15, especially for fair-complexioned persons who sunburn easily. These measures should aid in halting the upward trend in the incidence of skin cancer, including melanoma, which may be attributed to increasing sunlight exposures from changing clothing styles and leisure time activities of the population (Marks, 1995). Special efforts are needed to protect infants and children, since NMSC risks are related to cumulative lifetime exposures and vulnerability appears greatest in early life (Marks et al, 1990).

There is widespread concern that exposures to UV radiation will increase if the stratospheric ozone layer is modified by chlorofluorocarbon emissions and certain other pollutants, and international cooperation will be needed if regulatory measures are to be effective. In addition, it is important to protect against the hazards of UV exposures from artificial sources, including sun lamps, tanning salons, and certain industrial operations such as welding, and to be wary of the potential enhancement of UV damage by photosensitizing and immunosuppressive agents. Steps should also be taken to limit unnecessary exposures to ionizing radiation, polycyclic hydrocarbons, and inorganic arsenic, although their contributions to the skin cancer burden of the population may be limited.

Since skin tumors are easily visible and accessible, screening and educational programs for high-risk individuals will help ensure the early detection and treatment of precancerous lesions and skin cancer (Kopf et al, 1995; Rhodes, 1995). Regular examinations are especially recommended for individuals with a history of skin cancer or multiple keratoses, severely sun-damaged skin, genetic predisposition or immunologic impairment, and significant exposure to chemical carcinogens or ionizing radiation (Preston and Stern, 1992). In addition, high-dose oral retinoids have been found to be effective in the prevention of new skin cancers among patients with xeroderma pigmentosum (Kraemer et al,

1988). However, chemoprevention with high-dose retinoids is toxic and low-dose isotretinoin was not effective in preventing new tumors arising among patients previously treated for basal cell cancers (Tangrea et al, 1992). By focusing on groups at high risk of skin cancer, it should be possible to further investigate the potential benefits of dietary modification, chemopreventive measures, and other interventions (Greenberg et al, 1990; Black et al, 1994).

REFERENCES

AMERICAN CANCER SOCIETY. 1995. Cancer Facts and Figures 1995. Atlanta, GA, American Cancer Society.

ARMSTRONG BK. 1994. Stratospheric ozone and health. Int J Epidemiol 23:873–885.

AUBRY F, MACGIBBON B. 1985. Risk factors of squamous cell carcinoma of the skin: A case–control study in the Montreal region. Cancer 55:907–911.

BINGHAM E, TROSSET RP, WARSHAWSKY D. 1979. Carcinogenic potential of petroleum hydrocarbons: A critical review of the literature. J Environ Pathol Toxicol 3:483–563.

BLACK HS, HERD JA, GOLDBERG LH, et al. 1994. Effect of a low-fat diet on the incidence of actinic keratosis. N Engl J Med 330:1272–1275.

BLUM HF. 1976. Ultraviolet radiation and skin cancer: In mice and men. Photochem Photobiol 24:249–254.

BOOTSMA D. 1993. The genetic defect in DNA repair deficiency syndromes. Eur J Cancer 29A:1482–1488.

BRASH DE, RUDOLPH JA, SIMON JA, et al. 1991. A role for sunlight in skin cancer: UV-induced p53 mutations in squamous cell carcinoma. Proc Natl Acad Sci USA 88:10124–10128.

BROWN KG, BOYLE KE, CHEN CW, GIBB HJ. 1989. A dose–response analysis of skin cancer from inorganic arsenic in drinking water. Risk Anal 9:519–528.

CAMAIN R, TUYNS AJ, SARRAT H, et al. 1972. Cutaneous cancer in Dakar. J Natl Cancer Inst 48:33–49.

CHUANG TY, POPESCU NA, SU WP, CHUTE CG. 1990. Squamous cell carcinoma: A population-based incidence study in Rochester, Minn. Arch Dermatol 126:185–188.

CHUTE CG, CHUANG TY, BERGSTRALH EJ, SU WPD. 1991. The subsequent risk of internal cancer with Bowen's disease. JAMA 266:816–819.

CLEAVER JE, KRAEMER KH. 1995. Xeroderma pigmentosum and Cockayne syndrome. *In* Scriver CR, Beaudet AL, Sly WS, Valle D (eds): The Metabolic and Molecular Bases of Inherited Disease. New York, McGraw-Hill, Inc., pp. 4393–4419.

COEBERGH JW, NEUMANN HA, VRINTS LW, et al. 1991. Trends in the incidence of nonmelanoma skin cancer in the SE Netherlands 1975–1988: A registry-based study. Br J Dermatol 125:353–359.

CZARNECKI D, ZALCBERG J, MEEHAN C, et al. 1992. Familial occurrence of multiple nonmelanoma skin cancer. Cancer Genet Cytogenet 61:1–5.

CZARNECKI DB, LEWIS A, NICHOLSON I, TAIT B. 1991. Multiple nonmelanoma skin cancer associated with HLA DR7 in southern Australia. Cancer 68:439–440.

DEVESA SS, BLOT WJ, STONE BJ, et al. 1995. Recent cancer trends in the United States. J Natl Cancer Inst 87:175–182.

DOLL R, VESSEY MP, BEASLEY RW, et al. 1972. Mortality of gasworkers: Final report of a prospective study. Br J Indust Med 29:394–406.

EUVRARD S, CHARDONNET Y, POUTEIL-NOBLE C, et al. 1993. Association of skin malignancies with various and multiple carcinogenic and noncarcinogenic human papillomaviruses in renal transplant recipients. Cancer 72:2198–2206.

EVERALL JD, DOWD PM. 1978. Influence of environmental factors excluding ultraviolet radiation on the incidence of skin cancer. Bull Cancer (Paris) 65:241–248.

FARNDON PA, DEL MASTRO RG, EVANS DGR, KILPATRICK MW. 1992. Location of gene for Gorlin syndrome. Lancet 339:581–582.

FEARS TR, SCOTTO J. 1983. Estimating increases in skin cancer morbidity due to increases in ultraviolet radiation exposure. Cancer Invest 1:119–126.

FEARS TR, SCOTTO J, SCHNEIDERMAN MA. 1977. Mathematical models of age and ultraviolet effects on the incidence of skin cancer among whites in the United States. Am J Epidemiol 105:420–427.

FLEMING MD, HUNT JL, PURDUE GF, SANDSTAD J. 1990. Marjolin's ulcer: A review and reevaluation of a difficult problem. J Burn Care Rehabil 11:460–469.

GALLAGHER RP, HILL GB, BAJDIK CD, et al. 1995a. Sunlight exposure, pigmentary factors, and risk of nonmelanocytic skin cancer: I. Basal cell carcinoma. Arch Dermatol 131:157–163.

GALLAGHER RP, HILL GB, BAJDIK CD, et al. 1995b. Sunlight exposure, pigmentary factors, and risk of nonmelanocytic skin cancer: II. Squamous cell carcinoma. Arch Dermatol 131:164–169.

GALLAGHER RP, MA B, MCLEAN DI, et al. 1990. Trends in basal cell carcinoma, squamous cell carcinoma, and melanoma of the skin from 1973 through 1987. J Am Acad Dermatol 23:413–421.

GILES GG, MARKS R, FOLEY P. 1988. Incidence of non-melanocytic skin cancer treated in Australia. BMJ 296:13–17.

GLASS AG, HOOVER RN. 1989. The emerging epidemic of melanoma and squamous cell skin cancer. JAMA 262:2097–2100.

GOLDBERG GI, EISEN AZ, BAUER EA. 1988. Tissue stress and tumor promotion: Possible relevance to epidermolysis bullosa. Arch Dermatol 124:737–741.

GORLIN RJ. 1987. Nevoid basal-cell carcinoma syndrome. Medicine 66:98–113.

GOUDIE DR, YUILLE MAR, LEVERSHA MA, et al. 1993. Multiple self-healing squamous epitheliomata (ESS1) mapped to chromosome 9q22-q31 in families with common ancestry. Nature Genetics 3:165–169.

GREEN AC, BATTISTUTTA D. 1990. Incidence and determinants of skin cancer in a high-risk Australian population. Int J Cancer 46:356–361.

GREENBERG ER, BARON JA, STUKEL TA, et al. 1990. A clinical trial of beta-carotene to prevent basal-cell and squamous-cell cancers of the skin. New Engl J Med 323:789–795.

GREENE MH, FRAUMENI JF JR. 1979. The hereditary variant of malignant melanoma. *In* Clark WH, Goldman LI, Mastrangelo MJ (eds): Human Malignant Melanoma. New York, Grune and Stratton, pp. 139–166.

HALDER RM, BANG KM. 1988. Skin cancer in blacks in the United States. Dermatol Clin 16:397–405.

HALDER RM, BRIDGEMAN-SHAH S. 1995. Skin cancer in African Americans. Cancer 75:667–673.

HALL J, ENGLISH DR, ARTUSO M, et al. 1994. DNA repair capacity as a risk factor for non-melanocytic skin cancer: A molecular epidemiological study. Int J Cancer 58:179–184.

HARTEVELT MM, BAVINCK JN, KOOTTE AM, et al. 1990. Incidence of skin cancer after renal transplantation in the Netherlands. Transplantation 49:506–509.

HENDRICKS NV, BERRY CM, LIONE JG, et al. 1959. Cancer of the scrotum in wax pressmen. AMA Arch Ind Hyg 19:524–529.

HOFFMAN JS. 1987. Assessing the Risks of Trace Gases that Can Modify the Stratosphere. Vol 1: Executive Summary, Office of Air and Radiation. Washington, D.C., U.S. Environmental Protection Agency, pp. ES 1–64.

HOLLOWAY L. 1992. Atmospheric sun protection factor on clear days: Its observed dependence on solar zenity angle and its relevance to the shadow rule for sun protection. Photochem Photobiol 56:229–234.

HOOVER R, FRAUMENI JF JR. 1973. Risk of cancer in renal transplant recipients. Lancet 2:55–57.

HSUEH YM, CHENG GS, WU MM, et al. 1995. Multiple risk factors associated with arsenic-induced skin cancer: Effects of chronic liver disease and malnutrional status. Br J Cancer 71:109–114.

HUNTER DJ, COLDITZ GA, STAMPFER MJ, et al. 1992. Diet and risk of basal cell carcinoma of the skin in a prospective cohort of women. Ann Epidemiol 2:231–239.

INTERNATIONAL AGENCY FOR RESEARCH ON CANCER. 1980. IARC: Monographs on the Evaluation of Carcinogenic Risk of Chemical to Man, Vol. 23, Some Metals and Metallic Compounds. Lyon, pp 39–141.

INTERNATIONAL AGENCY FOR RESEARCH ON CANCER. 1992. Solar and Ultraviolet Radiation. IARC Monogr Eval Carcinog Risks Hum 55. Lyon, International Agency for Research on Cancer.

KALDOR J, SHUGG D, YOUNG B, et al. 1993. Non-melanoma skin cancer: Ten years of cancer-registry-based surveillance. Int J Cancer 53:886–891.

KAPLAN RP. 1987. Cancer complicating chronic ulcerative and scarifying mucocutaneous disorders. Adv Dermatol 2:19–46.

KARAGAS MR, STUKEL TA, GREENBERG ER, et al. 1992. Risk of subsequent basal cell carcinoma and squamous cell carcinoma of the skin among patients with prior skin cancer. JAMA 267:3305–3310.

KELFKENS G, DE GRUIJL FR, VAN DER LEUN JC. 1990. Ozone depletion and increase in annual ultraviolet radiation dose. Photochem Photobiol 52:819–823.

KIPLING MD, WALDRON HA. 1976. Polycyclic aromatic hydrocarbons in mineral oil, tar, and pitch, excluding petroleum pitch. Prev Med 5:262–278.

KINLEN L. 1982. Immunosuppressive therapy and cancer. Cancer Surv 1:565–583.

KOPF AW, SALOPEK TG, SLADE J, et al. 1995. Techniques of cutaneous examination for the detection of skin cancer. Cancer 75:684–690.

KRAEMER KH, DIGIOVANNA JJ, MOSHELL AN, et al. 1988. Prevention of skin cancer in xeroderma pigmentosum with the use of oral isotretinoin. N Engl J Med 318:1633–1637.

KRAEMER KH, LEE MM, ANDREWS AD, LAMBERT WC. 1994. The role of sunlight and DNA repair in melanoma and nonmelanoma skin cancer: The xeroderma pigmentosum paradigm. Arch Dermatol 130:1018–1021.

KRAEMER KH, LEE MM, SCOTTO J. 1987. Xeroderma pigmentosum: Cutaneous, ocular, and neurological abnormalities in 830 published cases. Arch Dermatol 123:241–250.

KRICKER A, ARMSTRONG BK, ENGLISH DR. 1994. Sun exposure and non-melanocytic skin cancer. Cancer Causes Control 5:367–392.

KRICKER A, ARMSTRONG BK, ENGLISH DR, HEENAN PJ. 1991. Pigmentary and cutaneous risk factors for non-melanocytic skin cancer: A case–control study. Int J Cancer 48:650–662.

KRIPKE ML. 1994. Ultraviolet radiation and immunology: Something new under the sun. Cancer Res 54:6102–6105.

KUNE GA, BANNERMAN S, FIELD B, et al. 1992. Diet, alcohol, smoking, serum β-carotene, and vitamin A in male nonmelanocytic skin cancer patients and controls. Nutr Cancer 18:237–244.

LAYCOCK HT. 1948. The "kang cancer" of North-West China. BMJ 1:982.

LEE JA, YONGCHAIYUDHA S. 1971. Incidence of and mortality from malignant melanoma by anatomical site. J Natl Cancer Inst 47:253–263.

LINDQVIST C. 1979. Risk factors in lip cancer: A questionnaire survey. Am J Epidemiol 109:521–530.

LOBO DV, CHU P, GREKIN RC, BERGER TG. 1992. Nonmelanoma skin cancers and infection with the human immunodeficiency virus. Arch Dermatol 128:623–627.

MARKS R. 1995. An overview of skin cancers: Incidence and causation. Cancer 75:607–612.

MARKS R, JOLLEY D, LECTSAS S, FOLEY P. 1990. The role of childhood exposure to sunlight in the development of solar keratoses and non-melanocytic skin cancer. Med J Aust 152:62–66.

MARKS R, STAPLES M, GILES GG. 1993. Trends in non-melanocytic skin cancer treated in Australia: The second national survey. Int J Cancer 53:585–590.

MILLER DL, WEINSTOCK MA. 1994. Nonmelanoma skin cancer in the United States: Incidence. J Am Acad Dermatol 30:774–778.

MULAY DM. 1963. Skin cancer in India. Natl Cancer Inst Monogr 10:215–223.

NATIONAL INSTITUTES OF HEALTH. 1991. Summary of the Consensus Development Conference on Sunlight, Ultraviolet Radiation, and the Skin. J Am Acad Dermatol 24:608–612.

NATIONAL RESEARCH COUNCIL. 1990. Committee on the Biological Effects of Ionizing Radiations (BEIR V): Health Effects of Exposure to Low Levels of Ionizing Radiation. Washington, D.C., National Academy Press, pp. 325–327.

PARTENEN T, BOFFETTA P. 1994. Cancer risk in asphalt workers and roofers: Review and meta-analysis of epidemiologic studies. Am J Ind Med 26:721–740.

PARTANEN T, PUKKALA E, VAINIO H, et al. 1994. Increased incidence of lung and skin cancer in Finnish silicotic patients. J Occup Med 36:616–622.

PRESTON DS, STERN RS. 1992. Nonmelanoma cancers of the skin. N Engl J Med 327:1649–1662.

PUKKALA E, NOKSO-KOIVISTO P, ROPONEN P. 1992. Changing cancer risk pattern among Finnish hairdressers. Int Arch Occup Environ Health 64:39–42.

RHODES AR. 1995. Public education and cancer of the skin: What do people need to know about melanoma and nonmelanoma skin cancer? Cancer 75:613–636.

RIES LAG, HANKEY BF, EDWARDS BK. 1990. Cancer statistics review 1973–87. NIH Publication 90–2789. Washington, D.C., U.S. Department of Health and Human Services.

SCOTTO J. 1986. Nonmelanoma skin cancer—UVB effects. *In* Titus JG (ed): Effects of Changes in Stratospheric Ozone and Global Climate, Vol. 2: Stratospheric Ozone. Washington, D.C., U.S. Environmental Protection Agency, pp. 33–61.

SCOTTO J, COTTON G, URBACH F, et al. 1988. Biologically effective ultraviolet radiation: Surface measurements in the United States, 1974 to 1985. Science 239:762–764.

SCOTTO J, FEARS TR. 1987. The association of solar ultraviolet and skin melanoma incidence among Caucasians in the United States. Cancer Invest 5:275–283.

SCOTTO J, FEARS TR, FRAUMENI JF JR. 1983. Incidence of Nonmelanoma Skin Cancer in the United States. DHEW Publ. No. (NIH) 83-2433. Washington, D.C., U.S. Government Printing Office.

SCOTTO J, FEARS TR, GORI GB. 1976a. Measurements of Ultraviolet Radiation in the United States and Comparisons with Skin Cancer Data. DHEW (NIH) 76-1029. Bethesda, National Cancer Institute.

SCOTTO J, FEARS TR, GORI GB. 1976b. Ultraviolet exposure patterns. Environ Res 12:228–237.

SCOTTO J, NAM JM. 1980. Skin melanoma and seasonal patterns. Am J Epidemiol 111:309–314.

SCOTTO J, PITCHER H, LEE JAH. 1991. Indications of future decreasing trends in skin-melanoma mortality among whites in the United States. Int J Cancer 49:490–497.

SHORE RE. 1990. Overview of radiation-induced skin cancer in humans. Int J Radiat Biol 57:809–827.

SIRINAVIN C, TROWBRIDGE AA. 1975. Dyskeratosis congenita: Clinical features and genetic aspects. Report of a family and review of the literature. J Med Genet 12:339–354.

SOBER AJ, BURSTEIN JM. 1995. Precursors to skin cancer. Cancer 75:645–650.

SPRINGATE JE. 1986. The nevoid basal cell carcinoma syndrome. J Pediatr Surg 21:908–910.

STERN RS, LAIRD N. 1994. The carcinogenic risk of treatments for severe psoriasis. Cancer 73:2759–64.

STRICKLAND PT, VITASA BC, WEST SK, et al. 1989. Quantitative carcinogenesis in man: Solar ultraviolet B dose dependence of skin cancer in Maryland watermen. J Natl Cancer Inst 81:1910–1913.

STRONG LC. 1977. Theories of pathogenesis: Mutation and cancer. *In* Mulvihill JJ, Miller RW, Fraumeni JF Jr (eds): Genetics of Human Cancer. New York, Raven Press, pp. 401–415.

SVINDLAND HB. 1980. Kangri cancer in the brick industry. Contact Dermatitis 6:24–26.

TANGREA JA, EDWARDS BK, TAYLOR PR, et al. 1992. Long-term therapy with low-dose isotretinoin for prevention of basal cell carcinoma: A multicenter clinical trial. J Natl Cancer Inst 84:328–332.

TYRING SK. 1993. Human papillomaviruses in skin cancer. Cancer Bull 45:212–219.

UNITED NATIONS ENVIRONMENT PROGRAMME ENVIRONMENTAL EFFECTS PANEL. 1990. Environmental effects of ozone depletion. Nairobi, United Nations Environment Programme.

UNITED NATIONS SCIENTIFIC COMMITTEE ON THE EFFECTS OF ATOMIC RADIATION. 1994. Sources and Effects of Ionizing Radiation. (UNSCEAR 1994 Report to the General Assembly. New York, United Nations, p. 30.

URBACH F. 1971. Geographic distribution of skin cancer. J Surg Oncol 3:219–234.

WALLBERG P, SKOG E. 1991. The incidence of basal cell carcinoma in an area of Stockholm County during the period 1971–1980. Acta Derm Venereol (Stockh) 71:134–137.

WANG HH, MACMAHON B. 1979. Mortality of pesticide applicators. J Occup Med 21:741–744.

WEI Q, MATANOSKI GM, FARMER ER, et al. 1993. DNA repair and aging in basal cell carcinoma: A molecular epidemiology study. Proc Natl Acad Sci USA 90:1614–1618.

WEI Q, MATANOSKI GM, FARMER ER, et al. 1994a. DNA repair related to multiple skin cancers and drug use. Cancer Res 54:437–440.

WEI Q, MATANOSKI GM, FARMER ER, et al. 1994b. Vitamin supplementation and reduced risk of basal cell carcinoma. J Clin Epidemiol 47:829–836.

WEI Q, MATANOSKI GM, FARMER ER, et al. 1994c. DNA repair and susceptibility to basal cell carcinoma: A case–control study. Am J Epidemiol 140:598–607.

WEINSTOCK MA. 1993. Nonmelanoma skin cancer mortality in the United States, 1969 through 1988. Arch Dermatol 129:1286–1290.

WEINSTOCK MA. 1994a. Epidemiology of nonmelanoma skin cancer: Clinical issues, definitions, and classification. J Invest Dermatol 102:4S–5S.

WEINSTOCK MA. 1994b. Epidemiologic investigation of nonmelanoma skin cancer mortality: The Rhode Island follow-back study. J Invest Dermatol 102:6S–9S.

WHITAKER CJ, LEE WR, DOWNES JE. 1979. Squamous cell skin cancer in the North-west of England, 1967–69, and its relation to occupation. Br J Ind Med 36:43–51.

WITKOP CJ, QUEVADO WC, FITZPATRICK TB, KING RA. 1989. Albinism. *In* Scriver CR, Beaudet AL, Sly WS, Valle D (eds): The Metabolic Basis of Inherited Disease, 6th ed. New York, McGraw-Hill pp. 2905–2947.

YIANNIAS JA, GOLDBERG LH, CARTER-CAMPBELL S, et al. 1988. The ratio of basal cell carcinoma to squamous cell carcinoma in Houston, Texas. J Dermatol Surg 14:886–889.

YUSPA SH. 1994. The pathogenesis of squamous cell cancer: Lessons learned from studies of skin carcinogenesis. Cancer Res 54:1178–1189.

YUSPA SH, DLUGOSZ AA. 1991. Cutaneous carcinogenesis: natural and experimental. *In* Goldsmith L (ed): Physiology, Biochemistry and Molecular Biology of the Skin. New York, Oxford University Press, pp. 1365–1402.

ZIEGLER A, JONASON AS, LEFFELL DJ, et al. 1994. Sunburn and p53 in the onset of skin cancer. Nature 372:773–776.

61 Cancers in children

WONG-HO CHOW
MARTHA S. LINET
JONATHAN M. LIFF
RAYMOND S. GREENBERG

In the United States, less than 1% of all cancers occur in children under 15 years of age (Young et al, 1978). According to recent national estimates, over 7500 cancers are diagnosed annually among children (Bleyer, 1990; Miller et al, 1993). During the past four decades, there has been a dramatic decrease in mortality for many types of childhood cancer (Young et al, 1986; Miller et al, 1993). The notable decline in mortality has been accompanied by improvements in survival primarily due to treatment advances (Steinhorn and Gloeckler-Ries, 1988). In spite of this clinical progress, however, cancer remains the second most common cause of death among children in the United States, trailing only accidents (Boring et al, 1994).

Aside from the importance of cancer as a cause of mortality in childhood, research on the epidemiology of malignancies in children has been stimulated by the recognition that genetic factors (Knudson, 1971) and prenatal exposures (Stewart et al, 1958; MacMahon, 1962; Herbst et al, 1971) can influence the risk of developing these diseases. Data from case-control studies reported in the past couple of decades also have suggested that environmental (pesticides, ionizing and nonionizing radiation), parental occupational (petrochemical and hydrocarbon, metal, and pesticide), and medical (prenatal x-rays, chemotherapy, and other medications) exposures may increase risk. In this chapter, an overview of the epidemiology of cancer in children is presented. The initial sections focus on the patterns of disease occurrence and the latter sections include summaries of specific research findings on suspected risk factors.

The authors thank Ms. Diane Irwin of Information Management Services, Inc., for computer programming and graphics support, Dr. Susan Devesa for helpful suggestions in development of the figures, and Dr. Alisa Goldstein for reviewing the genetics section of this chapter.

CLASSIFICATION

Cancers that arise in the pediatric age group differ from those that occur among adults with respect to the distributions of anatomic sites of involvement, as well as the predominant histological patterns. For example, malignancies of epithelial tissues are common among adults but occur rarely among children. Conversely, tumors in young persons often are composed of embryonal cell types (ie, morphologically similar to fetal cells), which are uncommon among malignancies of adults. With these distinctions in mind, it is not surprising that nosological schemes developed for the categorization of adult cancers are not ideally suited to the classification of childhood cancers. A diagnostic grouping scheme has been developed for pediatric cancer (Birch and Marsden, 1987) as an adaptation of the standard *International Classification of Disease for Oncology* (ICD-O) (World Health Organization, 1976). In this modified system, 12 major diagnostic categories are specified as follows:

1. Leukemia
2. Lymphomas and other reticuloendothelial neoplasms
3. Central nervous system and miscellaneous intracranial and intraspinal neoplasms
4. Sympathetic and allied nervous system tumors
5. Retinoblastoma
6. Renal tumors
7. Hepatic tumors
8. Malignant bone tumors
9. Soft tissue sarcomas
10. Germ cell, trophoblastic, and other gonadal neoplasms
11. Carcinomas and other malignant epithelial neoplasms
12. Other and unspecified malignant neoplasms

Distributed among these 12 major categories are 40 subgroups. For example, under the major heading of leukemias, there are five subgroups: acute lymphocytic leukemia, other lymphoid leukemia, acute nonlymphocytic leukemia, chronic myeloid leukemia, and other and unspecified leukemia.

Although this classification scheme was introduced as recently as 1987, it was quickly incorporated as the basis for classification of malignancies in the benchmark volume *International Incidence of Childhood Cancer* (Parkin et al, 1988a). It is likely, therefore, to continue to be considered the standard nosological scheme for epidemiological research on pediatric cancers, and consequently it is employed throughout this chapter.

DEMOGRAPHIC PATTERNS

Incidence

There are slightly less than 15 per 100,000 diagnosed childhood cancer cases occurring annually among children under 15 years of age in the United States, and an estimated 200,000 incident cases throughout the world (Parkin et al, 1988a; Bleyer, 1990; Miller et al, 1993). The most commonly diagnosed malignancy in this age group in the United States and many other industrialized countries is leukemia (constituting about one third of childhood neoplasms), followed by central nervous system malignancies (19%), neuroblastoma (18%), lymphomas (12%) and others (about 20%). Lymphomas are the second most common malignancy after leukemias in several Latin American and Asian countries, whereas in many African nations, lymphomas are the most commonly reported neoplasms among children.

The volume *International Incidence of Childhood Cancer* (Parkin et al, 1988a) presents the most recent comprehensive information available in a standardized format on the worldwide variation of childhood malignancies among several efforts of this type (Miller, 1974; Munoz, 1976; Breslow and Langholz, 1983; West, 1984). The most recent summary of trend data can be found in Draper and coworkers (1994). To enable comparisons among populations, Parkin and coworkers (1988a) sought data from the collaborating registries for all malignancies diagnosed among children aged 0–14 during 1970–1979, or as close as possible to that time period.

International comparisons of incidence rates are subject to potential biases from lack of uniformity in completeness of case identification and in accuracy of population estimates, disparities in access to medical care, variation in diagnostic practices, histopathologic classification, and in coding schemes used, and differences in the proportion of cases designated as other and not otherwise specified (NOS) (Stiller and Draper, 1982; Mattson and Wallgren, 1984; Storm, 1988; Alexander et al, 1989; Draper et al, 1994). Also, findings based on small numbers should be considered tentative until additional cases substantiate a clear pattern. Data described below and shown in the accompanying figures were generally from older, larger, and more established population-based registries with rates based on high-quality census survey information, and usually derived from a minimum of 20 cases (Parkin et al, 1988a; Miller et al, 1993). Data are presented for all childhood cancers combined and for four of the most common childhood cancers (leukemia, lymphoma, CNS neoplasms, and neuroblastoma). Descriptive information for other childhood malignancies is based on literature review.

Total Childhood Cancer. Compared with the notable geographic variation in incidence rates observed internationally for most adult malignancies, differences in total childhood cancer rates among the 22 populations shown are relatively small (Fig. 61–1). Age-adjusted rates vary approximately twofold (ranging from 86.3 to 164.1 per million for boys and from 54.5 to 130.4 per million for girls), with the greatest variation among Asian populations. Rates are high among Hispanics in Costa Rica and Los Angeles, but low to mid-level

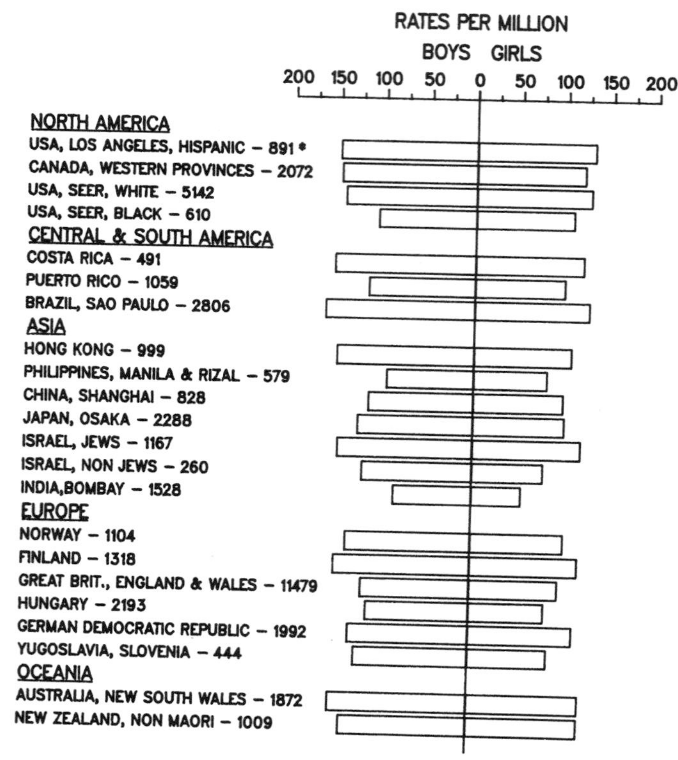

FIG. 61–1. International childhood total cancer incidence rates, age-adjusted to world standard, circa 1970–1979. (From Parkin et al., 1988a.)

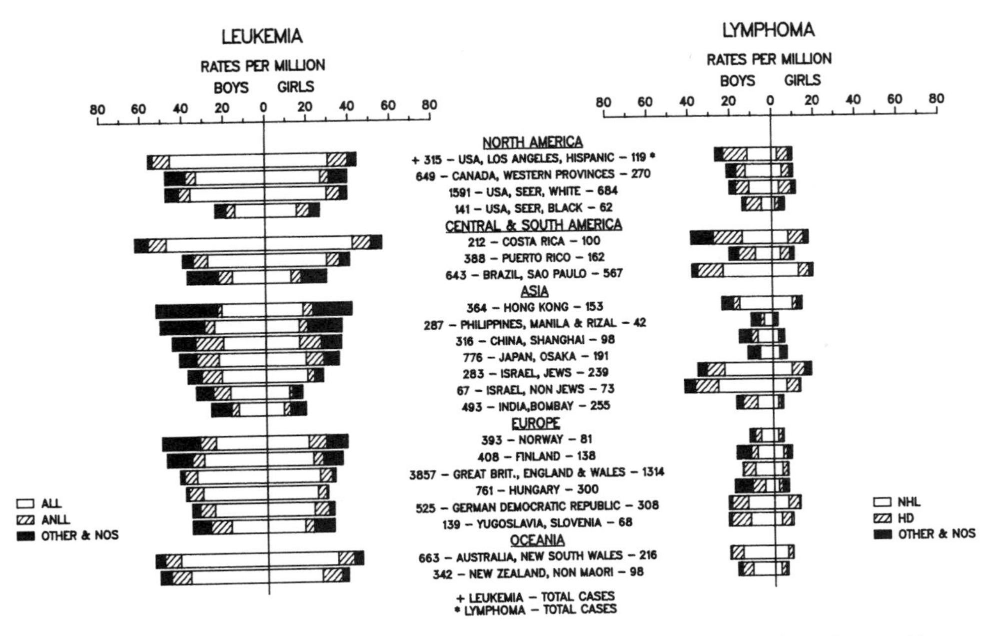

FIG. 61–2. International childhood leukemia and lymphoma incidence rates, age-adjusted to world standard, by cell type, circa 1970–1979. (From Parkin et al., 1988a.)

among other Hispanic populations such as Puerto Ricans. For virtually all populations, rates are higher among boys than girls, with male-to-female ratios generally ranging from 1.1 to 1.4:1. In general, incidence is higher among whites than blacks, with a white-to-black incidence ratio of 1.2 for both males and females (Miller et al, 1993). In contrast with the incidence in adults, epithelial tumors in children are rare; elevated incidence of these malignancies among children parallels high incidence areas for adults (Parkin et al, 1988b; Parkin et al, 1992).

Leukemia and Lymphoma. The patterns of age-adjusted rates for leukemia and lymphoma are generally similar in most of the developed countries, although in general the total leukemia rates are substantially higher than the total lymphoma rates (1.5- to three-fold higher for most boys and two- to six-fold higher for most girls) (Fig. 61–2). In contrast, the lymphoma/leukemia ratios are higher in developing countries than in industrialized countries, with the five highest ratios in Africa and the Middle East (Parkin et al, 1988a).

Among children, acute lymphoblastic leukemia (ALL) is the commonest form in most countries. Rates are highest in Costa Rica, among U.S. Hispanic males in Los Angeles, and in Australia; low rates occur among Bombay Indians, Israeli non-Jews and U.S. blacks. Incidence is quite uniform among Far East Asian populations. Acute nonlymphoblastic leukemia (ANLL) is an uncommon leukemia type in children. Similar to ALL, rates for ANLL are relatively high among Hispanics and low among Bombay Indians, but unlike ALL, ANLL rates are similar among whites and blacks in the United States and vary substantially among Far East Asians.

In general, ALL rates are highest among children under age five, with a notable peak in incidence between the ages of two and four in many populations, followed by a decline in rates with increasing age (Fig. 61–3). Rates for girls are lower in each group than those for boys (male to female ratios ranging from 1.1 to 1.4:1), except among U.S. blacks (whose male to female ratio is 0.9). Acute nonlymphoblastic leukemia rates are highest among infants and similar for boys and girls, but lower and more uniform than those for ALL at all ages (Linet and Devesa, 1991).

Lymphoma is the predominant malignancy among children in Uganda, Nigeria, other countries in Africa,

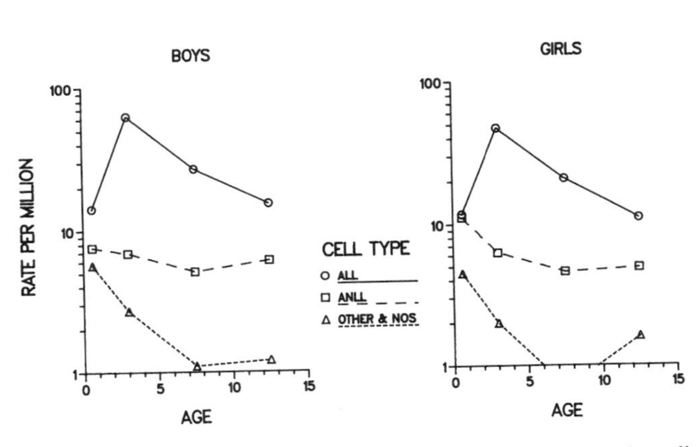

FIG. 61–3. Age-specific variation in leukemia incidence rates by cell type in England and Wales, 1971–1980. (From Parkin et al., 1988a.)

and in Papua, New Guinea (Parkin et al, 1988b). In Latin America and several countries in Asia, malignant lymphomas are the second most common malignancy among children after leukemias. Of the two major types of lymphomas, incidence (age-adjusted) of non-Hodgkin's lymphoma (NHL) is higher than that of Hodgkin's disease (HD) among children in most countries. High rates of NHL are found in Sao Paulo, Brazil, and among Jews and non-Jews in Israel (Fig. 61–2), whereas low rates are observed in the Philippines, Hungary, and among blacks in the United States. The international patterns for Hodgkin's disease rates are similar to those for NHL.

Burkitt's lymphoma is rare in Western countries; age-adjusted rates in most populations in Europe, North and South America, and Oceania are less than one per million (Parkin et al, 1988a). The rate among U.S. whites is estimated as two per million, which is higher than the corresponding incidence for blacks in the United States (Stiller and Parkin, 1990a). Burkitt's lymphoma accounts for a higher frequency (ranging from 2.9% to 9.3%) of all childhood cancers in North Africa, Middle Eastern and western Asian populations, and is the commonest type of childhood cancer in Papua, New Guinea (Stiller and Parkin, 1990a).

The age-specific patterns for total lymphoma in most populations differ from those observed for total leukemia, in that rates for the former are generally highest among children in the oldest age group whereas leukemia rates are highest among the youngest children. There is also substantially greater variation in the age-specific patterns for lymphoma among populations, although the rates for girls in each age group are distinctly lower than those for boys. (Male to female ratios generally range from 1.8 to 3.5:1). In children younger than 10, NHL rates are substantially higher than those for HD (Fig. 61–4). Hodgkin's disease is rare among infants and young children, but rates rise rapidly during childhood and become similar to those for NHL by ages 10–14. Among populations in industrialized countries, HD incidence is low in childhood compared with that in young adults (Stiller and Parkin, 1990a). In most populations, Burkitt's lymphoma is extremely rare in infants, increasing to a peak incidence at ages 1–4 in North Africa, western Asia, and among Israeli Jews (Stiller and Parkin, 1990a). In high-incidence tropical regions of Africa, the highest frequency occurs at ages 5–9, whereas rates appear uniform at all ages among children in industrialized countries. Burkitt's lymphoma occurs more commonly in boys than in girls, with male to female ratios ranging from 1.5 to 2.5:1 in tropical Africa, North Africa, and western Asia. Higher ratios are found in Europe (3.5) and the United States (5.0).

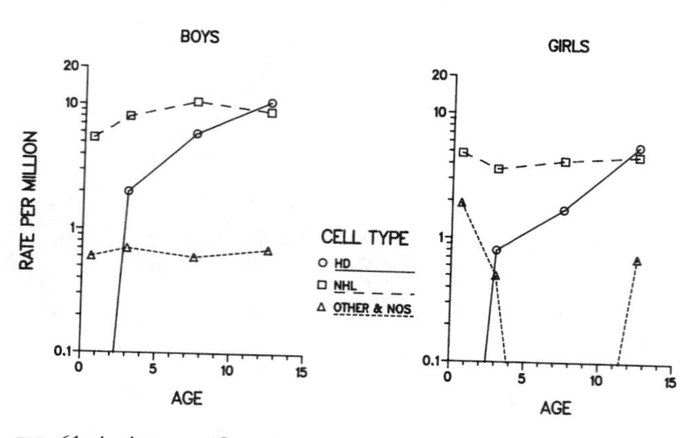

FIG. 61–4. Age-specific variation in lymphoma incidence rates by cell type in England and Wales, 1971–1980. (From Parkin et al., 1988a.)

Central Nervous System Tumors. Interpretation of geographic differences in the occurrence of central nervous system (CNS) malignancies is particularly problematic because (1) ascertainment and pathological classification are variable from region to region; (2) the distinction between benign and malignant may be unclear for some childhood intracranial tumors; and (3) there may be a substantial proportion diagnosed without biopsy (Zulch, 1979; Birch et al, 1980; Stevens et al, 1991). In Europe, North America, Australia, and Japan, CNS tumors are the second most common childhood cancer after leukemia (Parkin et al, 1988b). The greatest variation in rates for CNS tumors is seen among Asians, who also demonstrate notable differences in the proportions of other and not otherwise specified (NOS) (Fig. 61–5). Even in England and Wales, where the proportion of other and NOS for many childhood cancers is relatively low, incidence rates for CNS tumors undesignated by type are high.

Incidence of CNS neoplasms, all types combined, does not vary much by age in about 40% of the population; rates are highest among children5–9 years old in another 40%; and rates decline slightly with age in the remainder. The male to female differences are smaller than those for lymphomas or leukemias, with the ratio generally ranging from 0.9 to 1.3:1. Glioma, consisting of astrocytoma, ependymoma, and other glial tumors, is the commonest form of CNS neoplasia in most countries. Rates are highest for Caucasians in North America, Scandinavia, and Oceania, mid-level among Hispanics in Central and South America, and lowest among most Far Eastern Asians and non-Jews in Israel. Age-adjusted and age-specific rates (at all ages) for glioma were substantially higher than those for medulloblastoma. The male to female ratio for glioma is close to 1:1, whereas boys have higher rates of medulloblastoma at all ages than do girls. The age-specific patterns are generally similar for glioma and medulloblastoma, although there is a steeper decline with age for medulloblastoma (Fig. 61–6).

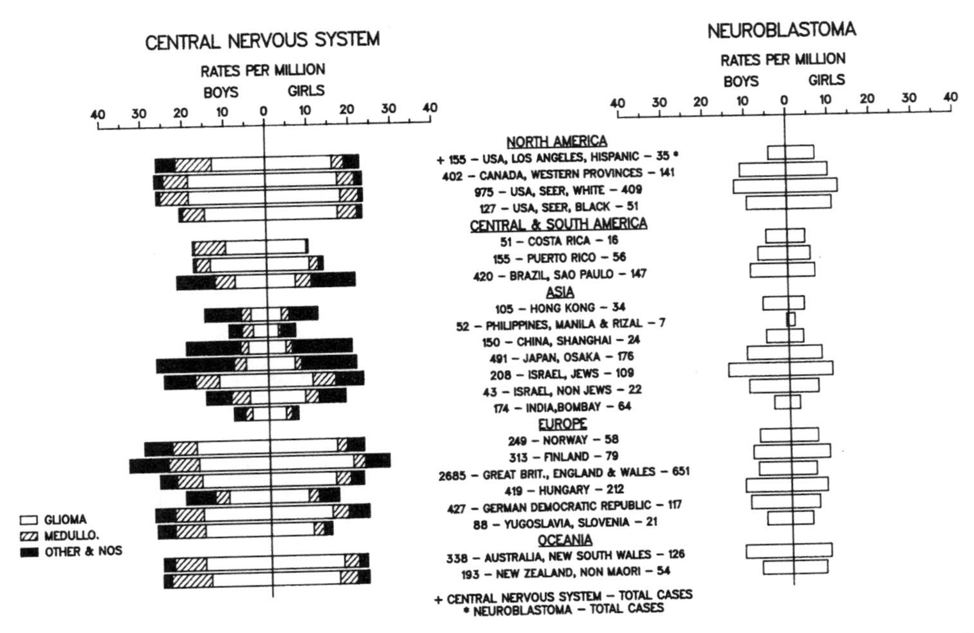

FIG. 61–5. International childhood central nervous system and neuroblastoma incidence rates, age-adjusted to world standard, by cell type, circa 1970–1979. (From Parkin et al., 1988a.)

Neuroblastoma. Incidence rates for neuroblastoma are highest among Caucasians of both sexes in North America and among Israeli Jews; high rates for boys are also observed in Hungary and Australia, and elevated incidence for girls among blacks in the United States. The higher age-adjusted incidence among U.S. whites than blacks is due to a higher rate among children diagnosed under age five (Davis et al, 1987). For virtually all registries and both sexes, neuroblastoma rates are highest in infancy, then decline dramatically with age (Parkin et al, 1988a) as seen for England and Wales (Fig. 61–7). Similar to the pattern observed for CNS tumors, the male to female ratio generally ranges from 0.9 to 1.4:1, but the male predominance is notable primarily among children diagnosed under age five (Davis et al, 1987).

Wilms' Tumor. Wilms' tumor is the most common malignant kidney tumor in all regions with approximately threefold variation in incidence (Parkin et al, 1988a; Stiller and Parkin, 1990b). Highest rates are observed among blacks in the United States, and lowest among Asians in Shanghai, the Philippines, and Japan. In the United States, females have a slightly higher rate than males in all ethnic groups (Breslow et al, 1994). Stiller and Parkin (1990b) have suggested that the variation in patterns of incidence along ethnic rather than geographic lines implies a greater likelihood that genetic predisposition is important in etiology.

Retinoblastoma. Annual age-adjusted incidence rates for retinoblastoma in white populations is estimated to be

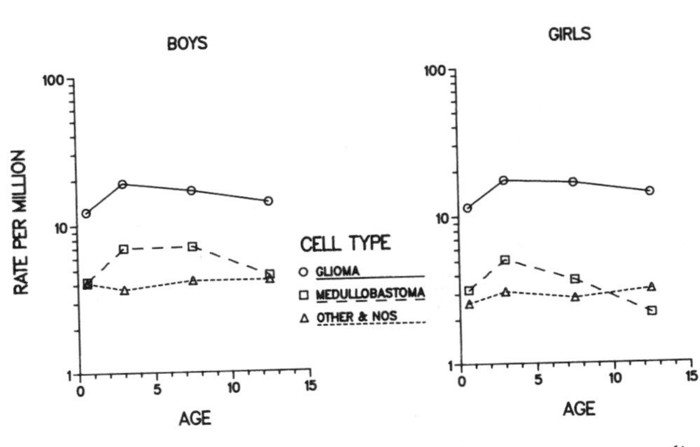

FIG. 61–6. Age-specific variation in central nervous system malignancy incidence rates by cell type in England and Wales, 1971–1980. (From Parkin et al., 1988a.)

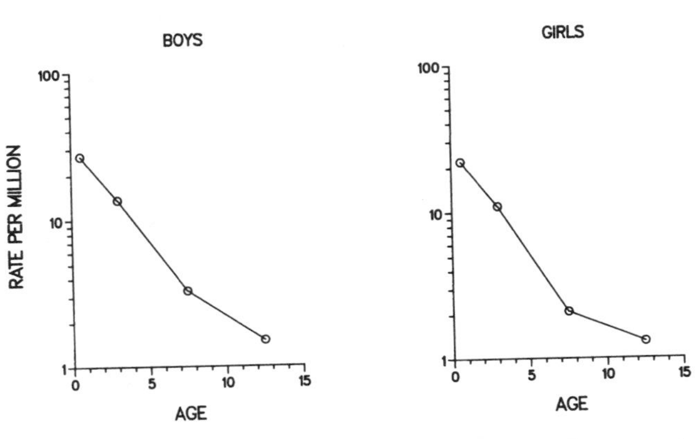

FIG. 61–7. Age-specific variation in neuroblastoma incidence rates in England and Wales, 1971–1980. (From Parkin et al., 1988a.)

3–5 per million (Parkin et al, 1988a; 1988b). Rates are higher among U.S. blacks (5.1 per million) than whites (4.0 per million) in the SEER Program (Parkin et al, 1988b). High rates also are reported in Sao Paulo, Brazil, and in Osaka, Japan, and Bombay, India. Although most registries do not separately designate cases as unilateral versus bilateral (the latter are believed to be characterized by an autosomal dominant mode of inheritance), the limited information available suggests that the international variation is primarily due to differences in incidence of unilateral disease (Parkin et al, 1988b).

Sarcomas. Most bone tumors in children are osteosarcomas or the less common Ewing's sarcomas (Parkin et al, 1988a, b; 1993a). High incidence rates for osteosarcomas occur in Sao Paulo, Brazil, and Turin, Italy, and among U.S. blacks, while low rates are reported in Osaka, Japan, in Bombay, India, and in Hungary. In the United States, incidence is higher in blacks than whites in most age groups other than infants (Parkin et al, 1988a, b; 1993a). Age-specific incidence is very low in the first 5 years, then increases during adolescence. Rates are higher in girls aged 10–14 than in boys of the same age, but postpubertal boys (age 15 and older) have higher rates than girls, a finding ascribed to the association of osteosarcoma with hormonal effects on bone growth (Miller, 1981; Parkin et al, 1988b). Approximately 80% of cases occur in the long bones of the leg, followed by about 12% in the long bones of the arm (Parkin et al, 1993a).

High rates of Ewing's sarcoma are observed among white populations in Europe and North America (rates ranging from 1.5–3.0 per million), and very low rates among blacks in the United States (0.3 per million) and in Far East Asians (0.3–0.5 per million) (Glass and Fraumeni, 1970; Li et al, 1980; Parkin et al, 1988a, b; 1993a). Incidence increases with age throughout childhood, during which rates are similar in males and females. In Ewing's sarcoma, in contrast with osteosarcoma, approximately 38% of cases have tumor in the long bones of the lower limb, 18% have pelvic neoplasms, 17% have malignancies in the upper limb, 13% in the ribs, and the remainder in the spine, skull or jaw. Chondrosarcomas account for less than 5% of bone cancers in most populations (Parkin et al, 1993a).

The majority of childhood soft tissue sarcomas are rhabdomyosarcomas or fibrosarcomas. Among North American and European whites, incidence of rhabdomyosarcomas ranges from 3 to 5 per million, whereas incidence is lower in blacks in the United States (Parkin et al, 1988a;b). The highest age-specific incidence occurs at ages 0–4 and the male to female ratio generally ranges from 1.2 to 1.5:1. In the United States, blacks have slightly higher rates of fibrosarcomas than whites, and rates generally range from 0.8 to 2.0 per million. Incidence increases with age throughout childhood; rates are similar in boys and girls. In East Africa, Kaposi's sarcoma constitutes 25%–50% of childhood soft tissue sarcomas (Parkin et al, 1988b).

Other Tumors. Incidence of hepatoblastoma appears to be quite uniform internationally, with age-adjusted rates among children ranging from 0.5 to 1.5 per million. Rates are highest among those aged 0–4. Hepatocellular carcinoma is uncommon in childhood, but shows substantially more geographic variation than hepatoblastoma. Incidence of hepatocellular carcinoma is high in eastern Asia and Latin America. The highest frequency appears to be in Papua, New Guinea, and Bulawayo, Zimbabwe. Most cases occur in persons aged 10–14 (Parkin et al, 1988a;b); this tumor is rare among adolescents.

Germ cell, trophoblastic, and other gonadal tumors are rare. The highest rates of gonadal tumors occur in East Asian countries (Parkin et al, 1988a;b). Germ cell tumors are slightly more frequent in gonadal sites than other anatomic regions. In boys, peak incidence for gonadal germ cell tumors is among those aged 0–4, whereas in girls most cases occur between the ages of 10–14. Germ cell tumors at nongonadal sites occur most frequently in children of both sexes under age five.

Survival

The survival trends in the United States for white children with cancer have shown dramatic improvement over time (Bleyer, 1993). The overall 5-year relative survival for all childhood cancers increased from 54% in 1973 to 71% in 1985 (Miller et al, 1993). When changes in survival are considered by type of malignancy, however, substantial variation is observed. In evaluating the most recent survival statistics using population-based data from the Survival Epidemiology and End Results (SEER) Program, which comprises several city and state registries covering approximately 10% of the U.S. population, the most favorable prognosis is for patients with Wilms' tumor, who currently have a 88% relative probability of surviving for 5 years. Among children with leukemias or lymphomas, survival varies further by diagnostic subgroup. For example, the 5-year relative survival rate for children with Hodgkin's disease is 88%, compared with 68% for non-Hodgkin's lymphomas. Children with acute lymphocytic leukemia have a 72% 5-year relative survival rate, whereas the corresponding rate for those with acute myeloid leukemia is 31% (Miller et al, 1993). Although the total number of black children with cancer in the SEER areas is small, leading to imprecise estimates of survival, black children generally have experienced a poorer survival from cancers (Szklo et al, 1978; Steinhorn and Myers, 1981; Steinhorn and Gloeckler-Ries, 1988; Miller et al, 1993). In Great Britain, there were also highly significant improvements in survival during 1954–1985 for many major diagnostic groups of childhood malignancies (Birch et al, 1988; Stiller and Bunch, 1990).

Mortality

Interpretation of childhood cancer mortality data is complicated by (1) inadequate specification of subtypes on death certificates, (2) changes in classification as designated in the International Classification of Diseases (ICD) revisions, which have occurred about every 10 years, (3) limitations of the ICD as a classification system for childhood malignancies as noted above, (4) misclassification of cancer types, and (5) notable changes over time in rates for competing causes of mortality.

Because incidence rates in general provide better estimates of risk than do mortality rates, international mortality data are not presented in detail. For the period prior to the 1960s, when incidence data were less frequently collected, the description of time trends will focus on mortality patterns; incidence data for the 1960s and later will be considered in the discussion of more recent trends.

Time Trends

Mortality. Between 1911–1915 and 1951–1955, leukemia mortality in Great Britain increased fourfold (Court Brown and Doll, 1961; Adelstein and White, 1976). There was a similar increase in rates during 1920–1940 in the United States, although part of this was ascribed to improvements in diagnostic ascertainment (Gilliam and Walter, 1958; Gilliam and MacMahon, 1960). In Great Britain, leukemia mortality rates began to decrease during the 1960s, falling approximately 50% during the subsequent two decades (Adelstein and White, 1976; Draper et al, 1982). Rates also declined dramatically among children in all age groups during the past three decades in the United States and many other countries (Bailar, 1990). Between 1950 and 1989, U.S. rates declined more than 60%, from approximately 80 per million to just over 30 per million (Miller and McKay, 1984; Young et al, 1986; Miller et al, 1993).

In the United States, the rate of decrease in total leukemia death rates among white children was greater for the youngest children, whose mortality was higher in 1950–1954 than that among older children, but lower in 1984–1986 (Linet and Devesa, 1991). Dramatic declines in rates were observed also for childhood Hodgkin's disease (to a lesser extent for non-Hodgkin's lymphoma), and for brain, bone, and renal cancers (Miller and McKay, 1984; Young et al, 1986).

The peak occurrence of ALL at ages 2–4 has been postulated to be a relatively recent development; it was relatively uncommon until the 1920s in Great Britain, until the 1940s in U.S. whites, and more recently among blacks in the United States and among Japanese children (Court Brown and Doll, 1961; Fraumeni and Miller, 1967; Bowman et al, 1984; Kato et al, 1985). Mortality data are generally not very useful for clarifying this issue, because leukemia subtypes frequently are not specified on death certificates. Long-term population-based incidence data to evaluate this hypothesis generally are not available. Within populations, an inverse relationship has been described between childhood lymphoma and ALL; industrialized countries have relatively higher incidence of ALL and substantially lower incidence of lymphoma, whereas in many African and other developing nations, lymphoma is the most common childhood malignancy and rates of ALL are substantially lower (Greenberg and Schuster, 1985). It has been hypothesized that a decline in childhood malignant lymphoma and a corresponding rise in ALL (together with emergence of the early childhood peak at ages 2–4) parallels industrialization and improvements in public health (Greaves and Chan, 1986). For example, a decrease in lymphoma in Israel has been accompanied by an increase in ALL over a relatively short time period as living standards improved (Ramot and Magrath, 1982).

Incidence. Data for the United States during 1969–1971 through 1987–1989 are shown in Tables 61–1 through 61–4 (SEER Program unpublished data, 1992). There is no clear pattern of an increase in incidence of total leukemia (Table 61–1) and no evidence of any striking change for the lymphomas (Table 61–2). Primary CNS tumors may be increasing slightly since the early 1980s among children aged 0–4 and those 5–9, but the pattern in the oldest children is not clear. There is no apparent change in rates for neuroblastoma.

Increases in childhood leukemia have been noted in Connecticut among boys aged 0–4 (van Hoff et al, 1988), but not in the larger composite of five geographic areas (including Atlanta, Connecticut, Detroit, Iowa, and San Francisco–Oakland) shown in Tables 61–1 through 61–4. Leukemia rates among young boys in Connecticut were noted to be lower in the past and higher during recent years than those of the larger population in the five geographic areas (Devesa et al, 1987). Incidence of acute leukemia increased among children aged 0–9 in Denmark from the 1940s until about 1970, then declined (Hansen et al, 1983). Leukemia rose among boys 0–4 in Great Britain during 1968–1976 (Stiller and Draper, 1982), although rates were still lower than those observed in the aggregated five geographic areas within the United States (Linet and De-

TABLE 61–1. *Trends in Childhood Leukemia, All Types Combined Incidence among Whites of Both Sexes in Five Geographic Areas* of the United States, 1969–1971 through 1987–1989*

	Ages							
	0–4		*5–9*		*10–14*		*Total*	
Years	*No.*	*Rate*[a]	*No.*	*Rate*	*No.*	*Rate*	*No.*	*Rate*[b]
1969–1971	228	73.4	125	34.6	98	25.5	451	42.8
1975–1977	168	69.1	99	34.2	73	21.5	340	40.0
1978–1980	154	65.1	86	33.2	70	23.4	310	39.2
1981–1983	152	62.0	85	36.9	64	23.3	301	39.4
1984–1986	182	72.5	71	30.4	71	29.0	324	42.4
1987–1989	193	75.9	90	37.2	52	22.9	335	43.5

*Atlanta, Connecticut, Detroit, Iowa, San Francisco–Oakland.
[a]Per million person-years.
[b]Per million person-years, age-adjusted using the 1970 U.S. Standard Source: Devesa et al, 1987 and unpublished SEER program data.

vesa, 1991). Using data from the first four volumes of *Cancer Incidence in Five Continents* (generally covering the years 1960–1977), Breslow and Langholz (1983) found no consistent change in incidence for leukemia, although there may have been a small increase in rates in Canada.

Despite the absence of changing rates for total leukemia during the past two decades in the United States (Linet and Devesa, 1991), acute lymphoblastic leukemia has steadily increased approximately 14% overall between 1973 and 1990 (Miller et al, 1993). One explanation is a reduction in the occurrence of untyped leukemia as a result of improved characterization of leukemia subtypes, since the specificity of action of chemotherapy agents for treating childhood acute lymphoblastic leukemia versus acute myeloid leukemia became apparent beginning in the mid-1970s (Miller, 1992).

Lymphomas increased slightly among boys only in Denmark, slowly rising during 1943–1947 to 1968–1972, then more rapidly during 1973–1977 to 1983–1984. A corresponding decline in rates for the leukemias during the same period may indicate that the apparent increase in lymphoma could be due to misclassification of leukemias as lymphomas (de Nully Brown et al, 1989). There was evidence for a 10% increase in Hodgkin's disease between 1970 and 1975 in the analysis of data from *Cancer Incidence in Five Continents,* particularly in the United States and the former German Democratic Republic (Breslow and Langholz, 1983). Table 61–2 shows no evidence of a continuing increase in the United States.

An apparent increase in brain and CNS tumors was observed in the data from *Cancer Incidence in Five Continents* (Breslow and Langholz, 1983), but the authors note that this may have reflected changes in reporting practices over time for these tumors. Increases were found also in Denmark (de Nully Brown et al, 1989), Sweden (Ericsson et al, 1978), and in Finland (Teppo et al, 1975). These and other investigators have suggested that the apparent increase in incidence for brain and CNS tumors may reflect improvements in diagnosis related to development of high-resolution imaging devices (de Nully Brown et al, 1989; Lannering et al, 1990).

Rates of neuroblastoma increased dramatically

TABLE 61–2. *Trends in Childhood Lymphoma, All Types Combined, Incidence among Whites of Both Sexes in Five Geographic Areas of the United States, 1969–1971 through 1987–1989*

	Ages							
	0–4		*5–9*		*10–14*		*Total*	
Years	*No.*	*Rate*[a]	*No.*	*Rate*	*No.*	*Rate*	*No.*	*Rate*[b]
1969–1971	14	4.5	58	16.0	57	14.8	129	12.2
1975–1977	15	6.2	42	14.5	90	26.5	147	16.4
1978–1980	17	7.2	38	14.7	82	27.4	137	17.0
1981–1983	15	6.1	39	16.9	65	23.6	119	16.1
1984–1986	12	4.8	33	14.1	69	28.2	114	16.4
1987–1989	16	6.3	41	16.9	55	24.2	112	16.4

*Atlanta, Connecticut, Detroit, Iowa, San Francisco–Oakland.
[a]Per million person-years.
[b]Per million person-years, age-adjusted using the 1970 U.S. Standard Source: Devesa et al, 1987 and unpublished SEER program data.

TABLE 61–3. *Trends in Childhood Primary Central Nervous System Malignancies, All Types Combined, Incidence among Whites of Both Sexes in Five Geographic Areas of the United States,* 1969–1971 through 1987–1989*

	Ages							
	0–4		5–9		10–14		Total	
Years	No.	Rate[a]	No.	Rate	No.	Rate	No.	Rate[b]
1969–1971	86	27.7	105	29.1	79	20.6	270	25.6
1975–1977	69	28.4	86	29.8	79	23.3	234	27.0
1978–1980	86	36.4	70	27.0	75	25.1	231	29.1
1981–1983	62	25.3	63	27.4	52	18.9	177	23.7
1984–1986	102	40.6	80	34.2	45	18.4	227	30.4
1987–1989	96	37.8	85	35.1	60	26.4	241	32.8

*Atlanta, Connecticut, Detroit, Iowa, San Francisco–Oakland.
[a]Per million person-years.
[b]Per million person-years, age-adjusted using the 1970 U.S. Standard Source: Devesa et al, 1987 and unpublished SEER program data.

among boys and girls in Denmark over the 40-year period 1943–1984, primarily due to an increase among infant boys in particular. A similar increase was not found internationally (Breslow and Langholz, 1983).

Socioeconomic Status

The relationship between social class and risk of cancer in children has been examined only to a limited extent. Most of the published work has focused on leukemia. In a 1985 review article, the findings of six studies were compared (Greenberg and Schuster, 1985). Although these studies were undertaken in a wide range of locales and time periods, the results consistently indicated that children with higher socioeconomic status were at increased risk of leukemia (Pinkel and Nefzger, 1959; Stewart et al, 1958; Browning and Gross, 1968; Fasal et al, 1971; Sanders et al, 1981; McWhirter, 1982).

There is far less information available on the association of socioeconomic status with risk of other pediatric cancers. A study of Hodgkin's disease in adolescents and young adults found case patients more likely to have better-educated mothers than control patients (Gutensohn and Cole, 1981). Paternal employment in managerial or professional occupations has been linked to risk of brain tumors, and more weakly to risk of Wilms' tumor among the offspring (Sanders et al, 1981). In contrast, neuroblastoma was inversely related to socioeconomic level based on per capita income in one investigation (Davis et al, 1987), and rhabdomyosarcoma was inversely related to parental education and family income in another study (Grufferman et al, 1982).

ENVIRONMENTAL EXPOSURES

Ionizing Radiation

Preconception Exposure

Medical. Paternal preconception diagnostic x-ray exposure has been linked with an elevated risk of leukemia

TABLE 61–4. *Trends in Childhood Neuroblastoma Incidence among Whites of Both Sexes in Five Geographic Areas* of the United States, 1969–1971 through 1987–1989*

	Ages							
	0–4		5–9		10–14		Total	
Years	No.	Rate[a]	No.	Rate	No.	Rate	No.	Rate[b]
1969–1971	96	30.9	14	3.9	6	1.6	116	11.0
1975–1977	75	30.8	11	3.8	6	1.8	92	11.1
1978–1980	76	32.1	11	4.2	4	1.3	91	11.5
1981–1983	73	29.8	9	3.9	3	1.1	85	10.6
1984–1986	91	36.2	9	3.9	2	0.8	102	12.4
1987–1989	78	30.7	10	4.1	3	1.3	91	11.0

*Atlanta, Connecticut, Detroit, Iowa, San Francisco–Oakland.
[a]Per million person-years.
[b]Per million person-years, age-adjusted using the 1970 U.S. Standard Source: Devesa et al, 1987 and unpublished SEER program data.

among offspring (Graham et al, 1966; Shu et al, 1988). In a subsequent study in Shanghai based on interviews with subjects' fathers (Shu et al, 1994), no association was observed for leukemia or other childhood cancers with paternal preconception diagnostic x-ray exposure. The positive association found in the earlier U.S. (Graham et al, 1966) and Shanghai (Shu et al, 1988) studies was ascribed to recall bias of the mothers who were the only respondents (Shu et al, 1994). In addition, paternal or maternal preconception pelvic x-ray exposure was not associated with Wilms' tumor or retinoblastoma in offspring (Bunin et al, 1987; 1989b).

Occupational. Increased leukemia incidence has been associated with father's preconception occupational exposure to radiation in some (Shu et al, 1988; Gardner et al, 1990; McKinney et al, 1991), but not all studies (Urquhart et al, 1991; Draper et al, 1993; Kinlen et al, 1993a; McLaughlin et al, 1993). Radiation-induced mutations of germ cell lines have been postulated to explain the observed excess leukemia among children of fathers employed in nuclear plants (Gardner et al, 1990; Greaves, 1990). Recent estimates from the Japanese atomic bomb data, however, suggest that humans may not be as sensitive to the genetic effects of radiation as extrapolation from laboratory animal data had previously suggested (Neel et al, 1990). Experimental studies also suggest that low doses and prolonged exposures, as might apply to nuclear plant workers, produce fewer mutations than do high doses and acute exposures, such as the atomic bomb exposure (Boice, 1990; Baverstock, 1991).

Prenatal Exposure

Leukemia. An increased risk of leukemia in children who were exposed to diagnostic irradiation in utero was first reported in 1956 (Stewart et al, 1956). That initial association was replicated later in an expanded case-control study (Stewart et al, 1958). Subsequently, a number of additional case-control studies were conducted to evaluate this hypothesis. Although two of these investigations revealed no leukemogenic effect (Polhemus and Koch, 1959; Murray et al, 1959), most other studies found a modest excess risk of leukemia following prenatal irradiation (Ford et al, 1959; MacMahon, 1962; Graham et al, 1966; Monson and MacMahon, 1984; Van Steensel-Moll et al, 1985a).

It has been postulated that the excess risk of leukemia among prenatally irradiated children may be related to gestational conditions requiring radiation examinations, rather than to the radiation per se (Burch, 1970). In an effort to address this criticism, a reanalysis of data presented in an early report was undertaken with stratification by the clinical reasons for antenatal irradiation (Stewart and Kneale, 1971). In each subgroup considered, gestational irradiation was found to increase the risk of leukemia in offspring. This relationship was further strengthened by an observed gradient of risk with increasing numbers of radiographic examinations (Stewart and Kneale, 1970). Other factors may modify the leukemogenic effect of prenatal irradiation, including the trimester of exposure (Graham et al, 1966; Stewart and Kneale, 1970; Gilman et al, 1988), race (Diamond et al, 1973) and the susceptibility of the fetus (Bross and Natarajan, 1974).

Cohort studies of prenatal exposure to diagnostic radiation were conducted in England (Court Brown et al, 1960) and the United States (Diamond et al, 1973), and a follow-up investigation was carried out in Japan among children exposed in utero to radiation from the atomic bomb blasts (Jablon and Kato, 1970; Kato, 1971). Only one of these investigations provided some support for the leukemogenesis hypothesis (Diamond et al, 1973). All three studies, however, yielded a small number of children with leukemia, and therefore a weak effect of prenatal irradiation could not be excluded. Further follow-up of the Japanese cohort exposed prenatally suggested that overall cancer risk may be increased in adult life (Yoshimoto et al, 1988). In contrast, no excess risk of leukemia or other heritable cancers has been observed among children who were born to atomic bomb survivors, but who were conceived after the bomb explosions (Yoshimoto, 1990; Yoshimoto et al, 1990).

Other cancers. Modest associations have been demonstrated in some studies between intrauterine irradiation and other childhood cancers, such as neoplasms of the central nervous system (MacMahon, 1962; Bithell and Stewart, 1975), osteosarcoma (Operskalski et al, 1987), nonheritable retinoblastoma (Bunin et al, 1989b), Wilms' tumors, neuroblastomas, and lymphomas (Bithell and Stewart, 1975). The level of the effects were smaller in later studies, paralleling reductions over time in the average radiation exposure per prenatal x-ray (Bithell and Stewart, 1975; Bithell and Stiller, 1988). After reviewing available data from Britain, Mole (1990) concluded that cancer rates among children increased significantly after prenatal exposure to diagnostic x-rays, and suggested that carcinogenesis by ionizing radiation may have no threshold.

Other investigations found no associations between in utero radiation exposure and neuroblastoma (Kramer et al, 1987), central nervous system tumors (Howe et al, 1989; Birch et al, 1990; Kuijten et al, 1990), bone and soft tissue sarcomas (Hartley et al, 1988a), testicular cancer (Swerdlow et al, 1982), and hepatoblastoma (Buckley et al, 1989b). The absence of an effect among children exposed in utero to atomic bomb radiation also argues against a causal relationship between prenatal radiation exposure and childhood cancer (MacMahon, 1989).

Twin studies. It has been suggested that twin studies may provide the best evidence of whether prenatal irradiation causes childhood cancer (Mole, 1974; Harvey et al, 1985). Historically, twins were more likely to be exposed to prenatal irradiation in order to confirm the twin status or to determine fetal position, as opposed to the major reasons for radiologic examination of singletons, namely, the evaluation of adverse medical conditions that potentially could predispose to cancer. In the Oxford Childhood Cancer Survey (Mole, 1974), the risk of developing leukemia and solid cancers in twins exposed to radiation in utero relative to nonexposed twins was greater than the corresponding risk ratio in singleton births. In a case-control study based on linkage of records between the Connecticut twin and tumor registries, a 1.6-fold excess risk of leukemia and a threefold excess of other childhood cancer in twins was associated with prenatal exposure to radiation (Harvey et al, 1985). It has been argued, however, that these data did not support a causal relationship because of methodological limitations, such as small numbers of subjects and uncertainties about other gestational indications for radiography (MacMahon, 1985). After considering potential confounding factors—including obstetric complications, drug use during pregnancy, previous miscarriages, length of pregnancy, maternal age and social class—a record-linkage case-control study nested within a national cohort of Swedish twin births (Rodvall et al, 1990), however, still found a small excess of cancer, particularly leukemias, among children irradiated in utero. The excess risk was observed primarily among children born before 1960 when x-ray techniques were changed to lower the radiation exposure. In contrast, data from most cohort studies have not shown increased risks of childhood cancer among twins relative to singletons (Windham et al, 1985; Inskip et al, 1991; Rodvall et al, 1992), although the expected excesses generally were small (Rodvall et al, 1992).

Because other diagnostic techniques not employing ionizing radiation are replacing prenatal x-rays (Mettler and Moseley, 1985), from a public health perspective the issue of leukemogenesis from intrauterine irradiation could become inconsequential (MacMahon, 1985). Comparison of data collected in the 1963 and 1980 National Natality Surveys, however, indicated that the prevalence of pelvimetry in the United States actually increased by 37% (Kaczmarek et al, 1989). Future surveys should continue to monitor the use of pelvimetry in this and other countries.

Postnatal Exposure. The carcinogenic effect of postnatal irradiation is more clearly established than the effect of in utero exposure. Moderate to heavy doses of radiation treatments in children have been shown to increase the risk of leukemia and other neoplasms (Stewart et al, 1958; Polhemus and Koch, 1959; Murray et al, 1959; Graham et al, 1966; Ron and Modan, 1984; Ron et al, 1988a; Nishi and Miyake, 1989). From the experience of atomic bomb survivors in Hiroshima and Nagasaki, it appears that age at exposure to radiation is an important determinant of the subsequent risk of developing acute leukemias. Young children were found to have had particularly high risk ratios for the development of leukemias (Ichimaru et al, 1978).

Cancers other than leukemia also can be induced by postnatal radiation exposure. Similar to leukemia, the risk of solid tumors is modified greatly by age of exposure. An investigation of Japanese atomic bomb survivors observed a particularly high risk among persons who were less than 10 years of age at the time of the bombing (Jablon and Kato, 1972).

Therapeutic irradiation. Cancer risk following therapeutic irradiation has been well documented. It has been suggested that children with prior histories of allergic or infectious disorders are especially susceptible to the leukemogenic effects of therapeutic radiation (Bross and Natarajan, 1974). To date, this finding of synergy between the leukemogenic effect of irradiation and host susceptibility has not been evaluated adequately.

Among infants who were irradiated for thymic enlargement, the risk of thyroid cancer was estimated to be 100 times greater than the risk generally expected among children (Hempelmann et al, 1975). The incidence of thyroid malignancies for exposed females was over twice as high as the rate for exposed males. Among the irradiated children, most thyroid cancers were diagnosed before 20 years of age. Among subjects for whom an estimated dose of irradiation to the thyroid was available, a dose-response relationship was demonstrated (Hempelmann et al, 1975).

In a large clinical series of persons irradiated for treatment of tinea capitis (ringworm of the scalp), four times as many head and neck cancers were observed among irradiated children as would have been expected (Modan et al, 1974). The greatest excesses in observed numbers of cancers were found for primary cancers of the brain, parotid, and thyroid. The interval between first irradiation and detection of these malignancies ranged from four to 21 years, with a median interval of 11 years. In a subsequent study of over 10 thousand persons who were irradiated for tinea capitis during childhood between 1948 and 1960, a nearly fivefold risk of thyroid carcinoma was observed relative to an unirradiated matched population, and a nearly threefold risk increase compared to unexposed siblings (Ron and Modan, 1980). All of the malignancies were diagnosed during childhood or young adulthood. In subsequent follow-up of this cohort, the risk was found to be higher among females and among persons who were irradiated at age 5 or younger (Ron and Modan, 1984). Further follow-up of this cohort until 1986 with revised dosimetry found a fourfold increase of thyroid cancer and twofold excess of benign thyroid tumors associated with an estimated thyroid dose of 9 cGy (Ron et al, 1989). A linear dose-response relation was estimated.

The incidence of benign and malignant tumors of the brain and nervous system also was evaluated in this cohort of children irradiated for treatment of tinea capitis. A sevenfold excess risk of all tumors was associated with radiation therapy for tinea capitis. The risk of malignant neoplasms of the head and neck in irradiated children was almost fivefold greater than that of the comparison groups (Ron et al, 1988b). The pattern of cancer mortality over time was bimodal, with an early peak of leukemia deaths within a few years of exposure and an excess of deaths due to solid tumors about 15 years after irradiation (Ron et al, 1988a).

Having had five or more full-mouth dental x-rays was associated with a more than twofold risk of childhood brain tumors in a matched case-control study (Preston-Martin et al, 1982). A significant excess of brain tumors in children also was associated with diagnostic x-rays to the skull at least 5 years prior to diagnosis in another study (Howe et al, 1989). The authors, however, suggested that this association was likely due to early symptoms of brain tumors that were not yet diagnosed. No association with x-rays to the skull or dental x-rays was detected in a subsequent case-control study of childhood brain cancers (McCredie et al, 1994b).

While parent-reported neonatal diagnostic x-ray exposure was associated with a twofold risk of childhood cancer in a case-control study, no excess was found when only x-ray information documented in the medical records was examined (Hartley et al, 1988b). Still other studies found no association between childhood exposure to medical or dental x-rays and astrocytomas (Kuijten et al, 1990) or osteosarcomas in children (Operskalski et al, 1987).

Second primary cancer. Second primary cancers following radiation therapy for initial neoplasms also have been investigated among children (Robison, 1996). Children who have had an initial tumor are at a greatly increased risk of a second primary cancer (Mike et al, 1982; Li et al, 1983; Tucker et al, 1984; Tsunematsu et al, 1985; Hawkins et al, 1987; Tucker et al, 1987; Breslow et al, 1988b; Hawkins, 1990; Jankovic et al, 1991; Eguiguren et al, 1991; Nygaard et al, 1991; Olsen et al, 1993; Dopfer and Niethammer, 1993). Although some children with multiple primary cancers may have a genetic predisposition to these diseases (Farwell and Flannery, 1984a; Cullen, 1991; Malkin et al, 1992), a substantial proportion of the second primary cancers may be induced by cancer treatments, including radiation therapy given for the initial tumor. Genetic factors also may interact with radiation treatment to further increase the risk of a second cancer. It has been shown that children with the hereditary form of retinoblastoma are particularly sensitive to the carcinogenic effect of radiation (Draper et al, 1986; Eng et al, 1993), and the excess risks of a second primary cancer may extend into adulthood (Eng et al, 1993).

In a nested case-control study within a cohort of children with a variety of initial tumors, including retinoblastoma, Ewing's sarcoma, rhabdomyosarcoma, Wilms' tumor, and Hodgkin's disease, a nearly threefold risk of bone cancer has been estimated following radiation therapy for the initial tumor, with a dose-response reaching 40-fold risk after doses to the bone of more than 6000 rad (Tucker et al, 1987). It has been observed that girls have a greater risk than boys to develop a second primary cancer following radiation treatment for Hodgkin's disease (Tarbell et al, 1993). In other studies, excess brain tumors were found after cranial irradiation for leukemia (Jankovic et al, 1991; Nygaard et al, 1991; Neglia et al, 1991). A variety of second cancers have been reported following treatment for Wilms' tumor (Li et al, 1983; Breslow et al, 1988b). Increased incidence of thyroid cancer also was revealed among children treated with high doses of radiation for Wilms' tumor, neuroblastoma, and Hodgkin's disease (Tucker et al, 1984).

Radioactive fallout. The possible leukemogenic effect of radioactive fallout has been studied in children. In an ecological analysis, it was suggested that children from counties in Utah with high exposure to fallout from the testing of nuclear weapons had excessive death rates from leukemia (Lyon et al, 1979). These results, however, may have been influenced by lack of information on individual exposure levels and the possibility of confounding effects (Land, 1979). Subsequently, a similar study was conducted to test the possible relation between childhood leukemia and atomic radiation fallout, using cancer mortality data from the U.S. National Center for Health Statistics between 1950 and 1978 (Land et al, 1984). No pattern of temporal or geographic variation in cancer mortality supportive of this association was detected. The authors further suggested that the results of the original ecological study (Lyon et al, 1979) were spurious because of the extremely low mortality of childhood leukemia in southern Utah for the pre-exposure reference years between 1944 and 1949.

A subsequent study was conducted to compare cancer mortality among residents born during the peak fallout period in a three-county region in southwestern Utah with reasonably uniform fallout deposition with rates in the remainder of the state (Machado et al, 1987). No cancer mortality excess was found in southwestern

Utah, except for a nearly threefold elevated rate of leukemia deaths among children. In addition, a subsequent case-control study among Utah residents reported a small dose-response relation between estimated bone marrow radiation dose from fallout deposition and leukemia deaths at all ages (Stevens et al, 1990). The greatest excess risk was found for acute leukemia among persons receiving high doses before age 20 and dying before 1964. The study population was confined to persons connected to the Mormon church so that accurate residential histories during the fallout period could be ascertained from church records.

In an ecological study correlating leukemia mortality in the United States with radiation fallout from worldwide nuclear tests, Archer (1987) observed an increase of acute myeloid leukemia among children a few years after the peaks in fallout. Elevated leukemia mortality among residents of states with high strontium^{90} also was reported. There was no association, however, between childhood leukemia incidence trends and estimated peak exposure from fallout in Scotland (Hole et al, 1993) or in England and Wales, Norway, and Denmark (Darby and Doll, 1987). In a later investigation conducted in five Nordic countries with nearly complete cancer registration, the same investigators estimated a 10% excess risk of leukemia among children exposed to high level of radiation from fallout relative to children with medium level of exposure (Darby et al, 1992). Risk of leukemia among children estimated to have low exposure, however, was similar to those with high exposure. Overall, recent investigations in the United States and Europe (Archer, 1987; Machado et al, 1987; Stevens et al, 1990; Darby et al, 1992) seem to suggest a small increase in childhood leukemia among populations exposed to radiation from fallout due to nuclear weapons testing. Because of the uncertainties involved in retrospective estimation of the level of radiation from fallout in various geographic areas and, in most cases, the lack of information on individual exposure and confounding factors, caution must be invoked in drawing inferences regarding the impact of radioactive fallout on leukemia risk.

Proximity to nuclear plants. A number of studies were conducted in order to investigate the occurrence of childhood leukemia around several nuclear plants in Britain, including the Sellafield nuclear reprocessing plant near Seascale in West Cumbria (Black, 1984) and the Dounreay plant near Thurso (Heasman et al, 1987), the atomic weapons research establishments in West Berkshire (Roman et al, 1987), and the nuclear power station at Hinkley Point in Somerset (Ewings et al, 1989). These studies were carried out, in part, to address public concerns that childhood leukemia rates might have been elevated around these nuclear facilities.

Follow-up studies in Seascale revealed that the excess of leukemia was confined to children born in Seascale (Gardner et al, 1987a), because risk was not increased among children born elsewhere but attending school there (Gardner et al, 1987b). An increased risk of retinoblastoma in children of former residents of Seascale also has been suggested (Morris et al, 1993). A subsequent case-control study suggested that paternal preconception radiation exposure during employment at the Sellafield plant might explain the observed cluster of childhood leukemia cases in Seascale (Gardner et al, 1990), although this finding was not confirmed by other additional studies (Draper et al, 1993; Kinlen et al, 1993a; Kinlen, 1993; Parker et al, 1993). After considering the level of radiation exposure and the estimated mutagenic effect, it was concluded that the childhood leukemia cluster in Seascale was not likely due to paternal germ cell injury from radiation (Abrahamson, 1990; Evans, 1990; Watson, 1991). Paternal employment was not found to be a risk factor in a similar investigation at the Dounreay plant (Urquhart et al, 1991). Darby and Doll (1987) had concluded that the elevated incidence of leukemia in young persons around Dounreay could not be explained by radiation exposure levels resulting from the radioactive discharges from the plant.

Significantly elevated numbers of leukemias and non-Hodgkin's lymphomas were observed among children residing in the area proximate to the Hinkley Point nuclear plant a few years after the power station began operations, compared with the national rates of these malignancies (Ewings et al, 1989). The authors, however, determined that radioactive waste disposal from the power station contributed only a small fraction of the total environmental ionizing radiation exposure. In West Berkshire, a subsequent case-control study found an elevated incidence of leukemia among children under 5 years of age whose fathers were monitored for external radiation exposure. The monitored doses were low, however, and the authors therefore concluded that factors other than fathers' exposure to external radiation might be related to cancer in their offspring (Roman et al, 1993). A case-control study in Ontario, Canada, also found no association with paternal employment in nuclear facilities and leukemia in offspring (McLaughlin et al, 1993b).

In studies of geographic variation of leukemia and non-Hodgkin's lymphoma in England and Wales, no elevation in risk was observed with increasing proximity to nuclear installations (Cook-Mozaffari et al, 1989a; Bithell et al, 1994). It is also of interest to note that childhood leukemia clusters have been observed in many geographic locations and are not confined to areas surrounding nuclear facilities (Alexander et al, 1990;

Cartwright, 1992). Increased childhood leukemia and lymphoma rates also have been observed in sites where nuclear facilities were planned but never built (Cook-Mozaffari et al, 1989b; Bithell et al, 1994). In addition, most of the reported clusters involve small numbers of cases (Beral, 1990). One interpretation of a detailed review of the evidence concerning radiation discharge from nuclear facilities and leukemia clusters in Britain (MacMahon, 1992) has suggested that all of the clusters appeared to result from selection of study areas based on prior information on disease occurrence, arbitrary identification of geographic boundaries or time periods, or chance.

Other hypotheses on the apparent clustering of leukemias and other childhood cancers near nuclear installations are being examined, including those of viral origin (Kinlen, 1988) and natural background sources of radiation (Hatch and Susser, 1990). It also has been proposed that in order to gain new insight into the risk associated with radiation exposure among persons residing near nuclear facilities, new techniques in molecular genetics and epidemiology should be used to examine preneoplastic endpoints, such as the rate and type of somatic mutations (Morris, 1994).

Studies of leukemias among young persons residing near nuclear facilities in France (Viel and Richardson, 1990; Hill and Laplanche, 1990), Israel (Sofer et al, 1991), Ontario, Canada (McLaughlin et al, 1993a) and the United States (Clapp et al, 1987; Jablon et al, 1991) found no excess risk. Although no overall increase in risk was observed among children residing near nuclear power plants in Germany, children under five years of age and those residing within 5 kilometers of a nuclear plant were found to have an elevated risk of acute leukemia (Michaelis et al, 1992). Greater excesses of leukemia, however, were found in regions in West Germany near projected installations than in areas near installed facilities.

Overall, to date there is no convincing evidence linking childhood leukemia and other cancers to radiation exposure from emissions at nuclear facilities. Currently, children from many European countries and areas in the former Soviet Union, who might have been exposed to radioactive discharges from the Chernobyl nuclear power plant accident in the Ukraine, are under surveillance for increased incidence of leukemia and lymphoma in a large, multi-registry study coordinated by the International Agency for Research on Cancer (Parkin et al, 1993b; Linet and Boice, 1993). Readers interested in the issue of clusters of leukemia around nuclear plants are referred to a book that contains the main research articles on this topic over the past decade (Beral et al, 1993).

Other environmental radiation. In North Carolina, increased childhood cancer mortality rates, especially for leukemias, were found in counties with high average groundwater radon concentrations (Collman et al, 1991). Internationally, mean indoor radon concentrations also have been correlated with childhood cancer incidence (Henshaw et al, 1990). These associations, however, were not confirmed in two small case-control studies (Stjernfeldt et al, 1987; Wakefield and Kohler, 1991). Further investigations will provide greater understanding of the total sources of radiation exposure, particularly in view of new evidence that low doses of alpha particles, a large proportion of which could come from decay of radon gas, may induce cell mutation in some circumstances (Cartwright, 1992; Kadhim et al, 1992).

Extremely Low Frequency Electromagnetic Fields

In 1979, Wertheimer and Leeper reported that childhood cancer mortality in Denver was significantly increased among children aged 18 and under who resided near high-tension electrical power lines. These investigators found statistically significant two- to three-fold excesses of leukemia and primary brain neoplasms among children whose residences (at death and also at birth) were characterized as high current configuration, based on a combination of wiring pattern and distance between the nearest distribution or transmission power line and the residence. Several subsequent case-control studies and one cohort study among children have assessed cancer risk in relation to extremely low frequency electromagnetic field (ELF-EMF) 50 or 60 Hertz exposures (Fulton et al, 1980; Tomenius, 1986; Savitz et al, 1988; Coleman et al, 1989; Myers et al, 1990; London et al, 1991; Feychting and Ahlbom, 1993; Olsen et al, 1993; Verkasalo et al, 1993).

Some (Tomenius, 1986; Savitz et al, 1988; London et al, 1991) of the studies incorporated assessment of field strength within residences, including spot (Savitz et al, 1988; London et al, 1991; Feychting and Ahlbom, 1993) and 24-hour (London et al, 1991) measurements. Others included measurements taken immediately outside the front entrance (Tomenius, 1986). The highest measurement levels of residential ELF-EMF exposure were not associated with significantly elevated risks of leukemia (Tomenius, 1986; Savitz et al, 1988; London et al, 1991) or brain tumors (Tomenius, 1986; Savitz et al, 1988), nor were risks significantly increased for these malignancies when the data were pooled (National Radiological Protection Board, 1992). For all childhood cancers combined, risk was not significantly elevated among children in the highest exposure category in Denver (Savitz et al, 1988); the significant increase in risk for all childhood neoplasms in Stockholm (Tomenius, 1986) is difficult to interpret because the data are reported by number of affected dwellings (with a variable number of dwellings per subject) and not by number of affected cases or controls. Because the studies of Savitz and coworkers and Tomenius are not comparable in the outcome considered, it is also difficult to interpret a pooled-risk estimate.

Three recent studies in Scandinavia utilized an exposure assessment methodology that differed from prior studies. Residential exposures were estimated from annual average flow of current in proximate power lines and other historical estimates based on load flow and other power data obtained from electric utilities (Feychting and Ahlbom, 1993; Olsen et al, 1993; Verkasalo et al, 1993). In Sweden, borderline or significantly elevated risks of childhood leukemia were observed among children with historically estimated annual exposures greater than 0.2 or 0.3 microtesla, respectively, although the findings were based on seven cases with these estimated high exposure levels out of a total of 38 leukemia cases (Feychting and Ahlbom, 1993). Neither lymphoma nor brain tumors were associated with elevated historical ELF-EMF exposures. The Danish study demonstrated significant associations of historical estimated exposures with all childhood cancers and with Hodgkin's disease, but these findings were derived from small numbers of highly exposed cases (10 children with all types of cancer, three with Hodgkin's disease) among a large number of childhood cancer cases (1677 children with cancers of all types, 247 with malignant lymphoma) (Olsen et al, 1993) and controls evaluated. Investigators in Finland examined cancer risk among 68,300 boys and 66,500 girls and identified 140 cancers (Verkasalo et al, 1993). No excesses of cancers of any type were associated with historical estimates of high magnetic field exposure, with the possible exception of brain tumors among boys; the male brain tumor increase was based on five or seven brain tumor cases, depending on the criteria used to define high magnetic field exposure, with three of the five or seven tumors arising in one patient with neurofibromatosis considered by the investigators as three separate primary tumors. When the three Scandinavian studies are considered all together, the findings do not demonstrate consistency overall or by specific type of childhood malignancy, and are limited by small numbers of subjects in high exposure categories.

In addition to the original report by Wertheimer and Leeper, three (Fulton et al, 1980; Savitz et al, 1988; London et al, 1991) subsequent studies also utilized the Wertheimer-Leeper wire coding classification in the exposure assessment. In the first population-based study in Denver, Wertheimer and Leeper (1979) reported a 2.2-fold increase for all cancers, and odds ratios of 3.0 and 2.4 for leukemia and brain tumors, respectively, among children residing in high wire code configuration residences compared to those living in homes characterized by low wire code configurations. The second Denver (Savitz et al, 1988) and Los Angeles (London et al, 1991) population-based studies revealed 50%–60% increased risks for leukemia among children living in high current configuration homes compared with risk among those in low current configuration residences, whereas the hospital-based study in Rhode Island (Fulton et al, 1980) found no excess. Nevertheless, the pooled risk for the three studies was determined to be statistically significant (National Radiological Protection Board, 1992). Similar to Wertheimer and Leeper (1979), Savitz and coworkers (1988) found significantly increased risks of brain neoplasms and all cancers combined among children residing in high current configuration homes.

Distance from ELF-EMF sources, such as overhead power lines and electric substations, was reported in the earlier European studies (Tomenius, 1986; Coleman et al, 1989; Myers et al, 1990) and a study described in abstract form only from Taiwan (Lin and Lu, 1989). No significant increase of leukemia (Tomenius, 1986; Coleman et al, 1989; Myers et al, 1990) or all cancers (Tomenius, 1986; Lin and Lu, 1989; Myers et al, 1990) was found among children residing within 50 meters (informally designated as analogous to classification in the high current configuration category in the paper by Coleman et al) of these sources of ELF-EMF exposures. Pooled results also showed little indication of an association for distance from ELF-EMF sources either for leukemia or for all cancers combined. A borderline excess of brain tumors was reported by Tomenius, but this finding is difficult to interpret because the outcome was proportions of exposed dwellings rather than proportions of exposed subjects. Lin and Lu (1989) observed no increase in brain tumor risk.

In summary, although high current configuration homes were significantly associated with increased risk of leukemia, brain tumors, and all cancers, and residences within 50 meters of ELF-EMF sources were linked with borderline increased risk of brain tumors, these findings were based on only three studies (Tomenius, 1986; Savitz et al, 1988; London et al, 1991) in addition to the original Wertheimer and Leeper (1979) report. The major contributions of the three recent Scandinavian studies include efforts to utilize more information to estimate historical exposures, to expand the residential magnetic field exposure assessment to include longer proportions of the subjects' lifetimes, and to enlarge the size of the study population; none of the three investigations included comprehensive direct exposure measurements. As pointed out in a recent systematic evaluation of the literature by Washburn and coworkers (1994), the available data is problematic both in quality and quantity, and the nature and/or magnitude of any potential risk remains unknown. Substantially larger childhood leukemia and brain tumor studies are needed, with comprehensive exposure assessment components, and subjects chosen from diverse populations with a wide range of magnetic field exposure levels. Such research efforts also should include comparable metrics to facilitate future meta-analyses, and detailed evaluation of all potential confounders.

Prenatal Ultrasound

Diagnostic ultrasonography was introduced into obstetric practice in the early 1970s. There is relatively little information available on the long-term health effects of antenatal exposure to ultrasound. Findings from several case-control studies have shown no overall association between intrauterine ultrasonography and subsequent risk of leukemia or other cancers in children (Kinnier Wilson and Waterhouse, 1984; Cartwright et al, 1984; Hartley et al, 1988a; Buckley et al, 1989b; Birch et al, 1990; Shu et al, 1994), although one of these investigations revealed a statistically significant excess of antenatal ultrasound exposure among children aged 6 or older at diagnosis (Kinnier Wilson and Waterhouse, 1984). In that study, the estimated risk ratio associated with obstetric ultrasound among children aged 6 or older was 4.6 for leukemia and 2.7 for solid tumors. This may have been a chance association, however, since effect modification by age was not observed in the other studies (Cartwright et al, 1984; Hartley et al, 1988a; Buckley et al, 1989b; Birch et al, 1990; Shu et al, 1994).

Viral Infections

Prenatal Exposure. In 1972, a strong association was reported between in utero infection with influenza and the subsequent risk of childhood leukemia (Fedrick and Alberman, 1972). Weaker but still statistically significant leukemogenic effects were found for gestational influenza infections by other investigators (Bithell et al, 1973; Hakulinen et al, 1973; Austin et al, 1975). In two of these studies (Fedrick and Alberman, 1972; Bithell et al, 1973), information on exposure to influenza was obtained by maternal interview; in two other studies (Hakulinen et al, 1973; Austin et al, 1975), ecological measures of exposure were employed. Negative findings were reported from several other ecological studies of this question (Leck and Steward, 1972; McCrea Curnen et al, 1974; Randolph and Heath, 1974). If prenatal exposure to influenza is associated with increased risk of leukemia in children, the preponderance of evidence indicates that it is probably a weak risk factor. Since influenza is a fairly common exposure, however, even a modest effect on the risk of leukemia in children may have important implications for prevention.

Other gestational viral infections, such as those caused by herpesviruses (chicken pox or cytomegalovirus) (Adelstein and Donovan, 1972; Bithell et al, 1973; Fine et al, 1985) and rubella (Bithell et al, 1973) have been associated with elevated risk of cancer during childhood. In an exploratory analysis, an increased risk of Wilms' tumor was found among mothers who had vaginal infection during pregnancy (Bunin et al, 1987). Maternal infection during pregnancy, however, was not linked to cancer in offspring in several other investigations (Blot et al, 1980; Operskalski et al, 1987; Hartley et al, 1988a; Buckley et al, 1989b; Birch et al, 1990; Giuffre et al, 1990).

Postnatal Exposure

Childhood diseases and vaccination. An excess risk of leukemia or lymphoma was observed among children exposed to viral infections during the perinatal period or early infancy (McKinney et al, 1987; Hartley et al, 1988b). Germ cell tumors (Hartley et al, 1988b) and hepatoblastoma (Buckley et al, 1989b) also were associated with perinatal infection and increased frequency of childhood illness. The authors of one of these studies suggested that recall bias and early manifestations of the tumor might have accounted for the observed association (Buckley et al, 1989b). No association with childhood illnesses was reported for other childhood cancers (Hartley et al, 1988a; Birch et al, 1990).

A 40% reduction in risk of acute lymphocytic leukemia was observed in the Netherlands for children who were hospitalized with infectious diseases during the first year of life (van Steensel-Moll et al, 1986). A mild reduction in risk was also associated with other more common childhood infections, such as measles, chickenpox, mumps, rubella, otitis media, and common colds. Chance, however, could not be excluded as an explanation for these findings. In this study, cases also were less likely than controls to have received usual vaccinations; a risk reduction of 70% was estimated for those children reported as being vaccinated. A protective effect of childhood immunizations also was found in several other case-control studies (Grufferman et al, 1982; Kneale et al, 1986; Hartley et al, 1988b). Other investigators found a reduced risk of leukemia associated with bacillus Calmette-Guérin (BCG) vaccination and a combined history of measles or measles vaccination (Haro, 1986; Nishi and Miyake, 1989). These observations, however, were not consistent with those of an earlier controlled trial that found no reduction of leukemia among children receiving BCG (Comstock et al, 1975; Snider et al, 1978).

Infants who were breast-fed for more than 6 months had a significantly reduced risk of childhood cancer, particularly lymphoma (Davis et al, 1988). The authors postulated that inadequate exposure to the immunological benefits of human milk could affect an infant's response to infection and render the child more susceptible to malignancies. A protective effect of breast-feeding, however, was not observed in several other investigations (Van Duijn et al, 1988; Magnani et al, 1988; Hartley et al, 1988b; Bunin et al, 1989b; Birch et al, 1990).

A case-control study of Hodgkin's disease in persons aged 15 to 39 years found a reduced risk to be associated with a larger number of siblings, a later birth order and residence in multiple-family homes (Gutensohn and Cole, 1981). Case patients also had fewer playmates, better-educated mothers, and a higher rate of infectious mononucleosis compared with controls. The authors suggested that childhood environments that decrease or delay early exposure to infections may increase the risk of Hodgkin's disease, with age at infection as an effect modifier.

Leukemia clusters. The observed clustering of some childhood leukemia cases could result from the effect of an underlying infectious agent. Greaves (1988) suggested that protection from general infections and, therefore, antigenic challenge during infancy may increase the risk of leukemia. Kinlen (1988), examining population statistics and leukemia incidence and mortality rates, hypothesized that leukemia represented a rare response to a common infection. He and his colleagues speculated that the normal immune response to a common infection within a community could be disturbed by a change in population structure and social contact, such as an influx of new immigrants to a previously isolated susceptible population, or convergence of a large number of people of different origins, particularly with large numbers of children and increased social contact (Kinlen et al, 1990; Kinlen et al, 1991; Kinlen et al, 1993b). Alexander and colleagues (1990) also reported a higher incidence of leukemia in isolated communities. It has been suggested that birth order, which can affect age of exposure to infection, should be considered in evaluation of the potential link between childhood infection and leukemia (MacMahon, 1992a). The hypothesis of a protective effect of infection early in life was supported by a case-control study that found a significant reduction in the risk of leukemia among children who attended day care during infancy (Petridou et al, 1993).

The infection-related hypothesis of leukemia etiology also was supported by several investigations of leukemia clustering (Morris, 1990; Alexander, 1992; Alexander et al, 1992). It should be noted, however, that apparent space-time leukemia clusters also could arise from common-source environmental exposures other than infectious agents. Evaluation of leukemia clusters also requires a clear definition of the underlying population distribution, and the proposed timing of the exposures, which may be difficult to characterize (Linet, 1985; Alexander et al, 1990). Methodological issues involving studies of leukemia clusters near nuclear plants in the United Kingdom have been discussed elsewhere (Beral, 1990; MacMahon, 1992b). Finally, it should be noted that no specific infectious agents have been identified in these studies, nor have leukemogenic mechanisms been proposed.

Other infectious agents. In a comparative serological study of populations with high (Greenland Eskimos) and low (Danes) incidence rates of nasopharyngeal carcinoma, exposure to Epstein-Barr virus was linked with the occurrence of nasopharyngeal cancer in children (Melbye et al, 1984). In a prospective study of children less than 8 years of age in Uganda, children with high antibody titers to Epstein-Barr viral capsid antigens were found to be at increased risk of Burkitt's lymphoma, and risk rose with increasing levels of viral capsid antigen antibodies (de-The et al, 1978; Geser et al, 1982). The evidence etiologically linking Epstein-Barr virus with Burkitt's lymphoma has been reviewed elsewhere (de-The, 1985). Similarly, higher serum titers to Epstein-Barr virus were found in Hodgkin's disease patients compared with controls (Bogger-Goren et al, 1983). Young hemophilia patients (aged 10 to 39) who were exposed to human immunodeficiency virus had a 38-fold risk of developing non-Hodgkin's lymphoma relative to the general population (Rabkin et al, 1992). A potential etiologic role of hepatitis B virus infection in the development of childhood hepatocellular carcinoma also has been suggested (Leuschner et al, 1988; Giacchino et al, 1991; Pontisso et al, 1991). A greater number of sexual partners and a history of *Chlamydia trachomatis* infection was associated with cervical intraepithelial neoplasia in female adolescents (aged 14–19 years) referred to a colposcopy clinic, compared with controls referred to a gynecology clinic (Moscicki et al, 1989). The observed association, in part, may be due to the differences in the type of patients referred to these two clinics.

Drugs and Chemicals

Prenatal Exposure

Medication. In experimental studies, many carcinogens have been shown to be more potent against fetuses than adult animals (Napalkov, 1986). Excess risks of acute nonlymphocytic leukemia (Robison et al, 1989), retinoblastoma (Bunin et al, 1989b), and astrocytoma

(Kuijten et al, 1990) were observed among children whose mothers used antinausea medications during pregnancy, although these findings were not supported by two other case-control studies (McKinney et al, 1985; Birch et al, 1990). Increased risk of childhood brain and nervous system malignancies also was linked with maternal use of neurally active drugs, including sedatives and sleeping pills such as barbiturates, during pregnancy in some studies (Gold et al, 1978; Van Steensel-Moll et al, 1985a; Kramer et al, 1987; Schwartzbaum, 1992), but not in others (Goldhaber et al, 1990; Kuijten et al, 1990; McCredie et al, 1994a). Prenatal exposure to anticonvulsants also was not linked to childhood cancers (Gilman et al, 1989; Olsen et al, 1990). In another investigation, an association was found between childhood brain tumors and maternal use of sodium pentothal for general anesthesia, but not with other types of barbiturates (Preston-Martin et al, 1982). An exploratory population-based case-control study, linking childhood leukemia cases and controls with a standardized data collection of certain pregnancy-related medical information on all live-born children in Sweden, suggested that an excess risk of this neoplasm was associated with the use of nitrous oxide anesthesia during delivery, and treatment of newborns with supplemental oxygen (Zack et al, 1991). No association was found with mothers' use of general or dental anesthesia during pregnancy or at delivery in other studies (Birch et al, 1990; McCredie et al, 1994a and 1994b). Pethidine given during labor was associated with cancer among offspring in one study (Gilman et al, 1989), but not another (Golding et al, 1992). Overall, there is no consistent evidence linking maternal use of neurally active medications and cancers in offspring.

Medications used for infection during pregnancy were associated with a more than threefold risk of childhood cancer in a nested case-control study of Swedish twins (Rodvall et al, 1990). It was impossible, however, to distinguish between the effects of the infection versus the medication used for treatment, although a nonsignificant and less than twofold risk was associated with a history of prenatal infection in this study. In a study of Wilms' tumor, a twofold risk was associated with use of antibiotics, but no excess risk was linked to a history of infection during pregnancy (Olshan et al, 1993). Associations were reported for maternal use of marijuana during pregnancy and subsequent occurrence of childhood astrocytoma (Kuijten et al, 1990) and acute nonlymphocytic leukemia (Robison et al, 1989).

N-nitroso compounds. In a case-control study of childhood brain tumors (Preston-Martin et al, 1982; Preston-Martin and Henderson, 1984), elevated odds ratios ranging from 1.5 to 3.4 were associated with maternal use of nitrosamine-containing substances or precursors of *N*-nitroso compounds, such as burning incense, sidestream cigarette smoke, facial cosmetics, diuretics or antihistamines, and maternal consumption of cured meats. In another case-control study, a nearly twofold risk of astrocytoma was related to maternal consumption of cured meat during pregnancy (Kuijten et al, 1990). Furthermore, the risk increased with the amount of cured meat consumed. In this study, no association with other nitrosamine-containing substances was found. Several subsequent case-control studies also reported an association between maternal consumption of preserved meat, such as hot dogs and cured meats, and risk of acute lymphocytic leukemia, brain tumors, astrocytic glioma, and other childhood cancers (Bunin et al, 1994; McCredie et al, 1994a; Sarasua and Savitz, 1994). Paternal intake of hot dogs was suggested as a risk factor for childhood leukemia in another study (Peters et al, 1994). These findings may be explained in part by residual confounding by socioeconomic status, however.

A study in which the relationship between *N*-nitroso compounds and childhood brain cancer was examined led to the detection of a significant excess risk only for beer consumption by the mother during pregnancy (Howe et al, 1989). Association between selected types of brain tumors and maternal intake of dimethynitrosamine was examined, but the results were inconclusive (Bunin et al, 1993; Bunin et al, 1994). Although a more than twofold risk of tumor was found among children whose mothers used nitrosatable drugs during pregnancy, no specific tumor type was in excess (Olshan and Faustman, 1989). Hepatoblastoma was not linked to nitrosamine exposure in another study (Buckley et al, 1989b).

Other drugs and chemicals. Frequent alcohol consumption during pregnancy was found to increase the risk of neuroblastoma in offspring (Kramer et al, 1987). Another study reported an association between maternal alcohol consumption during pregnancy and risk of acute myeloid leukemia among children who were diagnosed at age two or younger (Severson et al, 1993). Several studies of other childhood cancers, however, revealed no association with maternal alcohol consumption (Van Steensel-Moll et al, 1985a; Buckley et al, 1989b; Birch et al, 1990; Kuijten et al, 1990). Other in utero exposures implicated as potential risk factors for neuroblastoma included maternal use of diuretic drugs, nonprescription pain relievers, and hair coloring products (Kramer et al, 1987; Schwartzbaum, 1992). These findings were not supported in a later study of childhood brain cancers (McCredie et al, 1994a). Use of hair coloring products, tea drinking, and hypertension during pregnancy were related to Wilms' tumor in offspring in one report (Bunin et al, 1987), but not another (Olshan et al, 1993). Use of multiple vitamins and high consumption of fruits and vegetables during pregnancy, on the other hand, was found to reduce the risk of retinoblastoma and primitive neuroectodermal brain tumors (Bunin et al, 1989b; Bunin et al, 1993; McCredie et al, 1994a). Additional work is needed to better characterize these purported associations, with respect to the timing and intensity of exposures during pregnancy, and interactive effects with other carcinogens. To the extent possible, the accuracy of self-reported exposures, such as prescription drug use during pregnancy, also should be validated.

Postnatal Exposure

Barbiturates. It has been reported that children who were treated with barbiturates had a more than twofold increased risk of subsequent brain tumors (Gold et al, 1978). The authors of this study concluded that the greater exposure to barbiturates of these children was not related to prediagnostic symptoms of brain tumors. In a separate case-control study in Los Angeles (Preston-Martin et al, 1982), however, no association between childhood brain tumors and the use of barbiturates was detected after exclusion of subjects who had used barbiturates for epilepsy. Both of these studies were based on relatively small numbers of exposed children, and thus a weak association could not be excluded with confidence. In another case-control study of central nervous system tumors, risk associated with barbiturate use during childhood was examined, with exposures ascertained from medical records for members of a group health plan (Goldhaber et al, 1990). The most common indication for barbiturate use for both cases and controls was gastrointestinal disorders. An apparent dose-response effect disappeared when history of epilepsy was taken into account. Even after adjustment for epilepsy, however, a 40% excess risk was found for childhood barbiturate use. The authors concluded that barbiturate use for epilepsy due to undiagnosed brain tumors explained some, but not all, of the observed association. Further investigation was recommended, however, because of the small residual risk observed in this study.

Antibiotics. The use of certain antibiotics in children has been associated with the occurrence of leukemia. In a population-based case-control study in Shanghai, China (Shu et al, 1987; Shu et al, 1988), treatment with chloramphenicol increased the risk of leukemia more than twofold relative to untreated children. Moreover, the risk of leukemia was observed to rise with increased use of chloramphenicol; an odds ratio of almost 10-fold was estimated for those who had used this medication for more than 10 days. An elevated risk of acute nonlymphocytic leukemia also was demonstrated with the use of syntomycin, an antibiotic pharmacologically related to chloramphenicol (Shu et al, 1987; Shu et al, 1988).

An association was reported in another study between antibiotics received soon after birth and rhabdomyosarcoma (Hartley et al, 1988a). Chance variation could not be ruled out, however. In another study, no association was observed between medication use during childhood and subsequent occurrence of central nervous system tumors (Birch et al, 1990).

Growth hormone. There have been several case reports of acute leukemia arising in growth hormone–treated children (Komp et al, 1977; Watanabe et al, 1988; Delemarre-Van de Waal et al, 1988). With the increased availability and use of growth hormone for treatment of a variety of disorders, heightened concern has been raised about a possible leukemogenic effect (Delamarre-Van de Waal et al, 1988; Ritzén, 1993). To address this issue, an international workshop was convened to review known leukemia cases since 1959 among growth hormone–treated patients in Europe, North America, Japan, and Australia (Fisher et al, 1988). While the relative risk of development of leukemia among growth hormone-treated children was estimated to be about two, the absolute risk was determined to be only about one in 2400 children treated for an average duration of 10 years.

A subsequent international survey of children with growth hormone deficiency who developed leukemia, preleukemia, or histiocytosis revealed that a large proportion of these subjects had other medical or genetic risk factors associated with increased risk of leukemia. Among those with no known risk factors, the observed incidence was not significantly higher than that expected in the general population (Ritzén, 1993). In a cohort of 6284 recepients of pituitary-derived human growth hormone between 1963 and 1985, a greater than twofold significant relative risk of leukemia was observed. However, five of the six subjects who developed leukemia had antecedent cranial tumors, and four were treated with radiotherapy (Fradkin et al, 1993). Therefore, there is insufficient evidence to implicate growth hormone therapy as a risk factor for childhood leukemia.

Chemotherapy. Certain chemotherapy regimens used for treatment of cancer may increase the risk of a subsequent cancer among children. Children who had received chemotherapy were shown to have an increased frequency of variant erythrocytes that are thought to be the result of somatic cell mutations, suggesting a genotoxic effects of chemotherapeutic agents (Hewitt and Mott, 1992). In one nested case-control study, treatment with alkylating agents increased the risk of a subsequent bone sarcoma by nearly fivefold, with the risk increasing as cumulative drug exposure rose (Tucker et al, 1987). The carcinogenic effect of alkylating agents was independent of those of radiation therapy. Alkylating agents also were implicated in another study of second cancers following Hodgkin's disease among children (Meadows et al, 1989). A specific type of alkylating agent, cyclophosphamide, was linked to second cancers after treatment for hereditary retinoblastoma in one study (Draper et al, 1986), but no association with subsequent cancer was found in studies of acute lymphoid leukemia (Pui et al, 1989; Neglia et al, 1991). On the other hand, children who received another antineoplastic drug, epipodophyllotoxin, for treatment of acute lymphoblastic leukemia had an excess risk of a subsequent acute myeloid leukemia (Pui et al, 1989, 1991; Kreissman et al, 1992; Winick et al, 1993). Elevated risks were confined to the subgroup of children treated with this agent at least weekly, but not among those who were treated less frequently (Pui et al, 1991). Risk of secondary acute myeloid leukemia or myelodysplastic syndrome in children treated for a solid tumor, however, was relatively low compared with risks reported for adults (Pui et al, 1990).

Vitamin K. A cohort study with small number of cases reported a more than twofold risk of childhood cancer associated with drugs received during the neonatal period (Golding et al, 1990). The drug category, however, included a variety of apparently unrelated items, with vitamin K being the most commonly used medication. In a subsequent case-control study that specifically examined the risk associated with vitamin K, a drug routinely administered to newborns to prevent hemorrhagic disease, only children who received vitamin K intramuscularly had a twofold excess risk of cancer; the risk was somewhat higher for leukemia than for other childhood cancers (Golding et al, 1992). Oral administration of vitamin K was not linked to childhood cancer in this study.

To further examine this issue, a nationwide cohort of nearly 1.4 million full-term births born in Sweden between 1973 and 1989 were followed until January 1, 1992, for cancer incidence using linked registries (Ekelund et al, 1993). In this study, childhood cancer risk was not elevated after intramuscular administration of vitamin K compared with that after oral administration. Studies of childhood leukemia and other cancer incidence in Denmark and the United States also did not show elevated risk among children born in time periods when intramuscular administration of vitamin K to newborns was an accepted practice (Miller, 1992; Olsen et al, 1994). In addition, no excess risk was observed in a nested case-control study using data from the Collaborative Perinatal Project (Klebanoff et al, 1993). The overall evidence therefore does not support an association between intramuscular administration of vitamin K and cancer in children (Hilgartner, 1993; Draper and McNinch, 1994).

Diet and vitamins. Vitamins generally have been shown to have a protective effect against childhood cancer. Long-term use (more than one year) of cod liver oil formulations containing vitamins A and D was estimated to reduce the risk of acute leukemia in children by 60% to 70% (Shu et al, 1988). Although there is limited experimental evidence to support a protective role of vitamins A and D against leukemia (Koeffler, 1985, 1986), additional epidemiological research is needed to confirm these findings. Intake of fruit or juice was found to be protective of childhood brain tumors in some studies (Howe et al, 1989; McCredie et al, 1994b), but no association was found in other studies of astrocytic glioma (Bunin et al, 1994) or leukemia (Peters et al, 1994). On the other hand, high intake of hot dogs and hamburgers has been linked to childhood leukemia and brain tumors (Peters et al, 1994; Sarasua and Savitz, 1994), although these findings need to be replicated in studies with careful attention to potential confounders.

Other environmental exposures. The carcinogenic effect of exposure to pesticides in children has been evaluated in a variety of studies. A series of five cases of neuroblastoma has been reported among children who were exposed to chlordane (Infante et al, 1978). In a case-control study, it was found that children with brain tumors or other malignancies were more likely than controls to have been exposed to insecticides (Gold et al, 1979). This finding has been replicated in some (Lowengart et al, 1987; Buckley et al, 1989a; Schwartzbaum et al, 1991), but not all subsequent studies (Preston-Martin et al, 1982; Howe et al, 1989). Exposure to pesticides also has been linked to other childhood cancers, including rhabdomyosarcoma (Grufferman et al, 1982) and Wilms' tumor (Olshan et al, 1993). Another study (Savitz and Feingold, 1989), using traffic density as a marker of potential exposure to motor vehicle exhaust, found excess risks of cancer for children residing at high traffic density areas. The greatest elevated risk was found for childhood leukemias. For all of these studies, the important shortcoming is limitation of exposure assessment to interview-derived information and lack of validation with measured levels of pesticides as well as the difficulty in collecting data on individual chemical agents (Copeland et al, 1977; Greenberg and Shuster, 1985).

Maternal Hormones

Diethylstilbestrol (DES) formerly was used by some obstetricians to treat pregnant women, with the intent of preventing spontaneous abortions (Boston Collaborative Drug Surveillance Program, 1973). In 1971, a strong association was reported between in utero exposure to DES and the subsequent occurrence in the exposed offspring of clear-cell adenocarcinoma of the vagina, a rare malignancy in young women (Herbst et al, 1971). The youngest observed age at onset of this neoplasm was 7 years old (Herbst, 1981), the oldest was 34, with a median age of 19 years at diagnosis (Melnick et al, 1987). The risk of clear-cell adenocarcinoma of the vagina from birth through age 34 years was estimated to be one case per 1000 exposed female progeny. The incidence rate rose sharply at age 15, with a peak of occurrence between ages 17 and 22 (Melnick et al, 1987). In a case-control comparison, the estimated risk ratio of vaginal clear-cell adenocarcinoma was higher for offspring whose mothers began using DES before the 12th week of pregnancy. Maternal history of at least one prior spontaneous abortion also further elevated the risk of this cancer among women prenatally exposed to DES (Herbst et al, 1986).

The potential carcinogenic effect of DES among males exposed in utero remains inconclusive. Although an association between prenatal exposure to DES and subsequent risk of testicular cancer in young males was observed in one study (Henderson et al, 1979), this finding was not supported by another investigation (Schottenfeld et al, 1980).

Use of sex hormones (predominantly oral contraceptives) 3 months prior to or during pregnancy has been associated with a more than twofold elevated risk of neuroblastoma in the offspring (Kramer et al, 1987). In another setting, increased risk of childhood leukemia was related to maternal use of drugs to maintain the pregnancy, including hormones, medications for threatened abortion, and drugs that inhibit early labor (Van Steensel-Moll et al, 1985a). Maternal use of sex hormones during pregnancy was not related to other childhood cancers (Operskalski et al, 1987; Hartley et al, 1988a; Buckley et al, 1989b; Olshan et al, 1993; McCredie et al, 1994a).

Parental Smoking

A case-control study in Sweden reported a greater than 50% increase in risk of cancer among children born to mothers who smoked 10 or more cigarettes per day while pregnant (Stjernfeldt et al, 1986). This study, however, was criticized for the selection of children with diabetes mellitus as controls and lack of adjustment for confounding factors (Dahlquist and Wall, 1986). Several subsequent studies also reported an association between maternal smoking and childhood cancer (Golding et al, 1990), including Ewing's sarcoma (Winn et al, 1992), neuroblastoma (Schwartzbaum, 1992), brain tumors (Filippini et al, 1994), lymphomas and certain types of leukemias (John et al, 1991; Schwartzbaum et al, 1991). Prenatal exposure to paternal smoke also had been reported to increase childhood cancer risk, independent of maternal smoking (John et al, 1991; Filippini et al, 1994; McCredie et al, 1994a).

On the other hand, data from the Inter-Regional Epidemiological Study of Childhood Cancer in England (McKinney and Stiller, 1986) and the Children's Cancer Study Group in the United States (Buckley et al, 1986; Severson et al, 1993) did not support the association between maternal smoking during pregnancy and cancer in children. In addition, a Swedish record-linkage cohort study of nearly one-half million children found no association between maternal smoking at 2–3 months of pregnancy and cancers, including solid tumors and hematopoietic malignancies, in the offspring (Pershagen et al, 1992). Other studies also detected no excess risk of childhood cancer (Forsberg and Kallen, 1990), including Wilms' tumor (Olshan et al, 1993), brain tumors (Howe et al, 1989; Kuijten et al, 1990; Gold et al, 1993; McCredie et al, 1994a), and leukemia (Van Steensel-Moll et al, 1985a), in relation to prenatal exposure to maternal or paternal cigarette smoke. Thus, a definitive conclusion cannot be reached on the potential carcinogenic effect of the antenatal exposure to maternal cigarette smoke. It is also difficult, if not impossible, to separate the effect of prenatal exposure and postnatal sidestream smoke exposure in homes where parents smoke. A study that examined passive exposure to parental cigarette smoke found no association with childhood brain tumors (Gold et al, 1993).

Parental Occupation

Hydrocarbon-related Work. Since Fabia and Thuy (1974) reported a link between paternal work in hydrocarbon-related occupations and fatalities from cancer in young children, increasing attention has been directed toward research on the association between parental occupation and risk of cancer in children. This topic also has been the subject of several review articles (Arundel and Kinnier-Wilson, 1986; Savitz and Chen, 1990; O'Leary et al, 1991; Kuijten and Bunin, 1993).

In the study of Fabia and Thuy (1974), hydrocarbon-related occupations were considered to include service station attendants, motor vehicle mechanics, machinists, miners, lumberman, painters, dyers, and cleaners. Subsequent studies have linked paternal work in gas stations, automobile or truck repair, and aircraft maintenance with infant leukemia (Vianna et al, 1984). Fathers who held jobs as machinists and welders and mothers who were laundry/dry cleaner owners also were associated with excess risk of Wilms' tumor and other cancers in offspring (Bunin et al, 1989c; Olsen et al, 1991). The Wilms' tumor risk was strongest when the fathers started work as machinists or welders prior to conception, as compared with those who held these jobs only during the mother's pregnancy or after birth of the child (Bunin et al, 1989c).

A study examining specific paternal occupational exposures found an increased risk of leukemia with exposure to chlorinated solvents, spray paint, dyes or pigments, methylethylketone, and cutting oil (Lowengart et al, 1987). Other studies also have reported associations between paternal exposure to hydrocarbons and cancer in children, including benzene with childhood leukemia (McKinney et al, 1991), solvents and petroleum products with acute nonlymphocytic leukemia (Buckley et al, 1989a), petroleum products, paints or pigments with hepatoblastoma (Buckley et al, 1989b), and paternal exposures to paint during the postnatal period with astrocytoma (Kuijten et al, 1992). Interestingly, the study of astrocytoma did not reveal an excess risk for children of chemical and petroleum workers with high exposures (Kuijten et al, 1992). Chance variation could explain the discrepant findings in this study, however.

Although the risk for total childhood cancers was not elevated when paternal exposure to all combined hydrocarbons was examined (Feingold et al, 1992), a statistically nonsignificant increased risk of acute lymphocytic leukemia was observed for paternal exposures to aniline, benzene, and petroleum/coke pitch/tar. An excess risk of brain cancer also was found in relation to potential exposure to creosote (Feingold et al, 1992). Another case-control study revealed an excess risk of intracranial malignancies among children born to fathers who worked in jobs with moderate-to-heavy exposure to aromatic and aliphatic hydrocarbons (Wilkins and Sinks, 1990).

The positive associations between hydrocarbon-related paternal occupations and childhood cancers summarized above are not universally supported in all studies. No associations were observed between hydrocarbon-related paternal occupations and childhood cancer in case-control studies carried out in Finland (Hakulinen et al, 1976), the Netherlands (van Steensel-Moll et al, 1985b), China (Shu et al, 1988), Canada (Howe et al, 1989), and the United States (Kwa and Fine, 1980; Zack et al, 1980; Gold et al, 1982; Shaw et al, 1984; Johnson et al, 1987; Nasca et al, 1988; Bunin et al, 1990). An expanded version of the Finnish study (Hakulinen et al, 1976), however, indicated that children of painters were at increased risk of all malignancies. The Finnish group also found an association between paternal work in machine repair and brain tumors in the offspring, as well as leukemia in children of fathers who drove motor vehicles. A case-control study in the United States (Johnson et al, 1987) revealed an increased risk of tumors of the nervous system in children of printers, graphic arts workers and chemical and petroleum workers, but no association was detected for other hydrocarbon exposures. A recent Norwegian study (Kristensen and Andersen, 1992) also found no excess cancer among children born to a cohort of male printing workers. The small size of the study and the lack of an independent assessment of completeness of record linkage, however, limited the inferences that could be drawn from this study (Annegers and Johnson, 1992).

Metal-related Work. Paternal employment in lead-related occupations was found to increase the risk of Wilms' tumor (Kantor et al, 1979). The authors of that study included in the category of lead-exposed workers fathers employed in the following jobs: drivers, motor vehicle mechanics, service station attendants, welders, solderers, metallurgists, and scrap metal workers. It should be noted that there is considerable overlap between the occupations that were defined as lead-related and those previously described as hydrocarbon-related. A significant excess risk was observed for children of fathers employed in the manufacture of iron and metal structures, and as machinists or smiths (Olsen et al, 1991). An increased risk of Wilms' tumor also was found among children of machinists and welders in another study (Bunin et al, 1989c). The association between paternal exposure to lead compounds and Wilms' tumor was not confirmed in another investigation, however (Wilkins and Sinks, 1984a,b).

Other studies have suggested a link between paternal exposure to metals and cancers in children (Feingold et al, 1992), including an association between lead and acute nonlymphocytic leukemia (Buckley et al, 1989a), between metals and hepatoblastoma (Buckley et al, 1989b), and between metal-related jobs and brain cancer (Wilkins and Koutras, 1988; Wilkins and Sinks, 1990). In another study, a greater than expected incidence of childhood solid tumors also was observed among residents near a smelter (Alexander et al, 1991).

Radiation-related Work. Increased risk of childhood leukemia has been associated with father's occupational exposure to radiation (Gardner, 1991; McKinney et al, 1991). A case-control study among young persons residing near the Sellafield nuclear plant found an association between leukemia incidence and father's recorded external radiation dose during preconception employment (Gardner et al, 1990). Another British study in three high-incidence areas also demonstrated an excess risk of leukemia among children whose fathers were exposed to occupational radiation during the preconceptional and/or the gestational period (McKinney et al, 1991). In the Oxford Survey of Childhood

Cancers (Sorahan and Roberts, 1993), paternal exposure to radionuclides, but not external radiation, was associated with risk of childhood cancer. Transmission of radiation-induced mutations in germ cell lines has been suggested as an explanation for the observed excess of leukemia in offspring (Gardner et al, 1990; Greaves, 1990), although a causal link and a mechanism for leukemogenesis has not yet been established (Greaves, 1990). Reasonable doubt about a causal explanation was raised by the observation that the excess risk of leukemia among children residing near another nuclear facility in Scotland was unrelated to parental employment at this plant, or father's estimated radiation exposure (Urquhart et al, 1991).

Other Paternal Occupations. While childhood brain cancer has been linked to paternal jobs with moderate-to-heavy exposures to nonionizing electromagnetic field radiation exposures (Wilkins and Sinks, 1990), another study found inconclusive evidence regarding these associations (Nasca et al, 1988). Excess brain and other nervous system malignancies were reported among children of fathers employed as electricians, or electrical and electronics workers (Spitz and Johnson, 1985; Wilkins and Koutras, 1988; Johnson and Spitz, 1989; Kuijten et al, 1992). These occupations were thought to involve potential electromagnetic field exposure (Spitz and Johnson, 1985; Johnson and Spitz, 1989), although these workers also may be exposed to other potential carcinogens, such as hydrocarbons. A subsequent case-control study, using similar classifications for occupational exposure to electromagnetic field, also observed a weak association between paternal exposure and neuroblastoma in offspring (Wilkins and Hundley, 1990). No association was observed between neuroblastoma and paternal employment in jobs in the electronics industry or occupations with exposure to electricity or electromagnetic fields (Bunin et al, 1990).

Paternal employment in agriculture or occupational exposure to pesticides was associated with increased childhood cancer risk in some studies (Buckley et al, 1989a; Hemminki et al, 1981; Wilkins and Koutras, 1988; Wilkins and Sinks, 1990; Winn et al, 1992), but not in others (Fabia and Thuy, 1974; Sanders et al, 1981; Spitz and Johnson, 1985). Excess risks have been observed for exposures that occurred in the preconception or gestational period (Wilkins and Koutras, 1988; Wilkins and Sinks, 1990) or postnatally (Buckley et al, 1989a).

Other paternal occupations also have been implicated in occurrence of childhood cancer, including medical and dental professions (Olsen et al, 1991), work in pulp and paper manufacturing (Johnson et al, 1987; Nasca et al, 1988; Kuijten et al, 1992) and exposures to wood dust (McKinney et al, 1991). In a case-control study of brain cancer carried out among children living in Los Angeles (Peters et al, 1981), risk factors included maternal occupational chemical exposures and paternal exposures to solvents, as well as paternal employment in the aircraft industry. The association with employment in the aircraft industry was supported by some subsequent investigations (Hicks et al, 1984; Vianna et al, 1984; Lowengart et al, 1987), but not by others (Olshan et al, 1986; Nasca et al, 1988).

Maternal Occupation. It has been suggested that children with malignant disease were more likely to be born to mothers who worked in pharmacies, bakeries, and factories (Hemminki et al, 1981). In another case-control study, increased risks of leukemia were found for children whose mothers worked as physicians, pharmacists, or pharmaceutical manufacturing workers (Shu et al, 1988). Risk of Wilms' tumor and osteogenic and soft tissue sarcomas also was associated with mothers' employment in medical and dental care (Olsen et al, 1991). In addition, mothers of case patients were more likely to have worked during pregnancy in the chemical industry and/or related occupations with exposure to benzene, gasoline, pesticides, and related agents (Shu et al, 1988). Other studies reported excess cancers in children of mothers who worked as nurses, physicians, pharmacists, or hairdressers (Olsen et al, 1991; Kuijten et al, 1992), or in the food industry (McKinney et al, 1991). Implicated maternal occupational exposures include benzene, petroleum products, pesticides, paints or pigments, metals, soot, sawdust, and organic dusts (van Steensel-Moll et al, 1985b; Buckley et al, 1989a, b; Infante-Rivard et al, 1991; Feingold et al, 1992). Elsewhere, it was found that the risk of leukemia was related to maternal employment in personal service industries, but not to specific occupational exposures (Lowengart et al, 1987).

It is difficult to reach firm conclusions from the research on parental occupations and risk of cancer in children. A large number of studies have involved broad categories of employment, often abstracted from data collected for other purposes, such as birth certificates. Specific exposures, if presented, often are based upon estimates from linkage of job title with industrial hygiene survey data. The estimated exposures for a job title may vary from survey to survey (Linet et al, 1987). Relatively few data have been collected on actual levels of exposure in most childhood cancer case-control studies. Also, in many job settings, exposure to multiple agents occur. Although it is important to establish parental exposures in relation to the timing of a pregnancy—preconceptional, gestational, or postnatal period—few studies are large enough to delineate separate effects of these highly correlated exposure periods. Advances in biomolecular techniques, such as the identification of different germline mutations and markers for exposure in affected children, may bring new insight into research on the relation of parental occupational exposures and childhood cancer. Although some general patterns of association are evident from the current literature, the number of discrepant findings is too great to allow firm conclusions.

HOST FACTORS

Genetic Factors

Hereditary factors associated with an increased risk of cancer have been described in several review articles (Mulvihill, 1975; Mulvihill, 1977; Swift, 1982; Lynch, 1982; Littlefield, 1984; Strong, 1984; Knudson, 1986; Ponder, 1990). About 200 different types of genetic disorders have been described for which such a relationship may exist (Mulvihill, 1977), but the evidence for many of these associations has been no more substantial than case reports.

The hereditary clinical syndromes for which the evidence of an excess cancer risk in children is most persuasive include ataxia-telangiectasia, Fanconi's anemia, Bloom's syndrome, Li-Fraumeni syndrome, neurofibromatosis, and Down syndrome.

Ataxia-telangiectasia. Ataxia-telangiectasia (AT) is generally believed to be inherited recessively, although it has been suggested that this disorder may not always follow a Mendelian recessive inheritance pattern (Taylor, 1992; Woods et al, 1990). Patients with AT show a variety of chromosomal abnormalities, with translocation involving chromosomes 7 and 14 being the most common features (McKusick, 1992; Taylor, 1992). An AT gene has been mapped to chromosome 11q22-q23 by genetic linkage analysis (Gatti et al, 1988). The cytogenetic abnormalities of AT predisposing to cancer have been reviewed in detail elsewhere (McKusick, 1992; Taylor, 1992). The majority of cancers occurring in these patients are lymphoid leukemias and lymphomas. A small number of other cancers also are observed, including tumors of the stomach, liver, breast, uterus, and ovary, and central nervous system tumors (Swift, 1982; Morrell et al, 1986; Swift et al, 1987; Pippard et al, 1988; Taylor, 1992). Family members of patients with this disorder also have been reported to have greater than expected numbers of many of these same cancers (German et al, 1979; Swift et al, 1987; Pippard et al, 1988).

Fanconi's Anemia. Children with Fanconi's anemia, an autosomal recessive syndrome, are at increased risk of developing myelomonocytic leukemia (Schroeder et al, 1979), but family members of patients with this condition have not been found to have an overall excess of cancer deaths (Swift et al, 1980). Similarly, there is no conclusive evidence of an excess cancer risk among relative of persons with Bloom's syndrome (Swift, 1982), another autosomal recessive disorder, although acute leukemias and lymphomas have been observed with unusual frequency among homozygotic children (German et al, 1979). Wilms' tumor also has been reported in patients with Bloom's syndrome (Cairney et al, 1987).

Neurofibromatosis. Children with neurofibromatosis, an autosomal dominant syndrome, are at increased risk of developing a wide variety of malignancies, most of which are of neural-crest origin, such as ganglioneuroma, meningioma, and neurofibroma (Swift, 1982; Schneider et al, 1986; Blatt et al, 1986; Sorensen et al, 1986; Matsui et al, 1993). Other cancers also have been reported in excess, including myelogenous leukemia and soft tissue sarcomas (Bader and Miller, 1978; Matsui et al, 1993). It has been estimated that children with neurofibromatosis have a more than 16-fold excess risk of cancer (Narod et al, 1991). The defective gene causing von Recklinghausen neurofibromatosis (NF1) is on chromosome 17, at band q11.2 (Seizinger et al, 1987a; Cawthon et al, 1990). Molecular studies of malignant tumors from patients with NF1 suggest that the NF1 gene functions as a tumor suppressor in neural-crest tumors (Skuse et al, 1989; Glover et al, 1991). Shannon and colleagues (1994) found that in bone marrow cells in five of 11 children with NF1 who developed myeloid disorders, the normal allele was deleted and the NF1 allele was inherited from a parent with NF1. In contrast, no allelic loss of the NF1 gene was detected in 25 children with myeloid disorders who did not have NF1. These results suggest that the NF1 gene also may function as a tumor-suppressor in malignant myeloid diseases in children (Shannon et al, 1994; Brodeur, 1994). The NF1 gene also regulates the activity of *ras*, a family of proto-oncogenes (Shannon et al, 1994; Brodeur, 1994). Mutations of the *ras* gene have been demonstrated in children with myelogenous leukemia (Vogelstein et al, 1990; Miyauchi et al, 1994). In a follow-up study of a nationwide cohort of 84 patients with NF1 and 128 of their relatives established in Denmark in 1944, malignant neoplasms or benign central nervous system tumors occurred in 45% of the probands by 1983 (Sorenson et al, 1986).

The defective gene causing the bilateral acoustic form of neurofibromatosis (NF2) is on chromosome 22 (Rouleau et al, 1987; Wertelecki et al, 1988; Rouleau et al, 1993). A loss of alleles on chromosome 22 has been observed in acoustic neuromas, meningiomas, and neurofibromas (Seizinger et al, 1987b, c).

Li-Fraumeni Syndrome. Families with the Li-Fraumeni syndrome have been described as including a proband with a soft tissue sarcoma diagnosed early in life, and at least two other close relatives with cancers diagnosed before age 45 (Li and Fraumeni, 1969a; Li et al, 1988). This rare autosomal dominant syndrome is characterized by an unusually high incidence of sarcomas in children and young adults, premenopausal breast cancer, and a variety of other neoplasms, including brain tumors, leukemias, and adrenocortical carcinomas (Li and Fraumeni, 1969a, b; Li and Fraumeni, 1982; Li et al, 1988; Malkin et al, 1990; Srivastava et al, 1990). It has been estimated that 5% to 10% of children with soft tissue sarcomas belong to families with the Li-Fraumeni syndrome (Birch et al, 1984; Williams and Strong, 1985). Inherited mutations in the p53 tumor-suppressor gene were first described in families with this syndrome (Malkin et al, 1990; Srivastava et al, 1990; Levine, 1992). In a study of DNA sequence of the entire coding region of the p53 gene in 12 families with classic Li-Fraumeni syndrome, mutations in the germ cell line was found in six of the families. Among these six families, five included young children with rhabdomyosarcoma and three included infants with adrenal cortical carcinoma (Birch et al, 1994). In other studies, mutations of the p53 gene in the germ cell line also have been observed among some children and young adults with a second primary cancer (Malkin et al, 1992) and patients with sarcoma (Toguchida et al, 1992; McIntyre et al, 1994). Since persons with an inherited p53 mutation do not necessarily have a cancer diagnosed at an early age (Toguchida et al, 1992; Malkin et al, 1992; Levine, 1992) and families with Li-Fraumeni syndrome may not have mutations in the p53 germ cell line (Birch et al, 1994), other genetic and/or environmental factors may affect the cancer risk in Li-Fraumeni families, or alter the cancer risk among carriers of a mutant p53 gene (Malkin et al, 1992; Levine, 1992).

Down Syndrome. The incidence of acute leukemia among children with Down syndrome is 20 to 30 times that of other children (Fong and Brodeur, 1987; Robison and Neglia, 1987; Mili et al, 1993a, b). The age-specific proportions of lymphoblastic and nonlymphoblastic cell types are similar to those of leukemia patients without Down syndrome. This association has been studied epidemiologically, clinically, and cytogenetically for many years, and the reader is referred to detailed literature reviews (Fong and Brodeur, 1987; Robison and Neglia, 1987). Although the link is well established, the mechanism is not yet understood. Trisomy 21 is the common cytogenetic abnormality identified in leukemia cells of Down syndrome patients (Fong and Brodeur, 1987). It has been suggested that mutant oncogenes, including the Hu-*ets*-2 oncogene located at q21.1-q22.3 on chromosome 21, may be associated with hematopoietic dysregulation and acute leukemia (Miller and Miller, 1990).

Other Familial Cancer Syndromes. Children with other dominantly inherited syndromes, including basal cell nevus syndrome (also known as Gorlin syndrome) (Lorenz and Fuhrmann, 1978) and multiple endocrine neoplasia syndrome type 1 (MEN1) and type 2 (MEN2) (Freier et al, 1977; Girvan and Holliday, 1987; Eng et al, 1994), also are at increased cancer risk. Linkage studies recently have mapped the basal cell nevus syndrome to chromosome 9q22.3-9q31 (Gailani et al, 1992; Goldstein et al, 1994). The gene for MEN1 was mapped to chromosome 11q13 (Larsson et al, 1988; Bale et al, 1989) and for MEN2 to chromosome 10q11 (Gardner et al, 1993; Mole et al, 1993; Mulligan et al, 1993).

Childhood cancers that follow autosomal dominant patterns of inheritance, but are not manifestations of a hereditary clinical syndrome with multiple features include retinoblastoma, Wilms' tumor, and neuroblastoma.

Retinoblastoma. It has been estimated that 40% of retinoblastoma cases are attributable in part to autosomal dominant germ cell mutations (Knudson, 1971). Others have estimated that nearly 50% of retinoblastomas are genetic in origin if unilateral cases with a family history or new germ cell mutations also are included (Narod et al, 1991). The development of retinoblastoma involves loss of both alleles at a single locus, mapped to the long arm of chromosome 13 (Ponder, 1988). Children with the hereditary form of retinoblastoma have been shown to have inherited the loss of one copy of the gene in the germ cell line (Hansen and Cavenee, 1988). Chromosomal abnormalities involving 13q also have been identified in some patients with retinoblastoma and other developmental defects (Knudson et al, 1976; Wilson et al, 1977; Meadows et al, 1985; Draper et al, 1986; Bunin et al, 1989a). The hereditary form of retinoblastoma is characterized by an earlier age at onset and a greater likelihood of multiple foci of involvement including an increased probability of bilateral disease (Knudson, 1971) and an increased risk of development of second tumors (Jensen and Miller, 1971; Knudson, 1971; Draper et al, 1986). Children born to survivors of hereditary retinoblastoma also have an elevated risk of developing this disease compared with children born to survivors of unilateral retinoblastoma with no family history of the disease. In one study, 23 of 52 offspring of heritable retinoblastoma survivors and none of the 94 offspring of nonheritable retinoblastoma survivors developed retinoblastoma (Hawkins et al, 1989).

Wilms' Tumor. Unlike retinoblastoma, familial Wilms' tumor is rare, making up 1–2.4% of all cases (Bonaïti-Pellié et al, 1992; Coppes et al, 1994). An apparent autosomal dominant pattern of inheritance was reported (Knudson and Strong, 1972), although genes responsible for the transmission of the familial form of Wilms' tumor have not been identified (Coppes et al, 1994). On the other hand, remarkable progress has been made in the identification of genetic mutations involved in the development of sporadic Wilms' tumor (Haber and Housman, 1992; Slater and Mannens, 1992; Koo and Hensle, 1993; Coppes and Williams, 1994). The deletion of the short arm of one of the two chromosomes 11 in patients with Wilms' tumor and aniridia provided the first indication of involvement of this region of chromosome 11 (Riccardi et al, 1978). A Wilms' tumor suppressor gene was identified on the short arm of chromosome 11 at band p13 subsequently (Bonetta et al, 1990; Call et al, 1990; Gessler et al, 1990). However, a deletion on the short arm of chromosome 11 also has been observed in children who do not develop Wilms' tumor (Riccardi et al, 1978). Thus, additional events appear to be necessary for the development of Wilms' tumor beyond a sporadic or inherited cytogenetic defect on chromosome 11 (Riccardi et al, 1978; Li, 1982). Genomic imprinting, featuring the preferential retention of the paternal rather than the maternal allele, also has been proposed as a mechanism in Wilms' tumor development (Schroeder et al, 1987; Reik and Surani, 1989; Ponder, 1990).

Patients with sporadic aniridia are more likely to develop bilateral Wilms' tumor than patients without this anomaly (Miller et al, 1964). Other congenital defects, such as hemihypertrophy, genitourinary abnormalities, and cardiac septal defects also have been linked to Wilms' tumor (Stiller et al, 1987; Breslow et al, 1988a; Bonaïti-Pellié et al, 1992). In one study, congenital anomalies were found in five of 11 patients with bilateral Wilms' tumor, and in only three of 76 patients of the unilateral disease (Bond, 1975). Bilateral Wilms' tumor tends to occur at an earlier age than the unilateral form (Breslow et al, 1988a; Narod et al, 1991).

Patients with Beckwith-Wiedemann syndrome (BWS) are predisposed to a number of embryonal tumors, most commonly Wilms' tumor, but also adrenocortical carcinoma, hepatoblastoma, and rhabdomyosarcoma (Sotelo-Avila and Gooch, 1976). Although most cases are sporadic, pedigrees of BWS with evidence for autosomal dominant inheritance have been reported (Niikawa et al, 1986). The BWS gene was mapped to chromosome 11p15 by genetic linkage analysis (Koufos et al, 1989; Ping et al, 1989). Evidence for genomic imprinting has been shown (Henry et al, 1991; Weksberg et al, 1993).

Neuroblastoma. Some children with neuroblastoma have been found to have deletions of the short arm of chromosome 1 and amplification of the N-*myc* protooncogene (Brodeur et al, 1977; Haag et al, 1981; Schwab et al, 1984; Brodeur, 1990). Although some patterns of tumor occurrence have suggested an autosomal dominant inheritance, the proportion of neuroblastomas due to hereditary factors is estimated to be small, probably less than 1% (Kushner et al, 1986; Brodeur and Fong, 1989; Narod et al, 1991). Other evidence for a role of heredity in neuroblastoma includes the observation of familial clustering (Chatten and Voorhess, 1967; Pegelow et al, 1975) and its development in multiple generations within families (Knudson and Strong, 1972).

Family History

Relatives of children who were diagnosed with primitive neuroectodermal tumor were found to have an excess risk of childhood cancers, including brain tumors, leukemia, lymphoma, and sarcoma (Kuijten et al, 1993). An increased risk associated with a family history of cancer also has been reported for other childhood malignancies (Miller, 1971; Draper et al, 1977; Farwell and Flannery, 1984b; Strong et al, 1987). On the other hand, no association with family history of cancer was observed in other studies (Bondy et al, 1991; Gold et al, 1994; McCredie et al, 1994a). Risk of childhood brain tumors was not increased with the number of relatives affected with a variety of cancers common in the Li-Fraumeni syndrome (Gold et al, 1994).

In addition, relatives of brain tumor patients also were more likely to have had a history of birth defects or other medical conditions, such as seizures and febrile convulsions (Kuijten et al, 1993; Gold et al, 1994). Potential recall bias should be considered in interpreting these findings.

Birth Characteristics

Possible associations have been evaluated between risk of cancer during childhood, particularly leukemia, and several pregnancy and/or birth-related factors. Such factors have included maternal age, history of maternal fetal loss, birth weight, and birth order.

Maternal Age. The association between advanced maternal age (generally age 35 or older) and the risk of childhood leukemia in offspring has been noted for several decades (Manning and Carroll, 1957; Stewart et al, 1958; MacMahon and Newill, 1962; Kaye et al, 1991). The association with leukemia was found not due to a birth cohort effect (Stark and Mantel, 1967), and was stronger among males (Fasal et al, 1971). Other investigations, however, revealed either a statistically nonsignificant association (Shaw et al, 1984; Robison et al, 1987) or no association of childhood leukemia with advanced maternal age (van Steensel-Moll, 1985a; Zack et al, 1991).

Similarly, evidence regarding maternal age and other childhood cancers is inconclusive. Associations between advanced maternal age and rhabdomyosarcoma, astrocytoma, sporadic heritable retinoblastoma, and testicular cancer have been reported (Grufferman et al, 1982; Swerdlow et al, 1982; Bunin et al, 1989b; Emerson et al, 1991), although some are not statistically significant (Swerdlow et al, 1982; Bunin et al, 1989b). In a hospital-based study (Greenberg, 1983), an inverse association between risk of neuroblastoma and maternal age was observed, and in a population-based study incidence was higher in mothers under age 20 or older than 34 years of age at birth (Carlsen, 1986). Other studies found no association between maternal age and a variety of childhood malignancies (Johnson and Spitz, 1985; Neglia et al, 1988; Birch et al, 1990; Kuijten et al, 1990; Rodvall et al, 1990; Matsunaga et al, 1990; Ghali et al, 1992). A study of Wilms' tumor suggested that in hereditary cases the mothers were significantly older than their controls, but no association with maternal age was observed for sporadic cases (Bunin et al, 1987).

Maternal Pregnancy History. A history of miscarriage or stillbirth has been associated with a small increase in risk of cancer in offspring, including leukemias, astrocytomas, and rhabdomyosarcomas (van Steensel-Moll et al, 1985a; Rodvall et al, 1990; Kaye et al, 1991; Emerson et al, 1991; Ghali et al, 1992). In another study of childhood testicular cancer, an association was observed for a history of stillbirth, but not miscarriage (Swerdlow et al, 1982). Elsewhere a reduced risk of cancer was observed among children whose mothers had a history of miscarriage or stillbirth (Hartley et al, 1988a; Neglia et al, 1988; Kuijten et al, 1990). Still other studies of childhood cancer have revealed no association with miscarriage or stillbirth (Bunin et al, 1987; Bunin et al, 1989b; Birch et al, 1990; Zack et al, 1991). Overall, there is no conclusive evidence that a history of adverse reproductive outcomes is related to cancer in offspring.

Birth Order. For firstborn children, an elevated risk of leukemia, particularly the lymphocytic and blast cell varieties, was reported in one study (Stewart et al, 1958) and confirmed by others (MacMahon and Newill, 1962; Stark and Mantel, 1967). No association was observed in other investigations, however (Fasal et al, 1971; Shaw et al, 1984; Robison et al, 1987; Shu et al, 1988; Kaye et al, 1991). Weak and statistically nonsignificant associations with birth order have been found for childhood brain tumors (Gold et al, 1979), neuroblastoma (Greenberg, 1983) and rhabdomyosarcoma (Grufferman et al, 1982). In another study, a significantly elevated risk of brain tumor was found only among firstborn children of mothers age 30 or older at birth of the patient (Emerson et al, 1991). Other investigations have observed either no association (Neglia et al, 1988; Bunin et al, 1989b; Ghali et al, 1992; McCredie et al, 1994b) or a reduced risk among firstborn children (Swerdlow et al, 1982; Howe et al, 1989). Thus, there is no compelling evidence for a connection between birth order and risk of childhood cancer.

Birth Weight. Several investigators have documented a tendency toward elevated birth weight among children who later developed leukemia (Fasal et al, 1971; Hirayama, 1980; Daling et al, 1984). This association appears to be stronger in girls than boys (Fasal et al, 1971; Daling et al, 1984) and among children diagnosed with leukemia during the first years of life (Hirayama, 1980; Daling et al, 1984; Robison et al, 1987). Other studies have indicated no association between birth weight and childhood leukemia (Shaw et al, 1984; Kaye et al, 1991; Zack et al, 1991).

A significant association between higher birth weight and childhood brain tumor, especially astrocytomas, has been reported by a number of investigators (Gold et al, 1979; Kuijten et al, 1990; Emerson et al, 1991). Two others (Greenberg, 1983; Daling et al, 1984) found a tendency toward heavier birth weights in children who subsequently developed neuroblastoma. The latter finding was not confirmed in a birth certificate study (Johnson and Spitz, 1985; Johnson and Spitz, 1986) that found the reverse—elevated neuroblastoma risks for preterm and low-weight full-term infants. A subsequent study also found no association between malignant brain tumors and birth weight (McCredie et al, 1994b). Another investigation, although observing no association with childhood cancer overall (Hartley et al, 1988b) or soft tissue sarcomas (Hartley et al, 1988a), found a significantly lower mean birth weight among children diagnosed with bone cancer, and in particular Ewing's sarcoma (Hartley et al, 1988a, b). Wilms' tumor was associated with heavy birth weight in two reports (Daling et al, 1984; Bunin et al, 1987), but not another (Olshan et al, 1993). No association with birth weight was observed in other studies of childhood cancers (Grufferman et al, 1982; Neglia et al, 1988; Bunin et al, 1989b; Howe et al, 1989; Birch et al, 1990; Forsberg and Kallen, 1990; Ghali et al, 1992). Although it is possible that extreme birth weights may be linked to increased risk of certain childhood cancers (Olshan, 1986), there is no conclusive evidence to suggest an association between birth weight and childhood cancer overall.

PREVENTION

It is difficult to identify prevention measures, because etiologic factors for childhood cancer are not well understood. For families whose offspring are likely to be at high risk for the few congenital disorders linked with childhood malignancies, genetic counseling may be helpful. Progress in identifying genetic markers for such predisposing conditions should also be a high priority.

Clearly, it would be prudent to limit diagnostic x-ray exposures in women of childbearing age who have discontinued or are not using birth control measures, who are attempting to become pregnant, or who are known to be pregnant. In the absence of greater knowledge about the role of pregnancy-related medications or other treatments in carcinogenesis, it would also be sound clinical practice to limit, to the extent feasible, any such medications, treatments, or anesthetic agents not critically important for the health of the mother.

Similarly, x-ray exposures, medications, and related medical exposures should also be limited to the extent possible among children and not used or given unless important in maintaining the child's health. For children diagnosed with cancer, the potential benefits of cytotoxic agents and radiotherapy must be weighed, and the lowest clinically effective doses should be used.

In the absence of consistent findings about the role of parental occupational exposures in the occurrence of cancer among their offspring, it is difficult to recommend avoidance of specific agents, although minimization of occupational ionizing radiation (including preconceptional period exposures for both parents), hydrocarbon-related, and metal exposures would clearly be prudent.

Postnatal environmental exposures consistently linked with increased risk of childhood cancer (eg, ionizing radiation, pesticides, and others) should be limited to the extent possible. If use of agents such as pesticides is necessary, then children's exposure should be minimized by prevention of contact with such exposures.

Transmission of specific infectious agents implicated in carcinogenesis should be prevented through prophylactic vaccination (eg, against hepatitis B virus) or minimized by education of older children to limit sexual spread or transmission via intravenous drug use. In addition to all the other medical benefits of breast-feeding for 6 months or longer, this activity should be encouraged for the possible reduction in risk of childhood lymphoma, except among those mothers who test positive for the HIV viruses.

FUTURE RESEARCH

The publication in 1988 of the most comprehensive, standardized international data (Parkin et al, 1988a) available to date on childhood cancer incidence from population-based cancer registries is a landmark event for the field of childhood cancer epidemiology. These data are particularly valuable because they follow the diagnostic grouping scheme recently developed by Birch and Marsden (1987) for pediatric cancer. The data have provided an important starting point to consider and further evaluate international and within-population variation in age-adjusted and age-specific cancer rates for all cancers combined and for specific cancer types by sex, race or ethnic group, and histologic type. Geographic, sociodemographic, and race or ethnic group differences in specific cancer incidence rates should provide clues to environmental etiologic factors, and should point to populations among whom analytic studies can be most productive in elucidating causal factors. In populations with longstanding high-quality cancer registries, complete ascertainment and certification of deaths, and accurate census data, time trends in incidence, mortality, and survival can be monitored in an ongoing fashion.

Childhood cancer is not a single entity and undoubtedly is a consequence of a variety of endogenous as well as exogenous factors. Case reports and analytic studies of familial aggregation and congenital and cytogenetic abnormalities associated with childhood cancer indicate the important role of host factors in predisposition to many of these diseases. Both population-based epidemiological studies with methodologically rigorous genetic components and detailed investigations of families with two or more members affected by childhood cancer, and/or those with hereditary syndromes that include an elevated childhood cancer risk, will be critical in clarifying the role of host and environmental factors in childhood cancer etiology. These kinds of investigations are also crucial for identifying children at greatest risk, so that early detection and effective treatment can be implemented. Advances in molecular genetics also should be incorporated within both types of studies to elucidate mechanisms of cancer development, and to help determine which markers are sensitive and specific enough to be used eventually to identify high-risk families and children.

Analytic studies have begun to address the role of environmental factors in cancer causation in children either independently or in conjunction with genetic factors. The compelling evidence of the role of diethylstilbestrol in inducing cancers transplacentally underscores the need to examine prenatal events. Early efforts to evaluate parental occupational exposures, medications used during pregnancy, and other medical-related exposures associated with increased risk of childhood cancer occurrence have produced inconsistent findings. Future efforts will require the clear specification of individual agents, and incorporation of pilot-tested methods for measuring and validating past exposures. Although two of the three cohort investigations and several case-control studies showed no excess of childhood leukemia or other cancers among children exposed in utero to diagnostic x-rays, many studies have revealed a 1.5- to 2.0-fold increased risk. Yet, concern has begun to decline because it was believed that such exposures were disappearing. The continuing importance of intrauterine diagnostic irradiation is highlighted by indications (Kaczmarek et al, 1989) that, contrary to these assumptions, the frequency of pelvimetry has not declined according to recent U.S. national survey results. Therefore, investigation of the unintended effects of pelvimetry as well as other diagnostic procedures should be continued.

The potential impact of postnatal exposures on carcinogenesis in the young also is most clearly established for therapeutic irradiation. Continued investigation of the role of environmental sources of man-made and natural background ionizing radiation, nonionizing extremely low frequency electromagnetic field radiation exposures, pesticides and other chemical agents, as well as immunologic and nutritional status is warranted. In these studies, too, accurate quantitative and qualitative characterization of the exposures is essential. Use of appropriate measurements, medical and other types of preexisting records (to validate past exposure information), in addition to parental interviews, often will be necessary to obtain such information.

Epidemiological research on cancer in children is subject to methodological impediments related to the rarity of these diseases and the fairly weak associations with most of the identified risk factors. In order to achieve sufficient statistical power for analytical investigations and to evaluate the importance of the timing of many types of exposures (preconception, gestational, or postnatal), the use of large samples obtained through multicenter studies will be increasingly necessary. Inferences about purported risk factors remain controversial because of criticisms regarding potential biases in the selection of subjects and the collection of data. Failure to give adequate attention to the timing of potentially carcinogenic exposures and the role of confounding variables has characterized many earlier studies. For future research to resolve these controversies and advance the understanding of childhood cancer, attention must be given to such methodological concerns.

REFERENCES

ABRAHAMSON S. 1990. Childhood leukemia at Sellafield. Radiat Res 123:237–238.

ADELSTEIN AM, DONOVAN JW. 1972. Malignant disease in children whose mothers had chickenpox, mumps, or rubella during pregnancy. Br Med J 4:629–631.

ADELSTEIN A, WHITE T. 1976. Leukemia 1911–1973: cohort analysis. Popul Trends 3:9–13.

ALEXANDER FE. 1992. Space-time clustering of childhood acute lymphoblastic leukaemia: indirect evidence for a transmissible agent. Br J Cancer 65:589–592.

ALEXANDER F, MCKINNEY PA, CARTWRIGHT RA. 1991. The pattern of childhood and related adult malignancies near Kingston-upon-Hull. J Public Health Med 13:96–100.

ALEXANDER FE, MCKINNEY PA, MONCRIEFF KC, et al. 1992. Residential proximity of children with leukaemia and non-Hodgkin's lymphoma in three areas of Northern England. Br J Cancer 65:583–588.

ALEXANDER F, RICKETTS TJ, MCKINNEY PA, et al. 1989. Cancer registration of leukaemias and lymphomas: results of a comparison with a specialist registry. Community Med 11:81–89.

ALEXANDER FE, RICKETTS TJ, MCKINNEY PA, et al. 1990. Community lifestyle characteristics and risk of acute lymphoblastic leukaemia in children. Lancet 336:1461–1465.

ANNEGERS JF, JOHNSON CC. 1992. Studying parental occupation and childhood cancer. (Editorial). Epidemiology 3:1–2.

ARCHER VE. 1987. Association of nuclear fallout with leukemia in the United States. Arch Environ Health 42:263–271.

ARUNDEL SE, KINNIER-WILSON LM. 1986. Parental occupations and cancer: a review of the literature. J Epidemiol Community Health 40:30–36.

AUSTIN DF, KARP S, DWORSKY R, et al. 1975. Excess leukemia in cohorts of children born following influenza epidemics. Am J Epidemiol 101:77–83.

BADER JL, MILLER RW. 1978. Neurofibromatosis and childhood leukemia. J Pediatr 92:925–929.

BAILAR JC. 1990. Death from all cancers: trends in sixteen countries. In: *Trends in Cancer Mortality in Industrial Countries,* Davis DL, Hoel D (eds). New York: The New York Academy of Sciences, pp 49–57.

BALE SJ, BALE AE, STEWART K, et al. 1989. Linkage analysis of multiple endocrine neoplasia type 1 with INT2 and other markers on chromosome 11. Genomics 4:320–322.

BAVERSTOCK KF. 1991. DNA instability, paternal irradiation and leukaemia in children around Sellafield. Int J Radiat Biol 60:581–595.

BERAL V. 1990. Childhood leukemia near nuclear plants in the United Kingdom: the evolution of a systematic approach to studying rare disease in small geographic areas. Am J Epidemiol 132:563–568.

BERAL V, ROMAN E, BOBROW M, EDS. 1993. Childhood Cancer and Nuclear Installations. London: BMJ Publishing Group.

BIRCH JM, HARTLEY AL, MARSDEN HB, et al. 1984. Excess risk of breast cancer in the mothers of children with soft tissue sarcomas. Br J Cancer 49:325–331.

BIRCH JM, HARTLEY AL, TEARE MD, et al. 1990. The Inter-Regional Epidemiological Study of Childhood Cancer (IRESCC): case-control study of children with central nervous system tumors. Br J Neurosurg 4:17–26.

BIRCH JM, HARTLEY AL, TRICKER KJ, et al. 1994. Prevalence and diversity of constitutional mutations in the p53 gene among 21 Li-Fraumeni families. Cancer Res 54:1298–1304.

BIRCH JM, MARSDEN HB. 1987. A classification scheme for childhood cancer. Int J Cancer 40:620–624.

BIRCH JM, MARSDEN HB, MORRIS JONES PH, et al. 1988. Improvements in survival from childhood cancer: results of a population based survey over 30 years. Br Med J 296:1372–1376.

BIRCH JM, MARSDEN HB, SWINDELL R. 1980. Incidence of malignant disease in childhood: a 24-year review of the Manchester Children's Tumor Registry. Br J Cancer 42:215–223.

BITHELL JF, DRAPER GF, GORBACH PD. 1973. Association between malignant disease in children and maternal virus infections. Br Med J 1:706–708.

BITHELL JF, DUTTON SJ, DRAPER GJ, NEARY NM. 1994. Distribution of childhood leukemia and non-Hodgkin's lymphomas near nuclear installations in England and Wales. Br Med J 309:501–505.

BITHELL JF, STEWART AM. 1975. Pre-natal irradiation and childhood malignancy: a review of British data from the Oxford Study. Br J Cancer 31:271–287.

BITHELL JF, STILLER CA. 1988. A new calculation of the carcinogenic risk of obstetric x-raying. Stat Med 7:857–864.

BLACK D. 1984. Investigation of the possible increased incidence of cancer West Cumbria. London: Her Majesty's Stationery Office.

BLATT J, JAFFE R, DEUTSCH M, et al. 1986. Neurofibromatosis and childhood tumors. Cancer 57:1225–1229.

BLEYER WA. 1990. The impact of childhood cancer on the United States and the world. CA 40:355–367.

BLEYER WA. 1993. What can be learned about childhood cancer from "Cancer Statistics Review 1973–1988." Cancer 71:3229–3236.

BLOT WJ, DRAPER G, KINLEN L, et al. 1980. Childhood cancer in relation to prenatal exposure to chickenpox. Br J Cancer 42:342–344.

BOGGER-GOREN S, ZAIZOV R, VOGEL R, et al. 1983. Clinical and virological observations in childhood Hodgkin's disease in Israel. Isr J Med Sci 19:989–991.

BOICE JD. 1990. Studies of atomic bomb survivors: understanding radiation effects (Editorial). JAMA 264:622–623.

BONAÏTI-PELLIÉ C, CHOMPRET A, TOURNADE MF, et al. 1992. Genetics and epidemiology of Wilms' tumor: The French Wilms' Tumor Study. Med Pediatr Oncol 20:284–291.

BOND JV. 1975. Bilateral Wilms' tumors: age at diagnosis, associated congenital anomalies, and possible pattern of inheritance. Lancet 2:482–484.

BONDY ML, LUSTBADER ED, BUFFLER PA, et al. 1991. Genetic epidemiology of childhood brain tumors. Genet Epidemiol 8:253–267.

BONETTA L, KUEHN SE, HUANG A, et al. 1990. Wilms tumor locus on 11p13 defined by multiple CpG island-associated transcripts. Science 250:994–997.

BORING CC, SQUIRES TS, TONG T, et al. 1994. Cancer Statistics, 1994. Atlanta, Georgia: American Cancer Society.

BOSTON COLLABORATIVE DRUG SURVEILLANCE PROGRAM. 1973. Diethylstilbestrol in pregnancy. Cancer 31:573–577.

BOWMAN WP, PRESBURY G, MELVIN SL, et al. 1984. A comparative analysis of acute lymphocytic leukemia in white and black children: presenting clinical features and immunological markers. In: *Pathogenesis of Leukemias and Lymphomas: Environmental Influences.* Magrath IT, O'Conor GT, Ramot B (eds). New York: Raven Press, pp 169–177.

BRESLOW NE, BECKWITH JB, CIOL M, et al. 1988a. Age distribution of Wilms' tumor: report from the National Wilms' Tumor Study. Cancer Res 48:1653–1657.

BRESLOW NE, LANGHOLZ B. 1983. Childhood cancer incidence: geographical and temporal variations. Int J Cancer 32:703–716.

BRESLOW NE, NORKOOL PA, OLSHAN A, et al. 1988b. Second malignant neoplasms in survivors of Wilms' Tumor: a report from the National Wilms' Tumor Study. J Natl Cancer Inst 80:592–595.

BRESLOW N, OLSHAN A, BECKWITH JB, et al. 1994. Ethnic variation in the incidence, diagnosis, prognosis, and follow-up of children with Wilms' tumor. J Natl Cancer Inst 86:49–51.

BRODEUR GM. 1990. Neuroblastoma: clinical significance of genetic abnormalities. Cancer Surv 9:673–688.

BRODEUR GM. 1994. The NF1 gene in myelopoiesis and childhood myelodysplastic syndromes. N Engl J Med 330:637–639.

BRODEUR GM, FONG CT. 1989. Molecular biology and genetics of human neuroblastoma. Cancer Genet Cytogenet 41:153–174.

BRODEUR GM, SEKHON GS, GOLDSTEIN MN. 1977. Chromosomal aberrations in human neuroblastomas. Cancer 40:2256–2263.

BROSS IDJ, NATARAJAN N. 1974. Risk of leukemia in susceptible children exposed to preconception, in utero, and postnatal radiation. Prev Med 3:361–369.

BROWNING D, GROSS S. 1968. Epidemiological studies of acute childhood leukemia: a survey of Cuyahoga County, Ohio. Am J Dis Child 116:576–585.

BUCKLEY JD, HOBBIE WL, RUCCIONE K, et al. 1986. Re: Maternal smoking during pregnancy and the risk of childhood cancer. Lancet 2:519–520.

BUCKLEY JD, ROBINSON LL, SWOTINSKY R, et al. 1989a. Occupational exposures of parents of children with acute nonlymphocytic leukemia: a report from the Childrens Cancer Study Group. Cancer Res 49:4030–4037.

BUCKLEY JD, SATHER H, RUCCIONE K, et al. 1989b. A case-control study risk factors for hepatoblastoma: a report from the Childrens Cancer Study Group. Cancer 64:1169–1176.

BUNIN GR, EMANUEL BS, MEADOWS AT, et al. 1989a. Frequency of 13q abnormalities among 203 patients with retinoblastoma. J Natl Cancer Inst 81:370–374.

BUNIN GR, KRAMER S, MARRERO O, et al. 1987. Gestational risk factors for Wilms' tumor: results of case-control study. Cancer Res 47:2972–2977.

BUNIN GR, KUIJTEN RR, BOESEL CP, et al. 1994. Maternal diet and risk of astrocytic glioma in children: a report from the Childrens Cancer Group. Cancer Causes Control 5:177–187.

BUNIN GR, KUIJTEN RR, BUCKLEY JD, et al. 1993. Relation between maternal diet and subsequent primitive neuroectodermal brain tumors in young children. N Engl J Med 329:536–541.

BUNIN GR, MEADOWS AT, EMANUEL BS, et al. 1989b. Pre- and postconception factors associated with sporadic heritable and nonheritable retinoblastoma. Cancer Res 49:5730–5735.

BUNIN GR, NASS CC, KRAMER S, et al. 1989c. Parental occupation and Wilms' tumor: results of a case-control study. Cancer Res 49:725–729.

BUNIN GR, WARD E, KRAMER S, et al. 1990. Neuroblastoma and parental occupation. Am J Epidemiol 131:776–780.

BURCH PRJ. 1970. Prenatal radiation exposure and childhood cancer. Lancet 2:1189.

CAIRNEY AEL, ANDREWS M, GREENBERG M, et al. 1987. Wilms tumor in three patients with Bloom syndrome. J Pediatr 111:414–416.

CALL KM, GLASER T, ITO CY, et al. 1990. Isolation and characterization of a zinc finger polypeptide gene at the human chromosome 11 Wilms' tumor locus. Cell 60:509–520.

CARLSEN NLT. 1986. Epidemiological investigations on neuroblastomas in Denmark 1943–1980. Br J Cancer 54:977–988.

CARTWRIGHT RA. 1992. Leukemia clusters around nuclear facilities in Britain. Cancer Causes Control 3:393–394.

CARTWRIGHT RA, MCKINNEY PA, HOPTON PA, et al. 1984. Ultrasound examinations in pregnancy and childhood cancer. Lancet 2:999–1000.

CAWTHON RM, WEISS R, XU G, et al. 1990. A major segment of the neurofibromatosis type 1 gene: cDNA sequence, genomic structure, and point mutations. Cell 62:193–201.

CHATTEN J, VOORHESS ML. 1967. Familial neuroblastoma: report of a kindred with multiple disorders, including neuroblastomas in four siblings. N Engl J Med 277:1230–1236.

CLAPP RW, COBB S, CHAN CK, WALKER B JR. 1987. Re: leukemia near Massachusetts nuclear power plant. Lancet 2:1324–1325.

COLLMAN GW, LOOMIS DP, SANDLER DP. 1991. Childhood cancer mortality and radon concentration in drinking water in North Carolina. Br J Cancer 63:626–629.

COLEMAN MP, BELL CMJ, TAYLOR HL, et al. 1989. Leukaemia and residence near electricity transmission equipment: a case-control study. Br J Cancer 60:793–798.

COMSTOCK GW, MARTINEZ I, LIVESAY VT. 1975. Efficacy of BCG vaccination in prevention of cancer. J Natl Cancer Inst 54:835–839.

COOK-MOZAFFARI PJ, DARBY SC, DOLL R, et al. 1989a. Geographical variation in mortality from leukemia and other cancers in England and Wales in relation to proximity to nuclear installations, 1969–78. Br J Cancer 59:476–485.

COOK-MOZAFFARI PJ, DARBY SC, DOLL R. 1989b. Cancer near potential sites of nuclear installations. Lancet 2:1145–1147.

COPELAND KT, CHECKOWAY H, MCMICHAEL AJ, et al. 1977. Bias due to misclassification in the estimation of relative risk. Am J Epidemiol 105:488–495.

COPPES MJ, WILLIAMS BRG. 1994. The molecular genetics of Wilms tumor. Cancer Invest 12:57–65.

COURT BROWN WM, DOLL R. 1961. Leukaemia in childhood and young adult life: trends in mortality in relation to aetiology. Br Med J 1:981–988.

COURT BROWN WM, DOLL R, HILL AB. 1960. Incidence of leukemia after exposure to diagnostic radiation in utero. Br Med J 2:1539–1545.

CULLEN JW. 1991. Second malignant neoplasms in survivors of childhood cancer. Pediatrician 18:82–89.

DAHLQUIST G, WALL S. 1986. Re: maternal smoking during pregnancy and the risk of childhood cancer. Lancet 2:519.

DALING JR, STARZYK P, OLSHAN AF, et al. 1984. Birth weight and the incidence of childhood cancer. J Natl Cancer Inst 72:1039–1041.

DARBY SC, DOLL R. 1987. Fallout, radiation doses near Dounreay, and childhood leukemia. Br Med J 294:603–607.

DARBY SC, OLSEN JH, DOLL R, et al. 1992. Trends in childhood leukaemia in the Nordic countries in relation to fallout from atmospheric nuclear weapons testing. Br Med J 304:1005–1009.

DAVIS MK, SAVITZ DA, GRAUBARD BI. 1988. Infant feeding and childhood cancer. Lancet 2:365–368.

DAVIS S, ROGERS MAM, PENDERGRASS TW. 1987. The incidence and epidemiologic characteristics of neuroblastoma in the United States. Am J Epidemiol 126:1063–1074.

DELEMARRE-VAN DE WAAL HA, ODINK RJH, GRAUW TJ, et al. 1988. Re: leukaemia in patients treated with growth hormone. Lancet 1:1159.

DE NULLY BROWN P, HERTZ H, OLSEN JH, et al. 1989. Incidence of childhood cancer in Denmark 1943–1984. Int J Epidemiol 18:546–555.

DE-THÈ G. 1985. Epstein-Barr virus and Burkitt's lymphoma worldwide: the causal relationship revisited. IARC Sci Publ 60:165–176.

DE-THÈ G, GESER A, DAY NE, et al. 1978. Epidemiological evidence for a causal relationship between Epstein-Barr virus and Burkitt's lymphoma: results of the Uganda prospective study. Nature 274:756–761.

DEVESA SS, SILVERMAN DT, YOUNG JL, JR. 1987. Cancer incidence and mortality trends among whites in the United States, 1947–84. J Natl Cancer Inst 79:701–745.

DIAMOND EL, SCHMERLER H, LILIENFELD AM. 1973. The relationship of intra-uterine radiation to subsequent mortality and development of leukemia in children. Am J Epidemiol 97:283–313.

DOPFER R, NIETHAMMER D. 1993. Report on the international workshop of the Kind Philipp Foundation on late effects after bone marrow transplantation in childhood malignancies. Pediatr Hematol Oncol 10:63–84.

DRAPER GJ, BIRCH JM, BITHELL JF, et al. 1982. Childhood Cancer in Britain: Incidence, Survival and Mortality. London: HMSO.

DRAPER GJ, HEAF MM, KINNIER-WILSON LM. 1977. Occurrence of childhood cancers among sibs and estimation of familial risks. J Med Genet 14:81–90.

DRAPER GJ, KROLL ME, STILLER CA. 1994. Childhood cancer. In: *Trends in Cancer Incidence and Mortality*, Doll R, Fraumeni JF Jr, Muir CS (eds). Cancer Surveys 19/20. New York: Cold Spring Harbor Laboratory Press, pp 493–517.

DRAPER G, MCNINCH A. 1993. Vitamin K for neonates: the controversy. Br Med J 308:867–868.

DRAPER GJ, SANDERS BM, KINGSTON JE. 1986. Second primary neoplasms in patients with retinoblastoma. Cancer 53:661–671.

DRAPER GJ, STILLER CA, CARTWRIGHT RA, et al. 1993. Cancer in Cumbria and in the vicinity of the Sellafield nuclear installation, 1963–90. Br Med J 306:89–94.

EGUIGUREN JM, RIBEIRO RS, PUI C-H, et al. 1991. Secondary non-Hodgkin's lymphoma after treatment for childhood cancer. Leukemia 5:908–911.

EKELUND H, FINNSTRÖM O, GUNNARSKOG J, et al. 1993. Administration of vitamin K to newborn infants and childhood cancer. Br Med J 307:89–91.

EMERSON JC, MALONE KE, DALING JR, et al. 1991. Childhood brain tumor risk in relation to birth characteristics. J Clin Epidemiol 44:1159–1166.

ENG C, LI FP, ABRAMSON DH, et al. 1993. Mortality from second tumors among long-term survivors of retinoblastoma. J Natl Cancer Inst 85:1121–1128.

ENG C, STRATTON M, PONDER B, et al. 1994. Familial cancer syndromes. Lancet 343:709–713.

ERICSSON JLE, KARNSTROM L, MATTSON B. 1978. Childhood cancer in Sweden, 1958–1974. Acta Paediatr Scand 67:425–432.

EVANS HJ. 1990. Ionising radiation from nuclear establishments and childhood leukemias—an enigma. Bio Essays 12:541–549.

EWINGS PD, BOWIE C, PHILLIPS MJ, et al. 1989. Incidence of leukemia in young people in the vicinity of Hinkley Point nuclear power station, 1959–86. Br Med J 299:289–293.

FABIA J, THUY TD. 1974. Occupation of father at time of birth of children dying of malignant diseases. Br J Prev Soc Med 28:98–100.

FARWELL J, FLANNERY JT. 1984a. Second primaries in children with central nervous system tumors. J Neurooncol 2:371–375.

FARWELL J, FLANNERY JT. 1984b. Cancer in relatives of children with nervous-system neoplasms. N Engl J Med 311:749–753.

FASAL E, JACKSON EW, KLAUBER MR. 1971. Birth characteristics and leukemia in childhood. J Natl Cancer Inst 47:501–509.

FEDRICK J, ALBERMAN EA. 1972. Reported influenza in pregnancy and subsequent cancer in the child. Br Med J 2:485–488.

FEINGOLD L, SAVITZ DA, JOHN EM. 1992. Use of a job-exposure matrix to evaluate parental occupation and childhood cancer. Cancer Causes Control 3:161–169.

FEYCHTING M, AHLBOM A. 1993. Magnetic fields and cancer in children residing near Swedish high-voltage power lines. Am J Epidemiol 138:467–481.

FINE PEM, ADELSTEIN AM, SNOWMAN J, et al. 1985. Longterm effects of exposure to viral infections in utero. Br Med J 290:509–511.

FISHER DA, JOB J-C, PREECE M, et al. 1988. Re: leukemia in patients treated with growth hormone. Lancet 1:1159–1160.

FILIPPINI G, FARINOTTI M, LOVICU G, et al. 1994. Mothers' active and passive smoking during pregnancy and risk of brain tumours in children. Int J Cancer 57:769–774.

FONG C-T, BRODEUR GM. 1987. Down's syndrome and leukemia: epidemiology, genetics, cytogenetics and mechanisms of leukemogenesis. Cancer Genet Cytogenet 28:55–76.

FORD DD, PATERSON JCS, TREUTING WL. 1959. Fetal exposure to diagnostic x-rays, and leukemia and other malignant diseases in childhood. J Natl Cancer Inst 22:1093–1104.

FORSBERG J-G, KALLEN B. 1990. Pregnancy and delivery characteristics of women whose infants develop child cancer. APMIS 98:37–42.

FRADKIN JE, MILLS JL, SCHONBERGER LB, et al. 1993. Risk of leukemia after treatment with pituitary growth hormone. JAMA 270:2829–2832.

FRAUMENI JF, JR, MILLER RW. 1967. Epidemiology of human leukemia: recent observations. J Natl Cancer Inst 38:593–605.

FREIER DT, THOMPSON NW, SISSON JC, et al. 1977. Dilemmas in the early diagnosis and treatment of multiple endocrine adenomatosis, type II. Surgery 82:407–413.

FULTON JP, COBB S, PREBLE L, et al. 1980. Electrical wiring configurations and childhood leukemia in Rhode Island. Am J Epidemiol 111:292–296.

GAILANI MR, BALE SJ, LEFFELL DJ, et al. 1992. Developmental defects in Gorlin Syndrome related to a putative tumor suppressor gene on chromosome 9. Cell 69:111–117.

GARDNER E, PAPI L, EASTON D, et al. 1993. Genetic linkage studies map the multiple endocrine neoplasia type 2 loci to a small interval on chromosome 10q11.2. Hum Molecular Genet 2:241–246.

GARDNER MJ. 1991. Father's occupational exposure to radiation and the raised level of childhood leukemia near the Sellafield nuclear plant. Environ Health Perspect 94:5–7.

GARDNER MJ, HALL AJ, DOWNES S, et al. 1987a. Follow-up study of children born to mothers resident in Seascale, West Cumbria (birth cohort). Br Med J 295:222–227.

GARDNER MJ, HALL AJ, DOWNES S, et al. 1987b. Follow up study of children born elsewhere but attending schools in Seascale, West Cumbria (schools cohort). Br Med J 295:819–822.

GARDNER MJ, SNEE MP, HALL AJ, et al. 1990. Results of the case-control study of leukemia and lymphoma among young people near Sellafield nuclear plant in West Cumbria. Br Med J 300:423–429.

GATTI RA, BERKEL I, BODER E, BRAEDT G, et al. 1988. Localisation of an ataxia telangiectasia gene to chromosome 11q22–23. Nature 336:577–580.

GERMAN J, BLOOM D, PASSARGE E. 1979. Bloom's syndrome. VII. Progress report for 1978. Clin Genet 15:361–367.

GESER A, DE-THE G, LENOIR G, et al. 1982. Final case reporting from the Ugandan prospective study of the relationship between EBV and Burkitt's lymphoma. Int J Cancer 29:397–400.

GESSLER M, POUSTKA A, CAVENEE W, et al. 1990. Homozygous deletion in Wilms' tumours of a zinc-finger gene identified by chromosome jumping. Nature 343:774–778.

GHALI MH, YOO K-Y, FLANNERY JT, et al. 1992. Association between childhood rhabdomyosarcoma and maternal history of still births. Int J Cancer 50:365–368.

GIACCHINO R, NAVONE C, FACCO F, et al. 1991. HB-DNA-related hepatocellular carcinoma occurring in childhood: report of three cases. Dig Dis Sci 36:1143–1146.

GILLIAM AG, MACMAHON B. 1960. Geographic distribution and trends of leukemia in the United States. Acta Unio Int Contra Cancrum 16:1623–1628.

GILLIAM AG, WALTER WA. 1958. Trends of mortality from leukemia in the United States, 1921–55. Public Health Rep 73:773–784.

GILMAN EA, KINNEAR-WILSON LM, KNEALE GW, et al. 1989. Childhood cancers and their association with pregnancy drugs and illnesses. Paediatr Perinat Epidemiol 3:66–94.

GILMAN EA, KNEALE GW, KNOX EG, et al. 1988. Pregnancy x-rays and childhood cancers: effects of exposure age and radiation dose. J Radiol Prot 8:3–8.

GIRVAN DP, HOLLIDAY RL. 1987. Pediatric implications of multiple endocrine neoplasia. J Pediatr Surg 22:806–808.

GIUFFRE R, LICCARDO G, PASTORE FS, et al. 1990. Potential risk factors for brain tumors in children. Childs Nerv Syst 6:8–12.

GLASS AG, FRAUMENI JF JR. 1970. Epidemiology of bone cancer in children. J Natl Cancer Inst 58:1267–1270.

GLOVER TW, STEIN CK, LEGIUS E, et al. 1991. Molecular and cytogenetic analysis of tumors in von Recklinghausen neurofibromatosis. Genes Chromosom Cancer 3:62–70.

GOLD EB, DIENER MD, SZKLO M. 1982. Parental occupations and cancer in children: a case-control study and review of the methodologic issues. J Occup Med 24:578–584.

GOLD E, GORDIS L, TONASCIA J, et al. 1978. Increased risk of brain tumors in children exposed to barbiturates. J Natl Cancer Inst 61:1031–1034.

GOLD E, GORDIS L, TONASCIA J, et al. 1979. Risk factors for brain tumors in children. Am J Epidemiol 109:309–319.

GOLD EB, LEVITON A, LOPEZ R, et al. 1993. Parental smoking and risk of childhood brain tumors. Am J Epidemiol 137:620–628.

GOLD EB, LEVITON A, LOPEZ R, et al. 1994. The role of family history in risk of childhood brain tumors. Cancer 73:1302–1311.

GOLDHABER MK, SELBY JV, HIATT RA, et al. 1990. Exposure to barbiturates in utero and during childhood and risk of intracranial and spinal cord tumors. Cancer Res 50:4600–4603.

GOLDING J, GREENWOOD R, BIRMINGHAM K, et al. 1992. Childhood cancer, intramuscular vitamin K, and pethidine given during labor. Br Med J 305:341–346.

GOLDING J, PATERSON M, KINLEN LJ. 1990. Factors associated with childhood cancer in a national cohort study. Br J Cancer 62:304–308.

GOLDSTEIN AM, STEWART C, BALE AE, et al. 1994. Localization of the gene for the Nevoid Basal Cell Carcinoma Syndrome. Am J Hum Genet 54:765–773.

GRAHAM S, LEVIN ML, LILIENFELD AM, et al. 1966. Preconception, intrauterine and postnatal irradiation as related to leukemia. NCI Monogr 19:347–371.

GREAVES MF, CHAN LC. 1986. Is spontaneous mutation the major "cause" of childhood acute lymphoblastic leukemia? Br J Haematol 64:1–13.

GREAVES MF. 1988. Speculations on the cause of childhood acute lymphoblastics leukemia. Leukemia 2:120–125.

GREAVES MF. 1990. The Sellafield childhood leukemia cluster: are germline mutations responsible? Leukemia 4:391–396.

GREENBERG RS. 1983. The Population Distribution and Possible Determinants of Neuroblastoma in Children (Dissertation). Chapel Hill, University of North Carolina.

GREENBERG RS, SHUSTER JL, JR. 1985. Epidemiology of cancer in children. Epidemiol Rev 7:22–48.

GRUFFERMAN S, WANG HH, DELONG ER, et al. 1982. Environmental factors in the etiology of rhabdomyosarcoma in childhood. J Natl Cancer Inst 68:107–113.

GUTENSOHN N, COLE P. 1981. Childhood social environment and Hodgkin's disease. N Engl J Med 304:135–140.

HAAG MM, SOUKUP SW, NEELY JE. 1981. Chromosome analysis of a human neuroblastoma. Cancer Res 41:2995–2999.

HABER DA, HOUSMAN DE. 1992. Role of the WT1 gene in Wilms' tumour. Cancer Surv 12:105–117.

HAKULINEN T, HOVI L, KARKINEN-JAAKELAINEN M, et al. 1973. Association between influenza during pregnancy and childhood leukemia. Br Med J 4:265–267.

HAKULINEN T, SALONEN T, TEPPO L. 1976. Cancer in the offspring of fathers in hydrocarbon-related occupations. Br J Prev Soc Med 30:138–140.

HANSEN MF, CAVENEE WK. 1988. Retinoblastoma and the progression of tumor genetics. Trends Genet 4:125–128.

HANSEN NE, KARLE H, JENSEN OM. 1983. Trends in the incidence of leukemia in Denmark, 1943–77: an epidemiologic study of 14,000 patients. J Natl Cancer Inst 71:697–701.

HARO AS. 1986. The effect of BCG-vaccination and tuberculosis on the risk of leukemia. Dev Biol Stand 58 (part A): 433–449.

HARTLEY AL, BIRCH JM, MCKINNEY PA, et al. 1988a. The Inter-Regional Epidemiological Study of Childhood Cancer (IRESCC): case control study of children with bone and soft tissue sarcomas. Br J Cancer 58:838–842.

HARTLEY AL, BIRCH JM, MCKINNEY PA, et al. 1988b. The Inter-Regional Epidemiological Study of Childhood Cancer (IRESCC): past medical history in children with cancer. J Epidemiol Community Health 42:235–242.

HARVEY EB, BOICE JD, HONEYMAN M, et al. 1985. Prenatal x-ray exposure and childhood cancer in twins. N Engl J Med 312:541–545.

HATCH M, SUSSER M. 1990. Background gamma radiation and childhood cancers within ten miles of a US nuclear plant. Int J Epidemiol 19:546–552.

HAWKINS MM. 1990. Second primary tumors following radiotherapy for childhood cancer. Int J Radiat Oncol Biol Phys 19:1297–1301.

HAWKINS MM, DRAPER GJ, KINSTON JE. 1987. Incidence of second primary tumors among childhood cancer survivors. Br J Cancer 56:339–347.

HAWKINS MM, DRAPER GJ, SMITH RA. 1989. Cancer among 1348 offspring of survivors of childhood cancer. Int J Cancer 43:975–978.

HEASMAN MA, URQUHART JD, BLACK RJ, et al. 1987. Leukaemia in young persons in Scotland: a study of its geographical distribution and relationship to nuclear installations. Health Bull 45:147–151.

HEMMINKI K, SALONIEMI I, SALONEN T, et al. 1981. Childhood cancer and parental occupation in Finland. J Epidemiol Community Health 35:11–15.

HEMPELMANN LH, HALL WJ, PHILLIPS M, et al. 1975. Neoplasms in persons treated with x-rays in infancy: fourth survey in 20 years. J Natl Cancer Inst 55:519–530.

HENDERSON BE, BENTON B, JING J, et al. 1979. Risk factors for cancer of the testis in young men. Int J Cancer 23:598–609.

HENRY I, BONAITI-PELLIÉ C, CHEHENSSE V, et al. 1991. Uniparental paternal disomy in a genetic cancer-predisposing syndrome. Nature 351:665–667.

HENSHAW DL, EATOUGH HP, RICHARDSON RB. 1990. Radon as a causative factor in induction in myeloid leukemia and other cancers. Lancet 335:1008–1012.

HERBST AL. 1981. Clear cell adenocarcinoma and the current status of DES-exposed females. Cancer 48:484–488.

HERBST AL, ANDERSON S, HUBBY MM, et al. 1986. Risk factors for the development of diethystilbestrol-associated clear cell adenocarcinoma: a case-control study. Am J Obstet Gynecol 154:814–822.

HERBST AL, ULFELDER H, POSKANZER DC. 1971. Adenocarcinoma of the vagina: association of maternal stilbestrol therapy with tumor appearance in young females. N Engl J Med 284:878–881.

HEWITT M, MOTT MG. 1992. The assessment of in vivo somatic mutations in survivors of childhood malignancy. Br J Cancer 66:143–147.

HICKS N, ZACK M, CALDWELL GG, et al. 1984. Childhood cancer and occupational radiation exposure in parents. Cancer 53:1637–1643.

HILGARTNER MW. 1993. Vitamin K and the newborn. New Engl J Med 329:957–958.

HILL C, LAPLANCHE A. 1990. Overall mortality and cancer mortality around French nuclear sites. Nature 347:755–757.

HIRAYAMA T. 1980. Descriptive and analytical epidemiology of childhood malignancy in Japan. In: *Recent Advances in Management of Children with Cancer*, Kobayashi N (ed). Tokyo, The Children's Cancer Association of Japan, pp 27–43.

HOLE DJ, GILLIS CR, SUMMER D. 1993. Childhood cancer in birth cohorts with known levels of strontium-90. Health Rep 5:39–43. (Statistics Canada, Cat. 82-003)

HOWE GR, BURCH JD, CHIARELLI AM, et al. 1989. An exploratory case-control study of brain tumors in children. Cancer Res 49:4349–4352.

ICHIMARU M, ISHIMARU T, BELSKY JL. 1978. Incidence of leukemia in atomic bomb survivors belonging to a fixed cohort in Hiroshima and Nagasaki 1950–1971: radiation dose, years after exposure, age at exposure and type of leukemia. J Radiat Res (Tokyo) 19:262–282.

INFANTE PF, EPSTEIN SS, NEWTON WA, JR. 1978. Blood dyscrasias and childhood tumors and exposure to chlordane and heptachlor. Scand J Work Environ Health 4:137–150.

INFANTE-RIVARD C, MUR P, ARMSTRONG B, et al. 1991. Acute lymphoblastic leukaemia among Spanish children and mothers' occupation: a case-control study. J Epidemiol Community Health 45:11–15.

INSKIP PD, HARVEY EB, BOICE JD, et al. 1991. Incidence of childhood cancer in twins. Cancer Causes Control 2:315–324.

JABLON S, KATO H. 1970. Childhood cancer in relation to prenatal exposures to A-bomb radiation. Lancet 2:1000–1003.

JABLON S, KATO H. 1972. Studies of the mortality of A-bomb survivors. 5. Radiation dose and mortality 1950–1970. Radiat Res 50:649–698.

JABLON S, HRUBEC Z, BOICE JD, JR. 1991. Cancer in populations living near nuclear facilities. JAMA 265:1403–1408.

JANKOVIC M, MASERA G, CRISTIANI ML, et al. 1991. Brain tumors as second malignancies in children treated for acute lymphoblastic leukemia. Neurooncol 66:365–369.

JENSEN RD, MILLER RW. 1971. Retinoblastoma: epidemiologic characteristics. N Engl J Med 285:307–311.

JOHN EM, SAVITZ DA, SANDLER DP. 1991. Prenatal exposure to parents' smoking and childhood cancer. Am J Epidemiol 133:123–132.

JOHNSON CC, ANNEGERS JF, FRANKOWSKI RF, et al. 1987. Childhood nervous system tumors—an evaluation of the association with paternal occupational exposure to hydrocarbons. Am J Epidemiol 126:605–613.

JOHNSON CC, SPITZ MR. 1985. Neuroblastoma: case-control analysis of birth characteristics. J Natl Cancer Inst 74:789–792.

JOHNSON CC, SPITZ MR. 1986. Re: prematurity and risk of childhood cancer. J Natl Cancer Inst 76:359.

JOHNSON CC, SPITZ MR. 1989. Childhood nervous system tumours: an assessment of risk associated with paternal occupations involving use, repair or manufacture of electrical and electronic equipment. Int J Epidemiol 18:756–762.

KACZMAREK RG, MOORE RM JR, KEPPEL KG, et al. 1989. X-ray examinations during pregnancy: National Natality Surveys, 1963 and 1980. Am J Public Health 79:75–77.

KADHIM MA, MACDONALD DA, GOODHEAD DT. 1992. Trauma of chromosomal instability after plutonium alpha-particle irradiation. Nature 355:738–740.

KANTOR AF, MCCREA CURNEN MG, MEIGS JW, et al. 1979. Occupations of fathers of patients with Wilms' tumor. J Epidemiol Community Health 33:253–256.

KATO H. 1971. Mortality in children exposed to the A-bombs while in utero, 1945–1969. Am J Epidemiol 93:435–442.

KATO I, TAJIMA K, HIROSE K, et al. 1985. A descriptive epidemiologic study of hematopoietic neoplasms in Japan. Jpn J Clin Oncol 15:347–364.

KAYE SA, ROBISON LL, SMITHSON WA, et al. 1991. Maternal reproductive history and birth characteristics in childhood acute lymphoblastic leukemia. Cancer 68:1351–1355.

KINLEN L. 1988. Evidence for an infective cause of childhood leukaemia: comparison of a Scottish New Town with nuclear reprocessing sites in Britain. Lancet 2:1323–1327.

KINLEN LJ. 1993. Can paternal preconceptional radiation account for the increase of leukemia and non-Hodgkin's lymphoma in Seascale? Br Med J 306:1718–1721.

KINLEN LJ, CLARKE K, BALKWILL A. 1993a. Paternal preconceptional radiation exposure in the nuclear industry and leukemia and non-Hodgkin's lymphoma in young people in Scotland. Br Med J 306:1153–1158.

KINLEN LJ, CLARKE K, HUDSON C. 1990. Evidence from population mixing in British New Towns 1946–85 of an infective basis for childhood leukemia. Lancet 336:577–582.

KINLEN LJ, HUDSON CM, STILLER CA. 1991. Contacts between adults as evidence for an infective origin of childhood leukemia: an explanation for the excess near nuclear establishments in West Berkshire. Br J Cancer 64:549–554.

KINLEN LJ, O'BRIEN F, CLARKE K, et al. 1993b. Rural population mixing and childhood leukemia: effects of the North Sea oil industry in Scotland, including the area near Dounreay nuclear site. Br Med J 306:743–748.

KINNIER WILSON LM, WATERHOUSE JAH. 1984. Obstetric ultrasound and childhood malignancies. Lancet 2:997–999.

KLEBANOFF MA, READ JS, MILLS JL, SHIONO PH. 1993. The risk of childhood cancer after neonatal exposure to vitamin K. N Engl J Med 329:905–908.

KNEALE GW, STEWART AM, KINNIER WILSON LM. 1986. Immunizations against infectious diseases and childhood cancers. Cancer Immunol Immunother 21:129–132.

KNUDSON AG, JR. 1971. Mutation and cancer: statistical study of retinoblastoma. Proc Natl Acad Sci U S A 68:820–823.

KNUDSON AG, JR. 1986. Genetics of human cancer. Ann Rev Genet 20:231–251.

KNUDSON AG, JR, MEADOWS AT, NICHOLS WW, et al. 1976. Chromosomal deletion and retinoblastoma. N Engl J Med 295:1120–1123.

KNUDSON AG, JR, STRONG L. 1972. Mutation and cancer: a model for Wilms' tumor of the kidney. J Natl Cancer Inst 48:313–323.

KOEFFLER HP. 1985. Vitamin D: myeloid differentiation and proliferation. Haematol Blood Transf 29:409–417.

KOEFFLER HP. 1986. Human acute myeloid leukemia lines: models of leukemogenesis. Semin Hematol 23:223–236.

KOMP D, ROGOL A, SABIO H. 1977. Possible effects of growth hormone on development of acute lymphoblastic leukemia. Lancet 2:434–435.

KOO HP, HENSLE TW. 1993. Molecular biology of Wilms' tumor. Urol Clin North Am 20:323–331.

KOUFOS A, GRUNDY P, MORGAN K, et al. 1989. Familial Wiedemann-Beckwith syndrome and a second Wilms tumor locus both map to 11p15.5. Am J Hum Genet 44:711–719.

KRAMER S, WARD E, MEADOWS AT, et al. 1987. Medical and drug risk factors associated with neuroblastoma: a case-control study. J Natl Cancer Inst 78:797–804.

KREISSMAN SG, GELBER RD, COHEN HJ, et al. 1992. Incidence of secondary acute myelogenous leukemia after treatment of childhood acute lymphoblastic leukemia. Cancer 70:2208–2213.

KRISTENSEN P, ANDERSEN A. 1992. A cohort study on cancer incidence in offspring of male printing workers. Epidemiology 3:6–10.

KUIJTEN RR, BUNIN GR. 1993. Risk factors for childhood brain tumors. Cancer Epidemiol Biomark Prev 2:277–288.

KUIJTEN RR, BUNIN GR, NASS CC, et al. 1990. Gestational and familial risk factors for childhood astrocytoma: results of a case-control study. Cancer Res 50:2608–2612.

KUIJTEN RR, BUNIN GR, NASS CC, et al. 1992. Parental occupation and childhood astrocytoma: results of a case-control study. Cancer Res 52:782–786.

KUIJTEN RR, STROM SS, RORKE LB, et al. 1993. Family history of cancer and seizures in young children with brain tumors: a report from the Childrens Cancer Group. Cancer Causes Control 4:455–464.

KUSHNER BH, GILBERT F, HELSON L. 1986. Familial neuroblastoma. Cancer 57:1887–1893.

KWA SL, FINE LJ. 1980. The association between parental occupation and childhood malignancy. J Occup Med 22:792–794.

LAND CE. 1979. The hazards of fallout or of epidemiologic research? N Engl J Med 300:431–432.

LAND CE, MCKAY FW, MACHADO SG. 1984. Childhood leukemia and fallout from the Nevada nuclear tests. Science 223:139–144.

LANNERING B, MARKY I, NORDBORG C. 1990. Brain tumors in childhood and adolescence in West Sweden 1970–1984. Cancer 66:604–609.

LARSSON C, SKOGSEID B, OBERG K, et al. 1988. Multiple endocrine neoplasia type 1 gene maps to chromosome 11 and is lost in insulinoma. Nature 332:85–87.

LECK I, STEWARD JK. 1972. Incidence of neoplasms in children born after influenza epidemics. Br Med J 4:631–634.

LEUSCHNER I, HARMS D, SCHMIDT D. 1988. The association of hepatocellular carcinoma in childhood with hepatitis B virus infection. Cancer 62:2363–2369.

LEVINE AJ. 1992. The p53 tumor-suppressor gene (Editorial). N Engl J Med 326:1350–1352.

LI FP. 1982. Cancers in children. In: *Cancer Epidemiology and Prevention*, Schottenfeld D, Fraumeni JF, Jr (eds). Philadelphia: W.B. Saunders, pp 1012–1024.

LI FP, FRAUMENI JF, JR. 1969a. Soft-tissue sarcomas, breast cancer, and other neoplasms: a familial syndrome? Ann Intern Med 71:747–752.

LI FP, FRAUMENI JF, JR. 1969b. Rhadomyosarcoma in children: epidemiologic study and identification of a familial cancer syndrome. J Natl Cancer Inst 43:1365–1373.

LI FP, FRAUMENI JF, JR. 1982. Prospective study of a family cancer syndrome. JAMA 247:2692–2694.

LI FP, FRAUMENI JF, JR, MULVIHILL JJ, et al. 1988. A cancer family syndrome in twenty-four kindreds. Cancer Res 48:5358–5362.

LI FP, TU JT, LIU FS, et al. 1980. Rarity of Ewing's sarcoma in China. Lancet 1:1255–1258.

LI FP, YAN JC, SALLAN S, et al. 1983. Second neoplasms after Wilms' tumor in childhood. J Natl Cancer Inst 71:1205–1209.

LIN SR, LU PY. 1989. An epidemiologic study of childhood cancer in relation to residential exposure to electromagnetic fields. Abstract from DOE/EPRI 'Contractors' meeting, Portland, Oregon.

LINET MS. 1985. The Leukemias: Epidemiological Aspects. Monographs in Epidemiology and Biostatistics. New York: Oxford University Press.

LINET MS, BOICE JD. 1993. Radiation from Chernobyl and risk of childhood leukemia. Eur J Cancer 29A:1–3.

LINET MS, DEVESA SS. 1991. Descriptive epidemiology of childhood leukaemia. Br J Cancer 63:424–429.

LINET MS, STEWART WF, VAN NATTA M, et al. 1987. Comparison of methods for determining occupational exposure in a case-control interview study of chronic lymphocytic leukemia. J Occup Med 29:136–141.

LITTLEFIELD JW. 1984. Genes, chromosomes, and cancer. J Pediatr 104:489–494.

LONDON SJ, THOMAS DC, BOWMAN JD, et al. 1991. Exposure to residential electric and magnetic fields and risk of childhood leukemia. Am J Epidemiol 134:923–937.

LORENZ R, FUHRMANN W. 1978. Familial basal cell nevus syndrome. Hum Genet 44:153–163.

LOWENGART RA, PETERS JM, CICIONI C, et al. 1987. Childhood leukemia and parents' occupational and home exposures. J Natl Cancer Inst 79:39–46.

LYNCH HT. 1982. Hereditary factors in childhood cancer. Paediatrician 11:205–221.

LYON JL, KLAUBER MR, GARDNER JW, et al. 1979. Childhood leukemias associated with fallout from nuclear testing. N Engl J Med 300:397–402.

MACHADO SG, LAND CE, MCKAY FW. 1987. Cancer mortality and radioactive fallout in southwestern Utah. Am J Epidemiol 125:44–61.

MACMAHON B. 1962. Prenatal x-ray exposure and childhood cancer. J Natl Cancer Inst 28:1173–1191.

MACMAHON B. 1985. Prenatal x-ray exposure and twins. N Engl J Med 312:576–577.

MACMAHON B. 1989. Some recent issues in low-exposure radiation epidemiology. Environ Health Perspect 81:131–135.

MACMAHON B. 1992a. Is acute lymphoblastic leukemia in children virus-related? Am J Epidemiol 136:916–924.

MACMAHON B. 1992b. Leukemia clusters around nuclear facilities in Britain. Cancer Causes Control 3:283–288.

MACMAHON B, NEWILL VA. 1962. Birth characteristics of children dying of malignant neoplasms. J Natl Cancer Inst 28:231–244.

MAGNANI C, PASTORE G, TERRACINI B. 1988. Re: infant feeding and childhood cancer. Lancet 2:1136.

MALKIN D, JOLLY KW, BARBIER N, et al. 1992. Germ line mutations of the p53 tumor-suppressor gene in children and young adults with second malignant neoplasms. N Engl J Med 326:1309–1315.

MALKIN D, LI FP, STRONG LC, et al. 1990. Germ line p53 mutations in a familial syndrome of breast cancer, sarcomas, and other neoplasms. Science 250:1233–1238.

MANNING MD, CARROLL BE. 1957. Some epidemiological aspects of leukemia in children. J Natl Cancer Inst 19:1087–1094.

MATSUI I, TANIMURA M, KOBAYASHI N, et al. 1993. Neurofibromatosis type 1 and childhood cancer. Cancer 72:2746–2754.

MATSUNAGA E, MINODA K, SASAKI MS. 1990. Parental age and seasonal variation in the births of children with sporadic retinoblastoma: a mutation-epidemiologic study. Hum Genet 84:155–158.

MATTSON B, WALLGREN J. 1984. Completeness of registration in the Swedish Cancer Registry. Non-notified cancer recorded on death certificates in 1978. Acta Radiol (Oncol) 23:305–131.

MCCREA CURNEN MG, VARMA AAO, CHRISTINE BW, et al. 1974. Childhood leukemia and maternal infectious disease during pregnancy. J Natl Cancer Inst 53:943–947.

MCCREDIE M, MAISONNEUVE P, BOYLE P. 1994a. Antenatal risk factors for malignant brain tumours in New South Wales children. Int J Cancer 56:6–10.

MCCREDIE M, MAISONNEUVE P, BOYLE P. 1994b. Perinatal and early postnatal risk factors for malignant brain tumours in New South Wales children. Int J Cancer 56:11–15.

MCINTYRE JF, SMITH-SORENSEN B, FRIEND SH, et al. 1994. Germline mutations of the p53 tumor suppressor gene in children with osteosarcoma. J Clin Oncol 12:925–930.

MCKINNEY PA, ALEXANDER FE, CARTWRIGHT RA, PARKER L. 1991. Parental occupations of children with leukaemia in West Cumbria, North Humberside, and Gateshead. Br Med J 302:681–687.

MCKINNEY PA, CARTWRIGHT RA, SAIN JMT, et al. 1987. The Interregional Epidemiological Study of Childhood Cancers (IRESCC): a case-control study of aetiological factors in leukemia and lymphoma. Arch Dis Child 62:279–287.

MCKINNEY PA, CARTWRIGHT RA, STILLER CA, et al. 1985. Inter-Regional Epidemiological Study of Childhood Cancer (IRESCC): childhood cancer and the consumption of Debendox and related drugs in pregnancy. Br J Cancer 52:923–929.

MCKINNEY PA, STILLER CA. 1986. Re: Maternal smoking during pregnancy and the risk of childhood cancer. Lancet 2:519.

MCKUSICK VA. 1992. Mendelian Inheritance in Man. 10th Edition. Baltimore: The Johns Hopkins University Press.

MCLAUGHLIN JR, CLARKE EA, NISHRI D, ANDERSON TW. 1993a. Childhood leukemia in the vicinity of Canadian nuclear facilities. Cancer Causes Control 4:51–58.

MCLAUGHLIN JR, KING WD, ANDERSON TW, et al. 1993b. Paternal radiation exposure and leukemia in offspring: the Ontario case-control study. Br Med J 307:959–966.

MCWHIRTER WR. 1982. The relationship of incidence of childhood lymphoblastic leukemia to social class. Br J Cancer 46:640–645.

MEADOWS AT, BAUM E, FOSSATI-BELLANI F, et al. 1985. Second malignant neoplasms in children: an update from the late effects study group. J Clin Oncol 3:532–538.

MEADOWS AT, OBRINGER AC, MARRERO O, et al. 1989. Second malignant neoplasms following childhood Hodgkin's disease: treatment and splenectomy as risk factors. Med Pediatr Oncol 17:477–484.

MELBYE M, EBBESEN P, LEVINE PH, et al. 1984. Early primary infection and high Epstein-Barr virus antibody titers in Greenland Eskimos at high risk for nasopharyngeal carcinoma. Int J Cancer 34:619–623.

MELNICK S, COLE P, ANDERSON D, et al. 1987. Rates and risks of diethylstilbestrol-related clear-cell adenocarcinoma of the vaginal and cervix: an update. N Engl J Med 316:514–516.

METTLER FA, MOSELEY RD. 1985. Medical Effects of Ionizing Radiation. Orlando, Grune & Stratton.

MICHAELIS J, KELLER B, HAAF G, KAATSCH P. 1992. Incidence of childhood malignancies in the vicinity of West German nuclear power plants. Cancer Causes Control 3:255–263.

MIKE V, MEADOWS AT, D'ANGIO GJ. 1982. Incidence of second malignant neoplasms in children: results of an international study. Lancet 2:1326–1331.

MILI F, KHOURY MJ, FLANDERS WD, et al. 1993a. Risk of childhood cancer for infants with birth defects. I. Record-linkage study, Atlanta, Georgia, 1968–1988. Am J Epidemiol 137:629–638.

MILI F, LYNCH CF, KHOURY MJ, et al. 1993b. Risk of childhood cancer for infants with birth defects. II. Record-linkage study, Iowa, 1983–1989. Am J Epidemiol 137:639–644.

MILLER BA, RIES LAG, HANKEY BF, et al, eds. 1993. SEER Cancer Statistics Review: 1973–1990, National Cancer Institute. NIH Pub. No. 93-2789.

MILLER DR, MILLER LP. 1990. Acute lymphoblastic leukemia in children: an update of clinical, biological, and therapeutic aspects. Crit Rev Oncol Hematol 10:131–164.

MILLER RW. 1971. Deaths from childhood leukemia and solid tumors among twins and other sibs in the United States, 1960–1967. J Natl Cancer Inst 46:203–209.

MILLER RW. 1974. Childhood cancer epidemiology: two international activities. NCI Monogr 40:71–74.

MILLER RW. 1981. Contrasting epidemiology of childhood osteosarcoma, Ewing's tumor, and rhabdomyosarcoma. NCI Monogr 56:9–15.

MILLER RW. 1992. Vitamin K and childhood cancer. Br Med J 305:1016.

MILLER RW. 1992. Childhood leukemia and neonatal exposure to lighting in nurseries. Cancer Causes Control 3:581–582.

MILLER RW, FRAUMENI JF, JR, MANNING MD. 1964. Association of Wilms' tumor with aniridia, hemihypertrophy and other congenital malformations. N Engl J Med 270:922–927.

MILLER RW, MCKAY FW. 1984. Decline in U.S. childhood cancer mortality, 1950 through 1980. JAMA 251:1567–1570.

MIYAUCHI J, ASADA M, SASAKI M, et al. 1994. Mutations of the N-ras gene in juvenile chronic myelogenous leukemia. Blood 83:2248–2254.

MODAN B, BAIDATZ D, MART H, et al. 1974. Radiation-induced head and neck tumours. Lancet 1:277–279.

MOLE RH. 1990. Childhood cancer after prenatal exposure to diagnostic x-ray examinations in Britain. Br J Cancer 62:152–160.

MOLE RH. 1974. Antenatal irradiation and childhood cancer: causation or coincidence? Br J Cancer 30:199–208.

MOLE SE, MULLIGAN LM, HEALEY CS, et al. 1993. Localisation of the gene for multiple endocrine neoplasia type 2A to a 480 kb region in chromosome band 10q11.2. Hum Molecular Genet 2:247–252.

MONSON RR, MACMAHON B. 1984. Prenatal X-ray exposure and cancer in children. In: *Radiation Carcinogenesis: Epidemiology and Biological Significance,* Boice JD, Fraumeni JF (eds). New York: Raven Press.

MORRELL D, CROMARTIE E, SWIFT M. 1986. Mortality and cancer incidence in 263 patients with ataxia-telangiectasia. J Natl Cancer Inst 77:89–92.

MORRIS JA. 1994. Childhood cancer around nuclear installations. Eur J Cancer Prev 3:15–21.

MORRIS JA, BUTLER R, FLOWERDEW R, et al. 1993. Retinoblastoma in children of former residents of Seascale. Br Med J 306:650.

MORRIS V. 1990. Space-time interactions in childhood cancers. J Epidemiol Comm Health 44:55–58.

MOSCICKI A-B, WINKLER B, IRWIN CE, SCHACHTER J. 1989. Differences in biologic maturation, sexual behavior, and sexually transmitted disease between adolescents with and without cervical intraepithelial neoplasia. J Pediatr 115:487–493.

MULLIGAN LM, KWOK JWJ, HEALEY CS, et al. 1993. Germ-line mutations of the RET proto-oncogene in multiple endocrine neoplasia type 2A. Nature 363:458–460.

MULVIHILL JJ. 1975. Congenital and genetic diseases. In: *Persons at High Risk of Cancer,* Fraumeni JF Jr (ed). New York: Academic Press, pp 3–37.

MULVIHILL JJ. 1977. Genetic repertory of human neoplasia. In: *Genetics of Human Cancer,* Mulvihill JJ, Miller RW, Fraumeni JF (eds). New York: Raven Press, pp 137–143.

MUNOZ N. 1976. Geographical distribution of childhood tumors. Tumori 62:145–156.

MURRAY R, HECKEL P, HEMPELMANN LH. 1959. Leukemia in children exposed to ionizing radiation. N Engl J Med 261:585–589.

MYERS A, CLAYDEN AD, CARTWRIGHT RA, et al. 1990. Childhood cancer and overhead powerlines: A case-control study. Br J Cancer 60:1008–1013.

NAPALKOV NP. 1986. Prenatal and childhood exposure to carcinogenic factors. Cancer Detect Prev 9:1–7.

NAROD SA, STILLER C, LENOIR GM. 1991. An estimate of the heritable fraction of childhood cancer. Br J Cancer 63:993–999.

NASCA PC, BAPTISTE MS, MACCUBBIN PA, et al. 1988. An epidemiologic case-control study of central nervous system tumors in children and parental occupational exposures. Am J Epidemiol 128:1256–1265.

NATIONAL RADIOLOGICAL PROTECTION BOARD. 1992. Electromagnetic Fields and the Risk of Cancer. Report of an Advisory Group on Non-ionizing Radiation. Vol 3. No 1. Chilton, Didcot, Oxon, National Radiological Protection Board.

NEEL JV, SCHULL WJ, AWA AA, et al. 1990. The children of parents exposed to atomic bombs: estimates of the genetic doubling dose of radiation for humans. Am J Hum Genet 46:1053–1072.

NEGLIA JP, MEADOWS AT, ROBISON LL, et al. 1991. Second neoplasms after acute lymphoblastic leukemia in childhood. N Engl J Med 325:1330–1336.

NEGLIA JP, SMITHSON WA, GUNDERSON P, et al. 1988. Prenatal and perinatal risk factors for neuroblastoma: a case-control study. Cancer 61:2202–2206.

NIIKAWA N, ISHIKIRIYAMA S, TAKAHASHI S, et al. 1986. The Wiedemann-Beckwith syndrome: pedigree studies on five families with evidence for autosomal dominant inheritance with variable expressivity. Am J Med Genet 24:41–55.

NISHI M, MIYAKE H. 1989. A case-control study of non-T cell acute lymphoblastic leukemia of children in Hokkaido, Japan. J Epidemiol Community Health 43:352–355.

NYGAARD R, GARWICZ S, HALDORSEN T, et al. 1991. Second malignant neoplasms in patients treated for childhood leukemia. Acta Pediatr Scand 80:1220–1228.

O'LEARY LM, HICKS AM, PETERS JM, et al. 1991. Parental occupational exposures and risk of childhood cancer: a review. Am J Ind Med 20:17–35.

OLSEN JH, BOICE JD JR, FRAUMENI JF JR. 1990. Cancer in children of epileptic mothers and the possible relation to maternal anticonvulsant therapy. Br J Cancer 62:996–999.

OLSEN JH, BROWN P DEN, SCHULGEN G, et al. 1991. Parental employment at time of conception and risk of cancer in offspring. Eur J Cancer 27:958–965.

OLSEN JH, GARWICZ S, HERTZ H, et al. 1993. Second malignant neoplasms after cancer in childhood or adolescence. Br Med J 307:1030–1036.

OLSEN JH, HERTZ H, BLINKENBERG K, VERDER H. 1994. Vitamin K regimens and incidence of childhood cancer in Denmark. Br Med J 308:895–896.

OLSHAN AF. 1986. Wilms' tumor, overgrowth, and fetal growth factors: a hypothesis. Cancer Genet Cytogenet 21:303–307.

OLSHAN AF, BRESLOW NE, DALING JR, et al. 1986. Childhood brain tumors and paternal occupation in the aerospace industry. J Natl Cancer Inst 77:17–19.

OLSHAN AF, BRESLOW NE, FALLETTA JM, et al. 1993. Risk factors for Wilms tumor—Report from the National Wilms Tumor Study. Cancer 72:938–944.

OLSHAN AF, FAUSTMEN EM. 1989. Nitrosatable drug exposure during pregnancy and adverse pregnancy outcome. Int J Epidemiol 18:891–899.

OPERSKALSKI EA, PRESTON-MARTIN S, HENDERSON BE, et al. 1987. A case-control study of osteosarcoma in young persons. Am J Epidemiol 126:118–126.

PARKER L, CRAFT AW, SMITH J, et al. 1993. Geographical distribution of preconceptional radiation doses to fathers employed at the Sellafield nuclear installation, West Cumbria. Br Med J 307:966–971.

PARKIN DM, CARDIS E, MASUYER E, et al. 1993b. Childhood leukemia following the Chernobyl accident: the European Childhood Leukemia—Lymphoma Incidence Study (ECLIS). Eur J Cancer 29A:87–95.

PARKIN DM, MUIR CS, WHELAN SL, et al. 1992. Cancer Incidence in Five Continents. Vol 6, Lyon, France: IARC Scientific Publications No. 120.

PARKIN DM, STILLER CA, DRAPER GJ, et al (eds). 1988a. International Incidence of Childhood Cancer. IARC Scientific Publication No. 87. Lyon, International Agency for Research on Cancer (IARC).

PARKIN DM, STILLER CA, DRAPER GJ, et al. 1988b. The international incidence of childhood cancer. Int J Cancer 42:511–520.

PARKIN DM, STILLER CA, NECTOUX J. 1993a. International variations in the incidence of childhood bone tumors. Int J Cancer 53:371–376.

PEGELOW CH, EBBIN AJ, POWARS D, TOWNER JW. 1975. Familial neuroblastoma. J Pediatr 87:763.

PERSHAGEN G, ERICSSON A, OTTERBLAD-OLAUSSON P. 1992. Maternal smoking in pregnancy: does it increase the risk of childhood cancer? Int J Epidemiol 21:1–5.

PETERS JM, PRESTON-MARTIN S, LONDON SJ, et al. 1994. Processed meats and risk of childhood leukemia. Cancer Causes Control 5:195–202.

PETERS JM, PRESTON-MARTIN S, YU MC. 1981. Brain tumors in children and occupational exposure of parents. Science 213:235–236.

PETRIDOU E, KASSIMOS D, KALMANTI M, et al. 1993. Age of exposure to infections and risk of childhood leukemia. Br Med J 307:774.

PING AJ, REEVE AE, LAW DJ, et al. 1989. Genetic linkage of Beckwith-Wiedemann syndrome to 11p15. Am J Hum Genet 44:720–723.

PINKEL D, NEFZGER D. 1959. Some epidemiological features of childhood leukemia in the Buffalo, NY, area. Cancer 12:351–358.

PIPPARD EC, HALL AJ, BARKER DJP, et al. 1988. Cancer in homozygotes and heterozygotes of ataxia-telangiectasia and xeroderma pigmentosum in Britain. Cancer Res 48:2929–2932.

POLHEMUS DW, KOCH R. 1959. Leukemia and medical radiation. Pediatrics 23:453–461.

PONDER B. 1988. Gene losses in human tumours. Nature 335:400–402.

PONDER BAJ. 1990. Inherited predisposition to cancer. Trends Genet 6:213–218.

PONTISSO P, BASSO G, PERILONGO G, et al. 1991. Does Hepatitis B virus play a role in primary liver cancer in children of Western countries? Cancer Detect Prev 15:363–368.

PRESTON-MARTIN S, HENDERSON BE. 1984. N-Nitroso compounds and human intracranial tumors. In: *N-Nitroso Compounds: Occurrence, Biological Effects and Relevance to Human Cancer,* O'Neill IK, von Borstel BC, Miller CT, et al (eds). IARC Scientific Publication No. 57. Lyon, IARC, pp 887–894.

PRESTON-MARTIN S, YU MC, BENTON B, et al. 1982. N-Nitroso compounds and childhood brain tumors: a case-control study. Cancer Res 42:5240–5245.

PUI C-H, BEHM FG, RAIMONDI SC, et al. 1989. Second acute myeloid leukemia in children treated for acute lymphoid leukemia. N Engl J Med 321:136–142.

PUI C-H, HANCOCK ML, RAIMONDI SC, et al. 1990. Myeloid neoplasia in children treated for solid tumours. Lancet 336:417–421.

PUI C-H, RIBEIRO RC, HANCOCK ML, et al. 1991. Acute myeloid leukemia in children treated with epipophyllotoxins for acute lymphoblastic leukemia. N Engl J Med 325:1682–1687.

RABKIN CS, HILGARTNER MW, HEDBERG KW, et al. 1992. Incidence of lymphomas and other cancers in HIV-infected and HIV-uninfected patients with hemophilia. JAMA 267:1090–1094.

RAMOT B, MAGRATH I. 1982. Hypothesis: the environment is a major determinant of the immunologic subtype of lymphoma and acute lymphoblastic leukaemia in children. Br J Haematol 52:183–189.

RANDOLPH VL, HEATH CW, JR. 1974. Influenza during pregnancy in relation to subsequent childhood leukemia and lymphoma. Am J Epidemiol 100:399–409.

REIK W, SURANI MA. 1989. Genomic imprinting and embryonal tumours. Nature 338:112–113.

RICCARDI VM, SUJANSKY E, SMITH AC, et al. 1978. Chromosomal imbalance in the aniridia-Wilms' tumor association: 11p interstitial deletion. Pediatrics 61:604–610.

RITZÉN EM. 1993. Does growth hormone increase the risk of malignancies? Horm Res 39:99–101.

ROBISON LL. 1996. Second primary cancers after childhood cancer. Br Med J 312:861–862.

ROBISON LL, BUCKLEY JD, DAIGLE AE, et al. 1989. Maternal drug use and risk of childhood nonlymphoblastic leukemia among offspring. Cancer 63:1904–1911.

ROBISON LL, CODD M, GUNDERSON P, et al. 1987. Birth weight as a risk factor for childhood acute lymphoblastic leukemia. Pediatr Hematol Oncol 4:63–72.

ROBISON LL, NEGLIA JP. 1987. Epidemiology of Down syndrome and childhood acute leukema. In: *Oncology and Immunology of Down Syndrome*, McCoy EE, Epstein CJ (eds). New York: Alan Liss, pp 19–32.

RODVALL Y, HRUBEC Z, PERSHAGEN G, et al. 1992. Childhood cancer among Swedish twins. Cancer Causes Control 3:527–532.

RODVALL Y, PERSHAGEN G, HRUBEC Z, et al. 1990. Prenatal x-ray exposure and childhood cancer in Swedish twins. Int J Cancer 46:362–365.

ROMAN E, BERAL V, CARPENTER L, et al. 1987. Childhood leukemia in the West Berkshire and Basingstoke and North Hampshire District Health Authorities in relation to nuclear establishments in the vicinity. Br Med J 294:597–602.

ROMAN E, WATSON A, BERAL V, et al. 1993. Case-control study of leukemia and non-Hodgkin's lymphoma among children aged 0-4 years living in West Berkshire and North Hampshire health districts. Br Med J 306:615–621.

RON E, MODAN B. 1980. Benign and malignant thyroid neoplasms after childhood irradiation for tinea capitis. J Natl Cancer Inst 65:7–11.

RON E, MODAN B. 1984. Thyroid and other neoplasms following childhood scalp irradiation. In: *Radiation Carcinogenesis: Epidemiology and Biological Significance*, Boice JD, Jr, Fraumeni JF, Jr (eds). New York: Raven Press.

RON E, MODAN B, PRESTON D, et al. 1989. Thyroid neoplasia following low-dose radiation in childhood. Radiat Res 120:516–531.

RON E, MODAN B, BOICE JD. 1988a. Mortality after radiotherapy for ringworm of the scalp. Am J Epidemiol 127:713–725.

RON E, MODAN B, BOICE JD, et al. 1988b. Tumors of the brain and nervous system after radiotherapy in childhood. N Engl J Med 319:1033–1039.

ROULEAU GA, MEREL P, LUTCHMAN M, et al. 1993. Alteration in a new gene encoding a putative membrane-organizing protein causes neuro-fibromatosis type 2. Nature 363:515–521.

ROULEAU GA, WERTELEVKI W, HAINES JL, et al. 1987. Genetic linkage of bilateral acoustic neurofibromatosis to a DNA marker on chromosome 22. Nature 329:246–248.

SANDERS BM, WHITE GC, DRAPER GJ. 1981. Occupations of fathers of children dying from neoplasms. J Epidemiol Community Health 35:245–250.

SARASUA S, SAVITZ DA. 1994. Cured and broiled meat consumption in relation to childhood cancer: Denver, Colorado. Cancer Causes Control 5:141–148.

SAVITZ DA, CHEN J. 1990. Parental occupation and childhood cancer: review of epidemiologic studies. Environ Health Perspect 88:325–337.

SAVITZ DA, FEINGOLD L. 1989. Association of childhood cancer with residential traffic density. Scand J Work Environ Health 15:360–363.

SAVITZ DA, WACHTEL H, BARNES FA, et al. 1988. Case-control study of childhood cancer and exposure to 60-Hz magnetic fields. Am J Epidemiol 128:21–38.

SCHNEIDER M, OBRINGER AC, ZACKAI E, et al. 1986. Childhood neurofibromatosis: risk factors for malignant disease. Cancer Genet Cytogenet 21:347–354.

SCHNITZER B, NISHIYAMA RH, HEIDELBERGER KP, et al. 1973. Hodgkin's disease in children. Cancer 31:560–567.

SCHOTTENFELD D, WARSHAUER ME, SHERLOCK S, et al. 1980. The epidemiology of testicular cancer in young adults. Am J Epidemiol 112:232–246.

SCHROEDER TM, POHLER E, HUFNAGL HD, et al. 1979. Fanconi's anemia: terminal leukemia and "Forme fruste" in one family. Clin Genet 16:260–268.

SCHROEDER WT, CHAO LY, DAO DD, et al. 1987. Nonrandom loss of maternal chromosome 11 alleles in Wilms tumors. Am J Hum Genet 40:413–420.

SCHWAB M, VARMUS HE, BISHOP JM, et al. 1984. Chromosome localization in normal human cells and neuroblastomas of a gene related to c-myc. Nature 308:288–291.

SCHWARTZBAUM JA. 1992. Influence of the mother's prenatal drug consumption on risk of neuroblastoma in the child. Am J Epidemiol 135:1358–1367.

SCHWARTZBAUM JA, GEORGE SL, PRATT CB, et al. 1991. An exploratory study of environmental and medical factors potentially related to childhood cancer. Med Pediatr Oncol 19:115–121.

SEIZINGER BR, ROULEAU GA, OZELUIS LF, et al. 1987a. Genetic linkage of von Recklinghausen neurofibromatosis to the nerve growth factor receptive gene. Cell 49:589–594.

SEIZINGER BR, ROULEAU G, OZELIUS LJ, et al. 1987b. Common pathogenetic mechanism for three tumor types in bilateral acoustic neurofibromatosis. Science 236:317–319.

SEIZINGER BR, DE LAMONTE S, ATKINS L, et al. 1987c. Molecular genetic approach to human meningioma—loss of genes on chromosome 22. Proc Natl Acad Sci USA 84:5419–5423.

SEVERSON RK, BUCKLEY JD, WOODS WG, et al. 1993. Cigarette smoking and alcohol consumption by parents of children with acute myeloid leukemia: an analysis within morphological subgroups—a report from the Childrens Cancer Group. Cancer Epidemiol Biomark Prev 2:433–439.

SHANNON KM, O'CONNELL P, MARTIN GA, et al. 1994. Loss of the normal NF1 allele from the bone marrow of children with type 1 neurofibromatosis and malignant myeloid disorders. N Engl J Med 330:597–601.

SHAW G, LAVEY R, JACKSON R, AUSTIN D. 1984. Association of

childhood leukemia with maternal age, birth order, and paternal occupation: a case-control study. Am J Epidemiol 119:788–795.

SHU XO, GAO YT, BRINTON LA, et al. 1988. A population-based case-control study of childhood leukemia in Shanghai. Cancer 62:635–644.

SHU XO, GAO YT, LINET MS, et al. 1987. Chloramphenicol use and childhood leukemia in Shanghai. Lancet 2:934–937.

SHU XO, JIN F, LINET MS, et al. 1994. Diagnostic X-ray and ultrasound exposure and risk of childhood cancer. Br J Cancer 70:531–536.

SKUSE GR, KOSCIOLEK BA, ROWLEY PT. 1989. Molecular genetic analysis of tumors in von Recklinghausen neurofibromatosis: loss of heterozygosity for chromosome 17. Genes Chromosom Cancer 1:36–41.

SLATER RM, MANNENS MMAM. 1992. Cytogenetics and molecular genetics of Wilms' tumor of childhood. Cancer Genet Cytogenet 61:111–121.

SNIDER DE, COMSTOCK GW, MARTINEZ I, et al. 1978. Efficiency of BCG vaccination in prevention of cancer: an update. J Natl Cancer Inst 60:785–788.

SOFER T, GOLDSMITH JR, NUSSELDER I, et al. 1991. Geographical and temporal trends of childhood leukemia in relation to the nuclear plant in the Negev, Israel, 1960–1985. Public Health Rev 92:191–198.

SORAHAN T, ROBERTS PJ. 1993. Childhood cancer and paternal exposure to ionizing radiation: preliminary findings from the Oxford Survey of Childhood Cancers. Am J Ind Med 23:343–354.

SORENSEN SA, MULVIHILL JJ, NIELSEN A. 1986. Long-term follow-up of von Recklinghausen neurofibromatosis: survival and malignant neoplasms. N Engl J Med 314:1010–1015.

SOTELO-AVILA C, GOOCH WM, III. 1976. Neoplasms associated with the Beckwith-Wiedemann syndrome. Perspect Pediatr Pathol 3:255–272.

SPITZ MR, JOHNSON CC. 1985. Neuroblastoma and paternal occupation: a case-control analysis. Am J Epidemiol 121:924–929.

SRIVASTAVA S, ZOU ZQ, PIROLLO K, et al. 1990. Germ-line transmission of a mutated p53 gene in a cancer-prone family with Li-Fraumeni syndrome. Nature 348:747–749.

STARK CR, MANTEL N. 1967. Temporal-spatial distribution of birth dates for Michigan children with leukemia. Cancer Res 27:1749–1755.

STEINHORN SC, GLOECKLER RIES L. 1988. Improved survival among children with acute leukemia in the United States. Biomed Pharmacother 42:675–682.

STEINHORN SC, MYERS MH. 1981. Progress in the treatment of childhood acute leukemia. Med Pediatr Oncol 9:333–337.

STEVENS MCG, CAMERON AH, MUIR KR, et al. 1991. Descriptive epidemiology of primary central nervous system tumours in children: a population-based study. Clin Oncol (R Coll Radiol) 3:323–329.

STEVENS W, THOMAS DC, LYON JL, et al. 1990. Leukemia in Utah and radioactive fallout from the Nevada test site: a case-control study. JAMA 264:585–591.

STEWART A, KNEALE GW. 1970. Radiation dose effects in relation to obstetric x-rays and childhood cancer. Lancet 1:1185–1188.

STEWART A, KNEALE GW. 1971. Prenatal radiation exposure and childhood cancer. Lancet 1:42–43.

STEWART A, WEBB J, GILES D, et al. 1956. Malignant disease in childhood and diagnostic irradiation in utero. Lancet 2:447.

STEWART A, WEBB J, HEWITT D. 1958. A survey of childhood malignancies. Br Med J 1:1495–1508.

STILLER CA, BUNCH KJ. 1990. Trends in survival for childhood cancer in Britain diagnosed 1971–85. Br J Cancer 62:806–815.

STILLER CA, DRAPER GJ. 1982. Trends in childhood leukemia in Britain, 1968–1978. Br J Cancer 45:543–548.

STILLER CA, LENNOX EL, KINNIER-WILSON LM. 1987. Incidence of cardiac septal defects in children with Wilms' tumour and other malignant diseases. Carcinogenesis 8:129–132.

STILLER CA, PARKIN DM. 1990a. International incidence of childhood lymphomas. Paediatr Perinatal Epidemiol 4:302–324.

STILLER CA, PARKIN DM. 1990b. International variations in the incidence of childhood renal tumours. Br J Cancer 62:1026–1030.

STJERNFELDT M, BERGLUND K, LINDSTEN J, et al. 1986. Maternal smoking during pregnancy and risk of childhood cancer. Lancet 1:1350–1352.

STJERNFELDT M, SAMNELSSON L, LUDVIGSSON J. 1987. Radiation in dwellings and cancer in children. Pediatr Hematol Oncol 4:55–61.

STORM HH. 1988. Completeness of cancer registration in Denmark 1943–1966 and efficacy of record linkage procedures. Int J Epidemiol 17:44–48.

STRONG LC. 1984. Genetics, etiology and epidemiology of childhood cancer. In: *Clinical Pediatric Oncology*, 3rd edition, Sutow WW, Vietti TJ, Fernbach DJ (eds). St. Louis: CV Mosby Co, pp 14–41.

STRONG LC, STINE M, NORSTED TL. 1987. Cancer in survivors of childhood soft tissue sarcoma and their relatives. J Natl Cancer Inst 79:1213–1220.

SWERDLOW AJ, STILLER CA, KINNIER WILSON LM. 1982. Prenatal factors in the aetiology of testicular cancer: an epidemiological study of childhood testicular cancer deaths in Great Britain, 1953–73. J Epidemiol Community Health 36:96–101.

SWIFT M. 1982. Single gene syndromes. In: Cancer Epidemiology and Prevention, Schottenfeld DF, Fraumeni JF, Jr (eds). Philadelphia: WB Saunders, pp 475–482.

SWIFT M, CALDWELL RJ, CHASE C. 1980. Reassessment of cancer predisposition of Fanconi anemia heterozygotes. J Natl Cancer Inst 65:863–867.

SWIFT M, REITNAUER PJ, MORRELL D, CHASE CL. 1987. Breast and other cancers in families with ataxia-telangiectasia. N Engl J Med 316:1289–1294.

SZKLO M, GORDIS L, TONASCIA J, et al. 1978. The changing survivorship of white and black children with leukemia. Cancer 42:59–65.

TARBELL NJ, GELBER RD, WEINSTEIN HJ, MAUCH P. 1993. Sex differences in risk of second malignant tumors after Hodgkin's disease in childhood. Lancet 341:1428–1432.

TAYLOR AMR. 1992. Ataxia telangiectasia genes and predisposition to leukemia, lymphoma and breast cancer. Br J Cancer 66:5–9.

TEPPO L, SALONEN T, HAKULINEN T. 1975. Incidence of childhood cancer in Finland. J Natl Cancer Inst 55:1065–1067.

TOGUCHIDA J, YAMAGUCHI T, DAYTON SH, et al. 1992. Prevalence and spectrum of germline mutations of the p53 gene among patients with sarcoma. N Engl J Med 326:1301–1308.

TOMENIUS L. 1986. 50-Hz electromagnetic environment and the incidence of childhood tumors in Stockholm County. Bioelectromagnetics 7:191–207.

TSUNEMATSU Y, WATANABE S, INOUE R, et al. 1985. Multiple primary malignancies in childhood cancer. Jpn J Clin Oncol 15(Suppl 1):223–233.

TUCKER MA, D'ANGIO GJ, BOICE JD, et al. 1987. Bone sarcomas linked to radiotherapy and chemotherapy in children. N Engl J Med 317:588–593.

TUCKER MA, MEADOWS AT, BOICE JD JR, et al. 1984. Cancer risk following treatment of childhood cancer. In: *Radiation Carcinogenesis: Epidemiology and Biological Significance*, Boice JD Jr, Fraumeni JF Jr. (eds). New York: Raven Press, pp 211–224.

URQUHART JD, BLACK RJ, MUIRHEAD MJ, et al. 1991. Case-control study of leukemia and non-Hodgkin's lymphoma in children in Caithness near the Dounreay nuclear installation. Br Med J 302:687–692.

VAN DUIJN CM, VAN STEENSEL-MOLL HA, VAN DER DOES-VD BERG A, et al. 1988. Re: Infant feeding and childhood cancer. Lancet 2:796–797.

VAN HOFF J, SCHYMURA M, CURNEN MGM. 1988. Trends in the incidence of childhood and adolescent cancer in Connecticut, 1935–1979. Med Pediatr Oncol 16:78–87.

VAN STEENSEL-MOLL HA, VALKENBURG HA, VANDENBROUCKE JP, et al. 1985a. Are maternal fertility problems related to childhood leukemia? Int J Epidemiol 14:555–560.

VAN STEENSEL-MOLL HA, VALKENBURG HA, VAN ZANEN GE. 1985b. Childhood leukemia and parental occupation: a register-based case-control study. Am J Epidemiol 121:216–224.

VAN STEENSEL-MOLL HA, VALKENBURG HA, VAN ZANEN GE. 1986. Childhood leukemia and infectious diseases in the first year of life: a register-based case-control study. Am J Epidemiol 124:590–594.

VERKASALO PK, PUKKALA E, HONGISTO MY, et al. 1993. Risk of cancer in Finnish children living close to power lines. Br Med J 307:895–899.

VIANNA NJ, KOVASZHAY B, POLAN A, et al. 1984. Infant leukemia and paternal exposure to motor vehicle exhaust fumes. J Occup Med 26:679–682.

VIEL JF, RICHARDSON ST. 1990. Childhood leukemia around the LaHague nuclear waste reprocessing plant. Br Med J 300:580–581.

VOGELSTEIN B, CIVIN CI, PREISINGER AC, et al. 1990. RAS gene mutations in childhood acute myeloid leukemia: a Pediatric Oncology Group study. Genes Chromosom Cancer 2:159–162.

WAKEFIELD M, KOHLER JA. 1991. Re: indoor radon and childhood cancer. Lancet 338:1537–1538.

WASHBURN EP, ORZA MJ, BERLIN JA, et al. 1994. Residential proximity to electricity transmission and distribution equipment and risk of childhood leukemia, childhood lymphoma, and childhood nervous system tumors: systematic review, evaluation, and meta-analysis. Cancer Causes Control 5:299–309.

WATANABE S, TSUNEMATSU Y, FUJIMOTO J, et al. 1988. Re: leukemia in patients treated with growth hormone. Lancet 1:1159.

WATSON GM. 1991. Leukemia and paternal radiation exposure. Med J Australia 154:483–487.

WEKSBERG R, TESHIMA I, WILLIAMS BRG, et al. 1993. Molecular characterization of cytogenetic alterations associated with the Beckwith-Wiedemann syndrome (BWS) phenotype refines the localization and suggests the gene for BWS is imprinted. Hum Molecular Genet 2:549–556.

WERTELECKI W, ROULEAU GA, SUPERNEAU DW, et al. 1988. Neurofibromatosis 2: clinical and DNA linkage studies of a large kindred. N Engl J Med 319:278–283.

WERTHEIMER N, LEEPER E. 1979. Electrical wiring configurations and childhood cancer. Am J Epidemiol 109:273–284.

WEST R. 1984. Childhood cancer mortality: international comparisons 1955–74. World Health Stat Q 37:98–127.

WILKINS JR, HUNDLEY VD. 1990. Paternal occupational exposure to electromagnetic fields and neuroblastoma in offspring. Am J Epidemiol 131:995–1008.

WILKINS JR III, KOUTRAS RA. 1988. Paternal occupation and brain cancer in offspring: a mortality-based case-control study. Am J Ind Med 14:299–318.

WILKINS JR III, SINKS TH. 1984b. Occupational exposures among fathers of children with Wilms' tumor. J Occup Med 26:427–435.

WILKINS JR III, SINKS T. 1990. Parental occupation and intracranial neoplasms of childhood: results of a case-control interview study. Am J Epidemiol 132:275–292.

WILKINS JR III, SINKS TH JR. 1984a. Paternal occupation and Wilms' tumour in offspring. J Epidemiol Community Health 38:7–11.

WILLIAMS WR, STRONG LC. 1985. Genetic epidemiology of soft tissue sarcomas in children. In: *Familial Cancer*, Miller H, Weber W (eds). Basel, Switzerland: S. Karger, pp 151–153.

WILSON MG, EBBIN AJ, TOWNER JW, et al. 1977. Chromosomal anomalies in patients with retinoblastoma. Clin Genet 12:1–8.

WINDHAM GC, BJERKEDAL T, LANGMARK F. 1985. A population-based study of cancer incidence in twins and in children with congenital malformations or low birth weight, Norway, 1967–1980. Am J Epidemiol 121:49–56.

WINICK NJ, MCKENNA RW, SHUSTER JJ, et al. 1993. Secondary acute myeloid leukemia in children with acute lymphoblastic leukemia treated with etoposide. J Clin Oncol 11:209–217.

WINN DM, LI FP, ROBISON LL, et al. 1992. A case-control study of the etiology of Ewing's sarcoma. Cancer Epidemiol Biomark Prev 1:525–532.

WOODS CG, BUNDEY SE, TAYLOR AMR. 1990. Unusual features in the inheritance of ataxia telangiectasia. Hum Genet 84:555–562.

WORLD HEALTH ORGANIZATION. 1976. International Classification of Diseases for Oncology. Geneva, WHO.

YOSHIMOTO Y. 1990. Cancer risk among children of atomic bomb survivors: a review of RERF epidemiologic studies. JAMA 264:596–600.

YOSHIMOTO Y, KATO H, SCHULL WJ. 1988. Risk of cancer among children exposed in utero to A-bomb radiations, 1950–84. Lancet 2:665–669.

YOSHIMOTO Y, NEEL JV, SCHULL WJ, et al. 1990. Malignant tumors during the first 2 decades of life in the offspring of atomic bomb survivors. Am J Hum Genet 46:1040–1052.

YOUNG JL JR, GLOECKLER REIS L, SILVERBERG E, et al. 1986. Cancer incidence, survival, and mortality for children younger than age 15 years. Cancer Suppl 58:598–602.

YOUNG JL JR, HEISE HW, SILVERBERG E, et al. 1978. Cancer Incidence, Survival and Mortality for Children Under 15 years of Age. ACS Professional Education Publication. New York, American Cancer Society.

ZACK M, CANNON S, LOYD D, et al. 1980. Cancer in children of parents exposed to hydrocarbon-related industries and occupations. Am J Epidemiol 111:329–336.

ZACK M, ADAMI H-O, ERICSON A. 1991. Maternal and perinatal risk factors for childhood leukemia. Cancer Res 51:3696–3701.

ZULCH KG. 1979. Histological Typing of Tumors of the Central Nervous System. International Histological Typing of Tumors. Geneva: World Health Organization.

62 Multiple primary cancers

DAVID SCHOTTENFELD

Since the earliest case reports of Billroth (1889), multiple primary cancers have been described with increasing frequency. Warren and Gates (1932) offered as criteria for classifying multiple primaries that the tumors must present a definite picture of malignancy, each must be distinct, and the probability of one being a metastasis of the other must be excluded.

The classification by Moertel (1966) distinguished cancers of multicentric origin from those arising in different tissues or organs. The multicentric origin of cancer has been documented repeatedly within a single organ, in paired organs, and in the contiguous epithelial tissues ("field cancerization") shared by different organs (Slaughter et al, 1953). The multifocal clinical presentation of a malignant tumor within a particular organ may arise from a single cell (monoclonal) or have a multicellular (multiclonal) origin. Fialkow (1974) proposed that a neoplasm developing as the result of rare random events would be expected to have a monoclonal origin, whereas if malignant transformation occurs in many contiguous cells simultaneously, the resulting tumors might be expected to be multiclonal. The clonality of a multicentric cancer of the same histopathology may be determined by the generic nature of the inducing agent and its interaction with genetic susceptibility characteristics (Hsu et al, 1991).

A more complex issue is whether the individual with one cancer of a particular organ and morphology has an increased, decreased, or unaltered risk of incurring a second primary cancer of a different organ or tissue of the same or different morphology. If the subsequent incidence or risk of developing a second primary cancer is decreased significantly, then it may be inferred that the presence of one cancer for various reasons is accompanied by inherent resistance or protection. If, on the other hand, the incidence of a second primary is increased significantly, then it may be inferred that (1) shared etiologic factors are operating in the pathogenesis of both neoplasms; (2) agents used in the treatment of the index cancer are oncogenic; or (3) a random event or spurious association is the more likely interpretation. Additional criteria for judging the biological plausibility of a common pathogenesis for cancers of two or more organ sites would be the demonstration of mutually excessive occurrences of multiple primary cancers and epidemiological features that are common to the organ sites. The identification of specific and predictive patterns of multiple primary cancers should facilitate the targeting of long-term early detection methods or chemopreventive interventions, and provide potential leads for establishing causal mechanisms.

METHODOLOGY

While observations on prevalence and proportional frequencies of specific combinations of multiple primary cancers are of historical interest, they do not enable as precise a determination of relative risk as when this is based upon incidence within a cohort of patients with a particular index cancer. In order to determine whether various combinations of second primary cancers are occurring more frequently than might be expected on the basis of chance, the observed number of site-specific cancers are summarized in relation to the person-years of observation subsequent to the diagnosis of the index cancer. The expected number of second primary cancers is derived by multiplying the person-years at risk, which are stratified by age, sex, and calendar period, by age-, sex-, and calendar period–specific incidence rates for cancers of all and selected sites of a population-based cancer registry (Schoenberg, 1977). A unique advantage of a cohort study that is developed from a population-based cancer registry, as distinguished from one in which the patients are derived from one or more hospital cancer registries, is that the observed and expected numbers of second primary cancers are derived from the same reference population. One cautionary note would be that because cancer patients are under closer medical surveillance than the general population, the diagnosis of a second primary cancer may be subject to lead-time bias, or detected before the tumor would have become clinically diagnosed in the usual medical practice setting. This may result in an inflated standardized incidence ratio (SIR) within the first few years after the index cancer diagnosis.

The denominator, person-years, increases either with longer follow-up or with selection of a larger sample, and treats equivalently the exposure time of five persons for 1 year, one person for 5 years, or 10 persons for 6 months. As a measure of risk of second primary cancers, this index of incidence density would be appropriate for a homogeneous cohort of cancer patients experiencing a constant risk per unit of person-time (Sheps, 1966). If this were not the case, then an actuarial or life-table method of survival analysis would be more appropriate.

Since the probability of a subsequent or metachronous primary cancer (ie, a primary cancer diagnosed at least 2 months after the initial cancer diagnosis) is relatively small, the number of primary cancers can be expected to follow a Poisson distribution. The statistical significance of the standardized ratio of the observed to the expected number of cancers can be tested readily (Bailar and Ederer, 1964).

The cornerstone of epidemiological research on cohorts with multiple primary cancers is precise morphologic classification. The same histopathologic criteria and methods of case ascertainment should be employed uniformly in the study group, who have previously developed the index cancer, and in the comparison population. Misclassification is likely to be more common when multiple tumors of the same morphology occur in contiguous tissues. For example, in a study of multiple primary cancers of the upper digestive system, recurrent carcinoma may be distinguished from a subsequent primary carcinoma within adjacent tissues by demonstrating clear margins of resection for the previous primary and in situ foci of origin for the subsequent primary. Cytogenetic studies and identification of cell surface markers may facilitate identification of independent clones of malignant cells, for example, within the hematopoietic and lymphopoietic systems. Clinically apparent metachronous primary cancers should be distinguished from the latent in situ cancers that are discovered through cytologic screening and the occult or incidental cancers that are discovered at necropsy (Schottenfeld, 1977).

As summarized by Flannery and colleagues (1985), the rules for coding multiple primary cancers in the Connecticut Tumor Registry are:

1. A single neoplasm of one type of histology, or of mixed histology, is considered a single primary cancer even if the lesion extends into different anatomic areas.
2. A lesion of the same histology as the initial cancer, diagnosed in the same anatomic site of the index primary but after an interval of at least 2 months, is considered a separate primary unless stated to be recurrent or metastatic.
3. Multicentric foci within the same primary site are considered as a single primary cancer. Synchronous (ie, <2 months) multiple primary lesions of the same histology occurring in different organs are considered to be independent primary cancers unless stated to be metastatic.
4. Multiple neoplasms of different types of histology within a single organ are considered separate primary cancers whether occurring simultaneously or metachronously.
5. If only one histologic type is reported and if paired organs are involved within 2 months of diagnosis, a determination must be made as to whether the patient has one, with metastasis to the contralateral organ, or two independent primary cancer(s). This determination is generally made by the pathologist based on whether areas of in situ cancer are seen in each paired organ. An exception to this rule is that involvement of both ovaries in which only a single histology is reported is generally considered to be a single primary cancer.

One bias that may operate in the selection of cases for study from major cancer treatment centers is the "healthy person-years" bias, which is defined as the cancer-free interval between primary diagnosis and treatment and referral to a specialized center, in which the preceding person-years at risk for a study subject inflate the calculation of the expected number of cancers. In effect, these patients must survive to enable subsequent referral. The difficulty arises because of the interpretation of selection factors in patients who were treated previously or who presented with recurrence of their disease.

If one decides to include referral patients and to accumulate patient-years at risk in the development of subsequent primary cancers from the date of diagnosis or date of first treatment, then "healthy person-years at risk" would be selected into the study. One can adjust for this by accumulating patient-years of observation from the date first seen at the referral institution. Such individuals should be considered as late entries into follow-up after an appropriate interval of time that is equivalent to the period from diagnosis or first treatment to the date first seen at the referral center. Although "healthy person-years" can be accounted for with such an approach, one cannot disregard the implications of ignoring previous treatment factors, which may have intrinsic oncogenic potential.

As suggested previously, use of person-years at risk may not always be appropriate in studies of multiple primaries, because a major assumption of the approach requires that the risk following a putative causal exposure remains constant over time. The standard approach in which all person-years of observation are allocated to a single exposure category, such as a course of treatment, fails to take into account the transient nature of the exposure. Misclassification results from such an approach because all person-years at risk are assigned to a single treatment classification. A method of analysis should be employed that allocates person-years of exposure to different treatment categories as a patient's course of treatment changes, and that takes into account the interval since initial exposure and the different degrees of censoring among treatment groups (Brody and Schottenfeld, 1980).

Pasternack and Shore (1977) have reviewed methodologic approaches in allocating person-years in studies of cancer risk following exposure to suspect environmental carcinogens in which transient exposure dose levels are encountered. Modifications of standard life-table analyses using techniques appropriate for analyzing transient levels of exposure as suggested by Turnbull and colleagues (1974) and Mantel and Byar (1974) provide a means of analyzing longitudinal data in which cohorts of patients who have received different intensities and combinations of therapy can be identified. The use of multiple entry and exit life tables in such studies will permit patients to be entered or withdrawn from each relevant treatment interval.

The statistical techniques that are used to compare the observed actuarial survival and cancer-specific survival in patients with varying distributions of prognostic factors can be adopted to adjust for variables that may influence the cumulative probability of developing multiple primary cancers (Hankey and Myers, 1971; Myers and Axtell, 1973). An implicit assumption of the life-table method is that subjects who are censored as losses, withdrawals, or transfers, and subjects who remain under observation, are similar with respect to the probability of developing multiple primary cancers. Tests of significance, such as the Mantel-Haenszel summary chi-square (Mantel, 1966), the log-rank chi-square (Peto and Pike, 1973), or the generalized Wilcoxon test (Gehan, 1965), which are used in survival analysis or estimating cumulative probability, involve similar assumptions about censored observations. When there are unequal patterns of censoring in the data, other nonparametric procedures (Breslow, 1970) with less restrictive assumptions regarding patterns of censoring are preferred when testing for significant differences between cumulative probabilities.

The development of regression models for survival analysis has made it possible to examine time-dependent dose-response relationships, control for confounding by age, sex, race, calendar period and other potential prognostic or risk factors, and explore interactions among putative causal factors. Regression models proposed for survival functions generally involve the assumption of proportional hazard. One such model introduced by Cox (1972) has had wide application in the analysis of survival data. The assumption of proportional hazard implies that the probability of fatality or some end point for an individual is a constant multiple of a baseline risk level at all times. Thus, although the instantaneous risk may change with time, the ratio of risks or relative risk is assumed to be constant.

In studies concerned with the potential carcinogenic effects of various modalities or agents used in anti-cancer therapy, the internal comparison of subgroups of patients is more informative than comparisons with an external reference population. Assuming that the cohort of cancer patients has been assembled, and that the multiple primary cancer cases have been diagnosed at specific points in time, other epidemiological design options include the nested case-control study or case-control within a cohort study.

PREVALENCE AND INCIDENCE

In one of the earliest studies by Warren and Gates (1932) of 1078 autopsies on cancer patients, 40 patients (3.7%) had either occult or clinically apparent secondary primary cancers. In a subsequent report by Warren and Ehrenreich (1944) of 2829 autopsies, it was estimated that the prevalence was 6.8%. Hajdu and Hajdu (1968) employed the criteria of Warren and Gates in their autopsy study of 3321 patients and reported that 5.3% of patients had second primary cancers, after excluding multicentric cancers of the same or paired organs. Berg and Foote (1971) reviewed 5636 autopsies on cancer patients and reported that 3.1% of patients had occult second primary cancers, after excluding symptomatic and multicentric multiple primaries. In women, the age-specific prevalence of occult second primaries did not exceed 2.0% between 20 and 59 years, and then increased to 3.6% at 60 to 69, to 4.8% at 70 to 79, and to 7.0% at 80 years and older. In men, the prevalence varied between 1.0 and 2.1% between 20 and 59 years and then increased to 5.8% at 60 to 69, to 9.4% at 70 to 79, and to 16.5% at 80 years and older.

In a review of 37,580 patients at the Mayo Clinic (Moertel et al, 1961), 5.1% of patients manifested clinically apparent multiple primary cancers; 2.8% manifested cancers in different organs or tissues. In a review of 41,341 cancer patients at the Memorial Sloan-Kettering Cancer Center (Schottenfeld and Berg, 1975), the average annual incidence of clinically apparent second primary cancers in different organs or tissues was 10.9 per 1000 per year; after excluding metachronous skin cancers (3.0 per 1000 per year), the incidence of metachronous cancers in other organs and tissues, including melanoma, was 7.9 per 1000 per year.

The average annual incidence of subsequent primary cancers (excluding nonmelanotic skin cancers) observed in residents of Connecticut with a previous primary can-

TABLE 62–1. *Examples of Hereditary Phenotypes Associated with Multiple Primary Neoplasms: Autosomal Dominant Traits*

Disorder	*Associated Neoplasms*	*Chromosomal Regional Assignment*	*Clinical and Molecular Features*
Familial adenomatous polyposis	Adenocarcinomas of large intestine	5q21 deletion	Frequency of mutant gene in general population is 1:10,000. Multiple adenomatous polyps; some families exhibit osteomas, fibromas, lipomas, epidermal cysts (Gardner's syndrome).
Multiple endocrine neoplasia, types 2A and 2B	2A: medullary thyroid carcinoma, pheochromocytoma, parathyroid adenoma. Tissues derived from neuroectoderm.	10q11 RET oncogene	Medullary thyroid carcinoma develops from parafollicular calcitonin-secreting C cells of thyroid; polyclonal hyperplasia occurs in the germline cells of the various endocrine tissues as an initial event; one or more subsequent genetic events (eg, deletions at loci on chromosomes 1, 3, 11, 13, 17, and 22) associated with clonal tumor progression.
	2B: medullary thyroid carcinoma, pheochromocytoma, marfanoid habitus, mucosal neuromas, ganglioneuromatosis of small and large intestine	10q11	
Nevoid basal cell carcinoma	Basal cell carcinomas of skin, medulloblastoma, ovarian fibroma	9q31	Increased sensitivity to UV and ionizing radiation; multiple nevi, skeletal abnormalties, jaw cysts, exostoses.
Neurofibromatosis type 1 (NF1)	Multiple peripheral neurofibromas. Neurofibrosarcoma, glioma and astrocytoma of brain; glioma of optic nerve; acute leukemia, pheochromocytoma, duodenal carcinoid, neuroblastoma, rhabdomysarcoma, Wilms' tumor.	17q11	NF1 appears to function as a tumor-suppressor gene interacting with ras oncogene product (GTPase) that regulates cell growth in neuronal tissue; cafe-au-lait spots; fibromatous skin tumors; Lisch nodules (iris hamartomas); about 50% of patients are new mutants. Incidence of about 1/3,000.
Neurofibromatosis type 2 (NF2)	Bilateral acoustic neuromas, meningioma, astrocytoma, ependymoma, neurofibroma(s) and neurofibrosarcoma(s) or malignant schwannoma(s) of dorsal spinal nerve root(s) and/or cranial nerves.	22q12	Penetrance exceeds 95% at age 50 years; earlier age at onset when disease inherited from mother; about 50% of patients are new mutants. Incidence of about 1/37,000. NF2 gene product designated merlin or schwannomin, proposed to link cytoskeletal components with cell membrane proteins.

cer of any site was almost 12.0 per 1000; the average annual incidence of metachronous cancers in men was 15.0 per 1000, and in women, 10.3 per 1000. Individuals with a previous primary cancer had a relative risk of 1.29 ($P<0.01$) of developing a metachronous primary cancer when compared to individuals in the general population without an antecedent primary cancer. The incidence rates within the resident population included both multicentric multiple primaries and multiple primaries in different organs or tissues (Schoenberg, 1977).

CAUSAL MECHANISMS

Familial Predisposition

Between 5% and 10% of the 3000 known or suspected single-gene, inherited syndromes in humans have neoplasia as a prominent phenotypic feature (McKusick, 1988). More commonly, familial cancers or conditions predisposing to cancer are inherited in an autosomal dominant fashion (Table 62–1), although there are notable examples of autosomal recessive and X-linked segregation (Table 62–2). The single-gene disorders are often distinguished by their Mendelian pattern of inheritance, which is more readily demonstrable in large family pedigrees accompanied by high penetrance or expression of the mutant gene, earlier onset or "anticipation" of disease when compared with the usual clinical course in the general population, and the frequent occurrence of multiple primary cancers.

Familial predisposition to cancer is viewed in general to be associated with a germline mutation ("first hit") of a putative autosomal tumor suppressor gene in all embryonic cells. Malignant transformation occurs with a "second hit" in the remaining homologous wild-type allele at the locus of the tumor suppressor gene in the same somatic cell (Knudson, 1986). The tumor suppressor gene model would suggest that predisposition to heredofamilial cancers is a dominant condition,

TABLE 62–2. *Examples of Hereditary Phenotypes Associated with Multiple Primary Neoplasms: Autosomal Recessive Traits*

Disorder	*Associated Neoplasms*	*Chromosomal Regional Assignment*	*Clinical and Molecular Features*
Xeroderma pigmentosum	Multiple squamous cell and basal cell skin cancers; melanomas; sarcomas; squamous cell carcinomas, oral cavity and pharynx. Increased risk of cancers in other organ sites (eg, lung, uterus, brain) has been described.	?	Incidence of about 1/70,000. Sensitivity to UV radiation and genotoxic chemicals associated with defective DNA endonuclease, and excision and repair of thymine dimers; nine complementation subgroups of patients with defective unscheduled DNA synthesis. Dryness, atrophy, actinic keratoses, freckling and mottled pigmentation of skin appear early, often in childhood.
Ataxia-telangiectasia	Non-Hodgkin's lymphoma, acute lymphocytic leukemia, stomach cancer; heterozygous carrier (about 1% of general population) predisposed to breast cancer (women)	11Q22-23	Sensitivity to ionizing radiation; DNA repair defects (5 complementation groups); cerebellar ataxia, telangiectasia, growth retardation, immunoglobulin deficiencies.
Bloom syndrome	Non-Hodgkin's lymphoma, acute lymphocytic leukemia, gastrointestinal carcinoma	?	High frequency of sister chromatid exchange and chromosome breakage; low birth weight, dwarfism, malar hypoplasia; butterfly rash of face exacerbated by sunlight sensitivity; immune dysfunction and chronic respiratory and gastrointestinal infections.
Fanconi's anemia	Acute myelomonocytic leukemia, oropharyngeal squamous carcinoma, hepatocellular carcinoma usually following androgenic anabolic steroid therapy for aplastic anemia.	?	Highly sensitive to genotoxic agents; high frequency of chromosome breakage; short stature, radial hypoplasia, hyper- and hypo-pigmentation of skin.

whereas the actual mechanism of tumor development in a specific cell is recessive, or that tumors appear only when both copies of the gene are inactivated. The mechanism for the loss of the wild-type homologous allele in a somatic cell may involve an independent point mutation; chromosomal deletion as a result of nondisjunction and duplication of the mutant chromosome; loss of the normal chromosome with a remaining mutant monosomic chromosome; or mitotic recombination. Tumor suppressor genes have been implicated in several Mendelian forms of cancer including retinoblastoma, Wilms' tumor of the kidney, familial adenomatous polyposis of the large intestine, neurofibromatosis type 1, Li-Fraumeni syndrome, and the Beckwith-Wiedemann syndrome. In the context of the more common nonheritable (sporadic) forms of cancer, deletion or ablation of tumor suppressor genes removes their essential modulating or regulatory action on somatic cell proliferation and tumor progression (Squire and Phillips, 1992).

Retinoblastoma, an embryonal malignant neoplasm of the eye with an incidence of 1 in 20,000 births is a prototypic disease of familial predisposition to cancer caused by a germline mutation of a tumor suppressor gene, which has been cloned, in chromosomal region 13q14. It occurs in hereditary and nonhereditary forms. The nonhereditary cases, 60% of incident tumors, are unifocal and unilateral, with an average age at clinical diagnosis beyond 24 months but before 5 years of age, when the embryonic retinoblast cells have terminally differentiated into mature photoreceptor cells. The remaining 40% of cases are of the hereditary form, usually multifocal and bilateral (80%) with clinical presentation before 18 months of age. In most families the penetrance of the germline mutation is at least 90%, and it is inherited as an autosomal dominant trait. Approximately three fourths of the hereditary cases are due to new mutations in the germline, and thus these probands may not describe a family history of retinoblastoma in prior generations. Infants who survive with heritable retinoblastoma have an increased cumulative risk, ranging from 10% to 30%, of developing second primary tumors, in particular osteogenic sarcomas, soft tissue sarcomas, and melanomas. The osteogenic sarcomas originate in both irradiated and nonirradiated areas, suggesting that inactivation of the retinoblastoma locus, which encodes a specific nuclear phosphoprotein, is an important genetic event in the development of retinoblastoma and osteogenic sarcoma (Friend et al, 1986). Structural abnormalities of the RB1 locus have been identified in osteogenic and soft tissue sarcomas, and a variety of adult-onset cancers, including breast, urinary bladder, lung (small cell carcinoma) and glioblastoma, underscoring the importance of this tumor suppressor gene in the regulation of normal somatic cell proliferation (Cordon-Cardo et al, 1992).

The Li-Fraumeni syndrome is a familial cancer syndrome with an autosomal dominant pattern of inheritance in which there is a varied spectrum of mesenchymal and epithelial tumors, and multiple primary neoplasms, expressed in children and young adults (Li and Fraumeni, 1969; Li et al, 1988). The various cancers include soft tissue sarcoma, osteosarcoma, breast cancer, brain tumor, leukemia, and adrenocortical carcinoma (Table 62–3). The penetrance of the rare Li-Fraumeni cancer syndrome gene (gene frequency = 0.00002) is estimated to be 50% by age 30 years and 90% by age 60 years (Strong et al, 1992). It has been suggested that 5% to 10% of children with soft tissue sarcomas belong to families with the Li-Fraumeni syndrome (Malkin et al, 1992). Follow-up of the previously reported families, as well as the identification of additional families, has broadened the spectrum of tumors to include lung, melanoma, pancreas, uterine cervix, prostate, and gonadal germ cell. In some of these instances it is difficult, in the absence of a specific cytogenetic or molecular linkage marker, to distinguish those tumors that occur in families but are due to sporadic, stochastic events in a somatic cell, from those due to genetic predisposition. Germline point mutations have been identified in the p53 gene on the short arm of chromosome 17, 17p13.1, in families with the Li-Fraumeni syndrome. The base-pair missense mutations in general have involved substitutions of amino acids between codons 242 and 258. Sporadic somatic cell mutations in the p53 tumor suppressor gene have been identified in 70% of colon cancers, 30% to 50% of breast cancers, 50% of non–small cell lung cancers and 100% of small cell lung cancers (Levine, 1992). Studies in transgenic mice, where missense mutation of the p53 gene is associated with an elevated incidence of cancer, emphasize the presumed importance of the p53 protein in negatively regulating the G1 phase of cell cycle replication (Lavigueur et al, 1989). Negative regulation or blocking of progression of the cell cycle in the G1 or gap phase between mitosis and DNA synthesis may result in repair or apoptosis of cells with accumulated genetic and epigenetic alterations that are prone to malignant transformation. The study by Toguchida and colleagues (1992) suggests that sarcoma patients with a germline p53 mutation, with or without the Li-Fraumeni syndrome, are at increased risk of second primary cancers after exposure to cytotoxic chemotherapy or ionizing radiation.

TABLE 62–3. *Li-Fraumeni Cancer Family Syndrome: Distribution of Types of Cancer in 24 Families**

Type	*Number of Patients*	*Number with Second Primary Cancers*[a]	*Percent of Total Cancers*
Brain	14	1	9.3
Leukemia	9		6.0
Breast	36	3	23.8
Sarcoma	55	7	36.4
Soft tissue	(32)	(5)	—
Bone	(23)	(2)	—
Adrenocortical	4		2.6
Lung	7		4.6
Stomach	2		1.3
Other	24	3	15.9
Total	151	21	100.0

*923 members of 24 families.
[a]Six patients had second primaries associated with radiotherapy.
Source: Li FP, et al, 1988.

The autosomal dominant familial Beckwith-Wiedemann syndrome (BWS) is associated with multiple malformations of increased growth (eg, macroglossia, enlarged kidneys and other internal organs, hemihypertrophy of the extremities) and increased predisposition to cancers in childhood (eg, Wilms' tumor, gonadoblastoma, adrenocortical carcinoma, hepatoblastoma, rhabdomyosarcoma, neuroblastoma, and pancreatic carcinoma). The genetic locus for Wilms' tumor, the most common tumor associated with the BWS, has been identified by genetic linkage and molecular studies to reside within the chromosomal band 11p13. A second Wilms' tumor locus has been suggested by loss of heterozygosity studies to be located at 11p15.5, presumably the origin of a tumor suppressor gene, which appears to be the same location for the BWS. The pleiotropic manifestations in BWS may be related to the overexpression of the insulin-like growth factor 2 (IGF-2) gene located on chromosome 11p15.5. The sporadic and familial forms of BWS appear to be an example of genomic imprinting where through an epigenetic mechanism, differential expression or repression of an allele occurs depending on its parental origin. Various genetic mechanisms for genomic imprinting have been suggested, such as (1) reciprocal balanced chromosomal translocation; (2) uniparental disomy; or (3) preferential transmission of paternal or maternal susceptibility alleles (Reik, 1992). The molecular mechanism for genomic imprinting may be related to gene-specific differences in DNA methylation, whereby a specific allele in a methylated state would be inactive and the unmethylated allele active transcriptionally (Barlow, 1993).

Relatively rare monogenic syndromes characterized by deficiencies in DNA-excision and repairing enzymes, DNA synthesis, chromosomal instability, immune dysfunction and/or dysregulation of organ tissue growth are predisposing to malignant neoplasia in multiple organs or multiple clonal tumors in a specific organ. The autosomal recessive, "chromosome instability syndromes" include ataxia-telangiectasia, Fanconi's anemia, and Bloom syndrome. In addition to spontaneous chromosomal aberrations, the lymphocytes and skin fibroblasts of patients with these syndromes demonstrate in vitro hypersensitivity to chemical and physical genotoxic agents (Cohen and Levy, 1989; Little et al, 1989).

Xeroderma pigmentosum, an autosomal recessive inherited syndrome involving hypersensitivity to ultraviolet irradiation and an increased risk of multiple primary skin cancers of various histopathologic types, has served as a model for understanding how defective DNA-excision-repair may be associated with predisposition to cancer. Xeroderma pigmentosum is characterized by both clinical and genetic heterogeneity in that there are at least nine different potentially defective genetically determined DNA-excision-repair complementation groups, and variability in the spectrum of neurological symptoms and age of onset, type, and multiplicity of cancers (Kraemer et al, 1984, 1987).

Genetically determined clinical disorders, or even more subtle metabolic dysfunctional phenotypes, can be demonstrated to alter susceptibility to environmental mutagens. The carcinogenic process may be viewed as a complex and dynamic interaction of environment and heredity. Examples of increased susceptibility to the mutagenic and carcinogenic effects of ionizing radiation include the monogenic disorders characterized by chromosomal fragility, or in retinoblastoma, the nevoid basal cell carcinoma syndrome or the Li-Fraumeni syndrome. Epidermodysplasia verruciformis (EV), an autosomal recessively inherited condition, is associated with multiple skin cancers as a result of infection with human papillomavirus (HPV), mainly HPV 5 or related HPV genomes. The malignant transformation of keratotic lesions in EV is related to increased susceptibility to the genotoxic effects of exposure to other co-carcinogens such as ultraviolet radiation or ionizing radiation in conjunction with systemic depression of cell-mediated immunity (Lowy, 1995).

Adult-onset cancers may exhibit a familial and hereditary pattern, characterized by earlier onset when compared with sporadic disease, in conjunction with multiclonal tumors within a single organ, bilaterality, and/or multiple primary cancers in different organs. According to the Knudson model (Knudson, 1971), the hereditary and sporadic components of a type-specific cancer involve the same genomic changes. These general comments are applicable to the familial patterns of breast and ovarian cancers.

Family history, age at diagnosis, and the presence or absence of bilateral breast cancer impact significantly on the relative risk or lifetime cumulative incidence of breast cancer in first-degree female relatives. In a population-based study of patients from the Los Angeles County Cancer Surveillance Program, the cumulative risk of breast cancer approached 50% in family members when both the mother and sister were affected with bilateral breast cancer of premenopausal onset (Ottman et al, 1986). Four inherited patterns of breast cancer have been identified:

1. Li-Fraumeni syndrome.
2. Cowden disease or the multiple hamartoma syndrome with lesions of the skin and oral cavity that occur in association with benign and malignant thyroid tumors, and breast cancer, often bilateral, in approximately 50% of women before 50 years of age.
3. Familial, site-specific breast cancer, presumably genetically heterogeneous, where the susceptibility allele in a particular pedigree segregates in an autosomal dominant pattern.
4. Familial breast/ovarian cancer syndrome characterized by an autosomal dominant pattern of susceptibility to both carcinoma of the breast (usually bilateral) and ovary, where one susceptibility locus, BRCA1, occurring in about 1 in 800 women, resides within the region on chromosome 17Q21-22 (Lynch and Lynch, 1992; Ford et al, 1994). Carriers of the susceptibility allele, thought to be a tumor supressor gene, are at greater relative risk than noncarriers at all ages, with extremely elevated relative risks at younger ages. The genetic locus or loci associated with chromosome 17 may be predictive of 25%–50% of breast cancer occurring before age 35 years. The cumulative lifetime risk of breast cancer for a woman who carries the allele has been estimated to be around 85%, compared with 11% in the general United States population; by age 50 years, the BRCA1 mutation is associated with a risk of 50%, with 2% in the general population (Easton et al, 1993; Evans et al, 1994). A second early-onset breast cancer susceptibility locus has been linked to 13q12-13 (Wooster et al, 1994).

It has been suggested that 5% of all incident breast cancer cases in the United States are transmitted as an autosomal dominant trait from either the maternal or paternal lineage in a particular pedigree (Hall et al, 1990; Schwartz et al, 1985). Hereditary syndromes involving ovarian carcinoma include the breast/ovarian cancer syndrome; the autosomal dominant site-specific ovarian carcinoma syndrome; and the Lynch cancer family syndrome type II, which is characterized by an autosomal dominant inheritance pattern, and manifested by adenocarcinoma of the large intestine (nonpolyposis syndrome or limited number of polyps) with predominance in the proximal colon, multiple primary colon cancers, and other adenocarcinomas, particularly of the ovary, endometrium, breast, stomach, pancreas, urinary tract, and biliary tract (Lynch and Lynch, 1992).

TOBACCO, ALCOHOL, AND NUTRITION

Patients with an antecedent or index primary epidermoid carcinoma in the upper aerodigestive tract (ie, oral cavity and pharynx, esophagus, larynx, lung and bronchus) are at increased risk of developing metachronous primary cancers in the contiguous aerodigestive tract mucosal tissues. Multicentric squamous cell carcinomas or "field cancerization" developing in the aerodigestive tract is an important determinant of therapeutic failure following treatment of the index primary cancer (Slaughter et al, 1953; Strong et al, 1984). The cumulative incidence of metachronous multiple primary cancers in the aerodigestive tract within 10 years after treatment of the index primary cancer has been reported variously between 5% and 40%, or between 0.5% and 3.5% per year (Winn and Blot, 1985).

Using the data collected from nine population-based cancer registries in the United States, Day and Blot (1992) reviewed the incidence of second primary cancers in patients with cancer of the oral cavity and pharynx. The relative risks of a second primary cancer in the upper aerodigestive tract ranged from 4 to 30, and were highest for metachronous oral and esophageal primary cancers. The increased risks persisted even after 10 years following the diagnosis of the index primary cancer. The incidence density or rate of occurrence per 1000 patients per year of metachronous second primary cancers in the aerodigestive tract in the cohort with an index primary cancer of the oral cavity and pharynx was lung, 10.1; buccal cavity and pharynx, 9.1; esophagus, 3.8; and larynx, 1.4 (Day and Blot, 1992). Patients who are currently smoking at the time of diagnosis of the index primary of the aerodigestive tract are at significantly greater risk, approximately fourfold, when compared with former smokers, for a second aerodigestive tract cancer (Day et al, 1994).

The bidirectional or mutual nature of elevated risks for multiple primary cancers in the upper aerodigestive tract may be attributed to common causal associations with cumulative consumption levels of tobacco and alcohol (Schottenfeld et al, 1974; Schottenfeld and Berg, 1975; Schottenfeld, 1992). The recent study by Nam and colleagues (1992) provided preliminary evidence that the risk of nasopharyngeal carcinoma in low-risk countries, where the annual incidence is less than 1 per 100,000, may be enhanced by tobacco smoking and alcohol consumption. Overall, the upper aerodigestive tract is the anatomic setting for approximately 70% of metachronous primary cancers experienced by patients in whom the index primary was located in the oral cavity, pharynx, esophagus, larynx, or lung.

Epidemiological studies have demonstrated that the ingestion of alcohol increases independently the risk of epidermoid carcinomas of the upper aerodigestive tract (LaVecchia and Negri, 1989). A proposed schematic summary of putative mechanisms for the carcinogenic actions of ethanol is presented in Figure 62–1. Of biological and public health significance is the demonstration of potentiation of risk by the supra-additive or multiplicative interaction of increasing levels of exposure to both tobacco and alcohol (International Agency for Research on Cancer [IARC], 1988). For oral and pharyngeal cancer, joint exposure to tobacco and alcohol resulted in odds ratios that were 2–2.5 times those expected if the effects of alcohol and tobacco were only additive (Rothman and Keller, 1972). For laryngeal cancer, Flanders and Rothman (1982) concluded that the interaction of alcohol and tobacco increased the risk about 50% more than the increase predicted if the effects were only additive. The subsites within the upper aerodigestive tract exhibiting interaction with previous ethanol exposure are the floor of mouth, hypopharynx, supraglottis, and esophagus (Blot et al, 1988). Combined exposures to alcohol and tobacco in the United States account for 75%–85% of the incident cancers of the oral cavity, pharynx, larynx, and esophagus.

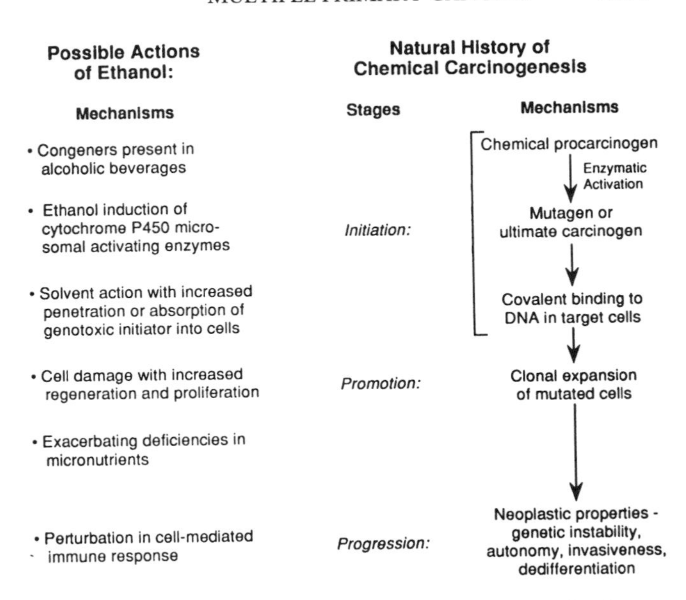

FIG. 62–1. Carcinogenic or co-carcinogenic mechanisms of action attributed to ethanol; its metabolite, acetaldehyde; or to toxic derivatives or contaminants. (Source: Schottenfeld, 1992.)

A number of nutritional factors are thought to be important as modifiers of aerodigestive tract carcinogenesis. In the United States, nutritional deficiencies are commonly associated with, or exacerbated by, excessive alcohol ingestion. The potential interactions of deficiencies in essential micronutrients and exogenous genotoxic agents may give rise to altered mucosal integrity, enzyme and metabolic dysfunction, and morphologic abnormalities in specific target organs (Micozzi, 1989).

Vitamin A and its provitamin, beta-carotene, are needed for normal growth and differentiation of epithelial tissues, presumably mediated by regulating gene expression and transcription. Deficiency of vitamin A leads to a loss of mucociliary epithelium in the respiratory tract and its replacement by metaplastic squamous epithelium. The antioxidant micronutrients, such as the carotenoids and vitamin C, serve to trap free radicals and reactive oxygen molecules, which are generated endogenously. Free radicals are highly reactive and attack the nucleic acids in DNA, denature proteins, and cause peroxidation of cell membrane polyunsaturated lipids (Peto et al, 1981; Krinsky and Deneke, 1982; Garewal, 1991).

Vitamin C, ascorbic acid, is a water-soluble antioxidant that, in addition to trapping free radicals and reactive singlet oxygen molecules, blocks the formation of carcinogenic *N*-nitroso compounds. The substrate or precursors for these compounds may be derived from tobacco, foods, and food additives (eg, nitrite-cured meats and salted, pickled, or smoked fish or meat); alcoholic beverages; or pharmaceuticals. The primary dietary sources of vitamin C are fruits and vegetables, especially citrus fruits, green leafy vegetables, tomatoes, and potatoes (Mirvish, 1975; Block, 1991).

Vitamin A in food may occur as preformed vitamin A, namely, retinol and retinol esters derived from animal foods, or as provitamin A carotenoids derived from plant foods, which can be converted to vitamin A. There are other naturally occurring carotenoids in fruits and vegetables, however—for example, lutein, lycopene, and canthaxanthin—that are not precursors of vitamin A, but are effective antioxidants and efficient scavengers of reactive oxygen molecules. Foods such as green and orange-yellow vegetables are a rich source of carotenoids, in addition to vitamin C, calcium, dietary fiber, indoles, flavonoids, and isothiocyanates.

Infrequent consumption of fresh fruits and vegetables was noted in populations throughout the world at increased risk for esophageal cancer. In a study of black males with esophageal cancer in the United States, food frequency consumption at the lowest tertile for vegetables and fruits, and of nutrient sources of vitamin C, was associated with twofold increases in relative risk after adjusting for tobacco and ethanol consumption (Ziegler et al, 1981). Of five case-control studies that estimated vegetable sources for total dietary carotenoids or vitamin A, three detected an inverse association with esophageal cancer (Tuyns et al, 1987; Decarli et al, 1987; Graham et al, 1990). Case-control studies have provided support for a protective effect of vitamin C, of dietary carotenoids, of fresh citrus fruits, or of green leafy vegetables, on the relative risk of oral and pharyngeal cancers. Smoking- and alcohol-adjusted odds ratios for low consumption of dietary vitamin C or of fresh fruits, as compared with high consumption levels, have ranged from 1.7 to 2.5 in studies of patients with oral and pharyngeal cancers (McLaughlin et al, 1988).

Animal and epidemiological studies have provided the rationale for developing and testing chemopreventive agents, generally composed of natural or synthetic analogues of micronutrients, that may inhibit or reverse the carcinogenic process. The various mechanisms of action expressed by chemopreventive agents include (1) inducing metabolic detoxification of proximate or ultimate carcinogens; (2) scavenging reactive singlet oxygen molecules and free radicals; and (3) inducing epithelial cell differentiation and reversing preneoplastic morphologic lesions (Wattenberg, 1985; Boone et al, 1990). In a controlled clinical trial conducted in patients who were disease-free after undergoing primary treatment for squamous cell carcinoma of the oral cavity, pharynx, or larynx, the random assignment of patients to receive daily oral isotretinoin (13-cis-retinoic acid) resulted, after a median follow-up of 32 months, in the cumulative incidence of second primary cancers of 24% in the placebo group, as compared with 4% in the treatment group (Hong et al, 1990).

BREAST, OVARY, AND ENDOMETRIUM: A MULTIPLEX INTERACTION

Women with breast cancer exhibit a threefold to fourfold excess risk of contralateral breast cancer (Schottenfeld and Berg, 1971; Prior and Waterhouse, 1978; Hislop et al, 1984). Of the 3571 nonsynchronous second primary cancers, namely those diagnosed 1 year or later after the diagnosis of the index primary, occurring between 1935 and 1982 in Connecticut among 36,068 breast cancer patients, 47% were cancers of the contralateral breast (Harvey and Brinton, 1985). The risk of a second primary breast cancer is increased in women (1) when the index primary breast cancer is classified as lobular carcinoma; (2) with a prior history of biopsy for benign breast disease; or (3) when there is a history of breast cancer, endometrial cancer, or ovarian cancer in a first-degree relative (Horn and Thompson, 1988; Bernstein et al, 1992). Harris and colleagues (1978) estimated that in breast cancer patients without a family history, the incidence of contralateral breast cancer was about 1% per year; in breast cancer patients with a mother or sister with breast cancer, the average annual incidence was increased to about 3% per year. Among breast cancer patients who received radiotherapy for the index primary breast cancer, the increased relative risk (1.59) of contralateral breast cancer due to scatter radiation exposure was experienced only by the subset of women who survived for at least 10 years and were less than 45 years of age at the time of treatment (Boice et al, 1992).

Previous studies of multiple primary cancers have described mutual increases in relative risks for cancers of the breast, ovary, and uterine corpus (Schoenberg, 1977; Schottenfeld and Berg, 1971). In the cohort of women in Connecticut with an initial breast cancer, the relative risk of a metachronous primary carcinoma of the ovary during more than 10 years of follow-up was increased to 1.7; in the cohort of women with an initial cancer of the ovary, the relative risk of a metachronous primary breast cancer was increased to 1.8 during the 5-year interval after the diagnosis of the first primary, and then declined (1.2) over the next 5-year interval (Harvey and Brinton, 1985). The interactive effect of age at diagnosis is illustrated in Table 62–4, where the subcohort of women with breast cancer diagnosed before 45 years of age exhibited increases in relative risk for second primary cancers of the ovary (2.6) and colon (1.6); in the subcohort of women with breast cancer diagnosed after 55 years of age, the most significant increase in relative risk was for a second primary cancer of the uterine corpus (1.5). In the studies by Annegers and Malkasian (1981), Bailar (1963), MacMahon and Austin (1969), and Schoenberg and colleagues (1969), the enhanced relative risk of breast cancer in patients with an initial primary carcinoma of the uterine corpus was within the range of 1.3 to 2.0.

The multiplex and interactive causal mechanisms for the mutual increases in risk of developing second primary cancers of the breast, ovary, and endometrium may be inferred by comparing the distribution of established epidemiological risk factors for each organ site (Table 62–5). In a genetic epidemiological case-control study of patients with ovarian cancer, diagnosed between the ages 20–54 years, a significant risk factor was a family history in a first-degree relative of breast, colorectal, or endometrial carcinoma; the risk associations with a family history of breast (odds ratio = 2.3) or endometrial carcinoma (odds ratio = 2.7) were most significantly increased in the subgroup of ovarian cancer cases classified as endometrioid carcinoma (Schildkraut and Thompson, 1988b). Familial and reproductive risk factors (ie, parity and lactation) associated with ovarian cancer appear to be more strongly associated with breast cancer in premenopausal women (Pike, 1987). Conditions associated with reduced cumulative frequency of ovarian cyclical activity and/or inhibition of pituitary secretion of gonadotropins, namely multiple pregnancies, long-term oral contraceptive use, and delayed menarche and early menopause, are associated with reduced risks of ovarian and endometrial cancers (Whittemore et al, 1992; Lesko et al, 1991).

In contrast to the protective effects demonstrated for combination oral contraceptives in studies of endometrial and ovarian cancer patients, the oral contraceptives do not protect against breast cancer (Institute of Medicine, 1991; Weinstein et al, 1991; Thomas, 1993). Indeed, epidemiological studies of breast cancer patients under 45 years of age have suggested that protracted exposure to oral contraceptives after menarche and before the first pregnancy may be associated with an increased risk of breast cancer of at least 50% (McPherson et al, 1987; Miller et al, 1989; UK National Case-Control Study Group, 1989). In perimenopausal women, circadian ovarian and pituitary interactions are accompanied by decreasing circulating estrogens and rising gonadotropins in conjunction with relatively more frequent anovular cycles; during this interval, exposure to oral contraceptives would supplement the decreasing endogenous levels of estrogens and may increase the subsequent risk of breast cancer in susceptible women (Henderson et al, 1988). Estrogen replacement

TABLE 62–4. *Observed (O) and Expected (E) Numbers of Second Primary Cancers by Interval (Years) after Diagnosis of Initial Breast Cancer, Connecticut Cancer Registry, 1935–1982*

	Interval (yr) after Diagnosis														
Females <45 yr:	<1			1–4			5–9			10+			Total		
SECOND PRIMARY CANCER SITE	O	E	O/E	O	E	O/E	O	E	O/E	O	E	O/E	O	E	O/E
Breast	61	4.19	14.6[a]	194	19.82	9.8[a]	113	20.94	5.4[a]	150	50.5	3.0[a]	518	95.42	5.4[a]
Ovary	2	0.68	2.9	12	3.18	3.8[a]	8	3.49	2.3	20	8.83	2.3[a]	42	16.18	2.6[a]
Corpus uteri	0	0.44	0.0	0	2.62	0.0	6	3.94	1.5	19	15.13	1.3	25	22.13	1.1
Cervix uteri	1	1.16	0.9	6	4.31	1.4	6	3.61	1.7	6	6.06	1.0	19	15.13	1.3
Colon	0	0.49	0.0	7	2.54	2.8[a]	2	3.38	0.6	30	18.26	1.6[a]	39	24.66	1.6[a]
Females 55+ yr:	<1			1–4			5–9			10+					
SECOND PRIMARY CANCER SITE	O	E	O/E	O	E	O/E	O	E	O/E	O	E	O/E	O	E	O/E
Breast	112	49.48	2.3[a]	349	157.73	2.2[a]	221	95.41	2.3[a]	167	75.50	2.2[a]	849	377.86	2.2[a]
Ovary	9	8.46	1.1	21	26.57	0.8	25	15.52	1.6[a]	16	11.15	1.4	71	61.65	1.2
Corpus uteri	14	13.00	1.1	56	40.76	1.4[a]	50	23.17	2.2[a]	21	15.60	1.3	141	92.48	1.5[a]
Cervix uteri	7	5.72	1.2	17	16.79	1.0	6	8.89	0.7	5	5.78	0.9	35	37.14	0.9
Colon	24	30.88	0.8	97	102.96	0.9	80	68.23	1.2	96	62.26	1.5[a]	297	264.16	1.1

[a] $P<0.05$
Source: Harvey and Brinton, 1985.

TABLE 62–5. *Distribution of Risk Factors for Cancers of the Breast, Ovary, and Endometrium*

Risk Factor	*Breast*	*Ovary*	*Endometrium*
MENSTRUATION			
Early age at menarche	+	+/?	+/?
Early age at natural (or surgical) menopause	–	–[a]	–
Late age at natural menopause	+	?	+
Years between menarche and menopause, excluding pregnancies, lactation-months, and/or duration of OC use	+	+	+
PREGNANCY			
Married, never pregnant	+	+	+
Early age, first full-term pregnancy	–	O	O
Multiple full-term pregnancies	–	–	–
Late age (>35 yr) first full-term pregnancy	+	?	O
Late age (>35 yr) last full-term pregnancy	+	?	–
Cumulative number of lactating months	–/?	–	O
FAMILY HISTORY			
Organ-specific	+	+	+
Multiple organ primary cancers: ovary, breast, endometrium, colon	+	+	+
OBESITY: EXCESS AVERAGE WEIGHT, WEIGHT GAIN, AND/OR CENTRAL VS PERIPHERAL OBESITY			
Premenopausal women	–	?	+
Postmenopausal women	+	?	+
ORAL CONTRACEPTIVE STEROIDS			
Estrogen/Progestin <45 yrs	+/?	–	–
Estrogen/Progestin 45+ yrs	O/?	–	–
ESTROGEN REPLACEMENT THERAPY			
Without Progestin	+/?	?	+
With Progestin	+/?	?	–[b]
NUTRITION			
Fat (total, saturated)	+/?	+/?	+/?
Calories	+/?	+/?	+/?
Fruits and vegetables	–/?	–/?	–/?
TOBACCO	O	O	–
ETHANOL	+	O	O
PHYSICAL ACTIVITY	–/?	–/?	–/?

+ = Increased risk
– = Decreased risk
O = No relationship established based upon adequate data
? = Insufficient information; equivocal or conflicting data
+/? } = May be associated with increased (or decreased) risk, although studies may be conflicting, or suggest that the association may be limited to one or more subgroups of women
–/? }

[a]In addition to hysterectomy, tubal sterilization may substantially reduce the risk of ovarian cancer (Hankinson et al, 1993).

[b]Reduction in risk toward 1.0.

therapy without progesterone supplementation in perimenopausal and postmenopausal women increases the risk of endometrial cancer approximately sixfold (Jick et al, 1993). There has been no demonstrable risk of ovarian cancer associated with unopposed exogenous estrogens; however, postmenopausal women who have used estrogens for at least 10–15 years, have experienced a 25%–30% increased risk of breast cancer (Grady and Ernster, 1991).

The endocrine interactions in the pathogenesis of breast, ovarian, and endometrial cancer underscore the complexity and heterogeneity of time-dependent pathophysiological events. Target tissues responsive to estrogen hormones contain high-affinity receptor proteins. Steroid receptors for estrogens, progesterone, glucocorticoids, vitamin D, retinoids and thyroid hormone constitute a "super-family" of ligand-activated transcriptional factors that bind with DNA. An important difference between breast and endometrium is the mechanism of action of progesterone and synthetic progestins. The administration of progestins inhibits the proliferation of endometrial epithelial cells by promoting differentiation to secretory cells, downregulating both estradiol and progesterone receptors in endometrial cells, and inducing the estrogen steroid metabolizing enzymes, estradiol dehydrogenase and 20-alpha-hydroxy steroid dehydrogenase. The antagonistic effects of progestins on the stimulatory effects of estrogens are evident in normal and neoplastic endometrial tissues, and are consistent with the protective effects of combination oral contraceptives demonstrated in epidemiological studies. However, as suggested by epidemiological investigations, the effect of estrogen plus progestin does not appear to have the same protective effect for breast cancer (Ewertz, 1988; Bergkvist et al, 1989; Kaufman et al, 1991). In the normal breast, it is during the luteal or progesterone-dominant phase rather than the follicular phase of the menstrual cycle, when the size and mitotic activity of ductal and lobular epithelium increase.

When compared with endometrial and breast carcinomas, ovarian carcinomas contain a significantly lower frequency and concentration of estrogen and progesterone receptors. The ovarian cells that respond to and produce estradiol, progesterone, and androgen are the thecal and granulosa stromal cells, while 80%–90% of ovarian cancers arise from the surface epithelial cells. The mechanism for the protective effect of combined oral contraceptives, or multiple events of pregnancy, on ovarian cancer appears to be different from that for endometrial cancer. The study of Godwin and colleagues (1992) provides an experimental model of the molecular basis for malignant transformation of ovarian epithelium. Namely, repeated ovulation, as suggested originally by Fathalla (1971), traumatizes the epithelium, which induces cycles of proliferative repair that may be accompanied by an expanding population of daughter cells susceptible to genetic alteration and neoplastic conversion.

The risks of endometrial cancer in premenopausal and postmenopausal women, and of breast cancer in postmenopausal women, are significantly increased in relation to obesity as measured by increased age-specific weight, weight gain during adult life, increased body mass index, or in the distribution of excessive body fat (Brinton and Swanson, 1992; Shu et al, 1992). Measures of obesity are not associated with the risk of ovarian cancer or appear to be protective in breast cancer diagnosed in women under age 50 years (Table 62–5). Excess body fat in premenopausal women may be accompanied by an increasing frequency of anovulatory cycles and increased concentration of bioavailable testosterone, but would have minimal influence on mean serum concentration of estrogen (estradiol) of ovarian origin in menstruating women (Henderson et al, 1988).

In postmenopausal women, significantly increased weight and body mass index are associated with increased production, particularly in the adrenal gland, of androgen (ie, androstenedione), which is converted in adipose tissue to estrone, and concomitant decreased synthesis of sex hormone–binding globulin (Fig. 62–2). Adipose tissue is the primary extraovarian site for estrone production through the action of an aromatase enzyme (MacDonald et al, 1978). Women with increased body mass, or in whom the preponderance of excessive fat is distributed on the trunk and subscapular region, when compared with women of lesser body weight or fat deposition, have relatively higher levels of endogenous estrogen and testosterone, and lower levels of sex hormone–binding globulin and progesterone. Increased bioavailability of estrogens occurs in women who are taller and heavier, consume a relatively high fat diet, and excrete lower amounts of estrogens in the feces (Adlercreutz et al, 1994). A unifying hypothesis that requires future investigation is that in the setting of relatively higher levels of endogenous bioavailable estrogens and androgens in postmenopausal obese women, the risks of endometrial and breast cancer are enhanced (Barbosa et al, 1990; Prentice et al, 1990).

LATE EFFECTS OF TREATMENT

There is experimental (Dedrich and Morrison, 1992) and epidemiological evidence for the carcinogenic toxicity of antineoplastic agents. The carcinogenic potential of chemotherapeutic agents, in particular the DNA-alkylating agents (Table 62–6), may be enhanced when administered in conjunction with ionizing radiation (Kaldor and Lasset, 1991). The chemotherapeutic activ-

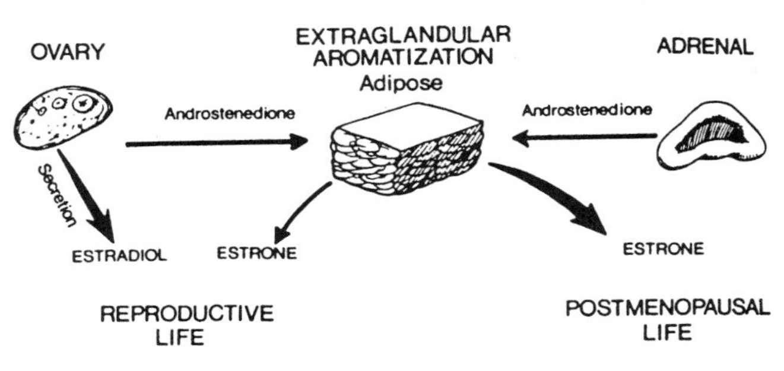

FIG. 62–2. The metabolism of circulating estrogens in women during the reproductive and postmenopausal years of life. (Source: Carr and MacDonald, 1983.)

TABLE 62–6. *Evidence for Carcinogenicity of Antineoplastic Chemotherapeutic Agents*

Mechanism of Action	*Name*	*Evidence for Carcinogenicity*	
		Animal	*Human*
Alkylation	Busulfan	L	S
	Chlorambucil	S	S
	Cyclophosphamide	S	S
	Melphalan	S	S
	Methyl-CCNU	L	S
	CCNU	S	I
	BCNU	S	I
	Cisplatin	S	I
	Dacarbazine	S	I
	Mitomycin C	S	I
	Nitrogen mustard	S	I
	Procarbazine	S	I
	Thio-TEPA	S	S
	Isophosphamide	L	ND
Mitosis inhibition	Vinblastine	I	I
	Vincristine	I	I
Antimetabolite	5-Fluorouracil	I	I
	6-Mercaptopurine	I	I
	Methotrexate	I	I
DNA intercalation and strand breakage	Actinomycin D	L	I
	Adriamycin	S	I
DNA strand breakage	Bleomycin	I	I

S = Sufficient evidence for carcinogenicity
L = Limited evidence for carcinogenicity
I = Insufficient evidence for carcinogenicity
ND = No data for evaluation
Source: International Agency for Research on Cancer (1981; 1986).

ity and toxicity of such DNA-alkylating compounds as nitrogen mustard, cyclophosphamide, melphalan, procarbazine, and the nitrosoureas are mediated through perturbation of the fundamental mechanisms concerned with cell replication and differentiation. The capacity of these agents to alter normal mitosis, cellular function and terminal differentiation provides the basis for therapeutic efficacy, mutagenicity and potential carcinogenicity. There is preliminary evidence that cancer patients who develop chemotherapy-induced second primary cancers have significantly less efficient DNA-repair capacity than patients undergoing the same treatment but not developing second primary cancers (Bohr, 1992).

HODGKIN'S DISEASE

The determination of the risks of second primary acute leukemias, non-Hodgkin's lymphomas, carcinomas, and other sarcomas in patients with Hodgkin's disease is based upon the assessment of the long-term sequelae of various treatment regimens, inherent features of the natural history of a malignant lymphoma, predisposing genetic or altered host immune factors, exposure to other environmental lifestyle risk factors, and target tissue susceptibilities. The risk-benefit evaluation of a therapeutic agent or regimen should take into account the likely outcome of the disease if untreated, and whether or not alternative methods of treatment are more efficacious without incurring serious long-term adverse effects (Canellos et al, 1992).

In comparison with the clinical reports of patients with Hodgkin's disease treated and evaluated before 1970, the relative risk or cumulative actuarial or absolute risk of acute nonlymphocytic leukemia (ANLL) has been observed to increase significantly in cohorts studied during the past 25 years. Concurrently, the innovative use of high-dose extended field or total nodal radiation therapy and/or cyclical multidrug chemotherapy have improved significantly the survival rates in patients with advanced stages (III and IV) of Hodgkin's disease. Overall, 70% to 75% of all advanced-stage patients are now potentially curable.

The cumulative actuarial risk of ANLL at 10 years after treatment for Hodgkin's disease is generally estimated to vary between 2% and 3.5%; the relative risk of ANLL in relation to antecedent combination chemotherapy is increased 10-fold to more than 100-fold (Kaldor and Lasset, 1991; Henry-Amar and Dietrich, 1993). The observed number of leukemias does not exceed the expected number, in general, among patients who have received intensive radiotherapy without chemotherapy. The incidence of ANLL is elevated within 2 years after the initiation of chemotherapy, peaks around 5 to 7 years, and then declines. A myelodysplastic or preleukemic phase is observed in at least 70% of patients who develop therapy-related ANLL. This contrasts with de novo ANLL, in which only 20% of patients have a similar prodromal syndrome (Levine and Bloomfield, 1992). Cytogenetic studies in therapy-related preleukemia/ANLL patients show a predominance of hypodiploid cell lines because of partial or total deletions of chromosomes 5 and/or 7 (Rowley et al, 1977). Similar cytogenetic lesions are frequently observed in preleukemic/leukemic patients following a history of occupational exposure to benzene (Mitelman et al, 1981).

An elevated risk of ANLL has also been established in patients treated with alkylating and other classes of cytotoxic agents, with or without radiation therapy, for ovarian cancer, breast cancer, small cell lung cancer, and multiple myeloma (Tucker and Fraumeni, 1987; Pedersen-Bjergaard et al, 1985; Sagman et al, 1992). Curtis and colleagues (1992) reported in a nested case-control study that after adjuvant therapy with cyclophosphamide, methotrexate, and 5-fluorouracil (CMF) in women with breast cancer, the subsequent excess risk of ANLL over a 10-year period was estimated to be 4.76 per 10,000 person-years. Whereas the relative risk of ANLL and the myelodysplastic syndrome after CMF was increased to 8.7 (95% C.I., 4.3–17.8), joint exposure to CMF and ionizing radiation elevated the risk to 17.4 (95% C.I., 6.4–47.0). However, the odds of dying of breast cancer in premenopausal women treated with CMF was reduced by 25%–30%. The increased incidence of ANLL in patients with small cell lung cancer, although attributed to therapy, may also be influenced by genetic (Whang-Peng et al, 1988) or environmental factors such as cigarette smoking (McLaughlin et al, 1989).

In a survey of over 1500 patients with Hodgkin's disease treated at one university medical center from 1968–1985, Tucker and colleagues (1988) reported that the actuarial risk for all second primary cancers at 15 years was increased to 17.6%, compared with the risk of 2.6% in the general population. The cumulative risk at 15 years was elevated for leukemia (3.3% ± 0.6%), non-Hodgkin's lymphoma (1.6% ± 0.7%), and solid tumors (13.2% ± 3.1%). In the follow-up study of 1939 patients with Hodgkin's disease who were admitted to two major treatment centers in the Netherlands, the 20-year cumulative risk of second primary cancers was 20.0% (95% CI, 16.6%–24.0%), and the absolute risk was 63 excess cancers per 10,000 patients per year (van Leeuwen et al, 1994). The cumulative risk at 20 years was elevated for leukemia and the myelodysplastic syndrome (4.0%); solid tumors, in particular lung, connective tissue, melanoma, uterine cervix, and ovary (13.1%); and non-Hodgkin's lymphoma (4.1%). The relative risk for non-Hodgkin's lymphoma has been reported to be increased throughout all intervals of follow-up and not associated with a specific type of treatment (van Leeuwen et al, 1994; Tucker, 1993). A substantial proportion of these lymphomas involved the gastrointestinal tract or retroperitoneum. The relative risk for solid tumors was increased over all intervals of follow-up and in relation to radiotherapy and/or chemotherapy. Many of the soft tissue and bone sarcomas, and carcinomas, developed within the irradiated areas. The median interval of diagnosis of bone sarcoma or melanoma was less than 10 years, whereas for carcinomas, the relative and attributable risks increased significantly after 10 years following initial treatment of Hodgkin's disease. The observed excess risk for lung cancer developed in individuals who were cigarette smokers. Women with Hodgkin's disease who underwent radiation therapy in which a portion of the breast was in the radiation treatment field experienced a fourfold increase in relative risk of breast cancer (Curtis and Boice, 1988). The relative risk of developing breast cancer was greatest in young women exposed to ionizing radiation before 20 years of age (relative risk = 39), and decreased with increasing age at exposure (Shapiro and Mauch, 1992).

Immunologic impairment in the patients with Hodgkin's disease may play a role in the subsequent development of non-Hodgkin's lymphoma, lung cancer, and cutaneous melanoma. The degree of immunologic dysfunction of both T cells and B cells may be related to the stage of disease, histopathologic type of Hodgkin's lymphoma, peripheral lymphocyte count, and antineoplastic therapy. Similar patterns for metachronous primary mesenchymal and epithelial neoplasms have been described in patients with chronic lymphocytic leukemia, or in renal transplant recipients treated with immunosuppressive drugs to prevent graft rejection (Davis et al, 1987; Travis et al, 1992). In immunocompromised patients with AIDS, or in individuals undergoing organ transplantation, the increased risk of immunoblastic lymphomas appears to be associated with a B-cell lymphoproliferative disorder induced by reactivated Epstein-Barr virus infection (Kinlen, 1992).

REFERENCES

Adlercreutz H, Gorbach SL, Goldin BR, et al. 1994. Estrogen metabolism and excretion in Oriental and Caucasian women. J Natl Cancer Inst 86:1076–1082.

Alper JC. 1991. Genetic disease predisposing to malignancy. In: *Cancer of the Skin,* Friedman RJ, Rigel DS, Kopf AW, Harris MN, Baker D (eds). Philadelphia: W.B. Saunders Co., pp 101–113.

Amos CI, Shaw GL, Tucker MA, Hartge P. 1992. Age at onset for familial epithelial ovarian cancer. JAMA 268:1896–1899.

Annegers JF, Malkasian GD. 1981. Patterns of other neoplasia in patients with endometrial carcinoma. Cancer 48:856–859.

Bailar JC. 1963. The incidence of independent tumors among uterine cancer patients. Cancer 16:842–853.

Bailar JC, Ederer F. 1964. Significance factors for the ratio of a Poisson variable to its expectation. Biometrics 20:639–643.

Barbosa JC, Shultz TD, Filley SJ, Nieman DC. 1990. The relationship among adiposity, diet, and hormone concentrations in vegetarian and nonvegetarian postmenopausal women. Am J Clin Nutr 51:798–803.

Barlow DP. 1993. Methylation and imprinting: from host defense to gene regulation? Science 260:309–310.

Berg JW, Schottenfeld D, Ritter F. 1970. Incidence of multiple primary cancers. III. Cancers of the respiratory and upper digestive system as multiple primary cancers. J Natl Cancer Inst 44:263–274.

Berg JW, Foote FW. 1971. The prevalence of latent cancers in cancer patients. Arch Pathol 91:183–186.

Bergkvist L, Adami HO, Persson I., et al. 1989. The risk of breast cancer after estrogen and estrogen-progestin replacement. N Engl J Med 321:293–297.

Bernstein JL, Thompson WD, Risch N, Holford TR. 1992a. Risk factors predicting the incidence of second primary breast cancer among women diagnosed with a first primary breast cancer. Am J Epidemiol 136:925–936.

Bernstein JL, Thompson WD, Risch N, Holford TR. 1992b. The genetic epidemiology of second primary breast cancer. Am J Epidemiol 136:937–948.

Billroth CAT. 1889. Die allgemeine chirurgische pathologie und therapie. Berlin: G. Reimer, p 908.

Block G. 1991. Vitamin C and cancer prevention: the epidemiologic evidence. Am J Clin Nutr 53:270S–272S.

Blot WJ, McLaughlin JK, Winn DM, et al. 1988. Smoking and drinking in relation to oral pharyngeal cancer. Cancer Res 48:3282–3287.

Bohr VA. 1992. Intragenomic DNA repair: molecular and clinical considerations. In: *Late Effects of Treatment For Childhood Cancer,* Green DM, D'Angio GJ (eds). New York: Wiley-Liss, pp 103–111.

Boice JD, Harvey EB, Blettner M, et al. 1992. Cancer in the contralateral breast after radiotherapy for breast cancer. N Engl J Med 326:781–785.

Boivin JF, O'Brien K. 1988. Solid cancer risk after treatment of Hodgkin's disease. Cancer 61:2541–2546.

Boone CW, Kelloff GJ, Malone WE. 1990. Identification of candidate cancer chemopreventive agents and their evaluation in animal models and human clinical trials: a review. Cancer Res 50:2–9.

Breslow N. 1970. A generalized Kruskal-Wallis test for comparing K samples subject to unequal patterns of censorship. Biometrika 57:579–594.

Breslow NE, Norkool PA, Olshan A, et al. 1988. Second malignant neoplasms in survivors of Wilms' tumor: a report from the National Wilms' Tumor Study. J Natl Cancer Inst 80:592–595.

Brinton LA, Swanson CA. 1992. Height and weight at various ages and risk of breast cancer. Ann Epidemiol 2:597–609.

Brody RS, Schottenfeld D. 1980. Multiple primary cancers in Hodgkin's disease. Semin Oncol 7:187–201.

Canellos GP, Anderson JR, Propert KJ, et al. 1992. Chemotherapy of advanced Hodgkin's disease with MOPP, ABVD, or MOPP alternating with ABVD. N Engl J Med 327:1478–1484.

Carr BR, MacDonald PC. 1983. Estrogen treatment of postmenopausal women. In: *Advances in Internal Medicine* (Volume 28), Stollerman GH (ed). Chicago: Year Book Medical, pp 491–508.

Cohen MM, Levy HP. 1989. Chromosome instability syndromes. Adv Hum Genet 18:43–149.

Coleman CN. 1986. Secondary malignancy after treatment of Hodgkin's disease: an evolving picture. J Clin Oncol 4:821–824.

Cordon-Cardo C, Dalbagni G, Richon VM. 1992. Significance of the retinoblastoma gene in human cancer. Princ Pract Oncol Updates 6:1–9.

Cox DR. 1972. Regression models and life-tables. J Royal Statist Soc B 34:187–220.

Curtis RE, Hoover RN, Kleinerman RA, Harvey EB. 1985. Second cancer following cancer of the female genital system in Connecticut, 1935–82. NCI Monogr 68:113–137.

Curtis RE, Boice JD Jr. 1988. Second cancers after radiotherapy for Hodgkin's disease. N Engl J Med 319:244–245.

CURTIS RE, BOICE JD JR, STOVALL M, et al. 1992. Risk of leukemia after chemotherapy and radiation treatment for breast cancer. N Engl J Med 326:1745–1751.

DAVIS JW, WEISS NS, ARMSTRONG BK. 1987. Second cancers in patients with chronic lymphocytic leukemia. J Natl Cancer Inst 78:91–94.

DAY GL, BLOT WJ. 1992. Second primary tumors in patients with oral cancer. Cancer 70:14–19.

DAY GL, BLOT WJ, SHORE RE, et al. 1994. Second cancers following oral and pharyngeal cancers: role of tobacco and alcohol. J Natl Cancer Inst 86:131–137.

DECARLI A, LIATI P, NEGRI E, et al. 1987. Vitamin A and other dietary factors in the etiology of esophageal cancer. Nutr Cancer 10:29–37.

DEDRICK RL, MORRISON PF. 1992. Carcinogenic potency of alkylating agents in rodents and humans. Cancer Res 52:2464–2467.

DEVATHAIRE F, FRANCOIS P, SCHWEISGUTH O, et al. 1988. Irradiated neuroblastoma in childhood as potential risk factor for subsequent thyroid tumor. Lancet 2:455–459.

DICIOCCIO RA, PIVER S. 1992. The genetics of ovarian cancer. Cancer Invest 10:135–141.

DRAPER GJ, SANDERS BM, KINGSTON JE. 1986. Second primary neoplasms in patients with retinoblastoma. Br J Cancer 53:661–671.

EASTON DF, BISHOP DT, FORD D, CROCKFORD GP, AND THE BREAST CANCER LINKAGE CONSORTIUM. 1993. Genetic linkage analysis in familial breast and ovarian cancer: results from 214 families. Am J Hum Genet 52:678–701.

EVANS DGR, FENTIMAN IS, MCPHERSON K, et al. 1994. Familial breast cancer. Br Med J 308:183–187.

EWERTZ M. 1988. Influence of non-contraceptive exogenous and endogenous sex hormones on breast cancer risk in Denmark. Int J Cancer 42:832–838.

FARWELL J, FLANNERY JT. 1984. Cancer in relatives of children with central nervous system neoplasms. N Engl J Med 311:749–753.

FATHALLA MF. 1971. Incessant ovulation—a factor in ovarian neoplasia? Lancet 2:163.

FIALKOW PJ. 1974. The origin and development of human tumors studied with cell markers. N Engl J Med 291:26–35.

FLANDERS WD, ROTHMAN KJ. 1982. Interaction of alcohol and tobacco in laryngeal cancer. Am J Epidemiol 115:371–379.

FLANNERY JT, BOICE JD JR, DEVESA SS, et al. 1985. Cancer registration in Connecticut and the study of multiple primary cancers, 1935–1982. NCI Monogr 68:13–24.

FORD D, EASTON DF, BISHOP DT, et al. 1994. Risks of cancer in BRCA1-mutation carriers. Lancet 343:692–695.

FRIEND SH, BERNARDS R, ROGELJ S, et al. 1986. A human DNA segment with properties of the gene that predisposes to retinoblastoma and osteosarcoma. Nature 323:643–646.

GARBER JE, GOLDSTEIN AM, KANTOR AF, et al. 1991. Follow-up study of twenty-four families with Li-Fraumeni syndrome. Cancer Res 51:6094–6097.

GAREWAL HS. 1991. Potential role of beta-carotene in prevention of oral cancer. Am J Clin Nutr 53:294S–297S.

GEHAN EA. 1965. A generalized Wilcoxon test for comparing arbitrarily singly censored samples. Biometrika 52:203–223.

GODWIN AK, TESTA JR, HANDEL LM, et al. 1992. Spontaneous transformation of rat ovarian surface epithelial cells: association with cytogenetic changes and implications of repeated ovulation in the etiology of ovarian cancer. J Natl Cancer Inst 84:592–601.

GRADY D, ERNSTER V. 1991. Invited commentary: does postmenopausal hormone therapy cause breast cancer? Am J Epidemiol 134:1396–1400.

GRAHAM S, MARSHALL J, HAUGHEY B, et al. 1990. Nutritional epidemiology of cancer of the esophagus. Am J Epidemiol 131:454–467.

HAJDU SI, HAJDU EO. 1968. Multiple primary malignant tumors. J Am Geriatr Soc 16:16–26.

HALL JM, LEE MK, NEWMAN B, et al. 1990. Linkage of early-onset familial breast cancer to chromosome 17Q21. Science 250:1684–1689.

HANKEY BF, MYERS MH. 1971. Evaluating differences in survival between two groups of patients. J Chron Dis 24:523–531.

HANKINSON SE, HUNTER DJ, COLDITZ GA, et al. 1993. Tubal ligation, hysterectomy, and risk of ovarian cancer: a prospective study. JAMA 270:2813–2818.

HARRIS RE, LYNCH HT, GUIRGIS HA. 1978. Familial breast cancer: risk to the contralateral breast. J Natl Cancer Inst 60:955–960.

HARVEY EB, BRINTON LA. 1985. Second cancer following cancer of the breast in Connecticut, 1935–82. NCI Monogr 68:99–112. (NIH publication no. 85-2714)

HAWKINS MM, DRAPER GJ, KINGSTON JE. 1987. Incidence of second primary tumors among childhood cancer survivors. Br J Cancer 56:339–347.

HENDERSON BE, ROSS RK, BERNSTEIN L. 1988. Estrogens as a cause of human cancer: The Richard and Hinda Rosenthal Foundation Award Lecture. Cancer Res 48:246–253.

HENRY-AMAR M, DIETRICH P-Y. 1993. Acute leukemia after the treatment of Hodgkin's disease. Hemat/Oncol Clin N America 7:369–387.

HISLOP TG, ELWOOD JM, COLDMAN AJ, et al. 1984. Second primary cancers of the breast: incidence and risk factors. Br J Cancer 49:79–85.

HONG WK, LIPPMAN SM, ITRI LM, et al. 1990. Prevention of second primary tumors with isotretinoin in squamous cell carcinoma of the head and neck. N Engl J Med 323:795–801.

HORN PL, THOMPSON D. 1988. Risk of contralateral breast cancer: associations with factors related to initial breast cancer. Am J Epidemiol 128:309–323.

HSU TC, SPITZ MR, SCHANTZ SP. 1991. Mutagen sensitivity: a biological marker of cancer susceptibility. Cancer Epidemiol Biom Prev 1:83–89.

INSTITUTE OF MEDICINE. 1991. Oral Contraceptives and Breast Cancer. National Academy Press, Washington, DC.

INTERNATIONAL AGENCY FOR RESEARCH ON CANCER. 1981. Some Antineoplastic and Immunosuppressive Agents. IARC Monographs on the Evaluation of Carcinogenic Risks to Humans Vol 26. Lyon: World Health Organization.

INTERNATIONAL AGENCY FOR RESEARCH ON CANCER. 1986. Schmähl D, Kaldor JM (eds). Carcinogenicity of Alkylating Cytostatic Drugs (Number 78) Lyon: World Health Organization.

INTERNATIONAL AGENCY FOR RESEARCH ON CANCER. 1988. Alcohol Drinking, IARC Monographs on the Evaluation of Carcinogenic Risks to Humans. Vol 44. Lyon: World Health Organization.

JEFFREY PK. 1990. Tobacco smoke-induced lung disease. In: *The Metabolic and Molecular Basis of Acquired Disease,* Cohen RD, Lew R, Alberti K, Denman AM (eds). London: Bailliere, Tindall, pp 466–495.

JICK SS, WALKER AM, JICK H. 1993. Estrogens, progesterone, and endometrial cancer. Epidemiol 4:20–24.

KALDOR JM, DAY NE, CLARKE A, et al. 1990a. Leukemia following Hodgkin's disease. N Engl J Med 322:7–13.

KALDOR JM, DAY NE, PETTERSSON F, et al. 1990b. Leukemia following chemotherapy for ovarian carcinoma. N Engl J Med 322:1–6.

KALDOR JM, LASSET C. 1991. Cytotoxic chemotherapy for cancer. In: *Cancer Risk After Medical Treatment,* Coleman MP (ed). New York: Oxford University Press, pp 50–70.

KANTARJIAN HM, KEATING MJ. 1987. Therapy-related leukemia and myelodysplastic syndrome. Semin Oncol 14:435–443.

KAUFMAN DW, PALMER JR, DE MOUZON J, et al. 1991. Estrogen replacement therapy and the risk of breast cancer: results from case-control surveillance study. Am J Epidemiol 134:1375–1385.

KAYE SA, FOLSOM AR, SOLER JT, et al. 1991. Associations of body mass and fat distribution with sex hormone concentrations in postmenopausal women. Int J Epidemiol 20:151–156.

KINGSTON JE, HAWKINS MM, DRAPER GJ, et al. 1987. Patterns of multiple primary tumors in patients treated for cancer during childhood. Br J Cancer 56:331–338.

KINLEN L. 1992. Immunosuppressive therapy and acquired immunological disorders. Cancer Res (Suppl) 52:5474s–5476s.

KNUDSON AG. 1986. Genetics of human cancer. Annu Rev Genet 20:231–251.

KRAEMER KH, LEE MM, SCOTTO J. 1984. DNA repair protects against cutaneous and internal neoplasia: evidence from xeroderma pigmentosum. Carcinogenesis 5:511–514.

KRAEMER KH, LEE MM, SCOTTO J. 1987. Xeroderma pigmentosum, cutaneous, ocular, and neurologic abnormalities in 830 published cases. Arch Dermatol 123:241–250.

KRINSKY NI, DENEKE SM. 1982. Interaction of oxygen and oxyradicals with carotenoids. J Natl Cancer Inst 69:205–209.

KUSHNER BH, ZAUBER A, TAN CTC. 1988. Second malignancies after childhood Hodgkin's disease. Cancer 62:1364–1370.

LAVECCHIA C, NEGRI E. 1989. The role of alcohol in esophageal cancer in non-smokers, and the role of tobacco in non-drinkers. Int J Cancer 43:784–785.

LAVIGUEUR A, MALTBY V, MOCK D, et al. 1989. High incidence of lung, bone, and lymphoid tumors in transgenic mice overexpressing mutant alleles of the p53 oncogene. Mol Cell Biol 9:3982–3991.

LESKO SM, ROSENBERG L, KAUFMAN DW, et al. 1991. Endometrial cancer and age at last delivery: evidence for an association. Am J Epidemiol 133:554–559.

LEVINE AJ. 1992. The p53 tumor-suppressor gene. N Engl J Med 326:1350–1351.

LEVINE EG, BLOOMFIELD CD. 1992. Leukemias and myelodysplastic syndromes secondary to drug, radiation, and environmental exposure. Semin Oncol 19:47–84.

LI FP, FRAUMENI JF, JR. 1969. Soft-tissue sarcomas, breast cancer, and other neoplasms: a familial syndrome? Ann Intern Med 71:747–752.

LI FP, FRAUMENI JF JR, MULVIHILL JJ, et al. 1988. A cancer family syndrome in twenty-four kindreds. Cancer Res 48:5358–5362.

LI FP. 1988. Cancer families: human models of susceptibility to neoplasia—the Richard and Hinda Rosenthal Foundation award lecture. Cancer Res 48:5381–5386.

LIEBER CS. 1988. Biochemical and molecular basis of alcohol-induced injury to liver and other tissues. N Engl J Med 319:1639–1650.

LITTLE JB, NICHOLS WW, TROILO P, et al. 1989. Radiation sensitivity of cell strains from families with genetic disorders predisposing to radiation-induced cancer. Cancer Res 49:4705–4714.

LOWY DR. 1995. Human papillomaviruses and epithelial cancer. In: Mukhtar H (ed.) Skin Cancer: Mechanisms and Human Relevance. Boca Raton, CRC Press, 351–358.

LYNCH HT, LYNCH JF. 1992. Hereditary ovarian carcinoma. Hematol Oncol Clin North Am 6:783–811.

MACDONALD PC, EDMAN CD, HEMSELL DL, et al. 1978. Effect of obesity on conversion of plasma androstenedione to estrone in postmenopausal women with and without endometrial cancer. Am J Obstet Gynecol 130:448–455.

MACMAHON B, AUSTIN JH. 1969. Association of carcinomas of the breast and corpus uteri. Cancer 23:275–280.

MAKUCH R, SIMON R. 1979. Recommendations for the analysis of the effect of treatment on the development of second malignancies. Cancer 44:250–253.

MALKIN D, JOLLY KW, BARBIER N, et al. 1992. Germline mutations of the p53 tumor-suppressor gene in children and young adults with second malignant neoplasms. N Engl J Med 326:1309–1315.

MANTEL N. 1966. Evaluation of survival data and two rank order statistics arising in its consideration. Cancer Chemother Rep 50:163–170.

MANTEL N, BYAR DP. 1974. Evaluation of response-time data involving transient states: an illustration using heart transplant data. J Am Stat Assoc 69:81–86.

MCKUSICK VA. 1988. Mendelian Inheritance in Man. Catalogs of Autosomal Dominant, Autosomal Recessive, and X-Linked Phenotypes, 8th Edition. Baltimore: The John Hopkins University Press.

MCLAUGHLIN JK, GRIDLEY G, BLOCK G, et al. 1988. Dietary factors in oral and pharyngeal cancer. J Natl Cancer Inst 80:1237–1243.

MCLAUGHLIN JK, HRUBEC Z, LINET MS, et al. 1989. Cigarette smoking and leukemia. J Natl Cancer Inst 81:1262–1263.

MCPHERSON K, VESSEY MP, NEIL A, et al. 1987. Early contraceptive use and breast cancer: results of another case-control study. Br J Cancer 56:653–660.

MEADOWS AT. 1988. Risk factors for second malignant neoplasms: report from the Late Effects Study Group. Bull Cancer 75:125–130.

MICOZZI MS. 1989. Foods, micronutrients, and reduction of human cancer. In: *Nutrition and Cancer Prevention: Investigating the Role of Micronutrients,* Moon TE, Micozzi MS (eds). New York: Marcel Dekker, pp 213–241.

MIKE V, MEADOWS AT, D'ANGIO GJ. 1982. Incidence of second malignant neoplasms in children: results of an international study. Lancet 2:1326–1331.

MILLER DR, ROSENBERG L, KAUFMAN D, et al. 1989. Breast cancer before age 45 and oral contraceptive use: new findings. Am J Epidemiol 129:269–280.

MIRVISH SS. 1975. Blocking the formation of *N*-nitroso compounds with ascorbic acid in vitro and in vivo. Ann N Y Acad Sci 258:175–180.

MITELMAN F, NILSSON PG, BRANDT L, et al. 1981. Chromosome pattern, occupation, and clinical features in patients with acute nonlymphocytic leukemia. Cancer Genet Cytogenet 4:197–214.

MOERTEL CG, DOCKERTY MB, BAGGENSTOSS AH. 1961. Multiple primary malignant neoplasms. I. Introduction and presentation of data. II. Tumors of different tissues or organs. Cancer 14:221–237.

MOERTEL CG. 1966. Multiple Primary Malignant Neoplasms: Their Incidence and Significance. New York, Springer-Verlag.

MOERTEL CG. 1977. Multiple primary malignant neoplasms: historical perspectives. Cancer 40(suppl): 1786–1792.

MYERS MH, AXTELL LM. 1973. Statistical procedures for evaluating survival in Hodgkin's disease. Natl Cancer Inst Monogr 36:555–559.

NAM J, MCLAUGHLIN JK, BLOT WJ. 1992. Cigarette smoking, alcohol, and nasopharyngeal carcinoma: a case-control study among U.S. whites. J Natl Cancer Inst 84:619–622.

NAROD SA, FEUNTEUN J, LYNCH HT, et al. 1991. Familial breast-ovarian cancer locus on chromosome 17Q 12-Q23. Lancet 338:82–83.

OBE G, RISTOW H. 1977. Acetaldehyde but not alcohol induces sister chromatid exchanges in Chinese hamster cells in vitro. Mutat Res 56:211–213.

OTTMAN R, PIKE MC, KING M-C, et al. 1986. Familial breast cancer in a population-based series. Am J Epidemiol 123:15–21.

PARAZZINI F, RESTELLI C, LAVECCHIA C, et al. 1991. Risk factors for epithelial ovarian tumors of borderline malignancy. Int J Epidemiol 20:871–877.

PASTERNACK BS, SHORE RE. 1977. Statistical methods for assessing risk following exposure to environmental carcinogens. In: Whittemore A (ed) Environmental Health: Quantitative Methods Philadelphia, Society for Industrial and Applied Mathematics, pp 49–71.

PEDERSEN-BJERGAARD J, OSTERLIND K, HANSEN M, et al. 1985. Acute non-lymphocytic leukemia, preleukemias and solid tumors following intensive chemotherapy of small cell carcinoma of the lung. Blood 66:1393–1397.

PETO R, PIKE MC. 1973. Conservation of the approximation sum (O-E)2 /E in the log-rank test for survival data or tumor incidence data. Biometrics 29:579–584.

PETO R, DOLL R, BUCKLEY JD, et al. 1981. Can dietary beta-carotene materially reduce cancer rates? Nature 290:201–208.

PIKE MC. 1987. Age-related factors in cancers of the breast, ovary, and endometrium. J Chronic Dis 40(Suppl):59S-69S.

PRENTICE R, THOMPSON D, CLIFFORD C, et al. 1990. Dietary fat reduction and plasma estradiol concentration in healthy postmenopausal women. J Natl Cancer Inst 82:129–134.

PRIOR P, WATERHOUSE JA. 1978. Incidence of bilateral tumors in a population-based series of breast cancer patients. I. Two approaches to an epidemiologic analysis. Br J Cancer 37:620–634.

REIK W. 1992. Imprinting in leukemia. Nature 359:362–363.

ROTHMAN K, KELLER AZ. 1972. The effect of joint exposure to alcohol and tobacco on risk of cancer of the mouth and pharynx. J Chron Dis 25:711–716.

ROWLEY JD, GOLOMB H., VARDIMAN J. 1977. Nonrandom chromosomal abnormalities in acute non-lymphocytic leukemia in patients treated for Hodgkin's disease and non-Hodgkin's lymphomas. Blood 50:759–770.

SAGMAN U, LISHNER M, MAKI E, et al. 1992. Second primary malignancies following diagnosis of small-cell lung cancer. J Clin Oncol 10:1525–1533.

SCHILDKRAUT JM, THOMPSON WD. 1988a. Relationship of epithelial ovarian cancer to other malignancies within families. Genet Epidemiol 5:355–367.

SCHILDKRAUT JM, THOMPSON WD. 1988b. Familial ovarian cancer: a population-based case-control study. Am J Epidemiol 128:456–466.

SCHOENBERG BS, GREENBERG RA, EISENBERG H. 1969. Occurrence of certain multiple primary cancers in females. J Natl Cancer Inst 43:15–32.

SCHOENBERG BS, MYERS MH. 1977. Statistical methods for studying multiple primary malignant neoplasms. Cancer 40(suppl):1982–1988.

SCHOENBERG BS. 1977. Multiple Primary Malignant Neoplasms: The Connecticut Experience, 1935–1964. New York: Springer-Verlag.

SCHOTTENFELD D, BERG J. 1971. Incidence of multiple primary cancers. IV. Cancers of the female breast and genital organs. J Natl Cancer Inst 46:161–170.

SCHOTTENFELD D, GANTT RC, WYNDER EL. 1974. The role of alcohol and tobacco in multiple primary cancers of the upper digestive system, larynx, and lung: a prospective study. Prev Med 3:277–293.

SCHOTTENFELD D, BERG JW. 1975. Epidemiology of multiple primary cancers. In: *Cancer Epidemiology and Prevention: Current Concepts,* Schottenfeld D (ed). Springfield: Charles C. Thomas, pp 416–434.

SCHOTTENFELD D. 1977. Concluding commentary for the international workshop on multiple primary cancers. Cancer (supplement) 40:1982–1985.

SCHOTTENFELD D. 1992. The etiology and prevention of aerodigestive tract cancers. In: *The Biology and Prevention of Aerodigestive Tract Cancers,* Newell GR, Hong WK (eds). New York: Plenum, pp 1–19.

SCHWARTZ AG, KING M-C, BELLE SH, et al. 1985. Risk of breast cancer to relatives of young breast cancer patients. J Natl Cancer Inst 75:665–668.

SHAPIRO CL, MAUCH PM. 1992. Radiation-associated breast cancer after Hodgkin's disease: risks and screening in perspective. J Clin Oncol 10:1662–1665.

SHEPS MC. 1966. On the person years concept in epidemiology and demography. Milbank Mem Fund Quart 44:69–91.

SHORE RE, WOODWARD ED, HEMPELMANN LH. 1984. Radiation-induced thyroid cancer. In: *Radiation Carcinogenesis: Epidemiology and Biological Significance,* Boice JD Jr, Fraumeni JF Jr (eds). New York: Raven Press, pp 131–141.

SHU XO, BRINTON LA, ZHENG W, et al. 1992. Relation of obesity and body fat-distribution to endometrial cancer in Shanghai, China. Cancer Res 52:3865–3870.

SLAUGHTER DP, SOUTHWICK HW, SMEJKAL W. 1953. "Field cancerization" in oral stratified squamous epithelium: clinical implications of multicentric origin. Cancer 6:963–968.

SQUIRE J, PHILLIPS RA. 1992. Genetic basis of cancer. In: *The Basic Science of Oncology,* Tannock IF, Hill RP (eds). New York: McGraw-Hill, pp 41–60.

STRONG LC, STINE E, NORSTED TL. 1987. Cancer in survivors of childhood soft tissue sarcoma and their relatives. J Natl Cancer Inst 79:1213–1220.

STRONG LC, WILLIAMS WR, TAINSKY MA. 1992. The Li-Fraumeni syndrome: from clinical epidemiology to molecular genetics. Am J Epidemiol 135:190–199.

STRONG MS, INCZE J, VAUGHAN CW. 1984. Field cancerization in the aerodigestive tract: its etiology, manifestation and significance. J Otolaryngol 13:1–6.

THOMAS DB. 1993. Oral contraceptives and breast cancer. J Natl Cancer Inst 85:359–364.

TOGUCHIDA J, YAMAGUCHI T, IAYTON SH, et al. 1992. Prevalance and spectrum of germline mutations of the p53 gene among patients with sarcoma. N Engl J Med 326:1301–1308.

TRAVIS LB, CURTIS RE, HANKEY BF, et al. 1992. Second cancers in patients with chronic lymphocytic leukemia. J Natl Cancer Inst 84:1422–1427.

TUCKER MA, FRAUMENI JF JR. 1987. Treatment-related cancers after gynecologic malignancy. Cancer 60:2117–2122.

TUCKER MA, D'ANGIO GJ, BOICE JD, et al. 1987. Bone sarcomas linked to radiotherapy and chemotherpy in children. N Engl J Med 317:588–593.

TUCKER MA, MEADOWS AT, BOICE JD, et al. 1987. Leukemia after therapy with alkylating agents for childhood cancer. J Natl Cancer Inst 78:459–464.

TUCKER MA, COLEMAN CN, COX RS, et al. 1988. Risk of second cancers after treatment for Hodgkin's disease. N Engl J Med 318:76–81.

TUCKER MA. 1993. Solid second cancers following Hodgkin's disease Hemat/Oncol Clin N America 7:389–400.

TURNBULL BW, BROWN BW, HU M. 1974. Survivorship analysis of heart transplant data. J Am Stat Assoc 69:74–80.

TUYNS AJ, RIBOLI E, DOORNBOS G, et al. 1987. Diet and esophageal cancer in Calvados (France). Nutr Cancer 9:81–92.

UK NATIONAL CASE-CONTROL STUDY GROUP. 1989. Oral contraceptive use and breast cancer risk in young women. Lancet 1:973–982.

VALAGUSSA P, SANTORO A, FOSSATI-BELLANI F, et al. 1986. Secondary acute leukemia and other malignancies following treatment for Hodgkin's disease. J Clin Oncol 4:830–837.

VAN LEEUWEN FE, KLOKMAN WJ, HAGENBEEK A, et al. 1994. Second cancer risk following Hodgkin's disease: a 20-year follow-up study. J Clin Oncol 12:312–325.

WARREN S, GATES O. 1932. Multiple primary malignant tumors: a survey of the literature and statistical study. Am J Cancer 16:1358–1414.

WARREN S, EHRENREICH T. 1944. Multiple primary malignant tumors and susceptibility to cancer. Cancer Res 4:554–570.

WATTENBERG LW. 1985. Chemoprevention of cancer. Cancer Res 45:1–8.

WEINSTEIN AL, MAHONEY MC, NASCA PC, et al. 1991. Breast cancer risk and oral contraceptive use: results from a large case-control study. Epidemiology 2:353–358.

WHANG-PENG J, LEE EC, MINNA JD. 1988. Deletion of 3 (p14p23) in secondary erythroleukemia arising in long-term survivors of small-cell lung cancer. J Natl Cancer Inst 80:1253–1255.

WHITTEMORE AS, HARRIS R, ITNYRE J. 1992. Collaborative Ovarian Cancer Group: Characteristics relating to ovarian cancer risk: collaborative analysis of 12 U.S. case-control studies. IV. The pathogenesis of epithelial ovarian cancer. Am J Epidemiol 136:1212–1220.

WINN DM, BLOT WJ. 1985. Second cancers following cancers of the buccal cavity and pharynx in Connecticut, 1935–1982. NCI Monogr 68:25–48.

WOOSTER R, NEUHAUSEN SL, MANGION J, et al. 1994. Localization of a breast cancer susceptibility gene, BRCA2, to chromosome 13q12-13. Science 265:2088–2090.

ZIEGLER RG, MORRIS LE, BLOT WJ, et al. 1981. Esophageal cancer among black men in Washington, D.C. II. Role of nutrition. J Natl Cancer Inst 67:1199–1206.

PART V | Cancer Prevention and Control

63 Principles and applications of cancer prevention

DAVID SCHOTTENFELD

It is axiomatic that the least costly illness, measured in terms of human suffering or the required medical and social services, is the illness which does not occur. The principles and applications of preventive oncology have evolved from a foundation of epidemiologic research. The National Cancer Act of 1971 embraced cancer control activities which, through research and development, were to prevent as many cancers as possible, cure patients who develop cancer, and rehabilitate treated patients. As Breslow (1979) emphasized, however, the precise steps by which cancer control research discoveries were to be incorporated into preventive medical and therapeutic practices remained to be developed and evaluated.

The year 2000 objectives are focusing on goals in cancer prevention and control that will achieve substantial reductions in cancer incidence, mortality, and morbidity (U.S. Department of Health and Human Services, 1991). The National Cancer Institute (NCI) has estimated that by effectively applying health educational measures to target high-risk behaviors for the more common cancers, promoting screening and early detection of breast and uterine cervical cancers, and facilitating access to currently available methods of cancer treatment, up to a 50% reduction in cancer mortality could be achieved (U.S. Department of Health and Human Services, 1991). Total eradication of cancer by curative and preventive interventions would ultimately result in a gain of about 2.5 years in average life expectancy in the general population, but for the one in four Americans who would have died of cancer, the gain in life expectancy would range from 10 to 15 years.

In 1992 there were 520,578 certified cancer deaths in the United States which accounted for 23.9% of all deaths in this country (Kochanek and Hudson, 1994). By comparison, diseases of the heart represented 33% of all deaths. Assuming the continuity of current trends, it is anticipated that beyond the year 2000, in part because of declining mortality due to cardiovascular and cerebrovascular diseases, cancer will emerge as the leading cause of death in the United States and in other industrialized nations (Sondik, 1988; Cole and Amoateng-Adjepong, 1994).

Reductions in cancer incidence, potentially achievable through elimination or amelioration of major risk factors prevalent in the population, will ultimately have an impact on site-specific mortality trends. From 1975–1979 to 1987–1991 in the United States, when combining all sites, age-standardized cancer incidence rates increased 18.6% among white men and 12.4% among white women; concurrently, cancer mortality increased 3.1% and 6.3%, respectively (Devesa et al, 1995). Five-year relative survival rates for all cancer sites combined increased from 49.3% for patients diagnosed in 1974–1976 to 53.0% for patients diagnosed in 1983–1989 (Miller et al, 1993). In a population-based survey in 1987 of U.S. adults 18 years of age and older, the prevalence of cancer (excluding nonmelanoma skin cancers) in women was estimated to be 4,412 per 100,000 and in men, 1,930 per 100,000. From the sample survey it was projected that in 1987 there were 5.7 million adults who were cancer survivors, or 3.3% of the adult population. Increasing incidence rates for site-specific cancers and/or advances in cancer treatment will almost certainly increase future cancer prevalence rates (Byrne et al, 1992). Janerich (1984) predicted for the year 2030 that there would be 1.5 million incident invasive cancer cases; more recently, based on census population and NCI Surveillance, Epidemiology and End Results (SEER) cancer incidence projections, Polednak (1994) estimated that there would be 2.1 million incident invasive cancer cases in the year 2030.

In the United States during the period 1973–1990, the major site-specific increases in cancer incidence among those under 65 years of age were due to melanoma, non-Hodgkin's lymphoma, and cancers of the prostate, lung (female), testis, liver (including intrahepatic bile duct), kidney and renal pelvis, and thyroid (female). Concurrently, there were significantly decreasing incidence trends for stomach, pancreas, cervix uteri (invasive), and corpus uteri. For the subgroup 65 years and over, the significantly increasing incidence trends were exhibited for melanoma, non-Hodgkin's lymphoma, and cancers of the lung, prostate, brain, kidney and renal pelvis, liver (including intrahepatic bile duct), breast, esophagus, and ovary. Significantly decreasing trends were demonstrated for Hodgkin's lymphoma, and cancers of the stomach and cervix uteri (invasive) (Table 63–1).

With global incidence of approximately 6.4 million invasive cancers per year, the most common cancers worldwide are attributed to stomach, lung, upper aerodigestive tract, breast, uterine cervix, and liver. The global incidence of lung cancer is increasing by about 0.5% per year, while that of stomach cancer is decreasing by approximately 2% per year. Cancers of the upper aerodigestive tract account for about one-third of all global incident cancers. The international variations in cancer incidence patterns—fivefold for all sites combined and more than 100-fold for such sites as liver, melanoma, and nasopharynx—provide a strategic framework for cancer prevention and control research (Table 63–2).

TABLE 63–1. *Age-Adjusted Average Annual Cancer Incidence Rates per 100,000 and Percent Change (1973–1990) by Age (under 65, 65 and over), Selected Primary Cancer Sites, United States**

Site	*Incidence*	*Percent Change 1973–1990*
UNDER 65		
Prostate	22.7	+110.9
Melanoma	8.7	+79.4
Non-Hodgkin's Lymphoma	8.1	+68.8
Lung (female)	21.3	+64.4
Testis	4.8	+51.3
Liver	1.5	+31.7
Kidney and renal pelvis	4.8	+29.5
Thyroid (female)	6.0	+29.6
Brain	4.8	+12.9
Breast	37.3	+12.4
Stomach	3.2	−20.6
Pancreas	3.5	−21.0
Cervix uteri (invasive)	5.8[a]	−31.7
Corpus and uterus NOS	12.5	−43.5
65 AND OVER		
Lung (female)	203.7	+182.0
Melanoma	31.6	+119.5
Prostate	884.1	+79.5
Non-Hodgkin's lymphoma	67.5	+62.0
Brain	19.6	+58.2
Kidney and renal pelvis	41.8	+38.7
Liver	15.8	+37.4
Breast	261.9	+37.0
Thyroid (female)	9.4	+15.7
Esophagus	21.2	+24.5
Lung (male)	501.5	+19.4
Ovary	56.7	+18.8
Urinary bladder (invasive and in situ)	108.8	+13.7
Larynx	20.6	+12.8
Multiple myeloma	27.5	+12.1
Leukemias	50.8	−11.5
Stomach	50.5	−26.6
Hodgkin's	4.0	−26.6
Cervix uteri (invasive)	17.7[a]	−45.0

*From Miller et al, 1993, SEER Cancer Statistics Review 1973–1990.

[a]Cervix uteri (invasive) is presented for <50, 50+ ages.

PHASES OF CANCER CONTROL RESEARCH

The testing and validation of cancer prevention and control interventions generally involves a multistep process that begins with the formulation of a hypothesis (Cullen, 1990). The interventions to be evaluated may be concerned with screening and early detection, health education and health-promoting behavior, chemoprevention, multidisciplinary treatment, or rehabilitation that affects quality of life. A second phase after hypothesis formulation is the development and testing of the research protocol with respect to feasibility, acceptability, reliability, accuracy, and potential adverse effects. After validation of the experimental methodology and measurement instruments, efficacy of the preventive intervention is evaluated based on controlled observational (i.e., case–control, cross-sectional or prospective) or experimental (i.e., randomized controlled trial) research designs that are structured in selected or targeted populations. Subsequent phases of cancer prevention or management research studies are designed to have an impact on defined populations and are then ultimately implemented as an established public health program. A population may be defined with respect to demographic characteristics, disease-specific incidence or mortality, lifestyle or environmental risk factors, or genetic susceptibility factors.

ECONOMICS OF CANCER PREVENTION

In assessing the preventive benefits of an intervention geared towards individuals at high risk of cancer, compared with a community- or population-based intervention, Rose (1992) has reminded us of the "prevention paradox"—namely, that preventive measures that significantly benefit a population (i.e., mortality, incidence, morbidity) may provide minimal benefits for individuals. The high-risk approach aims to "label" or identify individuals with increased probability of disease, and then to lower their risk by reducing high-risk

TABLE 63–2. *Worldwide Variation in Site-Specific, Age-Adjusted Cancer Incidence Rates (per 100,000), in Males (M) and Females (F), 1985–1989**

Site	*Sex*	*High (H) Population*	*Rate*	*Low (L) Population*	*Rate*	*Ratio H/L*
All Sites	M	Brazil, Porto Alegre	420.8	India, Madras	93.9	4.48
Brain and nervous system	M	Sweden	10.7	Peru, Trujillo	0.6	17.83
Breast	F	USA, San Francisco Bay Area	104.2	China, Qidong	9.5	10.97
Cervix uteri	F	Peru, Trujillo	54.6	Israel, non-Jews	2.6	21.00
Colon	M	USA, Hawaii: Japanese	37.2	India, Madras	1.5	24.80
Corpus uteri	F	USA, San Francisco Bay Area: white	22.2	China, Qidong	0.4	55.50
Esophagus	M	France, Calvados	26.5	USA, Filipino	0.6	44.17
Gallbladder	F	Peru, Trujillo	12.9	China, Qidong	0.4	32.25
Hodgkin's disease	M	USA, Connecticut: white	4.4	USA, Los Angeles: Filipino	0.2	22.00
Kidney and renal pelvis	M	France, Bas Rhin	15.2	France, Martinique	0.5	30.40
Liver and intrahepatic bile duct	M	China, Qidong	89.9	Netherlands, Maastricht	0.8	112.38
Lung	M	New Zealand: Maori	119.1	India, Madras	8.5	14.01
Lung	F	New Zealand: Maori	62.2	India, Madras	1.4	44.43
Melanoma	M	Australian Capital Territory	28.9	Japan, Osaka	0.2	144.50
Nasopharynx	M	Hong Kong	28.5	Ecuador, Quito	0.1	285.00
Non-Hodgkin's lymphomas	M	USA, San Francisco Bay Area: white	17.4	India, Madras	2.6	6.69
Oral Cavity	M	France, Bas Rhin	13.4	China, Qidong	0.3	44.67
Ovary	F	Iceland	16.6	Mali, Bamako	1.0	16.60
Pancreas	M	USA, Alameda: black	13.7	India, Ahmedabad	0.7	19.57
Prostate	M	USA, Atlanta: black	102.0	China, Tianjin	1.2	85.00
Stomach	M	Japan, Yamagata	93.3	India, Ahmedabad	2.1	44.43
Testis	M	Denmark	8.4	USA, SEER:[2] Black	0.7	12.00
Thyroid	F	USA, Hawaii: Filipino	24.2	China, Qidong	0.7	34.57
Urinary bladder	M	USA, Connecticut: white	26.1	USA, Los Angeles: Filipino	1.8	14.50

*Rates are adjusted to standard world population.
Source: Parkin et al, Cancer Incidence in Five Continents, Volume VI (1992).

behaviors or exposures, treating precursor conditions, or by chemopreventive methods. The population-based strategy aims to shift the distribution of a risk factor (e.g., use of tobacco, dietary fat, obesity, regular exercise, or screening for breast cancer) in the direction of enhanced health promotion. These two strategic approaches are not mutually exclusive, however, and at the foundation of the paradox is that most risk factors cannot be interpreted as dichotomous but rather function along a continuum or quantitatively. In addition, there is the important distinction between relative and attributable risk, and the observation that the risk of disease is not usually restricted to individuals with extreme values for a given risk factor. Those individuals with extreme values will exhibit a significantly increased relative risk when compared with individuals at the lowest level for a particular risk factor. However, more individuals in the population will be distributed between the extreme values for a risk factor, and they will account for a substantial proportion of cases, presumably because of the multifactorial etiology of cancer.

How should the allocation of resources for cancer preventive services be evaluated or justified? Net health benefits may be expressed in terms of the number of added years of life, perhaps adjusted for quality, as a result of early intervention in the natural history of a specific neoplasm. The basis for such a determination or extrapolation would usually be an experimental randomized trial or controlled observational study. Net benefits would be compared with net costs, which would include the costs of diagnostic and treatment services, minus the cost savings as a result of illness prevention. As emphasized by Russell (1986; 1993), preventive services may incur increases in medical expenditures and should not be justified or offered solely on the basis of anticipated medical cost-saving. The investment in a prevention program, with a rationale emanating from scientific research, would be justified if it were demonstrated to promote health, extend life, and reduce suffering, when compared with an alternative application of resources.

In cost–benefit analysis as applied to disease prevention and health promotion, the benefits of transferring limited resources into a prevention program are compared with competing opportunity costs. The concept of opportunity cost pertains to assigning priority to a particular program but at the same time foregoing the potential benefits of a competing program with a different objective. The measure of benefit depends on the societal value assigned to life-years gained for specific groups of individuals. A related economic and social issue is that the value of any cost or benefit changes when projected over time. Because preventive interventions are designed to achieve future benefits, the current monetary value of allocated resources or expenditures will be altered at some future date. The process of discounting converts future benefits or costs into its present value. The optimal discount rate (4–6%) may be explored through sensitivity analysis and represents a social opportunity cost, or the rate of return on public sector activities. The current value of the costs and benefits may be derived from the formula (Cohen and Henderson, 1988):

$$\text{Present value} = \frac{\text{Current dollar amount}}{(1 + r)^n}$$

where r = rate of discount and n = number of years before realizing benefits.

Cost-effectiveness analysis differs from cost–benefit analysis in that the discounted costs of alternative programs are compared with respect to efficiency and effectiveness in achieving a specified outcome or objective. Rather than assigning monetary values to differing or competing health objectives, where the emphasis is on the value of the return on an investment of public funds, cost-effectiveness analysis expresses benefits in units of effectiveness, such as the cost per year of life saved or death averted. In this context, the cost-effective value of a specific preventive intervention is measured in comparison with an alternative program designed to achieve the same objective. Cost-effectiveness analysis of a primary or secondary cancer prevention program is more readily achieved and generalizable under a uniform health care system. Cost-effectiveness analyses have also been applied to nonmedical interventions as, for example, in the assessment of regulatory policies limiting exposures to specific occupational and environmental carcinogens (Warner, 1995).

Economic and ethical considerations in assessing the efficacy of screening for cancer in apparently healthy people are analogous to the methods required in evaluating the safety, effectiveness, and efficiency of any medical intervention. The potential benefits of screening may be broadly translated into individual gains in years of productive life and reassurances about current "wellness," in addition to advancements in clinical and biological understanding of the natural history of a neoplastic disease process. Where the aim is to insure an appropriate use of health care resources, a public policy decision would assign priority to a program that achieves the equitable distribution of maximum benefits and minimum opportunity costs (Donaldson, 1994).

In illustrating the application of cost-effectiveness analysis to breast cancer screening in women 65–74 years of age, the costs would include direct costs of the screening test, follow-up costs for diagnostic (biopsy) procedures and treatment for those who are true positives, follow-up costs for those who are false positives and for complications from procedures associated with the screening, and estimated net costs (or savings) as a consumer of health services resulting from changes in life expectancy and productivity. Measurable or projected savings subtracted from costs include the savings of diagnostic and therapeutic procedures that are avoided as a result of the effectiveness of the intervention. A study by the Office of Technology Assessment (1987) examined the cost-effectiveness of screening of women 65–74 years of age with clinical and mammographic examinations. Assuming a constant unit charge of $50 for a biennial screening examination during the years 1990 to 2020, and discounting at 5% the costs and life-years saved in terms of 1984 dollars, the cost-effectiveness ratio was estimated to range from $13,000 to $35,000 per life-year saved. It has been difficult to assess the independent cost-effectiveness ratio for physical examinations and the incremental value of screening mammography. The cost-effectiveness ratio will be affected by unit screening and diagnostic costs, number of cancers detected compared to the number of screening examinations, and the proportion of false positives. Efficiency is enhanced by screening high-risk populations, and by careful consideration of the costs and benefits of the interval or frequency of screening (e.g., biennial vs. annual) and the projected life expectancy of the individual (Brown, 1992; Oddone et al, 1992).

Periodic screening for breast and uterine cervical cancer is currently an insurance entitlement for elderly women under Medicare. As was demonstrated for breast cancer screening, Pap testing for cervical cancer in elderly women at 3-year intervals will achieve limited average gains (16 days) in life extension; the cost per year of life saved, when compared with no screening for women 65–74 years of age, was estimated to be $2,254 (Fahs et al, 1992). Annual screening would achieve approximately a 15% increase in life-years, or 6,800 life-years per one million elderly women, but at a cost of almost $40,000 per year of life saved. Costs in relation to screening efficiency and effectiveness are enhanced in targeting high-risk, previously underserved populations.

MINORITY POPULATIONS

An important national goal of *Healthy People 2000* is to redress the inequities in general health status that cur-

TABLE 63–3. *Age-Adjusted Cancer Incidence and Mortality Rates per 100,000, and Five-Year Relative Survival Rates (Persons Diagnosed During 1983–89), U.S. Whites and Blacks, Males and Females, All Cancer Sites, 1990*

	Male			*Female*		
	Whites	*Blacks*	*Ratio Black/White*	*Whites*	*Blacks*	*Ratio Black/White*
Incidence	464.9	556.3	1.20	348.1	334.4	0.96
Mortality	214.7	323.4	1.50	140.5	169.7	1.21
Five-year relative survival (%)	49.6	34.4	0.69	59.1	44.7	0.76

rently exist among racial and ethnic minority populations. African-Americans comprise the largest minority group, consisting of first and second generation descendants and foreign-born immigrants, and numbering more than 30 million, or 12% of the U.S. population. African-American men currently have a 20% higher age-adjusted rate of cancer incidence than U.S. white men when combining all sites; the age-adjusted cancer incidence rate (all sites combined) for African-American women is slightly less than for U.S. white women (Table 63–3). The disparity between African-American men and white men and all women is more apparent for cancer mortality and survival rates. The determinants of excessive mortality among African-Americans are highly correlated with socioeconomic status (Otten et al, 1990; Sorlie et al, 1992). Economic disparities are expressed in terms of social conditions, such as nutrition, housing, employment and the safety of the working environment, and the affordability and quality of medical care. Excessive risks in cancer mortality, after adjusting for age and income, may in addition be due to differences in the distribution of epidemiologic risk factors or in attitudes and practices with respect to screening and detection of early stage disease. In a study of the relationship of personal factors (i.e., smoking, alcohol, body mass index, elevated cholesterol, diabetes, and blood pressure) and income as independent predictors of excess mortality (all causes) among African-Americans aged 35–54 years, when compared with U.S. whites, Otten et al (1990) noted that controlling for income accounted for one-third to almost 60% of the elevated mortality risks in this age-group; however, about one-third of the excess in mortality could not be accounted for by the six personal risk factors and their colinear relationship with income. Major risk factors for cancer such as cigarette smoking, obesity, and a sedentary lifestyle are more prevalent among African-Americans with low levels of education and income (Centers for Disease Control and Prevention, 1992).

Specific sites for which there were significantly increased risks for African-Americans included cervix uteri, esophagus, larynx, liver and intrahepatic bile duct, non-small cell lung, multiple myeloma, oral cavity and pharynx, pancreas, prostate and stomach. It is also instructive to note those sites for which African-Americans were at significantly reduced risk: corpus uteri, melanoma, non-Hodgkin's lymphoma, ovary, testis, thyroid, and urinary bladder (Table 63–4). While total cancer incidence increased 14–20% among African-Americans between 1975 and 1991, the increase in lung cancer incidence among men and the decrease in incidence of invasive uterine cervix cancer among women

TABLE 63–4. *Comparison of Age-Adjusted, Site-Specific Cancer Incidence Rates (per 100,000) in U.S. Whites and Blacks, 1990**

	Incidence		
Site	*Black*	*White*	*Black/White Ratio*
All (invasive)	423.1	392.3	1.08
Breast (female)	95.8	112.7	0.85
Cervix uteri	14.3	7.9	1.81
Colon and rectum	52.9	47.4	1.12
Corpus uteri (including uterus NOS)	14.5	22.7	0.64
Esophagus	11.5	3.6	3.19
Hodgkin's disease	2.7	3.0	0.90
Kidney and renal pelvis	8.8	8.9	0.99
Larynx	8.3	4.4	1.89
Liver and intrahepatic bile duct	5.3	2.4	2.21
Lung	74.7	57.2	1.31
Small cell	8.3	9.7	0.86
Non-small cell	66.3	47.5	1.40
Melanoma (skin)	0.9	12.0	0.08
Multiple myeloma	8.9	3.8	2.34
Non-Hodgkin's lymphoma	10.8	15.5	0.70
Oral cavity and pharynx	14.3	10.5	1.36
Ovary	10.2	15.0	0.68
Pancreas	12.3	8.2	1.50
Prostate	163.6	128.5	1.27
Stomach	11.7	6.2	1.89
Testis	0.5	5.2	0.10
Thyroid	3.1	4.7	0.66
Urinary bladder	10.1	17.9	0.56

*Based on data from the Surveillance Epidemiology and End Results (SEER) program, Cancer Statistics Review, 1973–1990. Rates are age-adjusted based on the 1970 U.S. standard population.

TABLE 63–5. *Comparison of Age-Adjusted, Site-Specific Cancer Incidence Rates (per 100,000) by Racial and Ethnic Groups, U.S. Males, 1980–1985**

	Whites		*Chinese*		*Japanese*		*Filipinos*		*Hawaiians*		*Hispanics*		*Native American*	
	Rate	*Rate Ratio*	*Rate*	*Rate Ratio*	*Rate*	*Rate Ratio*	*Rate*	*Rate Ratio*	*Rate*	*Rate Ratio*	*Rate*	*Rate Ratio*	*Rate*	*Rate Ratio*
All sites	404.1	1.00[a]	292.7	0.72	303.6	0.75	242.0	0.60	398.9	0.99	265.5	0.66	184.5	0.46
Colon	40.3	1.00	33.6	0.83	42.1	1.04	24.0	0.60	25.8	0.64	17.9	0.44	8.4	0.21
Esophagus	4.9	1.00	6.1	1.24	5.6	1.14	4.9	1.00	15.1	3.08	2.9	0.59	1.9	0.39
Kidney	10.3	1.00	4.9	0.48	6.1	0.59	4.6	0.45	6.9	0.67	8.7	0.84	9.2	0.89
Liver	2.7	1.00	19.5	7.22	7.1	2.63	10.2	3.78	9.8	3.63	4.3	1.59	4.5	1.67
Lung	82.1	1.00	61.2	0.76	48.4	0.59	39.9	0.49	108.2	1.32	32.2	0.39	14.2	0.17
Melanoma (skin)	9.8	1.00	0.4	0.04	1.5	0.15	1.2	0.12	1.6	0.16	1.6	0.16	2.2	0.22
Nasopharynx	0.6	1.00	13.9	23.17	1.4	2.33	2.9	4.83	1.5	2.50	0.9	1.50	0.5	0.83
Non-Hodgkin's lymphoma	13.0	1.00	10.2	0.78	9.2	0.71	9.8	0.75	10.9	0.84	6.9	0.53	4.7	0.36
Oral cavity and pharynx	11.8	1.00	6.2	0.53	6.0	0.51	6.8	0.58	10.1	0.86	5.2	0.44	1.7	0.14
Pancreas	11.2	1.00	8.7	0.78	9.9	0.88	7.9	0.71	10.6	0.95	12.4	1.11	9.0	0.80
Prostate	77.3	1.00	32.5	0.42	45.7	0.59	47.4	0.61	59.6	0.77	71.5	0.92	45.5	0.59
Stomach	11.5	1.00	14.5	1.26	38.6	3.36	9.6	0.83	40.4	3.51	20.8	1.81	26.1	2.27
Testis	4.2	1.00	1.9	0.45	1.3	0.31	0.5	0.12	2.6	0.62	3.0	0.71	1.8	0.43
Thyroid	2.3	1.00	4.5	1.96	6.2	2.70	6.8	2.96	7.4	3.22	2.9	1.26	2.3	1.00
Urinary bladder	30.2	1.00	13.9	0.46	12.5	0.41	6.0	0.20	10.6	0.35	10.9	0.36	3.6	0.12

*Based on data from the SEER program (New Mexico, San Francisco, and Hawaii). Rates are age-adjusted based on the 1970 United States standard population.

[a]Referent group for rate ratios is whites (1.00).

were more prominent trends than among U.S. whites. As noted for white men, lung cancer incidence in African-American men declined after 1975 among those aged 35–54 but increased among older men; cancer mortality rates (all sites combined) generally declined among African-Americans under age 55 and increased at older ages (Devesa et al, 1995). The decline in cancer mortality among younger cohorts over the past 15–20 years may be attributed to the availability and utilization of improving treatment and preventive services. Lung and prostate cancer mortality are jointly responsible for more than half of the excess cancer mortality among African-American men, and breast and uterine cervix cancer mortality account for approximately one-third of the excess in cancer mortality among African-American women.

The higher rate of lung cancer mortality among African-American men is associated with a higher tobacco smoking prevalence, preference for high-tar and mentholated cigarettes, and a lower likelihood of smoking cessation; by contrast, the odds of heavy smoking are diminished among African-Americans, when compared with whites (Novotny et al, 1988). African-Americans tend to start smoking at a later age, prefer high-nicotine, high-tar, and mentholated cigarettes across various socioeconomic subgroups, and exhibit a pattern of more intense nicotine dependency, even while smoking less each day, than U.S. (non-Hispanic) whites (Royce et al, 1993; Coultas et al, 1994).

The population of the United States includes other minority groups of diverse racial (genetic, biologic, and geographic) and ethnic (sociocultural) origins, and patterns of health, disease, and illness. In the 1990 U.S. Census, minority groups other than African-Americans constituted about 12% of the population, or 30 million people. During the 10-year period 1980–1990, while the non-Hispanic white population increased by 6%, Asians-Pacific Islanders increased by 108%, Hispanics increased by 53%, Native Americans, 38%, and African-Americans by 13%. The minority populations tend to be younger than the non-Hispanic whites and to have a smaller proportion of elderly. The effects of race and ethnicity on site-specific patterns of cancer incidence are mediated through a complex web of lifestyle, socioeconomic, cultural, and genetic determinants (Tables 63–5, 63–6). Language or communication and employment skills influence the process and degree of psychosocial acculturation and ultimately have an impact on health behavior, access to health care, and preventive practices.

The heterogeneity and dynamic transitioning of cancer incidence patterns in generations of minority racial and ethnic groups are providing challenging opportunities for the epidemiologic study of potential causal mechanisms and the targeting of cancer control inter-

TABLE 63–6. *Comparison of Age-Adjusted, Site-Specific Cancer Incidence Rates (per 100,000) by Racial and Ethnic Groups, U.S. Females, 1980–1985**

	Whites		*Chinese*		*Japanese*		*Filipinos*		*Hawaiians*		*Hispanics*		*Native American*	
	Rate	*Rate Ratio*	*Rate*	*Rate Ratio*	*Rate*	*Rate Ratio*	*Rate*	*Rate Ratio*	*Rate*	*Rate Ratio*	*Rate*	*Rate Ratio*	*Rate*	*Rate Ratio*
All sites	316.1	1.00[a]	242.2	0.77	214.0	0.68	202.6	0.64	344.1	1.09	220.4	0.70	168.8	0.53
Gallbladder	1.6	1.00	1.0	0.63	1.7	1.06	1.8	1.13	1.3	0.81	7.1	4.44	17.1	10.69
Lung	29.7	1.00	27.6	0.93	13.2	0.44	17.9	0.60	45.8	1.54	15.6	0.53	4.6	0.15
Breast	91.5	1.00	58.7	0.64	57.1	0.62	45.6	0.50	104.6	1.14	50.9	0.56	25.6	0.28
Cervix uteri	8.8	1.00	10.5	1.19	5.8	0.66	10.8	1.23	14.5	1.65	17.1	1.94	20.0	2.27
Corpus uteri (including uterus NOS)	27.1	1.00	18.2	0.67	17.6	0.65	11.0	0.41	28.0	1.03	11.2	0.41	5.2	0.19
Ovary	14.1	1.00	10.3	0.73	8.5	0.60	9.7	0.69	13.2	0.94	11.3	0.80	8.9	0.63
Thyroid	5.5	1.00	6.9	1.25	6.6	1.20	17.3	3.15	13.7	2.49	7.9	1.44	6.1	1.11

*Based on data from the SEER program (New Mexico, San Francisco, and Hawaii). Rates are age-adjusted based on the 1970 United States standard population.
[a]Referent group for rate ratios is whites (1.00).

ventions. Compared with other racial and ethnic groups, non-Hispanic whites were, with few exceptions, at higher risk of melanoma, non-Hodgkin's lymphoma, and cancers of the breast, corpus uteri, ovary, testis, and urinary bladder. Chinese-Americans experienced elevated rates for cancers of the nasopharynx and liver, whereas Japanese-Americans were at higher risk than non-Hispanic whites for cancers of the stomach, colon, and thyroid. Filipino-American women and men had an elevated risk for thyroid cancer, whereas Hawaiian-Americans demonstrated increased incidence rates for cancers of the lung, esophagus, liver, breast, uterine corpus, stomach, and thyroid. Native Americans (American Indians) experienced about half the overall cancer incidence of non-Hispanic whites, but were distinguished by elevated rates for cancers of the liver and bile ducts, gallbladder, stomach, and uterine cervix.

The age-adjusted incidence of lung cancer among Native American men of the Southwest was 17% that of the rate registered among non-Hispanic white men (Table 63–5). Although absolute and relative risks for Native Americans were low, lung cancer rates in New Mexico had increased from 1958 to 1982 by 104% for men and by 163% for women. Although smoking prevalence rates had increased during this interval, a substantial proportion of the increment among men was attributable to exposure to radon progeny by workers in uranium mines (Samet et al, 1988). In the north central United States, where the prevalence of smoking among Native Americans was higher than in the Southwest and comparable to that of the general population, lung cancer mortality increased fivefold (25×10^{-5}) but was only one-half the rate for non-Hispanic whites (Coultas et al, 1994).

Hispanic Americans residing in New Mexico were at an elevated risk for cancers of the liver, stomach, and uterine cervix. South Florida Hispanic women of Caribbean origin were at significantly lower risk than non-Hispanic whites for cancers of the oral cavity, esophagus, colon, lung, breast, ovary, urinary bladder, non-Hodgkin's lymphoma and melanoma; the rates for Hispanic women were significantly higher than those for non-Hispanic white women for cancers of the liver, gallbladder, and uterine cervix (Trapido et al, 1994). The currently observed lower rates of lung cancer among Hispanics appear to be consistent with differences in tobacco smoking prevalence rates between Hispanics and non-Hispanic whites. Hispanics are a diverse cultural group, numbering approximately 22 million, or 9% of the total population, with origins in Mexico, Cuba, Puerto Rico, and Central and South America. In future surveillance reports of white and black Hispanic-Americans, who are increasing at five times the rate of non-Hispanic U.S. whites, it will be important to distinguish cancer incidence and mortality patterns based on characteristics of race, country of birth for the population at risk and their parents, length of residence in the United States, and population-based prevalence rates of behavioral risk factors.

CHEMOPREVENTION

Chemoprevention is an emerging translational concept in cancer control that involves the use of selected synthetic, chemical, or natural agents to reverse, suppress, or prevent the carcinogenic process. The theoretical foundation for evaluating the therapeutic efficacy of chemopreventive pharmaceutical agents and antioxidant micronutrients is "multistep, multistage carcinogenesis", and "field cancerization." The development of a malignant tumor involves multiple stages that include initiation; promotion, which may lead ultimately to the appearance of a benign tumor; neoplastic transformation; and progression, with advancing steps of malignancy. The transitions between successive stages are enhanced or inhibited by different types of agents. DNA-damaging agents initiate the carcinogenic process and affect the stage of tumor progression by activating cellular protooncogenes, ablating the modulating mechanisms of tumor suppressor genes, and dysregulating cyclin kinases and related genes. The increasing heterogeneity and autonomy that is exhibited in the progression stage is accompanied by karyotypic instability and frequently gene amplification. Alterations in the fidelity of DNA and chromosome replication and of DNA repair represent perturbations of endogenous mechanisms that may potentiate tumor initiation and progression. In addition to the multiple genetic mutations in carcinogenesis, there are epigenetic distortions that occur in signal transduction, gene expression, gene imprinting, and differentiation which play a critical role in promotion and provide mechanistic pathways of action by specific chemopreventive agents. Field cancerization advances the concept that upon exposure to a carcinogen, a contiguous "field" of tissue is conditioned for the development of malignant cells. This would be applicable, for example, to the upper aerodigestive, lower urinary, anogenital (female), cutaneous, and mammary tissues, where multiple primary cancers are commonly observed.

Candidate chemopreventive agents are (1) compounds that reduce the endogenous synthesis of carcinogens (e.g., ascorbic acid and alpha-tocopherol which block in vivo formation of nitrosamines); (2) compounds that reduce rate and amount of absorption of carcinogenic chemicals (e.g., dietary fiber, substances that bind fatty and bile acids); (3) chemicals that alter the metabolism of carcinogens or the generation of free radicals and activated forms of oxygen (e.g., isothiocyanates in cruciferous vegetables, retinoids, and carotenoids); (4) chemicals that inhibit the covalent binding of carcinogens to DNA (e.g., flavonoids, which are present in vegetables and fruits); (5) dietary substances that inhibit tumor formation by unknown mechanisms (e.g., organosulfur compounds in garlic and onions, various protease inhibitors, and polyphenols in green tea); and (6) chemicals that inhibit tumor promotion and cell proliferation (e.g., estrogen hormone agonist inhibitors such as progestins, tamoxifen, and 4-(hydroxyphenyl) retinamide). Examples of other antiproliferative pharmaceutical agents include piroxicam (a nonsteroidal anti-inflammatory), 2-difluoromethylornithine (an inhibitor of ornithine decarboxylase), oltipraz (which maintains reduced glutathione pools and is structurally related to dithiolthiones that have been identified in cruciferous vegetables), and ellagic acid (which inhibits the formation of electrophilic covalent DNA adducts such as with diol-epoxides and O^6-methylation of guanine in DNA) (Kelloff et al, 1990).

Chemopreventive agents are being evaluated in patients with preneoplastic lesions (e.g., dysplasia, oral leukoplakia, adenomatous polyps, Barrett's esophagus, etc.), or after a previous primary cancer, in persons identified as part of a high-risk group (e.g., family history, xeroderma pigmentosum, heavy smoker, etc.), or in the general population where the cancer occurs with anticipated high frequency (e.g., prostate cancer in U.S. men over age 50, esophageal/gastric cardia cancer in Linxian, China). An ethical issue in chemoprevention trials of uncertain efficacy is that even mild toxicity in healthy subjects may be unacceptable. In the evaluation of chemopreventive compounds, a three-tiered approach is used to determine efficacy, safety and toxicity in humans. Phase I trials determine the dose-related safety and patterns of toxicity of pharmaceuticals and include pharmacokinetic studies. Phase II trials are limited-scale, short-term evaluations of biological activity, determined by measuring effects on surrogate or intermediate end points in the carcinogenic process. An intermediate end point is a biological event that takes place between carcinogenic exposure and the development of cancer. Phase III testing involves a large-scale controlled experimental trial usually comparing a new agent with a placebo and involving long-term follow-up in thousands of subjects (Ederer et al, 1993; Church et al, 1993; Kelloff et al, 1995). Factorial designs allow for the randomized testing of more than one agent to achieve more than one therapeutic goal in the same population. A "run-in" feasibility phase of 2 to 4 months may serve to enhance long-term participation and limit the potential bias of noncompliance.

The end point of a trial may be the incidence of cancer or an intermediate event, such as a premalignant lesion (e.g., dysplasia) or a biochemical or molecular marker. A specific predictive biomarker, for example, of genotoxicity or abnormal proliferation, should be responsive to the pharmacologic action of the agent and expressed differently in neoplastic or high-risk preneoplastic tissue, when compared with background spontaneous events in normal tissue in the same organ site (Lippman et al, 1994). Potential intermediate end point biomarkers that are being evaluated in clinical trials include, for example, aneuploidy, DNA adducts, *p53* mutations, *ras* mutations, and cell surface carbohydrate antigens. A review of suggested candidate biomarkers for investigation and validation in chemoprevention studies of aerodigestive tract tumorigenesis listed (1) general genomic markers (e.g., micronuclei, DNA content, chromosomal alterations; (2) specific genetic markers (e.g., *ras, myc, erb* oncogene alterations; *p53, rb, 3p* tumor suppressor genes; Src family; retinoic acid receptors); (3)

proliferation markers (e.g., mitotic frequency, thymidine labeling index, nuclear antigens (PCNA, DNA-polymerase α), polyamines, ornithine decarboxylase; (4) differentiation markers (e.g., cytokeratins, involucrin); and (5) cell loss markers for apoptosis (e.g., Bcl-2 expression, in situ end labeling of fragmented DNA) (Shin et al, 1994).

The Alpha-Tocopherol, Beta-Carotene Cancer Prevention Study was a randomized double-blind, placebo-controlled prevention trial with a total of 29,133 participants that was undertaken in Finland to determine whether supplementation with daily alpha-tocopherol (50 mg), beta-carotene (20 mg), or both, would reduce the incidence of lung cancer in male smokers 50 to 69 years of age (Alpha-Tocopherol, Beta-Carotene Cancer Prevention Study Group, 1994). Compliance with the four-armed protocol was estimated to be at least 80% and comparable for each subgroup. After 5 to 8 years of dietary supplementation, no reduction in lung cancer incidence was observed in any of the intervention subgroups. In fact, by the end of the study, the incidence of lung cancer among the men who received beta-carotene alone (57.2×10^{-4} person-years) was significantly higher than the incidence in the placebo group (47.7×10^{-4} person-years). There was no apparent confounding of results by prior cigarette smoking history or spontaneous smoking cessation after the initiation of the trial. The daily dose of beta-carotene used in the trial increased the median baseline blood levels more than ten-fold; however, the daily dose of alpha-tocopherol used increased the median baseline blood levels by only 50%.

Previous epidemiologic studies have suggested that higher intake of vegetables and fruits was associated with 40–50% reduction in smoking-age-gender–adjusted relative risk of lung cancer of various cell types (Bjelke, 1975; Byers et al, 1987; LeMarchand et al, 1989). Although beta-carotene is one of the few carotenoids converted to retinol (vitamin A) in vivo, its mechanism of inhibition of carcinogenesis may be due to "quenching" or neutralizing of free radicals or of reactive oxygen species that are generated endogenously, and to regulation of gene expression and transcription. Free radicals, such as superoxide anion and the hydroxyl radical, are highly reactive and attack the nucleic acids in DNA, denature proteins, and cause peroxidation of cell membrane lipids. The existence of other potentially anticarcinogenic substances in vegetables and fruits—including other antioxidant, non-provitamin A carotenoids (e.g., lutein, lycopene), selenium, ascorbic acid, dithiolthiones, indoles, isothiocyanates, allium compounds, isoflavones, saponins, and plant sterols—underscores the potential pitfall of interpreting the epidemiologic data narrowly as favoring a single nutrient or biochemical mechanism. The results of the Finnish trial do not disprove the potential benefits of supplemental dietary interventions, other than with beta-carotene, in conjunction with other health-promoting actions such as smoking cessation. The modulating effects of natural or synthetic chemopreventive agents, particularly if they have an impact on early stages of cancer induction, may require many years before they are demonstrable. In the nutrition intervention trial in Linxian, China, however, supplementation with beta-carotene (15mg/day), vitamin E (30mg/day), and selenium (50μg/day) was associated with a 21% reduction in stomach cancer mortality. The reduction in risk was first apparent after about 30 months and was sustained over a period of 63 months. Linxian provided an optimal setting in that there was a large, stable population with baseline nutrient deficiencies and an extraordinarily high incidence of stomach cancer (Blot et al, 1993).

PRIMARY CARE SETTING

The challenge for cancer control practitioners is to apply effectively and efficiently the technologies that serve to alter high-risk behaviors and ensure early detection and curative intervention before the usual presentation of illness symptoms. During a given year, approximately three out of four Americans visit a physician and average about 3 office or clinic visits (National Center for Health Statistics, 1988). The opportunity for providing preventive services in the medical care setting would appear to be potentially achievable but requires consideration of economic, organizational, and conceptual barriers. In a survey of physicians' attitudes and practices conducted by the American Cancer Society (1990), 78% reported following or exceeding the guidelines for breast physical exams, 37% adhered to mammography guidelines, 55% administered the Pap test, and 48% the digital rectal exam. Screening sigmoidoscopy is performed or recommended in patients over age 50 years by 34% of primary care physicians (Schoen et al, 1995). Physicians' self-reports in general have not been validated by a review of medical records, and may have overestimated the extent of adherence with the guidelines. Even when physicians agree with the guidelines for specific preventive interventions, this may not be sufficient for compliance. Continuing medical education programs have not been generally effective in sustaining changes in physician behavior, unless they were designed to provide new diagnostic and communication skills and alter the office practice environment, including the activities of office staff (Cohen et al, 1994). Technical skills training would address how to incorporate a physician and patient reminder system for preventive examinations and services into the medical office practice setting.

Studies of potential deterrents of optimal use of cancer screening tests have described the determining role of physicians who may, for various reasons, not recommend, provide, or facilitate access to screening examinations. The lack of physician advocacy of cancer screening in clinical practice may be due to disagreement with or confusion about prevention guidelines, concerns about safety and efficacy of testing and patient compliance, absence of economic incentives, or logistical barriers arising from limited resources in a particular geographic area. Screening practices may also vary in relation to the patient's age, race, health insurance status, and the nature of pre-existing medical conditions. Prior studies have identified similar motivational barriers to physician involvement in primary and secondary cancer prevention and control activities, which have included (1) a relatively low frequency of cancer in primary care settings; (2) competing priorities for treating illness complaints; (3) confusion about indications for and implementation of counseling (e.g., smoking cessation, weight reduction, familial history) or screening examinations; and (4) lack of positive reinforcement from office staff (Williams and Williams, 1987; Nutting, 1986; Orlandi, 1987). We may assume that physician behavior will be significantly influenced by financial incentives. A carefully rationalized strategy for providing periodic cancer preventive services will be effectively implemented in the ambulatory practice setting when health insurance sources of reimbursement are available. As stated previously, the justification for investing in a comprehensive cancer prevention program should not be anticipation of cost-saving, but rather as a means of promoting health and extending productive life.

PREVENTION THROUGH LEGISLATION

It is the responsibility of government to protect the public from exposures to known or suspected carcinogens occurring in the workplace, ambient environment, tobacco products, foods, pharmaceuticals, medical devices, and other consumer products.

Tobacco

Tobacco use in the United States has been estimated to contribute directly to 30.5% of total cancer mortality; the corresponding attributable proportion for all cancer deaths in women was estimated to be 21.5% and in men, 45%. Lung cancer has displaced coronary heart disease as the leading cause of excess mortality among smokers in the 1990s in the United States (Shopland et al, 1991). Tobacco control in the United States has evolved since the publication of the Surgeon General's report in 1964 on the health consequences of smoking (U.S. Department of Health, Education, and Welfare, 1964). Smoking prevalence in adult men had declined substantially from 52% in 1965 to 28% in 1991; during this period, the prevalence of smoking in adult women declined from 34% to 24%. During the 1991 survey, there were 43 million persons who were classified as former smokers. A variety of interventions have been advocated to influence smoking cessation and smoking initiation: school-based health education programs; reducing minors' access to tobacco products; developing and enacting clean indoor air policies and laws; restricting or eliminating advertising directed toward persons aged < 18 years; and increasing tobacco excise taxes. In 1991 the prevalence of smoking was highest among persons 25–44 years of age (30%), and lowest for those 65 years of age and over (13%). Even though the sale of tobacco products to minors is illegal in 46 states, compliance with these laws is poorly enforced, and there are about one million new smokers each year who are children and adolescents (Morbidity and Mortality Weekly Report, 1994; Novotny, 1992).

In the United States, the advertising ban on tobacco products on radio and television (electronic media) for manufacturers (Public Health Cigarette Smoking Act of 1969) went into effect in January 1971. However, although advertising in the electronic media ceased, cigarette advertising in magazines and newspapers and on billboards increased significantly; from 1975 to 1990, when measured in the context of 1975 dollars, annual expenditures on cigarette advertising and promotional events increased more than threefold.

In 1989, U.S. legislation banned smoking on domestic airline flights. Subsequently, in 1993 the U.S. Environmental Protection Agency (EPA) classified environmental tobacco smoke as a class A human carcinogen that was responsible for approximately 3,000 lung cancer deaths each year in nonsmokers.

While smoking prevalence rates have been gradually declining in North America and Western Europe, they have been rising at about 2% per year in Eastern European and Asian countries. The Japanese market, for example, was opened to foreign cigarette manufacturers in 1986, and from 1986 through 1991, smoking prevalence rates among Japanese women increased from 8.6% to 18.2%; in 1991, 27% of Japanese women 20–29 years of age were smokers, which was comparable to the prevalence reported in U.S. white women. About one-third of all cancer deaths in developed countries are attributed to the use of tobacco; during the 1990s, the attributable fraction in males was estimated to be 47% and in females, 14% (Peto et al, 1992).

In a comprehensive review of international regulatory action to control the global tobacco epidemic, Roemer (1993) described legislative initiatives that controlled advertising, sponsorship, and promotion; required health warnings and statements of tar and nicotine contents; classified tobacco as a harmful substance; restricted sales; restricted smoking in public places, as when using public transportation, and/or at the workplace; and recommended stringent tax and price policies. In general, a policy of increasing taxes was designed to promote the production of low-tar and low-nicotine cigarettes and to enable funds to be allocated for health education and smoking cessation programs or for tobacco-related research. Increasing taxes on tobacco has generally resulted in decreased consumption. A 10% increase in the price of cigarettes has resulted in a 4% decrease in adult consumption and a 14% decrease in teenage consumption (Warner, 1986; MacKenzie et al, 1994). Regulation of the addicting and carcinogenic potential of tobacco by controlling nicotine and tar yield has been beneficial. In the American Cancer Society Prospective Study, Stellman and Garfinkel (1986) concluded that by doubling the cigarette tar yield, the risk of dying of lung cancer would increase 40%, independently of the amount smoked or depth of inhalation.

Occupational and Environmental Safety and Health

Many of the chemical agents currently viewed as human carcinogens were originally identified by epidemiologic and animal studies as workplace exposures (Schottenfeld and Haas, 1981). However, toxic substances originating in the workplace may escape into the air, soil, and ground and surface water. Ambient contamination can occur as a result of industrial processing, accidents, or the improper disposal of toxic substances and hazardous wastes. Numerous laws have been enacted and amended in response to concerns regarding hazardous materials and wastes (Table 63–7). The Occupational Safety and Health Act (1970) created the federal Occupational Safety and Health Administration (OSHA), which was assigned to the Department of Labor. The OSH Act was to control risks by setting specific safety and hygiene standards and exposure limits, and by requiring record keeping and hazard communication to workers. The Act also allowed individual states to enact laws that could assume responsibility for part or all of the federal OSHA functions.

Other laws were enacted to regulate substances in the environment and disposal of hazardous materials. These laws included the Clean Air Act, Clean Water Act, Toxic Substance Control Act (TSCA), and the Resource Conservation and Recovery Act. The TSCA regulates hazardous chemicals currently in existence and determines the risks of chemicals that are to be introduced. It also mandates that the EPA maintain and publish a listing of chemicals manufactured or processed in the United States. Manufacturers are required to report to the EPA about uses, amounts produced, byproducts, number of exposed workers, and adverse effects on human health and the environment of any chemical; for manufacturers and processors of new chemicals, the EPA requires a 90-day notice prior to manufacturing or use. The EPA has the authority to regulate or prohibit use, production, processing, distribution, or disposal of a chemical.

TABLE 63–7. *Occupational and Environmental Safety Legislation in the United States**

Agency	*Status (year[s] of enactment)*
Department of Labor	
Occupational Safety and Health Administration (OSHA)	Occupational Safety and Health Act (1970) (established National Institute for Occupational Safety and Health [NIOSH]
Mine Safety and Health Administration (MSHA)	Mine Safety and Health Act (1977)
Environmental Protection Agency (EPA)	Clean Air Act (1963, 1970, 1974, 1977) Clean Water Act (1972) Safe Drinking Water Act (1974) Resource Conservation and Recovery Act (1976) Federal Insecticide, Fungicide, and Rodenticide Act (1948, 1972, 1975, 1978) Toxic Substances Control Act (1976) Superfund Amendment and Reauthorization Act (1986) Comprehensive Environmental Response, Compensation, and Liability Act (1981)
Food and Drug Administration (FDA)	Federal Food, Drug, and Cosmetic Act (1906, 1938, 1960, 1962, 1968) (Delaney Clause [1958] for food additives that caused cancer on animal testing)
Consumer Product and Safety Commission	Federal Hazardous Substances Act (1960, 1981) Consumer Product Safety Act (1972, 1981)

*As of January 1, 1992.

Regulatory decisions on toxic or hazardous substances are guided by the methodology of risk assessment. The objective of risk assessment is to characterize the potential adverse health effects of human exposures to environmental hazards. Risk assessment also includes characterization of the uncertainties inherent in inferring the extent of risk under given conditions of exposure. The multistep components of risk assessment address at least four elements:

1. *Hazard identification* is based on methods of causal inference, which include epidemiologic and/or animal experimental studies, short-term in vitro testing

TABLE 63–8. *Chemicals and Industrial Processes Associated with Human Lung Cancer**

Agent	*Human Target Organs*	*Epidemiology*	*Toxicology*
Arsenic	Lung Skin Urinary tract	Over 95% of arsenic produced in the United States is by-product of copper, lead, zinc and tin ore smelting. Excess lung cancer reported in association with use and production of inorganic trivalent arsenic-containing pesticides. Dose–response trends have been validated by measuring concentrations in air and urine. Joint action with tobacco smoking appears to be more than additive and less than multiplicative. Latency of 10–35 years.	No satisfactory animal model. In tissue culture system: chromosomal aberrations inhibition of DNA repair increased sister chromatid exchanges
Asbestos	Lung Mesothelium or serosa of pleura, pericardium, and peritoneum ?GI tract ?Larynx	Various workers in asbestos industries at increased risk: miners, millers, textile, insulation, shipyard, cement. Average latency period of 25–30 years for carcinoma of lung. Length of interval varies with type of fiber, exposure intensity and duration, and host factors. Dose–response relationship is approximately linear in form across mid- to upper levels of exposure. Relative risk of lung cancer appears to decrease following cessation of exposure. Synergistic relationship with cigarette smoking, which is more than additive and close to multiplicative. Asbestos exposure in the U.S. accounts for approximately 5% of lung cancer deaths in men.	Asbestos minerals are divided into: a) the amphiboles, including amosite, crocidolite, anthophyllite, and tremolite; b) serpentine class which is represented by chrysotile. All types of commercial asbestos fibers are carcinogenic in mice, rats, hamsters and rabbits; after inhalation, or intrapleural and intraperitoneal administration, cancers of the lung and bronchus, and/or mesotheliomas have been induced.
Bis (chloromethyl) ether, and chloromethyl methyl ether	Lung	Used in manufacture of ion exchange resins, polymers, plastics; tumor cell type was primarily (85%) small-cell (oat-cell) carcinoma. Changes in industrial process from open-kettle to closed, hermetically isolated systems in 1971 have markedly reduced exposure and were accompanied by declining risk of lung cancer. Increasing risk with increasing intensity and duration of exposure.	Highly carcinogenic in rodents by inhalation, skin application, or subcutaneous injection. BCME is a more potent carcinogen than CMME.
Chromium and compounds	Lung Nasal and paranasal sinuses	Used in metal alloys, electroplating, lithography magnetic tapes, paint pigments, cement, rubber, photoengraving, composition floor covering, and as oxidant in synthesis of organic chemicals. Excess risk, threefold and higher, was demonstrated for all cell types of lung cancer in the chromate-producing industry, particularly during 1930–1945. Risks in other occupational settings, with lower intensity exposures, have not been consistently or substantially increased.	Epidemiologic and experimental data implicate hexavalent and not trivalent chromium compounds.
Nickel and compounds	Lung Nasal and paranasal sinuses Larynx	Used in electroplating, manufacturing of steel and other alloys, ceramics, storage batteries, electric circuits, petroleum refining, and oil hydrogenation. Risk associated with earliest stage of refining, involving heavy exposure to dust from relatively crude ore. In some nickel refineries, high levels of PAHs, arsenic, or other agents may have contributed to increased risks. In mining for nickel, workers may be exposed to asbestos.	Animal studies indicate that nickel compounds can produce local sarcomas by injection, and pulmonary tumors by inhalation and intratracheal instillation. Several forms of nickel may be carcinogenic, and include oxides, sulfites, and soluble nickel.
Polycyclic aromatic hydrocarbons (PAHs)	Lung Skin and scrotum Urinary bladder	Chemicals may result from ferrochromium production, and smelting of nickel-containing ores; aluminum production, iron and steel founding, coke production, and coal gasification; coal tars, coal tar pitches, untreated mineral oils, soot from combustion and diesel engine exhausts.	PAHs result from pyrolysis or incomplete combustion of organic compounds.

(continued)

TABLE 63–8. (*Continued*)

Agent	*Human Target Organs*	*Epidemiology*	*Toxicology*
	In relation to coke oven emissions, risk of lung cancer is highest in workers on the topside of coke ovens. Among the most heavily exposed, lifetime risk could reach 40%.	Benzo(a)pyrene-DNA adducts, a marker of PAH exposure, have been detected in the blood samples of coke oven workers.	
Radon	Lung	Increased risks of lung cancer have been observed among underground miners in North America, Europe, and Asia, and quantitatively related to the inhalation of radon daughter products.	Dose of high LET alpha particles to individual cells will vary with respiratory dynamics, thickness of the epithelial cell and overlapping mucous layers, and the clearance rate of absorbed radioactive particles.
		Although small-cell cancers predominate, all cell types are affected.	Cellular DNA damage depends on the type of radiation, amount of energy deposited per volume of tissue, the rate at which the energy is deposited, and the time over which a given dose is accumulated.
		Radiation and cigarette smoking are interactive with relative risks somewhat less than multiplicative.	
		Exposure levels in miners associated with elevated risks generally exceeded 100 working level months (about 0.5Gy).	
		Linear non-threshold dose–response. For the same cumulative dose, prolonged exposures at low dose rates appear more hazardous than shorter exposures at higher dose rates.	
Vinyl chloride	Liver (angiosarcoma) Lung Brain ? Lymphoreticular	Principal use is in production of plastics, packaging materials, and vinyl asbestos floor tiles.	Inhalation of vinyl chloride monomer and polyvinyl chloride in experimental animals causes pulmonary fibrosis and adenomas, skin appendage tumors, and osteochondromas.
		A review of 12 cohort studies of men employed at synthetic or polyvinyl chloride polymerization plants reported SMRs for lung cancer indicating an overall observed-to-expected lung cancer ratio of 1.12 (95% confidence interval from 1.0 to 1.2).	

*Agents are those classified as known carcinogens (Group 1) by the International Agency for Research on Cancer.

(e.g., mutagenicity), and structure–activity correlations for putative toxic agents.

2. *Dose–response assessment* is an analysis of the relationship of incidence of adverse health outcome(s) to dose intensity and cumulative exposure levels, absence or presence of a demonstrable dose threshold, and modifying personal risk factors.

3. *Exposure assessment* describes the intensity, duration, temporal variability, and route(s) of exposure and patterns of distribution in human populations.

4. *Risk characterization* estimates the incidence of adverse effects and the variability or uncertainty of such estimates, based on the assessments of exposure and dose–response.

The limitations of risk assessment are apparent when there is wide disparity in the predictions of risk based on different statistical models, which may be attributed in part to the lack of empirical or epidemiological verification of any model and the uncertainties inherent in extrapolating from an animal species to humans or from high-dose to low-dose exposure levels. *Low-dose extrapolation* describes the fitting of mathematical dose–response models to data at high doses where increases in tumor incidence in experimental animals or humans can be readily measured, and then estimating risks from exposures to low doses where epidemiologic or animal data are lacking or inconsistent. The various statistical models that have been developed attempt, with arguable

TABLE 63–9. *Major Environmental (Non-occupational) Causes of Human Cancer: Strategic Targets for Prevention and Control*

Agent	*Site(s) of Cancer*	*Commentary*
Tobacco	Oral cavity, pharynx, larynx, esophagus, lung and bronchus, pancreas, kidney parenchyma, pelvis, ureter, urinary bladder	Risks are also associated with uterine cervix, stomach (cardia), leukemia, myeloma(?), colorectal adenoma and carcinoma, anogential carcinomas (male and female). Tobacco smoking accounts for about 40% of all cancer deaths in men and 20% in women in the U.S. For smokers of 1–2 packs per day, relative risks (point estimates) compared to non-smokers range as follows: lung and bronchus (10), larynx (8), mouth and pharynx (4), esophagus (3), urinary bladder (2), pancreas (2). Degree of risk correlated with duration of smoking, number of cigarettes smoked, depth of inhalation, tar content. Pipe and cigar smokers are at increased risk for oral cavity, pharynx, larynx, esophagus. Smokeless tobacco (chewing tobacco and snuff) is associated with oral cancer, particularly gingivobuccal mucosa. Environmental tobacco smoke in lifetime non-smokers is associated with 30–70% increased risk of lung cancer, with dose–response effect; approximately 3,000 lung cancer deaths per year in the U.S. among non-smokers. Cessation of smoking is associated with gradual decline in risk, approaching but not equivalent to the risk in the never smoker.
Alcohol	Oral cavity, pharynx, esophagus, larynx, liver Possible association with breast and colorectal cancers	Accounts for 3%–5% of all cancer deaths in USA. Combined exposure with tobacco accounts for 75–85% of oral and pharyngeal, and of esophageal cancers in the U.S. Alcohol effects are more prominently associated with supraglottic (extrinsic larynx) than glottic (intrinsic larynx) cancers. Cirrhosis potentiates risk of liver cancer (hepatocellular carcinoma). Possible mechanisms of carcinogenic action include: Local cytotoxicity affecting mucosal permeability Presence of low levels of carcinogens in alcoholic beverages (e.g., fusel oils, polycyclic aromatic hydrocarbons, nitrosamines); Induction of microsomal enzymes that activate pro-carcinogens in remote and target tissues; Alcoholic liver injury may affect important mechanisms of chemical detoxification; Nutritional deficiencies (e.g., vitamins A, C, riboflavin, and iron) give rise to altered mucosal integrity, enzyme and metabolic dysfunction, and morphologic abnormalities Decreased immune responsiveness
Ionizing radiation	Bone marrow, breast, and thyroid tissues are the most radiosensitive. Lung, connective tissue, and bone represent other important target tissues. All other exposed sites are potentially at risk.	Approximately 5% of all cancer deaths in the U.S., the upper limit depending on estimate of lung cancer deaths attributable to domestic radon exposure. Radiation-induced leukemias (excluding chronic lymphocytic leukemia) appear after minimal latency interval of 2–4 years, peaking at 6–8 years, and declining to approximate normal in 25 years. Radiation-induced carcinomas have minimal latency of 5–10 years. Temporal distribution is consistent with age- and site-specific incidence curve of background in population; thus radiation superimposed on underlying risk pattern. Genetic factors may affect susceptibility, e.g., retinoblastoma, Li-Fraumeni syndrome, ataxia telangiectasia, Gorlin syndrome (nevoid basal cell carcinoma syndrome). Regulatory agencies generally assume linear nonthreshold dose–response curve. Indoor radon accounts for over 50% of all radiation exposures received by general population, and based on extrapolations from high-dose miner studies, may cause between 5,000 and 20,000 lung cancer deaths per year in the U.S. Tobacco smoke is interactive with alpha particles resulting in biologic synergy.
Ultraviolet (solar) radiation	Skin: melanoma, and squamous and basal cell carcinomas	Accounts for 10% of all cancer cases and 2% of all cancer deaths. Of major concern are the u.v.-B radiations (290–320 nm). Skin cancer is predominantly a disease of the white race and is rare in deeply pigmented ethnic and racial groups.

(continued)

TABLE 63–9. (*Continued*)

Agent	Site(s) of Cancer	Commentary
		In nonmelanoma skin cancer, lesions occur primarily on parts of the body with direct chronic exposure; outdoor workers are at greater risk than indoor workers; incidence is greatest in areas of high exposure intensity and is inversely correlated with latitude. Solar etiology of malignant melanoma is more consistent with intermittent intense exposures beginning in childhood, accompanied by acute episodes of blistering or erythema, rather than gradual tanning, and development of junctional nevi. Melanoma incidence is not correlated with outdoor work, is particularly high in upper managerial and professional employment categories, and, in contrast with squamous carcinoma of the skin, is not significantly age-dependent. Host factors, such as familial dysplastic nevus syndrome, and other genetic conditions such as xeroderma pigmentosum with defective DNA repair enzymes, albinism, and acquired immune dysfunction, may serve as predisposing or enhancing characteristics in melanoma.
Exogenous estrogen	Endometrium, breast	Peak incidence of endometrial adenocarcinoma in the mid 1970s among U.S. white women, 45–64 years of age, attributed to estrogen replacement therapy. FDA warning issued in 1976 accompanied by 30% decline in incidence by 1990; declining incidence and mortality due to changing regimen among post-menopausal women that combined lower level estrogen with progestogen. Combination oral contraceptives are effectively chemopreventive in reducing risk of endometrial cancer (and ovarian cancer); odds ratios around 0.50. Based on several cohort studies, cumulative exposure to estrogen (or estrogen plus progestogen), generally over a period exceeding 10 years, associated with 15% to 50% increase in relative risk of breast cancer in post-menopausal women. Preliminary studies have suggested that hormone supplementation may reduce risk of colon cancer. Oral contraceptives (estrogen plus progestogen) have been associated with increased risks of invasive cancers of the uterine cervix and vagina. Protective effect of oral contraceptives not evident for breast cancer, and may be associated with elevated risks in subgroups of women during reproductive years. Prenatal estrogen exposure, including non-steroidal DES, associated with increased risk of clear-cell adenocarcinoma of vagina; putative risk factor for germ cell neoplasms of the testis and ovary.
INFECTIOUS AGENTS		
Epstein-Barr (EBV)	Lymphomas [African Burkitt's (90% or greater), other non-Hodgkin's (10%-15%), Hodgkin's disease (about 50%)], Nasopharyngeal carcinoma	Infectious agents account for 5% of all cancers in the U.S. Probably closer to 10% worldwide, but up to 20% in areas of Asia and Africa. Enhanced cancer risks due to the persistence and reactivation of viral agents in immunosuppressed (genetic or acquired) patients. Previous infectious mononucleosis associated with 3-fold increased risk of Hodgkin's disease. Association of EBV demonstrated in T-cell non-Hodgkin's lymphomas.
Hepatitis B and C	Hepatocellular carcinoma	Exposure to aflatoxin, particularly in Asia and African countries, accompanied by liver tumor cell mutation at codon 249 of *p53*, appears to be interactive with hepatitis B virus.
Human immunodeficiency (HIV)	Kaposi's sarcoma, non-Hodgkin's lymphoma, carcinomas of anus and oral cavity	
Human T-lymphotropic virus	T-cell leukemia/lymphoma	Human retrovirus infection endemic in areas of Japan, Caribbean and Melanesia.
Human papillomavirus (HPV types 16, 18; also types 31, 33, etc.)	Uterine cervix, vagina, vulva, anus, penis	Preliminary studies suggest that HPV may be a co-factor in a subset of proliferative and invasive squamous carcinomas of the upper aerodigestive tract. Increased risk of skin cancer in patients with autosomal dominant, inherited epidermodysplasia verruciformis, associated with impaired cell-mediated immunity, and HPV types 5, 8 infection.

(continued)

TABLE 63–9. *Major Environmental (Non-occupational) Causes of Human Cancer: Strategic Targets for Prevention and Control (Continued)*

Helicobacter pylori	Stomach (adenocarcinoma of antrum or body of stomach) with atrophic gastritis and intestinal metaplasia; B-cell lymphoma	Stomach cancer incidence declining in most countries. Reduction in incidence and mortality accompanied by improvement in living standards and food-preservation technology. *H. pylori* is a causal agent for chronic atrophic gastritis, a precursor of gastric carcinoma. Prevalence of infection with *H. pylori* is positively correlated with stomach cancer mortality rates in countries throughout the world. Increased prevalence at older age; among blacks, Hispanics, and Orientals; and generally a higher prevalence at younger ages in association with lower socioeconomic status. In developing countries, 80% of children are infected. Odds ratios range from 2.7 to 12. *H. pylori* is a putative causal factor in gastric mucosal–associated lymphoid tumors, including poorly differentiated non-Hodgkin's lymphoma. Antimicrobial therapy with bismuth salts, metronidazole, and amoxicillin or tetracycline, has eradicated the organism in 60–90% of patients.
Trematodes: Schistosoma haematobium	Urinary bladder	High incidence in Northern Africa and Middle East where schistosomiasis is endemic. Squamous cell carcinoma predominates in non-trigone areas of urinary bladder in association with squamous metaplasia; male predominance, with age at diagnosis about 10–20 years younger than transitional cell carcinoma of urinary bladder in western countries. Urinary concentrations of tryptophan metabolites and beta-glucuronidase increased.
Liver flukes: Opisthorchis viverrini Clonorchis sinensis	Cholangiocarcinoma	Endemic in Southeast Asia. Associated with adenomatous hyperplasia and squamous metaplasia of bile and pancreatic ducts. Clonorchiasis and opisthorchiasis acquired by human ingestion of raw or inadequately cooked fish.
Diet (deficiencies and/or excesses)	Oral cavity, esophagus, stomach, colon, pancreas, gall bladder and biliary, lung, larynx, prostate, breast, endometrium, uterine cervix, ovary, etc.	International comparisons of site-specific cancer mortality, "experiments of nature" provided by migrant studies, and case–control and cohort studies have suggested that a substantial etiologic fraction of some of the major cancer sites in the U.S. may be attributable to dietary factors. Thus it has been estimated that through dietary modifications, the U.S. might ultimately achieve a 35% reduction in cancer mortality. Various nutrition hypotheses have been concerned with excess in dietary fat and/or energy consumption, and/or the role of obesity, with respect to incidence of cancers in the colon, endometrium, breast, and prostate; or with deficiencies in fresh fruits and vegetables with respect to risk of various gastrointestinal and respiratory tract cancers. Cooking practices, particularly at high temperatures, may generate polycyclic hydrocarbons, heterocyclic aromatic amines, and other potentially carcinogenic compounds.
Pollution	Respiratory, large intestine, urinary bladder	Pollutants in urban air have long been suspected in the etiology of lung cancer, with fossil fuel combustion products, especially polycyclic hydrocarbons, being of concern. Some studies have suggested that tobacco smoke may interact with carcinogens in the ambient atmosphere, or that neighborhood communities may be affected by airborne pollutants from industrial sources. Interest has also centered on contaminants in drinking water, since several halogenated organic compounds (trihalomethanes) produced during chlorination are carcinogenic or mutagenic on laboratory tests. Levels of these compounds in surface drinking water have been positively correlated with mortality rates for cancers of the urinary bladder and large bowel. Case–control and cohort studies have not in most instances adequately controlled for confounding and other sources of bias, and have not satisfactorily estimated historical exposures to waterborne mutagens or organic chlorination by-products. The attributable risk has been difficult to estimate with any precision, but probably does not exceed 1–2%. The U. S. Environmental Protection Agency is requiring that total trihalomethane levels be maintained at or below 100μ g/L (ppb).

validity, *not* to underestimate any serious risks, to accommodate biological mechanisms of carcinogenesis, and to incorporate dose–response points of data that are available and verifiable. Regulatory agencies have generally utilized linearized, non-threshold dose–response models for assessing risks at low exposures (e.g., the "one-hit model" and the "multistage model"). The "probit model" assumes that there are individual tolerance levels to environmental carcinogens that are log-normally distributed. The probit and logit models result in S-shaped dose–response curves and lower estimates of cancer risk than the linear one-hit model at low doses (Crump, 1994). The theoretical assumption of no threshold in risk assessment limits the probability that a sufficiently low level of exposure will be without elevated risk of developing cancer in a lifetime or that there is an acceptable minimal exposure level. A biological argument in favor of the no-threshold linearized model is the irreversible self-replicating lesion of somatic cell mutation that may occur after a single exposure to a genotoxic agent.

In principle, it may not be possible to prove or disprove the existence of an absolute threshold. Of further concern in low-dose, intraspecies extrapolation is that a variety of factors may affect an individual's dose–incidence curve in response to a mutagen or procarcinogen, including genetically determined metabolic or pharmacokinetic mechanisms for detoxification and activation and the capacity for DNA repair. Of additional significance would be interactive exposures to other chemical or physical agents with genotoxic, co-carcinogenic, promoting, or inhibiting properties. The choice of a linear/non-linear, threshold/non-threshold model must consider each agent individually and assess all relevant clinical, epidemiological, and animal toxicological data.

In contrast to the hundreds of chemicals that have been observed to possess tumorigenic activity in laboratory animals, the International Agency for Research on Cancer (IARC) listed approximately 25 occupational chemicals and manufacturing processes that were probably carcinogenic to humans (International Agency for Research on Cancer, 1987). The IARC was created by the World Health Assembly in 1965 and has as one of its essential missions the identification and quantification of cancer risks to humans. For an agent to be classified as category I, namely, causally related to cancer in humans, the strength of the evidence is based on epidemiological studies (Table 63–8). The term "carcinogenic risk" in future IARC Monographs will be based on the evidence in human studies and in experimental animals, and will include research data on mechanisms of action using biological samples and animal models.

FUTURE DIRECTIONS

Most human cancers are "triggered" or propagated by exposures to environmental agents that are associated with lifestyle choices (Table 63–9) (Henderson et al, 1991). Multistep carcinogenesis is the cumulative expression of various exogenous and endogenous factors which evoke molecular and cellular responses in the exposed host that are under genetic control. The ultimate outcome of exposures to toxic chemical, physical, and biological agents will depend on competitive gene–enzyme interactions that effect activation (phase I enzymes) or detoxification (phase II enzymes) of mutagens or procarcinogens (Wolf et al, 1994; Shaw et al, 1995), on immunocompetence (Kinlen, 1992), and on the integrity of endogenous mechanisms for neutralizing free radicals or repairing lesions in DNA (Wiencke et al, 1991; Marx, 1994; Cleaver, 1994; Olden, 1994). A future challenging direction in cancer prevention and control will be the application of technology for identifying genotypic and phenotypic markers of cancer susceptibility and predicting levels or degrees of individual lifetime risks for specific types of cancer. Individuals may then be counseled about actions they should take to reduce their susceptibility or expression of risk (Austoker, 1994; Hoskins et al, 1995; Andrews et al, 1994).

REFERENCES

AMERICAN CANCER SOCIETY. 1990. 1989 Survey of physicians' attitudes and practices in early cancer detection. Cancer 40:77–101.

ANDREWS LB, FULLARTON JE, HOLTZMAN NA, MOTULSKY AG (editors). 1994. Assessing Genetic Risks: Implications for Health and Social Policy. Washington, D.C., National Academy Press.

AUSTOKER J. 1994. Cancer prevention in primary care. Current trends and some prospects for the future—II. BMJ 309:517–520.

BJELKE E. 1975. Dietary vitamin A and human lung cancer. Int J Cancer 15:561–565.

BLOT WJ, LI J-Y, TAYLOR PR, et al. 1993. Nutrition intervention trials in Linxian, China: supplementation with specific vitamin/mineral combinations, cancer incidence, and disease-specific mortality in the general population. J Natl Cancer Inst 85:1483–1492.

BRESLOW L. 1979. A History of Cancer Control in the United States, 1946–1971. Introductory Materials. DHEW Publication No. (NIH) 79-1516. Atlanta, National Institues of Health.

BROWN ML. 1992. Economic considerations in breast cancer screening of older women. J Gerontol 47:51–58.

BYERS TE, GRAHAM S, HAUGHEY BP, et al. 1987. Diet and lung cancer risk: Findings from the western New York diet study. Am J Epidemiol 125:351–363.

BYRNE J, KESSLER LG, DEVESA SS. 1992. The prevalence of cancer among adults in the United States: 1987. Cancer 69:2154–2159.

CENTERS FOR DISEASE CONTROL AND PREVENTION. 1992. Chronic Disease in Minority Populations. Atlanta, Centers for Disease Control and Prevention.

CHURCH TR, EDERER F, MANDEL JS, et al. 1993. Estimating the duration of ongoing prevention trials. Am J Epidemiol 137:797–810.

CLEAVER JE. 1994. It was a very good year for DNA repair. Cell 76:1–4.

COHEN SJ, HALVORSON HW, GOSSELINK CA. 1994. Changing physician behavior to improve disease prevention. Prev Med 23:284–291.

COHEN DR, HENDERSON JB. 1988. Health, Prevention, and Economics. Oxford, Oxford University Press.

COLE P, AMOATENG-ADJEPONG Y. 1994. Cancer prevention: accomplishments and prospects. Am J Pub Health 84:8–10.

COULTAS DB, GONG H JR, GRAD R, et al. 1994. Respiratory diseases in minorities of the United States. Am J Respir Crit Care Med 149:S93–S131.

CRUMP KS. 1994. Use of mechanistic models to estimate low-dose cancer risks. Risk Anal 14:1033–1038.

CULLEN JW. 1990. Phases in cancer control: Intervention research. *In* Hakama M, Beral V, Cullen JW, Parkin DM (eds): Evaluating Effectiveness of Primary Prevention of Cancer. Lyon, IARC Scientific Publications, pp. 1–11.

DEVESA SS, BLOT WJ, STONE BJ, et al. 1995. Recent cancer trends in the United States. J Natl Cancer Inst 87:175–182.

DONALDSON C. 1994. Using economics to assess the place of screening. J Med Screening 1:124–129.

EDERER F, CHURCH TR, MANDEL JS. 1993. Sample sizes for prevention trials have been too small. Am J Epidemiol 137:787–796.

FAHS M, MANDELBLATT J, SCHECHTER C, et al. 1992. The costs and effectiveness of cervical cancer screening in the elderly. Ann Intern Med 117:520–527.

U.S. DEPARTMENT OF HEALTH AND HUMAN SERVICES. 1991. Healthy People 2000: National Health Promotion and Disease Prevention Objectives. DHHS Publication No. (PHS) 91-50212. Washington, DC, U.S. Government Printing Office.

HENDERSON BE, ROSS RK, PIKE MC. 1991. Toward the primary prevention of cancer. Science 254:1131–1138.

HOSKINS KF, STOPFER JE, CALZONE KA, et al. 1995. Assessment and counseling for women with a family history of breast cancer: A guide for clinicians. JAMA 273:577–585.

INTERNATIONAL AGENCY FOR RESEARCH ON CANCER. 1987. Overall evaluations of carcinogenicity. IARC Monog Eval Carcinog Risks Hum. An Updating of IARC Monogr Vol 1–42, Suppl. 7.

JANERICH DT. 1984. Forecasting cancer trends to optimize control strategies. J Natl Cancer Inst 72:1317–1321.

KELLOFF GJ, JOHNSON JR, CROWELL JA, et al. 1995. Approaches to the development and marketing approval of drugs that prevent cancer. Cancer Epidemiol Biomarkers Prev 4:1–10.

KELLOFF GJ, MALONE WF, BOONE CW, et al. 1990. Progress in applied chemoprevention research. Semin Oncol 17:438–455.

KINLEN LJ. 1992. Immunosuppression and cancer. *In* Vainio H, Magee PN, McGregor DB, McMichael AJ (eds): Mechanisms of Carcinogenesis in Risk Identification. Lyon, International Agency for Research on Cancer (IARC), pp. 237–253.

KOCHANEK KD, HUDSON BL. 1994. Advance report of final mortality statistics, 1992. Monthly Vital Statistics Report; vol 43 no 6, suppl. Hyattsville, Maryland; National Center for Health Statistics.

LEMARCHAND LL, YOSHIZAWA CN, KOLONEL LN, et al. 1989. Vegetable consumption and lung cancer risk: A population-based case–control study in Hawaii. J Natl Cancer Inst 81:1158–1164.

LIPPMAN SM, BENNER SE, HONG WK. 1994. Cancer chemoprevention. J Clin Oncol 12:851–873.

MACKENZIE TD, BARTECCHI CE, SCHRIER RW. 1994. The human costs of tobacco use. N Engl J Med 330:975–980.

MARX J. 1994. DNA repair comes into its own. Science 266:728–730.

MILLER BA, RIES LAG, HANKEY BF, et al. 1993. SEER Cancer Statistics Review: 1973–1990. National Cancer Institute NIH Pub. No. 93-2789. Bethesda, National Cancer Institute.

MORBIDITY AND MORTALITY WEEKLY REPORT. 1994. Surveillance for Selected Tobacco—Use Behaviors—United States, 1900–1994.43/ No. SS-3:1–43. Washington, DC, U.S. Government Printing Office.

NATIONAL CENTER FOR HEALTH STATISTICS. 1988. Health, United States 1987. DHHS Publication No. (PHS) 88-1232. Washington, DC: U.S. Government Printing Office.

NOVOTNY TE. 1992. The public health practice of tobacco control: Lessons learned and directions for the states in the 1990s. Annu Rev Public Health 13:287–318.

NOVOTNY TE, WARNER KE, KENDRICK JS, et al. 1988. Smoking by blacks and whites: socioeconomic and demographic differences. Am J Public Health 78:1187–1189.

NUTTING PA. 1986. Health promotion in primary medical care: Problems and potential. Prev Med 15:537–548.

ODDONE EZ, FEUSSNER JR, COHEN HJ. 1992. Can screening older patients for cancer save lives? Clin Geriatr Med 8:51–67.

OFFICE OF TECHNOLOGY ASSESSMENT. 1987. Breast cancer screening for Medicare beneficiaries: effectiveness, costs to Medicare and medical resources required. Washington, D.C.; U.S. Government Printing Office.

OLDEN K. 1994. Mutagen hypersensitivity as a biomarker of genetic predisposition to carcinogenesis. J Natl Cancer Inst 86:1660–1661.

ORLANDI MA. 1987. Promoting health and preventing disease in health care settings: An analysis of barriers. Prev Med 16:1–12.

OTTEN MW, TEUTSCH SM, WILLIAMSON DF, et al. 1990. The effect of known risk factors on the excess mortality of black adults in the United States. JAMA 263:845–850.

PARKIN DM, MUIR CS, WHELAN SL, GAO Y-T, FERLAY J, POWELL J (EDS). 1992. Cancer Incidence In Five Continents. Volume VI. Lyon, IARC Scientific Publications.

PETO R, LOPEZ AD, BOREHAM J, et al. 1992. Mortality from tobacco in developed countries: indirect estimation from national vital statistics. Lancet 339:1268–1278.

POLEDNAK AP. 1994. Projected numbers of cancers diagnosed in the US elderly population, 1990 through 2030. Am J Public Health 84:1313–1316.

ROEMER R. 1993. Legislative Action to Combat the World Tobacco Epidemic. Second ed. Geneva, World Health Organization.

ROSE G. 1992. The Strategy of Preventive Medicine. Oxford, Oxford University Press.

ROYCE JM, HYMOWITZ N, CORBETT K, et al. 1993. Smoking cessation factors among African Americans and whites. Am J Public Health 83:220–226.

RUSSELL LB. 1986. Is prevention better than cure? Washington, D.C. Brookings Institution.

RUSSELL LB. 1993. The role of prevention in health reform. New Engl J Med 329:352–354.

SAMET JM, WIGGINS CL, KEY CR, et al. 1988. Mortality from lung cancer and chronic obstructive pulmonary disease in New Mexico, 1958–82. Am J Public Health 78:1182–1186.

SCHOEN RE, WEISSFELD JL, KULLER LH. 1995. Sigmoidoscopy use among primary care physicians. Prev Med 24:249–254.

SCHOTTENFELD D, HAAS JF. 1981. Carcinogens in the workplace. *In* Sax IN (ed): Cancer Causing Chemicals. New York, VanNostrand Reinhold Company, pp. 14–27.

SHAW GL, FALK RT, DESLAURIERS J, et al. 1995. Debrisoquine metabolism and lung cancer risk. Cancer Epidemiol Biomarkers Prev 4:41–48.

SHIN DM, HITTELMAN WN, HONG WK. 1994. Biomarkers in upper aerodigestive tract tumorigenesis: A review. Cancer Epidemiol Biomarkers Prev 3:697–709.

SHOPLAND DR, EYRE HJ, PECHACEK TF. 1991. Smoking-attributable cancer mortality in 1991: Is lung cancer now the leading cause of death among smokers in the United States? J Natl Cancer Inst 83:1142–1148.

SONDIK EJ. 1988. Progress in cancer prevention and control. *In* Maulitz RC (ed): Unnatural Causes: The Three Leading Killer Diseases in America. New Brunswick, NJ; Rutgers University Press, pp. 111–134.

SORLIE P, ROGOT E, ANDERSON R, et al. 1992. Black-white mortality differences by family income. Lancet 340:346–350.

STELLMAN SD, GARFINKEL L. 1986. Smoking habits and tar levels in a new American Cancer Society prospective study of 1.2 million men and women. J Natl Cancer Inst 76:1057–1063.

ALPHA-TOCOPHEROL, BETA CAROTENE CANCER PREVENTION STUDY GROUP (THE). 1994. The effect of vitamin E and beta carotene on the incidence of lung cancer and other cancers in male smokers. N Engl J Med 330:1029–1035.

TRAPIDO EJ, CHEN F, DAVIS K, et al. 1994. Cancer in South Florida Hispanic women. Arch Intern Med 154:1083–1089.

U.S. DEPARTMENT HEALTH, EDUCATION, WELFARE. 1964. Smoking and Health Report of the Advisory Committee to the Surgeon General of the Public Health Service. PHS Pub No. (HEW) 1103. Washington, DC, U.S. Government Printing Office.

U.S. DEPARTMENT OF HEALTH AND HUMAN SERVICES. 1991. Healthy People 2000. National Health Promotion and Disease Prevention Objectives. DHHS Publ No. 91-50212.

WARNER KE. 1986. Smoking and health implications of a change in the federal cigarette excise tax. JAMA 255:1028–1032.

WARNER KE. 1995. Public policy issues. *In* Greenwald P, Kramer BS, Weed DL (eds): Cancer Prevention and Control. New York, Marcel Dekker, pp. 451–472.

WIENCKE JK, WRENSCH MR, MIIKE R, et al. 1991. Individual susceptibility to induced chromosome damage and its implications for detecting genotoxic exposures in human populations. Cancer Res 51:5266–5269.

WILLIAMS PA, WILLIAMS M. 1987. Barriers and incentives for primary care physicians in cancer prevention and detection. Cancer 60:1970–1978.

WOLF RC, SMITH AD, FORMAN D. 1994. Metabolic polymorphisms in carcinogen metabolizing enzymes and cancer susceptibility. Br Med Bull 50:718–731.

64 Health education and health promotion in cancer prevention

NOREEN M. CLARK
MARSHALL H. BECKER

We have three goals in this chapter. First, to present two current theories of importance in developing health promotion and health education interventions. These theories explain why people will undertake actions to prevent the onset of cancer; they also suggest how education can be designed to increase both motivation and the ability to take action. Second, to provide examples of the theories as they relate to cancer prevention, using as an illustration breast self-examination. We will show how effective health promotion efforts are based on the theories. Third, to discuss how the behavior of health care providers can influence patients' behavior. We will outline ways in which provider and patient encounters can be managed to best encourage and enable patients to undertake cancer-prevention actions.

THE HEALTH BELIEF MODEL

Central to the design of successful health education and promotion programs is an understanding of *why* people behave as they do when confronting illness or a potential health problem. The Health Belief Model (HBM) posits that there are several primary categories of influence: how susceptible individuals feel in relation to the illness, how serious they perceive it to be, and the relative benefit they see in taking a preventive or curative action given the costs of taking that action. The HBM, as discussed by Rosenstock (1974), Becker (1974b), and others (Kirscht, 1974; Maiman and Becker, 1974), has its origins in psychological theories of decision making. The model, developed in the early 1950s by a group of social psychologists at the U.S. Public Health Service, was an attempt to understand the "widespread failure of people to accept disease preventives or screening tests for the early detection of asymptomatic disease" (Rosenstock, 1974). Later the model was applied to patients' responses to symptoms, and to compliance with prescribed medical regimens (Kirscht, 1974; Becker, 1974b). The basic components of the model are derived from a well-established body of psychological and behavioral theory (Lewin, 1951), whose various models hypothesize that behavior depends mainly upon two variables: (1) the value placed by an individual on a particular goal and (2) the individual's estimate of the likelihood that a given action will achieve that goal. In the context of health-related behavior, the variables are (1) the desire to avoid illness (or if ill to get well) and (2) the belief that a specific health action will prevent or ameliorate illness. The model is depicted in Figure 64–1.

The HBM has four dimensions:

1. *Perceived susceptibility*. This concept postulates that we vary widely in our feelings of personal vulnerability to a disease (including resusceptibility if already ill, belief in the diagnosis, and susceptibility to illness in general); it refers to our subjective perception of the risk of contracting a disease.

2. *Perceived severity*. Feelings concerning the seriousness of contracting an illness or leaving it untreated also vary from person to person; this dimension includes evaluations of both medical/clinical consequences (e.g., death, disability, and pain) and possible social consequences (eg, effects of the conditions on work, family life, and social relations).

3. *Perceived benefits*. While acceptance of personal susceptibility to an illness also believed to be serious is held to produce a force leading to behavior, it does not define the particular course of action that is likely to be taken; this is hypothesized to depend upon beliefs regarding the effectiveness of the various actions available in reducing the disease threat. Thus, even if we are "sufficiently threatened," we would not be expected to accept the recommended health action unless it was perceived as feasible and efficacious.

4. *Perceived barriers*. The potential negative aspects of a particular health action may act as impediments to undertaking the recommended behavior. A kind of cost-benefit analysis is thought to occur wherein we weigh the action's effectiveness against perceptions that it may be expensive, dangerous (e.g., have side effects or iatro-

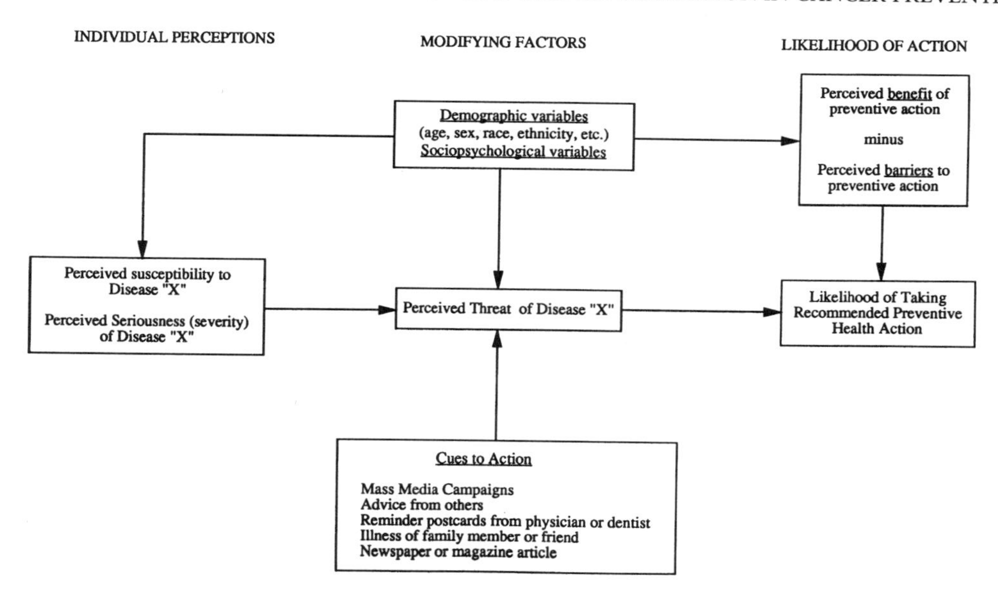

FIG. 64–1. Basic elements of the Health Belief Model. (Reproduced by permission of *Medical Care*.)

genic outcomes), unpleasant (eg, painful, difficult, upsetting), inconvenient, time consuming, and so forth.

Rosenstock (1974) summarized these dimensions as follows: "the combined levels of susceptibility and severity provides the energy or force to act, and the perception of benefits (less barriers) provides a preferred path of action." However, some stimulus is necessary to trigger the decision-making process. This "cue to action" might be internal (eg, a symptom) or external (eg, mass communications, interpersonal interactions, a reminder from a health care provider). Finally, it is assumed that demographic, sociopsychological, and structural variables affect our perceptions and thus indirectly influence health-related behavior.

The HBM is a psychosocial model. It is limited to accounting for as much of the variance in individuals' health-related actions as can be explained by their attitudes and beliefs. The model is predicted on the premises that "health" is a highly valued concern or goal for most individuals, and that "cues to action" are widely prevalent. It is clear that in some situations these conditions are not satisfied and other forces influence health actions as well. For example, some behaviors have a substantial habitual component obviating any psychosocial decision making (toothbrushing is one example). Further, some behaviors are undertaken for nonhealth reasons (eg, dieting to look more attractive). Finally, where economic or environmental factors prevent individuals from taking a preferred course of action, the model may not suffice. Nonetheless, an impressive body of research has linked Health Belief Model dimensions to health actions (French et al, 1992; Janz and Becker, 1984; Petosa and Jackson, 1991).

SOCIAL COGNITIVE THEORY

Social cognitive theory, as discussed by Bandura (1977a,b, 1982, 1986), has received a significant amount of attention as a basis for understanding health behavior. Indeed, some have commented that social cognitive theory and the Health Belief Model are highly complementary (Becker and Rosenstock, 1987; Rosenstock et al, 1988). The Health Belief Model predicts a given health behavior on the basis of beliefs and how seriously needed or costly one perceives an action to be; it does not attempt to describe how these beliefs come into existence. Social cognitive theory emphasizes the mechanisms of change—how one might come to believe certain things about his or her health and take actions as a result of these beliefs. One can envision using the two theories to design different elements of cancer-prevention education. The HBM can discern the content of health promotion or health education programs; that is, identify what will be persuasive and likely to predispose individuals to action given their beliefs. Social cognitive theory can illuminate the processes that need to be incorporated into education to bring an individual to the new behavior.

Social cognitive theory is based on the notion of reciprocal determinism. Bandura (1986) has stated that in the social cognitive view, "people are neither driven by inner forces nor automatically shaped and controlled by external stimuli." Human functioning is explained by a model in which behavior, cognitive and other personal factors, and environmental events are interacting determinants of each other. Individual personal factors engender behavior through which one acts on the environment; in turn, changes in the environment modify personal factors and subsequent behavior. In addition, one's own capacity to self-regulate is an important source for changing personal factors. We are able to self-observe, self-evaluate, and give ourselves "feedback" about our own behavior. In social cognitive theory, the environment that is most influential in shaping behavior is the social environment, which provides people with models of behavior, cues to action, feedback, reinforcement, and rewards. The reciprocal nature of the model has been diagrammed in Figure 64–2.

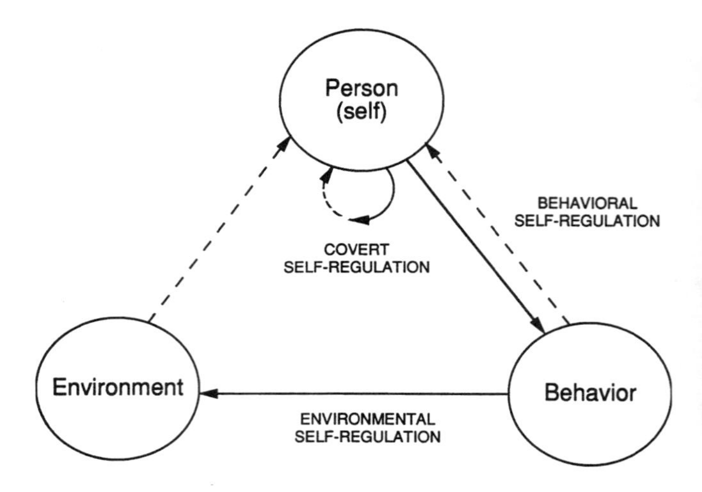

FIG. 64–2. Reciprocal determinants of self-regulated functioning. (From "A social cognitive view of self-regulated academic learning" by B.J. Zimmerman, 1989, *Journal of Educational Psychology*, 81, p. 330. Copyright 1989 by the American Psychological Association. Adapted by permission.)

Cognitive events are central in social cognitive theory. While strict behaviorists downplay cognitive events as influences on behavior (Skinner, 1974), social cognitive theory accepts that cognitive aids are fundamental in learning, and that cognition has a causal influence on action. The ability to anticipate a consequence is a cognitive function that significantly influences behavior. One behaves in a specific way in order to achieve a specific consequence of the behavior. The consequence is the reinforcement of the behavior. When the consequence is rewarding—even on an intermittent basis—one is likely to continue to behave in the same way in hopes of attaining the consequence once again. Our cognitive ability to integrate experience over time enables us to anticipate that under a given set of circumstances, we are likely (though not always certain) to achieve the reward (consequence). We anticipate an outcome, arrange the social and physical environment to enhance the potential for reaching it, observe and evaluate our own behavior, and draw some conclusions about it (self-reaction). One of the most important self-reactions we can have, related to trying a new behavior or continuing an old one, is believing that we are competent at it. Our feeling of self-efficacy (our confidence that we can successfully carry out the task) is an important determinant of behavior.

In anticipating an outcome we have two types of expectancies that the behavior will produce the outcome we want and that we can perform the behavior as needed to achieve that outcome. Figure 64–3 illustrates how expectations function. For example, for a woman (person) to practice breast self-examination (behavior) for health reasons (outcome), she must believe both that BSE will benefit her health (outcome expectation) and that she is capable of conducting it properly (efficacy expectation).

Five capabilities described by Bandura enable individuals to anticipate outcomes and shape their own behavior in the effort to attain outcomes. The first is symbolizing capability. This capacity obviates the need to experience every behavior on a trial and error basis. Symbols enable people "to process and transform transient experiences into internal models that serve as guides for future action" (Bandura, 1986). Symbols enable people to communicate both intrapersonally and with others at any distance in time and space.

As Bandura points out (1977b), the fact that people base actions on thought does not mean that the thought is always rational. The symbolic formulation of experience may be based on poor judgment, or missampling, or misreading of events. Nonetheless, thoughts as symbolic representations of experience are a primary influence on behavior.

Forethought is another capability. Most behavior, being purposive, is regulated by forethought. People anticipate the likely consequences of their potential actions, set goals, and plan courses of action. Through forethought, people motivate themselves and guide their actions, as Bandura says, "anticipatorily."

We have, as well, a capability for vicarious experience. We learn by observation; from this, we generalize rules for generating and regulating behavioral patterns without having to form them gradually by trial and error (which can be both tedious and dangerous). Models of behavior allow us to shortcut the acquisition process. Models are powerful influences on thought patterns, values, attitudes, or styles of behavior (Bandura, 1986).

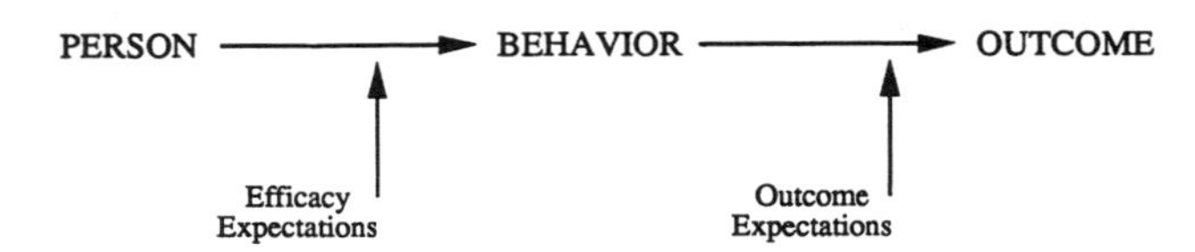

FIG. 64–3. The relation of efficacy and outcome expectations. From "Social Learning Theory" by A. Bandura, 1977, Englewood Cliffs, NJ: Prentice-Hall. Figure used with permission.

The process of modeling requires attending to the modeled behavior; retaining patterns of the behavior in symbolic form (visual or verbal), and motor reproduction (ie, turning symbolic representations into appropriate actions). Innovative patterns of behavior can emerge through modeling, an idea that helps to explain differences in behavior between parent and child. People enact those things from among the many they learn on the basis of whether or not they value the anticipated outcome.

We are also capable of self-regulating our behavior and of being self-reflective. These capabilities have been described as carried out through three subprocesses (Clark and Zimmerman, 1990; Zimmerman, 1994). First is self-observation, the ability to watch ourselves in action. Second is self-evaluation, the ability to judge the success of our behavior given some criterion (much human behavior is motivated by internal standards). Third is self-reaction, the ability to draw some conclusions about our experiences and ourselves given self-evaluation. As noted above, feeling efficacious is a self-reaction. Self-efficacy, it should be noted, is not a generalized state; one feels efficacious about a specific behavior. As stated by Bandura (1986), "by arranging facilitative environmental conditions, recruiting cognitive guides and creating incentives for their own efforts, people make causal contributions to their own motivation and actions. . . . Reflective self-consciousness . . . enables people to analyze their experiences and to think about their own thought processes. By reflecting on their varied experiences and on what they know, they can derive generic knowledge about themselves and the world around them."

HEALTH BELIEFS AS PREDICTORS OF BREAST SELF-EXAMINATION

In the course of their lives, one in nine women will develop breast cancer (American Cancer Society, 1994; USDHHS, 1994). Although prospects for the clinical management of breast cancer have improved significantly over the years, the condition continues to have a serious psychosocial impact on women (Glanz and Lerman, 1992). Several studies posit that early detection of breast cancer leads to a good outcome (Henderson and Cancellos, 1980), and the American Cancer Society has stated that with early detection and treatment, breast cancer survival rates for women after 5 years is almost 100% (Smith and Hailey, 1988) when the cancer is localized in the breast. Of the three available approaches to detecting breast cancer (clinical examination, mammography, and self-exam), breast self-examination (BSE) seems most feasible for the largest number of women; the other procedures are inconvenient, time consuming, and costly. Although BSE has drawbacks, it has been called the most effective mass approach to early detection and continues to be widely recommended (Janz et al, 1989/90; Mayer and Solomon, 1992; O'Malley and Fletcher, 1987; Pennypacker et al, 1982). Of course, once a lump is detected, clinical examination and mammography are required to confirm the finding. Studies have suggested that although approximately 90% of American women are aware of BSE as a preventive measure, only 25%–35% actually examine their breasts on a monthly basis (Weinberg et al, 1982; NIH, 1980; Amsel et al, 1985; Shelley, 1983).

According to the HBM, a woman will practice BSE if she believes that she is susceptible to breast cancer, believes that the disease is serious, and believes that the benefit of deterring serious illness through early detection is greater than the "costs" or "barriers" to her of conducting the exam. Several studies related to BSE have illustrated the relation of beliefs and behavior in cancer prevention. Examples are summarized in Table 64–1.

In the main these studies describe the intricacies of the relation between beliefs and preventive behavior. In general, beliefs have been shown to account for only part of the variance in the practice of BSE. Although the variance is not always great, health beliefs are important variables if for no other reason than they are modifiable—they can be influenced by the health professional. Data from the Walker and Glanz (1986) study (see Table 1), for example, illustrate that encouragement from a health care provider is an important influence on the practice of BSE. The health professional can be persuasive in convincing individuals about their susceptibility to serious disease. Obviously, some characteristics that research has associated with BSE are not amenable to change on the part of the health care provider (eg, marital status, available social support, general level of self-esteem). However, health beliefs, especially the level of a person's vulnerability to a cancer risk and the benefits of the recommended practice, are topics that can easily be addressed in even limited physician-patient encounters. It is clear from the findings of the summarized studies that most women have anxiety about breast cancer and most believe that BSE is a beneficial practice, and that the beliefs auguring against practice may vary according to age. The extent of the benefit may not be understood by many, and this is an important topic for health professional counseling. An individual's degree of vulnerability may also be misunderstood and deserves attention from health professionals. As we will discuss below, however, it is important not to unduly raise anxiety levels about breast cancer or any serious health threat. The listener, to be persuaded, must feel

TABLE 64–1. *Studies of the Health Belief Model (HBM) in Breast Self-Examination (BSE)*

Study	*Purpose*	*Subjects*	*Data Collection*	*Findings*
Strauss et al (1987)	Assess perceived: severity of breast cancer; susceptibility to breast cancer lumps; benefits of BSE; barriers to practice; lack of confidence; overreliance on physician; and forgetting	59 women with previous breast cancer; 33 women with previously treated benign breast lumps; 80 women in general population with no history of breast disease	Mailed questionnaires	Women with breast cancer history: higher rates of BSE, more proficient in BSE, perceived cancer as less threatening, and were less likely to forget; women with no history perceived less susceptibility to cancer; all groups believed in BSE
Mamon and Zapka (1986)	Correlates of frequency of breast self-examination	869 college women	Questionnaire	Confidence in ability to perform BSE was the influential factor in performance; susceptibility contributed 19% of the variance in BSE
Champion (1992)	BSE probability and barriers according to age	322 women (35–44 years, 45–54, and 55 and older)	Questionnaire	Beliefs about barriers and self-confidence predicted BSE in women 45–54; for younger women all HBM elements predicted BSE
Stillman (1977)	Perceived benefits/susceptibility	122 women in suburban Connecticut without history of breast cancer (20–59 years)	Questionnaire	Modest relationship of BSE and health beliefs; women 40 to 60, most frequent practice of BSE
Hallal (1982)	Health beliefs, health locus of control, and self-concept predicting BSE	207 women	Questionnaire	Overall self-esteem was best predictor of BSE; perceived benefits also significant
Walker and Glanz (1986)	Influences on practice of BSE	264 female students, faculty, and staff in university community	Questionnaire	All HBM predictors significant; strongest predictor was physician encouragement, followed by personal belief in BSE and receiving instruction
Owens et al (1987)	Factors associated with attending breast screening units	406 urban women in the United Kingdom: 183 at breast screening unit; 182 at hospital clinic; 41 at outpatient clinic, aged 17–76	Questionnaire/screening exam	Health beliefs had little effect on choosing to attend screening units but did relate to BSE
Calnan and Moss (1984)	HBM predicting attendance at breast exam classes	678 women in large city in the United Kingdom	Questionnaire/screening exam	Women who reported use of preventive health care and those feeling more susceptible were more likely to attend screening; older women more compliant with BSE schedule
Calnan (1984)	Distinguish between women who attended screening and those who attended self-exam classes based on HBM	825 women in health district in Midlands in England invited to attend BSE; 561 women in southern England invited to breast screening	Questionnaires	While overall variance from HBM was low, health belief variables were among best discriminators of BSE
Calnan and Rutter (1986)	Comparison of screening attenders and non-attenders	278 women who attended BSE class, 262 invited but did not attend, 594 in another control community	Questionnaire/screening classes	HBM elements predicted behavior in BSE; relation between behavior and dimensions of belief not as strong as expected and complex
Hirshfield-Bartek (1982)	Beliefs among those with recurrence of cancer; benefits of BSE; barriers to performing BSE	25 women with a prior history of breast cancer who had received radiation therapy, 29–76 years of age	Questionnaire	All women saw the practice as highly beneficial; susceptibility beliefs influenced the frequency of BSE
Fletcher et al (1989)	Women's current BSE practice and variables relevant to accuracy and frequency	300 women 40–68 years of age in a general medicine group practice, predominantly nonwhite with less than a high school education	Home interview and use of silicone breast models	Correct identification of lumps associated with susceptibility beliefs

vulnerable enough to take an action but not be overcome with fear to the point of inaction. Rosenstock and others (1988) have advised that fear-arousing messages must be accompanied by problem-solving strategies that are within the capability of the patient. In the case of BSE, the fear associated with cancer can by allayed with the reassuring message that early detection and treatment leads to a positive prognosis in many cases.

These studies also make clear that women's experiences give rise to their health beliefs. Women with a history of cancer may not see themselves as more vulnerable, yet they view breast exam as more beneficial than do women without this history. Further, women with confidence in their own ability to perform BSE effectively will be much more likely to practice it. This point—the confidence of the individual to undertake a new behavior—is a principle shared by the HBM and social cognitive theory. We have made the point that the HBM provides the content of teaching related to cancer-preventive behavior. In the case of BSE, the constructs of perceived susceptibility, seriousness, costs, and benefits of the practice seem central. Let us turn now to an examination of studies in which constructs from social cognitive theory have been utilized in interventions to change health behavior. We will use examples from studies of aspects of social cognitive theory to answer the questions: how does a person come to believe that she is vulnerable to cancer, a most serious illness and that performing BSE is more beneficial than the costs associated with it?

SOCIAL COGNITIVE THEORY IN BSE EDUCATION

If a goal of cancer prevention is to get as many women as possible to practice BSE on a regular basis, it follows that a significant amount of education is necessary to reach the unaware, the unconvinced, and those without requisite skills. Social cognitive theory has given rise to several strategies for teaching (Clark and Zimmerman, 1990; Parcel and Baranowski, 1982). Given the learning mechanisms described at the beginning of this chapter, it is possible to construct conditions and interventions that best enable people to learn. Intervention studies illustrating several social cognitive learning strategies that may be particularly relevant for cancer prevention education are summarized in Table 64–2 (the trials are controlled unless otherwise indicated).

These studies suggest that six principles from social cognitive theory may be especially pertinent: reduction of anxiety; verbal persuasion; modeling; and self-regulation and its related components, self-efficacy and self-reinforcement. In one sense, social cognitive theory views anxiety as "noise" in the system. When one is engaged in the process of learning, anxiety is dysfunctional. It reduces the learner's capacity to self-regulate, to attend to symbols and cues in the environment, and to receive feedback. Applying this principle in BSE education requires that a woman's fears be allayed to the extent that she can attend to instruction and be capable of carrying out BSE at home on her own. Fears can emanate from many quarters. For example, a woman may view finding a lump as catastrophic (here her health beliefs come into play), or she may be afraid or embarrassed when touching herself. Anxiety reduction will be necessary to move her to the desired behavior. Reassuring messages from the health professional and the opportunity to rehearse BSE and receive feedback in a safe and encouraging environment appear to be important elements of BSE education.

Learning vicariously by virtue of observing models in the social environment is a powerful vehicle for change. Health professionals can provide models of BSE behavior in a number of ways. One way is demonstrating correct practice; another is alluding to successful cases—those instances where self-examination by women like the intended learner has averted serious illness.

Verbal persuasion is another way that those in the social environment of the learner can influence behavior. By using symbols, giving feedback, and providing cues for action, instructors (in this case health professionals) can begin to influence the way in which the learner anticipates outcomes and views her own capabilities. Believing a desired outcome will emanate from the behavior (for example, that BSE will deter catastrophe) and that one is self-efficacious (able to practice BSE in the desired way) is instrumental to change.

The feeling of self-efficacy is a reaction deriving from self-regulation. When learners have the opportunity to observe themselves (eg, rehearse BSE with an instructor and subsequently note how they carry it out at home), make judgments using given criteria (eg, assess their performance against the ideal provided by the health professional), and give themselves positive feedback (eg, judge that they are meeting the criteria—in part from being verbally commended by the health professional), they are more likely to continue to engage in BSE.

Reinforcement of behavior is considered instrumental in social cognitive descriptions of change. When the consequence of behavior is rewarding or reinforcing to an individual, he or she is much more likely to attempt the behavior again. Rewards can come from the environment but, as the studies reviewed in Table 64–2 suggest, the most important reward is self-reinforcement. As part of their reaction to their own behavior, individuals will reward themselves (eg, by silently congratulating themselves on their own performance or noting their feeling of security when no abnormalities are found during a breast self-exam) or will rearrange contingencies in the environment to obtain a reward (eg, treating

TABLE 64–2. *Breast Self-Examination (BSE) Intervention Studies in Social Cognitive Theory*

Study	*Purpose*	*Subjects*	*Data Collection*	*Findings*
Edwards (1980)	BSE instruction using model and three supplements: group 1, guided practice; group 2, self-monitoring instruction; group 3, peer support	130 women attending 24 cancer screening clinics	Pre/post questionnaire	BSE increased in all groups after 6 months; self-monitoring group, most frequent BSE
Grady (1984)	Examine the utility of self-monitoring versus external cues to action for BSE (ie, reminder postcards and combination of both)	189 women from medical group practices	Pre/post interview	After 6 months 15% of those in the control group always did BSE, 22% in the self-management condition, 33% in cues only group, and 41% in combination instruction
Mayer et al (1987)	Compare mailed prompts with face-to-face prompts to action for BSE	151 women employees of a Veterans Administration medical center	Pre/post questionnaire	Personal contact group practiced BSE more frequently; however, over 6 months was not sufficient to maintain BSE
Craun and Deffenbacher (1987)	Evaluate effectiveness of combination approaches to teaching BSE, including (1) information, (2) demonstration, (3) prompts	227 female college students	Pre/post questionnaire	At 6 months 70% of prompt groups practiced BSE versus 48% in other groups; all groups, including control, increased BSE
Grady (1988)	Examine self-monitoring with rewards versus prompts for BSE	153 women aged 21–77 in medical group practices	Pre/post questionnaire	Small external rewards effective in maintaining BSE; self-reward effective for those (only half) who used it
Kenney et al (1986)	Intervention to increase self-efficacy through group and individual instruction	73 university students	Pre/post class questionnaire (with comparison group)	Intervention group increased in correct performance and confidence; however, overall frequency of BSE low
Dorsay et al (1988)	Test intervention based on role models and rehearsal	459 Kaiser Foundation Health Plan members, mean age 44.5	Pre/post class questionnaire (no control)	Positive effect on frequency and quality of BSE; women with greater increases in frequency tended to be older
Gravell et al (1985); Mamon and Zapka (1985)	Intervention involving role modeling to increase communication about BSE among mothers, daughters, sisters, and friends: (1) education in classroom, (2) education through campus organization	1682 women in a large university	Pre/post questionnaire	At 6 months, women in both types of education more likely to practice BSE and be more proficient; more likely to have communicated about BSE with other women
Baker (1989)	Combined elements of HBM and social cognitive theory in education and workbook	194 women in community-based senior programs	Pre/post questionnaire (with comparison group)	Intervention group at 3 months had higher quality BSE and increased perception of susceptibility, benefits of BSE, and self-efficacy to perform; comparison group also increased in latter two variables

themselves to a special gift for keeping to the examination schedule). Health professionals can contribute to reinforcement for a preventive behavior such as BSE by verbally praising women who practice it.

Compliance with breast self-examination recommendations has, in general, been low; however, it has been noted that a number of cognitive and behavioral factors subsumed under the rubrics of social cognitive and health belief theory help to explain why this is the case (Pinto and Fuqua, 1991). Subsequent to their review of training in BSE, Pinto and Fuqua (1991) concluded that although individual cases are idiosyncratic, in general, low levels of adherence are associated with a weak belief in the benefits of BSE and early detection, and a low-level appraisal of one's competence to perform the exam. Combining principles from both HBM and social cognitive theory should significantly increase the effectiveness of patient education.

HOW HEALTH PROFESSIONALS CAN ENCOURAGE PREVENTIVE BEHAVIOR

One infers from social cognitive theory and the HBM that health professionals who use modeling and verbal persuasion, who assist individuals to engage in self-regulation, and who directly address health beliefs are likely to have an influence on the behavior of their patients. Getting women to accurately carry out BSE seems fundamental to the prevention effort. While carefully performed BSE may avoid the development of some advanced-stage breast cancers, the way it is currently practiced by many women may produce little or no benefit (Newcomb, et al, 1991). The health care provider is key in the learning process.

It has been suggested (Siminoff, 1989) that when cancer is the subject, the communication process between physician and patient shares most of the general features of the standard doctor-patient interaction but is burdened with additional problems. Discussing cancer is emotionally charged; stigma and fear are associated with both diagnosis and treatment (Sontag, 1978). The medical information having to do with cancer is complex, and the course of disease and benefits of treatment are uncertain (Hoy, 1985; Frei, 1982; National Cancer Institute, 1987).

Siminoff (1989) has suggested that health professionals have four goals for the communication process: *cognitive outcomes*, or the patient's recall and understanding of what the health professional has said and why the information is important; *affective outcomes*, or the reduction of patient anxiety and the satisfaction of health provider and patient with the encounter; *behavioral outcomes*, or the patient's adherence to the proposed regimen; and *clinical outcomes*, or the actual prevention of disease or improvement in the patient's condition. There is a voluminous literature related to health professional–patient communication, most of it relevant to cancer communication and education. In general, in this literature, patient recall of information has been used to assess the quality of an interaction with the health professional (Inui and Carter, 1985; Meisel and Roth, 1983). However, as the theories discussed above illustrate, behavior change is a complex problem. Assessing success of education by measuring the amount of information a patient can remember is bound to be an inadequate, if not misleading, procedure (Tuckett et al, 1985). Most studies have shown that patient recall of information about cancer diagnosis and treatment is low (Mitchell et al, 1977; Goldberg and Cullen, 1980; Morrow et al, 1978; Robinson and Merav, 1976; Robinson, 1986; Jones et al, 1983; Rimer et al, 1983; Dodd, 1982), both with regard to knowing what treatment entails (Cassileth et al, 1980) and to knowing the risks or benefits of treatment (Muss et al, 1979; Morrow et al, 1978).

The problems associated with recall as a measure of successful communication includes the complication of distinguishing what the patient remembers and what the health professional actually said (or didn't say). In a study of a large group of physicians seeing women with breast cancer, Liberati (1986) found that the characteristics of their patients influenced the type and level of information the physicians provided. Younger and more-educated women were much more likely to be given thorough information. In addition, age, education, and size of the breast tumor were each independent significant predictors of the quality of the information received. Greiner and Weiler (1983) found that over half the breast cancer patients being treated with primary radiation therapy in their study were told by surgeons that no alternative to mastectomy existed.

Wu and Perlman (1988) found among hospitalized cancer patients on a general medicine service that treatment rationale was the topic most frequently communicated to them by their health providers, followed by benefit, risk, and treatment alternatives. Nonetheless, shared understanding between provider and patient related to any of these topics never exceeded 60%. Taylor (1988) examined communication patterns of breast cancer surgeons and demonstrated that, rather than tailor their communications to the individual patient, physicians routinized them.

A number of studies have shown that educational interventions for situations in which cancer is a concern can increase knowledge and decrease emotional distress (Rainey, 1985), improve depression and decrease the level of life disruption (Jacobs et al, 1983), reduce functional limitations, decrease anxiety, and increase compliance (Molleman et al, 1984; Jacobs et al, 1983;

Greenfield et al, 1985; Speedling and Rose, 1985; Wartman et al, 1983; Roter, 1977).

What specific things can a health care provider do to improve communication and assist patients to follow recommended preventive therapies such as BSE? A comprehensive look at the problem of patient compliance or adherence to the recommendations of health professionals was taken by Becker (1985). After reviewing over 100 studies of provider-patient interaction, he derived a series of actions that are most likely to improve patient understanding and behavior related to preventive and curative practices. These recommended actions for health care providers included the following:

Increasing Patient Knowledge

This includes providing more information about details of the prescribed therapy (eg, length of time and frequency with which a therapy is to be followed), avoiding medical jargon, and providing important points in writing to reinforce the oral communication.

Modifying Regimen Characteristics

This includes adjusting the therapeutic recommendation to make it less complex, of shorter duration, less dependent on alteration of the patient's lifestyle, and less inconvenient and expensive. The therapy can be made less complex by four actions: avoiding the routine prescription of nonessential steps in the prescribed procedure or variations in scheduling; emphasizing the necessity of adherence to particularly critical aspects of the regimen (ie, setting priorities in recognition that only those recommendations of highest priority are likely to be carried out); breaking the recommended procedure into less complex steps than can be implemented sequentially; and minimizing inconvenience and forgetfulness by matching the regimen schedule to the patient's daily activities (ie, tailoring the procedure to fit the individual's lifestyle).

Addressing Health Beliefs and Self-Efficacy

This includes consideration of the extent to which the patient considers herself or himself susceptible to cancer, considers cancer a serious illness, and sees benefits or costs in the recommended procedure(s). It also includes recognition of the fact that patients often make inferences from incidents during history taking or the physical workup or other elements of the encounter with the health professional that influence their confidence in the provider's determinations. Confidence may wane, for example, when the physician appears to pay insufficient attention to the presenting complaint. Similarly, patients may have difficulty being candid with the health professional—but knowing that they have not confided complete information, they may subsequently consider the physician's diagnosis and recommendations as inaccurate or incomplete. Finally, some information may be too painful to accept. A disease such as cancer gives rise to a variety of fears and anxieties. To offset these eventualities, the health provider can try to set a nonthreatening and safe environment for the patient interaction, can model being open in discussion by engaging in candid (and respectful) communication with the patient, can verbally reinforce the feelings of self-efficacy of a patient to perform a procedure or carry out a recommendation, and can be verbally persuasive in describing the benefits of the treatment given the costs.

Influencing the Treatment Experience

This includes altering the treatment experience to optimize the potential for adherence. One way to modify the treatment experience is the contingency contract, wherein both parties (health professional and patient) set a goal, describe the obligations of each party in reaching it, and establish a time limit for achievement. Several studies have shown the utility of writing out these contracts (Janz et al, 1984; Lowe and Lutzker, 1979). In addition, other personnel in the office, clinic, or hospital can be involved in providing clarification and reinforcement of the provider's educational messages.

Influencing the Doctor-Patient Relationship

This includes improving the nature and process of the communication between health professional and patient. For example, studies have illustrated that impersonality and brevity negatively affect patient behavior (Coe and Wessen, 1965; Becker and Maiman, 1975). Physician communication patterns that are rejecting, controlling, disagree completely with the patient, or fail to provide feedback are strongly associated with patients' failure to adhere to advice (Davis, 1968; Francis et al, 1969). Better compliance with recommendations is found when the health care professional is friendly, understands the patient's perspective, elicits and meets patient's expectations for the visit and addresses his or her concerns, provides responsive information about the situation and progress, expresses sincere concern and sympathy, and provides clear explanations for findings and recommendations. The professional's orientation has been shown to be a factor in adherence to therapy. Schulman (1979) found that physicians with an active patient orientation (ie, who considered their patients as active participants in the treatment process) were much more likely to have patients that followed their advice. Glanz (1979) showed that professionals who were more predisposed toward actively influencing their patients, and used more influence strategies to involve patients in counseling sessions, had patients with more appropriate health beliefs and compliance behaviors.

Improving Ways of Providing Care

This includes providing increased support and clearer expectations for the patient throughout the care system. Such things as definite appointments, better monitoring, home visits, continuity of care, have all been shown to be associated with better adherence by patients to professional recommendations (Becker, 1985).

Enlisting Family and Social Support

Social support appears to be particularly important for recommendations that are long-term in nature, and that require continuous action on the part of the patient. A family's own health beliefs influence the patient's adherence. Similarly, when the family's normal roles and patterns are compatible with demands of the patient's regimen, or when family members can easily make needed changes, adherence to recommendations is stronger. Becker (1985) has posited that given our current concern with chronic conditions and the concomitant shift in emphasis from direct medical care to continuous patient self-management, the effect of the family and other social support systems on the patient's adherence is likely to be of tremendous importance, with many possibilities for substantial positive or negative impacts.

No discussion of cancer-related health promotion and health education can conclude without reference to the individual's right *not* to follow health education and medical recommendations. Weintraub (1976) has used the term "intelligent noncompliance" to describe the clinical situation where a prescribed procedure or therapy is purposely not taken and the patient's reason for noncompliance appears valid when analyzed dispassionately (eg, when the patient experiences substantial adverse reactions or side effects, or when the course of the health problem changes and the recommendations are no longer relevant). Physicians rarely assess their patients' compliance behaviors, even ones as pertinent to cancer prevention as breast self-examination or cessation of smoking. Failure to assess patient behavior over time may result both in a weakening of patient confidence in the health care provider and in the mistaken belief on the part of the professional that the patient is following recommendations. A knowledgeable and active health care provider will have more educated and active patients with regard to cancer-preventing behaviors.

REFERENCES

AJZEN I, FISHBEIN M. 1980. Understanding attitudes and predicting social behavior. Englewood Cliffs, NJ: Prentice-Hall.

AMERICAN CANCER SOCIETY. 1994. Cancer Facts & Figures—1994. New York: American Cancer Society.

AMSEL Z, GROVER PL, BALSHEM AM. 1985. Frequency of breast self-examination practice as a function of physician reinforcement. Patient Educ Counsel 7:147–155.

BAKER JA. 1989. Breast self-examination and the older woman: field testing an educational approach. Gerontologist 29(3):405–407.

BANDURA A. 1977a. Self-efficacy: toward a unifying theory of behavioral change. Psychol Rev 84:191–215.

BANDURA A. 1977b. Social Learning Theory. Englewood Cliffs, NJ: Prentice-Hall.

BANDURA A. 1982. Self-efficacy mechanism in human agency. Am Psychol 37:122–147.

BANDURA A. 1986. Social Foundations of Thought and Action: A Social Cognitive Theory. Englewood Cliffs, NJ: Prentice-Hall.

BECKER MH. 1974a. The health belief model and sick role behavior. Health Educ Monogr 2:409–419.

BECKER MH, ed. 1974b. The health belief model and personal health behavior. Health Educ Monogr 2:324–508.

BECKER MH. 1985. Patient adherence to prescribed therapies. Med Care 23(5):539–555.

BECKER MH, MAIMAN LA. 1975. Sociobehavioral determinants of compliance with health and medical care recommendations. Med Care 13:10.

BECKER MH, ROSENSTOCK IM. 1987. Comparing social learning theory and the health belief model. Adv Health Educ Promotion 2:245–249.

CALNAN M. 1984. The health belief model and participation in programmes for the early detection of breast cancer: a comparative analysis. Soc Sci Med 19(8):823–930.

CALNAN MW, MOSS S. 1984. The health belief model and compliance with education given at a class in breast self-examination. J Health Soc Behav 25:198–210.

CALNAN MW, MOSS S, CHAMBERLAIN J. 1984. Explaining attendance at a class teaching breast self-examination. Patient Educ Counsel 6(2):83–90.

CALNAN M, RUTTER DR. 1986. Do health beliefs predict health behaviour? An analysis of breast self-examination. Soc Sci Med 22(6):673–678.

CASSILETH BR, VOLCKMAR D, GOODMAN RL. 1980. The effect of experience on radiation therapy patients' desire for information. Int J Radiat Oncol Biol Phys 6:493–496.

CHAMPION VL. 1992. Relationship of age to factors influencing breast self-examination practice. Health Care Women Int 13(1):1–9.

CLARK N, ROSENSTOCK I, HASSAN H, WASILEWSKI Y, EVANS D, FELDMAN C, MELLINS R. 1988. The effect of health beliefs and feelings of self-efficacy on self-management behavior of children with a chronic disease. Pat Couns Educ 11(2):131–139.

CLARK N, ZIMMERMAN BJ. 1990. A social cognitive view of self-regulated learning about health. Health Educ Res 5(3):371–379.

COE RM, WESSEN A. 1965. Social-psychological factors influencing the use of community health resources. Am J Public Health 55:1024.

CRAUN AM, DEFFENBACHER JL. 1987. The effects of information, behavioral rehearsal, and prompting on breast self-exams. J Behav Med 10(4):351–356.

DAVIS MS. 1968. Variations in patients' compliance with doctors' advice: an empirical analysis of patterns of communication. Am J Public Health 58:274.

DODD MJ. 1982. Cancer patients' knowledge of chemotherapy: Assessment and informational interventions. Oncol Nurs Forum 9(3):39–44.

DORSAY RH, CUNEO WD, SOMKIN CP, TEKAWA IS. 1988. Breast self-examination: improving competence and frequency in a classroom setting. Am J Public Health 78(5):520–522.

EDWARDS V. 1980. Changing breast self-examination behavior. Nurs Res 29(5):301–306.

FISHBEIN M, AJZEN I. 1975. Belief, attitude, intention and behavior; an introduction to theory and research. Reading, Mass: Addison-Wesley.

FLETCHER SW, MORGAN TM, O'MALLEY MS, EARP JAL, DEGNAN D. 1989. Is breast self-examination predicted by knowledge, attitudes, beliefs, or sociodemographic characteristics? Am J Prev Med 5(4):207–215.

FRANCIS W, KORSCH BM, MORRIS MH. 1969. Gaps in doctor-patient communication: patients' response to medical advice. N Engl J Med 280:535.

FREI E. 1982. The national cancer program. Science 217:600–606.

FRENCH BN, KURCZYNSKI TW, WEAVER MT, PITUCH MJ. 1992. Evaluation of the Health Belief Model and decision making regarding amniocentesis in women of advanced maternal age. Health Educ Q 19(2):177–186.

GLANZ K. 1979. Dietitians' effectiveness and patient compliance with dietary regimens. J Am Diet Assoc 75:631.

GLANZ K, LERMAN C. 1992. Psychosocial impact of breast cancer: a critical review. Ann Behav Med 14(3):204–212.

GOLDBERG RJ, CULLEN LO. 1980. Factors important to psychosocial adjustment to cancer: a review of the evidence. Soc Sci Med 20(8):803–807.

GRADY KE. 1984. Cue enhancement and the long-term practice of breast self-examination. J Behav Med 7(2):191–204.

GRADY KE, GOODENOW C, BORKIN JR. 1988. The effect of reward on compliance with breast self-examination. J Behav Med 11(1):43–57.

GRAVELL J, ZAPKA JG, MAMON JA. 1985. Impact of breast self-examination planned educational messages on social network communications: an exploratory study. Health Educ Q 12(1):51–64.

GREENFIELD S, KAPLAN S, WARE JE JR. 1985. Expanding patient involvement in care: effects on patient outcomes. Ann Intern Med 102(4):520–528.

GREINER L, WEILER C. 1983. What do women know about breast cancer treatment choices? Am J Nurs 83(11):1570.

HALLAL JC. 1982. The relationship of health beliefs, health locus of control, and self concept to the practice of breast self-examination in adult women. Nurs Res 31(3):137–142.

HENDERSON I, CANCELLOS G. 1980. Cancer of the breast: the past decade. N Engl J Med 302:17.

HIBBARD JH. 1983. Sex differences in health and illness orientation. Int Q Community Health Educ 84(4):95–104.

HIBBARD JH, POPE CR. 1987. Women's roles, interests in health and health behavior. Women Health, 12:67–85.

HIRSCHFIELD-BARTEK J. 1982. Health beliefs and their influence on breast self-examination practices in women with breast cancer. Oncol Nurs Forum 9(3):77–81.

HOY AM. 1985. Breaking bad news to patients. Br J Hosp Med 34(2):96–99.

INUI TS, CARTER WB. 1985. Problems and prospects for health services research on provider-patient communication. Med Care 23:521–538.

JACOBS C, ROSS RD, WALKER IM, STOCKDALE FE. 1983. Behavior of cancer patients: a randomized study of the effects of education and peer support groups. Am J Clin Oncol 6(3):347–353.

JANZ NK, BECKER MH. 1984. The health belief model: a decade later. Health Educ Q 11(1):1–47.

JANZ NK, BECKER MH, ANDERSON LA, MARCOUX BC. 1989/90. Interventions to enhance breast self-examination practice: a review. Public Health Rev 17(2-3):89–163.

JANZ NK, BECKER MH, HARTMAN PE. 1984. Contingency contracting to enhance patient compliance: a review. Patient Educ Counsel 5:165.

JONES WL, DAYAL HH, GROVER PL, et al. 1983. Research in cancer patient education and compliance. Prog Clin Biol Res 120:467–481.

KENNEY E, HOVELL MF, DOCKTER B, CHIN L, MEWBORN CR. 1986. Training breast self-examination to competence: assessment of an education program. J Psychosom Obstet Gynaecol 5:65–79.

KIRSCHT JP. 1974. The health belief model and illness behavior. Health Educ Monogr 2:387–408.

LEWIN K. 1951. The nature of field theory. In: Psychological Theory, Marx MH (ed). New York: Macmillan.

LIBERATI A. 1986. What doctors tell patients with breast cancer about diagnosis and treatment. Br J Cancer 54:319–326.

LOWE K, LUTZKER JR. 1979. Increasing compliance to a medical regimen with a juvenile diabetic. Behav Ther 10:57.

MAIMAN LA, BECKER MH. 1974. The health belief model: origins and correlates in psychological theory. Health Educ Monogr 2:336–353.

MAMON JA, ZAPKA JG. 1985. Improving frequency and proficiency of breast self-examination: effectiveness of an education program. Am J Public Health 75(6):618–624.

MAMON JA, ZAPKA JG. 1986. Breast self-examination by young women: I. Characteristics associated with frequency. Am J Prev Med 2(2):61–69.

MAYER JA, DUBBERT PM, SCOTT RR, DAWSON BL, EKSTRAND ML, FONDREN TG. 1987. Breast self-examination: the effects of personalized prompts on practice frequency. Behav Ther 2:135–146.

MAYER JA, SOLOMON LJ. 1992. Breast self-examination skill and frequency: a review. Ann Behav Med 14(3):189–196.

MEISEL A, ROTH LH. 1983. Toward an informed discussion of informed consent: a review and critique of the empirical studies. Ariz Law Rev 25(2):265–346.

MITCHELL GW, GLICKSMAN AS. 1977. Cancer patients: knowledge and attitudes. Cancer 40:61–66.

MOLLEMAN E, KRABBENDAM PJ, ANNYAS AA, et al. 1984. The significance of the doctor-patient relationship in coping with cancer. Soc Sci Med 18(6):475–480.

MORROW G, GOOTNICK J, SCHMALE A. 1978. A simple technique for increasing cancer patients' knowledge of informed consent to treatment. Cancer 42:793–799.

MUSS HB, WHITE DR, MICHIELUTTE R, et al. 1979. Written informed consent in patients with breast cancer. Cancer 43:1549–1556.

NATIONAL CANCER INSTITUTE. 1987. Division of Cancer Prevention and Treatment: Annual Report. Bethesda, MD, National Cancer Institute.

NEWCOMB PA, WEISS NS, STOUR BE, SCHOLES D, YOUNG BE, VOIGHT LF. 1991. Breast self-examination in relation to the occurrence of advanced breast cancer. J Natl Cancer Inst 83(4):260–265.

NIH. 1980. A Measure of Progress in Public Understanding: National Survey on Breast Cancer. DHHS Publ. No. NIH 82-2305. Washington DC: US Government Printing Office.

O'MALLEY MS, FLETCHER SW. 1987. Screening for breast cancer with breast self-examination. JAMA 257(16):2197–2203.

OWENS RG, DALY J, HERON K, LEINSTER SJ. 1987. Psychological and social characteristics of attenders for breast screening. Psychol Health 1:303–313.

PARCEL GS, BARANOWSKI T. 1982. Social learning theory and health education. Health Educ 12(3):14–18.

PENNYPACKER HS, BLOOM HS, CRISWELL EL, NEELAKANTAN P,

GOLDSTEIN MK, STEIN GH. 1982. Toward an effective technology of instruction in breast self-examination. Int J Mental Health 11:98–116.

PETOSA R, JACKSON K. 1991. Using the Health Belief Model to predict safer sex intentions among adolescents. Health Educ Q 18(4):463–476.

PINTO B, FUQUA RW. 1991. Training breast self examination: research review and critique. Health Educ Q 18(4):495–516.

RAINEY LC. 1985. Effects of preparatory patient education for radiation oncology patients. Cancer 56(5):1056–1061.

RIMER B, JONES WL, KEINTZ MK, et al. 1983. Informed consent: a crucial step in patient education. Health Educ Q 10(1):30–42.

ROBINSON G, MERAV A. 1976. Informed consent: recall by patients tested postoperatively. Ann Thorac Surg 22(3):209–212.

ROBINSON G. 1986. The treating physician's view of informed consent: observations made in a retrospective study. Conn Med 50(12):818–819.

ROSENSTOCK IM. 1974. Historical origins of the health belief model. Health Educ Monogr 2:332.

ROSENSTOCK IM, STRECHER MJ, BECKER MH. 1988. Social learning theory and the health belief model. Health Educ Q 15:175–183.

ROTER DL. 1977. Patient participation in the patient-provider interaction: the effects of patient question-asking on the quality of interaction, satisfaction, and compliance. Health Educ Monogr 5(4):281–315.

SCHULMAN BA. 1979. Active patient orientation and outcomes in hypertensive treatment: application of a socio-organizational perspective. Med Care 17:267.

SHELLEY JF. 1983. Inadequate transfer of breast cancer self-detection technology. Am J Public Health 73:1317–1320.

SIMINOFF LA. 1989. Cancer patient and physician communication: progress and continuing problems. Ann Behav Med 11(3):108–112.

SKINNER BF. 1974. About Behaviorism. New York: Vintage Books.

SMITH PC, HAILEY BJ. 1988. Compliance with instructions for regular breast self-examination. The Journal of Compliance in Health Care, 3(2):151–161.

SONTAG S. 1978. Illness as Metaphor. New York: Farrar, Straus, and Giroux.

SPEEDLING EJ, ROSE DN. 1985. Building an effective doctor-patient relationship: from patient satisfaction to patient participation. Soc Sci Med 21(2):115–120.

STILLMAN MJ. 1977. Women's health beliefs about breast cancer and breast self-examination. Nurs Res 26(2):121–127.

STRAUSS LM, SOLOMON LJ, COSTANZA MC, WORDEN JK, FOSTER RS. 1987. Breast self-examination practices and attitudes of women with and without a history of breast cancer. J Behav Med 10(4):337–349.

STRECHER VJ, DEVELLIS BM, BECKER MH, ROSENSTOCK IM. 1986. The role of self-efficacy in achieving health behavior change. Health Educ Qu 13:73–92.

TAYLOR KM. 1988. Telling bad news: physicians and the disclosure of undesirable information. Sociol Health Illness 10(2):109–132.

TROTTA P. 1980. Breast self-examination: factors influencing compliance. Oncol Nurs Forum 7:13–17.

TUCKETT DA, BOULTON M, OLSON C. 1985. A new approach to the measurement of patients' understanding of what they are told in medical consultations. J Health Soc Behav 26:27–38.

USDHHS. 1994. Health United States 1993. (PHS:94-1232) PHS/CDC/National Center for Health Statistics.

WALKER LR, GLANZ K. 1986. Psychosocial determinants of breast self-examination. Am J Prevent Med 2(3):169–178.

WARTMAN SA, MORLOCK LL, MALITZ FE, PALM EA. 1983. Patient understanding and satisfaction as predictors of compliance. Med Care 21(9):886–891.

WEINBERG AD, SPIKER CA, INGERSOLL RW, HOERSTING SR. 1982. Public knowledge and attitudes toward cancer: their roles in health decisions and behaviors. Health Values 6:19–26.

WEINTRAUB M. 1976. Intelligent noncompliance and capricious compliance. In: Patient Compliance, Lasagna L (ed). New York: Futura Publishing Company, pp 39–47.

WU WC, PERLMAN RA. 1988. Consent in medical decision-making. J Gen Intern Med 3:9–14.

ZIMMERMAN BJ. 1994. Dimensions of academic self-regulation: a conceptual framework for education. In: Self-Regulation of Learning and Performance, Schunk DH, Zimmerman BJ (eds). Hillsdale, NJ: Erlbuan Associates, pp 3–21.

65 Intervention studies

JULIE E. BURING
CHARLES H. HENNEKENS

During the past several decades, numerous observational analytic epidemiologic studies have provided data concerning alterable determinants of cancer risk. Cessation of cigarette smoking and reduction of heavy alcohol consumption are the two most reliably known as well as leading avoidable causes of U.S. cancer deaths, with cigarettes known to be directly responsible for 30% and alcohol about 3% of all cancer deaths each year (Doll and Peto, 1981). Recently, however, evidence has been accumulating that has raised the possibility that diet may be implicated in as many as 35% of all deaths from cancer (Doll and Peto, 1981).

As such data on diet as well as other potential risk factors for cancer continue to accumulate from case–control and cohort studies, as well as from basic research designed to elucidate the underlying biologic mechanisms, intervention studies, or clinical trials, are assuming increasing importance (Greenwald et al, 1993; Greenwald, 1994). The clinical trial may be viewed as a special type of prospective cohort study, in which the investigator allocates the exposure. The primary advantage of this design is that when exposures are allocated at random in a sample of sufficiently large size, intervention studies have the potential to provide a degree of assurance about the validity of a result that is simply not possible with any observational design strategy (Hennekens and Buring, 1987).

The 10- to 20-fold increase in risk of lung cancer attributable to cigarette smoking (U.S. Department of Health and Human Services [DHHS], 1982), or even the approximately threefold increase of laryngeal cancer associated with heavy alcohol consumption (Rothenberg et al, 1987), is easily detectable from case–control and cohort studies. However, the postulated effects of many dietary and other risk factors are small to moderate in size, on the order of 30–50%. While reductions in risk of this magnitude for a disease as common as cancer can be extremely important from a clinical or public health perspective, such effects are very difficult to establish reliably from observational studies because they may easily be as large as the amount of uncontrolled confounding or bias inherent in these designs. In such circumstances, a randomized trial is the only design which can provide reliable evidence to address such questions.

In this chapter, we discuss issues in the design, conduct, and analysis of intervention studies in cancer prevention.

TYPES OF CANCER PREVENTION TRIALS

Intervention studies can be generally classified into three major types: secondary prevention, primary prevention, and community trials. *Secondary prevention* (or therapeutic) trials are conducted among patients with a particular disease to determine the ability of an agent or procedure to diminish symptoms, prevent recurrence, or decrease risk of death from that disease. For example, to evaluate the efficacy of radical mastectomy compared with a more limited procedure to prevent recurrence in breast cancer, early breast cancer patients were randomized to undergo radical mastectomy, simple mastectomy or more limited resection with concomitant radiation therapy (Fisher et al, 1985a,b). Similarly, trials have been carried out to determine the ability of antioxidant vitamins to prevent recurrence of basal- and squamous-cell carcinoma (Greenberg et al, 1990) and colorectal adenomas (Greenberg et al, 1994).

A *primary prevention* (or preventive) *trial* is conducted among those who are disease free at enrollment to determine whether an agent or procedure reduces the risk of subsequently developing that outcome. Such trials can be conducted either among apparently healthy individuals at usual risk of developing the disease, or among those already recognized to be at high risk because of the presence of known risk factors.

An example of the former trial is the Physicians' Health Study, a primary prevention trial of subjects at usual risk, which has tested whether supplementation with beta-carotene decreases the incidence of cancers of epithelial cell origin in a population of apparently healthy male physicians, who were free of cancer at entry (Hennekens and Eberlein, 1985). With respect to prevention studies among high-risk subjects, a trial of vitamin E and beta-carotene has been completed among a population of middle-aged men in Finland who were at high baseline risk for lung cancer due to cigarette smoking history (Alpha-Tocopherol, Beta Carotene Cancer Prevention Study Group, 1994). Similarly, a trial of beta-carotene and retinol has been conducted among individuals at high risk for lung cancer due to occupational asbestos exposure and/or a history of cigarette smoking (Omenn et al, 1988). Cancer prevention trials of high-risk individuals may also involve assessment of whether an intervention can halt, slow, or even reverse the progression of a premalignant condition, such as dysplasia, into a frank malignancy (Stich et al, 1984a,b).

The third type of intervention study, the *community trial*, involves allocating entire populations to receive or not receive a particular intervention program. For example, to evaluate the effectiveness of various approaches to encourage smoking cessation, a trial in California assigned one town to receive a mass media campaign urging smoking cessation, one town to offer smokers counselling for smoking cessation, and a third town to receive no special intervention (U.S. DHHS, 1982).

UNIQUE PROBLEMS OF INTERVENTION STUDIES

Unlike observational analytic study designs in which the investigator is a passive observer, in the intervention study there is active assignment of participants to a particular agent or procedure. Consequently, intervention studies pose unique problems of ethics, feasibility, and costs. For reasons of both ethics and feasibility, there must be sufficient doubt about the efficacy of an intervention to allow withholding it from half of the subjects at the same time as there is sufficient belief in its potential to justify exposing the other half. It would be unethical either to administer an exposure known to be harmful, such as cigarette smoking, or to prevent or limit access to an agent of proven value. On the other hand, in instances where there is truly insufficient evidence in either direction, it may be considered unethical not to conduct a randomized trial.

The widespread adoption of practices by either the general public or the medical community in the absence of adequate information on which to base a sound policy decision can adversely affect the feasibility of conducting a randomized trial. For example, the standard choice of the radical mastectomy for breast cancer, introduced by William Halsted in the early twentieth century, was based on the clinical impression that removal of the breast as well as surrounding lymph nodes and muscles would reduce risks of recurrence or spread. It was only in the 1970s that this hypothesis was formally tested in randomized trials that showed no differences in mortality for early breast cancer patients receiving the radical mastectomy, simple mastectomy, or removal of the lump with radiation therapy (Fisher et al, 1985a,b). Similarly, in recent years, usage of vitamin supplements in the U.S. has increased from 26.1% in the early 1970s (Block et al, 1988) to 57.6% in 1985 (U.S. Department of Agriculture, 1985). Such widespread use of vitamins can make the conduct of any randomized trial of the possible chemopreventive effects of vitamins much less feasible, since it may become difficult to find a sufficiently large population of individuals willing to forego their use for the duration of a trial. Thus, in practical terms, it is generally optimal to conduct a randomized trial when a potentially promising agent or procedure is first identified rather than after it gains widespread acceptance and becomes standard practice.

Finally, as regards costs, intervention studies have traditionally been substantially more expensive than observational investigations. The need for study personnel to evaluate and treat subjects individually and to monitor them carefully through periodic and extensive examinations at a hospital or clinic has undoubtedly contributed to high costs, which have been on the order of $3,000 to $15,000 per randomized participant. In recent years, however, attention has begun to focus on the possibility of conducting large trials with streamlined protocols that have been carefully designed to minimize time and expense (Hennekens, 1984; Yusuf et al, 1984; Peto et al, 1993; Buring et al, 1994). In such circumstances, the cost of conducting an efficiently designed intervention study should be no greater than for observational studies of comparable sample sizes.

ISSUES IN THE DESIGN AND CONDUCT OF INTERVENTION STUDIES

There are a number of methodologic considerations that must be addressed in the design and conduct of intervention studies, including the selection of an appropriate study population; allocation of the treatment regimens; maintenance and assessment of compliance; achieving complete and uniform rates of ascertainment of outcomes; and the use of a factorial design.

Selection of the Study Population

The *reference population* for a clinical trial, or the group to whom the investigators expect the results of the particular trial to be applicable, may include all human beings if it seems likely that the study findings are universally applicable. Conversely, the reference population may necessarily be restricted by geography, age, sex, or some other characteristic that is thought to modify the existence or magnitude of the effects observed in the trial. Thus the reference population represents the scope of the public health impact of the intervention.

The *experimental population* is the actual group within which the trial is conducted. While it is usually preferable that this group not differ from the reference population in such a way that generalizations can't be drawn to the latter, the primary consideration in the design of the trial should always be to obtain a valid result. The selection of the experimental population is crucial to achieving that aim and involves consideration of several important issues. First, it is essential to determine whether the proposed experimental population is sufficiently large to achieve the necessary sample size for the trial. Analogously, it is essential to choose an experimental population who will experience a sufficient number of outcomes of interest to permit meaningful comparisons between interventions within a reasonable period of time. For cancer trials, this may involve selecting individuals at increased risk of developing the outcome of interest on the basis of baseline characteristics or health habits, such as age, sex, cigarette smoking, occupational exposures, or the presence of premalignant conditions.

An additional concern is the selection of a population from whom complete and accurate follow-up information can be obtained for the duration of the trial. The Physicians' Health Study, for example, has been conducted among male physicians in the U.S. who were 40 to 84 years of age at entry (Hennekens and Eberlein, 1985). This population represents a group of individuals who are less mobile and easier to trace than members of the general population, are particularly well aware of their medical history and health status, and can report such information with a high degree of accuracy. In fact, after an average of 5 years of follow-up, 99.7% of the participants were still providing complete follow-up information, and mortality data were available for every physician randomized into the trial (Steering Committee of the Physicians' Health Study Research Group, 1989). In contrast, a trial conducted among a highly mobile group or among a group of infirm elderly subjects who would be required to make frequent clinic visits would likely result in low follow-up rates, which would render the findings uninterpretable.

Since male physicians constitute a highly select subgroup of the population, a potential limitation of their use as the study population in the Physicians' Health Study is that the trial findings will not be directly relevant to the population at large. The participants in the trial did report a more favorable baseline health profile than the general U.S. population, and their subsequent mortality rate was substantially lower than expected, based on rates among white males in the U.S. (Steering Committee, 1989). Nevertheless, while the baseline disease risks of U.S. male physicians may be lower than those of a more representative population, there is no reason to believe that any trial findings concerning the effects of aspirin and beta-carotene would be materially different among the general population of U.S. men. However, the precise benefit-to-risk ratio for these agents may differ for certain population subgroups, such as women, in whom it would be desirable to obtain direct evidence. For this reason, a large-scale trial is, in fact, now underway testing the benefits and risks of low-dose aspirin and vitamin E among a population of female health professionals (Buring, 1992a,b).

In some cases, two populations may differ so greatly that the results of a trial carried out in one may have no relevance to the other. For example, a trial of vitamin and mineral supplements was recently completed in a rural region in northcentral China (Blot et al, 1993). This area suffers from one of the world's highest rates of esophageal and gastric cancer, and nutritional intake of several micronutrients is very low. Participants in the trial who were randomized to a combined regimen of beta-carotene, vitamin E, and selenium experienced a significantly lower risk of gastric cancer than those who did not receive this supplement combination. However, because baseline intake of these nutrients is so low among this population, it remains uncertain whether these results have any relevance to populations with adequate nutritional intake.

Those who are eventually determined to be both willing and eligible to enroll in a trial comprise the actual study population, and they are often a relatively small and very select subgroup of the experimental population. It is well recognized that those who participate in an intervention study are very likely to differ from nonparticipants in ways that may affect the rate of development of the outcomes under investigation (Friedman et al, 1985). Among all who are eligible, those willing to participate tend to experience lower morbidity and mortality than those who do not, regardless of the hypothesis under study, as well as the actual treatment to which they are assigned (Horwitz and Wilbeck, 1971; Wilhelmsen et al, 1976). Volunteering is likely to be associated with age, sex, socioeconomic status, education, and other, less well defined correlates of health consciousness that might significantly influence subsequent morbidity and mortality. Whether the subgroup of participants is representative of the entire experimental population will not affect the validity of the results of a trial conducted among that group. It may, however, affect the ability to generalize those results to either the experimental or the reference population. If it is possible to obtain baseline data and/or to ascertain outcomes for subjects who are eligible but unwilling to participate, such information is extremely valuable to assess the presence and extent of differences between participants and nonparticipants in a particular trial. This will aid in the judgment of whether the results observed among trial participants are generalizable to the reference population.

Allocation of Study Regimens

Since participants and nonparticipants may differ in important ways related to the outcome under investigation, allocation to the various treatment options takes place after potential subjects have been determined to be eligible and have expressed a willingness to participate. To maximize the probability that the groups receiving the different interventions will be comparable, this allocation should be made at random. Random assignment implies that each individual has the same chance of receiving each of the possible interventions and that the probability that a given subject will receive a particular assignment is independent of the probability that any other participant will receive the same assignment. When the frequency of developing the outcome under investigation is expected to vary appreciably among subgroups of the study population, such as for men and women, or when the response to an intervention is likely to differ markedly between subjects, such as those with different stages of disease, the efficiency of the study may be increased by ensuring that treatment groups are balanced with respect to such characteristics. This is achieved through the use of blocked randomization, in which every participant is classified with respect to each such variable before allocation and then randomized within that subgroup. The use of blocking has particular relevance when the study size is limited (Peto et al, 1976, 1977).

Randomization offers a number of unique advantages relative to other methods of allocation. First, if it is done properly, no one involved in either deciding whether a potential subject is eligible to enter the trial or assigning participants to an intervention group will know the assigned treatment group in advance. Thus the potential for bias in allocation of treatment is removed, and investigators can be confident that observed differences are not due to the selection of particular patients to receive a given intervention. Other allocation schemes that can be predicted, such as alternate allocation or allocation by day of the week, always have the potential for manipulation, leading to a serious imbalance in the treatment groups with respect to factors affecting the outcome under study.

Another advantage of randomization is that on average, the study groups will be comparable with respect to all variables except for the interventions being studied. The larger the sample size, the more successful the randomization process will usually be in distributing these factors equally among the treatment groups. This feature is important because all baseline characteristics that affect risk and differ between the study groups could potentially confound the relationship between exposure and disease. While those potential confounders that are known or suspected can be taken into account in the analysis of data from a trial, there is no way other than randomization to control the influence of unknown confounding variables. Consequently, randomization can provide a degree of assurance about the comparability of the study groups that is simply not possible in any observational study design.

Maintenance and Assessment of Compliance

By definition, an intervention study requires the active participation and cooperation of the study subjects. After agreeing to participate, subjects may deviate from the protocol for a variety of reasons: these include development of side effects, failure to take the medication or perform new behaviors, or simply withdrawal of consent after randomization. Those who were randomized to one group may choose to obtain the alternative intervention on their own initiative. In addition, there may be instances where participants cannot comply, such as when they develop a condition that requires or contraindicates a particular therapy. Consequently, the problem of achieving and maintaining a high rate of compliance is a serious issue in the design and conduct of all clinical trials. For cancer prevention trials in particular, where extended periods of follow-up are usually necessary to test the hypothesis adequately, it is essential that this problem be carefully considered. This is because the extent of noncompliance in any trial is related to the length of time that participants are expected to adhere to the intervention.

There are a number of strategies to try to enhance compliance among the participants in a trial. One of the most important is the selection of a population of individuals who are both interested and reliable. Other ways of attempting to increase compliance include frequent contact with participants by home or clinic visit, telephone, or mail; the use of calendar packs of study medication, in which each pill is labelled with the day it is to be taken; and the use of incentives such as evaluations not ordinarily available from the participants' usual source of health care.

Monitoring compliance is important because noncompliance will decrease the statistical power of a trial to detect any true effect of the intervention (Buring and Hennekens, 1985). Thus, the interpretation of any trial result must take into account the degree of adherence to the assigned intervention in all groups. To the extent that either participants in the alternative treatment group receive the intervention under study or those in the active group do not actually adhere to their assigned regimen, the two groups will become more similar. Consequently, a true effect of an intervention may not be detected when the degree of noncompliance is high. The need to monitor compliance as objectively as possible may pose logistic difficulties. Often the only practical way to assess compliance is by self-report. In trials of pharmacologic agents, it is often useful to validate self-reports by pill counts of unused medication or the use of biochemical markers. For example, a number of standardized laboratory methods have been established for assessing individual nutrient status for many micronutrients, including retinol, beta-carotene, alpha-tocopherol, vitamins B6, B12, and C, folic acid, and selenium (Reynolds, 1985). Because of individual variability in dietary intake and absorption of these nutrients, however, estimates obtained from biochemical assays to corroborate compliance will always need to be interpreted with caution (Baron, 1985).

Selection of Proper Dose

In cancer prevention trials of pharmacologic or nutritional agents, the selection of a proper dose is an important design consideration. Many of the most promising cancer prevention interventions are vitamins, minerals, and other non-nutritive constituents of vegetables and fruits that trial participants are already consuming at varying levels through individual dietary practices. In observational studies of these dietary factors, subjects are often divided into quintiles based on their level of intake of the exposure of interest. Comparisons are usually then made between the highest and lowest quintiles. In contrast, in a randomized trial testing antioxidant vitamins in cancer prevention, for example, intake among placebo group subjects will reflect the distribution of intakes among the general population, not the lowest intake category. Therefore, in order to achieve sufficient differences in intake between the treatment and comparison groups, the active treatment groups need to be given doses high enough to put subjects into the top few percentiles of intake, not merely the top quintile. At the same time, trials of antioxidant vitamins, as well as of any other agent, must utilize doses that will not cause any real or perceived adverse effects that might lower compliance.

Ascertainment of Outcomes

The primary objective in the ascertainment of outcomes is to ensure that results are not biased by the collection of more complete or accurate information from one or another of the study groups. In addition to this need for uniformity in ascertainment of outcome is the requirement for complete follow-up of all randomized subjects. When outcomes for a proportion of study subjects are not identified but that proportion is similar for all treatment groups, the smaller the losses, the greater the likelihood that the magnitude of a bias will be small. On the other hand, if the proportion of outcomes that are not ascertained is large or differs among the study groups, the result could be an under- or overestimate or even, by chance, reflect the true effect. To avoid this situation, where it is not possible to know the magnitude or direction of the bias, it is crucial to keep the number of individuals lost to follow-up to an absolute minimum.

The required duration of treatment and follow-up, or the interval that elapses between allocation to the intervention and ascertainment of outcome, is related to the length of the latency period for the outcome under investigation. In general, the longer the duration of follow-up required, the more difficult it will be to achieve complete information, because people are more likely to move, change jobs, change their names, or lose touch with the study organization. For trials that have mortality as an endpoint, the availability of the U.S. National Death Index has enabled researchers, at the very least, to assess the vital status on every individual entered into a trial (Stampfer et al, 1984).

The potential for observation bias in ascertainment of outcome can exist in an intervention study in that knowledge of a participant's treatment status might, consciously or not, influence the identification or reporting of relevant events. The likelihood of such bias is directly related to the subjectivity of the outcomes under study. If the outcome being considered is total mortality, observation bias is unlikely, since the fact of death is objective and indisputable and cannot be affected by knowledge of a person's treatment regimen. In contrast, ascertainment of a specific cause of death may be less clear-cut and thus may be influenced by a clinician's knowledge of treatment assignment.

One approach to minimize observation bias is to keep the study participants and/or the investigators blinded, as far as possible, to the identity of the interventions until data collection has been completed. In a double-blind design, neither the participants nor the investigators know to which treatment group an individual has been assigned. The ability to conduct a double-blind trial is dependent on having treatment and comparison programs that are as nearly identical as possible. Consequently, in many trials, especially of drug therapies, the comparison group is assigned to receiving a placebo, an inert agent indistinguishable from the active treatment. By making it extremely difficult, if not impossible, to differentiate between the treatment and comparison groups, the use of a placebo will minimize bias in the ascertainment of subjective disease outcomes as well as side effects. Unfortunately, such trials are usually more complex and difficult to conduct than trials using an open design. Procedures must be established for immediate unblinding of a participant's physician in the event of serious side effects or other clinical emergencies in which this information seems relevant. Moreover, in some circumstances, it is not possible to blind both the participants and the investigators to the allocated treatment regimen. It is very difficult to design a double-blind trial for the evaluation of programs involving substantial changes in lifestyle, such as exercise, cigarette smoking cessation, or diet. In such circumstances, a single-blind or unblinded trial may be necessary. In a single-blind design, the investigator but not the participant is aware of the intervention being received, while in an unblinded or open trial, both the subject and the investigator know to which study group the individual has been assigned.

Single-blind as well as open trials are both simpler to execute than double-blind studies. While they tend to be more acceptable both to physicians randomizing patients and to participants, such designs also impose special problems. Subjects aware that they are not on the new or experimental program may become dissatisfied, resulting in differential compliance and/or loss to follow-up. Moreover, as discussed earlier, knowledge of the intervention to which the participant has been assigned raises the potential for observation bias in the reporting of side effects or assessment of outcomes. Thus, when a double-blind design is not possible, it is imperative that special precautions be taken to reduce the potential for observation bias. Objective criteria should be used, and the study groups should be followed with equal intensity by independent examiners who are unaware of the subjects' treatment status.

Use of a Factorial Design

Given the cost and feasibility issues in intervention studies, one approach to improve efficiency is to test two or more hypotheses simultaneously in a factorial design (Byar; Byar and Piantados, 1985). In a 2×2 factorial design, subjects are first randomized to treatments A or B to address one hypothesis, and then within each treatment group there is further randomization to treatments α or β to evaluate a second question. For example, the Physicians' Health Study has utilized a 2×2 factorial design to evaluate two primary prevention questions: 1) whether 325 mg of aspirin (Bufferin, supplied by Bristol-Myers Products) taken every other day reduces cardiovascular mortality, and 2) whether 50 mg of beta-carotene (Lurotin, supplied by BASF, AG) taken on alternate days reduces cancer incidence (Stampfer et al, 1985). Participants in the trial were first randomized into two groups, one receiving aspirin and the other aspirin placebo. Each of these groups was then randomized to receive either beta-carotene or its placebo. Thus participants in the trial were allocated to one of four possible regimens: aspirin alone, beta-carotene alone, both active agents, or both placebos. Similarly, the Women's Health Study is employing this design in order to assess the balance of benefits and risks of vitamin E (600 IU on alternate days, supplied by the Natural Source Vitamin E Association) and low-dose aspirin (100 mg on alternate days, supplied by Miles, Inc.) on cancer and cardiovascular disease among approximately 40,000 US female health professionals (Buring and Hennekens, 1992a,b).

The principal advantage of the factorial design is its ability to answer two or more questions in a single trial for only a marginal increase in cost. When the Physicians' Health Study was being planned in the late 1970s, there was a large body of sound evidence from laboratory research, observational epidemiologic studies, and secondary prevention trials supporting the hypothesis that aspirin might be effective in the primary prevention of cardiovascular disease. At that time, the beta-carotene hypothesis was much less mature, and it seemed unlikely that the available data would justify mounting a large-scale chemoprevention trial. Coupling these two research questions in a factorial design made it possible to address both questions in a single trial without loss of sensitivity or major increase in cost. Such an approach is a particularly attractive option for cancer chemoprevention trials, where there may be many promising but unproven hypotheses of interest (Sestelli and Dell, 1985).

Ideally, additional treatments in a factorial design should not complicate trial operations, materially affect eligibility requirements, or cause side effects that could lead to poor compliance or losses to follow-up. In addition, the possibility of an interaction between treatment regimens must be considered. Fortunately, such interactions tend to affect the magnitude of observed treatment effects rather than changing their direction from benefit to harm or vice versa. Moreover, while the possibility of interactions could be viewed as a potential limitation of a factorial trial, this design is in fact the only way to identify their existence. This is of potential importance particularly in the evaluation of the chemoprevention potential of micronutrients, which often are available to the general public in combinations.

In the cancer prevention trial carried out in Linxian, China, nine different vitamin and minerals were tested (Blot et al, 1993). However, the trial used only a partial factorial design in which the agents were grouped into four different vitamin/mineral combination. The trial found a significant 21% reduction in risk of gastric cancer among those assigned to the combined regimen of beta-carotene, vitamin E, and selenium. However, because of the use of combined groups, it was not possible to distinguish the relative contributions of the three agents to the observed effect.

STOPPING RULES FOR EARLY TERMINATION OF TRIALS

In the design phase of any trial, it is necessary to establish guidelines for deciding whether the trial should be modified or terminated before originally scheduled. To assure that the welfare of participants is protected, interim results should be monitored by a group that is independent of the investigators conducting the trial. If the data indicate a clear and extreme benefit on a primary end point, or if one treatment is clearly harmful, then early termination of the trial must be considered.

A variety of sophisticated statistical methods are available for monitoring accumulating trial data. As a general rule, the first requirement for even considering modification or early termination of an ongoing trial is the observation of an extreme finding that is so highly statistically significant that it is virtually impossible to arise by chance alone (Armitage, 1975; Friedman et al, 1985; Peto et al, 1976; Pocock, 1977; Peto, 1982). While a statistical test should not normally form the sole basis for a decision to stop or continue a trial, it can alert those responsible for data monitoring to the possibility that there may be cause for concern. The observed association must then be considered in the context of the totality of evidence, which includes possible biological mechanisms, results from other randomized trials and, to a lesser extent, observational studies; as well as an assessment of how the observed association would affect the overall risk-to-benefit ratio of the intervention. Similarly, the specific statistical criterion used to trigger this process cannot be specified exactly for all trials. In fact, there are many different views of what constitutes sufficient proof that an observed association in interim data does not represent a temporary, random fluctuation. Some investigators feel that this criterion should not be equally stringent for beneficial and harmful effects, or with respect to anticipated and unanticipated findings. Whatever the specific guideline, however, the aim is to achieve a balance between protecting participants against real harm and minimizing the risk of stopping or modifying the trial in error (Armitage, 1975; Coronary Drug Project Research Group, 1981; DeMets et al, 1984; Friedman et al, 1985; Peto et al, 1976; Pocock, 1977).

SAMPLE SIZE AND STATISTICAL POWER

Although sample size must be addressed early in the planning stage of any analytic epidemiologic investigation, it has particular importance in intervention studies. Observational analytic study designs can most reliably study large effects, so that the sample may be moderate in size and still yield a reliable result. In contrast, a trial must have a sufficient sample size to have adequate statistical power or ability to detect reliably the small to moderate but clinically important differences between treatment groups that are most likely to occur. Trials of inadequate sample size are particularly prone to being misinterpreted as demonstrating that an intervention has no effect when in fact the trial was not capable of providing an informative null result.

Consequently, even if an investigator feels confident that an intervention will have a large benefit (i.e., a 50% or greater reduction in the primary outcome), it is far preferable to design the trial to test the more likely small to moderate benefits (i.e., 10–20% reduction) than to anticipate a larger effect and have no ability to detect the more plausible but smaller differences.

In designing clinical trials, investigators often devote considerable time and effort to increasing the total number of participants enrolled. However, while recruitment of a sufficient number of subjects is certainly important, the absolute number of individuals enrolled is less critical a factor to the statistical power of the trial than the number of end points they will contribute. In addition, the ability of a trial to detect a postulated difference between treatment groups, if one truly exists, is also dependent on the difference in compliance between the treatment groups.

Accumulating Adequate Numbers of Endpoints

To accumulate sufficient numbers of endpoints, two major strategies can be considered: selecting a high-risk population for study and ensuring an adequate duration of follow-up.

Selection of a High-Risk Study Population. A primary strategy to ensure the accumulation of an adequate number of endpoints is to select individuals at increased risk of developing the outcomes of interest. With respect to the general population, a simple but important criterion for this selection is age. Since the frequency of most chronic diseases rises substantially with increasing age, the impact of this factor can be dramatic. For example, in a cancer prevention trial, 10,000 men aged 45 to 54 followed for 4 years would experience only about 82 cancer deaths, while a comparable group of men aged 55 to 74 followed for 4 years would yield about 627 fatal malignancies (National Center for Health Statistics, 1988). Other risk factors on which selection of a study population might be based include sex, occupation, geographic area, or one or more medical or lifestyle variables, such as cigarette smoking or alcohol consumption.

In addition, the collection of baseline data can be planned to permit the identification of particular subgroups who might experience different effects of an intervention. For example, in the Physicians' Health Study, participants provided prerandomization blood specimens. These will be analyzed for baseline levels of retinol, carotene, and retinol-binding protein, thereby increasing the sensitivity of the trial to identify which particular subgroup of doctors, if any, stands to benefit most from dietary supplementation with beta-carotene (Hennekens and Eberlein, 1985). A large trial such as the Physicians' Health Study, which randomized 22,071 participants, could easily demonstrate a 30% reduction in total cancer incidence related to beta-carotene if such an effect exists, but would not have sufficient power to detect a significant difference between treatment groups if the overall effect were only 10%. However, it is possible that a small but clinically important 10% overall reduction in cancer incidence would result from a much larger effect confined exclusively to that subgroup of doctors who had low carotene or retinol levels at entry. This important public health finding could easily be picked up, given the ability to stratify participants by baseline levels of these parameters, and future public health recommendations could be aimed at that particular subgroup. Conversely, if there is no true effect of beta-carotene supplementation on cancer incidence, this strategy would in fact produce a more convincing and informative null result. In such a circumstance, it could be stated that no significant overall effect was observed, and in addition, that no effect of supplementation was apparent regardless of initial blood levels.

Adequate Duration of Treatment and Follow-up. The planned length of follow-up for any trial should take into account the likelihood that the actual rate of accrual of endpoints will be less than projected. This situation is not unusual in clinical trials and may occur for reasons beyond the control of the investigators. First, as discussed earlier, those who volunteer to participate are a self-selected group who also tend to experience generally lower morbidity and mortality rates than those who do not take part, regardless of the hypothesis under study or the treatment allocated at random (Horowitz and Wilbeck, 1971; Wilhelmsen et al, 1976). They may also tend to adopt healthier practices irrespective of the specific intervention being studied (Kuller, 1985). Moreover, there may be secular changes in disease rates during the course of the trial, sometimes as great as that postulated as attributable to the intervention being studied.

In cancer prevention trials, a particularly important consideration in determining the duration of treatment and follow-up is the postulated mechanism by which the intervention exerts its effects as well as the latency period for the cancer outcome of interest. For example, the analogy from observational studies with cessation of smoking and risk of lung cancer (Doll and Peto, 1978) suggests that interventions such as micronutrient supplements are likely to require at least several years of treatment before any decrease in risk begins to become apparent and perhaps a decade or more before the effect becomes maximal. In the Finnish trial of beta-carotene and vitamin E, conducted among middle-aged male smokers, there was no apparent benefit of either agent on lung cancer, the primary trial endpoint. In fact, those assigned to beta-carotene experienced an 18% higher risk, a finding greatly at variance with the totality of available evidence suggesting a possible benefit. However, the 6-year duration of treatment and follow-up may simply have been inadequate to yield a clearly detectable reduction in lung cancer, which is a multistage process that often proceeds over a decade or more (Hennekens et al, 1994).

Every effort should be made during the planning phase to choose an adequate length of follow-up. Nonetheless, the emergence of new evidence on mechanisms, changes in rates of disease within the general population, and even, on occasion, the failure to achieve a sufficient sample size or accrue sufficient endpoints within the trial itself may raise the question of increasing the duration of the study beyond the planned period of follow-up. Any such decision should be made as early in the trial as possible to maintain scientific credibility and avoid any implication that the change in design was based on last-minute efforts to achieve statistical significance (Friedman et al, 1985).

The Effect of Compliance

The second major factor influencing the power of a trial to detect a true difference between treatment groups is compliance. The effect of noncompliance is to make the intervention and comparison subjects more alike, which decreases the ability of the trial to detect any true differences between the groups. In fact, the power of a trial is proportional to the square of the difference in compliance between the study groups.

One strategy to maximize compliance that has been used relatively infrequently to date but which could have wide applicability in intervention studies is the implementation of a run-in or "wash-out" period prior to actual randomization. In this approach, all participants receive either the active treatment or placebo for a number of weeks or months before the formal randomization to a treatment group. This permits potentially eligible participants who have difficulty adhering to the intervention program or those perceiving adverse effects to withdraw before randomization without affecting the validity of the study (Buring and Hennekens, 1985; Hennekens, 1984; Omenn et al, 1988). The chief reason for adopting this strategy is that the largest proportion of subjects who eventually become noncompliant tend to do so in the first months following initiation of the intervention. While the total sample size of randomized subjects will be lower if a run-in is implemented, any corresponding increase in power and efficiency (as well as decreased costs in following a smaller number of more cooperative people) make this a particularly attractive option for primary prevention trials, where it is not necessary for an intervention to begin during or immediately following an acute event.

The actual format of the run-in period for a particular trial will depend on the hypotheses being tested. In studies of behavioral interventions, an appropriate test of willingness and ability to comply with the study protocol might consist of attendance at multiple screening visits, completion of forms or records similar to those that would be used in the actual trial, or willingness to undergo any laboratory procedures that might be required. In trials testing pill-taking regimens, the postulated mechanisms of action as well as the frequency of side effects should be taken into account in determining the regimen to implement during a run-in. For example, in the Physicians' Health Study, since the postulated beneficial effects of aspirin are acute and side effects common, it was desirable to expose all willing and eligible subjects to active aspirin during the run-in. As regards beta-carotene, however, its possible beneficial effects are postulated to be cumulative and side effects minimal, so that it was optimal to use carotene placebo. Thus the 33,223 initially willing and eligible physicians were sent calendar packs containing active aspirin and beta-carotene placebo. After approximately 18 weeks, the participants were sent questionnaires, and individuals who reported side effects or a desire to discontinue participation, as well as those who developed an exclusion criterion or even those who wished to continue but whose compliance was judged to be inadequate, were excluded from the trial before randomization. This left a total of 22,071 physicians, proven good compliers, who were then randomized into the trial (Hennekens, 1984).

ISSUES IN THE ANALYSIS AND INTERPRETATION OF DATA

The fundamental comparison in an intervention study is between the rate of the outcome of interest in the treated group and the corresponding rate in the comparison group. As for any analytic epidemiologic study, the roles of chance, bias, and confounding must be evaluated as possible alternative explanations of the findings. However, the unique design features of intervention studies have special implications for their analysis and interpretation.

As regards chance, a sufficient sample size addresses this issue in a manner analogous to any observational analytic design. Moreover, randomization minimizes the potential for bias in the allocation of participants to treatment group, and bias in the observation of outcomes of interest can be minimized by using blind or double-blind procedures. With respect to confounding, randomization tends to distribute both known and unknown confounders evenly among the treatment groups. If the sample size is large, this comparability is virtually guaranteed. However, with a small sample size or even, in the rare instance, as a result of the play of chance in a large sample, randomization may not always result in groups that are alike with respect to every factor except the treatment under study. Consequently, one important early step in the analysis of any clinical trial is to compare the relevant characteristics of the randomized treatment and comparison groups to assure that balance was achieved. This comparison should always be presented as one of the first tables in the report of the study findings. If such imbalances do, by chance, occur, it is possible to adjust for them in the data analysis using a variety of statistical techniques (Hennekens and Buring, 1987.

One major question that often arises in clinical trials is the question of which subjects to include in the analysis. Some investigators remove from the analysis randomized subjects who either were determined to be ineligible after randomization or who did not comply with the study protocol. While it may be particularly appealing, intuitively, to eliminate those who become noncompliant, the exclusion of any randomized subjects from the analysis can lead to biased results. For a number of reasons, it is unwarranted and incorrect to perform a fundamental analysis that compares the outcome rates of only those individuals who actually received that treatment with only those who did not.

First, in most trials, perfect compliers represent only a fraction of the total study population. As with losses to follow-up, noncompliance may be related to factors that also affect the risk of the outcome under study, and failure to analyze data on all randomized participants could introduce bias. A second limitation in evaluating data on only those subjects who comply with the study regimen is that such an analysis does not address the actual research question being posed in an intervention study—whether the *offering* of a treatment program is of benefit. While one wishes to study the actual effect of the treatment, randomization is on the basis of the offering of the treatment, so data must be analyzed on this basis to preserve the power of randomization. It is only the entire groups allocated by randomization that are truly comparable. Once participants are randomized to a treatment group, their subsequent health experience must be assessed and analyzed along with all others in that group, regardless of whether they comply with their assigned regimen. This methodologic issue emphasizes the need to maintain high compliance with their assigned regimen among all study participants. It is also important to keep in mind that if a particular regimen is so difficult and uncomfortable that it is likely to be accepted and used by only a small proportion of the reference population, it may not be practical to recommend its use, no matter how effective the actual treatment may be.

Thus, in all circumstances, the optimal comparison for estimating the true potential benefit of the intervention program is to analyze by intention to treat—in other words, "once randomized, always analyzed." For this reason, it is imperative to maintain high levels of compliance, keep losses to follow-up to a minimum, and to collect complete information on all randomized subjects (Peto et al, 1976; May et al, 1981). Those who are no longer complying with the study regimen should continue to provide all follow-up information whenever possible, or at the very least, their vital status should be ascertained. Subsequent analyses can certainly be performed based on that subgroup of participants who actually received their assigned treatment. However, if this is done, while it is possible to perform analyses that achieve balance in the distribution of known confounders, it is impossible to regain the control of unknown confounders that had been achieved originally through randomization.

The need to perform randomized comparisons in the analyses of data from a trial is equally important when subgroups are identified on the basis of characteristics other than compliance. Investigators are often tempted to examine differences in treatment effects among those with various baseline characteristics, such as age, prognostic factors, or previous medical history. In general, the caveats needed to compare subgroups defined *a priori* by baseline characteristics are far less than those required when comparisons are made on the basis of variables chosen after randomization, such as compliance. As regards the former, a minor concern involves a loss of statistical power because only subgroups of the total number of randomized subjects are being compared. A greater concern, however, is to ensure adequate control of variables that may no longer be distributed at random among the subgroups. With respect to analyses of subgroups defined *a posteriori* on the basis of information accumulated after randomization, they can only raise data-derived hypotheses, not test particular research questions.

CONCLUSION

The ultimate goal of all the methodologies discussed in this chapter is to allow an intervention study to clearly refute or prove the hypotheses being tested. Large-scale randomized trials that can be conducted at low cost per subject enrolled are crucial to the advancement of knowledge concerning any postulated small to moderate effects in cancer prevention. However, in an area of research where there are a number of hypotheses that are both promising and unproven, it is essential that each trial be properly designed and conducted so as to obtain either a definitive positive result on which public policy can be based, or a null result that is truly informative.

REFERENCES

Alpha-Tocopherol, Beta Carotene Cancer Prevention Study Group. 1994. The effect of vitamin E and beta carotene on the incidence of lung cancer and other cancers in male smokers. N Engl J Med 330:1029–1035.

Armitage P. 1975. Sequential Medical Trials, 2nd ed. New York; John Wiley and Sons.

Aspirin after myocardial infarction. 1980. Lancet 1:1172.

Baron JA. 1985. Compliance issues/biological markers. *In* Sestili MA, Dell JG (eds): Chemoprevention Clinical Trials. Problems and Solutions, 1984. NIH Publ. No. 85-2715. Hyattsville, MD; U.S. Department of Health and Human Services.

Block G, Cox C, Madans J, Schreiber GB, Licitra L, Melia N. 1988. Vitamin supplement use, by demographic characteristics. Am J Epidemiol 127:297–309.

Blot WJ, Li J-Y, Taylor PR, Guo W, Dawsey S, Wang G-Q, Yang CS, Zheng S-F, Gail M, Li G-Y, Yu Y, Liu B-q, Tangrea J, Sun Y-h, Liu F, Fraumeni JF, Zhang Y-H, Li B. 1993. Nutrition intervention trials in Linxian, China: Supplementation with specific vitamin/mineral combinations, cancer incidence, and disease-specific mortality in the general population. J Natl Cancer Inst 85:1483–1492.

Buring JE, Hennekens, CH. 1985. Sample size and compliance in randomized trials. *In* Sestili MA, Dell JG (eds): Chemoprevention Clinical Trials. Problems and Solutions, 1984. NIH Publ. No. 85-2715. Hyattsville, MD; U.S. Department of Health and Human Services.

Buring JE, Hennekens CH, for the Women's Health Study Research Group. 1992a. The Women's Health Study: Summary of the study design. J Myocardial Ischemia 4:27–29.

Buring JE, Hennekens CH, for the Women's Health Study Research Group. 1992b. The Women's Health Study: Rationale and background. J Myocardial Ischemia 4:30–40.

Buring JE, Jonas MA, Hennekens CH. 1994. Large and simple randomized trials. Background paper #3 associated with the OTA report, "Identifying Health Technologies That Work: Searching for Evidence." Office of Technology Assessment, Congress of the United States, Washington DC.

Byar DP. 1985. Sample size considerations for prevention studies. *In* Sestili MA, Dell JG, (eds): Chemoprevention Clinical Trials. Problems and Solutions, 1984. NIH Publ. No. 85-2715. Hyattsville, MD; U.S. Department of Health and Human Services.

Byar DP, Piantadosi S. 1985. Factorial designs for randomized clinical trials. Cancer Treat Rep 69:1055–1063

Coronary Drug Project Research Group. 1981. Practical aspects of decision making in clinical trials: The Coronary Drug Project as a case study. Control Clin Trials 1:363–376.

DeMets DL, Hardy R, Friedman LM, Lan KKG. 1984. Statistical aspects of early termination in the Beta-Blocker Heart Attack Trial. Control Clin Trials 5:362–372.

Doll R, Peto R. 1978. Cigarette smoking and bronchial carcinoma: dose and time relationships among regular smokers and lifelong non-smokers. J Epidemiol Commun Health 32:303–313.

DOLL R, PETO R. 1981. The Causes of Cancer. Oxford; Oxford University Press.

FISHER B, BAUER M, MARGOLESE R, POISSON R, PILCH Y, REDMOND C, FISHER E, WOLMARK N, DEUTSCH M, MONTAGUE E, SAFFER E, WICKERHAM L, LERNER H, GLASS A, SHIBATA H, DECKERS P, KETCHAM A, OISHI R, RUSSELL I. 1985a. Five-year results of a randomized clinical trial comparing total mastectomy and segmental mastectomy with or without radiation in the treatment of breast cancer. N Engl J Med 312:665–673.

FISHER B, REDMOND C, FISHER ER, BAUER M, WOLMARK N, WICKERHAM L, DEUTSCH M, MONTAGUE E, MARGOLESE R, FOSTER R. 1985b. Ten-year results of a randomized clinical trial comparing radical mastectomy and total mastectomy with or without radiation. N Engl J Med 312:674–681.

FRIEDMAN LM, FURBERG CD, DEMETS DL. 1985. Fundamentals of Clinical Trials, 2nd ed. Littleton, MA, PSG.

GREENBERG ER, BARON JA, STUKEL TA, STEVENS MM, MANDEL JS, SPENCER SK, ELIAS PM, LOWE N, NIERENBERG DW, BAYRD G, et al. 1990. A clinical trial of beta carotene to prevent basal-cell and squamous-cell cancers of the skin. N Engl J Med 323:789–795.

GREENBERG ER, BARON JA, TOSTESON TD, FREEMAN DH, BECK GJ, BOND JH, COLACCHIO TA, COLLER JA, FRANKL HD, HAILE RW, MANDEL JS, NIERENBERG DW, ROTHSTEIN R, SNOVER DC, STEVENS MM, SUMMERS RW, VAN STOLK RU, for the Polyp Prevention Study Group. 1994. A clinical trial of antioxidant vitamins to prevent colorectal adenomas. N Engl J Med 331:141–147.

GREENWALD P. 1994. Experience from clinical trials in cancer prevention. Ann Med 26:73–80.

GREENWALD P, MALONE WF, CERNY ME, STERN HR. 1993. Cancer prevention research trials. Adv Cancer Res 71:1–23.

HENNEKENS CH. 1984. Issues in the design and conduct of clinical trials. J Natl Cancer Inst 73:1473–1476.

HENNEKENS CH, BURING JE. 1987. Epidemiology in Medicine. Boston, Little, Brown and Company.

HENNEKENS CH, BURING JE, PETO R. 1994. Antioxidant vitamins—benefits not yet proved. N Engl J Med 330:1080–1081.

HENNEKENS CH, EBERLEIN K. 1985. A randomized trial of aspirin and beta-carotene among U.S. physicians. Prev Med 14:165–168.

HORWITZ D, WILBECK E. 1971. Effect of tuberculosis infection on mortality risk. Am Rev Respir Dis 104:643–655.

KULLER LH. 1985. Pilot studies. *In* Sestili MA, Dell JG (eds): Chemoprevention Clinical Trials. Problems and Solutions, 1984. NIH Publ. No. 85-2715. Hyattsville, MD, U.S. Department of Health and Human Services.

MAY GS, DEMETS DL, FRIEDMAN LM, FURBERG C, PASSAMANI E. 1981. The randomized clinical trial: bias in analysis. Circulation 64:669–673.

NATIONAL CENTER FOR HEALTH STATISTICS. 1988. Health, United States, 1987. DHHS Publ. No. (PHS) 88-1231. Washington, DC, U.S. Govt. Printing Office.

OMENN GS, GOODMAN GE, KLEINMAN GD, ROSENSTOCK L, BARNHART S, GEIGL P, THOMAS DB, KALMAN D, LUND B, PRENTICE RL, HENDERSON MM. 1988. The role of intervention studies in ascertaining the contribution of dietary factors in lung cancer. Ann N Y Acad Sci 534:575–583.

PETO R. 1982. Statistics of cancer trials. *In* Halnan KE (ed): Treatment of Cancer. London, Chapman and Hall.

PETO R, COLLINS R, GRAY R. 1993. Large-scale randomized evidence: Large, simple trials and overviews of trials. Ann N Y Acad Sci 703:314–340.

PETO R, PIKE MC, ARMITAGE P, BRESLOW NE, COX DR, HOWARD SV, MANTEL N, MCPHERSON K, PETO J, SMITH PG. 1976. Design and analysis of randomized clinical trials requiring prolonged observation of each patient. I. Introduction and design. Br J Cancer 34:585–612.

PETO R, PIKE MC, ARMITAGE P, BRESLOW NE, COX DR, HOWARD SV, MANTEL N, MCPHERSON K, PETO J, SMITH PG. 1977. Design and analysis of randomized clinical trials requiring prolonged observation of each patient. II. Analyses and examples. Br J Cancer 35:1–38.

POCOCK SJ. 1977. Group sequential methods in the design and analysis of clinical trials. Biometrika 64:191–199.

REYNOLDS RD. 1985. Laboratory monitoring for nutritional status. *In* Sestili MA, Dell JG (eds): Chemoprevention Clinical Trials. Problems and Solutions, 1984. NIH Publ. No. 85–2715. Hyattsville, MD; U.S. Department of Health and Human Services.

ROTHENBERG R, NASCA P, MIKL J, BURNETT W, REYNOLDS B. 1987. Cancer. *In* Amler RW, Cull HB (eds): Closing the Gap: The Burden of Unnecessary Illness. New York, Oxford University Press.

SESTILI MA, DELL JG, EDS. 1985. Chemoprevention Clinical Trials. Problems and Solutions, 1984. NIH Publ. No. 85–2715. Hyattsville, MD; U.S. Department of Health and Human Services.

STAMPFER M, BURING JE, WILLETT W, ROSNER B, EBERLEIN K, HENNEKENS CH. 1985. The 2×2 factorial design: its application to a randomized trial of aspirin and beta-carotene in US physicians. Stat Med 4:111–116.

STAMPFER MJ, WILLETT WC, SPEIZER FE, DYSERT DC, LIPNICK R, ROSNER B, HENNEKENS CH. 1984. Test of the National Death Index. Am J Epidemiol 119:837–839.

STEERING COMMITTEE OF THE PHYSICIANS' HEALTH STUDY RESEARCH GROUP. 1989. Final report from the aspirin component of the ongoing Physician's Health Study. N Engl J Med 321:129–135.

STICH HF, ROSIN MP, VALLEJERA MO. 1984a. Reduction with vitamin A and beta-carotene administration of the proportion of micronucleated buccal mucosal cells in Asian betel nut and tobacco chewers. Lancet 2:1204–1206.

STICH HF, STICH W, ROSIN M, VALLEJERA M. 1984b. Use of the micronucleus test to monitor the effect of vitamin A, beta-carotene and canthaxanthin on the buccal mucosa of betal nut/tobacco chewers. Int J Cancer 34:745–750.

U.S. DEPARTMENT OF AGRICULTURE. 1985. Nationwide Food Consumption Survey: Continuing Survey of Food Intakes by Individuals. Women 19–50 Years and Their Children 1–5 Years. Nutrition Monitoring Division Report No. 85–1. Hyattsville, MD; Human Nutrition Information Service.

U.S. DEPARTMENT OF HEALTH AND HUMAN SERVICES. 1982. The Health Consequences of Smoking. Cancer. A Report of the Surgeon General. Rockville, MD; Office on Smoking and Health.

WILHELMSEN L, LJUNGBERG S, WEDEL H, WERKO L. 1976. A comparison between participants and non-participants in a primary preventive trial. J Chron Dis 29:331–339.

YUSUF S, COLLINS R, PETO R. 1984. Why do we need some large, simple randomized trials? Stat Med 3:409–420.

66 Fundamental issues in screening for cancer

ANTHONY B. MILLER

Ideally, the control of cancer should be achievable—either by preventing the disease from occurring or, if it does occur, by curing those who develop it by appropriate treatment. Complete success from one of these approaches would make the other obsolete. However, at present it seems unlikely that either will be completely successful; they will continue to complement each other, while for a number of cancer sites, another approach to cancer control may prove to be appropriate and complementary to one or both of the other approaches. Such an approach is screening.

Screening was defined by the United States Commission on Chronic Illness (1957) as: "the presumptive identification of unrecognized disease or defect by the application of tests, examinations or other procedures that can be applied rapidly."

A screening test is not intended to be diagnostic. Rather, a positive finding will have to be confirmed by special diagnostic procedures.

Because of the deep-rooted belief among physicians that "early diagnosis" of disease is beneficial, many regard screening as bound to be effective. However, for a number of reasons this is not necessarily so, as shown by the failure of screening for lung cancer using sputum cytology or chest x-rays to reduce mortality from the disease (Prorok et al, 1984). It is the purpose of this chapter to attempt to define some of the fundamental issues that are relevant to the consideration of screening for cancer control, to discuss some of the solutions to these issues, to describe approaches to evaluating the efficacy of screening before it can be accepted as an established cancer control measure for any cancer site, and to briefly consider the extent to which programs proposed or under way for some major cancer sites comply with these criteria.

I am indebted to my colleagues on the Core Committee of the Project on Evaluation of Screening for Cancer (Jocelyn Chamberlain, Nick Day, Matti Hakama, and Phil Prorok) over the period 1980–1993 for many useful discussions that have helped to sharpen my understanding of screening for cancer.

THE ETHICS OF SCREENING

In general medical practice the special nature of the relationship between patient and physician has dictated the need to build up a core of ethical principles that govern this relationship. Further, it is generally accepted that additional issues arise when a patient becomes the subject of a research investigation that is superimposed upon his or her search for and receipt of appropriate medical care. It was not initially appreciated, however, that screening opened up a completely new spectrum of issues, possibly requiring more restrictive boundaries of ethical behavior than those applied in usual medical care. For example, when a patient goes to see a physician for relief of a symptom or treatment of an established condition, the physician is required to exercise his or her skills only to the extent that knowledge is currently available, while doing what is possible with available expertise and appropriate assistance to help the patient. Treatment may be offered without any implied guarantee that it is necessarily efficacious or will do more than just temporarily relieve the symptoms of which the patient complains. Thus the physician promises to do his or her best for the patient; there is no implied promise that the patient will be cured.

In screening, however, those who are approached to participate are not patients and most of them do not become patients. The screener believes that as a result of screening the health of the community will be better. He or she does not necessarily intend to imply that the condition of every individual will be better. However, screening is often promoted as if it implies a benefit to everyone who is screened. In fact, in some circumstances individuals included in a screening program may be placed at a disadvantage, as will subsequently be discussed. At the very least, therefore, those planning to introduce a screening program should be in a position to guarantee overall benefit to the community and a minimum of risk that certain individuals may be disadvantaged by the program. It was the inability to guarantee overall benefit and lack of disadvantage for those screened that led to the proscription of mammography in women under the age of 50 in the Breast Cancer Detection Demonstration Projects (Beahrs et al, 1979).

A second ethical issue, which is directed more to the obligations for appropriate care in the community than toward individuals, concerns how limited resources are equitably distributed across the whole community to obtain maximum benefit. Under certain circumstances the offer of screening could diminish the total level of health in a community. This may be a particular problem for developing countries by diverting resources intended for routine health care into screening. Thus, resources diverted to a cancer screening project, which might be regarded as prestigious, especially if involving high technology, could lower the resources available for other more pressing but also more mundane health problems. Although several screening programs have been proposed for developing countries, there is a particular need for caution and care in order to ensure that they do not overbalance the health care system in the area in which they are introduced. Even in technically advanced countries the same issue could arise. Indeed, one of the considerations that has been reflected in the controversy as to whether routine breast cancer screening for women under the age of 50 should be adopted is the high cost of the procedures involved if screening is extended over the total community (Eddy et al, 1988).

Screening programs, therefore, carry an ethical responsibility as least as great as that for medical practice in that approaches to participate are made to ostensibly healthy people. Indeed, the burden of proof for efficacy of the procedures and the necessity to avoid harm are greater than may be required for diagnostic or therapeutic procedures carried out when a patient presents with symptoms to a physician. In screening, the physician or public health worker initiates the process and he or she bears the onus of responsibility to be certain that benefit will follow.

GENERAL PRINCIPLES GOVERNING THE INTRODUCTION OF SCREENING

The principles that should govern the introduction of screening programs have been reviewed during international workshops on screening in cancer held under the auspices of the International Union Against Cancer (UICC) (Miller, 1978; Miller et al, 1990; Prorok et al, 1984). These will now be considered.

The Disease Should Be an Important Health Problem

This principle was reformulated in the earlier UICC workshop as "The disease should be common and should be the cause of substantial mortality and/or morbidity." In practical terms this means that the disease prevalence should be high and the consequences of the disease dire. However, it is important to recognize that the life expectancy of a screened population may be changed little even if the program is successful. In most technically advanced countries, even if all cancer were to be eradicated, the effect of other competing causes of death is such that life expectancy would be increased only by about 2 1/2 years. Thus expectations that screening for a single cancer site would significantly lower mortality from all causes of death considered together are unrealistic. Nevertheless, screening for cancers of the breast and cervix may prove to be worthwhile in these countries because of the predilection of these diseases for younger women and the greater economic importance of reducing deaths at younger ages. Cancer of the colon and rectum tends to affect an older population more at risk of death from other causes so that premature mortality is less than for breast cancer. This is even more marked for cancer of the prostate. Thus the prima facie basis for introducing screening for these two latter cancers is less.

There may be certain circumstances when the major benefit from screening may follow not from the reduction of mortality, but from reduction of morbidity consequent upon the diagnosis of a cancer in a more treatable phase in its natural history. This could mean that the extent of treatment required and the possibility that treatment may be debilitating or mutilating would be much less. Such advantages may be difficult to quantify in other than economic terms; however, as they may be considerable in psychological terms to individuals, and to communities in the lowering in the requirements for extensive rehabilitation services, they should not be overlooked.

The Disease Should Have a Detectable Preclinical Phase (DPCP)

It is important to recognize that this principle is *not* "The disease should have a precancerous phase." In practice, for many cancers, including breast cancer, the DPCP is largely asymptomatic invasive cancer, as there is some reason to doubt that all, or even a majority, of the in situ breast cancers found on mammography screening would progress in the absence of screening. For cervix cancer, on the other hand, the DPCP probably includes the whole range from dysplasia through to occult invasive cancer. The important aspect of the DPCP is that it is detectable by the screening test(s) used. However, it seems clear from the different levels of effectiveness estimated for breast and cervix cancer, that a cancer in which the main component of the DPCP is invasive, even though asymptomatic, will have a lower order of effectiveness for screening than a cancer in which the main component of the DPCP is indeed a precancerous precursor.

The Natural History of the Condition Should Be Known

Ideally such a requirement implies that it is known at what stage in the disease process progression, metastases, and death can no longer be prevented. If such information was available and the stage that the development of the disease had reached in individuals was determinable, it would be possible to decide precisely when a screening test should be applied in order to achieve maximum benefit and minimal overutilization of resources. Unfortunately it seems unlikely that knowledge will be accumulated to be able to determine the natural history of disease in individuals in such a precise fashion. It is recognized that the progression of clinically detected disease from the point of diagnosis to cure, if possible, or to death varies substantially in different individuals. It seems almost certain that the distribution of rates of growth of preclinically detectable disease that might be identified by screening is equally wide. Thus, although an objective for research on screening has to be to determine the extent of the distribution of the sojourn times of the DPCP (the period when the preclinical phase of the disease is detectable), in considering the introduction of screening programs and the scheduling of tests within programs it is necessary to balance benefits with costs.

It should also not necessarily be assumed that disease processes are inevitably progressive. For cancer of the cervix, for example, it has been determined that in situ carcinoma may undergo regression in a large proportion of cases (Boyes et al, 1982; Miller, Knight, and Narod, 1991). In breast cancer it also seems likely that many early or minimal in situ cancers may not progress either. Such conclusions have substantial implications with regard to the optimum frequency of screening examinations. Designing a program directed to those lesions that, in the absence of screening, will progress and more rapidly escape curability will be the appropriate approach if such lesions can be identified. Designing a program that maximizes the detection of cases that have a good prognosis, but that in the absence of screening may be unlikely to progress to death, will waste resources. Such a situation seems possible for mammography screening for breast cancer (Miller, 1994).

The Disease Should Be Treatable, and There Should Be a Recognized Treatment for Lesions Identified following Screening

In the early UICC workshop there were two recommendations relevant to treatment:

> There should be evidence of the effectiveness of treatment of lesions discovered as a result of screening in reducing mortality and the level of improvement expected should be stated,

and secondly,

> There should be reasonable expectation that recommendations for the appropriate management of the lesions discovered from a screening program will be complied with both by the individual with the lesion and by the physician responsible for his (or her) health care.

Underlying these recommendations was the concern that programs should only be set up when there were adequate facilities for treating lesions discovered as a result of screening and functioning referral systems for securing such treatment. This unfortunately has not been true for all programs introduced for screening for cancer, particularly in some developing countries. There is obviously no point in establishing a screening program and identifying lesions that should be treated if the facilities are not available, or the infrastructure for referral, confirmation of diagnosis, and treatment is not in place. In general this is not a problem for technically advanced countries, although unfortunately problems allied to these have occurred. Thus on occasions it has not been certain whether or not lesions identified as a result of screening should be regarded as truly malignant. Indeed, it has to be recognized that when lesions are first identified in a screening program, information may not be available as to their appropriate treatment, and special studies may be required. Otherwise, errors in terms of observation rather than treatment on the one hand or too extensive treatment on the other are possible. In prostate cancer screening, for example, if too radical treatment is applied in the elderly to the latent or good-prognosis prostate cancers that may be identified in a screening program, the morbidity in terms of incontinence and impotence, and even the mortality from treatment, could offset any benefit from the earlier detection of lesions with truly malignant potential (Chodak and Schoenberg, 1989; Miller, 1991c).

A different sort of difficulty could arise when, as a result of screening, lesions are diagnosed earlier in their natural history, but in spite of this, death is still inevitable. If this is so—if all available screening methods will not succeed in diagnosing more lesions before they have metastasized widely and are outside the range of current therapy—then screening to detect such lesions is not worthwhile. The studies of screening for lung cancer suggest this is a condition not amenable to screening, probably for this reason (Prorok et al, 1984).

The Screening Test to Be Used Should Be Acceptable and Safe

In general this implies a noninvasive test with high validity. Other criteria of a good screening test include ease of use and relatively low cost. These principles and various approaches to assessing validity will now be discussed.

THE VALIDITY OF A SCREENING TEST

Two measures suffice to describe the validity of screening tests: sensitivity and specificity. Sensitivity is defined as the ability of a test to detect all those with the disease in the screened population. This is expressed as the proportion of those with the disease in whom a screening test gives a positive result. Specificity is defined as the ability of a test to correctly identify those free of the disease in the screened population. This is expressed as the proportion of people free of the disease in whom the screening test gives a negative result. These two terms may be further expressed in terms of test results as follows: sensitivity is calculated as the true positives divided by the sum of the true positives and false negatives and expressed as a percentage; specificity is calculated as the true negatives divided by the sum of the true negatives and the false positives and expressed as a percentage.

In practice, difficulties with these measures arise over defining a positive result from the test as well as distinguishing the true positives from the false positives among those who test positive, and the true negatives from the false negatives among those who test negative. A relatively imperfect test of a quantitative, continuously distributed measurement can be artificially given a very high sensitivity by setting the boundary between negative and positive to incorporate a high proportion of those who are eventually found to have the disease in the positive category, but at a substantial cost in terms of low specificity. Conversely the same test can be made to appear highly specific, but it will then become insensitive if the boundary between positive and negative is shifted in the opposite direction.

If the test result is expressed in a quantitative form so that the boundaries between what is defined as positive and negative can be varied at will, it is possible to plot a receiver operating characteristic (ROC) curve (Swets et al, 1979). What is plotted is the sensitivity in the vertical axis and 1-specificity in the horizontal axis. The point on the curve that is chosen as optimal is that furthest from the 45° diagonal. ROC curves are most easily derived for blood tests, but have also been applied to mammography, by varying the extent to which different mammographic abnormalities were regarded as an indication of suspicion of malignancy (Goin and Haberman, 1982). Such curves cannot be applied to a test with a dichotomous outcome. Further they imply a similar weight to sensitivity and specificity, which as discussed below may not be ideal.

The position of the boundaries that are set between what is regarded as disease and non-(or benign) disease can also considerably influence the numerical values placed on sensitivity and specificity. This arises because of uncertainty as to what truly constitutes an abnormality in the context of a screening program. In order to come to such a decision it is essential that the conditions identified as a result of screening should have a known natural history. However, as has already been pointed out, such knowledge may not be available at the initiation of a screening program and may only be obtained as a result of careful study of findings from screening programs.

Nevertheless, the definition as to what constitutes disease is crucial in order to determine sensitivity and specificity. Most people have a clear idea as to what they regard as disease in terms of that which surfaces in standard medical practice. Cancers in general present with recognizable characteristics in symptomatic individuals. By definition, screening is conducted on asymptomatic individuals, so that many cancers that are identified through screening are likely to be at an early stage and may not have the generally recognized clinical characteristics of relatively advanced disease. This difficulty should theoretically be overcome by having clearly defined histological definitions of cancer. However, histology only imperfectly characterizes behavior, and this is even more true for the DPCP. One hope for the future is that some of the markers for prognosis currently being evaluated, such as markers of oncogene expression or other markers of DNA change, may serve to identify those precancerous or in situ components of the DPCP that are likely to progress.

A common error in evaluating potential screening tests is to determine the sensitivity by utilizing the experience of the test in relation to people who have clinical disease. A test that may appear to be highly sensitive under these circumstances may later be found to be much less sensitive when its ability to detect the DPCP is evaluated. In the screening context, therefore, sensitivity and specificity may vary according to whether they are estimated for early invasive carcinomas, in situ cancers, or precancerous lesions, and both should be determined in active screening programs. To do so for specificity is very much easier than for sensitivity. This is because the diagnostic process put in train by a positive screening test generally fairly rapidly identifies those who have the disease and thus distinguishes the true from the false positives. As under most circumstances the proportion of those who have the disease in relation to the total population screened is low, a very good approximation to specificity is obtained by calculating the proportion of all those who tested negative of the sum of the test negatives and false positives. Including the unidentified false negatives in the numerator and denominator of this expression will in practice introduce little error.

Sensitivity is, however, a difficult measure to determine initially in a screening program. The reason for this is that the false negatives are not immediately apparent, as there is no justification to retest all the test negatives just to identify a few false negatives. Only by following the total population who screened negative is it eventually possible to identify those who had the disease at the time the test was administered but were not so identified through definitive diagnostic tests. This is facilitated if test materials are retained; for example, cervical smears or mammograms originally classed negative can be reassessed for those who are found to have disease at the next scheduled screen, or who develop disease during the interval between screens. Such reassessments should preferably be made blind to avoid bias. We have used just such an approach in the assessment of the sensitivity of the "reader error" for cervical cancer screening (Boyes et al, 1981) and in the assessment of the sensitivity of mammography in a trial of breast cancer screening (Baines et al, 1986, 1988).

When test materials cannot be retained, however, such as in the assessment of the sensitivity of physical examination as a screening test for breast cancer, and for what we have called the "taker error and the biological component" of false negatives in cervical cytology—that is, disease that was indeed present but was not incorporated in the smear or for some reason did not exfoliate—a direct identification of false negatives will not be possible. A usual approach is to assume that interval cancers occurring within a certain period are false negatives, an approach we were forced to use in estimating the sensitivity of physical examination in our breast screening trial (Baines et al, 1989). However a possibly more satisfactory approach is to assess the expected detection rate of disease on screening after repeated screens, assuming that most of the false negatives had by then been identified, and to regard the excess disease above this level at the second screen as a measure of the false negatives at the first screen. As a result of such an approach it was determined that the taker and biological component of false negatives was approximately equal to the directly measured reader error, so that the level of sensitivity for cervical cytology approximated 78% (Miller, 1981).

Two recommendations were made in the early UICC workshop with regard to the validity of screening tests. First,

> The sensitivity and specificity of the screening tests to be used should have been evaluated and their expected values stated,

and second,

> There should be an acceptable program of quality control to ensure that the stated levels of sensitivity and specificity are attained and maintained.

The second of these recommendations raises the issue of the problems that can arise in a screening program if adequate quality is not maintained. Quality control involves issues that concern not only the validity of the screening test but also its safety. There is, for example, the need to ensure that radiation exposure does not drift upwards in a mammography screening program. Quality control embraces issues that involve the training of those who will actually administer and read screening tests, their supervision, and the introduction of procedures to check actively on the extent to which those testing positive or negative are misclassified. In general, their consideration falls outside the scope of this chapter.

It is to be emphasized, however, that quality may also suffer because of overwork and boredom. One of the reasons why it was felt desirable to recommend changing the frequency of examination for most women in cervical cytology screening programs in Canada was to avoid repetitive rescreening of normal women, with the flooding of laboratories with unnecessary and unrewarding work (Task Force, 1976). Indeed, the Task Force that made these recommendations was at some pains to describe the mechanisms for ensuring appropriate quality control in cytology laboratories. It is relevant that these requirements had to be reemphasized more than a decade later (Miller et al, 1991). That such issues are not simple was underlined by considerations in our group of observer variation in mammography reading (Boyd et al, 1982). Relevant to breast cancer screening programs is not only the accuracy with which abnormalities are identified, but if identified, the extent to which appropriate recommendations are made on their management. Our experience suggested that including a category of "probably benign" in a screening mammography report increases the extent of observer variation. Readers differ substantially in the extent they use this category, the extent to which they recommend special observation of individuals placed in this category, and the extent to which they recommend biopsy. Dual reading helps to increase specificity, without much, if any, loss of sensitivity. This permits the simplification of recommendations into two groups, "suspicious of malignancy" and "satisfactory (normal)" examination, and results in far greater consistency. Further, it is compatible with the appropriate separation of findings from screening tests into the probably abnormal (test positive) and probably normal (test negative) dichotomy. The probably abnormal group is subjected to diagnostic tests in the normal way. That this approach to use of screening mammography was accepted with difficulty in North America, including our own National Breast Screening Study (NBSS), was due to an initial tendency for most radiologists to regard mammography as a diagnostic rather than a screening test, largely because the great majority of those who moved into screening had had prior experience with diagnostic mammography. They accepted with considerable reluctance the processes necessary in a screening situation. One result was a greater use of biopsy as a diagnostic test in North America than that reported from Europe (McLelland and Pisano, 1992), where more use was made of diagnostic mammography subsequent to screening mammography (often called by European radiologists "complete" mammography) with a consequent reduction in biopsies and a much lower benign to malignant ratio.

Most commentators in the past, when considering the relative weight to be placed on sensitivity and specificity for screening programs for cancer, have tended to encourage high sensitivity at the cost of relatively low specificity, as it was felt important to attempt to avoid missing individuals who truly had malignant disease. One vigorous exponent of this view for breast cancer screening was Moskowitz, who coined the term "aggressive screening," as only by such an approach did he feel that the "minimal" breast cancers with an excellent prognosis would be identified (Moskowitz et al, 1976). However, there continues to be little evidence that such cancers are really responsible for the mortality reduction following breast cancer screening. Rather, there is much evidence that the early diagnosis of more advanced disease results in the benefit (Miller, 1987, 1994). A disadvantage of Moskowitz's policy was a high benign to malignant ratio, and low specificity of the screen. This, as pointed out earlier in the UICC workshop (Miller, 1978) is probably unwise. Although the objective of screening for cancer is to identify disease in the DPCP before it gets to the stage of escaping from curability, if a test is made so sensitive that it picks up lesions that would never have progressed in that individual's lifetime, there will be substantial additional costs for diagnosis and treatment (this is one consequence of the "overdiagnosis" bias, which is more fully discussed in relation to survival of cases following screen detection in a later section of this chapter). There is no point in identifying through screening a cancer that would never have presented clinically, and little point (other than less radical therapy) in identifying early a cancer that would have been cured anyway if it had presented clinically. Similarly the cancers that result in death, even after screen identification and subsequent treatment, only result in greater observation time and no benefit to the screenee. It is only the cancers that result in death in the absence of screening, but that are cured following treatment after screen detection, from which the real benefit of a screening program derives. Hence, if high "sensitivity" is largely based on finding more good-prognosis cancers, but results in lowering specificity, the program will incur much greater costs without corresponding benefit.

The process measure, as distinct from a measure of validity, that most clearly expresses this difficulty is the predictive value of a positive screen. This is defined as the proportion of those who test positive who truly have the disease. This measure is influenced not only by the sensitivity and specificity of the test, especially the latter, but by the prevalence of disease in the population, whereas sensitivity and specificity are invariant with regard to disease prevalence. In Tables 66–1 and 66–2 examples are given illustrating the particular importance of disease prevalence and specificity in arriving at a high predictive value for a positive test. If tests are administered under circumstances that incur a low predictive value positive, then not only may costs be high in terms of correctly identifying those who are falsely positive, but also the potential hazard may be high, as an individual classified as positive falsely derives no benefit and potentially a substantial risk from the associated diagnostic procedures. A test with a low predictive value positive rapidly enters into disrepute.

To complete discussion of process measures, the predictive value negative should be defined. This is the proportion of those who test negative who are truly free of the disease. This measure, like sensitivity, is dependent on identifying the false negatives and therefore is rarely determined, being of little operational value. In practice, however, it is usually high.

TABLE 66–1. *Hypothetical Initial Screen**

	Disease		
Test	*Present*	*Absent*	*Total*
LOW PREVALENCE			
Positive	124	3,993	4,117
Negative	41	95,842	95,883
Total	165	99,835	100,000
	(Predictive value positive test = 3%)		
HIGH PREVALENCE			
Positive	1,240	3,934	5,174
Negative	410	94,416	94,826
Total	1,650	98,350	100,000
	(Predictive value positive test = 24%)		

*Parameters: sensitivity 75%; specificity 96%.

TABLE 66–2. *Effect on Predictive Value of Positive Test of Modifying Parameters*

		Predictive Value (%)	
Sensitivity (%)	*Specificity (%)*	*Low Prevalence*	*High Prevalence*
75	96	3	24
75	99	11	56
100	96	4	30
100	99	14	63

As Day (1985) has pointed out, because of the difficulty in identifying false negatives, and because of the overdiagnosis bias, the usual approach to defining sensitivity is not ideal, or in some circumstances particularly biologically meaningful. He suggested an alternative measure of sensitivity that can be derived if the expected incidence of disease in the absence of screening can be determined, ideally from the control group in a randomized trial, but sometimes in population-based programs from historical data or data from comparable unscreened populations. The method basically computes the extent a program is successful in reducing the expected incidence in the absence of screening occurring as interval cancers. The lower the proportion of expected incidence occurring as interval cancers (cancers not diagnosed as a result of screening and presenting clinically between screens) the greater the sensitivity.

THE ACCEPTABILITY OF THE TEST

One of the desirable attributes of a good screening test is that it should be acceptable to the population to which screening is offered and acceptable to those who will administer the test. In general, cervical cytology screening programs have found acceptance with women and their physicians, except for those who tend to be at highest risk for the disease. This results in lower effectiveness of programs than would be the case if all women were to be included. This lack of acceptance is largely related to lower socio-economic status, where presumably other health concerns take precedence over a long-term preventive maneuver such as screening.

Breast cancer screening has encountered different problems over acceptability, though this varies substantially in different countries, ranging from the 90% acceptance with screening invitations in Sweden (Tabar et al, 1985) to the difficulties with both physicians' and women's compliance in the United States (Howard, 1987). Even without an economic barrier, in Canada, recruitment into a screening trial ran into difficulties due to multiple concerns, including concerns over radiation (Baines et al, 1984).

Screening for colorectal cancer also has its own difficulties, particularly in the inevitable distaste of individuals for a procedure that involves manipulation of feces. In a number of pilot programs, therefore, the return rates for Hemoccult slides have been low, though they have been better in well-organized studies (Chamberlain and Miller, 1988).

A screening test, therefore, has to be acceptable to the population in its widest sense. The test should be simple and as far as possible easily administered. It should involve procedures that are not unacceptable, and its use should not have unpleasant or potentially hazardous implications. There are also economic advantages in a test being administered or read by allied health professionals, such as use of technologists in initial screening of cervical cytology slides (Anderson, 1985), or the use of nurses to perform breast examinations (Bassett, 1985; Miller et al, 1991).

POPULATION TO BE INCLUDED IN SCREENING PROGRAMS

For a screening program to be successful, the population to be included should be one in which it is known that the disease has a high prevalence. This will not only encourage a high predictive value for a positive test, it will tend to promote higher quality of performance and assessment of results of screening tests, and will result in lower costs per case detected. Thus in all screening programs it is desirable to attempt to include only those who are at high risk for the disease. This approach was recognized by the Canadian Task Force on Cervical Cytology Screening Programs (1976), who carefully defined those whom it believed were at such low risk for the disease that they need not be included in cervical cytology screening programs, thus defining the remaining "at risk" population on whom major efforts should be concentrated to bring them into screening programs. Although at that time we defined a high-risk subgroup on which special concentration was justified, this approach was not continued by the reconvened Task Force (1982), nor by a subsequent National Workshop (Miller et al, 1991) when recommendations were developed directed to the total "at-risk" population; in part this was because we recognized that identifying high-risk women is not easy in practice, even though the risk groups for cervical cancer are well defined.

For other cancers, however, the known risk factors, apart from age, may not suffice to adequately distingish between those who should be considered for inclusion in screening programs compared to those who should not. For breast screening programs, for example, although some discrimination using risk factors has been achieved (Shapiro et al, 1971; Schechter et al, 1986) this has not been sufficient to justify selection on this basis alone. However, age is an important predictor of risk, and for breast cancer in technically advanced countries, all women in the appropriate age group can be regarded as at high risk. Thus for breast cancer currently, it seems unlikely that any program could justify routine screening of women under the age of 40, while screening women aged 40–49 may not be cost-effective (Eddy et al, 1988). For colon cancer screening, concentration on even older age groups would be necessary to have an acceptable detection rate (Miller, 1986b).

One possible approach to concentrating on the relevant segment of the population for screening might be to administer a prescreening test, especially if for a marker for a factor necessary in the causation of the disease. Such a test can be envisaged for human papilloma virus infection as a prescreen for cancer of the cervix though a difficulty here could be lack of systemic evidence of the disease so that a blood test, even if developed, could be falsely negative in too high a proportion of those with evidence of virus infection in the smear. This could be overcome if a highly sensitive test for evidence of infection could be applied to smears. Such approaches would have to be carefully evaluated, however. Thus it is possible that cancers occurring in people identified as being at risk by a prescreening test might behave in a different way from other cancers, and this could affect the success of the program. If, for example, the prescreening test tended to concentrate people with precursors of slowly growing cancers, then the major benefit from a screening program might be lost by allowing those with the tendency to develop more rapidly progressive disease to escape from screening.

Hakama (1986) has pointed out that in programs that attempt to select for screening on the basis of risk, there will usually be cases occurring in the unscreened group. Another consequence of such programs, however, will be reduced numbers of false positives (in absolute terms), which with the increased prevalence of the disease will result in a higher predictive value positive of the screen. Hakama (1984) coined the terms program sensitivity and program specificity, which help in understanding the effects of screening concentrating on high risk (Table 66–3). The more a program concentrates on "high-risk" groups, the lower the program sensitivity, as more and more cases will occur in unscreened people (the PFN, or program false negatives of Table 66–3). Conversely, however, the program specificity will increase because of the increase in healthy people unscreened (the PTN or program true negatives of Table 66–3) with a reduction in the costs of screening. However, because the reduction in program sensitivity will result in a reduction in the overall effectiveness of the program, for most cancers, because of the imprecision by which high-risk groups are identified, the overall result of such an approach will be unacceptable.

One other approach to using risk factors is to help determine the optimal periodicity of rescreening. Once again, however, much of the necessary research is incomplete, and we do not know how appropriate such an approach may be. It will probably be necessary to calculate the marginal cost-effectiveness of extending screening from high- to low-risk groups (ie, the additional cost for such an extension of screening related to the increase in effectiveness of the screening) in order to make the necessary policy decisions.

TABLE 66–3. *Sensitivity and Specificity of the Test and the Program*

Attendance for Screening	*Screening Test*	*True State*	
		Cancer	*Healthy*
Yes	Positive	STP	SFP
Yes	Negative	SFN	STN
No	—	PFN	PTN
Test sensitivity	= STP/STP + SFN		
Program sensitivity	= STP/STP + SFN + PFN		
Test specificity	= STN/STN + SFP		
Program specificity	= STN + PTN/STN + PTN + SFP		

Abbreviations: STP = Screen true positive; SFN = Screen false negative; SFP = Screen false positive; STN = Screen true negative; PFN = Program false negative; PTN = Program true negative.

A number of recommendations have been made on these issues (Miller, 1978):

1. The target population should be clearly defined and selected in such a way that given the likely sensitivity and specificity of the test, an acceptable predictive value will be obtained.
2. As far as possible, the target population should be limited to those at particular risk of the disease to give a reasonable prevalence of detection, where such individuals at risk can be identified.
3. There should be a reasonable expectation of reaching the target population and of achieving reasonable compliance in response to invitations for attendance. The expected level of compliance should be stated.

DIAGNOSIS AND TREATMENT OF THE DISCOVERED LESIONS

As a screening test is not diagnostic, inevitably the success of the program will ultimately depend upon the extent those identified as being abnormal on the test accept the procedures offered to them for further evaluation, and the effectiveness of the therapy offered.

A number of areas may create difficulties. For example, in the initial phases of many breast cancer screening programs, it was necessary to demonstrate to the general community of medical practitioners that the abnormalities identified were indeed of importance and that they required care and expertise to biopsy. Indeed in the absence of skills in diagnosis and management, there can be unnecessary biopsy (potentially reducible by the use of diagnostic mammography and fine needle aspiration biopsies) as well as failure to excise the lesion when biopsy is performed. This is part of the spectrum of problems that arise over the fact that lesions may be identified in screening programs whose biological features, natural history, and other characteristics may be in doubt. The screening participants may require special education programs so that they understand the diagnostic process to reduce as far as possible one of the major adverse consequences of screening, the anxiety accompanying the identification of an abnormality, as well as ensuring that they comply with the recommendations for management. There may even be major disagreements over the histological interpretation of the excised lesions, with uncertainties over the borderline between benign and malignant. Thus the public and the professionals at all levels in a screening program may require education and/or retraining dependent on their responsibilities. One mechanism to reduce difficulties in the professional area that should be encouraged is the provision of special diagnostic and treatment centers where the necessary expertise in diagnosis and management can be concentrated and where the necessary facilities are available (Miller and Tsechovski, 1987). Such centers could be regionally based, serving a number of screening centers.

In the early UICC Workshop the following recommendations were made on these issues (Miller, 1978):

> 4. There should be a reasonable expectation that recommendations for further diagnostic evaluation will be complied with in individuals who have a positive test.
>
> 5. There should be an agreed-upon policy on classification of borderline abnormalities and also on their management and policy on recommendations for their follow-up.
>
> 6. There should be a reasonable expectation that recommendations for appropriate management of lesions discovered from a screening program will be complied with both by the individual with the lesion and by the physician responsible for his (or her) health care.

EVALUATION OF SCREENING PROGRAMS

A number of issues have to be noted when evaluating screening programs. Almost invariably individuals with disease identified as a result of screening will have a longer survival time than those diagnosed in the normal way. Four biases associated with screening explain this. The first is "lead time," defined as the interval between the time of detection by screening and the time at which the disease would have been diagnosed in the absence of screening. In other words, it is the period by which screening advances the diagnosis of the disease. For example, if as a result of screening, the average point of diagnosis is advanced by one year, then inevitably cases diagnosed by screening will survive one year longer even if there is no long-term benefit. It is important to recognize that the lead time for different cases will vary, depending in part on the timing of the screening test in relation to the duration of the DPCP in that case, as well as the rapidity of progression of the DPCP in that individual. Thus there will be a distribution of lead times (Morrison, 1985). The lead time for fatal cases will be fairly short, but in at least one study some have been identified as having a lead time of one or more years following mammography screening (Miller et al, 1992b).

The determination of lead time is complex, but models have been developed that do so providing there are control data that permit comparison of screen detection with that expected (Walter and Day, 1983).

Differential lead time can be an important factor in comparing the outcome among cases detected by different screening modalities, making it almost impossible to make a comparison based on survival, unless it is possible to estimate and correct for differential lead time (Walter and Stitt, 1987).

The second bias that accounts for improved survival of screen-detected cases is "length-biased sampling." This relates to the fact that individuals who have rapidly progressive disease will tend to develop symptoms that cause them to consult physicians directly. Thus only less rapidly progressive cases are likely to remain to be detected by screening. Yet the former have a poorer and the latter a better prognosis, hence the improved survival of screen-detected cases, over and above lead time. This bias is most likely to operate at the initiation of a screening program, at the first or prevalent screen. It is related to the well-known prevalence-incidence bias in other situations. However, length bias will affect the type of cases detected at rescreening, with the more rapidly progressive cancers diagnosed in the intervals between screens. Hence in evaluating the total impact of programs, the interval cases must be identified and taken into consideration as well as the screen-detected cases.

The third bias that can artifactually improve survival is selection bias. Those who enter screening programs are volunteers, and almost invariably more health conscious than those who decline to enter. This means that they are likely, even in the absence of screening, to have a better outcome from their disease than the overall rates in the general population. This has clearly influenced the survival of those who entered our National Breast Screening Study, for example (Miller et al, 1992 a,b).

The fourth bias is overdiagnosis bias. Simply, it means that some lesions identified and counted as cancers would not have presented clinically in those individuals during their lifetimes in the absence of screening. It is, in practice, an extreme example of lead and length bias. It is difficult to obtain absolute confirmation of the existence of this bias, though it seems very likely that it is at least in part an explanation for the substantial excess of cancers found in some breast screening studies, such as appears to have happened in the mammography-containing arms of our National Breast Screening Study (Miller et al, 1992a,b).

The only design that effectively eliminates the effect of all these biases is the randomized controlled trial (Prorok et al, 1984), but only if mortality from the disease (ie, deaths related to the person-years of observation) is used as the end point, rather than survival. Survival could be used in a randomized controlled trial only under special circumstances. These are that there is good evidence because of the equivalence in cumulative numbers of cases during the relevant period of observation that there is no overdiagnosis bias; and that the start of the period of observation of the cases is taken as the date of randomization, as that will eliminate differential lead time. This is the approach that will be used in a study of breast self-examination in Russia, where it will not be possible to follow all entrants to determine their alive or dead status at the end of the trial (Russian Federation/World Health Organization Study, 1993). Length bias and selection bias are not issues, the latter having been equally distributed by the randomization, and the former by having started at the same point in time, and by including all cases that occur during follow-up in the evaluation.

Outside a randomized trial, if the screening test detects a precursor, reduction in incidence of the clinically detected disease can be expected and evaluated. This effect has been well demonstrated in the Nordic countries in relation to screening for cancer of the cervix (Hakama, 1982). If the screening test does not detect a precursor, or even if it does but the main yield is invasive cancer, then incidence can be expected to increase initially following the introduction of screening, and substantially and persistingly while screening continues if overdiagnosis bias is an important feature of case detection. Under such circumstances, when reduction in incidence cannot be anticipated, and improvement in survival cannot be relied on because of the biases already discussed, the only valid outcome for assessment of results of a screening program is mortality from the disease in the total population offered screening in comparison with the mortality that would be expected in the same population if screening had not been offered.

As already emphasized the design of choice for evaluation of changes in mortality is the randomized controlled trial. This can either be an efficacy trial, based on the randomization of the screening test, which answers the biologically relevant question as to whether mortality is reduced in those screened, or an effectiveness trial. An effectiveness trial is based on the randomization of invitations to attend for screening, and more nearly replicates the circumstances that may eventually pertain in practice in a population. Both those who accept the invitation as well as those who refuse will have to be included in the assessment of outcome. Thus it tests the impact of introducing screening in a population. Some trials of this type involve randomization by cluster.

If for some reason randomization is believed inappropriate, a second-best method is the quasi-experimental study in which screening is offered in some areas, and unscreened areas as comparable as possible are used for comparison purposes. However, this design is not a cheap and easy way out but demands the same methodological accuracy as required for randomized trials. Further, in view of the substantially larger populations that may have to be studied than in randomized trials, it may prove to be more expensive than the preferred design. In addition, difficulties in analysis may ensue if the baseline mortality in the comparison areas differ (UK Trial of Early Detection of Breast Cancer Group, 1988).

Nevertheless, ethical issues may preclude the utilization of randomized trials, particularly for programs that were introduced before the necessity of utilizing trials as far as possible for evaluation was appreciated. This has been the case for screening for cancer of the cervix and even for some breast cancer screening studies. One approach under these circumstances is to compare the mortality in defined populations before and after the introduction of screening programs, preferably with data available on the trends in acceptance of screening so that changes in mortality can be correlated with the mortality trends. Such a correlation study will be strengthened if other data that could be related to changes in the outcome variable are entered into a multivariate analysis (Miller et al, 1976).

A case-control study of screening is another approach that can be used to evaluate programs that were introduced sufficiently long before the study that an effect can be expected to have occurred. Case-control studies depend on comparing the screen histories of the cases with the histories of comparable controls drawn from the population from which the cases arose. Individuals with early-stage disease, if sampled, would be eligible as a control if the date of diagnosis was not earlier than that of the case, as diagnosis of disease truncates the screening history. However, a bias would arise if advanced disease is compared only with early-stage disease, as the latter is likely to be screen detected, though this is just a function of the screening process, not its efficacy (Weiss, 1983). Cases have to reflect the end points used to evaluate screening—that is, those that would be expected to be reduced by screening. Thus, cases are often deaths from the disease or advanced disease as a surrogate for deaths, or if a precursor of the disease is detected through screening, incident cases in the population. If incident cases are screen-detected, the controls should be drawn from those screened in the same program; if the cases are not screen-detected, the controls should be population based (Sasco et al, 1986).

One difficulty with case-control studies of screening is that they may be affected by selection bias, as the health conscious may select themselves for screening. This may be difficult to correct in the analysis, though such a correction should be attempted if the relevant data on risk factors for the disease (confounders) are available. Such a bias may not be a problem, however, if it can be demonstrated that the incidence of cancer in those who declined the invitation to the screening program is similar to that expected in an unscreened population.

It is now recognized, however, that even if data are available on risk factors for disease, control for them may not result in avoiding the effect of selection bias. For breast cancer, for example, experience in studies in Sweden and the United Kingdom, where case-control studies were performed within trials, show that although those who refuse invitations for screening show a breast cancer incidence similar to that of controls, their breast cancer mortality experience is worse than that of controls. This means that the estimate of the effect of screening in such case-control studies will show a greater effect than could be expected in the total population (Miller et al, 1990; Moss, 1991).

In addition to assessing effectiveness of screening, case-control studies may also be of use to assess other aspects of screening programs. For example, a method has been proposed for estimation of the natural history of preclinical disease from screening data based on case-control methodology (Brookmeyer et al, 1986).

The cohort study design may also provide an estimate of the effect of screening, an approach in which the mortality from the cancer of interest in an individually identified and followed screened group (the cohort) is compared to the mortality experience in a control population, often derived from the general population. This approach has been used to evaluate the mortality experience in the U.S. Breast Cancer Detection Demonstration Project (Morrison et al, 1988) and in a cohort of women in Finland included in a breast self-examination program (Gastrin et al, 1994). In these studies it has to be recognized that those recruited into a screening program are initially free of the disease of interest; therefore, it is not appropriate to apply population mortality rates for the disease to the person-years experience of the study cohort. Rather, as is required in estimating the sample size required for a controlled trial of screening, it is first necessary to determine the expected incidence of the cases of interest, then apply to that expectation the expected case-fatality rate from the disease to derive the expectation for the deaths (Moss et al, 1987). In practice, a cohort study of screening suffers from the same problem of selection bias as for case-control studies, so the results have to be interpreted with caution.

Indirect indicators of effectiveness are often desired in evaluating screening programs, especially ones that would predict subsequent mortality. Compliance with screening, and rate of screen detection, as well as the ratio of prevalence and incidence, can be indicators of potentially effective screens (Day, 1989). The cumulative prevalence (not the percentage distribution) of advanced disease is one such measure, though the extent to which it reflects subsequent mortality needs further evaluation (Prorok et al, 1984). However, it became clear in our National Breast Screening Study that failure of mammography screening to reduce the cumulative prevalence of advanced (Stage 2 or more) disease was an accurate indicator of failure to reduce breast cancer mortality (Miller et al, 1992 a,b). Nevertheless, case detection frequency, numbers of small tumors, and stage shift in percentages of the total should not be used as indicators of effectiveness, because they potentially reflect all four screening biases.

One important evaluation issue is the determination of risk versus benefit for those who participate. As discussed earlier, those who achieve benefit in the screening program are those in whom screening identifies disease at the point in its natural history when cure is possible with effective treatment, but who would not have been cured if the disease had been allowed to progress and present in the normal way. Those individuals with true positive tests who would have been cured following treatment if their disease had been allowed to present normally may have some reduced morbidity, but will have the disadvantage of a longer observation period for their disease. However those with disease identified by screening that would never have presented in their lifetime, and those who will inevitably die whether screen-detected or not, will be disadvantaged by the program. All false positives will also be disadvantaged, the extent of hazard depending on the risks of the test and the cost and inconvenience as well as the risks of the diagnostic investigations that are prescribed following the positive test. False negatives will also be disadvantaged if they fail to take early action after the development of symptoms of the disease because of the false reassurance they received from the screening. The true negatives will be rightly reassured, however, achieving the benefit for which most people attend screening, namely the assurance that they do not have the disease. No one has yet adequately computed these costs and benefits for screening programs, except possibly for breast cancer screening (Eddy et al, 1988).

ORGANIZED SCREENING PROGRAMS

There are a number of features of effective screening programs that are largely related to good organization. Indeed there is good evidence, at least for cancer of the cervix, that unorganized or opportunistic screening programs, which depend on the willingness of individuals to volunteer for screening, and the extent to which their physicians offer screening, often to low-risk women, are far less successful (Hakama et al, 1985).

Hakama and colleagues (1985) defined certain essential elements of organized programs. These are:

1. The target population has been identified.
2. The individual women are identifiable.
3. Measures are available to guarantee high coverage and attendance, such as a personal letter of invitation.
4. There are adequate field facilities for performing the screening tests.
5. There is an organized quality control program on performing and reading the tests.
6. Adequate facilities exist for diagnosis and for appropriate treatment of confirmed neoplastic lesions.
7. There is a carefully designed and agreed referral system, an agreed link between the participant, the screening center and the clinical facility for diagnosis of an abnormal screening test, for management of any abnormalities found and for providing information about normal screening tests.
8. Evaluation and monitoring of the total program is organized in terms of incidence and mortality rates among those attending, among those not attending, at the level of the total target population. Quality control of the epidemiological data should be established.

Although these elements are present in many European screening programs, especially in the Nordic countries, and contribute greatly to their success, several elements are missing from programs elsewhere, especially those largely based on the private medical care system in North America. In Canada, there are opportunities for introducing some of them, such as the first three, and these were recommended by the two Canadian Task Forces on cervical cancer screening (1976, 1982). Unfortunately, in Canada, none of the provincial health care authorities except Manitoba and British Columbia (the latter having accepted from the beginning the need for centralized laboratory services) have taken the initiative to establish such programs. However, following a National Workshop, there is hope that organized programs for cervical cancer screening may be introduced in Canada (Miller et al, 1991).

I have already referred to the differences between the European and North American approach to the organization of diagnosis and management of positives in breast screening programs, accounting for the substantial difference in the benign to malignant ratios reported for biopsy. It seems probable that unless programs are organized on the lines recommended by Hakama and coworkers (1985), they will be more costly and less effective than they could be. Again, an attempt is being made in Canada to replicate the organization of breast cancer screening that is proving successful in some of the Nordic countries and in the United Kingdom (Workshop Group, 1988).

ECONOMICS OF SCREENING

Space does not permit a detailed evaluation of the various principles that have to be considered in assessing the economics of screening. The interested reader is referred to reviews by Simpson (1984) and Neuhauser (1985). In brief, it is necessary to determine the costs of the test and the subsequent diagnostic tests. Also should be included are the costs associated with any hazard of the test as well as the costs of overtreatment. Balancing these costs may be reduced costs of therapy of the primary condition, reduced costs associated with less expenditure on the treatment of advanced disease, and the economic value of the additional years of life gained. The latter is often disputed, if not regarded with some distaste, so that often what is computed is the cost per year of life saved. Critical may be the marginal costs of additional tests in relation to the benefit, especially when considerations of the frequency of rescreening arise.

Part of the difficulty in complete economic assessments is that costs are often incurred early, while benefits flow later, so that for proper comparisons of such costs they have to be discounted to the present day. Additional complexity ensues if attempts are made to assess quality of life in economic terms, while the calculations rarely attempt an economic assessment of the fact that if a death is prevented by screening, the relevant individual will inevitably die of some other condition, and that death could be more costly.

It is likely that economic assessments will increasingly guide policy decisions in the future, so it behooves those interested in evaluation of screening to collect the necessary data. Although some economic assessments have suggested that cost-effective programs are achievable, for example programs of breast cancer screening using single-view mammography in Sweden (Jonsson et al, 1988), others have suggested that programs may not be cost-effective; for example, breast cancer screening programs for younger women in the United States (Eddy et al, 1988).

SCREENING FOR MAJOR CANCER SITES

In this section, I shall summarize my major conclusions on the appropriateness of screening for several major cancer sites. I shall draw heavily on the deliberations of the UICC project on screening (Prorok et al, 1984; Hakama et al, 1985; Chamberlain et al, 1986; Day et al, 1986; Miller et al, 1990) and will compare their recommendations for screening with those of the American Cancer Society (1980; 1983; Mettlin et al, 1993) and recommendations from the U.S. National Cancer Institute (Greenwald and Sondik, 1986; Early Detection Branch, 1987; Kaluzny et al, 1994) (see Table 66–4).

Screening for Lung Cancer

Both the UICC project (Prorok et al, 1984) and the American Cancer Society (1980) concluded that screening with sputum cytology and/or chest x-rays could not be recommended. The conclusive nature of the negative evidence from the three American controlled trials was such that the National Cancer Institute working guidelines (Early Detection Branch, 1987) does not discuss screening for this site. However, there has been concern that screening using annual chest radiography has never been properly evaluated, and therefore this will be reexamined in a large study evaluating screening for a number of cancer sites (Prorok et al, 1991).

Screening for Breast Cancer

The UICC project concluded that mass screening for breast cancer can reduce mortality from the disease (Day et al, 1986). Both single-view mammography alone and double-view mammography combined with physical examination are effective as screening modalities. Current data are insufficient to determine whether appreciable extra benefit in terms of mortality reduction derives from adding physical examination to mammography, or from double-view as distinct from single-view mammography. Furthermore, at that time it was not clear whether mammography adds appreciable extra benefit to screening by physical examination, a question raised by the working group to review the uncontrolled U.S. Breast Cancer Detection Demonstration Projects (Beahrs et al, 1979) and under investigation in the Canadian National Breast Screening Study (NBSS) in women aged 50–59 on entry to the study (Miller et al, 1981; 1992b). These questions are often regarded as answered by analyses of modalities of detection on screening, or by analyses of relative sensitivity of different screening tests. However, as emphasized earlier in this chapter, case-finding is not equivalent to mortality reduction.

An update led to little change (Miller et al, 1990). It was concluded that "Screening for breast cancer by mammography every 1 to 3 years can reduce breast can-

TABLE 66–4. *Summary of Screening Recommendations for Major Cancer Sites*

Site	*UICC*[a]	*A C S*[b]	*N C I*[c]	*N C I*[d]
Stomach	NR (except Japan)	NR	NR	NR
Colon, rectum	NR	FOBT every year. Sigmoidoscopy (pref. flexible) every 3–5 years from age 50. Annual rectal exam from age 40.	NR	FOBT every year. Sigmoidoscopy every 3–5 years from age 50. Annual rectal exam from age 40.
Lung	NR	NR	NR	NC
Breast	Ma +/− Px every 2 years age 50–69	Px every year from age 40. Ma every 1–2 yrs from age 40, every year from age 50. BSE every month.	Ma + Px every year from age 50	Px with each periodic exam. Ma every year from age 50[e]. BSE every month.
Cervix	Smear every 3 years from age 25–64	Annual smear from age 18. After 3 neg. smears, less frequently at discretion of physician.[f]	Smear every 3 years from age 20–70	Annual smear from age 18. After 3 neg. smears, less frequently at discretion of physician.
Prostate	NR	Annual rectal exam, plus PSA from age 50.[g]	NR	Annual rectal exam from age 40.

Abbreviations: NR = No recommendation; NC = Not considered; FOBT = Fecal occult blood test; Ma = mammography; Px = physical examination; PSA = prostate-specific antigen; BSE = breast self-examination.

[a]Prorok et al, 1984; Hakama et al, 1985; Chamberlain et al, 1986; Day et al, 1986; Miller et al, 1990.

[b]American Cancer Society, 1980, 1983.

[c]Greenwald and Sondik, 1986.

[d]Early Detection Branch, 1987.

[e]As modified, see Kaluzny et al, 1994.

[f]Fink, 1988.

[g]Mettlin et al, 1993.

cer mortality substantially in women age 50–69. In women under age 50 there is little evidence of a benefit, at least in the first 10 years after screening is initiated. The cost-effectiveness of screening every 2–3 years by mammography for women aged 50–70 compares well with many other medical procedures."

The American Cancer Society (ACS) guidelines for the cancer-related checkup have tended to be regarded as the basis for standards of care. They are updated periodically as new evidence becomes available. The ACS maintains that the guidelines are intended to help individual physicians and patients select the best early detection protocol for their needs. Nevertheless, they have in practice been interpreted as guidelines for screening.

The ACS guidelines for breast cancer detection are that every woman should be urged to practice breast self-examination every month from the age of 20, that women should have a breast physical examination every 3 years from the age of 20 and every year from the age of 40, and that mammography should be given every 1 to 2 years from 40 to 49 and every year from the age of 50 (Table 66–4). These guidelines are similar to those of the American College of Radiology (1982), and the working guidelines of the National Cancer Institute (Early Detection Branch, 1987). However, the U.S. Preventive Services Task Force (1989) did not recommend mammography screening for women aged 40–49, and the National Cancer Institute has now accepted that the scientific evidence does not confirm efficacy of screening in women age 40–49 (Kaluzny et al, 1994).

The initial reports of the first randomized trial of breast cancer screening, the Health Insurance Plan (HIP) trial, provided no evidence that breast cancer screening was effective in women aged 40–49 (Shapiro et al, 1971). The long-term follow-up of the HIP trial, however, appeared to suggest similar benefit in all age groups at 18 years after entry (Chu et al, 1988; Shapiro et al, 1988). Nevertheless, the main reason for an apparent reduction of mortality in women aged 40–49 appears to be a poorer survival of stage I cancers in the control group of the trial than both the screen-detected cancers and the non–screen-detected cancers in the study group (Miller, 1991a), suggesting the apparent benefit is an artifact, and not an effect of mammography.

The higher than expected survival of the screen-detected cancers in the Breast Cancer Detection Demonstration Project (BCDDP) (Seidman et al, 1987) led some commentators to assume a benefit from screening. However, it is not appropriate to rely on survival analyses to assume a benefit, because of the biases associated with survival following screening. Negative evidence came from an analysis of breast cancer mortality in the BCDDP comparing the observed numbers of deaths with those expected (Morrison et al, 1988), which showed little evidence of a benefit from screening in the 40–49 age group.

Subsequently, the evidence that has accrued on breast cancer screening in this age group has come from outside the United States. A Swedish overview analysis combined the data from the two-county, Malmö, Stockholm, and Gothenberg trials by age at entry (Nystrom et al, 1993). This suggested a beneficial effect of mammography screening: Beginning about 10 years after initiation of screening, the relative risk (RR) was 0.87 (95% confidence intervals [CI] 0.63–1.20), thus not statistically significant.

In the UK trial (UK Trial of Early Detection of Breast Cancer Group, 1993) women from the age of 45 were recruited. The relative risk at 10 years for women aged 45–49 on entry was 0.74 (95% CI 0.54–1.01), a finding of borderline significance. However, the UK "trial" was not randomized, but based on a geographic comparison.

One of the suggestions made to explain a lack of effect of the European studies is that they evaluated mammography every 2 years, often using single-view mammography, and that screening every year with two-view mammography is necessary for effectiveness in women aged 40–49 (Kopans, 1992). The evidence from the Canadian National Breast Screening Study (NBSS), however, does not support this view.

The NBSS is an individually randomized trial of over 50,000 volunteers aged 40–49. In the mammography plus physical examination group, double-view mammography was used, given every year, combined with good physical examinations and the teaching of breast self-examination. The controls received usual care in the community, after a single physical examination and the teaching of breast self-examination. The 7-year results show no evidence of any benefit from the mammography screening in terms of reduction in mortality from breast cancer (Miller et al, 1992a).

In women over the age of 50 nearly all trials have shown a benefit from screening by mammography alone or with physical examination (Fletcher et al, 1993). However, in the NBSS a different question was asked for women aged 50–59: What is the contribution of mammography over and above screening with physical examination? We concluded that screening of women aged 50–59 with yearly mammography in addition to physical examination detected considerably more node-negative and small breast cancers than screening with physical examination alone, but had no impact on mortality from breast cancer in the period of observation up to 7 years from entry (Miller et al, 1992b).

An independent team have reviewed the data from all available screening trials (Fletcher et al, 1993). Of the indicators of mammography quality, only for the percentage node negative is the NBSS slightly inferior to another trial. For all other trials and all other parameters the NBSS was either equivalent to the best (the sensitivity of mammography), or superior to all others (the ratio of prevalence of cancers detected at the first screen compared to expected incidence and the percentage of in situ cancers detected on screening). The team concluded that for women aged 40–49, randomized controlled trials of breast cancer screening show no benefit 5–7 years after entry. At 10–12 years, benefit is uncertain and, if present, marginal; thereafter, it is unknown. It was this conclusion that eventually led to the NCI change (Kaluzny et al, 1994).

Although the assumption has been made that sensitivity of mammography in the 1990s is superior to that of mammography in the 1980s, the detection rates by age on screening achieved in the current breast screening programs do not support this. It is therefore by no means certain that even earlier diagnosis than achieved in the reported trials will result in benefit; all that may be achieved may be the earlier detection of good-prognosis cancers, the poor-prognosis cances still being fatal even though lead time has been gained. However, modern mammography, with the ready application of coned-down (magnification) views of suspect abnormalities, has improved the specificity of screening, and thus reduction of unnecessary biopsies.

New large screening trials are likely to be futile. Benefit seems likely to require an improvement in therapy to improve the prognosis of women with poor-prognosis cancers, but in that case the improvement will also be available for the non–screen-detected cancers, and there could still be no additional benefit from screening (Miller, 1993).

Many groups (eg, Miller and Bulbrook, 1982; Day et al, 1986; Miller and Tsechovski, 1987), have emphasized the importance of high-quality mammography and the necessity for the skills to be available to localize and diagnose the impalpable lesions found on mammography. The UICC project (Day et al, 1986; Miller et al, 1990) considered that screening every 2 years in women over the age of 50 is satisfactory, but if screening is to be given in younger women, the interval may need to be shorter. These conclusions are reflected in the Swedish and Canadian programs (National Board of Health and Welfare, 1986; Workshop Group, 1989), though in the United Kingdom the program is restricted to women aged 50–69, and given (as single-view mammography) every 3 years (Working Group, 1987). These approaches to initiation of programs are quite different from those advocated by the American Cancer Society (1980, 1983) and recently defended (Mettlin and Smart, 1994), and appear to represent a different emphasis when programs are directed to general population groups.

The other screening test for which we currently have little evidence of effectiveness is breast self-examination (BSE). Several studies are ongoing that may eventually provide the evidence needed (Day et al, 1986). Clearly only BSE has the potential to improve the outlook for interval cancers, while its teaching has probably gone some way to diminish false reassurance in the NBSS. The World Health Organization has concluded that only BSE has the potential to provide early diagnosis of breast cancer in many parts of the world (Miller et al, 1985). Two case-control studies have shown no overall benefit in the reduction of advanced disease (Muscat and Huncharek, 1991; Newcomb et al, 1991), but one suggested benefit in BSE compliers (Newcomb et al, 1991). A cohort study of BSE compliers in Finland has, however, suggested a benefit in reducing breast cancer mortality (Gastrin et al, 1994).

Screening for Cancer of the Cervix

The UICC project concluded that screening for cancer of the cervix was effective in reducing the incidence and mortality from the disease, but that for maximal effectiveness attention needed to be paid to the organizational aspects of screening (Hakama et al, 1985; Miller et al, 1990). It is the organized programs that have shown the greatest effect, while using less resources than the unorganized programs. Essential elements of an organized program were summarized above.

An element of the organization of cervical cancer screening programs that has caused great controversy has been the optimal frequency of rescreening and the appropriate ages to initiate and stop screening. The UICC project had the benefit of the availability of the results of an IARC study based on the records of a number of screening programs in Europe and Canada (IARC Working Group on Cervical Cancer Screening, 1986). Starting at age 25 and stopping at age 64 with 3-year intervals gives 90% of the maximal protection and requires only 13 tests a lifetime. Even screening starting at age 20 with annual screens gives only just over 90% protection yet requires 45 tests per woman. Thus the marginal yield in a population from annual compared to triennial screening is minimal. This is of course the same conclusion reached by David Eddy through the application of his model (Eddy, 1980) which underlay the original American Cancer Society's recommendation for triennial repeat screening (American Cancer Society, 1980). It is therefore unfortunate that the Society changed its guidelines (Fink, 1988) as did the National Cancer Institute (Early Detection Branch, 1987), without any scientific evidence to support the change. The difficulty with this type of change, even in a wealthy country, is that it places emphasis on rescreening of women already in programs, while the emphasis needs to shift to bring women who are poorly screened, or not screened at all, into programs, if failures of screening policies are to be avoided (Task Force, 1976; Chamberlain, 1986). In Canada, a National Workshop reinforced the appropriateness of triennial screening, in the context of an organized program with high-quality laboratory services (Miller et al, 1991).

Another aspect of cervical cancer screening requires more attention. There are substantial costs associated with the management of the large numbers of cases of mild and moderate dysplasia found as a result of cervical cytology. It has been well demonstrated that there is massive overdiagnosis of carcinoma in situ of the cervix, and even more so for dysplasia, especially mild dysplasia (Miller, Knight, and Narod, 1991). Until there is a marker that enables us to identify the lesions that if untreated would progress, it is necessary to ensure appropriate management of all lesions detected, but this does not have to be immediate ablation. Time is on the physician's side, and cytologic surveillance is certainly appropriate for mild dysplasia (cervical intraepithelial neoplasia [CIN] I) until it is clearer whether the lesion will regress spontaneously (Miller et al, 1991).

Screening for Gastric Cancer

Screening programs for gastric cancer were introduced in Japan over 20 years ago (Chamberlain et al, 1986). The screening test used has gradually been standardized and now comprises a photoflourographic barium meal technique with six standard views. In Finland, screening using an immunological test on gastric juice has been conducted in one area (Hakama and Pukkala, 1988).

The UICC project concluded that considerable observational evidence had accumulated, including time trend analyses and one case-control study, that the widespread application of screening in Japan had contributed to a fall in mortality, though its contribution is probably small in relation to that resulting from falling incidence (Chamberlain et al, 1986; Miller et al, 1990). In view of the uncertainty over its effectiveness, screening for gastric cancer in countries other than Japan cannot at present be recommended as public health policy. In the United States, no organization advocates screening for gastric cancer (Table 66–4).

Screening for Large Bowel Cancer

In contradistinction to gastric cancer screening, a number of controlled trials of colorectal cancer screening have been conducted or are in progress. The earliest evaluated rigid sigmoidoscopy as part of a multiphasic health screen. Although a reduction in mortality from colorectal cancer was seen in the study group, this was probably due to chance and not due to the effect of sigmoidoscopy (Selby et al, 1988).

There is now further evidence to support sigmoidoscopy as possibly appropriate for colorectal cancer screening. This evidence has come from two case-control studies (Newcomb et al, 1992; Selby et al, 1992). An interesting feature of one (Selby et al, 1992) was that there appeared to be benefit from sigmoidoscopy, lasting for up to 10 years. However, it is known that such studies cannot eliminate the effect of selection bias, so that benefit may have been overestimated. This is why there is a new trial evaluating the effect of flexible sigmoidoscopy (Prorok et al, 1991).

All the other trials are evaluating the effect of the fecal occult blood test (FOBT). Of these, two, both in the United States, have reported mortality results. One of these, in New York, evaluated the effect of the addition of the FOBT to routine sigmoidoscopic screening (Flehinger et al, 1988). The trial was not randomized and the results are difficult to interpret (Miller, 1991b). In patients who were already attending the Strang clinic, no effect of adding FOBT tests to sigmoidoscopy was seen in mortality reduction from colorectal cancer (Winawer et al, 1993). In the first-time attenders, although compliance was difficult to secure with repeat attendance, a reduction in colorectal cancer mortality in the screened group was seen, which was of borderline statistical significance.

The other trial, in Minnesota, used the FOBT alone, annually in one group, biennially in another. A decision was taken to resume screening in that trial (stopped by design a few years ago) (Mandel et al, 1988). Recently evidence has accrued that annual but not biennial fecal occult blood tests reduce mortality from colorectal cancer after about a 10-year period (Mandel et al, 1993). This was achieved at a substantial cost in terms of false-positive results.

It is clear, especially from the Minnesota trial, that a major difficulty with screening using the FOBT is lack of specificity, especially if the test is rehydrated. Further, there seems to be a lack in sensitivity for adenomas. The evidence for this is somewhat indirect but relates to the postulated adenoma-cancer sequence. If an appreciable proportion of cancers arise from adenomas, and if the FOBT is capable of detecting adenomas, a reduction in incidence of colorectal cancer should be seen following FOBT screening, yet this has so far not been seen in the trials (Chamberlain et al, 1986; Miller et al, 1990).

It is difficult to be enthusiastic about the possibility that screening for colorectal cancer could make an important impact on mortality from the disease, especially with the older ages of most of those affected, and the low specificity of the FOBT. The ongoing European trials should provide answers to some of the remaining uncertainties over the FOBT, but results cannot be expected for 4 to 5 years. In the meantime, it is important to obtain further evidence on the efficacy of sigmoidoscopy, as in the current NCI Prostate-Lung-Colorectal-Ovarian cancer screening trial.

Screening for Prostate Cancer

Screening for prostate cancer using the digital rectal examination is recommended by the American Cancer Society and in the early detection guidelines of the National Cancer Institute (Table 66–4). It is not clear, however, that this is a valid screening test. Other screening tests under consideration include the prostate-specific antigen and trans-rectal ultrasound, though the latter may be of more value as a diagnostic test (Miller et al, 1990).

There are many obstacles in the way of an effective screening program for a disease that is a relatively unimportant cause of premature mortality. Not only has an acceptable and valid screening test to be available, but an acceptable and effective treatment for the preclinical lesions found as a result of screening (Miller et al, 1990). This is analogous to the situation for bladder cancer screening (Prorok et al, 1984). This problem is particularly acute for prostate cancer because of the increasing frequency of latent prostate carcinoma with increasing age and the not inappreciable morbidity and mortality of the radical procedures usually used to treat prostate cancer. There is no question that even when these problems are solved, it will be necessary to establish the effectiveness of screening programs for prostate cancer by well-designed randomized trials, before a recommendation on public health policy could be developed (Miller et al, 1990).

The crucial distinction between screening and normal medical diagnosis and care is that the encounter is not originated by the individual who is the subject of screening; rather, the provider of screening initiates the process (Miller, 1988). The screener believes that as a result of screening, the health of the community will be better. It is not possible to be certain that the health of everyone offered screening will be better, but at the very least the screener has an obligation to reduce to the minimum the possibility that individuals will receive harm. Clearly these conditions cannot yet be met for screening for prostate cancer, and therefore screening for this condition should only be offered in the context of a properly designed randomized trial with validly constituted informed consent forms. Such trials will have to be completed before a recommendation on including screening in programs of cancer control could be developed. We must be at least a decade away from such a recommendation.

Other Sites

The UICC project has considered screening for bladder and mouth cancer (Prorok et al, 1984), screening for endometrial and ovarian cancer (Hakama et al, 1985; Miller et al, 1990), screening for esophagus and liver cancer (Chamberlain et al, 1986) and screening for melanoma, neuroblastoma, and nasopharyngeal carcinoma (Miller et al, 1990). For none of these conditions is screening recommended as public health policy. In the majority of instances this is because of the absence of a valid screening test; but for oral cancer and melanoma, the issue is the lack of documented effectiveness of screening—especially, in the case of oral cancer, from developing countries where the disease is sufficiently common to propose programs based on inspection of the mouth by allied health professionals. Oral examination as part of the periodic health examination is recommended by the National Cancer Institute (Early Detection Branch, 1987), though no guidance is offered on how to ensure that those most at risk for the disease can be persuaded to accept such examinations, a difficulty identified by the UICC project as a major barrier to consideration of screening for oral cancer in Europe or North America (Prorok et al, 1984). The Early Detection Branch (1987) also recommends testicular self-examination and routine palpation of the testicles as part of the periodic health examination. However, no data relevant to the evaluation of screening for this site uncontaminated by screening biases are offered in support of this recommendation.

Prospects for the Future

There are a number of obstacles to a major contribution of screening to cancer control (Miller, 1986a). These include an unfavorable natural history of many cancers, in particular lung cancer; poor organization of screening programs; poor compliance of those at risk, sometimes exacerbated by economic barriers as, for example, mammography for breast cancer; as well as the non-availability of a valid and effective screening test. One class of screening test that is under development could be based on monoclonal antibodies; such tests are being considered for ovarian cancer, for example (Hakama et al, 1985; Miller et al, 1990). However, there would have to be available sensitive diagnostic tests to localize the very small cancers that might be detected, unless the screening test was sufficiently developed that it served both functions, as by linkage for diagnosis to a radiolabelled antibody.

In considering the potential contribution of screening to reduction in cancer mortality by the year 2000, only screening for cancer of the breast and cervix were judged likely to make an impact, and even the relatively small impact envisaged (a 3% reduction in overall cancer mortality) would require substantial increases in the proportion of women being screened (Greenwald and Sondik, 1986). For the other sites, it seems unlikely that any major impact will be achieved before the year 2000. However, even the impact envisaged must be regarded as temporary palliation, as for continued effect, screening programs have to be continued indefinitely. Thus it is a less optimal approach to the control of cancer than primary prevention. Nevertheless, primary prevention may require many decades to achieve its full potential. Pending this, screening, which offers a fairly rapid return from appropriate investment, should remain part of our armamentarium for cancer control.

CONCLUSION

In conclusion, there are a number of fundamental issues that have to be resolved when considering cancer control by screening. The general principles that govern the introduction of screening programs include: (1) the disease should be an important health problem; (2) the disease should have a detectable preclinical phase; (3) the natural history of the lesions identified by screening should be known; (4) there should be an effective treatment for such lesions; and (5) the screening test should be acceptable and safe.

The other issues range from ethics to economics. Critical issues include the population to be included in screening programs and whether or not it is possible to introduce an organized screening program. It cannot necessarily be assumed that a screening program for cancer will benefit the population to which it is applied. Not only do ethics demand that only programs with proven effectiveness be widely disseminated, it is also necessary to ensure that the program is continually monitored to confirm that effectiveness is maintained. Further, the benefits derived from the program must be clearly shown to exceed the costs, both in terms of ill health induced by the test and accompanying procedures, and in economic terms.

In spite of these caveats, screening carries the potential for a fairly rapid and important impact on cancer mortality, often exceeding what can currently be anticipated from other approaches to cancer control. Hence the current interest in and expectation from existing and potential programs of cancer screening will be maintained—even though for only two sites, breast and cervix, can an important impact be expected by the year 2000.

REFERENCES

AMERICAN CANCER SOCIETY. 1980. Guidelines for the cancer-related check-up. Recommendations and rationale. CA 30:193–240.

AMERICAN CANCER SOCIETY. 1983. Mammography Guidelines 1983: Background statement and update of cancer-related checkup guidelines for breast cancer detection in asymptomatic women age 40 to 49. CA 33:255.

AMERICAN COLLEGE OF RADIOLOGY. 1982. New ACR guidelines on mammography. ACR Bull 38:6–7.

ANDERSON GH. 1985. Cervical cytology. In: Screening for Cancer, Miller AB (ed). Orlando, Fla: Academic Press, pp 87–103.

BAINES CJ. 1984. Impediments to recruitment in the Canadian National Breast Screening Study: response and resolution. Controlled Clin Trials 5:129–140.

BAINES CJ, MCFARLANE DV, MILLER AB, et al. 1988. Sensitivity and specificity for first screen mammography in 15 NBSS centres. J Can Assoc Rad 39:273–276.

BAINES CJ, MILLER AB, BASSETT AA, et al. 1989. Physical examination; evaluation of its role as a single screening modality in the Canadian National Breast Screening Study. Cancer 63:160–166.

BAINES CJ, WALL C, MILLER AB, et al. 1986. Sensitivity and specificity of first screen mammography in a Canadian National Breast Screening Study. Radiology 160:295–298.

BASSETT AA. 1985. Physical examination of the breast and breast self-examination. In: Screening for Cancer, Miller AB (ed). Orlando, Fla: Academic Press pp 271–291.

BEAHRS OH, SHAPIRO S, SMART C, et al. 1979. Report of the working group to review the National Cancer Institute, American Cancer Society Breast Cancer Detection Demonstration Projects. J Natl Cancer Inst 62:640–709.

BOYD NF, WOLFSON C, MOSKOWITZ M, et al. 1982. Observer variation in the interpretation of Xeromammograms. J Natl Cancer Inst 68:357–363.

BOYES DA, MORRISON B, KNOX EG, et al. 1981. A cohort study of cervical cancer screening in British Columbia. Clin Invest Med 5:1–29.

BROOKMEYER R, DAY NE, MOSS S. 1986. Case-control studies for estimation of the natural history of preclinical disease from screening data. Stat Med 5:127–138.

CHAMBERLAIN J. 1986. Reasons that some screening programmes fail to control cervical cancer. In: Screening for Cancer of the Uterine Cervix, Hakama M, Miller AB, Day NE (eds). IARC Scientific Publications no 76. Lyon: International Agency for Research on Cancer, pp 161–168.

CHAMBERLAIN J, DAY NE, HAKAMA M, et al. 1986. UICC workshop of the project on evaluation of screening programmes for gastrointestinal cancer. Int J Cancer 37:329–334.

CHAMBERLAIN J, MILLER AB, EDS. 1988. Screening for gastrointestinal cancer. Toronto: Hans Huber.

CHODAK GW, SCHOENBERG HW. 1989. Progress and problems in screening for carcinoma of the prostate. World J Surg 13:60–64.

CHU KC, SMART CR, TARONE RE. 1988. Analysis of breast cancer mortality and stage distribution by age for the Health Insurance Plan clinical trial. J Natl Cancer Inst 80:1125–1132.

DAY NE. 1985. Estimating the sensitivity of a screening test. J Epidemiol Community Health 39:364–366.

DAY NE. 1989. Quantitative approaches to the evaluation of screening programs World J Surg 13:3–8.

DAY NE, BAINES CJ, CHAMBERLAIN J, et al. 1986. UICC project on screening for cancer: report of the workshop on screening for breast cancer. Int J Cancer 38:303–308.

EARLY DETECTION BRANCH. 1987. Working guidelines for early cancer detection. Bethesda, Division of Cancer Prevention and Control, National Cancer Institute.

EDDY D. 1980. Screening for Cancer: Theory, Analysis, and Design. Englewood Cliffs, NJ: Prentice Hall.

EDDY DM, HASSELBLAD V, MCGIVNEY W, et al. 1988. The value of mammography screening in women under age 50 years. JAMA 259:1512–1519.

FINK DJ. 1988. Change in American Cancer Society checkup guidelines for early detection of cervical cancer. CA 38:127–128.

FLEHINGER BJ, HERBERT E, WINAWER SJ, et al. 1988. Screening for colorectal cancer with fecal occult blood test and sigmoidoscopy: preliminary report of the colon project of Memorial Sloan-Kettering Cancer Center and PMI-Strang Clinic. In: Screening for Gastrointestinal Cancer, Chamberlain J, Miller AB (eds). Toronto: Hans Huber, pp 9–16.

FLETCHER SW, BLACK W, HARRIS R, et al. 1993. Report of the international workshop on screening for breast cancer. J Natl Cancer Inst 85:1644–1656.

GASTRIN G, MILLER AB, TO T, et al. 1994. Incidence and mortality from breast cancer in the Mama program for breast screening in Finland, 1973–1986. Cancer 73:2168–2174.

GOIN JE, HABERMAN JD. 1982. Comments on the logistic function in ROC analysis: applications to breast cancer detection. Meth Inf Med 21:26–30.

GREENWALD P, SONDIK EJ, EDS. 1986. Cancer control objectives for the nation: 1985–2000. NCI Monogr No. 2.

HAKAMA M. 1982. Trends in the incidence of cervical cancer in the Nordic countries. In: Trends in Cancer Incidence, Magnus K (ed). Washington, DC: Hemisphere Publ, pp 279–292.

HAKAMA M. 1984. Selective screening by risk groups. In: Screening for Cancer, Prorok PC, Miller AB (eds). UICC Technical Report Series, Vol 78. Geneva, International Union Against Cancer, pp 71–79.

HAKAMA M. 1986. Cervical cancer: risk groups for screening. In: Screening for Cancer of the Uterine Cervix, Hakama M, Miller AB, Day NE (eds). IARC Scientific Publications no 76. Lyon, International Agency for Research on Cancer, pp 213–216.

HAKAMA M, CHAMBERLAIN J, DAY NE, et al. 1985. Evaluation of screening programmes for gynaecological cancer. Br J Cancer 52:669–673.

HAKAMA M, PUKKALA E. 1988. Evaluation of an immunological screening for stomach cancer. In: Screening for Gastrointestinal Cancer, Chamberlain J, Miller AB (eds). Toronto: Hans Huber pp 71–75.

HOWARD J. 1987. Using mammography for cancer control: an unrealized potential. CA 37:33–48.

IARC WORKING GROUP ON CERVICAL CANCER SCREENING. 1986. Summary chapter. In: Screening for Cancer of the Uterine Cervix, Hakama M, Miller AB, Day NE (eds). IARC Scientific Publications No. 76. Lyon: International Agency for Research on Cancer, pp 133–142.

JONSSON E, HAKANSSON S, TABAR L. 1988. Cost of mammography screening for breast cancer: Experiences from Sweden. In: Screening for Breast Cancer, Day NE, Miller AB (ed). Toronto: Hans Huber, pp 113–115.

KALUZNY AD, RIMER B, HARRIS R. 1994. The National Cancer Institute and guideline development: lessons from the breast cancer screening controversy. J Natl Cancer Inst 86:901–903.

KOPANS DB. 1992. Response (Letter). J Natl Cancer Inst 84:1367–1368.

MANDEL JS, BOND J, SNOVER D, et al. 1988. The University of Minnesota's colon cancer control study: design and progress to date. In: Screening for Gastrointestinal Cancer, Chamberlain J, Miller AB (eds). Toronto: Hans Huber, pp 17–24.

MANDEL JS, BOND JH, CHURCH TR, et al. 1993. Reducing mortality from colorectal cancer by screening for fecal occult blood. N Engl J Med 328:1365–1371.

MCLELLAND R, PISANO ED. 1992. The politics of mammography. Radiol Clin North Am 30:235–241.

METTLIN C, JONES G, AVERETTE H, et al. 1993. Defining and updating the American Cancer Society guidelines for the cancer-related checkup: prostate and endometrial cancers. CA 43:42–46.

METTLIN C, SMART CR. 1994. Breast cancer detection guidelines for women aged 40–49 years: rationale for the American Cancer Society reaffirmation of recommendations. CA 44:248–255.

MILLER AB, ED. 1978. Screening in cancer: a report of the UICC International Workshop in Toronto. UICC Technical Report Series, Volume 40. Geneva, International Union Against Cancer.

MILLER AB. 1981. An evaluation of population screening for cervical cancer. In: Advances in Clinical Cytology, Koss LG, Coleman DV (eds). London: Butterworths, pp 64–94.

MILLER AB. 1986a. Screening for cancer: issues and future directions. J Chron Dis 39:1067–1077.

MILLER AB. 1986b. Principles of screening for colorectal cancer. Front Gastrointest Res 10:35–45.

MILLER AB. 1987. Early detection of breast cancer. In: *Breast Diseases*, Harris JR, Henderson IC, Hellman S, et al (eds). Philadelphia: Lippincott pp 122–134.

MILLER AB. 1988. The ethics, the risks and the benefits of screening. Biomed Pharmacother 42:439–442.

MILLER AB. 1991a. Is routine mammography screening appropriate for women 40–49 years of age? Am J Prev Med 7:55–62.

MILLER AB. 1991b. Colorectal cancer screening (Letter). J Natl Cancer Inst 83:1111–1112.

MILLER AB. 1991c. Issues in screening for prostate cancer. In: *Cancer Screening*, Miller AB, et al (eds). Cambridge: Cambridge University Press, pp 289–293.

MILLER AB. 1993. Implications of the National Breast Screening Study. Can J Oncol 3:189–192.

MILLER AB. 1994. Screening for cancer: is it time for a paradigm shift? Ann R Coll Phys Surg Can 27:353–355.

MILLER AB. 1992. Control of cancer of the cervix by exfoliative cytology screening. In: Gynecologic Oncology, Second Ed, Coppleson M, Monaghan JM, Morrow CP, Tattersall MHN (eds). London: Churchill Livingstone, Vol 1, pp 543–555.

MILLER AB, ANDERSON G, BRISSON J, et al. 1991. Report of a National Workshop on Screening for Cancer of the Cervix. Can Med Assoc J, 145:1301–1325.

MILLER AB, BAINES CJ, TO T, WALL C, et al. 1992a. Canadian national breast screening study: 1. Breast cancer detection and death rates among women age 40–49 years. Can Med Assoc J 147:1459–1476.

MILLER AB, BAINES CJ, TO T, WALL C, et al. 1992b. Canadian national breast screening study: 2. Breast cancer detection and death rates among women age 50–59 years. Can Med Assoc J 147:1477–1488.

MILLER AB, BAINES CJ, TURNBULL C. 1991. The role of the nurse-examiner in the National Breast Screening Study. Can J Public Health 82:162–167.

MILLER AB, BULBROOK RD. 1982. Screening, detection and diagnosis of breast cancer. Lancet 1:1109–1111.

MILLER AB, CHAMBERLAIN J, DAY NE, HAKAMA M, PROROK PC. 1990. Report on a workshop of the UICC project on evaluation of screening for cancer. Int J Cancer 46:761–769.

MILLER AB, CHAMBERLAIN J, TSECHOVSKI M. 1985. Self-examination in the early detection of breast cancer: a review of the evidence, with recommendations for further research. J Chron Dis 38:527–540.

MILLER AB, HOWE GR, WALL C. 1981. The national study of breast cancer screening. Clin Invest Med 4:227–258.

MILLER AB, KNIGHT J, NAROD S. 1991. The natural history of cancer of the cervix, and the implications for screening policy. In: *Cancer Screening*, Miller AB et al (eds). Cambridge: Cambridge University Press, pp 141–152.

MILLER AB, LINDSAY J, HILL GB. 1976. Mortality from cancer of the uterus in Canada and its relationship to screening for cancer of the cervix. Int J Cancer 17:602–612.

MILLER AB, TSECHKOVSKI M. 1987. Imaging technologies in breast cancer control: summary report of a world health organization meeting. AJR Am J Roentgenol 148:1093–1094.

MORRISON AS. 1985. Screening in Chronic Disease. Oxford: Oxford University Press, pp 48–63.

MORRISON AS, BRISSON J, KHALID N. 1988. Breast cancer incidence and mortality in the breast cancer detection demonstration project. J Natl Cancer Inst 80:1540–1547.

MOSKOWITZ M, PEMMARAJU S, FIDLER JA, et al. 1976. On the diagnosis of minimal breast cancer in a screenee population. Cancer 37:2543–2552.

MOSS SM. 1991. Case-control studies of screening. Int J Epidemiol, 20:1–6.

MOSS S, DRAPER GJ, HARDCASTLE JD, CHAMBERLAIN J. 1987. Calculation of sample size in trials of screening for early diagnosis of disease. Int J Epidemiol 16:104–110.

MUSCAT JE, HUNCHAREK MS. 1991. Breast self-examination and extent of disease: a population-based study. Cancer Detect Prevent 15:155–159.

NATIONAL BOARD OF HEALTH AND WELFARE. 1986. Mammographic screening for early detection of breast cancer. Guidelines from the National Board of Health and Welfare of Sweden, No 1986:3 Stockholm.

NEWCOMB PA, NORFLEET RG, STORER BE, et al. 1992. Screening sigmoidoscopy and colorectal cancer mortality. J Natl Cancer Inst 84:1572–1575.

NEWCOMB PA, WEISS NS, STORER BE, et al. 1991. Breast self-examination in relation to occurrence of advanced breast cancer. J Natl Cancer Inst 83:260–265.

NEUHAUSER D. 1985. Economic aspects of screening. In: *Screening for Cancer*, Miller AB (ed). Orlando, Fla: Academic Press, pp 49–57.

NYSTRÖM L, RUTQVIST LE, WALL S, et al. 1993. Breast cancer screening with mammography: overview of Swedish randomized trials. Lancet 341:973–978.

PREVENTIVE SERVICES TASK FORCE. 1989. Guide to clinical preventive services. Washington, DC, Department of Health and Human Services pp 26–31.

PROROK PC, BYAR DP, SMART CR, et al. 1991. Evaluation of screening for prostate, lung and colorectal cancers: the PLC trial. In: Cancer Screening, Miller AB, et al (eds). Cambridge: Cambridge University Press, pp 300–320.

PROROK PC, CHAMBERLAIN J, DAY NE, et al. 1984. UICC workshop on the evaluation of screening programmes for cancer. Int J Cancer 34:1–4.

RUSSIAN FEDERATION/WORLD HEALTH ORGANIZATION STUDY. 1993. Study of the role of breast self-examination in the reduction of mortality from breast cancer. Eur J Cancer 29A:2039–2046.

SASCO AJ, DAY NE, WALTER SD. 1986. Case-control studies for the evaluation of screening. J Chron Dis 39:399–405.

SCHECHTER MT, MILLER AB, BAINES CJ, et al. 1986. Selection of women at high risk of breast cancer for initial screening. J Chron Dis 39:253–260.

SEIDMAN H, GELB SK, SILVERBERG E, et al. 1987. Survival experience in the Breast Cancer Detection Demonstration Project. CA 37:258–290.

SELBY JV, FRIEDMAN GD, COLLEN MF. 1988. Sigmoidoscopy and mortality from colorectal cancer: the Kaiser Permanente multiphasic evaluation study. J Clin Epidemiol 41:427–434.

SELBY J, FRIEDMAN GCD, QUESENBERRY CP JR, et al. 1992. A case-control study of screening sigmoidoscopy and mortality from colorectal cancer. N Engl J Med 326:653–657.

SHAPIRO S, STRAX P, VENET L. 1971. Periodic breast cancer screening in reducing mortality from breast cancer. JAMA 215:1777–1785.

SHAPIRO S, VENET W, STRAX P, et al. 1988. Current results of the breast cancer screening randomized trial: the Health Insurance Plan (HIP) of Greater New York study. In: Screening for Breast Cancer, Day NE, Miller AB (eds). Toronto: Hans Huber, pp 3–15.

SIMPSON P. 1984. Economic aspects of screening. In: Screening for Cancer, Prorok PC, Miller AB (eds). UICC Technical Report Series, Vol 78. Geneva, International Union Against Cancer, pp 81–93.

SWET JA. 1979. ROC analysis applied to the evaluation of medical imaging technologies. Invest Radiol 14:109–121.

TABAR L, FAGERBERG CJG, GAD A, et al. 1985. Reduction in mortality from breast cancer after mass screening with mammography: randomized trial from the breast cancer screening working group of the Swedish National Board of Health and Welfare. Lancet 1:829–832.

TASK FORCE. 1976. Cervical cancer screening programs: The Walton Report. Can Med Assoc J 114:1003–1033.

TASK FORCE. 1982. Cervical cancer screening programs: summary of the 1982 Canadian task force report. Can Med Assoc J 127:581–589.

UK TRIAL OF EARLY DETECTION OF BREAST CANCER GROUP. 1988. First results on mortality reduction in the UK Trial of Early Detection of Breast Cancer. Lancet 2:411–416.

UK TRIAL OF EARLY DETECTION OF BREAST CANCER GROUP. 1993. Breast cancer mortality after 10 years in the UK Trial of Early Detection of Breast Cancer. Breast 2:13–20.

WALTER SD, DAY NE. 1983. Estimation of the duration of a preclinical disease state using screening data. Am J Epidemiol 118:865–886.

WALTER SD, STITT LW. 1987. Evaluating the survival of cancer cases detected by screening. Stat Med 6:885–900.

WEISS NS. 1983. Control definition in case-control studies of the efficacy of screening and diagnostic testing. Am J Epidemiol 116:457–460.

WINAWER SJ, FLEHINGER BJ, SCHOTTENFELD D, MILLER DG. 1993. Screening for colorectal cancer with fecal occult blood testing and sigmoidoscopy. J Natl Cancer Inst 85:1311–1318.

WORKING GROUP. 1987. Breast cancer screening: report to the Health Ministers of England, Wales, Scotland and Northern Ireland. London: H.M. Stationery Office.

THE WORKSHOP GROUP. 1989. Reducing deaths from breast cancer in Canada. Can Med Assoc J, 141:199–201.

67 Environmental regulation and policy making

LESTER B. LAVE

Chapters fourteen through twenty-seven examine the environmental and genetic factors associated with cancer. According to Doll and Peto (1981), Henderson and coworkers (1991), and Ames and coworkers (1995), the majority of current human cancers could be prevented by getting people to change their diet and stop using tobacco. Cancer is only one, and not the most important, reason for eating a more healthful diet (National Research Council, 1989a). Inasmuch as people say that preventing cancer and other disease is important to them—and there is a general consensus on how to accomplish this—why don't we do what we know will work?

If cancer prevention were the public's only concern, or even the most important goal, the U.S. National Cancer Institute's (1986) goal of reducing cancer deaths by half before the end of the century would be achieved easily. For example, Ames and coworkers (1995) point out that the Seventh-Day Adventists, "who generally do not smoke, drink heavily, or eat much meat but do eat a diet rich in fruits and vegetables..." have about half the cancer mortality of the general population. Few Americans are attracted to this lifestyle, even with the promise of halving their cancer incidence.

In contrast to the often-expressed desire to eliminate, or at least lower, cancer incidence, consumers, businesses, and governments seek other goals, such as pleasure, profits, and security. We seem to want cancer prevention as long as it doesn't interfere with other goals.

Legislation and regulation to lower cancer incidence is more complicated than discovering what is carcinogenic and eliminating exposure. People get pleasure from smoking cigarettes, from eating diets high in fats, and from other cancer-causing behavior. People like the low prices that are associated with producing goods and services without care for the exposure of workers or the environmental discharge of carcinogens. People like the appearance, flavor, and relative nonperishability of hot dogs and other nitrite-preserved meat despite the cancer risk. Getting people to change their behavior is difficult, as more than three decades of attempting to eliminate smoking have shown (Fielding, 1991). Reducing the exposure of workers and the public to environmental toxicants has proved difficult, as two decades of regulation have shown (Lave and Upton, 1988; Mendeloff, 1988; U.S. Environmental Protection Agency, 1990; Pierce, 1991).

Society finds it both impossible and undesirable to eliminate human exposure to environmental carcinogens. Regulation to reduce cancer incidence is complicated by the need to balance the pleasures and other social benefits from various behaviors with the cancer incidence arising from that behavior. Eliminating exposure to carcinogens is impossible because the vast majority of the carcinogens in our diet are natural constituents of the food (Ames and Gold, 1990; Scheuplein, 1990; Ames et al 1995). Reducing exposure to the extent technically feasible is undesirable because people would have to give up habits they value more than the risk of getting cancer (even when the risk is not small, as from cigarettes and sun bathing). For example, even after saccharin was shown to cause bladder cancer in rats—and people were informed of the risks—most people elected to continue consuming diet drinks (National Research Council, 1978, 1979).

If society wanted to reduce exposure to environmental carcinogens as much as is technically (and economically) feasible, a chapter on regulation would be short. These issues are complicated precisely because people want to eliminate risk without compromising pleasure; they want the variety, convenience, and low prices associated with current practices without their risks.

Rather than eliminating exposures, a balance must be struck between risks and benefits. Balancing requires quantification of at least the risks (Lave, 1981; National Research Council, 1983). In order to improve government management of environmental risks, each president from Nixon onward has required that regulatory agencies do some sort of balancing of risks and benefits. The most specific requirement was Reagan's Executive Order 12291, which requires a formal benefit-cost analysis of every major rule.

This chapter describes the interface between science and regulation; the regulatory process focuses on scientific uncertainties and disagreement over public goals. What determines the headline story and much of congressional opinion is the newsworthy event, even though this may have nothing to do with sensible public policy concerning prevention. However, the Administrative Procedure Act requires a deliberate pace in proposing, getting comment on, and implementing regulations. This process and the judicial review that follows gives much more attention to the underlying science and careful analysis. My purpose is not only to provide scientists with information about why seemingly simple actions seem to take forever, or never get done, but to show how they can help to facilitate translating scientific discoveries into effective regulatory policy.

The next section explores the nature of individual preferences and spillover effects. Then safety goals are examined. The following two sections deal with the methods used to estimate risks qualitatively and quantitatively and then manage them. Then there is a section illustrating the estimation and management of risks with several controversial examples, and finally a conclusion.

INDIVIDUAL PREFERENCES REGARDING RISK

Because regulation requires a balancing between the desires for satisfaction, fulfillment, and so on and the desire to lower cancer incidence, this section begins with attitudes toward risk. How much risk of cancer in the future is an individual willing to tolerate in order to eat better-tasting food today?

Normally, people accept life-threatening risks only if they are not aware of what they are doing or if they perceive themselves to be getting something worth the risk. Thus, with an occasional exception, needless health and safety risks are undesirable, and often unintended, consequences of activities (Fischhoff et al, 1981). The person who took up smoking didn't desire lung cancer, but the undesired consequence of the action seemed remote while the benefits of smoking were immediate. The plant spewing toxic chemicals into the environment is disposing of the material at least (private) cost; the plant manager regrets any health risks or environmental degradation that results. Human activities, including all production and consumption activities, generate increased health and safety risks as an undesired side effect. In the past two decades, however, people throughout the world—especially those with high income—have been willing to give up some desired activities and consumption in order to lower risks and improve environmental quality.

Often the risks are personal and their consequences known, at least qualitatively. For example, deciding to sunbathe is now known to most Americans to increase the risk of skin cancer. People who go to the Caribbean in the winter and get a sunburn know they are increasing their risk. When later diagnosed with skin cancer, individuals might protest that they didn't know precisely how dangerous the behavior was, but they certainly knew that they had increased their risk of skin cancer to some degree.

When the risks are personal and the consequences are known, society generally allows each individual to make a personal decision, as with sunbathing. Often society will attempt to provide additional information and regulate the safety of a product (the dose of x-rays or the carcinogenic contaminants in food), but the decision to eat peanut butter (with some aflatoxin contamination) is fundamentally personal. Not everyone agrees on which decision ought to be personal, as explored below.

Some decisions involve risks to others, and often the risks are so diffuse that there is no way to identify the individual who will be harmed. For example, diesel emissions from trucks increase cancer risks (Watson et al, 1988). But who is damaged and the extent of damage are unknown. In some instances, the victims are known; for example, people who installed asbestos insulation and later developed mesothelioma. In most cases, the victims may never be known; for example, those getting lung cancer from diesel truck emissions.

People tend to assign lower value to "statistical lives" than to identified ones (Schelling, 1968). If Baby Jane falls into an abandoned mine, society will go to great lengths to rescue her, even after it is likely she has died. The public is adamant, although somewhat less so, when a automobile model has a safety defect. Although no one knows who will be injured or killed, there is certainty that someone will be and we will know who the victim was when the inevitable crash occurs. One stage more removed from Baby Jane is exposure to some environmental toxicant, if there is uncertainty about how many (or even whether) people will be injured and we will never know whether anyone was harmed. For example, exposure to radon in buildings can lead to lung cancer, but there is no way of knowing whether a particular victim incurred the cancer from radon exposure (Axelson, 1991; Upton et al, 1992; National Research Council, 1988).

When the production or consumption decisions of Jones impose risk on Smith, without Smith's consent, there is an "externality,"—for example, Jones' buying a diesel car. Unless something is done to force Jones to get Smith's consent or to take account of the risks to Smith, in optimizing his personal decisions Jones will not be optimizing society's interests. The most direct way to internalize the externality is to require Jones to get Smith's permission before the production or consumption can take place. Jones might, for example, change the production or consumption process to remove, or at least decrease, the risk to Smith. Or Jones might get Smith to accept the increased risk by compensating Smith, who can then take other actions to lower other risks or increase consumption.

One indirect way of internalizing the risk is to proscribe inherently dangerous activities, such as keeping Siberian tigers or smoking in public places. For some inherently dangerous activities, the law allows the individual to engage in them but warns that the owner does so at his own risk. For ordinary activities, such as operating an automobile, someone who is injured must first prove that the owner's car caused the injury and then prove that the owner was operating the car in an unsafe fashion. For an inherently dangerous activity, such as keeping tigers, a victim need merely prove that he was injured by the tigers; the law assumes that having the tigers is inherently unsafe. This doctrine of "strict liability" warns the individual keeping tigers that he must pay for any damage the tigers do without the need for the victim to prove that the risk was unreasonable (Baram, 1982).

Another indirect way to lower risk is to "regulate" the way in which activities can be conducted. For example, automobiles must be manufactured with seat belts, steel mills must have air pollution control equipment, and automobile occupants must wear their seat belts (Graham, 1988; Evans, 1990, 1994). Until recently, most Americans didn't want the government to tell them what they must or must not do. They believed that workers and consumers should be vigilant in protecting their own interests.

During this century, particularly during the past two decades, the public has become more conscious of health and safety risks and increasingly has sought to reduce them. The result has been myriad new regulations of health and safety risks (Asch, 1988). Regulators have banned some products, for example, three-wheeled all-terrain vehicles and asbestos insulation. They have changed the design of other products, such as the distance between slats in baby cribs and the design of automobile dashboards, to eliminate protruding objects and cushion hard surfaces. They have banned production facilities, such as beehive coke ovens. Regulations are rarely cost-effective; for example, the Environmental Protection Agency (EPA) regulates some sources of benzene exposure at costs that translate into hundreds of millions of dollars per leukemia prevented (Lutter and Morall, 1994).

SETTING SAFETY GOALS

Managing health and safety risks requires answering the question: "How safe is safe enough?" Either a quantitative safety goal or a process is required. Decisions will be inconsistent if the goal is vague. Although attempts have been made by Congress and several regulatory agencies to set risk goals, the results are not sufficient to guide decisions.

Congress has hesitated to set quantitative safety goals. For example, the Food, Drug, and Cosmetic Act directs the Food and Drug Administration (FDA) to ban "unreasonable risks." Who can argue that "unreasonable" risks should be tolerated? The problem is that what is unreasonable will depend on the individual, circumstances, and the time. For example, guidelines for tolerable concentrations of toxic substances in the workplace have continually been lowered during the past fifty years; almost all of the occupational guidelines are considered insufficiently stringent to serve as guidelines for public exposure. Banning "unreasonable risks" gives great flexibility to the regulatory agency; there is little they must do and little they are precluded from doing. Such a vague safety goal seems designed to protect Congress against criticism of ineffectual legislative initiative rather than to provide guidance to the regulatory agency.

Occasionally Congress has specified safety goals implicitly by setting detailed regulations. For example, Congress set specific automobile emissions standards in the 1970 Clean Air Act and got even more specific in the 1990 Clean Air Act, specifying the sulfur dioxide reduction, a list of toxic pollutants, and a specific time table for substantial abatement of these pollutants. The most celebrated congressional decision concerning risk was the Delaney clause inserted into the Food, Drug, and Cosmetic Act in 1958: In ordering the FDA to ban carcinogenic food additives, Congress made it clear that they desired an extreme safety goal—eliminating the risk of getting cancer from food additives.

Congress cannot specify detailed regulations with success. The whole point of creating regulatory agencies was to create bodies that had the time and expertise to carry out Congress' directives. Congress doesn't have the time or knowledge to set detailed regulations. Unfortunately, Congress finds it easier to respond to public criticism by specifying an end result rather than taking the time to be thoughtful about such a difficult subject as specifying a safety goal so that the agency can carry out Congress' wishes.

Without congressional guidance or explicit policy, agencies make inconsistent decisions about how safe is safe enough (Milvy, 1986; Byrd and Lave, 1987; Whipple, 1987; Travis and Hattemer-Fry, 1988). The courts have suggested that agencies must first find that a risk is nontrivial (not *de minimis*) before it can consider regulation. Unfortunately, there is no working definition of what is a *de minimis* risk.

Because Congress provided them only vague guidance, several regulatory agencies have decided they would manage risks better if they had quantitative safety goals. Unfortunately, there is no agreement among agencies. As shown in Table 67–1, safety goals for protecting the public from cancer vary by a factor of 600. Using risk-analysis methods that it considered to be conservative, the FDA decided that a risk of less than one additional cancer per 1 million people exposed over their lifetimes constituted a trivial risk. The FDA determined that so small a risk is beneath its notice.

The U.S. Environmental Protection Agency (1989) went through a rule-making process, asking for public comment, to set a safety goal. It proposed four possible rules: (1) a goal of no more than one additional cancer per million individuals exposed, (2) a goal of no more than one additional cancer per 10,000 individuals exposed, (3) a goal of no more than one additional cancer per year among those at risk, or (4) no quantitative standard. After sifting through public comment, the EPA embraced all four rules. The agency said that it would like to reduce cancer risks to one in 1 million, but that wasn't presently possible. It said that, ordinarily, it would act on risks greater than one in 10,000. It also said that, ordinarily, it would act in cases where more than one additional cancer each year was expected. Finally, it said that none of these standards would prevent the EPA from acting as it deemed necessary in specific cases. In other words, the EPA rule provides little or no guidance to individuals and companies.

The Nuclear Regulatory Commission (NRC) set a safety standard that the mortality rate increase no more than 0.1% among the population living around a nuclear reactor. This goal was based on the lowest population death rate, that for young girls. This goal is equivalent to about 300–600 deaths per million people exposed. Thus, the NRC goal sets a lower standard of safety than even the EPA's proposal of one death in 10,000.

The California agency implementing Proposition 65 has set a safety level of one death in 100,000.

Only one of these safety levels is offered with any justification: The NRC goal is related to the lowest death rate observed among any group in the population. All the other goals are expected to be intuitively appealing.

Byrd and Lave (1987) and Cross and coworkers (1991) have proposed that a risk be deemed "trivial" if it could not be observed in an epidemiology study. They argue that a risk that society could never be sure exists is trivial. Weinberg (1972) coined the term "trans-science" for issues that could not be resolved by scientific theory and experiments. Thus, Byrd and Lave are proposing that nontrivial risks must be large enough to be above the trans-science threshold.

TABLE 67–1. *Agency Risk Goals*

Agency	Cancers per 1 Million Lifetimes
FDA	1
EPA	1–10
Nuclear Regulatory Commission	300–600
California Proposition 65	10

TABLE 67–2. *Expected Deaths among 1 Million Americans*

Cancer deaths	190,000
Cancer incidence	350,000
FDA risk goal	350,001
Total deaths	1,000,000

One way to put these safety goals into perspective is shown in Table 67–2. Consider 1 million Americans born in 1992. Eventually, all of them will die. The only questions are when they will die, and of what. About 30%–35% of them will be expected to have cancer and about 19% can be expected to die of cancer. Thus, the FDA considers that increasing the number of cancers from 350,000 to 350,001 would be a trivial increase.

Doll and Peto (1981) estimate that about one third of cancers are due to cigarette smoking and one third to diet. Environmental exposure to carcinogens causes perhaps 1%–2% of cancers. Certainly, there is a good deal of judgment in the Doll and Peto estimates. However, they are remarkably similar to estimates based on toxicology (Gough, 1990). Gough also finds that the EPA would be able to regulate away less than 1% of cancers. Henderson and coworkers (1991) confirm the Doll and Peto estimates.

Americans could reduce their likelihood of getting cancer by more than 50% just by not smoking and by eating a more healthful diet. Government actions to discourage smoking and limit exposure of nonsmokers to cigarette smoke have probably prevented more cancers than all the laws regulating toxic chemicals. If the government can undertake actions that would lower cancer incidence from 350,000 per million Americans to perhaps half that level, why are so many resources and so much attention being devoted to toxic chemicals in the environment and so little to smoking cessation and improving diet?

These facts have not been ignored by health professionals. Public health and other health professionals lobby for smoking cessation. The U.S. National Cancer Institute (1986) has set a goal of halving the number of cancer deaths in the United States by the end of the century. Their report focuses on smoking prevention and changing diet; environmental carcinogens are not even mentioned. Although the misallocation of resources is not as bad as it was a decade ago, it is still shameful.

By using a safety goal of no more than one additional cancer per million people, the FDA is wasting resources and misleading the public. Even a safety goal three orders of magnitude less stringent is likely to be lost in the noise of individual habits and exposures. Good management calls for focusing on the most important risks and using cost-effectiveness in managing them. This doesn't mean that carcinogenic chemicals in the environment should be forgotten, but it does mean that former EPA Administrator O'Reilly was correct in asking Congress for the ability to shift EPA resources toward more cost-effective programs.

Equity

Society is concerned not only with the average level of risk, but also with the distribution of risks (Been, 1994). When some localities or individuals face relatively high risks, this violates social notions of equity. The result might be rejection of some programs because of the inequities. An alternative is to compensate those at high risk or the victims (Cross, 1989).

Equity concerns extend to risks over time. Society doesn't want to ignore those who will be injured, or whose injury will be manifested in the future. How can decisions consider cancers in future years at the same time as current cancers? This issue is especially important for many cancers because of their latency period of several decades. Cropper and coworkers (1994) report an experiment in which they asked members of the public about the trade-off between saving a life several decades in the future compared to saving a life now. Most people answered that saving people today was much more important, in part because advances in research might cure a cancer that was not manifested for 30 years.

A particularly difficult and contentious issue has been finding sites for hazardous facilities (Kleindorfer and Kunreuther, 1994). Even when the risk is calculated to be small, those living near a prospective hazardous facility do not want to accept the additional risk. Social equity issues enter because society doesn't want to impose risks on any group against their will. The result has been the near impossibility of finding sites for facilities that discharge even small amounts of toxic chemicals into the environment.

MANAGING A REDUCTION IN CANCER INCIDENCE

How much cancer results from environmental exposures? Ames and colleagues (1995) estimate that 35% of cancer deaths in the United States are due to tobacco use, 30% (20%–40%) due to diet, and 5% to alcohol (4%–6%). Thus, a substantial fraction of cancer deaths may be impacted by individual lifestyle decisions.

These estimates are a refinement of those offered by Doll and Peto (1981) and Henderson and coworkers (1991). These studies reflect agreement among most epidemiologists that exposures to carcinogenic chemicals, ionizing radiation, and other agents produced by humans is responsible for less than 5% of human cancers.

Nonetheless, public attention has been focused on these agents, rather than on smoking, diet, and alcohol. Congress has responded with stringent environmental laws. The EPA has responded to the laws, and all environmental regulations currently cost the U.S. economy about $150 billion per year. Are the gains commensurate with the costs? Using EPA data, Gough (1990) estimates that no more than 6500 cancers per year in the United States would be prevented if the EPA were able to eliminate all chemicals it is investigating or regulating. This number is less than 1% of the annual incidence of cancers.

A less sanguine view comes from the finding of Davis and colleagues (1994) that the incidence of some cancers has been rising in the United States and other countries (Hoel et al, 1992). After eliminating smoking-related cancers, the investigators still find the incidence and mortality rates due to cancer have been rising since 1973, in contrast to a sharp drop in cardiovascular disease. Although the analysis doesn't pinpoint the cause(s) of the cancer increase, there is certainly the possibility that it is due to carcinogenic agents generated by humans and discharged into the environment.

METHODS FOR ESTIMATING HEALTH AND SAFETY RISKS

Management requires balancing risks and benefits, which requires quantifying risks. This section introduces the methods used to quantify both health and safety risks.

Health Risks

Isolating the causes of chronic disease is inherently more difficult than identifying the cause of a traumatic event. The chronic disease is caused by exposure over a long period of time. Myriad insults, or the interaction among insults, might be the causes or aggravating factors.

Epidemiology. Epidemiologic studies of putative toxic agents have consisted of the analysis of disease-specific incidence patterns, and more formal analytic methods including cohort and case-control studies.

Epidemiologic research is inherently challenging, time consuming, and expensive. Epidemiologists are concerned with inferring risks of exposures, sometimes 40 years in the past. For example, exposure to asbestos among shipyard workers from 1940 to 1945 has been shown to elevate the risk of lung cancer, but no measurements were taken of worker exposure (Royal Commission, 1984; Weill and Hughes, 1986; Mossman et al, 1990). Even after the example of asbestos, it is hard to establish the carcinogenic effects of other man-made fibers (Enterline, 1991). When the chronic disease essentially never occurs in the absence of a particular toxicant—for example, angiosarcoma of the liver from vinyl chloride monomer (Doniger, 1978)—isolating the cause is much easier than if the disease can be caused by multiple toxicants; for example, lung cancer might be caused by cigarette smoke, radon, asbestos—even by someone else's cigarette smoke (Greenberg et al, 1991; Stone, 1992).

The differences in genetic susceptibility among individuals, differences in lifestyles and consumption habits and differences in exposure to myriad toxicants mean that relatively large samples are required in order to draw a confident conclusion. The result is that only about three dozen substances have been shown to be human carcinogens by epidemiologists (IARC 1987). The current emphasis on prevention results in suspected carcinogens being banned or exposures being minimized; as a result epidemiologists may be limited in their ability to demonstrate whether a new agent has caused or will cause cancer in humans.

Toxicology. Toxicology is the science studying poisons. The father of toxicology, Paracelsus, wrote that any substance is toxic in high enough doses and no substance is a poison in a sufficiently small dose (Gallo et al, 1987). Thus, toxicology is focused on finding the nature of the health effects and at what dose they occur.

Toxicology is a laboratory-based science. Although occasionally humans are used as subjects, rodents or other laboratory animals are generally the subjects used to develop models for human effects. In some cases the models are extremely simple, as with the assumption that any substance causing an increase in tumors (benign or malignant) in a mammalian species should be regarded as a human carcinogen. Nature is generally more complicated than these simple assumptions; research on the mechanisms of action has made progress (Clayson, et al, 1990). For example, *d*-limonene is a chemical that gives lemons their special flavor. It also causes kidney tumors in male rats (Detrich and Swenberg, 1991). But toxicologists were surprised that it didn't cause tumors in female rats or other rodents. The carcinogenic nature of *d*-limonene has great health and economic significance because it is used in almost all soft drinks and in many other foods; large quantities of citrus fruit with *d*-limonene are consumed by people. An intensive investigation revealed that the male rat has a hormone that reacts with *d*-limonene to produce a carcinogen. As the female rat, mouse, and human don't have this hormone, there is no evidence that *d*-limonene would be carcinogenic in humans.

The classic National Toxicology Program rodent cancer bioassay is a relatively simple test. Sixteen groups of 50 animals are used: both sexes of two rodent species (usually rats and mice) are exposed at either the maximum tolerated dose (MTD), one half the MTD, one quarter the MTD, or zero dose (the control group). The animals are exposed to the test chemical beginning a few weeks after weaning and for the next 50 weeks, at which time they are sacrificed. An extensive pathological examination is made of each animal to determine if there are tumors. The test attempts to determine if there are more tumors in the test animals than in the controls. The biological plausibility of the results is the primary basis for accepting or rejecting statistically significant results. For example, does the number of tumors rise with the dose?

This lifetime rodent bioassay has been the focus of much criticism (Lave and Omenn, 1986; Lave et al, 1988; Ames and Gold, 1990; Rall, 1991; Ames and Gold, 1991). Ames and Gold charge that using the MTD results in promotion of cancer, leading to a result different than would be obtained if lower doses, such as those experienced by humans, were used. Lave and coworkers (1988) argue that the test isn't likely to predict human carcinogenicity better than much less expensive and time-consuming in vitro tests. Salsburg (1977) charges that the method of analysis overstates the statistical significance of the tests, leading to the conclusion that most chemicals tested give rise to a "statistically significant" increase in tumors.

The two largest challenges in toxicology are (1) devising an animal model that will predict human responses, and (2) predicting human responses at low doses versus those at high doses. Both challenges require knowing the mechanisms of action, the way the chemicals are metabolized and detoxified, and the way the chemicals arrive at the target organ. Great progress has been made in toxicology during the past decade with regard to carcinogenesis. Toxicologists now routinely examine pharmacokinetics and mechanisms of action rather than just counting tumors in the rodents (National Research Council, 1987). They are willing to classify some chemicals as rodent carcinogens, but comment that these are not likely to be human carcinogens. Methods now exist to determine that some chemicals have thresholds in causing cancer.

Carcinogenic Risk Analysis. In contrast to the analysis of what caused existing diseases, carcinogenic risk analysis attempts to determine the causes of cancer and the dose-response relationship (National Research Council,

1983; Travis, 1987). For example, ionizing radiation is a known human carcinogen (National Research Council, 1980, 1988). Carcinogenic risk analysis attempts to estimate the incidence of cancer that would be expected from low levels of exposure.

Prevention requires determining which agents are likely to be human carcinogens and then preventing or at least mitigating exposure. Thus, toxicologists work with in vivo and in vitro test systems to discover probable human carcinogens.

Because of its preventive nature, risk analysis relies more on toxicology with its animal experiments and analysis of chemical structure than on epidemiology with its analysis of the incidence of disease in humans. In the past two decades, toxicology has taken over from epidemiology the principal role of identifying possible risks to humans (National Research Council, 1983).

While there are many charges and countercharges, the preventive approach is firmly anchored in current regulation. No one wants to return to the "bad old days" when carcinogenicity was discovered by counting human cancers. However, current analysis involves needless controversy.

Epidemiology and toxicology are not competitors. Rather, they are different approaches and each has its comparative advantages. Test strategies need to identify the comparative advantages of each approach and to use each appropriately (Lave and Omenn, 1986).

Although risk analysis was designed to be conservative, to overstate risk, there is no proof that it does so in all cases. Bailar and coworkers (1989) find data indicating that risk analysis is not necessarily conservative. Graham and colleagues (1988) explore many of the conservative biases in risk analysis showing that often risk analysis would be expected to overstate the risk by several orders of magnitude. However, no one can guarantee that risk analysis is biased in showing greater risk in any particular case.

Safety Risks

Trauma occurs when the normal operation of a system fails, resulting in an undesired event, for example, a car crash or boiler explosion. Risk analysts attempt to discover the consequences of various deviations from normal operation and the causes of the deviations.

Investigation of Individual Crashes. Crash investigators examine undesired events to discover their cause. For example, The National Transportation Safety Board (NTSB) investigates all aircraft, train, and commercial bus crashes. The investigation team attempts to determine the cause of the crash and what might have prevented it. For aircraft crashes, the most frequent cause is pilot error; often, however, new procedures and instruments will be prescribed to avoid this situation or to prevent future crashes—for example, radar that automatically warns a pilot that another aircraft is near.

Just as the NTSB attempts to determine the causes of air crashes, so police attempt to determine the causes of fatal highway crashes. For example, the National Highway Transportation Safety Administration gathers data on all fatal automobile crashes (the Fatal Accident Reporting System [FARS] and a sample of nonfatal automobile crashes (National Accident Severity System [NASS] to determine the causes and describe the crash. The methods used tend to be informal, based on experience. After a fatal crash, the investigator attempts to determine speed, weather and other environmental conditions, experience and other attributes of the driver, and possible failure of some mechanical part or system.

Statistical Analysis of Crashes. A more systematic investigation of crashes involves statistical analysis of databases tabulating individual crashes; for example, the FARS and NASS data (Evans, 1990). These statistical investigations seek factors that are common to many crashes. Unlike the investigation of individual crashes, these statistical endeavors attempt to quantify the effects of a given risk factor, such as a driver having a high level of alcohol in his blood.

One difficulty with investigating individual crashes is that there is little or no ability to discover patterns and subtle or contributing causes. The NTSB seeks to discover the cause of each crash and how to prevent it. There is no mechanism for determining that one cause is common and another rare; thus, there is no way to focus prevention efforts on the common causes.

Unless there are data on the underlying incidence of causes, the statistical analysis has difficulty in isolating the conditions of concern (Evans, 1990). For example, suppose the FARS data showed that 100 drivers over age 69 were killed in night crashes. If older drivers were as likely to be on the road at night as during the day, this result would have no significance. However, if only 400 older drivers had been out on the road at night during this period, the statistic would imply that older drivers are at extraordinarily high risk when they drive at night. Evans develops extremely clever ways to utilize data where the population at risk is not known. For example, to estimate whether women are more likely than men to be killed in a crash of equal force, he selects crashes in which either a driver, passenger, or both were killed. For crashes with female drivers and male passengers, he calculates the ratio of killed drivers to killed passengers. He calculates the same ratio for male drivers and male passengers. In dividing the first ratio by the second, he derives an estimate of the fatality risk of female relative to males, controlling for driving frequency and speed.

Event-Tree and Fault-Tree Analyses. In contrast to these two methods used to determine the cause of a crash, event-tree and fault-tree analyses seek to estimate factors leading to a crash before it occurs (Linnerooth-Bayer and Wahlstrom, 1991). For example, Rasmussen and colleagues attempted to isolate all causes of failure in the operation of a nuclear power reactor that would result in immediate or later injury to workers or the public (U.S. Nuclear Regulatory Commission, 1975, 1978; Rasmussen, 1981). They first identified the events that would release a large amount of radioactive material from its prescribed location in the reactor, those that would breach the containment vessel for the reactor, and those that would scatter millions of curies of radioactivity to the environment.

The Reactor Safety Study proved to be extremely controversial (U.S. Nuclear Regulatory Commission, 1978). Critics disagreed with the failure probabilities assigned to individual components (for example, cooling pumps), claimed that some failure modes had not been identified or analyzed (for example, fire due to a technician inspecting wiring with a candle), and claimed that safety had been overestimated due to "common mode" failure. The painstaking process of specifying each event sequence leading to catastrophe and estimating the likelihood of each event is extraordinarily difficult and inherently arbitrary.

It may not be possible to engineer complicated systems that have expected failure rates of 1/100,000 per year or smaller. For example, Perrow (1984) argues that large, tightly coupled systems are inherently subject to high failure rates because of the interconnections. If Perrow is correct and there was a significant increase in the size or tight-connectedness of industrial facilities, there should be an increase in the proportion of losses in catastrophic events, compared to minor mishaps. From 1974 through 1988, Wulff (1991) found no increase in the proportion of fire loss due to the ten largest fires, implying that both major and minor fire losses seem to be increasing in proportion.

Even if systems could be built that are safe, it may not be possible to demonstrate their safety, even if millions of years of operating experience can be accumulated. Equipment is constantly being modified to take advantage of new materials, new designs, and new manufacturing processes. Even small differences in components change their reliability. Thus, even if a new model is designed to fail no more often than once every million hours, rather than once every hundred thousand hours for previous models, there may never be sufficient experience with this model to demonstrate the level of reliability has increased.

For example, Resendiz-Carrillo and Lave (1987) attempt to estimate the likelihood of a flood that would cause catastrophic failure of a dam. The event is believed to have less than a 1 in 10,000 likelihood of occurring each year. Unfortunately, for U.S. locations, less than 100 years of data are available on the largest flood each year. Alternative, equally plausible, functional forms for the frequency distribution give return periods that differ by several orders of magnitude. It is hardly surprising that a 10,000-year event cannot be estimated with confidence from 67 years of data. However, the return period for all the functional forms is greater than 10,000 years. Thus, contrary to expert judgment, the design safety criterion appears to be satisfied for this dam and no safety improvements were required.

RISK MANAGEMENT TOOLS

A fundamental question to be answered is whether the goal is to reduce risks or to optimize them. The former is much easier than the latter. However, attempting to reduce all risks makes no sense. All activities involve risk. Lowering all risks in a setting can only be done at the cost of eliminating the activity or spending inordinate amounts of resources—for example, eliminating carcinogens from the food supply.

In some cases, Congress enacted legislation that seeks to lower risks, no matter what costs are incurred; for example, the Delaney clause in the Food, Drug, and Cosmetic Act bans adding carcinogens to food (Lave, 1981). More generally, Congress has written statutes that ask for some balancing of the costs and benefits of risk reduction—for example, the Federal Insecticide, Fungicide, and Rodenticide Act that instructs the EPA to balance the good of a pesticide against its harm. Risk analysis is the primary mechanism for quantifying risk and therefore is a necessary step in optimizing safety.

Even when, as in the Delaney clause, Congress desires only the reduction of risk, no matter what the consequences, the analysis is difficult. For example, some essential nutrients may be potential carcinogens (Scheuplein, 1990; Ames et al, 1995). A current theory of carcinogenicity is that even a single molecule of a carcinogen conveys a tiny risk of developing cancer. Thus, for a region where these nutrients were absent from the diet, the Delaney clause would prevent adding them to food, with the probable result being a serious increase in disease or death.

Although regulatory actions are well intended, they may not improve public health and safety. The development of risk analysis in the 1970s was an attempt to quantify the risks associated with a situation of concern. Despite limitations and its inability to solve all problems, quantitative risk analysis has been helpful for policy decisions and even patient care (Lave, 1987; Graham et al, 1988). For example, screening tests sometimes convey some risk to the patient; for example, x-rays for mammography. The risk analysis permits a careful examination of the risks and benefits of the procedure.

Risk Management Tools

Risk Perception and Communication. Labeling and the provision of information more generally are the focus of many efforts at increasing health and safety (Hadden, 1986; Viscusi and Magat, 1987; Viscusi, 1992). For example, California's Proposition 65 requires that products be labeled if they present a nontrivial risk of cancer or birth defects (Roberts, 1989). Alcoholic beverages and cigarettes contain prominent warnings. For cigarettes and whiskey, there is no adjustment that the manufacturer can make that will obviate the need for labeling. However, for other products manufacturers have changed the formulation of the product in order to avoid a warning label. For example, Gillette changed the formulation of Liquid Paper to eliminate a solvent that is a carcinogen. While there is controversy about the extent to which warning labels on cigarette and liquor containers deter consumption, there is no doubt that reformulating products lowers exposures.

The Occupational Safety and Health Administration has mandated labeling when carcinogenic chemicals are used; they require warning posters (Mendeloff, 1988). Similarly, Congress inserted a provision in the Superfund Amendments and Reauthorization Act requiring plants to report their total discharges of more than 600 toxic chemicals each year. These reports are made available to the public and were the source of extensive media coverage. To avoid malpractice suits, physicians are advised to inform patients fully about the possible risks of a treatment regimen. Numerous requirements have been established for informing people of health and safety risks directly or through labeling products. Although it is far from clear that all or even most people understand these warnings, they provide significant information.

If labels and other warning are to work, more must be known about how people perceive risks and what they want to know in their decision making (Slovic, 1987; National Research Council, 1989b; Morgan, et al, 1992; Morgan 1993). For example, people give more attention to, and tend to exaggerate the risks of, nuclear reactors and airline crashes compared to the more dangerous coal-fired power plants and automobile crashes. In the midst of the public concern over asbestos, the *New York Times* reported that buildings with asbestos were hard to sell or to rent (Berg, 1988). Public perceptions are a concern in many areas (Farhar, 1994).

Risk-Risk Analysis. Another class of decisions involves both risk from the action and risk from not taking the action. For example, fungicides, all of which are toxic to some degree, can impede the growth on grain of some fungi that produce carcinogens. Thus, spraying fungicides on grain conveys some risk to the consumer but helps to prevent other risks. Still another example stems from the high injury and death rate for construction work. Increasing the amount of construction in order to increase a facility's safety has the effect of increasing the injury and death of workers. For example, the danger of accidental release of radiation from light-water reactors might be reduced by building a containment shield around the entire reactor to supplement the containment already present. Such an addition would cost billions of dollars and lead to a minuscule drop in the risk of inadverent releases of radiation. The deaths that might result from the construction would be expected to be greater than the cancers saved by lowering slightly the danger of breech of containment.

Some analysts have attempted to estimate the dollar trade-offs (Wildavsky, 1980; Kenney, 1990, 1994; Viscusi, 1994). This tool provides a brake on extreme safety programs that have lost their focus in the pursuit of safety no matter what the consequences.

Benefit-Cost Analysis. A more general tool than risk-risk analysis is benefit-cost analysis. This tool considers all the consequences of a proposed action, not just the health and safety risks. In Section 812 of the 1990 Clean Air Act, Congress required the EPA to do retrospective and prospective analyses of the benefits and costs of abating air pollution. Congress went on record as desiring a quantification and valuation of risks and other benefits from regulation as well as the costs; such information is an essential input to good decisions. Unfortunately, benefit-cost analysis is a demanding tool. It requires quantification of health effects from exposure to toxicants. This quantification is controversial for cancer, air pollution, and other health effects (Lave and Seskin, 1977; Schwartz, 1992).

Design Standards. If a press can crush the arms of the operator, an obvious remedy is to require a design change to prevent the trauma (Baram, 1982). For example, the press can be fitted with a switch that doesn't permit the press to close until both hands of the operator are on the switch. When individuals who have worked as safety consultants or worked for firms making safety equipment become regulators, they are tempted to specify the solution in the regulation. If a GT model 407b switch will stop the operator from being injured, why not require it to be used?

Design standards are the norm for environmental regulation. Congress ordered the EPA to set technology standards for the "Best Available Control Technology," and so on. In general the EPA specifies a particular technology, thus setting a design standard.

Design standards often are not efficient or effective. A cheaper switch might fulfill the same function, or a guard that pushes the operator's hand out of the press might be as effective but be cheaper or lead to less productivity loss. Even for design standards that are efficient at the time they are promulgated, technological progress is likely to produce more efficient solutions in response to this stated need.

Design standards are inflexible; the standard must be changed whenever there is a new technology. Perhaps the most important point is that there are dozens of different types of presses and types of applications. No one solution is likely to work well in all applications. If so, a design standard that works well in one circumstance will be ineffective or inefficient in another.

For example, the Nuclear Regulatory Commission spells out detailed procedures that must be followed in using radioactive byproduct materials in medicine (Paperiello, 1993). These procedures are essentially design standards. The radiation safety officer and medical staff are not free to design alternative procedures that would give greater safety or increase productivity at the current safety level.

Design standards appear to be simple and direct, with little need for arguing about the details. However, often the argument about the detail is necessary to discover the best current solution and to allow new solutions to emerge.

Performance Standards. Performance standards specify what is to be accomplished and leave it to the individual responsible for compliance to come up with a solution. For example, a design standard might require the press to be designed so that it prevents injury to the operator's hands. How that is done is up to the designer. As another example, the National Highway Transportation Safety Administration required that occupants of automobiles must be protected in crashes without having to buckle their seat belts (Graham, 1988). Auto manufacturers then came up with several ways to meet the standard, including air bags, seat belts on a motorized system in the ceiling, and fixed passive belts. There has been great controversy about the effectiveness, cost, and potential dangers of each system, but the standard spurred a search for superior technology that a design standard, such as an air bag requirement, would have cut off.

EPA sometimes sets performance rather than design (technology) standards. For example, the New Source Performance Standard for coal-burning power plants was specified to be emissions of no more than 1.2 pounds of sulfur dioxide per 1 million BTU of energy from coal. This performance standard allows utilities the flexibility to select low-sulfur coal, coal gasification, or other options instead of flue gas desulfurization.

Performance standards give more flexibility to producers. In doing so, they can enable producers to achieve the standards at lower cost. For example, Tietenberg (1992, p403) estimates substantial difference in implementation cost between design (technology-based) and performance standards.

The problem with performance standards is that the regulators have to specify precisely the outcome they desire. For example, the National Ambient Air Quality Standards specify that the concentration of sulfur dioxide cannot exceed a certain level. The cheapest way of meeting this standard in many cases is to build a tall stack to carry away the sulfur emissions. The tall stack ensures that the sulfur will not reach ground level in the immediate area, and so the performance standard is satisfied. However, tall stacks turn a local problem into a regional problem (Raufer and Feldman, 1987; Regens and Rycroft, 1988). They send the sulfur oxides to other areas, allowing the sulfur to remain in the atmosphere longer so that it is transformed into sulfates, and do nothing to decrease the sulfur loading in the atmosphere. The performance standard worked, but it created a problem that might be worse than the one it sought to alleviate.

Regulatory Frameworks

Health and safety issues are highly emotional ones (Fischhoff, et al., 1981; Efron, 1984; Epstein, 1978; Whelan, 1985; National Research Council, 1989b). When Congress has attempted to grapple with food safety or toxic substances in the environment, it has found itself in "no win" debates (Merrill, 1978; Miller and Skinner, 1984; Consumers Research, 1989; Hutt, 1978; Hutt and Merrill, 1991). On the one hand, health and safety advocates demand stringent standards. On the other hand, manufacturers claim that it isn't feasible to achieve the most stringent standards and that moderately stringent standards are expensive to attain. Manufacturers may also point out that regulation is not cost-effective, with vast resources being devoted to one area, such as toxic waste dumps, while almost no resources go to much more important environmental problems, such as radon in buildings (U.S. Environmental Protection Agency, 1987, 1990; California Environmental Protection Agency, 1994).

Congress has learned that it cannot please the advocates on either side, or hope to educate the public quickly about the nature of the trade-offs and uncertainties. Consequently, Congress typically charges a regulatory agency with responsibility for handling a problem, but often withholds a large part of the authority necessary to accomplish the task. More importantly, Congress enacts legislation with contradictory instructions to the regulatory agency. For example, the Occupational Safety and Health Administration is charged with protecting the worker over his or her working lifetime so that there is no diminution in function (Mendeloff, 1988). The OSHA is also charged with not promulgating regulations unless they are "feasible" in both an economic and technical sense.

Congress can be seen as providing some rough guidelines to the regulator (Lave, 1981). In particular, Congress has specified a number of frameworks for use in legislation. In choosing a framework for a particular bill, Congress implicitly specifies how the regulatory agency is to act.

A first framework used by Congress is "no risk"—for example, the Delaney clause. The instruction to the FDA is clear, simple, and leaves no doubt about what Congress desired.

A second framework specified by Congress is "risk-risk" analysis. As noted above, when the FDA ponders whether to license a drug, they understand that almost all drugs have undesirable side effects in some people. Thus, almost all drugs pose a risk. However, there can be no benefit from the drug without taking the risk. Thus, the FDA examines the risk of taking the drug and attempts to balance that against the risk of not having access to the drug. Where death is likely to result without intervention, and where no less toxic drug is available, the FDA is willing to license known carcinogens, as for chemotherapy for cancer.

A third framework is "technology-based standards." As described above, the language of the clean air and water pollution acts state that a company must install the "best available control technology" (BACT) or "best practical technology" (BPT), or that its control technology must meet "new source performance standards" (NSPS) or achieve the "least achievable emissions rate" (LAER). None of the phrases can be taken literally; all involve a trade-off between cost and level of control. For example, NSPS is more stringent than BACT but less stringent than LAER. Deciding among control technologies involves judgments about what trade-off between control and costs is reasonable and what technologies are "available." BACT requires that the technology be demonstrated on a commercial scale—thus availability isn't an issue. However, the trade-off between control and cost is assumed to be at a reasonable level; that is, it cannot cost 10 times as much to get 1% additional control as it has cost to get the control up to this point. In contrast, LAER implies a willingness to spend much more to get additional control. The term also implies that the technology need not be fully proven at a commercial scale.

These technology-based standards have put the EPA and the Office of Management and Budget (OMB) continually in conflict. The EPA interprets the various phrases as implying more control while OMB interprets them as implying greater consciousness of cost. Congress has tended to stay out of the conflict, save for direct interventions in favor of some plant in a particular congressional district.

The fourth framework used by Congress is "cost-effectiveness" analysis. This framework assumes that a goal is specified and instructs the regulatory agency to achieve this goal at least cost. This framework was refined for the military as a way of suboptimizing, given the defense mission. Having specified the defense mission, cost-effectiveness analysis is used to decide what mix of weapons systems will achieve this mission at least cost. The Nuclear Regulatory Commission has also used this framework in regulating exposures to ionizing radiation. "As low as reasonably achievable" is interpreted to mean that companies should continue to abate exposure to ionizing radiation as long as the cost per rem averted is less than $1,000 (Pochin, 1983). Lutter and Morrall (1994) and others have calculated the cost-effectiveness of saving lives or preventing cancers. They find an enormous range of values, indicating that society is not saving all the "inexpensive lives" and is allocating resources to saving extremely expensive lives.

The fifth framework is "risk-benefit analysis" (Starr, 1969). Congress asks the regulatory agency to weigh the benefits of a technology against its risks. The difference between the risk-benefit and risk-risk frameworks is that the latter includes only health risks while the former includes the whole range of benefits, rather than being limited to health. For example, a risk-benefit analysis of electricity generation would seek to weigh the additional risks to health against all of the benefits of having the electricity, from health benefits to greater enjoyment from television.

The sixth framework, "benefit-cost analysis," attempts to evaluate the full social benefits and full social costs in deciding what regulatory action to take. Benefit-cost analysis differs from risk-benefit analysis by considering all the social costs, not just health costs. As noted above, in the 1990 Clean Air Act Congress joined many presidents (such as Ronald Reagan in Executive Order 12291) in explicitly requiring a full quantification of the benefits and costs of regulations.

These frameworks are arrayed in terms of increasing difficulty in getting the data required for the analysis, in terms of the amount of analysis required, and in terms of the difficulty of required value judgments. The Delaney clause is simple to apply, requires only one datum, and requires no value judgments from the regulatory agency. At the other end of the spectrum is benefit-cost analysis, which requires full-scale analysis and quantification of every aspect of the decision. All of the aspects must not only be quantified, they must be translated into a common metric: dollars. Not only is the analysis difficult, it requires myriad value judgments about what is important and how much society values each aspect. Benefit-cost analysis is extremely difficult to do well. Even for the best analysis, differences in values can lead to opposite conclusions. Congress provided the value judgment in the Delaney clause (no cancer risk from food additives); Congress offered no guidance to the EPA in requiring it to find values for the benefit-cost analysis of the Clean Air Act.

Decentralized Regulation

Scholars have long recognized that centralized command and control regulation (hereafter called simply "regulation") is far from the perfect solution to complicated issues. Regulation is a blunt instrument. Formulating a new regulation takes years and thousands of professional work hours. Guarantees of due process mean that those with a stake in the issue get many chances to change the outcome; failing that, they can delay promulgation of the regulation and then delay its enforcement by legal and political challenges. Regulation is not capable of optimizing nor is it capable of dealing with "less important" issues—it is simply too costly and clumsy.

Recognition of these facts has tended to promote the search for alternatives to centralized regulation, such as insurance or the legal system (Huber and Litan, 1991). Each of these alternatives has received vast criticism for being inefficient, costly, or not getting at the central issues. While this criticism may be true, often it is irrelevant. Regulation is also inefficient, costly, and often focuses on the wrong issues. What is relevant is finding which alternative or combination of alternatives manages to achieve the social goals best. In some cases, the legal system or arbitration is likely to lead to superior outcomes.

Economists have discussed the use of market incentives to solve environmental problems for almost a century (Pigou, 1920; Baumol and Oates, 1975). Particularly in the last two decades, economists have asserted that market incentives will speed compliance as well as lessening the cost (Kneese and Schultze, 1975; Stavins, 1988; Hahn and Hester, 1989; Hahn and Hird, 1991, Hahn and May, 1994; Howe, 1994; Macauley et al, 1992; U.S. General Accounting Office, 1993; Reshovsky and Stone, 1994).

A particular nonmarket alternative that is receiving a great deal of attention focuses on improving enforcement. The use of "market incentives" can simplify enforcement and even simplify setting the regulatory goals (Gruenspecht and Lave, 1991). For example, a great deal of work has been done to relate the quantity of emissions of air pollutants to the resulting ambient air quality (Portney, 1990). A target air quality is set, and this quality goal is then translated into a target emissions level. For standard regulation, current emissions levels are estimated. Abatement targets are established and regulations are designed to reduce emissions to these targets.

For example, if current emissions are 500 and the target emissions level is 100, 80% abatement is required. A technology-based standard could be specified to attain this abatement level. However, the emissions estimate might be wrong or the technologies might not give 80% abatement. An alternative approach would be to establish discharge licenses for emissions of 100. These discharge licenses could be sold or given to current polluters as a proportion of their emissions. Anyone emitting more than his discharge licenses would be shut down or given a large fine.

The advantage of the discharge licenses is that the regulators don't have to estimate current emissions levels or find what technology or regulations will reduce emissions an average of 80%. A second advantage should be ease of enforcement. Regulators can be challenged on their estimates of current emissions or their estimates about what regulations will achieve 80% abatement. These challenges make it less likely that a judge will insist that a polluter really adhere to the regulations or be forced to shut down or pay a large fine. The use of discharge licenses chops two important, controversial steps from the regulatory process.

Similarly, if there is a determination that sulfur oxide emissions cost society $0.50 per pound, an effluent fee of $0.50 per pound could be set. No determination needs to be made of the inventory of current emissions or some target emissions goal set. Enforcement consists simply of measuring total sulfur oxide emissions from each polluter and charging $0.50 per pound.

The case for economic incentives is usually made on the ground that they are cost-effective; that is, they provide the agreed-upon amount of abatement at the lowest cost. For example, if the discharge license approach is taken, these discharge licenses can be bought and sold. The market determines the value of a license to discharge one pound of sulfur dioxide per day. If a firm can abate pollution for less than the cost of this discharge license, it will do so. If a firm cannot cover its costs, including the cost of the abatement and discharge license, it will go out of business and sell its discharge licenses. The system provides flexibility for firms to minimize their costs, given the emissions goals.

Similarly, effluent fees provide a strong incentive to provide the "proper" (in the sense of least costly) level of emissions. Firms will abate emissions as long as that is the least-cost means of lowering their costs; pay an effluent fee; or go out of business if the business is so marginal that it cannot cover its pollution control costs. At $500 per ton of sulfur dioxide, the typical coal-burning utility would abate 90%–95% of sulfur oxide emissions for this effluent fee, and pay the effluent fee for the remainder. At this effluent fee, some firms, such as old foundries, would cease to operate. In theory, this effluent fee would be efficient in the sense of producing the greatest amount of pollution abatement at the least cost.

A current example is the use of effluent fees for reducing the production of chlorofluorocarbons (CFCs) (Orlando, 1990). In addition to legislation phasing out the production of CFCs, Congress imposed a fee of about $1 per pound on the producer. The precise fee is related to the ozone-destroying potential of each CFC aerosol (Orlando, 1990).

An example of the use of marketable discharge allowances is the 1990 Clean Air Act. In order to abate sulfur dioxide, an emissions limit is set for each electricity generation plant (Goldburg and Lave, 1992). Plants that abate more than the target are allowed to sell the additional allowances to plants that have not abated the target amount. The result is additional flexibility that is estimated to lower the cost of abating sulfur dioxide by more than 20% compared to centralized command and control regulation.

CASE STUDIES OF MANAGING HEALTH AND SAFETY RISKS

To illustrate the conceptual frameworks, three examples are presented. One example is an accident where the effect is immediate. The other two concern a chronic disease where the effect does not occur for two or more decades after initial exposure.

Managing Food-Borne Carcinogens

As discussed above, toxic substances, particularly carcinogenic chemicals in food, have elicited great concern from Americans (Cross, et al, 1991; Lave and Upton, 1988). Food is an especially emotional issue (Hutt, 1978; Merrill, 1978; Hutt and Merrill, 1991).

Congress specified a "no-risk" framework for carcinogenic food additives (the Delaney clause). The U.S. Food and Drug Administration revolted against the Delaney clause where the resulting risks were trivially small (*Public Citizen v Young*, 1987). The courts ordered the FDA to rescind its exemption because the plain language of the Delaney clause shows that Congress wanted no carcinogenic food additives.

Because some essential nutrients are potential carcinogens and there are many natural carcinogens in food, the no-risk framework would eliminate much of the food supply and increase disease. Thus, it is not reasonable to apply the no-risk framework to all foods; it is possible, although not very sensible, to apply the framework only to food additives.

"Technology-based standards" have been used to require a particular control device or process. For example, the best available machinery could be used to separate nuts and grains contaminated with aflatoxin so they are not consumed by people. Another possible interpretation is that carcinogens cannot be present in detectable amounts in food. Congress actually wrote this interpretation into the Food, Drug, and Cosmetic Act. However, as analytical chemistry has been able to detect ever more minuscule amounts, this interpretation has come to mean that no amount of the carcinogen can be present.

All of the other frameworks require some quantification of the risk of carcinogenicity. This means that the carcinogenic potency of the chemical must be estimated as well as the number of people exposed at each level. The former can be estimated from the rodent bioassay; the latter is estimated from discharges of the chemical into the environment, dispersion modeling via air or water, possible biological reconcentration, and then human exposure.

Once the number of human cancers has been estimated, risk-risk analysis would weight the number of cancers against the health effects of having more expensive, less available food or of denying some essential minerals. For the essential minerals that are carcinogens, the decision would presumably permit people to consume the required amount, but no more. In a time or place when food was in short supply, foods with small risks of causing cancer would be tolerated.

The risk-benefit framework would compare the estimated number of cancers to the benefit from being exposed. For example, the FDA sets a tolerance level for aflatoxin in peanuts and peanut products by some sort of informal risk-benefit calculus. Peanuts are a cheap source of protein and a popular food. Setting a stringent tolerance level would mean that much of the peanut crop could not be available for human consumption, raising the price of peanuts and peanut products. The FDA permits rich desserts to be sold despite the heart disease and cancer risks. The judgment is that consumers choose the benefits of consumption over the risks of disease.

A cost-effectiveness analysis would have the FDA set the aflatoxin tolerance level at a point where the cost per cancer prevented was about the same as cancer prevention decisions for other carcinogenic substances. Since many of these substances are not in food, FDA,

EPA, OSHA and other agencies would have to coordinate their decisions.

A benefit-cost analysis would set the tolerance level at the point where the incremental benefit was just equal to the incremental cost (assuming that, in the neighborhood of this standard, more stringent standards increase incremental cost and decrease incremental benefit).

Note that the "no-risk" and technology-based standard frameworks requires much less information and analysis than the other decision frameworks; the only relevant attribute is whether the substance is a carcinogen. All of the other frameworks require a quantification of the disease resulting from exposure. The risk-risk framework trades off the disease risk from exposure to the health risk from not having the food. The risk-benefit and cost-effectiveness frameworks require still more information. For the former, benefits must be described so that risks can be traded off against benefits. For the latter, the cost per cancer prevented must be estimated for a number of programs to set the abatement level. Benefit-cost analysis requires the greatest amount of data and analysis because the benefits and costs must be described, quantified, and translated into dollars in order to determine the abatement level at which incremental benefits equal incremental costs.

The nonregulatory alternatives provide a rich array of approaches. A believer in the free market could decide to provide consumers with information or decide to tax the aflatoxin level in food. A lawyer would specify a tort-liability approach. There is an extremely heavy burden of analysis in attempting to decide which of the regulatory or nonregulatory frameworks to use. In few cases should anyone attempt to examine the full menu of possibilities. For better or worse, when Congress chooses a regulatory or nonregulatory framework, it is making an important decision, even if it doesn't specify an explicit health, safety, and environmental goal.

Interpreting Test Information

An important issue has to do with which tests should be used to determine whether a chemical is a carcinogen. The general answer from toxicologists is that the test that is most accurate should be selected. In fact, neither the most accurate nor the least-cost test is necessarily the best (Lave and Omenn, 1986; Lave et al, 1988).

Shown in Figure 67–1 is a simplified representation of the testing decision. The chemical either is or is not a carcinogen (the simplification doesn't change the nature of the conclusions); the test is either positive or negative. The test would be perfect if it was positive whenever the chemical was a carcinogen and negative whenever the chemical was not. Unfortunately, there

Test Result	True Biological Activity: Carcinogen	True Biological Activity: Noncarcinogen	
Positive	True Positive 8	False Positive 36	44 test Postitves
Negative	False Negative 2	True Negative 54	56 test Negatives
	10	90	

c: Cost of testing each chemical: $1 million
x: Social cost of a false positive: $1 million
bx: Social cost of a false negative: $10 million

Social Cost: Classify all chemicals as noncarcinogens: 10 bx : $100 million
Social Cost: Classify all chemicals as carcinogens: 90 x : $90 million
Social Cost: Test and classify according to test: 100c + 2bx + 36x : $156 million

For Ames test, c = $2,000, 55% sensitivity, 45% specificity
Test: $0.2 + 40.5 + 45 = $85.7

FIG. 67–1. Information value of lifetime rodent bioassay.

are false negatives and false positives, instances where the test is negative for a carcinogen or positive for a noncarcinogen.

Assume that the cost of testing a chemical is c, the social cost of a false positive is x and the social cost of a false negative is bx. Now suppose that the a priori likelihood this chemical is a carcinogen is 0.1 and that the test is 80% sensitive and 60% specific. If so, there will be 0.02 false negatives and 0.36 false positives.

The social cost of testing 100 chemicals of this sort is $100c + 36x + 2bx$. The social cost of classifying all chemicals as noncarcinogens without testing (the policy prior to the preventive approach) is $10bx$. The social cost of classifying all chemicals as carcinogens without testing is $90x$. Whether to test is determined by the alternative with the lowest social cost. For example, if the cost of testing were $1 million (the cost of a lifetime rodent bioassay), the cost of a false positive were $1 million and the cost of a false negative were $10 million, the cost of the three alternatives in millions of dollars would be: Test, 100 + 36 + 20 = 156. Don't test, noncarcinogens = 100. Don't test, carcinogens = 90. Because "don't test, and classify all chemicals as carcinogens" has the least cost under these assumptions, it is the dominant strategy.

An alternative test could be compared to the rodent bioassay; knowing the other test's cost, sensitivity, and specificity, society ought to select the test with the lowest social cost. For example, an Ames test costs $2,000 and is perhaps 55% sensitive and 45% specific. The cost of the three alternatives is: Test, 0.2 + 40.5 + 45 = 85.7. Don't test, noncarcinogen = 100. Don't test, carcinogen = 90. In this case, the Ames test has the lowest social cost. Even though it is less sensitive and less specific than the lifetime rodent bioassay, its test cost is low enough to offset the decreased accuracy.

These calculations can be done for other proposed tests or for chemicals whose costs of misclassification or likelihood of carcinogenicity are different. For example, for chemicals with a 0.5 likelihood of being carcinogens, "don't test, carcinogen" is likely to be the best alternative.

Highway Safety

About 45,000 Americans are killed on highways each year. Highway crashes are the leading cause of death of children and young adults. Since 1965, when Congress passed the Highway Transportation Safety Act and created the National Highway Transportation Safety Administration (NHTSA) to administer the law, the United States has displayed a high level of concern for highway safety (Graham, 1988).

One of the major issues has been the effect of automobile size and weight on safety (Evans, 1990, 1994; Graham, 1988). In reaction to the OPEC oil embargo and sharp increase in petroleum prices, Congress enacted fuel economy standards for automobiles in 1975. The standard required that the average new car sold in 1985 would have to get 27.5 miles per gallon, almost double the 1974 average. As a result, automobiles were "downsized," becoming both lighter and smaller.

Data on two-car crashes have shown that lighter, smaller cars are much more likely to involve a fatality in a crash. However, the data don't allow control for vehicle speed and other factors. It is known that smaller, lighter cars tend to be driven by young adults who are more likely to be involved in crashes and to drive at greater speeds.

A further controversy involved the assertion that Detroit didn't design cars that stressed safety. Rather, the cars were designed for speed or attractive appearance, with little consideration for safety. Safe cars could be designed, even light cars could be designed to be safe.

Evans (1990) finds that cars that weigh 500–900 kilograms are much more likely to result in the death of the driver or passengers in a crash than would a car weighing 1800–2400 kg. This is especially true in a collision between cars of different sizes. In a crash between cars of these two size classes, the driver in the lighter car is 16.5 times more likely to be killed than the driver of the heavier car. If both cars in a collision weigh 1800–2400 kg, the likelihood that the occupants will be killed is 3.5 times as great as if the car were hit by a 500–900 kg car. Finally, if two small cars collide, the occupants are twice as likely to be killed as if they were in two large cars that collided. Thus, Evans demonstrates that being in a car with greater mass in a crash is highly beneficial.

If Congress had written a "no-risk" decision framework into traffic safety law, all motor vehicles would be banned. Even though society regrets the 45,000 premature deaths each year, everyone appears to agree that having the freedom and access of automobiles is worth it.

Some individuals believe that wearing a safety belt would increase their chance of being injured in a crash—for example, in slowing their exit from a burning car after a crash. A risk-risk analysis shows that seat belts do occasionally increase risk, but that in general they are extremely helpful.

A technology-based standard decision framework would lead to adding all safety devices that appears to offer any increase in safety. The result would be an extremely expensive vehicle that was clumsy and fuel inefficient.

Risk-benefit analysis would examine the nonhealth consequences of wearing a seat belt. If the belt were uncomfortable or difficult to buckle or unbuckle, the benefit of the belt might be negative.

A cost-effectiveness framework would attempt to save lives at least cost, whatever the safety device. The NHTSA analysis suggests that improved traffic signals, increasing seat belt use, and other activities are more cost-effective that adding additional safety devices to cars. However, for cars already equipped with seat belts, it is highly cost-effective to get people to buckle their belts.

Benefit-cost analysis attempts to quantify both benefits and costs and set incremental benefit equal to incremental cost. This framework requires a dollar estimate for the social value of preventing a premature death. While there is little agreement on this figure, benefit-cost analysis has provided some insights (Viscusi, 1993). For example, seat belts have a high net benefit when they are worn. But at the usage rate in the early 1980s (about 10%), the safety devices were not worth having. At the same time, with seat belts in all cars, the cheapest way of increasing highway safety is to increase belt usage. This was done by nearly all states imposing mandatory belt use laws and campaigning to increase belt use, a highly successful (and cost-effective) campaign.

CONCLUSION

The formal analysis of risks to health and safety has contributed much to decreasing risks (Breyer, 1993). An array of analytic tools are available to address a wide variety of concerns. The further development of these tools and their application in improving the management of health and safety risks has much to offer the nation.

REFERENCES

AMES BN, GOLD LS. 1990. Too many rodent carcinogens: mitogenesis increases mutagenesis. Science 249:970–971.

AMES BN, GOLD LS. 1991. Reply to Rall. Science 251:11–12.

AMES BN, GOLD LS, WILLETT WC. 1995. The causes and prevention of cancer. Proc Natl Acad Sci 92:5258–5265.

ASCH P. 1988. Consumer Safety and Regulation: Putting a Price on Life and Limb, New York: Oxford University Press.

AXELSON O. 1991. Occupational and environmental exposures to radon: cancer risks. In Ommen G, Fielding J, Lave L (eds). Annu Rev Public Health 12:235–256.

BAILAR JC, III, CROUCH EAC, SHAIKH R, SPIEGELMAN D. 1989. One-hit models of carcinogenesis: conservative or not? Risk Anal 8:485–497.

BARAM MS. 1982. Alternatives to Regulation, Lexington: Lexington Books.

BAUMOL W, OATES W. 1975. The Theory of Environmental Policy. Englewood Cliffs, NJ: Prentice Hall.

BEEN V. 1994. Locally undesirable land uses in minority neighborhoods: disproportionate siting or market dynamics? Yale Law J 13:1383.

BERG EN. 1988. Asbestos buildings go begging; now harder to sell, lease, or finance. New York Times, 137, 25.

BREYER S. 1993. Breaking the Vicious Circle: Toward Effective Risk Regulation. Cambridge: Harvard University Press.

BYRD DM, III, LAVE LB. 1987. Significant risk is not the antonym of de minimis risk. In De Minimis Risk, Contemporary Issues in Risk Analysis, Vol. 2, Chris Whipple (ed). New York: Plenum pp 41–60.

CALIFORNIA ENVIRONMENTAL PROTECTION AGENCY. 1994. Toward the 21st Century: Planning for the Protection of California's Environment, California Comparative Risk Project, Sacramento, CA.

CLAYSON DB, MUNRO IC, SHUBIK P, SWENBERG JA, eds. 1990. Progress in Predictive Toxicology. New York: Elseview Science Publishers.

CONSUMERS RESEARCH. 1989. Does everything cause cancer? 72:11.

CROPPER ML, AYDEDE SK, PORTNEY PR. 1994. Preferences for life saving programs: how the public discounts time and age. J Risk Uncertainty 8:243–265.

CROSS FB. 1989. Environmental Induced Cancer and the Law: Risks, Regulation, and Victim Compensation, New York: Quorum Books.

CROSS FB, BYRD DM III, LAVE LB. 1991. Discernible Risk—a proposed standard for significant risk in carcinogen regulation. Admin Law Rev 43:61–88.

DAVIS DL, DINSE GE, HOEL DG. 1994. Decreasing cardiovascular disease and increasing cancer among whites in the United States from 1973 through 1987. JAMA 271:431–437.

DETRICH DR, SWENBERG JA. 1991. The presence of a 2μ-globulin is necessary for d-limonene promotion of male rat kidney tumors. Cancer Res 51:3512–3521.

DOLL R, PETO R. 1981. The cause of cancer: quantitative estimates of avoidable risks of cancer in the United States today. J Nat Cancer Inst 66:1193–1308.

DONIGER D. 1978. The Law and Policy of Toxic Substances Control: A Case Study of Vinyl Chloride. Baltimore: Johns Hopkins.

EFRON E. 1984. The Apocalyptics: How Environmental Politics Controls What We Know About Cancer. New York: Simon and Schuster.

ENTERLINE PE. 1991. Carcinogenic effects of man-made vitreous fibers. In: G. Ommen, J. Fielding, and L. Lave (eds), Annu Rev Public Health 12:459–480.

EPSTEIN S. 1978. The Politics of Cancer. San Francisco: Sierra Club Books.

EVANS L. 1990. Traffic Safety and the Driver, New York: Van Nostrand-Reinhardt.

EVANS L. 1994. Small cars, big cars: what is the safety difference? Chance 7:9–16.

FARHAR BC. 1994. Trends in US public perceptions and preferences on energy and environmental policy. In Socolow R, Anderson D, Harte J (eds). Annual Review of Energy and the Environment 19:211–239.

FIELDING J. 1991. Smoking control at the workplace. In: Ommen G, Fielding J, Lave L (eds). Annu Rev Public Health 12:209–234.

FISCHHOFF B, LICHTENSTEIN S, SLOVIC P, DERBY SL, KEENEY RL. 1981. Acceptable Risk. New York: Cambridge University Press.

GALLO M, GOCHFELD M, GOLDSTEIN BD. 1987. Biomedical aspects of environmental toxicology. In: Lave L, Upton A (eds). Toxic Chemicals, Health, and the Environment. Baltimore: Johns Hopkins.

GOUGH M. 1990. How much cancer can EPA regulate away? Risk Anal 10:1–6.

GRAHAM JD. 1988. Preventing Automobile Injury: New Findings for Evaluation Research. Dover, MA: Auburn House.

GRAHAM JD, GREEN LC, ROBERTS MJ. 1988. In Search of Safety: Chemicals and Cancer Risk. Cambridge, MA: Harvard University Press.

GREENBERG RA, BAUMAN KE, STRETCH VJ, KEYES LL, GLOVER LH, HALEY NJ, STEDMAN HC, LODA FA. 1991. Passive smoking during the first year of life. Am J Public Health 81:850–853.

GRUENSPECHT HK, LAVE LB. 1991. Increasing the efficiency and effectiveness of environmental decisions: benefit-cost analysis and effluent fees: a critical review. J Air Waste Management Assoc 41:680–693.

HADDEN SG. 1986. Read the Label: Reducing Risk by Providing Information. Boulder, CO: Westview Press.

HAHN RW, HESTER GL. 1989. Marketable permits: lessons for theory and practice. Ecol Law Q 16:361–406.

HAHN RW, HIRD JA. 1991. The costs and benefits of regulation: review and synthesis. Yale J Reg 8:233–278.

HAHN RW, MAY CA. 1994. The behavior of the allowance market: theory and evidence. Electricity J 7:28–36.

HENDERSON BE, ROSS RK, PIKE MC. 1991. Toward the primary prevention of cancer. Science 254:1131–1138.

HOEL DG, DAVIS DL, MILLER AB, et al. 1992. Trends in cancer mortality in 15 industrialized countries, 1969–1986. J Natl Cancer Inst 84:313–320.

HOWE CW. 1994. Taxes vs. tradeable discharge permits: a review in the light of U.S. and European experience. Environ Resource Econ 4:151–170.

HUBER PW, LITAN RE, EDS. 1991. The Liability Maze: The Impact of Liability Law on Safety and Innovation. Washington, DC: Brookings Institution.

HUTT PB. 1978. Food Regulation. FDC Law J 33:505–592.

HUTT PB, MERRILL RA. 1991. Food and Drug Law. Westbury NY: The Foundation Press.

IARC. 1987. Monographs on the Evaluation of Carcinogenic Risks of Chemicals to Humans, Overall Evaluations of Carcinogenicity. An Updating of IARC Monographs, vols 1–42. Lyon: International Agency for Research on Cancer.

KEENEY RL. 1990. Mortality risks induced by economic expenditures. Risk Anal 10:147–159.

KEENEY RL. 1994. Mortality risks induced by the cost of regulation. J Risk Uncertainty 8:95–110.

KLEINDORFER PR, KUNREUTHER HC. 1994. Siting of hazardous facilities. In: Pollock S, Rothkopf M, Barnett A (eds). Operations Research and the Public Sector, Amsterdam: North Holland, pp 403–440.

KNEESE AV, SCHULTZE CL. 1975. Pollution, Prices, and Public Policy. Washington, DC: Brookings Institution.

LAVE LB. 1981. The Strategy of Social Regulation. Brookings Institution, Washington, DC.

LAVE LB. 1987. Health and safety risk analysis: information for better decisions. Science 236:291–295.

LAVE LB, ENNEVER FK, ROSENKRANZ HS, OMENN GS. 1988. Information value of the rodent bioassay. Nature 336:631–633.

LAVE LB, OMENN GS. 1986. Cost-effectiveness of short-term tests of carcinogenicity. Nature 324:329–334.

LAVE L, SESKIN E. 1977. Air Pollution and Human Health. Baltimore: Johns Hopkins University Press.

LAVE LB, UPTON AC EDS. 1988. Toxic Chemicals, Health, and the Environment. Baltimore: Johns Hopkins University Press.

LINNEROOTH-BAYER J, WAHLSTROM B. 1991. Applications of probabilistic risk assessments: the selection of appropriate tools. Risk Anal 11:249–254.

LUTTER R, MORALL JF III. 1994. Health-health analysis: a new way to evaluate health and safety regulation. J Risk Uncertainty 8:43–66.

MACAULEY MK, BOWES MD, PALMER KL. 1992. Using Economic Incentives to Regulate Toxic Substances. Washington: Resources for the Future.

MENDELOFF JM. 1988. The Dilemma of Toxic Substance Regulation. Cambridge, MA: MIT Press.

MERRILL RA. 1978. Regulating Carcinogens in Food: A Legislator's Guide to the Food Safety Provisions of the Federal Food, Drug, and Cosmetic Act. Mich Law Rev 77:171–50.

MILLER SA, SKINNER K. 1984. The nose of the camel: the paradox of food standards. FDC Law J 39:99–108.

MILVY P. 1986. A general guideline for management of risk from carcinogens. Risk Anal 6:60–80.

MORGAN MG. 1993. Risk analysis and management. Sci Am July: 32–41.

MORGAN MG, FISCHHOFF B, BOSTROM A, LAVE L, ATMAN CJ. 1992. Communicating risk to the public. Environ Sci Technol 26:2048–2056.

MOSSMAN BT, BIGNON J, CORN M, SEATON A, GEE JBL. 1990. Asbestos: scientific developments and implications for public policy. Science 247:294–301.

NATIONAL RESEARCH COUNCIL. 1978. Saccharin: Technical Assessment of Risks and Benefits. Washington: National Academy Press.

NATIONAL RESEARCH COUNCIL. 1979. Food Safety Policy, Washington: National Academy Press.

NATIONAL RESEARCH COUNCIL. 1980. The Effects on Populations of Exposures to Low Levels of Ionizing Radiation. Washington: National Academy Press.

NATIONAL RESEARCH COUNCIL. 1983. Risk Assessment in the Federal Government: Managing the Process. Washington: National Academy Press.

NATIONAL RESEARCH COUNCIL. 1987. Pharmacokinetics in Risk Assessment: Drinking Water and Health, Volume 8. Washington, National Academy Press.

NATIONAL RESEARCH COUNCIL. 1988. Health Risks of Radon and Other Internally Deposited Alpha-Emitters (BEIR IV). Washington: National Academy Press.

NATIONAL RESEARCH COUNCIL. 1989a. Diet and Health: Implications for Reducing Chronic Disease Risk. Washington: National Academy Press.

NATIONAL RESEARCH COUNCIL. 1989b. Improving Risk Communication. Washington, DC: National Academy Press.

ORLANDO GA. 1990. Understanding the Excise Tax on Ozone-Depleting Chemicals. Tax Exec 359–363.

PAPERIELLO CJ. 1993. Internal Management Review of the U.S. Nuclear Regulatory Commission's Program for the Medical Use of By-product Material: Findings and Reccomendations. Washington: U.S. Nuclear Regulatory Commission.

PERROW C. 1984. Normal Accidents. New York: Basic Books.

PIERCE JP. 1991. Progress and problems in international public health efforts to reduce tobacco usage. In: Ommen G, Fielding J, Lave L (eds). Annu Rev Public Health 12:383–400.

PIGOU AC. 1920. The Economics of Welfare. London: Macmillan.

POCHIN E. 1983. Nuclear Radiation: Risks and Benefits. New York: Oxford University Press.

PORTNEY PP. 1990. Public Policies for Environmental Protection. Washington, D.C., Resources for the Future.

PUBLIC CITIZEN V. YOUNG, SUPRA. 1987. 831 F.2d at 1123 U.S. Court of Appeals for the District of Columbia Circuit, October 23, 1987.

RALL DP. 1991. Comment on Ames and gold. Science 251:10–11.

RASMUSSEN NC. 1981. The application of probabilistic risk assessment techniques to energy technologies. In: Hollander JM, Simmons MK, Wood DO (eds). Annu Rev Energy. Palo Alto, CA: Annual Reviews, pp 123–138.

RAUFER RK, FELDMAN SL. 1987. Acid Rain and Emissions Trading: Implementing a Market Approach to Pollution Control. Totowa, NJ: Towman and Littlefield.

REGENS JL, RYCROFT RW. 1988. The Acid Rain Controversy. Pittsburgh, PA: University of Pittsburgh.

RESENDIZ-CARRILLO D, LAVE LB. 1987. Optimizing spillway capacity with an estimated distribution of floods. Water Resources Res 23 2043–2049.

RESHOVSKY JD, STONE SE. 1994. Market incentives to encourage household waste recycling: paying for what you throw away. J Policy Anal Management 13:120–139.

ROBERTS L. 1989. A corrosive fight over California's toxics law. Science 243:306–309.

ROYAL COMMISSION ON MATTERS OF HEALTH AND SAFETY, CANADA. 1984. Report on Matters of Health and Safety Arising from the Use of Asbestos in Ontario. Toronto: Ontario Ministry of Government Services.

SALSBURG DS. 1977. Use of statistics when examining lifetime studies in rodents to detect carcinogenicity. J Toxicol Hum Health 3.

SCHELLING TC. 1968. The life you save may be your own. In: Chase S (ed). Problems in Public Expenditure Analysis. Washington: Brookings.

SCHWARTZ J. 1992. Particulate air pollution and daily mortality: a synthesis. Public Health Rev 56:204–213.

SCHEUPLEIN RJ. 1990. Perspectives on toxicological risk—an example: food-borne carcinogenic risk. In: Clayson DB, Munro IC, Shubik P, Swenberg JA (eds). Progress in Predictive Toxicology, New York: Elseview Science Publishers.

SLOVIC P. 1987. Perception of Risk. Science 236:280–286.

STARR C. 1969. Social benefits versus technological risk. Science 165:1232–1238.

STAVINS RN, ED. 1988. Project 88: Harnessing Market Forces to Protect Our Environment—Initiatives for the New President, A Public Policy Study Sponsored by Senator Timothy E. Wirth, Colorado and Senator John Heinz, Pennsylvania. Washington, DC.

STONE R. 1992. Bad News on Second-Hand Smoke. Science 257:607.

TIETENBERG T. 1992. Environmental and Natural Resource Economics. New York: HarperCollins.

TRAVIS CC, ED. 1987. Risk Analysis. New York: Plenum.

TRAVIS CC, HATTEMER-FREY HA. 1988. Determining an acceptable level of risk. Environ Sci Tech 22:873–876.

UPTON AC, SHORE RE, HARLEY NH. 1992. The Health Effects of Low-Level Ionizing Radiation. In: Omenn G, Fielding J, Lave L (eds). Annu Rev Public Health 13:127–150.

U.S. ENVIRONMENTAL PROTECTION AGENCY. 1987. Unfinished Business: A Comparative Assessment of Environmental Problems,

Washington: U.S. Environmental Protection Agency (EPA-450/1-85-001).

U.S. Environmental Protection Agency. 1989. Final rule on risk goals. Fed Reg 54:38,044–58.

U.S. Environmental Protection Agency. 1990. Reducing Risk: Setting Priorities and Strategies for Environmental Protection, Report of the Relative Risk Reduction Strategies Committee, Science Advisory Board, SAB-EC-90-021.

U.S. Food and Drug Administration. 1993. Toxicological Principles for the Safety Assessment of Direct Food Additives and Color Additives Used in Food, Washington, DC.

U.S. General Accounting Office. 1993. Implications of Using Pollution Taxes to Supplement Regulation, GAO/RCED-93-13, February, Washington, DC: USGAO.

U.S. National Cancer Institute. 1986. Cancer Control Objectives for the Nation: 1985–2000, Bethesda, MD: National Cancer Institute.

U.S. Nuclear Regulatory Commission. 1975. Reactor Safety Study: WASH 1400, Washington: Government Printing Office.

U.S. Nuclear Regulatory Commission. 1978. Risk Assessment Review Group Report, NUREG/CR 0400, Washington: Government Printing Office.

Viscusi WK. 1992. Fatal Tradeoffs: Public and Private Responsibilities for Risk. New York: Oxford University Press.

Viscusi WK. 1993. The value of risks to life and health. J Econ Lit XXXI: 1912–1946.

Viscusi WK. 1994. Risk-risk analysis, J Risk Uncertainty 8:5–18.

Viscusi WK, Magat WA. 1987. Learning About Risk: Consumer and Worker Responses to Hazard Information. Cambridge, MA: Harvard University Press.

Watson AY, Bates R, Kennedy D, eds. 1988. Air Pollution, the Automobile, and Public Health. Washington: National Academy Press.

Weill H, Hughes JM. 1986. Asbestos as a public health risk: disease and policy. In: Breslow L, Fielding J, Lave L, (eds), Annu Rev Public Health 7:171–192, Palo Alto, CA: Annual Reviews.

Weinberg AM. 1972. Science and trans-science. Minerva 10:202–222.

Whelan EM. 1985. Toxic Terror. Ottawa, IL: Jameson Books.

Whipple C. 1987. De Minimis Risk. New York: Plenum.

Wildavsky A. 1980. Richer is Safer. Public Interest 60:23–39.

Wulff P. 1991. More Large Accidents Through Complexity? Risk Anal 11:249–253.

Index

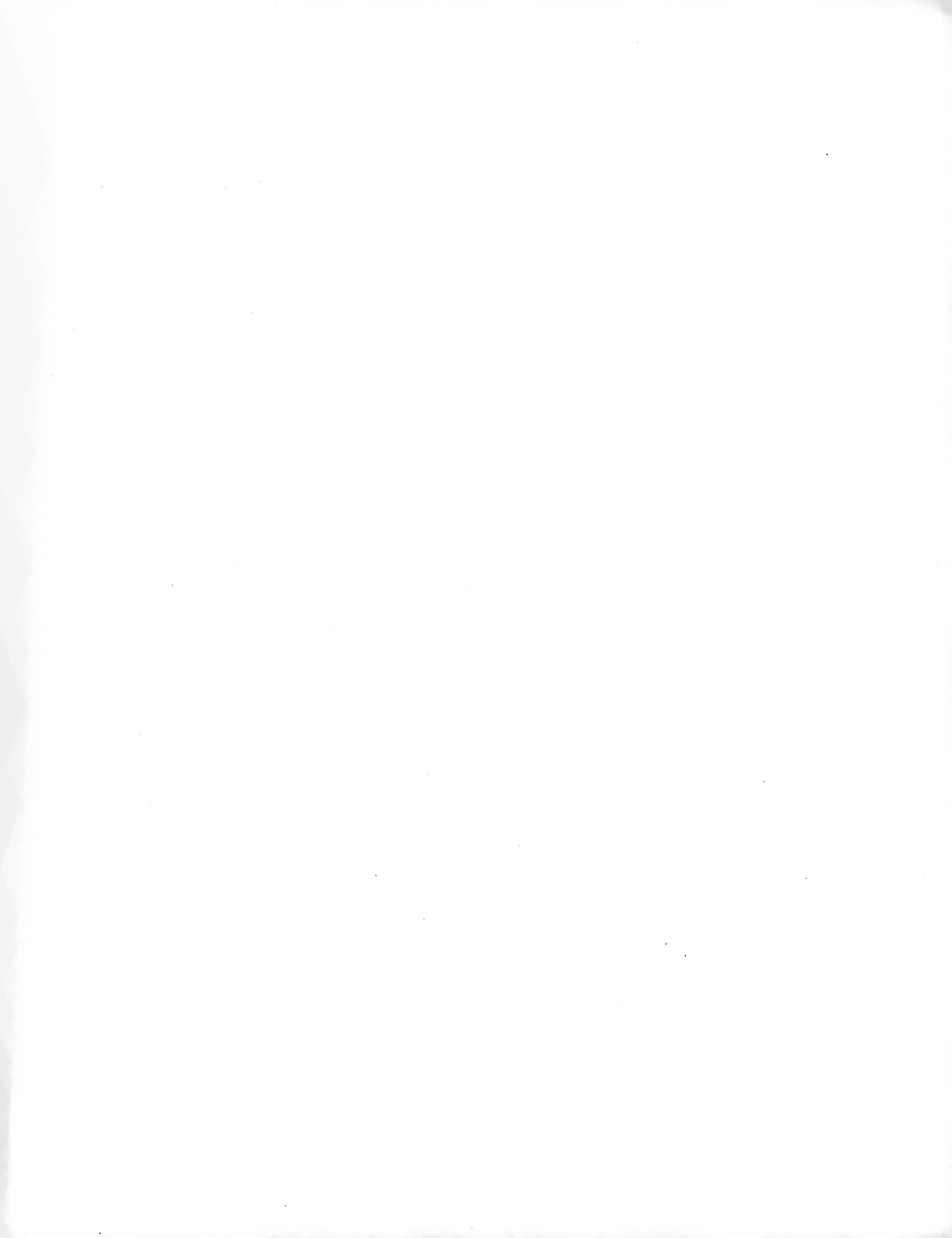